SUBSTANCE ABUSE

A Comprehensive Textbook

Fourth Edition

SUBSTANCE ABUSE

A Comprehensive Textbook

Fourth Edition

Editors

Joyce H. Lowinson, M.D.

Professor Emeritus of Psychiatry
Albert Einstein College of Medicine of Yeshiva University
Adjunct Faculty The Rockefeller University
New York, New York

Pedro Ruiz, M.D.

Professor and Vice Chairman
Department of Psychiatry and Behavioral Sciences
The University of Texas Medical School
Houston, Texas

Robert B. Millman, M.D.

Saul P. Steinberg Distinguished Professor of Psychiatry and Public Health
Cornell University Medical College
Director, Division of Substance Abuse Services
New York Hospital-Payne Whitney Psychiatry Clinic
New York, New York

John G. Langrod, A.C.S.W., C.A.S.A.C., L.C.S.W., Ph.D.

Director of Admissions and Evaluation
Division of Substance Abuse
Albert Einstein College of Medicine of Yeshiva University
Bronx, New York

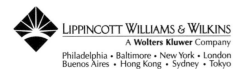

LIPPINCOTT WILLIAMS & WILKINS
A **Wolters Kluwer** Company
Philadelphia • Baltimore • New York • London
Buenos Aires • Hong Kong • Sydney • Tokyo

Acquisitions Editor: Charles W. Mitchell
Developmental Editor: Joyce Murphy
Production Editor: David Murphy
Manufacturing Manager: Ben Rivera
Marketing Manager: Sharon Zinner
Compositor: TechBooks
Printer: Quebecor World—Versailles

© **2005 by LIPPINCOTT WILLIAMS & WILKINS**
530 Walnut Street
Philadelphia, PA 19106 USA
LWW.com

Printed in the USA

First Edition, 1981; Second Edition, 1992; Third Edition, 1997

Library of Congress Cataloging-in-Publication Data
Substance abuse : a comprehensive textbook / editors, Joyce H. Lowinson . . . [et al.]. — 4th ed.
    p. ; cm.
  Includes bibliographical references and index.
  ISBN: 0-7817-3474-6
  1. Substance abuse.   2. Substance abuse—Treatment.   3. Substance abuse—Social aspects.
4. Substance abuse—United States.   I. Lowinson, Joyce H.
  [DNLM: 1. Substance-Related Disorders.   WM 270 S941 2004]
RC564.S826   2004
362.29—dc22

                              2004019274

Care has been taken to confirm the accuracy of the information presented and to describe generally accepted practices. However, the authors, editors, and publisher are not responsible for errors or omissions or for any consequences from application of the information in this book and make no warranty, expressed or implied, with respect to the currency, completeness, or accuracy of the contents of the publication. Application of this information in a particular situation remains the professional responsibility of the practitioner.

    The authors, editors, and publisher have exerted every effort to ensure that drug selection and dosage set forth in this text are in accordance with current recommendations and practice at the time of publication. However, in view of ongoing research, changes in government regulations, and the constant flow of information relating to drug therapy and drug reactions, the reader is urged to check the package insert for each drug for any change in indications and dosage and for added warnings and precautions. This is particularly important when the recommended agent is a new or infrequently employed drug.

    Some drugs and medical devices presented in this publication have Food and Drug Administration (FDA) clearance for limited use in restricted research settings. It is the responsibility of the health care provider to ascertain the FDA status of each drug or device planned for use in their clinical practice.

                                              10 9 8 7 6 5 4 3 2 1

We wish to dedicate this work to Drs. Vincent Dole and Marie Nyswander, who through their pioneering efforts and dedication brought the substance abuse treatment field to the high level that it is today.

We also want to thank our families, spouses, children, relatives, friends and patients for their support and inspiration, which helped to once again bring this work to a successful conclusion.

Preface

The fourth edition of *Substance Abuse: A Comprehensive Textbook* serves as a continuing response to society's growing recognition of the prevalence of alcohol and drug use, abuse, and dependence and of their profound impact not only upon people's health but on almost every other aspect of life. This volume also draws upon and makes available to practicioners and students in this field the very latest information resulting from the remarkable growth of basic and applied research, treatment, epidemiology, pharmacology, policy, as well as other areas related to substance abuse. This volume also draws upon knowledge and expertise required not only of health professionals, but of social service; law enforcement; judicial, legal, and correctional personal; as well as of economists, ethicists, and governmental and private administrative staff. Thus the transmission of such knowledge has been a determining factor in the organization of this text.

The principle objective of this edition are therefore quite ambitious. As was the case with the previous editions, our goal is to provide the most authoritative and comprehensive resource on the subject of substance abuse and its related areas. This book continues to serve as the definitive text for students in all related professional disciplines and also continues to be a source of information and knowledge for scientists and clinicians working in the field of drug, alcohol, and other addictions. This work is useful to other health care professionals, particularly those involved in the delivery of primary care services as well as workers in related fields who require an overview of particular areas or detailed discussions of specific scientific, clinical, or administrative subjects. Since scientists and researchers must anticipate the questions that clinicians are posing, and policymakers must understand how treatments work, this volume translates data across disciplines in order to facilitate research, treatment, and policy development.

This textbook provides state-of-the-art presentations by top experts and practicioners in their respective areas. For example, chapters on the clinical evaluation of patients with alcohol and substance abuse disorders in all their diversity not only offer guidelines for optimal patient care including appropriate treatment placement, but also contributes to the development of programs of excellence.

The section regarding treatment of the acute sequelae of various drugs, as well as the intervention in the management of various types of withdrawal symptoms, has been considerably expanded and updated. Discussions of basic scientific and clinical research developments (which are becoming clinically relevant at an ever-increasing rate) constitute integral parts of the sections on pharmacology and on treatment of the various substance abuse syndromes.

We have retained the sections on sociology, evaluation, and treatment of specific populations because patterns of abuse and treatment approaches change with the passage of time. We have added much new information on the relation of psychopathology to substance abuse as well as changes in psychiatric diagnoses. Based on the above, we have presented the most effective methods and programs for treating, dually diagnosed patients—mentally ill chemical abusers (MICAs). We have updated the diagnostic sections by presenting the DSM IV-R, which has been further developed since the previous edition of our book.

New chapters include studies of other addictive/compulsive behaviors related to cybernet abuse, hoarding, gambling, sex, and cults. Since numerous characteristics and dynamics of these behaviors are similar to the behaviors of patients presenting with substance abuse and dependency problems, some addictive behaviors such as gambling and sex have been discussed in conjunction with the abuse of drugs and alcohol. We have also updated the section on religious approaches to treatment in view of recent court decisions that require that patients be offered secularly oriented treatment and that they not be coerced into religiously oriented modalities. This issue has become important because of recent successful initiatives to fund faith-based treatments, including religiously oriented correctional facilities.

In view of the increased application of cognitive/behavioral therapies (CBTs) in the treatment of substance abuse and related behaviors, we have updated the chapters on the history, indications, and methodologies of these therapies and present combination pharmacotherapy and cognitive behavioral approaches. Combining CBT with medications has proved to be particularly effective. The section on policy, and issues such as demand and supply reduction, legalization, decriminatization, and harm reduction are covered in considerable detail, since reliance on interdiction has not had a great deal of success.

The face of the health care system has changed remarkably in recent years. In the name of cost containment, managed care companies through the application of capitation payment formulas and increasing reliance on health maintenance organizations, are forcing both practicioners and patients involved in the substance abuse and psychiatric treatment systems to accept significant change which has in many respects been detrimental to both. This problem has been compounded by an unwillingness or inability of the United States Congress to approve parity legislation. We have therefore, included in this edition separate chapters on health insurance systems, managed care, and their historical antecedents, as well as likely future developments and consequences. The health care system, in general, and behavioral health care, in particular, are facing serious restrictions in their funding and practices. How can service providers working in these systems continue to serve patients of lower and middle socioeconomic levels who have serious substance abuse problems requiring long-term, highly intensive care, and cannot currently afford to pay for it?

Specific treatment approaches and goals such as detoxification, attainment and maintenance of abstinence, relapse-prevention, and psychotherapeutic and pharmacotherapeutic regimens have been updated and are described in considerable detail in this volume. Many therapists and treatment programs have become more sophisticated, more effective, and perhaps more humane than in the past. Unfortunately, some programs continue to zealously advance and protect their therapeutic regimens while often disparaging methods based on other etiological models. Important therapeutic modalities do not necessarily share identical objectives. For example, rehabilitation programs based on a 12-step system require abstinence as their main objective. What then do proponents of these programs think about maintenance programs using medications such as methadone, LAAM, buprenorphine, naltrexone, disulfiram, and acamprosate? Conflict between abstinence-oriented programs and those that value function and espouse harm-reduction techniques is destructive and not in the best interest of the field. It is startling and humbling to recall that few of these programs are over 30 years old, and thus barely out of their adolescence.

Each patient or client develops problems in unique ways and forms a unique relation to the substance of choice. Common sense dictates that treatment must be tailored and respond to the needs of each individual. Therapists must try to learn as much as possible about patients and their problems in order to match them with the most effective, least expensive treatments or to develop new, more effective treatments that integrate several strategies.

Whenever possible, chapters dealing with treatment modalities provide process and outcome data that are designed to improve workers' evaluative and referral capabilities. New and alternative programs now in development often combine elements of conventional modalities into interesting hybrids. These new programs need room to change and expand. Referral agents unfortunately are all too often motivated to send patients to those modalities that reflect their own belief systems, and therapists often treat patients according to their own philosophies. We expect that eclectic and needs-based treatment will become the wave of the future. We therefore hope and expect that this volume will continue to contribute to the development of more rationally based treatment approaches.

We have presented the latest developments in the field of pharmacotherapy in the treatment of substance abusing patients. Major changes have occurred with the removal of LAAM from the marketplace throughout the world. This occurred because there were reports of cardiotoxicity among some patients taking this medication. Specifically, there occurred a prolongation of the QT intervals in electrocardiograms taken on these patients. This situation places some patients at risk for cardiac arrythmias. Since the medication was "black-boxed" in the Physicians Desk Reference (PDR) in the United States and other countries, the medication was taken off the market. It should be noted however, that other medication such as tricyclic antidepressants have been reported to have similar effects, but they continue to be prescribed. This may be one of the reasons the buprenorphine has proved to be attractive, and its use has now been introduced in the United States and throughout the world. This new medication and its application is discussed extensively in this volume. One of the advantages of LAAM was that it was difficult to test for—this proved especially appealing to employed patients.

Despite our expectations, the size of this volume remains similar to that of its predecessors. We have, however, endeavored to reduce redundancy and to present information in an understandable, clear, and crisp style. We trust that we have succeeded in this endeavor without reducing the richness of detail, language, and graphics.

We are deeply grateful to the many distinguished contributors who made this volume possible. Our charge to them was quite rigorous, and we believe that they have more than satisfied our expectations. Our work could not have been successful without the invaluable assistance and support of our editors, Charles Mitchell and Joyce Murphy, project manager, Stephanie Lentz at TechBooks, and others too numerous to mention. We hope that we have met the expectations of our readers, for they will be the final judges.

Joyce H. Lowinson, M.D.
Pedro Ruiz
John Langrod
Robert Millman

Contributors

James T. Abel M.A., M.S.W.
Director, Chemical Dependency Service
Albert Einstein College of Medicine
Division of Substance Abuse
Bronx, New York

Nassima Ait-Daoud M.D.
Assistant Professor
Department of Psychiatry
The University of Texas Health
Science Center at San Antonio
South Texas Addiction Research &
Technology (START) Center
San Antonio, Texas

Charles R. Albrecht III
Johns Hopkins University/Sinai Hospital Program in
Internal Medicine
Baltimore, Maryland

Robert M. Anthenelli M.D.
Associate Professor
Department of Psychiatry
University of Cinnati College of Medicine
Director, Substance Dependence Program
Cincinnati Veterans Affairs Medical Center
Cincinnati, OH

Julia H. Arnsten M.D., M.P.H.
Assistant Professor
Departments of Medicine, Epidemiology and Social
Medicine, and Department of Psychiatry and
Behavioral Sciences
Albert Einstein College of Medicine
Bronx, New York

Sudie Back Ph.D.
Department of Psychiatry
Yale University School of Medicine
New Haven, Connecticut

James B. Bakalar JD
Lecturer in Law
Department of Psychiatry
Harvard Medical School
Boston, Massachusetts

Steven L. Batki M.D.
Professor and Research Director
Department of Psychiatry
SUNY Upstate Medical University
Syracuse, New York

Sheila B. Blume M.D.
Clinical Professor of Psychiatry
Department of Psychiatry
State University of New York at StonyBrook
StonyBrook, New York

Stephen Boehm, II Ph.D.
Postdoctoral Fellow
The University of Texas at Austin
Waggoner Center for Alcohol and Addiction Research
Austin, Texas

Gilbert J. Botvin M.D.
Professor of Public Health
Weill Medical College of Cornell University
New York, New York

Bruna Brands Ph.D
Assistant Professor
Clinical Research Department Centre for Addictions
and Mental Health
Department of Pharmacology
University of Toronto
Toronto, Ontario, Canada

Nancy M. Brehm Ph.D.
Practicing Psychologist, Psycholanalytic Institute
New Orleans, Louisiana

Margaret K. Brooks J.D.
New Perspectives
Montclair, New Jersey

Lawrence S. Brown Jr, M.D., M.P.H.
Senior Vice President
Addiction Research and Treatment Corporation
Brooklyn, New York

Betty J. Buchan M.D.
Vice President of Research at Operation PAR
Tampa, Florida

Milton Earl Burglass M.D., M.P.H.
formerly, Zinberg Center for Addiction Studies
Harvard Medical School
Cambridge, Massachusetts

Ron Burks Ph.D.
Clinical Director
Wellspring Retreat and Resource Center
Albany, OH

Robert P. Cabaj M.D.
Associate Professor
Department of Psychiatry
University of California, San Francisco
San Francisco, California

John S. Cacciola Ph.D.
Senior Scientist
The Treatment Research Institute
Philadelphia, Pennsylvania

Kathleen Carrol Ph.D.
Professor, Department of Psychiatry
Yale University School of Medicine
New Haven, Connecticut

Grace Chang M.D., M.P.H.
Associate Professor, Department of Psychiatry
Harvard Medical School, Brigham and
  Women's Hospital
Boston, Massachusetts

John N. Chappel M.D.
Professor Emeritus of Psychiatry,
  Department of Psychiatry
University of Nevada
Reno, Nevada

Domenic A. Ciraulo M.D.
Professor and Chairman
Division of Psychiatry
Boston University School of Medicine
Boston, Massachusetts

Chinazo Cunningham M.D.
Assistant Professor
Department of Internal Medicine
Albert Einstein College of Medicine
Bronx, New York

Eugenia Curet Ph.D., C.A.S.A.C., L.C.S.W.
Administrative Director
The Adolescent Development Program
Cornell Medical College
Department of Public Health and Pediatrics
New York, New York

Dennis C. Daley Ph.D.
Associate Professor
Department of Psychiatry
University of Pittsburgh
Chief, Addiction Medicine Services
Western Psychiatric Institute and Clinic
Pittsburgh, Pennsylvania

David A. Deitch Ph.D.
Professor of Clinical Psychiatry
Department of Psychiatry
University of California
San Diego, La Jolla, California

Katherine A. DeLaune
Fellow, Substance Abuse Research Center
Department of Psychiatry and Behavioral Sciences
University of Texas Mental Sciences Institute
Houston, Texas

Sylvia J. Dennison M.D.
Associate Professor
Department of Psychiatry
Chief, Division of Addiction Services
University of Illinois at Chicago
Chicago, Illinois

Don C. Des Jarlais Ph.D
Professor, Epidemiology and Social Medicine
Albert Einstein College of Medicine
Director of Research, Baron Edmond de Rothschild
  Chemical Dependency
Beth Israel Medical Center
New York, New York

Lance M. Dodes M.D.
Assistant Clinical Professor of Psychiatry
Harvard Medical School
Training and Supervising Analyst
Boston Psychoanalytic Institute
Boston, Massachusetts

Ernest Drucker Ph.D.
Professor, Epidemiology and Social Medicine
Albert Einstein College of Medicine
Director of Public Health and Policy Research
Epidemiology and Social Medicine
Montefiore Medical Center
Bronx, New York

Joel A. Dvoskin Ph.D.
Assistant Professor, Department of Psychiatry
University of Arizona College of Medicine
Tucson, Arizona

Elyse R. Eisenberg M.D.
Research Physician, Pharmacologic Research
Division Haight Ashbury Free Clinics, Inc.
San Francisco, California

Everett H. Ellinwood, Jr. M.D.
Professor, Department of Biological Psychiatry
Duke University Medical Center
Durham, North Carolina

Paul F. Engelhart M.A., M.S.
Chief Program Officer
Catholic Charities–Diocese of Rockville Center
Hicksville, New York

Mathea Falco J.D.
President, Drug Strategies
San Francisco, California

David J. Farabee Ph.D.
Research Psychologist
University of California at Los Angeles
   Drug Abuse Research Center
Los Angeles, California

Francisco Fernandez M.D.
Professor and Chairman
Department of Psychiatry University of South Florida
Tampa, Florida

Loretta P. Finnegan M.D., Ph.D.
Medical Advisor for the Director
Office of Research on Women's Health
US Department of Health and Human Services
National Institutes of Health
Bethesda, Maryland

Edward F. Foulks M.D.
Professor
Department of Psychiatry
Tulane University School of Medicine
New Orleans, Louisiana

Samuel R. Friedman Ph.D.
National Development and Research Institute, Inc
New York, New York

Paul J. Fudala Ph.D.
Associate Professor of Pharmacology in Psychiatry
University of Pennsylvania School of Medicine
Philadelphia, Pennsylvania

Marc Galanter M.D.
Professor
Department of Psychiatry
NYU School of Medicine
Director, Division of Alcoholism and Drug Abuse
NYU Medical Center
New York, New York

Gantt P. Galloway Pharm.D.
Assistant Professor
Department of Clinical Pharmacy
University of California, San Francisco
Chief of Pharmacologic Research, Research
   Education and Training Section
Haight-Ashbury Free Clinics
San Francisco, California

Steven R. Gambert M.D.
Professor of Medicine
Department of Medicine
Johns Hopkins University School of Medicine
Baltimore, Maryland

Eliot L. Gardner Ph.D.
National Institute of Health
National Insitute on Drug Abuse
Behavioral Neuroscience Research Branch
Bethesda, Maryland

Walter Ginter C.M.A.
Vice President
National Alliance of Methadone Advocates
New York, New York

Stuart Gitlow M.D., M.P.H.
Medical Director
Nantucket Family and Children's Service
Nantucket, Massachusetts

Jane Glick M.S.W., C.S.W.
Social Worker
Social Work Services
New York Presbyterian Hospital
   Columbia-Presbyterian Campus
New York, New York

Mark S. Gold M.D.
Distinguished Professor
McKnight Brain Institute
Departments of Psychiatry
Neuroscience Community Health and Family
   Medicine
Chief, Division of Addiction Medicine
Gainesville, Florida

Howard H. Goldman M.D., Ph.D.
Professor of Psychiatry
University of Maryland School of Maryland
Baltimore, Maryland

Andrew Golub Ph.D.
Principal Investigator
National Development and Research Institutes, Inc
New York, New York

Aviel Goodman M.D.
Director
Minnesota Institute of Psychiatry
St. Paul, Minnesota

Carolyn Goodman Ed.D
Assistant Clinical Professor Emeritus
Albert Einstein College of Medicine of Yeshiva
*   University*
Founder and Director, PACE
Bronx Psychiatric Center
Bronx, New York

Marc Gourevich M.D.
Director, Division of General Internal Medicine
NYU School of Medicine
Department of Medicine
New York, New York

Robert A. Greenstein M.D.
Behavioral Health Service
Mental Health Clinic
VA Medical Center
Philadelphia, Pennsylvania

Kenneth W. Griffin Ph.D., M.P.H.
Associate Professor
Department of Public Health
Cornell University Medical College
New York, New York

Roland R. Griffiths Ph.D.
Professor
Department of Psychiatry & Behavioral Sciences
Department of Neuroscience
Johns Hopkins University School of Medicine
Baltimore, MD

Lester Grinspoon M.D.
Associate Professor of Psychiatry
Harvard Medical School
Boston, Massachusetts

Charles S. Grob M.D.
Professor
Department of Psychiatry and Pediatrics
UCLA School of Medicine, Los Angeles
Director, Division of Child & Adolescent Psychiatry
Harbor–UCLA Medical Canter
Torrance, CA

Holly C. Hagan Ph.D., M.P.H.
Clinical Assistant Professor of Epidemiology
University of Washington School of Public Health
*   and Community Medicine*
Seattle, Washington

David A. Halperin MD
Deceased

Ji-Sheng Han M.D.
Professor
Neuroscience Research Institute
Peking University
Beijing, China

Melanie S. Harned M.D.
Research Fellow
Department of Psychiatry
Harvard Medical School
Boston, Massachusetts

R. Adron Harris Ph.D.
Professor
Department of Neurobiology
University of Texas
Austin, Texas

Nancy A. Haug Ph.D.
Postdoctoral Fellow
Department of Psychiatry
University of California, San Francisco
San Francisco, California

Anthony Heath Ph.D.
Director, Division of Behavioral Sciences
McHeal Family Practice Residency Program
Berwyn, Illinois

Allen W. Heinemann Ph.D.
Professor
Physical Medicine & Rehabilitation
Feinberg School of Medicine, Northwest University
Director, Center for Rehabilitation Outcome
*   Research*
Rehabilitation Institute of Chicago
Chicago, Illinois

Ronald Hopson Ph.D.
Department of Psychology and School of Divinity
Howard University
Washington, DC

Arthur T. Horvath Ph.D.
Center for Cognitive Therapy, La Jolla, California
*   and President*
S.M.A.R.T Recovery
Mentor, Ohio
President
Practical Recovery Service
La Jolla, California

Robert L. Hubbard Ph.D.
Center Director
Institute for Community-Based Research
National Development & Research Institutes
Raleigh, North Carolina

James A. Inciardi Ph.D.
Professor and Director
Center for Drug and Alcohol Studies
University of Delaware
Newark, Delaware

William S. Jacobs M.D.
Clinical Assistant Professor
University of Florida
Departments of Psychiatry and Anesthesiology
Gainesville, Florida

Jerome H. Jaffe M.D.
Clinical Professor
Institute of Psychiatry and Human Behavior
University of Maryland School of Medicine
Baltimore, Maryland

Daniel C. Javitt M.D.
Professor of Psychiatry
New York University
Nathan Kline Institute
Orangeburg, New York

Bruce D. Johnson Ph.D.
Director, Institute of Special Populations Research
National Development and Research Institute
New York, New York

Bankole A. Johnson M.D.
Wurzbach Distinguished Professor of Psychiatry and
*   Pharmacology*
Department of Psychiatry
The University of Texas Health Science Center at San
*   Antonio*
The South Texas Addiction Research and Technology
*   (START) Center*
San Antonio, Texas

Steven Jonas M.D., M.P.H., M.S.
Professor of Preventive Medicine
School of Medicine
Stony Brook University
Stony Brook, New York

Herman Joseph Ph.D.
Adjunct Faculty
The Rockefeller University
Research Scientist, Bureau of Methadone Policy and
*   Planning*
New York State Ofice of Alcoholism and Substance
*   Abuse Services*
New York, New York

Patti Juliana M.S.W., A.C.S.W., L.C.S.W.,
D.S.W., [cand]
Director of Clinical Services
Divison of Substance Abuse
Albert Einstein College of Medicine of Yeshiva
*   University*
Bronx, New York

Laura M. Juliano Ph.D.
Assistant Professor
Department of Psychology
American University
Washington, DC

Ari D. Kalechstein Ph.D.
Associate Research Psychologist
David Geffen School of Medicine at UCLA
Los Angeles, California

Stephen R. Kandall MD
Professor (Retired)
Department of Pediatrics and Neonatology
Albert Einstein College of Medicine–Beth Israel
*   Medical Center*
Bronx, New York

Edward J. Khantzian M.D.
Clinical Professor
Department of Psychiatry
Harvard Medical School
Boston, Massachusetts
Associate Chief
Department of Psychiatry
Tewksbury Hospital
Tewksburg, Massachusetts

Mark D. Kilgus M.D.
Medical Director
Woodridge Hospital
Johnson City, Tennessee

George R. King Ph.D.
Assistant Professor
Department of Psychology
Texas Christian University
Fort Worth, Texas
Research Associate Professor
Pharmacology and Neuroscience
UNT Health Science Center
Fort Worth, Texas

Herbert D. Kleber M.D.
Professor
Department of Psychiatry
Columbia University
College of Physicians and Surgeons
Director, Division on Substance Abuse
New York State Psychiatric Institute
New York, New York

Clifford M. Knapp Ph.D.
Assistant Professor of Psychiatry
Boston University School of Medicine
Clinical Director of Psychopharmacology
Medication Development Research Unit
Veterans Administration Medical Center
*   Outpatient Clinic*
Boston, Massachusetts

Thomas R. Kosten M.D.
Professor of Psychiatry
Yale University School of Medicine and VA
*   Connecticut Healthcare System*
West Haven, Connecticut

Igor Koutsenok M.D.
Associate Director
Addiction Training Center
University of California San Diego
San Diego, California

John G. Langrod A.C.S.W., C.A.S.A.C.,
L.C.S.W., Ph.D.
Director of Admissions and Evaluation
Division of Substance Abuse
Albert Einstein College of Medicine of
*   Yeshiva University*
Bronx, New York

William B. Lawson M.D., Ph.D.
Professor and Chairman
Department of Psychiatry, Howard University
Washington, DC

Bruce S. Liese Ph.D.
Professor of Family Medicine and Psychiatry
University of Kansas Medical Center
Kansas City, Kansas

Show W. Lin M.D.
Assistant Professor of Clinical Psychiatry
Department of Psychiatry
University of Cincinnati College of Medicine
Associate Chief, Substance Dependence Program
Cincinnati Veterans Affairs Medical Center
Cincinnati, Ohio

Walter Ling M.D.
Professor
Department of Psychiatry and Biobehavioral
*   Sciences*
University of California at Los Angeles
Los Angeles, California

Joyce H. Lowinson M.D.
(Retired)
Professor Emeritus of Psychiatry
*   and Executive Director*
Albert Einstein College of Medicine of
*   Yeshiva University*
Adjunct Faculty, The Rockefeller University
New York, New York

Charles Madray
Addiction Research and Treatment Corporation
Brooklyn, New York

Jorge Maldonado M.D.
Staff Psychiatrist
Alamo Mental Health Group
San Antonio, Texas

Kasia Malinowska-Semprucht M.S.W.
DPH [Cand]
Director, International Harm Reduction
Development of the Open Society Institute
New York, New York

Ira J. Marion M.A.
Executive Director
Division of Substance Abuse
Albert Einstein College of Medicine of
*   Yeshiva University*
Bronx, New York

G. Alan Marlatt Ph.D.
Professor of Psychology
Director, Addictive Behaviors Research Center
Department of Psychology
University of Washington
Seattle, Washington

David Marsh M.D.
Medical Director, Addiction, HIV and
*   Aboriginal Health*
Vancouver Coastal Health
Clinical Associate Professor, Department of
*   Health Care and Epidemiology*
Faculty of Medicine
University of British Columbia
Vancouver, British Columbia, Canada

Karin Marsolais
Associate Coordinator
PSATTC University of California
San Diego, California

Charles O. Matthews Ph.D.
NIDA Fellow on Co-occurring Disorders
Department of Mental Health Law and Policy
Louis de la Parte Florida Mental Institute
University of South Florida
Tampa, Florida
Clinical Psychologist
Mental Health & Biobehavioral Science
*   Service/Psychology*
James A. Haley Veterans Hospital
Tampa, Florida

Dennis McCarty Ph.D.
Professor
Department of Public Health and
*   Preventive Medicine*
Oregon Health and Science University
Portland, Oregon

Jennifer McNeely M.D.
Albert Einstein College of Medicine
Formerly Senior Research Associate,
*   Linda Smith Center*
Bronx, New York

Gerard Meenan M.S.
Chief Toxicologist
MetLife Insurance Testing Laboratory
Elmsford, New York

John P. Morgan M.D.
Professor of Pharmacology
The City University of New York Medical School
The City College of New York
New York, New York

John P. Muffler Ed. D.
Pastor
South Presbyterian Church
Yonkers, NY

Sheigla Murphy Ph.D.
Director
Center for Substance Abuse Studies
Institute for Scientific Analysis
San Francisco, California

David F. Musto M.A., M.D.
Professor of Child Psychiatry and
*   History of Medicine*
Yale University
New Haven, Connecticut

Edgar P. Nace M.D.
Professor of Clinical Psychiatry
Department of Psychiatry
University of Texas Southwestern Medical School
Dallas, Texas

Ethann Nadelman J.D., Ph.D.
Executive Director, Drug Policy Alliance
New York, New York

Lisa M. Najavits Ph.D.
Associate Professor
Department of Psychiatry
Harvard Medical School
Boston, Massachusetts

Robert G. Newman M.P.H., M.D.
Executive Director, Baron Edmond de Rothschild
*   International Center for Advancement of Addiction*
*   Treatment*
Beth Israel Medical Center
Professor of Epidemiology and Population Health
Professor of Psychiatry
Albert Einstein College of Medicine
New York, New York

R.L. Norman Ph.D.
Research Associate
New York State Office of Alcoholism and Substance
*   Abuse Services*
New York, New York

Mgr. William B. O'Brien
President, Daytop Village, Inc.
New York, New York

Eugene Oscapella J.D.
Barrister and Solicitor
President, Oscapella and Associates Consulting Ltd.
Ottawa, Canada

Steven D. Passik Ph.D.
Director
Symptom Management and Palliative Care Program
Markey Cancer Center
Associate Professor of Medicine and
*   Behavioral Science*
University of Kentucky
Lexington, Kentucky

Richard Payne M.D.
Director
Insitute On Care at the End of Life
Duke University
Durham, North Carolina

J. Thomas Payte M.D.
Medical Director
Drug Dependence Associates
San Antonio, Texas

Robert N. Pechnick Ph.D.
Associate Director of Research
Department of Psychiatry
Cedars-Sinai Medical Center
Thalians Mental Health Center
Los Angeles, California

Fernando B. Perfas D.S.W.
Director of Special Projects
Daytop Village, Inc.
New York, New York

Roger H. Peters Ph.D.
Professor and Associate Chair
Department of Mental Health Law and Policy
Louis de la Porte Florida Mental Health Institute
University of South Florida
Tampa, Florida

Edmond H. Pi M.D.
Professor and Executive Chairman
Department of Psychiatry and Human Behavior
Charles R. Drew University of Medicine and Science
Los Angeles, California

Russel E. Poland Ph.D
Professor
Department of Psychiatry
University of California Los Angeles
Director of Research
Department of Psychiatry
Cedars-Sinai Medical Center
Los Angeles, California

Russell K. Portenoy Ph.D.
Professor
Department of Neurology
Albert Einstein College of Medicine
Bronx, New York
Chairman, Department of Pain Medicine and
*   Palliative Care*
Beth Israel Medical Center
New York, New York

Beny J. Primm M.D.
Executive Director
Addiction Research and Treatment Corporation
Brooklyn, New York

Andres J. Pumariega M.D.
Professor and Director
Child and Adolescent Psychiatry
Psychiatry and Behavioral Sciences Department
East Tennessee State University
Johnson City, Tennessee

Purva M. Rawal B.A., Ph.D.
Postdoctoral Fellow
Division of Clinical Psychology
Institute for Health Services Research and
*   Policy Studies*
Feinberg School of Medicine
Northwestern University
Chicago, Illinois

Martin Repetto M.D., Ph.D.
Department of Psychiatry
University of Florida
Gainesville, Florida

James T. Richardson J.D., Ph.D.
Director, Judicial Studies Program
Professor of Sociology and Judicial Studies
University of Nevada, Reno
Reno, Nevada

Leonardo Rodriguez M.D.
Addiction Psychiatry Fellow
Department of Psychiatry
University of Florida
Gainesville, Florida

Marsha Rosenbaum Ph.D.
Director
Drug Policy Alliance
San Francisco, California

Neil L. Rosenberg M.D.
Deceased

Bruce J. Rounsaville M.D.
Professor
Department of Psychiatry
Yale University School of Medicine
Director
New England Mental Illness Research Education and
*   Clinical Center*
VA Connecticut Healthcare
West Haven, Connecticut

Pedro Ruiz M.D.
Professor and Vice Chairman
Department of Psychiatry and Behavioral Sciences
The University of Texas Medical School
Houston, Texas

Ethan Russo M.D.
Neurologist
Clinical Assistant Professor
University of Washington School of Medicine
Seattle, Washington
Adjunct Associate Professor
Department of Pharmacy
University of Montana
Missoula, Montana

Edward A. Salsitz M.D.
Associate Professor of Medicine
Beth Israel Medical Center
New York, New York

Sally Satel M.D.
Lecturer
Department of Psychiatry
Yale University School of Medicine
New Haven, Connecticut

Martin Schechter M.D.
Director, Department of Healthcare and
*   Epidemiology*
Faculty of Medicine
University of British Columbia
Vancouver, British Columbia, Canada

Joy M. Schmitz Ph.D.
Professor
Department of Psychiatry and Behavioral Sciences
University of Texas Medical School
Houston, Texas

Tony Scro M.S.
Grievance Coordinator
National Alliance of Methadone Advocates
New York, New York

Peter A. Selwyn M.D., M.P.H.
Professor and Chairman
Department of Family Medicine Community Health
Albert Einstein College of Medicine
Chairman
Department of Family Medicine
Montefiore Medical Center
Bronx, New York

Richard B. Seymour M.A.
Director, Haight Ashbury Publications
Editor in Chief, Journal of Psychoactive Drugs
  and International Addictions Infoline
San Francisco, California

Charles W. Sharp Ph.D.
(Retired)
Associate Director for Special Programs
Division of Preclinical Research
National Insitute on Drug Abuse
Rockville, Maryland

Eric Simon Ph.D.
Professor of Psychiatry and Pharmacology
New York University School of Medicine
New York, New York

Zili Sloboda Sc.D.
Institute of Health and Social Policy
The University of Akron
Akron, Ohio

David E. Smith M.D.
Founder and Medical Director
Haight Asbury Free Clinics, Inc.,
Medical Director, State of California Alcohol and
  Drug Programs
San Francisco, California

James L. Sorensen Ph.D.
Professor
Department of Psychiatry
University of California
San Francisco, California

M. Duncan Stanton Ph.D.
Professor of Psychiatry
University of Rochester School of Medicine
  and Dentistry
Division of Family Programs
Strong Memorial Hospital
Rochester, New York

Jodi Star M.D.
Assistant Professor
McKnight Brain Institute
Department of Psychiatry
Gainesville, Florida

Zebulon Taintor M.D.
Professor and Vice Chair
Department of Psychiatry
New York University Medical School
New York, New York

Douglas V. Talbott M.D.
Medical Director Emeritus
Talbott Recovery Campus
Atlanta, Georgia

Hermano Tavares M.D., Ph.D.
Post-doctoral Fellow
Department of Psychiatry
University of Calgary
Calgary, Alberta, Canada

Alan Trachtenberg M.D.
Assistant Clinical Professor
Department of Psychiatry
Cornell-Weill Medical College
New York, New York
Director
Recovery Center
Department of Psychiatry
Lincoln Medical and Mental Health Center
Bronx, New York

John W. Tsuang M.D.
Associate Clinical Professor
Department of Psychiatry
UCLA School of Medicine
Los Angeles, California

J. Thomas Ungerleider M.D.
Professor, Emeritus of Psychiatry
UCLA School of Medicine
Los Angeles, California

C. Fernando Valenzuela Ph.D.
Assistant Professor
Department of Neurosciences
University of New Mexico School of Medicine
Albuquerque, New Mexico

Wilfred G. van Gorp Ph.D.
Professor of Psychiatry
Columbia University
New York, New York

Karl G. Verebey Ph.D.
Director
Clincal Laboratory
Ammon Analytical
Hollside, New Jersey

Arnold M. Washton Ph.D.
Private Practice
Addiction Psychology
New York, New York

Sandra Welch M.D.
Professor
Department of Pharmacology and Toxicology
Virginia Commonwealth University
Richmond, Virginia

Donald R. Wesson M.D.
Consultant
CNS Medications Development
Oakland, California

Joseph J. Westermeyer M.D., M-PH., Ph.D.
Professor
Department of Psychiatry
University of Minnesota
Minneapolis, Minnesota

Philip O. Wilson Ph.D.
Addictionologist
Talbott Recovery Campus
Atlanta, Georgia

Charles Winick Ph.D.
Professor, Emeritus of Sociology
CUNY Graduate School
New York, New York

Alex Wodak M.D.
Director, Alcohol and Drug Service
St. Vincents Hospital
Sydney, Australia

Joycelyn Sue Woods M.A.
President
National Alliance of Methadone
  Advocates
New York, New York

George E. Woody M.D.
Professor of Psychiatry
Department of Psychiatry
University of Pennsylvania School
  of Medicine
Philadelphia, Pennsylvania

Garrett J. Zelen M.D.
Private Practice
Los Angeles, California

Monica L. Zilberman M.D., Ph.D.
Post-Doctoral Fellow
Department of Psychiatry
University of Calgary
Calgary, Alberta, Canada

Stephen R. Zukin M.D.
Director, Clinical Research
Neuroscience Astrazeneca
Wilmington, Delaware

Contents

V. Evaluation and Early Treatment

VI. Treatment Approaches

XII. Other Populations

XIII. Models of Prevention

XIV. Training and Education

XV. Policy Issues

CHAPTER 1

Historical Perspectives

DAVID F. MUSTO

The last three decades of the nineteenth century saw far-reaching transformations in American life. With immigration from all parts of Europe and from Asia, the population expanded greatly and became heterogeneous in speech, religion, and way of life. Many of the immigrants, unprepared to join the agricultural sector of the economy, crowded into the growing cities, which soon began to exhibit today's familiar urban problems. With the industrial revolution, large enterprises grew and attained a new level of economic power; with the construction of the railroads, vast areas of the West were opened for settlement and exploitation of the timber and mineral resources. In social terms, the geographic dispersal of the population that occurred as many moved west spelled the end of the once close-knit family. In political terms, these changes terminated the hegemony of the Protestant, North European group that had controlled the affairs of the nation through the Civil War.

The variety of social ills that inevitably attended these rapid changes in all aspects of life gave rise to a spirit of reform that ran through American culture from the mid-nineteenth century to 1920. This reformist or "progressive" impulse stemmed largely from the fear of social disorder among the same middle- and upper-class citizens whose political and economic power was increasingly insecure. Rapid transformation seemed to threaten the heart of American life. While most reforms of the Progressive Era (1890–1917) were aimed at curing the disorder itself, some movements naturally responded to specific evils that seemed to result from the upheaval (1). Increasingly, crime and immorality were blamed on easily obtained narcotics

and alcohol. This goal of moral uplift of the underprivileged was shared by Progressive Era temperance activists, political reformers, and crusaders against the indiscriminate use of psychoactive substances such as opium and cocaine.

THE BACKGROUND OF PROGRESSIVE ERA REFORMS

Alcohol and the Prohibition Movement

Alcohol had been the object of recurrent prohibition crusades in the nineteenth century, and as the Progressive Era developed, some sociologists began to speculate that alcohol abuse was actually the result, rather than the cause, of poverty. However, alcohol seemed to exacerbate almost all the evils of a disorderly society. Even if it could not be wholly blamed for economic failure, it certainly did not help. Alcohol lowered efficiency and productivity and, in the eyes of the reformers, increased all the evils of the urban scene: prostitutes worked in and around saloons; alcohol apparently made men more susceptible to the influence of corrupt city bosses; and it broke up families and invited violence. It reduced the chances for freedom, prosperity, and happiness and did not contribute to the virtue and enlightened character of an electorate needed by a democracy.

Furthermore, alcohol worsened the situation of Protestant Christianity. Not only was the saloon associated with Catholic immigrants, but it also seemed to make people incapable of responding to evangelical Protestantism (2). If it made a person unconcerned about something as urgent as salvation, then surely it would make that person oblivious to public concerns. Democratization, therefore, made it even more important that the saloon be abolished. Extending the powers of the landless class, in itself, posed quite a threat to stability; drunken masses would constitute an intolerable danger (3).

1

With the final temperance movement that led to the adoption in 1919 of the Eighteenth Amendment, the nation moved toward implementation of a prohibition justified on moral, religious, and scientific grounds (4). It is quite likely that by 1919 a majority of Americans believed that liquor prohibition would be a great benefit in reducing poverty, crime, broken families, lost work time, and immorality. Eventually, every state except Rhode Island and Connecticut ratified the amendment.

Narcotics, Cocaine, and Cannabis

By the end of the nineteenth century, the narcotics problem was also worrying reform-minded legislators, health professionals, and the laity. Opium in its crude form had been imported into North America from the time of the earliest European settlements. Various medicines were made from it. Alcohol extracts of crude opium included laudanum and paregoric, and opium was mixed with other drugs in patent medicines, among the most popular of which was Dover's Powder, originating in England in the eighteenth century. American statistics on opium imports were not kept until the 1840s, but from that time on, domestic consumption rose rapidly until the mid-1890s, when the annual importation of crude opium leveled off at about a half million pounds (5). After passage of federal laws in 1914 strictly limiting importation of opium, the import statistics became less helpful in estimating national consumption, and smuggling became a greater problem. Yet, statistics for the pre-World War I period provide good evidence that a steady increase of opium use in the United States occurred in the nineteenth century and that when the twentieth century began, there was already a substantial consumption of the drug for medicinal and nonmedicinal purposes. State laws regulating the availability of narcotics were first enacted around the time of the Civil War, and many states attempted to control the drugs by the 1890s.

Several major technologic and chemical advances made the most powerful ingredients in opium available in pure, cheap form. In the first decade of the nineteenth century, morphine was isolated from opium, and by 1832, American pharmaceutical manufacturers were preparing morphine from imported crude opium. Codeine was isolated in 1832, and this less-addicting substance became a common form of manufactured derivative, particularly after morphine and heroin were severely restricted in the United States after World War I (6,7). Heroin, a trade name of the Bayer Company for diacetylmorphine, was introduced commercially in 1898, with the hope that acetylation of the morphine molecule would reduce its side effects while maintaining its effectiveness in suppressing the cough reflex. A similar hope was entertained the next year for acetylation of salicylic acid, a mild analgesic with undesirable side effects, which was then marketed as Aspirin, the Bayer trademark for sodium acetylsalicylate. Heroin, of course, proved to be at least as addictive as morphine and eventually ousted morphine as the drug of choice among American drug habitués (8). The increasing use of heroin in this period is an example of the effectiveness of three innovations adopted by nineteenth-century industrial enterprises: manufacturing, rapid distribution, and effective marketing techniques.

Coca leaves, in their indigenous growth areas in South America, were known to have stimulant properties and had been used for centuries by natives. Coca's unusual properties were popularized in Europe and America in the mid-nineteenth century, and an alcohol extract of the leaves, which contained some of the active stimulant cocaine, often appeared under the name "wine of coca." In the 1880s, pure cocaine became more easily available because of advances in manufacturing technology, and it was immediately praised, especially in the United States. Its stimulating and euphoric properties were touted for athletes, workers, and students, and bottlers of popular soda drinks, and easily obtained "tonics" added cocaine to obtain a stimulant effect. Medical uses were soon discovered, and worldwide experimentation established cocaine as an anesthetic for the surface of the eye and as a block to pain stimuli when injected near a nerve. The stimulant properties were bothersome side effects of cocaine when used as an anesthetic, but within a few decades, satisfactory substitutes were developed that were considered less habituating, such as procaine in 1905. Cocaine was also convenient for shrinking nasal and sinus membranes, and it became one of the early effective remedies for "hay fever," allergies, and sinusitis. As an over-the-counter remedy for hay fever or "nasal catarrh," in powder form to be sniffed or as a spray, cocaine began to be criticized as misused or carelessly dispensed for mere pleasure or dissipation.

In the period from about 1895 to 1915, cocaine became associated in the popular and medical press with southern blacks' hostility toward whites. Vicious crimes said to have been perpetrated by blacks were commonly attributed to the effects of cocaine. In efforts to pass antinarcotic legislation, this association was repeated by federal officials and spokesmen for the health professions, although direct evidence for such a close and specifically racial association was wanting or even contradictory (9). Eighty years ago, cocaine was considered a typically "Negro" drug, whereas opiates, and specifically heroin, were described as characteristically "white," illustrating the influence of social tensions and racial stereotypes on interpretation of the narcotics problem.

Cannabis, or marihuana, in the form of "reefers" or "joints," seems to have been unfamiliar in the United States until the twentieth century, yet there has been a long-standing fear of hashish, a concentrated and powerful form of cannabis. Hashish was known from its use as an esoteric and perilous drug popular in the Middle East and from the description of its bizarre effects by literary figures who experimented with it in the mid-nineteenth century (10).

PROGRESSIVE ERA FOOD AND DRUG REFORMS (1898–1906)

Faced with what they perceived as social breakdown associated with the pernicious effects of drugs and alcohol, reformers turned to the federal government. In the period leading to the Progressive Era, state and local laws were losing credibility as effective measures to control distribution and consumption of both alcohol and psychoactive drugs. The failure was usually ascribed to the patchwork-quilt character of laws below the federal level of government (11). But federal action was limited by the few constitutional bases for laws that would affect abuses. Other than the tariff, the federal government was restricted mostly to regulating interstate commerce and levying taxes. Police and health powers, obviously the most appropriate for combating addiction and illicit drugs, were the province of the states. For example, the United States Public Health Service and its antecedent agencies were limited to dealing with communicable diseases and gathering and disseminating such medical information as vital statistics and public health advice; they could not provide direct delivery of health services except to their legal wards, chiefly the Merchant Marine and American Indians (12). The armed services excepted, federal police agencies included alcohol tax agents, members of the Coast Guard, and customs and immigration officers. Therefore, there was little precedent for federal regulation of dangerous drugs, and no federal policing agency could easily add this burden to its current duties. As a result, the range of activities that were left to an individual's or company's sense of fair play was remarkably large. In the nineteenth century, federal law did not require the labeling of drugs on over-the-counter proprietaries. Thus, these patent medicines could contain any amount of, say, morphine without acknowledgment, and could even aver that the potion contained no morphine. The percentage of alcohol in some popular remedies was higher than that in many cocktails today. Claims that a proprietary could cure cancer, tuberculosis, or any other ailment were legally unchallengeable; no tests of efficacy, purity, or standardization were required. In addition, newspapers, the primary source of information for most Americans, were chary of offending their advertisers, and many papers had contracts with proprietary manufacturers that would become invalid with the enactment of any state law requiring disclosure of contents or any modification of advertising claims (13).

Hence, it is not surprising that no federal law requiring content information and some accuracy of claims was enacted until 1906, when public concern reached a pitch sufficient to propel the government to resort to its power over interstate commerce to enact such a measure. The law, the Pure Food and Drug Act, contained some of the earliest federal provisions affecting narcotics; if any over-the-counter remedy in interstate commerce contained an opiate, cannabis, cocaine, or chloral hydrate, the label was required to state its contents and percentage. The effect of this simple measure apparently was to reduce the amount of such drugs in popular remedies and also to hurt their sales, although other proprietaries flourished. The Proprietary Association of America, dismayed at the accusation of being "dopers," favored strict limitation of dangerous drugs in their products and ostracized manufacturers who continued to put such drugs as cocaine in "asthma cures."

Although a step had been taken to warn proprietary users of the amount of dangerous drugs in the remedies, still nothing had been done to bring under control another target of reform: "dope doctors" and pharmacists who purveyed opiates and cocaine to anyone who asked for them. The percentage of such deviants in each profession was not large, but they took advantage of the broad authority given to all licensed pharmacists and physicians to use their professional judgment in the delivery of medicines and services, and the dominance of the state in the licensing of the health professions seemed unassailable by the federal government. In addition to purchasing drugs from professional miscreants, one could order them from mail-order houses. How to rectify this promiscuous distribution of narcotics presented another difficult constitutional problem for federal action.

TOWARD PROHIBITION OF NARCOTIC DRUGS (1909–1919)

The Shanghai Commission and the Smoking Opium Act (1909)

Several bills directed at the traffic in narcotics had been introduced into Congress before 1908, but federal legislation was accomplished only after President Theodore Roosevelt convened the Shanghai Opium Commission in 1909 to aid the Chinese Empire in its desire to stamp out opium addiction, particularly opium smoking (14). The measure, intended more as evidence of America's good faith in convening the commission than as an adequate weapon against American narcotic abuse, was modest and limited. Called The Smoking Opium Exclusion Act, it outlawed importation of opium prepared for smoking (15). Its passage while the Shanghai Commission was in session under the chairmanship of an American, the Right Reverend Charles H. Brent, Episcopal bishop of the Philippine Islands, was designed to show the delegates of other nations that the United States was willing to take steps to aid control of world opium traffic. American delegates reported back to the State Department that the announcement of the act's passage was met with an impressive response from the other 12 nations represented.

The American delegates, however, and indeed the departments most closely associated with narcotic policy planning—State, Treasury, and Agriculture—were aware that the legislation against smoking opium was but the first step in controlling a national problem described as serious and threatening to progress. The nation needed a law that more closely controlled sales of over-the-counter remedies, excessive or careless prescribing of narcotics, and other avenues of easy access to narcotics. The question, of course, was how the federal government could accomplish this by constitutional means. Both the power to regulate interstate commerce and to levy taxes provided some basis for federal narcotics control. The State Department, which coordinated domestic legislation and planning until 1914, eventually opted for the latter, reasoning that by using tax administration, all narcotics could be traced, not just drugs shipped from one state to another.

The first of the administration's proposed bills, drafted in 1909, provided for extremely harsh penalties and was intricately detailed but without exemption for proprietaries that contained very small amounts of the narcotics (16). The effect of such bills would have been to make the handling of narcotic preparations so risky and complicated for retail outlets that the whole narcotic traffic would fall into the hands of physicians. The physicians would be limited only by their good judgment and by restrictions that state legislatures might enact (e.g., record keeping, prohibiting the refilling of narcotic prescriptions, or maintaining addicts) (17).

Such tough proposals met with opposition from the rank and file of the drug trades, proprietary manufacturers, and some members of Congress who feared, among other things, that such a precedent might be extended to alcohol. Before the Webb-Kenyon Act was passed over President Taft's veto in 1913 and upheld by the Supreme Court, it was legal to live in a dry state, purchase liquor from a wet state, and have it delivered via interstate commerce.

The Hague Treaty (1912)

While domestic debate continued among the specific interests affected by the proposed narcotic legislation, the United States continued its campaign to regulate the international traffic in narcotics. Because the Shanghai Commission was not empowered to draft a treaty (the delegates could only make recommendations), American diplomats sought a second meeting for the preparation of an international treaty. After much persuasion and repeated setbacks, the Netherlands, at America's request, convened the International Opium Conference at The Hague in December 1911. Again, Bishop Brent, head of the American delegation, was chosen to preside, and after weeks of debate and compromise, the delegates signed The Hague Opium Convention in January 1912 (5). The title is somewhat misleading; the treaty also sought to control cocaine. An American and Italian suggestion that cannabis be included was not accepted.

The Hague Treaty emphasized enactment of legislation in each nation to control the production of crude substances, their manufacture into pharmaceutical products, and their distribution within the nation and abroad (18). The United States government believed that its people were extravagant consumers of opiates; federal publications reported that the country was, by far, the largest consumer of opium per capita among Western nations. In the words of the State Department's opium commissioner, Dr. Hamilton Wright, "Uncle Sam is the worst drug fiend in the world," consuming, he claimed, more opium per capita than the fabled opium-using Chinese (19). The thought within the State Department was that if the nations that grew opium and coca enacted strict legislation in the spirit of the treaty, the American problem would be greatly reduced, perhaps would even vanish. The challenge was to persuade other nations to have a "correct" view of narcotic use and to enforce legislation in accord with this view.

Yet the stern international measures envisaged by such reformers as Dr. Wright were not adopted before World War I. The Hague Treaty was not airtight; its vague phrases did not compel the ratifying nations to enact strict laws to reduce narcotic distribution to solely medical purposes. Moreover, American domestic legislation, now promoted as the American implementation of The Hague Treaty, was still hampered by doctrines of states' rights and constitutional interpretation, to say nothing of the competing interests of physicians, pharmacists, and manufacturers of proprietary medicines.

The Harrison Act (1914)

In 1913, the administration of President Woodrow Wilson drafted legislation grounded in its constitutional taxation power. It was hoped that the new measure would, at the very least, bring into the open the vast narcotic traffic so that the states could take appropriate health and police measures or step up enforcement of existing laws. At the most, Wright hoped the Harrison Act, as the legislation was called, would be recognized as the fulfillment of an international obligation in accord with Article VI of the Constitution and thus take precedence over the rights of states. If this were the case, the general phraseology of the Harrison Bill, such as requiring the prescription of narcotics "in good faith," could be interpreted broadly and would allow prosecution of "dope doctors," other malpracticing professionals, and peddlers.

The measure passed the House of Representatives relatively easily but slowed down in the Senate and did not finally pass into law until December 1914. It was to come into effect on March 1, 1915 (20). In its final form, the act allowed proprietary medicines to include small amounts of narcotics, and physicians were not required to keep records of medicines dispensed while they personally attended a patient. Legitimate purveyors of opiate and cocaine preparations were required to register with the Bureau of Internal

Revenue and obtain a tax stamp, for which they paid one dollar per year. Detailed record keeping was required for most transactions, and legal possession by a consumer was made dependent on a physician's or dentist's prescription. Individual consumers were forbidden to register (21). But when federal personnel sought to arrest the dope doctors for prescribing, they discovered that many federal district court judges thought the action was an infringement of state police powers. In 1916, a crucial Supreme Court interpretation, known as the first *Jin Fuey Moy* decision, held that it was beyond federal powers to prohibit narcotics possession by anyone to whom the Treasury Department had refused registration, such as a peddler or addict (22).

Not until the height of the war effort—and in the midst of a zealous drive to rid the nation of perceived threats to its integrity and security—was a successful campaign mounted to strengthen the Harrison Act to prevent health professionals from dispensing narcotics to persons whose only problem was addiction itself.

DRUG CONTROL IN A PERIOD OF DIMINISHING USE (1919–1962)

Size and Symbolism of the Addiction Problem

The true size of the drug abuse problem in the early decades of the twentieth century (Dr. Wright's hyperbole not withstanding) was a matter of public debate, much as it is today. Whereas the Public Health Service in rather sober studies published in 1915 and 1924 argued that there were probably never more than a quarter million habitual users of opiates and cocaine in the nation, the Treasury Department assessed the number at slightly more than one million, who were described as moral wretches for the most part (23,24). New York City officials claimed that heroin addicts were responsible for huge numbers of crimes and estimated that in 1924, the remarkable figure of 75% of all crimes were committed by addicts (25). In 1919, the mayor of New York City linked heroin with anarchism and political bombings (26)—and his was not an isolated opinion. There was fear in the nation about several groups that were considered extreme domestic threats: socialists, members of the Industrial Workers of the World, Bolsheviks, and addicts (27). The image of the addict as immoral and criminal, a belief dating back among respectable writers and observers well into the nineteenth century, made them an obvious target for serious social reformers, as well as for ambitious politicians and bureaucrats. If one accepted that they numbered more than 1 million in a nation of 100 million, stern action and uncompromising control seemed entirely justified. Nevertheless, this sentiment coexisted with experiments in public-health-based addiction management and medical theories of addiction as a treatable disease. When the results of attempts at treatment proved disappointing, faith in treatment waned, and

the punitive model of drug abuse control won, as it were, by default.

Maintenance Clinics (1912–1925)

Beginning in 1912 in Jacksonville, Florida, 40-odd clinics were established in various parts of the country to supply addicts with maintenance doses of narcotics in what were designed to be controlled conditions. The clients were usually those too poor or socially marginal to have access to private physicians. A relatively small percentage of the nation's addicts were enrolled in these clinics, particularly if one accepted the extravagant estimate of more than a million addicts for the whole nation. It is likely that the number of addicts registered at any one time in maintenance clinics did not exceed 5,000 (28). The average age of patrons was about 30 years, and they had usually been addicts for at least several years before joining the clinic. Some clinics were operated by police departments (e.g., New Haven) and others by health departments (e.g., Atlanta), and attitudes toward the clinics varied from one city to another. Some were clearly operated under political patronage and for a profit. In a few instances, as in Albany, New York, both cocaine and morphine were dispensed.

An exception to the policy of almost all these clinics, which was to maintain addicts indefinitely on morphine, was the clinic operated in 1919 and 1920 by the New York City Department of Health. Here heroin was used to entice addicts into a detoxification and rehabilitation program. After almost a year of operation, the city ended its experiment. It found that almost all addicts, even if detoxified, returned to heroin after release from six weeks of hospital treatment. The Health Department concluded that restriction of availability by the police and federal agents was necessary if addiction was to be effectively diminished. About 7,500 persons registered at the clinic, and almost all received gradually decreasing doses of heroin; 10% were younger than age 19 years (29).

Adoption of a Federal Antimaintenance Policy

Given the inadequacy and variety of state laws, there seemed no way to control physicians and pharmacists—even though the unethical percentage was small—other than by imposition of federal authority. If a physician could exercise judgment as to when and whom to maintain in an opiate habit, it was certain that some physicians would be unscrupulous, thus spreading the habit and reaping a profit. Therefore, in addition to reforms in the medical and pharmaceutical professions, the goal of the federal government was to restrict that breadth of medical judgment by law. The undertaking was hazardous, for such federal encroachment on medicine was unprecedented; the physician would be allowed to maintain an opiate addict only if approved by a local narcotics agent. These exceptions would be chiefly iatrogenically addicted and middle-class patients. (One should keep in mind that some observers believed that physicians created about half of American opiate addiction.)

In 1918, partly to counteract the *Jin Fuey Moy* decision, the Treasury Department established a Special Committee on Narcotics Traffic. The committee helped persuade Congress to pass strengthening legislation in February 1919 (30). Then, aiding the government effort, the Supreme Court, in two fundamental interpretations of the act, rejected by a vote of five to four the argument that it was legal to maintain an addict by prescription if the addict had no problem except addiction (31). To carry out the strict Supreme Court ruling that addiction maintenance be severely limited in the United States, a Narcotics Division was established in the Treasury Department in December 1919. It was part of the newly formed Prohibition Unit of the Internal Revenue Bureau, which had been created to enforce liquor prohibition. Its first head was Levi G. Nutt, a pharmacist from Ohio who had risen in the ranks of the tax unit. He now oversaw about 150 narcotic agents scattered across the nation.

Addiction Disease and Law Enforcement

One result of antimaintenance law enforcement, which was backed by leading physicians and such reformers as Dr. Alexander Lambert, president of the American Medical Association (AMA) in 1919, was a curious decline in the respectability of a certain medical theory that would have admitted maintenance as a rational therapy response: the immunochemical theory of opiate addiction. This happened because both reformers and government agents feared maintenance and were disgusted by the subterfuges some health professionals used to justify a profitable trade. Their fear and disgust extended to suspicion of any justification for maintenance. Supplying drugs to an addict came to be considered a form of medical malpractice that endangered society by perpetuating criminal and immoral persons in their esoteric pleasures.

In the immunologic reasoning that was popular among some addiction experts prior to 1919, the argument ran that ingestion of, say, morphine stimulated the formation of antibodies, like those produced against smallpox virus, or of antitoxins, like those produced against the toxins of the diphtheria bacterium. Such theories were popular explanations for illnesses in the late nineteenth and early twentieth centuries, and in many cases, saved lives. With regard to addiction, and according to several competent and respected clinicians, the theory held that maintenance doses of an opiate would be required to bring an addict's physiology into balance with the level of antibodies or antitoxins present. If too little opiate were administered, the body would begin to experience withdrawal symptoms as a result of the action of unneutralized antibodies or antitoxins; if too much opiate were administered, the body

would experience the physiologic effects of opiates. According to Dr. Ernest Bishop of New York, the amount of opiate required to balance an individual's physiology could be determined with great precision, and the addict would remain a fully normal person only so long as this exact dose was maintained. However, Dr. Bishop did not rule out cure in some instances by various popular medical regimens (32).

The intimate link between this scientific theory and its implications for public policy made its adherents suspect. Those who practiced medicine in accordance with the theory could be indicted and convicted of violating the laws defining what was legitimate medical practice as interpreted by 1919 Supreme Court decisions. When Dr. A. G. DuMez of the Hygienic Laboratory (now the National Institutes of Health), one of the leading addiction experts of the United States Public Health Service, published his endorsement of some of the immunologic experiments in 1919, he was asked by the AMA's Committee on Addiction to retract his statement, which he did, in part, by qualifying his previous endorsement (33,34). Within two years, the question of the cause of addiction was so controversial that the Surgeon General of the Public Health Service wrote the president of the Louisiana State Board of Health to advise that the phrase "physiological balance" was too controversial to be included in a description of narcotic treatment and the enforcement problem (14).

It was soon demonstrated that immunologic substances could not be found in the blood; the adherents of "addiction disease" caused by a simple and easily detectable immunologic process were evidently in error. Yet the intense political nature of the addiction question and the fear of addicts, whose numbers were very likely overestimated, had an impact on the exchange of scientific information and medical practice. At the level of social planning, maintenance was judged poor public policy, and it was to be eliminated if at all possible. This decision might, indeed, have been the correct one, but the suddenness of implementation and the emotionally charged attitude toward addicts and their maintainers caused policy to collide dramatically with research and medical opinion.

The events of 1919 spelled the eventual end of the clinic experiment and of the concept of addiction as a health problem. Maintenance of nonmedical addicts had become illegal, even if records were carefully kept and a physician examined every patient and tried to keep the drug down to a minimum. By 1925, all the clinics known to the Narcotics Division had been closed.

The rapidity with which opinion on controversial questions like addiction and narcotics can be crystallized is one of the most interesting features of narcotic control in the United States. To resist the closure of maintenance was difficult; the new policy ensued from the anger, scapegoating, fatigue, and frustration of the lawmakers because a simple answer to addiction was still not available. The burden for the next several decades would rest on law enforcement to prevent illegal access to narcotic supplies. The hope for a simple medical cure had been dashed.

Fear of Federal Control on the Part of Health Professions

Court decisions continued to restrict what remained of a physician's right to maintain an addict. Procedures used by agents to get information led to hostility and suspicion, but the reason that enforcement personnel used such methods as informers was that they had repeatedly encountered determined profit-making physicians whose concern for the welfare of their patients and the community was nil. A further disagreement between the federal government and the medical profession arose from a question even more fundamental than maintenance: Did the federal government have the right to interfere with medical practice and exempt certain classes of patients from a doctor's judgment? The medical profession came out of the social agitation associated with World War I with a fear that the federal government would enter into "state medicine" or compulsory health insurance. After 1920, the AMA greatly resisted the various federal measures concerning health, such as the Sheppard-Towner Act for Maternal and Child Care, which was to be financed by matching grants to the states. The medical profession fought such federal intervention with great vigor and generally with success (35).

Yet the Harrison Act remained a thorn in the side of professional medicine. If it was constitutional for government to say who could be maintained or not, a precedent was set for further incursions into medical practice. A similar problem for the AMA was the Willis-Campbell Act of 1921, which limited a physician's prescriptions for alcohol to a fairly modest number and placed other restrictions on the kind and amount of alcohol that could be prescribed. Hence, physicians were disturbed at the Harrison and Willis-Campbell Acts in part not because they wanted to maintain addicts or become saloonkeepers (although at times a few seemed quite willing to do just that), but because they were fearful of where this unprecedented use of federal power in the health fields might lead.

Narcotic Drugs Import and Export Act (1922)

After the outlawing of addiction maintenance, a series of federal statutes in the 1920s sought to fill gaps in the federal control of narcotics. The first, the Narcotic Drugs Import and Export Act of 1922, permitted only crude narcotics to enter the United States; American drug companies would manufacture them into pure substances (36). Any subsequently manufactured foreign narcotic product in the United States, like Swiss morphine or German cocaine, was illegal. Intricate restrictions were placed on American export and transshipment of narcotics because it was feared that a great deal of morphine was arriving in China, via Japan, in this manner or that it was being smuggled back into the United States after export to Canada or Mexico. Finally, the Federal Narcotic Control Board, composed of the secretaries of Treasury, Commerce, and State, was established to authorize legitimate imports and exports.

Restrictions on Heroin (1924)

In the mid-1920s, the United States attempted to obtain international sanctions against the manufacture of heroin, which by then was considered the most dangerous narcotic, particularly for adolescents. Most of the crime in New York City was blamed on heroin, including daring bank robberies, senseless violence, and murders. The danger of heroin was exaggerated by respectable antinarcotic reformers in order to inform the American people of its peril. One excellent example is the educational campaign of Captain Richmond Pearson Hobson, a hero of the Spanish-American War, former congressman, and ardent Prohibitionist, who directed his speaking and organizational talents against narcotics shortly after the Eighteenth Amendment's ratification. Captain Hobson was wont to warn women who habitually used any particular face powder to have it checked for heroin, lest they become addicted. He claimed that one dose of heroin was addictive, and that an ounce of heroin could addict 2,000 persons. He blamed a national crime wave on heroin, claiming that it was a stimulant to senseless violence. He desired that a compilation of such warnings be sent into every American home and requested Congress to print 50 million copies of his eight-page brochure, "The Peril of Narcotics" (37). The pamphlet was not printed, but a revised version of his message was printed in the Congressional Record and distributed by sympathetic congressmen (38). Hobson represents a popularizer of heroin dangers who disseminated grossly erroneous information on addiction that tended to alarm the public while providing a convenient explanation for unrelated, serious social problems.

In 1924, partly to encourage other nations to regulate narcotics and partly to assist in the American fight against addiction, Congress prohibited importation of crude opium into the United States for the manufacture of heroin (39). The author of this legislation, Representative Stephen Porter of Pittsburgh, chairman of the House Foreign Affairs Committee, took the leading congressional role in the international negotiations and planning for domestic control of narcotics in the 1920s.

Federal Narcotic Farms (1929)

Porter's second major effort was to provide for two "narcotic farms" where addicts could be treated as sick individuals and detoxified, and where they could perhaps assist investigators in the search for a cure (40). A factor in this legislation was that federal prisons were becoming jammed with Harrison Act violators, most of whom were also addicts. Congress had to build either two new prisons or two treatment centers. Thus came into being the Lexington, Kentucky, and Fort Worth, Texas, narcotic hospitals operated by the United States Public Health Service. This legislation also provided for the Public Health Service Narcotics Division, which evolved into the present National Institute of Mental Health (NIMH) and National Institute on Drug Abuse (NIDA).

The Federal Bureau of Narcotics (1930)

Finally, Representative Porter sought to establish in the Treasury Department an independent narcotics agency. The Narcotics Division had accompanied the Prohibition Unit when the latter was raised to the rank of bureau in 1927, and although still subordinate and headed by an assistant commissioner, it was gradually expanding. In 1930, shortly before his death, Porter shepherded through Congress the act creating the Federal Bureau of Narcotics (FBN) (41). When the Prohibition Bureau moved from the Treasury Department to the Justice Department in the mid-1920s, the Narcotics Division remained behind, but its head, Levi G. Nutt, was not to become the first commissioner of narcotics. Nutt's son and son-in-law were implicated by a federal grand jury in "indiscreet" dealings with the recently slain New York narcotics underworld figure, Arnold Rothstein (42). Nutt was transferred from his post a week after the filing of the grand jury's report, which also touched on his own activities and those of the New York district office. Assistant Prohibition Commissioner Harry J. Anslinger was picked from the international control section of the Prohibition Bureau to take temporary charge of the Narcotics Division.

Anslinger had not been deeply involved with narcotics; his training was in the foreign service and in international negotiations to cut off rum running. To Representative Porter, however, he seemed the ideal candidate. Accustomed to what Porter likely regarded as foreign wiles and ulterior motives in areas of American moral concern, he could ably represent the United States in its struggle, dating back to 1906, to achieve international control of narcotics traffic. The medical aspect of the question seemed secondary, for if smuggling could be ended, the narcotics problem would take care of itself.

Thus began the 32-year tenure of Commissioner Anslinger. Most of the enforcement questions had been settled: maintenance was illegal; the image of the heroin addict was well-publicized by such spokesmen as Captain Hobson; and a national system of agents was established with fairly well-defined styles of enforcement, although there was the eternal integrity problem in the agents' dealings with smugglers. The most profound effect on narcotics enforcement in the immediate future was not new policies but the Depression, which drastically reduced the FBN's budget, led to detailed scrutiny of even its telephone bills by Congress, and probably helped ex-

plain the parsimony characteristic of the Anslinger tenure. Even in the 1960s, the Bureau made a fetish of a low budget.

The Marihuana Problem (1930–1937)

Commissioner Anslinger's first major issue appeared even as he took office—a quickly burgeoning fear centered in the Southwest about a plant grown and used by Mexicans who had poured into the region as farm laborers in the prosperous 1920s. This drug or plant was known as locoweed, marihuana, or, more scientifically, cannabis. As the fear of marihuana grew, so did the belief that it stimulated violence and was being slyly sold to American school children. In the early 1930s, the FBN tried to minimize these fears and suggested that state laws were the appropriate response. The Uniform State Narcotic Drug Act proposed in 1932 included marihuana regulations as an option for state legislation; the Bureau thought it had found the solution. The plant grew in the United States, so the best response would be from local government, not from an agency that had its eyes on the smuggling of drugs from Turkey, France, Bolivia, China, and Siam.

Yet, recalled Anslinger, the Treasury Department decided to make marihuana use a federal offense, more as a gesture to the fearful Southwest than as a comprehensive and probably effective plan for marihuana control. The Department's bill was modeled on the National Firearms Act, which was declared constitutional by the Supreme Court in March 1937. In April, Treasury representatives went before Congress to ask for a similar "transfer tax" and licensing system for marihuana. Congress passed the Marihuana Tax Act of 1937 without dissent, and by October it was in effect (43). Opposition to the act in committee came from an AMA representative, Dr. William C. Woodward, who stated that this was an area of state concern, and that it should not become one more example of federal encroachment on the medical profession.

In the enforcement of the act, the Bureau described marihuana as a fearsome substance, but played down any suggestion that it was a problem out of control. The apparent goal was to make the drug unattractive, but not to create a panic over claims that it was widely disseminated to school children (10).

Adoption of Mandatory Minimum Sentences (1951–1956)

World War II brought narcotic use, particularly opiates, to a low point. Control over the growth of opium poppies had been sought in 1942 by the Opium Poppy Control Act (44). There was other legislation at this time to resolve technical problems, strengthen penalties, and include synthetic narcotics, such as meperidine, under federal regulations (45). At the close of hostilities, however, the FBN anticipated a resumption of illicit world narcotic trade. The Bureau looked back to World War I when, it was claimed, there had been a postwar upsurge. Consequently, when there was a rise in addiction among ghetto youth in Chicago and New York City in the late 1940s, and authorities noted a lower age among those sent to prisons or narcotic hospitals, the Bureau asked Congress for stronger penalties. The variability in judges' sentences and disposition of cases—a short sentence or probation for a trafficker the Bureau might have spent years trying to convict—led to the proposal to take sentencing of certain offenders out of the hands of judges. Also, a mandatory sentence might deter the potential trafficker or even the drug user.

Such legislation was introduced by Representative Hale Boggs and enacted in 1951 (46). In 1956, after Senate hearings chaired by Senator Price Daniel, the death penalty was allowed at the jury's discretion in some instances of heroin sales (47). This was the peak of punitive legislation against drug addiction in the United States. In a half century, the federal response to dangerous drugs had advanced from requiring accurate labeling of narcotics in over-the-counter remedies (but with no limit on how much could be present) to the possibility of the death penalty or, at least, a mandatory sentence for conveying heroin to a minor (regardless of the quantity of heroin).

Voices were raised against such harsh measures, but they were not very effective in modifying the course of events up to 1956. The American Bar Association (ABA) questioned the wisdom of mandatory minimum sentences, and a joint ABA-AMA committee began to examine the narcotics question with a philosophy far different from that embodied in the Boggs-Daniel acts. Staff of the committee looked at the British experience, in which legal heroin maintenance was available to the several hundred known addicts, and wondered whether some similar system would be suitable for the United States (48). Presidential and congressional confidence in various forms of psychological and chemical treatment flourished and was expressed in such national projects as the Community Mental Health Center program of 1963. Narcotic maintenance programs reappeared, using the synthetic narcotic methadone. The police effort to make narcotic supplies scarce—which seemed so reasonable to progressive medical leadership in 1919—began to seem crude, ineffective, and conducive to gross malfeasance. A turning point in the national approach to narcotics was again at hand.

DRUG CONTROL IN A PERIOD OF RISING USE (1962–1980)

Medical and Psychological Response to Addiction (1962–1970)

After Anslinger announced his retirement in 1962—a sign of hope to those wanting to see some form of maintenance or at least less reliance on mandatory prison sentences—President John F. Kennedy called the White House Conference on Narcotics and Drug Abuse (49). Its participants represented the various conflicting points of view; after the conference was over, the President's Advisory Commission on Narcotics and Drug Abuse considered how to carry out the spirit of reexamination and make specific recommendations. The Commission's *Final Report*, published in 1963, marks a definite, if small, shift from the trend to see all "narcotics" as equal in the sight of the law. There was a suggestion that psychological treatment might be useful and that some variations in prison sentencing, such as civil commitment, might prove effective against addiction (50).

In the 1960s, the appearance of psychedelic substances, such as lysergic acid diethylamide (LSD), and the quick rise in marihuana use drew attention to the varieties of drugs available and abusable. Further studies of marihuana suggested that it was less dangerous than had been assumed in the early 1930s, and the fact that millions of individuals were estimated to have used it in the 1960s also suggested that marihuana was not so very dangerous in moderate use. Other drugs, like amphetamines and barbiturates, became as popular in the streets as they had previously been common in middle-class homes. The number of heroin addicts began to rise, and the nation perceived itself under attack by a "drug culture" linked by many observers to a youth "counter-culture."

Both the legislative and executive branches of the government began to respond to the drug problem in ways that reflected, at the same time, concern about increasing drug use and changing opinions on the nature of drugs and the best ways to prevent abuse. The Drug Abuse Amendments of 1965 created the Bureau of Drug Abuse Control in the Department of Health, Education, and Welfare to address diversion and misuse of barbiturates and amphetamines; and the Narcotic Addict Rehabilitation Act of 1966 approved civil commitment as an alternative to prison for addicted drug offenders (51,52).

The high hopes held for civil commitment of drug addicts were not to be realized. At first such commitment seemed in keeping with advanced notions of psychological and milieu treatment, but it was modified to guarantee that the addict would remain for treatment. Yet the cost and length of treatment, as well as the dismal success rate, brought this apparently more sophisticated form of confinement into question. Civil commitment may also have conflicted with the legal rights of the individual: An addict could be confined for several years, not for a crime but because he or she had a disease. These many difficulties with civil commitment caused a shift from optimism in the Advisory Commission's report of 1963 to a close questioning of the concept in the report of the President's Commission on Law Enforcement and the Administration of Justice in 1967 (53).

Reorganization of the Federal Drug Control Bureaucracy

In response to political and social pressures similar to those that had prompted the transfer of the Prohibition Unit from the Treasury Department to the Justice Department in the late 1920s, the Federal Bureau of Narcotics was joined with the Bureau of Drug Abuse and Control in 1968 and moved to Justice under the name, Bureau of Narcotics and Dangerous Drugs (BNDD).

When Richard Nixon took office as president in 1969, his advisors saw almost immediately that narcotics control offered an opportunity to make good on Nixon's campaign promise to reduce crime (54). The first major legislative initiative of the Nixon administration was the Comprehensive Drug Abuse Prevention and Control Act of 1970, which brought together and rationalized all previous drug legislation under the interstate commerce powers of the federal government. The new law also established schedules that differentiated among the various drugs of abuse and formed the basis for a new penalty structure that abandoned mandatory minimum sentences (55).

In the spring of 1971, President Nixon issued an executive order that established the Special Action Office for Drug Abuse Prevention (SAODAP), a White House office that was meant to oversee the prevention and treatment programs of a host of cabinet departments and agencies. SAODAP was given statutory existence through the Drug Abuse Office and Treatment Act of 1972 (56). That same year a special unit in aid of local law enforcement called the Office of Drug Abuse Law Enforcement (ODALE) was also established through executive order, as was the Office of National Narcotics Intelligence (ONNI). The expenditure of the Bureau of Narcotics and Dangerous Drugs in fiscal year 1972 was more than $60 million, a remarkable amount when compared with the FBN expenditures in 1962 of about $4 million.

In 1973, ODALE and ONNI were combined with BNDD to form the Drug Enforcement Administration. Also in 1973, the National Institute on Drug Abuse (NIDA) evolved from SAODAP and the Division of Narcotics and Drug Abuse to the National Institute of Mental Health (NIMH). To date, the Drug Enforcement Agency (DEA) and the NIDA have pursued the law enforcement and drug research components of national drug policy (16).

Methadone Maintenance

Perhaps the most fundamental change in narcotics control of this period was the widespread use of methadone maintenance in control and treatment of narcotic addiction. The technique, begun in the 1960s, was given enthusiastic support by the Nixon administration, in no small measure because of its apparent effectiveness in reducing addict crime. Methadone is a long-acting synthetic narcotic that was developed in Germany during World War II.

It is given orally to lessen or even eliminate the desire for heroin. Some of the similarities between the use of and theoretical justification for methadone maintenance now and morphine maintenance in the World War I period are obvious, and both have encountered some of the same practical problems.

Some experts say that methadone may be required by a hard-core addict indefinitely; that is, it does not end narcotic addiction but makes it more socially acceptable or feasible. This policy runs counter to an old theme in American attitudes, namely, that addiction should be stopped, not catered to. As realized a half century ago, however, a maintenance system, if deployed across the nation, is difficult to regulate, and diversion of supplies to nonaddicts can be a problem. One objection to the old maintenance clinics was the enormous profits garnered by some individuals who operated them; the implication was that profits stimulated the distribution of narcotics and the temptation to recruit new customers. Another problem was the failure of neat scientific explanations, such as Dr. Bishop's theory that a patient in precise opiate maintenance balance is quite normal. This did not work out so conveniently in practice. Maintenance, which was legal, for example, in New York State in 1918 and 1919, eventually led to abuses among health professionals and, in times of national fear, made the thousands of addicts scapegoats for social problems. Legal maintenance systems can thus become unpalatable or abhorred. They are sensitive to public pressure and political influences, and their existence is precarious, especially when the public believes that addiction itself is the cause of immorality, criminal behavior, and loss of productivity.

Changing Mores, Changing Laws

Gerald R. Ford brought a markedly different political style to the White House in August 1974. The new president wanted to distance himself from Nixon's heated antidrug rhetoric and from his management style that had concentrated power in the White House at the expense of the cabinet departments. To these ends, Ford adamantly resisted congressional attempts to institute an Office of Drug Control Policy in the White House to continue SAODAP-style oversight functions. He did sign amendments to the Drug Abuse Office and Treatment Act of 1972 that mandated establishment of such a body in the Executive Office of the President, but did not seek appropriations to fund it.

In March 1975, in the face of what appeared to be a worsening drug situation, the administration ordered a comprehensive study of the nature and extent of drug use and directions for future remedial policy. The study, known as the *White Paper on Drug Abuse,* was published in September 1975, and set a new tone for drug abuse policy in the years to come. It recognized that the "total elimination of drug abuse is unlikely, but government actions can contain the problem and limit its adverse effects," a view that presaged the "harm reduction" argument of today. It also established antidrug priorities: "All drugs are not equally dangerous, and all drug use is not equally destructive. . . . Priority in both supply and demand reduction should be directed toward those drugs which inherently pose a greater risk—heroin, amphetamines (particularly when used intravenously), and mixed barbiturates" (57).

In the end, Ford turned away from the spirit of the *White Paper* and, in an attempt to bolster his chances in the 1976 presidential elections, resorted to the law-and-order approach to narcotics control that still paralleled the sentiments of an ever-narrowing majority of voters. In April 1976, he introduced the Narcotic Sentencing and Seizure Act of 1976, which tried to revive the concept of mandatory minimum sentences for drug-trafficking offenses, and established cabinet committees for drug policy oversight and coordination. Whatever the merits of the bill, Ford was defeated, and the trend toward greater toleration of drug use and less emphasis on control of abuse through law enforcement accelerated.

The election of Jimmy Carter was most welcome to those who supported profound revision of the laws governing possession and use of recreational drugs, particularly marihuana. Carter appointed Dr. Peter Bourne as his special assistant for health issues and decided after some delay to implement the legislation establishing the Office of Drug Abuse Policy with Dr. Bourne as its head. Dr. Bourne set a tone of accommodation to the view that possession of marihuana in small amounts for personal use ought to be decriminalized as a step toward wiser and more just use of law-enforcement resources. Dr. Bourne was also of the opinion, as he wrote in August 1974, that "Cocaine. . . is probably the most benign of illicit drugs currently in widespread use. At least as strong a case could be made for legalizing it as for legalizing marihuana. Short-acting—about 15 minutes—not physically addicting, and acutely pleasurable, cocaine has found increasing favor at all socioeconomic levels in the last year" (58). But the career of Dr. Bourne dramatically illustrates that toleration of recreational drug use would not become characteristic of more than a vocal minority of Americans.

Bourne served the Carter administration from January 1977 until July 1978. During this time, drug policy continued to focus on the international aspects of the heroin problem and on domestic control of barbiturates and amphetamines. The Drug Strategy Council was revitalized and published national strategies for the duration of the administration. Bourne was able to report an apparent reversal of the 1974 and 1975 trends that had indicated a worsening heroin situation: Overdose death rates were declining, as were heroin prices and purity. In early 1977, President Carter decided to advocate decriminalization of marihuana in accordance with a trend that was being acted on by state legislatures throughout the nation. This was startling evidence of the profound change in attitudes toward drug consumption that had taken place since the 1960s. But in July 1978, Dr. Bourne resigned because of allegations that he had written a fraudulent prescription for methaqualone for a member of his staff and that he himself had used cocaine—an accusation that Bourne denied; the Carter administration was suddenly in no position to appear soft on the drug issue. Although not obvious to most observers at the time, the wave of toleration that had been rising since the 1960s had crested, and both public opinion and public policy were about to change course.

THE NEW WAR ON DRUGS (1980 TO THE PRESENT)

Cocaine and Drug Intolerance

As the 1980s opened, cocaine use became more common but seemed to be characteristic of an economic elite who preferred to sniff or inject it. But by the middle of the decade, the method of consuming cocaine was shifting to smoking. Cocaine hydrochloride had to be converted to a base form for successful volatilizing. At first, smokers would use a "free-base kit," a dangerous method involving open flames and ether, often purchased at a drug paraphernalia store or "head shop." Then, about 1985, drug dealers began distributing "crack" to the streets of America's large urban centers. "Crack" was a rock-like base form of cocaine that could be volatilized easily without requiring any preliminary ether treatment. The extraordinary blood levels of cocaine one could achieve by inhaling cocaine fumes from "crack," and its availability in units costing only a few dollars, greatly expanded the cocaine market among poor and minority populations. Accompanying the "crack epidemic" were turf wars in urban areas as sellers competed for territory. Through the latter part of the decade, the street price drifted lower until eventually, in terms of equivalent value, crack sold for less than cocaine had on New York City streets prior to the Harrison Act of 1914 (59).

The arrival of crack, coupled with the overdose deaths of well-known youthful sports stars, combined with growing political pressure from anxious and angry parents, contributed to a new sense of national crisis over the cocaine problem. From the historian's perspective, the shift in attitude was rapid, widespread, and profound. The perception of cocaine for many moved from that of a safe, nonaddictive tonic to that of a feared substance linked to ruined careers and families. The stereotypic "coke head"—anxious, fearful, paranoid, hyperactive, and out of touch with others—may be the most fear-producing drug image to the American public. Perhaps the change in attitude is so striking because the initial image of cocaine was so optimistic (60). The fear of cocaine as well as popular and, at times, expert opinion that cocaine use would continue unabated unless legislators took drastic action spurred Congress and President Reagan into dramatic attacks on the drug problem.

In the fall of 1986, shortly before congressional elections, the executive and legislative branches of the federal government competed to enact the most severe laws against drug use. Billions were authorized by the Anti-Drug Abuse Act of 1986, although much less was later appropriated by Congress (61). Many observers, especially those within the treatment community, believed that the actual impact and funding of the law was a discouraging anticlimax to the promises and expectations that had accompanied its passage.

In 1988, as the presidential election approached, the fear of cocaine was reflected in enormous media coverage. Democrats and Republicans were each expressing outrage over drugs and drug use, neither side wanting to appear less determined than its opponent. An emphasis on law enforcement, so characteristic of the decline phase of the earlier wave of drug use, was most clearly demonstrated by the competition between the two major presidential contenders in which the Democratic candidate proposed greatly expanding the number of DEA agents, a stance in favor of law enforcement that eloquently illustrated the great change that had taken place in American attitudes since the Carter–Ford campaign. In 1976, the candidates had vied with one another as to which would be more understanding of casual or recreational use of what were considered to be "soft" drugs.

The 1988 Anti-Drug Abuse Act, like the one passed two years earlier, authorized substantial sums for treatment, but about two-thirds of funding went to law enforcement (62). Also, the 1988 act targeted the casual user much more prominently, with provisions such as fines for possession of personal amounts of drugs. An indication that the concern over drugs was expanding to include alcohol was the 1988 act's provision that a year after enactment, every bottle of beverage alcohol manufactured in the United States would have to carry a warning label.

One of the most significant provisions of the 1988 law was its Title I, known as the National Narcotics Leadership Act. Reaching back to the 1972 Drug Abuse Office and Treatment Act and the 1974 amendments to it, this title again established an Office of National Drug Control Policy (ONDCP) in the Executive Office of the President and with it the position of Director of National Drug Control Policy—the so-called "drug czar." The legislation also included a requirement that the executive branch provide a comprehensive national strategy with guidelines to measure its success. A series of federal strategies have been published since September 1989, including the latest one, put out by the George W. Bush White House in February 2002.

CONCLUSION

We can now look back on nearly four decades of continuous and widespread exposure to illicit drugs. Those who have lived through this most recent "drug epidemic" can testify to the remarkable change in attitude toward drugs since the 1970s. When we recall Jerry Rubin's claim in 1970 that "marijuana makes each person God," Timothy Leary's recommendation to youth to "turn on, tune in, and drop out," and a *Time* magazine cover in 1981 attractively exhibiting cocaine in a martini glass, we know that a shift in social norms has taken place. Legislatively, we have moved from softening of antidrug laws in the 1970s to renewing their severity since the late 1980s.

Our society has been through two "experiments in nature" regarding cocaine in the United States: twice (once beginning in the 1880s and again around 1970) a young population with no deeply held antagonism to the drug or even information about it has been exposed to the euphoric effects of cocaine. In each instance, 15–20 years passed before the nation started to change its mind on the value and risks of cocaine.

An important difference between the earlier cocaine problem and the present one is that the first anticocaine laws came as public attitudes turned against the drug, while in the current episode, severe anticocaine laws were on the statute books at the very beginning of the new infatuation. The result has been a much longer controversy over control of cocaine and the efficacy of legal restrictions than was the case early in the twentieth century.

Debate over legalization of drugs received public prominence during the current wave of drug use, both as drug toleration was quickly rising—in the mid-1970s—and as drug toleration was rapidly falling—in the late 1980s. The dominant argument for legalizing or "decriminalizing" cocaine, marihuana, and opiates in each case reflects the shift in the public's assumptions about drugs. In the 1970s, the argument was commonly made that the drugs were relatively safe, especially when compared with alcohol or tobacco; in the recent controversy, the argument has seldom been made that a drug like cocaine is safe, but rather that availability of a cheaper product would end turf wars and allow the dollars spent on interdiction to be spent improving conditions in the inner city. Comparison with alcohol and tobacco seems to have diminished as the public has become increasingly alarmed at these two legal substances.

Crime reduction was a core goal of the Nixon administration's broad campaign against drugs. Interestingly, property crime has fallen since 1980 by about 63%. Violent crime has fallen by 48% in the past 10 years. Curiously, neither side in the drug debate makes much mention of these astounding statistics, which imply that much progress has been made toward the goal of the original impetus for national drug strategies.

The rise of acquired immune deficiency syndrome (AIDS) adds another dimension to drug abuse control; the epidemic is now spreading most rapidly among intravenous drug users, many of whom engage in both needle sharing and unprotected sex. Here the debate about relaxing legal restrictions has centered on the wisdom of distributing sterile syringes and needles, condoms, and methadone without many of the elaborate regulations now controlling this opioid. The full social and medical impact of AIDS lies in the future, but it would not be surprising if the stress of these concerns—as happened in the history of other chronic, often fatal diseases, such as tuberculosis—tended toward restrictive public policies (63).

Change in the perception of alcohol over the past 10 years is another marker of evolving attitudes toward psychoactive substances of all kinds. More people now regard alcohol as a dangerous substance, rather than as a beverage to be used in moderation with meals and on festive occasions. In 1984, the federal government required states to raise the drinking age to 21 years or lose a part of highway taxes; in 1989, as noted, all beverage alcohol had to carry warning labels; the federal government has pressured states to lower the driving under the influence level to 0.08% for those older than age 21 years, and to 0.02% for those younger than age 21 years. In the past, antagonism to alcohol has led, over three or four decades, to extreme restrictions, which, in turn, were followed by a backlash against alcohol's tarnished image. For almost 50 years following repeal of national prohibition in 1933, it was difficult to discuss the problems associated with alcohol consumption without being accused of sympathy with discredited prohibitionists. Now the mood has changed, and the task will be to see whether this time the nation can establish a sustainable alcohol policy that will not be swept aside in frustration and resentment.

Recent legislation bearing on drug abuse control attempts once again to make the consequences of violating drug laws more dire. The Violent Crime Control and Law Enforcement Act of 1994 enhanced penalties for drug trafficking in prisons and drug-free zones, allowed the president to declare a violent crime or drug emergency in a specific area on request of the state or local executive, and amended the National Narcotics Leadership Act of 1988 to strengthen ONDCP (64).

The question for public policy is the degree to which a growing reliance on law enforcement will be balanced by availability of treatment and sustained support for research.

REFERENCES

1. Clark N. *Deliver us from evil: an interpretation of American prohibition.* New York: WW Norton, 1976:29.
2. Beecher L. Six sermons on the nature, occasions, signs, evils and remedy of intemperance, 4th ed. 1828. In: Musto DF, ed. *Drugs in America: a documentary history.* New York: New York University Press, 2002:44–86.
3. Timberlake JH. *Prohibition and the Progressive Movement.* Cambridge, MA: Harvard University Press, 1963.
4. Sinclair A. *Era of excess: a social history of the Prohibition Movement.* New York: Harper & Row, 1962:36–49.
5. Terry CE, Pellens M. *The opium problem.* New York: Bureau of Social Hygiene, 1928:50–51, 929–937.
6. Sonnedecker G. Emergence of the concept of opiate addiction. 1. *J Mon Pharm* 1962;6:275.
7. Sonnedecker G. Emergence of the concept of opiate addiction. 2. *J Mon Pharm* 1963;7:27.
8. Musto DF, ed. *One hundred years of heroin.* Westport, CT: Auburn House, 2002.
9. Wright H. Report on the international opium commission and on the opium problem as seen within the United States and its possession. In: 61st Congress, 2nd Session. *Opium problem: message from the President of the United States, February 21, 1910.* Senate document no. 377. Washington, DC: Government Printing Office, 1910:49.
10. Musto DF. The Marihuana Tax Act of 1937. *Arch Gen Psychiatry* 1972; 26:101–108.
11. Wilbert MI, Motter MG. *Digest of laws and regulations in force in the United States relating to the possession, use, sale, and manufacture of poisons and habit-forming drugs.* Public Health Bulletin no. 56. Washington, DC: US Government Printing Office, 1912.
12. Dupree AH. *Science in the federal government: a history of policies and activities to 1940.* Cambridge, MA: Harvard University Press, 1957:267–270.
13. Young JH. *The toadstool millionaires: a social history of patent medicines in America before federal regulation.* Princeton, NJ: Princeton University Press, 1961.
14. Taylor AH. *American diplomacy and the narcotics traffic, 1900–1939: a study in international humanitarian reform.* Durham, NC: Duke University Press, 1969:48–81.
15. United States 60th Congress. Public law no. 221. An act to prohibit the importation and use of opium for other than medicinal purposes. Approved February 9, 1909.
16. Musto DF. *The American disease: origins of narcotic control,* 3rd ed. New York: Oxford University Press, 1999:41–42.
17. State of Massachusetts, Acts of 1914, Chapter 694. An act to regulate the sale of opium, morphine and other narcotic drugs. Approved June 22, 1914.
18. Renborg BA. *International drug control: a study of international administration by and through the League of Nations.* Washington, DC: Carnegie Endowment for International Peace, 1947:15–17.
19. Wright H. Uncle Sam is the worst drug fiend in the world. *New York Times* 1911;March 12:(sect 5):12.
20. United States 63rd Congress. Public law no. 233. To provide for the registration of, with collectors of internal revenue, and to impose a special tax upon all persons who produce, import, manufacture, compound, deal in, dispense, sell, distribute, or give away opium or coca leaves, their salts, derivatives or preparations. Approved December 17, 1914.
21. United States Treasury Department. Treasury decision no. 2172. March 9, 1915.
22. *United States vs. Jin Fuey Moy,* 241 U.S. 394 (1916).
23. Kolb L, DuMez AG. The prevalence and trend of drug addiction in the United States and factors influencing it. *Public Health Rep* 1924;39:1179.
24. United States Treasury Department. *Traffic in narcotic drugs.* Washington, DC: US Government Printing Office, 1919.
25. Kuhne G. Statement of Gerhard Kuhne, head of Identification Bureau, New York City Department of Correction.

In: *Conference on narcotic education: hearings before the Committee on Education of the House of Representatives, December 16, 1925.* Washington, DC: US Government Printing Office, 1926:175.

26. Mayor appoints drug committee. *New York Times* 1919; May 27:9.

27. Murray RK. *Red scare: a study of national hysteria, 1919–1920.* Minneapolis: University of Minnesota, 1955.

28. Federal Bureau of Narcotics. *Narcotic clinics in the United States.* Washington, DC: US Government Printing Office, 1955.

29. Hubbard SD. New York City narcotic clinic and differing points of view on narcotic addiction. *New York City Department of Health Monthly Bulletin* 1920;Jan:45–47.

30. United States 65th Congress. Public law no. 254, sections 1006 to 1009. An act to provide revenue, by paying special taxes for every person who imports, manufactures, produces, compounds, sells, deals in, dispenses or gives away opium. Approved February 24, 1919.

31. *Webb et al. vs. United States,* 249 U.S. 96 (1919); *United States vs. Doremus* 249 U.S. 86 (1919).

32. Bishop ES. The narcotic drug problem. New York: Macmillan, 1920. Partially reprinted in David F. Musto, ed., *Drugs in America: a documentary history.* New York: New York University Press, 2002:265–270.

33. American Medical Association, House of Delegates. Report of the committee on the narcotic drug situation in the United States. *JAMA* 1920;74:1326.

34. DuMez AG. Increased tolerance and withdrawal phenomena in chronic morphinism. *JAMA* 1919;72:1069.

35. Burrow JG. *AMA, voice of American medicine.* Baltimore: Johns Hopkins University Press, 1963.

36. United States 67th Congress. Public law no. 227. To amend the act of February 9, 1909, as amended, to prohibit the importation and use of opium for other than medicinal purposes. Approved May 26, 1922.

37. United States Senate, Committee on Printing. *Use of narcotics in the United States, June 3, 1924.* Washington, DC: US Government Printing Office, 1924.

38. Hobson RP. The peril of narcotic drugs. *Congressional Record* 1925; Feb 18:4088–4091.

39. United States 68th Congress. Public law no. 274. Prohibiting the importation of crude opium for the purpose of manufacturing heroin. Approved June 7, 1924.

40. United States 70th Congress. Public law no. 672. To establish two United States narcotic farms for the confinement and treatment of persons addicted to the use of habit-forming narcotic drugs who have been convicted of offenses against the United States. Approved January 19, 1929.

41. United States 71st Congress. Public law no. 357. To create in the Treasury Department a Bureau of Narcotics. Approved June 14, 1930.

42. United States House of Representatives, Committee on Ways and Means. *Bureau of Narcotics: presentment and report by the Grand Jury on the subject of the narcotic traffic.* Filed February 19, 1930. Washington, DC: US Government Printing Office, 1930;Feb 19:73–77.

43. United States 75th Congress. Public law no. 238. To impose an occupational excise tax upon certain dealers in marihuana, to impose a transfer tax upon certain dealings in marihuana. Approved August 2, 1937.

44. United States 77th Congress. Public law no. 797. Opium poppy control act of 1942. Approved December 12, 1942.

45. Udell GG, compiler. *Opium and narcotic laws.* Washington, DC: US Government Printing Office, 1968.

46. United States 82nd Congress. Public law no. 255. To amend the penalty provision applicable to persons convicted of violating certain narcotic laws. Approved November 2, 1951.

47. United States 84th Congress. Public law no. 728. Narcotic control act of 1956. Approved July 18, 1956.

48. Joint Committee of the American Bar Association and the American Medical Association on Narcotic Drugs. *Interim and final reports. Drug addiction: crime or disease?* Bloomington, IN: Indiana University Press, 1961.

49. *Proceedings of the White House Conference on Narcotic and Drug Abuse.* Washington, DC: US Government Printing Office, 1962.

50. President's Advisory Commission on Narcotics and Drug Abuse. *Final report.* Washington, DC: US Government Printing Office, 1963.

51. United States 89th Congress. Public law no. 89–74. Drug abuse control amendment act of 1965. Approved February 1965.

52. United States 89th Congress. Public law no. 793. Narcotic addict rehabilitation act of 1966. Approved November 8, 1966.

53. President's Commission on Law Enforcement and the Administration of Justice. *The challenge of crime in a free society.* Washington, DC: US Government Printing Office, 1967:228–229.

54. Musto DF, Korsmeyer P. *The quest for drug control: politics and federal policy in a period of increasing substance abuse, 1963–1981.* New Haven, CT: Yale University Press, 2002.

55. United States 91st Congress. Public law no. 513. Comprehensive drug abuse prevention and control act of 1970. Approved October 27, 1970.

56. United States 92nd Congress. Public law no. 92–255. Drug abuse office and treatment act of 1972. Approved March 21, 1972.

57. Domestic Council on Drug Abuse Task Force. *White paper on drug abuse.* Washington, DC: US Government Printing Office, 1975:97–98.

58. Bourne PG. The great cocaine myth. *Drugs and Drug Abuse Education Newsletter* 1974;5:5.

59. Musto DF. Illicit price of cocaine in two eras: 1908–1914 and 1982–1989. *Conn Med* 1990;54:321–326.

60. Musto DF. America's first cocaine epidemic. *Wilson Q* 1989;13:59–64.

61. United States 99th Congress. Public law no. 570. Anti-drug abuse act of 1986. Approved October 27, 1986. For summary, see *Congressional Quarterly Wkly Rep* 1986;44(Oct 25):2699–2707.

62. United States 100th Congress. Public law no. 690. Anti-drug abuse act of 1988. Approved November 18, 1988. For summary, see *Congressional Quarterly Wkly Rep* 1988;46(Nov 19):3145–3151.

63. Musto DF. Quarantine and the problem of AIDS. *Milbank Q* 1986;64[Suppl 1]:97–117.

64. United States 103rd Congress. Public law no. 103–322. Violent crime control and law enforcement act of 1994. Approved September 13, 1994.

CHAPTER 2

Epidemiology

CHARLES WINICK AND R.L. NORMAN

Epidemiology, the distribution and determinants of disease occurrence involving alcohol, tobacco, and other drugs (ATOD), plays an increasingly important role in planning and programs involving substance use, abuse, and dependence (1).

DATA COLLECTION TECHNIQUES

Surveys

Since 1971, the National Household Survey on Drug Abuse (NHSDA) has been the leading source on incidence and prevalence of ATOD. The NHSDA uses an interactive, bilingual, computer-assisted home interview with a sample of some 72,000 persons older than age 12 years (2). It is sponsored by the Substance Abuse and Mental Health Services Administration.

Beginning in 1975, and supported by the National Institute on Drug Abuse, the University of Michigan has annually conducted Monitoring the Future (MTF), the primary source for data on ATOD use by elementary and high school students. Its probability sample in 2001 included 16,800 eighth graders, 14,300 tenth graders, and 13,300 twelfth graders. MTF uses self-report questionnaires administered in the schools (3).

Every 5 years, the National Institute on Alcohol Abuse and Alcoholism sponsors the National Alcohol Survey, conducted by the Alcohol Research Group, University of California at Berkeley. In 1995, 4,925 household interviews were conducted. The 2000 survey was conducted by telephone (4).

The Behavioral Risk Factor Surveillance System (BRFSS) is an annual state-based telephone survey of the adult civilian population sponsored by the Centers for Disease Control and Prevention (CDC). The Youth Risk Behavior Survey (YRBS) is also conducted by CDC, with a sample size of 12,000 to 16,000, every 2 years. States can implement their own versions of the survey.

Each state has an office that coordinates substance abuse activities, including licensing treatment providers and personnel. To help make informed decisions on resources needed for various services, the state typically conducts epidemiologic investigations, which may include studies of prices, quality, and availability of illegal drugs. Some states conduct studies of special situations, such as the effects of the September 11, 2001 terrorist attacks, on levels of illicit drug use.

All probability sample surveys must consider how to reach hidden populations of illegal users or persons oth-

erwise difficult to interview. Various forms of purposive sampling or ethnography-based techniques are used to locate hidden populations, such as noninjecting heroin users (5). Nonprobability sampling approaches include targeted sampling, key informant sampling, snowball sampling, and respondent-driven sampling. A feasibility study to estimate the size of the hard core drug-using population in Cook County, Illinois, concluded that there were about three times more users than could be identified by traditional surveys (6).

One broad-based contributor to epidemiology is the Community Epidemiology Work Group (CWEG), which observed its twenty-fifth birthday in 2001 (7). This group of epidemiologists from 21 sentinel urban areas meets biannually to assess drug abuse patterns, enhanced with information from many community-based sources. The presentations from each meeting, including information on substance purity, prices and distribution, are widely disseminated.

Drug Abuse Warning Network

In 2000, the Drug Abuse Warning Network (DAWN) had a sample of 466 general hospitals with 24-hour emergency departments, in 21 key metropolitan areas (8). Episodes reportable to DAWN by its participating hospitals may result from chronic or unexpected reactions to prescription, over-the-counter, or illicit drugs. Neither accidental ingestion nor reactions that do not have any intent of abuse is included. Up to four substances can be recorded or "mentioned" for each episode. Reports from DAWN appear twice yearly. In 2001 episodes, the substances most often reported were cocaine/crack (29%), heroin/morphine (16%), marihuana/hashish (16%), and methamphetamine/speed (2%) (9).

Fatalities directly or indirectly related to drug misuse or abuse are reported by a DAWN sample of coroners or medical examiners (ME) in 27 metropolitan areas. MEs may use circumstantial evidence and/or toxicologic analysis.

Arrestee Drug Abuse Monitoring

The Arrestee Drug Abuse Monitoring (ADAM) system is a probability-based urinalysis measure of the extent of drug use in people who have been arrested. Succeeding the Drug Use Forecasting (DUF) program, established in 1987 by the National Institute of Justice, ADAM became fully implemented in 2000 with 38 sites (10).

Urinalysis is used to detect marihuana, cocaine, methamphetamine, opiates, and phencyclidine (PCP). Urinalysis completion rates were above 85% in most of the reporting sites. Most participants were arrested for offenses not directly related to drug use.

Among adult male arrestees, a mean of 65% tested positive for recent use of a listed drug. Median arrestee rates for specific drugs were: cocaine (30%), methamphetamine (5%), opiates (6%), and marihuana (40%) (10). Binge drinking for the previous 30 days was reported by a median 56.7%.

ADAM data collection was terminated in December 2003. Previous DVF and ADAM data are available at the University of Michigan's Inter-University Consortium for Political and Social Research. The Department of Justice is considering future ADAM-related studies.

Substance Use As Epidemic

The concept of the epidemic has been adapted from social medicine in order to help clarify the spread of specific substances of abuse (11,12). One study using ADAM data suggests that drug epidemics usually follow a natural course, with movement from incubation to expansion, plateau, and decline (13). The crack/cocaine epidemic had its incubation from 1979 to 1981, expansion from 1982 to 1986, plateau from 1987 to 1989, and decline from 1990 to 1996.

Marihuana's latest cycle of ADAM popularity, especially among youths, started its incubation phase around 1992, expanded in the years to 1996, and was on a plateau through 2000 (14). Such generalizations must take into account the local nature of drug epidemics, differential use by age, criminal justice involvement, period and cohort effects, and the difficulties of measuring illegal or concealed behavior. Differences between substance use by arrestees and the mainstream population must also be considered.

Earlier studies had traced the movement of heroin through a community (15). Long-term studies of drug cycles provide a necessary historical context (16). Such studies may report on relatively parallel movement of different mood modifying substances, like the general decline in consumption of both alcohol and illicit drugs that began around 1980–1981 and has continued to the present.

Drug Users in Prison

A major reason for the increase in prison and jail inmates from 645,713 in 1983 to 2,078,570 in 2003 is the number of drug abusers who are arrested and convicted under state or federal statutes, usually for possession or trafficking. The number of prosecutions and length of sentences have been steadily increasing. During 2000 in federal courts, the mean sentence for persons convicted of drug felonies was 75.6 months, compared with 63.0 months for all violent felonies (17). Much of the increase in the federal prison population and the prison budget increase since 1986 was a result of mandatory minimum sentencing for drug offenders (18–20). By 2000, drug offenders were 56.9% of the federal prison population and 21% of the 1,206,400 adults serving time in state prisons (21,22).

By the end of 2002, approximately 15% of the country's prisons had established treatment programs for inmates who had been drug abusers. Correctional treatment situations sometimes attempt to have followup aspects, which may or may not be residential. These programs tend to be variants of the therapeutic community approach (23,24).

Users and Treatment Programs

More than 18 million alcohol users and 5 million illicit drug users need treatment. More than 11,000 treatment providers annually handle more than 1.6 million admissions. Because people may come for treatment more than once in a year, the number of admissions is more than the number of persons admitted annually. In a year, a treatment slot turns over an average of perhaps three times. More than 900,000 clients are treated on any given day, with greater than 83% in outpatient counseling settings (25). Pharmacotherapy and short- and long-term residential approaches are the other major formats for treatment.

Approximately 200,000 heroin addicts are currently in methadone maintenance programs. Recent liberalization of the methadone maintenance procedures and the 2002 approval by the Food and Drug Administration of buprenorphine and buprenorphine-naloxone in treating heroin addicts should substantially increase the number of opiate addicts in pharmacologic treatment, with more office-based service (26).

Different parts of the country have very different treatment needs. Thus, the most primary treatment admissions for cocaine/crack in 2001 were in Atlanta (70.3%), followed by Philadelphia (48.1%), with the lowest in Newark (9.0%) (27). However, Newark had the highest primary heroin treatment admissions (83.8%).

The Substance Abuse and Mental Health Services Administration's Treatment Episode Data Set (TEDS) represents 76% of admissions to all known substance abuse treatment providers. Based on the TEDS data for the period 1992–1995, some generalizations can be made (28). Admissions for combined drug and alcohol abuse are more common than those for either substance alone. Admitted clients are more male, black, educationally disadvantaged, unmarried, and young than the U.S. population.

TEDS 1995 admissions reflect a high rate of self referrals for heroin (69%) and a high rate of referral by the criminal justice system for marihuana (49%), PCP (47%), and alcohol-only (46%). Public assistance was the major source of income for heroin abusers (33%) and for smoked cocaine (26%) and nonsmoked cocaine (20%) abusers.

In 1999, four substances represented 91% of all TEDS admissions: alcohol (47%), opiates (16%), cocaine (14%), and marihuana/hashish (14%). Polydrug use characterized 54% of admissions (29). Whether the user will get treatment depends on a range of factors. For many users, problems are likely to become salient between three to five years after beginning significant levels of use.

SOME DIMENSIONS

Sociodemographic Factors

Rates of use of illicit drugs in 2000 for persons age 12 years and older was 6.4% for blacks, 6.4% for whites, and 5.3% for Hispanics (30). The Native American/Alaska Native rate was highest (12.6%) and the Asian rate was lowest (2.7%). These rates are inconsistent with the rates at which these racial/ethnic groups appear in treatment or prison. In 1999, there were 78,018 DAWN mentions for blacks and 56,730 for whites, and TEDS admissions for crack were 58% black (8,29).

In 2001 in state prisons, the increasing number of drug offenses represented 27% of the growth among black inmates, 15% of the growth among white inmates, and 7% of the growth among Hispanic inmates (31). Among the factors that might be contributing to the overrepresentation of blacks are their relative use of publicly financed treatment facilities, patterns of enforcement, and features of the federal sentencing guidelines relating to crack.

Another ethnic/racial difference is that although blacks have lower ATOD use rates in adolescence, their rates equal or exceed those of whites in adulthood (32). This paradox is probably, at least in part, the result of later initiation into, and lower rates of quitting, substance use. Another difference is that Hispanics could have an earlier age for starting marihuana than other groups (33). The use of ATOD may have different functions for specific subgroups, and both risk and protective factors relevant to such use could operate differently across ethnic/racial subgroups (34).

Education is inversely correlated with illicit drug use rates, with college graduates having the lowest rate of current use (4.2%). Adults who did not complete high school had a 6.3% rate (30).

The Life Cycle and Substance Use

For 2000, use of any illicit drug for various age groups in the previous month was 3% for ages 12 to 13 years, 9.8% for those ages 14 to 15 years, 16.4% for ages 16 to 17 years, 15.9% for ages 18 to 25 years, dropping to 4.2% for ages 26+ years (30). The peak subgroup was ages 18 to 20 years, with 19.6%; overall, 49% of current illicit drug users were younger than age 26 years.

Pharmacokinetics and pharmacodynamics provide information on how age impacts on drug use. For the first 6 months of 2001, DAWN reported episodes at a rate per 100,000 of the general population of 206 for persons ages 35 to 44 years, 110 for those ages 45 to 54 years, and 23 for those age 55 years and older (8). NHSDA reported rates of illicit drug use declining consistently in persons older than age 44 years, but above 2% for adults in their fifties (30). The illicit drugs most popular with persons older than age 55 years were marihuana and psychotherapeutics used nonmedically. In 2000, 38% of adults over 55, or 21 million people, had past-month alcohol use. More than 5 million were binge alcohol users. Among persons over 55, whites had higher rates of past-month illicit drug use than did Hispanics, and higher past-month alcohol use than either blacks or Hispanics. The highest older-age illicit drug use was found among those aged 55 to 59 years (35).

Birth cohorts with high rates of illicit drug use in their younger years usually have, when compared to other cohorts, higher rates as they age. The 50% illicit drug use rate among those age 35 to 54 years in 2000—the "baby boomers"—was significantly higher than among older adults (13%). It can be expected that the large number of "boomers" and their higher prevalence of illicit drug use will lead to an increase in use as the younger group enters older adulthood (35).

Users of licit substances may try, without treatment, to stop their use of a substance on which they are dependent. Although two-thirds of the country's 47 million adult smokers want to quit, only some 2.5% succeed in doing so each year (25). Similar statistics are not available for the large number of regular users of alcohol and/or illicit substances who may to try to end their dependency without formal treatment. Perhaps half the persons meeting the American Psychiatric Association criteria for alcoholism can cease drinking without outside help (36).

The concept of "maturing out" of narcotic addiction helped to focus attention on the life cycle of substance use. This is a complex process and different subgroups appear to have different rates of loosening and/or maintaining their ties to a substance. These rates are often associated with the economy, age, gender, role, the life cycle of substance use, shifts in the popularity of substances, and other factors (37,38).

Gender Differences

Men have a higher rate than women of most kinds of illicit substance use; the difference increases with age and degree of involvement. Male high school seniors, college students, and young adults generally use illicit substances more frequently and heavily than their female counterparts. However, in 2000, among young people ages 12 to 17 years, the rate of current illicit drug use was not significantly different for boys (9.8%) and girls (9.5%) (30). Men are generally more likely than women to report smoking a tobacco product in the previous month. Men consume more alcohol and have more alcohol-related problems than women. In 1990 and 1995, 6% of men and 2% of women were alcohol dependent (39).

College Students

College students reflect usage rates that are about average for high school graduates of their age for many illicit drugs, but represent lower rates for cocaine, crack/cocaine, heroin, and amphetamines (40). Some 39% of college students engage in heavy drinking. Weekend drinking tends to characterize college students, with daily drinking found in 3.6%.

Pregnant Women

Some 3.3% of pregnant women ages 15 to 44 years used an illicit substance in the preceding month, compared with

7.7% of women in the general population (30). Pregnant women ages 15 to 17 years used at a 12.9% rate. Some 18.6% of pregnant women smoked cigarettes, compared to 29.8% of nonpregnant women of the same age. Pregnant cocaine users are likely to use alcohol, marihuana, and tobacco, and probably receive little prenatal care.

The use of most substances—except tobacco—usually decreases during pregnancy. Alcohol use among pregnant women has declined in the last two decades, although substantial deficits can be found in children born with fetal alcohol syndrome.

Comorbidity

The recent availability of data on mental health problems of substance users has led to new interest in such users, who are identified as either dual diagnosis or mentally ill chemical abusers (MICA).

In a national survey of psychiatric comorbidity, some 8% were drug dependents at some time in their lives and 1.8% were dependent in the previous year (41). A study with a new instrument designed to identify mental health problems in substance abusers found that the majority of clients in a therapeutic community had mental health problems at some point in their lives (42).

Analysis of the NHSDA data for the period 1994–1996, based on a mental health checklist, found that 13% of adolescents ages 12 to 17 years had emotional problems and 17% had behavioral problems. The severity of these problems is associated with the likelihood of substance abuse (43).

A number of therapeutic community programs have been developed to treat dual-diagnosis cases, some with considerable success (44).

Occupational Substance Abuse

Some 15.4% of unemployed adults, 6.3% of full-time employed adults, and 7.8% of part-time employed adults were current illicit drug users in 2000 (30). Of the 11.8 million adult illicit drug users, 77% were employed full- or part-time.

The recession of the early 1990s led to reconsideration of studies showing how mental illness and alcoholism were inversely related to the state of the economy (45). Increased use of illicit drugs may characterize some people who experience role deprivation because they have lost the anchorages provided by work (46).

A survey of U.S. military personnel worldwide found that their rates of illicit drug use were significantly lower (2.6%) than the rates among civilians (10.7%) (47). Military personnel exhibited significantly higher rates of heavy alcohol use (14.2%) than their civilian counterparts (9.9%). Differences in military and civilian heavy alcohol use were largest for men ages 18 to 25 years. Nearly all military personnel had been tested for drugs since joining the military.

Mortality and the Acquired Immune Deficiency Syndrome

Approximately one-fourth of the deaths in the United States each year can be attributed to illicit drug use, alcohol, and tobacco (25). Such deaths may be identified as either drug related, induced, involved, or detected.

The DAWN mortality component reports on deaths associated with drug abuse. Indirect causes of drug-related death may involve collateral diseases, such as hepatitis or AIDS among injecting drug users, violence related to illegal drug sales, and automobile and other accidents. In North America and Western Europe, 25% to 50% of human immunodeficiency virus (HIV) infections are from injecting drug users, which accounts for more than 30% of U.S. AIDS cases (48).

Drug-related deaths frequently involve illicit drugs combined with alcohol. Almost 16,000 deaths annually have been attributed to illicit drug use in recent years. About one in five drug deaths is a suicide. Tobacco causes about 430,700 deaths annually (25). Alcohol is credited with more than 100,000 deaths annually.

SUBSTANCES

Heroin and Other Opiates

Heroin of relatively high purity and low cost has become widely available in recent years. Intranasal sniffing and smoking, to a lesser extent in some geographic areas, are more frequent than injecting drug users (49). Younger and more suburban and rural residents appear to be trying heroin.

Another development since the 1990s has been an increase in "cutting" heroin, for example, adulteration (adding pharmacologically active or psychoactive substances like quinine) and dilution (adding inert substances like lactose) (50). The adulterants may be added by marketers to ease the absorption of heroin into the mucous membranes of intranasal users.

There are at least 600,000 regular heroin users in the United States. In recent years, the number of new users annually has been estimated to be between 135,000 and 190,000 persons.

Most parts of the country report problems with opiates other than heroin, for example, oxycodone (OxyContin and Percocet), hydrocodone (Vicodin, Lortab, or Lorcet), hydromorphone (Dilaudid), and codeine, which are among the pharmaceuticals that have been diverted to illicit use.

Marihuana

Eight states, including California, permit some use of medical marihuana but the U.S. government has a zero-tolerance policy, so that federal laws conflict with some state laws. Marihuana was used in 2000 by 76% of current illicit drug users, with 59% of current drug users consuming only marihuana (30). It is widely available in most parts of the country. Since 1990, along with a decline in stigma, there has been some increase in its use, along with substantial increases in arrests, DAWN mentions, and treatment admissions. Treatment admissions for primary abuse of marihuana in large cities range between 20.5% and 32.3% (8) of all drug abuse admissions.

Marihuana was formerly a significant nexus of the gateway theory of substance abuse, which suggested that young people started with illicit substances like cigarettes, beer, wine, and spirits, and then used marihuana, after which some moved to other illicit substances such as heroin or cocaine. Recently, there is a tendency to view it as more likely to be a terminus rather than a gateway (51).

Cocaine/Crack

Cocaine and crack have been stabilizing and trending down since the 1990s. Cocaine can be smoked in the form of crack crystals, sniffed, taken intravenously, or mixed with other drugs. Past-month use of cocaine in 2000 was 0.5% among persons older than age 12 years, down from 0.7% in 1999 (30). In 2001, substantially more patients entering treatment had been taking crack rather than powder cocaine. Cocaine mentions by DAWN have remained high.

Club Drugs

Methylenedioxymethamphetamine (MDMA), usually referred to as "ecstasy," is the leading club drug, which is used by young persons at dances, nightclubs, musical performances, after-hours clubs, and extended dance gatherings ("raves"). They can also be found in many non-club casual settings. Clandestine laboratories in Belgium or Holland produce much of the world's supply of this stimulant and low-level hallucinogenic drug. It is usually ingested orally via tablet or less often, in capsule form.

Ecstasy pills are widely available and often sold with brand names. Users consider it a safe drug, although occasional deaths have been reported by DAWN. Other club drugs are flunitrazepam (Rohypnol), the veterinary anesthetic ketamine, and gamma hydroxybutyrate (GHB).

Forensic analysis has found that the active ingredients in the pills and capsules sold as ecstasy are not exclusively MDMA. MDMA is a Schedule I drug, with no recognized medical use. DAWN mentions of MDMA have been increasing (9).

Methamphetamine

Western cities report a high percentage of primary methamphetamine treatment admissions in recent years. Prices of "ice" are down, purity is high, and supplies appear plentiful. Methamphetamine mentions in DAWN are increasing slowly. TEDS data suggest that the proportion of admissions for methamphetamine problems increased from 3% to 5% between 1994 and 1999 (28). Smoking (35%), injection (29%), and inhalation (25%) are among the methods of ingestion.

Alcohol

In a typical recent year, almost half (46.6%) of Americans age 12 years and older, or 104 million persons, were current drinkers of alcohol and heavy drinking (5 or more drinks on the same occasion on at least 5 different days in the past 30 days) characterized 5.6% (12 million people) (30). Binge drinking (5 or more drinks on the same occasion at least once in the previous 30 days) and heavy drinking are highest in those ages 18 to 25 years, with the peak rate at age 21 years. The 10% of the population that drinks the most heavily consumes half of the alcohol in this country.

Per capita sales data indicate that alcohol consumption per person decreased from 2.76 gallons per person in 1981 to 2.17 gallons in 1995 (52). The decline in alcohol use facilitates the recognition of problems. Thus, more drunkenness was reported in 1995 than in 1979, although the number of drinks required to be "drunk" declined from 8.2 to 6.3.

Subjective measures of drunkenness can predict social consequences and harm as effectively as the more objective "5+" measures (53). Because almost half of American current drinkers report drunkenness at least once during the last year, systematic use of subjective measures is a current research area.

Frequent heavy drinking has decreased among whites in practically all sociodemographic groups (54). Among blacks and Hispanics, the abstention rate has increased, but frequent heavy drinking has remained stable. The frequent heavy drinkers' rates are noteworthy because they are associated with problem incidence.

Driving under the influence of alcohol (DUI) remains frequent, especially among white and Hispanic men (55). More than one-fifth of white (22%) and Hispanic (21%) men who drove in the previous year were drunk enough to be in trouble if stopped by police. However, the men's actual arrest rate for DUI is only 1% of the whites and 4% of the Hispanics.

Ethnicity, socioenvironmental factors, and alcohol consumption are interrelated. Binge alcohol use is least likely among Asians and most likely in Native Americans. In all ethnic groups, being male and consumption of 10 or more drinks per week are significant risk factors for drinking and driving problems. Underage current alcohol use rates are approximately similar in metropolitan areas of all sizes.

In 1982, 53% of fatal auto accidents, or 22,246 deaths, were linked to a blood alcohol level of at least 0.08. This figure declined to 34% of fatal auto accidents, or 14,421 deaths, by 1997, but increased to 35% of fatal auto accidents and 14,953 deaths in 2001 (56).

Intimate partner violence is a significant problem in the United States, and 30% to 40% of the men and 27% to 34% of the women who perpetrated violence against their partners were drinking at the time of the event (57).

Tobacco

In 2000, 65.5 million Americans age 12 years and older reported current use of a tobacco product, a prevalence rate of 29.3% (30). Of these, 55.7 million (24.9%) smoked cigarettes. After age 25 years, cigarette smoking rates generally declined, reaching 19.1% for persons ages 60 to 64 years. Whites are more likely to be heavy smokers than are blacks or Hispanics.

Although there was a dramatic increase in teen smoking in the early 1990s, in the latter half of the 1990s there was a decline that has continued into the beginning of the new century. Since peak levels in the mid-1990s, the 30-day prevalence of smoking has dropped by 42% in eighth grade, 30% in tenth grade, and 19% in twelfth grade (58).

ROLE OF EPIDEMIOLOGIC INDICATORS

Substance abuse programs increasingly require measurements of the extent to which their objectives are being achieved. Explicit goals, major objectives, targets, and measures to track progress toward targets are necessary steps in the process (59). Epidemiologic measurements, based on triangulation of different approaches, are essential vehicles for local, state, and federal programs, as well as the voluntary sector.

REFERENCES

1. American Psychiatric Association. *Diagnostic criteria from DSM–IV.* Washington, DC: Author, 1994:108–112.
2. Office of Applied Studies. *Development of computer-assisted interviewing procedures for the National Household Survey on Drug Abuse.* Rockville, MD: Department of Health and Human Services, 2001.
3. Johnston LD, O'Malley PM, Bachman JG. *Monitoring the future: overview of key findings 2001.* Rockville, MD: Department of Health and Human Services, 2002.
4. Midanik LT, Greenfield TK, Rogers JD. Reports of alcohol-related harm: telephone versus face-to-face interviews. *J Stud Alcohol* 2001;62:74–78.
5. Sifaneck SJ, Heaigus A. The ethnographic accessing, sampling and screening of hidden populations: heroin sniffers in New York City. *Addict Res Theory* 2001;9:519–543.
6. Abt Associates. *A plan for estimating the number of "hardcore" drug users in the United States.* Washington, DC: Office of National Drug Control Policy, 1997.
7. Community Epidemiology Work Group. *Epidemiologic trends in drug abuse advance report.* Bethesda, MD: National Institute on Drug Abuse, 2001:Jun.
8. Office of Applied Studies. *Emergency department trends from the Drug Abuse Warning Network: preliminary estimates January–June 2001 with revised estimates.* Rockville, MD: Department of Health and Human Services, 2002.
9. Community Epidemiology Work Group. *Epidemiologic trends in drug abuse advance report.* Bethesda, MD: Department of Health and Human Services, 2001:Dec.
10. Taylor BG, Fitzgerald N, Hunt D, et al. *ADAM preliminary 2000 findings on drug use and drug markets.* Washington DC: National Institute of Justice, 2001.
11. Rogers E. *The diffusion of innovations.* New York: Free Press, 1982.
12. Chambers CD, Harter MT. The epidemiology of narcotics abuse among blacks in the United States: 1935–1980. In: Brill L, Winick C, eds. *Yearbook of substance use and abuse.* New York: Human Sciences Press, 1985:307–343.
13. Golub AL, Johnson BD. *Crack's decline: some surprises across US cities.* Washington DC: National Institute of Justice Research in Brief, 1997.
14. Golub AL, Johnson BD. *The rise of marihuana as the drug of choice among youthful adult arrestees.* Washington, DC: National Institute of Justice Research in Brief, 2001.
15. de Alarcon R. The spread of heroin abuse in a community. *Bull Narc* 1969;21:17–22.
16. Musto DF. *The American disease: origins of narcotic control,* 3d ed. New York: Oxford University Press, 1999.
17. Bureau of Justice Statistics. *Federal criminal case processing 2000, with trends 1982–2000.* Washington, DC: US Department of Justice, 2001;Nov:12.
18. Bureau of Justice Statistics. *Prisoners in 1996.* Washington, DC: US Department of Justice, 1997.
19. Executive Office of the President. *Budget of the United States Government, fiscal year 2002.* Washington, DC: US Government Printing Office, 2001:134.
20. Bureau of Justice Statistics. *Sourcebook of criminal justice statistics 1996.* Washington, DC: US Government Printing Office, 1997:20.
21. Bureau of Justice Statistics. *Sourcebook of criminal justice statistics 2000.* Washington, DC: US Government Printing Office, 2001:526.
22. Harrison PM, Beck AJ. *Bureau of Justice statistics. Prisoners in 2001.* Washington DC: US Department of Justice, 2002;Jul:12–13.
23. Graham WF, Wexler WF. The Amity therapeutic community program at Donovan Prison. In: De Leon G, ed. *Community as method.* Westport, CT: Praeger, 1997:69–86.
24. Lockwood D, Inciardi JA, Butzin CA, et al. The therapeutic community continuum in corrections. In: De Leon G, ed. *Community as method.* Westport, CT: Praeger, 1977:87–96.
25. Robert Wood Johnson Foundation. *Substance abuse, the nation's number one health problem: key indicators for policy.* Princeton, NJ: Robert Wood Johnson Foundation, 2001.
26. Markel H. For addicts, relief may be an office visit away. *New York Times* 2002 Oct 27:4.
27. Community Epidemiology Work Group. *Epidemiologic trends in drug abuse, highlights and executive summary.* Bethesda, MD: National Institute on Drug Abuse, 2001;Dec:3.
28. Office of Applied Studies. *National admissions to substance abuse treatment services, the Treatment Episode Data Set (TEDS) 1992–1995.* Rockville, MD: US Department of Health and Human Services, 1997.
29. Office of Applied Studies. *Treatment Episode Data Set (TEDS) 1994–1999.* Rockville, MD: US Department of Health and Human Services, 2001.
30. Office of Applied Studies. *Summary of*

findings from the 2000 National House-hold Survey on Drug Abuse. Rockville, MD: US Department of Health and Human Services, 2001.

31. Bureau of Justice Statistics. *Prisoners in 2001.* Washington, DC: US Department of Justice, 2002:Jul.

32. Department of Health and Human Services. *Prevalence of substance use among racial and ethnic subgroups in the United States 1991–1993.* Rockville, MD: Office of Applied Studies, 1998.

33. Sussman S, Stacy AW, Dent CW, et al. Marihuana use: current issues and new research directions. *J Drug Issues* 1996;26:695–733.

34. Resnicow K, Soler R, Braithwaite RL. Cultural sensitivity in substance use prevention. *J Commun Psychol* 2000; 28:270–290.

35. National Household Survey on Drug Abuse. *The NHSDA report.* Rockville, MD: Office of Applied Studies, 2001; Nov:23.

36. Institute of Medicine. *Broadening the base of treatment for alcohol problems.* Washington DC: National Academy Press, 1990:152–156.

37. Winick C. Maturing out of narcotic addiction. *Bull Narc* 1962;14:1–7.

38. Prins EH. *Maturing out: an empirical study of personal histories and processes in hard-drug addiction.* Rotterdam, Holland: Van Gorcum, 1995.

39. Caetano R, Greenfield TK. *Trends in DSM-IV alcohol dependence: 1990 and 1995. US national alcohol surveys.* Berkeley, CA: Alcohol Research Group, 1997.

40. Johnston LD, O'Malley PM, Bachman JG. *National survey results on drug use: college students and young adults ages 19–40, 2000.* Rockville, MD: Department of Health and Human Services, 2001.

41. Kessler RC, McGonagle KA, Zhao S, et al. Lifetime and 12-month prevalence of *DSM–III–R* psychiatric disorders in the United States. *Arch Gen Psychiatry* 1994;51:8–19.

42. Carroll JFX, McGonley JJ. A screening form for identifying mental health problems in alcohol/other drug dependent persons. *Alcohol Treat Q* 2001;19:33–47.

43. Office of Applied Studies. *The relationship between mental health and substance abuse among adolescents.* Rockville MD: Department of Health and Human Services, 1999.

44. Sacks S, De Leon G, Bernhardt AI, et al. A modified therapeutic community for homeless mentally ill chemical abusers. In: De Leon G, ed. *Community as method.* Westport, CT: Praeger, 1997;19–38.

45. Brenner MH. *Mental illness and the economy.* Cambridge, MA: Harvard University Press, 1973.

46. Winick C. A theory of drug dependence based on role, access to and attitudes toward drugs. In: Lettieri DJ, Sayers M, Pearson H, eds. *Theories on drug abuse.* Rockville, MD: National Institute on Drug Abuse, 1980:225–236.

47. Bray RM, Sanchez RP, Ornstein ML, et al. *1998 Department of Defense survey of health-related behaviors among military personnel.* Research Triangle Park, NC: Research Triangle Institute, 1999.

48. Center for Drug Use and HIV Research. *International trends.* New York: National Development and Research Institute, 2002:Summer.

49. Andrade X, Sifaneck SJ, Neaigus A. Dope sniffers in New York City: an ethnography of heroin markets and patterns of use. *J Drug Issues* 1999;29:271–298.

50. Furst RT. The re-engineering of heroin: an emerging heroin "cutting" trend in New York City. *Addict Res* 2000;8:357–379.

51. Zimmer L, Morgan JP. *Marihuana myths, marihuana facts.* New York: The Lindesmith Center, 1997.

52. Midanik LT, Greenfield TK. Trends in social consequences and dependence symptoms in the United States: The National Alcohol Surveys 1984–1995. *Am J Public Health* 2000;90: 53–56.

53. Midanik LT. Drunkenness, feeling the effects and 5 + measures. *Addiction* 1999; 94;887–897.

54. Caetano R, Clark CL. Trends in alcohol consumption patterns among whites, blacks, and Hispanics. *J Stud Alcohol* 1998;59:659–668.

55. Caetano R, Clark CL. Hispanics, blacks, and whites driving under the influence of alcohol: results from the 1995 National Alcohol Survey. *Accid Anal Prev* 2000;32:57–64.

56. Wald ML. Deaths mounting again in war on drunk driving. *New York Times* 2002 Oct 22:C22.

57. Caetano R, Schaefer J, Cunradi CB. Alcohol-related intimate partner violence among white, black, and Hispanic couples in the United States. *Alcohol Res Health* 2001;25: 58–65.

58. Johnston LD, O'Malley PM, Bachman JF. *National results on adolescent drug use, overview of key findings 2001.* Bethesda, MD: National Institute on Drug Abuse, 2002.

59. Office of National Drug Control Policy. *Performance measures of effectiveness: a system for assessing the performance of the national drug control strategy.* Washington, DC: US Government Printing Office, 1998.

CHAPTER 3

U.S. Federal Drug Policy

MATHEA FALCO

Americans rank alcohol and drug abuse as the nation's most serious public health problem, ahead of cancer, heart disease, and depression (1). Four of five police chiefs rank drug and alcohol abuse as the top problem in their communities, ahead of gun availability and gang activity (2,3). Federal government estimates put the national economic costs of alcohol and other drug abuse at nearly $375 billion annually—a burden shared by individuals, businesses, and all levels of government. Direct medical expenses and lost economic productivity as a result of smoking-related illness and premature death cost another $170 billion each year (4).

Illegal drug use cuts across all economic and ethnic groups. Of the 16 million Americans who admit using drugs at least once a month, 75% are white and the majority are employed. Among young adults age 18 to 21 years, 1 in 5 reports using illicit drugs at least once a month (5). Direct experience with drug addiction is also widespread, although rarely discussed publicly.

This deep concern about drugs has made drug policy a top priority for decades. Since 1980, taxpayers have spent more than $500 billion on federal, state, and local antidrug efforts. This amount—some $21 billion a year—is more than the federal government spends annually for all biomedical research, including research on heart disease, cancer, and acquired immune deficiency syndrome (AIDS) (6,7).

FEDERAL REGULATION OF PSYCHOACTIVE DRUGS

Since the early decades of the twentieth century, the federal government has imposed regulatory controls over psychoactive drugs that officials believe threaten the public health because of their abuse potential. The most notable of these drugs have traditionally been heroin, cocaine, and marijuana, although amphetamines, barbiturates, and methaqualone also periodically dominate federal drug control concerns. Amphetamine abuse, for example, reached epidemic proportions in the 1960s, when the axiom "speed kills" ultimately turned a generation away from the drug, only to reappear as a major problem in the mid-1990s (8).

The federal Controlled Substances Act is the legal framework that differentiates permissible medical drug use from prohibited drug abuse.[a] For example, drugs regulated in Schedule II of the Act (such as cocaine and amphetamines) are deemed to have limited prescribed uses but severe abuse potential; those drugs regulated in Schedule I (heroin and marijuana, for example) are determined to have no permitted medical use as well as great abuse potential. Although the Act gives the Food and Drug Administration (FDA) an advisory role, the Drug Enforcement Administration (DEA) ultimately determines how restrictively to schedule a particular drug.

This regulatory intersection of psychopharmacology and enforcement is sometimes caught up in larger political concerns. A striking example is the persistent policy debate over the medical use of marijuana. The FDA recommended more than a decade ago that marijuana be transferred to Schedule II so that the drug could be prescribed for certain conditions, such as glaucoma, severe chronic pain, and appetite loss associated with chemotherapy and AIDS. Although the DEA administrative judge upheld the FDA recommendation, DEA has not modified marijuana's legal status. Arguing that other drugs can effectively be prescribed for these conditions, DEA administrators assert that even limited medical use of marijuana will encourage increased nonmedical use by implicitly endorsing the drug's safety.

Whatever the pharmacologic merits of these arguments concerning medical marijuana, it is clear that politics predominate. Despite the federal prohibition, 36 states have adopted laws that permit patients with certain conditions to use marijuana with a physician's approval. While the vast majority of Americans oppose the legalization or decriminalization of marihuana (9), most believe that the drug should be medically available (10).

In California, whether to permit medical use of marijuana was decided by voter referendum in November 1996. The legislation allows seriously ill patients to use marijuana in their medical treatment, exempting them from the state's criminal marijuana laws. In the years since the California voters approved this initiative, the federal government has threatened doctors with federal criminal prosecution if they advise their patients about the medical uses of marijuana. In addition, the Department of Justice has prosecuted several individuals who grow marijuana for medicinal purposes as major traffickers, despite the provisions of the state law making medical marijuana use legal. The federal government claims that federal drug laws govern, not state laws. However, in July 2003, the U.S. Court of Appeals for the Ninth Circuit found that doctors have the right to recommend marijuana to their patients because states, not the federal government, have the power to regulate the practice of medicine. This landmark issue will ultimately be decided by the U.S. Supreme Court.

In 1996, voters in Arizona approved by referendum new legislation that requires that nonviolent drug offenders arrested for possession or use must receive drug treatment instead of jail time for their first and second offenses. (The law also allows doctors to prescribe marijuana and other drugs for medicinal use "when it becomes legal to do so under federal law." This has not yet happened.) An evaluation of the impact of the new law after its first year found that 2,600 nonviolent offenders had been diverted into treatment, saving Arizona taxpayers $2.56 million. In its second year, the law saved more than $6 million in prison costs. Of the offenders completing the program, 75% tested drug-free.

In 2000, California voters approved a referendum similar to the Arizona measure: nonviolent drug offenders arrested for possession or use receive drug treatment rather than incarceration. The California measure also appropriated additional funds ($120 million annually) to support treatment services. During the law's first year of implementation, drug possession admissions to prison per 1,000 arrests fell by 30% compared to the year 2000. The estimated savings to California taxpayers over 5 years is $1.5 billion.

Several other states have considered initiatives expanding permissible marijuana use, including for medical purposes; however, these have generally not succeeded.

The political intensity surrounding the medical marijuana issue suggests the larger landscape of federal drug policy, which seeks to protect Americans from illicit drugs by reducing drug availability (supply control) and by reducing demand for drugs through prevention and treatment.

---

[a] The Controlled Substances Act, 21 U.S.C. §§ 801ff., was originally passed as Title II of the Comprehensive Drug Abuse Prevention and Control Act of 1970.

FEDERAL ANTIDRUG SPENDING TARGETS ILLEGAL DRUGS

In 2003, the federal antidrug budget exceeded $19 billion. These funds were targeted against illegal drugs, primarily heroin, marijuana, cocaine, and amphetamines. Every cabinet department had a substantial antidrug program, ranging from $9 billion in the Justice Department to $40 million in the Department of Agriculture. In 1988, Congress created the Office of National Drug Control Policy (ONDCP) to coordinate this multibillion dollar, multiagency federal effort. The ONDCP director, known as the "drug czar," is also responsible for developing the national drug strategy.

Alcohol and Tobacco

The legal drugs alcohol and tobacco, which cannot legally be sold to minors, are generally not considered part of federal drug control policy. Although these two drugs account for more than 500,000 deaths a year in the United States, they have traditionally been addressed as public health issues, quite separate from the government's "war on drugs." This distinction has begun to erode in recent years. In August 1996, President William Clinton approved the FDA's assertion of regulatory authority over tobacco. Powerful industry interests mounted legal challenges to this initiative, and in March 2000, the U.S. Supreme Court ruled 5 to 4 that Congress had not yet given the FDA jurisdiction to regulate tobacco products or related marketing practices (11–14). Although the Court found that "tobacco use, particularly among children and adolescents, poses perhaps the single most significant threat to public health in the United States," it determined that Congress had precluded the FDA from asserting jurisdiction to oversee tobacco products or their marketing to minimize health harms. According to the Supreme Court, Congress must adopt new legislation that expressly provides FDA (or another federal agency) this authority. To date, the tobacco industry has successfully resisted congressional efforts to legislate tough regulatory powers for the FDA over tobacco.

Adolescent smoking and drinking are addressed as part of federal drug policy in the context of adolescent drug prevention efforts. About a third of the government's limited drug prevention budget goes toward school and community programs to curtail youthful substance abuse, which predominantly consists of smoking, drinking, and marijuana use. Despite these efforts, alcohol use remains widespread among young teenagers. In 2002, 1 in 5 eighth-grade students reported regular drinking (i.e., had a drink at least once in the past 30 days) while 1 in 7 reported having been drunk at least once in the previous month. Two-thirds of high school seniors say they know a peer with a drinking problem (7).

More than 1 million teens become regular smokers each year, even though they cannot legally purchase tobacco. By twelfth grade, 1 in 4 students smokes. Advertising plays a critical role in encouraging teens to smoke. In 2001, the tobacco industry spent $11.22 billion for advertising and promotions, much of it directed toward young people. Nicotine addiction is acquired early: 95% of all adult smokers began smoking before the age of 19 years (15).

FEDERAL DRUG STRATEGY CONCENTRATES ON REDUCING SUPPLIES

The federal drug budget has grown more than tenfold since 1981, when President Ronald Reagan radically changed the focus of drug policy. Under previous Republican and Democratic administrations, prevention and treatment—efforts to reduce the demand for drugs—received at least as much funding as supply control initiatives. President Richard Nixon, faced with a heroin epidemic among U.S. personnel serving in the Vietnam War, actually devoted 75% of his drug budget to treatment during the early 1970s (16).

President Reagan, promising to end the "evil scourge" of drugs, more than doubled drug enforcement funding from 1981 to 1986. Reagan believed that the nation's borders could effectively be sealed against foreign drugs in much the same way Americans could be protected from the missiles of the "evil empire" (the former Soviet Union) by the Strategic Defense Initiative. At the same time, federal funding for prevention, education, and treatment was substantially cut. From 1981 to 1985, prevention and education programs received an average of $23 million a year, less than 1% of the total federal drug budget (17). These cuts in demand-reduction programs undermined the basic premise of earlier U.S. drug policy: that a reduction in illicit supplies would force addicts into treatment and prevent potential new users from trying drugs.

The primary concentration on supply control strategies has continued under both Republican and Democratic presidents, whose antidrug budgets have generally allocated two-thirds of all funding to enforcement, interdiction, and source country programs. In part, these spending decisions reflect political pressures to appear "tough" on drugs, particularly in election years, when voter concerns are more loudly expressed. At the same time, Americans are increasingly concerned about drug treatment. Because of inadequate funding both at the federal and state levels, as well as shrinking insurance coverage, only 1 in 4 addicts can get treatment.

The imbalance of the federal drug budget, which strongly favors enforcement, has been widely criticized in recent years. In 2003, the George W. Bush administration radically changed the way in which the drug budget is calculated with the result that spending for treatment appears to have achieved a balance with spending for enforcement. For more than two decades, the drug budget provided a comprehensive summary of antidrug spending by all Federal agencies. However, the new format specifically excludes billions of dollars spent for incarcerating drug offenders as well as other drug enforcement costs. Because these amounts (about $8 billion a year) are no longer attributed to federal drug spending, the overall budget looks far more balanced between supply reduction (law enforcement) and demand reduction (prevention and treatment). In addition, the budget now includes several hundred million dollars for treatment of alcohol abuse, which has never before been part of the federal drug budget.

Both Republican and Democratic administrations have been criticized for devoting the majority of resources to enforcement—usually two-thirds of total spending—with much smaller amounts going for prevention and treatment. The new Bush administration approach does not actually reduce spending for drug enforcement and incarceration of drug offenders; it simply does not include these costs in its reporting of the federal drug budget. The result is that the proposed 2004 drug budget of $11 billion appears to be split almost evenly between supply and demand reduction efforts. If traditional accounting methods were used, the proposed drug budget would actually be almost $20 billion, two-thirds of which is allocated for supply reduction.

Supply side drug strategies reflect the long-standing popular view that other countries are largely responsible for America's drug problems. This view has deep historic roots dating back a hundred years. When the first drug laws were adopted early in this century, immigrant groups and minorities were linked in the public mind with drug abuse: opium was associated with Chinese laborers in the West, cocaine with blacks in the South, and marihuana with Mexican immigrants in the Southwest. These drugs were seen as foreign threats to America's social fabric, undermining traditional moral values and political stability (8, pp. 5–6).

Blaming foreigners for America's recurring drug epidemics continues to have powerful political appeal. Getting Mexican and Bolivian farmers to stop growing opium and coca seems easier than curbing America's demand for heroin and cocaine. The argument also seems logically compelling: If there were no drugs coming in, there would be no drug problem. Even if some drugs got through, reduced supplies should drive up drug prices, cutting drug abuse within the United States. Unfortunately, the experience of the past two decades has demonstrated that supply control efforts themselves cannot reduce America's drug problems.

The Supply Side Scorecard

Since 1981, American taxpayers have spent more than $150 billion on federal efforts to reduce illicit drug supplies and availability through enforcement, interdiction, and international programs. Yet heroin and cocaine in the United States are more available at cheaper prices than ever before (6). Over the last decade, worldwide opium production has more than doubled, while coca production has also doubled (18). Heroin now sells for less than half its 1981 street price, and heroin purity exceeds 85% in many cities, compared with only 7% purity in 1981. Cocaine prices have dropped by half (19). High school seniors nationwide report that crack is as easy to obtain now as it was during the height of the crack epidemic in 1987, and that heroin is significantly easier to get now.

The "new" heroin epidemic widely described by the popular press in the mid-1990s primarily involved affluent professionals, high-fashion figures, and rock stars. Driven in large part by the ready availability of high-quality, cheap heroin, this epidemic has since spread to all levels of society, including small towns where heroin was virtually unknown. However, the "new" heroin is so pure that it can be snorted or smoked, avoiding the dangers of human immunodeficiency virus (HIV) infection and unsightly track marks involved with intravenous heroin use. Like powder cocaine two decades ago, heroin seems to offer the seductive illusion of a relatively safe, intensely pleasurable high. Unfortunately, the "new" heroin causes overdose deaths from snorting or smoking just as the old heroin did from mainlining. From 1989 to 1998, heroin overdoses in the United States almost tripled (20).

U.S. International Drug Control Policy

A top priority of U.S. drug control efforts is to keep illegal drugs out of the country and to curtail illegal drug production and trafficking in other parts of the world. U.S. policy is carried out both bilaterally, where assistance is provided directly to foreign governments, and multilaterally through the United Nations and regional organizations, such as the Organization of American States (OAS). The United States is a signatory to all the major international drug treaties, including the 1961 Single Convention on Narcotic Drugs, the 1976 Convention on Psychotropic Substances, and the 1988 Vienna Convention Against Illicit Traffic in Narcotic Drugs and Psychotropic Substances, which provide an international legal framework that binds signatory countries to adopt measures to implement various drug control measures.

The governmental structure of U.S. international drug control efforts has changed with the creation of the Department of Homeland Security in response to the terrorist attacks of September 11, 2001. Two major agencies charged with border interdiction, the Customs Service and the Coast Guard, have been incorporated into the new department, where the focus is primarily on protecting the U.S. from terrorism. It is still too soon to know how this reorganization will affect the interdiction of drugs, although some observers believe that heightened security at airports and border check points will result in increased seizures. (Alternatively, drug traffickers may develop new routes that bypass checkpoints.)

In many ways, America's war on terrorism has subsumed the war on drugs. In addition to the bureaucratic reorganization of drug interdiction agencies, the government now actively links terrorism to drug trafficking, particularly in terms of public perception. A striking example of this change came just after 9/11, when the drug czar's office announced a new series of costly antidrug advertisements aimed at youth. The central message of these ads was that users of illicit drugs were in effect supporting terrorists, on the theory that some terrorist groups (such as the FARC in Colombia) used drug money to buy weapons. One widely used ad suggested that a teen who smoked marijuana on the weekend should feel responsible indirectly for the murder of judges in Colombia. Public response to this campaign was overwhelmingly negative, in large part because teens generally found the ads ridiculous, and experts were concerned that this lack of credibility would undermine other prevention efforts. By the end of 2002, the drug czar's office had terminated the ads.

The great majority of the U.S. international drug control budget, which was $1.1 billion in 2003, supports drug enforcement efforts with foreign governments, targeting drug production and trafficking. Drug-eradication programs, which usually involve aerial spraying of herbicides on illicit drug crops by local officials with U.S. assistance, are also an important priority. In addition to enforcement and crop eradication, a portion of the $2.3 billion spent on interdiction (in 2003) supports international efforts to disrupt drug transit routes and to seize drug shipments and financial assets. Since 1988, total federal spending for international drug control, including interdiction, has exceeded $30 billion.

The primary targets for U.S. international control efforts are in Latin America: Mexico, a major source of heroin and marijuana for the U.S. market; Colombia, which now produces more than half the heroin consumed in the United States and almost all the cocaine; and to a much lesser extent, Peru and Bolivia which have traditionally grown coca and are important, although currently much reduced, sources for cocaine. A much smaller portion of U.S. international efforts are directed against opium and heroin coming from Pakistan and Afghanistan, as well as from Southeast Asia's Golden Triangle.

U.S. international drug eradication efforts have sometimes had unanticipated political consequences. A recent example is Bolivia, which has been a major producer of coca for decades. Although there is a limited legal market for Bolivian coca—both for indigenous coca chewing and for Coca Cola syrup that uses coca without cocaine—the big demand is from the illicit international cocaine traffic. During the 1990s, U.S. pressure intensified on a series of Bolivian governments to curtail coca production. This pressure, accompanied by hundreds of millions of dollars in U.S. foreign assistance, appeared to be working, because Bolivian coca production dropped dramatically in the late 1990s. However, faced with the loss of their only reliable cash crop and no effective crop substitutes, coca growers, known as cocaleros, became increasingly vocal about their grievances. The cocaleros, who now have considerable political power after years of protest, currently threaten the stability of the already fragile Bolivian government. Meanwhile, illegal coca production is again increasing.

Structural Flaws in Supply Side Strategy

In the past three decades, drug production has expanded rapidly into every region of the world. Poor farmers who do not have solid alternative sources of income have strong economic incentives to grow drug crops even under difficult circumstances. If one production area is wiped out, crops can easily be replaced. In the early 1990s, for example, a coca fungus in one region of Peru pushed cultivation into more remote, previously uncultivated areas. In the Central Asian republics of the former Soviet Union, opium became an important new source of revenue after the fall of the Soviet Union. In Kyrgyzstan, for example, a pound of opium brought $400 in 1994—two-thirds of the per capita gross national product (GNP).

Hard drugs are an easy way to generate hard currency, particularly in countries where foreign reserves are low. In early 2003, a North Korean defector, in testimony before the U.S. Senate, reported that the North Korean government is overseeing the production and export of thousands of pounds of heroin and methamphetamine each month to bolster the country's failing foreign currency reserves. The cash-strapped dictatorship is relying on illicit drug production and trafficking to finance its costly nuclear weapons program.

The economics of drug cultivation make sustained worldwide reductions in supply very unlikely. Moreover, the American market does not need to depend on foreign drug supplies. Many psychoactive drugs, such as amphetamines, lysergic acid diethylamide (LSD), and methylenedioxymethamphetamine (MDMA), are produced illicitly within the United States. Marijuana has also become a major crop in this country, despite its illegality: at least a third of all marijuana consumed here is domestically cultivated (6).

America's drug requirements can be supplied from a relatively small growing area and transported in a few airplanes. Although the United States has large numbers of illicit drug users, Americans actually consume a relatively small portion of total worldwide drug production— approximately 5% of all heroin and about 33% of all cocaine production. A 35-square-mile poppy field (about half the area of Washington, DC) can supply the American heroin market for a year, while annual cocaine demand can be met from coca fields covering about 300 square miles (less than one-quarter of the size of Rhode Island).

Three Boeing 747 cargo planes could transport the nation's annual cocaine supply of 260 metric tons; 3 much smaller DC-3A planes could carry the annual 13-metric-ton heroin supply. Given the country's long, porous borders and the high volume of cross-border air, sea, and land traffic, interdiction has not proved successful in markedly reducing drug availability within the United States.

Most important, however, is that the price structure of the drug market severely limits any impact interdiction efforts might have. The largest drug profits are made at the street level, not in foreign poppy or coca fields or on the high seas. The RAND Corporation estimates that the total cost of growing, refining, and smuggling cocaine to the United States accounts for less than 12% of retail prices. The cost of producing and importing heroin accounts for an even smaller fraction of the retail price (21). Even if the United States were able to intercept half the cocaine coming from South America—or eradicate half the coca crop—the price of cocaine in cities would increase by only 5%. With cocaine prices at record lows, such a minor increase would be unlikely to affect consumption. It is ironic that the street price of a gram of illicit cocaine is now lower than the price of a gram of legal, medicinal cocaine, according to the Office of National Drug Control Policy.

DEMAND REDUCTION SHOWS GREATER PROMISE

Recent history offers an important lesson: the steepest declines in illicit drug use occurred during a period when drug availability was rapidly increasing. For example, in 1985, 5.75 million Americans reported using cocaine during the past month. By 1991, when cocaine prices hit new lows, only 2.37 million Americans reported cocaine or crack use within the past month (22). This sharp drop reflected growing public awareness that cocaine is harmful as well as a change in social attitudes, particularly among Americans most responsive to health concerns.

Since 1992, however, public tolerance for drug use has increased; a majority of both teenagers and adults view drugs as less harmful than they did a decade ago (23). During the same period, marijuana use among eighth graders has more than doubled. The link between social attitudes and drug use is clear: as public acceptance of drugs increases, so does use, particularly among young people.

PREVENTION REMAINS LOW PRIORITY IN FEDERAL POLICY

Despite the encouraging results of a wide range of prevention initiatives, including antitobacco and antidrug advertising, prevention remains the lowest policy priority. The federal government, as well as most states and cities, spend less than 15% of their total antidrug budgets on prevention. In the fiscal year 2003 federal drug budget, prevention programs received $2.47 billion, compared to $12.89 billion for domestic law enforcement, interdiction, and international efforts to curtail the supply of drugs.

For officials whose horizons are often defined by election cycles, prevention may seem too long-term an investment to provide immediate political returns. The impact of prevention is difficult to capture visually, particularly in 30-second segments on the evening news. The results of good programs may require years to develop, and are often measured in negative terms, when something—such as smoking or using drugs—doesn't happen. Drug seizures or arrests of drug dealers provide far more graphic demonstrations that officials are responding to voter concerns about drug abuse.

Although many Americans strongly support prevention, they often do not have a clear understanding of what actually works. Prevention research, which has received even lower funding priority than prevention itself, is often difficult for nonspecialists to interpret. Findings are generally published in academic journals, which lag behind the research by several years and which are intended for scholarly rather than lay audiences. As a result, the case for prevention in the public arena often lacks a sound research basis, leaving prevention funding vulnerable to rapid shifts in political direction.

Extensive studies over the past two decades have documented the cost-effectiveness of early prevention and education efforts. For example, two thoroughly evaluated school curricula, Life Skills Training (LST) and Students Taught Awareness and Resistance (STAR), reduce new smoking and marijuana use by half and drinking by one-third (24). The cost of these programs ranges between $15 and $35 per pupil, including classroom materials and teacher training. By contrast, the average cost for 1 year of outpatient drug treatment is about $7,500; for residential treatment, about $16,500; and for incarceration, about $27,500.

Unfortunately, many of the programs currently being used in classrooms across the country do not cover the essential elements of prevention. Moreover, many have not been evaluated using pretest, posttest control group designs that measure actual reductions in tobacco, drug, and alcohol use. Some programs that have been adequately evaluated, like LST, STAR, and Project Alert, have produced promising behavioral results. However, without subsequent booster sessions, these results disappear within several years. Nonetheless, any delay in starting to smoke, drink, and use drugs is beneficial, because children gain time to develop social competence and strength to resist peer and media influences to smoke, drink, and use drugs.

Families, communities, and the media shape the larger social context in which children make decisions about alcohol, tobacco, and drug use. Prevention is most effective when school lessons are reinforced by a clear, consistent message that teen alcohol, tobacco, and drug use is harmful, unacceptable, and illegal.

TREATMENT WORKS BUT IS OFTEN UNAVAILABLE

Although the public is skeptical about the efficacy of drug treatment, two-thirds of Americans support treatment rather than incarceration as a primary approach to nonviolent drug offenders (25). Numerous long-term, large-scale studies report that treatment works—particularly for addicts who remain in treatment for 1 year or longer (26, p. 135). Yet since the early 1980s, treatment has also been a far lower priority of federal drug policy than drug enforcement. As a result, only 1 in 4 of the nation's addicts can obtain treatment unless they can pay for private care. In many states, managed care is further eroding treatment availability as insurers reduce coverage for drug treatment (27,28).

Treatment is effective in reducing the social, health, and lost productivity costs related to drug addiction. A major study in 1994, the California Drug and Alcohol Treatment Assessment, found that $1 invested in alcohol and drug treatment saved taxpayers $7.14 in future costs (29). Providing treatment to all addicts in the United States would save more than $150 billion in social costs over the next 15 years, while requiring $21 billion in treatment costs (30). In 2003, the federal drug budget allocated $3.8 billion to treatment, less than one-third the amount devoted to supply control efforts.

DRUG ABUSE IS PERVASIVE AMONG CRIMINAL OFFENDERS

In 2000, approximately 2 million people were incarcerated in the United States with an additional 4 million under the jurisdiction of the criminal justice system. At the time of arrest, on average, two-thirds of arrestees nationwide (regardless of crime) tested positive for an illegal drug (31). Without treatment, 9 of 10 incarcerated criminals return to crime and drugs after prison, and the majority are rearrested within 3 years (26, p. 184).

Treatment is cost-effective even for seriously addicted criminal offenders. A 1994 RAND Corporation study found that $34 million invested in treatment would reduce cocaine use as much as an expenditure of $246 million for domestic law enforcement (30). Extensive studies show that treatment of drug offenders does work. Therapeutic communities inside prisons reduce recidivism by a third to a half after inmates return to society. The most effective programs are extremely rigorous, demanding far more from offenders than passive incarceration, and they cost only $5,000 to $8,000 a year per inmate (26, pp. 177–180).

Yet treatment for criminals is scarce. Less than 5% of federal prisoners with drug abuse problems participate in intensive treatment programs (32). In addition, more than 75% of all state prison and county jail inmates are drug abusers, but only 10% receive any help. Even these numbers are inflated, because most prison treatment—which consists of drug education and occasional counseling—is ineffective, according to the General Accounting Office (GAO) (33,34).

Within prisons, priority should be given to treating offenders with serious heroin and cocaine problems, because they are responsible for the largest proportion of predatory crimes. Intensive residential drug treatment, which has proven effective in reducing recidivism among this group, is the most cost-effective approach according to the Institute of Medicine. The Institute of Medicine estimates that there are at least 250,000 prison inmates and 750,000 offenders on probation and parole who need this kind of intensive treatment (26, p. 235).

Treatment should also be provided for parolees. Community supervision programs for offenders on parole or probation—regardless of their offense—usually fail unless drug treatment is provided (35). The more intensive and structured the treatment, the more likely it is to be effective. But because the number of treatment programs of any sort are woefully inadequate, offenders must compete with noncriminal addicts for limited treatment space. Since 1992, every major city has created special drug courts to provide immediate treatment for drug offenders. (In 2003, there were an estimated 1,000 drug courts operating in every state in the country.) These programs have shown good results, with an annual treatment cost per offender of $2,500 to $4,000. But in most cities, drug offenders generally do not get treatment, although many would participate if treatment were available.

POLARIZED DEBATE OVER FEDERAL POLICY

The public debate over drug policy, unlike many other areas of government action, is often polarized by deeply felt moral and philosophical differences. Some people advocate tougher drug enforcement and more prisons, while others urge legalization of drugs. This debate affects a wide range of issues involving the treatment of addicts and drug offenders (36). One example of the "get tougher" view is legislation adopted by Congress in August 1996, making anyone convicted of a drug-related felony (possession, use, or distribution) ineligible for welfare (Aid for Families with Dependent Children) and food stamps.

The history of methadone maintenance treatment in this country has been seriously affected by the debate over policy. Developed more than 30 years ago as a legal synthetic narcotic, methadone has proved effective in reducing heroin use, increasing productivity, and curtailing criminal activity from the first day of treatment. Methadone maintenance has a significant effect on the spread of HIV/AIDS, hepatitis B and C, tuberculosis, and sexually transmitted diseases (37). The National Institute on Drug Abuse found that weekly heroin use among outpatients receiving methadone decreased by 69%, criminal activity decreased by 52%, and employment increased by 24% (38).

Despite the extensive evidence of methadone's efficacy as a treatment of last resort for heroin addicts, methadone maintenance remains quite limited as a treatment modality. In 2000, about 108,000 of the estimated 810,000 heroin addicts in the United States received methadone (39). In March 2001, a new regulatory system was established for methadone treatment for the purpose of making it more accessible. This change reflected recommendations by the National Academy of Science's Institute of Medicine in 1995 that the federal government expand the availability of methadone treatment and simplify regulations governing dosage levels and take-home medication (40).

The government's reluctance to expand methadone availability reflects broader political questions concerning treatment. Some officials (particularly in Congress) argue that methadone simply substitutes one narcotic for another and does not produce abstinence, which should be the goal of treatment. In this view, making methadone more readily available would discourage addicts from becoming abstinent, as well as deflect federal funds from drug-free treatment programs. On the other hand, many clinicians and researchers argue that methadone, the most extensively studied treatment modality in our history, should be allowed to play a larger role in reducing drug abuse and drug-related HIV infection—even if methadone-maintained addicts never achieve abstinence.

In 2002, the FDA approved a new drug for heroin treatment—buprenorphine (Buprenex), a partial opiate agonist that blocks withdrawal and craving without producing a strong narcotic high. Patients can get the drug privately at a doctor's office; about 2,000 physicians have been certified to prescribe it (under Schedule III of the Controlled Substances Act). Each physician is permitted to treat up to 30 patients. Available in pill form, buprenorphine may signal a new approach to addiction that expands narcotic treatment to physicians' offices and gives private practitioners a primary role in opiate treatment for the first time in many decades.

Needle-exchange programs, designed to provide clean injection equipment to intravenous drug users, continue to be controversial despite proven public health benefits. The percentage of AIDS cases attributed to injecting drug use accounts for one-third of all AIDS cases nationwide. Drug use accounts for two-thirds of AIDS cases among women and more than half of all pediatric AIDS cases (41). In an effort to reduce HIV transmission by drug users, needle-exchange (or clean-needle distribution) programs now operate in more than 60 cities across the country, although they are illegal in most states. The mayors of San Francisco and Los Angeles have declared states of emer-gency, which permit these programs to continue despite California law.

Since 1988, Congress has prohibited the use of federal funds to directly support needle-exchange programs, largely because officials feared that these programs might encourage addiction by making needles easier to obtain and by tacitly communicating social approval of drug use. According to language adopted by Congress in 1992, the ban on federal funds for needle-exchange programs is to remain in effect "unless the Surgeon General of the United States determines that such programs are effective in preventing the spread of HIV and do not encourage the use of illegal drugs." Despite the ban on direct support, Congress has permitted the use of federal funds to conduct demonstration and research projects that involve the provision of needles (42).

Studies in a number of cities—including a comprehensive evaluation commissioned by the U.S. Centers for Disease Control and Prevention—found that needle-exchange programs reduce the spread of HIV and hepatitis B without increasing drug use (43). In 1995, after a 2-year review mandated by Congress, the National Academy of Sciences explicitly recommended that the Surgeon General rescind the prohibition against applying any federal funds to support needle exchange programs (44). The American Medical Association, the American Academy of Pediatrics, and many other scientific organizations supported this recommendation. However, neither the Clinton administration nor the Bush administration acted on this recommendation. In contrast, countries with very strict drug laws, such as China, Iran, and Indonesia, have recently sanctioned needle-exchange programs in an effort to check the rapid rise of HIV/AIDS and hepatitis infections from shared needles, particularly among young people. Although this is a very new approach for countries where enforcement has long dominated drug policy, the AIDS epidemic has forced governments to turn to public health measures designed to reduce at least some of the harms related to intravenous drug use.

FEDERAL POLICY RESISTANT TO NEW DIRECTIONS

There are a number of reasons why federal drug policy continues to concentrate primarily on supply control rather than demand reduction. Bureaucratic inertia plays a considerable role; despite quite different political rhetoric under Republican and Democratic administrations, the policy remains essentially unchanged. In part, this reflects the interests of the many agencies involved in maintaining their share of the ever-larger federal drug budget, including personnel, equipment, and operating funds. More significant, however, is the historical legacy of the early drug laws and the traditional view of the nation's drug problem as predominantly criminal and foreign in origin.

As discussed earlier, Americans have traditionally blamed other countries for "supplying" domestic drug abusers. Recent history provides a number of dramatic examples of how this view affects policy. In the late 1960s, President Richard Nixon sealed a major border crossing point with Mexico in an effort to force the Mexican government to take action against marihuana and heroin production. At the same time, a U.S. Senator publicly threatened to bomb Istanbul, Turkey, if the Turkish government did not curtail illegal opium production used in the infamous "French Connection" heroin traffic. Since then, U.S. officials have issued similar threats against other drug-producing countries, most recently in Latin America. In 1989, President George Bush invaded Panama and transported then-dictator General Manuel Noriega to the United States for trial because of his role in drug trafficking. (Notwithstanding Noriega's departure, Panama remains a major cocaine transshipment site. According to the U.S. Department of State (18), Panama is "ideal for narcotics smuggling and illicit financial transactions" and "has not yet developed the resources or expertise to interdict narcotics on a consistent basis.")

In 1996, President Clinton "decertified" Colombia for inadequate antidrug cooperation, which effectively meant the cutoff of U.S. aid (except for drug-control aid) and U.S. opposition to World Bank and other multilateral development loans (45).[b] However, 3 years later, under a newly elected president, Colombia became the third largest recipient of U.S. foreign assistance in the world (after Egypt and Israel), receiving $1.3 billion in U.S. aid over a 3-year period for a major offensive against coca cultivation and cocaine trafficking. Known as "Plan Colombia," this campaign is directed at heavily armed rebel groups at war with the Colombian government that finance their insurgency with money from the drug trade.

Although U.S.-supported foreign campaigns against drugs can produce temporary declines in supplies, they do not last. In the past three decades, the opium eradication programs in Mexico and Turkey were the only successes, and these were very short-lived. In both cases, other suppliers quickly filled the production gap. Within 5 years, Mexico resumed its major illegal production role, while Turkey became prominent in drug trafficking (confining its opium production to the legal pharmaceutical market).

In Colombia, when the Medellin cartel was broken up and its leaders killed by government forces in 1989 and 1990, cocaine prices in the United States temporarily increased (because of interrupted supplies). However, within 6 months, prices declined to their original levels as other trafficking groups (particularly the Cali cartel) took over the Medellin business (46).[c] Colombia is now the single largest supplier of both heroin and cocaine for the U.S. market.

In addition to viewing other countries as the source for domestic drug abuse problems, Americans have traditionally looked to drug enforcement as the primary means to curb addiction and to protect citizens from drug offenders. The underlying assumption has been that the threat of jail is sufficient deterrence to keep people from using, buying, and selling illegal drugs. While the prospect of a criminal record is undoubtedly an effective deterrent for many Americans, it does not prevent everyone from trying drugs, as the rising use of marijuana and synthetic drugs like ecstasy (MDMA) among young teenagers demonstrates. And people who are already addicted are often not responsive to threats of punishment, because much of their lives focus on finding the next fix. Nor does time behind bars change addictive behavior for most drug offenders, judging from the high recidivism rates.

Yet arrest, prosecution, and incarceration provide tangible proof that the government is "doing something" about drugs. Sizable drug seizures also provide concrete evidence of official vigilance, more easily understood than lengthy treatment and prevention programs that measure progress over years rather than months.

Recently, Americans have begun questioning whether this approach actually produces positive results, including lower rates of addiction, less drug crime, and safer schools and neighborhoods. A small mountain of cocaine seized by Customs officials projects a powerful image of enforcement effectiveness on the nightly news; however—as many communities have discovered—these seizures don't necessarily translate into less cocaine or fewer addicts on their streets. Indeed, the experience of the past two decades suggests that drug enforcement has its greatest impact at the street level when police are involved with communities in driving out drug dealers (36,47). A nationwide survey of police chiefs reported that they believe (by a margin of two to one) that reducing drug and alcohol abuse

---

[b] For a discussion of the annual process by which the president must certify whether or not other countries are cooperating with U.S. antidrug efforts, see reference 45. Subject to domestic political concerns, as well as competing foreign policy interests, the certification process is a dubious gauge of antidrug cooperation, even as it provokes resentment toward the United States, especially in Latin America. Moreover, certification's exclusive focus on international drug control perpetuates the notion that supply rather than demand is at the heart of America's drug problem.

[c] For a discussion of fluctuations in illicit drug prices over time, see reference 47, Table 4. Apparently as a consequence of the 1989 crackdown in Colombia, the U.S. retail price per pure gram of cocaine rose by about $50 in 1990. However, in 1991, the average price receded to the low levels of the late-1980s, and dropped still lower in 1992 and 1993. The continued low U.S. prices in the early 1990s occurred despite the fungal infestation of Peruvian coca, which resulted in an estimated 30% reduction in cocaine production from 1992 to 1993. Prices did not rise, in part, because cocaine suppliers stockpile supplies in anticipation of shortages.

is a more effective strategy for combating violent crime than longer prison sentences for criminals (2). There is a remarkable consensus among those who are directly involved in dealing with drug addiction and drug crime: new approaches are needed if lasting solutions are to be found.

Despite the urgent need for more effective strategies, research receives approximately 5% of the drug budget, which is used primarily for treatment studies. Only $50 million of the $1 billion research budget is used to evaluate drug enforcement and interdiction, which in 2003 constituted two-thirds of total antidrug spending (6). While enforcement must be an important part of any comprehensive national drug strategy, it cannot, by itself, solve the nation's drug abuse problems, as experience has demonstrated.

In the rapid buildup of drug enforcement since 1981, funding decisions have been driven largely by political pressures rather than research or empirical evidence. The Clinton administration experience provides an excellent example. Responding to Republican attacks on his drug-fighting record, President Clinton requested interdiction funding that increased by nearly 20% from fiscal 1995 to fiscal 1997, while requested funding for prevention fell by 22% over the same period. Clinton's budget increases for interdiction ignored the findings of a major National Security Council policy review in 1993 that concluded that interdiction had not succeeded in slowing the flow of cocaine into this country.[d] But the political stakes of changing policy direction are high. Republicans in Congress tried to eliminate the ONDCP, contending that its budget would be better spent on interdiction than on coordinating the multiagency federal antidrug effort (19, pp. 123). Although Clinton succeeded in having ONDCP's budget restored (under threat of a presidential veto), he also moved to increase supply side spending, particularly interdiction. As a result, the Clinton administration's drug budget from 1993 to 2001 looked very much like the drug budgets of the previous decade, with more than two-thirds of the funds supporting enforcement, interdiction, and source country programs.

TOWARD A MORE EFFECTIVE FEDERAL DRUG POLICY

The political obstacles facing any real change in policy direction are formidable. Nationwide surveys, however, indicate that the American people are more pragmatic and less ideologic about drug policy than the polarized political debate suggests. Hart polls in 1995 and 1996 found that the public and the nation's police chiefs strongly favor a balanced approach, with an equal emphasis on reducing demand through education, prevention, and treatment (1,2). The surveys convey above all that Americans want programs that work.

Yet most people do not have a clear sense of what does work to reduce drug abuse and drug crime. Nor do most officials know the results of recent research on prevention, treatment, and law enforcement. The information is often difficult to obtain and ambiguous, without sharply defined findings or apparent practical relevance. Indeed, our present knowledge could best be described as possible indicators for a map, pointing in promising directions, rather than a blueprint for a perfect strategy.

But we do know a great deal more about what works than we did in the late 1960s, when the current "war on drugs" began. Some of this knowledge has come from research; much has come from experience. From 1977 to 1981, the author was Assistant Secretary of State for International Narcotics Matters, responsible for designing and implementing many of the source-country programs still operating today. At the time, crop eradication and income substitution (to assist opium and coca farmers develop alternative livelihoods) seemed a promising approach to reducing illicit drug cultivation in underdeveloped countries. In the 1970s, these programs were largely experimental, but later administrations expanded them significantly. From 1984 to 1994, for example, the United States provided nearly $2 billion in economic, police, and military aid to Bolivia, Peru, and Colombia (48). Despite this considerable effort, annual coca production nearly doubled over the course of the decade; after apparently leveling off in the early 1990s, more land was under coca and opium poppy cultivation in 1995 than ever before, setting new records for potential yields of cocaine and heroin.[e]

Despite continuing U.S. pressure, governments have been unwilling or unable to sustain drug-eradication campaigns. According to State Department figures, from 1989 through 1996, less than 3.5% of the Andean coca cultivation was eradicated. Any reductions in cultivation have been temporary and symbolic, because new plantings continue to expand. For example, from 1987 to 1993, the Bolivian government used $49 million in U.S. foreign aid to pay farmers to pull up 25,000 hectares of coca. During the same period, however, farmers planted more than 37,000 hectares of new coca (51). Ironically, this well-intended U.S. aid program became little more than a coca support

---

[d] Presidential Decision Directive (PDD) 14, issued November 1993, called for a controlled shift in focus of cocaine interdiction operations from the transit zones to source countries, on the theory that it is more effective to attack drugs at the source of production rather than once they are in transit to the United States.

[e] The International Narcotics Control Strategy Report (49), published annually since 1987 by the U.S. State Department, is regarded as more authoritative than any other report on illicit drug production, but its estimates are generally considered conservative and have displayed inexplicable inconsistencies over time. (Because the information sources and technology used to make the estimates are classified, the government's methodology cannot be evaluated independently.)

program for Bolivian farmers. It has had no impact on America's cocaine problem.

At the same time that the inherent limitations of U.S. international supply control efforts have become apparent, research on prevention, treatment, and community-based law enforcement has pointed out new directions for effective action. The current laws provide sufficient flexibility for a major shift away from supply control strategies toward demand-reduction initiatives. Law enforcement still has an important role to play, particularly in helping citizens restore the fabric and the safety of their communities. But the effectiveness of drug enforcement spending has to be subject to the same scrutiny as prevention and treatment, so that our tax dollars support programs that measurably reduce addiction and crime.

The experience of many Western countries is instructive, despite considerable cultural differences between those countries and ours. In the past decade, many European governments have modified previously strict laws prohibiting drug sales and possession. Spain and Italy decriminalized marijuana in the 1990s; Portugal in 2001; and Luxembourg and Belgium in 2002. The Netherlands has tolerated drug use since the late 1970s, and now is making heroin maintenance available on a limited basis. (The Scandinavian countries are the exception, retaining very tough drug laws.) Regardless of the legal framework, most European countries give priority to demand reduction. Arrest and imprisonment are a last resort, reserved for dealers and addicts who repeatedly reject treatment. Social and health services, as well as drug treatment, are readily available and prevention is the primary strategy for reducing drug abuse (52).

Despite strong opposition from the Bush administration, Canada has also moved to decriminalize possession of small amounts of marijuana. Although they are technically illegal, safe injection sites now operate in Vancouver, supervised by medical staff that provides free needles, swabs, and sterile water for cooking heroin and cocaine.

Similar facilities operate in Australia, Germany, Switzerland, and the Netherlands. In a notable break with U.S. drug policy, the Canadian government now takes the view that drug use and addiction are primarily health concerns rather than criminal justice issues.

In the United States, we have made considerable progress against occasional drug use, particularly of cocaine. However, the number of hard-core drug users (heroin and cocaine) has increased from 600,000 a decade ago to nearly 1 million in 2002. This trend is marked among young adults. The number of 18- to 25-year-olds who reported using heroin in the last month jumped to 67,000 in 2001 from 26,000 in 2000, according to the National Household Survey.

Health concerns and social attitudes play a powerful role in shaping drug-taking behavior, as changes in adult cocaine, tobacco, and marijuana use show. Studies show that prevention programs, reinforced by community efforts, can substantially reduce new drug and alcohol use among schoolchildren. Treatment also can be effective. Extensive research has found that 3 of 4 addicts can learn to live without drugs if treatment is structured and sustained for 1 year or longer, and if meaningful alternatives are available (25, pp. 14–15). Within the criminal justice system, treatment can reduce recidivism among drug offenders by a third to a half (25 , p. 184).

How do we translate this knowledge into federal drug policy so that federal spending priorities reflect the lessons learned from earlier approaches? Unless we are to remain prisoners of our past failures, drug policy should not be left solely to elected officials as it traditionally has been. Citizen coalitions, teachers, police, civic leaders, parents—all must play an active role in making sure the reality they experience in their homes, schools, and communities shapes the future direction of drug policy. The medical and scientific communities, too, must increase their involvement— their work lies at the heart of finding lasting solutions to America's drug problems.

REFERENCES

1. Roper ASW. *Social education survey.* Princeton, NJ: Author, 2001.
2. Peter D. Hart Research Associates. *Drugs and crime across America: police chiefs speak out.* Washington, DC: Drug Strategies and Police Foundation, 1996:2, 11–12.
3. Dieter RC. *On the front line: law enforcement views on the death penalty.* Washington, DC: Death Penalty Information Center, 1995:3–6.
4. Office of National Drug Control Policy. *The economic costs of drug abuse in the United States, 1992–1998.* 2001 Sep. GPO, Washington D.C.
5. U.S. Department of Health and Human Services. *Preliminary estimates from the National Household Survey on Drug Abuse, 1990–1994.* Washington, DC: US Government Printing Office, 1995.
6. Office of National Drug Control Policy. *The national drug control strategy: FY 2004, budget summary.* Washington, DC: US Government Printing Office, 2003.
7. Johnston LD, O'Malley PM, Bachman JG. *Monitoring the future: national survey results on drug use, 1975–2002.* Bethesda, MD: National Institute on Drug Abuse, 2003.
8. Musto DF. *The American disease,* 2nd ed. New York: Oxford University Press, 1987.
9. Maguire K, Pastore AL, eds. *Sourcebook of criminal justice statistics 1994.* Washington, DC: US Department of Justice, 1995:196–197.
10. Grinspoon L, Bakalar J. Marijuana as medicine. A plea for reconsideration *JAMA* 1995;23:1875–1876.
11. Bartecchi CE, MacKenzie TD, Schrier RW. The global tobacco epidemic. *Sci Am* 1995;272(5):44–51.
12. Ferraro T. The tobacco lobby. *Multinational Monitor* 1992;Jan/Feb:19–22.
13. Kluger R. *Ashes to ashes: America's hundred year cigarette war, the public health, and the unabashed triumph of Philip Morris.* New York: Knopf, 1996.
14. Massing M. How to win the tobacco war. *New York Review of Books* 1996;Jul 11:32–36.

15. Lynch BS, Bonnie RJ, eds. *Growing up tobacco free: preventing nicotine addiction in children and youths.* Washington, DC: National Academy Press, 1994.
16. Baum D. *Smoke and mirrors: the war on drugs and the politics of failure.* Boston: Little, Brown, 1996:56–57.
17. Falco M. Toward a more effective drug policy. In: University of Chicago Legal Forum, ed. *Toward a rational drug policy.* Chicago: University of Chicago Press, 1994:11–24.
18. Bureau for International Narcotics and Law Enforcement Affairs. *International narcotics control strategy report (INCSR), March 2002.* Washington, DC: US Department of State, 2002.
19. Falco M. U.S. drug policy: addicted to failure. *Foreign Policy* 1996;102:124–130.
20. CDC Compressed mortality data. Available from http://wonder.cdc.gov. Last accessed March 29, 2004.
21. Reuter P, Crawford G, Cave J. *Sealing the borders: The effects of increased military participation in drug interdiction.* Santa Monica, CA: RAND Corporation, 1988.
22. National Institute on Drug Abuse. *National household survey on drug abuse: main findings 1985 and 1991.* Washington, DC: US Department of Health and Human Services, 1988, 1992.
23. U.S. Department of Health and Human Services. *National survey results on drug abuse from the Monitoring the Future study, 1992–2001.* Washington, DC: US Government Printing Office, 2002.
24. Botvin GJ, Baker E, Dusenbury L, et al. Preventing adolescent drug abuse through a multimodal cognitive-behavioral approach: results of a 3-year study. *J Consult Clin Psych* 1992;58:437–446.
25. Peter Hart Research Associates. *Americans look at the drug problem.* Washington, DC: Drug Strategies, 1995.
26. Gerstein DR, Harwood HJ, eds. *Treating drug problems.* Washington, DC: National Academy Press, 1992.
27. U.S. Bureau of Labor Statistics. *Employee benefits in medium and large private establishments, 1993.* Washington, DC: US Government Printing Office, 1994.
28. Drug Strategies. *Investing in the workplace: how business and labor address substance abuse.* Washington, DC: Author, 1996:11–19.
29. *Evaluating recovery services: the California drug and alcohol treatment assessment (CALDATA), executive summary.* Sacramento, CA: Department of Alcohol and Drug Programs, 1994.
30. Rydell CP, Everingham SS. *Controlling cocaine: supply versus demand programs.* Santa Monica, CA: RAND Corporation, 1994.
31. Bureau of Justice Statistics (BJS). *Substance abuse and treatment, state and federal prisoners. Jan. 1999; BJS, Prisoners in 2001.* Jul 2002. GPO, Washington D.C.
32. National Institute of Corrections. *Intervening with substance-abusing offenders: a framework for action: The report of the National Task Force on Correctional Substance Abuse Strategies.* Washington, DC: US Government Printing Office, 1991.
33. U.S. General Accounting Office. *Drug treatment: despite new strategy, few federal inmates receive treatment.* Washington, DC: US Government Printing Office, 1991.
34. U.S. General Accounting Office. *Drug treatment: state prisons face challenges in providing services.* Washington, DC: US Government Printing Office, 1991.
35. Petersilia J, Turner S. *Evaluating intensive supervision probation/parole programs: results of a nationwide experiment.* Washington, DC: National Institute of Justice, 1991.
36. Falco M. *The making of a drug-free America: programs that work.* New York: Times Books, 1994:175–188.
37. McLellan AT, Arndt IO, Woody GE, et al. The effects of psychosocial services in substance abuse treatment. *JAMA* 1993;269:1953–1959; N.Y. State Committee of Methadone Program Administrators. *Regarding methadone treatment.* New York: 1997:6, 9, 10.
38. ONDCP. *Consultation document on methadone/LAAM.* GPO, Washington, DC: 1998 Sep 29.
39. U.S. Department of Health and Human Services. *Treatment episode data set (TEDS): 1992–2000.* 2003 (Jan.).
40. Rettig RA, Yarmolinsky A, eds. *Federal regulation of methadone treatment.* Washington, DC: National Academy Press, 1995.
41. U.S. Department of Health and Human Services. *HIV/AIDS surveillance report.* Atlanta: Centers for Disease Control and Prevention, 1995.
42. U.S. General Accounting Office. *Needle exchange programs: research suggests promise as an AIDS prevention strategy.* Washington, DC: US Government Printing Office, 1993.
43. Lurie P, Reingold AL. *The public health impact of needle exchange programs in the United States and abroad.* San Francisco, CA: University of California, 1993.
44. Normand J, Vlahov D, Moses LE, eds. *Preventing HIV transmission: the role of sterile needles and bleach.* Washington, DC: National Academy Press, 1995:1–8.
45. Falco M. Passing grades: branding nations won't resolve the U.S. drug problem. *Foreign Affairs* 1995;74(5):15–20.
46. Abt Associates. *What America's users spend on illegal drugs, 1988–1993.* Washington, DC: Office of National Drug Control Policy, 1995:18.
47. Kleiman MAR, Smith KD. State and local drug enforcement. In search of a strategy. In: Tonry M, Wilson JQ, eds. *Drugs and crime.* Chicago: University of Chicago Press, 1990:69–108.
48. U.S. Agency for International Development. *Congressional presentations, fiscal years 1984–1994.* Washington, DC: US Government Printing Office, 1985–1995.
49. Bureau for International Narcotics and Law Enforcement Affairs. *International narcotics control strategy reports (INCSRs), 1987–1996.* GPO, Washington D.C.
50. Reuter P. The mismeasurement of illegal drug markets: the implications of its irrelevance. In: Pozo S, ed. *Exploring the underground economy.* Kalamazoo, MI: W.E. Upjohn Institute, 1996:20–42.
51. Lee R. The economics of cocaine capitalism. *Cosmos* 1996;Jun:58–64.
52. Leuw E. Drugs and drug policy in the Netherlands. In: Tonry M, ed. *Crime and justice: a review of research.* Chicago: University of Chicago Press, 1991:71–93.

Determinants of Substance Abuse and Dependence

CHAPTER 4

Genetic Factors in the Risk for Substance Use Disorders

SHOW W. LIN AND ROBERT M. ANTHENELLI

More than a decade ago, the *New York Times* reported that, "scientists (had) link(ed) alcoholism to a specific gene, . . . opening the window of hope for prevention of a deadly disease." Although the accuracy of the finding on which the headline was based is controversial (1,2), the story remains historically significant.

Sixty years ago there were those who doubted they would ever read such a headline (3). As our understanding of alcoholism (i.e., alcohol dependence) and other substance use disorders has advanced, so, too, have our ideas about their patterns of transmission. For instance, the moralistic idea of alcoholism as a characterologic weakness has given way to the more contemporary view of the condition as a debilitating, heterogeneous group of disorders with multifactorial origins. The importance of environmental, developmental, and social factors championed by Jellinek and others in the 1940s has had to share the stage with a growing body of evidence supporting a genetic vulnerability to the disorder. All are important. No one headline tells the whole story, and it is the interaction of genes, environment and developmental influences that ultimately predict vulnerability to substance use disorders (4,5).

This updated chapter reviews the role of genetic factors in the risk for alcohol, tobacco, and other drug dependence. Because the preponderance of data are from studies on alcohol and tobacco, these drugs are emphasized. Reflecting the clinical nature of this text and the authors' area of expertise, this chapter focuses primarily on human genetic aspects of substance disorders. Interested readers may wish to pursue more comprehensive reviews of the animal and preclinical literature (6,7).

GENETIC INFLUENCES IN ALCOHOLISM

Traditionally, the search for genetic influences in any complex disorder begins with studies of families, twins, and adoptees affected with the condition (8). These investigations can provide preliminary evidence on the probable importance of genetic factors and serve as the foundation for subsequent research. The following sections briefly review the results of more than four decades of family, twin, and adoption studies in alcoholism. Although these investigations are not unanimous in their results, when taken together, they provide compelling evidence for the importance of genetic influences in this disorder and indicate that 40% to 60% of the variance in heritability of alcoholism can be attributed to genetic factors (9).

Family, Twin, and Adoption Studies of Alcoholism

Family Studies

For centuries, philosophers, writers, and clergy have commented on the familial nature of alcoholism. Plutarch's assertion that "drunks beget drunkards" was based on anecdotal observation alone, and it was not until the last few decades that this contention came under careful scientific scrutiny (10). The basic design for family studies of any complex illness is to compare the risk for developing the disorder in relatives of probands (individuals manifesting the phenotype or trait) with the rate for relatives of control groups or for the general population (8).

Numerous studies have found that rates of alcoholism are substantially higher in relatives of alcoholics than in relatives of nonalcoholics, with children of alcoholics demonstrating a four- to fivefold increased risk for developing the disorder (7,11). This increased risk appears to be relatively specific for alcoholism, with most family studies showing an increased rate for the disorder among relatives of alcoholic probands, while the same group does not show higher rates of other mental disorders, such as schizophrenia or bipolar disorder (12,13).

Although family studies provide preliminary evidence that alcoholism might be inherited, in themselves, they are inconclusive. Familial aggregation might also reflect the shared social and developmental influences of being raised in the same environment by biologic parents. To disentangle these factors, other approaches are required.

Twin Studies

Research with twins evaluates the relative contributions of genetic and environmental factors by comparing the similarity or concordance rates for illness in pairs of monozygotic twins with those of dizygotic twins. The twin study design allows researchers to estimate the contribution of genetic and environmental effects to the individual's liability for alcoholism and other substance use disorders. The liability identified in twin research generally has three components: (a) additive genetic effects; (b) common environmental effects shared by twins (e.g., intrauterine environment, parental upbringing); and (c) specific, nonshared environmental experiences (14). Identical twin pairs who share all of their genes should show higher concordance rates for gene-transmitted disorders than should fraternal twin pairs, who like ordinary siblings, generally share only half of their genes. On the other extreme, environmentally influenced disorders should show no difference between monozygotic and dizygotic twin pairs so long as both types of twins were exposed to the same childhood environment.

Several major twin studies have directly addressed the concordance rates for alcoholism in identical versus fraternal twins. The first of these was conducted in Sweden where Kaij found that the concordance rate for alcoholism in male monozygotic pairs was greater than that for dizygotic twins (approximately 60% vs. 39%) (15). Interestingly, the discrepancy between concordance rates increased in proportion to the severity of alcoholism in these male twin pairs, favoring a genetic diathesis. A Veterans Administration twin register study in the United States revealed a similar higher concordance rate for identical male twin pairs (16) as did two other smaller studies (17,18).

These findings were further corroborated by Prescott et al. in a population-based sample of twins in the United States (19); however, not all studies agree (20).

While results among male-male twin pairs had consistently demonstrated that genetic factors were important in the etiology of alcoholism in men, results in women were initially less consistent. Thus, several smaller twin studies found no (18,20) or relatively little (17) genetic influence in females compared to males. However, in a large sample of female same-sex twin pairs in the United States, Kendler et al. reported that the concordance for alcoholism was greater in monozygotic than in dizygotic twin pairs (21). These results were corroborated in a study of Australian twin pairs that found that genetic factors play as important a role in determining alcoholism risk in women as in men (22). Thus, the vast majority of twin studies support the notion that alcoholism is genetically influenced and that heritable factors are important in the vulnerability for the disorder in both men and women.

Adoption Studies

Perhaps the most convincing way to separate genetic from environmental effects is to study individuals who were separated soon after birth from their biologic relatives and who were raised by nonrelative adoptive parents (23). This can be done through classical adoption studies or through a half-sibling approach.

There have been several half-sibling and adoption studies evaluating the possibility that alcoholism, at least in part, has genetic determinants. Regarding the half-sibling approach, Schuckit and colleagues evaluated a group of individuals who had been raised apart from their biologic parents but who had either a biologic or surrogate parent with alcoholism (24). Subjects who had a biologic parent with severe alcohol problems were significantly more likely to have alcoholism themselves than if their surrogate parent were alcoholic.

Over the last two decades, several adoption studies in Denmark, Sweden, and the United States have yielded similar results. In Denmark, Goodwin and coworkers found that the sons of alcoholics were about four times more likely to be alcoholic than were sons of nonalcoholics, and that being raised by either nonalcoholic adoptive parents or by biologic parents did not affect this increased risk (25). Furthermore, although the sons of alcoholics were found to be at highest risk for developing alcoholism, they were no more likely to have other psychiatric disorders than were sons of nonalcoholics (23,25). As with some of the twin studies cited above, results for women in the Copenhagen Adoption Study were not significant, but the sample size for women was too small to reach any firm conclusions about potential gender differences in genetic vulnerability. Similar results were found in another large study done in Stockholm, Sweden, where Cloninger and colleagues showed significantly higher rates of alcohol abuse in adopted-out sons of biologic fathers registered with alcohol problems (26). Data from two smaller-scale adoption studies in Iowa, confirmed the results of the larger European studies (27,28); however, Cadoret et al. did find important genetic influences in female adoptees (29). In fact, only one study, by Roe, has found contrary results (30), and most authors agree that the disparity probably reflects methodologic problems in its design (e.g., small sample size and lack of rigorous diagnostic criteria for alcohol problems in the parents) or differences in the sub-populations of twins studied (10,23,31).

In summary, the combination of family, twin, and adoption studies strongly suggests that genetic determinants play an important part in the etiology of alcoholism for both men and women.

THE SEARCH FOR GENETICALLY MEDIATED MARKERS OF ALCOHOLISM

The results of family, twin, and adoption studies offered ample support for genetic factors to justify a search for what might be inherited to increase the risk for this disorder. However, before such a search can be optimally conducted, it is important to consider several major factors that obscure our ability to identify the genetic factors that predispose to alcoholism.

Clinical and Etiologic Heterogeneity

First, when studying complex disorders like alcoholism and other kinds of drug dependence, it is essential to realize that one's diagnosis rests at the clinical syndrome level and that it is likely that many different pathways or etiologies can lead to this combination of symptoms and signs (32,33). As a result of this etiologic heterogeneity and the likelihood that multiple different genes are involved for each of the various pathways that may lead to the broad clinical phenotype of alcoholism, consideration of the sample in which the genetic analyses are conducted is of paramount importance.

Comorbidity with Other Psychiatric Disorders

A second, related consideration is that life problems from excessive use of alcohol or other drugs may coexist with other disorders in the same patient. In fact, at least 30% of alcoholic men have evidence of preexisting disorders (34), and this figure soars to 60% to 70% among alcoholic women (35). For instance, 70% of men with antisocial personality disorder (ASPD) have secondary alcohol problems during the course of their disorder (34), and during the manic phase of bipolar illness, approximately 50% of patients develop severe ethanol-related difficulties (36). The phenotypic variations between these groups of "alcoholics" having two disorders are obvious. If these men and women carry genetic factors related to their ASPD or

mania, it could be difficult to identify specific inherited influences related to the alcohol dependence.

Subtypes of Alcoholism

Currently, several overlapping approaches are in use to categorize alcoholics into various clinical phenotypes or subgroups based on family history, age of onset, clinical symptoms, and personality traits (23,37–39). Although each of these methods has its strengths and limitations, the validity of any one method over the others has not yet been established (40,41). Reviewed in detail elsewhere (42), the underlying philosophy behind their use is an attempt to better define subsets of alcoholics who are at increased risk for developing the disorder.

Among the many different subtype classifications currently under study, one theory proposed by Cloninger, Bohman, and Sigvardsson and their colleagues gained much popularity (26,31,38,43,44). Using a discriminate function analysis of their large sample of Swedish adoptees, this group initially proposed two forms of alcoholism (types 1 and 2) that could be distinguished on the basis of the biologic parents' pattern of alcohol abuse and the degree to which postnatal environmental factors affected the inheritance of susceptibility to alcoholism (26,43). Combining results from a variety of personality, clinical, and neuropsychopharmacologic studies with the genetic epidemiologic findings, these authors elaborated on this theory, expanding its original focus on the importance of gene–environment interactions in alcoholism.

Type 1, or "milieu-limited," alcoholism, thought to predominate among female alcoholics and their male relatives, was hypothesized to be characterized by loss of control of drinking after the age of 25 years, pronounced environmental reactivity to drinking, minimal associated criminality, and "passive–dependent personality traits" marked by high degrees of harm avoidance, reward dependence, and low levels of novelty seeking as measured by Cloninger's Tridimensional Personality Questionnaire (TPQ) (38). In contrast, the "male-limited," or type 2, subgroup was postulated to have an inheritance pattern less dependent on environmental factors for phenotypic expression and an earlier age of onset, more associated criminal behavior, and a triad of personality traits that run opposite those of the prototypic "milieu-limited" alcoholic (31,38,45). This group later refined their theory to include a *third* class of alcoholism, which they call "antisocial behavior disorder with alcohol abuse" (31,45,46).

Babor and colleagues (39) used an empirical clustering technique and described a subgrouping scheme for alcoholics that included type A and type B alcoholics, named after the Roman gods Apollo and Bacchus. Type A alcoholics are characterized by later age-at-onset, fewer childhood risk factors, less-severe dependence, fewer alcohol-related problems, and less psychopathologic dysfunction.

Type B alcoholics typically exhibit an early onset of alcohol-related problems; higher levels of childhood risk factors and familial alcoholism; greater severity of dependence; multiple substance use; a long-term treatment history; greater psychopathologic dysfunction; and greater life stress (39,47). The type A/B dichotomy was replicated in another large sample of alcohol-dependent subjects even after the exclusion of individuals with ASPD and those with an onset of alcohol dependence before age 25 years, further supporting this subtyping method's potential usefulness (48).

In summary, the search for what is inherited in the predisposition toward alcoholism is challenging because alcoholism is a clinically and etiologically heterogeneous disorder. Moreover, because of the comorbidity between alcoholism and certain other psychiatric disorders, studies that do not adequately control for this increased variability may yield spurious genetic associations. Furthermore, among the broad clinical phenotype of alcoholics, subgroups may exist who differ in the degree of genetic susceptibility.

Intermediate Phenotypes

Before the explosion in molecular genetics research took place (see Molecular Genetic Studies on pg. 37), the search for vulnerability factors for alcoholism focused on identifying endophenotypes or intermediate phenotypes that might be associated with the predisposition toward the disease. These are neurobiologic or neurobehavioral characteristics associated with alcoholism whose manifestation may be more closely linked to gene expression than the broad clinical phenotype of alcoholism itself (49). The focus of many older articles (32,50) and book chapters (51) dedicated to the topic of the genetics of alcoholism, these intermediate phenotypes remain relevant because they may represent some of the endstage pathophysiologic processes through which genetic factors influence susceptibility to the disease. Because of space limitations, only some of these phenotypic markers are discussed here, and interested readers may seek more detailed reviews of these broad phenotypes elsewhere (49,52).

Electrophysiologic Markers

Electrophysiologic measurements of brain activity have been demonstrated as potentially promising neurobiologic markers that might be associated with the predisposition toward alcoholism, at least among some subgroups of individuals (53,54). Event-related brain potentials (ERPs) have been used extensively to study information processing in both long-term abstinent alcoholics as well as in unaffected high- and low-risk populations who differ by having the presence or absence of a family history of alcoholism, respectively (32). The amplitude of one important component of the ERP, the positive wave observed at 300 to 500 milliseconds after a rare but expected stimulus (P3), has been demonstrated to be significantly decreased in about one-third of the sons of alcoholic fathers, when compared with controls (53,55). Although some studies do not agree with these results (56,57), differences probably reflect variations in the studies' designs, including the sample population chosen. Begleiter and Porjesz have proposed that such ERP anomalies may reflect brain disinhibition and/or hyperexcitability (impulsivity) that is critically involved in the vulnerability toward alcohol dependence (49). In addition to this elicited brain-wave marker, a second approach has relied on measurements of the power of wave forms on the background cortical electroencephalogram (EEG) (32). Male alcoholics and their sons might demonstrate a decreased amount of slow-wave (e.g., alpha wave) activity at baseline when compared with controls (58,59). Similarly, Ehlers and Schuckit reported that sons of alcoholics differ from lower-risk, matched controls at baseline on the amount of activity in one part of the frequency range of alpha waves (i.e., men with a positive family history of alcoholism had more energy in the fast alpha range than did controls) (60,61).

Low Level of Response to Alcohol

Schuckit et al. and others have documented differences in the response to alcohol between high-risk and control populations. Otherwise healthy groups of 18- to 25-year-old sons of primary alcoholic men were selected as higher-risk, or family history positive (FHP), subjects who were then compared with controls comprised of lower-risk, family history negative (FHN) individuals. Each FHP–FHN matched pair was carefully evaluated at baseline and then observed for 3 to 4 hours after consuming placebo or the equivalent of 3 to 5 drinks of beverage alcohol.

After drinking the alcohol, the two family history groups developed similar patterns of blood alcohol concentrations over time, making it unlikely that group differences depended on the rate of absorption or metabolism of ethanol (32,62). However, a major consistent difference between FHP and FHN subjects was in the intensity of their subjective feelings of intoxication after imbibing alcohol (62–64). Using an analogue scale and asking subjects to rate the intensity of different aspects of intoxication, FHP men rated themselves as significantly less intoxicated than did their FHN matched controls after drinking ethanol (62–64). This decreased intensity of reaction to alcohol among FHP men was also observed for at least one measure of motor performance; the level of sway in the upper body (65). Furthermore, following the ethanol challenge, FHP men also exhibited less-intense change in the levels of cortisol and prolactin, two hormones shown to be altered after ethanol (66,67).

Schuckit et al. hypothesized that a decreased intensity of reaction to lower doses of alcohol might make it more difficult for susceptible individuals to discern when they are becoming drunk at low enough blood levels to be able to stop drinking during an evening. Without this feedback, and especially in the setting of a heavy drinking society, predisposed individuals may be inclined to drink more and, thus run an increased risk for subsequent alcohol-related life problems (12). Consequently, these investigators conducted a follow-up study; interviewers blind to the initial family history and the determination of the level of response to alcohol located all 453 subjects an average of 8.2 years after the time of their initial evaluation (68,69). The data revealed that the family history groups had been correctly identified, and that the sons of alcoholics had a threefold increased risk for alcohol dependence. The results also demonstrated a strong and significant relationship between a low level of response to alcohol and the future development of alcoholism.

These studies demonstrate some important attributes regarding genetic influences in the alcoholism risk. First, a family history of alcoholism is associated with increased risk for this disorder among people of diverse socioeconomic classes. Second, it is likely that there are multiple roads into the heightened alcohol risk, with, for example, some individuals developing their alcoholism in part through very high levels of impulsivity, others increasing their risk for alcoholism through a low level of response to alcohol in the context of a heavy drinking society, and so on (52,70). Third, it is unlikely that any single gene explains the alcoholism risk, but rather it is multiple genes interacting with environment.

Molecular Genetic Studies

With the advent of modern molecular genetic techniques blossoming over the past two decades, more recent efforts have targeted identifying genes that influence susceptibility to alcoholism. Although the details of the molecular genetic techniques used to identify such genetic markers are beyond the scope of this chapter, briefly, they involve the meticulous dissection of deoxyribonucleic acid (DNA) into specific nucleotide (e.g., the building blocks of DNA) patterns called markers or microsatellites (for details see references) (54,71,72). Such markers are then analyzed to determine whether there is *linkage* between the marker and the phenotype (i.e., the marker is transmitted along with the disease in families) or whether there is an *association* between the polymorphism and the phenotype (73,74) (i.e , a given marker allele is more common among those individuals with the disease in a population). Indeed, such genetic strategies have been used extensively in the large multicenter effort entitled the Collaborative Study on the Genetics of Alcoholism (COGA) Study (75).

A number of candidate genes for alcohol dependence have been proposed thus far; interested readers are urged

to see other recent reviews of this topic to appreciate the full breadth of this massive research effort (7,9). Because genes encoding the alcohol-metabolizing enzymes are the only genes consistently demonstrated to contribute to alcoholism susceptibility, these genes are highlighted.

Alcohol Dehydrogenase and Aldehyde Dehydrogenase

Blood alcohol concentration (BAC) and an individual's subjective response to alcohol represents a complex interaction of pharmacokinetic and pharmacodynamic effects of ethanol in the brain and body. There is a large degree of interindividual variation, as a function of genetic, gender, and ethnic influences, in how one responds to alcohol that involves the drug's absorption, distribution, metabolism, and elimination. Alcohol dehydrogenase (ADH) and aldehyde dehydrogenase (ALDH) are the major enzymes involved in the degradation of ethanol; ADH catabolizes alcohol to acetaldehyde, which ALDH breaks down to acetate and water (76–78). Numerous studies have found that allelic variants of ADH and ALDH genes play an important role in influencing the metabolism of alcohol and that these polymorphisms are associated with the risk for developing alcohol dependence.

ALDH is the major enzyme that catabolizes acetaldehyde in the liver and other organs. There are many ALDH gene families distributed on several different chromosomes (79). Family 2 genes (ALDH 2) have been the most well-studied genes regarding an association with alcohol dependence. This family of genes encodes mitochondrial enzymes that oxidize acetaldehyde. ALDH 2 has a deficient allelic variant (ALDH 2*2), when compared with the wild-type of ALDH 2 (ALDH 2*1). The ALDH 2*2 variant gene is found in approximately 50% of the Asian population (80–82). Individuals with the ALDH 2*2 variant typically experience aversive responses (e.g., facial flushing, tachycardia, and a burning sensation in the stomach) to alcohol consumption as a result of the accumulation of acetaldehyde. Several studies demonstrate the protective effect of ALDH 2*2 gene carriers from developing alcohol dependence (83–85).

The association between polymorphisms in ADH genes (located on chromosome 4) and alcohol dependence is not as robust as for ALDH genes. The variant allele ADH 2*2 (more recently renamed the ADH1B*2 allele) encodes a high-activity enzyme involved in the oxidation of ethanol to acetaldehyde (9). Interestingly, it has been found that having the combination of the ADH 2*2 and ALDH 2*2 gene variants was associated with the lowest risk for alcoholism (84). Taken together, then, there is compelling evidence that the interaction between a genetically controlled alcohol-metabolizing enzyme system and environmental factors (such as attitudes about drinking and drunkenness) appears to contribute significantly to the lower alcoholism risk among a subgroup of Asians (86).

Dopaminergic System

As alluded to at the beginning of this chapter, the first report of an "alcoholism gene" occurred in 1990, when Blum et al. reported that he and his colleagues had identified a gene—an allele of the D2 dopamine receptor (DRD2)—that appeared to be implicated in severe cases of alcoholism (87). The finding had good face validity because the mesolimbic dopamine reward circuit in the brain has been repeatedly demonstrated to play a major role in ethanol's rewarding producing effects (88,89). The subject of much debate with studies both finding (1,73,90–94) and not finding (2,95–98) an association with alcoholism, the DRD2 controversy remains relevant because it heralded the advent of modern molecular genetic approaches to this complex genetic disease. Interestingly, there is also some evidence to implicate the DRD2 gene in other substance use disorders, leading some investigators to label it a potential "reward gene," as discussed subsequently in this chapter (see Tobacco section on pg. 40 and cocaine section on pg. 41) (90).

Ebstein et al. (99) reported an association between a polymorphism of the dopamine D4 receptor (DRD4) and the novelty seeking subscale as measured by Cloninger's TPQ (38). That report, along with other confirmatory results (100) published in the same journal issue, provided the first replicated association between a specific genetic polymorphism and a personality trait that has been linked with alcoholism and other substance use disorders (99). Although the subjects in this study were nonalcoholic normal controls, it is intriguing that a personality trait believed to predict an increased risk for alcoholism might have heritable components. Studies examining the associations among the DRD1 gene polymorphism (affecting the dopamine D1 receptor) (101,102) and the dopamine D3 gene (affecting dopamine D3 receptors) (103–105) and alcoholism have yielded inconsistent and generally negative results.

GABAergic System

γ-Aminobutyric acid (GABA) receptor genes, that encode the $GABA_A$ and $GABA_B$ receptors that bind GABA (the human brain's major inhibitory neurotransmitter), have also been identified as promising candidate genes for alcoholism (7,9). *In vitro* studies have found that ethanol potentiates GABAergic neurotransmission (106), and preclinical studies in experimental animals have determined that GABA plays an important role in alcohol's brain depressant behavioral effects (107). In particular, $GABA_A$ receptor genes located on chromosomes 4 and 15 have been associated with intermediate phenotypes linked with the alcoholism risk such as the aforementioned electrophysiological markers (108) and the low level of response to alcohol (109,110).

Serotonergic System

As described in greater detail below in our discussion of the genetics of tobacco dependence, serotonin dysfunction has also been repeatedly implicated in both preclinical (111,112) and clinical (113,114) studies examining the vulnerability for alcoholism. As a result, a growing number of studies have evaluated candidate genes that encode various components (i.e., the serotonin transporter and serotonin receptor subtypes that modulate serotonergic neurotransmission) of the serotonergic system. Reviewed in greater detail elsewhere (7,9), there is controversial support for an association between alcoholism and genetic polymorphisms on chromosome 17 that encode the serotonin transporter (115,116); however, not all studies agree (117,118).

In summary, advances in molecular genetics and an explosion of studies in this field in the last decade have added important information to our understanding of the genetic factors associated with the susceptibility to alcoholism. Many potential candidate genes have been identified that might be associated with the risk for the disorder; we highlighted only a few of these as examples of the findings accumulating from this massive search. What is clear is that many genes likely influence the vulnerability for alcoholism and that different combinations of genes are likely to be more or less salient for each endophenotype associated with the disorder. Certain genes (e.g., the ALDH 2*2 gene) may provide protection against developing serious alcohol-related problems, while others (e.g., the DRD2 gene) might predispose certain individuals to alcoholism and other substance use disorders that are discussed next.

GENETIC INFLUENCES IN TOBACCO AND OTHER DRUG DEPENDENCE

This section focuses on nicotine dependence because of its high prevalence, associated morbidity and mortality, and the relative preponderance of genetic studies, when compared with other categories of illicit drugs. Genetic influences on other drugs of abuse (cocaine and other stimulants, opioids, and cannabinoids) are discussed subsequently.

Nicotine/Tobacco Dependence

The prevalence of tobacco smoking in the United States steadily declined following the Surgeon General's 1964 report that definitively linked cigarette smoking to health problems (119). However, in the last decade, the rate of decline of cigarette smoking among U.S. adults has slowed. In 2000, approximately 23% of adults in the United States were current smokers; this was a decline from 25% in 1993 (120). Cigarette smoking is still the leading preventable cause of death each year in the United States, with more than 400,000 deaths being attributed to tobacco smoking (121). Smoking-related illnesses cost the nation more than $150 billion annually and, somewhat alarmingly, every day nearly 5,000 young people under the age of 18 years try their first cigarette. Thus, searching for the genetic and environmental factors that contribute to the initiation and persistence of cigarette smoking is of paramount importance in the prevention and treatment of nicotine dependence. This section reviews the role of genetic factors in the initiation and maintenance of tobacco smoking, and organizes this literature into population versus molecular genetics studies.

Family, Twin, and Adoption Studies of Tobacco Dependence

Family Studies

In contrast to the large literature on family studies in the genetics of alcoholism, there are fewer studies examining the familial transmission of tobacco smoking. Initiation of cigarette smoking is strongly associated with parental and sibling smoking; thus the prevalence of smoking among teenagers is two to four times higher in individuals whose parents or siblings smoke (122). For example, Hughes reported that individuals whose parents smoked during the probands' adolescence were more likely to be smokers (52%) than were individuals whose parents did not smoke during the subjects' adolescence (20%) (122). In the Collaborative Study on the Genetics of Alcoholism, Bierut et al. found that siblings of habitual smoking probands had a roughly twofold (relative risk = 1.77) elevated risk of becoming smokers when compared with siblings of nonsmoking probands (123). However, as stated previously, family studies have difficulty disentangling genetic from environmental factors because the study subjects involved lived together and shared the same environment. For this reason, more recent studies examining the genetic influences on cigarette smoking have focused on twin pairs raised in the same or mixed families, and on combined twin and adoption studies, in order to tease out more precisely the relative contributions of genetic and environmental factors that lead to the initiation and perpetuation of tobacco use (124,125).

Twin Studies

Twin studies are a very powerful tool to explore the relative contributions of genetic factors in the etiology of nicotine dependence. Monozygotic twins share the same genetic makeup, while dizygotic twins share only approximately 50% of their genes. Taken together, results of several twin studies indicate that there is a significant genetic influence on the development and continuation of habitual cigarette smoking. Carmelli et al. compared male monozygotic and dizygotic twins in the genetic influence on smoking. They found that the concordance rate for smoking was significantly higher in monozygotic twins than among the dizygotic twins across all three categorizations (i.e., among never, former, and current smokers) of smokers they examined (126). Interestingly, the data also suggested that genetic factors appear to influence an individual's ability to quit smoking; monozygotic twins were more likely than dizygotic twins to be concordant for quitting smoking (rate ratio = 1.24).

As alluded to earlier, recent studies on the genetics of cigarette smoking not only focus on nicotine dependence itself, but also investigate the related process of initiating tobacco smoking behavior (127–131). Parsing the relative genetic contributions to the various component behaviors that ultimately contribute to tobacco addiction (i.e., initiation, amount smoked, continuation), it appears that approximately 50% of the initiation of smoking behavior is genetically influenced, while persistence of smoking and amount smoked have approximately a 70% genetic contribution (132). Heath et al. retrospectively analyzed 3,810 adult Australian twin pairs on age-at-onset of smoking to determine the role of genetic and environmental factors in the onset of smoking (129). For female twins and younger male twins, the onset of smoking was strongly influenced by genetic factors. Kendler et al., studying female twins on smoking initiation and nicotine dependence, suggested that heritable factors played an important etiologic role in both smoking initiation and nicotine dependence (131). However, while the liabilities to smoking initiation and nicotine dependence were highly correlated, they were not identical, suggesting that both independent and common genetic factors may underlie these behaviors.

Even though the twin study design is a powerful tool in the study of genetic factors in nicotine dependence, studies have found that monozygotic twins co-socialized more, spent more time together, and shared peer groups more closely than dizygotic twins (133,134). Thus, based on these studies, the higher concordance rate of monozygotic twins could be inflated as a consequence of the co-socialization (shared environment), requiring other population genetic techniques be used.

Adoption Studies

Adoption studies provide another powerful tool to disentangle the environmental and genetic contributions to tobacco smoking. An older adoption study found that parental and child smoking was significantly correlated among biologically related pairs, but was not correlated among adoptive parents and adoptees (135). These results were extended in a more recent analysis of the Danish Adoption Register, where it was demonstrated that adoptees' smoking status was strongly associated with their biologic full-siblings' smoking status (124). Another novel approach is to combine both twin and adoption designs by examining concordance rates in twins reared together versus those reared apart. Consistent with results from regular twin studies, both male monozygotic twins reared together and reared apart had higher correlations in smoking behavior, when compared with their dizygotic twin counterparts. However, the monozygotic twins reared together exhibited greater concordance rates in smoking than monozygotic twins reared apart, providing further evidence that the rearing environment and genes interact to influence an individual's risk to be a smoker (136).

Molecular Genetic Studies

The evidence to date has been very consistent with respect to the significance of genetic contributions to smoking initiation and tobacco dependence. As was the case for alcoholism, the more daunting task is to determine the genes responsible for nicotine dependence susceptibility. As with other addictive disorders, the inheritance of tobacco smoking is most likely polygenic and multifactorial, involving a complex web of genetic, environmental and developmental influences. Indeed, the severity of the disorder may reflect on how many different genes are involved.

The search for genetic factors contributing to nicotine dependence susceptibility is focused primarily on genetic variations (polymorphisms) between smokers and nonsmokers. A variety of potential candidate genes are implicated that affect multiple aspects of nicotine metabolism and other components of the mesolimbic brain reward system that includes various neurotransmitters, receptors, and transporters as briefly described in the next four subsections.

Dopaminergic System

Much attention is focused on the mesolimbic dopamine system as playing an important role in mediating the vulnerability for tobacco dependence. There are five categories of dopamine receptor subtypes labeled D1 to D5. Since the first report of an association of the A1 allele of the dopamine D2 receptor (DRD2) gene with alcoholism described previously (137), the DRD2 gene has been intensively studied in other substance use disorders, including nicotine dependence. Both past and current cigarette smokers were found to have a significantly higher prevalence of the A1 allele of the DRD2 than did nonsmoking controls (138). Moreover, the prevalence of the A1 allele increased progressively from nonsmokers to past smokers to active smokers. Another study found a significantly higher A1 allele frequency (48.7%) of the DRD2 in smokers who made unsuccessful quit attempts, when compared with controls (25.9%) (139). Spitz et al. suggested that smokers had significantly higher B1 allele frequency of

the DRD2 gene than nonsmokers (140). In addition, subjects with the A1 allele had significant inverse associations between the prevalence of the A1 allele and (a) the age-at-onset of smoking and (b) the number of attempts at quitting smoking. However, other studies have not found any increase in A1 allele frequency when comparing smokers with nonsmokers (141), raising concerns that population stratification in some case-control studies might have influenced the results.

How may the A1 allele DRD2 polymorphism influence the risk for developing and maintaining tobacco dependence? Some studies have found that subjects carrying the A1 allele in the DRD2 gene have significantly reduced D2 receptor density (142), as indexed by a lower mean relative glucose metabolic rate on positron emission tomography testing (143). Thus, it has been hypothesized that patients may use nicotine (and other drugs of abuse) to compensate for a deficiency of their dopaminergic system. Many other polymorphisms have also been found in genes encoding other dopamine receptors, some of which have been associated with tobacco smoking (144–146).

Lerman et al. compared the dopamine transporter (SLC6A3) and the DRD2 genes in a group of smokers and nonsmokers and found that individuals with allele 9 of the SLC6A3 gene (SLC6A3-9) were significantly less likely to be smokers, especially when this polymorphism was found in combination with the A2 allele of the DRD2 genotype (147). Sabol et al. replicated this finding (148). Thus, it has been hypothesized that the presence of the A2 allele of the DRD2 gene may be negatively associated with tobacco smoking or might yield a protective effect against smoking.

Serotonergic System

The brain's serotonergic system is involved in regulating a variety of functions that includes mood, sleep, appetite, aggression, and sexual behavior. Several studies have found that nicotine increases central nervous system (CNS) serotonin release and that acute nicotine withdrawal is marked by a relative depletion in central serotonin (149,150). After serotonin is released into the synaptic cleft from terminals of serotonergic neurons, it is promptly taken back up into the presynaptic neuron via the actions of serotonin transporter (5-HTT). Thus, the function of the 5-HTT has a marked impact on the magnitude and duration of serotonin neurotransmission. Two functional alleles of the serotonin transporter-linked polymorphic region (5-HTTLPR) have been identified and labeled the long (L) and short (S) types (151,152). The S-type allele decreases the transcriptional activity of the 5-HTT gene, as compared to the L-type allele, and subsequently decreases the function of the 5-HTT. An association between tobacco smoking and the S allele of the 5-HTTLPR was reported (153). However, another study failed to confirm this finding (154). Another study found that if the short (s/s or s/1) genotype interacted with neuroticism, then the rate of nicotine intake, nicotine dependence, and smoking motivation was higher in s carriers than in those individuals carrying the homozygous long (1/1) genotype (155).

To our knowledge, there are no published reports of an association between cigarette smoking and the multiple serotonin-receptor-subtype polymorphisms.

Polymorphic variants in the gene encoding the protein involved with serotonin synthesis are also implicated in tobacco smoking behavior. Tryptophan hydroxylase (TPH) is the enzyme that performs the initial and rate-limiting step in the production of serotonin from tryptophan. Individuals with the A/A genotype of the TPH gene were found to have started smoking earlier than other genotypes; however, there was no association of TPH alleles with subjects' current smoking status (156). Interestingly, Sullivan et al. also found that TPH markers were significantly associated with the onset of smoking initiation (157).

Cytochrome P450 Enzyme System

The cytochrome P450 enzyme system plays important roles in the metabolism of drugs and other xenobiotic agents. Nicotine is metabolized through polymorphic CYP2A6 to its major breakdown product, cotinine (158,159). Recent studies found that individuals carrying inactive alleles of the CYP2A6 gene have decreased nicotine metabolism, increased cotinine levels in urine, and were less likely to become tobacco smokers. Moreover, individuals carrying these alleles smoked fewer cigarettes if they do smoke (160,161).

Nicotinic Acetylcholine Receptors

Nicotine is the major addictive ingredient in tobacco smoke (132). Nicotine activates the nicotinic acetylcholine receptors (nAChRs) and stimulates dopamine release in the mesolimbic brain reward system. nAChRs are widely distributed in the CNS and peripheral nervous system. These receptors are excitatory, ligand-gated channels and are comprised of five subunits. Twelve subunit genes have been identified and labeled α_2 to α_{10} and β_2 to β_4 (162–164). The properties of these receptors depend on the various composition of these subunit combinations. Much of our current understanding about the structure and function of nAChRs comes from studies carried out in other species, such as mice, and information concerning human nicotinic receptors and nicotine addiction is still relatively limited in the literature. In animal studies, nicotine stimulates dopamine release in the ventral striatum of wild-type mice, but not in mice lacking the β_2 subunit (i.e., in so-called β_2 knock-out mice). Picciotto et al. suggested that the β_2 subunit may be involved in mediating the reinforcing properties of nicotine (165,166). While the clinical implications of these finding remain unclear, genetic variants of nAChR subunits, especially those involving the α_7

subunit (167), have been used in the study of cognitive and attentional deficits associated with schizophrenia and Alzheimer disease.

Other Drugs of Abuse

Before embarking on a brief synopsis of the genetic influences implicated in other categories of drug abuse, some general comments bear mentioning. First, as for nicotine dependence where we focused on genetic factors involved in the initiation of smoking behavior versus those involved in the development of nicotine dependence, a few studies have examined the related process of making the transition from substance use to heavy use to abuse and on to dependence in male-male twin pairs (168,169). In general, these twin studies found that genetic factors play a significant role in these transitions from drug initiation to dependence. Second, many studies have found that personality variables such as sensation seeking play a salient role in the prediction of both substance abuse and dependence (170–172). Thus, in searching for genes that contribute to the risk of developing substance use disorders, genes affecting personality traits have received considerable consideration.

Cocaine and Other Stimulants

Population genetic studies of cocaine users and addicts found that cocaine use, and especially cocaine abuse and dependence in women, is substantially influenced by genetic factors. A study suggested that twin resemblance for liability to cocaine use was a result of genetic and familial–environmental factors, while twin resemblance for cocaine abuse and dependence was solely a result of genetic factors (173).

Cocaine inhibits the reuptake of dopamine and other monoamines via its blockade effects at monoamine transporters. This results in an acute accumulation of extracellular dopamine in the synapse. Although a growing preclinical literature exists, there is relatively limited information available about genetic variants affecting dopamine transporter function and cocaine dependence in humans. Regarding dopamine receptor subtypes, Comings et al. reported that the dopamine D3 (DRD3) receptor gene may play a modest role in the susceptibility to cocaine dependence (174), a finding that corroborates results obtained in animals (175). Allelic variants in the DRD2 gene have also been associated with cocaine dependence (176). However, as was the case for the DRD2 gene and alcoholism, other reports have been unable to replicate this finding (177).

Cocaine and other stimulants also affect serotonin reuptake, prompting some interest in exploring genetic variants in the serotonergic system and their relation to stimulant dependence. To date, these studies have yielded mostly negative results. For example, Patkar et al. found that polymorphisms in the serotonin transporter gene were not associated with cocaine dependence among African American subjects (178,179), and another group reported no association between single-nucleotide polymorphisms in the serotonin B1 receptor gene and cocaine abuse or dependence (180).

Opiates

Opiates are involved in many physiologic functions throughout the body and the opioidergic system also plays an important role in the modulation of pain. Opioid medications are used primarily in the treatment of pain, and opiate use and abuse has been described for centuries. The μ opioid receptor is one of several opioid receptors characterized and is the primary site of drug action. A polymorphism at position 118 (A118G) of the μ receptor gene has been found which changes the receptor's ability to bind opioid ligands, especially β-endorphin. It has been suggested that this single-nucleotide polymorphism may be implicated in the development or protection from opioid addiction (181,182). However, not all studies have been able to replicate this association (183,184).

Oral opioid analgesics (e.g., oxycodone, hydrocodone, and codeine) are common medications prescribed for pain. Although relatively rare in occurrence, some patients become addicted to these oral opioids to the extent that they fulfill the *Diagnostic and Statistical Manual of Mental Disorders, 4th Edition* (*DSM–IV*) diagnosis of opioid dependence. These oral opiates are metabolized by CYP2D6 to morphine in order to exert their analgesic effects. Individuals with two nonfunctional alleles of CYP2D6 (2D6*3 and 2D6*4) are poor metabolizers of these oral opiate drugs. Intriguingly, Tyndale et al. found no poor metabolizers in a sample of opioid dependent subjects, and suggested that the CYP2D6 defective genotype may provide pharmacogenetic protection against developing opiate dependence (185).

Cannabinoids

Marijuana is the most commonly used illicit drug in the United States, with data from the 2002 National Survey on Drug Use and Health indicating that roughly 14.6 million Americans used marijuana in the past month. Lynskey et al., studying Australian twins, found that genetic factors were important determinants for the risk of developing cannabis dependence among men, but results among women were less certain (183). However, Kendler et al. found that heavy use of cannabis, as well as cannabis abuse and dependence, were largely attributable to genetic factors, with heritabilities ranging from 62% to 79% in female twins (186). Another study by these same authors also demonstrated that cannabis use appears to be substantially influenced by genetic factors (187).

There are at least two cannabinoid receptors: CB1 primarily located in the CNS, and CB2 located strictly in the periphery (188). Studies on the relationships among substance use disorders and genetic variants in the cannabinoid receptor gene (CNR1) are in progress and have, to date, provided conflicting results (189,190).

In summary, genetic factors play an important role in the initiation (in tobacco studies) and persistence of substance dependence. The search for candidate genes that contribute to the risk of developing and maintaining substance use disorders is still in its early stages. The task of identifying such genes is made more arduous because it is likely that variation in substance-dependence susceptibility results not only from genotypic differences and environmental influences, but also from their interactions (5). Thus, genetic factors are background sources of variance that can be minimized or exaggerated by environmental factors before the phenotype (substance dependence) can be expressed.

CONCLUSIONS AND IMPLICATIONS

In the introduction to this chapter, we alluded to the work being done in molecular genetics and the search for "the gene for alcoholism." One purpose of this chapter has been to provide the reader with much of the small print apt to be left out in headlines. As described, much work has preceded and followed the preliminary molecular genetic studies that once captured the news. We have organized more than four decades of diverse findings into a format that is understandable and illustrative of the promise of this line of research, while not minimizing the complexity of the issues at hand.

In many ways, the "window of hope" offered by better understanding of the probable genetic influences of alcoholism has already been opened and does not depend solely on identifying gene(s) at a molecular level. The clinical, societal, and research implications of this body of work have already emerged, with results from family, twin, and adoption studies helping to shape programs aimed at preventing the illness by educating children at high risk for alcoholism, tobacco dependence, and other drug use disorders early on, allowing them to modify their drinking and drug use patterns. Individuals already suffering from the disorder are being matched to more appropriate therapies using the information obtained in studies of alcoholic subtypes. Pharmacogenetic approaches are offering a powerful new tool to match specific elements of an individual's complex genetic blueprint (e.g., allelic variants in genes encoding various neurotransmitter receptors or transporters) with targeted pharmacotherapies to which that person may optimally respond. The stigma once associated with the view of substance dependence as a "moral weakness" is fading with the accumulation of evidence supporting the importance of biologic factors. The studies pointing to the importance of gene-environment interactions have demonstrated the need for cooperation among researchers in different disciplines, and they highlight the fact that unitary hypotheses arguing exclusively for any one approach are inadequate in explaining these heterogeneous disorders. It is hoped that such a coordinated effort might provide insights into how the disorder is transmitted and might expand our knowledge about the biologic basis of the inherited factors.

ACKNOWLEDGMENTS

Dr. Anthenelli's work is supported by the National Institute on Alcohol Abuse and Alcoholism grant # RO1 AA013307 and by the Veterans Affairs Research Service.

REFERENCES

1. Noble EP. The D2 dopamine receptor gene: a review of association studies in alcoholism and phenotypes. *Alcohol* 1998;16(1):33–45.
2. Gelernter J, Kranzler H. D2 dopamine receptor gene (DRD2) allele and haplotype frequencies in alcohol dependent and control subjects: no association with phenotype or severity of phenotype. *Neuropsychopharmacology* 1999;20(6):640–649.
3. Goodwin DW. The gene for alcoholism. *J Stud Alcohol* 1989;50:397–398.
4. Rutter M. The interplay of nature, nurture, and developmental influences. The challenge ahead for mental health. *Arch Gen Psychiatry* 2002;59:996–1000.
5. Gunzerath L, Goldman D. G × E: a NIAAA workshop on gene–environment interactions. *Alcohol Clin Exp Res* 2003;27(3):540–562.
6. Schumann G, Spanagel R, Mann K. Candidate genes for alcohol dependence: animal studies. *Alcohol Clin Exp Res* 2003;27(5):880–888.
7. Enoch MA, Goldman D. Molecular and cellular genetics of alcohol addiction. In: Davis KL, Charney D, Coyle JT, et al., eds. *Neuropsychopharmacology: the fifth generation of progress.* Philadelphia: Lippincott Williams & Wilkins, 2002:1413–1423.
8. Pardes H, Kaufmann CA, Pincus HA, et al. Genetics and psychiatry: past discoveries, current dilemmas, and future directions. *Am J Psychiatry* 1989;164(4):435–443.
9. Dick DM, Foroud T. Candidate genes for alcohol dependence: a review of genetic evidence from human studies. *Alcohol Clin Exp Res* 2003;27(5):868–879.
10. Goodwin DW. Alcoholism and genetics: the sins of the fathers. *Arch Gen Psychiatry* 1985;42:171–174.
11. Cotton NS. The familial incidence of alcoholism. *J Stud Alcohol* 1979;40:1:89–116.
12. Schuckit MA. Biological vulnerability to alcoholism. *J Consult Clin Psychol* 1987;55:1–9.
13. Schuckit MA. Genetic and clinical implications of alcoholism and affective disorder. *Am J Psychiatry* 1986;143:140–147.
14. Prescott CA, Kendler KS. Twin study design. *Alcohol Health Res World* 1995;19:200–205.
15. Kaij L. *Studies on the etiology and sequels of abuse of alcohol.* Lund: University of Lund Press, 1960.
16. Hrubec Z, Omenn GS. Evidence of genetic predisposition to alcoholic cirrhosis and psychosis: twin concordances for alcoholism and its biological end points by zygosity among male veterans. *Alcohol Clin Exp Res* 1981;5:207–215.
17. Pickens RW, Svikis DS, McGue M, et al. Heterogeneity in the inheritance of alcoholism. *Arch Gen Psychiatry* 1991;48:19–28.
18. McGue M, Pickens RW, Svikis DS. Sex and age effects on the inheritance of alcohol problems: a twin study. *J Abnorm Psychol* 1992;101:3–17.
19. Prescott CA, Kendler KS. Genetic and environmental contributions to alcohol abuse and dependence in a population-based sample of male twins. *Am J Psychiatry* 1999;156(1):34–40.
20. Gurling HM, Oppenheim BE, Murray RM. Depression, criminality and psychopathology associated with alcoholism: evidence from a twin study. *Acta Genet Med Gemellol (Roma)* 1984;33:333–339.
21. Kendler KS, Heath AC, Neale MC, et al. A population-based twin study of alcoholism in women. *JAMA* 1992;268:1877–1882.
22. Heath AC, Bucholz KK, Madden PA, et al. Genetic and environmental contributions to alcohol dependence risk in a national twin sample: consistency of findings in women and men. *Psychol Med* 1997;27(6):1381–1396.
23. Goodwin DW. Familial alcoholism: a separate entity? *Substance Alcohol Actions/Misuse* 1983;4:129–136.
24. Schuckit MA, Goodwin DW, Winokur GA. A study of alcoholism in half-siblings. *Am J Psychiatry* 1972;128:1132–1136.
25. Goodwin DW. Alcoholism and heredity. *Arch Gen Psychiatry* 1979;36:57–61.
26. Cloninger CR, Bohman M, Sigvardsson S. Inheritance of alcohol abuse: cross-fostering analysis of adopted men. *Arch Gen Psychiatry* 1981;38:861–868.
27. Cadoret RJ, Cain CA, Grove WM. Development of alcoholism in adoptees raised apart from alcoholic biologic relatives. *Arch Gen Psychiatry* 1980;37:561–563.
28. Cadoret RJ, Troughton E, O'Gorman TW. Genetic and environmental factors in alcohol abuse and antisocial personality. *J Stud Alcohol* 1987;48:1–8.
29. Cadoret RJ, O'Gorman TW, Troughton E, et al. Alcoholism and antisocial personality: interrelationships, genetic and environmental factors. *Arch Gen Psychiatry* 1985;42:161–167.
30. Roe A. The adult adjustment of children of alcoholic parents raised in foster homes. *J Stud Alcohol* 1994;5:378–393.
31. Cloninger CR, Sigvardsson S, Reich T, et al. Inheritance of risk to develop alcoholism. In: Braude MC, Chao HM, eds. *Genetic and biological markers in drug abuse and alcoholism.* NIDA Research Monograph 66. U.S. Dept. of Health and Human Services, Rockville, MD. 1986:86–96.
32. Anthenelli RM, Schuckit MA. Genetic studies on alcoholism. *Int J Addict* 1990;25:81–94.
33. McHugh PR, Slavney PR. *The perspectives of psychiatry.* Baltimore: Johns Hopkins University Press, 1983.
34. Helzer JE, Pryzbeck TR. The co-occurence of alcoholism with other psychiatric disorders in the general population and its impact on treatment. *J Stud Alcohol* 1988;49:219–224.
35. Kessler RC, Crum RM, Warner LA, et al. Lifetime co-occurence of DSM–III–R alcohol abuse and dependence with other psychiatric disorders in the national comorbidity survey. *Arch Gen Psychiatry* 1997;54:313–321.
36. Strakowski SM, DelBello MP, Fleck DE, et al. The impact of substance abuse on the course of bipolar disorder. *Biol Psychiatry* 2000;48(6):477–485.

37. Schuckit MA. The clinical implications of primary diagnostic groups among alcoholics. *Arch Gen Psychiatry* 1985;42:1043–1049.

38. Cloninger CR. Neurogenetic adaptive mechanisms in alcoholism. *Science* 1987;236:410–416.

39. Babor TF, Hofmann M, DelBoca FK, et al. Types of alcoholics. I: evidence for an empirically derived typology based on indicators of vulnerability and severity. *Arch Gen Psychiatry* 1992;49:599–608.

40. Penick EC, Powell BJ, Nickel EJ, et al. Examination of Cloninger's type I and type II alcoholism with a sample of men alcoholics in treatment. *Alcohol Clin Exp Res* 1990;14:623–629.

41. Anthenelli RM, Smith TL, Irwin MR, et al. A comparative study of criteria for subgrouping alcoholics: the primary/secondary diagnostic scheme versus variations of the type 1/type 2 criteria. *Am J Psychiatry* 1994;151:10:1468–1474.

42. Epstein EE, Labouvie E, McCrady BS, et al. A multi-site study of alcohol subtypes: classification and overlap of unidimensional and multi-dimensional typologies. *Addiction* 2002;97(8):1041–1053.

43. Bohman M, Sigvardsson S, Cloninger CR. Maternal inheritance of alcohol abuse: cross-fostering analysis of adopted women. *Arch Gen Psychiatry* 1991;38:965–969.

44. von Knorring L, von Knorring AL, Smigan L, et al. Personality traits in subtypes of alcoholics. *J Stud Alcohol* 1987;48:523–527.

45. Bohman M, Cloninger R, Sigvardsson S, et al. The genetics of alcoholisms and related disorders. *J Psychiatr Res* 1987;21:4:447–452.

46. Devor EJ, Cloninger CR. Genetics of alcoholism. *Annu Rev Genet* 1989;23:19–36.

47. Anthenelli RM, Tabakoff B. The search for biochemical markers. *Alcohol Health Res World* 1995;19:176–181.

48. Schuckit MA, Tipp JE, Smith TL, et al. An evaluation of type A and B alcoholics. *Addiction* 1995;90:1189–1203.

49. Begleiter H, Porjesz B. What is inherited in the predisposition toward alcoholism? A proposed model. *Alcohol Clin Exp Res* 1999;23(7):1125–1135.

50. Schuckit MA. A clinical model of genetic influences in alcohol dependence. *J Stud Alcohol* 1994;55:5–17.

51. Anthenelli RM, Schuckit MA. Genetics. In: Lowinson JH, Ruiz P, Millman RB, et al., eds. *Substance abuse: a comprehensive textbook,* 2nd ed. Baltimore: Williams & Wilkins, 1992:39–50.

52. Schuckit MA. Vulnerability factors for alcoholism. In: Davis KL, Charney D, Coyle JT, et al., eds. *Neuropsychopharmacology: the fifth generation of progress.* Philadelphia: Lippincott Williams & Wilkins, 2002:1399–1411.

53. Begleiter H, Porjesz B, Bihari B, et al. Event-related brain potentials in boys at risk for alcoholism. *Science* 1984;227:1493–1496.

54. Begleiter H. The collaborative study on the genetics of alcoholism. *Alcohol Health Res World* 1995;19:228–236.

55. Hesselbrock V, O'Connor S, Tasman A, et al. Cognitive and evoked potential indications of risk for alcoholism in young men. In: Kuriyamam K, Takada A, Ishii H, eds. *Biomedical and social aspects of alcohol and alcoholism.* Amsterdam: Elsevier Science Publishers, 1988.

56. Polich J, Bloom FE. Event-related brain potentials in individuals at high and low risk for developing alcoholism: failure to replicate. *Alcohol Clin Exp Res* 1988;12:368–373.

57. Hill SY, Steinhauer SR, Zubin J, et al. Event-related potentials as markers for alcoholism risk in high density families. *Alcohol Clin Exp Res* 1988;12:368–373.

58. Pollock VE, Volavka J, Goodwin DW. The EEG after alcohol administration in men at risk for alcoholism. *Arch Gen Psychiatry* 1983;40:857–861.

59. Volavka J, Pollock VE, Gabrielli WF, et al. *The EEG in persons at risk for alcoholism. Currents in alcoholism.* New York: Grune & Stratton, 1982.

60. Ehlers CL, Schuckit MA. Evaluation of EEG alpha activity in sons of alcoholics. *Neuropsychopharmacology* 1991;4:199–205.

61. Ehlers CL, Phillips E. EEG low-voltage alpha and alpha power in African American young adults: relation to family history of alcoholism. *Alcohol Clin Exp Res* 2003;27(5):765–772.

62. Schuckit MA. Subjective responses to alcohol in sons of alcoholics and control subjects. *Arch Gen Psychiatry* 1984;41:879–884.

63. Schuckit MA. Reactions to alcohol in sons of alcoholics and controls. *Alcohol Clin Exp Res* 1988;12:465–470.

64. Schuckit MA, Gold EO. A simultaneous evaluation of multiple markers of ethanol/placebo challenges in sons of alcoholics. *Arch Gen Psychiatry* 1988;45:211–216.

65. Schuckit MA. Ethanol-induced changes in body sway in men at high alcoholism risk. *Arch Gen Psychiatry* 1985;42:375–379.

66. Schuckit MA, Gold E, Risch C. Serum prolactin levels in sons of alcoholics and control subjects. *Am J Psychiatry* 1987;144:854–859.

67. Schuckit MA. Differences in plasma cortisol after ethanol in relatives of alcoholics and controls. *J Clin Psychiatry* 1984;45:374–379.

68. Schuckit MA. A long-term study of sons of alcoholics. *Alcohol Health Res World* 1995;19:172–175.

69. Schuckit MA, Smith TL. An 8-year follow-up of 450 sons of alcoholic and control subjects. *Arch Gen Psychiatry* 1996;53:202–210.

70. Anthenelli RM, Schuckit MA. Genetics. In: Lowinson JH, Ruiz P, Millman RB, et al., eds. *Substance abuse: a comprehensive textbook,* 3rd ed. Baltimore: Williams and Wilkins, 1997:41–51.

71. Mullan M. Alcoholism and the "new genetics." *Br J Addict* 1989;84:1433–1440.

72. Goldman D. Identifying alcoholism vulnerability alleles. *Alcohol Clin Exp Res* 1995;19:824–831.

73. Cloninger CR. D2 dopamine receptor gene is associated but not linked with alcoholism. *JAMA* 1991;266:1833–1834.

74. Parsian A, Todd RD, Devor EJ, et al. Alcoholism and alleles of the human D2 dopamine receptor locus. *Arch Gen Psychiatry* 1991;48:655–666.

75. Begleiter H, Reich T, Nurnberger J Jr, et al. Description of the Genetic Analysis Workshop 11 Collaborative Study on the Genetics of Alcoholism. *Genet Epidemiol* 1999;17[Suppl 1]:S25–S30.

76. Neumark YD, Friedlander Y, Thomasson HR, et al. Association of the ADH2*2 allele with reduced ethanol consumption in Jewish men in Israel: a pilot study. *J Stud Alcohol* 1998;59(2):133–139.

77. Yoshida A, Rzhetsky A, Hsu LC, Chang C. Human aldehyde dehydrogenase gene family. *Eur J Biochem* 1998;251(3):549–557.

78. Caballeria J. Current concepts in alcohol metabolism. *Ann Hepatol* 2003;2(2):60–68.

79. Vasiliou V, Bairoch A, Tipton KF, et al. Eukaryotic aldehyde dehydrogenase (ALDH) genes: human polymorphisms, and recommended nomenclature based on divergent evolution and chromosomal mapping. *Pharmacogenetics* 1999;9(4):421–434.

80. Goedde HW, Agarwal DP, Fritze G, et al. Distribution of ADH2 and ALDH2 genotypes in different populations. *Hum Genet* 1992;88(3):344–346.

81. Goedde HW, Harada S, Agarwal DP. Racial differences in alcohol sensitivity: a new hypothesis. *Hum Genet* 1979;51(3):331–334.

82. Agarwal DP. Genetic polymorphisms of alcohol metabolizing enzymes. *Pathol Biol* 2001;49(9):703–709.

83. Peng GS, Yin JH, Wang MF, et al. Alcohol sensitivity in Taiwanese men with different alcohol and aldehyde dehydrogenase genotypes. *J Formos Med Assoc* 2002;101(11):769–774.

84. Chen CC, Lu RB, Chen YC, et al. Interaction between the functional polymorphisms of the alcohol-metabolism genes in protection against alcoholism. *Am J Hum Genet* 1999;65(3):795–807.

85. Ramchandani VA, Bosron WF, Li TK. Research advances in ethanol metabolism. *Pathol Biol* 2001;49(9):676–682.

86. Wall TL, Ehlers CL. Genetic influences affecting alcohol use among Asians. *Alcohol Health Res World* 1995;19:184–189.

87. Blum K, Noble EP, Sheridan PJ, et al. Allelic association of human dopamine D2 receptor gene in alcoholism. *JAMA* 1990;263:2055–2060.

88. McBride WJ, Murphy JM, Lumeng L, et al. Serotonin, dopamine and GABA involvement in alcohol drinking of selectively bred rats. *Alcohol* 1990;7:199–205.

89. Koob GF, Rassnick S, Heinrichs S, et al. Alcohol, the reward system and dependence. *EXS* 1994;71:103–114.

90. Noble EP. Polymorphisms of the D2 dopamine receptor gene and alcoholism and other substance use disorders. *Alcohol* 1994;35–43.

91. Noble EP, Blum K, Ritchie T, et al. Allelic association of the D2 dopamine receptor gene with receptor-binding characteristics in alcoholism. *Arch Gen Psychiatry* 1991;48:648–654.

92. Limosin F, Gorwood P, Loze JY, et al. Male limited association of the dopamine receptor D2 gene TaqI a polymorphism and alcohol dependence. *Am J Med Genet* 2002;112(4):343–346.

93. Connor JP, Young RM, Lawford BR, et al. D(2) dopamine receptor (DRD2) polymorphism is associated with severity of alcohol dependence. *Eur Psychiatry* 2002;17(1):17–23.

94. Noble EP, Zhang X, Ritchie TL, et al. Haplotypes at the DRD2 locus and severe alcoholism. *Am J Med Genet* 2000;96(5):622–631.

95. Goldman D, Brown GL, Albaugh B, et al. D2 receptor genotype and linkage disequilibrium and function in Finnish, American Indian and U.S. Caucasian patients. In: Gershon ES, Cloninger CR, eds. *Genetic approaches to mental disorders*. Washington DC: American Psychiatric Press, 1994:327–344.

96. Bolos AM, Dean M, Lucas-Derse S, et al. Population and pedigree studies reveal a lack of association between the dopamine D2 receptor gene and alcoholism. *JAMA* 1990;264:3156–3160.

97. Edenberg HJ, Foroud T, Koller DL, et al. A family-based analysis of the association of the dopamine D2 receptor (DRD2) with alcoholism. *Alcohol Clin Exp Res* 1998;22:505–512.

98. Blomqvist O, Gelernter J, Kranzler HR. Family-based study of DRD2 alleles in alcohol and drug dependence. *Am J Med Genet* 2000;96(5):659–664.

99. Ebstein RP, Novick O, Umansky R, et al. Dopamine D4 receptor (D4DR) rcon III polymorphism associated with the human personality trait of novelty seeking. *Nat Genet* 1996;12:78–80.

100. Benjamin J, Greenberg B, Murphy DL, et al. Population and familial association between the D4 dopamine receptor gene and measures of Novelty seeking. *Nat Genet* 1996;12:81–84.

101. Thompson M, Comings DE, Feder L, et al. Mutation screening of the dopamine D1 receptor gene in Tourette's syndrome and alcohol-dependent patients. *Am J Med Genet* 1998;81(3):241–244.

102. Sander T, Harms H, Podschus J, et al. Dopamine D1, D2 and D3 receptor genes in alcohol dependence. *Psychiatr Genet* 1995;5(4):171–176.

103. Gorwood P, Limosin F, Batel P, et al. The genetics of addiction: alcohol-dependence and D3 dopamine receptor gene. *Pathol Biol (Paris)* 2001;49(9):710–717.

104. Lee MS, Ryu SH. No association between the dopamine D3 receptor gene and Korean alcohol dependence. *Psychiatr Genet* 2002;12(3):173–176.

105. Parsian A, Chakraverty S, Fisher L, et al. No association between polymorphisms in the human dopamine D3 and D4 receptors genes and alcoholism. *Am J Med Genet* 1997;74(3):281–285.

106. Aguayo LG, Peoples RW, Yevenes GE, et al. GABA(A) receptors as molecular sites of ethanol action. Direct or indirect actions. *Curr Top Med Chem* 2002;2(8):869–885.

107. McBride WJ, Li TK. Animal models of alcoholism: neurobiology of high alcohol-drinking behavior in rodents. *Crit Rev Neurobiol* 1998;12(4):339–369.

108. Porjesz B, Begleiter H, Wang K, et al. Linkage and linkage disequilibrium mapping of ERP and EEG phenotypes. *Biol Psychol* 2002;61:229–248.

109. Schuckit MA, Mazzanti C, Smith TL, et al. Selective genotyping for the role of 5-HT2A, 5-HT2C, and GABA alpha 6 receptors and the serotonin transporter in the level of response to alcohol: a pilot study. *Biol Psychiatry* 1999;45(5):647–651.

110. Wilhelmsen KC, Schuckit M, Smith TL, et al. The search for genes related to a low-level response to alcohol determined by alcohol challenges. *Alcohol Clin Exp Res* 2003;27(7):1041–1047.

111. Yoshimoto K, McBride WJ, Lumeng L, et al. Alcohol stimulates the release of dopamine and serotonin in the nucleus accumbens. *Alcohol* 1991;9:17–22.

112. Roberts AJ, McArthur RA, Hull EE, et al. Effects of amperozide, 8-OH-DPAT, and FG 5974 on operant responding for ethanol. *Psychopharmacology (Berl)* 1998;137(1):25–32.

113. Anthenelli RM, Maxwell RA, Geracioti TD Jr, et al. Stress hormone dysregulation at rest and following serotonergic stimulation among alcohol-dependent men with extended abstinence and controls. *Alcohol Clin Exp Res* 2001;25(5):692–703.

114. Heinz A, Mann K, Weinberger DR, et al. Serotonergic dysfunction, negative mood states, and response to alcohol. *Alcohol Clin Exp Res* 2001;25(4):487–495.

115. Sander T, Harms H, Dufeu P, et al. Serotonin transporter gene variants in alcohol-dependent subjects with dissocial personality disorder. *Biol Psychiatry* 1998;43(12):908–912.

116. Hammoumi S, Payen A, Favre JD, et al. Does the short variant of the serotonin transporter linked polymorphic region constitute a marker of alcohol dependence? *Alcohol* 1999;17(2):107–112.

117. Kranzler H, Lappalainen J, Nellissery M, et al. Association study of alcoholism subtypes with a functional promoter polymorphism in the serotonin transporter protein gene. *Alcohol Clin Exp Res* 2002;26(9):1330–1335.

118. Edenberg HJ, Reynolds J, Koller DL, et al. A family-based analysis of whether the functional promoter alleles of the serotonin transporter gene HTT affect the risk for alcohol dependence. *Alcohol Clin Exp Res* 1998;22(5):1080–1085.

119. Rigotti NA. Clinical practice. Treatment of tobacco use and dependence. *N Engl J Med* 2002;346(7):506–512.

120. Niaura R, Abrams DB. Smoking cessation: progress, priorities, and prospectus. *J Consult Clin Psychol* 2002;70(3):494–509.

121. McGinnis JM, Foege WH. Actual causes of death in the United States. *JAMA* 1993;270(18):2207–2212.

122. Hughes JR. Genetics of smoking: a brief review. *Behav Ther* 1986;17:335–345.

123. Bierut LJ, Dinwiddie SH, Begleiter H, et al. Familial transmission of substance dependence: alcohol, marijuana, cocaine, and habitual smoking. *Arch Gen Psychiatry* 1998;55:982–988.

124. Osler M, Holst C, Prescott E, et al. Influence of genes and family environment

on adult smoking behavior assessed in an adoption study. *Genet Epidemiol* 2001;21(3):193–200.

125. Boomsma DI, Koopmans JR, Van Doornen LJ, et al. Genetic and social influences on starting to smoke: a study of Dutch adolescent twins and their parents. *Addiction* 1994;89(2):219–226.

126. Carmelli D, Swan GE, Robinette D, et al. Genetic influence on smoking—a study of male twins. *N Engl J Med* 1992;327(12):829–833.

127. Heath AC, Madden PA, Martin NG. Statistical methods in genetic research on smoking. *Stat Methods Med Res* 1998;7(2):165–186.

128. Griesler PC, Kandel DB, Davies M. Ethnic differences in predictors of initiation and persistence of adolescent cigarette smoking in the National Longitudinal Survey of Youth. *Nicotine Tob Res* 2002;4(1):79–93.

129. Heath AC, Kirk KM, Meyer JM, et al. Genetic and social determinants of initiation and age at onset of smoking in Australian twins. *Behav Genet* 1999;29(6):395–407.

130. Heath AC, Martin NG, Lynskey MT, et al. Estimating two-stage models for genetic influences on alcohol, tobacco or drug use initiation and dependence vulnerability in twin and family data. *Twin Res* 2002;5(2):113–124.

131. Kendler KS, Neale MC, Sullivan P, et al. A population-based twin study in women of smoking initiation and nicotine dependence. *Psychol Med* 1999;29(2):299–308.

132. Stolerman IP, Jarvis MJ. The scientific case that nicotine is addictive. *Psychopharmacology (Berl)* 1995;117(1):2–10.

133. Kendler KS, Heath A, Martin NG, et al. Symptoms of anxiety and depression in a volunteer twin population. The etiologic role of genetic and environmental factors. *Arch Gen Psychiatry* 1986;43(3):213–221.

134. Kendler KS, Gardner CO Jr. Twin studies of adult psychiatric and substance dependence disorders: are they biased by differences in the environmental experiences of monozygotic and dizygotic twins in childhood and adolescence? *Psychol Med* 1998;28(3):625–633.

135. Hall W, Madden P, Lynskey M. The genetics of tobacco use: methods, findings and policy implications. *Tob Control* 2002;11:119–124.

136. Kendler KS, Thornton LM, Pedersen NL. Tobacco consumption in Swedish twins reared apart and reared together. *Arch Gen Psychiatry* 2000;57(9):886–892.

137. Blum K, Noble EP, Sheridan PJ, et al. Association of the A1 allele of the D2 dopamine receptor gene with severe alcoholism. *Alcohol* 1991;8(5):409–416.

138. Noble EP, St Jeor ST, Syndulko K, et al. D2 dopamine receptor gene and cigarette smoking: a reward gene? *Med Hypotheses* 1994;42:257–260.

139. Comings DE, Ferry L, Bradshaw-Robinson S, et al. The dopamine D2 receptor (DRD2) gene: a genetic risk factor in smoking. *Pharmacogenetics* 1996;6(1):73–79.

140. Spitz MR, Shi H, Yang F, et al. Case-control study of the D2 dopamine receptor gene and smoking status in lung cancer patients. *J Natl Cancer Inst* 1998;90(5):358–363.

141. Singleton AB, Thomson JH, Morris CM, et al. Lack of association between the dopamine D2 receptor gene allele DRD2*A1 and cigarette smoking in a United Kingdom population. *Pharmacogenetics* 1998;8(2):125–128.

142. Pohjalainen T, Rinne JO, Nagren K, et al. The A1 allele of the human D2 dopamine receptor gene predicts low D2 receptor availability in healthy volunteers. *Mol Psychiatry* 1998;3(3):256–260.

143. Noble EP, Gottschalk LA, Fallon JH, et al. D2 dopamine receptor polymorphism and brain regional glucose metabolism. *Am J Med Genet* 1997;74(2):162–166.

144. Lerman C, Caporaso N, Main D, et al. Depression and self-medication with nicotine: the modifying influence of the dopamine D4 receptor gene. *Health Psychol* 1998;17(1):56–62.

145. Sullivan PF, Neale MC, Silverman MA, et al. An association study of DRD5 with smoking initiation and progression to nicotine dependence. *Am J Med Genet* 2001;105(3):259–265.

146. Shields PG, Lerman C, Audrain J, et al. Dopamine D4 receptors and the risk of cigarette smoking in African-Americans and Caucasians. *Cancer Epidemiol Biomarkers Prev* 1998;7(6):453–458.

147. Lerman C, Caporaso NE, Audrain J, et al. Evidence suggesting the role of specific genetic factors in cigarette smoking. *Health Psychol* 1999;18(1):14–20.

148. Sabol SZ, Nelson ML, Fisher C, et al. A genetic association for cigarette smoking behavior. *Health Psychol* 1999;18(1):7–13.

149. Mihailescu S, Palomero-Rivero M, Meade-Huerta P, et al. Effects of nicotine and mecamylamine on rat dorsal raphe neurons. *Eur J Pharmacol* 1998;360(1):31–36.

150. Ribeiro EB, Bettiker RL, Bogdanov M, et al. Effects of systemic nicotine on serotonin release in rat brain. *Brain Res* 1993;621(2):311–318.

151. Eichhammer P, Langguth B, Wiegand R, et al. Allelic variation in the serotonin transporter promoter affects neuromodulatory effects of a selective serotonin transporter reuptake inhibitor (SSRI). *Psychopharmacology (Berl)* 2003;166(3):294–297.

152. Mancama D, Kerwin RW. Role of pharmacogenomics in individualising treatment with SSRIs. *CNS Drugs* 2003;17(3):143–151.

153. Ishikawa H, Ohtsuki T, Ishiguro H, et al. Association between serotonin transporter gene polymorphism and smoking among Japanese males. *Cancer Epidemiol Biomarkers Prev* 1999;8(9):831–833.

154. Lerman C, Shields PG, Audrain J, et al. The role of the serotonin transporter gene in cigarette smoking. *Cancer Epidemiol Biomarkers Prev* 1998;7(3):253–255.

155. Lerman C, Caporaso NE, Audrain J, et al. Interacting effects of the serotonin transporter gene and neuroticism in smoking practices and nicotine dependence. *Mol Psychiatry* 2000;5(2):189–192.

156. Lerman C, Caporaso NE, Bush A, et al. Tryptophan hydroxylase gene variant and smoking behavior. *Am J Med Genet* 2001;105(6):518–520.

157. Sullivan PF, Jiang Y, Neale MC, et al. Association of the tryptophan hydroxylase gene with smoking initiation but not progression to nicotine dependence. *Am J Med Genet* 2001;105(5):479–484.

158. Benowitz NL, Jacob P III, Jones RT, et al. Interindividual variability in the metabolism and cardiovascular effects of nicotine in man. *J Pharmacol Exp Ther* 1982;221(2):368–372.

159. Cashman JR, Park SB, Yang ZC, et al. Metabolism of nicotine by human liver microsomes: stereoselective formation of trans-nicotine N′-oxide. *Chem Res Toxicol* 1992;5(5):639–646.

160. Tyndale RF, Sellers EM. Genetic variation in CYP2A6-mediated nicotine metabolism alters smoking behavior. *Ther Drug Monit* 2002;24(1):163–171.

161. Raunio H, Rautio A, Gullsten H, et al. Polymorphisms of CYP2A6 and its practical consequences. *Br J Clin Pharmacol* 2001;52(4):357–363.

162. Elgoyhen AB, Johnson DS, Boulter J, et al. Alpha 9: an acetylcholine receptor with novel pharmacological properties expressed in rat cochlear hair cells. *Cell* 1994;79(4):705–715.

163. Lindstrom J. Neuronal nicotinic acetylcholine receptors. *Ion Channels* 1996;4:377–450.

164. Elgoyhen AB, Vetter DE, Katz E, et al. Alpha10: a determinant of nicotinic

cholinergic receptor function in mammalian vestibular and cochlear mechanosensory hair cells. *Proc Natl Acad Sci USA* 2001;98(6):3501–3506.

165. Picciotto MR, Zoli M, Rimondini R, et al. Acetylcholine receptors containing the beta2 subunit are involved in the reinforcing properties of nicotine. *Nature* 1998;391(6663):173–177.

166. Picciotto MR, Zoli M, Changeux JP. Use of knock-out mice to determine the molecular basis for the actions of nicotine. *Nicotine Tob Res* 1999;1[Suppl 2]:S121–S125.

167. Waldo MC, Adler LE, Leonard S, et al. Familial transmission of risk factors in the first-degree relatives of schizophrenic people. *Biol Psychiatry* 2000;47(3):231–239.

168. Kendler KS, Karkowski LM, Neale MC, et al. Illicit psychoactive substance use, heavy use, abuse, and dependence in a US population-based sample of male twins. *Arch Gen Psychiatry* 2000;57(3):261–269.

169. Tsuang MT, Lyons MJ, Harley RM, et al. Genetic and environmental influences on transitions in drug use. *Behav Genet* 1999;29(6):473–479.

170. Martin CS, Clifford PR, Clapper RL. Patterns and predictors of simultaneous and concurrent use of alcohol, tobacco, marijuana, and hallucinogens in first-year college students. *J Subst Abuse* 1992;4(3):319–326.

171. Brook JS, Whiteman M, Finch S, et al. Mutual attachment, personality, and drug use: pathways from childhood to young adulthood. *Genet Soc Gen Psychol Monogr* 1998;124(4):492–510.

172. Kosten TA, Ball SA, Rounsaville BJ. A sibling study of sensation seeking and opiate addiction. *J Nerv Ment Dis* 1994;182(5):284–289.

173. Kendler KS, Prescott CA. Cocaine use, abuse and dependence in a population-based sample of female twins. *Br J Psychiatry* 1998;173:345–350.

174. Comings DE, Gonzalez N, Wu S, et al. Homozygosity at the dopamine DRD3 receptor gene in cocaine dependence. *Mol Psychiatry* 1999;4(5):484–487.

175. Vorel SR, Ashby CR Jr, Paul M, et al. Dopamine D3 receptor antagonism inhibits cocaine-seeking and cocaine-enhanced brain reward in rats. *J Neurosci* 2002;22(21):9595–9603.

176. Noble EP, Blum K, Khalsa ME, et al. Allelic association of the D2 dopamine receptor gene with cocaine dependence. *Drug Alcohol Depend* 1993;33(3):271–285.

177. Gelernter J, Kranzler H, Satel SL. No association between D2 dopamine receptor (DRD2) alleles or haplotypes and cocaine dependence or severity of cocaine dependence in European- and African-Americans. *Biol Psychiatry* 1999;45(3):340–345.

178. Patkar AA, Berrettini WH, Hoehe M, et al. No association between polymorphisms in the serotonin transporter gene and susceptibility to cocaine dependence among African-American individuals. *Psychiatr Genet* 2002;12(3):161–164.

179. Patkar AA, Berrettini WH, Hoehe M, et al. Serotonin transporter (5-HTT) gene polymorphisms and susceptibility to cocaine dependence among African-American individuals. *Addict Biol* 2001;6(4):337–345.

180. Cigler T, LaForge KS, McHugh PF, et al. Novel and previously reported single-nucleotide polymorphisms in the human 5-HT(1B) receptor gene: no association with cocaine or alcohol abuse or dependence. *Am J Med Genet* 2001;105(6):489–497.

181. Bond C, LaForge KS, Tian M, et al. Single-nucleotide polymorphism in the human mu opioid receptor gene alters beta-endorphin binding and activity: possible implications for opiate addiction. *Proc Natl Acad Sci USA* 1998;95(16):9608–9613.

182. Szeto CY, Tang NL, Lee DT, et al. Association between mu opioid receptor gene polymorphisms and Chinese heroin addicts. *Neuroreport* 2001;12(6):1103–1106.

183. Kranzler HR, Gelernter J, O'Malley S, et al. Association of alcohol or other drug dependence with alleles of the mu opioid receptor gene (OPRM1). *Alcohol Clin Exp Res* 1998;22(6):1359–1362.

184. Franke P, Wang T, Nothen MM, et al. Nonreplication of association between mu-opioid-receptor gene (OPRM1) A118G polymorphism and substance dependence. *Am J Med Genet* 2001;105(1):114–119.

185. Tyndale RF, Droll KP, Sellers EM. Genetically deficient CYP2D6 metabolism provides protection against oral opiate dependence. *Pharmacogenetics* 1997;7:375–379.

186. Kendler KS, Prescott CA. Cannabis use, abuse, and dependence in a population-based sample of female twins. *Am J Psychiatry* 1998;155(8):1016–1022.

187. Kendler KS, Neale MC, Thornton LM, et al. Cannabis use in the last year in a US national sample of twin and sibling pairs. *Psychol Med* 2002;32(3):551–554.

188. Ameri A. The effects of cannabinoids on the brain. *Prog Neurobiol* 1999;58(4):315–348.

189. Comings DE, Muhleman D, Gade R, et al. Cannabinoid receptor gene (CNR1): association with i.v. drug use. *Mol Psychiatry* 1997;2(2):161–168.

190. Heller D, Schneider U, Seifert J, et al. The cannabinoid receptor gene (CNR1) is not affected in German i.v. drug users. *Addict Biol* 2001;6(2):183–187.

CHAPTER 5

Brain-Reward Mechanisms

ELIOT L. GARDNER

Among the social and medical ills of the twentieth century, substance abuse ranks as one of the most devastating and costly. Although totally accurate data on the cost to society are difficult to arrive at, well-informed estimates of the yearly cost to just the United States alone are in the range of $250–300 billion (1,2). Of course, substance abuse is not new. Descriptions of it are as old as the written word, with a particularly ancient one to be found in *Genesis* 9:20–23, in which Noah is described as becoming drunk with wine and found lying in a drunken stupor in his tent. At present, though, this age-old human scourge has taken on a new and frightening dimension with the realization that intravenous cocaine and heroin use now constitute the principal vector for the spread of acquired immunodeficiency syndrome (AIDS) in North America and Europe (3–5).

A question obviously arises: Why do human beings initiate and persist in such an obviously self-destructive and aberrant behavior as substance abuse? As with all aberrant behavior patterns, compulsive drug-seeking and drug-taking pose two fundamental questions, one for the scientist and one for the clinician. For the scientist, the question is, "What causes and perpetuates such patently self-destructive behavior?" For the clinician, the question is, "How can such behavior be modified or curbed to the ultimate benefit of the patient?" In the absence of purely accidental or fortuitous discoveries of effective treatment methods for pathologic drug-seeking and drug-taking, the scientific question becomes paramount, because from an understanding of the causes of drug self-administration can come rational hypothesis-driven treatment modalities.

Obviously, the causes of substance abuse are complex and multifactorial, including profoundly important social, economic, and educational factors. On the other hand, why is it that laboratory animals, on whom social, economic, and educational variables are inoperative, voluntarily (indeed, avidly) self-administer the same drugs that human beings use and abuse (6–9), and will not self-administer other drugs? This argues compellingly for a profoundly important biologic basis for substance abuse. Also, that laboratory animals will voluntarily self-administer these same drugs into highly selective and specific brain loci, but not into others, argues that this core of basic biologic causation for substance abuse is neurobiologic in nature.

Historically, explanatory postulates of the neurobiologic motivating forces behind the specific behavioral pattern of substance abuse have tended to parallel the more general explanatory postulates put forth by neurobehavioral theorists for the motivating forces behind all behavior. Early general theories of motivation, especially those of the nineteenth century, posited that behavior results primarily from subconscious "instincts" coded in the brain that impel certain behaviors to occur (10). Other early general theories of motivation, especially those popular during the first four decades of the twentieth century, posited that it is the activation of internal homeostatic brain mechanisms (e.g., hunger) that "drive" behavior (e.g., eating) to occur (10). Thus, both concepts hold that behavior is primarily the result of activation of internal neuropsychobiologic states within the organism, and the resulting behavior serves to relieve or reduce such internal activation. In quite parallel fashion, early explanations for substance abuse posited that compulsive drug users have a preexisting "psychic" disturbance (the so-called addict personality) that impels drug-taking behavior (11). Such "instinct-satisfaction" or "drive-reduction" theories do not explain why certain behaviors are preferred over others with presumably equivalent "instinct-satisfaction" or "drive-reduction" value (e.g., why some foods are preferred over others), and the postulation of a precoded "heroin drive" or "cocaine drive" in the central nervous system has seemed far-fetched to even the most dyed-in-the-wool instinct or drive-reduction theorists. There is also an displeasing element of circularity to such concepts, i.e., a drug addict uses drugs because the addict has a predisposition to do so. True in some cases, no doubt, but hardly a richly satisfying explanation of the underlying neurobiologic or psychobiologic mechanisms. During the middle decades of the twentieth century, an alternative explanation came to dominate motivational theory in both psychology and psychiatry. This view, termed "reinforcement theory" (10,12), explains behavior in terms of contingent associations between initially random behavioral elements and environmental stimuli. That is, if certain environmental stimuli ("reinforcers") are contingently paired with behavior, the future probability of that same behavior increases. Thus, reinforcement theory holds that behavior is primarily the result of the presence of salient environmental stimuli, which act on the central nervous system in such a way as to alter the future probability of behavior occurring in their presence (10,12). The "reinforcement theory" explanation for substance abuse posits that compulsive substance abusers use drugs because these same drugs have been positive reinforcers on previous occasions. Again, as with "instinct" and "drive-reduction" theories, there is a displeasing circularity to such an explanation, i.e., a drug addict uses drugs because drugs were previously "reinforcing." All very true in most cases, no doubt, but because reinforcement theory makes no attempt to describe the neurophysiologic processes that occur in the presence of reinforcers, the "reinforcement" explanation for substance abuse is as unsatisfying with respect to underlying neurobiologic or psychobiologic substrates and mechanisms as are "instinct" and "drive-reduction" explanations. Seemingly more germane to these issues is the notion of "incentive stimulation" or "incentive motivation," a more modern concept in motivational theory (10). This view attempts to describe reinforcers as having the ability to activate internal sensory or affective processes within the organism that are inherently pleasurable or rewarding (i.e., subjectively pleasant), and which then organize and influence behavior to occur (10,13–15). For example, if an organism ingests heroin or cocaine and finds that pleasure or reward ensues, the likelihood of future ingestion of heroin or cocaine increases. This position is, of course, strikingly close to the "common sense" hedonistic explanation for motivation which, as Young (13) notes, "implies that subjective feelings of pleasantness and unpleasantness influence behavior."

That drugs of abuse are positive reinforcers is clear. As early as 1940, it was demonstrated by Spragg's pioneering work (16) that laboratory animals will voluntarily engage in behaviors that lead to the injection of habit-forming drugs. Indeed, in Spragg's studies chimpanzees would drag the researcher to the cupboard where the morphine, syringes, and needles were stored, and voluntarily assume the proper position to receive the injections. In 1962, Weeks (6) demonstrated that animals will voluntarily self-administer habit-forming drugs if placed in a laboratory setting in which the animal's response on a manipulandum activates an automatic infusion system, which delivers a preset amount of drug through a surgically implanted venous catheter. Thus, the human researcher is totally out of the loop; drug delivery or nondelivery is totally under the voluntary control of the animal. This work set the stage for the now widely used paradigm of drug self-administration in laboratory animals as a tool for studying drug-induced reinforcement processes. One important ancillary result of the discovery of voluntary drug self-administration in animals is that it turned scientific attention away from hypothetical internal states within substance abusers (i.e., the "addict" personality) that supposedly "drove" them to abuse drugs, and focused attention instead on the drugs themselves, and on the common neuropharmacologic properties they might possess that make them positive reinforcers for man and animal alike.

As already noted, "incentive motivation" theory holds that positive reinforcers activate internal neural processes that are inherently pleasurable or rewarding (10,13–15). The study of the nature of these inherently pleasurable or rewarding neural processes activated by positive reinforcers was advanced dramatically in 1954 with the seminal discovery by Olds and Milner that laboratory animals will voluntarily (indeed, avidly) self-administer electrical stimulation delivered through electrodes deep in the brain (17). This finding was of great importance for many reasons. First, such brain stimulation appears to act precisely as other positive reinforcers, and selectively strengthens any behavior linked contingently to it (17). Second, the finding that only a limited number of brain sites support such brain stimulation reward (18) strongly implies that there are anatomically specific circuits in the brain dedicated to the neural mediation of reward or pleasure (19–21). Third, that electrical stimulation of brain-reward sites can also evoke natural consummatory behaviors such as eating and drinking (22–26) implies that such electrical stimulation activates neural systems involved in natural reward and motivation.

Evidence that habit-forming drugs might derive their rewarding properties by activating such brain-reward circuits was presented less than 3 years after the discovery of the brain-stimulation reward phenomenon (27), and has been amply confirmed in the more than five decades since. This acute enhancement of brain-reward mechanisms now appears to be the single essential pharmacologic commonality of abusable substances, and the hypothesis that abusable substances act on these brain mechanisms to produce the subjective reward that constitutes the reinforcing "high" or "rush" or "hit" sought by substance abusers is, at present, the most compelling hypothesis available on the neurobiology of substance abuse (28–31).

The remainder of this chapter addresses various aspects of this unifying conception of the neural nature of the positive reinforcement engendered by self-administration of abusable substances.

DRUG REWARD MODELS: SELF-ADMINISTRATION OF ABUSABLE SUBSTANCES BY LABORATORY ANIMALS

As stated previously, until approximately 30 years ago, the standard explanation for compulsive substance abuse emphasized predisposing internal drives (e.g., the "addict" personality) within the substance abuser that drove the abuser to abuse drugs. Additionally, there was a second aspect to the standard 1950s and 1960s explanation for substance abuse—that substance abusers, driven to drug use by predisposing internal states, soon become caught up in a vicious cycle of drug administration, tolerance, physical dependence, withdrawal, and readministration. Driven by this vicious cycle, the substance abuser was believed to self-administer abusable substances primarily to ward off the unpleasant consequences of withdrawal. The emphasis of this explanatory rubric was thus negative—to ward off the negative physical consequences of drug withdrawal. No emphasis was placed on the possibility that abusable substance might have powerful positively reinforcing properties.

It was the demonstration that laboratory animals will voluntarily (often avidly) self-administer abusable substances (6–9) that decisively reoriented scientific attention onto the positively rewarding properties of the drugs themselves.

Self-Administration Paradigm

Abusable substances can be self-administered by laboratory animals using a variety of administration routes. The intravenous, intramuscular, intraperitoneal, and intracerebral injection routes have all been used, as have the oral ingestion, intragastric, and inhalation routes. The typical drug self-administration paradigm uses the intravenous route in laboratory animals surgically implanted with chronic indwelling intravenous catheters (6–9,32,33). Most typically rats (34,35) or rhesus monkeys (36–40) are used, although other mammalian species have also been successfully used (41–43). Strikingly, animals will self-administer abusable substances in the absence of tolerance, physical dependence, withdrawal, or, indeed, any prior history of drug taking. The importance of this fact can hardly be overstated because it clearly shows that drug-taking behavior cannot be explained simply in terms of the ability of abusable drugs to ameliorate the withdrawal discomfort associated with abstinence from prior administration of such drugs. In addition, the use of operant conditioning procedures shows that animal behavior can be controlled by abusable substances in much the same manner that food or water can control the behavior of a hungry or thirsty animal (39), with the obvious caveats that drugs can produce nonspecific increases or decreases in motoric behavior and that under certain operant schedules of drug self-administration (e.g., low fixed-ratio schedules) successive doses may cumulate rapidly within the body, resulting in limitations on rate of response (32). With ratio schedules of operant reinforcement, responding by laboratory animals for drug self-administration has been demonstrated for cocaine (39,44–47), amphetamines (39,43,48–54), other stimulants (55,56), caffeine (36), opiates (6,36,41,45,57–64), ethanol (65–66), sedative-hypnotics (36,44,67–70), dissociative anesthetics (71,72), and other abusable substances (9,33). With interval schedules of operant reinforcement, responding by laboratory animals for drug self-administration has been demonstrated for cocaine (47,73–77), opiates (78–81), ethanol (80,82,83), sedative–hypnotics (70), and other abusable substances (9,33). As with human substance abuse, drug self-administration in laboratory animals is profoundly influenced by the subject's previous experience with drugs and by the environmental context in which the drug administration takes place (32).

Typically, operant responding for drug self-administration in laboratory animals is compared against operant responding on a control manipulandum that does not deliver drug administration, or against operant responding for saline or vehicle administration. For some abusable substances, acquisition of operant responding for self-administration is rapid and facile—the catheterized laboratory animal is simply placed into the operant chamber and allowed to explore. Normal curiosity and exploratory behavior soon result in an initially random response on the manipulandum that delivers a drug injection. With the appropriate drug, dose, and reinforcement contingency, the animal experiences a subjective reward, with resulting "self-shaping" of behavior to the motor response that delivers the drug. Self-administration of the abusable substance ensues, with a characteristic learning curve and characteristic asymptotic self-administration behavior. For other abusable substances (presumably substances with a lower initial reward efficacy), such "self-learning" does not result in reliable self-administration behavior. In such cases, other experimental procedures are followed to obtain reliable self-administration behavior. These procedures include (a) training the animal first to respond for a traditional reinforcer such as food and then substituting the drug reinforcer for the food (60); (b) training the animal first to respond for another drug with presumably higher initial reward efficacy and then substituting the drug under investigation for the original drug (52,65,84); (c) deliberately shaping the animal's operant behavior toward the manipulandum that delivers drug administration (55); (d) using noncontingent drug administration during the initial stages of the animal's exposure to the drug self-administration situation (85); (e) using an aversive stimulus such as foot-shock to initiate the operant responding for drug administration (38); (f) using food or water deprivation to encourage responding on the drug-administering manipulandum (86); and (g) first making the animal physically dependent upon the drug by programmed drug delivery and then allowing the animal to respond for drug injections after the termination of programmed delivery (6). Some authorities argue that the use of such procedures constitute less-rigorous demonstrations that a drug can serve as a reinforcer (33). Such arguments are debatable. So long as the final drug self-administration behavior is reliably higher than operant responding on a control manipulandum that does not deliver drug administration, or higher than operant responding for saline or vehicle administration, the laboratory "tricks" used to initiate or facilitate initial operant responding for drug reinforcement would seem more related to initial reward efficacy, which can have significant pharmacokinetic, as well as pharmacodynamic, components, than to basic reinforcement value. No matter how the drug self-administration is initiated, it can easily be determined whether the contingent drug administration is truly reinforcing the operant behavior by simply disabling the drug delivery system or substituting saline or vehicle for the active drug and seeing whether behavioral extinction (cessation of responding) occurs. If the drug is serving as a reinforcer, extinction ensues. If the drug is not serving as a reinforcer, the behavior continues unabated. Extinction of drug-reinforced responding follows a highly characteristic pattern that is essentially identical to extinction of food- or water-reinforced behavior—an initial increase in response rate (frustrative nonreward behavioral augmentation), followed by decreased responding, and, ultimately, total cessation of responding. Recent demonstrations that extinction of responding for direct intracranial electrical brain-stimulation reward follows the same highly characteristic behavioral pattern as extinction of drug-reinforced responding (87; see also later discussion of this point, in section entitled "Electrical Brain-Stimulation Reward Paradigm") are an important element of the argument that drug self-administration activates the same brain-reward mechanisms activated by electrical brain-stimulation reward.

Characteristic Patterns of Drug Intake in the Self-Administration Paradigm

Patterns of drug intake in the self-administration paradigm in laboratory animals vary with drug class (33) and are provocatively similar to intake patterns seen in humans. With unlimited access to opiates, self-administration is quite uniform and constant, characterized by moderate and measured self-administration of modest doses without voluntary abstinence periods (36,88). In contrast, unlimited self-administration of stimulants (cocaine, amphetamines, methylphenidate, caffeine) is characterized by alternating periods of drug-intake and drug-abstinence (36,50,52,89–91). During drug-intake periods the self-administration behavior often reaches frenzied levels, accompanied by characteristic dopaminergic behavioral stereotypies, markedly reduced food and water intake, and total lack of sleep. During drug-abstinence periods, a semblance of normal eating, drinking, and sleeping returns. The alternating drug-intake and drug-abstinence periods can continue for months, and markedly resemble the alternating binge and abstinence pattern of human stimulant abuse (92). Unlimited ethanol self-administration in animals is also characterized by alternating binge and abstinence periods (65). Unlimited barbiturate and dissociative anesthetic (e.g., phencyclidine) self-administration in animals is characterized by maximum self-administration of available drug, without abstinence periods (36,68,93). Unlimited benzodiazepine self-administration is characterized by very modest intake patterns (68). Given the right reinforcement schedule and dose, nearly all intravenously self-administered drugs can be consumed by laboratory animals to the point of toxicity and/or death (36,52,65,88). The death rate from unlimited stimulant self-administration is very high; that from opiates, ethanol, and barbiturates is very much lower although still significant. When drug availability is limited to a preset daily session, drug intake tends to be stable from session to session. Within each session, drug intake pattern varies with drug class. Opiate self-administration is measured and steady, while stimulant self-administration is characterized by "mini-binges" at the start of test sessions followed by more measured self-administration for the remainder of the session. With different doses available during different test sessions, drug intake appears to be regulated by the animal to produce fairly uniform actual drug intake over a broad range of doses, a phenomenon that has been interpreted as supporting the concept that laboratory animals self-administer drugs to maintain a constant blood and brain level (94).

Modelling Drug Appetitiveness in Laboratory Animals: Drug Self-Administration Under Progressive-Ratio Reinforcement Schedules

The self-administration paradigm in animals can be modified to assess the relative appetitive value of different addicting drugs. One such modification is the "progressive ratio" self-administration paradigm (95,96), in which the amount of work an animal has to expend to receive a single intravenous injection is progressively increased in ratio fashion (e.g., one lever-press for the first injection, two lever-presses for the second injection, four lever-presses for the third injection, eight lever-presses for the fourth injection, etc.). In any such progressive-ratio run, there comes a point where the animal simply gives up and abruptly stops lever-pressing (the "Oh hell, this ain't worth it anymore" point), the so-called "breakpoint." By comparing breakpoints between different classes of addicting drugs, one can establish hierarchies of appetitiveness. Such hierarchies closely resemble those observed in humans (e.g., cocaine extremely appetitive, morphine moderately appetitive, benzodiazepines marginally appetitive). Of course, there are individual differences amongst animals just as there are amongst humans. But cocaine is so appetitive to most laboratory animals that, if given continuous access, they will spend most of their waking hours self-administering the drug and will self-administer it to the point of starvation and death, even if hundreds or thousands of lever-presses are needed to obtain one dose of the drug (50,89,97). The parallels to the extreme appetitiveness of crack cocaine in vulnerable humans is striking.

Essential Commonalities of Substances Self-Administered by Laboratory Animals

Although *Chemical Abstracts* lists millions of different known chemicals, the number of chemicals voluntarily self-administered by laboratory animals is only a tiny fraction of that number—no more than a few score compounds (8,9,33). Also, the chemicals voluntarily self-administered by laboratory animals differ quite strikingly from each other in chemical structure and pharmacologic class. The following questions obviously arise: (a) What do these self-administered compounds have in common? and (b) What distinguishes these compounds from the millions of other known compounds? The answers appear to be threefold. First, although there are inexplicable exceptions (33), by and large the substances that are voluntarily self-administered by laboratory animals are the same ones that human beings also voluntarily self-administer (8,9,33,98–102), and by and large the same drugs that are eschewed by animals are also eschewed by humans. Second, virtually all adequately studied abusable substances (including opiates, cocaine, amphetamines, dissociative anesthetics, barbiturates, benzodiazepines, alcohol, and marihuana) enhance brain-stimulation reward or lower brain-reward thresholds in the mesotelencephalic dopamine (DA) system (28–31,103–113). Third, virtually all adequately studied abusable substances enhance basal neuronal firing and/or basal neurotransmitter release in reward-relevant brain circuits (105,114–124). These essential commonalities of substances self-administered by laboratory animals are important elements in the theory that drug self-administration activates the same brain-reward mechanisms activated by electrical brain-stimulation reward and that these brain-reward mechanisms include a mesotelencephalic DA component that runs through the medial forebrain bundle. In this last regard, it is compelling that animals voluntarily self-administer the DA reuptake blockers bupropion, mazindol, and nomifensine (55,125–130), as well as 1-{2-[bis(4-fluorophenyl)methoxy]ethyl}-4-(3-phenylpropyl) piperazine (GBR 12909), a highly selective DA reuptake blocker (131,132). It is similarly compelling in this regard that animals also voluntarily self-administer direct DA receptor agonists such as apomorphine and piribedil (84,133–136).

An interesting variant of the drug self-administration paradigm in laboratory animals is one in which the drug infusion is automatically delivered and the animal can voluntarily respond to terminate the infusion (137). Just as the voluntarily self-administration paradigm assesses the positive reward of drugs, this voluntary termination-of-infusion paradigm assesses the negative reward value or aversive property of drugs. Interestingly, some drugs do act as negative reinforcers in this paradigm (137,138). Provocatively, most drugs that act as negative reinforcers in this paradigm, and may thus be inferred to have negative reward value, are DA antagonists such as chlorpromazine and perphenazine (137,138). Most humans find such drugs dysphorigenic (139,140). These findings are additional important elements in the theory that the brain-reward mechanisms activated by drug self-administration include a crucial DA component.

Alteration of Drug Self-Administration by Pharmacologic or Neurobiologic Manipulations

One of the many approaches used to unravel the neuroanatomic, neurophysiologic, and neurochemical substrates of drug-induced reward has been to attempt to alter systemic drug self-administration in laboratory animals by pharmacologic manipulations or specific brain lesions. Obviously, when attempting to alter drug self-administration by administering another pharmacologic

agent, one has to be alert to the possibility of nonspecific drug effects on behavior. Thus, a compound could theoretically inhibit an animal's lever-pressing or bar-pressing for drug injections simply by being so powerful a sedative as to inhibit all motor behavior in a nonspecific fashion. The key, then, to inferring a specific effect on drug-induced reward is to look for specific effects on behavior maintained by drug reward (33). Thus, pharmacologic manipulations that augment the reinforcing properties of a self-administered drug will selectively suppress drug responding (similar to increasing the unit dose of the self-administered drug) without altering other behaviors, whereas pharmacologic manipulations that diminish the reinforcing properties of a self-administered drug will selectively increase drug responding (to compensate for the reduced effectiveness of the self-administered drug) without altering other behaviors. A manipulation that completely abolishes the reinforcing value of a self-administered drug should produce characteristic extinction of drug-reinforced responding—an initial increase in response rate (frustrative nonreward behavioral augmentation) followed by decreased responding and, finally, cessation of responding. Not unexpectedly, administration of opiate antagonists (e.g., naloxone, naltrexone) to animals self-administering morphine or heroin produces characteristic extinction of the drug responding (57,81,141–143). Provocatively, antibodies to morphine also produce a partial extinction-like increase in heroin intake (144).

Pharmacologic challenges that specifically disrupt individual neurotransmitter systems can obviously yield important information on the neurochemical substrates of drug-induced reward. In the many reports in which such neurotransmitter-specific pharmacologic manipulations have been paired with drug self-administration in laboratory animals, a striking common thread stands out: Pharmacologic challenges that disrupt brain DA systems interfere with the reward value of self-administered drugs. Thus, α-methyl-para-tyrosine (αMPT), a DA synthesis inhibitor, initially produces a partial-extinction-like increase in cocaine or amphetamine self-administration, followed by full extinction of the self-administration behavior as the αMPT dose increases (145–147). Similarly, gradually increasing doses of the DA antagonist pimozide produce an initial dose-dependent increase in self-administered amphetamine intake, followed at higher doses by cessation of self-administration (148). The stereoisomers (+)butaclamol (possessing potent DA antagonism) and (−)butaclamol (devoid of DA antagonism) have also been used to assess DA substrates of drug-induced reward (149). In these studies, (+)butaclamol produced partial and then complete extinction of amphetamine self-administration while (−)butaclamol had no effect on amphetamine self-administration (149). Similar patterns of increased drug self-administration after low-dose DA blockers followed by decreased drug self-administration after higher doses have also been reported from a large number of laboratories for animals self-administering a wide range of abusable substances, including cocaine, amphetamine, and morphine (133,142,150–163). In contrast, noradrenergic blockers have no effect on drug self-administration in laboratory animals (147,149,150,153,155). In humans, DA antagonists and DA synthesis inhibitors blunt the euphorigenic effects of at least some abusable substances (164–167).

Another approach to pharmacologic manipulation of drug self-administration in laboratory animals is the administration of neurotransmitter-specific agonists. The rationale for this approach is that of substitution: just as noncontingent administration of amphetamine temporarily decreases amphetamine self-administration, so, too, a neurotransmitter-specific agonist that activates the same brain-reward substrates should temporarily decrease drug self-administration. Such, in fact, is the case. Noncontingent administrations of the DA agonists apomorphine or piribedil dose-dependently decrease amphetamine self-administration (84).

A further approach to elucidating the neurochemical substrates of drug-induced reward is to study the effect on drug self-administration of selective lesions, induced either surgically or pharmacologically, of specific neurotransmitter systems in the brain. Obviously, such studies also help to elucidate the neuroanatomic substrates of drug-induced reward. Such studies typically are of two types: (a) studies of the effects of brain lesions on stable, previously acquired drug self-administration, and (b) studies of the effects of brain lesions on acquisition of drug self-administration (168). In such studies, the use of neurotransmitter-specific neurotoxins to produce the desired lesion is generally preferable to nonneurotransmitter-specific knife cuts, electrolytic lesions, or thermocoagulative lesions (168). When the catecholamine-specific neurotoxin 6-hydroxydopamine (6-OHDA) is used to selectively lesion the DA-rich nucleus accumbens, cocaine self-administration is disrupted but self-administration of the direct DA receptor agonist apomorphine in the same animals is unaffected (169). Similarly, when 6-OHDA is used to lesion the DA-rich ventral tegmental area, cocaine self-administration is disrupted, but apomorphine self-administration is unaffected (170). 6-OHDA lesions of other brain sites do not affect cocaine self-administration (168–170). These data argue that cocaine self-administration is critically dependent upon a highly specific subset of the DA wiring of the mammalian brain—the mesolimbic DA system, which originates in the ventral tegmental area and projects importantly to the nucleus accumbens (171). In animals with 6-OHDA lesions of either of these two DA loci, the extent of 6-OHDA-induced DA depletion in the nucleus accumbens is highly predictive of duration of curtailment of cocaine self-administration. The greater the DA deple-

tion, the longer the animal takes to recover drug self-administration behavior; animals with the greatest DA loss (more than 90%) often fail to recover at all (168). 6-OHDA lesions of the nucleus accumbens also block acquisition of amphetamine self-administration (172). Heroin and morphine self-administration in laboratory animals have been similarly demonstrated to be critically dependent upon the functional integrity of the mesolimbic DA system (173–175). It is compelling that the mesolimbic DA system constitutes a critical component of the reward system of the mammalian brain (29,31,104,105; see, in section entitled "Neuroanatomy and Neurochemistry of Brain-Stimulation Reward"). In this regard, the previously reviewed data suggest that functional blockade, either pharmacologically induced or lesion-induced, of brain-reward substrates is the important commonality of manipulations blocking systemic drug self-administration. Thus, studies in which alteration of drug self-administration has been achieved by pharmacologic or neurobiologic manipulations are important elements in the theory that drug self-administration activates the same brain-reward mechanisms activated by electrical brain-stimulation reward and that these brain-reward mechanisms include the mesolimbic DA subsystem that runs through the medial forebrain bundle.

UNDERLYING NEUROBIOLOGY OF DRUG REWARD: ELECTRICAL SELF STIMULATION OF BRAIN-REWARD CIRCUITS

Electrical Brain-Stimulation Reward Paradigm

To study electrical brain-stimulation reward, animals are first surgically implanted with chronic indwelling intracranial stimulating electrodes in specific brain loci, allowed to recover from the surgery, and then trained to self-administer the rewarding electrical stimulation by bar-pressing or lever-pressing in a standard operant chamber. The training techniques typically used are essentially identical to those employed to train animals for drug self-administration (see, in section entitled "Self-Administration Paradigm"). Acquisition of lever-pressing for brain-stimulation reward is very rapid, with high asymptotic operant levels. Volitional self-administration of the rewarding electrical stimulation, often termed intracranial self-stimulation, is easily maintained by simple operant schedules of reinforcement. The reward engendered by such stimulation, and the brain substrates that support it, have been much studied and well characterized over the last 50 years (176–178). With electrodes in the proper brain loci, such direct brain-stimulation reward is intensely powerful. Hungry animals ignore food to get it and thirsty animals ignore water to get it, in strikingly similar fashion to the way in which cocaine self-administering animals ignore food and water during a drug binge.

Animals even endure pain to reach the lever that delivers brain-stimulation reward. Response rates of animals self-stimulating for electrical brain reward are extremely high, often in excess of 100 lever-presses per minute. In short, electrical brain-stimulation reward is one of the most powerful rewards known to biology, rivaled only by the reward engendered by the most powerful self-administered drugs (e.g., cocaine). The few human studies of electrical stimulation of brain-reward areas confirm this, the human experience being one of intense subjective pleasure or euphoria (179).

With simple operant schedules of reinforcement, lever-pressing for electrical brain-stimulation reward extinguishes essentially immediately upon termination of the reward, without the normal frustrative nonreward increase in responding that characterizes the early stages of extinction to lever-pressing for food, water, or drug reward. For many years, this was a major conundrum, with some workers arguing that this distinction between electrical brain-stimulation reward and drug self-administration reward implied that different brain substrates are activated by the two types of reward. However, Lepore and Franklin, in an extremely important piece of work, showed that the rapid extinction of brain-stimulation reward behavior on low-ratio reinforcement schedules is essentially an artifact of the immediacy of the electrical brain-stimulation reward and of the operant behavioral schedules typically used in brain-stimulation reward studies (87). The paradigm developed by Lepore and Franklin, called "self-administration of brain-stimulation," delivers rewarding electrical brain stimulation in a manner deliberately designed to mimic the pharmacokinetics of drug self-administration as closely as possible. The animal's first response on the brain-stimulation reward lever turns on the brain stimulator, which then stays permanently on for the duration of the test session to deliver a continuous train of biphasic pulse-pairs of rewarding stimulation. However, the frequency of the pulse-pairs decreases with time, in much the same way that brain and blood levels of a self-administered drug decrease with time. Successive lever-presses increase the stimulation frequency by a preset amount. Because for any given set of electrical stimulation parameters (pulse-width, current, etc.) there is a range of stimulation frequencies that is optimally rewarding, animals in this paradigm typically lever-press enough times to bring the frequency into the optimal range, and then wait while it slowly decays (in much the same fashion that animals on drug self-administration wait for drug reward to decay after taking a few "hits"). When the stimulation frequency has decayed enough to bring it out of the rewarding range, the animals typically take a few more "hits" on the lever to once again bring the stimulation back up to the optimal range. In this paradigm, which so deliberately models the pharmacokinetics of drug self-administration, extinction is essentially identical to extinction of drug-reinforced behavior, complete

with an initial frustrative nonreward increase in responding followed by a slow decrease and ultimate cessation of responding. The importance of this "self-administration of brain-stimulation" paradigm can hardly be overstated, for it shows that once the "pharmacokinetics" of electrical brain-stimulation reward are made to emulate those of drug reward, the difference between the two reward paradigms disappears. In view of these developments, the hypothesis that drug-reward and brain-stimulation reward activate the same brain-reward substrates appears more compelling than ever.

Neuroanatomy and Neurochemistry of Brain-Stimulation Reward

The neuroanatomic substrates of direct electrical brain-stimulation reward were initially unclear. Early anatomic mapping studies of the brain for positive brain-stimulation reward sites, carried out in the 1950s and 1960s, demonstrated that electrical brain reward could be elicited in laboratory rats, cats, and monkeys from a wide variety of brainstem, midbrain, and forebrain loci, including the ventral tegmental area; substantia nigra; hypothalamus; medial forebrain bundle; septum; amygdala; neostriatum; nucleus accumbens; ventral forebrain olfactory nuclei; and portions of the cingulate cortex and frontal cortex (17,180–185). Such a hodgepodge of sensory, motor, limbic, midbrain, diencephalic, and cortical domains made little sense at the time, although even the early workers noted that the vast majority of brain sites positive for electrical brain-stimulation reward correspond to the aggregate of ascending and descending tracts that comprise the medial forebrain bundle, the nuclei and projections of which extend from brainstem to cortex. Then, in the mid 1960s, pioneering Scandinavian neuroanatomists began to illuminate the monoaminergic anatomy of the brain using the newly developed neurotransmitter mapping technique of histofluorescence microscopy (186–189). A striking correspondence was noted between sites positive for brain-stimulation reward and the mesotelencephalic DA system, the major portions of which are carried through the medial forebrain bundle from the ventral mesencephalon to the limbic and cortical forebrain (171).

Guided by this anatomic correspondence, workers in many laboratories began to study the effects of pharmacologic manipulation of DA neurotransmission on brain-stimulation reward. In 1969, the author and his colleagues found that selective inhibition of tyrosine hydroxylase profoundly inhibited brain reward in monkeys, but that selective inhibition of DA-β-hydroxylase did not, prompting the postulation that brain reward was critically dependent upon the functional integrity of DA neurotransmission. In 1972, Crow suggested that direct activation of the cell bodies or axons of the mesolimbic and mesostriatal DA systems was rewarding, and that DA was the crucial neurotransmitter of at least one major reward system in the brain (190). In 1980, Corbett and Wise, using movable electrodes to map brain-reward substrates in the ventral mesencephalon, showed that brain-stimulation reward thresholds were a function of the density of DA elements surrounding the electrode tip (191). Also compelling is that DA blockade disrupts brain-stimulation reward at all brain sites adequately tested (192–194), and that, following DA denervation that abolishes neostriatal brain-stimulation reward, direct electrical brain reward can be restored in the denervated neostriatum by DA reinnervation from embryonic substantia nigra transplants (195). From these studies, and literally hundreds of other experiments (summarized in references 31, 105, 194, and 196–198), it has become abundantly clear that brain reward is, in fact, critically dependent upon the functional integrity of DA neurotransmission within the mesotelencephalic DA systems, with the mesolimbic DA system constituting a particularly important focal point within these brain-reward systems. Compellingly, DA blockade mimics the effect of decreasing the electrical intensity of the rewarding brain stimulation (193).

However, the original supposition of many researchers that electrical brain-stimulation reward directly activates the DA fibers of the medial forebrain bundle appears contrary to the preponderance of evidence. This evidence derives in large part from the studies of Gallistel, Yeomans, Shizgal, and their colleagues (199–203), which argue persuasively on electrophysiologic grounds that the primary medial forebrain bundle substrate directly activated by electrical brain-stimulation reward is a myelinated, caudally running fiber system whose neurons have absolute refractory periods of 0.5 to 1.2 msec and local potential decay time-constants of approximately 0.1 msec. Because none of these neurophysiologic properties agrees with those of the ascending mesotelencephalic DA neurons of the medial forebrain bundle, Wise and his colleagues argue that the DA neurons cannot be the "first-stage" reward neurons preferentially activated by electrical brain-stimulation reward, but must, instead, constitute a crucial "second-stage" anatomic convergence within the reward circuitry of the brain, upon which the "first-stage" neurons (those preferentially activated by rewarding electrical stimulation) synapse to form an "in series," reward-relevant neural circuit (29,104,105). It is on this "second-stage" DA convergence—with its DA cell bodies in the ventral tegmental area and DA axon terminals in the nucleus accumbens (29,104,105)—that abusable substances appear to act to enhance brain reward and produce the euphorigenic effects that constitute the "high" or "rush" sought by substance abusers (29–31,104,105,194; see, in section entitled "Effects of Abusable Substances on Brain-Stimulation Reward"). Furthermore, it seems likely that only a small subset of these DA neurons are specialized for carrying reward-relevant information (105). Although apparently preferentially activated by abusable substances, these DA substrates also appear capable of direct activation by electrical brain-stimulation reward under proper conditions of electrical stimulation (204).

Efforts have been directed toward determining (a) the neuroanatomic site(s) of origin of the non-DA rostrocaudally conducting "first-stage" reward neurons within the medial forebrain bundle, and (b) whether a single, anatomically defined set of "third-stage" reward neurons carries the pleasure/reward neural signal even further (i.e., beyond the mesolimbic DA terminal loci that the "second-stage" DA caudorostrally-conducting medial forebrain bundle reward neurons project to), and, if so, to which neuroanatomic site(s).

With respect to the first question, it has been clear for almost two decades (on the basis of electrophysiologic studies employing anodal block [205]) that the majority of "first-stage" non-DA medial forebrain bundle reward neurons conduct their pleasure/reward neural signals caudally along axons projecting from the area of the lateral hypothalamus to the ventral tegmental area. This has led to the hypothesis that a majority of "first-stage" reward neurons arise rostral to the lateral hypothalamus and send their descending neuronal projections to the ventral tegmental area (205). To test this hypothesis, several research groups studied the role of descending medial forebrain bundle neurons in electrical brain stimulation reward by damaging their various nuclei of origin. Lesions of a number of the descending inputs to the medial forebrain bundle have been found to not degrade the reward efficacy of medial forebrain bundle electrical brain-stimulation reward. Thus lesions of the amygdala (206), dorsomedial hypothalamus (207), frontal cortex (208,209), medial preoptic area (210), medial septal area (210), or vertical limb of the diagonal band of Broca (210) produce no permanent or substantial effect on frequency or current thresholds for electrical brain stimulation reward in the medial forebrain bundle at the level of the lateral hypothalamus. Such lesion data can be reconciled with the hypothesis that "first-stage" non-DA reward neurons descend in the medial forebrain bundle if it is assumed that such "first-stage" neurons arise in one or several anterior medial forebrain bundle nuclei spared by such lesions—in particular, the rostral bed nuclei of the medial forebrain bundle, including the anterior lateral hypothalamus, horizontal limb of the diagonal band of Broca, interstitial nucleus of the stria medullaris, lateral preoptic area, magnocellular preoptic nucleus, olfactory tubercle, substantia innominata, and ventral pallidum (211–214). Shizgal and his colleagues, using electrophysiologic and behavioral methods for inferring anatomic linkage between rewarding brain-stimulation sites (201) and using lesion studies, reported that psychophysical collision effects are obtained for electrical brain-stimulation reward sites in the anterior lateral hypothalamus and the ventral tegmental area (213) and that sufficiently large lesions of the anterolateral medial forebrain bundle produce substantial and/or permanent elevations in brain reward thresholds at posterior medial forebrain bundle sites (212). This strongly suggests that descending "first-stage" reward neurons directly link the anterolateral medial forebrain bundle and the ventral tegmental area and that these axons may constitute a fairly heterogeneous population arising in a number of separate anterior bed nuclei of the medial forebrain bundle. Further, descending medial forebrain bundle axons arising from several of these anterior bed nuclei possess neural excitability properties closely matching behaviorally derived estimates for the "first-stage" reward neurons of the medial forebrain bundle (214). Thus the best current judgment is that the non-DA rostrocaudally conducting "first-stage" medial forebrain-bundle reward neurons originate diffusely within the anterior bed nuclei of the medial forebrain bundle (anterior lateral hypothalamus; horizontal limb of the diagonal band of Broca; interstitial nucleus of the stria medullaris; lateral preoptic area; magnocellular preoptic nucleus; olfactory tubercle; substantia innominata; and ventral pallidum), presumably constituting an anatomic convergence of disparate neurally encoded information critical to the set point of hedonic tone. On the other hand, and stressing what they believe to be the extremely disparate neuroanatomic nature of this reward system, Gallistel and colleagues (215) argued that the "first-stage" reward neurons are extensively collateralized bipolar neurons with both their cell bodies and the majority, if not all, of their terminals located in the midbrain. They base this argument on the facts that (a) as noted earlier, forebrain lesions and knife cuts that transect most major medial forebrain bundle projection systems are remarkably ineffective in reducing the rewarding efficacy of medial forebrain bundle electrical brain-stimulation reward (210); (b) nearly complete destruction of the medial forebrain bundle rostral to the brain-stimulation site by as little as less than 1.0 mm often fails to alter both the efficacy of electrical brain-stimulation reward and the number of neurons in the population of reward-relevant fibers at the site of stimulation (the latter ascertained by quantitative psychophysical methods), while destruction caudal to the site of stimulation often significantly attenuates reward efficacy and substantially reduces the population of fibers carrying the reward signal (215); and (c) anodal electrical brain-stimulation reward to the ventral tegmental area blocks cathodal electrical brain-stimulation reward to the lateral hypothalamus, but not vice versa (205). This rather extreme view of the location, morphology, and distribution of the "first-stage" reward neurons implies that these neurons are distributed over so broad a midbrain region as to extend well beyond the conventionally defined borders of the medial forebrain bundle.

With respect to the second question, it is now clear that a "third-stage" reward pathway does exist, carrying the pleasure/reward neural signal beyond the nucleus accumbens, i.e., beyond the mesolimbic DA terminal loci to which the "second-stage" DA caudorostrally conducting medial forebrain bundle reward neurons project. Furthermore, it is clear that this "third-stage" pathway uses the endogenous opioid peptide enkephalin as its primary neurotransmitter and projects anatomically to the ventral pallidum. Anatomic mapping and tracing studies show clearly that a major efferent pathway for nucleus accumbens output signals projects to the ventral pallidum, and that this pathway is enkephalinergic (216–219). Electrophysiologic studies (220) show that a large majority of nucleus accumbens output neurons are opiate-sensitive and naloxone-blockable, tending to confirm that this is the major efferent pathway of the accumbens and tending to confirm its opioid peptidergic nature. This nucleus accumbens output pathway is known to be critical for expression of reward-related and incentive-related behaviors (as is the next-following transsynaptic pathway from the ventral pallidum to the pedunculopontine tegmental nucleus [221]). Manipulations of this nucleus accumbens–ventral pallidum pathway have clear effects on brain-stimulation reward and reward-driven behaviors. For example, lesions of this pathway significantly reduce both cocaine and opiate intravenous self-administration (222,223). Such lesions also significantly attenuate acquisition of a drug-conditioned cue (place) preference (219). Very importantly, endogenous opioid release is selectively seen in the ventral pallidum as a consequence of rewarding electrical brain stimulation in other parts of the reward axis (e.g., ventral tegmental area [224]). Equally importantly, opioid microinjections into the ventral pallidum alter electrical brain-stimulation reward in an anatomically site-specific manner (225,226). Provocatively, there are mutually reciprocal anatomic interconnections between the ventral pallidum, nucleus accumbens, and ventral tegmental area (227), which appear functionally relevant to the set-point of DA reward functions within the reward circuitry (228). Another nucleus accumbens output pathway—the medium spiny output neurons which use γ-aminobutyric acid (GABA) as a neurotransmitter—has been postulated on extremely good neuroanatomic, neurochemical, and neuropharmacologic grounds to constitute another brain-reward, final, common, output path (229–231). In fact, Carlezon and Wise (231) have a very plausible model of drug-induced reward in which the critical event is inhibition of the GABAergic medium spiny output neurons in nucleus accumbens. However, because GABA appears to be co-localized with the opioid neuropeptide enkephalin in at least a portion of the medium spiny projection pathway from nucleus accumbens to pallidum and from nucleus accumbens to ventral tegmental area (218,232–238) (as well as apparently being co-localized with the opioid neuropeptide dynorphin and the nonopioid neuropeptide Substance P in a major portion of the medium spiny projection pathway from nucleus accumbens to ventral tegmental area [232,233,235,236]), this suggestion may well be fully congruent with the earlier-noted hypothesis that the "third-stage" reward neurons are coextensive with at least a portion of the

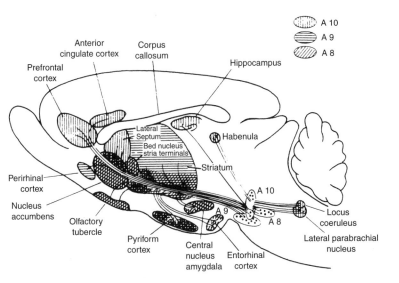

FIG. 5.1. The mesotelencephalic dopamine (DA) circuitry of the mammalian (laboratory rat) brain. The primary brain-reward-relevant portion appears to be a subset of the mesolimbic projections originating in the ventral tegmental area (DA nucleus "A10") and terminating in the nucleus accumbens. From Cooper JR, Bloom FE, Roth RH. *The biochemical basis of neuropharmacology*, 5th ed. New York: Oxford University Press, 1986:266, with permission.

enkephalinergic pathway from nucleus accumbens to ventral pallidum.

A number of additional circuits synapse onto the "first-stage," "second-stage," or "third-stage" elements of this brain-reward system, to apparently regulate and modulate the overall set-point of hedonic tone. The neurotransmitters of some of these additional circuits are known—including opioid peptides, serotonin, glutamate, and GABA (see later discussion in section entitled "DA Reward Synapse and Modulatory Mechanisms acting on the DA Reward System").

Figure 5.1 illustrates some of the DA circuitry of the forebrain involved in these reward mechanisms.

Effects of Abusable Substances on Brain-Stimulation Reward

For studying the effects of abusable substances on these brain-reward mechanisms in the laboratory, a number of paradigms of electrical brain-stimulation reward have been used (see references 105 and 239 for reviews and discussions). Unfortunately, most early studies (1950s, 1960s, and early 1970s) used simple response-rate measures for brain-stimulation of fixed voltage or current and fixed stimulation frequency. Such response-rate studies were inadequate on many grounds, not the least being that some abusable substances are strong sedative–hypnotics and others are strong psychomotor stimulants. Such compounds may spuriously produce depressed or enhanced responding for brain-reward in a simple response-rate paradigm simply as a result of nonspecific motor effects. Consequently, much of the early literature dealing with the effects of abusable substances on brain reward is either difficult to interpret or, worse, leads to incorrect conclusions. For these reasons, attention has shifted to threshold measures, response-pattern analyses, choice measures, "curve-shift" rate-frequency function measures analogous

to the dose–response paradigm of traditional pharmacology, and a host of other conceptually similar, but operationally very distinct, brain-stimulation reward paradigms (see references 105 and 239 for excellent discussions and comparisons amongst these paradigms). The author's laboratory has used a number of variants of the decremental titrating-threshold brain-reward paradigm, commonly known in the brain-reward literature as the "autotitration" paradigm, which was developed by Stein and Ray (240). In one of the autotitration variants used (110,111,113,241–244), the animal presses a "reward" lever to self-administer a brief (300 msec) train of rewarding brain stimulation, which automatically decreases in intensity with each successive lever-press. When this decremental stimulation passes through the threshold for activating the underlying neural substrate of reward, the animal presses a "reset" lever, which does not deliver any brain reward, but resets the brain-reward intensity back to its initial level. By analyzing "reset" values, measure of the activation threshold (in microamperes of delivered current) of the neural system subserving brain reward is obtained, which is independent of response rate and thus independent of the incidental sedation or psychomotor stimulation produced by many abusable drugs. In another autotitration variant (245,246), the "reset" of brain-reward intensity back to initial level is not controlled by a second lever, but rather by a time-delay circuit, which triggers only when the animal stops responding on the "reward" lever for a preset length of time (e.g., 5 seconds). Because animals will respond for even marginally rewarding brain stimulation rather than none at all, this paradigm tends to give a more accurate measure of true threshold rather than threshold of a preferred range. Using these paradigms, the author has studied the effects on brain-stimulation reward of a wide range of abusable substances, including cocaine, amphetamines, opiates, barbiturates, ketamine, phencyclidine, benzodiazepines, alcohol, nicotine, and marihuana (110,111,113,242–244). In every case, robust enhancement of brain-stimulation reward is seen. Similar robust enhancement of brain-stimulation reward by representative compounds from virtually every class of abusable substance has also been reported from other laboratories (for reviews see references 29–31, 103, 194, and 239; see also references 110, 193, and 247–263).

Arguing persuasively for the view that all abusable substances act by facilitating a common brain-reward substrate is the finding that abusable substances of different pharmacologic classes (e.g., opiates and stimulants) have a synergistic effect on brain-stimulation reward thresholds when coadministered (249,260).

Arguing persuasively for the view that facilitation of brain-reward mechanisms is closely related to abuse potential are findings with the class of compounds known variously as opiate partial agonists or mixed agonist–antagonists. This class, synthesized in large measure as part of a deliberate effort to develop effective narcotic analgesics with little or no abuse potential, contains some compounds that appear to possess no abuse potential and others that do possess abuse potential (264). Amongst this class, the brain-stimulation reward paradigm discriminates nicely between those compounds having abuse potential and those devoid of it. For example, the abusable substance pentazocine lowers brain-reward thresholds whereas other mixed agonist–antagonists lacking abuse potential (e.g., cyclazocine, nalorphine) do not (257).

An intriguing finding is that brain-stimulation reward undergoes an age-related decline (253,254), which is reversed by a single dose of d-amphetamine (253). It is tempting to conclude that this age-related decline in central reinforcement mechanisms may correlate with age-related decline in central DA function (265), which is temporarily restored by acute amphetamine.

A striking finding of many different laboratories is that DA antagonists, such as neuroleptics, inhibit electrical brain-stimulation reward of the medial forebrain bundle and associated DA loci (i.e., raise brain-reward thresholds) in a manner that appears diametrically opposite to the enhancement of brain-stimulation reward (lowering of brain-reward thresholds) produced by substances of abuse. This is a very robust and replicable finding, first reported 40 years ago by Stein and his colleagues (240,248) and replicated many times since in a number of different laboratories (266–268; see also reference 198 for a review of related studies and a theoretical formulation of the role of DA antagonism in anhedonia). Such findings, coupled with the findings that animals volitionally terminate infusions of DA antagonists, and taken in the overall context of the findings already described that DA agonists are volitionally self-administered and enhance electrical brain-stimulation reward, are important elements in the theory that electrical brain-stimulation reward activates the same DA brain-reward substrates activated by drug self-administration, and that these substrates include the mesolimbic DA reward systems of the medial forebrain bundle.

For some abusable substances, the dose range within which electrical brain-stimulation reward enhancement is seen is relatively narrow. Phencyclidine and ketamine, for example, produce brain-reward enhancement within a comparatively narrow range of low doses, but inhibit brain reward, in neuroleptic-like fashion, at higher doses (243). The author has suggested that this low-dose brain-reward-enhancement, high-dose brain-reward-inhibition phenomenon in laboratory animals is homologous with the "low-dose good-trip," "high-dose bad-trip" phenomenon reported by street users of these drugs.

Provocatively, the author (110,111,242,243,250,269) and others (259,270,271; see also references 29 and 104) have found that the brain-reward enhancement produced by abusable substances (including compounds in such different classes as opiates, amphetamines, cocaine, ethanol, barbiturates, benzodiazepines, phencyclidine, and ketamine) is in every case significantly attenuated by the opiate antagonists naloxone or naltrexone. Interestingly, naloxone not only attenuates the low-dose enhancement of brain-stimulation reward produced by ketamine and phencyclidine, but also attenuates the high-dose inhibition of brain reward produced by these same drugs. Equally provocatively, naloxone is reported to augment neuroleptic-induced inhibition of brain-stimulation reward (268). In view of the naloxone-induced attenuation of the brain-stimulation reward enhancement produced by all known classes of abusable substances, it would appear that there exists an important anatomic and functional interrelationship between the crucial drug-sensitive "second-stage" DA fibers of the reward system (29–31,105,194) and endogenous opioid peptide circuitry, and furthermore, that this interrelationship is important for the brain-reward enhancement produced by all substances of abuse, not just opiates, and hence for their abuse liability. Anatomically, there are many brain loci where such a functional interaction between reward-relevant DA neurons and endogenous opioid peptide neurons could take place. Cell bodies, axons, and synaptic terminals of endogenous opioid peptidergic neurons are found in veritable profusion throughout the extent of the reward-relevant mesotelencephalic DA circuitry (272,273). The author (274) and others (275,276) have shown that endogenous opioid peptide neurons synapse directly onto mesotelencephalic DA axon terminals, forming precisely the type of axoaxonic synapses one would expect of a system designed to modulate the flow of reward-relevant neural signals through the DA circuitry. In addition to the DA axon terminal regions (e.g., nucleus accumbens), other possible sites of DA-opioid peptide functional interaction include the DA cell body region of the ventral tegmental area (197) and transsynaptic modulation via afferents to the ventral mesencephalon from the region of the locus coeruleus (29), although there does not appear to be direct synaptic interaction between coerulear noradrenergic efferent projections and either the "first-stage" or "second-stage" reward neurons in the ventral tegmental area. As noted above, there are excellent reasons for believing that opioid peptidergic (enkephalinergic) "third-stage" reward neurons project from the nucleus accumbens to the ventral pallidum (216–226), thus carrying the neural reward signal one synapse further. Additional evidence for believing that this is so includes the facts that (a) the author has shown (242) that naloxone significantly attenuates the enhanced brain-stimulation reward induced by chronic pharmacologic upregulation of DA receptors in the mesolimbic DA system, suggesting that a crucial naloxone-blockable endogenous opioid peptide link lies efferent to the upregulated DA receptors; and (b) the author has also shown (277) that naloxone significantly modulates behavioral responses induced by direct postsynaptic DA-receptor agonists in animals in whom the presynaptic DA fiber system has been destroyed by selective lesions of the DA mesotelencephalic system, again implicating a crucial naloxone-sensitive endogenous opioid peptide link efferent to the ascending DA mesotelencephalic DA system. Although some workers believe that the synaptic interaction in the nucleus accumbens between the "second-stage" DA reward neurons and the "third-stage" enkephalinergic neurons is an indirect one (i.e., mediated through interneurons), there is reason to believe that at least a portion of the "second-stage" DA reward neurons may synapse directly onto the "third-stage" endogenous opioid peptide neurons. Pickel et al. have demonstrated, using double-label electron microscopy, that a portion of the ascending mesotelencephalic DA fibers synapse directly onto endogenous opioid peptide neurons (278). A similar suggestion, again on the basis of ultrastructural evidence, had previously been made by Kubota et al. (279).

It seems, therefore, on the basis of the best presently available data, that likely sites for the interaction of abusable substances with endogenous brain opioid mechanisms that functionally modulate the intensity of reward signals carried through the DA reward system are the ventral tegmental area, the nucleus accumbens, and the ventral pallidum.

CRITICAL NEUROANATOMY OF DRUG REWARD: INTRACRANIAL MICROINJECTION OF ABUSABLE SUBSTANCES

Although it is possible to infer anatomic sites of drug reward from studies such as those just described, there are other more direct ways of studying the neuroanatomy of drug-induced reward. Two such ways involve direct intracranial microinjections of abusable substances, in the first case coupled with the electrical brain-stimulation reward paradigm, and in the second case coupled with self-administration methodologies.

Effects of Intracranial Microinjections of Abusable Substances on Electrical Brain-Stimulation Reward

When making intracranial microinjections of chemical substances to infer localized sites of action within the brain, a number of potentially serious methodological considerations arise, including the dangers of misinterpretation of data because of diffusion of the injected substance, local anesthesia within the injection site, and nonspecific irritation within the injection site. Also, local pressure effects and high local concentrations of the injected substance can be problematic. For a review of these and other important methodological considerations that apply to paradigms using direct intracranial microinjections, the interested reader is directed to reviews by Routtenberg (280), Bozarth (281), and Broekkamp (282). With due regard for these methodological considerations, direct intracranial microinjections of abusable substances can be combined with electrical intracranial self-stimulation methods to infer the local site(s) of rewarding effects. Using these techniques, Broekkamp and colleagues found that the focal area for morphine's enhancing effects on electrical brain-stimulation reward lies within the ventral tegmental area and caudal hypothalamus (283,284), with microinjections into the ventral tegmental area producing more immediate enhancement than microinjections into the caudal hypothalamus (285). In these studies, the latency time for enhancement of brain-stimulation reward was highly correlated with distance from the DA cells of the ventral mesencephalic DA nuclei that give rise to the mesotelencephalic DA fibers of the medial forebrain bundle (r = 0.83, p < 0.0001) (282,285). These data are compelling, given the evidence already reviewed from other experimental paradigms and approaches for a focal role of the "second-stage" DA neurons of the mesotelencephalic DA system in mediating drug-induced reward. Using similar methods, Broekkamp and colleagues found that the focal area for amphetamine's enhancing effects on electrical brain-stimulation reward lies within the nucleus accumbens and neostriatal forebrain DA terminal projection loci of the "second-stage" mesotelencephalic DA reward-relevant systems (286). Microinjections of DA antagonists into these same DA terminal projection loci inhibit brain-stimulation reward (284,287), with the DA axon terminals in the nucleus accumbens playing the most crucial role in hedonic set-point as measured by electrical brain-stimulation reward (287). Wise and colleagues (288,289) and Fibiger and colleagues (290) confirmed that the ventral tegmental area is the crucial anatomic site for augmentation of electrical brain-stimulation reward by opiates (288,290), while the nucleus accumbens is the crucial anatomic site for augmentation of electrical brain-stimulation reward by amphetamine (289). Opiate-induced augmentation of electrical brain stimulation in the ventral tegmental area appears to be mediated by μ and δ opioid receptors, but not by κ receptors (288).

Intracranial Self-Administration of Abusable Substances

A direct way to study the neuroanatomy of drug-induced reward is to meld intracranial microinjection technology with the self-administration paradigm, so that animals are allowed to work for direct intracranial self-administration of abusable substances into discrete brain loci. Although conceptually simple, this is actually a very difficult laboratory paradigm (for reviews see references 280, 281, and 291–293). As noted by Olds (20), early work with intracranial self-administration was almost universally methodologically flawed. Even with sophisticated microinjection technologies (294), many conceptual and interpretational problems remain. For example, it is difficult with microinjection procedures (which must perforce be kept to sufficiently small volumes and forces as to preclude nonspecific neuronal effects) to duplicate the close time-link between behavioral response and reinforcement that occurs with natural rewards, and virtually impossible to duplicate the immediacy of electrical brain-stimulation reward. Because a reinforcement delay of only a few seconds is often enough to disrupt operant behavior (295,296), this is a serious concern. Similarly, issues of drug diffusion, anatomic specificity, pharmacologic specificity, and the multiple and distinct physiologic systems activated by most drugs pose major methodological and conceptual problems. Also, as noted by Bozarth in his many insightful reviews of intracranial self-administration (281,291), the fact that a given brain site does not support self-administration does not eliminate that site as a reward locus, because competing behaviors (e.g., sedation) produced by the drug injection may mask the reward behavior. Additionally, and again as noted by Bozarth (281), successful intracranial self-administration only identifies a site as being involved in the initiation of drug reward, not necessarily in the complex and multistepped neurophysiologic components of the overall subjective experience of drug-induced reward or pleasure. In spite of the many methodological and interpretational problems that accrue to it, the paradigm's seeming face validity has made it appealing to researchers studying the neurobiology and neuroanatomy of drug-induced reward, and a number of laboratories have succeeded in overcoming most of the paradigm's problems and generating provocative and compelling data.

Thus, animals will voluntarily self-administer microinjections of amphetamine into the nucleus accumbens and prefrontal cortex (297–299), both of which are mesolimbic DA terminal projection loci, but not into other brain sites. Similarly, cocaine is voluntarily self-administered into the prefrontal cortex (300). Morphine is self-administered into the ventral tegmental area (301,302), lateral hypothalamus (303,304), and nucleus accumbens (305), all of which are either nuclei or terminal projection loci of the mesolimbic DA system (171), but not into other brain sites. Other opioids, both synthetic and endogenous, are also self-administered intracranially. Fentanyl is self-administered into the ventral tegmental area (306), met-enkephalin is self-administered into the nucleus accumbens (307), and the met-enkephalin analogue d-ala^2-met-enkephalinamide is self-administered into the lateral hypothalamus (308). A related and conceptual derivative of these kinds of studies is the finding by Britt and Wise that microinjections of a hydrophilic opioid antagonist with limited diffusion characteristics (diallyl-normorphinium bromide) into the ventral tegmental area blocks intravenous opiate self-administration (309). Ethanol is self-administered into the ventral tegmental area, but—provocatively—only by animals with a genetic predisposition to high oral ethanol self-administration and not by animals with a genetic predisposition to ethanol abstinence (310). Phencyclidine is self-administered into the nucleus accumbens, and within that structure, preferentially self-administered into the "shell" subportion of nucleus accumbens as compared to the "core" subportion (231) (see later discussion of the apparent specialization of the "shell" subportion of nucleus accumbens for brain, in sections entitled "In Vivo Brain Microdialysis Studies" and "DA Reward Synapse and Modulatory Mechanisms Acting on the DA Reward system"). Interestingly, the phencyclidine (PCP)-related drugs MK-801 (dizocilpine) and CPP [3-(($\pm$)2-carboxypiperazinyl)propyl-1-phosphate], which share PCP's actions on excitatory amino acid receptor (N-methyl-D-aspartate [NMDA]) functions but not its direct DA reuptake blocking actions, are also self-administered preferentially into the accumbens "shell," suggesting that at least some of the rewarding effects of PCP-like dissociative anesthetics may be mediated through NMDA receptors on reward neurons or reward-modulating neurons (231).

An important theme in such intracranial microinjection studies, already alluded to, is the ability of such approaches to yield data showing which brain loci are responsible for the initiation of each separate and individual pharmacologic action of any given abusable substance. So, for example, the analgesic effect of opiates is mediated by local action on opioid peptidergic circuits within the periaqueductal and periventricular gray matter of the brainstem (311,312), the thermoregulatory effect by action in the preoptic area (313), while the rewarding effects appear mediated by action on the nuclei, tracts, and terminal projection loci of the mesolimbic DA system. Very importantly, physical dependence upon opiates has been shown by microinjection studies to be mediated by action on brainstem loci anatomically distinct and far removed from the mesolimbic DA loci mediating opiate-induced reward (314), and repeated morphine injections into the mesolimbic DA loci critical for drug reward utterly fail to produce physiologic dependence (314).

Despite the difficulties that the intracranial self-administration paradigm poses, completed studies add persuasively to the hypothesis that the "second-stage" DA neurons of the mesotelencephalic DA system play a focal and essential role in mediating drug-induced reward.

CRITICAL NEUROCHEMISTRY OF DRUG REWARD: *IN VIVO* BRAIN CHEMISTRY MEASUREMENTS DURING ADMINISTRATION OF ABUSABLE SUBSTANCES

If the ascending mesotelencephalic DA systems play the crucial role in drug-induced brain-reward that researchers in the field currently ascribe to them, one would expect abusable substances to act, at least indirectly or transsynaptically, in a DA-agonist-like fashion in these systems. For many years, this crucial derivative of the theory was untestable. However, two techniques were developed that allow for *in vivo* real-time measurements of neurotransmitter release in discrete brain loci of living (indeed, in many cases, conscious, freely moving) animals. These techniques are *in vivo* brain microdialysis and *in vivo* brain voltametric electrochemistry (315,316). Both of these paradigms have proven themselves to be valid and sensitive ways of measuring real-time neurotransmitter release in extremely discrete loci of the living brain, and both of these paradigms have now been applied to the question of which neurotransmitter substrates are activated by administration of abusable substances. Additionally, classical *in vivo* single-neuron electrophysiologic recording techniques have also been applied to the same question. There is also an extensive literature on the use of push–pull cannula perfusion (317) for studying the effects of abusable substances on *in vivo* neurotransmitter release in forebrain reward-relevant loci (318,319), but this literature is not separately reviewed here, because the push–pull cannula perfusion technique is conceptually, and even methodologically, analogous to *in vivo* brain microdialysis and the effects of abusable substances on DA in forebrain reward loci as determined by *in vivo* push–pull perfusion are essentially identical to those determined by *in vivo* brain microdialysis.

Paradigms of *In Vivo* Brain Microdialysis and *In Vivo* Brain Voltammetric Electrochemistry

Although *in vivo* brain microdialysis (320–323) is conceptually similar to the much older push–pull cannula paradigm (317), it is technologically superior. For *in vivo* microdialysis studies, a microdialysis probe (324) is fabricated from miniature stainless steel and dialysis tubing

and surgically implanted, by standard stereotaxic technique, into the desired brain locus. A pump is used to drive buffered Ringer solution (similar in ionic constituents and concentrations to the extracellular fluid of the brain) through the probe at a slow rate. At the tip of the probe, located in the brain site to be measured, extracellular neurotransmitters and metabolite molecules dialyze across the membrane and are carried out of the probe in the buffered Ringer solution to an analytical biochemistry apparatus. Typically, the analytic biochemistry apparatus is a high-performance liquid chromatograph with electrochemical detection, although other analytic devices can also be used. If high-performance liquid chromatography with electrochemical detection is used, the neurotransmitters and metabolites in the dialysate are first separated by reverse-phase column chromatography and the eluting species are then measured with an electrochemical detector. The *in vivo* sensitivity of this paradigm is excellent, allowing detection of basal DA release in even diffusely innervated DA terminal projection loci (e.g., prefrontal cortex). The selectivity of the paradigm is also excellent, because of the excellent separation of chemical species afforded by the chromatography columns. Time resolution is typically on the order of one measurement every 5 or 10 minutes, although much shorter sampling times (1 minute or less) are possible with microbore chromatography techniques (322).

In vivo brain voltammetric electrochemistry (316,317, 322,325–327) is based upon the fortuitous chemical coincidence that many neurotransmitters of interest (in the present instance, DA) and their metabolites are capable of electrooxidation. Such oxidation yields an oxidation current that can be measured using electrodes and apparatus essentially identical to that used in axon-conduction voltage-clamp measurements of traditional neurophysiology. The neurotransmitter molecules are identified by their characteristic oxidation potential, their characteristic electrochemical signatures (e.g., the shape of the voltammogram when performing fast cyclic voltammetry [322] or the characteristic oxidation-reduction ratios when performing high-speed chronoamperometry [322]), and by altering the physical–chemical nature of the electrode working surface, at which the electrochemical reactions take place, to produce electrodes with high selectivity for specific molecules (322,328). For *in vivo* voltammetric electrochemistry studies, a "working" electrode (so-called because the electrochemical reactions "work" at its surface) is fabricated, typically from carbon fibers and miniature glass tubing, and then calibrated for selectivity and sensitivity and characterized for response time. This working electrode is then surgically implanted, by standard stereotaxic technique, into the desired brain locus. At the same time, reference and auxiliary electrodes are implanted, typically at the brain surface. Electrochemical measurements are then begun, and continued for the duration of the experiment. The *in vivo* sensitivity of this paradigm is good, and the time resolution of high-speed versions (fast cyclic voltammetry, high-speed chronoamperometry) is excellent, allowing 10 to 20 independent measurements of neurotransmitter efflux per second (322).

Both *in vivo* brain microdialysis and *in vivo* brain voltammetric electrochemistry are markedly superior to older *in vitro* and *ex vivo* neurochemical paradigms, because they are real-time paradigms allowing correlations between neurochemistry and ongoing behavior, and because they eliminate the artifactual elevations in extracellular neurotransmitter concentrations seen at death with *in vitro* and *ex vivo* paradigms (329). In their most sophisticated usages, both *in vivo* brain microdialysis and *in vivo* brain voltammetric electrochemistry are carried out in awake animals to obviate artifacts introduced by anesthesia.

In Vivo Brain Microdialysis Studies

Using *in vivo* brain microdialysis, a number of laboratories have shown that cocaine produces a robust enhancement of extracellular DA in the neostriatal and nucleus accumbens terminal projection areas of the reward-relevant mesotelencephalic DA system (117,330–339). This enhancement of time-course of DA is more pronounced in the nucleus accumbens than in other forebrain DA loci (330), and is dose-dependent (339). The time-course measured in forebrain DA loci after cocaine administration closely mirror the extracellular levels of cocaine itself in the same loci (331,335,340). The DA-enhancing effect is seen whether the cocaine is exogenously administered by the experimenter or self-administered by the animal (332,333). Relative reelevation of extracellular DA evoked by cocaine, rather than absolute amount of extracellular DA evoked by cocaine, may be the critical factor correlating with cocaine self-administration, because animals self-administering cocaine who had lengthy previous repeated exposure to the drug show lower cocaine-induced enhancement of extracellular DA than animals self-administering cocaine who had no previous exposure to the drug (332,333). Thus, repeated use of cocaine over extended time periods may reduce the reward threshold, i.e., the required amount of extracellular DA necessary for reward (332), perhaps because of the development of DA receptor supersensitivity (341,342), which amplifies the reward signal. Alternatively, repeated cocaine use over extended time periods may result in decreased reward from the same amount of cocaine self-administered in the future, which would agree with some human reports, in which some cocaine users state that they continually "chase the first high" and never successfully reachieve it. In animals repeatedly given cocaine so as to evoke cocaine sensitization (343,344), enhanced DA efflux is observed in both the nucleus accumbens and neostriatum (335,338), with cross-sensitization to methamphetamine (334). The enhanced DA efflux seen with cocaine sensitization may

be in part accounted for by increased local concentrations of cocaine in relevant brain sites (335), a finding that gains special significance in view of reports that DA synthesis rate appears to decrease in cocaine sensitization (345–347). Cocaine's enhancing effects on extracellular DA in reward-relevant forebrain DA loci are blocked by tetrodotoxin, which prevents action potentials by blocking voltage-dependent Na^+ channels, indicating that cocaine's effects on forebrain DA reward neurons require the functional integrity of those neurons, which is congruent with cocaine's actions as a specific inhibitor of the reuptake of neuronally released DA from the synaptic cleft (348,349).

Combining *in vivo* microdialysis and drug self-administration, Pettit and Justice (339) showed that animals intravenously self-administering cocaine adopt a paced and measured pattern of self-infusion which, after an initial burst of responding to produce a loading dose of cocaine and quickly elevated extracellular DA levels in the nucleus accumbens, maintains extracellular DA levels in the nucleus accumbens at significantly elevated, stable levels that oscillate within a relatively constrained range. Thus, animals volitionally self-administering cocaine appear to regulate their self-infusion behavior so as to deliberately titrate a specific, set, stable level of extracellular DA in the reward-critical DA terminal projection fields of the nucleus accumbens (see later discussions for additional experiments using combined drug self-administration and *in vivo* neurochemistry or *in vivo* electrophysiology, in section entitled "In Vivo Brain Chemistry Measurements in Brain Reward Circuits During Self-Administration of Abusable Substances, as Assessed by Microdialysis, Voltammetric Electrochemistry, and Electrophysiology").

Amphetamine also produces a robust enhancement of extracellular DA in reward-relevant neostriatal and nucleus accumbens DA terminal projection areas as measured by *in vivo* microdialysis (117,123,323,330,349–357), with stronger effect in the nucleus accumbens than in other forebrain DA loci (330,350). When the amphetamine is microinjected directly into the DA reward loci, instead of administered systemically, the enhancing effect on extracellular DA is extremely strong (352,357). Neither abolition of action potentials by tetrodotoxin nor depletion of vesicular DA pools by reserpine has any significant effect on amphetamine's extracellular DA-enhancing effects in reward loci. On the other hand, inhibition of DA synthesis by αMPT or inhibition of the membrane-bound DA uptake carrier by nomifensine effectively inhibits amphetamine's effect on extracellular DA in forebrain reward loci. Thus, amphetamine acts as a presynaptic DA releaser, in contrast to cocaine's reuptake blockade mechanism, but does not release DA by action-potential-dependent exocytosis (123,353,355). Rather, amphetamine appears to preferentially release DA from the newly synthesized DA pool, probably via a DA-carrier-mediated mechanism (123,353,356). In animals given chronic amphetamine so as to produce amphetamine sensitization, a significantly increased DA efflux to amphetamine challenge is seen, but with no effect on basal DA efflux (355). 3,4-Methylenedioxymethamphetamine (MDMA), the amphetamine analogue known by the street name "ecstasy," also robustly enhances extracellular DA levels in forebrain terminal loci of the reward-relevant mesotelencephalic DA system in freely moving animals (358). This report also underscores the importance of doing these types of experiments in awake rather than anesthetized animals, as the same authors report that MDMA decreases extracellular DA levels in anesthetized animals (359).

Morphine also produces robust dose-dependent enhancement of extracellular DA in reward-relevant neostriatal and nucleus accumbens DA terminal loci as measured by *in vivo* microdialysis (123,330,360–362). This effect is duplicated by other μ opiate receptor agonists, including methadone, levorphanol, and fentanyl (115,360), and by the μ-selective opioid peptide agonist [D-Ala^2,methyl-Phe^4,Gly^5-ol]-enkephalin (DAMGO) (362,363). This effect is antagonized by low-dose naloxone and by the irreversible μ receptor antagonist β-funaltrexamine (360). DAMGO-enhanced extracellular DA in the nucleus accumbens is antagonized by the highly specific μ opioid antagonist D-Pen-Cys-Tyr-D-Trp-Orn-Thr-Pen-Thr-NH$_2$ (363), which does not itself affect basal DA levels. The δ-selective opioid peptide agonist [D-Pen^2,D-Pen^5]-enkephalin (DPDPE) also enhances extracellular DA in the nucleus accumbens when microinjected intracerebroventricularly (363), and the highly specific δ opioid antagonist N-allyl$_2$-Tyr-Aib-Aib-Phe-Leu-OH (ICI 174,864), which by itself has no effect on extracellular DA, blocks DPDPE's DA-enhancing effects (363). Provocatively, κ opiate receptor agonists (bremazocine, tifluadom, U-50,488, and the dynorphin derivative N-CH$_3$-Tyr-Gly-Gly-Phe-Leu-Arg-N-CH$_3$-Arg-D-Leu-NHC$_2$H$_5$ [E-2078]), which are *aversive* rather than appetitive to animals (364,365), have been shown to *inhibit* rather than stimulate DA efflux in forebrain reward loci (330,360). That this inhibition of DA efflux is mediated by endogenous κ opioid receptor mechanisms is buttressed by the finding that the selective κ opioid receptor antagonist norbinaltorphimine attenuates E-2078's inhibition of DA efflux in nucleus accumbens (363). The enhancing effect on DA efflux of morphine and other μ opiate receptor agonists is significantly stronger in the nucleus accumbens than in the neostriatum (330,360). The enhanced DA efflux in nucleus accumbens is also seen with direct microinjection of μ opioid agonist into the ventral tegmental area, nucleus of origin of the mesolimbic DA reward neurons projecting to nucleus accumbens (362). Studies with tetrodotoxin show that opiate-agonist-induced enhancement of DA efflux in nucleus accumbens is action-potential-dependent (123,363). Selective 5-hydroxytryptamine receptor type 3 (5-HT$_3$) antagonism, either systemically administered or microinjected directly into the ventral tegmental area, antagonizes morphine's enhancement of DA release in nucleus accumbens (361,362).

Microinjections of baclofen, an agonist of the GABA$_B$ receptor, directly into the ventral tegmental area, blocks μ opiate-agonist-induced enhancement of DA release in nucleus accumbens (366), suggesting that activation of GABA$_B$ receptors on DA perikarya inhibits DA reward functions.

It should be noted that these *in vivo* microdialysis findings of opiate-induced enhancement of extracellular DA are in line with findings of opiate-induced enhancement of DA release *in vivo* as inferred from measurements of 3-methoxytyramine in discrete brain loci (see reference 367 for a review).

It should also be noted that there is a remarkable correlation between the specific doses of μ, δ, and κ opioid agonists found to cause DA enhancement or inhibition in the nucleus accumbens (363) and the specific doses of μ, δ, and κ opioid agonists found to cause appetitive or aversive effects (364,365) in the conditioned place preference paradigm of reward (see, in section entitled "DA Reward Mechanisms and the Conditioned Place Preference (cue Preference) Animal Model of Drug Seeking").

Nicotine enhances extracellular DA levels in both nucleus accumbens and neostriatum (120,330,368), with more pronounced effects in nucleus accumbens (120,330). Muscarinic cholinergic agonists and antagonists are without effect on DA efflux in forebrain reward loci (368). Nicotine's enhancing effect on DA efflux is blocked by 5-HT$_3$ antagonists (362). Alcohol also enhances extracellular DA levels in both nucleus accumbens and neostriatum with more pronounced effects in nucleus accumbens (115,119,310,330). This effect of alcohol is dose-dependent; low and moderate doses enhance DA efflux while the highest dose produces a biphasic effect—initial inhibition of DA release followed (as the high dose begins to wear off, as assessed by independent measures) by facilitation of DA efflux (119). The mechanism of action by which alcohol enhances DA efflux is not known, but some clues to its action may be that alcohol appears to potentiate L-dopa's augmentation of brain DA (369), and that low-dose γ-butyrolactone and low-dose apomorphine each block alcohol's enhancing effects on DA efflux (119). The abusable dissociative anesthetic phencyclidine also enhances extracellular DA levels in both nucleus accumbens (370) and neostriatum (114) after either systemic administration (114) or local intracranial microinjection (369), with preferential effects in the nucleus accumbens (371). Barbiturates, including pentobarbital, phenobarbital, and barbital, enhance extracellular DA levels in both nucleus accumbens and neostriatum, with more pronounced effects in nucleus accumbens (115). This effect of barbiturates is dose-dependent; low doses enhance DA efflux, whereas high doses inhibit it (115). Δ^9-Tetrahydrocannabinol, the psychoactive constituent of marihuana and hashish, also enhances extracellular DA levels in nucleus accumbens (372), neostriatum (373,374), and medial prefrontal cortex (375)—all DA terminal fields of the reward-relevant mesotelencephalic

DA system. This effect is calcium-dependent and tetrodotoxin-sensitive (372).

As noted by DiChiara, Imperato, and coworkers (330,376), a common theme runs through all of these studies: drugs that are abused by humans and self-administered by laboratory animals act to produce enhanced extracellular DA levels in the terminal projection loci of the reward-relevant mesotelencephalic DA system, with the nucleus accumbens as a focal and extremely sensitive site of this action. Within the nucleus accumbens, drugs of abuse (cocaine, amphetamine, morphine) preferentially increase extracellular DA in the "shell" subportion of nucleus accumbens as compared to the "core" subportion (376), congruent with the suggestion that the "shell" subportion of nucleus accumbens is specialized for mediating brain reward functions (see reference 231 and later discussions to this point, in section entitled "DA Reward Synapse and Modulatory Mechanisms Acting on the DA Reward System"). Interactions have been noted between the enhanced DA produced in nucleus accumbens by abusable substances and normal biologic reward functions apparently mediated by the nucleus accumbens (377).

Given naloxone's ability to block the brain-reward–enhancing effects of a wide range of abusable substances as assessed in the already discussed electrical brain-stimulation reward paradigm, it would be interesting to know if naloxone similarly blocks the DA-enhancing effects of abusable substances as assessed with the *in vivo* brain microdialysis paradigm. This has been tested for opiates (115) and for Δ^9-tetrahydrocannabinol (372); in both cases, low doses of naloxone effectively block the enhancing effects on extracellular DA levels.

In Vivo Brain Voltammetric Electrochemistry Studies

Unfortunately, early *in vivo* brain voltammetric electrochemical techniques were flawed by an inability to distinguish between catecholamines and ascorbic acid (378–381), and between indoles and uric acid (382–384). Because ascorbate levels far exceed DA levels in forebrain DA terminal loci, and because at least some abusable substances (e.g., amphetamines) produce a profound elevation of brain ascorbate levels (380,381,385), this was a source of confounding in many early studies. Another major source of difficulty also attended early *in vivo* brain voltammetric electrochemical studies: with the combination of some early electrodes and the slow voltammetric scanning techniques used in many early studies, DA measurements were confounded by the electrocatalytic regeneration of DA in the presence of ascorbic acid (386,387). Also, many early *in vivo* brain voltammetric electrochemical techniques were unable to distinguish DA from 3,4-dihydroxyphenylacetic acid (DOPAC) (for a discussion, see reference 388). For these and other reasons, many early reports of enhanced DA release by abusable substances, assessed voltammetrically, are either erroneous or very difficult to interpret. However, *in vivo* voltammetric laboratory techniques have been improved by the development of neurotransmitter-selective recording procedures (322) involving, among other things, alterations of electrode working surfaces to impart high selectivity for specific molecules and use of molecule-specific electrochemical signatures. With these newer techniques, studies of the effects of abusable substances on extracellular DA in forebrain reward loci are less questionable.

Using these newer voltammetric techniques, cocaine has been shown to robustly augment extracellular DA in both the nucleus accumbens and neostriatum (389–391). The effect is seen both with systemic cocaine administration (389,390) and with local cocaine microinjections directly into DA terminal regions (391). The effect is seen on both electrical- and K^+-stimulated DA release (389–391), but not on basal extracellular DA levels (391). Cocaine's augmentation of the extracellular DA electrochemical signal differs qualitatively from the augmentation produced by other monoamine uptake inhibitors (390,391), suggesting that cocaine's mechanism of action may differ from that of other reuptake blockers (e.g., nomifensine). Cocaine's augmentation of extracellular DA in these studies is similar to its action in brain-slice preparations using voltammetric electrochemical recordings (392). When cocaine is given chronically, both DA reuptake and electrically stimulated (by stimulation of the medial forebrain bundle) DA release in the nucleus accumbens are robustly augmented (393). This augmentation is temporary, disappearing after 10 days of abstinence from cocaine, and may represent neuronal compensatory responses to prolonged uptake blockade of synaptic DA by cocaine (393).

Amphetamine also augments extracellular DA in forebrain reward loci as measured by *in vivo* brain voltammetric electrochemistry (394–407). This amphetamine-induced DA augmentation is seen in both mesolimbic (400,403,407) and neostriatal (394–402,405,406) reward-relevant DA terminal projection fields. A significant rostrocaudal gradient in amphetamine-induced extracellular DA augmentation is seen in the neostriatum (406), the DA increase being highest in rostral neostriatum (more than 800% of predrug levels) and lowest in the most caudal neostriatum (425% of predrug levels). A similar rostrocaudal gradient in amphetamine-evoked extracellular DA in the neostriatum is seen with *in vivo* brain microdialysis measurements (406). The amphetamine analogue MDMA ("ecstasy") also robustly enhances extracellular DA levels in forebrain terminal loci of the reward-relevant mesotelencephalic DA system in awake, freely moving animals as measured by *in vivo* brain voltammetric electrochemistry (408). This effect of MDMA is dose-dependent and is seen in both nucleus accumbens and neostriatum (408). Methylphenidate similarly enhances extracellular DA in reward-relevant mesolimbic forebrain DA loci as assessed by *in vivo* brain electrochemistry (407).

In vivo brain voltammetric electrochemistry has been used less than other approaches to study opiate effects on DA release in forebrain reward loci. The extant studies do, however, appear to reveal a pattern of enhanced DA release. Thus, acute morphine administration produces robustly enhanced extracellular DA in the nucleus accumbens (409,410) and a biphasic effect—early enhancement of extracellular DA followed by later inhibition—in the neostriatum (409–411). The biphasic pattern of enhancement and inhibition seen with voltammetric electrochemistry in the neostriatum after acute morphine is strikingly similar to the biphasic effect of morphine on reward-relevant mesostriatal DA neurons as assessed by single-neuron electrophysiologic recording studies (412) and by electrical brain-stimulation reward approaches (110). Acute morphine also produces a robust enhancement ($\approx$100% increase) of the DA metabolite homovanillic acid (HVA) in nucleus accumbens (411). When administered systemically for 2 days in a row, morphine produces increased DA release in nucleus accumbens after a single repeated administration (413), suggesting that DA turnover mechanisms may be altered early in the course of chronic opiate administration. Fentanyl produces a robust ($\approx$150%) increase in neostriatal DOPAC (414). The δ-selective opioid neuropeptide agonist [D-Ala^2,D-Pro^5]-enkephalin appears to be without effect on DA in nucleus accumbens, but inhibits DA release in the neostriatum (415). Provocatively, the κ opiate receptor agonist dynorphin-(1-13), which has the aversive properties common to κ agonists in animals rather than the appetitive properties seen with μ or δ agonists (364,365), produces a profound and long-lasting *inhibition* rather than stimulation of DA efflux in the neostriatum as determined with *in vivo* voltammetric electrochemistry (416).

In awake, freely moving animals, caffeine and theophylline enhance extracellular DA levels in neostriatum as assessed by *in vivo* voltammetric electrochemistry (417). These effects are dose-dependent; low doses enhance DA efflux whereas high doses inhibit it (417). Noteworthily, the DA-enhancing effects of caffeine and theophylline are seen only in awake, unanesthetized animals;—in anesthetized animals, all doses inhibit DA efflux (417), stressing once again the importance of doing these types of *in vivo* experiments in awake, unanesthetized animals, because the high doses of anesthetics needed to produce immobilizing anesthesia are known to inhibit forebrain DA release signals as measured by *in vivo* voltammetric electrochemistry (418) (see also the earlier mention of this point with respect to *in vivo* brain microdialysis). Alcohol produces a robust enhancement of extracellular DA in reward-relevant forebrain DA loci as measured by *in vivo* voltammetric electrochemistry (419,420). The effect is seen in both the nucleus accumbens and neostriatum (419,420), and is seen in both anesthetized (419) and freely moving, unanesthetized (420) animals. Both DA release and DA metabolism are enhanced (419), and these

effects are significantly antagonized by pretreatment with the calcium channel blocker nifedipine (419). Provocatively, the same dose of nifedipine that blocks alcohol-induced enhancement of DA metabolism and release in forebrain reward loci also blocks animal preference for alcohol, as determined by relative intake of alcohol versus water in a free-choice situation (419), suggesting that alcohol's rewarding properties may involve calcium-channel mechanisms modulating DA release in forebrain reward loci. The abusable dissociative anesthetic phencyclidine also enhances extracellular DA levels in neostriatum after local intracranial microinjection, as measured by *in vivo* voltammetric electrochemistry (421). The phencyclidine analogue MK-801 markedly enhances DA metabolism in the nucleus accumbens at intraperitoneal doses as low as 0.1 mg/kg, as measured by *in vivo* voltammetric electrochemistry (422). Studies of benzodiazepine action on DA function in reward-relevant brain loci using *in vivo* voltammetric electrochemistry have been interpreted as indicating that benzodiazepines inhibit DA function. Thus, 10 mg/kg diazepam significantly reduces DOPAC levels in striatum (423) and 10 mg/kg flurazepam significantly reduces the normal nocturnal rise in both HVA levels and the DOPAC/DA ratio in nucleus accumbens (424,425). However, several points regarding these studies must be made. First, the doses of benzodiazepines administered were massive, and because it is well established that, for some drugs of abuse, low doses enhance DA efflux in reward-relevant DA brain loci whereas high doses inhibit it (see earlier discussion of this point), the benzodiazepine doses may simply have been out of the DA-enhancing range. Second, many of these studies (423–425) measured DA efflux inferentially (on the basis of DOPAC and HVA levels) rather than directly, and it is well established on the basis of *in vivo* brain microdialysis studies that some drugs of abuse increase extracellular DA while *simultaneously* decreasing DOPAC and HVA. Third, the pattern of benzodiazepine-induced changes in DOPAC and HVA reported in these studies is strikingly amphetamine-like. Fourth, low-dose benzodiazepines augment food consumption and induce spontaneous eating in many species (426–436), behaviors known to correlate with DA efflux in reward-relevant forebrain DA loci (117) and to even be mediated by the same neural fibers mediating electrical brain-stimulation reward (437,438). In addition, this low-dose benzodiazepine-induced feeding is blocked by naloxone (431,434) and appears identical to the augmented feeding induced by low-dose barbiturates (427,433). For all these reasons, it does not appear to this reviewer that claims based on *in vivo* voltammetric electrochemistry that benzodiazepines inhibit DA function in brain-reward loci can at this point be considered definitive. Δ^9-Tetrahydrocannabinol, the psychoactive constituent of marihuana and hashish, enhances extracellular DA levels in reward-relevant forebrain DA loci as measured by *in vivo* voltammetric electrochemistry (374).

Thus, the same common theme can be seen in these *in vivo* voltammetric electrochemistry studies as previously noted in the *in vivo* brain microdialysis studies—substances that are abused by humans and self-administered by laboratory animals act to produce enhanced extracellular DA levels in the terminal projection loci of the reward-relevant mesotelencephalic DA system, with the nucleus accumbens as a focal and extremely sensitive site of this action.

In Vivo Electrophysiologic Studies

Clearly, one of the ways in which abusable substances can enhance extracellular DA release in reward-relevant brain loci is to increase the firing rate of reward-relevant DA neural fibers of the mesotelencephalic DA system. Thus, classical *in vivo* single-neuron electrophysiologic recording techniques can also be applied to the question of activation of reward-relevant DA neural systems in the brain by abusable substances. There is, in fact, a large literature on this topic, and the present review must therefore be selective.

Equally clearly, enhancement of presynaptic DA neuronal firing in reward-relevant DA circuits would not be an appropriate mechanism of action for abusable substances acting directly on presynaptic DA release and/or reuptake (e.g., cocaine, amphetamines). In fact, because of compensatory neural feedback, autoreceptor-mediated, and/or enzymatic regulatory mechanisms, many such substances would be expected to inhibit presynaptic DA neural firing while enhancing overall synaptic function in reward-relevant DA synapses. Thus, single-neuron microelectrode recording studies show that cocaine inhibits presynaptic DA neural firing (439) while enhancing extracellular DA in reward-relevant DA forebrain synapses (117,330–339,389–393) and enhancing the normal postsynaptic electrical effects of DA synaptic functioning in reward loci (440). Similarly, the acute inhibitory effect of amphetamine on the firing rate of mesotelencephalic DA neurons is well documented (441–444), but the overall net effect of amphetamine is one of enhanced DA synaptic action in reward-relevant DA synapses (117,123,323,330,349–357,394–407). Interestingly, dose–response analyses of the electrophysiologic effects of amphetamine on the activity of dopaminoceptive cells (i.e., neurons efferent to the ascending DA reward neurons) in forebrain reward loci reveal qualitative as well as quantitative changes in response to amphetamine (445–446). At low doses (less than 2.5 mg/kg), amphetamine dose-dependently increases synaptic DA levels and dose-dependently enhances the normal postsynaptic electrical effects of the dopaminoceptive cells, while dose-dependently inhibiting the firing rate of the presynaptic DA neurons. At high doses (greater than 2.5 mg/kg), however, a qualitative change occurs such that the dopaminoceptive cells become profoundly activated

in the absence of further changes in synaptic DA levels (319,445,446).

Opiate-induced enhancement of the firing of reward-relevant mesotelencephalic DA neurons is well established (116,118,121,122,412,447–452). Mesolimbic DA neurons originating in the ventral tegmental area and projecting to nucleus accumbens are preferentially sensitive to this opiate-induced activation (448). Opiate action on the firing rate of reward-relevant mesotelencephalic DA neurons is heterogeneous; some DA neurons are activated by opiates, whereas others are inhibited (412,450,451). This dual action, with some DA reward neurons activated and some inhibited by opiates, may well constitute the neural substrate for the observation that electrical brain-stimulation reward is enhanced by opiates in some brain-reward loci, but inhibited in others (110), and also for the observation that extracellular DA is enhanced by opiates in some reward-relevant forebrain DA terminal loci, but inhibited in others (409–411). While the action of μ opiate receptor agonists on the firing rate of mesotelencephalic DA neurons in reward-relevant brain loci is primarily an activating one, κ opiate receptor agonists (which have aversive rather than appetitive properties in animals [364,365]) inhibit the firing rates of these same neurons (452). The neural mechanisms by which opiates activate the firing rates of DA neurons in reward-relevant loci appear relatively straight forward. Although direct excitatory action mediated via either axoaxonic receptors or axosomatodendritic receptors cannot be ruled out, in view of the presence of endogenous opioid peptide receptors on the axon terminals of mesotelencephalic DA neurons (274–276), and direct excitatory effects of opiates on nerve membranes (453,454) the basic underlying mechanism appears to be disinhibition. Opiates acting via the μ receptor produce inhibitory effects on nerve membranes (455–457). Therefore, μ opiate receptor activation on the tonically inhibitory GABAergic neurons that synapse on the second stage, DA reward neurons in the ventral tegmental area serves to activate the mesolimbic DA reward neurons through a disinhibitory mechanism (458,459).

Nicotine also acutely activates mesotelencephalic DA neurons, as measured by single-neuron electrophysiologic recording techniques (460). The activating effect is dose-dependent within the range of 50 to 500 μg/kg administered intravenously. The same range of doses was more than three times as effective on mesolimbic DA neurons as on mesostriatal DA neurons, and all nicotine-induced activation of DA neurons was prevented or reversed by intravenous mecamylamine, implicating the involvement of nicotinic cholinergic receptors in mediating this neural activation (460). These results suggest that nicotine shares with other abusable substances the characteristic of being selectively effective in activating mesolimbic DA neurons that originate in the ventral tegmental area and project to the nucleus accumbens

(460). Alcohol also enhances the firing rates of meso-telencephalic DA neurons in reward-relevant brain loci (461). The effects of phencyclidine and phencyclidine analogues on DA neuronal firing rates are interesting. When administered directly onto mesotelencephalic DA neurons, phencyclidine inhibits spontaneous DA neuronal firing in a manner similar to local applications of DA itself (462–466). When administered systemically, both phencyclidine itself and the phencyclidine analogue N-[1-(2-thiophenyl)cyclohexyl]piperidine (TCP) elicit dose-dependent biphasic effects on the firing rate of identified mesotelencephalic DA neurons (464,467). At low doses, an activation of DA neuron firing rate is seen, followed by inhibition at higher doses (464,467). When administered systemically, the phencyclidine analogue MK-801 activates DA neurons in a manner equipotent to that of phencyclidine itself (468). Diazepam, the prototypical benzodiazepine, markedly excites mesolimbic DA neurons in the ventral tegmental area when administered intravenously (469). This excitation is reversed by the benzodiazepine antagonist Ro 15–1788. The same doses of diazepam potently inhibit non-DA substantia nigra–pars reticulata-like neurons in the ventral tegmental area, suggesting that benzodiazepines act directly on these non-DA cells to produce inhibition of neuronal activity and a disinhibition of the ventral tegmental area mesolimbic DA neurons (469). Curiously, at the doses tested, chlordiazepoxide and flurazepam did not mimic diazepam's potent activating effect on DA neurons (469).

In Vivo Brain Chemistry Measurements in Brain Reward Circuits During Self-Administration of Abusable Substances, as Assessed by Microdialysis, Voltammetric Electrochemistry, and Electrophysiology

As already noted, a number of research groups have combined self-administration techniques with *in vivo* microdialysis, *in vivo* voltammetric electrochemistry, and *in vivo* electrophysiology techniques for direct measurements of the functioning of the "second-stage" DA reward neurons (which, as noted earlier, appear to be the principal substrates for the reward-enhancing properties of abusable substances) during behaviorally separate subcomponents of volitional self-administration of abusable substances.

Using *in vivo* microdialysis techniques several research groups have reported that nucleus accumbens extracellular DA levels are elevated during cocaine self-administration (333,335,339,470–473). A relatively consistent picture emerges from these experiments. First, nucleus accumbens DA is contingently elevated by individual cocaine reinforcements during cocaine self-administration. Second, regardless of dosing regimen, nucleus accumbens DA levels are tonically elevated by a very large amount (200% to 800%) at the beginning of cocaine self-administration,

and then for the duration of the drug-taking session fluctuate phasically—in a reinforcement-contingent fashion—within a relatively constrained range at the upper end of the large tonic elevation. Third, these phasic DA fluctuations are time-locked to the drug reinforcements. Fourth, when the drug amount received by the animal per reinforcement is varied, greater DA elevations and longer interresponse times follow injections of higher doses. Fifth, animals appear to regulate their drug-taking behavior so as to deliberately titrate a given level of extracellular DA within the reward-critical nucleus accumbens DA synapses. Sixth, the absolute amount of DA within the nucleus accumbens extracellular space does not appear to be the critical factor correlated with the self-administration behavior; rather, relative DA increases against the baseline of tonic elevation appear to be the critical factor. Seventh, the phasic DA fluctuations appear consistent with the multiple infusion pharmacokinetics of cocaine. Eighth, animals also appear to titrate drug-taking behavior so as to avoid aversive effects. Taken as a whole, these data strongly suggest that—during volitional drug-taking behavior—the rewarding properties of cocaine are primarily mediated by extracellular DA levels in the reward synapses of the nucleus accumbens. This conclusion is strongly congruent with the finding that microinjections of DA antagonists into the nucleus accumbens, but not into other brain areas, block voluntary intravenous cocaine self-administration in laboratory animals (290).

Using *in vivo* microdialysis techniques, Wise and colleagues reported that nucleus accumbens extracellular DA levels are elevated during opiate (heroin) self-administration (470,474). Dworkin et al. have reported that while noncontingent intravenous heroin administration produced dose-dependent increases in nucleus accumbens extracellular DA, response-contingent heroin self-administration did not (475). The reason for this difference from the findings of Wise and colleagues (470,474) is not apparent to this reviewer.

Also using *in vivo* microdialysis, Koob et al. reported that nucleus accumbens extracellular DA levels are elevated during voluntary ethanol self-administration (476). Provocatively, dose–effect functions revealed significantly steeper slopes for the DA-enhancing effects of ethanol in rats of the alcohol-preferring P strain than in genetically heterogeneous nonpreferring Wistar rats.

Studies using *in vivo* voltammetric electrochemistry techniques for measuring extracellular nucleus accumbens DA during drug self-administration are strangely at variance with those studies, just cited, using *in vivo* brain microdialysis techniques (470). Thus, Wise, Kiyatkin, Gratton, and Stein have reported that electrochemical signals presumably reflecting extracellular DA in nucleus accumbens rise phasically to a peak immediately prior to each cocaine or heroin self-administration, and then fall immediately after each self-administered intravenous drug injection (470,477–482). This pattern of electrochemical changes is 180 degrees out of phase with the findings from the *in vivo* microdialysis studies. The reasons for this variance are not apparent. Suggestions range from overstimulation of the DA neurons resulting in temporary depolarization inactivation to the temporary DA neuronal inhibition seen electrophysiologically in a subpopulation of nucleus accumbens neurons in animals working for food or drug reward (in this section under the findings of the Schultz, Woodward, and Koob laboratories, respectively) to fundamental methodological flaws in the electrochemical technique that might permit other electrooxidizable molecules to be mistaken for DA. In truth, the electrochemistry findings are a conundrum. As Wise has noted, "... since the voltammetric data that have been collected thus far show changes that are out of phase with the predictions of ... current theories regarding the role of dopamine in addiction [and, as noted above, with *in vivo* microdialysis data], further studies with, and further refinements of, *in vivo* neurochemical methods are of major importance" (470 at p. 341).

Using *in vivo* single-neuron electrophysiologic recording techniques, many research groups have studied the responses of DA neurons in the ventral tegmental area and nucleus accumbens (as well as other reward-related forebrain loci) to rewarding and reward-associated stimuli. The findings of three such groups will be mentioned here, as they are representative of the findings, the interpretations given to such findings, and the methodological and interpretational problems that accrue to such experiments. Schultz and his colleagues (483–490) have found that individual DA neurons in both the ventral tegmental area and the nucleus accumbens are selectively activated during different components of a rewarded go–no go task in monkeys. Some DA neurons appear to signal the expectancy activated by the first instruction in each trial; others appear to signal the expectancy activated by specific visual trigger stimuli during each trial; others appear to signal preparation for movement or movement inhibition; others appear to signal the expectancy activated by conditioned stimuli associated with reward; and still others appear to signal the actual receipt of reward. The responses of some of the DA neurons that appear to signal reward expectancy were particularly interesting (484). These DA neuronal activations preceded the delivery of reward, were time-locked to the subsequent reward, and disappeared within a few trials when reward was omitted. Also, changes in the appetitive value of the reward modified the magnitude of these DA neuronal activations, suggesting a relationship between the DA neuronal signaling and the hedonic value of the expected reward (484). In the ventral mesencephalon, DA neurons signaling some aspect of reward or reward-associated stimuli were significantly more numerous in the ventral tegmental area than in adjacent DA loci (487). Because many of the reward-associated DA neurons identified in these experiments responded to reward during learning, but not after the task was learned (at which time the same neurons responded

to the conditioned, reward-predicting, stimulus), it would seem that DA neurons play an especially important role in reward-driven learning (488). Schultz and colleagues also hypothesize that many DA neurons may serve to signal the presence of high-priority reward-related stimuli (489), while others may serve to signal errors in reward-prediction (490).

Coupling single-neuron electrophysiologic recording from the nucleus accumbens with voluntary intravenous cocaine self-administration in rats, Woodward and colleagues (491) have reported that approximately 20% of nucleus accumbens neurons exhibit altered firing rates in the few seconds prior to the rat's emission of the learned behavioral act (lever-pressing) that activated the cocaine infusion apparatus (anticipatory neural responses) while approximately 50% of nucleus accumbens neurons exhibit altered firing rates in the few minutes after the rat's emission of the learned behavioral act that activated the cocaine infusion apparatus (postcocaine neural responses). Approximately two-thirds of the neurons showing anticipatory responses also showed postcocaine responses. Neurophysiologically, the anticipatory responses were of two types: anticipatory excitatory responses (increased neuronal firing) and anticipatory inhibitory responses (decreased neuronal firing). The postcocaine responses were similarly of two types: postcocaine excitatory responses and postcocaine inhibitory responses. Behaviorally, the anticipatory responses were of two types: "orienting-related" anticipatory responses (sustained alterations in neuronal firing with an onset centered around self-generated interruption of cocaine-induced behavioral stereotypy and orientation toward the lever) and "lever-pressing-related" anticipatory responses (alterations in neuronal firing with a tight temporal relation to the sequences of movements directly related to lever-pressing for the next cocaine infusion). Very importantly, anticipatory-like neuronal activity was not observed during similar movements unrelated to lever-pressing for cocaine. Woodward and colleagues hypothesize that the "orienting-related" anticipatory responses reflect neural "... trigger systems activated by a motivation to obtain reward," while the "lever-pressing-related" anticipatory responses reflect the "... transformation of internal motivational states into components of a sustained motor plan to acquire reward (in this case, presumably a euphoric state elicited by cocaine)" (491 at p. 1239). Behaviorally, the postcocaine neuronal responses (especially postcocaine inhibition) were predictive of cocaine readministration: "The ramp-like return to baseline firing rates of some neurons ... during postcocaine inhibition proved to be a good predictor of the next lever-press" (491 at p. 1240). Furthermore, higher cocaine doses produced longer periods of postcocaine inhibition that coincided with a longer self-administration interval, with the return to baseline firing rates of such neurons providing an accurate predictor of subsequent drug self-administration. Systemic administration of D_1 or D_2 DA receptor antagonists typically produced extinction of cocaine-taking behavior, and blocked the postcocaine inhibitory response of neurons that had anticipatory responses. Neither DA antagonist modified anticipatory neural responses, nor did they affect postcocaine inhibitory responses in neurons that did not show anticipatory responses. All together, these findings suggest that the role of nucleus accumbens neural circuitry in drug-taking behavior may be twofold: (a) an initiation or trigger mechanism (represented by the anticipatory neuronal responses), which—considering that the anticipatory responses were not affected by DA receptor antagonists—may derive from neural signals carried by non-DA afferents to the nucleus accumbens; and (b) a reward mechanism per se, directly activated by drug reinforcement (represented by the postcocaine responses) which—considering that the postcocaine inhibitory response of neurons with anticipatory responses was blocked by DA receptor antagonists—presumably involves a DA substrate.

Koob and colleagues (492) have coupled single-neuron electrophysiological recording from the nucleus accumbens with voluntary intravenous heroin self-administration in rats, and observed postheroin neuronal inhibitory responses similar to the postcocaine inhibitory responses observed by Woodward et al. (491). These neuronal inhibitory responses seemed clearly related to the drug-induced reward event, because nonrewarded behavioral responses (similar in behavioral topology to the heroin-reward behavioral responses) did not produce event-related neuronal inhibitory responses in the nucleus accumbens.

Taken together, such studies of concurrent *in vivo* microdialysis or *in vivo* single-neuron electrophysiology during volitional self-administration of abusable substances (or during volitional self-administration of other hedonically salient rewards) present a compelling argument for the intimate involvement of ventral tegmental area and nucleus accumbens DA neural circuits in the regulation of hedonic tone and in drug-induced reward (as well as in other reward-associated neural processes, such as reward expectancy and anticipation, that may well be involved in such clinically crucial phenomena as drug craving). As noted, the *in vivo* voltammetric electrochemistry studies are inexplicably at variance with the *in vivo* microdialysis studies.

PERTURBATIONS OF THE DOPAMINERGIC BRAIN REWARD SYSTEM LEADING TO INCREASED VULNERABILITY TO DRUG-TAKING BEHAVIOR

DA Reward Synapse and Modulatory Mechanisms Acting on the DA Reward System

From many of the separate strands of evidence reviewed here, inferences may be made regarding the neuroanatomy, neurophysiology, neurochemistry, and neuropharmacol-

ogy of the pleasure/reward circuitry of the brain and of the crucial "second-stage" DA link within this pleasure/reward circuitry, which apparently constitutes the primary neuropharmacologic site of action wherein abusable substances act to produce their intensely rewarding effects, and perhaps also wherein are encoded some neural aspects of substance abuse vulnerability and craving. First, the "first-stage" neurons of the reward system appear to originate within the anterior bed nuclei of the medial forebrain bundle, and project caudally within the medial forebrain bundle in a moderately fast-conducting, myelinated, heavily collateralized and diffuse neural system, of unknown neurotransmitter type(s), to synapse within the somatodendritic zone of DA cell bodies in the ventral tegmental area. Second, these DA neurons of the ventral tegmental area constitute the "second-stage" neurons of the reward system. Third, the ventral tegmental area that gives rise to these "second-stage" DA reward neurons is heavily innervated, and neurophysiologically modulated (in some cases transsynaptically), by numerous synaptic inputs including GABAergic, glutamatergic, serotonergic, noradrenergic, opioid peptidergic (including enkephalinergic, endorphinergic, and dynorphinergic systems [see also references 493–516]), cholecystokinergic (517–524), and neurotensinergic (525–533) neural systems. Fourth, the "second-stage" DA reward neurons project rostrally within the medial forebrain bundle to synapse in the nucleus accumbens. Fifth, these "second-stage" DA reward neurons constitute a critical locus for the addictive pharmacologic actions of abusable substances. Sixth, within the region of their axonal terminal projections in the nucleus accumbens, these "second-stage" reward neurons are heavily innervated, and neurophysiologically modulated (in some cases, transsynaptically), by numerous synaptic inputs including GABAergic, glutamatergic, serotonergic, opioid peptidergic, cholecystokinergic (518,522,534–540), and neurotensinergic (527,530,541–545) neural systems. Seventh, the most crucial reward synapses within the nucleus accumbens may be defined by their intra-accumbens locations and their synaptic connectivities—i.e., within the accumbens shell, in reward-relevant synaptic plexuses containing an opioid-DA axoaxonic link, a DA-opioid presynaptic–postsynaptic link, and neural inputs from limbic cortex and amygdala (409,546–562). Eighth, from the nucleus accumbens, additional "third-stage" reward-relevant neurons, some of them opioid peptidergic and/or GABAergic, appear to carry the reward signal further, to or via the ventral pallidum (216–238). Ninth, the profuse, complex, and reciprocal neural interconnections between the ventral tegmental area, nucleus accumbens, ventral pallidum, amygdala, and bed nuclei of the medial forebrain bundle appear to be critically involved in regulating the functional set-point for hedonic tone (216–238,546–567). In all of this complex neuronal computational machinery, the DA link between ventral tegmental area and nucleus accumbens seems central and crucial for drug-induced alterations in hedonic tone.

Although previously alluded to, it warrants reemphasis that the drug-sensitive DA "second-stage" component of the reward circuitry appears to be under the modulatory control of a wide variety of other neural systems, including GABAergic, glutamatergic, serotonergic, noradrenergic, and neuropeptide neurotransmitter and neuromodulatory mechanisms (see also 29,241,568–586), and theoretically an even wider variety of transsynaptic modulatory influences on the brain-reward systems are possible. Furthermore, it appears that the functioning of the reward system, and its sensitivity to abusable substances, can be altered by directly manipulating these other neurotransmitter systems that synaptically interconnect with the DA substrates (241,587–595), as well as by manipulating the DA substrates directly.

Genetically Imparted DA Reward Perturbations Leading to Increased Vulnerability to Drug-Taking Behavior

For many drugs of abuse, genetic differences influence both drug preferences and propensity for drug self-administration (596–600). Mouse strains that show high ethanol preference and high ethanol self-administration appear to generalize this increased vulnerability to other drugs of abuse, such as nicotine and opiates (597,601,602). This suggests that some inbred animal strains may have a generalized vulnerability to the rewarding effects of abusable drugs. The Lewis rat strain is particularly interesting in this regard. Lewis strain rats have a high vulnerability for both ethanol and cocaine oral self-administration (601,603). Furthermore, Lewis rats also (a) learn cocaine or opiate self-administration more readily, (b) work harder for cocaine or opiate self-administration, and (c) cue-condition for cocaine or opiates more readily, all in comparison to other rat strains (603–605). The author and his coworkers found that the brain-reward–enhancing property of Δ^9-tetrahydrocannabinol, the addictive substance in marihuana and hashish, is much more pronounced in Lewis rats than in other strains, as measured both by direct electrical brain-stimulation reward and by *in vivo* brain microdialysis of synaptic DA overflow in nucleus accumbens DA reward loci (606–609). This suggests that a basal dysfunction in DA regulation within the DA forebrain reward system may constitute a genetic vulnerability to the phenotypic polydrug preferences shown by Lewis rats (609). Congruent with this hypothesis, Nestler et al. reported basal differences in DA neurotransmitter synthesis, transport, and release, as well as DA-dependent receptor, second messenger, and immediate early gene function in DA reward neurons in Lewis rats as compared to other rat strains (605,610). Compellingly, the same dysfunctional differences in DA neurotransmitter synthesis, transport, and release, as well as DA-dependent receptor, second messenger, and immediate early gene function in DA reward neurons, can be induced by chronic drug administration in genetically nonvulnerable rats, and

this results in the same behavioral phenotype of polydrug preference as seen in the genetically vulnerable Lewis rats (605).

Genetic contributions also appear to play a role in drug-abuse vulnerability at the human level (603). Family, twin, and adoption studies all support a substantial genetic component in drug-abuse vulnerability and ongoing drug dependence (reviewed in reference 611). Identifying genetic factors in drug-abuse vulnerability is crucial to understanding addiction and, possibly, to identifying clinical subpopulations who may respond differently to potential pharmacotherapies. Linkage analysis in well-defined pedigrees is a powerful approach for studying single-gene disorders (612). However, for complex inherited traits, association studies, which are statistical correlations between an inherited condition and polymorphisms occurring in strong candidate genes, may be a superior approach (613,614). Because drug-abuse vulnerability does not follow clear mendelian patterns of inheritance, most genetic studies on drug abuse are association studies. Considering the wealth of data demonstrating the importance of DA in brain-reward mechanisms, polymorphisms in genes that regulate DA neurotransmission are candidates as genetic vulnerability factors for drug abuse (615). The DA D_2 and D_4 receptors and the DA transporter are some of the candidate genes previously analyzed. An allelic association to Taq I restriction fragment length polymorphisms (RFLPs) located in the D_2 receptor gene was found in alcoholics and drug abusers in some studies (616–619). These results are controversial, because negative association and linkage studies have also been reported (620,621). However, a meta-analysis conducted on published studies supports a positive association to the D_2 Taq A1 and B1 alleles (619). One problem with these polymorphisms is that they are generated by nonfunctional intronic mutations. Consequently, if the DA D_2 gene is involved in drug abuse vulnerability, the Taq polymorphisms must be in linkage disequilibrium with functional alterations located elsewhere in the gene. So far, none have been found. A variable numbers of tandem repeats (VNTR) polymorphism in the 3' untranslated region of the DA transporter gene, which has been linked to attention deficit hyperactivity disorder, shows a weak association in alcoholics who have specific aldehyde dehydrogenase-2 genotypes and in cocaine-induced paranoia (622–625). However, another association study in polysubstance abusers was negative (626). An association with attention deficit hyperactivity disorder would be interesting, because a high percentage of children and adolescents with this condition become substance abusers. However, the VNTR polymorphism is nonfunctional and, so far, no significant alterations in the gene have been found that could explain the positive linkage and association findings. A VNTR in the third cytoplasmic loop of the DA D_4 gene has been reported to be associated with both alcoholism and novelty-seeking behavior (627,628). The DA D_4 gene differs from other DA candidate genes analyzed so far in that the polymorphism is functionally significant, as differences in clozapine binding have been found in the 4 and 7 repeat polymorphisms (629). Additional evidence that the DA D_4 polymorphism is functionally significant is its association with the behavioral trait of thrill-seeking (627,628). No association to the DA D_4 gene was detected in a study conducted on alcoholics (630). The DA D_3 receptor gene has a common missense mutation that leads to a serine $\rightarrow$ glycine substitution (631), but thus far no significant association has been reported in drug or alcohol abusers (632).

Yet another DA-related candidate gene polymorphism for drug abuse vulnerability has emerged as a strong possibility—a codon 108/158 catechol-O-methyltransferase gene polymorphism. Catechol-O-methyltransferase plays an important role in regulating DA neurotransmission by inactivating synaptic DA (633). A single gene encodes membrane-bound and soluble forms of the enzyme, which differ by a 50-amino-acid hydrophobic N-terminal anchoring sequence present in the membrane-bound form (634). A common enzyme activity polymorphism exists in humans that results in a three- to fourfold variation in enzymatic activity (635–639). Approximately 25% of whites express a low activity form of the enzyme, another 25% have a high activity variant, and 50% display an intermediate level of activity (638,639). To identify the genetic basis of this enzymatic variability, Lachman and colleagues screened the catechol-O-methyltransferase gene by deoxyribonucleic acid (DNA) sequence analysis of polymerase chain reaction (PCR)-amplified genomic fragments, to identify allelic forms of the gene. They found a G $\rightarrow$ A transition at codon 158 of membrane-bound catechol-O-methyltransferase (corresponding to codon 108 of soluble catechol-O-methyltransferase) that results in a valine to methionine substitution. In retrospect, the two alleles were evident from a comparison of the two catechol-O-methyltransferase complementary deoxyribonucleic acid (cDNA) sequences published several years previously (640,641). In collaboration with Uhl and colleagues at the National Institute on Drug Abuse, Lachman and colleagues found a significant increase in the frequency of catechol-O-methyltransferase 158[val], the high activity allele, in substance abusers (both opiate preferring and cocaine preferring). This finding is consistent with the hypothesis that blunted DA reward system function enhances vulnerability to drug abuse—as Schuckitt (642) found for ethanol-responsiveness in alcoholics and sons of alcoholics—because expression of the high activity catechol-O-methyltransferase variant would magnify the decrease in DA. These data suggest that the DA-related codon 108/158 polymorphism could be a factor in genetic vulnerability to drug abuse.

Taking some of these concepts even further, Blum and colleagues (643) postulated the existence of a generalized "reward-deficiency syndrome," subsuming a large class of addictive, impulsive, and compulsive disorders (including drug abuse/dependence and nonchemical [behavioral] addictions) under a common rubric and positing that they have a common genetic basis. They postulate that all these disorders are connected by a common biologic substrate—an alteration in the brain system that provides positive reinforcement (positive hedonic tone) for specific behaviors. They further postulate that "reward-deficiency syndrome" results from a basal dysfunction of DA brain-reward mechanisms. Evidence cited in support of this hypothesis includes the following facts: (a) drugs of abuse (which produce augmented hedonic tone) have one major commonality—they augment DA function as a final common neuropharmacologic action, particularly in the DA mesocorticolimbic system so vital for the regulation of reward functions; (b) molecular biologic, electrophysiologic, and neurochemical studies show considerable differences in the DA reward systems of drug-preferring versus nonpreferring genetic strains of rats (see also references 644 and 645); and (c) alcoholics, cocaine addicts, compulsive gamblers, and patients with obesity (a majority being compulsive eaters) or attention deficit hyperactivity disorder are reported to possess the A1 D_2 receptor allele (646–650). The number of D_2 receptors in A1 carriers may be 20% to 30% lower than those lacking the A1 genotype (648). Also, the likelihood that an individual possesses the A1 genotype increases dramatically when two or more of the clinical conditions noted under (c) above are found to coexist. Furthermore, animal studies show that DA agonists can decrease the consumption/self-administration of various drugs of abuse or reduce drug craving, and that animals deliberately bred for high ethanol preference have decreased brain DA function (651–653). In addition, alcoholics possessing the A1/A1 genotype are more responsive to DA agonist therapy (e.g., bromocriptine) for treatment of alcohol craving (654). Provocatively, a predictive model based on Bayes' theorem of probability suggests that an individual with the A1 allele for the D_2 receptor has a 74% chance of developing one of the disorders that comprises the "reward-deficiency syndrome" (643). In sum, the "reward-deficiency syndrome" theory holds that addictive, impulsive, and compulsive disorders may have a common genetic basis—DA hypoactivity in reward pathways.

DA Reward Mechanisms and Vulnerability to Drug-Taking Behavior

Whether increased vulnerability to drug-taking behavior is imparted genetically or by other factors, the bulk of the currently available evidence suggests a central role for aberrations of brain DA reward function in imparting such vulnerability. Thus, animals bred for high ethanol self-administration have lower densities of DA receptors, lower extracellular DA levels, and lower DA innervation density in DA forebrain reward areas than do animals bred for ethanol avoidance (652,653). Notably, the lower DA innervation densities were found only in DA limbic cortex and the shell of the nucleus accumbens (653). There were no differences in DA innervation densities between ethanol-preferring and non–ethanol-preferring rats in other major DA mesolimbic brain loci (653). Moreover, the subpopulation of DA neurons in the ventral tegmental area that project to the nucleus accumbens was found to be smaller (as shown by horseradish peroxidase tracing and immunocytochemical double staining) in the ethanol-preferring as compared to the non–ethanol-preferring rats (653). In outbred heterogeneous rat strains, propensity to drug self-administration is also correlated with aberrant DA reward-system function (655–657). Glick and colleagues found that low to moderate DA levels are positively correlated with cocaine self-administration rates, whereas moderate to high DA levels are negatively correlated with self-administration rates (656). They also found that DA release in the medial prefrontal cortex appears to be an important predictor of initiation of drug-taking (657). They suggest that " . . . normal variability in drug-seeking behavior is at least in part attributable to individual differences in the activity of brain DA systems." Differentiating between initiation and maintenance of drug-taking behavior, they conclude that the nucleus accumbens is a "critical component" in both mechanisms (656). Piazza, Le Moal, Simon, and colleagues report that individual differences in locomotor responses to novelty are predictive of differences in rats' tendencies to begin amphetamine self-administration, and that endogenous variations in brain DA systems mediating both stress and drug reward are responsible for individual differences in propensity to engage in drug-taking behavior (655,658,659). Interestingly, they report that animals showing high DA responses to cocaine challenge have an increased vulnerability for cocaine self-administration (655).

DA Reward Mechanisms and Relapse to Drug-Taking Behavior

The phenomenon of drug "priming"—the ability of a "priming" drug dose to reinstate previously extinguished drug taking (660) has been extensively (and very profitably, in terms of data gathered and hypotheses generated) studied in animals as a model of relapse to drug taking, primarily by Stewart and her colleagues (661–666). In this paradigm, the ability of drugs (or other stimuli, including stressors and drug-associated environmental cues) to reestablish extinguished drug-taking habits in laboratory animals is measured. As noted by Stewart and Wise (664), "the most potent stimulus for renewed responding that has been demonstrated in this model is a free 'priming' injection of the training drug; a priming injection of the training drug can re-establish extinguished habits much as a single drink, cigarette, or injection are thought to reestablish such habits in detoxified ex-addicts." Provocatively, such priming injections can be successfully given intravenously or directly into component parts of the brain-reward circuitry—most cru-

cially the ventral tegmental area or nucleus accumbens (665,666), but not into other brain loci. Equally provocatively, cross-priming (from one class of abusable substances to another) has been demonstrated. Thus, priming doses of morphine reinstate cocaine self-administration (665) and priming doses of amphetamine or the DA agonist bromocriptine reinstate heroin-trained responding (666,667). In this reviewer's opinion, such cross-priming between drugs of different classes speaks powerfully to the existence of common neurobiologic and common neuropharmacologic substrates for the actions of abusable substances within the DA reward circuitry of the brain, as detailed in previous sections of this chapter. Importantly, the drugs and doses known to reinitiate drug self-administration in both humans and animals are drugs and doses known to increase DA function within the brain's reward circuitry, as detailed earlier in this chapter. Thus, acute administration of DA-mimetic compounds precipitates relapse to drug-taking, just as acute heroin precipitates clinical relapse in human opiate abusers, and just as a single cigarette precipitates relapse to smoking in former nicotine addicts.

Stress is also a precipitant of relapse to drug taking at the human level, and consequently has been extensively studied in several animal models of drug self-administration, including fixed ratio reinforcement, progressive ratio reinforcement, and the drug reinstatement model noted in the previous paragraph. Working in this area, Shaham and colleagues shown that stress (a) increases opiate self-administration and opiate preferences in animals (668); (b) increases opiate appetitiveness as assessed by self-administration performance and breakpoints on progressive ratio reinforcement schedules (669,670); (c) enhances the reinforcing efficacy of drug self-administration (670); (d) provokes relapse to drug-taking behavior (671,672); and (e) provokes relapse to drug-seeking behavior (672). Provocatively, Shaham and Stewart report (672) that the same parameters of stress that acutely reinstate drug-seeking behavior also increase DA overflow in the nucleus accumbens in drug-naive animals, implicating a common DA-mediated neurobiologic substrate in drug-induced and stress-induced relapse to drug-taking behavior. Similarly, DA overflow in the nucleus accumbens was increased by systemic injections of morphine, an effect that was reversed by an injection of naltrexone given 40 minutes later to induce opiate withdrawal. As noted, an interpretation of these results is that stressors can reinstate drug-taking behavior by activating neural systems in common with those activated by drugs of abuse. Again, the crucial role of the DA reward system of the brain appears evident. At the same time, an extensive body of research implicates noradrenergic-mediated and corticotropin-releasing-factor (CRF)-mediated brain circuits in stress-triggered relapse to drug-seeking and drug-taking behaviors, a body of work so extensive as to be quite beyond the scope of the present review.

DA Reward Mechanisms and Drug Craving

DA Reward Mechanisms and the Conditioned Place Preference (Cue Preference) Animal Model of Drug Seeking

Drug craving is widely accepted to be a major component of drug addiction and dependence (673–679). Drug and/or alcohol addicts frequently report intense and/or prolonged yearning for additional drug or alcohol while in either voluntary or enforced abstinence periods, and a causal relation between such yearnings and drug or alcohol readministration has been suggested by many observers (674,676–679). Thus, craving is typically experienced by chronic substance abusers when they have been deprived of drug for a period of time. By definition, then, animal models of craving must differ from the acute-administration and self-administration paradigms detailed earlier. Because craving at the human level is often elicited by sensory stimuli previously associated with drug taking, various conditioning paradigms have been used to model craving in laboratory animals. One of the most widely used is conditioned place preference (680–682) (also referred to as conditioned cue preference). In this paradigm, animals are tested (when free of drug) to determine whether they prefer an environment in which they previously received drug or an environment in which they previously received saline or vehicle. If the animal, in the drug-free state, consistently chooses the environment previously associated with drug delivery, the inference is drawn not only that the drug was appetitive but also that the appetitive hedonic value was coded in the brain and is accessible during the drug-free state, which, if not craving per se, would appear to be closely related to craving. The questions that obviously arise are: (a) Is craving coded in the same neural circuitry as drug-induced reward? and (b) Do pharmacologic manipulations and/or lesions of the reward-relevant DA circuitry alter conditioned place preferences induced by abusable substances? With respect to the first question, many workers have, out of simple regard for parsimony, posited that craving is coded in the reward circuitry of the forebrain, and some have even posited that craving results directly from a functional deficiency of DA in the reward-relevant DA circuitry (676). With respect to the second and closely related question, it is now quite clear, on the basis of much work (reviewed in reference 682), that pharmacologic manipulations or lesions of the mesotelencephalic DA system profoundly alter place conditioning of abusable substances, and that the mesotelencephalic DA system almost certainly serves as an important substrate for the central encoding in the brain of the hedonic value imparted by abusable substances. Furthermore, and very provocatively, White and Hiroi showed (546,547,683,684) that different aspects of conditioned hedonic value appear to depend upon different neurochemically specific DA substrates. Specifically, in amphetamine place conditioning, the newly synthesized DA pool appears to subserve the neural encoding of hedonic value, while the vesicular DA pool appears crucial for the behavioral expression or readout of that previously encoded hedonic value (546,547,683). Furthermore, while systemically administered D_1 and D_2 DA antagonists blocked both acquisition and expression of conditioned place preference for amphetamine, selective D_1 antagonism was significantly more effective at blocking behavioral expression or readout of previously encoded hedonic value than D_2 antagonists. Also, preconditioning and postconditioning lesions of the lateral amygdaloid nucleus impaired the conditioned place preference for amphetamine. It is concluded on the basis of these experiments that the behavioral expression or readout of conditioned incentive stimuli for amphetamine (i.e., the animal homologue of amphetamine craving) is mediated by a DA neural system that involves the vesicular DA pool and the D_1 DA receptor in the nucleus accumbens and the lateral amygdaloid nucleus (546,547,683). These workers also demonstrated that the ventral pallidum is involved in the acquisition of amphetamine-conditioned place preference but not its behavioral expression or readout (685). If the conditioned place preference paradigm validly models drug-conditioned incentive stimuli, as many believe, we may be well and truly understanding the neurochemical substrates for the craving that substance abusers feel when confronted visually with syringes, needles, crack vials, smoking pipes, or even the street corner where they normally buy their illicit drugs.

DA Reward Mechanisms During Chronic Drug Administration and Withdrawal

In contrast to the clear-cut and agreed-on effects of acute administration of addicting drugs on brain-reward mechanisms cited previously, the effects of chronic administration of abuse-prone drugs on reward mechanisms are less clear-cut. With respect to neurochemical indices (*in vivo* brain microdialysis measures of DA overflow in forebrain reward loci), a clear difference appears to exist between the effects of continuous administration (or intermittent high-dose treatment, which presumably produces continuous intoxication) and the effects of intermittent low-dose treatment, which presumably produces intermittent phasic stimulation. With intermittent low doses of psychostimulants (cocaine, amphetamines), "reverse tolerance" or "sensitization" of DA overflow in forebrain reward loci is seen upon subsequent psychostimulant rechallenge (335,338,355,686–692). Similar psychostimulant neurochemical sensitization has also been reported with self-administered, rather than exogenous, dosing (693). This sensitization may extend to basal DA overflow as well as to drug-challenge-evoked DA overflow (687,694). Similar sensitization of DA overflow in forebrain-reward loci has been reported for opiates (695,696) and many other classes of abused drugs. With chronic continuous or intermittent high-dose psychostimulant treatment, decreased DA synthesis is seen (347), and, in withdrawal from such dose regimens, depletion of basal extracellular DA in such brain-reward loci as nucleus accumbens (697–699). When cocaine is administered to emulate human "binges," decreased basal and cocaine-stimulated DA levels are reported (700). Reward-related functional and behavioral sequelae have also been reported. With continuous treatment or intermittent treatment with high doses, acute tolerance to cocaine's rewarding effects develops (701,702), and withdrawal from the continuous intoxication produced by frequent low-dose cocaine or amphetamine produces elevations in brain-stimulation reward thresholds (703–710). In opiate withdrawal from chronic dosing regimens (either abstinence withdrawal or precipitated withdrawal), a pattern of decreased DA levels in forebrain reward loci (particularly nucleus accumbens) similar to that seen in withdrawal from continuous or high-dose intermittent psychostimulant administration is seen (711–715). Clear reward-related functional and behavioral sequelae are also seen in opiate withdrawal (i.e., elevated electrical brain-reward thresholds [716,717]). Also, opiate withdrawal produces conditioned cue aversion (715,716,718–726). Furthermore, opiate self-administration increases significantly in withdrawal, and the increase correlates with severity of withdrawal (671,727,728). Significantly, the neural mechanisms underlying this withdrawal-produced presumptive negative hedonic tone or dysphoria may involve the nucleus accumbens (718,719), just as the acute-drug-induced positive hedonic tone may. Congruent with these findings from a variety of paradigms, DA depletion of the nucleus accumbens and elevation in brain-reward thresholds have been proposed as neural substrates for postdrug-use anhedonia and drug craving (676,718,729). Very importantly, because DA depletion, unlike other withdrawal symptoms (730), offers a withdrawal symptom common to psychostimulants, opiates, and ethanol, it may offer a long-sought common denominator for addiction (731). Adding credence to this possibility are findings from studies in which animals are allowed to self-administer intravenous cocaine or heroin and *in vivo* DA neurochemistry is concomitantly monitored in nucleus accumbens by brief-sampling-time microdialysis (470,471,474). In these studies, noted earlier in this chapter, both tonic and phasic alterations in nucleus accumbens DA levels are observed as a function of drug self-administration. At the beginning of each self-administration session, an enormous tonic elevation in nucleus accumbens DA occurs after the first "loading" doses of self-administered drug. This tonic DA elevation plateaus quickly, and is then followed by small but significant phasic fluctuations that correlate very tightly with voluntary self-administration. Nucleus accumbens DA decreases prior to, and appears to predict, each drug self-administration, whereas nucleus accumbens DA increases immediately after each drug self-administration, and appears to correlate with behavioral indices of satiation.

DA Reward Mechanisms and "Opponent Process" Theory of Drug Craving

From the previously cited evidence, and from "opponent process" theory (732,733), Koob and his colleagues proposed an opponent process theory of the motivation for drug taking (718,729,734). This theory is based on the negative reinforcement (i.e., relief from aversive stimuli) that drug-taking in the face of the dysphoria and anhedonia imputed from this evidence entails. The theory holds that drug reinforcers arouse both positive (appetitive, pleasurable) and negative (aversive, dysphoric) hedonic processes in the brain, and that these processes oppose one another in a simple dynamic system. The time-dynamics and tolerance patterns of the two processes are hypothesized to differ. The positive hedonic processes are hypothesized to be simple, stable, of short latency and duration, to follow the reinforcer closely, and to develop tolerance rapidly. The negative hedonic processes are hypothesized to be of longer latency and duration (thus, they increase and decay more slowly), and to be resistant to the development of tolerance. Thus, if self-administration of an abusable drug is frequently repeated, two correlated changes in hedonic tone are postulated to occur. First, tolerance to the euphoric effects of the drug develops, while at the same time the withdrawal or abstinence syndrome becomes more intense and of longer duration (615,718,729,734). Thus, the positive reinforcing properties of the drug diminish while the negative reinforcing properties (relief of withdrawal-induced anhedonia) strengthen. Koob and colleagues propose that not only are the positive reinforcing properties of abusable drugs mediated by drug effects in the nucleus accumbens, but that opponent processes within these same brain-reward circuits become sensitized during the development of dependence and thus become responsible for the aversive stimulus properties of drug withdrawal, and ultimately for the negative reinforcement processes that come, in this view, to dominate the motivation for chronic drug abuse. Thus, brain DA reward mechanisms, and the regulatory neural mechanisms controlling them, are conceptualized to dominate not only the positively reinforcing acute "hit," "rush," or "high" resulting from early administration, but also the negatively reinforcing properties that develop with chronic drug use and that are important in the maintenance of drug habits. Koob and colleagues have postulated that endogenous opioid peptide mechanisms intrinsic to, and synaptically interacting with, the DA reward circuitry of the forebrain are critically involved in this opponent process motivation for drug dependence and addiction. (Such negative hedonic processes within the reward-encoding circuitry of the brain must differ from the aversive physical abstinence symptoms produced by drug withdrawal, which are mediated by non–reward-related neural circuitry involving the periaqueductal gray, locus coeruleus, medial thalamus, and the diencephalic-mesencephalic juncture [314,735,736].) Congruent with this concept, the author has gathered evidence—using both *in vivo* electrical brain-stimulation reward and *in vivo* brain voltammetric electrochemistry—suggesting that drug administration does evoke both positive and negative affective/hedonic processes within the pleasure/reward DA circuitry of the forebrain (110,410,411,737). Medial brain-reward DA circuitry, originating in the ventral tegmental area and projecting through the medial portions of the medial forebrain bundle to the nucleus accumbens, appears uniquely sensitive to the brain-reward enhancing properties of addicting drugs (110,737). With electrodes in the medial portions of the reward circuitry, opiates enhance brain-stimulation reward, this enhancement dissipates as time passes following each daily injection, and tolerance to this brain-reward enhancement develops with repeated daily morphine injections (110). With electrodes in the lateral portions of the reward circuitry, opiates inhibit brain-stimulation reward (are dysphorigenic), this inhibition dissipates as time passes following each daily injection, and a progressive augmentation of this brain reward inhibition develops with repeated daily injections (110,737). Both the medial and lateral loci are DA-mediated (246,738–740). Thus, these two anatomic domains (medial and lateral) within the DA reward circuitry of the ventral forebrain respond to drug administration in a manner consistent with the predicted behavior of the "positive hedonic processes" and "negative hedonic processes" of Koob et al. Using *in vivo* voltammetric electrochemistry, we have seen that some DA reward neurons respond to drug administration by inhibition of DA overflow while other DA neurons within the same circuitry (but anatomically distinct) respond to drug administration by enhancement of DA overflow (410,411,737). Congruent with these observations are electrophysiologic data showing that some DA reward neurons respond to opiate administration by inhibiting their firing (741) rather than by the enhanced firing (116,742) normally seen. This, in turn, is congruent with reports from Woodward et al. and from Schultz et al., reviewed earlier, concerning the heterogeneity of response patterns of reward-related DA neurons in nucleus accumbens.

Also congruent with some of these concepts are (a) the findings of Aston-Jones (743) that nucleus accumbens DA neural mechanisms are not only important in the acute rewarding effects of abusable substances, but also important in drug withdrawal, with the latter effects mediated by DA D_2 receptors; and (b) the findings of van der Kooy and colleagues that DA neural mechanisms are involved in the motivational effects produced by opiate withdrawal (744–746).

However, as the author has argued (737), simple "opponent process" conceptions seem unlikely, on the preponderance of presently available evidence, to constitute fully satisfactory explanations of the undoubtedly complex neurobiologic phenomena subsumed under the term "craving." Also, given that the presently available data generated with the "reinstatement" paradigm of relapse to drug-seeking behavior indicate that only a drug "priming"

injection or environmental stress—but not withdrawal-induced anhedonia—provoke relapse to drug-taking in drug-taking-extinguished animals, one is left with the following conundrum: (a) opponent process neural mechanisms seem to exist, either directly within the DA reward circuitry or intimately connected to it synaptically (or both); (b) such opponent process mechanisms may well mediate some aspects of anhedonia or dysphoria; (c) such opponent process mechanisms appear to be triggered by withdrawal from addictive drug use; but (d) there is no present evidence that such withdrawal-triggered dysphoric opponent neural processes provoke relapse to drug-seeking behavior in animal models such as the reinstatement paradigm of relapse to drug self-administration.

CONCLUSION

A summary description of the role of brain-reward mechanisms in substance abuse may be derived from all the evidence cited in this chapter.

First, it appears that abusable substances have two fundamental commonalities: (a) that they are voluntarily self-administered by nonhuman mammals, and (b) that they acutely enhance brain-reward mechanisms. From this latter property presumably derives their euphorigenic potency, their appeal to nonhuman mammals, and the "hit," "rush," or "high" sought by the human substance abuser. Second, the reward circuits of the brain, upon which abusable substances act to enhance brain reward, include "first-stage," "second-stage," and "third-stage" components. The "first-stage" component comprises descending, myelinated, moderately fast conducting neurons that run caudally within the medial forebrain bundle and are preferentially activated by direct electrical brain-stimulation reward. These "first-stage" fibers synapse into the ventral mesencephalic nuclei containing the cell bodies of the ascending mesotelencephalic DA system, the axons of which run rostrally through the medial forebrain bundle to limbic and cortical projection areas. These mesotelencephalic DA neurons constitute the "second-stage" fibers of the reward system, and form a crucial drug-sensitive component of the reward circuitry, which appears preferentially activated neurochemically and/or electrophysiologically by abusable substances to enhance brain reward. The mesolimbic DA fibers terminating in the nucleus accumbens, and most especially in the nucleus accumbens "shell," appear to be the most crucial reward-relevant component of the ascending mesotelencephalic DA system. From the nucleus accumbens, "third-stage" reward-relevant neurons, some of them enkephalinergic and/or GABAergic, appear to carry the reward signal further, to or via the ventral pallidum. Third, abusable substances appear to act on or synaptically close to these DA fibers to produce their reward-enhancing actions, possibly via an opioid peptidergic mechanism. This DA component appears crucial for drug self-administration, and self-administration can be attenuated by manipulating these

DA substrates. Fourth, different classes of abusable substances appear to act on these DA reward substrates at different anatomic levels and via different sites of action on or near the DA neurons. Fifth, this crucial drug-sensitive DA component of the reward system is functionally modulated by a wide variety of other neurotransmitter-specific neural systems (including GABAergic, glutamatergic, serotonergic, noradrenergic, enkephalinergic, endorphinergic, dynorphinergic, cholecystokinergic, and neurotensinergic neural systems), which appear importantly involved in setting the level of hedonic tone carried through the DA reward system. Drug self-administration can be attenuated (at least in laboratory animals) by manipulating these other neurotransmitter systems that modulate the DA reward system. Sixth, complex reciprocal neural interconnections between the "first-stage," "second-stage," and "third-stage" reward neurons also appear to be importantly involved in regulating the functional set-point for hedonic tone, and (at least in laboratory animals) manipulating these neural interconnections can alter drug taking-behavior. Seventh, perturbations in the neural substrates of the DA reward system (genetically imparted or otherwise) may be capable of altering vulnerability to drug-taking behavior. Eighth, relapse to drug-seeking or drug-taking behavior triggered by reexposure to drug appears to involve reactivation of DA reward-linked substrates. Ninth, the subjective experience of drug craving itself may also involve activation of DA reward-linked substrates. A clinically relevant derivative of such considerations is that pharmacotherapeutic interventions to alter drug reward, drug craving, or even preexisting drug vulnerabilities could conceivably target an exceedingly wide range of neurotransmitter systems that synaptically modulate the reward circuitry.

The admittedly incomplete picture of the reward systems of the mammalian brain painted in the present chapter, and drug interaction therewith, is illustrated in Figure 5.2. It will be instructive for the reader to compare Figures 5.1 and 5.2 and to note therefrom how little we yet know about the functional anatomy of the brain, as compared to the static anatomy. It will also be obvious to the reader that Figure 5.2 represents a *reductio ad minima* approach to the anatomy, chemistry, pharmacology, and function of the reward systems of the mammalian brain. It will be remarkable, indeed, if the anatomy of brain reward, and the actions of abusable substances thereon, turn out to be as simple as that sketched in this chapter and as simple as shown in Figure 5.2. At the same time, knowledge does accumulate from year to year, and it will be equally instructive for the reader to compare Figure 5.2 in the present chapter with Figure 5.2 from the same chapter in the second edition of this textbook (747). It will be obvious from such a comparison that we have learned a great deal more about the underlying neuroanatomy, neurochemistry, and neuropharmacology of brain reward mechanisms than was known or even conjectured 12 years ago. Of course, more complex and comprehensive conjectural pictures of the re-

ward apparatus of the mammalian brain, and of abusable drug action on these systems, have been presented. Although some such schemes are arguably less defensible, at our present limited state of knowledge, than the deliberately simplified picture painted in the present chapter, the interested reader is referred to them (748–756).

What, then, is the actual role of the ascending DA reward-relevant neuron and the seemingly crucial DA synapse to which it feeds? No suggestion appears yet to have bettered Wise's hypothesis that "the dopamine junction represents a synaptic way station for messages signaling the rewarding impact of a variety of normally powerful rewarding events. It seems likely that this synapse lies at a critical junction between branches of the sensory pathways which carry signals of the intensity, duration, and quality of the stimulus, and the motivational pathways where these sensory inputs are translated into the hedonic messages we experience as pleasure, euphoria or 'yumminess'" (194 at p. 94). However, as noted repeatedly in this chapter, it has become clear in the years since Wise's suggestion, that the encoding of hedonic tone by the DA reward system of the brain is far more complex and subtle than was realized as recently as a decade ago, incorporating nuances of anticipatory and conditioned reinforcement as well as anhedonia/dysphoria, craving, and (some) neural mechanisms underlying both preexisting vulnerability to drug taking and relapse to previously extinguished drug taking.

Finally, the question arises as to the biologic purposes these brain-reward systems evolved to serve. No one, after all, seriously believes that they emerged during the eons of evolution simply so that modern *Homo sapiens* could inject themselves with chemicals. What purposes, then, did these brain-reward systems evolve to serve? As Wise has noted (194 at p. 94), most workers believe that addictive drugs act on brain circuits that evolved to subserve the normal reinforcement functions of the central nervous system, for example, in reinforcing such biologically essential behaviors as feeding, as postulated more than 55 years ago in the pioneering ideas of Hebb (757), and as more recently stated in the eloquent writings of Goldstein (758). In fact, one of the oldest observations in the research literature on electrical stimulation of the brain is that stimulation in brain-reward areas can also evoke natural consummatory behaviors such as feeding and other species-typical biologically essential behaviors (22–25). Furthermore, the directly activated neural substrates of stimulation-induced feeding and brain-stimulation reward in the lateral hypothalamus and ventral tegmental area appear identical in terms of refractory periods, conduction velocities, and medial–lateral and dorsal–ventral alignment of the nerve fibers subserving the two stimulation-induced effects (feeding and reward), suggesting strongly that the same fibers mediate both effects (437,438). It is intriguing in this regard to note that the same mesotelencephalic DA circuits that appear to subserve the reward induced by abusable drugs are also biochemically activated, in a manner seemingly

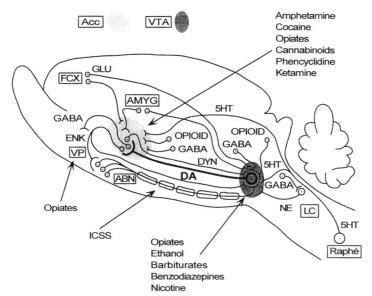

FIG. 5.2. Diagram of the brain-reward circuitry of the mammalian (laboratory rat) brain, with sites at which various abusable substances appear to act to enhance brain-reward and thus to induce drug-taking behavior and possibly drug-craving. ABN, anterior bed nuclei of the medial forebrain bundle; Acc, nucleus accumbens; AMYG, amygdala; DA, subcomponent of the ascending mesolimbic dopaminergic system that appears preferentially activated by abusable substances; DYN, dynorphinergic outflow from the nucleus accumbens; ENK, enkephalinergic outflow from the nucleus accumbens; FCX, frontal cortex; GABA, GABAergic inhibitory fiber systems synapsing upon the locus coeruleus noradrenergic fibers, the ventral tegmental area, and the nucleus accumbens, as well as the GABAergic outflow from the nucleus accumbens; GLU, glutamatergic neural systems originating in frontal cortex and synapsing in both the ventral tegmental area and the nucleus accumbens; 5HT, serotonergic (5-hydroxytryptamine) fibers, which originate in the anterior raphe nuclei and project to both the cell body region (ventral tegmental area) and terminal projection field (nucleus accumbens) of the DA reward neurons; ICSS, descending, myelinated, moderately fast conducting component of the brain-reward circuitry that is preferentially activated by electrical intracranial self-stimulation; LC, locus coeruleus; NE, noradrenergic fibers, which originate in the locus coeruleus and synapse into the general vicinity of the ventral mesencephalic DA cell fields of the ventral tegmental area; Opioid, endogenous opioid peptide neural systems synapsing into both the ventral tegmental DA cell fields and the nucleus accumbens DA terminal projection loci; Raphé, brainstem serotonergic raphe nuclei; VP, ventral pallidum; VTA, ventral tegmental area.

identical to the DA activation produced by abusable drugs, by natural rewards (117,759–762). Other more complex interactions between the DA reward system and natural rewards have also been reported (377). Is it possible, then, that some substance abusers have a defect in their ability to capture reward and pleasure from everyday experience, as postulated by some clinicians (763–765) and as postulated by Blum and colleagues (643) in the context of their formulation of "reward-deficiency syndrome"? Interestingly, this very concept—of a basal hypofunctionality in brain mechanisms subserving normal reward and pleasure functions—was originally postulated (albeit in rather elementary form) by Dole and his colleagues nearly 40 years ago during the development of methadone maintenance therapy for heroin addiction (766,767). If these conceptions have merit, they have profound implications: (a) our goals are not only to acutely rescue addicts from the clutches of their addictions, but also, more importantly, to restore their reward systems to a level of functionality

that will enable them to "get off" on the real world; and (b) pharmacotherapeutic interventions for clinical treatment of substance abuse that are predicated on blockade of brain reward functions are doomed to failure.

ACKNOWLEDGMENTS

Preparation of this chapter, and the development of concepts contained herein, was supported by the Intramural Research Program of the National Institute on Drug Abuse, the Aaron Diamond Foundation, the Russell Sage Foundation, the Old Stones Foundation, the Norwegian Research Council, the Norwegian Institute for Alcohol and Drug Research, the Norwegian Directorate for the Prevention of Alcohol and Drug Problems, and by funds from the New York State Office of Alcohol and Substance Abuse Services. The author is indebted to William Paredes for his tireless assistance; to Dr. Joyce H. Lowinson for her unwavering support; and to Dr. Roy A. Wise for inspiration, for clear thinking, for pioneering and continuing contributions to the study of brain-reward mechanisms, and for frequently discerning a path where others see only impenetrable jungle. Work from the author's laboratory cited in this chapter was supported by the U.S. Public Health Service under research grants DA-01560, DA-02089, and DA-03622 from the National Institute on Drug Abuse, research grant NS-09649 from the National Institute of Neurological Disorders and Stroke, research grant AA-09547 from the National Institute on Alcohol Abuse and Alcoholism, and research grant RR-05397 (Biomedical Research Support Grant) from the National Institutes of Health; by U.S. National Science Foundation research grant BNS-86-09351; by the U.S. Air Force Aeromedical Division, under research projects 6893-02-005 and 6893-02-039; by research grants and fellowships from the Natural Sciences and Engineering Research Council of Canada; by the Julia Sullivan Medical Research Fund; and by very generous research grant and fellowship support from the Aaron Diamond Foundation of New York City. This chapter is dedicated to Dr. Vincent P. Dole—physician, innovator, scientist, teacher, and humanitarian nonpareil.

REFERENCES

1. Lierman TL, ed. *Building a healthy America.* New York: Mary Ann Liebert, 1987.
2. Rice DP, Kelman S, Miller LS. Estimates of economic costs of alcohol and drug abuse and mental illness, 1985 and 1988. *Public Health Rep* 1991;106:280–292.
3. D'Aquila RT, Williams AB. Epidemic human immunodeficiency virus (HIV) infection among intravenous drug users (IVDU). *Yale J Biol Med* 1987;60:545–567.
4. Guinan ME, Hardy A. Epidemiology of AIDS in women in the United States: 1981 through 1986. *JAMA* 1987;257:2039–2042.
5. Des Jarlais DC, Friedman SR, Stoneburner RL. HIV infection and intravenous drug use: critical issues in transmission dynamics, infection outcomes, and prevention. *Rev Infect Dis* 1988;10:151–158.
6. Weeks JR. Experimental morphine addiction: method for automatic intravenous injections in unrestrained rats. *Science* 1962;138:143–144.
7. Schuster CR, Thompson T. Self administration of and behavioral dependence on drugs. *Annu Rev Pharmacol* 1969;9:483–502.
8. Griffiths RR, Bigelow CE, Liebson I. Experimental drug self-administration: generality across species and type of drug. *NIDA Res Monogr* 1978;20:24–43.
9. Brady JV, Lucas SE. Testing drugs for physical dependence potential and abuse liability. *NIDA Res Monogr* 1984;52.
10. Bindra D, Stewart J, eds. *Motivation,* 2nd ed. Baltimore: Penguin, 1971.
11. Jaffe JH. Drug addiction and drug abuse. In: Goodman LS, Gilman A, eds. *The pharmacological basis of therapeutics,* 3rd ed. New York: Macmillan, 1965:285–311.
12. Skinner BF. *The behavior of organisms: an experimental analysis.* New York: Appleton-Century-Crofts, 1938.
13. Young PT. The role of affective processes in learning and motivation. *Psychol Rev* 1959;66:104–125.
14. Pfaffmann C. The pleasures of sensation. *Psychol Rev* 1960;67:253–268.
15. Young PT. *Motivation and emotion: a survey of the determinants of human and animal activity.* New York: Wiley, 1961.
16. Spragg SDS. Morphine addiction in chimpanzees. *Comp Psychol Monogr* 1940;15(7):1–132.
17. Olds J, Milner P. Positive reinforcement produced by electrical stimulation of septal area and other regions of rat brain. *J Comp Physiol Psychol* 1954;47:419–427.
18. Olds ME, Olds J. Approach-avoidance analysis of rat diencephalon. *J Comp Neurol* 1963;120:259–295.
19. Olds J. Pleasure centers in the brain. *Sci Am* 1956;195(4):105–116.
20. Olds J. Hypothalamic substrates of reward. *Physiol Rev* 1962;42:554–604.
21. Olds ME, Olds J. Drives, rewards and the brain. In: Newcomb TM, ed. *New directions in psychology.* New York: Holt, Rinehart & Winston, 1965:329–410.
22. Miller NE. Motivational effects of brain stimulation and drugs. *Fed Proc* 1960;19:846–853.
23. Margules DL, Olds J. Identical "feeding" and "rewarding" systems in the lateral hypothalamus of rats. *Science* 1962;135:374–375.
24. Hoebel BG, Teitelbaum P. Hypothalamic control of feeding and self-stimulation. *Science* 1962;135:375–377.
25. Coons EE, Levak M, Miller NE. Lateral hypothalamus: learning of food-seeking response motivated by electrical stimulation. *Science* 1965;150:1320–1321.
26. Hoebel BG. Feeding and self-stimulation. *Ann N Y Acad Sci* 1969;157:758–778.
27. Killam KF, Olds J, Sinclair J. Further studies on the effects of centrally acting drugs on self-stimulation. *J Pharmacol Exp Ther* 1957;119:157.
28. Kornetsky C. Brain-stimulation reward: a model for the neuronal bases for drug-induced euphoria. *NIDA Res Monogr Ser* 1985;62:30–50.
29. Wise RA. Action of drugs of abuse on brain reward systems. *Pharmacol Biochem Behav* 1980;13[Suppl 1]:213–223.
30. Wise RA. Neural mechanisms of the reinforcing action of cocaine. *NIDA Res Monogr Ser* 1984;50:15–33.
31. Wise RA, Bozarth MA. Brain substrates for reinforcement and drug self-administration. *Prog Neuropsychopharmacol* 1981;5:467–474.
32. Spealman RD, Goldberg SR. Drug self-administration by laboratory animals: control by schedules of reinforcement. *Annu Rev Pharmacol Toxicol* 1978;18:313–339.
33. Yokel RA. Intravenous self-administration: response rates, the effects of pharmacological challenges, and drug preferences. In: Bozarth MA, ed. *Methods of assessing the reinforcing properties of abused drugs.* New York: Springer-Verlag, 1987:1–33.
34. Weeks JR. Long-term intravenous infusion. In: Meyers RD, ed. *Methods in psychobiology.* New York: Academic Press, 1972:2;155–168.
35. Smith SG, Davis WM. A method for chronic intravenous drug administration in the rat. In: Ehrenpreis S, Neidle A, eds. *Methods in narcotics research.* New York: Marcel Dekker, 1975:3–32.
36. Deneau G, Yanagita T, Seevers MH. Self-administration of psychoactive substances by the monkey: a measure of psychological dependence. *Psychopharmacologia* 1969;16:30–48.
37. Yanagita T, Deneau GA, Seevers MH. Evaluation of pharmacologic agents in the monkey by long-term intravenous

self or programmed administration. *Excerpta Med Int Congr Ser* 1965;87:453–457.

38. Findley JD, Robinson WW, Peregrino L. Addiction to secobarbital and chlordiazepoxide in the rhesus monkey by means of a self-infusion preference procedure. *Psychopharmacologia* 1972;26:93–114.

39. Goldberg SR. Comparable behavior maintained under fixed-ratio and second-order schedules of food presentation, cocaine injection or *d*-amphetamine injection in the squirrel monkey. *J Pharmacol Exp Ther* 1973; 186:18–30.

40. Stretch R, Gerber GJ. A method for chronic intravenous drug administration in squirrel monkeys. *Can J Physiol Pharmacol* 1970;48:575–581.

41. Jones BE, Prada JA. Relapse to morphine use in dog. *Psychopharmacologia* 1973;30:1–12.

42. Smith JM, Renault PF, Schuster CR. A mild restraint and chronic venous catheterization system for cats. *Pharmacol Biochem Behav* 1975;3:713–715.

43. Balster RL, Kilbey MM, Ellinwood EH Jr. Methamphetamine self-administration in the cat. *Psychopharmacologia* 1976;46:229–233.

44. Goldberg SR, Hoffmeister F, Schlichting UU, et al. A comparison of pentobarbital and cocaine self-administration in rhesus monkeys: effects of dose and fixed-ratio parameter. *J Pharmacol Exp Ther* 1971;179:277–283.

45. Downs DA, Woods JH. Codeine- and cocaine-reinforced responding in rhesus monkeys: effects of dose on response rates under a fixed-ratio schedule. *J Pharmacol Exp Ther* 1974;191: 179–188.

46. Pickens R, Thompson T. Cocaine-reinforced behavior in rats: effects of reinforcement magnitude and fixed ratio size. *J Pharmacol Exp Ther* 1968; 161:122–129.

47. Goldberg SR, Kelleher RT. Behavior controlled by scheduled injections of cocaine in squirrel and rhesus monkeys. *J Exp Anal Behav* 1976;25:93–104.

48. Schlichting UU, Goldberg SR, Wuttke W, et al. *d*-Amphetamine self-administration by rhesus monkeys with different self-administration histories. *Excerpta Med Int Congr Ser* 1971;220:62–69.

49. Pickens R, Meisch R, McGuire LE. Methamphetamine reinforcement in rats. *Psychonomic Sci* 1967;8:371–372.

50. Pickens R, Harris WC. Self-administration of *d*-amphetamine by rats. *Psychopharmacologia* 1968;12:158–163.

51. Balster RL, Schuster CR. A comparison of *d*-amphetamine, *l*-amphetamine and methamphetamine self-administration in rhesus monkeys. *Pharmacol Biochem Behav* 1973;1:167–172.

52. Yokel RA, Pickens R. Self-administration of optical isomers of amphetamine and methylamphetamine by rats. *J Pharmacol Exp Ther* 1973; 187:27–33.

53. Risner ME. Intravenous self-administration of *d*- and *l*-amphetamine by dog. *Eur J Pharmacol* 1975;32:344–348.

54. Götestam KG, Andersson BE. Self-administration of amphetamine analogues in rats. *Pharmacol Biochem Behav* 1975;3:229–233.

55. Johanson CE, Schuster CR. A choice procedure for drug reinforcers: cocaine and methylphenidate in the rhesus monkey. *J Pharmacol Exp Ther* 1975;193:676–688.

56. Griffiths RR, Winger G, Brady JV, et al. Comparison on behavior maintained by infusions of eight phenylethylamines in baboons. *Psychopharmacology (Berl)* 1976;50:251–258.

57. Weeks JR, Collins RJ. Factors affecting voluntary morphine intake in self-maintained addicted rats. *Psychopharmacologia* 1964;6:267–279.

58. Hoffmeister F, Schlichting UU. Reinforcing properties of some opiates and opioids in rhesus monkeys with histories of cocaine and codeine self-administration. *Psychopharmacologia* 1972;23:55–74.

59. Collins RJ, Weeks JR. Relative potency of codeine, methadone and dihydromorphinone to morphine in self-maintained addict rats. *Naunyn Schmiedebergs Arch Pharmacol* 1965; 249:509–514.

60. Talley WH, Rosenblum I. Self-administration of dextropropoxyphene by rhesus monkeys to the point of toxicity. *Psychopharmacologia* 1972;27:179–182.

61. Smith SG, Werner TE, Davis WM. Effect of unit dose and route of administration on self-administration of morphine. *Psychopharmacology (Berl)* 1976;50:103–105.

62. Werner TE, Smith SG, Davis WM. A dose-response comparison between methadone and morphine self-administration. *Psychopharmacology (Berl)* 1976;47:209–211.

63. Schuster CR, Balster RL. Self-administration of agonists. In: Kosterlitz HW, Collier HOJ, Villarreal JE, eds. *Agonist and antagonist actions of narcotic analgesic drugs.* Baltimore: University Park Press, 1973:243–254.

64. Moreton JE, Roehrs T, Khazan N. Drug self-administration and sleep-wake activity in rats dependent on

morphine, methadone, or 1-alpha-acetylmethadol. *Psychopharmacology (Berl)* 1976;47:237–241.

65. Winger GD, Woods JH. The reinforcing property of ethanol in the rhesus monkey. I. Initiation, maintenance and termination of intravenous ethanol-reinforced responding. *Ann N Y Acad Sci* 1973;215:162–175.

66. Woods JH, Ikomi F, Winger G. The reinforcing property of ethanol. In: Roach MK, McIsaac WM, Creaven PJ, eds. *Biological aspects of alcohol.* Austin, TX: University of Texas Press, 1971:371–388.

67. Winger G, Stitzer ML, Woods JH. Barbiturate-reinforced responding in rhesus monkeys: comparisons of drugs with different durations of action. *J Pharmacol Exp Ther* 1975;195:505–514.

68. Yanagita T, Takahashi S. Dependence liability of several sedative-hypnotic agents evaluated in monkeys. *J Pharmacol Exp Ther* 1973;185:307–316.

69. Davis JD, Lulenski GC, Miller NE. Comparative studies of barbiturate self-administration. *Int J Addict* 1968;3: 207–214.

70. Kelleher RT. Characteristics of behavior controlled by scheduled injections of drugs. *Pharmacol Rev* 1975;27:307–323.

71. Balster RL, Johanson CE, Harris RT. Phencyclidine self-administration in the rhesus monkey. *Pharmacol Biochem Behav* 1973;1:167–172.

72. Moreton JE, Meisch RA, Stark L, Thompson T. Ketamine self-administration by the rhesus monkey. *J Pharmacol Exp Ther* 1977;203:303–309.

73. Pickens R, Thompson T. Characteristics of stimulant drug reinforcement. In: Thompson T, Pickens R, eds. *Stimulus properties of drugs.* New York: Appleton, 1971:177–192.

74. Pickens R, Thompson T. Simple schedules of drug self-administration in animals. In: Singh JM, Miller L, Lal H, eds. *Drug addiction. Experimental pharmacology.* Mount Kisco, NY: Futura, 1972;1:107–120.

75. Goldberg SR, Kelleher RT. Reinforcement of behavior by cocaine injections. In: Ellinwood EH Jr, Kilbey MM, eds. *Cocaine and other stimulants.* New York: Plenum, 1977:523–544.

76. Balster RL, Schuster CR. Fixed-interval schedule of cocaine reinforcement: effect of dose and infusion duration. *J Exp Anal Behav* 1973;20:119–129.

77. Dougherty J, Pickens R. Fixed-interval schedules of intravenous cocaine presentation in rats. *J Exp Anal Behav* 1973;20:111–118.

78. Woods JH, Schuster CR. Reinforcement properties of morphine, cocaine and SPA as a function of unit dose. *Int J Addict* 1968;3:231–237.

79. Schuster CR, Woods JH. The conditioned reinforcing effects of stimuli associated with morphine reinforcement. *Int J Addict* 1968;3:223–230.

80. Carney JM, Llewellyn ME, Woods JH. Variable interval responding maintained by intravenous codeine and ethanol injections in the rhesus monkey. *Pharmacol Biochem Behav* 1977;5:577–582.

81. Thompson T, Schuster CR. Morphine self-administration, food-reinforced and avoidance behaviors in rhesus monkeys. *Psychopharmacologia* 1964;5:87–94.

82. Anderson WW, Thompson T. Ethanol self-administration in water-satiated rats. *Pharmacol Biochem Behav* 1974;2:447–454.

83. Meisch RA, Thompson T. Ethanol as a reinforcer: an operant analysis of ethanol dependence. In: Singh JM, Lal H, eds. *Drug addiction,* vol. 3. *Neurobiology and influences on behavior.* Miami, FL: Symposia Specialists, 1974;3:117–133.

84. Yokel RA, Wise RA. Amphetamine-type reinforcement by dopaminergic agonists in the rat. *Psychopharmacology (Berl)* 1978;58:289–296.

85. Lyness WH, Friedle NM, Moore KE. Increased self-administration of *d*-amphetamine after destruction of 5-hydroxytryptaminergic neurons. *Pharmacol Biochem Behav* 1980;12:937–941.

86. Lang WJ, Latiff AA, McQueen A, et al. Self-administration of nicotine with and without a food delivery schedule. *Pharmacol Biochem Behav* 1977;7:65–70.

87. Lepore M, Franklin KBJ. Modelling drug kinetics with brain stimulation: dopamine antagonists increase self-stimulation. *Pharmacol Biochem Behav* 1992;41:489–496.

88. Harrigan SE, Downs DA. Self-administration of heroin, acetylmethadol, morphine, and methadone in rhesus monkeys. *Life Sci* 1978;22:619–624.

89. Johanson CE, Balster RL, Bonese K. Self-administration of psychomotor stimulant drugs: the effects of unlimited access. *Pharmacol Biochem Behav* 1976;4:45–51.

90. Risner ME, Jones BE. Self-administration of CNS stimulants by dog. *Psychopharmacologia* 1975;43:207–213.

91. Risner ME, Jones BE. Characteristics of unlimited access to self-administered stimulant infusions in dogs. *Biol Psychiatry* 1976;11:625–634.

92. Kramer JC, Fischman VS, Littlefield DC. Amphetamine abuse: pattern and effects of high doses taken intravenously. *JAMA* 1967;201:305–309.

93. Yanagita T, Takahashi S. Development of tolerance to and physical dependence on barbiturates in rhesus monkeys. *J Pharmacol Exp Ther* 1970;172:163–169.

94. Yokel RA, Pickens R. Drug level of *d*- and *l*-amphetamine during intravenous self-administration. *Psychopharmacologia* 1974;34:255–264.

95. Roberts DC, Bennett SA. Heroin self-administration in rats under a progressive ratio schedule of reinforcement. *Psychopharmacology (Berl)* 1993;111:215–218.

96. Roberts DC. Self-administration of GBR 12909 on a fixed ratio and progressive ratio schedule in rats. *Psychopharmacology (Berl)* 1993;111:202–206.

97. Bozarth MA, Wise RA. Toxicity associated with long-term intravenous heroin and cocaine self-administration in the rat. *JAMA* 1985;254:81–83.

98. Weeks JR, Collins RJ. Screening for drug reinforcement using intravenous self-administration in the rat. In: Bozarth MA, ed. *Methods of assessing the reinforcing properties of abused drugs.* New York: Springer-Verlag, 1987:35–43.

99. Brady JV, Griffiths RR, Hienz RD, et al. Assessing drugs for abuse liability and dependence potential in laboratory primates. In: Bozarth MA, ed. *Methods of assessing the reinforcing properties of abused drugs.* New York: Springer-Verlag, 1987:45–85.

100. Meisch RA, Carroll ME. Oral drug self-administration: drugs as reinforcers. In: Bozarth MA, ed. *Methods of assessing the reinforcing properties of abused drugs.* New York: Springer-Verlag, 1987:143–160.

101. Amit Z, Smith BR, Sutherland EA. Oral self-administration of alcohol: a valid approach to the study of drug self-administration and human alcoholism. In: Bozarth MA, ed. *Methods of assessing the reinforcing properties of abused drugs.* New York: Springer-Verlag, 1987:161–171.

102. Yanagita T. Prediction of drug abuse liability from animal studies. In: Bozarth MA, ed. *Methods of assessing the reinforcing properties of abused drugs.* New York: Springer-Verlag, 1987:189–198.

103. Esposito RU, Kornetsky C. Opioids and rewarding brain stimulation. *Neurosci Biobehav Rev* 1978;2:115–122.

104. Wise RA, Bozarth MA. Brain reward circuitry: four circuit elements "wired" in apparent series. *Brain Res Bull* 1984;12:203–208.

105. Wise RA, Rompre P-P. Brain dopamine and reward. *Annu Rev Psychol* 1989;40:191–225.

106. Reid LD. Tests involving pressing for intracranial stimulation as an early procedure for screening likelihood of addiction of opioids and other drugs. In: Bozarth MA, ed. *Methods of assessing the reinforcing properties of abused drugs.* New York: Springer-Verlag, 1987:391–420.

107. Olds J, Travis RP. Effects of chlorpromazine, meprobamate, pentobarbital and morphine on self-stimulation. *J Pharmacol Exp Ther* 1960;128:397–404.

108. Olds ME. Facilitatory action of diazepam and chlordiazepoxide on hypothalamic reward behavior. *J Comp Physiol Psychol* 1966;62:136–140.

109. Olds ME. Comparative effects of amphetamine, scopolamine, chlordiazepoxide and diphenylhydantoin on operant and extinction behaviour with brain stimulation and food reward. *Neuropharmacology* 1970;9:519–532.

110. Nazzaro JM, Seeger TF, Gardner EL. Morphine differentially affects ventral tegmental and substantia nigra brain reward thresholds. *Pharmacol Biochem Behav* 1981;14:325–331.

111. Nazzaro JM, Gardner EL, Bridger WH, et al. Pentobarbital induces a naloxone-reversible decrease in mesolimbic self-stimulation thresholds. *Soc Neurosci Abstr* 1981;7:262.

112. Herberg LJ, Rose IC. The effect of MK-801 and other antagonists of NMDA-type glutamate receptors on brain-stimulation reward. *Psychopharmacology (Berl)* 1989;99:87–90.

113. Gardner EL, Paredes W, Smith D, et al. Facilitation of brain stimulation reward by Δ^9-tetrahydrocannabinol. *Psychopharmacology (Berl)* 1988;96:142–144.

114. Chen J, Gardner EL. *In vivo* brain microdialysis study of phencyclidine on presynaptic dopamine efflux in rat caudate nucleus. *Soc Neurosci Abstr* 1988;14:525.

115. Di Chiara G, Imperato A. Preferential stimulation of dopamine release in the nucleus accumbens by opiates, alcohol, and barbiturates: studies with transcerebral dialysis in freely moving rats. *Ann N Y Acad Sci* 1986;473:367–381.

116. Gysling K, Wang RY. Morphine-induced activation of A10 dopamine neurons in rats brains. *Brain Res* 1983;277:119–127.

117. Hernandez L, Hoebel BG. Food reward and cocaine increase extracellular dopamine in the nucleus accumbens as measured by microdialysis. *Life Sci* 1988;42:1705–1712.

118. Hommer DW, Pert A. The action of opiates in the rat substantia nigra: an electrophysiological analysis. *Peptides* 1983;4:603–608.
119. Imperato A, Di Chiara G. Preferential stimulation of dopamine release in the nucleus accumbens of freely moving rats by ethanol. *J Pharmacol Exp Ther* 1986;239:219–228.
120. Imperato A, Mulas A, Di Chiara G. Nicotine preferentially stimulates dopamine release in the limbic system of freely moving rats. *Eur J Pharmacol* 1986;132:337–338.
121. Kalivas PW, Widerlov E, Stanley D, et al. Enkephalin action on the mesolimbic system: a dopamine-dependent and a dopamine-independent increase in locomotor activity. *J Pharmacol Exp Ther* 1983;227:229–237.
122. Kalivas PW, Duffy P, Dilts R, et al. Enkephalin modulation of A10 dopamine neurons: a role in dopamine sensitization. *Ann N Y Acad Sci* 1988;537:405–414.
123. Westerink BHC, Tuntler J, Damsma G, et al. The use of tetrodotoxin for the characterization of drug-enhanced dopamine release in conscious rats studied by brain dialysis. *Naunyn Schmiedebergs Arch Pharmacol* 1987;336:502–507.
124. Wise RA, Bozarth MA. A psychomotor stimulant theory of addiction. *Psychol Rev* 1987;94:469–492.
125. Wilson MC, Schuster CR. Mazindol self-administration in the rhesus monkey. *Pharmacol Biochem Behav* 1976;4:207–210.
126. Bergman J, Madras BK, Johnson SE, et al. Effects of cocaine and related drugs in nonhuman primates. III. Self-administration by squirrel monkeys. *J Pharmacol Exp Ther* 1989;251:150–155.
127. Woods JH, Katz JL, Medzihradsky F, et al. Evaluation of new compounds for opioid activity: 1982 annual report. *NIDA Res Monogr Ser* 1983;43:457–511.
128. Winger G, Woods JH. Comparison of fixed-ratio and progressive-ratio schedules of maintenance of stimulant drug-reinforced responding. *Drug Alcohol Depend* 1985;15:123–130.
129. Risner ME, Silcox DL. Psychostimulant self-administration by beagle dogs in a progressive-ratio paradigm. *Psychopharmacology (Berl)* 1981;75:25–30.
130. Corwin RL, Woolverton WL, Schuster CR, et al. Anorectics: effects on food intake and self-administration in rhesus monkeys. *Alcohol Drug Res* 1987;7:351–361.
131. van der Zee P, Koger HS, Gootjes J, et al. Aryl 1,4-dialk(en)yl-piperazines as selective and very potent inhibitors of dopamine uptake. *Eur J Med Chem* 1980;15:363–370.
132. Heikkila RE, Manzino L. Behavioral properties of GBR 12909,GBR 13069 and GBR 13098: specific inhibitors of dopamine uptake. *Eur J Pharmacol* 1984;103:241–248.
133. Gill CA, Holz WC, Zirkle CL, et al. Pharmacological modification of cocaine and apomorphine self-administration in the squirrel monkey. In: Denker P, Radouco-Thomas C, Villeneuve A, et al. eds. *Proceedings of the Tenth Congress of the Collegium Internationale Neuropsychopharmacologium.* New York: Pergamon Press, 1978:1477–1484.
134. Woolverton WL, Goldberg LI, Ginos JZ. Intravenous self-administration of dopamine receptor agonists by rhesus monkeys. *J Pharmacol Exp Ther* 1984;230:678–683.
135. Baxter BL, Gluckman MI, Stein L, et al. Self-injection of apomorphine in the rat: positive reinforcement by a dopamine receptor stimulant. *Pharmacol Biochem Behav* 1974;2:387–391.
136. Davis WM, Smith SG. Catecholaminergic mechanisms of reinforcement: direct assessment by drug self-administration. *Life Sci* 1977;20:483–492.
137. Hoffmeister F, Wuttke W. Psychotropic drugs as negative reinforcers. *Pharmacol Rev* 1975;27:419–428.
138. Kandel DA, Schuster CR. An investigation of nalorphine and perphenazine as negative reinforcers in an escape paradigm. *Pharmacol Biochem Behav* 1977;6:61–71.
139. Baldessarini RJ. Drugs and the treatment of psychiatric disorders. In: Gilman AG, Goodman LS, Rall TW, et al, eds. *Goodman and Gilman's the pharmacological basis of therapeutics,* 7th ed. New York: Macmillan, 1985:387–445.
140. Rech R. Neurolepsis: anhedonia or blunting of emotional reactivity? *Behav Brain Sci* 1982;5:72–73.
141. Downs DA, Woods JH. Fixed-ratio escape and avoidance-escape from naloxone in morphine-dependent monkeys: effects of naloxone dose and morphine pretreatment. *J Exp Anal Behav* 1975;23:415–427.
142. Ettenberg A, Pettit HO, Bloom FE, Koob GF. Heroin and cocaine intravenous self-administration in rats: mediation by separate neural systems. *Psychopharmacology (Berl)* 1982;78:204–209.
143. Goldberg SR, Hoffmeister F, Schlichting U, et al. Aversive properties of nalorphine and naloxone in morphine-dependent rhesus monkeys. *J Pharmacol Exp Ther* 1971;179:268–276.
144. Killian A, Bonese K, Rothberg RM, et al. Effects of passive immunization against morphine on heroin self-administration. *Pharmacol Biochem Behav* 1978;9:347–352.
145. Baxter BL, Gluckman MI, Scerni RA. Apomorphine self-injection is not affected by alpha-methylparatyrosine treatment: support for dopaminergic reward. *Pharmacol Biochem Behav* 1976;4:611–612.
146. Pickens R, Meisch RA, Dougherty JA Jr. Chemical interactions in methamphetamine reinforcement. *Psychol Rep* 1968;23:1267–1270.
147. Wilson MC, Schuster CR. Aminergic influences on intravenous cocaine self-administration by rhesus monkeys. *Pharmacol Biochem Behav* 1974;2:563–571.
148. Yokel RA, Wise RA. Increased lever pressing for amphetamine after pimozide in rats: implications for a dopamine theory of reward. *Science* 1975;187:547–549.
149. Yokel RA, Wise RA. Attenuation of intravenous amphetamine reinforcement by central dopamine blockade in rats. *Psychopharmacology (Berl)* 1976;48:311–318.
150. de Wit H, Wise RA. Blockade of cocaine reinforcement in rats with the dopamine receptor blocker pimozide, but not with the noradrenergic blockers phentolamine or phenoxybenzamine. *Can J Psychol* 1977;31:195–203.
151. Herling S, Woods JH. Chlorpromazine effects on cocaine-reinforced responding in rhesus monkeys: reciprocal modification of rate-altering effects of the drugs. *J Pharmacol Exp Ther* 1980;214:354–361.
152. Johanson CE, Kandel DA, Bonese K. The effects of perphenazine on self-administration behavior. *Pharmacol Biochem Behav* 1976;4:427–433.
153. Risner ME, Jones BE. Role of noradrenergic and dopaminergic processes in amphetamine self-administration. *Pharmacol Biochem Behav* 1976;5:477–482.
154. Risner ME, Jones BE. Characteristics of b-phenethylamine self-administration by dog. *Pharmacol Biochem Behav* 1977;6:689–696.
155. Risner ME, Jones BE. Intravenous self-administration of cocaine and norcocaine by dogs. *Psychopharmacology (Berl)* 1980;71:83–89.
156. Stretch R. Discrete-trial control of cocaine self-injection behaviour in squirrel monkeys: effects of morphine, naloxone, and chlorpromazine. *Can J Physiol Pharmacol* 1977;55:778–790.
157. Wilson MC, Schuster CR. The effects of chlorpromazine on psychomotor stimulant self-administration in the

rhesus monkey. *Psychopharmacologia* 1972;26:115–126.

158. Wilson MC, Schuster CR. The effects of stimulants and depressants on cocaine self-administration behavior in the rhesus monkey. *Psychopharmacologia* 1973;31:291–304.

159. Davis WM, Smith SG. Noradrenergic basis for reinforcement associated with morphine action in nondependent rats. In: Singh JM, Lal H, eds. *Drug addiction, vol. 3. Neurobiology and influences on behavior.* Miami, FL: Symposia Specialists, 1974:155–168.

160. Hanson HM, Cimini-Venema CA. Effects of haloperidol on self-administration of morphine in rats. *Fed Proc* 1972;31:503.

161. Roberts DCS, Vickers G. Atypical neuroleptics increase self-administration of cocaine: an evaluation of a behavioral screen for antipsychotic activity. *Psychopharmacology (Berl)* 1984;82:135–139.

162. de la Garza R, Johanson CE. Effects of haloperidol and physostigmine on self-administration of local anesthetics. *Pharmacol Biochem Behav* 1982;17:1295–1299.

163. Woolverton WL. Effects of a D1 and D2 dopamine antagonist on the self-administration of cocaine and piribedil by rhesus monkeys. *Pharmacol Biochem Behav* 1986;24:531–535.

164. Jönsson LE, Gunne LM, Änggard E. Effects of alpha-methyltyrosine in amphetamine-dependent subjects. *Pharmacol Clin* 1969;2:27–29.

165. Jönsson L, Änggard E, Gunne L. Blockade of intravenous amphetamine euphoria in man. *Clin Pharmacol Ther* 1971;12:889–896.

166. Jönsson LE. Pharmacological blockade of amphetamine effects in amphetamine dependent subjects. *Eur J Clin Pharmacol* 1972;4:206–211.

167. Gunne LM, Änggard E, Jönsson LE. Clinical trails with amphetamine-blocking drugs. *Psychiat Neurol Neurochir* 1972;75:225–226.

168. Roberts DCS, Zito KA. Interpretation of lesion effects on stimulant self-administration. In: Bozarth MA, ed. *Methods of assessing the reinforcing properties of abused drugs.* New York: Springer-Verlag, 1987:87–103.

169. Roberts DCS, Corcoran ME, Fibiger HC. On the role of ascending catecholamine systems in self-administration of cocaine. *Pharmacol Biochem Behav* 1977;6:615–620.

170. Roberts DCS, Koob GF. Disruption of cocaine self-administration following 6-hydroxydopamine lesions of the ventral tegmental area in rats. *Pharmacol Biochem Behav* 1982;17:901–904.

171. Moore RY, Bloom FE. Central catecholamine neuron systems: anatomy and physiology of the dopamine systems. *Annu Rev Neurosci* 1978;1:129–169.

172. Lyness WH, Friedle NM, Moore KE. Destruction of dopaminergic nerve terminals in nucleus accumbens: effect on *d*-amphetamine self-administration. *Pharmacol Biochem Behav* 1979;11:553–556.

173. Glick SD, Cox RS, Crane AM. Changes in morphine self-administration and morphine dependence after lesions of the caudate nucleus in rats. *Psychopharmacologia* 1975;41:219–224.

174. Bozarth MA, Wise RA. Heroin reward is dependent on a dopaminergic substrate. *Life Sci* 1981;29:1881–1886.

175. Spyraki C, Fibiger HC, Phillips AG. Attenuation of heroin reward in rats by disruption of the mesolimbic dopamine system. *Psychopharmacology (Berl)* 1983;79:278–283.

176. Rolls ET. *The brain and reward.* Oxford: Pergamon Press, 1975.

177. Routtenberg A. The reward system of the brain. *Sci Am* 1978;239(5):154–164.

178. Olds ME, Fobes JL. The central basis of motivation: intracranial self-stimulation studies. *Annu Rev Psychol* 1981;32:523–574.

179. Heath RG. Pleasure response of human beings to direct stimulation of the brain: physiologic and psychodynamic considerations. In: Heath RG, ed. *The role of pleasure in behavior.* New York: Hoeber, 1964:219–243.

180. Bursten B, Delgado JMR. Positive reinforcement induced by intracerebral stimulation in the monkey. *J Comp Physiol Psychol* 1958;51:6–10.

181. Wilkinson HA, Peele TL. Intracranial self-stimulation in cats. *J Comp Neurol* 1963;121:425–440.

182. Briese E, Olds J. Reinforcing brain stimulation and memory in monkeys. *Exp Neurol* 1964;10:493–508.

183. Valenstein ES. The anatomical locus of reinforcement. *Prog Physiol Psychol* 1966;1:149–190.

184. Wetzel MC. Self-stimulation's anatomy: data needs. *Brain Res* 1968;10:287–296.

185. Routtenberg A, Malsbury C. Brainstem pathways of reward. *J Comp Physiol Psychol* 1969;68:22–30.

186. Dahlström A, Fuxe K. Evidence for the existence of monoamine-containing neurons in the central nervous system: I. Demonstration of monoamines in the cell bodies of brainstem neurons. *Acta Physiol Scand* 1964;62[Suppl 232]:1–80.

187. Fuxe K. Evidence for the existence of monoamine neurons in the central nervous system: IV. Distribution of monoamine nerve terminals in the central nervous system. *Acta Physiol Scand* 1965;64[Suppl 247]:37–85.

188. Andén N-E, Dahlström A, Fuxe K, et al. Ascending monoamine neurons to the telencephalon and diencephalon. *Acta Physiol Scand* 1966;67:313–326.

189. Ungerstedt U. Stereotaxic mapping of the monoamine pathways in the rat brain. *Acta Physiol Scand* 1971;82[Suppl 367]:1–48.

190. Crow TJ. A map of the rat mesencephalon for electrical self-stimulation. *Brain Res* 1972;36:265–273.

191. Corbett D, Wise RA. Intracranial self-stimulation in relation to the ascending dopaminergic systems of the midbrain: a moveable electrode mapping study. *Brain Res* 1980;185:1–15.

192. Mogenson GJ, Takigawa M, Robertson A, et al. Self-stimulation of the nucleus accumbens and ventral tegmental area of Tsai attenuated by microinjections of spiroperidol into the nucleus accumbens. *Brain Res* 1979;171:247–259.

193. Zarevics P, Setler PE. Simultaneous rate-independent and rate-dependent assessment of intracranial self-stimulation: evidence for the direct involvement of dopamine in brain reinforcement mechanisms. *Brain Res* 1979;169:499–512.

194. Wise RA. The dopamine synapse and the notion of "pleasure centers" in the brain. *Trends Neurosci* 1980;3:91–95.

195. Fray PJ, Dunnett SB, Iversen SD, et al. Nigral transplants reinnervating the dopamine-depleted neostriatum can sustain intracranial self-stimulation. *Science* 1983;219:416–420.

196. Wise RA. Brain dopamine and reward. In: Cooper SJ, ed. *Theory in psychopharmacology.* New York: Academic Press, 1981;1:103–122.

197. Fibiger HC, Phillips AG. Mesocorticolimbic dopamine systems and reward. *Ann N Y Acad Sci* 1988;537:206–215.

198. Wise RA. Neuroleptics and operant behavior: the anhedonia hypothesis. *Behav Brain Sci* 1982;5:39–53.

199. Gallistel CR. Self-stimulation in the rat: quantitative characteristics of the reward pathway. *J Comp Physiol Psychol* 1978;92:977–998.

200. Gallistel CR, Shizgal P, Yeomans J. A portrait of the brain for self-stimulation. *Psychol Rev* 1981;88:228–273.

201. Shizgal P, Bielajew C, Corbett D, Skelton R, Yeomans J. Behavioral methods for inferring anatomical linkage between rewarding brain stimulation sites. *J Comp Physiol Psychol* 1980;94:227–237.

202. Yeomans JS. The absolute refractory periods of self-stimulation neurons. *Physiol Behav* 1979;22:911–919.

203. Yeomans JS, Matthews GG, Hawkins

RD, et al. Characterization of self-stimulation neurons by their local potential summation properties. *Physiol Behav* 1979;22:921–929.

204. Yeomans JS. Two substrates for medial forebrain bundle self-stimulation: myelinated axons and dopamine axons. *Neurosci Biobehav Rev* 1989;13:91–98.

205. Bielajew C, Shizgal P. Evidence implicating descending fibers in self-stimulation of the medial forebrain bundle. *J Neurosci* 1986;6:919–929.

206. Waraczynski MA, Ng Cheong Ton JM, et al. Failure of amygdaloid lesions to increase the threshold for self-stimulation of the lateral hypothalamus and ventral tegmental area. *Behav Brain Res* 1990;40:159–168.

207. Waraczynski MA, Conover K, Shizgal P. Rewarding effectiveness of caudal MFB stimulation is unaltered following DMH lesions. *Physiol Behav* 1992;52:211–218.

208. Colle LM, Wise RA. Opposite effects of unilateral forebrain ablations on ipsilateral and contralateral hypothalamic self-stimulation. *Brain Res* 1987;407:285–293.

209. Ikemoto S, Panksepp J. The relationship between self-stimulation and sniffing in rats: does a common brain system mediate these behaviors? *Behav Brain Res* 1994;61:143–162.

210. Waraczynski MA. Basal forebrain knife cuts and medial forebrain bundle self-stimulation. *Brain Res* 1988;438:8–22.

211. Geeraedts LMG, Nieuwenhuys R, Veening JG. Medial forebrain bundle of the rat: III. Cytoarchitecture of the rostral (telencephalic) part of the medial forebrain bundle bed nucleus. *J Comp Neurol* 1990;294:507–536.

212. Murray B, Shizgal P. Attenuation of medial forebrain bundle reward by anterior lateral–hypothalamic lesions. *Behav Brain Res* 1996;75:33–47.

213. Murray B, Shizgal P. Behavioral measures of conduction velocity and refractory period for reward-relevant axons in the anterior LH and VTA. *Physiol Behav* 1996;59:643–652.

214. Murray B, Shizgal P. Physiological measures of conduction velocity and refractory period for putative reward-relevant MFB axons arising in the rostral MFB. *Physiol Behav* 1996;59:427–437.

215. Gallistel CR, Leon M, Lim BT, et al. Destruction of the medial forebrain bundle caudal to the site of stimulation reduces rewarding efficacy but destruction rostrally does not. *Behav Neurosci* 1996;110:766–790.

216. Heimer L, Zahm DS, Churchill L, et al. Specificity in the projections patterns of accumbal shell and core in the rat. *Neuroscience* 1991;41:89–125.

217. Mogenson GJ, Swanson LW, Wu M. Neural projections from nucleus accumbens to globus pallidus, substantia innominata, and lateral preoptic–lateral hypothalamic area: an anatomical and electrophysiological investigation in the rat. *J Neurosci* 1983;3:189–202.

218. Kalivas PW, Churchill L, Klitenick MA. GABA and enkephalin projection from the nucleus accumbens and ventral pallidum to the ventral tegmental area. *Neuroscience* 1993;57:1047–1060.

219. McAlonan GM, Robbins TW, Everitt BJ. Effects of medial dorsal thalamic and ventral pallidal lesions on the acquisition of a conditioned place preference: further evidence for the involvement of the ventral striatopallidal system in reward-related processes. *Neuroscience* 1993;52:605–620.

220. Chrobak JJ, Napier TC. Opioid and GABA modulation of accumbens-evoked ventral pallidal activity. *J Neural Transm Gen Sect* 1993;93:123–143.

221. Inglis WL, Dunbar JS, Winn P. Outflow from the nucleus accumbens to the pedunculopontine tegmental nucleus: a dissociation between locomotor activity and the acquisition of responding for conditioned reinforcement stimulated by *d*-amphetamine. *Neuroscience* 1994;62:51–64.

222. Hubner CB, Koob GF. The ventral pallidum plays a role in mediating cocaine and heroin self-administration in the rat. *Brain Res* 1990;508:20–29.

223. Robledo P, Koob GF. Two discrete nucleus accumbens projection areas differentially mediate cocaine self-administration in the rat. *Behav Brain Res* 1993;55:159–166.

224. Stein EA. Ventral tegmental self-stimulation selectively induces opioid peptide release in rat CNS. *Synapse* 1993;13:63–73.

225. Johnson PI, Stellar JR, Paul AD. Regional reward differences within the ventral pallidum are revealed by microinjections of a mu opiate receptor agonist. *Neuropharmacology* 1993;32:1305–1314.

226. Johnson PI, Stellar JR. Comparison of delta opiate receptor agonist induced reward and motor effects between the ventral pallidum and dorsal striatum. *Neuropharmacology* 1994;33:1171–1182.

227. Klitenick MA, Deutsch AY, Churchill L, et al. Topography and functional role of dopaminergic projections from the ventral mesencephalic tegmentum to the ventral pallidum. *Neuroscience* 1992;50:371–386.

228. Anagnostakis Y, Spyraki C. Effect of morphine applied by intrapallidal microdialysis on the release of dopamine in the nucleus accumbens. *Brain Res Bull* 1994;34:275–282.

229. Sesack SR, Pickel VM. Prefrontal cortical efferents in the rat synapse on unlabelled neuronal targets of catecholamine terminals in the nucleus accumbens septi and on dopamine neurons in the ventral tegmental area. *J Comp Neurol* 1992;320:145–160.

230. Self DW, Nestler EJ. Molecular mechanisms of drug reinforcement and addiction. *Annu Rev Neurosci* 1995;18:463–495.

231. Carlezon WA Jr, Wise RA. Rewarding actions of phencyclidine and related drugs in nucleus accumbens shell and frontal cortex. *J Neurosci* 1996;16:3112–3122.

232. Graybiel AM. Neurotransmitters and neuromodulators in the basal ganglia. *Trends Neurosci* 1990;13:244–254.

233. Gerfen CR. The neostriatal mosaic: multiple levels of compartmental organization. *Trends Neurosci* 1992;15:133–139.

234. Kawaguchi Y, Wilson CJ, Augood SJ, et al. Striatal interneurones: chemical physiological and morphological characterization. *Trends Neurosci* 1995;18:527–535.

235. Smith AD, Bolam JP. The neural network of the basal ganglia as revealed by the study of synaptic connections of identified neurons. *Trends Neurosci* 1990;13:259–265.

236. Bolam JP, Bennett BD. Microcircuitry of the neostriatum. In: Ariano MA, Surmeier DJ, eds. *Molecular and cellular mechanisms of neostriatal function.* New York: R.G. Landes, 1995:1–19.

237. Sesack SR, Pickel VM. Ultrastructural relationships between terminals immunoreactive for enkephalin, GABA, or both transmitters in the rat ventral tegmental area. *Brain Res* 1995;672:261–275.

238. Maneuf YP, Mitchell IJ, Crossman AR, et al. On the role of enkephalin cotransmission in the GABAergic striatal efferents to the globus pallidus. *Exp Neurol* 1994;125:65–71.

239. Esposito RU, Porrino LJ, Seeger TF. Brain stimulation reward: measurement and mapping by psychophysical techniques and quantitative 2-[^{14}C]deoxyglucose autoradiography. In: Bozarth MA, ed. *Methods of assessing the reinforcing properties of abused drugs.* New York: Springer-Verlag, 1987:421–445.

240. Stein L, Ray OS. Brain stimulation reward "thresholds" self-determined in rat. *Psychopharmacologia* 1960;1:251–256.

241. Nazzaro JM, Gardner EL. GABA antagonism lowers self-stimulation

thresholds in the ventral tegmental area. *Brain Res* 1980;189:279–283.

242. Seeger TF, Nazzaro JM, Gardner EL. Selective inhibition of mesolimbic behavioral supersensitivity by naloxone. *Eur J Pharmacol* 1980;65:435–438.

243. Nazzaro JM, Seeger TF, Gardner EL. Naloxone blocks phencyclidine's dose-dependent effects on direct brain reward thresholds. In: *Proceedings of world conference on clinical pharmacology and therapeutics.* London: British Pharmacological Society, 1980:949.

244. Gardner EL, Paredes W, Seeger TF, et al. Mesolimbic DA antagonism by 5HT₃ receptor blockade. In: *Book of abstracts. World Psychiatric Association regional symposium: the research and clinical interface for psychiatric disorders, October 13–16, 1988, Washington, DC.* Washington, DC: American Psychiatric Association, 1988:222.

245. Gardner EL. An improved technique for determining brain reward thresholds in primates. *Behav Res Methods Instrum* 1971;3:273–274.

246. Seeger TF, Gardner EL. Enhancement of self-stimulation behavior in rats and monkeys after chronic neuroleptic treatment: evidence for mesolimbic supersensitivity. *Brain Res* 1979;175:49–57.

247. Esposito RU, Kornetsky C. Morphine lowering of self-stimulation thresholds: lack of tolerance with long-term administration. *Science* 1977;195:189–191.

248. Stein L. Effects and interactions of imipramine, chlorpromazine, reserpine, and amphetamine on self-stimulation: possible neurophysical basis of depression. In: Wortis J, ed. *Recent advances in biological psychiatry.* New York: Plenum Press, 1962;4:297–311.

249. Seeger TF, Carlson KR. Amphetamine and morphine: additive effects on ICSS threshold. *Soc Neurosci Abstr* 1981;7:974.

250. Seeger TF, Carlson KR, Nazzaro JM. Pentobarbital induces a naloxone-reversible decrease in mesolimbic self-stimulation threshold. *Pharmacol Biochem Behav* 1981;15:583–586.

251. Cassens GP, Mills AW. Lithium and amphetamine: opposite effects on threshold of intracranial reinforcement. *Psychopharmacologia* 1973;30:283–290.

252. Kelly K, Reid LD. Addictive agents and intracranial stimulation: morphine and thresholds for positive intracranial reinforcement. *Bull Psychonomic Soc* 1977;10:298–300.

253. Lewis MJ. Age related decline in brain stimulation reward: rejuvenation by amphetamine. *Exp Aging Res* 1983;7:225–234.

254. Lewis MJ, Phelps RW. A multifunctional on-line brain stimulation system: investigation of alcohol and aging effects. In: Bozarth MA, ed. *Methods of assessing the reinforcing properties of abused drugs.* New York: Springer-Verlag, 1987:463–478.

255. Marcus R, Kornetsky C. Negative and positive intracranial reinforcement thresholds: effects of morphine. *Psychopharmacologia* 1974;38:1–13.

256. Esposito RU, McLean S, Kornetsky C. Effects of morphine on intracranial self-stimulation to various brain stem loci. *Brain Res* 1979;168:425–429.

257. Kornetsky C, Esposito RU. Euphorigenic drugs: effects on the reward pathways of the brain. *Fed Proc* 1979;38:2473–2476.

258. Esposito RU, Motola AHD, Kornetsky C. Cocaine: acute effects on reinforcement thresholds for self-stimulation behavior to the medial forebrain bundle. *Pharmacol Biochem Behav* 1978;8:437–439.

259. Esposito RU, Perry W, Kornetsky C. Effects of d-amphetamine and naloxone on brain stimulation reward. *Psychopharmacology (Berl)* 1980;69:187–191.

260. Hubner CB, Bain GT, Kornetsky C. Morphine and amphetamine: effect on brain stimulation reward. *Soc Neurosci Abstr* 1983;9:893.

261. Atrens DM, Von Vietinghoff-Reisch F, Der-Karabetian A, et al. Modulation of reward and aversion processes in the rat diencephalon by amphetamine. *Am J Physiol* 1974;226:874–880.

262. Liebman JM, Butcher LL. Comparative involvement of dopamine and noradrenaline in rate-free self-stimulation in substantia nigra, lateral hypothalamus and mesencephalic central gray. *Naunyn Schmiedebergs Arch Pharmacol* 1974;284:167–194.

263. Phillips AG, Fibiger HC. Dopaminergic and noradrenergic substrates of positive reinforcement: differential effects of d- and l-amphetamine. *Science* 1973;179:575–577.

264. Jaffe JH, Martin WR. Opioid analgesics and antagonists. In: Gilman AG, Goodman LS, Rall TW, Murad F, eds. *Goodman and Gilman's the pharmacological basis of therapeutics,* 7th ed. New York: Macmillan, 1985:491–531.

265. Marshall JF, Rosenstein AJ. Age-related decline in rat striatal dopamine metabolism is regionally homogeneous. *Neurobiol Aging* 1990;11:131–137.

266. Franklin KBJ. Catecholamines and self-stimulation: reward and performance effects dissociated. *Pharmacol Biochem Behav* 1978;9:813–820.

267. Esposito RU, Faulkner W, Kornetsky C. Specific modulation of brain stimulation reward by haloperidol. *Pharmacol Biochem Behav* 1979;10:937–940.

268. Esposito RU, Perry W, Kornetsky C. Chlorpromazine and brain-stimulation reward: potentiation of effects by naloxone. *Pharmacol Biochem Behav* 1981;15:903–905.

269. Gardner EL, Paredes W, Smith D, et al. Facilitation of brain stimulation reward by Δ⁹-tetrahydrocannabinol is mediated by an endogenous opioid mechanism. *Adv Biosci* 1989;75:671–674.

270. Lorens SA, Sainati SM. Naloxone blocks the excitatory effect of ethanol and chlordiazepoxide on lateral hypothalamic self-stimulation behavior. *Life Sci* 1978;23:1359–1364.

271. Kornetsky C, Bain G, Reidl EM. Effects of cocaine and naloxone on brain stimulation reward. *Pharmacologist* 1981;23:192.

272. Khachaturian H, Lewis ME, Schäfer MK-H, et al. Anatomy of the CNS opioid systems. *Trends Neurosci* 1985;8:111–119.

273. Mansour A, Khachaturian H, Lewis M, et al. Anatomy of CNS opioid receptors. *Trends Neurosci* 1988;11:308–314.

274. Gardner EL, Zukin RS, Makman MH. Modulation of opiate receptor binding in striatum and amygdala by selective mesencephalic lesions. *Brain Res* 1980;194:232–239.

275. Pollard H, Llorens C, Bonnet JJ, et al. Opiate receptors on mesolimbic dopaminergic neurons. *Neurosci Lett* 1977;7:295–299.

276. Pollard H, Llorens C, Schwartz JC, et al. Localization of opiate receptors and enkephalins in the rat striatum in relationship with the nigrostriatal dopaminergic system: lesion studies. *Brain Res* 1978;151:392–398.

277. Hirschhorn ID, Hittner D, Gardner EL, et al. Evidence for a role of endogenous opioids in the nigrostriatal system: influence of naloxone and morphine on nigrostriatal dopaminergic supersensitivity. *Brain Res* 1983;270:109–117.

278. Pickel VM, Chan J. Ultrastructural basis for interactions between opioid peptides and dopamine in rat striatum. *Soc Neurosci Abstr* 1989;15:810.

279. Kubota Y, Inagaki S, Kito S, et al. Ultrastructural evidence of dopaminergic input to enkephalinergic neurons in rat neostriatum. *Brain Res* 1986;367:374–378.

280. Routtenberg A. Intracranial chemical injection and behavior: a critical review. *Behav Biol* 1972;7:601–641.

281. Bozarth MA. Intracranial self-administration procedures for the assessment of drug reinforcement. In: Bozarth MA, ed. *Methods of assessing the reinforcing properties of abused drugs.* New York: Springer-Verlag, 1987:173–187.

282. Broekkamp CLE. Combined microinjection and brain stimulation reward methodology for the localization of reinforcing drug effects. In: Bozarth MA, ed. *Methods of assessing the reinforcing properties of abused drugs.* New York: Springer-Verlag, 1987:479–488.

283. Broekkamp CLE, van den Bogaard JH, Cools AR, et al. Separation of inhibiting and stimulating effects of morphine on self-stimulation behavior by intracerebral microinjections. *Eur J Pharmacol* 1976;36:443–446.

284. Broekkamp CLE, van Rossum JM. The effect of microinjections of morphine and haloperidol into the neostriatum and the nucleus accumbens on self-stimulation behavior. *Arch Int Pharmacodyn Ther* 1975;217:110–117.

285. Broekkamp CLE, Phillips AG, Cools AR. Facilitation of self-stimulation behavior following intracerebral microinjections of opioids into the ventral tegmental area. *Pharmacol Biochem Behav* 1979;11:289–295.

286. Broekkamp CLE, Pijnenburg AJJ, Cools AR, et al. The effect of microinjections of amphetamine into the neostriatum and nucleus accumbens on self-stimulation behavior. *Psychopharmacology (Berl)* 1975;42:179–183.

287. Stellar JR, Corbett D. Regional neuroleptic microinjections indicate a role for nucleus accumbens in lateral hypothalamic self-stimulation reward. *Brain Res* 1989;477:126–143.

288. Jenck F, Gratton A, Wise RA. Opioid receptor subtypes associated with ventral tegmental facilitation of lateral hypothalamic brain stimulation reward. *Brain Res* 1987;423:34–38.

289. Colle LM, Wise RA. Effects of nucleus accumbens amphetamine on lateral hypothalamic brain stimulation reward. *Brain Res* 1988;459:361–368.

290. Phillips AG, Broekkamp CL, Fibiger HC. Strategies for studying the neurochemical substrates of drug reinforcement in rodents. *Prog Neuropsychopharmacol Biol Psychiatry* 1983;7:585–590.

291. Bozarth MA. Opiate reward mechanisms mapped by intracranial self-administration. In: Smith JE, Lane JD, eds. *Neurobiology of opiate reward processes.* Amsterdam: Elsevier North Holland Biomedical Press, 1983:331–359.

292. Myers RD. Methods for chemical stimulation of the brain. In: Myers RD, ed. *Methods in psychobiology.* New York: Academic Press, 1972;1:247–280.

293. Myers RD. *Handbook of drug and chemical stimulation of the brain.* New York: Van Nostrand Reinhold, 1974.

294. Bozarth MA, Wise RA. Electrolytic microinfusion transducer system: an alternative method of intracranial drug application. *J Neurosci Methods* 1980;2:273–275.

295. Renner KE. Delay of reinforcement: a historical review. *Psychol Bull* 1964;61:341–361.

296. Tarpy RM, Sawabini FL. Reinforcement delay: a selective review of the last decade. *Psychol Bull* 1974;81:984–997.

297. Phillips AG, Mora F, Rolls ET. Intracerebral self-administration of amphetamine by rhesus monkeys. *Neurosci Lett* 1981;24:81–86.

298. Monaco AP, Hernandez L, Hoebel BG. Nucleus accumbens: site of amphetamine self-administration. Comparison with the lateral ventricle. In: Chronister RB, DeFrance JF, eds. *Neurobiology of the nucleus accumbens.* Brunswick, ME: Haer Institute, 1981:338–343.

299. Hoebel BG, Monaco AP, Hernandez L, et al. Self-injection of amphetamine directly into the brain. *Psychopharmacology (Berl)* 1983;81:158–163.

300. Goeders NE, Smith JE. Cortical dopaminergic involvement in cocaine reinforcement. *Science* 1983;221:773–775.

301. Bozarth MA, Wise RA. Intracranial self-administration of morphine into the ventral tegmental area in rats. *Life Sci* 1981;28:551–555.

302. Bozarth MA, Wise RA. Localization of reward-relevant opiate receptors. *NIDA Res Monogr Ser* 1982;41:158–164.

303. Stein EA, Olds J. Direct intracerebral self-administration of opiates in the rat. *Soc Neurosci Abstr* 1977;3:302.

304. Olds ME. Hypothalamic substrate for the positive reinforcing properties of morphine in the rat. *Brain Res* 1979;168:351–360.

305. Olds ME. Reinforcing effects of morphine in the nucleus accumbens. *Brain Res* 1982;237:429–440.

306. van Ree JM, De Wied D. Involvement of neurohypophyseal peptides in drug-mediated adaptive responses. *Pharmacol Biochem Behav* 1980;13[Suppl 1]:257–263.

307. Goeders NE, Lane JD, Smith JE. Self-administration of methionine enkephalin into the nucleus accumbens. *Pharmacol Biochem Behav* 1984;20:451–455.

308. Olds ME, Williams KN. Self-administration of d-ala^2-met-enkephalinamide at hypothalamic self-stimulation sites. *Brain Res* 1980;194:155–170.

309. Britt MD, Wise RA. Ventral tegmental site of opiate reward: antagonism by a hydrophilic opiate receptor blocker. *Brain Res* 1983;258:105–108.

310. McBride WJ, Murphy JM, Gatto GJ, et al. CNS mechanisms of alcohol self-administration. *Alcohol Alcohol Suppl* 1993;2:463–467.

311. Pert A, Yaksh T. Sites of morphine induced analgesia in the primate brain: relation to pain pathways. *Brain Res* 1974;80:135–140.

312. Part A, Yaksh T. Localization of the antinociceptive action of morphine in primate brain. *Pharmacol Biochem Behav* 1975;3:135–138.

313. Teasdale JAP, Bozarth MA, Stewart J. Body temperature responses to microinjections of morphine in brain sites containing opiate receptors. *Soc Neurosci Abstr* 1981;7:799.

314. Bozarth MA, Wise RA. Anatomically distinct opiate receptor fields mediate reward and physical dependence. *Science* 1984;244:516–517.

315. Justice JB Jr, ed. *Voltammetry in the neurosciences: principles, methods, and applications.* Clifton, NJ: Humana Press, 1987.

316. Marsden CA, ed. *Measurement of neurotransmitter release in vivo. IBRO handbook series: Methods in the neurosciences,* vol. 6. New York: Wiley, 1984.

317. Myers RD, Knott PJ, eds. Neurochemical analysis of the conscious brain: voltammetry and push–pull perfusion. *Ann N Y Acad Sci* 1986;473.

318. Leviel V, Guibert B. Involvement of intraterminal dopamine compartments in the amine release in the cat striatum. *Neurosci Lett* 1987;76:197–202.

319. Kuczenski R. Dose response for amphetamine-induced changes in dopamine levels in push–pull perfusates of rat striatum. *J Neurochem* 1986;46:1605–1611.

320. Imperato A, Di Chiara G. Transstriatal dialysis coupled to reverse phase high performance liquid chromatography with electrochemical detection: a new method for the study of the *in vivo* release of endogenous dopamine and metabolites. *J Neurosci* 1984;4:966–977.

321. Johnson RD, Justice JB Jr. Model studies for brain dialysis. *Brain Res Bull* 1983;10:567–571.

322. Gardner EL, Chen J, Paredes W. Overview of chemical sampling techniques. *J Neurosci Methods* 1993;48:173–197.

323. Zetterström T, Sharp T, Marsden CA, et al. In vivo measurement of dopamine and its metabolites by intracerebral dialysis: changes after *d*-amphetamine. *J Neurochem* 1983;41:1769–1773.

324. Paredes W, Chen J, Gardner E. A miniature microdialysis probe: a new simple construction method for making a chronic, removable and recyclable probe. *Curr Separations* 1989;9:94.

325. Adams RN, Marsden CA. Electrochemical detection methods for monoamine measurements *in vitro* and *in vivo*. In: Iversen LL, Iversen SS, Snyder SH, eds. *Handbook of psychopharmacology*. New York: Plenum, 1982;15:1–74.

326. Stamford JA. *In vivo* voltammetry: promise and perspective. *Brain Res Rev* 1985;10:119–135.

327. Schenk JO, Adams RN. Chronoamperometric measurements in the central nervous system. In: Marsden CA, ed. *Measurement of neurotransmitter release in vivo. IBRO handbook series: Methods in the neurosciences,* vol. 6. New York: Wiley, 1984:193–208.

328. Gerhardt GA, Oke AF, Nagy G, et al. Nafion-coated electrodes with high selectivity for CNS electrochemistry. *Brain Res* 1984;290:390–395.

329. Vulto AG, Sharp T, Ungerstedt U. Rapid post-mortal increase in extracellular concentration of dopamine in the rat brain as assessed by intra-cranial dialysis. *Soc Neurosci Abstr* 1985;11:1207.

330. Di Chiara G, Imperato A. Drugs abused by humans preferentially increase synaptic dopamine concentrations in the mesolimbic system of freely moving rats. *Proc Natl Acad Sci U S A* 1988;85:5274–5278.

331. Hurd YL, Kehr J, Ungerstedt U. In vivo microdialysis as a technique to monitor drug transport: correlation of extracellular cocaine levels and dopamine overflow in the rat brain. *J Neurochem* 1988;51:1314–1316.

332. Hurd YL, Weiss F, Koob G, et al. Cocaine reinforcement and extracellular dopamine overflow in rat nucleus accumbens: an *in vivo* microdialysis study. *Brain Res* 1989;498:199–203.

333. Hurd YL, Weiss F, Koob G, et al. The influence of cocaine self-administration on *in vivo* dopamine and acetylcholine neurotransmission in rat caudate-putamen. *Neurosci Lett* 1990;109:227–233.

334. Akimoto K, Hamamura T, Kazahaya Y, et al. Enhanced extracellular dopamine level may be the fundamental neuropharmacological basis of cross-behavioral sensitization between methamphetamine and cocaine—an *in vivo* dialysis study in freely moving rats. *Brain Res* 1990;507:344–346.

335. Pettit HO, Pan H-T, Parsons LH, et al. Extracellular concentrations of cocaine and dopamine are enhanced during chronic cocaine administration. *J Neurochem* 1990;55:798–804.

336. Nomikos GG, Damsma G, Wenkstern D, et al. In vivo characterization of locally applied dopamine uptake inhibitors by striatal microdialysis. *Synapse* 1990;6:106–112.

337. Church WH, Justice JB Jr, Byrd LD. Extracellular dopamine in rat striatum following uptake inhibition by cocaine, nomifensine and benztropine. *Eur J Pharmacol* 1987;139:345–348.

338. Akimoto K, Hamamura T, Otsuki S. Subchronic cocaine treatment enhances cocaine-induced dopamine efflux, studied by *in vivo* intracerebral dialysis. *Brain Res* 1989;490:339–344.

339. Pettit HO, Justice JB Jr. Dopamine in the nucleus accumbens during cocaine self-administration as studied by *in vivo* microdialysis. *Pharmacol Biochem Behav* 1989;34:899–904.

340. Nicolaysen LC, Pan H, Justice JB Jr. Extracellular cocaine and dopamine concentrations are linearly related in rat striatum. *Brain Res* 1988;456:317–323.

341. Goeders NE, Kuhar MJ. Chronic cocaine administration induces opposite changes in dopamine receptors in the striatum and nucleus accumbens. *Alcohol Drug Res* 1987;7:207–216.

342. Memo M, Pradhan A, Hanbauer I. Cocaine-induced supersensitivity of striatal dopamine receptors: role of endogenous calmodulin. *Neuropharmacology* 1981;20:1145–1150.

343. Post RM, Rose H. Increasing effects of repetitive cocaine administration in the rat. *Nature* 1976;260:731–732.

344. Shuster L, Yu G, Bates A. Sensitization to cocaine stimulation in mice. *Psychopharmacology (Berl)* 1977;52:185–190.

345. Trulson ME, Ulissey MJ. Chronic cocaine administration decreases dopamine synthesis rate and increases [³H]spiroperidol binding in rat brain. *Brain Res Bull* 1987;19:35–38.

346. Kalivas PW, Duffy P, DuMars LA, et al. Behavioral and neurochemical effects of acute and daily cocaine administration in rats. *J Pharmacol Exp Ther* 1988;245:485–492.

347. Brock JW, Ng JP, Justice JB Jr. Effect of chronic cocaine on dopamine synthesis in the nucleus accumbens as determined by microdialysis perfusion with NSD-1015. *Neurosci Lett* 1990;117:234–239.

348. Van Rossum J, Van Schoot J, Hurkman J. Mechanism of action of cocaine and amphetamine in the brain. *Experientia* 1982;18:229–230.

349. Reith MEA, Meisler BE, Sershen H, et al. Structural requirements for cocaine congeners to interact with dopamine and serotonin uptake sites in mouse brain and to induce stereotyped behavior. *Biochem Pharmacol* 1986;35:1123–1129.

350. Sharp T, Zetterström T, Ljungberg T, et al. A direct comparison of amphetamine-induced behaviours and regional brain dopamine release in the rat using intracerebral dialysis. *Brain Res* 1987;401:322–330.

351. Wood PL, Kim HS, Marien MR. Intracerebral dialysis: direct evidence for the utility of 3-MT measurements as an index of dopamine release. *Life Sci* 1987;41:1–5.

352. Hernandez L, Lee F, Hoebel BG. Simultaneous microdialysis and amphetamine infusion in the nucleus accumbens and striatum of freely moving rats: increase in extracellular dopamine and serotonin. *Brain Res Bull* 1987;19:623–628.

353. Butcher SP, Fairbrother IS, Kelly JS, et al. Amphetamine-induced dopamine release in the rat striatum: an *in vivo* microdialysis study. *J Neurochem* 1988;50:346–355.

354. Zetterström T, Sharp T, Collin AK, et al. *In vivo* measurement of extracellular dopamine and DOPAC in rat striatum after various dopamine-releasing drugs: implications for the origin of extracellular DOPAC. *Eur J Pharmacol* 1988;148:327–334.

355. Robinson TE, Jurson PA, Bennett JA, et al. Persistent sensitization of dopamine neurotransmission in ventral striatum (nucleus accumbens) produced by prior experience with (+)-amphetamine: a microdialysis study in freely moving rats. *Brain Res* 1988;462:211–222.

356. Westerink BH, Hofsteede RM, Tuntler J, et al. Use of calcium antagonism for the characterization of drug-evoked dopamine release from the brain of conscious rats determined by microdialysis. *J Neurochem* 1989;52:722–729.

357. Hoebel BG, Hernandez L, Schwartz DH, et al. Microdialysis studies of brain norepinephrine, serotonin, and dopamine release during ingestive behavior: theoretical and clinical implications. *Ann N Y Acad Sci* 1989;575:171–191.

358. Hiramatsu M, Cho AK. Enantiomeric differences in the effects of 3,4-methylenedioxymethamphetamine on extracellular monoamines and metabolites in the striatum of freely-moving rats: an *in vivo* microdialysis study. *Neuropharmacology* 1990;29:269–275.

359. Gazzara RA, Takeda H, Cho AK, et al. Inhibition of dopamine release by methylenedioxymethamphetamine is mediated by serotonin. *Eur J Pharmacol* 1989;168:209–217.

360. Di Chiara G, Imperato A. Opposite effects of mu and kappa opiate agonists on dopamine release in the nucleus accumbens and in the dorsal caudate of

freely moving rats. *J Pharmacol Exp Ther* 1988;244:1067–1080.

361. Imperato A, Angelucci L. 5-HT₃ receptors control dopamine release in the nucleus accumbens of freely moving rats. *Neurosci Lett* 1989;101:214–217.

362. Carboni E, Acquas E, Frau R, et al. Differential inhibitory effects of a 5-HT₃ antagonist on drug-induced stimulation of dopamine release. *Eur J Pharmacol* 1989;164:515–519.

363. Spanagel R, Herz A, Shippenberg TS. The effects of opioid peptides on dopamine release in the nucleus accumbens: an *in vivo* microdialysis study. *J Neurochem* 1990;55:1734–1740.

364. Mucha RF, Herz A. Motivational properties of kappa and mu opioid receptor agonists studied with place and taste preference conditioning. *Psychopharmacology (Berl)* 1985;86:274–280.

365. Shippenberg TS, Bals-Kubik R, Herz A. Endogenous opioids and reinforcement: role of multiple opioid receptor types and dopamine. *NIDA Res Monogr Ser* 1988;90:40.

366. Kalivas PW, Duffy P, Eberhardt H. Modulation of A10 dopamine neurons by gamma-aminobutyric acid agonists. *J Pharmacol Exp Ther* 1990;253:858–866.

367. Wood PL, Altar CA. Dopamine release *in vivo* from nigrostriatal, mesolimbic, and mesocortical neurons: utility of 3-methoxytyramine measurements. *Pharmacol Rev* 1988;40:163–187.

368. Damsma G, Westerink BH, de Vries JB, et al. The effect of systemically applied cholinergic drugs on the striatal release of dopamine and its metabolites, as determined by automated brain dialysis in conscious rats. *Neurosci Lett* 1988;89:349–354.

369. Cashaw JL, Geraghty CA, McLaughlin BR, et al. Effect of acute ethanol administration on brain levels of tetrahydropapaveroline in L-dopa-treated rats. *J Neurosci Res* 1987;18:497–503.

370. Hernandez L, Auerbach S, Hoebel BG. Phencyclidine (PCP) injected in the nucleus accumbens increases extracellular dopamine and serotonin as measured by microdialysis. *Life Sci* 1988;42:1713–1723.

371. Carboni E, Imperato A, Perezzani I, et al. Amphetamine, cocaine, phencyclidine and nomifensine increase extracellular dopamine concentrations preferentially in the nucleus accumbens of freely moving rats. *Neuroscience* 1989;28:653–661.

372. Chen J, Paredes W, Li J, et al. Δ⁹-Tetrahydrocannabinol produces naloxone-blockable enhancement of presynaptic basal dopamine efflux in nucleus accumbens of conscious, freely-moving rats as measured by in-

tracerebral microdialysis. *Psychopharmacology (Berl)* 1990;102:156–162.

373. Ng Cheong Ton JM, Gardner EL. Effects of delta-9-tetrahydrocannabinol on dopamine release in the brain: intracerebral dialysis experiments. *Soc Neurosci Abstr* 1986;12:135.

374. Ng Cheong Ton JM, Gerhardt GA, et al. Effects of Δ⁹-tetrahydrocannabinol on potassium-evoked release of dopamine in the rat caudate nucleus: an *in vivo* electrochemical and *in vivo* microdialysis study. *Brain Res* 1988;451:59–68.

375. Chen J, Paredes W, Lowinson JH, et al. Δ⁹-Tetrahydrocannabinol enhances presynaptic dopamine efflux in medial prefrontal cortex. *Eur J Pharmacol* 1990;190:259–262.

376. Pontieri FE, Tanda G, Di Chiara G. Intravenous cocaine, morphine, and amphetamine preferentially increase extracellular dopamine in the "shell" as compared with the "core" of the rat nucleus accumbens. *Proc Natl Acad Sci U S A* 1995;92:12304–12308.

377. Pothos EN, Creese I, Hoebel BG. Restricted eating with weight loss selectively decreases extracellular dopamine in the nucleus accumbens and alters dopamine response to amphetamine, morphine, and food intake. *J Neurosci* 1995;15:6640–6650.

378. Brazell MP, Marsden CA. Intracerebral injection of ascorbate oxidase—effect on *in vivo* electrochemical recordings. *Brain Res* 1982;249:167–172.

379. Mueller K. *In vivo* voltammetric recording with Nafion-coated carbon paste electrodes: additional evidence that ascorbic acid release is monitored. *Pharmacol Biochem Behav* 1986;25:325–328.

380. Ewing AG, Alloway KD, Curtis SD, et al. Simultaneous electrochemical and unit recording measurements: characterization of *d*-amphetamine and ascorbic acid on neostriatal neurons. *Brain Res* 1983;261:101–108.

381. Salamone JD, Hambry LS, Neill DB, et al. Extracellular ascorbic acid increases in striatum following systemic amphetamine. *Pharmacol Biochem Behav* 1984;20:609–612.

382. Crespi F, Sharp T, Maidment N, et al. Differential pulse voltammetry: *in vivo* evidence that uric acid contributes to the indole oxidation peak. *Neurosci Lett* 1083;43:203–207.

383. Mueller K, Palmour R, Andrews CD, et al. *In vivo* voltammetric evidence of production of uric acid by rat caudate. *Brain Res* 1985;335:231–235.

384. Haskett C, Mueller K. The effects of serotonin depletion on the voltammetric response to amphetamine. *Pharmacol Biochem Behav* 1987;28:381–384.

385. Mueller K, Haskett C. Effects of

haloperidol on amphetamine-induced increases in ascorbic acid and uric acid as determined by voltammetry *in vivo*. *Pharmacol Biochem Behav* 1987;27:231–234.

386. Dayton MA, Ewing AG, Wightman RM. Response of microvoltammetric electrodes to homogeneous catalytic and slow heterogeneous charge-transfer reactions. *Anal Chem* 1980;52:2392–2396.

387. Echizen M, Freed CR. Factors affecting *in vivo* electrochemistry: electrode-tissue interactions and the ascorbate amplification effect. *Life Sci* 1986;39:77–89.

388. Gonon F, Buda M, Cespuglio R, et al. *In vivo* electrochemical detection of catechols in the neostriatum of anesthetized rats: dopamine or DOPAC? *Nature* 1980;286:902–904.

389. Stamford JA, Kruk ZL, Millar J. Stimulated limbic and striatal dopamine release measured by fast cyclic voltammetry: anatomical, electrochemical and pharmacological characterisation. *Brain Res* 1988;454:282–288.

390. Stamford JA, Kruk ZL, Millar J. Dissociation of the actions of uptake blockers upon dopamine overflow and uptake in the rat nucleus accumbens: *in vivo* voltammetric data. *Neuropharmacology* 1989;28:1383–1388.

391. Gerhardt GA, Gratton A, Rose GM. *In vivo* electrochemical studies of the effects of cocaine on dopamine nerve terminals in the rat neostriatum. *Physiol Bohemoslov* 1988;37:249–257.

392. Kelly RS, Wightman RM. Detection of dopamine overflow and diffusion with voltammetry in slices of rat brain. *Brain Res* 1987;423:79–87.

393. Ng JP, Hubert GW, Justice JB Jr. Increased stimulated release and uptake of dopamine in nucleus accumbens after repeated cocaine administration as measured by *in vivo* voltammetry. *J Neurochem* 1991;56:1485–1492.

394. Forni C, Nieoullon A. Electrochemical detection of dopamine release in the striatum of freely moving hamsters. *Brain Res* 1984;297:11–20.

395. Nieoullon A, Forni C, El Ganouni S. Contribution to the study of nigrostriatal dopaminergic neuron activity using electrochemical detection of dopamine release in the striatum of freely moving animals. *Ann N Y Acad Sci* 1986;473:126–134.

396. Gazzara RA, Fisher RS, Howard-Butcher S. The ontogeny of amphetamine-induced dopamine release in the caudate-putamen of the rat. *Devel Brain Res* 1986;28:213–220.

397. Stamford JA, Kruk ZL, Millar J. Measurement of stimulated dopamine release in the rat by *in vivo* voltammetry:

the influence of stimulus duration on drug responses. *Neurosci Lett* 1986; 69:70–73.

398. Knott PJ, Brannan TS, Andrews CD, et al. Drug, stress, and circadian influences on dopaminergic neuronal function in the rat studied by voltammetry and chronoamperometry. *Ann N Y Acad Sci* 1986;473:493–495.

399. Gazzara RA, Howard-Butcher S. A developmental study of amphetamine-induced dopamine release in rats using *in vivo* voltammetry. *Ann N Y Acad Sci* 1986;473:527–529.

400. Hughes CW, Pottinger HJ. Chronic CNS recording with *in vivo* electrochemistry in rats: monitoring biogenic amine release in behavioral and pharmacological models of depression. *Ann N Y Acad Sci* 1986;473:530–534.

401. Lane RF, Blaha CD, Hari SP. Electrochemistry *in vivo*: monitoring dopamine release in the brain of the conscious, freely moving rat. *Brain Res Bull* 1987;19:19–27.

402. Gonzalez-Mora JL, Sanchez-Bruno JA, Mas M. Concurrent on-line analysis of striatal ascorbate, dopamine and dihydroxyphenylacetic acid concentrations by *in vivo* voltammetry. *Neurosci Lett* 1988;86:61–66.

403. Gonon FG. Nonlinear relationship between impulse flow and dopamine released by rat midbrain dopaminergic neurons as studied by *in vivo* electrochemistry. *Neuroscience* 1988;24:19–28.

404. May LJ, Kuhr WG, Wightman RM. Differentiation of dopamine overflow and uptake processes in the extracellular fluid of the rat caudate nucleus with fast-scan *in vivo* voltammetry. *J Neurochem* 1988;51:1060–1069.

405. Forni C, Brundin P, Strecker RE, et al. Time-course of recovery of dopamine neuron activity during reinnervation of the denervated striatum by fetal mesencephalic grafts as assessed by *in vivo* voltammetry. *Exp Brain Res* 1989;76:75–87.

406. Yamamoto BK, Pehek EA. A neurochemical heterogeneity of the rat striatum as measured by *in vivo* electrochemistry and microdialysis. *Brain Res* 1990;506:236–242.

407. Suaud-Chagny M-F, Buda M, Gonon FG. Pharmacology of electrically evoked dopamine release studied in the rat olfactory tubercle by *in vivo* electrochemistry. *Eur J Pharmacol* 1989;164:273–283.

408. Yamamoto BK, Spanos LJ. The acute effects of methylenedioxymethamphetamine on dopamine release in the awake-behaving rat. *Eur J Pharmacol* 1988;148:195–203.

409. Gardner EL. Cannabinoid interaction with brain reward systems—The neurobiological basis of cannabinoid abuse. In: Murphy LL, Bartke A, eds. *Marijuana/cannabinoids: neurobiology and neurophysiology.* Boca Raton, FL: CRC Press, 1992:275–335.

410. Broderick PA, Gardner EL, van Praag HM. *In vivo* electrochemical evidence for an opiate-induced modulation of dopaminergic and serotonergic systems in rat striatum. Paper presented at meetings of American College of Neuro-Psychopharmacology, San Juan, Puerto Rico, 1983.

411. Broderick PA. *In vivo* electrochemical studies of rat striatal dopamine and serotonin release after morphine. *Life Sci* 1985;36:2269–2275.

412. Ostrowski NL, Paul I, Drnach M, et al. Changes in locomotor activity and in the discharge rates of midbrain dopamine neurons with repeated administrations of low doses of morphine. *Soc Neurosci Abstr* 1983;9:280.

413. Broderick PA, Phelan FT. Neurochemical aspects of morphine tolerance in the freely moving and behaving animal: voltammetric studies. *Prog Clin Biol Res* 1990;328:501–506.

414. Milne B, Quintin L, Pujol JF. Fentanyl increases catecholamine oxidation current measured by *in vivo* voltammetry in the rat striatum. *Can J Anaesth* 1989;36:155–159.

415. Broderick PA, Gardner EL, van Praag HM. *In vivo* electrochemical and behavioral evidence for specific neural substrates modulated differentially by enkephalin in rat stimulant stereotypy and locomotion. *Biol Psychiatry* 1984;19:45–54.

416. Broderick PA. Striatal neurochemistry of dynorphin-(1–13): *in vivo* electrochemical semidifferential analyses. *Neuropeptides* 1987;10:369–386.

417. Morgan ME, Vestal RE. Methylxanthine effects on caudate dopamine release as measured by *in vivo* electrochemistry. *Life Sci* 1989;45:2025–2039.

418. Ford AP, Marsden CA. Influence of anaesthetics on rat striatal dopamine metabolism *in vivo*. *Brain Res* 1986;379:162–166.

419. Engel JA, Fahlke C, Hulthe P, et al. Biochemical and behavioral evidence for an interaction between ethanol and calcium channel antagonists. *J Neural Transm* 1988;74:181–193.

420. Signs SA, Yamamoto BK, Schechter MD. *In vivo* electrochemical determination of extracellular dopamine in the caudate of freely-moving rats after a low dose of ethanol. *Neuropharmacology* 1987;26:1653–1656.

421. Gerhardt GA, Pang K, Rose GM. *In vivo* electrochemical demonstration of the presynaptic actions of phencyclidine in rat caudate nucleus. *J Pharmacol Exp Ther* 1987;241:714–721.

422. Serrano A, D'Angio M, Scatton B. NMDA antagonists block restraint-induced increases in extracellular DOPAC in rat nucleus accumbens. *Eur J Pharmacol* 1989;162:157–166.

423. Crespi F, Keane PE. The effect of diazepam and Ro 15–1788 on extracellular ascorbic acid, DOPAC and 5-HIAA in the striatum of anesthetized and conscious freely moving rats, as measured by differential pulse voltammetry. *Neurosci Res* 1987;4:323–329.

424. Brose N, O'Neill RD, Boutelle MG, et al. Dopamine in the basal ganglia and benzodiazepine-induced sedation. *Neuropharmacology* 1988;27:589–595.

425. Brose N, O'Neill RD, Boutelle MG, et al. The effects of anxiolytic and anxiogenic benzodiazepine receptor ligands on motor activity and levels of ascorbic acid in the nucleus accumbens and striatum of the rat. *Neuropharmacology* 1989;28:509–514.

426. Randall LO, Schallek W, Heise GA, et al. The psychosedative properties of methaminodiazepoxide. *J Pharmacol Exp Ther* 1960;129:163–197.

427. Soubrié P, Kulkarni S, Simon P, et al. Effets des anxiolytiques sur la prise de nourriture de rats et de souris placés en situation nouvelle ou familière. [The effects of anxiolytics on feeding behavior in rats and mice in novel or familiar environments.] *Psychopharmacologia* 1975;45:203–210.

428. Cooper SJ. Benzodiazepines as appetite-enhancing compounds. *Appetite* 1980;1:7–19.

429. Cooper SJ. A microgram dose of diazepam produces specific inhibition of ambulation in the rat. *Pharmacol Biochem Behav* 1985;22:25–30.

430. Poschel BPH. A simple and specific screen for diazepam-like drugs. *Psychopharmacologia* 1971;19:193–198.

431. Stapleton JM, Lind MD, Merriman VJ, et al. Naloxone inhibits diazepam induced feeding in rats. *Life Sci* 1979;24:2421–2426.

432. Wise RA, Dawson V. Diazepam-induced eating and lever pressing for food in sated rats. *J Comp Physiol Psychol* 1974;86:930–941.

433. Anderson-Baker WC, McLaughlin CL, Baile CA. Oral and hypothalamic injections of barbiturates, benzodiazepines and cannabinoids and food intake in rats. *Pharmacol Biochem Behav* 1979;11:487–491.

434. Britton DR, Britton KT, Dalton D, et al. Effects of naloxone on anti-conflict and hyperphagic actions of diazepam. *Life Sci* 1981;29:1297–1302.

435. Cole SO. Combined effects of chlordiazepoxide treatment and food deprivation on concurrent measures of feeding and activity. *Pharmacol Biochem Behav* 1983;18:369–372.
436. Della-Fera MA, Baile CA, McLaughlin CL. Feeding elicited by benzodiazepine-like chemicals in puppies and cats: structure-activity relationships. *Pharmacol Biochem Behav* 1980;12:195–200.
437. Gratton A, Wise RA. Comparisons of refractory periods for medial forebrain bundle fibers subserving stimulation-induced feeding and brain stimulation reward: a psychophysical study. *Brain Res* 1988;438:256–263.
438. Gratton A, Wise RA. Comparisons of connectivity and conduction velocities for medial forebrain bundle fibers subserving stimulation-induced feeding and brain stimulation reward. *Brain Res* 1988;438:264–270.
439. Pitts DK, Marwah J. Cocaine modulation of central monoaminergic neurotransmission. *Pharmacol Biochem Behav* 1987;26:453–461.
440. Peterson SL, Olsta SA, Matthews RT. Cocaine enhances medial prefrontal cortex neuron response to ventral tegmental area activation. *Brain Res Bull* 1990;24:267–273.
441. Bunney BS, Walters JR, Roth RH, et al. Dopaminergic neurons: effect of antipsychotic drugs and amphetamine on single cell activity. *J Pharmacol Exp Ther* 1973;185:560–571.
442. Bunney BS. The electrophysiological pharmacology of midbrain dopaminergic systems. In: Horn AS, Korf J, Westerink BHC, eds. *The neurobiology of dopamine.* New York: Academic Press, 1979:417–452.
443. Rebec GV. Electrophysiological pharmacology of amphetamine. *Monogr Neural Sci* 1987;13:1–33.
444. Chiodo LA. Dopamine-containing neurons in the mammalian central nervous system: electrophysiology and pharmacology. *Neurosci Biobehav Rev* 1988;12:49–91.
445. Rebec GV, Segal DS. Dose-dependent biphasic alterations in the spontaneous activity of neurons in the rat neostriatum produced by *d*-amphetamine and methylphenidate. *Brain Res* 1978;150:353–366.
446. Rebec GV, Alloway KD, Curtis SD. Apparent serotonergic modulation of the dose-dependent biphasic response of neostriatal neurons produced by *d*-amphetamine. *Brain Res* 1981;210:277–289.
447. Iwatsubo K, Clouet DH. Effects of morphine and haloperidol on the electrical activity of rat nigrostriatal neurons. *J Pharmacol Exp Ther* 1977;202:429–436.
448. Matthews RT, German DC. Electrophysiological evidence for excitation of rat ventral tegmental dopamine neurons by morphine. *Neuroscience* 1984;11:617–625.
449. Nowycky MC, Walters JR, Roth RH. Dopaminergic neurons: effect of acute and chronic morphine administration on single cell activity and transmitter metabolism. *J Neural Transm* 1978;42:99–116.
450. Hakan RL, Henriksen SJ. Systemic opiate administration has heterogeneous effects on activity recorded from nucleus accumbens neurons *in vivo*. *Neurosci Lett* 1987;83:307–312.
451. Henriksen SJ, Hakan RL. Responses of nucleus accumbens neurons to systemically and locally administered opiates provide evidence for dopamine (DA)-dependent and DA-independent circuitry underlying opiate self-administration. *Adv Biosci* 1989;75:675–678.
452. Walker JM, Thompson LA, Frascella J, et al. Opposite effects of mu and kappa opiates on the firing-rate of dopamine cells in the substantia nigra of the rat. *Eur J Pharmacol* 1987;134:53–59.
453. Crain SM, Shen K-F, Chalazonitis A. Opioids excite rather than inhibit sensory neurons after chronic opioid exposure of spinal cord–ganglion cultures. *Brain Res* 1988;455:99–109.
454. Crain SM, Shen K-F. Dual excitatory and inhibitory opioid modulation of the action potential duration of mouse dorsal root ganglion neurons in cultures. *Adv Biosci* 1988;75:189–192.
455. North RA. Opioid receptor types and membrane ion channels. *Trends Neurosci* 1986;9:114–117.
456. Nicoll RA, Siggins GR, Ling N, et al. Neuronal actions of endorphins and enkephalin among brain regions: a comparative microiontophoretic study. *Proc Natl Acad Sci U S A* 1977;74:2584–2588.
457. Duggan AW, North RA. Electrophysiology of opioids. *Pharmacol Rev* 1984;35:219–281.
458. Finnerty EP, Chan SHH. Morphine suppression of substantia nigra zona reticulata neurons in the rat: implicated role for a novel striato-nigral feedback mechanism. *Eur J Pharmacol* 1979;18:37–56.
459. Kelley AE, Stinus L, Iversen SD. Interaction between d-ala-met-enkephalin, A₁₀ dopaminergic neurons and spontaneous behavior in the rat. *Behav Brain Res* 1980;1:3–24.
460. Mereu G, Yoon KW, Boi V, et al. Preferential stimulation of ventral tegmental area dopaminergic neurons by nicotine. *Eur J Pharmacol* 1987;141:395–399.
461. Mereu GP, Fadda F, Gessa GL. Ethanol stimulates the firing-rate of nigral-dopaminergic neurones in anaesthetized rats. *Brain Res* 1984;292:63–69.
462. Johnson SW, Haroldsen PE, Hoffer BJ, et al. Presynaptic dopaminergic activity of phencyclidine in rat caudate. *J Pharmacol Exp Ther* 1984;229:322–332.
463. Johnson SW, Palmer MR, Freedman R. Effects of dopamine on spontaneous and evoked activity of caudate neurons. *Neuropharmacology* 1983;22:843–851.
464. Freeman AS, Bunney BS. The effects of phencyclidine and N-allylnormetazocine on midbrain dopamine neuronal activity. *Eur J Pharmacol* 1984;104:287–293.
465. Marwah J. Candidate mechanisms underlying phencyclidine-induced psychosis: an electrophysiological, behavioral, and biochemical study. *Biol Psychiatry* 1982;17:155–198.
466. Kirch DG, Palmer MR, Egan M, et al. Electrophysiological interactions between haloperidol and reduced haloperidol, and dopamine, norepinephrine and phencyclidine in rat brain. *Neuropharmacology* 1985;24:375–379.
467. Rouillard C, Chiodo LA, Freeman AS. The effects of the phencyclidine analogs BTCP and TCP on nigrostriatal dopamine neuronal activity. *Eur J Pharmacol* 1990;182:227–235.
468. Steinfels GF, Tam SW, Cook L. Electrophysiological effects of selective sigma-receptor agonists, antagonists, and the selective phencyclidine receptor agonist MK-801 on midbrain dopamine neurons. *Neuropsychopharmacology* 1989;2:201–208.
469. O'Brien DP, White FJ. Inhibition of non-dopamine cells in the ventral tegmental area by benzodiazepines: relationship to A10 dopamine cell activity. *Eur J Pharmacol* 1987;142:343–354.
470. Wise RA. *In vivo* estimates of extracellular dopamine and dopamine metabolite levels during intravenous cocaine or heroin self-administration. *Semin Neurosci* 1993;5:337–342.
471. Wise RA, Newton P, Leeb K, et al. Fluctuations in nucleus accumbens dopamine concentration during intravenous cocaine self-administration in rats. *Psychopharmacology (Berl)* 1995;120:10–20.
472. Pettit HO, Justice JB Jr. Effect of dose on cocaine self-administration behavior and dopamine levels in the nucleus accumbens. *Brain Res* 1991;539:94–102.

473. Parsons LH, Koob GF, Weiss F. Serotonin dysfunction in the nucleus accumbens of rats during withdrawal after unlimited access to intravenous cocaine. *J Pharmacol Exp Ther* 1995;274:1182–1191.

474. Wise RA, Leone P, Rivest R, Leeb K. Elevations of nucleus accumbens dopamine and DOPAC levels during intravenous heroin self-administration. *Synapse* 1995;21:140–148.

475. Hemby SE, Martin TJ, Co C, et al. The effects of intravenous heroin administration on extracellular nucleus accumbens dopamine concentrations as determined by *in vivo* microdialysis. *J Pharmacol Exp Ther* 1995;273:591–598.

476. Weiss F, Lorang MT, Bloom FE, et al. Oral alcohol self-administration stimulates dopamine release in the rat nucleus accumbens: genetic and motivational determinants. *J Pharmacol Exp Ther* 1993;267:250–258.

477. Gratton A, Wise RA, Kiyatkin EA. Chronoamperometric measurements of dopamine levels in rat nucleus accumbens during cocaine self-administration. *Soc Neurosci Abstr* 1992;18:1076.

478. Gratton A, Wise RA. Drug- and behavior-associated changes in dopamine-related electrochemical signals during intravenous cocaine self-administration in rats. *J Neurosci* 1994;14:4130–4146.

479. Kiyatkin EA, Stein EA. Biphasic changes in mesolimbic dopamine signal during cocaine self-administration. *Neuroreport* 1994;5:1005–1008.

480. Kiyatkin EA, Stein EA. Fluctuations in nucleus accumbens dopamine during cocaine self-administration behavior: an *in vivo* electrochemical study. *Neuroscience* 1995;64:599–617.

481. Kiyatkin EA, Wise RA, Gratton A. Drug- and behavior-associated changes in dopamine-related electrochemical signals during intravenous heroin self-administration in rats. *Synapse* 1993;14:60–72.

482. Kiyatkin EA. Behavioral significance of phasic changes in mesolimbic dopamine-dependent electrochemical signal associated with heroin self-administration. *J Neural Transm* 1994;96:197–214.

483. Apicella P, Ljungberg T, Scarnati E, Schultz W. Responses to reward in monkey dorsal and ventral striatum. *Exp Brain Res* 1991;85:491–500.

484. Schultz W, Apicella P, Scarnati E, et al. Neuronal activity in monkey ventral striatum related to the expectation of reward. *J Neurosci* 1992;12:4595–4610.

485. Ljungberg T, Apicella P, Schultz W. Responses of monkey dopamine neurons during learning of behavioral reactions. *J Neurophysiol* 1992;67:145–163.

486. Apicella P, Scarnati E, Ljungberg T, et al. Neuronal activity in monkey striatum related to the expectation of predictable environmental events. *J Neurophysiol* 1992;68:945–960.

487. Schultz W, Apicella P, Ljungberg T. Responses of monkey dopamine neurons to reward and conditioned stimuli during successive steps of learning a delayed response task. *J Neurosci* 1993;13:900–913.

488. Mirenowicz J, Schultz W. Importance of unpredictability for reward responses in primate dopamine neurons. *J Neurophysiol* 1994;72:1024–1027.

489. Schultz W. Behavior-related activity of primate dopamine neurons. *Rev Neurologique* 1994;150:634–639.

490. Mirenowicz J, Schultz W. Preferential activation of midbrain dopamine neurons by appetitive rather than aversive stimuli. *Nature* 1996;379:449–451.

491. Chang JY, Sawyer SF, Lee RS, et al. Electrophysiological and pharmacological evidence for the role of the nucleus accumbens in cocaine self-administration in freely moving rats. *J Neurosci* 1994;14:1224–1244.

492. Henriksen SJ, Callaway CW, Negus SS, et al. Properties of neurons recorded in the rodent nucleus accumbens, *in vivo*: relationship to behavioral state and heroin self-administration. *Soc Neurosci Abstr* 1992;18:373.

493. Herz A, Shippenberg TS, Bals-Kubik R, et al. Opiatsucht. Pharmakologische und biochemische Aspekte. [Opiate addiction. Pharmacologic and biochemical aspects]. *Arzneimittel-Forschung* 1992;42:256–259.

494. Dauge V, Kalivas PW, Duffy T, et al. Effect of inhibiting enkephalin catabolism in the VTA on motor activity and extracellular dopamine. *Brain Res* 1992;599:209–214.

495. Johnson SW, North RA. Opioids excite dopamine neurons by hyperpolarization of local interneurons. *J Neurosci* 1992;12:483–488.

496. Klitenick MA, DeWitte P, Kalivas PW. Regulation of somatodendritic dopamine release in the ventral tegmental area by opioids and GABA: an *in vivo* microdialysis study. *J Neurosci* 1992;12:2623–2632.

497. Heidbreder C, Gewiss M, Lallemand S, et al. Inhibition of enkephalin metabolism and activation of mu- or delta-opioid receptors elicit opposite effects on reward and motility in the ventral mesencephalon. *Neuropharmacology* 1992;31:293–298.

498. Spanagel R, Herz A, Shippenberg TS. Opposing tonically active endogenous opioid systems modulate the mesolimbic dopaminergic pathway. *Proc Natl Acad Sci U S A* 1992;89:2046–2050.

499. Yoshida M, Yokoo H, Tanaka T, et al. Facilitatory modulation of mesolimbic dopamine neuronal activity by a μ-opioid agonist and nicotine as examined with in vivo microdialysis. *Brain Res* 1993;624:277–280.

500. Noel MB, Wise RA. Ventral tegmental injections of morphine but not U-50, 488H enhance feeding in food-deprived rats. *Brain Res* 1993;632:68–73.

501. Devine DP, Leone P, Wise RA. Mesolimbic dopamine neurotransmission is increased by administration of μ-opioid receptor antagonists. *Eur J Pharmacol* 1993;243:55–64.

502. German DC, Speciale SG, Manaye KF, et al. Opioid receptors in midbrain dopaminergic regions of the rat. I. Mu receptor autoradiography. *J Neural Transm* 1993;91:39–52.

503. Speciale SG, Manaye KF, Sadeq M, et al. Opioid receptors in midbrain dopaminergic regions of the rat. II. Kappa and delta receptor autoradiography. *J Neural Transm* 1993;91:53–66.

504. Bals-Kubik R, Ableitner A, Herz A, et al. Neuroanatomical sites mediating the motivational effects of opioids as mapped by the conditioned place preference paradigm in rats. *J Pharmacol Exp Ther* 1993;264:489–495.

505. Devine DP, Leone P, Pocock D, et al. Differential involvement of ventral tegmental mu, delta and kappa opioid receptors in modulation of basal mesolimbic dopamine release: *in vivo* microdialysis studies. *J Pharmacol Exp Ther* 1993;266:1236–1246.

506. Mansour A, Fox CA, Burke S, et al. Mu, delta, and kappa opioid receptor mRNA expression in the rat CNS: an in situ hybridization study. *J Comp Neurol* 1994;350:412–438.

507. Devine DP, Wise RA. Self-administration of morphine, DAMGO, and DPDPE into the ventral tegmental area of rats. *J Neurosci* 1994;14:1978–1984.

508. Unterwald EM, Rubenfeld JM, Kreek MJ. Repeated cocaine administration upregulates kappa and mu, but not delta, opioid receptors. *Neuroreport* 1994;5:1613–1616.

509. Singh J, Desiraju T, Nagaraja TN, et al. Facilitation of self-stimulation of ventral tegmentum by microinjection of opioid receptor subtype agonists. *Physiol Behav* 1994;55:627–631.

510. Phillips GD, Robbins TW, Everitt BJ. Mesoaccumbens dopamine-opiate interactions in the control over behaviour by a conditioned reinforcer. *Psychopharmacology (Berl)* 1994;114:345–359.

511. Badiani A, Leone P, Noel MB, et al. Ventral tegmental area opioid mechanisms and modulation of ingestive behavior. *Brain Res* 1995;670:264–276.

512. Noel MB, Wise RA. Ventral tegmental injections of a selective μ or δ opioid enhance feeding in food-deprived rats. *Brain Res* 1995;673:304–312.

513. Badiani A, Leone P, Stewart J. Intra-VTA injections of the mu-opioid antagonist CTOP enhance locomotor activity. *Brain Res* 1995;690:112–116.

514. Mansour A, Fox CA, Burke S, et al. Immunohistochemical localization of the cloned mu opioid receptor in the rat CNS. *J Chem Neuroanat* 1995;8:283–305.

515. Klitenick MA, Wirtshafter D. Behavioral and neurochemical effects of opioids in the paramedian midbrain tegmentum including the median raphe nucleus and ventral tegmental area. *J Pharmacol Exp Ther* 1995;273:327–336.

516. Noel MB, Gratton A. Electrochemical evidence of increased dopamine transmission in prefrontal cortex and nucleus accumbens elicited by ventral tegmental μ-opioid receptor activation in freely behaving rats. *Synapse* 1995;21:110–122.

517. Derrien M, Durieux C, Dauge V, et al. Involvement of D_2 dopaminergic receptors in the emotional and motivational responses induced by injection of CCK-8 in the posterior part of the rat nucleus accumbens. *Brain Res* 1993;617:181–188.

518. Hamilton ME, Freeman AS. Effects of administration of cholecystokinin into the VTA on DA overflow in nucleus accumbens and amygdala of freely moving rats. *Brain Res* 1995;688:134–142.

519. Markowski VP, Hull EM. Cholecystokinin modulates mesolimbic dopaminergic influences on male rat copulatory behavior. *Brain Res* 1995;699:266–274.

520. Rompré PP, Boye SM. Opposite effects of mesencephalic microinjections of cholecystokinin octapeptide and neurotensin-(1-13) on brain stimulation reward. *Eur J Pharmacol* 1993;232:299–303.

521. Rasmussen K, Czachura JF, Stockton ME, et al. Electrophysiological effects of diphenylpyrazolidinone cholecystokinin-B and cholecystokinin-A antagonists on midbrain dopamine neurons. *J Pharmacol Exp Ther* 1993;264:480–488.

522. Tanaka J, Kariya K, Ushigome A, et al. CCK activates excitatory ventral tegmental pathways to the posterior nucleus accumbens. *Neuroreport* 1994;5:2558–2560.

523. Ladurelle N, Durieux C, Roques BP, et al. Different modifications of the dopamine metabolism in the core and shell parts of the nucleus accumbens following CCK-A receptor stimulation in the shell region. *Neurosci Lett* 1994;178:5–10.

524. Rasmussen K, Howbert JJ, Stockton ME. Inhibition of A9 and A10 dopamine cells by the cholecystokinin-B antagonist LY262691: mediation through feedback pathways from forebrain sites. *Synapse* 1993;15:95–103.

525. Angulo JA, McEwen BS. Molecular aspects of neuropeptide regulation and function in the corpus striatum and nucleus accumbens. *Brain Res Brain Res Rev* 1994;19:1–28.

526. Nicot A, Rostene W, Berod A. Neurotensin receptor expression in the rat forebrain and midbrain: a combined analysis by in situ hybridization and receptor autoradiography. *J Comp Neurol* 1994;341:407–419.

527. Atoji Y, Watanabe H, Yamamoto Y, et al. Distribution of neurotensin-containing neurons in the central nervous system of the dog. *J Comp Neurol* 1995;353:67–88.

528. Nicot A, Rostene W, Berod A. Differential expression of neurotensin receptor mRNA in the dopaminergic cell groups of the rat diencephalon and mesencephalon. *J Neurosci Res* 1995;40:667–674.

529. Jiang ZG, Pessia M, North RA. Neurotensin excitation of rat ventral tegmental neurones. *J Physiol* 1994;474:119–129.

530. Steinberg R, Brun P, Souilhac J, et al. Neurochemical and behavioural effects of neurotensin vs [D-Tyr^{11}]neurotensin on mesolimbic dopaminergic function. *Neuropeptides* 1995;28:43–50.

531. Steinberg R, Brun P, Fournier M, et al. SR 48692, a non-peptide neurotensin receptor antagonist differentially affects neurotensin-induced behaviour and changes in dopaminergic transmission. *Neuroscience* 1994;59:921–929.

532. Faure MP, Nouel D, Beaudet A. Axonal and dendritic transport of internalized neurotensin in rat mesostriatal dopaminergic neurons. *Neuroscience* 1995;68:519–529.

533. Mercuri NB, Stratta F, Calabresi P, et al. Neurotensin induces an inward current in rat mesencephalic dopaminergic neurons. *Neurosci Lett* 1993;153:192–196.

534. Kariya K, Tanaka J, Nomura M. Systemic administration of CCK-8S, but not CCK-4,enhances dopamine turnover in the posterior nucleus accumbens: a microdialysis study in freely moving rats. *Brain Res* 1994;657:1–6.

535. Li XM, Hedlund PB, Fuxe K. Cholecystokinin octapeptide in vitro and ex vivo strongly modulates striatal dopamine D_2 receptors in rat forebrain sections. *Eur J Neurosci* 1995;7:962–971.

536. Corwin RL, Jorn A, Hardy M, et al. The CCK-B antagonist CI-988 increases dopamine levels in microdialysate from the rat nucleus accumbens via a tetrodotoxin- and calcium-independent mechanism. *J Neurochem* 1995;65:208–217.

537. Ladurelle N, Roques BP, Dauge V. The transfer of rats from a familiar to a novel environment prolongs the increase of extracellular dopamine efflux induced by CCK8 in the posterior nucleus accumbens. *J Neurosci* 1995;15:3118–3127.

538. Morino P, Mascagni F, McDonald A, et al. Cholecystokinin corticostriatal pathway in the rat: evidence for bilateral origin from medial prefrontal cortical areas. *Neuroscience* 1994;59:939–952.

539. Morency MA, Quirion R, Mishra RK. Distribution of cholecystokinin receptors in the bovine brain: a quantitative autoradiographic study. *Neuroscience* 1994;62:307–316.

540. Josselyn SA, Vaccarino FJ. Interaction of CCK$_B$ receptors with amphetamine in responding for conditioned rewards. *Peptides* 1995;16:959–964.

541. Wagstaff JD, Bush LG, Gibb JW, et al. Endogenous neurotensin antagonizes methamphetamine-enhanced dopaminergic activity. *Brain Res* 1994;665:237–244.

542. Diaz J, Levesque D, Griffon N, et al. Opposing roles for dopamine D_2 and D_3 receptors on neurotensin mRNA expression in nucleus accumbens. *Eur J Neurosci* 1994;6:1384–1387.

543. Ikemoto K, Satoh K, Maeda T, et al. Neurochemical heterogeneity of the primate nucleus accumbens. *Exp Brain Res* 1995;104:177–190.

544. Brun P, Steinberg R, Le Fur G, et al. Blockade of neurotensin receptor by SR 48692 potentiates the facilitatory effect of haloperidol on the evoked *in vivo* dopamine release in the rat nucleus accumbens. *J Neurochem* 1995;64:2073–2079.

545. Diaz J, Levesque D, Lammers CH, et al. Phenotypical characterization of neurons expressing the dopamine D_3 receptor in the rat brain. *Neuroscience* 1995;65:731–745.

546. Hiroi N, McDonald RJ, White NM. Involvement of the lateral nucleus of the amygdala in amphetamine and food conditioned place preferences (CPP). *Soc Neurosci Abstr* 1990;16:605.

547. Hiroi N. *A pharmacological and neuroanatomical investigation of the conditioned place preference produced by*

amphetamine [Dissertation]. Montreal, Quebec: McGill University; 1990.

548. Hiroi N, White NM. The lateral nucleus of the amygdala mediates expression of the amphetamine-produced conditioned place preference. *J Neurosci* 1991;11:2107–2116.

549. White NM, Hiroi N. Amphetamine conditioned cue preference and the neurobiology of drug-seeking. *Semin Neurosci* 1993;5:329–336.

550. White NM, Hiroi N. Preferential localization of self-stimulation sites in striosomes/patches of rat caudate-putamen. *Soc Neurosci Abstr* 1995;21:2079.

551. Ragsdale CW Jr, Graybiel AM. Fibers from the basolateral nucleus of the amygdala selectively innervate striosomes in the caudate nucleus of the cat. *J Comp Neurol* 1988;269:506–522.

552. Ragsdale CW Jr, Graybiel AM. Compartmental organization of the thalamostriatal connection in the cat. *J Comp Neurol* 1991;311:134–167.

553. Ragsdale CW Jr, Graybiel AM. A simple ordering of neocortical areas established by the compartmental organization of their striatal projections. *Proc Natl Acad Sci U S A* 1990;87:6196–6199.

554. Gerfen CR. The neostriatal mosaic: striatal patch-matrix organization is related to cortical lamination. *Science* 1989;246:385–388.

555. Berendse HW, Galis-de Graaf Y, Groenewegen HJ. Topographical organization and relationship with ventral striatal compartments of prefrontal corticostriatal projections in the rat. *J Comp Neurol* 1992;316:314–347.

556. Groenewegen HJ, Room P, Witter MP, et al. Cortical afferents of the nucleus accumbens in the cat, studied with anterograde and retrograde transport techniques. *Neuroscience* 1982;7:977–995.

557. Phillipson OT, Griffiths AC. The topographic order of inputs to nucleus accumbens in the rat. *Neuroscience* 1985;16:275–296.

558. Christie MJ, Summers RJ, Stephenson JA, et al. Excitatory amino acid projections to the nucleus accumbens septi in the rat: a retrograde transport study utilizing D[³H]aspartate and [³H]GABA. *Neuroscience* 1987;22:425–439.

559. Borg JS, Deutsch AY, Zahm DS. Afferent projection to the nucleus accumbens core and shell in the rat. *Soc Neurosci Abstr* 1991;17:454.

560. Kelley AE, Domesick VB, Nauta WJH. The amygdalostriatal projection in the rat—an anatomical study by anterograde and retrograde tracing methods. *Neuroscience* 1982;7:615–630.

561. McDonald AJ. Topographical organization of amygdaloid projections to the caudatoputamen, nucleus accumbens,

and related striatal-like areas of the rat brain. *Neuroscience* 1991;44:15–33.

562. Robinson TG, Beart PM. Excitant amino acid projections from rat amygdala and thalamus to nucleus accumbens. *Brain Res Bull* 1988;20:467–471.

563. Price JL, Amaral DG. An autoradiographic study of the projections of the central nucleus of the amygdala. *J Neurosci* 1981;1:1242–1259.

564. Haber SN, Groenewegen HJ, Grove EA, et al. Efferent connections of the ventral pallidum: evidence of a dual striato pallidofugal pathway. *J Comp Neurol* 1985;235:322–335.

565. Oades RD, Halliday GM. Ventral tegmental (A10) system: neurobiology. 1. Anatomy and connectivity. *Brain Res* 1987;434:117–165.

566. Gonzales C, Chesselet MF. Amygdalonigral pathway: an anterograde study in the rat with Phaseolus vulgaris leucoagglutinin (PHA-L). *J Comp Neurol* 1990;297:182–200.

567. Canteras NS, Simerly RB, Swanson LW. Connections of the posterior nucleus of the amygdala. *J Comp Neurol* 1992;324:143–179.

568. de Belleroche JS, Bradford HF. Presynaptic control of the synthesis and release of dopamine from striatal synaptosomes: a comparison between the effects of 5-hydroxytryptamine, acetylcholine, and glutamate. *J Neurochem* 1980;35:1227–1234.

569. Chesselet MF. Presynaptic regulation of neurotransmitter release in the brain: facts and hypothesis. *Neuroscience* 1984;12:347–375.

570. Hetey L, Drescher K. Influence of antipsychotics on presynaptic receptors modulating the release of dopamine in synaptosomes of the nucleus accumbens of rats. *Neuropharmacology* 1986;25:1103–1109.

571. Tricklebank MD. Interactions between dopamine and 5HT₃ receptors suggest new treatment for psychosis and drug addiction. *Trends Pharmacol Sci* 1989;10:127–129.

572. Westfall TC, Titternary V. Inhibition of the electrically induced release of [³H]dopamine by serotonin from superfused rat striatal slices. *Neurosci Lett* 1982;28:205–209.

573. Bissette G, Nemeroff CB. Neurotensin and the mesocorticolimbic dopamine system. *Ann N Y Acad Sci* 1988;537:397–404.

574. Hervé D, Tassin JP, Studler JM, et al. Dopaminergic control of ¹²⁵I-labelled neurotensin binding site density in corticolimbic structures of the rat brain. *Proc Natl Acad Sci U S A* 1986;83:6203–6207.

575. Hökfelt T, Everitt BS, Theodorsson-Norheim E, et al. Occurrence of

neurotensin-like immunoreactivity in subpopulations of hypothalamic, mesencephalic, and medullary catecholamine neurons. *J Comp Neurol* 1984;222:543–559.

576. Kelley AE, Cador M. Behavioral evidence for differential neuropeptide modulation of the mesolimbic dopamine system. *Ann N Y Acad Sci* 1988;537:415–434.

577. Kelley AE, Stinus L, Iversen SD. Behavioural activation induced in the rat by substance P infusion into ventral tegmental area: implication of dopaminergic A10 neurones. *Neurosci Lett* 1979;11:335–339.

578. Kalivas PW, Jennes L, Miller JS. A catecholaminergic projection from the ventral tegmental area to the diagonal band of Broca: modulation by neurotensin. *Brain Res* 1985;326:229–238.

579. Nemeroff CB, Cain ST. Neurotensin-dopamine interactions in the CNS. *Trends Pharmacol Sci* 1985;6:201–205.

580. Palacios JM, Kuhar MJ. Neurotensin receptors are located on dopamine-containing neurones in rat midbrain. *Nature* 1981;294:587–589.

581. Pernow B. Substance P. *Pharmacol Rev* 1983;35:85–141.

582. Phillips AG, Blaha CD, Fibiger HC, et al. Interactions between mesolimbic dopamine neurons, cholecystokinin, and neurotensin: evidence using *in vivo* voltammetry. *Ann N Y Acad Sci* 1988;537:347–361.

583. Pickel VM, Joh TH, Chan J. Substance P in the rat nucleus accumbens: ultrastructural localization in axon terminals and their relation to dopaminergic afferents. *Brain Res* 1988;444:247–264.

584. Quirion R, Chiueh CC, Everist HD, et al. Comparative localization of neurotensin receptors on nigrostriatal and mesolimbic dopaminergic terminals. *Brain Res* 1985;327:835–839.

585. Studler J-M, Kitagbi P, Tramu G, et al. Extensive co-localization of neurotensin with dopamine in rat mesocortico-frontal dopaminergic neurons. *Neuropeptides* 1988;11:95–100.

586. Voigt MM, Wang RY, Westfall TC. The effects of cholecystokinin on the *in vivo* release of newly synthesized [³H]dopamine from the nucleus accumbens of the rat. *J Neurosci* 1985;5:2744–2749.

587. Amit Z, Sutherland EA, Gill K, et al. Zimeldine: a review of its effects on ethanol consumption. *Neurosci Biobehav Rev* 1984;8:35–54.

588. Gill K, Amit Z, Ögren SO. The effects of zimelidine on voluntary ethanol consumption: studies on the mechanism of action. *Alcohol* 1985;2:343–347.

589. Le Bourhis B, Uzan A, Aufrere G, et al. Effets de l'indalpine, inhibiteur

spécifique de la récapture de la sérotonine sur la dépendance comportementale à l'éthanol et sur la prise volontaire d'alcool chez le rat. [Effects of indalpine, a specific serotonin reuptake inhibitor, on ethanol behavioral dependence and voluntary alcohol consumption in the rat]. *Ann Pharm Fr* 1981;39:11–20.

590. Leccese AP, Lyness WH. The effects of putative 5-hydroxytryptamine receptor active agents on *d*-amphetamine self-administration in controls and rats with 5,7-dihydroxytryptamine medial forebrain bundle lesions. *Brain Res* 1984;303:153–162.

591. Murphy JM, Waller MB, Gatto GJ, et al. Monoamine uptake inhibitors attenuate ethanol intake in alcohol-preferring (P) rats. *Alcohol* 1985;2:349–352.

592. Naranjo CA, Sellers EM, Lawrin MO. Modulation of ethanol intake by serotonin uptake inhibitors. *J Clin Psychiatry* 1986;47(4)[Suppl]:16–22.

593. Rockman GE, Amit Z, Carr G, et al. Attenuation of ethanol intake by 5-hydroxytryptamine uptake blockade in laboratory rats: I. involvement of brain 5-hydroxytryptamine in the mediation of the positive reinforcing properties of ethanol. *Arch Int Pharmacodyn Ther* 1979;241:245–259.

594. Yu DSL, Smith FL, Smith DG, et al. Fluoxetine-induced attenuation of amphetamine self-administration in rats. *Life Sci* 1986;39:1383–1388.

595. Zabik JE, Roache JD, Sidor R, et al. The effects of fluoxetine on ethanol preference in the rat. *Pharmacologist* 1982;24:204.

596. Cannon DS, Carrell LE. Rat strain differences in ethanol self-administration and taste aversion. *Pharmacol Biochem Behav* 1987;28:57–63.

597. George FR. Genetic and environmental factors in ethanol self-administration. *Pharmacol Biochem Behav* 1987;27:379–384.

598. Li TK, Lumeng L. Alcohol preference and voluntary alcohol intakes of inbred rat strains and the National Institutes of Health heterogeneous stock of rats. *Alcoholism* 1984;8:485–486.

599. Ritz MC, George FR, DeFiebre CM, et al. Genetic differences in the establishment of ethanol as a reinforcer. *Pharmacol Biochem Behav* 1986;24:1089–1094.

600. Suzuki T, George FR, Meisch RA. Differential establishment and maintenance of oral ethanol reinforced behavior in Lewis and Fischer 344 inbred rat strains. *J Pharmacol Exp Ther* 1988;245:164–170.

601. George FR, Meisch RA. Oral narcotic intake as a reinforcer: genotype x environment interaction. *Behav Genet* 1984;14:603.

602. Khodzhagel'diev T. Formirovanie vlecheniia k nikotinu u myshei linii C57BL/6 i CBA. [Development of nicotine preference in C57BL/6 and CBA mice.] *Biull Eksp Biol Med* 1986;101:48–50.

603. George FR, Goldberg SR. Genetic approaches to the analysis of addiction processes. *Trends Pharmacol Sci* 1989;10:78–83.

604. Kosten TA, Miserendino MJ, Chi S, et al. Fischer and Lewis rat strains show differential cocaine effects in conditioned place preference and behavioral sensitization but not in locomotor activity or conditioned taste aversion. *J Pharmacol Exp Ther* 1994;269:137–144.

605. Nestler EJ. Molecular mechanisms of drug addiction in the mesolimbic dopamine pathway. *Semin Neurosci* 1993;5:369–376.

606. Gardner EL, Lowinson JH. Marijuana's interaction with brain reward systems: update 1991. *Pharmacol Biochem Behav* 1991;40:571–580.

607. Chen J, Paredes W, Lowinson JH, et al. Strain-specific facilitation of dopamine efflux by Δ^9-tetrahydrocannabinol in the nucleus accumbens of rat: an *in vivo* microdialysis study. *Neurosci Lett* 1991;129:136–140.

608. Gardner EL, Paredes W, Smith D, et al. Strain-specific facilitation of brain stimulation reward by Δ^9-tetrahydrocannabinol in laboratory rats. *Psychopharmacology (Berl)* 1988; 96[Suppl]:365.

609. Lepore M, Liu X, Savage V, et al. Genetic differences in Δ^9-tetrahydrocannabinol-induced facilitation of brain stimulation reward as measured by a rate-frequency curve-shift electrical brain stimulation paradigm in three different rat strains. *Life Sci* 1996;25:PL365–372.

610. Guitart X, Beitner-Johnson D, Marby DW, et al. Fischer and Lewis rat strains differ in basal levels of neurofilament proteins and their regulation by chronic morphine in the mesolimbic dopamine system. *Synapse* 1992;12:242–253.

611. Uhl GR, Elmer GI, Labuda MC, et al. Genetic influences in drug abuse. In: Bloom FE, Kupfer DJ, eds. *Psychopharmacology: the fourth generation of progress.* New York: Raven Press, 1995:1793–1806.

612. Krugylak L, Lander ES. High resolution genetic mapping of complex traits. *Am J Hum Genet* 1995;56:1212–1223.

613. Lander ES, Schork NJ. Genetic dissection of complex traits. *Science* 1994;265:2037–2048.

614. Elston RC. Linkage and association to genetic markers. *Exp Clin Immunogenet* 1995;12:129–140.

615. Koob GF, Bloom F. Cellular and molecular mechanisms of drug dependence. *Science* 1988;242:715–723.

616. Blum K, Noble E, Sheridan PJ, et al. Allelic association of human dopamine D_2 receptor gene in alcoholism. *JAMA* 1990;263:2055–2060.

617. Smith SS, O'Hara BF, Persico AM, et al. Genetic vulnerability to drug abuse: the D_2 dopamine receptor Taq I B1 restriction fragment length polymorphism appears more frequently in polysubstance abusers. *Arch Gen Psychiatry* 1992;49:723–727.

618. Noble EP. The D_2 dopamine receptor gene: a review of association studies in alcoholism. *Behav Genet* 1993;23:119–129.

619. Uhl G, Blum K, Noble E, Smith S. Substance abuse vulnerability and D_2 receptor genes. *Trends Neurosci* 1993;16:83–88.

620. Bolos AM, Dean M, Lucas-Derse S, et al. Population and pedigree studies reveal a lack of association between the dopamine D_2 receptor gene and alcoholism. *JAMA* 1990;264:3156–3160.

621. Suarez BK, Parsian A, Hampe CL, et al. Linkage disequilibria at the D_2 dopamine receptor locus (DRD2) in alcoholics and controls. *Genomics* 1994;19:12–20.

622. Vandenbergh DJ, Persico AM, Hawkins AL, et al. Human dopamine transporter gene (DAT1) maps to chromosome 5p15.3 and displays a VNTR. *Genomics* 1992;14:1104–1106.

623. Cook EH, Stein MA, Krasowski MD, et al. Association of attention deficit disorder and the dopamine transporter gene. *Am J Human Genet* 1995;56:993–998.

624. Muramatsu T, Higuchi S. Dopamine transporter gene polymorphism and alcoholism. *Biochem Biophys Res Commun* 1995;211:28–32.

625. Gelernter J, Kranzler HR, Satel SL, et al. Genetic association between dopamine transporter protein alleles and cocaine-induced paranoia. *Neuropsychopharmacology* 1994;11:195–200.

626. Persico AM, Vandenbergh DJ, Smith SS, et al. Dopamine transporter gene polymorphisms are not associated with polysubstance abuse. *Biol Psychiatry* 1993;34:265–267.

627. Ebstein EP, Novick O, Umansky R, et al. Dopamine D4 receptor (D4DR) exon III polymorphism associated with the human personality trait of novelty seeking. *Nat Genet* 1996;12:78–80.

628. Benjamin J, Li L, Patterson C, et al. Population and familial association between the D4 dopamine receptor gene

and measures of novelty seeking. *Nat Genet* 1996;12:81–84.

629. Van Tol HHM, Wu CM, Guan HC, et al. Multiple dopamine D4 receptor variants in the human population. *Nature* 1992;358:149–152.

630. Adamson MD, Kennedy J, Petronis A, et al. DRD4 dopamine receptor genotype and CSF monoamine metabolites in Finnish alcoholics and controls. *Am J Med Genet* 1995;60:199–205.

631. Lannfelt L, Sokoloff P, Martes M-P, et al. Amino acid substitution in the dopamine D-3 receptor as a useful marker to investigating psychiatric disorders. *Psychiatr Genet* 1992;2:249–256.

632. Rietschel M, Nöthen MM, Lannfelt L, et al. A serine to glycine substitution at position 9 in the extracellular N-terminal part of the dopamine D_3 receptor protein: no role in the genetic predisposition to bipolar affective disorder. *Psychiatr Res* 1993;46:253–259.

633. Axelrod J, Tomchick R. Enzymatic *O*-methylation of epinephrine and other catechols. *J Biol Chem* 1958;233:702–705.

634. Tenhunen J, Salminen M, Lundstrom K, et al. Genomic organization of the human catechol-*O*-methyltransferase gene and its expression from two distinct promoters. *Eur J Biochem* 1994;223:1049–1054.

635. Weinshilboum RM, Raymond FA. Inheritance of low erythrocyte catechol-*O*-methyl transferase activity in man. *Am J Hum Genet* 1977;29:125–135.

636. Scanlon PD, Raymond FA, Weinshilboum RA. Catechol-*O*-methyl transferase: thermolabile enzyme in erythrocytes of subjects homozygous for the allele for low activity. *Science* 1979;203:63–65.

637. Spielman RS, Weinshilboum RM. Genetics of red cell COMT activity: analysis of thermal stability and family data. *Am J Med Genet* 1981;10:279–290.

638. Aksoy S, Klener J, Weinshilboum RM. Catechol-*O*-methyltransferase pharmacogenetics: photoaffinity labelling and Western blot analysis of human liver samples. *Pharmacogenetics* 1993;3:116–122.

639. Boudikova B, Szumlanski C, Maidak B, et al. Human liver catecholamine-*O*-methyltransferase pharmacogenetics. *Clin Pharmacol Ther* 1990;48:381–389.

640. Bertocci B, Miggiano V, Da Prada M, et al. Human catechol-*O*-methyltransferase: cloning and expression of the membrane associated form. *Proc Natl Acad Sci U S A* 1991;88:1416–1420.

641. Lundstrom K, Salminen M, Jalanko A, et al. Cloning and characteriza-tion of human placental catechol-*O*-methyltransferase cDNA. *DNA Cell Biol* 1991;10:181–189.

642. Schuckitt MA. Low level of response to alcohol as a predictor of future alcoholism. *Am J Psychiatry* 1994;151:184–189.

643. Blum K, Cull JG, Braverman ER, Comings DE. Reward deficiency syndrome. *Am Sci* 1996;84:132–145.

644. Minabe Y, Emori K, Ashby CR Jr. Significant differences in the activity of midbrain dopamine neurons between male Fischer 344 and Lewis rats: an *in vivo* electrophysiological study. *Life Sci* 1995;56:PL135–PL141.

645. Beitner-Johnson D, Guitart X, Nestler EJ. Dopaminergic brain reward regions of Lewis and Fischer rats display different levels of tyrosine hydroxylase and other morphine- and cocaine-regulated phosphoproteins. *Brain Res* 1991;561:146–149.

646. Comings DE, Comings BG, Muhleman G, et al. The dopamine D_2 receptor locus as a modifying gene in neuropsychiatric disorders. *JAMA* 1991;266:1793–1800.

647. Blum K, Sheridan PJ, Wood RC, et al. Dopamine D2 receptor gene variants: association and linkage studies in impulsive-addictive-compulsive behaviour. *Pharmacogenetics* 1995;5:121–141.

648. Noble EP, Blum K, Ritchie T, et al. Allelic association of the D_2 receptor gene with receptor-binding characteristics in alcoholism. *Arch Gen Psychiatry* 1991;48:648–654.

649. Noble EP, St Jeor ST, Ritchie T, et al. D2 dopamine receptor gene and cigarette smoking: a reward gene? *Med Hypotheses* 1994;42:257–260.

650. Noble EP, Blum K, Khalsa ME, et al. Allelic association of the D_2 dopamine receptor gene with cocaine dependence. *Drug Alcohol Depend* 1993;33:271–285.

651. Dyr W, McBride WJ, Lumeng TK, et al. Effects of D1 and D2 dopamine receptor agents on ethanol consumption in the high-alcohol-drinking (HAD) line of rats. *Alcohol* 1993;10:207–212.

652. McBride WJ, Chernet JE, Dyr W, et al. Densities of dopamine D2 receptors are reduced in CNS regions of alcohol preferring P rats. *Alcohol* 1993;10:387–390.

653. Zhou FC, Zhang JK, Lumeng L, et al. Mesolimbic dopamine system in alcohol-preferring rats. *Alcohol* 1995;12:403–412.

654. Lawford BR, Young RM, Rowell JA, et al. Bromocriptine in the treatment of alcoholics with the D_2 dopamine receptor A1 allele. *Nat Med* 1995;1:337–341.

655. Rouge-Pont R, Piazza PV, Kharouby M, et al. Higher and longer stress-induced increase in dopamine concentrations in the nucleus accumbens of animals predisposed to amphetamine self-administration. A microdialysis study. *Brain Res* 1993;602:169–174.

656. Glick SD, Raucci J, Wang S, et al. Neurochemical predisposition to self-administer cocaine in rats: individual differences in dopamine and its metabolites. *Brain Res* 1994;653:148–154.

657. Glick SD, Merski C, Steindorf S, et al. Neurochemical predisposition to self-administer morphine in rats. *Brain Res* 1992;578:215–220.

658. Piazza PV, Deminiere JM, Le Moal M, et al. Factors that predict individual vulnerability to amphetamine self-administration. *Science* 1989;245:1511–1513.

659. Piazza PV, Rouge-Pont R, Deminiere JM, et al. Individual vulnerability to amphetamine self-administration is correlated with dopaminergic activity in frontal cortex and nucleus accumbens. *Soc Neurosci Abstr* 1990;16:585.

660. Gerber GJ, Stretch R. Drug-induced reinstatement of extinguished self-administration behavior in monkeys. *Pharmacol Biochem Behav* 1975;3:1055–1061.

661. de Wit H, Stewart J. Drug reinstatement of heroin-reinforced responding in the rat. *Psychopharmacology (Berl)* 1983;79:29–31.

662. Stewart J. Conditioned and unconditioned drug effects in relapse to opiate and stimulant drug self-administration. *Prog Neuropsychopharmacol Biol Psychiatry* 1983;7:591–597.

663. Stewart J, de Wit H. Reinstatement of drug-taking behavior as a method of assessing incentive motivational properties of drugs. In: Bozarth MA, ed. *Methods of assessing the reinforcing properties of abused drugs.* New York: Springer-Verlag, 1987:211–227.

664. Stewart J, Wise RA. Reinstatement of heroin self-administration habits: morphine prompts and naltrexone discourages renewed responding after extinction. *Psychopharmacology (Berl)* 1992;108:79–84.

665. Stewart J. Reinstatement of heroin and cocaine self-administration behavior in the rat by intracerebral application of morphine in the ventral tegmental area. *Pharmacol Biochem Behav* 1984;20:917–923.

666. Stewart J, Vezina P. A comparison of the effects of intra-accumbens injections of amphetamine and morphine on reinstatement of heroin intravenous self-administration behavior. *Brain Res* 1988;457:287–294.

667. Wise RA, Murray A, Bozarth MA. Bromocriptine self-administration and

bromocriptine-reinstatement of cocaine-trained and heroin-trained lever pressing in rats. *Psychopharmacology (Berl)* 1990;100:355–360.

668. Shaham Y, Alvares K, Nespor SM, et al. Effect of stress on oral morphine and fentanyl self-administration in rats. *Pharmacol Biochem Behav* 1992;41:615–619.

669. Shaham Y, Klein LC, Alvares K, et al. Effect of stress on oral fentanyl consumption in rats in an operant self-administration paradigm. *Pharmacol Biochem Behav* 1993;46:315–322.

670. Shaham Y, Stewart J. Exposure to mild stress enhances the reinforcing efficacy of intravenous heroin self-administration in rats. *Psychopharmacology (Berl)* 1994;114:523–527.

671. Shaham Y. Immobilization stress-induced oral opioid self-administration and withdrawal in rats: role of conditioning factors and the effect of stress on "relapse" to opioid drugs. *Psychopharmacology (Berl)* 1993;111:477–485.

672. Shaham Y, Stewart J. Stress reinstates heroin-seeking in drug-free animals: an effect mimicking heroin, not withdrawal. *Psychopharmacology (Berl)* 1995;119:334–341.

673. Jaffe JH. Current concepts of addiction. *Res Publ Assoc Res Nerv Ment Dis* 1992;70:1–21.

674. O'Brien CP, Childress AR, McLellan AT, et al. A learning model of addiction. *Res Publ Assoc Res Nerv Ment Dis* 1992;70:157–177.

675. Kreek MJ. Rationale for maintenance pharmacotherapy of opiate dependence. *Res Publ Assoc Res Nerv Ment Dis* 1992;70:205–230.

676. Dackis CA, Gold MS. New concepts in cocaine addiction: the dopamine depletion hypothesis. *Neurosci Biobehav Rev* 1985;9:469–477.

677. Gawin FH, Kleber HD. Abstinence symptomatology and psychiatric diagnosis in cocaine abusers. *Arch Gen Psychiatry* 1986;43:107–113.

678. Vaillant GE. What can long-term follow-up teach us about relapse and prevention of relapse in addiction? *Br J Addict* 1988;83:1147–1157.

679. Hoffmann NG, Miller NS. Perspectives of effective treatment for alcohol and drug disorders. *Psychiatr Clin North Am* 1993;16:127–140.

680. van der Kooy D. Place conditioning: a simple and effective method for assessing the motivational properties of drugs. In: Bozarth MA, ed. *Methods of assessing the reinforcing properties of abused drugs.* New York: Springer-Verlag, 1987:229–240.

681. Bozarth MA. Conditioned place preference: a parametric analysis using systemic heroin injections. In: Bozarth MA, ed. *Methods of assessing the reinforcing properties of abused drugs.* New York: Springer-Verlag, 1987:241–273.

682. Phillips AG, Fibiger HC. Anatomical and neurochemical substrates of drug reward determined by the conditioned place preference technique. In: Bozarth MA, ed. *Methods of assessing the reinforcing properties of abused drugs.* New York: Springer-Verlag, 1987:275–290.

683. Hiroi N, White NM. The reserpine-sensitive dopamine pool mediates (+)-amphetamine-conditioned reward in the place preference paradigm. *Brain Res* 1990;510:33–42.

684. Hiroi N, White NM. The amphetamine conditioned place preference: differential involvement of dopamine receptor subtypes and two dopaminergic terminal areas. *Brain Res* 1991;552:141–152.

685. Hiroi N, White NM. The ventral pallidum area is involved in the acquisition but not expression of the amphetamine conditioned place preference. *Neurosci Lett* 1993;156:9–12.

686. Pettit HO, Pettit AJ. Disposition of cocaine in blood and brain after a single pretreatment. *Brain Res* 1994;651:261–268.

687. Parsons LH, Justice JB Jr. Serotonin and dopamine sensitization in the nucleus accumbens, ventral tegmental area, and dorsal raphe nucleus following repeated cocaine administration. *J Neurochem* 1993;61:1611–1619.

688. Kalivas PW, Duffy P. Time course of extracellular dopamine and behavioral sensitization to cocaine. I. Dopamine axon terminals. *J Neurosci* 1993;13:266–275.

689. Wolf ME, White FJ, Hu XT. MK-801 prevents alterations in the mesoaccumbens dopamine system associated with behavioral sensitization to amphetamine. *J Neurosci* 1994;14:1735–1745.

690. Wolf ME, White FJ, Nassar R, et al. Differential development of autoreceptor subsensitivity and enhanced dopamine release during amphetamine sensitization. *J Pharmacol Exp Ther* 1993;264:249–255.

691. Horger BA, Valadez A, Wellman PJ, et al. Augmentation of the neurochemical effects of cocaine in the ventral striatum and medial prefrontal cortex following preexposure to amphetamine, but not nicotine: an *in vivo* microdialysis study. *Life Sci* 1994;55:1245–1251.

692. Paulson PE, Robinson TE. Amphetamine-induced time-dependent sensitization of dopamine neurotransmission in the dorsal and ventral striatum: a microdialysis study in behaving rats. *Synapse* 1995;19:56–65.

693. Hooks MS, Duffy P, Striplin C, et al. Behavioral and neurochemical sensitization following cocaine self-administration. *Psychopharmacology (Berl)* 1994;115:265–272.

694. Weiss F, Paulus MP, Lorang MT, et al. Increases in extracellular dopamine in the nucleus accumbens by cocaine are inversely related to basal levels: effects of acute and repeated administration. *J Neurosci* 1992;12:4372–4380.

695. Schrater PA, Russo AC, Stanton TL, et al. Changes in striatal dopamine metabolism during the development of morphine physical dependence in rats: observations using *in vivo* microdialysis. *Life Sci* 1993;52:1535–1545.

696. Spanagel R, Shippenberg TS. Modulation of morphine-induced sensitization by endogenous kappa opioid systems in the rat. *Neurosci Lett* 1993;153:232–236.

697. Imperato A, Mele A, Scrocco MG, et al. Chronic cocaine alters limbic extracellular dopamine: neurochemical basis for addiction. *Eur J Pharmacol* 1992;212:299–300.

698. Parsons LH, Smith AD, Justice JB Jr. Basal extracellular dopamine is decreased in the rat nucleus accumbens during abstinence from chronic cocaine. *Synapse* 1991;9:60–65.

699. Robertson MW, Leslie CA, Bennett JP Jr. Apparent synaptic dopamine deficiency induced by withdrawal from chronic cocaine treatment. *Brain Res* 1991;538:337–339.

700. Maisonneuve IM, Kreek JM. Acute tolerance to the dopamine response induced by a binge pattern of cocaine administration in male rats: an *in vivo* microdialysis study. *J Pharmacol Exp Ther* 1994;268:916–921.

701. Emmett-Oglesby MW, Lane JD. Tolerance to the reinforcing effects of cocaine. *Behav Pharmacol* 1992;3:193–200.

702. Fischman MW, Schuster CR, Javaid J, et al. Acute tolerance development to the cardiovascular and subjective effects of cocaine. *J Pharmacol Exp Ther* 1985;235:677–682.

703. Kokkinidis L, Zacharko RM, Predy PA. Post-amphetamine depression of self-stimulation responding from the substantia nigra: reversal by tricyclic antidepressants. *Pharmacol Biochem Behav* 1980;13:379–383.

704. Kokkinidis L, McCarter BD. Post-cocaine depression and sensitization of brain-stimulation reward: analysis of reinforcement and performance effects. *Pharmacol Biochem Behav* 1990;36:463–471.

705. Barrett RJ, White DK. Reward system depression following chronic amphetamine: antagonism by haloperidol. *Pharmacol Biochem Behav* 1980; 13:555–559.

706. Cassens G, Actor C, Kling M, et al. Amphetamine withdrawal: effects on threshold of intracranial reinforcement. *Psychopharmacology (Berl)* 1981;73:318–322.

707. Leith NJ, Barrett RJ. Amphetamine and the reward system: evidence for tolerance and post-drug depression. *Psychopharmacology (Berl)* 1976;46:19–25.

708. Simpson DM, Annau Z. Behavioral withdrawal following several psychoactive drugs. *Pharmacol Biochem Behav* 1977;7:59–64.

709. Wise RA, Munn E. Withdrawal from chronic amphetamine elevates baseline intracranial self-stimulation thresholds. *Psychopharmacology (Berl)* 1995;117:130–136.

710. Frank RA, Martz S, Pommering T. The effect of chronic cocaine on self-stimulation train-duration thresholds. *Pharmacol Biochem Behav* 1988;29:755–758.

711. Pothos E, Rada P, Mark GP, et al. Dopamine microdialysis in the nucleus accumbens during acute and chronic morphine, naloxone-precipitated withdrawal and clonidine treatment. *Brain Res* 1991;566:348–350.

712. Crippens D, Robinson TE. Withdrawal from morphine or amphetamine: different effects on dopamine in the ventral-medial striatum studied with microdialysis. *Brain Res* 1994;650:56–62.

713. Rossetti ZL, Hmaidan Y, Gessa GL. Marked inhibition of mesolimbic dopamine release: a common feature of ethanol, morphine, cocaine and amphetamine abstinence in rats. *Eur J Pharmacol* 1992;221:227–234.

714. Acquas E, Di Chiara G. Depression of mesolimbic dopamine transmission and sensitization to morphine during opiate abstinence. *J Neurochem* 1992;58:1620–1625.

715. Spanagel R, Almeida OF, Bartl C, et al. Endogenous κ-opioid systems in opiate withdrawal: role in aversion and accompanying changes in mesolimbic dopamine release. *Psychopharmacology (Berl)* 1994;115:121–127.

716. Schulteis G, Markou A, Gold LH, et al. Relative sensitivity of multiple indices of opiate withdrawal: a quantitative dose-response analysis. *J Pharmacol Exp Ther* 1994;271:1391–1398.

717. Schaefer GJ, Michael RP. Changes in response rates and reinforcement thresholds for intracranial self-stimulation during morphine withdrawal. *Pharmacol Biochem Behav* 1986;25:1263–1269.

718. Koob GF, Stinus L, Le Moal M, et al. Opponent process theory of motivation: neurobiological evidence from studies of opiate dependence. *Neurosci Biobehav Rev* 1989;13:135–140.

719. Stinus L, Le Moal M, Koob GF. Nucleus accumbens and amygdala are possible substrates for the aversive stimulus effects of opiate withdrawal. *Neuroscience* 1990;37:767–773.

720. Kelsey JE, Arnold SR. Lesions of the dorsomedial amygdala, but not the nucleus accumbens, reduce the aversiveness of morphine withdrawal in rats. *Behav Neurosci* 1994;108:1119–1127.

721. Nader K, Bechara A, Roberts DC, et al. Neuroleptics block high- but not low-dose heroin place preferences: further evidence for a two-system model of motivation. *Behav Neurosci* 1994;108:1128–1138.

722. Kosten TA. Clonidine attenuates conditioned aversion produced by naloxone-precipitated opiate withdrawal. *Eur J Pharmacol* 1994;254:59–63.

723. Higgins GA, Nguyen P, Sellers EM. The NMDA antagonist dizocilpine (MK801) attenuates motivational as well as somatic aspects of naloxone precipitated opioid withdrawal. *Life Sci* 1992;50:PL167–PL172.

724. Harris GC, Aston-Jones G. Beta-adrenergic antagonists attenuate somatic and aversive signs of opiate withdrawal. *Neuropsychopharmacology* 1993;9:303–311.

725. Higgins GA, Nguyen P, Joharchi N, et al. Effects of 5-HT$_3$ receptor antagonists on behavioural measures of naloxone-precipitated opioid withdrawal. *Psychopharmacology (Berl)* 1991;105:322–328.

726. Mucha RF. Is the motivational effect of opiate withdrawal reflected by common somatic indices of precipitated withdrawal? A place conditioning study in the rat. *Brain Res* 1987;418:214–220.

727. Dai S, Corrigall WA, Coen KM, et al. Heroin self-administration by rats: influence of dose and physical dependence. *Pharmacol Biochem Behav* 1989;32:1009–1015.

728. Young GA, Moreton JE, Meltzer LT, et al. 1-alpha-acetylmethadol (LAAM), methadone and morphine abstinence in dependent rats: EEG and behavioral correlates. *Drug Alcohol Depend* 1977;2:141–148.

729. Markou A, Koob GF. Postcocaine anhedonia: an animal model of cocaine withdrawal. *Neuropsychopharmacology* 1991;4:17–26.

730. Kalant H. Comparative aspects of tolerance to, and dependence on, alcohol, barbiturates, and opiates. In: Gross MM, ed. *Alcohol intoxication and withdrawal.* New York: Plenum Press, 1977:169–186.

731. Wise RA. The role of reward pathways in the development of drug dependence. *Pharmacol Ther* 1987;35:227–263.

732. Solomon RL. The opponent process theory of acquired motivation. *Am Psychol* 1980;35:691–712.

733. Solomon RL, Corbit JD. An opponent-process theory of motivation: I. Temporal dynamics of affect. *Psychol Rev* 1974;81:119–145.

734. Koob GF, Markou A, Weiss F, et al. Opponent process and drug dependence: neurobiological mechanisms. *Semin Neurosci* 1993;5:351–358.

735. De Vry J, Donselaar I, Van Ree JM. Intraventricular self-administration of heroin in the rat: reward seems dissociated from analgesia and physical dependence. *Eur J Pharmacol* 1989;161:19–25.

736. Wei E, Loh HH, Way EL. Brain sites of precipitated abstinence in morphine dependent rats. *J Pharmacol Exp Ther* 1973;185:108–115.

737. Gardner EL, Lowinson JH. Drug craving and positive/negative hedonic brain substrates activated by addicting drugs. *Semin Neurosci* 1993;5:359–368.

738. Gardner EL, Walker LS, Paredes W. Clozapine's functional mesolimbic selectivity is not duplicated by the addition of anticholinergic action to haloperidol: a brain stimulation study in the rat. *Psychopharmacology (Berl)* 1993;110:119–124.

739. Eichler AJ, Antelman SM, Fisher AE. Self-stimulation: site-specific tolerance to chronic dopamine receptor blockade. *Soc Neurosci Abstr* 1976;2:440.

740. Ettenberg A, Wise RA. Non-selective enhancement of locus coeruleus and substantia nigra self-stimulation after termination of chronic dopaminergic receptor blockade with pimozide in rats. *Psychopharmacol Commun* 1976;2:117–124.

741. Ostrowski NL, Hatfield CB, Caggiula AR. The effects of low doses of morphine on the activity of dopamine-containing cells and on behavior. *Life Sci* 1982;31:2347–2350.

742. Matthews RT, German DC. Electrophysiological evidence for excitation of rat ventral tegmental area dopaminergic neurons by morphine. *Neuroscience* 1984;11:617–626.

743. Harris GC, Aston-Jones G. Involvement of D2 dopamine receptors in the nucleus accumbens in the opiate withdrawal syndrome. *Nature* 1994;371:155–157.

744. Bechara A, Harrington F, Nader K, et al. Neurobiology of motivation: double dissociation of two motivational

mechanisms mediating opiate reward in drug-naive versus drug-dependent animals. *Behav Neurosci* 1992;106:798–807.

745. Nader K, Bechara A, Roberts DCS, et al. Neuroleptics block high- but not low-dose heroin place preferences: further evidence for a two-system model of motivation. *Behav Neurosci* 1994;108:1128–1138.

746. Bechara A, Nader K, van der Kooy D. Neurobiology of withdrawal motivation: evidence for two separate aversive effects produced in morphine-naive versus morphine-dependent rats by both naloxone and spontaneous withdrawal. *Behav Neurosci* 1995;109:91–105.

747. Gardner EL. Brain reward mechanisms. In: Lowinson JH, Ruiz P, Millman RB, et al, eds. *Substance abuse: a comprehensive textbook,* 2nd ed. Baltimore: Williams & Wilkins, 1992:70–99.

748. Smith JE, Dworkin SI. Neurobiological substrates of drug self-administration. *NIDA Res Monogr Ser* 1986;71:127–145.

749. Goeders NE, Smith JE. Intracranial self-administration methodologies. *Neurosci Biobehav Rev* 1987;11:319–329.

750. Alheid GF, Heimer L. New perspectives in basal forebrain organization of special relevance for neuropsychiatric disorders: the striatopallidal, amygdaloid, and corticopetal components

of substantia innominata. *Neuroscience* 1988;27:1–39.

751. Heimer L, de Olmos J, Alheid GF, et al. "Perestroika" in the basal forebrain: opening the border between neurology and psychiatry. *Prog Brain Res* 1991;87:109–165.

752. Fibiger HC, Phillips AG, Brown EE. The neurobiology of cocaine-induced reinforcement. *Ciba Found Symp* 1992;166:96–111.

753. Koob GF. Neural mechanisms of drug reinforcement. *Ann NY Acad Sci* 1992;654:171–191.

754. Amalric M, Koob GF. Functionally selective neurochemical afferents and efferents of the mesocorticolimbic and nigrostriatal dopamine system. *Prog Brain Res* 1993;99:209–226.

755. Koob GF. Neurobiological mechanisms in cocaine and opiate dependence. *Res Publ Assoc Res Nerv Ment Dis* 1992;70:79–92.

756. Koob GF. Drugs of abuse: anatomy, pharmacology and function of reward pathways. *Trends Pharmacol Sci* 1992;13:177–184.

757. Hebb DO. *The organization of behavior: a neuropsychological theory.* New York: Wiley, 1949.

758. Goldstein A, *Addiction:* From Biology to Drug Policy, 2nd ed. New York: Oxford Univ. Press, 2001.

759. Damsma G, Pfaus JG, Wenkstern D, et al. Sexual behavior increases dopamine transmission in the nucleus accumbens

and striatum of male rats: comparison with novelty and locomotion. *Behav Neurosci* 1992;106:181–191.

760. Wilson C, Nomikos GG, Collu M, et al. Dopaminergic correlates of motivated behavior: importance of drive. *J Neurosci* 1995;15:5169–5178.

761. Wenkstern D, Pfaus JG, Fibiger HC. Dopamine transmission increases in the nucleus accumbens of male rats during their first exposure to sexually receptive female rats. *Brain Res* 1993;618:41–46.

762. Maldonado-Irizarry CS, Swanson CJ, Kelley AE. Glutamate receptors in the nucleus accumbens shell control feeding behavior via the lateral hypothalamus. *J Neurosci* 1995;15:6779–6788.

763. Gawin FH, Kleber HD. Abstinence symptomatology and psychiatric diagnosis in cocaine abusers. *Arch Gen Psychiatry* 1986;43:107–113.

764. Siegel RK. Cocaine smoking. *J Psychoactive Drugs* 1982;14:321–337.

765. Weiss RD, Mirin SM, Michael JL, et al. Psychopathology in chronic cocaine abusers. *Am J Drug Alcohol Abuse* 1986;12:17–29.

766. Dole VP, Nyswander ME, Kreek MJ. Narcotic blockade. *Arch Intern Med* 1966;118:304–309.

767. Dole VP. Implications of methadone maintenance for theories of narcotic addiction. *JAMA* 1989;261:1879–1880.

CHAPTER 6

Psychodynamics

EDWARD J. KHANTZIAN, LANCE DODES, AND NANCY M. BREHM

Substance use disorders are one of the foremost public and mental health problems of our time. Despite the unrelenting and deadly progression associated with drug/alcohol use and abuse, individuals who are enmeshed with substances remain powerfully driven to persist in such behaviors. This chapter discusses the perplexing psychological issues of what it is in the nature of people that causes them to succumb to, maintain, and relapse to the use of alcohol and drugs, despite the devastating consequences. As the foregoing chapters amply demonstrate, there are numerous perspectives, and determinants that grow out of these perspectives, to explain why substances of abuse can become so compelling. This chapter adopts a psychodynamic perspective, one that examines the inner emotional

terrain and the psychological organization and structures of an individual, to explore the psychological compulsion to use and become dependent upon addictive drugs. Our opinion is that it is a neglected but important perspective, but it need not, and should not, compete with other perspectives.

During the past several decades, important shifts have occurred in psychodynamic thinking about substance abuse (1–12). This chapter first summarizes early psychoanalytic theories about addiction, which primarily emphasized the use of drugs as a regressive, pleasurable adaptation. Following recent developments in psychodynamic thinking, it then explores the gradual shift in emphasis to a view of substance abuse as a progressive response to psychological suffering and related problems with self-regulation. These deficiencies include impaired self-care, vulnerabilities in self-development and self-esteem, troubled self-object relations, and affect deficits. Early theories had viewed addictive behavior as seeking early infantile pleasure. In contrast, a contemporary psychodynamic perspective views addiction as an adaptive effort for survival. The chapter then considers treatment implications, based on current theory and practice.

EARLY PSYCHOANALYTIC THEORIES OF ADDICTION

Early psychoanalytic theories of addictive behavior were congruent with the emergent theory at the beginning of the twentieth century. Thus it is not surprising that libidinal factors, aggressive drives, and a topographic model of the mind (i.e., conscious vs. unconscious) of the mind were emphasized.

Freud viewed masturbation as the primary addiction. Addiction to alcohol, morphine, and tobacco served as substitute compulsions to satisfy infantile pleasurable drives (13,14).

Abraham (15) stressed the role of alcohol in reducing sexual inhibitions in men. Rado (16) emphasized the "elatant" effect of drugs to alter depressed moods. He suggested that an understanding of addiction came from the recognition that the strength of the impulse to use a substance was more important than the substance in determining whether or not an individual became an addict. Anticipating more recent theory, he believed that drugs relieved a "tense depression."

In contrast to the emphasis on libidinal and erotic aspects of addiction, Glover (17) focused primarily on aggression and sadism as the factors most pivotal in addiction, viewing the addict's obsessional involvement with drugs as a progressive and successful defense against paranoid-sadistic tendencies and psychosis. Clearly, Glover's view of addiction as a progressive rather than a regressive adaptation marked the onset of a new perspective in psychodynamic formulations of addiction.

Expanding on Glover's ideas, Knight (18) described alcoholism as "regressive acting out of unconscious libidinal and sadistic drives" (p. 234) toward an overindulgent mother, and as progressive attempts at the solution of the conflict such drives evoked. Fenichel (19) saw alcoholism as a maladaptive defense mechanism employed in order to resolve neurotic conflict, particularly between dependence and the expression of anger. Balint (20) characterized the alcoholic as achieving "inner harmony" from the effect of intoxication.

DEVELOPMENT OF CONTEMPORARY THEORIES OF PSYCHOANALYSIS

As early psychodynamic formulations of addiction paralleled early psychoanalytic theory, more recent psychoanalytic understanding of addictive vulnerability has drawn on advances in contemporary psychoanalysis, which places emphasis on developmental, structural (ego/self), and object relations theory, as well as the centrality of affects (21–37). A detailed review of modern psychoanalytic theory is beyond the scope of this chapter. For a better appreciation of modern psychodynamic theory as it pertains to substance use disorders, the reader is referred to works by Levin, Walant, and Director (38–41). In what follows,

we draw on these more contemporary psychodynamic paradigms to explain the operative factors that make the powerful, repetitive drive to use and relapse to drugs so compelling.

Psychological Suffering

Whether addictive behavior is rooted in unbearable affects or confusion or absence of feelings (5,9), or whether patients with substance use disorders struggle with a sense of helplessness and enfeeblement (6,42), or by feelings of rage, shame, and interpersonal isolation (12,41), there are abundant clinical observations and studies to support the significant role of human psychological suffering in addictive disorders. Addicted individuals, if asked, frequently indicate that their pursuit and use of drugs make them feel "normal," "calm," "relaxed," "alive," "energized," and "not anxious—overwhelmed—[or] out of control." What such individuals indicate, and what contemporary psychodynamic theorists draw from clinical experience, suggests that substance use disorders are an attempt at self-correction. In one view of this, addictive behaviors become a special adaptation to compensate for inadequate or overdrawn defenses to regulate relationships, sense of self/self-respect, intense (and often undifferentiated) emotions, and compulsive/impulsive behaviors. Contemporary theory attempts to unravel the psychodynamic underpinnings of the suffering entailed in substance use disorders and how individuals resort to addictive behaviors to relieve their suffering.

Psychoanalytic ideas pertaining to this hypothesis first appeared in the writings of Gerard and Kornetsky (43,44) and Chein et al. (45). They emphasized that adolescents "use drugs adaptively to cope with overwhelming (adolescent) anxiety in anticipation of adult roles in the absence of adequate preparation, models and prospects" (cited in Khantzian, 3, p. 1261). Chein et al. (45) stated that addiction was "adaptive and functional"; that is, narcotics are used to help one cope and interact with one's emotions and the outside world.

Wieder and Kaplan (46) developed this perspective further by emphasizing that "the dominant conscious motive for drug use is not the seeking of 'kicks,' but the wish to produce pharmacologically a reduction in distress that the individual cannot achieve by his own psychic efforts" (p. 403). For some drug users, the substance functions in the same way as an external object. The choice of a specific drug depends on the interaction between the idiosyncratic meaning and the physical effect of the drug "with the particular conflicts and defects in a person's psychic structure" (46, p. 428). Therefore, drugs are not selected indiscriminately; they are chosen to act as "structural prostheses."

Based on the work of Wieder and Kaplan and the problems associated with adaptation and the ego function of addicts, Milkman and Frosch (47) tested the hypothesis that the self-selections of specific drugs are related to a preferred defensive style. Using the Bellack and Hurvich Interview and Rating Scale for Ego Functioning, they compared heroin and amphetamine addicts in drugged and nondrugged conditions. Their preliminary findings supported the hypothesis that heroin addicts prefer the calming and dampening effects of opiates; opiates also seemed to strengthen the addicts' tenuous defenses while simultaneously reinforcing their tendencies toward withdrawal and isolation. Conversely, amphetamine addicts used the stimulating action of these drugs to induce an inflated sense of self-worth and a defensive style involving active confrontation of their environment.

The work of Wurmser (12,48) and Khantzian (49–51) suggested that the excessive emphasis on the regressive effects of narcotics in the early psychoanalytic and some of the contemporary studies was unwarranted. Wurmser and Khantzian considered the specific pharmacologic action of opiates as a progressive effect whereby regressive states may actually be reversed. Wurmser's work suggested that narcotics are used adaptively by narcotic addicts to compensate for defects in affect defense, particularly against feelings of rage, shame, and abandonment. In his early work, Khantzian (1,49) stressed the use of narcotics in the service of drive defense. Narcotics act to reverse regressive states by their direct antiaggression action and serve to counteract the disorganizing influences of rage and aggression on the ego. Further expansion of these views led to a "self-medication" hypothesis, which focused on the use of heroin and cocaine dependence as an attempt to alleviate emotional suffering (3). Addicts, for the most part, do not choose drugs randomly to alleviate the painful affect states and underlying psychiatric disorders. Rather, drugs are chosen because an individual discovers a specific psychopharmacologic action, which helps alleviate the individual's suffering (3,4). Weissman et al. (52), McLellan et al. (53), Rounsaville et al. (54,55), Khantzian and Treece (56), and Blatt et al. (57) have documented the evidence of underlying psychiatric disorders that supports a self-medication hypothesis of addictive disorders. These researchers produced diagnostic findings documenting the co-occurrence of depression, personality disorder, and alcoholism. More recent studies further elaborate on the relationship between psychiatric disorders, in particular mood disorders, and substance use disorders (58–62). In addition, there is evidence that when psychiatric disorders are treated, mood improves significantly and there is a trend for diminished reliance on substances of abuse (63–72).

Recently, more emphasis has been placed on understanding addiction as "self-medication" to alleviate suffering, with less emphasis on severe psychopathology (5). For example, pain-relieving properties of the opiates help the user modulate disturbing, rageful feelings that are the source of much suffering in their lives, feelings that may originate in past experiences in which they were

victims, perpetrators, or both (3). The sedative–hypnotics can help tense, emotionally restricted individuals to experience walled-off affect and to overcome related fears concerning closeness, dependency, and intimacy (4,5). Cocaine, because of its energizing and activating properties, appeals to both high-energy and low-energy individuals. It can help overcome feelings of fatigue and the depletion states associated with depression or boredom (12,73), and persons with high-energy may be attracted to cocaine because it increases feelings of self-esteem and frustration tolerance (46) or augments a preferred hyperactive style and amplifies feelings of self-sufficiency (74). Paradoxically, stimulants also calm the restlessness and hyperactivity in individuals who suffer with attention deficit disorder (3,4).

In an update of the self-medication hypothesis, Khantzian (4) focused on subjective states of distress that are often as confusing and elusive as they are painful and unbearable. These states of subjective distress are involved in three areas not previously considered, namely (a) depressive affect in nicotine dependence, (b) self-medication of negative symptoms in schizophrenia, and (c) self-medication of psychic numbing and flooding involved in posttraumatic stress disorder (PTSD).

Dodes (6) suggested that addiction is a response to feelings of helplessness that are experienced by addicts as a narcissistic injury. In his view, addiction is an active behavior that reverses the feeling of helplessness and restores a sense of internal power by controlling and regulating one's affective state (something that drugs are particularly well-suited to do). At the same time, addictive behavior is an expression of the narcissistic rage that inevitably accompanies such states of helplessness. Indeed, Dodes suggested that the defining "addictive" qualities of addiction—its intensity and its limitless disregard of ordinary considerations—are a result of the expression of this underlying narcissistic rage as a central factor in addiction.

Dodes (7) expanded this theory by viewing addictions as a subset of compulsions. The action of using a drug is seen as a displacement or substitution for more direct action to correct the addict's helplessness and express the addict's rage: "Thus the addiction contains within it a superego prohibition expressed in the (unconscious) requirement to displace the narcissistic imperative for mastery to the addictive behavior" (7, p. 821). Dodes notes that compulsions may be defined following Fenichel, as "intense ideas that have to be thought about (or acted upon); their persistence represents the energy of some other associatively connected impulsive idea that has been warded off" (19, p. 268). When addictive behavior is seen as the expression of an idea that must be acted on (the enraged impulse to reassert mastery against helplessness) and as an action that must be taken in displacement because of the need to ward off the direct expression of this feeling, then addiction can be understood to be a subset of compulsions. This hypothesis is significant because it suggests the treatability of addictions with a psychodynamic approach that has been accepted for many years for compulsions. This view also allows many compulsions to be better understood as true addictions. In considering the implications of this hypothesis for treatment, the therapist can reframe the impulse for the patient as a healthy drive for mastery of helplessness, but displaced. The drive can be seen as "a drive for life" that can help alleviate the feelings of shame and helplessness that are so painful for the abuser.

Wurmser (42) conceptualizes substance abuse as an artificial affective defense, suggestive of a "primary phobia about "being closed in, captured, or trapped by structures and limitations, and any type of closeness" (p. 93). He suggests that the compulsive search of the addict for the addictive object (alcohol, drugs, etc.) is a mirror image of the usual avoidant behavior of the phobic. This external addictive object serves as a narcissistic protector against the primary phobia, becoming highly overvalued. Internally, a defense of narcissism is developed that produces "grandiosity, haughtiness, and withdrawal from the external world." This defense is experienced by others as ruthlessness and coldness, who then punish the addict's perceived haughtiness with humiliation and shame. In Wurmser's view, splitting, fragmentation, and massive depersonalization can occur. The limiting functioning of the superego is experienced as restricting and suffocating, reenacting the primary phobia. The protecting self-care functions of the superego are pathologized into new constricting structures.

SELF-REGULATORY DEFICIENCIES

A main framework for understanding substance abuse emphasizes self-regulatory deficiencies, encompassing deficits in self-care, self-development and self-esteem, self-object relationships, and affects. The ego must serve as a signal and guide in protecting the self against realistic, external dangers and against instability and chaos in internal emotional life (75). It follows that many substance abusers, as a consequence of deficits in self-regulation, experience painful and confusing emotions, troubled behaviors, poor self-esteem, stormy relationships or isolated existences (75).

Wilson et al. (76) proposed a hierarchic model of opiate addiction based on failures in self-regulation, using the hierarchic (multimodal) epigenetic theory of self-organization, originally proposed by Gedo and Goldberg and associates (77–82). Using the Scale for Failures in Self-Regulation to measure verbal and nonverbal manifestation in self-regulation failures in addicts, their study showed that addicts have significantly greater difficulties in self-regulation than do normal subjects.

Zinberg (27) offered a slightly different perspective regarding self-regulation in the addict. Building on the ideas of Rapaport (26), Zinberg emphasized the imbalance of the addict's ego, and the inability of the addict to maintain ego

autonomy as a consequence of their dependency on drugs, the artificial drives the drugs engender, and their social isolation.

Impairments in Self-Care

Many patients who are drug dependent show a disregard of possible dangers to their well-being, including the use of abusive substances. The inability to provide self-care is associated with a set of ego functions related to "signal-anxiety, reality-testing, judgment, and synthesis" (75, p. 165). The addict's disregard of self is not primarily the result of unconscious motivations of self-destructiveness but the "result of failures to adopt and internalize these functions from the caring parents in early and subsequent phases of development" (2, p. 193). Many problems in self-care are apparent in the histories of substance abusers prior to the use of a drug or subsequently even after long periods of abstinence.

Another deficit related to problems in self-care is the inability of addicts to soothe and calm themselves especially when stressed, and, conversely, the inability to be active in situations that call for activity when their well-being depends on it (75,83,84). This vulnerability is thought to be related to difficulties the child has in internalizing the caring functions of the mother (2).

Empiric research by Shedler and Block (85) provided support for the hypotheses of inadequate internalization of caring functions as a cause of substance abuse. They found that psychological differences between frequent drug users, experimenters, and abstainers in an adolescent population correlated with the type of parenting each group received. Mothers of frequent drug users were described as "relatively cold, unresponsive, and underprotective. They appear to give their children little encouragement, while, conjointly, they are pressuring and overly interested in their children's 'performance'" (85, p. 641).

Vulnerabilities in Self-Development and Self-Esteem

Basing his work on Jacobson's concept of self and object (86), Kernberg (87) described four stages of human development, culminating in object constancy. Kernberg believed that the alcoholic developed a pathologic "grandiose self," which is refueled by alcohol. This entitled "grandiose self" perceives that the self is perfect and the object is loving, and any other perceptions are denied. Alcoholics then use rigid and primitive defenses of splitting, denial, and projection to keep from their awareness the bad self or inadequate self at all costs. Alcoholics views alcohol use as a means to counter or overcome their rigid and overdrawn defenses.

Kohut (32–34) describes a continuum in the development of a sense of self, fragmentation at one end of the continuum and a cohesive enduring sense of self at the other. The latter confers a sense of well being and self-esteem extending into adulthood and assures a capacity for self-soothing and a realistic appreciation of self/other needs and capacities. Kohut (34) hypothesized that the substance abuser does not internalize the functions of the self-object, which results in "fragmentation of the self that the addict tries to counteract by his addictive behavior" (p. 197).

More recently, Goldberg and associates (88) considered a range of behaviors as addictive in nature, which serve to ward off painful affects and dysphoria. They consider such conduct as narcissistic behavioral disorders (as opposed to narcissistic personality disorders) in which parts of self are warded off to preserve self-cohesion.

From his observations of patients in treatment, Khantzian (2) reported shifting bipolar affects experienced in therapeutic relationships. Most of the time, patients show difficulties in having their needs met and are compliant, cooperative, and passive. Occasionally, however, they lapse into opposite attitudes of intrusiveness and demandingness, which reveal an enormous sense of narcissistic entitlement.

Wurmser (12) speculated that compulsive drug users try "to reestablish an omnipotent position where either their self is grandiose and without limitations" or where the other person, "the archaic self-object," is treated as all-giving and is required to live up to the highest ideals. When limitations are imposed, the painful affects of rage, shame, and abandonment are experienced. Rage ensues when the ideal self or the ideal world collapses. Shame is experienced because of discrepancies between the limited, disappointing self and the grandiose, ideal self. The feelings of abandonment become devastating when the self-objects are not as all-giving as expected. "The importance of narcotics . . . lies in their effect of reducing or even eliminating these three basic affects," Wurmser wrote (12, p. 833).

This overt grandiose self can be isolated both affectively and cognitively from an existing, enfeebled self who has chronic feelings of poor self-esteem, such as is frequently found in addicts (38). Substance abusers do not develop a sufficient capacity for self-love and self-esteem. They do not enjoy confidence in themselves or their abilities and have difficulty feeling valued in the world (84). The effects of drugs and alcohol interact with the painful feelings of inadequacies and related defenses, and momentarily alleviate their pain or improve how they feel about themselves.

In addition, addicts cannot retain narcissistic supplies from external sources to maintain their fragile self-esteem (11). The only continuously available source is drugs. Hence, the addict craves drugs for their effect of maintaining a sense of self-worth and of dissipating feelings of depletion. This is a never-ending process. Krystal likened it to a "baby [who] constantly regurgitates and swallows the contents of the stomach" (11, p. 186), demonstrating possibly the precursor "of an inability to retain the yearned for supplies [of affection] that we see in drug-dependent patients and in bulimia" (p. 186).

Troubled Self-Object Relations

Deficits in self-development and self-esteem in substance abusers may cause major problems in relationships (5,84). "As much as they need others to know how they feel, they often fear and distrust their dependency, disavow their needs, and act in counterdependent ways" (84, p. 264). They can be experts in disguising their needs for nurturance, although these needs can be excessive. They may be at the mercy of their "significant other" or external world to supply self-esteem, but at the same time may be paralyzed in asking for validation. They tend to go to either extreme, totally depending on and being subservient to the other, or isolating themselves (4).

Over the past decade illuminating works by Walant (40) drawing on Winnicott (89), and Flores (90) drawing on Bowlby (91), and Director (41) have helped to appreciate the troubled infrastructure of substance abusers' self-object relationships.

Deficits in Affect Tolerance

Deficits in affect tolerance have an important relationship to the craving for drugs or alcohol. Sashin (92) has described substance abusers problems with affect regulation as being too porous, allowing the contents (e.g., rage and anger) to pour out uncontrollably; as overly restrictive and sealed, thus constricting experiences and communication; or as depleted, resulting in emptiness (84).

Another developmental line involves the desomatization of affects. Affects that are experienced only as physiologic experiences are overwhelming and experienced as very dangerous (10,93). Krystal and Raskin (9) believed that the drug abuser lives in constant dread of reexperiencing the traumatic feelings that occurred preverbally: "These persons function as though they have an unconscious memory of the danger of trauma" (p. 33). The use of drugs is seen as an attempt to shore up the defense against reexperiencing the chaos: "The patient may be caught in a involuntary, compulsive need to repeat the pattern of selectively retained excessive reaction to a specific affect or to the alexithymic undifferentiated affect pattern" (94, p. 74). The continued pattern of working himself into an unbearable state drives the addictive person to search for a substance that will give relief.

In attempting to understand why a user continues, beyond physiologic addictive factors, despite chronic suffering from their abuse (physical deterioration, psychological regression, and an internal world of chaos), Khantzian and Wilson (95) speculated that the abuser feels some means of control in the active behavior of using. Thus the suffering experienced from the drug or alcohol is more bearable because it is something the user understands and controls. Krystal (11) adopted the term *alexithymia*, originally used by Sifneos (96) and Nemiah (97), to describe the condition of substance-abusing patients who could not verbalize what they were feeling. These patients cannot tell whether they are "sad, tired, hungry, or ill." Paradoxically, these patients can display intense affects in brief moments (11).

McDougall (98) described a similar inability to display affect in some of her patients. She used the term *disaffected* to describe the lifeless emotional experience that these patients bring into analysis. She hypothesized that their "narcissistic economy and the incapacity to contain and elaborate affective experience" was caused not only by mothers' being out of touch with their babies' needs but also squelching any outburst of spontaneous affective display. To maintain the frozen quality of their affects, she hypothesized these patients drown their feelings in alcohol, bulimic bouts, or drug abuse. If the affects are allowed to be felt, there is danger of feeling overwhelmed and of psychosomatic regression. Consequently, an attempt to avoid intense feelings might greatly stimulate the use of substance abuse (99).

In summary, the vulnerabilities of affect tolerance exhibited by addicts may involve attempts to block feelings, not connect their affect with cognition, and therefore not feel at all, or be frozen without fantasy or metaphor.

TREATMENT IMPLICATIONS

The goal of treatment is to first attend to the immediate need for containment and comfort (i.e., the destructive behaviors and self-disregulation), and second to attend to the more long-term goals of self-understanding and transformations in personality and the deficits and conflicts in ego/self structures that predispose to addictive behaviors.

Initial Treatment Stage—Stabilization

Where loss of control is the danger and stabilization is the therapeutic task, the therapist must fulfill a special role initially as a caretaker. The patient must be provided with hope that relief from being overwhelmed will occur and with the expectation that comfort and containment can be achieved. Thus hope and expectation gradually become the "regulator[s] of [the] inner state" (22).

In the initial stage of treatment, the therapist's role may need to be expanded to that of a "primary care therapist" (100). The primary care therapist is concerned about the early tasks of treatment. The initial concern of the therapist is to often help the patient gain control over the use of alcohol or other drugs (75,101). As a start, the therapist should take an extensive drug and developmental history. This includes an empathic investigation to discover when the abuse first began, where the substance was used, the pattern and progression of use that developed, and how internal feeling states were changed (102). Through the telling of his or her own life story, the alcoholic or drug abuser begins to be gently confronted with the deleterious consequences of the abused substance. At the same time, the therapist builds a therapeutic alliance through concern for the addict's suffering.

The therapist and the patient carefully evaluate the severity of the substance abuse and the immediate and long-term steps whereby control can be achieved (100). Some patients may need immediate hospitalization in order not to place themselves or others in a dangerous situation. However, many do not need this level of intervention. The therapist and patient can begin immediately in a therapeutic mode. The need for control rather than abstinence should be emphasized: "Keeping the focus on control allows a strategy to develop that avoids premature insistence on permanent abstinence, or an equally untenable permissive acceptance of uncontrolled drinking" (75, p. 173).

Dodes (103) has pointed out that the "therapist's caring concern" may either immediately or gradually be internalized by the patient, thus allowing a "nucleus" of internal self-regulation to develop control or abstinence to occur (103). This internalization may be possible through an immediate identification with the therapist as an "idealized object" or even an aggressive object. However, drinking may continue to occur. Therapy may proceed in spite of this so long as the drinking is intermittent and does not either prevent the therapy from usefully continuing, or create a crisis in the person's life. By continuing the treatment, versus interrupting it, Dodes noted that the factors interfering with abstinence or control can be explored. If drinking continues and is destructive, however, there may be a need for hospitalization, day treatment, or interruption of therapy.

During the initial stage of therapy, where control is of paramount importance, many addicted individuals have found the use of self-help groups such as Alcoholics Anonymous (AA) and Narcotics Anonymous (NA) to provide a network of relationships that is supportive (100). Mack views the function of AA as providing the individual with a framework of "self-governance" in a social context (104). Alternatively, Dodes (105) describes AA and its "higher power" as being used as transitional objects, whose omnipotence substitutes for the power against helplessness sought through addictive behavior, and now lost in abstinence. AA and NA are frequently inappropriate for patients, particularly those who suffer from intense shame and anxiety or whose personality makes it untenable to accept the AA/NA message of "surrender—belief in a higher power," and the like (106). Indeed, as Dodes has noted, the idea of "surrendering" is antithetical to many addicts, for psychologically sound reasons. This factor, plus the risk to people in AA of being shamed if they don't "get with the program" indicate that 12-step programs should be prescribed judiciously and on an individualized basis; they should not be assumed to be the proper treatment for addiction for all individuals (107).

During the initial phases of therapy, the therapist must also make a careful evaluation of whether to use "adjunctive pharmacological agents" and other treatment strategies to help the patient achieve and maintain control (100). For example, methadone maintenance can be effective not only in the achievement of biologic homeostasis for narcotic addicts, but also in the management of their painful feelings of aggression and rage. The use of Antabuse and naltrexone and other monitoring procedures, such as the screening of urine, may be useful in selected cases.

Some patients may not require ongoing therapy. However, most will benefit from understanding the psychological factors that led to their addictive behavior. The psychotherapy for people with addictions proceeds like any other psychodynamic therapy, because people with addictions are just as capable of insight and self-understanding as anyone else (Dodes, 107,108). Dodes has emphasized the value in therapy of identifying the moments when addicts first have the thought of repeating an addictive behavior (107). These thoughts always precede the action itself—sometimes by a long time. Once those moments are identified, it is often possible for the person to recognize the precipitant for which the person's addictive act is a restorative response. According to Dodes, these precipitants are in general situations that arouse a sense of intolerable helplessness. The particular type of situation, and why it is associated with a helplessness that feels intolerable, is highly individualized and is always of great psychological importance to that person. Through identifying these precipitants, the patient comes to know the psychological purpose of his addictive behavior—the specific issues whose associated helplessness the patient is attempting to reverse through the displaced act of an addictive behavior. Beyond this, understanding the psychology of the patient's addiction allows the patient to know the most important emotional issues for himself in general, because the factors that drive addictive behavior are inevitably intertwined with the rest of a person's emotional life. Indeed, Dodes has noted this fact as a reason to not separate addiction treatment from the rest of psychotherapy—addictions are part of a person's psychology, not a separate entity. Hence they deserve our best efforts at psychological insight rather than being isolated as problems whose treatment should be referred elsewhere (107).

Building Internal Self-Regulation

A phased treatment approach appreciates and addresses initial needs for abstinence, safety, and comfort, and, subsequently, the psychotherapeutic understanding and modification of self-regulation vulnerabilities. The role of the primary care therapist in early phases of treatment helps the patient to appreciate shared and real concerns for stabilization and control. The patient may be encouraged to use 12-step groups in order to benefit from the containing and transforming influences that they supply. Subsequently, individual and group psychotherapy provide therapeutic contexts for the unfolding of patients' characterologic defenses and underlying self-regulation vulnerabilities, as well as internalization of self-regulating capacities for better affect management, self-other relations, and self-care that otherwise have been absent or underdeveloped (5,101,106,109). Khantzian (110) recently explored in more detail how group therapy serves as a corrective for these defenses and vulnerabilities in substance abusers. Kaufman (111) focused on the benefits of psychotherapy for "the addicted person" and emphasized the importance of integrating 12-step and psychotherapy approaches.

In addressing narcissistic characteristics of substance abuser, Derby (112) describes difficulties therapists encounter in surviving the interpersonal exploitation, grandiosity, and lack of empathy a substance abuser can exhibit. Derby believes that this behavior can quickly be interpreted by the therapist as sociopathic. The use of contracts (so many AA meetings, urine tests, etc.), which are useful with the sociopathic population, are doomed to failure with the substance abuser because this patient may respond with "rage, inadequacy, shame, and emptiness." The substance abuser may have difficulty in finding words for expressing these feelings because of hyposymbolization and isolation of affect. Derby emphasizes the importance of the therapist's countertransference in the treatment of addicts. Preset ideas about addicts must be abandoned, and the therapist must be open to each individual story without countertransferential feelings of moral judgment.

Internalizing Self-Care Functions

Self-care functions may be internalized as the result of the care and concern of the therapist (106). It is more useful for the therapist to talk about the inability of substance abusers to take care of themselves than to emphasize the destructiveness of their behavior. For those patients who have a significant self-care deficit, the therapist needs to explore developmental deficiencies and defects that do not allow danger to be anticipated and to help the patient understand that this disability is correctable (106). Modified dynamic group therapy is especially helpful in the internalization of self-care functions (109).

Some patients may benefit from alternatives for self-soothing rather than the use of alcohol or drugs. The auxiliary use of acupuncture, meditation, exercise, pharmacotherapy, hypnosis, and the like may, in selected cases, help to relieve emotional suffering or irritability.

Repairing Self-Deficits and Enhancing Self-Esteem

The control of inner tension, establishing and prioritizing personal goals, and giving up illusions about oneself and others are therapeutic goals that help to repair self-deficits and enhance self-esteem (113). The establishment of a caring relationship in therapy creates a "holding environment" in which optimal frustration allows for acquisition of psychological skills. An environment of excessive frustration or disappointment which may have been present in the past, may have created an atmosphere in which learning these skills could not take place, and thus became the root of self-deficits. The circumstances surrounding the origins of self-deficits must also be understood (113). For instance, it is often important to uncover identifications with primary caretakers, such as parents, who also had an addiction.

Maintaining Mature Self-Object Relationships

Those substance abusers who disavow their needs for attachment by grandiose illusions about themselves typically keep themselves in functional and actual psychological isolation (84). When the addict begins to view the therapist as a "transformational other" who is powerful enough to separate the addict from the addict's drug or alcohol, feelings of idealization and love may be expressed toward the therapist (40). Self-help groups or group psychotherapy can often be used to give human support and contact or appropriate reality testing (109).

Identifying Affect

Krystal (114) suggested specific technical modifications to help those patients who have difficulties in the identification of affect. The therapist takes an active role in teaching the patient "what affect responses are and how one uses them to one's advantage" (114, p. 371). Because many of the feelings are experienced somatically in this subgroup, the therapist must understand the intense discomfort that feelings create and help the patient begin to contain them appropriately. "Affect-naming and verbalization must be encouraged; supplying (to the patient) the words and names of emotions is a slow task, because verbalization represents just one half of the task. The other half consists in desomatization" (114, p. 371). A bridge must be built between the affective and cognitive components. The feeling must become attached to the story.

Finally, the therapist helps the addict to develop his or her capacity to fantasize. Wolff (115) suggested the use of play as a technique in helping the patient who is deprived of feelings. Using Winnicott's (31) hypothesis that the patient must learn to play before the patient can use psychotherapy, Wolff stressed the use of creative play, in which fantasies are encouraged and feelings, desires, and bodily sensations are explored.

CONCLUSIONS

The psychology of substance abuse, as formulated from a psychodynamic perspective, focuses on understanding addictions as adaptive attempts to alleviate emotional suffering and repair self-regulatory deficiencies. Treatment emphasizes the development of an understanding of the emotional factors that lie behind and produce addiction as a restorative response. This is fostered by mutual understanding of the addict's suffering, gradual toleration, and modulation of painful feelings, learning of psychological skills to care for and nurture the self, and the adoption of a reality not based on childhood illusions. Our greatest source of knowledge is our patients. We learn by listening attentively to the uniqueness of their stories.

REFERENCES

1. Khantzian EJ. Opiate addiction: a critique of theory and some implications for treatment. *Am J Psychother* 1974;28:59–74.
2. Khantzian EJ. The ego, the self and opiate addiction: theoretical and treatment considerations. *Int Rev Psychoanal* 1978;5:189–198.
3. Khantzian EJ. The self-medication hypothesis of addictive disorders: a focus on heroin and cocaine [special article]. *Am J Psychiatry* 1985;142:1259–1264.
4. Khantzian EJ. The self-medication hypothesis of substance use disorders: a reconsideration and recent applications. *Harv Rev Psychiatry* 1997;4:231–244.
5. Khantzian EJ. Self-regulation vulnerabilities in substance abusers: treatment implications. In: Dowling S, ed. *The psychology and treatment of addictive behaviors.* Madison, CT: International University Press, 1995:17–41.
6. Dodes LM. Addiction, helplessness, and narcissistic rage. *Psychoanal Q* 1990;59:398–419.
7. Dodes LM. Compulsion and addiction. *J Am Psychoanal Assoc* 1996;44:815–836.
8. Johnson B. Three perspectives on addiction. *J Am Psychoanal Assoc* 1999;791–815.
9. Krystal H, Raskin HA. *Drug dependence aspects of ego function.* Detroit: Wayne State University Press, 1970.
10. Krystal H. Trauma and affects. *Psychoanal Study Child* 1978;33:81–116.
11. Krystal H. *Integration and self-healing: affect, trauma, alexithymia.* Hillsdale, NJ: Analytic Press, 1988.
12. Wurmser L. Psychoanalytic considerations of the etiology of compulsive drug use. *J Am Psychoanal Assoc* 1974;22:820–843.
13. Freud S. Three essays on the theory of sexuality. In: Strachey J. ed. *Standard edition.* London: Hogarth Press, 1955;7:125–245 (original work published in 1905).
14. Freud S. *The complete letters of Sigmund Freud to Wilhelm Fliess.* Cambridge, MA: Harvard University Press, 1985:287. Masson JM, translator/editor.
15. Abraham K. The psychological relation between sexuality and alcoholism. In:

Selected papers of Karl Abraham. New York: Basic Books, 1964:80–89 (original work published in 1908).

16. Rado S. The psychoanalysis of pharmacothymia. *Psychoanal Q* 1933;2:1–23.

17. Glover E. On the etiology of drug addiction. In: *On the early development of mind.* New York: International Universities Press, 1956:187–215.

18. Knight RP. The dynamics and treatment of chronic alcohol addiction. *Bull Menninger Clin* 1937;1:233–250.

19. Fenichel O. *The psychoanalytic theory of neurosis.* New York: WW Norton, 1945:375–386.

20. Balint M. *The basic fault: therapeutic aspects of regresssion.* New York: Brunner Mazel, 1968.

21. Freud S. Remembering, repeating, and working-through. In: Strachey J. ed. *Standard edition.* London: Hogarth Press, 1955;12:145–156 (original work published in 1914).

22. Pine F. *Drive ego, object, and self: a synthesis for clinical work.* New York: Basic Books, 1990.

23. Freud A. *The ego and the mechanisms of defense.* Vol II. New York: International Universities Press, 1966.

24. Brenner C. *Mind in conflict.* Madison, CT: International Universities Press, 1982.

25. Hartmann H. *Ego psychology and the problem of adaptation.* New York: International Universities Press, 1958 (original work published in 1939).

26. Rapaport D. The theory of ego autonomy: a generalization. In: Gill M, ed. *The collected papers of David Rapaport.* New York: Basic Books, 1967:722–744 (original work published in 1957).

27. Zinberg NE. Addiction and ego function. *Psychoanal Stud Child* 1975; 30:567–588.

28. Freud A. A psychoanalytic view of developmental psychopathology. In: *The writings of Anna Freud.* New York: International Universities Press, 1981;8:57–74 (original work published in 1974).

29. Klein M. *Contributions to psychoanalysis.* London: Hogarth Press, 1948 (original work published 1921–1945).

30. Fairbairn WRD. A revised psychopathology of the psychoses and psychoneuroses. *Int J Psychoanal* 1941; 22:250–279.

31. Winnicott DW. The capacity to be alone. In: *The maturational processes and the facilitating environment.* Madison, CT: International Universities Press, 1965:29–36 (original work published in 1958).

32. Kohut H. *The analysis of the self.* New York: International Universities Press, 1971.

33. Kohut H. Thoughts on narcissism and narcissistic rage. *Psychoanal Stud Child* 1972;27:364–400.

34. Kohut H. *The restoration of the self.* New York: International Universities Press, 1977.

35. Spitz RA. *No and yes.* New York: International Universities Press, 1957.

36. Mahler MS. Notes on the development of basic moods: the depressive affect. In: Loewenstein RM, Newman LM, Schur M, et al., eds. *Psychoanalysis: a general psychology.* New York: International Universities Press, 1966:152–168.

37. Mahler MS, Pine F, Bergman A. *The psychological birth of the human infant.* New York: Basic Books, 1975.

38. Levin JD. *Treatment of alcoholism and other addictions.* Northvale, NJ: Jason Aronson, 1987.

39. Levin JD. *Therapeutic strategies for treating addiction: from slavery to freedom.* Northvale, NJ: Jason Aronson, 2001.

40. Walant KB. *Creating the capacity for attachment: treating addictions and the alienated self.* Northvale, NJ: Jason Aronson, 1995.

41. Director L. The value of relational psychoanalysis in the treatment of chronic drug and alcohol use. *Psychoanal Dialog* 2002;12:551–579.

42. Wurmser L. Psychology of compulsive drug use. In: Wallace B, ed. *The chemically dependent—phases of treatment and recovery.* New York: Brunner/Mazel, 1992.

43. Gerard DL, Kornetsky C. Adolescent opiate addiction: a case study. *Psychiatr Q* 1954;28:367–380.

44. Gerard DL, Kornetsky C. Adolescent opiate addiction: a study of control and addict subjects. *Psychiatr Q* 1955;29:457–486.

45. Chein I, Gerard DL, Lee RS, et al. *The road to H.* New York: Basic Books, 1964.

46. Wieder H, Kaplan EH. Drug use in adolescents: psychodynamic meaning and pharmacogenic effect. *Psychoanal Stud Child* 1969;24:399–431.

47. Milkman H, Frosch WA. On the preferential abuse of heroin and amphetamine. *J Nerv Ment Disord* 1973; 156:242–248.

48. Wurmser L. Methadone and the craving for narcotics; observations of patients on methadone maintenance in psychotherapy. In: *Proceedings of the Fourth National Methadone Conference, San Francisco, 1971.* New York: National Association for the Prevention of Addiction to Narcotics, 1972:525–528.

49. Khantzian EJ. A preliminary dynamic formulation of the psychopharmaco-

logic action of methadone. In: *Proceedings of the Fourth National Methadone Conference, San Francisco, 1971.* New York: National Association for the Prevention of Addiction to Narcotics, 1972.

50. Khantzian EJ. An ego-self theory of substance dependence: a contemporary psychoanalytic perspective. In: Lettieri DJ, Sayers M, Pearson HW, eds. *Theories on drug abuse.* NIDA research monograph 30. Rockville, MD: National Institute on Drug Abuse, 1980:29–33.

51. Khantzian EJ. Psychological (structural) vulnerabilities and the specific appeal of narcotics. *Ann N Y Acad Sci* 1982;398:24–32.

52. Weissman MM, Slobetz F, Prusoff B, et al. Clinical depression among narcotic addicts maintained on methadone in the community. *Am J Psychiatry* 1976;133:1434–1438.

53. McLellan AT, Woody GE, O'Brien CP. Development of psychiatric illness in drug abusers. *N Engl J Med* 1979;201:1310–1314.

54. Rounsaville BJ, Weissman MM, Crits-Cristoph K, et al. Diagnosis and symptoms of depression in opiate addicts: course and relationship to treatment outcome. *Arch Gen Psychiatry* 1982;39:151–156.

55. Rounsaville BJ, Weissman MM, Kleber H, et al. Heterogeneity of psychiatric diagnosis in treated opiate addicts. *Arch Gen Psychiatry* 1982;39:164–166.

56. Khantzian EJ, Treece C. *DSM-III* psychiatric diagnosis of narcotic addicts: recent findings. *Arch Gen Psychiatry* 1985;42:1067–1071.

57. Blatt SJ, Berman W, Bloom-Feshback S, et al. Psychological assessment of psychopathology in opiate addiction. *J Nerv Ment Dis* 1984;172:156–165.

58. Brady K, Anton R, Ballenger JC, et al. Cocaine abuse among schizophrenic patients. *Am J Psychiatry* 1990; 147:1164–1167.

59. Flynn PM, Luckey JW, Brown BS, et al. Relationship between drug preference and indicators of psychiatric impairment. *Am J Drug Alcohol Abuse* 1995;21:153–166.

60. Serper MR, Alpert M, Richardson NA, et al. Clinical effects of recent cocaine use on patients with acute schizophrenia. *Am J Psychiatry* 1995;152:1464–1469.

61. Aharonovich E, Nguyen HT, Nunes EV. Anger and depressive states among treatment-seeking drug abusers: testing the psychopharmacological specificity hypothesis. *Am J Addict* 2001;10:327–334.

62. Hasin D, Liu X, Nunes E, et al. Effects of major depression on remission and

relapse of substance dependence. *Arch Gen Psychiatry* 2002;59:375–380.

63. Cornelius JR, Salloum IM, Eliler JG, et al. Fluoxetine in depressed alcoholics: a double-blind, placebo-controlled trial. *Arch Gen Psychiatry* 1997;54:700–705.

64. Greenfield SJ, Weiss RD, Muenz LR, et al. The effect of depression on return to drinking: a prospective study. *Arch Gen Psychiatry* 1998;55:259–265.

65. Mason BJ, Kocsis JH, Ritvo CE, et al. A double-blind, placebo-controlled trial of desipramine for primary alcohol dependence stratified on the presence or absence of major depression. *JAMA* 1996;275:761–767.

66. McGrath PJ, Nunes EV, Stewart JW, et al. Imipramine treatment of alcoholics with major depression: a placebo-controlled clinical trial. *Arch Gen Psychiatry* 1996;53:232–240.

67. Nunes EV, Quitkin FM. Treatment of depression in drug dependent patients; effects on mood and drug use. In: Onken LS, Blaine JD, Horton M, eds. *Treatment of drug dependent individuals with comorbid mental disorders.* NIDA Research Monograph No. 172. Rockville, MD: National Institute on Drug Abuse, 1997:61–85.

68. Nunes EV, Quitkin FM, Stewart JW, et. al. Imipramine treatment of opiate-dependent patients with depressive disorders. *Arch Gen Psychiatry* 1996;55: 153–160.

69. Petrakis I, Carroll KM, Nich C, et al. Fluoxetine treatment of depressive disorders in methadone-maintained opioid addicts. *Drug Alcohol Depend* 1998;50:221–226.

70. Roy A. Placebo-controlled study of sertraline in depressed recently abstinent alcoholics. *Biol Psychiatry* 1998;44: 633–637.

71. Roy Byrne PP, Pages KP, Russo JE, et al. Nefazodone treatment of major depression in alcohol-dependent patients: a double-blind, placebo-controlled trial. *J Clin Psychopharmacol* 2000;20:129–136.

72. Willens TE, Biederman J, Millstein RB, et al. Risk for substance use disorders in youths with child-adolescent onset bipolar disorders. *J Am Acad Child Adolesc Psychiatry* 1999;38:680–685.

73. Khantzian EJ. Self-selection and progression in drug dependence. *Psychiatry Dig* 1975;10:19–22.

74. Khantzian EJ. Impulse problems in addiction: cause and effect relationships. In: Wishnie H, ed. *Working with the impulsive person.* New York: Plenum, 1979:97–112.

75. Khantzian EJ. Some treatment implications of the ego and self disturbances in alcoholism. In: Bean MH, Zinberg NE, eds. *Dynamic approaches to the understanding and treatment of alcoholism.* New York: Macmillan, 1981:163–193.

76. Wilson A, Passik SD, Faude J, et al. A hierarchical model of opiate addiction. Failures of self-regulation as a central aspect of substance abuse. *J Nerv Ment Dis* 1989;177:390–399.

77. Gedo JE, Goldberg A. *Models of the mind: a psychoanalytic theory.* Chicago: University of Chicago Press, 1973.

78. Gedo JE. *Beyond interpretation: toward a unified theory of psychoanalysis.* New York: International Universities Press, 1979.

79. Gedo JE. *Psychoanalysis and its discontents.* New York: International Universities Press, 1984.

80. Gedo JE. *Conflict in psychoanalysis: essays in history and method.* New York: Guilford Press, 1986.

81. Wilson A, Passik S, Faude J. Self-regulation and its failures. In: Masling J, ed. *Empirical studies in psychoanalytic theory.* Hillsdale, NJ: Erlbaum, 1996:149–214.

82. Wilson A, Malatesta C. Affects and the compulsion to repeat: Freud's repetition compulsion revisited. *Psychoanal Contemp Thought* 1989;12:265–312.

83. Khantzian EJ, Mack JE. Self-preservation and the care of the self: ego instincts reconsidered. *Psychoanal Stud Child* 1983;28:209–232.

84. Khantzian EJ. Self-regulation and self-medication factors in alcoholism and the addictions: similarities and differences. In: Galanter M, ed. *Recent developments in alcoholism.* New York: Plenum, 1990;8:255–270.

85. Shedler J, Block J. Adolescent drug use and psychological health. *Am Psychol* 1990;45:612–630.

86. Jacobson E. *The self and the object world.* New York: International Universities Press, 1964.

87. Kernberg O. *Borderline conditions and pathological narcissism.* New York: Jason Aronson, 1975.

88. Goldberg A, ed. *Errant selves: a casebook of misbehavior.* Hillsdale, NJ: The Analytic Press, 2000.

89. Winnicott DW. *Playing and reality.* London: Tavistock, 1971.

90. Flores PJ. Addiction as an attachment disorder: implications for group therapy. *Int J Group Ther* 2001;51:63–81.

91. Bowlby J. *Attachment and loss: vol. 2. Separation and anxiety and anger.* New York: Basic Books, 1973.

92. Sashin JI. Affect tolerance: a model of affect-response using catastrophe theory. *J Soc Biol Struct* 1985;8:175–202.

93. Freud S. Cited in Stern MM. Fear of death and neurosis. *J Am Psychoanal Assoc* 1968;16:3–31.

94. Krystal H. Disorders of emotional development in addictive behavior. In: Dowling S, ed. *The psychology and treatment of addictive behavior.* Madison, CT: International Universities Press, 1995.

95. Khantzian EJ, Wilson A. Substance dependence, repetition and the nature of addictive suffering. In: Wilson A, Gedo JE, eds. *Hierarchical concepts in psychoanalysis.* New York: Guilford Press, 1993:263–283.

96. Sifneos P. Clinical observations on some patients suffering from a variety of psychosomatic diseases. Proceedings of the 7th European Conference on Psychosomatic Research, Rome, September 11–16, 1967. *Acta Med Psychosom* 1967:452–458.

97. Nemiah JC. The psychological management and treatment of patients with peptic ulcer. *Adv Psychosom Med* 1970;6:169–173.

98. McDougall J. The. "dis-affected" patient; reflections on affect pathology. *Psychoanal Q* 1984;53:386–409.

99. Berger LS. *Substance abuse as symptom—a psychoanalytic critique of treatment approaches and the cultural beliefs that sustain them.* Hillsdale, NJ: Analytic Press, 1991.

100. Khantzian EJ. The primary care therapist and patient needs in substance abuse treatment. *Am J Drug Alcohol Abuse* 1988;14:159–167.

101. Dodes LM, Khantzian EJ. Individual psychodynamic psychotherapy with addicts. In: *Clinical textbook of addiction disorders.* London: Guilford Press, 1991:391–405.

102. Khantzian EJ. Psychotherapeutic interventions with substance abusers—the clinical context. *J Subst Abuse Treat* 1985;2:83–88.

103. Dodes LM. Abstinence from alcohol in long-term individual psychotherapy with alcoholics. *Am J Psychother* 1984;36:248–256.

104. Mack JE. Alcoholism AA, the governance of the self. In: Bean MH, Zinberg NE, eds. *Dynamic approaches to the understanding and treatment of alcoholism.* New York: Free Press, 1981:163–188.

105. Dodes, LM. The psychology of combining dynamic psychotherapy and Alcoholics Anonymous. *Bull Menninger Clin* 1988;52:283–293.

106. Khantzian EJ. A contemporary psychodynamic approach to drug abuse treatment. *Am J Drug Alcohol Abuse* 1986;12:213–222.

107. Dodes LM. *The heart of addiction.* New York: HarperCollins, 2002.

108. Dodes LM. Psychotherapy is useful,

often essential, for alcoholics. *Psychodynamic Lett* 1991;1:4–7.

109. Khantzian EJ, Halliday KS, McAuliffe WE. *Addiction and the vulnerable self: modified dynamic group therapy for substance abusers.* New York: Guilford Press, 1990.

110. Khantzian EJ. Reflections on group treatments as corrective experiences for addictive vulnerability. *Intl J Group Psychother* 2001;51:11–20.

111. Kaufman E. *The psychotherapy of addicted persons.* New York: Guilford Press, 1994.

112. Derby K. Some difficulties in the treatment of character-disordered addicts. In: Wallace BC, ed. *The chemically dependent—phases of treatment and recovery.* New York: Brunner/Mazel, 1992.

113. Gedo JE. *The mind in disorder: psychoanalytic models of pathology.* Hillsdale, NJ: Analytic Press, 1988.

114. Krystal H. Alexithymia and the effectiveness of psychoanalytic treatment. *Int J Psychoanal Psychother* 1983;9:353–378.

115. Wolff HH. The contribution of the interview situation to the restriction in fantasy and emotional experience in psychosomatic patients. *Psychother Psychosom* 1977;28:58–67.

CHAPTER 7

Sociocultural Issues

BRUCE D. JOHNSON AND ANDREW GOLUB

Substance use takes place within an evolving sociocultural environment that mediates which substances are available, their desirability, and their acceptability. Accordingly, the drugs to which persons are exposed and their reactions to them are strongly influenced by the person's place in the prevailing society. Not all performance-enhancing or recreational substance use is defined as deviant or illegal. And despite legal prohibitions, illicit drug use is widespread in American society. The 2001 National Survey on Drug Use and Health (NSD4H, formerly National Household Survey on Drug Abuse [NHSDA]) indicated that about 94 million people (42% of the population) aged 12 years and older had used an illicit drug in their lifetime, about 28 million (12.5%) used an illicit drug in the past year, and 16 million (7%) used an illicit drug in the past month (1). Even more persons reported consuming two legal substances, alcohol and tobacco. Moreover, the NSDUH does not ask about use of caffeine that is consumed in coffee, tea, and sodas, often explicitly as a pick-me-up. Use of caffeine is still widespread and broadly accepted despite a growing awareness of its potential for abuse (see Chapter 24).

Marijuana is the most common illicit drug NSDUH respondents reported using. Relatively fewer persons reported trying crack or heroin. These drugs are commonly referred to as "hard drugs" because they are broadly perceived as potentially causing greater health problems, as having greater potential for dependence, and as potentially leading to undesirable social behaviors. (The scientific literature supporting this perspective is reviewed in other chapters.) The use of crack and heroin has been widespread and even the norm within some subpopulations, particularly among impoverished persons in the inner-city. Illicit drug use in the inner city is especially important because this behavior and its attendant activities are often viewed by many as the core of "the drug problem." Poor inner-city minorities are typically the most likely to come to the attention of law enforcement, public drug treatment, other public mental health service providers, and welfare agencies. This chapter discusses the harsh circumstances of inner-city life that magnify drug-related social problems, describes the sociocultural processes that underlie the emergence and course of drug eras, and recounts the natural history of recent shifts in drug use both in the general population and in inner-city communities.

MULTIPLE SOCIAL CRISES IN THE INNER CITY

A major phenomenon of the modern city is the reality of the visibly poor living near rich or middle-income people. The stark contrast between the "haves" and "have nots" is the result of a legacy of separation and disadvantage further exacerbated by recent structural shifts in American society. In particular, "ghettoization" increased during the 1970s and 1980s. Inner-city neighborhoods comprised mainly of low-income, welfare, and poor people from minority (Hispanic and African American) backgrounds have expanded in geographic area and population size (2–5). The more successful and stable working people tended to move out of these ghettos, leaving behind the poorest and least successful (6). Such neighborhoods have a conspicuous absence of small businesses that create entry-level jobs and economic opportunities for youths and young adults (7–9). Even outside of inner-city ghettos, similar trends have had a great impact on the lives of low-income people and families (10). Multiple social crises continue to persist in employment, housing, family composition, and education—setting a framework for the patterns of drug abuse and use chronicled in this chapter.

During the 1970s, but especially in the 1980s and 1990s, American cities experienced a continued catastrophic decline in manufacturing and other labor-intensive industries that provide unskilled "working-class" jobs with steady employment and low but adequate incomes. When and if new jobs were created, they tended to require advanced education or skills (11,12). Other new jobs tended to be in fast food or other service industries, paying a near-minimum wage, which was far less than needed to live (13,14). The result was that many minority males, especially, were unlikely to have any legal employment and many became "discouraged workers" who were "out of the labor force" (7,15). The end result has been the marginalization of working-class and middle-class people, white and minority, who have limited access to legal jobs, diminished income and purchasing power, little access to affordable housing, and little financial support (16).

By 1960, many structurally sound housing units provided low-cost housing to working families living in the inner city. While the costs of maintaining and renovating such buildings climbed, rental income or income for maintenance did not increase substantially. Therefore, large segments of the low-cost housing stock deteriorated or were abandoned during the 1960s and 1970s, particularly in inner-city neighborhoods (17,18). In the 1980s and 1990s, real estate values in most major metropolitan areas soared. Affordable housing rose beyond the economic reach of much of the population (19), while funds for subsidized housing were reduced by more than 90% in the 1980s (20,21).

Important shifts also occurred in family structure, particularly among minorities. The proportion of African American children living in mother-only families increased from 30% to 51% between 1970 and 1985. Almost 90% of African American children will experience poverty if the family is headed by a single woman younger than age 30 years (8). Poor families headed by single women will likely be without adequate financial support for housing, so they must live with other relatives, in public shelters, or in very deteriorated buildings (14,22). Even when a household is maintained, several different family members, relatives, and unaffiliated persons may reside in or be "couch persons" who contribute little to and consume much of the minimal financial resources provided by public transfers for the household head and children (23–25).

Other crises compound the difficulties faced by inner-city residents and low-income persons. The Personal Responsibility and Work Opportunity Reconciliation Act of 1996 mandated that persons receiving welfare be required to work 35 hours a week. Many welfare recipients found their opportunities for legal employment, when available, rarely paid much more than welfare (26–30). High school dropouts rarely find employment, and even high school graduates are fortunate to find jobs paying much above the minimum wage (31,32). Inner-city hospitals have closed or reduced services. Health care and preventive health clinic services have been cut back (33). Youth recreation and service programs have been reduced. State mental health institutions have released large numbers of clients into communities with marginal support services (34–36). Child abuse and neglect have increased (especially because parental drug abuse is now defined as neglect). Transfer payments, such as home relief, Tempo-

rary Assistance to Needy Families (TANF, formerly Aid to Families with Dependent Children [AFDC]), and Supplemental Security Income (SSI) have declined in purchasing power. The nearly complete absence of public transfer payments to young adults (especially males ages 18 to 25 years) without childcare responsibilities systematically impoverishes those who cannot obtain employment or training stipends. Homicide became a leading killer of young African American men about 1990 (7,8,37,38); however, such early deaths had declined substantially by 2000 (39).

A sizable proportion of inner-city households can be categorized as severely distressed—not simply experiencing a few temporary social problems, but enduring the impact of multiple and continual social crises level conditions (14,25,40,41). In such households, income from legal employment is usually unstable and insufficient to pay for family members' rent, food, and clothing. Transfer payments are always inadequate. Only a few people in the family or kin network can support marginally adequate housing. Family or kin without housing or shelter descend continuously upon such households, sleeping and eating "free" to themselves but at high cost to the householder's marginal budget (42,43). Youths growing up in such households have no place to study and little time or support to do so. Facing many distractions, they do poorly in marginal inner-city schools (44). The household head is frequently a maternal figure. She is likely to be a grandmother or older aunt to the children who either replaces or accompanies the birth mother (45). Economic contributions to the family by the children's father or male partners of the household's head are rare. At various times, family members or kin experience serious illness, mental health problems, drug or alcohol abuse, jail or prison, child abuse or neglect, or death by injury or disease (24,40,41). A situation has arisen that socializes many people into a cycle of deviant behaviors, helps to perpetuate learned helplessness, and maintains the disenfranchisement of poor people and their communities within the larger society (23–25). While households with multiple problems are most numerous and persistent in the inner cities and ghettos of major American cities, households throughout American society experience similar problems. Usually such households have slightly more resources (income, family members, access to help) to resolve issues privately (9) or they need limited assistance from publicly funded programs.

Individuals from severely distressed households routinely come to the attention of various social programs, including drug treatment. As adults, these persons often need "habilitation" rather than "rehabilitation" to establish conventional practices and behaviors and to acquire the ability to contribute to the legitimate economic system. A vast array of ongoing efforts to control or improve inner-city conditions have been affected by constrictions imposed by legislation, funding, and professional staff practices, as well as by client perceptions of their needs and expectations of services. As a result, staff typically reach only a fraction of the population and provide targeted services according to the problem they are mandated to resolve, falling far short of addressing the complex of multiple problems that individual clients present.

THE NATURAL HISTORY OF RECENT DRUG ERAS

Overall, widespread use of illicit drugs emerged in the 1960s as the first members of the baby boom came of age and developed their own distinctive subcultural identities with associated behaviors. Since then, evolving tastes in the face of a changing sociohistorical context has led to five distinct nationwide drug eras: marihuana, heroin, powdered cocaine, crack cocaine, and blunts. The popularity of other illicit drugs—methamphetamine (46) and methylenedioxymethamphetamine (MDMA) (47,48)—has been highly limited regionally and/or subculturally.

These drug eras are identified as historical periods during which a new drug or "innovative" mode of use (e.g., heroin use, or crack use as an innovative mode of cocaine administration) becomes institutionalized within segments of the population (49–52). Typically, four phases to a drug era can be distinguished (51). First is the *incubation phase* in which some "pioneers" begin use, refine innovations, and develop relatively standard patterns of use and/or selling practices. This usually takes place within a highly specific social context as the "in" thing to do, without anticipation of creating a larger drug era. The *expansion phase* occurs when the pioneers "initiate" or "turn on" larger numbers of users to the new drug or mode of consumption, usually those with other illicit drug use experience. The *plateau phase* occurs when most of those at highest risk for becoming regular users have had the opportunity to do so, leading to a leveling of the overall prevalence. Subsequently, a steady flow of new initiates continues as many adolescents first coming of age choose to use whichever drug is currently popular. The *decline phase* represents a shift in a drug's popularity, especially among adolescents first coming of age as proportionately fewer of them even try the drug. Nevertheless, because many older users of a specific drug/modality will persist in their habits, the overall prevalence of use will decline only slowly with time.

This section traces the course of five major drug eras both within inner-city, multiply disadvantaged, high-risk populations, and within the general population. The occurrence of these drug eras, as well as their timing, intensity, significance, and concomitance of social problems, differs among these populations. Moreover, there is growing evidence that general population surveys tend to systemically exclude many of the most serious drug abusers that tend to come in contact with public agencies (53,54). The analysis of trends within the general population uses data from two programs: (a) the NSDUH, which has collected data

from a representative sample of all households intermittently starting in 1971 and annually since 1990 (55), and (b) the Monitoring the Future (MTF) program, which has collected annual survey data from a representative sample of high school seniors since 1975 (56). The analysis of trends within the inner city is based on data from the Arrestee Drug Abuse Monitoring (ADAM) program (formerly the Drug Use Forecasting [DUF] program), which has interviewed arrestees and obtained urine samples to test for drugs from about 30 sites since 1987 (57,58). The ADAM findings are location specific. This chapter presents findings for ADAM-Manhattan and provides citations to publications that provide more detailed analyses, including examination of variation across locations. Illicit drug use and abuse have always been widespread in New York City. These users have often been trendsetters and suppliers to the nation's Northeast.

Figures 7.1 and 7.2 indicate the lifetime use of marihuana, cocaine, crack, and heroin reported by the NSDUH and ADAM-Manhattan (New York) respondents age 25 years and older, respectively. This serves to identify those birth cohorts most affected by the five major drug eras, referred to as *drug generations*. The subsequent analyses presented in this chapter examine when members of each drug generation initiated use. Use of each drug (but especially crack and heroin) was much more common among Manhattan arrestees than in the general population. Marihuana use grew in popularity and achieved particularly high levels among each birth cohort born since 1950, both within the general population (approximately

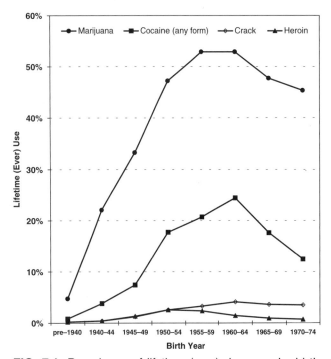

FIG. 7.1. Prevalence of lifetime (ever) drug use by birth year among NSDUH 1995–1998 respondents age 25 years and older.

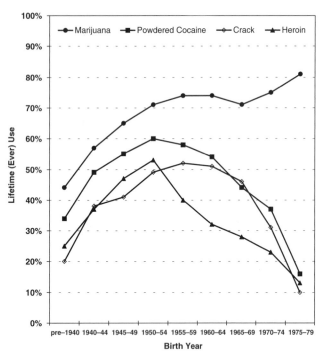

FIG. 7.2. Prevalence of lifetime (ever) drug use by birth year among ADAM-Manhattan 1987–2001 arrestees age 25 years and older.

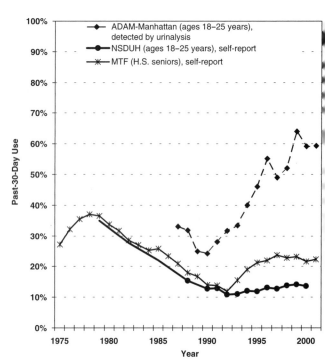

FIG. 7.3. Prevalence of past-30-day marihuana use among young adults (ages 18 to 25 years) and high school seniors, NSDUH 1979–2000, ADAM-Manhattan 1987–2001, and MTF 1975–2001.

50%, Fig. 7.1) and among arrestees (above 70%, Fig. 7.2). Heroin use was never particularly common within the general population, but reached a peak among those born in the period 1950–1954 (2.6%, Fig. 7.1). Heroin use was much more common (approximately 50%, Fig. 7.2) among Manhattan arrestees, especially those born in the period 1945–54. Cocaine use (in any form) rose in the general population to peak at over 20% (Fig. 7.1) among persons born in the period 1955–1964; within this population crack use never exceeded 4%. Powdered cocaine use peaked among arrestees born in the period 1950–1954 (60%, Fig. 7.2). Crack use peaked among arrestees born in the period 1955–1964 (above 50%).

Marihuana Era (1965–1979)

Marihuana use emerged in the 1960s as the post-World War II baby boom came of age, along with youthful rebellion and calls for social changes. Eras of use of lysergic acid diethylamide (LSD) and other psychedelics, amphetamines, and barbiturates occurred parallel to the marihuana era, with important increases during the 1970s, peaking around 1979, and declining in the 1980s (56).

A study of marihuana initiation over time using the NSDUH 1991–1993 data found that initiation grew over the 1960s and 1970s achieving a peak level in 1978, and steadily declined thereafter (59). The NSDUH data further indicates that prevalence of past-30-day marihuana use among young adults (ages 18 to 25 years) declined

from 35% in 1979 to a temporary low of 11% in 1992 (Fig. 7.3; the discussion of the marihuana/blunts era, in "Marihuana/Blunts Era (1990–2000s)" below, describes marihuana use in the 1990s). The prevalence of past-30-day use among high school seniors closely paralleled the trend in the general population, declining from a peak 37% in 1978 to 12% by 1992 (Fig. 7.3).

A variety of other research shows that marihuana use became institutionalized and widespread among American youths and young adults in the 1970–1990 period. Longitudinal research (60–64) shows that sizable proportions of people who initiated marihuana use and became regular users in the 1970s remained persistent users during the 1980s, especially those who did not settle into conventional adult roles (e.g., marriage, steady employment). Marihuana is a common secondary drug (along with alcohol and cigarettes) used by most drug abusers. Virtually all users of other illegal drugs also use marihuana, and regular marihuana use is common among abusers of other drugs (62,65). It is the most frequently used illicit drug by the nation's numerous intermittent and recreational drug users.

Heroin Injection Era (1965–1973)

Even at its peak, heroin use has always been rare within the general population; generally less than 2% of NSDUH respondents reported any lifetime heroin use, and less than 0.5% reported heroin use in the past 30 days in most surveys (56,66). The heroin and crack eras have been centered among inner-city youths. Within these social environs, heroin users have tended to use frequently. Many would organize their lives' activities around obtaining money for the next fix, obtaining the drugs, injecting at least once a day (42). This discussion focuses on heroin trends in inner-city New York; similar heroin epidemics have been documented for other cities (67–70), although the timing and intensity years may not be as well-documented as for New York City.

Heroin was known among white ethnics and a relatively small number of jazz musicians prior to the 1950s. Heroin use began to spread among males in Harlem during the 1950s (71,72). Among young men in Manhattan, heroin use increased from 3% in 1963 to a peak of 20% in 1972, and the decline phase began in 1974, as only 13% used heroin (73,74). A conservative estimate placed the number of active heroin abusers in New York City during the 1975 to 1995 period at about 150,000, excluding persons in methadone maintenance (75,76). The impact of this spike in the popularity of heroin was most pronounced among youths coming of age during this period, early baby boomers born during the years 1945–1954 (73). Half of all Manhattan-arrestees born during the years 1945–1954 reported having used heroin (Fig. 7.2). Many became addicted within 2 years. Persons addicted during this heroin era primarily consume heroin (often mixed with cocaine powder as a speedball) via intravenous injection.

Less than half of all heroin users persisted in their addiction for more than a few years (77). However, others continued to use throughout adulthood, constituting a large population with special needs that would be hard to ignore. These individuals became a continual target for the criminal justice system because of their persistent use of illicit drugs and their crimes to support their habits (78). Their continuing need for treatment and addiction-related health problems, especially human immunodeficiency virus (HIV), greatly affected public health programs (79).

In response to this heroin era, the foundations of the current drug treatment system were established during the late 1960s and early 1970s. Methadone maintenance expanded from fewer than 100 clients to about 20,000 clients between 1965 and 1974; by 1975, the number of readmissions to methadone exceeded new (not previously known) heroin abusers (see Chapter 39). Most therapeutic communities were established by the early 1970s, as were most outpatient drug-free programs (80). Federal- and state-sponsored "civil" and "criminal" commitment programs begun in the 1960s placed heroin abusers in prison-like facilities with mandated aftercare programs. They were found to be very expensive, rehabilitated few, and were closed in the midst of fiscal crises during the 1970s (81). The criminal commitment program in California was modestly successful in interrupting runs of heroin addic-

tion, but methadone treatment was more successful at reducing criminality (82,83).

The drug treatment system that evolved between 1965 and 1980 was focused primarily on rehabilitation of heroin abusers. In the early 1980s, approximately 75% of those admitted to public drug treatment programs had heroin as their primary drug of abuse, but this was to change in the mid-1980s. One piece of "good news" in inner-city New York's hard-drug scene is that declining proportions of youths reaching adulthood after 1975 initiated or became regular users of heroin (Fig. 7.2); a definite norm against any heroin use—and especially against heroin injection—become widespread among arrested persons born after 1970 (78). Compared to their counterparts 20 years earlier (e.g., those born during the years 1950–1959 and who were often their parents), the birth cohort born during the years 1970–1975 "turned off" to heroin (or more precisely not "turned on" to heroin) and developed strong norms against heroin use, especially against injection drug use (52,84).

Powdered Cocaine Era (1974–1985)

As with marihuana, the use of powdered cocaine (cocaine hydrochloride) was uncommon prior to 1965. As of 1972, only 3% of the general population reported having ever used cocaine (85). This rate grew to 12% by the early 1980s. The proportion of those who used cocaine in the past 30 days increased from 0.2% in 1972 to approximately 3% in the first half of the 1980s (85). This rate subsequently declined to 0.7% in 1994, and was at about the same level by 2001 (55). Among high school seniors, past-30-day cocaine use increased from 2% in 1975 to a peak of 6.7% in 1985, and declined to under 2% by 1990 (56). Interestingly, since 1985 about half of all high school seniors reported that cocaine is easily available in their community (56). Despite perceived availability, the prevalence of recent use suggests that the cocaine era has been in decline.

Most cocaine use among students and the general population (including middle-income and upper-income groups) involved snorting (nasal inhalation) of cocaine powder (62,65). Virtually all cocaine users were (or had been) regular marihuana users and regular consumers of alcohol. Longitudinal research indicates that substantial proportions of marihuana users from the 1970s initiated cocaine use and became regular users in the 1980s (62). Relatively smaller proportions injected cocaine or smoked crack (65,86–88). Whereas, substantial portions of the general population from some birth years tried cocaine use, many fewer tried crack (Fig. 7.1). Particularly among white cocaine users, a variety of informal norms defining cocaine as a "recreational" drug effectively limited its use to weekends, parties, and social occasions (86–88).

Cocaine and the Freebase Era (1975–1984)

Cocaine snorting (nasal inhalation) became popular among increasingly larger proportions of nonheroin drug users in the inner city. From 1975 to 1983, cocaine gained a reputation as a "status drug" that was relatively innocuous; large numbers of inner-city drug users were snorting cocaine when they could afford its high price in the 1970s. In New York, "after-hours clubs" became a gathering place for cocaine users and dealers (88). By 1980, powdered cocaine sellers outnumbered heroin sellers by two to one. By 1984, 43% of all Manhattan arrestees tested positive for cocaine, while only 22% were positive for heroin; more than half of the latter were also positive for cocaine (89) and were probably "speedballers" (90).

"Freebasing" emerged on the West Coast (91) but began to spread to New York in the early 1980s. This process converts adulterated cocaine hydrochloride powder into alkaloidal cocaine or "freebase." Cocaine freebase is not water soluble and cannot be conveniently snorted or injected. When the freebase is heated at low temperatures and the fumes inhaled, the user becomes euphoric within seconds. The high from freebase lasts less than 20 minutes and is followed by rapid dysphoria in which the user feels worse than usual, often leading to further use in a vain attempt to regain that high or at least avoid feeling down (43,91,92). Freebasing became increasingly popular in New York from 1980 to 1984; many after-hours clubs became "base houses" where cocaine could be purchased and someone would "cook it up" or "base it" (23,93). Although some base houses were in transitional areas, most were located in minority, low-income neighborhoods and run by minority owners (93,94).

Crack Era (1985–1989)

In 1984 and 1985, New York officials saw dealers selling vials containing what users called "crack" (95–98)—also frequently called "rock" and sold in baggies on the West Coast. Crack is cocaine freebase packaged in retail form, typically in a small plastic vial (about the size of a perfume sample) with a watertight cap. The asking price in 1985 was $20 for a standard vial containing several chunks of freebase. Prices, vial shapes, and the amount provided changed frequently, but most importantly, the price for a standard dose of one or two small chunks of freebase dropped dramatically to about $3 to $5 in the late 1980s and early 1990s (23). The ease of use, strong high, accessible price per use, cachet of cocaine, and subcultural social norms facilitated the expansion in crack use during the mid-1980s. Many users became obsessed with their crack habits. They would buy several vials at a time or return to purchase crack multiple times over the course of use during a typical day. The major limitation facing users was money to support their habits (43,93).

Crack use exploded during the years 1984 to 1986 in New York, Miami, Detroit, Washington, DC, and elsewhere, quickly dominating illicit drug markets in many inner-city neighborhoods (95–98). While crack selling was based predominantly in inner-city neighborhoods and among minorities, crack use and crack sellers had spread to virtually all neighborhoods of the New York City region by the late 1980s (99). The history of the crack era has been documented with some precision in New York (51,100) and other ADAM sites (101): the expansion phase lasted from 1984–1986, the plateau phase lasted from 1986–1989, the decline phase began in 1990 and continued thereafter. In particular, among ADAM-Manhattan arrestees, the 1955–1969 birth cohort had the highest rates of detected cocaine use (over 60%) and may be considered the "crack generation" in New York City (101). They were joined, however, by very sizable proportions of older birth cohorts and heroin injectors that had equally high levels of detected cocaine use. This mass of crack users had an immediate and enduring impact on the criminal justice system, drug treatment programs, life in the inner-city, and the broader society.

The crack era contributed a major expansion to the existing drug abuse and sales patterns in inner-city communities (23,102). Recent research (99,102–107) suggested several major findings about the crack era. Almost no drug neophytes "turned on" to crack as their first drug. The vast majority of crack abusers had prior histories of regular illicit use of marihuana or cocaine powder, and a sizable proportion were heroin injectors (104,108). Such drug abusers tended to "add" crack to their already existing patterns of drug consumption. Apparent remission in their "old drugs" probably occurred because they expended most of their funds for crack. Two-thirds of crack abusers consumed crack on a daily basis and more than half used crack four or more times daily; more than half of the crack abusers used more than $1,000 per month of crack (102). By contrast, about a third of heroin injectors used heroin daily, but few used heroin four or more times daily. In short, crack was used more intensively (higher frequencies and expenditures, especially among daily users) than were heroin and cocaine powder.

Crack abusers were significantly different from other drug user subgroups on many dimensions. They generally had the highest proportions of people involved in and receiving high incomes from drug sales and other criminality. Among crack abusers, crack use greatly exceeded the cost and frequency of use of the other drugs that they also consumed. Crack abusers had higher frequencies of and cash incomes from other crimes (robbery, burglary, thefts, etc.) than did cocaine powder users. By 1988, crack had become the most frequently sold and lucrative drug in the street drug market (102). Crack selling became the most common crime and generated the largest cash income for all illicit drug user subgroups studied. Crack sales generated higher cash incomes than did the sales of heroin, cocaine powder, or marihuana, or the commission of other crimes (robbery, burglary, thefts, etc.). Crack use did not greatly increase violence among drug abusers; rather, persons who were already violent (robbers, assaulters, etc.) tended to become crack abusers and spent large amounts on crack (105,109). Many people who became crack abusers between 1985 and 1989 were children of alcoholics or heroin abusers, or were otherwise abused or neglected in childhood (110,111), and came from severely distressed households or families (23,25,40,41,112).

Overall, during the crack era, a substantial expansion in the number of daily drug abusers occurred. In New York City, a substantial proportion of an estimated 150,000 persistent heroin injectors appeared to have added crack abuse and sale to their daily activities. A relatively smaller proportion (probably less than 20%) of recreational cocaine snorters (who avoided heroin) became crack abusers (65,113). But because recreational cocaine snorters were so numerous, substantial numbers became crack abusers. While precise estimates are not available, the U.S. Senate Committee on the Judiciary (113) estimated that New York State had 434,000 cocaine/crack addicts in 1988. This report estimated that 2.2 million people were cocaine addicts nationally; a RAND report (109) estimates approximately 2.5 million monthly or more frequent users of cocaine. Among reported daily users, most were crack users who consume the majority of the total volume of cocaine.

Beginning in early 1990, a variety of indicators suggested that the crack era entered the decline phase (100,101,114,115). Most centrally, persons born since 1970 have been increasingly less likely to use crack, especially those disadvantaged persons that tend to sustain arrests (Fig. 7.2). The vast majority of young Manhattan-arrestees were detected as recent cocaine users in 1987 (100); in contrast, less than 10% of young arrestees in the 2000s were detected as cocaine users (84). For many of these youths, not using crack or heroin was an act of resilience in the face of the degraded lifestyles they observed among members of their community (52). "Crack-head" became one of the most disparaging and stigmatized names on the streets (116). Some who were actively abusing crack in the late 1980s were able to desist, at least for longer periods of time, often with the support of treatment programs (117,118). Nevertheless, it is clear that many persons affected by the crack era (especially those born during the years 1955–1969) persisted throughout the 1990s and will likely continue to do so into the future.

Marihuana/Blunts Era (1990–2000s)

In the 1990s, marihuana use reemerged as the illicit drug-of-choice of a new generation, especially among those persons who tend to sustain arrests (119). The previous marihuana era associated with the youth subcultures of the 1960s was in decline and marihuana use had reached

a low in 1992 (Fig. 7.3). Among persons aged 18 to 25 years in the general population, past-30-day marihuana use increased modestly from 11% in 1992 to 13% to 14% in the late 1990s, an increased level far below the peak 37% recorded back in the late 1970s. Among high school seniors, past-30-day use increased more substantially from 12% in 1992 to 21% to 24% in the late 1990s. Among Manhattan-arrestees aged 18 to 25 years, marihuana use detected by urinalysis increased dramatically from 24% in 1990 up to 59% to 63% during the period 1999–2001. These trends suggest that the expansion phase of this new marihuana era started first and had a much larger impact among inner-city arrestees. By the end of the 1990s, all three surveys recorded elevated but rather steady levels of marihuana use suggesting this new marihuana era had entered its plateau phase. We refer to this recent drug-use trend as the marihuana/blunts era based on reports that marihuana was increasingly smoked in a blunt (an inexpensive cigar in which the tobacco filler is replaced with marihuana) as well as evidence on T-shirts and in rap music celebrating blunts and establishing the symbolic importance of this drug consumption practice (52,120,121).

In the early 2000s, persons born since 1970 have largely avoided heroin, cocaine, and crack. At this point, available data suggest that no "new" drug, such as methamphetamine, or consumption technique, such as heroin smoking, has "replaced" heroin or crack. This stands in direct contradiction to the "gateway hypothesis" (122). A vast literature has documented that drug use tends to pass through a sequence of stages from (a) nonuse to use of (b) alcohol and/or tobacco, and then to (c) marihuana and (d) other drugs such as cocaine, crack, and heroin. Not all persons progress to the highest stages, but persons who do use substances at one stage rarely progress to use of those associated with higher stages. A naïve application of this gateway hypothesis would suggest that a new era of hard drug use (such as crack or heroin) is imminent (123).

Recent evidence greatly questions whether the widely observed gateway phenomenon could be the result of a biopharmacologic linkage (119,124); rather, the observed gateway sequence would appear to be an artifact of age-graded subcultural expectations regarding the availability and significance of various substances. Alcohol and tobacco are widely available and legally consumed by adults within our culture. This may explain their role as the first substances used. Marihuana use is often initiated in the mid-teens. Use of crack and heroin is more broadly frowned on, considered dangerous, and is less common. Initiation tends to take place in the late teens and early twenties by a few individuals. However, this pathway did not appear to exist before the 1960s. Few persons born before World War II used marihuana, powdered cocaine, crack or heroin (Figs. 7.1 and 7.2). Moreover, the emergence of the marihuana/blunts era has not been accompanied by an increase in other drugs. Youths that initiated marihuana use in the 1990s were substantially much less likely to progress to cocaine, crack, and heroin than were preceding birth cohorts at the same age (124).

IMPACT OF DRUG ERAS ON PUBLIC AGENCIES

In addition to affecting patterns of drug abuse, drug sales, and nondrug criminality by users, these drug eras have had a substantial impact on the drug treatment system, the criminal justice system, and the health care system. The major social response has been primarily punitive—with substantial increases in arrests and jail or prison sentences (some with mandatory minimums), but with few increases in drug treatment.

Drug Treatment

The drug treatment system has been impacted substantially (Fig. 7.4). During the late 1970s in New York City (125) approximately 25,000 admissions (90% for heroin)

for drug abuse treatment occurred annually. The number of heroin admissions declined during the 1980s to about 15,000 in 1991, and increased modestly through the 1990s to about 23,000 in 2001 (126).

Beginning in 1984, cocaine as the primary drug of abuse at admission began to increase substantially; it rose from about 2,000 in 1983, to more than 8,000 in 1986, to 13,000 in 1991, to 17,000 in 1997, to 14,000 in 2001. Most of these cocaine admissions were for crack abuse although several were for cocaine snorting (117,118,125,126). These figures do not include the numerous cocaine and crack abusers with concurrent alcohol abuse problems who seek treatment at alcohol treatment programs or attend meetings of Alcoholics Anonymous and Narcotics Anonymous. Virtually all drug treatment programs indicate that they routinely cannot admit the many crack abusers who seek help. The need for crack treatment by crack abusers without heroin addiction greatly exceeds the available slots. At drug-free residential and outpatient programs, approximately 80% of admissions listed cocaine or crack as the primary drug of abuse (125).

Unfortunately, two decades of research has not developed effective treatments for cocaine. Scientific efforts

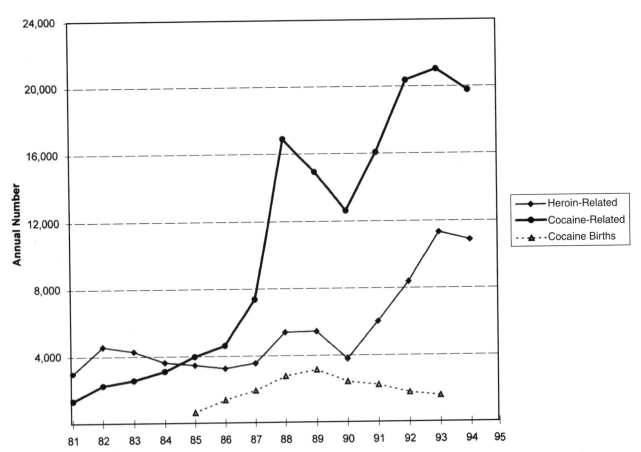

FIG. 7.4. Changes in the number of heroin and cocaine-related emergency room mentions and births to women using cocaine in New York City, 1981–1994. (Reproduced with permission from Frank B, Galea J. Current drug abuse trends in New York city. Community epidemiological trends in drug abuse: Community epidemiological work group. Vol. II proceedings. Rockville, MD: National Institute on Drug Abuse, 1996.)

to develop a cocaine antagonist (like naltrexone for opiates or Antabuse for alcohol) or a long-acting substitute (like methadone for heroin) have had little success (see Chapters 16 and 17). Only a few crack detoxification programs have been established (110,111), and these appear to have little or no measurable effect in preventing relapse to cocaine and crack abuse.

The 1990s and early 2000s also experienced a large influx of marihuana/blunt users into drug treatment programs. Treatment admissions for marijuana increased steadily from about 1,000 in 1991 to 13,000 in 2001 (126). Most marihuana/blunt users do not voluntarily seek drug treatment, rather they are referred by the criminal justice system as an alternative to incarceration for commission of some felony offenses. Unfortunately, no marihuana-specific treatments are available to address youths and young adults who are marihuana dependent (but have no cross addictions to heroin or crack). While regularly referred by courts, only modest proportions of marihuana/blunts users actually enroll and even fewer are retained in drug treatment.

Hence, a crying need exists for new treatment approaches that are even modestly effective in helping crack abusers "come off" crack or blunts smokers to "give up" marihuana—most importantly—in preventing relapse to regular crack abuse or marihuana dependency. In the absence of such new approaches, a significant expansion of the treatment system is essential, but unlikely in the current political climate. Significantly, after 20 years of development, another opiate agonist, buprenorphine, has been approved for office-based treatment of heroin and opiate addiction (127–129). Such an investment to improve crack and marihuana treatment needs rival the investment made by society in the criminal justice system to arrest, jail, and imprison crack and marihuana abusers.

The Criminal Justice System

The public and politicians demanded a harsh approach to reducing drug use and the open-air markets. In New York City (as elsewhere), police developed special task forces to "crack down" on crack dealers. Operation Pressure Point (1983–1986) was instituted to "take back" the streets from heroin and cocaine dealers (130). Tactical Narcotic Teams (1987–1990) consisted of roving squads designed to make numerous buy–bust arrests of dealers, especially crack sellers. Community policing (1991–1995) now focuses on drug sellers and "quality of life" crimes (like prostitution, trespassing, shoplifting, and fare beating) (131,132). The number of heroin arrests increased from about 17,000 in 1987, to 24,000 in 1990, to 33,000 in 1994 (125). Cocaine and crack arrests nearly doubled from 28,600 in 1986 to 54,000 in 1989, and then declined to 40,200 in 1995 and to 32,000 in 2001 (126). Heroin-related arrests increased from 24,000 in 1991 to 38,000 in 1995, but declined to about 33,000 in 2000. Marijuana-related arrests soared from about 5000 in 1991 to 60,000 in 2000 (126) as

quality-of-life policing was implemented (131,132). Such mass arrest strategies as a means of controlling drug selling remain politically popular, but the effectiveness of this strategy remains unresolved (39,130,133–135).

The criminal justice system's intensive focus on crack was not limited to law enforcement (136). A comparison of arrestees charged with a crack offense from 1986 to 1988 with arrestees charged with a cocaine powder offense in 1983 and 1984 found the crack arrestees were more likely to receive jail and prison sentences (137). However, this discrepancy disappeared in the late 1980s and early 1990s (138). The most substantial impact has occurred within the correctional system. Most of the dramatic rise in correctional populations in the mid-1980s was as a result of convictions for drug sales (139,140), primarily crack. Prison populations grew from 196,007 in 1969 to 315,974 in 1980 (141). The population continued to grow to 739,980 by 1990. It surpassed a million by year end 1994 and reached 1.35 million by 2001. The imprisonment rate increased from 139 in 1980 to 470 per 100,000 U.S. residents.

The jail population increased as well, from 183,998 in 1980, to 405,320 in 1990, and to 631,240 in 2001. More than 1.96 million people were in jails and prisons at the end of 2001 (141). The number of probationers increased from 1,118,097 in 1980, to 2,670,234 in 1990, to 3,932,751 in 2001. The number of parolees also increased, from 220,438 in 1980, to 531,407 in 1990 to 731,147 in 2001 (141). The annual percentage increases accelerated sharply between 1987 and 1989, when more than 100,000 additional persons were added to each system: prison, jail, probation, and parole. More than 6.6 million persons were under criminal supervision or incarcerated in 2001, compared with less than 2 million in 1980. During each year, 1980 to 1995, the average increase in prison populations was between 6% and 13% above the prior year. Only after 1995, did the annual increase slow to approximately 2% to 4%.

Much of the growth in criminal justice populations is a result of convictions for drug crimes. The proportion of drug offenders rose from 8% to 26% between 1980 and 1994, forcing down the proportion imprisoned for violent and property crimes. Especially in federal prisons, the proportion serving sentences for drug crimes increased from 25% to 60% (139,140,143). A careful analysis of this increase indicated that much of the increase was a consequence of mandatory sentences imposed on crack sellers possessing more than 5 g of crack, almost all of whom were African American. Indeed, the U.S. Sentencing Commission (144) recommended that penalties for crack sales be set equal to those for cocaine powder (where 500 g must be sold to invoke 5-year mandatory minimum penalties). To maintain the political appearance of being "tough" on crack sellers, however, Congress voted, and President Clinton signed, legislation to maintain the current harsh mandatory penalties for sales involving only 5 g of crack—and the penalties remain unchanged in the 2000s.

In 1989, 25% of all young African American males were under criminal justice supervision (jail, prison, parole, or probation); this figure reached 33% in 1994 (145,146), and 46% in 2001 (an additional 16% were Hispanics) (147). Most data show that minorities are disproportionately arrested and incarcerated for drug offenses. Popular support for the "incarceration" solution to the crack and drug problem proved very expensive. In 1980, the nation's corrections (jail and prison) costs were about $9 billion; this rose to $49 billion by 2001, a fivefold increase (142).

Public Health System

Heroin and crack abuse continue to have a substantial impact on the public health and social service delivery system in New York City and elsewhere. Figure 7.4 shows that the number of emergency room mentions for heroin in New York declined slightly in the early 1980s and rose to about 5,000 per year in the last years of the 1980s, but doubled to about 10,000 in 1995 (125) and has remained relatively constant through 2001 (149). The number of cocaine-related emergency room mentions, however, increased much more dramatically from 1,324 in 1981, to 3,102 in 1984, to 14,925 in 1989, with further increases to about 20,000 in the period 1992–1998 (125), but declined to about 14,000 in the period 1999–2001 (149).

The number of births in which cocaine use by the mother was detected rose from 628 in 1985 to 3,168 in 1989, but has since declined to fewer than 500 by 2001 (125,126). The number of children placed in foster care in New York City more than quadrupled in the last half of the 1980s, and remained high thereafter. In many other areas of the public health system, crack abusers and their chronic problems have placed major strains.

The AIDS epidemic is directly linked to the heroin epidemic of the early 1970s. The numerous heroin addicts who shared needles and routinely went to shooting galleries in the 1970s and 1980s became major carriers and transmitters of HIV and acquired immune deficiency syndrome (AIDS) (150). Thousands have died from AIDS-related illnesses. Along the way, they may transmit HIV to their sexual partners and, among needle-using women, transmit HIV to their children (150, see Chapters 57 to 60). In a similar fashion, increasing evidence suggests that cocaine and crack may decrease immune system function and increase the speed of dying from AIDS-related illnesses. Moreover, some new (and yet unanticipated) disaster like AIDS could possibly emerge among crack abusers within the next several years. In short, the public health consequences of the crack era are likely to continue in the future.

illicit drug-of-choice changes over time. More centrally, the impact of drug use in a person's life is strongly mediated by the person's social position. Illicit drug abuse is associated with particularly widespread devastation in disadvantaged inner-city communities. Members of these communities have limited social capital, resources to draw upon when their lives are stressed by crisis. Consequently, drug use often leads these persons into contact with the criminal justice system, leads them to public drug treatment programs, and complicates their family's relationship with public welfare programs. This comorbidity of drug abuse with other social problems suggests that the negative impact of illicit drug use, and, possibly, the use itself might be reduced by addressing broader social problems. Members of these communities have suffered from ghettoization and marginalization. Perhaps drug abuse control programs (law enforcement, prevention, and treatment) have also suffered a policy ghettoization, being forced to focus nearly exclusively on a single behavior (drug abuse), its punishment and treatment. In this manner, their potential impact in persons' lives has been marginal at best.

From a sociocultural perspective, there are encouraging and discouraging processes in place. The persistence of multiple inner-city crises in employment opportunity, education, housing, family formation, health, crime, and drugs has had cumulative negative effects. Members of the crack era cohort are middle-age adults in the 2000s and now constitute a major segment of the inner-city communities. These inner-city adults are poorly prepared for conventional adult roles such as parenthood. These crack abusers and their descendants will prove to be one of the major problem populations confronting drug/alcohol treatment programs, the criminal justice system, and many other agencies in the 2000s. Almost no efforts at substantial reform are underway as politicians remain "tough" on crack (133,151,152). Breakthroughs in treatment of heroin and crack abuse have yet to materialize.

There is some hope for the future with regard to recent trends in illicit drug abuse in the inner-city with the emergence of the marihuana/blunts cohort of persons born since 1970. These youths, who are growing up in severely distressed households, have largely avoided heroin injection and crack smoking. Their consumption of blunts and alcohol is associated with less criminality and problem behavior in young adulthood than was evident among their predecessors during the heroin injection and crack eras (52). However, these blunt-smoking youths have many deficits and face numerous challenges to establishing conventional lifestyles and to have the potential for becoming productive members of society.

CONCLUSION

Drug abuse and its attendant problems are embedded within a complex evolving sociocultural context. The

ACKNOWLEDGMENTS

This article draws important insights from several research grants supported by the National Institute on

Drug Abuse (5 T32 DA07233–19; 1 R01 DA05126–08; 5R01 DA09339-03, 5 R01 DA09056-08; 1 R01 DA/CA13690-01), the Arrestee Drug Abuse Monitoring program (OJP-98C-003;OJP-2001-C-003), the National Institute of Justice (95-IJ-CX0028; 99-IJ-CX0020; 98-IJ-CX-K012; 2000-7353-NY-IJ), and the Robert Wood Johnson Foundation Substance Abuse Policy Research Program (037864). Additional support was provided by National Development and Research Institutes.

Points of view and the opinions in this paper do not necessarily represent the official positions of the United States government, the funding agencies that supported this work, or the National Development and Research Institutes.

The authors wish to thank Drs. Blanche Frank and Rozanne Marel of the New York State Office of Alcohol and Substance Abuse Services for collecting, maintaining, and providing the epidemiologic data on drug abuse for three decades; these data are included in Fig. 7.4.

REFERENCES

1. Substance Abuse and Mental Health Services Administration. Office of Applied Studies. *Results from the 2001 National Household Survey on Drug Abuse, Vol. 3: detailed tables.* Rockville, MD: US Department of Health and Human Services, 2002. Available at www.samhsa.gov.
2. Hughes MA. *Concentrated deviance or isolated deprivation? The "underclass" idea reconsidered.* Report prepared for the Rockefeller Foundation. Princeton, NJ: Princeton University, Princeton Urban and Regional Research Center, 1988.
3. Jargowsky PA. *Poverty and place ghettos, barrios, and the American city.* New York: Russell Sage Foundation, 1997.
4. Massey D, Denton N. *American apartheid: segregation and the making of the underclass.* Cambridge, MA: Harvard University Press, 1993.
5. Ricketts E, Sawhill I. Defining and measuring the underclass. *J Policy Anal Manage* 1988;7(2):316–325.
6. Wilson WJ. *The truly disadvantaged.* Chicago: University of Chicago Press, 1988.
7. Jaynes GD, Robin WM Jr. *A common destiny: blacks and American society.* Washington, DC: National Academy Press, 1989.
8. Gibbs TJ, ed. *Young, black, and male in America: an endangered species.* Dover, MA: Auburn House, 1988.
9. Sullivan M. *Getting paid.* New Brunswick, NJ: Rutgers University Press, 1989.
10. Sandefur GD, Tienda M. *Divided opportunities: minorities, poverty, and social policy.* New York: Plenum Press, 1988.
11. Kazis R, Miller MS. *Low-wage workers in the new economy.* Washington, DC: Urban Institute Press, 2001.
12. Saegert S, Thompson JP, Warren MR. *Social capital and poor communities.* New York: Russell Sage Foundation, 2001.
13. Johnson J. *Getting by on the minimum: the lives of working class women.* New York: Routledge, 2002.
14. Edin K, Lein L. *Making ends meet: how single mothers survive welfare and low-wage work.* New York: Russell Sage Foundation, 1997.
15. Larson TE. Employment and unemployment of young black males. In: Gibbs JT, ed. *Young, black, and male in America: an endangered species.* Dover, MA: Auburn House, 1988:97–125.
16. Danziger S, Haveman RH, eds. *Understanding poverty.* Cambridge, MA: Harvard University Press, 2002.
17. Hartman C, ed. *Housing crisis: what is to be done?* Boston: Routledge and Kegan, 1983.
18. Hartman C, Keating D, Le Gates R. *Displacement: how to fight it.* Berkeley, CA: National Housing Law Project, 1986.
19. Tucker W. *The excluded Americans. Homelessness and housing politics.* San Francisco: Laissez Faire Books, 1989.
20. Downs A. *Rental housing in the 1980s.* Washington, DC: Brookings Institute, 1983.
21. Sanjek R. *Federal housing programs and their impact on homelessness.* New York: National Coalition for the Homeless, 1986.
22. Smith JP. Poverty and the family. In: Sandefur GD, Tienda M, eds. *Divided opportunities. Minorities, poverty, and social policy.* New York: Plenum Press, 1988:141–192.
23. Johnson BD, Williams T, Dei K, et al. Drug abuse in the inner city: impact on hard drug users and the community. In: Tonry M, Wilson JQ, eds. *Drugs and crime.* Chicago: University of Chicago Press, 1990;13:9–67.
24. Dunlap E. Inner-city crisis and drug dealing: portrait of a drug dealer and his household. In: MacGregor S, ed. *Crisis and resistance: social relations and economic restructuring in the city.* London: University of Minnesota and Edinburgh Press, 1995:114–131.
25. Dunlap E, Johnson BD, Golub A, et al. Intergenerational transmission of conduct norms for drugs, sexual exploitation and violence: a case study. *Br J Criminol* 2002;42:1–20.
26. Card DE, Blank RM. *Finding jobs work and welfare reform.* New York: Russell Sage Foundation, 2000.
27. Loprest PJ. Making transition from welfare to work: successes but continuing concerns. In: Weil A, Finegold K, eds. *Welfare reform the next act.* Washington, DC: Urban Institute Press, 2002:17–23.
28. Moffitt R, Ver Ploeg M, eds. *National Research Council (U.S.), and Panel on Data and Methods for Measuring the Effects of Changes in Social Welfare Programs. Evaluating welfare reform in an era of transition.* Washington, DC: National Academy Press, 2001.
29. Weil A, Finegold K, eds. *Welfare reform the next act.* Washington, DC: Urban Institute Press, 2002.
30. Meyer BD, Holtz-Eakin D. *Making work pay: the earned income tax credit and its impact on America's families.* New York: Russell Sage, 2002.
31. Glasgow D. *The black underclass.* New York: Vintage Books, 1981.
32. Reed RJ. Education and achievement of young black males. In: Gibbs JT, ed. *Young, black, and male in America: an endangered species.* Dover, MA: Auburn House, 1988:37–96.
33. Health problems of inner-city poor reach crisis point. *New York Times* 1990 Dec 24:1,24.
34. Bachrach L. *The homeless mentally ill: an analytic review of the literature.* Washington, DC: Alcohol and Drug Abuse and Mental Health Administration, 1984.
35. Burt MR. *Helping America's homeless emergency shelter or affordable housing?* Washington, D.C: Urban Institute Press, 2001.
36. Hope M, Young J. *The faces of homelessness.* Lexington, MA: Lexington Books, 1986.
37. Brunswick AF. Young black males and substance use. In: Gibbs JT, ed. *Young,

black, and male in America: an endangered species. Dover, MA: Auburn House, 1988:166–187.

38. Dembo R. Young black males and delinquency. In: Gibbs JT, ed. *Young, black, and male in America: an endangered species.* Dover, MA: Auburn House, 1988:129–165.

39. Blumstein A, Wallman J, eds. *The crime drop in America.* New York: Cambridge, 2000.

40. Dunlap E, Johnson BD. The setting for the crack era: macro forces, micro consequences (1960–92). *J Psychoactive Drugs* 1992;24(3):307–321.

41. Dunlap E, Johnson BD. Family/resources in the development of a female crack seller career: case study of a hidden population. *J Drug Issues* 1996;26(1):175–198.

42. Johnson BD, Goldstein P, Preble E, et al. *Taking care of business: the economics of crime by heroin abusers.* Lexington, MA: Lexington Books, 1985.

43. Johnson BD, Hamid A, Sanabria H. Emerging models of crack distribution. In: Mieczkowksi T, ed. *Drugs and crime: a reader.* Boston: Allyn and Bacon, 1991:56–78.

44. Duncan GJ, Brooks-Gunn J, eds. *Consequences of growing up poor.* New York: Russell Sage Foundation, 1997.

45. Dunlap E, Johnson BD, Tourigny SC. Dead tired and bone weary: Grandmothers as caregivers in drug-affected inner-city households. *Race and Society* 2000;3:143–163.

46. Feucht TE, Kyle GM. *Methamphetamine use among adult arrestees: findings from the Drug Use Forecasting (DUF) Program.* NCJ 161842. National Institute of Justice Research in Brief, 1996. Washington, DC.

47. Golub A, Johnson BD, Sifaneck S, et al. Is the U.S. experiencing an incipient epidemic of *hallucinogen use? Substance Use and Misuse* 2001;36(12):1699–1729.

48. Hunt D. *Rise of hallucinogen use.* NCJ 166607. National Institute of Justice Research in Brief, 1997. Washington, DC.

49. Becker HS. History, culture, and subjective experience: an exploration of the social bases of drug-induced experiences. *J Health Soc Behav* 1967;8:163–176.

50. Musto D. Historical perspectives on alcohol and drug abuse. In: Lowinson J, Ruiz P, Millman R, et al, eds. *Substance abuse: a comprehensive textbook,* 2nd ed. Baltimore: Williams & Wilkins, 1992:2–14.

51. Golub A, Johnson BD. The crack epidemic: empirical findings support a hypothesized diffusion of innovation process. *Socio-Economic Planning Sciences* 1996;30(3):221–231.

52. Johnson BD, Golub A, Dunlap E. The rise and decline of hard drugs, drug markets and violence in New York City. In: Blumstein A, Wallman J, eds. *The crime drop in America.* New York: Cambridge, 2000:164–206.

53. Wright D, Gfroerer J, Epstein J. The use of external data sources and ratio estimation to improve estimates of hard-core drug use from the NHSDA. In: Harrison L, Hughes A, eds. *The validity of self-reported drug use: improving the accuracy of survey estimates. NIDA Research Monograph 167, NIH Publication No. 97—4147.* Rockville, MD: National Institute on Drug Abuse, 1997:477–497.

54. Golub A, Johnson BD. The misuse of the "gateway theory" in U.S. policy on drug abuse control: a secondary analysis of the muddled deduction. *Int J Drug Policy* 2002;13(1):5–19.

55. Substance Abuse and Mental Health Services Administration. *2000 National Household Survey on Drug Abuse: public use file codebook, main study.* DHHS Publication No. (SMA) 01–3514. Rockville, MD: US Department of Health and Human Services, 2002. Available at www.icpsr.umich.edu.

56. Johnston LD, O'Malley PM, Bachman JG. *Monitoring the Future: national survey results on drug use, 1975–2001, vol. 1: secondary school students.* NIH Publication No. 02-5106. Bethesda, MD: US Department of Health and Human Services, 2002.

57. Arrestee Drug Abuse Monitoring Program. *1999 Annual report on drug use among adult and juvenile arrestees.* NCJ 181426. Washington, DC: National Institute of Justice, 2000.

58. Hunt D, Rhodes W. *Methodology guide for ADAM.* Washington, DC: National Institute of Justice, 2001.

59. Johnson RA, Gerstein DR, Ghadialy R, et al. *Trends in the incidence of drug use in the United States, 1919-1992.* Rockville, MD: US Department of Health and Human Services, 1996.

60. Elliott DB, Huizinga D, Menard S. *Multiple problem youth: delinquency, substance use, and mental health problems.* New York: Springer-Verlag, 1989.

61. Kandel DB, Yamaguchi K. Job mobility and drug use: an event history analysis. *Am J Sociology* 1987;92:836–878.

62. Kandel DB, Murphy D, Karus D. Cocaine use in young adulthood: patterns of use and psychosocial correlates. In: Kozel NJ, Adam EH, eds. *Cocaine use in America: epidemiologic and clinical perspectives. NIDA Research Mono-*

graph no. 61. Rockville, MD: National Institute on Drug Abuse, 1985:76–110.

63. Yamaguchi K, Kandel DB. Patterns of drug use from adolescence to young adulthood. Sequences and predictors of progression. *Am J Public Health* 1984;74:668–681.

64. Johnson BD. *Marihuana users and drug subcultures.* New York: Wiley-Interscience, 1973.

65. Frank B, Morel R, Schmeidler J, et al. Cocaine and crack use in New York State. New York: Division of Substance Abuse Services, 1988.

66. Johnston LD, O'Malley PM, Backman JG. *National survey results on drug use from the Monitoring the Future study, 1975–1994, vol. II: secondary school students.* Rockville, MD: National Institute on Drug Abuse, 1995.

67. Hunt LG, Chambers CD. *The heroin epidemics: a study of heroin use in the U.S., 1965–75 (part II).* Holliswood, NY: Spectrum, 1976.

68. Rittenhouse JD, ed. *The epidemiology of heroin and other narcotics.* NIDA Research Monograph no. 16. Rockville, MD: National Institute on Drug Abuse, 1977.

69. Hunt L. *Heroin epidemics: a quantitative study of current empirical data.* Washington, DC: Drug Abuse Council, 1978.

70. Hughes PH. *Behind the walls of respect: community experiments in heroin addiction control.* Chicago: University of Chicago Press, 1977.

71. Brown C. *Manchild in the promised land.* New York: Signet Books, 1965.

72. Haley A. *Autobiography of Malcolm X.* New York: Signet Books, 1965.

73. Clayton RR, Voss HL. *Young men and drugs in Manhattan: a causal analysis.* Rockville, MD: National Institute on Drug Abuse, 1981.

74. Boyle J, Brunswick AF. What happened in Harlem? Analysis of a decline in heroin use among a generation unit of urban black youth. *J Drug Issues* 1980;10:109–130.

75. Frank B. An overview of heroin trends in New York City. *Mt. Sinai J Med* 2001;67(5):340–346.

76. Frank B, Schmeidler J, Johnson BD, et al. Seeking the truth in heroin indicators: the case of New York City. *Drug Alcohol Depend* 1978;3:345–358.

77. Johnson BD. Once an addict, seldom an addict. *Contemp Drug Probl* 1978;Spring:35–53.

78. Johnson BD, Thomas G, Golub A. Trends in heroin use among Manhattan arrestees from the heroin and crack eras. In: Inciardi JA, Harrison LD, eds. *Heroin in the age of crack cocaine.*

Thousand Oaks, CA: Sage 1998;109–130.

79. Hser YI, Hoffman V, Grella CE, et al. A 33-year follow-up of narcotics addicts. *Arch Gen Psychiatry* 2001;58:503–508.

80. Brecher EM. *Licit and illicit drugs.* Boston: Little, Brown, 1972.

81. Anglin MD, ed. Special issue: a social policy analysis of compulsory treatment for opiate dependence. *J Drug Issues* 1988;18(4).

82. McGlothlin WH, Anglin MD, Wilson BD. Narcotic addiction and crime. *Criminology* 1978;16:293–315.

83. Anglin MD, Hser Y. Treatment of drug abuse. In: Tonry M, Wilson JQ, eds. *Drugs and crime.* Chicago: University of Chicago Press, 1990.

84. Golub A, Johnson BD. *Trends in heroin use and injection and disclosure of heroin use among ADAM-Manhattan arrestees 1987–2001.* Paper presented at the American Society of Criminology Annual Meeting, Chicago, IL, November 2002.

85. Substance Abuse, Mental Health Services Administration. Office of Applied Studies. *National household survey on drug abuse: population estimates 1994.* Washington, DC: US Department of Health and Human Services, 1995.

86. Zinberg N. *Drugs, set, and setting.* New Haven: Yale University Press, 1984.

87. Spotts JV, Shontz FC. *Cocaine users: a representative case approach.* New York: Free Press, 1980.

88. Williams T. *The cocaine culture in after hours clubs.* New York: City University of New York; 1978(thesis).

89. Wish ED, Brady E, Cuadrado M. *Drug use and crime of arrestees in Manhattan. Paper presented at the 47th meeting of the Committee on Problems of Drug Dependence.* New York: Narcotic and Drug Research, 1984.

90. Sanchez JE, Johnson BD. Woman and the drug-crime connection: crime rates among drug-abusing women at Rikers Island. *J Psychedelic Drugs* 1987;19:200–216.

91. Seigel RK. Cocaine smoking. *J Psychoactive Drugs* 1982;14:277–359.

92. Van Dyke C, Byck R. Cocaine. *Sci Am* 1983;246:128–141.

93. Williams T. *The cocaine kids.* New York: Addison-Wesley, 1989.

94. Williams T. *The crack house.* Reading, MA: Addison-Wesley, 1991.

95. Johnson BD, Golub A, Fagan J. Careers in crack, drug use, drug distribution, and nondrug criminality. *Crime and Delinquency* 1995;41:275–295.

96. Brody J. Crack: a new form of cocaine. *New York Times* 1985 Nov 29:1.

97. Kids and cocaine: an epidemic strikes middle America. *Newsweek* 1986;Mar 17:58–65.

98. Crack and crime. *Newsweek* 1986;Jun 16:15–22.

99. Belenko S, Fagan J. *Crack and the criminal justice system.* New York: New York City Criminal Justice Agency, 1987.

100. Golub A, Johnson BD. A recent decline in cocaine use among youthful arrestees in Manhattan (1987—1993). *Am J Public Health* 1994;84:1250–1254.

101. Golub AL, Johnson BD. *Crack's decline: some surprises across U.S. cities.* NCJ 165707. National Institute of Justice Research in Brief, 1997. Washington, DC.

102. Johnson BD, Natarajan M, Dunlap E, et al. Crack abusers and noncrack abusers: profiles of drug use, drug sales, and nondrug criminality. *J Drug Issues* 1994;24:117–141.

103. Fagan J, Chin K. Social processes of initiation into crack. *J Drug Issues* 1991;21:313–344.

104. Fagan J, Chin K. Initiation into crack and cocaine: a tale of two epidemics. *Contemp Drug Probl* 1989;16:579–618.

105. Fagan J, Chin K. Violence as regulation and social control in the distribution of crack. In: De La Rosa M, Lambert E, Gropper B, eds. *Drugs and violence.* NIDA Research monograph no. 103. Rockville, MD: National Institute on Drug Abuse, 1991:8–43.

106. Fagan J, ed. *Special issues on crack cocaine. Contemp Drug Probl* 1989;16(4) and 1990;17(1).

107. Frank B, Morel R, Schmeidler J, et al. *Illicit substance use among Hispanics in New York State.* New York: Division of Substance Abuse Services, 1988.

108. Golub A, Johnson BD. Cohort differences in drug use pathways to crack among current crack abuser in New York City. *Crim Just Behav* 1994;21:403–422.

109. Rydell CP, Everingham SS. *Controlling cocaine: supply vs demand programs.* Santa Monica, CA: Rand Drug Policy Research Center, 1994.

110. Wallace B. Crack addiction: treatment and recovery issues. *Contemp Drug Probl* 1990;17:79–120.

111. Wallace B. *Crack cocaine: a practical treatment approach for the chemically dependent.* New York: Bruner/Mazel, 1991.

112. Dunlap E. Impact of drugs on family life and kin networks in the inner-city African-American single-parent household. In: Harrell A, Peterson G, eds. *Drugs, crime, and social isolation: barriers to urban opportunity.* Washington, DC: Urban Institute Press, 1992:181–207.

113. U.S. Senate Committee on the Judiciary. *Hardcore cocaine addicts: measuring—and fighting—the epidemic. A staff report.* Washington, DC: US Government Printing Office, 1990.

114. New York reports a drop in crack traffic. *New York Times* 1990 Dec 27:B1, B4.

115. Johnson BD, Dunlap E, Hamid A. Changes in New York's crack distribution scene. In: Vamos P, Corriveau P, eds. *Drugs and society to the year 2000.* Montreal: Portage Program for Drug Dependencies, 1992:360–364.

116. Furst RT, Johnson BD, Dunlap E, et al. The stigmatized image of the "crack head": a sociocultural exploration of a barrier to cocaine smoking among a cohort of youth in New York City. *Deviant Behav* 1999;20:153–181.

117. Rainone G, Frank B, Kott A, et al. *Crack users in treatment.* New York: Division of Substance Abuse Services, 1987.

118. Simeone R. *The problem of crack in New York City.* New York: Division of Substance Abuse Services, 1989.

119. Golub A, Johnson BD. *The rise of marijuana as the drug of choice among youthful arrestees.* NCJ 187490. National Institute of Justice Research in Brief, 2001. Washington DC.

120. U.S. Department of Health and Human Services. *Youth use of cigars: Patterns of use and perceptions of risk.* Washington, DC: 1999. Published by U.S. Department of Health and Human Services, Publication number OEI-06098-0030.

121. Sifaneck SJ, Kaplan CD, Dunlap E, et al. 2003. Blunts and blowtjes: cannabis use practices in two cultural settings and their implications for secondary prevention. *Free Inquiry in Creative Sociology;* 31:1–11.

122. Kandel DB, ed. *Stages and pathways of drug involvement: examining the gateway hypothesis.* New York: Cambridge, 2002.

123. Gfroerer JC, Epstein JF. Marijuana initiates and their impact on future drug abuse treatment need. *Drug Alcohol Depend* 1999;54:229–237.

124. Golub A, Johnson BD. Variation in youthful risk of progression from alcohol/tobacco to marijuana and hard drugs across generations. *Am J Pub Health* 2001;91(2):225–232.

125. Frank B, Galea J. *Current drug abuse trends in New York City. Community epidemiological trends in drug abuse: community epidemiological work group. Vol. II proceedings.* Rockville, MD: National Institute on Drug Abuse, 1996.

126. Marel R, Galea J, Robertson KA, et al. *Drug use trends in New York City.* New York State Office of Alcoholism

and Substance Abuse Services, 2002. Albany, NY.

127. Johnson BD, Rosenblum A, Kleber H. *A new opportunity to expand treatment for heroin users in New York City: public policy challenges for bringing buprenorphine into drug treatment programs and general medical practice.* White paper submitted to New York City Department of Health and Mental Hygiene, National Development and Research Institutes, Inc., January 18, 2003.

128. U.S. Food and Drug Administration. Subutex (buprenorphine hydrochloride) and Suboxone tablets (buprenorphine hydrochloride and naloxone hydrochloride) 2002. Available at: http://www.fda.gov/cder/drug/mfopage/subutex_suboxone/dcfault.htm.

129. Substance Abuse and Mental Health Services Administration. *Buprenorphine is new medical treatment.* News release. December 12, 2002. Available at www.icpsr.umich.edu.

130. Zimmer L. *Operation Pressure Point: the disruption of street-level trade on New York's Lower East Side.* Occasional paper from the Center for Research in Crime and Justice. New York: University School of Law, 1987.

131. Bratton WJ, Knobler P. *Turnaround: how America's top cop reversed the crime epidemic.* New York: Random House, 1998.

132. Maple J, Mitchell C. *The crime fighter: how you can make your community crime free.* New York: Broadway, 1999.

133. Brownstein HH. *The rise and fall of a violent crime wave: crack cocaine and the social construction of a crime problem.* Guilderland, NY: Harrow and Heston, 1998.

134. Kleiman MAR, Smith KD. State and local drug enforcement: in search of a strategy. In: Tonry M, Wilson JQ, eds. *Drugs and crime.* Chicago: University of Chicago Press, 1990;13:68–108.

135. Moore M. Supply reduction and law enforcement. In: Tonry M, Wilson JQ, eds. *Drugs and crime.* Chicago: University of Chicago Press, 1990;13:109–159.

136. Belenko S. The impact of drug offenders on the criminal justice system. In: Weisheit RA, ed. *Drugs, crime, and the criminal justice system.* Cincinnati, OH: Anderson, 1990:27–78.

137. Belenko S, Fagan J, Chin K. Criminal justice responses to crack. *J Res Crime Delinquency* 1991;28:55–74.

138. Belenko S. *Crack and the evolution of anti-drug policy.* Westport, CT: Greenwood, 1993.

139. Austin J, McVey A. The impact of the war on drugs. *Focus* [newsletter]. San Francisco: National Council on Crime and Delinquency, December 1989.

140. Join Together Policy Panel. *Fixing a failing system. National policy recommendations. How the criminal justice system should work with communities to reduce substance abuse.* Boston: Join Together (Boston University School of Public Health), 1996.

141. U.S. Bureau of Justice Statistics. Source book of Criminal Justice Statistics, 30th Edition. 2004. Available at: http://www.albany.edu/sourcebook

142. Bureau of Justice Statistics. *Prisoners in 1994.* Washington, DC: US Government Printing Office, 1995.

143. Meierhoefer BS. *The general effect of mandatory minimum prison terms: a longitudinal study of federal sentences imposed.* Washington, DC: Federal Judicial Center, 1992.

144. Mauer M. *Young black men and the criminal justice system: a growing national problem.* Washington, DC: The Sentencing Project, 1990.

145. Mauer M. *Young black Americans and the criminal justice system: five years later.* Washington, DC: The Sentencing Project, 1995.

146. King RS, Mauer M. *Distorted priorities: drug offenders in state prisons.* Washington, DC: The Sentencing Project 2002. Available at http://sentencingproject.org.

147. Bureau of Justice Statistics. *Justice expenditure and employment 2001.* Washington, DC: Government Printing Office, 2002.

148. Drug Abuse Warning Network. 2003. Available at http://dawninfo.samhsa.gov.

149. Turner CF, Miller HG, Moses LE. *AIDS, sexual behavior, and intravenous drug use.* Washington, DC: National Research Council, 1989.

150. Reuter P. Hawks ascendant: the punitive trend in American drug policy. *Daedalus* 1992;121(3):15–52.

151. Reuter P. On the consequences of toughness. In: Lazear E, Krauss M, eds. *Searching for alternatives.* Stanford, CA: Hoover Institution, 1991:138–164.

Substances of Abuse

CHAPTER 8

Alcohol: Neurobiology

STEPHEN L. BOEHM II, C. FERNANDO
VALENZUELA, AND R. ADRON HARRIS

Alcoholism is one of the most costly diseases afflicting persons in the United States today. It has often been described as a chronically relapsing disorder in which the alcoholic compulsively consumes alcohol at the expense of all other "normal" behaviors. The circumstances that lead to this compulsive alcohol intake are complex and include psychosocial, environmental, genetic, and neurobiologic factors. This chapter focuses on the neurobiologic actions of alcohol. Historically, it was believed that alcohol produced its effects in the brain through perturbation of neuronal membrane lipids (1). However, it is now widely accepted that alcohol directly interacts with neuronal proteins. The following pages discuss the various neurotransmitter receptor systems implicated in these interactions. We then turn to several new and novel neurobiologic techniques in the study of alcoholism, and discuss two promising animal model systems of alcohol abuse and dependence.

NEURONAL TARGETS OF ALCOHOL ACTION

Ligand-Gated Ion Channels

Members of the superfamily of ligand-gated ion channels mediate fast synaptic chemical neurotransmission in the central nervous system (CNS) (reviewed in reference 2). These channels are multi-subunit structures that open in response to a specific neurotransmitter and selectively conduct cations or anions from the extracellular to the intracellular neuronal compartments, thereby

altering the excitability of the cell on which they reside. Inhibitory control of brain function is exerted via anion conducting ion channels, whereas excitatory tone is a result of cation selective channels. The anion-conducting ligand-gated ion channels are the type-A γ-aminobutyric acid (GABA$_A$; see Fig. 8.1A) and the glycine receptors, both of which conduct chloride ions. The cation-conducting ligand-gated ion channels are the N-methyl-D-aspartate (NMDA; see Fig. 8.1B), α-amino-3-hydroxy-5-methylisoxazole-4-propionate (AMPA), kainate, nicotinic acetylcholine (nACh), and the 5-hydroxytryptamine type 3 (5-HT$_3$) receptors. NMDA, AMPA, kainate, and nACh receptors conduct sodium, potassium, and calcium, whereas 5-HT$_3$ receptors conduct only sodium and potassium. Evidence suggests that alcohol (ethanol) interacts with each of these receptor types, altering the ease with which ions pass through their respective receptor channels.

GABA$_A$ Receptor System

In the 1980s, a number of laboratories found that drugs (e.g., GABA$_A$ agonists, uptake inhibitors) that augment GABAergic function enhance behavioral actions of ethanol, and drugs (e.g., GABA$_A$ antagonists, synthesis inhibitors) that inhibit GABAergic function reduce ethanol behaviors. Furthermore the Long-Sleep/Short-Sleep (LS/SS) mice, selectively bred to differ in genetic sensitivity to the hypnotic effects of ethanol, were found to differ in their behavioral sensitivities to GABAergic drugs (3). In 1986, three different research groups directed by Adron Harris, Steven Paul, and Maharaj Ticku, demonstrated that intoxicating concentrations (5 to 50 mmol/L) of ethanol enhanced the function of GABA$_A$ receptors using chloride flux assays (4–6). A detailed discussion of this literature is beyond the scope of this section, but is covered in reviews (7–9), and in earlier editions of this book.

More recent behavioral studies continue to implicate the GABA$_A$ receptor system in the behavioral actions of

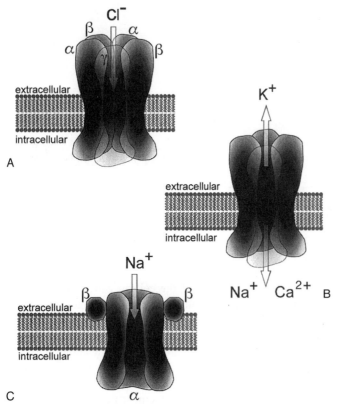

FIG. 8.1. Ligand- and voltage-gated ion channels. **A:** Representative pentameric ligand-gated ion channel: GABA$_A$ receptor complex. Five subunits come together to form an ion pore. When bound by an agonist, the channel opens and chloride ions (Cl$^-$) are allowed passage through the pore. **B:** Representative tetrameric ligand-gated ion channel: N-methyl-D-aspartate (NMDA) receptor complex. Four subunits are arranged to form an ion pore. Activation by an agonist results in channel opening, and the movement of sodium (Na$^+$) and calcium (Ca^{2+}) ions into the cell, and potassium (K$^+$) ions out of the cell. **C:** Representative voltage-gated ion channel: sodium channel. The functional channel is composed of three subunits, although the α subunit alone forms the ion pore. In response to a neuronal depolarization, sodium channels open allowing the passage of Na$^+$ into the cell.

ethanol, including stimulation of motor activity (10), discriminative stimulus (11), and rewarding and aversive effects (12). A great deal of data suggests that the GABA$_A$ receptor system plays an important role in influencing alcohol consumption. Inverse agonists and antagonists at the benzodiazepine receptor site on the GABA$_A$ receptor/chloride channel complex decrease alcohol consumption in rats (13,14). Genetic deletion of the δ subunit of the GABA$_A$ receptor also results in decreases in alcohol consumption, as well as reduced anticonvulsant effects of ethanol (15). Benzodiazepine receptor antagonism of α_1 subunit-containing GABA$_A$ receptors in the medial and ventral pallidum decreases alcohol consumption in alcohol-preferring P rats, selectively bred to genetically

differ in ethanol preference (16), and intrahippocampal infusion of an α_5 subunit-specific benzodiazepine receptor inverse agonist antagonizes ethanol seeking behaviors (17).

Electrophysiologic studies have been conducted using brain primary cultures, acutely prepared tissue slices as well as *in vivo* preparations. Ethanol potentiation of GABA$_A$ receptor function has been observed in a variety of primary cultures, including rat dorsal root ganglion neurons (18,19) and chick embryo cerebral cortical neurons (20). Reynolds et al. (21) examined acutely dissociated neurons from rat neocortical slices and primary cultures of chick, mouse, and rat brain regions and demonstrated that a concentration of 1 to 50 mmol/L ethanol potentiated GABA$_A$ responses in some cells from each brain region studied. Aguayo (22), studying GABA$_A$-activated chloride currents in cultured mouse hippocampal and cortical neurons, found ethanol effects similar to those of Reynolds and Prasad (20). Whole-cell patch-clamp recordings showed a biphasic effect of ethanol with a maximal effect at a concentration of 10 mmol/L, and less potentiation using 80 mmol/L ethanol. On the single-channel level, ethanol enhanced the frequency of GABA-mediated channel opening events, the mean open time, percentage open time, frequency of opening bursts, and mean burst duration; in contrast, the mean closed time was decreased (23).

A number of studies have identified factors important for ethanol enhancement of neuronal GABA$_A$ receptor function. In an attempt to explain discrepancies in the literature regarding alcohol effects on hippocampal GABA$_A$ receptors, Weiner et al. (24) undertook a study of GABA$_A$ receptor sensitivity to ethanol in subpopulations of rat hippocampal CA1 pyramidal neurons. Electrical stimulation adjacent to the stratum pyramidale activated different populations of GABA$_A$ receptors in a single CA1 neuron than stimulation within the stratum lacunosum-moleculare. Stimulation at the former site resulted in GABA$_A$ responses with greater sensitivity to the enhancing effects of a concentration of 40 to 160 mmol/L ethanol, suggesting that ethanol sensitivity of GABA$_A$ receptors can vary not only among brain regions, but also among different receptors within the same neuron. Local application of GABA to the somatic regions of rat cerebral cortical neurons in brain slices also demonstrated cell-site specificity of ethanol enhancement of GABA$_A$ receptor function (25). Furthermore, Dunwiddie and colleagues showed that ethanol enhancement of GABAergic inhibitory postsynaptic currents produced by stimulation of proximal hippocampal CA1 synapses in mice and rats was correlated with their genetic sensitivity to alcohol measured *in vivo* (26). A recent study of the central amygdala nucleus showed that ethanol (11 to 66 mmol/L) enhances GABAergic neurotransmission by actions at both pre- and postsynaptic sites (27). Thus, the GABA$_A$ synapses in this region are particularly sensitive to ethanol, which may be related to the role of the amygdala in reinforcing actions of ethanol (28).

Weiner et al. (29) examined the molecular mechanisms responsible for ethanol enhancement of GABA$_A$ currents in hippocampal CA1 neurons. Ethanol (10 to 50 mmol/L) potentiated GABA$_A$-mediated inhibitory postsynaptic currents with a requirement for the presence of intracellular adenosine triphosphate (ATP); in contrast, diazepam enhancement did not require ATP. The link between protein kinase C (PKC) activity and ethanol sensitivity of GABA$_A$ receptors was also made in several studies (29,30), demonstrating that brain-slice preparation techniques with elevated PKC activity increased GABA$_A$ receptor sensitivity to ethanol. The importance of PKC activity was also underscored by our finding (31) that null mutant mice lacking the γ isoform of PKC displayed decreased sensitivity to ethanol-induced hypothermia and duration of loss of righting reflex. Furthermore, ethanol did not enhance GABA-mediated chloride influx into brain microsacs prepared from these PKCγ knock-out mice.

Wan et al. (32) identified another factor important for ethanol enhancement of GABA$_A$ receptor function in CA1 hippocampal pyramidal cells. They found that blockade of G-protein coupled GABA$_B$ receptors using the selective antagonist CGP-35348 greatly enhanced the responses of GABA$_A$ receptors to ethanol, and postulated that concurrent synaptic activation of GABA$_B$ and GABA$_A$ receptors obscures enhancement by ethanol at the latter site. β-Adrenergic receptor activation also appears to play an important role in permitting ethanol's enhancing effects on GABA receptor function, at least in cerebellar Purkinje neurons (33–35). This was shown to occur via β-adrenergic receptor stimulation of the cyclic adenosine monophosphate (cAMP)/protein kinase A second messenger system (36).

Several groups have not found ethanol enhancement of GABA$_A$ receptor-mediated currents. Ethanol did not potentiate GABA-activated currents in rat locus coeruleus brain slice preparations (37). Despite seeing ethanol inhibition of an NMDA-activated current, White et al. (38) also found no enhancement of a GABA-mediated chloride current by 10 to 100 mmol/L ethanol in isolated adult rat sensory neurons. Ming et al. (39) found no effects of ethanol (up to 300 mmol/L) on either NMDA or GABA responses in cultured cortical neurons. It is of interest to note that an early study (40) indicated that ethanol blocked hippocampal long term potentiation (LTP) solely by inhibition of NMDA receptors, but recent, more detailed, studies conclude that both NMDA and GABA$_A$ receptor systems are required for this action of ethanol (41).

Many studies have been published on the effects of ethanol and other intoxicant/anesthetics on GABA receptors composed of defined subunits and we have reviewed this area (8,9,42). In brief, studies of the sub-

unit combinations most commonly found in brain do not show marked differences in alcohol sensitivity when tested in *Xenopus* oocytes. All of these receptor combinations are enhanced by ethanol, but concentrations of 25 to 100 mmol/L are required. The only marked deviation in alcohol action that we have found was in the inhibition of the GABA$_C$ rho1 subunit (43). A recent study reported that $\alpha_4\beta_2\delta$ GABA$_A$ receptors expressed in *Xenopus* oocytes are very sensitive to alcohol, with concentrations as low as 1 to 3 mmol/L ethanol significantly enhancing GABAergic currents (44). This receptor subunit combination is found in high concentrations in the hippocampus. Another recent study found that concentrations of ethanol as low as 9 mmol/L markedly enhanced the function of GABA$_A$ ($\alpha_1\beta_2\gamma_2$) receptors in HEK293 cells if the experiments were performed in the presence of a low, subthreshold, concentration of a neurosteroid (45).

For a more in depth review of GABA$_A$ receptor systems and alcohol sensitivity, the reader is referred to earlier editions of this book.

Glycine Receptor Systems

Glycine receptors constitute the major inhibitory neurotransmitter receptor system in the brainstem and spinal cord, but are also found in significant numbers in higher brain regions such as the olfactory bulb, midbrain, cerebellum, and cerebral cortex (46). Enhancement of glycine receptor function would be consistent with some behavioral actions of ethanol observed *in vivo*. For example, ethanol-induced loss of righting reflex in mice is augmented by the intracerebroventricular administration of glycine, as well as by its precursor serine (47). This effect is blocked by the glycine receptor antagonist strychnine. Studies performed on genetically altered mice also implicate glycine receptors as important targets of alcohol actions. Homanics and colleagues recently showed that the hypnotic effects of ethanol were altered in *spastic* and *spasmodic* mice bearing dysfunctional glycine receptors (48). Furthermore, a transgenic mouse bearing a glycine receptor that, *in vitro*, shows ethanol inhibition of receptor function, is less sensitive to ethanol in behavioral measures, including loss of righting reflex, anticonvulsant activity (strychnine seizures), and motor incoordination (49).

Compared to the abundance of data available for GABA$_A$ receptors, fewer investigators have examined ethanol effects on glycine receptors. Electrophysiologic studies showed that ethanol enhances glycine receptor function in mouse and chick embryonic spinal neurons in a concentration-dependent manner (50,51). The glycine EC$_{50}$ is decreased by 100 mmol/L ethanol with no effect on the maximal glycinergic currents (52); that is, as with GABA$_A$ receptor, ethanol left-shifts glycine concentration-response curves. Furthermore, concentrations of ethanol that enhance glycine receptor function in mouse spinal cord neurons (10 to 200 mmol/L) have no effect on membrane lipid order (53). Studies using dissociated ventral tegmental area (VTA) dopamine neurons, cells thought to be important for ethanol's reinforcing effects, also demonstrate ethanol enhancement of glycine receptor function (54). Finally, ethanol increases glycine-mediated chloride uptake into rat brain synaptoneurosomes (55).

Mascia et al. (56) demonstrated ethanol enhancement of the function of glycine receptors of defined composition expressed in *Xenopus* oocytes. Concentrations as low as 10 mmol/L ethanol were effective, especially when lower concentrations of glycine were tested. Homomeric α_1 receptors were more sensitive to low concentrations of ethanol than were α_2 receptors, and this difference in ethanol sensitivity was attributed to a difference between the two at amino acid 52, the amino acid responsible for the *spasmodic* phenotype in mice (56). Corroborating this finding, Eggers et al. (57) found that glycine receptors from juvenile hypoglossal motoneurons (expressing primarily the α_1 glycine receptor isoform) showed greater ethanol enhancement than neonatal glycine receptors that express the α_2 isoform. Particularly in the α_1-containing glycine receptors, ethanol enhanced the amplitudes of miniature and evoked inhibitory postsynaptic potentials, suggesting that it was having a postsynaptic effect at these receptors. The degree of ethanol enhancement may also depend on the expression system. Valenzuela et al. (58) found that glycine receptors transiently transfected in HEK293 cells, or stably transfected into Ltk⁻ cells, were less sensitive to ethanol than receptors expressed in oocytes.

NMDA Receptor Systems

The NMDA receptor system represents the major excitatory neurotransmitter system in the mammalian (CNS). Early behavioral studies suggested that ethanol reduced NMDA-induced seizures (59,60) and hyperalgesia (61) in rodents. The sedative effects of ethanol were greatly increased by NMDA antagonists (62–64), and noncompetitive NMDA receptor antagonists produced ethanol-like effects in rats trained to discriminate ethanol from vehicle (65). Moreover, NMDA antagonists attenuate the development of rapid and chronic tolerance to the motor incoordinating and hypothermic effects of ethanol in rats (66–69), effects that have been associated with their ability to block learning processes thought to have a role in tolerance mechanisms (70,71).

Efforts to create genetically altered mice that lack functional NMDA receptors were only recently successful. Targeted disruption of the NMDA receptor NR1 subunit gene in mice resulted in death shortly after birth (72), and mice in which the NR2B subunit gene was deleted died perinatally (73). Consequently, determining the effects on ethanol sensitivity in these mutant mice was not possible. However, a recent study showed that mice expressing a mutated form of the NR1 subunit that alters affinity for the coagonist, glycine, exhibit reduced sensitivity to ethanol's motor incoordinating and anxiolytic effects, but not ethanol intake (74).

Consistent with its behavioral effects, electrophysiologic studies show that acute ethanol exposure inhibits NMDA receptor function. Ethanol dose-dependently inhibited NMDA-stimulated calcium uptake in rat cerebellar granule cells and dissociated brain cells from newborn rats (75–77). Moreover, ethanol inhibited NMDA-induced currents in rat hippocampal neurons and dissociated adult rat dorsal root ganglia (38,78), and decreased open-channel probability and mean open time in cultured rat hippocampal neurons at concentrations greater than 86 mmol/L (79). However, it should be noted that lower ethanol concentrations had no effect, or even increased, the frequency of channel openings. Ethanol has also been found to inhibit NMDA-dependent excitatory postsynaptic potentials in adult rat hippocampal slices (80,81).

Ethanol has had similar effects on NMDA receptor systems when tested using the *Xenopus* oocyte expression system. Ethanol inhibited NMDA-gated currents in *Xenopus* oocytes expressing hippocampal or cerebellar rat brain messenger ribonucleic acid (mRNA) (82). Experiments with recombinant receptors expressed in *Xenopus* oocytes demonstrated that ethanol inhibits NMDA receptors in a manner that is dependent on subunit composition and phosphorylation factors. Differentially spliced variants of NMDA receptor NR1 subunits vary in their sensitivity to ethanol (83), and heteromeric NMDA receptors containing the NR1/2A or NR1/2B subunits are more sensitive to the inhibitory actions of ethanol than receptors containing NR1/2C or NR1/2D subunits (84–86). In addition to subunit composition, evidence also suggests that other factors such as PKC-dependent phosphorylation might modulate the ethanol sensitivity of NMDA receptors (87). More in-depth discussions of the effects of ethanol on native and recombinant NMDA receptors are available for the interested reader (88,89).

AMPA and Kainate Receptor Systems

A number of studies have demonstrated that AMPA and kainate receptor systems are sensitive to alcohol (75,78,80). Several studies using the *Xenopus* oocyte expression system showed that alcohol inhibits these receptors (82,90), and electrophysiologic studies in cortical (91), striatal (92,93), and hippocampal (94–96) neurons corroborated these findings. Moreover, for at least kainate receptors, the degree of alcohol inhibition appears to depend on agonist concentration and subunit composition (90,97), and may involve both PKC-dependent and -independent mechanisms (97). Recent work suggests that alcohol may inhibit the AMPA receptor by stabilizing the desensitized state (91).

Several recent reports implicate AMPA and kainate receptor systems in the behavioral actions of alcohol. For example, a recent investigation suggested that alcohol might enhance the excitability of pyramidal neurons by indirectly inhibiting the kainate receptor-dependent drive of GABAergic interneurons in the hippocampus (98). These authors proposed that this mechanism could, in part, explain the facilitatory effects on memory seen following administration of low alcohol doses. Another study showed that glutamate systems other than the NMDA receptor system (i.e., AMPA and kainate) play a role in alcohol withdrawal hyperexcitability because alcohol withdrawal *in vivo* leads to increased activity of these systems in hippocampal CA1 neurons (99). Interestingly, pharmacologic studies seem to support this latter finding because systemic kainate administration reduces the behavioral signs of alcohol withdrawal in rats (100), and increases the latency and amount of kainate necessary to induce seizures in alcohol withdrawn mice (101). Thus, whereas AMPA and kainate receptor systems appear to be important mediators of alcohol sensitivity, future studies will be necessary to more fully elucidate the mechanisms by which alcohol interacts with these receptor systems.

Nicotinic Acetylcholine Receptor Systems

Behavioral studies suggest a role for nACh receptors in the mediation of alcohol sensitivity, and a number of these have focused on its involvement in ethanol's sedative and/or hypnotic effects (102,103). Nevertheless, nicotine was also shown to alter the locomotor stimulant effects of ethanol (104). Moreover, the nACh receptor channel blocker, mecamylamine, partially counteracts these effects, as well as attenuates the associated ethanol-induced increases in rat nucleus accumbens dopamine (105). These results imply a role for these receptors in the modulation of ethanol's reinforcing and/or motivational effects (106). However, despite the recent development of a number of different nACh-receptor mutant mice (107), to date there are no published reports on the ethanol sensitivity of these potentially important animal models.

Consistent with the behavioral literature, *in vitro* studies demonstrate that ethanol potentiates nACh receptor function. Ethanol potentiated nACh receptor-mediated currents in cultured rat cortical neurons (108), when expressed in HEK293 cells (109), and when recombinant receptors were expressed in *Xenopus* oocytes (110). For a recent review of this literature, see Narahashi et al. (111).

5-HT₃ Receptor Systems

A growing literature implicates the 5-HT₃ receptor system in mediating alcohol sensitivity. A number of behavioral studies show that antagonists of these receptors attenuate alcohol preference drinking (112–115). Transgenic mice that overexpress 5-HT₃ receptors in the forebrain, resulting in chronic enhancement of receptor function, exhibited reduced ethanol intake (116) and enhanced sensitivity to alcohol-potentiation of 5-HT₃ receptor currents in dissociated forebrain neurons (117). Moreover, ethanol (25 to 100 mmol/L) potentiated 5-HT₃ receptor-mediated currents in neuroblastoma cells (118) and nodose ganglion neurons (119). Recent experiments with recombinant 5-HT₃ receptors expressed in *Xenopus* oocytes yielded similar results (120). The reader is referred to Lovinger (121) for a more detailed review of 5-HT₃ receptors and alcohol sensitivity.

G Protein-Coupled Receptor Systems

Alcohol interacts with a number of G protein-coupled receptor systems, important for neuronal signal transduction (Fig. 8.2). The family of G protein-coupled receptors are activated by a myriad of ligands, including the amines (dopamine, norepinephrine, 5-hydroxytryptamine [5-HT or serotonin], acetylcholine), amino acids (glutamate, GABA), peptides and proteins (vasopressin, oxytocin), nucleosides (adenosine), and fatty acid and phospholipid derivatives. These receptors couple to one or more classes of heterotrimeric G proteins formed by α, β, and γ subunits, and are grouped into four subfamilies, based on their subunit homology. Members of the G_s subfamily stimulate adenylyl cyclase, whereas members of the G_i subfamily have a variety of effects, including inhibition of adenylyl cyclase and inhibition of calcium channels. Finally, the G_q subfamily stimulates phospholipase C_β.

Dopamine Receptor Systems

A number of addictive substances are thought to be reinforcing because they activate the mesolimbic dopamine pathway (primarily projections from the VTA to the nucleus accumbens), enhancing dopamine release in the nucleus accumbens. Evidence suggests that alcohol may have similar effects on the system. Early biochemical studies showed that alcohol increases the synthesis and release (turnover) of dopamine (see reference 122 for a review). Moreover, later studies demonstrated that systemically administered alcohol produces a significant increase in dopamine release in the nucleus accumbens (123). Electrophysiologic studies supported these findings by showing that the firing rate of VTA dopamine neurons increased after systemic or *in vitro* administration of alcohol

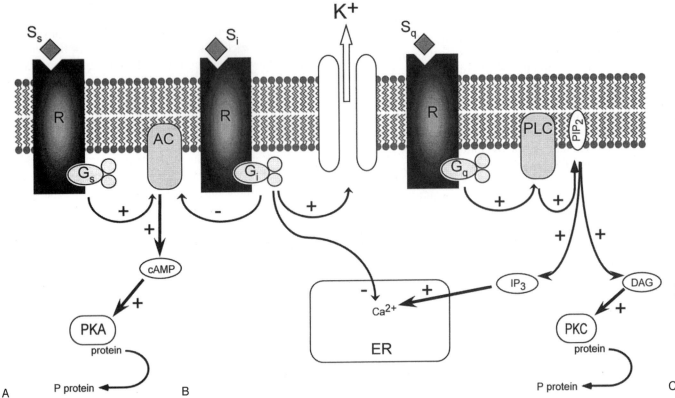

FIG. 8.2. G protein-coupled receptor systems. **A:** G_s-coupled systems. The binding of an agonist (S_s) results in activation of adenylyl cyclase (AC) through a stimulatory G protein-coupled mechanism (G_s). This results in enhanced cyclic adenosine monophosphate (cAMP) formation, stimulating protein kinase A (PKA) phosphorylation of various intracellular proteins. **B:** G_i-coupled systems. The binding of an agonist (S_i) results in inhibition of AC, and thus reduced cAMP formation. PKA phosphorylation of proteins is inhibited through this mechanism. Moreover, G_i also interacts with inwardly rectifying potassium channels, enhancing efflux of K^+, and with intracellular calcium stores, inhibiting the release of Ca^{2+} from the endoplasmic reticulum (ER). These effects further hyperpolarize the cell, making action potential generation less likely. **C:** G_q-coupled systems. The binding of agonist (S_q) results in activation of phospholipase C (PLC) through a stimulatory G protein-coupled mechanism (G_q). PLC catalyzes the conversion of phosphatidylinositol bisphosphate (PIP_2), leading to release of inositol triphosphate (IP_3) and diacylglycerol (DAG). DAG activates protein kinase C (PKC) phosphorylation of various intracellular proteins, whereas IP_3 stimulates the release of intracellular Ca^{2+} from the ER.

(124,125); more recently Brodie and colleagues demonstrated that this increased excitability occurs through a direct excitatory cellular activation (126,127). Finally, a compelling study showed that alcohol self-administration increased the release of dopamine in the rat nucleus accumbens, an effect that was greater in alcohol-preferring (P) rats (compared to Wistar rats), and that was not observed following self-administration of saccharine (128).

Studies have demonstrated a potential connection between dopamine receptors and the alcohol reinforcement (reviewed in reference 129). Several groups have found small reductions in the number of D2 receptors in several limbic structures, including the nucleus accumbens, in P and Sardinian ethanol-preferring rats (130–132), and at least in Sardinian ethanol-preferring rats, the number of D1 receptors was also reduced (133). Pharmacologic studies

support these findings. Systemic administration of nonspecific dopamine agonists decreased alcohol consumption in P rats (134,135), and self-administration in several rat populations, including P and Wistar rats (134,136,137). Furthermore, microinjection of nonspecific, as well as specific, D2/D3 dopamine agonists into the nucleus accumbens increased reinforced responding to alcohol (138). Administration of D1 receptor antagonists in studies examining alcohol's reinforcing properties has produced somewhat equivocal results (134,139–141), likely a result of the involvement of more than one dopamine receptor subtype. Nevertheless, the dopamine agonist studies suggest that these drugs may substitute for alcohol's stimulating effects on the mesolimbic dopamine pathway. See Samson et al. (141) for a more in depth review of this literature.

Although contradicting, lesion studies using the neurotoxin 6-hydroxydopamine also suggest that mesolimbic dopamine systems have a role in the control of ethanol reinforcement. This neurotoxin causes degeneration of dopaminergic and noradrenergic neurons. One study suggested that these lesions decrease alcohol preference in rats (142), whereas several others have shown that 6-hydroxydopmaine lesions enhance alcohol intake (143–146). More recently, Rassnick et al. (146) found that 6-hydroxydopamine lesions of the nucleus accumbens have no affect on alcohol self-administration in rats. It is not immediately clear why the above studies do not agree. However, possibilities include the use of different rat strains and experimental paradigms. Finally, in an interesting study, Lança (147) showed that intrastriatal transplantation of fetal dopaminergic grafts reduced voluntary alcohol intake in rats.

Studies using genetically altered mice have also pointed to the importance of dopamine receptor systems in alcohol sensitivity. Null mutation of the D4 receptor gene resulted in exaggerated sensitivity to alcohol's locomotor stimulant effects (148), and deletion of the D2 receptor gene resulted in reduced sensitivity to alcohol's locomotor stimulant and motor incoordinating effects, as well as reduced alcohol preference drinking in two-bottle choice procedure (149). Moreover, overexpression of the D2 receptor gene via adenoviral vector delivery to the nucleus accumbens in rats also reduced alcohol preference drinking (150). Disruption of the D1 receptor gene also resulted in reduced alcohol preference drinking in a two-bottle choice paradigm (151). Mice lacking the D3 receptor gene exhibited more severe alcohol withdrawal following chronic access to an alcohol-liquid diet (152). Finally, mice made deficient for the dopamine transporter exhibited reduced alcohol preference drinking in a two-bottle choice paradigm (153). Thus, taken together, the available data suggest that dopamine receptor systems play an important role in alcohol reinforcement mechanisms, as well as in sensitivity to a number of alcohol's behavioral effects.

5-HT Receptor Systems

5-HT receptors exert a wide variety of actions, including inhibition of neurotransmitter release, increase in phosphoinositide turnover, and decrease or increase in cAMP levels (154). One class of 5-HT receptors, the 5-HT$_3$ receptors, are ligand-gated ion channels, and their involvement in alcohol's actions was discussed in a previous section entitled "Neuronal Targets of Alcohol Action, Diganel-Gated Ion channels, *5-HT$_3$ Receptor Systems*." 5-HT receptor systems have been implicated in modulating a number of alcohol's actions, including reinforcement and tolerance.

The role of 5-HT receptor systems in modulating alcohol intake has been reviewed (113,155). LeMarquand et al.

(113) summarized studies examining alcohol intake after several manipulations that increase or decrease serotonergic function. The majority of the studies support the hypothesis that an increase in serotonergic function leads to a decrease in alcohol consumption. In these studies, serotonin function was increased by means of brain or peripheral injections of serotonin or its precursors, serotonin uptake inhibitors, serotonin releasers, or serotonin agonists. Conversely, the majority of the studies do not support the hypothesis that a decrease in serotonergic function leads to an increase in alcohol consumption. Serotonin function was decreased by means of serotonergic neurotoxins, electrolytic lesioning of serotonergic pathways, serotonin receptor antagonists, and serotonin uptake enhancers. The reasons for these apparent inconsistencies can be related to experimental factors such as the doses, times of exposure, and animal species used (122). Nevertheless, these, and other studies examining the effects of serotonergic drugs on alcohol discrimination suggest that serotonin may play a role in alcohol reinforcement.

A number of studies demonstrating a link between alcohol and 5-HT receptor systems have been performed using the alcohol-preferring P, and nonpreferring NP rats. Wong et al. (156) found that 5-HT$_{1A}$ receptors were more abundant in membranes isolated from the cortical areas of P, but not NP rats. Levels of 5-HT$_2$ receptors were also reduced in several brain regions of P, but not NP rats (157). Finally, the serotonin content and density of serotonin immunoreactive fibers appear to be reduced in the forebrain, and dorsal and medial raphe nuclei of P rats (158,159).

Genetically altered mice have also been used to investigate the role of 5-HT receptor systems and alcohol sensitivity. An early study suggested that 5-HT$_{1B}$ null mutant mice consumed more alcohol in a two-bottle choice drinking study (160). Whereas at least one study has corroborated these findings (161), many have not agreed (162–165). Although the reasons for these discrepancies are not immediately clear, possibilities include differing experimental testing paradigms, as well as issues surrounding the genetic backgrounds of the mutant mice. Studies with 5-HT$_{1B}$-deficient mice also implicate this receptor in the meditation alcohol's motor incoordinating effects (160,166), and although these mice have not been specifically tested, pharmacologic investigations suggest a role for this receptor in the mediation of alcohol-enhanced aggression in mice (167,168).

Pharmacologic studies also implicate 5-HT$_{1A}$ receptors in the mediation of alcohol sensitivity. These studies reveal a role for this serotonin receptor in alcohol's reinforcing (169), hypothermic and sedative (170), and aggression-enhancing effects (171). Mice lacking the 5-HT$_{1A}$ receptor subtype are available. However, to date, there are no published reports on the alcohol sensitivity of these mice.

Consistent with the above behavioral studies suggesting that 5-HT receptor systems play a role in the modulation alcohol intake, a number of electrophysiologic and neurochemical studies have demonstrated that serotonin modulates the activity of dopamine neurons (172,173). Microdialysis experiments revealed that alcohol stimulates serotonin release in the nucleus accumbens (123,174). It was shown that serotonergic neurons projecting from the anterior raphe nuclei make synaptic connections with dopaminergic neurons in the VTA (175). Moreover, microinjections of serotonin into the VTA enhance dopamine release in the nucleus accumbens (176). It is possible that this effect may occur via 5-HT$_3$ receptors because agonists of these receptors increase (177), whereas antagonists decrease (174), dopamine release in the nucleus accumbens. Consequently, 5-HT receptor systems might be important mediators of alcohol's effects on dopamine neurotransmission. For further details on the role of 5-HT$_3$ receptors on alcohol reinforcement, see Grant (155) and LeMarquand et al. (113).

Adenosine Receptor Systems

Adenosine is believed to serve as a neuromodulator rather than a neurotransmitter. Whereas specific neurons containing adenosine have not been identified, its levels appear sufficient to activate adenosine receptors on neuronal membranes (178). Four subtypes of adenosine receptors have been identified; activation of A$_1$ receptors produces inhibition of adenylyl cyclase activity, activation of A$_{2a}$ and A$_{2b}$ receptors stimulates this activity, and activation of A$_3$ receptors activates phospholipase C (178,179).

Although a handful of studies investigated alcohol's actions on adenosine-stimulated adenylyl cyclase activity (see below), most of the evidence for an interaction between alcohol and adenosine receptor systems comes from behavioral studies. In mice, adenosine antagonists reduced the sedative and motor incoordinating effects of alcohol, whereas agonists and adenosine uptake inhibitors enhanced these responses to alcohol (180). Furthermore, similar effects were seen when these compounds were administered intracerebroventricularly (181). In another study, adenosine agonists or antagonists were chronically administered to mice, and the motor incoordinating effect of alcohol was measured. In animals that received caffeine or isobutylmethylxanthine (but not theophylline), adenosine receptors were upregulated, and sensitivity to alcohol's motor-impairing effects were enhanced (182). Whereas these data point to the importance of adenosine receptor systems in mediating alcohol's motor incoordinating effects, studies with LS and SS mice do not support such a conclusion. LS mice were more sensitive to the sedative actions of an adenosine agonist, and the excitatory actions of an adenosine antagonist than were SS mice. However, no difference in the number or electrophysiologic responses of adenosine receptors in the hippocampus were detected (7). Moreover, it should also be pointed out that some of the methylxan-

thine adenosine receptor antagonists that have been used to link adenosine receptor systems to alcohol's motor incoordinating effects may also antagonize its sedative effects.

Recent behavioral studies demonstrate that the adenosine A$_1$ and A$_{2A}$ receptor subtypes are particularly important in the mediation of alcohol sensitivity. A$_1$ receptor antisense oligodeoxynucleotides blocked alcohol's motor incoordinating effects when they were microinjected into the striatum (183) or the cerebellum (184) of rats; the specific antisense oligodeoxynucleotides used did not alter normal motor control. Furthermore, Dar showed that intrastriatal infusion of two different A$_1$ receptor antagonists and an A$_1$ receptor agonist, dose-dependently attenuated and potentiated, respectively, alcohol-induced motor incoordination. More recently, he demonstrated that functional antagonism between striatal NMDA and adenosine A$_1$ receptors modulates sensitivity to alcohol's motor incoordinating effects (185). Finally, two recent investigations using adenosine A$_{2A}$ receptor-deficient mice implicated this receptor subtype in the mediation of alcohol preference drinking using a two-bottle choice procedure and alcohol withdrawal seizures. These studies demonstrated that mice lacking A$_{2A}$ receptors exhibit greater alcohol preference drinking (186) and reduced sensitivity to alcohol withdrawal seizures (187). Thus, adenosine receptor systems appear to be important for at least several behavioral effects of alcohol.

Biochemical studies have attempted to determine the mechanism(s) by which adenosine receptor systems might influence alcohol sensitivity. For example, one study showed that alcohol enhances cAMP responses to adenosine in cultured human lymphocytes and neuroblastoma X glioma (NG 108-15) cells (188,189). Effects were detectable at 50 mmol/L alcohol, a concentration that could be achieved at the synapse. However, this effect may not be specific for adenosine receptors as alcohol enhances the cAMP responses to a number of stimulatory agonists, likely by targeting G$_s$ directly (190). Experiments show that a selective adenosine receptor antagonist or agonist can block the ethanol-induced inhibition of potassium-stimulated glutamate release in near-term fetal guinea pig hippocampus (191). Consequently, alcohol could have direct or indirect effects on the function of the adenosine A$_1$ receptor. A more specific action of alcohol on adenosine receptor systems has also been proposed. In NG 108-15 and S49 lymphoma cells, alcohol (100 to 200 mmol/L) increased the accumulation extracellular adenosine (192–194). The authors proposed that alcohol enhancement of adenylyl cyclase in the cell lines was a consequence of the presence of increased extracellular adenosine, which secondarily activated A$_2$ receptors and increased cAMP and/or protein kinase A activity. This mechanism could account for the ability of adenosine to increase behavioral responses to alcohol. Interestingly, recent work by Yao and colleagues (195) supports a role for adenosine A$_2$ and dopamine D2 receptor stimulated PKA signaling in the regulation of voluntary alcohol consumption. These authors showed that R-(−)-N-propylnorapomorphine (D2 agonist) and alcohol produce synergistic PKA translocation and cAMP regulatory element-mediated gene expression, at concentrations that have no effect on their own. Furthermore, they showed that A₂ or D2 receptor antagonists, pertussis toxin, the cAMP inhibitor Rp-cAMP, or overexpression of dominant-negative peptides that sequester $G_s\beta\gamma$ dimmers prevent this synergy, and that overexpression of the $G_s\beta\gamma$ inhibitor peptides in the nucleus accumbens reduced sustained alcohol intake. Thus the available evidence appears to support a role for adenosine receptor systems in alcohol sensitivity at the cellular level, and the control of alcohol intake at the behavioral level.

Arginine Vasopressin Systems

Arginine vasopressin (AVP), primarily synthesized in the hypothalamic and extrahypothalamic areas, exerts a number of actions on neuroadaptive processes (learning and memory) in the CNS. Interestingly, AVP also appears to have a role in maintaining alcohol tolerance, even in the absence of further alcohol intake (196,197). AVP maintains tolerance to the sedative, hypothermic, and motor-impairing effects of alcohol in mice, and to the motor-impairing effects of alcohol in rats (196–198). Moreover, it inhibits the locomotor stimulant effects of alcohol in mice (199). The action of AVP on tolerance is mediated by AVP receptors in the brain, as its effect was observed after intracerebroventricular administration of doses that did not have detectable peripheral effects (200). Furthermore, pharmacologic studies indicate that V₁ receptors, coupled to polyphosphoinositide metabolism and increases in intracellular calcium, mediate this effect (201).

The mechanism by which AVP modulates the loss of tolerance may involve effects on neurotransmitter release. In mice, depletion of norepinephrine after tolerance had been developed (this depletion did not affect expression of tolerance [202]) blocked the ability AVP to maintain tolerance (203). More recent autoradiographic studies demonstrated that 6-hydroxydopamine treatment that blocked the effect of AVP on tolerance also reduced the number of V₁ receptors in the lateral septum (204). These data suggest that a portion of septal AVP receptors are localized on the terminals of catecholaminergic neurons. AVP may act at these presynaptic terminals to directly modulate the release of norepinephrine (and/or dopamine). Although a direct effect of AVP on the release of norepinephrine in hippocampal slices could not be demonstrated (205), similar experiments have not yet been done with tissue from the lateral septum.

In rats, serotonergic systems also appear to interact with AVP in the maintenance of alcohol tolerance. Specifi-

cally, an AVP analogue could no longer maintain tolerance in animals in which the dorsal serotonergic afferent pathways to the hippocampus had been chemically denervated (206). Intracerebroventricular injection of 5,7-dihydroxytryptamine into mice, which destroys serotonergic terminals from the raphe to the forebrain, impaired the ability of AVP to maintain tolerance, and continuous infusion of serotonin or a selective agonist for 5-HT₂ receptors was able to restore AVP's effects (207).

In addition to the postulated presynaptic action of AVP in maintaining alcohol tolerance, data suggest an intriguing postsynaptic action of the peptide that may affect the rate of loss of tolerance. When administered intracerebroventricularly, AVP was found to increase expression of the immediate early gene c-fos in the lateral septum and hippocampus via action at V₁ receptors (208,209). Furthermore, when antisense oligonucleotides of arginine vasopressin were intracerebroventricularly administered to ethanol-tolerant mice, elevated c-fos mRNA levels in the lateral septum were attenuated, as was the subsequent maintenance of tolerance (210). Hence, if the effect of AVP on c-fos expression is important for the maintenance of tolerance, the available data suggest that its site of action may be the lateral septum (208).

Most of the studies examining the ability of AVP to maintain tolerance examined the effect of administered peptide. However, there is also some evidence that endogenous AVP plays a role in the normal maintenance of ethanol tolerance. For example, intracerebroventricular administration of V₁ receptor antagonists increased the rate of loss of alcohol tolerance in mice, presumably by blocking the action of the endogenous peptide (201). In another study, Pittman and colleagues (211) reported that alcohol tolerance did not develop in AVP-deficient Brattleboro rats (212). However, tolerance was measured 48 hours after the animals were removed from an alcohol vapor chamber, so it is possible that they had developed tolerance but had lost it more rapidly than controls.

Adenylyl Cyclase-Coupled Systems

In addition to its effects at the receptor level, the available evidence suggests that alcohol may directly stimulate adenylyl cyclase-coupled systems. Alcohol stimulated basal- and dopamine-stimulated adenylyl cyclase activity in mouse striatum, cerebellum, and cerebral cortex in one study (213), and β-adrenergic receptor-coupled adenylyl cyclase activity in mouse cerebral cortex in another (214). These investigators proposed that, in addition to its actions at the receptors, alcohol was also acting at the levels of the coupled G proteins, and the adenylyl cyclase itself. Indeed, behavioral studies have suggested that alcohol may produce its sedative and motor incoordinating effects via actions on adenylyl cyclase-coupled systems (215–217).

Similar results have been seen in cultured neuronal and nonneuronal cells. Alcohol enhanced the adenosine receptor-induced increase in cAMP levels in neuroblastoma X glioma NG 108-15 cells (188) and similar results were observed in another neuroblastoma clonal cell line (218). In one study using mutant S49 cells lacking the α_s subunit of G_s, alcohol had little effect on guanine nucleotide- and fluoride-stimulated adenylyl cyclase activity (219), suggesting that G_s plays an important role in alcohol enhancement of agonist-stimulated adenylyl cyclase activity. Interestingly, mutant mice with targeted disruption of $G_{s\alpha}$ exhibit reduced alcohol preference drinking and are more sensitive to alcohol's sedative effects, whereas mutant mice overexpressing constitutively active $G_{s\alpha}$ are less sensitive to the sedative effects of alcohol (220).

Despite the above evidence supporting alcohol enhancement of adenylyl cyclase systems, not all studies using cultured cell lines agree. Chik and Ho (221) did not see enhancement of norepinephrine-induced stimulation of cAMP levels. One possible explanation for these opposite results might be that the alcohol sensitivity depends on the specific class of adenylyl cyclase present. Indeed, Yoshimura and Tabakoff (222) measured the effects of alcohol on various isoforms of adenylyl cyclase expressed in human embryonic kidney cells, and alcohol alone did not enhance adenylyl cyclase activity. However, in the presence of prostaglandin E_1, generation of cAMP was enhanced in adenylyl cyclase types II, IV, V, and VI, with the greatest enhancement in the type VII isoform. Recent behavioral studies support these findings, because mutant mice that overexpress the type VII isoform are less sensitive to alcohol's motor incoordinating effects (223). These results indicate that ethanol preferentially interacts with some, but not all, isoforms of adenylyl cyclase, and that this could be important for determining the mechanism of action of alcohol in the CNS. Interestingly, adenylyl cyclase type VII-dependent signaling is important for the modulation of the alcohol sensitivity of $GABA_A$ receptors (34).

Phospholipase C-Coupled Systems

Early studies did not support the notion that alcohol alters phosphoinositide (PI) turnover in murine brain (224,225). However, it was later shown that alcohol inhibits neurotensin- and bradykinin-stimulated PI turnover (226). More recently, it was shown that alcohol affects the function of G_q protein-coupled receptors such as $5-HT_{2c}$ and muscarinic type 1 (227). Alcohol produced a dose-dependent inhibition of currents evoked by 5-HT and acetylcholine in Xenopus oocytes expressing these receptors, and the 5-HT responses were blocked by a specific inhibitor of protein kinase C. Considered along with the behavioral and neurochemical evidence of altered alcohol sensitivity in PKCγ and PKCϵ null

mutant mice (31,228,229), the available evidence supports the contention that at least some classes of phospholipase C-coupled systems are sensitive to alcohol.

Voltage-Gated Ion Channels

A depolarization that initiates an action potential produces transient changes in neuronal membranes, altering the permeability of ions. These permeability changes occur because of the orchestrated opening and closing of voltage-gated ion channels, which propagate the electrical message along the axon. Several different voltage-gated ion channels have been discovered, including calcium, sodium (Fig. 8.1C), and potassium channels, and each of these is sensitive to alcohol.

Calcium Channels

Three main types of voltage-gated calcium channels (VGCC) are found in neurons: the T type (small conductance and transient fast current), N type (neuronal type, intermediate conductance, and transient fast current), and L type (large conductance and long-lasting slow current) (2). The first evidence implicating VGCC in alcohol sensitivity was a study showing that the intracerebroventricular administration of calcium increased sensitivity to the sedative effects of alcohol in SS, but not LS, mice, and that these behavioral responses were correlated with enhanced electrophysiologic responses to alcohol (230). More recent work shows that administration of nitrendipine and V-conotoxin, blockers of VGCC, enhanced the motor-incoordinating and sedative effects of alcohol (231,232). These effects are in line with biochemical studies of the effect of ethanol on calcium flux through VGCC in various brain membrane preparations (reviewed in reference 233). In general, alcohol (>50 mmol/L) inhibits calcium entry into synaptosomal preparations over very short depolarization times (233).

Electrophysiologic evidence for an effect of alcohol on VGCC has been sparse. It was suggested that most of the data obtained in electrophysiologic studies could be explained by an alcohol-induced increase in intracellular calcium, inhibiting inward calcium flux (234). High concentrations of alcohol (350 to 700 mmol/L) increased resting intracellular calcium in synaptosomal preparations (235,236), and it was postulated that this effect could account for alcohol's ability to stimulate neurotransmitter release and inhibit calcium influx (235). Alcohol was also found to inhibit VGCC in Aplysia-cultured abdominal ganglion neurons, although high concentrations (>100 mmol/L) were necessary to produce this effect (237). These data are consistent with other work in cultured neuroblastoma and neuroblastoma X glioma cells indicating that alcohol (>30 mmol/L) inhibited calcium flux through VGCC (238). Interestingly, it has been reported that G_i might be involved in the alcohol inhibition of

L-type calcium channels in undifferentiated pheochromo-cytoma cells (239).

Whereas some of the above data suggest that inhibition of calcium flux may play a role in the sedative effects of alcohol, there is no clear behavioral correlate for this effect. However, L-type calcium channels have been implicated in the neuroadaptive processes following *in vivo* alcohol exposure. A detailed discussion of these studies is beyond the scope of this chapter, but can be found in the prior edition of this text.

Sodium Channels

Much less is known about the effects of alcohol on the function of other voltage-gated ion channels. In rodent brain synaptosomes, high concentrations of alcohol (>350 mmol/L) inhibited batrachotoxin- and veratridine-stimulated sodium uptake (reviewed in reference 240). Kukita and Mitaku (241) showed that high concentrations of various aliphatic alcohols produced an irreversible suppression of sodium currents in squid giant axons. However, this effect appeared to be the result of denaturation of the sodium channels. Finally, Krylov and colleagues (242) recently showed that application of alcohol (10 to 100 mmol/L) results in the attenuation of reversal potentials in rat spinal ganglia tetrodotoxin-sensitive and -resistant sodium channels.

Potassium Channels

Potassium channels also appear to be sensitive to alcohol. Low concentrations of alcohol inhibited a voltage-dependent potassium channel in CA1 hippocampal pyramidal neurons (243). Anantharam et al. (244) and Yamakura et al. (245) examined the effects of alcohol on many different classes of voltage-gated potassium channels expressed in *Xenopus* oocytes. Although there were some differences in the sensitivity of the channels to high concentrations of alcohol (>200 mmol/L), none of the potassium channels examined were particularly sensitive to low concentrations of alcohol. An exception appears to be the large-conductance, calcium-activated potassium channels in neurohypophysial terminals (246). These channels are involved in the control of hypophyseal hormone release, and alcohol increases their activity by altering channel gating (246,247). Thus, alcohol's inhibitory effects on the release of hormones such as arginine vasopressin and oxytocin could, in part, be a result of neuronal hyperpolarization produced by its actions at these potassium channels.

Recent work is producing interesting insights into the interaction between potassium channels and alcohols (248). Concentrations of alcohol between 17 and 170 mmol/L selectively inhibited a cloned noninactivating potassium channel from *Drosophila*. Competition experiments among alcohols and site-directed mutagenesis experiments indicate that the alcohols act on a discrete site, possibly a putative hydrophobic pocket, in the potassium channel.

Evidence recently surfaced suggesting that the G protein-activated inwardly rectifying potassium (GIRK) channels are sensitive the alcohol. Two different groups demonstrated that when expressed in *Xenopus* oocytes, alcohol activated GIRK1, GIRK2, and GIRK4 channels (but not inwardly rectifying potassium channels) at pharmacologically relevant concentrations (249,250). Moreover, these actions occurred in the absence of interactions with G proteins. Kobayashi et al. (249) also showed that weaver mutant mice possessing a missense mutation in the GIRK2 channel exhibited reduced sensitivity to alcohol's analgesic effects. Consistent with these findings, GIRK2 null mutant mice were recently generated, and also exhibit reduced sensitivity to alcohol's analgesic effects (251), as well as enhanced alcohol preference drinking in a two-bottle choice procedure, increased sensitivity to alcohol's locomotor stimulant properties, reduced sensitivity to alcohol's anxiolytic effects, attenuated alcohol withdrawal severity, and reduced alcohol conditioned place preference and taste aversion (252,253).

Finally, it should be pointed out that one other study has also provided evidence that voltage-gated potassium channels mediate alcohol sensitivity. Whereas either mutation alone had no observable effect, double-mutant mice lacking the voltage-gated potassium channels Kv3.1 and Kv3.3 were more sensitive to alcohol's motor incoordinating effects (254). Thus, taken together, voltage-gated potassium channels appear to be important neuronal targets for alcohol.

NEUROTROPHIC FACTORS

Neurotrophic factors are growth factors important for the development and/or maintenance of the nervous system (255). The list of neurotrophic factors includes fibroblast growth factor (FGF), epidermal growth factor (EGF), insulin and insulin-related growth factor (IGF), platelet-derived growth factor (PDGF), vascular endothelial growth factor (VEGF), glial-derived neurotrophic factor (GDNF), and the neurotrophins. The neurotrophins include nerve-derived growth factor (NGF), brain-derived neurotrophic factor (BDNF), and neurotrophins 3 and 4/5. Neurotrophic factors bind to one of six classes of tyrosine kinase-coupled receptors designated as the EGF (class I), IGF (class II), PDGF (class III), FGF (class IV), eph (class V; orphan receptor), and Trk (class VI) family of receptors (255). In most cases, binding of the growth factors to their receptors produces conformational changes that lead to the activation of the receptor's intrinsic tyrosine kinase activity and autophosphorylation of tyrosine residues (256). These autophosphorylated tyrosine residues act as docking sites for the binding and activation of proteins containing *src* homology-2 (SH_2) domains

(255,256). The list of SH_2-domain-containing proteins that are activated by neurotrophic factor receptors include the *src* family of tyrosine kinases, phosphatidylinositol 3-kinase, ras-guanosine triphosphatase (GTPase)-activating protein (GAP), protein tyrosine phosphatase 1D, phospholipase $C\gamma$ ($PLC\gamma$), and several adaptor proteins (Shc, Grb2, Nck) involved in the ras signal transduction cascade (255,256). Numerous studies suggest that neurotrophic factors may influence sensitivity to alcohol's neurotoxic effects, as well as maintain functional tolerance to alcohol.

A growing body of experimental evidence indicates that ethanol interacts with the NGF-coupled signaling systems. Ethanol administration *in ovo* to chick embryos decreases choline acetyltransferase activity of both brain and spinal cord, an effect reversed by concomitant administration of NGF (or EGF) (257). Moreover, ethanol increased cholinergic and decreased GABAergic neuronal expression in cultures from chick embryo cerebral hemispheres (258). The ethanol-induced decrease in GABAergic neuronal expression was blocked by NGF, whereas the NGF-induced increase in cholinergic neuronal expression was affected by ethanol (258). NGF was also shown to ameliorate ethanol-induced toxicity in cultured dorsal root ganglion neurons (259), dissociated septal neuronal cultures from fetal rats (260), and cultured cerebellar granule cells (261). In addition, recent evidence suggests that NGF's protective effects may (as well as those of FGF-2 and IGF-1), in part, occur via activation of the nitric oxide-mediated pathway, resulting in downstream activation of cyclic guanosine monophosphate (cGMP)-dependent protein kinases (262). Consequently, NGF appears to exert protective actions against the neurotoxic actions of ethanol in different neuronal populations. Similar neuroprotective effects have been reported for GDNF (263,264) and BDNF (263).

Other investigators found that NGF (and FGF) can enhance the neurotoxic effects of ethanol. Messing et al. (265) found that ethanol potentiated NGF- and FGF-induced neurite outgrowth in cultured neurons derived from pheochromocytomas (PC12 cells). These authors postulate that ethanol alters the normal functioning or development of the nervous system by increasing the growth of neural processes and disturbing synaptic organization. Recent work by the same group further elucidated the mechanism of action of ethanol on neurite outgrowth in growth factor-treated PC12 cells. Ethanol increased NGF- and FGF-induced activation of mitogen-activated protein (MAP) kinases, which relays trophic signals from membrane growth factor receptors to the nucleus (266). This increase in growth factor-activated MAP kinase activity was blocked by downregulation of the isoforms β, δ, and ϵ of PKC. Consequently, ethanol appears to enhance growth factor-dependent signal transduction downstream of growth factor receptors, and its effects seem to involve other signaling molecules such as PKC.

The effects of alcohol on insulin and IGF-coupled signaling systems in the brain have also been studied. Resnicoff et al. (267,268) showed that alcohol inhibited IGF-1-induced proliferation of cultured fibroblasts and blocked IGF-1 receptor tyrosine autophosphorylation, tyrosine phosphorylation of insulin receptor substrate 1, and the association of phosphatidylinositol 3-kinase. A similar inhibitory effect of alcohol on insulin-induced tyrosine phosphorylation of insulin receptor substrate 1 was found by Xu et al. (269), along with an alcohol-induced inhibition of insulin-stimulated neuronal thread protein gene expression in a primitive neuroectodermal tumor cell line. Conversely, others have shown that alcohol enhances the stimulatory effects of insulin and IGF-1 on deoxyribonucleic acid (DNA) synthesis in fibroblasts (270). More work is required to determine the reasons for the discrepancies between the results of these studies.

Several studies have used mutant mice to investigate the interaction between neurotrophic factors and alcohol sensitivity. In one study, 4-day-old mice overexpressing NGF were found to exhibit reduced sensitivity to Purkinje cell loss following a 2-day exposure to alcohol vapor inhalation (261). Moreover, 7-day-old mice made deficient for the BDNF gene exhibited enhanced sensitivity to alcohol's neurotoxic effects on Purkinje cells following a 2-day exposure to alcohol vapor inhalation (271). Future studies with similar mutant models will no doubt shed considerable light on the interactions between neurotrophic factors and alcohol's neurotoxic effects.

Neurotrophic factors may also influence the maintenance of functional tolerance to alcohol. Szabó and Hoffman (272) fed mice an alcohol-containing liquid diet, and measured the effects of BDNF, neurotrophin-3, and neurotrophin-4/5 on the maintenance of tolerance to the sedative effects of alcohol. Following cessation of the liquid diet, vehicle-injected controls gradually lost tolerance to alcohol. However, each of the above neurotrophic factors, when injected intracerebroventricularly, maintained tolerance to alcohol's sedative effects. These results demonstrate that certain neurotrophic factors may also modulate neuroadaptation to some of alcohol's effects.

In summary, several lines of experimental evidence suggest that some neurotrophic factor-dependent signaling systems are sensitive to alcohol. These factors might protect neuronal cells against alcohol's neurotoxic effects, or help to maintain tolerance to alcohol's effects. Because these factors are important during the development of the CNS, the interaction between ethanol and neurotrophic factors might be of special importance in the pathogenesis of the fetal alcohol syndrome. In addition, alcohol's effects on these neurotrophic signaling systems might also be important in the adult brain because they produce short- and long-term modulatory effects on neuronal signaling and synaptic plasticity (273–275). However, it should be noted that not all neurotrophic factors appear to be sensitive to alcohol. Indeed, some of the above studies also measured the effects of alcohol on the PDGF receptor system (267–269,276) and found no effect. Thus future research needs to determine the precise role of specific neurotrophic factors in the actions of alcohol in the developing and mature nervous system.

NOVEL TARGETS OF ALCOHOL ACTION

Endogenous Opioids

The notion that endogenous opiate systems have a role in the reinforcing or other actions of alcohol is inherently attractive because of the numerous studies demonstrating the reinforcing and/or addictive properties of opiates. An interaction between alcohol and opioid receptor systems could indicate common mechanisms mediate the reinforcing mechanisms of both drugs. A number of approaches have provided evidence that alcohol's effects on brain opiate systems might play a role in reinforcement.

Three major subtypes of opiate receptors (μ, κ, and δ) have been identified to date (reviewed in reference 277), and the effects of alcohol on the binding of ligands at each have been extensively investigated and reviewed elsewhere (190). Alcohol has selective effects on the binding of opiate receptor ligands. In mouse striatal tissue, alcohol had a biphasic effect on dihydromorphine binding to μ opiate receptors: lower concentrations of alcohol (50 mmol/L) increased binding, whereas higher concentrations (200 mmol/L) inhibited binding (278). Alcohol inhibited the binding of (2-D-Ala, 5-D-Leu)-enkephalin to striatal δ opiate receptors (278). The striatal δ receptors were more sensitive to alcohol's inhibitory effects than were the μ receptors. Similar effects were seen in whole rat brain (279). However, in mouse frontal cortex, alcohol had an approximately equal inhibitory effect on ligand binding to μ and δ opiate receptors, whereas binding to κ receptors was unaffected by alcohol (280).

Investigations into the effects of alcohol on opiate peptide dynamics are difficult to perform. Because of the relatively complex mechanisms for synthesis and release of endogenous opiates, the results obtained so far are equivocal. Studies by Herz and colleagues (289) indicated that acute alcohol treatment of rats result in increased striatal levels of methionine enkephalin. However, Ryder et al. (282) found that administration of a higher dose of alcohol in rats did not alter levels of leucine enkephalin. Alcohol was found to reduce β-endorphin precursor proopiomelanocortin (POMC) mRNA and reduced β-endorphin release in cultured rat pituitary and transformed pituitary cells (283). Interestingly, alcoholics are reported to exhibit reduced CSF levels of β-endorphin (284), and possibly lower CSF levels of enkephalin (285) when sober.

An interesting series of pharmacogenetic studies demonstrated that there are differences between the brain and pituitary β-endorphin systems of the high-alcohol drinking Alko-alcohol (AA) and low-alcohol-drinking Alko-nonalcohol (ANA) rats, implicating opioid systems in alcohol reinforcement mechanisms. POMC mRNA or β-endorphin–like peptide levels were significantly higher in some brain regions of the AA rats than in ANA rats (286). Moreover, voluntary alcohol consumption in the AA rats was reduced by intracerebroventricular injections of a selective μ-receptor antagonist (287), and spontaneous in vivo hypothalamic release of β-endorphin was higher in AA than in ANA rats (288). However, alcohol-induced increases in β-endorphin were similar in both rat lines.

More recent pharmacologic studies have suggested a role for opioid receptor systems in the modulation of alcohol reinforcement mechanisms. Both selective (for the μ- and δ-opioid receptors) and nonselective opioid receptor antagonists reduced measures of alcohol reinforcement (289,290). Moreover, alcohol consumption, alcohol-reinforced operant responding, and alcohol-stimulated locomotion were each reduced in μ-receptor null mutant mice (291,292). In contrast to predictions made by the antagonist studies, alcohol self-administration was increased in δ-opioid receptor-deficient mice (293). However, these mice were also more anxious, and self-administration of alcohol may have reversed this phenotype. Taken together, these data suggest that opioid systems play an important role in alcohol reinforcement mechanisms. Indeed, alcohol increases extracellular endorphins in the nucleus accumbens (294), and microinjections of opioid receptor antagonists (295) and μ-receptor antisense oligonucleotides (296) into the nucleus accumbens reduce voluntary alcohol drinking. Furthermore, both systemic (297) and site-specific (298) injection of opioid receptor antagonists attenuated nucleus accumbens dopamine, implicating this effect in the reduction of alcohol intake following administration of these drugs (299). It should be noted that one study suggested mechanisms other than those directly involving nucleus accumbens dopamine contribute to the suppressive effects of opioid receptor antagonists (300). Thus, the mechanisms by which alcohol increases nucleus accumbens endorphin levels, and by which opioid antagonists reduce voluntary alcohol intake, remain to be elucidated.

The importance of the opioid system in alcohol reinforcement and dependence is underscored by the approval of naltrexone (Depade, ReVia) (opioid receptor antagonist) for the treatment of alcoholism. A double-blind, placebo-controlled clinical trail with 70 male alcohol-dependent patients demonstrated that naltrexone significantly reduced craving, as well as the number of days during which alcohol was consumed. Moreover, naltrexone reduced the number of relapse events in the alcohol treated group (301). Several other groups have come to similar conclusions (302,303). A more recent study reported that naltrexone treatment reduced the "high" produced by alcohol, as well as the amount of alcohol consumed during the first drinking episode (304). The authors concluded "the lower alcohol consumption by the naltrexone-treated subjects may have resulted from naltrexone's blockage of the pleasure produced by alcohol." Thus, blockade of the opioid system appears to reduce the reinforcing or euphoric effects of alcohol. However, it should be noted that naltrexone neither blocked nor delayed relapse in a recent report by Krystal and colleagues (305), although this result is likely a consequence of differences in the age and severity of the alcoholic patients. Nevertheless, naltrexone is the first clinically approved pharmacologic agent capable of blocking the reinforcing properties of alcohol.

Endocannabinoids

To date, two different subtypes of cannabinoid receptors have been identified. Of these, the CB_1 receptor is found predominantly in the CNS, whereas the CB_2 receptor is found in immune cells. Endogenous cannabinoids that act at the CB_1 receptor subtype appear to play a role in the mechanisms of alcohol reinforcement and tolerance/dependence (see reference 306 for a review).

Administration of a CB_1 cannabinoid receptor antagonist decreased voluntary alcohol intake in mice (307) and alcohol-preferring sP (Sardinian Preferring) rats (308), and an agonist at the same receptor subtype increased voluntary alcohol intake in sP rats (309). Moreover, CB_1 receptors were shown to exert control over appetitive and consummatory aspects of alcohol intake (310). In a recent report, mutant mice lacking the CB_1 receptor exhibited both reduced voluntary alcohol consumption, and reduced alcohol-induced dopamine release in the nucleus accumbens (311). However, Racz and colleagues (312) observed increased voluntary alcohol consumption following null mutation of the CB_1 receptor gene. The reasons for these contrasting results are not immediately clear, but may be related to the very different two-bottle choice procedures used. Nevertheless, these studies suggest that CB_1 receptors may also modulate alcohol intake, and that this effect may occur via modulation of the mesolimbic dopamine projection.

Evidence also suggests a role for CB_1 receptors in alcohol tolerance and dependence. Chronic alcohol exposure increased the levels of anandamide, an endogenous cannabimimetic compound, in neuroblastoma cells (313), and chronic alcohol exposure in mice resulted in downregulation of CB_1 receptor expression and agonist-stimulated function (313). Moreover, alcohol withdrawal symptoms were absent in CB_1-receptor null mutant mice, as was stress-induced enhancement of alcohol preference drinking (311). Thus, while the available evidence points to its participation in the modulation of alcohol reinforcement, tolerance, and dependence, future work will be necessary to elucidate the specific mechanisms by which the cannabinoid receptor system influences these neuroadaptive processes.

Neuropeptide Y

Known to play a role in food consumption (314), neuropeptide Y (NPY) was recently implicated in the regulation of ethanol intake. Thiele and colleagues (315) showed that null mutation of the NPY gene resulted in increased, whereas overexpression resulted in decreased, voluntary alcohol consumption. Interestingly, null mutant and overexpressing mice also displayed reduced, and enhanced, sensitivity to alcohol's sedative effects, respectively (315), and these responses (alcohol intake and sedation) were associated with the NPY Y1 receptor subtype (316). However, it should be mentioned that other studies have associated the Y2 receptor with alcohol self-administration (317), and the Y5 receptor with alcohol-induced sedation (318). Intraventricular administration of NPY decreases alcohol drinking in alcohol-preferring P rats (319), and both P and the high alcohol drinking (HAD) rats exhibited reduced levels of NPY in the central nucleus of the amygdala (320). Thus, NPY appears to inhibit voluntary alcohol intake, and possibly other alcohol-related behaviors. However, not all studies agree. At least in alcohol nonpreferring NP and outbred rats, NPY did not alter alcohol intake (319,321,322), and microinjections of NPY into the paraventricular nucleus of the hypothalamus increased (not decreased) alcohol intake (323). The reasons for these inconsistent data are not immediately clear, but may depend on the site specificity of NPY, or on the ability of NPY to modulate stress responses in different genetic animal models. Regardless, these data demonstrate the importance of NPY in the mechanisms mediating excessive alcohol consumption.

Two studies also suggest a role for NPY in alcohol withdrawal mechanisms. A recent report demonstrated that NPY expression levels are attenuated in several rat cortical, amygdaloid, and hypothalamic structures 24 hours following alcohol withdrawal (324). These changes were observed in the absence of any significant changes in NPY expression levels immediately after chronic alcohol exposure. In another study, Woldbye and colleagues (325) found that the behavioral signs of alcohol withdrawal in rats were reduced by intracerebroventricular administration of NPY. Thus the available evidence suggests that NPY may also be an important mediator of alcohol withdrawal severity.

Corticotrophin-Releasing Factor

Stress is believed to be a major factor influencing drug-seeking behavior, including that of alcohol. Indeed, research shows that social, emotional, and physical stress facilitates the acquisition, as well as increases self-administration, of alcohol in rodents and nonhuman primates (326–328). Moreover, stressful stimuli elicit reinstatement (see below: Animal models of Alcoholism, Reinstatement) in animals in which alcohol self-administration was extinguished (329). Taken together, these studies support a role for stress in the development and maintenance of alcohol addiction.

Early on it was believed that stress-induced drug administration was solely mediated by the hypothalamic–pituitary–adrenal (HPA) axis. In response to acute stressors, corticotrophin-releasing factor (CRF) is synthesized and released by the paraventricular nucleus, increasing the production and release of the stress hormone corticosterone from the adrenal glands. Acute alcohol administration is known to stimulate CRF secretion from the paraventricular nucleus, elevating serum corticosterone levels (330). Interestingly, a number of behavioral studies demonstrate that corticosterone administration enhances voluntary alcohol consumption, suggesting a role for the HPA axis in alcohol reinforcement mechanisms (331–334). However, evidence has begun to accumulate suggesting that a separate and distinct CRF system exists in the central nucleus of the amygdala (CeA), and that this system may exert an independent role on the interaction between addictive behaviors and stress (335). A high density of CRF immunoreactive cells and receptors can be found in the CeA, and the CRF neurons in this brain structure have been implicated in modulating emotional and behavioral responses to stressful stimuli (336,337). Examples of this modulation can be found in studies showing that immobilization stress elevates extracellular CRF levels in the CeA (338,339), and that microinjection of a CRF receptor antagonist attenuates the behavioral signs of social and environmental stressor-induced anxiety (340,341). Given the alcohol sensitivity of CRF receptors in the paraventricular nucleus and the apparent importance of both CRF receptor systems in mediating behavioral and emotional responses to stress, researchers have begun to investigate the alcohol sensitivity of CRF neurons in the CeA.

Anxiety and emotional stress are common symptoms of the alcohol withdrawal syndrome, and one possibility is that CRF neurons in the CeA modulate the emotional stress and anxiety experienced during alcohol withdrawal. Consistent with this possibility, a microdialysis study showed that extracellular CRF levels in the CeA were elevated during alcohol withdrawal (342). Furthermore, another study showed that functional antagonism of CRF neurotransmission in the CeA reduces aversive and anxiety-like behavior during alcohol withdrawal (343). Interestingly, activation of CRF neurotransmission in the CeA is not only implicated in the modulation of the emotional stress and anxiety experienced during alcohol withdrawal, but may also play a role in the neuroadaptive changes responsible for the development of compulsive drug-seeking behavior. Indeed, the reward deficits and "dysphoria" indicated by measurement of brain-stimulation reward thresholds (344) are a common consequence of withdrawal from abused drugs (345).

A number of mutant mouse models of the CRF receptor system have been developed, and several of these have been tested for alcohol sensitivity. Lee et al. (346) developed mutant mice lacking functional CRF type 1 receptors (CRFR1), and showed that although alcohol still elicited CRF release from the paraventricular nucleus, corticosterone secretion from the adrenal glands was blunted. CRFR1 null mutant mice were also developed by Sillaber and colleagues (347), and these mice were tested for stress-induced voluntary alcohol intake. Both social defeat stress and forced swim stress significantly increased voluntary alcohol intake among the CRFR1-deficient mice, without altering the alcohol consumption of wild-type controls. Finally, a recent report examined alcohol preference drinking, locomotor stimulation, and conditioned place preference in mutant mice lacking CRF (348). These mice ingested nearly twice as much alcohol, exhibited a blunted locomotor stimulant response, and failed to display a conditioned place preference to a 2 g/kg alcohol dose; mutant mice did develop a conditioned place preference to a 3 g/kg alcohol dose. Thus, in addition to its role in mediating alcohol's affects on emotional stress and anxiety, studies using null mutants suggest that the CRF receptor system is also an important player in the mediation of alcohol sensitivity, in particular its reinforcing properties.

α-Synuclein

One of the first links between alcoholism and α-synuclein came in a report by Mayfield et al. (349). Using microarray analysis techniques (see below, in section entitled New Techniques in the Study of Alcoholism, Microarray Analysis of Gene Expression) to assess differences in gene expression, these authors showed that expression of α-synuclein was differentially regulated in the frontal and motor cortices of postmortem alcoholics. α-Synuclein is expressed at presynaptic nerve terminals throughout the central nervous system (350–352), and is thought to inhibit dopamine synthesis by interacting with tyrosine hydroxylase (353). However, the precise role of α-synuclein in the regulation of dopamine systems remains unclear. Nevertheless, a more recent study has corroborated the findings of Mayfield and colleagues (349) using inbred rat models of high (iP) and low (iNP) alcohol preference drinking. This study showed that the lines differed in α-synuclein protein levels in both the hippocampus and caudate-putamen (354). Moreover, the authors went on to show that the α-synuclein gene mapped to a region of rat chromosome 4 that overlapped with a quantitative trait locus (see below, in section entitled New Techniques in the Study of Alcoholism, Gene Mapping by Quantitative Trait Loci Analysis) for alcohol preference drinking in the iP and iNP rat lines. Thus, this protein would appear to be a new and exciting player in the regulation of alcohol intake. Additional studies are necessary to establish the exact nature of this role.

ALTERNATIVE IDEAS IN ALCOHOL NEUROBIOLOGY

Acetaldehyde

Acetaldehyde is produced by alcohol dehydrogenase and other enzymatic processes, representing the first step of alcohol metabolism. An unanswered question is whether any of the actions produced by alcohol are actually caused by acetaldehyde. Acetaldehyde has aversive (or toxic) peripheral effects. Indeed, in some Oriental populations, lower genetic alcohol dehydrogenase activity results in higher-than-normal blood ethanol concentrations of acetaldehyde, resulting in nausea, headache, and palpitations (355). Individuals exhibiting this phenotype consume less alcohol than those exhibiting normal aldehyde dehydrogenase activity (356). However, in addition to these peripheral effects, evidence has accumulated suggesting that this biologically active compound may have a role in producing some of alcohol's CNS effects (357). For example, acetaldehyde may modulate or augment some of alcohol's actions, including its reinforcing effects, or may react with other endogenous substances, such as dopamine, to form other biologically active compounds which produce these effects. Support for this possibility was bolstered by studies demonstrating that alcohol can be oxidized to acetaldehyde in brain, perhaps by the enzyme catalase (358,359).

Acetaldehyde has been implicated in the modulation of several of alcohol's actions, including its hypnotic, locomotor stimulant, and reinforcing effects. Zimatkin et al. (360,361) showed that the degree of acetaldehyde accumulation in brain correlates with the hypnotic effects of alcohol in rats. Moreover, another study showed that whereas stimulated catalase activity reduces sensitivity to alcohol's hypnotic effects in mice, treatment with the catalase inhibitor 3-amino-1,2,3-triazole increased sensitivity to these effects, presumably by limiting the accumulation of acetaldehyde (362). Correa and colleagues (363) saw similar results with regard to alcohol-induced locomotion; whereas increased catalase activity enhanced sensitivity to alcohol's locomotor stimulant effects, treatment with the catalase inhibitor attenuated these effects in a dose-dependent manner.

Behavioral studies also suggest that acetaldehyde might have some reinforcing value. Three early studies reported intraventricular self-administration of acetaldehyde by rats (364–366), and one of these went on to demonstrate a relationship between acetaldehyde self-administration and voluntary alcohol consumption (366). Another study demonstrated positive place conditioning immediately following intraventricular infusions of acetaldehyde (367).

Several years later it was shown that brain catalase activity positively correlated with voluntary alcohol consumption (368,369), and that the catalase inhibitor 3-amino-1,2,4-triazole reduced voluntary alcohol consumption (358).

Although not in agreement, recent studies have also examined the reinforcing properties of acetaldehyde. Quertemont and De Witte (370) showed that rats readily develop an acetaldehyde-conditioned place preference using olfactory cues as the conditioning stimulus. In another study, rats readily self-administered acetaldehyde into the posterior ventral tegmental area (371), a region that was previously shown to support self-administration of alcohol (372). However, a recent report by Quertemont and Grant (373) demonstrates that rats do not develop discriminative stimulus effects similar to those of alcohol, an unexpected result if acetaldehyde is indeed responsible for alcohol's reinforcing actions, or other effects. Moreover, whereas administration of acetaldehyde alters dopamine and other monoamine levels in the nucleus accumbens, these changes are opposite those observed following alcohol administration (374). Thus, future work will be necessary to fully characterize the reinforcing or other actions of acetaldehyde.

Salsolinol is formed by the condensation of dopamine with acetaldehyde. The available evidence suggests that salsolinol may also be an important mediator of some of alcohol's actions. Two different studies show that salsolinol levels rise in the striatum and limbic structures following forced alcohol intake (375,376). Moreover, studies also indicate that intracerebroventricular administration of salsolinol increases alcohol consumption in rats (377,378). More recently, evidence suggests that compared to naive alcohol nonpreferring (NP) rats, naive alcohol-preferring (P) rats exhibited lower levels of salsolinol in the nucleus accumbens. Furthermore, chronic alcohol intake increased the accumbal levels of salsolinol to levels similar to the NP rats, suggesting that P rats may prefer alcohol in order to "normalize" their salsolinol levels (379). In support of this contention, P rats self-administered more salsolinol to the shell of the nucleus accumbens than vehicle, achieving tissue levels approximately equal to those seen following chronic ethanol consumption (379). Thus, salsolinol may, indeed, play a role in mediating alcohol reinforcement. However, the mechanisms involved will have to wait further investigation.

Finally, it should be noted that one study examined the effects of acetaldehyde using the *Xenopus* oocyte expression system (380). Ten different ligand gated ion channels (glycine, α_1 homomeric; GABA$_A$, $\alpha_1\beta_2\gamma_{2S}$; GABA$_C$, ρ_1 homomeric; 5-HT$_{3A}$; NMDA, NR1A/NR2A; AMPA, GluR1/GluR2; kainate, GluR6/KA2; and nicotinic acetylcholine, $\alpha_4\beta_2$, $\alpha_4\beta_4$, $\alpha_2\beta_4$), as well as the inwardly rectifying potassium channel GIRK2 and the dopamine transporter, were studied to determine whether the central actions of alcohol could be attributed to acetaldehyde. Of these, only glycine receptor-mediated current was altered by acetaldehyde application; high concentrations of acetaldehyde enhanced glycine receptor currents. None of the other ligand-gated ion channels were affected by acetaldehyde, nor was GIRK2 current or dopamine uptake by the dopamine transporter.

Acetate

Several lines of evidence suggest that acetate, the primary by-product of alcohol catabolism, may also mediate some effects of alcohol in the CNS (381). Though the data are not in full agreement, one possible mechanism for these effects may involve adenosine. Adenosine is produced during the conversion of acetate to acetyl coenzyme A (CoA). Indeed, evidence suggests that adenosine is produced by astrocytes following the application of acetate (382,383). Consequently, some of alcohol's effects may be attributable to the production of adenosine. Partial support for this idea come from behavioral studies showing that alcohol and acetate produced similar effects on motor coordination and anesthetic potency tests, and that the effects of acetate and alcohol were blocked and partially blocked, respectively, by the adenosine receptor antagonist 8-phenyltheophylline (384). However, acetate inhibited locomotor activity in mice, whereas alcohol enhanced it. Moreover, whereas the locomotor effects of acetate were blocked by 8-phenyltheophylline, those of alcohol were enhanced. In another study, Cullen and Carlen (385) demonstrated that acetate, alcohol, and adenosine each produced similar hyperpolarizing effects in rat hippocampal dentate granule cells, and that these effects were blocked by 8-phenyltheophylline. It should be noted, however, that other effects of adenosine cannot be induced by acetate in hippocampal CA1 pyramidal neurons (386).

NEW TECHNIQUES IN THE STUDY OF ALCOHOLISM

Gene Mapping by Quantitative Trait Loci Analysis

Risk for developing alcohol abuse and dependence is influenced by environmental and genetic factors, as well as by their interaction. Alcoholism is considered a complex trait. This means that many different genes influence one's individual risk of developing this disorder. Over the past decade, techniques have been developed to map the many chromosomal regions that contain these genes. Referred to as quantitative trait loci (QTL) analysis, these techniques aim to identify novel genes influencing genetic risk for alcoholism.

The basic premise of QTL analysis is simple (387). The researcher starts by measuring a specific phenotype within a population. Next, the population is genotyped at 100 or more marker loci distributed throughout the genome. The researcher then compares the genotype (at each marker

locus) of each individual animal with its phenotypic score. The idea is to identify animals of one genotype that score differently on the phenotypic trait than animals of another genotype. If such animals are found, a QTL is detected and mapped to the chromosomal region containing the associated marker loci.

To date a number of significant QTLs for different alcohol-related traits have been identified in mice and rats. Most of these have recently been reviewed by Crabbe et al. (388) and Crabbe (389), and include QTLs for acute alcohol-withdrawal severity, alcohol reinforcement (alcohol preference drinking, conditioned taste aversion, conditioned place preference, locomotor stimulation, and locomotor sensitization), sedation (loss of righting reflex), hypothermia, and motor incoordination. Moreover, a number of candidate genes are known to reside within the regions spanned by these QTLs. For example, a QTL for acute alcohol withdrawal contains the $GABA_A$ α_1, γ_2, and α_6 subunit genes (390), and a QTL for alcohol preference drinking contains the dopamine D2 and 5-HT$_{1B}$ receptor genes (391–393). However, the specific genes responsible for the QTLs are difficult to identify. This is because the initial mapping of QTLs usually occurs with a resolution of 10 to 30 cM (388), a region containing hundreds of genes. Thus, the researcher must narrow the region spanned by the QTL.

Congenic strains are currently being used to narrow the QTL-spanning region, thereby eliminating irrelevant candidate genes. A congenic strain is produced by repeatedly backcrossing animals with the desired QTL sequence onto another recipient genetic background (i.e., placing the alleles for one strain onto the genetic background of a second strain). Continued backcrossing narrows the QTL-spanning region considerably, because only those congenics possessing the desired phenotype are backcrossed. This process reduces the amount of donor genome contained within the chromosomal region of interest, significantly reducing the number of possible candidate genes. This approach has recently been used to narrow the spanning region for an alcohol withdrawal QTL to less than 1 cM (394). Moreover, because fewer than 20 genes exist in this region, the authors have identified a strong candidate gene that codes for *Mpdz,* a member of family of intracellular proteins thought to couple ligands with their receptors, thereby facilitating intracellular signaling. This protein is known to interact with several 5-HT receptor subtypes, including the 5-HT$_{2A}$, 5-HT$_{2B}$, and 5-HT$_{2C}$ receptors. Thus, although progress toward identifying alcohol sensitive genes via QTL analysis has been slow, an exciting future would appear to lie ahead.

Microarray Analysis of Gene Expression

The use of microarray analysis in the study of alcoholism was reviewed by Lewohl et al. (395) and Rahman and Miles (396). Using several different experimental paradigms, sustained alcohol exposure was shown to alter the expression of many genes, including some coding for neurotransmitter receptors, hormones and their receptors, signaling molecules, molecular chaperones, transcription factors, and cytokines (397). It is not currently known whether alcohol has a direct affect on these genes, or an indirect effect that involves many systems. For example, changes in transcription factor activation or in second messenger systems may initiate gene-expression cascades (i.e., the concentration of cAMP is altered by both acute and chronic alcohol exposure [188], which may change the expression of cAMP-dependent genes). Alternatively, activation or suppression of alcohol responsive transcription factors may also result in changes in gene expression (397).

The kinds of complex changes detailed above are difficult to detect by measuring the expression of only a few genes (such as with Northern blot), but are well suited for microarray analysis. Microarrays (gene chips) are silicon or glass slides on which partial or complete complementary deoxyribonucleic acid (cDNA) sequences are immobilized. They allow rapid and detailed analysis of thousands of transcripts simultaneously, and provide a means by which direct comparison of the relative expression of genes between samples can be made. Because of the large number of genes that can be analyzed in each experiment, it is possible to generate gene expression profiles of changes in cellular pathways, and not just expression changes in individual genes.

To date, only a few papers investigating alcohol dependence have been published using this very new and exciting technique. Thibault et al. (398) used microarray analysis to study the expression of about 6000 genes in SH-SY5Y neuroblastoma cells that had been chronically exposed to alcohol and found that dopamine β-hydroxylase gene, as well as other genes involved in norepinephrine metabolism, were differentially regulated. Furthermore, these authors found that dibutyryl-cAMP and alcohol similarly regulate the same set of genes, suggesting that cAMP-signaling systems may have a role in mediating alcohol's effects. Our laboratory has used microarray analysis to investigate the expression of 4000 to 10,000 genes in the frontal and motor cortices of human alcoholics (349,395,399). These studies used postmortem tissue samples from alcoholic subjects, and found pronounced changes in the expression of myelin-related genes, as well as in those involved in protein trafficking. The expression of cAMP-signaling genes were also differentially regulated.

Microarray analysis has also been used to investigate gene expression in animal models of alcohol sensitivity. Xu and colleagues (400) examined differential expression of nearly 20,000 genes in the brains of inbred Long-Sleep and Short-Sleep selected mouse lines and found that 41 genes were differently regulated. Microarray analysis was also used to investigate the expression of more than 5000 genes in the dorsal hippocampus of rats that had been exposed to either 12% alcohol or tap water for 15 months (401). Notable alcohol-sensitive genes in this study included some that were involved in protein trafficking.

Despite the power of microarray techniques to identify new and novel alcohol-sensitive genes, they do have some problems. Because of the number of genes on the chip, and hence the vast number of statistical comparisons, researchers must interpret their findings with some caution; the more statistical comparisons that are run, the greater the risk of identifying a gene that is not really differently regulated. Thus, researchers often confirm genes detected through microarray with other techniques (Northern blot, Western blot, or reverse transcriptase polymerase chain reaction [RT-PCR]) to more precisely identify regulated genes. Nevertheless, just as with QTL, microarray analysis appears to be a bright spot in research aimed at identifying neuronal pathways important in alcohol use and abuse.

Animal Models of Alcoholism

Nonhuman primates voluntarily develop excessive alcohol consumption when given free access to beverage alcohol (402). However, it is difficult to obtain high alcohol consumption in rodents unless drinking is forced (e.g., schedule-induced polydipsia, liquid diet). This section reviews progress in obtaining excessive alcohol consumption in rodents.

Alcohol Deprivation Effect

The phrase alcohol deprivation effect was first used by Sinclair and Senter (403) to describe the temporary increase in alcohol consumption after periods of abstinence in rats. Rats were first trained to consume alcohol using a two-bottle-choice drinking procedure, and then the alcohol solution was removed for varying periods of time. Upon reintroduction of the alcohol solution, the authors observed a temporary increase in alcohol intake that returned to normal after about 48 hours. Since the work of Sinclair and Senter (403), the alcohol deprivation effect has been observed in a number of other studies using rats, mice, monkeys, and human social drinkers, and using both two-bottle-choice and operant alcohol self-administration procedures (404). Studies show that the alcohol deprivation effect is dependent upon the duration of the abstinence period, and that it can be observed repeatedly following cycles of alcohol deprivation (404).

Recent evidence suggests that the alcohol deprivation effect may result from an enhanced reinforcing value of alcohol. Using a progressive ratio schedule of reinforcement, Spanagel and Holter (405) found that alcohol deprivation leads to higher break point values for alcohol. In a progressive ratio schedule, the fixed ratio requirements for obtaining the reinforcer are increased with each subsequent session to determine the maximum effort that a particular subject will emit for that reinforcer. The highest response requirement emitted by a particular subject is defined as the break point (406), and with regard to drug self-administration, the higher the break point for a drug, the higher its reinforcing efficacy (407). Moreover, the break point is correlated with the dose of self-administered drug, and receptor antagonists reduce break point values. Thus the results of Spanagel and Holter (405) appear to suggest that the reinforcing properties of alcohol may be enhanced by the alcohol deprivation effect.

The mechanisms underlying the alcohol deprivation effect are not clear. The deprivation phenomenon has been observed following abstinence from other abused drugs, and other consummatory behaviors, including salt and saccharine consumption, and social and sexual activity (404). Moreover, genetic susceptibility to the alcohol deprivation effect also appears to differ, even among rat lines that were selected for high alcohol intake. Whereas the alcohol deprivation effect was observed in alcohol-preferring P rats using both two-bottle-choice and operant procedures (408,409), it was not seen in Alko-alcohol (AA) rats (409,410). Furthermore, whereas the alcohol deprivation effect was limited to the first hour of alcohol intake and was not dependent on the length of the deprivation period in Sardinian alcohol-Preferring (sP) rats, the alcohol deprivation effect was only observed after repeated cycles of deprivation in high alcohol drinking (HAD) rats (411). Thus, much work remains to determine the mechanisms that mediate the alcohol deprivation phenomenon.

On a final note, the alcohol deprivation effect is a suggested animal model of relapse to alcohol (405,412) in part because it is a relatively simple behavioral manipulation with a reliable effect on alcohol self-administration. Furthermore, the enhancement in alcohol-seeking behavior seen after the deprivation parallels the priming effect of alcohol seen in humans (404), giving the model good predictive validity. However, Lê and Shaham (404) point out that the abstinence period is not under the control of the animal, and that while the model is used to characterize relapse following reexposure to the drug, human motivation to seek alcohol is antecedent to drug exposure. Thus, the alcohol-deprivation model may not provide us with much information on the factors that precede alcohol relapse in human alcoholics.

Reinstatement

Reinstatement describes the resumption of extinguished lever-pressing behavior observed following presentation of drug or nondrug stimuli (413). In this model, animals are trained to self-administer alcohol by pressing a lever in an operant chamber. Following the training phase, the alcohol-reinforced responding is extinguished by substituting vehicle for alcohol, or by simple discontinuation of alcohol delivery. After the lever-pressing behavior is

extinguished, the capacity of noncontingent alcohol (drug priming) or nondrug cues to reestablish alcohol-seeking behavior under extinction conditions is measured (404). Although it has been argued that it does not mimic conditions that lead to periods of abstinence in humans, the reinstatement model has good predictive validity because conditions thought to cause relapse and craving in human alcoholics reliably reinstate drug-seeking behavior in animal models (404). Indeed, a recent report suggests that rodent models of alcohol abuse and dependence, the alcohol-preferring (P) rats, are more sensitive to olfactory cue-induced reinstatement of alcohol-seeking behavior than are their nonpreferring (NP) counterparts (414). Thus, the model appears to offers a means by which to study the neurobiology underlying drug relapse.

As mentioned above, alcohol priming and exposure to nondrug cues are two means by which to reinstate noncontingent responding on the previously reinforced lever. Alcohol priming involves presentation of a pharmacologically relevant dose of alcohol after the alcohol-reinforced responding has been extinguished. Alcohol priming was first demonstrated by Chiamulera et al. (415). However, the priming dose of alcohol was not sufficient to produce pharmacologic effects on its own, and it therefore was more likely caused by other conditioned cues. More recently, Lê et al. (329) demonstrated that noncontingent priming with alcohol reinstates alcohol-seeking behavior after 4 to 8 days of extinction. Moreover, two studies demonstrated alcohol priming of noncontingent behavior when tests for reinstatement were conducted intermittently between the training days (416,417). However, recent data suggest that alcohol priming may require concurrent presentation of alcohol-associated cues (329,418). Consequently, the pharmacologic effects of a priming dose of alcohol are less likely to reinstate noncontingent lever pressing if the priming dose is administered in an alternative environment form that in which alcohol-reinforced responding was established (i.e., in the lever pressing chamber).

Recent work demonstrated that alcohol-associated cues or stimuli reinstate alcohol-seeking behavior. When Katner and colleagues (419) trained rats to lever press for alcohol or water, each fluid was paired with an auditory discriminative stimulus. During the extinction phase, lever pressing did not result in alcohol or water presentation, and the discriminative stimuli were not presented. Although reintroduction of the auditory cues that were associated with alcohol or water presentation did not reinstate alcohol-seeking behavior, presentation of the smell of alcohol (olfactory cue) modestly reinstated noncontingent responding on the previously alcohol-reinforced lever (419). A subsequent study used the smell of alcohol to signal its presentation, and achieved similar results (420). Moreover, whereas use of compound auditory/visual stimuli alone was unsuccessful, the addition of water in the dipper successfully reinstated alcohol-seeking behavior

(417), as did auditory cues previously associated with foot-shock stress (421). Thus, the available evidence suggests that alcohol- and stress-associated cues can reinstate alcohol-seeking behavior. However, not all cues are created equal. For example, olfactory cues such as the smell of alcohol are more effective conditioned stimuli than are audio or visual cues, unless these cues are associated with stressful stimuli. In other words, exposure to more salient stimuli may block the ability of less salient stimuli from becoming effective conditioned cues (422).

Recently a number of neurotransmitter/receptor systems were implicated in mediating reinstatement of alcohol-seeking behavior. Microinjections of a 5-HT$_{1A}$ receptor antagonist, as well as small amounts of CRF, into the median raphe nucleus, reinstated noncontingent responding for alcohol (423). Moreover, the same study also demonstrated that microinjections of a CRF receptor antagonist into the same brain region blocked the reinstatement of alcohol-seeking behavior normally seen in response to intermittent foot shock. Thus, the available evidence suggests that serotonin and CRF receptor systems likely have a role in reinstatement. Evidence also supports the involvement of endogenous opioid receptor systems. Naltrexone reduced the ability of alcohol-related cues to reinstate of alcohol-seeking behavior (424). However, allowing the animals to experience multiple withdrawals from alcohol reversed this effect. GABA$_A$ receptor systems may also have a role because the administration of allopregnenolone, a positive allosteric modulator at this receptor, also reinstated alcohol-seeking behavior (425). Finally, a recent study demonstrated involvement of dopamine receptor systems (426). Both D1 and D2 receptor antagonists dose dependently attenuated the reinstatement of alcohol-seeking behavior to an olfactory cue (the smell of alcohol). Thus, it appears that the reinstatement model may indeed provide useful information about the various neurotransmitter receptor systems underlying alcohol relapse, and will be a key model in the study of alcohol neurobiology in the future.

SUMMARY

During the past decade, neurobiology has made tremendous advances in our understanding of alcohol's actions on the brain. However, key questions regarding the precise sites of alcohol's action remain unanswered. Here we briefly discuss what we have learned and what questions remain. Notable discoveries are that alcohol, like other drugs of abuse, increase the firing and dopamine release of VTA dopamine neurons. This action is likely critical for the reinforcing aspects of alcohol, but the neurochemical and biophysical mechanisms responsible for this effect remain to be elucidated. The reductionist approach of searching for alcohol sensitive synaptic receptors has been successful, and the ligand-gated ion channels (i.e., GABA$_A$, glycine, NMDA, 5-HT$_3$, and nACh receptors) have emerged as likely sites of alcohol action. However, the molecular mechanisms by which alcohol affects the function of these receptors are not clear. There is considerable evidence that protein phosphorylation either determines or modifies the actions of alcohol on some of these receptors, but questions regarding alcohol interactions with protein kinases and phosphatases remain. Furthermore, in addition to the voltage-gated ion channels, G protein-coupled receptor systems have also been shown to be sensitive to alcohol. Now that these actions of alcohol have been identified in isolated systems, the challenge is to determine which sites are important for specific electrophysiologic and behavioral actions of alcohol.

In conclusion, alcohol has widespread and complex neurobiologic actions. How can neurobiology establish a causal relationship between neurochemical or electrophysiologic changes and behavior for a drug with such diverse actions? Perhaps the most powerful approach would employ a combination between molecular and behavioral genetics. Behavioral actions of alcohol such as voluntary intake, intoxication, tolerance, and physical dependence have been successfully studied in mice and rats, and recent advances in molecular genetics make it feasible to identify specific genes that regulate these actions of alcohol. Indeed, strategies that incorporate the use of genetically altered mutant mice, QTL, and microarray analyses, offer new and innovative ways of linking specific proteins to the behavioral actions of alcohol. Once specific genes (proteins) are identified, the relationship of the corresponding human genes to alcoholism can be determined, leading to the potential discovery of new therapeutic interventions. Thus, it appears that alcohol research is entering a synergistic phase in which rapid advances in molecular and biophysical analysis of brain function will be combined with molecular genetic analysis of animal models to answer some of the long-standing questions regarding the neurobiology of alcohol action.

REFERENCES

1. Goldstein DB. Pharmacological aspects of physical dependence on ethanol. *Life Sci* 1976;18:553–561.
2. Hille B. *Ionic channels of excitable membranes,* 2nd ed. Sunderland, MA: Sinauer, 1992:1–170.
3. Martz A, Deitrich RA, Harris RA. Behavioral evidence for the involvement of γ-aminobutyric acid in the actions of ethanol. *Eur J Pharmacol* 1983;89:53–62.
4. Allan AM, Harris RA. Gamma-aminobutyric acid and alcohol actions: neurochemical studies of Long Sleep and Short Sleep mice. *Life Sci* 1986;39:2005–2015.
5. Suzdak PD, Schwartz RD, Skolnick P, et al. Ethanol stimulates

γ-aminobutyric acid receptor-mediated chloride transport in rat brain synaptoneurosomes. *Proc Natl Acad Sci U S A* 1986;83:4071–4075.

6. Ticku MK, Lowrimore P, LeHoullier P. Ethanol enhances GABA-induced 36Cl-influx in primary spinal cord cultured neurons. *Brain Res Bull* 1986;17:128–136.

7. Deitrich RA, Dunwiddie TV, Harris RA, et al. Mechanism of action of ethanol: initial central nervous system actions. *Pharmacol Rev* 1989;41:491–537.

8. Mihic SJ, Harris RA. Alcohol actions at the GABA_A receptor/chloride channel complex. In: Deitrich RA, Erwin VG, eds. *Pharmacological effects of ethanol on the nervous system.* Boca Raton, FL: CRC Press, 1995:51–72.

9. Harris RA. Ethanol actions on multiple ion channels: which are important? *Alcohol Clin Exp Res* 1999;23:1563–1570.

10. Palmer AA, McKinnon CS, Bergstrom HC, et al. Locomotor activity responses to ethanol, other alcohols, and GABA-_A acting compounds in forward- and reverse-selected FAST and SLOW mouse lines. *Behav Neurosci* 2002;116:958–967.

11. Shelton KL, Grant KA. Discriminative stimulus effects of ethanol in C57BL/6J and DBA/2J inbred mice. *Alcohol Clin Exp Res* 2002;26:747–757.

12. Chester JA, Cunningham CL. Modulation of corticosterone does not affect the acquisition or expression of ethanol-induced conditioned place preference in DBA/2J mice. *Pharmacol Biochem Behav* 1998;59:67–75.

13. June HL, Torres L, Cason CR, et al. The novel benzodiazepine inverse agonist RO19—4603 antagonizes ethanol motivated behaviors: neuropharmacological studies. *Brain Res* 1998;784:256–275.

14. June HL, Zuccarelli D, Torres L, et al. High-affinity benzodiazepine antagonists reduce responding maintained by ethanol presentation in ethanol-preferring rats. *J Pharmacol Exp Ther* 1998;284:1006–1014.

15. Mihalek RM, Bowers BJ, Wehner JM, et al. GABA_A-receptor delta subunit knockout mice have multiple defects in behavioral responses to ethanol. *Alcohol Clin Exp Res* 2001;25:1708–1718.

16. Harvey SC, Foster KL, McKay PF, et al. The GABA_A receptor alpha1 subtype in the ventral pallidum regulates alcohol-seeking behaviors. *J Neurosci* 2002;22:3765–3775.

17. June HL, Harvey SC, Foster KL, et al. GABA_A receptors containing α5 subunits in the CA1 and CA3 hippocampal fields regulate ethanol-motivated behaviors: an extended ethanol reward circuitry. *J Neurosci* 2001;21:2166–2177.

18. Nishio M, Narahashi T. Ethanol enhancement of GABA-activated chloride current in rat dorsal root ganglion neurons. *Brain Res* 1990;518:283–286.

19. Nakahiro M, Arakawa O, Narahashi T. Modulation of gamma-aminobutyric acid receptor-channel complex by alcohols. *J Pharmacol Exp Ther* 1991;259:235–240.

20. Reynolds JN, Prasad A. Ethanol enhances GABAA receptor-activated chloride currents in chick cerebral cortical neurons. *Brain Res* 1991;564:138–142.

21. Reynolds JN, Prasad A, MacDonald JF. Ethanol modulation of GABA receptor-activated Cl- currents in neurons of the chick, rat and mouse central nervous system. *Eur J Pharmacol* 1992;224:173–181.

22. Aguayo LG. Ethanol potentiates the GABA_A-activated Cl- current in mouse hippocampal and cortical neurons. *Eur J Pharmacol* 1990;187:127–130.

23. Tatebayashi H, Motomura H, Narahashi T. Alcohol modulation of single GABA(A) receptor-channel kinetics. *Neuroreport* 1998;9:1769–1775.

24. Weiner JL, Gu C, Dunwiddie TV. Differential ethanol sensitivity of subpopulations of GABAA synapses onto rat hippocampal CA1 pyramidal neurons. *Neurophysiol* 1997;77:1306–1312.

25. Soldo BL, Proctor WR, Dunwiddie TV. Ethanol selectively enhances the hyperpolarizing component of neocortical neuronal responses to locally applied GABA. *Brain Res* 1998;800:187–197.

26. Poelchen W, Proctor WR, Dunwiddie TV. The *in vitro* ethanol sensitivity of hippocampal synaptic gamma-aminobutyric acid(A) responses differs in lines of mice and rats genetically selected for behavioral sensitivity or insensitivity to ethanol. *J Pharmacol Exp Ther* 2000;295:741–746.

27. Roberto M, Madamba SG, Moore SC, et al. Ethanol increases GABAergic transmission at both pre- and postsynaptic sites in rat central amygdala neurons. *Proc Natl Acad Sci U S A* 2003;100:2053–2058.

28. Roberts DD, Lewis SD, Ballou DP, et al. Reactivity of small thiolate anions and cysteine-25 in papain toward methyl methanethiosulfonate. *Biochemistry* 1986;25:5595–5601.

29. Weiner JL, Zhang L, Carlen P. Potentiation of GABA_A-mediated synaptic current by ethanol in hippocampal CA1 neurons: possible role of protein kinase C. *J Pharmacol Exp Ther* 1994;268:1388–1395.

30. Weiner JL, Valenzuela CF, Watson PL, et al. Elevation of basal protein kinase C activity increases ethanol sensitivity of GABA_A receptors in rat hippocampal CA1 pyramidal neurons. *J Neurochem* 1997;68:1949–1959.

31. Harris RA, McQuilkin SJ, Paylor R, et al. Mutant mice lacking the gamma isoform of protein kinase C show decreased behavioral actions of ethanol and altered function of gamma-aminobutyrate type A receptors. *Proc Natl Acad Sci U S A* 1995;92:3658–3662.

32. Wan FJ, Berton F, Madamba SG, et al. Low ethanol concentrations enhance GABAergic inhibitory postsynaptic potentials in hippocampal pyramidal neurons only after block of GABA_B receptors. *Proc Natl Acad Sci U S A* 1996;93:5049–5054.

33. Lin AM, Freund RK, Palmer MR. Ethanol potentiation of GABA-induced electrophysiological responses in cerebellum: requirement for catecholamine modulation. *Neurosci Lett* 1991;122:154–158.

34. Lin AM, Freund RK, Palmer MR. Sensitization of gamma-aminobutyric acid-induced depressions of cerebellar Purkinje neurons to the potentiative effects of ethanol by beta adrenergic mechanisms in rat brain. *J Pharmacol Exp Ther* 1993;265:426–432.

35. Yang X, Knapp DJ, Criswell HE, et al. Action of ethanol and zolpidem on gamma-aminobutyric acid responses from cerebellar Purkinje neurons: relationship to beta-adrenergic receptor input. *Alcohol Clin Exp Res* 1998;22:1655–1661.

36. Freund RK, Palmer MR. Beta adrenergic sensitization of gamma-aminobutyric acid receptors to ethanol involves a cyclic AMP/protein kinase A second-messenger mechanism. *J Pharmacol Exp Ther* 1997;280:1192–1200.

37. Osmanovic SS, Shefner SA. Enhancement of current induced by superfusion of GABA in locus coeruleus neurons by pentobarbital, but not ethanol. *Brain Res* 1990;517:324–329.

38. White G, Lovinger DM, Weight FF. Ethanol inhibits NMDA-activated current but does not alter GABA-activated current in an isolated adult mammalian neuron. *Brain Res* 1990;507:332–336.

39. Ming Z, Knapp DJ, Mueller RA, et al. Differential modulation of GABA- and NMDA-gated currents by ethanol and isoflurane in cultured rat cerebral cortical neurons. *Brain Res* 2001;920:117–124.

40. Morrisett RA, Swartzwelder HS. Attenuation of hippocampal long-term potentiation by ethanol: a patch-clamp

analysis of glutamatergic and GABAergic mechanisms. *J Neurosci* 1993;13:2264–72.

41. Schummers J, Browning MD. Evidence for a role for GABA$_A$ and NMDA receptors in ethanol inhibition of long-term potentiation. *Brain Res Mol Brain Res* 2001;94:9–14.

42. Yamakura T, Bertaccini E, Trudell JR, et al. Anesthetics and ion channels: molecular models and sites of action. *Annu Rev Pharmacol Toxicol* 2001;41:23–51.

43. Mihic SJ, Harris RA. Inhibition of rho1 receptor GABAergic currents by alcohols and volatile anesthetics. *J Pharmacol Exp Ther* 1996;277:411–416.

44. Sundstrom-Poromaa I, Smith DH, Gong QH, et al. Hormonally regulated alpha(4)beta(2)delta GABA$_A$ receptors are a target for alcohol. *Nat Neurosci* 2002;5:721–722.

45. Akk G, Steinbach JH. Low doses of ethanol and a neuroactive steroid positively interact to modulate rat GABA$_A$ receptor function. *J Physiol* 2003;546:641–646.

46. Betz H. Glycine receptors: heterogeneous and widespread in the mammalian brain. *Trends Neurosci* 1991;14:458–461.

47. Williams KL, Ferko AP, Barbieri EJ, et al. Glycine enhances the central depressant properties of ethanol in mice. *Pharmacol Biochem Behav* 1995;50:199–205.

48. Quinlan JJ, Ferguson C, Jester K, et al. Mice with glycine receptor subunit mutations are both sensitive and resistant to volatile anesthetics. *Anesth Analg* 2002;95:578–582.

49. Findlay GS, Wick MJ, Mascia MP, et al. Transgenic expression of a mutant glycine receptor decreases alcohol sensitivity of mice. *J Pharmacol Exp Ther* 2002;300:526–534.

50. Aguayo LG, Pancetti FC. Ethanol modulation of the gamma-aminobutyric acid$_A$- and glycine-activated Cl- current in cultured mouse neuron. *J Pharmacol Exp Ther* 1994;270:61–69.

51. Celentano JJ, Gibbs TT, Farb DH. Ethanol potentiates GABA- and glycine-induced chloride currents in chick spinal cord neurons. *Brain Res* 1988;455:377–380.

52. Aguayo LG, Tapia JC, Pancetti FC. Potentiation of the glycine-activated Cl-current by ethanol in cultured mouse spinal neurons. *J Pharmacol Exp Ther* 1996;279:1116–1122.

53. Tapia JC, Aguilar LF, Sotomayor CP, et al. Ethanol affects the function of a neurotransmitter receptor protein without altering the membrane lipid phase. *Eur J Pharmacol* 1998;354:239–244.

54. Ye JH, Tao L, Ren J, et al. Ethanol potentiation of glycine-induced responses in dissociated neurons of rat ventral tegmental area. *J Pharmacol Exp Ther* 2001;296:77–83.

55. Engblom AC, Akerman KE. Effect of ethanol on gamma-aminobutyric acid and glycine receptor-coupled Cl– fluxes in rat brain synaptoneurosomes. *J Neurochem* 1991;57:384–390.

56. Mascia MP, Mihic SJ, Valenzuela CF, et al. A single amino acid determines differences in ethanol actions on strychnine-sensitive glycine receptors. *Mol Pharmacol* 1996;50:402–406.

57. Eggers ED, O'Brien JA, Berger AJ. Developmental changes in the modulation of synaptic glycine receptors by ethanol. *J Neurophysiol* 2000;84:2409–2416.

58. Valenzuela CF, Cardoso RA, Wick MJ, et al. Effects of ethanol on recombinant glycine receptors expressed in mammalian cell lines. *Alcohol Clin Exp Res* 1998;22:1132–1136.

59. Kulkarni SK, Mehta AK, Ticku MK. Comparison of anticonvulsant effects of ethanol against NMDA-, kainic acid-, and picrotoxin-induced convulsions in rats. *Life Sci* 1990;46:481–487.

60. Sharma AC, Thorat SN, Nayar U, et al. Dizocilpine, ketamine and ethanol reverse NMDA-induced EEG changes and convulsions in rats and mice. *Indian J Physiol Pharmacol* 1991;35:111–116.

61. Meller ST, Dykstra C, Pechman PS, et al. Ethanol dose-dependently attenuates NMDA-mediated thermal hyperalgesia in the rat. *Neurosci Lett* 1993;54:137–140.

62. Daniell LC. The noncompetitive N-methyl-D-aspartate antagonists, MK-801, phencyclidine and ketamine, increase the potency of general anesthetics. *Pharmacol Biochem Behav* 1990;36:111–115.

63. Daniell LC. Effect of CGS 19755, a competitive N-methyl-D-aspartate antagonist, on general anesthetic potency. *Pharmacol Biochem Behav* 1991;40:767–769.

64. Wilson WR, Bosy TZ, Ruth JA. NMDA agonists and antagonists alter the hypnotic response to ethanol in LS and SS mice. *Alcohol* 1990;7:389–395.

65. Grant KA, Colombo G. Discriminative stimulus effects of ethanol: effect of training dose on the substitution of N-methyl-D-aspartate antagonists. *J Pharmacol Exp Ther* 1993;264:1241–1247.

66. Khanna JM, Wu PH, Weiner JL, et al. NMDA antagonist inhibits rapid tolerance to ethanol. *Brain Res Bull* 1991;26:643–645.

67. Khanna JM, Kalant H, Shah G, et al. Effects of (+)MK-801 and ketamine on rapid tolerance to ethanol. *Brain Res Bull* 1992;28:311–314.

68. Khanna JM, Mihic SJ, Weiner J, et al. Differential inhibition by NMDA antagonists of rapid tolerance to, and cross-tolerance between, ethanol and chlordiazepoxide. *Brain Res* 1992;574:251–256.

69. Khanna KM, Shah G, Weiner J, et al. Effect of NMDA receptor antagonists on rapid tolerance to ethanol. *Eur J Pharmacol* 1993;230:23–31.

70. Szabó G, Tabakoff B, Hoffman PL. The NMDA receptor antagonist dizocilpine differentially affects environment-dependent and environment-independent ethanol tolerance. *Psychopharmacology (Berl)* 1994;113:511–517.

71. Rafi-Tari S, Kalant H, Liu JF, et al. Dizocilpine prevents the development of tolerance to ethanol-induced error on a circular maze test. *Psychopharmacology (Berl)* 1996;125:23–32.

72. Forrest D, Yuzaki M, Soares HD, et al. Targeted disruption of NMDA receptor 1 gene abolishes NMDA response and results in neonatal death. *Neuron* 1994;13:325–338.

73. Kutsuwada T, Sakimura K, Manabe T, et al. Impairment of suckling response, trigeminal neuronal pattern formation, and hippocampal LTD in NMDA receptor epsilon 2 subunit mutant mice. *Neuron* 1996;16:333–344.

74. Kiefer F, Jahn H, Koester A, et al. Involvement of NMDA receptors in alcohol-mediated behavior: mice with reduced affinity of the NMDA R1 glycine binding site display an attenuated sensitivity to ethanol. *Biol Psychiatry* 2003;53:345–351.

75. Hoffman PL, Moses F, Tabakoff B. Selective inhibition by ethanol of glutamate-stimulated cyclic GMP production in primary cultures of cerebellar granule cells. *Neuropharmacology* 1989;28:1239–1243.

76. Dildy JE, Leslie SW. Ethanol inhibits NMDA-induced increases in intracellular Ca^{2+} in dissociated brain cells. *Brain Res* 1989;499:383–387.

77. Rabe CS, Tabakoff B. Glycine site-directed agonists reverse the actions of ethanol at the N-methyl-D-aspartate receptor. *Mol Pharmacol* 1990;38:753–757.

78. Lovinger DM, White G, Weight FF. Ethanol inhibits NMDA-activated ion current in hippocampal neurons. *Science* 1989;243:1721–1724.

79. Lima-Ladman MTR, Albuquerque EX. Ethanol potentiates and blocks NMDA-activated—single channel currents in rat hippocampal pyramidal cells. *FEBS Lett* 1989;247:61–67.

80. Lovinger DM, White G, Weight FF. NMDA receptor-mediated synaptic excitation selectively inhibited by ethanol in hippocampal slice from adult rat. *J Neurosci* 1990;10:1372–1379.

81. Morrisett RA, Martin D, Oetting TA, et al. Ethanol and magnesium ions inhibit N-methyl-D-aspartate-mediated synaptic potentials in an interactive manner. *Neuropharmacology* 1991; 30:1173–1178.

82. Dildy-Mayfield JE, Harris RA. Comparison of ethanol sensitivity of rat brain kainate, dl-a-amino-3-hydroxy-5-methyl-4-isoxolone propionic acid and N-methyl-D-aspartate receptors expressed in *Xenopus oocytes*. *J Pharmacol Exp Ther* 1992;262:487–494.

83. Koltchine V, Anantharam V, Wilson A, et al. Homomeric assemblies of NM-DAR1 splice variants are sensitive to ethanol. *Neurosci Lett* 1993;152:13–16.

84. Kuner T, Schoepfer R, Korpi ER. Ethanol inhibits glutamate-induced currents in heteromeric NMDA receptor subtypes. *Neuroreport* 1993;5:297–300.

85. Chu B, Anantharam V, Treistman SN. Ethanol inhibition of recombinant heteromeric NMDA channels in the presence and absence of modulators. *J Neurochem* 1995;65:140–148.

86. Mirshahi T, Woodward JJ. Ethanol sensitivity of heteromeric NMDA receptors: effects of subunit assembly, glycine and NMDAR1 Mg^{2+}-insensitive mutants. *Neuropharmacology* 1995;34:347–355.

87. Snell LD, Tabakoff B, Hoffman PL. Involvement of protein kinase C in ethanol-induced inhibition of NMDA receptor function in cerebellar granule cells. *Alcohol Clin Exp Res* 1994;18:81–85.

88. Woodward JJ. Inotropic glutamate receptors as sites of action for ethanol in the brain. *Neurochem Int* 1999;35:107–113.

89. Allgaier C. Ethanol sensitivity of NMDA receptors. *Neurochem Int* 2002; 41:377–382.

90. Dildy-Mayfield JE, Harris RA. Acute and chronic ethanol exposure alters the function of hippocampal kainate receptors expressed in Xenopus oocytes. *J Neurochem* 1992;58:1569–1572.

91. Möykkynen T, Korpi ER, Lovinger DM. Ethanol inhibits alpha-amino-3-hydyroxy-5-methyl-4-isoxazolepropionic acid (AMPA) receptor function in central nervous system neurons by stabilizing desensitization. *J Pharmacol Exp Ther* 2003;306:546–555.

92. Teichberg VI, Tal N, Goldberg O, et al. Barbiturates, alcohols, and the CNS excitatory neurotransmission: specific effects of the kainate and quisqualate receptors. *Brain Res* 1984;292:285–292.

93. Lovinger DM. High ethanol sensitivity of recombinant AMPA-type glutamate receptors expressed in mammalian cells. *Neurosci Lett* 1993;159:83–87.

94. Martin D, Tayyeb MI, Swartzwelder HS. Ethanol inhibition of AMPA and kainate receptor-mediated depolarization of hippocampal are CA1. *Alcohol Clin Exp Res* 1995;19:1312–1316.

95. Weiner JL, Dunwiddie TV, Valenzuela CF. Ethanol inhibition of synaptically evoked kainate responses in rat hippocampal CA3 pyramidal neurons. *Mol Pharmacol* 1999;56:85–90.

96. Crowder TL, Ariwodola OJ, Weiner JL. Ethanol antagonizes kainate receptor-mediated inhibition of evoked GABA$_A$ inhibitory postsynaptic currents in the rat hippocampal CA1 region. *J Pharmacol Exp Ther* 2002;303:937–944.

97. Dildy-Mayfield JE, Harris RA. Ethanol inhibits kainate responses of glutamate receptors expressed in *Xenopus oocytes*: role of calcium and protein kinase C. *J Neurosci* 1995;15:3162–3171.

98. Carta M, Ariwodola OJ, Weiner JL, et al. Alcohol potently inhibits the kainate receptor-dependent excitatory drive of hippocampal interneurons. *Proc Natl Acad Sci U S A* 2003;100:6813–6818.

99. Molleman A, Little HJ. Increases in non-N-methyl-D-aspartate glutamatergic transmission, but no change in γ-aminobutyric acid$_B$ transmission, in CA1 neurons during withdrawal from *in vivo* chronic ethanol treatment. *J Pharmacol Exp Ther* 1995;272:1035–1041.

100. Matsumoto I, Davidson M, Otsuki M, et al. Decreased severity of ethanol withdrawal behaviors in kainic acid-treated rats. *Pharmacol Biochem Behav* 1996;55:371–378.

101. Becker HC, Veatch LM, Diaz-Granados JL. Repeated ethanol withdrawal experience selectively alters sensitivity to different chemoconvulsant drugs in mice. *Psychopharmacology (Berl)* 1998;139:145–153.

102. Erickson CK, Burnam WL. Cholinergic alteration of ethanol-induced sleep and death in mice. *Agents Actions* 1971;21:8–13.

103. Graham DT, Erickson CK. Alteration of ethanol-induced CNS depression: ineffectiveness of drugs that modify cholinergic transmission. *Psychopharmacology (Berl)* 1974;34:173–180.

104. Blomquist O, Soderpalm B, Engel JA. Ethanol-induced locomotor activity: involvement of central nicotinic acetylcholine receptors? *Brain Res Bull* 1992;29:173–178.

105. Blomquist O, Engel JA, Nissbrandt H, et al. The mesolimbic dopamine-activating properties of ethanol are antagonized by mecamylamine. *Eur J Pharmacol* 1993;249:207–213.

106. Söderpalm B, Ericson M, Olausson P, et al. Nicotinic mechanisms involved in the dopaminergic activating and reinforcing properties of ethanol. *Behav Brain Res* 2000;113:85–96.

107. Picciotto MR, Caldarone BJ, Brunzell DH, et al. Neuronal nicotinic acetylcholine receptor subunit knockout mice: physiological and behavioral phenotypes and possible clinical implications. *Pharmacol Ther* 2001;92:89–108.

108. Aistrup GL, Marszalec W, Narahashi T. Ethanol modulation of nicotinic acetylcholine receptor currents in cultured cortical neurons. *Mol Pharmacol* 1999;55:39–49.

109. Zuo Y, Aistrup GL, Marszalec W, et al. Dual action of n-alcohols on neuronal nicotinic acetylcholine receptors. *Mol Pharmacol* 2001;60:700–711.

110. Cardoso RA, Brozowski SJ, Chavez-Noriega LE, et al. Effects of ethanol on recombinant human neuronal nicotinic acetylcholine receptors expressed in Xenopus oocytes. *J Pharmacol Exp Ther* 1999;289:774–780.

111. Narahashi T, Aistrup GL, Marszalec W, et al. Neuronal nicotinic acetylcholine receptors: a new target site of ethanol. *Neurochem Int* 1999;35:131–141.

112. Fadda F, Garau B, Marchei F, et al. MDL 72222, a selective 5-HT3 receptor antagonist, suppresses voluntary ethanol consumption in alcohol-preferring rats. *Alcohol Alcohol* 1991;26:107–110.

113. LeMarquand D, Pihl RO, Benkelfat C. Serotonin and alcohol intake, abuse, and dependence: findings of animal studies. *Biol Psychiatry* 1994;36:395–421.

114. Sellers EM. Biobehavioural basis of pharmacologic treatment of alcohol dependence. *Alcohol Alcohol Suppl* 1994;2:517–521.

115. Tomkins DM, Le AD, Sellers EM. Effect of the 5-HT3 antagonist ondansetron on voluntary ethanol intake in rats and mice maintained n a limited access procedure. *Psychopharmacology (Berl)* 1995;117:479–485.

116. Engel SR, Lyons CR, Allan AM. 5-HT$_3$ receptor over-expression decreases ethanol self administration in transgenic mice. *Psychopharmacology (Berl)* 1998;140:243–248.

117. Sung K-W, Engel SR, Allan AM, et al. 5-HT3 receptor function and potentiation by alcohols in frontal cortex neurons from transgenic mice overexpressing the receptor. *Neuropharmacology* 2000;39:2346–2351.

118. Lovinger DM. Ethanol potentiation of

5-HT$_3$ receptor-mediated ion current in NCB-20 neuroblastoma cells. *Neurosci Lett* 1991;122:57–60.

119. Lovinger DM, White G. 5-Hydroxy-tryptamine$_3$ receptor-mediated ion current in neuroblastoma cells and isolated adult mammalian neurons. *Mol Pharmacol* 1991;40:263–270.

120. Machu TK, Harris RA. Alcohols and anesthetics enhance the function of 5-hydroxytryptamine$_3$ receptors expressed in *Xenopus* laevis. *J Pharmacol Exp Ther* 1994;271:898–905.

121. Lovinger DM. 5-HT3 receptors and the neural actions of alcohols: an increasingly exciting topic. *Neurochem Int* 1999;35:125–130.

122. Hoffman PL, Tabakoff B. Ethanol's action on brain biochemistry. In: Tarter RE, van Thiel DH, eds. *Alcohol and the brain: chronic effects.* New York: Plenum Press, 1985:19–68.

123. Imperato A, Di Chiara G. Preferential stimulation of dopamine release in the nucleus accumbens of freely moving rats by ethanol. *J Pharmacol Exp Ther* 1986;239:219–228.

124. Gessa GL, Muntoni F, Collu M, et al. Low doses of ethanol activate dopaminergic neurones in the ventral tegmental area. *Brain Res* 1985;348:201–203.

125. Brodie MS, Shefner SA, Dunwiddie TV. Ethanol increases the firing rate of dopamine neurons of the rat ventral tegmental area *in vitro. Brain Res* 1990;508:65–69.

126. Brodie MS, Pesold C, Appel SB. Ethanol directly excites dopaminergic ventral tegmental area reward neurons. *Alcohol Clin Exp Res* 1999;23:1848–1852.

127. Brodie MS, Appel SB. Dopaminergic neurons in the ventral tegmental area of C57Bl/6J and DBA/2J mice differ in sensitivity to ethanol excitation. *Alcohol Clin Exp Res* 2000;24:1120–1124.

128. Weiss F, Lorang MT, Bloom FE, et al. Oral alcohol self-administration stimulates dopamine release in the rat nucleus accumbens: genetic and motivational determinants. *J Pharmacol Exp Ther* 1993;267:250–258.

129. Nevo I, Hamon M. Neurotransmitter and neuromodulatory mechanisms involved in alcohol abuse and alcoholism. *Neurochem Int* 1995;26:305–336.

130. Korpi ER, Sinclair JD, Malminen O. Dopamine D$_2$ receptor binding in striatal membranes of rat lines selected for differences in alcohol-related behaviors. *Pharmacol Toxicol* 1987;61:94–97.

131. Stefanini E, Frau M, Garau MG, et al. Alcohol-preferring rats have fewer dopamine D$_2$ receptors in the limbic system. *Alcohol Alcohol* 1992;27:127–130.

132. McBride WJ, Chernet E, Dyr W, et al. Densities of dopamine D$_2$ receptors are reduced in CNS regions of alcohol-preferring P rats. *Alcohol* 1993;10:387–390.

133. De Montis MG, Gambarana C, Gessa GL, et al. Reduced [^{3}H]SCH 23390 binding and DA-sensitive adenylyl cyclase in the limbic system of ethanol-preferring rats. *Alcohol Alcohol* 1993;28:397–400.

134. Dyr W, McBride WJ, Lumeng L, et al. Effects of D$_1$ and D$_2$ dopamine receptor agents on ethanol consumption in the high-alcohol-drinking (HAD) line of rats. *Alcohol* 1993;10:207–212.

135. Weiss F, Mitchiner M, Bloom FE, et al. Free-choice responding for ethanol versus water in alcohol preferring (P) and unselected Wistar rats is differentially modified by naloxone, bromocriptine, and methysergide. *Psychopharmacology (Berl)* 1990;101:178–186.

136. Samson HH, Tolliver GA, Schwarz-Stevens K. Oral ethanol self-administration: a behavioral pharmacological approach to CNS control mechanisms. *Alcohol* 1990;7:187–191.

137. Koob GF, Weiss F. Pharmacology of drug self-administration. *Alcohol* 1990;7:193–197.

138. Hodge CW, Samson HH, Haraguchi M. Microinjections of dopamine agonists in n. accumbens increase ethanol reinforced responding. *Pharmacol Biochem Behav* 1992;43:249–254.

139. Pfeffer AO, Samson HH. Haloperidol and apomorphine effects on ethanol reinforcement in free feeding rats. *Pharmacol Biochem Behav* 1988;29:343–350.

140. Morgenroth VH, Walters JR, Roth RH. Dopaminergic neurons—alteration in the kinetic properties of tyrosine hydroxylase after cessation of impulse flow. *Biochem Pharmacol* 1976;25:655–661.

141. Samson HH, Tolliver GA, Haraguchi M, et al. Alcohol self-administration: role of mesolimbic dopamine. *Ann N Y Acad Sci* 1992;654:242–253.

142. Brown ZW, Amit Z. The effects of selective catecholamine depletions by 6-hydroxydopamine on ethanol preference in rats. *Neurosci Lett* 1977;5:333–336.

143. Lê AD, Khanna JM, Kalant H, et al. Effect of modification of brain serotonin. *(5-HT),* norepinephrine (NE) and dopamine (DA) on ethanol tolerance. *Psychopharmacology (Berl)* 1981;75:231–235.

144. Lê AD, Khanna JM, Kalant H, et al. The effect of lesions in the dorsal, median and magnus raphe nuclei on the development of tolerance to ethanol. *J Pharmacol Exp Ther* 1981;218:525–529.

145. Quarfordt SD, Kalmus GW, Myers RD. Ethanol drinking following 6-OHDA lesions of nucleus accumbens and tuberculum olfactorium of the rat. *Alcohol* 1991;8:211–217.

146. Rassnick S, Stinus L, Koob GF. The effects of 6-hydroxydopamine lesions of the nucleus accumbens and the mesolimbic dopamine system on oral self-administration of ethanol in the rat. *Brain Res* 1993;623:16–24.

147. Lança AJ. Reduction of voluntary alcohol intake in the rat by modulation of the dopaminergic mesolimbic system: transplantation of ventral mesencephalic cell suspensions. *Neuroscience* 1994;58:359–369.

148. Rubinstein M, Phillips TJ, Bunzow JR, et al. Mice lacking dopamine D4 receptors are supersensitive to ethanol, cocaine, and methamphetamine. *Cell* 1997;90:991–1001.

149. Phillips TJ, Brown KJ, Burkhart-Kasch S, et al. Alcohol preference and sensitivity are markedly reduced in mice lacking dopamine D$_2$ receptors. *Nat Neurosci* 1998;1:610–615.

150. Thanos PK, Volkow ND, Freimuth P, et al. Overexpression of dopamine D2 receptors reduces alcohol self-administration. *J Neurochem* 2001;78:1094–1103.

151. El-Ghundi M, George SR, Drago J, et al. Disruption of dopamine D1 receptor gene expression attenuates alcohol-seeking behavior. *Eur J Pharmacol* 1998;353:149–158.

152. Narita M, Soma M, Tamaki H, et al. Intensification of the development of ethanol dependence in mice lacking dopamine D$_3$ receptor. *Neurosci Lett* 2002;324:129–132.

153. Savelieva KV, Caudle WM, Findlay GS, et al. Decreased ethanol preference and consumption in dopamine transporter female knock-out mice. *Alcohol Clin Exp Res* 2002;26:758–764.

154. Hoyer D, Clarke DE, Fozard JR, et al. International union of pharmacology classification of receptors for 5-hydroxytryptamine (serotonin). *Pharmacol Rev* 1994;46:157–203.

155. Grant KA. The role of 5-HT$_3$ receptors in drug dependence. *Drug Alcohol Depend* 1995;38:155–171.

156. Wong DT, Reid LR, Li TK, et al. Greater abundance of serotonin$_{1A}$ receptor in some brain areas of alcohol-preferring (P) rats compared to nonpreferring (NP) rats. *Pharmacol Biochem Behav* 1993;46:173–177.

157. McBride WJ, Chernet E, Rabold JA, et al. Serotonin-2 receptors in the CNS of alcohol-preferring and nonpreferring rats. *Pharmacol Biochem Behav* 1993;46:631–636.

158. Zhou FC, Bledsoe S, Lumeng L, et al.

Reduced serotoninergic immunoreactivity fibers in the forebrain of alcohol-preferring rats. *Alcohol Clin Exp Res* 1994;18:571–579.

159. Zhou FC, Pu CF, Murphy J, et al. Serotoninergic neurons in the alcohol preferring rats. *Alcohol* 1994;11:397–403.

160. Crabbe JC, Phillips TJ, Feller DJ, et al. Elevated alcohol consumption in null mutant mice lacking 5-HT1B serotonin receptors. *Nat Genet* 1996;14:98–101.

161. Risinger FO, Bormann NM, Oakes RA. Reduced sensitivity to ethanol aversion in mice lacking 5-HT1B receptors. *Alcohol Clin Exp Res* 1996;20:1401–1405.

162. Crabbe JC, Wahlsten D, Dudek BC. Genetics of mouse behavior: Interactions with laboratory environment. *Nature* 1999;284:1670–1672.

163. Risinger FO, Doan AM, Vickrey AC. Oral operant ethanol self-administration in 5-HT1b knockout mice. *Behav Brain Res* 1999;102:211–215.

164. Bouwknecht JA, Hijzen TH, van der Gugten J, et al. Ethanol intake is not elevated in male 5-HT$_{1B}$ receptor knockout mice. *Eur J Pharmacol* 2000;403:95–98.

165. Gorwood P, Aissi F, Batel P, et al. Reappraisal of the serotonin 5-HT1B receptor gene in alcoholism: of mice and men. *Brain Res Bull* 2002;57:103–107.

166. Boehm SL II, Schafer GL, Phillips TJ, et al. Sensitivity to ethanol-induced motor incoordination in 5-HT1B receptor null mutant mice is task-dependent: Implications for behavioral assessment of genetically altered mice. *Behav Neurosci* 2000;114:401–409.

167. Fish EW, Faccidomo S, Miczek KA. Aggression heightened by alcohol or social instigation in mice: reduction by the 5-HT$_{1B}$ receptor agonist CP-94, 253. *Psychopharmacology (Berl)* 1999;146:391–399.

168. de Almeida RMM, Nikulina EM, Faccidomo S, et al. Zolmitriptan-a 5-HT$_{1B/D}$ agonist, alcohol, and aggression in mice. *Psychopharmacology (Berl)* 2001;157:131–141.

169. Risinger FO, Boyce JM. 5-HT1A receptor blockade and the motivational profile of ethanol. *Life Sci* 2002;71:707–715.

170. Popova NK, Ivanova EA. 5-HT$_{1A}$ receptor antagonist p-MPPI attenuates acute ethanol effects in mice and rats. *Neurosci Lett* 2002;322:1–4.

171. Miczek KA, Hussain S, Faccidomo S. Alcohol-heightened aggression in mice: attenuation by 5-HT1A receptor agonists. *Psychopharmacology (Berl)* 1998;139:160–168.

172. Blandina P, Goldfarb J, Craddock-Royal B, et al. Release of endogenous dopamine by stimulation of 5-hydroxytryptamine$_3$ receptors in rat striatum. *J Pharmacol Exp Ther* 1989;251:803–809.

173. Richardson BP, Engel G, Donatsch P, et al. Identification of serotonin M-receptor subtypes and their specific blockade by a new class of drugs. *Nature* 1985;316:126–131.

174. Yoshimoto K, McBride WJ, Lumeng L, et al. Alcohol stimulates the release of dopamine and serotonin in the nucleus accumbens. *Alcohol* 1991;9:17–22.

175. Herve D, Pickel VM, Joh TH, et al. Serotonin axon terminals in the ventral tegmental area of the rat: fine structure and synaptic input to dopaminergic neurons. *Brain Res* 1987;435:71–83.

176. Guan XM, McBride WJ. Serotonin microinfusion into the ventral tegmental area increases accumbens dopamine release. *Brain Res Bull* 1989;23:541–547.

177. Jiang LH, Ashby CR, Dasser RJ, et al. The effect of intraventricular administration of the 5-HT$_3$ receptor agonist 2-methylserotonin on the release of dopamine in the nucleus accumbens: an *in vivo* chroniculometric study. *Brain Res* 1990;513:156–160.

178. Dunwiddie TV. The physiological role of adenosine in the central nervous system. *Int Rev Neurobiol* 1985;27:63–139.

179. Olah ME, Stiles GL. Adenosine receptor subtypes: characterization and therapeutic regulation. *Annu Rev Pharmacol Toxicol* 1995;35:581–606.

180. Dar MS, Mustafa SJ, Wooles WR. Possible role of adenosine in the CNS effects of ethanol. *Life Sci* 1983;33:1363–1374.

181. Dar MS. Central adenosinergic system involvement in ethanol-induced motor incoordination in mice. *J Pharmacol Exp Ther* 1990;255:1202–1209.

182. Dar MS, Wooles WR. Effect of chronically administered methylxanthines on ethanol-induced motor incoordination in mice. *Life Sci* 1986;39:1429–1437.

183. Phan TA, Gray AM, Nyce JW. Intrastriatal adenosine A1 receptor antisense oligodeoxynucleotide blocks ethanol-induced motor incoordination. *Eur J Pharmacol* 1997;323:R5–7.

184. Dar MS, Mustafa SJ. Acute ethanol/cannabinoid-induced ataxia and its antagonism by oral/systemic/intracerebellar A1 adenosine receptor antisense in mice. *Brain Res* 2002;957:53–60.

185. Dar MS. Mouse cerebellar adenosine-glutamate interactions and modulation of ethanol-induced motor incoordination. *Alcohol Clin Exp Res* 2002;26:1395–1403.

186. Naassila M, Ledent C, Daoust M. Low ethanol sensitivity and increased ethanol consumption in mice lacking adenosine A2A receptors. *J Neurosci* 2002;22:10487–10493.

187. El Yacoubi M, Ledent C, Parmentier M, et al. Absence of the adenosine A(2A) receptor or its chronic blockade decrease ethanol withdrawal-induced seizures in mice. *Neuropharmacol* 2001;40:424–432.

188. Gordon AS, Collier K, Diamond I. Ethanol regulation of adenosine receptor-stimulated cAMP levels in a clonal neural cell line: An in vitro model of cellular tolerance to ethanol. *Proc Natl Acad Sci U S A* 1986;83:2105–2108.

189. Nagy LE, Diamond I, Gordon A. Cultured lymphocytes from alcoholic subjects have altered cAMP signal transduction. *Proc Natl Acad Sci U S A* 1988;85:6973–6976.

190. Hoffman PL, Tabakoff B. Ethanol and guanine nucleotide binding proteins: a selective interaction. *FASEB J* 1990;4:2612–2622.

191. Reynolds JD, Brien JF. The role of adenosine A1 receptor activation in ethanol-induced inhibition of stimulated glutamate release in the hippocampus of the fetal and adult guinea pig. *Alcohol* 1995;12:151–157.

192. Nagy LE, Diamond I, Collier K, et al. Adenosine is required for ethanol-induced heterologous desensitization. *Mol Pharmacol* 1989;36:744–748.

193. Krauss SW, Ghirnikar RB, Diamond I, et al. Inhibition of adenosine uptake by ethanol is specific for one class of nucleoside transporters. *Mol Pharmacol* 1993;44:1021–1026.

194. Sapru MK, Diamond I, Gordon AS. Adenosine receptors mediate cellular adaptation to ethanol in NC108-15 cells. *J Pharmacol Exp Ther* 1994;271:542–548.

195. Yao L, Arolfo MP, Dohrman DP, et al. $\beta\gamma$ dimers mediate synergy of dopamine D2 and adenosine A2 receptor-stimulated PKA signaling and regulate ethanol consumption. *Cell* 2002;109:733–743.

196. Hoffman PL, Ritzmann RF, Walter R, et al. Arginine vasopressin maintains ethanol tolerance. *Nature* 1978;276:614–616.

197. Lê AD, Kalant H, Khanna JM. Interaction between des-9-glycinamide-[8-Arg]vasopressin and serotonin on ethanol tolerance. *Eur J Pharmacol* 1982;80:337–345.

198. Hoffman PL, Tabakoff B. Neurohypophyseal peptides maintain tolerance to the incoordinating effects of ethanol. *Pharmacol Biochem Behav* 1984;21:539–543.

199. Chiu J, Kalant H, Le DA. Vasopressin opposes locomotor stimulation

by ethanol, cocaine and amphetamine in mice. *Eur J Pharmacol* 1998;355:11–17.

200. Hung C-R, Tabakoff B, Melchior CL, et al. Intraventricular arginine vasopressin maintains ethanol tolerance. *Eur J Pharmacol* 1984;106:645–648.

201. Szabó G, Tabakoff B, Hoffman PL. Receptors with V_1 characteristics mediate the maintenance of ethanol tolerance by vasopressin. *J Pharmacol Exp Ther* 1988;247:536–541.

202. Tabakoff B, Ritzmann RF. The effects of 6- hydroxydopamine on tolerance to and dependence on ethanol. *J Pharmacol Exp Ther* 1977;203:319–332.

203. Hoffman PL, Melchior CL, Tabakoff B. Vasopressin maintenance of ethanol tolerance requires intact brain noradrenergic systems. *Life Sci* 1983;32:1065–1071.

204. Ishizawa H, Tabakoff B, Mefford IN, et al. Reduction of arginine vasopressin binding sites in mouse lateral septum by treatment with 6-hydroxydopamine. *Brain Res* 1990;507:189–194.

205. Hagan JJ, Balfour DJK. Lysine vasopressin fails to alter. (3H)noradrenaline uptake or release from hippocampal tissue in vitro. *Life Sci* 1983;32:2517–2522.

206. Speisky MB, Kalant H. Site of interaction of serotonin and desglycinamide-arginine vasopressin in maintenance of ethanol tolerance. *Brain Res* 1985;326:281–290.

207. Wu PH, Liu JF, Lança AJ, et al. Selective involvement of central 5-HT2 receptors in the maintenance of tolerance to ethanol by arginine. (8)-vasopressin. *J Pharmacol Exp Ther* 1994;270:802–808.

208. Rathna Giri P, Dave JR, Tabakoff B, et al. Arginine vasopressin induces the expression of c-fos in the mouse septum and hippocampus. *Mol Brain Res* 1990;7:131–137.

209. Hoffman PL. Neuroadaptive functions of the neuropeptide arginine vasopressin. *Ann N Y Acad Sci* 1994;739:168–175.

210. Szabó G, Mácsai M, Schek E, et al. The effect of vasoactive intestinal polypeptide and pituitary adenylate cyclase activating polypeptide on tolerance to morphine and alcohol in mice. *Ann N Y Acad Sci* 1998;865:566–569.

211. Pittman QJ, Rogers J, Bloom FE. Arginine vasopressin deficient Brattleboro rats fail to develop tolerance to the hypothermic effects of ethanol. *Regul Pept* 1982;4:33–41.

212. Schmale H, Ivell R, Breindl M, et al. The mutant vasopressin gene from diabetes insipidus (Brattleboro) rats is transcribed but the message is not efficiently translated. *EMBO J* 1984;3:3289–3293.

213. Rabin RA, Molinoff PB. Activation of adenylate cyclase by ethanol in mouse striatal tissue. *J Pharmacol Exp Ther* 1981;216:129–134.

214. Saito T, Lee JM, Tabakoff B. Ethanol's effects on cortical adenylate cyclase activity. *J Neurochem* 1985;44:1037–1044.

215. Dar MS. Mouse cerebellar $GABA_B$ participation in the expression of acute ethanol-induced ataxia and in its modulation by the cerebellar adenosinergic A_1 system. *Brain Res Bull* 1996;41:53–59.

216. Dar MS. Mouse cerebellar adenosinergic modulation of ethanol-induced motor incoordination: possible involvement of cAMP. *Brain Res* 1997;749:263–274.

217. Froehlich JC, Wand GS. Adenylyl cyclase signal transduction and alcohol-induced sedation. *Pharmacol Biochem Behav* 1997;58:1021–1030.

218. Stenstrom S, Richelson E. Acute effect of ethanol on prostaglandin E_1-mediated cyclic AMP formation by a murine neuroblastoma clone. *J Pharmacol Exp Ther* 1982;221:334–341.

219. Rabin RA, Molinoff PB. Multiple sites of action of ethanol on adenylate cyclase. *J Pharmacol Exp Ther* 1983;227:551–556.

220. Wand G, Levin M, Zweifel L, et al. The cAMP-protein kinase A signal transduction pathway modulates consumption and sedative effects of ethanol. *J Neurosci* 2001;21:5297–5303.

221. Chik CL, Ho AK. Ethanol reduces norepinephrine-stimulated melatonin synthesis in rat pinealocytes. *J Neurochem* 1992;59:1280–1286.

222. Yoshimura M, Tabakoff B. Selective effects of ethanol on the generation of cAMP by particular members of the adenylyl cyclase. *Alcohol Clin Exp Res* 1995;19:1435–1440.

223. Hoffman PL, Yagi T, Tabakoff B, et al. Transgenic and gene "knockout" models in alcohol research. *Alcohol Clin Exp Res* 2001;25:60S–66S.

224. Hoffman PL, Moses F, Luthin GR, et al. Acute and chronic effects of ethanol on receptor-mediated phosphatidylinositol 4,5-bisphosphate breakdown in mouse brain. *Mol Pharmacol* 1986;30:13–18.

225. Gonzales RA, Theiss C, Crews FT. Effects of ethanol on stimulated inositol phospholipid hydrolysis in rat brain. *J Pharmacol Exp Ther* 1986;237:92–98.

226. Smith TL. The effects of acute exposure to ethanol on neurotensin and guanine-nucleotide-stimulation of phospholipase C activity in intact N1E-115 neuroblastoma cells. *Life Sci* 1990;47:115–119.

227. Sanna E, Dildy-Mayfield JE, Harris RA. Ethanol inhibits the function of 5-hydroxytryptamine type 1c and muscarinic M1 G protein-linked receptors in *Xenopus* oocytes expressing brain mRNA: role of protein kinase C. *Mol Pharmacol* 1994;45:1004–1012.

228. Bowers BJ, Wehner JM. Ethanol consumption and behavioral impulsivity are increased in protein kinase Cγ null mutant mice. *J Neurosci* 2001;21:RC180.

229. Proctor WR, Poelchen W, Bowers BJ, et al. Ethanol differentially enhances hippocampal $GABA_A$ receptor-mediated responses in protein kinase C gamma (PKC gamma) and PKC epsilon null mutant mice. *J Pharmacol Exp Ther* 2003;305:264–270.

230. Palmer MR, Morrow EL, Erwin VG. Calcium differentially alters behavioral and electrophysiological responses to ethanol in selectively bred mouse lines. *Alcohol Clin Exp Res* 1987;11:457–463.

231. Dolin SJ, Little HJ. Are changes in neuronal calcium channels involved in ethanol tolerance? *J Pharmacol Exp Ther* 1989;250:985–991.

232. Brown LM, Sims JS, Randall P, et al. V-conotoxin increases sleep time following ethanol injection. *Alcohol* 1993;10:159–162.

233. Leslie SW. Sedative-hypnotic drugs: interaction with calcium channels. *Alcohol Drug Res* 1986;6:371–377.

234. Carlen PL, Wu PH. Calcium and sedative-hypnotic drug actions. *Int Rev Neurobiol* 1988;29:161–189.

235. Daniell LC, Brass EP, Harris RA. Effect of ethanol on intracellular ionized calcium concentrations in synaptosomes and hepatocytes. *Mol Pharmacol* 1987;32:831–837.

236. Shah J, Pant HC. Spontaneous calcium release induced by ethanol in the isolated rat brain microsomes. *Brain Res* 1988;474:94–99.

237. Treistman SN, Wilson A. Effects of chronic ethanol on currents carried through calcium channels in *Aplysia*. *Alcohol Clin Exp Res* 1991;15:489–493.

238. Twombly DA, Herman MD, Kye CH, et al. Ethanol effects on two types of voltage-activated calcium channels. *J Pharmacol Exp Ther* 1990;254:1029–1037.

239. Mullikin-Kilpatrick D, Mehta ND, Hildebrandt JD, et al. G_i is involved in ethanol inhibition of L-type calcium channels in undifferentiated but not differentiated PC-12 cells. *Mol Pharmacol* 1995;47:997–1005.

240. Sanna E, Harris RA. Neuronal ion channels. *Recent Dev Alcohol* 1994;11:169–186.

241. Kukita F, Mitaku S. Kinetic analysis of the denaturation process by alcohols of sodium channels in squid giant axon. *J Physiol* 1993;463:523–543.

242. Krylov BV, Vilin YY, Katina IE, et al. Ethanol modulates the ionic permeability of sodium channels in rat sensory neurons. *Neurosci Behav Physiol* 2000;30:331–337.

243. Moore SD, Madamba SG, Siggins GR. Ethanol diminishes a voltage-dependent K^+ current, the M-current, in CA1 hippocampal pyramidal neurons *in vitro*. *Brain Res* 1990;516:222–228.

244. Anantharam V, Bayley H, Wilson A, et al. Differential effects of ethanol on electrical properties of various potassium channels expressed in oocytes. *Mol Pharmacol* 1992;42:499–505.

245. Yamakura T, Lewohl JM, Harris RA. Differential effects of general anesthetics on G protein-coupled inwardly rectifying and other potassium channels. *Anesthesiology* 2001;95:144–153.

246. Dopico AM, Lemos JR, Treistman SN. Ethanol increases the activity of large conductance, Ca^{2+}-activated K^+ channels in isolated neurohypophysial terminals. *Mol Pharmacol* 1996;49:40–48.

247. Dopico AM, Anantharam V, Treistman SN. Ethanol increases the activity of Ca^{++}-dependent K^+ (mslo) channels: functional interaction with cytosolic Ca^{++}. *J Pharmacol Exp Ther* 1998;284:258–268.

248. Covarrubias M, Vyas TB, Escobar L, et al. Alcohols inhibit a cloned potassium channel at a discrete saturable site. Insights into the molecular basis of general anesthesia. *J Biol Chem* 1995;270:19408–19416.

249. Kobayashi T, Ikeda K, Kojima H, et al. Ethanol opens G-protein-activated inwardly rectifying K+ channels. *Nat Neurosci* 1999;2:1091–1097.

250. Lewohl JM, Wilson WR, Mayfield RD, et al. G-protein-coupled inwardly rectifying potassium channels are targets of alcohol action. *Nat Neurosci* 1999;2:1084–1090.

251. Blednov YA, Stoffel M, Alva H, et al. A pervasive mechanism for analgesia: activation of GIRK2 channels. *Proc Natl Acad Sci U S A* 2003;100:277–282.

252. Blednov YA, Stoffel M, Chang SR, et al. Potassium channels as targets for ethanol: studies of G-protein-coupled inwardly rectifying potassium channel 2 (GIRK2) null mutant mice. *J Pharmacol Exp Ther* 2001;298:521–530.

253. Hill KG, Alva H, Blednov YA, et al. Reduced ethanol-induced conditioned taste aversion and conditioned place preference in GIRK2 null mutant mice. *Psychopharmacology (Berl)* 2003;169:108–114.

254. Espinosa F, McMahon A, Chan E, et al. Alcohol hypersensitivity, increased locomotion, and spontaneous myoclonus in mice lacking the potassium channels Kv3.1 and Kv3.3. *J Neurosci* 2001;21:6657–6665.

255. Weiner HL. The role of growth factor receptors in central nervous system development and neoplasia. *Neurosurgery* 1995;37:179–194.

256. Heldin C-H. Dimerization of cell surface receptors in signal transduction. *Cell* 1995;80:213–223.

257. Brodie C, Kentroti S, Vernadakis A. Growth factors attenuate the cholinotoxic effects of ethanol during early neuroembryogenesis in the chick embryo. *Int J Dev Neurosci* 1991;9:203–213.

258. Brodie C, Vernadakis A. Ethanol increases cholinergic and decreases GABAergic neuronal expression in cultures derived from 8-day-old chick embryo cerebral hemispheres: interaction of ethanol and growth factors. *Dev Brain Res* 1992;65:253–257.

259. Heaton MB, Paiva M, Swanson DJ, et al. Modulation of ethanol neurotoxicity by nerve growth factor. *Brain Res* 1993;620:78–85.

260. Heaton MB, Paiva M, Swanson DJ, et al. Responsiveness of cultured septal and hippocampal neurons to ethanol and neurotrophic substances. *J Neurosci Res* 1994;39:305–318.

261. Heaton MB, Mitchell JJ, Paiva M. Overexpression of NGF ameliorates ethanol neurotoxicity in the developing cerebellum. *J Neurobiol* 2000;45:95–104.

262. Bonthius DJ, Karacay B, Dai D, et al. FGF-2, NGF, IGF-1, but not BDNF, utilize a nitric oxide pathway to signal neurotrophic and neuroprotective effects against alcohol toxicity in cerebellar granule cell cultures. *Dev Brain Res* 2003;140:15–28.

263. Bradley DM, Beaman FD, Moore DB, et al. Neurotrophic factors BDNF and GDNF protect embryonic chick spinal cord motoneurons from ethanol neurotoxicity *in vivo*. *Dev Brain Res* 1999;112:99–106.

264. McAlhany RE Jr, West JR, Miranda RC. Glial-derived neurotrophic factor (GDNF) prevents ethanol-induced apoptosis and JUN kinase phosphorylation. *Dev Brain Res* 2000;119:209–216.

265. Messing RO, Henteleff M, Park JJ. Ethanol enhances growth factor-induced neurite formation in PC12 cells. *Brain Res* 1991;565:301–311.

266. Roivainen R, Hundle B, Messing RO. Ethanol enhances growth factor activation of mitogen-activated protein kinases by a protein kinase C-dependent mechanism. *Proc Natl Acad Sci U S A* 1995;92:1891–1895.

267. Resnicoff M, Sell C, Ambrose D, et al. Ethanol inhibits the autophosphorylation of the insulin-like growth factor 1 receptor and the IGF-1-mediated proliferation of 3T3 cells. *J Biol Chem* 1993;268:21777–21782.

268. Resnicoff M, Rubini M, Barsega R, et al. Ethanol inhibits insulin-like growth factor-1-mediated signaling and proliferation of C6 glioblastoma cells. *J Clin Invest* 1994;71:657–662.

269. Xu YY, Bhavani K, Wands JR, et al. Ethanol inhibits insulin receptor substrate-1 tyrosine phosphorylation and insulin-stimulated neuronal thread protein gene expression. *Biochem J* 1995;310:125–132.

270. Tomono M, Kiss Z. Ethanol enhances the stimulatory effects of insulin and insulin-like growth factor-1 on DNA synthesis in NIH 3T3 fibroblasts. *Biochem Biophys Res Commun* 1995;208:63–67.

271. Heaton MB, Madorsky I, Paiva M, et al. Influence of ethanol on neonatal cerebellum of BDNF gene-deleted animals: analysis of effects on Purkinje cells, apoptosis-related proteins, and endogenous antioxidants. *J Neurobiol* 2002;51:160–176.

272. Szabó G, Hoffman PL. Brain-derived neurotrophic factor, neurotrophin-3 and neurotrophin-4/5 maintain functional tolerance to ethanol. *Eur J Pharmacol* 1995;287:35–41.

273. Valenzuela CF, Kazlauskas A, Brozowski SJ, et al. Platelet-derived growth factor is a novel modulator of type A γ-aminobutyric acid-gated ion channels. *Mol Pharmacol* 1995;48:1099–1107.

274. Valenzuela CF, Xiong Z, MacDonald JF, et al. Platelet-derived growth factor (PDGF) induces a long-term inhibition of NMDA receptor function. *J Biol Chem* 1996;271:16151–16159.

275. Lo DC. Neurotrophic factors and synaptic plasticity. *Neuron* 1995;15:979–981.

276. Valenzuela CF, Harris RA. Effects of ethanol on PDGF receptor-dependent signal transduction. *Alcohol Clin Exp Res* 1995;19[Suppl]:32A.

277. Knapp RJ, Malatynska E, Collins N, et al. Molecular biology and pharmacology of cloned opioid receptors. *FASEB J* 1995;9:516–525.

278. Tabakoff B, Hoffman PL. Alcohol interactions with brain opiate receptors. *Life Sci* 1983;32:197–204.

279. Hiller JM, Angel JM, Simon EJ. Characterization of the selective inhibition of the delta subclass of opioid binding sites by alcohols. *Science* 1981;214:468–469.

280. Khatami S, Hoffman PL, Shibuya T, et al. Selective effects of ethanol on

opiate receptor subtypes in brain. *Neuropharmacology* 1987;26:1503–1507.

281. Seizinger BR, Bovermann K, Maysinger D, et al. Differential effects of acute and chronic ethanol treatment on particular opioid peptide systems in discrete regions of brain and pituitary. *Pharmacol Biochem Behav* 1983;18:361–369.

282. Ryder S, Straus E, Lieber CS, et al. Cholecystokinin and enkephalin levels following ethanol administration in rats. *Peptides* 1981;2:223–226.

283. Dave JR, Tabakoff B, Hoffman PL. Ethanol withdrawal seizures produce increased c-fos mRNA in mouse brain. *Mol Pharmacol* 1990;37:367–371.

284. Genazzani AR, Nappi G, Facchinetti F, et al. Central deficiency of β-endorphin in alcohol addicts. *J Clin Endocrinol Metab* 1982;55:583–586.

285. Borg S, Kvande H, Rydberg U, et al. Endorphin levels in human cerebrospinal fluid during alcohol intoxication and withdrawal. *Psychopharmacology (Berl)* 1982;78:101–103.

286. Gianoulakis C, De Waele JP, Kiianmaa K. Differences in the brain and pituitary β-endorphin system between the alcohol-preferring AA and alcohol avoiding ANA rats. *Alcohol Clin Exp Res* 1992;16:453–459.

287. Hyytia P. Involvement of μ-opioid systems in alcohol drinking by alcohol preferring rats. *Pharmacol Biochem Behav* 1993;45:697–701.

288. De Waele JP, Kiianmaa K, Gianoulakis C. Spontaneous and ethanol-stimulated in vitro release of β-endorphin by the hypothalamus of AA and ANA rats. *Alcohol Clin Exp Res* 1994;18:1468–1473.

289. Herz A. Endogenous opioid systems and alcohol addiction. *Psychopharmacology (Berl)* 1997;129:99–111.

290. Gianoulakis C. Influence of the endogenous opioid system on high alcohol consumption and genetic predisposition to alcoholism. *J Psychiatry Neurosci* 2001;26:304–318.

291. Roberts AJ, McDonald JS, Heyser CJ, et al. μ-Opioid receptor knockout mice do not self-administer alcohol. *J Pharmacol Exp Ther* 2000;293:1002–1008.

292. Hall FS, Sora I, Uhl GR. Ethanol consumption and reward are decreased in μ-opiate receptor knockout mice. *Psychopharmacology (Berl)* 2001;154:43–49.

293. Roberts AJ, Gold LH, Polis I, et al. Increased ethanol self-administration in delta-opioid receptor knockout mice. *Alcohol Clin Exp Res* 2001;25:1249–1256.

294. Olive MF, Koenig HN, Nannini MA, et al. Stimulation of endorphin neurotransmission in the nucleus accumbens by ethanol, cocaine, and amphetamine. *J Neurosci* 2001;21:RC184.

295. Heyser CJ, Roberts AJ, Schulteis G, et al. Central administration of an opiate antagonist decreases oral ethanol self-administration in rats. *Alcohol Clin Exp Res* 1999;23:1468–1476.

296. Myers RD, Robinson DE. Mmu and D2 receptor antisense oligonucleotides injected in nucleus accumbens suppress high alcohol intake in genetic drinking HEP rats. *Alcohol* 1999;18:225–233.

297. Benjamin D, Grant ER, Pohorecky LA. Naltrexone reverses ethanol-induced dopamine release in the nucleus accumbens in awake, freely moving rats. *Brain Res* 1993;621:137–140.

298. Acquas E, Meloni M, Di Chiara G. Blockade of delta-opioid receptors I the nucleus accumbens prevents ethanol-induced stimulation of dopamine release. *Eur J Pharmacol* 1993;230:239–241.

299. Gonzales RA, Weiss F. Suppression of ethanol-reinforced behavior by naltrexone is associated with attenuation of the ethanol-induced increase in dialysate dopamine levels in the nucleus accumbens. *J Neurosci* 1998;18:10663–10671.

300. Koistinen M, Tuomainen P, Hyytia P, et al. naltrexone suppresses ethanol intake in 6-hydroxydopamine-treated rats. *Alcohol Clin Exp Res* 2001;25:1605–1612.

301. Volpicelli JR, Alterman AI, Hayashida M, et al. Naltrexone in the treatment of alcohol dependence. *Arch Gen Psychiatry* 1992;49:876–880.

302. O'Malley SS, Jaffe AJ, Chang G, et al. Naltrexone and coping skills therapy for alcohol dependence. A controlled study. *Arch Gen Psychiatry* 1992;49:881–887.

303. Anton RF, Moak DH, Waid LR, et al. Naltrexone and cognitive behavioral therapy for the treatment of outpatient alcoholics: results of a placebo-controlled trial. *Am J Psychiatry* 1999;156:1758–1764.

304. Volpicelli JR, Watson NT, King AC, et al. Effect of naltrexone on alcohol "high" in alcoholics. *Am J Psychiatry* 1995;152:613–615.

305. Krystal JH, Cramer JA, Krol WF, et al. Naltrexone in the treatment of alcohol dependence. *N Engl J Med* 2001;345:1734–1739.

306. Basavarajappa BS, Hungund B. Neuromodulatory role of the endocannabinoid signaling system in alcoholism: an overview. *Prostaglandins Leukot Essent Fatty Acids* 2002;66:287–299.

307. Arnone M, Maruani J, Chaperon F, et al. Selective inhibition of sucrose and ethanol intake by SR 141716, an antagonist of central cannabinoid (CB1) receptors. *Psychopharmacology (Berl)* 1997;132:104–106.

308. Colombo G, Agabio R, Fa M, et al. Reduction of voluntary ethanol in take in ethanol preferring sP rats by the cannabinoid antagonist SR-141716. *Alcohol Alcohol* 1998;33:126–130.

309. Colombo G, Serra S, Brunetti G, et al. Stimulation of voluntary ethanol intake by cannabinoid receptor agonists in ethanol-preferring sP rats. *Psychopharmacology (Berl)* 2002;159:181–187.

310. Freedland CS, Sharpe AL, Samson HH, et al. Effects of SR141716A on ethanol and sucrose self-administration. *Alcohol Clin Exp Res* 2001;25:277–282.

311. Hungund BL, Szakall I, Adam A, et al. Cannabinoid CB1 receptor knockout mice exhibit markedly reduced voluntary alcohol consumption and lack alcohol-induced dopamine release in the nucleus accumbens. *J Neurochem* 2003;84:698–704.

312. Racz I, Bilkei-Gorzo A, Toth ZE, et al. A critical role for the cannabinoid CB_1 receptors in alcohol dependence and stress-stimulated ethanol drinking. *J Neurosci* 2003;23:2453–2458.

313. Basavarajappa BS, Hungund B. Downregulation of cannabinoid receptor agonist-stimulated [35S]GTPγS binding in synaptic plasma membrane from chronic ethanol exposed mouse. *Brain Res* 1999;815:89–97.

314. Kalra SP, Dube MG, Sahu A, et al. Neuropeptide Y secretion increases in the paraventricular nucleus in association with increased appetite for food. *Proc Natl Acad Sci U S A* 1991;88:10931–10935.

315. Thiele TE, Marsh DJ, Ste Marie L, et al. Ethanol consumption and resistance are inversely related to neuropeptide Y levels. *Nature* 1998;396:366–369.

316. Thiele TE, Koh MT, Pedrazzini T. Voluntary alcohol consumption is controlled via the neuropeptide Y Y1 receptor. *J Neurosci* 2002;22:RC206.

317. Thorsell A, Rimondini R, Heilig M. Blockade of central neuropeptide Y (NPY) Y2 receptors reduces ethanol self-administration in rats. *Neurosci Lett* 2002;332:1–4.

318. Thiele TE, Miura GI, Marsh DJ, et al. Neurobiological responses to ethanol in mutant mice lacking neuropeptide Y or the Y5 receptor. *Pharmacol Biochem Behav* 2000;67:683–691.

319. Badia-Elder NE, Stewart RB, Powrozek TA, et al. Effect of neuropeptide Y (NPY) on oral ethanol intake in Wistar alcohol-preferring (P), and -nonpreferring (NP) rats. *Alcohol Clin Exp Res* 2001;25:386–390.

320. Hwang BH, Zhang JK, Ehlers CL, et al. Innate differences of neuropeptide Y

(NPY) in hypothalamic nuclei and central nucleus of the amygdala between selectively bred rats with high and low alcohol preference. *Alcohol Clin Exp Res* 1999;23:1023–1030.

321. Slawecki CJ, Betancourt M, Walpole T, et al. Increases in sucrose consumption, but not ethanol consumption, following ICV NPY administration. *Pharmacol Biochem Behav* 2000;66:591–594.

322. Katner SN, Slawecki CJ, Ehlers CL. Neuropeptide Y administration into the amygdala does not affect ethanol consumption. *Alcohol* 2002;28:29–38.

323. Kelley SP, Nannini MA, Bratt AM, et al. Neuropeptide-Y in the paraventricular nucleus increases ethanol self-administration. *Peptides* 2001;22:515–522.

324. Roy A, Pandey S. The decreased cellular expression of neuropeptide Y protein in rat brain structures during ethanol withdrawal after chronic ethanol exposure. *Alcohol Clin Exp Res* 2002;26:796–803.

325. Woldbye DPD, Ulrichsen J, Haugbl S, et al. Ethanol withdrawal in rats is attenuated by intracerebroventricular administration of neuropeptide Y. *Alcohol Alcohol* 2002;37:318–321.

326. Nash J Jr, Maickel RP. The role of the hypothalamic-pituitary-adrenocortical axis in post-stress-induced ethanol consumption by rats. *Prog Neuropsychopharmacol Biol Psychiatry* 1988;12:653–671.

327. Higley JD, Hasert MF, Suomi SJ, et al. Nonhuman primate model of alcohol abuse: effect of early experience, personality, and stress on alcohol consumption. *Proc Nat Acad Sci U S A* 1991;88:7261–7265.

328. Mollenauer S, Bryson R, Robinson M, et al. EtOH self-administration in anticipation of noise stress in C57BL/6J mice. *Pharmacol Biochem Behav* 1993;46:35–38.

329. Lê AD, Quan B, Juzytch W, et al. Reinstatement of alcohol-seeking by priming injections of alcohol and exposure to stress in rats. *Psychopharmacology (Berl)* 1998;135:169–174.

330. Rivier C. Alcohol stimulates ACTH secretion in the rat: mechanisms of action and interactions with other stimuli. *Alcohol Clin Exp Res* 1996;20:240–254.

331. Fahlke C, Hard E, Hansen S. Facilitation of ethanol consumption by intracerebroventricular infusions of corticosterone. *Psychopharmacology (Berl)* 1996;127:133–139.

332. Lamblin F, DE Witte P. Adrenalectomy prevents the development of alcohol preference in male rats. *Alcohol* 1996;13:233–238.

333. Fahlke C, Hansen S. Effect of local intracerebral corticosterone implants on alcohol intake in the rat. *Alcohol Alcohol* 1999;34:851–861.

334. Fahlke C, Eriksson CJ. Effect of adrenalectomy and exposure to corticosterone on alcohol intake in alcohol-preferring and alcohol-avoiding rat lines. *Alcohol Alcohol* 2000;35:139–144.

335. Weiss F, Ciccocioppo R, Parsons LH, et al. Compulsive drug-seeking behavior and relapse. Neuroadaptation, stress, and conditioning factors. *Ann N Y Acad Sci* 2001;937:1–26.

336. Dunn AJ, Berridge CW. Physiological and behavioral responses to corticotropin-releasing factor administration: I CRF a mediator of anxiety or stress responses? *Brain Res Rev* 1990;15:71–100.

337. Koob GF, Heinrichs SC, Menzaghi F, et al. Corticotropin releasing factor, stress and behavior. *Semin Neurosci* 1994;6:221–229.

338. Merlo Pich E, Lorang MT, Yeganeh M, et al. Increase of extracellular corticotropin-releasing factor-like immunoreactivity levels in the amygdala of awake rats during stress and ethanol withdrawal as measured by microdialysis. *J Neurosci* 1995;18:5439–5447.

339. Merali Z, McIntosh J, Kent P, et al. Aversive and appetitive events evoke the release of corticotropin-releasing hormone and bombesin-like peptides at the central nucleus of the amygdala. *J Neurosci* 1998;18:4758–4766.

340. Heinrichs SC, Merlo Pich E, Miczek KA, et al. Corticotropin-releasing factor reduces emotionality in socially defeated rats via direct neurotropic action. *Brain Res* 1992;581:190–197.

341. Swiergiel AH, Takahashi LK, Kalin NH. Attenuation of stress-induced behavior by antagonism of corticotropin-releasing factor receptors in the central amygdala in the rat. *Brain Res* 1993;623:229–234.

342. Merlo Pich E, Lorang M, Yeganeh M, et al. Increase of extracellular corticotropin releasing factor-like immunoreactivity levels in the amygdala of awake rats during restraint stress and ethanol withdrawal as measured by microdialysis. *J Neurosci* 1995;5439–5447.

343. Rassnick S, Heinrichs SC, Britton KT, et al. Microinjection of a corticotropin-releasing factor antagonist into the central nucleus of the amygdala reverses anxiogenic-like effects of ethanol withdrawal. *Brain Res* 1993;605:25–32.

344. Macey DJ, Basso AM, Rivier J, et al. Corticotropin releasing factor (CRF) decreases brain stimulation reward in the rat. *Soc Neurosci Abstr* 1997;23:521.

345. Koob GF. Stress, corticotropin-releasing factor, and drug addiction. *Ann N Y Acad Sci* 1999;897:27–45.

346. Lee S, Smith GW, Vale W, et al. Mice that lack corticotropin-releasing factor (CRF) receptors type 1 show a blunted ACTH response to acute alcohol despite up-regulated constitutive hypothalamic CRF gene expression. *Alcohol Clin Exp Res* 2001;25:427–433.

347. Sillaber I, Rammes G, Zimmermann S, et al. Enhanced and delayed stress-induced alcohol drinking in mice lacking functional CRH1 receptors. *Science* 2002;296:931–933.

348. Olive MF, Mehmert KK, Koenig HN, et al. A role for corticotropin-releasing factor (CRF) in ethanol consumption sensitivity, and reward as revealed by CRF-deficient mice. *Psychopharmacology (Berl)* 2003;165:181–187.

349. Mayfield RD, Lewohl JM, Dodd PR, et al. Patterns of gene expression are altered in the frontal and motor cortices of human alcoholics. *J Neurochem* 2002;81:802–813.

350. Maroteaux L, Campanelli JT, Scheller RA. Synuclein: a neuron-specific protein localized to the nucleus and presynaptic nerve terminal. *J Neurosci* 1988;8:2804–2815.

351. Iwai A, Masliah E, Yoshimoto M, et al. The precursor protein of non-A beta component of Alzheimer's disease amyloid is a presynaptic protein of the central nervous system. *Neuron* 1995;14:467–475.

352. Mori F, Tanji K, Yoshimoto M, et al. Immunohistochemical comparison of alpha- and beta-synuclein in adult rat central nervous system. *Brain Res* 2002;941:118–126.

353. Perez RG, Waymire JC, Line E, et al. A role for alpha-synuclein in the regulation of dopamine biosynthesis. *J Neurosci* 2002;22:3090–3099.

354. Liang T, Spence J, Liu L, et al. α-Synuclein maps to a quantitative trait locus for alcohol preference and is differentially expressed in alcohol-preferring and -nonpreferring rats. *Proc Natl Acad Sci U S A* 2003;100:4690–4695.

355. Enomoto N, Takase S, Yasuhara M, et al. Acetaldehyde metabolism in different aldehyde dehydrogenase-2 genotypes. *Alcohol Clin Exp Res* 1991;15:141–144.

356. Higuchi S, Muramatsu T, Shigemori K, et al. The relationship between low Km aldehyde dehydrogenase phenotype and drinking behavior in Japanese. *J Stud Alcohol* 1992;53:170–175.

357. Hunt WA. Role of acetaldehyde in the actions of ethanol on the brain-a review. *Alcohol* 1996;13:147–151.

358. Aragon CM, Amit Z. The effect

of 3-amino-1,2,4-triazole on voluntary ethanol consumption: evidence for brain catalase involvement in the mechanism of action. *Neuropharmacology* 1992;31:709–712.

359. Gill K, Menez JF, Lucas D, et al. Enzymatic production of acetaldehyde from ethanol in rat brain tissue. *Alcohol Clin Exp Res* 1992;16:910–905.

360. Zimatkin SM, Liopo AV, Satanovskaya VI, et al. Relationship of brain ethanol metabolism to the hypnotic effect of ethanol. II: studies in selectively bred rats and mice. *Alcohol Clin Exp Res* 2001;25:982–988.

361. Zimatkin SM, Liopo AV, Satanovskaya VI, et al. Relationship of brain ethanol metabolism to the hypnotic effect of ethanol. II: studies in outbred animals. *Alcohol Clin Exp Res* 2001;25:976–981.

362. Correa M, Sanchis-Segura C, Aragon CMG. Influence of brain catalase on ethanol-induced loss of righting reflex in mice. *Drug Alcohol Depend* 2001;65:9–15.

363. Correa M, Sanchis-Segura C, Aragon CMG. Brain catalase activity is highly correlated with ethanol-induced locomotor activity in mice. *Physiol Behav* 2001;73:641–647.

364. Amit Z, Brown ZW, Rockman GE. Possible involvement of acetaldehyde, norepinephrine and their tetrahydroisoquinoline derivatives in the regulation of ethanol self-administration. *Drug Alcohol Depend* 1977;2:495–500.

365. Brown ZW, Amit Z, Rockman GE. Intraventricular self-administration of acetaldehyde, but not ethanol, in naïve laboratory rats. *Psychopharmacology (Berl)* 1979;64:271–276.

366. Brown ZW, Amit Z, Smith B. Intraventricular self-administration of acetaldehyde and voluntary consumption of ethanol in rats. *Behav Neural Biol* 1980;28:150–155.

367. Smith BR, Amit Z, Splawinsky J. Conditioned place preference induced by intraventricular infusions of acetaldehyde. *Alcohol* 1984;1:193–195.

368. Aragon CM, Sternklar G, Amit Z. A correlation between voluntary ethanol consumption and brain catalase activity in the rat. *Alcohol* 1985;2:353–356.

369. Amit Z, Aragon CMG. Catalase activity measured in rats naïve to ethanol correlates with later voluntary ethanol consumption: possible evidence for a biological marker system of ethanol intake. *Psychopharmacology (Berl)* 1988;95:512–515.

370. Quertemont E, De Witte P. Conditioned stimulus preference after acetaldehyde but not ethanol injections. *Pharmacol Biochem Behav* 2001;68:449–454.

371. Rodd-Henricks ZA, Melendez RI,
Zaffaroni A, et al. The reinforcing effects of acetaldehyde in the posterior ventral tegmental area of alcohol-preferring rats. *Pharmacol Biochem Behav* 2002;72:55–64.

372. Rodd-Henricks ZA, McKinzie DL, Murphy JM, et al. Regional heterogeneity for the intracranial self-administration of ethanol within the ventral tegmental area of female Wistar rats. *Psychopharmacology (Berl)* 2000;149:217–224.

373. Quertemont E, Grant KA. Role of acetaldehyde in the discriminative stimulus effects of ethanol. *Alcohol Clin Exp Res* 2002;26:812–817.

374. Ward RJ, Colantuoni C, Dahchour A, et al. Acetaldehyde-induced changes in the monoamine and amino acid extracellular microdialysate content of the nucleus accumbens. *Neuropharmacology* 1997;36:225–232.

375. Sjoquist B, Liljequist S, Engel J. Increased salsolinol levels in rat striatum and limbic forebrain following chronic ethanol treatment. *J Neurochem* 1982;39:259–262.

376. Haber H, Roske I, Rottmann M, et al. Alcohol induces formation of morphine precursors in the striatum of rats. *Life Sci* 1997;60:79–89.

377. Myers RD, Melchior CL. Alcohol drinking: abnormal intake caused by tetrahydropapaveroline in brain. *Science* 1977;196:554–556.

378. Duncan C, Deitrich RA. A critical evaluation of tetrahydroisoquinoline-induced ethanol preference in rats. *Pharmacol Biochem Behav* 1980;13:265–281.

379. McBride WJ, Li T-K, Deitrich RA, et al. Involvement of acetaldehyde in alcohol addiction. *Alcohol Clin Exp Res* 2002;26:114–119.

380. Mascia MP, Maiya R, Borghese CM, et al. Does acetaldehyde mediate ethanol action in the central nervous system? *Alcohol Clin Exp Res* 2001;25:1570–1575.

381. Carmichael FJ, Israel Y, Crawford M, et al. Central nervous system effects of acetate: contribution to the central effects of ethanol. *J Pharmacol Exp Ther* 1991;259:403–408.

382. Gonthier B, Eysseric H, Soubeyran A, et al. Free radical production after exposure of astrocytes and astrocytic C6 glioma cells to ethanol. Preliminary results. *Free Radic Res* 1997;27:645–656.

383. Waniewski RA, Martin DL. Preferential utilization of acetate by astrocytes is attributable to transport. *J Neurosci* 1998;18:5225–5233.

384. Israel Y, Orrego H, Carmichael FJ. Acetate-mediated effects of ethanol. *Alcohol Clin Exp Res* 1994;18:144–148.

385. Cullen N, Carlen PL. Electrophysiolog-
ical actions of acetate, a metabolite of ethanol, on hippocampal dentate granule neurons: interactions with adenosine. *Brain Res* 1992;588:49–57.

386. Brundege JM, Dunwiddie TV. The role of acetate as a potential mediator of the effects of ethanol in the brain. *Neurosci Lett* 1995;186:214–218.

387. Phillips TJ, Belknap, JK. Complex-trait genetics: emergence of multivariate strategies. *Nat Rev Neurosci* 2002;3:478–485.

388. Crabbe JC, Phillips TJ, Buck KJ, et al. Identifying genes for alcohol and drug sensitivity: recent progress and future directions. *Trends Neurosci* 1999;22:173–179.

389. Crabbe JC. Alcohol and genetics: new models. *Am J Med Gen* 2002;114:969–974.

390. Buck KJ, Metten P, Belknap JK, et al. Quantitative trait loci involved in genetic predisposition to acute alcohol withdrawal in mice. *J Neurosci* 1997;17:3946–3955.

391. Phillips TJ, Crabbe JC, Metten P, et al. Localization of genes affecting alcohol drinking in mice. *Alcohol Clin Exp Res* 1994;18:931–941.

392. Phillips TJ, Belknap JK, Buck KJ, et al. Genes on mouse chromosomes 2 and 9 determine variation in ethanol consumption. *Mamm Genome* 1998;9:936–941.

393. Belknap JK, Richards SP, O'Toole LA, et al. Short-term selective breeding as a tool for QTL mapping: ethanol preference drinking in mice. *Behav Genet* 1997;27:55–66.

394. Fehr C, Shirley RL, Belknap JK, et al. Congenic mapping of alcohol and pentobarbital withdrawal liability loci to a <1 centimorgan interval of murine chromosome 4: identification of Mpdz as a candidate gene. *J Neurosci* 2002;22:3730–3738.

395. Lewohl JM, Dodd PR, Mayfield RD, et al. Application of DNA microarrays to study human alcoholism. *J Biomed Sci* 2001;8:28–36.

396. Rahman S, Miles MF. Identification of novel ethanol-sensitive genes by expression profiling. *Pharmacol Ther* 2001;92:123–134.

397. Miles MF. Alcohol's effects on gene expression. *Alcohol Health Res World* 1995;19:237–243.

398. Thibault C, Lai C, Wilke N, et al. Expression profiling of neural cells reveals specific patterns of ethanol-responsive gene expression. *Mol Pharmacol* 2000;52:1593–1600.

399. Lewohl JM, Wang L, Miles MF, et al. Gene expression in human alcoholism: microarray analysis of frontal cortex. *Alcohol Clin Exp Res* 2000;24:1873–1882.

400. Xu Y, Ehringer M, Yang F, et al. Comparison of global brain gene expression profiles between inbred long-sleep and inbred short-sleep mice by high-density gene array hybridization. *Alcohol Clin Exp Res* 2001;25:810–818.

401. Saito M, Smiley J, Toth R, et al. Microarray analysis of gene expression in rat hippocampus after chronic ethanol treatment. *Neurochem Res* 2002;27:1221–1229.

402. Shelton KL, Young JE, Grant KA. A multiple schedule model of limited access drinking in the cynomolgus macaque. *Behav Pharmacol* 2001; 12:559–573.

403. Sinclair JD, Senter RJ. Increased preference for ethanol in rats following alcohol deprivation. *Psychosom Sci* 1967;8:11–16.

404. Lê AD, Shaham Y. Neurobiology of relapse to alcohol in rats. *Pharmacol Ther* 2002;94:137–156.

405. Spanagel R, Holter SM. Pharmacological validation of a new animal model of alcoholism. *J Neural Transm* 2000;107:669–680.

406. Hodos W. Progressive ratio as a measurement of reward strength. *Science* 1961;134:943–944.

407. Richardson NR, Roberts DC. Progressive ratio schedules in drug self-administration studies in rats: a method to evaluate reinforcing efficacy. *J Neurosci Methods* 1996;66:1–11.

408. McKinzie DL, Nowak KL, Yorger L, et al. The alcohol deprivation effect in the alcohol-preferring P rat under free-drinking and operant access conditions. *Alcohol Clin Exp Res* 1998;22:1170–1176.

409. Sinclair JD, Li TK. Long and short alcohol deprivation: effects on AA and P alcohol-preferring rats. *Alcohol* 1989;6:505–509.

410. Hilakivi L, Eriksson CJ, Sarviharju M, et al. Revitalization of the AA and ANA rat lines: effects on some line characteristics. *Alcohol* 1984;1:71–75.

411. Rodd-Henricks ZA, McKinzie DL, Murphy JM, et al. The expression of an alcohol deprivation effect in the high-alcohol-drinking replicate rat lines is dependent on repeated deprivations. *Alcohol Clin Exp Res* 2000;24:747–753.

412. Li TK. Clinical perspectives for the study of craving and relapse in animal models. *Addiction* 2000;95:S55–S60.

413. Stewart J, de Wit H. Reinstatement of drug-taking behavior as a method of assessing incentive motivational properties of drugs. In: MA Bozarth, ed. *Methods of assessing the reinforcing properties of abused drugs.* New York: Springer-Verlag, 1987:211–227.

414. Ciccocioppo R, Angeletti S, Weiss F. Long-lasting resistance to extinction of relapse reinstatement induced by ethanol-related stimuli: role of genetic ethanol preference. *Alcohol Clin Exp Res* 2001;25:1414–1419.

415. Chiamulera C, Valerio E, Tessari M. Resumption of ethanol-seeking behaviour in rats. *Behav Pharmacol* 1995;6:32–39.

416. Bienkowski P, Kostowski W, Koros E. The role of drug-paired stimuli in extinction and reinstatement of ethanol-seeking behaviour in the rat. *Eur J Pharmacol* 1999;374:315–319.

417. Bienkowski P, Koros E, Kostowski W, et al. Reinstatement of ethanol seeking in rats: behavioral analysis. *Pharmacol Biochem Behav* 2000;66:123–128.

418. Lê AD, Poulos CX, Harding S, et al. Effects of naltrexone and fluoxetine on alcohol self-administration and reinstatement of alcohol seeking induced by priming injections of alcohol and exposure to stress. *Neuropsychopharmacology* 1999;21:435–444.

419. Katner SN, Magalong JG, Weiss F. Reinstatement of alcohol-seeking behavior by drug-associated discriminative stimuli after prolonged extinction in the rat. *Neuropsychopharmacology* 1999;20:471–479.

420. Katner SN, Weiss F. Ethanol-associated olfactory stimuli reinstate ethanol-seeking behavior after extinction and modify extracellular dopamine levels in the nucleus accumbens. *Alcohol Clin Exp Res* 1999;23:1751–1760.

421. Liu X, Weiss F. Stimulus conditioned to foot-shock stress reinstates alcohol-seeking behavior in an animal model of relapse. *Psychopharmacology (Berl)* 2003;168:184–191.

422. Kamin LJ. Predictability, surprise, attention and conditioning. In: Campbell BA, Church RM, eds. *Punishment and aversive behavior.* New York: Appleton-Century-Crofts, 1969:279–296.

423. Lê AD, Harding S, Juzytsch W, et al. The role of corticotropin-releasing factor in the median raphe nucleus in relapse to alcohol. *J Neurosci* 2002;22:7844–7849.

424. Ciccocioppo R, Lin D, Martin-Fardon R, et al. Reinstatement of ethanol-seeking behavior by drug cues following signal versus multiple ethanol intoxication in the rat: Effects of naltrexone. *Psychopharmacology (Berl)* 2003;168:208–215.

425. Nie H, Janak PH. Comparison of reinstatement of ethanol- and sucrose-seeking by conditioned stimuli and priming injections of allopregnanolone after extinction in rats. *Psychopharmacology (Berl)* 2003;168:222–228.

426. Liu X, Weiss F. Reversal of ethanol-seeking behavior by D1 and D2 antagonists in an animal model of relapse: Differences in antagonist potency in previously ethanol-dependent versus nondependent rats. *J Pharmacol Exp Ther* 2002;300:882–889.

CHAPTER 9

Alcohol: Clinical Aspects

BANKOLE A. JOHNSON, MD, PHD
AND NASSIMA AIT-DAOUD, MD

HISTORY AND DEFINITION

For more than 200 years, the medical profession has attempted to define alcoholism. As early as 1784, Benjamin Rush recognized that a key component of alcoholism is an inability to control the urge to drink (1), and among the earliest descriptions of delirium tremens were those proposed independently by Pearson and Sutton in 1813 (2). René-Théophile Hyacinthe Laennëc, writing in 1802 to 1803, while still a medical student, described the "tawny" appearance of the liver of an alcoholic, later termed *Laennec's cirrhosis* (3,4). The importance of moderate drinking, promulgated by individuals such as Sir William Osler (1849–1919), gave rise to the temperance movement, which he went on to describe as "becoming a characteristic for Americans" (3). This movement enshrined the pre-Darwinian concept of *degenerationism,* whereby a multitude of moral vices such as alcoholism (but also strokes, epilepsy, and dementia, among others) were passed on to succeeding generations until the family line became extinct. While this provided for a "medicalization" of the alcoholism concept and a focus on the individual rather than the disease itself, it also brought about futile attempts at eradication such as the prohibition movement in the United States. It was not until 1954, in a World Health Organization report, that Griffith Edwards turned attention back to the pharmacologic effects of alcohol as the critical factor in the disease process (5). This notion gained ground and was expanded in the writings of Jellinek, who linked the features of tolerance and adaptation to the "craving" to drink excessively (6).

Nowadays, our characterization of the alcoholism disease is based on the understanding that it is a multifactorial, chronic disease that might be brought about by a mixture of genetic, biologic, social, cultural, and environmental factors. It is evident that alcoholism is not a homogeneous disease but consists of subtypes, each with varying degrees of biologic and psychosocial antecedents (7–10). Standardized nomenclatures, such as the *Diagnostic and Statistical Manual of Mental Disorders,* 4th edition, text revision (*DSM–IV–TR*), define the core features of alcoholism, which encompass the concepts of tolerance, withdrawal, and reinstatement after a period of abstinence (11). The *DSM–IV–TR* is widely used throughout the world, and the term *alcohol dependence* is used in favor of *alcoholism* to remove emphasis on the individual but instead focus on the concept of disease. In this chapter, however, the terms are used interchangeably. Table 9.1 lists the *DSM–IV–TR* criteria for alcohol dependence.

EPIDEMIOLOGY

Alcoholism is a major cause of morbidity and mortality in the United States and worldwide. In the United States and worldwide (12), alcohol dependence ranks third and fifth, respectively, with respect to disease impact. Globally, the disease impact of alcoholism is greatest in regions with the highest per-capita consumption such as Latin America, and is smallest in regions like the Middle East where drinking levels are relatively low. In the United States, there are 8 million individuals dependent on alcohol (13). An additional 5.6 million American citizens abuse alcohol (13). Not only is the disease prevalence for alcoholism high, but it also tends to run in families. More than half of American adults have a close family member who is dependent on alcohol (14), and greater than 25% of children younger than age 18 years have knowledge of a relative with alcoholism (15). Society pays a high price for the consequences of alcoholism. In all, alcohol abuse costs the nation about $185 billion per annum—more than $600 for every man, woman, and child living in the United States (16).

Alcoholism is associated with a range of physical and mental disorders. Perhaps the best known disease associated with alcoholism is liver cirrhosis. In the United States, about 900,000 individuals have liver cirrhosis; of

TABLE 9.1. *DSM–IV-TR Diagnostic criteria for alcohol dependence*

A maladaptive pattern of alcohol use, leading to clinically significant impairment or distress, as manifested by 3 or more of the following, occurring at any time within the same 12-month period:

A. Tolerance, as defined by either of the following:
   1. A need for markedly increased amounts of alcohol to achieve intoxication or desired effect
   2. A markedly diminished effect with continued use of the same amount of alcohol
B. Withdrawal, as manifested by either of the following:
   1. The characteristic withdrawal syndrome for alcohol
   2. Alcohol, or a closely related substance, is taken to relieve or avoid withdrawal symptoms
C. Alcohol is often taken in larger amounts or over a longer period than was intended.
D. There is a persistent desire or unsuccessful effort to cut down or control alcohol use.
E. A great deal of time is spent in activities necessary to obtain alcohol, use alcohol, or recover from its effects.
F. Important social, occupational, or recreational activities are given up or reduced because of alcohol use.
G. Alcohol use is continued despite knowledge of having a persistent or recurrent physical or psychological problem that is likely to have been caused or exacerbated by alcohol (e.g., continued drinking despite recognition that an ulcer was worsened by alcohol consumption).

Specify whether:
   With physiological dependence: evidence of tolerance or withdrawal (i.e., either item 1 or 2 is present).
   Without physiological dependence: no evidence of tolerance or withdrawal (i.e., neither item 1 nor 2 is present).
Course specifiers:
   Early full remission
   Early partial remission
   Sustained full remission
   Sustained partial remission
   On agonist therapy
   In a controlled environment

Adapted with permission from the *Diagnostic and Statistical Manual of Mental Disorders, 4th ed., text revision.* Copyright 2000. American Psychiatric Association.

these, more than 20,000 die each year. Approximately 33% of all cases of liver cirrhosis are associated with alcohol abuse or dependence. Recent statistics suggest that women have an increasing rate of liver cirrhosis as a consequence of their growing trend to drink at levels comparable to men (17,18). Cancer of the oropharynx, the prevalence of which is associated with the extent of tissue exposure to alcohol, is on the increase (19). Local gastrointestinal effects of alcohol include chronic gastritis, and excessive drinking increases the risk of both rectal and pancreatic cancer (19,20). Women receiving hormone replacement therapy who drink may be at increased risk of breast cancer; however, it does not appear that alcohol intake is associated with prostate or endometrial cancers.

Mental disorders appear to be commonly associated with alcohol dependence; however, it is often difficult to determine which is the primary or preceding disorder. The risk of mental disease appears to be correlated with the amount of alcohol consumed, and the intake of more than 29 drinks per week can double the risk of mental disease. Individuals with affective and anxiety disorders have high rates of alcohol dependence. For instance, rates of alcohol dependence are as high as 60% among those with bipolar disorder. Excessive drinking undoubtedly aggravates concurrent Alzheimer's or multiinfarct dementia. Nevertheless, in practice, it is often difficult to differentiate these dementias from a supervening or underlying alcohol dementia (16).

Excessive and binge drinking episodes increase the risk of a multitude of injuries that can occur from the operation of heavy machinery, vehicle accidents, fires, and falls (21,22). No level of drinking can be considered "safe" because the risk of injury correlates predictably with the amount of alcohol-related performance impairment. Aggressive behavior and related traumatic injuries also become more likely if alcohol is consumed 6 hours or less prior to the incident.

In general, mortality rates are increased when drinking levels rise. For instance, a 25-nation European study showed that a rise of 1 L per capita in alcohol consumption was associated with a 1% rise in all causes of morbidity; the converse was true for decreases in drinking. Interestingly, there appears to be a protective effect of light or moderate drinking on the development of coronary heart disease; hence, mortality rates for abstainers approach those of heavy drinking. Mortality rates for those drinking 6 or more drinks per day exceed 154 and 130 per 100,000 for men and women, respectively (23,24).

In sum, alcoholism is an important disease worldwide, and it contributes substantially to the health care costs of most nations. Alcoholism is associated with a range of physical and mental disorders and is a leading cause of traumatic injuries in the Western world. Per-capita drinking levels appear to be a reasonable barometer for measuring the impact of alcoholism on a nation's health. There are, however, some protective effects of temperate drinking at reducing mortality rates from coronary heart disease.

DRINKING THROUGH THE AGES AND NATURAL HISTORY

In recent times, there has been no improvement in the epidemic patterns of underage drinking, even though there appears to have been a slight decrease in alcohol con-

sumption among those older than age 12 years from 72.9% in 1979 to 63.7% in 2001 (25). From the 2000 National Household Survey on Drug Abuse report, it can be seen that the average age at which drinking starts among those between 12 years and 20 years of age is 14 years (26). Furthermore, a person who starts drinking before the age of 15 years is about four times more likely to develop alcohol dependence—these rates increase with earlier ages of drinking onset (27). Thus, the most important factor that predicts progression into adulthood is an early age of onset of drinking problems (28), and the delay of drinking until adulthood reduces the risk of lifetime alcohol dependence. Nevertheless, not all cases of early problem drinking progress into adulthood. Only in approximately 20% to 30% of people who have early alcohol problems does this progress into adulthood (29,30). Children who drink alcohol frequently have prior behavioral problems, especially conduct disorder (31,32). Among adolescents, it appears that the symptoms of depression and anxiety often precede alcohol abuse (33,34).

While there is a long-held belief that alcohol dependence is a chronic unremitting disorder, the research evidence does not entirely bear this out. Indeed, data from the influential longitudinal studies of Vaillant and colleagues (35–38), Temple, Fillmore, and coworkers (29,39,40), and national surveys (41,42) suggest that alcohol dependence is a chronic remitting disorder, with those who develop the disease in middle age showing the greatest stability of lifetime disease. Those who develop alcohol dependence early (i.e., younger than age 30 years) experience considerable variations in symptoms and appear to have "bouts" of disease as they get older, rather than persistent disease. Individuals who develop alcohol dependence after the age of 50 years tend to decrease their drinking as they get older. Importantly, however, the proportion of the elderly (i.e., older than age 65 years) who are dependent on alcohol continues to rise in the United States. Generally, the proportion of elderly women with at-risk drinking is 12%, compared with 10% for elderly men (16).

ETHNICITY, GENDER, PLACE OF RESIDENCE, AND RELIGION

Drinking patterns differ between men and women, as well as between ethnic and racial groups. Overall, whites have the highest alcohol consumption levels, followed by Hispanics and then blacks. Despite a number of earlier references to epidemic drinking levels among Native Americans, this does vary tremendously between tribes. The trend toward reduced drinking with age is not uniform across ethnic groups. White men peak first (age 18 to 25 years), followed by Hispanic and black men, with peak ages between 26 years and 30 years. Interestingly, however, Hispanic men tend to maintain heavy drinking patterns acquired as adults even as they become elderly. The high levels of drinking persistence among Hispanic men are associated with elevated levels of partner abuse, and this subgroup may soon exert the heaviest burden of care on society for alcohol problems (43). Women are drinking more. In 1940, men, compared with women, were more than twice as likely to be dependent on alcohol; nowadays, the proportion is approaching parity. Those who live in cities and suburbs, compared with those who reside in rural areas, have the higher rates of alcohol dependence. Jews, Episcopalians, and Baptists living in rural areas exhibit low rates of alcohol dependence when compared with the general population (16).

CLINICAL PICTURE

The presentation of alcoholism is often multifaceted. Although there is no typical pattern that describes the progression of an individual from excessive drinking to alcohol dependence, and an exhaustive description that encompasses every heavy drinker is not possible, certain features appear to be dominant themes as the disease progresses. In the early phases of the disease process, the most obvious feature is excessive or binge drinking to the point of intoxication. Some alcohol-dependent individuals ascribe their desire to drink to be motivated by emotional factors such as dysthymic mood or negative affect and, sometimes, elation. In others, there is the description of what may be loosely termed as "craving" or a hard-to-suppress urge to drink. Some of the individuals whom we have attended frequently describe this desire as a "thirst which must be quenched." Contemporary research has, however, found it difficult to accurately describe what constitutes craving, and from the extensive literature that has developed on trying to reach an accepted definition, no consensus has emerged. Nevertheless, a large proportion of heavy drinkers are unable to provide a plausible explanation of what triggered the use of increasing amounts of alcohol. Increasingly, heavy drinking onset is not wholly precipitated by underlying emotional circumstances but out of a peer culture of drinking in school, in college, with friends, or with workmates. In these circumstances, there is some concealment of a heavy drinking pattern for the individual as the group norm of accepted levels of alcohol consumption has been set upwards. For some, there is a high level of exposure to drinking situations (e.g., working as a bartender), and the progression to heavier drinking patterns is not easily noticed. Increased *tolerance* to alcohol may drive a rise in consumption to maintain the same pharmacologic effect.

Once the bouts of drinking to *intoxication* become an embedded behavioral pattern, the likelihood that the individual will develop alcohol-related problems tends to increase. Typically, there are increasing days of sick leave taken from work, interpersonal relationships begin to break down, and driving while intoxicated not only leads to legal problems but increases the risk of traumatic injury. Heavy drinking may become associated with "blackouts" with amnesia for events the night before, and "hangovers" on waking the next morning may become a common event. By this time, the chronic drinker's performance is generally impaired, he or she may appear to be more forgetful, and there is increasing neglect of comportment and attention to hygiene. Also, the chronic drinker may describe feelings of guilt, remorse, or disgust following drinking. These symptoms lead to concealment of drinking, with alcoholic beverages being hidden in the home, and drinking alone becomes a more frequent endeavor. To offset feelings of guilt and remorse, a new pattern of drinking to provide "relief" emerges. This "relief" may involve not only the temporary suspension of guilt and anxiety, but also an attempt to reduce insomnia or daytime nervousness. Drinking then becomes the paramount activity, irrespective of the cost to personal relationships, psychosocial well-being, or society at large. An ingrained pattern of heavy drinking over many months can establish the physical features of the alcohol-dependence syndrome, which become most marked with drinking cessation. That is, at this juncture, drinking cessation triggers symptoms of autonomic hyperactivity, which can include nervousness and tremulousness, and can develop into symptoms associated with greater neurologic impairment such as delirium tremens. "Relief drinking" may occur to avoid withdrawal symptoms that arise from temporary periods of abstinence.

On physical examination and laboratory testing, there are no pathognomonic features of alcoholism. There are, however, a range of signs and symptoms that should be sought in an established drinker or, if found, should increase the physician's suspicion that the patient may have an alcohol problem. It is important to remember that the alcohol-dependent individual can present in almost any medical setting. Below is a summary of some of the more notable features that may be detected by physical examination or simple laboratory tests—none of these features alone should be taken to confirm (except fetal alcohol syndrome) or exclude a diagnosis of alcohol abuse or dependence.

Features Detectable by Physical Exam or Laboratory Tests

Skin and Muscle

Many skin conditions are exacerbated by heavy alcohol consumption. Exposure to sunshine leading to erythematous eruptions without blistering may be a sign of erythropoietic protoporphyria. Psoriasis vulgaris and acne rosacea (red nose) are also commonly found. Rarely, hepatic porphyrias can be triggered by alcohol and result in skin eruptions—porphyria cutanea tarda—which are characterized by bullous erosions, blistering, crusting, and scarred healing with hyperpigmentation or depigmentation, especially to the face, side of the neck, and back of the hands (44). Palmar erythema (red palms) may be seen, and with the onset of alcoholic liver disease, there may be spider nevi (angiomas of interlaced red blood vessels). Myopathy can be a rare complication of alcoholism.

Eyes

Arcus senilis may be present as a result of increased blood lipid levels in heavy drinkers. However, this sign is so ubiquitous as to not be of much diagnostic use. Rarely, prominent eye signs can be manifested in individuals with chronic severe alcoholism such as ophthalmoplegia and nystagmus, which are features of Wernicke's encephalopathy. However, patients with this condition are unlikely to present in general practice.

Limbs

Tremulousness may be noticed as an early sign of alcohol withdrawal but is more likely to be associated with anxiety or a benign nonessential tremor. Sometimes, individuals with chronic alcoholism may present with peripheral neuropathy as a consequence of deficiencies of vitamin B_{12}, thiamin, or both. Asterixis or "liver flap" may be seen in individuals with established alcoholic liver disease.

Cardiovascular System

Excessive drinkers may present with hypertension. Although the etiology of most cases of hypertension is unknown, the possibility that heavy drinking may be involved should be considered. Arrhythmias are uncommon, but infrequently an individual may report having "butterflies in the chest" (i.e., bouts of atrial fibrillation) associated with heavy drinking episodes. When this occurs while on vacation, it is referred to as the *holiday heart syndrome*. Rare cardiac complications include cardiomyopathy.

Gastrointestinal System

Excessive drinking can bring about a range of gastrointestinal disorders. Enlarged salivary glands can occur. Also, heavy drinkers may describe episodes of reflux esophagitis with a burning or persistent raw feeling in the throat, and retching from vomiting can produce *Mallory-Weiss tears* to the esophagus and the vomiting of frank red blood. Rarely, long-standing esophagitis may predispose the individual to esophageal cancer. Generally, individuals with alcoholism have higher rates of oropharyngeal cancer than the general population. Stomach ulcers and gastritis are common; the patient may complain of dark stools, and intestinal malabsorption is possible. Diarrhea often signals the involvement of the colon; colonic polyps and rectal cancer are rare possibilities. The liver may be enlarged and easily palpated under the right costochondral margin, but it is usually nontender. Tenderness and pain in the upper abdominal cavity of an excessive drinker should lead to the suspicion of acute pancreatitis, typically with calcification.

Endocrine System

Heavy alcohol consumption can exacerbate hypoactivity of a number of endocrine organs such as the thyroid, hyperthyroid, and pancreas, and should be considered as a complicating factor in individuals with these conditions who are not improving or who are treatment resistant.

Rheumatic and Immune System

With the onset of alcoholic liver disease, most alcoholics develop autoantibodies to smooth muscle, mitochondria, and nuclei, perhaps because of the cytosolic proteins modified by alcohol's metabolites. Therefore, drinkers tend to experience a reduction in symptoms of autoimmune diseases such as systemic lupus erythematosus and rheumatoid arthritis. Heavy drinking may, however, precipitate attacks of gout, and less commonly there may be signs of osteoporosis and myopathy. Heavy drinkers are more susceptible to infections caused by an increase in the CD4:CD8 ratio; however, this would be difficult to distinguish from other conditions that may increase liability to infections (45).

Erythropoiesis

Anemias are common and should be examined for clinically by inspecting the lower eyelids and the bed of the finger nails. Typically these are macrocytic; however, sideroblastic anemia also can occur. Microcytic anemia is typically associated with blood loss from ulcers or cancers. Thrombocytopenia can be a rare complication of alcoholism.

Mammary Glands

Chronically heavy-drinking women are at increased risk of breast cancer.

Central Nervous System

Impairment of cognitive function is a common complaint among chronic heavy drinkers. Of these, the specific deficit of Korsakoff's syndrome, which is detailed below, needs to be tested for by the examination of short-term memory. Dementias caused by alcohol may complicate those of other etiologies, particularly those of the Alzheimer's and multiinfarct type. Rare and complex neurologic disorders, such as central pontine myelinosis, also are associated with chronic heavy alcohol consumption.

Fetal Development

Alcohol and its metabolite acetaldehyde can have serious effects on the developing fetus. High levels of alcohol consumption in pregnant mothers can produce spontaneous abortion and *in utero* death. Infants born to mothers who drank heavily during pregnancy may suffer from fetal alcohol syndrome. Fetal alcohol syndrome can include severe mental retardation, small head, short stature, facial deformity (absent philtrum, flattened nasal bridge, and an epicanthal eye fold), syndactyly, and atrial septal defect.

Laboratory Tests

Laboratory tests may provide evidence that increases the physician's suspicion about the possibility that the patient may be a heavy drinker. Laboratory tests can also provide evidence to substantiate a history of heavy drinking. A complete blood count may lead to the finding of anemia, typically macrocytic, but it also could be microcytic or sideroblastic. Triglyceride levels are typically elevated. Abnormal liver function tests are common, particularly elevation of the enzyme, γ-glutamyl transferase (GGT). Bilirubin and uric acid levels also may be raised. Recently, measurement of percent carbohydrate-deficient transferrin (CDT) level, a carrier protein, was approved by the Food and Drug Administration (FDA) as a marker of heavy drinking. Research evidence suggests that serial measurements of the combination of CDT and GGT are the best biochemical method in a particular individual to characterize heavy drinking behavior (46). Raised mean corpuscular volume (MCV) is a traditional measure of heavy drinking; however, its predictive power is low. Knowledge that heavy drinking may result in the derangement of multiple biochemical and hematologic measures has been used over the last two decades to develop the early detection of alcohol consumption (EDAC) score. The short version of the EDAC score compiles 13 tests—Na, Cl, K, bilirubin ratio, total protein, cholesterol, high-density lipoprotein, albumin, GGT, aspartate aminotransferase, MCV, white blood cell count, and monocytes. More specific biochemical markers of recent heavy alcohol consumption are under development (47).

COMPLICATIONS OF ALCOHOLISM

Alcoholism affects practically all organ systems in the body at different stages of the natural history of the disease. One method for categorizing the medical complications of alcoholism is to describe its acute, chronic, and withdrawal effects.

Acute Effects

The acute effects of alcohol depend on the time course of drinking. During the initial period of up to 30 minutes after ingesting even small amounts of alcohol (ascending

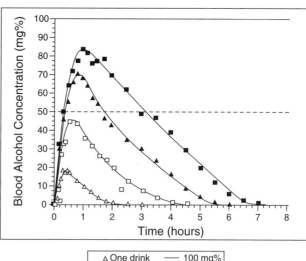

FIG. 9.1. Alcohol metabolism. Blood alcohol concentration after the rapid consumption of different amounts of alcohol by eight adult, fasting, male subjects. Blood alcohol concentration decreases by 15% every hour (one standard drink* per hour). Females have less body water so a smaller volume of distribution. *One standard drink is defined as 0.35 L of beer, 0.15 L of wine, or 0.04 L of 80-proof liquor. (From the National Institute on Alcohol Abuse and Alcoholism. *Alcohol Alert* No. 35, PH 371: *Alcohol Metabolism*. Bethesda, MD: National Institute on Alcohol Abuse and Alcoholism, January 1997 with permission.)

curve), there is typically mood elevation, which is then followed by sedative and anxiolytic effects. Additionally, the blood alcohol concentration (BAC) reached is practically a direct function of the amount ingested. Figure 9.1 shows typical BAC curves after the ingestion of varying amounts of alcohol.

As Table 9.2 demonstrates, depending upon the BAC reached, there are various consequences of intoxication. The acute consumption of large amounts of alcohol can lead to profound respiratory depression (especially if combined with tranquilizers), followed by coma and death. However, there is tremendous interindividual variation as to the BAC level that will result in death. Rare acute complications of alcohol dependence include alcohol-induced psychotic disorder and Wernicke's encephalopathy. *Alcohol-induced psychotic disorder* usually occurs in the presence of active drinking, but also has been described during withdrawal. It is characterized by the acute onset of visual and auditory hallucinations, and schizophreniform-like delusions of a persecutory nature. A distinguishing feature between alcoholic hallucinosis and delirium tremens is that the former occurs in clear consciousness. Typically, alcohol-induced psychotic disorder lasts about 10 to 15 days. *Wernicke's encephalopathy*

TABLE 9.2. *Alcohol intoxication*

- Most common alcohol-induced disorder
- Reversible

DSM–IV–TR diagnostic criteria

A. Recent ingestion of alcohol
B. Clinically significant maladaptive behavior or psychological changes (e.g., inappropriate sexual or aggressive behavior, mood lability, impaired judgment, impaired social or occupational functioning) that developed during, or shortly after, alcohol ingestion
C. One (or more) of the following signs, developing during, or shortly after, alcohol use:
   1. Slurred speech
   2. Incoordination
   3. Unsteady gait
   4. Nystagmus
   5. Impairment in attention or memory
   6. Stupor or coma
D. The symptoms are not due to a general medical condition and are not better accounted for by another mental disorder.

Possible sequelae of various blood alcohol concentration (BAC) levels

- BAC of 0.03 mg% → Euphoria
  - 0.05 mg% → Mild coordination problems
  - 0.1 mg% → Ataxia (5–6 drinks in a 2-hour period)
  - 0.2 mg% → Confusion
  - >0.3 mg% → Coma and death

Adapted in part from the *Diagnostic and Statistical Manual of Mental Disorders, 4th ed., text revision.* Copyright 2000. American Psychiatric Association.

TABLE 9.3. *Alcohol-induced amnestic disorder*

Diagnostic criteria for substance-induced persisting amnestic disorder

A. The development of memory impairment as manifested by impairment in the ability to learn new information or the inability to recall previously learned information.
B. The memory disturbance causes significant impairment in social or occupational functioning and represents a significant decline from a previous level of functioning.
C. The memory disturbance does not occur exclusively during the course of a delirium or a dementia and persists beyond the usual duration of alcohol intoxication or withdrawal.
D. There is evidence from the history, physical examination, or laboratory findings that the memory disturbance is etiologically related to the persisting effects of alcohol use.

Wernicke-Korsakoff syndrome

- Wernicke's encephalopathy
  - Abrupt onset
  - Truncal ataxia
  - Ophthalmoplegia
  - Mental confusion
- Korsakoff's syndrome
  - Severe anterograde amnesia *(memory is not transferred from short- to long-term memory storage)*
  - Retrograde amnesia
  - Cognitive deficits
- Etiology is based on thiamin deficiency

Adapted in part from the *Diagnostic and Statistical Manual of Mental Disorders, 4th ed., text revision.* Copyright 2000. American Psychiatric Association.

is a life-threatening condition, and individuals with this disorder are typically managed in an intensive care unit, where fluid and electrolyte support and assisted mechanical ventilation, if needed, can be provided. Table 9.3 lists the clinical characteristics of Wernicke's encephalopathy.

Chronic Effects

Although these have mostly been described above, two disorders merit emphasis. Perhaps the best known chronic effect of heavy drinking is liver disease, which can manifest in two forms: *fatty liver* and *liver cirrhosis*. While the former may progress to the latter, the relationship between the two conditions is not direct. Chronic alcoholism also tends to be associated with malabsorption and multiple vitamin B deficiencies, which typically present as *peripheral neuropathy*. A third disorder, *Korsakoff's syndrome*, is also a chronic condition brought about by the deficiency of thiamin. Korsakoff's syndrome is associated with damage to the mamillary bodies, and its most striking feature is short-term memory impairment. Because individuals with

this disorder often confabulate to fill in memory gaps, diagnosis of this condition is often missed if memory is not specifically tested in the mental state examination. A striking illustration of this condition is a patient with Korsakoff's syndrome who presents to the physician with his wife. The physician is unaware of the patient's condition or the circumstances that have precipitated the visit. On greeting the physician, the patient proceeds to discuss a baseball game that happened a few years earlier, and his wife, not being interested in baseball, seizes this opportunity to leave the consultation and go to the restroom. When the patient's wife returns a few minutes later, the patient stands up and greets his wife as if this is the first time that they had met that day, and he cannot recall that she had been in the room with him a few minutes earlier. Table 9.3 lists the other clinical features of Korsakoff's syndrome.

Alcohol Withdrawal

Chronic heavy drinkers who abstain from alcohol for more than a few hours can experience *withdrawal* symptoms.

These withdrawal symptoms can vary widely in intensity and typically start with tremulousness and signs of sympathetic overactivity such as palpitations and sweating. At its most extreme, alcohol withdrawal can produce the syndrome of *delirium tremens,* occurring about 24 to 48 hours postalcohol cessation, which is characterized by clouding of consciousness, phonemes (auditory and vivid visual hallucinations, typically of the persecutory type), and seizures. Rarely, individuals may experience seeing animals or people of small or diminished size, often in amusing guises; these are termed *Lilliputian hallucinations* (48). However, a more common and disturbing hallucination is that associated with the sensation of insects crawling over the skin (*tactile hallucinations*). The mortality rate from delirium tremens is approximately 5% to 15% (49). Typically, the signs and symptoms of alcohol withdrawal have a progressive nature from mild to severe. Therefore, in clinical practice it is difficult to determine whether a person will have severe symptoms a day later if at present only mild symptoms are in evidence. Thus, individuals who begin to develop withdrawal symptoms that appear to be progressing need to be monitored closely. On the other hand, it is reasonable to expect that a chronic heavy drinker with confirmed abstinence for more than 72 hours with mild and nonprogressing withdrawal symptoms is unlikely to experience severe withdrawal symptoms from this episode a day or two later.

COMORBIDITY

Alcohol dependence often occurs contemporaneously with other addictive and psychiatric disorders. Among addictive disorders, the highest association rates of alcoholism are with nicotine dependence. For example, in sample sizes ranging from 103 to 1010, surveys of both inpatient and outpatient treatment participants for alcohol dependence showed an 86% to 97% smoking rate among males, and an 82% to 92% rate among females (50–56). More recently, Batel and colleagues (57) noted a 91.5% prevalence rate of nicotine dependence among 325 outpatients attending an alcohol clinic, using *DSM–III–R* criteria for both disorders. Cigarettes and alcohol consumed and severity ratings for both disorders were also positively related. Comorbid alcohol dependence with smoking has important treatment implications. In one of the largest epidemiologic surveys addressing this question (N = 2115), Zimmerman and colleagues (58) noted that current heavy drinkers made the fewest cessation attempts and had the least success, whereas alcohol abstainers quit smoking most often. DiFranza and Guerrera (59) observed a smoking cessation rate of 7% in a nonrandomized case control study of alcoholics who received no formal treatment for nicotine dependence, compared with 49% in nonalcoholic controls.

Alcoholism also occurs commonly with addiction to narcotics. For example, up to 89% of cocaine-dependent individuals are also dependent on alcohol (60). Prevalence estimates of alcohol misuse among cocaine-dependent individuals are twice as high as for opiates. Alcoholism is associated with greater severity of cocaine dependence, and increased alcohol misuse commonly follows the establishment of cocaine dependence (61,62). Misuse of other psychostimulants, sedatives (e.g., benzodiazepines, barbiturates, and marihuana), and hallucinogenic drugs also occurs commonly against a background of alcohol abuse or dependence.

An interesting feature of the comorbidity of alcoholism with other addictive disorders is that the association is greatest for those with the youngest age of onset of problem drinking. This raises the possibility that such individuals either may be particularly prone to inheriting a range of addictive or impulse dyscontrol disorders or may come from a familial or psychosocial background that encourages substance use, or both. Another feature of individuals with alcohol dependence who abuse or are dependent on other addictive drugs is the finding that their comorbidity is the result of using the effects of one drug to modulate the adverse effects of the other. For instance, it is not unusual for cocaine users to report the use of alcohol as a sedative to "smooth out" the excessive psychomotor stimulation from taking cocaine. Research is ongoing to determine the relative merits of phased versus concurrent treatment for comorbid alcoholism and other addictive disorders.

Individuals with alcohol dependence also tend to have high rates of comorbidity with other psychiatric disorders. Of these, the more notable association appears to be with alcoholism and a variety of affective and anxiety-related disorders. For example, between 33% and 67% of individuals with alcohol dependence also have major depression, and up to 60% of people with bipolar disorder either abuse or are dependent on alcohol. Rates of alcohol abuse and dependence are high among those with anxiety (63) or posttraumatic stress disorder (64). Antisocial personality disorder is common among those who develop problem drinking early in life (8,10), and tends to develop a few years before the problem drinking (65), leading to the proposition that antisocial personality disorder is the primary disorder in such individuals. Rates of alcohol abuse and dependence are also elevated among individuals with schizophreniform disorders. While it is premature to posit an overarching theory that might explain the co-occurrence of alcoholism and other psychiatric disorders, it is tempting to speculate that these conditions might be related through dimensional constructs that affect impulse dyscontrol.

TREATMENT

The treatment of alcohol-related disorders is appraised in this section by first reviewing the management of their sequelae followed by the treatment of alcohol dependence *per se.*

The acute effects of alcohol are seldom treated as the symptoms tend to subside with time. Nevertheless, it is sometimes important to intervene medically, especially if there is a risk of profound respiratory depression. In this instance, flumazenil (a benzodiazepine antagonist) has been used to reverse alcohol-related respiratory suppression and coma. Typically, this treatment is administered on highly supervised medical units, where supportive therapy (which may include assisted mechanical ventilation) is available. Similarly, the treatment of Wernicke's syndrome is a medical emergency requiring treatment on a highly supervised medical unit. The mainstay of treatment for Wernicke's syndrome is intravenous hydration and thiamin. Magnesium sulfate is often a component of treatment to reduce the potential for seizures. The mortality rate from Wernicke's encephalopathy may exceed 50%, even in specialized centers.

The chronic sequelae of alcohol dependence are typically managed in medical settings and are designed specifically to address the secondary disorder(s). For example, the treatment for alcohol-induced malabsorption leading to vitamin B deficiency disorders is, of course, to administer the appropriate vitamin supplements, usually for a period of several months. Of the other conditions, Korsakoff's syndrome deserves special mention because it may be mostly reversible in some cases with appropriate treatment. It is important to administer thiamin at appropriate doses (100 mg/day) for at least 6 months, and in some cases, continued improvements have been seen with medication administration periods of up to 1 year or more.

The treatment of alcohol withdrawal depends on its severity. Individuals with mild withdrawal symptoms are typically treated with small doses of the long-acting benzodiazepine, chlordiazepoxide, for no more than a few days. Severe withdrawal syndromes, especially those complicated by neuropsychiatric disorders such as delirium tremens and seizures, require hospitalization. As a rough guide, individuals withdrawing from alcohol with clinical institute withdrawal assessment for alcohol scale–revised (CIWA-Ar) (66) scores of less than 12 can often be managed as outpatients, but those above this threshold may require hospitalization; however, this decision should be based also upon clinical condition, taking the particular characteristics of each individual into consideration. Individuals with CIWA-Ar scores of less than 8 do not usually require medication aids for the treatment of withdrawal symptoms. Table 9.4 contains a proposed schedule for the inpatient treatment of alcohol withdrawal.

The treatment of alcohol dependence *per se* usually starts with the individual's recognition that he or she needs treatment for the disorder. Unfortunately, because of the prevailing societal stigma of alcohol dependence, most people with alcohol dependence need to be confronted by a family member, friend, or health worker for them to present for treatment. New methods using a more em-pathetic approach, by highlighting the negative consequences of drinking to the patient and allowing the patient to move into advanced stages of readiness for change, show better success in getting individuals with alcohol dependence to seek treatment (67). Once this has been accomplished, the next hurdle involves determining the treatment setting. Although some alcohol-dependent individuals with low levels of motivation and severely impaired lifestyles may require long-term rehabilitation, there is growing awareness that most people can be treated as outpatients. Consideration of the particular clinical needs of each alcohol-dependent individual, as well as that individual's personal circumstances, should ensure appropriate treatment placement. Irrespective of treatment setting, the modalities of available treatment are a variety of psychosocial treatments either alone or with the addition of pharmacotherapy.

Perhaps the best known psychosocial intervention for individuals dependent upon alcohol has been referral to Alcoholics Anonymous. This psychosocial treatment is, however, better described as 12-step facilitation. Basically, the treatment formalizes 12 steps through which the alcohol-dependent individual needs to progress to initiate recovery. The hallmark of treatment is that drinkers admit that they are powerless over alcohol, appraise their morals, admit the nature of their wrongs, make a list of everyone they have harmed, and make plans to make amends to those people. Cognitive-behavioral therapy also is a common treatment for alcohol dependence. The key to improvement is to teach the addicted individual cognitive and behavioral skills for changing the drinking behavior. For instance, addicted individuals are taught to identify "high-risk" situations that would increase craving and relapse, and they learn and rehearse strategies for coping with these situations. Motivational enhancement therapy uses the addicted individual's own desire for change as the treatment vehicle. A landmark study comparing the relative effectiveness of 12-step facilitation, cognitive-behavioral therapy, and motivational enhancement therapy found them to be equally useful (68,69). Therefore, the choice between any of these therapies should probably be made based on physician or referrer and patient preference. Importantly, there is a growing and compelling literature on the use of brief interventions (70) for the treatment of alcohol dependence. These have the advantage of being more easily delivered by nonspecialized staff in generic settings; however, some authorities have questioned their suitability for those with severe lifestyle impairment or a high chronicity of disease. Nevertheless, brief interventions are proving useful and effective in a variety of treatment settings.

In the last decade, there has been growing interest in the use of pharmacotherapies for the treatment of alcohol dependence. Disulfiram (Antabuse) is perhaps the most widely used medication in the United States. Disulfiram works by inhibiting aldehyde dehydrogenase,

TABLE 9.4. *Inpatient management of severe alcohol withdrawal symptoms*

1. Supportive and preventive medications:
   - Thiamin 100 mg p.o. q.d. (alternative is 100 mg i.m. for 3 days if patient has significant emesis; then p.o.)
   - Multivitamins 1 p.o. q.d.
   - Folate 1 mg p.o. q.d.
   - Haldol 0.5–2.0 mg p.o./i.m. q 4 h p.r.n. for hallucinations
   - Phenergan 25 mg p.o./i.m. q 6 h p.r.n. for severe nausea or vomiting
   - Disalcid (salsalate) 500 mg p.o. t.i.d. with meals p.r.n. for severe pain
   - Magnesium sulfate 1 g i.m. four times for 2 days if there is a history of seizure
2. Benzodiazepines:
   The best method of using benzodiazepines is p.r.n. dosing combined with tapering the dose. Chlordiazepoxide is indicated in most cases. P.r.n. dosing should be adjusted according to the CIWA-Ar score. Below is a method that may be used for tapering benzodiazepines used in treating alcohol withdrawal. The combined benzodiazepine dose per day should not exceed 250 mg of chlordiazepoxide, 100 mg of diazepam, or 12 mg of lorazepam. Patients may have different response levels, and medication dose should be adjusted for the need of each patient.

	Chlordiazepoxide (Librium)	Diazepam (Valium)	Lorazepam (Ativan)
Day 1	50 mg p.o. now, then 25 mg q 6 h from time of first dose	10 mg p.o. now, then 10 mg q 6 h from time of first dose	2 mg now, then 2 mg q 6 h from time of first dose
Day 2	25 mg p.o. t.i.d.	10 mg p.o. t.i.d.	2 mg p.o. t.i.d.
Day 3	25 mg p.o. b.i.d.	10 mg p.o. b.i.d.	2 mg p.o. b.i.d.
Day 4	10 mg p.o. b.i.d.	5 mg p.o. b.i.d.	1 mg p.o. b.i.d.
Day 5	5 mg p.o. b.i.d.	2 mg p.o. b.i.d.	0.5 mg p.o. b.i.d.
Day 6	5 mg p.o. q.d.	2 mg p.o. q.d.	0.5 mg p.o. q.d.
Day 7	Discharge	Discharge	Discharge

Lorazepam is preferred if significant hepatic damage (i.e., elevation of total bilirubin levels) is present. Lorazepam is preferred due to its short half-life and the absence of active metabolites, which, in the case of impaired hepatic clearance, decreases the risk of medication accumulation and excessive sedation. Elevation of transaminases and GGT up to 3–4 times the upper limit of normal does *not* exclude the use of chlordiazepoxide.

Diazepam doses are provided if the patient is dependent on both alcohol and opiates; then, the physician can just prescribe a single benzodiazepine for both the alcohol and opiate withdrawal.

3. Adjunctive agents:
   - Anticonvulsants such as carbamazepine have been widely used in practice to decrease the severity of withdrawal symptoms. When compared to benzodiazepine such as oxazepam, carbamazepine was shown to reduce emotional distress and allow a faster recovery and discharge better than benzodiazepine (79). Carbamazepine use was also associated with less neurocognitive adverse reactions such as memory loss and drowsiness. Nausea and vomiting are common side effects of carbamazepine. Carbamazepine augmentation also should be considered in individuals with a previous history of seizures. Other anticonvulsants that are being evaluated for the treatment of alcohol withdrawal symptoms include valproate and topiramate.
   - α Agonists such as clonidine may be used to decrease the severity of the withdrawal symptom by reducing sympathetic overactivity.
   - β Blockers such as atenolol and propranolol may also help to reduce signs of sympathetic overactivity, particularly tachycardia and hypertension.

thereby preventing the metabolism of alcohol's primary metabolite, acetaldehyde; this leads to the production of a range of unpleasant side effects, such as nausea, vomiting, flushing, sympathetic overactivity, and palpitations, if drinking is initiated. However, disulfiram is only effective in those with a high level of motivation and a supportive partner to help ensure that it is taken—just the sort of alcohol-dependent individuals who are likely to abstain on their own (71). In 1995, the μ-opioid antagonist, naltrexone (Depade, ReVia; 50 mg/day), was approved by the FDA for the treatment of alcohol dependence. Naltrexone presumably works at maintaining abstinence by reducing the craving for alcohol. In Europe, acamprosate (Aotal) is widely used for the treatment of alcohol dependence. Importantly, however, the FDA did not approve acamprosate for use in the United States because its efficacy was not demonstrated in a recent multicenter United States trial. Other promising medications are in development for the treatment of alcohol dependence. For instance, the serotonin-3 antagonist, ondansetron (Zofran; 4 μg/kg), has shown promise in a double-blind, randomized clinical trial as a treatment for early onset alcoholism (72), and findings from an open-label clinical trial consistent with this study were published recently (73). Early onset alcoholics differ from those of late onset by having greater familial disease predisposition, serotonergic dysregulation, and a range of antisocial behaviors (10,74). The combination of ondansetron and naltrexone may be even more effective for the treatment of early onset alcoholism than either alone (75,76). Selective serotonin reuptake inhibitors may be effective as a treatment for late onset alcoholism (77). Finally, a recent double-blind trial showed that the anticonvulsant, topiramate (Topamax; up to 300 mg/day), appears to be an effective treatment for alcoholism (78). Further clinical trials are ongoing to continue the development of topiramate for the treatment of alcohol dependence. Importantly, all these pharmacotherapies are being developed as adjuncts to psychosocial treatments of varying intensities, and the ultimate goal is to develop therapies that optimize the combination of pharmacotherapy and psychosocial treatment.

Despite the marked advances in alcoholism treatment, some individuals with alcohol dependence will go through several periods of alternating sobriety and relapse before attaining the ultimate goal of sustained sobriety. Therefore, treatment(s) that convert an individual's heavy drinking to nonpathologic levels may be a practical short-term goal.

While there is always the risk of relapse when alcohol-dependent individuals remain exposed to drinking, even at very low levels, there may be some advantages to a harm reduction approach. For instance, it may enable the skilled practitioner time to work progressively with the patient who cannot immediately achieve abstinence, and allow for milestones of recovery to be mutually decided. Also, it may enable a flexible management approach to helping dependent individuals who are initially ambivalent about seeking treatment, and provide more time for the development of a therapeutic alliance, prior to setting stringent goals. Even when there is rapid reduction in harmful drinking patterns, the skilled practitioner should remain engaged, and use the improvements to motivate the individual toward achieving the ultimate goal of abstinence. It may well be that the notable achievements in the reduction of heavy drinking and maintenance of abstinence seen with the short-term administration of pharmacotherapies can be sustained if long-term treatment is provided. Indeed, this would appear to be likely unless there is resistance to the continuing efficacy of pharmacotherapy over time. Presently, this is an intense area of research for our group and others in the field.

CONCLUSIONS

In summary, there is increasingly new knowledge about the pathophysiology of alcoholism, and how a multitude of biologic, psychosocial, sociocultural, and environmental factors influence the alcoholism disease. The complexity of the potential sequelae of alcohol dependence means that a variety of physicians, and not only psychiatrists, as well as a range of treatment settings, are needed to provide a comprehensive level of care. Treatments for alcohol dependence are becoming even more effective, and developments in the neurosciences have promulgated important advances in the use of pharmacotherapies for the treatment of alcohol dependence.

ACKNOWLEDGMENTS

We thank the National Institute on Alcohol Abuse and Alcoholism for its support of Professor Bankole Johnson (grants N01 AA 01016, R01 AA 010522-10, and R01 AA 012964-03) and Assistant Professor Nassima Ait-Daoud (grant K23 AA 00329-01). We also are grateful to Robert H. Cormier, Jr., for his assistance with manuscript preparation.

REFERENCES

1. Mann K, Hermann D, Heinz A. One hundred years of alcoholism: the twentieth century. *Alcohol Alcohol* 2000;35:10–15.
2. Kielhorn FW. Zur Geschichte des Alkoholismus: Pearson, Sutton und das Delirium tremens. *Suchtgefahren* 1988;34:111–114.
3. Millikan LE. History and epidemiology of alcohol use and abuse. *Clin Dermatol* 1999;17:353–356.
4. Nuland S. *Doctors. Special edition.* Birmingham, AL: Gryphon Editions, 1988.
5. Edwards G. Withdrawal symptoms and alcohol dependence: fruitful mysteries. *Br J Addict* 1990;85:447–461.
6. Jellinek EM. *The disease concept of*

alcoholism. New Haven, CT: Hillhouse Press, 1960.

7. Cloninger CR, Bohman M, Sigvardsson S. Inheritance of alcohol abuse: cross-fostering analysis of adopted men. *Arch Gen Psychiatry* 1981;38:861–868.

8. Schuckit MA, Tipp JE, Smith TL, et al. An evaluation of type A and B alcoholics. *Addiction* 1995;90:1189–1203.

9. Bucholz KK, Heath AC, Reich T, et al. Can we subtype alcoholism? A latent class analysis of data from relatives of alcoholics in a multicenter family study of alcoholism. *Alcohol Clin Exp Res* 1996;20:1462–1471.

10. Johnson BA, Cloninger CR, Roache JD, et al. Age of onset as a discriminator between alcoholic subtypes in a treatment-seeking outpatient population. *Am J Addict* 2000;9:17–27.

11. American Psychiatric Association. *Diagnostic and statistical manual of mental disorders,* 4th ed., text revision. Washington, DC: Author, 2000.

12. Murray CJ, Lopez AD. Regional patterns of disability-free life expectancy and disability-adjusted life expectancy: Global Burden of Disease Study. *Lancet* 1997;349:1347–1352.

13. Grant BF, Harford TC, Chou P, et al. Prevalence of *DSM–IV* alcohol abuse and dependence: United States. *Alcohol Health Res World* 1992;18:243–248.

14. Dawson DA, Grant BF. Family history of alcoholism and gender: their combined effects on *DSM–IV* alcohol dependence and major depression. *J Stud Alcohol* 1998;59:97–106.

15. Grant BF. Estimates of U.S. children exposed to alcohol abuse and dependence in the family. *Am J Public Health* 2000;90:112–115.

16. U.S. Department of Health and Human Services. *10th special report to the U.S. Congress on alcohol and health.* Bethesda, MD: National Institutes of Health, National Institute on Alcohol Abuse and Alcoholism, 2000.

17. Parrish KM, Dufour MC, Stinson FS, et al. Average daily alcohol consumption during adult life among decedents with and without cirrhosis: the 1986 National Mortality Followback Survey. *J Stud Alcohol* 1993;54:450–456.

18. Naveau S, Giraud V, Borotto E, et al. Excess weight risk factor for alcoholic liver disease. *Hepatology* 1997;25:108–111.

19. Doll R, Forman D, La Vecchia D, et al. Alcoholic beverages and cancers of the digestive tract and larynx. In: Verschuren PM, ed. *Health issues related to alcohol consumption.* Washington, DC: International Life Sciences Institute Press, 1993:125–166.

20. Seitz H, Poschl G. Alcohol and gastroin-testinal cancer: pathogenic mechanisms. *Addict Biol* 1997;2:19–33.

21. Hurst PM, Harte D, Frith WJ. The Grand Rapids dip revisited. *Accid Anal Prev* 1994;26:647–654.

22. Cherpitel CJ. Epidemiology of alcohol-related trauma. *Alcohol Health Res World* 1992;16:191–196.

23. Thun MJ, Peto R, Lopez AD, et al. Alcohol consumption and mortality among middle-aged and elderly U.S. adults. *N Engl J Med* 1997;337:1705–1714.

24. Her M, Rehm J. Alcohol and all-cause mortality in Europe 1982–1990: a pooled cross-section time-series analysis. *Addiction* 1998;93:1335–1340.

25. Johnston LD, O'Malley PM, Bachman JG. *Ecstasy use among American teens drops for the first time in recent years, and overall drug and alcohol use also declines in the year after 9/11* [press release]. Ann Arbor, MI: University of Michigan News and Information Services, 2002.

26. Office of Applied Studies. *National household survey on drug abuse, 2000.* Ann Arbor, MI: University Consortium for Political and Social Research, 2001.

27. DeWit DJ, Adlaf EM, Offord DR, et al. Age at first alcohol use: a risk factor for the development of alcohol disorders. *Am J Psychiatry* 2000;157:745–750.

28. Kilbey MM, Downey K, Breslau N. Predicting the emergence and persistence of alcohol dependence in young adults: the role of expectancy and other risk factors. *Exp Clin Psychopharmacol* 1998;6:149–156.

29. Fillmore KM, Midanik L. Chronicity of drinking problems among men: a longitudinal study. *J Stud Alcohol* 1984;45:228–236.

30. Grant BF. Prevalence and correlates of alcohol use and *DSM–IV* alcohol dependence in the United States: results of the National Longitudinal Alcohol Epidemiologic Survey. *J Stud Alcohol* 1997;58:464–473.

31. Donovan JE, Jessor R, Jessor L. Problem drinking in adolescence and young adulthood: a follow-up study. *J Stud Alcohol* 1983;44:109–137.

32. Jessor R. Problem-behavior theory, psychosocial development, and adolescent problem drinking. *Br J Addict* 1987;82:331–342.

33. Rohde P, Lewinsohn PM, Seeley JR. Psychiatric comorbidity with problematic alcohol use in high school students. *J Am Acad Child Adolesc Psychiatry* 1996;35:101–109.

34. Kessler RC, Crum RM, Warner LA, et al. Lifetime co-occurrence of *DSM–III–R* alcohol abuse and dependence with other psychiatric disorders in the National Comorbidity Survey. *Arch Gen Psychiatry* 1997;54:313–321.

35. Vaillant GE. Natural history of male psychological health: VIII. Antecedents of alcoholism and "orality." *Am J Psychiatry* 1980;137:181–186.

36. Vaillant GE, Gale L, Milofsky ES. Natural history of male alcoholism. II. The relationship between different diagnostic dimensions. *J Stud Alcohol* 1982;43:216–232.

37. Vaillant GE. Natural history of male alcoholism. V: is alcoholism the cart or the horse to sociopathy? *Br J Addict* 1983;78:317–326.

38. Vaillant GE. A long-term follow-up of male alcohol abuse. *Arch Gen Psychiatry* 1996;53:243–249.

39. Temple MT, Fillmore KM. The variability of drinking patterns and problems among young men, age 16–31: a longitudinal study. *Int J Addict* 1985;20:1595–1620.

40. Fillmore KM, Hartka E, Johnstone BM, et al. A meta-analysis of life course variation in drinking. *Br J Addict* 1991;86:1221–1267.

41. Grant BF, Dawson DA. Age at onset of alcohol use and its association with *DSM–IV* alcohol abuse and dependence: results from the National Longitudinal Alcohol Epidemiologic Survey. *J Subst Abuse* 1997;9:103–110.

42. Dawson DA, Grant BF, Chou SP, et al. Subgroup variation in U.S. drinking patterns: results of the 1992 National Longitudinal Alcohol Epidemiologic Study. *J Subst Abuse* 1995;7:331–344.

43. Caetano R, Kaskutas LA. Changes in drinking patterns among whites, blacks and Hispanics, 1984–1992. *J Stud Alcohol* 1995;56:558–565.

44. Grassegger A. Skin. In: Zernig G, Saria A, Kurz M, et al., eds. *Handbook of alcoholism.* Boca Raton, FL: CRC Press, 2000:243–250.

45. Schirmer M, Wiedermann C, Konwalinka G. Immune system. In: Zernig G, Saria A, Kurz M, et al., eds. *Handbook of alcoholism.* Boca Raton, FL: CRC Press, 2000:225–229.

46. Javors M, Johnson B. Current status of carbohydrate deficient transferrin, total serum sialic acid, sialic acid index of apolipoprotein J, and serum beta-hexosaminidase as markers for alcohol consumption. *Addiction* 2003;98[Suppl 2]:45–50.

47. Javors MA, Bean P, King TS, et al. Biochemical markers for alcohol consumption. In: Johnson BA, Ruiz P, Galanter M, eds. *Handbook of clinical alcoholism treatment.* Baltimore, MD: Lippincott Williams & Wilkins, 2003:62–79.

48. Lishman WA. *Organic psychiatry: the psychological consequences of cerebral disorder,* 2nd ed. Oxford: Blackwell Scientific, 1987:514–515.

49. Erwin WE, Williams DB, Speir

WA. Delirium tremens. *South Med J* 1998;91:425–432.

50. Dreher KF, Fraser JG. Smoking habits of alcoholic out-patients. I. *Int J Addict* 1967;2:259–270.

51. Ayers J, Ruff CF, Templer DI. Alcoholism, cigarette smoking, coffee drinking and extraversion. *J Stud Alcohol* 1976;37:983–985.

52. Walton RG. Smoking and alcoholism: a brief report. *Am J Psychiatry* 1972;128:1455–1456.

53. Kozlowski LT, Jelinek LC, Pope MA. Cigarette smoking among alcohol abusers: a continuing and neglected problem. *Can J Public Health* 1986;77: 205–207.

54. Burling TA, Ziff DC. Tobacco smoking: a comparison between alcohol and drug abuse inpatients. *Addict Behav* 1988;13:185–190.

55. Burling TA, Reilly PM, Moltzen JO, et al. Self-efficacy and relapse among inpatient drug and alcohol abusers: a predictor of outcome. *J Stud Alcohol* 1989;50:354–360.

56. Bien TH, Burge R. Smoking and drinking: a review of the literature. *Int J Addict* 1990;25:1429–1454.

57. Batel P, Pessione F, Maitre C, et al. Relationship between alcohol and tobacco dependencies among alcoholics who smoke. *Addiction* 1995;90:977–980.

58. Zimmerman RS, Warheit GJ, Ulbrich PM, et al. The relationship between alcohol use and attempts and success at smoking cessation. *Addict Behav* 1990; 15:197–207.

59. DiFranza JR, Guerrera MP. Alcoholism and smoking. *J Stud Alcohol* 1990; 51:130–135.

60. Miller NS, Gold MS, Belkin BM. The diagnosis of alcohol and cannabis dependence in cocaine dependence. *Adv Alcohol Subst Abuse* 1990;8:33–42.

61. Gorelick DA. Alcohol and cocaine: clinical and pharmacological interac-

tions. *Recent Dev Alcohol* 1992;10:37–56.

62. Carroll KM, Rounsaville BJ, Bryant KJ. Alcoholism in treatment-seeking cocaine abusers: clinical and prognostic significance. *J Stud Alcohol* 1993;54:199–208.

63. Burns L, Teesson M. Alcohol use disorders comorbid with anxiety, depression and drug use disorders. Findings from the Australian National Survey of Mental Health and Well Being. *Drug Alcohol Depend* 2002;68:299–307.

64. Breslau N, Davis GC, Schultz LR. Posttraumatic stress disorder and the incidence of nicotine, alcohol, and other drug disorders in persons who have experienced trauma. *Arch Gen Psychiatry* 2003;60:289–294.

65. Bahlmann M, Preuss UW, Soyka M. Chronological relationship between antisocial personality disorder and alcohol dependence. *Eur Addict Res* 2002;8:195–200.

66. Sullivan JT, Sykora K, Schneiderman J, et al. Assessment of alcohol withdrawal: the revised clinical institute withdrawal assessment for alcohol scale (CIWA-Ar). *Br J Addict* 1989;84:1353–1357.

67. Prochaska JO, DiClemente CC. Stages of change in the modification of problem behaviors. *Prog Behav Modif* 1992;28:183–218.

68. Project MATCH Research Group. Project MATCH (Matching Alcoholism Treatment to Client Heterogeneity): rationale and methods for a multisite clinical trial matching patients to alcoholism treatment. *Alcohol Clin Exp Res* 1993;17:1130–1145.

69. DiClemente CC, Jordan L, Marinilli A, et al. Psychotherapy in alcoholism treatment. In: Johnson BA, Ruiz P, Galanter M, eds. *Handbook of clinical alcoholism treatment.* Baltimore, MD: Lippincott Williams & Wilkins, 2003: 102–110.

70. Edwards G, Orford J, Egert S, et al. Alcoholism: a controlled trial of "treat-

ment" and "advice." *J Stud Alcohol* 1977;38:1004–1031.

71. Ait-Daoud N, Johnson BA. Medications for the treatment of alcoholism. In: Johnson BA, Ruiz P, Galanter M, eds. *Handbook of clinical alcoholism treatment.* Baltimore, MD: Lippincott Williams & Wilkins, 2003:119–130.

72. Johnson BA, Roache JD, Javors MA, et al. Ondansetron for reduction of drinking among biologically predisposed alcoholic patients: a randomized controlled trial. *JAMA* 2000;284:963–971.

73. Kranzler HR, Pierucci-Lagha A, Feinn R, et al. Effects of ondansetron in early-versus late-onset alcoholics: a prospective, open-label study. *Alcohol Clin Exp Res* 2003;27:1150–1155.

74. Johnson BA, Ait-Daoud N. Neuropharmacological treatments for alcoholism: scientific basis and clinical findings. *Psychopharmacology* 2000;149:327–344.

75. Johnson BA, Ait-Daoud N, Prihoda TJ. Combining ondansetron and naltrexone effectively treats biologically predisposed alcoholics: from hypotheses to preliminary clinical evidence. *Alcohol Clin Exp Res* 2000;24:737–742.

76. Ait-Daoud N, Johnson BA, Prihoda TJ, et al. Combining ondansetron and naltrexone reduces craving among biologically predisposed alcoholics: preliminary clinical evidence. *Psychopharmacology* 2001;154:23–27.

77. Pettinati HM, Volpicelli JR, Kranzler HR, et al. Sertraline treatment for alcohol dependence: interactive effects of medication and alcoholic subtype. *Alcohol Clin Exp Res* 2000;24:1041–1049.

78. Johnson BA, Ait-Daoud N, Bowden CL, et al. Oral topiramate for treatment of alcohol dependence: a randomised controlled trial. *Lancet* 2003;361:1677–1685.

79. Stuppaeck CH, Pycha R, Miller C, et al. Carbamazepine versus oxazepam in the treatment of alcohol withdrawal: a double-blind study. *Alcohol Alcohol* 1992;27:153–158.

CHAPTER 10
Opiates: Neurobiology

ERIC J. SIMON

Since the previous edition of this book there have been a number of major developments in the area of the biology of the opiate drugs, in particular in our understanding of the endogenous opioid system. A very important advance was the cloning of the three major types of opioid receptors, which happened just prior to the publication of the previous edition and was summarized. This section has been appropriately updated. The availability of the genes for the opioid receptors and endorphins has led to further advances in our understanding of opioid receptor structure and function. There were also discoveries in the area of signal transduction, set into motion by opioid receptor activation, and these will be discussed. Finally, a novel receptor has been discovered, closely related to the three classical opioid receptors, but with different functions and its own endogenous ligand.

The demonstration of receptors for the opiate narcotic analgesics in animal and human central nervous systems, followed by the discovery that the body produces its own opiate-like substances, was hailed as a major breakthrough in neuroscience. It was widely felt that these discoveries would lead to an understanding of the biochemical basis of analgesia and pain regulation, as well as narcotic addiction. The molecular basis of narcotic addiction is still not understood in spite of the strides made in information concerning the endogenous opioid system and other neurotransmitter systems likely to be of importance. However, progress is being made and is summarized.

This chapter is a review of the current status of our knowledge of the biology of the endogenous opioid system and provides a summary of some of its postulated functions with emphasis on the question of its possible relevance to narcotic addiction. Finally, it provides some speculations as to where the field may be going in the next few years and how it may ultimately benefit clinical medicine, in particular our ability to prevent and treat narcotic addiction.

DISCOVERY OF OPIOID RECEPTORS AND ENDOGENOUS OPIOID PEPTIDES

Opium, an extract derived from the poppy, *Papaver somniferum*, is one of the oldest medications known. Its psychological effects and usefulness in relieving pain and diarrhea were already known to the ancient Sumerians (4000 BC) and Egyptians (2000 BC). The main active ingredient of opium is the alkaloid morphine, which is still the most effective and widely used analgesic drug for severe and chronic pain. The numerous pharmacologic activities of morphine have long fascinated scientists, who have attempted to understand the mechanisms that underlie these activities. The most interesting actions of morphine and related drugs are those affecting the central nervous system (CNS), such as the control of pain, mood changes, and the phenomena of tolerance and physical and psychological dependence, which develop following chronic drug intake and which together make up the major undesirable side effect of the opiate drugs, namely, narcotic addiction.

In the 1940s and 1950s, a very active synthetic program was mounted by the pharmaceutical industry, in an attempt to produce a nonaddictive analgesic. This goal has, unfortunately, not been achieved to this day, but this program did result in the synthesis of a large number of clinically effective medications, many of which are still in use. The work also yielded a number of scientific findings, which gave rise to the hypothesis that opiate drugs must bind to highly specific sites or receptors on nerve cells in order to exert most of their effects. This hypothesis was based on the observation that many of the pharmacologic effects of these drugs, including analgesia, exhibit considerable stereospecificity; i.e., the levorotatory enantiomer is usually active, and the dextrorotatory form is essentially inactive. In 1973, our laboratory (1) and two others (2,3) simultaneously published biochemical evidence for the existence of stereospecific binding sites for opiates in animal brain. This was quickly followed by our finding that such sites also exist in human brain (4). It is now generally accepted that these binding sites are receptors that mediate various pharmacologic effects of the opiate drugs.

The important finding that specific receptors for opiate drugs exist in every vertebrate species, and even in some invertebrate species, led to yet another exciting discovery. Scientists posed the questions: Why are such receptors so widespread? and Why have they survived eons of evolution? This led to the postulate that they must have endogenous functions, suggesting that endogenous opiate-like ligands are likely to exist in the central nervous system and, perhaps, elsewhere in the body. An exhaustive study of the known neurotransmitters and neurohormones failed to reveal any that exhibited high affinity for the newly found receptors. This stimulated a number of laboratories to begin the tedious work of trying to isolate from animal brain a novel substance with the appropriate characteristics. In 1974–1975, John Hughes and the late Hans Kosterlitz (5) and Terenius and Wahlstrom (6) reported the detection of substances that exhibited opiate-like (opioid) activity in brain extracts. Success in purifying and characterizing the structure of endogenous molecules with opioid activity was first achieved by Hughes and Kosterlitz and their coworkers (7). These substances proved to be two closely similar pentapeptides, Tyr-Gly-Gly-Phe-Met and Tyr-Gly-Gly-Phe-Leu, which they named methionine and leucine enkephalin (Greek for "in the brain"), respectively. Since then, at least eight peptides with opioid activity have been found, including the endorphins, derived from the previously known pituitary hormone β-lipotropin, of which the most important is β-endorphin (8,9). Dynorphin (10) is a very potent opioid peptide with Leu-enkephalin at its N-terminal. It is a very basic peptide; i.e., it contains many basic amino acids, such as lysine and arginine, and is clearly not derived from β-lipotropin.

Because these opioid peptides are thought to be the natural ligands of the opiate receptors, the latter have been renamed *opioid* receptors, a term used throughout the rest of this review. The name *endorphin* was first suggested by the author of this chapter in 1975, as a useful generic term for all peptides with endogenous opiate-like activity (see footnote in reference 11). It is a contraction of "endogenous" and "morphine" (the terminal "e" was dropped at the suggestion of Avram Goldstein to conform to nomenclature for peptides). This term is used interchangeably with the more cumbersome term *endogenous opioid peptides* throughout this review.

It should be mentioned that two laboratories have found that authentic morphine and codeine exist in animal CNS (12,13). The significance of the presence of these alkaloids, formerly thought to be the products of plants only, remains to be determined. It has not yet been proven that these molecules are indeed synthesized by animal cells.

OPIOID PEPTIDES

A considerable body of knowledge has accumulated regarding the pharmacology and molecular biology of the opioid peptides, which knowledge is summarized in this section.

The complexity of the endogenous opioid system is considerably greater than originally suspected. At least eight or nine endogenous peptides with opioid activity are known, and, as is discussed later, in section entitled Multiple Receptors, Properties, and Distribution, there are also multiple types of receptors.

The techniques of molecular biology have permitted some order to be established among the many opioid peptides known. As shown in Figure 10.1, it is now clear that all of the known opioid peptides are derived from three large precursor proteins—proopiomelanocortin, proenkephalin, and prodynorphin—each of which is encoded by a separate gene. As discussed below and depicted in Figure 10.2, the structures of the genes are also known.

The discovery of proopiomelanocortin (POMC) (14,15) was of considerable importance, not only for opioid research, but also for the entire field of biology. It was the first protein precursor found to give rise to several different

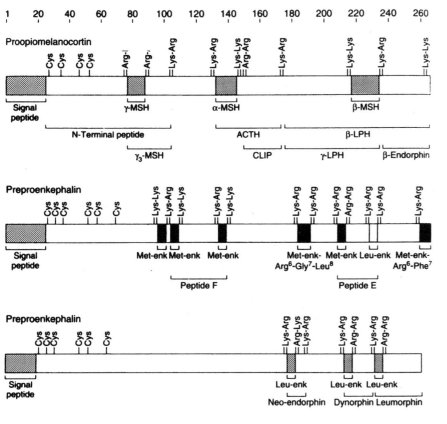

FIG. 10.1. Diagrammatic representation of structures of opioid peptide precursors, Met-enkephalin (Met-enk), Leu-enkephalin (Leu-enk), signal peptides, and MSH units are shown. Cysteine and dibasic acid residues are shown above, and major peptides derived from each precursor are shown below each diagram. CLIP, corticotropin-like intermediate lobe peptide; LPH, lipotropin; MSH, melanocyte-stimulating hormone. From Imura H, Kato Y, Nakai Y, et al. Endogenous opioids and related peptides: from molecular biology to clinical medicine. The Sir Henry Dale lecture for 1985. *J Endocrinol* 1985;107:147–157, with permission.

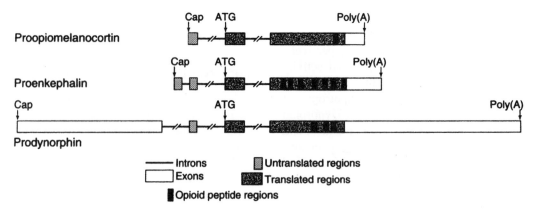

FIG. 10.2. Opioid peptide gene family. *Cap*, start of transcription; *ATG*, start of translation; *Poly(A)*, start of polyadenylation; and *solid bars*, opioid peptide regions, i.e., Met-enkephalin and/or Leu-enkephalin. From Höllt V. In: Almeida OFX, Shippenberg TS, eds. *Neurobiology of opioids*. Heidelberg: Springer-Verlag, 1991;12:Fig. 1, with permission.)

and seemingly unrelated biologically active peptides. In addition to being the precursor of the endorphins, POMC gives rise to adrenocorticotropin (ACTH) and a family of melanocyte-stimulating hormones (a-, β-, and γ-MSH), as indicated by its name coined by the late Sidney Udenfriend. The intermediate lobe of the pituitary is the major source of POMC, and β-endorphin is the major opioid peptide derived from this precursor. It exists mainly in the pituitary gland and the CNS.

POMC was the first of the opioid peptide precursors to be sequenced (16). As shown in Figure 10.2, its gene structure has also been determined, and it contains three expressed sequences (these are the translated regions of the deoxyribonucleic acid [DNA], called *exons* for short) and two intervening sequences (these are sequences called *introns* for short, which are often quite long and which are "spliced out" and therefore no longer present in mature messenger ribonucleic acid [mRNA]). POMC is the primary gene product, which is subsequently processed into the various biologically active peptides. Pairs of basic amino acids (in rare cases, a single basic amino acid) border each biologically active peptide present in the precursor proteins and are the targets for proteolytic cleavage by "processing" enzymes. The extent and nature of the processing vary from tissue to tissue. A number of the processing enzymes are known and have been cloned and thoroughly characterized.

Proenkephalin was first discovered in bovine adrenal cortex, where enkephalin biosynthesis was elucidated by Udenfriend and collaborators (17). It has been cloned and sequenced from bovine and human tissues (18). It contains one copy of Leu-enkephalin, four copies of Met-enkephalin, and two copies of C-terminal-extended Met-enkephalin peptides, a heptapeptide and an octapeptide. The gene coding for proenkephalin contains four exons and five introns.

Prodynorphin, the last of the opioid peptide precursors to be characterized (19,20), has been isolated from various mammalian tissues, including brain and spinal cord, pituitary and adrenal glands, and reproductive organs. All of the opioid peptides derived from this protein, dynorphin A and B and α- and β-neoendorphin, are C-terminal extensions of Leu-enkephalin. The prodynorphin gene has four exons and three introns (21).

There is considerable similarity between the three precursors and between their genes. They contain almost the same total number of amino acids. All have several opioid peptides contained largely in the C-terminal half of the molecule and, as stated, framed by pairs of basic amino acids. They all possess a cysteine-rich N-terminal sequence preceded by similarly sized signal peptides. There is considerable amino acid sequence homology, which in the case of proenkephalin and prodynorphin exceeds 50%. The genes also exhibit similarity in the placement and size of their respective introns and exons. All this evidence has given rise to the hypothesis that the three genes have developed from a common ancestor gene by gene duplication in the course of evolution.

All of the opioid peptides produce a variety of pharmacologic effects when injected intraventricularly. These effects include analgesia, respiratory depression, and a wide variety of behavioral changes, including the production of a rigid catatonia. It is evident that they are remarkably similar to the opiate drugs in the types of changes they produce. The peptides do not pass very efficiently through the blood–brain barrier, but a number of effects, particularly on memory and learning, have been reported for systemically administered opioid peptides (22). Presumably only very tiny amounts of the peptides are required to penetrate into the CNS. The actions of the enkephalins tend to be short-lived, probably as a result of their rapid destruction by peptidases. Several peptidases capable of hydrolyzing enkephalins have been studied in detail by a number of laboratories. Inhibitors of these enzymes cause analgesia (23), presumably by conserving the brain's enkephalins. The longer-chain peptides tend to be more stable and produce effects of long duration. Thus, β-endorphin can produce analgesia that can last 3 to 4 hours. All of the responses to endogenous opioids are readily reversed by opiate antagonists, such as naloxone and naltrexone.

The distribution of the major opioid peptides, enkephalins, β-endorphin, and dynorphin A, has been mapped in rat brain by the powerful technique of immunocytochemistry (for a review see reference 24). It was found that many groups of cell bodies throughout the brain and spinal cord contain and probably produce enkephalins. Dynorphins also seem to be produced in a considerable number of cell groups. This is in contrast to β-endorphin, which is found in cell bodies of only two brain areas, the arcuate nucleus of the hypothalamus and the nucleus tractus solitarius of the brainstem. All of the peptides seem to be moved to nerve terminals in many regions by means of axonal transport.

MULTIPLE OPIOID RECEPTORS, PROPERTIES AND DISTRIBUTION

When opioid receptors were first demonstrated, it was thought that only a single type existed. However, this idea quickly changed, based on there being multiple opioid peptides, some of which may be neurotransmitters. It is a well-known fact that the classical neurotransmitters tend to have more than one receptor each. The first definitive evidence for multiple opioid receptors was obtained by Martin and coworkers (25,26), who studied the pharmacology of morphine and its congeners in chronic spinal dogs. Their findings appeared to be consistent with the existence of at least three types of opioid receptors, which they named μ (for morphine), κ (for ketocyclazocine), and σ (for SKF-10047, N-allyl-normetazocine). These drugs exhibited quite different pharmacologic profiles and were unable to replace each other in the suppression of withdrawal symptoms in dogs treated chronically with one of them. Separate receptors appeared to be the simplest explanation. Experiments in whole animals, *in vitro* bioassay systems, and binding studies in cell membrane preparations continue to confirm the existence of the receptor types postulated by Martin and coworkers.

The discovery of the enkephalins by Hughes and Kosterlitz led to the postulate of another receptor type with preference for these opioid pentapeptides. The first evidence for this came from work in Kosterlitz's laboratory with isolated organ systems (27). Enkephalins were much less effective than morphine in inhibiting electrically evoked contractions of the isolated guinea pig ileum, whereas the reverse was true in the isolated mouse vas deferens. The enkephalin-preferring receptor that seemed to predominate in the latter tissue was named δ (for *deferens*, because there is no Greek equivalent of the letter v). Further support for this hypothesis came from competition binding studies and from the finding that the receptors in the

mouse vas deferens were significantly more resistant to naloxone than those in the guinea pig ileum; i.e., ten times as much naloxone was required for the same degree of reversal of opioid inhibition of contraction. The receptors that predominate in the guinea pig ileum were similar to Martin's μ receptor and were therefore assumed to be the same receptor type.

Since then several additional types of receptors have been postulated, most notably a specific receptor for β-endorphin called ϵ (28) and another receptor for the enkephalins, different from β receptors, called ι (29), because it seemed to predominate in intestines. Subtypes of receptors, such as μ_1 and μ_2, β_1 and β_2, and κ_1 and κ_2, have also been suggested. Space does not permit discussion of these additional, less-well-established opioid receptors, but this should not be interpreted to mean that they may not be real and of considerable importance. The σ receptor is very interesting but is perhaps not truly an opioid receptor, because actions mediated via this receptor are not reversed by the opiate antagonist naloxone, an operational definition of opioid receptors that is widely accepted. There is considerable evidence suggesting that the σ receptors are binding sites for another abused drug, phencyclidine, also known as "angel dust" or PCP (30).

The most recently discovered receptor is not really an opioid receptor, although it has very high amino acid homology with the opioid receptor family and especially with the κ receptor; it is called the ORL-1 receptor. An endogenous peptide that appears to be the natural ligand for this receptor has also been identified (31,32). It has been called orphanin FQ, because ORL-1 had been for some time an "orphan" receptor in search of a ligand. The ligand has also been called nociceptin, because receptor activation alters nociception. The ORL-1 receptors do not bind opioid peptides or opiate drugs. This system is widely distributed in the brain and spinal cord. Its activation produces hyperalgesia in most instances, although analgesia and no effect on pain have also been reported. In a recent review (33), the authors suggest that the reason for the discrepancy in results is that the system is inhibitory for many different neurons in the CNS, which includes inhibition of excitatory as well as inhibitory neurons. The nociceptin system may have a wide range of actions, but its functions are not yet understood and even its role in nociception is still not clear. It is thought probable that this system interacts with the more classical endogenous opioid system. The system is under intensive study and is likely to be of considerable importance.

The rest of this section concentrates on the three major and best-studied types of opioid receptors, μ, δ, and κ. The fine mapping of the three major types of opioid receptors in rat brain was accomplished primarily by the technique of autoradiography (34,35), using radiolabeled highly selective ligands (see below). All three major types of opioid receptors are widely distributed throughout the gray areas of the brain and spinal cord, with limbic and limbic-associated areas tending to have the highest levels. While there is some overlap, the μ, δ, and κ receptors show quite distinct localizations, suggesting that they are likely to be different molecular species rather than different forms of a single receptor, a hypothesis that has been proven (see section on receptor cloning).

Two other opioid peptides with very high selectivity and affinity for μ opioid receptors were recently reported. Zadina and coworkers call them endomorphin 1 and endomorphin 2. They were isolated from bovine and human brain and are proposed to be the endogenous ligands of the μ opioid receptors. They mediate many of the functions known to result from the activation of μ opioid receptors. However, it should be noted that no precursor protein or gene has so far been discovered for these peptides. It is therefore not yet proven that they are indeed endogenous opioid peptides (for reviews see references 36–38).

Distribution of opioid receptors in other species, including human brain (4), has also been studied. The distribution tends to be quite similar from species to species. There are, however, some interesting and poorly understood species differences. An example is the cerebellum, which is high in μ receptors in the guinea pig, high in κ receptors in the rabbit, and virtually devoid of any opioid receptors in the rat. All types of opioid receptors bind their ligands stereospecifically and with affinities in the nanomolar range.

The naturally occurring peptides have a preference for a particular receptor type but are not highly selective. It is postulated that enkephalins are endogenous ligands for δ receptors and dynorphins are endogenous ligands for κ receptors, whereas there are several candidates for the μ receptor, including β-endorphin and morphine. Even the enkephalins have significant affinity at this receptor, which could serve as a second or "iso" receptor for them. More work is needed to establish definitively which peptides (or natural alkaloids) go with which receptors.

The lack of selectivity of the natural opioid peptides presented serious problems for the characterization of the different types of opioid receptors and led to a major effort by organic chemists to synthesize analogues that are highly selective ligands for the three major types. This quest has met with considerable success. Highly specific agonists are now available. For the μ site, there is a gly-ol derivative of D-Ala^2-enkephalin, called DAMGO ([D-Ala^2,methyl-Phe^4,Gly^5-ol]-enkephalin) (39) for δ, there are the dipenicillamine analogues of enkephalin, DPDPE ([D-Pen^2,D-Pen^5]-enkephalin) and DPLPE (40) and hexapeptides called DTLET, DSLET ([D-serine^2]-D-leucine-enkephalin-threonine) and DSBuLET (41); for κ receptors, there are stable derivatives of dynorphin (42,43) and nonpeptide derivatives synthesized by scientists at the Upjohn Company, called U 50,488H and U 69,593 (44,45). All the compounds discussed so far are agonists, but specific antagonists have also become available for all three receptor types. For μ receptors, cyclic derivatives of somatostatin are highly selective antagonists (46). For δ receptors, a peptide synthesized at Imperial Chemical Industries (ICI) (47) and a derivative of naltrexone called naltrindole (48) serve as selective antagonists, while a "double-headed" molecule called *nor-binaltorphimine* (49) proved effective in antagonizing effects mediated via κ receptors.

A most surprising and intriguing finding was the natural existence in unexpected places of highly selective ligands. Thus, selective ligands for μ opioid receptors were found in casein hydrolysates (50) called casomorphin and in frog skin (51) named dermorphin. Several δ-receptor-selective agonists, called deltorphins, were also isolated from frog skin (52).

CLONING OF OPIOID RECEPTORS

Although cloning was briefly alluded to in the discussion of the sequencing of the genes that encode the opioid peptide precursor proteins, a brief explanation of precisely what cloning is and what it can do is deemed appropriate for the diverse readership of this book. As explained in the next paragraph, it is merely a more rapid and convenient way to obtain the amino acid sequence of a protein by sequencing the DNA that encodes it.

The opioid receptors, like the peptide precursors, are protein molecules; i.e., they are long chains of amino acids. In nature, 20 different amino acids exist of which all proteins are composed. It is the amino acid sequence or primary structure that confers uniqueness on each protein. The amino acid sequence dictates the three-dimensional structure, i.e., the way the protein is folded and displayed in the cell, which in large measure is responsible for the unique function of a protein, such as that of an enzyme, receptor, or ion channel. To understand the structure and function of a protein, therefore, it is essential to know its amino acid sequence. After the classical work of Fred Sanger in Cambridge, England, who sequenced the short protein, insulin, it became evident that direct sequencing of very large proteins is very tedious and labor-intensive. It proved much easier to sequence the DNA of the gene encoding the protein and to use the genetic code to translate the nucleotide triplets or codons into amino acids. This has the additional advantage of providing the sequence for the coding region of the gene as well as of the protein and facilitates obtaining the sequence of the entire gene. The reverse, obtaining the DNA sequence from the amino acid sequence, would be much more difficult because the genetic code is "degenerate;" i.e., in many cases there are as many as four to six codons (nucleotide triplets) that encode the same amino acid.

The technique, which has become known as cloning, consists of isolating the mRNA from an appropriate source. The mRNA is converted to its complementary

DNA (cDNA) by the enzyme, reverse transcriptase. The cDNA is isolated and sequenced. Cloning can also be done with genomic DNA, but using cDNA is easier because the mRNA from which it is made has been processed to remove the large, confusing introns that are almost always present in the gene. Pieces of the cDNA are placed into a vector (DNA that can replicate, such as phage or plasmid DNA). The vector is introduced into bacteria (a strain of *Escherichia coli* is most commonly used), which are grown into colonies. This step is the cloning, because it results in bacterial colonies or clones that contain the gene in question, and these can be greatly amplified by simply growing large amounts of the bacteria from the appropriate clone. Usually an antibiotic resistance gene is introduced into the vector and the bacteria are grown in the antibiotic, so that only resistant bacteria, the ones that have received the desired DNA, survive and form colonies. A suitable analytical method is required to determine the desired DNA to be sequenced. If a portion of the sequence is known, hybridization of the clones with a labeled oligonucleotide probe, prepared from the known sequence, can be used for identification. If not, expression cloning can be used, in which the DNA is transferred to an appropriate mammalian cell (*Xenopus oocytes* have also been used) capable of expressing the gene product. The presence of the gene product, the protein encoded by the gene, is detected by measuring a function, such as receptor binding, enzymatic activity, or ion channel function or by selection with a specific antibody against the protein. If the gene is expressed, the DNA is amplified, purified, and sequenced.

For several years, many laboratories, including ours, tried hard, but in vain, to clone and sequence DNA-encoding opioid receptors. It was usually done by purifying the receptor (in our case the μ receptor) and obtaining a short amino acid sequence from the purified protein, translating it into its nucleotide sequence, and labeling it with a radioisotope. This labeled probe was then used to recognize the clones containing the gene by hybridization with the appropriate DNA. For various reasons, too complex to discuss here, this did not succeed. Expression cloning proved successful in two laboratories. In this technique, pieces of DNA, a "cDNA library," are transfected into mammalian cells and assayed for expression of the receptor, i.e., for opioid ligand binding. Positive cells have received the cDNA encoding the receptor, which can be isolated and sequenced. Kieffer et al. (53) and Evans et al. (54), using this approach simultaneously and independently, succeeded in cloning the δ opioid receptor from a neuroblastoma X glioma hybrid cell line, NG 108–15. Since that time, based on the expected similarity between opioid receptor types, all three major opioid receptors have been sequenced from several species, including humans (for a review of this field read reference 55). It is noteworthy that, as this is being written, 12 years after the first opioid receptor was cloned, no subtypes of μ, δ, or κ receptors, nor any other opioid receptors, have been cloned. This may simply mean that they are sufficiently different to have so far escaped detection. It could also signify that the subtypes and other types, postulated on the basis of pharmacology, are not encoded by separate genes but are modifications of the cloned proteins, which occurred after protein synthesis, i.e., so-called posttranslational modifications. Such posttranslational changes include the addition of sugars (glycosylation), of phosphate groups (phosphorylation), or of lipids (lipidation).

When the large introns present in raw transcribed RNA are spliced out to form mature mRNA, some differences in the type and number of exons left in for translation can occur. This gives rise to slightly different proteins, called *splice variants*. Thus, receptor subtypes could result from splice variants of the three opioid receptor genes currently known. A considerable number of such splice variants, by now at least 10, have been isolated, for the μ opioid receptor gene, primarily in the laboratories of Hoellt (56) and Pasternak (57,58). Interestingly, none have been found to be pharmacologically identical to the postulated opioid receptor subtypes or postulated types, beyond μ, δ, and κ. The physiologic role of these splice variants is currently under intensive study.

WHAT HAS BEEN LEARNED FROM KNOWLEDGE OF PROTEIN AND GENE STRUCTURES?

The availability of the complete amino acid sequences of all three major types of opioid receptors and knowledge of the structure of the genes encoding these receptors have already led to considerable progress in our understanding of how these receptors function. It has long been postulated that opioid receptors belong to the large family of receptors that can couple to guanine nucleotide-regulatory proteins (G proteins). However, it was only after the amino acid sequence and protein structure was known that this could be definitively established. The signal generated when an opioid agonist binds to its receptor is transduced and propagated via G proteins and second messenger systems. This is discussed in somewhat more detail later in this chapter, in section entitled Mechanisms of Opioid Action. Structurally, the hypophobicity profile of the opioid receptors suggests that these proteins traverse the cell membrane seven times, a characteristic of all G protein-coupled receptors. This structure has been most thoroughly studied with rhodopsin, the vision protein, a prototypical member of this group, whose "ligand" happens to be light.

A great deal has been learned about the nature of the opioid binding site on the receptor by mutating the cDNA so as to change or delete one or more amino acids in the protein and transfecting the mutated DNA into suitable cells for expression. These techniques are known as deletion and site-directed mutation analyses. Another clever technique, widely used now, is the creation of cDNA that gives rise to molecules that are hybrids between two receptors, e.g., molecules that are part μ and part δ receptor. These new receptors are called chimeras, after the Greek mythological monster with the head of a lion, the body of a she-goat, and the tail of a dragon. Studies of these chimeras permit analysis, for example, of what region confers ligand specificity for one or the other type of receptor and which region is responsible for signal transduction by a particular activated receptor. A detailed discussion of these studies is not possible in this chapter. Suffice it to say that the ligand binding site, even for relatively hydrophilic ligands, is not on the outer surface of the cell membrane, as had been expected, but deep inside the rather hydrophobic (fatty) membrane itself. When this was first discovered for the β-adrenergic receptor, a member of the same family, it was a great surprise to scientists in this field. For readers who wish to know more about this fascinating area of research, excellent reviews have appeared (55,59–61).

One of the most powerful techniques made possible by cloning and knowing the DNA sequence of a gene under study is gene targeting. It involves inactivation or "knockout" of a gene, usually in a mouse, and determining how the absence of the protein, no longer produced by the targeted gene, affects the phenotype of the mouse, termed a *knockout mouse*. This technique does have limitations that need to be kept in mind. If the gene is crucial for fetal survival or development, it will be lethal early in the life and no studies will be possible. When an adult mouse does develop in absence of a gene, there may be other genes that can make proteins that compensate for the absence of the product of the inactivated gene. Once these cautions are kept in mind, a great deal can be learned from knockout mice. Mice have been prepared in which any one or two of the three known opioid receptor genes were inactivated. Most recently, mice were produced lacking all three opioid receptors. All of these mice show normal development and appear to grow into normal adults. It requires careful testing to find changes in behavioral phenotype. To provide one example of what can be learned, there was always a controversy as to whether antinociception is a characteristic of μ receptor activation by μ ligands and by cross-reaction of δ and κ ligands with the μ receptor, or whether each of the three opioid receptors is able to produce analgesia. This has now been definitively settled. The activation of each of the three types of opioid receptors can result in analgesia. Another example of the power of this tool is the recent confirmation of the earlier suggestion by pharmacologic studies that the opioid and cannabinoid systems interact. Thus, knockout mice demonstrate that the opioid system plays a role in cannabinoid antinociception and tolerance (62). For further information on the knowledge gained by the use of knockout mice deprived of one or more genes coding for proteins of the endogenous opioid system, please refer to the excellent reviews by

Kieffer (63,64). It should be mentioned that another powerful novel molecular technique is gene transfer, the introduction of an altered or novel gene into a cell or animal and observing its effects on the phenotype.

PURIFICATION OF OPIOID RECEPTORS

Isolation and purification of opioid receptors is an important endeavor. Only by studying isolated, highly purified receptor proteins and their structures will we obtain answers to many important questions about their functions. For example, much can be learned about the structure of a protein and its posttranslational modifications (phosphorylation, glycosylation, lipidation, etc.) by the use of modern physical chemical techniques, such as mass spectrometry. It has also been possible, although difficult, to crystallize pure proteins and establish their precise three-dimensional structure and location of each atom by the powerful technique of x-ray diffraction. I briefly summarize progress in the area of receptor purification, especially because it is one in which my laboratory has pioneered.

The first purification to apparent homogeneity of a μ opioid binding site was reported from our laboratory almost 20 years ago (65). The starting tissue was a membrane fraction prepared from bovine striatum. The major purification step was affinity (also called biospecific) chromatography on a column in which a derivative of naltrexone was coupled to agarose beads. Because only opioid receptors bind to this matrix with high affinity, this step resulted in 3000- to 5000-fold purification. A second step made use of our finding that the receptors are glycoproteins containing the sugar N-acetylglucosamine (66) and involved absorption of the receptor on a wheat germ lectin column specific for this sugar and subsequent elution by competition with high concentrations of N-acetylglucosamine. The purified protein showed a single band with a molecular weight of 65 kDa on sodium dodecyl sulfate-polyacrylamide gel electrophoresis (SDS-PAGE). Its specific binding activity (15,000 pmol/mg protein) is close to the theoretical value for a pure protein of this size. Purification to homogeneity of μ receptors has since been reported by Cho et al. (67) and Ueda et al. (67a) The purification method developed in our laboratory is still in use in many laboratories including our own.

The δ receptor has been purified by Klee and coworkers (68) from NG 108–15 neuroblastoma X glioma hybrid cell cultures known to contain high levels of only this receptor type. This purification was done by affinity-labeling the receptor with an irreversible, δ-selective ligand, (^{3}H)-3-methylfentanylisothiocyanate, called *superFIT*. The purified protein showed a single band on SDS-PAGE with a molecular weight of 58 kDa. The amount of superFIT bound per mg protein was in agreement with the expected theoretical value. This purified δ receptor is covalently bound to superFIT and is therefore inactive. The purification of active β binding sites has been reported (69).

The purification of κ sites has been reported from frog brain (Simon, 1987 #827) and from human placenta (Ahmed, 1989 #7). To the best of my knowledge, this receptor has not yet been purified from mammalian nervous system. A useful affinity chromatography column to facilitate κ receptor purification has been constructed using the antagonist *nor*-binaltorphimine (70).

RECONSTITUTION OF μ OPIOID RECEPTORS IN ARTIFICIAL MEMBRANES

The μ opioid receptor protein we have purified is capable of binding opioid antagonists with high affinity, but it has very low affinity for agonists. This is not surprising, because it is well known that receptors of this family must be coupled to G proteins to bind agonists with high affinity. We have reported (71,72) our success in reconstituting our purified opioid receptor in lipoprotein particles or liposomes (sometimes referred to as artificial membranes) and to recouple it with various highly purified isoforms of G proteins. The coupled receptor, in this system containing only pure proteins and a defined phospholipid, is now able to bind agonists with high affinity, comparable to that of the native, membrane-bound receptor. Moreover, the binding is highly selective for μ agonists, as compared to δ or κ agonists.

G proteins all contain an enzymatic activity, namely an enzyme that hydrolyzes guanosine 5'-triphosphate (GTP) to guanosine 5'-diphosphate (GDP), called GTPase. This enzyme is known to be stimulated when a receptor coupled to the G protein is activated by an agonist ligand. We showed in the same study that when μ agonists bind to the purified, reconstituted μ receptor, GTPase is stimulated up to 100%. This stimulation is again highly specific for μ agonists, and no stimulation is seen with either δ or κ agonists. These experiments constitute proof that we have indeed purified a μ opioid receptor. We have now cloned the bovine μ opioid receptor (73) and have shown that the cloned receptor is identical to the one we purified.

FUNCTIONS OF ENDOGENOUS OPIOIDS AND THEIR RECEPTORS

Table 10.1 represents the major functions in which the endogenous opioid system has been implicated in the literature. It is evident that the opioid system may play a role in a wide variety of physiologic and pharmacologic phenomena, although the evidence in some cases is still quite preliminary. Our interest is, of course, primarily in the behavioral effects of the opiates, but actions on the autonomic nervous system and the endocrine system are of considerable importance, especially because these systems are known to interact with the CNS. A relatively

TABLE 10.1. *Functions in which endorphins have been implicated*

Behavioral and mood changes
Supraspinal and spinal analgesia
Stress-induced analgesia
Euphoria and dysphoria
Sedation
Locomotor activity
Tolerance
Withdrawal signs
Appetite suppression
Anticonvulsant activity
Mental disorders
Endocrine system
ACTH-cortisol release
Prolactin release
GH release
ADH inhibition
LH and testosterone inhibition
Autonomic effects
Mydriasis
Miosis
Smooth muscle motility
Body temperature
Respiratory depression
Heart rate
Blood pressure
Endotoxic and hemorrhagic shock
Spinal cord injury
Immune system
Monocyte and leukocyte chemotaxis
Mitogen-induced proliferation
Antibody production
Natural killer activity

GH, growth hormone; ADH, antidiuretic hormone; and LH, luteinizing hormone.

recent discovery is the cross-talk between the immune system and the CNS in which the endorphins appear to play a role. This is an exciting research area, because it has the potential to explain many aspects of diseases that are now poorly understood, such as the effect of stress in exacerbating many diseases, as well as increasing the susceptibility to diseases.

One caveat that should be kept in mind is that changes seen in or produced by endogenous opioids may be important, but such changes need not signify primary involvement of this system. The observed changes could be a secondary or tertiary consequence of some other perturbation of the nervous system. Because of limitations of space and in deference to the central theme of this book, I discuss only two possible functions, namely the control of pain and the development of addictive behavior: tolerance and physical and psychic dependence. Before beginning a discussion of these functions, it is appropriate to summarize the current ideas about how the receptors propagate the signal generated by ligand binding, which ultimately results in the observed pharmacologic or physiologic effects.

MECHANISMS OF OPIOID ACTION

From a biochemical viewpoint, the opioid peptides are thought to exert their actions at neuronal synapses as either neurotransmitters or neuromodulators. It is likely that the peptides act as neurotransmitters, i.e., by altering (generally decreasing) the transsynaptic potential, when their receptors are localized presynaptically. On the other hand, evidence suggests that many opioid receptors are localized postsynaptically. In this case, the peptides modulate the release of a neurotransmitter, which can be one of the classical amines, such as acetylcholine, norepinephrine, or serotonin, or another peptide, such as substance P or neurotensin.

An interesting series of experiments performed by Schoffelmeer and coworkers (74) points to a possible functional difference between opioid receptor types with respect to modulation of transmitter release. These workers found that activation of μ receptors in cortical slices from rat brain led to inhibition of norepinephrine release, activation of δ receptors in striatal slices inhibited acetylcholine release, and the activation of κ receptors inhibited the release of striatal dopamine. Each of these effects seemed to be quite specifically manifested by a particular type of receptor, suggesting a different function for each type.

As stated earlier, it is now definitely established that all three major types of opioid receptors are coupled to G proteins. The early results were obtained in cell cultures, but more recent results show this to be true in the brain. This area of investigation has been reviewed (75). The G proteins, in turn, can couple the receptors either to second messenger systems or directly to ion channels. It is thought that the slower effects of opioids may be exerted via an inhibition of the enzyme adenylate cyclase, which synthesizes the second messenger, cyclic adenosine 3',5'-monophosphate (cAMP). The level of cAMP affects the activity of an enzyme that is able to phosphorylate proteins (cAMP-activated protein kinase A). The phosphorylation of synaptic proteins would have relatively immediate effects. It is also possible that other proteins that act on gene expression can be phosphorylated, resulting in a downregulation or upregulation of gene transcription. This could be responsible for some of the very-long-lasting changes produced by opiates.

It is a widely held view that many of the long-term effects of opiates are the result of somatic cell changes in gene expression. The signaling system that has been implicated in gene regulation is the mitogen-activated protein (MAP) kinase cascade. The phosphorylation of kinases in this pathway results in changes in gene expression in many situations. It was thought until only a few years ago that this pathway was activated only by hormone and growth factor receptors, which contain an intrinsic tyrosine kinase. However, in 1995, it was shown that G protein-coupled receptors (GPCRs) were able to activate this pathway (76,77). This was quickly followed by the finding that opioid receptors are no exception (78,79). It has long been established that the phosphorylation of one or more receptor tyrosine residues is a prerequisite for the activation of the MAP kinase cascade. For some of the GPCRs it was demonstrated that this was accomplished by a cross-phosphorylation of tyrosine residues in a tyrosine kinase receptor, when the GPCR is activated (80,81). However, Dr. Kramer, of our laboratory, was the first to show that in the case of opioid receptors, tyrosine phosphorylation can, in fact, occur in the opioid receptor protein itself (82). Experiments in which he mutated tyrosines in the carboxyl tail of the δ opioid receptor (83) indicated that two tyrosine residues accounted for virtually all of the phosphorylation and that they are required for activation of MAP kinase. These results are likely to be of considerable value in our gaining an understanding of the long-term, probably genetic, changes that lead to drug abuse and recidivism from drug abuse.

The rapid effects of opioids are most likely a result of direct action of activated opioid receptors on ion channels. It was established that the μ and δ opioid receptors open potassium channels (84), which results in reduction of calcium conductance. The activation of κ receptors was found to reduce calcium conductance by closing calcium channels (85). It was recently found that all three types of opioid receptors can act by both mechanisms; i.e., they can open potassium channels or close calcium channels (86,87).

PAIN AND ITS MODULATION

Inasmuch as it was work on the opiate analgesics that led to the discovery of the endorphins and their receptors, it was natural to postulate that the endogenous opioid system may be involved in endogenous pain modulation as well as in analgesia. This notion was supported by the finding that all CNS regions, known to be implicated in the conduction and dampening of pain impulses, have high levels of opioid receptors. The application of opiates was found to inhibit selectively the firing of nociceptive neurons in the substantia gelatinosa of the spinal cord (88). Moreover, as mentioned earlier, the intraventricular injection of all opioid peptides produces analgesia. These findings were sufficiently suggestive to encourage further work in this area.

Many early experiments involved attempts to demonstrate that nondrug-induced types of analgesia could be reversed by naloxone. If successful, this would suggest the involvement of endorphin release onto their receptors. Akil and coworkers (89) showed partial reversal by naloxone of analgesia induced by electrical brain stimulation in rats. Such reversal was also observed in human patients with chronic pain in whom stimulation of the periaqueductal gray area provided effective pain relief for prolonged periods (90). Acupuncture and electroacupuncture are also reversed by opiate antagonists (91,92), and some provocative studies in humans (93) suggest that the endogenous opioids may also play a role in placebo-induced analgesia, which is effective in approximately 30% of subjects tested.

It was postulated that pain thresholds could be related to receptor occupancy by endorphins. If so, the administration of opiate antagonists should lower pain thresholds. Such an effect has been surprisingly difficult to demonstrate in animals or humans. Jacob et al. (94) demonstrated a lowering of the pain threshold in rats in carefully controlled experiments, with a hot plate used as a source of thermal pain.

More direct evidence for the release of opioid peptides during analgesia has been obtained. Using indwelling intraventricular cannulae, Akil et al. (95) observed a large increase in the amount of β-endorphin released into the cerebrospinal fluid of terminal cancer patients after analgesia caused by stimulation of electrodes implanted in the central gray region of the brain. These workers (96) also found an increased release of enkephalins during pain stimulation, although this increase was much less robust (about twofold), which is not surprising in view of the instability of these peptides.

A study by Han and coworkers (97) in Beijing, China, indicates release of endorphin during electroacupuncture in rats. Using radioimmunoassays, these workers found that low-frequency electroacupuncture resulted in the release of enkephalins into spinal perfusate, whereas high-frequency stimulation led to release of dynorphin A. The injection of antibodies to either enkephalins or dynorphin blocked analgesia produced at the appropriate frequencies. These studies suggest that δ (or μ) receptors may be involved at low frequency, whereas κ receptors play a predominant role at high frequencies. This raises the interesting question as to which types of opioid receptors play a role in pain modulation.

Once it was pretty clear that endogenous opioid peptides are released during antinociception, the question of whether preservation of endorphins could lead to analgesia was appropriately asked. Dr. Bernard Roques in Paris synthesized very powerful peptidase inhibitors which dramatically protect enkephalins from degradation. In animals (23,98) these inhibitors produce analgesia and they are now in clinical trial in humans.

It is now widely accepted that all three of the major receptor types are involved in analgesia, but some evidence that they may be implicated in different kinds of pain is also becoming available. Thus, most reports suggest that supraspinal analgesia may be mediated via μ rather than δ or κ receptors (99,100). However, lest this finding be taken too seriously, I hasten to add that there are also reports of supraspinal analgesia mediated via δ (101) and κ (102) receptors.

At the spinal level, analgesia against thermal pain stimuli seems to be mediated by both μ and δ mechanisms, whereas κ receptors seem to preferentially mediate analgesia against chemically induced visceral pain (103).

An interesting approach to the pharmacologic treatment of pain is suggested by a large body of work performed mainly in the laboratory of Crain. These researchers observed in animals that the effectiveness of opiate drugs is significantly enhanced by very small doses of an antagonist. Their evidence suggests that the activation of opioid receptors can lead to stimulatory as well as inhibitory effects. The stimulatory receptors appear to have very high ligand affinity. They suggest that the very low doses of antagonist block specifically the stimulatory effects, which normally partially antagonize the analgesic effects of opiates. Such combinations are currently in clinical trial. For more information see reference 104.

It is evident that much is yet to be learned regarding the mechanisms underlying analgesia and endogenous pain modulation. However, the evidence that suggests that the endogenous opioid system is involved in at least some of these mechanisms is quite impressive. The reader is referred to a recent review of this important area (105).

NARCOTIC ADDICTION

There were, and continue to be, great expectations that the discovery of the endogenous opioid system would lead to major advances in our understanding of the molecular mechanism of drug addiction. Virtually all of the work leading to the discoveries of opioid receptors and endogenous opioid peptides was supported by grants from the National Institute on Drug Abuse (NIDA) and was therefore directed toward learning about the biochemical basis of drug addiction. NIDA is still the largest supporter of research in this area. Although the molecular basis of drug addiction has yet to be elucidated, there has been much progress toward this goal since the earlier edition of this book. Moreover, some possible reasons why progress has not been more rapid can be suggested. Early work on possible changes in the number or properties of opioid receptors after chronic morphine administration was negative (106,107). However, this work was carried out before it became known that there are a number of different types and subtypes of receptors. It is evident that these experiments had to be redone on individual receptor types.

One report details such experiments for μ receptors (108). Some subtle changes in binding of the highly selective μ ligand, DAMGO, were observed, namely a decrease in the number of high-affinity binding sites, which resulted in a small change in total receptor number. A more striking, and perhaps more important, finding was the loss of the normal sensitivity of these receptors toward inhibition by GTP and its analogues. This could be construed as confirmation of earlier reports suggesting that uncoupling of receptors from G proteins may be a mechanism of tolerance development rather than changes that occur at the binding sites.

Considerable evidence suggests that tolerance can develop selectively to a given receptor type with little cross-tolerance toward the others. Such studies were first carried out on the isolated mouse vas deferens (109), but similar results in whole animals have also been obtained (110).

When animals are treated chronically with opiate antagonists such as naloxone or naltrexone, there is an upregulation, i.e., an increase in the number of opioid receptors in many brain areas (86–89,111–114). This has been observed for all three types of opioid receptors, although the extent tends to vary from one brain region to another (115). Downregulation of receptors because of chronic treatment with agonists has been more difficult to demonstrate, but some reports have appeared (for reviews of opioid receptor regulation, see references 116 and 117). Another theory suggested that the chronic administration of opiate drugs would lead to a decrease in the synthesis and/or release of endorphins. Efforts to show changes in the levels of these peptides were negative. Clearly, these experiments should be repeated for all of the endogenous opioids now known. Recent studies suggest that such changes in endorphin metabolism do occur but require more sophisticated experiments than were available when the earlier experiments were done.

When the processing of the precursor of β-endorphin, POMC, was examined, it was found to give rise to two major species: β-endorphin, which contains 31 amino acids, and β-endorphin$_{1-27}$, which has had its four C-terminal amino acids removed. These peptides exist in brain regions of naive rats in a ratio of 1:1 to 1.5:1. When this ratio was examined in rats made tolerant to and dependent on morphine (treated for 3 days with subcutaneous morphine pellets) (118), it was found to be almost 2:1 in favor of β-endorphin$_{1-27}$. This subtle change could not be observed with the usual rapid procedures, such as radioimmunoassays, but required sophisticated separation techniques, such as high-performance liquid chromatography (HPLC). It is made more intriguing by the finding (119) that the shorter form of β-endorphin seems to be an antagonist capable of reversing many of the effects of β-endorphin. It is evident that this result can give rise to interesting hypotheses regarding the mechanism of tolerance and/or dependence.

An additional important result was obtained in the same laboratory, showing that the biosynthesis of β-endorphin is, in fact, reduced in chronically morphinized rats. This was determined by demonstrating a reduction in the amount of mRNA for POMC present in the cells of the hypothalamus of morphine-treated rats. The reason why this is not reflected in the peptide level is that peptide release is closely coupled to synthesis and that a decrease in release compensates for the reduced production. This pseudo-feedback inhibition by the exogenous

drugs could also play a role in the effects produced by chronic opiates.

It was observed very early (120) that tolerance and physical dependence develops to pharmacologic doses of the opioid peptides. Cross-tolerance with synthetic and natural opiates has also been shown. This should not, however, be interpreted to mean that we develop tolerance and dependence to our endogenous opioid peptides. They are sequestered and released as needed in very small quantities, which may be the body's way to prevent the formation of tolerance to and dependence on its own substances.

There is abundant literature that suggests that many of the symptoms of opiate withdrawal are the result of interactions between the opioid and other neurotransmitter systems. This has been studied in detail for the noradrenergic system. Gold et al. (121) treated human heroin addicts with clonidine (Catapres), an α_2-noradrenergic agonist, in a double-blind, placebo-controlled study. They found that clonidine eliminated or reduced many objective signs and subjective symptoms of withdrawal for 4 to 6 hours in all addicts. In an open pilot study, the patients did well on clonidine for periods of 1 week. All of the patients had been addicted to opiates for 6 to 10 years and had been on methadone for 6 to 60 months at the time of the study. This clinical study is an interesting and successful followup of the basic research on interactions between the opioid and the noradrenergic system in the locus ceruleus, which is summarized next.

The failure to demonstrate good correlation between effects of chronic opiates and changes in opioid receptor binding prompted scientists to look for changes in the postreceptor cascade of events. The pioneering paper was that of Collier and Roy (122), who showed that morphine and other opiates inhibit cAMP formation in rat brain homogenates. This was followed quickly by another important paper by Sharma et al. (123), who demonstrated a similar inhibition in NG 108–15 cells in culture. They went on to show that chronic opiate treatment of NG 108–15 cells leads to a compensatory increase in adenylyl cyclase, which blunts the inhibition of the enzyme by opiates (tolerance?) and leads to an overshoot in cAMP production on antagonist-precipitated withdrawal (dependence?). These findings stimulated considerable work in a number of laboratories. In particular, a detailed study of acute and chronic effects of opiates on signal transduction has been carried out in the locus ceruleus. This brain region was chosen based on evidence for interaction between the opioid and noradrenergic systems, summarized above. The most important impetus was the seminal electrophysiologic research of Aghajanian and coworkers (124–126), indicating an important role for this region in opiate tolerance and withdrawal. In a series of important papers, it was shown by Nestler and colleagues that chronic morphine causes a compensatory increase in all of the components of the cAMP signal transduction pathway, including

G proteins, adenylyl cyclase, cAMP-dependent protein kinase, and several protein substrates for this kinase. Some of these protein substrates have been identified in the locus ceruleus and other brain regions of chronically morphinized rats (127). Increased phosphorylation was found for tyrosine hydroxylase (128), an important enzyme in the synthesis of catecholamines, and for myelin basic proteins (129), components of myelin. It is evident that alteration in this important signaling pathway could account for tolerance and many features of opiate dependence. Changes in the phosphorylation of proteins that can regulate gene transcription (transcription factors) could lead to even longer term effects by changing the level of gene expression for certain proteins. This would explain very early findings that tolerance development was attenuated by inhibitors of protein and nucleic acid synthesis (130) and could explain effects in chronic opiate users that appear to last months or even years, including the high rate of recidivism. Excellent reviews of these studies are in the literature (131,132). For a general review of the importance of signal transduction in opioid dependence, see reference 133.

A very important observation was made by Trujillo and Akil (134,135), who found that tolerance and physical dependence were dramatically reduced when MK-801, a noncompetitive antagonist at the N-methyl-D-aspartate (NMDA) glutamate receptor, was administered to rats along with chronic morphine. Excitatory amino acid receptors and, in particular, this glutamate receptor have a crucial function in brain development, long-term potentiation, and learning. The Pasternak and Inturrisi laboratories (136,137) have shown that competitive antagonists of the NMDA receptor also attenuate tolerance. They also found that this effect appears to be mediated via the gaseous neurotransmitter, nitrous oxide (NO), because inhibitors of the enzyme NO synthase also profoundly reduce tolerance to opiates. These investigators found (136) that the NMDA receptor seems to be involved in the development, as well as the maintenance, of tolerance; i.e., antagonists also reverse established tolerance, whereas the Akil group did not find reversal of established tolerance. The reason for this discrepancy is not known, but there are a number of important differences in the way the experiments were performed. Moreover, the NMDA antagonists exert behavioral effects of their own, which, according to Akil, could compete with and thus mask the withdrawal symptoms.

Two mechanisms of tolerance development have been defined. Pharmacologic (nonassociative) tolerance is a direct physiologic response to chronic drug treatment. Associative or behavioral tolerance is the result of conditioning, i.e., learning of associations between drug effects and environmental cues. It is interesting that several laboratories (see, for example, references 138 and 139) found that NMDA antagonists inhibit pharmacologic tolerance but do not seem able to inhibit associative tolerance (135). This is surprising in view of the well-known role of excitatory amino acid receptors in memory, including previous evidence that MK-801 interferes with some types of learning.

An investigation of the anatomic site at which NMDA receptor antagonists exert their effect on tolerance and dependence led to a surprising finding. Tolerance was found to be inhibited at the spinal level by Kest et al. (140), who used intrathecal administration. Moreover, studies in spinalized rats (141,142) provided evidence that inhibition at the spinal level was sufficient to inhibit tolerance to morphine analgesia. This suggests that the NMDA receptors, which are crucial for tolerance development, are located in the spinal cord. Excellent reviews of the role of excitatory amino acid receptors in the development of tolerance and physical dependence have been published (143–145).

Finally, a brief mention should be made of a recent hypothesis based on research by Sadee and coworkers and recently confirmed and expanded in our laboratory (HK Kramer et al., manuscript in preparation). It suggests that the dramatic increase in the proportion of constitutively active opioid receptors during chronic opiate treatment may play an important role in the development of tolerance and physical dependence. Constitutive receptors are defined as receptors that are active without having to bind a ligand. They exhibit greatly increased inverse agonist activity of opioid antagonists, which is the usual way to test for such receptors. This dramatic increase in inverse agonist activity after chronic opiate exposure also suggests an explanation for the well-known fact that relatively small doses of naloxone are highly effective in reversing heroin overdose toxicity in addicts.

CONCLUDING COMMENTS

It is evident that there have been many major developments in this field since the appearance of earlier editions. Because of limitations in both space and the author's expertise, many developments had to be given short shrift or left out altogether. This overview gives the interested reader an idea of the state of the art in many aspects of this exciting area of research and provides comprehensive reviews and original papers for those who wish more in-depth information. This research domain continues to be an extremely active one and findings in this area impinge on many other areas of neuroscience.

One important area I did not discuss is the research using self-administration and investigator-initiated administration of opiates in animals ranging from rats to monkeys. A great deal has been learned from these studies about the brain areas responsible for the hedonistic aspects of drug use. The mesolimbic dopamine system, which consists of dopaminergic neurons in the ventral tegmentum and the regions to which they project, particularly the nucleus accumbens, has emerged as an important system for the reinforcing effects of opiates and other drugs of abuse. A review of this research can be found in the review by Bodnar (146) and aspects of this field are covered in this book in Chapter 5, "Brain-Reward Mechanisms," by Dr. Eliot Gardner.

It is difficult and probably foolish to try to predict the future. However, I cannot resist making a few comments. There is considerable optimism that an understanding of the biochemistry and physiology of the endogenous opioid system will permit a more rational approach to the synthesis of medication for the treatment and prevention of drug addiction. It is also quite likely that the design of nonaddictive analgesic agents will be facilitated by the knowledge of the structures and functions of the different types of opioid receptors and their endogenous ligands. If one of the receptors is found to mediate analgesia but to have little or no role in addiction, ligands could be tailor-made for it. The κ receptor is currently the favorite candidate for this approach. However, drugs with decreased psychotomimetic side effects need to be synthesized, if this approach is to be useful clinically.

As stated earlier, analgesia can be produced by raising the level of endogenous enkephalins, which is deemed unlikely to be highly addictive. Powerful inhibitors of the enkephalin-splitting enzymes, synthesized in Dr. Bernard Roques' laboratory in Paris, are currently in clinical trial.

There is an increasing number of indications for the involvement of the endogenous opioid system in the chronic effects of opiate drugs. The hopes of scientists that the discoveries of opioid receptors and their endogenous ligands will give us important answers about the molecular mechanisms involved in narcotic addiction are higher than ever. The reasons for the relatively slow progress in our understanding of the molecular mechanism of drug abuse are becoming clear. It is a very complex process involving not only the endogenous opioid system but many other neurotransmitter and neuropeptide systems and their signal transduction cascades. Our understanding of these processes is nevertheless improving rapidly, and there many of us feel that we can see the light at the end of the tunnel.

The multitude of functions attributed to the endorphins makes it probable that they are brain chemicals, rivaling in importance the "classical" neurotransmitters. In fact, this seems to be true of a large number of neuropeptides, the study of which was greatly revitalized by the discovery of the endorphins.

No disease involving genetic alterations of the opioid peptides or their receptors has yet been discovered. However, it is tempting to predict that such diseases will eventually be found. Hereditary insensitivity to pain is a candidate for such a genetic defect, although the evidence is still sparse. Addictive disorders could prove to involve genetic and/or environmentally induced changes in the endogenous opioid machinery or elsewhere, and there are signs pointing to this. A very active area of research is the characterization of single-amino-acid mutations present in the human genome, which seem to be silent, i.e., produce no discernible change in phenotype. Such mutants are known as single nucleotide polymorphisms (SNPs) and are very common. They are being examined very carefully in a number of laboratories to determine whether such SNPs present in genes encoding proteins of the endogenous opioid and related systems might alter an individual's susceptibility to becoming addicted to opiates.

The question of whether there is a common mechanism for all addictive disorders is intriguing and much debated. Although the evidence to sustain this idea is still not yet very convincing, there is ever-increasing evidence for the involvement of the endogenous opioid system in other addictions, including alcohol, cannabinoids, and cocaine. The alterations in the signaling systems also seem to be quite similar for various drugs of abuse. A common mechanism of addictions and compulsive behaviors remains a very viable hypothesis. Much of the evidence for such common mechanisms underlying drug abuse is summarized in the two reviews by Nestler (131,132).

The methadone maintenance program, conceived and started by Vincent Dole and Marie Nyswander and now used worldwide for the treatment of heroin addiction, came out of the sound application of receptor theory and pharmacokinetics to the problem of drug abuse. The day when all types of drug abuse and compulsive behaviors can be prevented and successfully treated may not yet be around the corner, but the very active research effort in this area and the progress made during the past three decades provide reasons for optimism.

ACKNOWLEDGMENTS

The research performed in the author's laboratory was supported by grant DA-00017 from the National Institute on Drug Abuse. The long-standing support by NIDA is gratefully acknowledged.

REFERENCES

1. Simon EJ, Hiller JM, Edelman I. Stereospecific binding of the potent narcotic analgesic ³H-etorphine to rat brain homogenate. *Proc Natl Acad Sci U S A* 1973;70:1947–1949.
2. Terenius L. Stereospecific interaction between narcotic analgesics and a synaptic plasma membrane fraction of rat cerebral cortex. *Acta Pharmacol Toxicol* 1973;32:317–320.
3. Pert CB, Snyder SH. Opiate receptor: demonstration in nervous tissue. *Science* 1973;179:1011–1014.
4. Hiller JM, Pearson J, Simon EJ. Distribution of stereospecific binding of the potent narcotic analgesic etorphine in the human brain: predominance in the limbic system. *Res Commu Chem Pathol Pharmacol* 1973;6:1052–1062.
5. Hughes J. Isolation of an endogenous compound from the brain with

properties similar to morphine. *Brain Res* 1975;88:295–308.

6. Terenius, L, Wahlstrom, A. Inhibitor(s) of narcotic receptor binding in brain extracts and cerebrospinal fluid. *Acta Pharmacol Toxicol* 1974;35[Suppl 1]:55.

7. Hughes J, Smith TW, Kosterlitz HW, et al. Identification of two related pentapeptides from the brain with potent opiate agonist activity. *Nature* 1975;258:577–579.

8. Bradbury AF, Smyth DG, Snell CR, et al. C-fragment of lipotropin has a high affinity for brain opiate receptors. *Nature* 1976;260:793–795.

9. Cox BM, Goldstein A, Li CH. Opioid activity of a peptide, beta-lipotropin-(61–91) derived from beta-lipotropin. *Proc Natl Acad Sci U S A* 1976;73:1821–1823.

10. Goldstein A, Tachibana S, Lowney LI, et al. Dynorphin-(1-13), an extraordinarily potent opioid peptide. *Proc Natl Acad Sci U S A* 1979;76:6666–6670.

11. Goldstein A, Goldstein JS, Cox BM. A synthetic peptide with morphine-like pharmacological action. *Life Sci* 1975;17:1643–1654.

12. Donnerer J, Oka K, Brossi A, et al. Presence and formation of codeine and morphine in the rat. *Proc Natl Acad Sci U S A* 1986;83:4566–4567.

13. Goldstein A, Barrett RW, James IF, et al. Morphine and other opiates from beef brain and adrenal. *Proc Natl Acad Sci U S A* 1985;82:5203–5207.

14. Mains RE, Eipper BA, Ling N. Common precursor to corticotropins and endorphins. *Proc Natl Acad Sci U S A* 1977;74:3014–3018.

15. Roberts JL, Herbert E. Characterization of a common precursor to corticotropin and beta-lipotropin: cell-free synthesis of the precursor and identification of corticotropin peptides in the molecule. *Proc Natl Acad Sci U S A* 1977;74:4826–4830.

16. Nakanishi S, Inoue A, Kita T, et al. Nucleotide sequence of cloned cDNA for bovine corticotropin beta-lipotropin precursor. *Nature* 1979;278:423–428.

17. Udenfriend S, Kilpatrick DL. Proenkephalin and the products of its processing: chemistry and biology. In: Udenfriend S, Meienhofer JS, eds. *The peptides,* vol. VI. New York: Academic Press, 1984;6:25–68.

18. Comb M, Seeburg PH, Adelman J, et al. Primary structure of the human Met-and Leu-enkephalin precursor and its mRNA. *Nature* 1982;295:663–666.

19. Kakidani H, Furutani Y, Takahashi H, et al. Cloning and sequence analysis of cDNA for porcine beta-neoendorphin/dynorphin precursor. *Nature* 1982;298:245–248.

20. Civelli O, Douglass J, Goldstein A, et al. Sequence and expression of the rat prodynorphin gene. *Proc Natl Acad Sci U S A* 1985;82:4291–4294.

21. Horikawa S, Takai T, Toyosato M, et al. Isolation and structural organization of the human preproenkephalin B gene. *Nature* 1983;306:611–614.

22. Martinez JL, Weinberger SB, Schulteis G. Enkephalins and learning and memory: a review of evidence for a site of action outside the blood-brain barrier. *Behav Neural Biol* 1988;49:192–221.

23. Fournie Zaluski MC, Chaillet P, Bouboutou R, et al. Analgesic effects of kelatorphan, a new, highly potent inhibitor of multiple enkephalin degrading enzymes. *Eur J Pharmacol* 1984;102:525–528.

24. Watson SJ, Akil H, Khachaturian H, et al. Opioid systems: anatomical, physiological and clinical perspectives. In: Hughes J, Collier HOJ, Rance MJ, et al, eds. *Opioids past, present and future.* London: Taylor & Francis, 1984:145–178.

25. Gilbert PE, Martin WR. The effects of morphine- and nalorphine-like drugs in the nondependent morphine-dependent and cyclazocine-dependent chronic spinal dog. *J Pharmacol Exp Ther* 1976;198:66–82.

26. Martin WR, Eades CG, Thompson JA, et al. The effects of morphine- and nalorphine-like drugs in the nondependent and morphine-dependent chronic spinal dog. *J Pharmacol Exp Ther* 1976;197:517–532.

27. Lord JAH, Waterfield AA, Hughes J, et al. Endogenous opioid peptides: multiple agonists and receptors. *Nature* 1977;267:495–499.

28. Schulz R, Faase E, Wuster M, et al. Selective receptors for beta-endorphin on the rat vas deferens. *Life Sci* 1979;24:843–850.

29. Oka T. Enkephalin receptor in the rabbit ileum. *Br J Pharmacol* 1980;68:193–195.

30. Zukin SR, Zukin RS. Specific 3H-phencyclidine binding in rat central nervous system. *Proc Natl Acad Sci U S A* 1979;76:5372–5376.

31. Meunier J, Mollereau C, Toll L, et al. Isolation and structure of the endogenous agonist of opioid receptor-like ORL1 receptor. *Nature* 1995;377:532–535.

32. Reinscheid RK, Nothacker HP, Bourson A, et al. Orphanin FQ: a neuropeptide that activates an opioid-like G protein-coupled receptor. *Science* 1995;270:792–797.

33. Heinricher MM. Orphanin FQ/nociceptin: from neural circuitry to behavior. *Life Sci* 2003;73:813–822.

34. Mansour A, Khachaturian H, Lewis ME, et al. Autoradiographic differentiation of mu, delta and kappa opioid receptors in the rat forebrain and midbrain. *J Neurosci* 1987;7:2445–2464.

35. Tempel A, Zukin RS. Neuroanatomical patterns of the mu, delta and kappa opioid receptors of rat brain as determined by quantitative *in vitro* autoradiography. *Proc Natl Acad Sci U S A* 1987;84:4308–4312.

36. Okada Y, Tsuda Y, Bryant SD, et al. Endomorphins and related opioid peptides. *Vitam Horm* 2002;65:257–279.

37. Zadina JE. Isolation and distribution of endomorphins in the central nervous system. *Jpn J Pharmacol* 2002;89:203–8.

38. Zadina JE, Martin-Schild S, Gerall AA, et al. Endomorphins: novel endogenous mu-opiate receptor agonists in regions of high mu-opiate receptor density. *Ann N Y Acad Sci* 1999;897:136–144.

39. Handa BK, Lane AC, Lord JAH, et al. Analogues of beta-LPH 61–64 possessing selective agonist activity at mu opiate receptors. *Eur J Pharmacol* 1981;70:531–540.

40. Mosberg HI, Hurst R, Hruby VJ, et al. *Bis*-penicillamine enkephalins possess highly improved specificity toward delta opioid receptors. *Proc Natl Acad Sci U S A* 1983;80:5871–5874.

41. Delay-Goyet P, Seguin C, Gacel G, et al. ^{3}H-(D-Ser2(O-tert-butyl),Leu5) enkephalyl-Thr6 and (D-Ser2(O-tert-butyl),Leu5)enkephalyl-Thr6(O-tert-butyl), two new enkephalin analogs with both a good selectivity and a high affinity toward delta-opioid binding sites. *J Biol Chem* 1988;263:4124–4130.

42. Gairin JE, Mazarguil H, Alvinerie P, et al. Synthesis and biological activities of dynorphin A analogues with opioid antagonist properties. *J Med Chem* 1986;29:1913–1917.

43. Goldstein A, Nestor JJ Jr, Naidu A, et al. "DAKLI": a multipurpose ligand with a high affinity and selectivity for dynorphin (kappa) binding sites. *Proc Natl Acad Sci U S A* 1988;85:7375–7379.

44. Lahti RA, Mickelson MM, McCall JM, et al. 3H-U-69,593 a highly selective ligand for the opioid kappa receptor. *Eur J Pharmacol* 1985;109:281–284.

45. Von Voigtlander PF, Lahti RA, Ludens JH. U 50,488H; a selective and structurally novel non-mu (kappa) opioid agonist. *J Pharmacol Exp Ther* 1983;224:7–12.

46. Gulya K, Pelton JT, Hruby VJ, et al. Cyclic somatostatin octapeptide analogues with high affinity and selectivity toward mu opioid receptors. *Life Sci* 1986;30:2221–2229.

47. Cotton R, Giles MG, Miller L, et al. ICI 174864: a highly selective antagonist

for the opioid delta receptor. *Eur J Pharmacol* 1984;97:331–332.

48. Portoghese PS, Sultana M, Takemori AE. Naltrindole, a highly selective and potent non-peptide delta opioid receptor agonist. *Eur J Pharmacol* 1988;146:185–186.

49. Portoghese PS, Lipowski AW, Takemori AE. Binaltorphimine and nor-binaltorphimine, potent and selective kappa-opioid receptor antagonists. *Life Sci* 1987;40:1287–1292.

50. Chang K, Killian S, Hazum E, et al. Morphiceptin: a potent and specific agonist for morphine (mu) receptors. *Science* 1981;212:75–77.

51. Broccardo M, Erspamer V, Falconieri Erspamer G, et al. Pharmacological data on dermorphins, a new class of potent opioid peptides from amphibian skin. *Br J Pharmacol* 1981;73:625–631.

52. Erspamer V, Melchiorri P, Falconieri-Erspamer G, et al. Deltorphins: A family of naturally occurring peptides with high affinity and selectivity for delta opioid binding sites. *Proc Natl Acad Sci U S A* 1989;86:5188–5192.

53. Kieffer BL, Befort K, Gaveriaux-Ruff C et al. The delta-opioid receptor: Isolation of a cDNA by expression cloning and pharmacological characterization. *Proc Natl Acad Sci U S A* 1992;89:12048–12052.

54. Evans CJ, Keith DEJ, Morrison H, et al. Cloning of a delta opioid receptor by functional expression. *Science* 1992;258:1952–1955.

55. Minami M, Satoh M. Molecular biology of the opioid receptors: structures, functions and distributions. *Neurosci Res* 1995;23:121–145.

56. Koch T, Schulz S, Pfeiffer M, et al. C-terminal splice variants of the mouse mu-opioid receptor differ in morphine-induced internalization and receptor resensitization. *J Biol Chem* 2001;276:31408–31414.

57. Pasternak GW. Insights into mu opioid pharmacology the role of mu opioid receptor subtypes. *Life Sci* 2001;68:2213–2219.

58. Pasternak GW. The pharmacology of mu analgesics: from patients to genes. *Neuroscientist* 2001;7:220–231.

59. Law PY, Wong YH, Loh HH. Mutational analysis of the structure and function of opioid receptors. *Biopolymers* 1999;51:440–455.

60. Knapp RJ, Malatynska E, Collins N, et al. Molecular biology and pharmacology of cloned opioid receptors. *FASEB J* 1995;9:516–525.

61. Meng F, Hoversten MT, Thompson RC, et al. A chimeric study of the molecular basis of affinity and selectivity of the κ and the δ opioid receptors potential role

of extracellular domains. *J Biol Chem* 1995;270:12730–12736.

62. Maldonado R, Valverde O. Participation of the opioid system in cannabinoid-induced antinociception and emotional-like responses. *Eur Neuropsychopharmacol* 2003;13:401–410.

63. Kieffer B. Opioids: first lesson from knockout mice. *Trends Pharmacol Sci* 1999;20:19–26.

64. Kieffer B, Gaveriaux-Ruff C. Exploring the opioid system by gene knockout. *Prog Neurobiol* 2002;66:285–306.

65. Gioannini TL, Howard AD, Hiller JM, et al. Purification of an active opioid binding protein from bovine striatum. *J Biol Chem* 1985;260:15117–15121.

66. Gioannini TL, Foucaud B, Hiller JM, et al. Lectin binding of solubilized opiate receptors: evidence for their glycoprotein nature. *Biochem Biophys Res Commun* 1982;105:1128–1134.

67. Cho TM, Hasegawa J, Ge BL, et al. Purification to apparent homogeneity of a mu-type opioid receptor from rat brain. *Proc Natl Acad Sci U S A* 1986;83:4138–4142.

67a. Ueda H, Harada H, Misawa H, et al. Purified opioid mu receptor is of a different molecular size than delta and kappa receptors. *Neurosci Lett* 1987;75:339–344.

68. Simonds WF, Burke TR Jr, Rice KC, et al. Purification of the opiate receptor of NG 108–15 neuroblastoma glioma hybrid cells. *Proc Natl Acad Sci U S A* 1985;82:4974–4978.

69. Loukas S, Merkouris M, Panetsos F, et al. Purification to homogeneity of an active opioid receptor from rat brain by affinity chromatography. *Proc Natl Acad Sci U S A* 1994;91:4574–4578.

70. Song ZH, Barbas DP, Portoghese PS, et al. Isolation of kappa opioid receptor with an aminoethyl-nor-binaltorphimine (AE-norBNI) affinity column. *Prog Clin Biol Res* 1990;328:69–72.

71. Gioannini TL, Fan LQ, Hyde L, et al. Reconstitution of a purified mu-opioid binding protein in liposomes: selective, high affinity, GTP-gammaS-sensitive mu-opioid agonist binding is restored. *Biochem Biophys Res Commun* 1993;194:901–908.

72. Fan LQ, Gioannini TL, Wolinsky TD, et al. Functional reconstitution of a highly purified mu-opioid receptor protein with purified G-proteins in liposomes. *J Neurochem* 1995;65:2537–2542.

73. Onoprishvili I, Andria M, Vilim F, et al. The bovine mu-opioid receptor: cloning of cDNA and pharmacological characterization of the receptor expressed in mammalian cells. *Mol Brain Res* 1999;73:129–137.

74. Schoffelmeer ANM, Rice KC, Jacobson AE, et al. Mu, delta and kappa receptor-mediated inhibition of neurotransmitter release and adenylate-cyclase activity in rat brain slices: studies with fentanyl isothiocyanate. *Eur J Pharmacol* 1988;154:169–178.

75. Childers SR. Opioid receptor-coupled second messenger systems. In: Herz A, Akil H, Simon EJS, eds. *Opioids I: handbook of experimental pharmacology*, vol. 104/I. Heidelberg: Springer-Verlag, 1993:189–208.

76. Koch WJ, Hawes BE, Allen LF, et al. Direct evidence that G_i-coupled receptor stimulation of mitogen- activated protein kinase is mediated by G beta gamma activation of p21ras. *Proc Natl Acad Sci U S A* 1994;91:12706–12710.

77. Crespo P, Cachero TG, Xu N, et al. Dual effect of beta-adrenergic receptors on mitogen-activated protein kinase. Evidence for a beta gamma-dependent activation and a G alpha s-cAMP-mediated inhibition. *J Biol Chem* 1995;270:25259–25265.

78. Li LY, Chang KJ. The stimulatory effect of opioids on mitogen-activated protein kinase in Chinese hamster ovary cells transfected to express mu-opioid receptors. *Mol Pharmacol* 1996;50:599–602.

79. Gutstein HB, Rubie EA, Mansour A, et al. Opioid effects on mitogen-activated protein kinase signaling cascades. *Anesthesiology* 1997;87:1118–1126.

80. van Biesen T, Hawes BE, Luttrell DK, et al. Receptor-tyrosine-kinase- and G beta gamma-mediated MAP kinase activation by a common signalling pathway (see comments). *Nature* 1995;376:781–784.

81. Daub H, Weiss FU, Wallasch C, et al. Role of transactivation of the EGF receptor in signalling by G-protein- coupled receptors. *Nature* 1996;379:557–560.

82. Kramer HK, Andria ML, Esposito DH, et al. Tyrosine phosphorylation of the delta-opioid receptor: Evidence for its role in mitogen-activated protein kinase activation and receptor internalization. *Biochem Pharmacol* 2000;60:781–792.

83. Kramer HK, Andria ML, Kushner SA, et al. Mutation of tyrosine 318 (Y318F) in the delta opioid receptor attenuates tyrosine phosphorylation, agonist-dependent receptor internalization and mitogen-activated protein kinase activation. *Mol Brain Res* 2000;79:55–66.

84. North RA, Williams JT, Surprenant A, et al. Mu and delta receptors belong to a family of receptors that are coupled to potassium channels. *Proc Natl Acad Sci U S A* 1987;84:5487–5491.

85. Gross RA, Macdonald RL. Dynorphin A selectively reduces a large transient

(N-type) calcium current of mouse dorsal root ganglion neurons in cell culture. *Proc Natl Acad Sci U S A* 1987; 84:5469–5473.

86. North RA. Opioid actions on membrane ion channels. In: Herz AS, ed. *Opioids.* Berlin: Springer-Verlag, 1993:773–797.

87. Grudt TJ, Williams JT. Opioid receptors and the regulation of ion conductances. *Rev Neurosci* 1995;6:279–286.

88. Duggan AW, Hall JG, Headley PM. Suppression of transmission of nociceptive impulses by morphine: selective effects of morphine administered in the region of the substantia gelatinosa. *Br J Pharmacol* 1977;61:65–67.

89. Akil H, Mayer DJ, Liebeskind JC. Antagonism of stimulation-produced analgesia by naloxone, a narcotic antagonist. *Science* 1976;191:961–962.

90. Richardson DE, Akil H. Pain reduction by electrical brain stimulation in man. Part II: chronic self administration in the periaqueductal gray matter. *J Neurosurg* 1984;47:184–194.

91. Pomeranz B, Chiu D. Naloxone blockade of acupuncture analgesia: endorphin implicated. *Life Sci* 1976;19:1757–1762.

92. Mayer DJ, Price DD, Rafii A. Antagonism of acupuncture analgesia in man by the narcotic antagonist naloxone. *Brain Res* 1977;121:368–372.

93. Levine JD, Gordon NC, Fields HL. The mechanism of placebo analgesia. *Lancet* 1978;2:654–657.

94. Jacob JJ, Tremblay EC, Colombel MC. Facilitation de reactions nociceptives par la naloxone chez la souris et chez le rat. *Psychopharmacology (Berl)* 1974;37:217–219.

95. Akil H, Richardson ED, Barchas JD, et al. Appearance of beta-endorphin-like immunoreactivity in human ventricular cerebrospinal fluid upon analgesic electrical stimulation. *Proc Natl Acad Sci U S A* 1978;75:5170–5172.

96. Akil H, Richardson DE, Hughes J, et al. Enkephalin-like material elevated in ventricular cerebrospinal fluid of pain patients after analgesic focal stimulation. *Science* 1978;201:463–464.

97. Han JS, Xie GX, Zhou ZF. Acupuncture mechanisms in rabbits studied with micro-injection of antibodies against beta-endorphin, enkephalin and substance P. *Neuropharmacology* 1984;23:1–5.

98. Le Guen S, Mas Nieto M, Canestrelli C, et al. Pain management by a new series of dual inhibitors of enkephalin degrading enzymes: long-lasting antinociceptive properties and potentiation by CCK2 antagonist or methadone. *Pain* 2003;104:139–48.

99. Chaillet P, Coulaud A, Zajac JM, et al.

100. The mu rather than the delta subtype of opioid receptors appears to be involved in enkephalin induced analgesia. *Eur J Pharmacol* 1984;101:83–90.

100. Wood PL, Rackham A, Richard J. Spinal analgesia: comparison of the mu agonist morphine and the kappa agonist ethylkjetocyclazocine. *Life Sci* 1981;28:2119–2125.

101. Porreca F, Heyman JS, Mosberg HI, et al. Role of mu and delta receptors in the supraspinal and spinal analgesic effects of (D-Pen2,D-Pen5)enkephalin in the mouse. *J Pharmacol Exp Ther* 1987;241:389–393.

102. Carr KD, Bonnet KA, Simon EJ. Mu and kappa opioid-agonists elevate brain stimulation threshold for escape by inhibiting aversion. *Brain Res* 1982;245:389–393.

103. Yaksh TL. Multiple spinal opiate receptor systems in analgesia. In: Kruger L, Liebeskind JS, eds. *Advances in pain research and therapy.* New York: Raven Press, 1984:197–215.

104. Crain SM, Shen KF. Antagonists of excitatory opioid receptor functions enhance morphine's analgesic potency and attenuate opioid tolerance/dependence liability. *Pain* 2000; 84:121–131.

105. Inturrisi CE. Clinical pharmacology of opioids for pain. *Clin J Pain* 2002;18:S3–S13.

106. Bonnet KA, Hiller JM, Simon EJ. The effects of chronic opiate treatment and social isolation on opiate receptors in the rodent brain. In: Kosterlitz HWS, ed. *Opiates and endogenous opioid peptides.* Amsterdam: Elsevier Press, 1976:335–343.

107. Klee WA, Streaty RA. Narcotic receptor sites in morphine dependent rats. *Nature* 1974;248:61–63.

108. Werling LL, McMahon PN, Cox BM. Selective changes in mu opioid receptor properties induced by chronic morphine exposure. *Proc Natl Acad Sci U S A* 1989;86:6393–6397.

109. Schulz R, Wuster M, Herz A. Pharmacological characterization of the epsilon-opiate receptor. *J Pharmacol Exp Ther* 1980;216:604–606.

110. Schulz R, Wuster M, Herz A. Differentiation of opiate receptors in the brain by the selective development of tolerance. *Pharmacol Biochem Behav* 1981;14:75–79.

111. Lahti RA, Collins RJ. Chronic naloxone results in prolonged increases in opiate binding sites in brain. *Eur J Pharmacol* 1978;51:185–186.

112. Zukin RS, Sugarman JR, Fitz-Syage ML, et al. Naltrexone-induced opiate receptor supersensitivity. *Brain Res* 1982;245:285–292.

113. Tempel A, Zukin RS, Gardner EL. Su-

persensitivity of brain opiate receptor subtypes after chronic naltrexone treatment. *Life Sci* 1982;31:1401–1404.

114. Yoburn BC, Shah S, Chan K, et al. Supersensitivity to opioid analgesics following chronic opioid antagonist treatment: relationship to receptor selectivity. *Pharmacol Biochem Behav* 1995;51:535–539.

115. Morris BJ, Millan MJ, Herz A. Antagonist-induced opioid receptor upregulation. II. regionally specific modulation of mu, delta and kappa binding sites in rat brain revealed by quantitative autoradiography. *J Pharmacol Exp Ther* 1988;247:729–736.

116. Von Zastrow M. Opioid receptor regulation. *Neuromolecular Med* 2004;5:51–58.

117. Law PY, Wong YH, Loh HH. Molecular mechanisms and regulation of opioid receptor signaling. *Annu Rev Pharmacol Toxicol* 2000;40:389–430.

118. Bronstein DM, Przewlocki R, Akil H. Effect of morphine treatment on pro-opiomelanocortin systems in rat brain. *Brain Res* 1990;519:102–111.

119. Hammonds RGH Jr, Nicolas P, Li CH. Beta-endorphin (1–27) is an antagonist of beta-endorphin analgesia. *Proc Natl Acad Sci U S A* 1984;81:1389–1390.

120. Wei E, Loh HH. Physical dependence on opiate-like peptides. *Science* 1976;193:1262–1263.

121. Gold M, Redmond DEJ, Kleber HD. Clonidine blocks acute opiate withdrawal symptoms. *Lancet* 1978;2:599–600.

122. Collier HO, J, Roy AC. Morphine-like drugs inhibit the stimulation by E prostaglandins of cyclic AMP formation by rat brain homogenate. *Nature* 1974;248:24–27.

123. Sharma SK, Klee WA, Nirenberg M. Dual regulation of adenylate cyclase accounts for narcotic dependence and tolerance. *Proc Natl Acad Sci U S A* 1975;72:3092–3096.

124. Rasmussen K, Beitner-Johnson D, Krystal DB, et al. Opiate withdrawal and the rat locus coeruleus: behavioral, electrophysiological and biochemical correlates. *J Neurosci* 1990;10:2308–2317.

125. Aghajanian GK. Tolerance of locus coeruleus neurones to morphine and suppression of withdrawal response by clonidine. *Nature* 1978;276:186–188.

126. Aghajanian GK, Wang YY. Common alpha-2 and opiate effector mechanisms in the locus coeruleus: intracellular studies in brain slices. *Neuropharmacology* 1987;26:789–800.

127. Guitart X, Nestler EJ. Identification of morphine-and cyclic AMP-regulated phosphoproteins (MARPP's) in the locus coeruleus and other regions of rat

brain: regulation by acute and chronic morphine. *J Neurosci* 1989;9:4371–4387.

128. Guitart X, Hayward M, Nisenbaum LK, et al. Identification of MARPP-58, a morphine-and cyclic AMP-regulated phosphoprotein of 58 kDa, as tyrosine hydroxylase: evidence for regulation of its expression by chronic morphine in the rat locus coeruleus. *J Neurosci* 1990;10:2649–2659.

129. Guitart X, Nestler EJ. Identification of MARPP-14–20, morphine- and cyclic AMP-regulated phosphoproteins of 14–20 kD, as myelin basic proteins. Evidence for their acute and chronic regulation by morphine in rat brain. *Brain Res* 1990;516:57–65.

130. Cox BM, Osman OH. Inhibition of the development of tolerance to morphine in rats by drugs which inhibit ribonucleic acid or protein synthesis. *Br J Pharmacol* 1970;38:157–170.

131. Nestler EJ. Molecular neurobiology of addiction. *Am J Addict* 2001;10:201–217.

132. Nestler EJ, Malenka RC. The addicted brain. *Sci Am* 2004;290:78–85.

133. Tso PH, Wong YH. Molecular basis of opioid dependence: role of signal regulation by G-proteins. *Clin Exp Pharmacol Physiol* 2003;30:307–316.

134. Trujillo KA, Akil H. Inhibition of morphine tolerance and dependence by the NMDA receptor antagonist MK-801. *Science* 1991;251:85–87.

135. Trujillo KA, Akil H. Inhibition of opiate tolerance by non-competitive N-methyl-D-aspartate receptor antagonists. *Brain Res* 1994;633:178–188.

136. Elliott K, Minami N, Kolesnikov YA, et al. The NMDA receptor antagonists, LY274614 and MK-801, and the nitric oxide synthase inhibitor, NG-nitro-L-arginine, attenuate analgesic tolerance to the mu-opioid morphine but not to kappa opioids. *Pain* 1994;56:69–75.

137. Tiseo PJ, Cheng J, Pasternak GW, et al. Modulation of morphine tolerance by the competitive N-methyl-D-aspartate receptor antagonist LY274614: assessment of opioid receptor changes. *J Pharmacol Exp Ther* 1994;268:195–201.

138. Marek P, Ben-Eliyahu S, Vaccarino AL, et al. Delayed application of MK-801 attenuates development of morphine tolerance in rats. *Brain Res* 1991;558:163–165.

139. Ben-Eliyahu S, Marek P, Vaccarino AL, et al. The NMDA receptor antagonist MK-801 prevents long-lasting non-associative morphine tolerance in the rat. *Brain Res* 1992;575:304–308.

140. Kest B, Mogil JS, Shamgar B-E, et al. The NMDA receptor antagonist MK-801 protects against development of morphine tolerance after intrathecal administration. *Proc West Pharmacol Soc* 1993;36:307–310.

141. Gutstein HB, Trujillo KA. MK-801 inhibits the development of morphine tolerance at spinal sites. *Brain Res* 1993;626:332–334.

142. Gutstein HB, Trujillo KA, Akil H. Does MK-801 inhibit the development of morphine tolerance in the rat at spinal sites? *Anesthesiology* 1992;77:A737.

143. Siggins GR, Martin G, Roberto M, et al. Glutamatergic transmission in opiate and alcohol dependence. *Ann N Y Acad Sci* 2003;1003:196–211.

144. Trujillo KA, Akil H. Excitatory amino acids and drugs of abuse: a role for N-methyl-D-aspartate receptors in drug tolerance, sensitization and physical dependence. *Drug Alcohol Depend* 1995;38:139–154.

145. Trujillo KA. The neurobiology of opiate tolerance, dependence and sensitization: mechanisms of NMDA receptor-dependent synaptic plasticity. *Neurotox Res* 2002;4:373–391.

146. Bodnar RJ, Hadjimarkou MM. Endogenous opiates and behavior: 2001. *Peptides* 2002;23:2307–2365.

CHAPTER 11
Opiates: Clinical Aspects

CLIFFORD M. KNAPP, PhD, DOMENIC A. CIRAULO, MD, AND JEROME JAFFE, MD

This chapter summarizes the pharmacology of opioid drugs and then relates this pharmacology to the phenomenon of repetitive opioid use and complications of such use.

OPIOID ACTIONS

Opioid drugs exert their actions by binding to receptors on the cell membranes of neurons and certain other cells, such as white blood cells (1). Three major types of opioid receptors have been identified (μ, δ, and κ), which appear to subserve different physiologic functions. While the physiologic role of each of the three receptor types is not yet fully known, it does appear that μ and δ receptors are involved in systems that influence mood, reinforcing effects, respiration, pain, blood pressure, and endocrine and gastrointestinal function (2). κ Receptors, when activated, can produce endocrine changes and analgesia. In contrast to μ and δ agonists, which are self-administered by animals under experimental conditions, pure κ receptor agonists are not. Instead, κ agonists appear to produce aversive effects in animals (3) and dysphoria, rather than euphoria, in human subjects (4).

Three opioid receptor genes have been identified: the MOR, DOR, and KOR genes that encode for the μ, δ, and κ receptors, respectively. Although pharmacologic evidence suggests that subtypes of the three basic opioid receptors exist, distinct genes for these subtypes have not been isolated. However, variations in opioid receptor proteins may arise from two sources, namely alternate pathways in the splicing of opioid receptor messenger ribonucleic acids (mRNAs) and allelic variants, that is, variations in the nucleotide sequences in particular opioid receptor genes. Several putative splice variants of the human μ opioid receptor have been identified (5,6). These include a variant described as the μ_3 *receptor,* which is expressed in vascular tissue and leukocytes and is sensitive to morphine but not the opioid peptide metenkephalin (5). An example of a polymorphism of the human opioid receptor MOR (also called *OPRM1*) gene is one that involves substitution of aspartate for asparagine in amino acid sequence of the receptor protein at position 40 (the $A_{+118}G$ polymorphism). There is some evidence that there are differences in the pharmacologic properties of the different variants of this biallelic polymorphism. The A/G (asparagine40aspartate)

TABLE 11.1. *Selectivities of opioid analgesics for opioid receptor classes*

Drugs	μ	δ	κ
Buprenorphine	Partial agonist		Antagonist
Butorphanol	Partial agonist		Agonist
Fentanyl	Agonist		
Levorphanol	Agonist		
Morphine	Agonist		Weak agonist
Nalbuphine	Antagonist		Agonist
Pentazocine	Partial agonist		Agonist
Sufentanil	Agonist	Weak agonist[a]	Weak agonist

[a]Weak agonist indicates a low affinity for the receptor.
Adapted from Reisine T, Pasternak G. Opioid analgesics and antagonists. In: Hardman JG, Limbird LE, Molinoff RW, et al., eds. *Goodman and Gilman's the pharmacologic basis of therapeutics*, 9th ed. New York: McGraw-Hill, 1995:521–556; and Gutstein HB, Akil H. Opioid analgesics. In: Hardman JG, Limbird LE, eds. *Goodman and Gilman's the pharmacological basis of therapeutics*, 10th ed. New York: McGraw-Hill, 2001:569–620.

variant of the $A_{+118}G$ polymorphism binds to the opioid peptide β-endorphin with three times greater affinity than does the more common A/A variant (7). Also, plasma cortisol levels were significantly greater following challenge with the opioid antagonist, naloxone (Narcan), in subjects with A/G or G/G variants of this polymorphism than in those with the A/A variants (8).

Opioid drugs are defined and categorized in terms of their capacity to bind and activate the various opioid receptor types (see Table 11.1). Those that bind and activate a receptor are *agonists* at that receptor. Those that bind but do not activate a receptor function as *antagonists* at that receptor. Opioids can differ greatly in their relative affinity for the various receptor types. They can also differ in their intrinsic activity in that they may bind very well to a receptor, but may produce less than full receptor activation. A partial agonist at a receptor can, under some circumstances, act as an antagonist at that same receptor (2). For example, after surgical procedures involving the potent μ agonists, fentanyl (Sublimaze) and sufentanil (Sufenta), respiratory depression can be reversed by naloxone, an antagonist that binds preferentially at the μ receptor. However, naloxone-induced reversal of respiratory depression can be accompanied by a reversal of analgesic actions or sometimes by acute opioid withdrawal. It is also possible to use a partial μ agonist such as buprenorphine (Buprenex) to alleviate fentanyl respiratory depression (2). By displacing fentanyl, buprenorphine alleviates severe respiratory depression but continues to exert some μ agonist activity, including analgesia.

Until the latter part of the twentieth century, the opioids commonly abused were prototypic μ agonists exerting preferential binding at the μ receptor and acting as full agonists. Most of the opioids that are readily available, legally or illegally, are prototypical μ agonists, partial μ agonists, or mixed agonist–antagonists. The latter are agents exerting some agonist actions at κ receptors and either antagonist or weak agonist actions at μ and δ

receptors. Opioid agonists and antagonists have been developed that act much more specifically at the δ and κ receptors, but these are not currently in clinical use (2). Some of the available agents also bind to a σ receptor. Because binding to a σ receptor is not antagonized by naloxone, it is no longer thought of as an opioid receptor. It was once believed that the dysphoric and hallucinatory effects seen with some agonist–antagonists were a result of actions at the σ receptor, but with the recognition that κ activation can produce dysphoric effects, the significance of σ binding is now uncertain (2,4).

Opioid receptors are found throughout the brain and spinal cord, in neural plexuses in the gastrointestinal tract and other parts of the autonomic nervous system, and on white blood cells. Not surprisingly, opioid drugs have diverse actions on many organ systems. The most prominent effects, and the effects for which the opioids are most commonly prescribed, are exerted on the central nervous system (CNS) and the gastrointestinal tract.

Acting in the CNS, the opioids produce analgesia, a sense of tranquillity and decreased sense of apprehension, and a suppression of the cough reflex. These are the CNS actions for which they are prescribed. However, opioids also can produce nausea, vomiting, depression of respiration, constriction of the pupils, alterations in temperature regulation, and a variety of changes in the neuroendocrine system. These are the generally unwanted side effects that clinicians as well as illicit users of the drugs try to avoid (2).

Effects of opioids on pain and anticipation of pain and distress can be profound. At high enough doses, indifference to pain is sufficient to permit major surgery, but the profound respiratory depression that accompanies this level of opioid effect requires mechanical support of respiration (9). More commonly, however, opioids are used as analgesics in much lower doses, such as 10 mg of morphine or 1.5 mg of hydromorphone (Dilaudid). At such doses the analgesia is marked but there is no loss of consciousness, and other senses and cognition are generally unaffected. The use of opioids in treatment of acute and chronic pain is discussed at length in Chapter 55. This chapter focuses on those other effects of opioids that are, in all likelihood, the reason that they are self-administered by individuals who are not in pain.

Even at analgesic doses, opioids produce changes in mood and feeling. Typically, among medical patients, these are described as decreased anxiety, drowsiness, and a sense of tranquillity (2). There appear to be significant differences among individuals in the way they feel when they take opioids. Postaddict volunteers usually experience an elevation of mood and increased sense of self-esteem (i.e., euphoria). Others given the same dose may complain of a sense of confusion and drowsiness, which they experience as unpleasant (10,11). Such dysphoric responses are aggravated by opioid-induced nausea, but it is not the nausea that causes the dysphoria. Heroin addicts who do not have a high tolerance sometimes experience nausea and vomiting along with a sense of euphoria. As is discussed further below, it is likely that repeated opioid use is motivated by a desire to reexperience this sense of euphoria. The complex of euphoria and decreased concern with anticipated problems is often referred to as a "high." When μ agonist opioids are self-administered intravenously (or, sometimes, when heroin or opium is smoked) there is a sharp and rapid increase in brain opioid levels that produces a distinct, intense, and generally pleasurable sensation often referred to by heroin addicts as a "flash" or "rush." Some users liken the feeling to sexual orgasm. Because "rush" is not experienced with a slower onset of opioid action (through oral or subcutaneous routes) addicts may persist in intravenous use despite its risks (12). Descriptions of "rush" can be surprisingly varied (13).

For some individuals, opioids appear to have the capacity to ameliorate certain varieties of depression, to control anxiety, to reduce anger, and to blunt paranoid feelings and ideation (14,15). Chapter 6 discusses at greater length the notion that some individuals take opioids as a form of self-medication for emotions that are otherwise abnormally painful. The neural mechanisms by which opioids produce reinforcing effects in animals and, presumably, their mood-elevating effects in humans are discussed below briefly and also more extensively in Chapter 5. μ Opioids inhibit the activity of the locus coeruleus, the principal clustering of noradrenergic neurons in the brain. Activity in these neurons is associated with subjective symptoms and autonomic signs of anxiety (16). The antianxiety actions of opioids are probably partly a result of their capacity to inhibit locus coeruleus activity. The significance of this action is that α_2-adrenergic agonists, which can also inhibit the locus coeruleus, can be used to control signs of opioid withdrawal (see in section entitled Managing Opioid Physical Dependence).

Included among the many other effects opioids produce through their CNS action are suppression of the cough re-

flex (which makes them useful antitussives) and effects on the neuroendocrine system. Most of these neuroendocrine effects, such as the inhibition of gonadotropin-releasing hormone (which results in decreased luteinizing hormone [LH] and follicle-stimulating hormone [FSH] and, ultimately, in decreased testosterone levels in males and disturbed menstrual function in females) are unwanted side effects (2). The opioid inhibition of corticotropin-releasing factor (CRF) results in decreased adrenocorticotropic hormone (ACTH) and decreased levels of cortisol. It is conceivable that for some individuals the inhibition of CRF is useful in dealing with anxiety or stress.

μ Agonist opioids have many effects on the gastrointestinal system, such as slowing the passage of food in the stomach, small intestine, and large intestine. Because of this action, opioid drugs are still key therapeutic agents in the treatment of diarrhea. Drugs such as diphenoxylate (the main active ingredient in Lomotil) and loperamide (Imodium) are actually specialized opioids. The latter can be sold without special controls because very little of it gets into the CNS and therefore it acts primarily on the gut. Because little tolerance develops to this gut-slowing effect, patients with chronic pain given large doses of opioids are often constipated, as are heroin addicts if their supply is uninterrupted over long periods. (Opioid withdrawal generally produces cramps and diarrhea.) Former addicts maintained on methadone also typically have problems with constipation. Mixed agonist–antagonists (such as pentazocine [Talwin], butorphanol [Stadol], and nalbuphine [Nubain]) and κ agonists have less-prominent constipating effects.

Some opioids, such as morphine, produce histamine release, which is associated with vasodilatation of skin vessels and itching. The nose scratching that is seen when addicts are quite intoxicated is probably related, in part, to this effect. However, pruritus is also seen with opioids that do not release histamine and may, therefore, be related to opioid effects on neurons (2). The effects of most opioids on the cardiovascular system are not prominent except under special circumstances; one of these is hypovolemia, in which opioids can aggravate shock. However, in rare instances levo-alpha-acetylmethadol (LAAM) may produce prolongation of the QT interval and cardiac arrhythmias including torsades de pointes (17).

Opioids also have effects on the bladder; they tend to increase sphincter tone and decrease the voiding reflexes; in this way, they can increase the likelihood of urinary retention (1). The effects of opioids on the immune system are discussed in Chapter 54.

SOME CLINICAL IMPLICATIONS OF DIFFERENCES IN DRUG DISPOSITION

In the United States, there are at least 20 drugs available that have opioid actions; additional opioids are available in other countries (2). As already mentioned, many of these drugs may be thought of as prototypic μ agonists; some have actions on other receptors as well, or act preferentially at other receptors. However, differences in receptor activity profiles are not the only clinically important way in which specific drugs differ. They may also differ in the way they are absorbed, metabolized, and eliminated by the body. For example, some opioids, such as sufentanil, may be metabolized so rapidly that they are of limited use as oral analgesics but are quite useful when given intravenously in managing anesthesia for major surgery (18). In contrast, LAAM (Orlaam), with a half-life of 2 days, is very slowly cleared from the body, as are its active metabolites noracetylmethadol and dinoraceacetyl-methadol, whose half-lives are 2 and 4 days, respectively. These slow rates of elimination allow LAAM to be administered as infrequently as three times a week as a maintenance agent for opioid dependence (1).

Conjugation with glucuronide is a major route of metabolism for several opioid agents including morphine, codeine, and buprenorphine. Recent evidence indicates that the glucuronidation of opioid drugs is catalyzed by several isoforms of the enzyme UDPglucuronyltransferase. The glucuronidation of morphine can be catalyzed by several UDP-glucuronyltransferase isoforms, including UGT2B7 (19), UGT2B1 (20), UGT1A3 (21), and UGT2B9 (22). The closely related isoforms, UGT2B7 (19) and UGT2B9 (22), mediate the glucuronidation of codeine. The conjugation of buprenorphine with glucuronide is mediated by UGT2B1 and by UGT1.1 (20), an isoform that does that does not readily catalyze the glucuronidation of morphine. The clinical significance of the finding that different isoforms of the glucuronyltransferase enzyme may be involved in the metabolism of different opioid drugs remains to be determined.

The glucuronidation of morphine involves its conversion to either morphine-3-glucuronide, and to a lesser extent, morphine-6-glucuronide (23). Formation of the morphine-6-glucuronide in the human liver can be inhibited by dextromethorphan (24), while that of the 3 position glucuronide can be blocked by oxazepam (Serax) in the human liver (24) and by ranitidine (Zantac) in guinea pig hepatocytes (25). Morphine-6-glucuronide is a more potent analgesic agent than morphine and may contribute significantly to the analgesic effects of morphine treatment (26). Renal insufficiency can lead to a reduction in the clearance rate of morphine-6-glucuronide and the resultant high concentrations of this compound may have toxic effects (27). The meperidine metabolite, normeperidine, may also accumulate to produce toxicity in patients with renal dysfunction (28). Normeperidine has no analgesic activity but can induce seizures (2,29) and cause serious problems, such as twitching, tremors, and mental confusion (29). Problems can also arise when excessive amounts of meperidine (Demerol) are used, as in meperidine addiction, a problem occasionally seen among physi-

cians, nurses, and other medical personnel with access to meperidine. In these cases it is not unusual for the problem to come to notice because the user has a grand mal seizure as a consequence of the build-up of normeperidine (12).

In some instances, the drug administered is actually quite inactive as an opioid, and only when it is metabolized by the body, does it become able to readily attach to and activate opioid receptors (a prodrug). At least two examples are relevant to problems of drug dependence. The most obvious is the case of heroin (diacetylmorphine). Heroin is not itself a potent μ agonist; but, because it is more lipid soluble than morphine, it can more rapidly enter the brain, where it is converted to 6-mono-acetyl-morphine and morphine. In the brain, heroin and morphine produce virtually identical effects because heroin acts primarily as morphine and 6-mono-acetyl-morphine (2). Very little heroin is detected in the urine of heroin addicts; what is excreted is morphine. Heroin may be preferred by addicts because they value the rapid onset of effects, which may be linked to the sensation of "rush."

Codeine is also primarily a prodrug. Codeine (3-methoxy-morphine, or morphine-3-methyl ether) does not bind significantly to opioid receptors. However, in the body, a small percentage of codeine is converted to morphine, which then may produce its characteristic effects (2). Codeine is valuable clinically because it is well-absorbed when given by mouth and is not deactivated by the liver as it is absorbed into the bloodstream. Individuals taking codeine for medical purposes usually will have traces of morphine in their urine.

DRUG INTERACTIONS

The metabolism of codeine is catalyzed by cytochrome P450 enzymes as is the biotransformation of several of other opioids. The cytochrome P450 enzymes are produced by 12 different gene families, 3 of which, CYP1, CYP2, and CYP3, may play a major role in drug metabolism in humans. These families are further divisible into several subfamilies, each of which is to some extent selective for the drug reactions they catalyze.

Many compounds may selectively inhibit the activity of different isoforms of the cytochrome P450 enzymes. Some of these enzyme inhibitors may be substrates of specific enzymes; that is, their transformation is catalyzed by that enzyme, and they inhibit metabolism through competitive inhibition. Other compounds inhibit enzymes but are not substrates of these enzymes. These inhibitors may reduce enzyme activity by mechanisms such as noncompetitive inhibition.

The cytochrome enzyme CYP3A4 has been implicated as playing a major role in the metabolism of several opioids, including alfentanil (30,31), buprenorphine (32), fentanyl (33), LAAM (34), methadone (Dolophine) (35), sufentanil (33), and tramadol (Ultram) (36). This enzyme mediates the dealkylation of buprenorphine, an action that is inhibited by the CYP3A4 inhibitor, ketoconazole (32). The oxidative *N*-dealkylation of alfentanil, fentanyl, and sufentanil are all catalyzed by CYP3A4. Severe respiratory depression has occurred when fentanyl levels were markedly elevated after the administration of the CYP3A4 inhibitor, ritonavir (Norvir) (37). Several agents. including troleandomycin (Tao), midazolam (Versed), ketoconazole (Nizoral), and nefazodone (Serzone) may inhibit CYP3A4 from catalyzing the biotransformation of alfentanil (38,39).

CYP3A4 plays a major role in the biotransformation of methadone into its main metabolite, EDDP (2-ethylidene-1,5-dimethyl-3,3-diphenenylpyrrolidine). Inhibitors of CYP3A, including troleandomycin, ketoconazole, and fluvoxamine (Luvox) (40), can readily block the formation of EDDP from methadone (34,41,42). Administration of ciprofloxacin, a CYP3A4 inhibitor, has produced marked respiratory depression when administered to a patient being treated with methadone (43). Plasma levels of methadone may be elevated by a number of CYP3A4 inhibitors, including fluconazole (Diflucan) (44) and fluvoxamine (45). However, two inhibitors of CYP3A, ritonavir (46,47) and nelfinavir (Viracept) (48), paradoxically decrease methadone plasma concentrations via an unknown mechanism. The administration of substances that produce an induction of the CYP3A enzyme may produce a reduction in plasma methadone concentrations that, in turn, may lead to withdrawal in maintenance therapy patients. This can occur after the administration of the CYP3A inducer rifampin (49–51). Table 11.2 lists other drugs that induce this enzyme.

In addition to CYP3A4, the biotransformation of methadone may be metabolized by several other enzymes, including CYP2C9 and CYP2C19 (42). The role played by the CYP2D6 enzyme in the metabolism of methadone remains unclear (52). Administration of either paroxetine (Paxil) (53) or fluoxetine (Prozac) (45), which are both inhibitors of CYP2D6, can produce elevations in the plasma concentrations of the active enantiomer (i.e., the R– enantiomer) of methadone.

The biotransformation of codeine is catalyzed by the hepatic cytochrome CYP2D6 enzyme. This enzyme also catalyzes the transformation of hydrocodone into hydromorphone (Dilaudid) (54) and oxycodone (Oxycontin)

TABLE 11.2. *Agents (reference) that may decrease methadone plasma concentration through the induction of CYP3A4 enzymes*

Amprenavir (Agenerase) (126)
Efavirenz (Sustiva) (127–129)
Nevirapine (Viramune) (129–130)
Phenobarbital (131)
Phenytoin (Dilantin) (132,133)
Rifampicin (Rifadin) (49–51)
Spironolactone (Aldactone) (134)

into oxymorphone (Numorphan). Small subpopulations of individuals are poor metabolizers of these drugs as compared to most of the population who extensively metabolize these agents. Poor metabolizers of codeine will obtain less analgesia from a given dose of codeine (55,56) than will extensive metabolizers of these agents. A deficiency in the ability of individuals to metabolize codeine may result from polymorphisms of the CYP2D6 genes which lead to altered enzyme activity (57,58). Genotypes can be determined by challenging subjects with a pharmacologic probe such as dextromethorphan, which is mostly metabolized by CYP2D6. Between 4 to 10% of the white population are poor metabolizers of dextromethorphan (59).

Quinidine can inhibit the activity of CYP2D6 and the administration of this drug has the potential to reduce the analgesic potency of codeine and related compounds. Quinidine may inhibit the metabolism of tramadol (Ultram) which is also dependent on CYP2D6 for its biotransformation into an active metabolite (36). The rate of biotransformation of tramadol, codeine, and related compounds metabolized by CYP2D6 may also be decreased by fluoxetine and paroxetine (60).

Other pharmacokinetic interactions may also have clinical importance. Propoxyphene (Darvon), which is structurally related to methadone, can inhibit the metabolism of carbamazepine (Tegretol) (61). Symptoms associated with carbamazepine toxicity were greater in patients between 65–85 years of age, who are treated concurrently with carbamazepine and propoxyphene (62). The metabolism of meperidine is increased by either phenytoin (63) or phenobarbital (64) treatment, resulting in increased normeperidine levels (65). Chronic carbamazepine treatment can lead to an increase in the rate at which tramadol is metabolized. Finally, the clearance of zidovudine (Retrovir) is reduced by both acute and chronic methadone administration (66). This action may result, in part, from the inhibition of the glucuronidation of zidovudine by methadone (67).

P-glycoprotein may mediate the transportation of opioids across the blood brain barrier. In mutant mice with the gene for P-glycoprotein deleted, the analgesic effects of morphine, methadone, and fentanyl are greater than they are in wild-type mice (68,69). The administration of either verapamil (Calan) or cyclosporin (Sandimmune), which are P-glycoprotein inhibitors, increases the analgesic potency of morphine in mice (68,69). In addition to cyclosporin and verapamil, numerous drugs may inhibit P-glycoprotein–mediated transport, including quinidine, ketoconazole, lovastatin (Mevacor), and erythromycin (70). Whether the administration of these inhibitors to humans will increase the effects of morphine, fentanyl, or methadone remains to be determined. In one study, the administration of the P-glycoprotein inhibitor valspodar to healthy subjects attenuated rather than enhanced the effects of a low dose of morphine on reaction time, while it did not significantly alter morphine-induced decreases in respiratory rate (71).

Certain opioid-related drug interactions do not involve the factors that regulate drug pharmacokinetics. Many central nervous system depressants, including barbiturates, benzodiazepines, propofol (Diprivan), and neuroleptics, may potentiate the sedative actions of opioids. The administration of either meperidine or tramadol to patients being treated with monoamine oxidase inhibitors (MAOIs) such as phenelzine (Nardil) or tranylcypromine (Parnate) can cause toxic reactions to occur. These reactions may result from alterations in cerebral serotonin levels and in the case of tramadol also norepinephrine levels. The administration of meperidine to a patient being treated with an MAOI may lead to hypertension, excitement, hyperreflexia, hyperthermia, and tachycardia (72). This reaction may progress to coma and sometimes death. The administration of tramadol may increase the risk of seizures in patients also being treated with tricyclic antidepressants, cyclobenzaprine (Flexeril), promethazine (Phenergan), selective serotonin reuptake inhibitors (e.g., fluoxetine, sertraline [Zoloft], paroxetine), and neuroleptic agents.

HOW CAN THE ACTIONS OF OPIOIDS EXPLAIN CONTINUED OPIOID USE?

For more than a century, three major hypotheses have been put forth to account for continued opioid use (73). The first is that after a period of opioid use (for whatever reason), people become physically dependent and continue use to avoid the distress of withdrawal. The characteristics of opioid dependence are described below and in Chapter 35. A second hypothesis is that people continue to use opioids because they like the effects (e.g., euphoria) produced. Although many behavioral psychologists reject words such as *liking* or *euphoria,* preferring terms such as *positive reinforcing effects* to explain repeated drug taking in the absence of physical dependence, in practice, volunteers in laboratories studying opioid effects are asked to answer to questions such as, "How much do you 'like' the drug's effects?" and "How 'high' do you feel?" The third major hypothesis is that, for some people, even on initial use, opioids alleviate some preexisting dysphoric or painful affective state. Hence, for these individuals, opioid use is repeated not because of a desire for euphoria but to relieve some psychological distress that is not being caused by withdrawal; that is, it is used for self-medication. This latter notion is discussed at length in Chapter 6.

Over the years there have been a number of elaborations, variations, and combinations of these three basic hypotheses, each with different implications for the understanding and management of opioid dependence. For example, it has been postulated that euphoria is an atypical response to opioids that occurs primarily in individuals with psychopathology (74). Continued opioid seeking and opioid use despite societal prohibitions against such use was viewed, in part, as a manifestation of the antecedent psychopathology that caused the individual to experience euphoria initially. Another variation is that psychopathology is the basis for both the initial experimentation and the initial experience of euphoria, but that after repeated use the avoidance of withdrawal becomes the major motivation for continued use (74). Other recent variations on these themes are that individuals who respond positively to opioids have some neurophysiologic deficit, (e.g., deficient endorphins) that is corrected by exogenous opioids (15), or that repeated use of opioids (for whatever reason) produces a relatively permanent dysfunction in some biologic system (e.g., an endogenous opioid system), such that normal mood and function require the continuous use of exogenous opioids (75).

While there is some comfort in the hypothesis that only a limited percentage of the population will experience opioid euphoria and, therefore, be vulnerable to opioid dependence, the proportion of the population that is vulnerable must be quite large. When heroin was widely available to U.S. Army personnel in Vietnam, 42% of enlisted men experimented with opioids and, of these, about half became physically dependent. Of those who tried it at least five times, 73% became physically dependent. Interestingly, the characteristics that predicted who would become dependent in Vietnam were not the same as the characteristics that predicted who would relapse to opioids after return to the United States (76).

One of the most significant advances in understanding how opioids can lead to sustained drug-using behavior and relapse to opioid use after a period of withdrawal has been the recognition that both drug effects and drug withdrawal phenomena can become linked through learning to environmental cues and internal mood states (77–79). Because the concept of learned or conditioned craving tends to amplify and extend both the motivating effects of opioid withdrawal and their positive reinforcing actions, it is presented here not as a distinct hypothesis about continued opioid use, but as a process that should be considered whatever the initial or primary motives for use may have been.

There is little question that opioid withdrawal produces dysphoria and significant distress (see in section entitled Physical Dependence (Neuroadaptation) and Tolerance) and that avoidance of opioid withdrawal can be a major motive for continuing opioid use if there is a significant degree of physical dependence (12,75). However, avoidance of withdrawal does not readily explain relapse once acute and protracted withdrawal phenomena have abated. Consequently, much current work focuses on how the acute effects of drugs come to have so much value for the individual that other values are subordinated to the goal of obtaining and using opioids, and on how emotions and environmental cues reevoke the distress of withdrawal or the memory of opioid euphoria or opioid reduction of dysphoria. Chapter 6 considers the issues at greater length.

OPIOID REINFORCEMENT AND OTHER DRUGS

As described in Chapter 5, there has been a remarkable increase in knowledge about the neurophysiologic substrates of the positive reinforcing actions of opioid drugs. Multiple lines of evidence point to a critical role for dopaminergic neurons originating in the ventral tegmental area and ascending to the nucleus accumbens and frontal cortex. μ-Agonist opioids appear to increase activity in this system, with a resultant increase in dopamine release in the nucleus accumbens. In contrast, κ agonists tend to have either no effect or to decrease dopamine release (2). Cocaine and amphetamines, although acting on different receptors, also produce increases in dopamine release at the nucleus accumbens. On the basis of such findings, it is postulated that cocaine and opioids (as well as certain other commonly abused drugs) share a common pathway that is critical for their reinforcing actions (80,81). These common actions on dopaminergic pathways may account for the well-known synergistic effects of opioids and agents such as cocaine and amphetamines that induce euphoric effects by releasing or inhibiting reuptake of dopamine. Addicts frequently inject heroin and cocaine simultaneously (a "speedball") and claim that the euphoria is in some way more intense or satisfying than with either agent alone. Opioids and amphetamines are also synergistic in producing both analgesia and euphoria. It is interesting that the combinations do not produce additive side effects or toxicity. The combination of morphine and amphetamine produces more analgesia and more euphoria, but fewer unwanted side effects, than morphine alone (82,83). Addicts have long recognized that opioids can ameliorate some of the anxiogenic effects of cocaine. In mice, μ-agonist opioids can significantly attenuate the lethality of cocaine, an effect that is antagonized by naloxone (84).

PHYSICAL DEPENDENCE (NEUROADAPTATION) AND TOLERANCE

Physical dependence is usually defined as an altered state of biology induced by a drug, such that when the drug is withdrawn (or displaced from its receptors by an antagonist), a complex set of biologic events (withdrawal or abstinence phenomena) ensue that are typical for that drug (or class of drugs) and that are distinct from a simple return to normal function (2,12). So defined, physical dependence may develop within a single cell (e.g., a neuron in a culture), a complex of cells (e.g., the spinal cord), or the whole organism. Physical dependence can be observed with a number of classes of pharmacologic agents that have psychoactive effects, including opioids, CNS depressants, nicotine, as well as with drugs that are not ordinarily thought of as psychoactive agents (12).

The type of physical dependence induced by opioids is one of the most thoroughly studied, in part because the

clinical manifestations of the opioid withdrawal syndrome are easily measured, and in part because the availability of specific antagonists, such as naloxone, have facilitated research in human and infrahuman species.

Recent research has shed new light on the mechanisms involved in the development of opioid tolerance and dependence. Stimulation of opioid receptors located on critical cells such as those located in the locus coeruleus produces a decrease in cell firing. This effect reflects cellular hyperpolarization that results from both the activation of potassium channels and the inhibition of slowly depolarizing sodium channels (85). These actions occur in conjunction with a decrease in intracellular cyclic adenosine monophosphate (cAMP) levels. Following chronic exposure to opioids, potassium channel currents become reduced while cAMP pathways become upregulated, which leads to an increase in the phosphorylation of slowly depolarizing sodium channels. These events cause cells to become hyperexcitable (85).

Experiments with transgenic mice have implicated the transcription factor, cAMP response element-binding (CREB) protein as being critical in the changes produced by chronic opioid treatment (86). Symptoms of opioid withdrawal are markedly less in mice missing two CREB proteins. The actions of CREB protein may result from its effects on key signaling proteins. Phosphorylated CREB protein alters transcription in several genes by binding to the cAMP response element (CRE) (87). In mice, during naloxone-precipitated withdrawal from morphine, CRE-mediated transcription appears to be increased in several brain regions linked to opioid-induced changes in reward system activity and mood regulation including the nucleus accumbens, the amygdala, and the bed nucleus of the stria terminalis (88). The basic cellular mechanisms underlying opioid dependence are considered in greater detail in Chapter 10.

Substantial evidence exists that N-methyl-D-aspartate (NMDA) receptors are involved in the development of opioid-induced tolerance and dependence (89). Morphine tolerance and dependence are attenuated in mutated mice in which the GluRϵ1 NMDA receptor subunit has been deleted (90). Administration of the NMDA-antagonist dextromethorphan blocks the development of morphine tolerance and dependence in rats (91). Opioids may alter the activity of NMDA receptors by activating protein kinase C (92). This enzyme phosphorylates the NMDA receptor, which leads to an increase in the permeability of the receptor to calcium.

The acute administration of the NMDA antagonist memantine decreases the severity of naloxone-induced withdrawal in morphine-dependent addicts (93). This may be explained by possible increases in brain NMDA receptor activity during the development of opioid dependence. This is suggested by evidence from the mouse that chronic morphine administration produces an increase in GluRϵ1 NMDA receptor subunits in several brain regions, including the periaqueductal gray matter, the ventral tegmental area, and the nucleus accumbens (90).

The biologic changes responsible for opioid physical dependence begin as soon as opioid receptors are activated by opioid agonists. With prototypical μ-opioid agonists such as morphine, some degree of physical dependence can be induced in nontolerant human volunteers by single doses of opioids in the same dose range used for analgesia (15 to 30 mg). The low degree of physical dependence induced in this way is of little clinical significance, and withdrawal symptoms are not typically seen when opioids are given briefly for acute pain. However, even this degree of physical dependence can easily be demonstrated by administering a specific antagonist such as naloxone. Subjects given up to 10 mg of naloxone 6 hours after a dose of morphine (18 to 30 mg/70 kg body weight) report nausea and other feelings of dysphoria and exhibit yawning, sweating, tearing, and rhinorrhea (94). Animals previously made physically dependent on opioids and then withdrawn appear to become physically dependent more rapidly upon a second exposure to opioids, and it is likely that this is also the case with humans who were previously dependent. Certainly, *tolerance* to opioids can develop quite rapidly in opioid users, and in experiments with volunteers the dose of morphine can be increased from ordinary clinical doses (e.g., 60 mg/day) to 500 mg per day over as short a period as 10 days (12).

Although the characteristics of the opioid withdrawal syndrome produced by a variety of available μ-opioid agonists are all qualitatively similar, they can differ considerably with respect to the time of onset of symptoms, peak intensity, time to peak intensity, and duration of signs and symptoms (12). The signs and symptoms of the opioid withdrawal syndrome used as criteria for diagnosing this syndrome are presented in by the *Diagnostic and Statistical Manual of Mental Disorders*, 4th edition, text revision (*DSM–IV–TR*) (95). These symptoms include dysphoric mood, nausea, vomiting, muscle aches, tearing, rhinorrhea, pupil dilation, sweating, diarrhea, and insomnia, and must occur after the cessation of chronic opioid use or following the administration of an opioid antagonist. In general, the time course and intensity of the opioid withdrawal syndrome are related to how quickly the specific agonist is removed from its receptors. Drugs such as heroin, morphine, and hydromorphone have relatively short biologic half-lives (2 to 3 hours). When these drugs are stopped after a period of chronic use, the receptors are cleared relatively quickly. The onset of observable withdrawal is typically within 8 to 12 hours, and the acute syndrome reaches peak intensity within 48 hours and then begins to subside over a period of about 5 to 7 days. With drugs such as methadone or LAAM, which have half-lives after chronic administration ranging from 16 hours to more than 60 hours and are sequestered in body tissues, observable withdrawal may not develop until 36 to 48 hours or more after the last dose, peak intensity may not develop

until the fourth to sixth day, and some signs may persist for more than 14 days. When naloxone is used to displace methadone from its receptors, the onset of withdrawal is within minutes and a brief (30 to 60 minutes) but severe syndrome develops (12). As the naloxone is excreted, the methadone that is still in the body again binds to the receptors and withdrawal subsides.

However, in considering the older literature on the characteristics of the syndromes produced by drugs such as heroin, morphine, methadone, and buprenorphine, it is important to recognize that most of this classic work (just described) was carried out at the Addiction Research Center at Lexington, Kentucky, where the primary instrument used for measuring withdrawal intensity was the Himmelsbach scale. This scale focused exclusively on observable physiologic or behavioral signs such as blood pressure, pulse, temperature, lacrimation, pupillary size, sweating, piloerection, vomiting, diarrhea, and insomnia. No weight was given to more subjective manifestations of opioid withdrawal such as anxiety, drug craving, depression, irritability, muscle cramps, backache, bone pains, and general dysphoria (96). Hence, with certain μ agonists, the onset of peak severity and duration of withdrawal when described by the Himmelsbach scale may not always truly reflect the time course of dysphoria, craving, or sense of need for withdrawal relief experienced by a drug user. Two examples of this discrepancy are seen with methadone and buprenorphine. While it is generally reported that the withdrawal from methadone is milder yet more protracted than that of heroin and morphine, this generality does not necessarily reflect the subjective sense of distress (muscle aches, bone pains, dysphoria, depression) that drug addicts may experience during withdrawal. These symptoms are measurable using symptom checklists. When account is taken of these symptoms, withdrawal after cessation of methadone is found to develop in some drug-dependent individuals less than 24 hours after the last dose, and in some individuals, it persists for weeks. Buprenorphine is a partial μ agonist, but it binds quite firmly to the receptors. Buprenorphine is associated with little or no withdrawal phenomena when these are measured by the Himmelsbach scale (97,98); but by using a symptom checklist, withdrawal (although generally not severe) is easily measurable starting about 30 to 48 hours after the last dose, and the onset and time course of the syndrome generally correlate with subjects' sense of wanting something (a drug) to alleviate the discomfort. The experienced subjects in the studies rated the intensity of buprenorphine withdrawal as less than that which they had experienced with other opioid drugs such as heroin and methadone (98).

Protracted Abstinence

It has been long recognized that, after the more obvious and measurable manifestations of opioid withdrawal have subsided, many previously physically dependent individuals continue to experience unwanted feelings ranging from a vague sense of not feeling normal to more easily described symptoms of depression and abnormal responses to stressful situations. In two prospective studies in which former heroin users were stabilized on opioids (in one study the drug was morphine, in the second, methadone), there continued to be deviations from baseline on several physiologic measures (respiration, temperature, etc.) for up to 24 weeks after withdrawal. These were associated with feelings of decreased self-esteem, anxiety, and other indices of psychological disturbances (99,100). These physiologic and psychological deviations from baseline have been referred to frequently as the *protracted abstinence syndrome,* and it is postulated that this state contributes to relapse following withdrawal (75). Patients who have successfully participated in methadone maintenance programs often complain of protracted abstinence symptoms even when withdrawal was carried out quite slowly. In many cases, there is also a return of thoughts about opioid use (drug hunger). The biologic basis for protracted opioid abstinence is largely unexplored. Among the factors complicating the study of this phenomenon is the high prevalence of other psychiatric disorders (e.g., affective disorders, antisocial personality) among those who become heroin dependent (see Chapters 9 and 36). Hence, the appearance of depression, anxiety, or irritability during the weeks following withdrawal cannot usually be attributed exclusively to opioid withdrawal.

Receptor Specificity of Tolerance and Physical Dependence

It is also of clinical significance that the phenomena of tolerance and physical dependence appear to be relatively receptor specific. Hence, induction of tolerance to a μ agonist such as morphine will induce some degree of tolerance to other μ agonists such as hydromorphone, levorphanol, and methadone but little cross-tolerance to drugs acting primarily at κ receptors (1). However, tolerance to μ agonists is generally accompanied by μ agonist physical dependence and therefore any effort to abruptly substitute a κ agonist with either no action or antagonistic actions at the μ receptor will generally be associated with varying degrees of withdrawal. However, if such an agent were available, it might be possible to use a drug that has μ as well as δ and κ actions, thereby exerting analgesic effects through the non-μ receptors. Conversely, if tolerance develops to a relatively selective κ agonist, substitution of an opioid with actions at other receptors might still yield analgesia. Because clinically available opioids have somewhat different profiles of relative receptor affinity, some patients may respond better to one than to another and cross-tolerance is often incomplete. Yet the cross-tolerance between methadone and other μ agonists is such that patients maintained on methadone doses of 60 to 100 mg orally report little or no euphoria from a dose of heroin up to 25 mg.

While the currently available opioids may exhibit preferential binding to one or another of the receptor types (e.g., morphine and methadone bind preferentially to μ receptors), at very high doses even these drugs may begin to exert some of their effects through other receptors to which they bind with lesser affinity.

Some available agents categorized as agonist–antagonists (such as butorphanol, nalbuphine, and pentazocine) appear to exert either weak agonist or antagonist actions at the μ receptor, but their actions at other receptors, such as κ, render them useful analgesics. However, if such agents are administered to individuals dependent on a μ agonist such as morphine or heroin, it may displace the more potent agonists and precipitate μ agonist withdrawal. In general, these agonist–antagonists have lower abuse potential than prototypical μ agonists, probably because their actions at κ receptors are such that, when the dose is increased, most individuals begin to experience dysphoria rather than greater euphoria (1). However, when pentazocine (Talwin) is combined with the antihistamine tripelennamine (Ts and Blues—Talwin and blue-colored pyribenzamine tablets), the combination appears to be more euphorigenic than is either agent alone. Interestingly, in rats, combining tripelennamine with pentazocine or nalbuphine results in a significantly greater lowering of the threshold for electrical self-stimulation than do the opioids alone (101,102).

κ Agonist physical dependence has been studied in animals and appears to be distinct from μ agonist physical dependence, although there are some common elements (103). Physical dependence on relatively pure κ agonists has not been thoroughly studied in humans, in part because volunteers are reluctant to take high dosages because of the dysphoric effects. Physical dependence on nalorphine, an opioid with μ antagonist and κ agonist actions, has been studied in humans, and while there is a measurable syndrome when nalorphine is discontinued, and while the syndrome shares some features with morphine withdrawal, it is not characterized by drug-seeking behavior (104).

Buprenorphine is best characterized as a partial μ agonist. Given to nontolerant and nondependent volunteers, it is generally identified as an opioid drug and produces elevation of mood and other effects typical of morphine-like agents (97). Therefore, it is considered to have abuse potential and is subject to regulation under the Controlled Substances Act. However, it appears to exhibit a different slope for its dose–effect curve so that increasing doses do not produce comparable increases in euphoria or μ agonist toxicity (i.e., respiratory depression). At low levels of μ agonist physical dependence, buprenorphine can substitute for morphine or heroin in suppressing μ agonist withdrawal. However, at very high levels of μ agonist physical dependence it may not substitute completely or may precipitate withdrawal. Another interesting characteristic of buprenorphine is the tenacity with which it binds to the μ receptor. One consequence of this characteristic is that unusually high doses of naloxone are required to reverse effects of overdoses or to precipitate withdrawal (97). Buprenorphine is now approved as an alternative to methadone for opioid maintenance treatment (see below, in section entitled Managing Opioid Physical Dependence).

Managing Opioid Physical Dependence

There are many ways to deal with the development of opioid neuroadaptation (physical dependence). As is emphasized in Chapter 33, *physical dependence* and *addiction* are not (or should not be) interchangeable terms. When a patient with intractable pain becomes physically dependent, the situation should not evoke any sense of urgency about "getting the patient off narcotics." Ideally, in such a situation the issue is proper pain management, and withdrawal from opioids is undertaken only when there is some confidence that pain can be managed without opioid drugs. However, circumstances are not always ideal, and doctors are often pressured to withdraw patients from opioids even when there is no medical indication for doing so or no clear plan for alternative pain relief.

Treatment of individuals who are dependent on illicit opioids may involve either the use of maintenance therapies or medically managed withdrawal. Until recently, maintenance therapy relied solely on the use of methadone. Both LAAM and buprenorphine are approved for use as an opioid-maintenance agent. LAAM and its metabolites act as μ receptor agonists. The metabolites of LAAM have a much greater affinity for the μ receptor and have more agonist activity than does the parent compound (105). This may account for LAAM's slow onset of action. These compounds have comparatively long half-lives that allow LAAM to be administered as infrequently as three times a week. Withdrawal from LAAM is characterized by the slow onset of mild abstinence symptoms and a protracted course.

As an alternative to either methadone or LAAM maintenance regimens, buprenorphine may be used as a maintenance agent. The use of buprenorphine for opioid maintenance therapy is not restricted to approved treatment programs. Buprenorphine offers the advantage of a good safety profile, a lower potential for abuse than full μ receptor agonists, and an ability to block the reinforcing effects of other opioids. Because of its long duration of action and low toxicity, high doses of buprenorphine may be used for maintenance therapy when administered only three times a week (106). This drug is absorbed when administered sublingually. Sublingual tablets are available in two forms, those containing solely buprenorphine, as well as those that also contain naloxone to discourage diversion for parenteral use.

Many individuals, who have been maintained on methadone or other maintenance agents at some point, elect (or are pressured) to withdraw from maintenance opioid therapy. In each situation, the approach to withdrawal must take into account the current clinical situation of the patient (i.e., what specific opioid, for how long, at what dose, and for what reason), any associated medical or psychiatric problems, past experiences with withdrawal, the motives of the patient in seeking withdrawal, the available clinical resources, and the patient's social support network (see also Chapter 35).

The objective of medically managed withdrawal is to make the syndrome more tolerable for the individual. Hence, the technique selected often depends in part on how much discomfort the individual is willing to tolerate and the support system that is available. In a hospital situation, the standard method has been to substitute oral methadone for shorter-acting opioids such as morphine or heroin, then after a day or two of stabilization to reduce the methadone by approximately 20% per day. With few exceptions (e.g., medical personnel on very high doses of pure opioids), initial stabilization rarely requires more than 40 mg per day, usually given in divided doses. Because of the kinetics of methadone, with this approach some modest withdrawal discomfort begins about the third or fourth day and often persists for a number of days after the dose has been reduced to zero. Sedatives help to deal with the restless sleep and insomnia that often persist for many days or weeks. Because temptations to use opioids are typically fewer in a hospital than in an outpatient setting, patients are generally better able to tolerate some discomfort and craving in a hospital setting. Unfortunately, because of the costs of in-patient treatment, patients typically are discharged still experiencing low-level withdrawal and still having a relatively high craving for opioids. Relapse to opioids after brief in-hospital detoxification is quite high.

Hospital stays can be further shortened by managing withdrawal with clonidine (Catapier) (or other α_2-adrenergic agonists) (107–109). These agents act on autoreceptors, which inhibit locus coeruleus and other noradrenergic neurons that become hyperactive during μ opioid agonist withdrawal (12,16). Clonidine suppresses many of the autonomic signs and symptoms of withdrawal (e.g., nausea, vomiting, sweating, intestinal cramps, and diarrhea) (107–110), although it does little to alleviate the muscle aches, back pain, insomnia, and craving for opioids (112). By omitting the substitution of methadone, the duration of the acute heroin withdrawal syndrome is shortened. Clonidine can also be used to facilitate withdrawal from methadone. Clonidine is usually given orally, 0.1 to 0.3 mg every 6 hours up to a total of 2 mg in hospitalized patients, and 1.2 mg per day in outpatients. More experienced clinicians have given higher doses, but the sedation and marked hypotension associated with higher doses can make nursing care a problem.

Buprenorphine appears to be a very useful agent for managing opioid withdrawal. In contrast to clonidine, buprenorphine does not tend to produce marked decreases in blood pressure. Patients transferred to buprenorphine experience little or no withdrawal and craving is generally suppressed (111). Buprenorphine can then be discontinued or naltrexone treatment can be initiated. During acute detoxification of opioid dependent patients, including methadone dependent individuals, buprenorphine reduces subjective and physiologic withdrawal symptoms with an efficacy comparable or greater than that of clonidine (112,113).

Ultrarapid detoxification approaches have been developed that involve antagonist-precipitated opioid withdrawal using heavy sedation with short-acting benzodiazepines, (e.g., midazolam i.v.), followed by naloxone and naltrexone administration. It is been reported that with the ultrarapid detoxification approach, few or no withdrawal symptoms are observed when the effects of the benzodiazepine wear off. In short, the patient is able to tolerate naltrexone only hours after being dependent on opioids (114). Other studies indicate that patients will experience withdrawal symptoms for several days following ultrarapid detoxification (115). Pretreating patients with buprenorphine prior to ultrarapid detoxification may diminish the occurrence of persistent gastrointestinal adverse effects, such as nausea and vomiting, following the detoxification procedure (116).

In addition to the persistence of withdrawal symptoms, other disadvantages associated with ultrarapid detoxification include high cost and the risks associated with the induction of anesthesia or deep sedation. The long-term efficacy of ultrarapid withdrawal procedures has not been extensively studied, but some evidence suggests that this method fails to prevent relapse to heroin use in the majority of patients who have undergone ultrarapid withdrawal over 3- to 6-month time spans (115–117).

Rather than using the ultrarapid detoxification approach, some investigators have focused on the development of rapid detoxification procedures in which naltrexone is administered concurrently with medications that will reduce withdrawal symptoms in the conscious patient. Examples of this include the use of decreasing doses of buprenorphine with increasing doses of naltrexone (118) or α_2-adrenergic agonists such as either lofexidine or clonidine in combination with naltrexone (119,120). Administration of these drug combinations appears to reduce the duration and intensity of withdrawal symptoms to levels below those seen with single-agent treatment. Furthermore, if patients can be persuaded to continue taking naltrexone for a week after withdrawal, the probability of early relapse can be reduced.

Following successful withdrawal from opioids, the opioid antagonist naltrexone may be administered on a chronic basis to block the reinforcing effects of opioids during periods of relapse. It has been difficult to demonstrate the efficacy of naltrexone "maintenance" therapy (121). Noncompliance is a major problem associated with the use of naltrexone to maintain abstinence. The administration of naltrexone in long-lasting depot formulation is one approach used to address the issue of maintaining compliance with naltrexone therapy. These formulations can block heroin-induced mood-elevating effects for a period of 3 to 5 weeks (122).

There is evidence that the chronic administration of an opioid antagonist such as naltrexone produces an upregulation of opioid receptors. Following discontinuation of naltrexone there is increased sensitivity to opioid actions (123,124). In recently detoxified heroin addicts, this could result in an increased risk of overdosage if they experiment with opioids soon after naltrexone discontinuation.

The most common approach to opioid withdrawal for those who were heroin addicts is to stabilize the patient on relatively low doses of oral methadone (20 to 40 mg) and then, while the patient remains ambulatory in the community, to gradually reduce this dose to zero over a period of several weeks. For a number of years, treatment programs in the United States were obliged to withdraw heroin addicts who were not eligible for methadone maintenance within 21 days. The rate of relapse to heroin was exceedingly high. Clinical studies of the relative effects of different rates of withdrawal suggested that some patients were more likely to avoid relapse if methadone was reduced by very small increments of 1 to 3 mg per week over a period of up to 6 months (125). Federal regulations governing methadone programs were recently changed to allow for more flexible and extended periods of dose reduction and withdrawal.

In summary, there are a number of pharmacologic options and techniques available for withdrawing opioids from individuals who have become physically dependent. More recently, clinical research has focused on psychological and social support techniques for reducing the high rate of relapse following withdrawal (see Chapter 51). What remains to be learned is which pharmacologic approach, if any, combines best with which relapse prevention approach to yield the best long-term outcome.

OPIOID TOXICITY

When opioids are given orally under medical supervision, even prolonged periods of use appear to produce no major toxic effects on physiologic systems. However, in some individuals it is likely that prolonged exposure to opioids induces long-lasting adaptive changes that require continued administration of an opioid to maintain normal mood states and normal responses to stress. In contrast to the modest effects of medically supervised oral opioids, the toxic effects associated with unsupervised use of illicit, often contaminated, opioids by parenteral routes are severe and quite common. These toxic effects range from acute and sometimes fatal overdoses to a wide range of infections associated with shared or contaminated injection implements, to neurologic, muscular, pulmonary, and renal damage, the etiology of which is sometimes obscure. These toxic effects and medical complications are described in detail in Chapter 54. Opioid users are more likely than age-matched controls to die as a result of suicide or violence. Prior to the beginning of the human immunodeficiency virus (HIV) epidemic, mortality among illicit opioid users was two to three times higher than that of age- and gender-matched controls for older addicts, and 20-fold higher for younger addicts. However, because in some cities 50% of intravenous drug users are HIV seropositive, these older estimates of excess mortality among opioid users of 1.5% to 2% per year grossly understate the situation now emerging (12).

Acute opioid overdose is not uncommon among opioid addicts despite the remarkable tolerance that can develop to μ agonists such as morphine. For example, patients with terminal cancer may sometimes require doses in excess of 500 mg of morphine per hour intravenously. However, as noted in Chapter 55, a high degree of tolerance to opioids is not inevitable; many cancer patients can be managed for long periods without sharp escalation of dosage. This variability in the development of opioid tolerance, as well as the fluctuating levels of purity of illicit opioids, may help to explain why even opioid users with some degree of tolerance may experience severe opioid overdoses. Other factors that may contribute to overdosage is the tendency to combine other drugs such as alcohol or sedatives with opioids, or the return to opioid use shortly after a period of detoxification, which is associated with significant loss of acquired tolerance.

The characteristic signs of acute opioid toxicity include varying degrees of clouded consciousness (up to complete and unresponsive coma), severe respiratory depression, and markedly constricted (pinpoint) pupils. Often, there is pulmonary edema associated with the severe respiratory depression. While blood pressure is reduced by such doses of opioids, severe hypotension and cardiovascular collapse do not generally occur unless hypoxia is severe and prolonged. In such situations, the pupils may be dilated (12).

The first response should be to reestablish adequate ventilation and to administer an opioid antagonist such as naloxone. This should be given intravenously, if possible, with cautious increments to avoid precipitation of opioid withdrawal. Doses of less than 0.5 mg of naloxone are sometimes adequate to reverse respiratory depression, and the response is typically seen within 1 or 2 minutes of initial intravenous administration. Generally, if there is no substantial response to 5 to 10 mg of naloxone, there is little likelihood that the coma and respiratory depression are solely caused by opioid overdose. One possible exception is in the case of buprenorphine. As noted above, buprenorphine appears to bind firmly to receptors, so that if an overdose does occur, it is likely to require in excess of 10 mg of naloxone to antagonize its effects. Notably, this amount requires 25 ampules of naloxone. Mild degrees of pulmonary edema may clear when the respiratory rate is normalized. More severe pulmonary edema may require positive pressure ventilation.

Naloxone is a short-acting drug. If the opioid overdose is caused by an agent with a much longer half-life such as methadone, the patient may lapse back into coma when the naloxone is metabolized and the methadone still present reattaches to the receptors (12). In such instances, continued observation of the patient is called for. Alternatively, it may be possible to follow naloxone with a longer-acting antagonist such as naltrexone orally, recognizing that, unless used judiciously, naltrexone could precipitate severe withdrawal.

REFERENCES

1. Jaffe JH. Opioid-related disorders. In: Kaplan HI, Sadock BJ, eds. *Comprehensive textbook of psychiatry,* 6th ed. Baltimore, MD: Williams and Wilkins, 1995:842–863.
2. Jaffe JH, Martin WR. Opioid analgesics and antagonists. In: Gilman AG, Rall TW, Nies AS, et al, eds. *Goodman and Gilman's the pharmacological basis of therapeutics,* 8th ed. New York: Pergamon Press, 1990:485–521.
3. Woods JH, Winger G. Behavioral characterization of opioid mixed agonist-antagonists. *Drug Alcohol Depend* 1987;20:303–315.
4. Musacchio JM. The psychotomimetic effects of opiates and the sigma receptor. *Neuropsychopharmacology* 1990;3:191–200.
5. Cadet P, Mantione KJ, Stefano GB. Molecular identification and functional expression μ_3, a novel alternatively spliced variant of the human μ opiate receptor gene. *J Immunol* 2003;170:5118–5123.
6. Pan Y-X, Xu J, Mahurter L, Xu M, et al. Identification and characterization of two new human mu opioid receptor splice variants, hMOR-1O and hMOR-1X. *Biocem Biophys Res Commun* 2003;301:1057–1061.
7. Bond C, LaForge KS, Tian M, et al. Single-nucleotide polymorphism in the human mu opioid receptor gene alters beta-endorphin binding and activity: possible implications for opiate addiction. *Proc Natl Acad Sci USA* 1998;95:9608–9613.
8. Hernandez-Avila CA, Wand G, Luo X, et al. Association between the cortisol response to opioid blockade and the Asn40Asp polymorphism at the μ-opioid receptor locus (OPRM1). *Am J Med Genet* 2003;118B:60–65.
9. Marshall BE, Longnecker DE. General anesthetics. In: Gilman AG, Rall TW, Nies AS, et al, eds. *Goodman and Gilman's the pharmacological basis of therapeutics,* 8th ed. New York: Pergamon Press, 1990:311–331.
10. Lasagna L, Von Felsinger JM, Beecher HK. Drug-induced changes in man. 1. Observations on healthy subjects, chronically ill patients, and "postaddicts." *JAMA* 1955;157:1106–1120.
11. Von Felsinger JM, Lasagna L, Beecher HK. Drug-induced changes in man. 2. Personality and reactions to drugs. *JAMA* 1955;157:1113–1119.
12. Jaffe JH. Drug addiction and drug abuse. In: Gilman AG, Rall TW, Nies AS, et al, eds. *Goodman and Gilman's the pharmacological basis of*

therapeutics, 8th ed. New York: Pergamon Press, 1990:522–573.

13. Seecof R, Tennant FS. Subjective perceptions of the intravenous "rush" of heroin and cocaine in opioid addicts. *Am J Drug Alcohol Abuse* 1986;12:79–87.

14. McKenna GJ. Methadone and opiate drugs: psychotropic effect and self-medication. In: Verebey K, ed. *Opioids in mental illness: theories, clinical observations, and treatment possibilities.* New York: New York Academy of Sciences, 1982:44–55.

15. Gold MS, Pottash AC, Sweeney D, et al. Antimanic, antidepressant, and antipanic effects of opiates: clinical, neuroanatomical, and biochemical evidence. In: Verebey K, ed. *Opioids in mental illness: theories, clinical observations, and treatment possibilities.* New York: New York Academy of Sciences, 1982:141–150.

16. Redmond DE, Krystal JH. Multiple mechanisms of withdrawal from opioid drugs. *Annu Rev Neurosci* 1984;7:443–478.

17. European Agency for the Evaluation of Medicinal Products. *Evaluation of medicines for human use. EMEA public statement on the recommendation to suspend the marketing authorization for ORLAAM (levacetylmethadol) in the European Union.* Available at: http://www.emea.eu.int/pdfs/human/press/pus/877601en.pdf. Accessed October 2003.

18. Reisine T, Pasternak G. Opioid analgesics and antagonists. In: Hardman JG, Limbird LE, Molinoff RW, et al, eds. *Goodman and Gilman's the pharmacologic basis of therapeutics,* 9th ed. New York: McGraw-Hill, 1995:521–556.

19. Coffman BL, Rios GR, King CD, et al. Human UGT2B7 catalyzes morphine glucuronidation. *Drug Metab Dispos* 1997;25:1–4.

20. King CD, Rios GR, Green MD, et al. Comparison of stably expressed rat UGT1. 1 and UGT2B1 in the glucuronidation of opioid compounds. *Drug Metab Dispos* 1997;25:251–255.

21. Green MD, King CD, Mojarrabi B, et al. Glucuronidation of amines and other xenobiotics catalyzed by expressed human UDP-glucuronosyltransferase 1A3. *Drug Metab Dispos* 1998;26:507–512.

22. Green MD, Belanger G, Hum DW, et al. Glucuronidation of opioids, carboxylic acid-containing drugs, and hydroxylated xenobiotics catalyzed by expressed monkey UDP-glucuronosyltransferase 2B9 protein. *Drug Metab Dispos* 1997;25:1389–1394.

23. Hasselström J, Säwe J. Morphine pharmacokinetics and metabolism in humans: enterohepatic cycling and relative contribution of metabolites to active opioid concentrations. *Clin Pharmacokinet* 1993;24:344–354.

24. Wahlstrom A, Pacifici GM, Lindstrom B, et al. Human liver morphine UDP-glucuronyl transferase enantioselectivity and inhibition by opioid congeners and oxazepam. *Br J Pharmacol* 1988;94:864–870.

25. Aasmundstad TA, Morland J. Differential inhibition of morphine glucuronidation in the 3-and 6-position by ranitidine in isolated hepatocytes from guinea pig. *Pharmacol Toxicol* 1998;82:272–279.

26. Portenoy RK, Thaler HT, Inturrisi CE, et al. The metabolite morphine-6-glucuronide contributes to analgesia produced by morphine infusion in patients with pain and normal renal function. *Clin Pharmacol Ther* 1992;51:422–431.

27. Osborne RJ, Joel SP, Slevin ML. Morphine intoxication in renal failure: the role of morphine-6-glucuronide. *Br Med J* 1986;292:1548–1549.

28. Szeto HH, Inturrisi CC, Houde R, et al. Accumulation of normeperidine, an active metabolite of meperidine, in patients with renal failure. *Ann Intern Med* 1977;86:738–741.

29. Houde RW. Misinformation: side effects and drug interactions. In: Hill CS Jr, Fields WS, eds. *Advances in pain research and therapy,* 'vol. 11. *Drug treatment of cancer pain in a drug-oriented society.* New York: Raven Press, 1989:145–161.

30. Yun C-H, Wood M, Wood AJJ, et al. Identification of the pharmacogenetic determinants of alfentanil metabolism: cytochrome P-450 3A4. *Anesthesiology* 1992;77:467–474.

31. Kharasch ED, Russell M, Mautz D, et al. The role of cytochrome P450 3A4 in alfentanil clearance. *Anesthesiology* 1997;87:36–50.

32. Iribarne C, Picart D, Díeano Y, et al. Involvement of cytochrome P450 3A4 in N-dealkylation of buprenorphine in human liver microsomes. *Life Sci* 1997;60:1953–1964.

33. Tateishi T, Krivoruk Y, Ueng Y-F, et al. Identification of the human liver cytochrome P-450 3A4 as the enzyme responsible for fentanyl and sufentanil N-dealkylation. *Anesth Analg* 1996;82:167–172.

34. Moody DE, Alburges ME, Parker RJ, et al. The involvement of cytochrome P450 3A4 in the N-demethylation of L-alpha-acetylmethadol (LAAM), norLAAM, and methadone. *Drug Metab Dispos* 1997;25:1347–1353.

35. Iribarne C, Díeano Y, Bardou LG, et al.

Interaction of methadone with substrates of human hepatic cytochrome P450 3A4. *Toxicology* 1997;117:13–23.

36. Subrahmanyam V, Renwick AB, Walters DG, et al. Identification of cytochrome P-450 isoforms responsible for cis-tramadol metabolism in human liver microsomes. *Drug Metab Dispos* 2001;29:1146–1155.

37. Olkkaola KT, Palkama VJ, Neuvonen PJ. Ritonavir's role in reducing fentanyl clearance and prolonging its half-life. *Anesthesiology* 1999;91:681–685.

38. Bartowski RR, Goldberg ME, Larijani GE, et al. Inhibition of alfentanil metabolism by erythromycin. *Clin Pharmacol* 1989;46:99–102.

39. Labroo RB, Thummel KE, Kunze KL, et al. Catalytic role of cytochrome P4503A4 in multiple pathways of alfentanil metabolism. *Drug Metab Dispos* 1995;23:490–496.

40. Iribarne C, Picart D, Díeano Y, et al. *In vitro* interactions between fluoxetine or fluvoxamine and methadone or buprenorphine. *Fund Clin Pharmacol* 1998;12:194–199.

41. Iribarne C, Berthou F, Baird S, et al. Involvement of cytochrome P450 3A4 enzyme in the N-demethylation of methadone in human liver microsomes. *Chem Res Toxicol* 1996;9:365–373.

42. Foster DJR, Somogyi AA, Bochner F. Methadone N-demethylation in human liver microsomes: lack of stereoselectivity and involvement of CYP3A4. *Br J Clin Pharmacol* 1999;47:403–412.

43. Herrlin K, Segerdahl M, Gustafsson LL, et al. Methadone, ciprofloxacin, and adverse drug reactions. *Lancet* 2000;356:2069–2070.

44. Cobb MN, Desai J, Brown LS Jr, et al. The effect of fluconazole on the clinical pharmacokinetics of methadone. *Clin Pharmacol Ther* 1998;63:655–662.

45. Eap CB, Bertschy G, Powell K, et al. Fluvoxamine and fluoxetine do not interact in the same way with the metabolism of the enantiomers of methadone. *J Clin Psychopharmacol* 1997;17:113–117.

46. Geletko SM, Erickson AD. Decreased methadone effect after ritonavir initiation. *Pharmacotherapy* 2000;20:93–94.

47. Gerber JG, Rosenkranz S, Segal Y, et al. Effect of ritonavir/saquinavir on stereoselective pharmacokinetics of methadone: results of AIDS clinical trials group (ACTG) 401. *J Acquir Immune Defic Syndr* 2001;27:153–160.

48. Beauverie P, Taburet AM, Dessalles MC, et al. Therapeutic drug monitoring of methadone in HIV-infected patients receiving protease inhibitors. *AIDS* 1998;12:2510–2511.

49. Bending MR, Skacel PO. Rifampicin and methadone withdrawal. *Lancet* 1977;1:1211.

50. Kreek MJ, Garfield JW, Gutjahr CL, et al. Rifampin-induced methadone withdrawal. *N Engl J Med* 1976;294:1104–1106.

51. Holmes VF. Rifampin-induced methadone withdrawal in AIDS. *J Clin Psychopharmacol* 1990:10:443–444.

52. Eap CB, Buclin T, Baumann P. Interindividual variability of the clinical pharmacokinetics of methadone. *Clin Pharmacokinet* 2002;41:1153–1193.

53. Berge S, von Bardeleben U, Ladewig D, et al. Paroxetine increases steady-state concentrations of (R)-methadone in CYP2D6 extensive but not poor metabolizers. *J Clin Psychopharmacol* 2002;22:211–215.

54. Otton SV, Schadel M, Cheung SW, et al. CYP2D6 phenotype determines the metabolic conversion of hydrocodone to hydromorphone. *Clin Pharmacol Ther* 1993;54:463–472.

55. Sindrup SH, Brøsen K, Bjerring P, et al. Codeine increases pain thresholds to copper vapor laser stimuli in extensive but not poor metabolizers of sparteine. *Clin Pharamcol Ther* 1990;48:686–693.

56. Desmeules J, Gascon M-P, Dayer P, et al. Impact of environmental and genetic factors on codeine analgesia. *Eur J Clin Pharmacol* 1991;41:23–26.

57. Gaedigk A, Blum M, Gaedigk R, et al. Deletion of the entire cytochrome P450 CYP2D6 gene as a cause of impaired drug metabolism in poor metabolizers of the debrisoquine/sparteine polymorphism. *Am J Hum Genet* 1991;48:943–950.

58. Ingelman-Sundberg M, Oscarson, McLellan RA. Polymorphic human cytochrome P450 enzymes: an opportunity for individualized drug treatment. *TiPS* 1999;20:342–349.

59. Schmid B, Bircher J, Preisig R, et al. Polymorphic dextromethorphan metabolism: cosegregation of oxidative *O*-demethylation with debrisoquin hydroxylation. *Clin Pharmacol* 1985;38:618–24.

60. Ciraulo DA, RI Shader, Greenblatt DJ, et al. Basic concepts. In: Ciraulo DA, Shader RI, Greenblatt DJ, et al, eds. *Drug interactions in psychiatry,* 2nd ed. Baltimore, MD: Williams & Wilkins, 1995:1–28.

61. Ciraulo DA, Slattery M. Anticonvulsants. In: Ciraulo DA, Shader RI, Greenblatt DJ, et al, eds. *Drug interactions in psychiatry,* 2nd ed. Baltimore, MD: Williams & Wilkins, 1995:249–310.

62. Bergendal L, Friberg A, Schaffrath AM, et al. The clinical relevance of the interaction between carbamazepine and dextropropoxyphene in elderly patients in Gothenburg, Sweden. *Eur J Clin Pharmacol* 1997;53:203–206.

63. Pond SM, Kretschzmar KM. Effect of phenytoin on meperidine clearance and normeperidine formation. *Clin Pharmacol Ther* 1981;30:680–686.

64. Strambaugh JE, Wainer IW, Hemphill DM, et al. A potentially toxic drug interaction between pethidine (meperidine) and phenobarbitone. *Lancet* 1977;1:398–399.

65. Edwards DJ, Svensson CK, Visco JP, et al. Clinical pharmacokinetics of pethidine. *Clin Pharmacokinetics* 1982;7:421–433.

66. McCance-Katz EF, Rainey PM, Jatlow P, et al. Methadone effects on zidovudine disposition (AIDS clinical trials group 262). *J Acquir Immune Defic Syndr Hum Retrovirol* 1998;18:435–443.

67. Trapnell CB, Klecker RW, Jamis-Dow C, et al. Glucuronidation of 3′-azido-3′-deoxythymidine (zidovudine) by human liver microsomes: relevance to clinical pharmacokinetic interactions with atovaquone, fluconazole, methadone, and valproic acid. *Antimicrob Agents Chemother* 1998;42:1592–1596.

68. Zong J, Pollack GM. Morphine antinociception is enhanced in mdr1a gene-deficient mice. *Pharm Res* 2000;17:749–753.

69. Thompson SJ, Koszdin K, Bernards CM. Opiate-induced analgesia is increased and prolonged in mice lacking p-glycoprotein. *Anesthesiology* 2000;92:1392–1399.

70. Kim RB, Wandel C, Leake B, et al. Interrelationship between substrates and inhibitors of human CYP3A and p-glycoprotein. *Pharm Res* 1999;16:408–414.

71. Drewe J, Ball HA, Beglinger C, et al. Effect of P-glycoprotein modulation on the clinical pharmacokinetics and adverse effects of morphine. *Br J Clin Pharmacol* 2000;50:237–246.

72. Creelman WL, Ciraulo DA. Monoamine oxidase inhibitors. In: Ciraulo DA, Shader RI, Greenblatt DJ, et al, eds. *Drug interactions in psychiatry,* 2nd ed. Baltimore, MD: Williams & Wilkins, 1995:249–310.

73. Jaffe JH, Jaffe FK. Historical perspectives on the use of subjective effects measures in assessing the abuse potential of drugs. *Natl Inst Drug Abuse Res Monogr* 1989;92:43–72.

74. Kolb L. Pleasure and deterioration from narcotic addiction. *Mental Hygiene* 1925;9:699–724.

75. Dole V, Nyswander M. Heroin addiction—a metabolic disease. *Arch Intern Med* 1967;120:19–24.

76. Robins LN. Addict careers. In: DuPont RL, Goldstein A, O'Donnell J, eds. *Handbook on drug abuse.* Washington, DC: US Government Printing Office, 1979:325–336.

77. Childress AR, McLellan AT, O'Brien CP. Conditioned responses in a methadone population. *J Subst Abuse Treat* 1986;3:173–179.

78. Wikler A. *Opioid dependence: mechanisms and treatment.* New York: Plenum Press, 1980.

79. Meyer RE, Mirin SM. *The heroin stimulus: implication for a theory of addiction.* New York: Plenum Press, 1979.

80. Wise RA. The neurobiology of craving: implications for the understanding and treatment of addiction. *J Abnorm Psychol* 1988;2:118–132.

81. Koob GF, Bloom FE. Cellular and molecular mechanisms of drug dependence. *Science* 1988;242:715–723.

82. Forrest WH Jr, Brown BW Jr, Brown CR, et al. Dextroamphetamine with morphine for the treatment of postoperative pain. *N Engl J Med* 1977;296:712–715.

83. Jasinski DR, Preston K. Evaluation of mixtures of morphine and D-amphetamine for subjective and physiological effects. *Drug Alcohol Depend* 1986;17:1–13.

84. Witkin JM, Johnson RE, Jaffe JH, et al. The partial opioid agonist, buprenorphine, protects against lethal effects of cocaine. *Drug Alcohol Depend* 1991;27:177–184.

85. Hyman SE. Shaking out the cause of addiction. *Science* 1996;273:611–612.

86. Maldonado R, Blendy JA, Tzavara E, et al. Reduction of morphine abstinence in mice with a mutation in the gene encoding CREB. *Science* 1996;273:657–659.

87. Shaywitz AJ, Greenberg ME. CREB: a stimulus-induced transcription factor activated by a diverse array of extracellular signals. *Annu Rev Biochem* 1999;68:821–861.

88. Shaw-Lutchman TZ, Barrot M, Wallace T, et al. Regional and cellular mapping of cAMP response element-mediated transcription during naltrexone-precipitated morphine withdrawal. *J Neurosci* 2002;22:3663–3672.

89. Mao J. NMDA and opioid receptors: their interactions in antinociception, tolerance and neuroplasticity. *Brain Res Rev* 1999;30:289–304.

90. Inoue M, Mishina M, Ueda H. Locus-specific rescue of GluRε1 NMDA receptors in mutant mice identifies

the brain regions important for morphine tolerance dependence. *J Neurosci* 2003;23:6529–6536.

91. Mao J, Price DD, Caruso FS, et al. Oral administration of dextromethorphan prevents the development of morphine tolerance and dependence in rats. *Pain* 1996;67:361–368.

92. Chen L, Huang LY. Sustained potentiation of NMDA receptor-mediated glutamate responses through activation of protein kinase C by a mu opioid. *Neuron* 1991;7:319–326.

93. Bisaga A, Comer SD, Ward AS, et al. The NMDA antagonist memantine attenuates the expression of opioid physical dependence in humans. *Psychopharmacology* 2001;157:1–10.

94. Heishman SJ, Stitzer ML, Bigelow GE, et al. Acute opioid physical dependence in postaddict humans: naloxone dose effects after brief morphine exposure. *J Pharmacol Exp Ther* 1989;248:127–134.

95. American Psychiatric Association. *Diagnostic and statistical manual of mental disorders,* 4th ed., text revision. Washington, DC: Author, 2000.

96. Kolb L, Himmelsbach CK. Clinical studies of drug addiction. III. A critical review of withdrawal treatments with method of evaluating abstinence syndromes. *Am J Psychiatry* 1938;94:759–799.

97. Jasinski DR, Pevnick JS, Griffith JD. Human pharmacology and abuse potential of the analgesic buprenorphine. *Arch Gen Psychiatry* 1978;35:501–516.

98. Fudala PJ, Jaffe JH, Dax EM, et al. Use of buprenorphine in the treatment of opioid addiction. II. Physiologic and behavioral effects of daily and alternate-day administration and abrupt withdrawal. *Clin Pharmacol Ther* 1990;47:525–534.

99. Martin WR, Jasinski DR. Physiological parameters of morphine dependence in man—tolerance, early abstinence, protracted abstinence. *J Psychiatr Res* 1969;7:9–17.

100. Martin WR, Jasinski DR, Haertzen CA, et al. Methadone—a reevaluation. *Arch Gen Psychiatry* 1973;28:286–295.

101. Unterwald EM, Kornetsky C. Effects of concomitant pentazocine and tripelennamine on brain-stimulation reward. *Pharmacol Biochem Behav* 1984;21:961–964.

102. Unterwald EM, Kornetsky C. Effects of nalbuphine alone and in combination with tripelennamine on rewarding brain stimulation thresholds in the rat. *Pharmacol Biochem Behav* 1986;25:629–632.

103. Gmerek DE, Dykstra LA, Woods JH. Kappa opioids in rhesus monkeys. III.

Dependence associated with chronic administration. *J Pharmacol Exp Ther* 1987;242:428–436.

104. Martin WR, Fraser HF, Gorodetzky CW. Demonstration of tolerance and physical dependence on N-allyl-normorphine (nalorphine). *J Pharmacol Exp Ther* 1965;150:437–442.

105. Bertalmio AJ, Medzihradsky, Winger G, et al. Differential influence of N-dealkylation on the stimulus properties of some opioid agonists. *J Pharmacol Exp Ther* 1992;261:278–284.

106. Amass L, Kamien JB, Mikulich SK. Thrice-weekly supervised dosing with the combination buprenorphine-naloxone tablet is preferred to daily supervised dosing by opioid-dependent humans. *Drug Alcohol Depend* 2001; 61:173–181.

107. Washton AM, Resnick RG. Clonidine in opiate withdrawal: review and appraisal of clinical findings. *Pharmacotherapy* 1981;1:140–146.

108. Kleber HD, Topazian M, Gaspari J, et al. Clonidine and naltrexone in outpatient treatment of opioid withdrawal. *Am J Drug Alcohol Abuse* 1987;13:1–18.

109. Vining E, Kosten TR, Kleber HG. Clinical utility of rapid clonidine-naltrexone detoxification for opioid abusers. *Br J Addict* 1988;83:567–575.

110. Jasinski DR, Johnson RE, Kocher TR. Clonidine in morphine withdrawal. Differential effects on signs and symptoms. *Arch Gen Psychiatry* 1985;42:1063–1065.

111. Johnson RE, Cone EJ, Henningfield JE, et al. Use of buprenorphine in the treatment of opiate addiction. I. Physiologic and behavioral effects during a rapid dose induction. *Clin Pharmacol Ther* 1989;46:335–343.

112. Cheskin LJ, Fudala PJ, Johnson RE. A controlled comparison of buprenorphine and clonidine for acute detoxification from opioids. *Drug Alcohol Depend* 1994;36:115–121.

113. Janiri L, Mannelli P, Persico AM, et al. Opiate detoxification of methadone maintenance patients using lefetamine, clonidine, and buprenorphine. *Drug Alcohol Depend* 1994;36:139–145.

114. Loimer N, Lenz K, Schmid R, et al. Technique for greatly shortening the transition from methadone to naltrexone maintenance of patients addicted to opiates. *Am J Psychiatry* 1991;148:933–935.

115. Cucchia AT, Monnat M, Spagnoli J, et al. Ultra-rapid opiate detoxification using deep sedation with oral midazolam: short and long-term results. *Drug Alcohol Depend* 1998;52:243–250.

116. Bochud Tornay C, Favrat B, Monnat M, et al. Ultra-rapid opiate detoxification using deep sedation and prior oral buprenorphine preparation: long-term results. *Drug Alcohol Depend* 2003;69:283–288.

117. Lawental E. Ultra rapid opiate detoxification as compared to 30-day inpatient detoxification program—a retrospective follow-up study. *J Subst Abuse* 2000;11:173–181.

118. Umbricht A, Montoya ID, Hoover DR, et al. Naltrexone shortened opioid detoxification with buprenorphine. *Drug Alcohol Depend* 1999;56:181–190.

119. Gerra G, Zaimovic A, Giusti F, et al. Lofexidine versus clonidine in rapid detoxification. *J Subst Abuse Treat* 2001;21:11–17.

120. Buntwal N, Bearn J, Gossop M, et al. Naltrexone and lofexidine combination treatment compared with conventional lofexidine treatment for in-patient opiate detoxification. *Drug Alcohol Depend* 2000;59:183–188.

121. Kirchmayer U, Davoli M, Verster AD, et al. A systematic review on the efficacy of naltrexone maintenance treatment in opioid dependence. *Addiction* 2002;97:1241–1249.

122. Comer SD, Collins ED, Kleber HD, et al. Depot naltrexone: long-lasting antagonism of the effects of heroin in humans. *Psychopharmacology (Berl)* 2002;159:351–360.

123. Zukin RS, Sugarman JR, Fitz-Sayage ML, et al. Naltrexone-induced opiate receptor supersensitivity. *Brain Res* 1982;245:285–292.

124. Sicuteri F, Nicolodi M, Del Bene E, et al. Chronic naloxone improves migraine and modifies iris reactivity to morphine. *Biol Psychiatry* 1991;29:5035(abst).

125. Senay EC, Dorus DW, Goldberg F, et al. Withdrawal from methadone maintenance: rate of withdrawal and expectation. *Arch Gen Psychiatry* 1977;34:361–367.

126. Bart PA, Rizzardi PG, Gallant S, et al. Methadone concentrations are decreased by the administration of abacavir plus amprenavir. *Ther Drug Monit* 2001;23:533–535.

127. Marzolini C, Troillet N, Telenti A, et al. Efavirenz decreases methadone blood concentrations. *AIDS* 2000;14:1291–1292.

128. Clarke SM, Mulcahy FM, Tjia J, et al. The pharmacokinetics of methadone in HIV-positive patients receiving the non-nucleoside reverse transcriptase inhibitor efavirenz. *Br J Clin Pharmacol* 2001;51:213–217.

129. Pinzani V, Faucherre V, Peyriere H, et al. Methadone withdrawal symptoms

with nevirapine and efavirenz. *Ann Pharmacother* 2000;34:405–407.

130. Altice FL, Friedland GH, Cooney EL. Nevirapine-induced opiate withdrawal among injection drug users with HIV infection receiving methadone. *AIDS* 1999;13:957–962.

131. Lui S-J, Wang RIH. Case report

of barbiturate-induced enhancement of methadone metabolism and withdrawal syndrome. *Am J Psychiatry* 1984;141:1287–1288.

132. Finelli PF. Phenytoin and methadone tolerance. *N Engl J Med* 1976;294: 227(letter).

133. Tong TG, Pond SM, Kreek MJ, et al.

Phenytoin-induced methadone withdrawal. *Ann Intern Med* 1981;94:349–351.

134. Plummer JL, Gourlay GK, Cherry DA, et al. Estimation of methadone clearance: application in the management of cancer pain. *Pain* 1988;33:313–322.

CHAPTER 12

Cocaine and Crack: Neurobiology

MARTIN REPETTO AND MARK S. GOLD

The study of cocaine addiction is both exciting and instructive to the experienced professional and the layperson, despite the tragic and far-reaching consequences experienced by the victims (1–3). The course of addiction to cocaine is intense and can be measured in weeks and months, in contrast to years with alcohol and other drugs of abuse. As a result, clinicians and researchers can more easily study many of the principles that are generalizable to other forms of drug and alcohol addiction. The behavioral components identifiable in cocaine addiction are observable in virtually all forms of addiction: the drive for the drug, the intense preoccupation with acquiring the substance, the compulsive use despite adverse consequences, and the pattern of relapse. Finally, cocaine use stimulates its own taking without interference from satiety.

Perhaps the greatest legacy in the study of cocaine addiction has been the elucidation of several important neurochemical factors that appear to link the original drive for the drug in all addictive behaviors. The discovery that a number of neurotransmitters, residing in discrete brain sites, play a role in the initiation and propagation of cocaine addiction has changed the attitudes and perspectives of researchers and clinicians regarding the etiology and course of addictive diseases. The discovery of underlying neurologic mechanisms contributing to cocaine addiction has led to the acceptance that addiction is a true disease state with its own unique pathology (4–6), with or without a dramatic abstinence syndrome. Current research is focused on the cocaine-induced changes in brain metabolism, the impact of prenatal exposure to cocaine in brain development, the long-term effects of cocaine on the brain, and new treatments for cocaine dependence.

EPIDEMIOLOGY

Prevalence

The Annual Monitoring the Future surveys and other less formally structured sources of information show decreases in the lifetime, annual, monthly, and daily use of cocaine. Although the lifetime prevalence of illicit drugs use among twelfth graders decreased from its peak of 66% in 1982 to 40.7% in 1992, a gradual increase occurred during the 1990s. In the year 2001, the lifetime prevalence for the use of any illicit drug was 53.9%. This age group showed a similar increase in the lifetime prevalence of cocaine use. The peak lifetime use of cocaine by high school seniors decreased from 17.3% in 1985 to 5.9% in 1994. This tendency, however, changed in the following years, increasing to 8.2% in 2001.

Crack use also has decreased significantly among high school seniors between 1989 and 1990, but additional decreases have been difficult to demonstrate. Again, the lifetime prevalence for crack use had a mild increase from 3.0% in 1994 to 3.7% in 2001. In 2001, 2.1% of twelfth graders used crack in the last year and 1.1% in the past month.

The 1993 National Household Survey on Drug Abuse estimated that 4.5 million Americans age 12 years or older used cocaine in 1992, 1.3 million of whom used it at least monthly. Since then, the number of current cocaine users in the same age group has increased to 1.7 million Americans in 2001. An additional 406,000 people were current crack users in 2001.

Clinical experience and some governmental data suggest that most surveys underestimate the number of cocaine addicts in the United States. Surveying only 10 cities, the Department of Justice identified about 650,000 cocaine addicts through urine testing (7). In a study of 1,116 patients admitted for alcohol and drug treatment, 150 patients qualified for cocaine dependence, representing a 12% of the inpatient population (8,9). Cocaine abuse and dependence is a common problem that is often part of the increasing trend of polydrug abuse, which commonly includes alcohol, nicotine, marijuana, opiates, and/or cocaine. Cocaine and heroin users account for a major new group of persons with human immunodeficiency virus infection.

Patterns of Addictive Use

The patterns of cocaine use in particular vary, and no one stereotype prevails. Cocaine may be used continuously for days in "runs" or "binges" or at regular intervals when a paycheck is received (that is, only for a day or so every 2 weeks). Cocaine acquires a value greater than money and all resources are exhausted to satisfy the drive for the drug.

Cocaine users come from all social strata, all races, and both sexes. Demographically, cocaine addicts are usually young (12 to 39 years of age), dependent on at least three drugs (including alcohol), and predominantly male (75%). Many, if not most, have important comorbid psychiatric and addictive illnesses. Alcohol dependence is exceedingly common among cocaine users. In the Epidemiological Catchment Area Study, 84% of those with cocaine dependence were also alcohol dependent (10).

While the glamour of cocaine use of the late 1970s and early 1980s has subsided, it appears that the so-called recreational use has also lost some of its appeal. It is not known beyond the surveys already mentioned just how many individuals can and do use cocaine for "sport" or "pleasure" without significant abuse and addiction liability. However, there is clearly a substantial number of users who have tried cocaine once or more without serious consequence and who have now stopped as a result of education, prevention, or changes in attitudes. If 1 of every 2 Americans between the ages of 25 and 30 years has used cocaine, then the overwhelming majority have stopped on their own. What is certain is that the risk for developing cocaine addiction is substantial and the morbidity and mortality high (11,12).

Chen and Kandel (13) studied the relationship between different aspects of cocaine use such as intensity of use, route of administration, gender, and race. They found that higher rates of cocaine use favor the development of dependence. They also reported that female adolescents have a higher likelihood of becoming dependent on cocaine than do male adolescents because of their tendency to use higher quantities and their higher sensitivity to the effects of the drug. They also reported that African Americans have a higher risk of developing cocaine dependency than do white Americans. African Americans show a tendency to use cocaine more frequently and are more sensitive to the effects of the drug than whites. In addition, African Americans have a higher tendency to use intravenous injection and smoking as routes of cocaine administration. Regarding the route of administration, these authors found that the simultaneous use of intravenous administration and smoking increase the risk of developing cocaine dependence.

Cocaine and Alcohol (Cocaethylene)

Cocaine and alcohol are frequently combined. Researchers have clearly demonstrated that in the presence of two drugs of abuse, cocaine and alcohol, the body creates a third, cocaethylene. Thus, the effects observed in persons who combined ethanol and cocaine are the result of the interactions between these two substances and effects of cocaethylene. Interestingly, the combined effects of cocaine and ethanol vary depending on the order in which the substances are consumed. Additive myocardial depressant effects, not related to ischemia, but rather a direct toxic effect of cocaine plus ethanol, have similarly been reported (14). Small, "recreational" doses of cocaine produce coronary vasoconstriction and impair myocardial function. Ethanol has coronary vasoconstrictive and myocardial depressant effects as well. Additive effects on the nucleus locus coeruleus may also contribute to the panic and anxiety produced by cocaine and alcohol. Because cocaine is most often taken with other drugs such as alcohol, many of the findings that clinicians attribute to cocaine may in fact be caused by the combination of drugs. Ethanol plus cocaine appears to increase the period of time associated with cocaine-related increases in blood pressure. Such an interaction between cocaine and alcohol might increase the likelihood of small-vessel, intracerebral, ischemic infarcts.

In a single-photon emission computed tomography (SPECT) study, Gottschalk and Kosten (15) found that whereas cocaine produces significant changes in cerebral blood flow, these changes differ from those induced by the simultaneous use of cocaine and alcohol. Thus, while cocaine produces areas of hyper- and hypoperfusion, cocaine and alcohol users were more likely to show a decreased blood flow in the occipital and temporal areas and the cerebellum.

Ethanol use increases cocaine use and liking for cocaine, possibly by the association of combined use with cocaethylene production. In a recent study, nondependent cocaine users were chosen on the basis of ability to choose cocaine versus placebo. Thereafter they were pretreated with small social doses of alcohol and given choices of cocaine and money. Alcohol pretreatment significantly increased choice of cocaine (16) over the alternative reinforcer, money. Alcohol can make it particularly difficult to reduce or abstain from cocaine use.

Chronic cocaine abusers often experience persistent panic attacks or bouts of anxiety, which are reported to persist months after discontinuation of cocaine (17,18) These consequences may be linked to cocaine and alcohol use. Heuristically consistent with reports of cocaine kindling and cocaine modification of benzodiazepine receptor binding (19) and withdrawal "anxiety" in animals (20), combined use of cocaine and alcohol is quite common among cocaine users (21), with approximately 12 million combination users (22). While initially used by the addict to modify the anxiogenic effects of cocaine and reduce the likelihood of insomnia (23), upon withdrawal, anxiety is increased, and possibly prolonged well into abstinence (24).

The longer half-life of cocaethylene (2 hours compared with 38 minutes for cocaine), and additive effect of cocaethylene on the dopamine (DA) transporter (25), and the 40-fold greater affinity for the serotonin transporter may explain the occurrence of lethal heart attacks and stroke (18-fold increase in the risk of sudden death compared to cocaine alone [26]), the greater irritability, and the prolonged toxicity (27). In the case of simultaneous cocaine and alcohol withdrawal, symptoms of cocaine discontinuation can mask the clinical presentation of alcohol withdrawal. Thus, patients undergoing concurrent cocaine and alcohol withdrawal usually receive less oxazepam (Serax) than do patients with alcohol-only withdrawal, because of the decreased autonomic reaction (28).

Cocaine addiction is also common among heroin addicts; studies show ranges between 20% and 50% for concomitant cocaine addiction (29). Moreover, studies clearly show that alcohol is so commonly used that it is the first drug of abuse for cocaine addicts, followed closely by cannabis. Studies also show that people who have never used marijuana do not generally use cocaine. Early data from the National Institute of Drug Abuse suggested that if a person has used marijuana fewer than 10 times that person is not as likely to use cocaine as they are if marijuana has been used 100 times. Viewed conversely, 98% of cocaine addicts have used marijuana (30).

Preparations and Routes of Administration

Cocaine is known by names that reflect both appearance and effects. Coca paste is known as "base," "pasta," "pitillo," and "buscuso." The powdered crystalline form is known as "snow" and "coke," and the rock base form as "crack." Cocaine is an alkaloid that is found in the leaves of *Erythroxylon coca,* a tree or shrub indigenous to western South America. The fact that nearly all of the world's coca-producing countries are concentrated in one geographic area has led some to conclude cocaine eradication possible if the "Drug War" was viewed as an actual war. Abundant numbers of the plant are found in the wild state in Peru, Colombia, Ecuador, and Bolivia. Coca paste is prepared by dissolving dried coca leaves in a solution of kerosene or gasoline, alkaline bases, potassium permanganate, and sulfuric acid. The resultant coca paste contains not only cocaine but also adulterants, diluents, sulfates, and other coca alkaloids (31). The other forms of cocaine are prepared from coca paste: cocaine hydrochloride, by the mixture of hydrochloric acid and paste, and crack, by the mixture of bases and paste (32).

While clinical wisdom and some systematic studies have suggested that certain preparations of cocaine are more addictive, some notable exceptions make a generalization impossible at this time (33). The principal routes of administration are oral, intranasal, intravenous, and inhalation. The slang terms for these routes are, respectively, "chewing," "snorting," "mainlining," and "smoking." Oral absorption is the slowest, within 45 to 60 minutes. While there is evidence that routes with quicker and higher peak absorption of cocaine leads to greater intoxication and addiction rates, any of the routes of administration can lead to absorption of large and toxic amounts of cocaine, especially once the onset of regular and addictive use is established. The absorption patterns parallel the behavioral and subjective effects of cocaine. Most controlled studies report close correlation between the plasma levels of cocaine and the physiologic and behavioral effects. Also, the toxicities are believed to reflect the route of administration. There is sufficient evidence that acute administration follows differential effects on routes of cocaine administration, with greater toxicity for inhalation than for intravenous than for intranasal than for oral.

The purity of the preparations influences the rate and completeness of absorption of cocaine. In coca leaf chewing, the purity is 0.5%, and it is higher for the cocaine hydrochloride form taken via the oral or intranasal route, with a wide range of 20% to 80%. The purity for intravenous preparations and the smoked form also varies, from 7% to 100% for the former, and from 40% to 100% for the latter.

Orally consumed cocaine has an area under the curve, or total amount absorbed, equal to that of the intranasal route, with similar bioavailability of 20% to 30%. The loss of cocaine after oral absorption is a result of the first pass hepatic biotransformation, which metabolizes 70% to 80% of the dose. For oral absorption, the cocaine concentrations in the blood rise slowly such that at 10 to 15 minutes, levels are 30 to 50 ng/mL, with a peak of 160 ng/mL at about 60 minutes. The slow and more sloped peak blood level is thought to be responsible for the oral route's apparent low rate of addiction.

After intranasal absorption, the loss of cocaine is a result of the ionized form of cocaine's (cocaine HCl) poor penetration of biologic membranes, particularly the nasal mucosa; the vasoconstricting properties of cocaine limit its own passage into blood vessels. The onset of activity is within 3 to 5 minutes and the blood level peaks at 10 to 20 minutes, fading in 45 to 60 minutes. Because cocaine has a biologic half-life of 1 hour, repeated self-administrations are necessary to maintain an effect.

After i.v. injection, the entire bolus of cocaine is delivered to the vessel chamber and has a bioavailability of 100%. The limiting factor for i.v. cocaine concentration is the original purity of the injected sample. The onset of activity is within 30 seconds, with a duration of action of 10 to 20 minutes. The venous system must still be traveled, with the sequence being from the peripheral veins back to the heart and subsequently through the pulmonary system for ejection by the left ventricle to the brain.

Cocaine inhalation became popular because it produces the quickest and highest peak blood levels to the brain without the risks attendant to i.v. use. Freebase cocaine, whether in coca paste, freebase, or crack form, is much more volatile and lipid soluble than the leaf and powder forms. Because the freebase can be inhaled and thus delivered to the pulmonary bed, it is pumped by the heart directly into the brain. The bioavailability is low, at 6% to 32%, as a consequence of the pyrolysis that occurs on heating the cocaine for vaporization.

With all the routes of administration, chronic and repetitive use of cocaine produces high blood levels. In this regard, the various routes of administration tend to merge and clinical distinctions may be more difficult to make. One study found no significant differences among the routes of administration on several measures of behavioral effects, including paranoia and violence (34).

While cocaine has reliable effects, the state of the organism at the time of the cocaine challenge is an important, often neglected factor. Cocaine appears to produce its greatest effects when the user is not full from overeating or sexually exhausted from recent activity. Chronic food deprivation decreases extracellular DA in the nucleus accumbens, providing more motivation and reward for the animal who has learned how self-administer cocaine for DA release (35). Stress, anxiety, and fear may also increase the rewarding qualities of cocaine. Cocaine reward may also be influenced by genetic factors and *in utero* exposure.

Prenatal cocaine exposure led to a marked and stable enhancement of the rates of self-administration for all periods examined, suggesting that prenatal exposure to cocaine alters cocaine reinforcement properties for adults (36). Increases in DA in nucleus accumbens and other systems and serotonin systems in brain have been demonstrated for prenatally exposed animals.

What the host brings to the drug challenge may help us to ultimately explain pathologic attachment to drugs, and the relative aversion and resistance of others to the same drugs at the same time.

PHARMACOLOGY

Chemistry

Cocaine was the first local anesthetic to be discovered. The pure alkaloid was first isolated in 1860 by Niemann, who noted that it had a bitter taste and produced a peculiar effect on the tongue by making it devoid of sensation. Cocaine is an ester of benzoic acid and a nitrogen-containing base. Cocaine has the base structure of the synthetic local anesthetics. The structure contains hydrophilic tertiary amine and hydrophobic aromatic residue that are separated by an intermediate alkyl chain.

Neurophysiology

Cocaine's most important clinical action is its ability to impede the initiation or conduction of the nerve impulse by blocking the Na voltage-sensitive channels. Its most striking systemic effect is its stimulation of the central nervous system (CNS). Cocaine is a stimulant by means of its potentiation of the responses of sympathetically in-

nervated organs to norepinephrine and, to a lesser extent, epinephrine. Centrally, it inhibits the reuptake of norepinephrine, serotonin and dopamine.

The assumption that cocaine affinity for the DA transporter (DAT) is directly related to self-administration underlies the DA hypothesis of cocaine reward. According to this theory, the DA transporter serves as the primary means of removing DA from the synaptic cleft after its release; inhibition of this uptake results in an acute excess of DA in the synaptic cleft (1). Cocaine blocks DA uptake into presynaptic terminals and the acute systemic administration of cocaine transiently and dose-dependently increases the extracellular concentration of DA in the nucleus accumbens of rats (37–40) and is associated in humans with mood elevation and arousal.

The intensity of the cocaine's induced "high" is positively correlated to the proportion of DA transporter blockage (41). Chronic cocaine use upregulates the DA transporter in the ventromedial caudate nucleus, the putamen, and the nucleus accumbens. The failure of the dopamine system to adapt to the cocaine-induced changes in the DA transporter can have serious consequences. Patients presenting excited cocaine delirium, a sometimes fatal complication of cocaine intoxication, did not show DA transporter upregulation in postmortem studies (42).

While DA appears essential to cocaine reward, other evidence suggests that no single neurotransmitter is responsible for all of the clinical or experimental effects of cocaine. Serotonergic activation modulates the reward potency of both cocaine and amphetamines, and pharmacologic agents that activate dopaminergic systems without affecting the serotonergic systems do not produce typical self-administration as in addictive use by animals or humans. Correspondingly, pure serotonin agonists and antagonists that lack DA-stimulating properties do not produce reward behavior, further indicating that both systems are required for the expression of compulsive use of cocaine. Cocaine blockades the reuptake of serotonin and enhances its activity at different levels of the CNS. Research demonstrates that the behavioral manifestations of cocaine intoxication (i.e., agitation, aggression, impulsivity, and euphoria) are related to the drug's effects on the serotonergic system. Animal studies show that the administration of serotonin antagonists, either through intraperitoneal injections or through microinjections in the nucleus accumbens, decrease cocaine-induced hyperactivity (43). Moreover, the administration of serotonin (5-HT) agonists in the nucleus accumbens increases cocaine induced motor activity (44). Coincidentally, positron emission tomography (PET) studies show an increased binding capacity of the serotonin transporters in acutely abstinent patients. The increased binding capacity is consistent with an upregulation of the serotonin transporter in response to the cocaine-induced blockade of the system (45). Serotonin was found to play a role in cocaine induced impulsivity. For instance, 5-HT$_{1b}$ receptor knockout mice showed increased aggression and cocaine self-administration (46). In addition, impulsive and aggressive behavior correlates to buspirone (BuSpar)-induced changes in serotonin function in humans (47). Serotonin is also related to cocaine-seeking behavior. Serotonin depletion with tryptophan hydroxylase inhibitors reduces cocaine-seeking activity (48). Based on the clinical similarities between major depression and cocaine's abstinence depression, recent research focused on the biologic parallels between these two conditions. Similar to depression in humans, cocaine withdrawal in rats decreases serotonin levels in the CNS, decreases fenfluramine-induced adrenocorticotropic hormone (ACTH) and corticosterone release, and decreases prolactin response to stimulants (49).

Importantly, serotonin modulates the activity of other neurotransmitters in the nucleus accumbens, such as γ-aminobutyric acid (GABA) and dopamine. On the other hand, GABA modulates the dopaminergic activity in the ventral tegmental area (VTA). GABA$_B$ receptor stimulation with baclofen (Lioresal) in the VTA blockades the rewarding effects of brain self-stimulation (50). GABA agonists reduce the reinforcing effects of cocaine in animal models of cocaine dependence.

Cocaine also facilitates the release of norepinephrine, activates tyrosine hydroxylase, increases acutely the levels of neurotransmitters in synapses, and increases adrenergic β-cell populations and the inhibition of neurotransmitter release via action of autoreceptors on presynaptic sites. The net effect of the blockage is an increase in the amount of neurotransmitter available at the postsynaptic site for a putative enhanced effect at the postsynaptic sites. Cocaine does not directly activate opioid receptors but may indirectly influence these systems. Cocaine also affects neurotransmission in histamine, acetylcholine, and phenethylamine pathways (51).

Glutamate is an amino acid with excitatory properties. Glutamate is involved in the psychomotor response to stimulants (52). Experimental research shows cocaine-seeking behavior reinstatement increases firing activity in the hippocampal ventral subiculum activity, an area rich in glutamate neurons. In addition, whereas the administration of the glutamate antagonist kynurenate (KYN) in the VTA can prevent the reinstatement of cocaine seeking, the glutamate agonist N-methyl-D-aspartate (NMDA) enhances this type of conduct (53).

Problems exist with these hypotheses. Antidepressants characteristically affect the same neurotransmitter systems, as do cocaine and amphetamines, by inducing a presynaptic blockade of the reuptake of these neurotransmitters, but are not drugs of abuse. Neuroleptics block DA transmission at the postsynaptic site, but clinically do not stop cocaine use. While it is relatively clear that these neurotransmitters are required for these functions, and interactions between them or other systems appear important, there are limitations in our present knowledge and ability to link together all the phenomena in cocaine addiction.

Considerable animal and human data suggest that high-dose cocaine use over prolonged periods of time leads to sustained neurophysiologic changes in the brain that are responsible for mood-and-reward behavior. Studies of electrical and pharmacologic self-stimulation of brain sites for drive states provide a model for some of the behaviors witnessed in cocaine addiction. Chronic cocaine administration increases the threshold voltage required to elicit self-stimulation behavior in dopaminergic areas such as the nucleus accumbens. The increased voltage requirement indicates subsensitive or downregulated brain sites as responsible for compulsive use of cocaine. The dysregulation appears to represent a depletion of dopaminergic neurons that may also contribute to the anhedonia and depression during acute and subacute withdrawal in animals and humans following chronic cocaine stimulation (54).

Behavioral sensitization produced by repeated cocaine use is associated with enhanced response in caudate and nucleus accumbens. Such an important effect, which may explain cocaine binges, suggests that the DA transporter is induced by DA blockade during cocaine self-administration to produce compensatory increases in the DA uptake carrier (55).

Dopamine and Reward

Furthermore, the rewarding effects of cocaine self-administration are reduced by D1, D2, and D3 receptor antagonists but not by noradrenergic receptor antagonists (56). Self-administration of cocaine is reduced or eliminated following lesions of the dopaminergic innervation of the nucleus accumbens or lesions of nucleus accumbens cell bodies. In contrast, lesions of noradrenergic or dopaminergic terminals in the striatum or prefrontal cortex are without effect. Finally, evidence suggests that the DA receptors of the nucleus accumbens may function as part of a neuronal mechanism responsible for endogenous reward, which reinforces behaviors leading to natural stimuli such as food and water. Thus, operant conditioning experiments with animals indicate that the rewarding properties of food, water, or intracranial brain stimulation may depend on the nucleus accumbens DA receptor activation. Therefore, the rewarding properties of drugs that lead to excessive self-administration may result from the ability of one or a combination of compounds to activate this neural substrate for endogenous reward (57,58).

Recent data suggest that cocaine has many but not all of the same effects on DA systems as primary reinforcers. In a recent study, monkeys were trained to work to obtain intravenous cocaine and juice rewards. During these trials, the investigators recorded 62 neurons, with both cocaine and juice rewards producing characteristic changes. However, the neuronal release produced by rewards was independent—a response to one did not predict the other. The neural basis for cocaine reward does not appear to be the same as for juice. Signals generated for juice and cocaine reward are at least partially separable at the neuronal levels within the ventral striatum and cocaine does not act on the reward system in the same ways as a natural reward or reinforcer (59,60).

Moreover, individual differences in the release of dopamine in response to stress can affect cocaine use. Rats that show increased motor activity (i.e., grooming behavior) under stress exhibit higher rates of cocaine self-administration. The increase in stress reactivity was related to a decreased level of dopamine release in the substantia nigra, medial prefrontal cortex, and amygdala (61).

The Dopamine Depletion Hypothesis of Cocaine Dependence

The DA depletion hypothesis suggests that repetitive stimulation by cocaine and the subsequent chronic blockade of reuptake lead to a depletion of presynaptic DA stores. Because reuptake of DA is the principal source of DA for future release, a chronic blockade understandably would result in a relative decrease in DA transmission. A neuroadaptive mechanism of a nerve ending to the severing of its stimulation is an upregulation or enhanced sensitivity of the postsynaptic sites, hence, receptor supersensitivity (62).

The D2 receptor is an autoreceptor whose agonist action is to decrease the release of DA, and supersensitivity of this receptor would lead to decreased DA release, as suggested by animal studies. Other possible mechanisms for decreased DA function are neurotoxic degeneration of dopaminergic neurons, D1-receptor-mediated feedback innervation to the cell bodies of mesolimbic DA neurons, and multiple feedback loops involving serotonergic, noradrenergic, enkephalinergic, and GABAergic synapses. Relapse appears to be related to the DA system as well. The priming effects of cues in cocaine-seeking behavior can be mimicked by activation of the mesolimbic DA system. DA acts at two general classes of DA receptors, termed D1-like and D2-like, which are distinguished by structure, opposite modulation of adenylate cyclase, and differential localization. Priming ability of the D1-like and D2-like selective agonists was assessed by their ability to reinstate nonreinforced lever pressing (63). Priming effect was selectively induced by D2-like, but not D1-like, DA receptor agonists. Moreover the D1-like agonists prevented cocaine-seeking behavior induced by cocaine itself, whereas D2-like agonists enhanced this behavior. These recent data suggest that D1-like agonists may be useful pharmacotherapies for cocaine addiction.

These neurophysiologic changes have been understandably difficult to measure, and studies in animals have not always closely followed the long-term patterns of use that are frequently observed in cocaine addicts. However, in some studies of humans, decreased DA transmission has been documented. Both homovanillic acid, the principal metabolite of DA in humans, and prolactin, the hormone whose release is inhibited by DA, have been found in decreased amounts in humans who consumed cocaine chronically. Moreover, other studies show that transiently increased dopaminergic transmission is associated with recurrent desire to use cocaine.

The cocaine-DA hypothesis is supported by the following studies:

- Selective 6-hydroxydopamine lesions of DA terminals in the nucleus accumbens, but not in the caudate nucleus, abolish cocaine self-administration (64).
- Intra-accumbens administration of selective D1- and D2-antagonist drugs attenuate cocaine reinforcement in a dose-dependent manner (65).
- *In vivo* microdialysis has demonstrated that a single injection of cocaine increases the concentration of extracellular DA in the nucleus accumbens, with a maximal effect reached at peak-reported cocaine euphoria in humans at approximately 30 to 40 minutes postexposure (66). Other changes in dopaminergic neurotransmission may appear only after cocaine administration has been terminated, including persistently reduced DA metabolism and decreased DA synthesis. Postmortem binding to DA transporters in striatum is also reduced in humans with a history of cocaine abuse (67–69).
- Repeated i.v. administration of cocaine followed by its withdrawal persistently reduces the number of DA transporters in the nucleus accumbens, but not in the striatum (70).
- Adaptive regulation of DA transporter function appears to be more pronounced in the nucleus accumbens than striatum in chronic administration studies (71).
- Both decreased synthesis and concentrations of DA have been reported for cocaine in the nucleus accumbens and frontal cortex following chronic administration, with long-lasting decreases in extracellular DA in the nucleus accumbens after just 10 days of cocaine administration. The decreased density of D1-receptor binding sites in various areas of the brain have been reported to persist for at least 2 weeks after cocaine use (72).
- Weiss et al. (73) found a significant decrease in basal DA release as early as 2 to 4 hours after discontinuation of cocaine self-administration and demonstrated, in 1992, that the onset of the synaptic DA deficiency is greatly accelerated by sustained cocaine self-administration. These data support the Dackis and Gold 1985 hypothesis that cocaine craving and withdrawal are a result of a deficiency of mesolimbic DA, which could involve a depletion of intraneuronal DA pools or autoregulation of DA neurons, as suggested by intermittent cocaine modification administration studies (74,75).
- Bromocriptine is somewhat efficacious in acute cocaine withdrawal. Bromocriptine is a DA agonist that

is widely used without abuse in the treatment of infertility, amenorrhea–galactorrhea, and Parkinson disease. It also shows promise in reducing acute cocaine craving and withdrawal dysphoria (76–84).

- Prolactin is increased in chronic users (85–87).
- Some corresponding neurochemical data have been obtained from humans by brain imaging. Humans abstaining from cocaine for 10 days show decreased cerebral blood flow and changes in brain glucose metabolism in the frontal cortex, accompanied by significant decreases in DA D2 receptors in basal ganglia. The combined findings led these researchers to propose that a long-lasting deficit in dopaminergic neuronal function may occur in this group of patients (88).
- PET studies in humans and in nonhuman primates demonstrate cocaine binding to DA transporters *in vivo* at pharmacologic and subpharmacologic levels (89,90).
- Mice lacking the DA transporter lend evidence to the critical role of DA, specifically the DA's reuptake transporter, in the reinforcing and biochemical actions of cocaine. The transporter controls the levels of DA in the synapse by feedback after cocaine binding blocks reuptake. DA remains at very high concentrations in the synapse during cocaine intoxication. Giros and colleagues (91) studied a mouse strain in which the gene encoding the DA transporter was disabled by a knockout. Without functioning DA transporters, these mice do not respond to cocaine. Cocaine produced no changes in DA or behavior, demonstrating that the DA transporter is absolutely necessary for cocaine to produce its psychostimulant effects.

Toxicity

While there are general ranges for doses and blood levels that produce toxicity, considerable individual variation exists, so caution is urged in interpreting predicted conditions of use for the development of toxicity. The majority of the organ-specific toxicities are referable to the CNS and cardiovascular system; however, other organ systems may be involved. Cocaine produces its toxic effects directly and through metabolites, such as benzoylecgonine, or compounds, such as cocaethylene, although many toxic effects depend on cocaine's vasoactive properties on the CNS and peripheric terminals.

At the level of the CNS, cocaine lowers the seizure threshold, and seizures are the most common serious neurologic complication, followed by stroke from cerebral hemorrhage or infarction, ischemia of the spinal cord, hyperpyrexia, and coma from respiratory depression. Other less-common and less-severe symptoms are dizziness, headache, paresthesias, tremor, and syncope.

Cardiovascular toxicity includes cocaine-induced cardiac cell death, reduced oxygenation, myocarditis, high-output cardiac failure, dilated cardiomyopathy, aortic dissection, rhabdomyolysis with acute renal and hep-

atic failure, and disseminated intravascular coagulopathy. Cocaine increases plasminogen activator inhibitor activity, resulting in antifibrinolytic activity and an increased likelihood of coronary thrombosis and acute ischemia (92). Other less-severe, acute, cocaine-related symptoms are chest pain, shortness of breath, palpitations, and diaphoresis.

Gastrointestinal complaints include nausea, abdominal pain, and vomiting. Although infrequent, cocaine can produce a wide spectrum of gastrointestinal complications, including ischemic colitis, gastric ulcerations, retroperitoneal fibrosis, visceral infarction, intestinal ischemia, and gastrointestinal tract perforation (93).

Cocaine has an anorectic effect. The expression of cocaine- and amphetamine-regulated transcript (CART) messenger ribonucleic acid (mRNA) is related to decreased food intake (94).

Cocaine abuse can cause kidney damage through different mechanisms. Cocaine-induced agitation can cause rhabdomyolysis and secondary renal failure. Although cocaine-related renal infarction is unusual, clinical evidence shows that cocaine accelerates the development of renal failure in patients with malignant hypertension (95). Moreover, pathologic changes, such as arteriolosclerosis and glomeruli hyalinosis, are found more frequently in the kidneys of cocaine-dependent patients (96).

Relatively common head and throat complaints, especially from smoking, are throat tightness, hoarseness, and cough with production of black sputum. Nasal congestion and frank necrosis of the nasal septum commonly occur following chronic intranasal use of cocaine. More general constitutional symptoms and signs are weakness, chills, myalgias, fever, back pain, fatigue, and insomnia. Cocaine has been implicated in ischemia and infarction of many organs, especially the heart and brain, although ischemic small bowel, kidneys, and spleen also have been reported. Vasospasm, platelet activation, and accelerated atherosclerosis have been suggested as causing the increased incidence of cocaine-induced ischemia (97).

Traumatic injuries are frequently related to cocaine. A case review study of 634 injured motor vehicle accident patients admitted to a trauma center revealed that 22.6% had positive urine drug screens and that cocaine was the drug most frequently used (98). In addition, recent data indicate that cocaine-related injuries are an important cause of death among young adults (99). Cocaine use is associated with poor concentration and judgment, making accidents, injuries and exposure to human immunodeficiency virus (HIV) more common.

Neuroimaging studies demonstrate that cocaine causes abnormal cerebral blood flow. Several researchers (100,101) report that cocaine users present limited areas of decreased blood flow in the anterior frontal cortex, inferior parietal cortex, and basal ganglia. Although, the cortical blood flow abnormalities are reversible, basal ganglia deficits persist after abstinence (102).

ACUTE INTOXICATION

Psychological Effects

As a CNS stimulant, cocaine has many psychological effects that are predictable and similar to those of other stimulants such as amphetamines and caffeine. As with toxicity, psychological variations exist and are dependent on the user, environment, dose, and route of administration. Nonetheless, the intensity and duration of the acute manifestations correlate with the rate of increase and height of the peak blood level, and are subsequently reflected in brain concentrations. Crack smoking, which produces a faster rise and higher blood levels, results in earlier-onset and most prominent clinical psychological signs and symptoms. The dose and route of administration determine these pharmacokinetic parameters for cocaine absorption and distribution in the body. The acute psychological effects begin when cocaine reaches the brain, which occurs within seconds by any route of administration. The major psychological functions affected by cocaine are mood; cognition; drive states such as hunger, sex, and thirst; and consciousness. An immediate and intense euphoria, analogous to a sexual orgasm, occurs and may last seconds or minutes, depending on the dose, route of administration, and tolerance of the user. Other alterations arising from elevation in mood include giddiness, enhanced self-confidence, and a forceful boisterousness. The subsequent level of mood is milder euphoria mixed with anxiety, which can last for minutes, followed by a more protracted anxious state that persists for hours. During intoxication, a state virtually indistinguishable from hypomania or frank mania is typical. Thoughts race and the user speaks in a rapid, often pressured manner. The user is garrulous and grandiose with tangential and incoherent speech. Appetite is suppressed during the period of intoxication usually followed by a rebound increased appetite as the cocaine is eliminated. In low doses, the libido is stimulated and sexual performance in men is reported to be enhanced by a prolonged erection and a heightened orgasm. In high doses, spontaneous ejaculation and orgasm can occur. The level of sensory awareness is altered and hypervigilance is typical. The user may develop ideas of reference and other mental alterations. Insomnia is common. With increasing doses, acts and decisions of poor judgment and indiscretions are more common. Motor activity is increased, as are driven atypical behaviors. Cocaine restlessness and fidgety behavior are accompanied by a driven state of perpetual motion.

After taking cocaine, subjects reported positive effects, such as feelings of carefreeness, friendliness, high, liking the drug, increased motivation, and willingness to pay for more drug or to take it again.

Cognition is significantly impaired during acute cocaine intoxication. Recent research shows that low doses of cocaine can interfere with behavioral inhibition. For instance, using a stop signal task, Filmore and Rush (103) found that participants under the effects of cocaine have difficulties inhibiting their responses to a "stop" sign even on doses that were not high enough to affect their reaction times to the "go" signs. Neuropsychological testing of cocaine-dependent patients yield inconclusive results. Abstinent cocaine-dependent patients show difficulties completing the Trail Making Test that measures visual scanning, motor speed and agility and that is highly sensitive to brain injury (104). Cocaine-dependent patients also show problems in the Digit-Symbol Substitution test (psychomotor performance, sustained attention, and visuomotor coordination), arithmetic subtest of the Wechsler Adult Intelligence Scale, Revised (WAIS-R) test (working memory, concentration) (105,106).

Physiologic Effects

The acute physiologic effects result from sympathetic nervous discharge after cocaine releases norepinephrine, epinephrine, and DA. CNS stimulation lowers seizure threshold and causes other changes such as tremor, arousal electrographic changes, emesis, and hyperpyrexia. Activation of the cardiovascular system results in tachycardia, hypertension, and diaphoresis. Peripheral nervous system stimulation results in urinary and bowel delay and retention, muscular contractions, and cutaneous flushing.

Again, the magnitude and direction of the cocaine-induced behavioral and physiologic changes depend on many variables, including the dose used and individual characteristics of the person using the cocaine. Cocaine intoxication effects such as euphoria, increased pulse and blood pressure, and psychomotor activity are expected. Depressant effects such as sadness, bradycardia, decreased blood pressure, and decreased psychomotor activity are less common in naive users, but can be seen in chronic high-dose users.

CHRONIC INTOXICATION

Psychological Effects

Chronic, persistent, and regular use of cocaine by any route of administration has characteristic consequences that are commonly identified by the clinician who is informed about and alert to them. Chronic administration of cocaine produces and can easily be confused with virtually all of the psychiatric syndromes and disorders (i.e., mania, depression, eating disorders, schizophrenic syndromes, and personality disturbances). When cocaine is included in the differential diagnosis, urine testing is necessary. Tolerance and dependence can develop immediately to cocaine use and have been demonstrated at wide ranges of doses, particularly at higher doses. Withdrawal from chronic cocaine use also has a predictable and stereotypical, protracted psychological and physiologic course in some addicts.

The development of tolerance is reflected by the waning of some of the acute effects of intoxication, which become less intense and shorter in duration with continued and chronic use and are only partly overcome by escalation of the dose. The euphoria lessens with the onset of tolerance. An extremely interesting phenomenon is that most cocaine addicts recall that their very early trials of cocaine yielded the greatest and most satisfying euphoria, even greater than that experienced during a cocaine "run" or "binge" or following reinstitution of use after a period of prolonged abstinence. Most cocaine addicts will reliably choose cocaine over other drugs even if they say that they are not getting the quality of the high. They will also work to acquire and use it, suggesting that sensitization has occurred and also that some aspects of cocaine reward are not consciously appreciated. While not as dramatic as reported for methylenedioxymethamphetamine (MDMA or ecstasy), subsequent use of cocaine may produce less euphoria. Episodes of cocaine-induced euphoria typically are not as long, despite larger doses taken more frequently in shorter intervals. The euphoria diminishes even more with further cocaine use over months and years, despite increasingly higher doses—up to several grams of cocaine a day. In a sense, the cocaine addict continues to chase the original "high" with lesser results. Adverse psychological effects commonly follow chronic cocaine use, including anxiety and a depression with panic and hopelessness. Many of these effects may be a result of cocaine-induced changes in the brain, which are quite persistent.

Chronic cocaine abuse is associated with a number of very important long-lasting changes in the CNS. Neuropathologic changes include cerebrovascular events, lacunar events, DA transporter deficits, electroencephalogram (EEG) abnormalities, vasculitis, seizures, and decrements in neurobehavioral performance (107). In some cases, cocaine addiction induces a neuropsychiatric disease similar to Parkinson disease with cell loss and functional decrements related to the drug self-administration. The sensation of being out of control, accompanied by intense apprehension of impending doom, is a regular occurrence with addictive cocaine use and is indistinguishable from panic disorder. The subjective feelings of helplessness and hopelessness may lead to suicidal thinking and behavior in many cocaine addicts. The paranoid delusions are common and quite distressing to the addict, who mistakenly believes that others are "spying on him" or "out to get her," and who already may be suspicious because of the illicit nature of cocaine use and the sometimes devious means required to obtain it (108).

NEUROBIOLOGY OF COCAINE DEPENDENCE

Neurotransmitter Systems

Cocaine dependence was described as a disorder of the reward system. Cocaine produces an alternative sequence of positive (euphoria) and negative (craving) reinforcements that tend to perpetuate the addictive behavior (109).

The neurologic substrate for addiction is located in the limbic system. Within the limbic system is housed the biologically primitive circuitry for the drive states such as hunger, sex, and thirst, as well as mood and memory. Cocaine induces a highly intense stimulation of the limbic system that is misinterpreted as a major organismic event. The limbic system is composed of various centrally located structures loosely organized but richly interconnected by neuronal pathways that use certain neurotransmitters at the synapses.

Environmental factors can sensitize individuals to the effects of drugs. For instance, animal studies demonstrated that subjects exposed to early stressors such as maternal separation, have an increased motor responsiveness to cocaine. Early stressors sensitize the dopaminergic cells in the mesolimbic system that play a main role in reward. Clinical studies in humans are consistent with these findings. We know that physical or sexual abuse increase stress sensitivity (110). On the other hand, cocaine-dependent patients report a high incidence of physical abuse and also there is a high comorbidity between posttraumatic stress disorder (PTSD) and cocaine dependence (111).

After exposure, the interaction of positive and negative reinforcers facilitate the establishment of dependence. The cocaine-induced euphoria and feelings of well-being act as a positive reinforcer, whereas the cravings act as a negative reinforcer (109). The dependent patient balances between these two forces.

PET studies confirm the role of the limbic system in dependence, showing an increase of the cerebral blood flow in the amygdala and cingulate gyrus of cocaine-dependent patients exposed to visual cues of cocaine-use-related situations (112).

Cravings are frequently triggered by environmental cues that "remind" the patient the experience of drug use. Recent studies show an increased firing rate in the ventral subiculum of the hippocampus during the reinstatement of cocaine seeking behaviors (113).

The hypothalamic–pituitary–adrenal (HPA) axis also participates in the acquisition, maintenance, and reinstatement of cocaine abuse. The acquisition of cocaine self-administration in animal models is facilitated by stress-increased plasma levels of corticosterone. On the other hand, drugs that interfere with the secretion of corticosterone (i.e., benzodiazepines or ketoconazole) decrease on going to self-administration. In addition, elevated levels of corticosterone facilitate the reinstatement of cocaine self-administration after extinction (114).

Dopamine and the Mesolimbic System

The DA-containing neurons have cell bodies that are part of the ventral tegmentum and whose fibers project to "reward cells" located in the hippocampus and the nucleus accumbens to form the mesolimbic pathway. It has been clear for some time that the reinforcing effects of amphetamines and cocaine result from their ability to elevate synaptic concentrations of DA. Moreover, D2-receptor knockout mice fail to respond to the reinforcing action of opiates (115). The reduction in gene expression appears to be related to the reduction in transporter sites because both occur in the same anatomical pathway. This suggests that the regulation of uptake in the mesolimbic neuron is separate or different from that in nigrostriatal neurons.

Serotonin and the Dorsal Raphe Nuclei

The serotonergic neurons in the raphe nucleus were found to play an important role in cocaine reward. Although, the rewarding properties of cocaine have been related to its effects on the dopamine transporter system, the deletion of the genes encoding this system is insufficient to eliminate drug-conditioned behavior in rats. Interestingly, only rats with total deletion of the dopamine transport system and partial or complete deletion of the serotonin transport system become immune to the rewarding and reinforcement properties of cocaine (116). The administration of serotonin agonists in the raphe nucleus increases the rewarding effect of brain self-stimulation in rats (117). Recent research suggests that the reward activity of the raphe nucleus depends on the activation of the 5-HT$_{1A}$ somatodendritic receptors. This group of autoreceptors inhibits the release of serotonin in the raphe nucleus and participates in the rewarding actions of this system (118). The cocaine-induced elevation of serotonin could stimulate the 5-HT$_{1A}$ Somato-Dendritic receptors and modulates cocaine reward. Serotonin neurons in the raphe nucleus also participate in the regulation of cocaine-induced motor activity. For instance, the administration of serotonin antagonists in the dorsal raphe nucleus increased the number of head movements in Glaxo-Winstar rats following the administration of cocaine (119).

Norepinephrine and the Locus Coeruleus

Noradrenergic cell bodies are located in the pons near the fourth ventricle and project to various aspects of the limbic system and cerebral cortex. While these neurons are implicated in withdrawal from various drugs, including opiates and alcohol, and are stimulated during cocaine intoxication, they play only a permissive role in addictive behaviors (120).

Neuroimaging Studies

Using PET, Volkow (121) reported that chronic cocaine use disrupts the metabolic activity of the brain. Volkow and collaborators found that cocaine use significantly decreases DA D2 receptors and that this pattern persisted even after protracted withdrawal. The reduction in D2 receptors is associated with functional changes in the brain that involve among others areas the orbitofrontal cortex and the cingulate gyrus. Volkow postulated that the decreased activation of the orbitofrontal cortex could diminish the response to the rewarding effects of natural reinforcers and that cocaine use could be a way of overcoming this deficit (122).

Recent research in functional neuroimaging has focussed on the correlation between brain activity and different clinical aspects of cocaine addiction. For instance, cravings induced by visual cues have been related to the activation of the left lateral amygdala, lateral orbitofrontal cortex, and rhinal cortex and the right dorsolateral prefrontal cortex, and cerebellum (123). The poor impulse control and the compulsive consumption of the drug seen in cocaine-dependent patients was related to lower levels of D2 receptors in the orbitofrontal cortex and cingulate gyri (124,125).

TOLERANCE AND DEPENDENCE

Tolerance and dependence are best viewed as neuroadaptations to the presence of a foreign drug and are related on a continuum of neurochemical changes and clinical expression. Tolerance and dependence are not specific for addiction; they can develop after chronic treatment with drugs of abuse and other commonly prescribed medications. The overemphasis on the inclusion of tolerance and dependence for diagnosis has led to confusion, misdiagnosis, and underdiagnosis (126). In brief, tolerance is the adaptation of the brain to the effects of the drug and dependence is the de-adaptation to the absence of the drug. In the case of cocaine, tolerance develops to some of its central effects. Research indicates that tolerance is related to the reduction in the levels of dopamine and serotonin in the nucleus accumbens (127,128). Tolerance to the euphoria develops quickly and has been measured within 1 hour after a single intravenous dose, so that the dose must be escalated or the route and dose changed to experience desired effects of equal intensity. Moreover, chronic cocaine users become tolerant to the rewarding effects of cocaine (129). A small degree of tolerance to effects on heart rate and blood pressure develops during the infusion of cocaine over the course of 4 hours; however, it is unlikely that significant tolerance to its cardiovascular actions is usually achieved. Also, in controlled studies performed in the laboratory, cocaine addicts did not achieve tolerance to the paranoia induced by cocaine. In a large survey of 452 cocaine addicts, paranoia and suspiciousness actually worsened with increasing use of cocaine over time and with larger doses (130). What is clear, although not well documented in studies, is that cocaine addicts typically increase the dose of cocaine both throughout the natural history of their addiction over months and years and during a cocaine binge over days. It is not unusual to find in clinical practice cocaine addicts who have reached intranasal doses of 1 to 3 g per day or more, and many state that they would use more if their supply did not become exhausted. Tolerance does not seem to drive the use of cocaine. The adverse effects of, for example, anxiety, depression, financial expense, suicidal thinking, and disrupted lives increase as the euphoria decreases, so that tolerance would seem to be a rate-limiting factor at best.

WITHDRAWAL

Until the mid-1980s, cocaine use was not considered dangerous because it was not associated with an abstinence syndrome of any consequence (131–134). Such mythology only added to the widespread notion that cocaine was safe and nonaddicting. Organized psychiatry was not immune to the cocaine misinformation because current practice considered drugs to be addicting on the basis of the withdrawal syndrome produced upon discontinuation. Cocaine was clearly dangerous and also had an important discontinuation syndrome. Observations in humans (135) and, more recently, animal studies (136,137) support the concept of a sometimes subtle but important cocaine abstinence state (138).

The essential feature of cocaine withdrawal is the presence of a characteristic withdrawal syndrome that develops within a few hours to several days after the cessation of (or reduction in) cocaine use that has been heavy and prolonged. The withdrawal syndrome is characterized by the development of dysphoric mood accompanied by two or more of the following physiologic changes: fatigue; vivid and unpleasant dreams; insomnia or hypersomnia; increased appetite; and psychomotor retardation or agitation. Anhedonia and drug craving are often present, but are not part of the diagnostic criteria. These symptoms cause clinically significant distress or impairment in social, occupational, or other important areas of functioning (139).

A definite, stereotypical withdrawal syndrome is observed in some users following either long-term use or even a binge of a few days. On abrupt cessation, withdrawal can be accompanied by depression, anxiety, and craving for the drug that is soon followed by general fatigue and a need for sleep ("crash"). Upon initial awakening, hyperphagia, continued sleepiness, depression, and anhedonia ensue. Mood returns to normal over a period of days, although in some cases, dysphoria and anhedonia may persist for weeks. Craving for the drug may wax and wane over weeks in response to emotions and cocaine-related stimuli. Although these signs and symptoms meet the requirement for withdrawal and are similar to those of the withdrawal from other drugs, there are no consistent measurable or observable physiologic disruptions that require gradual withdrawal of the drug or pharmacologic intervention.

The occurrence of a withdrawal dysphoria with neurovegetative symptoms that occurs within hours after a binge is now generally accepted by cocaine users and psychiatrists as "the crash" (140,141). In human beings, the acute abstinence state is of variable intensity and symptomatology (142), but includes irritability, anxiety, and depression, which can, and often is, self-medicated with cocaine. Acute withdrawal symptoms ("a crash") are often seen after periods of repetitive high-dose use ("runs" or "binges"). These periods are characterized by intense and unpleasant feelings of lassitude and depression, generally requiring several days of rest and recuperation. Depressive symptoms with suicidal ideation or behavior can occur and are generally the most serious problems seen during "crashing" or other forms of cocaine withdrawal. A substantial number of individuals with cocaine dependence have few or no clinically evident withdrawal symptoms on cessation of use.

However, a more complicated three-phase abstinence symptomatology has been proposed to characterize cocaine withdrawal (140). The phases represent progression of signs and symptoms of withdrawal subsequent to cocaine cessation. The three phases are crash, withdrawal, and extinction. According to this model, the crash is exhaustion lasting from hours to 4 days and is associated with intense depression, agitation, anxiety, hypersomnolence, hyperphagia, and craving for cocaine. The withdrawal phase ranges from 1 to 10 weeks, with an absence of craving in the early weeks and a reemergence of craving in the middle weeks. Toward the end of withdrawal the symptoms of anhedonia, anergia, anxiety, and intense cocaine craving appear gradually. Extinction lasts indefinitely and consists of normal mood and recurrent craving for cocaine, either spontaneously or in response to cues.

Other studies have not supported the three-phase abstinence syndrome for cocaine. Two major studies (140,143) differed in that craving was greatest in the 24 hours before admission (day 1) and was associated with intense depression. No definite crash was observed, and mood states, craving, and sleep disturbances gradually, yet perceptibly, improved during the initial 4 weeks. In these studies, the withdrawal was most severe in the initial days and gradually subsided over the ensuing weeks before discharge without pharmacologic intervention. In general, cocaine withdrawal is neither acutely life-threatening nor problematic in a secure, locked environment, but relapse is easily provoked by a host of conditioned cues (143).

Withdrawal is also related to a dysregulation of the monoaminergic system, particularly dopamine and serotonin, associated with the anhedonia and depression observed during cocaine abstinence. For example, the administration of the dopamine agonist bromocriptine was found to reduce the elevation of intracranial self-stimulation that follows the discontinuation of cocaine in rats (144). In addition, recent research shows that cocaine has long-term effects on the serotonergic transmission. Animal models of cocaine withdrawal demonstrate a significant decrease in the behavioral responses to D-fenfluramine–induced serotonin release. Interestingly, this lack of response is not observed immediately after cocaine discontinuation, but after at least 2 days (145).

COCAINE AND CONDITIONING

Cocaine users describe intense craving for cocaine when cocaine is made available to them or merely when the word cocaine is uttered in conversation. Handling paper money or seeing a bill rolled may produce intense craving. Seeing people or places where cocaine was used, smelling cocaine, seeing a cocaine pipe, seeing a friend who used cocaine with them, hearing a song that they used cocaine to, and numerous other casual smells, sights, and sounds can trigger an intense reaction in the current user or the person who has used in the past but is now abstinent (146). Users report tasting cocaine, craving cocaine, sweating and experiencing shortness of breath, feeling faint, smelling cocaine, and feeling a little of the cocaine euphoria. All of these experiences contribute to cocaine taking and the persistence of cocaine dependence. In humans, even the presentation of cocaine paraphernalia after weeks or months of abstinence produces intense cravings and withdrawal-like symptoms (147,148). In experimental studies in humans, individuals with a history of cocaine use show greater physiologic reactivity in response to cocaine cues than do cocaine-naive individuals. The greater responses were also demonstrated to cocaine stimuli rather than powerful opiate cues. Cocaine-related stimuli elicit conditioned physiologic and subjective states in cocaine users (149).

COMPARISON BETWEEN AMPHETAMINE AND COCAINE

Amphetamine, cocaine, and methylphenidate have quite similar pharmacologic and clinical characteristics and are almost identical in their sympathetic properties. They differ mainly in onset of action and half-life. Amphetamine and cocaine are potent CNS stimulants that have almost equal reinforcing properties in self-administration studies in animals and humans. In rankings of toxicity from self-administration, both cocaine and amphetamines are more reinforcing than opiates, barbiturates, benzodiazepines, and alcohol. The patterns of addictive use for amphetamines and cocaine in humans are similar, and both drugs typically are taken in binges until either the sup-

ply of the drug or the user is exhausted. However, daily or weekly repetitive use of the drug consistently over months and weeks is also common. Amphetamines are often taken orally, but intravenous use is not uncommon among established addicts. With either route, the addiction is identifiable and not fixed in outward appearances. What is clear about the addictive pattern is that no route of administration, sequence, or interval is the rule for either drug, and a variety of patterns that depend on the user, supply, and purity of the drug is possible (150).

The effects of the drugs are so similar that cocaine users describe the euphoric effects of cocaine in terms that are almost indistinguishable from those used by amphetamine users. In laboratory studies, subjects familiar with cocaine cannot distinguish between the subjective effects of 16 mg of cocaine and a dose of 10 mg of dextroamphetamine when both are given intravenously. However, the duration of cocaine's effects are shorter than that of amphetamines, with a half-life of 1 hour for cocaine and 10 hours for amphetamines. As a result, addictive or repeated use may be more common with cocaine and the withdrawal syndrome may be more protracted with amphetamines. Otherwise, the toxicities from cocaine are clinically indistinguishable from those produced by amphetamines.

Clinically, while amphetamine use and addiction continues, their prevalence has not returned to the level of the 1960s, when both "street addicts" and "housewives" typified the greatest consumer of the drug. The largest sources of amphetamines remain physicians, illicit methamphetamine laboratories, and pharmaceutical manufacturers who legally produce and distribute them, whereas cocaine is imported chiefly from South America, albeit illegally. It also is not clear whether a diminished supply of cocaine would correspondingly increase the rate of amphetamine addiction (151). In the case of psychostimulants, rats will self-administer amphetamine and DA directly into the nucleus accumbens. Although cocaine is not self-administered into the nucleus accumbens, bilateral injections of DA-receptor antagonists into the nucleus accumbens or lesions of the mesoaccumbens DA system attenuate the reinforcing effects of intravenously self-administered cocaine. These studies provide strong evidence that DA receptors in the nucleus accumbens mediate the reinforcing effects of psychostimulants. A large body of evidence suggests that the reinforcing effects of drugs as diverse as psychostimulants and opiates are mediated by a common neurobiologic substrate. In particular, psychostimulants and opiates are thought to produce reinforcement by direct or indirect actions on the dopaminergic neurons in the ventral tegmental area or on their target neurons in the nucleus accumbens.

Cocaine and amphetamines induce the synthesis of CART, a mRNA that encodes a polypeptide with apparent neurotransmitter properties. CART is highly expressed in the nucleus accumbens after the administration of cocaine and amphetamines. After receiving CART, animals show behaviors similar to those induced by stimulants. The cocaine- and amphetamine-induced CART demonstrate that drugs actively interact with the deoxyribonucleic acid (DNA) modulating the expression of different genes (152).

NEUROTOXICITY

One new area of investigations is the role of persistent deficits produced by drug-related effects. The optimistic assertions that illicit drug use could be discontinued and the user would be able to return to normal is at odds with developmental theories that would assert that drug intoxication and addiction might interfere with normal development and further that drugs taken for their specific effects and target in the brain appear equally proficient at inducing changes in heart, brain, and other vital organs. Cocaine use is associated with increases in blood pressure that are much greater in small vessels in the brain. Cocaine increases the oxygen demands on the heart but decreases the available blood. Ischemic cerebrovascular accidents occur commonly in cocaine users and their significance extends beyond the PET scan deficits reported for addicts to persistent neuropsychological deficits. Abstinence may simply allow certain addicts to recognize that they cannot function at their premorbid level or that they cannot hit a curve ball as they did before cocaine. Volkow has reported that cocaine causes a decrease in the number of D2 receptors with corresponding decreases in brain metabolism, especially in the frontal cortex (153). These drug-induced changes apparently persist for many months or even years after abstinence. Such changes could underlie craving or the perception that the addict would be better, would feel and think better, if they only had their drug to use. The more cocaine is used, the more DA is released and available to act at DA receptors but the greater the need for animals to electrically self-stimulate pleasure systems when cocaine is no longer available. Similar findings suggesting acute and persisting anhedonia on withdrawal have been reported by Weiss for cocaine, alcohol, nicotine, and opiates (154). Once changes occur in neurotrophin, neurofilaments, glutamate receptors, and glial filaments, use becomes addiction as the brain is changed and trained. Exposure to conditioned cues, stress, D2 agonists, and so on, all make use more likely and driven. Cocaine-related ischemic strokes and gross anatomic changes, and also subtler ventral tegmental, nucleus accumbens cell, and nuclear program changes, produce neurotoxic consequences. This suggests that any short-term treatment approach is questionable with long-term abstinence assumed to be necessary for full return to premorbid functioning. While there are multiple DA receptors on the postsynaptic membrane that respond differently to different compounds and certainly serve different biologic functions, research (155) suggests that new pharmacotherapies target the D1-receptor system. D1-receptor agonists may dimin-

ish episodes of intense cocaine craving and reduce relapse in addicts who have stopped using the drug. D2 agonists, stress, and conditioned cues might increase cocaine seeking and drive to use.

Several researchers reported a decrease in gray-matter volume in the prefrontal lobe of polysubstance abusers, and in those who abuse cocaine, crack cocaine, and alcohol. This decrease in prefrontal volume is not an acute effect of the drug and can be observed even after 6 weeks of abstinence (156,157).

Adaptive changes are referred to as tolerance, or a reduction in the drug's effects after repeat administration, or the need to increase the dose to maintain the same effect. Addiction is a drug-induced brain change, which presumably can be studied in animals to generate neural change models, and once these changes are understood, new treatments can be tried in these animal models. Investigators look for the changes cocaine produces in the brain that cause addiction and possibly specific interactions between genetic and environmental factors that make certain animals or people more likely to become addicts.

COCAINE ADDICTION AS A DRIVE STATE

It has been suggested that humans and lower animals have an aberrant or "fourth" drive for drugs. It appears that the brain mechanisms for feeding account for self-intoxication, at least in lower animals. Studies of the neurobiology of the DA system confirm that the brain circuits that play a role in food-rewarded behavior are the brain circuits that play a role in drug-rewarded behavior. DA antagonists block the rewarding effects of food and water just as they block the self-administration of stimulants such as cocaine.

Recent studies using *in vivo* voltammetry and microdialysis make it possible to monitor the synaptic levels of brain DA in the nucleus accumbens of freely moving animals. The studies suggest that drugs of addiction have much more powerful effects on the mesolimbic DA system than do most natural rewards. Only very palatable foods and highly potent sex-related stimuli seem capable of activating the mesolimbic system with anywhere near the potency of ventral tegmentum-injected morphine or nucleus accumbens-injected amphetamine (158).

Dissociations of Addiction and Pharmacologic Dependence

Although the acute effects of a drug vary from one drug to the other, the underlying mechanisms of dependence are the same.

Opiates have two clearly established sites of reinforcing self-administration of drugs, namely, the ventral tegmental area of the dopaminergic cells and the nucleus accumbens, to which these cell project to form the mesolimbic pathway. The ventral tegmental cells contain opiate receptors, and the main output of the nucleus accumbens uses GABA as a neurotransmitter. These GABA neurons project to the pedunculopontine nucleus, which may be a final common pathway for addictive behavior, because lesions of this nucleus block the self-administration of both amphetamine and morphine (159).

Important neurochemical evidence for the dissociation of addiction from pharmacologic tolerance is obtained by the finding that classic opiate withdrawal signs do not occur in animals whose stimulation of the ventral tegmentum is terminated, whereas if the same morphine injections are given a few millimeters distant in the periaqueductal gray matter, the animals do develop physical dependence and hence do express withdrawal signs when the opiate injections are terminated or blocked. Other animal experiments support the finding that addictive behavior can be demonstrated with the very first injection of morphine (160,161).

This dissociation of addiction sites from pharmacologic to dependence sites can also be inferred from the relapse of an addict to a drug long after pharmacologic withdrawal has been completed. Relapse (162) to cocaine despite well-known and previously experienced adverse side effects cannot be explained by withdrawal. Moreover, the term reward behavior for addictive use of a drug is ill conceived, because the addict relapses and continues to use drugs after suffering a sometimes excruciating withdrawal. The negative, unpleasant, and unrewarding effects of the drug begin to far outweigh the pleasure derived, yet the addict continues to pursue the drug.

FAMILY HISTORY AND GENETIC STUDIES

In one prospective study of 56 cocaine addicts, the rate for familial alcoholism was 52% in male and 60% in female patients (163,164). In a later study of 31 cocaine addicts, 68% had a family history positive for alcoholism without a significant gender difference (165).

The prevalence of familial alcoholism among male alcoholics has been well documented in numerous studies. The rate of familial alcoholism is 50% according to most studies, while the rate for familial alcoholism among females is generally more variable, with prevalence rates above and below 50%. The prevalence of familial alcoholism was 50% among males and 80% among females in a retrospective study of 150 cocaine-dependent persons.

Persons with opiate dependence who have a parental history of alcoholism are more frequently diagnosed with concurrent alcoholism. In one study, 21.3% of those who had opiate and alcohol dependence had at least one parent with alcohol dependence. Persons with opiate dependence without the diagnosis of alcohol dependence (4,25) had a 12.5% rate of alcohol dependence in their families. The familial transmission of nonalcohol drug use and dependence in combination and for specific drug types has not been completely studied. In family members of drug addicts, rates for drug abuse or addiction range between 15% and 20%, and in family members of drug addicts with alcohol addiction, rates are approximately 25%. The rate for familial drug addiction in alcoholics only (without drugs) is lower (3%). The drugs in these studies were stimulants, opiates, cannabis, and barbiturates or benzodiazepines. Some familial studies show that the drug type in probands follows that of parents (166,167).

While several twin studies show that monozygotic twins are significantly more concordant for alcoholism than are dizygotic twins, only one study shows a similar twin difference for monozygotic twins for illicit drugs. Also, only one adoption study is available that examines the transmission of drugs from biologic parents to adopted-out offspring. This study shows that drug abuse in the adoptees was significantly more likely to be associated with drug abuse in the biologic parent than in the adoptive, nonbiologic parents (168–171).

The implications of these familial and genetic studies, and of the high rate of comorbidity of drugs with other drugs and alcohol, are that those addicted to alcohol and drugs have a generalized vulnerability to both alcohol and drugs. Whereas an alcoholic has an increased risk of developing drug dependence, often to cocaine, a drug-dependent or cocaine addict has an increased risk of developing alcohol dependence. The substitution of one drug for another and between alcohol and drugs, and the simultaneous and concurrent use of drugs and alcohol, compels investigators to search for common denominators on all levels, including biologic and environmental.

The role of the expression of dopamine receptors in substance abuse has been the focus of many genetic studies. Several control studies report an increased prevalence of the DRD2 A1 and B1 alleles in alcoholics and polysubstance abusers (172). However, recent family based studies failed to identify a relation between the DRD2 alleles and substance abuse (173,174).

PSYCHIATRIC COMORBIDITY

Comorbid psychiatric syndromes occur commonly in patients with cocaine dependence because (a) intoxication and withdrawal from cocaine and other drugs produce psychiatric syndromes; (b) both categories of disorders are common, and the chance of co-occurrence is high; and (c) the psychopathology of the disorders is greater when they are found together in the same individual. The Epidemiologic Catchment Area study reported that 47% of patients with either a diagnosis of schizophrenia or a schizophreniform disorder have also been diagnosed with some form of substance abuse. The lifetime prevalence for cocaine use among schizophrenics is between 15% and 50% (175).

There is confirmatory evidence that cocaine and other drugs can produce psychiatric syndromes through several pharmacologic and psychological mechanisms. Acute and chronic intoxication with stimulants, as well as withdrawal from depressants, can cause many symptoms of anxiety syndromes that are indistinguishable from phobias, obsessive-compulsiveness, panic, and generalized anxiety. Conversely, acute and chronic intoxication with depressants or withdrawal from stimulants can cause a severe and incapacitating depression indistinguishable from major depression from other causes (176–178).

Psychotic symptoms, particularly of the paranoid type, are produced during intoxication with stimulants and during withdrawal from depressants. For example, cocaine or amphetamine administration can result in hallucinations and delusions during intoxication. In contrast, alcohol and sedative–hypnotic administration can result in these same symptoms during withdrawal. Personality disturbances are less clear, but it is documented that chronic drug and alcohol use in an addictive fashion often leads to severe alterations in attitudes and behaviors in the addict. These frequently resemble antisocial, borderline, dependent, immature, and narcissistic personality disorders, and ameliorate or disappear with abstinence from drugs and alcohol, and especially with specific treatment of the addictive disorder (178,179). There is no familial and genetic evidence to support a high rate of primary anxiety or affective or psychotic disorders among drug addicts, including cocaine addicts and alcoholics. Familial, adoption, and twin studies have found these psychiatric disorders to be independent of drug and alcohol dependence. Moreover, the sociodemographics, early life course, and prognosis of drug addicts and alcoholics more closely resemble those observed for drug addiction and alcoholism than for those with the psychiatric disorders.

There are several Axis I diagnoses in the *Diagnostic and Statistical Manual of Mental Disorders-TR,* 4th ed. (2000) (*DSM–IV-TR*) that require the exclusion of drug and alcohol use diagnoses before the psychiatric diagnoses can be made. For instance, patients with comorbid cocaine dependence and depression show higher prevalence of antisocial personality disorder, and had more difficulties in remaining abstinent (180).

Treatment of Comorbid Psychiatric and Substance Abuse Disorders

Treatment intervention for psychiatric disorders in cocaine addicts usually can be applied only after abstinence has been achieved and treatment for the addictive disorder has been initiated. For those patients with psychiatric disorders and concurrent cocaine, drug, and/or alcohol dependence, specific pharmacologic therapies can be instituted when indicated for the psychiatric disorders. In general, the comorbid psychiatric disorder improves and the response to treatment is more efficacious with abstinence and specific treatment of the addictive disorder.

In general, the same pharmacologic approaches already mentioned can be used in the addicted patient with a psy-chiatric disorder, with notable exceptions. Specifically, antidepressants and antipsychotic medications with low anticholinergic and low sedative properties are preferred because of established abuse and addiction potential of medications with stronger anticholinergic and sedative effects. Importantly, the use of sedative–hypnotics and tranquilizers, including benzodiazepines, is to be avoided because of their clearly documented addictive potential, particularly in the high-risk population of alcoholics and drug addicts. Moreover, a poorly accepted clinical caveat is that alcoholics and drug addicts do not respond well to drug effects in their attempts to achieve and maintain abstinence, so that a conservative approach for all medications is strongly suggested (181,182).

Interactions between Addiction and Psychiatric Disorder

There is little direct evidence for the self-medication hypothesis that purports that addicts use because of underlying psychiatric disorders; the bulk of the evidence is to the contrary. Alcoholics and drug addicts use despite the adverse, toxic, and counter-therapeutic effects of addictive use of drugs and alcohol. In animal studies, cocaine is self-administered in spite of serious and often fatal adverse consequences. Rhesus monkeys and rats have been reported to continue to press a bar in order to receive injections of cocaine to the point of convulsions, inanition, exhaustion, and death. In these animals, the pursuit of cocaine itself and not some underlying psychological factors motivated this extraordinarily addictive cocaine use. The animals pursue cocaine for its pharmacologic effects, as no personality factors or underlying psychopathology has been identified in these experiments (183–185).

Clinical experience and controlled studies of human cocaine addicts bear out the findings in the animal studies. Stimulants and other drugs, including alcohol, have powerfully controlling effects on mind and behavior. The morbidity and mortality arising from cocaine addiction and the pursuit and self-administration of cocaine by humans are staggering.

Some authors have speculated that it is the poverty of inner-city conditions and the poverty of the addicts' social interactions that are the primary factors in drug use and addiction. However, laboratory animals find these drugs powerfully reinforcing whether they are raised in isolation or in groups, and regardless of whether they are experimentally stressed or coddled. Conditions of housing and stress can influence how rapidly animals learn to self-administer these drugs and whether they will learn to self-administer marginally effective doses. However, in most experiments with these animals and drugs, all healthy animals were reasonably quick to self-administer moderate intravenous doses of cocaine, heroin, and alcohol. The combination of a powerful reinforcing drug, and motivated goal-directed behavior aimed toward euphoria production, morbidly accelerated the addiction process. Just receiving the same amount of drug previously would not pose as great a threat.

COCAINE ADDICTION TREATMENTS

Neurobiologic Treatments

Throughout the 1980s addiction specialists and researchers responded to the increasing numbers of cocaine addicts who came to medical attention looking for treatment with a series of frantic efforts to find therapeutic modalities specific enough to "treat" cocaine abuse. Yet, at the same time, exactly what was to be treated remained an issue of considerable debate. Pharmacologic treatments were necessary for cocaine overdose; cocaine toxicity; to replace cocaine; to blunt or block the effects of cocaine; to support cocaine abstinence; to reduce cocaine dysphoria; or to produce nausea or vomiting when cocaine was taken. None were discovered (186).

No potential new treatment was more important than the development of medicine that could separate the cocaine urge from drug taking or alter the attachment of the addict for the drug. Naturally, progress came at a slow pace and without regard for the needs of the physicians and clinics. More effective management of acute cocaine intoxication; early diagnosis; urine and blood testing for cocaine and benzoylecgonine; the discovery of the uniquely toxic properties of cocaine when taken with alcohol; and the treatment of medical and psychiatric complications of cocaine have been important advances. All have combined to reduce cocaine-related morbidity and mortality. These and other efforts helped to dispel the notion so prevalent in the late 1970s and early 1980s that cocaine was a "safe" drug of abuse—an oxymoron if there ever was one. Significant progress has been made in the laboratory, enabling a clearer understanding of cocaine's effects on the brain and its relationship to the endogenous reinforcement systems. Significant progress has been made in understanding and targeting with psychopharmacologic agents for what patients describe as cocaine craving. Yet continued use of cocaine in the absence of craving has been reported.

Theories of cocaine abstinence and reward have led to large numbers of human clinical trials with a variety of disparate substances: amantadine (Symmetrel); bromocriptine (Parlodel); buprenorphine (Buprenex); bupropion (Wellbutrin); carbamazepine (Tegretol); desipramine (Norpramin); fluoxetine (Prozac); flupentixol; gepirone; imipramine (Tofranil); lithium; levodopa-carbidopa; maprotiline; methadone; methylphenidate (Ritalin); naltrexone (Revia); pergolide (Permax); phenelzine (Nardil); ritanserin; sertraline (Zoloft); trazodone; tryptophan; and tyrosine have all been reported or proposed as treatments. In general, all medications tried have been demonstrated to have some subjective effect on the cocaine experience or craving but do not alter or interfere with the natural history of cocaine dependence and use as assessed by testing or euphoria (187–192).

Bupropion was proposed as a possible therapeutic agent for cocaine dependence. A multicenter study reported that buspirone (BuSpar) was effective treating cocaine-dependent patients in a methadone maintenance program who also present with symptoms of depression (193). In addition, a clinical trial with bupropion that included cocaine-dependent patients with comorbid attention deficit hyperactivity disorder (ADHD) reported decreased cravings and increased abstinence (194). However, bupropion had no effects on the subjective effects of cocaine (195).

Pergolide, a D1/D2 agonist, was tested as a possible therapeutic agent for cocaine dependence. Although pergolide had no effects on self-administration, the drug was well tolerated. On the other hand, pergolide decreased not only the subjective responses to cocaine (i.e., high, stimulation, and pay for a dose) but it also decreased the cocaine-induced heart rate increase. Cocaine-dependent patients treated with pergolide reported increased cravings that were not associated with an increase in cocaine consumption (196).

The D1 agonist ABT-431 showed a profile similar to pergolide. However, in addition to decreased subjective reactions to cocaine, ABT-431 also decreased cravings for cocaine. These effects were largely overcome by higher doses of cocaine (197).

Dextroamphetamine (Dexedrine) is a stimulant that facilitates the release of biogenic amines in the CNS. Similar to the use of methadone in opiate dependencies, the stimulant dextroamphetamine was proposed as a treatment alternative for cocaine dependency. A double-blind, randomized, clinical trial found that after 12 weeks of dextroamphetamine therapy, cocaine-dependent patients reported a decrease in cocaine consumption and increased compliance with treatment (198).

Because cocaine is frequently consumed in combination with alcohol, research has focused on the possible use of disulfiram (Antabuse) in the treatment of cocaine dependence. The discontinuation of alcohol consumption would result in a decrease of the reinforcing effects of the alcohol-enhanced cocaine high. A double-blind, randomized, clinical trial studied the effects of disulfiram in combination with psychotherapy in the treatment of alcohol- and cocaine-abusing patients. Patients on disulfiram decreased their consumption of alcohol and cocaine (199). However, McCance-Katz and collaborators (200) found that disulfiram significantly increases cocaine-induced heart rate and blood pressure, questioning the medical safety of this treatment.

The use of the monoamine oxidase type B (MAO-B) inhibitor selegiline (Eldepryl) was proposed to be potentially beneficial for treating cravings during cocaine abstinence. Theoretically, selegiline could be helpful in restoring dopamine and dopamine receptors to normal levels. A double-blind, nonrandomized, crossover-design study found that selegiline does not modify the effects of cocaine on heart rate or blood pressure. The study concluded that, although there were no significant changes in subjective variables such as euphoria or rush, selegiline could be safely use in the treatment of cocaine dependence (201). A recent PET study found that patients treated with selegiline reported a 40% decrease in subjective euphoria and it was associated with significant changes in the amygdala's glucose consumption (202).

A new therapeutic approach focused on the development of an immune therapy to neutralize cocaine before it interacts with the CNS. An immunogenic agent was synthesized, conjugating cocaine with keyhole limpet hemocyanin (KLH). This product induces antibodies that interfere the analgesic and the rewarding actions of cocaine (203). Active immunization with the cocaine immunogen GNC-KLH prevented the reinstatement of cocaine self-administration following the exposure to a single dose of cocaine, but not under free cocaine availability conditions. The addition of the anticocaine immunoglobulin GNC92H2 in previously immunized animals significantly decreased the use of cocaine in free cocaine conditions (204). Using a different approach, Mets and colleagues (205) developed catalytic antibodies that hydrolyze cocaine, blocking its rewarding and toxic effects. The efficacy of these agents in humans still needs to be tested.

Serotonergic agents such as fluoxetine, ritanserin, and sertraline have effects on cocaine craving in humans, and on cocaine responding in animals, but generally only at doses that suppress behaviors maintained by food and other reinforcers (206). As one of the new avenues in pharmacotherapy for cocaine dependence, 5-HT agents have not been well studied. They may find a niche in the treatment of the patient with obsessive ruminations about cocaine, or they may simply go the way of desipramine. At this point it is safe to say that none of the currently available psychopharmacologic treatment approaches has shown the relative strength of cocaine reward and attachment. Animal and clinical studies showed promising results using GABA$_B$ agonist to reduce the reinforcing effects of cocaine. For instance, animals receiving baclofen (Lioresal) reduce cocaine self-administration in both fixed ratio and progressive ratio reinforcing schedules. In addition, GABA$_B$ antagonists inhibit the effect of baclofen on cocaine use. Studies in cocaine-dependent patients suggest similar results. Cocaine-dependent patients taking baclofen report less craving, cocaine use, and cue-induced craving (207). Available data suggest that a wide range of compounds can modify cocaine abuse. Developing safe and effective medications to treat cocaine abuse and dependence is an ongoing challenge (208).

New treatments for cocaine intoxication are currently being tested. Thus, the use of a recombinant butyryl-cholinesterase to accelerate the metabolism of cocaine was proposed as an alternative treatment for cocaine intoxication. Butyrylcholinesterase hydrolyzes cocaine into inactive compounds. Pretreatment with recombinant butyryl-cholinesterase before cocaine administration decreased cocaine plasma levels in animals. The clinical implications of these results are being investigated (209).

New behavioral models in animals (210,211) and the characterization of the cocaine receptor site on the DA transporter molecule appear to offer promise for identifying new treatments that might prevent relapse or cocaine euphoria. The fact that not all DA uptake inhibitors exert reinforcing properties similar to cocaine (212) suggests that once the neuronal DA transporter is purified and cloned, new nonaddicting pharmacologic treatments for human cocaine addicts might be developed. To date, the bulk of work has focused on the ability of pharmacologic agents to attenuate craving.

Behavioral Interventions

Physicians are frequently in a position to identify, treat, and refer cocaine addicts for further treatment. It has been reported that more than 50% of patients in psychiatric settings, including inpatients and outpatients, suffer from a drug or alcohol dependence. Moreover, it has been found that 25% to 50% of a general medical practice is made up of persons who are drug and alcohol dependent (213).

Several studies focus on predicting factors of treatment initiation and outcomes. Siegal et al. (214) reported that youth, legal problems, and a prior history of drug abuse treatment are associated with the initiation of the treatment. Interestingly, this study found no association between treatment initiation and either gender, ethnicity, education, employment, marital status, or duration of drug use. On the other hand, in a sample of 207 cocaine-dependent patients, Reiber et al. (215) found that the number of days of cocaine use in the 30 days before the initiation of treatment is the best predictor of treatment outcome.

Physicians can initiate an intervention through prompt and proper diagnosis and treatment in clinical practice. It is imperative to develop diagnostic skills that are focused on the behaviors and consequences of addiction and to become knowledgeable in the laboratory confirmation of use and addiction. The physician often may not be the primary caregiver, but frequently is involved through a particular specialty with the recovering drug addict. Because addiction often requires continuous treatment for an indefinite time, the physician will have many opportunities to continue to intervene in positive ways in the long-term treatment of addictive disorders (216). The clinical findings and natural history of cocaine dependence, the attachment of the user for the drug, and the power of the cocaine reward in shaping, conditioning, and modifying behavior have contributed to the current therapeutic approach, which combines a number of modalities. Current treatment strategies are not mutually exclusive, but always combine rehabilitative, psychodynamic, and behavioral approaches with pharmacologic treatment during the acute withdrawal period and during early abstinence. Pharmacologic agents have been successfully used to decrease abstinence complaints and to decrease early treatment dropout rates.

Recent behavioral techniques of relapse prevention based on principles of behavioral therapies have been employed. In this type of treatment, patients are encouraged to identify internal and external precipitants of drug urges, to restructure their lifestyles in order to engage in healthy activities and avoid drug-oriented situations, to understand in detail the process of relapse in order to avoid it, and to stop relapses early (in the "lapse" stage) before they cause severe problems. Also, patients are exposed to increasingly vivid reminders of their cocaine use, while concomitantly being taught various cognitive behavioral techniques and relaxation exercises in order to reduce conditioned craving and to learn alternative methods of dealing with their drug urges (217). Higgins and colleagues (16) reported on the use of a novel behavioral model of cocaine addiction treatment commonly called the incentive method. They gave patients an increasing incentive payment for each clean urine specimen with the possibility of earning $1,000 over a 3-month period. At the end of a 12-week study period more than 60% of patients achieved stable abstinence, which was two times greater than that achieved by patients treated without incentive payments. At the 1-year followup, these differences persisted. The contingency payments may not be a treatment per se, but may be a mechanism to keep the patient in treatment while behavioral treatment, including relapse prevention, are prescribed.

We have successfully used contingency approaches concurrently with other approaches in the treatment of physicians, health providers, and athletes. Five-year recovery and return to work among physicians is remarkable for all substances of abuse when physician-addicts are monitored by the state and required to attend a recovery support group such as Alcoholics Anonymous/Narcotics Anonymous, have randomized at least weekly urine monitoring, and have counselor and physician/psychiatrist evaluations (218). The mainstay of treatment for cocaine dependence remains psychological (219). Treatment for cocaine dependence and prevention of relapse has been tried for the past decade and has now evolved to include elements of relapse prevention, 12-step programs, and other therapies to stop drug use and reduce recidivism (220–223). Recovery is a process that begins with a break in denial, a learning process of breaking old habits, friendships, and "triggers" to the first desire to use cocaine, and leads to eventual new healthy patterns of living, shifting the locus of control from external to internal. Patients are encouraged to identify internal and external precipitants of drug urges and

to restructure their lifestyles to avoid drug situations and relapse in relapse prevention protocols, as compared with behavioral treatment that focuses on extinguishing conditioned craving responses. Community reinforcement, payment for abstinence, and relapse prevention are the three major types of cocaine treatment programs in widespread use in the United States.

All of the therapies, including behavioral techniques, psychotherapy, and abstinence-based approaches, use the goal of abstinence and promote participation in self-help groups such as Alcoholics Anonymous (AA), Narcotics Anonymous (NA), and Cocaine Anonymous (CA) in their treatment programs (224). Initially, some cocaine-dependent patients might need alcohol detoxification; others might need alcohol detoxification plus the nicotine patch. Others might be candidates for immediate antidepressant treatment. All might be candidates for 12-step fellowship and some might need some kind of psychotherapy. Many cocaine addicts also have comorbid medical disorders such as hepatitis or bronchitis, personality disorders such as antisocial personality disorder, other drug use, and a number of psychiatric disorders ranging from major depression and bipolar illness to eating disorders and anxiety disorders. As demonstrated in a recent study of alcoholics, vigorous treatment for nicotine dependence (225) is absolutely essential in preventing relapse morbidity and mortality.

Long-term treatment in self-help groups has arisen for specific drug types, such as CA and NA. These are similar to AA and suggest abstinence and adherence to a 12-step program of recovery from both alcohol and other drugs. Importantly, the principles of an abstinence-based treatment program that includes AA, CA, and NA will work for the alcoholic who has an additional drug dependence or the multiple-drug-dependent with an alcohol dependence diagnosis. The similarities in the treatment of the addictive disorders are greater than the differences, so that recovery by most cocaine addicts is possible in any of these groups (226–228).

SUMMARY

Cocaine addiction differs from opiate and other addictions in many important ways. Cocaine does not produce an opiate calming effect or brief euphoria, but is used in binges, frantically, until the supply or the user is exhausted. Satiety for cocaine is an oxymoron. Satiety for the drug does not exist or develop, and cocaine use can take place every 15 to 30 minutes for hours or days. Craving, lust, or desirous drive for cocaine is common. The euphoric effect is a function of host factors, blood concentration, rapidity, and rise of cocaine concentrations in brain DA systems. Prolonged blockade of the DA transporter by cocaine results in long-term adaptive changes that can markedly impair mesolimbic DA function and also induce a state of supersensitivity. Adaptive changes in G proteins and the cyclic adenosine monophosphate (cAMP) pathway were implicated by Nestler (229). Neurobiologic research may help us understand the complex relationship between cocaine addiction and major psychological, psychosocial, cognitive, and neurologic impairments, which persist long after detoxification. Those patients in need of the most intense medical and psychiatric evaluation are those who use by inhalation and intravenously (230). Scientific understanding of the mechanistic basis of the effects of cocaine is rudimentary and developing relevant and effective treatments slower than expected. Cocaine induces a complex state with alternating euphoria and dysphoria supporting binge use. Cocaine is taken whether the user defines the effect as positive or negative or both. Use of cocaine reinforces compulsive thinking about and use of cocaine, regardless of consequences. Cocaine addiction is a heterogeneous disorder where specialized treatments targeted to clinically distinct subgroups are desperately needed.

REFERENCES

1. Dackis CA, Gold MS. New concepts in cocaine addiction: the dopamine depletion hypothesis. *Neurosci Biobehav Rev* 1985;9:469–477.
2. Kleber HD. Cocaine abuse: historical, epidemiological and psychological perspectives. *J Clin Psychiatry* 1988;49[2 Suppl]:3–6.
3. Gold MS, Verebey K. The psychopharmacology of cocaine. *Psychiatr Ann* 1984;14:714–723.
4. Wise RA. The brain and reward. In: Liebman JM, Cooper SJ, eds. *The neuropharmacological basis of reward.* Oxford, England: Oxford University Press, 1989:377–424.
5. Gawin FH. Cocaine addiction, psychology, and neurophysiology. *Science* 1991;251:1580–1586.
6. Gawin FH, Ellinwood EH. Cocaine and other stimulants. *N Engl J Med* 1988;318:1173–1182.
7. Department of Justice. National Drug Threat Assessment 2004; http://www.usdoj.gov/ndic/pubs8/8731/8731p.pdf
8. Miller NS, Gold MS, Belkin BM. Family history and diagnosis of alcohol dependence in cocaine dependence. *Psychiatry Res* 1989;29:113–121.
9. Miller NS, Gold MS. Alcohol and other drug dependence and withdrawal characteristics. In: Gold MS, ed. *Alcohol.* New York: Plenum Books, 1991.
10. U.S. Department of Health and Human Services. *Drug abuse warning network, 1992.* Washington, DC: US Government Printing Office, 1993.
11. Gold MS. The cocaine epidemic: what are the problems, insights, and treatments? *Pharmacy Times* 1987;3:36–42.
12. Miller NS, Gold MS, Millman RB. Cocaine: general characteristics, abuse and addiction. *NY State J Med* 1989; 89:390–395.
13. Chen K, Kandel D. Relationship between extent of cocaine use and dependence among adolescents and adults in the United States. *Drug Alcohol Depend* 2002;68(1):65–85.
14. Uszenski RT, Gills RA, Schaer G. Additive myocardial depressant effects of cocaine and ethanol. *Am Heart J* 1992;124:1276–1283.
15. Gottschalk P, Kosten T. Cerebral perfusion defects in combined cocaine and alcohol dependence. *Drug Alcohol Depend* 2002;68(1):95–104.
16. Higgins ST, Roll JM, Bickel WK. Alcohol pretreatment increases preference for cocaine over monetary reinforcement. *Psychopharmacology* 1996;123:1–8.
17. Washton AM, Gold MS. Chronic cocaine abuse: evidence for adverse effects on health and functioning. *Psychiatr Ann* 1984;14:733–739.
18. Louie AK, Lannon RA, Keiter TA. Treatment of cocaine-induced panic disorder. *Am J Psychiatry* 1989; 146:40–44.
19. McAllister K, Goeders N, Dworkin S. Chronic cocaine modifies brain benzodiazepine receptor densities. *NIDA Res Monogr* 1988;81:101–108.
20. Wood DM, Lal H. Anxiogenic properties of cocaine withdrawal. *Life Sci* 1987;41:1431–1436.
21. Grant BF, Harford TC. Concurrent and simultaneous use of alcohol with cocaine: results of a national survey. *Drug Alcohol Depend* 1990;25:97–104.
22. Randall T. Cocaine, alcohol mix in body to form even longer lasting, more lethal drugs. *JAMA* 1992;267:1043–1044.
23. Sands BF, Ciraulo DA. Cocaine drug-interactions. *J Clin Psychopharmacol* 1992;12:49–55.
24. Prather PL, Lal H. Protracted withdrawal: sensitization of the anxiogenic response to cocaine in rats concurrently treated with ethanol. *Neuropsychopharmacology* 1992;6:23–29.
25. Hearn WL, Flynn DD, Hime GW. Cocaethylene: a unique cocaine metabolite displays high affinity for the dopamine transporter. *J Neurochem* 1991;56:698–701.
26. Rose S, Hearn WL, Hime GW. Cocaine and cocaethylene concentrations in human postmortem cerebral cortex. *Soc Neurosci Abst* 1990;11.6:14.
27. Fowler JS, Volkow ND, MacGregor RR, et al. Comparative PET studies of the kinetics and distribution of cocaine and cocaethylene in baboon brain. *Synapse* 1992;12:220–227.
28. Kampman KM, Pettinati H, Volpicelli J. Concurrent cocaine withdrawal alters alcohol withdrawal symptoms. *J Addict Dis* 2002;21(4):13–26.
29. Kosten TR, Rounsaville BJ, Kleber HD. Parental alcoholism in opioid addicts. *J Nerv Ment Dis* 1987;173:461–468.
30. Kandel DB, Raveis VH. Cessation of illicit drug use in young adulthood. *Arch Gen Psychiatry* 1989;46:109–116.
31. Verebey K, Gold MS. From coca leaves to crack: the effects of dose and routes of administration in abuse liability. *Psychiatr Ann* 1988;18:513–520.
32. Strang J, Edwards G. Cocaine and crack: the drug and the hype are both dangerous. *BMJ* 1989;299:337–338.
33. Smart RG. Crack cocaine use: a review of prevalence and adverse effects. *Am J Drug Alcohol Abuse* 1991;17:13–26.
34. VanDyke C, Ungerer J, Jatlow P, et al. Intranasal cocaine: dose relationship of psychological effects and plasma levels. *Int J Psychiatry Med* 1982;12:1–13.
35. Pothos EN, Hernandez L, Hoebel BG. Chronic food deprivation decreases extracellular dopamine in the nucleus accumbens: Implications for a possible neurochemical link between weight loss and drug abuse. *Obes Res* 1995;3:525s–529s.
36. Keller RW, LeFevre R, Raucci J, et al. Enhanced cocaine self-administration in adult rats prenatally exposed to cocaine. *Neurosci Lett* 1996;205:153–156.
37. Harris JE, Baldessarini RJ. Uptake of (3H)-catecholamines by homogenates of rat corpus striatum and cerebral cortex: effects of amphetamine and analogues. *Neuropharmacology* 1973;12:659–679.
38. Heikkila RE, Orlansky H, Cohen G. Studies on the distinction between uptake inhibition and release of [3H]-dopamine in rat brain and tissue slices. *Biochem Pharmacol* 1975;103:241–248.
39. Hurd YL, Kehr J, Ungerstedt U. *In vivo*

microdialysis as a technique to monitor drug transport: correlation of extracellular cocaine levels and dopamine overflow in the rat brain. *J Neurochem* 1988;51:1314–1316.

40. deWit H, Stewart J. Reinstatement of cocaine-reinforced responding in the rat. *Psychopharmacology* 1981;75:134–143.

41. Volkow ND, Wang GJ, Fowler JS, et al. Relationship between psychostimulant-induced "high" and dopamine transporter occupancy. *Proc Natl Acad Sci U S A* 1996;93(19):10388–10392.

42. Mash DC, Pablo J, Ouyang Q, et al. Dopamine transport function is elevated in cocaine users. *J Neurochem* 2002;81(2):292–300.

43. McMahon LR, Cunningham KA. Antagonism of 5-hydroxytryptamine(4) receptors attenuates hyperactivity induced by cocaine: putative role for 5-hydroxytryptamine(4) receptors in the nucleus accumbens shell. *J Pharmacol Exp Ther* 1999;291(1):300–307.

44. Filip M, Cunningham KA. Serotonin 5-HT(2C) receptors in nucleus accumbens regulate expression of the hyperlocomotive and discriminative stimulus effects of cocaine. *Pharmacol Biochem Behav* 2002;71(4):745–756.

45. Jacobsen LK, Staley JK, Malison RT, et al. Elevated central serotonin transporter binding availability in acutely abstinent cocaine-dependent patients. *Am J Psychiatry* 2000;157(7):1134–1140.

46. Brunner D, Hen R. Insights into the neurobiology of impulsive behavior from serotonin receptor knockout mice. *Ann N Y Acad Sci* 1997;836:81–105.

47. Moeller FG, Steinberg JL, Petty F, et al. Serotonin and impulsive/aggressive behavior in cocaine dependent subjects. *Prog Neuropsychopharmacol Biol Psychiatry* 1994;18(6):1027–1035.

48. Tran-Nguyen LT, Baker DA, Grote KA, et al. Serotonin depletion attenuates cocaine-seeking behavior in rats. *Psychopharmacology (Berl)* 1999;146(1):60–66.

49. Baumann MH, Rothman RB. Alterations in serotonergic responsiveness during cocaine withdrawal in rats: similarities to major depression in humans. *Biol Psychiatry* 1998;44(7):578–591.

50. Willick ML, Kokkinidis L. The effects of ventral tegmental administration of GABA$_A$, GABA$_B$ and NMDA receptor agonists on medial forebrain bundle self-stimulation. *Behav Brain Res* 1995;70(1):31–36.

51. Jaffe JH. Drug addiction and drug abuse. In: Gilman AG, Rall TW, Nies AS, et al., eds. Goodman and Gilman's *The pharmacological basis of therapeutics,* 8th ed. New York: Pergamon Press, 1990:522–573.

52. Rockhold RW. Glutamatergic involvement in psychomotor stimulant action. *Prog Drug Res* 1998;50:155–192.

53. Vorel SR, Liu X, Hayes RJ, et al. Relapse to cocaine-seeking after hippocampal theta burst stimulation. *Science* 2001;292(5519):1175–1178.

54. deWit H, Stewart J. Reinstatement of cocaine-reinforced responding in the rat. *Psychopharmacology* 1981;75:134–143.

55. Segal DS, Kuczenski R. Repeated cocaine administration induces behavioral sensitization and corresponding decreased extracellular dopamine response in caudate and accumbens. *Brain Res* 1996;577:351–355.

56. Koob GF, Vaccarino FJ, Amalric M, et al. Neural substrates for cocaine and opiate reinforcement. In: Fischer S, Raskin A, Uhlenhuth EH, eds. *Cocaine: clinical and behavioral aspects.* New York: Oxford University Press, 1987:80–108.

57. Gold MS. *Drugs of abuse: a comprehensive series for clinicians, vol. III. Cocaine.* New York: Plenum, 1993.

58. Gold MS. Clinical implications of the neurobiology of addiction. In: Miller NS, ed. *Principles of addiction medicine.* Chevy Chase, MD: American Society of Addiction Medicine, 1995;1(14):1–9.

59. Shidara M, Aigner TG, Richmond BJ. Neuronal signals in the monkey ventral striatum related to progress through a predictable series of trials. *J Neurosci* 1998;18(7):2613–2625.

60. Bowman EM, Aigner TG, Richmond BJ. Neural signals in the monkey ventral striatum related to motivation for juice and cocaine rewards. *J Neurophysiol* 1996;75:1061–1073.

61. Homberg JR, van den Akker M, Raaso HS, et al. Enhanced motivation to self-administer cocaine is predicted by self-grooming behaviour and relates to dopamine release in the rat medial prefrontal cortex and amygdala. *Eur J Neurosci* 2002;15(9):1542–1550.

62. Callahan PM, Appel JB, Cunningham KA. Dopamine D1 and D2 mediation of the discriminative stimulus properties of *d*-amphetamine and cocaine. *Psychopharmacology* 1991;103:50–55.

63. Self DW, Barnhart WJ, Lehman DA, et al. Opposite modulation of cocaine-seeking behavior by D1- and D2-like dopamine receptor agonists. *Science* 1996;271:1586–1589.

64. Roberts DC, Koob GF, Klonoff P, et al. Extinction and recovery of cocaine self-administration following 6-hydroxydopamine lesions of the nucleus accumbens. *Pharmacol Biochem Behav* 1980;12:781–787.

65. Robledo P, Maldonado LR, Koob GF. Role of dopamine receptors in the nucleus accumbens in the rewarding properties of cocaine. *Ann N Y Acad Sci* 1992;654:509–512.

66. Hernandez L, Hoebel BG. Food reward and cocaine increase extracellular dopamine in the nucleus accumbens as measured by microdialysis. *Life Sci* 1988;42:1705–1712.

67. Karoum F, Suddath RL, Wyatt RJ. Chronic cocaine and rat brain catecholamine. Long-term reduction in hypothalamic and frontal cortex dopamine metabolism. *Eur J Pharmacol* 1990;186:1–8.

68. Brock JW, Ng JP, Justice JB Jr. Effect of chronic cocaine on dopamine synthesis in the nucleus accumbens as determined by microdialysis perfusion with NSD-1015. *Neurosci Lett* 1990;117:234–239.

69. Hurd YL, Herkenham M. Molecular alteration in the neostriatum of human cocaine addicts. *Synapse* 1993;13:357–369.

70. Pilotte NS, Sharpe LG, Kuhar MJ. Withdrawal of repeated intravenous infusions of cocaine persistently reduces binding to dopamine transporters in the nucleus accumbens of Lewis rats. *J Pharmacol Exp Ther* 1994;269:963–969.

71. Izenwasser S, Cox BM. Inhibition of dopamine uptake by chronic cocaine and nicotine: tolerance to chronic treatments. *Brain Res* 1992;573:119–125.

72. Zahniser NR, Peris J, Dworkin LP, et al. Sensitization to cocaine in the nigrostriatal dopamine system. *NIDA Res Monogr* 1988;88:55–77.

73. Weiss F, Markou A, Lorang MT. Basal extracellular dopamine levels in the nucleus accumbens are decreased during cocaine withdrawal after unlimited-access self-administration. *Brain Res* 1992;593:314–318.

74. Weiss F, Hurd YL, Ungerstedt U, et al. Repeated cocaine administration potentiates the hypomotility effects of apomorphine. *Soc Neurosci Abstr* 1989;15:250.

75. Dackis CA, Gold MS. Bromocriptine as treatment of cocaine abuse. *Lancet* 1985;1(8438):1151–1152.

76. Nunes EV, McGrath PJ, Stewart JW, et al. Bromocriptine treatment for cocaine addiction. *Am J Addictions* 1992;2:169–172.

77. Moskovitz H, Brookoff D, Nelson L. A randomized trial of bromocriptine for cocaine users presenting to the emergency department. *J Gen Intern Med* 1993;8:1–4.

78. Giannini AJ, Bilet W. Bromocriptine therapy in cocaine withdrawal. *J Clin Pharmacol* 1987;27:267–270.

79. Dackis CA, Gold MS, Sweeney DR, et al. Single-dose bromocriptine reverses cocaine craving. *Psychiatry Res* 1987;20:261–264.

80. Giannini AJ, Folts DJ, Feather JN, et al. Bromocriptine and amantadine in cocaine detoxification. *Psychiatry Res* 1989;29:11–16.

81. Tennant FS, Sagherian A. A double-blind comparison of amantadine and bromocriptine for ambulatory withdrawal from cocaine dependence. *Arch Intern Med* 1987;147:109–112.

82. Kosten TR, Schumann B, Wright D. Bromocriptine treatment of cocaine abuse in patients maintained on methadone. *Am J Psychiatry* 1988;145: 381–382.

83. Bradberry CW, Roth RH. Cocaine increases extracellular dopamine in rat nucleus accumbens and ventral tegmental area as shown by *in vivo* microdialysis. *Neurosci Lett* 1989;103:97–102.

84. Eiler K, Schaefer MR, Salstrom D, Lowery R. Double-blind comparison of bromocriptine and placebo in cocaine withdrawal. *Am J Drug Alcohol Abuse* 1995 Feb;21(1):65–79.

85. Mendelson JH, Mello NK, Teoh SK, et al. Cocaine effects on pulsatile secretion of anterior pituitary, gonadal, and adrenal hormones. *J Clin Endocrinol Metab* 1989;69:1256–1260.

86. Krantzler HR, Wallington DJ. Serum prolactin level, craving, and early discharge from treatment in cocaine-dependent patients. *Am J Drug Alcohol Abuse* 1992;18:187–195.

87. Mello NK, Sarnyai Z, Mendelson JH, et al. Acute effects of cocaine on anterior pituitary hormones in male and female rhesus monkeys. *J Pharmacol Exp Ther* 1993;266:804–811.

88. Volkow ND, Mullani N, Gould KL, et al. Cerebral blood flow in chronic cocaine users: a study with positron emission tomography. *Br J Psychiatry* 1988;152:641–648.

89. Volkow ND, Hitzemann R, Wang GJ, et al. Long-term frontal brain metabolic changes in cocaine abusers. *Synapse* 1992;11:184–190.

90. Volkow ND, Fowler JS, Wang GJ, et al. Decreased dopamine D2 receptor availability is associated with reduced frontal metabolism in cocaine abusers. *Synapse* 1993;14:169–177.

91. Giros B, Jaber M, Jones SR, et al. Hyperlocomotion and indifference to cocaine and amphetamine in mice lacking the dopamine transporter. *Nature* 1996;379:606–612.

92. Moliterno DJ, Lange RA, Gerard RD, et al. Influence of intranasal cocaine on plasma constituents associated with endogenous thrombosis and thrombolysis. *Am J Med* 1994;96:492–496.

93. Linder JD, Monkemuller KE, Raijman I, et al. Cocaine-associated ischemic colitis. *South Med J* 2000;93(9):909–913.

94. Li HY, Hwang HW, Hu YH. Functional characterizations of cocaine- and amphetamine-regulated transcript mRNA expression in rat hypothalamus. *Neurosci Lett* 2002;323(3):203–206.

95. van der Woude FJ. Cocaine use and kidney damage. *Nephrol Dial Transplant* 2000;15(3):299–301.

96. Di Paolo N, Fineschi V, Di Paolo M, et al. Kidney vascular damage and cocaine. *Clin Nephrol* 1997;47(5):298–303.

97. Chen JC, Hsiang N, Morris C, et al. Cocaine-induced multiple vascular occlusions. *J Vasc Surg* 1996;23:719–723.

98. Orsay EM, Doan-Wiggins L, Lewis R, et al. The impaired driver: hospital and police detection of alcohol and other drugs of abuse in motor vehicle crashes. *Ann Emerg Med* 1994;24(1):51–55.

99. Marzuk PM, Tardiff K, Leon AC. Fatal injuries after cocaine use as a leading cause of death among young adults in New York City. *N Engl J Med* 1995;332:1753–1757.

100. Volkow ND, Mullani N, Gould KL, et al. Cerebral blood flow in chronic cocaine users: a study with positron emission tomography. *Br J Psychiatry* 1988;152:641–648.

101. Holman BL, Carvalho PA, Mendelson J, et al. Brain perfusion is abnormal in cocaine-dependent polydrug users: a study using technetium-99m-HMPAO and ASPECT. *J Nucl Med* 1991;32(6):1206–1210.

102. Holman BL, Mendelson J, Garada B, et al. Regional cerebral blood flow improves with treatment in chronic cocaine polydrug users. *J Nucl Med* 1993;34(5):723–727.

103. Fillmore MT, Rush CR. Impaired inhibitory control of behavior in chronic cocaine users. *Drug Alcohol Depend* 2002;66(3):265–273.

104. Berry J, van Gorp WG, Herzberg DS, et al. Neuropsychological deficits in abstinent cocaine abusers: preliminary findings after two weeks of abstinence. *Drug Alcohol Depend* 1993;32(3):231–237.

105. Beatty WW, Katzung VM, Moreland VJ, et al. Neuropsychological performance of recently abstinent alcoholics and cocaine abusers. *Drug Alcohol Depend* 1995;37(3):247–253.

106. O'Malley S, Adamse M, Heaton RK, et al. Neuropsychological impairment in chronic cocaine abusers. *Am J Drug Alcohol Abuse* 1992;18(2):131–144.

107. Cadet JL, Bolla KI. Chronic cocaine use as a neuropsychiatric syndrome: a

model for debate. *Synapse* 1996;22:28–34.

108. Siegal RK. Cocaine smoking disorders: diagnosis and treatment. *Psychiatr Ann* 1984;14:728–732.

109. Dackis CA, O'Brien CP. Cocaine dependence: a disease of the brain's reward centers. *J Subst Abuse Treat* 2001;21(3):111–117.

110. Heim C, Newport DJ, Bonsall R, et al. Altered pituitary–adrenal axis responses to provocative challenge tests in adult survivors of childhood abuse. *Am J Psychiatry* 2001;158(4):575–581.

111. Back S, Dansky BS, Coffey SF, et al. Cocaine dependence with and without post-traumatic stress disorder: a comparison of substance use, trauma history and psychiatric comorbidity. *Am J Addict* 2000;9(1):51–62.

112. Childress AR, Mozley PD, McElgin W, et al. Limbic activation during cue-induced cocaine craving. *Am J Psychiatry* 1999;156(1):11–18.

113. Vorel SR, Liu X, Hayes RJ, et al. Relapse to cocaine-seeking after hippocampal theta burst stimulation. *Science* 2001;292(5519):1175–1178.

114. Goeders NE. The HPA axis and cocaine reinforcement. *Psychoneuroendocrinology* 2002;27(1–2):13–33.

115. Elmer GI, Pieper JO, Rubinstein M, et al. Failure of intravenous morphine to serve as an effective instrumental reinforcer in dopamine D2 receptor knock-out mice. *J Neurosci* 2002;22(10):RC224.

116. Sora I, Hall FS, Andrews AM, et al. Molecular mechanisms of cocaine reward: combined dopamine and serotonin transporter knockouts eliminate cocaine place preference. *Proc Natl Acad Sci U S A* 2001;98(9):5300–5305.

117. Fletcher PJ, Tampakeras M, Yeomans JS. Median raphe injections of 8-OH-DPAT lower frequency thresholds for lateral hypothalamic self-stimulation. *Pharmacol Biochem Behav* 1995;52(1):65–71.

118. Harrison AA, Markou A. Serotonergic manipulations both potentiate and reduce brain stimulation reward in rats: involvement of serotonin-1A receptors. *J Pharmacol Exp Ther* 2001;297(1):316–325.

119. Herges S, Taylor DA. Involvement of serotonin in the modulation of cocaine-induced locomotor activity in the rat. *Pharmacol Biochem Behav* 1998;59(3):595–611.

120. Gold MS, Pottash ALC. Endorphins, locus coeruleus, clonidine, and lofexidine: a mechanism for opiate withdrawal and new nonopiate treatments. *Adv Alcohol Subst Abuse* 1981;3:33–51.

121. Volkow ND, Fowler JS, Wolf AP, et al. Metabolic studies of drugs of abuse. *NIDA Res Monogr* 1991;105:47–53.

122. Volkow ND, Fowler JS, Wang GJ. Imaging studies on the role of dopamine in cocaine reinforcement and addiction in humans. *J Psychopharmacol* 1999;13(4):337–345.

123. Bonson KR, Grant SJ, Contoreggi CS, et al. Neural systems and cue-induced cocaine craving. *Neuropsychopharmacology* 2002;26(3):376–386.

124. Volkow ND, Fowler JS, Wang GJ, et al. Decreased dopamine D2 receptor availability is associated with reduced frontal metabolism in cocaine abusers. *Synapse* 1993;14(2):169–177.

125. Goldstein RZ, Volkow ND, Wang GJ, et al. Addiction changes orbitofrontal gyrus function: involvement in response inhibition. *Neuroreport* 2001;12(11):2595–2599.

126. Miller NS, Dackis CA, Gold MS. The relationship of addiction, tolerance and dependence: a neurochemical approach. *J Subst Abuse Treat* 1987;4:197–207.

127. Weiss F, Hurd YL, Ungerstedt U, et al. Neurochemical correlates of cocaine and ethanol self-administration. *Ann N Y Acad Sci* 1992;654:220–241.

128. Parsons LH, Koob GF, Weiss F. Serotonin dysfunction in the nucleus accumbens of rats during withdrawal after unlimited access to intravenous cocaine. *J Pharmacol Exp Ther* 1995;274(3):1182–1191.

129. Ahmed SH, Koob GF. Transition from moderate to excessive drug intake: change in hedonic set point. *Science* 1998;282(5387):298–300.

130. Satel SL, Southwick SM, Gawin FH. Clinical features of cocaine-induced paranoia. *Am J Psychiatry* 1991;148:495–498.

131. Grinspoon L, Bakalar JB. Drug dependence: non-narcotic agents. In: Kaplan HI, Freedman AM, Sadock BJ, eds. *Comprehensive textbook of psychiatry*, 3rd ed. Baltimore: Williams & Wilkins, 1980.

132. Washton AM, Gold MS. Successful use of naltrexone in addicted physicians and business executives. *Adv Alcohol Subst Abuse* 1984;4(2):89–96.

133. Washton AM, Gold MS. Intranasal cocaine addiction. *Lancet* 1983;2(8363):1374.

134. Gold MS. Science sizes up cocaine. In: *Encyclopedia britannica, Medical and health annual*. Philip W. Goetz (ed.), Chicago, IL. 1987:184–203.

135. Dackis CA, Gold MS, Sweeney DR. The physiology of cocaine craving and "crashing." *Arch Gen Psychiatry* 1987;44(3):298–299.

136. Markou A, Koob GF. Post cocaine anhedonia: an animal model of cocaine withdrawal. *Neuropsychopharmacology* 1991;4:17–26.

137. Kokkindis L, McCarter BD. Post cocaine depression and sensitization of brain-stimulation reward: analysis of reinforcement and performance effects. *Pharmacol Biochem Behav* 1990;36:463–471.

138. Gold MS. Dopamine depletion hypothesis for acute cocaine abstinence: clinical observations, prolactin elevations, and persistent anhedonia/dysphoria. *Neuroendocrinol Lett* 1993;15(4):271.

139. *Diagnostic and statistical manual of mental disorders*, 4th ed. Washington, DC: American Psychiatric Association, 1994.

140. Gawin FH, Kleber HD. Abstinence symptomatology and psychiatric diagnosis in cocaine abusers: clinical observations. *Arch Gen Psychiatry* 1986;43:107–113.

141. Gold MS, Vereby K. The psychopharmacology of cocaine. *Psychiatr Ann* 1984;14:714–723.

142. Satel SL, Price LH, Palumbo JM, et al. Clinical phenomenology and neurobiology of cocaine abstinence: a prospective inpatient study. *Am J Psychiatry* 1991;148:1712–1716.

143. Weddington WW, Brown BS, Haertzen CA, et al. Changes in mood, craving, and sleep during short-term abstinence reported by male cocaine addicts. *Arch Gen Psychiatry* 1990;47:861–868.

144. Markou A, Koob GF. Bromocriptine reverses the elevation in intracranial self-stimulation thresholds observed in a rat model of cocaine withdrawal. *Neuropsychopharmacology* 1992;7(3):213–224.

145. Darmani NA. Deficits in D-fenfluramine-sensitive pool of brain 5-HT following withdrawal from chronic cocaine exposure. *Life Sci* 1997;61(26):2575–2582.

146. Gold MS. *800-COCAINE*. New York: Bantam, 1984.

147. Dackis CA, Gold MS. Addictiveness of central stimulants. *Adv Alcohol Subst Abuse* 1990;9:9–26.

148. Childress AR, McLellan AT, Ehrman RN, et al. Extinction of conditioned responses in abstinent cocaine or opioid users. *NIDA Res Monogr* 1987;76:189–195.

149. Ehrman RN, Robbins SJ, Childress AR, et al. Conditioned responses to cocaine-related stimuli in cocaine abuse patients. *Psychopharmacology* 1992;107:523–529.

150. Roache JD, Meisch RA. Drug self-administration in drug and alcohol addiction. In: Miller NS, ed. *Comprehensive handbook of drug and alcohol addiction*. New York: Marcel Dekker, 1991:625–640.

151. Miller NS. Amphetamines. In: Miller NS, ed. *Comprehensive handbook of drug and alcohol addiction*. New York: Marcel Dekker, 1991:427–435.

152. Kuhar MJ, Joyce A, Dominguez G. Genes in drug abuse. *Drug Alcohol Depend* 2001;62(3):157–162.

153. Volkow ND. *Imaging pharmacological actions of psychostimulants during drug addiction*. Paper presented at the Institute of Medicine Symposium on NeuroScience Research: Advancing our Understanding of Drug Addiction. Washington, DC, July 29, 1996.

154. Weiss F. *Neuroscience of addiction. the state of the science*. Paper presented at the Institute of Medicine Symposium on Neuroscience Research: Advancing our Understanding of Drug Addiction. Washington, DC, July 29, 1996.

155. Self DW, Barnhart WJ, Lehman DA, et al. Opposite modulation of cocaine-seeking behavior by D1- and D2-like dopamine receptor antagonists. *Science* 1996;271:1586–1589.

156. Liu X, Matochik JA, Cadet JL, et al. Smaller volume of prefrontal lobe in polysubstance abusers: a magnetic resonance imaging study. *Neuropsychopharmacology* 1998;18(4):243–252.

157. Fein G, Di Sclafani V, Cardenas VA, et al. Cortical gray matter loss in treatment-naive alcohol dependent individuals. *Alcohol Clin Exp Res* 2002;26(4):558–564.

158. DiChiara G, Imperato A. Drugs of abuse preferentially stimulate dopamine release in the mesolimbic system of freely moving rats. *Proc Natl Acad Sci U S A* 1988;85:5274–5278.

159. Bechara A, Vander Kooy D. The tegmental pedunculo-pontine nucleus: a brain stem output of the limbic system critical for the conditioned place preferences produced by morphine and amphetamine. *J Neurosci* 1989;9:3400–3409.

160. Bozarth MA, Wise RA. Anatomically distinct opiate receptor fields mediate reward and physical dependence. *Science* 1984;224:516–517.

161. Bozarth MA, Wise RA. Dissociation of the rewarding and physical dependence-producing properties of morphine. *NIDA Res Monogr* 1983;43:171–177.

162. Miller NS, Gold MS. Dissociation of "conscious desire" (craving) from and relapse in alcohol and cocaine dependence. *J Clin Psychiatry* 1994;6:99–106.

163. Miller NS, Belkin BM, Gold MS. Multiple addictions: cosynchronous use of

alcohol and drugs. *N Y State J Med* 1990;90:596–600.

164. Helzer JE, Przybeck TR. The co-occurrence of alcoholism with other psychiatric disorders in the general population and its impact on treatment. *J Stud Alcohol* 1988;49:219–224.

165. Miller NS. Comorbidity of psychiatric alcohol/drug disorders: interactions and independent status. *J Addict Dis* 1993;12(3):5–16.

166. Hill SY, Cloninger CR, Ayre FR. Independent familial transmission of alcoholism and opiate abuse. *Alcohol Clin Exp Res* 1977;1:335–342.

167. Meller WH, Rinehart R, Cadoret RJ, et al. Specific familial transmission in substance abuse. *Int J Addict* 1988;23:1029–1039.

168. Miller NS, Gold MS. Research approaches to inheritance to alcoholism. *Subst Abuse* 1988;9:157–163.

169. Pickens RW. Genetic vulnerability to drug abuse. *NIDA Res Monogr* 1988;89:41–51.

170. Pickens RW, Svikis DS, McGue M, et al. Heterogeneity in the inheritance of alcoholism: a study of male and female twins. *Arch Gen Psychiatry* 1991;48:19–28.

171. Cadoret RJ, Troughton E, O'Gorman TW, et al. An adoption study of genetic and environmental factors in drug abuse. *Arch Gen Psychiatry* 1986;43:1131–1136.

172. Noble EP. The D2 dopamine receptor gene: a review of association studies in alcoholism and phenotypes. *Alcohol* 1998;16(1):33–45.

173. Edenberg HJ, Foroud T, Koller DL, et al. A family-based analysis of the association of the dopamine D2 receptor (DRD2) with alcoholism. *Alcohol Clin Exp Res* 1998;22(2):505–512.

174. Blomqvist O, Gelernter J, Kranzler HR. Family-based study of DRD2 alleles in alcohol and drug dependence. *Am J Med Genet* 2000;96(5):659–664.

175. Buckley PF. Substance abuse in schizophrenia: a review. *J Clin Psychiatry* 1998;59[Suppl 3]:26–30.

176. Miller NS, Mahler JC, Belkin BM, et al. Psychiatric diagnosis in alcohol and drug dependence. *Ann Clin Psychiatry* 1991;3:79–89.

177. Gold MS. *The good news about depression.* New York: Villard Books, 1987.

178. Gold MS, Slaby AE. *Dual diagnosis in substance abuse.* New York: Marcel Dekker, 1991.

179. Schuckit MA. Alcoholism and other psychiatric disorders. *Hosp Community Psychiatry* 1983;34:1022–1027.

180. Schmitz JM, Stotts AL, Averill PM, et al. Cocaine dependence with and without comorbid depression: a comparison of patient characteristics. *Drug Alcohol Depend* 2000;60(2):189–98.

181. Dilsaver SC, Alessi NE. Antipsychotic withdrawal symptoms: phenomenology and pathophysiology. *Acta Psychiatr Scand* 1988;77:241–246.

182. Dilsaver SC, Greden JF, Snider RM. Antidepressant withdrawal syndromes: phenomenology and pathophysiology. *Int Clin Psychopharmacol* 1987;2(1):1–19.

183. Miller NS, Gold MS. Dependence syndrome: a critical analysis of essential features. *Psychiatr Ann* 1991;21:282–290.

184. Mayfield D. Psychopharmacology of alcohol. II. Affective tolerance in alcohol intoxication. *J Nerve Ment Dis* 1968;146:322–327.

185. Mayfield DG. Alcohol and effect: experimental studies. In: Goodwin DW, Erickson CK, eds. *Alcoholism and affective disorders.* New York: SP Medical and Scientific Books, 1979:99–107.

186. Leshner AI, Molecular mechanisms of cocaine addiction. *N Engl J Med* 1996;335:128–129.

187. Weiss SRB, Post RM, Aigner TG. Carbamazepine in the treatment of cocaine-induced disorders. In: Watson RR, ed. *Drug and alcohol abuse reviews: treatment of drug and alcohol abuse.* Totowa, NJ: Humana Press, 1992:149.

188. Berger P, Gawin F, Kosten TR. Treatment of cocaine abuse with mazindol. *Lancet* 1989;1:283.

189. Gawin FH, Riordan C, Kleber HD. Methylphenidate treatment of cocaine abusers without attention deficit disorder: a negative report. *Am J Drug Alcohol Abuse* 1985;11:193–197.

190. Jaffe JH, Witkin JM, Goldberg SR, et al. Potential toxic interactions of cocaine and mazindol. *Lancet* 1989;8654:111.

191. Kosten TR, Steinberg M, Diakogiannis IA. Crossover trial of mazindol for cocaine dependence. *Am J Addictions* 1993;2:161–164.

192. Shottenfeld RS, Pakes J, Ziedonis D, et al. Buprenorphine: dose-related effects on cocaine and opioid use in cocaine-abusing opioid-dependent humans. *Biol Psychiatry* 1993;34:66–74.

193. Margolin A, Kosten TR, Avants SK, et al. A multicenter trial of bupropion for cocaine dependence in methadone-maintained patients. *Drug Alcohol Depend* 1995;40(2):125–131.

194. Levin FR, Evans SM, McDowell DM, et al. Bupropion treatment for cocaine abuse and adult attention-deficit/hyperactivity disorder. *J Addict Dis* 2002;21(2):1–16.

195. Oliveto A, McCance-Katz FE, Singha A, et al. Effects of cocaine prior to and during bupropion maintenance in cocaine-abusing volunteers. *Drug Alcohol Depend* 2001;63(2):155–167.

196. Haney M, Foltin RW, Fischman MW. Effects of pergolide on intravenous cocaine self-administration in men and women. *Psychopharmacology (Berl)* 1998;137(1):15–24.

197. Self DW, Karanian DA, Spencer JJ. Effects of the novel D1 dopamine receptor agonist ABT-431 on cocaine self-administration and reinstatement. *Ann N Y Acad Sci* 2000;909:133–144.

198. Grabowski J, Rhoades H, Schmitz J, et al. Dextroamphetamine for cocaine-dependence treatment: a double-blind randomized clinical trial. *J Clin Psychopharmacol* 2001;21(5):522–526.

199. Carroll KM, Nich C, Ball SA, et al. Treatment of cocaine and alcohol dependence with psychotherapy and disulfiram. *Addiction* 1998;93(5):713–727.

200. McCance-Katz EF, Kosten TR, Jatlow P. Disulfiram effects on acute cocaine administration. *Drug Alcohol Depend* 1998;52(1):27–39.

201. Haberny KA, Walsh SL, Ginn DH, et al. Absence of acute cocaine interactions with the MAO-B inhibitor selegiline. *Drug Alcohol Depend* 1995;39(1):55–62.

202. Bartzokis G, Beckson M, Newton T, et al. Selegiline effects on cocaine-induced changes in medial temporal lobe metabolism and subjective ratings of euphoria. *Neuropsychopharmacology* 1999;20(6):582–590.

203. Ettinger RH, Ettinger WF, Harless WE. Active immunization with cocaine-protein conjugate attenuates cocaine effects. *Pharmacol Biochem Behav* 1997;58(1):215–220.

204. Carrera MR, Ashley JA, Zhou B, et al. Cocaine vaccines: antibody protection against relapse in a rat model. *Proc Natl Acad Sci U S A* 2000;97(11):6202–6206.

205. Mets B, Winger G, Cabrera C, et al. A catalytic antibody against cocaine prevents cocaine's reinforcing and toxic effects in rats. *Proc Natl Acad Sci U S A* 1998;95(17):10176–10181.

206. Kleven MS, Woolverton WL. Effects of three monoamine uptake inhibitors on behavior maintained by cocaine or food presentation in rhesus monkeys. *Drug Alcohol Depend* 1993;31:149–158.

207. Brebner K, Childress AR, Roberts DC. A potential role for GABA(B) agonists in the treatment of psychostimulant addiction. *Alcohol* 2002;37(5):478–484.

208. Mendelson JH, Mello NK. Management of cocaine abuse and dependence. *N Engl J Med* 1996;334:965–972.

209. Sun H, Shen ML, Pang YP, et al. Cocaine metabolism accelerated

by a re-engineered human butyryl-cholinesterase. *J Pharmacol Exp Ther* 2002;302(2):710–716.

210. Markou A, Koob GF, Bromocriptine reverses the elevation in intracranial self-stimulation thresholds observed in a rat model of cocaine withdrawal. *Neuropharmacology* 1992;7:213–224.

211. Markou A, Weiss F, Gold LH, et al. Animal models of drug craving. *Psychopharmacology* 1992;112:163–182.

212. Rothman RB. High-affinity dopamine reuptake inhibitors as potential cocaine antagonists: a strategy for drug development. *Life Sci* 1990;46: 17–21.

213. Whitlock EP. Alcohol screening in primary care. BMJ. 2003 Dec 20; 327(7429):E263-4; discussion E265.

214. Siegal H, Falck R, Wang J, et al. Predictors of drug abuse treatment entry among crack-cocaine smokers. *Drug Alcohol Depend* 2002;68(2):159–166.

215. Reiber C, Ramirez A, Parent D, et al. Predicting treatment success at multiple timepoints in diverse patient populations of cocaine-dependent individuals. *Drug Alcohol Depend* 2002;1;68(1):35–48.

216. Mersy DJ. Interventions for recovery in drug and alcohol addiction. In: Miller NS, ed. *Comprehensive handbook of drug and alcohol addiction.* New York: Marcel Dekker, 1991:1063–1078.

217. Schmitz JM, Oswald LM, Jacks SD, Rustin T, Rhoades HM, Grabowski J. Relapse prevention treatment for cocaine dependence: group vs. individual format. Addict Behav. 1997 May–Jun;22(3):405–18.

218. Gold MS, Pomm R, Kennedy Y, et al. 5-Year state-wide study of physician addiction treatment outcomes confirmed by urine testing. *Abstract Viewer/Itinerary Planner.* Washington, DC: Society for Neuroscience, 2001. Online. www.addiction&psychiatry. com

219. Dackis CA, Gold MS, Estroff TW. Inpatient treatment of addiction. In: Karasu TB, ed. *Treatments of psychiatric disorders. A task force report of the American Psychiatric Association.* Washington, DC: American Psychiatric Press, 1989;2:1359–1379.

220. Weiss RD, Mirin SM. *Cocaine.* Washington DC: American Psychiatric Press, 1987.

221. Washton AM. Nonpharmacologic treatment of cocaine abuse. *Psychiatr Clin North Am* 1986:563–571.

222. Foote J, Seligman M, Magura S, Handelsman L, Rosenblum A, Lovejoy M, Arrington K, Stimmel B. An enhanced positive reinforcement model for the severely impaired cocaine abuser. *J Subst Abuse Treat.* 1994 Nov–Dec;11(6):525–39.

223. Miller NS, Gold MS. The psychiatrist's role in integrating pharmacological and nonpharmacological treatments for addictive disorders. *Psychiatr Ann* 1992;22(8):436–440.

224. Chappel JN. The use of Alcoholics Anonymous and Narcotics Anonymous by the physician in treatment of drug and alcohol addiction. In: Miller NS, ed. *Comprehensive handbook of drug and alcohol addiction.* New York: Marcel Dekker, 1991:1079–1090.

225. Hurt RD, Offord KP, Croghan IT, et al. Mortality following inpatient addictions treatment. *JAMA* 1996;275:1097–1103.

226. Schulz JE. 12-Step programs in recovery for drug and alcohol addiction. In: Miller NS, ed. *Comprehensive handbook of drug and alcohol addiction.* New York: Marcel Dekker, 1991:1255–1274.

227. Gold MS. *The facts about drugs and alcohol,* 3rd ed. New York: Bantam Books, 1991.

228. Washton A, Gold MS. *Cocaine: a clinician's manual.* New York: Guilford Press, 1985.

229. Nestler, EJ. The molecular neurobiology of drug addiction. *Neuropsychopharmacology* 1994;11:77–87.

230. Mendelson JH, Mello NK. Management of cocaine abuse and dependence. *N Engl J Med* 1996;334:965–972.

CHAPTER 13

Cocaine and Crack: Clinical Aspects

MARK S. GOLD AND WILLIAM S. JACOBS

To the Incas of Peru, cocaine was a gift from the gods. In our own age, cocaine is seen by many to be a curse from the devil. Dr. Howard P. Rome, editorial director of *Psychiatric Annals,* commented that the ravages of cocaine "have added the fifth pale horseman as civilization hurtles toward its Apocalypse" (1).

Although cocaine abuse in this country had reached epidemic proportions, as early as 1990, the National Household Survey on Drug Abuse (NHSDA) found cause for hope. Data from that survey showed that the number of current cocaine users—people who had used the drug within the past 30 days—had decreased from 5.8 million in 1985 to 1.6 million in 1990. In 2001, rates were increasing again. An estimated 1.7 million Americans ages 12 years and older were current cocaine users and 406,000 were current crack users in 2001 (2). The NHSDA also found that cocaine use increased among young adults age 18 to 25 years, from 1.4% in 2000 to 1.9% in 2001. Unlike other drugs of abuse, where rates are higher among youth and young adults, only 40% of cocaine users were age 12 to 25 years in 2001.

According to the Monitoring the Future annual survey, the peak lifetime use of cocaine decreased from 17.3% in 1985 to 5.9% in 1994 among high school seniors. However, it later increased, and in 2001 was 8.2% (3). Crack use also decreased significantly among high school seniors between 1989 and 1990, but additional decreases have been difficult to demonstrate. The lifetime prevalence for crack use had a mild increase from 3.0% in 1994 to 3.7% in 2001. In 2003, 2.2% of twelfth graders used crack in the last year and 0.9% used crack in the past month (3).

Cocaine-related emergency room visits declined 26% between 1988 and 1990. To a significant degree, the decline can be attributed to widespread public education about the dangers of cocaine. Despite this early decline, cocaine was the most frequently reported drug in emergency room visits in 2001. The Drug Abuse Warning Network (DAWN) reported a significant increase in emergency department mentions between 2000 and 2001, from 174,881 to 193,034, respectively (4). In 2001, 24% of the emergency mentions were attributed to crack alone. Cocaine is consistently among the top three drugs mentioned in mortality data from DAWN. Cocaine and cocaine in combination with alcohol were the most commonly mentioned in suicide cases in 2001 (5).

The number of people using cocaine every day or every week rose during the late 1980s and early 1990s. We have reported on the role of early drug experimentation and intrauterine exposure in changing the risk profile of the person toward drug experimentation and dependence. We have reported on proteomic changes produced by stimulants which suggest short-term exposure changes the brain in important ways (ref 1). Occupational exposure has been ignored as a major environmental factor in cocaine and opiate use (ref 2). Studying physician addicts it is clear that drugs of abuse used in medical practice can, through second hand exposure, induce changes in the physicians' brains that makes their own drug use and dependence more likely. For anesthesiologists, opiate dependence is an occupational hazard as is cocaine for ENT physicians who use cocaine in their practice (ref 2). Prevention should include prevention of second hand exposure to drugs of abuse.

EPIDEMIOLOGY

The history of cocaine has been thoroughly discussed elsewhere (8–10). The relevant clinical issues related to cocaine's history have to do largely with the changes over time in dosage, route of administration, patterns of use, and the technology of cocaine production. The amount of cocaine ingested by the Incas was probably low. It is estimated that the average user chewed 60 g of coca leaves a day. Given that the alkaloid content of a coca leaf is approximately 0.5% to 0.7% and that only a portion of the alkaloid is absorbed in digestion, the total dosage would have been 200 to 300 mg over a 24-hour period (11).

Word about cocaine spread to Europe through reports first by explorers and later by naturalists and botanists (12). By 1860, essays about the virtues of cocaine inspired makers of wines and tonics to add the drug to their formulations. Within 15 years people could also buy snuff that contained pure cocaine and that was touted as a remedy for asthma and hay fever. These new cocaine preparations, doses, and routes of administration marked the first change in the pattern of cocaine use in more than 4,000 years (13). The established daily doses of cocaine ingested via these products would have ranged from about 225 to 1,620 mg—more than 5 to 8 times the cocaine intake of the coca chewer in Peru.

In 1884, Sigmund Freud published his essay "Uber Coca" (14) in which he advocated the therapeutic use of cocaine as a stimulant, an aphrodisiac, a local anesthetic, and a medicine for treating asthma, wasting diseases, digestive disorders, nervous exhaustion, hysteria, syphilis,

and even altitude sickness (15). Freud, who himself used cocaine in dosages of about 200 mg a day, recommended cocaine in oral doses of 50 to 100 mg as a stimulant and as a euphoriant in depressive states (16,17). For 90 years his essay was the only report that used controlled studies to document the effects of cocaine on humans (18).

Freud also prescribed cocaine to alleviate the symptoms of withdrawal from alcohol and morphine addiction. Because the addictive power of cocaine was not then recognized, some patients who used cocaine as a substitute for alcohol or morphine became addicted to cocaine instead. As these and other adverse consequences of cocaine use soon became apparent, Albrecht Ehrlenmeyer accused Freud of having unleashed "the third scourge of humanity," the other two being alcohol and opiates (18).

In America, during the mid-1880s, Atlanta druggist John Pemberton devised a patent medicine that contained two naturally occurring stimulants: cocaine and caffeine (19). Because it contained no alcohol, he advertised his product—eventually known as Coca-Cola—as an "intellectual beverage," a "temperance drink," and a "brain tonic" (20–22). Until 1903, Coca-Cola contained approximately 60 mg of cocaine per 8-ounce serving. The maker voluntarily removed cocaine from the formulation in response to public pressure and news reports about the dangers of cocaine.

The turn of the century thus also marked a turn in public attitudes about cocaine. The American Medical Association, seeking to raise the standards of medical practice, lobbied to curb the sales of patent medicines, including those containing cocaine. The Harrison Narcotic Act of 1914, which mistakenly listed cocaine as a narcotic, banned the use of cocaine in proprietary medications and tightened the restrictions on the manufacture and distribution of coca products (8).

As a result of these restrictions, and for other reasons, drug users turned to amphetamines and other centrally stimulating drugs that were developed beginning in the 1930s. These drugs easily substituted for cocaine because they cost less, were more widely available, and induced a sense of euphoria that lasted longer (22). They were also deadly. By the late 1960s, the drug-using subculture recognized the danger in amphetamines, as reflected in the contemporary slogan "speed kills." Eventually amphetamines were listed as Schedule II drugs (drugs with a high abuse potential and prescription limitations), making them much more difficult to obtain.

Stimulant abusers searching for a "safe" recreational euphoria soon rediscovered cocaine (23). In the early 1970s, cocaine abuse skyrocketed, especially among middle- and upper middle-class populations, where it became known as "the champagne of pharmaceuticals." The warnings of cocaine's dangers from the previous cocaine epidemic during the late nineteenth century had long been forgotten.

During the 1970s, cocaine was usually administered intranasally in a powder form. A typical user bought 1 g of cocaine for approximately $150 and snorted the drug from a tiny "coke spoon" or perhaps even a fingernail cultivated for the purpose. Such methods delivered between 5 and 10 mg of the drug. A "line" of cocaine inhaled through a straw delivered approximately 25 mg. Typical users would repeat the dose in both nostrils, thus taking between 10 and 50 mg of cocaine at a time (24).

The perception among users was that cocaine was safe and nonaddictive. Perception of safety appears necessary for widespread use of illicit drugs. Drugs of abuse tend to be viewed as safe until proven dangerous—the opposite burden of proof applied to new pharmaceuticals. The medical literature of the time did little to contradict this false perception. An article appearing in 1977 claimed that "aside from financial depletion, the main undesirable effects of 'social snorting' are nervousness, irritability, and restlessness from overstimulation" (25). The authors went on to state that cocaine may improve physical performance, cure stage fright, and fortify the body and mind without the risk of causing withdrawal syndrome marked by prolonged cravings for the drugs. The same authors, writing in the 1980 edition of the *Comprehensive Textbook of Psychiatry* (26), stated: "Used no more than two or three times a week, cocaine creates no serious problems. In daily and fairly large amounts, it can produce minor psychological disturbances. Chronic cocaine abuse usually does not appear as a medical problem."

People willing or prone to misuse drugs interpreted these and other similar statements from medical "experts" as a license to try, and then to use, cocaine freely. As the supply of cocaine rose, the price dropped and the amount of a typical dose increased.

A newer method called "freebasing" began in the late 1970s and became popular in the mid-1980s. Freebasing made cocaine "smokable," allowing rapid self-administration of high blood and brain levels without intravenous injection. Freebase enabled users to ingest a much higher doses than ever before (10).

Another "smokable" form of cocaine in the mid-1980s opened a tragic chapter in the history of the drug. Essentially mass-produced freebase cocaine, crack was low priced (as little as $2 a dose), making it available to younger users and sending the average age of the user spiraling downward. Crack made users feel more confident, more intelligent, more in control, and sexier. Smoked cocaine is rapidly addicting and produces medical effects previously seen only in long-term intranasal users (27). Kandel and Yamaguchi reported that crack smoking was the last drug in a long chain of substances used by youth, often after cocaine hydrochloride (28).

Crack differs from cocaine hydrochloride, the powdered form of cocaine, in several ways (27). Because it is smoked, the user feels a "high" in less than 10 seconds.

Conditioning can cause euphoria to be reported when the warm pipe touches the lips of the experienced user. In contrast, sniffing cocaine produces a high after a delay of 1 to 2 minutes. The feeling of euphoria from crack wears off after 5 to 15 minutes; the effects of snorted cocaine may last slightly longer. Another difference is that the user reports that the crack-induced euphoria is far more powerful than that created by powder. Pharmacokinetic studies of intranasal and intravenous cocaine administration are reviewed elsewhere (29). Following intranasal administration of 96 mg of cocaine, peak venous plasma levels of between 150 and 200 ng/mL are reached in 30 minutes. Intravenous administration of 32 mg produces peak venous plasma levels of 250 to 300 ng/mL after only 4 minutes. A similar rise in plasma levels occurs following the smoking of 50 mg of cocaine base (30). The levels of cocaine reaching the heart and brain after either smoking or intravenous administration are much greater and faster, peaking in seconds when arterial rather than venous sampling is done. Concurrent use of alcohol can increase blood levels of cocaine. The smoked drug is absorbed rapidly from the lungs to the heart and then to the brain, rather than passing incompletely and slowly through the nasal membrane on the long route to the brain. Cocaine smoking and intravenous use tend to be particularly associated with a rapid progression from use to abuse or dependence, often occurring over weeks to months. Intranasal use is associated with a more gradual progression, usually occurring over months to years. Cocaine is metabolized by cholinesterase present in plasma and liver into two metabolites, benzoylecgonine and ecgonine methyl ester, which are excreted and can be measured in urine for 36 hours or longer after last use. Dependence is commonly associated with a progressive tolerance to the desirable effects of cocaine, leading to increasing doses and/or changes in route of administration. With continuing use, there is a diminution of pleasurable effects as a consequence of tolerance and an increase in dysphoric effects. While reporting decreased pleasure, use continues unabated. It may even accelerate.

COCAINE USE TODAY

Surveys of callers to the National Helpline conducted from 1983 to 1989 identified some persistent shifts in the cocaine epidemic (31). For example, in 1983, the typical caller was a 31-year-old intranasal cocaine user, college educated, and employed with an income of more than $25,000. By 1989, the typical caller was less educated, unemployed, a non-intranasal user, and had an income of less than $25,000. Since 1989, these early findings have been replicated and it has become routine to consider crack the drug of abuse of the urban and poor populations, and to consider cocaine hydrochloride as the drug of abuse of the suburban and middle-class populations. Patients report that it is easy to find crack cocaine in any city at any time by simply finding the poorest neighborhoods or looking for a ghetto. While crack has been the focus of media reports, cocaine is linked to violence, irritable aggression, and even traffic accidents and dangerous driving. It is now clear that driving under the influence of intoxicating drugs other than alcohol may be an important cause of traffic injuries. Using a rapid urine test to identify reckless drivers who were under the influence of cocaine or marijuana (32), 59% of 150 subjects stopped for reckless driving and providing a urine specimen tested positive. A community survey conducted in the United States in 1991, reported that 12% of the population had used cocaine one or more times in their lifetime; 3% had used it in the last year; and less than 1% had used it in the last month. In 2001, an estimated 1.7 million (0.7%) of Americans aged 12 years or older were current cocaine users and 406,000 (0.2%) were current crack users (2). Clinical experience and some governmental data suggest that most surveys underestimate the number of cocaine addicts in the United States. Surveying only 10 cities, the Department of Justice identified about 650,000 cocaine addicts through urine testing (33).

As with amphetamines, cocaine dependence is associated with either of two patterns of self-administration: episodic or daily (or almost daily) use. Serious medical, social, and other consequences have been reported with daily use, episodic use, and even experimental use. Cocaine use separated by 2 or more days of nonuse is episodic. "Binges" are characterized by use that typically involve continuous high-dose use over a period of hours or days. Binges usually terminate only when cocaine supplies are depleted, or the user is so exhausted that they "pass out," or so experienced that they realize that a rest is necessary for neurotransmitter repletion and renewed feeling of cocaine's euphoric effects. In chronic daily use, there are generally no wide fluctuations in dose on successive days; rather, it is an increase in dose over time. Cocaine and crack use are reported to occur in all groups and among all demographic groups, at all levels of society.

Crack use is associated with binge use, addiction, urban decay, crime, and violence. Cocaine hydrochloride also causes these consequences. Just being shot appears to be associated with the presence of cocaine in the blood. Commission of a felony is similarly highly associated with the presence of cocaine or another illicit drug in the body of the perpetrator. Still, the association between crack, violence, and medical emergencies is compelling. A way of measuring the impact of cocaine and then crack use is by looking at changes in emergency room (ER) visits. Between 1976 and 1986 there was a 15-fold increase in the number of emergency room visits because of cocaine use and in the number of admissions to public treatment programs for cocaine use (34). These were cocaine hydrochloride effects. Cocaine-related ER visits jumped again by 86% in 1987, largely because of the invention and use of crack (35). In 1994, emergency room visits were rising again.

DAWN recently reported a significant increase in ER mentions of cocaine, from 174,881 in 2000 to 193,034 in 2001 (4). Nearly 1 in 4 drug-related ER visits involved some combination of drugs and alcohol (36). A 1988 survey by DAWN found that 1 of 4 cocaine-related ER visits was related to crack smoking, compared with 1 of 20 in the previous survey (37). In 2001, 24% of the emergency mentions continued to be attributed to crack. In 1989, cocaine was the number one cause of emergency room visits in Washington, DC, and New York, as well as in Atlanta, Baltimore, Chicago, Indianapolis, Detroit, Los Angeles, New Orleans, and many other cities (38). By 2001, cocaine was the most frequently reported drug in emergency room visits nationwide, with 76 visits per 100,000 population. Rates in some metropolitan areas far exceeded the national rates. Nine cities had double the national rate of cocaine emergency visits in 2001, and Atlanta, Chicago, and Philadelphia had rates triple the national rate.

Drug use is common among arrestees, and it has been reported that more than 70% of arrestees in major cities such as New York, Philadelphia, and Washington, DC, tested positive for one or more drugs, usually including cocaine (39). Recent cocaine use is associated with a range of adverse outcomes including reckless driving (32) and violent premature deaths, including homicides, suicides, and accidents (40). Autopsies revealed the presence of cocaine in more than 18% of motor vehicle fatalities in New York City between 1984 and 1987 (41). These data are consistent with the driving impaired report of Brookhoff (32). It is likely that the well-known direct effects of cocaine—feelings of alertness, euphoria, aggressiveness, irritability, psychotic distortions and increased risk-taking behavior—diminish a driver's ability to control the vehicle (34,42). It is evident that cocaine is a major cause of traumatic accidents (43). Cocaine and cocaine in combination with alcohol were the most commonly mentioned in suicide cases in 2001. Cocaine is consistently among the top three drugs mentioned in mortality data from DAWN (5).

Cocaine has changed society in other ways as well. It has changed professional and nonprofessional sports. It has altered the process by which businesses screen job candidates and has led to the development of employee assistance programs in the workplace. It has thwarted decades of progress in international diplomacy and threatened the relationships between our nation and other parts of the world.

The proportion of individuals abusing psychoactive substances, legal and illegal, remains at alarming levels in the United States. According to a comprehensive report by the Robert Wood Johnson Foundation (44), substance abuse is the number one health problem in the United States, with more deaths and disabilities from substance abuse than from any other preventable cause. The Robert Wood Johnson Foundation also reports a direct link between illicit drugs (including cocaine) and violent crime.

Our own recent reports correlate illicit drug use with carrying weapons and violence among sixth through twelfth grade students (45).

As a result of widespread education and prevention and the harsh reality that most Americans knew or could readily identify with a victim of the cocaine epidemic, self-reported perception of danger ("using cocaine once or twice") has increased throughout the 1980s and with it cocaine use fell. However, continued decreases in addictive use did not follow and recent use has rebounded since 1993. In summary, dramatic changes in the patterns of cocaine use, the typical dosage, and the route of administration have combined to produce a deadly epidemic of addiction to a drug once touted by medical experts as "safe." Experimental use has decreased in response to massive reeducation of the American people. However, addiction continues to be a major public health problem and rates of adolescent use may have begun a new upward trend.

COCAINE INTOXICATION AND ADDICTION

By claiming that cocaine was relatively harmless and dismissing the notion that the drug could be addictive, medical experts ignored Freud's own observation, published in an 1887 paper, that cocaine was "a far more dangerous enemy to health than morphine" (46). The result was that cocaine was essentially field-tested on the public, with deadly results.

Many people whose use of cocaine could be described as "moderate" or "recreational" claimed that cocaine was not addictive. A June 1990 survey of callers to the National Helpline found that even callers using cocaine once or twice a week (the "recreational" users) report severe problems stemming from their drug use. Cocaine is taken for the positive or expected cocaine intoxication state. Table 13.1 reproduces the criteria for cocaine intoxication listed in the *Diagnostic and Statistical Manual of Mental Disorders*, 4th ed. (*DSM–IV*). Acute intoxication with high doses of cocaine may be associated with rambling speech, headache, transient ideas of reference, and tinnitus. There may also be paranoid ideation, auditory hallucinations in a clear sensorium, and tactile hallucinations ("coke bugs"), which the user usually recognizes as effects of cocaine. Extreme anger with threats or acting out of aggressive behavior may occur. Mood changes such as depression, suicidal ideation, irritability, anhedonia, emotional lability, or disturbances in attention and concentration are common. After oral administration, cocaine concentrations in the blood rise slowly, peaking approximately 1 hour after ingestion. Behavioral effects of the drug tend to follow the same curve. In contrast, intranasal use produces a quicker onset of drug effects, shorter duration of action, and higher peak blood levels. Hence the addiction potential of intranasal cocaine abuse is higher than that of oral use, largely because of the more rapid onset of

TABLE 13.1. *Diagnostic criteria for cocaine intoxication*

A. Recent use of cocaine
B. Clinically significant maladaptive behavioral or psychological changes: euphoria or affective blunting; changes in sociability; hypervigilance; interpersonal sensitivity; anxiety, tension, or anger; stereotyped behaviors; impaired judgment; impaired social or occupational functioning that developed during or shortly after use of cocaine.
C. Two (or more) of the following, developing during, or shortly after, cocaine use:
  (1) tachycardia or bradycardia
  (2) pupillary dilation
  (3) elevated or lowered blood pressure
  (4) perspiration or chills
  (5) nausea or vomiting
  (6) evidence of weight loss
  (7) psychomotor agitation or retardation
  (8) muscular weakness, respiratory depression, chest pain, or cardiac arrhythmias
  (9) confusion, seizures, dyskinesias, dystonias, or coma
D. The symptoms are not due to a general medical condition and are not better accounted for by another mental disorder.

From American Psychiatric Association. 292.89 Cocaine intoxication. In: *Diagnostic and statistical manual of mental disorders*, 4th ed. Washington, DC: Author, 1994: 224–225, with permission.

pharmacologic effects. Today, we know that cocaine use leads to addiction. In 2000, 22.5% (0.7 million) of cocaine users met *DSM–IV* criteria for cocaine dependence or abuse (47).

Addiction Liability

Clearly, the addictive power of cocaine is deceptive. In fact, most users who deny that they are addicted cannot say no to cocaine if it is made available. Typically, addicts continue to seek the drug even though their lives are being destroyed. Cocaine must produce a state similar to a delusion in users. Loved ones see a fragile, sickly, imperiled addict; at the same time, the users say that they see nothing of the kind and are simply fine. Our past failure to recognize the delusionary and addictive power of cocaine is in part responsible for the cocaine epidemic (48).

A person's susceptibility to cocaine addiction depends to a large degree on the dose, duration, and route of administration. Anecdotal data suggest that cocaine smokers are twice as likely to fail to complete their treatment program as are intranasal abusers. Other elements that determine addiction susceptibility are (a) the psychological and physical changes brought about by drug use, (b) the degree of that change, (c) the speed of onset of the change, (d) the duration of change, and (e) the postdrug effects (49).

Cocaine tends to be less addictive if the dose is small, the peak plasma levels low, the onset of activity slow, the duration of action long, and the unpleasant withdrawal effects absent or very mild. If cocaine is taken by means of chewed coca leaves, through oral ingestion, or, to some extent, through intranasal use, consequences are generally slow to develop. Swallowing or snorting cocaine is an inefficient way of using the drug, because cocaine penetrates biologic membranes poorly. Hepatic biotransformation prevents 70% to 80% of the oral or intranasal dose from reaching the circulatory system (50).

Intravenous (i.v.) cocaine use ranks higher on the addiction potential scale than intranasal use. Given unlimited access to the drug, i.v. cocaine abusers will escalate the dose until they deteriorate physically and mentally. The onset of the i.v. cocaine "rush" is within 30 to 45 seconds, and the drug's effects last for 10 to 20 minutes. Peak blood levels can be more than twice those that occur following intranasal ingestion. What is more, 100% of an i.v. dose is delivered to the circulatory system, compared with 20% to 30% of an intranasal dose (49). For many reasons—pain of injection, difficulty of finding and using needles and syringes, risk of infectious disease—i.v. administration is less appealing to cocaine abusers than other administration methods.

Given the parameters that define addiction susceptibility, choosing to take cocaine in any smokable form has the highest addictive potential. Cocaine can be smoked as coca paste, as freebase, or as crack, which is freebase prepared by a different method. The popularity of crack compared with freebase is largely a product of marketing techniques that make small amounts of high-quality cocaine available at low prices and without having to undertake a dangerous chemical process to convert cocaine to a smokable form.

In actuality, smoking is not the most efficient system for delivering cocaine to the body; a significant portion of the drug dose is lost to pyrolysis. Nonetheless, the remaining dose produces potent effects. The resulting high is intense—some users describe it as "full-body orgasm." The onset is extremely rapid; only 8 to 10 seconds elapse before the user experiences the high. The concentration of the drug in the brain also occurs more rapidly than following i.v. use, resulting in greater behavioral effects.

Addiction implies goal-directed behavior aimed at finding and using cocaine to produce maximal euphoria. The user is not primarily focused on neural adaptation or withdrawal. Recent studies have tried to separate addiction from neural adaptation by comparing volitional self-administration from passive drug injections, which are involuntary. Not only does addiction develop in the former, but neurochemical changes appear maximized during the self-administration model. In a study of nonhuman primates, after only five sessions, cocaine self-administration reduced glucose utilization in several areas of the mesolimbic system, and metabolic activity was increased in the dorsolateral and dorsomedial prefrontal cortex and in the mediodorsal nucleus of the thalamus (51). Porrino and colleagues conclude that the involvement of areas of the brain that subserve working memory suggests that there may be strong associations between cocaine and the internal and external environment are formed from the very beginning of cocaine use. It is as if wanting to be high and finding and self-administering cocaine combine to produce maximal brain-rewarding and dependency-producing effects. Chronic self-administration of cocaine, but not passive receipt of the same doses at the same frequency, in yoked animals is associated with addiction and markedly elevated dopamine (DA) and serotonin levels. These brain neurochemical effects can be followed in the amygdala, suggesting altered neuronal activity in this brain area underlies drug-seeking behavior. The amygdala receives dopaminergic innervation from the ventral tegmental area and serotonergic innervation from the midbrain and pontine raphe, as well as extensive communication from the nucleus accumbens. Although the nucleus accumbens plays a critical role in the reinforcing properties of cocaine and other stimulants the amygdala might be involved in the acquisition of stimulus–reward associations or the motivational aspects of drug seeking (52). The danger and allure of the streets may actually increase the reinforcing potency of crack cocaine.

Also contributing to the addiction potential of crack is the fact that the effects of the drug last only 5 to 10 minutes. After the high is over, the crack user feels anxious, depressed, and paranoid. Such a rapid shift between the drug's positive and negative effects makes users crave another "hit" of the drug to restore the euphoria they felt just moments before. These cravings form a distinct part of the withdrawal syndrome associated with cocaine.

Withdrawal symptoms are the inverse of cocaine's effects. Most troubling to the clinician and addict is the dysphoria and drive for a cocaine remedy so typically reported by crack addicts. Removal of the withdrawal anhedonia by taking crack, is another positive reinforcer, adding to addiction liability of cocaine and crack. Cocaine withdrawal symptoms (Table 13.2) include decreased energy, dysphoric and anhedonic psychomotor retarded state with concurrent limited interest in the environment, and limited ability to experience pleasure. These symptoms are mildest immediately following cessation of cocaine use, but increase in intensity and remind the addict that this state is cocaine-reversible during the next 96 hours (50).

For years experts assumed cocaine was not addictive; however, *DSM–IV* now acknowledges that cocaine causes addiction and establishes criteria for dependence and for cocaine withdrawal (see Table 13.2).

NEUROBIOLOGIC EFFECTS OF COCAINE USE

For an extensive review of the neurobiology of cocaine see Chapter 12. Cocaine's addictive potential is the result

TABLE 13.2. *Diagnostic criteria for cocaine withdrawal*

A. Cessation of (or reduction in) cocaine use that has been heavy and prolonged.
B. Dysphoric mood and two (or more) of the following physiological changes, developing within a few hours to several days after Criterion A:
   (1) fatigue
   (2) unpleasant dreams
   (3) insomnia or hypersomnia
   (4) increased appetite
   (5) psychomotor retardation or agitation
C. The symptoms in Criterion B cause clinically significant distress or impairment in social, occupational, or other important areas of functioning.
D. The symptoms are not due to a general medical condition and are not better accounted for by another mental disorder.

From American Psychiatric Association. 292.0 Cocaine withdrawal. In: *Diagnostic and statistical manual of mental disorders*, 4th ed. Washington, DC: Author, 1994:225–226, with permission.

of the interaction of goal-directed volitional self-administration and profound drug-related effects on many of the most critical neurochemical systems of the brain. Although amphetamine has a number of direct DA-releasing and DA-storing vesicle effects, both amphetamine and cocaine produce positive reinforcement, blocking the reuptake of DA into the presynaptic neuron and causing an acute increase in synaptic DA availability. By preventing DA reuptake, greater concentrations of DA remain in the synaptic cleft with more DA available at the postsynaptic site for stimulation of receptors. The abnormally high levels of DA in the synapse inhibit the firing rate of dopaminergic cells. Numerous studies support the positive reinforcement effects associated with increased synaptic levels of DA. Recent laboratory research establishes that cocaine acts directly on the so-called reward pathways. These pathways are indirectly activated by pleasurable stimuli from other activities, including eating, drinking, and sex. So powerful is the direct stimulation provided by cocaine that sleep, safety, money, morality, loved ones, responsibility, and even survival become largely irrelevant to the cocaine user. In a sense, cocaine "short circuits" the process by which people normally achieve gratification and security (53). Cocaine access to primitive brain reward mechanisms appears to be the target of cocaine self-administration.

A primary effect of cocaine in the brain is to block the presynaptic reuptake of neurotransmitters, including serotonin, norepinephrine, and DA. Cocaine binds to the presynaptic transporter complexes inhibiting reuptake of DA, noradrenaline, and serotonin, prolonging monoamine neurotransmission. The reinforcing properties of cocaine are believed to be associated with enhanced dopaminergic neurotransmission in mesocorticolimbic pathways. Hence there is a surplus of these neurotransmitters at the postsynaptic receptor sites (54). This surplus, in turn, activates responses along the sympathetic nervous system, producing such effects as vasoconstriction and acute increases in heart rate and blood pressure (55,56). A receptor for cocaine has been identified in the brain and this receptor appears to be the cocaine binding site on the DA transporter on dopaminergic nerve terminals (57). By interfering with neurochemical activity, cocaine acts in many ways like a neuromodulatory neurotransmitter. Starting with the hypothesis that activation of DA systems in the mesocorticolimbic areas of the brain are responsible for the motor and reinforcing effects of cocaine, DA activation is essential in most, if not all, drug reinforcement (58). Petit (59) showed that the elevation of synaptic levels of DA in response to cocaine is augmented in the nucleus accumbens after repeated administration, explaining users' reports of continued and sometimes increasing euphoria early in a binge. Kalivas and Duffy (60) placed dialysis probes in the ventral tegmental area DA cell bodies that terminate in the nucleus accumbens; this gave evidence for a specific role for this neural structure in sensitization. Petit and Justice (61), using microdialysis in the nucleus accumbens, demonstrated that extracellular DA levels are increased during cocaine self-administration, with the behavior directed toward attaining specific, almost optimal, DA levels. DA levels attained were dose dependent and correlated with increased cocaine intake (62). DA neurons and DA release appear to demonstrate tolerance and diminished responses to chronic self-administration consistent with the notion of a functional DA deficit over time. By preventing DA reuptake, greater concentrations of DA remain in the synaptic cleft, with more DA available at the postsynaptic site for brain reinforcement, reward, or stimulation of specific salience supporting receptors. Cocaine reward or a particular drug experience is commonly explained by addicts in terms such as "hunger," "taste," and "sex." This may not be at all a coincidence. Users, by their choice of words and descriptions, may be confirming the similarities in critical brain sites for natural and drug reward. The nucleus accumbens and DA are critical in food, drinking, and sex reward (63,64), as well as drug reward.

More recently, investigators using a binge administration paradigm found that cocaine significantly lowers basal DA levels and alters the pattern but not the magnitude of the response to cocaine itself (65). Binge use is supported by the cocaine-DA connection. It is, therefore, well accepted that the mesolimbic and mesocortical dopaminergic systems are critical in the acute and binge reinforcing effects of cocaine and also cocaine-induced euphoria. Volkow and colleagues have characterized cocaine binding in the brain to a high-affinity on the DA transporter using positron emission tomography (PET)

TABLE 13.3. *Effects of cocaine*[a]

Generally enjoyable effects with great increase in
self-image. A rapid onset of "high" with the following
components:

1. Euphoria, seldom dysphoria
2. Increased sense of energy
3. Enhanced mental acuity
4. Increased sensory awareness (sexual, auditory,
   tactile, visual)
5. Decreased appetite (anorexia)
6. Increased anxiety and suspiciousness
7. Decreased need of sleep
8. Postponement of fatigue
9. Increased self-confidence, egocentricity
10. Delusions—dependence
11. Physical symptoms of a generalized sympathetic
    discharge

[a]Low to average doses (25–150 mg) (approximately 20–30
mg/line).

and tracer doses of [^{11}C]cocaine in the baboon *in vivo*
(66). At subpharmacologic doses, [^{11}C]cocaine binds
predominantly to a high-affinity site on the DA transporter.
Using PET and [^{11}C]cocaine, Volkow demonstrated cocaine binding to DA transporters *in vivo*. Because the
studies with [^{11}C]cocaine were done at subpharmacologic
levels of cocaine, [^{11}C]cocaine's binding to the DA transporter probably represented high-affinity sites. This may,
however, not be the only pharmacologically relevant binding site when cocaine is administered in behaviorally active, pharmacologic doses.

There is a wealth of evidence implicating DA in incentive motivational effects of drugs as well as of food, sex,
and other natural incentives (67–70). The treatment conundrum is how to have a treatment dose, power of therapy,
or incentives that can match the access and reinforcement
produced by cocaine.

The influence of cocaine use on the structure of neurons
in brain regions that contribute to its rewarding effects have
been studied in rat self-administration models. Robinson
and colleagues found that cocaine self-administration appears to alter patterns of synaptic connectivity within the
limbocortical circuitry, which may contribute to cocaine's
incentive motivational effects (71). They also found that
cocaine self administration may have neuropathologic effects in frontal areas of the brain that are involved in decision making and judgment. Both of these cocaine-induced
neuroadaptations may be involved in the development of
addiction.

Table 13.3 lists the basic effects of cocaine; Table 13.4
compares the drug's effects following different routes of
administration. The precise psychological and behavioral
effects depend on many factors: the purity of the drug,
route of administration, chronicity of use, the personality
and mental health of the user, past and present use of drugs
and alcohol, the environment in which the drug is used,
and other drugs taken simultaneously.

CLINICAL PHARMACOLOGY

The purer the drug, the greater its effects. As a rule, pure
cocaine is unavailable on the street. Instead, cocaine is usually adulterated with other substances such as mannitol,
lactose, or glucose to add weight, and caffeine, lidocaine,
amphetamines, quinine, or even heroin to add taste and
to provide additional central nervous system (CNS) stimulant effects (72). The typical concentration of cocaine
in street preparations ranges from 10% to 50%; rarely,
samples can contain as much as 70% cocaine. Both the
cocaine concentration and the adulterants affect the user's
response to the drug.

Whether a user enjoys or dislikes cocaine may depend on the individual's normal level of excitation,
which is controlled by the adrenergic system, the thyroid

TABLE 13.4. *Differential effects dependent on routes of cocaine administration*

Route	Mode	Action (sec)	"High" (min)	Dose (mg)	Peak plasma (ng/mL)	Purity (%)	Bioavailability absorbed
Oral	Coca leaf chewing	300–600	45–90	20–50	150	0.5–1	—
Oral	Cocaine HCl	600–1800		100–200	150–200	20–80	20–30
Intranasal	Cocaine HCl "Snorting"	120–180	30–45	5 × 30	150	20–80	20–30
Intravenous	Cocaine HCl	30–45	10–20	25–50 / >200	300–400 / 1,000–1,500	7–100 × 58	100
Smoking	Coca paste	8–10	5–10	60–250	300–800	40–85	6–32
Intrapulmonary	Freebase				250–1000	800–900	90–100
Crack						?	50–95

From Verebey K, Gold MS. From coca leaves to crack: the effects of dose and routes of administration in abuse
liability. *Psychiatr Ann* 1988;18:514, with permission.

hormone thyroxin, and other regulators (49). Certain people in their normal state are more subdued, while others are more excitable. Because cocaine stimulates the CNS, a person with a low level of arousal or excitement may be more likely to enjoy the changes in alertness and energy cocaine provides. On the other hand, people who are normally hyperexcited may feel uncomfortable and dysphoric, and may even develop paranoid psychosis as a consequence of the major sympathetic discharge triggered by cocaine.

Once consumed, cocaine triggers the series of physiologic responses that make up the natural "fight or flight" response to an impending threat. By affecting the release and reuptake of epinephrine, cocaine causes a shift in the blood supply from the skin and the viscera into the skeletal musculature. Oxygen levels rise, as do concentrations of sugar in the blood. After the acute dose of cocaine wears off, the user's body usually returns to its more normal state. Following chronic use, however, the body's reservoirs of neurotransmitters and hormones may be depleted. In addition, the drug may compromise the body's ability to regenerate these biochemicals. As a result, the chronic user may experience symptoms of withdrawal (48).

The cocaine-induced feeling of increased alertness is reported subjectively and can be confirmed by electroencephalogram and electrocardiogram recordings, which show a general desynchronization of brain waves after cocaine administration (73). Such desynchronization, which indicates arousal, occurs in the part of the brain that is thought to be involved in the regulation of conscious awareness, attention, and sleep. Despite the feeling of arousal, individuals using cocaine do not gain any particular superior ability or greater knowledge. Their sense of omnipotence is only an illusion; they tend to misinterpret their enhanced confidence and lowered inhibitions as signs of enhanced physical or mental acuity. The motivational symptoms of drug withdrawal are presumably mediated by molecular and cellular adaptations to chronic cocaine exposure but appear to occur in brain regions also associated with reinforcement. Cocaine is self-administered directly into the prefrontal cortex although dopaminergic innervation of this structure is not essential for maintaining intravenous self-administration.

The nucleus accumbens is a central hub in a functional circuit that allows drug reinforcement to occur through simultaneous activation of multiple reward sites and is considered a logical final common anatomic target for drugs acting on receptors in other reinforcing nuclei. The G-protein– cyclic adenosine monophosphate (cAMP) system in the nucleus accumbens is involved in acute drug reinforcement and is an important component of the adaptations that occur during chronic drug self-administration (74).

Through its impact on neurotransmitters, particularly DA, cocaine can affect sexual excitation. Cocaine used intravenously or in smokable form can produce sponta-

neous ejaculation without direct genital stimulation (75). In extreme cases, cocaine even replaces the sex partner. Tolerance to the sexual stimulation of cocaine develops rapidly, sometimes resulting in impotence or sexual frigidity. Cocaine use can therefore replace the natural sex drive, which, in turn, threatens long-term relationships and can disrupt family stability. In some cases, addicts trade sexual favors for crack. During a short period of time these persons may have sex with many partners, putting themselves and others at risk of infection (76).

By inactivating the feeding center located in the lateral hypothalamus, cocaine also supersedes the primary eating drive, thus leading to severe loss of appetite and loss of body weight. Cocaine is commonly used by women with and without primary eating disorders to curb appetite or lose weight. The cocaine user's decreased need for sleep may also result from the drug's effects on neurotransmitters, including serotonin, which at times functions as the "sleep transmitter."

Many clinical manifestations of cocaine intoxication are also found in cases of hyperthyroidism. Some of these manifestations include hypertension, hyperkinesis, sweating, rapid heartbeat, tremor, anxiety, and hyperthermia. Conversely, the cocaine "crash" following use shares many of the signs and symptoms with the hypothyroid state: low energy, depression, bradykinesia, weight gain, and hypersomnia. From such evidence, it can be assumed that cocaine activates the thyroid axis (77).

DA inhibits secretion of prolactin. Hyperprolactinemia is the endocrine abnormality most often reported in clinical studies of cocaine abusers (78), with clear elevations in prolactin observed during abuse and withdrawal (79–86) and in animals. Loss of interest in sex and poor sexual performance noted by cocaine addicts may be related to this DA-prolactin release from inhibition.

Another neuroendocrine abnormality related to the DA deficiency hypothesis is the study by Hollander (87), in which recently abstinent cocaine users had a 580% peak growth hormone response to apomorphine. Symptoms included gynecomastia, galactorrhea, and sexual dysfunctions such as infertility, impotence, and amenorrhea.

Laboratory evidence suggests that cocaine can cause adrenocortical hypertrophy, stimulating the release of high doses of cortisol in animals. It is possible that similar effects occur in humans. Hence another aspect of cocaine use may be its impact on the hypothalamic–pituitary–adrenal (HPA) axis (77). Goeders suggest that there are three or more general behavioral phases in the etiology of drug self-administration: acquisition, maintenance, and reinstatement (88). Corticosterone and corticotropin-releasing hormone (CRH), especially the CRH1 receptor, are critical for the stress- and cue-induced reinstatement of extinguished cocaine-seeking behavior, demonstrating an involvement of the HPA axis in the relapse to cocaine use as well (89). One recent review suggests that HPA-axis-suppressing medications are unlikely to completely block cocaine's reinforcing effects, but they may help to decrease the frequency of use by increasing the addict's resistance to stress-induced relapse (90).

Cocaine users report feeling more alert and more energetic. This reaction, in turn, produces a tremendous increase in self-confidence, self-image, and egocentricity; in some individuals this manifests as megalomania and feelings of omnipotence. Some groups, including athletes, salespeople, entertainers, musicians, and physicians, sometimes use cocaine to provide them with these effects, to enhance their energy, confidence, and "star image."

But there are limits to the degree to which CNS activity can be artificially stimulated. After chronic use, or following a prolonged binge, symptoms of depression, lack of motivation, sleeplessness, paranoia, irritability, and outright acute toxic psychosis may develop (48). States of severe transient panic accompanied by a terror of impending death can occur in persons with no preexisting psychopathologic conditions, as can paranoid psychoses (34,91,92). Because it affects the supply of acetylcholine, cocaine can lead to mental confusion and loss of coordination (93).

Clinicians focus on the rapidity of deterioration, addiction, and change. The tremendous attachment for cocaine and desire to repeat the pleasurable aspects of the cocaine experience and to counteract the depressive effects of the postcocaine crash can lead to compulsive chronic use of the drug. Such activity leads to a decrease or depletion in the neurotransmitter supply. The long-term results of such depletion include overt depression, dysphoria, hallucinatory experiences, and destructive antisocial behavior. More subtle changes in behavior include irritability, hypervigilance, psychomotor agitation, and impaired interpersonal relations (34). Cocaine is known to worsen the symptomatology of depression. People with major depression are likely to experience dysphoria after cocaine use, although in other individuals, cocaine acts like an antidepressant. Chronic cocaine use may lead to long-lasting and selective disruptions in serotonin pathways, which may be a neurochemical basis for mood changes that are commonly reported during cocaine withdrawal (94). Paranoia is another commonly seen product of cocaine abuse. In its ability to induce a state resembling functional paranoid psychosis, cocaine is similar to other central stimulants, including amphetamines (95).

Use of cocaine can also produce a psychotic syndrome characterized by paranoia, impaired reality testing, anxiety, a stereotyped compulsive repetitive pattern of behavior, and vivid visual, auditory, and tactile hallucinations such as the delusion that insects are crawling under the skin (84). Subjective and clinical data also show that cocaine can induce panic attacks (96).

A further complication of cocaine abuse is that many users ameliorate some of the unpleasant stimulating effects of the drug by concomitantly or subsequently ingesting sedating agents such as alcohol or marijuana (34,50).

The combined use of cocaine and alcohol is common, with reports of 62% to 90% of cocaine abusers also being concurrent ethanol abusers (97). Cocaine users report that concurrent ethanol use prolongs the "high" and attenuates a number of the unpleasant physical and psychological effects of cocaine. Cocaethylene, the ethyl ester of benzoylecgonine, is similar to cocaine in neurochemical and pharmacologic properties and behavioral effects. Cocaethylene binds to the DA transporter blocking DA uptake and increasing extracellular concentrations of DA in the nucleus accumbens; but unlike cocaine, it has little effect on the serotonin transporter. While similar to cocaine and having at least addictive effects on heart rate and reward, there are reports of increased lethality. Autopsies revealed that between 1984 and 1987, 56% of all drivers killed in traffic accidents in New York City had used either cocaine, alcohol, or both (41).

Cocaine memory of euphoria appears to peak immediately preceding cocaine self-administration and to be important in supporting a cocaine binge. Vivid, long-term memories of being high tend to persecute the drug abuser by invoking powerful cravings for the next high (34). Cocaine users describe intense craving for cocaine when cocaine is made available to them, or merely when the word cocaine is uttered in conversation. Seeing places or people where cocaine was used, smelling cocaine, seeing a cocaine pipe, seeing a friend who they used cocaine with, hearing a song that they used cocaine to, and numerous other casual smells, sights, and sounds can trigger an intense reaction in the user or the person who has used in the past but is now abstinent (98). Users report tasting cocaine, craving cocaine, sweating, feeling faint and short of breath, smelling cocaine, and feeling a little of the cocaine euphoria. All of these experiences contribute to cocaine taking and the persistence of cocaine dependence. In humans, even the presentation of cocaine paraphernalia after weeks or months of abstinence produces intense cravings and withdrawal-like symptoms (99,100). In experimental studies in humans, individuals with a history of cocaine use show greater physiologic reactivity in response to cocaine cues than do cocaine-naive individuals. The greater responses were also demonstrated to cocaine stimuli rather than to powerful opiate cues. Cocaine-related stimuli elicit conditioned physiologic and subjective states in cocaine users (101).

Many cocaine-dependent individuals also respond to drug cues in the human laboratory. They report increased craving for cocaine and have clear physiologic evidence of intense arousal. Such changes are being tested as treatment predictors and strategies for treatment itself. In a cue-reactivity protocol that concluded with relaxation exercises, patients who achieved abstinence were predicted by craving reported after relaxation training. Patients who subsequently initiated abstinence reported a reduction in cue-elicited craving to below baseline levels while those who did not succeed in treatment remained elevated (102).

As is discussed later in the section "Treatment of Cocaine Addiction," these cravings are one of the most difficult aspects in weaning addicts from cocaine.

MEDICAL COMPLICATIONS OF COCAINE ABUSE

The medical and psychiatric complications associated with cocaine use are so numerous (103) and severe that it would take an entire book to describe them completely. Benowitz (104) recently reviewed the organ toxicity of cocaine, including toxic paranoid psychosis, panic disorder, suicide, convulsions, cerebrovascular accidents, cardiotoxicity, and hepatotoxicity. Among the complications are cardiovascular effects, including arrhythmias and myocardial infarctions; respiratory effects, such as chest pain and respiratory failure; neurologic effects, such as seizure and headache; gastrointestinal complications, including abdominal pain and nausea; and many others. For the purposes of this chapter, a brief description of cocaine's far-ranging and troubling medical consequences must suffice.

Cardiovascular System

The first clinical report of cocaine abuse-associated cardiac toxicity appeared in 1978 (105). A review of the recent medical literature reveals that cocaine use has been linked to virtually every type of heart disease (106).

Cocaine produces a number of cardiovascular effects that may lead to the development of different forms of arrhythmia. Tachycardia often occurs within minutes of cocaine ingestion. Other forms of arrhythmia associated with cocaine use include sinus bradycardia, ventricular premature depolarization, ventricular tachycardia degenerating to defibrillation, and asystole. Crumb and Clarkson (107) suggest that cocaine may induce arrhythmias because it slows impulse conduction by blocking cardiac sodium channels. Tachycardia is also partly caused by cocaine's local anesthetic activity and by indirect stimulation of α receptors (108). One study found a greater acceleration in heart rate and blood pressure associated with cocaine smoking than with i.v. cocaine use (109).

Cocaine is known to elevate blood pressure through adrenergic stimulation. The pressor effects of cocaine continue to rise as dosage increases (110). The sudden increase in blood pressure may cause spontaneous bleeding in people with normal blood pressure and may underlie many incidents of cerebrovascular accidents associated with cocaine use (111).

Evidence suggests that cocaine can induce spasms in a number of vascular systems, including the coronary arteries (112). These spasms can produce myocardial infarction even in a person whose endothelium is otherwise intact (113). The pathologic changes in the vasculature, regardless of route of cocaine self-administration, that place individuals at high risk for a cardiovascular or cerebrovascular accident appear to include arteriolar thickening, increased perivascular deposits of collagen and glycoprotein, and inflammation (114).

Most of the case reports of cocaine-related cardiovascular toxicity involve myocardial infarctions, which may occur regardless of dosage level or route of administration (115). Cocaine increases myocardial oxygen consumption, but at the same time it interferes with the coronary circulation's ability to adjust to this increased demand by decreasing its resistance to blood flow. Cocaine users also frequently develop silent myocardial ischemia (116). This problem may also arise during the first weeks of withdrawal. So common is the incidence of myocardial infarction caused by cocaine that its occurrence in young patients who lack the usual coronary risk factors suggests a diagnosis of cocaine abuse (117).

In one study (118), whole-body timed distribution of pharmacologic doses of C-cocaine was studied in rats using quantitative autoradiographic microimaging. Rapid, intense uptake was seen in the brain, spinal cord, adrenals, and nuchal brown fat pad. Cocaine appears to bind in the brain to the DA transporter and, to a lesser extent, to transporters for norepinephrine and serotonin. Microvascular spasm may also be a major factor in producing thallium-201 defects in the presence of normal coronaries. In patients with nominal narrowing coronaries, cocaine-induced microvascular spasm may cause coronary thrombosis and infarction. The demonstration of cocaine binding in the heart and its time sequence is of relevance in understanding the cardiotoxicity of cocaine. Further support on the relevance of direct effect of cocaine on the heart is given by our studies showing decreased myocardial perfusion in naive anesthetized animals. These studies indicate that central effects are not essential in causing cardiovascular perturbations.

Cocaine addiction can accelerate coronary atherosclerosis. Cocaine use by patients with premature artery disease can exacerbate the problem and may result in death (119). Either directly or indirectly, cocaine may affect platelets, possibly causing them to form thrombi that can plug small vessels (120). Finally, long-term abuse of cocaine may lead to interstitial fibrosis and eventually to congestive heart failure (121). The cardiac effects of cocaine were previously treated with propranolol and may respond to the calcium channel blocker nitrendipine (77). The β blockers should be avoided in cocaine-induced myocardial infarction because the coronary spasm may worsen (122).

Myocardial infarction with normal coronary arteries is a syndrome that can result from several conditions, but cocaine users and cigarette smokers are more prone to develop this condition. Mechanisms causing this syndrome include coronary embolism; hypercoagulable states; oxygen imbalances; intense sympathetic stimulation; coronary vasospasm; coronary trauma; nonatherosclerotic coronary diseases; coronary thrombosis; and endothelial dysfunction. The clinical presentation is similar to that of myocardial infarction with coronary atherosclerosis, but this syndrome primarily affects individuals younger than 40.

Cocaine use is also associated with both acute renal failure and hypertension (HTN), and may lead to a chronic insidious form of renal failure. In one recent study of hemodialysis patients with and without a diagnosis of HTN-related end-stage renal disease (HTN-ESRD), a history of significant cocaine use before dialysis was reported by 28.5% of the patients (123). Diagnosis of HTN-ESRD was reported in 89.1% of cocaine users, as compared with 46.38% in nonusers (115). End-stage renal disease in patients without a clear cause of renal failure may be related to cocaine use. Renal infarction and aortic thrombus have been reported and are associated with nasal cocaine use (124).

Respiratory System

Smoking crack can induce severe chest pain or dyspnea (125). One explanation for this effect may be that cocaine significantly reduces the ability of the lungs to diffuse carbon monoxide (126). Often it is this symptom of chest pain that drives patients to seek medical attention.

Other respiratory effects of cocaine smoking include lung damage; pneumonia; pulmonary edema; cough; sputum production; fever; hemoptysis; pulmonary barotrauma; pneumomediastinum; pneumothorax; pneumopericardium; and diffuse alveolar hemorrhage (127–129). Cocaine inhalation can cause or contribute to asthma (130). Respiratory failure, resulting from cocaine-induced inhibition of medullary centers in the brain, may lead to sudden death (131). Chronic cocaine inhalation can cause progressive destruction of the hard palate, soft palate (132), septum, nasal cartilage, and can even progress to midfacial osteomyelitis (133).

Recently a new syndrome entered the medical terminology: "*crack lung*" (134). People with this condition present with the symptoms of pneumonia—severe chest pains, breathing problems, high temperatures. Chest x-rays reveal no evidence of pneumonia and the condition does not respond to standard treatments. The condition appears to be an eosinophilic pneumonitis with or without pleural effusions, which are also eosinophilic. Antiinflammatory drugs, specifically corticosteroids, may relieve symptoms of crack lung (135). The illness resolves with corticosteroid treatment. People with this syndrome may suffer oxygen starvation or loss of blood with potentially fatal results. Pneumomediastinum and bilateral pneumothorax have been recently reported (136).

Neurotoxicity

The spectrum of neuropathologic changes encountered in the brains of cocaine abusers is broad, but the major findings consist of ischemic and hemorrhagic stroke, subarachnoid and intracerebral hemorrhages and cerebral ischemia. Especially persons with underlying arteriovenous malformation or aneurysm are at risk for such events. In addition to pharmacologically induced vasospasm, vasculitis, impaired hemostasis and platelet function, and decreased cerebral blood flow appear to play a role. At the cellular level, abnormalities in the expression of transcription factors and changes of brain neurotransmitter systems have been reported (137).

As even Freud was aware, cocaine is an epileptogenic agent that can provoke generalized seizures, even after a single dose (18,138). With repeated administration, the ability of cocaine to produce clonic convulsions increases (139). This phenomenon, known as "*kindling*," may result from sensitization of receptors in the brain. Because seizure disorders can be unmasked or induced by cocaine's kindling effect on the brain, proper medical evaluation of patients must rule out epilepsy (77). In a recent study in mice, the effects of the endogenous cannabinoid anandamide and its analogues were compared to the CB1 agonist CP 55940 on cocaine-induced toxic symptoms. In this study, the CB1 agonists antagonized cocaine-induced convulsive seizures and cocaine-induced lethality (140).

Volkow et al. (141) studied postsynaptic DA receptor density in PET studies using (^{18}F)N-methylspiroperidol. Subjects abstinent for less than 1 week showed significantly lower values for uptake of the ligand in the striatum when compared to non–drug-using control subjects. The subjects abstinent for 4 to 5 weeks showed values comparable to normal. These findings suggest decreased density of postsynaptic DA receptors rather than a change in receptor affinity. Volkow also reported on the Swiss cheese, multiple, often silent, infarcts and neural change associated with cocaine and crack use.

Other researchers' work supports Volkow and indicates that cocaine significantly constricts the cerebral vasculature and can lead to ischemic brain infarction. Cocaine abuse significantly increases the risk of ischemic stroke, primarily through vasospasm of large cranial arteries or within the cortical microvasculature. Increased levels of extracellular dopamine mediate vasospasm. Studies show that dopamine-innervated neurons may regulate cerebral blood flow and regions of the brain that are dopamine-rich may be relatively specific targets for cocaine-induced cerebral ischemia. Dihydropyridine-class calcium channel antagonists inhibit cocaine-mediated dopamine release on neurons involved in vasospasm and the control of cortical circulation (142). Antithrombotic agents might also be useful in alleviating cocaine's neurotoxic effects, but because of the risk of spontaneous hemorrhage, their use is limited. A study comparing aspirin (a platelet aggregate inhibitor) against amiloride, a vasodilator, showed that following treatment, areas of hypoperfusion were improved with amiloride, unchanged with aspirin, and worsened with placebo in comparison to baseline levels. Platelet aggregation after adenosine diphosphate (ADP) showed no significant change during the month, but reduced regional cerebral blood flow (rCBF) significantly improved after a 1-month treatment with amiloride (Midamor) when compared with placebo and cocaine abstinence alone (143). Strickland et al. (144) investigated the long-term effects of intermittent or casual cocaine use in patients without symptoms of stroke or transient ischemic attack. Single-photon emission computed tomography with xenon-133 and (^{99m}Tc)hexamethylpropyleneamine oxime, magnetic resonance imaging, and selected neuropsychological measures were used to study cerebral perfusion, brain morphology, and cognitive functioning. Patients were drug free for at least 6 months before evaluation. All showed regions of significant cerebral hypoperfusion in the frontal, periventricular, and/or temporal–parietal areas. Deficits in attention, concentration, new learning, visual and verbal memory, word production, and visuomotor integration were observed. This study by Strickland and coworkers indicates that long-term cocaine use may produce sustained brain perfusion deficits and persistent neuropsychological compromise. Neurosurgeons have noted that cocaine adversely affects both the presentation of and outcome in patients with aneurysmal systemic arterial hypertension (SAH) who are undergoing treatment for this disease. The vasoactive properties of the drug appear to aggravate the already tenuous situation of SAH and increase both the occurrence and influence of cerebral vasospasm. The interpretation of the results of a large retrospective review indicate that cocaine use negatively affects outcome to such an extent that it should be considered equal to the presence of a major systemic illness (145). As noted, cocaine abuse is associated with intracranial hemorrhage. CNS stimulants such as cocaine can also cause tics, persistent mechanical repetition of speech or movement, ataxia, and disturbed gait, which may disappear after drug use is stopped (146). When high-dose users (2.2 g per day) are drug free for 6 months, they still show decreased brain function and decreased blood flow, suggesting that brain changes may persist long after cessation of use. Marijuana and cocaine are commonly used at the same time. While not entirely clear from anecdotal reports, marijuana may potentiate cocaine's effects. Smoking placebo, 1.24%, or 2.64% tetrahydrocannabinol (THC)-containing marijuana cigarettes followed by 0.9 mg/kg intranasal cocaine in a random design, marijuana pretreatment significantly reduced the latency to peak cocaine euphoria from 1.87 to 0.53 minutes, decreased the duration of dysphoric or bad effects, and increased peak cocaine levels and apparent bioavailability by area under the curve analysis when highest dose marijuana preceded cocaine (147). Marijuana-induced vasodilatation of the nasal mucosa attenuates the vasoconstrictive effects of cocaine and thus increases absorption (148).

A syndrome known as reversible posterior leukoencephalopathy, which is characterized by headache, visual disturbance, nausea, vomiting, depressed level of consciousness, convulsions and sometimes focal neurologic deficits has been reported in an habitual cocaine sniffer in the context of a hypertensive crisis (149). Patients with hypertensive crisis and cocaine abuse could have this syndrome and the diagnosis can be confirmed through neuroimaging.

Impact on Sexuality

Many users claim that cocaine is an aphrodisiac. Indeed, as mentioned earlier, the feeling of sexual excitement that sometimes accompanies cocaine use may be the result of its impact on the DA system and may produce spontaneous orgasm. Nonetheless, chronic cocaine abuse causes derangements in reproductive function including impotence and gynecomastia (148). These symptoms may persist for long periods, even after use of cocaine has stopped. Men who abuse cocaine chronically and in high doses may have difficulty maintaining an erection and ejaculating. Many men report experiencing periods when they completely lose interest in sex (11)—not surprising, perhaps, given the direct effects of cocaine on the primary reward systems of the brain.

In women, cocaine abuse has adverse effects on reproductive function, including derangements in the menstrual cycle function, galactorrhea, amenorrhea, and infertility (11). Some women who use cocaine report having greater difficulty achieving orgasm (150). To be detailed later, in the section entitled Cocaine and Pregnancy, children born to women who use cocaine during pregnancy are at high risk of congenital malformations and perinatal mortality (151).

Other Adverse Effects

Chronic cocaine abuse may induce persistent hyperprolactinemia (152), apparently because it disrupts DA's ability to inhibit prolactin secretion (153). This effect may continue for long periods even after a person has stopped using cocaine (77).

As a result of the drug's effects on the primary eating drive, many individuals who use cocaine compulsively lose their appetites and can experience significant weight loss (154).

Cocaine also produces hyperpyrexia, or extremely elevated body temperatures (54), which can contribute to the development of seizures, life-threatening cardiac arrhythmias, and death (155,156). This effect results from hypermetabolism combined with severe peripheral vasoconstriction and the impact of cocaine on the ability of the thalamus to regulate body heat (157). Experimental evidence suggests that treatment for hyperpyrexia may involve vigorous cooling of the body by immersing the trunk and the extremities in cold water (158).

Several investigators (159–161) implicate cocaine in the development of the muscle-wasting condition known as rhabdomyolysis. Why the drug should produce this effect is unclear. Roth and colleagues (162) suggest that it may arise as a result of arterial vasoconstriction, which can lead to tissue ischemia, or that it may be caused by a direct toxic effect of cocaine on muscle metabolism. A study of 39 patients with acute rhabdomyolysis found that onset was rapid and occurred in previously healthy individuals who used cocaine hydrochloride. A third of this group had acute renal failure, often together with severe hepatic dysfunction and disseminated intravascular coagulation. Seven patients became oliguric and eight required hemodialysis. Six of 13 patients with acute renal failure died, adding yet another fatal side effect to cocaine's already long list.

Sudden death from respiratory or cardiac arrest, myocardial infarction, and stroke are associated with cocaine use among young and otherwise healthy persons. These incidents are probably caused by the ability of cocaine to increase blood pressure, cause vasoconstriction, or alter the electrical activity of the heart. Seizures have been observed in association with cocaine use, as have palpitations and arrhythmias. Traumatic injuries because of disputes resulting in violent behavior are common, especially among persons who sell cocaine.

Different routes of cocaine administration can produce different adverse effects. Intranasal use can lead to sinusitis, loss of the sense of smell, atrophy of the nasal mucosa, nosebleeds, perforation of the nasal septum, problems with swallowing, and hoarseness (163,164). Ingested cocaine can cause severe bowel ischemia or gangrene as a consequence of vasoconstriction and reduced blood flow (165). Persons who inject cocaine have puncture marks and "tracks," most commonly on their forearms, as seen in those with opioid dependence. Human immunodeficiency virus (HIV) infection is associated with cocaine dependence as a result of the frequent intravenous injections and the increase in promiscuous sexual behavior. HIV seropositivity is associated with crack smoking without intravenous use. The clear association between the smoking of crack and high-risk sexual practices has been reported and linked to acceleration in the spread of the HIV virus (166). A study of 2,323 young adults age 18 to 29 years in cities from New York to Miami to San Francisco found a 15.7% HIV-positive rate among crack smokers and 5.2% among noncrack smokers. The prevalence of HIV was highest among crack-smoking women in New York (29.6%) and Miami (23.0%). Further analysis of 283 women who had sex in exchange for money or crack showed 30.4% were infected with HIV. Women who had had unprotected sex in exchange for money or drugs were as likely to be infected with the HIV virus as were men who had had recent anal sex with men. Cuts and burns on the lips from smoking crack cocaine are also associated with positive HIV serostatus, even after controlling for the amount of oral sex (167).

Other sexually transmitted diseases, hepatitis, tuberculosis, and other lung infections are also seen in cocaine abusers. Intravenous use is associated with diseases introduced by dirty needles contaminated with the blood of previous users, as well as with extra substances in the drug. The most common severe complications from i.v. cocaine use are bacterial or viral endocarditis, hepatitis, and acquired immune deficiency syndrome (AIDS) (168). Other conditions arising from parenteral cocaine use include cellulitis, cerebritis, wound abscess, sepsis, arterial thrombosis, renal infarction, and thrombophlebitis. As mentioned earlier, crack smoking can lead to the pneumonia-like symptoms of crack lung. Those who smoke cocaine are at increased risk for respiratory problems such as coughing, bronchitis, and pneumonitis as a consequence of irritation and inflammation of the tissues lining the respiratory tract. Deaths have occurred from all forms of cocaine (169,170).

Other medical complications include headache, thallium poisoning, retinal artery occlusion, dermatologic problems, and muscle and skin infarction. Ischemic finger necrosis and recent-onset Raynaud phenomenon are associated with cocaine abuse (171). Persons who lack the enzyme pseudocholinesterase are at risk for sudden death from cocaine use because the enzyme is essential for metabolizing the drug. Derlet and Albertson (103) found that 9.5% of patients attempted suicide with cocaine or as a result of cocaine intoxication. As mentioned previously, cocaine and cocaine in combination with alcohol were the most commonly mentioned in suicide cases in 2001 (5).

COCAINE AND PREGNANCY

One of the most troubling aspects of the cocaine epidemic, especially crack smoking, is its use by pregnant women. The available data have been at times conflicting and difficult to understand. Pregnancy increases a woman's susceptibility to the toxic cardiovascular effects of cocaine (172). Placental abruption, or premature separation of a normally implanted placenta, occurs in approximately 1% of pregnancies in women who use cocaine, making the drug a significant cause of maternal morbidity, as well as of fetal mortality (173). Women who use cocaine during pregnancy have a rate of spontaneous abortion even higher than that of heroin users (153).

Cocaine may produce toxic effects on the fetus at concentrations that are apparently nontoxic to the mother. The drug decreases blood flow to the uterus, increases uterine vascular resistance, and reduces fetal oxygen levels. The vasoconstriction, tachycardia, and increased blood pressure associated with cocaine use increase the risk of intermittent intrauterine hypoxia, preterm or precipitous labor, and placental abruption (174). Cocaine has a significant effect on the ability of fetal hearts to produce action potentials of normal rising velocity, amplitude, and duration (175). Cocaine can cause fetal cerebral infarction (153), growth retardation (176), and fetal death (177). In an interesting pilot study with implications for long-term development, cardiovascular effects of prenatal cocaine exposure in a small group of newborns were compared with a group of normal controls. Results from complete echocardiographic study indicated that the left ventricular (LV) posterior wall and septum were significantly thicker in the exposed group. In addition, the exposed group had significantly larger LV mass, suggestive of the LV hypertrophy found in adult cocaine users (178). The most noncontroversial finding regarding in utero cocaine exposure involves impaired somatic growth and decreased head circumference. Infant gestational age, birth weight, head circumference, and length were decreased, and the rate of low birth weight increased in the majority of studies of the offspring of cocaine-using women (179,180). Maternal cocaine use was also independently associated with reduced head circumference in a large, prospective survey in Boston. This finding was particularly compelling because all mothers received prenatal care. It seems clear that maternal cocaine use is related to lower infant birth weight and decreased head circumference (181). Results of a study of residential substance abuse treatment on pregnancy outcome in which 56% of the mothers were cocaine dependent showed that for every 10 weeks in treatment, birth weight was increased 340 g, estimated gestational age 1 week, average head circumference 0.8 cm, and mean birth length 1.8 cm. Thus, substance abuse treatment for pregnant women in the program increased fetal growth, which significantly decreased the risk for poor neonatal outcomes (182).

Experts have also argued over the prevalence of in utero cocaine exposure. The National Association for Perinatal Addiction Research and Education estimated that 11% of women studied in 36 hospitals had used illicit drugs during pregnancy. Several prospective surveys demonstrate a prevalence of drugs of abuse of 0.4% to 44% among pregnant patients. Study of the prevalence of intrauterine cocaine exposure revealed that meconium analysis was able to detect 2.68 times more instances of drug abuse in patients than could corresponding urine analysis. Lewis and coauthors' 25.8% prevalence rate compares with a 31% positive cocaine rate in other studies on urban patients and an 11.8% rate in the suburbs (183). While precise data are unavailable in many parts of the country, between 15% and 25% of babies are born with cocaine already in their system (184).

The syndrome associated with cocaine-addicted infants has been given the name "jittery baby" (177). In one series, 34 of 39 infants exposed to cocaine before birth displayed CNS irritability (185). Such children frequently present with such abnormalities as decreased birth weight, length, and head circumference, genitourinary malformations, and neurologic and behavioral impairments (153,186–188). Much of the early clinical research, giving rise to crack baby reports, was flawed by failing to consider the relative importance and frequency of polydrug use among pregnant women (189). In fact, a meta-analysis failed to confirm a number of cocaine-related effects in utero with the exception of low birth weight (190). Infants of substance-abusing mothers often have a decreased ventilatory response to carbon dioxide and a 5 to 10 times increased risk of sudden infant death syndrome (SIDS) (191). Chasnoff (192) reports that the incidence of SIDS in infants exposed to cocaine is 15%, more than three times that of infants exposed to heroin or methadone. Cocaine can be passed to infants through breast milk and can be found in milk up to 60 hours after the mother used the drug. Infants intoxicated by cocaine ingested via breast milk may present with hypertension, tachycardia, sweating, dilation of the pupils, and apnea (193).

Early studies of infants who were exposed prenatally to cocaine suggested that neurologic and developmental sequelae were common. One explanation of these findings is based on cocaine's action as a potent vasoconstrictor that causes decreased uterine and placental blood flow and that is related to fetal hypoxia in animal models. Cocaine readily crosses the placenta and can cause fetal cerebral vasoconstriction and ischemia directly. Cocaine-induced CNS malformations theoretically may result if the alteration in fetal cerebral blood flow occurs at a critical time in brain development. Cocaine also inhibits neurotransmitter reuptake, which theoretically may result if the alteration in fetal cerebral blood flow occurs at a critical time in brain development. Cocaine also inhibits neurotransmitter reuptake, which could result in long-lasting effects on CNS function. Several recent reviews of the effects of prenatal cocaine exposure suggest that caution is warranted in the interpretation of these early reports because of numerous methodologic weaknesses inherent in the study designs (194).

It is clear that a significant number of fetuses are exposed to cocaine in utero. Developmental consequences are likely. It is important to remember that historical accounts tend to minimize exposure. This "denial" is demonstrated by a recent study of 3,010 neonates. Although 11% of the women reported using illicit drugs during pregnancy, 31% of infants meconium tested positive for cocaine alone (195). A procedure to assess fetal exposure to cocaine based on liquid chromatography-mass spectrometry (LC-MS) has been described and validated in the range of 0.005 to 1.00 μg/g using 1 g of meconium per assay for determination of cocaine, benzoylecgonine, and cocaethylene in meconium obtained at birth (196). The results of hair analysis of specimens obtained from the newborn can also be performed and make it possible to confirm a fetal drug exposure, particularly when results obtained in other matrices are negative (197).

Cocaine's effects on the unborn and newborn may also be related to poor nutrition, poor hygiene, and neglect. Cocaine compromises the mother or any caregiver's ability to respond to the new baby through talking, eye contact, and tactile stimulation. Such disconnection and indifference to the infant's behavioral cues creates additional problems, because response is necessary for optimal intellectual and emotional infant development. It has been suggested that drug-dependent mothers are impaired in their ability to respond to their infants (180).

COCAINE AND OTHER PSYCHIATRIC DISORDERS

A patient who suffers from a psychiatric illness often appears more susceptible to stimulant toxicity and abuse. Some people with depression will experiment with cocaine, amphetamines, or even excessive caffeine and tobacco to lift themselves out of their fatigue, low energy, and disinterest in activities. They generally find that cocaine makes them no better, and sometimes makes them more depressed and hopeless. Recent use often appears temporarily related to depressive exacerbations and medication resistance. Surveys of people undergoing treatment for cocaine abuse reveal that at least half of a given patient population meet the diagnostic criteria for mood disorders (50,198). A similar incidence of depression can be seen among opiate addicts. However, 20% of cocaine abusers experience cyclic mood disorders such as bipolar disorders (manic-depressive illness) and cyclothymic disorder; the incidence of these conditions in opiate addicts is only 1%. Such findings suggest that people who experience mood swings prefer stimulants over other illicit drugs. Another commonly seen condition among cocaine patients is residual attention deficit hyperactivity disorder.

People with borderline personality disorder are likely to turn to mood-altering drugs for relief. They may use stimulants to induce feelings of pleasure, or depressants to reduce internal distress. Because these people are already on edge, use of stimulants and depressants may trigger a flare-up of anger or violence.

Perhaps more than those with any other personality disorder, people diagnosed as having antisocial personality disorder are prone to use mood-altering drugs. Alcohol is often the drug of choice in such individuals, but many also use cocaine or amphetamines or a combination of several drugs. People with this disorder are distressed, tense, unable to tolerate boredom, and agitated to the point of discomfort. Their use of drugs often removes any remaining inhibitions, increasing the risk of anger, violence, and actions that violate the rights or property of others. Because cocaine is by definition an illicit substance, use of the drug in itself constitutes a form of antisocial behavior.

Like a person with schizophrenia, a person in the throes of cocaine delirium may lose contact with reality and become confused and disoriented. Paranoia is a trait commonly seen in both schizophrenia and cocaine abuse. In both conditions the patient may experience auditory hallucinations. The delirium of cocaine usually dissipates within a few days, although some symptoms of delirium may persist for up to 1 year (199).

Many people with eating disorders—anorexia and bulimia—take diet pills containing amphetamines to suppress the appetite. Some of these people progress to using cocaine or illicitly acquired amphetamines, such as "crank" or "ice," the smokable version of methamphetamine. Over time they may become tolerant to these drugs and eventually dependent on them. In severe cases, use of amphetamines may lead to chronic intoxication and psychosis that resembles schizophrenia. Withdrawal produces symptoms that include fatigue and depression.

In a survey conducted by the National Helpline, 50% of callers reported experiencing cocaine-induced panic attacks. Treatment facilities specializing in panic and anxiety disorders also report that onset of panic attacks often begins with cocaine use (200). It appears that through the process of kindling—lowering the stimulation threshold of the brain—cocaine may increase the risk of panic. Over time, and following ingestion of large amounts of the drug, such reactions may occur spontaneously, without drug-induced stimulation. Panic reactions may persist even after use of cocaine has stopped.

As in other medical conditions, the results of treatment depend on a variety of factors. Persistent, untreated depression may compromise recovery. Moreover, abrupt cessation from cocaine use has been suggested with depressive symptoms (50). This is corroborated by the finding of high rates of depressive disorders among treatment-seeking cocaine abusers (201). Because serotonin uptake inhibitors are antidepressants (202), this type of agent is further suggested for treatment of depressive cocaine abusers.

Overall rates for active psychiatric disorders appear to be approximately 50% currently in cocaine abusers, and 75% to 85% lifetime. Some published literature and studies in progress report extremely high comorbidity for cocaine dependence. Such high rates of comorbidity may be related to poor outcome reported for cocaine treatment and numerous positive treatment reports that are tantalizing but difficult to replicate. The authors and other investigators have reported important associations between cocaine use and dependence and bipolar disorders, depression, marijuana abuse and dependence, and alcohol abuse and dependence (50,203). Some investigators have reported comorbidity of up to 25% for bipolar-spectrum illnesses (mania, hypomania, cyclothymia) in cocaine-dependent patients. Lifetime major depression is diagnosed in approximately 50% of patients, whereas dysthymia is diagnosed in another 25% to 50% (202,203). Rates for alcoholism are quite high, with as many as 60% having clear lifetime diagnoses. Marijuana use is common and may be related to cocaine pharmacokinetics. Marijuana and cocaine are commonly used at the same time. As described earlier in the chapter, marijuana may potentiate cocaine's effects (148).

Some clinicians suggest that a history of attention deficit hyperactivity disorder (ADHD) is common. Individuals with a cocaine dependence diagnosis often have temporary depressive symptoms that meet symptomatic and duration criteria for major depressive disorder if criterion D is not included. Cocaine-using patients give compelling histories consistent with repeated panic attacks, social phobic-like behavior, and generalized anxiety-like syndromes. Eating disorders are also commonly reported on the basis of pathologic starvation, satiety, or more traditional bulimia. Cocaine-induced psychotic disorder with delusions and hallucinations that resembles mania or schizophrenia, paranoid type, can occur and persist. More commonly, mental disturbances that occur in association with cocaine use resolve within hours to days after cessation of use.

Superstition and unusual behavior and thoughts are common. Individuals with cocaine dependence develop these "superstitions" as conditioned responses to cocaine-related stimuli and, unfortunately for them, they cannot successfully recognize the total number of such stimuli. They may say they feel better in Florida or give a history of seasonal affective changes, but really have so many associations that they are asking for a geographic cure. They may have extreme agitation, provoked nausea, provoked drive for the drug in the absence of a clear association with a sight or sound associated with the drug. Most common is their reaction to seeing, holding, or rolling paper money. These responses probably contribute to relapse, are difficult to extinguish, and typically persist long after detoxification is completed. Cocaine use disorders are often associated with other substance dependence or abuse, especially involving alcohol, marijuana, and benzodiazepines, which are often taken to reduce the anxiety and other unpleasant stimulant side effects of cocaine. Cocaine dependence may be associated with posttraumatic stress disorder, antisocial personality disorder, ADHD, and pathologic gambling. Cocaine addicts take alcohol and benzodiazepines in an effort to reduce the negative consequences of cocaine intoxication, but intravenous users commonly use cocaine in combination with heroin to produce a speedball effect that is described as better than either alone.

Mello and coworkers developed an animal model to evaluate the speedball phenomenon (204) in rhesus monkeys who simultaneously self-administer cocaine and heroin. Pretreatment with an opiate antagonist, quadazocine (0.1 mg/kg i.m.), had no effect on the discriminative stimulus effects of cocaine but antagonized the cocaine-like discriminative stimulus effects of heroin. Pretreatment with a DA antagonist, flupentixol (0.018 mg/kg), antagonized the discriminative stimulus effects of cocaine but did not affect the cocaine-like effects of heroin. The pharmacologic systems mediating the stimulus properties of cocaine and heroin in rhesus monkeys are not only distinct, but also functionally independent. The pharmacologic classification of cocaine as a stimulant and heroin

as an opiate tends to divert attention from exploration of the ways in which these drugs may have similar effects. This complex polydrug use is extremely compelling and further study may yield important information on the DA–endorphin–serotonin systems interplay in maximizing drug-induced brain reward. The addiction psychiatrist must always weigh the risk of withholding psychiatric treatment as one tries to establish a clear diagnosis and the propensity for relapse when comorbid psychopathology goes untreated.

TREATMENT OF COCAINE ADDICTION

The evaluation and initial treatment of cocaine-using patients is a complex, demanding, and sometimes confusing process (203). Thorough treatment requires the physician to integrate a range of medical, psychiatric, social, and drug-counseling services. Adding to the complexity is the need to address family issues and to anticipate the risk of relapse. Although the current success rate of drug-addiction treatment is less than is desired, new treatment strategies, including some pharmacologic interventions, offer hope for improving the outcome.

In recent years, many treatment facilities have adopted the chemical dependency model, which regards drug dependence as a primary condition—a disease unto itself— not a secondary problem arising from some other underlying psychopathology (205). Such programs take a multidisciplinary approach to drug treatment and provide a range of behavioral, cognitive, educational, and self-control techniques aimed at reducing drug cravings and the potential for relapse. Significantly, these programs also require patients to abstain from all drugs and to participate actively in 12-step programs such as Alcoholics Anonymous (AA) or Cocaine Anonymous (CA). The advantage in doing so is that patients learn to consider themselves as being continually at risk and in a recovering— rather than a recovered—state. They also learn to see themselves as chemically dependent, not crazy. Such a fundamental shift in perspective improves the chances that the patient will live a happy, healthy, and drug-free life.

Diagnosis

The first step in treatment, of course, is to diagnose the patient's condition accurately. Table 13.5 lists the clinical criteria for cocaine dependency (206). Of course, the clinical use of supervised urine testing for drugs, including cocaine, in diagnosis has been underused.

A diagnosis of cocaine withdrawal (see Table 13.2) can be made if the patient has stopped or reduced heavy use of the drug after a prolonged period (several days or longer) and experiences dysphoric mood (depression, irritability, anxiety) and fatigue, sleep disturbance, or psychomotor

TABLE 13.5. *Diagnostic criteria for cocaine dependency*

Loss of control
  Inability to stop using or refuse cocaine
  Failure to self-limit use
  Predictable or regular use
  Binges for 24 hours or longer
  Urges and cravings for cocaine
Exaggerated involvement
  Self-proclaimed need for cocaine
  Fear of distress without cocaine
  Feelings of dependency on cocaine
  Feelings of guilt about using cocaine and fear of being discovered
  Preference for cocaine over family, friends, and recreational activities
Continued use despite adverse effects
  Medical problems (e.g., fatigue, insomnia, headaches, nasal problems, bronchitis)
  Psychological problems (e.g., irritability, depression, loss of sex drive, lack of motivation, memory impairment)
  Social/interpersonal problems (e.g., loss of friends or spouse, job difficulties, social withdrawal, involvement in traffic accidents, excuse-making behavior)

From Washton AM, Gold MS, Pottash AC. Opiate and cocaine dependencies: techniques to help counter the rising tide. *Postgrad Med* 1985;77:293–300, with permission.

agitation persisting for at least 24 hours. Many patients report having "coke dreams" with themes involving the repeated pursuit or use of cocaine.

Other related diagnoses include cocaine delirium and cocaine delusional disorder. In the former, the patient develops delirium, marked by disorganized thinking, sensory misperceptions, and disorientation within 24 hours after drug use. Typically patients experience tactile or olfactory hallucinations. Affect is often labile. Because violent or aggressive behavior is common, especially after use of crack cocaine, restraint may be required. When the pharmacologic effects of cocaine have worn off, the delirium usually disappears.

The essential feature of cocaine delusional disorder involves the presence of persecutory delusions developing shortly after the use of cocaine. At first, the patient may experience the feelings of suspiciousness and curiosity as a source of pleasure or entertainment. In the later phases the suspiciousness, anxiety, and paranoia may provoke violent or aggressive behavior, often accompanied by hallucinations that further distort reality. Delusions may persist up to a year following use of cocaine.

In all cases, regardless of the exact diagnosis, toxicologic analysis of body fluids should be made to confirm the findings.

Inpatient versus Outpatient Care

The American Society of Addiction Medicine (ASAM) provides an accepted method for recommendations of level of intensity of treatment in its Patient Placement Criteria 2-R (PPC-2R). The ASAM PPC-2R provides two sets of guidelines, one for adults and one for adolescents, and five broad levels of care for each group. The PPC-2R uses information from six dimensions—(a) acute intoxication and/or withdrawal potential; (b) biomedical conditions and complications; (c) emotional/behavioral/cognitive conditions and complications; (d) readiness to change (formerly treatment acceptance/resistance); (e) relapse/continued use/continued problem potential; and (f) recovery environment—to determine the recommended level of care. The levels of care are Level 0.5, Early Intervention; Level I, Outpatient Treatment; Level II, Intensive Outpatient/Partial Hospitalization; Level III, Residential/Inpatient Treatment; and Level IV, Medically Managed Intensive Inpatient Treatment. Within these broad levels of service is a range of specific levels of care.

If circumstances permit, outpatient treatment is the preferred modality for delivery of care for several reasons. Many cocaine abusers can be treated as outpatients, because use of the drug usually can be stopped abruptly without medical risk or significant discomfort. The goal of treatment is to return the patient to a normal life; by definition there can be no "normal" life inside the hospital. The cost of outpatient treatment is lower (although some insurance companies may refuse to pay for care delivered in the outpatient setting). Many patients are more willing to accept help on an outpatient basis because it carries less of a social stigma and is less disruptive to daily life. Entering a hospital or a rehabilitation center as an inpatient with fewer privileges and liberties conveys an acceptance that the disease is an imminent danger to them. Perhaps the most important consideration, however, is that in all cases of substance abuse, outpatient care will eventually be needed, given the lifelong risk of relapse and the need for ongoing support (207). However, inpatient or residential treatment provides an ideal transition from drug use and dependency to abstinence and daily meetings.

When drug use is severe, or if outpatient care is not possible or has failed in the past, hospitalization is called for. Although not a complete listing, indications for inpatient care include the following:

1. Chronic crack, freebase, or intravenous use
2. Concurrent dependency on other addictive drugs or alcohol
3. Serious concurrent medical or psychiatric problems
4. Severe impairment of psychological or neurologic functioning
5. Insufficient motivation for outpatient treatment
6. Lack of family and social supports
7. Failure in outpatient treatment (208)

An important advantage of a treatment facility is removing patients from the environment—the home, the streets—that may be contributing to their drug use. Patients under round-the-clock supervision are unable (in most cases) to obtain illicit drugs. They can take daily advantage of the many types of therapy the hospital offers. Another advantage is that patients are available for full medical and psychiatric evaluations, which will reveal whether any coexisting problems, such as HIV infection, hepatitis, or clinical depression, exist (209). Many of these problems emerge, and can be properly evaluated, only after detoxification and during observation over a period of several drug-free days. Successful initial treatment in a residential setting may facilitate the integration and retention by the patient of outpatient and self-help meetings.

Treatment Strategies

Planning treatment requires a comprehensive assessment of the psychobiologic, social, and pharmacologic aspects of the patient's substance abuse. For many patients, cocaine use is the focus of their entire life. They become totally preoccupied with drug-seeking and drug-taking behaviors. They may have become accustomed to the mood changes invoked by cocaine and have forgotten what life without drugs is like. Thus they come to regard the drugged state as "normal" and may not believe any treatment is necessary. For this reason, they may refuse to acknowledge the need for help. Consequently, many patients enter treatment only under pressure from family, friends, employers, or the judicial system (201). In severe cases, the patient perceives such pressure to be a threat from "enemies," which only serves to reinforce drug-induced feelings of suspicion, persecution, and paranoia. For this and other reasons, families often need guidance in staging an intervention on a cocaine-abusing relative.

The initial contact with a patient may occur after the crash and during the withdrawal phase. The physician should take a complete family, medical, and forensic history, as well as a history of all drug use. However, information obtained from chemically dependent people can be incomplete or highly unreliable. For this reason the patient should undergo a thorough physical and dental examination. Chest x-rays and electrocardiograms may supply useful information and may help to reassure patients about their state of health. Any severe conditions or impending medical emergencies may necessitate transfer to the medical floor or hospital. One concern is that patients about to enter the hospital may ingest huge and potentially lethal doses of one or more drugs (207).

Immediately following the physical examination, blood and/or supervised urine samples should be collected and sent for analysis. If possible, a sample of the cocaine used by the patient should also be submitted to the laboratory. All subsequent urine collections should be supervised and taken first thing in the morning. Temperature and/or specific gravity should be measured to confirm that the sample has not been adulterated. Although expensive, gas chromatography-mass spectrography testing is many times more sensitive and specific than either thin-layer chromatography or immunoassay drug screens. Blood is the preferred sample for forensic purposes or to evaluate whether the person is under the influence at the time of the psychiatric exam (207). An analytical method for the simultaneous determination of cocaine and its major metabolites, ecgonine methyl ester and benzoylecgonine, in saliva (actually oral fluid) has been developed. These levels parallel thus found in plasma (208). Hair samples provide a long window of opportunity with each half inch of hair representing approximately 1 week of history. The National Institute of Standards and Technology currently provides a new standard reference material for drugs of abuse in human hair. SRM 2379 consists of hair spiked with cocaine, benzoylecgonine, cocaethylene, phencyclidine, amphetamine, and methamphetamine (210). Recent research has identified unique pyrolysis products of crack or burned cocaine as anhydroecgonine methylester and ecgonidine through gas chromatography-mass spectrometry that allow for the detection of crack use distinct from other cocaine use. A recent study suggests that crack use, as distinct from other cocaine use, can be detected in sweat, and that tamper-resistant patches are a promising new way to detect drugs of abuse, particularly those with short windows of detection in routine urine testing (211). Frequent laboratory testing is valuable because it eliminates the need to continually question the patient about current drug use, uncovers any drug use by the patient, and provides a strong motivation for the patient to remain drug free.

Medical Treatment of Withdrawal and Cocaine-Related Emergencies

As a rule, symptoms of cocaine withdrawal are not medically dangerous (212). Detoxification from cocaine requires no treatment other than abstinence (203). However, many patients find the symptoms of withdrawal intensely dysphoric, so much so that they feel driven to continue acquiring and using cocaine in order to fend off the symptoms. Any medical treatment that helps relieve withdrawal symptoms therefore improves the initial prognosis. A DA theory may explain drug reward, survival drive reward, symptoms or complaints common to acute drug withdrawal states (including cocaine withdrawal), and be a useful or predictor or model to identify potential new treatments. However, early in clinical trials it became quite clear that successful amelioration of withdrawal appears to be of limited clinical significance. Painless and symptomless cocaine withdrawal was often followed by relapse and readdiction, just as clonidine detoxification was followed by opiate relapse and success with the nicotine patch was followed by a return to smoking. New treatments directed at reversal of postabstinence craving—such as bromocriptine (Parlodel) or desipramine (Norpramin) (213–217) on cocaine abstinence—were based on the assumption that successful craving reduction would in some way reduce drug use or relapse. These and other recent treatments have been surprisingly ineffective at stopping relapse or cocaine-taking. They offered clinical support for the DA theory of abstinence and craving, but also convinced researchers that drug use and recidivism was clearly separable from drug withdrawal. More recently, researchers have focused the development of treatments on the direct prevention of further drug use as measured by urinalysis or tried to reduce the likelihood of relapse.

The choice of treatment for cocaine toxicity depends on the clinical signs and symptoms. Supportive therapy is the rule. Treating hyperthermia with vigorous body cooling may be a positive first step. Cardiac and neurologic status should be monitored closely, with medical strategies directed at providing symptom relief. Use of phenothiazines, especially chlorpromazine (Promapar, Thorazine), or of haloperidol (Haldol) is contraindicated for acute reactions because these drugs may lower the seizure threshold. Spontaneous cocaine-induced seizures can be treated with intravenous administration of 25 to 50 mg of a short-acting barbiturate such as pentobarbital sodium (Nembutal) (208).

Hospitalization with respiratory assistance and a life support system may be necessary in cases of severe cocaine overdose reaction. Treatment of overdose is often complicated by the presence of sedative-hypnotics, opiates, or alcohol, drugs that are frequently taken to mitigate the unpleasant effects of excessive cocaine use.

Typically, cocaine psychosis lasts for 3 to 5 days following cessation of use; if it persists for a longer period, or if the patient becomes increasingly difficult to manage, a reevaluation of the diagnosis is indicated and an antipsychotic medication such as haloperidol may be tried. Use of the newer "atypical" antipsychotics as monotherapy or in combination with benzodiazepines may also be helpful.

Long-Term Treatment of Cocaine Dependency

Patients with dependency problems usually experience the best outcome if treated by physicians, psychologists, and other caregivers who specialize in managing addictive disorders (208). In recent years, increasing demand for treatment has led to the burgeoning availability of specialized treatment centers in many parts of the country. Addiction specialists understand that animals and humans, whether bred for drug preference or not, whether dependent or drug naive, whether reared in Milan or Miami, self-administer drugs of abuse. The reinforcing properties of drugs are powerful motivational forces, which are preferred by the user to natural reinforcers. Addicts or

users in self-administration studies perform many difficult and time-consuming tasks to gain access to drugs. Drug users make active choices between the drug and work, spouse, friends, and other reinforcers. The drugs that stimulate their own taking and are positively reinforcing in animals do the same in humans. This relationship is so strong that drug self-administration in animals is now viewed as predictive of human drug abuse potential. The data derived from animal and human self-administration of abused drugs support the notion that drug reinforcement is the unifying feature of drug abuse and dependence. It is also true that drug abstinence is the behavioral and physical state "released" by the absence of the drug of abuse to which the chronic user has adapted. So, it is also positive reinforcement to reverse the negative hedonic state released by drug abstinence.

Addiction specialists focus on the motivational rather than the physical aspects of the withdrawal syndrome. Malaise, boredom, depression, anhedonia, decreased appetite, brain stimulation changes, increased behavioral responsiveness to stressors, and increases in reward thresholds are all part of the withdrawal syndrome. Human addicts report that they need cocaine to return to normal or simply to think straight after prolonged use. Musicians report a loss of creativity, authors report "writer's block," and others report a loss of color or brightness in their lives after abstinence. Reward and withdrawal mechanisms are associated with both positive and negative reinforcement in ways that are not easily separated clinically. The "good feeling" that is the goal of cocaine use usually involves both euphoria (positive reinforcement) and reversal of cocaine-absence dysphoria. In the past, the failure of cocaine addiction treatment was attributed to incomplete medical science and poor medical treatment options rather than to the positive drive of motivated behavior directed at the use of cocaine. While a desirable outcome over a period of many years was virtually unheard of following repeated detoxifications, it was remarkable how slow the medical profession was to recognize the implications of this observation. Rather than question the underlying assumption, which placed medical skills essential in the diagnosis and treatment of withdrawal at the center of the problem of addiction treatment, physicians seemed resigned to recycle addicted people through one emergency room or detoxification experience after another for what often proved to be an addiction-shortened lifetime.

Clinical Treatment Model

Whether it serves as the primary mode of care or as a sequel to hospitalization, a comprehensive outpatient program should include a range of treatment strategies. These include supportive counseling, drug education, peer support groups, and family meetings. Exercise therapy may also prove to be a helpful adjunct (201). For a period of time, caregivers should follow the patient on a daily basis. Severe depression may require psychotherapy and perhaps the use of medications. Regular telephone support should continue for several months. Many treatment centers offer ongoing group therapy sessions for patients and their families for a period of years following discharge.

In all cases, patients should be given frequent urine tests to screen for all drugs of abuse. Even in prisons and other criminal justice settings, urine testing is the most useful barometer of treatment outcome. The goal must be to achieve abstinence from mood-altering chemicals, including alcohol. Attaining this goal cannot be determined simply by asking the patient, family, or loved ones if the patient "is still using drugs." We should ask this question and look for drugs in the urine or other biologic specimens. There is no hope for effective treatment so long as the patient continues to use drugs. Personality problems, emotional difficulties, and psychiatric disorders should be addressed as they arise, but the chances of success are virtually nil unless the patient is drug free.

Another crucial element of long-term treatment is participation in a 12-step recovery program. In recent years the medical and psychiatric professions have come to recognize the significant contributions that AA and similar programs can make to the lives of substance abusers. Members draw strength and security from meeting with others who understand and share their concerns and can offer practical strategies for surviving "one day at a time." Any treatment program that does not embrace the 12-step approach and encourage patients to participate stands little chance of long-term success.

When considering the treatment of addictive disease, it is useful to recall that the use of medicines remains limited when compared to the role of medicines in many other mental disorders, including the affective and the anxiety disorders, the two diagnostic groupings that share with addiction the distinction of being the most prevalent classes of mental disorders. Although cognitive–behavioral approaches are effective in the treatment of affective and anxiety disorders, pharmacotherapy dominates the clinical management of these diseases. In contrast to the treatment of affective and anxiety disorders, when it comes to substance use disorders, pharmacotherapy plays a relatively minor role and 12-step programs, the most potent cognitive–behavioral approach, are ascendant.

In a recent study, the effectiveness and frequency of cognitive–behavioral therapy (CBT) counseling sessions was studied to evaluate CBT's effect on cocaine use and craving, retention, and psychiatric symptoms in cocaine-dependent patients (218). This study found that 12 weeks of CBT, whether it was twice a week, once a week, or biweekly, decreased by a small, but statistically significant amount, cocaine craving and use and psychiatric symptoms and retention was similar for all groups. The authors report that CBT is effective even when used on a less-intensive schedule (219). CBT depends on adequate cognitive functioning in patients, but prolonged cocaine use may impair cognitive functioning. Therefore, cognitive impairment may impede the ability of cocaine abusers to benefit from CBT. A study using the MicroCog computerized battery to assess cognitive performance at treatment entry was used to compare cognitive functioning between completers (patients remaining in treatment at least 12 weeks) and dropouts. The results indicated that treatment completers had demonstrated significantly better cognitive performance at baseline than had patients who dropped out of treatment. Cognitive domains that significantly distinguished between treatment completers and dropouts were attention, mental reasoning and spatial processing (220).

The dream of modern pharmacologic research is to find more specific and effective treatments that block ready access to the drug-induced effects of both the reward and the withdrawal pathways, without producing agonist effects or other effects. Naturally, antagonists that reverse the effects of cocaine and marijuana, like naloxone reverses the effects of opiates, are essential for emergency rooms and pharmacotherapies for relapse prevention. Relapse-preventing psychopharmacology is an important new addition to this phase. Medications that deny brain reward access to rewarding drugs of abuse rather than punish the addict for using are in the early phases of a dramatic change in the field of addiction medicine and addiction psychiatry (219).

Comorbid cocaine patients may represent up to 80% of patients with cocaine dependency according to studies reported at the 1995 meeting of the American Psychiatric Association. They need simultaneous and aggressive cocaine and psychiatric treatments. Patients need to find thorough treatment of their mental disorder, which will improve quality of life and reduce the risk for depression-related and anxiety-related relapses and suicides.

The 12-step programs use a unitary approach to addictive disease by largely disregarding the specific substances being used. AA takes a unitary view on addiction by making clear that staying sober means not only not drinking alcohol but also not using other brain-rewarding chemicals. Beyond not using alcohol or other drugs, AA works to change the addict's lifestyle to a better, less self-centered life (22).

Preventing Relapse

Despite progress in treatment for cocaine use, the risk of relapse is extremely high. As noted, the memory of cocaine euphoria is so powerful that it can produce overwhelming urges to revert to drug use. Patients whose lifestyles revolved around cocaine are susceptible to being reminded of the drug in surprising ways. For example, a patient who sees talcum powder, bread crumbs, or snow may be reminded of cocaine. Seeing cocaine-using friends or locations, smelling cocaine, or even hearing a song associated with cocaine use can trigger drug urges. The click of a cigarette lighter or the light from a match is enough to remind some patients of their cocaine-smoking habit. Apparently, almost any stimulus that has been repeatedly associated with obtaining and using cocaine can become a cocaine "reminder" (221). Gawin and Ellinwood (222) describe a four-step treatment approach to the extinction of cocaine cravings. In the first phase, patients are isolated from the events, objects, people, and locations that may provoke urges. Next, some of these stimuli are gradually reintroduced as mental images during psychotherapy sessions. Patients then discuss and rehearse strategies for managing the temptations arising from such provocation. In the third stage, patients reenter their former environments gradually and under the guidance of their caregivers. In the final phase of consolidation, patients continue to participate in self-help and aftercare groups, or resume treatment as necessary to counteract any recurring drug cravings.

Persistence of cocaine abstinence may be manifested in persistent dysphoria and cocaine self-administration. Recent data support persistent neural dysregulation in cocaine dependence. It is not uncommon for such persistent dysphoria or anxiety or panic symptoms to persist after discontinuation of cocaine and thus constitute a feature of the prolonged abstinence phase. We have seen patients who complain of panic attacks that continue for years.

Stress has long been thought to a precipitator of relapse. In animal models, the foot-shock stressor reliably reinstates extinguished cocaine-taking behavior. Corticotropin-releasing factor (CRF) is thought to play a role in the reinstatement of drug-seeking induced by stressors. Studies suggest that effective CRF receptor antagonists may be of use in the treatment of relapse to drug use (223). Ketoconazole, a cortisol synthesis inhibitor, reduces cocaine self-administration in rodents, but does not appear to reduce cocaine or opioid use in humans maintained on methadone (224).

Several groups that have studied prolactin as a marker of abnormal dopaminergic function report neurobiologic changes that persist after prolonged abstinence (225–231). One investigator (84) found persistent hyperprolactinemia in 14 male and 2 female cocaine abusers at admission and at inpatient day 28. Teoh et al. (232) also found that the relative duration and severity of hyperprolactinemia in abstinent cocaine addicts predicted enhanced risk of relapse.

Like our pioneering work (79), these studies suggest that cocaine-induced derangement of the dopaminergic system is consistent with decreased dopaminergic tone and consequent disinhibition of the DA-regulated prolactin system. Persistent abstinence manifested by continuing neural dysregulation and resultant dysphoria may be an unrecognized consequence of cocaine dependence.

Persistent neural compromise suggests that limitations may exist for the cocaine-dependent person even after abstinence. The mechanisms underlying cocaine-induced ischemic stroke are not well understood. Strategies for treatment do not exist. Generally these patients demonstrated multifocal areas of cortical hypoperfusion and scalloping of periventricular regions indicating that single-photon emission computed tomography (SPECT) is sensitive to perfusion abnormalities associated with cocaine use (233–236). Cerebral blood flow abnormalities and cognitive abnormalities may persist following extended periods of drug abstinence, particularly in chronic, long-term users. Moreover, there is evidence that there may be minimal recovery of some cognitive abilities following abstinence, especially recovery of short-term verbal memory deficits (237). These studies and clinical experience suggest that prolonged crack cocaine self-administration and cocaine hydrochloride use (238–240) are often accompanied by structural neuronal change and compromise that are not readily reversed.

Relapse prevention strategies developed according to a social learning theory model have been adapted to chemical dependency treatment that follows the disease model. Some of these techniques are helping the patient to recognize the warning signs of relapse; combating the powerful memories of euphoria; reinforcing the negative aspects of drugs; overcoming the desire to attempt to regain control over drug use; avoiding the people, places, and things that may trigger drug urges; preventing occasional "slips" from developing into full-blown binges; learning other ways to cope with dysphoric feelings that in the past may have led to drug use; and developing an array of pleasurable and rewarding alternatives to drugs (241). As the early preoccupation with withdrawal as the central focus of addictive disease was excessive, so, perhaps, today's dismissal of withdrawal as a major factor in addiction is an overreaction. If generally effective ways are found to treat the withdrawal symptoms resulting from the physiologic dependence on any substance, whether taken medically or nonmedically, such treatments might have broad application both in addiction treatment and in medical practice.

The most promising approach to treatment of cocaine abuse is one that recognizes the high risk of relapse and applies a range of cognitive and behavioral strategies, including a 12-step program, to minimize the risk. New treatment approaches include financial incentive motivation and cue-related relaxation have been reported and appear to offer some promise in prediction of high relapse potential patients and possibly in adding to what is the current approach to treatment. One study (242) confirmed that many cocaine-dependent individuals respond to drug cues in the laboratory with increased craving for cocaine and demonstrable physiologic arousal. In that study, Margolin et al. studied 19 patients in a cue–reactivity protocol that concluded with relaxation exercises. Self-reported craving and skin conductance levels were measured. Patients who achieved abstinence were predicted by craving reported after relaxation training. Patients who subsequently initiated abstinence reported a reduction in cue-elicited craving to below baseline levels, while those who did not succeed in treatment remained elevated.

The Future of Treatment for Cocaine Abuse/Dependence

New treatments must be assessed over long periods with regular, independent, urine and other testing to confirm efficacy. Recidivism is a major area for future research. Recidivism among cocaine patients is high; most treatment specialists acknowledge that they offer treatment, not a cure, for addiction. However, there is reason for hope. Perhaps a decade ago, only 10% to 20% of drug addicts recovered following treatment. More recently a study found that, on average, up to 80% of substance abusers treated for 3 months or longer had reduced their drug use significantly, and that fully 50% were still completely drug free 1 year after treatment ended (243). Some programs today report a success rate of 60% to 70%. However, most programs have a high initial dropout rate, and even patients who succeed in treatment with one program frequently may have benefited from previous attempts at treatment with different programs. Furthermore, a treatment program may have a different success rate with various types of drug users. For example, a program that helps a 40-year-old college-educated executive to recover may not succeed in treating a 19-year-old unemployed high school dropout. Five-year followup data on truly similar patients, with random assignment of treatment and confirmation by urine testing, are necessary to evaluate treatment success claims.

Most agents used to treat cocaine abuse target the DA system because of its role in reinforcement (244). However, serotonin (5-HT) has also been implicated in reinforcement (245) and is affected by cocaine. Acutely, cocaine increases DA and norepinephrine and also serotonergic activity by inhibiting uptake of neurotransmitter release in the synaptic cleft (246). When cocaine is used chronically, the increased neurotransmitter levels induced by cocaine cause an inhibition of transmitter synthesis (247). When chronic cocaine self-administration is stopped, DA in the DA system, and also the 5-HT system, may decrease synaptic transmitter levels (79). These changes may be related to cocaine craving and possibly relapse. In addition to DA treatments, pharmacologic treatment agents for cocaine craving might inhibit 5-HT uptake, like cocaine, but would be nonaddicting (248).

The 5-HT$_3$ antagonist ondansetron reduced the "rush" produced by cocaine (249) and the 5-HT$_2$ antagonist ritanserin reduces cocaine self-administration in rats. In one study, 25 cocaine-dependent males were exposed to cocaine craving cues, while their 5-HT levels were re-

duced by tryptophan depletion. Serotonin appeared to be related to cue-induced craving because the study found a decreased desire for cocaine stimulated by cue exposure (248).

Serotonergic agents have been used to treat other addictive disorders, such as alcoholism (250) and obesity (251). Fluoxetine, a 5-HT uptake inhibitor, is associated with reduced cocaine use among methadone-maintained patients (252) and may be tried (253,254). However, one recent study failed to support the role of fluoxetine even for treatment of patients meeting both *DSM–IV* diagnoses of cocaine dependence and major depressive disorder (253).

Animal studies suggest that preexposure to ($\pm$)3,4-methylenedioxymethamphetamine (MDMA) may facilitate acquisition of cocaine self-administration. MDMA is neurotoxic to 5-HT neurons and releases DA, both of which could contribute to MDMA facilitation of cocaine self-administration (254).

Some reports suggest that methylphenidate (Ritalin) reduces cocaine cravings in patients with attention deficit hyperactivity disorder, possibility because of its ability to stimulate the CNS. However, the abuse potential of methylphenidate and similar drugs severely limits their usefulness (255). The antidepressants bupropion (Wellbutrin) or trazodone (Desyrel), or the anticonvulsant carbamazepine (Tegretol), may be effective in relieving acute withdrawal symptoms and in maintaining abstinence from cocaine. The effects of cocaine have been examined prior to and during bupropion maintenance in nonopioid-dependent cocaine abusers; however, bupropion did not have a robust effect on the acute subjective or cardiovascular effects of cocaine (256).

Combinations of medications are often used to enhance treatment efficacy. The combination of bupropion and bromocriptine has been reported to result in significant reductions in self-reported cocaine use, with no significant change in proportion of urine toxicology tests positive for cocaine (257). Lack of patient compliance and the risk of extrapyramidal side effects may preclude the use of DA receptor neuroleptics, even though such drugs are known to block the euphoria caused by amphetamines. The efficacy of the treatment with the atypical antipsychotic olanzapine in cocaine abuse methadone patients has been studied. Consumption of cocaine was decreased or stopped in 53.2% of the patients and no withdrawal syndrome was observed in any patient. The results of this study suggest that for cocaine-abusing patients in a methadone maintenance program, olanzapine (Zyprexa) could be a useful treatment that does not induce any pharmacokinetic interaction with methadone (258,259). Another atypical antipsychotic, risperidone (Risperdal), a 5-HT (2)/DA (2) antagonist, has potential in treating cocaine addiction. It might have the ability to block cocaine-induced psychostimulant neurochemistry and behavior during acute studies while diminishing the withdrawal symptoms of cocaine during subacute studies (260). Risperidone pretreatment of cocaine-dependent volunteers may reduce the subjective "high" produced by cocaine (261).

In general, all medications tried have some subjective effect on the cocaine experience or craving, but do not alter or interfere with the natural history of cocaine dependence or euphoria (262). For example, lithium carbonate has been reported by some, but not others, to reduce the intensity of euphoria (263). While lithium is not currently used to treat cocaine dependence, the clinical utility of lithium in cocaine-abusing manic depressive or bipolar patients appears clear. A number of studies reported that desipramine reduced cocaine craving and it was thought to promote abstinence (264–267). Tricyclics such as desipramine seemed to be well suited to correct the catecholamine receptor supersensitivity that could accompany DA and norepinephrine depletion in chronic cocaine users. Yet as a treatment for cocaine dependence, it has been disappointing. Desipramine, imipramine (Tofranil), doxepin (Sinequan), and other tricyclics have been tried and while effects may be demonstrated for short periods, cocaine use and relapse are not prevented by such treatment. This was not as surprising to the basic researchers in the field who reported that desipramine has little or no effect on cocaine self-administration in animals (268) or humans (264,269). Desipramine was prescribed to large numbers of cocaine-dependent patients and has clearly been a disappointment as a promising pharmacotherapy. Still, this clinical experience may provide important clues regarding cocaine cues, craving, and euphoria. One recent review concluded that there is no current evidence supporting the clinical use of antidepressants in the treatment of cocaine dependence (270). Carbamazepine was believed to be an important treatment on the basis of animal models and reversal of cocaine-related kindling (271). Again, clinicians reported clinical success but double-blind and long-term studies with carbamazepine are as disappointing as for those with desipramine. A review of 5 studies of carbamazepine, with 455 people randomized, concluded that there is no current evidence supporting its clinical use in the treatment of cocaine dependence (272). This has been the pattern for cocaine-dependence treatment development, where many seemingly promising compounds from methylphenidate to mazindol were reported "to work" and ultimately failed as new treatments (273–279).

A recent study evaluated divalproex in subjects with cocaine dependence. Intensity and frequency of craving, as well as reported time using cocaine, decreased significantly, which indicates that it may be efficacious in the treatment of cocaine dependence (280).

Although recent studies found that disulfiram (Antabuse) reduced cocaine use in concomitant cocaine and alcohol abusers (281), Hameedi et al. (282) studied the effect of disulfiram pretreatment on the behavioral, physiologic, and pharmacologic effects of an acute dose of cocaine by using a double-blind, placebo-controlled, within-subject design. This study did not support the hypothesis that disulfiram affects cocaine-induced euphoria. They also showed that cocaine and disulfiram together increased nervousness and paranoia in three subjects, while not increasing heart rate and blood pressure more than cocaine alone. Unexpectedly, disulfiram also increased plasma cocaine levels, suggesting that disulfiram use in cocaine addicts may be problematic.

The use of dopamine agonists in the treatment of cocaine dependence has been extensively studied. A recent review reported that the clinical use of dopamine agonists in the treatment of cocaine dependence is not supported by current evidence (283).

Clinical trials of selegiline, and other indirect agents are underway and may prove helpful in cocaine abuse. Mazindol and methylphenidate have not proven effective. The results of animal studies suggest that tailoring based on genotype may improve responses (284). Selective D1 dopamine agonists represent a potential pharmacotherapy for the treatment of cocaine addiction. In a study of rats, a D1 agonist had the desired profile of a "methadone-like" compound for cocaine addiction (285). Further evidence for the usefulness of D1 agents in treatment of cocaine addiction is seen by the effects of ecopipam on maintenance (286). Dextroamphetamine sulfate was also studied recently and appeared to improve retention rates and decrease positive urine screens, suggesting it should be examined further (287).

Human trials with gamma-vinyl γ-aminobutyric acid (GVG), a selective and irreversible inhibitor of γ-aminobutyric acid (GABA)-transaminase, are currently being developed to examine the utility of GVG for the treatment of cocaine addiction (288,289). GVG (vigabatrin) is currently available around the world for the treatment of epilepsy and infantile spasms but is not approved for use in the United States (290). Inhibition of GABA-transaminase elevates human brain GABA concentration (291) via modulation of the $GABA_B$ receptor subtype (292). Animal studies show that GVG blocks drug- and cue-induced increases in nucleus accumbens and striatal dopamine; cocaine-induced self-administration; cocaine-induced lowering of brain-stimulation reward thresholds; expression and acquisition of cocaine-seeking behavior (conditioned place preference); and sensitization to cocaine. A small (n = 20) human clinical trial suggests that GVG in combination with psychosocial therapy offers a potential effective treatment for cocaine dependence (293).

There is evidence from research in animals and humans that the $GABA_B$ agonist baclofen (Lioresal) may have promise as a pharmacotherapy for cocaine addiction by reducing cocaine-evoked DA release in the shell of the nucleus accumbens in animals (294). However, data from Lile et al. demonstrates that acute administration of three clinically relevant baclofen doses (10, 20, 30 mg p.o.) did not influence the acute subject rated reinforcing behavioral effects of intranasal cocaine in humans (295).

Several immunotherapies are under development for cocaine and a cocaine vaccine has started human trials. The cocaine addiction immunotherapies have reduced relapse to drug use in animal model systems. To date, the active cocaine vaccine has few side effects and induces considerable antibody titers after active immunization in humans. Specific areas for immunotherapy may include treatment of drug overdose, prevention of brain or cardiac toxicity, and protection of a fetus during pregnancy in a drug abuser (296). Kuhar and colleagues suggest that other potential medications for cocaine abusers include 3-phenyltropane cocaine analogues, which could reduce drug-seeking and anticocaine catalytic antibodies, which could block the action of cocaine in the brain (297). Recent reports show that anticocaine catalytic monoclonal antibody 15A10 reduces the toxic effect of cocaine by increasing its breakdown to the systemically inert products ecgonine methylester and benzoic acid. An *in vivo* study in mice revealed the presence of antibody in blood up to 10 days following subcutaneous injections. These data demonstrate a potential for a sustained-release formulation of monoclonal antibody 15A10 for treatment of cocaine addiction (298).

Cocaine has humbled many researchers and research groups with its early and late recidivism, its persistent attachment of the user to the drug that is easily triggered by known and unrecognized environmental cues, and its willingness to "respond" to one or another experimental measure yet not stop continued use in clinical trials (299–309).

With continued understanding of the cellular basis for drug reward and the possibility that drug and other rewards are separable, new pharmacologic treatments that focus on the positive aspects of the drug-taking experience and that reduce drug reward and drug taking may be possible. While the brain produces neurotransmitters to maintain homeostasis, a drug like cocaine alters normal brain function to induce a sense of well-being. Repeated administration of cocaine causes the brain to function as if this new, drug-dependent, state was "normal." Our task in developing new and effective treatments is first to truly understand the effects of illicit drugs, then to establish a model for the abstinent state, and, finally, to provide a treatment that allows the person to feel safe and comfortable while permitting the brain the opportunity to return to its predrug normal state. Without an antidote to cocaine toxicity, it is doubtful that we will know enough about cocaine's effects to successfully undo them. It is hoped that cocaine treatment will soon evolve to match our treatment options for heroin.

The clinical findings and natural history of cocaine dependence, the attachment of the user to the drug, and the power of the cocaine reward in shaping, conditioning, and modifying behavior have contributed to the current therapeutic approach, which combines a number of modalities. Current treatment strategies are not one or another but are always a combined rehabilitation, psychodynamic, and behavioral with pharmacologic treatment during the acute withdrawal period and during early abstinence. Pharmacologic agents have been successfully used to decrease abstinence complaints and to decrease early treatment dropout rates. Pharmacologic agents have been used to reverse the acute abstinence-related inertia, dysphoria, and depression. Pharmacologic agents have also been used to reduce craving for cocaine with a hope that relapse might be prevented or made less likely. Finally, pharmacologic treatments have been given that were believed to modify cocaine's positive, rewarding effects to reduce relapse or the impact of a slip.

The mainstay of treatment for cocaine dependence remains behavioral. In treating physicians and celebrities addicted to cocaine, persistent abstinence can be achieved by contingent drug test-related contracting with swift consequences related to abstinence violation. For others, opposite reinforcement paradigms with monetary reward for abstinence have been successful. Community payment for abstinence or the "reinforcement approach" has shown more efficacy than traditional counseling or pharmacotherapies. Payment for abstinence by focusing on drug- and cocaine-free urines rather than a more amorphous outcome can succeed where standard drug-abuse counseling fails in retaining cocaine-dependent individuals in outpatient treatment. In one early study, a surprising 85% of patients completed 12 weeks of incentive treatment and 65% to 70% achieved 6 or more weeks of continuous cocaine abstinence across the two trials. By contrast, less than 45% of patients assigned to standard counseling completed 12 weeks of treatment. Higgins and colleagues (310) documented 6 or more weeks of continuous cocaine abstinence in only 5% to 10% of the nonincentive patients, results similar to those obtained by other clinicians trying to treat cocaine dependence. Their early work was followed by a random assignment test of incentives wherein patients earned vouchers exchangeable for retail items contingent on documentation of cocaine abstinence via urinalysis. Considering the widespread use of incentives in our capitalistic society the systematic use of incentives to foster cocaine abstinence may be warranted. Community reinforcement, payment for abstinence, and relapse prevention are the three major types of cocaine treatment programs in widespread use in the United States. A study by Higgins et al. (311) assessed whether incentives improved treatment outcome in ambulatory cocaine-dependent patients. They studied 40 cocaine-dependent adults randomly assigned to behavioral treatment with or without an added incentive program. The behavioral treatment was based on the community reinforcement approach and was provided to both groups. Subjects in the group with incentives received vouchers exchangeable for retail items contingent on submitting cocaine-free urine specimens during weeks 1 through 12 of treatment; the group without incentives received no vouchers during that period. The two groups were treated the same during weeks 13 to 24. In this important study, 75% of patients in the group with vouchers completed 24 weeks of treatment versus 40% in the group without vouchers. Average duration of continuous cocaine abstinence documented via urinalysis during weeks 1 to 24 of treatment were 11.7 ± 2.0 weeks in the group with vouchers versus 6.0 ± 1.5 weeks in the group without vouchers. At 24 weeks after treatment entry, the voucher group evidenced significantly greater improvement than the no-voucher group on the Addiction Severity Index (ASI) Drug scale, and only the voucher group showed significant improvement on the ASI Psychiatric scale. Their data support a greater role for incentives in cocaine relapse prevention.

Incentives delivered contingent on submitting cocaine-free urine specimens significantly improve treatment outcome in ambulatory cocaine-dependent patients. Standard treatment for cocaine dependence and prevention of relapse has been tried for the past decade and has now evolved to include elements of relapse prevention, 12-step programs, treatment of comorbid disorders, and other therapies to stop drug use and reduce recidivism. Recovery is a process that begins with a break in denial, a learning process of breaking old habits, friendships, and "triggers" to the first desire to use cocaine, and leading to eventual new healthy patterns of living centering the locus of control from an external one to an internal one. Patients are encouraged to identify internal and external precipitants of drug urges and to restructure their lives to avoid drug situations and relapse as compared with behavioral treatment, which focuses on extinguishing conditioned craving responses.

Mandatory Treatment

Two recent national studies (in the United States and England) reported what appear to be very poor 4- and 5-year outcomes for cocaine addiction. In the first study, 21% of the sample could not be located at the 5-year followup, 42% of the followup sample reported using cocaine in the past year, 25% admitted weekly use, and an additional 5% tested positive for use despite denying any use (312). At the time of followup, 17% of the patients were in drug treatment. In the second study of 4- and 5-year outcomes of addiction treatment in England, one-third of the sample used crack at admission and one-third of the sample used crack at followup—what appeared to be 100% relapse (313). Further examination revealed that among those who used crack at intake, more than half were no longer using it during followup, but about one-fourth of the noncrack users at intake were using crack at followup.

Cocaine addiction can be successfully treated, especially if the addict is a health professional. Mandatory,

monitored treatment for drug addiction can have long-term positive results. The Impaired Practitioners Program for the State of Florida, also known as Physician Resource Recovery Network (PRN) identifies, intervenes, and provides appropriate referral and case management for all physicians who are affected by chemical dependency/abuse. PRN follows individuals from evaluation through treatment, and then monitors their aftercare for 5 or more years. We recently examined 5-year outcomes data for 24 randomly selected Florida physicians who were monitored by PRN for substance abuse and dependence beginning in 1995 (314). During the monitoring phase (aftercare) each individual was required to attend a specialized monitoring group, was subject to randomized, at least weekly, urine monitoring, and was required to regularly attend a recovery support group program. Five-year recovery was documented by counselor reports, physician/psychiatrist evaluations, AA/NA attendance, return to work, and regular random urinalysis. Treatment setting varied widely. Regardless of setting of treatment, all had their urine testing and progress monitored and reported to the state. None were treated with methadone or other maintenance.

Physician recovery far exceeds rates reported for other patient groups. There was no statistically significant difference in outcome for M.D. crack/cocaine addicts as compared to opioid addicts or alcoholics. We found that after 5 years, 92% were drug free, had attended weekly meetings, had positive counselor and physician assessments, and returned to work (315). A recent study confirmed the importance of 12-step programs and lengthy aftercare. Crack cocaine abstinence for 18 months was significantly associated with frequent 12-step program attendance and having a longer period of aftercare (316).

While much is to be learned about the most effective approach for a particular patient, it does appear that cocaine addiction is a virulent disease where intensity of intervention and frequency of treatment contacts are important variables. All psychosocial treatments attempt to help patients understand their ambivalence to give up cocaine and clarify the importance of cocaine in the present problems. At the same time, the clinician and treatment program tries to reduce cocaine availability by encouraging patient avoidance of people, places, and things associated with the addiction. Active participation in a viable recovery group or program can reduce cocaine availability by supporting abstinence. The addict is encouraged to identify high-risk environments, feelings, and attitudes, and to prescribe a sponsor or group meeting rather than a relapse. Conditioned cues and cravings are identified in the context of the group meetings and the patient learns that an impulse does not mean an automatic action. In every drug challenge or potential use event, the user is asked to weigh the risks and benefits of a slip. Just coming to a daily treatment program is a lifestyle modification that can have a

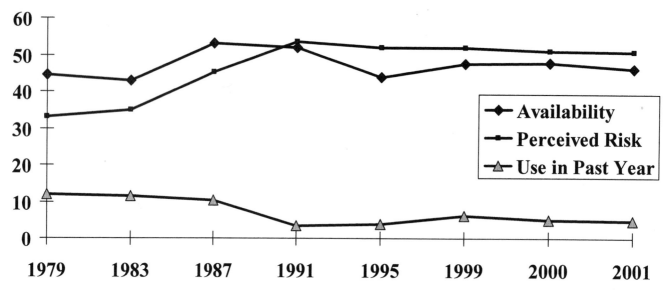

FIG. 13.1. Trends in cocaine availability, perceived risk, and use in past years for high school seniors.

very positive impact on recovery. Meetings provide an opportunity to learn and share with others and to develop new associates and coping skills. Finally, a slip does not automatically become a relapse and many intensive treatment programs manage such events by using them to prevent others. Recovery in such a model is very much like the recovery programs and attitudes commonly found in 12-step and other alcohol treatment programs—recovery is a marathon, not a sprint.

THE BEST TREATMENT IS PREVENTION

Cocaine dependence remains an intractable public health problem in the United States that contributes to many of our most disturbing social crises, including violent crime, unsafe streets, urban decay, accidents, unnecessary medical costs, the spread of infectious disease (e.g., AIDS, hepatitis, and tuberculosis), failures in school and work performance, and neonatal drug exposure. Every physician should realize that the experience of recent years has proved that effective education prevents drug abuse and results in abstinence. Beginning in the mid-1980s, America, under the influence of President and Mrs. Reagan, began to emphasize demand reduction through education. A wide

range of efforts based in schools, the community, the workplace, religious groups, and the family aimed at reducing drug use has resulted in a dramatic reduction of drug use. In addition, the Partnership for a Drug-Free America, an organization that uses many of this country's best advertising and marketing minds, has created a remarkable series of advertisements aimed at "unselling" drugs. These ads, in a direct and powerful manner, demystify and deglamorize drug use. These ads have helped to reduce drug use in general, but they have had an especially significant effect upon adolescents and children.

Education for prevention actually should begin before a child is conceived. Prospective parents should know the severe physical and mental side effects that may afflict their offspring if they use drugs prior to conception. After birth, drug education should begin at home and be reinforced by pediatricians and family physicians. A broad-based school program should start with kindergarten and end with college. Employers and governmental agencies must also share in this drug education program. Physicians should play a significant role in reducing the cocaine epidemic by never failing to consider the possibility of substance abuse in their patients and by inoculating their patients, especially their younger ones, with accurate information about this dangerous and deadly drug.

TABLE 13.6. *Recent trends in alcohol and drug use*

Substance	1985[a]	1992[a]	% Change
Alcohol	113,000,000	98,200,000	−13%
Cigarettes	60,000,000	54,000,000	−10%
Marijuana	18,000,000	9,000,000	−50%
Cocaine	6,000,000	1,300,000	−79%

[a]Current use (within previous 30 days) of drugs in the United States, 1985–1992.

Prevention and education are supported by a social climate where danger of cocaine is clear and social policies prohibit use on the basis of the hypothesis that safe use is an oxymoron. Dupont and Voth (315) reviewed current and historical trends in United States drug policy. They reported that a restrictive cocaine and other drug policy is a deterrent to drug use and helps reduce drug-related costs and societal problems. Although legalization or decriminalization of cocaine and other drugs might reduce some of the legal consequences of drug use, increased drug use would result and harmful consequences would far outweigh these initial benefits.

REFERENCES

1. Rome HP. Personal reflections—cocaine. *Psychiatr Ann* 1988;18(9):505.
2. Substance Abuse and Mental Health Services Administration. *Results from the 2001 National Household Survey on Drug Abuse: volume I. Summary of national findings* (Office of Applied Studies, NHSDA Series H-17, DHHS Publication No. SMA 02–3758). Rockville, MD: Author, 2002.
3. Johnston LD, O Malley PM, Bachman JG. *Monitoring the Future national survey results on drug use, 1975-2001. Volume I: secondary school students* (NIH Publication No. 02-5106). Bethesda, MD: National Institute on Drug Abuse, 2002.
4. Substance Abuse and Mental Health Services Administration, Office of Applied Studies. *Emergency Department Trends From the Drug Abuse Warning Network, Final Estimates.1994-2001* (DAWN Series D-21, DHHS Publication No. SMA 02–3635). Rockville, MD: Author, 2002.
5. Substance Abuse and Mental Health Services Administration, Office of Applied Studies. *Mortality data from the Drug Abuse Warning Network, 2000.* (DAWN Series D-19, DHHS Publication No. SMA 02–3633). Rockville, MD: Author, 2002.
6. Johnston LD, O Malley PM, Bachman JG. *National survey results on drug use from the Monitoring the Future study, 1975–1994.* Rockville, MD: National Institute on Drug Abuse, 1995.
7. *PRIDE survey, 1994–1995. National summary, United States, grades 6–12.* Bowling Green, KY: PRIDE, 1995.
8. Petersen RC. Cocaine: an overview. *NIDA Res Monogr* 1977;13:5–15.
9. Carroll E. Coca: the plant and its use. *NIDA Res Monogr* 1977;13:35–45.
10. Siegel RK. Cocaine smoking. *J Psychoactive Drugs* 1982;14:277–359.
11. Phillips J, Wynne RD. *Cocaine: The mystique and the reality.* New York: Avon Books, 1980.
12. Morimer WG. *Peru: history of coca, the "divine plant" of the Incas. With an introductory account of the Incas and of the Andean Indians of today.* New York: Vail, 1901; New York: AMS Press, 1978 (reprint).
13. Siegel RK. New patterns of cocaine use: changing dose and routes. *NIDA Res Monogr* 1985;61:204–220.
14. Freud S. Uber Coca [on cocaine]. In: Byck R, ed. *Cocaine papers.* New York: Stonehill Publishing, 1974:49–73.
15. Kleber HD. Introduction. Cocaine abuse: historical, epidemiological and psychological perspectives. *J Clin Psychiatry* 1988;49[Suppl 2]:3–6.
16. Freud S. On the general effects of cocaine (1885). *Drug Depend* 1970;5:15–17.
17. Jones E. The cocaine episode. In: Trilling L, Marcus S, eds. *The life and work of Sigmund Freud.* New York: Basic Books, 1953:52–67.
18. Byck R. *Cocaine papers: Sigmund Freud.* New York: Stonehill Publishing, 1974.
19. Louis JC, Yazijian HZ. *The cola wars.* New York: *Everest House Publishers,* 1980;13–38.
20. Graff H. The Coca-Cola conspiracy. *High Times* 1977;24:47–50, 76, 78.
21. Beattie GF. Soft drink flavours: their history and characteristics. *Perfumery and Essential Oil Record* 1956;47:437–442.
22. Estroff TW, Gold MS. Medical and psychiatric complications of cocaine abuse with possible points of pharmacological treatment. *Adv Alcohol Subst Abuse* 1986;5(1–2):61–76.
23. Van Dyke C, Byck R. Cocaine use in man. *Adv Alcohol Subst Abuse* 1983;3:1–24.
24. Siegel RK. Cocaine: recreational use and intoxication. *NIDA Res Monogr* 1977;13:119–136.
25. Grinspoon L, Bakalar JB. A kick from cocaine. *Psychology Today* 1977:41–42, 78.
26. Grinspoon L, Bakalar JB. Drug dependence: nonnarcotic agents. In: Kaplan HI, Freedman AM, Sadock BJ, eds. *Comprehensive textbook of psychiatry,* 3rd ed. Baltimore: Williams & Wilkins, 1980:1621
27. Gold MS. Crack abuse: its implications and outcomes. *Resident Staff Physician* 1987;33(8):45–53.
28. Kandel DB, Yamaguchi K. From beer to crack: developmental patterns of involvement in drugs. *Am J Public Health* 1993;83:851–855.
29. Johanson CE, Fischman MF. The pharmacology of cocaine related to its abuse. *Pharmacol Rev* 1989;41:3–52.
30. Foltin RW, Fischman MW. Smoked and intravenous cocaine in humans: acute tolerance, cardiovascular and subjective effects. *J Pharmacol Exp Ther* 1991;257:247–261.
31. Roehrich H, Gold MS. 800-COCAINE: origin, significance and findings. *Yale J Biol Med* 1988;61:149–155.
32. Brookoff D, Cook CS, Williams C, et al. Testing reckless drivers for cocaine and marijuana. *N Engl J Med* 1994;331:518–522.
33. US Dept of Justice National DNG Threat Assessment Product No. 2002–Q0317–001, Dec 2001.
34. Gawin FH, Ellinwood EH Jr. Cocaine and other stimulants. *N Engl J Med* 1988;318:1173–1182.
35. Adler J. Hour by hour crack. *Newsweek* 1988 Nov 28:64–79.
36. Miller NS, Mirin SM. Multiple drug use in alcoholics: practical and theoretical implications. *Psychiatr Ann* 1989;19:248–255.
37. National Institute on Drug Abuse. Cocaine tops list of drugs sending users to emergency rooms. *NIDA Notes* 1988:22–23.
38. National Institute on Drug Abuse. *Statistical series: semiannual report: trend data through July-December 1988.* Data from the Drug Abuse Warning Network, series G. 23:8ff. http://dawninfo.samnsa.gov
39. Wish ED, O'Neil JA. Drug use forecasting (DUF) research update. *US Department of Justice Newsletter,* September 1989.
40. Tardiff DP, Gross EM, Wu J, et al. Analysis of cocaine positive fatalities. *J Forensic Sci* 1989;34:53–63.
41. Marzuk PM, Tardiff K, Leon AC, et al. Prevalence of recent cocaine use among motor vehicle fatalities in New York City. *JAMA* 1990;263:250–256.
42. Lowenstein DH, Massa DM, Rowbotham MC, et al. Acute neurologic and psychiatric complications associated with cocaine abuse. *Am J Med* 1987;83:841–846.
43. Lindenbaum GA, Carroll SF, Daskal I, et al. Patterns of alcohol and drug abuse in an urban trauma center: the

increasing role of cocaine abuse. *J Trauma* 1989;29:1654–1658.

44. *Substance abuse. The nation's number one health problem.* The Robert Wood Johnson Foundation, 1993.

45. Gold MS, Gleaton TJ. Cocaine, marijuana, alcohol, violence. Results of annual high school survey. *Biol Psychiatry* 1995;37:627.

46. Brain PF, Coward GA. A review of the history, actions, and legitimate uses of cocaine. *J Subst Abuse* 1989;1:431–451.

47. Epstein JF. *Substance dependence, abuse, and treatment: findings from the 2000 National Household Survey on Drug Abuse* (NHSDA Series A-16, DHHS Publication No. SMA 02–3642). Rockville, MD: Substance Abuse and Mental Health Services Administration, Office of Applied Studies, 2002.

48. Gold MS, Verebey K. The psychopharmacology of cocaine. *Psychiatr Ann* 1984;140:714–723.

49. Verebey K, Gold MS. From coca leaves to crack: the effects of dose and routes of administration in abuse liability. *Psychiatr Ann* 1988;18:513–521.

50. Gawin FH, Kleber HD. Abstinence symptomatology and psychiatric diagnosis in cocaine abusers: clinical observations. *Arch Gen Psychiatry* 1986;43:107–113.

51. Porrino LJ, Lyons D, Miller MD, et al. Metabolic mapping of the effects of cocaine during the initial phases of self-administration in the nonhuman primate. *J Neurosci* 2002;22 (17):7687–7694.

52. Wilson JM, Nobrega JN, Corrigall WA, et al. Amygdala dopamine levels are markedly elevated after self—but not passive—administration of cocaine. *Brain Res* 1994;668:39–45.

53. Dunwiddie TV. Mechanisms of cocaine abuse and toxicity: an overview. *NIDA Res Monogr* 1988;88:185–198.

54. Ritchie JM, Greene NM. Local anesthetics. In: Gilman AG, Goodman LS, Rall TW, et al., eds. *Goodman and Gilman's the pharmacological basis of therapeutics,* 7th ed. New York: Macmillan, 1985:309–310.

55. Javaid J, Fischman MW, Schuster CR, et al. Cocaine plasma concentrations: relationship to physiological and subjective effects in humans. *Science* 1978;202:227–228.

56. Resnick R, Schuyten-Resnick E. Clinical aspects of cocaine: assessment of cocaine abuse behavior in man. In: Mulè SJ, ed. *Cocaine.* Boca Raton, FL: CRC Press, 1977.

57. Kuhar MJ, Ritz MC, Sharkey J. Cocaine receptors on dopamine transporters mediate cocaine-reinforced behavior. *NIDA Res Monogr* 1988;88:14–22.

58. Wise RA, Bozarth MA. A psychomotor stimulant theory of addiction. *Psychol Rev* 1987;94(4):469–492.

59. Petit Ho, Pan HT, Parsons LH, et al. Extracellular concentrations of cocaine and dopamine are enhanced during chronic cocaine administration. *J Neurochem* 1990;55:798–804.

60. Kalivas PW, Duffy P. Time course of extracellular dopamine and behavioral sensitization to cocaine. II. Dopamine perikarya. *J Neurosci* 1993;13:276–284.

61. Petit H, Justice J. Dopamine in the nucleus accumbens during cocaine self-administration as studied by *in vivo* microdialysis. *Pharmacol Biochem Behav* 1989;34:899–904.

62. Petit H, Justice JB. Effect of dose on cocaine self-administration behavior and dopamine levels in the nucleus accumbens. *Brain Res* 1991;539:94–102.

63. Yoshida M, Yokoo H, Mizoguchi Y, et al. Eating and drinking cause increased dopamine release in the nucleus accumbens and ventral tegmental area in the rat: measurement by *in vivo* microdialysis. *Neurosci Lett* 1992;139:73–76.

64. Hernandez L, Hoebel BG. Food reward and cocaine increase extracellular dopamine in the nucleus accumbens as measured by microdialysis. *Life Sci* 1988;42:1705–1712.

65. Maisonneuve IM, Ho A, Kreek MJ. Chronic administration of a cocaine "binge" alters basal extracellular levels in male rats: an *in vivo* microdialysis study. *J Pharmacol Exp Ther* 1995;272:652–657.

66. Volkow ND, Fowler JS, Logan J, et al. Carbon-11-cocaine binding compared at subpharmacological and pharmacological doses: a PET study. *J Nucl Med* 1995;36:1289–1297.

67. Robbins TW, Everitt BJ. Functions of dopamine in the dorsal and ventral striatum. *Semin Neurosci* 1992;4:119–127.

68. White NM, Milner PM. The psychobiology of reinforcers. *Annu Rev Psychol* 1992;43:443–471.

69. Wise RA, Rompre PP. Brain dopamine and reward. *Annu Rev Psychol* 1989;40:191–225.

70. Robinson TE, Berridge KC. The neural basis of drug craving: an incentive-sensitization theory of addiction. *Brain Res Rev* 1993;18:247–291.

71. Robinson TE, Gorny G, Mitton E, et al. Cocaine self-administration alters the morphology of dendrites and dendritic spines in the nucleus accumbens and neocortex. *Synapse* 2001;39(3):257–266.

72. Bastos ML, Hoffman DB. Detection and identification of cocaine, its metabolites and its derivatives. In: Mulé

SJ, ed. *Cocaine: chemical, biological, clinical, social and treatment aspects.* Boca Raton, FL: CRC Press, 1976:45.

73. Wallach MB, Gerson S. A neuropsychopharmacological comparison of *d*-amphetamine, L-DOPA and cocaine. *Neuropharmacology* 1971;10:743.

74. Self DW, Nestler EJ. Molecular mechanisms of drug reinforcement and addiction. *Annu Rev Neurosci* 1995;18:463–495.

75. Dimijian GG. Contemporary drug abuse. In: Goth A, ed. *Medical pharmacology, principles and concepts,* 7th ed. St. Louis: CV Mosby, 1974:313.

76. Sterk C. Cocaine, HIV seropositivity. *Lancet* 1988;1:1052–1053.

77. Dackis CA, Gold MS. Biological aspects of cocaine addiction. In: Volkow ND, Swann AC, eds. *Cocaine in the brain.* New Brunswick, NJ: Rutgers University Press, 1988.

78. Mello NK, Sarnyai Z, Mendelson JH, et al. Acute effects of cocaine on anterior pituitary hormones in male and female rhesus monkeys. *J Pharmacol Exp Ther* 1993;266:804–811.

79. Dackis CA, Gold, MS. New concepts in cocaine addiction: the dopamine depletion hypothesis. *Neurosci Biobehav Rev* 1985;9:469–477.

80. Kranzler HR, Wallington DJ. Serum prolactin level, craving and early discharge from treatment in cocaine-dependent patients. *Am J Drug Alcohol Abuse* 1992;18:187–195.

81. Krystal JH, Gawin F, Charney DS, et al. Clinical phenomenology and neurobiology of cocaine abstinence: a prospective inpatient study. *Am J Psychiatry* 1991;148:1712–1716.

82. Mello NK, Teoh SK, Ellingboe J, et al. Cocaine effects on pulsatile secretion of anterior pituitary, gonadal, and adrenal hormones. *J Clin Endocrinol Metab* 1989;69:1256–1260.

83. Mello NK, Sarnyai Z, Mendelson JH, et al. Acute effects of cocaine on anterior pituitary hormones in male and female rhesus monkeys. *J Pharmacol Exp Ther* 1993;266:804–811.

84. Teoh SK, Mendelson JH, Mello NK, et al. Hyperprolactinemia and risk for relapse of cocaine abuse. *Biol Psychiatry* 1990;28:824–828.

85. Krantzler HR, Wallington DJ. Serum prolactin level, craving, and early discharge from treatment in cocaine-dependent patients. *Am J Drug Alcohol Abuse* 1992;18:187–195.

86. Gold MS. *Cocaine.* New York: Plenum Medical Books, 1993.

87. Hollander E, Nunes E, DeCaria CM, et al. Dopaminergic sensitivity and cocaine abuse: response to apomorphine. *Psychiatry Res* 1990;33:161–169.

88. Goeders NE. The HPA axis and cocaine reinforcement. *Psychoneuroendocrinology* 2002;27(1–2):13–33.

89. Gurkovskaya O, Goeders NE. Effects of CP-154,526 on responding during extinction from cocaine self-administration in rats. *Eur J Pharmacol* 2001;432(1):53–56.

90. Winhusen T, Somoza E. The HPA axis in cocaine use: implications for pharmacotherapy. *J Addict Dis* 2001; 20(3):105–119.

91. Weinstein SP, Gottheil E, Smith RH, et al. Cocaine users seen in medical practice. *Am J Drug Alcohol Abuse* 1986;12:341–354.

92. Jeri FR, Sanchez CC, Del Pozo T, et al. Further experience with the syndromes produced by coca paste smoking. In: Jeri FR, ed. *Cocaine 1980.* Lima, Peru: Pacific Press, 1980.

93. Mulè SJ. The pharmacodynamics of cocaine abuse. *Psychiatr Ann* 1984;14: 724–727.

94. Haney M, Ward AS, Gerra G, et al. Neuroendocrine effects of D-fenfluramine and bromocriptine following repeated smoked cocaine in humans. *Drug Alcohol Depend* 2001;64(1):63–73.

95. Jaffee JH. Drug addiction and drug abuse. In: Gilman AG, Goodman LS, Rall TW, et al., eds. *Goodman and Gilman's the pharmacological basis of therapeutics,* 7th ed. New York: Macmillan, 1985:532–581.

96. Anthony JC, Tien AY, Petronis KR. Epidemiologic evidence on cocaine use and panic attacks. *Am J Epidemiol* 1989;129:543–549.

97. Jatlow P. Cocaethylene. Pharmacologic activity and clinical significance. *Ther Drug Monit* 1993;15:533–536.

98. Gold MS. *800-COCAINE.* New York: Bantam, 1984.

99. Dackis CA, Gold MS. Addictiveness of central stimulants. *Adv Alcohol Subst Abuse* 1990;9:9–26.

100. Childress AR, McLellan AT, Ehrman RN, et al. Extinction of conditioned responses in abstinent cocaine or opioid users. *NIDA Res Monogr* 1987;76:189–195.

101. Ehrman RN, Robbins SJ, Childress AR, et al. Conditioned responses to cocaine-related stimuli in cocaine abuse patients. *Psychopharmacology* 1992;107:523–529.

102. Margolin A, Avants K, Kosten TR. Cue-elicited cocaine craving and autogenic relaxation: association with treatment outcome. *J Subst Abuse Treat* 1994;11:549–552.

103. Derlet RW, Albertson TE. Emergency department presentation of cocaine intoxication. *Ann Emerg Med* 1989;18:115–119.

104. Benowitz NL. How toxic is cocaine? In: *Cocaine: scientific and social dimensions. Ciba Found Symp* 1992;166:125–148.

105. Benchimol A, Bartall H, Desser KB. Accelerated ventricular rhythm and cocaine abuse. *Ann Intern Med* 1978;88:519–520.

106. Karch SB, Billingham ME. The pathology and etiology of cocaine-induced heart disease. *Arch Pathol Lab Med* 1988;112:225–230.

107. Crumb WJ Jr, Clarkson CW. Characterization of cocaine-induced block of cardiac sodium channels. *Biophys J* 1990;57:589–599.

108. Jones LF, Tackett RL. Central mechanisms of action involved in cocaine-induced tachycardia. *Life Sci* 1990;46: 723–728.

109. Perez-Meyes M, DiGiuseppi S, Ondrusek G, et al. Free-base cocaine smoking. *Clin Pharmacol Ther* 1982; 32:459–465.

110. Foltin RW, Fischman MW, Pedroso JJ, et al. Repeated intranasal cocaine administration: lack of tolerance to pressor effects. *Drug Alcohol Depend* 1988;22:169–177.

111. Lichtenfeld PJ, Rubin DB, Feldman RS. Subarachnoid hemorrhage precipitated by cocaine snorting. *Arch Neurol* 1984;41:223–224.

112. Smith HWB, Lieberman HA, Brody SL, et al. Acute myocardial infarction temporally related to cocaine use. *Ann Intern Med* 1987;107:13–18.

113. Vitullo JC, Karam R, Mekhail N, et al. Cocaine-induced small vessel spasm in isolated rat hearts. *Am J Pathol* 1989;135:85–91.

114. Chow JM, Menchen SKL, Paul BD, et al. Vascular changes in the nasal submucosa of chronic cocaine addicts. *Am J Forensic Med Pathol* 1990;11:136–143.

115. Isner HM, Estes North AM III, Thompson PD, et al. Acute cardiac events temporally related to cocaine abuse. *N Engl J Med* 1986;315:1438–1443.

116. Wilkerson RD. Cardiovascular toxicity of cocaine. *NIDA Res Monogr* 1988;88:304–324.

117. Schachne JS, Roberts BH, Thompson PD. Coronary artery spasm and myocardial infarction associated with cocaine use. *N Engl J Med* 1984;310:1665–1666.

118. Som P, Oster ZH, Wans GJ, et al. Spatial and temporal distribution of cocaine and effects of pharmacological interventions: whole-body autoradiographic microimaging studies. *Life Sci* 1994;55:1375–1382.

119. Dressler FA, Malekzadeh S, Roberts WC. Quantitative analysis of amounts of coronary arterial narrowing in cocaine addicts. *Am J Cardiol* 1990;65(5):303–308.

120. Togna G, Tempesta E, Togna AR, et al. Platelet responsiveness and biosynthesis of thromboxane and prostacyclin in response in in vitro cocaine treatment. *Haemostasis* 1985;15:100–107.

121. Peng SK, French WJ, Pelikan PCD. Direct cocaine cardiotoxicity demonstrated by endomyocardial biopsy. *Arch Pathol Lab Med* 1989;113:842–845.

122. Tun A, Khan IA. Myocardial infarction with normal coronary arteries: the pathologic and clinical perspectives. *Angiology* 2001;52(5):299–304.

123. Norris KC, Thornhill-Joynes M, Robinson C, et al. Cocaine use, hypertension, and end-stage renal disease. *Am J Kidney Dis* 2001;38(3):523–528.

124. Mochizuki Y, Zhang M, Golestaneh L, et al. Acute aortic thrombosis and renal infarction in acute cocaine intoxication: a case report and review of literature. *Clin Nephrol* 2003;60(2):130–133.

125. Wiener MD, Putnam CE. Pain in the chest in a user of cocaine. *JAMA* 1987; 258:2087–2088.

126. Itkonen J, Schnoll A, Glassroth J. Pulmonary dysfunction in "freebase" cocaine users. *Arch Intern Med* 1984;144:2195–2197.

127. Hoffman CK, Goodman PC. Pulmonary edema in cocaine smokers. *Radiology* 1989;172:462–465.

128. Cregler LL, Mark H. Medical complications of cocaine abuse. *N Engl J Med* 1986;315:1495–1500.

129. Murray RJ, Albin RJ, Mergner W, et al. Diffuse alveolar hemorrhage temporally related to cocaine smoking. *Chest* 1988;93:427–429.

130. Rebhum J. Association of asthma and freebase smoking. *Ann Allergy* 1988;60:339–342.

131. Jonsson S, O'Meara M, Young JB. Acute cocaine poisoning: importance of treating seizures and acidosis. *Am J Med* 1983;75:1061–1064.

132. Monasterio L, Morovic GC. Midline palate perforation from cocaine abuse. *Plast Reconstr Surg* 2003;112 (3):914–915.

133. Talbott JF, Gorti GK, Koch RJ. Midfacial osteomyelitis in a chronic cocaine abuser: a case report. *Ear Nose Throat J* 2001;80(10):742–743.

134. Barden JC. Crack smoking seen as a peril to the lungs. *New York Times* 1989 Dec 24:19.

135. Strong DH, Westcott JY, Biller JA, et al. Eosinophilic "empyema" associated with crack cocaine use. *Thorax* 2003;58(9):823–824.

136. Maeder M, Ullmer E. Pneumomediastinum and bilateral pneumothorax as a complication of cocaine smoking. *Respiration* 2003;70(4):407.

137. Buttner A, Mall G, Penning R, et al. The neuropathology of cocaine abuse. *Leg*

Med (Tokyo) 2003;5[Suppl 1]:S240–S242.

138. Merriam AE, Medalia A, Levine B. Partial complex status epilepticus associated with cocaine abuse. *Biol Psychiatry* 1988;23:515–518.

139. Post RM, Kopanda RT, Black KE. Progressive effects of cocaine on behavior and central amine metabolism in the rhesus monkey: relationship to kindling and psychosis. *Biol Psychiatry* 1976;11:403–419.

140. Hayase T, Yamamoto Y, Yamamoto K. Protective effects of cannabinoid receptor ligands analogous to anandamide against cocaine toxicity. *Nihon Arukoru Yakubutsu Igakkai Zasshi* 2001;36(6):596–608.

141. Volkow ND, Fowler JS, Wolf AP, et al. Effects of chronic cocaine abuse on postsynaptic dopamine receptors. *Am J Psychiatry* 1990;147:719–724.

142. Johnson BA, Devous MD Sr, Ruiz P, et al. Treatment advances for cocaine-induced ischemic stroke: focus on dihydropyridine-class calcium channel antagonists. *Am J Psychiatry* 2001;158(8):1191–1198.

143. Kosten TR, Gottschalk PC, Tucker K, et al. Aspirin or amiloride for cerebral perfusion defects in cocaine dependence. *Drug Alcohol Depend* 2003;20:71(2):187–194.

144. Strickland TL, Mena I, Villanueva-Meyer J, et al. Cerebral perfusion and neuropsychological consequences of chronic cocaine use. *J Neuropsychiatry Clin Neurosci* 1993;5:419–427.

145. Howington JU, Kutz SC, Wilding GE, et al. Cocaine use as a predictor of outcome in aneurysmal subarachnoid hemorrhage. *J Neurosurg* 2003;99(2):271–275.

146. Estroff TW, Gold MS. Chronic medical complications of drug abuse. *Psychiatr Med* 1987;3:267–286.

147. Lukas SE, Sholar M, Kouri E, et al. Marijuana smoking increases plasma cocaine levels and subjective reports of euphoria in male volunteers. *Pharmacol Biochem Behav* 1994;48:715–721.

148. Ashley R. *Cocaine: its history, uses and effects.* New York: St. Martin's Press, 1975:240.

149. Rodriguez Gomez E, Rodriguez Gomez FJ, Merino MJ, et al. Reversible posterior leukoencephalopathy, severe hypertension, and cocaine abuse. *Nefrologia* 2001;21(3):305–308.

150. Smith DE, Wesson DR, Apter-Marsh M. Cocaine- and alcohol-induced sexual dysfunction in patients with addictive diseases. *J Psychoactive Drugs* 1984;16:359–361.

151. Chasnoff IJ, Burns WJ, Schnoll SH, et al. Cocaine use in pregnancy. *N Engl J Med* 1985;313:666–669.

152. Mendelson J, Teoh S, Lange U, et al. Hyperprolactinemia during cocaine withdrawal. *NIDA Res Monogr* 1988;81:67–73.

153. Mendelson JH, Mello NK, Teoh SK, et al. Cocaine effects on pulsatile secretion of anterior pituitary, gonadal, and adrenal hormones. *J Clin Endocrinol Metab* 1989;69:1256–1260.

154. Jonas JM, Gold MS. Cocaine abuse and eating disorders. *Lancet* 1986;1:390–391.

155. Roberts DCS, Quattrocchi E, Howland MA. Severe hyperthermia secondary to intravenous drug abuse. *Am J Emerg Med* 1984;2:373.

156. Loghmanee F, Tobak M. Fatal malignant hyperthermia associated with recreational cocaine and ethanol abuse. *Am J Forensic Med Pathol* 1986;7:246–248.

157. Goldfrank LR, et al., eds. *Toxicologic emergencies,* 3rd ed. Norwalk, CT: Appleton-Century-Crofts, 1986:477–486.

158. Gold MS. Medical implications of cocaine intoxication. *Alcoholism Addiction* 1989 (Oct):16.

159. Merigian KS, Roberts JR. Cocaine intoxication: hyperpyrexia, rhabdomyolysis, and acute renal failure. *J Toxicol Clin Toxicol* 1987;25:135–148.

160. Krohn KD, Slowman-Kovacs S, Leapman SB. Cocaine and rhabdomyolysis. *Ann Intern Med* 1988;208:639–640.

161. Doctora JS, Williams CW, Bennett CR, et al. Rhabdomyolysis in the acutely cocaine- intoxicated patient sustaining maxillofacial trauma: report of a case and review of the literature. *J Oral Maxillofac Surg* 2003;61(8):964–967.

162. Roth D, Alarcon FJ, Fernandez JA, et al. Acute rhabdomyolysis associated with cocaine intoxication. *N Engl J Med* 1988;319:673–677.

163. Schweitzer VG. Osteolytic sinusitis and pneumomediastinum: deceptive otolaryngologic complications of cocaine abuse. *Laryngoscope* 1986;96:206–210.

164. Vilensky W. Illicit and licit drugs causing perforation of the nasal septum. *J Forensic Sci* 1982;27:958–962.

165. Van Dyke C, Jatlow P, Ungerer J, et al. Oral cocaine: plasma concentrations and central effects. *Science* 1978;200:211–213.

166. Edlin BR, Irwin KL, Faruque S, et al. Intersecting epidemics-crack cocaine use and HIV infection among inner-city young adults. *N Engl J Med* 1994;331:1422–1427.

167. Theall KP, Sterk CE, Elifson KW, Kidder D. Factors associated with positive HIV serostatus among women who use drugs: continued evidence for expanding factors of influence. *Public Health Rep* 2003;118(5):415–424.

168. Kreek MJ. Multiple drug abuse patterns and medical consequences. In: Meltzer HY, ed. *Psychopharmacology: the third generation of progress.* New York: Raven Press, 1987:1600–1603.

169. Cregler LL, Mark H. Cardiovascular dangers of cocaine abuse. *Am J Cardiol* 1986;57:1185–1186.

170. Kosten TR, Kleber HD. Sudden death in cocaine abusers: relation to neuroleptic malignant syndrome. *Lancet* 1987;1(8543):1198–1199.

171. Balbir-Gurman A, Braun-Moscovici Y, Nahir AM. Cocaine-induced Raynaud's phenomenon and ischaemic finger necrosis. *Clin Rheumatol* 2001;20(5):376–378.

172. Woods JR Jr, Plessinger MA. Pregnancy increases cardiovascular toxicity to cocaine. *Am J Obstet Gynecol* 1990;162:529–533.

173. Pritchard JA, MacDonald PC, Gant NF. *Williams obstetrics. Norwalk, CT: Appleton-Century-Crofts,* 1985;395–407.

174. Finnegan L. The dilemma of cocaine exposure in the perinatal period. *NIDA Res Monogr* 1988;81:379.

175. Richards IS, Kulkarni AP, Bremner WF. Cocaine-induced arrhythmia in human foetal myocardium *in vitro*: possible mechanism for fetal death *in utero. Pharmacol Toxicol* 1990;66:150–154.

176. Hadeed AJ, Siegel SR. Maternal cocaine use during pregnancy: effect on the newborn infant. *Pediatrics* 1989;84:205–210.

177. Critchley HOD, Woods SM, Barson AJ, et al. Fetal death *in utero* and cocaine abuse. *Case report. Br J Obstet Gynecol* 1988;95:195–196.

178. Singer L, Arendt R, Minnes S. Neurodevelopmental effects of cocaine. *Clin Perinatol* 1993;20:245–261.

179. Bingol N, Fuchs M, Diaz V, et al. Teratogenicity of cocaine in humans. *J Pediatr* 1987;110:93–96.

180. Cherukuri R, Minkoff H, Feldman J, et al. A cohort study of alkaloidal cocaine (crack) in pregnancy. *Obstet Gynecol* 1989;72:145–151.

181. Zuckerman B, Amaro H, Bauchner H, et al. Depressive symptoms during pregnancy: relationship to poor health behaviors. *Am J Obstet Gynecol* 1989;160:1107–1111.

182. Little BB, Snell LM, Van Beveren TT, et al. Treatment of substance abuse during pregnancy and infant outcome. *Am J Perinatol,* 2003;20(5):255–262.

183. Lewis DE, Moore CM, Leikin JB, et al. Meconium analysis for cocaine: a validation study and comparison with paired urine analysis. *J Anal Toxicol* 1995;19:148–150.

184. Bateman DA, Heagarty MC. Passive freebase cocaine ("crack") inhalation by infants and toddlers. *Am J Dis Child* 1989;134:25–27.

185. Dobersczak TM, Shanzer S, Senie RT, et al. Neonatal neurologic and electroencephalographic effects of intrauterine cocaine exposure. *J Pediatr* 1988;113:354–358.

186. Zuckerman B, Frank DA, Hingson R, et al. Effects of maternal marijuana and cocaine use on fetal growth. *N Engl J Med* 1989;320:762–768.

187. Chasnoff IJ, Lewis DE, Squires L. Cocaine intoxication in a breast-fed infant. *Pediatrics* 1987;80:836–838.

188. Newald J. Cocaine infants: a new arrival at hospitals' step? *Hospitals* 1986;60(7):96.

189. Vidaeff AC, Mastrobattista JM. *In utero* cocaine exposure: a thorny mix of science and mythology. *Am J Perinatol* 2003;20(4):165–172.

190. Lutiger B, Graham K, Einarson TR, et al. Relationship between gestational cocaine use and pregnancy outcome: a meta-analysis. *Teratology* 1991;44:405–414.

191. Ward SLD, Schuetz S, Krishna V, et al. Abnormal sleeping ventilatory pattern in infants of substance-abusing mothers. *Am J Dis Child* 1986;140:1015–1020.

192. Chasnoff IJ. Perinatal effects of cocaine. *Contemp OB/GYN* 1987 (May):163–179.

193. Chasnoff IJ. Cocaine intoxication in an infant via maternal milk. *Pediatrics* 2004 (*in press*).

194. Hofkosh D, Pringle JL, Wald HP, et al. Early interactions between drug-involved mothers and infants. Within-group differences. *Arch Pediatr Adolesc Med* 1995;149(6):665–672.

195. Ostrea EM, Brady M, Gause S, et al. Drug screening of newborns by meconium analysis: a large-scale, prospective, epidemiologic study. *Pediatrics* 1992;89:107–113.

196. Pichini S, Pacifici R, Pellegrini M, et al. Development and validation of a liquid chromatography-mass spectrometry assay for the determination of opiates and cocaine in meconium. *J Chromatogr B Analyt Technol Biomed Life Sci* 2003;5;794(2):281–292.

197. Vinner E, Vignau J, Thibault D, et al. Neonatal hair analysis contribution to establishing a gestational drug exposure profile and predicting a withdrawal syndrome. *Ther Drug Monit* 2003;25(4):421–432.

198. Gold MS. Cocaine. In: *Medical and health annual.* Chicago: Encyclopedia Britannica, 1988:277–284.

199. Siegel RK. Cocaine smoking disorders: diagnosis and treatment. *Psychiatr Ann* 1984;14:728–732.

200. Gold MS. *The good news about panic, anxiety, and phobias.* New York: Villard Books, 1989.

201. Rounsaville BJ, Anton SF, Carroll K, et al. Psychiatric diagnosis of treatment seeking cocaine abusers. *Arch Gen Psychiatry* 1991;48:43–51.

202. Asberg M, Errikson B. The effects of serotonin re-uptake blockers on depression. *J Clin Psychiatry* 1986;41:23–35.

203. Gold MS, Estroff TW. The comprehensive evaluation of cocaine and opiate abusers. In: Hall RCW, Beresford TP, eds. *Handbook of psychiatric diagnostic procedures,* vol. 2. Spectrum Publications, 1985.

204. Mello NK, Negus SS, Scott E, et al. A primate model of polydrug abuse: cocaine and heroin combinations. *J Pharmacol Exp Ther* 1995;274:1325–1337.

205. Millman RB. Evaluation and clinical management of cocaine abusers. *J Clin Psychiatry* 1988;49[Suppl 2]:27–33.

206. Washton A, Gold MS, Pottash AC. Opiate and cocaine dependencies. *Postgrad Med* 1985;77:297.

207. Roehrich H, Gold MS. Emergency presentations of crack abuse. *Emerg Med Serv* 1988;17(8):41–44.

208. Campora P, Bermejo AM, Tabernero MJ, et al. Quantitation of cocaine and its major metabolites in human saliva using gas chromatography-positive chemical ionization-mass spectrometry (GC-PCI-MS). *J Anal Toxicol* 2003;27(5):270–274.

209. Dackis CA, Gold MS, Estroff TW. Inpatient treatment of addiction. In: *Treatments of psychiatric disorders: a task force report of the American Psychiatric Association.* Washington, DC: American Psychiatric Association, 1989:1359–1379.

210. Welch MJ, Sniegoski LT, Tai S. Two new standard reference materials for the determination of drugs of abuse in human hair. *Anal Bioanal Chem* 2003;376(8):1205–1211.

211. Liberty HJ, Johnson BD, Fortner N, et al. Detecting crack and other cocaine use with fastpatches. *Addict Biol* 2003;8(2):191–200.

212. Gold MS. Diagnosis and treatment of cocaine abuse-II. In: *Symposium of cocaine proceedings.* New York: American Psychiatric Association, 1982:3–4.

213. Roehrich H, Gold MS. Cocaine. In: Ciraulo DA, Shader RI, eds. *Clinical manual of chemical dependence.* Washington, DC: American Psychiatric Press, 1991:195–231.

214. Jonas JM, Gold, MS. The pharmacologic treatment of alcohol and cocaine abuse. *Psychiatr Clin North Am* 1992;15:179–190.

215. Gold MS. Cocaine (and crack): clinical aspects. In: Lowinson JH, Ruiz P, Millman RB, Langrod JG, eds. *Substance abuse: a comprehensive textbook,* 2nd ed. Baltimore: Williams & Wilkins, 1992:205–221.

216. Roehrich H, Dackis CA, Gold MS. Bromocriptine. *Med Res Rev* 1987;7(2):243–269.

217. Extein IL, Gold MS. The treatment of cocaine addicts: bromocriptine or desipramine. *Psychiatr Ann* 1988;18(9):535–537.

218. Covi L, Hess JM, Schroeder JR, et al. A dose-response study of cognitive behavioral therapy in cocaine abusers. *J Subst Abuse Treat* 2002;23(3):191.

219. Gold MS, Miller NS. The biology of addictive and psychiatric disorders. In: Miller NS, ed. *Treating coexisting psychiatric and addictive disorders.* Center City, MN: Hazelden, 1994:35–52.

220. Aharonovich E, Nunes E, Hasin D. Cognitive impairment, retention and abstinence among cocaine abusers in cognitive-behavioral treatment. *Drug Alcohol Depend* 2003;71(2):207–211.

221. Childress A, Ehrman R, McLellan AT, et al. Conditioned craving and arousal in cocaine addiction: a preliminary report. *NIDA Res Monogr* 1988;81:74–80.

222. Gawin F, Ellinwood E. Stimulants. In: Kleber HD, ed. *Treatment of psychiatric disorders: a task force report of the American Psychiatric Association.* Washington, DC: American Psychiatric Association, 1989:1218–1241.

223. Shaham Y, Erb S, Leung S, et al. CP-154,526, a selective, non-peptide antagonist of the corticotropin-releasing factor1 receptor attenuates stress-induced relapse to drug seeking in cocaine- and heroin-trained rats. *Psychopharmacology (Berl)* 1998;137(2):184–190.

224. Kosten TR, Oliveto A, Sevarino KA, et al. Ketoconazole increases cocaine and opioid use in methadone maintained patients. *Drug Alcohol Depend* 2002;66(2):173–180.

225. Mendelson JH, Teoh SK, Lange U, et al. Anterior pituitary, adrenal, and gonadal hormones during cocaine withdrawal. *Am J Psychiatry* 1988;145:1094–1098.

226. Teoh SK, Mendelson JH, Mello NK, et al. Hyperprolactinemia and risk for relapse of cocaine abuse. *Biol Psychiatry* 1990;28:824–828.

227. Swartz CM, Breen K, Leone F. Serum prolactin levels during extended cocaine abstinence. *Am J Psychiatry* 1990;147:777–779.

228. Lee MA, Bowers MM, Nash JF, et al. Neuroendocrine measures of dopaminergic function in chronic cocaine users. *Psychiatry Res* 1990;33:151–159.

229. Kranzler H, Wallington D. Serum prolactin, craving and early discharge

from treatment in cocaine-dependent patients. *Am J Drug Alcohol Abuse* 1992;18:187–196.

230. Hollander E, Nunes E, DeCaria C, et al. Dopaminergic sensitivity in cocaine abuse: response to apomorphine. *Psychiatry Res* 1990;33:161–169.

231. Mendelson JH, Teoh SK, Lange U, et al. Anterior pituitary, adrenal, and gonadal hormones during cocaine withdrawal. *Am J Psychiatry* 1988;145:1094–1098.

232. Teoh SK, Mendelson JH, Mello NK, et al. Hyperprolactinemia and risk for relapse of cocaine abuse. *Biol Psychiatry* 1990;28:824–828.

233. Miller BL, Cummings JL, Villanueva-Meyer J, et al. Frontal lobe degeneration: clinical, neuropsychological, and SPECT characteristics. *Neurology* 1991;41:1374–1382.

234. Tumeh S, Nagel JS, English RJ, et al. Cerebral abnormalities in cocaine abusers: demonstration by SPECT perfusion brain scintigraphy. *Radiology* 1990;176:821–824.

235. Volkow ND, Mullani N, Gould KL, et al. Cerebral blood flow in chronic cocaine users: a study with positron emission tomography. *Br J Psychiatry* 1988;152:641–648.

236. Holman BL, Moretti J-L, Hill TC. SPECT perfusion imaging in cerebrovascular disease. In: *Noninvasive imaging of cerebrovascular disease.* New York: Allan R Liss, 1989:147–162.

237. Manschreck TC, Margert L, Schneyer C, et al. Freebase cocaine and memory. *Compr Psychiatry* 1990;31:369–375.

238. Lichtenfeld PJ, Rubin DB, Feldman RS. Subarachnoid hemorrhage precipitated by cocaine snorting. *Arch Neurol* 1984;41:223–224.

239. Wojak JC, Flamm ES. Intracranial hemorrhage and cocaine abuse. *Stroke* 1987;18:712–715.

240. Kaye BR, Fainstat M. Cerebral vasculitis associated with cocaine abuse. *JAMA* 1987;258:2104–2106.

241. Washton AM. Nonpharmacologic treatment of cocaine abuse. *Psychiatr Clin North Am* 1986;9:563–571.

242. Margolin A, Avants K, Kosten TR. Cue-elicited cocaine craving and autogenic relaxation: association with treatment outcome. *J Subst Abuse Treat* 1994;11:549–552.

243. The White House. *National drug control strategy.* Washington, DC: Office of National Drug Control Policy, September 1989.

244. Wise RA. Catecholamine theories of reward: a critical review. *Brain Res* 1978;152:215–247.

245. Montgomery AM, Rose IC, Herberg LJ. 5-HT1A agonists and dopamine: the effects of 8-OH-SPAT and buspirone on brain stimulation reward. *J Neural Transm* 1991;83:139–158.

246. Cunningham KA, Lakokski JM. Electrophysiological effects of cocaine and procaine on dorsal raphe serotonin neurons. *Eur J Pharmacol* 1988;148:457–462.

247. Galloway MP. Regulation of dopamine and serotonin synthesis by acute administration of cocaine. *Synapse* 1990;6:63–72.

248. Satel SL, Krystal JH, Delgado PL, et al. Tryptophan depletion and attenuation of cue-induced craving for cocaine. *Am J Psychiatry* 1995;152:778–783.

249. Ye JH, Ponnudurai R, Schaefer R. Ondansetron: a selective 5-HT (3) receptor antagonist and its applications in CNS-related disorders. *CNS Drug Rev* 2001;7(2):199–213.

250. Naranjo CA, Kadlec KE, Sanhueza P, et al. Fluoxetine differentially alters alcohol intake and other consummatory behaviors in problem drinkers. *Clin Pharmacol Ther* 1990;47:490–498.

251. Shopsin B. Second generation antidepressants: a clinical pharmacotherapeutic research strategy. *Psychopharmacol Bull* 1981;17:33–35.

252. Batki SL, Manfredi LB, Sorensen JL, et al. Fluoxetine for cocaine abuse in methadone patients: preliminary findings. *NIDA Res Monogr* 1990;105:516–517.

253. Schmitz JM, Averill P, Stotts AL, et al. Fluoxetine treatment of cocaine-dependent patients with major depressive disorder. *Drug Alcohol Depend* 2001;63(3):207–214.

254. Fletcher PJ, Robinson SR, Slippoy DL. Pre-exposure to (±)3,4-methylenedioxy-methamphetamine (MDMA) facilitates acquisition of intravenous cocaine self-administration in rats. *Neuropsychopharmacology* 2001;25(2):195–203.

255. Herridge P, Gold MS. Pharmacological adjuncts in the treatment of opioid and cocaine addicts. *J Psychoactive Drugs* 1988;20:233–242.

256. Oliveto A, McCance-Katz FE, Singha A, et al. Effects of cocaine prior to and during bupropion maintenance in cocaine-abusing volunteers. *Drug Alcohol Depend* 2001;63(2):155–167.

257. Montoya ID, Preston KL, Rothman R, et al. Open-label pilot study of bupropion plus bromocriptine for treatment of cocaine dependence. *Am J Drug Alcohol Abuse* 2002;28(1):189–196.

258. Bano MD, Mico JA, Agujetas M, et al. Olanzapine efficacy in the treatment of cocaine abuse in methadone maintenance patients. Interaction with plasma levels. *Actas Esp Psiquiatr* 2001;29(4):215–220.

259. Sattar SP, Bhatia SC. Olanzapine for cocaine cravings and relapse prevention. *J Clin Psychiatry* 2003;64(8):969.

260. Broderick PA, Rahni DN, Zhou Y. Acute and subacute effects of risperidone and cocaine on accumbens dopamine and serotonin release using in vivo microvoltammetry on line with open-field behavior. *Prog Neuropsychopharmacol Biol Psychiatry* 2003;27(6):1037–1054.

261. Newton TF, Ling W, Kalechstein AD, et al. Risperidone pre-treatment reduces the euphoric effects of experimentally administered cocaine. *Psychiatry Res* 2001;102(3):227–233.

262. Meyer RE. New pharmacotherapies for cocaine dependence revisited. *Arch Gen Psychiatry* 1992;49:900–904.

263. Gawin FH, Kleber HD, Byck R, et al. Desipramine facilitation of initial cocaine abstinence. *Arch Gen Psychiatry* 1989;46:117–121.

264. Gawin FH, Byck R, Kleber HD. Desipramine augmentation of cocaine abstinence: initial results. *Clin Neuropharmacol* 1986;9[Suppl 4]:202–204.

265. Gawin FH, Kleber HD, Byck R, et al. Desipramine facilitation of initial cocaine abstinence. *Arch Gen Psychiatry* 1989;46:117–121.

266. Kosten TR. Pharmacotherapeutic interventions for cocaine abuse matching patients to treatments. *J Nerv Ment Dis* 1989;177:379–389.

267. Kosten TR. Pharmacotherapies for cocaine abuse: neurobiological abnormalities reversed with drug intervention. *The Psychiatric Times* 1993 Feb:25–27.

268. Mello NK, Lukas SE, Bree MP, et al. Desipramine effects on cocaine self-administration by rhesus monkeys. *Drug Alcohol Depend* 1990;26:103–116.

269. Fischman MW, Foltin RW, Nestadt G, et al. Effects of desipramine maintenance on cocaine self-administration by humans. *J Pharmacol Exp Ther* 1990;253:760–770.

270. Lima MS, Reisser AA, Soares BG, et al. Antidepressants for cocaine dependence. *Cochrane Database Syst* 2001;(4):CD002950.

271. Baptista T, Weiss SRB, Post RM. Carbamazepine attenuates cocaine-induced increases in dopamine in the nucleus accumbens: an *in vivo* dialysis study. *Eur J Pharmacol* 1993;236:39–42.

272. Lima AR, Lima MS, Soares BG, et al. Carbamazepine for cocaine dependence. *Cochrane Database Syst* 2001;(4):CD002023.

273. Weiss SRB, Post RM, Aigner TG. Carbamazepine in the treatment of cocaine-induced disorders: In: Watson RR, ed. *Drug and alcohol abuse reviews:*

treatment of drug and alcohol abuse. Totowa, NJ: Humana Press, 1992:149.

274. Gawin FH. Cocaine addiction: psychology and neurophysiology. *Science* 1991;251:1580–1586.

275. Berger P, Gawin F, Kosten TR. Treatment of cocaine abuse with mazindol. *Lancet* 1989;1:283.

276. Gawin FH, Riordan C, Kleber HD. Methylphenidate treatment of cocaine abusers without attention deficit disorder: a negative report. *Am J Drug Alcohol Abuse* 1985;11:193–197.

277. Jaffe JH, Witkin JM, Goldberg SR, et al. Potential toxic interactions of cocaine and mazindol. *Lancet* 1989;8654: 111.

278. Kosten TR, Steinberg M, Diakogiannis IA. Crossover trial of mazindol for cocaine dependence. *Am J Addictions* 1993;2:161–164.

279. Shottenfeld RS, Pakes J, Ziedonis D, et al. Buprenorphine: dose-related effects on cocaine and opioid use in cocaine-abusing opioid-dependent humans. *Biol Psychiatry* 1993;34:66–74.

280. Myrick H, Henderson S, Brady KT, et al. Divalproex loading in the treatment of cocaine dependence. *J Psychoactive Drugs* 2001;33(3):283–287.

281. Carroll K, Ziedonis M, O'Malley L, et al. Pharmacologic interventions for alcohol and cocaine abusing individuals: a pilot study of disulfiram vs. naltrexone. *Am J Addictions* 1993;2(1): 77–79.

282. Hameedi FA, Rosen MI, McCance-Katz EF, et al. Behavioral, physiological, pharmacological interaction of cocaine, disulfiram in humans. *Biol Psychiatry* 1995;37:560–563.

283. Soares BG, Lima MS, Reisser AA, et al. Dopamine agonists for cocaine dependence. *Cochrane Database Syst* 2001;(4):CD003352.

284. Kosten TR, George TP, Kosten TA. The potential of dopamine agonists in drug addiction. *Expert Opin Investig Drugs* 2002;11(4):491–499.

285. Self DW, Karanian DA, Spencer JJ. Effects of the novel D1 dopamine receptor agonist ABT-431 on cocaine self-administration and reinstatement. *Ann N Y Acad Sci* 2000;909:133–144.

286. Haney M, Ward AS, Foltin RW, et al. Effects of ecopipam, a selective dopamine D1 antagonist, on smoked cocaine self-administration by humans. *Psychopharmacology (Berl)* 2001;155(4):330–337.

287. Grabowski J, Rhoades H, Schmitz J, et al. Dextroamphetamine for cocaine-dependence treatment: a double-blind randomized clinical trial. *J Clin Psychopharmacol* 2001;21(5):522–526.

288. Kushner SA, Dewey SL, Kornetsky C. The irreversible gamma-aminobutyric acid (GABA) transaminase inhibitor gamma-vinyl-GABA blocks cocaine self-administration in rats. *J Pharmacol Exp Ther* 1999;290(2):797–802.

289. Dewey SL, Morgan AE, Ashby CR Jr, et al. A novel strategy for the treatment of cocaine addiction. *Synapse* 1998;30(2):119–129.

290. Manuchehri K, Goodman S, Siviter L, Nightingale S. A controlled study of vigabatrin and visual abnormalities. *Br J Ophthalmol* 2000;84(5):499–505.

291. Mattson RH, Petroff OAC, Rothman D, et al. Vigabatrin-effect on brain GABA levels measured by nuclear-magnetic-resonance spectroscopy. *Acta Neurol Scand* 1995;92:27–30.

292. Ashby CR, Rohatgi R, Ngosuwan J, et al. Implication of the GABA (B) receptor in gamma vinyl-GABA's inhibition of cocaine-induced increases in nucleus accumbens dopamine. *Synapse* 1999;31:151–153.

293. Brodie JD, Figueroa E, Dewey SL. Treating cocaine addiction: from preclinical to clinical trial experience with gamma vinyl GABA. *Synapse* 2003; 50:261–265.

294. Fadda P, Scherma M, Fresu A, et al. Baclofen antagonizes nicotine-, cocaine-, and morphine-induced dopamine release in the nucleus accumbens of rat. *Synapse* 2003;50(1):1–6.

295. Lile JA, Stoops WW, Allen TS, et al. Baclofen does not alter the reinforcing, subject-rated or cardiovascular effects of intranasal cocaine in humans. *Psychopharmacology (Berl)* 2003;171(4): 441–449.

296. Kosten TR, Biegel D. Therapeutic vaccines for substance dependence. *Expert Rev Vaccines* 2002;1(3):363–371.

297. Kuhar MJ, Carroll FI, Bharat N, et al. Anticocaine catalytic antibodies have no affinity for RTI compounds: implications for treatment. *Synapse* 2001; 41(2):176–178.

298. Homayoun P, Mandal T, Landry D, et al. Controlled release of anti-cocaine catalytic antibody from biodegradable polymer microspheres. *J Pharm Pharmacol* 2003;55(7):933–938.

299. Weiss RD. Relapse to cocaine abuse after initiating desipramine treatment. *JAMA* 1988;260:2545–2546.

300. Weiss RD, Mirin SM. Psychological and pharmacological treatment strategies in cocaine dependence. *Ann Clin Psychiatry* 1990;2:239–243.

301. Avants SK, Margolin A, Chang P, et al. Acupuncture for the treatment of cocaine addiction. Investigation of a needle puncture control. *J Subst Abuse Treat* 1995;12(3):195–205.

302. Kosten TA, Kosten TR, Gawin FH, et al. An open trial of sertraline for cocaine abuse. *Am J Addictions* 1992;1:349–353.

303. Kosten TA, Kosten TR. Pharmacological blocking agents for treating substance abuse. *J Nerv Ment Dis* 1991;179:583–592.

304. Kosten T, Silverman DG, Fleming J, et al. Intravenous cocaine challenges during naltrexone maintenance: a preliminary study. *Biol Psychiatry* 1992;32:543–548.

305. Mello NK, Mendelson JH, Bree MP, et al. Buprenorphine and naltrexone effects on cocaine self-administration by rhesus monkeys. *J Pharmacol Exp Ther* 1990;254:926–939.

306. Meert TF, Janssen PAJ. Ritanserin. A new therapeutic approach for drug abuse. Part 2. Effects on cocaine. *Drug Dev Res* 1992;25:39–53.

307. Ichikawa J, Meltzer HY. Amperozide. A novel antipsychotic drug, inhibits the ability of *d*-amphetamine to increase dopamine release *in vivo* in rat striatum and nucleus accumbens. *J Neurochem* 1992;58:2285–2291.

308. Markou A, Koob GF. Post cocaine anhedonia: an animal model of cocaine withdrawal. *Neuropsychopharmacology* 1991;4:17–26.

309. Gawin FH. Cocaine addiction: psychology and neurophysiology. *Science* 1991;251:1580–1586.

310. Higgins ST, Budney AJ, Bickel WK, et al. Achieving cocaine abstinence with a behavioral approach. *Am J Psychiatry* 1993;150:763–769.

311. Higgins ST, Budney AJ, Bickel WK, et al. Incentives improve outcome in outpatient behavioral treatment of cocaine dependence. *Arch Gen Psychiatry* 1994;51:568–576.

312. Simpson DD, Joe GW, Broome KM. A national 5-year follow-up of treatment outcomes for cocaine dependence. *Arch Gen Psychiatry* 2002;59(6):538–544.

313. Gossop M, Marsden J, Stewart D, et al. Changes in use of crack cocaine after drug misuse treatment: 4-5-year follow-up results from the National Treatment Outcome Research Study (NTORS). *Drug Alcohol Depend* 2002;66(1):21–28.

314. Gold MS, Pomm R, Kennedy Y, et al. *5-Year state-wide study of physician addiction treatment outcomes confirmed by urine testing.* San Diego, CA: Society for Neuroscience, November 13, 2001. Prog.# 668.1. Available at http://sfn.scholarone.com/itin2001.

315. DuPont RL, Voth EA. Drug legalization, harm reduction and drug policy. *Ann Intern Med* 1995;123:461–465.

316. Siegal HA, Li L, Rapp RC. Abstinence trajectories among treated crack cocaine users. *Addict Behav* 2002; 27(3):437–449.

CHAPTER 14

The Neurobiology of Marijuana

SANDRA P. WELCH, PhD

Cannabis, along with opium, is one of the oldest drugs in pharmaceutical use in the world (1). *Cannabis* use dates back more than 12,000 years (2). It was not only used for medicinal purposes, but also to make clothing and rope from the strong hemp fibers (3). The *cannabis* plant was introduced to the New World for non-pharmacologic purposes, as it was used in the Old World, about 1629. The ability of *cannabis* to survive and produce large amounts of fiber during the short growing season made hemp a valued commodity. The cultivation of *cannabis* became a major undertaking on farms and plantations (4). The warm, temperate and subtropical climates of the southern and southwestern United States produced a plant with less fiber and more psychoactive potency than that of the northern and midwestern areas. Once the pharmacologic properties of *cannabis* were realized, marijuana was included in the United States pharmacopoeia in 1850, and in the United States Dispensary in 1851. *Cannabis* tinctures were recommended for a variety of maladies, including gout, rheumatism, depression, and convulsions (5), and as treatment for constipation and malaria (6). It was the extensive work of O'Shaughnessy (7), an army physician in India, that lead to a compilation of potential uses for the plant that was published as a review on the use of *cannabis.* Most recent reviews on the medicinal uses of marijuana have alluded to O'Shaughnessy's early review because of the intriguing similarities between the conditions for which he reported therapeutic uses of *cannabis* and the much more sophisticated studies of its use today.

The complex physiologic activity of *Cannabis sativa,* has been documented anecdotally for centuries. However, its mechanism of action eluded scientists until recently and remains a subject of intense investigation. The question of the evolutionary significance and function of the presence of the endogenous cannabinoids (endocannabinoids) in the most basic of human functions remains a mystery with many scientific "detectives" sleuthing out the potential answers. Numerous developments have hastened investigations, such as the cloning of cannabinoid receptors and the development of antagonists, along with the ability to determine the localization of and activation of intracellular systems by cannabinoid receptors. Critical to the elucidation of mechanism of cannabinoids was the discovery, isolation and purification in 1965 of the major, psychoactive ingredient in marijuana,

Δ^9-tetrahydrocannabinol (THC) (8). Compounds structurally related to THC are referred to as *cannabinoids.* More than 400 chemicals are synthesized by the hemp plant, with approximately 60 being cannabinoids. Currently, scientists are merely on the "tip of the iceberg" in terms of cannabinoid physiology, with a wealth of information yet to be determined on the neurobiology of psychoactive cannabinoids.

CANNABINOID RECEPTORS

It was initially thought that because of the lipophilic nature of THC at room temperature, the central depressant effects of cannabinoids were mediated through the disruption of membrane ordering, similar to the mechanism of general anesthetics (9). Given that the cannabinoids have a high lipid/aqueous partition coefficient, it was hypothesized that these drugs produced their psychic effects by intercalating into biologic membranes, altering the activity of various enzymes (10). Consistent with this hypothesis is the finding by Gill et al. (11) that the cannabinoids increase membrane fluidization. Unlike the general anesthetics, a correlation has not been shown to exist between lipophilicity and potency for the cannabinoids (12). The absence of a correlation between lipophilicity and pharmacologic potency for the cannabinoids suggests that these drugs are not working nonspecifically at biologic membranes, but rather it suggests that the cannabinoids have a more specific, receptor-mediated action. Structure-activity relationship studies involving these compounds, primarily THC, resulted in several observations characteristic of receptor-mediated activities. Dewey et al. (13) demonstrated that the (+)*trans* isomer was more potent in several pharmacologic tests than the (−)*trans* isomer. Thus, stereoselectivity proved to be of greater importance than lipophilicity. Such selective activity is characteristic of receptor-mediated events. The (−)*trans* isomer of THC has 6 to 100 times more potency than the (+)*trans* isomer, depending on the pharmacologic test. In more recent studies, the enantiomeric purity of THC analogues synthesized in the Mechoulam laboratory were shown to have greater than 1000-fold stereoselectivity (14). Other crucial studies elucidating receptor-mediated effects of the cannabinoids were performed by Howlett, who, in numerous pioneering *in vitro* studies, revealed a distinct relationship between cannabinoid-induced attenuation of G protein-mediated cyclic adenosine monophosphate (cAMP) production and behavioral effects of the cannabinoids, as well as dose- and concentration-related pharmacologic effects of the cannabinoids (15–18). Herkenham et al. (19) demonstrated autoradiographically the specific areas of the brain in which cannabinoid receptors are localized, especially in those areas involved in nociceptive transmission, memory and learning, movement and ataxia, and hypothermia/cardiovascular control, as well as euphoria and mood modulation. Binding studies correlated with observed behavioral effects following cannabinoid administration.

Definitive evidence for a specific cannabinoid receptor became apparent when the first cannabinoid receptor (CB$_1$) was cloned from the rat (20,21). The CB$_1$ receptor is a G protein-coupled receptor, as predicted from Howlett's initial work, and is a member of the large G protein-coupled receptor (GPCR) superfamily of receptors of which the opioid receptors are also members. Messenger ribonucleic acid (mRNA) for the CB$_1$ receptor is found in regions of the brain that express cannabinoid receptors. Confirmation of the identity of the CB$_1$ clone occurred when adenylyl cyclase was inhibited upon exposure to THC in cells transfected with the clone. The human cannabinoid receptor was subsequently cloned and found to have almost identical homology to the rat receptor (22). Both the human and rat CB$_1$ receptors are saturable, high-affinity binding sites for cannabinoids, showing both stereoselectivity and structure–activity relationships (23). A splice variant of the cannabinoid CB$_1$ receptor, the cannabinoid CB$_{1A}$ receptor, has also been characterized (24). However, no pharmacologic relevance has been attributed to this splice variant.

Early studies were hampered by the lack of a selective antagonist. The discovery of an antagonist for the CB$_1$ receptor, SR141716A, was a major development in cannabinoid pharmacology (25). SR141716A selectively attenuates CB$_1$ receptor-mediated activity *in vivo* and *in vitro*. Investigations using CB$_1$ knock-out mice (mice with no gene for the CB$_1$ receptor) have provided evidence that the activation of CB$_1$ receptors is necessary for the elicitation of antinociception, decreased spontaneous activity and other psychopharmacologic effects (26–28). CB$_1$ receptors are also hypothesized to be required for the development of physical dependence to cannabinoids.

Given the large number of physiologic and pharmacologic effects of the cannabinoids, it was not surprising that a second cannabinoid receptor was cloned. The CB$_2$ receptor was first identified on splenic macrophages (21). A specific antagonist for the CB$_2$ receptor exists, SR144528 (29). Immunomodulatory effects of THC on macrophage function are abolished in CB$_2$ knockout mice shown to be devoid of CB$_2$ receptors (28). The effects of cannabinoids on the immune system are complex (30,31). For a recent review of immune function and the cannabinoid system see Berdyshev (32).

RECEPTOR SIGNALING

The majority of transmitters and hormones produce their biological effects via GPCRs (33), including cannabinoid (and opioid) receptors. G proteins transduce extracellular receptor activation into an intracellular response via effectors, including adenylyl cyclase, ion channels, and phospholipases (34), which regulate neuronal activity and genetic expression. G proteins in the brain include G$_s$

and G$_i$/G$_o$, both of which can be activated by cannabinoid receptors (35). G$_s$ stimulates adenylyl cyclase, whereas G$_i$/G$_o$ inhibit adenylyl cyclase and modulate ion channels.

The mechanism by which THC induces antinociception, following supraspinal administration, involves a decreased Ca^{2+} influx via the N-type Ca^{2+} channel (36). Intracellular Ca^{2+} concentrations are tightly regulated via sequestration into specific cellular compartments, the endoplasmic reticulum and active transport across the cell membranes (37). Upon neuronal stimulation, several voltage-sensitive Ca^{2+} channels allow for extracellular Ca^{2+} to enter the presynaptic terminal. This Ca^{2+} influx, in addition to release from intracellular sources, results in the initiation of processes associated with neurotransmitter release. THC decreases presynaptic Ca^{2+} influx (38). Mackie and Hille (36) found that in cultured neuroblastoma cells, cannabinoid receptors were coupled to N-type Ca^{2+} channels by G$_I$ proteins. From these studies, it is hypothesized that acute THC administration diminishes Ca^{2+} influx via the N-type Ca^{2+} channel. The result is a diminished Ca^{2+} influx on neurostimulation which prevents intracellular Ca^{2+} increases to levels necessary for efficient neurotransmitter release. Such activity is supported by the work of Turkanis and Karler (39), demonstrating THC-induced inhibition of neurotransmitter release.

The receptor–G protein-activation cycle has been well-characterized (34). The functional activity of G protein-coupled receptors can be measured directly using receptor-stimulated binding of the hydrolysis-resistant guanosine triphosphate (GTP) analogue, [^{35}S]GTPγS, in membranes and tissue sections (40). Previous studies using agonist-stimulated [^{35}S]GTPγS binding demonstrated cannabinoid receptor-activated G proteins in membrane homogenates and sections of brains from mouse (41), rat (42), guinea pig (43), and monkey (44). In addition, these studies showed cannabinoid receptor-stimulated G proteins in brain regions that show specific anatomic localization corresponding to appropriate receptor distribution and antagonist-reversible effects on G protein activation (42,43). Studies of G protein activation have been used to demonstrate cannabinoid receptor desensitization following chronic THC treatment (43), receptor efficiency, and agonist efficacy (45). Several intracellular events follow the activation of G proteins by the cannabinoids. GPCRs linked to a G$_{i/o}$ protein inhibit the activity of adenylyl cyclase, decrease levels of cAMP, and decrease activation of cAMP-dependent protein kinase A (PKA). However, a variety of other kinases have been linked to CB$_1$ receptor activation. For example, upon agonist binding to the CB$_1$ receptor, the $\beta\gamma$ subunit dissociates from the α subunit of the G$_{i/o}$ protein. The $\beta\gamma$ subunit is linked to activation of other cellular events, such as activation of tyrosine kinases (TKs). The next section presents a discussion of the modulation of protein phosphorylations by kinases that are cannabinoid sensitive.

Protein Phosphorylation

Protein phosphorylation is a critical component in the mechanism of action of GPCRs. The activity of several second messenger systems on protein phosphorylation alters both the acute and long-term effects of the cannabinoids (46). Mechanisms of tolerance and neuronal plasticity following long-term administration of the cannabinoids is discussed later, in the section entitled Tolerance. However, the mechanisms of tolerance are likely regulated by one or more of the following systems. The effects of cannabinoids on multiple families of kinases as discussed below indicates the importance of alterations in protein phosphorylation in the mechanism of action of cannabinoids.

- *Protein Kinase A*—Acute administration of THC decreases cAMP formation by inhibiting adenylyl cyclase and decreases PKA activity. Conversely, chronic cannabinoid exposure enhances adenylyl cyclase activity, increases cAMP levels and PKA activity in the same areas that CB_1 receptor downregulation is observed (i.e., cerebellum, striatum and cortex) (47). Thus the adenylyl cyclase cascade appears to become constitutively active during tolerance. Tolerance to the antinociceptive, cataleptic, hypothermic, and hypoactivity following can be reversed by, KT5720 an inhibitor of PKA(46). It also has been proposed that the inhibition of adenylyl cyclase and PKA activity may be involved in the CB_1-induced activation of focal adhesion kinases (FAK+) in hippocampal slices, an effect suggested to lead to modulation by cannabinoids of synaptic plasticity and learning processes (48).
- *Protein Kinase G*—The cannabinoid levonantradol, but not dextronantradol, decreases basal and isoniazid-induced increases in cyclic guanosine monophosphate (cGMP) (49). Thus, cannabinoids could alter cGMP formation (and thus cGMP-dependent protein kinase G [PKG], activity) in tolerance expression.
- *Protein Kinase C*—THC increases the activity of brain protein kinase C (PKC) *in vitro* (50). PKC appears to directly affect CB_1 receptors. Phosphorylation of the CB_1 receptor with PKC suppresses the modulation of calcium channels by cannabinoids (51). Neurotransmitters that activate PKC restore the neuronal excitability and synaptic activity inhibited by cannabinoids. Inhibition of PKC activity blocks the antinociceptive effect of THC (46).
- *Tyrosine Kinases*—CB_1 receptor activation of the $\beta\gamma$ subunit of G proteins can stimulate tyrosine kinases. One target of activation by the $\beta\gamma$ subunit are Src tyrosine kinases that activate Ras, which, in turn, activates mitogen-activated protein kinase (MAPK). Both CB_1 and CB_2 receptor stimulation increase the activation of MAPK (29) which becomes tyrosine-phosphorylated, an effect blocked by TK inhibitors (52). The Src tyrosine kinase inhibitor PP1 (52) reverses THC antinociceptive tolerance (46). Thus, TKs are likely to play a role in the development or expression of tolerance to cannabinoids.
- *Mitogen-Activated Protein Kinase*—THC, as well as the endocannabinoid anandamide, can activate the MAPK pathway, whereas the antagonist SR141716A inhibits this pathway (53–56). CB_1 receptor activation increases MAPK activity (52), and this effect, coupled with the inhibition of PKA, is the basis of a number of cannabinoid actions (57). In endothelial cells, MAPK activation appears to require PKC (58). MAPK is a complex system of not one, but numerous functionally linked kinases. The MAPK-linked kinases are abundantly expressed in neurons in the central nervous system (CNS), function in synaptic plasticity and memory, and are upregulated in inflammation (59). In addition, MAPK also phosphorylates a variety of proteins that alter cell function.

Other systems of cannabinoid-receptor signal-transduction pathways are proposed, such as the inositol phospholipid pathway. G-protein activation of phospholipase C leads to the cleavage of phosphatidylinositol-bisphosphate (PIP2) into inositol-triphosphate (IP3) and diacylglycerol (DAG). DAG activates PKC, and IP3 triggers calcium release from intracellular stores (60). Cannabinoids increase the activity of brain PKC *in vitro* (50). Phosphorylation of the CB_1 receptor by PKC attenuates N- and P/Q-type calcium currents and the inwardly rectifying potassium currents (51,61). Therefore, cannabinoid-induced activation of PKC decreases neuronal excitability and synaptic activity, decreases voltage-activated N-type calcium channel activity (36,62) and enhances hyperpolarization of cells via potassium channel activation (63).

The CB_2 receptor also is coupled to the G_i protein and inhibits adenylyl cyclase (64,65). However, evidence exists that the CB_2 receptor is not coupled to phospholipase C or to phospholipase D signal-transduction pathways, or to mobilization of intracellular Ca^{2+} stores, and does not inhibit voltage-gated Ca^{2+} currents or activate inwardly rectifying potassium channels.

Endocannabinoids

The first endogenous CB_1 ligand (endocannabinoid) to be discovered was arachidonylethanolamide (anandamide, AEA) (66). AEA is behaviorally similar to other psychoactive cannabinoids and cross-tolerance with other cannabinoids has been demonstrated (67–72). AEA is but one of a family of arachidonic acid derivatives that have cannabinoid-like effects (see references 3 and 73 for reviews). Another major endocannabinoid is 2-arachidonoylglycerol (2-AG) discovered by Mechoulam et al. (74) in canine gut along with endogenous substances known as *entourage proteins* that are released with and protect the degradation of 2-AG (75). For unknown reasons 2-AG levels are higher in the brain than are levels of AEA.

The synthetic pathways for AEA and 2-AG have been determined. The original hypothesis of the condensation of arachidonic acid with ethanolamine (76) would have required high micromolar concentrations of reactants. Di Marzo et al. (77) demonstrated the hydrolysis by phospholipase D of AEA from a precursor N-acylphosphatidylethanolamine in cultured neurons was a more likely mechanism for synthesis of AEA. The mechanisms underlying uptake of AEA and its metabolism to free arachidonic acid and ethanolamine have been also been the subject of considerable research (76,77). It is known that AEA is taken up into cells via an AEA transporter that remains to be cloned, although inhibitors of the transporter have been synthesized. The AEA transporter also transports 2-AG into cells (78) and is thought to be the first step in the termination of activity of both endocannabinoids. An AEA transporter inhibitor, AM404, has been synthesized and increases the duration of action of AEA (79). Fatty acid amide hydrolase (FAAH) was found in membrane fractions from brain (80), cloned (81), and shown to degrade intracellular AEA quickly, and to degrade 2-AG more slowly. A number of FAAH inhibitors have been synthesized and have been reviewed (82). FAAH-induced regulation of AEA activity appears to be the major regulation point in AEA signaling pathways. FAAH knockout mice exhibit antinociception, an effect correlated with increased endogenous AEA levels, leading to the hypothesis that FAAH inhibitors might serve therapeutically as analgesics (83).

Endocannabinoids bind both CB_1 and CB_2 receptors, decrease cAMP via inhibition of adenylyl cyclase, activate MAPK, and modulate calcium currents. In addition, Di Marzo et al. (73) showed that olvanil, an endocannabinoid, interacts with the vanilloid receptor 1 (VR1), a non-GPCR that is widely distributed in brain and spinal cord, heat-activated, and activated by the application of capsaicin, an ingredient in hot chili peppers. VR1 activation gates calcium entry to cells in particular sensory neurons (84), leading to nociception followed by rapid desensitization. AEA activation of VR1-mediated cardiovascular processes has also been shown (85). In addition to the potential interaction of endocannabinoids with VR1, other non–CB_1/non–CB_2-mediated effects of endocannabinoids have been reported. AEA produces antinociception in CB_1 knockout mice (mice devoid of the CB_1 receptor). Blockade of the effects of AEA and certain other endocannabinoids by SR141716A either has not been observed or requires heroic doses of SR141716A (86,87). In addition, no evidence of an interaction of exogenous THC-like cannabinoids with VR1 has been demonstrated. Such data are intriguing in that they suggest the presence of yet another cannabinoid receptor. The elucidation of distinct mechanisms by which the body produces and uses endocannabinoids in the modulation of nociception could have a potentially important impact on the design of new analgesics for clinical use.

NEUROPHARMACOLOGIC ACTIONS

Martin (88) developed the "tetrad" of tests for cannabinoid activity. In summary, cannabinoids are both stimulants and depressants and have both central and peripheral nervous system activity (89). Cannabinoids decrease spontaneous locomotor activity and a decrease response rates in behavioral tests. Cannabinoids also impair learning and memory in rodents and nonhuman primates. In addition, hypothermia (90), immobility (catalepsy), and antinociception are components of the tetrad. The mechanisms which underlie the tetrad-elucidated effects of cannabinoids are all pertussis toxin-sensitive (91), and thus are likely mediated via G protein activation. This chapter focuses on the antinociceptive (analgetic) effects of the cannabinoids and the mechanisms hypothesized to underlie such effects.

Analgesia

Recent reviews provide an insight into the analgetic effects of cannabinoids (92), as well as the neural substrates mediating such responses (93). Early experiments in human subjects indicate that THC is no more effective than codeine as an analgesic, but that it is a potent inducer of dysphoric side effects (94). In laboratory animals, a different profile of potency is observed. Cannabinoids are analgetic by several routes of administration (95–98) and in several analgesic tests, including thermal-, visceral-, inflammatory-, acute-, and chronic-pain models. Cannabinoid-induced antinociception appears to be produced by the inhibition of wide dynamic range neurons in the spinal cord dorsal horn (99). Endocannabinoids are apparently active components of chronic pain pathways as indicated by the hyperalgesic effects of SR141716A (100,101).

Cannabinoid–Opioid Interactions

Recently, the interaction of cannabinoids with opioids was extensively reviewed (102). Cannabinoids produce some pharmacologic effects similar to the opioids, such as sedation, hypothermia, inhibition of motor activity, and antinociception (103,104). Cannabinoids share a very similar binding distribution to the opioids throughout the brain and spinal cord. Thus, it is not surprising that a functional and anatomic interaction between the cannabinoids and opioids would occur. Several investigators provide convincing data that suggest a modulatory effect of the cannabinoids on the pharmacologic properties of the opioids. Early reports evaluating the cannabinoid–opioid interaction demonstrated that THC ameliorates naloxone (Narcan)-precipitated morphine withdrawal (105,106). Typically, only other μ opioid-selective drugs are expected to ameliorate this syndrome. Furthermore, certain pharmacologic effects of THC are antagonized by the opioid antagonists, naloxone (107) and chlornaltrexamine (108).

These early findings, which suggest the existence of a cannabinoid–opioid functional interaction, eventually led to studies designed to characterize this interaction at the level of the receptor (109).

Much of the recent work has focused on the interaction between the cannabinoids and κ opioids in the spinal cord. Two significant commonalties have been observed between the mechanisms involved in the mediation of cannabinoid and κ opioid agonist-induced analgesia. Both involve G_I-protein-mediated modulation of cAMP and are subject to κ opioid receptor antagonist attenuation. Bidirectional cross-tolerance between CI-977, a κ opioid agonist, and the cannabinoids, THC and CP55,940, in antinociceptive tests suggests a significant portion of the cannabinoid effect is κ opioid receptor mediated (110).

The dynorphins constitute a family of endogenous peptides for which the κ opioid receptors possess great affinity (111). Their distribution is widespread, but notably high in the spinal cord (112). Dynorphin A (1-17) is a pharmacologically active peptide derived from a prodynorphin precursor. It may be sequentially metabolized to smaller fragments such as dynorphin A (1-13) and dynorphin A (1-8). Dynorphin A (1-8) may be further metabolized to leucine enkephalin, a Δ opioid receptor agonist (113). The pharmacologic activities of the dynorphin peptides are complex. Whereas dynorphin A (1-17) produces antialgesic activity at low doses and antinociceptive activity at higher doses, smaller fragments such as dynorphin A (1-13) and dynorphin A (1-8) induce antinociception via the κ or μ opioid receptor, but lack the antialgesic properties of the larger dynorphin A (1-17) peptide (114–116). Observations suggest the involvement of dynorphin peptides, endogenous κ opioids (111), in THC-induced spinal antinociception (117–119). An increase in dynorphin A (1-17) levels during the initiation of THC induced-spinal antinociception has been shown (119). The temporal relationship between increased dynorphin A (1-17) concentration and the manifestation of spinal antinociception suggests that a THC-mediated release of dynorphin A (1-17) is responsible for the initiation of THC-induced spinal antinociception. κ Opioid antagonist-induced attenuation of THC-induced spinal antinociception suggests κ opioid receptor involvement throughout its time course (119). The attenuation of THC-induced antinociception and dynorphin A (1-17) release by SR141716A indicates both events are cannabinoid receptor mediated.

A unique aspect of THC-induced spinal antinociception in mice is THC–morphine synergy (120). This effect is diminished when dynorphin A metabolism is inhibited (121). Δ Opioid antagonists such as naltrindole fail to attenuate THC-induced spinal antinociception, but attenuate the synergistic antinociceptive effect of the THC–morphine combination. These findings demonstrate that dynorphin metabolism to a Δ opioid receptor ligand is critical to the enhancement of morphine-induced antinocicep-

tion by THC. Leucine enkephalin, a product of dynorphin A metabolism, is an endogenous Δ opioid receptor ligand (113). Leucine enkephalin produces a μ/Δ opioid synergism as described by Miaskowski et al. (122) and has been shown to underlie the synergistic activity, the naltrindole-sensitive enhancement, and peptidase-induced attenuation of the THC–opioid synergy.

Thus, acute administration of THC results in a CB_1-mediated release of dynorphin A (1-17). The early release of dynorphin A (1-17) is responsible for the initiation of spinal antinociception. The ensuing metabolism of dynorphin A (1-17) by endopeptidases results in the production of smaller dynorphin A peptides, such as dynorphin A (1-13) and dynorphin A (1-8) that are responsible for the antinociception late in the antinociceptive time course. The presence of leucine enkephalin, a metabolic product of dynorphin A (1-8) metabolism is required for the synergistic interaction of THC with morphine. Recent work with dynorphin, enkephalin, and κ opioid receptor knockout mice indicate that the antinociceptive effects of THC are attenuated (123). One explanation could be the functional coupling of the μ/Δ and μ/κ receptors that may lead to enhanced antinociceptive effects of opioids by the cannabinoids.

Interestingly, anandamide fails to demonstrate cross-tolerance to dynorphin peptides in antinociceptive tests (124). Administration of antisense to the κ opioid receptor, a technique used to modulate expression of the κ opioid receptor protein, attenuates THC and κ opioid-induced antinociception, but not that of anandamide (125). Anandamide-induced spinal antinociception is not attenuated by the κ opioid antagonist, nor-binaltorphimine dihydrochloride (nor-BNI), nor does anandamide enhance opioid-induced antinociception (126). Together, the studies reveal significant features concerning the mechanisms by which varied cannabinoids, representing distinct classes, induce antinociception. THC-induced antinociception involves a significant κ opioid contribution via dynorphin A. Anandamide-induced antinociception is mediated via a mechanism that does not employ the κ opioid system. Such a diversity of effects between anandamide and THC have been reported in other models (110).

In addition to producing a potent antinociceptive effect when administered intrathecally, THC produces other effects, including hypothermia (107) and decreased spontaneous activity (89). Experiments were conducted to determine if several of the observed physiologic and behavioral effects of THC are mediated in part through endogenous dynorphin release. The results of these experiments show that only the antinociceptive properties of THC are attenuated by dynorphin antisera without any effect on THC-induced changes in spontaneous activity, hypothermia, or catalepsy. This finding is significant because it (a) indicates that the action of endogenously released dynorphin is specifically contributing to the antinociceptive effects of THC and (b) correlates with the data previously obtained indicating that nor-BNI blocks only the antinociceptive effects of cannabinoids (110). Thus, the κ receptor appears to be involved only with the antinociceptive effects of the cannabinoids.

It is unlikely that THC-induced antinociception is totally caused by dynorphin release. The events that precede and follow dynorphin release, and are likely to modulate dynorphin release, have not yet been characterized. Cannabinoid-induced release of dynorphin most likely is a modulator of other "downstream" systems (possibly decreasing substance P release or calcitonin gene-related peptide [CGRP] release), which culminate in antinociception upon administration of cannabinoids. Substance P and related neurokinins are major mediators of nociceptive transmission in the spinal cord (127). Morphine and other opioids, as well as endogenous opioids, decrease the release of substance P (for reviews see references 128 and 129). In addition, chronic THC treatment increases substance P and enkephalin mRNAs concurrently in the same neurons in the caudate. Cannabinoid receptors colocalize with substance P receptors in the striatum (130), which is additional evidence for the interactions of the two systems. Recently, it was demonstrated that in CB_1 knockout mice, brain levels of substance P, dynorphin, and enkephalin are significantly increased. Thus, it is likely that the CB_1 receptor plays a role in the tonic regulation of these peptides (131). In summary, THC-induced release of endogenous κ opioid peptides plays a role in the production of THC-induced antinociception. The interaction of cannabinoids and opioids with similar downstream mediators of nociceptive transmission, such as substance P, provides evidence that it may be possible to enhance antinociception/analgesia by opioid–THC interactions without augmenting the side effects of either individual agent.

The clinical implications of the interplay of the cannabinoid and opioid systems may lead to the increased therapeutic potential for the use of the drugs in combination. The administration of low doses of THC in conjunction with low doses of morphine has been proposed as an alternative regimen for enhancing the pain-relieving effect of both THC and morphine without the side effects characteristic of either drug. Morphine is commonly given in oral preparation, primarily to ease chronic pain. However, continued administration of morphine can lead to tolerance and morphine-resistant pain, necessitating a steady increases in dosage that is potentially harmful to the patient. Also, high doses of morphine can have undesirable side effects, such as respiratory depression, constipation, and nausea (132). An extension of research using THC as an adjunct to other pain therapies is in keeping with the apparent goals stated by the Institute of Medicine (133), which recently affirmed the need for evaluation of cannabinoids as analgesics if they "have synergistic interactions with other analgesics" or if "... efficacy is enhanced in patients who have developed tolerance to opioids." By decreasing the dose of opioids administered, while maintaining antinociception by the adjunct administration of THC, one may be able to produce long-term antinociceptive effects at doses devoid of substantial side effects, while preventing the neuronal biochemical changes that accompany tolerance.

Tolerance

The precise mechanism of the development of tolerance is unknown. There is little evidence that chronic administration of cannabinoids alters disposition or metabolism of cannabinoids in the brain or periphery (134), suggesting that tolerance is pharmacodynamic in nature rather than a consequence of reduced bioavailability. Martin et al. (135), using dog and rat models, demonstrated that THC tolerance involves at best a minor pharmacokinetic component. That is to say, that tolerance does not involve altered absorption, distribution, metabolism, or excretion of THC.

A common pharmacodynamic response during tolerance development is modulation of the receptor protein. Cellular responses to exogenous agents maybe diminished or enhanced by increasing or decreasing receptor sensitivity, or availability. In the case of THC, receptor downregulation has been observed (134). Most of the research efforts to date have been directed toward receptor regulation by evaluation of receptor inactivation or desensitization, or on decreased receptor number (downregulation). The findings of studies investigating the relationship between cannabinoid receptor downregulation and behavioral tolerance to THC have been contradictory. In addition, tertiary signaling processes and plasticity of other neurotransmitter/neuromodulatory systems have been evaluated, such as those described above for the endogenous opioid system. Desensitization can involve a conformation change in the receptor, internalization of the receptor, uncoupling or the receptor from G proteins, or a combination of such processes. The process of downregulation includes loss of receptors from the membrane as evidenced by a decrease in receptor number in binding assays and/or changes in mRNA and protein levels for such receptors. Autoradiographic studies show that binding to the CB_1 receptor was decreased, with no apparent regional selectivity, suggesting a lack of involvement of neural circuitry, second messengers, or other intervening variables that might lead to differential effects. The reductions appear to be receptor-mediated. In chronically treated animals, a decrease in receptor number rather than a change in affinity was observed (134). Thus, there is not likely to be a conformational change in the receptor in chronically treated animals. In addition, Rodriguez de Fonseca et al. (136) found that the development of behavioral tolerance to THC occurred in conjunction with decreased cannabinoid binding in the striatal and limbic portions of the rat brain. Conversely, Romero et al. (137) reported increased binding following chronic administration of THC. Abood et al. (138) found neither increased cannabinoid binding nor mRNA levels in whole-brain homogenates. Previously discussed studies used specific brain regions. Thus, localized receptor regulation may occur during the development of cannabinoid tolerance.

The cannabinoid receptor is rapidly internalized following binding of an agonist. Internalization is not blocked by pretreatment with pertussis toxin and/or cholera toxin, suggesting activation of G proteins is not required for internalization. This pathway appears similar to that of the β_2-adrenergic receptor (139). Receptor internalization is highly dependent upon kinase-induced phosphorylation. The decreased responsiveness of the β_2-adrenergic receptor after stimulation with ligands appears to be a result of rapid cAMP-dependent PKA and G protein-coupled protein kinase (GRK) phosphorylation. In turn, GRK phosphorylation promotes β-arrestin binding and receptor internalization (140). Homologous desensitization to the inhibition of cAMP accumulation occurs during chronic cannabinoid exposure (141,142). A significant increase in cAMP levels and PKA activity in the same areas that CB_1 receptor downregulation is observed (i.e., cerebellum, striatum, and cortex) occurs in chronically THC-treated rats (47). CB_1 receptors appear to lose the ability to inhibit adenylyl cyclase, either through desensitization or switching to G_s protein stimulation. Thus, the adenylyl cyclase cascade appears to become constitutively active during tolerance (46).

There is indirect evidence that a variety of kinases, not just PKA and GRK, could be involved in the development of tolerance to cannabinoids. AEA and THC increase the activity of brain PKC in vitro (50). Phosphorylation of the CB_1 receptor with PKC suppresses the modulation of calcium channels by cannabinoids (51). However, application of neurotransmitters that stimulate the phosphoinositide (PI) cascade and activate PKC restores the neuronal excitability and synaptic activity inhibited by cannabinoids.

There is a bidirectional cross-tolerance noted between the κ opioids and THC, which implies that a common mechanism of tolerance may underlie both classes of drugs (125). Using direct measures of dynorphin release, it has been observed that acutely administered THC interacts with cannabinoid receptors in the outer lamina of the spinal cord. Activation of this cannabinoid receptor system results in an increase in spinal dynorphin A (1-17). With chronic THC administration, there is a measurable decrease in the ability of THC to release dynorphin A (1-17). Consequently, spinal dynorphin A (1-17) concentrations fail to reach levels necessary to affect nociception. Thus, the κ opioid system appears to play a role in the expression of tolerance to THC. Further evidence for the role of opioids in THC tolerance come from transgenic animal studies. In CB_1 knockout mice, the reinforcing effects of opioids are decreased (142). There are increases in prodynorphin and proenkephalin mRNA (precursors of dynorphins and enkephalins) following exposure to THC

(143). It is significant to note that the lack of behavioral tolerance to the low-dose combination of THC and morphine is accompanied by prevention of the development of biochemical correlates of tolerance observed with either drug alone, as quantified by changes in opioid and cannabinoid receptor proteins using Western immunoblotting techniques (144). Thus, an important potential clinical ramification of these studies is that combination cannabinoid/opioid treatment produces effective antinociception with reduced development of tolerance, and most likely dependence.

Physical Dependence

Animals develop tolerance to the effects of THC upon repeated exposure (145). Human chronic heavy cannabis users experience withdrawal symptoms on the abrupt cessation of cannabis use (146,147). The clinical features of *cannabis* dependence in humans need to be better defined. In animal studies, McMillan et al. (148) did not detect withdrawal symptoms following chronic administration of cannabinoids. However, the development of a specific cannabinoid antagonist led to the demonstration that a precipitated withdrawal syndrome could be elicited in animals treated chronically with THC. Studies in rats and mice chronically injected or infused with THC and then challenged with the antagonist SR141716A elicited behavioral signs such as head shakes, facial tremors, tongue rolling, biting, wet-dog shakes, eyelid ptosis, facial rubbing, paw treading, retropulsion, immobility, ear twitch, chewing, licking, stretching, and arched back (149,150). Subsequently, Aceto et al. (151) observed spontaneous withdrawal following abrupt cessation of chronic treatment with the synthetic cannabinoid WINN 55,212. These studies provide convincing evidence that cannabinoids can produce dependence in animals. In addition, several studies link withdrawal from cannabinoids with the opioid system. It appears that the opioid/endogenous opioid system may play a modulatory role in the severity of cannabinoid withdrawal signs because cannabinoid withdrawal is lessened in μ opioid-receptor knockout mice (152) and proenkephalin knockout mice (153). Conversely, in CB_1 knockout mice, the withdrawal effects from morphine are reduced (26). However, the relationship between these animal models and the abuse pattern of cannabinoids in humans remains to be understood.

SUMMARY

Advances into the pharmacology of the cannabinoids have been made in large part as a result of the cloning of receptors and the development of specific antagonists for those receptors. Many critical questions remain as to the role of the endocannabinoid system in human physiology and pathophysiology. Much controversy surrounds the use of THC or another cannabinoid analogue in a variety of disease states. As was evident from the ancient sources, cannabinoids appear to have a variety of potentially useful therapeutic effects, but are not devoid of undesirable side effects. If novel non-CB_1, non-CB_2 cannabinoid receptors were to be found, it certainly will become a therapeutic target. In addition, the increasing knowledge of the endocannabinoid system's role in tonic regulation of analgesia, cognition, food intake, and cardiovascular tone indicates that possible analogues of the endocannabinoids, or modulators of endocannabinoid pathways, may become

targets for drug development. The endocannabinoids and cannabinoid receptors are highly conserved phylogenically. For today's researcher remains the task of determining the reasons for the preservation of the cannabinoid system through both invertebrate and vertebrate evolution, and the roles such receptors, known and yet to be found, play in diseases, including addictive behaviors. The goal of novel therapeutic interventions is to decease the potential for tolerance and dependence to the cannabinoid drugs.

REFERENCES

1. Harris LS, Dewey WL, Razdan RK. Cannabis: its chemistry, pharmacology, and toxicology. In: *Handbook of experimental pharmacology.* New York: Springer-Verlag, 1977:371–429.
2. Abel EL. *A comprehensive guide to the cannabis literature.* Westport, CT: Greenwood Press, 1979.
3. Mechoulam R, Hanus L. A historical overview of chemical research on cannabinoids. *Chem Phys Lipids* 2000; 108:1–13.
4. Sloman L. *Reefer madness, a history of marijuana in America.* New York: Bobbs-Merrill, 1979.
5. Nahas G, Paris M. *Marijuana in science and medicine.* New York: Raven Press, 1984.
6. Grinspoon L, Bakalar JB. *Marihuana: the forbidden medicine.* New Haven, CT: Yale University Press, 1993.
7. O'Shaughnessy WB. On the preparation of Indian hemp or gunjah. *Transcripts of Medical Physicians Society* 1842;8:421–461.
8. Mechoulam R, Gaoni Y, Hashish IV. The isolation and structure of cannabinolic cannabidiolic and cannabigerolic acids. *Tetrahedron* 1965;21:1223–1229.
9. Paton WD, Pertwee RG. Effects of *cannabis* and certain of its constituents on pentobarbitone sleeping time and phenazone metabolism. *Br J Pharmacol* 1972;44:250–261.
10. Makriyannis A, Rapaka RS. The medicinal chemistry of cannabinoids: an overview. *NIDA Res Monogr* 1987;79:204–210.
11. Gill EW. The effects of cannabinoids and other CNS depressants on cell membrane models. *Ann N Y Acad Sci* 1976;281:151–161.
12. Thomas BF, Compton DR, Martin BR. Characterization of the lipophilicity of natural and synthetic analogs of Δ9-tetrahydrocannabinol and its relationship to pharmacological potency. *J Pharmacol Exp Ther* 1990;255:624–635.
13. Dewey WL, Martin BR, May EL.

Cannabinoid stereoisomers: pharmacological effects. In: Smith DF, ed. *CRC Handbook of stereoisomers: drugs in psychopharmacology.* Boca Raton, FL., CRC. 1984:317–326.
14. Martin BR. Compton DR. Thomas BF. et al. Behavioral, biochemical, and molecular modeling evaluations of cannabinoid analogs. *Pharmacol Biochem Behav* 1991;40:471–478.
15. Howlett AC. Inhibition of neuroblastoma adenylate cyclase by cannabinoid and nantradol compounds. *Life Sci* 1984;35:1803–1810.
16. Howlett AC, Qualy JM, Khachatrian LL. Involvement of G_i in the inhibition of adenylate cyclase by cannabimimetic drugs. *Mol Pharmacol* 1986;29:307–313.
17. Howlett AC, Johnson MR, Melvin LS, et al. Nonclassical cannabinoid analgesics inhibit adenylate cyclase: development of a cannabinoid receptor model. *Mol Pharmacol* 1988;33:297–302.
18. Howlett AC, Evans DM, Houston DB. The cannabinoid receptor. In: Murphy L, Burke A, eds. *Marijuana and cannabinoids: neurobiology and neurophysiology.* Boca Raton, FL., CRC, 1992:35–72.
19. Herkenham M, Lynn AB, DeCosta BR, et al. Characterization and localization of cannabinoid receptors in rat brain: a quantitative *in vitro* autoradiographic study. *J Neurosci* 1991;11:563–583.
20. Matsuda LA, Lolait SJ, Bowstein MJ, et al. Structure of a cannabinoid receptor and functional expression of the cloned cDNA. *Nature* 1990;346:561–564.
21. Munro S, Thomas KL, Abu-Shaar M. Molecular characterization of a peripheral receptor for cannabinoids. *Nature* 1993;365:61–65.
22. Gerard CM, Mollereau C, Vassart G, et al. Nucleotide sequence of a human cannabinoid receptor cDNA. *Nucleic Acids Res* 1990;18:7142.
23. Devane WA, Dysarz IFA, Johnson MR,

et al. Determination and characterization of a cannabinoid receptor in rat brain. *Mol Pharmacol* 1988;34:605–613.
24. Shire D, Carillon C, Kaghad M, et al. An amino-terminal variant of the central cannabinoid receptor resulting from alternative splicing. *J Biol Chem* 1995;270:3726–3733.
25. Rinaldi-Carmona M, Barth F, Heaulme M. et al. SR141716A, a potent and selective antagonist of the cannabinoid receptor. *Fed Eur Biochem Soc Lett* 1994;350:240–244.
26. Ledent C, Valverde O, Cossu G, et al. Unresponsiveness to cannabinoids and reduced addictive effects of opiates in CB_1 receptor knockout mice. *Science* 1999;283:401–404.
27. Zimmer A, Zimmer AM, Hohmann AG, et al. Increased mortality, hypoactivity, and hypoalgesia in cannabinoid CB_1 receptor knockout mice. *Proc Natl Acad Sci U S A* 1999;96:5780–5785.
28. Buckley NE, McCoy KL, Mezey E, et al. Immunomodulation by cannabinoids is absent in mice deficient for the cannabinoid CB(2) receptor. *Eur J Pharmacol* 2000;396:141–149.
29. Rinaldi-Carmona M, Barth F, Millan J, et al. SR 144528, the first potent and selective antagonist of the CB_2 cannabinoid receptor. *J Pharmacol Exp Ther* 1998;284:644–650.
30. Condie R, Herring A, Koh WS, et al. Cannabinoid inhibition of adenylate cyclase-mediated signal transduction and interleukin 2 (IL-2) expression in the murine T-cell line, EL4. IL-2. *J Biol Chem* 1996;31;27:13175–13183.
31. Kaminski NE, Koh WS, Yang KH, et al. Suppression of the humoral immune response by cannabinoids is partially mediated through inhibition of adenylate cyclase by a pertussis toxin-sensitive G-protein coupled mechanism. *Biochem Pharmacol* 1994;48:1899–1908.
32. Berdyshev EV. Cannabinoid receptors and the regulation of immune response. *Chem Phys Lipids* 2000;108(1–2):169–190.

33. Birnbaumer L, Abramowitz J, Brown AM. Receptor-effector coupling by G proteins. *Biochim Biophys Acta* 1990; 1031:163–224.

34. Gilman AG. G proteins: transducers of receptor-generated signals. *Ann Rev Biochem* 1987;56:615–649.

35. Childers SR, Breivogel CS. *Cannabis* and endogenous cannabinoid systems. *Drug Alcohol Depend* 1998;51:173–187.

36. Mackie K, Hille B. Cannabinoids inhibit N-type calcium channels in neuroblastoma glioma cells. *Proc Natl Acad Sci U S A* 1992;89:3825–3829.

37. Rasmussen H. The cycling of calcium as an intracellular messenger. *Sci Am* 1989;261:66–73.

38. Kambraci NM, Nastuk WL. Effects of delta 9-tetrahydrocannabinol on excitable membranes and neuromuscular transmission. *Mol Pharmacol* 1980;17:344–349.

39. Turkanis SA, Karler R. Changes in neurotransmitter release at a neuromuscular junction of the lobster caused by cannabinoids. *Neuropharmacology* 1988;22:737–742.

40. Sim LJ, Selley DE, Childers SR. *In vitro* autoradiography of receptor-activated G-proteins in rat brain by agonist-stimulated guanylyl 5′-[gamma[35S]thio]-triphosphate binding. *Proc Natl Acad Sci U S A* 1995;92:7242–7246.

41. Selley DE, Rorrer WK, Breivogel CS, et al. Agonist efficacy and receptor efficiency in heterozygous CB1 knockout mice: relationship of reduced CB1 receptor density to G-protein activation. *J Neurochem* 2001;77:1048–1057.

42. Sim LJ, Selley DE, Xiao R, et al. Differences in G-protein activation by mu and delta opioid, and cannabinoid, receptors in rat striatum. *Eur J Pharmacol* 1996;307:95–107.

43. Sim LJ, Childers SR. Anatomical distribution of mu, delta, and kappa opioid-and nociceptin/orphanin FQ-stimulated [35S]guanylyl-5′-O-(gamma-thio)-triphosphate binding in guinea pig brain. *J Comp Neurol* 1997;386:562–572.

44. Sim-Selley LJ, Daunais JB, Porrino LJ et al. Mu and kappa1 opioid-stimulated [35S]guanylyl-5′-O-(gamma-thio)-triphosphate binding in cynomolgus monkey brain. *Neuroscience* 1999;94:651–662.

45. Selley DE, Sim LJ, Xiao R, et al. mu-Opioid receptor-stimulated guanosine-5′-O-(gamma-thio)-triphosphate binding in rat thalamus and cultured cell lines: signal transduction mechanisms underlying agonist efficacy. *Mol Pharmacol* 1997;51:87–96.

46. Lee MC, Smith FL, Stevens DL, et al. The role of several kinases in mice tolerant to Δ9-tetrahydrocannabinol. *J Pharmacol Exp Ther* 2003;305:1–8.

47. Rubino T, Vigano D, Massi P, et al. Chronic delta-9-tetrahydrocannabinol treatment increases cAMP levels and cAMP-dependent protein kinase activity in some rat brain regions. *Neuropharmacology* 2000;39:1331–1336.

48. Derkinderen P, Toutant M, Burgaya F, et al. Regulation of a neuronal form of focal adhesion kinase by anandamide. *Science* 1996;273:1719–1722.

49. Leader JP, Koe BK, Weissman A. GABA-like actions of levonantradol. *J Clin Pharmacol* 1981;21:262S–270S.

50. Hillard CJ, Auchampach A. *In vitro* activation of brain protein kinase C by the cannabinoids. *Biochim Biophys Acta* 1994;1220:163–170.

51. Garcia DE, Brown S, Hille B, Mackie K. Protein kinase C disrupts cannabinoid actions by phosphorylation of the CB1 cannabinoid receptor. *J Neurosci* 1998;18:2834–2841.

52. Bouaboula M, Poinot-Chzel C, Bourrie B, et al. Activation of mitogen-activated protein kinases by stimulation of the central cannabinoid receptor CB1. *Biochem J* 1995;312:637–641.

53. Daub H, Wallasch C, Lankenau A. et al. Signal characteristics of G protein-transactivated EGF receptor. *EMBO J* 1997;16:7032–7044.

54. Wartmann M, Campbell D, Subramanian A, et al. The MAP kinase signal transduction pathway is activated by the endogenous cannabinoid anandamide. *FEBS Lett* 1995;13;359:133–136.

55. Liu J, Gao B, Mirshahi F, et al. Functional CB1 cannabinoid receptors in human vascular endothelial cells. *Biochem J* 2000;15:835–840.

56. Bouaboula M, Perrachon S, Milligan L, et al. A selective inverse agonist for central cannabinoid receptor inhibits mitogen-activated protein kinase activation stimulated by insulin or insulin-like growth factor 1. Evidence for a new model of receptor/ligand interactions. *J Biol Chem* 1997;272:22330–22339.

57. Melck D, Rueda D, Galve-Roperh I, et al. Involvement of the cAMP/protein kinase A pathway and of mitogen-activated protein kinase in the antiproliferative effects of anandamide in human breast cancer cells. *FEBS Lett* 1999;463:235–240.

58. Liu J, Gao B, Mirshahi F, et al. Functional CB1 cannabinoid receptors in human vascular endothelial cells. *Biochem J* 2000;346:835–840.

59. Jaffee BD, Manos EJ, Collins RJ, et al. Inhibition of MAP kinase kinase (MEK) results in an anti-inflammatory response *in vivo*. *Biochem Biophys Res Commun* 2000;268:647–651.

60. Chaudry A, Thompson RH, Rubin RP, et al. Relationship between Δ9-tetrahydrocannabinol-induced arachidonic acid release and secretagogue-evoked phosphoinositide breakdown and Ca2+ mobilization of exocrine pancreas. *Mol Pharmacol* 1988;34:543–548.

61. Zamponi GW, Bourinett E, Nelson D, et al. Crosstalk between G-proteins and protein kinase C mediated by the calcium channel α1 subunit. *Nature* 1997;385:442–446.

62. Caufield MP, Brown DA. Cannabinoid receptor agonists inhibit Ca Current in NG108–15 neuroblastoma cells via a pertussis toxin sensitive mechanism. *Br J Pharmacol* 1992;106:231–232.

63. Deadwyler SA, Hampson RE, Bennett BA, et al. Cannabinoids modulate potassium current in cultured hippocampal neurons. *Receptors Channels* 1993;1:121–134.

64. Schatz AR, Kessler FK, Kaminski NE. Inhibition of adenylate cyclase by delta 9-tetrahydrocannabinol in mouse spleen cells: a potential mechanism for cannabinoid-mediated immunosuppression. *Life Sci* 1992;51:PL25–PL30.

65. Felder CC, Joyce KE, Briley EM, et al. Comparison of the pharmacology and signal transduction of the human cannabinoid CB1 and CB2 receptors. *Mol Pharmacol* 1995;48:443–450.

66. Devane WA, Hanus L, Breuer A, et al. Isolation and structure of a brain constituent that binds to the cannabinoid receptor. *Science* 1992;258:1946–1949.

67. Pugh G Jr, Smith PB, Dombrowski DS, et al. The role of endogenous opioids in enhancing the antinociception produced by the combination of delta 9-tetrahydrocannabinol and morphine in the spinal cord. *J Pharmacol Exp Ther* 1996;279:608–616.

68. Fride E, Mechoulam R. Pharmacological activity of the cannabinoid receptor agonist, anandamide, a brain constituent. *Eur J Pharmacol* 1993;231:313–314.

69. Pertwee RG, Stevenson LA, Griffin G. Cross-tolerance between Δ9-THC and the cannabimimetic agents, CP 55,940, WIN 55,212–2 and anandamide. *Br J Pharmacol* 1993;110:1483–1490.

70. Welch SP, Dunlow LD, Patrick GS. Characterization of anandamide- and fluoroanandamide-induced antinociception and cross-tolerance to Δ9-THC following intrathecal administration to mice: blockade of Δ9-THC-induced antinociception. *J Pharmacol Exp Ther* 1995;273:1235–1244.

71. Vogel Z, Barg J, Levy R, et al. Anandamide, a brain endogenous compound, interacts specifically with cannabinoid receptors and inhibits adenylate cyclase. *J Neurochem* 1993;61:352–355.

72. Felder CC, Briley EM, Axelrod J, et al. Anandamide, an endogenous cannabimimetic eicosanoid, binds to the cloned human cannabinoids receptor and stimulates receptor-mediated signal transduction. *Cell Biol* 1993; 90:7656–7660.

73. Di Marzo V. Endocannabinoids and other fatty acid derivatives with cannabimimetic properties: biochemistry and possible physiopathological relevance. *Biochim Biophys Acta* 1998; 1392:153–75.

74. Mechoulam R, Ben-Shabat S, Hanus L, et al. Identification of an endogenous 2-monoglyceride, present in canine gut, that binds to cannabinoid receptors. *Biochem Pharmacol* 1995;50:83–90.

75. Ben-Shabat S, Fride E, Sheskin T, et al. An entourage effect: inactive endogenous fatty acid glycerol esters enhance 2-arachidonoyl-glycerol cannabinoid activity. *Eur J Pharmacol* 1998;353:23–31.

76. Deutsch DG, Chin SA. Enzymatic synthesis and degradation of anandamide, cannabinoid receptor agonist. *Biochem Pharmacol* 1993;46:791–796.

77. Di Marzo V, Fontana A, Cadas H, et al. Formation and inactivation of endogenous cannabinoid anandamide in central neurons. *Nature* 1994;372:686–691.

78. Piomelli D, Beltramo M, Glasnapp S, et al. Structural determinants for recognition and translocation by the anandamide transporter. *Proc Natl Acad Sci U S A* 1999;96:5802–5807.

79. Beltramo M, Stella N, Calignano A, et al. Functional role of high-affinity anandamide transport, as revealed by selective inhibition. *Science* 1997;277:1094–1097.

80. Desarnaud F, Cadas H, Piomelli D. Anandamide amidohydrolase activity in rat brain microsomes: identification and partial characterization. *J Biol Chem* 1995;270:6030–6035.

81. Cravatt BF, Giang DK, Mayfield SP, et al. Molecular characterization of an enzyme that degrades neuromodulatory fatty-acid amides. *Nature* 1996; 384:83–87.

82. Reggio PH, Traore H. Conformational requirements for endocannabinoid interaction with the cannabinoid receptors, the anandamide transporter and fatty acid amidohydrolase. *Chem Phys Lipids* 2000;108:15–35.

83. Cravatt BF, Demarest K, Patricelli MP, et al. Supersensitivity to anandamide and enhanced endogenous cannabinoid signaling in mice lacking fatty acid amide hydrolase. *Proc Natl Acad Sci U S A* 2001;98:9371–9376.

84. Szallasi A, Blumberg PM. Vanilloid (capsaicin) receptors and mechanisms. *Pharmacol Rev* 1999;51:159–212.

85. Zygmunt PM, Petersson J, Andersson DA, et al. Vanilloid receptors on sensory nerves mediate the vasodilator action of anandamide. *Nature* 1999;400:452–457.

86. Welch SP, Huffman JW, Lowe J. Differential blockade of the antinociceptive effects of centrally administered cannabinoids by SR141716A. *J Pharmacol Exp Ther* 1998;286:1301–1308.

87. Breivogel CS, Griffin G, Di Marzo V, et al. Evidence for a new G protein-coupled cannabinoid receptor in mouse brain. *Mol Pharmacol* 2001;60:155–163.

88. Martin BR. Characterization of the antinociceptive activity of intravenously administered Δ9-tetrahydrocannabinol in mice. In: Harvey DJ, ed. *Marihuana '84: proceedings of the Oxford symposium on cannabis.* Oxford, UK: IRL Press, 1985.

89. Dewey WL. Cannabinoid pharmacology. *Pharmacol Rev* 1986;38:151–175.

90. Compton DR, Rice KC, De Costa BR, et al. Cannabinoid structure-activity relationships: Correlation of receptor bonding and *in vivo* activities. *J Pharmacol Exp Ther* 1993;265:218–226.

91. Lichtman AH, Meng Y, Martin BR. Inhalation exposure to volatilized opioids produces antinociception in mice. *J Pharmacol Exp Ther* 1996;279:69–76.

92. Martin BR, Lichtman AH. Cannabinoid transmission and pain perception. *Neurobiol Dis* 1998;5:447–461.

93. Walker JM, Hohmann AG, Martin WJ, et al. The neurobiology of cannabinoid analgesia. *Life Sci* 1999;65:665–673.

94. Noyes R Jr, Brunk SF, Avery DA, et al. The analgesic properties of delta-9-tetrahydrocannabinol and codeine. *Clin Pharmacol Ther* 1975;18:84–89.

95. Yaksh TL. The antinociceptive effects of the intrathecally administered levonantradol and desacetyl levonantradol in the rat. *J Clin Pharmacol* 1981;21:334S–340S.

96. Gilbert PE. A comparison of THC, nantradol, nabilone, and morphine in the chronic spinal dog. *J Clin Pharmacol* 1981;21[8–9 Suppl]:311S–319S.

97. Lichtman AH, Martin BR. Spinal and supraspinal mechanisms of cannabinoid-induced antinociception. *J Pharmacol Exp Ther* 1991;258:517–523.

98. Welch SP, Stevens DL. Antinociceptive activity of intrathecally administered cannabinoids alone, and in combination with morphine, in mice. *J Pharmacol Exp Ther* 1992;262:10–18.

99. Hohmann AG, Tsou K, Walker JM. Cannabinoid suppression of noxious heat-evoked activity in wide dynamic range neurons in the lumbar dorsal horn of the rat. *J Neurophysiol* 1999;81:575–583.

100. Strangman NM, Patrick SL, Hohmann AG, et al. Evidence for a role of endogenous cannabinoids in the modulation of acute and tonic pain sensitivity. *Brain Res* 1998;813:323–328.

101. Richardson JD, Aanonsen L, Hargreaves KM. Antihyperalgesic effects of spinal cannabinoids. *Eur J Pharmacol* 1998;345:145–153.

102. Manzanares J, Corchero J, Romero J, et al. Pharmacological and biochemical interactions between opioids and cannabinoids. *Trends Pharmacol Sci* 1999;20:287–294.

103. Holtzman D, Lovell RA, Jaffe JH, et al. 1-delta-9-Tetrahydrocannabinol: neurochemical and behavioral effects in the mouse. *Science* 1969;163:1464–1467.

104. Sofia RD, Nalepa SD, Harakal JJ, et al. Anti-edema and analgesic properties of Δ9-tetrahydrocannabinol (THC). *J Pharmacol Exp Ther* 1973;186:646–655.

105. Bhargava HN. Effect of some cannabinoids on naloxone-precipitated abstinence in morphine-dependent mice. *Psychopharmacology* 1976;49:267–270.

106. Hine B, Torrelio M, Gershon S. Interactions between cannabidiol and delta9-THC during abstinence in morphine-dependent rats. *Life Sci* 1975;17:851–857.

107. Wilson RS, May EL. Analgesic properties of the tetrahydrocannabinols, their metabolites, and analogs. *J Med Chem* 1975;18:700–703.

108. Tulunay FC, Ayhan IH, Portoghese PS, et al. Antagonism by chlornaltrexamine of some effects of delta 9-tetrahydrocannabinol in rats. *Eur J Pharmacol* 1981;70:219–224.

109. Vaysse PJ, Gardner EL, Zukin RS. Modulation of rat brain opioid receptors by cannabinoids. *J Pharmacol Exp Ther* 1987;241:534–539.

110. Smith PB, Welch SP, Martin BR. Interactions between Δ9-tetrahydrocannabinol and kappa opioids in mice. *J Pharmacol Exp Ther* 1994;268:1381–1386.

111. Chavkin C, James I, Goldstein A. Dynorphin is a specific endogenous ligand for the kappa opioid receptor. 1992;215:413–415.

112. Basbaum AI, Fields HL. Endogenous pain control systems: brainstem spinal pathways and endorphin circuitry. *Annu Rev Neurosci* 1984;7:309–388.

113. Dixon DM, Traynor JR. Formation of [Leu5]-enkephalin from dynorphin A (1-8) by rat central nervous tissue

in vitro. J Neurochem 1990;54:1379–1385.

114. Fujimoto JM, Arts KS, Rady JJ, et al. Spinal dynorphin A (1-17): possible mediator of antianalgesic action. *Neuropharmacology* 1990;29:609–617.

115. Morris BJ, Herz A. Simultaneous down-regulation of Δ9-THC sites and up regulation of Δ9-THC sites following chronic agonist/antagonist treatment. *Adv Biol Sci* 1989;75:691–694.

116. Rady JJ, Fujimoto JM, Tseng LF. Dynorphins other than dynorphin lack spinal antianalgesic activity but do act on dynorphin A (1-17) receptors. *J Pharmacol Exp Ther* 1991;259:1073–1079.

117. Welch SP. Blockade of cannabinoid induced antinociception by norbinaltorphimine, but not n,n-diallyl-tyrosine-aib-phenylalanine-leucune, ICI 174864 or naloxone in mice. *J Pharmacol Exp Ther* 1993;265:633–640.

118. Welch SP. Blockade of cannabinoid-induced antinociception by naloxone benzoylhydrazone (NalBZH). *Pharmacol Biochem Behav* 1994;49:929–934.

119. Mason DJ, Welch SP. Cannabinoid modulation of dynorphin A: correlation to cannabinoid-induced antinociception, *Eur J Pharmacol* 1999;378:237–248.

120. Cichewicz DL, McCarthy EA. Antinociceptive synergy between delta(9) tetrahydrocannabinol and opioids after oral administration. *J Pharmacol Exp Ther* 2003; 304: 1010–1015.

121. Pugh GJ, Smith PB, Dombrowski DS, et al. The role of endogenous opioids in enhancing the antinociception produced by the combination of Δ9-THC and morphine in the spinal cord. *J Pharmacol Exp Ther* 1996;279:608–616.

122. Miakowski C, Taiwo YO, Levine JD. Kappa-and delta-opioid agonist synergize to produce potent analgesia. *Brain Res* 1990;509:165–168.

123. Zimmer A, Valjent E, Konig M, et al. Absence of delta-9-tetrahydrocannabinol dysphoric effects in dynorphin-deficient mice. *J Neurosci* 2001;21:9499–9505.

124. Welch SP, Dunlow LD, Patrick GS. Characterization of anandamide- and fluoroanandamide-induced antinociception and cross-tolerance to Δ9-THC following intrathecal administration to mice: blockade of Δ9-THC-induced antinociception. *J Pharmacol Exp Ther* 1995;273:1235–1244.

125. Rowen DW, Embrey JP, Moore CH, et al. Antisense oligodeoxynucleotides to the kappa₁ receptor enhance delta-9-THC-induced antinociceptive tolerance. *Pharmacol Biochem Behav* 1998;59:399–404.

126. Welch SP. Characterization of anandamide-induced tolerance: comparison to delta-9-THC-induced interactions with dynorphinergic systems. *Drug Alcohol Depend* 1997;45:39–45.

127. Nishiyama K, Kwak S, Murayama S, et al. Substance P is a possible neurotransmitter in the rat spinothalamic tract. *Neurosci Res* 1995;21:261–266.

128. Gao Z, Peet NP. Recent advances in neurokinin receptor antagonists. *Curr Med Chem* 1999;6:375–388.

129. Dray A, Rang H. The how and why of chronic pain states and the what of new analgesia therapies. *Trends Neurosci* 1998;21:315–317.

130. Mailleux P, Vanderhaeghen JJ. Delta-9-tetrahydrocannabinol regulates substance P and enkephalin mRNAs levels in the caudate-putamen. *Eur J Pharmacol* 1994;267:R1–R3.

131. Zimmer A, Zimmer AM, Hohmann AG, et al. Increased mortality, hypoactivity, and hypoalgesia in cannabinoid CB1 receptor knockout mice. *Proc Natl Acad Sci U S A* 1999;96:5780–5785.

132. Ellison NM, Lewis GO. Plasma concentrations following single doses of morphine sulfate in oral solution and rectal suppository. *Clin Pharm* 1984;3:614–617.

133. Joy J, Watson SJ, Benson JA, eds. *Intitute of Medicine (IOM), marijuana and medicine: assessing the science base.* Washington, DC: National Academic Press, 1999.

134. Oviedo A, Glowa J, Herkenham M. Chronic cannabinoid administration alters cannabinoid receptor binding in rat brain: a quantitative autoradiographic study. *Brain Res* 1993;616:293–302.

135. Martin BR, Dewey WL, Harris LS, et al. 3H-delta9-tetrahydrocannabinol tissue and subcellular distribution in the central nervous system and tissue distribution in peripheral organs of tolerant and nontolerant dogs. *J Pharmacol Exp Ther* 1976;196:128–144.

136. Rodriguez de Fonseca F, Gorriti MA, Fernandez-Ruiz JJ, et al. Down-regulation of rat brain cannabinoid binding sites after chronic delta 9-tetrahydrocannabinol treatment. *Pharmacol Biochem Behav* 1994;47:33–40.

137. Romero J, Garcia L, Fernandez-Ruiz JJ, et al. Changes in rat brain binding sites after acute or chronic exposure to their endogenous agonist, anandamide or delta 9-tetrahydrocannabinol. *Pharmacol Biochem Behav* 1995;51:731–737.

138. Abood ME, Sauss C, Fan F, et al. Development of behavioral tolerance to delta 9-THC without alteration of cannabinoid receptor binding or mRNA levels in whole brain. *Pharmacol Biochem Behav* 1993;46:575–579.

139. Garcia DE, Brown S, Hille B, et al. Protein kinase C disrupts cannabinoid actions by phosphorylation of the CB₁ cannabinoid receptor. *J Neurosci* 1998;18:2834–2841.

140. Seibold A, January BG, Friedman J, et al. Desensitization of beta₂-adrenergic receptors with mutations of the proposed G protein-coupled receptor kinase phosphorylation sites. *J Biol Chem* 1998;273:7637–7642.

141. Dill JA, Howlett AC. Regulation of adenylate cyclase by chronic exposure to cannabimimetic drugs. *J Pharmacol Exp Ther* 1988;244:1157–1163.

142. Howlett AC, Qualy JM, Khachatrian LL. Involvement of Gi in the inhibition of adenylate cyclase by cannabimimetic drugs. *Mol Pharmacol* 1986;29:307–313.

143. Corchero J, Avila MA, Fuentes JA, et al. Delta-9-tetrahydrocannabinol increases prodynorphin and proenkephalin gene expression in the spinal cord of the rat. *Life Sci* 1997;61:PL 39–43.

144. Cichewicz DL, Haller VL, Welch SP: Changes in opioid and cannabinoid receptor protein following short-term combination treatment with delta(9)-tetrahydrocannabinol and morphine. *J Pharmacol Exp Ther* 2001;297:121–127.

145. Compton DR, Dewey WL, Martin BR. *Cannabis* dependence and tolerance production. *Adv Alcohol Subst Abuse* 1990;9:129–147.

146. Jones RT, Benowitz N, Bachman J. Clinical studies of *cannabis* tolerance and dependence. *Ann N Y Acad Sci* 1976;282:221–239.

147. Haney M, Ward AS, Comer SD, et al. Abstinence symptoms following smoked marijuana in humans. *Psychopharmacology* 1999;141:395–404.

148. McMillan DE, Ford RD, Frankenheim JM, et al. Tolerance to active constituents of marihuana. *Arch Int Pharmacodyn Ther* 1972;198:132–144.

149. Tsou K, Patrick SL, Walker JM. Physical withdrawal in rats tolerant to delta 9-tetrahydrocannabinol precipitated by a cannabinoid receptor antagonist. *Eur J Pharmacol* 1995;280:R13–R15.

150. Aceto MD, Scates SM, Lowe JA, et al. Cannabinoid precipitated withdrawal by the selective cannabinoid receptor antagonist, SR 141716A. *Eur J Pharmacol* 1995;282:R1–R2.

151. Aceto MD, Scates SM, Martin BB. Spontaneous and precipitated withdrawal with a synthetic cannabinoid, WIN 55212—2. *Eur J Pharmacol* 2001;416:75–81.

152. Valverde O, Maldonado R, Valjent E, et al. Cannabinoid withdrawal syndrome is reduced in pre-proenkephalin knock-out mice. *J Neurosci* 2000;20: 9284–9289.

153. Valverde O, Maldonado R, Valjent E, et al. Cannabinoid withdrawal syndrome is reduced in pre-proenkephalin knock-out mice. *J Neurosci* 2000;20: 9284–9289.

CHAPTER 15

Marihuana: Clinical Aspects

LESTER GRINSPOON, JAMES B. BAKALAR, AND ETHAN RUSSO

The present generation of young people cannot remember when marihuana was an exotic weed with an aura of mythical power and mysterious danger. Although still illegal, it has become a commonplace part of the American social scene, used regularly by millions and occasionally used by millions more. A realistic view of this drug is now both more important and easier to achieve.

The use of marihuana reached a high point in the late 1970s and early 1980s, declined until the early 1990s, than began to rise slightly. In a 1978 National Institute on Drug Abuse (NIDA) survey, 37% of high school seniors said that they had smoked marihuana in the past 30 days. In 1989, that number fell to 17%, but by 2001, it had risen again to 22% (1). Trends at ages 18 to 25 years are similar. In 1969, 20% of high school seniors had used marihuana at least once; in 1979, 60% had; in 1989, 44%; and in 1994, 38%. Use in the past year reached a low of 22% in 1992 and rose to 30% in 1994. The perceived risk of regular marihuana use has also fallen slightly. In 1978, 35% of high school seniors said it was very risky; in 1986, 71%; in 1992, nearly 80%; in 1994, closer to 60%; and in 2001 it was 53% (2).

HISTORY

The earliest record of human *cannabis* use is a description of the drug in a Chinese compendium of medicines, the *Herbal of Emperor Shen Nung*, dated 2737 B.C. according to some sources, and 400 to 500 B.C. according to others. Marihuana was a subject of controversy even in ancient times. Some warned that the hemp plant lined the road to Hades, whereas others thought it led to paradise. Its intoxicating properties were known in Europe during the nineteenth century, and for a much longer time in South and Central America; thousands of tons of Indian hemp (the common name of the *Cannabis sativa* plant from which the drug is obtained) were produced for its commercially useful long bast fiber beginning in Jamestown, Virginia,

in 1611. Nevertheless, during the early American history of *cannabis*, nothing was known of its intoxicating properties.

In 1857, Fitz Hugh Ludlow (3), largely influenced by those members of the French romantic literary movement who belonged to *Le Club des Haschischins,* published *The Hasheesh Eater: Being Passages from the Life of a Pythagorean* and made a number of American literati aware of *cannabis'* euphoriant properties. Unlike his European counterparts, Ludlow did not use hashish but, rather, Tilden's Solution, one of a number of proprietary preparations of *Cannabis indica* (an alcoholic extract of *cannabis*), which he could obtain from his local apothecary. Ludlow established a link in the public mind, albeit a very narrow segment of it, between *cannabis* the medicine and *cannabis* the intoxicating drug. However, in the half-century from the publication of his book to the appearance, across the southern border, of what we now commonly call marihuana, grass, pot, or dope (all names for the dried and chopped flowering pistillate and staminate tops and leaves of the hemp plant), even this limited awareness all but completely vanished.

In any case, throughout history the principal interest in the hemp plant has been in its properties as an agent for achieving euphoria. In this country, it is almost invariably smoked, usually as a cigarette called a "joint" or "doobie"—but elsewhere the drug is often taken in the form of a drink or in foods such as candy. Recently, a new technology of *cannabis* vaporization was developed (4–6) that exploits the property that most of the plant's physiologically active constituents boil at a temperature below that at which the material burns (7). Thus, it becomes practical to administer *cannabis* vapor via the pulmonary route without throat or lung irritation or exposure to potential carcinogens from smoke.

Drug preparations from the hemp plant vary widely in quality and potency, depending on the type (there are possibly three species or, alternatively, various ecotypes of a single species), climate, soil, cultivation, and method of preparation. When the cultivated plant is fully ripe, a sticky, golden yellow resin with a minty fragrance covers its flower clusters and top leaves. The plant's resin contains the active substances, cannabinoids and essential oil terpenoids, which are produced by the plant in glandular trichomes (7). Preparations of the drug come in three grades, identified by Indian names. The cheapest and least potent, called *bhang,* is derived from the cut tops of uncultivated plants and has a low resin content. Much of the marihuana smoked in the United States, particularly a few years ago, was of this grade. *Ganja* is obtained from the unfertilized flowering tops and leaves of carefully selected, cultivated plants, and it has a higher quality and quantity of resin. The third and highest grade of the drug, called *charas* in India, is largely made from the resin itself, obtained from the tops of mature plants; only this version of the drug is properly called hashish. Hashish can also be smoked, eaten, or drunk. Recently, more potent and more expensive marihuana from Thailand, Hawaii, British Columbia, and California has become available in the United States. Some California growers have successfully cultivated an unpollinated plant by the early weeding out of male plants; the product is the much sought-after *sinsemilla*. Such new breeding and cultivation techniques have raised the tetrahydrocannabinol content of marihuana smoked in the United States over the last 20 years; although there are some extravagant claims made about the size of this increment, most authorities believe it has been modest (8,9). On average, street *cannabis* is not much more potent than it was in the 1960s.

The chemistry of the *cannabis* drugs is extremely complex and not completely understood. In the 1940s, it was determined that the active constituents are various isomers of tetrahydrocannabinol. The delta-9 form (hereafter called THC) has been synthesized and is believed to be the primary active component of marihuana. However, the drug's effects probably involve other components, such as cannabidiol, other cannabinoids, and terpenoids (7), and also depend on the form in which it is taken. There are more than 60 cannabinoids in marihuana and a number of them are thought to be biologically active. This activity is apparently mediated by the recently discovered receptors in the brain and elsewhere in the body that are stimulated by THC (10). This exciting discovery implied that the body produces its own version of cannabinoids for one or more useful purposes. The first of these cannabinoid-like neurotransmitters was identified in 1992 and named anandamide (*ananda* is the Sanskrit word for bliss) (11). Cannabinoid receptor sites occur not only in the lower brain but also in the cerebral cortex and the hippocampus.

The psychic effects of the drug have been described in a very extensive literature. Hashish long ago acquired a lurid reputation through the writings of literary figures, notably the group of French writers—Baudelaire, Gautier, Dumas père, and others—who formed *Le Club des Haschischins* in Paris in the 1840s. Their reports, written under the influence of large amounts of hashish, must be largely discounted as exaggerations that do not apply to moderate use of the drug. There is a story that hashish was responsible for Baudelaire's psychosis and death; the story overlooks the fact that he had relatively little experience with hashish, was in all probability actually writing about his experience with laudanum, and, moreover, had been an alcoholic and suffered from tertiary syphilis.

Bayard Taylor—the American writer, lecturer, and traveler best known for his translation of Goethe's *Faust*—

wrote one of the first accounts of a *cannabis* experience in terms that began to approach a clinical description. He tried the drug in a spirit of inquiry during a visit to Egypt in 1854. His narrative of the effects follows (12):

> The sensations it then produced were... physically of exquisite lightness and airiness—mentally of a wonderfully keen perception of the ludicrous in the most simple and familiar objects. During the half hour in which it lasted, I was at no time so far under its control that I could not, with the clearest perception, study the changes through which I passed. I noted with careful attention the fine sensations which spread throughout the whole tissue of my nervous fibers, each thrill helping to divest my frame of its earthly and material nature, till my substance appeared to me no grosser than the vapors of the atmosphere, and while sitting in the calm of the Egyptian twilight I expected to be lifted up and carried away by the first breeze that should ruffle the Nile. While this process was going on, the objects by which I was surrounded assumed a strange and whimsical expression.... I was provoked into a long fit of laughter.... [The effect] died away as gradually as it came, leaving me overcome with a soft and pleasant drowsiness, from which I sank into a deep, refreshing sleep.

Perhaps a better clinical account is that of Walter Bromberg, a psychiatrist, who described the psychic effects on the basis of his own experience and many observations and talks with people while they were under the influence of marihuana (13):

> The intoxication is initiated by a period of anxiety within 10 to 30 minutes after smoking, in which the user sometimes... develops fears of death and anxieties of vague nature associated with restlessness and hyperactivity. Within a few minutes he begins to feel more calm and soon develops definite euphoria; he becomes talkative... is elated, exhilarated... begins to have... an astounding feeling of lightness of the limbs and body... laughs uncontrollably and explosively... without at times the slightest provocation... has the impression that his conversation is witty, brilliant.... The rapid flow of ideas gives the impression of brilliance of thought and observation... [but] confusion appears on trying to remember what was thought... he may begin to see visual hallucinations... flashes of light or amorphous forms of vivid color which evolve and develop into geometric figures, shapes, human faces, and pictures of great complexity.... After a longer or shorter time, lasting up to two hours, the smoker becomes drowsy, falls into a dreamless sleep and awakens with no physiologic after-effects and with a clear memory of what happened during the intoxication.

Most observers confirm Bromberg's account as a composite, somewhat exaggerated, overinclusive description of marihuana highs. They find that the effects from smoking last from 2 to 4 hours, the effects from ingestion 5 to 12 hours. For a new user, the initial anxiety that sometimes occurs is alleviated if supportive friends are present. The intoxication heightens sensitivity to external stimuli, reveals details that would ordinarily be overlooked, makes colors seem brighter and richer, and brings out values in works of art that previously had little or no meaning to the viewer. It is as though the *cannabis*-intoxicated adult perceives the world with some of the newness, wonder, curiosity, and excitement of a child; the person's world becomes more interesting and details that had been taken for granted now attract more attention. The high also enhances the appreciation of music; many jazz and rock musicians have said that they perform better under the influence of marihuana, but this effect has not been objectively confirmed.

The sense of time is distorted: 10 minutes may seem like an hour. Curiously, there is often a splitting of consciousness, so that the smoker, while experiencing the high, is at the same time an objective observer of their own intoxication. The person may, for example, be afflicted with paranoid thoughts, yet at the same time be reasonably objective about them—laughing or scoffing at them and, in a sense, enjoying them. The ability to retain a degree of objectivity may explain why many experienced users of marihuana manage to behave in a perfectly sober fashion in public even when they are highly intoxicated.

Although the intoxication varies with psychological set and social setting, the most common response is a calm, mildly euphoric state in which time slows and sensitivity to sights, sounds, and touch is enhanced. The smoker may feel exhilaration or hilarity and notice a rapid flow of ideas with a reduction in short-term memory. Images sometimes appear before closed eyes; visual perception and body image may undergo subtle changes. It is dangerous to operate complex machinery, including automobiles, under the influence of marihuana, because it slows reaction time and impairs attention and coordination. There is uncertainty as to whether some impairment persists for several hours after the feeling of intoxication has passed (14,15).

Marihuana is sometimes referred to as a hallucinogen. Many of the phenomena associated with lysergic acid diethylamide (LSD) and LSD-type substances can be produced by *cannabis*, but only at very high dosage. As with LSD, the experience often has a wave-like aspect. Other phenomena commonly associated with both types of drugs are distorted perception of various parts of the body, spatial and temporal distortion, depersonalization, increased sensitivity to sound, synesthesia, heightened suggestibility, and a sense of thinking more clearly and having deeper awareness of the meaning of things. Anxiety and paranoid reactions are also sometimes seen as consequences of either drug. However, the agonizingly nightmarish reactions that even the experienced LSD user may endure are quite rare among experienced marihuana smokers, not simply because they are using a far less potent drug, but also because they have much closer and continuing control over the extent and type of reaction they wish to induce. Furthermore, *cannabis* has a tendency to produce

sedation, whereas LSD and LSD-type drugs may induce long periods of wakefulness and even restlessness. Unlike LSD, marihuana does not dilate the pupils or materially heighten blood pressure, reflexes, and body temperature. (On the other hand, it does increase the pulse rate, while lowering blood pressure.) Tolerance develops rapidly with LSD-type drugs but little with *cannabis*. Finally, marihuana lacks the potent consciousness-altering qualities of LSD, peyote, mescaline, psilocybin, and other hallucinogens; it is questionable whether in the doses ordinarily used in this country it can produce true hallucinations. These differences, particularly the last, cast considerable doubt on marihuana's credentials for inclusion among the hallucinogens.

HEALTH EFFECTS OF MARIHUANA USE

In recent years, the psychological and physical effects of long-term use have caused most concern. Studies are often conflicting and permit various views of marihuana's possible harmfulness. This complicates the task of presenting an objective statement about the issue.

One of the first questions asked about any drug is whether it is addictive or produces dependence. This question is hard to answer because the terms *addiction* and *dependence* have no agreed-to definitions. Two recognized signs of addiction are tolerance and withdrawal symptoms; these are rarely a serious problem for marihuana users. In the early stages, they actually become more sensitive to the desired effects. After continued heavy use, some tolerance to both physiologic and psychological effects develops, although it seems to vary considerably among individuals. Almost no one reports an urgent need to increase the dose to recapture the original sensation. What is called *behavioral tolerance* may be partly a matter of learning to compensate for the effects of high doses, and may explain why farm workers in some Third World countries are able to do heavy physical labor while smoking a great deal of marihuana (16).

A mild withdrawal reaction also occurs in animal experiments and possibly in some human beings who take high doses for a long time. The rarely reported mild symptoms are anxiety, insomnia, tremors, and chills, lasting for a day or two. It is unclear how common this reaction is; in a Jamaican study, heavy ganja users did not report abstinence symptoms when withdrawn from the drug. In any case, there is little evidence that the withdrawal reaction ordinarily presents serious problems to marihuana users or causes them to go on taking the drug. In a recent comprehensive review, *cannabis* withdrawal was seen as producing symptoms that were low level to nonexistent, with inconsistent onset and offset, with heterogeneous effects claimed with greatest support for transient agitation, appetite change, and sleep disturbance (17). In sum, the concept of *cannabis* withdrawal was considered unproven.

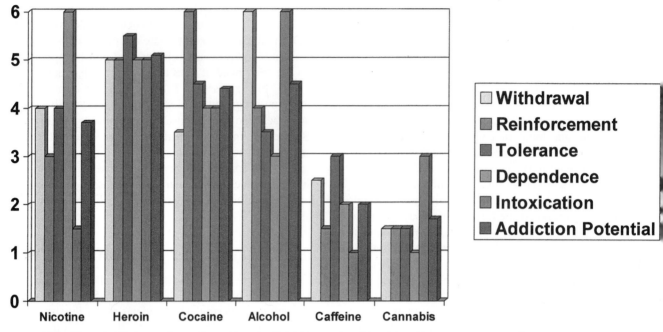

FIG. 15.1. Addiction ratings. From Henningfield, Benowitz. *New York Times* 1994 Aug 2:C3, with permission.

In a more important sense, dependence means an unhealthy and often unwanted preoccupation with a drug to the exclusion of most other things. People suffering from drug dependence find that they are constantly thinking about the drug, or intoxicated, or recovering from its effects. The habit impairs their mental and physical health and hurts their work, family life, and friendships. They often know that they are using too much and repeatedly make unsuccessful attempts to cut down or stop. These problems seem to afflict proportionately fewer marihuana smokers than users of alcohol, tobacco, heroin, or cocaine. Even heavy users in places like Jamaica and Costa Rica do not seem to be dependent in this damaging sense. Marihuana's capacity to lead to psychological dependence is not as strong as that of either tobacco or alcohol. Two experts from the University of California, San Francisco, and the National Institute on Drug Abuse independently compared the dependency potential of *cannabis*, alcohol, nicotine, caffeine, cocaine, and heroin (18,19). Cannabis was considered by both to carry the lowest overall risk (Fig. 15.1).

It is often difficult to distinguish between drug use as a cause of problems and drug use as an effect; this is especially true in the case of marihuana. Most people who develop a dependency on marihuana would also be likely to develop other dependencies because of anxiety, depression, or feelings of inadequacy. The original condition is likely to matter more than the attempt to relieve it by means of the drug. The troubled teenager who smokes *cannabis* throughout the school day certainly has a problem, and excessive use of marihuana may be one of its symptoms.

The idea has persisted that in the long run smoking marihuana causes some sort of mental or emotional deterioration. In three major studies conducted in Jamaica, Costa Rica, and Greece, researchers compared heavy long-term *cannabis* users with nonusers and found no evidence of intellectual or neurologic damage, no changes in personality, and no loss of the will to work or participate in society (20–22). The Costa Rican study showed no difference between heavy users (seven or more marihuana cigarettes a day) and lighter users (six or fewer cigarettes a day). Experiments in the United States show no effects of fairly heavy marihuana use on learning, perception or motivation over periods as long as 1 year (23–26).

On the other side are clinical reports of a personality change called the *amotivational syndrome*. Its symptoms are said to be passivity, aimlessness, apathy, uncommunicativeness, and lack of ambition. Some proposed explanations are hormone changes, brain damage, sedation, and depression. Because the amotivational syndrome does not seem to occur in Greek or Caribbean farm laborers, some writers suggest that it affects only skilled and educated people who need to do more complex thinking (21,22,27). However, there is no credible evidence that what is meant by this syndrome is related to any inherent properties of the drug rather than to different sociocultural adaptations on the part of the users.

The problem of distinguishing causes from symptoms is particularly acute here. Heavy drug users in our society are often bored, depressed, and listless, or alienated, cynical, and rebellious. Sometimes the drugs cause these states of mind, and sometimes they result from personality characteristics that lead to drug abuse. Drug abuse can be an excuse for failure, or a form of self-medication. Because of these complications and the absence of confirmation from controlled studies, the existence of an amotivational syndrome caused by *cannabis* use has to be regarded as unproved.

Much attention has also been devoted to the idea that marihuana smoking leads to the use of opiates and other illicit drugs—the stepping stone hypothesis, now commonly referred to as the gateway hypothesis, which was rejected after extensive study by the Institute of Medicine (28) and the Canadian Senate (29). In this country, almost everyone who uses any other illicit drug has smoked marihuana first, just as almost everyone who smokes marihuana has drunk alcohol first. Anyone who uses any given drug is more likely to be interested in others, for some of the same reasons. People who use illicit drugs, in particular, are somewhat more likely to find themselves in company where other illicit drugs are available. None of this proves that using one drug leads to or causes the use of another. Most marihuana smokers do not use heroin or cocaine, just as most alcohol drinkers do not use marihuana. The metaphor of stepping stones suggests that if no one smoked marihuana it would be more difficult for anyone to develop an interest in opiates or cocaine. There is no convincing evidence for or against this. What is clear is that at many times and places marihuana has been used without these drugs, and that these drugs have been used without marihuana.

Only the unsophisticated continue to believe that *cannabis* leads to violence and crime. Indeed, instead of inciting criminal behavior, *cannabis* may tend to suppress it. The intoxication induces a mild lethargy that is not conducive to any physical activity, let alone the commission of crimes. The release of inhibitions results in fantasy and verbal (rather than behavioral) expression. During the high, marihuana users may say and think things they would not ordinarily say and think, but they generally do not do things that are foreign to their nature. If they are not already criminals, they will not commit crimes under the influence of the drug.

Does marihuana induce sexual debauchery? This popular impression may owe its origin partly to writers' fantasies and partly to the fact that users in the Middle East once laced the drug with what they thought were aphrodisiacs. In actuality, there is little evidence that *cannabis* stimulates sexual desire or power. On the other hand, there are those who contend, with equally little substantiation, that marihuana weakens sexual desire. Many marihuana users report that the high enhances the enjoyment of sexual intercourse, and it has been an aid to tantric sexual meditation in India and Tibet since ancient times (30). This appears to be true in the same sense that the enjoyment of art and music is apparently enhanced. It is questionable, however, whether the intoxication breaks down barriers to sexual activity that are not already broken.

Does marihuana lead to physical and mental degeneracy? Reports from many investigators, particularly in Egypt and parts of the Orient, indicate that long-term users of the potent versions of *cannabis* are, indeed, typically passive, nonproductive, slothful, and totally lacking in ambition. This suggests that chronic use of the drug in its stronger forms may have debilitating effects, just as prolonged heavy drinking does. There is a far more likely explanation, however. Many of those who take up *cannabis* in these countries are poverty stricken, hungry, sick, hopeless, or defeated, seeking through this inexpensive drug to soften the impact of an otherwise unbearable reality. This also applies to many of the "potheads" in the United States. In most situations one cannot be certain which came first: the drug, on the one hand, or the depression, anxiety, feelings of inadequacy, or the seemingly intolerable life situation on the other. Numerous chronic use studies have failed to differentiate personality differences between *cannabis* users and nonusers.

There is a substantial body of evidence that moderate use of marihuana does not produce physical or mental deterioration. One of the earliest and most extensive studies of this question was an investigation conducted by the British government in India in the 1890s. The investigating agency, called the Indian Hemp Drugs Commission, interviewed some 800 people—including *cannabis* users and dealers, physicians, superintendents of mental asylums, religious leaders, and a variety of other authorities—and in 1894 published a report of more than 3,000 pages. It concluded that there was no evidence that moderate use of the *cannabis* drugs produced any disease or mental or moral damage, or that it tended to lead to excess any more than did the moderate use of whiskey (31,32).

In the LaGuardia study in New York City, an examination of chronic users who had averaged about seven marihuana cigarettes a day (a comparatively high dosage) over a long period (the mean was 8 years) showed that they had suffered no demonstrable mental or physical decline as a result of their use of the drug (33). The 1972 report of the National Commission on Marihuana and Drug Abuse (34), although it did much to demythologize *cannabis*, cautioned that, of people in the United States who used marihuana, 2% became heavy users and that these abusers were at risk, but it did not make clear exactly what risk was involved. Furthermore, since the publication of this report, several controlled studies of chronic heavy use have been completed that have failed to establish any pharmacologically induced harmfulness, including personality deterioration or the development of the so-called amotivational syndrome (21–26, 35–37). The most recent government-sponsored review of *cannabis*, *Marijuana and Medicine*, conducted by the Institute of Medicine, while cautious in its summary statement, found little documentation for most of the alleged harmfulness of this substance (28).

A common assertion made about *cannabis* is that it may lead to psychosis. The literature on this subject is vast, and it divides into all shades of opinion. Many psychiatrists in India, Egypt, Morocco, and Nigeria have declared emphatically that the drug can produce insanity; others insist that it does not. One of the authorities most often quoted in support of the indictment is Benabud of Morocco. He believes that the drug produces a specific syndrome called "*cannabis* psychosis." His description of the identifying symptoms is far from clear, however, and other investigators dispute the existence of such a psychosis. The symptoms said to characterize this syndrome are also common to other acute toxic states, including, particularly in Morocco, those associated with malnutrition and endemic infections. Benabud estimates that the number of kif (marihuana) smokers suffering from all types of psychosis is not more than 5 in 1,000 (38); this rate, however, is lower than the estimated total prevalence of all psychoses in populations of other countries. One would have to assume either (a) that there is a much lower prevalence of psychoses other than *cannabis* psychosis among kif smokers in Morocco or (b) that there is no such thing as a *cannabis* psychosis and the drug is contributing little or nothing to the prevalence rate for psychoses.

Bromberg, in a report of one of his studies, listed 31 patients whose psychoses he attributed to the toxic effects of marihuana. Of these 31, however, 7 patients were already predisposed to functional psychoses that were only precipitated by the drug, 7 others were later found to be schizophrenics, and 1 was later diagnosed as a manic-depressive (39). The Chopras in India, in examinations of 1,238 *cannabis* users, found only 13 users to be psychotic, which is about the usual prevalence of psychosis in the total population in Western countries (40). In the LaGuardia study, 9 of 77 people who were studied intensively had a history of psychosis; however, this high rate could be attributed to the fact that all those studied were patients in hospitals or institutions. Allentuck and Bowman, the psychiatrists who examined this group, concluded that "marihuana will not produce psychosis *de novo* in a well-integrated, stable person" (41).

A 1976 article by Thacore and Shukla revived the concept of the *cannabis* psychosis (42). The authors compared 25 people with what they call a paranoid psychosis precipitated by *cannabis* with an equal number of paranoid schizophrenics. The *cannabis* psychotics were described as patients in whom there had been a clear temporal relation between prolonged abuse of *cannabis* and the development of a psychosis on more than two occasions. All had used *cannabis* heavily for at least 3 years, mainly in the form of bhang, the weakest of the three preparations common in India (it is usually drunk as a tea or eaten in doughy pellets). In comparison with the schizophrenics, the *cannabis* psychotics were described as more panicky, elated, boisterous, and communicative; their behavior was said to be more often violent and bizarre, and their mental processes characterized by rapidity of thought and flight of ideas without schizophrenic thought disorder. The prognosis was said to be good; the symptoms could be easily relieved by phenothiazines and recurrence prevented by a decision not to use *cannabis* again. The syndrome was distinguished from an acute toxic reaction by the absence of clouded sensorium, confusion, and disorientation. Thacore and Shukla did not provide enough information to justify either the identification of their 25 patients' conditions as a single clinical syndrome or the asserted relation to *cannabis* use. They had little to say about the amount of *cannabis* used, except that relatives of the patients regarded it as abnormally large; they did not discuss the question of why the psychosis is associated with bhang rather than the stronger *cannabis* preparations ganja and charas. The meaning of "prolonged abuse on more than two occasions" in the case of men who were constant heavy *cannabis* users was not clarified, and the temporal relation between this situation and psychosis was not specified. Moreover, the *cannabis*-taking habits of the control group of schizophrenics were not discussed—a serious omission where use of bhang is so common. The patients described as *cannabis* psychotics were probably a heterogeneous mixture, with acute schizophrenic breaks, acute manic episodes, severe borderline conditions, and a few symptoms actually related to acute *cannabis* intoxication, mainly anxiety-panic reactions and a few psychoses of the kind that can be precipitated in unstable people by many different experiences of stress or consciousness change (42).

The explanation for such psychoses is that a person maintaining a delicate balance of ego functioning—so that, for instance, the ego is threatened by a severe loss, or a surgical assault, or even an alcoholic debauch—may also be overwhelmed or precipitated into a psychotic reaction by a drug that alters, however mildly, the person's state of consciousness. This concatenation of factors—a person whose ego is already overburdened in its attempts to manage a great deal of anxiety and to prevent distortion of perception and body image, plus the taking of a drug that, in some persons, promotes just these effects—may, indeed, be the last straw in precipitating a schizophrenic break. Of 41 first-break acute schizophrenic patients studied by Dr. Grinspoon at the Massachusetts Mental Health Center, it was possible to elicit a history of marihuana use in 6 (43). In 4 of the 6 patients, it seemed quite improbable that the drug could have had any relation to the development of the acute psychosis, because the psychosis was so remote in time from the drug experience. Careful history taking and attention to details of the drug experiences and changing mental status in the remaining two patients failed either to implicate or exonerate marihuana as a precipitant in their psychoses.

Our own clinical experience and that of others (44) suggests that *cannabis* may precipitate exacerbations in the psychotic processes of some schizophrenic patients at a time when their illnesses are otherwise reasonably well-controlled with antipsychotic drugs. In these patients, it is often difficult to determine whether the use of *cannabis* is simply a precipitant of the psychosis or whether it is an attempt to treat symptomatically the earliest perceptions of decompensation; needless to say, the two possibilities are not mutually exclusive. There is little support for the idea that *cannabis* contributes to the etiology of schizophrenia. And in one recently reported case, a 19-year-old schizophrenic woman was more successfully treated with cannabidiol (one of the cannabinoids in marihuana) than she had been with haloperidol (Haldol) (45).

A recent study from Sweden on schizophrenia is most suspect (46). The authors examined Swedish conscripts from 1969. This investigation seems to be an attempt to rehabilitate an extremely criticized study of the same cohort published in 1987 (47), which had been thoroughly criticized (48). In the current study, the authors claim that based on their data, up to 13% of schizophrenia incidence could be attributable to *cannabis*. This is an unsubstantiated allegation, given that only 1.4% of the conscripts that ever smoked *cannabis* wound up schizophrenic. Men of such age are at the critical time in development of the disorder. All of the eventual schizophrenics in the earlier study were recognized to have some psychiatric issue before they entered the service!

Another recent study examined a cohort of young New Zealanders for *cannabis* use versus development of adult psychosis (49). In this brief article, "controls" smoked *cannabis* zero to two times, while "*cannabis* users" took the drug "three times or more" by age 15 years and continued at some unspecified rate of intake by age 18 years. Supposedly smoking *cannabis* increased the incidence of psychosis in adults, and it was more likely the earlier they began. If *cannabis* were truly etiologic in the development of psychosis, it would be reasonable to expect some dose–response effect. That is not evident here in any respect.

Interestingly, *cannabis* may ameliorate certain symptoms of psychosis (50), including activation symptoms and subjective complaints of depression, anxiety, insomnia, and pain. It is noteworthy that levels of anandamide are elevated in the brains of schizophrenics (51).

Although there is little evidence for the existence of a *cannabis* psychosis, it seems clear that the drug may precipitate in susceptible people one of several types of mental dysfunction. The most serious and disturbing of these is the toxic psychosis. This is an acute state that resembles the delirium of a high fever. It is caused by the presence in the brain of toxic substances that interfere with a variety of cerebral functions. Generally speaking, as the toxins disappear, so do the symptoms of toxic psychosis. This type of reaction may be caused by any number of substances taken either as intended or inadvertent overdoses. The syndrome often includes clouding of consciousness, restlessness, confusion, bewilderment, disorientation, dream-like thinking, apprehension, fear, illusions, and hallucinations. It generally requires a rather large ingested dose of *cannabis* to induce a toxic psychosis. Such a reaction is apparently much less likely to occur when *cannabis* is smoked, perhaps because not enough of the active substances can be absorbed sufficiently rapidly, or possibly because the process of smoking modifies in some yet unknown way those cannabinoids that are most likely to precipitate this syndrome.

Some marihuana users suffer what are usually short-lived, acute, anxiety states, sometimes with and sometimes without accompanying paranoid thoughts. The anxiety may reach such proportions as properly to be called panic. Such panic reactions, although uncommon, probably constitute the most frequent adverse reaction to the moderate use of smoked marihuana. During this reaction, the sufferer may believe that the various distortions of bodily perceptions mean that the sufferer is dying or is undergoing some great physical catastrophe, and similarly the individual may interpret the psychological distortions induced by the drug as an indication of the sufferer's loss of sanity. Panic states may, albeit rarely, be so severe as to incapacitate, usually for a relatively short period of time. The anxiety that characterizes the acute panic reaction resembles an attenuated version of the frightening parts of an LSD or other psychedelic experience—the so-called bad trip. Some proponents of the use of LSD in psychotherapy assert that the induced altered state of consciousness involves a lifting of repression. Although the occurrence of a global undermining of repression is questionable, many effects of LSD do suggest important alterations in ego defenses. These alterations presumably make new percepts and insights available to the ego; some, particularly those most directly derived from primary process, may be quite threatening, especially if there is no comfortable and supportive setting to facilitate the integration of the new awareness into the ego organization. Thus, psychedelic experiences may be accompanied by a great deal of anxiety, particularly when the drugs are taken under poor conditions of set and setting; to a much lesser extent, the same can be said of *cannabis*.

These reactions are self-limiting, and simple reassurance is the best method of treatment. Perhaps the main danger to the user is that the user will be diagnosed as having a toxic psychosis. Users with this kind of reaction may be quite distressed, but they are not psychotic. The *sine qua non* of sanity, the ability to test reality, remains intact, and the panicked user is invariably able to relate the discomfort to the drug. There is no disorientation, nor are there true hallucinations. Sometimes this panic reaction is accompanied by paranoid ideation. The user may, for example, believe that the others in the room, especially if they are not well known, have some hostile intentions, or that someone is going to inform on the user, often to the police, for smoking marihuana. Generally speaking, these paranoid ideas are not strongly held, and simple reassurance dispels them. Anxiety reactions and paranoid thoughts are much more likely in someone who is taking the drug for the first time or in an unpleasant or unfamiliar setting, than in an experienced user who is comfortable with the surroundings and companions; the reaction is very rare where marihuana is a casually accepted part of the social scene. The likelihood varies directly with the dose and inversely with the user's experience; thus, the most vulnerable person is the inexperienced user who inadvertently (often precisely because the inexperienced user lacks familiarity with the drug) takes a large dose that produces perceptual and somatic changes for which the user is unprepared.

One rather rare reaction to *cannabis* is the flashback, or spontaneous recurrence of drug symptoms while not intoxicated. Although several reports suggest that this may occur in marihuana users even without prior use of any other drug (43), in general, it seems to arise only in those who have used more powerful hallucinogenic or psychedelic drugs. There are also some people who have flashback experiences of psychedelic drug trips while smoking marihuana; this is sometimes regarded as an extreme version of a more general heightening of the marihuana high that occurs after the use of hallucinogens. Many people find flashbacks enjoyable, but to others they are distressing. They usually fade with the passage of time. It is possible that flashbacks are attempts to deal with primary process derivatives and other unconscious material that has breached the ego defenses during the psychedelic or *cannabis* experience.

Rarely, but especially among new users of marihuana, there occurs an acute depressive reaction. It is generally rather mild and transient but may sometimes require psychiatric intervention. This type of reaction is most likely to occur in a user who has some degree of underlying depression; it is as though the drug allows the depression to be felt and experienced as such. Again, set and setting play an important part. Cannabis has been of benefit in mood stabilization in case reports from patients with bipolar disease (52).

Most recent research on the health hazards of marihuana concerns its long-term effects on the body. The main physiologic effects of *cannabis* are increased appetite, a faster heartbeat, and slight reddening of the conjunctiva. Although the increased heart rate could be a problem for people with cardiovascular disease, dangerous physical reactions to marihuana are almost unknown. No human being is known to have died of an overdose. By extrapolation from animal experiments, the ratio of lethal to effective (intoxicating) dose is estimated to be on the order of thousands to one.

Studies have examined the brain, the immune system, the reproductive system, and the lungs. Suggestions of long-term damage come almost exclusively from animal experiments and other laboratory work. Observations of marihuana users and the Caribbean, Greek, and other studies reveal little disease or organic pathology associated with the drug (21,22,27,53).

For example, there are several reports of damaged brain cells and changes in brain-wave readings in monkeys smoking marihuana, but neurologic and neuropsychological tests in Greece, Jamaica, and Costa Rica found no evidence of functional brain damage. A recent study of enrolled patients in the Compassionate Use Investigational New Drug Program in the United States also demonstrated no significant electroencephalograph (EEG) or P300 changes (54). Damage to white blood cells has also been observed in the laboratory, but again, its practical importance is unclear. Whatever temporary changes marihuana may produce in the immune system, they have not been found to increase the danger of infectious disease or cancer. If there were significant damage, we might expect to find a higher rate of these diseases among young people beginning in the 1960s, when marihuana first became popular. There is no evidence of that. Recent studies in human immunodeficiency virus (HIV) (55) and in the Missoula Chronic Use Study (54) also failed to demonstrate deleterious effects on white blood cell or CD4 counts.

The effects of marihuana on the reproductive system are a more complicated issue. In men, a single dose of THC lowers sperm count and the level of testosterone and other hormones. Tolerance to this effect apparently develops; in the Costa Rican study, marihuana smokers and controls had the same testosterone levels. Although the smokers in that study began using marihuana at an average age of 15 years, it had not affected their masculine development. There is no evidence that the changes in sperm count and testosterone produced by marihuana affect sexual performance or fertility.

In animal experiments, THC has also been reported to lower levels of female hormones and to disturb the menstrual cycle. When monkeys, rats, and mice are exposed during pregnancy to amounts of THC equivalent to a heavy human smoker's dose, stillbirths and decreased birth weight are sometimes reported in their offspring. There are also reports of low birth weight, prematurity, and even a condition resembling the fetal alcohol syndrome in some children of women who smoke marihuana heavily during pregnancy. The significance of these reports is unclear because controls are lacking and other circumstances make it hard to attribute causes. No endocrine changes were observed in the Missoula Chronic Use Study (54). To be safe, pregnant and nursing women should follow the standard conservative recommendation to avoid all drugs, including *cannabis*, that are not absolutely necessary. Nonetheless, evidence from a well-controlled study of *cannabis*-only smokers in Jamaica are supportive of a low risk to their children (56).

A well-confirmed danger of long-term, heavy marihuana use is its effect on the lungs. Smoking narrows and inflames air passages and reduces breathing capacity; damage to bronchial cells has been observed in hashish smokers. The possible side effects include bronchitis, emphysema, and lung cancer. Interestingly, one study failed to demonstrate emphysematous degeneration in *cannabis* smokers over time (57). Marihuana smoke contains the same carcinogens as tobacco smoke, usually in somewhat higher concentrations, at least in *cannabis* supplied by NIDA. THC may actually interfere with a key biochemical step in carcinogenesis (58). Marihuana is also inhaled more deeply and held in the lungs longer, which increases the danger (59,60). On the other hand, almost no one smokes 20 marihuana cigarettes a day. Marihuana of higher potency may reduce the danger of respiratory damage, because less smoking is required for the desired effect. There is now some experimental evidence demonstrating that high-potency THC cigarettes are smoked less vigorously than those of low potency; the user takes smaller and shorter puffs, inhaling less with each puff (61). Vaporization technology may also reduce risks (62).

It is hard to generalize about abuse or define specific treatments, because the problems associated with marihuana are so vague, and cause and effect so hard to determine. Marihuana smokers may be using the drug as a facet of adolescent exploration, to demonstrate rebelliousness, to cope with anxiety, to medicate themselves for early symptoms of mental illness, or, most commonly, simply for pleasure.

The complexity of the problem is illustrated by a most important long-term study by two Berkeley psychologists (63). Shedler and Block followed the progress of 101 San Francisco children of both sexes from ages 5 to 18 years, and gave them personality tests at 7, 11, and 18 years of age. By the end of the study, 68% had used marihuana and 39% had used it once a week or more; large minorities had also used cocaine, hallucinogens, and prescription stimulants and sedatives. Three main groups could be distinguished: 29 "abstainers" who had used no illicit drugs; 36 "experimenters" who had used marihuana no more than once a month and had tried at most one other drug; and 20 "frequent users" who had smoked marihuana at least once a week and had used at least one other drug. The other 16 fit into none of these categories and were not included in the study.

Striking personality differences among the three groups appeared in childhood, long before any drug use. The frequent users, as early as age 7 years, got along poorly with other children and had few friends. They found it difficult to think ahead and lacked confidence in themselves. They were untrustworthy and seemingly indifferent to moral questions. At age 11 years they were described as inattentive, uncooperative, and vulnerable to stress. At age 18 years, they were insecure, alienated, impulsive, undependable, self-indulgent, inconsiderate, and unpredictable in their moods and behavior; they overreacted to frustration; they felt personally inadequate, as well as victimized and cheated. They had lower high school grades than adolescents in the other two groups.

Abstainers, at age 7 years, were described as inhibited, conventional, obedient, and lacking in creativity. At age 11 years they were shy, neat, and orderly, eager to please, but lacking in humor, liveliness, and expressiveness. The terms that best described them at age 18 years were tense, overcontrolled, moralistic, anxious, and lacking in social

ease or personal charm. Their high school grades were average.

The happy mean, statistically, was found in the "experimenters." They were more likely to be warm, responsive, curious, open, active, and cheerful from the age of 7 years on. In the three broad categories of personal happiness, relations with others, and rational self-control, frequent users were doing worst and experimental users best. The authors pointed out that studies comparing moderate drinkers with alcoholics and abstainers have found similar personality differences.

To find some sources of these differences, the authors examined experiments conducted when the children were only 5 years old. Their parents' behavior was observed as they worked with the child on a laboratory task involving blocks and mazes. Mothers of both frequent users and abstainers tended to be cold and unresponsive. They gave their children little encouragement but insisted that they perform well; and the experience seemed unpleasant for both mother and child. Fathers of frequent users did not differ from fathers of experimenters, but abstainers' fathers were impatient, hypercritical, and domineering.

According to the authors, frequent drug users believe that they have nothing to look forward to and are therefore drawn to the immediate gratification provided by drugs. Their alienation and impulsiveness might have roots in their relationship with their mothers. The problems of abstainers are also serious, but they attract less attention, because they are less troublesome for society. Abstainers suppress their impulses to avoid feeling vulnerable, perhaps because they have internalized the attitudes of harsh, authoritarian fathers. Experimental users are the largest and most typical group. At least in the San Francisco area in the 1980s, reasonably inquisitive, open, and independent adolescents experimented with marihuana as part of growing up.

The inverted U-shaped relationship between the degree of drug use and psychological health suggests that the need for therapy would also describe such a curve. The fact that among the abstainers are to be found many individuals who could profit from psychotherapy is not relevant to this discussion of marihuana. The important question concerns the indications for therapy for those who comprise the other two arms of the curve. Given the current prevalence of drug use in our society, the developmentally appropriate propensity of adolescents to explore and experiment, and the relatively benign sequelae of such experimentation with *cannabis*, it is obvious that therapy is not properly indicated for young people who fit the description of the "experimenter."

It is appropriate to consider psychotherapy for the frequent adolescent users of marihuana. The picture that emerges is "one of a troubled adolescent who is interpersonally alienated, emotionally withdrawn, and manifestly unhappy, and who expresses his or her maladjustment through undercontrolled, overtly antisocial behavior"

(63). They are described as being "overreactive to minor frustrations, likely to think and associate to ideas in unusual ways, having brittle ego-defense systems, self-defeating, concerned about the adequacy of their bodily functioning, concerned about their adequacy as persons, prone to project their feelings and motives onto others, feeling cheated and victimized by life, and having fluctuating moods."

Obviously, psychotherapy is not inappropriate for individuals who exemplify this description. But it should be emphasized that this is not psychotherapy for marihuana abuse; it is therapy for the underlying psychopathology, one of whose symptoms is the abuse of *cannabis*. It is no more appropriate to see marihuana as the cause of the problem here than it is to see repetitive hand-washing as the cause of obsessive-compulsive disorder. The individual may be brought to psychiatric attention because of the hand-washing, but the therapy will address the underlying disorder. Becoming attached to *cannabis* is not so much a function of any inherent psychopharmacologic property of the drug as it is emotionally driven by the underlying psychopathology. Success in curtailing *cannabis* use requires dealing with that pathology.

MEDICINAL USES OF CANNABIS

Cannabis usage as a medicament is ancient, and it has included indications for headache (64,65), other types of pain (66), obstetric and gynecologic conditions (67), and psychiatric disorders (68,69).

The history of *cannabis* as a Western medicine begins in 1839, with a publication by W. B. O'Shaughnessy, a British physician working in Calcutta (70). He reported on the analgesic, anticonvulsant, and muscle relaxant properties of the drug. His paper generated a good deal of interest, and there followed more than 100 other papers in the Western medical literature from 1840 to the turn of the century. In the nineteenth century the drug was widely prescribed in the Western world for various ailments and discomforts, such as coughing, fatigue, rheumatism, asthma, delirium tremens, migraine headache, and painful menstruation. Although its use was already declining somewhat because of the introduction of synthetic hypnotics and analgesics, it remained in the United States Pharmacopoeia until 1941. The difficulties imposed on its use by the Marihuana Tax Act of 1937, as well as quality-control issues with uncertain supplies, completed its medical demise, and, from that time on, physicians allowed themselves to become ignorant about the drug.

The greatest advantage of *cannabis* as a medicine is its unusual safety. The ratio of lethal dose to effective dose is estimated on the basis of extrapolation from animal data to be about 20,000:1. Huge doses have been given to dogs without causing death, and there is no reliable evidence of death caused by *cannabis* in a human being. *Cannabis* also has the advantage of not disturbing any physiologic functions or damaging any body organs when it is used in therapeutic doses. It produces little physical dependence or tolerance; there has never been any evidence that medical use of *cannabis* has led to habitual use as an intoxicant.

Whole *cannabis* preparations have the disadvantages of instability, varying strength, and insolubility in water, which makes it difficult for the drug to enter the bloodstream from the digestive tract. The multitude of ingredients found in *cannabis* is also an opportunity, because it suggests the manufacture of different cannabinoids, synthetic or natural, with properties useful for particular purposes; some of these have now become available (66,71). One that is presently legally available for the treatment of nausea and vomiting of cancer chemotherapy and the acquired immune deficiency syndrome (AIDS) weight loss syndrome is dronabinol (Marinol), a synthetic THC. While it is not as useful medicinally as whole smoked marihuana, it is legally available as a Schedule III drug. Smoking generates quicker and more predictable results because it raises THC concentration in the blood more easily and predictably to the needed level. Also, it may be hard for a nauseated patient in chemotherapy to take oral medicine. But many patients dislike smoking or cannot inhale (69). Alternative-dosing approaches are discussed in several references (4,72–75).

There are many anecdotal reports of marihuana smokers using the drug to reduce postsurgery pain, headache, migraine, menstrual cramps, phantom limbs, and other kinds of pain. It is the case that *cannabis* acts by mechanisms different from those of other analgesics through the endocannabinoid pain mechanisms (66), and that *cannabis* may be more effective than opiates in neuropathic pain states. Again, some new synthetic derivatives might prove useful as an analgesic, but this is not an immediate prospect.

Because of reports that some people use less alcohol when they smoke marihuana, *cannabis* has been proposed as an adjunct to alcoholism treatment, but so far it has not been found useful (76–78). Most alcoholics neither want to substitute marihuana nor find it particularly helpful. But there might be some hope for use of marihuana in combination with disulfiram (Antabuse) (76). Certainly a *cannabis* habit would be preferable to an alcohol habit for anyone who could not avoid dependence on a drug but who was able to substitute one drug for another.

Approximately 20% of epileptic patients do not get much relief from conventional anticonvulsant medications. *Cannabis* has been explored as an alternative, at least since a case was reported in which marihuana smoking, together with the standard anticonvulsants phenobarbital and diphenylhydantoin (Dilantin), was apparently necessary to control seizures in a young epileptic man (79). Recent reports support the role of THC endocannabinoids in modulation of seizure threshold (80,81). Cannabidiol also demonstrates anticonvulsant properties (7,82). In one controlled study, cannabidiol in addition to prescribed anticonvulsants produced improvement in seven patients with grand mal seizures; three showed great improvement.

Of eight patients who received a placebo instead, only one improved (83).

Marihuana also reduces muscle spasm and tremors in some people who suffer from spastic disorders, including multiple sclerosis (84,85), cerebral palsy, and various causes of hemiplegia and quadriplegia, such as spinal cord injury or disease. Anecdotal reports of the use of *cannabis* for the relief of asthma abound. The antiasthmatic drugs that are available all have drawbacks—limited effectiveness or side effects. Because marihuana dilates the bronchi and reverses bronchial spasm, *cannabis* derivatives have been tested as antiasthmatic drugs. Smoking marihuana would probably not be a good way to treat asthma because of chronic irritation of the bronchial tract by tars and other substances in marihuana smoke, so recent research has sought a better means of administration. THC in the form of an aerosol spray has been investigated extensively (59,60). Other cannabinoids, such as cannabinol and cannabidiol, may be preferable to THC for this purpose. An interesting finding for future research is that cannabinoids may affect the bronchi by means of a different mechanism from that of the familiar antiasthmatic drugs. A promising new medical use for *cannabis* is treatment of glaucoma, the second leading cause of blindness in the United States. About a million Americans suffer from the form of glaucoma (wide angle) treatable with *cannabis*. Marihuana causes a dose-related, clinically significant drop in intraocular pressure that lasts several hours in both normal subjects and in those with the abnormally high ocular tension produced by glaucoma. Oral or intravenous THC has the same effect, which seems to be specific to *cannabis* derivatives rather than simply a result of sedation. *Cannabis* does not cure the disease, but it can retard the progressive loss of sight when conventional medication fails and surgery is too dangerous (86). A recent comprehensive review supports the use of cannabinoids as antioxidant protective agents in the development of vascular retinopathy of glaucoma, a process independent of intraocular pressure (87).

It remains to be seen whether topical use of THC or a synthetic cannabinoid in the form of eyedrops will be preferable to smoking marihuana for this purpose. So far THC eyedrops have not proved effective, and in 1981, the National Eye Institute announced that it would no longer approve human research using these eyedrops (76). Studies continue on certain synthetic *cannabis* derivatives and other natural cannabinoids (87). Smoking marihuana is a better way of titrating the dose than is the taking of an oral cannabinoid, and most patients seem to prefer it. Unfortunately, many patients, especially elderly ones, dislike the psychoactive effects of marihuana.

Cannabis derivatives have several minor or speculative uses in the treatment of cancer, and one major use. As appetite stimulants, marihuana and THC may help to slow weight loss in cancer patients (88), as they have in AIDS patients (55). THC has also retarded the growth of tumor cells in some animal studies, but results are inconclusive,

and another *cannabis* derivative, cannabidiol, seems to increase tumor growth (89). Possibly cannabinoids in combination with other drugs will turn out to have some use in preventing tumor growth. THC may promote apoptosis (programmed cell death) in some malignant cells (90). Limonene, a monoterpenoid component of *cannabis* resin, has similar activity on breast tumor cells (91). But the most promising use of *cannabis* in cancer treatment is the prevention of nausea and vomiting in patients undergoing chemotherapy. About half of patients treated with anticancer drugs suffer from severe nausea and vomiting. In 25% to 30% of these cases, the commonly used antiemetics do not work (69). The nausea and vomiting are not only unpleasant, but are a threat to the effectiveness of the therapy. Retching can cause tears of the esophagus and rib fractures, prevent adequate nutrition, and lead to fluid loss.

The antiemetics most commonly used in chemotherapy are prochlorperazine (Compazine) and the newer ondansetron (Zofran) and granisetron (Kytril). The suggestion that *cannabis* might be useful arose in the early 1970s when some young patients receiving cancer chemotherapy found that marihuana smoking, which was, of course, illegal, reduced their nausea and vomiting. In one study of 56 patients who got no relief from standard antiemetic agents, 78% became symptom free when they smoked marihuana (92). Previously unpublished state studies of smoked *cannabis* have demonstrated 70% to 100% relief of vomiting in some 748 chemotherapy patients (93).

Several of the most urgent medical uses of *cannabis* are for the treatment of the nausea and weight loss suffered by many AIDS patients. The nausea is often a symptom of the disease itself and a side effect of some of the medicines (particularly azidothymidine [zidovudine or AZT]). For many AIDS patients the most distressing and threatening symptom is cachexia. Marihuana will retard weight loss in most patients and even helps some regain weight (69).

A committee of the Institute of Medicine of the National Academy of Sciences remarked in a report in 1982 (28, p. 139):

> *Cannabis* shows promise in some of these areas, although the dose necessary to produce the desired effect is often close to one that produces an unacceptable frequency of toxic [undesirable] side effects. What is perhaps more encouraging... is that *cannabis* seems to exert its beneficial effects through mechanisms that differ from those of other available drugs. This raises the possibility that some patients who would not be helped by conventional therapies could be treated with *cannabis*.... It may be possible to reduce side effects by synthesizing related molecules that could have a more favorable ratio of desired to undesired actions; this line of investigation should have a high priority.

The committee recommended further research, especially in the treatment of nausea and vomiting in chemotherapy, asthma, glaucoma, and seizures and spasticity.

Under federal and most state statutes, marihuana is listed as a Schedule I drug: high potential for abuse, no currently accepted medical use, and lacking in accepted safety for use under medical supervision. It cannot ordinarily be prescribed and may be used only under research conditions. *Cannabis* was recently legalized for medical use in Canada and Holland, and liberalization of laws is proceeding in the United Kingdom and elsewhere in Western Europe.

The potential of *cannabis* as a medicine is yet to be realized, partly because of its reputation as an intoxicant, ignorance on the part of the medical establishment, and legal difficulties involved in doing the research (94). Recreational use of *cannabis* has affected the opinions of physicians about its medical potential in various ways. When marihuana was regarded as the drug of African Americans, Mexican Americans, and Bohemians, doctors were ready to go along with the Bureau of Narcotics, ignore its medical uses, and urge prohibition. For years the National Organization for the Reform of Marijuana Laws and other groups have been petitioning the government to change this classification. Now that marihuana has become so popular among a broad section of the population, we have been more willing to investigate its therapeutic value. Recreational use now spurs medical interest instead of medical hostility.

It is estimated that more than 70 million Americans have used *cannabis* and more than 10 million use it regularly. They use it not because they are driven by uncontrollable "reefer madness" craving, as some propaganda would lead us to believe, but because they have learned its value from experience. Yet almost all of the research, writing, political activity, and legislation devoted to marihuana has been concerned only with the question of whether it is harmful and how much harm it does. The only exception is the growing resurgence of interest in its usefulness as a medicine. But medicine represents only one category of marihuana use. The rest are sometimes grouped under the general heading of "recreational," but that is hardly an appropriate word to describe the many serious reasons for which people have learned to use *cannabis*. For example, many writers and artists have found that the *cannabis* high can be a catalyst to their creativity (95). Allen Ginsberg, writing while stoned, eloquently put it this way: ". . . the marihuana consciousness is one that, ever so gently, shifts the center of attention from habitual shallow purely verbal guidelines and repetitive secondhand ideological interpretations of experience to more direct, slower, absorbing, oc- casionally microscopically minute, engagement with sensing phenomena during the high moments or hours after one has smoked" (96). While many artists have learned to use *cannabis* as an aid to their creativity, many other users have discovered its capacity to catalyze the generation of ideas and insights, heighten the appreciation of music and art, or deepen emotional and sexual intimacy. (The reader who wishes to learn more about this is referred to the Uses of Marijuana Web Site [www.marihuana-uses.com], a collection of essays written by marihuana users who have found this drug useful as an enhancer of various capacities and experiences.)

This "enhancement" capacity is often underappreciated—not only by nonusers, but also by some users, especially young people who are primarily interested in promoting sociability and fun. Most of marihuana's powers of enhancement are subtle and not as immediately available as its capacity to lift mood or improve appetite and the taste of food. Many, if not most, people do not achieve a *cannabis* high during their first attempt or attempts because they have yet to learn to recognize the subtle changes in consciousness that comprise the marihuana experience. Similarly, the ability to make use of *cannabis* consciousness as an enhancer of various capacities appears to require both experience in achieving this state and learning how to make use of it.

The potential dangers of marihuana when taken for pleasure and enhancement, and its possible usefulness as a medicine are historically and practically interrelated issues—historically, because the arguments used to justify public and official disapproval of recreational use have had a strong influence on opinions about its medical potential; practically, because the more evidence accumulates that marihuana is relatively safe even when used as an intoxicant, the clearer it becomes that the medical requirement of safety is satisfied. Most recent research is tentative, and initial enthusiasm for drugs is often disappointed after further investigation. But it is not as though *cannabis* were an entirely new agent with unknown properties. Studies done during the past 10 years confirm a centuries-old promise. With the relaxation of restrictions on research and the further chemical manipulation of *cannabis* derivatives, this promise will eventually be realized. The weight of past and contemporary evidence will probably prove *cannabis* to be valuable in a number of ways as a medicine.

REFERENCES

1. Office of National Drug Control Policy. *Drug use trends*. Report No.: NCJ 190780. Washington, DC: Author, October 2002.
2. Substance Abuse and Mental Health Services Administration. *Results from the 2001 National Household Survey on Drug Abuse: vol. I. Summary of national findings*. Report No: Office of Applied Studies, NHSDA Series H-17. Rockville, MD: Author, 2002.
3. Ludlow FH. *The hasheesh eater: being passages form the life of a Pythagorean*. New York: Harper; 1857.
4. Gieringer DH. *Cannabis* "vaporization": a promising strategy for smoke harm reduction. *J Cannabis Ther* 2001;1(3–4): (in press).
5. Gieringer D. Why marijuana smoke harm reduction? Bulletin of the Multidisciplinary Association for Psychedelic Studies 1996;6(64–66).
6. Gieringer D. Waterpipe study. Bulletin of the Multidisciplinary Association

for Psychedelic Studies 1996;6:59–63.

7. McPartland JM, Russo EB. *Cannabis and cannabis extracts: Greater than the sum of their parts? J Cannabis Ther* 2001;1(3–4):103–132.

8. Mikuriya TH, Aldrich MR. *Cannabis* 1988. Old drug, new dangers. The potency question. *J Psychoactive Drugs* 1988;20(1):47–55.

9. El Sohly MA, Ross SA, Mehmedic Z, et al. Potency trends of delta9-THC and other cannabinoids in confiscated marijuana from 1980–1997. *J Forensic Sci* 2000;45(1):24–30.

10. Matsuda LA, Lolait SJ, Brownstein MJ, et al. Structure of a cannabinoid receptor and functional expression of the cloned cDNA. *Nature* 1990;346(6284): 561–564.

11. Devane WA, Hanus L, Breuer A, et al. Isolation and structure of a brain constituent that binds to the cannabinoid receptor. *Science* 1992;258(5090):1946–1949.

12. Ebin D. *The drug experience.* New York: Grove Press, 1961.

13. Bromberg W. Marihuana intoxication: a clinical study of *Cannabis sativa* intoxication. *Am J Psychiatry* 1934;91: 303.

14. Chait LD. Subjective and behavioral effects of marijuana the morning after smoking. *Psychopharmacology* 1990; 100:328–333.

15. Yeasavage JA, Leirer VO, Denari M, et al. Carry-over effects of marijuana intoxication on aircraft pilot performance: a preliminary report. *Am J Psychiatry* 1985;142:1325–1329.

16. Dreher MC. *Working men and ganja: marihuana use in rural Jamaica.* Philadelphia: Institute for the Study of Human Issues, 1982.

17. Smith NT. A review of the published literature into *cannabis* withdrawal symptoms in human users. *Addiction* 2002;97(6):621–632.

18. Hilts PJ. Is nicotine addictive? It depends on whose criteria you use. *New York Times* 1994 Aug 2:C3.

19. Mathre ML. Risk of dependence and addiction. In: Mathre ML, ed. *Cannabis in medical practice.* Jefferson, NC: McFarland, 1997.

20. Carter WE. *Cannabis in Costa Rica: a study of chronic marihuana use.* Philadelphia: Institute for the Study of Human Issues, 1980.

21. Rubin VD, Comitas L. *Ganja in Jamaica: a medical anthropological study of chronic marihuana use.* The Hague: Mouton, 1975.

22. Stefanis CN, Dornbush RL, Fink M. *Hashish: studies of long-term use.* New York: Raven Press, 1977.

23. Braude MC, Szara S. *Pharmacology of marihuana.* New York: Raven Press, 1976.

24. Culver CM, King FW. Neuropsychological assessment of undergraduate marihuana and LSD users. *Arch Gen Psychiatry* 1974;31:707–711.

25. Lessin PJ, Thomas S. Assessment of the chronic effects of marihuana on motivation and achievement: a preliminary report. In: Braude MC, Szara S, eds. *Pharmacology of marihuana.* New York: Raven Press, 1976.

26. Stefanis CN, Boulougouris J, Liakos A. Clinical and psychophysiological effects of *cannabis* in long-term users. In: Braude MC, Szara S, eds. *Pharmacology of marihuana.* New York: Raven Press, 1976.

27. Carter WE, Doughty PL. Social and cultural aspects of *cannabis* use in Costa Rica. *Ann N Y Acad Sci* 1976;282:2–16.

28. Joy JE, Watson SJ, Benson JA Jr. *Marijuana and medicine: assessing the science base.* Washington, DC: Institute of Medicine, 1999.

29. Canada S. *Cannabis: our position for a Canadian public policy. Report of the Senate Special Committee on Illegal Drugs.* Ottawa: Canada Senate; 2002 September. Available at: http://www.parl.gc.ca/Common/Committee_Sen RecentReps.asp?Language=E&Parl= 37&Ses=1

30. Aldrich MR. Tantric *cannabis* use in India. *J Psychedelic Drugs* 1977;9(3):227–233.

31. Solomon D, United States. The marihuana papers. Indianapolis: Bobbs-Merrill, 1966.

32. Commission IHD. *Report of the Indian Hemp Drugs Commission, 1893–94.* Simla: Government Central Printing Office, 1894.

33. New York (NY). Mayor's committee on marihuana, Wallace GB, Cunningham EV. *The marihuana problem in the city of New York; sociological, medical, psychological and pharmacological studies.* Lancaster, PA: The Jaques Cattell Press, 1944.

34. Abuse NCoMaD. *Marihuana: a signal of misunderstanding:* New American Library, 1972.

35. Beaubrun MH, Knight F. Psychiatric assessment of 30 chronic users of *cannabis* and 30 matched controls. *Am J Psychiatry* 1973;130(3):309–311.

36. Dornbush RL, Freedman AM. Chronic *cannabis* use: introduction. *Ann N Y Acad Sci* 1976;282:vii–viii.

37. Hochman JS, Brill NQ. Chronic marijuana use and psychosocial adaptation. *Am J Psychiatry* 1973;130(2):132–140.

38. Benabud A. Psychopathological aspects of the *cannabis* situation in Morocco: statistical data for 1956. *Bull Narc* 1957;9:2.

39. Bromberg W. Marihuana: a psychiatric study. *JAMA* 1939;113:4.

40. Murphy HBM. The *cannabis* habit: a review of the most recent psychiatric literature. *Addictions* 1966;13:3. [Citing Chopra RN, Chopra GS. The present position of hemp drug addiction in India. Indian Med Res Mem 1939;31.]

41. Allentuck S, Bowman KM. The psychiatric aspects of marihuana intoxication. *Am J Psychiatry* 1942;99:248.

42. Thacore VR, Shukla SR. *Cannabis* psychosis and paranoid schizophrenia. *Arch Gen Psychiatry* 1976;33(3):383–386.

43. Grinspoon L. *Marihuana reconsidered,* 2d ed. Cambridge, MA: Harvard University Press, 1977.

44. Treffert DA. Marijuana use in schizophrenia: a clear hazard. *Am J Psychiatry* 1978;135(10):1213–1215.

45. Zuardi AW, Morais SL, Guimaraes FS, et al. Antipsychotic effect of cannabidiol. *J Clin Psychiatry* 1995;56(10):485–486.

46. Zammit S, Allebeck P, Andreasson S, et al. Self-reported *cannabis* use as a risk factor for schizophrenia in Swedish conscripts of 1969: historical cohort study. *BMJ* 2002;325:1199–1203.

47. Andreasson S, Allebeck P, Engstrom A, et al. *Cannabis* and schizophrenia. A longitudinal study of Swedish conscripts. *Lancet* 1987;2(8574):1483–1486.

48. Zimmer LE, Morgan JP. *Marijuana myths, marijuana facts: a review of the scientific evidence.* New York: Lindesmith Center, 1997.

49. Arsenault L, Cannon M, Poulton R, et al. *Cannabis* use in adolescence and risk for adult psychosis: longitudinal prospective study. *BMJ* 2002;325:1212–1213.

50. Warner R, Taylor D, Wright J, et al. Substance use among the mentally ill: prevalence, Reasons for use, and effects on illness. *Am J Orthopsychiatry* 1994;64(1):30–39.

51. Leweke FM, Giuffrida A, Wurster U, et al. Elevated endogenous cannabinoids in schizophrenia. *Neuroreport* 1999;10(8):1665–1669.

52. Grinspoon L, Bakalar JB. The use of *cannabis* as a mood stabilizer in bipolar disorder: anecdotal evidence and the need for clinical research. *J Psychoactive Drugs* 1998;30(2):171–177.

53. Carter WE, Coggins WJ, Doughty PL, et al. *Chronic cannabis use in Costa Rica: a report by the Center for Latin American Studies of the University of Florida to the National Institute on Drug Abuse.* Gainesville, FL: University of Florida Press, 1976.

54. Russo EB, Mathre ML, Byrne A, et al. Chronic *cannabis* use in the Compassionate Investigational New Drug Program: an examination of benefits and

adverse effects of legal clinical *cannabis*. *J Cannabis Ther* 2002;2(1):3–57.

55. Abrams D, Leiser R, Hilton J, et al. Short-term effects of cannabinoids in patients with HIV-1 infection. In: *Symposium on the cannabinoids; 2002 July 13, Asilomar Conference Center*. Pacific Grove, CA: International Cannabinoids Research Society, 2002:58

56. Dreher MC, Nugent K, Hudgins R. Prenatal marijuana exposure and neonatal outcomes in Jamaica: an ethnographic study. *Pediatrics* 1994;93(2):254–260.

57. Tashkin DP, Simmons MS, Sherrill DL, et al. Heavy habitual marijuana smoking does not cause an accelerated decline in FEV1 with age. *Am J Respir Crit Care Med* 1997;155(1):141–148.

58. Roth MD, Marques-Magallanes JA, Yuan M, et al. Induction and regulation of the carcinogen-metabolizing enzyme CYP1A1 by marijuana smoke and delta (9)-tetrahydrocannabinol. *Am J Respir Cell Mol Biol* 2001;24(3):339–344.

59. Tashkin DP, Reiss S, Shapiro BJ, et al. Bronchial effects of aerosolized delta 9-tetrahydrocannabinol in healthy and asthmatic subjects. *Am Rev Respir Dis* 1977;115(1):57–65.

60. Tashkin DP, Shapiro BJ, Lee YE, et al. Effects of smoked marijuana in experimentally induced asthma. *Am Rev Respir Dis* 1975;112(3):377–386.

61. Heishman SJ, Stitzer ML, Yingling JE. Effects of tetrahydrocannabinol content on marijuana smoking behavior, subjective reports, and performance. *Pharmacol Biochem Behav* 1989;34(1):173–179.

62. Gieringer D. Medical use of *cannabis*: experience in California. In: Grotenhermen F, Russo E, eds. *Cannabis and cannabinoids: pharmacology, toxicology, and therapeutic potential*. Binghamton, NY: Haworth Press, 2001:153–170.

63. Shedler J, Block J. Adolescent drug use and psychological health: a longitudinal inquiry. *Am Psychologist* 1990;45:612–630.

64. Russo E. *Cannabis* for migraine treatment: the once and future prescription? An historical and scientific review. *Pain* 1998;76(1–2):3–8.

65. Russo EB. Hemp for headache: an in-depth historical and scientific review of *cannabis* in migraine treatment. *J Cannabis Ther* 2001;1(2):21–92.

66. Russo EB. Role of *cannabis* and cannabinoids in pain management. In: Weiner RS, ed. *Pain management: a practical guide for clinicians*, 6th ed. Boca Raton, FL: CRC Press, 2002.

67. Russo E. *Cannabis* treatments in obstet-

rics and gynecology: A historical review. *J Cannabis Ther* 2002;2(3–4):5–35.

68. Russo EB. *Handbook of psychotropic herbs: A scientific analysis of herbal remedies for psychiatric conditions*. Binghamton, NY: Haworth Press, 2001.

69. Grinspoon L, Bakalar JB. *Marihuana, the forbidden medicine*, revised and expanded ed. New Haven: Yale University Press, 1997.

70. O'Shaughnessy WB. On the preparations of the Indian hemp, or gunjah (*Cannabis indica*); their effects on the animal system in health, and their utility in the treatment of tetanus and other convulsive diseases. *Trans Med Physical Soc Bengal* 1838–1840:71–102,421–461.

71. Mechoulam R, Carlini EA. Toward drugs derived from *cannabis*. *Naturwissenschaften* 1978;65(4):174–179.

72. Grotenhermen F. Harm reduction associated with inhalation and oral administration of *cannabis* and THC. *J Cannabis Ther* 2001;1(3–4):133–152.

73. Grotenhermen F, Russo EB. *Cannabis and cannabinoids: pharmacology, toxicology and therapeutic potential*. Binghamton, NY: Haworth Press, 2002.

74. Jansen M, Terris R. One woman's work in the use of hashish in a medical context. *J Cannabis Ther* 2002;2(3–4):135–143.

75. Whittle BA, Guy GW, Robson P. Prospects for new *cannabis*-based prescription medicines. *J Cannabis Ther* 2001;1(3–4):183–205.

76. Roffman RA. *Marijuana as medicine*, 1st ed. Seattle: Madrona Publishers, 1982.

77. Rosenberg CM. The use of marihuana in the treatment of alcoholism. In: Cohen S, Stillman RC, eds. *The therapeutic potential of marihuana*. New York: Plenum Medical, 1976:173–182.

78. Rosenberg CM, Gerrein JR, Schnell C. *Cannabis* in the treatment of alcoholism. *J Stud Alcohol* 1978;39(11):1955–1958.

79. Consroe PF, Wood GC, Buchsbaum H. Anticonvulsant nature of marihuana smoking. *JAMA* 1975;234(3):306–307.

80. Wallace MJ, Martin BR, DeLorenzo RJ. Evidence for a physiological role of endocannabinoids in the modulation of seizure threshold and severity. *Eur J Pharmacol* 2002;452(3):295–301.

81. Wallace MJ, Blair RE, Razvi B, et al. CB1 receptor-dependent modulation of seizure frequency and duration in epileptic rats: implications for the endocannabinoid system in the treatment of epilepsy. In: *Symposium on the Cannabinoids; 2002 July 12, Asilomar Conference Center*. Pacific Grove, CA: International Cannabinoid Research Society, 2002:26.

82. Mechoulam R, Parker LA, Gallily R. Cannabidiol: an overview of some pharmacological aspects. *J Clin Pharmacol* 2002;42[11 Suppl]:11S–19S.

83. Cunha JM, Carlini EA, Pereira AE, et al. Chronic administration of cannabidiol to healthy volunteers and epileptic patients. *Pharmacology* 1980;21(3):175–185.

84. Petro DJ. Marihuana as a therapeutic agent for muscle spasm or spasticity. *Psychosomatics* 1980;21(1):81–85.

85. Petro DJ. *Cannabis* in multiple sclerosis: women's health concerns. *J Cannabis Ther* 2002;2(3–4):161–175.

86. Hepler RS, Rank IM, Petrus R. Ocular effects of marihuana smoking. In: Braude MC, Szara S, eds. *Pharmacology of marihuana*. New York: Raven Press, 1976.

87. Jarvinen T, Pate D, Laine K. Cannabinoids in the treatment of glaucoma. *Pharmacol Ther* 2002;95(2):203.

88. Regelson W, Butler JR, Schulz J, et al. Delta 9-tetrahydrocannabinol as an effective antidepressant and appetite-stimulating agent in advanced cancer patients. In: Braude MC, Szara S, eds. *Pharmacology of marihuana*, vol 2. New York: Raven Press, 1976:763–776.

89. White AC, Munson JA, Munson AE, et al. Effects of delta9-tetrahydrocannabinol in Lewis lung adenocarcinoma cells in tissue culture. *J Natl Cancer Inst* 1976;56(3):655–658.

90. Sanchez C, Galve-Roperh I, Canova C, et al. Delta-9 tetrahydrocannabinol induces apoptosis in C6 glioma cells. *FEBS Lett* 1998;436(1):6–10.

91. Vigushin DM, Poon GK, Boddy A, et al. Phase I and pharmacokinetic study of D-limonene in patients with advanced cancer. Cancer Research Campaign Phase I/II Clinical Trials Committee. *Cancer Chemother Pharmacol* 1998;42(2):111–117.

92. Vinciguerra V, Moore T, Brennan E. Inhalation marijuana as an antiemetic for cancer chemotherapy. *N Y State J Med* 1988;88(10):525–527.

93. Musty RE, Rossi R. Effects of smoked *cannabis* and oral delta-9-tetrahydrocannabinol on nausea and emesis after cancer chemotherapy: a review of state clinical trials. *J Cannabis Ther* 2001;1(1):29–42.

94. Abrams DI. Medical marijuana: tribulations and trials. *J Psychoactive Drugs* 1998;30(2):163–169.

95. Boon M. *The road of excess: a history of writers on drugs*. Cambridge, MA: Harvard University Press, 2002.

96. Ginsburg A. First manifesto to end the bringdown. In: Solomon D, ed. *The marijuana papers*. New York: Signet, 1966.

CHAPTER 16

Amphetamines and Other Stimulants

GEORGE R. KING AND EVERETT H. ELLINWOOD, JR.

The use of stimulant compounds has a long history. Chinese native physicians have been using the drug Ma-huang for more than 5,000 years. In 1887, Nagai found the active agent in Ma-huang to be ephedrine (1). Amphetamine proper was first synthesized in 1887 by Edeleau as part of a systematic program to manufacture aliphatic amines. Early investigations of the properties of amphetamine focused on the peripheral effects and found that amphetamine was a sympathomimetic agent with bronchodilator properties (1). Oddly, the central nervous system actions were not reported until approximately 1933, and this was closely followed by the first reports of amphetamine abuse. Amphetamines produce feelings of euphoria and relief from fatigue, may improve performance on some simple tasks, increase activity levels, and produce anorexia (1). The abuse liability of the amphetamines is thought to be primarily related to their euphorigenic effects.

This chapter reviews the literature regarding the use and abuse of the amphetamines. First, the basic behavioral neuropharmacology of the amphetamines is reviewed, followed by a brief discussion of the metabolism and toxic consequences of the amphetamines. Next, the epidemiology and economics of amphetamine use and abuse is discussed to put in context the social development and extent of abuse. The medical uses of amphetamine are then presented with a focus on the use of stimulants to treat attention deficit hyperactivity disorder. Following the review of medical uses, the literature regarding amphetamine abuse is also reviewed, and where appropriate, the physiologic and potential neurobiologic bases for such effects are discussed. Finally, the chapter presents a brief overview of some treatments of stimulant abuse.

PHARMACOLOGY

The present section describes the basic neurochemical, physiologic, and behavioral actions of acute and subchronic administration of amphetamines. The effects of chronic amphetamine administration are discussed under later sections entitled "Toxicity" and "Abuse." This section extensively examines the literature regarding high-dose effects in nonhumans, rather than extensively reviewing the low- to moderate-dose effects in humans. Unlike the causes and effects of many "natural" diseases, those of drug abuse are known (e.g., pharmacologic and toxic), and the results of animal experimentation allow for detailed research into these neurobiologic processes underlying the development of drug abuse.

Central Effects

Neurochemical

The amphetamines are indirect catecholamine agonists and administration results in the release of newly synthesized norepinephrine and dopamine (2–21). Several lines of evidence indicate that amphetamine acts on newly synthesized, versus stored, pools of catecholamines, by reversing the transporter, thereby reversing the transport of cytosolic neurotransmitter (22–24). First, reserpine pretreatment, which depletes stored catecholamines in synaptic vesicles, does not affect the central stimulating properties of amphetamine. Second, treatment with α-methyltyrosine inhibits the rate-limiting step of catecholamine biosynthesis and blocks the central stimulating properties of amphetamine (21,25). High doses of amphetamines will also decrease tyrosine hydroxylase (TH) activity in the neostriatum (26,27) and the substantia nigra (28).

In addition, high doses of amphetamines release 5-hydroxytryptamine and may affect serotonergic receptors (5,8,29,30). In much the same way that amphetamine affects TH activity, amphetamine also results in a decrease of tryptophan hydroxylase activity following acute administration (31–33). These synthesis-sensitive mechanisms are in contrast to other types of stimulants, such as methylphenidate and cocaine, which act through storage pools (but not on newly synthesized pools) of catecholamines.

Amphetamine administration also influences various neuropeptide systems (9). Peptidergic systems are associated with mesostriatal dopamine circuitry and are thought to play a modulatory role in dopaminergic activity. For example, substance P-containing neurons, whose cell bodies originate in the striatum, have terminal fields in the substantia nigra; Reid et al. (34) found that intranigral substance P injections result in striatal dopamine release. Furthermore, intranigral injections also result in increased locomotor activity (35); these locomotor-stimulating properties of substance P are blocked by mesostriatal 6-hydroxydopamine (6-OHDA) (35).

Neurotensin (NT) pathways also serve to modulate dopaminergic activity. First, in the rat brain, NT receptors are extensively colocalized with dopamine (36). It has been argued that NT preferentially activates somato-dendritic receptors, which inhibits terminal activity and neurotransmitter release (37). Given the modulatory effects of neuropeptides on dopaminergic functioning, one would expect that amphetamine would influence these systems. Hanson et al. (9) reported that 18 hours after five injections of amphetamine (15 mg/kg per injection; each injection separated by 6 hours), the levels of NT and substance P were elevated in the striatum. These changes in neuropeptide levels may mediate some of the behavioral effects to be described later (e.g., loss of baseline activity levels and anergia) of repeated doses of amphetamine.

Electrophysiologic

The systemic administration of amphetamines generally results in a dose-dependent depression of the firing rate of catecholaminergic neurons (38,39), and noradrenergic neurons in the locus ceruleus (40). This suppression of firing rate is caused by somatodendritic autoregulation. For example, Groves and colleagues have infused low doses of amphetamine into the substantia nigra pars compacta while simultaneously recording electrical activity (41–44). These authors found a dose-dependent inhibition of firing rate that lasted approximately 90 minutes. This result was not the result of a generalized neuronal suppression, because nondopaminergic neurons were not inhibited. Furthermore, lesions anterior to the substantia nigra attenuate this inhibitory effect (43,45,46); second, pretreatment with the synthesis blocker α-methyltyrosine also abolishes this effect (43,45), whereas these treatments do not abolish the inhibitory effects of the direct dopamine agonist apomorphine (38,46).

In contrast to the inhibitory effects of amphetamine on dopaminergic neurons in the substantia nigra, the effects of amphetamine in the neostriatum are biphasic (39,47,48). Low doses of amphetamine inhibit the firing rate of spontaneously active neostriatal neurons, while at higher doses there is an excitation of the firing rate. In the caudate putamen, administration of d-amphetamine results in a transient increase in the firing rate of dopaminergic neurons within the first 10 minutes and then a profound inhibition of the firing rate of these neurons (41). This dissociation of the effects of amphetamine on neostriatum and substantia nigra firing rates may underlie some of the behavioral effects of amphetamine described later, in the behavioral effects section.

Stimulants also have potent effects on electroencephalogram (EEG) recordings. Amphetamine accelerates and desynchronizes the EEG while also shifting the resting EEG toward higher frequencies. During sleep, the amplitude and duration of large delta waves are truncated (49). Furthermore, high-dose intravenous amphetamines and especially cocaine induce sinusoidal high-voltage waves of 20 to 50 Hz (i.e., spindling) in the olfactory and amygdaloid structures of rats (50), and cats (51,52).

Structure–Activity Relations

Amphetamine is a β-phenylisopropylamine. The critical structural components of amphetamine are an unsubstituted phenyl ring, the α-methyl group, the two-carbon side chain between the phenyl ring and the nitrogen, and the primary amino group (53). Research indicates that all the components are necessary for the typical biochemical and pharmacologic effects of amphetamine. Different structural modifications accentuate or attenuate various actions of the amphetamines and related compounds. These structure–activity relationships become ever more important in a culture in which tailor-made "designer" drugs increasingly include recreational drugs flowing from clandestine laboratories. The following section provides a brief description of the structure–activity relationships for the amphetamines and related compounds.

Dopamine

Amphetamine blocks the reuptake of and directly releases dopamine from newly synthesized pools. Unlike the reported differential affinity of the *dextro (d)* and *leva (l)* isomers of amphetamine for norepinephrine release and uptake, such stereospecificity does not seem to exist for the dopaminergic system (6,7,54,55); these researchers found that the d and l isomers were equipotent in inhibiting dopaminergic uptake from rat hypothalamic and corpus striatum synaptosomes.

Norepinephrine

Amphetamine blocks the reuptake of norepinephrine and also causes its release. The β-phenethylamine structure is critical for the actions of amphetamine; for example, increasing and/or decreasing the number of carbons between the phenyl ring and the nitrogen attenuates the effects of amphetamine on norepinephrine release and reuptake (53).

The α-methyl group also seems to be of importance in determining the activity of amphetamine on norepinephrine efflux. For example, the configuration of this group is responsible for the difference in the inhibitory dose 50 (ID_{50}) of d- and l-amphetamine (53); continued methylation in the α position to form phentermine and mephentermine extensively decreases the actions on norepinephrine uptake and release (53).

Serotonin

In general, the amphetamines do not have a strong effect on the serotonergic system. However, there are some exceptions to this general rule. For example, an early report by Pletscher et al. (56) indicated that p-chloro-N-methylamphetamine resulted in depleted serotonin (5-HT) and 5-hydroxyindoleacetic acid (5-HIAA) levels, while norepinephrine and dopamine levels were unchanged; similar results have been reported by Fuller et al. (57), Fuller and Molloy (58), and Moller-Nielsen and Dubnick (59). These results indicate that amphetamine derivatives with strong electron-withdrawing substituents on the phenyl ring affect the serotonergic system.

The 4-chlorinated derivatives of both amphetamine and methamphetamine have strong serotonergic depleting properties, and it appears that there must be at least a two-carbon chain between the phenyl ring and the nitrogen for such effects to occur (58,59). Both *p*-chloro-*N*-methylphenethylamine and *p*-chloromethamphetamine are potent depleters of serotonin, but *p*-chloro-α-methylbenzylamine is not (53).

Glutamate

Over the last decade, a considerable amount of research has focused on the effects of the amphetamines on glutamatergic systems. The results indicate that intracranial or systemic administration of the amphetamines produces glutamate release in the nucleus accumbens, striatal areas and the ventral tegmental area (VTA) (60–64). On the other hand, administration of amphetamine directly into the nucleus accumbens or VTA inhibits (or delays the onset of the increase in) glutamate release (62–65). Part of the reason for the focus on glutamatergic systems is the interest in stimulant sensitization (reverse tolerance), and the role of sensitization in drug abuse (see references 66 and 67 for recent reviews of this literature). Sensitization is an augmented behavioral and neurochemical response following repeated, intermittent stimulant administration. It is thought to be permanent, and may share some similarities to L-tryptophan (LTP), hence the interest in glutamate. A large body of research indicates that coadministration of the N-methyl-D-aspartate (NMDA) receptor antagonists MK-801 (63,68–76), ketamine (68), D-CPP-ene (73), and CPP (77) block the development of amphetamine sensitization.

CNS Stimulatory Effects

A primary effect of the amphetamines and related compounds is central nervous system (CNS) stimulation, which results in the characteristic activation of behavior. Early reports indicated that a two-carbon chain between the nitrogen and the phenyl ring was necessary for these stimulatory effects; Van der Shoot et al. (78) reported that two-carbon chain amphetamine derivatives increased the spontaneous locomotor activity of mice, whereas derivatives containing one to three or more carbon chains did not result in increased activity. These authors also reported that increasing the alkyl chain length on the amino group progressively decreased psychomotor stimulation. *N*-Dimethylation resulted in similar effects. These results would seem to indicate that the binding of an amino group to a secondary carbon seems to be necessary for the psychomotor stimulation produced by the amphetamines (53).

The α-methyl group also appears to be a critical determinant of stimulatory action: β-phenethylamine is minimally active, and phentermine is approximately half as active as amphetamine (53). Further evidence indicating the importance of the α-methyl group are results indicating that the *dextro* isomers of both amphetamine and methamphetamine are significantly more potent in stimulating behavior than are the *levo* isomers (19,54,55,79–81).

Behavioral Effects

The following section briefly reviews the immense literature regarding the major behavioral effects of acute and subchronic administration of amphetamines, and the possible neural substrates for these effects. These effects are locomotor stimulation, stereotypy induction, aggression, and anorexia.

Locomotion

Role of Dopamine: Acute Effects

Low doses of amphetamine result in increased locomotor activity, running, and forward motion associated with exploratory behaviors (82,83). Several lines of evidence indicate that this increase in locomotor activity is mediated by the mesolimbic dopaminergic system. First, Pijnenburg and van Rossum (84) found that dopamine injected into the nucleus accumbens increased locomotor activity, whereas intrastriatal injections did not increase activity. Second, this increase in locomotor activity is blocked by the administration of dopaminergic antagonists (85). Third, Thornburg and Moore (86) found that although blockage of dopamine synthesis by α-methyltyrosine inhibited the locomotor-stimulating effects of amphetamine, subsequent blockage of norepinephrine synthesis by the potent dopamine–β-hydroxylase inhibitor U-14,624 had no effect on this property of amphetamine. These results indicate that the locomotor-stimulating properties of amphetamine are selectively mediated by dopaminergic transmission.

Localization of the locomotor-stimulating properties of amphetamine to the mesolimbic system come from a variety of lesion studies. First, electrolytic (87) and 6-hydroxydopamine (88–90) lesions of the neostriatum fail to effect locomotion induced by amphetamine. Second, electrolytic lesions of the rostral hypothalamus, resulting in an interruption of mesolimbic dopaminergic input, reduce amphetamine-induced locomotion (91). Third, 6-OHDA lesions of the nucleus accumbens abolish the effects of amphetamine (90,92–96). Last, the locomotor stimulation produced by amphetamine injection into the nucleus accumbens is far more intense than the activity induced by amphetamine injection into the neostriatum (84,85).

Role of Dopamine: Chronic Effects

The effects of chronic stimulant (amphetamine and cocaine) administration on behavior and dopaminergic neurotransmission depend on the route and temporal pattern of administration. Daily intermittent injections induce enhanced locomotion and stereotypies (97–99), while the continuous infusion of an equivalent daily dose of cocaine induces tolerance to the behavioral effects of cocaine (97–100). These behavioral effects are associated with alterations in dopaminergic neurotransmission in several brain areas. Daily intermittent administration of stimulants induce augmented dopamine release in several brain areas (99,101–106). In contrast, the continuous administration of an equivalent daily dose of cocaine induces attenuated dopamine release in several brain areas (99,107,108).

Role of Serotonin

Although this research indicates that the locomotor properties are mediated by the mesolimbic dopamine system, several lines of evidence indicate that the serotonergic system plays an inhibitory modulating role on the effects of amphetamine. First, midbrain serotonergic raphe (91,109,110) or medial forebrain bundle lesions (111) enhance the locomotor-stimulating effects of amphetamine. Furthermore, administration of parachlorophenylalanine or 5,6- or 5,7-dihydroxytryptamine also enhances the locomotor-stimulating properties of the amphetamines (112–115). Therefore, the overall pattern of results indicates that increased serotonergic neurotransmission inhibits the locomotor-stimulating properties of amphetamines.

Role of Endogenous Opiates

Several reports indicate that endogenous opiate systems are important in the regulation of amphetamine-induced locomotion and dopamine release. For example, Schad et al. (116) recently reported that administration of naloxone, followed by amphetamine significantly reduced amphetamine-induced increase in extracellular dopamine in the nucleus accumbens and striatum and also attenuated the increase in locomotor activity elicited by amphetamine, suggesting that endogenous opiate systems are critical in modulating the behavioral and neurochemical effects of amphetamine. Similar behavioral results have been reported by Motles et al. (117).

Stereotypies

Acute Effects

High doses of amphetamines result in stereotyped behaviors that are representative for the respective species. These behaviors are continually repetitive acts that serve no apparent purpose (see, e.g., references 16 and 118). The stereotyped behavior elicited in the rat generally consists of sniffing, licking, biting, or gnawing (119). Although amphetamine will elicit all of these behaviors,

several lines of research indicate that they do not form a unitary package, to the extent that different behaviors seem to be under different neural control. First, at lower, stereotypy-inducing doses, the behavioral pattern consists mainly of sniffing and head and limb movements (91). At progressively higher doses, these behaviors are supplanted by biting, gnawing, and licking behaviors (91). Second, amantadine, phenylethylamine, and piribedil will induce only limb movements and sniffing but will not elicit the gnawing and biting behaviors (120–122). Third, biting and gnawing, but not limb movements and sniffing, are elicited by (f) (N-n-propylnorapomorphine (122). Fourth, amantadine inhibits biting while α-methylparatyrosine inhibits sniffing (122–124). Fifth, lesioning of different brain areas results in differential inhibition of various behaviors; Creese and Iversen (89) found that 6-OHDA lesions of the substantia nigra induced supersensitivity to sniffing caused by direct dopamine agonist treatment (i.e., apomorphine) but that the gnawing and biting components of the stereotypy were unaffected. On the other hand, 6-OHDA lesions of the caudate abolish the intense gnawing and biting components of the stereotypy (88,90). 6-OHDA lesions of the nucleus accumbens attenuate the sniffing component of the stereotypy while the biting/gnawing component is unaffected (88,90). The overall pattern of these results would seem to indicate that an intact caudate putamen is necessary for the development of the intense gnawing/biting portion of the stereotypy (122).

Chronic Effects

The effects of chronic amphetamine and cocaine administration depend, in part, on the dosing regime used. Use of a daily, intermittent dosing regime results in sensitization (i.e., an augmentation of the effects of amphetamine). Daily injections of amphetamine result in the preempting of locomotor stimulation by periods of intense, focused stereotypies (125–130). As the duration of amphetamine administration lengthens, tolerance to the dopamine effects of amphetamine develops and various "end-stage" behaviors appear; these behaviors are characterized by limb flicks, abortive grooming, increased startle responses to existent and nonexistent stimuli, and abnormal dystonic postures (50,51,131–135). In other words, animals progress from an initial stage in which they exhibit "exploratory, investigative," and repetitive movements, to a stage characterized by intense stereotypies interspersed with bizarre behavior. This behavior is unrelated to environmental cues and may consist of "bits and pieces" of earlier patterns and sequences of behavior that at one time served a purpose.

Social Behavior

Chronic amphetamine administration also has a profound effect on social behavior. For example, Schiorring (136) found that both acute and chronic amphetamine dosing resulted in extreme withdrawal from social activity in monkeys; social activity was replaced by stereotyped self-grooming or staring into space. Similar results on social behavior have been reported by Angrist and Gershon (137,138), Cole et al. (139), Ellinwood (140), Ellinwood et al. (141), and Ellinwood and Kilbey (142).

These results suggest increasing behavioral disintegration and social isolation during chronic amphetamine administration. The behavioral repertoire becomes increasingly restricted, and the animal becomes increasingly responsive to existent and nonexistent stimuli. In other words, the animal is increasingly losing contact with reality. Even months after withdrawal, a single moderate dose of amphetamine can reintroduce the original repertoire of intense bizarre behaviors that originally may have taken months to develop; thus, the behavior remains long-term in a residual latent state. At the abuse level, these latent behavioral residuals may include drug acquisition behaviors that become incorporated into the stereotyped patterns. In part, these acquisition residuals may provide the basis for the "greased slide" fall into intense drug-seeking behavior after reinitiation of human abusers to a single dose of amphetamines (51,126).

The neurobiologic basis for such effects is currently under investigation. The effects apparently are not the result of changes in the number or affinity of postsynaptic dopamine receptors, because studies using chronic low, moderate, or high doses of amphetamine have not demonstrated consistently or sufficiently large enough changes in these parameters of dopamine neurons to account for the effects (143–146). The effects also apparently do not result from changes in the pharmacokinetics of amphetamine (147–150).

Chronic amphetamine administration is, however, associated with decreased dopamine stores and TH activity (129,152–156). Although these studies consistently describe monoamine depletions in the striatum, no consistent depletions in the nucleus accumbens are reported; however, any mesoaccumbens depletions are of considerably smaller magnitude than those found in the caudate (157). In addition to the effects on dopaminergic functioning, a profound depletion of serotonin and tryptophan hydroxylase activity has also been reported, although it seems that this effect is more specific to methylamphetamine than to d- or l-amphetamine (31).

Aggression

The effects of amphetamine on aggressive behavior are complex and as yet poorly understood. However, as a general statement, the effects seem to depend on the dose, the environment, and the individual. Amphetamine use has been associated with the potential for sudden violent outbursts for quite a while; indeed, a common street warning of the 1960s and 1970s was "speed kills." Be-

cause this is such an important but controversial topic, the present section reviews the experimental and clinical literature regarding the effects of amphetamine on aggressive behavior.

Several murders and other violent offenses have been attributed to amphetamine intoxication (158–160). For example, Ansis and Smith (158) describe a case of a male who murdered two individuals and shot several others. This individual had been consuming amphetamines in increasing doses for 3 weeks. The individual developed paranoid delusions and killed these people in a blind rage. (A more complete discussion of amphetamine psychosis is presented below in the section entitled "Abuse.") Several surveys of prison inmates have also found that a large percentage of inmates and juvenile delinquents committed their crimes while intoxicated by amphetamines (161,162). Such findings led Ellinwood (133) to conclude that stimulants (including the amphetamines) have a specific association with violent behavior. Furthermore, Ellinwood (133) found that many homicides were committed because of misinterpretation or, more often, for hallucinatory delusional reasons; they were not simply a result of the violence of the drug marketplace. In other words, the homicides were a consequence of drug consumption.

Some experimental research in humans indicates that acute doses of amphetamine can increase aggressiveness in humans. For example, Cherek et al. (163) exposed humans to a competitive task involving money. As part of the task, subjects could deliver blasts of white noise or take money from a competitor. The results indicated that 5- and 10-mg doses increased the frequency of noise deliveries and the taking away of money, suggesting an increase in aggressive behavior. In contrast to these results, caffeine reduced the frequency of such aggressive behavior, indicating that the effects are specific to amphetamine (164).

In spite of this evidence indicating that amphetamine increases aggressive behavior, other evidence indicates that amphetamine can decrease aggressive behavior. Amphetamine treatment is used to treat aggression in children diagnosed with hyperkinesis and/or attention deficit hyperactivity disorder (165). This effect has been repeatedly confirmed in controlled, double-blind studies (166–167). Not all surveys of prison populations and juvenile delinquents report finding a relation between aggression or hostility and amphetamine abuse (168–170).

Anorexia

The amphetamines are potent anorectics and have been used clinically for such purposes for a long time (82,171). The evidence indicates that this effect of the amphetamines is mediated by dopaminergic neurotransmission. First, pretreatment with α-methyl-p-tyrosine reduces the anorectic effects of amphetamine in rats (21,172–178). Second, administration of α and β blockers (e.g., phentolamine, phenoxybenzamine piperoxan, yohimbine, tolazoline, propranolol, pindolol, and dichloroisoproterenol) has no effect on amphetamine-induced anorexia (173,179–181). Third, administration of dopamine antagonists such as haloperidol, pimozide, penfluridol, and spiroperidol reduces the anorectic effects of amphetamine (173,175–177,179,182–185). Fourth, lesions of the dopaminergic system with 6-OHDA attenuate amphetamine-induced anorexia (177,186–188).

More specifically, this anorectic effect of amphetamine is probably mediated by the lateral hypothalamus. For example, Glick (189) reported that lateral hypothalamic lesions result in an attenuation of the anorectic effects of amphetamine (186,190–192). Furthermore, bilateral lesions of the nigrostriatal dopaminergic system induce the same aphagic-adipsic syndrome as do lateral hypothalamic lesions (186,193). Nigrostriatal dopamine neurons pass through the internal capsule, which is adjacent to the lateral hypothalamus, and the results of studies involving lateral hypothalamic lesions could also be attributed to destruction of these dopaminergic neurons (82).

Although the preceding research indicates that the amphetamines probably work through a dopaminergic mechanism, several lines of evidence indicate that structurally related compounds such as fenfluramine (N-ethyl-α-methyl-3-trifluoromethyl-β-phenylethylamine, a ring-substituted phenylisopropylamine) seem to act via a serotonergic mechanism. First, the administration of 5-HT antagonists attenuates fenfluramine-induced anorexia (173,175,176,179,181,194–199). Second, administration of the 5-HT uptake inhibitor chlorimipramine reduces fenfluramine-induced anorexia (175,183,188–201). Third, serotonergic lesions (195) and lesions produced by 5-dihydroxytryptamine (202) attenuate the effects of fenfluramine-induced anorexia.

Elimination and Pharmacokinetics

There are two primary modes of eliminating the amphetamines from a biologic system: renal excretion and metabolism. Both may be important in understanding pathophysiology and treatment, especially the treatment of overdoses in which facilitation of excretion is important.

Renal Excretion

Amphetamine is a basic (pK$_a$ 9.90), highly lipid-soluble drug. Because amphetamine is a basic drug, a primary mode of elimination is excretion of the unchanged drug in the urine; indeed, in some instances, most of a dose of amphetamine may be excreted in this way (49). Renal excretion is strongly determined by the pH of the urine; with acidic urine (e.g., pH 5) approximately 99% of a dose of amphetamine is ionized by glomerular filtration, and only the remaining nonionized portion of the drug is reabsorbed into the circulatory system (203). Hence

a treatment of amphetamine overdose is to acidify the urine (1).

Metabolism

There are several metabolic pathways for the biotransformation of the amphetamines. One pathway is aromatic hydroxylation (1). Aromatic hydroxylation is apparently restricted to the 4' position, as no evidence for 2'- or 3'-hydroxylation has been obtained (204,205); this hydroxylation results in phenolic amines, which are subsequently excreted in the urine or conjugated with sulfate, and then excreted (204,206). Ring substitution (e.g., fenfluramine) of amphetamine blocks this metabolic pathway (1,204).

p-Hydroxyamphetamine, a major metabolite of this metabolic pathway, is also extremely biologically active. For example, p-hydroxyamphetamine is three times more potent in inhibiting noradrenaline uptake than is amphetamine (207). The hydroxylated metabolite is also a potent pressor agent (208). When p-hydroxyamphetamine is administered intracerebrally, it is also a locomotor stimulant (209).

A second metabolic pathway is β-hydroxylation. This process is carried out by the enzyme dopamine β-hydroxylase, which converts dopamine to norepinephrine, and it is apparently restricted to the primary amines (1,204). The metabolites resulting from β-hydroxylation have the hydroxyl group in the 1r-(−) configuration (1,204,210). This metabolic route is blocked by the second α-methyl group in the phentermine derivatives (1,204). When the ring hydroxylated metabolites (e.g., p-hydroxyamphetamine) undergo β-hydroxylation, p-hydroxynorephedrine is produced. p-Hydroxynorephedrine can be taken up into norepinephrine terminals and probably can act as a "false transmitter," thereby enhancing the effects of amphetamine (205,211,212).

By far, the most important metabolic pathways for the amphetamines are those involving oxidation of the nitrogen and its a carbons (i.e., N-dealkylation and deamination). Both reactions result in a primary amine and a carbonyl function (1). During N-dealkylation, the alkyl or arylalkyl groups on the nitrogen atom are removed by the microsomal mixed function oxidase system. The process requires metabolic oxygen and nicotinamide adenine dinucleotide phosphate-2 (NADPH$_2$) and results in equal portions of the primary amine and the aldehyde (1,204).

Deamination results in the excretion of the corresponding ketone, secondary alcohol, or benzoic acid, although the major metabolite excreted is benzoic acid (1). Ketone is formed via oxidation of the α-carbon and N-oxidation (204,213,214); hydroxylation of the α-carbon results in the formation of an unstable α-carinolamine, which decays to the ketone and ammonia (215). N-oxidation may contribute to the metabolism of amphetamine by an N-hydroxylation, which results in N-hydroxyamphetamine

(1,215,216). *N*-hydroxyamphetamine forms strong complexes with cytochrome P450 (217–220). This complex is then further oxidized to the nitro (221) or nitroso (222) compound. This nitro compound is then converted to a ketone via an oxidative process involving a hydrolytic step (204,223).

After chronic administration of amphetamines, the tissue and brain contents of *p*-hydroxyamphetamine and *p*-hydroxynorephedrine are not significantly different from those of saline-treated control subjects, indicating that the rate of removal of amphetamine is not affected by chronic administration (224). These results are consistent with other findings that indicate that the urinary ratio of unchanged amphetamine to hydroxylated metabolites is unaltered following chronic amphetamine administration (12). However, following chronic amphetamine administration, the uptake of (3)H-amphetamine into the pons medulla is accelerated (224); furthermore, chronic amphetamine treatment also accelerates the uptake of (3)H-norepinephrine in the pons medulla (225,226).

These results indicate that the metabolism of amphetamine is different from that of most other drugs. Chronic amphetamine administration does not seem to result in enzyme induction as indicated by the lack of an increase in the rate of removal, or the production of hydroxylated metabolites. However, during chronic administration, amphetamine and *p*-hydroxyephedrine may accumulate in a pool that could eventually disrupt cellular functioning (224). Finally, the brain and heart levels of amphetamine in chronically treated animals are significantly higher than those in control animals, and this difference may in part account for the sensitization often produced by chronic amphetamine administration (224).

Toxicity

The chronic high-dose abuse of amphetamines results in toxic pathophysiologic changes. The present section describes these toxic effects. Table 16.1 presents some of the toxic effects of high-dose and chronic amphetamine use.

Central Toxicities

General Mechanisms

The classical view of amphetamine neurotoxicity centers on necrotic cell death induced by free radical formation (reactive oxygen and nitrogen species; see reference 227 for a review). Briefly, amphetamine enters dopaminergic or serotonergic neurons via the respective transporter. Amphetamine then displaces vesicular and cytosolic neurotransmitter. Dopamine (DA) is metabolized by monoamine oxidase (MAO) into dihydroxyphenylacetic acid (DOPAC) and hydrogen peroxide (H_2O_2), or DA can be oxidized by molecular O_2 via auto-oxidative processes

TABLE 16.1. *Toxic consequences of high-dose and chronic use of psychomotor stimulants*

Pattern of use	Toxic consequence
High dose	Slowing of cardiac conduction
	Ventricular irritability
	Hypertensive episode
	Hyperpyrexic episode
	Central nervous system seizures and anoxia
Dose escalation	Hyperpyrexia
	Cardiovascular hypertension
	Slowing of cardiac conduction
Binge	Physical exhaustion resulting in impaired judgment and insight
	Development of psychotic ideation
	Potential for sudden violence
	Neurotransmitter depletion
	Neuronal destruction
	High-risk behaviors (e.g., needle sharing, automobile accidents, sexual promiscuity)
Chronic	Long-term neurotransmitter depletion
	Neuronal destruction
	Cerebrovascular damage
	Psychosis

Adapted from Gawin FH, Ellinwood EH. Cocaine and other stimulants. *N Engl J Med* 1988;318:1173; and Ellinwood EH, Lee TH. Dose- and time-dependent effects of stimulants. *NIDA Res Monogr Ser* 1989;94:323–340.

(228–230). Alternatively, the stimulation of NMDA receptors (via accumulation of synaptic glutamate levels, 231–234) results in Ca^{2+} influx into the neuron, where Ca^{2+}-calmodulin binding activates neuronal nitric oxide synthase (nNOS). nNOS produces nitric oxide (NO) and hence the reactive nitrogen species peroxynitrite (235). Cell necrosis occurs as a direct result of the production of these reactive oxygen and nitrogen species.

However, more recent research suggests that other mechanisms may be involved in the neurotoxicity of amphetamine. For example, research suggests that amphetamine may exert a neurotoxic effect by the induction of apoptosis (227). Amphetamine is a highly lipophilic compound that can pass the neuronal membrane. Amphetamine can then, either directly or indirectly, interfere with mitochondrial function. Again, because amphetamine is a cationic lipophilic molecule, it can enter the mitochondria, initiating one or more possible cascades. First, accumulation of amphetamine in the mitochondria will dissipate the electrochemical gradient that is established by the electron transport chain. The electrochemical gradient is critical for the maintenance of adenosine triphosphate (ATP) synthase and the maintenance of the mitochondrial membrane (236,237). Second, mitochondria store Ca^{2+}, which is pumped into the mitochondrial space via calcium adenosine triphosphatase (ATPase). Release of the Ca^{2+}, possibly by scenario one, through the permeability transition pore would result in apoptosis by the activation of cysteine proteases, caspases (particularly caspase-3) (238). Lastly, cytochrome c, a critical cofactor in complex IV of the excitotoxic cascade (ETC), is released from damaged mitochondria. Release of cytochrome c also starts an apoptotic cascade that will result in necrosis.

This brief review of amphetamine neurotoxicity indicates that amphetamine has multiple, not necessarily exclusive, mechanisms for inducing necrosis. The following sections describe some of the neurotoxic effects of amphetamine within specific neurotransmitter systems.

Dopamine

In contrast to the generalized effects on norepinephrine levels (see below), only dopamine levels in the caudate putamen were depressed, with other brain regions showing no effect in the subjects sacrificed 24 hours after the last injection. Furthermore, this depletion appeared to be permanent because the degree of dopaminergic depletion was the same in the subjects sacrificed 24 hours or 3 to 6 months after the last injection (see also reference 239). These results are consistent with the results of Tonge (240), who found depressed norepinephrine levels for up to 36 hours after chronic oral amphetamine intake in rats, and the results of Harris and Baldessarini (241), who found that chronic amphetamine intake depresses TH activity in the corpus striatum. These results indicate that chronic amphetamine administration is toxic to the dopamine system. The results are also consistent with Woolverton et al. (242) who demonstrated reduced DA and 5-HT levels in the caudate of rhesus monkeys 4 years after the cessation of methamphetamine administration. Melaga et al. (243) also reported reduced DA synthetic capacity for 6 months after 10 days of an escalating amphetamine dose. This reduction in synthetic capacity required 2 years to recover (244). Villemagne et al. (245) also recently reported a dose dependent inhibition of [^{11}C]WIN-35,428 binding by positron emission tomography (PET) scanning. This reduction in binding was confirmed by postmortem decreases in [^{3}H]WIN-35,428 binding, as well as reduced DA and DOPAC content in the caudate-putamen.

More recent work demonstrates extensive toxicities induced by chronic amphetamine administration. First, dopamine and tyrosine β-hydroxylase levels are reduced for extended periods following chronic amphetamine administration (246–248). Second, the number of dopaminergic uptake sites is reduced (247,248). Third, there is evidence of neuronal degeneration, chromatolysis, and decreased catecholamine histofluorescence (248,249). Fourth, the number of dopamine transporters is reduced. All apparent evidence indicates that these effects are more severe following continuous or high-dose administration regimes (157).

Norepinephrine

Chronic and high-dose amphetamine use induces substantive toxic alterations in central monoaminergic systems. In one set of experiments examining the toxicity of amphetamines, Seiden et al. (250) injected rhesus monkeys eight times daily (final dose: 3 to 6.5 mg/kg per injection) for 3 to 6 months and then assessed acute and residual withdrawal effects. Subjects sacrificed 24 hours after the final injection exhibited a depletion of norepinephrine in all brain regions examined (pons medulla, midbrain, hypothalamus, and frontal cortex). In the subjects sacrificed 3 to 6 months after the final injection, the brain norepinephrine levels were still depressed in the midbrain and the frontal cortex, but had returned to control levels in the hypothalamus and the pons medulla.

Serotonin

These changes are not restricted to catecholamine neurons. The amphetamines also produce toxic effects in the serotonergic system. Chronic methamphetamine administration induces long-term changes in tryptophan hydroxylase activity (246), as well as in 5-HT content and uptake sites (247). Recent research also suggests that the neurotoxicity is selective. Brown and Molliver (251) reported that methamphetamine results in region-specific changes in serotonergic systems: 14 days after methamphetamine administration there was damage to the serotonergic system in the caudate and the core of the nucleus accumbens, but there was no damage in the medial shell of the accumbens. Furthermore, Cass (252) reported that high-dose methamphetamine administration reduced evoked 5-HT efflux for 1 month after administration, and that evoked efflux had returned to normal levels by 6 months.

The clinical significance of these changes is unclear, because a nonstimulant, anorectic agent that has been extensively used clinically induces analogous changes. Fenfluramine produces long-lasting changes in 5-HT and 5-HIAA content in the rat brain (182,253–257). Chronic fenfluramine administration also results in decreased numbers of 5-HT uptake sites (256) and depresses tryptophan hydroxylase activity (257). Finally, fenfluramine also produces morphologic damage to the terminal fields of serotonergic neurons (258).

Cerebral Vasculature

Changes in cerebral vasculature have also been reported following chronic amphetamine administration. For example, Rumbaugh (259) reported that monkeys treated with methamphetamine for 1 year demonstrated extensive changes in the small arterioles and capillary beds; the changes were characterized by patchy areas of beading, vascular filling or nonfilling, and fragmentation of the vessels. Further changes included loss of neurons with increased numbers of glial cells, satellitosis, and micro-hemorrhage in the cerebellum and hypothalamus. Similar results were obtained with animals who were treated only with methamphetamine for 3 months. This pattern of results indicates that chronic amphetamine users are at a high risk for cerebrovascular damage. In addition, high-dose amphetamines, both experimentally and clinically, induce hypertensive episodes associated with cerebral hemorrhage. Indeed, several cases of death have been attributed to hemorrhages induced by chronic amphetamine use (see reference 260 for a review). These results indicate that the amphetamines are potentially highly toxic and can result in severe brain damage even after a short period of use.

Peripheral Toxicities

Cardiovascular Effects

The cardiovascular effects of amphetamine are prominent. Amphetamine raises both systolic and diastolic blood pressure, and heart rate is reflexively slowed (49). Tachycardia and cardiac arrhythmias are not uncommon following high doses of amphetamines (171). Catecholamines have the effect of sensitizing the myocardium to ectopic stimuli, thereby increasing the risk of fatal cardiac arrhythmias. There are recorded cases of myocardial lesions in chronic amphetamine users. These lesions may have served as ectopic arrhythmogenic sites during amphetamine intoxication, resulting in cardiac arrest and death (261).

Thermal Regulation

The amphetamines result in peripheral hyperthermia via activation of the sympathoadrenal system (262–264). However, the amphetamines produce hypothermia centrally, and this seems to be mediated by the activity of the anterior hypothalamus (264–266). Another major cause of amphetamine abuse-related death is hyperpyrexia (260). This effect is directly related to the catecholamine effects of amphetamine (171) and, if not fatal in and of itself, leads to a cascade of convulsions, coma, and cerebral hemorrhage.

MEDICAL USES OF AMPHETAMINES

As stated earlier, in the late 1960s, at the height of the amphetamine-abuse epidemic in the United States, there were approximately 31 million prescriptions for anoretic stimulant drugs, yet enough was legally manufactured for 8 billion pills. This lax legal and social attitude of prescription-and-supply regulation was followed in most industrial nations by very strict control. From 1969 to 1971, the U.S. government (a) markedly reduced the production of amphetamines by 80%; (b) alerted physicians to their dependence-producing effects; and (c) through

the Food and Drug Administration (FDA) rescheduled amphetamines to Schedule II. The pendulum has swung back to the point that potentially important clinical uses are being avoided by physicians. Pitts (267) lamented that the usefulness of amphetamines in treating medically ill (see references 82 and 268) and treatment-failure-depressed patients had been discounted to the point that physicians were afraid to even consider their use. To provide balance for the clinician, potential usefulness of amphetamines, other than the well-known FDA-approved indications for narcolepsy and attention deficit disorder, are discussed here. In the United States, there are only two FDA-approved indications for dextroamphetamine and methylphenidate—narcolepsy and attention deficit hyperactivity disorder—although amphetamines were used to treat other disorders in the past.

Treatment of Attention Deficit Hyperactivity Disorder

Diagnosis of Children

The diagnosis of attention deficit hyperactivity disorder (ADHD) is fairly common; ADHD is thought to affect 2% to 5% of elementary school children, with the diagnosis three to six times more common in boys than in girls (269,270). For a diagnosis, the symptoms should develop before the age of 7 years, and be present for at least 6 months. The disorder is characterized by frequent fidgeting, difficulties in focusing on classroom assignments, impulsivity, excessive talking and interruption of others, and repeated shifting from one activity to another (270,271). Some current research focuses on the disruption of cognitive and executive functions as a core feature in ADHD. As such, this research has begun to reexamine the role of noradrenergic systems, and the disruptions of noradrenergic systems in ADHD (see reference 272) for a review of this literature.

Diagnosis of Adults

The literature indicates that approximately 30% of children diagnosed with ADHD will still have ADHD at 18 years of age, and approximately 8% of children with ADHD will have ADHD at 26 years of age (see reference 273 for a review). In contrast to younger individuals, older individuals more typically present with disorganization and impulsivity rather than hyperactivity (274).

Stimulant Treatment of Attention Deficit Hyperactivity Disorder

Treatment of Children

The treatment of first choice for ADHD involves the use of psychostimulants, primarily methylphenidate (Ritalin), dextroamphetamine (Dexedrine), or pemoline (Cylert).

An excellent review of stimulant treatment of ADHD can be found in Shenker (275). Methylphenidate, the most common treatment, is a piperidine derivative structurally related to amphetamine, and is a milder central nervous system stimulant than amphetamine. Numerous studies indicate that methylphenidate is highly effective in increasing attentiveness, reducing hyperactivity and destructive behavior, and improving classroom behavior and academic performance (see references 276–279 for reviews). The improvements in behavior and academic performance seem to persist as long as the drug is taken, with the behavior problems returning upon cessation of methylphenidate (279–282). Dextroamphetamine and pemoline are second-line stimulants used to those individuals who may not respond to methylphenidate. These drugs are reported to be as effective as methylphenidate in the treatment of ADHD (283,284). For example, Pelham et al. (284) reported that, while dextroamphetamine and pemoline produced more consistent effects on behavioral improvement, methylphenidate induced better improvement in academic improvement.

Treatment of Adults

Several recent reports suggest that stimulants are also efficacious treatments for adult attention deficit disorder. For example, Matochik et al. (285) reported that both chronic (minimum of 6 weeks' treatment) methylphenidate and *d*-amphetamine decreased restlessness and improved attention, although neither drug had any effect on whole-brain metabolism (as measured by PET). These authors reported similar effects following an acute dose of *d*-amphetamine and methylphenidate. Similar results following chronic methylphenidate were reported by Spencer et al. (286) using a randomized, 7-week, placebo-controlled, crossover study of methylphenidate in 23 adult patients (see also reference 287 for similar results). Also, Wilens et al. (288) reported that amphetamine and methylphenidate, as well as pemoline and noradrenergic antidepressants, were all effective in treating ADHD in adults. However, the effects of amphetamine and methylphenidate were immediate and dose-dependent, while the effects of pemoline the antidepressants were delayed.

Side Effects in the Use of Stimulants to Treat Attention Deficit Hyperactivity Disorder

Considerable concern surrounds the use in hyperactivity or ADHD in children of methylphenidate and, to a lesser extent, amphetamine and pemoline because of their possible detrimental effects on general physical and emotional growth and central nervous system development. The U.S. FDA Psychopharmacology Pediatric Subcommittee reviewed the literature relevant to growth suppression by stimulants in the treatment of hyperkinetic syndrome. There is clear evidence of temporary retardation in growth in weight and a suggestion of temporary slowing of stature growth related to drug dose and absence of drug holidays during the prepubertal period (289–291). To allow for growth rebound, the importance of drug holidays is evident in children requiring higher doses and manifesting drug plateaus. ADHD is associated with a variety of comorbid conditions, one of which is later substance abuse (292–294). However, treatment of ADHD significantly decreases the risk of later developing a substance abuse disorder (293).

Nonstimulant-Based Treatments of Attention Deficit Hyperactivity Disorder

Several studies suggest that clonidine (Catapres) may be useful in the treatment of ADHD (276,295–298). Tricyclic antidepressants are effective in treating ADHD (see references 275 and 291 for a discussion), although their use is not generally recommended in treating ADHD; tolerance develops to their effects (299) and several deaths have been reported following tricyclic antidepressants treatment of ADHD (300). Lastly, the monoamine oxidase type A (MAO-A) inhibitors clorgyline and tranylcypromine (301), but not the monoamine oxidase type B (MAO-B) inhibitor deprenyl (302,303), are reported to be therapeutically beneficial in the treatment of ADHD.

Use of Stimulants as Anorectics

The effectiveness of stimulants as anorectics is well documented. In 1972, a study (304) using 206 anorectic drug trials, found in a meta-analysis of the data that these anorectic drugs were effective for weight loss at least out to 16 weeks of treatment. The problem with the use of anorectics, besides their abuse potential, is that only a small percentage maintain weight loss after cessation of anorectics for 1 year (305). Where possible, stimulants with lower abuse potential should be used. For example, chlorimipramine is an amphetamine congener that appears to work primarily on the serotonergic system without major psychostimulant effects (306).

More recently, Weintraub et al. (307) clearly demonstrated that, combined with behavioral therapy, sustained dosing of fenfluramine plus phentermine is effective in initiating and maintaining long-term weight loss. In a study extending out beyond 3 years, fenfluramine (60 mg) and phentermine (15 mg per day) were remarkably effective, when compared to placebo, in reducing weight and maintaining weight control. However, side effects resulted in this combination being removed from the market. In summary, this type of study indicates that, when a serotonergic releasing-type anorectic and a lower-abuse-potential catecholamine-type anorectic are combined, there is a sustained improvement in weight control.

Finally, with any clinical use of psychostimulants, careful history taking of previous drug misuse is warranted. We think that previous abusers of other stimulants should be excluded from treatment even when medically warranted.

Stimulant Treatment of Depression

In Europe, some countries have prohibited any use of stimulants. In 1968, an English report concluded that, with regard to the previous clinical use for depression, "amphetamines . . . have no place in the treatment of depression" (308). Several prominent psychopharmacologists in the late 1960s and 1970s concluded that the addictive properties and the cardiovascular and central nervous system (CNS) side effects of amphetamines outweighed the meager therapeutic effects in most psychiatric conditions (309,310). The reinterpretation of these older studies of depression by Satel and Nelson (311) and Chiarello and Cole (312) is still not resolved, but, on balance, there is no evidence to justify the use of stimulants as a first-line or routine treatment with the usual depression patient (313). In their careful review, Fawcett and Busch (313) concluded that in endogenous depressed patients, stimulants may be useful to potentiate other antidepressant medications when used judiciously by experienced clinicians. They warn, clearly, of side effects, but review a number of studies that conclude that augmentation with stimulants may be effective in treatment failure depressions.

Potential Therapeutic Niche in Medically Ill and Geriatric Depression

Satel and Nelson (311) reviewed five the placebo-controlled studies of methylphenidate in senile and chronic brain syndrome patients and found that four of these studies found methylphenidate superior to placebo in improving the energy, mental alertness, and competence in self-care; all of which are not necessarily depressive symptoms. Other patients who are reported to respond rapidly and effectively to stimulants are medically ill or poststroke depressed patients (313–315). More recently, case reports have appeared indicating that 65% to 85% of patients with human immunodeficiency virus (HIV)-related neuropsychiatric symptoms, including depression, show some to marked improvement (260,268,316).

ABUSE

Amphetamines have been abused almost since their introduction (158,317,318). For example, benzedrine inhalers were abused by a wide segment of the population (e.g., athletes, professionals, and students) during the 1930s to overcome fatigue and increase alertness (158). Amphetamines were routinely available to soldiers during World War II and the Vietnam War to keep soldiers alert during combat conditions (158). Indeed, Grinspoon and Hedblom (319) reported that from 1966 to 1969, soldiers consumed more amphetamines than did the combined to-

tals of British and American soldiers during World War II. The abuse of amphetamine undoubtedly results from its euphoric and psychomotor-stimulating properties. In 1994, emergency room visits involving cocaine reached a record high 142,000 with an additional 17,400 visits related to methamphetamine and other stimulants.

As a result, amphetamine epidemics have been reported in Japan (320), Sweden (321), and the United States (322). These epidemics are generally associated with increasing levels of violence and the development of a "speed culture" (319,323–326). These epidemics often start by introducing segments of the population to amphetamines for medical purposes (327,328), with a subsequent diversion of licit amphetamines to illicit markets (319,322,329).

In an individual, the development of stimulant abuse follows a developmental pattern that has been qualitatively described (318,330). This profile describes the behavioral pathologies that emerge during the active abuse and withdrawal phases. A description of the underlying structural and functional phases has only recently begun to be elucidated (described earlier). A description of the relationship between the neurobiologic changes and the behavioral pathologies that develop is one of the major tasks that remains in the analysis of drug abuse.

Table 16.2 illustrates the different phases of stimulant abuse, the symptoms and behaviors of abuse, and the toxic side effects associated with each phase. Drug effects relating to abuse should be considered in relation to three phases of the establishment of an abusive pattern: initiation, consolidation and maintenance, and withdrawal. Each phase has its own unique profile of mechanisms that are involved in the drug-effect reinforcement profile.

Initiation Phase

During the initial, single-dose phase, the acute reinforcing actions of amphetamine are determined by the pharmacologic effects (i.e., release of dopamine) and the resulting euphoria, increase in energy, and enhancement of vocational and social interactions that occur following consumption. The individual may initially increase the number of settings and occasions on which the drug is used (e.g., for studying, at parties). During this phase, conditioning occurs: settings in which the drug is consumed become associated with the euphoriant and energizing effects of the drug, and this is especially true for individuals using rapid routes of administration (such as intravenous or smoking). This conditioning process is critical for the development of drug urges and cravings that manifest themselves during withdrawal (330).

The initiation phase is primarily concerned with classical conditioning of drug cue or reinforcement properties (331). During the initiation phase, both anticipatory acts and the stimulus properties of the drug are gradually linked in appropriate classically and operantly conditioned sequences. Anticipatory acts may include

TABLE 16.2. *Phases of development of amphetamine abuse: factors mediating abuse dependence, proposed mechanisms*

Phase	Abuse dependence	Mechanism
Single dose	Conditioned cues High-dose rush	Mesolimbic dopamine release Classical conditioning Operant conditioning Enhancement of social/sexual activity Antifatigue properties
Dose escalation	Acute tolerance results in increasing dose and frequency of use	Rapid routes of administration, resulting in fast delivery to central nervous system with resulting dopamine release and euphoria Onset of neurotransmitter depletion
Binge	Compulsive frequent use that may be related to stereotypical patterns of use	Neurotransmitter depletion Neuronal destruction Impulsivity caused by serotonin depletion Conditioned urges and memories of drug effects Acute tolerance coupled Drug acquisition behaviors become stereotyped
Crash		
Early	Depression Agitation Anxiety High drug craving	Neurotransmitter depletion Dopaminergic autoreceptor supersensitivity Memories of drug effects and conditioned urges
Middle	Fatigue No drug craving Insomnia with a high desire for sleep	
Late	Hyperphagia Hypersomnolence	
Withdrawal		
Intermediate	Reemergence of conditioned drug urges and cravings	Conditioned drug urges and cravings Impulsivity caused by serotonin depletion
Late	Gradual extinction of conditioned drug urges and cravings	Extinction of urges Possible restoration of neurotransmitter functiong

Adapted from Gawin FH, Ellinwood EH. Cocaine and other stimulants. *N Engl J Med* 1988;318:1173, and Ellinwood EH, Lee TH. Dose- and time-dependent effects of stimulants. *NIDA Res Monogr Ser* 1989;94:323–340.

drug-seeking behaviors. Drug stimulus properties include not only the reinforcing efficacy of the drug but also the cascade of other discriminative or internally appreciated drug cues (e.g., subjective effects) associated with the consumption of the drug. In the drug-culture vernacular, drug cues are described by such terms as a "taste." An anticipatory taste in human drug users or abusers often leads to associated autonomic responses and urges. Current theoretical formulations of these responses also include anticipatory conditioned effects that are opposite to the drug effect, not unlike a mini-withdrawal episode.

Consolidation Phase

With prolonged, intermittent consumption, the user discovers that higher doses produce greater effects; the individual starts to consume higher doses regularly, if the resources are available. Indeed, before the development of tolerance, the euphoriant effects of stimulants are proportional to amphetamine plasma levels (332,333). However,

as stimulant use continues, tolerance to the euphoriant effects develops, and the individual starts to escalate the frequency and dose in an attempt to chase the "flash" or "rush" of amphetamine administration. During the high-dose transition phase, the individual resorts to rapid routes of administration such as smoking or intravenous administration. In spite of any tolerance that may have developed, these routes of administration result in a rapid rise in plasma amphetamine levels, which produces an intense euphoria (i.e., "flash").

The individual may start binging during this period. A binge is characterized by the repeated readministration of the drug, resulting in frequent mood swings. Binges typically last 12 to 18 hours, but may last as long as 2, 3, or even 7 days (318). Such binges are facilitated by acute tolerance; the effects of the drug diminish rapidly. Acute tolerance, coupled with the memory of the preceding "flash," produces the desire to reinstate the drug effect; this is accomplished by the repeated consumption of the drug. These euphoric states result in strong memories of the drug effects and in the conditioning of previously neutral stimuli to the drug effects.

During this high-dose period of binges, the individual comes to focus on the internally generated sensations produced by stimulant consumption (e.g., energy and euphoria). As a result, the chronic user withdraws from social activities and pursues the direct pharmacologic effects, including sensations as well as stereotyped noninteractive behaviors, of amphetamine. Over time, in high-dose regimes, these stereotyped behaviors disintegrate into remnants of the original behaviors. During this period, the pattern of acquisition and intake becomes stereotyped and restricted; the individual's behavior focuses on the purchase and consumption of amphetamine, and the number of settings in which amphetamine is consumed becomes progressively restricted. This is functionally similar to the development of intense stereotypies and the withdrawal from the earlier described social interactions in nonhumans.

Withdrawal Phase

Early Withdrawal Phase

At the end of a binge, the individual enters the "crash" phase, which is characterized by initial depression, agitation, anxiety, anergia, and high drug craving (318). The memories of the drug effects and the stimuli associated with these effects can result in the conditioned drug craving experienced during the early crash phase.

In the middle period of the crash phase, drug craving is replaced by fatigue, depression, loss of desire for the drug, and insomnia accompanied by an intense desire for sleep. During this time, the individual may use alcohol, benzodiazepines, or opiates to induce the desired sleep.

During the late period of the crash phase, hypersomnolence is followed by awakening in a hyperphagic state (318).

Intermediate Withdrawal Phase

Following the crash period, if individuals remain abstinent, they enter an intermediate withdrawal phase with effects that are generally opposite those of the drug: loss of physical and mental energy necessary to most naturally occurring incentive behaviors. During withdrawal, individuals experience fatigue, decreased mental energy, limited interest in the environment, and anhedonia. These symptoms gradually increase in intensity during the 12 to 96 hours following the crash phase (318). At this time, memories of euphoria induced by amphetamine consumption stand in marked relief to the anhedonia being experienced at the moment. This results in intense drug craving, and the individual is highly prone to relapse by starting another binge cycle. If the individual can remain abstinent for 6

to 18 weeks, the anhedonia and dysphoria attenuate, but may wax and wane over the next 6 to 9 months (318).

Late Withdrawal Phase

During the extinction phase, brief periods of drug craving can occur. The individual may experience conditioned combinations of stimulus properties of both the drug and withdrawal "hunger" effects in the form of "urges" or "cravings." These episodes of craving are triggered by conditioned stimuli (circumstances and objects) that were previously associated with the drug effects. If the individual experiences these cues without the associated drug effects, then the ability of these cues to elicit drug craving will diminish over time; over time the individual will experience less-intense drug cravings, which should lessen the probability of relapse (318).

Amphetamine Psychosis

During the phase of chronic, high-dose consumption of amphetamines, the individual may develop "amphetamine psychosis." The stimulant psychosis is more prevalent with amphetamine than with cocaine, probably because of the difficulty in sustaining high chronic levels of cocaine. This psychosis has several profiles. First, and most commonly, the individual develops paranoid ideation (334–336). This paranoia usually is accompanied by ideas of reference and an extremely well-formed delusional structure. The paranoid structure is facilitated by a heightened awareness of the environment, coupled with the increasing social isolation induced by amphetamine use (325,337). In the beginning there is an exploratory, pleasurable, vague suspiciousness in which the individual continually wants to look beneath the surface of things (i.e., from the original term *subspicio*), and the individual watches others intensely (325,335). Later there is a phase reversal in which the person feels that others are watching and following him or her (141). As consumption continues, the individual may overreact to stimuli in the peripheral field of vision and may start to hallucinate (141). This pattern of hyperreactivity to environmental stimuli may be functionally similar to the hyperstartle reaction described previously in animals. During the later stages of psychosis development, the individual may lose all insight and develop extremely well-structured delusions of persecution (337). These delusions, when coupled with the loss of insight, the exhaustion produced by a binge, or the coadministration of sedatives, and the hyperreactivity to stimuli can produce a confused, panicky, fugue-like state that can result in sudden acts of violence (141).

Another prominent aspect of amphetamine psychosis is the development of stereotyped behavior patterns that are more complex than those found in animals and that typically consist of activities that the individual normally engaged in and enjoyed doing. Many psychotic and

TABLE 16.3. *Proposed treatments for stimulant abuse: symptoms treated, possible mechanisms of treatment efficacy*

Treatment	Symptoms	Mechanism
Pharmacotherapy		
Dopamine agonist	Dysphoria-anergia	Increased dopaminergic activity
Classical antidepressants	Depression, craving, dysphoria	Provision of low-grade enhancement of "energy-activating" or affective tone
		Reduction of fantasy urges
Fluoxetine	Reinforcing efficacy	Increased serotonergic activity
	Residual impulsivity	
Behavioral		
Extinction	Conditioned urges and craving	Extinction of conditioned responses
Self-mastery	Relapse prevention	Self-mastery and control over urges and situations that can trigger use
Contingency contracting	Relapse prevention (drug-free urine tests)	Aversive consequences for failure to adhere to the conditions of the contract
		Positive consequences for adhering to the conditions of the contract
Increasing natural reinforcement density	Relapse prevention	Reduction of the reinforcing value of the drug

prepsychotic individuals engage in the repetitive disassembling and reassembling of radios, engines, and various gadgets (335). Although individuals engaged in such activities are aware that the behavior is meaningless and serves no purpose, they report being unable to stop and become irritable and anxious if forced to stop. Furthermore, during engagement in the activity, the individuals report feeling an exploratory pleasure; they do not feel anxious (337).

The clinical description of human stimulant abuse presents all indications of a progressive behavioral and personality disintegration of the individual. Initially, the individual consumes the drug for the euphoric feelings. However, as consumption progresses, the individual switches to rapid routes of administration and starts binging. With prolonged consumption, the individual starts withdrawing from social interactions, and bizarre, even paranoid, ideations start developing. With further consumption, the individual becomes increasingly exhausted, loses insight into their actions, and may become violent or increasingly psychotic.

TREATMENT OF AMPHETAMINE ABUSE

An enormous research effort is based on the assumption that an understanding of the rate-limiting mechanisms underlying stimulant reinforcement, residual withdrawal states, and toxic consequences would lead to effective treatment regimes. Although a great deal has been learned about the neurobiologic mechanisms underlying these aspects of high-dose stimulant use, the development of rational treatment strategies has lagged behind. There

is virtually no controlled treatment literature specifically regarding amphetamine abuse. However, the rise in cocaine abuse has resulted in a controlled treatment literature that can be applied to amphetamines. Table 16.3 presents the different types of pharmacological and behavioral therapies applied to amphetamine and cocaine abuse, along with possible mechanisms underlying their efficacy.

No specific medication has gained widespread acceptance as having broad clinical effectiveness in the treatment of stimulant dependence (338). Nevertheless, medications are useful in managing particular manifestations of dependence in selected patients. Potential indications for pharmacotherapy include treatment of comorbid psychiatric disorders, management of stimulant withdrawal and other drug-induced mental disorders, treatment of concurrent substance use disorders (e.g., alcohol dependence), and facilitation of initial abstinence.

Pharmacotherapy

Clinical evidence indicates that pharmacotherapy can be effective in the treatment of stimulant abuse, putatively by reversing or compensating for the long-term residual neuroadaptations produced by chronic abuse. Pharmacologic treatments of stimulant abuse generally rest on one of the following approaches: (a) blockade of the reinforcing actions of amphetamines, or (b) the provision of low-grade enhancement of "energy-activating" or affective tone with direct dopamine agonists, or with classical antidepressants. The latter approach is thought to reduce the "fantasy urges" that trigger use.

Dopamine Agonists

Dopamine agonists have been used to attenuate the anergia-dysphoria experienced during withdrawal from stimulants (e.g., cocaine). For example, several controlled, double-blind studies indicate that the dopamine agonists bromocriptine and amantadine alleviate the craving and dysphoria during cocaine withdrawal (339–342). Indeed, in the Tennant and Sagherian (342) report, three subjects indicated that bromocriptine almost completely eliminated the euphoric effects of cocaine during treatment.

Tricyclic Antidepressants

Tricyclic antidepressants were first used to treat the amphetamine withdrawal anergic state in the 1970s. For example, imipramine and desipramine were used during this period, based largely on clinical case studies, and were especially effective during the early weeks of withdrawal for the waxing and waning period of psychasthenia and anergia (343). However, during this era there were no controlled studies. Subsequently, amphetamine-abuse mini-epidemics have been scattered and sporadic, and most recent controlled studies have focused on cocaine abuse treatment (318). Of the numerous medications that have been evaluated in the treatment of cocaine dependence, the tricyclic antidepressant desipramine is the most extensively studied. In a double-blind, placebo-controlled, outpatient trial, desipramine (Norpramin) was found to be superior to placebo or lithium in facilitating initial abstinence from cocaine (344); however, there is a delay of 2 to 3 weeks in onset of medication effect, and outpatient dropout rates are very high during this period (344,345). Controlled studies examining the use of desipramine in the treatment of cocaine dependence in methadone-maintained opioid addicts failed to demonstrate superiority over placebo (338,346). In a 12-week trial of psychotherapy and pharmacotherapy (desipramine vs. placebo) in outpatients, with followup extending to 1 year, Carroll et al. (347,348) found that desipramine-treated subjects had less cocaine use at 6 weeks, but not at 12 weeks or at the 6- and 12-month followups. Desipramine appeared to be most effective in subjects with lower severity of dependence (347,348). The precise role of desipramine and other antidepressants in the treatment of cocaine dependence has yet to be established; they may help relieve severe withdrawal symptoms when these are present, and is probably useful in treating stimulant addicts with persistent depressive symptoms (see reference 349 for an animal model of this approach). Several other studies indicate that desipramine can be effective in attenuating the depressive symptoms and craving associated with cocaine withdrawal (350–353). Other potential new treatments proposed for cocaine addiction in other chapters would apply equally to amphetamine abuse; these include the administration of D1-receptor antagonists and low-dose flupentixol. However, the sporadic, area-specific rise and fall of amphetamine mini-epidemics make this type of research extremely difficult.

Behavioral Therapy

As stated earlier, drug abuse is a behavioral problem that is initially maintained and partly sustained by the euphoric and behavioral activating effects of the stimulants. In other words, drugs act as reinforcers to partly maintain drug-seeking and drug-taking behaviors. Thus, nonpharmacologic treatments of stimulant abuse can be derived from an understanding of the conditioning process.

Extinction

As described in the Initiation section, during the active abuse phase, the pharmacologic effects of amphetamine consumption (e.g., euphoria and behavioral activation) become associated with various environmental stimuli via the process of classical conditioning. During the withdrawal phase, exposure to these same stimuli can elicit drug craving and urges. These cravings and urges are conditioned responses that extinguish slowly and that are not systematically affected by detoxification or the simple passage of time (i.e., forgetting). Hence, one behavioral treatment is to accelerate the extinction of these conditioned responses by exposing the individual, in a laboratory or clinical setting, to drug-related stimuli in the absence of any drug effects. Over repeated exposures, the cravings and urges diminish. The therapist starts by having the individual create a hierarchy of stimuli that elicit craving and urges, and then successively exposes the patient to these stimuli; this is similar to systematic desensitization for anxiety and phobic disorders (354).

This type of treatment is used with some success in the treatment of cocaine and opiate abusers (355–357). The efficacy of this treatment depends on several factors. First, the stimuli used for extinction training must be stimuli that are very similar to those the individual actually experienced. For example, if the individual were an intravenous user of amphetamine, then the therapist could expose the abuser to a needle and syringe, or other related paraphernalia. However, the use of a pipe, as in the case of the ice or crack user, would be inappropriate because such items would not represent conditioned stimuli for that particular individual. Second, the efficacy depends on the degree of generalization of the extinction training from the laboratory or clinical setting to the individual's natural environment. This generalization can be maximized by appropriately selecting conditioned stimuli and by making the therapeutic setting as similar to the natural environment of the abuser as possible, or by conducting the training in as many different settings as possible.

Much of the current literature on desensitization focuses on the automatic processes involved in the stimulus properties of abuse (e.g., contiguous pairings, generalization) without considering the sense of self-mastery. There is a very meager literature on facilitating the stimulant abuser's development of strategies to cope with, adapt to, and master the autonomic–automatic conditioned responses that develop during the course of abuse. The authors' own work with abusers includes several steps in strategy development for the abuser, such as (a) extensively identifying conditioned cues and the internal responses generated by these cues; (b) prioritizing the potency of these stimuli (i.e., creating a stimulus hierarchy); (c) bringing these conditioned stimuli to the forefront of one's thinking so that one tries not to forget about them; (d) identifying mood-setting events that may set the stage for conditioned stimuli to become prepotent (e.g., domestic quarrels, job stress); (e) developing strategies for anticipating and confronting these events ahead of time; (f) setting sequential "stops" in the steps needed for drug acquisition; (g) systematic reviewing and diary charting of "near misses" every day; (h) developing self-mastery from these near misses; and (i) developing emergency procedures for seeking immediate help in stopping if the abuser succumbs to the urge to use the drug. Obviously, the strategy development requires an assessment of the individual's personality and ego assets, along with a tailoring of the strategies to the capabilities and circumstances of the individual abuser.

Contingency Contracting

In contingency contracting the abuser signs a "contract" stating that the abuser will perform certain behaviors; under the terms of some contracts, failure to perform these behaviors results in aversive consequences (e.g., the abuser's money being sent to the abuser's most disliked charity, the loss of a license to practice a profession); conversely, the fulfillment of the conditions of the contract may result in positive consequences (e.g., receiving money). Some behavioral contracts incorporate both positive and negative consequences.

Contingency contracts are commonly used in urine-monitoring programs (358). In this treatment procedure, the individual agrees to participate in a urine-monitoring program, and failure to provide either a drug-free urine or a scheduled urine sample results in an aversive consequence; this aversive consequence is obtained from the abuser's own statements (359,360). It is important that any positive or negative consequences be derived from the abuser's own statements; otherwise, they will not be optimally effective. This form of treatment will probably be effective only in the mild abuser, because individuals with more-severe abuse problems will be aware of their degree of craving and will probably be unable to abstain from the drug; hence, the severe abuser would never agree to the conditions of the contract (358).

Increasing Natural Reinforcement Density

Basic behavioral research indicates that the reinforcing value (efficacy) of an event is inversely related to the overall density of reinforcement in the environment. In other words, a given event will be a more potent reinforcer in a relatively impoverished environment, as compared with the same event in a relatively enriched environment (see, e.g., reference 361 for a review of this literature). Drug abuse is more likely to be found in lower socioeconomic conditions (325), where the number of available reinforcers are likely to be limited. Thus, drugs are more efficacious reinforcers under these conditions, as compared with higher socioeconomic strata. Furthermore, this analysis would predict that, as the abuse continues and the behavioral repertoire becomes increasingly focused on drug-seeking and drug-taking behaviors, the reinforcing efficacy of the drug increases independent of any concomitant neurochemical changes.

This analysis implies that one potential method of treating stimulant abusers is to reinstate former natural behaviors such as sports and nondrug social activities. This would increase the overall reinforcement density that the individual experiences, thereby decreasing the reinforcing efficacy of the drug. Indeed, Carroll et al. (362) found that both the acquisition and rate of cocaine self-administration in rats decreases simply by introducing a second response alternative that delivers a glucose-saccharin solution.

Much research must still be conducted on the treatment of amphetamine and stimulant abuse; our limited knowledge regarding the residual behavioral and neurochemical changes produced by chronic, high-dose stimulant abuse precludes any definitive statement regarding the most efficacious treatments for the abuser. However, effective treatments are likely to contain a behavioral component to reduce conditioned craving and teach the necessary strategic coping skills for dealing with the original environment that contributed to the development of the abuse. Pharmacotherapy is also likely to be an important component, especially in dealing with the craving and depressive symptoms that occur during withdrawal. Ultimately, any treatment package must be tailored to the specific needs and situations of the individual.

CONCLUSION

The consumption of amphetamines for nonmedical reasons probably occurs because of their euphoriant and psychomotor-stimulating properties. Chronic consumption of amphetamine results in the development of stereotyped behavior, paranoia, and possibly aggression. During the protracted withdrawal phase from amphetamine, individuals experience anhedonia and anergia. This may be the result of long-lasting, and possibly permanent, changes in the neurobiologic substrates that mediate reward (105). In addition to these effects, acute and chronic consumption of amphetamine can be highly toxic. Deaths from amphetamine overdose are not uncommon and are caused by hyperpyrexia, cardiac failure, convulsions, and cerebral hemorrhage.

The neurobiologic substrates that mediate the effects of amphetamine and normally occurring behaviors are beginning to be elucidated. The effects of amphetamine are probably mediated by the mesolimbic dopaminergic system. Chronic amphetamine use results in permanent depletions of dopamine from a variety of brain regions. This depletion may mediate some of the tolerance, anhedonia, and anergia experienced by amphetamine users. Furthermore, chronic amphetamine use results in changes in somatodendritic and terminal autoreceptor sensitivity, which may negatively affect natural reinforcers.

In addition to the effects on the dopaminergic system, methamphetamine also depletes the serotonergic system, which may have several functional effects. Examination of the clinical psychiatric literature indicates that depletion of the serotonin system is associated with impulsive behavior (i.e., disinhibition of behavior); for example, Linnoila et al. (363) found that violent offenders with a diagnosis of personality disorder associated with impulsivity had lower 5-HIAA levels than did other offenders. Relating the amphetamine abuse syndrome and the literature on serotonergic activity and impulsivity provides for an operating hypothesis that the lower serotonergic activity during chronic amphetamine consumption, and the resulting impulsivity (disinhibition of behavior) that may result from this depletion, may result in amphetamine abusers being more likely to relapse. Furthermore, if the individual relapses, consumption of amphetamines will have a greater reinforcing effect because of the absence of the normal inhibitory effects of the serotonergic system on dopamine release.

The likelihood of relapse and disinhibition is further enhanced by the presence of stimuli that were previously associated with drug consumption and drug effects, similar to effects found with the conditioned place preference paradigm. During withdrawal, these stimuli can elicit conditioned craving that further tends to result in relapse and resumption of the binge cycle.

The current federal effort to curb cocaine importation and use, coupled with the large profit margins associated with amphetamine production, may result in an increase in the number of individuals abusing amphetamines. The individual who is prone to drug abuse may see the use of amphetamines as an economical alternative to cocaine abuse. This may be especially true given that the effects of amphetamine last longer than the effects of cocaine. If this increase does occur, then one would expect to see an increase in the number of individuals admitted to hospital emergency rooms for the treatment of the physical and behavioral effects of acute and chronic amphetamine use.

ACKNOWLEDGMENTS

Preparation of this chapter was supported by NIDA grant 1-R29-DA08899 and 1-R01-DA10468, G. R. King, PhD, principal investigator, and grants DA14323, DA10327, and DA12768, E. H. Ellinwood principal investigator.

REFERENCES

1. Caldwell J. The metabolism of amphetamines and related stimulants in animals and man. In: Caldwell J, ed. *Amphetamines and related stimulants: chemical, biological, clinical, and social aspects.* Boca Raton, FL: CRC Press, 1980.
2. Carlsson A. Amphetamine and brain catecholamines. In: Costa E, Garattini S, eds. *Amphetamines and related compounds.* New York: Raven Press, 1970:289–299.
3. Carlsson A, Waldeck B. Effects of amphetamine, tyramine, and protriptyline on reserpine resistant amine-concentrating mechanisms of adrenergic nerves. *J Pharm Pharmacol* 1966;18:252–253.
4. Carlsson A, Lindqvist M, Dahlstroem A, et al. Effects of the amphetamine group on intraneuronal brain amines *in vivo* and *in vitro*. *J Pharm Pharmacol* 1965;17:521–524.
5. Chiueh CC, Moore KE. *In vivo* evoked release of endogenously synthesized catecholamines from the cat brain evoked by electrical stimulation and *d*-amphetamine. *J Neurochem* 1974;23:159–168.
6. Coyle JT, Snyder SH. Catecholamine uptake by synaptosomes in homogenates of rat brain: stereospecificity in different areas. *J Pharmacol Exp Ther* 1969;170:221–231.
7. Dingell JV, Owens ML, Norvich MR, et al. On the role of norepinephrine biosynthesis in the central action of amphetamine. *Life Sci* 1967;6:1155–1162.
8. Fuxe K, Ungerstedt U. Histochemical, biochemical and functional studies on central monoamine neurons after acute and chronic amphetamine administration. In: Costa E, Garattini S, eds. *Amphetamines and related compounds.* New York: Raven Press, 1970:257–288.
9. Hanson GR, Sonsalla P, Letter A, et al. Effects of amphetamine analogs on central nervous system neuropeptide systems. *NIDA Res Monogr Ser* 1989;94:259–269.
10. Herman ZS. Influence of some psychotropic and adrenergic blocking agents upon amphetamine stereotyped behavior in white rats. *Psychopharmacologia* 1967;11:136–142.
11. Javoy F, Hamon H, Glowinski J. Disposition of newly synthesized amines in cell bodies and terminals of central catecholaminergic neurons. I. Effect of amphetamine and thioproperazine on the metabolism of CA in the caudate nucleus, the substantia nigra and the ventromedial nucleus of the hypothalamus. *Eur J Pharmacol* 1970;10:178–188.
12. Lewander T. A mechanism for the development of tolerance to amphetamine in rats. *Psychopharmacologia* 1971;21:17–31.
13. Littleton JM. The interaction of dexamphetamine with inhibitors of noradrenaline synthesis in rat brain *in vivo*. *J Pharm Pharmacol* 1967;19:414–415.
14. Lundborg P. Amphetamine-induced release of ^{3}H-metaraminol from subcellular fractions of the mouse heart. *J Pharm Pharmacol* 1969;21:266–268.
15. Obianwu HO. Possible functional differentiation between the stores from

which adrenergic nerve stimulation, tyramine and amphetamine release noradrenaline. *Acta Physiol Scand* 1969; 75:92–101.

16. Randrup DB, Munkvad I. Pharmacology and physiology of stereotyped behavior. *J Psychiatric Res* 1974;11:1.

17. Rech RH. Antagonism of reserpine behavioral depression by *d*-amphetamine. *J Pharmacol Exp Ther* 1964;146:369–376.

18. Scheel-Krueger J. Comparative studies of various amphetamine analogues demonstrating different interactions with the metabolism of the catecholamines in the brain. *Eur J Pharmacol* 1971;14:47–59.

19. Svensson TH. The effect of inhibition of catecholamine synthesis on dexamphetamine induced central stimulation. *Eur J Pharmacol* 1970;12:161–166.

20. Von Voigtlander PF, Moore KE. Involvement of nigro-striatal neurons in the *in vivo* release of dopamine by amphetamine, amantadine and tyramine. *J Pharmacol Exp Ther* 1973;184:542–552.

21. Weissman A, Koe BK, Tenen SS. Antiamphetamine effects following inhibition of tyrosine hydroxylase. *J Pharmacol Exp Ther* 1966;151:339–352.

22. Seiden LS, Sabol KE, Ricuarte GA. Amphetamine: Effects on catecholamine systems and behavior. *Annu Rev Pharmacol Toxicol* 1993;32:639–677.

23. Kuczenski R, Segal DS, Cho AK, et al. Hippocampus norepinephrine, caudate dopamine and serotonin, and behavioral responses to the stereoisomers of amphetamine and methamphetamine. *J Neurosci* 1993;15:1308–1317.

24. Reith MEA, Li M-Y, Yan Q-S. Extracellular dopamine, norepinephrine and serotonin in the ventral tegmental area and nucleus accumbens of freely moving rats during intracerebral dialysis following systemic administration of cocaine and other uptake blockers. *Psychopharmacology (Berl)* 1997;134:309–317.

25. Joensson L-E, Gunne L-M, Aenggaerd E. Effects of alpha-methyltyrosine in amphetamine dependent subjects. *Pharmacol Clin* 1969;2:27.

26. Koda LY, Gibb JW. The effect of repeated doses of methamphetamine on adrenal and brain tyrosine hydroxylase. *Pharmacologist* 1971;13:253.

27. Koda LY, Gibb JW. Adrenal and striatal tyrosine hydroxylase activity after methamphetamine. *J Pharmacol Exp Ther* 1973;185:42–48.

28. Kogan FJ, Nichols WK, Gibb JW. Influence of methamphetamine on nigral and striatal tyrosine hydroxylase activity and on striatal dopamine levels. *Eur J Pharmacol* 1976;36:363–371.

29. Reid WD. Turnover rate of brain 5-hydroxytryptamine increased by *d*-amphetamine. *Br J Pharmacol* 1970; 40:483.

30. Weiner N. Pharmacology of central nervous system stimulants. In: Zarafonetis CJD, ed. *Drug abuse: proceedings of the international conference.* Philadelphia: Lea & Febiger, 1972:243–251.

31. Hotchkiss AJ, Gibb JW. Long-term effects of multiple doses of methamphetamine on tryptophan hydroxylase and tyrosine hydroxylase activity in rat brain. *J Pharmacol Exp Ther* 1980; 214:257–262.

32. Knapp S, Mandell AJ, Geyer MA. Effects of amphetamine on regional tryptophan hydroxylase activity and synaptosomal conversion of tryptophan to 5-hydroxytryptamine in rat brain. *J Pharmacol Exp Ther* 1974;189:676–689.

33. Peat MA, Warren PF, Gibb JW. Effects of a single dose of methamphetamine and iprindole on the serotonergic and dopaminergic system of the rat brain. *J Pharmacol Exp Ther* 1983;255:126–131.

34. Reid M, Herrera-Marschitz M, Hokfelt T, et al. Differential modulation of striatal dopamine release by intranigral injection of gamma-aminobutyric acid (GABA), dynorphin A and substance P. *Eur J Pharmacol* 1988;147:411–420.

35. Herrera-Marschitz M, Christensson-Nylander I, Sharp T, et al. Striatonigral dynorphin and substance P pathways in the rat. II. Functional analysis. *Exp Brain Res* 1986;64:193.

36. Quirion R, Chiueh C, Everist H, Pert A. Comparative localization of neurotensin receptors on nigrostriatal and mesolimbic dopaminergic terminal. *Brain Res* 1985;327:385–389.

37. Nemeroff C. The interaction of neurotensin with dopaminergic pathways in the central nervous system: basic neurobiology and implications for the pathogenesis and treatment of schizophrenia. *Psychoneuroendocrinology* 1986;11:15–37.

38. Bunney BS, Aghajanian GK, Roth RH. Comparison of the effects of L-dopa, amphetamine, and apomorphine on firing rate of rat dopaminergic neurons. *Nat New Biol* 1973;245:123–125.

39. Rebec GV, Segal DS. Dose-dependent biphasic alterations in the spontaneous activity of neurons in the rat neostriatum produced by *d*-amphetamine and methylphenidate. *Brain Res* 1978;150:353–366.

40. Graham AW, Aghajanian GK. Effects of amphetamine on single cell activity in a catecholamine nucleus, the locus coeruleus. *Nature* 1971;234:100–102.

41. Groves PM, Rebec GV. Changes in neuronal activity in the neostriatum and the reticular formation following acute or long-term amphetamine administration. In: Ellinwood E, Kilbey M, eds. *Cocaine and other stimulants.* New York: Plenum Press, 1977:269–301.

42. Groves PM, Wilson CJ, Young SJ, et al. Self-inhibition by dopaminergic neurons. *Science* 1975;190:522–529.

43. Groves PM, Young SJ, Wilson CJ. Self-inhibition by dopaminergic neurons: disruption by (+/−)-alpha-methyl-para-tyrosine pretreatment or anterior diencephalic lesions. *Neuropsychopharmacology* 1976;15:755–762.

44. Groves PM, Young SJ, Wilson CJ. Nigro-striatal relations and mechanisms of action of amphetamine. In: Butcher LL, ed. *Cholinergic-monoaminergic interactions in the brain.* New York: Academic Press, 1978:177–218.

45. Bunney BS, Aghajanian GK. Electrophysiological effects of amphetamine on dopaminergic neurons. In: Usdin E, Snyder SH, eds. *Frontiers in catecholamine research.* Oxford: Pergamon Press, 1973:957–962.

46. Bunney BS, Aghajanian GK. *d*-Amphetamine-induced inhibition of central dopaminergic neurons: mediation by a striato-nigral feedback pathway. *Science* 1976;192:391–393.

47. Groves PM, Rebec GV, Segal DS. The action of *d*-amphetamine on spontaneous activity in the caudate nucleus and reticular formation of the rat. *Behav Biol* 1974;11:33–47.

48. Rebec GV, Groves PM. Differential effects of the optical isomers of amphetamine on neuronal activity in the reticular formation and caudate nucleus of the rat. *Brain Res* 1975;83:301–318.

49. Weiner N. Norepinephrine, epinephrine, and the sympathomimetic amines. In: Gilman AG, Goodman LS, Rall TW, et al, eds. *Gilman and Goodman's the pharmacological basis of therapeutics.* New York: Macmillan, 1985:145–180.

50. Stripling JS, Ellinwood EH. Augmentation of the behavioral and electrophysiological response to cocaine by chronic administration in the rat. *Exp Neurol* 1977;54:546–564.

51. Ellinwood EH, Kilbey MM. Chronic stimulant models of psychosis. In: Hanin I, Usdin E, eds. *Animal models of psychiatry.* New York: Pergamon Press, 1977.

52. Ellinwood EH, Sudilovsky A, Nelson LM. Behavior, EEG analysis of chronic amphetamine effect. *Biol Psychiatry* 1974;8:169–176.

53. Biel JH, Bopp BA. Amphetamine: structure-activity relationships. In: Iversen LL, Iversen SD, Snyderman

SH, eds. *Handbook of psychopharmacology,* vol. 11. *Stimulants.* New York: Plenum Press, 1978:1–39.

54. Snyder SH, Taylor KM, Coyle JT, et al. The role of brain dopamine in behavioral regulation of the actions of psychotropic drugs. *Am J Psychiatry* 1970;127:199–207.

55. Taylor KM, Snyder SH. Amphetamine: differentiation by *d-* and *l*-isomers of behavior involving brain norepinephrine or dopamine. *Science* 1970;168:1487–1489.

56. Pletscher A, Bartholini G, Bruderer H, et al. Chlorinated arylalkylamines affecting the cerebral metabolism of 5-hydroxytryptamine. *J Pharmacol Exp Ther* 1964;145:334–350.

57. Fuller RW, Snoddy HD, Roush BW, et al. Further structure-activity studies on the lowering of brain 5-hydroxyindoles by 4-chloroamphetamine. *Neuropharmacology* 1973;12:33–42.

58. Fuller RW, Molloy BB. Recent studies with 4-chloroamphetamine and some analogues. In: Costa E, Gessa GL, Sandler M, eds. *Advances in biochemical psychopharmacology,* vol. 10. New York: Raven Press, 1974:195–205.

59. Moller-Nielsen I, Dubnick B. Pharmacology of chlorphentermine. In: Costa E, Garattini S, eds. *Amphetamines and related compounds.* New York: Raven Press, 1970:63–73.

60. Del Arco A, Gonzalez-Mora JL, Armas VR, et al. Amphetamine increases the extracellular concentration of glutamate in striatum of the awake rat: involvement of high-affinity transporter mechanism. *Neuopharmacol* 1999;38:943–954.

61. Reid MS, Hsu K, Berger SP. Cocaine and amphetamine preferentially stimulate glutamate release in the limbic system: studies on the involvement of dopamine. *Synapse* 1997;27:95–105.

62. Wolf ME, Xue CJ. Amphetamine and D1 dopamine receptor agonists produce biphasic effects on glutamate efflux in rat ventral tegmental area: modification by repeated amphetamine administration. *J Neurochem* 1998;70:198–209.

63. Wolf ME, Khansa MR. Repeated administration of MK-801 produces sensitization to its own locomotor stimulant effects but blocks sensitization to amphetamine. *Brain Res* 1991;562:164–168.

64. Xue CJ, Ng JP, Li Y, et al. Acute and repeated systemic amphetamine administration: effects on extracellular glutamate, aspartate, and serine levels in rat ventral tegmental area and nucleus accumbens. *J Neurochem* 1996:67:352–363.

65. Kalivas PW, Duffy P. Dopamine regulation of extracellular glutamate in the nucleus accumbens. *Brain Res* 1997;761:173–177.

66. Vanderschuren LJMJ, Kalivas PW. Alterations in dopaminergic and glutamatergic transmission in the induction and expression of behavioral sensitization: a critical review of preclinical studies. *Psychopharmacology (Berl)* 2000;151:99–120.

67. Wolf ME. The role of excitatory amino acids in behavioral sensitization to psychomotor stimulants. *Prog Neurobiol* 1998;54:679–720.

68. Karler R, Chaudhry IA, Calder LD, et al. Amphetamine behavioral sensitization and the excitatory amino acids. *Brain Res* 1990;537:76–82.

69. Karler R, Calder LD, Chaudhry IA, et al. Blockade of "reverse tolerance" to cocaine and amphetamine by MK-801. *Life Sci* 1989;45:599–606.

70. Kim H-S, Jang C-G. MK-801 inhibits methamphetamine-induced conditioned place preference and behavioral sensitization to apomorphine in mice. *Brain Res Bull* 1997;44:221–227.

71. Kim J-H, Vezin P. Metabotropic glutamate receptors are necessary for sensitization by amphetamine. *Neuroreport* 1998;9:403–406.

72. Li Y, Wolf ME. Can the "state-dependency" hypothesis explain prevention of amphetamine sensitization in rats by NMDA receptor antagonists? *Psychopharmacology (Berl)* 1999;141:351–361.

73. Ohmri T, Abekawa T, Muraki A, et al. Competitive and noncompetitive NMDA antagonists block sensitization to methamphetamine. *Pharmacol Biochem Behav* 1994;48:587–591.

74. Stewart J, Druhan JP. Development of both conditioning and sensitization of the behavioral activating effects of amphetamine is blocked by the non-competitive NMDA receptor antagonist, MK-801. *Psychopharmacology (Berl)* 1993;110:125–132.

75. Tolliver BK, Ho LB, Reid MS, et al. Evidence for dissociable mechanisms of amphetamine- and stress-induced behavioral sensitization: effects of MK-801 and haloperidol pretreatment. *Psychopharmacology (Berl)* 126:191–198.

76. Wolf ME, Jeziorski M. Coadministration of MK-801 with amphetamine, cocaine or morphine prevents rather than transiently masks the development of behavioral sensitization. *Brain Res* 1993;613:291–294.

77. Cador M, Bjijou Y, Cailhol S, et al. *d*-Amphetamine-induced behavioral sensitization; implication of a glutamatergic medial prefrontal cortex-ventral tegmental area innervation. *Neurosci* 1999;94:705–721.

78. Van der Shoot JB, Ariens EJ, Van Rossum JM, et al. Phenylisopropylamine derivatives, structure, and action. *Arzneimittelforschung* 1961;9:902–907.

79. Moore KE. Toxicity and catecholamine releasing activities of *d-* and *l-*amphetamine in isolated and aggregated mice. *J Pharmacol Exp Ther* 1963;142:6–12.

80. Roth LW, Richards RK, Shemano I, et al. A comparison of the analeptic, circulatory and other properties of *d-* and *l*-desoxyephedrine. *Arch Int Pharmacodyn Ther* 1954;98:362–368.

81. Van Rossum JM. Mode of action of psychomotor stimulant drugs. *Int Rev Neurobiol* 1970;12:309–383.

82. Ellinwood EH. Neuropharmacology of amphetamines and related stimulants. In: Caldwell J, ed. *Amphetamines and related stimulants: chemical, biological, clinical, and sociological aspects.* Boca Raton, FL: CRC Press, 1980:69–84.

83. Iversen SD. Neural substrates mediating amphetamine responses. In: Ellinwood E, Kilbey M, eds. *Cocaine and other stimulants.* New York: Plenum Press, 1975:31–45.

84. Pijnenburg AJJ, van Rossum JM. Stimulation of locomotor activity following injection of dopamine into the nucleus accumbens. *J Pharm Pharmacol* 1973;25:1003.

85. Pijnenburg AJJ, Honig WMM, van Rossum JM. Inhibition of d-amphetamine induced locomotor activity by injection of haloperidol into the nucleus accumbens of the rat. *Psychopharmacologia* 1975;41:87–95.

86. Thornburg JE, Moore KE. The relative importance of dopaminergic and noradrenergic neuronal systems for the stimulation of locomotor activity induced by amphetamine and other drugs. *Neuropharmacology* 1973;12:853.

87. Naylor RJ, Ollay JE. Modification of the behavioural changes induced by amphetamine in rats by lesions in the caudate nucleus, the caudate-putamen and the globus pallidus. *Neuropharmacology* 1974;11:91–99.

88. Asher IM, Aghajanian GK. 6-Hydroxydopamine lesions of olfactory tubercules and caudate nuclei: effect on amphetamine-induced stereotyped behaviour in rats. *Brain Res* 1974;82:1–12.

89. Creese I, Iversen SD. The role of forebrain dopamine systems in amphetamine induced stereotyped behaviour in the rat. *Psychopharmacologia* 1975;39:345–357.

90. Kelly PH, Seviour PW, Iversen SD. Amphetamine and apomorphine responses in the rat following 6-OHDA lesions of the nucleus accumbens

septi and corpus striatum. *Brain Res* 1975;94:507–522.

91. Costall B, Naylor RJ. Extrapyramidal and mesolimbic involvement with the stereotypic activity of *d*- and *l*-amphetamine. *Eur J Pharmacol* 1974;25:121–129.

92. Iversen SD, Kelly PH, Miller RJ, et al. Amphetamine and apomorphine responses in the rat after lesion of the mesolimbic or striatal dopamine neurones. *Br J Pharmacol* 1975;54:244P.

93. Joyce EM, Koob GF. Amphetamine-, scopolamine-, and caffeine-induced locomotor activity following 6-hydroxydopamine lesions of the mesolimbic dopamine system. *Psychopharmacology (Berl)* 1981;73:311–313.

94. Kelly P-H, Iversen SD. Selective 6-OHDA-induced destruction of mesolimbic dopamine neurons: abolition of psychostimulant induced locomotor activity in rats. *Eur J Pharmacol* 1976;40:45–56.

95. Swerdlow NR, Koob GF. Separate neural substrates of the locomotor-activating properties of amphetamine, heroin, caffeine and corticotropin releasing factor (CRF) in the rat. *Pharmacol Biochem Behav* 1985;23:303–307.

96. Vaccarino FJ, Amalric M, Swerdlow NR, et al. Blockade of amphetamine but not opiate induced locomotion following antagonism of dopamine function in the rat. *Pharmacol Biochem Behav* 1986;24:61–65.

97. King GR, Joyner C, Lee T, Kuhn C, et al. Intermittent and continuous cocaine administration: residual behavioral states during withdrawal. *Pharmacol Biochem Behav* 1992;43:243–248.

98. King GR, Joyner C, Lee TH, et al. Withdrawal from continuous or intermittent cocaine: effects of NAN-190 on cocaine-induced locomotion. *Pharmacol Biochem Behav* 1993;44:253–262.

99. King GR, Kuhn C, Ellinwood EH Jr. Dopamine efflux during withdrawal from continuous or intermittent cocaine. *Psychopharmacology (Berl)* 1993;111:179–184.

100. Reith MEA, Benuck M, Lajtha A. Cocaine disposition in the brain after continuous or intermittent treatment and locomotor stimulation in mice. *J Pharmacol Exp Ther* 1987;243:281–287.

101. Akimoto K, Hammamura T, Otsuki S. Subchronic cocaine treatment enhances cocaine-induced dopamine efflux studied by in vivo intracerebral dialysis. *Brain Res* 1989;490:339–344.

102. Kalivas PW, Duffy P. Effects of daily cocaine and morphine treatment on somatodendritic and terminal field DA release. *J Neurochem* 1988;50:1498–1504.

103. Kalivas PW, Duffy P, Dumars LA, et al. Behavioral and neurochemical effects of acute and daily cocaine administration in rats. *J Pharmacol Exp Ther* 1988;245:485–492.

104. Kalivas PW, Duffy P, Barrow J. Regulation of the mesocorticolimbic dopamine system by glutamic acid receptor subtypes. *J Pharmacol Exp Ther* 1989;251:378–387.

105. Kalivas PW, Duffy P. Effect of acute and daily cocaine treatment on extracellular dopamine in the nucleus accumbens. *Synapse* 1990;5:48–58.

106. Kalivas PW, Stewart J. Dopamine transmission in the initiation and expression of drug and stress induced sensitization of motor activity. *Brain Res Rev* 1991;16:223–244.

107. Chen N-H, Reith MEA. Dopamine and serotonin release-regulation autoreceptor sensitivity in A_9/A_{10} cell body and terminal areas after withdrawal of rats from continuous infusion of cocaine. *J Pharmacol Exp Ther* 1993;267:1445–1453.

108. Izenwasser S, Cox BM. Inhibition of dopamine uptake by cocaine and nicotine: tolerance to chronic treatments. *Brain Res* 1992;573:119–125.

109. Jacobs BL, Wise WD, Taylor KM. Is there a catecholamine-serotonin interaction in the control of locomotor activity? *Neuropharmacology* 1975;14:501–506.

110. Neill DB, Grant LD, Grossman SP. Selective potentiation of locomotor effects of amphetamine by midbrain raphe lesions. *Physiol Behav* 1972;9:655.

111. Green TR, Harvey JA. Enhancement of amphetamine action after interruption of ascending serotonergic pathways. *J Pharmacol Exp Ther* 1974;190:109.

112. Breese GR, Cooper Br, Mueller RA. Evidence for involvement of 5-hydroxytryptamine in the actions of amphetamine. *Br J Pharmacol* 1974;52:307–314.

113. Mabry PD, Campbell BA. Serotonergic inhibition of catecholamine-induced behavioral arousal. *Brain Res* 1973;49:381–391.

114. Neuberg J, Thut PD. Comparison of the locomotor stimulant mechanisms of the action of d-amphetamine and *d*-amphetamine plus L-dopa: possible involvement of serotonin. *Biol Psychiatry* 1974;8:139–150.

115. Swonger AK, Rech RH. Serotonergic and cholinergic involvement in habituation of activity and spontaneous alterations of rats in a Y maze. *J Comp Physiol Psychol* 1972;81:509–522.

116. Schad CA, Justice JB Jr, Holtzman SG. Naloxone reduces the neurochemical and behavioral effects of amphetamine but not those of cocaine. *Eur J Pharmacol* 1995;275(1):9–16.

117. Motles E, Tetas M, Gonzalez M. Effects of naloxone on the behaviors evoked by amphetamine and apomorphine in adult cats. *Prog Neuropsychopharmacol Biol Psychiatry* 1995;19(3):475–490.

118. Wallach MB. Drug-induced stereotyped behavior: similarities and differences. In: Ungerstedt E, ed. *Neuropsychopharmacology of monoamines and their regulatory enzymes.* New York: Raven Press, 1974:241–260.

119. Fog R. On stereotypy and catalepsy: studies on the effect of amphetamine and neuroleptics in the rat. *Acta Neurol Scand* 1972;48[Suppl]:50.

120. Braestrup C, Anderson H, Randrup A. The monoamine oxidase B inhibitor deprenyl potentiates phenylethylamine behaviour in rats without inhibition of catecholamine metabolite formation. *Eur J Pharmacol* 1975;34:181–189.

121. Costall B, Naylor RJ. The site and mode of action of ET-495 for the mediation of stereotyped behaviour in the rat. *Naunyn Schmiedebergs Arch Pharmacol* 1973;278:117–133.

122. Costall B, Naylor RJ. Mesolimbic and extrapyramidal sites for the mediation of stereotyped behaviour patterns and hyperactivity by amphetamine and apomorphine in the rat. In: Ellinwood E, Kilbey M, eds. *Cocaine and other stimulants.* New York: Plenum Press, 1975:47–76.

123. Cox B, Tha SJ. Effects of amantadine and L1-dopa on apomorphine and *d*-amphetamine induced stereotyped behaviour in rats. *Eur J Pharmacol* 1973;24:96–101.

124. Hackman, SJ. Pentikaeinen P, Neuroven RJ, et al. Inhibition of apomorphine gnawing compulsion by amantadine. *Experentia* 1973;29:1524–1525.

125. Browne RG, Segal DS. Metabolic and experiential factors in the behavioral response to repeated amphetamine. *Pharmacol Biochem Behav* 1977;6:545–552.

126. Lee TH, Ellinwood EH, Nishita JK. Dopamine receptor sensitivity changes with chronic stimulants. In: Kalivas W, Nemeroff CB, eds. *The mesocorticolimbic system.* New York: Academy of Sciences, 1988:324–329.

127. Rebec GV, Segal DS. Enhanced responsiveness to intraventricular infusion of amphetamine following repeated system administration. *Psychopharmacology (Berl)* 1979;62:101–102.

128. Segal DS. Behavioral and neurochemical correlates of repeated *d*-amphetamine administration. In: Mandell AJ, ed. *Advances in biochemical psychopharmacology,* vol. 13. New York: Raven Press, 1975.

129. Segal DS, Weinberger SB, Cahill J, et al. Multiple daily amphetamine

administration: behavioral and neurochemical alterations. *Science* 1980; 207:904–906.

130. Segal DS, Mandell AJ. Long-term administration of *d*-amphetamine: progressive augmentation of motor activity and stereotypy. *Pharmacol Biochem Behav* 1974;2:249–255.

131. Castellani S, Ellinwood EH, Kilbey MM. Behavioral analysis of chronic cocaine intoxication in the cat. *Biol Psychiatry* 1978;13:203–205.

132. Ellinwood EH Jr. Effect of chronic methamphetamine intoxication in rhesus monkeys. *Biol Psychiatry* 1971;3:25–32.

133. Ellinwood EH Jr. Amphetamine psychosis: individuals, settings, and sequences. In: Ellinwood EH, Cohen S, eds. *Current concepts in amphetamine abuse*. Rockville, MD: National Institute on Mental Health, 1972:143–157.

134. Ho BT, Taylor DL, Estevez VS, et al. Behavioral effects of cocaine: metabolic and neurochemical approach. In: Ellinwood E, Kilbey M, eds. *Cocaine and other stimulants*. New York: Plenum Press, 1977.

135. Post RM. Progressive changes in behavior and seizures following chronic cocaine administration: relationship to kindling and psychosis. In: Ellinwood E, Kilbey M, eds. *Cocaine and other stimulants*. New York: Plenum Press, 1977.

136. Schiorring E. Changes in individual and social behavior induced by amphetamine and related compounds. In: Ellinwood E, Kilbey M, eds. *Cocaine and other stimulants*. New York: Plenum Press, 1977:481

137. Angrist BM, Gershon S. The phenomenology of experimentally induced amphetamine psychosis: preliminary observations. *Biol Psychiatry* 1970;2:95–107.

138. Angrist BM, Gershon S. Some recent studies on amphetamine psychosis—unresolved issues. In: Ellinwood EH, Cohen S, eds. *Current concepts on amphetamine abuse*. Rockville, MD: National Institute on Mental Health 1972:193–204.

139. Cole JO, Freedman AM, Friedhoff AJ. *Psychopathology and psychopharmacology*. Baltimore: Johns Hopkins University Press, 1973.

140. Ellinwood EH Jr. Comparative methamphetamine intoxication in experimental animals. *Pharmakopsychiatr Neuropsychopharmakol* 1971;4:351–361.

141. Ellinwood EH, Sudilovsky A, Nelson LM. Evolving behavior in the clinical and experimental amphetamine (model) psychosis. *Am J Psychiatry* 1973;130:1088–1093.

142. Ellinwood EH Jr, Kilbey MM. Species differences in responses to amphetamine. In: Eleftheriou BE, ed. *Psychopharmacogenetics*. New York: Plenum Press, 1975:323–375.

143. Burt DR, Creese I, Snyder SH. Antischizophrenic drugs: chronic treatment elevates dopamine receptor binding in brain. *Science* 1977;196:326–328.

144. Conway PG, Uretsky NJ. Role of striatal dopaminergic receptors in amphetamine-induced behavioral facilitation. *J Pharmacol Exp Ther* 1982;221:650–655.

145. Nielsen EB, Nielsen M, Ellison G, Braestrup C. Decreased spiroperidol and LSD binding in rat brain after continuous amphetamine. *Eur J Pharmacol* 1981;66:149–154.

146. Nielsen EB, Nielsen M, Braestrup C. Reduction of (3)H-spiroperidol binding in rat striatum and frontal cortex by chronic amphetamine: dose response, time course, and role of sustained dopamine release. *Psychopharmacology (Berl)* 1983;81:81–85.

147. Eison MS, Eison AS, Ellison G. The regional distribution of *d*-amphetamine and local glucose utilization in rat brain during continuous amphetamine administration. *Exp Brain Res* 1981;43:281–288.

148. Eison MS, Ellison G, Eison AS. The regional distribution of amphetamine in rat brain is altered by dosage and by prior exposure to drug. *J Pharmacol Exp Ther* 1981;218:237–241.

149. Jori A, Caccia S, Dolfini E. Tolerance to anorectic drugs. In: Garattini S, Samanin R, eds. *Central mechanism of anorectic drugs*. New York: Raven Press, 1978:179–189.

150. Kuhn CM, Schanberg SM. Metabolism of amphetamine after acute and chronic administration to the rat. *J Pharmacol Exp Ther* 1978;207:544–554.

151. Orzi F, Dow-Edwards D, Jehle J, et al. Comparative effects of acute and chronic administration of amphetamine on local cerebral glucose utilization in the conscious rat. *J Cereb Blood Flow Metab* 1983;3:154–160.

152. Ellison G, Eison MS, Huberman HS, et al. Long-term changes in dopaminergic innervation of caudate nucleus after continuous amphetamine. *Science* 1978;201:276–278.

153. Ellison G, Morris W. Opposed stages of continuous amphetamine administration: parallel alterations in motor stereotypies and *in vivo* spiroperidol accumulation. *Eur J Pharmacol* 1981;74:207–214.

154. Ellison G, Rattan R. The late stage following continuous amphetamine administration to rats is correlated with altered dopamine but not serotonin. *Life Sci* 1982;31:771–777.

155. Schmidt CJ, Ritter JK, Sonsalla PK, et al. Role of dopamine in the neurotoxic effects of methamphetamine. *J Pharmacol Exp Ther* 1985;233:539–544.

156. Steranka LR, Sanders-Bush E. Long-term effects of fenfluramine on central serotonergic mechanisms. *Neuropharmacology* 1979;18:895–903.

157. Lee T, Ellinwood EH. Time-dependent changes in the sensitivity of dopamine neurons to low doses of apomorphine following amphetamine infusion: electrophysiological and biochemical studies. *Brain Res* 1989;483:17–29.

158. Ansis SF, Smith RC. Amphetamine abuse and violence. In: Smith DE, ed. *Amphetamine use, misuse, and abuse*. Boston: G.K. Hall, 1979:205–217.

159. Ellinwood EH Jr. Assault and homicide associated with amphetamine abuse. *Am J Psychiatry* 1971;127:90–95.

160. Siomopoulos V. Violence: the ugly facet of amphetamine abuse. *Illinois Med J* 1981;159:375–377.

161. Hemmi T. How we handled the problem of drug abuse in Japan. In: Sjoqvist F, Tottie M, eds. *Abuse of central stimulants*. Stockholm: Almquist and Wiksell, 1969:147–153.

162. Simonds JF, Kashani J. Drug abuse and criminal behavior in delinquent boys committed to training school. *Am J Psychiatry* 1979;136:1444–1448.

163. Cherek DR, Steinberg JL, Kelly TH. Effects of *d*-amphetamine on human aggressive behavior. *Psychopharmacology (Berl)* 1986;88:381–386.

164. Cherek DR, Steinberg JL, Baruchi JT. Effects of caffeine on human aggressive behavior. *Psychiatry Res* 1983;8:137–145.

165. Bradley C. The behavior of children receiving benzedrine. *Am J Psychiatry* 1937;94:577–585.

166. Arnold LE, Kirilcuk V, Corson SA, Corson EO. Levoamphetamine and dextroamphetamine: differential effect on aggression and hyperkinesis in children and dog. *Am J Psychiatry* 1973;130:165–170.

167. Conners CK. A teacher rating scale for use in drug studies with children. *Am J Psychiatry* 1969;126:152–156.

168. Gossop MR, Roy A. Hostility and drug dependence: its relation to specific drugs, and oral or intravenous use. *Br J Psychiatry* 1976;128:188–193.

169. Tinklenberg JR, Roth WT, Kopell BS, et al. *Cannabis* and alcohol effects on assaultiveness in adolescent delinquents. *Ann N Y Acad Sci* 1977;282:85–94.

170. Tinklenberg JR, Woodrow KM. Drug use among youthful assaultive and sexual offenders. In: Frazier SH, ed. *Aggression. Research Publication*

Association for Research in Nervous and Mental Disease. Baltimore: Williams & Wilkins, 1974;52:209–224.

171. Ellinwood EH, Rockwell WJK. Central nervous system stimulants and anorectic agents. In: Blackwell B, ed. *Meyler's side effects of drugs.* Amsterdam: Elsevier, 1988:1–26.

172. Abdallah AH. On the role of norepinephrine in the anorectic effect of *d*-amphetamine in mice. *Arch Int Pharmacodyn Ther* 1971;192:72–77.

173. Abdallah AH, Roby DM, Boeckler WH, et al. Role of dopamine in the anorexigenic effect of DITA, comparison with *d*-amphetamine. *Eur J Pharmacol* 1976;40:39–44.

174. Baez LA. Role of catecholamines in the anorectic effects of amphetamine in rats. *Psychopharmacologia* 1974;35:91–98.

175. Clineschmidt BV, McGuffin JC, Werner AB. Role of monoamines in the anorexigenic actions of fenfluramine, amphetamine, and *p*-chloromethamphetamine. *Eur J Pharmacol* 1974;27:313–323.

176. Frey H-H, Schulz R. On the central mediation of anorexigenic drug effects. *Biochem Pharmacol* 1973;22:3041–3049.

177. Heffner TG, Zigmond MJ, Stricker EM. Effects of dopaminergic agonists and antagonists on feeding in intact and 6-hydroxydopamine-treated rats. *J Pharmacol Exp Ther* 1977;201:386–399.

178. Holtzman SG, Jewett RE. The role of brain norepinephrine in the anorexic effects of dextroamphetamine and monoamine oxidase inhibitors in the rat. *Psychopharmacologia* 1971;22:151–161.

179. Kruk ZL, Smith LA, Zarrindast MR. Antagonism of responses to anorectics by selective receptor blockers. *Br J Pharmacol* 1976;58:468–469.

180. Mantegazza P, Naimzada KM, Riva M. Effects of propranolol on some activities of amphetamine. *Eur J Pharmacol* 1968;4:25–30.

181. Schmitt H. Influence d'agents interferant avec les catecholamines et la 5-hydroxytryptamine sur les effets anorexigenes de l'amphetamine et de la fenfluramine. *J Pharmacol (Paris)* 1973;4:285–294.

182. Clineschmidt BV, McGuffin JC, Pflueger AB, et al. A 5-hydroxytryptamine-like mode of anorectic action for 6-chloro-2-(1-piperazinyl]-pyrazine (MK-212). *Br J Pharmacol* 1978;62:579–589.

183. Clineschmidt BV, Zacchei AG, Totaro JA, et al. Fenfluramine and brain serotonin. *Ann N Y Acad Sci* 1978;305:222–241.

184. Kruk ZL. Dopamine and 5-hydroxy-tryptamine inhibit feeding in rats. *Nature* 1973;246:52–53.

185. Samanin R, Bendotti C, Bernasconi S, et al. Differential role of brain monoamines in the activity of anorectic drugs. In: Garattini S, Samanin R, eds. *Central mechanisms of anorectic drugs.* New York: Raven Press, 1977:233–242.

186. Fibiger HC, Zis AP, McGeer EG. Feeding and drinking deficits after 6-hydroxydopamine administration in the rat: similarities to the lateral hypothalamic syndrome. *Brain Res* 1973;55:135.

187. Hollister AS, Ervin GN, Cooper Br, Breese GR. The roles of monoamine neural systems in the anorexia induced by (+)-amphetamine and related compounds. *Neuropharmacology* 1975;14:715–723.

188. Samanin R, Bernassconi S, Garattini S. The effect of selective lesioning of brain catecholamine-containing neurons on the activity of various anorectics in the rat. *Eur J Pharmacol* 1975;34:373–375.

189. Glick SD. Brain damage and changes in drug sensitivity. In: Glick SD, Goldfarb J, eds. *Behavioral pharmacology.* St. Louis, MO: CV Mosby, 1976:97.

190. Blundell JE, Leshem MB. Central action of anorexic agents: effects of amphetamine and fenfluramine in rats with lateral hypothalamic lesions. *Eur J Pharmacol* 1974;28:81–88.

191. Carlisle HJ. Differential effects of amphetamine on food and water intake in rats with lateral hypothalamic lesions. *J Comp Physiol Psychol* 1964;58:47–54.

192. Russek M, Rodriguez-Zendejas AM, Teitelbaum P. The action of adrenergic anorexigenic substances on rats recovered from lateral hypothalamic lesions. *Physiol Behav* 1973;10:329–333.

193. Carey RJ, Goodall EB. Attenuation of amphetamine anorexia by unilateral nigral striatal lesions. *Neuropharmacology* 1975;14:827.

194. Barrett AM, McSharry L. Inhibition of drug-induced anorexia in rats by methysergide. *J Pharm Pharmcol* 1975;27:889–895.

195. Blundell JE, Latham CJ, Leshem MB. Biphasic action of a 5-hydroxytryptamine inhibitor on fenfluramine-induced anorexia. *J Pharm Pharmacol* 1973;25:492–494.

196. Funderburk WH, Hazelwood JC, Ruckart RT, et al. Is 5-hydroxytryptamine involved in the mechanism of action of fenfluramine? *J Pharm Pharmacol* 1971;23:468–470.

197. Garattini S, Buczko W, Jori A, et al. The mechanism of fenfluramine. *Postgrad Med J* 1975;51[Suppl 1]:27–35.

198. Garattini S, Bizzi A, De Gaetano G, et al. Recent advances in the pharmacology of anorectic agents. In: Howard I, ed. *Recent advances in obesity research.* London: Newman Publishing, 1975:354–367.

199. Jespersen S, Scheel-Kruger J. Evidence for a difference in mechanism of action between fenfluramine- and amphetamine-induced anorexia. *J Pharm Pharmacol* 1973;25:49–54.

200. Duhalt J, Boulanger M, Voisin C, et al. Fenfluramine and 5-hydroxytryptamine. Part 2: involvement of brain 5-hydroxytryptamine in the anorectic activity of fenfluramine. *Arzneimittelforschung* 1975;25:1758–1762.

201. Ghezzi D, Samanin R, Bernasconi S, et al. Effect of thymoleptics of fenfluramine-induced depletion of brain serotonin in rats. *Eur J Pharmacol* 1973;24:205–210.

202. Clineschmidt BV. 5,6-Dihydroxytryptamine: suppression of the anorexigenic action of fenfluramine. *Eur J Pharmacol* 1973;24:405.

203. Vree TB, Henderson PTH. Pharmacokinetics of amphetamines: *in vivo* and *in vitro* studies of the factors governing their elimination. In: Cadwell J, ed. *Amphetamines and related stimulants: chemical, biological, clinical, and social aspects.* Boca Raton, FL: CRC Press, 1980.

204. Caldwell J. Metabolism of amphetamines in mammals. *Drug Metab Rev* 1976;5:219.

205. Dring LG, Smith RL, Williams RT. The metabolic fate of amphetamine in man and other species. *Biochem J* 1970;116:425.

206. Sever PW, Dring LG, Williams RT. Urinary metabolites of *p*-hydroxyamphetamine in man, rat and guinea pig. *Xenobiotica* 1976;6:345.

207. Iversen LL. *The uptake and storage of noradrenaline in sympathetic nerves.* Cambridge: Cambridge University Press, 1967.

208. Gill JR, Mason DT, Bartter FC. Effects of hydroxyamphetamine (Paredrine) on the function of the sympathetic nervous system in normotensive subjects. *J Pharmacol Exp Ther* 1967;155:288.

209. Taylor WA, Sulser F. Effects of amphetamine and its hydroxylated metabolites on central noradrenergic mechanisms. *J Pharmacol Exp Ther* 1973;185:620.

210. Jenner P, Testa B. The influence of stereochemical factors on drug disposition. *Drug Metab Rev* 1973;2:117.

211. Goldstein M, Anagoste B. The conversion *in vivo* of *d*-amphetamine to *p*-hydroxynorephedrine. *Biochim Biophys Acta* 1965;107:166–168.

212. Lewander T. Displacement of brain and heart noradrenaline by *p*-hydroxyephedrine after administration of *p*-hydroxyamphetamine. *Acta Pharmacol Toxicol* 1971;29:20–32.

213. Caldwell J. Round table discussion on mechanisms of amphetamine deamination. In: Gorrod JW, ed. *Biological oxidation of nitrogen.* Amsterdam: Elsevier/North Holland, 1978:495

214. Wright J, Cho AK, Gal J. The role of *N*-hydroxyamphetamine in the metabolic deamination of amphetamine. *Life Sci* 1977;20:467.

215. Beckett AH, Al-Saraj S. The mechanism of oxidation of amphetamine enantiomorphs by liver microsomal preparations from different species. *J Pharm Pharmacol* 1972;24:174.

216. Castagnoli N Jr. Drug metabolism: review of principles and the fate of one-ring psychotomimetics. In: Iversen LL, Iversen SD, Snyderman SH, eds. *Handbook of psychopharmacology,* vol. 11. *Stimulants.* New York: Plenum Press, 1978:335–387.

217. Franklin MR. The formation of a 455 nm complex during cytochrome P-450-dependent *N*-hydroxyamphetamine metabolism. *Mol Pharmacol* 1974;10:975–985.

218. Franklin MR. Complexes of metabolites of amphetamines with hepatic cytochrome P-450. *Xenobiotica* 1974;5:133–142.

219. Franklin MR. Inhibition of the metabolism of *N*-substituted amphetamines by SKF 525-A and related compounds. *Xenobiotica* 1974;4:143–150.

220. James RC, Franklin MR. Comparisons of the formation of cytochrome P-450 complexes absorbing at 455 nm in rabbit and rat microsomes. *Biochem Pharmacol* 1975;24:835–838.

221. Cho AK, Wright J. Pathways of metabolism of amphetamine and related compounds. *Life Sci* 1978;22:363.

222. Mansuy D, Beaune P, Chottard JC, et al. The nature of the "455 absorbing complex" formed during cytochrome P-450 dependent oxidative metabolism of amphetamine. *Biochem Pharmacol* 1976;25:609–612.

223. Jonsson J. Hydroxylation of amphetamine to parahydroxyamphetamine by rat liver microsomes. *Biochem Pharmacol* 1974;23:3191.

224. Kuhn CM, Schanberg SM. Distribution and metabolism of amphetamine in tolerant animals. In: Ellinwood E, Kilbey M, eds. *Cocaine and other stimulants.* New York: Plenum Press, 1975:161–177.

225. Cook J, Schanberg SM. Effect of methamphetamine on norepinephrine metabolism in various regions of the brain. *J Pharmacol Exp Ther* 1975;194:87–93.

226. Thierry A, Javoy F, Glowinski S, et al. Effects of stress on the metabolism of norepinephrine, dopamine and serotonin in the central nervous system of the rat. I. Modification of norepinephrine turnover. *J Pharmacol Exp Ther* 1968;163:163–171.

227. Davidson C, Gow AJ, Lee TH, Ellinwood EH. Methamphetamine neurotoxicity: necrotic and apoptotic mechanisms and relevance to human abuse and treatment. *Brain Res Rev* 2001;36:1–22.

228. Bolanos JP, Almeida A, Stewart V, et al. Nitric oxide mediated mitochondrial damage in the brain: mechanisms and implications for neurodegenerative diseases. *J Neurochem* 1997;68:2227–2240.

229. Cubells JF, Rayport S, Rajendran G, et al. Methamphetamine neurotoxicity involves vacuolation of endocytic organelles and dopamine-dependent intracellular oxidative stress. *J Neurosci* 1994;14:2260.

230. Seiden LS, Ricaurte GA. Neurotoxicity of methamphetamine and related drugs. In: HY Meltzer ed. *Psychopharmacology: the third generation of progress.* New York: Raven Press, 1987:359–366.

231. Nash JF, Yamamoto BK. Methamphetamine neurotoxicity and striatal glutamate release: comparison to 3,4-methyl-enedioxymethamphetamin. *Brain Res* 1992;58:237–243.

232. Nash JF, Yamamoto BK. Effect of *d*-amphetamine on the extracellular concentrations of glutamate and dopamine in iprindole-treated rats. *Brain Res* 1993;627:1–8.

233. Stephans SE, Yamamoto BK. Methamphetamine-induced neurotoxicity: roles for glutamate and dopamine efflux. *Synapse* 1994;17:203–209.

234. Yamamoto BK, Zhu W. The effects of methamphetamine on the production of free radicals and oxidative stress. *J Pharmacol Exp Ther* 1998;287:107–114.

235. Beckman JS, Beckman TW, Chen J, et al. Apparent hydroxyl radical production by peroxynitrite: implications for endothelial injury from nitric oxide and supraoxide. *Proc Natl Acad Sci U S A* 1990;87:1620–1624.

236. Chance B, Williams GR. The respiratory chain and oxidative phosphorylation. *Adv Enzymol* 1956;17:65.

237. Lemasters JJ, Qian T, Bradham CA, et al. Mitochondrial dysfunction in the pathogenesis of necrotic and apoptotic cell death. *J Bioenerg Biomembr* 1999:31:305–319.

238. Murphy AN, Fiskum G, Beal MF. Mitochondria in neurodegneration: bioenergetic function in cell life and death. *J Cereb Blood Flow Metab* 1999;19:231–245.

239. Ricaurte GA, Seiden LS, Schuster CR. Further evidence that amphetamines produce long-lasting dopamine neurochemical deficits by destroying dopamine nerve fibers. *Brain Res* 1984;303:359–364.

240. Tonge SR. Noradrenaline and 5-hydroxytryptamine metabolism in six areas of rat brain during post-amphetamine depression. *Psychopharmacologia* 1974;38:181–186.

241. Harris E, Baldessarini R. Amphetamine-induced inhibition of tyrosine hydroxylation in homogenates of rat corpus striatum. *J Pharm Pharmacol* 1973;25:755–757.

242. Woolverton WL, Ricuarte GA, Forno LS, et al. Long-term effects of chronic methamphetamine administration in rhesus monkeys. *Brain Res* 1989;486:73–78.

243. Melaga WP, Quintana J, Raleigh MJ, et al. 6-[^{18}F]fluoro-L-DOPA-PET studies show partial reversibility of long-term effects of chronic amphetamine in monkeys. *Synapse* 1996;22:63–69.

244. Melaga WP, Raleigh MJ, Stout DB, et al. Ethological and 6-[^{18}F]fluoro-L-DOPA-PET profiles of long-term vulnerability to chronic amphetamine. *Behav Brain Res* 1997;84:259–268.

245. Villemagne V, Yuan J, Wong DF, et al. Brain dopamine neurotoxicity in baboons treated with doses of methamphetamine comparable to those recreationally abused by humans: evidence from [11C]WIN 35,428 positron emission tomography studies and direct *in vitro* determinations. *J Neurosci* 1998;18:419–427.

246. Hotchkiss AJ, Morgan ME, Gibb JW. The long-term effects of multiple doses of methamphetamine on neostriatal tryptophan hydroxylase, tyrosine hydroxylase, choline acetyltransferase and glutamate decarboxylase activities. *Life Sci* 1979;25:1373–1378.

247. Ricaurte GA, Schuster CR, Seiden LS. Long-term effects of repeated methylamphetamine administration on dopamine and serotonin neurons in the rat brain: a regional study. *Brain Res* 1980;193:153–163.

248. Ricaurte GA, Guillery RW, Seiden LS, et al. Dopamine nerve terminal degeneration produced by high doses of methylamphetamine in the rat brain. *Brain Res* 1982;235:93–103.

249. Duarte-Escalante O, Ellinwood EH Jr. Central nervous system cytopathological changes in cat with chronic methedrine intoxication. *Brain Res* 1970;21:151–155.

250. Seiden LS, Fischman MW, Schuster CR. Changes in brain catecholamines induced by long-term methamphetamine administration in rhesus monkeys. In: Ellinwood E, Kilbey M, eds. *Cocaine and other*

stimulants. New York: Plenum Press, 1977:179–185.

251. Brown P, Molliver ME. Dual serotonin (5-HT) projections to the nucleus accumbens core and shell: relation of the 5-HT transporter to the amphetamine-induced neurotoxicity. *J Neurosci* 2000;20:1952–1963.

252. Cass WA. Attenuation and recovery of evoked overflow of striatal serotonin in rats treated with neurotoxic dose of methamphetamine. *J Neurochem* 2000;74:1079–1085.

253. Harvey JA, McMaster SE. Fenfluramine: evidence for a neurotoxic action on a long-term depletion of serotonin. *Comm Psychopharmacol* 1975;1:217–228.

254. Harvey JA, McMaster SE. Cumulative neurotoxicity after chronic treatment with low dosages in the rat. *Comm Psychopharmacol* 1977;1:3–17.

255. Kleven MS, Schuster CR, Seiden LS. The effect of depletion of brain serotonin by repeated fenfluramine on neurochemical and anorectic effects of acute serotonin. *J Pharmacol Exp Ther* 1988;246:1–7.

256. Schuster CR, Lewis M, Seiden LS. Fenfluramine. neurotoxicity. *Psychopharmacol Bull* 1986;22:148–151.

257. Steranka LR. Long-term decreases in striatal dopamine 3,4-dihydroxyphenylacetic acid after a single injection of amphetamine: time-course and time-dependent interactions with amfonelic acid. *Brain Res* 1982;234:123–126.

258. Appel NM, De Souza EB. Fenfluramine selectively destroys serotonin terminals in brain. Immunocytological evidence. *Soc Neurosci* 1988;14:556.

259. Rumbaugh CL. Small vessel cerebral vascular changes following chronic amphetamine intoxication. In: Ellinwood E, Kilbey M, eds. *Cocaine and other stimulants.* New York: Plenum Press, 1977:241–251.

260. Kalant H, Kalant O. Death in amphetamine users: causes and rates. In: Smith DE, ed. *Amphetamine use, misuse, and abuse.* Boston: G. K. Hall, 1979:169–188.

261. Richards HGH, Stephens A. Sudden death associated with the taking of amphetamines. *Med Sci Law* 1973;13:35–38.

262. Gessa GL, Clay GA, Brodie BB. Evidence that hyperthermia produced by *d*-amphetamine is caused by peripheral action of the drug. *Life Sci* 1969;8:135–141.

263. Haefely W, Bartholini G, Pletscher A. Monoaminergic drugs: general pharmacology. *Pharmacol Ther* 1976;2:185–218.

264. Jellinek P. Dual effect of dexam-

phetamine on body temperature in the rat. *Eur J Pharmacol* 1971;15:389–392.

265. Jacob J, Snaudeau C, Michaud G. Actions de la noradrenaline, de la dopamine, de l'isopropyladrenaline et de la 5-hydroxytryptamine administre par voie intracisternale et souscutanee sur la temperature du rat eveille. *J Pharmacol (Paris)* 1971;2:401–422.

266. McCullough D, Milberg J, Robinson SM. A central site for the hypothermic effects of (+)-amphetamine sulfate and *p*-hydroxyamphetamine hydrobromide in mice. *Br J Pharmacol* 1970;40:219–226.

267. Pitts FN Jr. The use of dextroamphetamine in mentally ill depressed patients. *J Clin Psychiatry* 1982;43:438.

268. Holmes VF, Fernandez F, Levy JK. Psychostimulant response in AIDS-related complex patients. *J Clin Psychiatry* 1989;50(1):5–8.

269. Calia KA, Grothe DR, Elia J. Attention-deficit hyperactivity disorder. *Clin Pharm* 1990;9:632–642.

270. Henker B, Whalen CK. Hyperactivity and attention deficits. *Am Psychol* 1989;44:216–223.

271. Meller W, Lyle K. Attention deficit disorder in childhood. *Prim Care* 1987;14:745–759.

272. Biederman J, Spencer T. Attention-deficit/hyperactivity disorder (ADHD) as a noradrenergic disorder. *Biol Psychiatry* 1999;46:1234–1242.

273. Klein RG, Mannozza S. Long-term outcome of hyperactive children: a review. *J Am Acad Child Adolesc Psychiatry* 1991;30:383–387.

274. Pary R, Lewis S, Matuschka PR, et al. Attention-deficit/hyperactivity disorder: an update. *South Med J* 2002;95:743–749.

275. Shenker A. The mechanism of action of drugs used to treat attention-deficit disorder hyperactivity disorder: focus on catecholamine receptor pharmacology. In: Barness LA, ed. *Advances in pediatrics.* St. Louis: Mosby Year Book, 1992;39:337–382.

276. Hart-Santora D, Hart L. Clonidine in attention-deficit hyperactivity disorder. *Ann Pharmacol* 1992;26:37–39.

277. Saffer DJ. Major treatment considerations for attention-deficit hyperactivity disorder. *Curr Prob Pediatr* 1995;25:137–143.

278. Simeon JG, Wiggins DM. Pharmacotherapy for attention-deficit hyperactivity disorder. *Can J Psychiatry* 1993;38:443–448.

279. Vinson DC. Therapy for attention-deficit hyperactivity disorder. *Arch Fam Med* 1994;3:445–451.

280. Brown RT, Wynne ME, Borden KA, et al. Methylphenidate and cognitive therapy in children with attention deficit

disorder: a double-blind trial. *J Dev Behav Pediatr* 1986;7:163–174.

281. Horn WF, Ialongo NS, Pascoe JM, et al. Additive effects of psychostimulants, parent training, and self-control therapy with ADHD children. *J Am Acad Child Adolesc Psychiatry* 1991;30:233–240.

282. Ialongo NS, Horn WF, Pascoe JM, et al. The effects of a multimodal intervention with attention-deficit hyperactivity disorder children: a 9-month follow-up. *J Am Acad Child Adolesc Psychiatry* 1993;32:182–189.

283. Elia J, Borcherding BG, Rapoport JL, et al. Methylphenidate and dextroamphetamine treatments of hyperactivity: are there true nonresponders? *Psych Res* 1991;36:141–155.

284. Pelham WE, Greenslade KE, Vodde-Hamilton M, et al. Relative efficacy of long-acting stimulants on children with attention deficit-hyperactivity disorder: a comparison of standard methylphenidate, sustained-release methylphenidate, sustained-release dextroamphetamine, and pemoline. *Pediatrics* 1990;86:226–237.

285. Matochik JA, Liebenauer LL, King AC, et al. Cerebral glucose metabolism in adults with attention deficit hyperactivity disorder after chronic stimulant treatment. *Am J Psychiatry* 1994;151:658–664.

286. Spencer T, Wilens T, Biederman J, et al. A double-blind, crossover comparison of methylphenidate and placebo in adults with childhood-onset attention-deficit hyperactivity disorder. *Arch Gen Psychiatry* 1995;52:434–443.

287. Spencner T, Biderman J, Wilens T, et al. Efficacy of a mixed amphetamine salts compound in adults with attention-deficit/hyperactivity disorder. *Arch Gen Psychiatry* 2001;58:775–782.

288. Willens TE, Spencer TJ, Biederman J. A review of the pharmacotherapy of adults with attention-deficit/hyperactivity disorder. *J Atten Disord* 2002;5:189–202.

289. Dickinson LD, Lee J, Ringdah IC, et al. Impaired growth in hyperkinetic children receiving pemoline. *J Pediatr* 1979;94:538.

290. Roche AF, Lipman RS, Overall JE, et al. The effects of stimulant medication of growth of hyperkinetic children. *Pediatrics* 1979;63:847.

291. Safer JJ, Allen RP, Barr E. Growth rebound after termination of stimulant drugs. *J Pediatr* 1975;86:709.

292. Biederman J, Wilens TE, Mick E, et al. Does attention-deficit/hyperactivity disorder impact the developmental course of drug and alcohol abuse and dependence? *Biol Psychiatry* 1998;44:269–273.

293. Biederman J, Wilens TE, Mick E,

et al. Pharmacotherapy of attention-deficit/hyperactivity disorder reduces the risk for substance use disorder. *Pediatrics* 1999;104:e20.

294. Levin FR, Kleber HD. Attention-deficit hyperactivity disorder and substance abuse: relationships an implications for treatment. *Harv Rev Psychiatry* 1995;2:246–258.

295. Hunt RD. Treatment effects of oral and transdermal clonidine in relation to methylphenidate: an open pilot study in ADD-H. *Psychopharmacol Bull* 1987;23:111–114.

296. Hunt RD, Capper L, O'Connell P. Clonidine in child and adolescent psychiatry. *J Child Adolesc Psychopharmacol* 1990;1:87–102.

297. Hunt RD, Minderra RB, Cohen DJ. Clonidine benefits children with attention deficit disorder and hyperactivity: report of a double-blind placebo-crossover therapeutic trial. *J Am Acad Child Psychiatry* 1985;24:617–629.

298. Willens TE, Biederman J, Spencer T. Clonidine for sleep disturbances associated with attention-deficit hyperactivity disorder. *J Am Acad Child Adolesc Psychiatry* 1994;33:424–426.

299. Pliszka SR. Tricyclic antidepressants in the treatment of children with attention deficit disorder. *J Am Acad Child Psychiatry* 1987;26:127–132.

300. Riddle MA, Geller B, Ryan N. Another sudden death in a child treated with desipramine. *J Am Acad Child Psychiatry* 1993;32:792–795.

301. Zametkin AJ, Rapoport JL, Murphy DL, et al. Treatment of hyperactive children with monoamine oxidase inhibitors I. Clinical efficacy. *Arch Gen Psychiatry* 1985;42:962–966.

302. Zametkin AJ, Rapoport JL. Neurobiology of attention deficit disorder with hyperactivity: where have we come in 50 years? *J Am Acad Child Psychiatry* 1987;26:676–686.

303. Zametkin AJ, Rapoport JL. Noradrenergic hypothesis of attention deficit disorder with hyperactivity: a critical review. In: Meltzer HY, ed. *Psychopharmacology: the third generation of progress.* New York: Raven Press, 1987:837–842.

304. Scoville BA. Review of amphetamine-like drugs by the Food and Drug Administration. In: Bray GA, ed. *Obesity in perspective.* DHEW Publication No. NIH (75–707). Washington, DC: US Department of Health, Education and Welfare, 1975:441–443.

305. Stunkard A, McLaren-Hume M. The results of treatment for obesity. *Arch Intern Med* 1959;103:79–85.

306. Gotestam KG, Gunne L. Subjective effects of two anorexigenic agents, fenfluramine and AN 448, in amphetamine-dependent subjects. *Br J Addict* 1972;67:39–44.

307. Weintraub M, Sundaresan PR, Schuster B, et al. Long-term weight control study III (weeks 104 to 156). *Clin Pharmacol Ther* 1992;51:602–607.

308. Working Party of the British Medical Association. Control of amphetamine preparations. *Br J Psychiatry* 1968;114:572–573.

309. Hollister LE. Drugs for mental disorders of old age. *JAMA* 1975;6:195–198.

310. Wheatley D. Amphetamines in general practice: their use in depression and anxiety. *Semin Psychiatry* 1969;1:163–173.

311. Satel SL, Nelson JC. Stimulants in the treatment of depression: a critical overview. *J Clin Psychiatry* 1989;50(7):241–249.

312. Chiarello RJ, Cole JO. The use of psychostimulants in general psychiatry. *Arch Gen Psychiatry* 1987;44:286–295.

313. Fawcett JF, Busch KA. Stimulants in psychiatry. In: Schatzberg AF, Nemeroff CB, eds. *The American Psychiatric Press textbook of psychopharmacology.* Washington, DC: American Psychiatric Press, 1995:417–435.

314. Ayd FJ, Zohar J. Psychostimulant (amphetamine of methylphenidate) therapy for chronic and treatment-resistant depression. In: Zohar J, Belmaker RH, eds. New York: PMA Publishing, 1987:343–355.

315. Lazarus LW, Winemiller DR, Lingam VR, et al. Efficacy and side effects of methylphenidate for poststroke depression. *J Clin Psychiatry* 1992;53:447–449.

316. Angrist B, D'Hollosy M, Sanfilipo M, et al. Central nervous system stimulants as symptomatic treatments for AIDS-related neuropsychiatric impairment. *J Clin Psychopharmacol* 1992;12:268–272.

317. Blum K. *Handbook of abusable drugs.* New York: Gardner, 1984:306–312.

318. Gawin FH, Ellinwood EH. Cocaine and other stimulants. *N Engl J Med* 1988;318:1173.

319. Grinspoon L, Hedblom P. *The speed culture.* Cambridge, MA: Harvard University Press, 1975.

320. Kato M. Epidemiology of drug dependency in Japan. In: Zarafonetis CJD, ed. *Drug abuse: proceedings of an international conference.* Philadelphia: Lea & Febiger, 1972:67–72.

321. Goldberg L. Epidemiology of drug abuse in Sweden. In: Zarafonetis CJD, ed. *Drug abuse: proceedings of an international conference.* Philadelphia: Lea & Febiger, 1972:27–66.

322. Cho AK. Ice: a new dosage form of an old drug. *Science* 1990;249:631–634.

323. Chance MRA. A peculiar form of social behavior induced in mice by amphetamine. *Behaviour* 1946;1:60–70.

324. Chance MRA. Aggregation as a factor influencing the toxicity of sympathomimetic amines in mice. *J Pharmacol Exp Ther* 1946;87:214–219.

325. Ellinwood EH Jr. Amphetamine and stimulant drugs. In: *Drug use in America: problem in perspective. Second report, Marihuana and Drug Abuse Commission.* 1973:140–157.

326. Smith R. *The marketplace of speed: violence and compulsive methamphetamine abuse. Final report of the Amphetamine Research Project to the National Institute on Mental Health.* Washington, DC: National Institute on Mental Health, 1972.

327. O'Conner MM. The arrest of doctors, pharmacists, and other medical licentiates. In: Smith DE, ed. *Amphetamine use, misuse, and abuse.* Boston: G. K. Hall, 1979:297–302.

328. Smith R. The world of the Haight-Ashbury speed freak. *J Psychedelic Drugs* 1969:172–188.

329. Sadusk JR. Non-narcotic addiction: size and extent of the problem. *JAMA* 1966;196:707–709.

330. Ellinwood EH, Lee TH. Dose- and time-dependent effects of stimulants. *NIDA Res Monogr Ser* 1989;94:323–340.

331. Pavlov IP. *Conditioned reflexes.* New York: Dover Publications, 1970.

332. Fischman MW, Schuster CR, Resnekov L, et al. Cardiovascular and subjective effects of intravenous cocaine administration in humans. *Arch Gen Psychiatry* 1976;33:983–989.

333. Javaid JI, Fischman MW, Schuster CR, et al. Cocaine plasma concentration: effects in humans. *Science* 1978;202:227–228.

334. Connell PH. *Amphetamine psychosis. Maudsley monograph number 5.* London: Oxford University Press, 1958.

335. Ellinwood EH Jr. Amphetamine psychosis. I. Description of the individuals and process. *J Nerv Ment Disord* 1967;144:273.

336. Snyder SH. Catecholamines in the brain as mediators of amphetamine psychosis. *Arch Gen Psychiatry* 1972;27:169.

337. Davis JM, Schlemmer RF Jr. The amphetamine psychosis. In: Caldwell J, ed. *Amphetamines and related stimulants: chemical, biological, clinical, and sociological aspects.* Boca Raton, FL: CRC Press, 1980:161–173.

338. Shuckit MA. *Drug and alcohol abuse: a clinical guide to diagnosis and treatment,* 4th ed. New York: Plenum, 1995:118–144.

339. Dackis CA, Gold MS. Pharmacological

approaches to cocaine addiction. *J Subst Abuse Treat* 1985;2:139–145.

340. Dackis CA, Gold MS, Sweeney DR, et al. Single-dose bromocriptine reverses cocaine craving. *Psychiatry Res* 1987;20:261–264.

341. Giannini AJ, Baumgartel P, DiMarzio LR. Bromocriptine therapy in cocaine withdrawal. *J Clin Pharmacol* 1987;27:267–270.

342. Tennant FS Jr, Sagherian AA. Double-blind comparison of amantadine and bromocriptine for ambulatory withdrawal from cocaine dependence. *Arch Intern Med* 1987;147:109–112.

343. Ellinwood EH Jr. Amphetamine and cocaine. In: Jarvik ME, ed. *Psychopharmacology in the practice of medicine.* New York: Appleton-Century-Crofts, 1977:467–479.

344. Wilkins JN, Gorelick DA. Management of stimulant dependence and withdrawal. In: Miller NS, ed. *Principles of addiction medicine.* Chevy Chase, MD: American Society of Addiction Medicine, 1994:1–8.

345. Withers NW, Pulvirenti L, Koob GF, et al. Cocaine abuse and dependence. *J Clin Psychopharmacol* 1995;15:63–78.

346. Substance Abuse, Mental Health Services Administration. Reported by Associated Press, November 7, 1995.

347. Carroll KM, Rounsaville BJ, Gordon LT, et al. One-year follow-up of psychotherapy and pharmacotherapy for cocaine dependence. *Arch Gen Psychiatry* 1994;51:989–997.

348. Carroll KM, Rounsaville BJ, Gordon LT, et al. Psychotherapy and pharmacotherapy for ambulatory cocaine abusers. *Arch Gen Psychiatry* 1994;51:177–187.

349. Kokkinidis L, Zacharko RM, Predy PA. Post-amphetamine depression of self-stimulation responding from the substantia nigra: reversal by tricyclic antidepressants. *Pharmacol Biochem Behav* 1980;13:379–383.

350. Gawin FH, Kleber HD. Cocaine abuse treatment: open pilot trial with desipramine and lithium carbonate. *Arch Gen Psychiatry* 1984;41:321–327.

351. Giannini AJ, Malone DA, Giannini MC, et al. Treatment of depression in chronic cocaine and phencyclidine abuse with desipramine. *J Clin Pharmacol* 1986;26:211–214.

352. Tennant FS Jr, Rawson RA. Cocaine and amphetamine dependence treated with desipramine. *NIDA Res Monogr Ser* 1983;43:351–355.

353. Tennant FS Jr, Tarver AL. Double-blind comparison of desipramine and placebo in withdrawal from cocaine dependence. *NIDA Res Monogr Ser* 1984;55:159–163.

354. Bandura A. *Principles of behavior modification.* New York: Holt, Rinehart, and Winston, 1969.

355. Childress AR, McLellan AT, O'Brien CP. Abstinent opiate abusers exhibit conditioned craving. *Br J Addic* 1986;81:701–706.

356. Childress AR, McLellan AT, Ehrman R, et al. Extinction of conditioned responses in abstinent cocaine or opioid users. *NIDA Res Monogr Ser* 1987;76:189–195.

357. O'Brien CP, Childress AR, Arndt IO, et al. Pharmacological and behavioral treatments of cocaine dependence: controlled studies. *J Clin Psychiatry* 1988;49[Suppl]:17–22.

358. Hall WC, Talbert RL, Ereshefsky L. Cocaine abuse and its treatment. *Pharmacotherapy* 1990;10:47–65.

359. Kleber HD, Gawin FH. The spectrum of cocaine abuse and its treatment. *J Clin Psychiatry* 1984;45[12 Pt 2]:18–23.

360. Resnick RB, Resnick EB. Cocaine abuse and its treatment. *Psychiatr Clin North Am* 1984;7:713–728.

361. Davison M, McCarthy D. *The matching law: a research review.* Hillsdale, NJ: Erlbaum, 1988.

362. Carrol ME, Lac ST, Nygaard ST. A concurrently available nondrug reinforcer prevents the acquisition or decreases the maintenance of cocaine-reinforced behavior. *Psychopharmacology (Berl)* 1989;97:23–29.

363. Linnoila M, Virkkunen M, Scheinin M, et al. Low cerebrospinal fluid 5-hydroxyindoleacetic acid concentrations differentiates impulsive from nonimpulsive violent behavior. *Life Sci* 1983;33:2609–2614.

CHAPTER 17
Sedative–Hypnotics

DONALD R. WESSON, DAVID E. SMITH, WALTER LING, AND RICHARD B. SEYMOUR

Sedative–hypnotics are drugs and medications that have, as prominent pharmacologic effects, the ability to reduce anxiety or induce sleep. Medications that reduce anxiety without producing unwanted sedation are also called tranquilizers. Pharmacology alcohol and marihuana are classified as sedative-hypnotics; however, because alcohol and marihuana are also important drugs of abuse, alcohol and marihuana are usually treated separately. The sedative–hypnotics included in this chapter are prescription medications that are manufactured by pharmaceutical companies for treatment of medical disorders.

This chapter focuses on the benzodiazepines and newer sedative–hypnotics because they have largely replaced the short-acting barbiturates and older nonbarbiturate hypnotics in medical therapeutics. Abuse of older sedative–hypnotics has been greatly curtailed by controls on their availability, by the availability of new medications, and by changes in physician prescribing practices.

Some tricyclic antidepressants, such as amitriptyline, have sedation as a prominent side effect. Although not usually classified as sedative–hypnotics, they have properties that are sometimes used therapeutically as an alternative to classical sedative–hypnotics for treatment of insomnia. They are included in this chapter because they are prescription medications that are sometimes misused by drug addicts for their sedative effects.

Anticholinergics, commonly used to counteract the side effects of neuroleptic medication, can have sedative effects and some patients with schizophrenia take them in larger doses than prescribed. They are not widely abused, but are included here because alcoholics and other sedative–hypnotic abusers sometimes seek them for their sedative–hypnotic effects.

Sodium oxybate (also known as gamma hydroxybutyrate or GHB) is a sedative-hypnotic and a common drug of abuse. Sodium oxybate is now marketed for treatment of cataplexy associated with narcolepsy under the trade name Xyrem. Like alcohol, GHB abuse and dependence is often addressed separately from the sedative–hypnotics. Because both GHB and the benzodiazepine, Rohypnol, are called "date rape drugs," they may be associated in the public mind and in criminal law.

Although the use of sedative–hypnotics is ubiquitous in American society, mainstream society is ambivalent about the appropriate role of sedative–hypnotics. As a consequence, laws relating to sedative–hypnotics are complex, bewildering, and inconsistent. Alcohol is socially sanctioned as an intoxicant; marihuana—although still the focus of vigorous criminal prosecution and crop eradication in some states—is grudgingly tolerated; and medical prescription of sedative–hypnotics is increasingly subjected to controls (e.g., benzodiazepines have been put on triplicate prescription in New York, and because of its abuse, methaqualone has been removed from the American market).

Sedative–hypnotic abuse is often attributed to physicians' overprescribing. What constitutes overprescribing, however, is a complex judgment that is molded by beliefs about the cause and appropriate treatment of anxiety and insomnia. Because everyone has experienced anxiety or transient difficulty sleeping, almost everyone presumes expertise about the most appropriate treatment of these conditions. Most people formulate their ideas about appropriate use of sedative–hypnotics from their personal experience with them and from the experiences of family or friends. The unrecognized pitfall in their thinking is that people who have not experienced a pathologic anxiety disorder believe that everyone's anxiety is the same as theirs. For this reason, they may oppose treating anxiety or insomnia with medications.

Opposition to treating anxiety with tranquilizers also comes from psychotherapists. Psychotherapists with a psychodynamic orientation view anxiety as a secondary symptom of underlying psychopathology. Psychotherapeutic treatment is directed toward understanding and resolving the underlying reasons for anxiety. Because anxiety is a common symptom that causes people to seek psychotherapy, many psychodynamically oriented therapists oppose pharmacotherapy of anxiety because they are concerned that medication treatment will undermine their patients' motivation for psychotherapeutic work.

Drug abuse counselors also may oppose medication, particularly treatment with sedative–hypnotics. All mood-altering prescription medications are viewed as risky for a drug addict because the medication may trigger a return to drug-seeking behavior, particularly among recovering addicts who previously abused prescription medications. Even therapeutically prescribed medications that have little abuse potential in nondrug addicts, such as antidepressants, are viewed as risky because they may produce desirable sedative or stimulant effects in drug addicts and because it is easier to define a line of "complete abstinence" than to figure out which medications are or are not risky for a particular addict.

Within the context of recovery-oriented drug-abuse treatment, most counselors and nurses, and some physicians are themselves recovering addicts and alcoholics. Patients usually feel that the recovering addict or alcoholic is better able to understand their experience of addiction because "they have been there, and their knowledge does not just come from books." Furthermore, recovering treatment personnel provide a valuable role model and an affirmation that "recovery is possible." Recovering treatment personnel may, however, have difficulty with regard to use of medications. They may feel, for example, that their own recovery is jeopardized by patients who take medications that they may desire. If they did not use medications during their own early recovery, they may believe that medications are unnecessary or that the anxiety, mood, and sleep disturbances, common in early recovery, are events that the recovering addict needs to learn to cope with. Finally, many recovering addicts and alcoholics believe that physicians enabled their drug use or contributed to their relapse to drug use because they inappropriately prescribed psychotropic medications.

Although physicians may view disabling anxiety as a disease process, many people believe that physicians have been overly influenced by pharmaceutical companies' advertising that promotes all human misery and suffering as an illness amenable to pharmacologic treatment. Although few people would find moral value in withholding penicillin for pneumococcal pneumonia, many would view the pharmacotherapy of other people's anxiety objectionable from a moral perspective.

Pharmacologic Calvinism causes needless human suffering. Some people who could benefit from sedative–hypnotics do not seek medical treatment even when anxiety is disabling and treatment alternatives to medication are not accessible.

Physicians are often faulted for "giving in" to their patients' request (or demand) for sedative–hypnotics. Clinically experienced physicians know, however, that trying to talk some patients out of taking sedative–hypnotics is futile, even when the distress is because of family discord, grief, an intolerable life situation, or an acute loss. When a physician refuses a patient's request for sedative–hypnotic medication, the patient generally concludes that the physician does not understand the severity of the patient's distress and consults another physician. The physician–patient transaction is often further distorted by patients who are drug dependent (1).

Prescribing guidelines for therapeutic use of benzodiazepines is beyond the scope of this chapter. The benzodiazepines remain therapeutically useful, although some of the conditions for which they were commonly prescribed (such as treatment for panic attacks, generalized anxiety disorder, and insomnia) have been largely supplanted by other medications.

BENZODIAZEPINES

Benzodiazepine use and abuse continues to generate professional controversy, legislative hearings, and articles in the lay press. Because of psychiatrists' concerns about benzodiazepine dependence, the American Psychiatric Association formed a task force that reviewed the issue and published a report in book form (2). Legislative concern about benzodiazepines generally involves benzodiazepines' contribution to the cost of medical care or to benzodiazepine abuse and dependence.

Abuse is a difficult concept when applied to prescription medications. In common use, concepts of drug abuse, misuse, and addiction are deeply rooted in social values and attitudes and have been inconsistently encoded into laws. For example, moderate use of alcohol is widely sanctioned for adults; but public intoxication or driving with an alcohol blood level above 0.8 to 1 mg/100 mL is generally considered alcohol abuse. Any use of prescription medications to produce intoxication is generally considered abuse, although it would not necessarily qualify as "abuse" according to criteria of the *Diagnostic and Statistical Manual of Mental Disorders*, 4th ed., text revision (*DSM–IV–TR*) (3).

The term *misuse* is commonly applied to prescription sedative–hypnotics, but unlike abuse and dependence, *DSM–IV–TR* does not provide specific criteria for misuse. When medications are taken in higher doses or more frequently than prescribed, or taken by someone other than the person for whom the medication was prescribed, or taken for reasons other than what would normally be considered medical use, the behavior is generally considered misuse of the medication.

DSM–IV–TR defines abuse and dependence in terms of behavioral and physiologic consequences to the person taking the medication. The criteria for abuse and dependence apply as uniformly as possible across classes of drugs, and the criteria do not distinguish the source of the medication or the intended purpose for which it was taken. Furthermore, when most people, including physicians, speak of drug *dependence*, they are referring to *physical dependence*. *DSM–IV–TR* uses the term *dependence* to denote a more severe form of substance use disorder than *abuse*, and uses the specifier "with or without physiological dependence," to indicate whether or not the patient has significant physical dependence. Physiologic dependence is not required for a *DSM–IV–TR* diagnosis of "drug dependence." A diagnosis of substance dependence is only made when a patient has dysfunctional behaviors that are a result of the drug use.

The qualification that the dysfunctional behavior be the result of drug use is extremely important, but in a practical sense, is often difficult to establish with certainty. In considering the diagnosis of sedative–hypnotic dependence among patients who are being treated for an anxiety disorder, it is not always possible to ascertain with certainty whether the behavioral dysfunction is produced by the underlying psychiatric disorder or by the drug use. Different attribution is often the basis of disagreement among psychiatrists, patients, and patient families. A patient whose "panic attacks" are ameliorated by a medication may exhibit what may be interpreted as "drug-seeking behavior" if their access to the medication is threatened.

In a regulatory context, "benzodiazepine abuse" can mean many things: self-administration of a benzodiazepine to produce intoxication; or long-term prescription of benzodiazepines at therapeutic doses to patients who subsequently develop physical dependence on the benzodiazepines; or patients' escalating their dose of benzodiazepines beyond that prescribed by their physicians; or use of a benzodiazepine by heroin or cocaine addicts to self-medicate symptoms of heroin withdrawal or cocaine toxicity; or intentional benzodiazepine overdose in a suicide or suicide attempt.

Legislative hearings often use data from the National Institute on Drug Abuse's Drug Abuse Warning Network (DAWN). DAWN is a national reporting system that tabulates "mentions" of psychotropic medications and drugs from patients treated in participating emergency rooms. In DAWN, drug abuse is defined as "the nonmedical use of a substance to obtain its psychic effect, or the use of a drug because of drug dependence, or the use of a drug to commit suicide, or the use of a medication inconsistent with accepted medical practice."

Effective legislative strategies for reducing or preventing benzodiazepine abuse must focus on the different behaviors that are often lumped together in a general category of "benzodiazepine abuse." The various forms of benzodiazepine abuse delineated above differ in their risk to public health and social cost, and they need different prevention and treatment approaches.

Epidemiology of Benzodiazepine Abuse

The incidence and prevalence of benzodiazepine abuse depend on how abuse is defined. If any nonmedical use of a benzodiazepine is defined as abuse, then benzodiazepine abuse is common. If, however, *DSM–IV–TR* criteria are used, the prevalence of abuse is much lower.

Given the frequency with which benzodiazepines are prescribed, the rates of their abuse, even those such as alprazolam that are widely prescribed, is remarkably low (4). The abuse of benzodiazepines and other sedative–hypnotics is, however, a significant problem among some subgroups of patients, such as those on methadone maintenance (5–7). Benzodiazepine abuse, particularly flunitrazepam abuse, is associated with death of patients treated with buprenorphine (Buprenex) (8,9).

Benzodiazepines are generally not primary drugs of abuse; that is, they are rarely taken by themselves to produce intoxication. Most people who take benzodiazepines do so for anxiolysis or sleep induction. After chronic use, they may also be taking them to ameliorate benzodiazepine withdrawal symptoms. Some alcoholic and sedative–hypnotic abusers find the subjective effects of benzodiazepines desirable, but even among this population, benzodiazepines are rarely used alone to produce intoxication.

The subjective effects of benzodiazepines on nondrug addicts have similarities to alcohol. In a double-blind, crossover study (10), intravenous diazepam 0.12 mg/kg (or 72 mg in a 60-kg person), intravenous diazepam 0.20 mg/kg (or 120 mg in a 60-kg person), and alcohol 0.75 mg/kg (about three shots of 86-proof liquor) were compared on various subjective and performance measures. On the Subjective High Assessment Scale, a visual analogue scale, peak subjective "drug effects," "drunk" and "high," were not statistically different between the low-dose diazepam and the alcohol dose. The higher dose of diazepam produced statistically greater effects on most scales except "drunk" and "nauseated," and the higher dose of diazepam produced greater impairment on all measures of performance. In normal-subject challenge studies, benzodiazepines generally produce dose-dependent increases in self-report levels of sedation and fatigue (11).

Benzodiazepines are commonly self-administered by drug addicts, sometimes to ameliorate withdrawal from heroin, alcohol, or other drugs or to attenuate the side effects of cocaine or methamphetamine intoxication. Addicts may also combine benzodiazepines with heroin, marihuana, or alcohol to enhance their effects.

During the first half of the 1990s, flunitrazepam (Rohypnol) gained popularity among some adolescents, particularly in Florida and Texas, as a drug that could be taken at school without the telltale odor of alcohol or marihuana.

Flunitrazepam is an effective hypnotic marketed in many countries for treatment of insomnia. Although not marketed in the United States or Canada, 1- and 2-mg tablets of flunitrazepam are available by prescription in Mexico, in Central and South America, and in many countries in Europe, Asia, and Africa. Until 1996, small quantities of flunitrazepam could be brought legally into the United States, but flunitrazepam is now subject to confiscation by U.S. Customs. Flunitrazepam abuse is most visible in Florida and Texas, although sporadic reports from drug-abuse treatment clinics and police seizures of flunitrazepam in other areas suggest a broader distribution. Street names of flunitrazepam vary by region. In Florida, flunitrazepam is most often referred to as "roSHAY" or "roofies;" in Texas, it is often called "Roche." In the street-drug marketplace, deception is common, and many different kinds of tablets are being sold under these street names.

The popular media has given flunitrazepam abuse considerable attention in the United States. Newspapers and television coverage have focused on its use for "date rape." While the publicity is framed to warn women that men may slip flunitrazepam into their drinks, another potential result of the publicity is to instruct unscrupulous men in its use.

A study of "Roche" abuse along the Texas–Mexico border from Brownsville to Laredo found that flunitrazepam abuse was only one of many benzodiazepines being abused (12). Although users in the area prefer white tablets imprinted with Roche and the number 2, many were not specifically seeking Rohypnol. From users' descriptions of the tablets and from police seizures of tablets at schools, it appears that many users are taking Rivotril (the trade name for clonazepam marketed in Mexico), Lexotán (the trade name for bromazepam, another benzodiazepine-hypnotic marketed in Mexico), and Valium (the trade name for diazepam), which is different in appearance from the Valium marketed in the United States. There is a great deal of misinformation among users, school nurses, police, and drug-treatment personnel about what "Roche" tablets are. Many users believe that "Roche" is the name of the drug. Some thought that the tablets were animal tranquilizers. Many users who had heard about Rohypnol thought all white tablets imprinted with "Roche" and the number 2 were Rohypnol.

Medical Uses of Benzodiazepines

Benzodiazepines have many important medical uses. Treatment of anxiety disorders, short-term treatment of insomnia, treatment of seizure disorders, and preoperative sedation and anesthesia are the most common uses. From an addiction medicine perspective, it is easy to lose sight of their medical utility because addiction medicine specialists treat patients who often misuse or abuse benzodiazepines or patients who have developed a dependence on them.

Benzodiazepines are still among the most widely prescribed medications, although there has been a steady decline in their prescription worldwide because new medications have been introduced for the same purposes and because there is concern about their overuse, misuse, and abuse. Benzodiazepines have been subject to increasing control and, in New York, have been placed on triplicate status. Benzodiazepines have a significant advantage over the previously available sedative–hypnotics. The short- and intermediate-acting barbiturates, meprobamate and ethchlorvynol, are lethal if taken in excess of 10 times a single therapeutic dose. Benzodiazepines, on the other hand, are virtually nonlethal unless combined with alcohol or other drugs. Because children may accidentally overdose on prescription medications and because adults who overdose in suicide attempts often take everything in the family medicine cabinet, it is of significant public health benefit to have nonlethal medications in the family medicine cabinet.

Some patients with debilitating anxiety symptoms derive great benefit from benzodiazepine treatment, even from long-term treatment, and tolerance to the therapeutic effects and physical dependence do not inevitably occur.

Adverse Effects of Benzodiazepines

Separate from issues of addiction and dependence, the prescription of benzodiazepines can be associated with adverse effects that may bring patients to the attention of addiction specialists. Alprazolam (Xanax) is noteworthy because it is prescribed for treatment of panic attacks (13) and depression (14,15) in relatively high doses (4 to 10 mg per day) for extended periods of time. Initial clinical trials suggested few side effects or adverse events (16). With accumulated clinical experience, there have been case reports of alprazolam-released hostility (17–19), rebound insomnia (20), major depression (21), amnesia (22,23), and aggressive and violent behavior (24). Physical dependence can result when higher-than-usual therapeutic doses are used daily for about a month and when usual therapeutic doses are used for several months.

The prescription of psychotropic medications is malevolent only when medication robs a patient of the opportunity to develop a more satisfactory nonpharmacologic solution or when the patient develops drug dependence or other adverse effects that compound the patient's difficulties.

Benzodiazepine Abuse Potential

The abuse potential of a drug or medication is often used to refer to the likelihood that addicts will self-administer the drug or medication to produce intoxication. In laboratory self-administration models, abuse potential is often inferred from addicts' comparison of their liking of the drug compared to other established drugs of abuse or to placebo.

Liking of Drug by Addicts

Current and ex-drug abusers may have different subjective responses to psychoactive drugs than do nondrug abusers. The different response may have a biologic component, because altered response to benzodiazepines has been observed in children of alcoholics (25,26). The extent to which altered drug effects are learned, are the result of some genetically determined biochemical or receptor site differences, or are caused by perturbations of metabolism or receptor site function induced by long-term exposure to drugs is not well delineated. Whatever the cause, some drugs have desirable or reinforcing effects in people with current or past histories of alcohol and other drug abuse that are not present in nondrug abusers (27). Most nondrug abuser or nonanxious people do not like the effects of benzodiazepines and prefer placebo. Studies in ex-drug abusers generally show that benzodiazepines are reinforc-

ing, but less so than short-acting barbiturates. Of the benzodiazepines, addicts generally prefer diazepam or alprazolam (28,29) to other benzodiazepines. Outside the laboratory setting, the benzodiazepine actually used by addicts is determined both by preference and accessibility.

Value on the "Street-Drug" Black Market

Availability of a drug or medication on the street-drug black market establishes that it has value to the drug abuser, although its availability does not necessarily mean that the drug or medication is a drug of abuse. For example, the antihypertensive medication, clonidine (Clonapres), is effective in reducing opiate withdrawal symptoms and is sold on the street-drug black market. Clonidine is not used, however, to produce intoxication; opiate addicts use it to self-medicate opiate withdrawal symptoms when trying to reduce heroin use or when heroin is not available.

The uses of benzodiazepines by addicts are varied. Benzodiazepines are used by cocaine addicts to ameliorate anxiety and agitation induced by cocaine or methamphetamine abuse, or by heroin addicts to self-medicate opiate withdrawal symptoms. Patients on methadone maintenance may use benzodiazepines to enhance or "boost" the subjective effects of methadone or to produce intoxication.

Diazepam is commonly sold or traded on the street-drug black market. Current price on the West Coast is $1 or $2 for a 10-mg Valium tablet. More commonly available and used by methadone-maintained patients is clonazepam (Klonopin). Klonopin is popular, in part, because it is not readily detectable in the drug screens commonly used by methadone-maintained programs and because it is the only benzodiazepine still on the California state formulary. Street price ranges from $1 to $3 for a 2-mg clonazepam tablet.

OTHER SEDATIVE–HYPNOTICS

When the short-acting sedative–hypnotics such as secobarbital (Seconal) and pentobarbital (Nembutal) were commonly prescribed, they were often taken orally or by injection to produce intoxication. Intoxication with sedative–hypnotics is qualitatively similar to intoxication with alcohol. The desired effect is a state of *disinhibition* in which mood is elevated; self-criticism, anxiety, and guilt are reduced; and energy and self-confidence are increased. During intoxication, the mood is often labile and may shift rapidly from euphoria to sadness. The user does not always obtain the desired effects and, while intoxicated, may be irritable, hypochondriacal, anxious, and angry to the point of rage. Preexisting personality, expectations, and circumstances under which the drug is used all interact. Users' perception that a drug effect is pleasurable is partly learned and partly the pharmacology of the drug.

A person intoxicated on sedative–hypnotics commonly has an unsteady gait, slurred speech, sustained horizontal nystagmus, and poor judgment. Intoxication with sedative–hypnotics may produce an amnesia for events that occur while intoxicated that is similar to alcoholic blackouts. Amnesia appears particularly likely to occur with benzodiazepine intoxication.

Sedative–Hypnotic Withdrawal

The sedative–hypnotic withdrawal syndrome is a spectrum of signs and symptoms that occur after stopping or markedly reducing the daily intake of a sedative–hypnotic. Signs and symptoms do not always follow a specific sequence. Common signs and symptoms include anxiety, tremors, nightmares, insomnia, anorexia, nausea, vomiting, postural hypotension, seizures, delirium, and hyperpyrexia. The withdrawal syndrome is similar for all sedative–hypnotics, but the severity and time course depend on the particular sedative–hypnotic. With short-active medications such as pentobarbital, secobarbital, meprobamate, and methaqualone, withdrawal symptoms typically begin 12 to 24 hours after the last dose and peak in intensity between 24 and 72 hours after the last dose. If the patient has liver disease or is over the age of 65, symptoms may develop more slowly. With long-active medications such as phenobarbital, diazepam, and chlordiazepoxide (Librium), the withdrawal syndrome usually begins 24 to 48 hours after the last dose and peaks on the fifth to eighth day.

During untreated sedative–hypnotic withdrawal, the electroencephalogram may show bursts of high-voltage, slow-frequency activity that precede clinical seizure activity. The withdrawal delirium may include disorientation as to time, place, and situation, and auditory and visual hallucinations. The delirium generally follows a period of insomnia. Some patients may have only delirium, others only seizures, and some may have both delirium and seizures.

The classical studies of barbiturate withdrawal were conduced in the 1950s (30). In the early 1960s, Hollister et al. reported on experimental studies of the physical dependence-producing effects of high-dose chlordiazepoxide (31) and diazepam (32). Clinical case reports of withdrawal leave little doubt that a similar withdrawal syndrome is produced by methaqualone (33), ethchlorvynol (34), and meprobamate (35).

With the exception of buspirone (BuSpar), which apparently does not have a withdrawal syndrome, the other sedative–hypnotics listed in Table 17.1 can produce clinically significant withdrawal signs and symptoms when taken at two or more times the maximum therapeutic range for more than 1 month.

Low-Dose Benzodiazepine Withdrawal Syndromes

Many patients who have taken benzodiazepines in therapeutic doses for months to years can abruptly discontinue the drug without developing withdrawal symptoms. The symptoms for which the benzodiazepine was being taken often return or intensify. The return of symptoms is called *symptom reemergence* (or *recrudescence*). Patients' symptoms of anxiety, insomnia, or muscle tension abate during benzodiazepine treatment. When the benzodiazepine is stopped, symptoms return to the same level as before benzodiazepine therapy. The reason for making a distinction between symptom rebound and symptom recurrence is that symptom recurrence suggests persistence of the original symptoms, whereas symptom rebound suggests a transient withdrawal syndrome.

Other patients chronically taking similar amounts of a benzodiazepine in therapeutic doses develop symptoms ranging from mild to severe when the benzodiazepine is stopped or when the dosage is substantially reduced. Characteristically, patients tolerate a gradual tapering of the benzodiazepine until they are at 10% to 20% of their peak dose. Further reduction in benzodiazepine dose causes patients to become increasingly symptomatic. In addiction medicine literature, the low-dose benzodiazepine withdrawal syndrome may be called therapeutic-dose withdrawal, normal-dose withdrawal, or benzodiazepine discontinuation syndrome.

Many patients experience a transient increase in symptoms for 1 to 2 weeks after benzodiazepine withdrawal. The symptoms are an intensified return of the symptoms for which the benzodiazepine was prescribed. The transient form of symptom intensification is called *symptom rebound*. The term comes from sleep research in which "rebound insomnia" is commonly observed following sedative–hypnotic use. Symptom rebound lasts a few days to weeks following discontinuation of the benzodiazepine. Symptom rebound is the most common withdrawal consequence of prolonged benzodiazepine use.

A few patients experience a severe, protracted withdrawal syndrome that includes symptoms (e.g., paresthesias and psychosis) that were not present before. It is this latter withdrawal syndrome that has generated much of the concern about the long-term "safety" of the benzodiazepines when taken daily for months to years.

Protracted Benzodiazepine Withdrawal Syndrome

In some patients, protracted benzodiazepine withdrawal consists of relatively mild withdrawal symptoms such as mild to moderate anxiety, mood instability, and sleep disturbance. In others, however, the protracted withdrawal syndrome consists of increased sensitivity to light and sound, psychosis, and severe insomnia. The symptoms can be severe and disabling and last many months.

There is considerable controversy surrounding even the existence of this syndrome. The notion of a protracted withdrawal syndrome evolves primarily from the addiction medicine literature (36). Many symptoms are nonspecific and often mimic an obsessive-compulsive disorder with

TABLE 17.1. *Common sedative–hypnotics and their phenobarbital withdrawal equivalency*[a]

Generic name	Trade name(s)	Common therapeutic indication	Usual therapeutic dose range (mg/day)	Dose equal to 30 mg of phenobarbital for withdrawal (mg)
Barbiturates				
Butabarbital	Butisol	Sedative	45–120	100
Butalbital[b]	Fiorinal, Sedapap	Sedative/analgesic	100–300	100
Pentobarbital	Nembutal	Hypnotic	50–100	100
Secobarbital	Seconal	Hypnotic	50–100	100
Benzodiazepines				
Alprazolam	Xanax	Antianxiety	0.75–4	1
Chlordiazepoxide	Librium	Antianxiety	15–100	25
Clonazepam	Klonopin	Anticonvulsant	0.5–4	1
Clorazepate	Tranxene	Antianxiety	15–60	30
Diazepam	Valium	Antianxiety	4–40	10
Estazolam	ProSom	Hypnotic	1–2	1
Flumazenil	Romazicon	Antagonist	—	—
Flunitrazepam[c]	Rohypnol	Hypnotic	1–2	1
Flurazepam	Dalmane	Hypnotic	15–30	30
Lorazepam	Ativan	Antianxiety	1–16	16
Midazolam	Versed	Anesthesia	—	—
Oxazepam	Serax	Antianxiety	10–120	30
Quazepam	Doral	Hypnotic	15	15
Temazepam	Restoril	Hypnotic	7.5–30	15
Triazolam	Halcion	Hypnotic	0.125–0.5	0.125
Others				
Chloral hydrate	Nocte, Somnos	Hypnotic	250–1000	500
Ethchlorvynol	Placidyl	Hypnotic	500–1000	500
Meprobamate	Miltown	Antianxiety	1200–2400	1200
Zaleplon	Sonata	Hypnotic	5–20	5
Zolpidem	Ambien	Hypnotic	5–10	5

[a] Withdrawal equivalency is not the same as therapeutic equivalency; see text.
[b] Butalbital is an ingredient in many combination analgesics.
[c] Not marketed in the United States.

psychotic features. As a practical matter, it is often difficult in the clinical setting to separate symptom reemergence from protracted withdrawal. New symptoms such as paresthesias and increased sensitivity to sound, light, and touch are particularly suggestive of low-dose withdrawal.

The protracted benzodiazepine withdrawal has no pathognomonic signs or symptoms, and the broad range of nonspecific symptoms produced by the protracted benzodiazepine withdrawal syndrome also could be the result of agitated depression, generalized anxiety disorder, panic disorder, partial complex seizures, or schizophrenia. The time course of symptom resolution is the primary differentiating feature between symptoms generated by withdrawal and symptom reemergence. Symptoms from withdrawal gradually subside with continued benzodiazepine abstinence, whereas symptom reemergence does not.

The waxing and waning of symptom intensity from day to day is characteristic of the low-dose protracted benzodiazepine withdrawal syndrome. Patients are sometimes asymptomatic for several days; then, without apparent reason, they become acutely anxious. Often there

are concomitant physiologic signs, for example, dilated pupils, increased resting heart rate, and increased blood pressure. The intense waxing and waning of symptoms is important in distinguishing low-dose withdrawal symptoms from symptom reemergence.

Risk Factors for Low-Dose Withdrawal

Some drugs or medications may facilitate neuroadaptation by increasing the affinity of benzodiazepines for their receptors. Phenobarbital, for example, increases the affinity of diazepam to benzodiazepine receptors, and prior treatment with phenobarbital has been found to increase the intensity of chlordiazepoxide (45 mg per day) withdrawal symptoms (37). Patients at increased risk for development of the low-dose withdrawal syndrome are those with a family or personal history of alcoholism, those who use alcohol daily, and those who concomitantly use other sedatives. Case control studies suggest that patients with a history of addiction, particularly to other sedative–hypnotics, are at high risk for low-dose benzodiazepine dependence. The short-acting, high-milligram-potency benzodiazepines appear to produce a more intense low-dose withdrawal syndrome.

Pharmacologic Treatment of Withdrawal

The strategies for treating physical dependence on sedative–hypnotics involve gradual reduction of a sedative–hypnotic or substitution of an anticonvulsant medication that allows the physiologic readjustment to occur gradually. There are three basic strategies: (a) use gradually decreasing doses of the sedative–hypnotic; (b) substitute long-active barbiturate for the sedative–hypnotic of abuse and gradually withdraw the long-acting sedative–hypnotic (38–40); and (c) substitute an anticonvulsant such as carbamazepine (Tegretol) (41–45) or valproate (Depakeve) (46,47).

Abrupt discontinuation of a sedative–hypnotic in a patient who is physically dependent on it is not acceptable medical practice. Unlike opiate withdrawal, whose withdrawal symptoms are unpleasant but not life-threatening in an otherwise healthy patient, abrupt withdrawal of sedative–hypnotics can be fatal (35,48).

Withdrawal with the Drug of Dependence

The classical treatment of a sedative–hypnotic patient is a gradual withdrawal of the drug of dependence (30). While the method is sound from a pharmacologic point of view, it has some disadvantages. When the drug of dependence is a short-acting hypnotic, such as a short-acting barbiturate, patients may become intoxicated and disinhibited, resulting in behavior problems. Giving an addict their drug of abuse, even in a therapeutic context, is problematic.

A gradual taper of the drug of dependence is more often used in the context of therapeutic discontinuation of patients from long-acting sedative–hypnotics. With long-term benzodiazepine therapy, for example, physical dependence can develop in patients who do not have a substance abuse disorder. In this situation, gradual taper of the drug of dependence can be an appropriate therapeutic strategy.

Substitution of Phenobarbital

Phenobarbital substitution has a number of advantages over withdrawal from the drug of dependence. First, phenobarbital is long-acting, and small changes in blood levels of phenobarbital occur between doses, allowing the safe use of smaller daily doses. Second, phenobarbital is safer than the shorter-acting barbiturates, because the lethal dose of phenobarbital is many times higher than the toxic dose and the signs of toxicity (e.g., sustained nystagmus, slurred speech, and ataxia) are easy to observe. Third, phenobarbital intoxication does not usually produce disinhibition, so most patients view it as a medication, not as a drug of abuse. Finally, the phenobarbital technique can be applied to a broad range of sedative–hypnotics and with patients who abuse a mixture of alcohol and/or sedative–hypnotics.

The disadvantages to phenobarbital substitution are that the calculations for making the conversion between the drug or drugs of abuse are tedious, and 1% to 5% of patients treated with phenobarbital develop a rash.

Stabilization Phase

The substitution dose of phenobarbital is calculated by substituting 30 mg of phenobarbital for each hypnotic dose of the drug of abuse. Phenobarbital withdrawal conversion equivalence is not the same as therapeutic dose equivalency. The phenobarbital withdrawal equivalence is the amount of phenobarbital that can be substituted to prevent emergence of serious sedative–hypnotic withdrawal signs and symptoms.

For sedative–hypnotics that are not marketed as sleeping pills, the upper recommended therapeutic single dose is considered equivalent to the hypnotic dose. For medications markets primarily for treatment of insomnia, the lower recommended dose is considered a "hypnotic dose." The conversion is, at best, a clinical approximation and published tables sometimes show different withdrawal equivalent values for phenobarbital. Phenobarbital equivalents do, however, provide a clinically appropriate starting dose of phenobarbital that will usually prevent the emergence of medically serious withdrawal symptoms. Because phenobarbital has a long half-life, blood levels of phenobarbital will continue to increase even with a fixed daily dose. The key to successful clinical use of phenobarbital is careful monitoring of the patient before each dose. If signs of sedative–hypnotic intoxication occur (e.g., slurred speech, sustained nystagmus) the dose is adjusted downward; if symptoms of withdrawal occur (e.g., intense nightmares, muscle twitching, psychosis) the dose is increased.

Regardless of the computed dose, the maximum starting daily dose of phenobarbital should not exceed 500 mg per day. Table 17.1 shows the phenobarbital conversion for common sedative–hypnotics.

Although sedative–hypnotic abusers may exaggerate the number of pills that they are taking, the patient's history is the best guide to initial therapy. If the patient has overstated the amount of drug used, they will become intoxicated during the first few days of treatment. Intoxication is easily managed by omitting one or more doses of phenobarbital and adjusting the daily phenobarbital dose downward as described later under "Withdrawal Phase."

If, on initial evaluation, the patient is in acute sedative–hypnotic withdrawal and has had a withdrawal seizure, the initial dose of phenobarbital is administered by injection. If nystagmus, slurred speech, or ataxia develop 1 to 2 hours after the intramuscular dose, the patient is in no immediate danger from sedative–hypnotic withdrawal.

Patients are maintained on the initial calculated schedule of phenobarbital for 2 days. Patients who have neither signs of sedative–hypnotic withdrawal nor signs of phenobarbital intoxication are ready to begin phenobarbital withdrawal.

Withdrawal Phase

For inpatients the daily phenobarbital dose is decreased 30 mg per day unless the patient develops signs or symptoms of phenobarbital toxicity or sedative–hypnotic withdrawal. (Outpatient withdrawal generally proceeds more slowly.) If signs of phenobarbital toxicity appear, the daily phenobarbital dose is decreased by 50%, and the 30-mg-per-day withdrawal is continued from the reduced phenobarbital dose. If the patient has objective signs of sedative–hypnotic withdrawal, the daily phenobarbital dose is increased 50%, and the patient is restabilized before continuing the withdrawal.

Substitution of an Anticonvulsant

Protocols using carbamazepine or valproic acid (Depakote, Depakene) have been used clinically for treatment of sedative–hypnotic withdrawal. Both medications enhance γ-aminobutyric acid (GABA) function. Both are effective in suppressing benzodiazepine withdrawal symptoms. Neither carbamazepine nor valproic acid produce effects that sedative–hypnotic abusers find desirable.

The use of valproate as a withdrawal protocol was suggested in 1989 (46), and there are clinical case reports of its use in benzodiazepine withdrawal (47,49). Valproic acid in a dosage up to about 1200 mg per day is useful both in acute withdrawal and in treatment of persistent symptoms following withdrawal.

Carbamazepine is reported to be useful in benzodiazepine withdrawal (41,44,45,50–52) and in alcohol withdrawal (53–55). It is also useful in treating benzodiazepine withdrawal in benzodiazepine-dependent, methadone-maintained patients. Both carbamazepine and phenobarbital can increase the metabolism of methadone and require that the dose of methadone be adjusted.

In patients with seizure disorders (56), valproic acid appears to be better tolerated than carbamazepine.

Zolpidem

Zolpidem (Ambien) is an imidazopyridine hypnotic, chemically unrelated to the benzodiazepines. Although zolpidem is not chemically a benzodiazepine, its pharmacologic profile is similar to a benzodiazepine, and it binds to a subunit of the same GABA/benzodiazepine receptor as the benzodiazepines (57,58). Its sedative effects are reversed by the benzodiazepine antagonist flumazenil (59). Zolpidem is rapidly absorbed and has a short half-life ($T_{1/2} = 2.2$ hours). Its sedative effects are additive with alcohol. Like triazolam, zolpidem decreases brain metabolism of glucose (60).

Zolpidem has been extensively used in Europe, and only a few cases of abuse have been reported. A case report from Italy suggests that some patients increase dosage many times that prescribed and that zolpidem produces a withdrawal syndrome similar to that of other sedative–hypnotics (61). The case histories illustrated significant tolerance to zolpidem and the rapid production of withdrawal symptoms that might be expected from a potent, short-acting sedative–hypnotic.

Some investigators suggest that zolpidem does not produce tolerance or physical dependence (62). Mice were administered zolpidem or midazolam (both 30 mg/kg) by gastric intubation for 10 days. Animals treated with midazolam, but not zolpidem, showed tolerance to the drug's sedative effects and had a lowered seizure threshold after the drug was stopped. Furthermore, the benzodiazepine antagonist flumazenil precipitated withdrawal in the midazolam-treated animals, but not in those treated with zolpidem.

Studies with baboons suggest that zolpidem is reinforcing and that it produces tolerance and physical dependence (82). In a free-choice paradigm, baboons consistently self-administered zolpidem intravenously at higher rates than either the vehicle solution alone or triazolam. After 2 weeks of zolpidem self-administration, substitution of the vehicle solution alone resulted in suppression of food pellet intake, which the investigators interpreted as zolpidem withdrawal. Baboons trained to discriminate oral doses of either phenobarbital (10 mg/kg) or lorazepam (Ativan) (1.8 mg/kg) from placebo responded to zolpidem as though it were the active drug more than 80% of the time. In another experiment, animals developed tolerance to zolpidem-induced ataxia and sedation over 7 days of drug administration. The investigators concluded that the rates of self-administration of zolpidem were similar to pentobarbital and higher than those maintained by the 11 benzodiazepines that they had studied.

Zaleplon

Zaleplon (Sonata) is a pyrazolopyrimidine that the Food and Drug Administration (FDA) approved for marketing in the United States in 1999. Like zolpidem, it is chemically unrelated to the benzodiazepines and binds to the omega-1 receptor, which is a subunit of the (γ-aminobutyric acid–benzodiazepine [GABA-BZ]) receptor. Studies in baboons (63) and healthy volunteers with a history of drug abuse (64) suggest abuse potential similar to triazolam. Peak plasma concentration occurs about 1 hour following oral ingestion. It is rapidly metabolized with a half-life of about 1 hour. A study comparing memory and cognitive effects of triazolam, zolpidem, and zaleplon showed that zaleplon (10 or 20 mg) demonstrated no evidence of cognitive impairment 8.25 hours after the dose, whereas triazolam (0.25) and zolpidem (20 mg, recommended therapeutic dose is 5 to 10 mg) showed measurable cognitive impairment (65).

Buspirone

Buspirone is an anxiolytic that is not chemically or pharmacologically related to the benzodiazepines, barbiturates, or other sedative–hypnotics. Buspirone is not cross-tolerant with classical sedative–hypnotics and will not prevent acute benzodiazepine withdrawal signs and symptoms (66), even when the buspirone is begun 4 weeks before benzodiazepine withdrawal is initiated (67).

From the neuropharmacology of benzodiazepine withdrawal, buspirone appears to have clinical utility in benzodiazepine discontinuation (50).

Buspirone's anxiolytic effects take days to weeks to develop. Buspirone has been proposed as an alternative to benzodiazepines in postdetoxification treatment of anxiety in patients who are alcohol or sedative–hypnotic dependent (68–72).

TRICYCLIC ANTIDEPRESSANTS

Tricyclic antidepressants are not drugs of abuse, although they are misused in several ways. They are commonly involved in suicide attempts. Amitriptyline (Elavil) and other tricyclics have sedative and other mood-altering effects that some patients find desirable, and they may escalate their dose and develop toxicity (73). Methadone-maintained patients use amitriptyline or other antidepressants to "boost" the sedative effects of methadone. Tricyclic antidepressants sometimes become snared in the lexicon of drug abuse. For example, a case report of a woman who covertly took amitriptyline to induce seizures was reported as amitriptyline abuse (74).

Blood levels of desipramine may be increased in methadone-maintained patients, and smaller doses of tricyclics may be indicated when treating depression in methadone-maintained patients (75). Tricyclic antidepressants are commonly used in the treatment of cocaine abuse among methadone-maintained patients. Clinical trial of antidepressants in the treatment of cocaine abuse has shown mixed results, although improvement in cocaine abuse among depressed, methadone-maintained patients has been reported (76).

ANTICHOLINERGICS

Trihexyphenidyl (Artane) and benztropine (Cogentin) are commonly used to ameliorate neuroleptic-induced extrapyramidal symptoms. In a case series (n = 214) from a hospital in Israel, evidence for abuse of trihexyphenidyl was found in 6.5% of admissions for schizophrenia (77). Although anticholinergics in low doses can have sedative–hypnotic effects, a case report suggests that patients may abuse high doses of trihexyphenidyl for nonspecific stimulant or euphoric effects (78). Long-term abuse of trihexyphenidyl has been reported to produced impairment of memory and cognitive function, which clears after withdrawal of the medication (79). The frequency of benztropine abuse in severely mentally disturbed population has been reported to be as high as 30% (80), and treatment of benztropine abuse can require hospitalization (81).

CONCLUSION

The benzodiazepines remain valuable medications and their general safety in terms of overdose lethality remains unchallenged. Most of the controversy or difficulty with benzodiazepines revolves around (a) the neuroadaptive changes that may occur with chronic use; (b) their prescription to addicts in recovery and their use by addicts to self-medicate drug toxicity from cocaine and methamphetamine; (c) their use by opioid addicts to boost methadone or buprenorphine effects; and (d) their nonmedical use as incapacitating agents for robbery or date-rape. Physical dependence may occur in the context of chronic therapeutic benzodiazepine use and may be, but is not necessarily, associated with a substance abuse or dependence disorder as defined by DSM–IV–TR.

Some of the conditions for which benzodiazepines have been chronically prescribed—treatment of generalized anxiety disorder, pain attacks, and insomnia—have been supplanted by the selective serotonin reuptake inhibitors and newer hypnotics. Therapeutic use of benzodiazepines in treatment of psychiatric disorders is still evolving and beyond the scope of this chapter, which focuses on diagnosis and treatment of benzodiazepine abuse and dependence.

REFERENCES

1. Wesson DR, Smith DE. Prescription drug abuse. Patient, physician, and cultural responsibilities. *West J Med* 1990; 152(5):613–616.
2. American Psychiatric Association Task Force on Benzodiazepine Dependency. *Benzodiazepine dependency, toxicity, and abuse.* Washington, DC: American Psychiatric Association, 1990.
3. American Psychiatric Association. *Diagnostic and statistical manual of mental disorders,* 4th ed., text revision. Washington, DC: Author, 2000.
4. Sellers EM, Ciraulo DA, DuPont RL, et al. Alprazolam and benzodiazepine dependence. *J Clin Psychiatry* 1993;54 [Suppl 10]:64–75.
5. Barnas C, Rossmann M, Roessler H, et al. Benzodiazepines and other psychotropic drugs abused by patients in a methadone maintenance program: familiarity and preference. *Clin Neuropharmacol* 1992;15[Suppl 1 Pt A]:110A–111A.
6. Iguchi MY, Griffiths RR, Bickel WK, et al. Relative abuse liability of benzodiazepines in methadone maintained popu-
lations in three cities. *NIDA Res Monogr Ser* 1989;95:364–365.
7. DuPont RL, Saylor KE. Marijuana and benzodiazepines in patients receiving methadone treatment. *JAMA* 1989; 261(23):3409(letter).
8. Reynaud M, Tracqui A, Pettit G, et al. Six deaths linked to misuse of buprenorphine-benzodiazepine combinations. *Am J Psychiatry* 1998;155(3):448–449.
9. Kintz, P. Deaths involving buprenorphine: a compendium of French cases. *Forensic Sci Int* 2001;121(1–2):65–69.

10. Schuckit MA, Klein JL. Correlations between drinking intensity and reactions to ethanol and diazepam in healthy young men. *Neuropsychopharmacology* 1991;4(3):157–163.

11. Shader RI, Pary RJ, Harmatz JS, et al. Plasma concentrations and clinical effects after single oral doses of prazepam, clorazepate, and diazepam. *J Clin Psychiatry* 1984;45(10):411–413.

12. Calhoun SR, Wesson DR, Galloway GP, Smith DE. Abuse of flunitrazepam (Rohypnol) and other benzodiazepines in Austin and south Texas. *J Psychoactive Drugs* 1996;28(2):183–189.

13. Nightingale S. New indication for alprazolam. *JAMA* 1990;264(22):2863.

14. Rickels K, Feighner JP, Smith WT. Alprazolam, amitriptyline, doxepin, and placebo in the treatment of depression. *Arch Gen Psychiatry* 1985;42(2):134–141.

15. Kravitz HM, Fawcett J, Newman AJ. Alprazolam and depression: a review of risks and benefits. *J Clin Psychiatry* 1993;54[Suppl 20]:78–84.

16. Noyes RJ, DuPont RL, Pecknold J, et al. Alprazolam in panic disorder and agoraphobia: results from a multicenter trial II. Patient acceptance, side effects, and safety. *Arch Gen Psychiatry* 1988;45:422–428.

17. Rosenbaum JF, Woods SW, Groves JE, Klerman GL. Emergence of hostility during alprazolam treatment. *Am J Psychiatry* 1984;141(6):792–793.

18. Rapaport M, Braff DL. Alprazolam and hostility. *Am J Psychiatry* 1985;142(1):146(letter).

19. Gardner DL, Cowdry RW. Alprazolam-induced dyscontrol in borderline personality disorder. *Am J Psychiatry* 1985;142(1):98–100.

20. Kales A, Bixler EO, Vala-Bueno A, et al. Alprazolam: effects on sleep and withdrawal phenomena. *J Clin Pharmacol* 1987;27:508–515.

21. Lydiard RB, Laraia MT, Ballenger JC, Howell EF. Emergence of depressive symptoms in patients receiving alprazolam for panic disorder. *Am J Psychiatry* 1987;144(5):664–665.

22. Curran HV. Tranquillising memories: a review of the effects of benzodiazepines on human memory. *Biol Psychol* 1986;23(2):179–213.

23. Curran HV, Bond A, O'Sullivan G, et al. Memory functions, alprazolam and exposure therapy: a controlled longitudinal study of agoraphobia with panic disorder. *Psychol Med* 1994;24(4):969–976.

24. Brown CR. The use of benzodiazepines in prison populations. *J Clin Psychiatry* 1978;39(3):219–222.

25. Ciraulo DA, Sarid-Segal O, Knapp C, et al. Liability to alprazolam abuse in daughters of alcoholics. *Am J Psychiatry* 1996;153(7):956–958.

26. Ciraulo DA, Barnhill JG, Ciraulo AM, et al. Parental alcoholism as a risk factor in benzodiazepine abuse: a pilot study. *Am J Psychiatry* 1989;146:1333–1335.

27. Griffiths R, Roache J. Abuse liability of benzodiazepines. A review of human studies evaluating subjective and/or reinforcing effects. In: Smith D, Wesson D, eds. *The benzodiazepines: current standards for medical practice.* Hingham, MA: MTP Press, 1985:209–225.

28. Schmauss C, Apelt S, Emrich HM. The seeking and liking potentials of alprazolam. *Am J Psychiatry* 1988;145(1):128(letter).

29. Schmauss C, Apelt S, Emrich HM. Preference for alprazolam over diazepam. *Am J Psychiatry* 1989;146(3):408(letter).

30. Isbell H. Addiction to barbiturates and the barbiturate abstinence syndrome. *Ann Intern Med* 1950;33:108–120.

31. Hollister L, Motzenbecker E, Degan R. Withdrawal reactions from chlordiazepoxide (Librium). *Psychopharmacologia* 1961;2:63–68.

32. Hollister LE, Motzenbecker E, Degan R, et al. Diazepam in newly admitted schizophrenics. *Dis Nerv Syst* 1963;24(12):746–750.

33. Swartzburg M, Lieb J, Schwartz AH. Methaqualone withdrawal. *Arch Gen Psychiatry* 1973;29:46–47.

34. Flemenbaum A, Gunby B. Ethchlorvynol (Placidyl) abuse and withdrawal. *Dis Nerv Syst* 1971;32(3):188–192.

35. Swanson LA, Okada T. Death after withdrawal of meprobamate. *JAMA* 1963;184(10):780–781.

36. Ladner M. History of benzodiazepine dependence. *J Subst Abuse Treat* 1991;8:53–59.

37. Covi L, Lipman RS, Pattison JH, et al. Length of treatment with anxiolytic sedatives and response to their sudden withdrawal. *Acta Psychiatr Scand* 1973;49:51–64.

38. Smith DE, Wesson DR. A new method for treatment of barbiturate dependence. *JAMA* 1970;213(2):294–295.

39. Smith DE, Wesson DR. Phenobarbital technique for treatment of barbiturate dependence. *Arch Gen Psychiatry* 1971;24(1):56–60.

40. Vestal RE, Rumack BH. Glutethimide dependence: phenobarbital treatment. *Ann Intern Med* 1974;80(5):670.

41. Garcia-Borreguero D, Bronisch T, Apelt S, et al. Treatment of benzodiazepine withdrawal symptoms with carbamazepine. *Eur Arch Psychiatry Clin Neurosci* 1991;241(3):145–150.

42. Neppe VM, Sindorf J. Carbamazepine for high-dose diazepam withdrawal in opiate users. *J Nerv Ment Dis* 1991;179(4):234–235.

43. Roy-Byrne PP, Sullivan MD, Cowley DS, Ries RK. Adjunctive treatment of benzodiazepine discontinuation syndromes: a review. *J Psychiatr Res* 1993;27[Suppl 1]:143–153.

44. Ries R, Cullison S, Horn R, Ward N. Benzodiazepine withdrawal: clinicians' ratings of carbamazepine treatment versus traditional taper methods. *J Psychoactive Drugs* 1991;23(1):73–76.

45. Schweizer E, Rickels K, Case WG, Greenblatt DJ. Carbamazepine treatment in patients discontinuing long-term benzodiazepine therapy. Effects on withdrawal severity and outcome. *Arch Gen Psychiatry* 1991;48(5):448–452.

46. Roy-Byrne PP, Ward NG, Donnelly PJ. Valproate in anxiety and withdrawal syndromes. *J Clin Psychiatry* 1989;50[Suppl]:44–48.

47. Apelt S, Emrich HM. Sodium valproate in benzodiazepine withdrawal. *Am J Psychiatry* 1990;147(7):950–951(letter).

48. Fraser HF, Shaver MR, Maxwell ES, et al. A fatal termination of barbiturate abstinence syndrome in man. *J Pharmacol Exp Ther* 1952;106:387.

49. McElroy SL, Keck PE Jr, Lawrence JM. Treatment of panic disorder and benzodiazepine withdrawal with valproate. *J Neuropsychiatry Clin Neurosci* 1991;3(2):232–233(letter).

50. Rickels K, Case WG, Schweizer, et al. Benzodiazepine dependence: management of discontinuation. *Psychopharmacol Bull* 1990;26(1):63–68.

51. Ries RK, Roy-Byrne P, Ward NG, et al. Carbamazepine treatment for benzodiazepine withdrawal. *Am J Psychiatry* 1989;146(4):536–537.

52. Klein E, Uhde TW, Post RM. Preliminary evidence for the utility of carbamazepine in alprazolam withdrawal. *Am J Psychiatry* 1986;143:235–236.

53. Malcolm R, Ballenger JC, Sturgis ET, Anton R. Double-blind controlled trial comparing carbamazepine to oxazepam treatment of alcohol withdrawal. *Am J Psychiatry* 1989;146(5):617–621.

54. Stuppaeck CH, Barnas C, Hackenberg K, et al. Carbamazepine monotherapy in the treatment of alcohol withdrawal. *Int Clin Psychopharmacol* 1990;5(4):273–278.

55. Stuppaeck CH, Pycha R, Miller et al. Carbamazepine versus oxazepam in the treatment of alcohol withdrawal: a double-blind study. *Alcohol Alcohol* 1992;27(2):153–158.

56. Richens A, Davidson DL, Cartlidge NE, Easter DJ. A multicentre comparative trial of sodium valproate and carbamazepine in adult onset epilepsy. *J Neurol Neurosurg Psychiatry* 1994;57(6):682–687.

57. Byrnes JJ, Greenblatt DJ, Miller LG. Benzodiazepine receptor binding of non-benzodiazepines *in vivo*: alpidem, zolpidem and zopiclone. *Brain Res Bull* 1992;29(6):905–908.

58. Langer SZ, Arbilla S, Benavides J, Scatton B. Zolpidem and alpidem: two imidazopyridines with selectivity for omega 1- and omega 3-receptor subtypes. *Adv Biochem Psychopharmacol* 1990;46:61–72.

59. Lheureux P, Debailleul G, De WO, Askenasi R. Zolpidem intoxication mimicking narcotic overdose: response to flumazenil. *Hum Exp Toxicol* 1990; 9(2):105–107.

60. Piercey MF, Hoffmann WE, Cooper M. The hypnotics triazolam and zolpidem have identical metabolic effects throughout the brain: implications for benzodiazepine receptor subtypes. *Brain Res* 1991;554(1–2):244–252.

61. Cavallaro R, Regazzetti MG, Corelli G, Smeraldi E. Tolerance and withdrawal with zolpidem. *Lancet* 1993;342 (8867):374–375(letter; see comments).

62. Perrault G, Morel E, Sanger DJ, Zivkovic B. Lack of tolerance and physical dependence upon repeated treatment with the novel hypnotic zolpidem. *J Pharmacol Exp Ther* 1992;263(1):298–303.

63. Ator NA, Weets EM, Kaminski BJ, et al. Zaleplon and triazolam physical dependence assessed across increasing doses under a once-daily dosing regimen in baboons. *Drug Alcohol Depend* 2000;61(1):69–84.

64. Rush CR, Frey JM, Griffiths RR. Zaleplon and triazolam in humans: acute behavioral effects and abuse potential. *Psychopharmacology (Berl)* 1999;145(1): 39–51.

65. Troy SM, Lucki I, Unruh MA, et al. Comparison of the effects of zaleplon, zolpidem, and triazolam on memory, learning, and psychomotor performance. *J Clin Psychopharmacol* 2000;20(3):328–337.

66. Schweizer E, Rickels K. Failure of buspirone to manage benzodiazepine withdrawal. *Am J Psychiatry* 1986; 143(12):1590–1592.

67. Ashton CH, Rawlins MD, Tyrer SP. A double-blind, placebo-controlled study of buspirone in diazepam withdrawal in chronic benzodiazepine users. *Br J Psychiatry* 1990;157(7):232–238.

68. Bruno F. Buspirone in the treatment of alcoholic patients. *Psychopathology* 1989;22[Suppl 1]:49–59.

69. Kranzler HR, Burleson JA, Del Boa FK, et al. Buspirone treatment of anxious alcoholics. A placebo-controlled trial. *Arch Gen Psychiatry* 1994;51(9):720–731.

70. Malcolm R, Anton RF, Randall CL, et al. A placebo-controlled trial of buspirone in anxious inpatient alcoholics. *Alcohol Clin Exp Res* 1992;16:1007–1013.

71. Olivera AO, Servis S, Heard C. Anxiety disorders coexisting with substance dependence: treatment with buspirone. *Curr Ther Res* 1990;47:52–61.

72. Tollefson GD, Montague-Clouse J, Tollefson SL. Treatment of comorbid generalized anxiety in a recently detoxified alcoholic population with a selective serotonergic drug (buspirone). *J Clini Psychopharmacol* 1992;12:19–26.

73. Delisle JD. A case of amitriptyline abuse. *Am J Psychiatry* 1990;147(10):1377–1378(letter).

74. O'Rahilly S, Turner T, Wass J. Factitious epilepsy due to amitriptyline abuse. *Irish Med J* 1985;78(6):166–167.

75. Maany I, Dhopesh V, Amdt IO, et al. Increase in desipramine serum levels associated with methadone treatment. *Am J Psychiatry* 1989;146(12):1611–1613.

76. Ziedonis DM, Kosten TR. Pharmacotherapy improves treatment outcome in depressed cocaine addicts. *J Psychoactive Drugs* 1991;23(4):417–425.

77. Zemishlany Z, Aizenberg D, Weiner Z, Weizman A. Trihexyphenidyl (Artane) abuse in schizophrenic patients. *Int Clin Psychopharmacol* 1996;11(3):199–202.

78. Lo Y, Tsai SJ. Trihexyphenidyl abuse in schizophrenic patient: a case report. *Zhonghua Yi Xue Za Zhi (Taipei)* 1996;57(2):157–160.

79. Kajimura N, Mizuki Y, Kai S, et al. Memory and cognitive impairments in a case of long-term trihexyphenidyl abuse. *Pharmacopsychiatry* 1993;26(2):59–62.

80. Buhrich N, Weller A, Kevans P. Misuse of anticholinergic drugs by people with serious mental illness. *Psychiatr Serv* 2000;51(7):928–929.

81. Grace RF. Benztropine abuse and overdose–case report and review. *Adverse Drug React Toxicol Rev* 1997; 16(2):103–112.

82. Griffiths RR, Sannerud CA, Ator NA, Brady JV. Zolpidem behavioral pharmacology in baboons: self-injection, discrimination, tolerance and withdrawal. *J Pharmacol Exp Ther* 1992;260(3):1199–1208.

CHAPTER 18

Hallucinogens

ROBERT N. PECHNICK AND
J. THOMAS UNGERLEIDER

This chapter focuses on the major current and past hallucinogens of abuse: the prototype ergot hallucinogen lysergic acid diethylamide (LSD); other indolealkylamines such as psilocybin, psilocin, and dimethyltryptamine (DMT); and the phenethylamines, including mescaline and dimethoxy-methylamphetamine (DOM). Marihuana, phencyclidine (PCP), and methylenedioxymethamphetamine (MDMA or ecstasy), which are sometimes classified as hallucinogens, are covered in other chapters in this volume. Comprehensive reviews of hallucinogenic substances not covered in this chapter, such as the piperidyl benzilate esters, as well as the historical use of hallucinogens by other cultures, are available elsewhere (1–3).

At the present time, the "war on drugs" continues; however, the focus has begun to change with respect to the hallucinogens. First, there are now data indicating that the use of hallucinogens is on the rise, especially among adolescents. Thus, the trend of decreased use of the hallucinogens from the mid 1970s through the 1980s has begun to reverse. Moreover, in recent years the Internet has become a widely used source of information on hallucinogens (4), and a vehicle for obtaining the drugs (5). Second, although during the 1980s little research was conducted wherein humans were administered hallucinogens, over the last few years there has been a resurgence of clinical studies carried out under highly controlled conditions (6–15). The results obtained from controlled clinical studies should provide important and unbiased information, in contrast to some of the clinical data that previously have come from anecdotal information obtained from limited first-person accounts (16), "street pharmacologists," or from hospital emergency room records. Third, this resurgence in clinical research has taken place at the same time that there have been major advances regarding the possible mechanisms of action of the hallucinogens. For example, much more is now known about the effects of hallucinogens on the synthesis, release, and metabolism of indoleamines and catecholamines, and their interactions with specific pre- and postsynaptic receptor subtypes. Although in the past decade there had been an ever-widening discrepancy between our limited knowledge of the clinical pharmacology of the hallucinogens and information on their mechanisms of action obtained from preclinical studies, we now may be reaching a point where we can begin to develop a unified conceptual framework regarding the fundamental mechanisms underlying their pharmacologic effects in humans. This chapter reviews the current information on the clinical effects of the hallucinogens, potential mechanisms of action, and the pathophysiologic sequelae of their use. The reader also is directed to other reviews (11,17–19).

HISTORICAL PERSPECTIVE

To a large degree, the revolution in the drug abuse field that began in the United States in the mid-1960s and continues today came from concern over the use of hallucinogens, particularly LSD. A detailed consideration of these events provides a window to view how the widespread concern about drug abuse in the United States first began. Until the mid-1960s, the use of illicit drugs in the United States largely had been limited to specific populations or subcultures: heroin was used by those in the inner-city ghettos; marihuana was used by jazz musicians and Hispanic immigrants; and amphetamine and amphetamine analogues were originally used by women who had them prescribed for weight loss. Prescription antianxiety agents, including meprobamate and benzodiazepines such as chlordiazepoxide (Librium), also were commonly used at that time. Moreover, most Americans drank alcohol.

In the early 1960s, Timothy Leary, then a young psychology instructor at Harvard, began experimenting with hallucinogens, particularly LSD. He claimed that it provided instant happiness, enhanced creativity in art and music, facilitated problem-solving ability in school and at work, increased self-awareness, and might be useful as an adjunct to psychotherapy. Leary popularized this on college campuses, coining the phrase "turn on, tune in, drop out." When he was not reappointed to the faculty at Harvard, he became a highly publicized self-proclaimed martyr to his cause, and his followers began to proselytize for LSD. Leary's advocates organized their lifestyle around LSD and developed a subculture of fellow LSD users who shared this common interest. They would never give it to anyone without their knowledge, and they would not use other classes of drugs. For example, they would not smoke tobacco, use amphetamine or amphetamine-like psychostimulants or barbiturates, or even drink alcohol. Thus, very little polydrug abuse occurred among these LSD users. In contrast to later patterns of hallucinogen use, the early users of LSD were older; a study published in 1968 revealed that the average age of persons using and in difficulty from LSD was 21 years (20). At that time the quality of street LSD ("Owsley's acid" or "Stanley's stuff") was equivalent to that made by legitimate chemists at Sandoz Laboratories, the original manufacturer of the drug.

The lay press repeatedly kept "discovering" LSD and, in effect, advertising it. As publicity increased, subcultures experimenting with LSD began to emerge in many East and West Coast cities. Other hallucinogenic compounds, such as mescaline and psilocybin, began to be taken as well, although LSD remained the most widely used hallucinogen because it was the most readily available on the street. Musicians, rock music, the hippie lifestyle, and "flower children" were loosely joined with Leary's philosophy. There were highly publicized festivals celebrating LSD, such as "The Summer of Love" in the Haight-Ashbury district of San Francisco. Later, younger individuals began to experiment with LSD, and its use began to increase in all socioeconomic groups, particularly among middle-class and affluent youth. Moreover, many of these individuals also became active in various "protest" movements, speaking out against such governmental policies as the war in Vietnam, and about other national issues, such as civil rights and "free speech." About this time, various adverse reactions began to be recorded from medical centers around the country. The whole phenomenon continued to be widely publicized, and in many cases sensationalized (21), by the press. The populace reacted with anxiety and fear, worrying that many of the young would soon become "acidheads."

Eventually, many of the LSD users became involved in polydrug abuse, using other drugs besides hallucinogens. This included the extensive use of marihuana, hashish, and, in some cases, methamphetamine or even heroin. Various "street" substances, whose identity was frequently unknown, as well as combinations of drugs, were consumed. In addition, in the search for new drugs with different and improved characteristics, such as more or less euphoria, hallucinogenic activity or stimulant properties, longer or shorter duration of action, literally hundreds of so-called designer drugs were synthesized (e.g., DOM, MDMA, DMT).

Concern about drug abuse rose until it finally was perceived as one of the nation's most pressing problems, along with the economy and the war in Vietnam (22). The nation geared up to declare war on drug abuse, and the national drug abuse effort expanded from a relatively small research-oriented program under the National Institute of Mental Health (NIMH) to the then newly created National Institute on Drug Abuse (NIDA) and the National Institute on Alcohol Abuse and Alcoholism (NIAAA). Eventually a new "superagency," ADAMHA (Alcohol, Drug Abuse, and Mental Health Administration), was established to oversee NIDA, NIAAA, and NIMH. In 1995, the combined NIDA and NIAAA annual budgets rose to more than $654 million dollars, not including the Drug Enforcement Agency (DEA) or the Bureau of Alcohol, Tobacco, and Firearms, who also have considerable budgets that are directed toward drug abuse enforcement. More recently, ADAMHA was merged into the National Institutes of Health (NIH).

By the mid-1960s more than a thousand articles on LSD had appeared in the medical literature. Sandoz

Laboratories stopped distributing the drug in late 1966 because of the reported adverse reactions and the resulting public outcry. At that time, all of the existing supplies of LSD were turned over to the government, which was to make the drug available for legitimate and highly controlled research; however, research on humans essentially was discontinued. Although some of the hallucinogens originally were developed and studied for use in chemical warfare, the results of these experiments remain classified. Today, LSD, along with heroin and marihuana, remains classified as a Schedule I drug according to the Comprehensive Drug Abuse Prevention and Control Act of 1970. Legally, LSD is regarded as having no currently accepted medical use in the United States, a high potential for abuse, and to be unsafe even when administered by a physician. The therapeutic potential of LSD as an adjunct to psychotherapy, in the management of the dying patient, and in the treatment of alcoholism and neuropsychiatric illness such as obsessive-compulsive disorder remains unresolved (23–26). Nevertheless, "black market" LSD remains widely available on the street.

DEFINITIONS AND TERMINOLOGY

The term *hallucinogen* means "producer of hallucinations." Many drugs, when taken in sufficient quantity, are psychoactive and can cause auditory and/or visual hallucinations. Such hallucinations may be present as part of a delirium, accompanied by disturbances in judgment, orientation, intellect, memory, emotion, and level of consciousness (e.g., organic brain syndrome). Delirium also may result from drug withdrawal (e.g., sedative–hypnotic withdrawal or delirium tremens in alcohol). Hallucinogen, however, generally refers to compounds that alter consciousness without producing delirium, sedation, excessive stimulation, or intellectual or memory impairment as prominent effects. This label actually is inaccurate because true LSD-induced "hallucinations" are rare; what are commonly seen are illusory phenomena. An illusion is a perceptual distortion of an actual stimulus in the environment: to see someone's face seeming to be melting is an illusion; whereas to see a melting face when no face is present is a hallucination.

There are a variety of widely accepted synonyms for the hallucinogens, including the term psychedelic, which was coined in 1957 by Osmond in the hope of finding a nonjudgmental term (27). Unfortunately, those who use the term psychedelic are criticized as being "prodrug" much as those who use the term hallucinogen are accused of being "antidrug." Other suggested names include phantastica, psychotaraxic, psycholeptic, and psychotomystic (28–30). The term *psychotomimetic*, meaning "a producer of psychosis," also has been widely used. For a review of Lewin's (31) original terminology and a classification system for the hallucinogenic drugs, see Shulgin (1).

EPIDEMIOLOGY

The epidemiologic data on the use of hallucinogens centers on the use of LSD. Both the use of LSD and its availability decreased from the mid-1970s through the 1980s (32). These downward trends appear to be reversing beginning in the 1990s (19,33). In 1992 there was an increase in prevalence in the use of LSD by school-age children and young adults, but there are indications that since that time increases have continued only in high school students (33). In 1994, the annual prevalence rates for LSD use were 7% in high school students and 5% in college students, and the lifetime prevalence rates for LSD and hallucinogens were 3.7% and 2.2% for students in the eighth grade, and 13.8% and 7.4%, respectively, in young adults (33). There are ethnic differences in the use of hallucinogens; in the twelfth grade whites have a higher usage of LSD and hallucinogens than either blacks and Hispanics (33). Other studies have shown even higher rates of hallucinogen usage. For example, a random survey of Tulane University undergraduates in 1990 indicated that the number of students reporting having tried LSD was more than 17% (34).

Hallucinogens appear to be readily available on the street. In 1994, more than 24% of 18-year-olds said that they were "exposed" (friends using drug or around people using drug) to LSD, whereas 14% said that they were "exposed" to other hallucinogens (33). Aside from increases in prevalence and use of hallucinogens, there also have been changes in attitudes toward their use. Among high school students there has been a decrease in the proportions disapproving of LSD use and associating risk with its use; in contrast, older groups are more likely to perceive LSD as dangerous (33). These changes in attitude are likely linked to the increase in use in those age groups.

PATTERNS OF ABUSE

In the 1960s, LSD was used primarily by those interested in its ability to alter perceptual experiences (sight, sound, taste, and even feeling states). Much attention was paid to *set*, the expectation of what the drug experience would be like, and *setting*, the environment in which the drug was used. The early drug missionaries promulgated the erroneous notion that only good LSD "trips" would result if the prospective user ensured a number of preconditions before their drug experience. Those preconditions relating to set included:

- Being relaxed and largely stress/anxiety free;
- Having no major resentment or anger and no recent arguments at home, school or work; and
- Freeing up several days, often an entire weekend, for the drug experience and its aftermath.

Those preconditions relating to setting included:

- Having a close friend present as a sitter or guide for the experience;

- Being in quiet, comfortable surroundings, particularly outdoors, or sitting on soft, thick carpeting;
- Listening to pleasant sounds (originally, the sitar music of Ravi Shankar); and
- Reading reassuring passages (originally, from the *Tibetan Book of the Dead.*)

In more recent times users often attended concerts, dances ("raves"), or films (particularly psychedelic or brightly colored ones) during the drug experience. Use is rarely more than once weekly because tolerance to LSD and other hallucinogens occurs so rapidly (see "Effects of Chronic Use" below).

CHEMICAL CLASSIFICATION

The commonly abused hallucinogenic substances can be classified according to their chemical structure. Figure 18.1 shows the structures of these hallucinogens. Note that all of these drugs are organic compounds and some occur naturally.

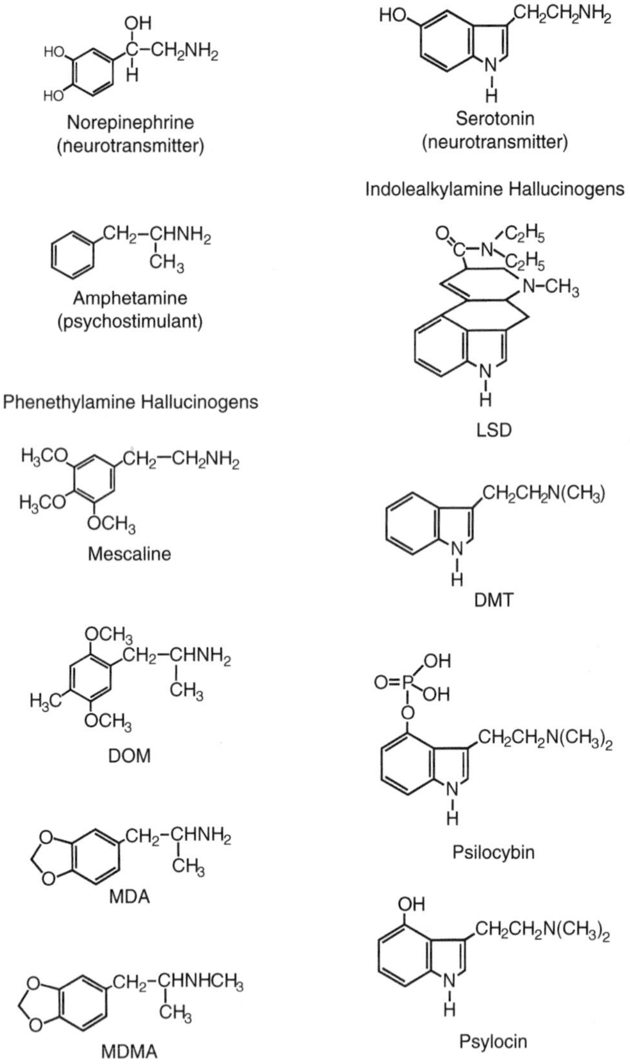

Indolealkylamines

All of the indole-type hallucinogens have structural similarities to the neurotransmitter serotonin (5-hydroxytryptamine [5-HT]), suggesting that their mechanism of action could involve the alteration of serotonergic neurotransmission.

Lysergic Acid Derivatives

Lysergic acid is one of the constituents of the ergot fungus that grows on rye. It has inadvertently been baked into bread, with profound mental changes occurring in those who consumed it (35). Because the presence of the diethylamide group is a prerequisite for hallucinogenic activity, it is not clear whether these reported epidemics actually were caused by ergot in the bread, or by some other related substances or (psychological) phenomena. LSD was first synthesized by Hofmann in 1938, and it was called LSD-25 because it was the twenty-fifth compound made in this series of experiments on ergot derivatives. In 1943, Hofmann accidentally ingested some of the compound, and soon had the first LSD "trip," a famous bicycle ride home from his laboratory. The seeds of the morning glory (*Ipomoea*) contain lysergic acid derivatives, particularly lysergic acid amide. Although they are packaged commercially, many varieties, such as Heavenly Blue and Pearly Gates, have been treated with insecticides, fungicides, and other toxic chemicals.

Substituted Tryptamines

Psilocybin and psilocin occur naturally in a variety of mushrooms that have hallucinogenic properties. The

FIG. 18.1. Structures of phenethylamine- and indolealkylamine-type hallucinogens.

most publicized is the Mexican or "magic" mushroom, *Psilocybe mexicana*, which contains both psilocybin and psilocin, as do some of the other *Psilocybe* and *Conocybe* species. DMT, although found in the psychoactive ayahuasca (15), is usually produced synthetically.

Substituted Phenethylamines

The substituted phenethylamine-type hallucinogens are structurally related to the catecholamine neurotransmitters dopamine, norepinephrine, and epinephrine.

Mescaline

Mescaline is a naturally occurring hallucinogen present in the peyote cactus (*Lophophora williamsii* or *Anhalonium lewinii*), which is found in the southwestern United States and northern Mexico. Peyote was used by the Indians in these areas in highly structured tribal religious rituals.

Phenylisopropylamines

The phenylisopropylamine hallucinogens DOM (or STP, from "serenity, tranquility and peace"), MDA (or "Eve"), and MDMA (or ecstasy) are synthetic compounds and are structurally similar to mescaline as well as the psychostimulant amphetamine. They have inaccurately been called "psychotomimetic amphetamines," and sometimes are referred to as "stimulant-hallucinogens." It should be pointed out that literally hundreds of analogues of the aforementioned compounds have been synthesized (16) and sometimes are found on the street, the so-called designer drugs.

ACUTE PSYCHOLOGICAL EFFECTS

The overall psychological effects of many of the hallucinogens are quite similar; however, the rate of onset, duration of action, and absolute intensity of the effects differ among the drugs. Moreover, the various hallucinogens vary widely in potency and the slope of the dose–response curve. Thus, some of the apparent qualitative differences among hallucinogens may be partly a result of the amount of drug ingested relative to its specific dose–response characteristics.

LSD is one of the most potent hallucinogens known, with behavioral effects occurring in some individuals after doses as low as 20 μg. In the past, typical street doses ranged from 50 to 300 μg; however, some anecdotal evidence indicates that today's street LSD is less potent, 20 to 80 μg. It should be pointed out that the reported street dose is often highly inaccurate.

Because of its high potency, LSD can be applied to paper blotters or the backs of postage stamps. The absorption of LSD from the gastrointestinal tract occurs rapidly, with drug diffusion to all tissues, including the brain. The onset of psychological and behavioral effects occurs approximately 60 minutes after oral administration and peaks 2 to 4 hours after administration, with a gradual return to the predrug state in 10 to 12 hours. Both Hofmann (36) and Hollister (2) have described the effects of LSD in great detail.

The first 4 hours are sometimes called a "trip." The subjective effects of LSD are dramatic (2), and can be divided into somatic (dizziness, paresthesias, weakness, and tremor), perceptual (altered visual sense and changes in hearing), and psychic (changes in mood, dream-like feelings, altered time sense, and depersonalization). The somatic symptoms usually occur first. Later, visual alterations are marked and sounds are intensified. Visual distortions and illusory phenomena occur, but true hallucinations are rare. Dream-like imagery may develop when the eyes are closed, and afterimages are prolonged. Sensory

input becomes mixed together, and synesthesia ("seeing" smells, "hearing" colors) is commonly reported. Touch is magnified and time is markedly distorted. Feelings of attainment of true insight are common, as is the experience of delusional ideation. Separating one object from another and self from environment becomes difficult, and depersonalization can develop. Emotions become intensified, and extreme lability may be observed, with rapid and extreme changes in affect. Several emotional feelings may occur at the same time. Performance on tests involving attention, concentration, and motivation is impaired. Several hours later, subjects sometimes feel that the drug is no longer active, but later they recognize that at that time they had paranoid thoughts and ideas of reference. This is a regular, but little publicized, aftereffect that finally dissipates 10 to 12 hours after the dose. From 12 to 24 hours after the trip there may be some slight let down or a feeling of fatigue. There is no immediate craving to take more drug to relieve this boredom; one trip usually produces "satiation" for some time. Memory for the events that occurred during the trip is quite clear.

DMT produces effects that are similar to those produced by LSD, but DMT is inactive after oral administration and must be injected, sniffed, or smoked. It has a rapid onset, almost immediately after intravenous administration, and a short duration of action, about 30 minutes (10). Because of its short duration of action, DMT was once known as the "businessman's LSD" (i.e., one could have a psychedelic experience during the lunch hour and be back at work in the afternoon). However, the sudden and rapid onset of a period of altered perceptions that soon terminates is disconcerting to some. DMT has never been a widely, steadily available or popular drug on the streets. The effects of ayahuasca, a psychoactive beverage that contains DMT, last about 4 hours (15).

In contrast to DMT, the effects of DOM have a very slow onset, but it has been reported to last more than 24 hours. Mescaline is approximately two to three orders of magnitude less potent than LSD, and its effects last about 6 to 10 hours, whereas the effects of psilocybin last about 2 hours (13).

AUTONOMIC AND OTHER EFFECTS

The hallucinogens also possess significant autonomic activity. LSD produces marked pupillary dilation, hyperreflexia, increases in blood pressure and body temperature, tremor, piloerection, and tachycardia. Some of these autonomic effects of the hallucinogens are variable and might be partly a result of the anxiety state of the user. DMT and ayahuasca also increases heart rate, pupil diameter, and body temperature (9,15). LSD also can cause nausea, and nausea and vomiting are especially noteworthy after the ingestion of mescaline or peyote. The hallucinogens also alter neuroendocrine function. For example, in humans, DMT elevates plasma levels of adrenocorticotropic hormone (ACTH), cortisol, and pro-lactin (9). Similarly, LSD (34) and the hallucinogen 1-(2,5-dimethoxy-4-iodophenyl)-2-aminopropane (DOI) (38) increase plasma glucocorticoids in the rat.

EFFECTS OF CHRONIC USE

A high degree of tolerance develops to the behavioral effects of LSD after repeated administration. Such behavioral tolerance develops very rapidly, after only several days of daily administration, and tolerance is also lost rapidly after the individual stops taking the drug for several days. Because of this rapid development of tolerance, LSD users usually limit themselves to taking the drug once or twice weekly (39). Cross-tolerance develops between LSD and other hallucinogens, such as mescaline and psilocybin, suggesting a similar mechanism of action. However, cross-tolerance does not develop to other classes of psychotropic agents that are thought to have different underlying mechanisms of action, such as amphetamine, phencyclidine, and marihuana. It should be pointed out that little tolerance develops to the various autonomic effects produced by the hallucinogens. There is no withdrawal syndrome after the cessation of the chronic administration of the hallucinogens.

MECHANISMS OF ACTION

The exact mechanisms of action of LSD and other hallucinogens still remain unclear. LSD affects the electrical activity of neurons in the locus ceruleus and certain cortical regions, and at a system level, these effects could change how the brain handles sensory information, as well as alter cognitive and perceptual processing (18). Although hallucinogenic drugs interact with several neurotransmitter systems (40), their ability to alter neurotransmission mediated by the neurotransmitter serotonin appears to be of critical importance (41,42). It is important to note that an ever-increasing number of serotonin receptors have been identified, and the terminology for these serotonin receptor families and subtypes is in a state of flux (43–45). Some of the receptors have been renamed and/or reclassified, and caution must be used in comparing results and conclusions drawn from older studies with the nomenclature currently used.

Early on it was noted that many hallucinogens, including LSD, were structurally similar to serotonin (see Fig. 18.1). Later, studies demonstrated that LSD could block the contractile effects of serotonin in isolated smooth-muscle preparations, suggesting that LSD might produce its psychic effects by having similar antagonist activity at central serotonergic synapses. However, it was found that brom-LSD, an LSD analogue that does not produce hallucinations, also has serotonergic antagonist activity. Thus, the mechanism of the hallucinogenic activity of LSD could not be explained solely by its direct serotonergic antagonist activity.

In 1961, Freedman (46) was the first to provide direct evidence that LSD acted upon serotonergic systems within the central nervous system. He found that LSD increases the levels of serotonin in rat brain, but decreases the levels of serotonin metabolites, whereas the nonhallucinogenic analogue brom-LSD failed to have the same effects. That brom-LSD does not produce hallucinatory phenomena, suggests that the hallucinogenic effects of LSD might be caused by LSD-induced decreases in serotonin turnover (synthesis and release) in the brain. Other evidence supporting the interaction of hallucinogens with serotonergic systems: (a) the chronic administration of monoamine oxidase inhibitors decreases the density of serotonin receptors and reduces the behavioral effects of LSD (47,48), and (b) treatments that decrease brain levels of serotonin (e.g., lesions, reserpine, parachloroamphetamine or other neurotoxins), upregulate postsynaptic serotonin receptors and increase the behavioral effects of LSD (41).

Aghajanian and coworkers (49) found that LSD inhibits the firing of serotonergic neurons in the dorsal raphe nucleus, most likely by interacting with presynaptic autoreceptors (50), now termed $5-HT_{1A}$ receptors. Other indole-type hallucinogens, such as psilocin and DMT, also produce this effect (50). A decrease in firing rate of serotonergic neurons would account for Freedman's (46) observation that LSD increases the levels of serotonin, but decreases the levels of serotonin metabolites. However, strong evidence refutes a direct linkage between the presynaptic effects of LSD and its hallucinogenic activity: (a) phenethylamine hallucinogens, such as mescaline, do not have the same inhibitory effects on the firing of serotonergic neurons (51); (b) there is no correlation between the activity of drugs at presynaptic $5-HT_{1A}$ receptors and their hallucinogenic activity (18); and (c) tolerance does not develop to the effects of the hallucinogens on neuronal firing, but behavioral tolerance rapidly develops after the repeated administration of hallucinogens (52). These findings suggest that interactions with presynaptic $5-HT_{1A}$ receptors cannot be the sole mechanism of action of the hallucinogens, and other factors must be involved.

Both indole- and phenethylamine-type hallucinogens bind to the serotonin $5-HT_{2A}$ receptor subtype (formerly called the $5-HT_2$ receptor) (53–58), where they act as agonists or partial agonists (56,58). This receptor subtype is found in high concentrations in cortical and limbic regions (59), and interactions with these receptors appear to underlie the mechanism of action of the hallucinogens. For example: (a) there are very high correlations between the binding affinities of both indolealkylamine- and phenethylamine-type hallucinogens for the $5-HT_{2A}$ receptor and their hallucinogenic activity in humans and their potency in behavioral studies in laboratory animals (53,58); (b) the chronic administration of LSD, but not the nonhallucinogenic analogue brom-LSD, decreases the density of 5-HT$_{2A}$ receptors, an effect associated with the development of tolerance to the behavioral effects of LSD (60); and (c) preclinical studies found that many of the effects of hallucinogens are blocked by 5-HT$_{2A}$ receptor antagonists (58,61).

Even though the interaction of hallucinogens with 5-HT$_{2A}$ receptors appears to be critical, other serotonergic receptor subtypes also might be involved. For example, interactions with the closely related 5-HT$_{2C}$ receptors (formerly called 5-HT$_{1C}$ receptors) might contribute to the psychoactive effects (55,62). Although apparently not critical for hallucinogenic activity, interactions with presynaptic 5-HT$_{1A}$ receptors might contribute to the effects of some hallucinogens. The differential interactions of the various hallucinogens with numerous sites and systems might underlie the qualitative differences between the drugs. However, the commonality of interactions with 5-HT$_{2A}$ receptors suggests that drugs that possess 5-HT$_{2A}$ receptor antagonist activity might be useful in blocking the behavioral effects of the hallucinogens in humans.

ADVERSE REACTIONS

Strassman (63) has characterized adverse reactions according to the temporal relationship between drug exposure and symptomatology, with acute and chronic reactions at the end of the continuum, and delayed (subsequent panic attacks) and intermittent (flashback phenomena) between the ends of the continuum. Although the existence of some of the acute adverse reactions is clear-cut and not subject to debate, some of the purported long-term adverse effects remain controversial. One of the problems is that many of the studies reporting long-term adverse reactions lack adequate predrug data.

Acute Adverse Reactions

Social factors, media presentations, and public fear have all shaped perceptions of the effects of LSD and other hallucinogens. A person's reaction to the effects of a drug may be felt to be either a pleasant or an unpleasant experience; a perceptual distortion or illusion may cause intense anxiety in one person and be a pleasant and amusing interlude in another. Individuals who place a premium on self-control, advance planning, and impulse restriction may do particularly poorly on LSD. Traumatic and stressful external events can precipitate an adverse reaction (e.g., being arrested and read one's rights in the middle of a pleasant experience may precipitate an anxiety reaction). Prediction of who will have an acute (or other) adverse reaction is unreliable (20), and the occurrence of multiple previous pleasurable LSD experiences renders no immunity from an adverse reaction. Adverse reactions have occurred after doses of LSD as low as 40 μg, and no adverse effects have been observed in some individuals after ingesting 2000 μg, although in general the hallucinogenic effects are dose-dependent. Thus, acute adverse behavioral reactions generally are not dose-related, but a function of personal predisposition, setting, and circumstance. Because of the perceptual distortions (and subsequent deficits in judgment), there is always the risk that self-destructive behavior will occur. Some of the adverse reactions that occur after ingesting hallucinogens can be caused by other contaminants in the product, such as strychnine, phencyclidine, or amphetamine. Once commonly reported by medical facilities (64), acute adverse LSD reactions are rarely seen today, yet the drug remains in use. Moreover, the paucity of users seeking emergency medical treatment may reflect increased knowledge of how to deal with such situations on the part of the "drug-using community," as well as a decrease in the doses of LSD currently used compared to those used in the past.

Acute anxiety or panic reactions, the so-called bad trip, are the most commonly reported acute adverse reactions. They usually wear off before medical intervention is sought; most LSD is metabolized and excreted within 24 hours, and acute panic reactions usually subside within this time frame. Depression with suicidal ideation can occur several days after LSD use (65).

Paranoid ideation, "hallucinations," and a confusional state (organic brain syndrome) are other commonly reported acute adverse reactions (66,67). Initially it was thought that LSD could replicate the signs and symptoms of schizophrenia in some subjects, and the induction of such a model psychosis could be used to study and potentially find a cure for this major psychiatric illness. These hopes did not materialize, as major differences have been found between hallucinogen-induced psychosis and the schizophrenic state (68). More recently, using single-photon emission computed tomography (SPECT), it was found that the administration of mescaline to controls produced a "hyperfrontal" pattern, whereas "hypofrontality" has been observed in schizophrenics (6). However, using positron emission tomography, Gouzoulis-Mayfrank et al. (12) found that psilocybin produced changes in glucose metabolism similar to those in acute schizophrenic patients.

Diagnostically, it is important to make a differential diagnosis between LSD psychosis and paranoid schizophrenia, particularly because patients, who in fact are paranoid, now often complain of being poisoned with LSD. A history of prior mental illness, a psychiatric examination that reveals the absence of an intact or observing ego, and auditory (rather than visual) hallucinations all suggest schizophrenia. Other drug-induced psychoses, including those from psychostimulants or PCP, must be ruled out. An organic brain syndrome in general speaks against LSD, especially when obtunded consciousness is present.

Toxicologic analysis of body fluids can be helpful in making the ultimate diagnosis, but supportive treatment must not be withheld. Atropine poisoning can be differentiated by the presence of prominent anticholinergic effects such as dry mouth and blurred vision. Patients with amphetamine psychosis often fail to differentiate their perceptual distortions from reality, whereas LSD users are aware of the difference.

In terms of adverse physiologic effects, LSD has a very high therapeutic index. An elephant was killed after the experimental administration of a massive dose relative to brain weight, 0.15 mg/kg, or approximately 300,000 μg of LSD (28). The lethal dose in humans has not been determined, and fatalities that have been reported usually are secondary to perceptual distortions with resultant accidental death (e.g., "flying" off a roof, merging with an oncoming automobile on the freeway) (69). Hemiplegia has been reported after taking LSD, possibly as a consequence of the production of vasospasm (70). More recently, a fibrotic inflammatory mass located in the mesentery was reported in a chronic LSD user (71), and multifocal cerebral demyelination was reported after the use of "magic mushrooms" (72). Although mescaline is often viewed as posing a minimal health risk, a case of fatal peyote ingestion associated with Mallory-Weiss lacerations, probably as a result of peyote-induced vomiting, has been reported (73).

Treatment of Acute Adverse Reactions

Treatment of the acute adverse reactions to hallucinogens first must be directed toward preventing the patient from physically harming self or others. Anxiety can be handled by means of interpersonal support and reassurance. Psychotherapeutic intervention consists of reassurance, placing the patient in a quiet room, and avoidance of physical intrusion until the patient begins to calm down. The use of a benzodiazepine, such as lorazepam (Ativan), also can be effective. The oral route can be used for administering such medication in mildly agitated patients; however, it can be difficult to convince severely agitated and/or paranoid patients to swallow a pill, in which case parenteral administration might be necessary. Severely agitated patients who fail to respond to a benzodiazepine may be given a neuroleptic agent. Caution must be used in administering neuroleptics because they can lower the seizure threshold and elicit seizures, especially if the hallucinogen has been cut with an agent that has convulsant activity, such as strychnine. Phenothiazines, such as chlorpromazine (Thorazine), given orally or intramuscularly can end an LSD trip and are effective in treating LSD-induced psychosis (29,74–76). Because anticholinergic crises can develop with chlorpromazine in combination with other drugs with anticholinergic activity (PCP and DOM), haloperidol (Haldol) is a safer drug to use when the true nature of the drug ingested is unknown. It has been suggested that a combination of intramuscular haloperidol and lorazepam is particularly effective in treating acute adverse reactions (77). Theoretically, selective 5-HT$_{2A}$ antagonists should block the effects of hallucinogens; however, other drugs with significant 5-HT$_{2A}$ antagonist activity (e.g., clozapine [Clozaril], olanzapine [Zyprexa], and risperidone [Risperdal]) also might be effective (18). Vollenweider et al. (13) found that the psychotomimetic effects of psilocybin are blocked by the 5-HT$_{2A}$ antagonists ketanserin and risperidone; however, haloperidol *increased* the psychotomimetic effects. It should be noted that there is some indication that risperidone might exacerbate flashbacks (78).

Drug Interactions

Drugs interactions involving the hallucinogens do not appear to be an important source of adverse reactions. There are reports that the effects of LSD are reduced after the chronic administration of monoamine oxidase inhibitors or selective serotonin reuptake inhibitor antidepressants such as fluoxetine (Prozac) (79–82), whereas the effects of LSD are increased after the chronic administration of lithium or tricyclic antidepressants (81,82).

Long-Term Adverse Effects

Chronic adverse reactions include psychoses, depressive reactions, acting out, paranoid states, and flashbacks (30,83). The use of LSD has been found to coincide with the onset of depression, suggesting its possible role in the etiology of some depression in the young (84). Flashbacks are a well-publicized adverse reaction. They now have been renamed "hallucinogen persisting perception disorder," and have specific diagnostic criteria (85). In the past, the use of variable definitions of what constitutes a flashback was a major problem (86); hopefully the establishment of specific diagnostic criteria will facilitate studying and understanding this problem. Only a small proportion of LSD and other hallucinogenic users experience flashbacks (87). They can occur spontaneously a number of weeks or months after the original drug experience, appear not to be dose-related, and can develop after a single exposure to the drug (88). During a flashback, the original drug experience is recreated complete with perceptual and reality distortion. Even a previously pleasant drug experience may be accompanied by anxiety when the person realizes that they have no control over its recurrence. In time, flashbacks decrease in intensity, frequency, and duration (although initially they usually last only a few seconds), whether treated or not. Flashbacks may or may not be precipitated by stressors or the subsequent use of other psychoactive drugs, such as psilocybin or marihuana. The administration of selective serotonin reuptake inhibitor antidepressants (89) and risperidone (78,90) is reported to initiate or exacerbate flashbacks in individuals with a history of LSD use. Flashbacks usually can be handled with psychotherapy. An anxiolytic or neuroleptic may be indicated, but probably is as much for the reassurance of the therapist as for the patient. Various pharmacologic agents, such as clonidine (Catapres) or clonazepam (Klonopin) (91), or drug combinations (e.g., fluoxetine and olanzapine) (92), have been found to be useful in the treatment of flashbacks. The exact mechanism underlying this phenomenon remains obscure. Individuals with flashbacks have a high lifetime incidence of affective disorder when compared to non–LSD-abusing substance abusers (67). LSD users have long-term changes in visual function (17,93–95). For example, a visual disturbance consisting of prolonged afterimages (palinopsia) has been found in individuals several years after the last reported use of LSD (96). Such changes in visual function might underlie flashbacks.

Psychosis can develop and persist after hallucinogen use, but it remains unclear whether hallucinogen use can "cause" long-term psychosis, or if it has a role in precipitating the onset of illness. For example, hallucinogens may have a variety of effects in a person who is genetically predisposed to schizophrenia: (a) they may cause the psychosis to manifest at an earlier age; (b) they may produce a psychosis that would have remained dormant if drugs had not been used; or (c) they may cause relapse in a person who has previously suffered a psychotic disorder (68). Although there is some evidence that prolonged psychotic reactions tend to occur in individuals with poor premorbid adjustment, a history of psychiatric illness and/or repeated use of hallucinogens, severe and prolonged illness has been reported in individuals without such a history (63).

There are few if any long-term neuropsychological deficits attributable to hallucinogen use (97). Chronic personality changes with a shift in attitudes and evidence of magical thinking can occur after the use of hallucinogens. There is always the risk that such thinking can lead to destructive behavior, in acute as well as chronic reactions. The effects of the chronic use of LSD must be differentiated from the effects of personality disorders, particularly in those who use a variety of drugs in polydrug abuse patterns. In some individuals with well-integrated personalities and with no previous psychiatric history, chronic personality changes have resulted from repeated LSD use. Personality changes that result from LSD use can occur after a single experience, unlike other classes of drugs (PCP, perhaps, excepted) (83). In addition, the hallucinogenic drugs interact in a variety of nonspecific ways with the personality, which may particularly impair the developing adolescent (74). The suggestibility that may come from many experiences with LSD may be reinforced by the social values of a particular subculture in which the drug is used. For example, if some of these subcultures embrace withdrawal from society, that is to say, a noncompetitive approach toward life, the person who "withdraws" after the LSD experience may be suffering from a side effect that represents more of a change in social values than a true drug effect. Treatment of chronic hallucinogen abuse can include psychotherapy on a long-term basis to determine what needs are being fulfilled by the use of the drug for this particular person. Twelve-step meetings also might be crucial for reinforcement of the decision to remain abstinent.

There is no generally accepted evidence of brain cell damage, chromosomal abnormalities, or teratogenic effects after the use of the indole-type hallucinogens and mescaline (63,98).

ACKNOWLEDGMENTS

The authors would like to thank Dr. Michael P. Bova for preparing the figure.

REFERENCES

1. Shulgin AT. Psychotomimetic drugs: structure-activity relationships. In: Iversen LL, Iversen SD, Snyder SH, eds. Handbook of psychopharmacology. New York: Plenum Press, 1978;11:243–333.
2. Hollister LE. Psychotomimetic drugs in man. In: Iversen LL, Iversen SD, Snyder SH, eds. Handbook of psychopharmacology. New York: Plenum Press, 1978;11:389–424.
3. Siegel RK. The natural history of hallucinogens. In: Jacobs BL, ed. Hallucinogens: neurochemical, behavioral, and clinical perspectives. New York: Raven Press, 1984:1–18.
4. Halpern JH, Pope HG Jr. Hallucinogens on the Internet: a vast new source of underground drug information. Am J Psychiatry 2001;158:481–483.
5. Al-Assmar SE. The seeds of the Hawaiian baby woodrose are a powerful hallucinogen. Arch Intern Med 1999;59:2090.
6. Hermle L, Fünfgeld M, Oepen G, et al. Mescaline-induced psychopathological, neuropsychological, and neurometabolic effects in normal subjects: experimental psychosis as a tool for psychiatric research. Biol Psychiatry 1992;32:976–991.
7. Hermle L, Spitzer M, Borchardt D, et al. Psychological effects of MDE in normal subjects. Neuropsychopharmacology 1993;8:171–176.
8. Gouzoulis E, von Bardeleben U, Rupp A, et al. Neuroendocrine and cardiovascular effects of MDE in healthy volunteers. Neuropsychopharmacology 1993;8:187–193.
9. Strassman RJ, Qualls CR. Dose-response study of N,N-dimethyltryptamine in humans. I. Neuroendocrine, autonomic and cardiovascular effects. Arch Gen Psychiatry 1994;51:85–97.
10. Strassman RJ, Qualls CR, Uhlenhuth EH, et al. Dose-response study of N,N-dimethyltryptamine in humans. II. Subjective effects and preliminary results of a new rating scale. Arch Gen Psychiatry 1994;51:98–108.
11. Strassman RJ. Hallucinogenic drugs in psychiatric research and treatment; perspectives and prospects. J Nerv Ment Dis 1995;183:127–138.

12. Gouzoulis-Mayfrank E, Schreckenberger M, Sabri O, et al. Neurometabolic effects of psilocybin, 3,4-methylenedioxyethylamphetamine (MDE) and d-methamphetamine in healthy volunteers. *Neuropsychopharmacology* 1999;20:565–581.

13. Vollenweider FX, Vollenweider-Scherpenhuyzen MFI, Babler A, et al. Psilocybin induces schizophrenia-like psychosis in humans via a serotonin-2 agonist action. *Neuroreport* 1998;9:3897–3902.

14. Vollenweider FX, Vontobel P, Hell D, et al. 5-HT modulation of dopamine release in basal ganglia in psilocybin-induced psychosis in man—a PET study with [^{11}C]raclopride. *Neuropsychopharmacology* 1999;20:424–433.

15. Riba J, Rodriguez-Fornells A, Urbano G, et al. Subjective effects and tolerability of the South American psychoactive beverage ayahuasca in healthy volunteers. *Psychopharmacology* 2001;154:85–95.

16. Shulgin A, Shulgin A. *PIHKAL: a chemical love story.* Berkeley, CA: Transform Press, 1991.

17. Abraham HD, Aldridge AM. Adverse consequences of lysergic acid diethylamide. *Addiction* 1993;88:1327–1334.

18. Aghajanian GK. Serotonin and the action of LSD in the brain. *Psychiatr Ann* 1994;24:137–141.

19. Schwartz RH. LSD: its rise, fall, and renewed popularity among high school students. *Pediatr Clin North Am* 1995;42:403–413.

20. Ungerleider JT, Fisher DD, Fuller MC, et al. The bad trip: the etiology of the adverse LSD reaction. *Am J Psychiatry* 1968;125:1483–1490.

21. Weil A. *Natural mind.* Boston: Houghton Mifflin, 1972:10

22. National Commission on Marijuana and Drug Abuse. *Appendices to marijuana: signal of misunderstanding, and drug abuse: problem in perspective.* Washington, DC: US Government Printing Office, 1972, 1973.

23. Magini M. Treatment of alcoholism using psychedelic drugs: a review of the program of research. *J Psychedelic Drugs* 1998;30:381–418.

24. Delgado PL, Moreno FA. Hallucinogens, serotonin and obsessive-compulsive disorder. *J Psychedelic Drugs* 1998;30:359–366.

25. Perrine DM. Hallucinogens and obsessive-compulsive disorder. *Am J Psychiatry* 1999;156(7):1123.

26. Grob CS. Psychiatric research with hallucinogens: what have we learned. In Grob CS, ed. *Hallucinogens, a reader.* New York: Jeremy P. Tarcher/Putnam, 2002:263–291.

27. Osmond H. A review of the clinical effects of psychotomimetic agents. *Ann N Y Acad Sci* 1957;66:418.

28. Cohen S. A quarter century of research with LSD. In: Ungerleider JT, ed. *The problems and prospects of LSD.* Springfield, IL: Charles C Thomas, 1972:20–45.

29. Cohen S. Psychotomimetics (hallucinogens) and cannabis. In: Clark WG, del Guidice J, eds. *Principles of psychopharmacology.* New York: Academic Press, 1978:357–371.

30. Shick JFE, Freedman DX. Research in non-narcotic drug abuse. In: Arieti S, ed. *American handbook of psychiatry.* New York: Basic Books, 1975;6:552–622.

31. Lewin L. *Phantastica: narcotic and stimulating drugs,* their use and abuse. 1931, E.P. Dutton and Company, New York. Translated from the second German edition by P.H.A. Wirth, Munich.

32. Johnston L. *Monitoring the Future—the national high school senior survey.* Washington, DC: National Institute of Drug Abuse, 1990.

33. Johnston LD, O'Malley PM, Bachman JG. *National survey results on drug use from the Monitoring the Future Study, Vol. II, 1975-1994.* NIH Publication 96-4027, Rockville, MD. National Institute on Drug Abuse, 1996.

34. Cuomo MJ, Dyment PG, Gammino VM. Increasing use of "ecstasy" (MDMA) and other hallucinogens on a college campus. *J Am Coll Health* 1994;42:271–274.

35. Fuller JG. *The day of St. Anthony's fire.* New York: Macmillan, 1968.

36. Hofmann A. Chemical, pharmacological and medical aspects of psychotomimetics. *J Exp Ment Dis* 1961;5:31–51.

37. Halaris AE, Freedman DX, Fang VS. Plasma corticoids and brain tryptophan after acute and chronic dosage of LSD. *Life Sci* 1975;17:1467–1472.

38. Nash FJ, Meltzer HY, Gudelsky GA. Selective cross-tolerance to 5-HT$_{1A}$ and 5-HT$_2$ receptor-mediated temperature and corticosterone responses. *Pharmacol Biochem Behav* 1989;33:781–785.

39. Ungerleider JT, Fisher DD. The problems of LSD and emotional disorders. *Calif Med* 1967;106:49–55.

40. Hamon M. Common neurochemical correlates to the action of hallucinogens. In: Jacobs BL, ed. *Hallucinogens: neurochemical, behavioral and clinical perspectives.* New York: Raven Press, 1984:143–169.

41. Freedman DX. Hallucinogenic drug research—if so, so what? Symposium summary and commentary. *Pharmacol Biochem Behav* 1986;24:407–415.

42. Jacobs BL. How hallucinogenic drugs work. *Am Sci* 1987;75:386–392.

43. Saxena PR. Serotonin receptors: subtypes, functional responses and therapeutic relevance. *Pharmacol Ther* 1995;66:339–368.

44. Humphrey PPA, Hartig PD. A proposed new nomenclature for 5-HT receptors. *Trends Pharmacol Sci* 1993;14:233–236.

45. Teitler M, Herrick-Davis K. Multiple serotonin receptor subtypes: molecular cloning and functional expression. *Crit Rev Neurobiol* 1994;8:175–188.

46. Freedman DX. Effects of LSD-25 on brain serotonin. *J Pharmacol Exp Ther* 1961;134:160–166.

47. Grof S, Dytrych Z. Blocking of LSD reaction by premedication with Niamid. *Act Nerv Super (Praha)* 1965;7:306.

48. Lucki I, Frazer A. Prevention of the serotonin syndrome in rats by repeated administration of monoamine oxidase inhibitors but not tricyclic antidepressants. *Psychopharmacology* 1981;77:205–211.

49. Aghajanian GK, Foote WE, Sheard MH. Lysergic acid diethylamide: sensitive neuronal units in the midbrain raphe. *Science* 1968;161:706–708.

50. Aghajanian GK, Sprouse JS, Rasmussen K. Physiology of the midbrain serotonin system. In: Meltzer HY, ed. *Psychopharmacology: the third generation of progress.* New York: Raven Press, 1987:141–149.

51. Trulson ME, Heym J, Jacobs BL. Dissociations between the effects of hallucinogenic drugs on behavior and raphe unit activity in freely moving cats. *Brain Res* 1981;215:275–293.

52. Trulson ME, Jacobs BL. Dissociations between the effects of LSD on behavior and raphe unit activity in freely moving cats. *Science* 1979;205:515–518.

53. Glennon RA, Titeler M, McKenney JD. Evidence for 5-HT$_2$ involvement in the mechanism of action of hallucinogenic agents. *Life Sci* 1984;35:2505–2511.

54. Lyon RA, Glennon RA, Titeler M. 3,4-Methylenedioxymethamphetamine (MDMA): stereoselective interactions at brain 5-HT$_1$ and 5-HT$_2$ receptors. *Psychopharmacology* 1986;88:525–526.

55. Titeler M, Lyon RA, Glennon RA. Radioligand binding evidence implicates the brain 5-HT$_2$ receptor as a site of action for LSD and phenylisopropylamine hallucinogens. *Psychopharmacology* 1988;94:213–216.

56. Sadzot B, Baraban JM, Glennon RA, et al. Hallucinogenic drug interactions at human 5-HT$_2$ receptors: implications for treating LSD-induced hallucinogens. *Psychopharmacology* 1989;98:495–499.

57. Pierce PA, Peroutka SJ. Hallucinogenic drug interactions with neurotransmitter receptor binding sites in human cortex. *Psychopharmacology* 1989;97:118–122.

58. Glennon RA. Do classical hallucinogens act as 5-HT$_2$ agonists or antagonists? *Neuropsychopharmacology* 1990;3: 509–517.

59. Pazos A, Cortes R, Palacios JM. Quantitative autoradiographic mapping of serotonin receptors in the rat brain. II. Serotonin-2 receptors. *Brain Res* 1985; 346:231–249.

60. Buckholtz NS, Zhou D, Freedman DX, et al. Lysergic acid diethylamide (LSD) administration selectively downregulates serotonin receptors in rat brain. *Neuropsychopharmacology* 1990;3: 137–148.

61. Glennon RA, Young R, Rosecrans JA. Antagonism of the effects of the hallucinogen DOM and the purported 5-HT agonist quipazine by 5-HT$_2$ antagonists. *Eur J Pharmacol* 1983;91:189–196.

62. Burris KD, Breeding M, Sanders-Bush E. (+)Lysergic acid diethylamide, but not its nonhallucinogenic congeners, is a potent serotonin 5-HT$_{1C}$ receptor agonist. *J Pharmacol Exp Ther* 1991;258:891–896.

63. Strassman RJ. Adverse reactions to psychedelic drugs: a review of the literature. *J Nerv Ment Dis* 1984;172:577–595.

64. Ungerleider JT, Fisher DD, Goldsmith SR, et al. A statistical survey of adverse reactions to LSD in Los Angeles County. *Am J Psychiatry* 1968;125:352–357.

65. Madden JS. LSD and post-hallucinogen perceptual disorder. *Addiction* 1994;86: 762–763.

66. Ungerleider JT. The acute side effects from LSD. In: Ungerleider JT, ed. *The problems and prospects of LSD.* Springfield, IL: Charles C Thomas, 1972:61–68.

67. Abraham HD, Aldridge AM. LSD: a point well taken. *Addiction* 1994;89:763.

68. Bowers MB Jr. The role of drugs in the production of schizophreniform psychoses and related disorders. In: Meltzer HY, ed. *Psychopharmacology: the third generation of progress.* New York: Raven Press, 1987:819–823.

69. Ungerleider JT, Fisher DD, Fuller MC. The dangers of LSD: analysis of seven months' experience in a university hospital's psychiatric service. *JAMA* 1966; 197:389–392.

70. Sobel J, Espinas O, Friedman S. Carotid artery obstruction following LSD capsule ingestion. *Arch Intern Med* 1971;127:290–291.

71. Berk SI, LeBlond RF, Hodges KB, et al. A mesenteric mass in a chronic LSD user. *Am J Med* 1999;107;188–198.

72. Spengos K, Schwartz A, Hennerici M. Multifocal cerebral demyelination after magic mushroom abuse. *J Neurol* 2000; 247;224–225.

73. Nolte KB, Zumwalt, RE. Fatal peyote ingestion associated with Mallory-Weiss lacerations. *West J Med* 1999;170; 328.

74. Miller D. The drug-dependent adolescent. In: Feinstein SC, Giovachini P, eds. *Adolescent psychiatry.* New York: Basic Books, pp. 70–97, 1973.

75. Neff L. Chemicals and their effects on the adolescent ego. In: Feinstein S, Giovacchini P, Miller A, eds. *Adolescent psychiatry.* New York: Basic Books, pp. 108–120, 1971.

76. Dewhurst K, Hatrick JA. Differential diagnosis and treatment of lysergic acid diethylamide-induced psychosis. *Practitioner* 1972;209:327–332.

77. Miller PL, Gay GR, Ferris KC, et al. Treatment of acute, adverse reactions: "I've tripped and I can't get down." *J Psychoactive Drugs* 1992;24:277–279.

78. Lerner AG, Shufman E, Kodesh A, et al. Risperidone-associated, benign transient visual disturbances in schizophrenic patients with a past history of LSD abuse. *Isr J Psychiatry Relat Sci* 2002;39:57–60.

79. Resnick O, Krus DM, Raskin M. LSD-25 action in normal subjects treated with a monoamine oxidase inhibitor. *Life Sci* 1964;3:1207–1214.

80. Strassman RJ. Human hallucinogen interactions with drugs affecting serotonergic neurotransmission. *Neuropsychopharmacology* 1992;7:241–243.

81. Bonson KR, Murphy DL. Alterations in responses to LSD in humans associated with chronic administration of tricyclic antidepressants, monoamine oxidase inhibitors or lithium. *Behav Brain Res* 1996;73:229–233.

82. Bonson KR, Buckholtz JW, Murphy DL. Chronic administration of serotonergic antidepressants attenuates the subjective effects of LSD in humans. *Neuropsychopharmacology* 1996;14:425–437.

83. Fisher DD. The chronic side effects from LSD. In: Ungerleider JT, ed. *The problems and prospects of LSD.* Springfield, IL: Charles C Thomas, 1972:69–80.

84. Abraham HD, Fava M. Order of onset of substance abuse and depression in a sample of depressed outpatients. *Comp Psychiatry* 1999;40:44–50.

85. American Psychiatric Association. *Diagnostic and statistical manual of mental disorders,* 4th ed. Washington, DC: Author, 1994.

86. Frankel FH. The concept of flashbacks in historical perspective. *Int J Clin Exp Hypn* 1994;42:321–335.

87. Shick JFE, Smith DE. An analysis of the LSD flashback. *J Psychedelic Drugs* 1970;3:13–19.

88. Levi L, Miller NR. Visual illusions associated with previous drug abuse. *J Clin Neuroophthalmol* 1990;10:103–110.

89. Markel H, Lee A, Holmes RD, et al. LSD flashback syndrome exacerbated by selective serotonin reuptake inhibitor antidepressants in adolescents. *J Pediatr* 1994:125:817–819.

90. Alcantara AG. Is the a role of alpha-2 antagonism in the exacerbation of hallucinogen-persisting perception disorder with risperidone. *J Clin Psychopharmacol* 1998;18:487–488.

91. Lerner AG, Gelkopf M, Skladman I, et al. Flashback and hallucinogen persisting perception disorder: clinical aspects and pharmacological treatment approach. *Isr J Psychiatry Relat Sci* 2002;39:92–99.

92. Aldurra G, Crayton JW. Improvement of hallucinogen persisting perception disorder by treatment with a combination of fluoxetine and olanzapine: case report. *J Clin Psychopharmacol* 2001;21:343–344.

93. Abraham HD. A chronic impairment of colour vision in users of LSD. *Br J Psychiatry* 1982;140:518–520.

94. Abraham HD, Wolf E. Visual function in past users of LSD: psychophysical findings. *J Abnorm Psychol* 1988;97:443–447.

95. Abraham HD, Duffy FH. EEG coherence in post-LSD visual hallucinations. *Psychiatry Res* 2001;107:151–163.

96. Kawasaki A, Purvin V. Persistent palinopsia following ingestion of lysergic acid diethylamide (LSD). *Arch Ophthalmol* 1996;114:47–50.

97. Halpern JH, Pope HG Jr. Do hallucinogens cause residual neuropsychological toxicity. *Drug Alcohol Depend* 1999;53:247–256.

98. Li J-H, Lin L-F. Genetic toxicology of abused drugs: a brief review. *Mutagenesis* 1998;13:557–565.

CHAPTER 19

Phencyclidine (PCP)

STEPHEN R. ZUKIN, ZILI SLOBODA, AND
DANIEL C. JAVITT

HISTORY

Phencyclidine (1-1(phenylcyclohexyl)piperidine; PCP; "angel dust") was developed by Parke-Davis under the trade name Sernyl during the 1950s in a research program targeting general anesthetics. In certain respects clinical trials in anesthesia were promising. Patients anesthetized with PCP did not manifest the depression of vital cardiovascular and respiratory functions typical of classical general anesthetic agents. In fact, the PCP-induced anesthetic state differed sharply from the state of relaxed sleep induced by barbiturates or opiates in nearly every respect (1–3). Patients appeared catatonic, displaying flat faces, open mouth, and fixed, sightless staring, with rigid posturing, and sometimes waxy flexibility. It was inferred that without overt loss of consciousness, patients were sharply dissociated from the environment. For this reason PCP and the related compounds cyclohexamine (1) and ketamine (4) were classified as "dissociative anesthetics."

Despite its physiologic advantages over traditional anesthetics, PCP was removed from the market in 1965 and officially limited thereafter to veterinary applications. Up to half of patients subjected to PCP anesthesia developed severe intraoperative reactions, including agitation and hallucinations (1–3). Many of these patients went on to develop psychotic reactions, which persisted beyond emergence from anesthesia, and in some cases persisted for an additional 12 to 240 hours (2,5). Qualitatively similar effects were observed when much lower doses of PCP were tried for chronic pain (5). As a result of these findings, PCP and cyclohexamine were abandoned for clinical use, although the shorter-acting and less-potent PCP-derivative ketamine did find a place in the anesthetic pharmacopoeia. The fact that drugs with such well-documented negative and aversive behavioral effects became widely abused during the 1970s is one of the most remarkable developments in psychopharmacology.

EPIDEMIOLOGY

The nature of phencyclidine and the characteristics of its abuse affect its epidemiologic features. Because it is water soluble, PCP is often adulterated and misrepresented on the street as THC (tetrahydrocannabinol, the principal psychoactive substance in marihuana), LSD (lysergic acid diethylamide), mescaline, psilocybin, amphetamine,

or cocaine. Because of this variability and the high frequency with which it is used in combination with other drugs, the user may not be aware of having ingested PCP. To add to the confusion, the street names for PCP vary considerably within and between regions of the country: angel dust, dust, crystal, cyclones, embalming fluid, wet, killer weed, mintweed, PeaCe Pill, goon, surfer, and as recently as 1994, Illy, crazy Eddie, Purple Rain, and Milk. Its abuse was first noted on the West Coast in 1965 (6). Its negative effects quickly made it an undesirable drug and it had limited popularity on the streets. Analyses of street samples collected on the West Coast between 1971 and 1974 found that, in about half of the PCP samples, PCP was mixed with other drugs. However, during the last half of the 1970s, almost 75% of the street samples were found to be pure PCP. It was originally ingested orally, but because the risk of overdose is greater with the oral form of the drug, it is now more commonly smoked or snorted, allowing the user more control of dosage. It has also been injected. Ethnographic studies of users of PCP in four metropolitan areas (7) found regional differences in first time use: snorting in Chicago and Philadelphia, smoking in Seattle, and both smoking and snorting in Miami.

Initial use is usually in a smoking form (about 1 to 100 mg of PCP per joint) in conjunction with marihuana, tobacco, or parsley. Chronic users may take from 100 mg to 1 g within a single 24-hour period. The effects last between 4 and 6 hours with a longer "coming down" period. It is most often used as a social drug, with other users. PCP is used by people from all socioeconomic backgrounds, with and without formal premorbid psychopathology. For those who become chronic users, PCP is generally a primary drug of choice. Studies of chronic users show persistent cognitive and memory problems, speech difficulties, mood disorders, loss of purposive activities, and weight loss, lasting a year or more after last use. Late-stage chronic use is associated with paranoia and violent behavior with auditory hallucinations (6).

Certain specific characteristics of PCP abuse render its study particularly difficult: episodic peaks of abuse, wide regional variations, media attention, public misconceptions, and sharp decline in use. However, a good epidemiologic picture of PCP use can be obtained by examining all the data sources together. The following sections will present the extent of PCP use in the United States over time and describe the characteristics of those persons who use PCP.

PCP "Epidemics"

The previously cited data sources suggest that there was an epidemic of phencyclidine use in the period between 1973 and 1979 and again, perhaps, between 1981 and 1984 (8–10). These increases in PCP use stimulated a number of scientific articles in professional journals, which examined the question of whether the epidemic was real or was a pseudoepidemic brought into being by exploitation of the most dramatic cases by the media (11). However, the national data systems, as well as many regional systems (12), support the increases in use in the late 1970s, but only the indicator data support the increases noted in the 1980s. By their very nature, indicator data represent legal or health problems associated with drug use; therefore, they are not good indicators of new users. Except, perhaps, for acute overdoses seen in the emergency room, those who represent the "statistics" in hospitals, the medical examiners' offices, drug abuse treatment, and jails are more likely to be intermediate or chronic users of drugs and as such represent the lag-end of an "epidemic."

Review of the National Household Survey on Drug Abuse (NHSDA) data for these periods indicate that in 1976 it was estimated that 9.5% of those age 18 to 25 years had ever used PCP; however, the estimates for 1977 and 1979 show increases to 13.9% and 14.5%, respectively. Estimates of PCP use for those age 12 to 17 years were 3.0% in 1976, 5.8% in 1977, and 3.9% in 1979. By 1982, these percentages began to decline significantly for both age groups (for those age 12 to 17 years it declined to 2.2%, and for those age 18 to 25 years it declined to 10.5%). For the 1985 and 1988 surveys, these figures were 1.1% and 1.2% for those age 12 to 17 years, and 5.6% and 4.4% for those age 18 to 25 years. Prior to 1985 survey data were reported for three age groups: age 12 to 17 years, age 18 to 25 years, and older than age 25 years. In 1985, the oldest group was divided into two groups, those age 26 to 34 years and those older than age 34 years. In that same year, the higher PCP use rates (10.6%) were noted for those age 26 to 34 years. Subsequently, although rates have always been highest within the 26- to 34-year-old age group, they have been decreasing.

As a source of information on young people, the Monitoring the Future study provides a better database for estimating the extent of "new" use of drugs specifically because of the age groups involved. PCP was added to the questionnaire in 1979. The percentage of high school seniors reporting use of PCP was 12.8% in 1979 and decreased over time to its lowest level of approximately 3% in 1987, where it remained stable through 1995 (2.7%) (13). Data are not available for the eighth and tenth graders.

During the same periods, increases were noted in the numbers of persons reported to DAWN (Drug Abuse Warning Network) for drug-related problems associated with PCP and in drug-abuse treatment admissions. The numbers of PCP-related emergency room mentions increased from 1,934 in 1974 to 4,993 in 1977; and from 9,877 in 1978 to a high of 10,288 in 1979 (14). After a decline to 5,840 in 1981, increases were again noted in 1982 and 1983 (8,067 and 9,782, respectively). Crider (15) points out that between 1973 and 1975, among treatment admissions, the rate of first-time users of PCP increased

more rapidly than was observed in the emergency room data system (3,420 in 1973; 4,240 in 1974; 7,180 in 1977; peaking at 9,130 in 1979; and declining to 1,270 by 1981). She attributes the observed increases to a change in route of administration from oral (tablet or capsule) to smoking (along with tobacco or marihuana). The subsequent decline in PCP use is thought to be the result of a number of activities aimed at making the population more aware of the abuse potential and dangers associated with PCP. At the same time, the drug was rescheduled in the Controlled Substances Act from Schedule III to Schedule II, restricting its availability. In addition, reporting on the production of the precursor drug, piperidine, was made a requirement in 1979. Finally, penalties for the possession of PCP with the intent to sell were increased. All of the activities were thought to be associated with the declines in use in the early 1980s. The increases that are noted in the DAWN system, for example, during the mid-1980s may actually represent a continuation of the "epidemic" from the late 1970s. This hypothesis is supported by the characteristics of the populations constituting those being seen in these agencies. First of all, they seem to come principally from Los Angeles, Washington, DC, and New York City. They are older and more likely to be African American. Finally, they seem to be using PCP in combination with alcohol and/or heroin (15).

Current Trends in PCP Use

Preliminary analyses of the 1994 NHSDA estimates that approximately 9 million people had used phencyclidine at least once in their lives, representing 4.3% of household residents age 12 years and older (16). The percent of persons reporting "lifetime" use of PCP has been increasing since 1985, when the estimate was 2.9%. Information available in detail from the 1993 NHSDA (17) shows higher rates of use estimated for persons between the ages of 26 and 34 years (8.2%) with the lowest rates reported for those 12 to 17 years of age (1.0%). About twice as many males (5.5%) report use as females (2.7%). Whites are more likely to use PCP (4.5%) than are other racial groups, with Hispanics reporting higher rates of use (3.2%) than African Americans (1.9%). Use tends to be greater in the western part of the country (5.9%). When lifetime use is compared across the six cities that were oversampled in the survey, these regional differences are underscored. In 1993, the city with the highest estimate of use was Denver with 6.5%. The next highest cities were Los Angeles (4.3%) and Washington, DC (4.2%). The city with the lowest percentage of use was Miami at 0.8%. These relationships have remained the same since 1991, with Denver having the highest percentage of users and Miami the lowest (18). Examination of these percentages by socioeconomic status shows that there are no differences in almost all the cities, except perhaps Chicago, where the percentage of users was somewhat higher for the middle and upper socioeconomic status populations (16–18).

These "lifetime" estimates provide a proxy assessment of cohort differences over time. For many illicit drugs, including PCP, changes in lifetime use patterns are associated with changes in perceptions of the "harmfulness" of their use and in reports as to the ease with which the drugs can be obtained. For PCP, the relationship between these perceptions and use have held steady. In 1994, 73% of those interviewed indicated that there were "great risks" associated with the use of PCP, even if tried once or twice. The percentage reporting that PCP was easy to obtain in 1994 was 29%. Lifetime estimates of use and for these measures of perception have not changed significantly over the last 6 years for the total population, within age groups, between sexes, among racial or ethnic groups, or by region of the country. However, when the data on perceptions of risk associated with PCP use are compared to reported use across age groups, it is difficult to assess the relationship of these measures. The group that has the lowest rates of use (those age 12 to 17 years) also has the fewest people who believe there is great risk associated with using PCP. Those who report the second lowest rate of use, those age 35 years and older, were the most likely to believe that PCP use poses great risk. Approximately 66% of those in the age group with the highest rates of use, those age 26 to 34 years, report that use is risky (16).

Annual prevalence, use within the year prior to survey, is a better estimate to use for public health programming because it represents the current picture of use. With this in mind, in 1994, 0.02%, or 478,000, people were estimated to have used PCP at least once in the prior year. Although involving a large number of cases, PCP use is dwarfed by annual rates of marihuana, cocaine, crack, and inhalant use (8.5%, 1.7%, 0.6%, and 1.1%, respectively) (16).

Earlier it was mentioned that since 1987 approximately 3% of high school seniors reported PCP use sometime in their lifetimes. The characteristics of the 1994 high school seniors who reported using PCP are similar to those mentioned above for the NHSDA: mostly male and from the northeast and western regions of the United States. When the members of the senior class of 1994 who reported use of PCP were asked about when they began its use, the mode was within the 2 to 3 years prior to interview (while in grades 10 and 11) (19). This survey also examines noncontinuation of drugs, defined as the proportion of people who ever tried a drug but do not continue to use it in the 12 months prior to the survey. In 1994, PCP ranked among the top seven most-often-discontinued drugs after inhalants (56%), heroin (50%), methamphetamine (47%), steroids (46%), tranquilizers (44%), and methaqualone (43%).

Although information on use is not available for the eighth and tenth graders, questions were included on their questionnaires as to perceptions regarding the difficulty in obtaining PCP. In 1994, approximately 18% of the eighth graders and 24% of the tenth graders thought that PCP was "fairly easy" or "very easy" to obtain, compared to 31% of the twelfth graders. Similar questions regarding marihuana elicited higher percentages for the eighth and tenth graders (49% and 75%, respectively) compared to 85% for twelfth graders. However, the proportion of eighth and tenth graders who thought PCP was easy to get was similar to those who thought heroin and crystal methamphetamine were easy to get (13).

Indicator Data

National data systems of indicators vary with regard to the specificity of the drug implication. Because DAWN was designed to ascertain emerging patterns of drug use it is a much better drug abuse surveillance indicator system. Reports from DAWN prior to 1989 were limited to sentinel cities and were not truly representative of the nation, although projected national estimates were made. Detailed national estimates are available for 1989 through 1993 when the system was based on a representative sample of hospitals. The ranking of PCP, relative to other drugs mentioned in the DAWN emergency room system, has changed from nineteenth in 1990 to twenty-seventh in 1991 and twenty-second in 1992 and 1993 (20,21). Throughout these years the cases were approximately 72% male, more than 40% in their mid-twenties, and approximately 40% to 43% African American. In 1990, 1991, and 1992, the percentages who were white were 26%, 29.6%, and 20.8%, and the percentages who were Hispanic were 16.4%, 35.5%, and 22.0%, respectively. The overall DAWN cases for these years are about half male, mostly white (approximately 60%), and between the ages of 26 and 34 years.

More than 38% of the PCP users reported that PCP was the only drug they had used prior to their admission to the emergency room, compared to 28% for all admissions. Approximately 33% of the DAWN PCP users reported that they used the drug for recreational reasons and about another 30% mentioned they were dependent, compared to total DAWN cases where approximately 33% mentioned dependence and more than 43% mentioned suicidal intent. For all 3 years, the same cities reported the highest numbers of emergency room admissions associated with PCP (in rank order): Los Angeles, Chicago, Washington, DC, New York City, San Francisco, Baltimore, and Philadelphia. These cities varied as to the race or ethnic groups involved, with African Americans and Hispanics more often mentioned for Los Angeles, New York City, and San Francisco; African Americans in Chicago; whites in Baltimore; and whites and African Americans in Philadelphia and Washington, DC.

The National Institute on Drug Abuse (NIDA) supports the Community Epidemiology Work Group (CEWG), which twice a year brings together drug-abuse researchers and program managers from 21 cities across the country to exchange data on drug use in their areas, including indicator data from the emergency rooms, medical examiners' offices, arrest records, and drug-abuse treatment facilities; information on price and purity of drugs seized; and other data for their communities. Through this mechanism it has been possible to identify emerging drug patterns as targets for study. In the meetings in June and December 1995, reports were made indicating a rebound of PCP use in emergency rooms in Washington, DC, Philadelphia, and New York City; among juvenile arrestees in Washington, DC, and Chicago; and among treatment admissions, particularly in conjunction with marihuana, in Miami (22,23). Future NHSDA and Monitoring the Future surveys will show whether these increases represent a significant trend.

NEUROBIOLOGY

Identification and Characterization of the PCP Receptor

The central nervous effects of PCP are initiated by binding of the drug to high-affinity PCP receptors whose existence in rat brain membranes was demonstrated in 1979 (24,25). PCP receptors are highly selective for drugs that elicit PCP-like effects on behavior, including PCP and related arylcyclohexylamines, the F-opioids, the dioxolanes (a class of dissociative anesthetics), and dizocilpine (MK-801) (24–31). Several classes of drugs not chemically derived from PCP, including the F-opiates (27,32–34), the dioxolane derivatives dexoxadrol and etoxadrol (29), and the anticonvulsant MK-801 (31), are active in the [^{3}H]PCP binding assay and exhibit PCP-like behavioral activity. All of these drugs mimic PCP in conditioned and unconditioned behavioral assays and generalize to PCP in the highly selective rat two-lever drug discriminative stimulus test. The relative potencies of these drugs in eliciting PCP-like behaviors are proportional to their potencies in competing for radioligand binding to the PCP receptor. More than 100 such derivatives have been so characterized. Drugs that exhibit PCP-like behavioral effects also block N-methyl-D-aspartate (NMDA)-activated channels in electrophysiologic assays. The rank order of potency of such drugs as channel blockers parallels their behavioral potencies and their potencies in binding to the PCP receptor. By contrast, a wide range of neurotransmitters, known agonists, and antagonists of other receptors (including the classical opiates and the psychotomimetic drugs LSD, THC, cocaine, and mescaline) are inactive in the PCP-binding assay and fail to elicit PCP-like behaviors or channel-blocking activity.

PCP–NMDA Receptor Interactions

Following the demonstration of PCP receptors, the next major advance in determining the molecular mechanism of PCP occurred in the early 1980s, with the demonstration that PCP receptor ligands potently inhibit neurotransmission mediated at NMDA-type glutamate receptors. NMDA receptors are one of several receptor types for the excitatory amino acid neurotransmitter glutamate. As opposed to other glutamate receptors, NMDA channels are permeable to Ca^{2+} along with Na^+. Following NMDA receptor activation, NMDA-mediated Ca^{2+} flux may lead to stimulation of calmodulin-dependent kinases, and activation of postsynaptic second messenger pathways (35). A unique functional property of the NMDA channel is that it is blocked in a voltage-dependent manner by the endogenous Mg^{2+} ion. The dual voltage and ligand dependence of NMDA receptors permits them to function in a Hebbian manner to integrate information from multiple input streams (36–38). One stream is represented as a modulation of presynaptic glutamate release; additional streams are reflected in modulation of resting membrane potential on the postsynaptic NMDA-bearing dendrites. Ca^{2+} flowing through open, unblocked NMDA channels may serve as the trigger for long-term potentiation, which, in turn, may represent the neurophysiologic substrate underlying learning and memory formation. In rodents, PCP and other NMDA antagonists lead to profound memory disturbances that are linked to inhibition of hippocampal long-term potentiation (39). Profound amnesia is also characteristic of both PCP psychosis and ketamine anesthesia.

Glycine Sensitivity of NMDA Receptor Activation

As opposed to most receptors, which require the presence of only a single neurotransmitter, NMDA receptors possess two distinct agonist binding sites, one for glutamate and other excitatory amino acids, and a second for glycine. Binding of both glycine and glutamate are required for NMDA receptor activation to occur, and, *in vitro*, total removal of glycine from the incubation medium prevents NMDA receptor activation by glutamate. From a technical viewpoint, therefore, glutamate and glycine should be considered coagonists at the NMDA receptor complex (40). However, the functional roles played by glutamate and glycine *in vivo* appear quite different. Thus, glutamate is released from presynaptic nerve endings in a pulsatile fashion and rapidly deactivated following release, as is the case for most classical neurotransmitters. In contrast, glycine in forebrain does not appear to be concentrated in presynaptic nerve endings nor released in response to electrical stimulation. Moreover, endogenous glycine levels are typically at or above the K_d (dissociation constant) of the NMDA-associated glycine site for these agents, indicating that activity-stimulated release of glycine is not required for neurotransmission. It has even been suggested that the glycine site may be saturated under normal brain conditions, and thus physiologically irrelevant, although this appears not to be the case (40). Instead, glycine appears to set the tonic level of NMDA excitability, determining the degree to which presynaptic glutamate release leads to postsynaptic excitation. Postsynaptic excitation, however, is triggered by presynaptic glutamate release. Functionally, therefore, glycine functions more similarly to a neuromodulator than a classical neurotransmitter. In addition to glycine, the NMDA-associated glycine site shows high affinity for D-serine, which may also serve as an endogenous NMDA agonist (41). The high affinity of the NMDA-associated glycine site for D-serine stands in contrast to the classical, strychnine-sensitive inhibitory glycine receptor found primarily in hindbrain, which binds D-serine with low affinity.

Use-Dependent Blockade

Because PCP mediates its effects at a binding site located within the NMDA channel, access of PCP to its site of action is affected by the degree of NMDA receptor activation. Opening of the NMDA channel facilitates access of PCP to its receptor, accelerating the rate at which PCP-induced blockade of NMDA receptor-mediated neurotransmission is observed. Thus, *in vitro*, NMDA currents show marked use-dependence, with greater use being associated with more rapid blockade over the course of seconds to minutes (42). However, the phenomenon of use-dependence appears to be true only over the course of minutes. When incubations are continued for several hours, significant PCP receptor occupancy is observed even in the absence of NMDA activation. The slow onset of closed channel blockade is most likely a result of the ability of PCP receptor ligands, all of which are highly lipophilic, to reach the NMDA channel by diffusion through the lipid bilayer (43).

Neurotoxicity

In the range of concentrations most associated with behavioral hyperactivity, PCP does not appear to cause significant long-lasting brain toxicity. At doses significantly above those used for behavioral studies (e.g., 5 to 50 mg/kg), however, PCP induces neuronal vacuolization, particularly in neurons in posterior cingulate/retrosplenial cortex (44). Similar vacuolization is observed following of administration of MK-801 (dizocilpine) and ketamine, indicating that the effect is probably NMDA receptor mediated. The effect is initially observed in layers III and IV of cortex. At lower doses (e.g., 5 mg/kg), the effect is transient, reaching peak levels approximately 12 hours after PCP or MK-801 administration and then resolving over 12 to 18 hours. Extremely large doses of drug, however, may lead to neuronal necrosis, which is apparent even 48 hours after drug administration. Although posterior cingulate/retrosplenial cortex appears most susceptible to the effects of PCP, other hippocampus and limbic brain regions may be affected at higher doses. Along with vacuolization, administration of high-dose PCP leads to elevation of glucose uptake (45), expression of heat shock protein (46),

and glial fibrillary acidic protein (47) in the affected regions. Vacuolization can be inhibited by prior administration of antipsychotic, anticholinergic, or γ-aminobutyric acid-(GABA)ergic agents, and is potentiated by administration of pilocarpine.

Behavioral Pharmacology

The behavioral effects of PCP in animals depend upon species (48). In rodents, PCP induces a characteristic syndrome of hyperactivity and stereotypies (48). These behavioral effects respond partially to treatment with neuroleptics (49), and may also be reversed by agents such as glycine that augment NMDA receptor-mediated neurotransmission (50). Because the serum half-life of PCP is shorter and the volume of distribution is larger, rodents typically require doses of PCP higher than those used clinically than in humans (51). Sensitization to the behavioral effects of PCP may occur following daily administration (52). In rodents, PCP may also inhibit social behavior. The effects of PCP on social behaviors are poorly reversed by typical or atypical antipsychotic agents (53).

PCP-induced hyperactivity in rodents is mediated at least in part by disruption of NMDA-mediated interaction with ascending midbrain dopamine systems (54). PCP-induced hyperactivity appears to be reflective of increased dopaminergic neurotransmission within nucleus accumbens, because this effect can be selectively inhibited by accumbens lesions (55–57). Other components of the PCP-induced behavioral syndrome (e.g., alterations in social behavior, stereotypies) persist even following accumbens lesion (57), however, suggesting that those behaviors may be mediated by other brain regions. In addition to being present in dopaminergic terminal fields, NMDA receptors are also present in substantia nigra (A9) and ventral tegmental area (A10). Glutamatergic innervation of substantia nigra from prefrontal cortex is a major determinant of dopaminergic activity levels and NMDA receptors appear to be the primary mediators of glutamate-induced stimulation of midbrain dopaminergic neurons (58). To the extent that NMDA receptors stimulate A9 and A10 neurons, PCP would, paradoxically, be expected to decrease dopaminergic outflow in striatum and accumbens. However, it has been found that direct application of PCP to A10 does not inhibit dopamine cell firing or alter dopamine release in accumbens, although it does prevent NMDA-induced neuronal activation (59). Thus, the predominant behavioral effects of PCP in rodents appear to be a result of its interactions within dopamine terminal fields rather than within dopaminergic midbrain nuclei.

In monkeys, doses of approximately 0.5 mg/kg PCP produce a tranquilization in which animals appear awake but unresponsive to the environment (60). At doses of 1.0 mg/kg, PCP induces a cataleptoid state in which animals show waxy flexibility and rigidity closely resembling catatonic schizophrenia. Doses of 2.5 mg/kg lead to stupor, 5.0 mg/kg to surgical anesthesia, and 15 mg/kg to convulsive seizures.

In both rats and monkeys, PCP administration also leads to profound disruption in learning and memory. In rodents, noncompetitive NMDA antagonists lead to disruptions in spatial delayed alteration performance, which can be reversed by dopamine (D2) receptor antagonists (61). Thus, in cortex, as in striatum, the effects of NMDA antagonists may, in part, reflect secondary dysregulation of dopaminergic neurotransmission. In monkeys, NMDA antagonists lead to impairments in learning and working memory performance that are not reproduced by amphetamine (62), indicating that the effect cannot be wholly attributed to increased dopaminergic neurotransmission. However, NMDA antagonists do lead to potentiation of the disruptive effects of amphetamine on learning in monkeys, indicating that interactions between the NMDA and dopamine systems may nevertheless be important.

Anatomic Localization

The anatomic localization of the PCP receptor in the rat brain has been determined by receptor autoradiography using [3H]PCP (63) and [3H]TCP ([3H]N-[1-(2-thienyl)cyclohexyl]piperidine) (64) as radioligands (Table 19.1). High densities of PCP receptors are found in anterior forebrain areas, including neocortex and olfactory

TABLE 19.1. *Densities of receptors labeled by [3H]TCP and [3H] (+)SKF-10,047*

| Region | Receptor densities (fmol/mg tissue) | |
	[3H]TCP site[a]	[3H](+)SKF-10,047 sites[b]
Hippocampus		
CA1	104	200
CA2	105	217
CA3	66	173
Dentate	111	200
Subiculum	84	—
Frontal cortex	83	134
Superior colliculus	65	134
Nucleus accumbens	52	100
Cerebellum	47	145
Locus ceruleus	46	140
Amygdala	42	—
Dorsomedial hypothalamus	40	162
Central gray	26	167
Substantia nigra	14	145
Pontine reticular nucleus	8	84
Globus pallidus	0	—
Corpus callosum	0	6

[a]See reference 25.
[b]See reference 127.

structures. The highest selective localization is observed in the dentate gyrus and the CA1 and CA2 subfields of the hippocampus. [3H]TCP binding displays low density in midbrain/pontine areas. White matter areas (including corpus callosum and anterior commissure), as well as certain gray matter areas (including globus pallidus, the ventral tegmental area, and some pontine and thalamic nuclei), show near background levels of [3H]TCP binding. Within the spinal cord [3H]TCP-labeled sites are localized primarily to laminae I and II in cervical and thoracic spinal segments. In lamina I the density of sites decreases along a rostral to caudal gradient (65). Autoradiographic evidence indicates that PCP receptors are located postsynaptically rather than presynaptically in the perforant path-dentate granule cell system of the adult rat (66). A phylogenetic study indicates that PCP receptors are old from an evolutionary standpoint, occurring in the neural tissue of a large number of animal species, including monkey, guinea pig, chicken, turtle, frog, goldfish, shark, planarian, and sea anemone, although their pharmacology in invertebrates is not congruent with that found in vertebrates (67).

Molecular Characterization of the PCP Receptor

On a molecular level, the NMDA receptor complex is heterooligomeric in structure, consisting of combinations of NMDAR1 and NMDAR2 subunits. NMDAR1 is the key subunit in the formation of the receptor complex (35). All functional NMDA receptor complexes contain a type 1 (NR1) subunit; complexes may also contain variable numbers of modulatory subunits (NR2A-D). The sensitivity of NMDA receptors to modulatory effects of glycine are conferred by residues within the NR1 subunit itself (68,69). Thus, in general, all functional NMDA receptor complexes should be sensitive to glycine. Eight variants of NMDAR1 (NMDAR1a–h) have been identified which reflect alternative messenger ribonucleic acid (mRNA) splicing. These clones have distinct sensitivities to agonists, antagonists, Zn^{2+}, and polyamines. Polyamines are also conferred by regulatory (NR2) subunits which are differentially expressed across brain regions (70). NMDA receptors are primarily postsynaptic in localization and occur on both projection and interneurons (71,72). In some brain regions, however, especially in target areas of the mesolimbic/mesocortical system, NMDA receptors may also be localized presynaptically and thus may regulate release of dopamine from presynaptic terminals (56,73,75). It has been suggested that such receptors consist solely of NR1 subunits and thus may have a different pharmacological profile from postsynaptic receptors (76).

Effects of PCP at Non-NMDA Receptor Molecular Targets

At doses at least tenfold higher than those at which it exerts its unique behavioral effects by blocking NMDA receptor-mediated neurotransmission, PCP also blocks presynaptic monoamine reuptake, thus directly increasing synaptic levels of dopamine and noradrenaline. Levels sufficient to block monoamine reuptake may be achieved during high-dose intoxication and may contribute to the stimulatory effects of PCP seen at those doses. Ketamine, even at high dose, fails to block monoamine transporters. This observation may contribute towards explaining the apparently lower incidence of episodes of extreme agitation and violence following ketamine, rather than PCP, intoxication. At doses associated with extremely high-dose intoxication, PCP blocks neuronal Na^+ and K^+ channels. Such effects may be relevant to the seizures observed following PCP overdose. PCP also interacts with a variety of other central nervous system (CNS) receptors including cholinergic, opiate, and γ-aminobutyric acid (GABA)/benzodiazepine receptors. However, the majority of such effects take place at concentrations that are not likely to be encountered in clinical situations.

PSYCHOPHARMACOLOGY

Pharmacokinetics

In practical terms, PCP must be considered an extremely potent compound among drugs of abuse. It is extremely lipid soluble and can reach significant brain levels upon administration via any one of several routes, including oral, inhalation, smoking, and topical (77). A typical street dose is about 5 mg (one pill, joint, or line) (see reference 103). Based upon the pharmacokinetics of PCP, such a dose would result in a serum PCP concentration between 0.01 and 0.1 μmole/L. Marked psychotic reactions have been observed associated with undetectably low serum concentrations (<0.02 μmole/L), while concentrations of >0.4 μmole/L induce gross impairment of consciousness. Abusers characteristically titrate their dose in an effort to maximize the "high" while avoiding unconsciousness. Failures of judgment or variations in purity of supplies often result in inadvertent overdose, which may lead to severe medical complications. Serum concentrations above 1.0 μmole/L are strongly associated with coma, seizures, respiratory arrest, and death (78,79). The highest recorded serum and cerebrospinal fluid concentrations are in the range of 1.0 to 2.0 μmole/L.

PCP manifests a volume of distribution of 6.2 L/kg (80). Its lipophilicity facilitates accumulation in fatty body tissues, including the brain (81,82). Mobilization of adipose stores, as with exercise, may release sequestered PCP, leading to "flashbacks" (81,82).

Metabolism is primarily hepatic, with renal secretion of hydroxylase metabolites (83). The pK_a of 8.5 implies that PCP is largely ionized while in the stomach or the urinary tract. In passing through the pyloric valve, PCP enters a nonacidic environment in the small intestine in which it becomes largely nonionized and readily absorbed across the mucosal membrane, whereupon enterohepatic recalculation can account for the fluctuating clinical course so often observed in intoxication.

Chemistry

A phenylcyclohexylamine, PCP is easily synthesized from the starting materials piperazine, cyclohexanone, and potassium cyanide. The synthesis proceeds through the intermediate 1-piperidinocyclohexanecarbonitrile (PC), which is reacted with phenylmagnesium bromide to form PCP (84). The simplicity of this reaction, which enables PCP to be synthesized with almost no training or equipment, suggests that a resurgence of PCP abuse may follow successful efforts to eliminate from the marketplace drugs of abuse derived from natural products. During the 1970s, analytic surveys of street samples revealed that a large portion of drugs marketed as THC, mescaline, and LSD were actually PCP (85). Another consequence of the ease of synthesis is the contamination of significant percentages of analyzed street samples of PCP by dangerously high amounts of residual PC (86). In physiologic saline, PC decomposes to hydrocyanic acid (87). When PC-contaminated PCP is smoked, approximately 58% of the PC breaks down to cyanide and organic by-products (88). Although devoid of PCP-like pharmacologic activity, PC is more acutely toxic and may be implicated in some PCP-related fatalities.

Psychotomimetic Effects

In normal volunteers, single, small, intravenous subanesthetic doses (0.05 to 0.1 mg/kg) of PCP acutely induced a psychotic state in which subjects became withdrawn, autistic, negativistic, and unable to maintain a cognitive set, and manifested concrete, impoverished, idiosyncratic, and bizarre responses to proverbs and projective testing. Some subjects showed catatonic posturing (89–95). These schizophrenia-like alterations in brain functioning went beyond the symptom level; thus, in formal studies of neuropsychological function, PCP induced a spectrum of specific disturbances in attention (96), perception (93–96), and symbolic thinking (92,96) strikingly similar to those seen in schizophrenia. The most severe impairment caused by PCP was observed in tests requiring selective attention and paired-association learning (89). An important clinical correlate of this data is that any person under the influence of even a small dose of PCP or a similar drug will have profound alterations of higher emotional functions affecting judgment and cognition, even in the absence of gross neurological findings.

In recompensated schizophrenic subjects, single low doses of PCP caused rekindling of presenting symptomatology lasting as long as 6 weeks, without evocation of any symptoms or signs not typical of the schizophrenic illness (90,91,93,97). An important clinical correlate of this data is that schizophrenics or preschizophrenics abusing a PCP-type drug run an extremely high risk of severe psychiatric morbidity.

The epidemic of PCP abuse during the 1970s yielded considerable data on psychotomimetic effects in other than experimental subjects. This literature cannot be used directly to ascertain risks because no firm evidence is available of what percentage of recreational PCP users sought or were brought to medical attention. However, it is striking that in retrospective studies of patients hospitalized for complications of PCP use, the PCP-intoxicated patients could not be distinguished from schizophrenics based upon presenting symptomatology (98,99).

Reinforcing Effects

Self-Administration

A series of studies established that experimental monkeys avidly self-administer large doses of PCP intravenously (100–102) and orally (103). In such studies the finding that the monkeys, given unlimited access to PCP, maintained nearly continuous intoxication distinguished abuse patterns of PCP from those of classical stimulants. In this respect the reinforcing properties of PCP resemble those of opiates and CNS depressants more than they resemble those of stimulants (104). Furthermore, as distinct from findings on opiate self-administration, monkeys self-administered doses of PCP high enough to cause marked behavioral effects (104). Given the similarities between behavioral effects of PCP in monkeys and humans, this research validates the clinical impression of avid human self-administration of PCP. PCP-like drugs stimulate brain reward areas, lowering the threshold for intracranial self-stimulation (105,106). Such effects define a classical profile for drugs abused by humans and are shared by other abused compounds, including opiates and benzodiazepines, despite their differing mechanisms of action.

Tolerance

In rats and monkeys, repeated administration of PCP on a daily or more frequent schedule leads to two- to fourfold rightward shifts in dose–response curves. The major determinant of this moderate tolerance appears to be biodispositional (107–109). Unlike the modest degree of tolerance observed upon intermittent dosing, it appears that much greater degrees of tolerance are induced by continuous self-administration (104). In human subjects, there is a paucity of scientific data on PCP tolerance, but tolerance has been observed in burn patients given repeated doses of ketamine for analgesia (110).

Dependence

After unlimited-access self-administration of PCP for 1 month or longer, severe signs of withdrawal reaction were observed in monkeys when the drug was discontinued.

These included vocalizations, bruxism, oculomotor hyperactivity, diarrhea, piloerection, somnolence, tremor, and seizures (111). Similarly severe reactions might be expected following binging upon PCP by human abusers.

In summary, primate research has established a compelling case that PCP is a strongly addictive drug. Despite a paucity of controlled studies of tolerance and dependence in humans, PCP must be considered comparable to classical drugs of abuse in this respect.

Clinical Toxicology

The range of clinical effects of PCP can be correlated with dose and serum PCP concentration (Fig. 19.1). The variety of effects of PCP are a result of its interaction with a variety of molecular target sites.

The highest-affinity target site is the CNS PCP/NMDA receptor, which would be the only system affected significantly at very low PCP doses. Serum PCP levels up to about 0.1 μmole/L would correspond with a clinical state manifesting psychotomimetic symptoms without overt physiologic disturbances of vital functions. Serum levels just higher than 0.1 μmole/L correspond to dissociative anesthesia. At still higher doses, as additional receptor sites are occupied, acute brain syndrome accompanied by prominent neurologic and cardiovascular complications ensues. Serum levels of 1.0 μmole/L and above are associated with coma and lethal complications. The PCP-induced organic mental syndrome and coma result from the summation of PCP's actions noncompetitively inhibiting the PCP/NMDA receptor, blocking the reuptake sites for catecholamines and indolamines, and blocking

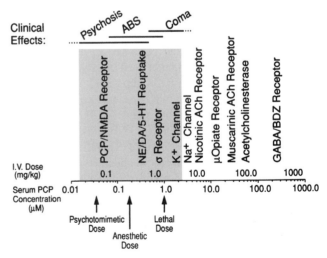

FIG. 19.1. Dose range of PCP effects. The relationship is shown among dose, serum concentration, molecular target sites, and clinical effects. The shaded area represents clinically relevant interactions. (From Javitt DC, Zukin SR. Recent advances in the phencyclidine model of schizophrenia. *Am J Psychiatry* 1991;148:1301–1308, with permission.)

sodium and potassium channels and nicotinic and muscarinic cholinergic receptors. Because it is not currently feasible to design and administer treatments specifically targeting each of the molecular sites at which PCP exerts its toxic effects, treatment must address each symptom cluster and organ system.

Measures to Reduce Systemic PCP Levels

Trapping of ionized PCP in the stomach has led to the suggestion of continuous nasogastric suction for PCP intoxication (112,113). However, such a strategy can be needlessly intrusive and can lead to complications such as electrolyte imbalances. The same principle can be more safely implemented by administration of activated charcoal, which binds PCP and diminishes the toxic effects of PCP in animals (114).

Trapping of ionized PCP in urine has led to the suggestion of urinary acidification as an aid to drug elimination. Current thinking (115) is that this strategy is ineffective and potentially dangerous, because only a small portion of PCP is excreted in urine; that metabolic acidosis itself carries significant risks; and that acidic urine would increase the risk of renal failure secondary to rhabdomyolysis (116,117).

Finally, the extremely large volume of distribution of PCP implies that neither hemodialysis nor hemoperfusion significantly promote drug clearance (115).

At present no drug functions as a "PCP antagonist." No drug will work for PCP as naloxone (Narcan) works for heroin because any compound binding to the PCP receptor, which is located within the ion channel of the NMDA receptor, would block NMDA receptor-mediated ion fluxes as does PCP itself. Recent progress in elucidation of NMDA receptor mechanisms suggests concepts that could lead to pharmacologic strategies promoting NMDA receptor activation, such as administration of glycine or polyamines (or derivatives or precursors of such substances). Increasing channel open time would promote dissociation of PCP from its binding sites. There is evidence that oral glycine in massive doses can antagonize PCP-induced behaviors in the mouse (118). However, no clinical trials of such strategies for PCP intoxication in humans have been carried out to date. Therefore, treatment must be supportive and directed at specific symptoms and signs of toxicity. It is important to remember that especially after oral administration, PCP levels may continue to rise unevenly over many hours or even days. Therefore, a prolonged period of clinical observation is mandatory before concluding that no serious or life-threatening complications will ensue.

Neurologic Toxicity

The majority of PCP-intoxicated patients manifest nystagmus, which may be horizontal, vertical, or rotatory

(119). Nystagmus is one of the crucial signs that can help distinguish PCP intoxication from a naturally occurring psychotic state. Coma can occur at any point during intoxication (120). There is a dose-dependent neuronal hyperexcitability ranging from increased deep tendon reflexes through opisthotonos to seizure states, generalized or focal, up to status epilepticus (119,121–123). Focal neurologic findings may arise on the basis of cerebral vasoconstriction (121,124). Seizures are managed with intravenous benzodiazepines (120).

Behavioral Toxicity

As noted earlier, a schizophrenia-like psychotic state can be observed after extremely low doses of PCP. In fact, such cognitive and emotional alterations are the threshold effects of this drug. The question of whether specific PCP-induced psychotic symptoms respond to treatment with neuroleptics has not been addressed. Clinically urgent behavioral complications of PCP abuse stem not from the "core" psychotic symptoms themselves but rather from behavioral disinhibition, which can be coupled with severe anxiety, panic, rage, and aggression. Such reactions are more common with somewhat higher doses, at which some degree of delirium, as well as neurologic symptoms and other medical derangements, can be observed. The behavioral manifestations can severely compromise the clinician's ability to treat the medical complications.

The disruption of sensory input by PCP causes unpredictable, exaggerated, distorted, or violent reactions to environmental stimuli. A cornerstone of treatment is therefore minimization of sensory inputs to PCP-intoxicated patients. Patients should be evaluated and treated in as quiet and isolated an environment as possible. Precautionary physical restraint is recommended by some authorities (115) with the risk of rhabdomyolysis balanced by the avoidance of violent or disruptive behavior.

Drug Treatment

Because no specific PCP antagonist is available, the goal of drug therapy for PCP-induced behavioral toxicity is sedation. This can be accomplished by using benzodiazepines or neuroleptics. There is no convincing evidence that either class of compounds is clinically superior to the other.

Benzodiazepines are effective via either oral or parenteral (intramuscular) routes. Diazepam (Valium) is effective via the oral route but may be poorly or erratically absorbed intramuscularly. Lorazepam (Ativan) may be given via either route of administration.

Haloperidol (Haldol) is the neuroleptic most commonly used for this indication. Because of the anticholinergic actions of PCP, neuroleptics with potent intrinsic anticholinergic properties should be avoided.

Autonomic Toxicity

Severe hyperthermia has been observed in PCP intoxication, which can arise in a delayed fashion and can be of fatal proportions (125,126). The anticholinergic properties of PCP can dose-dependently evoke a full spectrum atropine-like toxicity and can be managed accordingly when life-threatening.

Cardiovascular Toxicity

Mild hypertension may be seen even in minimal PCP intoxication. At higher doses hypertension may be severe and hypertensive crisis with CNS complications has been reported.

Rhabdomyolysis

This potentially devastating complication arises from multiple sources. First, PCP in high doses has a direct excitatory action upon the muscle end-plate. Second, the behavioral toxicity of high doses of PCP frequently leads to muscle trauma. This combination of factors can lead to severe rhabdomyolysis, myoglobinuria, and renal failure.

CONCLUSION

Phencyclidine stands as the prototype of a unique category of drugs—NMDA channel blockers—that have high abuse potential and severe adverse medical effects in the abuse situation. The epidemic of phencyclidine abuse in the late 1970s and early 1980s, in focusing scientific attention upon the basic mechanisms by which these drugs exert their singular combination of psychotomimetic, cognitive, and abuse-promoting effects, played a key role in advancing research in a major new area of neuroscience. Future scientific progress in elucidating mechanisms of NMDA receptor function may lead to specific pharmacotherapeutic approaches to treatment of PCP abuse and toxicity.

REFERENCES

1. Collins VJ, Gorospe CA, Rovenstine EA. Intravenous nonbarbiturate, non-narcotic analgesics: preliminary studies. I. Cyclohexylamines. *Anesth Analg* 1960;39:303–306.
2. Greifenstein FE, Yoskitake, J, DeVault M, et al. A study of 1-arylcyclohexylamine for anesthesia. *Anesth Analg* 1958;37:283–294.
3. Johnstone M, Evans V, Baigel S. Sernyl (Cl-395) in clinical anesthesia. *Br J Anaesth* 1958;31:433–439.
4. Corssen G, Domino EF. Dissociative anesthesia: further pharmacologic studies and first clinical experience with the phencyclidine derivative CI-581. *Anesth Analg* 1966;45:29–40.
5. Meyer JS, Greifenstein F, DeVault M. A new drug causing symptoms of sensory deprivation. *J Nerv Ment Dis* 1959; 129:54–61.
6. Petersen RC, Stillman RC. *Phencyclidine: a review.* National Institute on Drug Abuse publication no. 1980-0-341-166/614. Washington, DC: U.S. Government Printing Office, 1980.
7. Waldorf D, Beschner G. *PCP use. Services research notes.* Washington, DC: National Institute on Drug Abuse, 1979.
8. Fishburne PM, Cisin I. *National survey on drug abuse: main findings 1979.* National Institute on Drug Abuse publication no. (ADM) 80-976. Washington, DC: U.S. Government Printing Office, 1980.
9. Miller JD, Cisin I, et al. *National survey on drug abuse: main findings 1982.* National Institute on Drug Abuse publication no. (ADM) 83-1263. Washington, DC: U.S. Government Printing Office, 1983.
10. National Institute on Drug Abuse. *National survey on drug abuse: main findings 1985.* National Institute on Drug Abuse publication no. (ADM) 88-1586. Washington, DC: U.S. Government Printing Office, 1988.
11. Davis BL. The PCP epidemic: a critical review. *Int J Addictions* 1982;17 (7):1137–1155.
12. Newmeyer JA. The epidemiology of PCP use in the late 1970s. *J Psychedelic Drugs* 1980;12:211–215.
13. Johnston LD, Bachman JG, O'Malley PM. *National survey results on drug use from the Monitoring the Future study, 1975–1994. Volume I: secondary school students.* National Institute on Drug Abuse publication no. 95-4026. Washington, DC: U.S. Government Printing Office, 1995.
14. Hinkley S, Greenwood J. *Emergency room visits in DAWN projected to the nation. A report from the Drug Enforcement Administration.* Washington, DC: U.S. Government Printing Office, 1981.
15. Crider R. Phencyclidine: changing abuse patterns. *NIDA Res Monogr Ser* 1986;64.
16. Substance Abuse and Mental Health Services Administration, Office of Applied Studies. *National survey on drug abuse: population estimates 1994.* DHHS Publication No. (SMA) 95-33063. Washington, DC: U.S. Government Printing Office, 1995.
17. Substance Abuse and Mental Health Services Administration, Office of Applied Studies. *National survey on drug abuse: main findings 1993.* DHHS Publication No. (SMA) 95-3020. Washington, DC: U.S. Government Printing Office, 1995.
18. Substance Abuse and Mental Health Services Administration, Office of Applied Studies. *National survey on drug abuse: main findings 1992.* DHHS Publication No. (SMA) 94-3012. Washington, DC: U.S. Government Printing Office, 1994.
19. Release of national survey results on drug use from the Monitoring the Future study, 1995 [press release]. Washington, DC: National Institute on Drug Abuse, December 15, 1995.
20. Substance Abuse and Mental Health Services Administration, Office of Applied Studies. *Annual emergency room data 1992.* DHHS Publication No. (SMA) 94-2080. Washington, DC: U.S. Government Printing Office, 1994.
21. Substance Abuse and Mental Health Services Administration, Office of Applied Studies. *Annual emergency room data 1993.* DHHS Publication No. (SMA) 95-3019. Washington, DC: U.S. Government Printing Office, 1995.
22. National Institute on Drug Abuse. *Epidemiologic trends in drug abuse, community epidemiology work group, June 1995. Volume 1: highlights and executive summary.* National Institutes of Health publication no. 95-3990. Washington, DC: U.S. Government Printing Office, 1995.

23. National Institute on Drug Abuse. *Epidemiologic trends in drug abuse, community epidemiology work group, December 1995. Volume 1: highlights and executive summary.* National Institutes of Health publication no. 96-4128. Washington, DC: U.S. Government Printing Office, 1996.

24. Vincent JP, Kartalouski B, Geneste P, et al. Interaction of phencyclidine ("angel dust") with a specific receptor in rat brain membranes. *Proc Natl Acad Sci U S A* 1979;76:4678–4682.

25. Zukin SR, Zukin RS. Specific ^{3}H-phencyclidine binding in rat central nervous system. *Proc Natl Acad Sci U S A* 1979;76:5372–5376.

26. Holtzman SG. Phencyclidine-like discriminative effects of opioids in the rat. *J Pharmacol Exp Ther* 1980;214:614–619.

27. Holtzman SG. Phencyclidine-like discriminative stimulus properties of opioids in the squirrel monkey. *Psychopharmacology (Berl)* 1982;77:295–300.

28. Quirion R, Hammer RP Jr, Herkenham M, et al. Phencyclidine (angel dust) F "opiate" receptor: visualization by tritium-sensitive film. *Proc Natl Acad Sci U S A* 1981;78:5881–5885.

29. Hampton RY, Medzihradsky F, Woods JH, et al. Stereospecific binding of ^{3}H-phencyclidine in brain membranes. *Life Sci* 1982;30:3147–3154.

30. Mendelsohn LG, Kalra V, Johnson BG, et al. F opioid receptor: characterization and co-identity with the phencyclidine receptor. *J Pharmacol Exp Ther* 1985;233:597–602.

31. Sircar R, Rappaport M, Nichtenhauser R, et al. The novel anticonvulsant MK-801; a potent and specific ligand of the brain phencyclidine/F receptor. *Brain Res* 1987;435:235–240.

32. Zukin SR, Temple A, Gardner EL, et al. Interaction of [^{3}H](+)SKF-10,047 with brain F receptors: characterization and autoradiograph visualization. *J Neurochem* 1986;46:1032–1041.

33. Zukin SR. Differing stereospecificities distinguish opiate receptor subtypes. *Life Sci* 1982;31:1307–1310.

34. Holtzman SG. Phencyclidine-like discriminative stimulus properties of opioids in the squirrel monkey. *Psychopharmacology (Berl)* 1982;77:295–300.

35. Michaelis EK. Glutamate neurotransmission: characteristics of the NMDA receptors in mammalian brain. *Neural Notes* 1996;2:3–7.

36. Cotman CW, Monaghan DT, Ganong AH. Excitatory amino acid neurotransmission: NMDA receptors and Hebb-type synaptic plasticity. *Annu Rev Neurosci* 1988;11:61–80.

37. MacDermott AB, Mayer ML, Westbrook GL, et al. NMDA-receptor activation increases cytoplasmic calcium concentration in cultured spinal cord neurones. *Nature* 1985;321:519–522.

38. Mayer ML, MacDermott AB, Westbrook GL, et al. Agonist- and voltage-gated calcium entry in cultured mouse spinal cord neurons under voltage clamp measured using arsenazo III. *J Neurosci* 1987;7:3230–3244.

39. Morris RGM. Synaptic plasticity and learning: selective impairment of learning in rats and blockade of long-term potentiation in vivo by the N-methyl-D-aspartate receptor antagonist AP5. *J Neurosci* 1989;9:3040–3057.

40. Wood PL. The co-agonist concept: is the NMDA-associated glycine receptor saturated in vivo? *Life Sci* 1995;57:301–310.

41. Schell MJ, Molliver ME, Snyder SH. D-Serine, an endogenous synaptic modulator: localization to astrocytes and glutamate-stimulated release. *Proc Natl Acad Sci U S A* 1995;92:3948–3952.

42. Lerma J, Zukin RS, Bennett MV. Interaction of Mg^{2+} and phencyclidine in use-dependent block of NMDA channels. *Neurosci Lett* 1991;123:187–191.

43. Javitt DC, Zukin SR. Biexponential kinetics of [^{3}H]MK-801 binding: evidence for access to closed and open N-methyl-D-aspartate receptor channels. *Mol Pharmacol* 1989;35:387–393.

44. Olney JW, Labruyere J, Price MT. Pathological changes induced in cerebrocortical neurons by phencyclidine and related drugs. *Science* 1989;244:1360–1362.

45. Ellison G. The N-methyl-D-aspartate antagonists phencyclidine, ketamine, and dizocilpine as both behavioral and anatomical models of the dementias. *Brain Res Rev* 1995;20:250–267.

46. Sharp FR, Butman M, Aardalen K, et al. Neuronal injury produced by NMDA antagonists can be detected using heat shock proteins and can be blocked with antipsychotics. *Psychopharmacol Bull* 1994;30:555–560.

47. Fix AS. Pathological effects of MK-801 in the rat posterior cingulate/retrosplenial cortex. *Psychopharmacol Bull* 1994;30:577–582.

48. Chen G, Ensor CR, Russell D, et al. The pharmacology of 1-(1-phenylcychohexyl) piperidine-HCl. *J Pharmacol Exp Ther* 1959;127:240–250.

49. Jackson DM, Johansson C, Lindgren L-M, et al. Dopamine receptor antagonists block amphetamine and phencyclidine-induced motor stimulation in rats. *Pharmacol Biochem Behav* 1994;48:465–471.

50. Toth E, Lajtha E. Antagonism of phencyclidine-induced hyperactivity by glycine in mice. *Neurochem Res* 1986;11:393–400.

51. Owens SM, Hardwick WC, Blackall D. Phencyclidine pharmacokinetic scaling among species. *J Pharmacol Exp Ther* 1987;242:96–101.

52. Xu X, Domino EF. Phencyclidine-induced behavioral sensitization. *Pharmacol Biochem Behav* 1994;47:603–608.

53. Steinpreis RE, Sokolowski JD, Papnikolaou A, et al. The effects of haloperidol and clozapine on PCP- and amphetamine-induced suppression of social behavior in the rat. *Pharmacol Biochem Behav* 1994;47:579–585.

54. Irifune M, Shimizu T, Nomoto M, et al. Involvement of N-methyl-D-aspartate (NMDA) receptors in noncompetitive NMDA receptor antagonist-induced hyperlocomotion in mice. *Pharmacol Biochem Behav* 1995;51:291–296.

55. French ED, Vantini G. Phencyclidine-induced locomotor activity in the rat is blocked by 6-hydroxydopamine lesion of the nucleus accumbens: comparisons to other psychomotor stimulants. *Psychopharmacology (Berl)* 1984;82:83–88.

56. French ED, Pilapil C, Quirion R. Phencyclidine binding sites in the nucleus accumbens and phencyclidine-induced hyperactivity are decreased following lesions of the mesolimbic dopamine system. *Eur J Pharmacol* 1985;116:1–9.

57. Steinpreis RE, Salamone JD. The role of nucleus accumbens dopamine in the neurochemical and behavioral effects of phencyclidine: a microdialysis and behavioral study. *Brain Res* 1993;612:263–270.

58. Wang T, French ED. L-Glutamate excitation of A10 dopamine neurons is preferentially mediated by activation of NMDA receptors: extra-intracellular electrophysiological studies in brain slices. *Brain Res* 1993;627:299–306.

59. Wang T, O'Connor WT, Ungerstedt U, et al. N-methyl-D-aspartic acid biphasically regulates the biochemical and electrophysiological response of A10 dopamine neurons in the ventral tegmental area: *in vivo* microdialysis and in vitro electrophysiological studies. *Brain Res* 1994;666:255–262.

60. Chen GM, Weston JK. The analgesic and anesthetic effect of 1-(1-phenylcyclohexyl) piperidine-HCl on the monkey. *Anesth Analg* 1960;39:132–138.

61. Verma A, Moghaddam B. NMDA receptor antagonists impair prefrontal cortex function as assessed via spatial delayed alternation performance in rats:

modulation by dopamine. *J Neurosci* 1996;16:373–379.

62. Moersbaecher JM, Thompson DM. Effects of phencyclidine, pentobarbital, and d-amphetamine on the acquisition and performance of conditional discriminations in monkeys. *Pharmacol Biochem Behav* 1980;13:887–894.

63. Quirion R, Hammer RP Jr, Herkenham M, et al. Phencyclidine (angel dust)/ sigma "opiate" receptor: visualization by tritium-sensitive film. *Proc Natl Acad Sci U S A* 1981;78:5881–5885.

64. Sircar R, Zukin SR. Quantitative localization of [³H]TCP binding in rat brain by light microscopy autoradiography. *Brain Res* 1985;344:142–145.

65. Annonsen LM, Seybold VS. Phencyclidine and F receptors in rat spinal cord: binding characterization and quantitative auto radiography. *Synapse* 1989;4:1–10.

66. Bekenstein JW, Bennett JP Jr, Wooten GF, et al. Autoradiographic evidence that NMDA receptor-coupled channels are located postsynaptically and not presynaptically in the perforant path-dentate granule cell system of the rat hippocampal formation. *Brain Res* 1990;514:334–342.

67. Vu TH, Weissman D, London ED. Pharmacological characteristics and distributions of F- and phencyclidine receptors in the animal kingdom. *J Neurochem* 1990;54:598–604.

68. Hirai H, Kirsch J, Laube B, et al. The glycine binding site of the N-methyl-D-aspartate receptor subunit NR1: Identification of novel determinants of coagonist potentiation in the extracellular M3-M4 loop region. *Proc Natl Acad Sci U S A* 1996;93:6031–6036.

69. Wafford KA, Kathoria M, Bain CJ, et al. Identification of amino acids in the N-methyl-D-aspartate receptor NR1 subunit that contribute to the glycine binding site. *Mol Pharmacol* 1995;47:374–380.

70. Rock DM, MacDonald RL. Polyamine regulation of N-methyl-D-aspartate receptor channels. *Annu Rev Pharmacol Toxicol* 1995;35:463–482(review).

71. Huntley GW, Vickers JC, Morrison JH. Cellular and synaptic localization of NMDA and non-NMDA receptor subunits in neocortex: organizational features related to cortical circuitry, function and disease. *Trends Neurosci* 1994;17:536–542.

72. Landwehrmeyer GB, Standaert DG, Testa CM, et al. NMDA receptor subunit mRNA expression by projection neurons and interneurons in rat striatum. *J Neurosci* 1995;15:5297–5307.

73. Javitt DC. Negative schizophrenic symptomatology and the phencyclidine (PCP) model of schizophrenia. *Hillside J Clin Psychiatry* 1987;9:12–35.

74. Krebs MO, Desce JM, Kemel ML, et al. Glutamatergic control of dopamine release in the rat striatum: evidence for presynaptic N-methyl-D-aspartate receptors. *J Neurochem* 1991;56:81–85.

75. Koek W, Colpaert FC, Woods JH, et al. Glutamatergic control of dopamine release in the rat striatum: evidence for presynaptic N-methyl-D-aspartate receptors on dopaminergic nerve terminals. *J Neurochem* 1991;56:81–85.

76. Wang JK, Thukral V. Presynaptic NMDA receptors display physiological characteristics of homomeric complexes of NR1 subunits that contain the exon 5 insert in the N-terminal domain. *J Neurochem* 1996;66:865–868.

77. Burns RS, Lerner SE. Perspectives: acute phencyclidine intoxication. *Clin Toxicol* 1976;9:477–501.

78. Walberg CB, McCarron MM, Schulze BW. Quantitation of phencyclidine in serum by enzyme immunoassay: results in 405 patients. *J Anal Toxicol* 1983;7:106–110.

79. Pearce DS. Detection and quantitation of phencyclidine in blood by use of [²H₅]phencyclidine and select ion monitoring applied to non-fatal cases of phencyclidine intoxication. *Clin Chem* 1976;22:1623–1626.

80. Cook CE, Brine DR, Jeffcoat AR. Phencyclidine disposition after intravenous and oral doses. *Clin Pharmacol Ther* 1982;31:625–634.

81. James SH, Schnoll SH. Phencyclidine: tissue distribution in the rat. *Clin Toxicol* 1976;9:573–582.

82. Misra AL, Pontani RB, Bartolemeo J. Persistence of phencyclidine (PCP) and metabolites in brain and adipose tissue and implications for long-lasting behavioural effects. *Res Commun Chem Pathol Pharmacol* 1979;24:431–445.

83. Wong LK, Biemann K. Metabolites of phencyclidine. *Clin Toxicol* 1976;9:583–591.

84. Soine WH. Clandestine drug synthesis. *Med Res Rev* 1986;6(1):41–74.

85. Lerner SE, Burns RS. Phencyclidine use among youth: History, epidemiology, and chronic intoxication. *NIDA Res Monogr Ser* 1978;21:66–118.

86. Soine WH, Vincek WC, Agee DT, et al. Contamination of illicit phencyclidine with 1-piperidinocyclohexane-carbonitrile. *J Anal Toxicol* 1980;4:217–221.

87. Soine WH, Brady KT, Balster RL, et al. Chemical and behavioral studies of 1-piperidinocyclohexanecarbonitrile (PCC): evidence for cyanide as the toxic component. *Res Commun Chem Pathol Pharmacol* 1980;30(1):59–70.

88. Lue LP, Scimeca JA, Thomas BF, et al. Pyrolyte fate of piperidinocyclo-hexanecarbonitrile, a contaminant of phencyclidine during smoking. *J Anal Toxicol* 1988;12:57–61.

89. Bakker CB, Amini FB. Observations on the psychotomimetic effects of Sernyl. *Compr Psychiatry* 1961;2:269–280.

90. Luby ED, Cohen BD, Rosenbaum F, et al. Study of a new schizophrenomimetic drug Sernyl. *Arch Neurol Psychiatry* 1959;81:363–369.

91. Ban TA, Lohrenz JJ, Lehmann HE. Observations on the action of Sernyl–a new psychotropic drug. *Can Psychiatr Assoc J* 1961;6:150–156.

92. Davies BM, Beech HR. The effect of 1-arylcyclohexylamine (Sernyl) on twelve normal volunteers. *J Ment Sci* 1960;106:912–924.

93. Domino EF, Luby E. Abnormal mental states induced by phencyclidine as a model of schizophrenia. In: Domino EF, ed. *PCP (phencyclidine): historical and current perspectives.* Ann Arbor, MI: NPP Books, 1981:37–50.

94. Rodin EA, Luby ED, Meyer JS. Electroencephalographic findings associated with Sernyl infusion. *EEG Clin Neurophysiol* 1959;11:796–798.

95. Rosenbaum G, Cohen BD, Luby ED, et al. Comparisons of Sernyl with other drugs. *Arch Gen Psychiatry* 1959;1:651–656.

96. Cohen BD, Rosenbaum G, Luby ED, et al. Comparison of phencyclidine hydrochloride (Sernyl) with other drugs. *Arch Gen Psychiatry* 1961;6:79–85.

97. Itil T, Keskiner A, Kiremitci N, et al. Effect of phencyclidine in chronic schizophrenics. *Can Psychiatr Assoc J* 1967;12:209–212.

98. Erard R, Luisada PV, Peele R. The PCP psychosis: prolonged intoxication or drug-precipitated functional illness? *J Psychedelic Drugs* 1980;12:235–245.

99. Yesavage JA, Freeman AM III. Acute phencyclidine (PCP) intoxication: psychopathology and prognosis. *J Clin Psychiatry* 1978;44:664–665.

100. Balster RL, Johanson CE, Harris RT, Schuster CR. Phencyclidine self-administration in the rhesus monkey. *Pharmacol Biochem Behav* 1973;1:167–172.

101. Lukas SE, Griffiths RR, Brady JV, Wurster RM. Phencyclidine-analogue self-injection by the baboon. *Psychopharmacology (Berl)* 1984;83:316–320.

102. Risner ME. Intravenous self-administration of phencyclidine and related compounds in the dog. *J Pharmacol Exp Ther* 1982;221:627–644.

103. Carroll ME, Meisch RA. Oral phencyclidine (PCP) self-administration in rhesus monkeys: effects of feeding

conditions. *J Pharmacol Exp Ther* 1980;214:339–346.

104. Balster RL. Clinical implications of behavioral pharmacology research on phencyclidine. *NIDA Res Monogr Ser* 1986;64:148–161.

105. Nazzaro JM, Seeger TF, Gardner EL. Naloxone blocks phencyclidine's dose-dependent effects on direct brain reward thresholds. In: *Proceedings of World Conference on Clinical Pharmacology and Therapeutics.* London: British Pharmacological Society, 1980:949.

106. Herberg LJ, Rose IC. The effect of MK-801 and other antagonists of NMDA-type glutamate receptors on brain-stimulation reward. *Psychopharmacology (Berl)* 1989;99:87–90.

107. Woolverton WL, Balster RL. Tolerance to the behavioral effects of phencyclidine: importance of behavioral and pharmacological variables. *Psychopharmacology (Berl)* 1979;64:19–24.

108. Johnson KM, Balster RL. Acute and chronic phencyclidine administration: relationship between biodispositional factors and behavioral effects. *Subst Alcohol Actions Misuse* 1981;2:131–142.

109. Freeman AS, Martin BR, Balster RL. Relationship between the development of behavioral tolerance and the biodisposition of phencyclidine in mice. *Pharmacol Biochem Behav* 1984;20:373–377.

110. Carroll ME. PCP, the dangerous angel. In: Snyder SH, ed. *The encyclopedia of psychoactive drugs.* New York: Chelsea House, 1985.

111. Balster RL, Woolverton WL. Continuous access phencyclidine self-administration by rhesus monkeys leading to physical dependence. *Psychopharmacology (Berl)* 1980;70:5–10.

112. Aronow R, Done AK. Phencyclidine overdose: an emerging concept of management. *JACEP* 1978;7:56–59.

113. Done AK, Aronow R, Miceli JN. The pharmacokinetics of phencyclidine in overdosage and its treatment. *NIDA Res Monogr Ser* 1978;21:210–217.

114. Picchioni AL, Consroe PF. Activated charcoal—a phencyclidine antidote, or hog in dogs [Letter]. *N Engl J Med* 1979;300:202.

115. Baldridge EB, Bessen HA. Phencyclidine. *Emerg Med Clin North Am* 1990;8(3):541–550.

116. Bywaters EGL, Stead JK. The production of renal failure following injection of solutions containing myohaemoglobin. *Q J Exp Physiol* 1944;33:53–70.

117. Perri GC, Gorini P. Uraemia in the rabbit after injection of crystalline myoglobin. *Br J Exp Pathol* 1952;33:440–444.

118. Toth E, Lajtha A. Antagonism of phencyclidine-induced hyperactivity by glycine in mice. *Neurochem Res* 1986;11:393–400.

119. McCarron MM, Schulze BW, Thompson GA, et al. Acute phencyclidine intoxication: incidence of clinical findings in 1,000 cases. *Ann Emerg Med* 1981;10:237–242.

120. McCarron MM, Schulze BW, Thompson GA, et al. Acute phencyclidine intoxication: clinical patterns, complications, and treatment. *Ann Emerg Med* 1981;10:290–297.

121. Crosley CJ, Binet EF. Cerebrovascular complications in phencyclidine intoxication. *J Pediatr* 1979;94:316–318.

122. Kessler GF, Demers LM, Berlin C, et al. Phencyclidine and fatal status epilepticus [Letter]. *N Engl J Med* 1974;291:979.

123. Patel R, Connor G. A review of thirty cases of rhabdomyolysis-associated acute renal failure among phencyclidine users. *Clin Toxicol* 1986;23:547–556.

124. Altura BT, Altura BM. Phencyclidine, lysergic acid diethylamide, and mescaline: cerebral artery spasms and hallucinogenic activity. *Science* 1981;212:1051–1052.

125. Stine RJ. Heat illness. *JACEP* 1979;8:154–160.

126. Thompson TN. Malignant hyperthermia from PCP [Letter]. *J Clin Psychiatry* 1979;40:327.

127. Sircar R, Nichtenhauser R, Ieni JR, et al. Characterization and autoradiographic visualization of (+)-[3H]SKF10,047 binding in rat and mouse brain: further evidence for phencyclidine/"sigma opiate" receptor commonality. *J Pharmacol Exp Ther* 1986;237:681–688.

CHAPTER 20

Inhalants

CHARLES W. SHARP AND
NEIL L. ROSENBERG

Volatile substances are ubiquitous and varied. Numerous substances are currently abused, yet inhalation to produce euphoria can be traced to the ancient Greeks (1). With the advent of the use of anesthetics in the mid-1800s, chloroform and ether parties occurred, and these substances are still used (2,3). Another anesthetic, euphemistically called "laughing gas," accurately describes one of the recreational uses of another anesthetic, nitrous oxide, which also originated in the late 1800s. It is stated that the use of ether and nitrous oxide at parties initiated the use of these compounds as anesthetics (4). With the increased use of gasoline at the turn of the twentieth century, many more substances became available through the process of petroleum "cracking" and distillation, and were included in many types of solvents, cleaners, degreasers, and glues. These products can be found everywhere, in industry, in the workplace, and in the home. Thus it is not surprising that anyone could find a favorite intoxicating vapor to "get high on." These substances are a bargain when one compares the going price of a "toke" or a "hit" of marihuana or cocaine. With that in mind, this chapter reviews many of those substances now known to be commonly abused through inhalation of "unheated" vapors.

The practice of "sniffing," "snorting," "huffing," "bagging," or inhaling to get high describes various forms of inhalation. If the substance is glue or some other dissolved solid, the user will empty the can's contents (or a gas) into a plastic bag and then hold the bag to the nose and inhale ("bagging"). Another method is to soak a rag with the mixture and then stick the rag in the mouth and inhale the fumes ("huffing"). A simple but more toxic approach is to spray the substance directly into the oral cavities. This allows these abusers to be identified by various telltale clues, for example, organic odors on the breath or clothes, stains on the clothes or around the mouth, empty spray paint or solvent containers, and other unusual paraphernalia. These telltale clues may enable one to identify a serious problem of solvent abuse before it causes serious health problems or death.

EPIDEMIOLOGY

Prevalence

The prevalence of inhalant abuse continues to be a relatively unknown drug abuse issue, especially among adults. Inhalant use exists in both developed and in underdeveloped countries. England (5,6) and other countries are systematically evaluating the abuse of solvents (7–19). These reports continuously identify inhalant (solvent) abuse as a problem of serious proportion. In the United States, the pattern of inhalant abuse is exemplified by national studies, including the annual Monitoring the Future (MTF) (20), which primarily interviews public school and college students, and the National Household Survey on Drug Abuse (NHSDA) surveys (21), and by state surveys such as those conducted in New York (22) and Texas (23).

Although one often looks at large state or national surveys, these surveys do not clearly delineate many regions where there is a higher proportion of inhalant abuse, such as in some inner cities that include impoverished or ethnic minorities or other isolated communities, especially those of Native Americans (10). In some surveys, there appears to be an underrepresentation of African Americans in the solvent-abusing populations, but inhalants are abused by African Americans (22). Although Hispanic groups are often considered to be overrepresented in the solvent-abusing population, the large surveys generally do not show a much greater proportion of Hispanics than of the larger "Anglo American" population of the United States; however, relative to the population at large, this would represent a higher relative proportion. The extent of use in these groups is difficult to evaluate properly, because many of the inhalant-abuse individuals are not accessed by survey systems. To look at the regional problems of solvent abuse, Beauvais and Oetting extensively studied many Native American groups (10); Howard et al. (24) studied urban native Americans; others have studied Hispanic communities (25,26). Usually considered a problem more of youth than of adults, a New York study of transients reported a high use of inhalants in this group (22). Although the lifetime prevalence of inhalants by the household adult population in the state of New York was 2% to 4%, the lifetime use of "transients" was 15% to 18%. Cocaine use and heroin use (in New York City) were also higher in the group of transients (45% and 27%, respectively).

Individual states and the U.S. national government began to evaluate the extent of the problem of inhalant abuse in the late 1960s and early 1970s. Yearly surveys of the problem are now available on line (http://www.drugabusestatistics.samhsa.gov/, http://www.tcada.state.tx.us/, and http://www.vsareport.org/). The extent of use of inhalants can be compared (see earlier; reference 27) to that of cocaine or other stimulants (amphetamines or "uppers"); see Tables 20.1 and 20.2. (We have made an effort to compare data realizing the risks in doing this; the reader can read individual reports to best interpret this data.) In the national surveys, it is interesting to note that inhalant use is highest in junior high students, third only to cigarettes and alcohol. Although "lifetime use" of inhalants is often higher for youths younger than age 16 years (Table 20.1), the drop in lifetime use beyond this age raises several questions. Are some "heavy" users lost to the survey? Are the questions misinterpreted by young respondents (at either the eighth or twelfth grade level)? For example, could very young children think that "liking the smell" is the equivalent of "getting-high"? Is there a forgetfulness about this type of behavior, or a downgrading of this event in their conscious thinking as they mature?

TABLE 20.1. *Percentages reporting lifetime use of inhalants or cocaine among eighth and twelfth graders in the NHSDA, MTF, and Texas surveys in years 1988, 1994, and 2002*

	Lifetime use					
	Inhalants			Cocaine		
Current grade/age	1988	1994	2002	1988	1994	2002
MTF						
8th grade	—	19.9	17.1	—	3.6	4.3
12th grade	17.5	17.7	13.0	12.1	5.9	8.2
NHSDA						
8th grade	—	—	8.4	—	—	0.8
12th grade	—	—	8.5	—	—	5.1
12–17-year-olds	8.8	7.0	8.6	3.4	1.7	2.3
Texas						
8th grade	32	23.8	18.8	5.2	4.7	5.6
12th grade	25.5	14.5	15.4	11.6	8.3	12.7

TABLE 20.2. *Percentages reporting past month use of inhalants or cocaine among eighth and twelfth graders in the NHSDA, MTF, and Texas surveys in years 1988, 1994, and 2002*

	Past month use					
	Inhalants			Cocaine		
Current grade/age level	1988	1994	2002	1988	1994	2002
MTF						
8th grade	—	5.6	4.0	—	1.0	1.2
12th grade	3.0	2.7	1.7	3.4	1.5	2.1
NHSDA						
8th grade	—	—	0.9	—	—	0.0
12th grade	—	—	0.9	—	—	0.9
12–17-year-olds	2.0	1.6	1.0	1.1	0.3	0.4
Texas						
8th grade	9.4	7.1	8.2	2.7	1.4	2.0
12th grade	3.3	2.0	4.0	4.2	2.4	3.7

Some assign this change to a diminished "remembrance" of this event as "getting-high" for a number of reasons. Whatever the reason, there is still a high percentage of children who have ever used inhalants. With the increasing number of participants in the surveys, more interest has focused not only on "past year" experience but on "past month" use (Table 20.2). In either national survey, past month use is higher for inhalants than for cocaine (or stimulants) in the eighth grade (12- to 13-year-olds), but "past month use" of cocaine is comparable to inhalant use by the twelfth grade (16- to 17-year-olds) when a broader variety of drugs are available. Different but select cohorts seem to be those who abuse inhalants. Most importantly, these individuals may be those that are most in trouble in school or with the law and who have health problems as a result of their inhalant use.

Use of drugs for mind-altering purposes varies by substance and extent of use. It is still reasonable to say even today that more than 1 in 10 have used solvents/gases to get special feelings. Table 20.3 lists different types of inhalants surveyed in the NHSDA and Texas reports. This attempt to list two different tabulations is not for purposes of comparison (different groupings exist even in the same Texas survey) and comparisons should not be done. Nevertheless, it is interesting to see similarities in the two, as well as the trends over time, mimic those of inhalants in general. That is, with the exception of nitrous oxide. It is not evident by the categories of substances grouped; yet, one can interpolate from this data and other reports (see reference 28) that there is an increase in the use of the butane and propane gases, which replaced fluorocarbons as propellants for aerosols in the early 1980s. It is difficult, of course, to identify which volatile component is most desired in any aerosol. However, the popularity of "cigarette lighter gases" (which contain only these gases) during the 1980s and later, makes it clear that these gases are effective mind-altering substances. One substance worthy of note is nitrous oxide. Its use has been increasing in the young adult population (Table 20.3). This is also noted in the New York school survey (22). Just like ecstasy, it has been used at concerts and in various youthful party events. There is a great concern about any inhalation of gases/solvents by younger age groups (e.g., seventh and eighth graders) because of their lack of understanding of the problem, both what is meant by getting "high" and the resulting consequences of this habit. This emphasizes the need for increased education for children, especially their parents, about the nature and dangers of this problem.

One of the more grim statistics gathered regarding drug abuse relates to death. It is difficult to gather quantitative data on the number of deaths associated with inhalant use. Periodically, starting in 1970, Bass has attempted to obtain data related to deaths resulting from intentionally inhaling solvents/gases (29–31). Deaths caused by solvents/gases are identified by the Poison Control Centers and include accidental deaths, as well as those caused by the subject using the product to get high. Even though this data cannot be used to determine prevalence of deaths resulting from inhalation to get high, the Annual Report of the American Association of Poison Control Centers (32) lists many deaths caused by hydrocarbons, many of which are related to butane-caused deaths. This report includes only a fraction of the deaths relating to solvent abuse, as does the Drug Abuse Warning Network (DAWN), a nationwide data collection system that gathers data of deaths related to drugs of abuse, including inhalants (33). The deaths reported in the DAWN tabulations are far fewer than those reported in the daily newspapers and are only a limited number of those that can be attributed to inhalants. There are two other studies of "inhalant abuse" deaths, one for Virginia (28) and another for Texas (34). The deaths in Texas are neither limited to adolescents nor to the unemployed. The substances abused includes butane/propane gases (Virginia), as well as halogenated (fluoro- or

TABLE 20.3. *Percentage reporting use of different inhalants in their lifetime among different age groups in the NHSDA and Texas surveys in different years*

Current age group	NHSDA survey			Texas survey		
	1993	1997	2001	1994	2000	2001
Spray paint						
12–17-year-olds	1.0	2.2	2.0	—	—	—
18–25-year-olds	0.8	0.8	1.3	—	—	—
26–34-year-olds	0.6	0.2	0.3	—	—	—
35+ year-olds	0.1	0.3	—	—	—	—
8th grade	—	—	—	8.8	9.8	7.5
10th grade	—	—	—	6.4	6.9	6.6
12th grade	—	—	—	4.4	5.2	4.9
Correction fluid						
12–17-year-old	0.7	1.7	1.9	—	—	—
18–25-year-old	0.5	1.1	1.4	—	—	—
26–34-year-olds	0.3	0.4	0.5	—	—	—
35 + year-olds	—	0.1	—	—	—	—
8th grade	—	—	—	12.7	11.2	8.8
10th grade	—	—	—	8.4	6.8	5.7
12th grade	—	—	—	6.6	4.6	4.3
Gasoline						
12–17-year-olds	1.6	2.7	3.0	—	—	—
18–25-year-olds	1.5	1.8	2.5	—	—	—
26–34-year-olds	1.6	1.0	1.1	—	—	—
35+ year-olds	0.5	0.7	—	—	—	—
8th grade	—	—	—	7.7	7.1	4.8
10th grade	—	—	—	5.8	5.2	3.2
12th grade	—	—	—	3.5	3.5	3.9
Nitrous oxide						
12–17-year-olds	0.7	2.3	1.8	—	—	—
18–25-year-olds	4.7	6.6	9.3	—	—	—
26–34-year-olds	3.7	3.7	3.4	—	—	—
35+ year-olds	0.9	1.1	—	—	—	—
8th grade	—	—	—	—	5.0	4.4
10th grade	—	—	—	—	6.2	5.3
12th grade	—	—	—	—	6.3	8.1
Glue (plus other substances)						
12–17-year-olds	1.9	2.7	3.6	—	—	—
18–25-year-olds	1.3	1.8	2.1	—	—	—
26–34-year-olds	1.1	1.0	1.1	—	—	—
35+ year-olds	0.6	0.7	—	—	—	—
8th grade	—	—	—	7.9	6.8	5.1
10th grade	—	—	—	4.5	2.9	3.3
12th grade	—	—	—	3.4	2.9	2.7
Lighter gases						
12–17-year-olds	0.6	1.2	0.9	—	—	—
18–25-year-olds	0.7	1.0	1.0	—	—	—
26–34-year-olds	0.1	0.1	0.1	—	—	—
35+ year-olds	—	0.1	—	—	—	—
Aerosol sprays (not paint)						
12–17-year-olds	1.0	1.9	1.6	—	—	—
18–25-year-olds	0.3	1.3	1.6	—	—	—
26–34-year-olds	0.6	0.2	0.4	—	—	—
35+ year-olds	0.1	0.2	—	—	—	—
8th grade	—	—	—	5.3	5.8	10.2
10th grade	—	—	—	3.1	2.6	7.2
12th grade	—	—	—	2.1	1.7	4.7

chlorohydrocarbons) propellants/solvents (both states), as the causes of death. In another study (35), Anderson noted their concern about an increasing number of deaths caused by butane/propane gases in Great Britain. This group in England has been accumulating data on deaths related to inhalant abuse for three decades. They reported 63 in 1982, 117 in 1985, 152 in 1990 (the highest number), 122 in 1991, and 70 to 80 each year thereafter (19). Gas fuels currently account for approximately 50% of the inhalant-abuse deaths. They have not found a decrease in the number of deaths caused by gas fuels but there is a decrease in the other categories, including aerosols (mainly fluorocarbons), solvents in adhesives, other solvents (mainly trichloroethane), and glues (19). Most deaths are attributed to direct toxic effects (19,36), which include the cardiotoxic actions of butane, fluorocarbons, and other solvents/gases, inhalation of gastric contents, trauma, and suffocation (19,36). There are also other causes of death related to inhalation of these substances (e.g., running in front of a car during or after intoxication). Garriott et al. documented such occurrences in their compilation of similar data for the Dallas and San Antonio areas (37,38).

Sociocultural Factors

The bases for inhaling solvents are similar to those described over two decades ago by Cohen (39). These substances are widely available, are readily accessible, cheap, and legally obtained. The substances make the solvent abuser forget and relieve the solvent abuser's boredom. These substances provide a quick high, with a rapid dissipation of the high and with a minimal hangover. However, subjects who use inhalants heavily over short periods often complain of headache. Many solvent abusers, more than other drug users, are poor, come from broken homes, have lower self-esteem, and do poorly in school (40–42). Although these characteristics are often observed in black Americans, reports generally indicate a lower-than-expected use of inhalants in this population. Some Hispanic groups, especially recent immigrants from Latin American countries, and Native Americans on reservations have a higher percentage of inhalant users than the population as a whole. Difficulty with acculturation and strong peer influence enhance the entrance into inhalant use, as well as other drug use (27,42). The family atmosphere is often disruptive for the abuser and has been identified as less adjusted or more conflictual than for controls (43).

Oetting et al. (41) categorized those who use inhalants into three groups: (a) inhalant-dependent adults, (b) polydrug users, and (c) young inhalant users. Inhalant-dependent adults have the most serious health problems because they have used heavily for a long time; the young inhalant users are those for whom treatment is most desirable to keep them from progressing to the other groups and for whom there may be hope for successful intervention.

Although all inhalant abusers use other drugs or alcohol, the first group predominately use inhalants, even though other drugs are available. The second group infrequently uses inhalants primarily because they cannot get their drug of choice; their problems arise more from the use of other drugs and are less related to those outlined in this chapter. The young inhalant users, however, are in the experimentation period of solvents, having started with either tobacco, alcohol, or possibly even marihuana, as well as inhalants. Before any of this group matures into the first group, intervening behavioral modifications are very important (44).

One trait that is often associated with sniffers is disruptive behavior. Some report them to be more violent. In one carefully controlled study, the only aggressive feature that stood out was the self-directed aggression (40). Cognitive measures of these groups support the antisocial and self-destructive nature of inhalant abusers. At least two major studies found these groups to have lower Wechsler verbal scores; it remains unanswered as to whether these groups self-selected inhalant abuse because of these predilections or whether the deficiencies came about as the result of inhalant abuse (40). In some instances, examination of school records indicates that cognitive deficits probably occurred before inhalant use began. Although it is uncertain how they became dysfunctional, it is very likely that inhalants prevent their continued growth and development (41,44). For further reading on the nature of the problem, especially the social-cultural conditions, we refer the reader to other reviews of this area (27,42,44).

Substances Inhaled

Despite the widespread availability and inhalation of these substances, it was not until the 1950s that nationwide attention by reporters (45) and by judicial action focused on what was euphemistically called "glue sniffing." The term is still widely used today to describe a myriad of substances that now include special shoe polishes, glue, gasoline, thinners, solvents, aerosols (paint, cooking lubricant spray, deodorant, hair spray, electronic cleaners, and others), correction fluids, cleaning fluids, refrigerant gases (e.g., fluorocarbons and the newer incompletely halogenated replacements [46]), anesthetics, whippets (whipped cream propellants), room odorizers (organic nitrites), and even cooking or lighter gases. In this context, it is not unheard of to find children selling toluene obtained from large commercial drums or to see vendors distributing nitrous oxide in balloons filled from commercial cylinders of the gas that are easily transported in cars. It is important to keep in mind that there are many different chemicals in most of these different products, all of which have different physiologic effects and different toxicities, as well as different chemical properties. Sometimes, the substances are listed on the container with or without the proportion of each. Table 20.4 lists some of the possible substances found in different products.

TABLE 20.4. *Chemicals commonly found in inhalants*

Inhalant	Chemicals
Adhesives	
Airplane glue	Toluene, ethylacetate
Other glues	Hexane, toluene, methyl chloride, acetone, methyl ethyl ketone, methyl butyl ketone
Special cements	Trichloroethylene, tetrachloroethylene
Aerosols	
Paint sprays	Butane, propane, fluorocarbons, toluene,
Hair sprays	Butane, propane, chlorofluorocarbons (CFCs)
Deodorants, air fresheners	Butane, propane, CFCs
Analgesic spray	CFCs
Asthma spray	CFCs
Fabric spray	Butane, trichloroethane
Personal computer cleaners	Dimethyl ether, hydrofluorocarbons
Anesthetics	
Gaseous	Nitrous oxide
Liquid	Halothane, enflurane
Local	Ethyl chloride
Cleaning agents	
Dry cleaners	Tetrachloroethylene, trichloroethane
Spot removers	Xylene, petroleum distillates, chlorohydrocarbons
Degreasers	Tetrachloroethylene, trichloroethane, trichloroethylene
Solvents and gases	
Nail polish remover	Acetone, ethyl acetate, toluene
Paint remover	Toluene, methylene chloride, methanol, acetone, ethyl acetate
Paint thinners	Petroleum distillates, esters, acetone
Correction fluids and thinners	Trichloroethylene, trichloroethane
Fuel gas	Butane, isopropane
Cigar or cigarette lighter fluid	Butane, isopropane
Fire extinguisher propellant	Bromochlorodifluoromethane
Food products	
Whipped cream aerosols	Nitrous oxide
Whippets	Nitrous oxide
Room odorizers	
Poppers, fluids (Rush, Locker Room)	Isoamyl, isobutyl, isopropyl, or butylnitrite (now illegal) or cyclohexyl

No study to date answers the perplexing question: What attracts young people to certain specific substances/products? Some consider the odor, color, or type of product to be important; others believe that the feeling one gets is most important. Yet, it is difficult to say what substances are preferred. Rankings of ever used substances may put glue and gasoline at the top (NHSDA 12- to 17-year-olds in Table 20.3) or rank correction fluids at the top with glue, gasoline, and spray paint being the next most frequent (Texas eighth graders in Table 20.3). The restriction of the use of fluorocarbons in aerosols in 1980 has not abolished fluorocarbon-related deaths (19,32,47–49) in work-related accidents (50) and elsewhere. They may be less available, possibly because they are available only in the more expensive pressurized refrigerant replacement cans. However, there are still numerous deaths attributed to the inhalational abuse of these fluorocarbons, even the partially hydrogenated fluorocarbons (51). This is supported by reports of stealing of the refrigerant (fluorocarbon) gases from air conditioning units for inhalation purposes. The addictive nature of fluorocarbons is exemplified by cases of asthma inhalers who inhale beyond the point of medication (52). This is one of the few marketable forms of fluorocarbons (totally halogenated) present in substances used by the public, except for the pressurized refrigerant refillers for some air conditioner systems. This is because of the United States' banning the use of fluorocarbons as a propellant for most commercial aerosols at the onset of the 1980s because of atmospheric pollution. Another group of halocarbons, the chlorohydrocarbons present in correction fluids, are considered to be the cause of other deaths (53–55).

The use of the pure butane lighter and other "cooking" (including propane) gases available here and in England (19,56–58) in pressurized containers illustrates the desire for these gases, when present alone or in other aerosol products. It is indeed unusual that these very dangerous substances are inhaled, and it is hard to tell whether some deaths are a result of intentional or accidental "overexposure." This problem was identified in the United States in the Cincinnati region where the use of butane gas causes numerous deaths. Thus, Siegel and Wason sounded the alarm for this dangerous practice of inhaling fuel gases (59). Other cases continue to be reported (60,61). An additional problem of fire exists with this inhalant (62). The bottom line is that there are a variety of substances used, probably based more on availability than individual preference. Yet, sniffers seem to go out of their way to get their favorite, for example, Texas "shoe shine," or clear lacquer, or gold spray paints, or other local or current favorites. In some places, the fad may be limited to other inhalants such as nitrous oxide or gasoline.

Evans and Raistrick (63) summarized the "sniffer's" perception of this phenomena when they sniffed butane gas or toluene. Moods, thoughts, hallucinations (except tactile), and colors appeared similar under either compound. However, time passed slowly under butane and more rapidly under toluene. This one study indicates that butane may be an acceptable substitute for toluene (present in many inhalant-products), one of the most widely used substances, and be used for some time to come. More studies are needed to more clearly understand those factors most important to supporting and/or maintaining inhalant abuse. In an effort to reduce the undesired exposure to cooking gases, it is now mandatory to add thiols to some portable gas containers, such as propane tanks, and it has been suggested that thiols be added to all forms of gas containers similar to that added to our natural gas supply.

One study is notable because it evaluated the inhalation event and did not rely on retrospective evaluation (64). This was only possible because nitrous oxide is an approved anesthetic. The investigators measured moods over time at different doses resembling those of the "recreational user." They noted that the effects lasted only a couple of minutes, and word tests demonstrated that memory retention within 5 minutes of the event was reduced. Some users liked the effect, whereas others did not. Other studies have measured the neuropsychological effects of nitrous oxide on humans after lower 1-hour doses (65) or after anesthesia (66). The abuse of this substance may also be related to prior exposure in a medical situation. Reports discuss the use of nitrous oxide for anxiety reduction, especially for children in dental treatment (67,68); another report even suggests use of nitrous oxide for treatment of alcoholism (69), an untested and unapproved treatment.

Most tragically, deaths are still noted following abuse of this substance (70–73).

Even though most users focus on the inhalation of various commercial household products, many anesthetics, other than nitrous oxide, are often used for "pleasure" (74–76). The abuse of these substances by middle-class professionals demonstrates the diversity of the individuals that abuse inhalants and also points to a common physical property of most of these volatile agents. Almost all solvents produce anesthesia if sufficient amounts are inhaled; some of them are described in a detailed study (77). Although this is an important property of the agent, the ability to produce anesthesia has not been correlated with the extent of abuse of any given substance.

Because of the diversity and complex composition of the products, there are often incorrect identifications of the primary substance of inquiry. Toluene is often quoted as the substance involved when other substances are also present that may contribute to or be the primary substance at issue. This can best be visualized by the following example: Transmission fluid was reportedly abused in Florida and stated to contain toluene. However, there is no toluene in transmission fluid. However, there is toluene in "Transgo," a wax stripper, which is a substance of abuse in the same Florida area where transmission fluid is reportedly abused. When users are asked what substances they are abusing, it is easy to see how the above transliteration (misnomer) could easily occur, and a reporting error result. Also, some reports associating toluene with a particular syndrome may have missed the correct substance that is the cause of that syndrome. The best corroboration of the causative substance is a measure, when possible, of the substance in body fluids. Clues may be derived from containers, but that is often not helpful, because many products do not identify all the substances they contain and often only refer to some of the ingredients as "nontoxic" hydrocarbons. For example, one of the more toxic agents, hexane, affects the peripheral nervous system and has been identified in products that did not list it on the product's label. Only through an analysis of the products used (e.g., by quantitative gas chromatography) is it possible to determine most of the volatile solvents in a product with an incomplete label. This, of course, may be insufficient. The identification of one product used by the inhalant abuser may not reveal the toxicant (which may come from another product in the abuser's repertoire) that should be considered in the diagnosis of the health problem.

TOXICOLOGY OF INHALANT ABUSE

Acute Intoxication

Most commercial products that are inhaled contain several distinctly different solvents, each with its own unique toxicity. In addition, most inhalant abusers have inhaled a variety of products to excess before they appear in a

TABLE 20.5. *Signs that may develop during or shortly after inhalant use or exposure*

Initial intoxication
  Initial excitation
  Drowsiness, lightheadedness, disinhibition, and
    agitation
With increasing intoxication, individuals may develop
  Ataxia
  Dizziness
  Disorientation
  Incoordination
With extreme intoxications
  Signs of sleeplessness
  General muscle weakness
  Dysarthria
  Nystagmus and occasionally hallucinations
  Disruptive behavior
  Slurred speech
  Unsteady gait
  Lethargy
  Depressed reflexes and then stupor or coma may result

treatment facility. An exception would be a novice experiencing an overdose—usually resulting in anoxia and possibly death. However, the majority of inhalant abusers never reach a hospital or an outpatient facility.

To understand the solvent abuser, one can conceive of the intoxicated state as a quick "drunk," as many of the symptoms resemble alcohol intoxication. An evaluation of these individuals provides several symptoms, such as initial excitation turning to drowsiness, disinhibition, lightheadedness, and agitation (Table 20.5). With increasing intoxication, individuals may develop ataxia, dizziness, and disorientation. In extreme intoxications, they may show signs of sleeplessness, general muscle weakness, dysarthria, nystagmus, and, occasionally, hallucinations or disruptive behavior. Several hours after, especially if they have slept, they are likely to be lethargic, or hung over with mild to severe headaches. Chronic abuse is associated with more serious complications including weight loss, muscle weakness, general disorientation, inattentiveness, and lack of coordination.

Most reports have described the acute intoxication in heavy users of toluene vapors. Acute intoxication with toluene produces headache, euphoria, giddiness, and cerebellar ataxia. At lower levels (just over 200 parts per million [ppm]), fatigue, headache, paresthesia, and slowed reflexes appear (78). Exposure at levels approaching 1,000 ppm causes confusion or delirium, and euphoric effects appear at or above that level. Although solvent abusers have favorites, they often use an unpredictable array of solvents. Multiple components in the mixtures may enhance the net toxicity in a synergistic or additive manner. More specific syndromes and details of the clinical fea-

tures of the chronic inhalant abuser are described below and are related as closely as possible to specific substances.

Death can occur during the course of primary intoxication. When it does occur, it is usually the result of asphyxia, ventricular fibrillation, or induced cardiac arrhythmia following high exposures to various solvents. "Cerebral anoxia associated with VSA [volatile substance abuse] fatalities may be related to multiple factors including asphyxia, cerebral and pulmonary oedema, cardiac arrhythmias and arrest, terminal unconsciousness, hyperpyrexia and others" (reference 47, p. 194). It is not as evident, but the results of several cases link fibrillation and other cardiac insufficiencies to the use of halocarbons (3,53–55,79–85). These types of products range from anesthetics (halothane) used by hospital and other medical personnel to the more common solvents (fluorocarbons, dichloroethanes, trichloroethanes, tetrachloroethanes, trichloroethylene) contained in cleaning fluids and typing correction fluid solvents. Some cardiac arrhythmias have also been reported following abuse of substances containing toluene; this includes the only reported nonfatal respiratory arrest of an inhalant abuser (86). The concentration of toluene in the body that causes death has been estimated based on data from the deaths of painters by Hobara et al. (87).

Although not as common (excluding the propellant nitrous oxide), anesthetics are an abuse problem (2,74–76,88). Severe problems, even deaths, have resulted from the abuse of these compounds by medical professionals, especially nitrous oxide (72,73,89). It is well known that oxygen should be mixed with nitrous oxide when inhaled for several minutes to an hour. Apparatuses are available for this when it is being used as an anesthetic. However, in some instances (homes, food services, or the ophthalmologist's office where it may be used as a cryogen), there are usually no masks for mixing these gases, and death has occurred (72). Also, freezing of the lips to the cylinder may occur (90).

In evaluating any patient suspected of inhaling solvents either accidentally or to get "high," it is important to determine as precisely as possible not only the solvent(s) but also other contributing factors (including other drugs, such as alcohol, cigarettes, or marihuana, malnutrition, or respiratory irritants, such as fumes or viruses) before beginning treatment. These interrelating factors are often more important for some groups of inhalant abusers, in that they use more drugs, are less-well nourished, and live in more "polluted" areas than other types of drug abusers.

Recognition of and Criteria for Defining Neurotoxicity

The nervous system may be affected at many levels by organic solvents as well as other neurotoxic substances. As a general rule, resultant syndromes are diffuse in their manifestations (91). Because of their nonfocal presentation, neurotoxic disorders may be confused with metabolic, degenerative, nutritional, or demyelinating disease (91). This principle is illustrated in the setting of chronic toluene abuse, which clinically may resemble the multifocal demyelinating disease, multiple sclerosis, in the findings on neurologic examination (92–94). As a result, mild cases of intoxication may be very difficult to diagnose. The most reliable information comes from documented cases of massive exposure, and details of low-level exposure and presymptomatic diagnosis are vague at best.

In general, neurotoxic injuries rarely have specific identifying features on diagnostic tests such as computed tomography (CT), magnetic resonance imaging (MRI), or nerve conduction studies (91). Because many neurotoxic effects are reversible and some chronic neurotoxic injuries of the brain may not be associated with structural damage sufficiently large to be detected within the spatial resolution of current MRI scanners and imaging sequences, brain imaging studies are primarily used to rule-out other disorders. However, recent studies of chronic solvent inhalant abusers suggests that MRI may be the most sensitive and specific method of detecting the brain injury associated with the high dose setting of the inhalant abuser.

The most reliable information comes from documented cases of massive exposure (like that in the abuse setting); details of low-level exposure (like that which occurs in the occupational setting) and presymptomatic diagnosis are vague at best.

Acute, high-level exposure to most, if not all, solvents will induce short-lasting effects on brain function, most of which are reversible. Acute incidents that are irreversible probably act by producing secondary systemic effects such as cerebral hypoxia or a metabolic acidosis (95), and none of these acute incidents is proven to act by inducing an irreversible functional abnormality. In general, both acute high-level and low-level exposure to organic solvents are associated with full reversibility, and the acute toxicity with high-level exposure in no way predicts whether chronic low-level exposure will lead to an irreversible neurologic disease.

Chronic high-level exposure to organic solvents occurs only in the inhalant abuse setting, where levels several-thousand-fold higher than the occupational setting frequently occur. Chronic neurotoxic injury related to solvent abuse is slowly and incompletely reversible, and usually does not progress after cessation of exposure (93,94). Both acute and chronic neurotoxicity from organic solvents are functions predominantly related to the dose and duration of exposure.

There may be no relationship between the mechanism of acute neurotoxicity and the clinical manifestations of chronic neurotoxicity. For example, an acute effect of a particular organic solvent may be attributable to the parent compound, while a chronic effect may be associated with a metabolite of this compound. In addition, in several known cases, a solvent was reported to either diminish or potentiate the neurotoxic potency of a second solvent (96–98).

There is little or no apparent individual variability or altered susceptibility to the neurotoxic effects of either acute or chronic exposure to organic solvents. Except for other toxic exposures or illnesses that also cause neurologic sequelae, individuals will likely develop a similar clinical picture when exposed to solvents at equivalent doses for equivalent durations of time.

Chemical structure may predict, but not invariably predict, the neurotoxic effects. An example of this is seen with two closely related compounds: 2,5-hexanedione (the toxic metabolite of n-hexane) and 2,4-hexanedione. A fixed dose of 2,5-hexanedione produces axonal degeneration in a particular species that is very similar to that produced by hexane, whereas 2,4-hexanedione never produces these changes. Thus, a small but important change in the compound's structure elicits a change from a positive to a negative pharmacologic action.

TREATMENT OF THE INHALANT ABUSER

There is no accepted treatment approach for inhalant abusers. Many drug treatment facilities refuse treatment of the inhalant abuser, because many believe that inhalant abusers are resistant to treatment. One program that focusses solely on the comprehensive treatment of inhalant abusers, the International Institute for Inhalant Abuse (IIIA), based in Colorado, uses a three-phase model that allows for longer periods of treatment. Longer periods of treatment are needed to be able to address the complex psychosocial, economic, and biophysical issues of the inhalant abuser. When brain injury, primarily in the form of cognitive dysfunction, is present, the rate of progression in the treatment process is even slower.

The inhalant abuser typically does not respond to usual drug rehabilitation treatment modalities. Several factors may be involved, particularly in situations of the chronic abuser, where significant psychosocial problems may be present. Treatment becomes slower and progressively more difficult when the severity of brain injury worsens as abuse progresses through transient social use (experimenting in groups) to chronic use in isolation (Table 20.6).

Drug screening may be useful in monitoring inhalant abusers (99,100). Routine urine screens for hippuric acid, the major metabolite of toluene (101), performed two to three times weekly, will detect the high level of exposure to toluene usually seen in inhalant abusers. It should be noted that the metabolism of any one compound may be modified by the presence of another, either increased (following inducement by drugs, e.g., barbiturates) or decreased (benzene metabolism reduced in the presence of toluene) (102).

Neuroleptics and other forms of pharmacotherapy are usually not useful in the treatment of inhalant abusers. However, as alcohol is a common secondary drug of abuse

TABLE 20.6. *Clinical classification of inhalant abusers*

Transient social	Transient isolate
Short history of use	Short history of use
Use with friends	Use alone
Petty offenses while intoxicated	No legal involvement
Average intelligence	Average/above intelligence
Possible learning disabilities	No learning disabilities
10–16 years of age	10–16 years of age
Chronic social	Chronic isolate
Long history of use (>5 years)	Long history of use (>5 years)
Daily use with friends	Daily use alone
Legal involvement—misdemeanors	Legal involvement—assaults common
Poor social skills	Poor social skills
Ninth grade education	Ninth grade education
Brain damage	Brain damage
Mid-twenties to early thirties	Mid-twenties
Mental retardation prevalent	Preuse psychopathology prevalent

among inhalant abusers, a monitored program for alcohol abuse may be necessary.

NEUROLOGICAL SEQUELAE OF CHRONIC INHALANT ABUSE

Organic solvents are widely prevalent compounds and inadvertent exposure, primarily industrial, as well as volitional abuse occurs primarily by inhalation, with significantly less absorption occurring via skin or gastrointestinal routes. These compounds are highly lipophilic, which explains their distribution to organs rich in lipids (e.g., brain, liver, adrenal). Unexpired solvents absorbed by the tissues are then eliminated through the kidneys following metabolism of the solvents to more water soluble compounds. In addition, metabolism of some solvents may create additional compounds that are sometimes more toxic than the parent chemical (103–105).

Although most organic solvents produce nonspecific effects following absorption of extremely high concentrations (i.e., encephalopathy), a few produce relatively specific neurologic syndromes with low-level, chronic exposure. Table 20.7 lists those syndromes associated with organic solvent exposure. Most of the early animal studies, which served as the basis for the setting of tolerance levels in industry, used acute studies to measure the effects, often including high-level exposures that produced lethality. More recent experimental studies have focused on chronic low-level and/or high-level exposures to solvents that result in peripheral and central nervous system syndromes. Major neurotoxic syndromes occurring in individuals chronically exposed to select organic solvents include a peripheral neuropathy, ototoxicity, and an encephalopathy. Less commonly, a cerebellar ataxic syndrome, parkinsonism, or a myopathy may occur alone or in combination with any of these clinical syndromes. In some instances, solvents interact and cause synergistic effects, resulting in multifocal central and peripheral nervous system damage.

Compounds of Interest

The organic solvents described in detail below are not intended to be a complete listing of compounds with associated neurotoxicity. They represent those organic solvents that are more commonly associated with abuse or where clear neurotoxicity is associated with exposure.

n-*Hexane and Methyl Butyl Ketone*

These two organic solvents are classified together because both n-hexane and methyl butyl ketone (MBK) are metabolized to the same neurotoxin, 2,5-hexanedione (2,5-HD) and produce an identical clinical syndrome characterized by a peripheral neuropathy. Clinically, the peripheral neuropathy begins with symmetrical, distal sensory loss in

TABLE 20.7. *Major neurologic syndromes produced by organic solvents*

Encephalopathy
    Acute encephalopathy—nonspecific; high-level
      exposure
    Chronic encephalopathy—seen with repeated
      high-level exposure over years
Cerebellar ataxia
Peripheral neuropathy—distal axonopathy
Cranial neuropathy—primarily cranial nerves V and VII
Parkinsonism
Visual loss—optic neuropathy
Multifocal
    Central nervous system (e.g., toluene)
    Central and peripheral

the lower extremities, which may progress, if the abuse continues, and eventually produce distal motor weakness. Pathologically, the findings are that of a distal axonopathy, with the longest nerve fibers being preferentially affected.

2,5-HD is responsible for most, if not all, of the neurotoxic effects that follow exposure to n-hexane or MBK (106–110). Methyl ethyl ketone (MEK) alone produces neither clinical nor pathologic evidence of a peripheral neuropathy in experimental animals (106). The importance of MEK is related to a synergistic effect between MEK and MBK and between MEK and n-hexane detected in experimental animals and probably in humans (96–98,111). This potentiation of toxicity of one compound (MBK or n-hexane) by an otherwise nontoxic compound (MEK) underscores the difficulty with sorting out toxic effects of individual solvents contained within a mixture and suggests that occupational exposure to solvent mixtures should be minimized or avoided altogether.

Methyl Butyl Ketone

MBK had limited industrial use until the 1970s when it became more widely used as a paint thinner, clearing agent, and a solvent for dye printing. Soon afterward, numerous outbreaks of polyneuropathy associated with chronic exposure to MBK were being reported (112–116). Originally, MEK had been used as a solvent, followed by a mixture of MEK (90%)/methyl isobutyl ketone (10%). When the methyl isobutyl ketone was replaced by MBK (10%), reports of polyneuropathy began to appear in the literature. The route of exposure is usually inhalation, but exposure has also occurred by the oral route through ingesting contaminated food in work areas and by cutaneous contact.

The clinical syndrome is characterized by the insidious onset of an initially painless sensorimotor polyneuropathy, which begins several months after continued chronic exposure. Even following cessation of exposure, the neuropathy may develop or may continue to progress for up to 3 months. In severe cases, an unexplained weight loss may be an early symptom. Sensory and motor disturbance begins initially in the hands and feet, and sensory loss is primarily small fiber (i.e., light touch, pinprick, temperature) with relative sparing of large-fiber sensation (i.e., position and vibration). Electrophysiologic studies reveal axonal polyneuropathy, pathologically multifocal axonal degeneration and multiple axonal swellings, and neurofilamentous accumulation at paranodal areas (117). Overlying the axonal swellings, thinning of the myelin sheath occurs. These findings are typical of a distal axonopathy or "dying-back" neuropathy described in other toxic and metabolic causes of peripheral neuropathy.

Prognosis for recovery correlates directly with the intensity of the neurologic deficit before removal from toxic exposure, with mild to moderate residual neuropathy seen in the most severely affected individuals up to 3 years after exposure.

n-Hexane

Until the 1970s, n-hexane was considered an innocuous solvent. n-Hexane is used in the printing of laminated products, in the extraction of vegetable oils, as a diluent in the manufacture of plastics and rubber, in cabinet finishing, as a solvent in biochemical laboratories, and as a solvent for glues and adhesives.

Cases of n-hexane polyneuropathy have been reported both after occupational exposure (118) and after deliberate inhalation of vapors from products containing n-hexane, such as glues (119–127). Clinically and pathologically, the neuropathy occurring with n-hexane is that of a distal axonopathy (128), indistinguishable from that associated with MBK.

When glues have been analyzed in past reports of a polyneuropathy occurring after glue sniffing, n-hexane has been a major component of the products' composition (up to 50% by weight). Another major component of these glues has been toluene. However, polyneuropathy does not occur from inhalation of toluene alone, and in previous reports of n-hexane neuropathy, the neuropathy did not appear until the subject switched to a product containing n-hexane. In contrast to toluene, n-hexane does not usually induce significant signs of central nervous system (CNS) dysfunction, except with high-level exposures where an acute encephalopathy may occur.

Both clinical and experimental studies provide evidence of CNS effects from n-hexane. Experimental animal studies show n-hexane to cause axonal degeneration in the CNS (128,129). Clinically, cranial neuropathy, spasticity, and autonomic dysfunction occasionally occur (96). Abnormalities on electrophysiologic tests of CNS function, including electroencephalography, visual evoked responses, color vision testing, and somatosensory evoked responses, are also seen (130–132). In spite of these findings, clinical effects of chronic low-level exposure to n-hexane is restricted to the peripheral nervous system.

Toluene (Methyl Benzene)

Toluene is one of the most widely used solvents and is employed as a paint and lacquer thinner, as a cleaning and drying agent in the rubber and lumber industries, and in the motor and aviation fuels and chemical industries. It is a major component in many paints, lacquers, glues and adhesives, inks, and cleaning liquids. As with other solvents, inhalation is the major route of entry, although some absorption occurs percutaneously. Of all the solvents, toluene-containing substances seem to have the highest potential for abuse (133).

In 1961, Grabski (134) reported the first patient with persistent neurologic consequences of chronic toluene inhalation. Since then, many reports of neurotoxicity, often of a severe nature, have appeared in the literature (92–94,135–158).

Experience is still not sufficient to determine the incidence of chronic effects of toluene and other volatile hydrocarbons. The neurologic pattern, however, is very clearly delineated, with effects only on the CNS. Syndromes of persistent and often severe neurotoxicity include cognitive dysfunction (92–94,142,144,152, 153,155,159–161), cerebellar ataxia (92,94,134,137,141, 148,155,156), optic neuropathy (139,145,162), sensorineural hearing loss (139), and an equilibrium disorder (154). Most commonly, toluene neurotoxicity includes several of the above syndromes and with multifocal CNS involvement (92–94,149,152,153,155). Despite the many instances of "persistent" neurologic deficits, in only one study was abstinence documented prior to clinical evaluation (93). This point is of great importance, because some individuals will go into complete remission with prolonged abstinence (137,163).

In a study of 20 chronic abusers of spray paint, which almost entirely consisted of toluene, abstinence was documented for at least 1 month prior to evaluation (93). In those chronic solvent abusers, 65% showed neurologic impairment. This was a small and unselected sample, so the findings probably do not reflect the true prevalence of neurologic damage. However, there was a fairly consistent pattern of neurologic abnormality. As has been suggested, the CNS is selectively vulnerable. In fact, no peripheral neuropathy was found, and there is no convincing evidence that pure toluene or other aromatic hydrocarbons cause peripheral neuropathy. Aliphatic hydrocarbons such as n-hexane, as noted earlier, cause predominantly peripheral nerve damage.

Neurologic abnormalities varied from mild cognitive impairment to severe dementia, associated with elemental neurologic signs such as cerebellar ataxia, corticospinal tract dysfunction, oculomotor abnormalities, tremor, deafness, and hyposmia. Cognitive dysfunction was the most disabling and frequent feature of chronic toluene toxicity and may be the earliest sign of permanent damage. Dementia, when present, was typically associated with cerebellar ataxia and other signs (93). One patient had pyramidal and cerebellar signs without cognitive impairment. Oculomotor dysfunction, deafness, and tremor were seen only in severely affected individuals. Cranial nerve abnormalities were confirmed to olfactory and auditory dysfunction. Toluene-induced optic neuropathy, previously reported (145), was not reported in the larger studies (93,153) but was not specifically addressed. In a more recent study, visual evoked potential abnormalities were found in a large percentage of chronic toluene abusers and other drug-abusing controls (164).

Other investigators have found a similar syndrome after chronic exposure to toluene (92,94,137,148). Although some investigators emphasized the cerebellar disorder, they noted that most cases also showed impairment in a variety of cerebral functions. In one study, there was a similar pattern of cognitive impairment with neuro-

logic abnormality, but the individuals were studied as soon as 3 days after the last exposure, and there have been no data on long-term cognitive outcome long after cessation of prolonged toluene abuse. It should be noted, however, that many chronic toluene abusers have had no persistent cognitive impairment despite approximately calculated cumulative doses equivalent to those in individuals with cognitive impairment (93,153). This suggests either that the abuse histories obtained were inaccurate or that other factors possibly play a role in those individuals.

The clinical data suggest that the cognitive, cerebellar, corticospinal, and brainstem signs are caused by diffuse effects of toluene on the CNS. In one prior report of an autopsy of a chronic solvent abuser, there was prominent degeneration and gliosis of ascending and descending long tracts with cerebral and cerebellar atrophy (165). Unfortunately, as in most reports of toluene neurotoxicity, this patient was abusing many solvents contained in several different mixtures, so the effects of individual solvents could not be determined.

In the late 1980s, the first reports were published that began to look more closely at the pathophysiology of toluene inhalation (152,153). These studies used MRI and demonstrated for the first time that chronic abuse of toluene-containing substances caused diffuse CNS white matter changes (152,153). The first published report was based on the MRI findings of the brain in six individuals and the neuropathologic changes in one abuser not studied by MRI (152). All individuals abused the same toluene-containing mixture, which contained primarily toluene (61%) and methylene chloride (10%). MRI of the six individuals revealed the following abnormalities: (a) diffuse cerebral, cerebellar, and brainstem atrophy; (b) loss of differentiation in the gray and white matter throughout the CNS; and (c) increased periventricular white matter signal intensity on T2-weighted images. More recent MRI studies support these original observations (136,138,150,153,157,158).

More recent MRI studies in larger numbers of abusers have extended these earlier observations. Different studies from the United States (166), Japan (167), and Turkey (168) were published independently. MRI findings were similar in the three studies and extended the earlier studies by findings of diffuse white matter changes, thalamic hypointensity, and varying degrees of cerebral atrophy. Only the U.S. study had a comparison group of other drug abusers (primarily chronic cocaine abusers), which also exhibited significant neuropsychological abnormalities but fewer MRI abnormalities. Of interest in the U.S. study, there was a dose–response relationship between the inhalant abuse and the MRI changes, but no dose–response relationship was seen with neuropsychological measures. This suggests that additional detailed studies using additional MRI sequencing techniques may help to further define the pathophysiology of the neurologic effects of toluene abuse.

While MRI has been very useful in attempting to understand the central nervous system effects of toluene abuse, an additional study using the functional imaging technique of brain SPECT (single-photon emission computed tomography) was recently published (169). Although multifocal abnormalities were seen in all 10 patients studied, no distinct pattern of abnormalities emerged among the subjects. Based on this single study, SPECT does not seem to add to our understanding of the pathophysiology of the central nervous system effects of inhalant abuse. Future studies should focus on MRI, which not only demonstrates across all studies a consistent pattern of abnormality, but also demonstrates a dose–effect relationship and much greater spatial resolution than SPECT or its higher resolution functional imaging counterpart, PET (positron emission tomography).

Another study attempted to find correlation between the severity of the clinical involvement in 11 chronic toluene abusers and the findings on brainstem auditory evoked responses (BAERs) and MRI (153). Neurologic abnormalities, including cognitive, pyramidal, cerebellar, and brainstem findings, were seen in 4 of 11 individuals. MRI of the brain was abnormal in 3 of 11 individuals, and all 3 also had abnormalities on neurologic examination. Abnormalities on MRI were the same as those reported previously (152). BAERs were found to be abnormal in 5 of 11 individuals and were similar to those previously reported in toluene abusers (92,149). In this study (153), all three individuals with abnormal MRI scans and neurologic examinations also had abnormal BAERs. Of the five individuals with abnormal BAERs, however, two had normal neurologic examinations and MRI scans. This study suggests that BAERs may detect early CNS injury from toluene inhalation even at a time when neurologic examination and MRI scans are normal. These results suggested that BAERs may be a screening test to monitor individuals at risk from toluene exposure for early evidence of CNS injury. However, a more recent study (164) determined that while certain abnormalities on BAERs are very specific for effects of toluene abuse, they are too insensitive to observe in the usual clinical setting.

Neuropathology Section

The neuropathology of chronic inhalant abuse is poorly described, but recent studies have begun to shed some light on possible pathogenetic mechanisms. The first report of neuropathologic changes was in an individual who was primarily an abuser of paint thinner containing toluene (165). Closer examination of the case revealed that this individual abused many different volatile substances over more than a decade; consequently, the neuropathologic changes cannot be considered the result of just toluene. However, there were changes seen diffusely in the white matter that would correlate well with the MRI data. Rosenberg et al. (152) reported the neuropathologic findings in one individual who had only changes in the white matter, diffusely, again correlating with the MRI changes. The changes revealed diffuse, ill-defined myelin pallor, which was maximal in the cerebellar, periventricular, and deep cerebral white matter. Neurons were preserved throughout, axonal swelling or beading was not seen, gliosis was minimal, and occasional, scant perivascular macrophage collections were seen. These findings were supported in a more recent neuropathologic study (170). In this latter report, the neuropathologic and biochemical changes seen in the brains of chronic toluene abusers were identical with those seen in those with adrenoleukodystrophy (ALD). ALD is a rare X-linked disorder associated with accumulation of very-long-chain fatty acids in certain tissues, including brain (171). These findings suggest that toluene is a white matter toxin; the mechanism of action, however, needs to be explained.

A possible explanation for the effect of toluene on white matter was given by Unger et al. (157). In this study, the MRI spectroscopic characteristics of liposomes both with and without toluene embedded in the membrane of the liposome were described. The characteristics of the toluene liposomes suggest that there was increased water content, which was the same as the MRI characteristics in the brains of chronic toluene abusers. Their hypothesis is that toluene somehow changes the configuration of certain membrane lipoproteins, making them hydrophilic. Perhaps the gradual accumulation of water is only a marker for the molecular injury that occurs. This may also explain reports of some chronic toluene abusers who, following prolonged abstinence, will have gradual, though incomplete, improvement in their neurologic deficit. In other words, because neurons are not being destroyed and membrane components may be replaced over time, clinical improvement may be seen, even in the most severely affected individuals.

Although an exact dose–effect relationship cannot be drawn yet for chronic toluene exposure, it is clear that all severely affected individuals have had heavy and prolonged exposure. The lack of correlation between the type or duration of exposure and neurologic impairment may be a result of unreliable histories or other factors, such as genetic predisposition (unlikely) or hypoxemia resulting from "huffing" or "bagging." Nutritional factors and other concomitantly used substances may also be involved. Gradual resolution of acute toxicity and absence of withdrawal symptoms were probably due to slow elimination of toluene from the CNS.

Trichloroethylene

Trichloroethylene (TCE) is an important organic solvent used extensively in industry in metal degreasing, in extracting oils and fats from vegetable products, in cleaning optical lenses and photographic plates, in paints and enamels, in dry cleaning, and as an adhesive in the leather industry. Although its use in recent years has diminished somewhat as a result of concern that it could be a human carcinogen (172), the National Institute for Occupational Safety and Health (NIOSH) estimates the total number of individuals exposed to TCE to be in excess of 3.5 million (173).

TCE has been recognized for over 50 years as an industrial hazard with neurotoxic properties (174). It was once commonly used as an anesthetic agent despite early reports of toxicity (175–178). TCE was abandoned as an anesthetic agent, however, apparently not because of its toxicity, but because its anesthetic action was weak and eventually better agents became available (179). Clinical experience suggested that it was safe in minimal concentrations and useful, because at the time, it was one of the few nonexplosive agents that could supplement nitrous oxide and did not produce significant respiratory depression (179,180).

Its major neurologic manifestation is related to a slowly reversible trigeminal neuropathy (174–176,181–184), although involvement of other cranial nerves and peripheral nerves has also been described (174,185,186). The trigeminal neuropathy associated with TCE intoxication was recognized as characteristic and for a time intentional exposure was considered a useful treatment of trigeminal neuralgia (182). Cranial neuropathies after general anesthesia with TCE were noted more than 40 years ago (175,176,178). Of 13 cases of multiple cranial nerve palsies following general anesthesia, 2 were related to TCE anesthesia. Twenty-four to 48 hours after general anesthesia, individuals developed paresthesia around the lips that then spread to involve the entire trigeminal distribution bilaterally over the ensuing 2 to 3 days. Motor weakness also occasionally occurred in the trigeminal distribution, and other cranial nerves including facial (VII), optic (II) and other lower cranial nerves also became affected (174,175). Resolution of the trigeminal neuropathy occurs slowly in an "onion-peel" distribution, felt to be indicative of segmental or nuclear trigeminal involvement (174,186).

Most importantly, much of the earlier literature on the neurotoxicity of TCE includes observations that were most likely a result of decomposition products (e.g., dichloroacetylene) rather than TCE itself (176,178, 187,188). Dichloroacetylene, produced most prominently under alkali conditions, reacts violently with air to produce two noxious gases, phosgene and carbon monoxide (188). Dichloroacetylene disrupts the region of the brainstem where the trigeminal nucleus is located in experimental animals and is therefore probably responsible for the neurotoxic properties of TCE (189). Short-term exposure to narcotizing levels of TCE in the industrial setting has also been reported to induce a transverse myelopathy (190). This report is of interest because a transverse myelopathy can be experimentally induced in the rat with dichloroacetate, which is a possible metabolite

of TCE/dichloroacetylene (191). It has also been proposed that TCE activates latent herpes zoster virus in the trigeminal nerve ganglia—a location known to harbor the virus—as the cause of TCE "neurotoxicity" (192). Attempts to experimentally reproduce the neurotoxicity associated with the industrial use of TCE have not been successful with pure grades of TCE (193–196).

Little data are available on the neuropathologic changes after TCE exposure. A single autopsied case of an individual who died 51 days after industrial exposure to TCE and TCE decomposition products (probably dichloroacetylene) revealed bilaterally symmetric brainstem lesions (181). These changes were most prominent in the fifth nerve nuclei, spinal tracts, and nerve roots. The fifth nerves, both within and outside the brainstem, showed extensive myelin and axonal degeneration. Other neuropathologic changes were seen but were less prominent.

Although the higher level exposures to TCE and its decomposition products are well-described, reports of long-term, low-level exposure occurring in the industrial setting are relatively few. These reports have focused on neuropsychiatric and behavioral effects including a neurasthenic syndrome with subjective complaints of dizziness, headache, nausea, fatigue, anxiety, and insomnia (197–202). Although these disorders reportedly become more severe with length of employment and degree of exposure, the neurobehavioral and neuropsychological literature on the toxic effects of TCE is so fragmented and poorly documented that it is impossible to make any firm conclusions regarding the low-level, chronic exposure to TCE and its neurotoxic potential (203). Neurobehavioral disturbances to acute, high-level exposure include severe psychiatric presentations (204,205).

Several studies were performed to study the behavioral effects of single short-term exposure to TCE (201,206–209). These studies indicate that although fatigue and sleepiness occur in humans following exposure to TCE concentrations above 100 ppm for 2 hours, no deterioration in performance or manual dexterity occurs following exposure to levels up to 300 ppm. In one study, adverse effects on performance were seen at levels of 1,000 ppm, but no significant effects were seen at lower concentrations (210). In a frequently cited study, detrimental effects of 8 hours of exposure to TCE concentrations of 110 ppm were found on performing tests of perception, complex reaction time, memory, and manual dexterity (201). Others have been unable to replicate this study (206,209). In a study where subjects were exposed to TCE concentrations of 1,000 ppm and optokinetic nystagmus was measured, minimal effects were seen and found to persist for only up to 2 hours (210). Somewhat increased effects are seen when ethanol ingestion is added to the TCE exposure (207,208); ethanol will inhibit metabolism of TCE to its breakdown products, trichloroethanol and trichloroacetic acid, thereby increasing the TCE concentration in blood (211). In general, however, these studies show that the behavioral effects of ethanol are more pronounced than those of TCE.

Basic Animal Studies

Animals have proved valuable in resolving the basis of the *n*-hexane peripheral neuropathy. These laboratory-based studies have also clarified some of the apparent "toluene-induced" neurotoxicities (212–216). Early studies of Pryor et al. (214,217) were the first to demonstrate persistent irreversible midfrequency hearing loss by cued behavioral responses, BAERs, and pathology. Other studies (218–224) extended these findings. Hearing deficits are produced after as little as 2 weeks of exposure to 1,200 ppm or 1,400 ppm of toluene. This is attributed to cochlear dysfunction rather than the central conduction pathology found in the human studies noted above. Other studies from the Pryor group have measured a toluene-induced motor syndrome that is characterized by a widened landing foot splay and a short and widened gait that may relate to the cerebellar syndrome in humans (225). After the initial studies on toluene were observed, Pryor et al. conducted a broad ranged structure–activity study on other related solvents. This group was the first to identify a midfrequency hearing loss in rats after exposure to trichloroethylene similar to that observed for toluene exposure (226). Others have since corroborated these studies (218,227,228). Pryor has published a list (Table 20.8) of several solvents that produce this hearing loss, including trichloroethylene, ethylbenzene (but not benzene), and styrene (229). This neurotoxicity may be mostly periph-eral, that is, cochlear in origin. Other studies have since corroborated these findings (230–232). Based on these studies, the electronic structure of the solvent appears to be an important parameter of the basic solvent chemistry in producing this effect.

For producing this ototoxicity, the common feature of the most hazardous compounds is the presence of an unsaturation in the chemical structure, not dissimilar to that occurring in fatty acids. That is, the less saturated the chemical structure, the more toxic it is. Further work needs to be done to clarify the chemical and molecular basis of this toxicity. Niklasson and colleagues (233) also analyzed the effects of some of these compounds on the vestibular function and correlated the changes with nystagmus. In a related area, Mergler and Beauvais (234) studied olfactory responses to toluene.

Knowledge from other animal studies should assist in the delineation of many of these parameters. For example, hexane augments toluene toxicities (235), presumably through a reduction in the metabolism of toluene, which slows the elimination of toluene, the probable toxin. The reverse was found for the production of hexane neuropathies, as hexane metabolites, not hexane, are the toxins. Related studies of genetic differences in different inbred mice populations demonstrated in C57, but not CBA mice, an age-related hearing loss (236) that may indicate different rates of metabolism or other differences.

Methylene Chloride (Dichloromethane)

Methylene chloride is widely used in industry for paint stripping, as a blowing agent for foam, as solvent for degreasing, in the manufacture of photographic film, as the carrier in rapid-dry paints, and in aerosol propellants. It is also used in the diphasic treatment of metal surfaces, in the textile and plastics industry, and for extracting heat-sensitive edible fats and essential oils. It is estimated that nearly 100,000 individuals are exposed to methylene chloride in the workplace alone.

As with other solvents, methylene chloride has CNS depressant properties at high levels of exposure and may lead rapidly to unconsciousness and death (237–241). This has been reported both in industrial settings (237,239) and as a result of solvent inhalation abuse (240,241). A similar problem has also resulted from deliberate inhalation of the higher homologue dichloroethane (51).

Methylene chloride is generally considered safer than other chlorinated hydrocarbons and has not attracted the attention it deserves as a possible cause of chronic CNS dysfunction. Methylene chloride is metabolized to carbon monoxide (242–245); consequently, both its hypoxic effect and its narcotic actions must be considered with regard to its CNS-depressant effects. Carbon monoxide, at high levels, and other forms of cerebral hypoxia are known to cause permanent neurologic sequelae.

TABLE 20.8. *Hearing loss produced (or not) by different solvents*

Solvent	Hearing loss
Benzene	No
Toluene	Yes
Ethylbenzene	Yes
n-Propylbenzene	Yes
Isopropylbenzene (cumene)	No
Methoxybenzene	Yes
1,4-Dimethylbenzene (*p*-xylene)	Yes
1,2-Dimethylbenzene (*o*-xylene)	No
1,3-Dimethylbenzene (*m*-xylene)	No
Styrene	Yes
Monochlorobenzene	Yes
Carbon disulfide	Yes
Dichloromethane	No
Trichloroethane	No
Trichloroethylene	Yes
Tetrachloroethylene	No
Acetone	No
Methyl ethyl ketone	No
Ethyl alcohol	No
n-Hexane	No

The acute effects of exposure to methylene chloride have been studied in controlled experiments in humans (246–248). In one study, 11 healthy nonsmokers were exposed to levels of methylene chloride up to 1,000 ppm for 1–2 hours (246). Inhalation of methylene chloride at levels of 500 to 1,000 ppm for this length of time was followed promptly by a sustained (at 24 hours postexposure) elevation of carboxyhemoglobin. These levels never reached above 10% saturation, however. Visual evoked responses in the three subjects tested showed an increase in peak-to-peak amplitudes after 2 hours of exposure and a return to baseline 1 hour after termination of exposure. No untoward subjective symptoms occurred at levels of exposure below 1,000 ppm. At exposure to concentrations of 1,000 ppm, 2 of 3 subjects reported "mild lightheadedness," which promptly resolved after cessation of exposure.

The effects of methylene chloride exposure on three tests of cognitive function (reaction time, short-term memory, calculation ability) were tested in 14 normal subjects (247). Repeated tests at different exposures up to 3.5 g/m^3 methylene chloride showed no statistically significant impairment in performance, although at the highest exposure levels, a greater variation in the responses was obtained for reaction time than under control conditions.

Controlled exposure of normal volunteers for up to 24 hours to various concentrations (up to 800 ppm) of methylene chloride in five separate studies showed the following abnormalities: After 2.5 hours of exposure to 500 ppm, complaints of "general uneasiness" were noted. After 4 hours of exposure to 300 and 800 ppm, in only one experiment were mood rating scales noted to be significant for depression. There was no impairment of cognitive performance as measured by tests of short-term memory and calculation ability in any of these studies after 2.5 hours of exposure to methylene chloride at levels up to 1,000 ppm. Some impairment was noted in psychomotor performance and vigilance after 3 to 4 hours of exposure to 800 ppm.

Overall, studies of controlled human exposure to methylene chloride do not show effects of CNS toxicity, except at higher levels of exposure, and even then, the effects appear to be minimal and rapidly reversible. The one exception may be in those inhalant abusers described where methylene chloride is a major component of the compound that they are abusing (93,152,153). In this regard, a recent report on the oral ingestion emphasizes the problems occurring after deliberate high inhalation of methylene chloride (249). These include CNS depression, tachypnea, gastrointestinal injury and high carboxyhemoglobin.

There have been few attempts to address the issue of chronic exposure and permanent neurologic sequelae to methylene chloride. A group of 46 men working in a factory making acetate film reported an excess of neurologic symptoms, compared to a nonexposed referent group (250). These individuals were exposed to a methylene chloride:methanol (9:1) mixture, and methylene chloride concentrations were below 100 ppm. Although neu-

rologic symptoms were increased in the exposed group, no abnormalities were detected on neuropsychological tests. No evidence was found of long-term damage that could be attributed to exposure to methylene chloride. In a larger study to assess the potential chronic health effects of methylene chloride, no increase in the number of expected deaths resulting from diseases of the nervous system were seen among 1,013 workers chronically exposed to methylene chloride (251).

In summary, the evidence suggests that methylene chloride does not produce permanent neurological sequelae except with massive acute exposures that are associated with hypoxic encephalopathy. No evidence exists that chronic low-level exposure causes any long-term CNS injury.

1,1,1-Trichloroethane

1,1,1-Trichloroethane is widely used as an industrial degreasing solvent and, compared with other solvents, is less toxic, although several reports of severe toxicity and deaths exist in the literature (82,83,252,253). Its acute toxicity has made it unsuitable as a volatile anesthetic, and its use as a carrier in aerosols was abandoned in the United States in 1973.

In those cases where postmortem examination of the brain was undertaken, the pathologic changes suggested cerebral hypoxia either primary to CNS depressant effect (83) or secondary to cardiac or respiratory arrest (82,83). 1,1,1-Trichloroethane is postulated to act on either the autonomic nervous system (254) or on central sleep apnea (255). Chronic cardiac toxicity is also a possible mechanism of 1,1,1-trichloroethane toxicity (85).

There are several reports of the acute behavioral and neuropsychological changes occurring after voluntary exposure of humans to 1,1,1-trichloroethane (256–259). No impairment was indicated using a series of psychomotor tests and following several days of exposure to 500 ppm of 1,1,1-trichloroethane (256). In another study, no behavioral changes were measured after two 4.5-hour exposures to 450 ppm of 1,1,1-trichloroethane (257). Two studies demonstrated some performance deficits (258,259). In one study, after 3.5 hours of exposure to 0, 175, and 350 ppm of 1,1,1-trichloroethane, abnormalities were seen on some behavioral tests, most notably those tests concerned with attention and concentration and those concerned with analysis of grammatical statements (259). Overall, these studies suggest mild, if any, acute effects of exposure of individuals to levels of trichloroethane up to 500 ppm.

With regard to low-level, chronic exposure to 1,1,1-trichloroethane, a clinical, neurophysiological, and behavioral study of female workers chronically exposed to this agent at levels up to 1,000 ppm found no differences, compared to a reference solvent-unexposed group (260).

It appears that 1,1,1-trichloroethane is not associated with either acute or chronic neurotoxicity at levels below 1,000 ppm and that the only permanent neurologic sequelae are related to cerebral hypoxia after massive exposure. In contrast to trichloroethylene, equivalent doses of trichloroethane do not produce hearing loss when administered to rats (261).

Gasoline

Gasoline is a complex mixture of organic solvents and other chemicals and metals. The sniffing of gasoline is common among various solvent abusers, especially on some remote Native American reservations. Leaded gasoline is not now readily available in the United States but still presents a problem in some remote Indian villages. Although some CNS or peripheral neuropathies may occur as a result of the solvents in gasoline, other toxicities may result from tetraethyllead (or its metabolite triethyllead) (262–272). In cases where high lead levels were observed, various disorders were observed, including hallucinations and disorientation, dysarthria, chorea, and convulsions. The symptoms include moderate to severe ataxia, insomnia, anorexia, slowed peripheral nerve conduction, limb tremors, dysmetria, and sometimes limb paralysis. In most cases, the electroencephalogram (EEG) is normal, but in severe states, an abnormal to severely depressed cortical EEG is observed. In only one lethal case was any kidney damage noted; electrolytes are usually in the normal range. Because many of these symptoms in the early stages of the disease can be reversed by parenteral chelation therapy with ethylenediaminetetraacetic acid (EDTA), British anti-Lewisite (BAL) (dimercaprol), and/or penicillamine, it is important to check the serum lead levels in any chronic inhalant abuser to see if this treatment should be prescribed. This type of therapy has recently been reviewed for gasoline alkyllead additives. They did find it to be generally effective and discussed the complications surrounding the treatment of these individuals (273).

Alcohols and Solvents

One interesting phenomenon has been observed following the exposure to two or more solvents. Degreaser's flush was ascribed to a flushing of the face when occupational workers left their degreasing vats and drank alcohol after leaving work (274,275). Also, heavy drinking has been associated with toluene exposure (276). More recently, both humans and rats have been noted to be thirsty when exposed to toluene and alcohol (277,278). Also, animal studies have shown that solvents alter the metabolism of alcohol and prolong its action (99,279). This might explain the "flushing phenomenon" but may or may not relate to the psychological dependence of solvents or to the development of thirst. An attempt to study the acute effects of alcohol and toluene, at low exposures in human volunteers, failed to produce any interaction by their behavioral measures. This may be indicative that the inter-

action takes some time and/or high levels of exposure to develop. A recent laboratory study extended the studies of toluene-induced auditory toxicity described above. Campo et al. (280) showed an enhanced hearing loss in rats when ethanol is combined with toluene exposure. Again, both solvents given together are more hazardous than following administration only of each individual solvent.

Methanol neurotoxicity is well-known and exemplified by a recent case (281), where necrosis of the putamen region of the brain was noted. Recent studies of rats exposed to methanol have described the damage done to the retina and optic nerve (282). Methanol intoxication was identified in an individual intoxicated on a spray can of carburetor cleaner containing toluene (42%), methanol (23%), and methylene chloride (20%) (283). Although mild acidosis did occur, the main concern was the high blood level of methanol. Ethanol therapy was used to prevent formation of high levels of formic acid. The above mixture is abused and is very similar in composition to paint thinner; yet the repercussions of prolonged use are unclear.

Nitrous Oxide

Nitrous oxide is not an organic solvent, but it is an "inhalant" by definition. Nitrous oxide is a commonly used anesthetic and has been noted for some unusual toxicities. This substance is used as an anesthetic, as a propellant for whipped cream, and as an octane booster. As noted earlier, deaths often occur as a result of nitrous oxide "overexposure" in young people. Also, a neuropathy was first observed in medical personnel. Recently, three other cases of myelopathy were reported (284–286). In the early studies, it was shown that central and peripheral nerve damage resulted following high levels of N_2O exposure, even in the presence of adequate oxygen (287) and even in short-term use when nitrous oxide was used as an anesthetic (288). Patients with vitamin B_{12} deficiencies are especially sensitive (289). The symptoms include numbness and weakness in the limbs, loss of dexterity, sensory loss, and loss of balance. The neurologic examination indicates sensorimotor polyneuropathy. There is also a combined degeneration of the posterior and lateral columns of the cord that resembles vitamin B_{12} deficiencies (287). Studies focusing on the mechanism of action indicate that cobalamins (vitamin B_{12}) are inactivated by N_2O; more recent studies have focused on the methionine synthase enzyme that needs vitamin B_{12} to function (290). Vitamin B_{12} (or folinic acid) did not aid recovery from this disease in some patients (290,291), but did in others (292). In this regard, a report of a neuropathy in an undiagnosed "cobalamin-deficient" infant, which was exposed to nitrous oxide (293), is of interest. Another treatment approach, the use of dietary methionine might be helpful as indicated by studies in rats (294). Rehabilitation proceeds with abstinence from nitrous oxide exposure and is relative to the extent of neurologic damage. Recent reviews cover many of the medical aspects of the adverse effects of and the pros and cons of using nitrous oxide (290,295–298). Also, a recent report summarizes the basic mechanisms of actions of nitrous oxide (299). Despite the widespread distribution of this information (300) to the medical community and the reduced availability of pressurized cylinders, cases are still being observed (73,89).

In regard to the dependency of nitrous oxide, animal studies on selectively bred mice for alcohol dependence showed a cross-dependency on nitrous oxide (301). They also observed handling-induced convulsions shortly after cessation of nitrous oxide, which could be prevented by either alcohol or nitrous oxide. This might indicate a physical dependence on nitrous oxide that needs to be dealt with in the treatment of patients in this drug abuse state. Approaches to reducing alcohol consumption should also be considered during treatment.

PSYCHIATRIC DISTURBANCES IN ORGANIC SOLVENT ABUSE

Psychiatric disorders related to solvent abuse are rare, if existent. Ron (302) reviewed the subject and concluded that psychiatric morbidity is "highest in those referred to psychiatric hospitals and lowest in clinics dealing exclusively with volatile substance (VS) (solvent) abuse. The psychiatric diagnoses of these patients do not appear to differ in type or frequency from those given to well-matched populations of nonabusers, and there is little evidence to suggest that specific or persistent psychiatric disability results from this practice." On the other hand, there is little doubt that personality disorders of an antisocial type are common in VS abusers. In an earlier edition (27), Korman summarized an earlier study (303) of those admitted to a psychiatric emergency room as follows: "... inhalant users differed significantly from matched other drug users in that they displayed significantly more self-directed destructive behavior, as well as some degree of recent suicidal and homicidal behavior."

Other reports of older adult subjects (304,304a) observed that most of the patients had antisocial personality disorders. Although they were admitted for their drug dependency, especially on solvents (most for 5 to 13 years), they also used marihuana, alcohol, stimulants, and other drugs. They interpret this as indicative of the progression of the dependent state with age for a select group of solvent abusers. This chronically disturbed group was also refractory to treatment at this setting. Another study of psychiatric subjects did not identify any group of patients as being inhalant abusers, although 9% used inhalants and other drugs (305). Thus, they could not associate any disorder with the use of inhalants either because it does not exist or because they did not have the appropriate group of patients.

Only one report (306) has identified a personality disorder with inhalant abuse. In a group of 22 randomly selected subjects from a number of patients over a 5-year period, several were considered to have a personality devi-

ation on admission. These were subsequently diagnosed as substance abusers. These patients had inhaled a "toluene-based" glue daily for 2 years or more. Paranoid psychosis was diagnosed for 19 of the subjects; 3 patients had temporal lobe epilepsy. Family alcoholism, crime, and other negative life-styles were present, but no family history of hospitalization for severe mental illnesses was found. Another group studied whether drug abuse (including "glue") at age 11 years predicted the development of attention deficit hyperactivity disorder or depression 4 years later (307).

Some reports of single cases have identified a psychiatric illness associated with solvent overexposure from paints, glues and pure solvents, xylene, or trichlorohydrocarbons (148,308–311). Subjects showed mild tremors and ataxia, as well as disorientation, impaired attention and memory, and hallucinations. Subjects improved with time with supportive care and, in one case, with neuroleptics. However, only the latter case was identified as having irreversible schizophreniform psychosis (308).

Hallucinations are often associated with inhalant abuse (160,310,312). This seldom is seen or identified in studies of groups of inhalant abusers. Thus, this may be limited to some susceptible individuals or to a high degree of intoxication. One such case has been described to result from neurologic discharges that mimic a "crawling insect feeling" (264). One group was able to relate these hallucinations to abnormal EEG recordings (160). It is evident that a more comprehensive study of these conditions and/or individuals is needed. This issue is far from being resolved. Psychiatric conditions have been reviewed by Dinwiddie (313).

NONNERVOUS SYSTEM TOXICITY OF INHALANT ABUSE

Most of the adverse clinical effects of inhalant abuse are on the nervous system. There are, however, other significant adverse effects on other organ systems, including kidney, liver, lung, heart, and blood.

Renal Toxicity

Currently, spray paints are widely abused substances, at least in the United States. The abuse of these substances occurs not only among polydrug users but also by painters. The exposure to these and similar substances has resulted in the hospitalization of inhalant abusers for various kidney disorders (155,158,314–333). A 32-year-old woman, identified as having renal distal acidosis after sniffing spray paint (327), presented to the hospital with severe quadriparesis. These subjects often have associated gastrointestinal involvement, including nausea, vomiting, and severe abdominal cramps. Lauwerys et al. (334) reviewed the early reports on nephrotoxicity in humans.

In one of the early reports, Streicher et al. (155) examined several cases and described them in detail, eliciting the nature of distal renal acidosis in groups of paint and/or glue sniffers from the southwestern United States and Hawaii. Streicher et al. and others have noted the recurrence of renal dysfunction associated with solvent abuse; the disease state reappears in many individuals who return to their habit after release from the hospital. Their symptoms include hyperchloremic metabolic acidosis, hypokalemia, hypocalcemia, and other electrolyte imbalances. A recent case included quadriparesis and respiratory failure (332). Solvents usually cause a unique distal-type tubular acidosis, but proximal tubules are also affected. Although the distal tubule is responsible for the known electrolyte and metabolic imbalance, the proximal type is responsible for the wasting of amino acids and other proteins. In spite of this tubular damage being reversible, other organs, particularly brain, are the target of repetitive acidosis, plus a depletion of important amino acids. A slightly different kidney dysfunction, glomerulonephritis, has also been identified in workers using solvents (335), especially painters (328), and reviewed by Daniell et al. (318). In addition, an interstitial nephritis leading to renal failure was recently reported by Taverner et al. (329). Rhabdomyolysis is sometimes observed after exposure to solvents (336). All of these reports indicate that kidney dysfunction is a common toxicity noted for solvent abusers. Even of greater concern might be the diabetic who presents after an overdose of solvents. Solvent odors might cover up the "acetone breath" of the diabetic and prevent the identification of the condition and/or the basis of that acidosis if the patient is unconscious (337).

There are also reports that halohydrocarbons—chloroform and others (338), methylene chloride (339,340), trichloroethylene (341), methoxyflurane (342), and dichloropropane (343)—may contribute to, if not cause, renal damage. The nephrotic pathologic changes reported include tubular necrosis and calcification. The reversibility of these changes is unknown and is likely dependent on the extent of the damage. Others (344,345) observed signs of Goodpasture syndrome; also, bladder changes are correlated to toluene exposure (346).

Although toluene is often proposed as the toxic agent and is present in most of the substances abused by these subjects, there has been no animal data to verify that toluene is the primary agent, or even one of a group of substances, that can cause renal dysfunction. Recently, Batlle et al. (316) exposed the turtle bladder to high concentrations of toluene and observed a diminished hydrogen ion transport that had no affect on the sodium transport. Also, toluene did not reduce the pH gradient across the bladder. Efforts to reproduce these nephrotic changes in rodents have met with limited success. These studies indicate that hypocalcemia occurs only in a near-lethal situation (347).

Other animal studies have identified the nature of some of these nephrotic changes (338,341). Animal studies have also shown mild nephrotic changes following exposure to hydrocarbons (348). In most cases, more than one substance is present; this may indicate that the most severe nephrotic changes occur in the presence of two or more of these solvent compounds.

Thus several kinds of solvent mixtures are associated with either glomerulonephritis, distal renal tubular acidosis, or other nephrotic changes. Usually, these different kidney disorders do not occur in the same individual and may be related to individual and/or other environmental factors. Although metallic spray paints are frequently used by these subjects, they also use paint thinners, glue vapors, and other solvents. It would appear reasonable to conclude that toluene may account for some but not all of these renal abnormalities, which are likely caused by a combination of toxicants in these toluene products—possibly including the metals contained in the spray paint, such as cadmium and lead, which are known to be nephrotoxic (349), or concurrent alcohol use (320,350) and/or infections (328,351,352). As many cases of renal toxicity are being reported, it is important that individuals exposed to high doses of solvents be checked for renal changes and metabolic imbalance.

For most of these subjects, electrolyte repletion usually restores the kidney function and eliminates the muscle spasms, even in the more severely affected patients, in a few days. Lavoie et al. (323) cautioned the use of bicarbonate early for the treatment of these subjects. Correction of salt and electrolyte imbalance, including potassium, calcium, magnesium, and chloride, should be considered in the treatment of solvent abusers for muscle fatigue, even in the absence of more severe kidney disorders.

Renal Toxicity in Pregnancy

One must especially be alert for nephrotoxicity in pregnant women who abuse solvents (330,353–356). Numerous pregnant women have presented with renal tubular acidosis. In one report (353), 3 of 5 infants showed growth retardation. A similar case was reported where no known causative agent was identified (354). These women often, but not always, respond to treatment for their metabolic imbalance after 72 hours of treatment and abstinence of solvent abuse.

Hepatotoxicity

Chlorohydrocarbons (e.g., trichloroethylene, chloroform, halothane) have been known for years to produce hepatotoxicities (357). Several reports describe solvent-related toxicities (2,314,342,352,358–365). Any individual who is chronically exposed to these compounds would expect to develop hepatorenal toxicities, depending on the dose and length of exposure (358). Buring et al. (366) evaluated the effects of low levels of exposure measured retrospectively by several investigators. They concluded that there is increased risk for operating room personnel where these chlorohydrocarbon anesthetics are used. However, Brown and Gandolfi (342) have questioned whether liver toxicity occurs very often after use of halothane as an anesthetic. Shaw et al. (367) reviewed these rare occurrences and their etiologic factors. In addition, the situations where halothane hepatitis occurs were reviewed by Neuberger and Davis (368) who proposed a hypoxic model to explain those occurrences of hepatitis.

The recent increase in the inhalation of correction fluids for "pleasure," which contain trichloroethylene and trichloroethanes or tetrachloroethanes (369), increases the likelihood of observing more of these toxicities in inhalant abusers (370). Even during occupational use, exposure to chlorocarbons in poorly ventilated areas is considered to lead to hepatotoxicity. Nephronecrosis and/or hepatotoxicity were observed after exposure to mixtures containing methylene chloride and other solvents (339,360,371) and trichloroethane (344,372). Methylene chloride has been considered not to be hepatotoxic (340). However, a recent report may have identified an upper limit that may occur in inhalant abuse (360) where hepatotoxicity does occur. Ketones, including acetone, potentiate halocarbon hepatotoxicity (373). So far, there have been few inhalant abusers noted to have irreversible liver damage. This low incidence of liver damage so far noted for this group may be the result of a low rate of use of chlorinated solvents. However, the frequent heavy use of alcohol concurrently with inhalants should be of concern for this group, especially as they become older and have used these substances for many years. When these patterns of "drug" exposure are known, it would be advisable to conduct liver function tests. Animal studies of known hepatotoxins have measured reduction or repair under certain conditions (374,375).

A refrigerant gas, HCFC-123, was identified as hepatotoxic in a hospital worker (376). This is more readily metabolized than the previously used fully halogenated fluorocarbons and has been compared in toxicity to an analogue, halothane, which is used for anesthesia (377). Hepatocellular and other carcinomas are observed at high doses of trichloroethylene (341) and halothane (378). Anesthetic chlorinated hydrocarbons (halothane, trichloroethylene, chloroform) are also considered to be carcinogenic (379). Increased availability of trichloroethylene for drycleaning purposes could present more cases of nephrotic and hepatotoxic diseases, including cancer (380).

Pulmonary Toxicity

Despite the likelihood that solvents irritate the lungs, there are few cases noted where the pulmonary system is severely compromised. Solvents have, nevertheless, been noted to cause pulmonary hypertension, acute respiratory distress, increased airway resistance, and residual volume and restricted ventilation. A recent "outbreak of respiratory illness" was associated with changes in solvents/propellants of a leather conditioner (381). This product produced tachypnea, pulmonary edema and hemorrhage in rats. Respiratory problems would therefore be expected in inhalant abusers using these or similar products. In addition, increased airway resistance or residual volume may be more clearly noted following an exercise challenge (382). Additionally, response to an aerosolized bronchodilator is suggestive of an airway involvement perhaps induced by habitual inhalation of hydrocarbons. Smoking may have been a contributory factor in one study (383) and was not ruled out in the others. In studies of workers using waterproofing aerosols containing trichloroethane (384) or using a paint stripper (385), acute respiratory distress has been correlated with the chlorinated hydrocarbon exposure. Although solvents irritate the pulmonary system, it is not at all clear from the limited case studies reported, to date, how extensive or what types of pulmonary damage occur that can be primarily caused by solvent exposure and not to other inspired substances that are dissolved in the solvents. For example, a recent report of a homicidal case (a spray paint "sniffer") noted metallic deposition along with hemorrhagic alveolitis (386). It is uncertain how to generalize the impact of dual exposure of solvent and infection, but an animal study showed decreased pulmonary bacteriocidal activity after exposure to dichloroethylene (387).

Any change may be very slow in onset but most likely will be enhanced by the other substances volatilized along with the solvent (e.g., polystyrenes, tars) or used by the subject (e.g., tobacco and marihuana). Because of the potential for cause and augmentation by other substances, the amount of smoking should always be considered in any treatment of these individuals.

Cardiotoxicity

Many solvent abusers may die from direct or indirect cardiotoxic actions of solvents without note in any public or private record. More specifically, several recent reports identified ventricular fibrillation and cardiac arrest in hospitalized patients (85,388–396). Some of the subjects had inhaled trichloroethylene- (397) or trichloroethane-containing solvents (85,396) and were additionally compromised by anesthesia (e.g., halothane) (85). Fluorocarbons cause arrhythmias in animals (398). Chenoweth and colleagues showed that butane, hexane, heptane, gasoline, some anesthetics, and toluene also produce these arrhythmias (399). Recent reports (389–392) have linked glue sniffing to arrhythmias, myocarditis, and cardiac arrest. However, the linkage of arrhythmia to glue sniffing is not well supported by animal studies. Glues usually do not contain halocarbons but do contain toluene and other hydrocarbons. The somewhat different cardiotoxicities noted above are not all easily explained, but congenital or other environmental causes were not ruled out. Also, inhalant abusers are not likely to be resuscitated from cardiopulmonary arrest; however, a successful resuscitation from fluorocarbon overexposure has been reported (393). When this condition is observed, antiarrhythmic therapy should be used (85). Exercise and adrenaline exacerbate these cardiotoxicities, and efforts to minimize these situations should therefore be instituted. Also, anesthesia should not be induced in patients shortly after intoxication, and one should probably avoid the use of halogenated hydrocarbons in other circumstances where heavy solvent exposure is suspected.

Hematologic Toxicity

There are three areas of concern in regards to solvent inhalation and the hematopoietic system. First, methylene chloride exposure can increase the carboxyhemoglobin levels (241), a change that also occurs with cigarette smoking. The levels of carboxyhemoglobin may become sufficiently high to cause brain damage (400) or death (401). A second group of substances, the organic nitrites, produce methemoglobinemia and hemolytic anemia (402–405). A third substance, benzene, causes aplastic anemia, acute myelocytic leukemia, and other hematopoietic cancers (334,406–408). Benzene is present in thinners, varnish removers, and other solvents, and in varying proportions in gasoline.

One group of substances, the volatile liquid "amyl," "butyl," and cyclohexyl nitrites, deserve special discussion. During the late nineteenth and early twentieth centuries, amyl nitrite was used in clinical practice as a vasodilator to treat angina pectoris. Although this use of the drug is uncommon today, it is sometimes used for diagnostic purposes in echocardiogram examinations (409,410) and for cyanide poisoning (411). These drugs are not the typical solvents previously described; however, they are often included in the "inhalant abuse" category. As with nitrous oxide, different individuals (predominately homosexuals) are the primary abusers of isoamyl ("amyl"), isobutyl or butyl nitrites, propyl nitrites, cyclohexyl nitrites, and maybe others. They may use them for sphincter dilation and penile engorgement. Use by others for nonsexual purposes is unclear. One study could not correlate changes in regional blood flow with any psychological measures or somatic changes (412); also, isoamyl nitrite did not substitute for barbiturates, as do toluene and other solvents (413). These studies do not offer any explanation for why individuals become dependent on nitrites. However, the finding by Mathew et al. (412) that nitrites reduce anger, fatigue, and depression may offer a clue.

The nitrites are usually not considered toxic during inhalation because of syncope (fainting). However, Guss et al. (414) noted a dangerously high 37% methemoglobin level in a normal subject who had used isobutyl nitrite. This methemoglobinemia is the major identified toxicity and is the cause of several deaths (215). There is a specific treatment for nitrite overdose. The high and slowly reversible reduction of methemoglobin can be aided by the use of methylene blue (415). Organic nitrites also produce bradycardia (410), reduce killer cell activity (416),

produce allergic reactions (417), and are potentially carcinogenic (418).

Heavy organic nitrite use is a risk factor for the development of acquired immune deficiency syndrome (AIDS) (419,420) and of Kaposi sarcoma (421–424). The ability to produce nitrosamines has fueled the speculation that nitrites are carcinogenic (420,425,426). Yet, in contrast to sodium nitrite, organic nitrites produce methemoglobin instantly *in vitro* (427) and may therefore not be around long enough to produce nitrosamines. Thus, the rapid oxidation of organic nitrites by hemoglobin and the fact that detectable levels of organic nitrites in blood are noted only briefly after administration (428) may alter the outcome of carcinogenesis. While mutagenicity appears possible under special conditions, carcinogenicity is far from proven.

Organic nitrites also modulate the immune capacity of animals (429–431). Soderberg reviews the potential for nitrites to impair the immune system (432). In their studies, after inhalation exposure of mice for 14 days to isobutyl nitrite, there is a reduced capacity for the concanavalin A (but not lipopolysaccharide) stimulation of T-cell functions, an induction of cytotoxic T cells, a reduced tumoricidal activity, and an increased tumor incidence (433–436). He states (432) that nitrites may reduce immune capacity while augmenting viral growth and tumor growth.

In another case, related to trichloroethylene, hematopoietic effects were identified in a subject who used glue in his hobby; cessation of the symptoms occurred when he ceased his hobby (437).

NEONATAL SYNDROME

There is increasing evidence that solvent inhalation during pregnancy produces a "fetal solvent syndrome." There are numerous cases of infants of mothers who chronically abuse solvents (135,330,353–356,363,438–442) diagnosed with this syndrome. These mothers inhaled paint reducer (thinner?), solvent mixtures from paint sprays and drank various quantities of alcohol. Whether toluene alone (often noted as the major solvent), other solvent components, and/or these components in combination with alcohol or other environmental factors are responsible is still unsubstantiated by laboratory studies; yet toluene appears to be a major contributor. Toluene embryopathy is compared to the better recognized fetal alcohol syndrome (440). The infants present with growth retardation, some dysmorphic features, including microcephaly, as well as distal acidosis, aminoaciduria (135,355), ataxia, tremors, and slurred speech (439), and has been considered a human teratogen (441).

It is difficult to produce these abnormalities in rodents. Growth retardation occurred in rats with doses of toluene that produce fetal mortality without producing malformations (443,444), and an ataxic syndrome has been identified in young rats exposed to high levels of toluene throughout pregnancy (445). Lower doses of toluene produced "lower birth weight, delayed ontogeny of reflexes, increased motor activity" and "impaired cognitive function" (446); "gained less weight and performed more poorly on ... righting reflex, grip strength" (447,448); or with oral toluene, "growth retarded fetuses with smaller brain and caudate-putamen volumes" (449). Pregnant rats were exposed to a high level of trichloroethane (450). Some reduction in litter weight and behavioral measures were noted in the progeny.

Nitrous oxide (50% to 75% for 24 hours on day 8) produces some "major visceral and minor skeletal (fetal) abnormalities" (451). Surprisingly, these abnormalities are protected against by 0.27% halothane, but not by folinic acid. Also, animal fetal liver toxicities occur after administration of carbon tetrachloride (452) or malformations following chloroform (453). With so little knowledge and yet with all the potential dangers, it is very important that pregnant women not be exposed to very high concentrations of solvents/gases. It is encouraging to know that a critical prospective study of workers exposed to low levels of solvent showed no more abnormalities than the carefully matched controls (454). This does not, however, diminish the need for the avoidance of exposure of pregnant women to moderate or higher levels of solvents/gases.

ACKNOWLEDGMENT

Dr. Neil Rosenberg passed away suddenly during preparation of this chapter. Dr. Rosenberg, an active neurologist, was concerned about young people's drug habits' causing dementia prematurely. He focused not only on excessive voluntary exposure to solvents, but also on the use of other neurotoxic substances such as methamphetamine. He was a pioneer in the field of defining the neurologic manifestations of solvent abuse. To assist those in need, he and his wife, Cathy, founded the International Institute on Inhalant Abuse. He also devoted his energies through academic groups, including NIH and the American Academy of Neurology. More humbly, he traveled throughout the United States and Central and South America, educating people about the dangers of inhaling chemicals, and did extensive humanitarian work with poor people in Peru and other countries in Latin America, as well as with Native Americans in the northern hemisphere, always with the prime goal of diminishing solvent and other drug use.

REFERENCES

1. Carroll E. Notes on the epidemiology of inhalants. *NIDA Res Monogr* 1977;15:14–24.
2. Hutchens KS, Kung M. "Experimentation" with chloroform. *Am J Med* 1985;78:715–718.
3. Kringsholm B. Sniffing-associated deaths in Denmark. *Forensic Sci Int* 1980;15:215–225.
4. Smith TC, Cooperman LH, Wollman H. History and principles of anesthesiology. In: Goodman GA, Goodman LS, Gilman A, eds. *Goodman and Gilman's the pharmacological basis of therapeutics,* 6th ed. New York: Macmillan, 1980:258.
5. Flanagan RJ, Ives RJ. Volatile substance abuse. *Bull Narc* 1994;46(2):49–78.
6. Gilvary E, McCarthy S, McArdle P. Substance use among school children in the north of England. *Drug Alcohol Depend* 1995;37:255–259.
7. Kozel N, Sloboda Z, De La Rosa M. Epidemiology of inhalant abuse: an international perspective. Proceedings of a meeting. July 21–22, 1993. *NIDA Res Monogr* 1995;148:1–306.
8. Adelekan ML. Self-reported drug use among secondary school students in the Nigerian state of Ogun. *Bull Narc* 1989;41(1–2):109–116.
9. Alvarez FJ, Queipo D, Del Rio MC, et al. Patterns of drug use by young people in the rural community of Spain. *Br J Addict* 1989;84:647–652.
10. Beauvais F, Wayman JC, Thurman PJ, et al. Inhalant abuse among American Indian, Mexican American, and non-Latino white adolescents. *Am J Drug Alcohol Abuse* 2002;28(1):171–187.
11. Carlini-Cotrim B, Carlini EA. The use of solvents and other drugs among children and adolescents from a low socioeconomic background: a study in São Paulo, Brazil. *Int J Addict* 1988;23:1145–1156.
12. Cooke BR, Evans DA, Farrow SC. Solvent misuse in secondary school children—a prevalence study. *Community Med* 1988;10:8–13.
13. Diamond ID, Pritchard C, Choudry N, et al. The incidence of drug and solvent misuse among southern English normal comprehensive school children. *Public Health* 1988;102:107–114.
14. Levy SJ, Pierce JP. Drug use among Sydney teenagers in 1985 and 1986. *Community Health Stud* 1989;13:161–169.
15. Medina-Mora E, Ortiz A. Epidemiology of solvent/inhalant abuse in Mexico. In: Crider RA, Rouse BA, eds. Epidemiology of inhalant abuse: an update. *NIDA Res Monogr* 1988;85:140–171.
16. Pedersen W, Clausen SE, Lavik NJ. Patterns of drug use and sensation-seeking among adolescents in Norway. *Acta Psychiatry Scand* 1989;79:386–390.
17. Smart RG. Inhalant use and abuse in Canada. *NIDA Res Monogr* 1988;85:121–139.
18. Tapia-Conyer R, Cravioto P, De La Rosa B, et al. Risk factors for inhalant abuse in juvenile offenders: the case of Mexico. *Addiction* 1995;90:43–49.
19. Field-Smith ME, Bland JM, Taylor JC, et al. *Trends in deaths associated with abuse of volatile substances, 1971–2000. Report 15.* London: St. George's Hospital Medical School, 2002;July. Available at: http://www.vsareport.org/
20. Johnston LD, O'Malley PM, Bachman JG. *Monitoring the Future national survey results on drug use, 1994–2002.* National Institute on Drug Abuse, 2002. Available at: http://monitoringthefuture.org/
21. Substance Abuse and Mental Health Services Administration. *National Household Survey on Drug Abuse: population estimates 2001.* Washington, DC: U.S. Government Printing Office, 2002. Available at: http://www.aasamhsa.gov/centers/clearinghouse/clearinghouses.html
22. Johnson BD, Frank B, Marel R, et al. *Statewide household survey of substance abuse, 1986: illicit substance use among adults in New York State's transient population.* New York: New York State Division of Substance Abuse Services, 1988; and Rainone GR, Marel R.

The OASAS School Survey; alcohol and other drug use among 5th–12th grade students, 1998. New York: New York State Division of Substance Abuse Services, 1998.

23. Liu LY, Maxwell JC. *Texas school survey of substance use among students: grades 7–12, 1994.* Austin, TX: Texas Commission on Alcohol and Drug Abuse, 1995: March.

23a. Liu LY. *Texas School Survey of substance use among students: grades 7–12, 2002.* Austin, TX: Texas Commission on Alcohol and Drug Abuse (in press). Available at: http://www.tcada.state.tx.us/research/ May 2003.

24. Howard MO, Walker RD, Walker PS, et al. Inhalant use among urban American Indian youth. *Addiction* 1999;94: 83–95.

25. Padilla ER, Padilla AM, Morales A, et al. Inhalant, marijuana, and alcohol abuse among barrio children and adolescents. *Int J Addict* 1979;14:945–964.

26. Bernal B, Ardila A, Bateman JR. Cognitive Impairments in adolescent drug-abusers. *Int J Neurosci* 1994;75:203–212.

27. Sharp CW, Korman M. Volatile substances. In: Lowinson JH, Ruiz P, eds. *Substance abuse: clinical problems and perspectives.* Baltimore: Williams & Wilkins, 1981:233–255.

28. Bowen SE, Daniel J, Balster RL. Deaths associated with inhalant abuse in Virginia from 1987 to 1996. *Drug Alcohol Depend* 1999;53(3):239–245.

29. Bass M. Sudden sniffing death. *JAMA* 1970;212:2075–2079.

30. Bass M. Death from sniffing gasoline. *N Engl J Med* 1978;299:203.

31. Bass M. Abuse of inhalation anesthetics. *JAMA* 1984;251:604

32. Litovitz TL, Klein-Schwartz W, Rodgers GC, et al. 2001 *Annual report of the American Association of Poison Control Centers Toxic Exposure Surveillance System. Am J Emerg Med* 2002;20(5):391–452.

33. Office of Applied Sciences, Departmentt of Health and Human Services. *Mortality data from the Drug Abuse Warning Network, 2000.* Available at: http://www.aasamhsa.gov/oas/DAWN/mortality2k.pdf.

34. Maxwell JC. Deaths related to the inhalation of volatile substances in Texas: 1988–1998. *Am J Drug Alcohol Abuse* 2001;27(4):689–697.

35. Anderson HR. Increase in deaths from deliberate inhalation of fuel gases and pressurised aerosols [Letter]. *BMJ* 1990;301:41.

36. Shepherd RT. Mechanism of sudden death associated with volatile substance abuse. *Hum Toxicol* 1989;8:287–291.

37. Garriott J, Petty CS. Death from inhalant abuse: toxicological and pathological evaluation of 34 cases. *Clin Toxicol* 1980;16:305–315.

38. Garriott J. Death among inhalant abusers. *NIDA Res Monogr* 1992;129: 181–192.

39. Cohen S. Inhalant abuse: an overview of the problem. *NIDA Res Monogr* 1977;77:2–10.

40. Korman M, Matthews RW, Lovitt R. Neuropsychological effects of abuse of inhalants. *Percept Mot Skills* 1981;53:547–553.

41. Oetting ER, Edwards RW, Beauvais F. Social and psychological factors underlying inhalant abuse. *NIDA Res Monogr* 1988;85:172–203.

42. Howard MO, Jenson JM. Inhalant use among antisocial youth: prevalence and correlates. *Addict Behav* 1999;24:59–74.

43. Matthews RW, Korman M. Abuse of inhalants: motivation and consequences. *Psychol Rep* 1981;49:519–526.

44. Oetting ER, Webb J. Psychosocial characteristics and their links with inhalants, a research agenda. *NIDA Res Monogr* 1992;129:59–98; May PA, Del Vecchio AM. The three common behavioral patterns of inhalant/solvent abuse: selected findings and research issues. In: Beauvais F, Trimble J E, eds. *Drugs and society.* 1997;10(1/2):3–38.

45. Kerner K. Current topics in inhalant abuse. *NIDA Res Monogr* 1988;85:8–29.

46. Trochimowicz HJ. Development of alternative fluorocarbons. *NIDA Res Monogr* 1992;129:287–300.

47. al-Alousi LM. Pathology of volatile substance abuse: a case report and a literature review. *Med Sci Law* 1989;29:189–208.

48. Fitzgerald RL, Fishel CE, Bush LL. Fatality due to recreational use of chlorodifluoromethane and chloropenta-fluoroethane. *J Forensic Sci* 1993;38:477–483.

49. Groppi A, Polettini A, Lunetta P, et al. A fatal case of trichlorofluoromethane (Freon 11) poisoning. Tissue distribution study by gas chromatography-mass spectrometry. *J Forensic Sci* 1994;39:871–876.

50. Clark MA, Jones JW, Robinson JJ, et al. Multiple deaths resulting from shipboard exposure to trichlorotrifluoroethane. *J Forensic Sci* 1985;30:1256–1259.

51. Broussard LA, Brustowicz T, Pittman T, et al. Two traffic fatalities related to the use of dichloroethane. *J Forensic Sci* 1997;42:1186–1187.

52. Thompson PJ, Dhillon P, Cole P. Addiction to aerosol treatment: the asthmatic alternative to glue sniffing. *BMJ* 1983;287:1515.

53. King GS, Smialek JE, Troutman WG. Sudden death in adolescents resulting from the inhalation of typewriter correction fluid. *JAMA* 1985;253:1604–1606.

54. Macdougall IC, Isles C, Oliver JS, et al. Fatal outcome following inhalation of Tipp-Ex. *Scott Med J* 1987;32:55.

55. Troutman WG. Additional deaths associated with the intentional inhalation of typewriter correction fluid. *Vet Hum Toxicol* 1988;30:130–132.

56. Mathew B, Kapp E, Jones TR. Commercial butane abuse, a disturbing case. *Br J Addict* 1989;84:563–564.

57. Evans AC, Raistrick D. Patterns of use and related harm with toluene-based adhesives and butane gas. *Br J Psychiatry* 1987;150:773–776.

58. Siegel E, Wason S. Sudden death caused by inhalation of butane and propane. *N Engl J Med* 1990;323:1638.

59. Siegel E, Wason S. Sudden sniffing death following inhalation of butane and propane: changing trends. *NIDA Res Monogr* 1992;129:193–202.

60. Rohrig TP. Sudden death due to butane inhalation. *Am J Forensic Med Pathol* 1997;18:299–302.

61. Wheeler MG, Rozycki AA, Smith RP. Recreational propane inhalation in an adolescent male. *J Toxicol Clin Toxicol* 1992;30:135–139.

62. Huston BM, Lamm KR. Complications following butane inhalation and flash fire. *Am J Forensic Med Pathol* 1997;18(2):140–143.

63. Evans AC, Raistrick D. Phenomenology of intoxication with toluene-based adhesives and butane gas. *Br J Psychiatry* 1987;150:769–773.

64. Zacny JP, Coalson DW, Lichtor JL, et al. Effects of naloxone on the subjective and psychomotor effects of nitrous oxide in humans. *Pharmacol Biochem Behav* 1994;49:573–578.

65. Fagan D, Paul DL, Tiplady B, et al. A dose-response study of the effects of inhaled nitrous oxide on psychological performance and mood. *Psychopharmacology (Berl)* 1994;116:333–338.

66. Cheam EW, Dob DP, Skelly AM, et al. The effect of nitrous oxide on the performance of psychomotor tests. A dose-response study. *Anaesthesia* 1995;50: 764–768.

67. Veerkamp JS, Gruythuysen RJ, Hoogstraten J, et al. Anxiety reduction with nitrous oxide: a permanent solution? *ASDC J Dent Child* 1995;62:44–48.

68. Stach DJ. Nitrous oxide sedation: understanding the benefits and risks. *Am J Dent* 1995;8:47–50.

69. Daynes G. Nitrous oxide for alcohol withdrawal [Letter]. *S Afr Med J* 1994;84:708.

70. Winek CL, Wahba WW, Rozin L. Accidental death by nitrous oxide inhalation. *Forensic Sci Int* 1995;73:139–141.

71. DiMaio VJM, Garriott JC. Four deaths resulting from abuse of nitrous oxide. *J Forensic Sci* 1978;23:169–172.

72. Fraunfelder FT. Nitrous oxide warning. *Am J Ophthalmol* 1988;105:688.

73. Wagner SA, Clark MA, Wesche DL, et al. Asphyxial deaths from the recreational use of nitrous oxide. *J Forensic Sci* 1992;37:1008–1015.

74. Nordin C, Rosenqvist M, Hollstedt C. Sniffing of ethyl chloride—an uncommon form of abuse with serious mental and neurological symptoms. *Int J Addict* 1988;23:623–627.

75. Krause JG, McCarthy WB. Sudden death by inhalation of cyclopropane. *J Forensic Sci* 1989;34:1011–1012.

76. Jacob B, Heller C, Daldrup T, et al. Fatal accidental enflurane intoxication. *J Forensic Sci* 1989;34:1408–1412.

77. Eger EI II, Liu J, Koblin DD, et al. Molecular properties of the ideal inhaled anesthetic: studies of fluorinated methanes, ethanes, propanes, and butanes. *Anesth Analg* 1994;79:245–251.

78. Benignus VA. Health effects of toluene: a review. *Neurotoxicology* 1981;2:567–588.

79. Spencer JD, Raasch FO, Trefny FA. Halothane abuse in hospital personnel. *JAMA* 1976;235:1034–1035.

80. Yamashita M, Matsuki A, Oyama T. Illicit use of modern volatile anaesthetics. *Can Anaesth Soc J* 1984;31:76–79.

81. Nouchi T, Miura H, Kanayama M, et al. Fatal intoxication by 1,2-dichloroethane—a case report. *Int Arch Occup Environ Health* 1984;54:111–113.

82. Gresham GA, Treip CS. Fatal poisoning by 1,1,1-trichloroethane after prolonged survival. *Forensic Sci Int* 1983;23:249–253.

83. Jones RD, Winter DP. Two case reports of deaths on industrial premises attributed to 1,1,1-trichloroethane. *Arch Environ Health* 1983;38:59–61.

84. England A, Jones RM. Inhaled anaesthetic agents: from halothane to the present day. *Br J Hosp Med* 1992;48:254–257.

85. McLeod AA, Marjot R, Monaghan MJ, et al. Chronic cardiac toxicity after inhalation of 1,1,1-trichloroethane. *BMJ* 1987;294:727–729.

86. Cronk SL, Barkley DEH, Farrell MF. Respiratory arrest after solvent abuse. *BMJ* 1985;290:897–898.

87. Hobara T, Okuda M, Gotoh M, et al. Estimation of the lethal toluene concentration from the accidental death of painting workers. *Ind Health* 2000;38:228–231.

88. Allan AR, Blackmore RC, Toseland PA. A chloroform inhalation fatality—an unusual asphyxiation. *Med Sci Law* 1988;28:120–122.

89. Suruda AJ, McGlothlin JD. Fatal abuse of nitrous oxide in the workplace. *J Occup Med* 1990;32:682–684.

90. Rowbottom SJ. Nitrous oxide abuse [Letter]. *Anaesth Intensive Care* 1988;16:241–242.

91. Schaumburg HH, Spencer PS. Recognizing neurotoxic disease. *Neurology* 1987;37:276–278.

92. Lazar RB, Ho SU, Melen O, et al. Multifocal central nervous system damage caused by toluene abuse. *Neurology* 1983;33:1337–1340.

93. Hormes JT, Filley CM, Rosenberg NL. Neurologic sequelae of chronic solvent vapor abuse. *Neurology* 1986;36:698–702.

94. Fornazzari L, Wilkinson DA, Kapur BM, et al. Cerebellar, cortical and functional impairment in toluene abusers. *Acta Neurol Scand* 1983;67:319–329.

95. Rosenberg NL. Neurotoxicology. In: Sullivan JB, Krieger GR, eds. *Medical toxicology of hazardous materials.* Baltimore: Williams & Wilkins, 1992:145–153.

96. Altenkirch H, Wagner HM, Stoltenburg-Didinger G, et al. Potentiation of hexacarbon-neurotoxicity by methyl-ethyl-ketone (MEK) and other substances: clinical and experimental aspects. *Neurobehav Toxicol Teratol* 1982;4:623–627.

97. Altenkirch H, Mager J, Stoltenburg G, et al. Toxic polyneuropathies after sniffing a glue thinner. *J Neurol* 1977;214:137–152.

98. Saida K, Mendell JR, Weiss HS. Peripheral nerve changes induced by methyl n-butyl ketone and potentiated by methyl ethyl ketone. *J Neuropathol Exp Neurol* 1976;35:207–225.

99. Takahashi S, Kagawa M, Inagaki O, et al. Metabolic interaction between toluene and ethanol in rabbits. *Arch Toxicol* 1987;59:307–310.

100. Selden A, Hultberg B, Ulander A, et al. Trichloroethylene exposure in vapour degreasing and the urinary excretion of N-acetyl-beta-D-glucosaminidase. *Arch Toxicol* 1993;67:224–226.

101. Meulenbelt J, de Groot G, Savelkoul TJ. Two cases of acute toluene intoxication. *Br J Ind Med* 1990;47:417–420.

102. Plappert U, Barthel E, Seidel HJ. Reduction of benzene toxicity by toluene. *Environ Mol Mutagen* 1994;24:283–292.

103. Allen N. Solvents and other industrial organic compounds. In: Vinken PJ, Bruyn GW, eds. *Handbook of clinical neurology.* New York: Elsevier, 1979;36:361–389.

104. Goetz CG. Organic solvents. In: Goetz CG, ed. *Neurotoxins in clinical practice.* Jamaica, NY: Spectrum, 1985:65–90.

105. Spencer PS, Schaumburg HH. n-Hexane and methyl n-butyl ketone. In: Spencer PS, Schaumburg HH, eds. *Experimental and clinical neurotoxicology.* Baltimore: Williams & Wilkins, 1980:456–475.

106. Spencer PS, Schaumburg HH, Sabri MI, et al. The enlarging view of hexacarbon neurotoxicity. *Crit Rev Toxicol* 1980;7:279–356.

107. Graham DG, Carter AD, Boekelheide K. *In vitro* and *in vivo* studies of the molecular pathogenesis of n-hexane neuropathy. *Neurobehav Toxicol Teratol* 1982;4:629–634.

108. Perbellini L, Brugnone F, Gaffuri E. Neurotoxic metabolites of "commercial hexane" in the urine of shoe factory workers. *Clin Toxicol* 1981;18:1377–1385.

109. Backstrom B, Collins VP: The effects of 2,5-hexanedione on rods and cones of the retina of albino rats. *Neurotoxicology* 1992;13:199–202.

110. Ludolph AC, Spencer PS. Toxic neuropathies and their treatment. *Baillieres Clin Neurol* 1995;4(3):505–527.

111. Ichihara G, Saito I, Kamijima M, et al. Urinary 2,5-hexanedione increases with potentiation of neurotoxicity in chronic coexposure to n-hexane and methyl ethyl ketone. *Int Arch Occ Env Health* 1998;71:(2)100–104.

112. Menkes JH. Toxic polyneuropathy due to methyl n-butyl ketone. *Arch Neurol* 1976;33:309.

113. Billmaier D, Yee HT, Allen N, et al. Peripheral neuropathy in a coated fabrics plant. *J Occup Med* 1974;16:665–671.

114. McDonough JR. Possible neuropathy from methyl n-butyl ketone. *N Engl J Med* 1974;290:695.

115. Allen N, Mendell JR, Billmaier DJ, et al. Toxic polyneuropathy due to methyl n-butyl ketone: an industrial outbreak. *Arch Neurol* 1975;32:209–218.

116. Mallov JS. MBK neuropathy among spray painters. *JAMA* 1976;235:1455–1457.

117. Spencer PS, Schaumburg HH, Raleigh RL, et al. Nervous system degeneration produced by the industrial solvent methyl n-butyl ketone. *Arch Neurol* 1975;32:219–222.

118. Herskowitz A, Ishii N, Schaumburg H. n-Hexane neuropathy: a syndrome occurring as a result of industrial exposure. *N Engl J Med* 1971;285:82–85.

119. Gonzalez EG, Downey JA. Polyneuropathy in a glue sniffer. *Arch Phys Med Rehab* 1972;53:333–337.

120. Shirabe T, Tsuda T, Terao A, et al. Toxic polyneuropathy due to glue-sniffing:

report of two cases with a light and electron-microscopic study of the peripheral nerves and muscles. *J Neurol Sci* 1974;21:101–113.

121. Goto I, Matsumura M, Inove N, et al. Toxic polyneuropathy due to glue sniffing. *J Neurol Neurosurg Psychiatry* 1974;37:848–853.
122. Prockop LD, Alt M, Tison J. "Huffer's" neuropathy. *JAMA* 1974;229:1083–1084.
123. Korobkin R, Asbury AK, Sumner AJ, et al. Glue-sniffing neuropathy. *Arch Neurol* 1975;32:158–162.
124. Oh SJ, Kim JM. Giant axonal swelling in "huffer's" neuropathy. *Arch Neurol* 1976;33:583–586.
125. Towfighi J, Gonatas NK, Pleasure D, et al. Glue sniffer's neuropathy. *Neurology* 1976;26:238–243.
126. Dittmer DK, Jhamandas JH, Johnson ES. Glue-sniffing neuropathies. *Can Fam Physician* 1993;39:1965–1971.
127. Takeuchi Y. *n*-Hexane polyneuropathy in Japan: a review of *n*-hexane poisoning and its preventive measures. *Environ Res* 1993;62:76–80.
128. Schaumburg HH, Spencer PS. Degeneration in central and peripheral nervous systems produced by pure *n*-hexane: an experimental study. *Brain* 1976;99:183–192.
129. Frontali N, Amantini MC, Spagnolo A, et al. Experimental neurotoxicity and urinary metabolites of the C5-C7 aliphatic hydrocarbons used as glue solvents in shoe manufacture. *Clin Toxicol* 1981;18:1357–1367.
130. Issever H, Malat G, Sabuncu HH, et al. Impairment of colour vision in patients with *n*-hexane exposure-dependent toxic polyneuropathy. *Occup Med* 2002;52(4):183–186.
131. Seppalainen AM, Raitta C, Huuskonen MS. *n*-Hexane induced changes in visual evoked potentials and electroretinograms of industrial workers. *Electroencephalogr Clin Neurophysiol* 1979;47:492–498.
132. Mutti A, Ferri F, Lommi G, et al. *n*-Hexane-induced changes in nerve conduction velocities and somatosensory evoked potentials. *Int Arch Occup Environ Health* 1982;51:45–54.
133. Sharp CW, Beauvais F, Spence R. Inhalant abuse: a volatile research agenda. *NIDA Res Monogr* 1992;129.
134. Grabski DA. Toluene sniffing producing cerebellar degeneration. *Am J Psychiatry* 1961;118:461–462.
135. Arnold GL, Kirby RS, Langendoerfer S, et al. Toluene embryopathy: clinical delineation and developmental follow-up. *Pediatrics* 1994;93:216–220.
136. Ashikaga R, Araki Y, Miura K, et al. Cranial MRI in chronic thinner intox-

ication. *Neuroradiology* 1995;37:443–444.
137. Boor JW, Hurtig HI. Persistent cerebellar ataxia after exposure to toluene. *Ann Neurol* 1977;2:440–442.
138. Caldemeyer KS, Pascuzzi RM, Moran CC, et al. Toluene abuse causing reduced MR signal intensity in the brain. *AJR Am J Roentgenol* 1993;161:1259–1261.
139. Ehyai A, Freemon FR. Progressive optic neuropathy and sensorineural hearing loss due to chronic glue sniffing. *J Neurol Neurosurg Psychiatry* 1983;46:349–351.
140. Ikeda M, Tsukagoshi H. Encephalopathy due to toluene sniffing. Report of a case with magnetic resonance imaging. *Eur Neurol* 1990;30:347–349.
141. Kelly TW. Prolonged cerebellar dysfunction associated with paint-sniffing. *Pediatrics* 1975;56:605–606.
142. King MD. Neurological sequelae of toluene abuse. *Hum Toxicol* 1982;1:281–287.
143. King PJL, Morris JGL, Pollard JD. Glue sniffing neuropathy. *Aust N Z J Med* 1985;15:293–299.
144. Knox JW, Nelson JR. Permanent encephalopathy from toluene inhalation. *N Engl J Med* 1966;275:1494–1496.
145. Keane JR. Toluene optic neuropathy. *Ann Neurol* 1978;4:390.
146. Lolin Y. Chronic neurological toxicity associated with exposure to volatile substances. *Hum Toxicol* 1989;8:293–300.
147. Maas EF, Ashe J, Spiegel P, et al. Acquired pendular nystagmus in toluene addiction. *Neurology* 1991;41:282–285.
148. Malm G, Lying-Tunell U. Cerebellar dysfunction related to toluene sniffing. *Acta Neurol Scand* 1980;62:188–190.
149. Metrick SA, Brenner RP. Abnormal brainstem auditory evoked potentials in chronic paint sniffers. *Ann Neurol* 1982;12:553–556.
150. Ohnuma A, Kimura I, Saso S. MRI in chronic paint-thinner intoxication. *Neuroradiology* 1995;37:445–446.
151. Poungvarin N. Multifocal brain damage due to lacquer sniffing: the first case report of Thailand. *J Med Assoc Thai* 1991;74:296–300.
152. Rosenberg NL, Kleinschmidt-DeMasters BK, Davis KA, et al. Toluene abuse causes diffuse central nervous system white matter changes. *Ann Neurol* 1988;23:611–614.
153. Rosenberg NL, Spitz MC, Filley CM, et al. Central nervous system effects of chronic toluene abuse—clinical, brainstem evoked response and magnetic resonance imaging studies. *Neurotoxicol Teratol* 1988;10:489–495.
154. Sasa M, Igarashi S, Miyazaki T, et al. Equilibrium disorders with

diffuse brain atrophy in long-term toluene sniffing. *Arch Otorhinolaryngol* 1978;221:163–169.
155. Streicher HZ, Gabow PA, Moss AH, et al. Syndromes of toluene sniffing in adults. *Ann Intern Med* 1981;94:758–762.
156. Takeuchi Y, Hisanaga N, Ono Y, et al. Cerebellar dysfunction caused by sniffing of toluene-containing thinner. *Ind Health* 1981;19:163–169.
157. Unger E, Alexander A, Fritz T, et al. Toluene abuse: physical basis for hypointensity of the basal ganglia on T2-weighted MR images. *Radiology* 1994;193:473–476.
158. Xiong L, Matthes JD, Li J, et al. MR imaging of spray heads: toluene abuse via aerosol paint inhalation. *AJNR Am J Neuroradiol* 1993;14:1195–1199.
159. Berry JG, Heaton RK, Kirby MW. Neuropsychological deficits of chronic inhalant abusers. In: Rumack B, Temple A, eds. *Management of the poisoned patient.* Princeton, NJ: Science Press, 1977:9–31.
160. Channer KS, Stanley S. Persistent visual hallucination secondary to chronic solvent encephalopathy: case report and review of the literature. *J Neurol Neurosurg Psychiatry* 1983;46:83–86.
161. Tsushima WT, Towne WS. Effects of paint sniffing on neuropsychological test performance. *J Abnorm Psychol* 1977;86:402–407.
162. Muttray A, Wolters V, Jung D, et al. Effects of high doses of toluene on color vision. *Neurotoxicol Teratol* 1999;21(1):41–45.
163. Wiedmann KD, Power KG, Wilson JTL, et al. Recovery from chronic solvent abuse. *J Neurol Neurosurg Psychiatry* 1987;50:1712–1713.
164. Levisohn PM, Kramer RE, Rosenberg NL. Neurophysiology of chronic cocaine and toluene abuse. *Neurology* 1992;42[Suppl 3]:434(abst).
165. Escobar A, Aruffo C. Chronic thinner intoxication: clinicopathologic report of a human case. *J Neurol Neurosurg Psychiatry* 1980;43:986–994.
166. Rosenberg NL, Grigsby J, Dreisbach J, et al. Neuropsychologic impairment and MRI abnormalities associated with chronic solvent abuse. *J Toxicol Clin Toxicol* 2002;40(1):21–34.
167. Uchino A, Kato A, Yuzuriha T, et al. Comparison between patient characteristics and cranial MR findings in chronic thinner intoxication. *Eur Radiol* 2002;12:1338–1341.
168. Aydin K, Sencer S, Demir T, et al. Cranial MR findings in chronic toluene abuse by inhalation. *Am J Neuroradiol* 2002;23:1173–1179.
169. Kucuk NO, Kilic EO, Aysev A, et al. Brain SPECT findings in long-term

inhalant abuse. *Nucl Med Commun* 2000;21:769–773.

170. Kornfeld M, Moser AB, Moser HW, et al. Solvent vapor abuse leukoencephalopathy comparison to adrenoleukodystrophy. *J Neuropathol Exp Neurol* 1994;53:389–398.

171. Poser C. The dysmyelinating diseases. In: Joynt RJ, ed. *Clinical neurology.* Philadelphia: Lippincott-Raven, 1983:31–36.

172. Lloyd JW, Moore RM, Breslin P. Background information on trichloroethylene. *J Occup Med* 1975;17:603–605.

173. National Institute for Occupational Safety and Health. *Special occupational hazard review with control recommendations: trichloroethylene.* DHEW publication no. 78–130. Washington, DC: Department of Health, Education, and Welfare, 1978.

174. Feldman RG. Trichloroethylene. In: Vinken PJ, Bruyn GW, eds. *Handbook of clinical neurology. Intoxications of the nervous system, part I.* Amsterdam: North-Holland, 1979;36:457–464.

175. Humphrey JH, McClelland M. Cranial-nerve palsies with herpes following general anesthesia. *Br Med J* 1944;1:315–318.

176. McClelland M. Some toxic effects following trilene decomposition products. *Proc R Soc Med* 1944;37:526–528.

177. Enderby GEH. The use and abuse of trichloroethylene. *Br Med J* 1944;2:300–302.

178. Firth JB, Stuckey RE. Decomposition of trilene in closed circuit anaesthesia. *Lancet* 1945;1:814–816.

179. Atkinson RS. Trichloroethylene anesthesia. *Anesthesiology* 1960;21:67–77.

180. Hewer CL. Further observations on trichloroethylene. *Proc R Soc Med* 1943;36:463–465.

181. Buxton PH, Hayward M. Polyneuritis cranialis associated with trichloroethylene poisoning. *J Neurol Neurosurg Psychiatry* 1967;30:511–518.

182. Glaser MA. Treatment of trigeminal neuralgia with trichloroethylene. *JAMA* 1931;96:916–920.

183. Defalque RJ. Pharmacology and toxicology of trichloroethylene: a critical review of the world literature. *Clin Pharmacol Ther* 1961;2:665–688a.

184. Mitchell ABS, Parsons-Smith BG. Trichloroethylene neuropathy. *Br Med J* 1969;1:422–423.

185. Gwynne EI. Trichloroethylene neuropathy. *Br Med J* 1969;2:315.

186. Feldman RG, Mayer RM, Taub A. Evidence for peripheral neurotoxic effect of trichloroethylene. *Neurology* 1970;20:599–606.

187. Defalque RJ. The "specific" analgesic effect of trichloroethylene upon the trigeminal nerve. *Anesthesiology* 1961;22:379–384.

188. Waters EM, Gerstner HB, Huff JE. Trichloroethylene. I. An overview. *J Toxicol Environ Health* 1977;2:671–707.

189. Schaumburg HH, Spencer PS, Thomas PK. *Disorders of peripheral nerves.* Philadelphia: FA Davis, 1983.

190. Sagawa K. Transverse lesion of the spinal cord after accidental exposure to trichloroethylene. *Int Arch Arbeitsmed* 1973;31:257–264.

191. Spencer PS, Bischoff MC. Spontaneous remyelination of spinal cord plaques in rats orally treated with sodium dichloroacetate. *J Neuropathol Exp Neurol* 1982;41:373.

192. Cavanagh JB, Buxton PH. Trichloroethylene cranial neuropathy: is it really a toxic neuropathy or does it activate latent herpes virus? *J Neurol Neurosurg Psychiatry* 1989;52:297–303.

193. Adams EM, Spencer HC, Rowe VK, et al. Vapor toxicity of trichloroethylene determined by experiments on laboratory animals. *Arch Ind Hyg Occup Med* 1951;3:469.

194. Utesch RC, Weir FW, Bruckner JV. Development of an animal model of solvent abuse for use in the evaluation of extreme trichloroethylene inhalation. *Toxicology* 1981;19:169.

195. Tucker AW, Sanders VM, Barnes DW, et al. Toxicology of trichloroethylene in the mouse. *Toxicol Appl Pharmacol* 1982;62:351.

196. Dorfmueller MA, Henne SP, York RG, et al. Evaluation of teratogenicity and behavioral toxicity with inhalation exposure of maternal rats to trichloroethylene. *Toxicology* 1979;14:153.

197. Andersson A. Health dangers in industry from exposure to trichloroethylene. *Acta Med Scand* 1957;157[Suppl 323]:217–220.

198. Bardodej Z, Vyskocil J. Trichloroethylene metabolism and its effects on the nervous system as a means of hygienic control. *Arch Ind Health* 1956;13:581–592.

199. Grandjean E, Murchinger R, Turrian V, et al. Investigations into the effects of exposure to trichloroethylene in mechanical engineering. *Br J Ind Med* 1955;12:131–142.

200. Lilis R, Stanescu D, Muica N, et al. Chronic effects of trichloroethylene exposure. *Med Lav* 1969;60:595–601.

201. Salvini M, Binaschi S, Riva M. Evaluation of the psychophysiological functions in humans exposed to trichloroethylene. *Br J Ind Med* 1971;28:293–295.

202. Smith GF. Investigations of the mental effects of trichloroethylene. *Ergonomics* 1970;13:580.

203. Annau Z. The neurobehavioral toxicity of trichloroethylene. *Neurobehav Toxicol Teratol* 1981;3:417–424.

204. Todd J. Trichloroethylene poisoning with paranoid psychosis and Lilliputian hallucination. *Br Med J* 1954;7:439–440.

205. Harenko A. Two peculiar instances of psychotic disturbance in trichloroethylene poisoning. *Acta Neurol Scand* 1967;31[Suppl]:139–140.

206. Stewart RD, Dodd HC, Gay HH, et al. Experimental human exposure to trichloroethylene. *Arch Environ Health* 1970;20:64–71.

207. Ferguson RK, Vernon RJ. Trichloroethylene in combination with CNS drugs: effects on visual-motor tests. *Arch Environ Health* 1970;20:462–467.

208. Winneke G. Acute behavioral effects of exposure to some organic solvents—psychophysiological aspects. *Acta Neurol Scand* 1982;66[Suppl 92]:117–129.

209. Vernon RJ, Ferguson RK. Effects of trichloroethylene on visual-motor performance. *Arch Environ Health* 1969;18:894–900.

210. Kylin B, Axell K, Samuel HE, et al. Effect of inhaled trichloroethylene on the CNS: as measured by optokinetic nystagmus. *Arch Environ Health* 1967;15:49–52.

211. Muller G, Spassowski M, Henschler D. Metabolism of trichloroethylene in man. III. Interaction of trichloroethylene and ethanol. *Arch Toxicol* 1975;33:173–189.

212. Miyake H, Ikeda T, Maehara N, et al. Slow learning in rats due to long-term inhalation of toluene. *Neurobehav Toxicol Teratol* 1983;5:541–548.

213. Lorenzana-Jimenez M, Salas M. Neonatal effects of toluene on the locomotor behavioral development of the rat. *Neurobehav Toxicol Teratol* 1983;5:295–299.

214. Pryor GT, Dickinson J, Howd RA, Rebert CS. Transient cognitive deficits and high-frequency hearing loss in weanling rats exposed to toluene. *Neurobehav Toxicol Teratol* 1983;5:53–57.

215. Wood RW, Cox C. Acute oral toxicity of butyl nitrite. *J Appl Toxicol* 1981;1:30–31.

216. Rees DC, Knisely JS, Jordan S, et al. Discriminative stimulus properties of toluene in the mouse. *Toxicol Appl Pharmacol* 1987;88:97–104.

217. Rebert CS, Sorenson SS, Howd RA, et al. Toluene-induced hearing loss in rats evidenced by the brainstem auditory-evoked response. *Neurobehav Toxicol Teratol* 1983;5:59–62.

218. Niklasson M, Tham R, Larsby B, et al. Effects of toluene, styrene,

trichloroethylene, and trichloroethane on the vestibulo- and opto-oculo motor system in rats. *Neurotoxicol Teratol* 1993;15:327–334.

219. McWilliams ML, Chen GD, Fechter LD. Low-level toluene disrupts auditory function in guinea pigs. *Toxicol Appl Pharm* 2000;167(1):18–29.

220. Campo P, Lataye R, Cossec B, et al. Toluene-induced hearing loss: a mid-frequency location of the cochlear lesions. *Neurotox Teratol* 1997;19:129–140.

221. Lataye R, Campo P, Loquet G. Toluene ototoxicity in rats: assessment of the frequency of hearing deficit by electrocochleography. *Neurotoxicol Teratol* 1999;21:267–276.

222. Niklasson M, Stengard K, Tham R. Are the effects of toluene on the vestibular and opto-oculo motor system inhibited by the action of GABAB antagonist CGP 35348? *Neurotoxicol Teratol* 1995;17:351–357.

223. Nylen P, Hagman M, Johnson AC. Function of the auditory and visual systems, and of peripheral nerve, in rats after long-term combined exposure to *n*-hexane and methylated benzene derivatives. I. Toluene. *Pharmacol Toxicol* 1994;74:116–123.

224. Li HS, Johnson AC, Borg E, et al. Auditory degeneration after exposure to toluene in two genotypes of mice. *Arch Toxicol* 1992;66:382–386.

225. Pryor GT. A toluene-induced motor syndrome in rats resembling that seen in some solvent abusers. *Neurotoxicol Teratol* 1991;13:387–400.

226. Rebert CS, Day VL, Matteucci MJ, et al. Sensory-evoked potentials in rats chronically exposed to trichloroethylene: predominant auditory dysfunction. *Neurotoxicol Teratol* 1991;13:83–90.

227. Crofton KM, Zhao X. Mid-frequency hearing loss in rats following inhalation exposure to trichloroethylene: evidence from reflex modification audiometry. *Neurotoxicol Teratol* 1993;15:413–423.

228. Jaspers RM, Muijser H, Lammers JH, et al. Mid-frequency hearing loss and reduction of acoustic startle responding in rats following trichloroethylene exposure. *Neurotoxicol Teratol* 1993;15:407–412.

229. Pryor GT. Solvent-induced neurotoxicity: effects and mechanisms. In: Chang LW, Dyer RS, eds. *Principles of Neurotoxicity.* New York: Marcel Dekker, pp. 377–400, 1995.

230. Campo P, Lataye R, Loquet G, et al. Styrene-induced hearing loss: a membrane insult. *Hear Res* 2001;154:170–180.

231. Cappaert NLM, Klis SFL, Muijser H,

et al. Differential susceptibility of rats and guinea pigs to the ototoxic effects of ethyl benzene. *Neurotoxicol Teratol* 2002;24:503–510.

232. Fechter LD, Liu Y, Herr DW, et al. Trichloroethylene ototoxicity: evidence for a cochlear origin. *Toxicol Sci* 1998;42:28–35.

233. Niklasson M, Tham R, Larsby B, et al. Effects of toluene, styrene, trichloroethylene, and trichloroethane on the vestibulo- and opto-oculo motor system in rats. *Neurotoxicol Teratol* 1993;15:327–334.

234. Mergler D, Beauvais B. Olfactory threshold shift following controlled 7-hour exposure to toluene and/or xylene. *Neurotoxicology* 1992;13:211–215.

235. Nylen P, Hagman M, Johnson AC. Function of the auditory and visual systems, and of peripheral nerve, in rats after long-term combined exposure to *n*-hexane and methylated benzene derivatives. I. Toluene. *Pharmacol Toxicol* 1994;74:116–123.

236. Li HS, Johnson AC, Borg E, et al. Auditory degeneration after exposure to toluene in two genotypes of mice. *Arch Toxicol* 1992;66:382–386.

237. Moskowitz S, Shapiro H. Fatal exposure to methylene chloride vapor. *Arch Ind Hyg Occup Med* 1952;6:116–123.

238. Winek CL, Collum WD, Esposito F. Accidental methylene chloride fatality. *Forensic Sci Int* 1981;18:165–168.

239. Tariot PN. Delirium resulting from methylene chloride exposure: case report. *J Clin Psychiatry* 1983;44:340–342.

240. Sturmann K, Mofenson H, Caraccio T. Methylene chloride inhalation: an unusual form of drug abuse. *Ann Emerg Med* 1985;14:903–905.

241. Horowitz BZ. Carboxyhemoglobinemia caused by inhalation of methylene chloride. *Am J Emerg Med* 1986;4:48–51.

242. Stewart RD, Fisher TN, Hosko MJ, et al. Experimental human exposure to methylene chloride. *Arch Environ Health* 1972;25:342–348.

243. Kubic VL, Andres MW, Engel RR, et al. Metabolism of dihalomethanes to carbon monoxide. I. *In vivo* studies. *Drug Metab Dispos* 1974;2:53–57.

244. Ratney RS, Wegman DH, Elkins HB. *In vivo* conversion of methylene chloride to carbon monoxide. *Arch Environ Health* 1974;28:223–226.

245. Astrand I, Ovrum P, Carlsson A. Exposure to methylene chloride. I. Its concentration in alveolar air and blood during rest and exercise and its metabolism. *Scand J Work Environ Health* 1975;1:78–94.

246. Stewart RD, Fisher TN. Carboxyhemoglobin elevation after exposure to dichloromethane. *Science* 1972;176:295–296.

247. Gamberale F, Annwall G, Hultengren M. Exposure to methylene chloride. II. Psychological functions. *Scand J Work Environ Health* 1975;1:95–103.

248. Winneke G. The neurotoxicity of dichloromethane. *Neurobehav Toxicol Teratol* 1981;3:391–395.

249. Chang YL, Yang CC, Deng JF, et al. Diverse manifestations of oral methylene chloride poisoning: report of 6 cases. *J Toxicol Clin Toxicol* 1999;37(4):497–504.

250. Cherry N, Venables H, Waldron HA, et al. Some observations on workers exposed to methylene chloride. *Br J Ind Med* 1981;38:351–355.

251. Hearne FT, Grose F, Pifer JW, et al. Methylene chloride mortality study: dose-response characterization and animal model comparison. *J Occup Med* 1987;29:217–228.

252. Silverstein MA. Letter to the editor. *Arch Environ Health* 1983;38:252

253. McCarthy TB, Jones RD. Industrial gassing poisonings due to trichloroethylene, perchloroethylene, and 1,1,1-trichloroethane, 1961–80. *Br J Ind Med* 1983;40:450–455.

254. Kobayashi H, Hobara T, Kawamoto T, et al. Effect of 1,1,1-trichloroethane inhalation on heart rate and its mechanism: a role of autonomic nervous system. *Arch Environ Health* 1987;42:140–143.

255. Wise MG. Trichloroethane (TCE) and central sleep apnea: a case study. *J Toxicol Environ Health* 1983;11:101–104.

256. Stewart RD, Gay HH, Schaffer AW, et al. Experimental human exposure to methyl chloroform vapor. *Arch Environ Health* 1969;19:467–472.

257. Salvini M, Binaschi S, Riva M. Evaluation of the psychophysiological functions in humans exposed to the "threshold limit value" of 1,1,1-trichloroethane. *Br J Ind Med* 1971;28:286–292.

258. Gamberale F, Hultengren M. Methylchloroform exposure. II. Psychophysiological functions. *Work Environ Health* 1973;10:82–92.

259. Mackay CJ, Campbell L, Samuel AM, et al. Behavioral changes during exposure to 1,1,1-trichloroethane: time-course and relationship to blood solvent levels. *Am J Ind Med* 1987;11:223–239.

260. Maroni M, Bulgheroni C, Cassitto G, et al. A clinical, neurophysiological and behavioral study of female workers exposed to 1,1,1-trichloroethane. *Scand J Work Environ Health* 1977;3:16–22.

261. Pryor GT. Solvent-induced neurotoxicity: effects and mechanisms. In: Chang LW, Dyer RS, eds. *Handbook of*

toxicology. New York: Marcel Dekker, 1995.

262. Coodin FJ, Dawes C, Dean GW, et al. Riposte to "environmental lead and young children." *Can Med Asoc J* 1980;123:469–471.

263. Eastwell HD. Elevated lead levels in petrol "sniffers." *Med J Aust* 1985;143:563–564.

264. Goldings AS, Stewart RM. Organic lead encephalopathy: behavioral change and movement disorder following gasoline inhalation. *J Clin Psychiatry* 1982;43:70–72.

265. Goodheart RS, Dunne JW. Petrol sniffer's encephalopathy. A study of 25 patients. *Med J Aust* 1994;160:178–181.

266. Hansen KS, Sharp FR. Gasoline sniffing, lead poisoning, and myoclonus. *JAMA* 1978;240:1375–1376.

267. Prockop LD, Karampelas D. Encephalopathy secondary to abusive gasoline inhalation. *J Fla Med Assoc* 1981;68:823–824.

268. Reese E, Kimbrough RD. Acute toxicity of gasoline and some additives. *Environ Health Perspect* 1993;101[Suppl 6]:115–131.

269. Remington G, Hoffman BF. Gas sniffing as a form of substance abuse. *Can J Psychiatry* 1984;29:31–35.

270. Robinson RO. Tetraethyl lead poisoning from gasoline sniffing. *JAMA* 1978;241:1373–1374.

271. Tenenbein M, deGroot W, Rajani KR. Peripheral neuropathy following intentional inhalation of naphtha fumes. *Can Med Assoc J* 1984;131:1077–1079.

272. Valpey R, Sumi SM, Copass MK, et al. Acute and chronic progressive encephalopathy due to gasoline sniffing. *Neurology* 1978;28:507–510.

273. Burns CB, Currie B. The efficacy of chelation therapy and factors influencing mortality in lead intoxicated petrol sniffers. *Aust N Z J Med* 1995;25:197–203.

274. Pardys S, Brotman M. Trichloroethylene and alcohol: a straight flush. *JAMA* 1974;229:521–522.

275. Stewart RD, Hake CL, Peterson JE. "Degreasers' flush," dermal response to trichloroethylene and ethanol. *Arch Environ Health* 1974;29:1–5.

276. Antti-Poika M, Juntunen J, Matikainen E, et al. Occupational exposure to toluene: neurotoxic effects with special emphasis on drinking habits. *Int Arch Occup Environ Health* 1985;56:31–40.

277. Kira S, Ogata M, Ebara Y, et al. A case of thinner sniffing: relationship between neuropsychological symptoms and urinary findings after inhalation of toluene and methanol. *Ind Health* 1988;26:81–85.

278. Pryor GT, Howd RA, Uyeno ET, et al. Interactions between toluene and alcohol. *Pharmacol Biochem Behav* 1985;23:401–410.

279. Cunningham J, Sharkawi M, Plaa GL. Pharmacological and metabolic interactions between ethanol and methyl *n*-butyl ketone, methyl isobutyl ketone, methyl ethyl ketone, or acetone in mice. *Fundam Appl Toxicol* 1989;13:102–109.

280. Campo P, Lataye R, Cossec B, et al. Combined effects of simultaneous exposure to toluene and ethanol on auditory function in rats. *Neurotoxicol Teratol* 1998;20:321–332.

281. Kuteifan K, Oesterle H, Tajahmady T, et al. Necrosis and haemorrhage of the putamen in methanol poisoning shown on MRI. *Neuroradiology* 1998;40(3):158–160.

282. Eells JT, Henry MM, Lewandowski MF, et al. Development and characterization of a rodent model of methanol-induced retinal and optic nerve toxicity. *Neurotoxicology* 2000;21:321–330.

283. McCormick MJ. Methanol poisoning as a result of inhalational solvent abuse. *Ann Emerg Med* 1990;19:639–642.

284. Brett A. Myeloneuropathy from whipped cream bulbs presenting as conversion disorder. *Aust N Z J Psychiatry* 1997;31:131–132.

285. Pema PJ, Horak HA, Wyatt RH. Myelopathy caused by nitrous oxide toxicity. *Am J Neuroradiol* 1998;19:894–896.

286. Butzkueven H, King JO. Nitrous oxide myelopathy in an abuser of whipped cream bulbs. *J Clin Neurosci* 2000;7(1):73–75.

287. Layzer RB. Myeloneuropathy after prolonged exposure to nitrous oxide. *Lancet* 1978;2:1227–1230.

288. Kinsella LJ, Green R. "Anesthesia paresthetica": nitrous oxide-induced cobalamin deficiency. *Neurology* 1995;45:1608–1610.

289. Flippo TS, Holder WD Jr. Neurologic degeneration associated with nitrous oxide anesthesia in patients with vitamin B_{12} deficiency. *Arch Surg* 1993;128:1391–1395.

290. Nunn JF. Clinical aspects of the interaction between nitrous oxide and vitamin B_{12}. *Br J Anaesth* 1987;59:3–13.

291. Chanarin I. Nitrous oxide and the cobalamins. *Clin Sci* 1980;59:151–154.

292. Vishnubhakat SM, Beresford HR. Reversible myeloneuropathy of nitrous oxide abuse: serial electrophysiological studies. *Muscle Nerve* 1991;14:22–26.

293. Felmet K, Robins B, Tilford D, et al. Acute neurologic decompensation in an infant with cobalamin deficiency exposed to nitrous oxide. *J Pediatr* 2000;137(3):427–428.

294. Fujinaga M, Baden JM. Methionine prevents nitrous oxide-induced teratogenicity in rat embryos grown in culture. *Anesthesiology* 1994;81:184–189.

295. Brodsky JB, Cohen EN. Adverse effects of nitrous oxide. *Med Toxicol* 1986;1:362–374.

296. Gillman MA. Nitrous oxide has a very low abuse potential [Letter] (comment on *Addiction* 1994;89(7):831–839). *Addiction* 1995;90(3):439.

297. Jastak JT. Nitrous oxide and its abuse. *J Am Dent Assoc* 1991;122:48–52.

298. Louis-Ferdinand RT. Myelotoxic, neurotoxic and reproductive adverse effects of nitrous oxide. *Adverse Drug React Toxicol Rev* 1994;13:(4)193–206.

299. Fujinaga M, Maze M. Neurobiology of nitrous oxide-induced antinociceptive effects. *Mol Neurobiol* 2002;25:167–189.

300. Schwartz RH, Calihan M. Nitrous oxide: a potentially lethal euphoriant inhalant. *Am Family Pract* 1984;30:171–172.

301. Belknap JK, Laursen SE, Crabbe JC. Ethanol and nitrous oxide produce withdrawal-induced convulsions by similar mechanisms in mice. *Life Sci* 1987;41:2033–2040.

302. Ron MA. Volatile substance abuse: a review of possible long-term neurological, intellectual and psychiatric sequelae. *Br J Psychiatry* 1986;148:235–246.

303. Korman M, Semler I, Trimboli F. A psychiatric emergency room study of 162 inhalant users. *Addict Behav* 1980;5:143.

304. Dinwiddie SH, Zorumski CF, Rubin EH. Psychiatric correlates of chronic solvent abuse. *J Clin Psychiatry* 1987;48:334–337.

304a. Dinwiddie SH, Reich T, Cloninger CR. Solvent use and psychiatric comorbidity. *Br J Addict* 1990;85:1647–1656.

305. Fernandez-Pol B, Bluestone H, Mizruchi MS. Inner-city substance abuse patterns: a study of psychiatric inpatients. *Am J Drug Alcohol Abuse* 1988;14:41–50.

306. Byrne A, Kirby B, Zibin T, et al. Psychiatric and neurological effects of chronic solvent abuse. *Can J Psychiatry* 1991;36:735–738.

307. Henry B, Feehan M, McGee R, et al. The importance of conduct problems and depressive symptoms in predicting adolescent substance use. *J Abnorm Child Psychol* 1993;21:469–480.

308. Goldbloom D, Chouinard G. Schizophreniform psychosis associated with chronic industrial toluene exposure: case report. *J Clin Psychiatry* 1985;46:350–351.

309. Katzelnick DJ, Davar G, Scanlon JP. Reversibility of psychiatric symptoms in a chronic solvent abuser: a case

report. *J Neuropsychiatry Clin Neurosci* 1991;3:319–321.

310. Levy AB. Delirium induced by inhalation of typewriter correction fluid. *Psychosomatics* 1986;27:665–666.

311. Roberts FP, Lucas EG, Marsden CD, et al. Near-pure xylene causing reversible neuropsychiatric disturbance [Letter]. *Lancet* 1988;8605:273.

312. Chadwick OF, Anderson HR. Neuropsychological consequences of volatile substance abuse: a review. *Hum Toxicol* 1989;8:307–312.

313. Dinwiddie SH. Abuse of inhalants—a review. *Addiction* 1994;89:925–939.

314. Baerg RD, Kimberg DV. Centrilobular hepatic necrosis and acute renal failure in "solvent sniffers." *Ann Intern Med* 1970;73:713–720.

315. Bennett RH, Forman HR. Hypokalemic periodic paralysis in chronic toluene exposure. *Arch Neurol* 1980;37:673.

316. Batlle DC, Sabatini S, Kurtzman NA. On the mechanism of toluene-induced renal tubular acidosis. *Nephron* 1988;49:210–218.

317. Carlisle EJ, Donnelly SM, Vasuvattakul S, et al. Glue-sniffing and distal renal tubular acidosis: sticking to the facts. *J Am Soc Nephrol* 1991;1:1019–1027.

318. Daniell WE, Couser WG, Rosenstock L. Occupational solvent exposure and glomerulonephritis. *JAMA* 1988;259:2280–2283.

319. Gupta RK, van der Meulen J, Johny KV. Oliguric acute renal failure due to glue-sniffing. Case report. *Scand J Urol Nephrol* 1991;25:247–250.

320. Jone CM, Wu AH. An unusual case of toluene-induced metabolic acidosis. *Clin Chem* 1988;34:2596–2599.

321. Kamijima M, Nakazawa Y, Yamakawa M, et al. Metabolic acidosis and renal tubular injury due to pure toluene inhalation. *Arch Environ Health* 1994;49:410–413.

322. Kaneko T, Koizumi T, Takezaki T, et al. Urinary calculi associated with solvent abuse. *J Urol* 1992;147:1365–1366.

323. Lavoie FW, Dolan MC, Danzl DF, et al. Recurrent resuscitation and "no code" orders in a 27-year-old spray paint abuser (clinical conference). *Ann Emerg Med* 1987;16:1266–1273.

324. Marjot R, McLeod AA. Chronic non-neurological toxicity from volatile substance abuse. *Hum Toxicol* 1989;8:301–306.

325. Mizutani T, Oohashi N, Naito H. Myoglobinemia and renal failure in toluene poisoning: a case report. *Vet Hum Toxicol* 1989;31:448–450.

326. Nelson NA, Robins TG, Port FK. Solvent nephrotoxicity in humans and experimental animals. *Am J Nephrol* 1990;10:10–20.

327. Patel R, Benjamin J Jr. Renal disease associated with toluene inhalation. *Clin Toxicol* 1986;24:213–223.

328. Ravnskov U. Exposure to organic solvents—a missing link in poststreptococcal glomerulonephritis? *Acta Med Scand* 1978;203:351–356.

329. Taverner D, Harrison DJ, Bell GM. Acute renal failure due to interstitial nephritis induced by "glue-sniffing" with subsequent recovery. *Scott Med J* 1988;33:246–247.

330. Wilkins-Haug L, Gabow PA. Toluene abuse during pregnancy: obstetric complications and perinatal outcomes. *Obstet Gynecol* 1991;77:504–509.

331. Will AM, McLaren EH. Reversible renal damage due to glue sniffing. *Br Med J* 1981;283:525–526.

332. Kao KC, Tsai YH, Lin MC, et al. Hypokalemic muscular paralysis causing acute respiratory failure due to rhabdomyolysis with renal tubular acidosis in a chronic glue sniffer. *Clin Toxicol* 2000;38(6):679–681.

333. Caravati EM, Bjerk PJ. Acute toluene ingestion toxicity. *Ann Emerg Med* 1997;30(6):838–839.

334. Lauwerys R, Bernard A, Viau C, et al. Kidney disorders and hematotoxicity from organic solvent exposure. *Scand J Work Environ Health* 1985;11[Suppl 1]:83–90.

335. Harrison DJ, Thomson D, MacDonald MK. Membranous glomerulonephritis. *J Clin Pathol* 1986;39:167.

336. Anetseder M, Hartung E, Klepper S, et al. Gasoline vapors induce severe rhabdomyolysis. *Neurology* 1994;44:2393–2395.

337. Brown JH, Hadden DR, Hadden DS. Solvent abuse, toluene acidosis and diabetic ketoacidosis. *Arch Emerg Med* 1991;8:65–67.

338. Lock EA. Mechanism of nephrotoxic action due to organohalogenated compounds. *Toxicol Lett* 1989;46:93–106.

339. Miller L, Pateras V, Friederici H, et al. Acute tubular necrosis after inhalation exposure to methylene chloride. *Report of a case*. *Arch Intern Med* 1985;145:145–146.

340. Rioux JP, Myers RA. Methylene chloride poisoning: a paradigmatic review. *J Emerg Med* 1988;6:227–238.

341. Kimbrough RD, Mitchell FL, Houk VN. Trichloroethylene: an update. *J Toxicol Environ Health* 1985;15:369–383.

342. Brown BR, Gandolfi AJ. Adverse effects of volatile anaesthetics. *Br J Anaesth* 1987;59:14–23.

343. Pozzi C, Marai P, Ponti R, et al. Toxicity in man due to stain removers containing 1,2-dichloropropane. *Br J Ind Med* 1985;42:770–772.

344. Keogh AM, Ibels LS, Allen DH, et al. Exacerbation of Goodpasture's syndrome after inadvertent exposure to hydrocarbon fumes. *Br Med J* 1984;288:188.

345. Nathan AW, Toseland PA. Goodpasture's syndrome and trichloroethane intoxication. *Br J Clin Pharmacol* 1979;8:28406.

346. Yamamoto S, Mori NYH, Miyata M, et al. Neurogenic bladder caused by toluene abuse. *Acta Urol Jpn* 1992;38:459–462.

347. Pryor GT, Rebert CS. *Neurotoxicology of inhaled substances*. National Institutes on Drug Abuse Contract 271-90-7202 report. November 1992.

348. Short BG, Burnett VL, Cox MG, et al. Site-specific renal cytotoxicity and cell proliferation in male rats exposed to petroleum hydrocarbons. *Lab Invest* 1987;57:564–577.

349. Wedeen RP. Occupational renal disease. *Am J Kidney Dis* 1984;111:241–257.

350. Sarmiento Martinez J, Guardiola Sala JJ, et al. Renal tubular acidosis with an elevated anion gap in a "glue sniffer" [Letter]. *Hum Toxicol* 1989;8:139–140.

351. Yamaguchi K, Shirai T, Shimakura K, et al. Pneumatosis cystoides intestinalis and trichloroethylene exposure. *Am J Gastroenterol* 1985;80:753–757.

352. Farrell G, Prendergast D, Murray M. Halothane hepatitis. Detection of a constitutional susceptibility factor. *N Engl J Med* 1985;313:1310–1314.

353. Goodwin TM. Toluene abuse and renal tubular acidosis in pregnancy. *Obstet Gynecol* 1988;71:715–718.

354. Seoud M, Adra A, Khalil A, et al. Transient renal tubular acidosis in pregnancy. *Am J Perinatol* 2000;17:249–252.

355. Lindemann R. Congenital renal tubular dysfunction associated with maternal sniffing of organic solvents. *Acta Paediatr Scand* 1991;80:882–884.

356. Paraf F, Lewis J, Jothy S. Acute fatty liver of pregnancy after exposure to toluene. A case report. *J Clin Gastroenterol* 1993;17:163–165.

357. Stewart A, Witts LJ. Chronic carbon tetrachloride intoxication. 1944 [Classical article]. *Br J Ind Med* 1993;50:8–18.

358. Benjamin SB, Goodman ZD, Ishak KG, et al. The morphologic spectrum of halothane-induced hepatic injury: analysis of 77 cases. *Hepatology* 1985;5:1163–1171.

359. Clearfield HR. Hepatrenal toxicity from sniffing spot-remover (trichloroethylene). *Dig Dis* 1970;15:851–856.

360. Cordes DH, Brown WD, Quinn KM. Chemically induced hepatitis after inhaling organic solvents. *West J Med* 1988;148:458–460.

361. Dossing M. Occupational toxic liver damage. *J Hepatol* 1986;3:131–135.

362. Hakim A, Jain AK, Jain R. Chloroform ingestion causing toxic hepatitis. *J Assoc Physicians India* 1992;40:477.

363. Hodgson MJ, Furman J, Ryan C, et al. Encephalopathy and vestibulopathy following short-term hydrocarbon exposure. *J Occup Med* 1989;31:51–54.

364. McCunney RJ. Diverse manifestations of trichloroethylene. *Br J Ind Med* 1988;45:122–126.

365. McIntyre AS, Long RG. Fatal fulminant hepatic failure in a "solvent abuser." *Postgrad Med J* 1992;68:29–30.

366. Buring JE, Hennekens CH, Mayrent SL, et al. Health experiences of operating room personnel. *Anaesthesiology* 1985;62:325–330.

367. Shaw J, Brooks PM, McNeil JJ, et al. Modern inhalational anesthetic agents. *Med J Aust* 1989;150:95–102.

368. Neuberger J, Davis M. Advances in understanding of halothane hepatitis. *Trends Pharmacol Sci* 1983;Jan:19–20.

369. Ong CN, Koh D, Foo SC, et al. Volatile organic solvents in correction fluids: identification and potential hazards. *Bull Environ Contam Toxicol* 1993;50:787–793.

370. Greer JE. Adolescent abuse of typewriter correction fluid. *South Med J* 1984;77:297–298.

371. Mizutani K, Shinomiya K, Shinomiya T. Hepatotoxicity of dichloromethane. *Forensic Sci Int* 1988;38:113–128.

372. Hodgson MJ, Heyl AT, Van Thiel DH. Liver disease associated with exposure to 1,1,1-trichloroethane. *Arch Intern Med* 1989;149:1793–1798.

373. Plaa GL. Experimental evaluation of haloalkanes and liver injury. *Fundam Appl Toxicol* 1988;10:563–570.

374. Koporec KP, Kim HJ, MacKenzie WF, et al. Effect of oral dosing vehicles on the subchronic hepatotoxicity of carbon tetrachloride in the rat. *J Toxicol Env Health* 1995;44:(1)13–27.

375. Soni MG, Mangipudy RS, Mumtaz MM, et al. Tissue repair response as a function of dose during trichloroethylene hepatotoxicity. *Toxicol Sci* 1998;42:(2)158–165.

376. Omaehi T, Tanaka S, Sasaki K, et al. Acute and recurrent hepatitis induced by 2,2-dichloro-1,1,1-trifluoroethane (HCFC-123).

377. Keller DA, Lieder PH, Brock WJ, et al. 1,1,1-Trifluoro-2,2-dichloroethane (HCFC-123) and 1,1,1-trifluoro-2-bromo-2-chloroethane (halothane) cause similar biochemical effects in rats exposed by inhalation for five days. *Drug Chem Toxicol* 1998;21(4):405–415.

378. Redfern N. Morbidity among anaesthetists. *Br J Hosp Med* 1990;43:377–381.

379. Cohen EN. Inhalation anesthetics may cause genetic defects, abortions and miscarriages in operating room personnel. In: Eckenhoff JE, ed. *Controversy in anesthesiology.* Philadelphia: WB Saunders, 1979:47–57.

380. Mirza T, Gerin M, Begin D, et al. A study on the substitution of trichloroethylene as a spot remover in the textile industry. *Am Ind Hyg Assoc J* 2000;61:431–438.

381. Hubbs AF, Castranova V, Ma JYC, et al. Acute lung injury induced by a commercial leather conditioner. *Toxicol Appl Pharmacol* 1997;143:37–46.

382. Reyes de la Rocha S, Brown MA, Fortenberry JD. Pulmonary function abnormalities in intentional spray paint inhalation. *Chest* 1987;92:100–104.

383. Schikler KN, Lane EE, Seitz K, et al. Solvent abuse associated pulmonary abnormalities. *Adv Alcohol Subst Abuse* 1984;3:75–81.

384. Woo OF, Healey KM, Sheppard D, et al. Chest pain and hypoxemia from inhalation of a trichloroethane aerosol product. *J Toxicol Clin Toxicol* 1983;20:333–341.

385. Buie SE, Pratt DS, May JJ. Diffuse pulmonary injury following paint remover exposure. *Am J Med* 1986;81:702–704.

386. Engstrand DA, England DM, Huntington RW 3d. Pathology of paint sniffers' lung. *Am J Forensic Med Pathol* 1986;7:232–236.

387. Sherwood RL, O'Shea W, Thomas PT, et al. Effects of inhalation of ethylene dichloride on pulmonary defenses of mice and rats. *Toxicol Appl Pharmacol* 1987;91:491–496.

388. Boon NA. Solvent abuse and the heart [Editorial]. *BMJ* 1987;294:722.

389. Cunningham SR, Dalzell GWN, McGirr P, et al. Myocardial infarction and primary ventricular fibrillation after glue sniffing. *BMJ* 1987;294:739–740.

390. Wiseman MN, Banim S. "Glue sniffer's" heart? *BMJ* 1987;294:739.

391. Knight AT, Pawsey CG, Aroney RS, et al. Upholsterers' glue associated with myocarditis, hepatitis, acute renal failure and lymphoma. *Med J Aust* 1991;154:360–362.

392. Wernisch M, Paya K, Palasser A. Cardiovascular arrest after inhalation of leather glue. *Wien Med Wochenschr* 1991;141:71–74.

393. Brilliant LC, Grillo A. Successful resuscitation from cardiopulmonary arrest following deliberate inhalation of freon refrigerant gas. *Del Med J* 1993;65:375–378.

394. Wright MF, Strobl DJ. 1,1,1-Trichloroethane cardiac toxicity:

report of a case. *J Am Osteopath Assoc* 1984;84:285–288.

395. Ong TK, Rustage KJ, Harrison KM, et al. Solvent abuse. An anaesthetic management problem. *Br Dent J* 1988;164:150–151.

396. Wodka RM, Jeong EW. Cardiac effects of inhaled typewriter correction fluid [Letter]. *Ann Intern Med* 1989;110:91–92.

397. Mee AS, Wright PL. Congestive (dilated) cardiomyopathy in association with solvent abuse. *J R Soc Med* 1980;73:671–672.

398. Taylor GJ, Harris WS. Cardiac toxicity of aerosol propellants. *JAMA* 1970;214:81–85.

399. Chenoweth MB. Abuse of inhalation anesthetic drugs. *NIDA Res Monogr* 1977;15:102–111.

400. Barrowcliff DF, Knell AJ. Cerebral damage due to endogenous chronic carbon monoxide poisoning caused by exposure to methylene chloride. *J Soc Occup Med* 1979;29:12–14.

401. Manno M, Chirillo R, Daniotti G, et al. Carboxyhaemoglobin and fatal methylene chloride poisoning [Letter]. *Lancet* 1989;2(8657):274.

402. Wason S, Detsky AS, Platt OS, et al. Isobutyl nitrite toxicity by ingestion. *Ann Intern Med* 1980;92:637–638.

403. Brandes JC, Bufill JA, Pisciotta AV. Amyl nitrite-induced hemolytic anemia. *Am J Med* 1989;86:252–254.

404. Machabert R, Testud F, Descotes J. Methaemoglobinaemia due to amyl nitrite inhalation: a case report. *Hum Exp Toxicol* 1994;13:313–314.

405. Edwards RJ, Ujma J. Extreme methaemoglobinaemia secondary to recreational use of amyl nitrite. *J Accident Emerg Med* 1995;12:138–142.

406. Austin H, Delzell E, Cole, P. Benzene and leukemia. A review of the literature and a risk assessment. *Am J Epidemiol* 1988;127:419–439.

407. Snyder R, Kalf GF. A perspective on benzene leukemogenesis. *Crit Rev Toxicol* 1994;24:177–209.

408. Savitz DA, Andrews KW. Review of epidemiologic evidence on benzene and lymphatic and hematopoietic cancers. *Am J Ind Med* 1997;31:287–295.

409. Marwick TH, Nakatani S, Haluska B, et al. Provocation of latent left ventricular outflow tract gradients with amyl nitrite and exercise in hypertrophic cardiomyopathy. *Am J Cardiol* 1995;75:805–819.

410. Rosoff MH, Cohen MV. Profound bradycardia after amyl nitrite in patients with a tendency to vasovagal episodes. *Br Heart J* 1986;55:97–100.

411. Klimmek R, Krettek C. Effects of amyl nitrite on circulation, respiration and blood homeostasis in cyanide

poisoning. *Arch Toxicol* 1988;62:161–166.

412. Mathew RJ, Wilson WH, Tant SR. Regional cerebral blood flow changes associated with amyl nitrite inhalation. *Br J Addict* 1989;84:293–299.

413. Rees DC, Knisely JS, Balster RL, et al. Pentobarbital-like discriminative stimulus properties of halothane, 1,1,1-trichloroethane, isoamyl nitrite, flurothyl and oxazepam in mice. *J Pharmacol Exp Ther* 1987;241:507–515.

414. Guss DA, Normann SA, Manoguerra AS. Clinically significant methemoglobinemia from inhalation of isobutyl nitrite. *Am J Emerg Med* 1985;3:46–47.

415. Smith M, Stair T, Rolnick MA. Butyl nitrite and a suicide attempt. *Ann Intern Med* 1980;92:719–720.

416. Lotzova E, Savary CA, Hersh EM, et al. Depression of murine natural killer cell cytotoxicity by isobutyl nitrite. *Cancer Immunol Immunother* 1984;17:130–134.

417. Dax EM, Lange WR, Jaffe JH. Allergic reactions to amyl nitrite inhalation. *Am J Med* 1989;86:732.

418. Osterloh J, Goldfield D. Butyl nitrite transformation *in vitro*, chemical nitrosation reactions, and mutagenesis. *J Anal Toxicol* 1984;8:164–169.

419. Ostrow DG, DiFrancesico WJ, Chmiel JS, et al. A case-control study of human immunodeficiency virus type 1 seroconversion and risk-related behaviors in the Chicago MACS/CCS Cohort, 1984–1992 Multicenter AIDS Cohort Study. *Am J Epidemiol* 1994;142:875–883.

420. Burcham JL, Tindall B, Marmor M, et al. Incidence and risk factors for human immunodeficiency virus seroconversion in a cohort of Sydney homosexual men. *Med J Aust* 1989;150:634–639.

421. Newell GR, Adams SC, Mansell PWA, et al. Toxicity, immunosuppressive effects and carcinogenic potential of volatile nitrites: possible relationship to Kaposi's sarcoma. *Pharmacotherapy* 1984;4:284–291.

422. Seage GR, Mayer KH, Horsburgh CR Jr, et al. The relation between nitrite inhalants, unprotected receptive anal intercourse, and the risk of human immunodeficiency virus infection. *Am J Epidemiol* 1992;135:1–11.

423. Chesney MA, Barrett DC, Stall R. Histories of substance abuse and risk behavior. Precursors to HIV seroconversion in homosexual men. *Am J Public Health* 1998;88:113–116.

424. Moss AR, Osmond D, Bacchetti P, et al. Risk factors for AIDS and HIV seropositivity in homosexual men. *Am J Epidemiol* 1987;125:1035–1047.

425. Mirvish SS, Haverkos HW. Butyl nitrite in the induction of Kaposi's sarcoma in AIDS [Letter]. *N Engl J Med* 1987;317:1603.

426. Yamamoto M, Ishiwata H, Yamada T, et al. Studies in the guinea-pig stomach on the formation of *N*-nitrosomethylurea, from methylurea and sodium nitrite, and its disappearance. *Food Chem Toxicol* 1987;25:663–668.

427. Klimmek R, Krettek C, Werner HW. Ferrihaemoglobin formation by amyl nitrite and sodium nitrite in different species *in vivo* and *in vitro*. *Arch Toxicol* 1988;62:152–160.

428. Osterloh JD, Goldfield D. Uptake of inhaled *n*-butyl nitrite and *in vivo* transformation in rats. *J Pharm Sci* 1985;74:780–782.

429. Dunkel VC, Rogers-Back AM, Lawlor TE, et al. Mutagenicity of some alkyl nitrites used as recreational drugs. *Environ Mol Mutagen* 1989;14:115–122.

430. Lewis DM, Lynch DW. Toxicity of inhaled isobutyl nitrite in BALB/c mice: systemic and immunotoxic studies. *NIDA Res Monogr* 1988;83:50–58.

431. Jacobs RF, Marmer DJ, Steele RW, et al. Cellular immunotoxicity of amyl nitrite. *J Toxicol Clin Toxicol* 1983;20:421–449.

432. Soderberg LSF. Immunomodulation by nitrite inhalants may predispose abusers to AIDS and Kaposi's sarcoma. In: Sharp CW, ed. *Pharmaconeuroimmunology, a review. Advances in neuroimmunology.* Elmsford, NY: Pergamon Press, 1996.

433. Ratajczak HV, Thomas PT, House RV, et al. Local versus systemic immunotoxicity of isobutyl nitrite following subchronic inhalation exposure of female B6C3F1 mice. *Fund Appl Toxicol* 1995;27:177–184.

434. Soderberg LSF, Barnett JB. Inhaled isobutyl nitrite compromises T-dependent, but not T-independent antibody induction. *Int J Immunopharmacol* 1993;15:821–827.

435. Soderberg LSF, Barnett JB. Inhalation exposure to isobutyl nitrite inhibits macrophage tumoricidal activity and modulates inducible nitric oxide. *J Leukoc Biol* 1995;57:135–140.

436. Soderberg LSF. Increased tumor growth in mice exposed to inhaled isobutyl nitrite. *Toxicol Lett* 1999;104:35–41.

437. Pinkhas J, Cohen I, Kruglak J, et al. Hobby induced factor VII deficiency. *Haemeostasis* 1972;1:52–54.

438. Hersh JH, Podruch PE, Rogers G, et al. Toluene embryopathy. *J Pediatr* 1985;106:922–927.

439. Hersh JH. Toluene embryopathy: two new cases. *J Med Genet* 1989;26:333–337.

440. Pearson MA, Hoyme HE, Seaver LH, et al. Toluene embryopathy: delineation of the phenotype and comparison with fetal alcohol syndrome. *Pediatrics* 1994;93:211–215.

441. Wilkins-Haug L. Teratogen update: toluene. *Teratology* 1997;55:145–151.

442. Donald JM, Hooper K, Hopenhayn-Rich C. Reproductive and developmental toxicity of toluene: a review. *Environ Health Perspect* 1991;94:237–244.

443. Ono A, Sekita K, Ohno K, et al. Reproductive and developmental toxicity studies of toluene. I. Teratogenicity study of inhalation exposure in pregnant rats. *J Toxicol Sci* 1995;20:109–134.

444. Brown-Woodman PD, Webster WS, Picker K, et al. Embryotoxicity of xylene and toluene: an *in vitro* study. *Ind Health* 1991;29:139–152.

445. Pryor GT. Animal research on solvent abuse. *NIDA Res Monogr* 1992;129:233–258.

446. Hass U, Lund SP, Hougaard KS, et al. Developmental neurotoxicity after toluene inhalation exposure in rats. *Neurotox Teratol* 1999;21:349–357.

447. Jones HE, Balster RL. Inhalant abuse in pregnancy. *Obstet Gynecol Clin North Am* 1998;25(1):153–167.

448. Jones HE, Balster RL. Neurobehavioral consequences of intermittent prenatal exposure to high concentrations of toluene. *Neurotoxicol Teratol* 1997;19(4):305–313.

449. Gospe SM, Zhou SS. Prenatal exposure to toluene results in abnormal neurogenesis and migration in rat somatosensory cortex. *Pediatr Res* 2000;47(3):362–368.

450. Coleman CN, Mason T, Hooker EP, et al. Developmental effects of intermittent prenatal exposure to 1,1,1-trichloroethane in the rat. *Neurotoxicol Teratol* 1999;21(6):699–708.

451. Mazze RI, Fujinaga M, Baden JM. Halothane prevents nitrous oxide teratogenicity in Sprague-Dawley rats; folinic acid does not. *Teratology* 1988;38:121–131.

452. Cagen SZ, Klaassen CD. Hepatoxicity of carbon tetrachloride in developing rats. *Toxicol Appl Pharmacol* 1979;50:347–354.

453. Murray FJ, Schwetz BA, McBride JG, et al. Toxicity of inhaled chloroform in pregnant mice and their offspring. *Toxicol Appl Pharmacol* 1979;50:515–522.

454. Eskenazi B, Gaylord L, Bracken MB, et al. In utero exposure to organic solvents and human neurodevelopment. *Dev Med Child Neurol* 1988;30:492–501.

CHAPTER 21
Designer Drugs

JOHN P. MORGAN

"Designer" jeans all resemble Levi's. Similarly, "designer drugs" are imitative but not innovative. As a slogan, the phrase has notable media persistence because it provokes the image of a clever unaffiliated chemist in a hidden laboratory manipulating psychoactive chemicals toward new highs and dangers. However, most of the illegally designed drugs have been made by underground chemists simply following published syntheses. A search of the biomedical literature in 1996, using the subject heading *designer drug,* located papers almost always about methylenedioxymethamphetamine (MDMA or ecstasy). This chemical was first synthesized in 1910, and was patented by a pharmaceutical company in 1914 (1).

Until 100 years ago, only plants yielded psychoactive drug products. However, in the late nineteenth and early twentieth centuries, medicinal chemists began producing synthetic chemicals that could alter mood, change consciousness, induce pleasure, and modify unwanted feelings. Essentially all of the synthetic chemicals that have been used illicitly for psychoactivity (amphetamine, barbiturates, amyl nitrite, methaqualone) were initially made by pharmaceutical chemists seeking better treatments for disease. Sometime during their approved history, they were diverted for unsanctioned use. Additionally, some psychoactive chemicals never became commercial products. Illicit synthesis using methods published by pharmaceutical chemists always supplied the market for unsanctioned use. Among these are phencyclidine, lysergic acid diethylamide (LSD), 4-methylaminorex, and MDMA.

When Henderson (2) coined the term designer drug, he was characterizing successful attempts to produce fentanyl analogues that were legal, as well as potent and lucrative. The volume of use (and manufacture) of synthetic illegal drugs remains low in comparison to the ingestion of the botanical psychoactives cocaine, heroin, and cannabis; although it has been said that as much MDMA is now consumed in Great Britain as is marihuana (3). The products of illegal chemists are much feared. However, their output is modest. Since the 1992 edition of this book (4) only one new illicitly synthesized chemical, methcathinone, has become of any clinical importance. There is no evidence that difficult syntheses are undertaken underground and there is no evidence of increasing precision promoting bioavailability, distribution to the brain, or receptor tuning. The toxic opioid analogue MPTP (*N*-methyl-4-phenyl-1,2,3,6-tetrahydropyridine) is produced by careless management of temperature and pH during the attempted manufacture of MPPP (4′-methyl-α-pyrrolidinopropiophenone), as dis-

cussed later in this chapter. For a synthesized product to enter the illicit psychoactive market, it must produce a desired effect but should also be economical for clandestine manufacture. It must be easily made, and the precursors easily obtained.

The phrase controlled substance analogues could replace the confusing term designer drug, if any classification other than synthetic is needed. The Controlled Substances Act was amended to include the Controlled Substances Analogues Enforcement Act in 1986. According to this law, a controlled substance analogue to be classified as illegal is "substantially similar" to the chemical structure of an already controlled substance in Schedule I or II. Shulgin (5) believes that the phrase is essentially imprecise. Is a chemical substantially similar if it is an analogue; a homologue; or an isomer? Early decisions classified MDMA as "substantially similar" to methamphetamine. Some decisions evoke the pornography allusion of Supreme Court Justice Potter Stewart. No one can exactly define the standard but jurists and jurors know a "controlled substance analogue" when they see one.

The analysis that follows discusses only five important synthetic products (and a few analogues):

1. Congeners of the potent synthetic opioid fentanyl
2. The meperidine congener MPPP and its highly toxic contaminant MPTP
3. MDMA and some analogous phenethylamines
4. 4-Methylaminorex ("U4Euh") and its precedent analogue aminorex
5. Methcathinone (ephedrone), sometimes called "cat" or "jeff"

The section on MDMA is longer than all other discussions combined because its use is common, its market may be expanding, and toxicity is frequently reported.

OPIOID ANALOGUES

Opioid products are at the heart of the concern over controlled substance analogues. A number of congeners of the potent opioid fentanyl have appeared in illicit trade and were responsible for death in heroin injectors who were insufficiently tolerant. A meperidine analogue, 1-methyl-4-propionoxy-4-phenylpyridine (MPPP), was synthesized illicitly but because of preparation problems became contaminated with 1-methy-4-phenyl-1,2,3,6-tetrahydropyridine (MPTP). This drug causes a parkinsonian syndrome in humans and has become an important research tool in understanding pathology in the basal ganglion.

Fentanyl Analogues

In 1979, a series of unusual deaths occurred in Orange County, California. The fatalities occurred in heroin

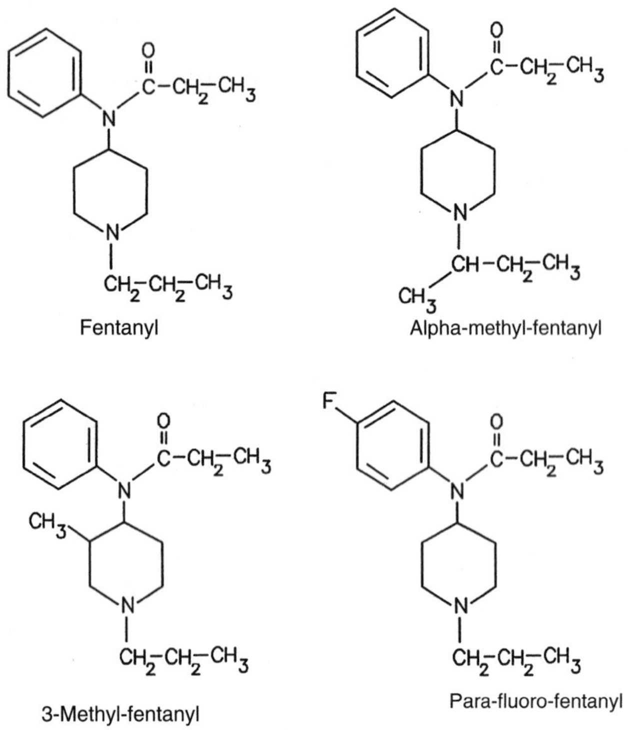

FIG. 21.1. Chemical structure of fentanyl, α-methyl-fentanyl, 3-methyl-fentanyl, and para-fluoro-fentanyl.

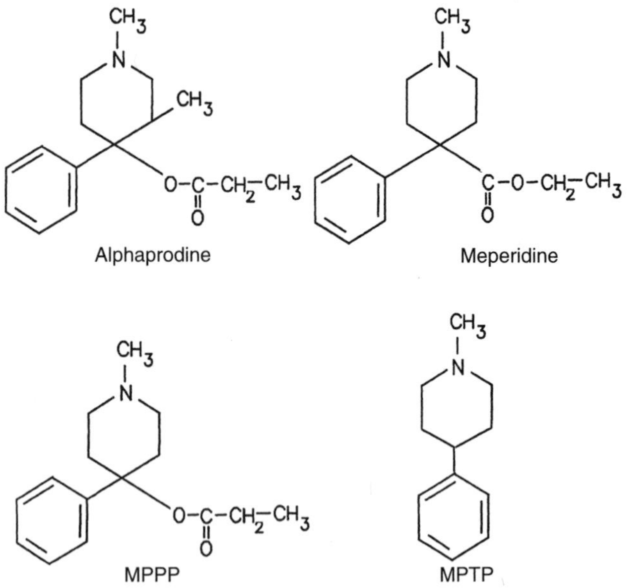

FIG. 21.2. Chemical structure of alphaprodine, meperidine, MPPP, and MPTP.

injectors and resembled heroin overdose but toxicologic analysis was negative. By the end of 1980, 15 such fatalities had been recorded. The toxin was later identified as an analogue of the legal opioid fentanyl α-methyl-fentanyl. It had been promoted in street sales as "China White" (sometimes a name for purported high-quality heroin). Between 1981 and 1984, at least three other analogues were identified in street drug samples and in the bodily fluids of overdose victims: α-methyl-acetyl-fentanyl, 3-methyl-fentanyl, and para-fluoro-fentanyl (Fig. 21.1). 3-Methyl-fentanyl (TMF) is approximately 6,000 times as potent as morphine. By the end of 1984, an apparent decline in use of these products had occurred as had the number of deaths, although perhaps 10 even more unusual analogues were identified. Writing in 1988, Henderson estimated that more than 100 deaths had occurred (only 3 outside California) (6).

However, TMF moved to the East Coast during 1988, and at least 16 overdose deaths occurred in and around Pittsburgh (7). TMF was not always identifiable as the sole cause of death but was detected in bodily fluids. The article describing the Pittsburgh deaths appeared in the *Journal of the American Medical Association* shortly after more deaths secondary to TMF were reported in *The New York Times*. The *Times* article described at least 17 deaths and a number of hospitalizations in New York City, Hartford, Connecticut, and Patterson, New Jersey (8).

Potency

Although it is likely that any marketed controlled substance analogue will be relatively potent, a potent opioid has particular dangerous significance. Many users of street heroin do not attain significant levels of tolerance even though previously low-quality, adulterated street heroin has improved. Additionally, "regular" injectors of heroin spend much time not using (9) and may often be susceptible to overdose with any potent material. It is not that fentanyl or its profoundly potent analogues cause a better high or more respiratory depression than heroin, it is that they do it in such a small volume of white powder.

MPTP

The illicit synthesis of the meperidine congener MPPP (Fig. 21.2) was effected as early as 1977 by a young man in Bethesda, Maryland. He developed Parkinson disease and the sequence was understood and described by Davis and his coworkers in 1979 (10).

MPPP, a close relative of meperidine, had previously been tested as an analgesic but possessed insufficient activity. The synthesis is particularly likely to be contaminated with the MPTP congener under conditions of inadequate control of temperature and pH. In 1982 in California, a number of injectors who had purchased "street heroin" developed parkinsonian symptoms and subsequent analysis of the product identified both MPTP and MPPP. The scientists who described this phenomenon reported that the description of the synthesis of MPPP had been carefully excised from journal pages in the Stanford Medical School

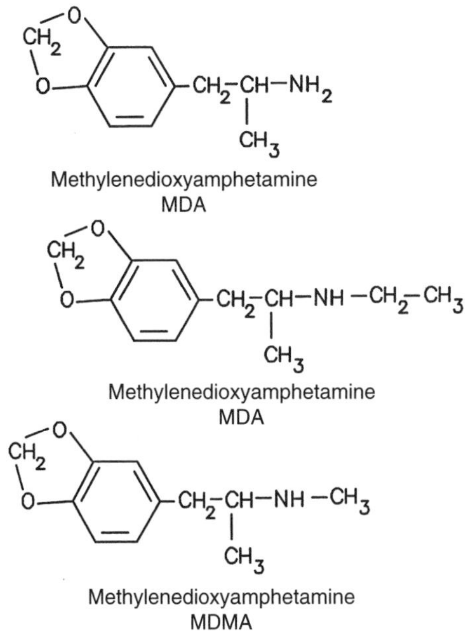

FIG. 21.3. Chemical structure of methylenedioxyamphetamine (MDA), methylenedioxyethylamphetamine (MDEA), and methylenedioxymethamphetamine (MDMA).

library (11). Primates given MPTP develop a parkinsonian syndrome secondary to destruction of dopaminergic neurons in the substantia nigra (12). MPTP may cause occupational Parkinson disease. One reported case involved a chemist who had conducted repeated synthetic reactions involving MPTP. Exposure may have occurred through accidental inhalation or skin contamination (13). Followup studies indicate that susceptibility to the toxicity is variable. All exposed to MPTP do not necessarily become ill. A review article in 1985 (14) estimated that of 300 exposed individuals, only 20 developed Parkinson disease.

Mechanism of Action

The neurotoxicity is not caused by MPTP itself but by a toxic metabolite. MPTP binds with high affinity to neural monoamine oxidase B and is converted to methylphenyldihydropyridine (MPP+). Interference with conversion by prior treatment with a monoamine oxidase inhibitor will prevent experimental toxicity. MPP+ is taken up by sensitive cells in the substantia nigra, reaches high intramitochondrial concentration, interferes with oxidative phosphorylation, and causes cellular death (15).

MDMA

MDMA and methylenedioxyamphetamine (MDA) (frequently referred to as designer amphetamines) were synthesized in 1910 (1) and patented by 1914 (Fig. 21.3). MDA was studied in humans as an appetite suppres-

sant in the 1950s and 1960s, but never marketed. It appeared as an illicit psychedelic in the late 1960s in the Haight-Ashbury district of San Francisco (16). Some early Canadian reports of serious toxicity may actually have involved paramethoxyamphetamine (PMA), an analogue believed to provoke severe hypertension (17). MDA was included in Schedule I of the (new) 1970 Controlled Substances Act. MDMA was ignored.

The author had an unusual personal experience in 1979 or 1980 involving the then largely unknown MDMA.

Two of my students approached me in 1979 or 1980 with two large, opaque white capsules. They had been purchased for $12 each at a party. The seller provided the students with an informational sheet I still possess. Copied from *Wet—The Magazine of Gourmet Bathing*, the article describes a drug called "XTC," identifying it as a close relative of MDA. The writer stated that some psychotherapists had found the drug useful, particularly in couples being counseled together, as a promoter of intimacy and communication. The article described the drug as legal under the Controlled Substance Act because of its chemical difference from MDA.

I told my student about reports of the hazards of MDA and also informed them that the claims in *Wet* were almost certain to be untrue, because claims regarding psychedelic exotica were frequently exaggerated. I was completely wrong. I sent a portion of the powder from one capsule for analysis. The first laboratory reported that the drug behaved as methamphetamine on thin-layer chromatography, but that this was not definitive. Later, a skilled analyst using gas chromatography and mass spectrometry identified the drug as "N-methylmethylenedioxyamphetamine." Unfortunately, I had given my students the news of the first analysis and one consumed the "methamphetamine" to stay awake for an all-night study session. He felt that it worked but not particularly well. A letter from Dr. A. T. Shulgin confirmed what *Wet* had published.

Shulgin and Nichols had referred to MDMA in 1978, describing the drug as producing an "easily managed" euphoria with emotional and sensual overtones (18). In correspondence, Shulgin described a group of psychotherapists who had begun to use the drug to facilitate therapeutic sessions and to promote communication and intimacy. This use of a phenethylamine psychedelic compound to assist psychotherapy had actually begun with MDA (19). Between 1978 and 1985, a network of such therapists and clients had grown in the United States. Most reports of the therapeutic outcome (admittedly uncontrolled) were positive. No serious toxicity occurred in these settings.

Two other recreational settings of use emerged by 1984. Groups of friends and invitees took the drug in small group social settings for fun and to enhance communication and intimacy. To some degree, this use related to the psychotherapeutic ideology. Later, a college-based urban party and dancing scene emerged (20). Large volumes of the drug were being manufactured in Boston, Arlington, Texas, and other cities. This casual and frequent use by young people attracted attention and, in 1984, the Drug Enforcement Agency (DEA) applied under the Controlled Substances Act to place MDMA in Schedule I on an emergency basis. Although there was evidence of widespread synthesis, marketing, and consumption, there was little evidence of harm. The only claim of toxicity presented by the DEA was a report of neurotoxic damage to rodent serotonergic brain cells not by MDMA but by MDA (21). There was significant legal opposition to the rescheduling by a group of psychotherapists and MDMA advocates who believed the drug to have legitimate value (22).

Effects

George Greer, a Santa Fe psychiatrist, had devised a protocol for MDMA use in therapy by 1983. He described administering the drug to 29 patients, usually beginning with 100 to 150 mg by mouth followed by an optional dose of 50 to 75 mg in 2 hours. His subjects reported positive feelings of closeness and an expanded perspective and insight into problematic conflicts or feelings (23). Other positive studies and reports were generated, including that of Liester et al. who questioned 20 psychiatrists who had previously taken MDMA (24). This report was also positive but listed some adverse effects, including a decreased desire to perform mental or physical work, decreased appetite, and trismus.

After 1986, when the drug was placed in Schedule I, use continued by young people in clubs. This early dance phenomenon (referred to as Acid House) evolved, particularly in Britain, Ireland, Western Europe, and later North America, into "raves." These are organized, large social events initially held in large warehouses—later in dance halls and clubs. Young people would often dance all night to recorded and programmed "house" music accompanied by light shows and computer-generated video images. The preferred drug was MDMA and dancers consumed uncertain amounts of the illicit material. This phenomenon continues in Europe and North America and accounts for what is apparently an enormous volume of consumption. The phenomenon of social contemplative small group use also continues—probably supplied by the same illicit market—although at a smaller volume (20).

Neuropharmacology

MDMA possesses a variety of psychoactive properties and interacts with a variety of neurotransmitters. It is a stimulant with amphetamine-like actions and users may, soon after ingestion, experience tachycardia, increased blood pressure, dry mouth, anorexia, diminished fatigue, mood elevation, and jaw clenching. Frank hallucinations are rarely, if ever, experienced. The desired effects, which may occur in any of the situations of use, include euphoria, heightened sensuality, enhanced feeling of closeness, affection, and comfort in communication. Many subjects report a remarkable diminution of self-consciousness and embarrassment. Adverse consequences (seldom causing major distress) include gait instability, jaw clenching, a distaste for mental or physical tasks, fatigue, and nausea. Some MDMA effects are mediated by displacement of dopamine and norepinephrine. In discrimination studies, MDMA will substitute for d-amphetamine in animals trained to distinguish that stimulant from saline. Most studies also point to serotonergic activity. MDMA displaces serotonin (5-HT) from nerve terminals but shows little affinity for postsynaptic 5-HT receptors. It seems very likely that the positive feelings reported by users have much to do with enhanced availability of serotonin at the synapse (25).

Neurotoxicity

MDMA produces, in many animal species, dose-related reductions in brain serotonin and 5-hydroxyindoleacetic acid (5-HIAA). There is diminution of 5-HT uptake sites and diminished activity of tryptophan hydroxylase—a necessary enzyme for serotonin synthesis. This neurotoxicity has been seen with other serotonin displacers, including MDA, methamphetamine, and the once widely prescribed appetite suppressant fenfluramine (26) (now no longer on the market). The toxic dose in many animal species is quite high compared to the "usual" human dose of 1.0 to 2.0 mg/kg. However, in some nonhuman primates, the toxic dose is closer to the recreational dose in humans. The dosage issues were closely examined in a 1995 review by Granquist (27). In nonhuman primates, the toxicity is usually produced by a course of intramuscular or subcutaneous injection. Typically, primates are given, by injection, 5 to 20 mg/kg twice per day for 4 days. Not only does this exceed the usual human dose (often taken as a single dose), but injection increases the likelihood of toxicity (28). One study in nonhuman primates administered 2.5 mg/kg by mouth once every 2 weeks for a total of eight doses over 4 months. In this study, there was no evidence of neurotoxic response in assays of 5-HT and 5-HIAA in a number of regions of the brain (27). Another study in primates (2.5 mg/kg for eight doses) produced decreases in 5-HT and 5-HIAA, but [^{3}H]paroxetine binding was not altered. Such a finding suggests (but does not prove) that 5-HT synaptic terminals were intact despite the decreases in neurotransmitter and metabolite concentrations (29). There have been few published studies assessing serotonergic functions in humans. One 1994 study comparing frequent users to controls identified a decrease of 32% in cerebrospinal fluid concentration of 5-HIAA. There were no other indications of neurotoxicity and these subjects also had significantly greater non-MDMA amphetamine experience than the controls. Extensive psychological testing in these users documented the "abnormalities" of decreased impulsivity and hostility (30). Another human study examined serum prolactin following injection of 1-tryptophan. This assessment of serotonergic function identified some diminution of prolactin blood levels but the study was preliminary and uncontrolled (31). A similar study measuring serum prolactin and cortisol after *d*-fenfluramine injection in a group of extremely frequent British users is planned (32). A dose-ranging National Institute on Drug Abuse (NIDA)-funded study in humans is largely completed (33). It assessed many important outcome variables, including pharmacokinetic and cardiovascular data, sleep encephalopathy, fenfluramine challenge, and a variety of neuroimaging studies (positron emission tomography [PET] and single-photon emission computed tomography [SPECT]).

General Toxicity

In England, there have been many reports of systemic toxic effects. These include reports of cardiac arrhythmia (34), aplastic anemia (35), and hepatotoxicity (36). There have been more frequent reports of a syndrome at raves that is probably related to extreme hyperthermia and dehydration. Some of these dancers underwent rhabdomyolysis, disseminated intravascular coagulation, renal failure, and death (34). It is generally believed that these disastrous clinical events are preventable by adequate hydration and adequate room cooling. Such advice is frequently provided to ravers. These serious consequences have been confined to England with no such reports in Holland or the United States.

Assays of MDMA

Some of the toxicities may relate to contamination and impurities in the illicit MDMA marketplace. A number of assays of MDMA preparations have been conducted and regular postings of assays and appearance of European products occur on the World Wide Web (see http://www.ecstasy.org). A recent survey of 22 American samples revealed that 8 had no MDMA at all, but 2 of these contained the MDMA analogue methylenedioxyethylamphetamine (MDE). This congener (also illegal) appears in European samples as well. Some American samples contained over-the-counter pharmaceuticals, including phenylpropanolamine, dextromethorphan, ephedrine guaifenesin, and caffeine. Unidentified fillers, binders, and "cuts" were included. Despite frequent claims (particularly in New York City), there were no American products containing heroin, ketamine, rat poison, or ground glass (37).

Nexus

The DEA has placed one other analogue, 4-bromo,3-4,dimethoxy-phenethylamine in Schedule I. This drug, often called *nexus* or *2-CB*, has MDMA-like properties in much lower doses (0.1 to 0.2 mg/kg) but is not widely distributed (38). 2-CB is also discussed in a remarkable and well-written novel, linking drug experience narratives to 179 distinct phenethylamines. This roman à clef also contains information on the synthesis of the drugs. The book has focused much attention (wanted and unwanted) on its authors—a medicinal chemist and his spouse. The title *PIHKAL* stands for "Phenethylamines I Have Known and Loved" (39).

4-METHYLAMINOREX (4MAM OR "U4Euh")

This compound was the first example of a controlled substance analogue stimulant. Currently, there is little evidence of widespread use, and its clinical importance is unassessed. The widespread availability of cocaine and synthetic methamphetamine may deter attempts to manufacture stimulant controlled substance analogues. 4-Methylaminorex has generally been sold in illicit markets as "U4Euh." This product was first synthesized by McNeil Laboratories in the 1960s and, like MDA, evaluated as an anorectic. It is illicitly synthesized from the widely available over-the-counter drug phenylpropanolamine. It is associated with one fatality and was moved to Schedule I by the DEA (40). This drug was never marketed, but a nonmethylated version (aminorex) was marketed in Europe as an appetite depressant in 1965. It was frequently associated with severe pulmonary hypertension and was withdrawn in 1968 (41). Reportedly, aminorex itself has recently appeared in illicit trade in America (42). Structurally, it most resembles the relatively mild prescription stimulant pemoline (Fig. 21.4). At oral doses of 10 to 20 mg, 4-MAM reportedly provokes a smooth episode of enhanced intellectual energy lasting 10 to 12 hours. Its advocates claim that work is facilitated not only without

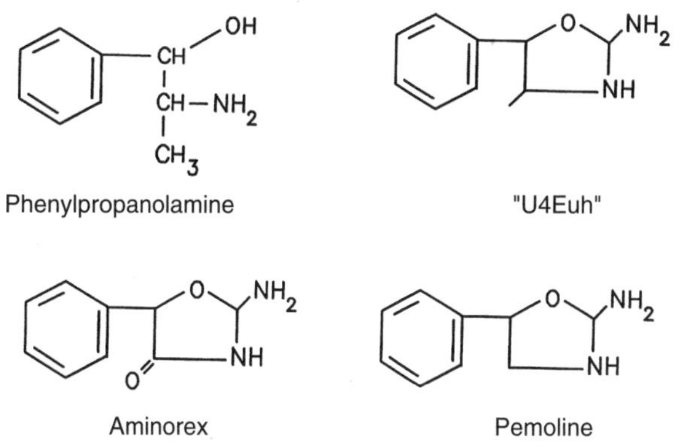

FIG. 21.4. Chemical structure of phenylpropanolamine, "U4Euh," aminorex, and pemoline.

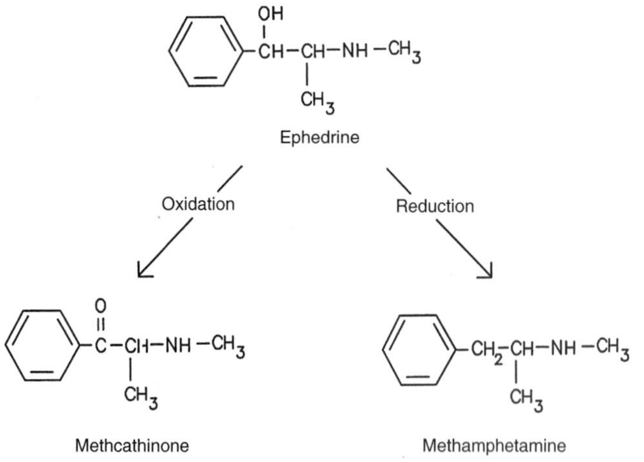

FIG. 21.5. Chemical structure of ephedrine, an oxidative precursor to methcathinone and a reductive precursor to methamphetamine.

agitation but with a diminution of anxiety. There is one published opinion that it should be carefully assessed in humans for potential benefits (43).

METHCATHINONE

A number of possible stimulant compounds appear in the khat plant (*Catha edulis*). It is now believed that cathinone is the chief active ingredient producing amphetamine-like effects when the leaves are chewed in the khat ceremony (44). In the 1950s, Parke-Davis conducted studies on an analogue of cathinone, methcathinone. There are no available human data but animal studies revealed a series of effects closely parallel to those of *d*-amphetamine. In 1987, Glennon et al. performed a number of behavioral studies confirming the stimulant actions of this product. Animals trained to discriminate *d*-amphetamine from saline would substitute methcathinone. Methcathinone, like amphetamine, displaces [³H]dopamine from rat cells in the caudate nucleus (45).

Methcathinone (called ephedrone) emerged as a marketed illicit drug in Russia. It was prominently used by heroin injectors in a "speedball" combination (46). Reportedly, Russian users would also use the drug alone in intravenous (IV) binges resembling a methamphetamine pattern first reported in the United States in the late 1960s.

The drug appeared in commerce in rural Michigan in 1991, reportedly having been manufactured in clandestine laboratories in the upper peninsula of that state. It was quickly placed into Schedule I of the Controlled Substances Act in 1992. Emerson and Cisek described four patients admitted to Michigan emergency rooms after episodes of IV use. These physicians also collected questionnaire data from 17 users in Michigan who sought the drug for its stimulant properties. Many were intranasal users. Snorting was followed by euphoria and excitement with enhancement of visual perception. Such use produced 5 to 8 hours of enhanced energy, feelings of toughness and invincibility, and increased sexual desire. Subsequent doses were said to push users from "speeding" to "tripping" with more visual effects and even hallucinations. Use was frequently accompanied by headaches, abdominal cramps, sweating, and tachycardia (47).

The drug is said to have spread from Michigan to other Midwestern states. Its appearance may lead to further restrictions on the availability of ephedrine—an oxidative precursor to "cat" and a reductive precursor to "ice" (Fig. 21.5).

CONCLUSION

It is unclear how often and with what impact synthetic chemicals will emerge onto the illicit psychoactive market. It is also unclear how toxic such products are likely to be. The assessment of toxicity is always difficult because of the overheated character of media and police reports when such products appear (48). Ten years after the emergence of "designer drugs," their continuing impact remains poorly defined.

REFERENCES

1. Mannich C, Jacobson W. Uber oxyphenylalkylamine und Dioxyphenylalkylamine. *Berl Dtsch Chem Ges* 1910;43:189.
2. Henderson GL. Designer drugs: past history and future prospects. *J Forensic Sci* 1988;33:569–575.
3. Karch S. Ecstasy in Europe. *Forensic Drug Abuse Advisor (FDAA)* 1995; 7:78.
4. Lowinson J, Ruiz P, Millman RB. *Substance abuse: a comprehensive textbook,* 2nd ed. Baltimore: Williams & Wilkins, 1992.
5. Shulgin AT. How similar is substantially similar? *J Forensic Sci* 1990;35: 10–12.
6. Henderson GL. Blood concentration of fentanyl and its analogs in overdose victims. *Proc West Pharmacol Soc* 1983;26:287–290.
7. Hibbs J, Perper J, Winek C. An outbreak of designer-drug related deaths in Pennsylvania. *JAMA* 1991;265:1011–1013.
8. Nieves E. Toxic heroin has killed 12, officials say. *The New York Times* 1991 Feb 4:B1–B2.
9. Johnson BD, Goldstein PJ, Preble E, et al. *Taking care of business: the economics of crime by heroin users.* Lexington, MA: Lexington Books, 1985.
10. Davis GC, Williams AS, Markey SP, et al. Chronic parkinsonism secondary to intravenous injection of meperidine analogues. *Psychiatry Res* 1979;1:249–254.
11. Langston JW, Ballard PA, Tetrud JW, et al. Chronic parkinsonism in human due to a product of meperidine-analogue synthesis. *Science* 1983;219: 979–980.
12. Burns RS, Chiueh CC, Markey SP,

et al. A primate model of parkinsonism: selective destruction of dopaminergic neurons in the pars compacta
of the substantia nigra by 1-methyl-4-
phenyl-1,2,3,6-tetrahydropyridine. *Proc
Natl Acad Sci U S A* 1983;80:4546–
4550.
13. Langston JW, Ballard PA. Parkinson's disease in a chemist working with
1-methyl-4-phenyl-1,2,3,6-tetrahydropy-
ridine. *N Engl J Med* 1983;309:
310.
14. Bianchine JR, McGhee B. MPTP and
parkinsonism. *Ration Drug Ther* 1985;
19:5–7.
15. D'Amato RJ, Lipman LP, Synder SH.
Selectivity of the parkinsonian neurotoxin MPTP: toxic metabolite MPP+
binds to neuromelanin. *Science* 1986;
231:987–989.
16. Meyers F, Rose A, Smith D. Incidents
involving the Haight-Ashbury population and some uncommonly used drugs.
J Psychedelic Drugs 1967–1968;1:140–
146.
17. Beck J. MDMA: the popularization and
resultant implications of a recently controlled psychoactive substance. *Contemp
Drug Probl* 1986;13:23–63.
18. Shulgin AT, Nichols D. Characterization of three new psychotomimetics.
In: Stillman RC, Willette RE, eds. *The
psychopharmacology of hallucinogens.*
New York: Pergamon Press, 1978.
19. Naranjo C, Shulgin AT, Sargent T. Evaluation of 3,4-methylenedioxyamphe-
tamine (MDA) as an adjunct to psychotherapy. *Medicine et Pharmacologia
Experimentalis* 1967;17:359–364.
20. Beck J, Rosenbaum M. *Pursuit of ecstasy: the MDMA experience. Worlds of
ecstasy: who uses ecstasy?* Albany, NY:
SUNY Press, 1994:27–55.
21. Ricaurte G, Bryan G, Strauss L, et al.
Hallucinogenic amphetamine selectively
destroys brain serotonin nerve terminals.
Science 1985;229:986–988.
22. Beck J, Rosenbaum M. Scheduling of
MDMA ("ecstasy"). In: Inciardi J, ed.
*The handbook of drug control in the
United States.* Westport, CT: Greenwood
Press, 1990.

23. Greer G. *MDMA: a new psychotropic
compound and its effect in humans.* Sante
Fe, NM: Author, 1983.
24. Liester MB, Grob CS, Bravo GL, et
al. Phenomenology and sequelae of 3,4-
methylenedioxymethamphetamine use.
J Nerv Ment Dis 1992;180:345–352.
25. Steele TD, McCann UD, Ricaurte GA.
3,4-Methylenedioxymethamphetamine
(MDMA, "ecstasy"): pharmacology and
toxicology in animals and human.
Addiction 1994;89:539–551.
26. Schuster C, Lewis M, Seiden L. Fenfluramine: neurotoxicity. *Psychopharmacol
Bull* 1988;22:148–151.
27. Granquist L. Neurochemical markers
and MDMA neurotoxicity. *Multidisciplinary Association for Psychedelic
Studies (MAPS) Newsletter* 1995;5:10–
13.
28. Ricaurte GA, DeLanney LE, Irwin I,
et al. Toxic effects of MDMA on central serotonergic neurons in the primate:
importance of route and frequency of administration. *Brain Res* 1988;446:165–
168.
29. Insel TR, Battaglia G, Johannessen
JN, et al. 3-4-Methylenedioxymetham-
phetamine ("ecstasy") selectively destroys brain serotonin terminals in Rhesus monkeys. *J Pharmacol Exp Ther*
1989;249:713–720.
30. McCann UD, Ridenour A, Shaham
Y, et al. Serotonin neurotoxicity after
(±)3,4-methylenedioxymethamphetami-
ne (MDMA, "ecstasy"): a controlled
study in humans. *Neuropsychopharmacology* 1994;10:129–138.
31. Price LH, Ricaurte GA, Krystal JH,
et al. Neuroendocrine and mood responses to intravenous L-tryptophan in
(±)3,4-methylenedioxymethamphetami-
ne (MDMA) users. *Arch Gen Psychiatry*
1989;46:20–22.
32. Jansen KLR. MDMA (ecstasy) studies at the Maudsley Hospital. *Multidisciplinary Association for Psychedelic
Studies (MAPS) Newsletter* 1996;6:7.
33. Grob C. Harbor-UCLA MDMA project
update Feb. *Multidisciplinary Association for Psychedelic Studies (MAPS)
Newsletter* 1995;5:2.

34. Henry J, Jeffreys K, Dawling S. Toxicity and deaths from 3,4-methylene-
dioxymethamphetamine ("ecstasy").
Lancet 1992;340:384–387.
35. Marsh JC, Abboudi ZH, Gibson FM,
et al. Aplastic anaemia following exposure to 3,4-methylenedioxymetham-
phetamine ("ecstasy"). *Br J Haematol*
1994;88:281–285.
36. O'Connor B. Hazards associated with the
recreational drug "ecstasy." *Br J Hosp
Med* 1994;52:507, 510–514.
37. Doblin R. MDMA analysis project.
*Multidisciplinary Association for Psy-
chedelic Studies (MAPS) Newsletter*
1996;6:11–13.
38. Karch S. Nexus banned by DEA. *Forensic Drug Abuse Advisor (FDAA)* 1994;
6:12.
39. Shulgin AT, Shulgin A. *PIHKAL: a
chemical love story.* Berkeley, CA:
Transform Press, 1991.
40. Davis FT, Brewster ME. A fatality involving "U4Euh," a cyclic derivative
of phenylpropanolamine. *J Forensic Sci*
1988;33:549–553.
41. Follath F. Drug-induced pulmonary hypertension? *Br Med J* 1971;1:265–266.
42. Karch S. Aminorex banned. *Forensic
Drug Abuse Advisor (FDAA)* 1994;6:
38.
43. Doblin R. 4-Methylaminorex. *Multidisciplinary Association for Psychedelic Studies (MAPS) Newsletter* 1996;
6:121.
44. Kalix P. Pharmacological properties of
the stimulant khat. *Pharmacol Ther*
1990;48:397–416.
45. Glennon RA, Yousif M, Naiman N,
et al. Methcathinone: a new and potent amphetamine-like agent. *Pharmacol
Biochem Behav* 1987;26:547–551.
46. Zhinge YK, Dovensky BS, Crossman
A, et al. Ephedrone: 2-methylamine-1-
phenylpropan-1-one (Jeff). *J Forensic
Sci* 1991;36:915–920.
47. Emerson TS, Cisek JE. Methcathinone:
a Russian designer amphetamine infiltrates the rural Midwest. *Ann Emerg Med*
1993;22:1897–1903.
48. Hettena S. Year of the cat. *Spin* 1995;10:
67–69, 90.

CHAPTER 22

MDMA

CHARLES S. GROB AND
RUSSELL E. POLAND

MDMA (3,4-methylenedioxymethamphetamine) is a novel psychoactive compound with structural similarities to both amphetamine and the psychedelic phenethylamine, mescaline. As was the case with the psychedelics three decades ago, MDMA has been at the center of a virulent controversy since the early 1980s, pitting proponents of its use as an adjunctive psychiatric treatment against those who argue that it poses a grave threat to public health and safety. By recapitulating the generational and cultural divides catalyzed by widespread use of lysergic acid diethylamide (LSD) and related compounds in the 1960s, the growing use of MDMA by young people has confounded and shifted debate from one examining the relative risks and benefits of a putative psychiatric treatment to questions addressing social control and protection of youth. Encompassing challenges to conventional cultural norms, defenses of social stability, and the inevitable media distortion and sensationalism, MDMA, as did psychedelics 30 years earlier, has become an issue of "more than medical significance" (126).

HISTORICAL BACKGROUND

MDMA was first synthesized in 1912 by chemists working for Merck Pharmaceuticals in Germany, who were attempting to create a new medication to stop bleeding. As an intermediate step in the synthesis of the styptic medication hydrastinine, MDMA itself was of little interest and was only included in the patent application as a secondary chemical compound. The Merck patent was approved in 1914, and has long since expired (81,174,176). In the early 1950s, as part of systematic U.S. Army Intelligence research on potential psychotropic drug applications to espionage and counterespionage endeavors, MDMA once again came to the attention of research pharmacologists. Allocated to the Edgewood Arsenal's Chemical Warfare Service, and provided the code name EA-1475, MDMA was administered to a variety of animals for standard median lethal dose (LD_{50}) screening. Plans to initiate human trials with MDMA were abandoned, however, following the tragic and untimely death in 1953 of a subject enrolled in a U.S. Army contract study at the New York State Psychiatric Institute who had received "forced injections" of EA-1298, or MDA (3,4-methylenedioxyamphetamine), an analogue and an active metabolite of MDMA (96). As a testimony to the capricious and often unethical "research" conducted under the auspices of U.S. intelligence

services during this period, one of the lead investigators of the fatal MDA study would later state, "We didn't know whether it was dog piss or what it was we were giving him" (105).

As with many of the powerful consciousness-altering compounds examined by the CIA and U.S. Army Intelligence, the 1960s witnessed a proliferation of information and interest in the phenethylamine psychedelics within the growing counterculture movement. MDA in particular enjoyed a brief period of popularity in the late 1960s and early 1970s, when it was euphemistically attributed the exotic name of the "love drug." MDMA, however, remained largely unknown to psychedelic enthusiasts and would not be examined until the mid-1970s when University of California Berkeley biochemist and toxicologist Alexander Shulgin, acting on the suggestion of a student who claimed to have successfully alleviated a severe stutter with the drug, synthesized and self-administered 120 mg of the compound (176). He would later describe MDMA as evoking "an easily controlled altered state of consciousness with emotional and sensual overtones, and with little hallucinatory effect" (175).

Highly impressed with the drug's apparent capacity to induce heightened states of empathic rapport, a critical component of successful psychotherapy, Shulgin introduced several psychiatrist and psychologist acquaintances to MDMA's unusual profile of action. Their responses, both to their own subjective experience, as well as responses from patients who had received the drug, were an unequivocal endorsement of MDMA's apparent capacity to facilitate the process of psychotherapy. For the remainder of the 1970s, a quiet underground of psychotherapists, particularly on the West Coast of the United States, conducted thousands of MDMA-augmented treatments with what at that time was still a legal and uncontrolled substance. Although, unfortunately, no methodological research was conducted to substantiate MDMA's alleged efficacy in alleviating psychological distress and modifying maladaptive personality structures, testimonials to its therapeutic range of action abounded. Unbridled enthusiasm for this novel, and as yet unsubstantiated, treatment was best summed up by a psychiatrist colleague of Shulgin's who told him, "MDMA is penicillin for the soul, and you don't give up penicillin, once you've seen what it can do" (176).

Sensitive to the fate suffered in the 1960s by proponents of psychiatric research and treatment with psychedelics once word of their highly unusual effects had been disseminated to the culture at large (65,68), knowledge of MDMA remained a tightly guarded secret among practitioners of its use and their patients for several years. By the early 1980s, however, word of MDMA had filtered out, abetted by media accounts of a new psychotherapeutic "miracle medicine" and the spread of an alternative recreational drug on some college campuses (particularly in California and Texas), where, for a period of time, MDMA replaced cocaine as the new drug of choice. First popularly called Adam during its early phase of use among psychotherapists, to signify "the condition of primal innocence and unity with all life" (1), it soon acquired the alternative appellation of "ecstasy," the name by which it is popularly known to this day. Indeed, the transformation of MDMA as "Adam" into MDMA as "ecstasy" appears to have been a marketing decision reached by an enterprising distributor searching for an alternative code name, who concluded that it would not be profitable to take advantage of the drug's most salient features. "Ecstasy was chosen for obvious reasons," this individual later reported, "because it would sell better than calling it 'Empathy.' 'Empathy' would be more appropriate, but how many people know what it means?" (48).

By 1984, with growing use on college campuses and increased media attention and embellishment, political pressure was placed on federal regulators to establish tight controls on what was still a legal drug. Consequently, in 1985 the U.S. Drug Enforcement Agency (DEA) convened hearings to determine the fate of MDMA. These highly publicized hearings achieved the unintended effect of further raising public awareness of MDMA, as well as interest in experimentation. Media accounts further polarized opinion, pitting enthusiastic claims of MDMA by proponents against dire warnings of unknown dangers to the nation's youth. Coverage of the MDMA scheduling controversy included a national daytime television talk show (the Phil Donahue program) highlighting the surprising disclosure by a prominent University of Chicago neuroscientist that recent (but as yet unpublished) research had detected "brain damage" in rats injected with large quantities of MDA, an analogue and metabolite of MDMA. Public debate was further confounded by the frequent confusion of MDMA with MPTP (N-methyl-4-phenyl-1,2,3, 6-tetrahydropyridine), a dopaminergic neurotoxin that had recently been revealed to have induced severe Parkinson-like disorders in users seeking synthetic heroin substitute highs. With growing concern over the dangers of new "designer drugs," public discussion took an increasingly discordant tone (11). In the spring of 1986, following a series of scheduling hearings on MDMA conducted by the DEA in several U.S. cities, the DEA administrative law judge presiding over the case determined on the weight of the evidence presented that there was sufficient indication for safe use under medical supervision and recommended Schedule III status (192). Not obliged to follow the recommendation of his administrative law judge, however, and expressing grave concerns that MDMA's growing abuse liability posed a serious threat to public health and safety, the DEA director overruled the advisement and ruled that MDMA be placed in the most restrictive category, Schedule I (95). Since then, with the exception of a 3-month period in early 1988 when it was briefly unscheduled as a result of a court challenge, MDMA has remained classified as a Schedule I substance.

In the years following the MDMA scheduling controversy, patterns of use have undergone a marked shift. With the failure to establish an official sanction for MDMA treatment, most psychotherapists who had used the drug adjunctively in their work ceased to do so, unwilling to violate the law and jeopardize their livelihoods through the use of a now illegal drug. In the wake of the highly publicized scheduling hearings, however, use among young people escalated. By the late 1980s, interest in MDMA had spread from the United States across the Atlantic to Europe, where it became the drug of choice at marathon dance parties called "raves." Beginning on the Spanish island of Ibiza, spreading across the continent, and then back to the United States, MDMA-catalyzed "raves" have drawn large numbers of young people, often attracting more than 10,000 individuals at a single event (161). Although use in the United States diminished in the early 1990s, by the end of the decade and into the new century its popularity surged. In Europe, and particularly the United Kingdom, MDMA use among young people has consistently maintained high levels for the past 15 years (23,160). With multiple illicit laboratories, including pharmaceutical manufacturers in former "Iron Curtain" countries, the European youth market appears to have become saturated with the drug in recent years (183).

EPIDEMIOLOGY

Although various estimates have been given on the extent of current illicit MDMA use in the United States and Western Europe, the exact prevalence remains unknown. Saunders (161) has stated that "millions" of young people in the United Kingdom have taken MDMA. A Harris Opinion Poll (75) for the BBC in Great Britain presented data that 31% of people between the ages of 16 and 25 years admitted to taking MDMA, most often at "dance clubs," and that 67% reported that their friends had tried the drug. In a survey of school children across the whole of England, 4.25% of 14-year-olds and, in another survey, 6.0% of those ages 14 and 15 years, were reported to have taken MDMA (161). The popular British press recently reported that an estimated 500,000 to 1,000,000 young people in Great Britain take MDMA every weekend (171,183). The "club" or "rave" scene in particular appears to be responsible for the explosive growth of MDMA in the United Kingdom (118), and has been described as developing into what many believe to be the "largest youth movement in British history" (10).

In the United States, reported use of ecstasy has increased significantly, doubling between 1998 and 2001. By the early twenty-first century, 12% of high school seniors admitted to having taken ecstasy (130). An interview study of Stanford University undergraduate students reported that 39% had taken MDMA at least once in their lives (140), while a Tulane University survey revealed that 24.3% of more than 1,200 students questioned had experimented with the drug (33). MDMA has been described as having the "greatest growth potential among all illicit drugs" in the United States, with tens of thousands of new users being introduced to the drug every month, particularly within the context of the "rave scene" (128). Over the last several years, however, public health concerns of MDMA taken as ecstasy have intensified, with a fivefold increase from 1998 to 2001 in emergency medical department mentions of patients reporting taking the drug shortly before admission (46).

POTENTIAL TREATMENT APPLICATIONS

Psychopharmacologic modification of psychotherapy is a treatment modality with prehistoric roots in the shamanic healing application of psychedelic plants within a societally sanctioned and ritualized context (19). Evidence has accumulated that the controlled use of psychedelics for therapeutic and initiatory purposes has played a vital role in aboriginal and preindustrial societies from before recorded history to the present (40,41,71). Indeed, over the last four decades, the advent of psychopharmacologic treatments has transformed the theory and practice of psychiatry; nevertheless, their impact upon psychotherapeutic technique and efficacy has been marginal (64). From 1950 to the mid-1960s, more than 1,000 professional papers were published in the clinical psychiatric literature in Europe and the United States describing the treatment of an estimated 40,000 patients with psychedelic substances (63), yet this era in the history of psychiatry has been virtually forgotten.

Beginning in the late 1970s, proponents of this form of drug-enhanced psychotherapy began to investigate the therapeutic potential of the still-legal MDMA. Compared to LSD, the prototype psychedelic of the twentieth century, MDMA was judged to possess distinct advantages as a therapeutic adjunct. MDMA was described as being a relatively mild, short-acting drug capable of facilitating heightened states of introspection and intimacy along with temporary freedom from anxiety and depression, yet without distracting alterations in perception, body image, and sense of self. Patients were reported as losing defensive anxiety, feeling more emotionally open and accessing feelings and thoughts not ordinarily available to them. Lasting improvement was often reported in patients' self-esteem, ability to communicate with significant others, capacity for achieving empathic rapport, interest in and capacity for insight, strengthened capacity for trust and intimacy, and enhanced therapeutic alliance (64).

A variety of treatment applications were explored prior to MDMA's scheduling in the mid-1980s, including the physical pain and emotional distress associated with severe medical illness, posttraumatic stress disorders, depression, phobias, addictions, psychosomatic disorders, and relationship (marital) problems (2,45,61,96). In reviewing their work with 80 patients treated with MDMA-

augmented psychotherapy, Greer and Tolbert (62) have noted long-lasting benefits in symptom reduction, particularly in diminishing the pathologic effects of prior traumatic experience, as well as sustained improvement in effective and empathic communication skills with family members. More recently, Riedlinger and Riedlinger (151) examined the putative rationale for treating suicidal depression with MDMA.

Unfortunately, before MDMA's value as a treatment modality could be subjected to a rigorous, methodological research evaluation in the United States, the drug was placed on Schedule I status. From the mid-1980s until the early twenty-first century, efforts to conduct clinical trials with MDMA were not permitted, although approved phase I investigations of physiologic and psychological effects in normal volunteers with prior MDMA experience were approved at three research centers in the United States (72,76,184,185). In 2002, a South Carolina study designed to assess safety and efficacy of MDMA in the treatment of chronic posttraumatic stress disorder was approved by the FDA; however, other necessary regulatory approvals have not as yet been received.

Consequently, because clinical patient populations have never been subjected to formal examination with MDMA, only anecdotal case reports are available for examination. In addition to accounts of treatment outcome, the experiences of long-term users of MDMA have also been systematically examined. One study (101), which subjected 20 psychiatrists with past personal histories of MDMA use to extensive semistructured interviews, reported that 85% had increased ability to interact with or be open with others, 80% had decreased defensiveness, 65% had decreased fear, 60% had decreased sense of separation or alienation from others, 50% had increased awareness of emotions, and 50% had decreased aggression. One-half of these psychiatrists with MDMA use experience also reported long-term improvement in social and interpersonal functioning.

In Europe, opportunities for more systematic study of MDMA treatment have been possible. Between 1988 and 1993, permission was granted by public health officials in Switzerland to several psychiatric clinicians, under the auspices of the Swiss Medical Society for Psycholytic Therapy, to treat patients with MDMA. Although authorities neglected to insist upon the implementation of prospective research designs, a retrospective analysis of treatment outcomes was recently conducted (57,58). One hundred and twenty-one former patients consented to examination, on average 2 years following termination of treatment. Patients (predominantly diagnosed with affective disorders, adjustment disorders, and personality disorders) had been engaged in long-term psychotherapy augmented with an average of 6.8 MDMA sessions over 3 years. Overall, 90.9% of patients reported to have experienced improved clinical status as a result of their prior treatment with MDMA, while 2.5% claimed to have clinically "deteriorated." Significant decreases were noted in self-administration of nicotine, alcohol, and cannabis in the years following MDMA treatment, and significant improvements were noted in self-acceptance, autonomy, and overall quality of life.

ADVERSE CLINICAL EFFECTS

When examining adverse effects of MDMA, it is important to distinguish between relatively benign, transient effects experienced by healthy, occasional users ingesting relatively moderate dosages versus more dangerous sequelae reported to occur in a small minority of individuals taking MDMA, often in the context of significant premorbid pathology, adverse settings, polysubstance use, and excessive dosing. Liester et al. (101) have reported in their evaluation of psychiatrists with past, personal use that common short-term side effects of MDMA were similar to effects induced by amphetamines, including trismus, bruxism, restlessness, anxiety, and decreased appetite. Other investigators have reported tachycardia, palpitations, dry mouth, and insomnia (61,142).

With substantial alterations in patterns of use over the past decade, from occasional use for therapeutic and spiritual purposes (187) to frequent, repeated ingestion at large rave dances, the reported risks have increased significantly (148). Although earlier investigations had concluded that MDMA was a drug with a relatively low potential for abuse (9,90,177,180) and where persistent use patterns were described as "extremely rare" (143), the likelihood of individuals frequently ingesting higher dosages of MDMA, often in association with other drugs or alcohol, appears to be increasing (160). Scientific investigations using state-of-the-art prospective methodologies have identified that MDMA possesses nonlinear pharmacokinetics (38). The implications of this important finding is that relatively small increases in the dose of MDMA ingested induce disproportionate increases in plasma concentrations of MDMA, thus exposing individuals to greater risk of developing acute toxicity.

Over the last several years an increasing number of reports of adverse effects attributed to recreational ecstasy have appeared in the medical literature in Europe and the United States. It is also critical to note that given the clandestine (and often amateur) context within which MDMA is manufactured for the escalating mass market, the available black market drug is often not necessarily what it is advertised as being (17,190). Besides escalating degrees of overt drug substitution, recreational ecstasy also often contains contaminants and adulterants (21,193). As was the case with psychedelics in the 1960s, following the transition over time from limited and legal use by relatively well-educated aficionados to mass market consumption for illicit and "recreational" purposes by youth, the purity and quality of MDMA has progressively declined, while the associated risks to the user have climbed.

The phenomenon of drug substitution of other and often more dangerous drugs for MDMA in ecstasy has become an increasing public health concern. Many surveys reveal that less than 50% of sampled ecstasy actually contains MDMA. Although some of this ersatz ecstasy has proved to be relatively innocuous, including aspirin and caffeine, significant degrees of more dangerous drug substitution have occurred (42,82,147,169,172,173). These adulterants have ranged from cocaine, methamphetamine, phencyclidine (PCP), hallucinogens (e.g., LSD), opiates, gamma hydroxybutyrate (GHB), ketamine and dextromethorphan (DXM) to paramethoxyamphetamine (PMA), a potent stimulant associated with a number of ecstasy fatalities (91,107). Indeed, the degree to which drug-substituted ecstasy has become increasingly common within recreational drug scenes is a serious predictor of relative risks youthful drug experimenters may incur.

Given the extent to which MDMA has been subject to widespread use and abuse in the past decade, it is somewhat surprising that more reports of serious adverse effects have not been reported (84,137,138,139,163). Particularly within a context of grave concerns raised over potential risks, fueled by media publicity and hyperbole, only a relatively small number of fatal reactions to the drug have made their way into the medical literature (28,29). Nevertheless, serious attention needs to be accorded the potential for catastrophic medical reactions, because they have occurred and are likely to continue, particularly to individuals with preexisting vulnerabilities (both medical and psychological) who take the drug under circumstances that accentuate the risks.

The first reports of fatalities associated with MDMA ingestion occurred in the United States in 1987. Dowling et al. (44) described five cases of individuals who had precipitously died; they had detected at postmortem positive toxicologic screens for MDMA or MDEA (N-ethyl-3,4-methylenedioxyamphetamine), an MDMA analogue. One of these cases was an individual who was electrocuted while under the influence of MDMA, whereas the other four were all associated with individuals who sustained fatal cardiovascular events. Three of these individuals apparently had preexisting severe cardiac or respiratory disease (atherosclerotic coronary artery disease, idiopathic hypertrophic cardiomyopathy, and bronchial asthma) that was felt to have played a primary role in their sudden death. Alcohol and drugs, in addition to MDMA, were also associated with the four cases of death induced by cardiovascular collapse. In two of these cases, alcohol use occurred shortly before death; in one case, alcohol along with a narcotic analgesic were found to be positive on postmortem toxicologic screen; and in one case, presence of a barbiturate was detected. Individuals who may be at heightened risk of life-threatening cardiac arrhythmias and associated cardiovascular collapse are those having underlying illnesses with heightened sensitivity to exogenous-induced adrenergic stimulation, such as ischemic heart disease, cardiac conduction defects, cardiomyopathy, and mitral valve prolapse (21,129). When MDMA is taken by such individuals with preexisting medical vulnerabilities, particularly in the presence of alcohol or other drugs, licit or illicit, the risks for life-threatening events are compounded. The development of prospective investigations on the effects of pure MDMA administered to human subjects has also yielded important information on the range of cardiovascular response. Studies in both the United States and Europe have reported that higher dosages of MDMA can induce marked increases in heart rate, blood pressure and myocardial oxygen consumption, thereby highlighting the heightened degree of risk for individuals with underlying cardiovascular vulnerabilities (98,108).

Several cases have also been reported over the last few years in the medical literature of severe cerebrovascular accidents apparently induced by MDMA. Manchanda and Connolly (104) described a young man who experienced a cerebral infarction after having consumed "several" MDMA tablets. Similarly, Rothwell and Grant (159) reported a young woman who had taken MDMA who subsequently sustained a cerebral venous sinus thrombosis after engaging in an extended period of prolonged dancing and associated dehydration. Preexisting neurologic vulnerabilities appear to accentuate the risks for devastating cerebrovascular events, as was the case of a young woman who had an intracerebral bleed from an aneurysm of the left posterior communicating artery shortly after ingesting 2.5 MDMA tablets (59). Associated polysubstance and alcohol use also appears to potentiate the dangers of MDMA use, inducing injury to central nervous system structures (182). Damage to subcortical structures through a mechanism of vasoconstriction brought on by enhanced serotonin neurotransmission has also been suggested as the pathogenesis of some strokes associated with MDMA (73).

With increasing use of MDMA, often of indeterminate quality and excessive quantity, cases of apparent hepatotoxicity have begun to emerge, particularly in Great Britain. Henry et al. (77) reported six young men and one young woman who had used MDMA within the previous few weeks who presented with jaundice, elevated bilirubin, and abnormal liver chemistries. Each was without a known history of heavy alcohol use, intravenous drug use, or evidence of infectious hepatitis. Dykhuizen et al. (47) also reported on three cases of idiosyncratic toxic hepatitis, presumably secondary to MDMA. Whether the liver damage in these cases was caused by an idiosyncratic reaction to MDMA or to some contaminant ingested along with it is not known (87). Although such case reports provoke the need to inquire about MDMA use histories in young people presenting with unexplained jaundice and hepatomegaly, they do appear to be extremely rare, even in the context of increasing usage of an often impure, illicit compound. Basic 28-day toxicologic studies in dogs and rats show no evidence of liver damage (56). Thus, the mechanism underlying the reported liver damage remains to be determined.

A severe medical complication of taking MDMA in the context of vigorous prolonged exercise, environmental crowding, lack of sufficient hydration, and high ambient temperature is the induction of a catastrophic hyperthermic reaction leading to disseminated intravascular coagulation (DIC), rhabdomyolysis, acute renal and hepatic failure, seizures and, on occasion, death (77). Virtually all of such reported cases have occurred in the rave dance club setting, and were associated with prolonged vigorous dancing in poorly ventilated environments and inadequate fluid replacement (148). Indeed, in some British rave dance halls, including settings where deaths from hyperthermia had occurred, access to water was often restricted by club management in order to increase the sales of soft drinks. In one particularly unscrupulous establishment, the water taps were reportedly turned off in the bathrooms while tap water was sold over the counter at the bar for the same price as beer (109).

While maintenance of adequate hydration is a critical component of harm reduction efforts, published case reports reveal that excessive consumption of fluids in association with MDMA administration may provoke severe and potentially fatal hyponatremia induced by the syndrome of inappropriate antidiuretic hormone secretion (SIADH) (80,110). A prospective study conducted in the United Kingdom demonstrated that the administration of a modest dose of MDMA induced significant elevations of antidiuretic hormone (vasopressin) in human research subjects (78). Several well-publicized deaths have occurred secondary to apparent water intoxication.

Given that the degree of MDMA use has climbed well into the millions, initially in Europe, and more recently in the United States, it is not surprising that cases of psychiatric disturbance have been reported. Reported adverse psychiatric events include panic disorder (112,136,189), paranoid psychoses (31,86,119,120), and depression (102,111). What is remarkable about many of these reports, apart from the surprisingly small numbers of presenting cases contrasted to the exceedingly large potential pool of (mostly young) individuals who have used MDMA, is the extremely high and frequent dosages of the drug that had been consumed by many of those individuals who had experienced adverse psychiatric sequelae (111,119,120,162,188). By the early twenty-first century, the Drug Abuse Warning Network (DAWN) in the United States reported that MDMA taken concomitantly with other dangerous drugs was becoming an increasingly dangerous phenomenon, accounting for 86% of all medical and psychiatric emergencies associated with MDMA. Indeed, alcohol was associated with almost half of all MDMA implicated medical and psychiatric emergencies, whereas cocaine was associated with nearly one-third of cases (46). Highlighting the often neglected self-medication model of substance abuse, recent research investigations have also clearly identified that the onset of mental disorders are far more likely to precede rather than to follow use of MDMA and related substances (100). In the face of significant premorbid psychopathology, and often in combination with other drugs or alcohol, frequent use of high-dose MDMA does appear to heighten risks for deterioration of psychiatric status. The evidence, however, for occasional, low-dose MDMA use, taken in controlled settings without additional drugs or alcohol by individuals with negative histories for psychiatric disorders, appears to be considerably lower.

An additional concern over the uncontrolled use of recreational MDMA has been the potential risks of dangerous interactions with prescription drugs. MDMA is metabolized primarily by the CYP2D6 and CYP3A4 hepatic systems (38,92). MDMA might influence or be influenced by other drugs metabolized by the same cytochrome P450 isozymes. Drugs also possessing prominent 2D6 metabolism, including the selective serotonin reuptake inhibitor (SSRI) antidepressants fluoxetine (Prozac) and paroxetine (Paxil), as well as the illicit drug cocaine, inhibit MDMA metabolism in human liver (146), thus posing the risk of impaired degradation and protracted exposure to high levels of MDMA. A life-threatening interaction was also reported in a young man infected with human immunodeficiency virus (HIV) between his treatment regimen of the protease inhibitors ritonavir (Norvir) and saquinavir (Fortovase), potent inhibitors of both CYP3A4 and CYP2D6, and recreational MDMA (74). Because 7% of whites are poor CYP2D6 metabolizers (13), these subjects might be at higher risk for development of drug interactions and toxic side effects.

NEUROTOXICITY

Since the mid-1980s, evidence has existed that MDMA and its analogues are capable of inflicting profound changes on brain serotonin systems in laboratory animals (92). Preclinical studies consistently demonstrate that MDMA causes an acute, but reversible, depletion of serotonin (121). Unlike other amphetamine-like compounds, which exert comparable effects on both serotonergic and dopaminergic neurons (168), MDMA's predominant target is the serotonin system (although dopamine systems also can be affected, particularly at high doses) (191).

Effects of serotonin systems in laboratory animals subjected to administration of large dosages of MDMA are divided into short-term and long-term effects. Some of the acute effects of MDMA, including the rapid release of intracellular serotonin, are presumed to mediate the behavioral and psychological profile observed in humans (72), whereas in animals, the neurotoxic effects are not manifested until days later (7). It would appear that neurotoxicity is not inextricably linked to the acute effects of the drug. Administration of fluoxetine prior to, or up to 6 hours after, MDMA administration blocks or attenuates the development of neurotoxicity (60), whereas some acute effects of MDMA (e.g., behavioral, neuroendocrine, and temperature) occur within minutes and peak within a few hours (20,72,125). The majority of work on MDMA has revolved around its neurotoxic effects and the mechanisms by which these effects are produced. Rats administered multiple doses of MDMA undergo serotonergic neurotoxic changes that can last for many months before neurochemical recovery occurs (7), although there can be considerable interanimal variability in the degree of neurotoxicity, as well as in the extent of recovery, from the same dosage regimen. In rats, neurotoxicity appears to be limited to axon terminals, with a relative sparing of cell bodies (8). Regeneration and sprouting of brain serotonin axonal projections do occur, yet may take up to a year to develop in rodents, and perhaps longer in nonhuman primates (155). The question of whether these axonal connections observed during recovery are "normal" or not, however, remains to be elucidated. In squirrel monkeys administered MDMA (5.0 mg/kg subcutaneously) twice daily for 4 consecutive days, profound reductions of brain serotonin, 5-hydroxyindoleacetic acid (5-HIAA), the primary metabolite of serotonin, and serotonin uptake sites, persist even at 18 months. Interestingly, the thalamus shows some recovery, while the hypothalamus shows an (apparent) overshoot in regeneration (3), suggesting that under some circumstances MDMA administration can lead to a lasting reorganization of ascending serotonin (5-HT) axon projections (52). A single oral dose of 5.0 mg/kg in primates, only two to three times higher than that usually taken by humans, produces thalamic and hypothalamic effects observed only at 2 weeks after administration (154). A no-effect level in monkeys has also been reported between 2.5 to 5.0 mg/kg (88). However, Ricaurte et al. (156) showed that administrations of injected MDMA (2.0 mg/kg 3 times at 3-hour intervals) produced marked reductions in measures of dopamine and serotonin. Despite the widespread damage to 5-HT neurons produced by high doses of the drug, initial studies found few functional consequences (55,97,158). However, more recent investigations indicate that long-term functional sequelae can be detected in animals (36,106,122,144,170) and, possibly, in humans (89,100,137,149,179). The mechanisms underlying MDMA-induced serotonin neurotoxicity are thought to occur by the uptake of MDMA into serotonin nerve terminals, causing an initial reduction of serotonin levels. A second phase of serotonin reduction follows, possibly as a consequence of the formation of neurotoxic metabolites (5) or by generation of free radicals (8,170), which causes degeneration of serotonin terminals (and in some cases axons) for weeks to months, depending upon the species and dosage regimen employed. Additional data indicate that dopamine also plays a role in the mechanism underlying the neurotoxic effects of MDMA on serotonin neurons (167), as does glutamate, because various NMDA (N-methyl-D-aspartate) antagonists can inhibit or attenuate MDMA induced neurotoxicity (60). Other compounds that modulate or prevent long-term serotonergic neurotoxic changes in laboratory animals administered MDMA include the serotonin reuptake inhibitors fluoxetine and citalopram (Celexa) (164,165), the serotonin antagonist ritanserin (166), the dopamine antagonist haloperidol (Haldol) (79), and the monoamine oxidase-B inhibitor 1-deprenyl (181), as well as the NMDA antagonists dizocilpine (27,79) and dextromethorphan (51). Furthermore, in addition to pure neurochemical modulators, temperature appears to be another variable in the mediation of MDMA neurotoxicity (50). Indeed, recent investigations demonstrate the critical role thermoregulatory mechanisms exert on the development of MDMA neurotoxicity, as relatively small changes in ambient temperature induce significant alterations in core temperature of MDMA-treated rats but do not affect core temperature of control saline-treated rats (103). Because MDMA neurotoxicity is evidently dependent upon high core temperatures, preventing the development of hyperthermic states in experimental animals will reduce the loss of serotonergic terminals (20).

Controversy exists over whether MDMA actually fits the precise definition of a neurotoxin. Contending that the term *neurotoxicity* has been too broadly applied, investigators have been influenced by their observations that standard techniques used to identify classic evidence of neuronal destruction, such as astrogliosis and silver degeneration staining, do not occur in animals treated with MDMA. Although known neurotoxins, such as bilirubin, cadmium, trimethyltin, the dopaminergic neurotoxin MPTP (*N*-methyl-4-phenyl-1,2,3,6-tetrahydropyridine), and the classic serotonergic neurotoxins *para*-chloramphetamine (PCA) and 5,7-dihydroxytryptamine (5,7-DHT) predictably induce a proliferation of enlarged astroglial cells, reactive gliosis is not reported in animals exposed to MDMA (85). Arguing that lower indices of serotonin should not necessarily be equated with the actual destruction of serotonin axons (the expected outcome in bona fide serotonin neurotoxicity) because assessments of serotonin are only indicative of the presence of the neurotransmitter in neurons, not the actual neuronal structures themselves, investigators have proposed an alternative model of neuromodulation, in which protein synthesis inhibition occurs as a natural extension of the pharmacological activity of the compounds (132–135).

Whereas multiple studies establish and reconfirm that MDMA provokes profound changes in brain serotonin systems of laboratory animals, evidence that functional or behavioral abnormalities are induced remain limited. Similarly, minimal data are available addressing the issue of whether normal function is restored following biochemical recovery. It has long been demonstrated that at least in some species serotonin and other monoaminergic neurons can undergo extensive regeneration following neurotoxin-induced degenerative change (14). As determined by immunocytochemical and autoradiographic techniques, regeneration of serotonin fibers occurs in the hypothalamus following serotonin lesions induced by the experimental neurotoxin 5,7-DHT. This reinnervation appears to be structurally normal (54). Although it is not known to what extent regenerated (or sprouted) fibers are able to reestablish original synaptic contacts (52), some data suggest that the observed patterns of reinnervation are abnormal (52). The degree to which such biochemical alterations affect functional normality is a question still awaiting elucidation. Indeed, it appears that it is the specific "damage" to serotonin fibers, (primarily serotonergic axonal terminals originating from the dorsal raphe), induced by neurotoxins causing significant declines in serotonin levels, that ultimately reactivate latent developmental signals in the brain. Most likely, this occurs at the genomic level, thus encouraging resprouting and regeneration along with the stimulation of an astrocytic growth factor (6). Whether the degenerative axonal changes associated with the phenomenon of serotonergic neurotoxicity is simply a prelude to what may eventually be recognized as a healthy and adaptive neuroplasticity response, or whether it is the substrate for what will eventuate in neuropsychiatric pathology, is not yet known.

MDMA is not the only drug known to induce long-standing effects on indices of serotonergic neurotransmission (12,18). However, the drug with the greatest relevance to MDMA in its effects on serotonergic function is fenfluramine. Marketed as an anorectic drug for the treatment of obesity, fenfluramine was administered to more than 50 million patients during a several-decade period (39). Fenfluramine has also been explored in controlled trials as a putative treatment for a variety of psychopathologic conditions, including infantile autism (157), attention deficit hyperactivity disorder (43), eating disorders (15), depression (186), and suicidal behavior (124). In spite of such a long history of clinical application without reports of adverse outcome, fenfluramine has come under increasing attack in recent years because preclinical investigations have identified that its effects on the brains of laboratory animals induce what has been described as serotonergic neurotoxicity (114). In rats, as well as nonhuman primates, fenfluramine causes long-standing depletions of regional brain 5-HT and 5-HIAA, changes very similar to those induced by MDMA. Indeed, some fenfluramine-induced neurotoxicity has been described as being the same as for MDMA-induced neurotoxicity (113). In the mid-1990s, a vigorous debate occurred at the FDA over approval of the more 5-HT–active optical isomer of fenfluramine, *d*-fenfluramine. Many of the same concerns over the long-term effects of serotonergic neurotoxicity as during the MDMA debates were raised; nevertheless, the decision of the FDA advisory panel was to recommend approval without restriction for the prescription drug *d*-fenfluramine. Although without the high public profile and notoriety of MDMA, fenfluramine is not itself lacking in potential for illicit use and abuse (99). Nevertheless, the government approval for the use of *d*-fenfluramine was no doubt influenced by the aggressive lobbying efforts of the pharmaceutical industry, a fact underscoring the intrusion of political and economic agendas into the realm of scientific policy. Although racemic and *d*-fenfluramine were ultimately removed by the FDA from the market over the question of possible cardiac valve injury, the role of fenfluramine as a putative serotonergic neurotoxin was not contributory to the decision.

As reviewed recently, efforts to extend the neurotoxicity hypothesis to human populations have met with mixed results (84,89,137–139,149). Measurements of neurotransmitter metabolites in the cerebrospinal fluid (CSF) of MDMA users were assessed in one early study as being within normal limits (141). A subsequent study (154), which reported lower levels of CSF 5-HIAA in MDMA users, is difficult to interpret because the control population employed was a group of patients with chronic back pain. Such a choice for the control group is suspect because of evidence that serotonergic mechanisms are involved in pain control (32,123) as well as the known association of increased levels of CSF 5-HIAA in patients suffering from chronic nonmalignant and malignant pain (24,30). Additional studies which reported serotonergic abnormalities in MDMA subjects (93,145), as reflected by abnormal neuroendocrine response to L-tryptophan and by mild to moderate cognitive impairment, need to be interpreted cautiously because of serious methodological concerns surrounding subject recruitment and assessment (66–70). The most methodologically sound retrospective evaluation of human MDMA users, although finding no differences between prolactin secretion induced by the L-tryptophan challenge test, did find significantly lower levels of cerebral spinal fluid 5-HIAA in MDMA users compared to controls (115). Surprisingly, however, and confounding expectations inferred by the neurotoxicity hypothesis, these same MDMA subjects with relatively low levels of CSF 5-HIAA were also assessed as having significantly lower scores on personality measures of impulsivity and hostility; opposite results were expected (53,178a,178b). Finally, a decrease in stage II sleep and sleep time has been reported in subjects with a history of MDMA (4). This is both an interesting and perplexing observation. Given the prominent role that serotonin plays in the regulation of both slow-wave and rapid eye movement (REM) sleep, one would have expected that these sleep electroencephalograph (EEG) measures might have been most affected by MDMA. In summary, most, if not all, of the observed changes reported thus far are compatible with a general effect of MDMA on serotonin neurotransmission independent of neurotoxicity, although the latter effect cannot be ruled out.

An additional area of controversy is the impact of MDMA use on mood and cognition, presumed clinical sequelae to suspected serotonin neurotoxicity. To accurately discern the degree to which MDMA will adversely impact long-term neuropsychological function, it is important for investigators to incorporate important critical lifestyle variables into their research methodologies. Regular users of MDMA most often take the drug at rave or club venues, which are marathon dance parties where a variety of drugs are ingested and participants often experience severe degrees of sleep and nutritional deprivation (34). It is also becoming increasingly apparent that more frequent and problematic users have had severe underlying psychopathology preceding their initiation to MDMA (100). One study conducted in the United Kingdom described persistent dysphoria and mild memory impairment experienced by rave participants during the week following their weekend of drug-fueled dancing (35). These "mid-week lows" were significantly more severe for MDMA users who were also regular users of cocaine and amphetamine. Only 2% of this MDMA-using subject cohort were not polysubstance users. A particularly confounding phenomenon is the increasing popularity among ravers of ketamine (Ketalar), a dissociative anesthetic, known to induce strong frontal lobe effects and cognitive dysfunction (37,49,83). Similarly, cannabis, which is consumed by a high proportion of recreational MDMA users, may also cause alterations in neuropsychological function, further challenging MDMA research methodologies (179). Unfortunately, many studies fail to adequately take into account the contributory role of other commonly used drugs when assessing the clinical effects of recreational MDMA use.

Over the past decade, MDMA neurotoxicity research in humans has become increasingly controversial, as methodologies and patterns of data analyses of high-profile investigations have been subjected to intense scrutiny and criticism (66,67,81,89). Well-publicized studies concluding that MDMA indubitably causes neuropsychological damage (16,117) often used poorly matched controls and minimized the contribution of serious polydrug use and lifestyle factors to outcome. Moreover, puzzling statistical manipulations and exclusion of critical data sets from publications have further obfuscated the veracity of such findings (127). While there is ample reason to remain concerned that individuals with serious underlying vulnerabilities for psychopathology who engage in extreme lifestyles that include excessive use of a variety of powerful psychoactive substances may be inducing neuropsychological injury to themselves, the unequivocal conclusion that all detected and anticipated pathologies must be attributed to MDMA use remains highly suspect.

The rapidly evolving field of brain imaging studies has also assumed prominence in world MDMA research (149). Unfortunately, methodological issues and data interpretation have again called into question highly sensationalized findings that MDMA users had sustained intractable serotonin neurotoxicity. Such studies, besides often entirely ignoring rampant drug substitution and the polymorphous nature of ecstasy itself, also routinely discount the significance of polydrug use histories as well as the fact that subjects were unarguably heavy users of MDMA itself (116). Furthermore, questions of experimental positron emission tomography (PET) scan technique, including the use of a serotonin ligand that had not been subjected to standard test–retest reliability, further complicate conclusions drawn from the data (22,89,94). Other investigations, examining cerebral blood flow through the use of coregistered brain single-photon emission computed tomography (SPECT) and magnetic resonance imaging (MRI), have found short-term reductions of blood flow followed by apparent return to normal over time (26). In addition, some (149,150), but not all (25,131), studies report reductions in brain n-acetyl aspartate, a marker of neuronal health. However, the magnitude of the n-acetyl aspartate reductions ($>10\%$) is too large to be accounted for solely by destruction of serotonin systems (150). Other factors, including polydrug use, might account for the findings.

Unfortunately, the question of MDMA's potential neurotoxicity in humans has been marked by unwelcome and excessive attention by the media. This has led not only to often sensationalized and distorted media reportage, but also to implicit and explicit pressures on scientific researchers to align their findings with conventional expectations. Needless to say, MDMA's role as a recreational drug for millions of young people worldwide is worrisome, particularly within the context of ill-prepared and vulnerable individuals consuming an illicitly manufactured and marketed drug of dubious quality in unpredictable and often dangerous settings. Nevertheless, for a true appreciation of MDMA's range of effects, it is imperative that objective investigations be conducted in a fair and honest scientific environment. Hopefully, the future will provide the opportunity for well-controlled and methodologically sound investigations to probe the full range of MDMA's effects, and begin to answer the as yet unanswered questions surrounding the drug's capacity to cause harm versus its innate potential under optimal conditions to facilitate beneficial outcomes.

REFERENCES

1. Adamson S, Metzner R. *Through the gateway of the heart: accounts of experiences with MDMA and other empathogenic substances.* San Francisco: Four Trees Publications, 1985.
2. Adamson S, Metzner R. The nature of the MDMA experience and its role in healing, psychotherapy, and spiritual practice. *Revision* 1988;10:59–72.
3. Ali SF, Newport GD, Scallet AC, et al. Oral administration or MDMA produces selective 5-HT depletion in the non-human primate. *Neurotoxicol Teratol* 1993;15:91–96.
4. Allen R, McCann U, Ricaurte G. Persistent effects of MDMA (ecstasy) in human sleep. *Sleep* 1993;16:560–564.
5. Axt KJ, Commins D, Seiden LS. Alphamethylparatyrosine prevents methylamphetamine induced formation of endogenous 5,6-DHT in rat hippocampus. *Soc Neurosci Ab* 1985;11:1193.
6. Azmitia EC, Whitaker-Azmitia, PM. Awakening, the sleeping giant: anatomy and plasticity of the brain serotonergic system. *J Clin Psychiatry* 1991; 52[Suppl]:4–16.
7. Battaglia G, Yeh SY, DeSouza EB. MDMA-induced neurotoxicity: parameters of degeneration and recovery of brain serotonin neurons. *Pharmacol Biochem Behav* 1988;29:269:274.
8. Baumgarten HG, Zimmermann B. Neurotoxic phenylalkylamines and indolealkylamines. In: Herken H, Hucho F, eds. *Selective neurotoxicity.* Berlin: Springer-Verlag, 1992:225–291.

9. Beck J. The public health implications of MDMA use. In: Peroutka SJ, ed. *The clinical, pharmacological, and neurotoxicological effects of the drug MDMA.* Boston: Kluwer, 1990:77–103.
10. Beck J. Ecstasy and the rave scene: historical and cross-cultural perspectives. *CEWG* 1993;Dec:424–431.
11. Beck J, Morgan PA. Designer drug confusion: a focus on MDMA. *J Drug Education* 1986;16:287–302.
12. Benwell ME, Balfour DJK, Anderson JM. Smoking-associated changes in the serotonergic systems of discrete regions of human brain. *Psychopharmacology (Berl)* 1990;102:68–72.
13. Bertilsson L, Dahl ML, Dalen P, et al. Molecular genetics of CYP2D6: clinical relevance with focus on psychotropic drugs. *Br J Clin Pharmacol* 2002;53:111–122.
14. Bjorklund A, Stenevi U. Regeneration of monoaminergic and cholinergic neurons in the mammalian central nervous system. *Physiol Rev* 1979;59:62–100.
15. Blouin AG, Blouin J, Perez EL, et al. Treatment of bulimia with fenfluramine and desipramine. *J Clin Psychopharmacol* 1988;8:261–269.
16. Bolla KI, McCann UD, Ricaurte GA. Memory impairment in abstinent MDMA ("ecstasy") users. *Neurology* 1998;51:1532–1537.
17. Bost RO. 3,4-Methylenedioxymethamphetamine (MDMA) and other amphetamine derivatives. *J Forensic Sci* 1988;22:576–587.

18. Bowers MB. Amitriptyline in man: decreased formation of central 5-hydroxyindoleacetic acid. *Clin Pharmacol Ther* 1974;15:167–170.
19. Bravo GL, Grob CS. Shamans, sacraments and psychiatrists. *J Psychoactive Drugs* 1989;21:123–128.
20. Broening HW, Bowyer JF, Slikker W. Age-dependent sensitivity of rats to the long-term effects of the serotonergic neurotoxicant ($\pm$) 3,4-methylenedioxymethamphetamine (MDMA) correlates with the magnitude of the MDMA-induced thermal response. *J Pharmacol Exp Ther* 1995;275:325–333.
21. Buchanan JF, Brown CR. Designer drugs: a problem in clinical toxicology. *Med Toxicol* 1988;3:1–17.
22. Buck A, Gucker P, Vollenweider FX, et al. Evaluation of serotonergic transporter using PET and 11C-(+)-McN-5652: assessment of methods. *J Cereb Blood Flow Metab* 2000;20:253–262.
23. Capdevila M. *MDMA o el extasis quimico.* Barcelona: Los Libros De La Liebre De Marzo, 1995.
24. Ceccherelli F, Costa C, Ischia S, et al. Cerebral tryptophan metabolism in humans in relation to malignant pain. *Funct Neurol* 1989;4:341–353.
25. Chang L, Ernst T, Grob CS, et al. Cerebral 1H MRS alterations in recreational 3,4-methylenedioxymethamphetamine (MDMA, "ecstasy") users. *J Magn Reson Imaging* 1999;10:521–526.

26. Chang L, Grob CS, Ernst T, et al. Effect of ecstasy (3,4-methlenedioxymethamphetamine [MDMA]) on cerebral blood flow: a coregistered SPECT and MRI study. *Psychiatry Res* 2000; 98:15–28.

27. Colado MI, Murray TK, Green AR. 5-HT loss in rat brain following 3,4-methylenedioxymethamphetamine (MDMA), *p*-chloroamphetamine and fenfluramine administration and effects of chlormethiazole and dizocilpine. *Br J Pharmacol* 1993;108:583–589.

28. Cole J, Sumnall H, Grob C. Sorted: ecstasy facts and fiction. *Psychologist* 2002;15:464–467.

29. Cole J, Sumnall H, Grob C. Where are the casualties? *Psychologist* 2002;15: 474.

30. Costa C, Ceccherelli F, Bettero A, et al. Tryptophan, serotonin and 5-hydroxyindoleacetic acid levels in human CSF in relation to pain. In: Schlossberger HG, Kochen W, Linzen B, et al, eds. *Progress in tryptophan and serotonin research.* New York: DeGruyter, 1984:413–416.

31. Creighton FJ, Black DL, Hyde CE. "Ecstasy" psychosis and flashbacks. *Br J Psychiatry* 1991;159:713–716.

32. Crisp T, Stafinsky JL, Boja JW, et al. The antinociceptive effects of 3,4-methylenedioxymethamphetamine (MDMA) in the rat. *Pharmacol Biochem Behav* 1989;34:497–501.

33. Cuomo MJ, Dyment PG, Gammino VM. Increasing use of "ecstasy" (MDMA) and other hallucinogens on a college campus. *J Am Coll Health Assoc* 1994;42:271–274.

34. Curran HV. *Is ecstasy (MDMA) neurotoxic?* Novartis Foundation, December 4, 1998.

35. Curran HV, Travill RA. Mood and cognitive effects of +3,4-methylenedioxymethamphetamine (MDMA, "ecstasy"'): weekend "high" followed by mid-week low. *Addiction* 1997;92:821–831.

36. Dafters RI, Lynch E. Persistent loss of thermoregulation in the rat induced by 3,4-methylenedioxymethamphetamine (MDMA or "ecstasy") but not by fenfluramine. *Psychopharmacology (Berl)* 1998;138:207–212.

37. Dalgarno PJ, Shewan D. Illicit use of ketamine in Scotland. *J Psychoactive Drugs* 1996;28:191–1999.

38. De La Torre R, Farre M, Ortuno J, et al. Non-linear pharmacokinetics of MDMA ("ecstasy") in humans. *J Clin Pharmacol* 2000;49:104–109.

39. Derome-Tremblay M, Nathan C. Fenfluramine studies. *Science* 1989;243: 991.

40. Dobkin de Rios, M. *Hallucinogens: cross-cultural perspectives.* Albuquer-que, NM: University of New Mexico Press, 1984.

41. Dobkin de Rios M, Grob CS. Hallucinogens, suggestibility and adolescence in cross-cultural perspective. *Yearbook Ethnomedicine* 1994;3:113–132.

42. Doblin R. MAPS MDMA analysis project. *MAPS* 1996;6:11–13.

43. Donnelly M, Rapoport JL, Potter WZ, et al. Fenfluramine and dextroamphetamine treatment of childhood hyperactivity: clinical and biochemical findings. *Arch Gen Psychiatry* 1989;46:205–212.

44. Dowling GP, McDonough ET, Bost RO. "Eve" and "ecstasy": a report of five deaths associated with the use of MDEA and MDMA. *JAMA* 1987;257: 1615–1617.

45. Downing J. The psychological and physiological effects of MDMA on normal volunteers. *J Psychoactive Drugs* 1986;18:335–339.

46. Drug Abuse Warning Network. Club drugs, 2001 update. *DAWN Rep* 2002; Oct:1–4.

47. Dykhuizen RS, Brunt PW, Atkinson P, et al. Ecstasy-induced hepatitis mimicking viral hepatitis. *Gut* 1995;36:939–941.

48. Eisner B. *Ecstasy: the MDMA story.* Berkeley, CA: Ronin Publishing, 1989.

49. Ellison G. The *N*-methyl-D-aspartate antagonists phencyclidine, ketamine and dizocilpine as both behavioral and anatomical models of dementias. *Brain Res Rev* 1995;20:250–267.

50. Fantegrossi WE, Godlewski T, Karabenick RL, et al. Pharmacological characterization of the effects of 3,4-methylenedioxymethamphetamine ("ecstasy") and its enantiomers on lethality, core temperature, and locomotor activity in singly housed and crowded mice. *Psychopharmacology (Berl)* 2003;166(3):202–211.

51. Finnegan KT, Skratt JJ, Irwin I, et al. The *N*-methyl-D-aspartate (NMDA) receptor antagonist, dextromethorphan, prevents the neurotoxic effects of 3,4-methylenedioxymethamphetamine (MDMA) in rats. *Neurosci Lett* 1990; 105:300–306.

52. Fischer C, Hatzidimitriou G, Wlos J, et al. Re-organization of ascending 5HT axon projections in animals previously exposed to the recreational drug MDMA ("ecstasy"). *J Neurosci* 1995;15:5476–5485.

53. Fishbein DH, Lozovsky D, Jaffe J. Impulsivity, aggression, and neuroendocrine responses to 5-HT stimulation in substance abusers. *Biol Psychol* 1989;25:1049–1066.

54. Frankfurt M, Azmitia E. Regeneration of 5-HT fibers in the rat hypothalamus following unilateral 5,7-DHT injection. *Brain Res* 1984;298:272–282.

55. Frederick DL, Ali SF, Alikker W, et al. Behavioral and neurochemical effects of chronic methylenedioxymethamphetamine (MDMA) treatment in rhesus monkeys. *Neurotoxicol Teratol* 1995;17:531–543.

56. Frith C, Chang L. Toxicity of methylenedioxymethamphetamine (MDMA) in the dog and rat. *Fundam Appl Toxicol* 1987;9:110–119.

57. Gasser P. Die psycholytische psychotherapie in der Schweiz (1988–1993). *Jahrbuch fur Transkulturelle Medizin und Psychotherapie* 1995;6: 143–162.

58. Gasser P. The psycholytic therapy in Switzerland from 1988–1993: a follow-up study. *MAPS Bulletin* 1995;5:3–7.

59. Gledhill JA, Moore DF, Bell D, et al. Subarachnoid hemorrhage associated with MDMA abuse. *J Neurol Neurosurg Psychiatry* 1993;56:1036–1037.

60. Green AR, Cross AJ, Goodwin GM. Review of the pharmacology and clinical pharmacology of MDMA ("ecstasy"). *Psychopharmacology (Berl)* 1995;119:247–260.

61. Greer G, Tolbert R. Subjective reports of the effects of MDMA in a clinical setting. *J Psychoactive Drugs* 1986;18:319–327.

62. Greer G, Tolbert R. The therapeutic use of MDMA. In: Peroutka SJ, ed. *Ecstasy: the clinical pharmacological and neurotoxicological effects of the drug MDMA.* Boston: Kluwer, 1990:21–35.

63. Grinspoon L, Bakalar JB. *Psychedelic drugs reconsidered.* New York: Basic Books, 1979.

64. Grinspoon L, Bakalar JB. Can drugs be used to enhance the psychotherapeutic process? *Am J Psychotherapy* 1986;40:393–404.

65. Grob CS. Psychiatric research with hallucinogens: what have we learned? *Yearbook Ethnomedicine* 1994;3:91–112.

66. Grob CS. Deconstructing ecstasy: the politics of MDMA research. *Addict Res* 2000;8:549–588.

67. Grob CS. The politics of ecstasy. *J Psychoactive Drugs* 2002;34:143–144.

68. Grob CS, ed. *Hallucinogens: a reader.* New York: Tarcher/Putnam, 2002.

69. Grob CS, Bravo GL, Walsh RN. Second thoughts on 3,4-methylenedioxymethamphetamine (MDMA) neurotoxicity. *Arch Gen Psychiatry* 1990;47: 288.

70. Grob CS, Bravo GL, Walsh RN, et al. The MDMA-neurotoxicity controversy: implications for clinical research with novel psychoactive drugs. *J Nerv Ment Dis* 1992;180:355–356.

71. Grob CS, Dobkin de Rios M.

Adolescent drug use in cross-cultural perspective. *J Drug Issues* 1992;22: 121–138.

72. Grob CS, Poland RE, Chang L, et al. Psychobiologic effects of 3,4-methylenedioxymethamphetamine in humans: methodological considerations and preliminary observations. *Behav Brain Res* 1996;73:103–107.

73. Hanyu S, Ikeguchi K, Imai H, et al. Cerebral infarction associated with 3,4-methylenedioxymethamphetamine ("ecstasy") abuse. *Eur Neurol* 1995; 35:173.

74. Harrington RD, Woodward JA, Hooton TM, et al. Life-threatening interactions between HIV-1 protease inhibitors and the illicit drugs MDMA and gamma-hydroxybutyrate. *Arch Intern Med* 1999;159:2221–2224.

75. Harris Research Center. Young peoples poll. London, January 1992.

76. Harris D, Baggott M, Jones RT, et al. MDMA pharmacokinetics and physiological and subjective effects in humans. *CPDD* 1999;59.

77. Henry JA, Jeffreys KJ, Dawling S. Toxicity and deaths from 3,4-methylenedioxymethamphetamine ("ecstasy"). *Lancet* 1992;340:384–387.

78. Henry JA, Fallon JK, Kicman AT, et al. Low-dose MDMA ("ecstasy") induces vasopressin secretion. *Lancet* 1998; 351:1784.

79. Hewitt KE, Green AR. Chlormethiazole, dizocilpine and haloperidol prevent the degeneration of serotonergic nerve terminals induced by administration of MDMA ("ecstasy"). *Neuropharmacology* 1994;33:1589–1595.

80. Holden R, Jackson MA. Near-fatal hyponatraeamic coma due to vasopressin over-secretion after "ecstasy" (3,4-MDMA). *Lancet* 1996;347:1052.

81. Holland J, ed. *Ecstasy: the complete guide.* Rochester, VT: Park Street Press, 2001.

82. Inciyan E. Ecsatsy's high-risk agenda. *The Guardian* 2000;Feb 24.

83. Jansen KLR. *Ketamine: dreams and realities* Sarasota, FL: MAPS, 2001.

84. Kalant H. The pharmacology and toxicology of "ecstasy" (MDMA) and related drugs. *CMAJ* 2001;165:917–928.

85. Kalia M, O'Callaghan JP, Miller DB, et al. Comparative study of fluoxetine, sibutramine, sertraline and dexfenfluramine on the morphology of serotonergic nerve terminals using serotonin immunohistochemistry. *Brain Res* 2000;858:92–105.

86. Kampen JV, Katz M. Persistent psychosis after a single ingestion of "ecstasy." *Psychosomatics* 2001;42:525–527.

87. Karch SB. *The pathology of drug abuse.* Boca Raton, FL: CRC Press, 1993:210–218.

88. Karel R. Fluoxetine may protect against MDMA neurotoxicity. *Psychiatric News* 1993;Aug 6.

89. Kish SJ. How strong is the evidence that brain serotonin neurons are damaged in human users of ecstasy? *Pharmacol Biochem Behav* 2002;71:845–855.

90. Korf D, Blanken P, Nabben T. *Een nieuwe wonderpil?* Amsterdam: Korf, 1991.

91. Kraner JC, McCoy DJ, Evans MA, et al. Fatalities caused by the MDMA-related drug paramethoxyamphetamine (PMA). *J Anal Toxicol* 2001;25:645–648.

92. Kreth KP, Kovar KA, Schwab M, et al. Identification of the human cytochromes P450 involved in the oxidative metabolism of "ecstasy" related designer drugs. *Biochem Pharmacol* 2000;59:1563–1571.

93. Krystal JH, Price LH, Opsahl C, et al. Chronic 3,4-methylenedioxymethamphetamine (MDMA) use: effects on mood and neuropsychological function? *Am J Drug Alcohol Abuse* 1992;18:331–341.

94. Kuikka JT, Ahonen AK. Toxic effect of MDMA on brain serotonin neurons [Letter]. *Lancet* 1999;353:1269.

95. Lawn JC. Schedules of controlled substances: scheduling of 3,4-methylenedioxymethamphetamine (MDMA) into schedule I. *Fed Reg* 1986;51:36552–36560.

96. Lee MA, Shlain B. *Acid dreams: the CIA, LSD and the sixties rebellion.* New York: Grove Weidenfeld, 1985.

97. LeSage M, Clark R, Poling A. MDMA and memory: the acute and chronic effects of MDMA in pigeons performing under a delayed-matching-to-sample procedure. *Psychopharmacology (Berl)* 1993;110:327–332.

98. Lester SJ, Baggott M, Welm S, et al. Cardiovascular effects of 3,4-methylenedioxymethamphetamine; a double-blind, placebo-controlled trial. *Ann Intern Med* 2000;133:969–973.

99. Levin A. Abuse of fenfluramine. *Br Med J* 1973;2:49.

100. Lieb R, Schuetz CG, Pfister H, et al. Mental disorders in ecstasy users: a prospective-longitudinal investigation. *Drug Alcohol Depend* 2002;68:195–207.

101. Liester MB, Grob CS, Bravo GL, et al. Phenomenology and sequelae of 3,4-methylenedioxymethamphetamine use. *J Nerv Ment Dis* 1992;180:343–352.

102. MacInness N, Handley SL, Harding GFA. Former chronic methylenedioxymethamphetamine (MDMA or ecstasy) users report mild depressive symptoms. *J Psychopharmacol* 2001;15:181–186.

103. Malberg JE, Seiden LS. Small changes

in ambient temperature cause large changes in 3,4-methylenedioxymethamphetamine (MDMA)-induced serotonin neurotoxicity and core body temperature in the rat. *J Neurosci* 1998; 18:5086–5094.

104. Manchanda S, Connolly MJ. Cerebral infarction in association with ecstasy abuse. *Postgrad Med J* 1993;69:874–879.

105. Marks J. *The search for the "Manchurian candidate."* New York: Dell, 1979.

106. Marston HM, Reid ME, Lawrence JA, et al. Behavioural analysis of the acute and chronic effects of MDMA treatment in the rat. *Psychopharmacology (Berl)* 1999;144:67–76.

107. Martin TL. Three cases of fatal paramethoxyamphetamine overdose. *J Anal Toxicol* 2001;25:649–651.

108. Mas M, Farre M, De La Torre R, et al. Cardiovascular and neuroendocrine effects and pharmacokinetics of 3,4-methylenedioxymethamphetamine in humans. *J Pharmacol Exp Ther* 1999; 290:136–145.

109. Matthews A, Jones C. Spate of British ecstasy deaths puzzles experts. *Int J Drug Policy* 1992;3:4

110. Maxwell DL, Polkey MI, Henry JA. Hyponatraemia and catatonic stupor after taking "ecstasy." *BMJ* 1993;307:1399.

111. McCann UD, Ricaurte GA. Lasting neuropsychiatric sequelae of (±)methylenedioxymethamphetamine ("ecstasy") in recreational users. *J Clin Psychopharmacol* 1991;11:302–305.

112. McCann UD, Ricaurte GA. MDMA ("ecstasy"), panic disorder: induction by a single dose. *Biol Psychiatry* 1992; 32:950–953.

113. McCann UD, Ricaurte GA. On the neurotoxicity of MDMA and related amphetamine derivatives. *J Clin Psychopharmacol* 1995;15:295–296.

114. McCann U, Hatzidimitriou G, Ridenour A, et al. Dexfenfluramine and serotonin neurotoxicity: further preclinical evidence that clinical caution is indicated. *J Pharmacol Exp Ther* 1994;269:792–798.

115. McCann UD, Ridenour BS, Shaham Y, et al. Serotonin neurotoxicity after (±)3,4-methylenedioxymethamphetamine (MDMA; "ecstasy"): a controlled study in humans. *Neuropsychopharmacology* 1994;10:129–138.

116. McCann UD, Szabo Z, Scheffel U, et al. Positron emission tomographic evidence of toxic effect of MDMA ("ecstasy") on brain serotonin neurons in human beings. *Lancet* 1998;352:1433–1437.

117. McCann UD, Mertl M, Eligulashvili V, et al. Cognitive performance in (+) 3,4-methylenedioxymethamphetamine

(MDMA, "ecstasy") users: a controlled study. *Psychopharmacology (Berl)* 1999;143:417–425.

118. McDermott P, Matthews A, O'Hare P, et al. Ecstasy in the United Kingdom: recreational drug use and subcultural change. In: Heather N, Wodak A, Nadelman E, et al., eds. *Psychoactive drugs and harm reduction: from faith to science.* London: Whurr Publishers, 1993.

119. McGuire PK, Cope H, Fahy TA. Diversity of psychopathology associated with use 3,4-methylenedioxymethamphetamine ("ecstasy"). *Br J Psychiatry* 1994;165:391–395.

120. McGuire P, Fahy T. Chronic paranoid psychosis after misuse of MDMA ("ecstasy"). *BMJ* 1991;302:697.

121. McKenna DJ, Peroutka SJ. Neurochemistry and neurotoxicity of 3,4-methylenedioxymethamphetamine. *J Neurochem* 1990;54:14–22.

122. Mechan AO, O'Shea E, Elliott JM, et al. A neurotoxic dose of 3,4-methylenedioxymethamphetamine (MDMA; ecstasy) to rats results in a long-term defect in thermoregulation. *Psychopharmacology (Berl)* 2001;155:413–418.

123. Messing RB, Fisher L, Phebus L, et al. Interaction of diet and drugs in the regulation of brain 5-hydroxyindoles and the response to painful electric shock. *Life Sci* 1976;18:707–714.

124. Meyendorff E, Jain A, Traskman-Bendz L, et al. The effects of fenfluramine on suicidal behavior. *Psychopharmacol Bull* 1986;22:155–159.

125. Nash FJ, Meltzer HY, Gudelsky GA. Elevation of serum prolactin and corticosterone concentrations in rat after administration of MDMA. *J Pharmacol Exp Ther* 1988;245:873–879.

126. Neill JR. "More than medical significance": LSD and American psychiatry 1953–1966. *J Psychoactive Drugs* 1987;19:39–45.

127. Nelson KT. MDMA and memory impairment: proven or not? *MAPS Bulletin* 1999;9(3):6–8.

128. Newmeyer JA. X at the crossroads. *J Psychoactive Drugs* 1993;25:341–342.

129. Nichols GR, Davis GJ, Corrigan CA, et al. Death associated with abuse of a "designer drug." *J Ky Med Assoc* 1990;88:601–603.

130. NIDA. *Monitoring the Future Study.* U.S. Department of Health and Human Services, National Institute on Drug Abuse, Bethesda, Md., 2002.

131. Obergriesser T, Ende G, Braus DF, et al. Hippocampal 1H-MRSI in ecstasy users. *Eur Arch Psychiatry Clin Neurosci* 2001;251:114–116.

132. O'Callaghan JP. Quantitative features

of reactive gliosis following toxicant-inducing damage to the CNS. *Ann N Y Acad Sci* 1993;679:195–210.

133. O'Callaghan JP. Commentary on article by Ricaurte and colleagues. *MAPS Bulletin* 1995;6(1):13.

134. O'Callaghan JP, Miller DB. Quantification of reactive gliosis as an approach to neurotoxicity assessment. *NIDA Res Monogr* 1993;136:188–212.

135. O'Callaghan JP, Miller DB. Neurotoxicity profiles of substituted amphetamines in the C57BL/6J mouse. *J Pharmacol Exp Ther* 1994;270:741–751.

136. Pallanti S, Mazzi D. MDMA (ecstasy) precipitation of panic disorder. *Biol Psychiatry* 1992;32:91–95.

137. Parrott AC. Human psychopharmacology of ecstasy (MDMA): a review of 15 years of empirical research. *Hum Psychopharmacol Clin Exp* 2001;1:557–577.

138. Parrott AC, Buchanan T, Scholey AB, et al. Ecstasy/MDMA attributed problems reported by novice, moderate and heavy recreational users. *Hum Psychopharmacol Clin Exp* 2002;17:309–312.

139. Parrott AC. Recreational Ecstasy/MDMA, the serotonin syndrome, and serotonergic neurotoxicity. *Pharmacol Biochem Behav* 2002;71:837–844.

140. Peroutka SJ. Incidence of recreational use of 3,4-methylenedioxymethamphetamine (MDMA, "ecstasy") on an undergraduate campus. *N Engl J Med* 1987;317:1542–1543.

141. Peroutka SJ, Pascoe N, Faull KF. Monoamine metabolites in the cerebrospinal fluid of recreational users of 3,4-methylenedimethoxymethamphetamine (MDMA; "ecstasy"). *Res Commun Subst Abuse* 1987;8:125–138.

142. Peroutka SJ, Newman H, Harris H. Subjective effects of 3,4-methylenedioxymethamphetamine in recreational users. *Neuropsychopharmacology* 1988;1:273–277.

143. Peroutka SJ. Ecstasy: a human neurotoxin? *Arch Gen Psychiatry* 1989;46:191.

144. Poland RE, Lutchmansingh P, McCracken JT, et al. Abnormal ACTH and prolactin responses to fenfluramine in rats exposed to single and multiple doses of MDMA. *Psychopharmacology (Berl)* 1997;131:411–419.

145. Price LH, Ricaurte GA, Krystal JH, et al. Neuroendocrine and mood responses to intravenous L-tryptophan in 3,4-methylenedioxymethamphetamine (MDMA) users. *Arch Gen Psychiatry* 1989;46:20–22.

146. Ramamoorthy Y, Ai-ming Y, Suh N, et al. Reduced (+)-3,4-methylene-

dioxymethamphetamine ("ecstasy") metabolism with cytochrome P450 2D6 inhibitors and pharmacogenetic variants *in vitro. Biochem Pharmacol* 2002;63:2111–2119.

147. Ramsey M, Partridge B, Byron C. Drug misuse declared in 1998: key results from the British Crime Survey. *Research Findings.* 1999;93:1–4.

148. Randall T. Ecstasy-fueled "rave" parties become dances of death for English youths. *JAMA* 1992;268:1505–1506.

149. Reneman L, Majoie CB, Schmand B, et al. Prefrontal N-acetylaspartate is strongly associated with memory performance in (abstinent) ecstasy users: preliminary report. *Biol Psychiatry* 2001;50:550–554.

150. Reneman L, Majoie CB, Flick H, et al. Reduced N-acetylaspartate levels in the frontal cortex of 3,4-methylenedioxymethamphetamine (ecstasy) users: preliminary results. *AJNR Am J Neuroradiol* 2002;23:231–237.

151. Riedlinger TJ, Riedlinger JE. Psychedelic and entactogenic drugs in the treatment of depression. *J Psychoactive Drugs* 1994;26:41–55.

152. Ricaurte G, Bryan G, Strauss L, et al. Hallucinogenic amphetamine selectively destroys brain serotonin nerve terminals. *Science* 1985;229:986–988.

153. Ricaurte GA, DeLanney LE, Irwin I, et al. Toxic effects of MDMA on 5-HT neurons in the primate: importance of route and frequency of administration. *Brain Res* 1988;446:165–168.

154. Ricaurte GA, Finnegan KT, Irwin I, et al. Aminergic metabolites in cerebrospinal fluid of humans previously exposed to MDMA: preliminary observations. *Ann N Y Acad Sci* 1990;600:699–708.

155. Ricaurte GA, Martello A, Katz JL, et al. Lasting effects of (±)3,4-methylenedioxy methamphetamine on central serotonergic neurons in non-primates. *J Pharmacol Exp Ther* 1992;261:616–622.

156. Ricaurte GA, Yuan J, Hatzidimitriou G, et al. Severe dopaminergic neurotoxicity in primates after a common recreational dose regimen of MDMA ("ecstasy"). *Science* 2002;297:2260–2263.

157. Ritvo ER, Freeman BJ, Geller E, et al. Effects of fenfluramine on fourteen autistic outpatients. *J Am Acad Child Psychiatry* 1983;222:549–558.

158. Robinson T, Castaneda E, Whishaw I. Effects of cortical serotonin depletion induced by 3,4-methylenedioxymethamphetamine (MDMA) on behavior, before and after additional cholinergic blockade. *Neuropsychopharmacology* 1993;8:77–85.

159. Rothwell PM, Grant R. Cerebral venous sinus thrombosis induced by "ecstasy." *J Neurol Neurosurg Psychiatry* 1993;56:1035.
160. Saunders N. *E for ecstasy*. London: Saunders, 1993.
161. Saunders N. *Ecstasy and the dance culture*. London: Saunders, 1995.
162. Schifano F, Magni G. MDMA ("ecstasy") abuse: psychopathological features and craving for chocolate: a case series. *Biol Psychiatry* 1994;36:763–767.
163. Schifano F, Oyefeso A, Webb L, et al. Review of deaths related to taking ecstasy, England and Wales, 1997–2000. *BMJ* 2003;326:80–81.
164. Schmidt CJ. Neurotoxicity of the psychedelic amphetamine, methylenedioxymethamphetamine. *J Pharmacol Exp Ther* 1987;240:1–7.
165. Schmidt CJ, Taylor VL. Depression of rat brain tryptophan hydroxylase following the acute administration of methylenedioxymethamphetamine. *Biochem Pharmacol* 1987;36:4095–4102.
166. Schmidt CJ, Abbate GM, Black CK, et al. Selective 5-HT2 receptor antagonists protect against the neurotoxicity of methylenedioxymethamphetamine in rats. *J Pharmacol Exp Ther* 1990;255:478–483.
167. Schmidt CJ, Sullivan CK, Fadayel GM. Blockade of striatal 5-hydroxytryptamine2 receptors reduces the increase in extracellular concentrations of dopamine produced by the amphetamine analogue 3,4-methylenedioxymethamphetamine. *J Neurochem* 1994;62:1382–1389.
168. Seiden LS, Ricaurte GA. Neurotoxicity of methamphetamine and related drugs. In: Meltzer HY, ed. *Psychopharmacology: the third generation of progress*. New York: Raven Press, 1987.
169. Sferios E. Report from DanceSafe: laboratory analysis program reveals DXM tablets sold as "ecstasy." *MAPS* 1999;9(4):47.
170. Shankaran M, Gudelsky GA. A neurotoxic regimen of MDMA suppresses behavioral, thermal and neurochemical responses to subsequent MDMA administration. *Psychopharmacology (Berl)* 1999;147:66–72.
171. Sharkey A. Sorted or distorted. *Guardian* 1996;Jan 26:2–4.
172. Shewan D, Dalgarno P, King LA. Tablets often contain substances in addition to, or instead of, ecstasy. *Lancet* 1996;313:423–424.
173. Sherlock K, Wolff K, Hay AWM, et al. Analysis of illicit ecstasy tablets: implications for clinical management in the accident and emergency department. *J Accid Emerg Med* 1999;16:194–197.
174. Shulgin AT. History of MDMA. In: Peroutka SJ, ed. *Ecstasy: the clinical, pharmacological and neurotoxicological effects of the drug MDMA*. Holland: Kluwer, 1990:1–20.
175. Shulgin AT, Nichols DE. Characterization of three new psychotomimetics. In: Stillman R, Willete R, eds. *The psychopharmacology of hallucinogens*. New York: Pergamon Press, 1978:74–83.
176. Shulgin A, Shulgin A. *PIHKAL*. Berkeley: Transform Press, 1991.
177. Siegel RK. MDMA: nonmedical use and intoxication. *J Psychoactive Drugs* 1986;18:349–354.
178a. Siever LJ, Coccaro EF, Zemishalny Z, et al. Psychobiology of personality disorders: pharmacologic implications. *Psychopharmacol Bull* 1987;23:333–336179.
178b. Siever LJ, Davis KL. A psychological perspective on personality disorders. *Am J Psychol* 1991;148:1647–1658.
179. Simon NG, Mattick RP. The impact of regular ecstasy use on memory function. *Addiction* 2002;97:1523–1529.
180. Solowij J, Lee N. *Survey of ecstasy (MDMA) users in Sydney*. Rozelle, New South Wales, Australia: New South Wales Health Department Research Grant Report Series DAD 1991:91.
181. Sprague JE, Nichols DE. The monoamine oxidase-B inhibitor 1-deprenyl protects against 3,4-methylenedioxymethamphetamine-induced lipid peroxidation and long-term serotonergic deficits. *J Pharmacol Exp Ther* 1995;273:667–673.
182. Squier MV, Jalloh S, Hilton-Jones D, Series H. Death after ecstasy ingestion: neuropathological findings. *J Neurol Neurosurg Psychiatry* 1995;58:756–764.
183. Sylvester R. Ecstasy: the truth. *Sunday Telegraph* 1995;Nov 19:24.
184. Tancer M, Schuster CR. Serotonin and dopamine system interactions in the reinforcing properties of psychostimulants: a research strategy. *MAPS* 1997;7(3):5–11.
185. Tancer M, Johanson CE. Subjective responses to MDMA and mCPP: a human dose run-up study. *CPDD* 1999;160.
186. Ward NG, Ang J, Pavinich G. A comparison of the acute effects of dextroamphetamine and fenfluramine in depression. *Biol Psychiatry* 1985;20:1090–1097.
187. Watson L, Beck J. New age seekers: MDMA use in spiritual pursuit. *J Psychoactive Drugs* 1991;23:261–270.
188. Winstock AR. Chronic paranoid psychosis after misuse of MDMA. *BMJ* 1991;302:1150–1151.
189. Whitaker-Azmitia PM, Aronson TA. "Ecstasy" (MDMA)-induced panic. *Am J Psychiatry* 1989;146:119.
190. Wolff K, Hay AWM, Sherlock K, et al. Contents of "ecstasy." *Lancet* 1996;346:1100–1101.
191. Yamamoto BK, Nash JF, Gudelsky GA. Modulation of methylenedioxymethamphetamine-induced striatal dopamine release by the interaction between serotonin and gamma-aminobutyric acid in the substantia nigra. *J Pharmacol Exp Ther* 1995;273(3):1063–1070.
192. Young F. *Opinion and recommended ruling, findings of fact, conclusions of law and decision of administrative law judge: submitted in the matter of MDMA scheduling*. U.S. Drug Enforcement Administration Docket No. 84–88, 22 May 1986.
193. Ziporyn T. A growing industry and menace: makeshift laboratory's designer drugs. *JAMA* 1986;256:3061–3063.

CHAPTER 23
Nicotine

JOY M. SCHMITZ AND
KATHERINE A. DELAUNE

Nicotine is one of the most widely abused substances in America. An estimated 25% of the U.S. population smokes, making nicotine addiction a critical public health problem in terms of morbidity, mortality, and economic costs to society. It is well documented that smoking substantially increases the risk of coronary heart disease, cancer, and more than 40 other medical diseases. Even in the face of negative health consequences, smokers continue to use tobacco and quit unsuccessfully, attesting to the high addictive potential of nicotine. In view of the pervasiveness and impact of this addiction, there has been great interest in advancing our understanding of the neurochemical actions of nicotine. Current scientific literature clearly establishes the actions of nicotine within the central nervous system that lead to acute positive reinforcement, the development of dependence, and withdrawal symptoms. Other factors that contribute considerably to nicotine's highly addictive potential include the efficient drug-delivery system of the cigarette, its high level of availability, the small number of legal and social consequences of tobacco use, and the sophisticated marketing and advertising methods used by tobacco companies. This chapter reviews the extent and impact of nicotine use, its addictive properties, and currently available pharmacologic and behavioral treatments.

EXTENT AND IMPACT OF NICOTINE USE

Prevalence

According to the Centers for Disease Control and Prevention (CDC), an estimated 46.5 million adults (23.3%) are current smokers (1). This represents a significant decline from rates reported in 1965 (42.4%), but little change from 1990 rates (25.5%) (see Fig. 23.1). The CDC's report highlights differences in smoking rates among certain demographic groups. Smoking prevalence is significantly higher among men (25.7%) than among women (21.0%). Among ethnic groups, Asians (14.4%) and Hispanics (18.6%) have the lowest smoking rates, while American Indians/Alaska Natives (36.0%) have the highest. Across education levels, rates are highest for adults who earned a General Educational Development (GED) diploma (47.2%) and lowest for those with advanced degrees (8.4%). Adults living below the poverty level (31.7%) have higher smoking rates than those at or above this income level (22.9%). Among age groups, persons age 18 to 44 years have the highest smoking rates and

those age 65 years or older, the lowest. An estimated 44.3 million adults (22.2%) are former smokers, and among current smokers, 70% report that they want to quit completely (1).

Health Consequences

Smoking is the leading cause of premature death in the United States, resulting in more than 440,000 deaths each year (2) (Fig. 23.2). Illness related to smoking costs the adult smoker an average of 13.2 (female) and 14.5 (male) years of life. Cigarette smoking significantly increases the risk of lung cancer, ischemic heart disease, chronic airway obstruction, and perinatal complications (2). The health benefits of quitting smoking are substantial, including a decreased risk of lung cancer, other cancers, cardiovascular disease, chronic lung disease, and infertility (3). Exposure to environmental tobacco smoke (ETS), a known human carcinogen, also increases the risk of cancer and is associated with the deaths of almost 40,000 nonsmokers each year (4). The economic costs of smoking are tremendous, with each pack of cigarettes sold in the United States resulting in costs of $7.18 in medical care expenses and lost productivity (2). Further, it is estimated that $75.5 billion is spent each year on smoking-related personal medical care.

NICOTINE AS AN ADDICTIVE DRUG

Addictive Properties

The majority of smokers use tobacco because they are addicted to nicotine. Nicotine is recognized as the primary compound in tobacco smoke that meets criteria for abuse potential and dependence (5). First, it has centrally mediated, psychoactive effects that are reliably discriminated from placebo (6,7). Second, nicotine produces pleasurable or euphoriant effects, as rated subjectively by smokers on drug "liking" scales (8). Third, nicotine functions as a positive reinforcer (see, e.g., references 6 and 9). Both animals and human smokers will self-administer nicotine over placebo (10). Fourth, tolerance to the effects of nicotine develops after repeated administration (11). Finally, an abstinence syndrome is observed when regular nicotine administration is discontinued (12).

Most smokers meet the diagnostic criteria for tobacco dependence, as specified in the 1994 *Diagnostic and Statistical Manual of Mental Disorders,* 4th ed. (*DSM–IV*) (13). These include (a) tolerance; (b) withdrawal; (c) used in larger amounts or over a longer period than intended; (d) persistent desire or unsuccessful efforts to cut down or quit; (e) a great deal of time spent using the substance; (f) giving up important social, occupational, or recreational activities because of substance use; and (g) continued use despite knowledge of medical problems related to use.

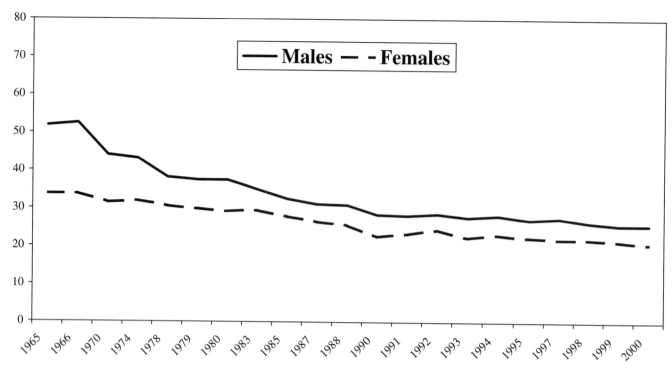

FIG. 23.1. Percentage of smoking prevalence among U.S. adults, 18 years of age and older, by gender, 1965–2000. (From Centers for Disease Control and Prevention (CDC). *MMWR Morb Mortal Wkly Rep* 2002, with permission.)

A host of smoking-related stimuli influence smoking reinforcement (14). Many of the behavioral and sensory components of the act of smoking provide cues that become reinforcing through their association with the pharmacologic effects of nicotine. Studies involving denicotinized tobacco cigarettes, that is, cigarettes that resemble normal cigarettes in taste, but deliver one-tenth of the nicotine, confirm the important role of non-nicotine factors in smoking reinforcement. For example, denicotinized cigarettes produce ratings of "liking and satisfaction" similar to regular cigarettes, and when smoked after a period of nicotine deprivation, may temporarily suppress cigarette withdrawal symptoms (15). Thus, the high abuse liability or "addictiveness" of cigarettes is partly influenced by non-nicotine sensory stimuli associated with smoking. Recent observations point to possible gender differences in the role of non-nicotine influences on smoking reinforcement. Women may be reinforced less by nicotine intake and more by other, non-nicotine factors, relative to men (14,16). Potential gender differences in the efficacy of nicotine are relevant in terms of treatments for smoking cessation, as discussed later in this chapter in the section titled "women".

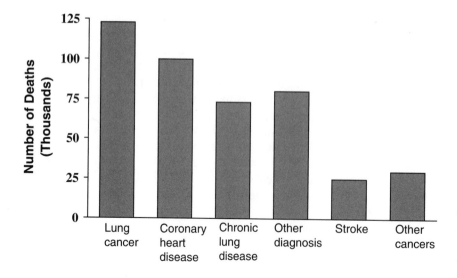

FIG. 23.2. Annual deaths attributable to smoking. (From Centers for Disease Control and Prevention (CDC). *MMWR Morb Mortal Wkly Rep* 1997;46:448–451, with permission.)

CHAPTER 23 NICOTINE / 389

A subpopulation of smokers (5% to 10%) appears to be resistant to nicotine dependence (termed *chippers* or occasional nondependent smokers). These individuals smoke fewer than five cigarettes per day for many years and stop smoking without experiencing withdrawal symptoms. Differences in smoking topography, or how cigarettes are smoked (e.g., intercigarette interval, puff number, interpuff interval) do not seem to account for the lack of dependence in tobacco chippers (17). Like dependent smokers, chippers absorb equal amounts of nicotine, eliminate nicotine at equal rates, and show similar cardiovascular responses to smoking (18,19). Thus, smoking patterns in chippers seem to be more influenced by situational factors than are the smoking patterns in dependent smokers (20).

Compared to cocaine, heroin, or alcohol, addiction to nicotine is far more common and the rate of progression from initial use to daily "addictive" levels of intake is considerably higher. Drug users rate perceived difficulty in quitting smoking as comparable to quitting other substances and, when attempts to quit are made, rates and patterns of relapse are similar across drugs (21). As presented in the next section, the neuropharmacologic actions of nicotine on the brain reward circuit are common to those for other drugs of abuse (22).

Determinants of Use

Neurochemical Actions

Actions of nicotine on the neurochemical system appear to be involved in mediating the acute positive reinforcing effects of nicotine. Nicotine activates nicotinic acetylcholine receptors (nAChRs) in the mesocorticolimbic dopaminergic system that projects from the ventral tegmental area (VTA) to the nucleus accumbens and the prefrontal cortex (23–25). Several nAChR subtypes have been identified, which differ in functional significance, distribution, and sensitivity to nicotine. It is the diversity of nAChRs that may explain the multiple effects of nicotine in humans. When activated, there is a cascade of reinforcing effects, particularly dopamine release (26). Experimentally, it has been shown that systemic administration of nicotine produces a dose-dependent increase in dopamine levels in the nucleus accumbens, whereas administration of mecamylamine, a nicotine antagonist, blocks nicotine-induced dopamine release (27). To date, the preponderance of data points to the critical role of the midbrain *dopamine* system in nicotine reinforcement processes. The increase in dopamine levels is a neurochemical effect shared by other drugs that also serve as positive reinforcers (25,28,29). It should be noted, however, that other neuronal pathways, including those involving glutamate (30), γ-aminobutyric acid (GABA) (31), opioid peptides (32), and serotonin (33), appear to contribute to the reinforcing properties of nicotine-induced dopaminergic neurotransmission.

Whereas initial acute nicotine exposure stimulates the nAChR, the effects of nicotine after chronic exposure appear paradoxical in that further exposure leads to receptor desensitization and inactivation (34). This is followed by an increase in the number of nAChRs, also known as receptor upregulation (35; for a review see reference 36). It is this type of neuroadaptation in the dopaminergic system following chronic administration of nicotine that marks the development of dependence. It has been hypothesized that nicotine addiction may involve self-medication to effectively control the number of functional nAChRs resulting from upregulation (37,38). Similarly, neuronal alterations involving dopamine appear to contribute to nicotine withdrawal symptomatology. Decreases in dopamine output in the nucleus accumbens have been observed during nicotine withdrawal (39–41). Additionally, upregulation of nicotine binding sites during cessation is thought to play a role in the intensity of the early withdrawal symptoms and the likelihood of relapse (41). Alterations in other neurotransmitter systems also may play a role in nicotine withdrawal (42).

In summary, preclinical studies have been useful in establishing some of the neuronal mechanisms related to the reinforcing effects of nicotine and chronic nicotine use. With increasing sophistication and specificity, these animal models have provided findings in accord with human models and thereby come increasingly close to capturing the complex behavior of human tobacco smoking (9).

Pharmacokinetic Dynamic Properties of Nicotine

Nicotine's pharmacokinetic properties also enhance its abuse potential. Inhaled nicotine is directly absorbed through the pulmonary capillaries into the pulmonary venous circulation and then to the left side of the heart. It is the arterial concentration of nicotine that first encounters the central nervous system and other tissues, driving acute pharmacologic effects. Peak arterial nicotine concentrations of up to 60 ng/mL during smoking have been reported (43–46). These high concentrations of nicotine in the arterial circulation produce a host of acute pharmacodynamic effects. In particular, nicotine induces release of epinephrine from the adrenal medulla, which acts, in part, to activate the sympathetic nervous system (10). Sympathomimetic effects of nicotine include heart rate acceleration, transient increase in blood pressure, increased cardiac output, and some constriction of blood vessels (47). Tolerance develops to some, but not all, of the cardiovascular effects of nicotine (48).

Additionally, the absorbed *dose* of nicotine is a determinant of its actions. In general, it has been shown that nicotine produces dose-related effects on cardiovascular, electroencephalographic, appetitive, emotional, and cognitive responses (8). Other variables that affect nicotine absorption and plasma concentrations during smoking include the interval between cigarettes, the frequency and degree of inhalation, and the nicotine content of the cigarette (49,50).

The *speed* at which a drug reaches the brain and central nervous system is critical to understanding its potential reinforcement and abuse liability (10). Rapid delivery systems have much higher abuse liability, or reinforcing efficacy, than slower delivering systems (51). Inhalation of nicotine via cigarette smoking produces the most rapid delivery of nicotine to the brain, with drug levels peaking within a few seconds of inhalation, similar to other drugs that have high abuse potential (41,52). Undeniably, the cigarette is an extremely efficient and highly engineered drug-delivery system. By inhaling, the smoker can get nicotine to the brain very rapidly with each puff. A typical smoker will take 10 puffs on a cigarette over a period of 5 minutes that the cigarette is lit. The acute effects of nicotine dissipate in a few minutes, causing the smoker to continue dosing frequently throughout the day to maintain the drug's pleasurable effects and prevent withdrawal. Thus, a person who smokes about 1.5 packs (30 cigarettes) daily gets 300 "hits" of nicotine to the brain each day across a variety of contexts. These rapid onset and offset effects of nicotine via inhaled tobacco smoke contribute considerably to its highly addictive nature.

In contrast to cigarette smoking, less-rapid release of nicotine, such as via transdermal nicotine, produces slower and lower peak arterial nicotine concentrations (53), resulting in a relatively steady level of nicotine and significantly less pharmacologic and behavioral reinforcement (54,55). Rate of nicotine absorption from other delivery systems, such as nicotine gum, nasal spray, and inhaler, is more rapid than the patch, but slower than with cigarette smoking. Of the different nicotine replacement systems, the nasal spray has a pharmacokinetic profile closest to cigarettes. After a single dose of 1 mg nicotine, the peak level is reached within 5 to 10 minutes. This rapid absorption rate also is associated with more intense subjective effects relative to other nicotine delivery systems (56). Thus, the delivery system, which controls the route and rate of nicotine dosing, is a critical determinant of the development of nicotine dependence.

At least 4,700 constituents of cigarette mainstream smoke have been identified, with more than 100,000 components still unidentified (57). Those constituents observed at higher concentrations (>1 μg) have been categorized into four groups: carbon monoxide; other vapor phase components (e.g., acetaldehyde, formaldehyde, nitrogen oxides); particulate matter or "tar;" and nicotine. These four components of cigarette smoke are delivered to the active smoker as a complex aerosol composed of semiliquid particles of combustion gases. A substantial literature supports the association between these components of cigarette smoke and risk for development or exacerbation of cardiovascular disease (for review, see reference 58).

Clinical Aspects of Tobacco Dependence

Development of Dependence

Only one-third to one-half of individuals who experiment with cigarette smoking become nicotine dependent (59). The development of dependence involves a progression through a series of stages. Initial use is largely driven by psychosocial motives or nonpharmacologic factors, whereas later use is motivated more by pharmacologic factors, including positive nicotine effects and withdrawal relief (60). More specifically, the stages of preparation, initial use or sampling, experimentation, regular smoking, and addiction have been described, although no accepted measurement of this classification scheme exists (61). Identifying which adolescents in the early stages will proceed to become established, dependent smokers has been the focus of considerable research. Beliefs and attitudes related to smoking appear to be important predictors of the transition from experimentation to established smoking (62), along with exposure to other smokers and perceived school performance. In a longitudinal study of 2,684 adolescents, Choi and colleagues (61) found that experimenters who were at highest risk to progress to later stages of smoking and nicotine dependence were those who lacked a firm commitment to abstain from smoking, associated with friends who smoke, and perceived their school performance as average or below. Similar findings have been reported in other prospective studies (see, e.g., references 63 and 64). There may be gender differences in determinants of smoking and nicotine dependence. Killen and colleagues (63) found that, for girls, a strong need for social interaction influences smoking development, whereas for boys, higher levels of depression symptoms are more influential. For girls, smoking onset and continuation may be influenced by concern for weight and body shape (63,65).

Vulnerability to nicotine dependence may be related to individual differences in sensitivity to nicotine, starting with initial exposure. Along these lines, two somewhat contrasting models have been put forth to explain why some people who experiment with tobacco go on to smoke regularly, whereas others do not. According to the "exposure" model of tolerance or dependence, more sensitive individuals, that is, those who encounter aversive effects on initial use, are less likely to engage in further experimentation, whereas people with less sensitivity to nicotine experience fewer unpleasant effects and, as a consequence, are more likely to continue (66). Social reinforcement, typically peer pressure, serves to further maintain early self-administration of nicotine. Beyond initial sensitivity, level of continued exposure to nicotine presumably leads to degree of tolerance and dependence. If the prevailing environment is facilitating or permissive of smoking, nicotine dependence is likely to develop.

In contrast, the "sensitivity" model of dependence proposes that dependent smokers are those who are constitutionally *more* sensitive to nicotine. For them, initial exposure to smoking produces aversive and rewarding effects, with continued exposure associated with a decrease in sensitivity as tolerance develops (67). Accumulating evidence favoring the sensitivity model of dependence includes research on the genetics of nicotine dependence. Twin studies conducted in the early 1980s consistently reported important genetic influences on the probability of smoking initiation and persistence (for a review, see reference 68). Heritability estimates for smoking initiation from various large sample twin studies fall within the range of 46% to 84%, with approximately 30% of the variance accounted for by shared environmental influences (68–71). Among those who become regular smokers, heritability estimates of 70% have been reported for smoking persistence, suggesting a more powerful genetic effect with little shared environmental influence for development of dependence. Genetic influences on smoking and dependence may arise from individual differences in response to nicotine. Specifically, initial nicotine sensitivity differs in selected mouse strains known to be genetically distinct (72,73). Thus, it appears that development of nicotine dependence is not simply the result of differential exposure to nicotine, but is also a consequence of preexisting differences in sensitivity to nicotine.

Dependence

Characteristic features of dependence include persistent use despite knowledge of medical problems related to smoking, withdrawal symptoms upon cessation of use, and unsuccessful efforts to stop (13). The majority of regular smokers meet the *DSM–IV* diagnostic criteria for tobacco dependence (74). Dependent smokers report desirable and useful effects derived from nicotine. For example, nicotine can alleviate stress and anxiety, facilitate learning and memory performance, and can function to control appetite and weight. These behavioral and subjective effects of smoking correspond strongly with the neuroregulatory actions of nicotine (75). For example, neuroregulatory mechanisms involving dopamine, norepinephrine, and β-endorphin mediate the pleasure and enhancement of pleasurable consequences of smoking, whereas mechanisms involving acetylcholine and norepinephrine mediate facilitation of task performance because of smoking (76,77). Thus dependent smokers smoke to produce a variety of effects that are positively, as well as negatively reinforcing.

Cotinine, the primary proximate metabolite of nicotine, is present in the blood of smokers in much higher levels than is nicotine. The half-life of cotinine is considerably longer than that of nicotine (average 16 hours vs. 2 hours) (55). Recent findings from a study of cotinine in abstinent cigarette smokers suggest that cotinine is behaviorally active. Keenan and colleagues (78) showed that cotinine, compared with placebo, produced significant changes in

(reversal of) subjective parameters of withdrawal, including restlessness, anxiety/tension, insomnia, sedation, and pleasantness. Whereas previously thought to have minimal pharmacologic activity (79,80), these data underscore the potentially important role of cotinine in the complex process of nicotine dependence.

Physical dependence is commonly measured by the demonstration of an abstinence syndrome characterized by signs and symptoms of withdrawal when regular drug use is discontinued. Abstinence from tobacco yields such an effect, as described in the following section.

Withdrawal

Diagnostic criteria for nicotine withdrawal according to the *DSM–IV* include at least four of the following signs occurring within 24 hours of abrupt cessation of nicotine use or reduction in the amount of nicotine use: (a) dysphoric or depressed mood; (b) insomnia; (c) irritability, frustration, or anger; (d) anxiety; (e) difficulty concentrating; (f) restlessness; (g) decreased heart rate; and (h) increased appetite or weight gain. Craving for nicotine, although no longer listed as a diagnostic criterion, is considered to be an important element in nicotine withdrawal. Craving and impaired concentration are two of the most frequently reported symptoms of nicotine withdrawal (12,81). It is well documented that nicotine deprivation can impair psychomotor and cognitive abilities (82,83) and that smoking reverses these performance deficits (84).

Traditional models of drug dependence posit withdrawal to be centrally involved in motivating drug use and relapse (see, e.g., reference 85). In support, a number of studies show a relationship between the presence and severity of nicotine withdrawal symptoms and the probability that a smoker attempting to quit will relapse (86–88). More recently, however, the withdrawal phenomenon has been challenged based on reported inconsistency in the interrelationship of dependence severity, withdrawal, and relapse. Smokers frequently do not identify withdrawal as precipitating relapse, and relapse often occurs long after cessation, when, presumably, withdrawal symptoms have abated (89). Using newer and more sensitive approaches to the study of withdrawal, Piasecki and colleagues showed that withdrawal profiles, consisting primarily of affect, urge, and sleep/energy dimensions, vary by individual and over time. Moreover, smokers having "atypical" withdrawal profiles, defined as those with unremitting symptoms peaking late after cessation, are more likely to relapse than other smokers having more common withdrawal patterns (90). Affective components of the withdrawal syndrome have shown the strongest relations with relapse (91–93). There is a robust link between depression, negative affect, and smoking relapse. That smokers exhibit higher rates of major depressive disorder than nonsmokers is established (94–96), as is the prediction that smokers with past depression will have greater withdrawal-related increases in anger and depression during the first week of quitting and be more likely to relapse (93). It is not so clear, however, whether negative affect in abstinent smokers constitutes a nicotine-induced withdrawal response or the emergence of an affective disorder. Thus, the effect of nicotine on mood and negative affect is complex and in need of further research.

Withdrawal symptoms are believed to be primarily caused by nicotine deprivation. Nevertheless, other nonpharmacologic factors of tobacco smoking, such as conditioning (97) and expectancy (98), influence aspects of behavior during nicotine withdrawal. Smoking denicotinized cigarettes can significantly reduce acute tobacco withdrawal symptoms and craving scores (15,82,99), pointing to the apparent contribution of sensory and environmental factors in nicotine withdrawal effects (100). That nicotine replacement strategies, which presumably suppress withdrawal, do not entirely correspond with their ability to produce abstinence (101) may be explained by the important role of factors other than nicotine in tobacco withdrawal.

TREATMENT OF NICOTINE ADDICTION

Given the substantial negative consequences of smoking, and the finding that 70% of smokers report wanting to quit (1), the goal of making effective treatment options available to all smokers has become a public health priority. In primary health care settings, however, fewer than one-third of smokers are asked about their smoking status, encouraged to quit, or offered assistance quitting smoking (102). This is unfortunate given the evidence that even brief smoking cessation interventions can be efficacious and cost-effective (103–105). To address this problem, the Agency for Health Care Policy and Research published *Treating Tobacco Use and Dependence Clinical Practice Guideline* (the *Guideline*) (103). The purpose of the *Guideline* is to identify effective smoking cessation interventions and provide treatment recommendations applicable to a wide array of clinical settings and patient populations. This is accomplished through a comprehensive, systematic review and meta-analysis of the smoking cessation literature, including only randomized, placebo-controlled trials. Recommendations from the *Guideline,* as well as other relevant findings, are reviewed below.

According to the *Guideline's* treatment model for clinical settings (see Fig. 23.3), tobacco use status (current, former, or never) should be assessed and documented for each patient. Current smokers should be advised to quit and their motivation to do so should be assessed. For those willing to make a quit attempt, counseling and/or pharmacotherapy should be used, either through a brief intervention or referral to more intensive treatment, keeping in mind that there is a strong dose–response relationship between treatment intensity and its effectiveness. Smokers unwilling to quit should be offered a brief motivational intervention designed to encourage a quit attempt. Recent quitters should receive an intervention to prevent relapse. No intervention is needed for never smokers or for those who have been abstinent for a long period of time.

Pharmacologic Interventions

The *Guideline* identified five first-line and two second-line smoking cessation pharmacotherapies. First-line pharmacotherapies are those that reliably increase long-term smoking abstinence rates; are safe and effective for the treatment of tobacco dependence; and are approved for this purpose by the U.S. Food and Drug Administration (FDA). These medications have been empirically tested for efficacy and are recommended, unless contraindicated for reasons such as pregnancy/breast-feeding or smoking fewer than 10 cigarettes per day. Second-line medications also have demonstrated efficacy but are not FDA-approved and therefore play a more limited role in treatment. Because there is greater concern about potential side effects, second-line pharmacotherapies should only be considered after first-line treatments have proven ineffective.

First-line pharmacotherapies include bupropion sustained release (Zyban) and four types of nicotine replacement therapy (NRT): nicotine gum, nicotine inhaler,

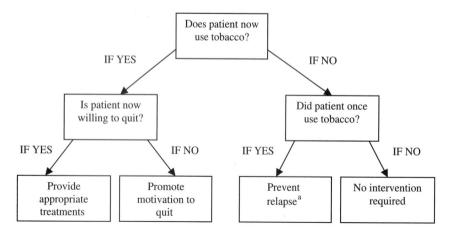

FIG. 23.3. Treatment model for tobacco use and dependence. [a]Relapse prevention interventions are not necessary in the case of the adult who has not used tobacco for many years. (From Fiore MC, Bailey WC, Cohen SJ, et al. *Treating tobacco use and dependence.* Rockville, MD: U.S. Department of Health and Human Services, Public Health Service, June, 2000, with permission.)

nicotine nasal spray, and nicotine patch. Second-line medications are clonidine (Catapres) and nortriptyline (Pamelor). These medications are described below, and their recommended usages are presented in Table 23.1. Tobacco users should be encouraged to use one or a combination of these medications. In addition, most studies reviewed by the *Guideline* combined medication with some type of counseling or behavioral intervention; therefore a multi-component approach is recommended.

Bupropion

Bupropion sustained release (SR) is the first non-nicotine FDA-approved medication for smoking cessation. Its mechanism of action is presumed to relate to its ability to block the reuptake of dopamine and norepinephrine, with no clinically significant effects on serotonin (106). The *Guideline* included results from multicenter studies comparing bupropion SR to placebo, with findings indicating that the medication approximately doubles long-term abstinence rates. More recent studies also support its efficacy. Gonzales et al. (107) evaluated smokers (n = 450) who had previously used bupropion in a smoking cessation attempt. Subjects received either bupropion SR 300 mg per day or placebo for 12 weeks. The bupropion group exhibited significantly higher continuous abstinence rates at 6 months post-quit (12%) than did the placebo group (2%). Hays and colleagues (108) examined 429 smokers who had recently quit smoking. All participants received bupropion SR 300 mg per day for the initial 7 weeks of the trial, then the same dosage or placebo for the next 38

weeks. Results indicate that bupropion, as compared to placebo, significantly improved abstinence rates for up to 18 months (47.7% vs. 37.7%).

Nicotine Replacement Therapy

Four different nicotine replacement products are FDA-approved medications for the treatment of tobacco dependence (see Table 23.1). Results, based on a review of 47 studies, indicate that nicotine gum, inhaler, nasal spray, and transdermal patch appear to be equally effective, with use of these products approximately doubling long-term abstinence rates when compared to placebo (103). Further, combination NRT (e.g., combining the patch with nicotine gum or nasal spray) appears to be more effective than use of a single form of NRT. Recent studies comparing preferences for these four products found that the nicotine patch was rated as less unpleasant than the other methods, but that smokers tend to quickly like whichever of the four they receive (109,110).

Clonidine

Clonidine is used primarily as an antihypertensive medication. The FDA has not approved its use as a smoking cessation medication, and no specific dose regimen for this purpose has been established. The five studies included in analyses for the *Guideline* revealed that clonidine approximately doubled abstinence rates when compared to placebo. The medication remains a second-line treatment because of dosing questions and the potentially high

TABLE 23.1. *Recommended pharmacotherapies for tobacco dependence*

Medication	Recommended dosage	Special considerations
First-Line medications Bupropion SR (Zyban) (prescription only)	Begin 1–2 weeks before quit date with a dose of 150 mg for 3 days, then increase to 300 mg for 7–12 weeks following quit date. Can be considered for maintenance therapy for up to 6 months at same dose.	Offer bupropion if there is a history of depression and/or weight concerns. Pregnant smokers should first be encouraged to quit without medication. *Contraindications:* history of seizure disorder or eating disorder; currently using another form of bupropion; use of an monoamine (MAO) inhibitor in past 14 days.
Nicotine replacement therapy (NRT)		NRT should be used with caution among certain cardiovascular patients. Pregnant smokers should first be encouraged to quit without medication.
Nicotine gum (over-the-counter only)	Gum is available in 2 mg and 4 mg (per piece) doses. For those smoking <25 cigarettes per day, the 2-mg dose is recommended; for >25 per day, the 4-mg dose is recommended. Gum should be used for up to 12 weeks, no more than 24 pieces per day. Dosage should be tailored to the individual patient.	Common side effects are mild and transient and include mouth soreness, hiccups, and jaw ache.

(continued)

TABLE 23.1. *(Continued)*

Medication	Recommended Dosage	Special Considerations
Nicotine inhaler (prescription only)	A dose from the inhaler consists of a puff or inhalation. Each cartridge delivers 4 mg of nicotine over 80 inhalations. Dosage of 6–16 cartridges per day for up to 6 months is recommended. Best effects are achieved by frequent puffing. Dosage should be tapered during final 3 months.	Common side effects include local irritation in the mouth and throat, coughing, and runny nose.
Nicotine nasal spray (prescription only)	A dose of nasal spray consists of 0.5 mg nicotine delivered to each nostril. Initial dosing should be 1–2 doses per hour, increasing as needed for symptom relief. Minimum recommended treatment is 8 doses per day, with no more than 40 per day. Therapy should last 3–6 months.	Most users report moderate to severe nasal irritation in the first 2 days of use, with some continuing for several weeks. Other common side effects include nasal congestion and transient changes in smell and taste. *Contraindications:* severe reactive airway disease.
Nicotine patch (transdermal; prescription and over-the-counter)	Dosage should be tailored to the individual based on severity of addiction. The patch should first be applied upon waking on the quit date. Recommended dosage on over-the-counter brands is typically 8 weeks, sometimes tapering the dosage after the first 4 weeks. 16- and 24-hour patches have been equally effective.	Up to 50% of patch users will have a local skin reaction that is typically mild but may worsen over the course of treatment. Another common side effect is insomnia.
Second-line medications		
Clonidine (Catapres) (oral or transdermal; prescription only)	Begin on or up to 3 days before quit date. Dosing in clinical trials has varied significantly, from 0.15–0.75 mg/day (oral) to 0.10–0.20 mg/day (transdermal), without a clear dose–response relation to cessation. Initial dosing is typically 0.10 mg/day and increases by 0.10 mg/day per week if needed. Dose duration has also varied across trials, ranging from 3–10 weeks.	Pregnant smokers should first be encouraged to quit without medication. Clonidine is an antihypertensive and can be expected to lower blood pressure in most patients. Failure to gradually reduce the dose over a period of 2–4 days may result in a rapid increase in blood pressure, agitation, confusion, and/or tremor. Common side effects include dry mouth, drowsiness, dizziness, and sedation.
Nortriptyline (Pomelor) (prescription only)	Begin 10–28 days before quit date. Clinical trials have initiated dosing at 25 mg/day, increasing gradually to a target dose of 75–100 mg/day. Duration in clinical trials has been approximately 12 weeks.	Pregnant smokers should first be encouraged to quit without medication. Nortriptyline is associated with limb reduction abnormalities. Use with extreme caution in cardiovascular patients because of risk of arrhythmias. Common side effects include sedation, dry mouth, blurred vision, urinary retention, lightheadedness, and shaky hands. Overdose may produce cardiotoxic effects.
Combination therapies		
Bupropion SR & NRT	Bupropion SR can be used in combination with NRT.	Combination therapies should be considered if a patient has a history of difficulty quitting and/or is unable to quit with a single medication.
Combination NRT	Combine the nicotine patch with a self-administered form of NRT (gum or nasal spray).	

Adapted from Fiore MC, Bailey WC, Cohen SJ, et al. *Treating tobacco use and dependence.* Rockville, MD: U.S. Department of Health and Human Services, Public Health Service, Agency for Health Care Policy and Research, 2000.

incidence of adverse events upon abrupt discontinuation of clonidine.

Nortriptyline

Nortriptyline, typically used as an antidepressant, does not have FDA approval for smoking cessation. It remains a second-line medication because of potential side effects and limited evidence to support its efficacy. Only two studies met criteria for inclusion in the *Guideline's* analyses, both showing improved outcome with nortriptyline versus placebo. More recently, Hall and colleagues (111) found no significant differences in abstinence rates between bupropion and nortriptyline, but both were more effective than placebo.

Other Nicotine Replacement Therapies

Since publication of the *Guideline,* several new methods of delivering NRT have been examined. Shiffman and colleagues (112) evaluated 2- and 4-mg nicotine lozenges and found both to significantly increase rates of smoking cessation compared to a placebo lozenge at 1 year postquit date. Wallstroem and colleagues (113) compared the nicotine sublingual tablet to placebo and found significant treatment effects at 6 months post-quit date (33% vs. 18%, respectively). Both of these NRT methods provide effective treatment alternatives for smokers.

Other Medications

A number of additional medications have been evaluated for use with smoking cessation; however, support for their efficacy is lacking. Naltrexone (ReVia) is an opioid antagonist approved by the FDA for treatment of opioid and alcohol dependence. Results of two placebo-controlled trials revealed no significant effect of naltrexone either alone (114) or when combined with the patch (115). Fluoxetine (Prozac), paroxetine (Paxil), and sertraline (Zoloft) are all selective serotonin reuptake inhibitors that have been tested in combination with NRT and/or behavioral treatments for smoking cessation. None is associated with a significant treatment effect (116–119). The *Guideline* also reviewed research on mecamylamine (a nicotine antagonist), diazepam (Valium) and buspirone (Buspan) (anxiolytics), and propranolol (Inderal) (a β–blocker), concluding that evidence was insufficient to recommend their use for smoking cessation.

Behavioral Interventions

The characteristics of behavioral interventions for smoking cessation vary widely. The *Guideline* examined four of these characteristics: advice to quit, intensity, treatment format, and type of clinician, as well as specific elements of various types of counseling and therapy. Recommendations based on these analyses are described below and are presented in Table 23.2.

TABLE 23.2. *Characteristics of behavioral interventions for smoking*

Treatment characteristic	Recommendation
Advice to quit smoking	All physicians and clinicians should strongly advise every patient who smokes to quit. Evidence shows that physician advice to quit increases abstinence rates and it is reasonable to believe that clinician advice should also be effective.
Intensity of clinical interventions	Every tobacco user should be offered at least a minimal intervention, whether or not referral to more intensive treatment is made. Evidence supports the efficacy of minimal interventions lasting 3 minutes or less for increasing abstinence rates. Intensive interventions are more effective than less-intensive interventions and should be used whenever possible. Four or more sessions of person-to-person treatment, with a session length of at least 10 minutes and a total contact time of 31–90 minutes per session, appears especially effective in increasing abstinence rates.
Treatment format	The following are effective and should be used in smoking cessation interventions: • Proactive telephone counseling • Group counseling • Individual counseling Interventions that are delivered in multiple formats increase abstinence rates and should be encouraged.
Type of clinician	Treatment delivered by a variety of clinician types (e.g., physician, psychologist, nurse, dentist) increases abstinence rates; therefore all clinicians should provide smoking cessation interventions. Whenever possible, treatment should be delivered by a combination of different types of clinicians, rather than one type of clinician.

Adapted from Fiore MC, Bailey WC, Cohen SJ, et al. *Treating tobacco use and dependence.* Rockville, MD: U.S. Department of Health and Human Services, Public Health Service, June, 2000.

TABLE 23.3. *Common components of effective behavioral treatments*

Treatment	Components
Practical counseling (problem solving training; coping skills training; relapse prevention)	• Identify high-risk situations that increase the risk of smoking • Develop and practice coping skills • Provide basic information about smoking and quitting
Intratreatment support (clinical management)	• Encourage the patient in the quit attempt • Communicate concern and caring • Encourage the patient to talk about the quitting process
Extratreatment support	• Train patient to solicit social support • Encourage support seeking • Arrange outside support for patient
Aversive smoking procedures (rapid smoking; rapid puffing; guided smoking)	• Patient performs procedure to point of discomfort, nausea, or vomiting • May constitute a health risk and should be conducted only with appropriate medical screening and monitoring, and only if other interventions have failed

Adapted from Fiore MC, Bailey WC, Cohen SJ, et al. *Treating tobacco use and dependence.* Rockville, MD: U.S. Department of Health and Human Services, Public Health Service, June, 2000.

Overall results revealed a strong dose–response relationship between treatment intensity (i.e., session length, total contact time, and number of sessions) and treatment effectiveness. However, evidence also indicated that physician advice to quit smoking significantly increases long-term abstinence rates, even with a modal intervention length of 3 minutes or less. Analysis of different treatment formats demonstrated that telephone, group, and individual counseling all improve smoking abstinence rates compared to no intervention; further, using multiple treatment formats increases abstinence rates as compared to use of a single format. A comparison of the effectiveness of different clinician types (e.g., physician, psychologist, nurse, dentist) revealed no significant differences in abstinence rates based on this factor. Also studied was the effectiveness of including multiple clinicians from different disciplines. Although nonsignificant, findings suggest that having a variety of clinician types participate in treatment may be more effective than utilizing a single clinician type.

Types of Behavioral Therapies

In a review of 62 studies examining the effectiveness of different types of counseling and behavioral therapy, 4 treatment types resulted in significant increases in abstinence rates as compared to no-contact control conditions (103): (a) providing practical counseling (e.g., skills training approaches); (b) providing intratreatment social support; (c) helping to increase social support outside of treatment; and (d) using aversive smoking procedures. Table 23.3 presents the common components of these treatment methods.

Alternative Behavioral Therapies

Several studies have examined the effectiveness of alternative interventions for smoking cessation, such as hyp-

nosis, physiologic feedback, exercise, and acupuncture. In the *Guideline,* data regarding hypnosis and physiologic feedback were insufficient to address the efficacy of these methods. Findings related to exercise and acupuncture are generally mixed. Marcus and colleagues (120), in a study of female smokers, combined a cognitive–behavioral smoking cessation intervention with a vigorous exercise program and compared this to the cessation program alone. They found that addition of the exercise component significantly increased continuous abstinence rates at end-of-treatment and at 3 and 12 months posttreatment. However, other evidence presented in the *Guideline* revealed no significant increase in abstinence rates as a result of exercise interventions. Results for acupuncture are similar. A study conducted by Bier and colleagues (121) found that acupuncture combined with education was significantly more effective at increasing end-of-treatment abstinence rates than either sham acupuncture with education or acupuncture alone; however, at 18 months posttreatment no differences between groups were apparent. In another study comparing stimulation of antismoking acupoints to stimulation of unrelated acupoints (122), the intervention resulted in reduced smoking rates, both at end of treatment and 8 months posttreatment. Again, however, results presented in the *Guideline* do not support the efficacy of acupuncture for smoking cessation. These findings suggest a need for further research in these areas.

Alternative Treatment Goals

Harm reduction has been recently suggested as an alternative treatment goal. Harm reduction strategies attempt to change, rather than eliminate, nicotine use so that its harmful effects are reduced. Smokers' views on such strategies are mixed. At least one study found that subjects viewed harm reduction as a more realistic goal than creating a smoke-free home (123). Smokers in methadone maintenance treatment expressed a desire to reduce their smoking if they had health concerns or doubted their ability to quit completely; however, others viewed complete cessation as the only acceptable goal (124).

Several methods for achieving harm reduction have been suggested, including decreased use of tobacco, use of low tar/nicotine cigarettes, or use of nicotine replacement products. However, there are concerns related to some methodologies. For example, smokers of reduced tar/nicotine cigarettes tend to engage in compensatory behaviors, such as smoking more cigarettes or inhaling more deeply (see, e.g., reference 125). Overall, a lack of published data on the efficacy of harm-reduction strategies makes it difficult to evaluate their potential benefits (103). (A more complete review of issues related to harm reduction is found in a special issue [Vol. 4, Supplement 2] of the journal *Nicotine and Tobacco Research*, 2002.)

Special Populations

Smoking and Depression

Much evidence supports an association between depressive symptomatology and smoking. Smokers exhibit higher rates of depression than do nonsmokers (126–128), and depressed, as compared to nondepressed, smokers experience greater difficulty quitting (129,130). Even subclinical levels of depression are associated with decreased latency to first cigarette following a quit attempt (131). Some pharmacotherapies, such as bupropion SR and nortriptyline, demonstrate efficacy for both smoking cessation and depression, and thus may be ideal for treating the depressed smoker. Attempts to establish the efficacy of other antidepressants for smoking cessation have generally been less successful, as previously discussed. However, Cornelius and colleagues (132), in their study of depressed, alcoholic smokers, observed a significant decrease in smoking over the course of treatment for those treated with fluoxetine when compared to placebo. The *Guideline* concludes that evidence is insufficient to determine whether depressed smokers benefit from behavioral treatment tailored to their symptoms, and few recent studies address this issue. In one study, Brown and colleagues (133) compared standard cognitive–behavioral therapy (CBT) for smoking cessation to a combination of standard CBT for smoking cessation plus CBT for depression in smokers with past major depressive disorder. Results indicated no overall group differences, but significantly higher abstinence rates in the combined treatment group for heavy smokers with recurrent, but not single episode, major depressive disorder. Clearly there is a need for further research in this area.

Smoking and Schizophrenia

Two recent studies examined the efficacy of bupropion in smokers with schizophrenia. George and colleagues (134) evaluated schizophrenic outpatients who received behavioral group therapy for smoking cessation and either bupropion SR 300 mg per day (n = 16) or placebo (n = 16) for 10 weeks. Bupropion SR significantly increased abstinence rates at end of treatment, but no group differences were apparent at 6 months posttreatment. In another study, Evins and colleagues (135) compared bupropion SR 150 mg per day (n = 9) to placebo (n = 9) in stabilized schizophrenic outpatients also receiving cognitive–behavioral treatment for smoking cessation. Bupropion was associated with significantly greater reduction in smoking at 6 months post-quit date.

Smoking and Other Chemical Dependence

Rates of smoking among abusers of other drugs are higher than those in the general population, with estimates ranging from 75% to 90% (127,136,137). Comorbidity is associated with increased health problems (138,139), as well as smoking and smoking cessation behaviors. Alcoholic smokers tend to smoke more heavily and experience less success achieving abstinence than their nonalcoholic counterparts (140,141). Despite the fact that nicotine continues to be one of the most common drugs of dependence among patients with alcohol and drug problems, and that many substance abusers express a desire to quit smoking (142), an optimal treatment for smoking cessation in this population has yet to be established. The *Guideline* recommends that smokers with comorbid chemical dependency should be treated with the same smoking cessation interventions proven to be effective in the general population. Available data indicate that patients can be treated for tobacco dependence concurrent to being treated for other chemical dependency (103), with little evidence of patients relapsing to other drugs when they stop smoking (143–145). However, results have been mixed in terms of smoking cessation efficacy. In a recent study by Gariti and colleagues (146) of substance use detoxification inpatients, a brief smoking cessation intervention combined with the nicotine patch resulted in a significant reduction in number of cigarettes smoked per day; however, the same was true for patients in the control group who received the patch and referral to an outpatient smoking program.

Women

Women tend to experience less success quitting smoking than do men (147). Clinical trials evaluated in the *Guideline* revealed that, although the same smoking cessation treatments are effective for both women and men, certain interventions (e.g., nicotine replacement therapy) are less efficacious in women. This may be related to the different stressors and barriers to quitting that women face. For example, women tend to have lower confidence in their ability to quit, a greater likelihood of depression, and greater weight control concerns, and thus may benefit from addressing such issues in treatment (148).

Studies show that women are not only more concerned about weight gain following quitting (149,150), but that they actually do gain more postcessation weight than do men (151). A number of interventions targeting these concerns have been evaluated. Perkins and colleagues (152) compared three adjunct treatments in women participating in group smoking-cessation therapy: (a) CBT aimed at reducing weight concerns and improving body image, in which dieting was discouraged; (b) weight control counseling with dieting; and (c) standard cessation counseling with no weight-related topics. CBT with no dieting resulted in significantly higher 12-month postquit abstinence rates than did standard counseling (21% vs. 9%), and weight control (13%) was not more effective than standard counseling. However, both weight control and CBT were associated with decreases in negative mood following quitting. In another study, Danielsson and colleagues (153) compared a very low-energy diet to no diet in women who had relapsed previously because of postcessation weight gain. All participants received nicotine gum and a combination of smoking cessation and weight-control counseling. The diet resulted in significantly higher abstinence rates at 1 year postquit date (28% vs. 16%).

Pregnant Women

Despite adverse effects of cigarette smoking on pregnancy outcomes, smoking cessation during pregnancy and postpartum relapse prevention remain significant treatment challenges. Evidence presented in the *Guideline* indicates that extended or augmented interventions should be offered to pregnant smokers whenever possible; in studies reviewed, these produced significantly higher rates of smoking cessation than did usual care conditions. The use of pharmacotherapy is recommended only if a pregnant woman is otherwise unable to quit and if the benefits of quitting outweigh the risks associated with the medication. Additional studies reveal some successful outcomes, but most report no treatment effects. Donatelle and colleagues (154) compared brief education for pregnant smokers to brief education combined with enhanced social support and financial incentives. The treatment group demonstrated significantly higher quit rates at both 8 months gestation and 2 months postpartum. In a study of smokers who quit during pregnancy, three treatments were compared: relapse prevention delivered pre- and postpartum, relapse prevention delivered prepartum only, and standard care. The pre- and postpartum intervention, as compared to the other groups, resulted in significantly higher abstinence rates at 6 and 8 weeks postpartum, but no differences were apparent at 12 months postpartum. Results from other studies are less encouraging. Comparisons of postpartum relapse prevention counseling to standard care (155,156), nicotine patch to placebo patch (157), and telephone counseling to self-help materials plus brief physician advice (158) all failed to demonstrate significant treatment effects. Taken together, these findings support the use of augmented behavioral interventions and suggest that increased social support, financial incentives, and relapse prevention counseling delivered both pre- and postpartum may be especially effective.

Adolescents

After increasing throughout most of the 1990s, smoking rates among adolescents have declined significantly since 1997, yet remain high (159). Findings from the National Youth Tobacco Survey indicate that current tobacco use ranges from 15.1% among middle school students to 34.5% among high school students (160). Each day in the United States more than 6,000 children and adolescents try their first cigarette (161). This represents a 30% increase between the years 1988 and 1996 in initiation of first use; over the same time period the incidence of first daily use has increased 50% (162). These statistics are made more disturbing by findings linking tobacco and other substance use. Teens who smoke are 3 times more likely than nonsmokers to use alcohol, 8 times more likely to use marijuana, and 22 times more likely to use cocaine (163).

Despite the fact that more than half of student smokers have expressed a desire to quit, most quit attempts are unsuccessful (160). These findings underscore the need to identify effective prevention and treatment programs for use with this population. The *Guideline* makes four recommendations based on available evidence: (a) clinicians should screen pediatric and adolescent patients, as well as their parents, for tobacco use, and they should strongly emphasize the need to abstain from tobacco use; (b) behavioral interventions with demonstrated efficacy for adults should be considered for children and adolescents after content is made developmentally appropriate; (c) bupropion SR and nicotine replacement therapy are also treatment options, given the lack of evidence that these medications are harmful for children; and (d) in pediatric settings, clinicians should offer advice and information regarding smoking cessation to parents to limit exposure of children to second-hand smoke (103).

CONCLUSIONS

Cigarette smoking, once referred to as a "habit," meets established medical criteria for drug dependence. Nicotine is the drug in tobacco that causes dependence or addiction, similar to the role of ethanol in alcoholic beverage consumption, or cocaine in coca leaf. Significant progress has been made in understanding the relationships among nicotine's behavioral, subjective, physiologic, and neuroregulatory effects. Moreover, this type of scientific research on nicotine dependence has led to improved techniques for reducing tobacco use. Based on a wealth of clinical trial data accumulated over the past decade, the efficacies and approval of five different pharmacotherapies have been established. These and other evidence-based treatments are recommended in a recent Public Health Service report (103) that provides a comprehensive and authoritative guide to the treatment of tobacco dependence. *Guideline* researchers conclude that first-line medications, including bupropion and nicotine replacement therapies, should be used in conjunction with behaviorally based counseling to produce optimal outcomes in smoking cessation. Despite the development of new medications and their increasing availability over the counter, treatment challenges remain. It has been suggested that as the proportion of smokers in the population declines, those who continue to smoke are likely to be those individuals who are most entrenched in their smoking behavior and, therefore, more difficult to treat (164). For example, the prevalence of smoking is declining slowest among individuals with comorbid psychiatric and substance abuse disorders, as well as among the poor and less-educated smokers (165). Thus, the need for brief, broad-based community interventions must be balanced against the need for more intensive and individualized smoking cessation treatments. With a changing population of smokers comes the pressing need to find new ways to help the most dependent smokers to quit.

ACKNOWLEDGMENTS

This research was supported in part by grants from the National Institute on Drug Abuse to Dr. Schmitz (DA08888), and from the National Institute on Alcohol Abuse and Alcoholism (AA11216). We thank Marc Mooney and Shelly Sayre for their helpful comments on an earlier version of the manuscript.

REFERENCES

1. Centers for Disease Control and Prevention. Cigarette smoking among adults—United States, 2000. *MMWR Morb Mortal Wkly Rep* 2002;51(29): 642–645.
2. Centers for Disease Control and Prevention. Annual smoking-attributable mortality, years of potential life lost, and economic costs—United States, 1995–1999. *MMWR Morb Mortal Wkly Rep* 2002;51(14):300–303.
3. Gotfredsen NS, Holst C, Prescott E, et al. Smoking reduction, smoking cessation, and mortality: a 16-year follow-up of 19,732 men and women from the Copenhagen Centre for Prospective Population Studies. *Am J Epidemiol* 2002;156:994–1001.
4. National Cancer Institute. *Health effects of exposure to environmental tobacco smoke: the report of the California Environmental Protection Agency.* Smoking and Tobacco Control Monograph 10, National Cancer Institute, Bethesda, Maryland, 1999.
5. U.S. Department of Health and Human Services. *The health consequences of smoking: nicotine addiction.* Rockville, MD: Office on Smoking and Health, Centers for Disease Control, 1988.
6. Henningfield J, Miyasato K, Jasinski D. Cigarette smokers self-administer intravenous nicotine. *Pharmacol Biochem Behav* 1983;19:887–890.
7. Henningfield J, Miyasato K, Jasinski DR. Abuse liability and pharmacodynamic characteristics of intravenous and inhaled nicotine. *J Pharmacol Exp Ther* 1985;234:1–12.
8. Henningfield JE, Nemeth-Coslett R. Nicotine dependence: interface between tobacco and tobacco-related disease. *Chest* 1988;93:37S–55S.
9. Rose JE, Corrigall WA, Nicotine self-administration in animals and humans: similarities and differences. *Psychopharmacology (Berl)* 1997;130:28–40.
10. Benowitz NL. Pharmacology of nicotine: addiction and therapeutics. *Annu Rev Pharmacol Toxicol* 1996;36:23–29.
11. Porchet HC, Benowitz NL, Sheiner LB, et al. Apparent tolerance to the acute effect of nicotine results in part from distribution kinetics. *J Clin Invest* 1987;80:1466–1471.
12. Hughes JR, Hatsukami D. Signs and symptoms of tobacco withdrawal. *Arch Gen Psychiatry* 1986;43(3):289–294.
13. American Psychiatric Association. *Diagnostic and statistical manual of mental disorders, 4th ed. (DSM-IV).* Washington, DC: American Psychiatric Association, 1994.
14. Perkins KA, Donny E, Caggiula AR. Sex differences in nicotine effects and self-administration: review of human and animal evidence. *Nicotine Tob Res* 1999;1:301–315.
15. Butschky MF, Bailey D, Henningfield JE, et al. Smoking without nicotine delivery decreases withdrawal in 12-hour abstinent smokers. *Pharmacol Biochem Behav* 1995;50:91–96.
16. Perkins KA. Sex differences in nicotine versus non-nicotine reinforcement as determinants of tobacco smoking. *Exp Clin Psychopharmacol* 1996;4:166–177.
17. Brauer LH, Hatsukami D, Hanson K, et al. Smoking topography in tobacco chippers and dependent smokers. *Addict Behav* 1996;21:233–238.
18. Shiffman S, Fischer LA, Zettler-Segal M, et al. Nicotine exposure in non-dependent smokers. *Arch Gen Psychiatry* 1990;47:333–336.
19. Shiffman S, Zettler-Segal M, Kassel J, et al. Nicotine elimination and tolerance in non-dependent cigarette smokers. *Psychopharmacology (Berl)* 1992;109:449–456.
20. Shiffman S, Kassel JD, Paty J, et al. Smoking typology profiles of chippers and regular smokers. *J Subst Abuse* 1994;6:21–35.
21. Maddux JF, Desmond DP. Relapse and recovery in substance abuse careers. *NIDA Res Monogr* 1986;72:49–71.
22. Picciotto MR. Common aspects of the action of nicotine and other drugs of abuse. *Drug Alcohol Depend* 1998;51:165–172.
23. Corrigall WA, Coen KM, Adamson KL. Self-administered nicotine activates the mesolimbic dopamine system through the ventral tegmental area. *Brain Res* 1994;653:278–284.
24. Nisell M, Nomikos GG, Svensson TH. Nicotine dependence, midbrain dopamine systems and psychiatric disorders. *Pharmacol Toxicol* 1995;76: 157–162.
25. Pontieri FE, Tanda G, Orzi F, et al. Effects of nicotine on the nucleus accumbens and similarity to those of addictive drugs. *Nature* 1996;382:255–257.
26. Pich EM, Pagliusi SR, Tessari M, et al. Common neural substrates for the addictive properties of nicotine and cocaine. *Science* 1997;275:83–86.
27. Nisell M, Nomikos GG, Svensson TH. Systemic nicotine induced dopamine

release in the rat nucleus accumbens is regulated by nicotinic receptors in the ventral tegmental area. *Synapse* 1994;16:36–44.

28. Nisell M, Marcus M, Nomikos GG, et al. Differential effects of acute and chronic nicotine on dopamine output in the core and shell of the rat nucleus accumbens. *J Neural Transm* 1997;104:1–10.

29. Pontieri FE, Passarelli F, Calo L, et al. Functional correlates of nicotine administration: Similarity with drugs of abuse. *J Mol Med* 1998;76:193–201.

30. Trujillo KA, Akil H. Excitatory amino acids and drugs of abuse: a role for *N*-methyl-aspartate receptors in drug tolerance, sensitization, and physical dependence. *Drug Alcohol Depend* 1995;38:139–154.

31. Kalivas PW, Churchill L, Klitenick MA. GABA and enkephalin projection from the nucleus accumbens and ventral pallidum to the ventral tegmental area. *Neuroscience* 1993;57:1047–1060.

32. Boyadjieva NI, Sarkar DK. The secretory response of hypothalamic β-endorphin neurons to acute and chronic nicotine treatments following nicotine withdrawal. *Life Sci* 1997;61:PL59–PL66.

33. Ribeiro EB, Bettiker RL, Bogdanov M, et al. Effects of systemic nicotine on serotonin release in rat brain. *Brain Res* 1993;621:311–318.

34. Corringer PJ, Bertrand S, Bohler S, et al. Critical elements determining diversity in agonist binding and desensitization on neuronal nicotinic acetylcholine receptors. *J Neurosci* 1998;18:648–657.

35. Perry DC, Davila-Garcia MI, Stockmeier CA, et al. Increased nicotinic receptors in brains from smokers: membrane binding and autoradiography studies. *J Pharmacol Exp Ther* 1999;289:1545–1552.

36. Wonnacott S. The paradox of nicotinic acetylcholine receptor upregulation by nicotine. *Trends Pharmacol Sci* 1990;11:216–219.

37. Dani JA, Heinemann S. Molecular and cellular aspects of nicotine abuse. *Neuron* 1996;16:905–908.

38. Koob GF, Sanna PP, Bloom FE. Neuroscience of addiction. *Neuron* 1998;21:467–476.

39. Hildebrand BE, Panagis G, Svensson TH, et al. Behavioral and biochemical manifestations of mecamylamine-precipitated nicotine withdrawal in the rat: role of nicotinic receptors in the ventral tegmental area. *Neuropsychopharmacology* 1999;21:560–574.

40. Fung YK, Schmid MJ, Anderson TM, et al. Effects of nicotine withdrawal on central dopaminergic systems. *Pharmacol Biochem Behav* 1996;53:635–640.

41. Mathieu-Kia AM, Kellogg SH, Butelman ER, et al. Nicotine addiction: insights from recent animal studies. *Psychopharmacology (Berl)* 2002;162:102–118.

42. Watkins SS, Stinus L, Koob GF, et al. Reward and somatic changes during precipitated nicotine withdrawal in the rat: central and peripheral mechanisms. *J Pharmacol Exp Ther* 2000;292:1053–1064.

43. Gourlay SG, Benowitz NL. Arteriovenous differences in plasma concentration of nicotine and catecholamines and related cardiovascular effects after smoking, nicotine nasal spray, and intravenous nicotine. *Clin Pharmacol Ther* 1997;62:453–463.

44. Henningfield JE, Stapleton JM, Benowitz NL, et al. Higher levels of nicotine in arterial than in venous blood after cigarette smoking. *Drug Alcohol Depend* 1993;33:23–29.

45. Armitage AK, Dollery CT, George CF, et al. Absorption and metabolism of nicotine from cigarettes. *Br Med J* 1975;4:313–316.

46. Moreyra AE, Lacy CR, Wilson AC, et al. Arterial blood nicotine concentration and coronary vasoconstrictive effect of low nicotine smoking. *Am Heart J* 1992;124:392–397.

47. Quillen JE, Rossen JD, Oskarsson HJ, et al. Acute effect of cigarette smoking on the coronary circulation: constriction of epicardial and resistance vessels. *J Am Coll Cardiol* 1993;22:642–647.

48. Porchet HC, Benowitz NL, Sheiner LB. Pharmacodynamic model of tolerance: application to nicotine. *J Pharmacol Exp Ther* 1988;244:231–236.

49. Benowitz NL. Pharmacology of nicotine: tolerance and kinetics. In: Henningfield JE, Stitzer ML, eds. *New developments in nicotine-delivery systems. Proceedings of a conference, Johns Hopkins University, September 24, 1990.* Ossining, NY: Cortlandt Communications, 1991:11–22.

50. Russell MAH, Jarvis M, Iyer R, et al. Relation of nicotine yield of cigarettes to blood nicotine concentrations in smokers. *Br Med J* 1980;280:972–976.

51. Henningfield JE, Keenan RM. Nicotine delivery kinetics and abuse liability. *J Consult Clin Psychol* 1993;61:743–750.

52. Quinn DI, Wodak A, Day RO. Pharmacokinetic and pharmacodynamic principles of illicit drug use and treatment of illicit drug users. *Clin Pharmacokinet* 1997;33:344–400.

53. Gorsline J. Nicotine pharmacokinetics of four nicotine transdermal systems. *Health Values* 1993;17:20–24.

54. Pickworth WB, Bunker EB, Henningfield JE. Transdermal nicotine: reduction of smoking with minimal abuse liability. *Psychopharmacology (Berl)* 1994;115:9–14.

55. McDonald JL, Olson BL. Pharmacodynamic and pharmacokinetic properties of nicotine from cigarettes, Nicorette, and NicoDerm. *Health Values* 1994;18:64–68.

56. Johansson CJ, Olsson P, Bende M, et al. Absolute bioavailability of nicotine applied to different nasal regions. *Eur J Pharmacol* 1991;41:585–588.

57. Green CR, Rodgman A. The Tobacco Chemists' Research Conference: a half century forum for advances in analytical methodology of tobacco and its products. *Recent Adv Tob Sci* 1996;22:131–304.

58. Smith CJ, Fischer TH. Particular and vapor phase constituents of cigarette mainstream smoke and risk of myocardial infarction. *Atherosclerosis* 2001;158:257–267.

59. McNeil AD. The development of dependence on smoking in children. *Br J Addict* 1991;86:589–592.

60. Russell MAH. The smoking habit and its classification. *Practitioner* 1974;212:791–800.

61. Choi WS, Pierce JP, Gilpin EA, et al. Which adolescent experimenters progress to established smoking in the United States. *Am J Prev Med* 1997;13:385–391.

62. Pierce JP, Choi WS, Gilpin EA, et al. Validation of susceptibility as a predictor of which adolescents take up smoking in the United States. *Health Psychol* 1996;15:355–361.

63. Killen JD, Robinson TN, Haydel KF, et al. Prospective study of risk factors for the initiation of cigarette smoking. *J Consult Clin Psychol* 1997;65:1011–1016.

64. Robinson TN, Killen JD, Taylor CB, et al. Perspectives on adolescent substance use: a defined poulation study. *JAMA* 1987;258:2072–2076.

65. French SA, Perry CL, Leon GR, et al. Weight concerns, dieting behavior, and smoking initiation among adolescents: a prospective study. *Am J Public Health* 1994;84:1818–1820.

66. Friedman LS, Lichtenstein E, Biglan A. Smoking onset among teens: an empirical analysis of initial situations. *Addict Behav* 1985;10:1–13.

67. Pomerleau OF, Collins AC, Shiffman S, et al. Why some people smoke and others do not: new perspectives. *J Consult Clin Psychol* 1993;61:723–731.

68. Heath AC, Madden PAF. Genetic influences on smoking behavior. In: Turner

JR, Cardon LR, Hewitt JK, eds. *Behavior genetic approaches in behavioral medicine.* New York: Plenum Press, 1995:45–66.

69. Medlund P, Cederlog R, Floderus-Myrhed B, et al. A new Swedish twin registry. *Acta Med Scand Suppl* 1977;600:1–11.

70. Heath AC, Martin NG. Genetic models for the natural history of smoking: Evidence for a genetic influence on smoking persistence. *Addict Behav* 1993;18:19–34.

71. True WR, Heath AC, Scherrer JF, et al. Genetic and environmental contributions to smoking. *Addiction* 1997;92:1277–1287.

72. Collins AC, Marks MJ. Chronic nicotine exposure and brain nicotinic receptors-influence of genetic factors. *Prog Brain Res* 1989;79:137–146.

73. Collins AC, Marks MJ. Progress towards the development of animal models of smoking-related behaviors. *J Addict Dis* 1991;10:109–126.

74. Hughes JR, Gust SW, Pechacek TF. Prevalence of tobacco dependence and withdrawal. *Am J Psychiatry* 1987;144:205–208.

75. Pomerleau OF. Nicotine dependence. In: Bolliger CT, Fagerstrom KO, eds. *The tobacco epidemic.* Basel: Karger, 1997:122–131.

76. Pomerleau OF, Pomerleau CS: Neuroregulators and the reinforcement of smoking: Towards a biobehavioral explanation. *Neurosci Biobehav Rev* 1984;8:503–513.

77. Hughes JR. Distinguishing withdrawal relief and direct effects of smoking. *Psychopharmacology (Berl)* 1991;104:409–410.

78. Keenan RM, Hatsukami DK, Pentel PR, et al. Pharmacodynamic effects of cotinine in abstinent cigarette smokers. *Clin Pharmacol Ther* 1994;55:581–590.

79. Benowitz NL, Kuyt F, Jacob P, et al. Cotinine disposition and effects. *Clin Pharmacol Ther* 1983;34:604–611.

80. Garcha HS, Goldberg SR, Reavill C, et al. Behavioural effects of the optical isomers of nicotine and nornicotine, and of cotinine, in rats. *Br J Pharmacol* 1986;88:289P.

81. Shiffman S, Paty JA, Gnys M, et al. Nicotine withdrawal in chippers and regular smokers: subjective and cognitive effects. *Health Psychol* 1995;14:301–309.

82. Gross TM, Jarvik ME, Rosenblatt MR. Nicotine abstinence produces content-specific Stroop interference. *Psychopharmacology (Berl)* 1993;110:333–336.

83. Snyder FR, Davis FC, Henningfield JE. The tobacco withdrawal syndrome: performance decrements assessed on a computerized test battery. *Drug Alcohol Depend* 1989;23:259–266.

84. Bell SL, Taylor RC, Singleton EG, et al. Smoking after nicotine deprivation enhances cognitive performance and decreases tobacco craving in drug abusers. *Nicotine Tob Res* 1999;1:45–52.

85. Wikler A. Dynamics of drug dependence: implications of a conditioning theory for research and treatment. *Arch Gen Psychiatry* 1973;28:611–616.

86. Killen JD, Fortmann SP. Craving is associated with smoking relapse: findings from three prospective studies. *Exp Clin Psychopharmacol* 1997;5:137–142.

87. Shiffman S, Engberg JB, Paty JA, et al. A day at a time: predicting smoking lapse from daily urge. *J Abnorm Psychol* 1997;106:104–116.

88. Swan GE, Ward MM, Jack LM. Abstinence effects as predictors of 28-day relapse in smokers. *Addict Behav* 1996;21:481–490.

89. Brandon TH, Tiffany ST, Obremski KM, et al. Postcessation cigarette use: the process of relapse. *Addict Behav* 1990;15:105–114.

90. Piasecki TM, Fiore MC, Baker TB. Profiles in discouragement: two studies of variability in the time course of smoking withdrawal symptoms. *J Abnorm Psychol* 1998;107:238–251.

91. West RJ, Hajek P, Belcher M. Severity of withdrawal symptoms as a predictor of outcome of an attempt to quit smoking. *Psychol Med* 1989;19:981–985.

92. Covey LS, Glassman AH, Stetner F. Depression and depressive symptoms in smoking cessation. *Compr Psychiatry* 1990;31:350–354.

93. Ginsberg D, Hall SM, Reus VI, et al. Mood and depression diagnosis in smoking cessation. *Exp Clin Psychopharmacol* 1995;3:389–395.

94. Breslau N, Kilbey M, Andreski P. Nicotine dependence, major depression, and anxiety in young adults. *Arch Gen Psychiatry* 1991;48:1069–1074.

95. Glassman AH, Helzer JE, Covey LS, et al. Smoking, smoking cessation, and major depression. *JAMA* 1990;264(12):1546–1549.

96. Kendler KS, Neale MC, MacLean CJ, et al. Smoking and major depression: a causal analysis. *Arch Gen Psychiatry* 1993;50:36–43.

97. Spiga R, Bennett RH, Schmitz J, et al. Effects of nicotine on cooperative responding among abstinent male smokers. *Behav Pharmacol* 1994;5:337–343.

98. Siegel S. Classical conditioning, drug tolerance and drug dependence. In: Smart RG, Glaser FB, Israel Y, et al., eds. *Research advances in alcohol and drug problems.* New York: Plenum Press, 1983:207–246.

99. Hasenfratz M, Baldinger B, Battig K. Nicotine or tar titration in cigarette smoking behavior? *Psychopharmacology (Berl)* 1993;112:253–258.

100. Rose JE, Behm FM, Levin ED. Role of nicotine dose and sensory cues in the regulation of smoke intake. *Pharmacol Biochem Behav* 1993;44:891–900.

101. Jorenby DE, Smith SS, Fiore MC, et al. Varying nicotine patch dose and type of smoking counseling. *JAMA* 1995;274:1347–1352.

102. Thorndike AN, Rigotti NA, Stafford RS, et al. National patterns in the treatment of smokers by physicians. *JAMA* 1998;279:604–608.

103. Fiore M, Bailey WC, Cohen SJ, et al. *Treating tobacco use and dependence clinical practice guideline.* Rockville, Maryland: U.S. Department of Health and Human Services, Public Health Service, June, 2000.

104. Glynn TJ, Manley WW, Pechacek TF. Physician-initiated smoking cessation program: The National Cancer Institute trials. *Prog Clin Biol Res* 1990;339:11–25.

105. Jaen CR, Strange KC, Tumiel LM, et al. Missed opportunities for prevention: smoking cessation counseling and the competing demands of practice. *J Family Pract* 1997;45(4):348–354.

106. Hurt RD, Sachs DP, Glover ED, et al. A comparison of sustained-release bupropion and placebo for smoking cessation. *N Engl J Med* 1997;337(17):1195–1202.

107. Gonzales DH, Nides MA, Ferry LH, et al. Bupropion SR as an aid to smoking cessation in smokers treated previously with bupropion: a randomized placebo-controlled study. *Clin Pharmacol Ther* 2001;69(6):438–444.

108. Hays JT, Hurt RD, Rigotti NA, et al. Sustained-release bupropion for pharmacologic relapse prevention after smoking cessation: a randomized, controlled trial. *Ann Intern Med* 2001;135(6):423–433.

109. West R, Hajek P, Foulds J, et al. A comparison of abuse liability and dependence potential of nicotine patch, gum, spray and inhaler. *Psychopharmacology (Berl)* 2000;149(3):198–202.

110. West R, Hajek P, Nilsson F, et al. Individual differences in preferences for and responses to four nicotine replacement products. *Psychopharmacology (Berl)* 2001;153(2):225–230.

111. Hall SM, Humfleet GL, Reus VI, et al. Psychological intervention and antidepressant treatment in smoking cessation. *Arch Gen Psychiatry* 2002;59(10):929–937.

112. Shiffman S, Dresler CM, Hajek P, et al. Efficacy of a nicotine lozenge for

smoking cessation. *Arch Intern Med* 2002;162(22):1267–1276.

113. Wallstroem M, Nilsson F, Hirsch J. A randomized, double-blind, placebo-controlled clinical evaluation of a nicotine sublingual tablet in smoking cessation. *Addiction* 2000;95(8):1161–1171.

114. Covey LS, Glassman AH, Stetner F. Naltrexone effects on short-term and long-term smoking cessation. *J Addict Dis* 1999;18(1):31–40.

115. Wong GY, Wolter TD, Croghan GA, et al. A randomized trial of naltrexone for smoking cessation. *Addiction* 1999;94(8):1227–1237.

116. Blondal T, Gudmundsson LJ, Tomasson K, et al. The effects of fluoxetine combined with nicotine inhalers in smoking cessation: a randomized trial. *Addiction* 1999;94(7):1007–1015.

117. Covey LS, Glassman AH, Stetner F, et al. A randomized trial of sertraline as a cessation aid for smokers with a history of major depression. *Am J Psychiatry* 2002;159(10):1731–1737.

118. Killen JD, Fortmann SP, Schatzberg AF, et al. Nicotine patch and paroxetine for smoking cessation. *J Consult Clin Psychol* 2000;68(5):883–889.

119. Niaura R, Spring B, Borrelli B, et al. Multicenter trial of fluoxetine as an adjunct to behavioral smoking cessation treatment. *J Consult Clin Psychol* 2002;70(4):887–896.

120. Marcus BH, Albrecht AE, King TK, et al. The efficacy of exercise as an aid for smoking cessation in women: a randomized controlled trial. *Arch Intern Med* 1999;159:1229–1234.

121. Bier ID, Wilson J, Studt P, et al. Auricular acupuncture, education, and smoking cessation: a randomized, sham-controlled trial. *Am J Public Health* 2002;92(10):1642–1647.

122. He D, Medbo JI, Hostmark AT. Effect of acupuncture on smoking cessation or reduction: an 8-month and 5-year follow-up study. *Prevent Med* 2001;33:364–372.

123. Gupta RK, Dwyer J. Focus groups with smokers to develop a smoke-free home campaign. *Am J Public Health Behav* 2001;25(6):564–571.

124. Richter KP, McCool RM, Okuyemi KS, et al. Patients' views on smoking cessation and tobacco harm reduction during drug treatment. *Nicotine Tob Res* 2002;4(S2):S175–S182.

125. Djordjevic MV, Stellman SD, Zang E. Doses of nicotine and lung carcinogens delivered to cigarette smokers. *J Natl Cancer Inst* 2000;92:106–111.

126. Acton GS, Prochaska JJ, Kaplan AS, et al. Depression and the stages of change for smoking in psychiatric outpatients. *Addict Behav* 2001;26(5):621–631.

127. Breslau N. Psychiatric comorbidity of smoking and nicotine dependence. *Behav Genet* 1995;25(2):95–101.

128. Scarinci IC, Thomas J, Brantley PJ, et al. Examination of the temporal relationship between smoking and major depressive disorder among low-income women in public primary care clinics. *Am J Health Promot* 2002;16(6):323–330.

129. Covey LS, Glassman AH, Stetner F. Cigarette smoking and major depression. *J Addict Dis* 1998;17(1):35–46.

130. Pomerleau CS, Brouwer RJN, Pomerleau CS. Emergence of depression during early abstinence in depressed and non-depressed women smokers. *J Addict Dis* 2001;20(1):73–80.

131. Niaura R, Britt DM, Shadel WG, et al. Symptoms of depression and survival experience among three samples of smokers trying to quit. Psychology of *Addict Behav* 2001;15(1):13–17.

132. Cornelius JR, Perkins KA, Salloum I, et al. Fluoxetine versus placebo to decrease the smoking of depressed alcoholic patients. *J Clin Psychopharmacol* 1999;19(2):183–184.

133. Brown RA, Kahler CW, Niaura R, et al. Cognitive–behavioral treatment for depression in smoking cessation. *J Consult Clin Psychol* 2001;69(3):471–480.

134. George TP, Vessicchio JC, Termine A, et al. A placebo-controlled trial of bupropion for smoking cessation in schizophrenia. *Biol Psychiatry* 2002;52(1):53–61.

135. Evins AE, Mays VK, Rigotti NA, et al. A pilot trial of bupropion added to cognitive behavioral therapy for smoking cessation in schizophrenia. *Nicotine Tob Res* 2001;3:397–403.

136. Hays LR, Farabee D, Miller W. Caffeine and nicotine use in an addicted population. *J Addict Dis* 1998;17(1):47–54.

137. Joseph AM. Nicotine treatment at the Drug Dependency Program of the Minneapolis VA Medical Center. A researcher's perspective. *J Subst Abuse Treat* 1993;10(2):147–152.

138. Bobo JK. Nicotine dependence and alcoholism epidemiology and treatment. *J Psychoactive Drugs* 1992;24(2):123–129.

139. Patkar AA, Sterling RC, Leone FT, et al. Relationship between tobacco smoking and medical symptoms among cocaine-, alcohol-, and opiate-dependent patients. *Am J Addict* 2002;11(3):209–218.

140. Bobo JK, McIlvain H, Gilchrist LD, et al. Nicotine dependence and intentions to quit smoking in three samples of male and female recovering alcoholics and problem drinkers. *Subst Use Misuse* 1996;31(1):17–33.

141. DiFranza JR, Guerrera MP. Alcoholism and smoking. *J Stud Alcohol* 1990;51(2):130–5.

142. Orleans CT, Hutchinson D. Tailoring nicotine addiction treatments for chemical dependency patients. *J Subst Abuse* 1993;10(2):197–208.

143. Bobo JK, McIlvain H, Lando H, et al. Effect of smoking cessation counseling on recovery from alcoholism: findings from a randomized community intervention trial. *Addiction* 1998;93(6):877–887.

144. Ellingstad TP, Sobell LC, Sobell MB, et al. Alcohol abusers who want to quit smoking: implications for clinical treatment. *Drug Alcohol Depend* 1999;54(3):259–265.

145. Kohn CS, Tsoh JY, Weisner CM. Changes in smoking status among substance abusers: baseline characteristics and abstinence from alcohol and drugs at 12-month follow-up. *Drug Alcohol Depend* 2003;69(1):61–71.

146. Gariti P, Alterman A, Mulvaney F, et al. Nicotine intervention during detoxification and treatment for other substance abuse. *Am J Drug Alcohol Abuse* 2002;28(4):671–679.

147. Wetter DW, Kenford SL, Smith SS, et al. Gender differences in smoking cessation. *J Consult Clin Psychol* 1999;67(4):555–562.

148. Etter JF, Prokhorov AV, Perneger TV. Gender differences in the psychological determinants of cigarette smoking. *Addiction* 2002;97(6):733–743.

149. Jeffery RW, Hennrikus DJ, Lando HA, et al. Reconciling conflicting findings regarding postcessation weight concerns and success in smoking cessation. *Health Psychol* 2000;19(3):242–246.

150. Meyers AW, Klesges RC, Winders SE, et al. Are weight concerns predictive of smoking cessation? A prospective analysis. *J Consult Clin Psychol* 1997;65(3):448–452.

151. Williamson DF, Anda, RF, Kleinman JC, et al. Smoking cessation and severity of weight gain in a national cohort. *N Engl J Med* 1991;324(11):739–745.

152. Perkins KA, Marcus MD, Levine MD, et al. Cognitive-behavioral therapy to reduce weight concerns improves smoking cessation outcome in weight-concerned women. *J Consult Clin Psychol* 2001;69(4):604–613.

153. Danielsson T, Rossner S, Westin A. Open randomised trial of intermittent very low energy diet together with nicotine gum for stopping smoking in women who gained weight in previous attempts to quit. *BMJ* 1999;319:490–494.

154. Donatelle RJ, Prows SL, Champeau D, et al. Randomised controlled trial using social support and financial incentives

for high risk pregnant smokers: Significant Other Supporter (SOS) program. *Tob Control* 2000;9(3):iii67–iii69.

155. Johnson JL, Ratner PA, Bottorff JL, et al. Preventing smoking relapse in postpartum women. *Nurs Res* 2000; 49(1):44–52.

156. Van't Hof SM, Wall MA, Dowler DW, et al. Randomised controlled trial of a postpartum relapse prevention intervention. *Tob Control* 2000;9[Suppl 3]:III64–III66.

157. Wisborg K, Henriksen TB, Jespersen LB, et al. Nicotine patches for pregnant smokers: a randomized controlled study. *Obstet Gynecol* 2000;96(6):967–971.

158. Ershoff DH, Quinn VP, Boyd NR,

et al. The Kaiser Permanente prenatal smoking-cessation trial: when more isn't better, what is enough? *Am J Prev Med* 1999;17(3):161–168.

159. Centers for Disease Control and Prevention. Trends in cigarette smoking among high school students—United States, 1991–2001. *MMWR Morb Mortal Wkly Rep* 2002;51(19):409–412.

160. Centers for Disease Control and Prevention. Youth Tobacco Surveillance—United States, 2000. *MMWR Morb Mortal Wkly Rep* 2001;50(SS04):1–84.

161. Centers for Disease Control and Prevention. Incidence and initiation of cigarette smoking—United States, 1965–1996. *MMWR Morb Mortal Wkly Rep* 1998;47(39):837–840.

162. Centers for Disease Control and Prevention. Incidence of initiation of smoking—United States, 1965–1996. *MMWR Morb Mortal Wkly Rep* 1998;47(39):837–840.

163. U.S. Department of Health and Human Services. *Preventing tobacco use among young people: a report of the surgeon general.* Atlanta, GA: U.S. Department of Health and Human Services, 1994.

164. Irvin JE, Hendricks PS, Brandon TH. The increasing recalcitrance of smokers in clinical trials II: pharmacotherapy trials. *Nicotine Tob Res* 2003;5:27–35.

165. Hughes JR. The future of smoking cessation therapy in the United States. *Addiction* 1996;91:1797–1802.

CHAPTER 24

Caffeine

LAURA M. JULIANO AND
ROLAND R. GRIFFITHS

Caffeine is the most widely used mood-altering drug in the world. Caffeine (1,3,7-trimethylxanthine) is found in more than 60 species of plants and is the best known member of the methylxanthine class of alkaloids. The dimethylxanthines, which include theophylline and theobromine, are structurally related compounds that are also found in various plants.

Caffeine, which has long been recognized for its mild stimulating effects, has been consumed in one form or another for thousands of years despite repeated attempts throughout history to ban its use on moral, economic, medical, or political grounds. Today, caffeine use remains ubiquitous. In fact, caffeine ingestion is woven so intricately into social customs and daily rituals that it is often not perceived as a drug, despite its well-documented pharmacologic effects. Moreover, common foods and other products often contain significant amounts of caffeine, although they may not be labeled as such. Thus, it is possible to significantly underestimate caffeine consumption and the role that it may play in one's daily subjective and behavioral experiences.

Behaviorally active doses of caffeine are consumed daily by a majority of adults in the United States. Caffeine is generally considered to be safe relative to classic drugs of dependence. However, caffeine is not a completely innocuous drug. Although there is a lack of agreement on whether caffeine should be formally considered a drug of clinical dependence, some behavioral features of caffeine use closely mirror those associated with classic drugs of dependence. Caffeine can produce tolerance and a characteristic withdrawal syndrome, and heavy use (>400 mg per day) is associated with increased risk for various health problems. Caffeine functions as a reinforcer and many habitual caffeine consumers report an inability to quit or reduce caffeine use despite a desire to do so (1). Caffeine can cause discrete psychopathology (e.g., caffeine intoxication, caffeine induced anxiety disorder), exacerbate existing psychopathology (e.g., anxiety, insomnia), and interfere with the efficacy of some medications (e.g., benzodiazepines). There is also some evidence that caffeine may interact with classic drugs of dependence. This chapter reviews empirical data on the pharmacologic, behavioral, and clinical effects of caffeine. The review concludes with a discussion of the clinical implications of caffeine and practical guidelines for modifying caffeine use.

HISTORY

Caffeine was first isolated from coffee in 1820 and tea in 1827, and its chemical structure was first characterized in 1875 (2). Caffeine has been ingested in one form or another throughout various parts of the world for thousands of years. Tea was first cultivated in China, coffee in Ethiopia, guarana, cocoa, and maté in South America, and kola nut in West Africa. The word coffee is believed to have been derived from the Arabic word "qahwa," which historically referred to wine. According to legend, coffee was discovered after an Arabian goatherd observed his goats eating berries and subsequently behaving in an energetic manner (3). The technique of roasting and grinding coffee beans for beverage preparation was developed in Arabia by the fourteenth century. With the development of world wide trade routes during the seventeenth and eighteenth centuries, caffeinated products spread rapidly from their indigenous environments to other parts of the world. The introduction of caffeine into societies, not unlike the introduction of other drugs such as tobacco, often inspired moral outrage and attempts to ban use. Failed efforts to suppress the use of caffeine-containing foods, usually in the form of coffee or tea, have been documented worldwide (including Arabia, Turkey, Egypt, England, France, and Prussia). In the late 1700s America protested a British tax on tea resulting in the Boston Tea Party in which shipments of tea were thrown into the Boston Harbor. The Continental Congress subsequently passed a resolution against tea consumption and over the course of a few years, coffee became the caffeinated beverage of choice in America (4). Today coffee is the second most valuable import in the United States (5).

In the late 1800s, entrepreneurs began selling flavored carbonated beverages with added caffeine. Original claims for promoting use of these products appealed directly to the stimulant pharmacology of caffeine (e.g., a 1907 advertisement for a cola beverage states: *It quickly relieves fatigue, destroys that "let down feeling" (don't care if tomorrow comes or not) that comes after dissipation of the mental or nervous forces*). In contrast, since 1981 the major manufacturers of soft drinks have denied that their products produce significant pharmacologic effects, while claiming that caffeine is added only as a flavor enhancer (6). Soft drink consumption has increased steadily over the last century and has become a significant source of caffeine use among individuals of all ages.

THERAPEUTIC USES

As a mild central nervous stimulant, caffeine is commonly taken as an energy and alertness enhancer. Studies clearly demonstrate that caffeine is effective at restoring performance that has been degraded by fatigue (7,8). Caffeine is also used to enhance athletic performance because of its ergogenic effects (9). There is evidence to suggest that caffeine functions as an analgesic adjuvant (10), and it is added to a wide variety of over-the-counter and prescription analgesics used to treat various types of pain including headache. Caffeine, a cerebral vasoconstrictor, is the most effective treatment for caffeine withdrawal headaches, which are likely caused by rebound cerebral vasodilation in response to the absence of caffeine. Likewise, prophylactic administration of caffeine prevents postsurgical caffeine-withdrawal headaches (11). Caffeine is used to treat neonatal apnea and has been administered prior to electroconvulsive therapy to increase seizure duration (12,13). Because of its lipolytic and thermogenic effects, caffeine is also used in some over-the-counter weight-loss preparations (12).

SOURCES OF CAFFEINE

Caffeine occurs naturally in a variety of plant-based products including coffee, tea, cocoa, kola nut, guarana, and maté. In addition to beverages made from these plants, significant amounts of caffeine may also occur in foods such as coffee ice cream, coffee yogurt, and dark chocolate.

In recent years, soft drinks and energy drinks made with guarana have become increasingly popular in the United States and elsewhere. Caffeine is added to cola and noncola soft drinks, as well as to other common food items, including gum, mints, water, and energy drinks. Caffeine is also added to thousands of prescription and over-the-counter medications, including stimulants, analgesics, weight-loss supplements, and nutritional supplements (14).

Table 24.1 lists the caffeine contents of many common foods and medications. In the United States, coffee and soft drinks are the major dietary sources of caffeine. The Food and Drug Administration limits the amount of caffeine that can be added to soft drinks to 0.2 mg per mL or 71 mg for a 12-oz serving. It is noteworthy, however, that energy drinks often contain significantly higher levels of caffeine than those permitted in soft drinks. Also, manufacturers are not required to list caffeine as an ingredient in products made with naturally occurring sources of caffeine (e.g., coffee, guarana, kola nut, maté). Products made from some of the less-well-recognized sources of caffeine can be a significant hidden source of caffeine exposure.

EPIDEMIOLOGY

Eighty percent to 90% of children and adults in North America report regular use of caffeinated products (5,15). Mean daily intake among adult caffeine consumers in the United States is approximately 280 mg, with higher daily intakes estimated in Denmark and the United Kingdom (14). Subgroups that have been identified as being heavy caffeine consumers include psychiatric patients, prisoners, smokers, alcoholics, and individuals with eating disorders (16). More than 50% of adults consume coffee every day, and drink an average of 3.3 cups per day (17). Approximately, 50% of caffeine consumers ingest caffeine from multiple sources (e.g., coffee and soft drinks) (15). Caffeinated soft drinks account for the vast majority of soft drink sales (6). In a recent survey of children up to 9 years old, soft drinks were the largest source of caffeine (18). A national survey found that 64% of children 6 to 12 years old and 83% of children 13 to 18 years old consume soft drinks within a 2-day period (19).

Figure 24.1 displays trends in annual per capita consumption of coffee, tea and soft drinks, the three major sources of caffeine consumption in the United States. Over the three decades shown, use of carbonated soft drinks more than doubled, while coffee consumption decreased by 25%. Tea consumption increased only slightly over this time period. The increasing trend in per-capita soft drink consumption is also reflected in the increasing consumption of soft drinks by children. From 1977 to 1996, daily consumption of soft drinks among 12- to 19-year-olds rose from 16 to 28 oz per day for boys and to 15 to 21 oz per day for girls (20).

Fourteen percent of adults with a lifetime history of caffeine use report stopping caffeine completely, usually

TABLE 24.1. *Caffeine content of common foods and medications*

Product	Serving size (volume or weight)	Typical caffeine content (in mg)	Range (in mg)
Coffee			
Brewed/drip	6 oz	100	77–150
Starbucks drip coffee	16 oz	400	
Espresso	1 oz	40	30–90
Starbucks espresso	1 oz	90	
Instant	6 oz	70	20–130
Decaffeinated	6 oz	4	2–9
Tea			
Brewed	6 oz	40	30–90
Instant	6 oz	30	10–35
Canned or bottled	12 oz	20	8–32
Soft drinks			
Typical caffeinated soft drink	12 oz	40	22–71.5
Jolt Cola	12 oz	71.5	
Mountain Dew/Diet Mountain Dew	12 oz	55	
Pepsi One	12 oz	55	
Surge	12 oz	51	
Mellow Yellow/Diet Mello Yellow	12 oz	51	
TAB	12 oz	47	
Diet Coke	12 oz	45	
RC Cola	12 oz	43.2	
Diet Sunkist	12 oz	42	
Sunkist	12 oz	41	
Dr. Pepper/Diet Dr. Pepper	12 oz	41	
Mr. Pibb/Diet Mr. Pibb	12 oz	40	
Pepsi-Cola	12 oz	38	
Diet Pepsi	12 oz	36	
Coke Classic	12 oz	34	
Cherry Coke	12 oz	34	
A&W Cream Soda	12 oz	29	
A&W Diet Cream Soda	12 oz	22	
Barq's Root Beer	12 oz	22	
7Up/Diet 7Up	12 oz	0	
Mug Root Beer	12 oz	0	
Sprite/Diet Sprite	12 oz	0	
Slice	12 oz	0	
Canada Dry Ginger Ale	12 oz	0	
Cocoa/hot chocolate	6 oz	7	2–10
Chocolate milk	6 oz	4	2–7
Chocolate			
Milk Chocolate Bar	1.5 oz	10	2–10
Dark Chocolate Bar	1.5 oz	30	5–35
Caffeinated water			
Typical amount	16.9 oz	60	50–200
Water Joe	16.9 oz	60	
Nitro Water	16.9 oz	56	
Buzzwater	16.9 oz	100 or 200	
Energy drinks			
Typical amount	8.4 oz	80	38–80
Red Bull	8.45 oz	80	
Sobe Adrenaline Rush	8.3 oz	86	
AMP	8.4 oz	75	
KMX	8.4 oz	38	
Coffee ice cream or yogurt	8 oz (1 cup)	50	8–85
Dannon Coffee Yogurt	8 oz	44.5	
Starbucks Coffee Ice Cream	8 oz	60	

(Continued)

TABLE 24.1. *(Continued)*

Product	Serving size (volume or weight)	Typical caffeine content (in mg)	Range (in mg)
Miscellaneous foods and beverages			
Starbucks bottled Frappuccino	9.5 oz	95	
Powerbar Tangerine Powergel	41 g	50	
Jolt Caffeinated gum	1 stick	33	
Penguin Peppermints	1 mint	7	
Stimulants			
Typical	1 tablet	100 or 200	75–350
Vivarin	1 tablet	200	
No-Doz	1 tablet	100 or 200	
Analgesics (over-the-counter and prescription)			
Typical	2 tablets	64 or 130	64–130
Anacin	2 tablets	64	
Excedrin	2 tablets	130	
Goody's Headache Powder	1 powder packet	32.5	
Fiorinal	2 tablets	80	
Darvon	1 tablet	32.4	
Weight-loss products/sports nutrition			
Typical	2–3 tablets	80–250	80–250
Metabolife 356	2 caplets	80	
Dexatrim Natural	1 caplet	80	
EAS Betalean	2 tablets	200	
Stacker 3	1 caplet	250	

1 fluid oz = 30 mL; 1 oz weight = 28 g; Serving sizes are based on commonly consumed portions, typical container sizes, or pharmaceutical instructions. Data are from the National Coffee Association (2001), National Soft Drink Association (2003), Center for Science in the Public Interest (2003), *Physicians Desk Reference* (2003), Barone and Roberts (1996; ref.14), Carrillo and Benitez (2000; ref. 26); Internet web sites for Hershey's Foods (2003), Water Joe (2003), Nitro Water (2003), Buzzwater (2003), Red Bull (2003), Lindt and Sprüngli AG (2001), AMP Energy Drink (2003), Powerbar (2003), Dexatrim (2003), Twinlab Corp (2001), Vivarin (2003), No-Doz (2003), Anacin (2003), Excedrin (2003); personal communication with Starbucks (2001, 2003), Ifive brands (Penguin peppermints) (2002), Jolt Gum (2003), Sobe (2003); and product labels for Goody's Headache Powder (2003), Metabolife 356 (2003), EAS Betalean (2003), Stacker 3 (2003).

because of health concerns or unpleasant side effects (15).

Estimating actual caffeine exposure in the population is challenging because in many widely used products, both the caffeine concentration and the serving sizes can vary over a wide range. For example, the amount of caffeine in a serving of coffee can range from 17 mg for a small 5-oz cup of instant coffee to 500 mg for a large 20-oz cup of drip coffee. Estimating caffeine exposure is also difficult because caffeine is present in such a vast number of products, and many consumers may be completely unaware of whether or not a given product contains caffeine.

GENETICS

Genetic factors account for some of the variability in the use and effects of caffeine. Monozygotic twins have more similar coffee consumption than dizygotic twins, with heritability coefficients for coffee drinking ranging between 36% and 51% (21,22). A study of female twins found that heavy caffeine use (>625 mg per day), total consumption, caffeine intoxication, tolerance, and withdrawal had greater co-occurrence in monozygotic twins than dizygotic twins, with heritabilities ranging between 35% and 77% (23). There is also evidence that common genetic factors underlie the use of caffeine, cigarette smoking, and alcohol (21,22).

PHARMACOKINETICS

After oral consumption, caffeine is rapidly and completely absorbed. Caffeine enters the brain rapidly, which accounts for the quick onset of mood-altering effects. Peak caffeine blood levels are generally reached in 30 to 45 minutes (24,25), but can be delayed by recent food consumption. Caffeine is highly lipid soluble and is widely distributed throughout all body tissues and fluids, including amniotic fluid, breast milk, and semen. Saliva caffeine concentrations are highly correlated with plasma caffeine concentrations and are often used as an alternative to measuring serum levels.

Caffeine metabolism is complex and more than 25 caffeine metabolites have been identified in humans (26). The primary metabolic pathways involve the P450 liver

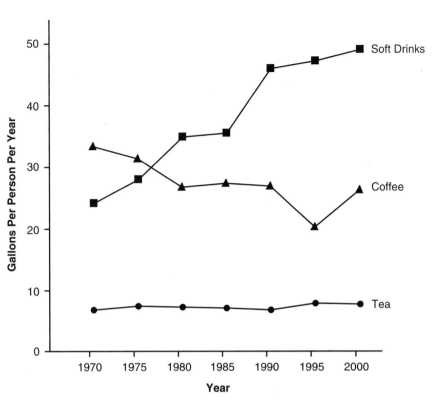

FIG. 24.1. Annual per capita consumption of the three major dietary sources of caffeine in the United States. (Adapted from the USDA/Economic Research Service 2002. *Food Consumption, Prices, and Expenditures, 1970–2000.*) Washington DC: USDA.

enzyme system, which carries out the demethylation of caffeine to three pharmacologically active dimethylxanthines: paraxanthine, theophylline, and theobromine (27). The half-life of caffeine is typically 4 to 6 hours; however, the rate of caffeine metabolism is quite variable among individuals and can vary more than tenfold in healthy adults (27). Tobacco smoking increases the metabolism of caffeine as a consequence of stimulation of liver enzymes, with smokers metabolizing caffeine about twice as fast as nonsmokers (28,29). Caffeine metabolism is slowed in pregnant women and in individuals with liver disease. The liver enzyme systems of infants are not fully developed until about 6 months of age and thus caffeine metabolism in infants is very slow, with a half-life of 80 to 100 hours (30,31). Numerous compounds decrease the rate of elimination of caffeine, including oral contraceptive steroids, cimetidine (Tagamet), and fluvoxamine (Luvox) (26,32). Caffeine decreases the rate of elimination of the antipsychotic clozapine (Clozaril) and the bronchodilator theophylline (Accurbron) (26). Significant differences in caffeine metabolism among animal species have been shown (33).

NEUROPHARMACOLOGY

Adenosine

Caffeine is structurally similar to adenosine an endogenous neuromodulator in both the central nervous system (CNS) and the periphery. The primary mechanism of ac-

tion of caffeine is believed to be competitive antagonism at A_1 and A_{2A} adenosine receptors. This is consistent with the observation that most of the effects of caffeine are opposite to those produced by adenosine (34). Adenosine receptors are members of the family of G protein-coupled receptors (35). Although there do not appear to be discrete adenosine pathways in the brain, A_1 and A_{2A} receptors are present in various brain regions. A_1 receptors are found in most brain regions, with the highest densities in the hippocampus, cerebellar cortex, cerebral cortex, and areas of the thalamus. The highest densities of A_{2A} receptors are found in dopamine-rich areas of the brain, including the caudate/putamen, nucleus accumbens, and the tuberculum olfactorium (36).

Adenosine plays a role in a number of central and peripheral nervous system functions. In the CNS, adenosine inhibits neurotransmitter release, reduces spontaneous neuronal firing, and has anticonvulsant activity. Behavioral manifestations of adenosine action include depression of locomotor activity and operant response rates. Adenosine also causes cerebral vasodilation, constricts bronchial smooth muscle, produces negative inotropic/chronotropic effects on the heart, and inhibits gastric secretions, lipolysis, and renin release (34).

It has also been suggested that adenosine functions as a sleep-inducing factor. It has been hypothesized that the accumulation of adenosine, triggered by energy depletion, decreases the activity of wakefulness-promoting cells, especially cholinergic cells in the basal forebrain, and in doing so increases sleep propensity (37,38).

All of these effects of adenosine are opposite to those produced by caffeine. For example, in the CNS, caffeine increases spontaneous neuronal firing, increases the turnover or levels of various neurotransmitters (e.g., acetylcholine, norepinephrine, dopamine, serotonin, glutamate and γ-aminobutyric acid [GABA]), has convulsant activity, and is a behavioral stimulant (34,39). Importantly, the relative potency of caffeine as an adenosine antagonist correlates with the relative potency of caffeine as a behavioral stimulant in rodents and monkeys (40,41). Such stimulant effects are abolished in A_{2A} receptor knockout mice (42), further suggesting that adenosine antagonism is a primary mechanism in the stimulant effects of caffeine.

Dopamine

Similar to classic stimulants such as amphetamine and cocaine, there is solid evidence that some of the behavioral effects of caffeine are mediated by dopaminergic mechanisms. Caffeine blocks the effects of adenosine at receptors that are colocalized and that functionally interact with dopamine receptors, thus stimulating dopaminergic activity (35). In preclinical studies, caffeine produced behavioral effects similar to classic dopaminergically mediated stimulants such as increased locomotor activity, increased rotational behavior, stimulant-like discriminative stimulus effects, and self-injection (43). Caffeine potentiates the behavioral effects of the dopaminergically mediated stimulants on these same behaviors. Furthermore, some of these effects can be blocked by dopamine receptor antagonists (43). Finally, one recent study showed that caffeine preferentially increased extracellular levels of dopamine in the shell of the nucleus accumbens, an effect caffeine shares with classic stimulants, as well as with a range of other drugs of abuse (44).

Other Mechanisms

Caffeine can also inhibit phosphodiesterase activity and mobilize intracellular calcium release (34). However, these effects are generally observed only at levels attained well above typical dietary doses. Nevertheless, it remains possible that these nonadenosine mechanisms may mediate some of the effects produced by high doses of caffeine, such as those associated with caffeine intoxication. For example, there are preclinical data that suggest that some of the cardiac and respiratory effects of caffeine may be mediated via inhibition of phosphodiesterase activity (34,41).

PHYSIOLOGIC EFFECTS

Caffeine produces effects on a wide variety of organ systems. At moderate dietary doses, caffeine increases blood pressure and tends to have no effect or to reduce heart rate (12,45). Caffeine-induced blood pressure increases tend to be small; however, such increases may be clinically significant for individuals with borderline hypertension (12,46,47). Both caffeinated and decaffeinated coffee contain lipids that significantly raise serum total and low-density lipoprotein (LDL) cholesterol. The highest levels of lipids are delivered from espresso, French press, mocha, Turkish, and boiled coffee (48). Instant coffees and those prepared by paper filtration contain much lower levels of these lipids.

Similar to the methylxanthine theophylline, caffeine dilates bronchial pathways (49,50). Caffeine is also a respiratory stimulant and has been used therapeutically to treat apnea in neonates and infants (12,13).

Caffeine stimulates gastric acid secretion (51) and colonic activity (52). There is no clear association of caffeine use with peptic or duodenal ulcers (12,53). Although coffee consumption exacerbates gastroesophageal reflux, this effect appears to be caused by coffee constituents other than caffeine (54).

Caffeine has a strong diuretic effect and increases urine volume 30% or more for several hours after caffeine ingestion (55). Caffeine also increases detrusor instability (i.e., unstable bladder) in patients with complaints of urinary urgency and detrusor instability (56,57). Perhaps related, chronic caffeine consumption was shown in one study to contributes to urinary incontinence in psychogeriatric patients (58).

Several studies show that caffeine causes increased urinary calcium excretion. It has been suggested that caffeine may have a negative effect on calcium balance, but the clinical significance of such an effect is unclear (59).

Caffeine produces dose-related thermogenic effects (60,61) and is ergogenic during exercise (9). Caffeine increases plasma epinephrine, norepinephrine, rennin, and free fatty acids (62–64). Some studies show that caffeine increases adrenocorticotropic hormone (ACTH) and cortisol levels (47,65,66).

Although caffeine has been shown to have mutagenic and carcinogenic effects in cultured cells *in vitro* at extremely high doses, it is consistently concluded that mutagenic and carcinogenic effects of caffeine are extremely unlikely to occur in humans (12,59).

Although findings are inconsistent and are difficult to interpret, maternal caffeine use may be associated with increased rate of spontaneous abortion (59,67,68) and lower birth weight (12,59).

SUBJECTIVE AND DISCRIMINATIVE STIMULUS EFFECTS

Acute doses of caffeine in the typical dietary dose range (i.e., 20 mg to 200 mg) produce a number of positive subjective effects, including increased well-being, happiness, energy, alertness, and sociability (69,70). These effects are qualitatively similar to those produced by amphetamine and cocaine. In caffeine consumers, such effects are most reliably demonstrated under conditions of caffeine abstinence. Positive subjective effects of caffeine have also been demonstrated in nonhabitual consumers (70).

Negative subjective effects typically emerge at higher doses. Acute doses of caffeine greater than 200 mg are associated with increased reports of anxiety, jitteriness, upset stomach, and insomnia (71). Individual differences in sensitivity and caffeine tolerance seem to play an important role in the likelihood and severity of negative subjective effects. Individuals with higher anxiety sensitivity, panic disorder, or general anxiety disorder tend to be particularly sensitive to the anxiogenic effects of caffeine (70,72). The negative subjective effects of caffeine tend to be relatively mild and short-lived. However, very high doses of caffeine are associated with clinically significant distress and psychopathology (e.g., caffeine intoxication), as discussed in later sections.

Several studies demonstrate that caffeine can function as a discriminative stimulus (i.e., caffeine can be discriminated from placebo under double-blind conditions) in humans, even at low dietary doses (i.e., 10 to 20 mg). Subjects in these studies generally report making the discrimination based on the subjective effects of caffeine. Positive subjective effects typically provide the basis for discrimination of low doses, whereas negative subjective effects are often reported as the basis for discrimination of high doses of caffeine (73).

Drug discrimination studies demonstrate both similarities and differences between caffeine and other stimulant drugs. For example, both caffeine and d-amphetamine produced cocaine-appropriate responding in a cocaine versus placebo discrimination study (74). Another study showed that caffeine produced dose-related partial generalization to d-amphetamine in d-amphetamine–trained subjects (75). In caffeine-trained subjects, methylphenidate and theophylline produced caffeine-appropriate responding (76,77). Individuals can be trained to reliably discriminate between caffeine and d-amphetamine (78).

CAFFEINE INTOXICATION

Caffeine intoxication is currently defined by the *Diagnostic and Statistical Manual of Mental Disorders,* 4th ed. (*DSM–IV*) by a number of symptoms and clinical features that emerge in response to excessive consumption of caffeine (Table 24.2) (79). The most common features of caffeine intoxication include nervousness, restlessness, insomnia, gastrointestinal upset, muscle twitching, tachycardia, and psychomotor agitation. Fever, irritability, tremors, sensory disturbances, tachypnea, and headaches have also been reported in response to excess caffeine use (16). *DSM–IV* diagnostic guidelines require that the diagnosis be dependent on recent consumption of at least 250 mg of caffeine, but much higher doses (>500 mg) are usually associated with the syndrome.

Although caffeine intoxication can occur in the context of habitual chronic consumption of high doses of caffeine,

TABLE 24.2. *Diagnostic criteria for caffeine intoxication (DSM–IV)*

A. Recent consumption of caffeine, usually in excess of 250 mg (e.g., more than 2 to 3 cups of brewed coffee)
B. Five (or more) of the following signs, developing during, or shortly after, caffeine use:

   (1) restlessness
   (2) nervousness
   (3) excitement
   (4) insomnia
   (5) flushed face
   (6) diuresis
   (7) gastrointestinal disturbance
   (8) muscle twitching
   (9) rambling flow of thought and speech
  (10) tachycardia or cardiac arrhythmia
  (11) periods of inexhaustibility
  (12) psychomotor agitation

C. The symptoms in Criterion B cause clinically significant distress or impairment in social, occupational, or other important areas of functioning.
D. The symptoms are not due to a general medical condition and are not better accounted for by another mental disorder (e.g., an Anxiety Disorder).

From the *Diagnostic and Statistical Manual of Mental Disorders*, 4th ed. (*DSM–IV*). Washington DC: American Psychiatric Association, 1994:213, with permission.

it most often occurs after consumption of large doses in infrequent caffeine users, or in regular users who have substantially increased their intake. High-dose intoxicating effects of caffeine are very unpleasant and are not usually sought out by users. Caffeine intoxication usually resolves spontaneously after caffeine use has ceased, consistent with the 4- to 6-hour half-life of caffeine. Treatment of caffeine intoxication may consist of short-term management and support of the patient until symptoms resolve. Although there are generally no long-lasting consequences of caffeine intoxication, caffeine can be lethal at very high doses (e.g., 5 to 10 g) and there are documented cases of suicide by caffeine overdose (80,81).

Individual differences in sensitivity to caffeine and tolerance most likely play a role in vulnerability to caffeine intoxication. It has been reported that caffeine intoxication can occur in chronic caffeine users with no prior apparent caffeine-related problems (82). Although the occurrence of individual symptoms of caffeine intoxication is fairly common (e.g., nervousness), caffeine intoxication serious enough to require medical attention is considered relatively rare (16).

Few studies have assessed the prevalence of caffeine intoxication, and most have evaluated selected populations and used ambiguous criteria (e.g., psychiatric inpatients). One general population survey found that 7% of respondents met *DSM–IV* criteria for caffeine intoxication (1).

CAFFEINE AND ANXIETY

The anxiogenic effects of caffeine are well established (83,84). Acute doses of caffeine generally greater than 200 mg have been shown to increase anxiety ratings in nonclinical populations (85), with higher doses sometimes inducing panic attacks (65,84).

Individuals with anxiety disorders tend to be particularly sensitive to the effects of caffeine. Experimental studies demonstrate that caffeine exacerbates anxiety symptoms in individuals with panic disorder and generalized anxiety disorder to a greater extent than healthy control subjects (72,86). Some survey studies found that individuals with anxiety disorders report less caffeine consumption than controls (87), however, not all individuals with anxiety problems naturally avoid caffeine (88). Abstention from caffeine has been shown to produce improvements in anxiety symptoms among individuals seeking treatment for an anxiety disorder (89). Interestingly, individuals with high caffeine consumption have greater rates of minor tranquilizer use (e.g., benzodiazepines) relative to those persons with low to moderate caffeine consumption (90), although the mechanism underlying this association has not been established.

The *DSM–IV* includes a diagnosis of caffeine-induced anxiety disorder (79). Caffeine-induced anxiety disorder is characterized by prominent anxiety, panic attacks, obsessions, or compulsions etiologically related to caffeine use. It is not necessary to meet full criteria for a *DSM–IV* anxiety disorder to qualify for a diagnosis of caffeine-induced anxiety disorder. The prevalence and incidence of caffeine-induced anxiety disorder is not known.

CAFFEINE AND SLEEP

It is well documented that caffeine increases wakefulness and inhibits sleep onset. Perhaps the most widely accepted therapeutic use of caffeine, which has been widely studied, is that caffeine increases wakefulness and decreases performance decrements produced by sleep deprivation (91). Of course, caffeine also has detrimental effects on planned sleep (i.e., insomnia). Caffeine ingested throughout the day or before bedtime has been shown to interfere with sleep onset, total time slept, sleep quality, and sleep stages (91). Because of caffeine's ability to disrupt sleep, researchers have used caffeine as a challenge agent in order to study insomnia in healthy volunteers (92). Caffeine's effects on sleep appear to be determined by a number of factors, including dose, the time between caffeine ingestion and attempted sleep, and individual differences in sensitivity and/or tolerance to caffeine (91). Caffeine's effects on sleep appear to be dose dependent, with greater amounts of caffeine causing greater sleep difficulties (93). The closer caffeine is taken to bedtime, the more likely it is to produce disruptive effects. However, 200 mg of caffeine taken

early in the morning has been shown to produce small but significant effects on the following night's total sleep time, sleep efficiency, and electroencephalogram (EEG) power spectra (94). Caffeine-induced sleep disturbance is greatest among nonconsumers; it is not clear, however, whether this difference is a result of an absence of acquired tolerance or to a preexisting population difference in sensitivity to caffeine (91,95,96). Although there is evidence for some tolerance to the sleep-disrupting effects of caffeine, tolerance appears to be incomplete and thus regular caffeine consumers may still be vulnerable to caffeine-related sleep problems (95,96).

In addition to caffeine's ability to disrupt sleep, there are reports of caffeine causing hypersomnia (97). Furthermore, acute abstinence after chronic caffeine consumption increases daytime sleepiness and increases nighttime sleep duration and quality (96,98).

The *DSM–IV* includes a diagnosis of caffeine-induced sleep disorder, which is characterized by a prominent sleep disturbance that is etiologically related to caffeine use (79). It is not necessary to meet full criteria for a *DSM–IV* sleep disorder to qualify for a diagnosis of caffeine-induced sleep disorder. Although caffeine is most often associated with insomnia, *DSM–IV* also recognizes hypersomnia caused by caffeine withdrawal. Caffeine-induced sleep disorder is diagnosed when symptoms of a sleep disturbance (e.g., insomnia) are greater than would be expected during caffeine intoxication or caffeine withdrawal. There are no specific data on the prevalence or incidence of caffeine-induced sleep disorder.

PERFORMANCE

Many studies have examined the effects of caffeine on human performance. Data support the conclusion that caffeine improves performance that has been degraded under conditions such as sleep deprivation, fatigue, prolonged vigilance, and caffeine withdrawal (12,99). Studies of the effects of caffeine on nondegraded performance are inconsistent. Although findings have varied, studies show that caffeine can improve attention, vigilance, reaction time, and psychomotor performance (100). However, the great majority of studies claiming to demonstrate performance-enhancing effects of caffeine are difficult to interpret because they do not account for the effects of caffeine withdrawal. That is, many studies compare the effects of caffeine versus placebo in chronic caffeine consumers who have abstained from caffeine, usually overnight. Under these conditions, improvements in performance after caffeine relative to placebo may reflect restoration of performance deficits caused by withdrawal, rather than a performance-enhancing effect of caffeine per se (12).

There is a growing body of literature on the effects of caffeine on exercise performance. Compared to placebo, caffeine increases endurance for long-term (30 to

60 minutes) exercise and improves speed and/or power output in simulated race conditions (9).

REINFORCEMENT

Caffeine functions as a reinforcer in humans (i.e., caffeine maintains self-administration or choice behavior). Controlled double-blind laboratory studies show that subjects will choose caffeine over placebo in double-blind choice procedures, as well as perform work or forfeit money in exchange for caffeine. When multiple self-administration opportunities are available within a day, doses as low as 25 mg are reinforcing (101,102). When self-administration is limited to once a day, then doses of 100 and 200 mg are reinforcing, while doses of 400 mg and greater tend to be avoided (103).

There is quite a bit of individual variability in the reinforcing effects of caffeine. Across studies, the overall incidence of caffeine reinforcement in normal caffeine users is approximately 40%, with a higher incidence (i.e., 80% to 100%) of reinforcement under conditions of repeated caffeine exposure (70). In choice studies, subjects who choose caffeine tend to report positive subjective effects, whereas those who choose placebo are more likely to report negative subjective effects (e.g., jitteriness) at low to moderate doses (104).

Caffeine physical dependence potentiates the reinforcing effects of caffeine. For example, caffeine consumers were more than twice as likely to show caffeine reinforcement if they reported caffeine withdrawal symptoms after drinking decaffeinated coffee (105). In studies in which caffeine physical dependence was experimentally manipulated, subjects are more than twice as likely to choose caffeine over placebo when they are physically dependent (106,107). There is also evidence that avoidance of caffeine withdrawal determines caffeine consumption to a greater extent than the positive effects of caffeine (107–109). Caffeine reinforcement also appears to be influenced by task requirements. That is, in a double-blind study, subjects chose caffeine over placebo when required to perform a vigilance task, but chose placebo over caffeine when required to engage in relaxation (110).

Recent studies have used a conditioned flavor preference paradigm as an indirect measure of caffeine reinforcement (111,112). Subjects who are repeatedly exposed to a novel flavored drink paired with caffeine tend to show increased ratings of drink pleasantness, whereas subjects receiving placebo-paired drinks show decreased ratings of drink pleasantness (113,114). It seems plausible that such conditioned flavor preferences in the natural environment play an important role in the development of consumer preferences for different types of caffeine-containing beverages.

In laboratory animals, studies of drug self-administration show that caffeine can function as a reinforcer under some conditions. In contrast to classic abused stimulants such as amphetamine and cocaine, caffeine self-administration is observed in animals under a relatively narrow range of conditions (71).

TOLERANCE

Tolerance refers to a decrease in responsiveness to a drug after repeated drug exposure. High doses of caffeine (750 to 1,200 mg per day spread throughout the day) administered daily produce "complete" tolerance (i.e., caffeine effects are no longer different from baseline or placebo) to some, but not all of the effects of caffeine. However, lower or typical dietary doses of caffeine produce incomplete tolerance. The degree of caffeine tolerance is likely to depend on a number of factors including dose, amount, and frequency of administration, as well as individual differences in elimination (115).

Controlled human laboratory studies demonstrate that complete tolerance develops to the subjective effects of high doses of caffeine (e.g., 300 mg t.i.d. for 18 days) (104) but not to lower doses (i.e., 200 mg b.i.d. for 7 days) (116). Likewise, studies show complete tolerance to blood pressure and other physiologic effects (plasma norepinephrine and epinephrine and plasma rennin activity) of high doses of caffeine (e.g., 250 mg t.i.d. for 4 days) (63), but only partial tolerance to blood pressure and middle cerebral artery velocity at somewhat lower doses (i.e., 200 mg b.i.d. for 7 days) (116). Substantial but incomplete tolerance has been shown to the sleep disruptive effects of high doses of caffeine (400 mg t.i.d. for 7 days) (117).

PHYSICAL DEPENDENCE AND WITHDRAWAL

Physical dependence on caffeine is demonstrated by the occurrence of a withdrawal syndrome (i.e., time-limited biochemical, physiologic, and behavioral disruptions) that occurs after cessation after a period of regular caffeine consumption. Caffeine withdrawal has been well-characterized (70,118). Table 24.3 lists commonly reported caffeine withdrawal symptoms compiled from more than 40 experimental caffeine withdrawal studies, the majority of which used double-blind procedures, and validated caffeine abstinence using biological measures.

Headache is the most common withdrawal symptom, with approximately 50% of regular caffeine users reporting headache by 24 hours of abstinence. Such headaches have been described as gradual in development, diffuse, and throbbing. Through adenosine antagonism, caffeine constricts cerebral blood vessels. Caffeine abstinence produces cerebral vasodilation and increased cerebral blood flow, an effect that may be potentiated by increased functional sensitivity to adenosine (which is a vasodilator) during caffeine withdrawal (73). Such vascular changes are a likely mechanism underlying caffeine withdrawal headache (119,120).

TABLE 24.3. *Symptoms of caffeine withdrawal in roughly decreasing order of incidence in blind studies*

Headache
Fatigue/lethargy
Drowsiness/sleepiness
Dysphoric mood (discontentedness)
Difficulty concentrating
Work difficulty/unmotivated
Irritability
Depression
Impairment on cognitive or behavioral performance tasks
Nausea or vomiting
Muscle aches or stiffness
Heavy feelings in arms and legs
Hot and cold spells

Other caffeine-withdrawal symptoms in roughly decreasing order of occurrence include fatigue, drowsiness, dysphoric mood, difficulty concentrating, work difficulty (lack of motivation), irritability, depression, and cognitive or behavioral task impairment. Occasionally, individuals experiencing caffeine withdrawal also report flu-like symptoms, which may include nausea or vomiting, muscle aches or stiffness, hot and cold spells, and heavy feelings in arms and legs (70).

In individuals reporting withdrawal symptoms, severity can range from mild to incapacitating. Also, there is variability in withdrawal severity, both within and across individuals. Significant disruptions of normal daily activities (e.g., work absence) upon caffeine abstinence have also been observed in clinical evaluations and experimental studies (70,121,122).

Withdrawal symptoms typically emerge 12 to 24 hours after the last dose of caffeine and tend to peak within 48 hours. Symptoms can persist from 2 days to 1 week or more (71). Caffeine withdrawal symptoms are usually alleviated quickly after caffeine reexposure. Caffeine withdrawal can be suppressed by caffeine doses well below the usual daily dose (e.g., 25 mg caffeine suppressed withdrawal after daily doses of 300 mg) (123). Caffeine withdrawal can occur after relatively short-term exposure to daily caffeine (e.g., 3 to 7 days of exposure) (123,124). The incidence and severity of caffeine withdrawal tends to increase as a function of daily maintenance dose (123). The daily caffeine dose necessary to produce withdrawal is surprisingly low, with significant withdrawal symptoms observed in individuals using as little as 100 mg caffeine per day (123,125).

In double-blind experimental studies, the incidence of caffeine withdrawal symptoms is usually greater than 50% (70,105,126). Retrospective survey studies have also been conducted to determine the frequency of caffeine withdrawal in the general population. In one population-based random digit-dialing survey study, 44% of caffeine users reported having stopped or reduced caffeine use for at least 24 hours in the past year. Of those, more than 40% reported experiencing one or more withdrawal symptoms. Interestingly, more than 70% of those who stopped or reduced caffeine as part of a permanent quit attempt reported withdrawal symptoms, and 24% reported headache and other symptoms that interfered with performance (1). In another study, 11% of caffeine users who were making an inquiry about participation in a clinical research trial reported that they had "problems or symptoms on stopping caffeine in the past," of which 25% reported that the problems were severe enough to interfere with normal activity (127). The number of individuals who actually experienced a period of caffeine abstinence was not ascertained.

Although most withdrawal research has been with adults, there is evidence that children and adolescents who use caffeine also experience caffeine withdrawal symptoms upon abstinence (128–132). It is possible that children may be even more susceptible to experiencing withdrawal episodes because they likely have less control over the regular availability of caffeine-containing products. More research is needed in this area.

The observations that caffeine withdrawal can cause clinically significant distress or functional impairment have resulted in the inclusion of caffeine withdrawal as an International Classification of Diseases (ICD)-10 diagnosis (133,134) and as a proposed diagnosis in *DSM–IV* (79,135). A growing body of research supports caffeine withdrawal as a discrete clinical syndrome. In the *DSM–IV*, caffeine withdrawal is defined by caffeine withdrawal symptoms (i.e., headache and one or more of the following: marked fatigue or drowsiness, marked anxiety or depression, nausea or vomiting), that cause "significant distress or impairment in social, occupational, or other important areas of functioning." The research literature on caffeine withdrawal has more than doubled since these diagnostic criteria were formulated in 1994. It is now clear that the *DSM–IV* criteria are conservative insofar as they exclude cases in which symptoms are experienced without headache, and they exclude several symptoms that have been repeatedly documented in recent studies, including dysphoric mood, difficulty concentrating, and irritability. To date, only one study has evaluated the incidence of caffeine withdrawal using *DSM–IV* criteria (1). This population-based survey found that 11% of those who had given up or reduced caffeine use in the past year met criteria for caffeine withdrawal. Among individuals who reported trying to stop caffeine use permanently, 24% met criteria for caffeine withdrawal.

CAFFEINE DEPENDENCE

Substance dependence is characterized by a cluster of cognitive, behavioral, and physiologic symptoms indicating that the individual continues use of a substance despite significant substance-related problems (79). It is important to make the distinction between physical dependence and a clinical diagnosis of substance dependence. Whereas the empirical evidence for the occurrence of caffeine physical dependence (reflected by withdrawal) is overwhelming, there is less information available about caffeine's ability to produce other clinically meaningful characteristics of a substance dependence syndrome. The *DSM–IV* presently excludes caffeine from its diagnostic schema for substance dependence. In contrast, the World Health Organization's ICD-10 recognizes a diagnosis of substance dependence caused by caffeine, using very similar diagnostic criteria as the *DSM–IV* (133). The rationale presented for excluding substance dependence on caffeine as a *DSM–IV* diagnosis was that although it had been established that caffeine produces physical dependence, there was insufficient information pertaining to other features of dependence, such as such as an inability to stop use and to continue use despite harm (135).

Since the publication of *DSM–IV*, four published studies have described adults and adolescents who report problematic caffeine consumption and fulfill *DSM–IV* substance-dependence criteria on caffeine (Table 24.4) (1,121,131,132). One investigation found that 16 of 99 individuals who self-identified as having psychological or physical dependence on caffeine met *DSM–IV* criteria for substance dependence on caffeine, when a restrictive set of four of the seven *DSM–IV* criteria that seemed most appropriate to problematic caffeine use were assessed (use despite harm, desire or unsuccessful efforts to stop, withdrawal, tolerance) (121). Interestingly, among those who met criteria for caffeine dependence, caffeine intake ranged from 129 mg to 2,548 mg, and the preferred caffeine vehicle was equally divided between coffee and soft drinks. Although there were few concurrent psychiatric disorders; 57% of those who met criteria for caffeine dependence had a history of alcohol abuse or dependence. Using the same four criteria, another study

identified adolescents who fulfilled diagnostic criteria for caffeine dependence (131,132). These studies, which represent a series of case reports, demonstrate that a clinically meaningful caffeine dependence syndrome does exist.

The one population-based survey to date suggests that when individuals in the general population are surveyed about their caffeine use, a surprisingly large proportion endorse substance-dependence criteria. In a random digit-dial telephone survey in which all seven *DSM–IV* criteria for substance dependence were assessed, 30% of caffeine users fulfilled diagnostic criteria by endorsing three or more dependence criteria. When the more restrictive set of four criteria were used, as in the studies described above, 9% met criteria for substance dependence. The most commonly reported symptom (56%) was persistent desire or unsuccessful efforts to cut down or control caffeine use (1).

The four *DSM–IV* criteria for substance dependence that appear to be most pertinent to a meaningful assessment of problematic caffeine use are (a) continued use despite knowledge of a persistent or recurrent physical or psychological problem that is likely to have been caused or exacerbated by the substance; (b) persistent desire or unsuccessful efforts to cut down or control substance use; (c) characteristic withdrawal syndrome or use of the substance to relieve or avoid withdrawal symptoms; and (d) tolerance as defined by a need for markedly increased amounts of the substance to achieve desired effect, or markedly diminished effect with continued use of same amount of substance. Although not assessed in the case report studies described above, an additional criterion may be relevant: (e) substance is often taken in larger amounts or over a longer period than was intended. The remaining two criteria would not seem to be relevant to a widely available, culturally accepted drug such as caffeine: (f) important social, occupational, or recreational activities are given up or reduced because of substance use; and (g) a

TABLE 24.4. *Prevalence of endorsement of DSM–IV criteria for substance dependence among caffeine users*

	General population	DSM–IV defined caffeine-dependent individuals	
	Adults (Hughes et al., 1998)[a]	Adults (Strain et al., 1998; ref. 121)[b]	Adolescents (Oberstar et al., 2002; ref. 132)[b]
Use despite harm	14%	94%	58%
Desire or unsuccessful efforts to stop	56%	81%	83%
Withdrawal	18%	94%	100%
Tolerance	8%	75%	92%
Used more than intended	28%	—	—
Give up activities to use	<1%	—	—
Great deal of time with the drug	50%	—	—

[a]Assessed all seven *DSM–IV* criteria for substance dependence.
[b]Assessed four *DSM–IV* criteria thought to be most pertinent to a meaningful assessment of problematic caffeine use.

great deal of time is spent in activities necessary to obtain the substance, use the substance, or recover from its effects. Furthermore, inclusion of the last criteria could trivialize the diagnosis of caffeine dependence (e.g., sipping coffee throughout the day).

More research is needed to determine the applicability of substance-dependence criteria to caffeine, the prevalence of the disorder, and the utility and clinical significance of the diagnosis. Meanwhile therapeutic assistance should be made available for those who feel that their caffeine use is problematic but have been unable to quit on their own. The Composite International Diagnostic Interview–Substance Abuse Module (CIDI-SAM), a well regarded structured interview focused on substance use disorders, contains a section for caffeine dependence according to *DSM–IV* and ICD-10 criteria (136,137).

CAFFEINE AND OTHER DRUGS OF DEPENDENCE

Tobacco Smoking and Nicotine

Epidemiologic studies show that cigarette smokers consume more caffeine than nonsmokers (138), and experimental studies show that cigarette smoking and coffee drinking covary temporally within individuals (139). Twin studies and patterns of consumption in drug abusers show co-occurrence of caffeine use and cigarette smoking (21,22,140). Although the administration of caffeine does not reliably increase cigarette smoking (141), one recent study showed that chronic consumption of dietary doses of caffeine increased the reinforcing and stimulant effects of intravenous nicotine (142). This latter finding is consistent with preclinical studies showing that chronic exposure to low doses of caffeine can facilitate the acquisition of nicotine self-administration, potentiate the stimulating effects of nicotine, and produced changes in brain dopaminergic activity consistent with caffeine increasing the reinforcing effects of nicotine (143).

Cigarette smoking significantly increases the rate of caffeine elimination, an effect that may partially explain increased caffeine use among smokers (29). Smoking abstinence produces substantial increases in caffeine blood levels among heavy caffeine consumers (144,145). It has been speculated that symptoms of caffeine intoxication caused by increased caffeine blood levels may interfere with smoking quit attempts and/or be misinterpreted as nicotine-withdrawal symptoms; however, the clinical significance of such an effect has not been demonstrated (146,147).

Alcohol

There is an association between heavy use and clinical dependence on alcohol and heavy use and clinical dependence on caffeine (140,148). Alcohol detoxification in alcoholics is associated with substantial increases in coffee consumption (149). In a study that identified individuals who met *DSM–IV* criteria for substance dependence on caffeine, 57% also had a lifetime history of alcohol abuse or dependence (121). Preclinical studies suggest that caffeine can promote alcohol self-administration (150). Although it is widely believed that caffeine can reverse the impairing effects of alcohol, animal and human studies have not shown this to be a reliable effect (151–153). The available data suggest that caffeine's reversal of impairment caused by alcohol is generally incomplete and inconsistent across different types of behavioral and subjective measures.

Benzodiazepines

Benzodiazepines are commonly used to treat anxiety disorders and insomnia. There is evidence from animal and human behavioral studies that suggests a mutually antagonistic relationship between benzodiazepines and caffeine (151). Although caffeine can interact at the benzodiazepine receptor (154), the lack of uniform antagonism across behavioral measures suggests that the antagonism is functional in nature (151,155,156).

One study showed that heavy caffeine users are almost twice as likely to use benzodiazepines than are low and moderate caffeine users (90). An important clinical implication is that, although individuals with anxiety disorders tend to use less caffeine than controls (86,87), caffeine use should be carefully evaluated when benzodiazepines are being considered for the treatment of anxiety and insomnia.

Cocaine

There is little epidemiologic data on the co-occurrence of caffeine and cocaine use. One study reported that the prevalence of caffeine use among cocaine abusers is lower than the general population (157). Interestingly, in that same study, cocaine users who consumed caffeine reported using less cocaine than those who do not regularly consume caffeine.

In animal studies, caffeine increases the acquisition of cocaine self-administration, reinstates responding previously maintained by cocaine, and potentiates the stimulant and discriminative stimulus effects of cocaine (43). In a human experimental study, caffeine produced cocaine-appropriate responding in a cocaine versus placebo discrimination study (74). The subjective effects of intravenous caffeine were reported as cocaine-like in one study (45), but not in another study (158). In one study intravenous caffeine administration produces a significant increase in craving for cocaine in cocaine abusers (45); however, oral administration of caffeine has not produced this effect (159). Although the documented interactions between caffeine and cocaine are interesting, the clinical importance has not been established.

CAFFEINE AND HEALTH

The possibility that caffeine may pose health risks is of great interest to the general public and scientific community, and has been the focus of numerous studies. A thorough review of the potential health implications of caffeine is beyond the scope of this chapter and is the focus of several scholarly books and reviews (12,59,160–162). There is no evidence for nonreversible pathologic consequences of caffeine use (e.g., cancer, heart disease, congenital malformations). In general, there is a lack of evidence to support the conclusion that moderate caffeine use causes significant health risk in healthy adults. However, some groups may be considered at risk for potential adverse health effects of caffeine including individuals with generalized anxiety disorder, panic disorder, primary insomnia, hypertension, and urinary incontinence; women who are pregnant or trying to become pregnant; and caffeine users who consume inadequate amounts of calcium. In addition, as discussed in more detail throughout this chapter, caffeine use can be associated with several distinct psychiatric syndromes: caffeine intoxication, caffeine withdrawal, caffeine dependence, caffeine-induced sleep disorder, and caffeine-induced anxiety disorder.

CLINICAL IMPLICATIONS

Given the wide range of symptoms produced by excessive caffeine use and withdrawal, as described throughout this chapter, caffeine use should be routinely assessed during medical and psychiatric evaluations. Caffeine use or intoxication should be assessed in individuals with complaints of anxiety, insomnia, headaches, palpitations, tachycardia, or gastrointestinal disturbance. Caffeine intoxication should be considered in the differential diagnosis of amphetamine or cocaine intoxication, mania, medication-induced side effects, hyperthyroidism, and pheochromocytoma. Likewise, caffeine withdrawal should be considered when patients present with headaches, fatigue, dysphoric mood, or difficulty concentrating. Caffeine withdrawal should be considered in the differential diagnosis of migraine or other headache disorders, viral illnesses, and other drug-withdrawal states.

Caffeine users who are instructed to refrain from all food and beverages prior to medical procedures may be at risk for experiencing caffeine withdrawal. Caffeine withdrawal has been identified as a cause of postoperative headaches, and caffeine supplements during surgery are effective in preventing withdrawal (163,164).

Caffeine interacts with a number of medications. Caffeine and benzodiazepine-like drugs (e.g., diazepam [Valium], alprazolam [Xanax], triazolam [Halcion]) are mutually antagonistic and thus caffeine use may interfere with the efficacy of benzodiazepines (151). Caffeine may also interfere with the metabolism of the antipsychotic clozapine as well as the bronchodilator theophylline to an extent that may be clinically significant (26). Case studies suggest that caffeine withdrawal may be associated with increased serum lithium concentrations and lithium toxicity (26). Numerous compounds decrease the rate of elimination of caffeine, including oral contraceptive steroids, cimetidine, and fluvoxamine (26,32).

IS CAFFEINE A DRUG OF ABUSE?

Caffeine is a widely used mood-altering drug that shares some features with classic drugs of abuse (e.g., use despite harm, difficulty stopping use, withdrawal, tolerance). Therefore, it is not surprising that caffeine is sometimes labeled a drug of abuse or addiction (3,12,165). Objections to this classification include the observations that caffeine is widely used, has relatively subtle psychological effects, produces less social and physical harm than classic drugs of abuse, and is less likely to be associated with craving. However, definitions of drug abuse and addiction are complex and controversial, as reflected in the not so distant debate about whether nicotine should be considered a drug of addiction (166,167). One approach to deciding if it is appropriate to label caffeine as a drug of abuse is an analysis of reinforcement and adverse effects (168). In this type of analysis, the relative abuse potential of a drug can be considered to be a multiplicative function of the degree of drug reinforcement and the degree of adverse effects. As discussed earlier, caffeine functions as a reinforcer under a more limited range of conditions than classic stimulant drugs of abuse, such as amphetamine. Caffeine produces some adverse psychological and physical effects; however, in contrast to classic drugs of abuse, life-threatening health risks from caffeine at usual dietary doses have not been conclusively demonstrated. Although caffeine has these two defining features of drugs of abuse, the modest reinforcing effects and modest adverse effects documented to date suggest that caffeine has a low abuse liability relative to classic drugs of abuse. However, this type of analysis would also predict that if future research were to demonstrate significant adverse effects of caffeine, societal perceptions of caffeine as a drug of abuse would be radically altered.

TREATMENT

Reduction or elimination of caffeine is advised for individuals who have caffeine-related psychopathology or when it is believed that caffeine is causing or exacerbating medical or psychiatric problems, or interfering with medication efficacy. A surprisingly large percentage of caffeine users in the general population (56%) report a desire or unsuccessful efforts to stop or reduce caffeine use (1).

There are no published reports of treatment interventions designed to assist individuals who would like to completely eliminate caffeine. Several reports suggest the efficacy of a structured caffeine reduction regimen (i.e., caffeine fading) for achieving substantial reductions of caffeine intake (169–172). For example, one study involving very heavy caffeine consumers found that a 4-week structured caffeine fading program was more effective than self-guided reduction in achieving a 5-cup-per-day goal of coffee or tea (171). A more recent study of patients recruited from a urinary continence clinic found that a 4-week reduction program with a consumption goal of <100 mg per day was effective at reducing caffeine intake, as well as urinary frequency and urgency outcomes (172).

Given the limited number of treatment strategies that have been evaluated for reducing or eliminating caffeine consumption, a reasonable approach is to draw from validated behavioral techniques used to treat dependence on other drugs (e.g., tobacco dependence). Effective behavior modification strategies include coping response training, self-monitoring, social support, and reinforcement for abstinence (173). Substance abuse treatment strategies, including relapse prevention (174) and motivational interviewing (175), could also be readily applied to the treatment of caffeine dependence. Providing a list of caffeine-containing products may help to increase awareness of sources of caffeine and should facilitate self-monitoring efforts. Some individuals may not readily accept the idea that caffeine is contributing to their problems (e.g., insomnia, anxiety). Such individuals should be encouraged to engage in a caffeine-free trial. There is some evidence that withdrawal symptoms may thwart quit attempts. Gradually reducing caffeine consumption may help attenuate withdrawal symptoms, although there has been no systematic research to determine the most efficacious reduction schedule. In general, reduction schedules over the course of 3 to 4 weeks are effective (169–172). No data about the

TABLE 24.5. *Guidelines for reducing or eliminating caffeine*

1. *Education*
   Patients should be educated about potential sources of caffeine. It may be useful to provide patients with a list of common caffeinated products (see Table 24.1). Some individuals may not be aware that caffeine is present in noncola beverages such as lemon-lime soft drinks and products made with guarana, maté, or kola nut.

2. *Self-monitoring*
   Caffeine use should be self-monitored using a food diary for 1 to 2 weeks to determine a baseline level. If a self-monitoring period is not feasible, treatment providers can determine a rough estimate of total caffeine consumption via self-report. Self-monitoring should also be continued during the caffeine-reduction phase of treatment.

3. *Calculate total daily caffeine consumption in mg*
   Calculate daily caffeine exposure in milligrams, taking into account the caffeine content of specific products, the serving sizes, and the number of servings.

4. *Determine a caffeine modification goal*
   Decide on a caffeine modification goal with the patient. Some individuals may be interested in completely eliminating caffeine, whereas others may want to reduce their caffeine consumption. Individuals who would like to continue to consume some amount of caffeine but who want to avoid experiencing withdrawal symptoms if they omit caffeine for a day, should be advised to consume no more than 50 mg per day.

5. *Generate a gradual reduction schedule*
   A gradual reduction schedule should help to prevent or alleviate caffeine withdrawal symptoms. A reasonable decrease would be 10% to 25% of the baseline dose every few days until the caffeine moderation or cessation goal is achieved. Patients should identify a noncaffeinated substitute for their usual caffeine-containing beverage. Caffeinated beverages can either be omitted to achieve the desire amount or can be mixed with decaffeinated beverages.

6. *Employ behavior modification techniques*
   Patients may benefit from behavior modification techniques that have been shown to be effective in the treatment of dependence on other substances (e.g., nicotine). Such strategies may include self-monitoring, coping response training, reinforcement for abstinence, identifying barriers to change, social support, and reframing withdrawal as a temporary inconvenience.

7. *Follow-up*
   Schedule a follow-up contact with the patient to check on the patient's progress.

probability of relapse is currently available, although relapse after caffeine reduction has been reported (82,176). Table 24.5 lists practical guidelines for reducing or ceasing caffeine use.

ACKNOWLEDGMENTS

Preparation of this review was supported, in part, by United States Public Health Service grant R01 DA03890 from the National Institute on Drug Abuse.

REFERENCES

1. Hughes JR, Oliveto AH, Liguori A, et al. Endorsement of *DSM-IV* dependence criteria among caffeine users. *Drug Alcohol Depend* 1998;52:99–107.
2. Arnaud MJ. Products of metabolism of caffeine. In: Dews PB, ed. *Caffeine.* Berlin: Springer-Verlag, 1984:3–38.
3. Austin G. Perspectives on the history of psychoactive substance use. In: *NIDA research issues.* Washington DC: US Government Printing Office, 1979:50–66.
4. Pendergrast M. *Uncommon grounds: the history of coffee and how it transformed our world.* New York: Basic Books, 1999.
5. Gilbert RM. Caffeine consumption. In: Spiller GA, ed. *The methylxanthine beverages and foods: chemistry, consumption, and health effects.* New York: Alan R. Liss, 1984:185–213.
6. Griffiths RR, Vernotica EM. Is caffeine a flavoring agent in cola soft drinks? *Arch Fam Med* 2000;9:727–734.
7. Penetar D, McCann UD, Thorne D, et al. Effects of caffeine on cognitive performance, mood, and alertness in sleep-deprived humans. In: Marriott B, ed. *Food components to enhance performance: an evaluation of potential performance enhancing food components for Operational Rations/Committee on Military Nutrition Research, Food and Nutrition Board, Institute of Medicine.* Washington DC: National Academy Press, 1994:407–431.
8. Patat A, Rosenzweig P, Enslen M, et al. Effects of a new slow release formulation of caffeine on EEG, psychomotor and cognitive functions in sleep-deprived subjects. *Hum Psychopharmacol* 2000;15:153–170.
9. Graham TE. Caffeine and exercise: metabolism, endurance and performance. *Sports Med* 2001;31:785–807.
10. Laska EM, Sunshine A, Mueller F, et al. Caffeine as an analgesic adjuvant. *JAMA* 1984;251:1711–1718.
11. Hampl KF, Schneider MC, Ruttimann U, et al. Perioperative administration of caffeine tablets for prevention of postoperative headaches. *Can J Anaesth* 1995;42:789–792.
12. James JE. *Understanding caffeine.* Thousand Oaks, CA: Sage Publications, 1997.

13. Tobias JD. Caffeine in the treatment of apnea associated with respiratory syncytial virus infection in neonates and infants. *South Med J* 2000;93:294–296.
14. Barone JJ, Roberts HR. Caffeine consumption. *Food Chem Toxicol* 1996;34:119–129.
15. Hughes JR, Oliveto AH. A systematic survey of caffeine intake in Vermont. *Exp Clin Psychopharmacol* 1997;5:393–398.
16. Strain EC, Griffiths RR. Caffeine use disorders. In: Tasman A, Kay J, Lieberman JA, eds. *Psychiatry.* Philadelphia: W.B. Saunders, 1997;779–794.
17. National Coffee Association of USA. *2000 National coffee drinking trends: consumption patterns from 1960 to present.* New York: National Coffee Association of USA, 2000.
18. Ahuja JKC, Perloff BP. Caffeine and theobromine intakes of children: results from CSFII 1994–1996, 1998. *Fam Econ Nutr Rev* 2001;13:47–51.
19. Harnack L, Stang J, Story M. Soft drink consumption among U.S. children and adolescents: nutritional consequences. *J Am Diet Assoc* 1999;99:436–441.
20. Jacobson MF. *Liquid candy: how soft drinks are harming American's health.* Center for Science in the Public Interest, Washington DC, 1998.
21. Swan GE, Carmelli D, Cardon LR. The consumption of tobacco, alcohol, and coffee in Caucasian male twins: a multivariate genetic analysis. *J Subst Abuse* 1996;8:19–31.
22. Swan GE, Carmelli D, Cardon LR. Heavy consumption of cigarettes, alcohol and coffee in male twins. *J Stud Alcohol* 1997;58:182–190.
23. Kendler KS, Prescott CA. Caffeine intake, tolerance, and withdrawal in women: a population-based twin study. *Am J Psychiatry* 1999;156:223–228.
24. Mumford GK, Benowitz NL, Evans SM, et al. Absorption rate of methylxanthines following capsules, cola and chocolate. *Eur J Clin Pharmacol* 1996;51:319–325.
25. Liguori A, Hughes JR, Grass JA. Absorption and subjective effects of caffeine from coffee, cola and capsules. *Pharmacol Biochem Behav* 1997;58:721–726.
26. Carrillo JA, Benitez J. Clinically significant pharmacokinetic interactions between dietary caffeine and medications. *Clin Pharmacokinet* 2000;39:127–153.

27. Denaro CP, Benowitz NL. Caffeine metabolism: Disposition in liver disease and hepatic-function testing. In: Watson RR, ed. *Drug and alcohol abuse reviews, vol. 2: liver pathology and alcohol.* Totowa, NJ: Humana Press, 1991:513–539.
28. May DC, Jarboe CH, VanBakel AB, et al. Effects of cimetidine on caffeine disposition in smokers and nonsmokers. *Clin Pharmacol Ther* 1982;31:656–661.
29. Parsons WD, Neims AH. Effect of smoking on caffeine clearance. *Clin Pharmacol Ther* 1978;24:40–45.
30. Aranda JV, Cook CE, Gorman W, et al. Pharmacokinetic profile of caffeine in the premature newborn infant with apnea. *J Pediatr* 1979;94:663–668.
31. Parsons WD, Neims AH. Prolonged half-life of caffeine in healthy term newborn infants. *J Pediatr* 1981;98:640–641.
32. Denaro CP, Brown CR, Wilson M, et al. Dose-dependency of caffeine metabolism with repeated dosing. *Clin Pharmacol Ther* 1990;48:277–285.
33. Bonati M, Latini R, Tognoni G, et al. Interspecies comparison of *in vivo* caffeine pharmacokinetics in man, monkey, rabbit, rat, and mouse. *Drug Metab Rev* 1984;15:1355–1383.
34. Daly JW. Mechanism of action of caffeine. In: Garattini S, ed. *Caffeine, coffee, and health.* New York: Raven Press, 1993:97–150.
35. Fredholm BB, Battig K, Holmen J, et al. Actions of caffeine in the brain with special reference to factors that contribute to its widespread use. *Pharmacol Rev* 1999;51:83–133.
36. Daly JW, Fredholm BB. Caffeine—an atypical drug of dependence. *Drug Alcohol Depend* 1998;51:199–206.
37. Porkka-Heiskanen T, Strecker RE, Thakkar M, et al. Adenosine: a mediator of the sleep-inducing effects of prolonged wakefulness. *Science* 1997;276:1265–1268.
38. Porkka-Heiskanen T, Alanko L, Kalinchuk A, et al. Adenosine and sleep. *Sleep Med Rev* 2002;6:321–332.
39. Shi D, Nikodijevic O, Jacobson KA,

et al. Chronic caffeine alters the density of adenosine, adrenergic, cholinergic, GABA, and serotonin receptors and calcium channels in mouse brain. *Cell Mol Neurobiol* 1993;13:247–261.

40. Snyder SH, Katims JJ, Annau A, et al. Adenosine receptors in the central nervous system: relationship to the central actions of methylxanthines. *Life Sci* 1981;28:2083–2097.

41. Howell LL, Landrum AM. Effects of chronic caffeine administration on respiration and schedule-controlled behavior in rhesus monkeys. *J Pharmacol Exp Ther* 1997;283:190–199.

42. El Yacoubi M, Ledent C, Menard JF, et al. The stimulant effects of caffeine on locomotor behaviour in mice are mediated through its blockade of adenosine A(2A) receptors. *Br J Pharmacol* 2000;129:1465–1473.

43. Garrett BE, Griffiths RR. The role of dopamine in the behavioral effects of caffeine in animals and humans. *Pharmacol Biochem Behav* 1997;57:533–541.

44. Solinas M, Ferre S, You ZB, et al. Caffeine induces dopamine and glutamate release in the shell of the nucleus accumbens. *J Neurosci* 2002;22:6321–6324.

45. Rush CR, Sullivan JT, Griffiths RR. Intravenous caffeine in stimulant drug abusers: subjective reports and physiological effects. *J Pharmacol Exp Ther* 1995;273:351–358.

46. Nurminen ML, Niittynen L, Korpela R, et al. Coffee, caffeine and blood pressure: a critical review. *Eur J Clin Nutr* 1999;53:831–839.

47. Lovallo WR, al'Absi M, Pincomb GA, et al. Caffeine and behavioral stress effects on blood pressure in borderline hypertensive Caucasian men. *Health Psychol* 1996;15:11–17.

48. Urgert R, Katan MB. The cholesterol-raising factor from coffee beans. *Annu Rev Nutr* 1997;17:305–324.

49. Becker AB, Simons KJ, Gillespie CA, et al. The bronchodilator effects and pharmacokinetics of caffeine in asthma. *N Engl J Med* 1984;310:743–746.

50. Duffy P, Phillips YY. Caffeine consumption decreases the response to bronchoprovocation challenge with dry gas hyperventilation. *Chest* 1991;99:1374–1377.

51. Cohen S, Booth GH Jr. Gastric acid secretion and lower-esophageal-sphincter pressure in response to coffee and caffeine. *N Engl J Med* 1975;293:897–899.

52. Rao SS, Welcher K, Zimmerman B, et al. Is coffee a colonic stimulant? *Eur J Gastroenterol Hepatol* 1998;10:113–118.

53. Aldoori WH, Giovannucci EL, Stampfer MJ, et al. A prospective study of alcohol, smoking, caffeine, and the risk of duodenal ulcer in men. *Epidemiology* 1997;8:420–424.

54. Wendl B, Pfeiffer A, Pehl C, et al. Effect of decaffeination of coffee or tea on gastro-oesophageal reflux. *Aliment Pharmacol Ther* 1994;8:283–287.

55. Wemple RD, Lamb DR, McKeever KH. Caffeine vs. caffeine-free sports drinks: effects on urine production at rest and during prolonged exercise. *Int J Sports Med* 1997;18:40–46.

56. Arya LA, Myers DL, Jackson ND. Dietary caffeine intake and the risk for detrusor instability: a case-control study. *Obstet Gynecol* 2000;96:85–89.

57. Creighton SM, Stanton SL. Caffeine: does it affect your bladder? *Br J Urol* 1990;66:613–614.

58. James JE, Sawczuk D, Merrett S. The effect of chronic caffeine consumption on urinary incontinence in psychogeriatric inpatients. *Psychology Health* 1989;3:297–305.

59. Nawrot P, Jordan S, Eastwood J, et al. Effects of caffeine on human health. *Food Addit Contam* 2003;20:1–30.

60. Astrup A, Toubro S, Cannon S, et al. Caffeine: a double-blind, placebo-controlled study of its thermogenic, metabolic, and cardiovascular effects in healthy volunteers. *Am J Clin Nutr* 1990;51:759–767.

61. Arciero PJ, Bougopoulos CL, Nindl BC, et al. Influence of age on the thermic response to caffeine in women. *Metabolism* 2000;49:101–107.

62. Patwardhan RV, Desmond PV, Johnson RF, et al. Effects of caffeine on plasma free fatty acids, urinary catecholamines, and drug binding. *Clin Pharmacol Ther* 1980;28:398–403.

63. Robertson D, Wade D, Workman R, et al. Tolerance to the humoral and hemodynamic effects of caffeine in man. *J Clin Invest* 1981;67:1111–1117.

64. Benowitz NL, Jacob P, Mayan H, et al. Sympathomimetic effects of paraxanthine and caffeine in humans. *Clin Pharmacol Ther* 1995;58:684–691.

65. Lin AS, Uhde TW, Slate SO, et al. Effects of intravenous caffeine administered to healthy males during sleep. *Depress Anxiety* 1997;5:21–28.

66. al'Absi M, Lovallo WR, McKey B, et al. Hypothalamic–pituitary–adrenocortical responses to psychological stress and caffeine in men at high and low risk for hypertension. *Psychosom Med* 1998;60:521–527.

67. Cnattingius S, Signorello LB, Anneren G, et al. Caffeine intake and the risk of first-trimester spontaneous abortion. *N Engl J Med* 2000;343:1839–1845.

68. Wen W, Shu X, Jacobs DR, et al. The associations of maternal caffeine consumption and nausea with spontaneous abortion. *Epidemiology* 2001;12:38–42.

69. Griffiths RR, Evans SM, Heishman SJ, et al. Low-dose caffeine discrimination in humans. *J Pharmacol Exp Ther* 1990;252:970–978.

70. Griffiths RR, Juliano LM, Chausmer AL. Caffeine pharmacology and clinical effects. In: Graham AW, Schultz TK, Mayo-Smith M, et al., eds. *Principles of addiction medicine,* 3rd ed. Chevy Chase, MD: American Society of Addiction Medicine, 2003:193–224.

71. Griffiths RR, Mumford GK. Caffeine—a drug of abuse? In: Bloom FE, Kupfer DJ, eds. *Psychopharmacology: the fourth generation of progress.* New York: Raven Press, 1995:1699–1713.

72. Boulenger JP, Uhde TW, Wolff EA 3rd, et al. Increased sensitivity to caffeine in patients with panic disorders. Preliminary evidence. *Arch Gen Psychiatry* 1984;41:1067–1071.

73. Griffiths RR, Mumford GK. Caffeine reinforcement, discrimination, tolerance, and physical dependence in laboratory animals and humans. In: Schuster CR, Kuhars MJ, eds. *Pharmacological aspects of drug dependence: toward an integrated neurobehavioral approach.* Heidelberg: Springer-Verlag, 1996;315–341.

74. Oliveto AH, McCance-Katz E, Singha A, et al. Effects of d-amphetamine and caffeine in humans under a cocaine discrimination procedure. *Behav Pharmacol* 1998;9:207–217.

75. Chait LD, Johanson CE. Discriminative stimulus effects of caffeine and benzphetamine in amphetamine-trained volunteers. *Psychopharmacology (Berl)* 1988;96:302–308.

76. Oliveto AH, Bickel WK, Hughes JR, et al. Pharmacological specificity of the caffeine discriminative stimulus in humans: effects of theophylline, methylphenidate and buspirone. *Behav Pharmacol* 1993;4:237–246.

77. Oliveto AH, Bickel WK, Hughes JR, et al. Caffeine drug discrimination in humans: acquisition, specificity and correlation with self-reports. *J Pharmacol Exp Ther* 1992;261:885–894.

78. Heishman SJ, Henningfield JE. Stimulus functions of caffeine in humans: relation to dependence potential. *Neurosci Biobehav Rev* 1992;16:273–287.

79. American Psychiatric Association. *Diagnostic and statistical manual of mental disorders,* 4th ed. Washington DC: American Psychiatric Association, 1994.

80. Serafin WE. Drugs used in the treatment of asthma. In: Wonsiewicz MJ, McCurdy P, eds. *The pharmacological*

basis of therapeutics. Hightstown, NJ: McGraw-Hill Publishers, 1996:659–682.

81. Bryant J. Suicide by ingestion of caffeine. *Arch Pathol Lab Med* 1981;105:685–686.

82. Greden JF, Pomerleau OF. Caffeine-related disorders and nicotine-related disorders. In: Kaplan HI, Sadock BJ, eds. *Comprehensive textbook of psychiatry IV.* Baltimore: Williams & Wilkins, 1995:799–810.

83. Greden JF. Anxiety or caffeinism: a diagnostic dilemma. *Am J Psychiatry* 1974;131:1089–1092.

84. Uhde TW. Caffeine provocation of panic: A focus on biological mechanisms. In: Ballenger JC, ed. *Neurobiology of panic disorder.* New York: Alan R. Liss, 1990:219–242.

85. Stern KN, Chait LD, Johanson CE. Reinforcing and subjective effects of caffeine in normal human volunteers. *Psychopharmacology (Berl)* 1989;98:81–88.

86. Lee MA, Cameron OG, Greden JF. Anxiety and caffeine consumption in people with anxiety disorders. *Psychiatry Res* 1985;15:211–217.

87. Rihs M, Muller C, Baumann P. Caffeine consumption in hospitalized psychiatric patients. *Eur Arch Psychiatry Clin Neurosci* 1996;246:83–92.

88. Eaton WW, McLeod J. Consumption of coffee or tea and symptoms of anxiety. *Am J Public Health* 1984;74:66–68.

89. Bruce MS, Lader M. Caffeine abstention in the management of anxiety disorders. *Psychol Med* 1989;19:211–214.

90. Greden JF, Procter A, Victor B. Caffeinism associated with greater use of other psychotropic agents. *Compr Psychiatry* 1981;22:565–571.

91. Snel J. Coffee and caffeine: sleep and wakefulness. In: Garattini S, ed. *Caffeine, coffee, and health.* New York: Raven Press, 1993;255–290.

92. Okuma T, Matsuoka H, Matsue Y, et al. Model insomnia by methylphenidate and caffeine and use in the evaluation of temazepam. *Psychopharmacology (Berl)* 1982;76:201–208.

93. Karacan I, Thornby JI, Anch M, et al. Dose-related sleep disturbances induced by coffee and caffeine. *Clin Pharmacol Ther* 1976;20:682–689.

94. Landolt HP, Werth E, Borbely AA, et al. Caffeine intake (200 mg) in the morning affects human sleep and EEG power spectra at night. *Brain Res* 1995;675:67–74.

95. Goldstein A. Wakefulness caused by caffeine. *Archiv fur Experimentelle Pathologic und Pharmakologic* 1964;248:269–278.

96. Goldstein A, Warren R, Kaizer S. Psychotropic effects of caffeine in man: I.

Individuals differences in sensitivity to caffeine-induced wakefulness. *J Pharmacol Exp Ther* 1965;149:156–159.

97. Regestein QR. Pathologic sleepiness induced by caffeine. *Am J Med* 1989;87:586–588.

98. James JE. Acute and chronic effects of caffeine on performance, mood, headache, and sleep. *Neuropsychobiology* 1998;38:32–41.

99. van der Stelt O, Snel J. Caffeine and human performance. In: Snel J, Lorist MM, eds. *Nicotine, caffeine, and social drinking.* Amsterdam, Netherlands: Harwood Academic Publishers, 1998:167–183.

100. Rogers PJ, Dernoncourt C. Regular caffeine consumption: a balance of adverse and beneficial effects for mood and psychomotor performance. *Pharmacol Biochem Behav* 1998;59:1039–1045.

101. Hughes JR, Hunt WK, Higgins ST, et al. Effect of dose on the ability of caffeine to serve as a reinforcer in humans. *Behav Pharmacol* 1992;3:211–218.

102. Liguori A, Hughes JR, Oliveto AH. Caffeine self-administration in humans: 1. Efficacy of cola vehicle. *Exp Clin Psychopharmacol* 1997;5:286–294.

103. Griffiths RR, Woodson PP. Reinforcing effects of caffeine in humans. *J Pharmacol Exp Ther* 1988;246:21–29.

104. Evans SM, Griffiths RR. Caffeine tolerance and choice in humans. *Psychopharmacology (Berl)* 1992;108:51–59.

105. Hughes JR, Oliveto AH, Bickel WK, et al. Caffeine self-administration and withdrawal: incidence, individual differences and interrelationships. *Drug Alcohol Depend* 1993;32:239–246.

106. Griffiths RR, Bigelow GE, Liebson IA, et al. Human coffee drinking: manipulation of concentration and caffeine dose. *J Exp Anal Behav* 1986;45:133–148.

107. Garrett BE, Griffiths RR. Physical dependence increases the relative reinforcing effects of caffeine versus placebo. *Psychopharmacology (Berl)* 1998;139:195–202.

108. Rogers PJ, Martin J, Smith C, et al. Absence of reinforcing, mood and psychomotor performance effects of caffeine in habitual non-consumers of caffeine. *Psychopharmacology (Berl)* 2003;167:54–62.

109. Schuh KJ, Griffiths RR. Caffeine reinforcement: the role of withdrawal. *Psychopharmacology (Berl)* 1997;130:320–326.

110. Silverman K, Mumford GK, Griffiths RR. Enhancing caffeine reinforcement by behavioral requirements following drug ingestion. *Psychopharmacology (Berl)* 1994;114:424–432.

111. Rogers PJ, Richardson NJ, Elli-

man NA. Overnight caffeine abstinence and negative reinforcement of preference for caffeine-containing drinks. *Psychopharmacology (Berl)* 1995;120:457–462.

112. Richardson NJ, Rogers PJ, Elliman NA. Conditioned flavour preferences reinforced by caffeine consumed after lunch. *Physiol Behav* 1996;60:257–263.

113. Yeomans MR, Spetch H, Rogers PJ. Conditioned flavour preference negatively reinforced by caffeine in human volunteers. *Psychopharmacology (Berl)* 1998;137:401–409.

114. Yeomans MR, Jackson A, Lee MD, et al. Expression of flavour preferences conditioned by caffeine is dependent on caffeine deprivation state. *Psychopharmacology (Berl)* 2000;150:208–215.

115. Shi J, Benowitz NL, Denaro CP, et al. Pharmacokinetic-pharmacodynamic modeling of caffeine: tolerance to pressor effects. *Clin Pharmacol Ther* 1993;53:6–14.

116. Watson J, Deary I, Kerr D. Central and peripheral effects of sustained caffeine use: tolerance is incomplete. *Br J Clin Pharmacol* 2002;54:400–406.

117. Bonnet MH, Arand DL. Caffeine use as a model of acute and chronic insomnia. *Sleep* 1992;15:526–536.

118. Griffiths RR, Woodson PP. Caffeine physical dependence: a review of human and laboratory animal studies. *Psychopharmacology (Berl)* 1988;94:437–451.

119. Couturier EG, Laman DM, van Duijn MA, et al. Influence of caffeine and caffeine withdrawal on headache and cerebral blood flow velocities. *Cephalalgia* 1997;17:188–190.

120. Jones HE, Herning RI, Cadet JL, et al. Caffeine withdrawal increases cerebral blood flow velocity and alters quantitative electroencephalography (EEG) activity. *Psychopharmacology (Berl)* 2000;147:371–377.

121. Strain EC, Mumford GK, Silverman K, et al. Caffeine dependence syndrome. Evidence from case histories and experimental evaluations. *JAMA* 1994;272:1043–1048.

122. Silverman K, Evans SM, Strain EC, et al. Withdrawal syndrome after the double-blind cessation of caffeine consumption. *N Engl J Med* 1992;327:1109–1114.

123. Evans SM, Griffiths RR. Caffeine withdrawal: a parametric analysis of caffeine dosing conditions. *J Pharmacol Exp Ther* 1999;289:285–294.

124. Driesbach RH, Pfeiffer C. Caffeine-withdrawal headache. *J Lab Clin Med* 1943;28:1212–1219.

125. Griffiths RR, Evans SM, Heishman SJ, et al. Low-dose caffeine physical

dependence in humans. *J Pharmacol Exp Ther* 1990;255:1123–1132.

126. Lader M, Cardwell C, Shine P, et al. Caffeine withdrawal symptoms and rate of metabolism. *J Psychopharmacol* 1996;10:110–118.

127. Dews PB, Curtis GL, Hanford KJ, et al. The frequency of caffeine withdrawal in a population-based survey and in a controlled, blinded pilot experiment. *J Clin Pharmacol* 1999;39:1221–1232.

128. Bernstein GA, Carroll ME, Dean NW, et al. Caffeine withdrawal in normal school-age children. *J Am Acad Child Adolesc Psychiatry* 1998;37:858–865.

129. Goldstein A, Wallace ME. Caffeine dependence in schoolchildren? *Exp Clin Psychopharmacol* 1997;5:388–392.

130. Hale KL, Hughes JR, Oliveto AH, et al. Caffeine self-administration and subjective effects in adolescents. *Exp Clin Psychopharmacol* 1995;3:364–370.

131. Bernstein GA, Carroll ME, Thuras PD, et al. Caffeine dependence in teenagers. *Drug Alcohol Depend* 2002;66:1–6.

132. Oberstar JV, Bernstein GA, Thuras PD. Caffeine use and dependence in adolescents: one-year follow-up. *J Child Adolesc Psychopharmacol* 2002;12:127–135.

133. World Health Organization. *The ICD-10 classification of mental and behavioural disorders: clinical descriptions and diagnostic guidelines.* Geneva: World Health Organization, 1992.

134. World Health Organization. *International statistical classification of diseases and related health problems,* 10th rev. Geneva: World Health Organization, 1992.

135. Hughes JR. Caffeine withdrawal, dependence, and abuse. In: American Psychiatric Association. *DSM-IV Sourcebook.* Washington DC: Author, 1994:129–134.

136. Cottler LB, Robins LN, Helzer JE. The reliability of the CIDI-SAM: a comprehensive substance abuse interview. *Br J Addict* 1989;84:801–814.

137. Compton WM, Cottler LB, Dorsey KB, et al. Comparing assessments of the *DSM-IV* substance dependence disorders using CIDI-SAM: a comprehensive substance abuse interview. *Br J Addict* 1996;84:801–814.

138. Swanson JA, Lee JW, Hopp JW. Caffeine and nicotine: a review of their joint use and possible interactive effects in tobacco withdrawal. *Addict Behav* 1994;19:229–256.

139. Emurian HH, Nellis MJ, Brady JV, et al. Event time—series relationship between cigarette smoking and coffee drinking. *Addict Behav* 1982;7:441–444.

140. Kozlowski LT, Henningfield JE, Keenan RM, et al. Patterns of alcohol, cigarette, and caffeine and other drug use in two drug abusing populations. *J Subst Abuse Treat* 1993;10:171–179.

141. Chait LD, Griffiths RR. Effects of caffeine on cigarette smoking and subjective response. *Clin Pharmacol Ther* 1983;34:612–622.

142. Jones HE, Griffiths RR. Oral caffeine maintenance potentiates the reinforcing and stimulant subjective effects of intravenous nicotine in cigarette smokers. *Psychopharmacology (Berl)* 2003;165:280–290.

143. Tanda G, Goldberg SR. Alteration of the behavioral effects of nicotine by chronic caffeine exposure. *Pharmacol Biochem Behav* 2000;66:47–64.

144. Brown CR, Jacob P 3rd, Wilson M, et al. Changes in rate and pattern of caffeine metabolism after cigarette abstinence. *Clin Pharmacol Ther* 1988;43:488–491.

145. Benowitz NL, Hall SM, Modin G. Persistent increase in caffeine concentrations in people who stop smoking. *BMJ* 1989;298:1075–1076.

146. Oliveto AH, Hughes JR, Terry SY, et al. Effects of caffeine on tobacco withdrawal. *Clin Pharmacol Ther* 1991;50:157–164.

147. Hughes JR, Oliveto AH. Coffee and alcohol intake as predictors of smoking cessation and tobacco withdrawal. *J Subst Abuse* 1993;5:305–310.

148. Istvan J, Matarazzo JD. Tobacco, alcohol, and caffeine use: a review of their interrelationships. *Psychol Bull* 1984;95:301–326.

149. Aubin HJ, Laureaux C, Tilikete S, et al. Changes in cigarette smoking and coffee drinking after alcohol detoxification in alcoholics. *Addiction* 1999;94:411–416.

150. Kunin D, Gaskin S, Rogan F, et al. Caffeine promotes ethanol drinking in rats. Examination using a limited-access free choice paradigm. *Alcohol* 2000;21:271–277.

151. White JM. Behavioral effects of caffeine coadministered with nicotine, benzodiazepines and alcohol. *Pharmacopsychoecologia* 1994;7:119–126.

152. Liguori A, Robinson JH. Caffeine antagonism of alcohol-induced driving impairment. *Drug Alcohol Depend* 2001;63:123–129.

153. Fillmore MT, Roach EL, Rice JT. Does caffeine counteract alcohol-induced impairment? The ironic effects of expectancy. *J Stud Alcohol* 2002;63:745–754.

154. Boulenger JP, Patel J, Marangos PJ. Effects of caffeine and theophylline on adenosine and benzodiazepine receptors in human brain. *Neurosci Lett* 1982;30:161–166.

155. Roache JD, Griffiths RR. Interactions of diazepam and caffeine: behavioral and subjective dose effects in humans. *Pharmacol Biochem Behav* 1987;26:801–812.

156. Oliveto AH, Bickel WK, Hughes JR, et al. Functional antagonism of the caffeine-discriminative stimulus by triazolam in humans. *Behav Pharmacol* 1997;8:124–138.

157. Budney AJ, Higgins ST, Hughes JR, et al. Nicotine and caffeine use in cocaine-dependent individuals. *J Subst Abuse* 1993;5:117–130.

158. Garrett BE, Griffiths RR. Intravenous nicotine and caffeine: subjective and physiological effects in cocaine abusers. *J Pharmacol Exp Ther* 2001;296:486–494.

159. Liguori A, Hughes JR, Goldberg K, et al. Subjective effects of oral caffeine in formerly cocaine-dependent humans. *Drug Alcohol Depend* 1997;49:17–24.

160. Spiller GA. *The methylxanthine beverages and foods: chemistry, consumption, and health effects.* New York: Alan R. Liss, 1984.

161. James JE. *Caffeine and health.* San Diego, CA: Academic Press, 1991.

162. Garattini S. *Caffeine, coffee, and health.* New York: Raven Press, 1993.

163. Weber JG, Ereth MH, Danielson DR. Perioperative ingestion of caffeine and postoperative headache. *Mayo Clin Proc* 1993;68:842–845.

164. Weber JG, Klindworth JT, Arnold JJ, et al. Prophylactic intravenous administration of caffeine and recovery after ambulatory surgical procedures. *Mayo Clin Proc* 1997;72:621–626.

165. Gilbert RM. Caffeine as a drug of abuse. In: Gibbins RJ, Israel Y, Kalant H, et al., eds. *Research advances in alcohol and drug problems.* New York: John Wiley, 1976:46–176.

166. Robinson JH, Pritchard WS. The role of nicotine in tobacco use. *Psychopharmacology (Berl)* 1992;108:397–407.

167. West R. Nicotine addiction: a reanalysis of the arguments. *Psychopharmacology (Berl)* 1992;108:408–410.

168. Griffiths RR, Lamb RJ, Ator NA, et al. Relative abuse liability of triazolam: experimental assessment in animals and humans. *Neurosci Biobehav Rev* 1985;9:133–151.

169. Bernard ME, Dennehy S, Keefauver LW. Behavioral treatment of excessive coffee and tea drinking: a case study and partial replication. *Behav Ther* 1981;12:543–548.

170. Foxx RM, Rubinoff A. Behavioral treatment of caffeinism: reducing excessive coffee drinking. *J Appl Behav Anal* 1979;12:335–344.

171. James JE, Stirling KP, Hampton

BA. Caffeine fading: behavioral treatment of caffeine abuse. *Behav Ther* 1985;16:15–27.

172. Bryant CM, Dowell CJ, Fairbrother G. Caffeine reduction education to improve urinary symptoms. *Br J Nurs* 2002;11:560–565.

173. U.S. Department of Health and Human Services, Public Health Service. Treating tobacco use and dependence. Rockville, MD: Author, 2000.

174. Marlatt GA, Gordon JR. *Relapse prevention: maintenance strategies in the treatment of addictive behaviors.* New York: Guilford Press, 1985.

175. Miller WR, Rollnick S. *Motivational interviewing: preparing people to change addictive behavior.* New York: Guilford Press, 1991.

176. James JE, Paull I, Cameron-Traub E, et al. Biochemical validation of self-reported caffeine consumption during caffeine fading. *J Behav Med* 1988;11:15–30.

CHAPTER 25

Anabolic–Androgenic Steroids

ELYSE R. EISENBERG AND
GANTT P. GALLOWAY

Humans have observed for millennia that the testes play a role in producing and maintaining male sexual characteristics. History records athletes and warriors since antiquity seeking to enhance their performance using both rituals and exogenous substances prior to the development of anabolic–androgenic steroids (AASs) (1,2). People from diverse cultures have sought to enhance virility by eating the testes of other species, and incorporating ingestion of the sexual organs in their medicinal practices. AASs have seen widespread use in modern times, with relatively few adverse events reported, and little long-term scientific study completed (3).

The hormonal nature of the action of the testes was demonstrated in 1849, and the endogenous AAS testosterone was isolated in 1935 (4). The first use of AASs as performance enhancers purportedly dates to World War II, when they were administered to German soldiers prior to combat (5). AASs were used for those injured in World War II and for concentration camp survivors to promote weight gain. Use in sports, which began in the 1940s, first brought AASs widespread public attention. During the Cold War, the intense international Olympics competition between Eastern Bloc and Chinese communist nations and Western democratic nations led to an official program of steroid development and use for athletes in the communist nations. Soviet weight lifters reportedly used steroids in the 1952 and 1956 Olympics. Because of limitations of analytic technology, testing of athletes for AAS use did not begin until the 1976 Olympic Games, when eight samples that had screened positive by a newly developed radioimmunoassay technique were confirmed by gas chromatography-mass spectroscopy (6). Additional notoriety accrued to AASs in 1988, when Ben Johnson, a world-record-holding runner, tested positive at the International Olympic Games, and lost his medal (7). That same year, survey results were published showing the lifetime prevalence of AAS usage to be 6.6% in male high school seniors in the United States (8). Classified documents recovered after the fall of the German Democratic Republic (GDR) in 1990 revealed a secret state program from 1966 to improve their national competitive athletic performance; this secret program consisted of sponsoring physicians and scientists in the development and administration of AASs and experimental drugs to several thousand GDR athletes annually, including minors of both sexes, to improve their athletic performance; medical and surgical interventions were required for deleterious side effects. Methods of administration were developed to prevent detection by international doping controls (9). In July 1991, when 42-year-old American football pro Lyle Alzado was diagnosed with inoperable brain cancer, he admitted he had secretly heavily abused AASs and other drugs since he was 20 years old. His announcement brought mainstream awareness to the potential risks of AAS abuse, even though his cancer proved to be lymphoma, metastatic to the brain, probably unrelated to AAS use (*Sports Illustrated*, July 1991). In 1994, 11 Peoples Republic of China athletes tested positive for AASs and were disqualified from the Asian Games in Hiroshima, and China has disqualified more than 2,000 of its own athletes from other competitions in preemptive testing for prohibited drugs. Long after the fact, former East German 1,500-meter swimming world-record-holder Jorg Hoffmann admitted taking an AAS for 3 years prior to winning the title in 1991. Subsequently, international conferences have been held to address the multiplicity of issues and enforcement procedures involving AASs and other performance-affecting drugs.

Key among these was the International Olympic Committee (IOC) World Conference on Doping in Sport in Lausanne in February 1999, whose proposal led to the establishment of the World Anti-Doping Agency (WADA) in November of that year. Other important summits included. The International Drugs in Sport Summit held in Sydney in 1999, and the Anti-Doping Convention of the Council of Europe, held in Strasbourg in 1989 (http://conventions.coe.int/Treaty/en/Treaties/Html/135.htm). Ultimately, the Intergovernmental Consultative Group on Anti-Doping, with 25 nations and additional representatives, met twice in an international summit in 2000 for the purpose of establishing uniform policies and testing procedures, and to support WADA. This summit produced important theme papers regarding coherent international standards, definitions, and testing guidelines for the Olympics and other athletic competitions (10). WADA is developing standard protocols for testing athletes for doping, granting accreditation to qualified laboratories for doping control analyses, including AASs, and publishing relevant news and information on prohibited substances on their web site (http://www.wada-ama.org/en/t1.asp). In October, 2003, the "designer steroid" tetrahydrogestrinone (THG) was detected in samples collected from athletes who competed in the 2003 U.S. Outdoor Track & Field Championships. Subsequently the test to detect THG, developed by the Catlin laboratory at UCLA, has been distributed to all WADA-accredited laboratories. The problem of AAS abuse is perceived to be of sufficient proportion and consequence that the January, 2004 United States of America's State of the Union Address contained this admonishment: "The use of performance-enhancing drugs like steroids in baseball, football, and other sports is dangerous, and it sends the wrong message—that there are shortcuts to accomplishment, and that performance is more important than character. So tonight I call on team owners, union representatives, coaches, and players to take the lead, to send the right signal, to get tough, and to get rid of steroids now" (delivered by President G.W. Bush). In February, 2004, the manufacturers of THG were indicted by the Federal Grand Jury. Meanwhile AAS abuse in and out of professional sports was discussed internationally and prominently in the publications of major news agencies.

A growing body of survey work (Table 25.1) confirms that illicit AAS use is no longer confined to elite and professional athletes. Male and female adolescents, amateur and recreational athletes, exercise enthusiasts, virility seekers, molestation victims, drug abusers, and people with personality disorders are among the wide spectrum of people abusing AASs around the world today.

This chapter uses the term anabolic–androgenic steroid to denote all steroids exhibiting myotrophic actions and that also promote the expression of male sexual characteristics in any ratio, and includes both endogenous animal or human hormones and synthetic derivatives of testosterone. The discovery of a new class of noncontrolled nonsteroidal androgen receptor agonists (11) promises new opportunities for research and therapeutics, as well as abuse.

Different types of steroids may be confused with AASs because the term *steroid* actually refers to a certain ring structure found in many organic chemical compounds, from pesticides to male and female hormones. In human biology and medicine, the term *steroids* encompasses glucocorticoids, mineralocorticoids, estrogens, progestins (12), and vitamin D. The actions of these other classes of steroids are distinct from, and, in some cases, opposed to those of AASs. Some users of illicit AASs are

surprisingly knowledgeable about the different types of steroids, steroid nomenclature, and endocrine physiology. They tend to refer to AASs by common street names such as "roids" or "juice."

PHYSIOLOGY AND PHARMACOLOGY

AASs affect somatic, sexual, and neural cell chemistry and function. Testosterone is produced in males by Leydig cells in the testes in response to luteinizing hormone, a gonadotropin secreted by the pituitary. Testosterone and its derivatives act directly on target cells, binding to an intracellular receptor. This androgen-receptor complex binds to chromosomes, leading to increases in the synthesis of specific messenger ribonucleic acids (mRNAs) and transcription to proteins (13). Expression of these protein products mediates the anabolic and androgenic effects of testosterone. The hormone 5α-dihydrotestosterone, produced by the action of 5α-reductase enzymes on testosterone, also produces these effects with a much greater potency. Intracellular 5α-reductase enzymes are limited to target tissues such as prostate, seminal vesicles, and pubic skin, serving to amplify the actions of testosterone in those tissues (14). Testosterone also is metabolized to estradiol, an estrogen, by aromatase enzymes. The role of endogenous estrogen in males remains unclear.

The complex mechanisms of action of AASs, particularly at supraphysiologic doses, include consequences of individual interactions with other steroid receptor systems, including those for estrogens, progestins, and glucocorticoids (15). AASs augment the release of growth hormone alpha (16).

The androgen and estrogen receptor binding profiles of AAS metabolites have, for the most part, not been defined. Human androgen receptor binding sites are under study. Androgen receptors were found in the soma, and densely in the nuclei, of cultured rat astrocytes and neurons, with less prevalence in glial cells (17).

Studies are elucidating the role of AASs in neurochemistry. A small short-term study of methyltestosterone in humans found decreases in cerebrospinal fluid (CSF) 3-methoxy-4-hydroxyphenylglycol levels and an increase in CSF 5-hydroxyindoleacetic acid (5-HIAA). CSF 5-HIAA levels significantly correlated with increases in "activation" symptoms (energy, sexual arousal, and diminished sleep). Chronic high-dose nandrolone decanoate in guinea pigs caused changes in the limbic regions of the brain involved with stress, behavioral responses, and reward. There were increased densities of c-Fos and Fos-related antigen-positive neurons in the central nucleus of the amygdala, and of Fos-related antigen-positive neurons in the frontal cortex, the shell of the nucleus accumbens, and the supraoptic nucleus (18). Chronic nandrolone administration increased dynorphin and Met-enkephalin-Arg(6)Phe(7) in rat hypothalamus, striatum and periaqueductal gray, brain regions involved in regulating emotions,

TABLE 25.1. *Prevalence of AAS use*

Ref. no.	Year	Location	Respondents	Timeframe	N	Prevalence
57	1984	IL US	weight lifters	lifetime	250 M and F, total	44%
8	1988	US	12th grade students	lifetime	3,403 M	6.6% M
458	1989	AR, US	11th grade students	lifetime	853 M, 914 F	11% M, 0.5% F
459	1990	OR, US	high school football players	current	191 M	1.1% M
459	1990	IL US	high school students	lifetime	1,028 M, 1,085 F	6.5% M, 2.5% F, 5.5% athletes, 2.4% non-athletes
30	1991	MI, US	weight lifters	lifetime	404 M, 45 F	12% M, 4% F
460	1992	AR, US	11th grade students	lifetime	672 M, 806 F	7.6% M, 1.5% F
58	1992	Western Cape, South Africa	high school seniors	lifetime	1,361 M and F, total	0.6% overall 1.2% M, 1.3% M sports participants
461	1992	WV, US	high school students	lifetime	3,900 M	5.3% M
462	1993	Scotland, UK	college students	lifetime	341 M, 292 F	4.4% M, 1.0% F
463	1993	CA, US	7th grade students	lifetime	782 M and F, total	4.7% M, 3.2% F
80	1993	GA, US	high school students	lifetime	962 M, 919 F	6.5% M, 1.9% F
466	1995	US	college students	past year	75,169 M and F, total	0.9%
65	1995	Falkenberg, Sweden	high school students	lifetime	688 M, 695 F	5.8% M
464	1995	MA, US	high school students	lifetime	1,501 M, 1,549 F	5.7% M, 1.7% F
30	1995	US	residents of households, age 12 and over	lifetime	7,950 M, 9,859 F	0.9% M, 0.2% F
465	1995	US	8th grade students 10th grade students 12th grade students	past year / lifetime	c. 17,300 c. 15,800 c. 15,400 M and F, total	1.8% M, 0.6% F 1.9% M, 0.4% F 2.1% M, 0.5% F 2.4%
32	1997	Australia	high school students	lifetime	13,355	3.2% M, 1.2% F
40	2002	MN, US	middle and high school students	past year	2,170 M, 2,174 F	M 5.4%, F 2.9%
38	2002	US	12th grade students	past year	12,900	3.8% M, 1.2% F

defensive reactions, and aggression (19). At higher levels, chronic daily nandrolone decanoate caused increased concentrations of β-endorphins in the ventral tegmental area, the reward center of the brain, suggesting a mechanism for AAS (and gateway to other drug) dependence (20). In addition, treated rats had increased aggression, less defensive immobility, and increased voluntary ethanol intake (21). Chronic supraphysiologic AAS in male rats causes elevations in choline acetyltransferase mRNA levels in spinal cord motor neurons (22). Other neurochemicals were not affected by administration of methyltestosterone (23). The impact of AASs in prepubertal female rats upon neuroendocrine regions involved with reproduction found potentiation of GABAergic activity in the ventromedial nucleus of the hypothalamus (VMN) similar to that of endoge-

nous androgens, and inhibition of GABAergic activity in the medial preoptic area in contrast to the potentiation by endogenous androgens (24).

Although testosterone is the major androgenic hormone, its clinical utility is limited by extensive hepatic first-pass liver metabolism and brief (10-minute) elimination half-life. Esterification of the 17β-hydroxyl group, alkylation of the 17α-position, modification of the steroid nucleus, and other alterations have been undertaken to increase the oral bioavailability, absorption half-life, elimination half-life, and ratio of anabolic-to-androgenic effects in synthetic and semisynthetic testosterone derivatives (25). 17-β-Esterification increases the lipophilicity of testosterone, increasing the absorption half-life when administered intramuscularly in oil. 17α-Alkylation slows hepatic metabolism and enhances bioavailability when testosterone is administered orally. However, this route has a high rate of hepatic toxicity, and causes a reversible but potentially fatal hepatorenal syndrome called cholestatic jaundice. Percutaneous delivery systems are now available which sidestep the problems associated with either oral or injection use.

The metabolism of testosterone to estradiol, 5α-dihydrotestosterone, and to the inactive metabolites androsterone and etiocholanolone, is well defined. The metabolism of 17β-esterified derivatives by rapid de-esterification to testosterone is also well defined. The metabolism of testosterone derivatives with modifications to the steroid nucleus, or 17α-alkyl substitutions, is considerably more complex; each of the dozens of compounds available has a separate pattern of biotransformation. 17-Epimerization (26) and 6β-hydroxylation (27,28) emerge as important pathways, although many other pathways contribute. (For more thorough reviews of AAS pharmacology and physiology, see references 13, 14, and 29.)

EPIDEMIOLOGY AND USAGE PATTERNS

Incidence and Prevalence

The spread of AAS use has been largely a silent phenomenon, yet the estimate from the United States Substance Abuse and Mental Health Services Administration (SAMHSA)'s National Household Drug Abuse Survey published in 1995 is that 1,084,000 Americans had ever used AASs and that 312,000 (29%) of those had AASs used in the prior year (30). The comparable figures for heroin use are 2,083,000 and 281,000 (13%), respectively; some people abuse both. AAS use is not confined to the United States; use is documented in the United Kingdom, Sweden, Belgium, Germany, China, Eastern Europe, and South Africa (see Table 25.1). Prevalence is higher in males than in females: lifetime estimates from population and school-based surveys are 1.8% to 11% in males and 0.2% to 3.2% in females in the United States. Athletes, particularly weight lifters, have a greater prevalence of use than do nonathletes everywhere, but the difference is surprisingly small in some studies, pointing to the importance of other factors in the decision to use AASs.

Data collection methods to assess steroid and other drug use in scientific and addiction medicine studies usually are by self-report, blinded correlated urine assay, or *other-witness* reports. One test of reliability of the self-report method done in 48 weight lifters found urine screen validating the self-report in 22 of 23 subjects, 15 participants reporting at least 1 drug that was not found in their urine, and AASs in the urine of 3 of 17 self-reported nonusers (31).

Accurate estimates of illicit AAS use outside the United States are rare. In 1997, a self-report survey of 13,355 representative Australian high school students found 213 (3.2%) of males and 74 (1.2%) of females with lifetime "ever" use of AASs (32). By 1998 in the United States, the lifetime prevalence rates for adolescent steroid use ranged between 2.6% and 12% among males, and between 0.5% and 2.8% for females (33,34). Studies to identify risk factors for onset and continued use of AAS by adolescents are underway (35). In a 1995 cross-sectional survey study of 2,088 eighteen-year-old high school graduates in Michigan, only 0.6% admitted to AAS use, and this was *not* associated with a desire for weight gain in the males; runners and swimmers were more likely than football players to have used AASs (36). However, a recent and comprehensive computerized and manual literature search of local, state, national, and international reports of illicit AAS use by American adolescents, that referenced risk factors, showed a different pattern. Male student athletes involved in weight lifting, football, and wrestling were more likely to use AASs than any other group, as well as to concurrently use other illicit drugs, alcohol, and tobacco (35). Australian adolescents had a different pattern of social and cultural factors associated with AAS abuse; their lifetime prevalence of AAS use was associated with 7 or more days of truancy versus no days of truancy for nonabusers in the last 2 weeks (odds ratio [OR] 17.7), and 6 or more nights of unsupervised recreation by AAS abusers versus 2 or fewer nights per week without supervision for nonusers (OR 8.4). AAS abuse among Australian adolescents also was associated with speaking only a non-English language at home (OR 7.75), Aboriginality (OR 3.4), male gender (OR 2.8), higher student income (OR 2.3), overseas born (OR 2.2), and low level of social support (OR 2.5). The risk factors for use within the previous past 1 month were identical, but these ORs were uniformly higher (32). By contrast, adult male elite Australian Rules Football League players were studied with randomized, unannounced, prospective urine testing at various times during the period 1990–1995, and no test was positive for steroids, caffeine, or diuretics (37).

Data show that AAS use is increasing among the group most physicians would be very unlikely to suspect or evaluate for AAS abuse: adolescent females in middle school (34) and high school. An important statistical analysis was undertaken in 1997 by Yesalis et al. to examine the trends in AAS use among male and female adolescents in the United States from 1989 to 1996. National, state, and local survey data were employed, including the Monitoring the Future study, the Youth Risk and Behavior Surveillance System, and the National Household Survey on Drug Abuse. State studies showed an overall decrease in teenage student lifetime AAS use rates from 1989 to 1994, although no tests of statistical significance were conducted. National data showed a significant decline in use by both males and females from 1989 to a nadir in 1991. This was followed by a stable rate of use among adolescent males only, from 1991 to 1994 in two of the three studies. The 2002 Monitoring the Future survey found the rate of use among adolescents to be increasing (38): 2.5% of eighth graders, 3.5% of tenth graders, and 4.0% of twelfth graders reported having ever used AASs. According to this annual survey, since 1991 there has been a 90% increase in AAS use among twelfth graders. Approximately 375,000 adolescent males and 175,000 adolescent females in public and private schools in the United States had used illicit AAS at least once (39). In Minneapolis in 2002, the Project EAT (Eating Among Teens) evaluated steroid use in 4,746 middle and high school students surveyed and examined them with anthropomorphic measurements. Steroid use reported among males was 5.4%, and among females was 2.9%. Among teenagers had the highest rate of use (40).

Reasons for Illicit Use

Direct pharmacologic actions of AASs result in euphoria and a subjective "high" in some individuals (41,42). Withdrawal symptoms, discussed at length below, (Dependence, Table 25.3) also can become important factors in continued use. Etiologic classifications of psychosocial factors, reality factors, and directly reinforcing effects are presented elsewhere (43). AASs seem to have a greater long-term effect on most users, rather than the immediate rush and alteration of mood, reward, or sense of well-being seen with other drugs of abuse (44). Yet some AAS users compulsively self-administer ever-increasing doses of AASs in the face of adverse consequences, are more likely to self-administer other drugs of abuse, and experience a withdrawal syndrome when AASs are discontinued. The highly addictive behavioral components of AAS use, i.e., use ritual, injection ritual, sensation, and peer approval, provide immediate rewards, are important factors in sustaining use, and probably contribute to the withdrawal syndrome.

Body builders generally start AAS use seeking psychological rewards from attention to, and admiration of, a muscular physique. Athletes use AASs seeking to improve their performance; this performance enhancement may be a result of objective effects of increased muscle mass, or because of subjective effects such as increased levels of aggression or increased confidence. Coaches and parents of adolescent athletes may encourage use of AASs (45,46). Law enforcement and corrections officers may use AASs seeking an intimidating physique and a fighting proficiency. Material benefits from use of AASs can include amateur and professional awards, achievement of new records, college athletic scholarships, lucrative employment opportunities with professional athletic teams, and advertising contracts for sports-related products and services. Female-to-male (FTM) transgendered individuals without access to appropriate medical care may self-medicate with AASs in an effort to increase secondary male characteristics and decrease female attributes.

Response to Assault

A study of 75 women weight lifters found 10 (13%) had been raped as teenagers or adults. Of these, nine (90%) began compulsively weight lifting and seven (70%) began using AASs or clenbuterol following the assault to improve their ability to defend themselves against men (47). Physically and sexually abused males, as well as females, may develop muscle dysmorphic disorder, and consequently abuse AASs (see also "Disorders of Body Image" below).

Personality Type

Clinical observations of AAS abusers' preoccupation with self and self-image led to investigations into personality characteristics of AAS abusers. All early studies examining personality and behavior of AAS abusers were done on male weight lifters; the presumption was that findings would generalize to the wider population, but there was no data to support that assertion (48). Recently, the first such study with women weight lifters reveals that findings in males do not apply to females. Women abusing AASs display several psychiatric syndromes not previously reported (47), including gender dysphoria, which is discussed at length throughout this article (see also "Disorders of Body Image" below).

In the first study examining personality traits in AAS abusers, Perry et al. compared rates of *Diagnostic and Statistical Manual of Mental Disorders,* 3rd ed. (*DSM–III*) defined personality disorders and traits in 20 AAS-using male weight lifters, versus 20 nonusing male weight lifter controls and 20 nonusing nonathletic male community controls (49). The AAS users had more personality disorders (85%) than either the nonusing weight lifters (50%), or the community controls (35%). A 27-fold higher incidence of personality disorders in the histrionic, narcissistic, antisocial, and borderline grouping was found in AAS users when compared to the community controls group, and a 9-fold higher incidence was found when compared to nonusing weight lifters (49). In a subsequent study of personality characteristics in adolescent males employing the same 3-group design with 24 subjects per group, no statistically significant differences between athletic users and nonusers were found, although trends toward greater forcefulness, greater impulsivity, and less cooperativeness, as measured by the Millon Adolescent Personality Inventory, were observed in the athletic users; similar trends were evident when comparing non-AAS–using athletes were compared to nonathletic, nonusing controls (50). The prevalence of antisocial personality disorder (ASPD) was ascertained in a study of 88 AAS-using athletes and 68 nonusing control athletes. A trend toward a higher incidence of ASPD as diagnosed with the Structured Clinical Interview for *Diagnostic and Statistical Manual of Mental Disorders,* 3rd ed., revised (*DSM–III–R*) found 9 (10%) of the AAS-users versus only 2 (3%) of the controls were diagnosed with ASPD (51). Porcerelli examined narcissism and empathy in 16 weight lifters who had used AASs and 20 weight lifters who had not used AASs. The AAS users had lower ratings of empathy and higher ratings on the three (of seven) dimensions of narcissism most associated with psychopathology: exploitativeness, exhibitionism, and entitlement (43). There is evidence that aggression and significant abnormal personality traits emerge in male bodybuilders who abuse AASs who had previously tested within normal limits (52,53). Most studies do not elucidate whether AAS use caused personality disorders, or if the personality disorders led to AAS use. Clinicians should be aware that both antisocial and narcissistic behaviors are relatively common in adult male bodybuilding AAS abusers.

Disorders of Body Image

Dissatisfaction with body image, specifically the perception of being too small or insufficiently muscular, is common in AAS users, and is associated with AAS dependence (41,54). In one study of males, bodybuilders were at greater risk than martial artists or runners for problems often seen in eating disorder patients: body dissatisfaction, thinness seeking, muscle bulk desiring, bulimia, self-esteem problems, depression, maturity fears, and perfectionism (54). One case report (55) and data from a comparison of 88 AAS-using male athletes and 68 nonusing male athletes (51) indicate that this dissatisfaction with body image reaches pathologic levels in some AAS users. This was observed in ten (11%) of the AAS users, but in none of the nonusers. The following description was given of this condition:

> Individuals with this disorder believed that they looked small and weak, even though they were large and muscular. They declined to be seen in public, refused invitations to the beach, or wore baggy sweat-clothes even in summer to avoid being seen as "small."

This disorder has been termed *reverse anorexia nervosa,* although it appears to meet diagnostic criteria for *body dysmorphic disorder.* Anorexia nervosa and bulimia nervosa were also diagnosed at high rates for males, 3 (3%) and 1 (1%), respectively, compared to the non-user group, 1 (1%) and 0, respectively, although neither of these differences reached statistical significance.

Disorders of body image associated with AASs are also found in women. The first significant psychiatric study of women weight lifters was done with 75 dedicated women athletes who were primarily from the Boston, Massachusetts area. Current or past AAS use was reported by 25 (33%) of the women. Unusual psychiatric syndromes reported by both the AAS users and nonusers included rigid dietary practices, and chronic dissatisfaction and preoccupation with their physiques that the authors classify as *eating disorder, bodybuilder type,* and *muscle dysmorphia,* respectively. Gender dysphoria, which leads some FTMs to exercise with weights to alter their physique toward the male, are expected to cluster in gymnasium, and such a cluster was found. Hypomanic symptoms were reported by 14 (56%) AAS users; depressive symptoms

during AAS withdrawal were reported by 10 (40%) AAS users. None of the reported symptom episodes met *Diagnostic and Statistical Manual of Mental Disorders,* 4th ed. (*DSM–IV*) criteria for hypomanic or major depressive episodes (56).

Sources for Abused Anabolic–Androgenic Steroids

Abused AASs are typically not acquired by prescription in the United States (57,58). In the United Kingdom, guidelines for prohibited substances banned in sports, including AASs, are found in The British National Formulary; a recent physician survey in West Sussex found that only 35% of respondents were aware of the guidelines, and that 12% of physicians incorrectly believed medical practitioners are allowed to prescribe AASs for nonmedical reasons (59). The 2001 National Collegiate Athletic Association (NCAA) survey of student athletes revealed that 32.1% of those who had used AASs had obtained them by prescription from a nonteam physician (60). The bulk of black market AASs is probably smuggled into the United States, although diversion of medications from veterinary clinics and suppliers also may occur. Small-scale importation of pharmaceutical AASs from Mexico (61), the Caribbean, and from offshore pharmacies marketing via the Internet is another source of supply for illicit use. Most people who sell AASs are themselves users of AASs and they often recruit new users at gymnasiums. The illicit market, which may include adulterated or counterfeit preparations, raises concerns about pharmacologic purity and biologic contamination; these concerns are particularly acute for injectable AASs. Table 25.2 lists AASs, their recommended doses and their abused doses. Dehydroepiandrosterone (DHEA) and numerous "proandrogens" are readily and cheaply available from the Internet and over the counter at "health food" and "natural food" stores. AASs or precursors are sometimes found as "contaminants" in supplements and in herbal and Chinese medicine remedies, and hence do not appear on the labels. A related development with abuse potential is a new class of noncontrolled nonsteroidal androgen agonists (11).

Patterns of Use

To obtain maximum increases in lean muscle mass, body weight, and strength, AAS abusers practice *stacking,* using three or more kinds of AASs, which may be administered by different routes. In an attempt to minimize deleterious side effects, abusers alternate between cycles of abuse and nonuse. Typical cycles may run 4 to 18 weeks on AASs and 1 month to 1 year off (41,49,57,62). Up to 99% of adult AAS users report having injected the drug, 82% report stacking three AASs during training, and 30% report having used seven or more (41,49,51,55,57,62–64). Injection is common even in adolescents (65).

TABLE 25.2. *Commercially available anabolic–androgenic steroids*

Generic names	Brand names	Route, recommended dosage	Abused doses and reference numbers
Boldenone undecenoate	Equipoise	veterinary only (horses: 0.5 mg/kg 1×/3 wks)	50–200 mg/wk (22,24,29,31)
Calusterone Dimethyttestosterone	—	—	—
Clostebol[b]	Clostene Steranabol Megagrisevit (multiingredient) Trofoseptine (multiingredient) Alfa-Trofodermin	i.m. 40 mg 2×/wk Topical	DNS (35)
Danazol[a,c] (a partial androgen agonist)	Cyclomen Danatrol Danazant Danocrine (U.S.) Danol Ladazol Mastodanatrol Winbanin	p.o. 100–800 mg/d	—
Dromostanolone[b] Drostanolone Methyldihydrotestosterone Propionate	Masterid Masteril Permastril	i.m. 100 mg 3×/wk	800 mg/wk (44)
Epitiostanol Ethylestrenol[b] Ethyloestrenol	— Orabolin	p.o. up to 4 mg/d	6–8 mg/d (68) 10–12 mg/d (31)
Fluoxymesterone[a,c]	Android-F Halotestin (U.S.) Halodrin (multiingredient)	p.o. 1–20 mg/d	—
Formebolone[b] Furazabol[b]	Esiclene Androfurazanol	p.o. 5–10 mg/d IM p.o. up to 3 mg/d i.m. 25 mg 1–2×/wk	
Mepitiostane Mesterolone[b]	Thioderon Mestoranum Proviron	p.o. p.o. 50–100 mg/d	25 mg/d(44) 350–700 mg/wk (34) DNS (24)
Methandrostenolone[b] Methandienone Methandienone	Metaboline (multiingredient)	p.o. 4 mg/d for 6 wks alternating with 2–4-wk drug-free periods	40 mg/d (48) 15 mg/d for 9 years (118) Mean, 28 mg/d in a group of 20 (22) 15 mg/d (119) 5–50 mg/d (36) 25–50 mg/d (44), 15–40 mg/d (29) DNS (25)
Methandiol Mestenediol Methylandrostenediol	Otormon F (multiingredient)	—	—
Methenolone[b] Methenolone Acetate Methenolone Enanthate	Primobolan Primobolan Depot Primobolan S AntiFocal N	p.o. (acetatate): up to 20 mg/d i.m. (enanthate): 100 mg/2–4 wks	100 mg/wk (34) 20 mg/wk (31) 200 mg/wk (44) 4 cc IM/wk (concentration unknown)(29)
Methenolone Enantate Methenolone Enanthate	(multiingredient) NeyChondrin (multiingredient)		

(continued)

TABLE 25.2. *(Continued)*

Generic names	Brand names	Route, recommended dosage	Abused doses and reference numbers
Methenolone Oenanthate	NeyGeront (multiingredient) NeyPulpin (multiingredient) NeyTumorin (multiingredient)		
Methyltestosterone[a,c]	Android-10, 25 (U.S.) Metandren Testomet Testovis Testred (U.S.) Virilon (U.S.) Multiingredient preparations: Eldec, Estratest, Estratest H.S., Mediatric, Mixogen, Pasuma, Premarin with Methyltestosterone Prowess, and Tylosterone	p.o. 10–50 mg/d	DNS (24)
Methyltestosterone[a,c]	Oreton Methyl (U.S.)	Buccal:5 to 25 mg/d	—
Mibolerone	Mibolerone	Veterinary only	—
Nandrolone[a,b] Nortestosterone in various salts and esters:	Activin Androlone-D Deca-Durabolin (U.S.)	i.m. 25–200 mg/1–4 wks	Mean dose 197 mg/wk (22) 100 mg/wk (31) 100–200 mg/wk (60) 100 mg/3d (48)
Cyclohexylpropionate Decanoate Hemisuccinate Laurate Phenylpropionate Sodium Sulfate Undecanoate	Deca-Durabol Durabolin (U.S.) Dynabolon Fherbolico Hybolin Decanoate Hybolin Improved (U.S.) Kabolin Keratyl Nandrobolic (U.S.) Nandrol Stenabolin Multiingredient preparations: Dexatopic Dinatrofon Docabolin Docabolina Trophobolene		100 mg/wk to 200 mg/d (44) 600 mg/wk to 200 mg/d (29) DNS (24,25,35,43,114)
Norclostebol Acetate	—	i.m.	—
Norethandrolone[b]	Nilevar	p.o. up to 30 mg/d	—
Oxandrolone[a]	Lonavar Oxandrin (U.S.)	p.o. 2.5 mg 2–4×/d	25 mg/d (25) Mean, 14 mg/d (22) 70–175 mg/wk (34) 25 mg/d (48) 12.5–15 mg/d (31) 20–40 mg/d (29)
Oxymetholone[a]	Adroyd Anadrol-50 (U.S.) Anapolon Oxitosona Plenastril	p.o.1–5 mg/kg/d	Mean, 46 mg/d (22) 250 mg/d (36) 100 mg/d (44)

(continued)

TABLE 25.2. *(Continued)*

Generic names	Brand names	Route, recommended dosage	Abused doses and reference numbers
Prasterone Sodium Sulfate	Multiingredient preparations:	i.m. 200 mg/4–6 wks	—
Prasterone Enanthate[b]	Gynodian Gynodian Depot		
Quinbolone[b]	Anabolicum Vister	p.o. up to 30 mg/d	—
Stanolone	Andractim	Topical	
Androstanolone	Gelovit	Sublingual	
Dihydrotestosterone	Ophtovitol (multiingredient)	Sublabial	
Stanozolol[a,b]	Stromba	p.o. initial dose of 2 mg 3×/d[c] maintenance dose of 2 mg/d[b]	30 mg/d to 250 mg/wk (44) 10 mg/d (36)
Androstanazole	Strombaject	p.o. 2.5 mg 3×/wk to 10 mg/d	DNS (22,31,35)
Methylstanazole	Winstrol (U.S.)	i.m. 50 mg every 2–3 wks	
Testosterone[a] transdermal patches	Testoderm (U.S.) Androderm (U.S.)	Transdermal: 4–6 mg/d	—
Testosterone[a] in aqueous suspension	Testandro (U.S.) Histerone (U.S.) Tesamone (U.S.)	i.m. 25–50 mg/2–3 wks	—
Testosterone[c] subcutaneous pellets	Testopel Pellets	Subcutaneous implantation: 150–450 mg/3–4 months	—
Testosterone esters[a,c]	Andro L.A. 200 (U.S.)	i.m. cypionate: 50–400 mg/ 2–4 wks	100 mg/3 days (17,22,24,101)
Acetate		Enanthate and propionate: 40–50 mg/2–4 wks to 100 mg 3×/wk	269–1400 mg/wk (17,22, 24,29, 36,48,101)
Cypionate	Andropository-200 (U.S.)		
Decanoate	Delatestryl (U.S.)		
Enanthate	Durathate-200 (U.S.)		
Hexahydrobenzoate	Everone 200 (U.S.)		
Hexahydrobenzylcorbonate	Andro-Cyp 100, 200		
Isocaproate	depAndro 100, 200 (U.S.)		
Phenylproplonate	Depotest 100, 200 (U.S.)		
Propionate	Depo-Testosterone (U.S.)		
Undecanoate	Duratest 100, 200 (U.S.) T-cypionate many other brand names, including combination products		
Trenbolone		Veterinary	76 mg/wk (34) Mean, 93 mg/3 days (22) 76 mg/wk (44)

[a]Dose information from Kastrup E, ed. *Facts and comparisons.* St. Louis: Facts and Comparisons, 1996.

[b]Dose information from Reynolds J, Paritt K, Parsons A, et al. eds., *Martindale: the extra pharmacopoeia.* 30th ed. London: The Pharmaceutical Press, 1993.

[c]Dose information from McEvoy G, ed. *AHFS 96 drug information.* Bethesda, MD: American society for Health-System Pharmacists, 1996.

Legend: DNS-abuse reported dose not stated; i.m.-intramuscular: p.o.-oral.

Bodybuilding and weight training are typically done in phases; AASs are commonly and heavily used during the muscle build-up phase, rather than during the training or maintenance phases that follow. Doses may range from 20 to 200 times the recommended daily medically prescribed dose. In some instances, the quest for maximal results leads to continuous administration. In other instances, periods of modest doses of a single AAS are interspersed between high-dose uses of many AASs. Cycles that involve building up to a peak dose and then tapering down are called *pyramids* (57). Administration of multiple steroids in increasing and tapering doses is known as *stacking the pyramid* (57). Users often meticulously plan and record their use of AASs, and may be able to give detailed histories of use. The patterns of cyclic use, variable doses, simultaneous use of multiple AASs that have differing physiologic effects, and use of grossly supratherapeutic doses makes extrapolations from therapeutic and experimental data problematic. Daily ingestion of over-the-counter (OTC) oral AAS precursors, such as DHEA, is a common practice among male and female bodybuilders and other athletes.

Other Drugs Used

Adolescent (66) and adult AAS users use alcohol, therapeutic drugs (including antiinflammatory drugs, muscle relaxants, and analgesics for pain), purportedly ergogenic or performance-enhancing drugs (including nutritionals, botanicals, and stimulants), illegal street drugs (marijuana and heroin), and tobacco (60,67,68). Additional drugs are used to minimize steroid side effects or to attempt to defeat testing for doping control.

AAS users also often consume prodigious amounts of dietary supplements, which may be associated with their own hazards (69). There are literally dozens of botanical and nutritional substances available in natural food stores, at gymnasium counters, and from the Internet that are touted to promote athletic stature and ability. Daily ingestion of OTC nutritional supplements, sometimes containing AASs, is a common practice among male and female bodybuilders and other athletes. A walk down the aisles of "health food and nutritional stores" reveals an enlarging cornucopia of biologically active, purportedly ergogenic and/or anabolic "supplements," for example, saponins derived from *Leuzea rhaponticum* sp. (70).

In Belgium, testing of 4,374 specimens from 1987 to 1994 found 5.8% to 8.9% of competitive bicyclists testing positive for prohibited substances. While the use of the stimulants methamphetamine, methylphenidate, and pemoline decreased, the Official Doping Laboratory of Flanders reported an increase in detection of prolintane, a central nervous system (CNS) stimulant, and codeine, as well as the anabolic steroids nandrolone and testosterone (71). The abused agents ephedrine, β adrenergics, human chorionic gonadotropin, antidepressants, and diuretics were recovered in biologic specimens from award-winning bodybuilders in France (72).

Psychoactive Drugs

Abuse of and dependence on other psychoactive drugs are prevalent among AAS users, although concerns about health and appearance may moderate such use. The data on concurrent substance abuse is highly variable with date, location, and other study factors. In a 1990 study of 20 AAS-using weight lifters, 7 (35%) were alcohol abusers, 2 (10%) were alcohol dependent, and 1 (5%) was a drug abuser; this compared to 13 (65%) alcohol abusers and 1 (5%) drug abuser in the control group of non–AAS-using weight lifters (49). In a 1988 convenience sample of 41

AAS users recruited from gymnasiums, 4 (9.8%) smoked cigarettes, 6 (14.6%) had past diagnoses of alcohol abuse or dependence, and 13 (31.7%) had prior diagnoses of other drug abuse or dependence, mostly marijuana (7 of 41, 17.1%) and cocaine (5 of 41, 12.2%), but none had current substance-abuse dependence, except for the nicotine dependence (62). Other studies have reported higher levels of substance abuse and dependence between cycles. One series of 23 AAS users included several subjects who only used psychoactive drugs between cycles (73). In another group of 88 athletes who used AASs, 28 (32%) had diagnoses of current substance abuse or dependence while off-cycle, but only 1 (1%) had a diagnosis of current substance abuse or dependence while on-cycle; in a comparison group of 68 nonusers, 15 (22%) had current substance abuse or dependence diagnoses (51). It is not clear from these data that abuse and dependence diagnoses for drugs other than AASs are any more common in AAS users than in the general population.

There is an association between overall tobacco use and AAS use among adolescent athletes. Professional athletes using and advertising "smokeless" tobacco products on television and in other media have long encouraged nicotine abuse among amateurs aspiring to greater ability (74,75, Christen, 1980 #1118), even though tobacco is ergolytic. Adolescent males and females may "try" buccal snuff (dip) (76), or chewing tobacco (67), and a percentage become chronic users; in an Alabama dental study, 8% of male athletes became chronic abusers of oral smokeless tobacco (77). A Louisiana study of high school males found that both white and African American males involved in athletics were 1.5 times more likely to use tobacco products than their peers. Higher-intensity sports are a significant predictor of smokeless tobacco use, but not of smoking behavior (78). West Virginia adolescent and adult males use smokeless tobacco at significantly greater rates than does the general population (79). AAS-abusing adolescents are more likely, rather than less, to use other drugs of abuse (68,80,81).

There is evidence that AAS abuse is a gateway or a risk indicator for opiate abuse (82). Some individuals choose opiates to increase pain tolerance, promote sleep, modulate stimulation from substances such as AAS, amphetamines, and ephedrine, or to seek euphoria.

Other Performance-Enhancing and Physique-Modifying Drugs

As discussed above, athletes who use AASs also may employ drugs from among a wide variety of psychomotor stimulants (83), including ephedrine, caffeine, phenylpropanolamine, pseudoephedrine, methoxyphenamine, cocaine, and methamphetamine (60,84,85). Although some of these may be abused for their psychoactive properties, this class of drugs is accepted by segments of the athletic community as performance enhancing, i.e., *ergonomic* or *ergogenic*.

Human growth hormone (hGH) is anabolic and is been used by AAS users (57,84,86). A lifetime hGH use prevalence of 5% was found in a survey of 224 male tenth grade students, suggesting that abuse of hGH may be widespread (87). A variety of substances purported to increase release of endogenous hGH are also abused, notably gamma hydroxybutyrate (88). Somatotropin and insulin-like growth factor I are anabolic; increased production of these hormones through gene therapy may be undertaken to increase athletic performance in the future (89). The β_2-adrenergic agonist clenbuterol was observed to increase the deposition rate of lean mass and to retard adipose gain in animal husbandry. Based on this information, clenbuterol entered into use by athletes as an anabolic agent (90). Other agents reportedly abused to enhance performance include salbutamol, deprenyl, β-adrenergic antagonists, levothyroxine, erythropoietin, and darbepoetin (84,85,91). An early example of botanicals employed to enhance performance is yohimbine bark. Yohimbine bark still is promoted as an alternative to AAS to enhance athletic, as well as male sexual, performance. As with many other OTC supplements and botanicals, there may be great variability in the actual yohimbine content of OTC yohimbine products (92).

Drugs to Evade Detection

The threat of disqualification for athletes found to use AASs led to the development and use of pharmacologic aids to evade detection. Detection of testosterone abuse is complicated by the fact that testosterone occurs endogenously. Therefore detection of testosterone abuse relies on the ratio of testosterone to epitestosterone. Normal ratios of testosterone to epitestosterone in urine are 1 to 2.5:1. Ratios of 6:1 or greater are considered positive for exogenous administration of testosterone; this has led some athletes to self-administer epitestosterone in combination with testosterone to attempt to defeat the test (85). Urinary concentrations of AASs are decreased by use of both probenecid and diuretics (85) (see "Screening, Diagnosis, and Testing" in "Evaluation and Treatment," below).

Drugs Taken to Ameliorate Side Effects

In a study of 100 male bodybuilders abusing AASs, 86% were using adjunctive medications to mitigate steroid-related side effects and withdrawal symptoms, as well as to enhance anabolic effects (93).

Diuretics are used by body builders to counter the fluid retention caused by AASs and to increase muscle definition—to create a more "ripped" or "cut up" look with increased definition of superficial vasculature, muscular shape, and muscular striations (50,64,84). Hemoconcentration with hematocrits of up to 71% has been reported in AAS abusers, possibly because of coadministration of diuretics that AASs users take to control secondary edema, increase muscle definition, and decrease

total weight; the resulting increase in blood viscosity may increase the risk for thromboembolic phenomena (64). Diuretic-induced electrolyte derangements, particularly of potassium, create a serious potential for dysrhythmias. Supplemental potassium may also be taken, leading to a risk of hyperkalemia, particularly when potassium-sparing diuretics are used (94,95).

Estrogenic effects of AASs and their metabolites can lead to gynecomastia. The partial estrogen antagonists tamoxifen (84,96,97) and clomiphene (98) are used to prevent and treat this complication of AAS abuse.

Human chorionic gonadotropin (hCG) stimulates androgen production by the interstitial cells of the testis. hCG is used to counter the profound suppression of production of endogenous testosterone and testicular atrophy caused by exogenous AASs. hCG is administered intramuscularly in doses from 3,000 USP units every week to 2,000 USP units every 2 days, either simultaneously with AASs or between cycles (49,57,62,64,85,96,98–100). hCG is one of the most common adjunctive medications used by AAS abusers. In one study, 17 of 53 (32%) AAS abusers also used hCG (84). hCG is used clinically to treat the hypogonadotrophic hypogonadism that results from AAS abuse (101).

The testosterone 5α-reductase inhibitor finasteride significantly reduces the level of dihydrotestosterone (DHT) in both serum and skin, where human androgen receptors are found, even at low doses (102,103). Because DHT in puberty is responsible for some male sexual characteristics of skin, it may have utility in preventing the emergence of male sexual characteristics in females abusing AASs, including facial hair and baldness, although there are significant teratogenicity concerns. Hence, doping tests for female athletes could include finasteride as an indirect indicator of AAS abuse.

CONSEQUENCES OF USE

Therapeutic Uses

The therapeutic utility of AASs was once limited because there were few indications for use and few patients with those indications. These medications now have an ever-expanding range of indications and patient populations who may benefit from them. They are employed in many fields of medicine for a variety of anabolic, endocrine, hematologic, psychiatric, oncologic, and other uses.

Classic uses of AASs are treatment of delayed puberty and primary and secondary hypogonadism in males. AASs have been recommended as adjuncts for treatment of hypogonadism caused by heroin and opioid abuse (104). Specific AASs have therapeutic utility in a variety of conditions that result in small stature. Oxandrolone has been employed successfully with hGH in the treatment of Turner syndrome (105–108) to increase final height, although this combination also has been reported to be ineffective in patients with Turner syndrome (109). In a case report of a male child with premature puberty treated with oxandrolone over 22 months for short stature, the height velocity increased above the 97th percentile. Discontinuation of the drug did not affect the height velocity (110). A healthy female child with short stature and early puberty was treated unsuccessfully with a gonadotropin-releasing hormone (GnRH) analogue alone and with a GnRH analogue plus growth hormone; with the addition of oxandrolone, a satisfactory rate of height progression was attained with little bone age progression (111).

There is continued interest in the therapeutic application of AASs to improve nutrition and lower-body muscle strength, and to promote weight gain. AASs, particularly oxandrolone, are widely used with varying success to treat cachexia in cancer patients, patients with chronic renal failure (112), human immunodeficiency virus (HIV)/acquired immune deficiency syndrome (AIDS) patients (113–116), and to improve stasis ulcer healing (117). There is also interest in their effectiveness for accelerated and improved wound healing in medical, renal (112), HIV, trauma, surgical, cachectic cancer, and burn patients, and in postmenopausal females (118–123). Some AASs up regulate transforming growth factor β_1 (124,125), which may increase collagen synthesis. Oxandrolone improved muscle protein metabolism in critically burned, cachectic children (126). Oxandrolone 20 mg per day did fail to show nutritional or clinical benefit in adult intensive care unit (ICU) patients with multiple traumas (127).

AASs are under investigation for treatment of lipodystrophy in HIV/AIDS patients taking protease inhibitors and nucleosides (128–129), although there is a 5-year cohort study of 221 patients indicating that AASs are associated with this condition (130). Tibolone and certain other AASs are used to ameliorate the lipodystrophy caused by protease inhibitors. Tibolone dramatically lowers triglycerides, and very-low-density lipoprotein (VLDL) cholesterol. However, it also adversely affects serum lipid profiles by lowering high-density lipoprotein (HDL) cholesterol, and apolipoprotein A-I (131,132) both in rats (133) and in humans (134–137).

Despite serious risks associated with long-term use (138,139), AASs are used, alone and in combination therapies, for short-term treatment of refractory anemia, especially aplastic anemia (140), anemia of chronic disease in renal failure (141–146), and Fanconi syndrome (147). Acute intermittent porphyria responds to AAS–GnRH analogue therapy (148).

Tibolone is often used to treat hormonally influenced conditions in women. Continuing research and therapeutic use of AASs, alone and in combination with calcium and vitamin D (149), or with estrogens, seek to treat the symptoms of menopause (150) and promote bone mineral density in postmenopausal women (151–153), and ovariectomized nonhuman primates (154). Tibolone is known to promote venous endothelial function (155)

and sometimes affect arterial resistance (156) in postmenopausal women, probably with minimal effect upon preexisting uterine myomas (157); these may be the mechanisms by which daily tibolone decreased endometrial thickness and uterine bleeding better than daily continuous estradiol plus norethisterone acetate (158) or other sex hormone regimens (159,160). Paradoxically tibolone sometimes is associated with an increased risk of uterine bleeding; up to 20% of postmenopausal women taking tibolone for symptom relief are reported to have uterine bleeding episodes (161,162). Tibolone (163) and other AASs have been used with benefit for the palliation of endometriosis in oophorectomized postmenopausal women. Danazol (Danocrine) also is given to reduce the size and complications of uterine leiomyomas. AASs are sometimes effective in palliation of carcinoma of the breast in women in combination chemotherapy in both induction and maintenance treatment phases, and helpful in recovery from certain effects of chemotherapy (164,165). Tibolone is not a pure androgen. The mechanisms of its effects are difficult to establish because of activity at estrogenic, progesterogenic, and androgenic receptors.

Miscellaneous Uses

17α-Alkylated AASs are useful in the short-term acute treatment of hereditary angioedema; AASs such as stanozolol and danazol are believed to increase the liver synthesis of C1 esterase inhibitor, and are administered before and after surgical and dental procedures to patients with hereditary or chronic angioedema (139,166,167). They are also used in the treatment of paroxysmal nocturnal hemoglobinuria (168). AASs are used to treat vitiligo in combination with thyroid hormone. The mechanism of repigmentation of affected skin involves increased α-melanocyte stimulating hormone, with consequent melanocyte proliferation and melanin production (169). Stanozolol proved highly effective therapy for a case of refractory aquagenic urticaria in an HIV patient in whom antihistamines had failed (170). Testosterone as sole therapy relieved severe suicidal depression in a previously untreated adult bilaterally cryptorchid male (171).

Investigational Uses

In distinguishing abuse from therapeutic use of AASs, the addiction physician should be aware of uses of AASs that are currently experimental. These include replacement therapy (172) with esterified testosterone in older men in whom serum testosterone concentrations decline—"male menopause"—and use as a component of male contraceptive regimens (173). The therapeutic goal is to maintain physiologic testosterone levels. Testosterone is used, rather than synthetic androgens. Oral 17α-alkylated androgens are hepatotoxic and are not used for androgen replacement therapy (ART). Androgen therapy is not indicated for male infertility or erectile dysfunction (174). Ongoing research with many AASs seeks to discover a safe and effective male contraceptive (173,175).

In a pilot study, ten boys with Duchenne muscular dystrophy had significant increases in muscle score and function with oxandrolone versus natural history of disease progression, equivalent to prednisone treatment (176). Although in the randomized, double-blinded study that followed oxandrolone did not show a significant increase in strength versus placebo, it caused significant improvement in averaged quantitative muscle tests without detrimental effects; hence oxandrolone is proposed as initial therapy to accelerate growth and slow the progression of weakness, prior to initiation of corticosteroid therapy (177). While AAS abusers seek to enhance muscle strength and function by systemic routes, direct local administration of AAS to selected muscles in sheep by osmotic pump is showing promise for the development of muscle grafts for cardiomyoplasty (178–180). Since World War II, AASs have been sought that might aid healing in severe muscle contusion; early work failed to answer the question, in part because of hepatic complications from orally active testosterone derivatives. In the modern era, research continues with a wide spectrum of AASs, and delivery systems, with promising results.

Efforts are underway to define the ability of AASs to modulate immunity or in stemming the progression of disease. There is more than one mechanism involved, and different AASs can impair or enhance the immune response. It appears that normal and moderately elevated levels of endogenous AASs are neutral or protective, whereas some synthetic AASs at doses used by addicts may impair immune function. Further research elucidating the immune effects of endogenous versus synthetic AASs, and how these effects differ by sex, is essential.

DHEA protects mice from lethal infections with bacteria, including *Enterococcus faecalis* and *Pseudomonas aeruginosa*, from viruses such as herpes simplex virus (HSV)-1 and HSV-2, coxsackievirus B4 (CVB4), and from the parasite *Cryptosporidium parvum*. Androstenediol (AED), derived from DHEA, is 100 times more effective than DHEA in increasing systemic resistance to CVB4. 7β-Hydroxylation of AED forms androstenetriol (AET), which is even more effective than AED in upregulating resistance to CVB4. DHEA, AED, and AET are not virucidal; their immunogenicity is at the host cellular level. *In vivo* their complex immune effects are similar (181); however, *in vitro* they differ widely. Only AET potentiates the cellular response, increases lymphocyte activation, and counters immunosuppression by hydrocortisone (181).

AASs may prevent or reverse the loss of antiviral immune function associated with aging. Treatment with AED restores youthful (3-month-old) antiviral immune function to 10-month-old mice, but not to 22-month-old mice, and protects 10-month-old mice against lethal influenza virus challenge (182). AASs antagonize corticosteroids, increase expression of interferon (IFN)-α mRNA, and decrease the expression of HSV-1 viral mRNA, prolong-

ing animals' lives (183). There is a protective influence of AASs against both gram-negative and gram-positive bacterial infections and lipopolysaccharide challenges; DHEA appears to mediate the blockade of toxin-induced production of pathophysiologic levels of tumor necrosis factor (TNF)-α and interleukin (IL)-1. AED usually has greater protective effects than DHEA; however, the AED effect is independent of TNF-α suppression, both *in vivo* and *in vitro* (184). Studies in mice show androstenetriol (AET) and androstenediol (AED) up regulate host immunity and increase survival to 60% to 70% after lethal radiation exposure by inducing rapid recovery of all hematopoietic precursors from the small number of surviving stem cells; AET augments IL-2, IL-3, IFN-γ levels, and counteracted hydrocortisone immune suppression (185). Immunity improved versus *Mycobacterium tuberculosis* (MTB) in mice treated with DHEA and its derivative AED by means of complex mechanisms involving ILs, TNF, and other cellular processes (186,187). Additionally, some AASs may decrease the production of antilysozyme by *Staphylococcus aureus* (188).

In contrast, synthetic AASs are often associated with impaired immune function. Nandrolone decanoate and stanozolol impaired mobility and mitogenic proliferation of rat lymphocytes (189), degrading the potential immune response. Oxymetholone, used medically for amelioration of anemias, had no impact on most parameters, and only at a high dose had effects: a 38% decrease in the spleen cell mixed leukocyte response, and a 15% decrease in cytotoxic T-cell activity, with no impairment of the host resistance to *Listeria monocytogenes* (190). Hughes investigated the impact on immunity in mice and humans by comparing endogenous AASs and sesame oil vehicle with the synthetic esterified derivatives nandrolone decanoate and oxymethenolone; only the esterified AASs significantly affected immune responses. These changes were inhibition of antibody production and direct induction of the inflammatory cytokines IL-1β (but not IL-2 or IL-10) and TNF-α from human peripheral blood lymphocytes. Nandrolone decanoate significantly inhibited IFN production *in vitro* in human and mouse cells, as well as the extrapituitary production of corticotropin in human peripheral blood lymphocytes following viral infection (191). Oral 17α-methyltestosterone (17-AMT) fed to female mice raised their circulating testosterone levels nearly tenfold; those mice infected with *Plasmodium chabaudi* malaria and fed 17-AMT died, whereas the 80% of infected mice fed a testosterone-free control diet developed protective immunity. Peritoneal cells of treated mice could not respond to an immune challenge by producing normal levels of oxygen intermediates. Other mice fed 17-AMT responded to heat-killed bacterial challenge with an increased serum TNF and suppressed splenic IL-10; there was no effect upon production of either IL-4 or IFN-γ (192). There is a case report of severe varicella (herpesvirus 2, "chickenpox") pneumonia in one AAS abuser (193).

AASs generally promote cell growth as previously discussed, and can enhance or inhibit myeloproliferation. *In vitro,* 17β-AED enhances myelopoiesis in oncogenic cell lines, but 17α-AED inhibits deoxyribonucleic acid (DNA) synthesis and cell proliferation, and can induce apoptosis (194). As an antineoplastic agent for potential chemotherapy, an androstanediol analogue showed promise in tissue culture, causing inhibition of human acute myeloid leukemia cell proliferation, with promotion of differentiation to macrophage-like cells (195).

AASs and AAS antagonists are used experimentally for gynecologic problems. Flutamide (Eulexin), a pure androgen receptor blocker, was employed to treat the hyperandrogenism, hyperinsulinemia, and dyslipidemia of polycystic ovary disease (PCOD) with results that underscore the potential negative effects of hyperandrogenism: the primary outcome was the change in the ratio of low-density lipoproteins (LDL) to HDL. Treatment with flutamide was associated with a significant decrease in the LDL-to-HDL ratio by 23%, in total cholesterol by 18%, in LDL by 13%, and in triglycerides by 23%. Flutamide treatment was also associated with a trend toward an increase in HDL by 14%. The effects on lipid profile were found regardless of obesity and were not associated with a change in weight. Furthermore, actions of flutamide on lipid metabolism were not associated with significant changes in circulating adrenaline or noradrenaline, glucose metabolism, or insulin sensitivity. Such beneficial effects, that are seen when an AAS antagonist is used to treat hyperandrogenism, provide additional evidence that AASs have serious adverse effects. This report demonstrates for the first time that treatment with the pure antiandrogen flutamide may improve the lipid profile, and that this effect may be a result of direct inhibition of androgenic actions (196).

The addition of AASs and vitamin D to a regimen of calcium supplementation given to postmenopausal women following hip fracture surgery was shown in a double-blind trial to prevent loss of muscle volume and reduce loss of bone mineral density (149). In a placebo-controlled trial in postmenopausal women, adding 2.5 mg of methyltestosterone to a regimen of 1.25 mg of esterified estrogen resulted in decreased body fat, increased lean body mass, and increased total body mass, as well as increased quality of life and sexual functioning (197), even though androgen in female animals depresses sexual activity (198). AAS formed part of an experimental regimen to treat severe premenstrual syndrome (199), and to suppress ovarian function in one case of menstruation-related hereditary pancreatitis (200).

One small study reported that methyltestosterone with esterified estrogen increased emotional well-being in postmenopausal females with cardiac "syndrome X": the triad of angina pectoris, abnormal exercise physiology testing, and clean coronary arteries (201). Some AASs may protect against vasoconstriction. Tibolone increases cardiac blood flow in ovariectomized sheep (202), just as it is thought to do in antianginal and cardioprotective fashion in postmenopausal women. Nandrolone causes relaxation of rat aortic ring-and-epithelium preparations pretreated with phenylephrine *in vitro* (203).

Effects on Athletic Performance

Today it is widely believed among the general public and among athletes that AASs increase lean muscle mass and strength for both men and women, and are necessary to attain the highest level of athletic achievement (204). AAS doping is a major issue in sports, as well as in animal competitions, such as horse racing. For many decades, the ability of AASs to promote weight gain by lean muscle growth in healthy adults was subject to divergent opinions from the athletic and medical communities. As late as 1977, the American College of Sports Medicine stated that AASs had no value in enhancing athletic performance (205). In 1984, the College acknowledged the potential effectiveness of AASs (206) and in 1987 stated that

1. Anabolic-androgenic steroids in the presence of an adequate diet can contribute to increases in body weight, often in the lean mass compartment.
2. The gains in muscular strength achieved through high-intensity exercise and proper diet can be increased by the use of anabolic-androgenic steroids in some individuals. (207)

The initial reluctance to acknowledge the effectiveness of AASs in enhancing athletic performance stemmed in part from the limitations of the clinical trials that had been conducted. Those early trials were often poorly controlled with respect to diet, level of exercise, and blinding, and employed doses of AASs much smaller than those used by competitive athletes. Small changes in percentage or hundredths of a second in a competition may make the difference between obscurity and world record setting performances. Such small changes require large sample sizes to detect. Review of the best clinical trials indicates that strength gains on the order of 5% can be achieved with doses of AASs that are modest compared to those often used illicitly (208).

The ability of AASs to increase strength and muscle mass but not aerobic performance is supported by a study of ultrastructural changes in muscle, in which fiber cross-sectional area increased but capillary density was unchanged (209). Similar effects are seen in horses (210). In rats injected with nandrolone decanoate and exercised, there was an increase in muscle mass, fast and slow twitches, and the amplitude and rate of recovery in K$^+$ contractures, and sensitivity to caffeine, as compared to controls (211). The myotrophic action of AASs at androgen receptors may be synergistic with AAS competitive antagonism at catabolism-mediating corticosteroid receptors (212,213). AASs may also enhance athletic performance through erythropoiesis (214) and psychological effects (25,215). Nandrolone laureate (19-nortestosterone) tested in horses improved muscle glycogen recovery following strenuous exercise (216).

Clearly the widespread use and popularity of AASs among athletes for performance enhancement without a rebound epidemic of reported serious health and legal problems suggests that many more people are benefitting from AAS use than are suffering because of it. It cannot yet be proven that the increased number of pulled and ruptured ligaments and related overpower injuries occurring among professional athletes are caused by AAS use, although animal studies are highly suggestive (217). Neither can it be proven that there is any real relationship between the number of new records and record salary levels and AAS use, because of a lack of data. Nonetheless statistics related in this chapter show that AASs and related nutritional supplements are seen and used by many as a way to shortcut the genetics, intense training, and discipline required to attain the highest individual personal athletic achievement.

Adverse Effects and Related Basic Science

Numerous behaviors, organs, tissues, and cellular functions are affected by AASs. Contraindications to therapeutic use of AASs are primary examples of serious risk factors, including androgen-sensitive epilepsy, migraine, sleep apnea, polycythemia, and congestive heart failure/fluid overload (174), for the abuser. Like other drugs of abuse, AASs appear to hold the promise of something desirable for the user, whereas for some, they instead negatively impact body, mind, emotions, and social stability. Society is negatively impacted as well. In 1993, self-reports by AAS users of various races and ages were significantly correlated with aggressive behavior and crimes against property (218). Competitive athletes are disqualified from competition when AAS use is discovered. Morbidity with negative impacts upon every organ system is reported, and numerous deaths have occurred from both medical and illegal AAS use.

Lipodystrophy

AASs are capable of producing marked adverse changes in serum lipids, with increases on the order of 35% in atherogenic LDL, decreases on the order of 60% in cardioprotective HDL (51,96,219–221), and increases in the total cholesterol-to-HDL ratio (131). There are case reports of AASs having adverse impacts on HDL cholesterol (222). The aromatizable 17β-esterified AASs, such as nandrolone, have much milder effects on serum lipid profiles (223,224). Tibolone, often prescribed to postmenopausal women, dramatically lowers triglycerides (33%) and, unlike many other AASs, VLDL cholesterol (43%) (131,132). It also lowers cardioprotective HDL cholesterol (18%) and lipoprotein(a) (132).

Physiologic levels of testosterone in males, whether from endogenous or exogenous sources, may not have adverse effects on serum lipids, but rather may be associated with higher HDL levels (225). In addition, a small study of six AAS-abusing male weight lifters found low serum total cholesterol levels (within the fifth percentile) and low plasma triglyceride levels in comparison with levels in nonabusing male weight lifters (131). Suppression of testosterone levels in males causes an increase in serum leptin, while AAS abuse causes an immediate suppression in leptin levels without a change in body fat mass (226).

Insulin Resistance

Hyperandrogenism is associated with insulin resistance (227). Hence, the impact of supraphysiologic doses of AASs on glucose metabolism is under study. A rise in fasting glucose levels seen in 17 adolescent Turner syndrome patients treated with oxandrolone in combination with growth hormone returned to levels seen in untreated controls after discontinuation of the drugs (228). Administration of methyltestosterone to euglycemic nonobese women to elucidate whether the androgen causes insulin resistance showed a direct positive association (227). In normal men, neither testosterone nor nandrolone adversely affected insulin-mediated glucose disposal, whereas high-dose nandrolone decanoate improved noninsulin-mediated glucose disposal (229).

Carcinogenesis

AASs have been implicated in carcinogenesis and the progression of human and animal carcinomas. Mutagenesis has been demonstrated with fluoxymesterone *in vitro* and *in vivo* (230). (See individual organ systems for carcinogenesis in relationship to other AASs.) There are clear increases in tissue proliferation, as well as cancerous tissue proliferation caused by AASs in animal models, such as increased papillomas in certain male and female mice exposed to dermal oxymetholone (231), although oxymetholone showed no evidence of genotoxicity in transgenic mice, human lymphocytes, Syrian hamster cells, or bacteria. Reports of carcinomas of the brain, breast, prostate, liver, biliary tract, pancreas, and testes are discussed by organ system in this section. (See also the beneficial effects of AASs employed in cancer treatment in "Therapeutic Uses" above.)

Vascular, Cardiac, and Hematologic Effects

Work to elucidate the mechanisms by which AASs may have adverse cardiovascular effects has been prompted by numerous case reports of unexpected cardiovascular events in AAS users. These have included myocardial infarctions (94,139,232–245); left ventricular hypertrophy (246); myocarditis with dilated cardiomyopathy (247); cardiac arrest with cardiomegaly and myocardial fibrosis and necrosis (95); cardiac arrest with cardiomegaly (248); cardiac tamponade (238); thrombophlebitis (113); peripheral arterial thrombosis (249); hemorrhagic cerebrovascular accident (242); ischemic cerebrovascular accident (250,251); severe lower limb ischemia caused by diffuse arterial thrombosis (250); and pulmonary embolism (252,253). The occurrence of many of these cases in young healthy individuals has raised concerns about the role of AASs and the mechanisms by which they might have deleterious effects on the cardiovascular system.

Both endogenous testosterone and abused AASs are implicated as significant risk factors but the causal relationship between AASs and the adverse cardiac and vascular events is difficult to establish (245). Coagulation abnormalities, serum lipid abnormalities (discussed above under "Lipodystrophy"), hypertension, and cardiomegaly (254) all are implicated. Adverse effects from coadministered diuretics may also increase these risks (see Diuretics, above Drugs taken to ameliorate side effects). Even young male athletes who abuse AASs have suffered cardiovascular sequelae. The mechanisms are under study (255,256) and are probably multiple and complex.

Thrombotic activity may be one of the causal mechanisms for the diverse spectrum of cardiovascular disease and accidents associated with steroid abuse. Thromboxane A (TXA) is a vasoconstrictor and platelet proaggregatory agent that is implicated in the pathogenesis of cardiovascular disease. Testosterone regulates the expression of human platelet TXA_2 receptors (257). Platelet activation is also increased in AAS users (258); however, increased fibrinolytic activity has also been reported (259).

Thrombosis can occur in weight lifters without evidence of atherosclerosis. Coagulation studies in male weight lifters confirmed AAS abusers had increased generation of both thrombin and plasmin compared to nonabusing weight-lifter controls. Results showed abnormally high concentrations in users compared to nonusers of products of coagulation: thrombin–antithrombin complexes (16% vs. 6%), prothrombin fragments F1 + F2 (44% vs. 24%), and D-dimers (9% vs. 0%). Higher antithrombin III and protein S activities (22% vs. 6% and 19% vs. 0%, respectively) occurred in users compared to nonusers. Nonusing weight-lifter controls had elevated levels of tissue plasminogen activator (t-PA) Ag and plasminogen activator inhibitor type 1 (PAI-1) in comparison with AAS-abusing weight lifters. The predictive value of these assays to any individual for a thrombotic event has not been studied (260).

Hypertension has long been identified as an adverse effect of AASs. Although a cause-and-effect relationship is supported by some work (261,262), other studies have not confirmed a direct relationship (84,263,264). AAS abuse by male bodybuilders during the build-up phase of train-

ing causes acute hyperhomocysteinemia, an independent risk factor for atherosclerosis and atherothrombosis (265). AASs cause endothelial dysfunction, a predisposing factor to atherogenesis (136). Weight lifters who abuse AASs have focally increased depositions of collagen in the myocardium not seen in nonabusing weight lifters (255). AAS dose-dependent apoptotic myocardial cell death has been shown in rats and is a possible mechanism for the ventricular remodeling, cardiomyopathy, and sudden cardiac death associated with AAS abuse (266). In contrast to the above factors that would be expected to increase cardiovascular risk, there are some indications that AASs can have salutary effects in cardiovascular disease (see Investigational Uses, above).

Hepatic and Biliary Tree

AASs are associated with a number of deleterious effects on the liver in humans and in other animals. Oral alkylated testosterones have caused primary biliary stasis, i.e., cholestatic jaundice, with consequent hepatorenal syndrome, a potentially fatal syndrome that has been reversed with full recovery (267,268). Chronic use of AASs may cause gross changes in the liver including hepatomegaly (95) and peliosis (269,270).

Are AAS-caused elevations in transaminases indications of disease? In one study, use of some AASs was shown to cause reversible doubling of aminotransferases, although the mechanism, (i.e., rhabdomyolysis versus hepatitis), was not elucidated (221). Elevated hepatic enzymes correlated with hepatic pathology has been demonstrated with supraphysiologic AASs in rats (271). There are a few case reports of AASs causing acute elevation of transaminases levels (96,272) and fatal hepatitis (273). These papers do not control for factors such as intense exercise, daily alcohol use, or gender, which can significantly impact test results (274). In fact, a recent case-controlled study comparing serum chemistry profiles from male elite bodybuilders using AASs (n = 15), male bodybuilders not using AASs (n = 10), patients with hepatitis (n = 49), and exercising and nonexercising medical students (n = 592), casts doubt on the relevance of AAS abuse to elevated hepatic transaminases: in all bodybuilders, levels of enzymes found both in skeletal muscle and liver (creatine kinase [CK], aspartate aminotransferase [AST], and alanine aminotransferase [ALT]) were abnormally elevated, but the nonmuscle enzyme, hepatic gamma-glutamyltranspeptidase (GGT), remained within the normal range. Patients with proven hepatitis who were not using steroids or lifting weights had elevations of all three hepatic enzymes—ALT, AST, and GGT—but not of the muscle enzyme CK. CK was elevated in all exercising groups. Only patients with viral hepatitis had elevated GGT (275). These results bring into question reports of AAS-induced hepatotoxicity in humans. Conclusive results would call for other studies, to distinguish liver from muscle damage (276), and for adequate assessment and control for alcohol, illness, medication, or other drug use history (274). When transaminases levels are elevated, the GGT and CK should be added to corroborate or clarify the etiology. When the GGT also is elevated, viral hepatitis testing is mandatory. If viral hepatitis is detected, it is advisable to screen the patient for exposure to HIV and, if indicated (i.e., positive history, presence of hepatitis B), sexually transmitted diseases.

AASs appear to increase the incidence of hepatic tumors in susceptible individuals. A case of hepatic adenomas with spontaneous hemorrhage was reported in a bodybuilder abusing AASs (277). Danazol in the presence of oversecretions of hGH and insulin-like growth factor I (IGF-I) is reported to have induced multiple hepatic adenomas in a female with acromegaly (278). There are other reports of hepatocellular carcinoma in AAS users; the tumors are often relatively benign compared to typical hepatocellular carcinoma (279–281). There is a case report of carcinoma of the ampulla of Vater in a female 39 months after the start of AAS therapy for aplastic anemia (282). Although 17α-alkylated AASs are implicated in these adverse hepatic effects, the possibility that other AASs, particularly in the high doses used illicitly, may be hepatotoxic cannot be excluded.

Musculoskeletal

Physicians treating professional athletic teams have noted a marked increase in the incidence of ruptured tendons and avulsions in their patients despite advanced training and nutrition regimens; some of these physicians acknowledge privately that they believe the enormous increase in muscle mass associated with illicit steroid abuse overwhelms tendons and ligaments, causing the injuries. Unfortunately, they are reluctant to report cases. These physicians have no direct proof or report from the players abusing steroids, and steroid use in professional sports remains taboo. There is a confidentiality and liability problem for these physicians because their affiliations with particular professional teams are public knowledge, as are the injuries of individual players on those teams. Nonetheless there are several case reports of tendon ruptures and avulsions in amateur AAS users (254,283,284). Simultaneous bilateral rupture of the quadriceps tendon is a usually rare injury that is often misdiagnosed (285), and which occurs in AAS abusers. Increased force from hypertrophied muscles, and abnormal tendon morphology each may play a role in increasing this risk (286). In rats, supraphysiologic stanozolol and nandrolone reversibly caused the Achilles tendon to lose elasticity, become stiffer than controls, to absorb less energy, and to fail with less elongation without detectable microfibril or biochemical changes (217). Electron microscopy of surgical specimens of ruptured ligaments from two AAS users compared to specimens from two nonusers shows no visible difference in collagen fibril ultrastructure (287). There is a case report of exertional rhabdomyolysis following AAS use (288).

Although being tall is typically a desired outcome for AAS users, those who are still growing may not attain their full stature because of premature closure of epiphyses (289). *In vivo* AASs caused differentiated skeletal muscle apoptosis in murine cells (290,291). Growth rates may be adversely affected by AASs in male rats, but enhanced in female rats given nandrolone decanoate (292), with increased IGF-I mRNA in female and high-dose-treated males (293). Supraphysiologic doses of nandrolone decanoate with and without exercise curtailed body weight gain, an effect not seen with stanozolol-treated or control group rats (189). Although the question has been raised, at least one study shows that androgens may have no impact on bone mineral density in adolescent females (294).

Immune Function, Exercise, and AASs

Animal studies of supraphysiologic doses of nandrolone decanoate and stanozolol with and without exercise promoted a redistribution of immune cells from thymus to spleen, impaired lymphocyte mobility, and inhibited the mitogen-induced proliferative response (approximately 90% inhibition for thymus-derived cells with nandrolone decanoate). High-intensity training alone reduced mobility and proliferation of lymphocytes with further impairment by AASs of some of the immune cell responses. Low-intensity training normalized the mobility and mitogen-induced proliferation of lymphocytes in AAS-treated rats (189). [See also sections above on Therapeutic Uses and Investigational Uses].

Complications and Infections Secondary to Injection Drug Use

Injection of AASs is common (80% in one sample [41]) and puts users at risk for a variety of complications from injection site infections to hepatitis or HIV infection. Three case reports are consistent with HIV infection from AAS injection (295–297). Although the risk of HIV transmission in adults appears to be low, based on the paucity of case reports and unanimous denial of sharing of injection equipment in two samples of 21 (96) and 39 (41) AAS injectors, the data from adolescents are alarming. Eighteen of 20 AAS-injecting high school students had shared needles in the preceding 30 days (80). An Australian study showed exposure to the hepatitis B and C viruses to be present among AAS abusers. However, factors such as imprisonment and age at first use of AAS, rather than steroid injecting per se, were statistically associated with viral exposure (298). A study of 149 AAS injectors in England enrolled from 1991 to 1996 showed only 2% with hepatitis B core antibody compared to intravenous heroin and amphetamine users who had a prevalence of 18% and 12%, respectively; none of the steroid injectors tested positive for anti-HIV (299). Further studies are needed to assess the risk of HIV transmission associated with injection of AASs and to assess the need for targeted HIV risk-reduction interventions. HIV risk-reduction programs and needle-exchange programs provide a model for instruction in safe-injection techniques, as well as offering sterile syringes, bleach, clean cotton balls, alcohol wipes, and other assistance to clients. Safe injection techniques include not sharing injection equipment or multidose vials. Other reported complications of AAS injection include hepatitis B infection (295), local infection with the atypical mycobacterium *M. smegmatis* (300), pseudotumor (301), knee joint sepsis, and radial nerve palsy (302).

Gynecomastia and Mastodynia in Men

Testosterone and other aromatizable AASs are metabolized in part to estradiol and other estrogen agonists. These estrogen agonists can lead to breast pain in men (84) and gynecomastia (50,51,97,99,254,303). Gynecomastia is one of the most frequently reported side effects of AAS abuse (93). Affected tissue contains both androgen and estradiol receptors (304). Gynecomastia is a sufficiently common and permanent adverse effect where staging criteria and techniques for surgical management have been presented (305,306).

Breast Health in Women

The impact of anabolic steroids on the female breast is an issue because AASs, especially tibolone, are used internationally to treat the symptoms of menopause and to prevent osteoporosis. At approved therapeutic doses, the consequences to breast tissue are probably minimal (307); however, long-term high-dose AAS abuse has not been well studied. Anabolic implants in female lambs caused breast cell autolysis and necrosis (308). In human breast cancer cell lines positive for androgen receptors, AASs show varied effects, with the growth of some cell lines promoted and the growth of others inhibited (309). Their role in the growth and progression of breast cancer is not well defined and is under study (310). *In vitro* 17α-AED inhibits breast cancer cell proliferation regardless of estrogen receptor positivity or negativity (311).

Male Genitourinary and Renal

AASs suppress gonadotropins, with variable effects on sexual interest, spontaneous erections, the prostate, the gonads, and fertility (312). Animal studies show a permanent loss of Leydig cells in the testes of adult males, but not pre- or peripubertal males, treated with testosterone propionate (313). Case reports of testicular atrophy in AAS users are common (50,63,99,314). Testicular atrophy has also been documented in a controlled study (51), and is an expected effect through negative feedback exerted by AASs on the testes. Azoospermia and oligospermia (315,316) may also follow AAS use, and may resolve spontaneously (317–319) or require gonadotropin treatment (316,320,321). Androgens are essential for normal

prostate physiology. Central prostate volume is responsive to AASs (322). Chronic use in monkeys leads to epithelial and stromal hyperplasia (323,324) and resultant increases may lead to bladder outflow obstruction (55,325). AASs may be cocarcinogens for adenocarcinoma of the prostate (326). The development and progression of prostate cancer may be positively influenced by AASs (327,328). Antiandrogen therapy and orchiectomy cause regression of prostatic cancer. Men with the highest normal levels of circulating testosterone had a 160% risk compared to other men tested. Testosterone induces prostate cancer in rats (329). The role of androgen receptors (330) and genetic mechanisms in normal function and carcinogenesis in the prostate are under investigation (324,327,331–333).

Renal failure has been reported, although the etiology was uncertain and possibly related to AAS-induced hypertension (334). A cluster of two cases of clear cell renal carcinoma are reported in 26-year-old male bodybuilders; one had a 6-year and the other a 20-month history of abusing multiple AASs in cyclic fashion, and no other known risk factors (335). This is a rare tumor in men younger than 30 years old. Testicular leiomyosarcoma, another extremely rare tumor to discover in a young man, was first reported in a 32-year-old with a 5-year history of use of Oral-Turinabol (4-chloro-1-dehydro-17α-methyltestosterone) that had ended 9 years before presentation (326).

Female Genitourinary

Uterine blood flow in ovariectomized ewes is significantly increased by tibolone, an AAS. This vascular response is mediated via an estrogen receptor-dependent, nitric oxide mechanism (202). Postmenopausal women treated with tibolone sometimes develop uterine bleeding; in one study of 47 consecutive cases, no anatomic pathologic cause for the uterine bleeding was found in the majority; however, endometrial polyp (11 patients), uterine fibroids (7 patients), thickened endometrium (6 patients), and carcinoma in situ (2 patients) were found in the other patients, further emphasizing the mandatory investigation of postmenopausal uterine bleeding, especially in the context of AAS use (161). Similar results are reported in other studies (162).

Raised levels of androgens have been implicated in epidemiologic studies of ovarian carcinogenesis, although the causal role and mechanisms are unknown. *In vitro* studies show that ovarian epithelial cells contain androgen receptors. The response of these cells to tibolone is increased DNA expression and a significant increase in proliferation with decreased cell death, important factors in the pathophysiology of ovarian cancer (336).

Virilization of Women

Supraphysiologic doses of AASs in women lead to virilization, although the effects and rate of development of changes vary with the drug and with the individual. Specifically, women taking AASs have been reported to have voice instability and deepening in both the projected speaking voice and the singing voice (337), clitoral hypertrophy (338), shrinking of the breasts, menstrual irregularities (339), nausea (339), and hirsutism (62,340,341). In contrast to the cosmetic side effects that occur in males, in females these side effects are largely irreversible. Conversely, an individual may abuse AASs without obvious side effects such as deepening of the voice or the appearance of acne.

Normal genetic and racial variants in women, including amount and distribution of body and facial hair, height, frame, vocal pitch, breast size, clitoral size, athletic ability, and mannerisms or behaviors can be mistaken as androgenized by culturally biased observers. There are additional examples of non-AAS causes of androgenization that could be mistaken for AAS abuse; these include hormone/antihormone therapies for breast cancer treatment, for various symptoms following natural or surgical menopause (342), polycystic ovary disease, thyroid disease, and anorexia.

FTM transsexuals treated by the City of San Francisco's Tom Waddell Clinic are oophorectomized and prescribed AASs. The AASs are administered as gel to the skin or by injection. In regions where standard medical care is not available for FTMs, many who self-medicate may use unregulated and nonstandardized DHEA purchased at natural food groceries and vitamin stores. Low-dose and intermittent AAS abuse by transgendered individuals may result in a confusing physical and psychological presentation, with a wide range of behaviors. Some FTMs who previously were living a dedicated lesbian lifestyle, report a new "fascination with the male form," resulting in a change in their sexual behavior to experimentation, or even promiscuity, with male sexual partners. Administration of AASs to lesbians or heterosexual women who are not psychologically FTM will not change their sexuality. Under medical management, non-AAS-abusing FTMs, both pre- and post-ovariectomy, will usually have been tapered up to a dose of testosterone ester, 200–250 mg IM, every two weeks adjusted up or down to attain physiologic male serum testosterone levels and to avoid undesirable side effects such as mood disturbances, 'roid rages', or other such limiting side effects of AASs. AAS-abusing FTMs may seek additional drug by seeing multiple physicians, claiming to have lost or broken their vials of medication, or by obtaining illegal drugs.

Dermatologic

Striae, acne, and balding are frequently reported stigmata of AAS abuse. Sebaceous gland hypertrophy, cysts, increased skin surface fatty acids, and increased cutaneous populations of *Propionibacterium acnes* put AAS abusers at increased risk for acne vulgaris (50,343,344); there is one case report of injection-related seeding and in-

fection of these bacteria causing spondylodiscitis in an AAS abuser. Acne is a common side effect of AASs, self-reported by 21 of 53 (40%) of AAS abusers in one series and 12 of 22 (55%) abusers in another study (63,84). Their high incidence makes cystic acne and pitting scars pertinent findings when screening for use of AASs.

Balding is under study. It occurs in both male and female AAS abusers and is believed to be a consequence of the gradual transformation of active large scalp epithelial hair follicles into smaller dermal vellus follicles via androgen receptors in the mesenchymal dermal papilla. Balding hair follicle cells contain a higher number of androgen receptors than do nonbalding cells (345). Other dermatologic effects of AAS abuse include linear keloids, striae, hirsutism, seborrheic dermatitis, and secondary infections, including furunculosis (95,343,346).

Central Nervous System Effects

Case reports of adverse effects to the central nervous system cover a wide spectrum of observations. The first case of secondary partial empty sella syndrome with significant pituitary gland atrophy from negative feedback inhibition was reported in an elite bodybuilder with a long history of exogenous abuse of growth hormone, testosterone, and thyroid hormone (347). AASs exert negative feedback on the hypothalamic–pituitary–gonadal axis and cause predictable depression in follicle-stimulating hormone, luteinizing hormone, and testosterone, unless testosterone is the exogenous AAS being administered (99,221,348). In rats, AASs at doses comparable to human abuse levels reversibly block sexual receptivity, and interrupt the neuroendocrine axis (349). The first case report of persistent hiccups in an elite bodybuilder abusing AASs discussed the hiccup reflex arc, and whether the brainstem is the steroid-responsive locus (350). There is a case report of permanent central vertigo in a 20-year-old male bodybuilder who abused three AASs for two courses (351). Insomnia in male AAS abusers is reported (352), although insomnia in postmenopausal females may improve with administration of AASs. Other central nervous system (CNS) effects are under investigation (353).

Other Physical Effects

AASs are associated with a wide variety of other adverse effects, including induction of an attack of coproporphyria (354), splenic peliosis and rupture (269), and aggravation of tics in Gilles de la Tourette syndrome (355). Fluid retention is commonly reported by AAS users (50,63,84) and largely drives their use of diuretics, as previously described. Alterations in thyroid function occur, most notably a decrease in thyroid-binding globulin, but the clinical significance is unclear (356). AASs cause adrenal hyperplasia, and elevated secretion of corticosterone and cortisol in treated female rats (357); the authors (357) conclude that AASs administered to animals are stressors that can adversely affect animal welfare. Unexplained increases in serum levels of medications metabolized by cytochrome P450 or cytochrome b5 may warrant investigation for AAS abuse in patients deemed at-risk; these enzymes decreased in rat liver in response to chronic AAS abuse (271).

Personality Disorders

Prospective controlled studies for the development of personality disorders in AAS abusers have not been done. Small studies evaluating AAS-abusing body builders/weight lifters with self-reported AAS-naïve matched controls, using self-reports and informants for retrospective assessment have been done. These studies concluded that AAS abusers have similar personality characteristics to controls before AAS use, but unlike controls, develop abnormal personality traits and disturbances which are attributed to AAS use (52).

Aggression

Endogenous testosterone has long been postulated as mediating aggressive behavior in males through brain AAS receptors. Aggression may be defined as a spectrum of behavior, from less fear or anticipatory anxiety all the way to explosive outbursts in humans and other animals (358). Animal studies show an increase in aggression in both males and females exposed to AASs, even at very low doses (359). Male hamsters given high-dose AASs during adolescence are significantly more aggressive, with increased intensity and frequency of biting (360). Neutering male rats and other pets is a well-known approach to cure the fighting and biting that may appear late in adolescence. In humans, self-report of aggression may be the only presentation of AAS misuse (361). Adolescents who abuse AASs have nearly triple the incidence of violent behavior. The abuse of alcohol, any illicit drug, or AAS was associated with significantly increased risk of carrying weapons and physically fighting in both males and females in a study of 12,272 high school students in public and private schools in all 50 of the United States (362). A Swedish attempt to screen male offenders jailed for violent crimes failed when nearly a quarter of the prisoners refused to cooperate; of the remaining 50, no one gave an AAS-positive urine, although 2 did claim to use AASs (363).

Many case reports lend credence to the hypothesis that exogenous AASs may increase aggressive behavior and violence (45,55,86,100,254,314,325,355,364,365). Explosive outbursts are well known among AAS abusers who refer to them as "roid rages." Violent behavior can occur in individuals with no prior history or other risk factors and may culminate in fatal and near-fatal outcomes (86).

Aggression and hostility are reported at high rates in a case series (e.g., 19 of 20 weight lifters 49).

Studies comparing AAS abusers to nonusing controls permit evaluation of actual drugs and doses of abuse, but random assignment is impossible. Careful selection of controls such as nonabusing athletes or bodybuilders is important because they may differ significantly from the general population. In a study of 46 male strength athletes (16 current users of anabolic steroids, 16 former users, and 14 nonusers) there was a trend toward higher self-ratings of impatience and belligerence in current users (366). The Profile of Mood States, Buss-Durkee Hostility Inventory, and subjective ratings of aggression and irritability were administered to 50 male weight lifters—12 current (within last 30 days) AAS users, 14 previous users, and 24 nonusers. Using Likert scales, current and former users reported greater aggression and irritability during periods of AAS use than was reported by controls. No differences in composite or individual scale scores from either the Profile of Mood States (POMS) or Buss-Durkee Hostility Inventory (former AAS users were not asked to use these instruments to rate their past moods), calling into question the sensitivity of these standard measures in this context (63).

Comparing on-cycle behavior with off-cycle behavior is a sensitive technique that can be embedded in studies that compare users with nonusers. POMS anger–hostility scores were higher in five on-cycle, adolescent, weight lifter AAS users than in 19 AAS users who were between cycles (50). Twenty-three AAS-using male strength-training athletes reported significantly more fights, verbal aggression, and violence toward their significant others when using AAS than when not using AAS, although when not using they did not differ from 14 nonusing control athletes (73).

Aggression from AASs can be assessed in prospective controlled trials in which AASs are administered to humans, although only a limited dose range has been tested. Another point of caution in interpreting these trials concerns blinding: the effectiveness of blinding is not reported in most trials, but in one placebo-controlled crossover trial of physiologic doses of testosterone, 12 of 13 subjects were able to break the blind (367). In an open-label trial, 30 subjects divided into 4 groups were administered testosterone enanthate 100 mg per week, testosterone enanthate 300 mg per week, nandrolone decanoate 100 mg per week, or nandrolone decanoate 300 mg per week for 6 weeks. Minnesota Multiphasic Personality Inventory hostility and aggression subscale scores increased compared to baseline, with greater increases in the high-dose groups (368). A small comparative study evaluated the effect of testosterone in 6 normal male volunteers. After achievement of steady state levels, neither physiologic (100 mg/week) nor supraphysiologic (250 or 500 mg/week) doses of testosterone cypionate led to an increase in aggressive driving in a simulator, or any increase in aggression as measured by the Buss-Durkee Hostility Inventory (369). Twenty healthy males without histories of AAS use were given 40 mg per day and then 240 mg per day of methyltestosterone in a double-blind inpatient trial. Irritability, mood swings, violent feelings, and hostility were greater during the high-dose period than at baseline (42).

The clear ability of high doses of AASs to promote aggression and irritability in some individuals raises several specific concerns. Although there are limited reports in the biomedical literature of sexual assault in connection with AAS use, increases in both aggression and libido have lead to concerns that AAS users may be likely to commit sexual assault (e.g., a report of an AAS user who was "irritable and "rough" with his wife, both physically and sexually) (45,98). Female sex partners of male AAS abusers may be at high risk for being assaulted (45,73). Abuse of AASs by law enforcement and corrections (86) personnel is of particular concern because individuals in these professions have an ongoing need for carefully measured levels of violent and aggressive behavior.

Sexuality and Gender Identity

AASs can have marked effects on sexual function. AASs are used therapeutically to increase libido for postmenopausal women, although animal studies show a decrease in sexual receptivity in oophorectomized females given AASs. There are many case reports of male AAS users experiencing increased libido (325), decreased libido (99), and impotence (99,314). In a study in which all 53 AAS-using bodybuilders attending one gymnasium were surveyed, 18 (34%) reported increased libido and 16 (30%) reported impotence (84). Both increases and decreases in libido were reported in a study comparing AAS-using athletes to nonusing athletes (63). Increased sexual arousal compared to baseline was demonstrated in males in a controlled inpatient trial of methyltestosterone, but other aspects of sexual function were not evaluated (42). A study of three groups of male bodybuilders (15 current AAS users, 15 former AAS users, and 15 who had never used AAS) who all had available sexual partners revealed higher levels of both erectile difficulties and orgasmic and coital frequency in current AAS users (98). Differences in dose, duration of use, and presence or absence of metabolites with estrogenic properties may account for the variable effects of AASs; evaluation of these factors will require further investigation. Different androgenic compounds at different doses will have differing effects on male sexual behavior and physiology, whether human or other species (353,370). In female rats tested with doses approximating those taken by human females abusing AASs, short-term administration of high doses of AASs disrupted female function, estrous cycles, and altered sexual receptivity (371). Women abusing AASs also may display nontraditional gender roles in a noncausal

relationship (47) (see Physiology and Pharmacology section, above). There is a case report of child sexual abuse by a female AAS abuser (372).

Anxiety, Mood Changes, and Psychotic Symptoms

Beyond aggression and libido changes, many other psychiatric effects of AAS use have been reported, including a variety of mood changes and slowed intellectual performance (366). When considering psychiatric effects of AASs, there are diagnoses for which organic causes, such as AAS use, are exclusion criteria. Per *DSM–IV* criteria, those diagnoses are then classified as substance-induced disorders. Abundant case reports exist of hypomania (373) and mania (86,374), along with reports of irritability, elation, recklessness, racing thoughts, and feelings of power and invincibility that did not clearly meet diagnostic criteria for hypomania or mania (55,86,100,355,364). One case of hypomania resolved 3 to 4 days after discontinuation of AAS use and recurred after resumption of AAS use, suggesting a causal relationship (373). Depressed mood (55,375) and major depression with psychotic features (376) also have been reported during periods of AAS use, as have paranoia, auditory, and tactile hallucinations (86).

In a series of 53 AAS-using body builders—the entire population of AAS-using regular attendees at one Swedish gymnasium—27 (51%) reported unspecified mood disturbances (84). Burnett et al. found on-cycle users (n = 5) to have higher depression, vigor, and total mood disturbance on the POMS than did 19 off-cycle users (50). In a study of 20 AAS-using athletes and 20 nonusing athletes, 14 (70%) of the AAS users reported increased frequency of depression while on-cycle, 14 reported an increase in paranoid thoughts while on-cycle, and 13 reported an increase in other psychotic symptoms while on-cycle, although the only psychiatric diagnoses per *DSM–III* were of *major depression, single episode* in one AAS user and two nonuser controls (49). Pope and Katz reported on a series of 41 AAS users: 5 (12.2%) had psychotic symptoms while on AASs, 4 (10%) had subthreshold psychotic symptoms while on AASs, but none had symptoms when off AASs (62). Five of these 41 subjects met criteria for manic episodes while on AASs, and an additional 8 met two of the first three *DSM–III–R* criteria (377) for mania. In a larger study examining psychiatric diagnoses, mood disorders were more common in male AAS users (n = 88) while they were on-cycle (23%) than while they were off-cycle (10%) or compared to male nonusers (N = 68, 6%) (51). These mood disorders experienced by AAS users while on-cycle were major depression (13%), hypomanic episode (10%), and manic episode (5%); a dose–response relationship was noted for each of these mood disorders. Psychotic symptoms were diagnosed in three (3%) of on-cycle users but not in any off-cycle users or nonusers.

Two prospective, controlled trials involving blinded administration of AASs also indicate that AASs can cause mood changes. Increased confidence in performance on a pegboard task was noted in subjects receiving nandrolone decanoate 300 mg per week or testosterone enanthate 100 mg or 300 mg per week (368). In Su et al.'s trial of administration of 0 mg, 40 mg, and then 240 mg per day of methyltestosterone, increases in euphoria, energy, and mood swings were noted; 1 of 20 subjects (5%) had an acute manic episode, and an additional subject had a hypomanic episode (42). There is a clear relationship, in at least some individuals, between mood changes and AASs; the ability of AASs to induce psychotic symptoms independent of mania has not been definitively established.

Cognitive Changes

Cognitive impairment, including distractibility, forgetfulness, and confusion has been demonstrated in controlled trials (42,366). Improvement in performance of a psychomotor task (a pegboard test) was noted in another controlled trial (368). While these changes are usually subtle, there may be significant impairment in a subset of AAS users (42).

Dependence

Acute anabolic steroid withdrawal symptoms usually include cravings and depression. In addition, visible changes are seen, including anxiety, aching, elevated blood pressure and heart rate, chills, piloerection, hot flashes, diaphoresis, nausea, anorexia, vomiting, irritability, and insomnia, all suggestive of central nonadrenergic hyperactivity (378).

Although abuse of AASs dates back several decades, the first reports of dependence did not emerge until the late 1980s (100,379). From these initial reports, a subsequent case report (55), and survey work by Brower et al. (41,375), it has become apparent that dependence on AASs per *DSM–III–R* (377) criteria is a real phenomenon. The full range of symptoms of dependence can exist, including loss of control, interference with other activities, and withdrawal symptoms (41) (Table 25.3). Although the data are sparse, dependence appears to be common in AAS users; in two studies of weight lifters, 6 of 8 (75%) (375) and 28 of 49 (57%) (41) respondents had three or more symptoms, as required for *DSM–III–R* diagnosis of dependence (377). Commonly reported symptoms during withdrawal include fatigue, depressed mood, and desire to take more AASs (Table 25.4). The depressed mood following discontinuation of AAS use may resolve within days (100) or may persist for more than a year (380). It is unclear whether persistent depression following withdrawal of high-dose AAS is a withdrawal phenomenon, an ongoing process triggered by withdrawal, or a recrudescence of depression obscured by AAS use. Prolonged depression following withdrawal of high-dose AAS has responded to fluoxetine in four cases (380); electroconvulsive therapy was used successfully in a fifth case that had not responded

to fluoxetine or desipramine with lithium augmentation (314).

The neurochemical basis of AAS withdrawal symptoms has not been fully elucidated. The opiate system is implicated based on a case report in which 0.2 mg of naloxone was administered to a patient in AAS withdrawal, eliciting a constellation of symptoms consistent with opiate withdrawal (379). The symptoms diminished after 4 hours and continued to resolve with clonidine (Catapres) treatment over the next 6 days, although on the seventh day the patient complained of craving, depression, and fatigue, and apparently relapsed. The role of clonidine in ameliorating these withdrawal symptoms is unclear because the time course of AAS withdrawal has not been defined. Rosse and Deutsch postulated a role for the benzodiazepine/γ-aminobutyric acid$_A$ receptor complex, citing tolerance

TABLE 25.3. *Symptoms of dependence reported by AAS using male weight lifters*

Symptom	Percentage
Withdrawal symptoms	84
More substance taken than intended	51
Large time expenditure on substance related activity	40
Continued AAS use despite problems caused or worsened by use	37
Social work, or leisure activities replaced by AAS use	29
Tolerance	18
Desire yet unable to cut down or control use	16
Frequent intoxication or withdrawal symptoms when expected to function or when physically hazardous	9
Substance used to relieve or avoid withdrawal symptoms	4

From Brower KJ, Blow FC, Young JP, et al. Symptoms and correlates of anabolic–androgenic steroid dependence. *Br J Addict* 1991;86(6):759–768, with permission.

TABLE 25.4. *Symptoms reported by male weight lifters during AAS withdrawal*

Symptom	Percentage
Desire to take more AASs	52
Fatigue	43
Dissatisfaction with body image	42
Depressed mood	41
Restlessness	29
Anorexia	24
Insomnia	20
Decreased libido	20
Headaches	20
Suicidal thoughts	4

From Brower KJ, Blow FC, Young JP, et al. Symptoms and correlates of anabolic–androgenic steroid dependence. *Br J Addict* 1991;86(6):759–768, with permission.

to the anticonvulsant effects of flurazepam (Dalmane) in mice chronically exposed to exogenous testosterone (381). While these observations provide a basis for further investigation, neither can be construed as indicating efficacy of any specific pharmacotherapy for AAS withdrawal.

EVALUATION AND TREATMENT

Screening, Diagnosis, and Testing

The prevalence of AAS use in competitive athletes, both male and female, is high enough that it should always be considered a possibility. Denial of use, or even negative testing, does not rule out steroid abuse, even in the context of national championships and the Olympics (204). Patients may not give their physician important history that would assist with diagnosis, treatment, and HIV risk reduction. For example, in 1997, of 1,004 gay male bodybuilders in London completing an anonymous, confidential questionnaire, more than 10% reported ever injecting AASs, but only 36% of those had reported their AAS injecting, highlighting the need to promote open communication from patients who may be reluctant to disclose potentially risky, illegal, or embarrassing behaviors (382).

Muscular hypertrophy and thin abdominal skin fold are among the most common findings in AAS abusers. Tight hamstrings and pectorals (383) or unusual injuries, for example, ruptured tendons, ligaments, or muscles; avulsions; or rhabdomyolysis, especially in the setting of minimal resistance exercise, should raise the question of recent AAS use. Unexplained low HDL cholesterol levels in athletic individuals may be a sign of steroid abuse (384). Pronounced acne in adults and extensive acne scarring are additional clues to a history of AAS abuse. Aggression may be a significant clinical indicator of AAS abuse (361). Some of the effects of AASs resolve upon discontinuation. In the Netherlands, weight lifters who had abused AASs but had attained 3 months of abstinence were compared to nonuser weight lifters. There were no differences seen in percentage of body fat or lipoprotein profiles. Former AAS users demonstrated the desired effects of AASs: larger bone-free lean body mass, larger circumferences of thorax, waist, upper arm and thigh and greater diameter of type I muscle fibers (385). In essence, only their unusual body conformation and evaluation of body composition by dual-energy x-ray absorptiometry (DEXA) (386) gave evidence of recent AAS abuse.

The combination of muscular hypertrophy with testicular atrophy in males, or with signs of virilization in women is strongly suggestive of AAS abuse. There is a wide range of normal variation in the human body, therefore clinicians must have an astute awareness of their own cultural and racial biases about masculine and feminine attributes, appearance, hair (color, quantity, and distribution), skin porosity, acne scarring, stature, and genital size and shape to avoid an incorrect diagnosis of AAS abuse. If one is unfamiliar with normal male pu-

berty, consultation with a pediatrician may be helpful, because normal males in puberty can present with breast buds, small testes, and cystic acne. The appearance of a breast mass in healthy adult males mandates a fine-needle aspiration; the otherwise rare cytologic finding of apocrine metaplasia in males who have not received legally prescribed AASs is a strong indication of AAS abuse (387). Hypertrichosis in many prepubertal females is a normal variant (388), particularly in noncaucasians. Just as it is possible to mistake unshaven legs in dark-haired women as "hirsutism," it is possible to miss AAS abuse in men or women who undergo electrolysis, laser or other hair removal, skin peels and retinoic acid therapy for acne, hair transplantation or amendment. To further confound a correct diagnosis, there are patients who alter their appearance in ways that mimic AAS abuse. An example is women who seek secondary male sexual characteristics without AASs. They grow male pattern hair by applying minoxidil to their faces and bodies, reduce body fat and increase muscle mass through exercise, and enlarge their clitorises by physical means. Endocrine disorders also may mimic AAS abuse; polycystic ovary disease and idiopathic hirsutism are highly relevant and treatable examples. Similarly, striae are found normally in some adolescents with rapid growth but poor nutrition, following treatment with high-dose corticosteroids, in people who are or were obese, and among women who have been pregnant. Pregnant women have endogenous AASs present in varying levels at different phases of pregnancy and are normally hyperandrogenic.

AASs can be delivered via multiple routes, including oral, intramuscular injection, adhesive patch, topical gel, or implant. An evaluation of possible AAS abuse should include a search for signs of injection in large muscles, and the pectoralis muscles, residual adhesive, and subcutaneous implants. Use of tobacco (especially smokeless tobacco) and illegal drugs is correlated with AAS abuse, and should raise the index of suspicion for AAS abuse. AAS abusers are more likely to use multiple drugs, including tobacco, engage in high-risk sexual behavior, engage in suicidal behavior, carry a weapon, and fight than nonusers. Best medical practice and public health practice include evaluating all steroid abusers for these potentially related risky behaviors, and treating as necessary, as summarized in Tables 25.5 and 25.6.

As with other drugs of abuse, laboratory analyses of biologic specimens for AASs can be helpful in both diagnosis and treatment. Most testing for AASs occurs in the context of athletic competition, where the object is to "level the playing field" by prohibiting a wide variety of performance-enhancing drugs. This rationale stands in contrast to testing in the workplace where the goal is to detect drug use associated with performance impairment. Ideally, results will be quickly obtainable from simple, rapid, sensitive, specific, and reproducible methodologies (389–391) that can be conducted on small aliquots of sample (392). Standards must be established for each type of

TABLE 25.5. *Signs of AAS abuse*

Musculoskeletal	
	Hypertrophied muscles, especially neck, shoulder, & thigh
Dermatologic	
	Deep glandular acne or pitting scars
	Striae
	Oily skin
	Needle punctures over large muscles
	Male pattern baldness in men and women[a]
	Hirsuitism in females[a]
Genitourinary	
	Testicular atrophy
	Prostatic hypertrophy
	Clitoral hypertrophy[a]
Chest	
	Gynecomastia in men
Abdomen	
	Heptatomegaly
Head and neck	
	Deep, unstable voice in women
	Enlarged larynx in women
Body as a whole	
	Edema
	Jaundice

[a]Hyperandrogenism of pregnancy also may cause this sign.

sample to be tested, for example, urine, serum, saliva, pigmented or unpigmented hair (72,393–396), or stool (397–401). In some contexts, it will be important that test methods detect rarely used, synthetic, or even never-marketed AASs, as well as those that are frequently abused (402). Tests must differentiate between normal variations in endogenous steroid and metabolite levels versus exogenous AASs (403–408). In athletic contexts, testing should be done without notice, at random, both during practice and during the regular season (409).

TABLE 25.6. *Common laboratory abnormalities in AAS abusers*

Elevated hemoglobin
Elevated hematocrit
Elevated low-density lipoprotein cholesterol
Depressed high-density lipoprotein cholesterol
Elevated[a] or depressed[b] serum testosterone
Decreased luteinizing hormone
Decreased follicle stimulating hormone
Urinary testosterone:epitestosterone ≥ 6[a]
Elevated serum estradiol[a]
Elevated alanine aminotransferase[c]
Elevated aspartate aminotransferase[c]
Elevated alkaline phosphatase
Elevated lactate dehydrogenase[c]

[a]In users of testosterone esters.
[b]In nonusers of testosterone esters or during withdrawal.
[c]May be elevated because of muscle damage from intense exertion or hepatic injury. Viral hepatic serologies, γ-glutamyltransferase, and creatine phosphokinase are often helpful to establish etiology.

Because the effects of AASs on musculature and health may persist for months after discontinuation, evaluation for past use may be desirable. In addition to direct assays for the presence of AASs, other tests may provide useful indirect evidence of AAS abuse; unexpectedly elevated hemoglobin and hematocrit (214), suppressed follicle-stimulating hormone (FSH), decreased luteinizing hormone (LH), increased acid phosphatase (322), and hyperlipidemia and hypertriglyceridemia (137), are examples of such indirect indicators of AAS abuse. (See "Hepatic and Biliary Tree" above for a discussion of liver function and muscle enzyme tests). For males who abuse synthetic AASs there may be profound and persistent suppression of endogenous testosterone production, lasting longer than 10 months in one case report (318); low, as well as high, levels of testosterone may therefore indicate abuse. The suppression of LH, and elevation of prostate specific antigen and prolactin seen in AAS-treated rhesus monkeys (323) suggest additional avenues for investigation of how past use may be assessed. Advances in gene therapy technology may make in possible to greatly increase endogenous production of testosterone. The potential for transfection of athletes with genes for performance-enhancing hormones, somatotropin, insulin-like growth factor I, and AASs presents a new challenge for doping-control experts and athletic officials (89). Should this become an issue, new testing methods will be needed to detect the stigmata of such genetic manipulation.

Highly sensitive and specific, rapid, reliable methods for AAS testing on small samples for minute concentrations of unknowns include gas chromatography-mass spectrometry/mass fragmentography (410), tandem mass spectrometry (397,411), high-pressure liquid chromatography (HPLC), and enzyme-linked immunoabsorbent assay (ELISA) (399). New testing methods are being developed (412–418). Because specimen collection sites may be at a great distance from AAS testing facilities, the specimen collection, preservation, and shipping conditions must be considered; for example, the use of dried capillary blood on filter paper, shipped through the mail, is highly effective and reproducible for nandrolone and testosterone level determinations by radioimmunoassay (419). Although testosterone is cleared relatively rapidly, other AASs may be detectable for a month or more after discontinuation (420). This prolonged half-life of some AASs needs to be considered when evaluating repeatedly positive results in those who deny current use. Metabolites of over-the-counter AAS precursors can be detected in urine, sometimes for 2 to 6 days (421).

Several points of caution need to be raised when considering which laboratory to employ and how to interpret test results. Even those laboratories that test for some AASs may not test for all of the dozens of different compounds that are abused (85,422), nor use techniques that detect picogram amounts, leading to the possibility of false-negative results. Inter- and intralaboratory reliability may be an issue. Researchers at the Biostatistics Branch of the U.S. National Cancer Institute sent split samples of serum to different laboratories to be tested for ten different endogenous AASs and AAS metabolites. There was poor reliability even within the same laboratory, with tests of different aliquots from the same blood sample usually yielding significantly different results (423).

Theoretically, one should consider variations in physiology and diet when interpreting results of tests for AASs. The normal ranges reported with results are established by tests on adults, and these AAS levels differ from those of the elderly. Pubertal, precocious pubertal, and other adolescent individuals have sex-steroid hormone levels considerably in excess of those of adults; *appropriate reference values must be determined and used* (424,425). Pregnant women (426) and normal non–AAS-abusing women who exercise heavily have elevated levels of endogenous AASs (426). When evaluating women who appear androgenized, it is important to remember that unlike acne (which is directly influenced by testosterone and not its 5α-reductase metabolites), hirsutism and baldness are conditions that are promoted by 5α-reductase activity, as well as responsiveness to 3α-androstanediol glucuronide (3α-diol G) *in the skin* of the individual. A correlation has not been shown between the serum level of 3α-diol G, and its skin level or activity. There are conflicting data for elevated 3α-diol G as a diagnostic indicator to confirm or clarify the clinical impression of endogenous androgenization. A case-controlled series showed this ovarian and adrenal androgen precursor to be elevated in both polycystic ovary disease (with or without hirsutism) and in idiopathic hirsutism (427). However, while a prospective study of hirsute women confirmed elevation of 3α-diol G in some hirsute women, no elevation was seen in the idiopathic hirsutism subgroup; in this latter study, serum testosterone, androstenedione, and DHEA sulfate were elevated in all hirsute women, compared to controls (428). Additionally, women with acne vulgaris had reduced levels of serum 3α-diol G proportionally to severity, and no elevations in the aforementioned serum androgens (429).

Animal-organ meats may contain significant amounts of *endogenous* AASs. Consuming boar skeletal muscle, liver, heart, kidney, or testis can result in positive urine tests for 17β-nortestosterone and 19-norsteroids (430,431). Policymakers need to be aware that some cultures consume both castrated and noncastrated male animals. It is unclear to what extent inadvertent dietary intake of *synthetic* AASs used in animal husbandry and persisting in animal tissues may affect humans (432,433) or lead to test results positive for those compounds (434).

Animal models provide additional information about AASs and tests for AASs (435). Illicit use of AASs and doping-control testing are issues in competitions involving animals, such as horse racing (436) and pigeon racing (398,399). Animal studies show a wide range of normal serum androgen profiles within species, varying with age of the animal, daylight photoperiod exposure, and season of the year (437). Variation in human male and female endogenous androgen levels under varying climactic conditions and diurnal photoperiods is unknown.

Treatment

Although it is estimated that there are more than 1 million AAS users in the United States, the percentage of those who receive treatment for dependence is minute. Controlled trials of psychosocial treatment for AAS dependence have not been reported and AAS users infrequently submit to substance abuse treatment programs (438). Nonetheless, tentative treatment recommendations can be made. These are based on treatment of other dependencies, the pharmacology of AASs, and the psychological characteristics of AAS users. Assessment of psychiatric status is essential; severe symptoms are an indication for inpatient treatment. AAS users may have a variety of relationship problems that merit therapy for the relationship with a qualified family or couples therapist. Because assault may occur in AAS users' relationships, it is important to interview the spouse separately and confidentially, and also to offer the spouse referral both to therapy and to appropriate recovery groups (for survivors of abuse, if indicated, and for partners of drug addicts). This is true in every relationship, both heterosexual and homosexual. Ongoing assessment of sexual function is indicated, as impotence and decreased libido may occur upon discontinuation of AASs (375) and diminished sexual function has reportedly led to relapse (99). Persistent decrease in an individual's sexual function relative to baseline, (i.e., prior to AAS use) is an indication for consultation with an endocrinologist. Depression is another common problem in AAS abstinence syndrome, and can lead to relapse. The recovering AAS addict should be evaluated for depression and treated accordingly.

Psychosocial treatment must include an understanding and acknowledgment of the motivation for continued use. Treatment approaches will differ for individuals whose use persists because of AAS-induced hypomania (an increase in confidence, energy, and self-esteem) or euphoria, versus those who continue to use because they experience depressed mood upon discontinuation, versus those who use it to enhance body image (particularly those with a distorted body image), versus those who use for performance enhancement. The nature and course of AAS withdrawal should be reviewed with the user. Conventional drug-abuse treatment is appropriate for those who abuse AASs for their mood-altering effects or who are dependent on additional substances. For people who are engrossed in the body-building culture or who are seeking increased athletic performance, realistic goals with respect to appearance and performance must be set, and a diet and exercise plan should be agreed upon to achieve these goals. Peer counseling by ex-bodybuilders and group support may be of particular value for these users. Nutritional counseling and consultation with a fitness expert may be helpful. Gymnasiums are a frequent locale for acquisition of AASs and need to be avoided until recovery is firmly established. Although a wide variety of individuals can deliver psychosocial treatment to AAS users, those who are physically fit or former AAS users will have certain advantages in terms of relating to the AAS abuser seeking treatment. For a more complete discussion of psychosocial treatment issues, see Corcoran and Longo (439).

The role of pharmacotherapy in treatment of AAS dependence is poorly defined. While depression, mania, and psychosis may be induced by AAS use or withdrawal, their etiology may be difficult to establish with certainty. Pharmacotherapy for psychiatric symptoms should be based on a consideration of the risks and benefits, including the potential side effects of the medications and the consequences of inaction, which may include problems with retention in treatment. Maintenance and controlled taper have not been reported as therapeutic modalities, and no routine pharmacotherapy is recommended.

PREVENTION

The development of interventions to reduce the initiation of AAS use is in its infancy. The primary force driving the illicit use of AASs appears to be a strong cultural value placed upon sports heroes, physical strength, and large, well-defined muscles, particularly for men, and physical competence and athletic achievement for all. Unless society sends a different message about physical beauty and athletic success, the demand and acceptance of AAS use is likely to persist (440). Hence it may be difficult for an adolescent to decline an offer of AASs, because AAS use may be seen as a way to achieve highly desired goals. It is important to direct educational programs both to parents and to student athletes, and to include a range of information about steroids, such as the risk of potential early epiphyseal closure in the adolescent skeleton (441,442), the association between body dysmorphia and initiation of steroid abuse, the high potential for addiction, and the nature of addiction in graphic detail.

Undefined factors, including legal regulation and education, reduced the overall lifetime anabolic steroid use rate among American adolescent males between 1989 and 1996, but not among adolescent females (39). Peer influ-

ence, Coaches' Rules, and NCAA policies on AASs and smokeless tobacco may be effective in reducing athletes' use of AASs and other substances of abuse (440,443,444). Adolescent male athletes with higher levels of alcohol and marijuana use, hostility, impulsivity, ruthlessness to win, dissatisfaction with their weight, greater tolerance of peer drug abuse, and less parental antidrug abuse influence had higher intent to use AASs and less ability to refuse an offer of AASs than did otherwise similar athletes despite education in nutrition and weight-training methods (445).

The association between AAS and tobacco use, especially among adolescents (218), and the association between smokeless tobacco use and certain sports, suggests that AAS abuse prevention programs may benefit from lessons learned regarding tobacco abuse prevention programs (79,446–450). Dispelling myths and providing sound scientific information about the effects of drugs used by athletes upon athletic performance provide a solid foundation for treatment, prevention, and relapse prevention: Alcohol, marijuana, smokeless tobacco, cocaine, caffeine, antihypertensives, diuretics, some antihistamines, and some antidepressants are ergolytic, not ergogenic agents (451). Unfortunately, the benefit of AASs with respect to muscular development raises the possibility that comprehensive and accurate information about AASs might serve to increase use. Hence, simply informing potential users of the risks of AASs may not be effective (321). In a randomized trial of high school football players of a balanced presentation discussing risks and benefits (N = 65), risks only (N = 70), and a control group (n = 57), only those in the balanced group increased their belief in adverse affects from AASs, although subjects in the risks only group decreased their belief in the benefits of AASs (452). There is a real possibility that interventions designed to prevent AAS use could have the opposite effect if applied to populations in which there is little familiarity with AASs. Controlled trials of interventions should be conducted in groups with different levels of familiarity with AASs (e.g., athletes vs. students who are not athletes), with AAS use as an outcome before those interventions are put into general practice.

The belief that there is peer acceptance of AAS use can be modified and dispelled to discourage students from AAS abuse. Adolescents Training and Learning to Avoid Steroids (ATLAS) is a prevention program whose components are a promotion of nutrition and strength training as alternatives to AAS abuse, drug refusal role play, and anti-AAS media campaigns (453). This intervention was tested in 3,207 high school football players in Portland, Oregon. After participating in the intervention, students had enhanced healthy behaviors, reduced impact from the factors that encourage AAS use, and lowered intent to use AASs. These changes were sustained over the period of 1 year (454,455). At season's end, both the intention to use and actual AAS use were significantly lower among students who participated in the study. Although AAS reduction no longer reached statistical significance at 1 year (p < 0.08), intentions to use AASs remained lower. A combined measure of alcohol, marijuana, amphetamines, and "narcotics" was reduced at 1 year, whether alcohol was included or excluded from the index. Other long-term effects included fewer students reporting drinking and driving; participants reported less sport supplement use and improved nutrition behaviors.

Prevention of transmission of hepatitis B, hepatitis C, and HIV should be addressed in AAS abusers. AAS abuse in adolescents or adults may be associated with risky behaviors, including sharing injection equipment (68,80,81) and engaging in unprotected sex. Prevention aimed at adult bodybuilders should cover all HIV risk-reduction topics. In a large London study of gay male bodybuilders, nearly 1 in 10 injected AASs or other fitness-enhancing drugs in 1999 (456), and 1 in 7 did so in 2000 (352), although none reported needle sharing in either study. However, the steroid users reported almost twice the incidence of unprotected intercourse with HIV-status-unknown partners than did nonusers. Hence, close surveillance of risk behaviors is recommended in this population. Gym-centered AAS-abusing communities are an appropriate venue for developing and testing risk-reduction interventions.

ACKNOWLEDGMENT

The authors gratefully acknowledge the research assistance of Michael Lim and Judith Rosen, MPH, and the encouragement and editorial suggestions of Donald Wesson, MD, with the original writing in 1995. We appreciate the extensive research and editorial assistance of Nicole Wolfe, BA, and acknowledge the editorial assistance of Basil Glew-Galloway on the current edition.

APPENDIX: INTERNET RESOURCES

1. Steroid abuse, a service of the National Institute on Drug Abuse: http://steroidabuse.org (accessed on 6/25/2004).
2. Doping control laboratories accredited by The World Anti-Doping Agency: http://www.wada-ama.org/en/t3.asp?p=41979 (accessed on 6/26/2004).
3. National Anti-Doping Agencies around the world: http://www.wada-ama.org/en/t2.asp?p=31224 (accessed on 6/26/2004).
4. The United States Anti-Doping Agency for Olympic sports in the U.S. http://www.usantidoping.org (accessed on 6/26/2004) includes the USADA Drug Reference Toll-Free Line http://www.usantidoping.org/line.htm) (accessed 6/26/2004).

REFERENCES

1. Applegate EA, Grivetti LE. Search for the competitive edge: a history of dietary fads and supplements. *J Nutr* 1997;127[5 Suppl]:869S–873S.
2. Inaba D, Cohen W. *Uppers, downers, all rounders.* Ashland, OR: CNS Publications, 2000.
3. Yesalis CE, Bahrke MS. Anabolic-androgenic steroids. Current issues. *Sports Med* 1995;19(5):326–340.
4. Kochakian CD. History of anabolic-androgenic steroids. In: Lin G, Erinoff L, eds. *Anabolic steroid abuse.* Rockville, MD: National Institute on Drug Abuse, 1990:29–59.
5. Wade N. Anabolic steroids: doctors denounce them, but athletes aren't listening. *Science* 1972;176:1399–1403.
6. Hatton C, Catlin D. Detection of androgenic anabolic steroids in urine. *Clin Lab Med* 1987;7:655–668.
7. Marshall E. The drug of champions. *Science* 1988;242:183–184.
8. Buckley WE, Yesalis CE, Freidl K, et al. Estimated prevalence of anabolic steroid use among male high school seniors. *JAMA* 1988;260:3441–3445.
9. Franke WW, Berendonk B. Hormonal doping and androgenization of athletes: a secret program of the German Democratic Republic government. *Clin Chem* 1997;43(7):1262–1279.
10. Anonymous. Summit theme papers. Theme 2: drug testing discussion paper. International Summit Drugs In Sport Pure Performance, 1999. Available at: http://pandora.nla.gov.au/parchive/2000/S2000-Nov-30/www.drugsinsport.isr.gov.au/section_3/DrugFINALnew.html (accessed 6/25/04).
11. Dalton JT, Mukherjee A, Zhu Z, et al. Discovery of nonsteroidal androgens. *Biochem Biophys Res Commun* 1998;244(1):1–4.
12. Higgins G. Adonis meets Addison: another potential cause of occult adrenal insufficiency [Letter]. *J Emerg Med* 1993;11(6):761–762.
13. Wilson J. Androgen abuse by athletes. *Endocrine Rev* 1988;9(2):181–199.
14. Winters S. Androgens: endocrine physiology and pharmacology. In: Lin G, Erinoff L, eds. *Anabolic steroid abuse.* Rockville, MD: National Institute on Drug Abuse, 1990:113–130.
15. Jänne O. Androgen interaction through multiple steroid receptors. In: Lin G, Erinoff L, eds. *Anabolic steroid abuse.* Rockville, MD: National Institute on Drug Abuse, 1990:178–186.
16. Genazzani AD, Gamba O, Nappi L, et al. Modulatory effects of a synthetic steroid (tibolone) and estradiol on spontaneous and GH-RH-induced GH secretion in postmenopausal women. *Maturitas* 1997;28(1):27–33.
17. Hosli E, Jurasin K, Ruhl W, et al. Colocalization of androgen, estrogen and cholinergic receptors on cultured astrocytes of rat central nervous system. *Int J Dev Neurosci* 2001;19(1):11–19.
18. Johansson-Steensland P, Nyberg F, Chahl L. The anabolic androgenic steroid, nandrolone decanoate, increases the density of Fos-like immunoreactive neurons in limbic regions of guinea-pig brain. *Eur J Neurosci* 2002;15(3):539–544.
19. Johansson P, Hallberg M, Kindlundh A, Nyberg F. The effect on opioid peptides in the rat brain, after chronic treatment with the anabolic androgenic steroid, nandrolone decanoate. *Brain Res Bull* 2000;51(5):413–418.
20. Johansson P, Ray A, Zhou Q, et al. Anabolic androgenic steroids increase beta-endorphin levels in the ventral tegmental area in the male rat brain. *Neurosci Res* 1997;27(2):185–189.
21. Johansson P, Lindqvist A, Nyberg F, Fahlke C. Anabolic androgenic steroids affects alcohol intake, defensive

behaviors and brain opioid peptides in the rat. *Pharmacol Biochem Behav* 2000;67(2):271–279.

22. Blanco CE, Popper P, Micevych P. Anabolic–androgenic steroid-induced alterations in choline acetyltransferase messenger RNA levels of spinal cord motoneurons in the male rat. *Neuroscience* 1997;78(3):873–882.

23. Daly RC, Su TP, Schmidt PJ, et al. Cerebrospinal fluid and behavioral changes after methyltestosterone administration: preliminary findings. *Arch Gen Psychiatry* 2001;58(2):172–177.

24. Jorge-Rivera JC, McIntyre KL, Henderson LP. Anabolic steroids induce region- and subunit-specific rapid modulation of GABA(A) receptor-mediated currents in the rat forebrain. *J Neurophysiol* 2000;83(6):3299–3309.

25. Kleiner SM. Performance-enhancing aids in sport: health consequences and nutritional alternatives. *J Am Coll Nutr* 1991;10(2):163–176.

26. Schanzer W, Opfermann G, Donike M, 17-Epimerization of 17 alpha-methyl anabolic steroids in humans: metabolism and synthesis of 17 alpha-hydroxy-17 beta-methyl steroids. *Steroids* 1992;57(11):537–550.

27. Kammerer RC, Merdink JL, Jagels M, et al. Testing for fluoxymesterone (Halotestin) administration to man: identification of urinary metabolites by gas chromatography-mass spectrometry. *J Steroid Biochem* 1990;36(6):659–666.

28. Schanzer W, Horning S, Donike M. Metabolism of anabolic steroids in humans: synthesis of 6 beta-hydroxy metabolites of 4-chloro-1,2-dehydro-17 alpha-methyltestosterone, fluoxymesterone, and methandienone. *Steroids* 1995;60(4):353–366.

29. Wilson J. Androgens. In: Hardman JG, Limbird LL, Molinoff PB, Ruddon RW, Gilman AG, eds. *Goodman & Gilman's the pharmacological basis of therapeutics*. New York: McGraw-Hill, 1996;1441–1457.

30. Substance Abuse and Mental Health Services Administration. *National household survey on drug abuse: population estimates 1994*. Washington, DC: U.S. Department of Health and Human Services, 1995.

31. Ferenchick GS. Validity of self-report in identifying anabolic steroid use among weightlifters. *J Gen Intern Med* 1996;11(9):554–556.

32. Handelsman DJ, Gupta L. Prevalence and risk factors for anabolic-androgenic steroid abuse in Australian high school students. *Int J Androl* 1997;20(3):159–164.

33. Bahrke MS, Yesalis CE, Brower KJ. Anabolic–androgenic steroid abuse and performance–enhancing drugs among adolescents. *Child Adolesc Psychiatr Clin N Am* 1998;7(4):821–838.

34. Faigenbaum AD, Zaichowsky LD, Gardner DE, Micheli LJ. Anabolic steroid use by male and female middle school students. *Pediatrics* 1998; 101(5):E6.

35. Bahrke MS, Yesalis CE, Kopstein AN, Stephens JA. Risk factors associated with anabolic-androgenic steroid use among adolescents. *Sports Med* 2000;29(6):397–405.

36. Drewnowski A, Kurth CL, Krahn DD. Effects of body image on dieting, exercise, and anabolic steroid use in adolescent males. *Int J Eat Disord* 1995;17(4):381–386.

37. Hardy KJ, McNeil JJ, Capes AG. Drug doping in senior Australian rules football: a survey for frequency. *Br J Sports Med* 1997;31(2):126–128.

38. Johnston LD, O'Malley PM, Bachman JG. *The Monitoring the Future national survey results on adolescent drug use: overview of key findings 2002*. NIH Publication No. 03—5374. 2003, Bethesda, MD: National Institute on Drug Abuse.

39. Yesalis CE, Barsukiewicz CK, Kopstein AN, Bahrke MS. Trends in anabolic-androgenic steroid use among adolescents. *Arch Pediatr Adolesc Med* 1997;151(12):1197–1206.

40. Irving LM, Wall M, Neumark-Sztainer D, Story M. Steroid use among adolescents: findings from Project EAT. *J Adolesc Health* 2002;30(4):243–252.

41. Brower KJ, Blow FC, Young JP, Hill EM. Symptoms and correlates of anabolic-androgenic steroid dependence. *Br J Addict* 1991;86(6):759–768.

42. Su TP, Pagliaro M, Schmidt PJ, et al. Neuropsychiatric effects of anabolic steroids in male normal volunteers. *JAMA* 1993;269(21):2760–2764.

43. Porcerelli JH, Sandler BA. Narcissism and empathy in steroid users. *Am J Psychiatry* 1995;152(11):1672–1674.

44. Yesalis CE, Wright JE, Lombardo JA. [Anabolic steroids in athletes.] *Wien Med Wochenschr* 1992;142(14):298–308.

45. Schulte HM, Hall MJ, Boyer M. Domestic violence associated with anabolic steroid abuse [Letter]. *Am J Psychiatry* 1993;150(2):348.

46. Salva PS, Bacon GE. Anabolic steroids: interest among parents and nonathletes. *South Med J* 1991;84(5):552–556.

47. Gruber AJ, Pope HG Jr. Compulsive weight lifting and anabolic drug abuse among women rape victims. *Compr Psychiatry* 1999;40(4):273–277.

48. Bahrke MS, Yesalis CE 3rd. Weight training. A potential confounding factor in examining the psychological and behavioural effects of anabolic–androgenic steroids. *Sports Med* 1994;18(5):309–318.

49. Perry PJ, Andersen KH, Yates WR. Illicit anabolic steroid use in athletes. A case series analysis. *Am J Sports Med* 1990;18(4):422–428.

50. Burnett KF, Kleiman ME. Psychological characteristics of adolescent steroid users. *Adolescence* 1994;29(113):81–89.

51. Pope HJ, Katz DL. Psychiatric and medical effects of anabolic-androgenic steroid use. A controlled study of 160 athletes. *Arch Gen Psychiatry* 1994;51(5):375–382.

52. Cooper CJ, Noakes TD, Dunne T, et al. A high prevalence of abnormal personality traits in chronic users of anabolic-androgenic steroids. *Br J Sports Med* 1996;30(3):246–250.

53. Galligani N, Renck A, Hansen S. Personality profile of men using anabolic androgenic steroids. *Horm Behav* 1996;30(2):170–175.

54. Blouin AG, Goldfield GS. Body image and steroid use in male bodybuilders. *Int J Eat Disord* 1995;18(2):159–165.

55. Hays LR, Littleton S, Stillner V. Anabolic steroid dependence [Letter]. *Am J Psychiatry* 1990;147(1):122.

56. Gruber AJ, Pope HG Jr. Psychiatric and medical effects of anabolic-androgenic steroid use in women. *Psychother Psychosom* 2000;69(1):19–26.

57. Frankle M. Use of androgenic anabolic steroids by athletes [Letter]. *JAMA* 1984;252(4):482.

58. Schwellnus MP, Lambert MI, Todd MP, Juritz JM. Androgenic anabolic steroid use in matric pupils. A survey of prevalence of use in the western Cape. *S Afr Med J* 1992;82(3):154–158.

59. Greenway P, Greenway M. General practitioner knowledge of prohibited substances in sport. *Br J Sports Med* 1997;31(2):129–131.

60. Green GA, Uryasz FD, Petr TA, Bray CD. NCAA study of substance use and abuse habits of college student-athletes. *Clin J Sport Med* 2001;11(1):51–56.

61. Shepherd M, McKeithan K. *Examination of the type and amount of pharmaceutical products being declared by U.S. residents upon returning to the U.S. from Mexico at the Laredo, Texas border crossing*. Austin, TX: The University of Texas, Report February 28, 1996.

62. Pope H, Katz D. Affective and psychotic symptoms associated with anabolic steroid use. *Am J Psychiatry* 1988;145(4):487–490.

63. Bahrke MS, Wright JE, Strauss RH, Catlin DH. Psychological moods and

subjectively perceived behavioral and somatic changes accompanying anabolic-androgenic steroid use. *Am J Sports Med* 1992;20(6):717–724.

64. Hickson JF Jr, Johnson TE, Lee W, Sidor RJ. Nutrition and the precontest preparations of a male bodybuilder. *J Am Diet Assoc* 1990; 90(2):264–267.

65. Nilsson S. Androgenic anabolic steroid use among male adolescents in Falkenberg. *Eur J Clin Pharmacol* 1995;48(1):9–11.

66. Gomez JE. Performance-enhancing substances in adolescent athletes. *Tex Med* 2002;98(2):41–46.

67. Green T. The risks to athletes of smokeless tobacco use. *J Mass Dent Soc* 1994;43(4):57–60.

68. DuRant RH, Escobedo LG, Heath GW. Anabolic-steroid use, strength training, and multiple drug use among adolescents in the United States. *Pediatrics* 1995;96[1 Pt 1]:23–28.

69. Pearl JM. Severe reaction to "natural testosterones": how safe are the ergogenic aids? [Letter]. *Am J Emerg Med* 1993;11(2):188–189.

70. Gadzhieva RM, Portugalov SN, Paniushkin VV, Kondrat'eva II. [A comparative study of the anabolic action of ecdysten, leveton and Prime Plus, preparations of plant origin.] *Eksp Klin Farmakol* 1995;58(5):46–48.

71. Delbeke FT. Doping in cyclism: results of unannounced controls in Flanders (1987–1994). *Int J Sports Med* 1996;17(6):434–438.

72. Dumestre-Toulet V, Cirimele V, Ludes B, et al. Hair analysis of seven bodybuilders for anabolic steroids, ephedrine, and clenbuterol. *J Forensic Sci* 2002;47(1):211–214.

73. Choi PY, Pope HJ. Violence toward women and illicit androgenic-anabolic steroid use. *Ann Clin Psychiatry* 1994;6(1):21–25.

74. Glover ED, Christen AG, Henderson AH. Just a pinch between the cheek and gum. *J Sch Health* 1981;51(6):415–418.

75. Christen AG, McDaniel RK, Doran JE. Snuff dipping and tobacco chewing in a group of Texas college athletes. *Tex Dent J* 1979;97(2):6–10.

76. Green T. Breaking the link between snuff and athletes. *Penn Dent J (Phila)* 1995;62(2):13–19.

77. Creath CJ, Shelton WO, Wright JT, et al. The prevalence of smokeless tobacco use among adolescent male athletes. *J Am Dent Assoc* 1988;116(1):43–48.

78. Davis TC, Arnold C, Nandy I, Bocchini JA, et al. Tobacco use among male high school athletes. *J Adolesc Health* 1997;21(2):97–101.

79. Horn KA, Maniar SD, Dino GA, et al. Coaches' attitudes toward smokeless tobacco and intentions to intervene with athletes. *J Sch Health* 2000;70(3):89–94.

80. DuRant RH, Rickert VI, Ashworth CS, et al. Use of multiple drugs among adolescents who use anabolic steroids. *N Engl J Med* 1993;328(13):922–926.

81. Durant RH, Ashworth CS, Newman C, Rickert VI. Stability of the relationships between anabolic steroid use and multiple substance use among adolescents. *J Adolesc Health* 1994;15(2):111–116.

82. Arvary D, Pope HG Jr. Anabolic–androgenic steroids as a gateway to opioid dependence. *N Engl J Med* 2000;342(20):1532.

83. Jones AR, Pichot JT. Stimulant use in sports. *Am J Addict* 1998;7(4):243–255.

84. Lindstrom M, et al. Use of anabolic-androgenic steroids among body builders—frequency and attitudes. *J Intern Med* 1990;227(6):407–411.

85. Benzi G. Pharmacoepidemiology of the drugs used in sports as doping agents. *Pharmacol Res* 1994;29(1):13–26.

86. Pope HJ, Katz DL. Homicide and near-homicide by anabolic steroid users. *J Clin Psychiatry* 1990;51(1):28–31.

87. Rickert VI, Pawlak-Morello C, Sheppard V, Jay MS. Human growth hormone: a new substance of abuse among adolescents? *Clin Pediatr (Phila)* 1992;31(12):723–726.

88. Galloway GP, Frederick SL, Staggers FE Jr, et al. Gamma-hydroxybutyrate: an emerging drug of abuse that causes physical dependence. *Addiction* 1997;92(1):89–96.

89. Friedmann T, Koss JO. Gene transfer and athletics- an impending problem. *Mol Ther* 2001;3(6):819–820.

90. Prather ID, Brown DE, North P, Wilson JR. Clenbuterol: a substitute for anabolic steroids? *Med Sci Sports Exerc* 1995;27(8):1118–1121.

91. Gareau R, Audran M, Baynes RD, et al. Erythropoietin abuse in athletes. *Nature* 1996;380:113.

92. Betz JM, White KD, der Marderosian AH. Gas chromatographic determination of yohimbine in commercial yohimbe products. *J AOAC Int* 1995;78(5):1189–1194.

93. Evans NA. Gym and tonic: a profile of 100 male steroid users. *Br J Sports Med* 1997;31(1):54–58.

94. Appleby M, Fisher M, Martin M. Myocardial infarction, hyperkalaemia and ventricular tachycardia in a young male body-builder. *Int J Cardiol* 1994;44(2):171–174.

95. Luke JL, Farb A, Virmani R, Sample RH. Sudden cardiac death during exercise in a weight lifter using anabolic androgenic steroids: pathological and toxicological findings. *J Forensic Sci* 1990;35(6):1441–1447.

96. Morrison CL. Anabolic steroid users identified by needle and syringe exchange contact. *Drug Alcohol Depend* 1994;36(2):153–155.

97. Salaman J. Misuse of anabolic drugs [Letter]. *BMJ* 1993;306(6869):62.

98. Moss HB, Panzak GL, Tarter RE. Sexual functioning of male anabolic steroid abusers. *Arch Sex Behav* 1993;22(1):1–12.

99. Bickelman C, Ferries L, Eaton RP. Impotence related to anabolic steroid use in a body builder. Response to clomiphene citrate. *West J Med* 1995;162(2):158–160.

100. Brower KJ, Blow FC, Beresford TP, Fuelling C. Anabolic-androgenic steroid dependence. *J Clin Psychiatry* 1989;50(1):31–33.

101. Gill GV. Anabolic steroid induced hypogonadism treated with human chorionic gonadotropin. *Postgrad Med J* 1998;74(867):45–46.

102. Drake L, Hordinsky M, Fiedler V, et al. The effects of finasteride on scalp skin and serum androgen levels in men with androgenetic alopecia. *J Am Acad Dermatol* 1999;41(4):550–554.

103. Castello R, Tosi F, Perrone F, et al. Outcome of long-term treatment with the 5 alpha-reductase inhibitor finasteride in idiopathic hirsutism: clinical and hormonal effects during a 1-year course of therapy and 1-year follow-up. *Fertil Steril* 1996;66(5):734–740.

104. Danniell HW. Narcotic-induced hypogonadism during therapy for heroin addiction. *J Addict Dis* 2002;21(4):47–53.

105. Haeusler G, Frisch H, Schmitt K, et al. Treatment of patients with Ullrich-Turner syndrome with conventional doses of growth hormone and the combination with testosterone or oxandrolone: effect on growth, IGF-I and IGFBP-3 concentrations. *Eur J Pediatr* 1995;154(6):437–444.

106. Haeusler G, Schmitt K, Blumel P, et al. Growth hormone in combination with anabolic steroids in patients with Turner syndrome: effect on bone maturation and final height. *Acta Paediatr* 1996;85(12):1408–1414.

107. Haeusler G, Schmitt K, Blumel P, et al. Insulin, insulin-like growth factor-binding protein-1, and sex hormone-binding globulin in patients with Turner's syndrome: course over age in untreated patients and effect of therapy with growth hormone alone and in combination with oxandrolone. *J Clin Endocrinol Metab* 1996;81(2):536–541.

108. Joss EE, Mullis PE, Werder EA, et al. Growth promotion and Turner-specific bone age after therapy with

growth hormone and in combination with oxandrolone: when should therapy be started in Turner syndrome? *Horm Res* 1997;47(3):102–109.

109. Cacciari E, Mazzanti L. Final height of patients with Turner's syndrome treated with growth hormone (GH): indications for GH therapy alone at high doses and late estrogen therapy. Italian Study Group for Turner Syndrome. *J Clin Endocrinol Metab* 1999;84(12):4510–4515.

110. Doeker B, Muller-Michaels J, Andler W. Induction of early puberty in a boy after treatment with oxandrolone? *Horm Res* 1998;50(1):46–48.

111. Hermanussen M. Growth promotion by oxandrolone in a girl with short stature and early pubertal development treated with growth hormone and gonadotropin-releasing hormone-analogue. A case study. *Acta Paediatr* 1995;84(10):1207–1210.

112. Johansen KL, Mulligan K, Schambelan M. Anabolic effects of nandrolone decanoate in patients receiving dialysis: a randomized controlled trial. *JAMA* 1999;281(14):1275–1281.

113. Buntzel J, Kuttner K. [Value of megestrol acetate in treatment of cachexia in head-neck tumors.] *Laryngorhinootologie* 1995;74(8):504–507.

114. Darnton SJ, Zgainski B, Grenier I, et al. The use of an anabolic steroid (nandrolone decanoate) to improve nutritional status after esophageal resection for carcinoma. *Dis Esophagus* 1999;12(4):283–288.

115. Gruzdev BM, Ivannikov EV, Gorbacheva ES. [Anabolic therapy in patients with HIV infections.] *Ter Arkh* 1999;71(11):35–37.

116. Hengge UR, Baumann M, Maleba R, et al. Oxymetholone promotes weight gain in patients with advanced human immunodeficiency virus (HIV-1) infection. *Br J Nutr* 1996;75(1):129–138.

117. Cioroiu M, Hanan SH. Adjuvant anabolic agents: a case report on the successful use of oxandrolone in an HIV-positive patient with chronic stasis ulceration. *J Wound Ostomy Continence Nurs* 2001;28(4):215–218.

118. Demling R, DeSanti L. Closure of the "non-healing wound" corresponds with correction of weight loss using the anabolic agent oxandrolone. *Ostomy Wound Manage* 1998;44(10):58–62, 64, 66 passim.

119. Demling RH. Comparison of the anabolic effects and complications of human growth hormone and the testosterone analog, oxandrolone, after severe burn injury. *Burns* 1999;25(3):215–221.

120. Demling RH. Oxandrolone, an anabolic steroid, enhances the healing of a cutaneous wound in the rat. *Wound Repair Regen* 2000;8(2):97–102.

121. Demling RH, DeSanti L. Oxandrolone, an anabolic steroid, significantly increases the rate of weight gain in the recovery phase after major burns. *J Trauma* 1997;43(1):47–51.

122. Demling RH, DeSanti L. The rate of restoration of body weight after burn injury, using the anabolic agent oxandrolone, is not age dependent. *Burns* 2001;27(1):46–51.

123. Demling RH, Orgill DP. The anticatabolic and wound healing effects of the testosterone analog oxandrolone after severe burn injury. *J Crit Care* 2000;15(1):12–17.

124. Falabella AF. American Academy of Dermatology 1998 Awards for Young Investigators in Dermatology. The anabolic steroid stanozolol upregulates collagen synthesis through the action of transforming growth factor-beta1. *J Am Acad Dermatol* 1998;39[2 Pt 1]:272–273.

125. Falanga V, Greenberg AS, Zhou L, et al. Stimulation of collagen synthesis by the anabolic steroid stanozolol. *J Invest Dermatol* 1998;111(6):1193–1197.

126. Hart DW, Wolf SE, Ramzy PI, et al. Anabolic effects of oxandrolone after severe burn. 201;233(4):556–564.

127. Gervasio JM, Dickerson RN, Swearingen J, et al. Oxandrolone in trauma patients. *Pharmacotherapy* 2000;20(11):1328–1334.

128. Gold J, Batterham M. Nandrolone decanoate; use in HIV-associated lipodystrophy syndrome: a pilot study. *Int J STD AIDS* 1999;10(8):558.

129. Currier JS. How to manage metabolic complications of HIV therapy: what to do while we wait for answers. *AIDS Read* 2000;10(3):162–169; discussion 171–174.

130. Tsiodras S, Mantzoros C, Hammer S, Samore M. Effects of protease inhibitors on hyperglycemia, hyperlipidemia, and lipodystrophy: a 5-year cohort study. *Arch Intern Med* 2000;160(13):2050–2056.

131. Dickerman RD. McConathy WJ, Zachariah NY. Testosterone, sex hormone-binding globulin, lipoproteins, and vascular disease risk. *J Cardiovasc Risk* 1997;4(5-6):363–366.

132. Farish E, Barnes JF, Fletcher CD, et al. Effects of tibolone on serum lipoprotein and apolipoprotein levels compared with a cyclical estrogen/progestogen regimen. *Menopause* 1999;6(2):98–104.

133. Frisch F, Sumida KD. Temporal effects of testosterone propionate injections on serum lipoprotein concentrations in rats. *Med Sci Sports Exerc* 1999;31(5):664–669.

134. Castelo-Branco C, Casals E, Figueras F, et al. Two-year prospective and comparative study on the effects of tibolone on lipid pattern, behavior of apolipoproteins AI and B. *Menopause* 1999;6(2):92–97.

135. Castro Cabezas M, van Loon D, de Hiep HJ, Meuwissen OJ. [A patient with an unexplained low level of high density lipoprotein cholesterol.] *Ned Tijdschr Geneeskd* 1997;141(4):200–202.

136. Ebenbichler CF, Sturm W, Ganzer H, et al. Flow-mediated, endothelium-dependent vasodilatation is impaired in male body builders taking anabolic-androgenic steroids. *Atherosclerosis* 2001;158(2):483–490.

137. Jockenhovel F, Bullmann C, Schubert M, et al. Influence of various modes of androgen substitution on serum lipids and lipoproteins in hypogonadal men. *Metabolism* 1999;48(5):590–596.

138. Chu K, Kang DW, Kim DE, Roh JK. Cerebral venous thrombosis associated with tentorial subdural hematoma during oxymetholone therapy. *J Neurol Sci* 2001;185(1):27–30.

139. Cicardi M, Castelli R, Zingale LC, Agostoni A. Side effects of long-term prophylaxis with attenuated androgens in hereditary angioedema: comparison of treated and untreated patients. *J Allergy Clin Immunol* 1997;99(2):194–196.

140. Yuan A, Liu C, Huang X. [Treatment of 34 cases of chronic aplastic anemia using prepared Rehmannia polysaccharide associated with stanozolol.] *Zhongguo Zhong Xi Yi Jie He Za Zhi* 1998;18(6):351–353.

141. Teruel JL, Aguilera A, Marcen R, et al. Androgen therapy for anaemia of chronic renal failure. Indications in the erythropoietin era. *Scand J Urol Nephrol* 1996;30(5):403–408.

142. Gascon A, Belvis JJ, Berisa F, Iglesias E. Nandrolone decanoate may be an adjuvant therapy to augment haemoglobin response today? *Nephrol Dial Transplant* 1999;14(9):2257–2258.

143. Gascon A, Belvis JJ, Berisa F, Iglesias E, et al. Nandrolone decanoate is a good alternative for the treatment of anemia in elderly male patients on hemodialysis. *Geriatr Nephrol Urol* 1999;9(2):67–72.

144. Gaughan WJ, Liss KA, Dunn SR, et al. A 6-month study of low-dose recombinant human erythropoietin alone and in combination with androgens for the treatment of anemia in chronic hemodialysis patients. *Am J Kidney Dis* 1997;30(4):495–500.

145. Geary CG, Harrison CJ, Philpott NJ,

et al. Abnormal cytogenetic clones in patients with aplastic anaemia: response to immunosuppressive therapy. *Br J Haematol* 1999;104(2):271–274.

146. Johansen KL. The role of nandrolone decanoate in patients with end stage renal disease in the erythropoietin era. *Int J Artif Organs* 2001;24(4):183–185.

147. Frikha M, Mseddi S, Elloumi M, et al. [Fanconi disease: study of 43 cases in southern Tunisia.] *Arch Pediatr* 1998;5(11):1200–1205.

148. Castelo-Branco C, Vicente JJ, Vanrell JA. Use of gonadotropin-releasing hormone analog with tibolone to prevent cyclic attacks of acute intermittent porphyria. *Metabolism* 2001;50(9):995–996.

149. Hedstrom M, Sjoberg K, Brosjo E, et al. Positive effects of anabolic steroids, vitamin D and calcium on muscle mass, bone mineral density and clinical function after a hip fracture. A randomised study of 63 women. *J Bone Joint Surg Br* 2002;84(4):497–503.

150. Berendsen HH, Weekers AH, Kloosterboer HJ. Effect of tibolone and raloxifene on the tail temperature of oestrogen-deficient rats. *Eur J Pharmacol* 2001;419(1):47–54.

151. Barrett-Connor E, Young R, Notelovitz M, et al. A two-year, double-blind comparison of estrogen-androgen and conjugated estrogens in surgically menopausal women. Effects on bone mineral density, symptoms and lipid profiles. *J Reprod Med* 1999;44(12):1012–1020.

152. Berning B, van Kuijk C, Kuiper JW, et al. Increased loss of trabecular but not cortical bone density, 1 year after discontinuation of 2 years hormone replacement therapy with tibolone. *Maturitas* 1999;31(2):151–159.

153. Watts NB, Notelovitz M, Timmons MC, et al. Comparison of oral estrogens and estrogens plus androgen on bone mineral density, menopausal symptoms, and lipid-lipoprotein profiles in surgical menopause. *Obstet Gynecol* 1995;85(4):529–537.

154. Huang RY, Miller LM, Carlson CS, Chance MR. Characterization of bone mineral composition in the proximal tibia of cynomolgus monkeys: effect of ovariectomy and nandrolone decanoate treatment. *Bone* 2002;30(3):492–497.

155. Ceballos C, Ribes C, Amado JA, et al. Venous endothelial function in postmenopausal women after six months of tibolone therapy. *Maturitas* 2001;39(1):63–70.

156. Doren M, Rubig A, Coelingh Bennink HJ, Holzgreve W. Resistance of pelvic arteries and plasma lipids in postmenopausal women: comparative study of tibolone and continuous combined

estradiol and norethindrone acetate replacement therapy. *Am J Obstet Gynecol* 2000;183(3):575–582.

157. Gregoriou O, Vitoratos N, Papadias C, et al. Effect of tibolone on postmenopausal women with myomas. *Maturitas* 1997;27(2):187–191.

158. Doren M, Rubig A, Coelingh Bennink HJ, Holzgreve W. Impact on uterine bleeding and endometrial thickness: tibolone compared with continuous combined estradiol and norethisterone acetate replacement therapy. *Menopause* 1999;6(4):299–306.

159. Hanggi W, Bersinger N, Altermatt HJ, Birkhauser MH. Comparison of transvaginal ultrasonography and endometrial biopsy in endometrial surveillance in postmenopausal HRT users. *Maturitas* 1997;27(2):133–143.

160. Hammar M, Christau S, Nathorst-Boos J, et al. A double-blind, randomised trial comparing the effects of tibolone and continuous combined hormone replacement therapy in postmenopausal women with menopausal symptoms. *Br J Obstet Gynaecol* 1998;105(8):904–911.

161. Ginsburg J, Prelevic GM. Cause of vaginal bleeding in postmenopausal women taking tibolone. *Maturitas* 1996;24(1–2):107–110.

162. Habiba M, Ramsay J, Akkad A, Hart DM, al-Azzawi F. Immunohistochemical and hysteroscopic assessment of postmenopausal women with uterine bleeding whilst taking tibolone. *Eur J Obstet Gynecol Reprod Biol* 1996;66(1):45–49.

163. Fedele L, Bianchi S, Raffaelli R, Zanconato G. Comparison of transdermal estradiol and tibolone for the treatment of oophorectomized women with deep residual endometriosis. *Maturitas* 1999;32(3):189–193.

164. Chang AY, Putt M, Pandya KJ, et al. Induction chemotherapy of dibromodulcitol, Adriamycin, vincristine, tamoxifen, and Halotestin with methotrexate in metastatic breast cancer: an Eastern Cooperative Oncology Group Study (E1181). *Am J Clin Oncol* 1998;21(1):99–104.

165. Falkson G, Gelman RS, Pandya KJ, et al. Eastern Cooperative Oncology Group randomized trials of observation versus maintenance therapy for patients with metastatic breast cancer in complete remission following induction treatment. *J Clin Oncol* 1998;16(5):1669–1676.

166. Glovsky MM. C1 esterase inhibitor transfusions in patients with hereditary angioedema. *Ann Allergy Asthma Immunol* 1998;80(6):439–440.

167. Sanchez Palacios A, Schamann Medina F, Garcia Marrero JA. Chronic

angioedema. Three relevant cases. *Allergol Immunopathol (Madr)* 1998;26(4):195–198.

168. Ben-Ami H, Edoute Y. [Paroxysmal nocturnal hemoglobinuria.] *Harefuah* 1998;134(3):178–180, 247.

169. Ichimiya M. Immunohistochemical study of ACTH and alpha-MSH in vitiligo patients successfully treated with a sex steroid-thyroid hormone mixture. *J Dermatol* 1999;26(8):502–506.

170. Fearfield LA, Gazzard B, Bunker CB. Aquagenic urticaria and human immunodeficiency virus infection: treatment with stanozolol. *Br J Dermatol* 1997;137(4):620–622.

171. Ehrenreich H, Halaris A, Ruether E, et al. Psychoendocrine sequelae of chronic testosterone deficiency. *J Psychiatr Res* 1999;33(5):379–387.

172. Bagatell C, Bremner W. Androgens in men—uses and abuses. *N Engl J Med* 1996;334(11):708–714.

173. Cummings DE, Kumar N, Bardin CW, et al. Prostate-sparing effects in primates of the potent androgen 7alpha-methyl-19-nortestosterone: a potential alternative to testosterone for androgen replacement and male contraception. *J Clin Endocrinol Metab* 1998;83(12):4212–4219.

174. Conway AJ, Handelsman DJ, Lording DW, et al. Use, misuse and abuse of androgens. The Endocrine Society of Australia consensus guidelines for androgen prescribing. *Med J Aust* 2000;172(5):220–224.

175. Behre HM, Kliesch S, Lemcke B, et al. Suppression of spermatogenesis to azoospermia by combined administration of GnRH antagonist and 19-nortestosterone cannot be maintained by this non-aromatizable androgen alone. *Hum Reprod* 2001;16(12):2570–2577.

176. Fenichel G, Pestronk A, Florence J, et al. A beneficial effect of oxandrolone in the treatment of Duchenne muscular dystrophy: a pilot study. *Neurology* 1997;48(5):1225–1226.

177. Fenichel GM, Griggs RC, Kissel J, Kramer TI, et al. A randomized efficacy and safety trial of oxandrolone in the treatment of Duchenne dystrophy. *Neurology* 2001;56(8):1075–1079.

178. Chekanov VS, Tchekanov GV, Rieder MA, et al. Force enhancement of skeletal muscle used for dynamic cardiomyoplasty and as a skeletal muscle ventricle. *ASAIO J* 1995;41(3):M499–M507.

179. Czesla M, Mehlhorn G, Fritzsche D, Asmussen G. Cardiomyoplasty–improvement of muscle fibre type transformation by an anabolic steroid (methenolone). *J Mol Cell Cardiol* 1997;29(11):2989–2996.

180. Fritzsche D, Krakor R, Asmussen G, et al. Anabolic steroids (methenolone) improve muscle performance and hemodynamic characteristics in cardiomyoplasty. *Ann Thorac Surg* 1995;59(4):961-969; discussion 969–970.

181. Loria RM, Padgett DA, Huynh PN. Regulation of the immune response by dehydroepiandrosterone and its metabolites. *J Endocrinol* 1996;150[Suppl]:S209–S220.

182. Padgett DA, MacCallum RC, Loria RM, Sheridan JF. Androstenediol-induced restoration of responsiveness to influenza vaccination in mice. *J Gerontol A Biol Sci Med Sci* 2000;55(9):B418–B424.

183. Daigle J, Carr DJ. Androstenediol antagonizes herpes simplex virus type 1-induced encephalitis through the augmentation of type I IFN production. *J Immunol* 1998;160(6):3060–3066.

184. Ben-Nathan D, Padgett DA, Loria RM. Androstenediol and dehydroepiandrosterone protect mice against lethal bacterial infections and lipopolysaccharide toxicity. *J Med Microbiol* 1999;48(5):425–431.

185. Loria RM, Conrad DH, Huff T, Carter H, et al. Androstenetriol and androstenediol. Protection against lethal radiation and restoration of immunity after radiation injury. *Ann N Y Acad Sci* 2000;917:860–867.

186. Hernandez-Pando R, De La Luz Streber M, Orozco H, et al. The effects of androstenediol and dehydroepiandrosterone on the course and cytokine profile of tuberculosis in BALB/c mice. *Immunology* 1998;95(2):234–241.

187. Hernandez-Pando R, Pavon L, Orozco EH, et al. Interactions between hormone-mediated and vaccine-mediated immunotherapy for pulmonary tuberculosis in BALB/c mice. *Immunology* 2000;100(3):391–398.

188. Ivanov IuB, Cherkasova SV, Kuzmin MD, Konstantinova OD. [The effect of steroid hormone preparations on the persistence and growth characteristics of staphylococci.] *Zh Mikrobiol Epidemiol Immunobiol* 1997(4):92–95.

189. Ferrandez MD, de la Fuente M, Fernandez E, Manso R. Anabolic steroids and lymphocyte function in sedentary and exercise-trained rats. *J Steroid Biochem Mol Biol* 1996;59(2):225–232.

190. Karrow NA, McCay JA, Brown R, et al. Oxymetholone modulates cell-mediated immunity in male B6C3F1 mice. *Drug Chem Toxicol* 2000;23(4):621–644.

191. Hughes TK, Fulep E, Juelich T, Smith EM, Stanton GJ. Modulation of immune responses by anabolic andro-genic steroids. *Int J Immunopharmacol* 1995;17(11):857–863.

192. Mossmann H, Benten WP, Galanos C, et al. Dietary testosterone suppresses protective responsiveness to *Plasmodium chabaudi* malaria. *Life Sci* 1997;60(11):839–848.

193. Johnson AS, Jones M, Morgan-Capner P, et al. Severe chickenpox in anabolic steroid user. *Lancet* 1995;345 (8962):1447–1448.

194. Huynh PN, Loria RM. Contrasting effects of alpha- and beta-androstenediol on oncogenic myeloid cell lines *in vitro*. *J Leukoc Biol* 1997;62(2):258–267.

195. He Q, Jiang D. A novel aminosteroid is active for proliferation inhibition and differentiation induction of human acute myeloid leukemia HL-60 cells. *Leuk Res* 1999;23(4):369–372.

196. Diamanti-Kandarakis E, Mitrakou A, Raptis S, et al. The effect of a pure antiandrogen receptor blocker, flutamide, on the lipid profile in the polycystic ovary syndrome. *J Clin Endocrinol Metab* 1998;83(8):2699–2705.

197. Dobs AS, Nguyen T, Pace C, Roberts CP. Differential effects of oral estrogen versus oral estrogen-androgen replacement therapy on body composition in postmenopausal women. *J Clin Endocrinol Metab* 2002;87(4):1509–1516.

198. Frye CA, Bayon LE. Mating stimuli influence endogenous variations in the neurosteroids 3alpha,5alpha-THP and 3alpha-Diol. *J Neuroendocrinol* 1999;11(11):839–847.

199. Di Carlo C, Palomba S, Tommaselli GA, et al. Use of leuprolide acetate plus tibolone in the treatment of severe premenstrual syndrome. *Fertil Steril* 2001;75(2):380–384.

200. Heinig J, Simon P, Weiss FU, et al. Treatment of menstruation-associated recurrence of hereditary pancreatitis with pharmacologic ovarian suppression. *Am J Med* 2002;113(2):164.

201. Adamson DL, Webb CM, Collins P. Esterified estrogens combined with methyltestosterone improve emotional well-being in postmenopausal women with chest pain and normal coronary angiograms. *Menopause* 2001;8(4):233–238.

202. Zoma W, Baker RS, Lang U, Clark KE. Hemodynamic response to tibolone in reproductive and nonreproductive tissues in the sheep. *Am J Obstet Gynecol* 2001;184(4):544–551.

203. Glusa E, Graser T, Wagner S, Oettel M. Mechanisms of relaxation of rat aorta in response to progesterone and synthetic progestins. *Maturitas* 1997;28(2):181–191.

204. Curry LA, Wagman DF. Qualitative description of the prevalence and use of anabolic androgenic steroids by United States powerlifters. *Percept Mot Skills* 1999;88(1):224–233.

205. American College of Sports Medicine. Position statement on the use and abuse of anabolic-androgenic steroids in sports. *Med Sci Sports* 1977;9:11–13.

206. American College of Sports Medicine. Position stand on the use and abuse of anabolic-androgenic steroids in sports. *Am J Sports Med* 1984;12:13–18.

207. American College of Sports Medicine. Position stand on the use of anabolic-androgenic steroids in sports. *Med Sci Sports Exercise* 1987;19(5):534–539.

208. Elashoff JD, Jacknow AD, Shain SG, Braunstein GD. Effects of anabolic-androgenic steroids on muscular strength. *Ann Intern Med* 1991;115(5):387–393.

209. Kuipers H, Peeze Binkhorst FM, Hartgens F, et al. Muscle ultrastructure after strength training with placebo or anabolic steroid. *Can J Appl Physiol* 1993;18(2):189–196.

210. Hyyppa S, Karvonen U, Rasanen LA, et al. Androgen receptors and skeletal muscle composition in trotters treated with nandrolone laureate. *Zentralbl Veterinarmed A* 1997;44(8):481–491.

211. Joumaa WH, Leoty C. Differential effects of nandrolone decanoate in fast and slow rat skeletal muscles. *Med Sci Sports Exerc* 2001;33(3):397–403.

212. Mayer M, Rosen F. Interaction of glucocorticoids and androgens with skeletal muscle. *Metabolism* 1977;27:937–962.

213. Raaka B, Finnerky M, Samuels H. The glucocorticoid antagonist 17 alpha-methyltestosterone binds to the 10S glucocorticoid receptor and blocks antagonist-mediated disassociation of the 10S oligomer to the 4S deoxyribonucleic acid-binding sub-unit. *Mol Endocrinol* 1989;3:322–341.

214. Jockenhovel F, Vogel E, Reinhardt W, Reinwein D. Effects of various modes of androgen substitution therapy on erythropoiesis. *Eur J Med Res* 1997;2(7):293–298.

215. Smith DA, Perry PJ. The efficacy of ergogenic agents in athletic competition. Part I: Androgenic-anabolic steroids. *Ann Pharmacother* 1992;26(4):520–528.

216. Hyyppa S. Effects of nandrolone treatment on recovery in horses after strenuous physical exercise. *J Vet Med A Physiol Pathol Clin Med* 2001;48(6):343–352.

217. Inhofe PD, Grana WA, Egle D, Min KW, Tomasek J. The effects of anabolic steroids on rat tendon. An ultrastructural, biomechanical, and biochemical analysis. *Am J Sports Med* 1995;23(2):227–232.

218. Yesalis CE, Kennedy NJ, Kopstein

AN, Bahrke MS. Anabolic-androgenic steroid use in the United States. *JAMA* 1993;270(10):1217–1221.

219. Glazer G. Atherogenic effects of anabolic steroids on serum lipid levels. A literature review. *Arch Intern Med* 1991;151(10):1925–1933.

220. Bausserman LL, Saritelli AL, Herbert PN. Effects of short-term stanozolol administration on serum lipoproteins in hepatic lipase deficiency. *Metabolism* 1997;46(9):992–996.

221. Inigo MA, Arrimadas E, Arroyo D. [Forty-three cycles of anabolic steroid treatment studied in athletes: the uses and secondary effects.] *Rev Clin Esp* 2000;200(3):133–138.

222. Heim J, Polard E. [HDL breakdown in an athlete taking anabolic steroids.] *Presse Med* 1996;25(9):458.

223. Glazer G, Suchman AL. Lack of demonstrated effect of nandrolone on serum lipids. *Metabolism* 1994;43(2):204–210.

224. Bagatell CJ, Bremner WJ. Androgen and progestogen effects on plasma lipids. *Prog Cardiovasc Dis* 1995;38(3):255–271.

225. Barrett CE. Testosterone and risk factors for cardiovascular disease in men. *Diabetes Metab* 1995;21(3):156–161.

226. Hislop MS, Ratanjee BD, Soule SG, Marais AD. Effects of anabolic-androgenic steroid use or gonadal testosterone suppression on serum leptin concentration in men. *Eur J Endocrinol* 1999;141(1):40–46.

227. Diamond MP, et al. Effects of methyltestosterone on insulin secretion and sensitivity in women. *J Clin Endocrinol Metab* 1998;83(12):4420–4425.

228. Joss EE, Zurbrugg RP, Tonz O, Mullis PE. Effect of growth hormone and oxandrolone treatment on glucose metabolism in Turner syndrome. A longitudinal study. *Horm Res* 2000;53(1):1–8.

229. Hobbs CJ, Jones RE, Plymate SR. Nandrolone, a 19-nortestosterone, enhances insulin-independent glucose uptake in normal men. *J Clin Endocrinol Metab* 1996;81(4):1582–1585.

230. Dhillon VS, Singh J, Singh H, Kler RS. *In vitro* and *in vivo* genotoxicity of hormonal drugs. VI. Fluoxymesterone. *Mutat Res* 1995;342(3–4):103–111.

231. Holden HE, Stoll RE, Blanchard KT. Oxymetholone: II. Evaluation in the Tg-AC transgenic mouse model for detection of carcinogens. *Toxicol Pathol* 1999;27(5):507–512.

232. Fisher M, Appleby M, Rittoo D, Cotter L. Myocardial infarction with extensive intracoronary thrombus induced by anabolic steroids. *Br J Clin Pract* 1996;50(4):222–223.

233. Godon P, Bonnefoy E, Guerard S, et al. [Myocardial infarction and anabolic steroid use. A case report.] *Arch Mal Coeur Vaiss* 2000;93(7):879–883.

234. Goldstein DR, Dobbs T, Krull B, Plumb VJ. Clenbuterol and anabolic steroids: a previously unreported cause of myocardial infarction with normal coronary arteriograms. *South Med J* 1998;91(8):780–784.

235. Hourigan LA, Rainbird AJ, Dooris M. Intracoronary stenting for acute myocardial infarction (AMI) in a 24-year-old man using anabolic androgenic steroids. *Aust N Z J Med* 1998;28(6):838–839.

236. Mewis C, Spyridopoulos I, Kuhlkamp V, Seipel L. Manifestation of severe coronary heart disease after anabolic drug abuse. *Clin Cardiol* 1996;19(2):153–155.

237. Nawroth PP, Bartsch P, Kasperk C, et al. [Thoracic pain in a power athlete.] *Internist (Berl)* 1997;38(10):984–988.

238. Parssinen M, Kujala U, Vartiainen E, et al. Increased premature mortality of competitive powerlifters suspected to have used anabolic agents. *Int J Sports Med* 2000;21(3):225–227.

239. Toyama M, Watanabe S, Kobayashi T, et al. Two cases of acute myocardial infarction associated with aplastic anemia during treatment with anabolic steroids. *Jpn Heart J* 1994;35(3):369–373.

240. Ferenchick GS, Adelman S. Myocardial infarction associated with anabolic steroid use in a previously healthy 37-year-old weight lifter. *Am Heart J* 1992;124(2):507–508.

241. McNutt RA, Ferenchick GS, Kirlin PC, Hamlin NJ. Acute myocardial infarction in a 22-year-old world class weight lifter using anabolic steroids. *Am J Cardiol* 1988;62:164.

242. Kennedy MC, Corrigan AB, Pilbeam ST. Myocardial infarction and cerebral haemorrhage in a young body builder taking anabolic steroids [Letter]. *Aust N Z J Med* 1993;23(6):713.

243. Kennedy C. Myocardial infarction in association with misuse of anabolic steroids. *Ulster Med J* 1993;62(2):174–176.

244. Lyngberg KK. [Myocardial infarction and death of a body builder after using anabolic steroids.] *Ugeskr Laeger* 1991;153(8):587–588.

245. Fineschi V, Baroldi G, Monciotti F, et al. Anabolic steroid abuse and cardiac sudden death: a pathologic study. *Arch Pathol Lab Med* 2001;125(2):253–255.

246. Dickerman RD, McConathy WJ, Schaller F, Zachariah NY. Echocardiography in fraternal twin bodybuilders with one abusing anabolic steroids. *Cardiology* 1997;88(1):50–51.

247. Schollert PV, Bendixen PM. [Dilated cardiomyopathy in a user of anabolic steroids.] *Ugeskr Laeger* 1993;155(16):1217–1218.

248. Dickerman RD, Schaller F, Prather I, McConathy WJ. Sudden cardiac death in a 20-year-old bodybuilder using anabolic steroids. *Cardiology* 1995;86(2):172–173.

249. Falkenberg M, Karlsson J, Ortenwall P. Peripheral arterial thrombosis in two young men using anabolic steroids. *Eur J Vasc Endovasc Surg* 1997;13(2):223–226.

250. Laroche GP. Steroid anabolic drugs and arterial complications in an athlete—a case history. *Angiology* 1990;41(11):964–969.

251. Akhter J, Hyder S, Ahmed M. Cerebrovascular accident associated with anabolic steroid use in a young man. *Neurology* 1994;44(12):2405–2406.

252. Robinson RJ, White S. Misuse of anabolic drugs [Letter]. *Br Med J* 1993;306(6869):61.

253. Siekierzynska-Czarnecka A, Polowiec Z, Kulawinska M, Rowinska-Zakrzewska E. [Death caused by pulmonary embolism in a body builder taking anabolic steroids (metanabol).] *Wiad Lek* 1990;43(19–20):972–975.

254. Visuri T, Lindholm H. Bilateral distal biceps tendon avulsions with use of anabolic steroids. *Med Sci Sports Exerc* 1994;26(8):941–944.

255. Di Bello V, Giorgi D, Bianchi M, et al. Effects of anabolic-androgenic steroids on weight-lifters' myocardium: an ultrasonic videodensitometric study. *Med Sci Sports Exerc* 1999;31(4):514–521.

256. Welder AA, Robertson JW, Fugate RD, Melchert RB. Anabolic-androgenic steroid-induced toxicity in primary neonatal rat myocardial cell cultures. *Toxicol Appl Pharmacol* 1995;133(2):328–342.

257. Ajayi AA, Mathur R, Halushka PV. Testosterone increases human platelet thromboxane A2 receptor density and aggregation responses. *Circulation* 1995;91(11):2742–2747.

258. Ferenchick G, Schwartz D, Ball M, Schwartz K. Androgenic-anabolic steroid abuse and platelet aggregation: a pilot study in weight lifters. *Am J Med Sci* 1992;303(2):78–82.

259. Ansell JE, Tiarks C, Fairchild VK. Coagulation abnormalities associated with the use of anabolic steroids. *Am Heart J* 1993:367–371.

260. Ferenchick GS, Hirokawa S, Mammen EF, Schwartz KA. Anabolic-androgenic steroid abuse in weight lifters: evidence for activation of the

hemostatic system. *Am J Hematol* 1995;49(4):282–288.

261. Kuipers H, Wijnen JA, Hartgens F, Willems SM. Influence of anabolic steroids on body composition, blood pressure, lipid profile and liver functions in body builders. *Int J Sports Med* 1991;12(4):413–418.

262. Riebe D, Fernhall B, Thompson PD. The blood pressure response to exercise in anabolic steroid users. *Med Sci Sports Exerc* 1992;24(6):633–637.

263. Pascual J, Teruel JL, Marcen R, Liano F, Ortuno J. Blood pressure after three different forms of correction of anemia in hemodialysis. *Int J Artif Organs* 1992;15(7):393–396.

264. Thompson PD, Sadaniantz A, Cullinane EM, et al. Left ventricular function is not impaired in weight-lifters who use anabolic steroids. *J Am Coll Cardiol* 1992;19(2):278–282.

265. Ebenbichler CF, Kaser S, Bodner J, et al. Hyperhomocysteinemia in bodybuilders taking anabolic steroids. *Eur J Intern Med* 2001;12(1):43–47.

266. Zaugg M, Jamali NZ, Lucchinetti E, et al. Anabolic-androgenic steroids induce apoptotic cell death in adult rat ventricular myocytes. *J Cell Physiol* 2001;187(1):90–95.

267. Alvaro D, Piat C, Francia C, et al. Ultrastructural features of danazol-induced cholestasis: a case study. *Ultrastruct Pathol* 1996;20(5):491–495.

268. Harkin KR, Cowan LA, Andrews GA, et al. Hepatotoxicity of stanozolol in cats. *J Am Vet Med Assoc* 2000;217(5):681–684.

269. Hirose H, Ohishi A, Nakamura H, et al. Fatal splenic rupture in anabolic steroid-induced peliosis in a patient with myelodysplastic syndrome. *Br J Haematol* 1991;78(1):128–129.

270. Gunji T, Ohnishi S, Hippo Y, et al. [A case of severe drug-induced peliosis hepatis with radiologically confirmed healing.] *Nippon Shokakibyo Gakkai Zasshi* 1998;95(12):1378–1381.

271. Boada LD, Zumbado M, Torrres S, et al. Evaluation of acute and chronic hepatotoxic effects exerted by anabolic-androgenic steroid stanozolol in adult male rats. *Arch Toxicol* 1999;73(8-9):465–472.

272. Wood P, Yin JA. Oxymetholone hepatotoxicity enhanced by concomitant use of cyclosporin A in a bone marrow transplant patient. *Clin Lab Haematol* 1994;16(2):201–204.

273. Tsukamoto N, Uchiyama T, Takeuchi T, et al. Fatal outcome of a patient with severe aplastic anemia after treatment with methenolone acetate. *Ann Hematol* 1993;67(1):41–43.

274. Grunenberg R, Banik N, Kruger J. [Alanine aminotransferase (ALAT,

GPT): a reevaluation of exclusion limits for blood donors.] *Infusionsther Transfusionsmed* 1995;22(3):145–151.

275. Dickerman RD, Pertusi RM, Zachariah NY, et al. Anabolic steroid-induced hepatotoxicity: is it overstated? *Clin J Sport Med* 1999;9(1):34–39.

276. Pertusi R, Dickerman RD, McConathy WJ. Evaluation of aminotransferase elevations in a bodybuilder using anabolic steroids: hepatitis or rhabdomyolysis? *J Am Osteopath Assoc* 2001;101(7):391–394.

277. Bagia S, Hewitt PM, Morris DL. Anabolic steroid-induced hepatic adenomas with spontaneous haemorrhage in a bodybuilder. *Aust N Z J Surg* 2000;70(9):686–687.

278. de Menis E, Tramontin P, Conte N. Danazol and multiple hepatic adenomas: peculiar clinical findings in an acromegalic patient. *Horm Metab Res* 1999;31(8):476–477.

279. Friedl K. Reappraisal of the health risks associated with high doses of oral and injectable androgenic steroids. *NIDA Res Monogr Ser* 1990;102:142–177.

280. Goldman B. Liver carcinoma in an athlete taking anabolic steroids. *J Am Osteopath Assoc* 1985;85:56.

281. Creagh T, Rubin A, Evans D. Hepatic tumours induced by anabolic steroids in an athlete. *J Clin Pathol* 1988;41:441–443.

282. Fujino Y, Ku Y, Suzuki Y, et al. Ampullary carcinoma developing after androgenic steroid therapy for aplastic anemia: report of a case. *Surgery* 2001;129(4):501–503.

283. Stannard JP, Bucknell AL. Rupture of the triceps tendon associated with steroid injections. *Am J Sports Med* 1993;21(3):482–485.

284. Liow RY, Tavares S. Bilateral rupture of the quadriceps tendon associated with anabolic steroids. *Br J Sports Med* 1995;29(2):77–79.

285. Faergemann C, Laursen JO. [Simultaneous bilateral rupture of the quadriceps tendon.] *Ugeskr Laeger* 1998;160(9):1329–1330.

286. Laseter JT, Russell JA. Anabolic steroid-induced tendon pathology: a review of the literature. *Med Sci Sports Exerc* 1991;23(1):1–3.

287. Evans NA, Bowrey DJ, Newman GR. Ultrastructural analysis of ruptured tendon from anabolic steroid users. *Injury* 1998;29(10):769–73.

288. Braseth NR, Allison EJ Jr, Gough JE. Exertional rhabdomyolysis in a body builder abusing anabolic androgenic steroids. *Eur J Emerg Med* 2001;8(2):155–157.

289. Moore W. Anabolic steroid use in

adolescence. *JAMA* 1988;260:3484–3486.

290. Abu-Shakra S, Alhalabi MS, Nachtman FC, et al. Anabolic steroids induce injury and apoptosis of differentiated skeletal muscle. *J Neurosci Res* 1997;47(2):186–197.

291. Abu-Shakra SR, Nachtman FC. Anabolic steroids induce skeletal muscle injury and immediate early gene expression through a receptor-independent mechanism. *Ann N Y Acad Sci* 1995;761:395–399.

292. Bisschop A, Gayan-Ramirez G, Rollier H, et al. Effects of nandrolone decanoate on respiratory and peripheral muscles in male and female rats. *J Appl Physiol* 1997;82(4):1112–1118.

293. Gayan-Ramirez G, Rollier H, Vanderhoydonc F, et al. Nandrolone decanoate does not enhance training effects but increases IGF-I mRNA in rat diaphragm. *J Appl Physiol* 2000;88(1):26–34.

294. Bertelloni S, Baroncelli GI, Sorrentino MC, et al. Androgen-receptor blockade does not impair bone mineral density in adolescent females. *Calcif Tissue Int* 1997;61(1):1–5.

295. Sklarek HM, Mantovani RP, Erens E, et al. AIDS in a bodybuilder using anabolic steroids [Letter]. *N Engl J Med* 1984;311:1701.

296. Scott M, Scott M Jr. HIV infection associated with injections of anabolic steroids [Letter]. *JAMA* 1989;262:207–208.

297. Henrion R, Mandelbrot L, Delfieu D. Contamination par le VIH à la suite d'injections d'anabolisants [Letter]. *Presse Med* 1992;21(5):218.

298. Aitken C, Delalande C, Stanton K. Pumping iron, risking infection? Exposure to hepatitis C, hepatitis B and HIV among anabolic-androgenic steroid injectors in Victoria, Australia. *Drug Alcohol Depend* 2002;65(3):303–308.

299. Crampin AC, Lamagni TL, Hope VD, et al. The risk of infection with HIV and hepatitis B in individuals who inject steroids in England and Wales. *Epidemiol Infect* 1998;121(2):381–386.

300. Plaus WJ, Hermann G. The surgical management of superficial infections caused by atypical mycobacteria. *Surgery* 1991;110(1):99–103.

301. Khankhanian NK, Hammers YA, Kowalski P. Exuberant local tissue reaction to intramuscular injection of nandrolone decanoate (Deca-Durabolin)—a steroid compound in a sesame seed oil base—mimicking soft tissue malignant tumors: a case report and review of the literature. *Mil Med* 1992;157(12):670–674.

302. Evans NA. Local complications of self administered anabolic steroid

injections. *Br J Sports Med* 1997; 31(4):349–350.

303. Spiga L, Gorrini G, Ferraris L, Odaglia G, Frassetto G. [Unilateral gynecomastia induced by the use of anabolic steroids. A clinical case report.] *Minerva Med* 1992;83(9):575–580.

304. Calzada L, Torres-Calleja J, Martinez JM, Pedron N. Measurement of androgen and estrogen receptors in breast tissue from subjects with anabolic steroid-dependent gynecomastia. *Life Sci* 2001;69(13):1465–1469.

305. Reyes RJ, Zicchi S, Hamed H, et al. Surgical correction of gynaecomastia in bodybuilders. *Br J Clin Pract* 1995;49(4):177–179.

306. Babigian A, Silverman RT. Management of gynecomastia due to use of anabolic steroids in bodybuilders. *Plast Reconstr Surg* 2001;107(1):240–242.

307. Colacurci N, Mele D, De Franciscis P, et al. Effects of tibolone on the breast. *Eur J Obstet Gynecol Reprod Biol* 1998;80(2):235–238.

308. Blanco A, Moya L, Flores R, Aguera E, Monterde JG. Effects of anabolic implants of oestradiol alone or in combination with trenbolone acetate on the ultrastructure of mammary glands in female lambs regarding their interference in prolactin secretion. *J Vet Med A Physiol Pathol Clin Med* 2002;49(1):13–17.

309. Birrell SN, Bentel JM, Hickey TE, et al. Androgens induce divergent proliferative responses in human breast cancer cell lines. *J Steroid Biochem Mol Biol* 1995;52(5):459–467.

310. Gingras S, Moriggl R, Groner B, Simard J. Induction of 3beta-hydroxysteroid dehydrogenase/delta5-delta4 isomerase type 1 gene transcription in human breast cancer cell lines and in normal mammary epithelial cells by interleukin-4 and interleukin-13. *Mol Endocrinol* 1999;13(1):66–81.

311. Huynh PN, Carter WH Jr, Loria RM. 17 alpha androstenediol inhibition of breast tumor cell proliferation in estrogen receptor-positive and -negative cell lines. *Cancer Detect Prev* 2000;24(5):435–444.

312. Anderson RA, Martin CW, Kung AW, et al. 7Alpha-methyl-19-nortestosterone maintains sexual behavior and mood in hypogonadal men. *J Clin Endocrinol Metab* 1999;84(10):3556–3562.

313. Feinberg MJ, Lumia AR, McGinnis MY. The effect of anabolic–androgenic steroids on sexual behavior and reproductive tissues in male rats. *Physiol Behav* 1997;62(1):23–30.

314. Allnutt S, Chaimowitz G. Anabolic steroid withdrawal depression: a case report [Letter]. *Can J Psychiatry* 1994;39(5):317–318.

315. Anderson RA, Wallace AM, Wu FC. Comparison between testosterone enanthate-induced azoospermia and oligozoospermia in a male contraceptive study. III. Higher 5 alpha-reductase activity in oligozoospermic men administered supraphysiological doses of testosterone. *J Clin Endocrinol Metab* 1996;81(3):902–908.

316. Anonymous. Male infertility due to anabolic steroids. *Prescrire Int* 1999; 8(40):54.

317. Sorensen MB, Ingerslev HJ. [Azoospermia in 2 body-builders after taking anabolic steroids.] *Ugeskr Laeger* 1995;157(8):1044–1045.

318. Boyadjiev NP, Georgieva KN, Massaldjieva RI, Gueorguiev SI. Reversible hypogonadism and azoospermia as a result of anabolic–androgenic steroid use in a bodybuilder with personality disorder. *A case report. J Sports Med Phys Fitness* 2000;40(3):271–274.

319. Gazvani MR, Buckett W, Luckas MJ, et al. Conservative management of azoospermia following steroid abuse. *Hum Reprod* 1997;12(8):1706–1708.

320. Turek PJ, et al. The reversibility of anabolic steroid-induced azoospermia. *J Urol* 1995;153(5):1628–1630.

321. Anshel MH, Russell KG. Examining athletes' attitudes toward using anabolic steroids and their knowledge of the possible effects. *J Drug Educ* 1997;27(2):121–145.

322. Jin B, Turner L, Walters WA, Handelsman DJ. The effects of chronic high dose androgen or estrogen treatment on the human prostate [corrected]. *J Clin Endocrinol Metab* 1996;81(12):4290–4295.

323. Jeyaraj DA, Udayakumar TS, Rajalakshmi M, et al. Effects of long-term administration of androgens and estrogen on rhesus monkey prostate: possible induction of benign prostatic hyperplasia. *J Androl* 2000;21(6):833–841.

324. Collins AT, Robinson EJ, Neal DE. Benign prostatic stromal cells are regulated by basic fibroblast growth factor and transforming growth factor-beta 1. *J Endocrinol* 1996;151(2):315–322.

325. Wemyss HS, Hamdy FC, Hastie KJ. Steroid abuse in athletes, prostatic enlargement and bladder outflow obstruction—is there a relationship? *Br J Urol* 1994;74(4):476–478.

326. Froehner M, Fischer R, Leike S, et al. Intratesticular leiomyosarcoma in a young man after high dose doping with Oral-Turinabol: a case report. *Cancer* 1999;86(8):1571–1575.

327. Collett GP, Betts AM, Johnson MI, et al. Peroxisome proliferator-activated receptor alpha is an androgen-responsive gene in human prostate and is highly expressed in prostatic adenocarcinoma. *Clin Cancer Res* 2000;6(8):3241–3248.

328. Gann PH, Hennekens CH, Ma J, et al. Prospective study of sex hormone levels and risk of prostate cancer. *J Natl Cancer Inst* 1996;88(16):1118–1126.

329. Noble R. The development of prostatic adenocarcinoma in Nb rats following prolonged sex hormone administration. *Cancer Res* 1977;37:1929–1933.

330. Zhu W, Zhang JS, Young CY. Silymarin inhibits function of the androgen receptor by reducing nuclear localization of the receptor in the human prostate cancer cell line LNCaP. *Carcinogenesis* 2001;22(9):1399–1403.

331. Guillemette C, Hum DW, Belanger A. Specificity of glucuronosyltransferase activity in the human cancer cell line LNCaP, evidence for the presence of at least two glucuronosyltransferase enzymes. *J Steroid Biochem Mol Biol* 1995;55(3–4):355–362.

332. Zhang S, Murtha PE, Young CY. Defining a functional androgen responsive element in the 5' far upstream flanking region of the prostate-specific antigen gene. *Biochem Biophys Res Commun* 1997;231(3):784–788.

333. Wu AH, Whittemore AS, Kolonel LN, et al. Lifestyle determinants of 5alpha-reductase metabolites in older African American, white, and Asian American men. *Cancer Epidemiol Biomarkers Prev* 2001;10(5):533–538.

334. Hartung R, Gerth J, Funfstuck R, Grone HJ, Stein G. End-stage renal disease in a bodybuilder: a multifactorial process or simply doping? *Nephrol Dial Transplant* 2001;16(1):163–165.

335. Bryden AA, Rothwell PJ, O'Reilly PH. Anabolic steroid abuse and renal-cell carcinoma. *Lancet* 1995; 346(8985):1306–1307.

336. Edmondson RJ, Monaghan JM, Davies BR. The human ovarian surface epithelium is an androgen responsive tissue. *Br J Cancer* 2002;86(6):879–885.

337. Baker J. A report on alterations to the speaking and singing voices of four women following hormonal therapy with virilizing agents. *J Voice* 1999;13(4):496–507.

338. Copeland J, Peters R, Dillon P. Anabolic–androgenic steroid dependence in a woman. *Aust N Z J Psychiatry* 1998;32(4):589.

339. Anonymous. Tibolone: new preparation. Menopausal symptoms: oestrogen-progestogen combinations are still the reference treatment. *Prescrire Int* 2002;11(59):79–82.

340. Gerritsma EJ, Brocaar MP, Hakkesteegt MM, Birkenhager JC. Virilization of the voice in post-menopausal women due

to the anabolic steroid nandrolone decanoate (Deca-Durabolin). The effects of medication for one year. *Clin Otolaryngol* 1994;19(1):79–84.

341. Strauss R, Liggett M, Lanese R. Anabolic steroid use and perceived effects in ten weight-trained woman athletes. *JAMA* 1985;253:2871–2873.

342. Albertazzi P, Natale V, Barbolini C, et al. The effect of tibolone versus continuous combined norethisterone acetate and oestradiol on memory, libido and mood of postmenopausal women: a pilot study. *Maturitas* 2000;36(3):223–229.

343. Scott M, Scott AM. Effects of anabolic-androgenic steroids on the pilosebaceous unit. *Cutis* 1992;50(2):113–116.

344. Merkle T, Landthaler M, Braun FO. [Acne conglobata-like exacerbation of acne vulgaris following administration of anabolic steroids and vitamin B complex-containing preparations.] *Hautarzt* 1990;41(5):280–282.

345. Hibberts NA, Howell AE, Randall VA. Balding hair follicle dermal papilla cells contain higher levels of androgen receptors than those from non-balding scalp. *J Endocrinol* 1998;156(1):59–65.

346. Scott M, Scott M, Scott AM. Linear keloids resulting from abuse of anabolic androgenic steroid drugs. *Cutis* 1994;53(1):41–43.

347. Dickerman RD, Jaikumar S. Secondary partial empty sella syndrome in an elite bodybuilder. *Neurol Res* 2001;23(4):336–338.

348. Broeder CE, Quindry J, Brittingham K, et al. The Andro Project: physiological and hormonal influences of androstenedione supplementation in men 35 to 65 years old participating in a high-intensity resistance training program. *Arch Intern Med* 2000;160(20):3093–3104.

349. Blasberg ME, Langan CJ, Clark AS. The effects of 17 alpha-methyltestosterone, methandrostenolone, and nandrolone decanoate on the rat estrous cycle. *Physiol Behav* 1997;61(2):265–272.

350. Dickerman RD, Jaikumar S. The hiccup reflex arc and persistent hiccups with high-dose anabolic steroids: is the brainstem the steroid-responsive locus? *Clin Neuropharmacol* 2001;24(1):62–64.

351. Bochnia M, Medras M, Pospiech L, Jaworska M. Poststeroid balance disorder—a case report in a body builder. *Int J Sports Med* 1999;20(6):407–409.

352. Bolding G, Sherr L, Elford J. Use of anabolic steroids and associated health risks among gay men attending London gyms. *Addiction* 2002;97(2):195–203.

353. Clark AS, Harrold EV, Fast AS. Anabolic-androgenic steroid effects on the sexual behavior of intact male rats. *Horm Behav* 1997;31(1):35–46.

354. Lane PR, Massey KL, Worobetz LJ, et al. Acute hereditary coproporphyria induced by the androgenic/anabolic steroid methandrostenolone (Dianabol). *J Am Acad Dermatol* 1994:308–312.

355. Leckman JF, Scahill L. Possible exacerbation of tics by androgenic steroids [Letter]. *N Engl J Med* 1990;322(23):1674.

356. Deyssig R, Weissel M. Ingestion of androgenic-anabolic steroids induces mild thyroidal impairment in male body builders. *J Clin Endocrinol Metab* 1993;76(4):1069–1071.

357. Illera JC, Silvan G, Blass A, Martinez MM, Illera M. The effect of clenbuterol on adrenal function in rats. *Analyst* 1998;123(12):2521–2524.

358. Agren G, Thiblin I, Tirassa P, Lundeberg T, Stenfors C. Behavioural anxiolytic effects of low-dose anabolic androgenic steroid treatment in rats. *Physiol Behav* 1999;66(3):503–509.

359. Bronson FH, Nguyen KQ, De La Rosa J. Effect of anabolic steroids on behavior and physiological characteristics of female mice. *Physiol Behav* 1996;59(1):49–55.

360. Harrison RJ, Connor DF, Nowak C, et al. Chronic anabolic-androgenic steroid treatment during adolescence increases anterior hypothalamic vasopressin and aggression in intact hamsters. *Psychoneuroendocrinology* 2000;25(4):317–338.

361. Copeland J, Peters R, Dillon P. Anabolic–androgenic steroid use disorders among a sample of Australian competitive and recreational users. *Drug Alcohol Depend* 2000;60(1):91–96.

362. Dukarm CP, Byrd RS, Auinger P, Weitzman M. Illicit substance use, gender, and the risk of violent behavior among adolescents. *Arch Pediatr Adolesc Med* 1996;150(8):797–801.

363. Isacsson G, Garle M, Ljung EB, Asgard U, Bergman U. Anabolic steroids and violent crime—an epidemiological study at a jail in Stockholm, Sweden. *Compr Psychiatry* 1998;39(4):203–205.

364. Dalby JT. Brief anabolic steroid use and sustained behavioral reaction [Letter]. *Am J Psychiatry* 1992;149(2):271–272.

365. Kennedy MC, Lawrence C. Anabolic steroid abuse and cardiac death. *Med J Aust* 1993;158(5):346–348.

366. Bond AJ, Choi PY, Pope HG Jr. Assessment of attentional bias and mood in users and non-users of anabolic-androgenic steroids. *Drug Alcohol Depend* 1995;37(3):241–245.

367. Tenover JS. Effects of testosterone supplementation in the aging male. *J Clin Endocrinol Metab* 1992; 75:1092–1098.

368. Hannan CJ Jr, Friedl KE, Zold A, et al. Psychological and serum homovanillic acid changes in men administered androgenic steroids. *Psychoneuroendocrinology* 1991;16(4):335–343.

369. Ellingrod VL, Perry PJ, Yates WR, et al. The effects of anabolic steroids on driving performance as assessed by the Iowa Driver Simulator. *Am J Drug Alcohol Abuse* 1997;23(4):623–636.

370. Clark AS, Fast AS. Comparison of the effects of 17 alpha-methyltestosterone, methandrostenolone, and nandrolone decanoate on the sexual behavior of castrated male rats. *Behav Neurosci* 1996;110(6):1478–1486.

371. Clark AS, Blasberg ME, Brandling-Bennett EM. Stanozolol, oxymetholone, and testosterone cypionate effects on the rat estrous cycle. *Physiol Behav* 1998;63(2):287–295.

372. Driessen M, Muessigbrodt H, Dilling H, Driessen B. Child sexual abuse associated with anabolic androgenic steroid use. *Am J Psychiatry* 1996;153(10):1369.

373. Freinhar J, Alvarez W. Androgen-induced hypomania. *J Clin Psychiatry* 1985;46(8):354–355.

374. Dean CE. Prasterone (DHEA) and mania. *Ann Pharmacother* 2000;34(12):1419–1422.

375. Brower KJ, Eliopulos GA, Blow FC, et al. Evidence for physical and psychological dependence on anabolic androgenic steroids in eight weight lifters. *Am J Psychiatry* 1990;147(4):510–512.

376. Pope H, Katz D. Bodybuilder's psychosis [Letter]. *Lancet* 1987 April; 1(8537):863.

377. American Psychiatric Association. *Diagnostic and statistical manual of mental disorders,* 3rd ed., revised. Washington, DC: American Psychiatric Association, 1987.

378. Kashkin K, Kleber H. Hooked on hormones? An anabolic steroid addiction hypothesis. *JAMA* 1989;262:3166–3170.

379. Tennant F, Black D, Voy R. Anabolic steroid dependence with opioid-type features [Letter]. *N Engl J Med* 1988;319:578.

380. Malone DJ, Dimeff RJ. The use of fluoxetine in depression associated with anabolic steroid withdrawal: a case series. *J Clin Psychiatry* 1992;53(4):130–132.

381. Rosse R, Deutsch F. Hooked on hormones [Letter]. *JAMA* 1990;263:2048–2049.

382. Elford J, Bolding G, Maguire M, Sherr L. Do gay men discuss HIV risk

reduction with their GP? *AIDS Care* 2000;12(3):287–290.

383. Giorgi A, Weatherby RP, Murphy PW. Muscular strength, body composition and health responses to the use of testosterone enanthate: a double blind study. *J Sci Med Sport* 1999;2(4):341–355.

384. Gebhardt DO. [A patient with an unexplained low level of high-density-lipoprotein cholesterol.] *Ned Tijdschr Geneeskd* 1997;141(13):651–652.

385. Hartgens F, Kuipers H, Wijnen JA, Keizer HA. Body composition, cardiovascular risk factors and liver function in long-term androgenic-anabolic steroids using bodybuilders three months after drug withdrawal. *Int J Sports Med* 1996;17(6):429–433.

386. Hartgens F, Van Marken Lichtenbelt WD, Ebbing S, et al. Body composition and anthropometry in bodybuilders: regional changes due to nandrolone decanoate administration. *Int J Sports Med* 2001;22(3):235–241.

387. Fowler LJ, Smith SS, Snider T, Schultz MR. Apocrine metaplasia in gynecomastia by fine needle aspiration as a possible indicator of anabolic steroid use. A report of two cases. *Acta Cytol* 1996;40(4):734–738.

388. Gryngarten M, Bedecarras P, Ayuso S, et al. Clinical assessment and serum hormonal profile in prepubertal hypertrichosis. *Horm Res* 2000;54(1):20–25.

389. Barron D, Barbosa J, Pascual JA, Segura J. Direct determination of anabolic steroids in human urine by online solid-phase extraction/liquid chromatography/mass spectrometry. *J Mass Spectrom* 1996;31(3):309–319.

390. Bowers LD, Segura J. Anabolic steroids, athletic drug testing, and the Olympic Games. *Clin Chem* 1996;42(7):999–1000.

391. Zhang XX, Li J, Gao J, Sun L, Chang WB. Determination of doping methyltestosterone by capillary electrophoresis immunological analysis with thermally reversible hydrogel and laser-induced fluorescence. *Electrophoresis* 1999;20(10):1998–2002.

392. Brind J, Borofsky N, Chervinsky K, et al. A simple, differential extraction method for the simultaneous direct radioimmunoassay of androgens and androgen glucuronides in human serum. *Steroids* 1996;61(7):429–432.

393. Cirimele V, Kintz P, Ludes B. Testing of the anabolic stanozolol in human hair by gas chromatography-negative ion chemical ionization mass spectrometry. *J Chromatogr B Biomed Sci Appl* 2000;740(2):265–271.

394. Deng XS, Kurosu A, Pounder DJ. Detection of anabolic steroids in head hair. *J Forensic Sci* 1999;44(2):343–346.

395. Gaillard Y, Vayssette F, Balland A, Pepin G. Gas chromatographic-tandem mass spectrometric determination of anabolic steroids and their esters in hair. Application in doping control and meat quality control. *J Chromatogr B Biomed Sci Appl* 1999;735(2):189–205.

396. Gaillard Y, Vayssette F, Pepin G. Compared interest between hair analysis and urinalysis in doping controls. Results for amphetamines, corticosteroids and anabolic steroids in racing cyclists. *Forensic Sci Int* 2000;107(1–3):361–379.

397. De Brabander HF, Batjoens P, Courtheyn D, et al. Comparison of the possibilities of gas chromatography-mass spectrometry and tandem mass spectrometry systems for the analysis of anabolics in biological material. *J Chromatogr A* 1996;750(1–2):105–114.

398. Hagedorn HW, Zankl H, Grund C, Schulz R. [Detection of doping compounds in the racing pigeon.] *Berl Munch Tierarztl Wochenschr* 1996;109(9):344–347.

399. Hagedorn HW, Zankl H, Grund C, Schulz R. Excretion of the anabolic steroid boldenone by racing pigeons. *Am J Vet Res* 1997;58(3):224–227.

400. Hold KM, Borges CR, Wilkins DG, et al. Detection of nandrolone, testosterone, and their esters in rat and human hair samples. *J Anal Toxicol* 1999;23(6):416–423.

401. Hold KM, Wilkins DG, Crouch DJ, et al. Detection of stanozolol in hair by negative ion chemical ionization mass spectrometry. *J Anal Toxicol* 1996;20(6):345–349.

402. Catlin DH, Ahrens BD, Kucherova Y. Detection of norbolethone, an anabolic steroid never marketed, in athletes' urine. *Rapid Commun Mass Spectrom* 2002;16(13):1273–1275.

403. Aguilera R, Catlin DH, Becchi M, et al. Screening urine for exogenous testosterone by isotope ratio mass spectrometric analysis of one pregnanediol and two androstanediols. *J Chromatogr B Biomed Sci Appl* 1999;727(1–2):95–105.

404. Aguilera R, Chapman TE, Starcevic B, et al. Performance characteristics of a carbon isotope ratio method for detecting doping with testosterone based on urine diols: controls and athletes with elevated testosterone/epitestosterone ratios. *Clin Chem* 2001;47(2):292–300.

405. Ayotte C, Goudreault D, Charlebois A. Testing for natural and synthetic anabolic agents in human urine. *J Chromatogr B Biomed Appl* 1996;687(1):3–25.

406. Coutts SB, Kicman AT, Hurst DT, Cowan DA. Intramuscular adminis-

tration of 5 alpha-dihydrotestosterone heptanoate: changes in urinary hormone profile. *Clin Chem* 1997;43(11):2091–2098.

407. Galan Martin AM, Marino JI, Garcia de Tiedra MP, et al. Determination of nandrolone and metabolites in urine samples from sedentary persons and sportsmen. *J Chromatogr B Biomed Sci Appl* 2001;761(2):229–236.

408. Garle M, Ocka R, Palonek E, Bjorkhem I. Increased urinary testosterone/epitestosterone ratios found in Swedish athletes in connection with a national control program. Evaluation of 28 cases. *J Chromatogr B Biomed Appl* 1996;687(1):55–59.

409. Epstein S, Eliakim A. Drug testing in elite athletes—the Israeli perspective. *Isr Med Assoc J* 1999;1(2):79–82.

410. Impens S, De Wasch K, De Brabander H. Determination of anabolic steroids with gas chromatography-ion trap mass spectrometry using hydrogen as carrier gas. *Rapid Commun Mass Spectrom* 2001;15(24):2409–2414.

411. Joos PE, Van Ryckeghem M. Liquid chromatography-tandem mass spectrometry of some anabolic steroids. *Anal Chem* 1999;71(20):4701–4710.

412. Bean KA, Henion JD. Direct determination of anabolic steroid conjugates in human urine by combined high-performance liquid chromatography and tandem mass spectrometry. *J Chromatogr B Biomed Sci Appl* 1997;690(1–2):65–75.

413. Bowers LD, Borts DJ. Separation and confirmation of anabolic steroids with quadrupole ion trap tandem mass spectrometry. *J Chromatogr B Biomed Appl* 1996;687(1):69–78.

414. Bowers LD, Borts DJ. Evaluation of selected-ion storage ion-trap mass spectrometry for detecting urinary anabolic agents. *Clin Chem* 1997;43[6 Pt 1]:1033–1039.

415. Gonzalo-Lumbreras R, Izquierdo-Hornillos R. Optimization of the high-performance liquid chromatographic separation of a complex mixture containing urinary steroids, boldenone and bolasterone: application to urine samples. *J Chromatogr B Biomed Sci Appl* 2000;742(1):47–57.

416. Gonzalo-Lumbreras R, Izquierdo-Hornillos R. High-performance liquid chromatographic optimization study for the separation of natural and synthetic anabolic steroids. Application to urine and pharmaceutical samples. *J Chromatogr B Biomed Sci Appl* 2000;742(1):1–11.

417. Gonzalo-Lumbreras R, Pimentel-Trapero D, Izqierdo-Hornillos R. Solvent and solid-phase extraction of natural and synthetic anabolic steroids

in human urine. *J Chromatogr B Biomed Sci Appl* 2001;754(2):419–425.

418. Yoon JM, Lee KH. Gas chromatographic and mass spectrometric analysis of conjugated steroids in urine. *J Biosci* 2001;26(5):627–634.

419. Howe CJ, Handelsman DJ. Use of filter paper for sample collection and transport in steroid pharmacology. *Clin Chem* 1997;43[8 Pt 1]:1408–1415.

420. Segura J, Pichini S, Peng SH, de la Torre X. Hair analysis and detectability of single dose administration of androgenic steroid esters. *Forensic Sci Int* 2000;107(1–3):347–359.

421. De Cock KJ, Delbeke FT, Van Eenoo P, et al. Detection and determination of anabolic steroids in nutritional supplements. *J Pharm Biomed Anal* 2001;25(5–6):843–852.

422. Choi MH, Chung BC. N-isobutyloxycarbonylation for improved detection of 3′-hydroxystanozolol and its 17-epimer in doping control. *Analyst* 2001;126(3):306–309.

423. Fears TR, Ziegler RG, Donaldson JL, et al. Reproducibility studies and interlaboratory concordance for androgen assays of male plasma hormone levels. *Cancer Epidemiol Biomarkers Prev* 2002;11(8):785–789.

424. Wudy SA, Homoki J, Teller WM. [Gas chromatography-mass spectrometry determination of plasma 5 alpha-androstane-3 alpha,17 beta-diol and 5 alpha-androstane-3 alpha,17 beta-diol glucuronide in children with premature and normal puberty.] *Klin Padiatr* 1996;208(6):334–338.

425. Wudy SA, Wachter UA, Homoki J, Teller WM. 5 Alpha-androstane-3 alpha, 17 beta-diol and 5 alpha-androstane-3 alpha, 17 beta-diol-glucuronide in plasma of normal children, adults and patients with idiopathic hirsutism: a mass spectrometric study. *Eur J Endocrinol* 1996;134(1):87–92.

426. Van Eenoo P, Delbeke FT, de Jong FH, De Backer P. Endogenous origin of norandrosterone in female urine: indirect evidence for the production of 19-norsteroids as by-products in the conversion from androgen to estrogen. *J Steroid Biochem Mol Biol* 2001;78(4):351–357.

427. Falsetti L, Rosina B, De Fusco D. Serum levels of 3alpha-androstanediol glucuronide in hirsute and non hirsute women. *Eur J Endocrinol* 1998;138(4):421–424.

428. Joura EA, Sator MO, Geusau A, et al. [The clinical value of 3 alpha-androstanediol-glucuronide in hirsute women.] *Wien Klin Wochenschr* 1997;109(23):919–921.

429. Joura EA, Geusau A, Schneider B, Soregi G, Huber JC. Serum 3 alpha-androstanediol-glucuronide is decreased in nonhirsute women with acne vulgaris. *Fertil Steril* 1996;66(6):1033–1035.

430. Le Bizec B, Gaudin I, Monteau F, et al. Consequence of boar edible tissue consumption on urinary profiles of nandrolone metabolites. I. Mass spectrometric detection and quantification of 19-norandrosterone and 19-noretiocholanolone in human urine. *Rapid Commun Mass Spectrom* 2000;14(12):1058–1065.

431. De Wasch K, Le Bizec B, De Brabander H, et al. Consequence of boar edible tissue consumption on urinary profiles of nandrolone metabolites. II. Identification and quantification of 19-norsteroids responsible for 19-norandrosterone and 19-noretiocholanolone excretion in human urine. *Rapid Commun Mass Spectrom* 2001;15(16):1442–1447.

432. Maghuin-Rogister G. [The use of anabolic hormones and growth promoters in meat production and its consequences to man.] *J Pharm Belg* 1995;50(5):455–460.

433. Ruiter A. EuroResidue III. Third conference on residues of veterinary drugs in food. *Z Lebensm Unters Forsch* 1996;203(3):F1.

434. Kicman AT, Cowan DA, Myhre L, et al. Effect on sports drug tests of ingesting meat from steroid (methenolone)-treated livestock. *Clin Chem* 1994:2084–2087.

435. Clouet AS, Le Bizec B, Montrade MP, et al. Identification of endogenous 19-nortestosterone in pregnant ewes by gas chromatography-mass spectrometry. *Analyst* 1997;122(5):471–474.

436. Dehennin L, Bonnaire Y, Plou P. Human nutritional supplements in the horse: comparative effects of 19-norandrostenedione and 19-norandrostenediol on the 19-norsteroid profile and consequences for doping control. *J Chromatogr B Analyt Technol Biomed Life Sci* 2002;766(2):257–263.

437. Frungieri MB, Gonzalez-Calvar SI, Bartke A, Calandra RS. Influence of age and photoperiod on steroidogenic function of the testis in the golden hamster. *Int J Androl* 1999;22(4):243–252.

438. Clancy GP, Yates WR. Anabolic steroid use among substance abusers in treatment. *J Clin Psychiatry* 1992;53(3):97–100.

439. Corcoran JP, Longo ED. Psychological treatment of anabolic-androgenic steroid-dependent individuals. *J Subst Abuse Treat* 1992;9(3):229–235.

440. Yesalis CE, Bahrke MS. Doping among adolescent athletes. *Baillieres Best Pract Res Clin Endocrinol Metab* 2000;14(1):25–35.

441. Al-Ismail K, Torreggiani WC, Munk PL, Nicolaou S. Gluteal mass in a bodybuilder: radiological depiction of a complication of anabolic steroid use. *Eur Radiol* 2002;12(6):1366–1369.

442. Albanese A, Stanhope R. Predictive factors in the determination of final height in boys with constitutional delay of growth and puberty. *J Pediatr* 1995;126(4):545–550.

443. Bower BL, Martin M. African American female basketball players: an examination of alcohol and drug behaviors. *J Am Coll Health* 1999;48(3):129–133.

444. Yesalis CE, Bahrke MS, Wright JE. Societal alternatives to anabolic steroid use. *Clin J Sport Med* 2000;10(1):1–6.

445. Elliot D, Goldberg L. Intervention and prevention of steroid use in adolescents. *Am J Sports Med* 1996;24[6 Suppl]:S46–S47.

446. Chakravorty B, Ahmed A, Buchanan RJ. Midproject findings from a study of the National Collegiate Athletic Association's policy on smokeless tobacco use. *Subst Use Misuse* 2000;35(10):1431–1441.

447. Epps RP, Lynn WR, Manley MW. Tobacco, youth, and sports. *Adolesc Med* 1998;9(3):483–490, vi.

448. Escher SA, Tucker AM, Lundin TM, Grabiner MD. Smokeless tobacco, reaction time, and strength in athletes. *Med Sci Sports Exerc* 1998;30(10):1548–1551.

449. Gingiss PL, Gottlieb NH. A comparison of smokeless tobacco and smoking practices of university varsity and intramural baseball players. *Addict Behav* 1991;16(5):335–340.

450. Hilton JF, Walsh MM, Masouredis CM, et al. Planning a spit tobacco cessation intervention: identification of beliefs associated with addiction. *Addict Behav* 1994;19(4):381–391.

451. Eichner ER. Ergolytic drugs in medicine and sports. *Am J Med* 1993;94(2):205–211.

452. Goldberg L, Bents R, Bosworth E, et al. Anabolic steroid education and adolescents: do scare tactics work? *Pediatrics* 1991;87(3):283–286.

453. Goldberg L, Elliot DL, Clarke GN, et al. The Adolescents Training and Learning to Avoid Steroids (ATLAS) prevention program. Background and results of a model intervention. *Arch Pediatr Adolesc Med* 1996;150(7):713–721.

454. Goldberg L, Elliot D, Clarke GN, et al. Effects of a multidimensional anabolic steroid prevention intervention. The Adolescents Training and Learning

to Avoid Steroids (ATLAS) Program. *JAMA* 1996;276(19):1555–1562.

455. Goldberg L, MacKinnon DP, Elliot DL, et al. The adolescents training and learning to avoid steroids program: preventing drug use and promoting health behaviors. *Arch Pediatr Adolesc Med* 2000;154(4):332–338.

456. Bolding G, Sherr L, Maguire M, Elford J. HIV risk behaviours among gay men who use anabolic steroids. *Addiction* 1999;94(12):1829–1835.

457. Goldberg L, Bosworth EE, Bents RT; Trevisan L. Effect of an anabolic steroid education program on knowledge and attitudes of high school football players. *J Adolesc Health Care* 1990;11(3):210–214.

458. Johnson MD, Jay MS, Shoup B,

Rickert VI. Anabolic steroid use by male adolescents. *Pediatrics* 1989 Jun;83(6):921–924.

459. Terney R, McLain LG. The use of anabolic steroids in high school students. *Am J Dis Child* 1990;144(1):99–103.

460. Komoroski EM, Rickert VI. Adolescent body image and attitudes to anabolic steroid use. *Am J Dis Child* 1992;146(7):823–828.

461. Whitehead R, Chillag S, Elliott D. Anabolic steroid use among adolescents in a rural state. *J Fam Pract* 1992;35(4):401–405.

462. Williamson DJ. Misuse of anabolic drugs [Letter]. *BMJ* 1993; 306(6869):61.

463. Radakovich J, Broderick P, Pickell G. Rate of anabolic-androgenic steroid

use among students in junior high school [published erratum appears in *J Am Board Fam Pract* 1993;6(6):616]. *J Am Board Fam Pract* 1993;6(4):341–345.

464. Middleman AB, Faulkner AH, Woods ER, et al. High-risk behaviors among high school students in Massachusetts who use anabolic steroids. *Pediatrics* 1995;96[2 Pt 1]:268–272.

465. Johnston L, O'Malley P, Bachman J. National survey results from the Monitoring the Future Study 1975–1994. Rockville, MD: National Institute on Drug Abuse, 1995.

466. Meilman PW, Crace RK, Presley CA, Lyerla R. Beyond performance enhancement: polypharmacy among collegiate users of steroids. *J Am Coll Health* 1995;44(3):98–104.

CHAPTER 26

Prescription Opiate Abuse

WALTER LING, DONALD R. WESSON, AND DAVID E. SMITH

Concurrently, with worldwide concern about the undertreatment of pain and the underuse of opioids in pain treatment, there is renewed concern about opiate addiction and opiate overdose deaths. The Joint Commission on Accreditation of Hospitals and Organizations has emphasized the need for better assessment and management of pain and has integrated this into the new accreditation standards, which consider pain as the fifth vital sign to be assessed whenever other vital signs are measured. The need to provide better pain control is also highlighted by the introduction of clinical practice guidelines for the management of both acute and cancer pain (developed by the U.S. Health and Human Services), as well as by the recent National Institutes of Health (NIH) program announcement, "The Management of Chronic Pain." Closely related to this chain of events, the pharmaceutical industry has introduced various sustained-release opioid formulations (e.g., oxycodone [OxyContin] and morphine sulfate [MS Contin]). It is ironic that one of the most powerful tools available to physicians for relieving patients' suffering has become a source of adverse medical and social issues.

Although the clinical limitations in the use of opioids are their side effects like constipation, sedation, and confusion, most health professionals and the general public are most concerned about the potential of opiates to pro-

duce addiction. Until recently, experts in pain management and drug addiction rarely communicated and each group maintained a separate point of view. Pain-management physicians rightly concern themselves with alleviation of pain and have traditionally underestimated addiction in the practice of pain treatment with opioids. Patients who developed problems of opioid abuse and addiction were often simply dismissed from further care. Addiction specialists, on the other hand, do not see the pain patients whose quality of life is vastly improved by opioids. Instead, they see failed patients from pain-treatment facilities. As a result, an issue that should have been one of common concern has been one of mutual neglect. Pain specialists, in their desire to provide adequate pain relief with opioids, have understated the problem of addiction and addiction specialists demonstrate a reluctance to using opioids in treating pain except in rare circumstances (1). Both groups draw their conclusions from scant data and both suffer as a result. What is needed is communication between pain and addiction specialists to develop a mutual understanding of the issues and to explore what is known and unknown as it relates to the treatment of both addiction and pain. This chapter discusses some of these pertinent issues.

DEFINITIONS OF SOME TERMS

To begin a meaningful dialogue, there must be some understanding of what is meant by some of the commonly used terms in addiction medicine (2).

Misuse generally refers to patients' incorrect use of a medication, such as taking it for other than the intended use, taking other than the prescribed amount, and taking it more frequently or for longer than prescribed. Misuse may also refer to the behavior of a physician, such as prescribing a medication for the wrong ailment, prescribing a dose that is too high, or prescribing the medication for longer than is necessary. "Off-label" prescribing, when the prescription is supported by common medical practice, research, or rational pharmacologic reasoning, would not be considered misuse. When referring to patient behavior, it is not certain whether *misuse* should be positioned at one end of a scale that ends with abuse or if it should be a distinct and separate phenomenon in itself.

Abuse is a term that varies widely depending on the context of its use and who is defining it. The U.S. Drug Enforcement Administration (DEA) defines *drug abuse* as the use of a Schedule II through Schedule V drug in a manner or amount that is inconsistent with the medical or social pattern of a culture. Drug abuse also refers to the use of prescription medications beyond "the scope of sound medical practice." Abuse and misuse often overlap when referring to prescription medication. A posting on the National Institute on Drug Abuse (NIDA) InfoFacts web site maintains that, "The misuse of prescribed medications may be the most common form of drug abuse among the elderly." Regarding prescription pain relievers, the same document equates misuse with any nonmedical use and cites the 1999 National Household Survey on Drug Abuse, which indicated that 2.6 million people "misused pain relievers." The American Psychiatric Association's *Diagnostic and Statistical Manual,*4th ed. text revision (*DSM–IV–TR*) defines abuse as "a maladaptive pattern of substance use, leading to clinically significant impairment or distress as manifested by one or more behaviorally based criteria" (3).

The medical profession, concerned primarily with clinical issues, has adopted a definition relevant to its own practices, but which may not be relevant for parents worrying about their children using prescribed medications recreationally. Law enforcement agencies are concerned with street diversion and maintaining the law and have little concern about clinical criteria. The Food and Drug Administration (FDA), as the drug-approval agency, is concerned with safety and efficacy, and proper labeling to prevent the adverse consequences from misuse. Ultimately, the issues of misuse and abuse need to be addressed in the context of both intended and unintended consumer populations.

Addiction, as defined in a public policy statement issued by the American Society of Addiction Medicine (ASAM), is considered, " . . . a primary, chronic, neurobiological disease, with genetic, psychosocial, and environmental factors influencing the development and manifestations. It is characterized by behaviors that include one or more of the following: impaired control over drug use, compulsive use, continued use despite harm, and craving" (4). Although this definition relates specifically to the use of drugs or medications, the term is often applied to other "undesirable" behaviors, such as gambling, that may also result in serious adverse medical or social consequences. The term is considered prejudicial and even derogatory in some contexts. Surprisingly, it appears in the names of both the American Society of Addiction Medicine and American Academy of Addiction Psychiatry.

Dependence has, in various iterations of the American Psychiatric Association's *Diagnostic and Statistical Manual*, replaced the term "addiction." Although more "politically correct," this lack of consistency continues to cause confusion. Opioid dependence, as defined in the latest version of the *DSM–IV–TR,* is a set of behaviors that differ from physical dependence on opiates, which is a neurobiologic adaptation that occurs with chronic exposure. Many people, including physicians, equate one term with the other, and the distinction is often lost. But opiate dependence in the addiction field is more than taking a large quantity of opiates; it is behaving like an opiate addict. A patient who takes a prescribed opiate on a regular basis may become physically dependent on the medication but is hardly an addict unless the patient's behavior meets the *DSM–IV–TR* diagnostic criteria for opiate dependence. It is often unclear whether the behaviors of patients, especially those receiving opiates for treatment of pain, are indicative of addiction.

Pseudoaddiction is a term used to describe drug-seeking behaviors iatrogenically produced in pain patients by inadequate pain treatment (5). Here the preoccupation with and pursuit of opiate medication is driven, first and foremost, by the patient's experience of pain relief and not the drug's mood-altering effects. Pseudoaddiction was described as occurring in three phases beginning with inadequate prescribing of analgesics to meet the needs of the pain patient (phase 1); leading to the patient's escalation of analgesic demands and behavioral changes, often exaggerated, to convince others of the severity of their pain and need for more medication (phase 2); which, in turn, results in a crisis of mistrust between the patient and the health care team (phase 3). In this context, it was emphasized that pseudoaddiction is preventable if a patient's report of pain is accepted as valid and the patient trusts that caregivers will use reasonable efforts to control it. Preventing pseudoaddiction requires rational use of opiates. Pseudoaddiction now refers to a broad spectrum of patient behaviors that are indicative of pain but erroneously interpreted as addiction.

RECENT TRENDS IN PRESCRIPTION OPIOID ABUSE

Recent media stories and data from such official sources as the National Household Survey on Drug Abuse suggest increased nonmedical use and abuse of prescription drugs. At issue is whether this is simply a reflection of increased medical use of opioids in response to the increasing use of opiates by pain physicians. In a study of the trends in the medical use and abuse of opiate analgesics from 1990 to 1996, Joranson and colleagues concluded that while there is an increase in the use of opioid analgesics, there is not a corresponding increase in the rate of abuse; consequently, the increased medical use of opiate analgesics for the treatment of pain did not appear to contribute to an increase in opiate analgesic abuse (6). A subsequent survey (2), however, found a significant increase in abuse of hydrocodone and oxycodone products since the period covered by the Joranson survey. Moreover, while the proportion of hydrocodone and oxycodone abuse relative to their availability remained relatively stable from 1994 to 1999, there has been a disproportionate rise since 2000 in the ratio of oxycodone abuse relative to its availability. This comes in the wake of reports describing a sharp rise in OxyContin-related deaths and lawsuits. More intriguing perhaps is what relationship, if any, this has with the more recent reports of increased methadone abuse and overdose deaths after more than 30 years of relatively safe clinical use in treatment of opiate addiction. A number of questions beg for answers. For example, has the wide availability of OxyContin and the subsequently reported problems of abuse and deaths resulted in more methadone being prescribed for pain patients with or without prior opioid exposure? Who are the people dying from overdose? Are they addicts or pain patients? Is it pain physicians or addiction specialists who prescribe methadone for these patients? Do they understand the special pharmacology of methadone? What proportion of those dying from methadone overdose were patients receiving oxycodone products before being prescribed methadone? (7)

EQUIANALGESIC DOSE OF METHADONE TO OTHER OPIATES IN CHRONIC DOSING

For almost four decades, addiction specialists have used methadone for the treatment of opiate dependence and a safe dosing regimen has been established for these patients, who are mostly heroin abusers. Overdose deaths from methadone, while an occasional happening, had not been a serious clinical issue. The recent sudden rise in reported methadone overdose deaths suggests that the patients may be different. Perhaps many of these new patients are abusers of prescribed opiates and their sensitivity to methadone differs from street heroin addicts. Although physicians specializing in the treatment of cancer pain frequently employ opioid rotation, they recognize that switching to methadone requires special knowledge of the pharmacology of methadone because methadone must be introduced in considerably lower doses than the current high dose of other opioids; this information may not be known to most primary care physicians and some addiction specialists (8,9).

The authors recommend caution and careful titration in transferring patients to methadone who were previously exposed to high doses of other opiates, noting that most published conversion tables are based on acute single-dose studies and not applicable to the clinical situation on hand. Low-dose methadone may appear to be almost equipotent to morphine but it could be five to ten times as potent in patients with prior high-dose morphine exposure. A

similar scenario probably exists with patient exposed to other opiates, such as oxycodone.

OPIOID PRESCRIPTION ABUSE AND ADDICTION IN PAIN PATIENTS

One cannot consider the increase in prescription opiate abuse without putting the matter in the context of the increased use of opiates for the treatment of pain. This issue has not been adequately studied. The impression that the risks of abuse and addiction are negligible in pain patients given an opiate is based on very little, if any, data. One of the most often cited references in this regard, based on the Boston Collaborative Drug Surveillance Project (10), which found only 4 cases of addiction in 11,828 nonaddict patients receiving opiate during an inpatient hospital stay, is a single paragraph letter to the editor. Another frequently quoted study (11), which surveyed the management of pain during débridement in burn units, asserts that not a single case of iatrogenic addiction could be demonstrated from the experience of 181 health care respondents with an average experience of more than 6 years on a burn unit and representing knowledge accumulated from at least 10,000 hospitalized burn patients. These are both inpatient reports and lack follow up. What is certain is that most physicians simply avoid prescribing opiate-containing analgesics to pain patients.

Nearly everyone interested in the subject matter has a favorite list of behaviors purporting to differentiate pain patients from addicts but there are still no research-based predictors to differentiate pain patients who are at risk of addiction from those who are not. In a study of 20 patients attending a pain clinic who had both chronic pain and substance abuse and who are receiving chronic opioid treatment, Dunbar and Katz found that 9 of the patients were abusing their medication and most who were not abusing were actively involved in recovery efforts (12). The study does not directly bear on the relative risks of prescribing opiates to patients with opiate addiction. In fact, more than half of the patients had alcohol as their primary drug of abuse. What the study did suggest is that patients, even alcoholics, with no history of opioid addiction are at no great risks of becoming addicted with short-term opioid exposure and those who do have a history of addiction would benefit from active recovery efforts while receiving such medications. Compton and colleagues used a 42-item behavioral check list to rate the likelihood of drug abuse as confirmed by an experienced psychiatrist using the *DSM–IV* criteria in a group of 50 chronic pain patients receiving opiates whose physicians were concerned about their having a problem with drug abuse (13). Three items accurately described more than 90% of the patients with drug abuse, one of which was the patient's own belief of having such a problem and the others being a preferred route of administration and a tendency to increase the dose or frequency of the medications. It is unclear how each of these three characteristics contribute to the overall predictive value, but it appears that the first alone would have been overwhelmingly predictive. More recently, Passik and colleagues applied an aberrant drug-seeking behavioral checklist based on input from pain and addiction specialists to a group of 388 chronic pain patients (14). Fifty-five percent of the patients demonstrated none of the behaviors and some 45% had an average of 1.5 (standard deviation [SD]: ±2.7) of a possible 29 items. Less than 4% of the patients had abused alcohol or street drugs or had contact with the street drug culture. Other aberrant behaviors occurred in as many as 18% of the patients. Some items on the behavioral checklist are so aberrant that their presence was virtually synonymous to abuse, but they occur rarely. Those that occur more commonly also have much lower predictive value. It is difficult to draw firm conclusions about these studies insofar as the predictive value of such checklists is concerned. In reality, some patients being treated with opiates for chronic pain do become problems to themselves and their treating physicians when their behavior suggests either prescription drug abuse or inadequate pain control. Unfortunately, physicians and patients do not always agree, and distinguishing addiction from pseudoaddiction is not always easy. An added complicating factor may be the recent realization that chronic opioid administration itself may induce a state of hyperalgesia. This requires a rethinking and adjustments in managing chronic pain patients with opiates and an open and trusting relationship between physicians and their patients.

A consensus statement from the American Society of Addiction Medicine (ASAM), the American Academy of Pain Medicine, and the American Pain Society approves the use of chronic opioid therapy for treatment of chronic nonmalignant pain. However, in defining terms used in the addiction field, it defines addiction in the course of prolonged opioid therapy for pain as "impaired control, craving and compulsive use, and continued use despite negative physical, mental, and or social consequences" (4). But the pattern of behavior as defined may also reflect undertreatment of pain and can only be adequately assessed when pain is under adequate control, which may or may not always be achievable. In the end, it is a matter of clinical judgment that may well include the use of additional opioids or other medications. One way to gauge the adequacy of pain control is to consider whether the use of added opiates has resulted in improvement in functional restoration, improvement in physical capacity, psychological well-being, family and other social interactions, and health care resource use. These benefits need to be weighed against the appearance of adverse effects such as unwanted daytime sedation, mental confusion, constipation, and other side effects. In an attempt to define prescription opiate abuse in chronic pain patients, Chabal and colleagues formulated a list of five behaviors, the presence of three or more of which was said to indicate prescription drug abuse: (a) overemphasis on opioid issues during pain

clinic visit that persists beyond the third treatment session; (b) pattern of early refills (three or more) or dose escalation in the absence of acute changes in medical condition; (c) multiple phone calls or visits to request more opiates or refills, or to discuss problems associated with opioid prescription; (d) pattern of prescription problems such as lost, spilled, or stolen medication; and (e) supplemental sources of opiates obtained from multiple providers, emergency rooms, or illegal sources (15). The authors found, in a group of 403 patients in a Veterans Administration (VA) pain clinic, that 21 of 76 patients who had used opiates for longer than 6 months met 3 or more of these criteria. However, a history of opioid or alcohol abuse was not predictive of addiction during chronic opioid treatment. Thus, although a pattern of aberrant behavior may be grounds for caution, a history of opioid abuse need not necessarily preclude a patient from successful treatment with an opiate.

PAIN IN ADDICTED AND OTHER PATIENTS CHRONICALLY MAINTAINED ON OPIOIDS

What little information we have about the pain experience of addicted patients has largely come from observations of patients on methadone maintenance. There is some general impression among pain clinicians that significant tolerance to the analgesic effects of opioids does not develop in pain patients receiving opioids chronically, and there are certainly many patients whose pain appears to be adequately managed for extended periods with stable doses of opioids, as are patients on methadone maintenance. Guidelines have been developed for managing pain in these patients, mostly based on clinical folklore and clinical experience, with little experimental data. One survey in several methadone clinics suggests that a significant portion of patients on methadone maintenance complain of moderate to severe pain with an average duration of 10 years (16). Moreover, almost half of these patients believe that prescription opioids had led to their opioid addiction. Compared to patients on methadone maintenance without pain, methadone-maintained patients with pain are more disabled, less employed, suffer more medical and psychiatric illnesses, and use more prescribed and nonprescribed medications (16). A more recent survey involving methadone maintained patients and addicts in residential substance abuse treatment programs appeared to confirm these earlier findings that chronic pain is prevalent among patients in substance abuse treatment, especially in methadone-maintained patients, and is associated with functional impairment (17).

Among pain clinicians, there is a general consensus that methadone-maintained patients require more, not less, opioids for treatment of acute pain and that they are some of the most undertreated pain patients. Recent studies show methadone-maintained patients to be significantly hyperalgesic and highly tolerant to the analgesic effects of added morphine (18). It is perhaps not coincidental that the length of methadone maintenance treatment appears to correlate with severity of pain (17). This remains one of the most understudied areas in pain and addiction, and one that calls for further study. Animal studies suggest that hyperalgesia may be universal to all chronic opioid exposure. It remains to be seen in humans whether the context under which chronic opioid exposure occurs, (i.e., pain versus addiction) the specific opioid used, the length and dose of exposure, makes a difference. What is clear is that managing pain in these patients continues to present enormous challenges; ways must be found to overcome or bypass opioid-induced hyperalgesia if adequate pain management in these patients is to be achieved. Some recent work shows promise in the use of N-methyl-D-aspartate (NMDA) receptor antagonists, substance P antagonists, and the combination of opioid agonists with ultralow doses of opioid antagonists, but most are still in the early stages of clinical development (19). At present, most recommendations and guidelines remain embedded in the clinical experience, common sense, and sound judgment of clinicians.

ABUSE LIABILITY AND DIVERSION OF PRESCRIPTION OPIOIDS

Prescription opiate abuse relates to the intrinsic abuse liability of the prescribed opiate and its diversion from the intended route of distribution. Abuse liability is correlated with ease of extraction and modification to produce the desired psychological effect while its potential for diversion relates to how readily it is redirected from the prescribed route. Abusability is, therefore, associated with certain pharmacologic properties. A medication tends to be more readily abusable if it has a rapid onset and short duration of action, is highly potent, and is smokable or easily ingested. Some medications are intrinsically more abusable than others. Dilaudid (hydromorphone) tablets for example, can be easily dissolved in a small amount of water and injected. OxyContin tablets (a controlled-release oral formulation of oxycodone) can be crushed to defeat its controlled release properties and then snorted, or dissolved in solution and injected. At times, the specific "black box warning" on the labeling of a medication becomes a recipe for abuse. Finally, a brand name drug, which carries a higher street value, is more subject to abuse than is a generic preparation.

Prevention of diversion of prescribed drugs depends mostly on legal controls, such as the use of triplicate prescriptions, computerized records of prescribing and sales, tracking of the prescriptions written by physicians, and field investigations of pharmacies and physicians. However, such data must be interpreted in the clinical context. Methadone clinics are the main source of street methadone, which has been bought and consumed by heroin addicts, many of whom use it to self-medicate symptoms of opiate withdrawal when they are trying to reduce their opioid tolerance or to bridge periods of time when their preferred opiate of abuse is not available. Still, the amount of methadone diverted in this manner is insignificant compared to the total amount prescribed, and there is no evidence that such diversion has resulted in a significant number of new cases of opioid addiction. Methadone is also prescribed in treatment of pain, and until recently, there was little evidence that diversion of methadone from pain management was occurring on any substantial scale. However, the recent reports of oxycodone and methadone abuse and overdose suggest that the scene may be changing.

OPIOIDS WITH ABUSE POTENTIAL AND HOW THEY ARE ABUSED

All prescription opiates have some abuse liability. This section provides an annotated discussion of selected opioids used in the treatment of pain.

Buprenorphine

Buprenorphine (Buprenex, Suboxone, Subutex), a partial opioid agonist, has been available in the United States since the mid-1980s in an injectable formulation (Buprenex) for the treatment of moderate pain. In many other countries, it is marketed as a 0.3- or 0.4-mg sublingual tablet (Temgesic, Buprigesic, Norphin, Pentorel Tidigesic).

In October 2002, the Food and Drug Administration (FDA) approved two sublingual formulations of buprenorphine for the treatment of opiate dependence. One formulation, Subutex, contains only buprenorphine (either 2 mg or 8 mg); the other, Suboxone contains 2 mg or 8 mg buprenorphine combined with naloxone in a 4:1 ratio, which may reduce its potential for intravenous use (also see the discussion of pentazocine below). Buprenex was a Schedule V narcotic until 2002, when it was reclassified to Schedule III along with Suboxone and Subutex. To date, buprenorphine has not been a common drug of abuse in the United States.

Fentanyl Transdermal Patches

Fentanyl transdermal patches (Duragesic), which deliver fentanyl through the skin for up to 72 hours, are marketed for patients who require continuous analgesia for the treatment of pain. The patch is distributed in four sizes, containing 2.5, 5, 7.5, and 10 mg of fentanyl.

As with the injectable formulation of fentanyl (Sublimaze), abuse of Duragesic has been reported primarily, but not exclusively, in health professionals, who extract the fentanyl from the patch and inject it (20). Abusers also have chewed (21), ingested (22), and inhaled (23) the contents of the patch. Even after a patch has been used for 3 days, it still contains sufficient fentanyl to be abused (24). In a case of fatal fentanyl poisoning, a funeral home employee was able to extract a lethal amount of fentanyl from a patch removed from a body (25).

Meperidine

Meperidine (Demerol) is primarily a drug of abuse among heath professionals. It is an unusual opiate because one of its metabolites, normeperidine, can produce seizures.

Methadone

In methadone-maintenance clinics, methadone generally is dispensed in prepared individual doses, usually mixed with a juice-flavored drink. The purpose of combining methadone with the juice is to discourage its abuse by intravenous injection. The stringent distribution system for methadone used in opiate addiction treatment is meant to discourage diversion.

Methadone also is prescribed for the treatment of pain. Until recently, there was little evidence that diversion of methadone from pain management was occurring on any substantial scale. Newspaper reports, such as one from Florida, of methadone overdose deaths in patients who had been switched from OxyContin to methadone, suggest that physicians not familiar with methadone may put patients at risk (26).

Most diverted methadone is bought and consumed by heroin addicts, many of whom use it to self-medicate symptoms of opiate withdrawal when they are trying to reduce their opioid tolerance or to bridge periods of time when their preferred opiate of abuse is not available. There is no evidence that street diversion of methadone from methadone clinics has resulted in new cases of opioid addiction in a significant number of addicts.

Pentazocine

In the 1970s and early 1980s, intravenous abuse of pentazocine (Talwin) tablets in combination with a blue-colored antihistamine tablet tripelennamine known as "T's and Blues," became common in the midwestern states (27,28). Factors that contributed to its widespread abuse included its placement outside Schedule II (so that its prescribing was not captured by triplicate prescriptions and other state monitoring programs) and to the wrongly held belief on the part of physicians that the drug was not abusable. Talwin also was widely abused by drug-addicted physicians because it could be prescribed in large quantities without being detected by monitoring systems. At one point, Talwin abuse became such a serious problem that the manufacturer considered removing the drug from the market. Its use was salvaged by reformulation of the drug to include the antagonist naloxone (Talwin Nx). When Talwin Nx is taken as directed, the user experiences only

the pentazocine effect because naloxone is not well absorbed through oral ingestion. However, if a tablet is dissolved and injected, the naloxone blocks the opiate effects of the pentazocine; in an opiate-dependent user, this would precipitate acute opiate withdrawal. The replacement of Talwin with the Talwin Nx tablet formulation reduced the abuse of T's and Blues to an insignificant level (28). This is a good example of how changing a drug's formulation can reduce its intrinsic abuse liability without seriously compromising its therapeutic utility.

Oxycodone

OxyContin, which has been marketed in the United States since 1995, is a Schedule II controlled released oral tablet formulation of oxycodone. (Oxycodone is available in immediate–release tablets in combination with aspirin or acetaminophen under trade names such as Percodan and Percocet. The immediate-release tablets contain 2.5 to 10 mg of oxycodone.) OxyContin was designed for the treatment of chronic pain patients who require continuous dosing. Its formulations range from 10 mg (the upper dose of the immediate-release products) to 80 mg (2). Taken orally, OxyContin tablets release their contents over about 12 hours. However, the controlled-release mechanism is destroyed if the tablets are crushed; the entire contents then become immediately available, and can be abused by snorting, ingesting, or injecting (3). Addicts' interest in OxyContin relates largely to its high oxycodone content in comparison with the immediate-release forms.

Data from the Drug Abuse Warning Network (DAWN) indicate an increase in the "abuse" of oxycodone (29). The number of oxycodone emergency department mentions increased from 3,369 in the first half of 1999 to 5,261 in the first half of 2000. (It should be noted that mentions of oxycodone do not necessarily equal mentions of OxyContin because oxycodone also is an ingredient in more than 50 pharmaceutical formulations.)

Cases of oxycodone addiction and overdose deaths, particularly in the Northeast and mid-Atlantic states, have generated widespread controversy, as well as lawsuits against physicians and the manufacturer. In fact, abuse of OxyContin raises many complex issues about the marketing of new drug technologies and the relationship between drug abuse and the treatment of pain. Should the pharmaceutical company be held liable when a product is not used in the appropriate medical context? Does aggressive marketing by a pharmaceutical company contribute to physician "overprescription" or street diversion? What is the role of the pharmaceutical company in training physicians to use new formulations of its medications? What is the role of medical schools in training students to manage pain and addiction? These questions are not new or unique to OxyContin, but the current controversy surrounding Oxy-Contin has renewed public attention to them.

PRESCRIBING OPIATES TO PATIENTS WITH PAIN AND ADDICTION

The general principles of good medical practice apply equally to prescribing for addicted patients and those at high risk of becoming addicted. There are, however, some specific areas of practice worthy of special attention when prescribing opioids to patients with pain and addiction.

Medical Records

The importance of keeping detailed and legible medical records cannot be overemphasized. In the event of a legal challenge, detailed medical records documenting what was done and why are the foundations of the physician's defense. A written treatment plan with measurable treatment goals is a key document. The plan should define goals related to pain management and goals related to minimizing and managing the risk of addiction. The treatment plan should be updated as new information becomes available. Generally, the treatment plan should be negotiated with the patient and signed by both the patient and the treating physician to indicate agreement on the goals and procedures. (It is best not to label these as treatment "contracts" because of the legal connotation.) A copy of the treatment plan should be provided to the patient and all other care providers.

Some documents that may be included in the medical records are the following:

- Diagnostic assessments: history, physical examination, laboratory tests ordered, and their results
- Actual copies of, or references to, medical records of past hospitalizations or treatment by other providers
- The treatment plan
- Signed consent for treatment or procedures
- Signed authorization for release of information to other treatment providers
- Documentation of discussions with and consultation reports from other health care providers
- Medications prescribed and the patient's response to them, including any adverse events

Medication Management

It is good practice for one physician to prescribe all psychotropic medications to a given patient. An addiction medicine specialist may or may not be the primary prescribing physician, depending on the nature of the patient's pain, the pathophysiology, and the status of any addictive disorder. Current management of pain, particularly neuropathic pain, often involves the use of ancillary medications, and the prescribing physician should be familiar with both opioid and adjuvant analgesics to effectively manage such pain (30).

Patients should be encouraged to use one pharmacy to fill all their prescriptions. This can aid in identifying possible drug interactions and in tracking the amount of medication being consumed.

Postmarketing Monitoring for Abuse

The FDA is now able to require that a pharmaceutical manufacturer that markets a drug with abuse liability must conduct postmarketing surveillance for such abuse, as it did in 1995 when it granted approval of tramadol (Ultram) (31). Similarly, the FDA added a requirement of postmarketing surveillance to its approval of sublingual buprenorphine (Subutex and Suboxone).

Consultations

Whenever the best clinical course is not clear or the patient's response is not as expected, consultation with another physician should be obtained. Generally, the results of the consultation should be discussed with the consulting physician and a written consultation report added to the patient's medical record.

Addiction medicine specialists and pain specialists often can provide better patient care by combining their expertise in the management of pain patients who are in recovery or in patients with an active substance abuse disorder. An addiction medicine specialist may be called upon to determine whether a patient is abusing pain medications or other drugs or is dependent on them (according to *DSM–IV–TR* diagnostic criteria). Such a determination requires an understanding of both addictive and pain behaviors. Table 26.1 may be helpful in clarifying the diagnosis. Although the distinction may be difficult, some behaviors occur only in patients with substance-abuse disorders. These include administering medications in other than the prescribed routes (as by crushing and injecting oxycodone tablets), and continued use of alcohol or other drugs after repeated physician warnings to the contrary. While addiction medicine specialists generally label such behaviors as addiction, pain specialists, who are reluctant to use the term "addiction" (32), commonly label these behaviors as "aberrant" (14).

Managing Patients with Active Addiction

Where and how best to manage patients who are actively abusing alcohol and other drugs and who also are in need of medical management with an abusable medication often is a contentious issue because of the clash in treatment philosophies between pain management programs and addiction treatment programs. There are no simple answers. The treating physicians must determine which intervention takes precedence. At times, it is adequate control of pain, but at other times adequate pain control cannot be achieved without first addressing the patient's addiction. Too often, treatment options and settings are limited. It is an area requiring more research and collaboration between specialists from both fields.

TABLE 26.1. *Comparison of DSM–IV criteria applied to nonaddicted chronic pain patients using opioids and opioid-abusing patients*

Diagnostic criteria[a] (Dependence requires meeting 3 or more criteria)	Pain patients	Opioid abusers
1. Tolerance, as defined by either of the following:		
(a) A need for markedly increased amounts of the substance to achieve intoxication of desired effect	Patient may require some increase in dose over time to accommodate for tolerance	May require progressive increases because patient is seeking mood effects of opiates as much or more than pain relief
(b) Markedly diminished effect with continued use of the same amount of the substance	May require some increase in dose over time to achieve continued pain relief	Much greater tolerance for mood effects than generally required for pain control
2. Withdrawal, as manifested by either of the following:		
(a) The characteristic withdrawal syndrome	May occur when opioids are stopped abruptly	Usually occurs and patient is unable or unwilling to tolerate withdrawal symptoms
(b) The same (or a closely related) substance is taken to relieve or avoid withdrawal symptoms	Rarely occurs with patient consulting primary treating physician	Patient often self-medicate without consulting with physician; withdrawal symptoms often precipitate frantic drug-seeking behavior
3. The substance is often taken in larger amounts or over a longer period of time than intended	Patient is able to ration medication between planned visits to prescribing physician	Episodes of intoxication and inability to ration medication use consistently; often calls for refills between visits with falsified reasons for needing refill (e.g., lost medication, it fell in the toilet)
4. There is a persistent desire or unsuccessful efforts to reduce or control substance use	May want to decrease or stop use, but when pain becomes worse with medication reduction agrees to continue	Repeatedly vacillates between use and wanting to stop; relapses to drug use after taper
5. A great deal of time is spent in activities necessary to obtain the substance, use the substance or recover from its effects	May spend large amounts of time going for treatment of pain; is generally cooperative with physicians about pursing nonopiate pain-control strategies	Time is consumed with drug-related activities
6. Important social, occupational, or recreational activities are given up or reduced because of substance use	Activities may be decreased primarily because of pain; may participate in more activities while on opioid medication	Activities not related to drug use cease to be a priority
7. The substance use is continued despite knowledge of having a persistent or recurrent physical or psychological problem that is likely to have been caused or exacerbated by the substance	May continue medication despite concerns about addiction expressed by family or friends, but will generally want to stop or reduce medication when it produces new physical or psychological problems	Will continue drug use despite adverse relationship, employment, or health consequences; often unable to be aware of cause and effect relationship between drug use and adverse consequences

[a]Criteria from table Source, p. 197.
American Psychiatric Association. *Diagnostic and statistical manual of mental disorders,* 4th ed., text revision. Washington, DC: American Psychiatric Association, 2000.

PHYSICIANS AND PRESCRIPTION DRUG ABUSE

Certain physicians are more prone than others to be involved in prescription drug diversion and abuse. Smith devised a classification of such physicians and presented it at a 1980 White House Conference on Prescription Drug Abuse; the definitions subsequently were adopted in a report of the American Medical Association (33,34). The classification is commonly referred to as the "four Ds": the "dated," the "duped," the "disabled," and the "dishonest" (4).

"Dated" physicians are those who have not kept up with changing standards of practice; "duped" physicians are those easily manipulated by addicts—perhaps because of their own gullibility, discomfort in confronting patients, or pride. While any physician occasionally can be manipulated or taken in by an addict's story, the duped physician has a recurring pattern of acquiescing to demands of patients and prescribing drugs in excessive amounts or for longer than necessary. "Disabled" physicians are those whose judgment is impaired by their own illness or alcohol or drug use (see the discussion of health care professionals as a special risk group below).

The physicians in these three categories are making a good faith effort to practice sound medicine, but their execution is flawed. They generally respond well to remedial and rehabilitative interventions. Dated and duped physicians, for example, are appropriate candidates for education and training to improve their practice procedures and skills, while disabled physicians often recover under the supervision of a physician health and effectiveness program.

"Dishonest" physicians (also known as "script doctors"), on the other hand, willfully prescribe controlled drugs for other than medical purposes—drugs that they know will be abused. Such physicians are not practicing good faith medicine but are using their medical licenses as a franchise to deal drugs. Organized medicine agrees that such physicians are not candidates for reeducation or rehabilitation and should be prosecuted to the full extent of the law (33).

Health Care Professionals as a Special Risk Group

Health care workers, because of their occupational access to opioids, constitute an unusually high-risk group

for opioid abuse. While the abuse of fentanyl (Sublimaze) by anesthesiologists (35) and the abuse of meperidine (Demerol) by nurses (36) have long been recognized, abuse of prescriptions by some other groups is less-well recognized. For example, the increased use of opioids in hospices has given many nurses relatively uncontrolled access to large quantities of high-potency prescription opioids. Large-animal veterinarians also have unmonitored access to large quantities of opioids. Physicians with drug-abuse problems may have ultraconservative or overly liberal prescribing habits because they fear drawing attention to themselves, or as a result of carelessness from impaired judgment.

FUTURE DIRECTIONS

A chapter such at this is not to suggest that pain specialists ought to become addictionologists or that addiction medicine specialists should become experts in pain management. However, each group must learn to appreciate the roles and contributions of the other group as well as the pitfalls and problems in the other's practice. The recent observation that chronic exposure to opiates itself may induce a state of hyperalgesia may require rethinking about opiate-addicted patients and pain patients chronically treated with opiates. It may well be that the way these patients come to be taking opiates chronically may be different but their underlying neurophysiologic adaptations and manifestations at the neurocircuitry level may be the same. That is to say, they may suffer from the same neuropathology and that perhaps their clinical manifestations are different only because of their different life experience, which would include their interaction with their physicians. The manner in which life experiences modify biology and in which biology determines subsequent behavior and life experience, may have more common threads among this diverse group of patients than has generally been assumed. It appears that the issue of opiate-induced hyperalgesia and ways to overcome it is an area of interest to both groups of physicians. Additional research in this area will influence both our thinking and our approach to the care of our respective patients. In the meantime, patients still require treatment by both pain specialists and addiction specialists. The sharing of information between the two groups can be beneficial to both groups of physicians and their patients.

REFERENCES

1. Passik SD. Responding rationally to recent report of abuse/diversion of OxyContin. *J Pain Symptom Manage* 2001;21(5):359.
2. Zacny J, Bigelow G, Compton P, et al. College on Problems of Drug Dependence taskforce on prescription opioid non-medical use and abuse: posi-

tion statement. *Drug Alcohol Depend* 2003;69(3):215–232.
3. American Psychiatric Association. *Diagnostic and statistical manual of mental disorders,* 4th ed., text revision. Washington, DC: American Psychiatric Association, 2000.
4. ASAM Public Policy Committee. Def-

initions related to the use of opioids for the treatment of pain. 2001. www. ASAM.ORG/Pain/definitions2.pdf
5. Weissman DE, Haddox JD. Opioid pseudoaddiction—an iatrogenic syndrome. *Pain* 1989;36(3):363–366.
6. Joranson DE, Ryan KM, Gilson AM, et al. Trends in medical

use and abuse of opioid analgesics. *JAMA* 2000;283(13):1710–1714.

7. Cone EJ, et al. Oxycodone involvement in drug abuse deaths: a DAWN-based classification scheme applied to an oxycodone postmortem database containing over 1000 cases. *J Anal Toxicol* 2003;27(2):57–67; discussion 67.

8. Anderson R, et al. Accuracy in equianalgesic dosing conversion dilemmas. *J Pain Symptom Manage* 2001;21(5):397–406.

9. Pereira J, et al. Equianalgesic dose ratios for opioids. A critical review and proposals for long-term dosing. *J Pain Symptom Manage* 2001;22(2):672–687.

10. Porter J, Jick H. Addiction rare in patients treated with narcotics [Letter]. *N Engl J Med* 1980;302(2):123.

11. Perry S, Heidrich G. Management of pain during débridement: a survey of U.S. burn units. *Pain* 1982;13(3):267–280.

12. Dunbar SA, Katz NP. Chronic opioid therapy for nonmalignant pain in patients with a history of substance abuse: report of 20 cases. *J Pain Symptom Manage* 1996;11(3):163–171.

13. Compton P, Darakjian J, Miotto K. Screening for addiction in patients with chronic pain and "problematic" substance use: evaluation of a pilot assessment tool. *J Pain Symptom Manage* 1998;16(6):355–363.

14. Passik SD, et al. A pilot survey of aberrant drug-taking attitudes and behaviors in samples of cancer and AIDS patients. *J Pain Symptom Manage* 2000;19(4):274–286.

15. Chabal C, et al. Prescription opiate abuse in chronic pain patients: clinical criteria, incidence, and predictors. *Clin J Pain* 1997;13(2):150–155.

16. Jamison RN, Kauffman J, Katz NP. Characteristics of methadone maintenance patients with chronic pain. *J Pain Symptom Manage* 2000;19(1):53–62.

17. Rosenblum A, et al. Prevalence and characteristics of chronic pain among chemically dependent patients in methadone maintenance and residential treatment facilities. *JAMA* 2003;289(18):2370–2378.

18. Doverty M, et al. Hyperalgesic responses in methadone maintenance patients. *Pain* 2001;90(1–2):91–96.

19. Mao J. Opioid-induced abnormal pain sensitivity: implications in clinical opioid therapy. *Pain* 2002;100(3):213–217.

20. DeSio JM, et al. Intravenous abuse of transdermal fentanyl therapy in a chronic pain patient. *Anesthesiology* 1993;79(5):1139–1141.

21. Arvanitis ML, Satonik RC. Transdermal fentanyl abuse and misuse [Letter]. *Am J Emerg Med* 2002;20(1):58–59.

22. Purucker M, Swann W. Potential for Duragesic patch abuse. *Ann Emerg Med* 2000;35(3):314.

23. Marquardt KA, Tharratt RS. Inhalation abuse of fentanyl patch. *J Toxicol Clin Toxicol* 1994;32(1):75–78.

24. Marquardt KA, Tharratt RS, Musallam NA. Fentanyl remaining in a transdermal system following three days of continuous use. *Ann Pharmacother* 1995;29(10):969–971.

25. Flannagan LM, Butts JD, Anderson WH. Fentanyl patches left on dead bodies—potential source of drug for abusers. *J Forensic Sci* 1996;41(2):320–321.

26. Associated Press. Researchers link prescription methadone, rise in overdose deaths. *Naples (FL) Daily News* Oct. 4, 2002.

27. Poklis A. Pentazocine/tripelennamine (T's and blues) abuse: a five-year survey of St. Louis, Missouri. *Drug Alcohol Depend* 1982;10(2–3):257–267.

28. Senay EC. Clinical experience with T's and B's. *Drug Alcohol Depend* 1985;14(3–4):305–312.

29. Office of National Drug Control Policy (ONDCP). *Drug policy information clearinghouse fact sheet.* 2002 www.whitehousedrugpolicy.gov/publication/factsht/oxycontin/index

30. Farrar JT, Portenoy RK. Neuropathic cancer pain: the role of adjuvant analgesics. *Oncology (Huntingt)* 2001;15(11):1435–1442, 1445.

31. Cicero TJ, et al. A postmarketing surveillance program to monitor Ultram (tramadol hydrochloride) abuse in the United States. *Drug Alcohol Depend* 1999;57(1):7–22.

32. Hung CI, et al. Meperidine addiction or treatment frustration? *Gen Hosp Psychiatry* 2001;23(1):31–35.

33. Council on Scientific Affairs. Drug abuse related to prescribing practice. *JAMA* 1982;247:864–866.

34. Wesson DR, Smith DE. Prescription drug abuse. Patient, physician, and cultural responsibilities. *West J Med* 1990;152(5):613–616.

35. Ward CF, Ward GC, Saidman LJ. Drug abuse in anesthesia training programs. A survey: 1970 through 1980. *JAMA* 1983;250(7):922–925.

36. Hoover RC, McCormick WC, Harrison WL. Pilferage of controlled substances in hospitals. *Am J Hosp Pharm* 1981;38(7):1007–1010.

Related Compulsive and Addictive Behaviors

CHAPTER 27

Eating Disorders

MARK S. GOLD AND JODI STAR

Addiction research has enhanced our ability to understand the common brain mechanisms involved in pain, appetite, drug reinforcement, and sexual behaviors. The definition of addiction has gone through considerable evolution. The focus in the past was that addiction results as a means of avoiding the distress of withdrawal. Addiction was inadvertent or somehow passive or an unintended consequence of pernicious agents. This model for addiction had a potent impact on both theory and treatment by putting a bizarre emphasis on neuroadaptation. Thus, by emphasizing abstinence symptomatology and treating withdrawal, we thought we understood addiction and its treatment. Treatment of addiction was often considered the same as or equivalent to treating withdrawal. Unfortunately, astounding success in the development of antiwithdrawal agents did little to improve treatment outcomes. The high rates of relapse after this "treatment" have led many to believe that positive reinforcement may be more active, purposeful, and important than anything else in the process of addiction and the persistence of relapse (1).

The brain's reinforcing pathways share common mesocorticolimbic projections, also known as the medial forebrain bundle. The brain does not seem to differentiate whether licit or illicit drugs provoke the reward, by extreme environmental manipulations, or by fasting. This much-studied area of the brain, which includes the ventral tegmental area (VTA) and the nucleus accumbens (nAC), is considered the neural center modulating positive rein-

forcement (2). Feeding, sex, and other survival behaviors are reinforced or made more likely by events occurring within the VTA and nAC. The central neurotransmitter involved in these events is dopamine (DA), although many other neurotransmitters modulate the effects of DA and the development of addiction.

Intracerebral microdialysis enables the study of neurotransmitters in the nAC and other localized brain regions in awake, freely moving and behaving animals (3–6). An increase in the extracellular level of DA in the nAC, a major target of the mesolimbic dopaminergic system (MDS) (7), during ingestion of food has been reported by numerous authors (8–13). This is quite similar to the result produced by cocaine or after other drug self-administration (14). This suggests that there is a relationship between food intake and the activity of the MDS just as it has been suggested that there is a relationship between reward (13), illicit drug reinforcement (14–16), self-stimulation and sexual behavior (17–19), and MDS dopaminergic activity.

Eating behavior is complex but it appears that the MDS is activated by food reward. Food is reported to be addicting or extremely rewarding by some patients who complain of compulsive candy, potato chip, or other food consumption. In animals, it appears that food reward depends in part on its palatability or the hedonic component related to the sensory properties of foods (15,16). When animals are offered a more palatable diet, most animal species eat more and become obese (17–19). Passive drug administration is not addicting whereas active goal-directed behavior seeking and using drugs for euphoria production is addicting. Being stuffed with cake is a markedly different experience than sneaking around and raiding the refrigerator after midnight. Host factors, such as genetic vulnerability at conception or acquired *in utero* or early in life, will play an important role in determining the pathologic reward produced by drugs, food, or some micronutrient, thus underlying the acquisition of a pathologic attachment we call addiction, binge eating, or obesity.

Consumption of food and water and copulative behavior increase the extracellular level of DA in conscious and freely moving animals. Many studies of addictive drugs including cocaine, ethanol, opiates, and nicotine also show such increases in DA within the nAC following their administration (20). We believe that this primitive reward system is central to the development of both eating disorders and addiction. The numerous associations between eating disorders and drug addictions, including a high comorbidity and recidivism, genetic linkage, and common neurobiologic pathways, modification of drug reward by eating or starvation lead us to consider the possibility that binge-eating disorders represent a drug-free autoaddiction for a significant subset of the addiction-prone. In others, it is a trigger leading to a drug or alcohol relapse. At other times, it is an apparent result of alcohol or drug abstinence. Mesolimbic DA activity is but one common thread attributing rewarding properties of both food and illicit drugs.

DRUG REWARD

The mesocorticolimbic dopaminergic system is thought to act as an interface between the midbrain and forebrain (21). It seems to function as a modulator, integrating emotion into directed behavior (22). Drug reward also confers importance or significance upon certain behaviors and not others. Many studies demonstrate that species-specific survival drives (feeding, drinking, and copulation) are reinforced or given salience through this system. Many studies of substance abuse disorders in animal models demonstrate that the addictive nature of these drugs is mediated by their direct effect upon this reward system (1,23). All drugs of abuse are self-administered by animals and man. Cocaine is self-administered to death in paradigms where use and access are unlimited (24). However, the most convincing evidence that drugs access this primitive system is that they decrease the amount of brain stimulation required to motivate baseline responding (25). Drug use motivates repetition of the behavior and creates a feeling of satisfaction like that produced by completion of a biologic imperative or normal survival behavior. Drug use produces the same sense of accomplishment and may be seen by the addict as tantamount to survival. The normal survival behaviors become less compelling as they are bypassed by the normal reinforcement system (26). In many instances, cocaine addicts stop eating, drinking, washing, talking, and interacting with others and look like patients with a primary eating disorder (27). The studies of divergent drugs of abuse from heroin to nicotine to cocaine all involve the VTA–nAC dopaminergic system; thus it is thought to be

the core neuroanatomy for addiction medicine and central to brain control of any goal-directed rewarding behavior (28).

Primary Reinforcers

Feeding, like drinking and copulation, is considered a specific species-survival behavior reinforced through the medial forebrain bundle. These survival behaviors are *primary reinforcers;* that is, they have a direct effect upon the medial forebrain bundle. Drugs of abuse are also primary reinforcers. Feeding within the arena of eating is also a primary reinforcer. But normal feeding behavior and eating disorders differ in the purpose they serve. Feeding behavior is typically a response to hunger. Hunger may have been a more important reason to eat in our past than it is in the United States today. Hunger is likely generated by depletion of nutrient and energy stores. The reward generated by feeding, paired with the state of hunger and its resolution into satiety, thus positively reinforces feeding behavior in a state of hunger. Studies show that a state of hunger via food deprivation in rats actually enhances the reward effect of feeding. A state of hunger also potentiates illicit drug reward. In this sense, hunger and craving could be seen as secondary reinforcers paired with the primary reward generated by feeding. Eating or the use of cocaine produces satiation. In this sense, illicit drugs acquire the organismic significance attributed to food. They become an acquired primary drive equated with survival. Feeding is a behavior that promotes survival of the health and thus, survival of the organism. This ultimately translates into a greater chance of survival of the species.

Neurobiology of Feeding

The neurobiology of feeding involves a complex interplay of peripheral afferent signaling, central modulation, and nutrient composition. This is a dynamic process of hunger, feeding, satiation, and satiety. The similar effect of food reward and addictive drugs on these regulatory systems may help to explain the relationship between substance abuse and eating disorders. It is becoming apparent that eating and drug disorders share a common neuroanatomic and neurochemical basis (29). The latter may access brain reward through exogenous, illicit drugs and the former through dietary and environmental manipulations. Understanding this relationship of substance abuse and eating disorders will allow us to create more effective and focused treatment strategies.

The concepts of hunger, satiation, and satiety have variable definitions. They may also be dependent on one's culture and the availability of food. In cultures without starvation and where few individuals eat in response to hunger, eating disorders appear much more common. Hunger can be thought of as both a physiologic drive to eat and as a perceived desire to eat. Satiation is generally recognized as the process that ends eating behavior. Satiety, then, is the state after the completion of eating behavior in which further eating is inhibited. Eating disorders and obesity may be divided into related groups that affect either aspect of the eating process.

While the precise physiologic mechanisms regulating feeding behavior have not been fully described, research studying the role of various neurotransmitters and neuropeptides has contributed to a greater understanding of this complex process. The overall regulation of feeding includes central nervous system (CNS) integration of peripheral afferent signals; reward; endocrine responses; energy states; drive and mood states; micronutrient intake and supply; neurotransmitter responses; and efferent motor commands. These compose a coordinated system assuring the organism's metabolic needs in the face of more global environmental factors. Our interest focuses on how disruptions in this system give rise to self-perpetuating, maladaptive behaviors. Furthermore, once established, the primitive reward systems seem to function to preserve these maladaptive behaviors. We will mainly consider the role of neurotransmitter systems in the pathogenesis of eating disorders and their similarity with substance abuse disorders.

NEUROBIOLOGY OF EATING DISORDERS AND REWARD

The defined teleology of eating disorders has changed considerably during this century. Early studies on eating disorders including obesity were primarily defined in psychological terms as the consequence of emotional upheaval, displacement of other psychological drives, or as the means to satisfy some unfulfilled psychological need. In the latter half of this century, the focus changed more toward physiologic mechanisms arising from work studying the effects of hypothalamic lesions and their subsequent effect upon feeding behavior and weight change. More recently, the physiologic mechanisms regulating feeding, diet, and weight have been under increasing scrutiny, particularly in light of the unfortunate trends of the increasing prevalence of eating disorders in industrialized nations. The definitive work in this area stems from the results of studies where microinjections of drugs are delivered to specific brain foci. Microdialysis studies of neurotransmitters in conjunction with the microinjection studies have allowed unprecedented access to brain mechanisms and a new understanding of the neurochemistry of addictive and eating disorders. Recently, many new neuropeptides have been discovered with crucial roles in regulating feeding. Furthermore, advances in neuroimaging and immunochemistry have also added to the evolving renaissance of neurobiologic understanding (30).

NEUROPEPTIDES

Many studies of brain lesions, microinjection of drugs, neuropeptides, and microdialysis studies of neurotransmitter levels in freely moving and behaving animals indicate that the control of feeding behavior can be localized to the hypothalamus. The paraventricular nucleus (PVN) seems to be the part of the hypothalamus that is most critical to this process. Lesions of these areas cause obesity, increased parasympathetic tone, and hyperphagia (31).

A significant amount of data suggests that eating disorders represent dysregulations in the neurotransmitter pathways involving DA, serotonin (5-HT), endogenous opioids, and other neuropeptides. The role of the dopaminergic system in eating disorders links them with the pathway of brain reward in which all the classical addictions appear to converge. This reality seems obvious considering the common desire for a cigarette or coffee after a good meal and the stereotypical use of alcohol before sex and a cigarette afterward. Patients in early alcoholism recovery begin eating ice cream and potato chips, bingeing at night. They note that this behavior calms them down. It seems likely that one of the stimulatory peptides is involved in the release of driven eating. Still, eating is much more complex, involving numerous stimulatory and inhibitory peptides and messengers. Table 27.1 lists some of the major neuropeptides involved in regulating appetite and feeding.

Of the inhibitory neuropeptides, neurotensin (NT) has a known important relationship with DA. In the mesencephalon, NT-containing neurons originate in the VTA and terminate in the substantia nigra pars compacta (SNC), the nAC, the caudate putamen, prefrontal cortex, and the central median amygdala. In the diencephalon NT is found within the zona incerta and the median eminence.

NT and DA are both colocalized in neuronal projections from the VTA to the SNC, the prefrontal cortex and within the tuberoinfundibular DA system, particularly the median eminence (32). The importance of NT is evinced through the studies of the effects of cocaine administration and withdrawal on the NT system. Chronic cocaine administration and withdrawal seem to disrupt the normal NT–DA interactions at the nerve cell bodies and terminals. Cocaine-induced increased NT binding in the prefrontal cortex and the SNC may be a result of selective depletion of NT from NT–DA nerve terminals as a result of upregulation of postsynaptic NT receptors. This is analogous to the enhancement of DA binding. Because peptides are not conserved after uptake, as are monoamines, NT is lost more readily than DA in the prefrontal cortex. Thus chronic administration of cocaine may selectively deplete NT from VTA projections to the prefrontal cortex and SNC without markedly affecting levels of DA or the reinforcing effects associated with enhanced DA levels (33).

It is believed that DA, norepinephrine, and 5-HT are all involved in eating and satiety. Recently, there has

TABLE 27.1. *Neuropeptides that regulate food intake and affect eating and energy expenditure*

Stimulate feeding decrease energy expenditure	Inhibit feeding increase energy expenditure
Neuropeptide Y	Serotonin
Galanin	Insulin
Dynorphin	Neurotensin
β-Endorphin	Corticotrophin-releasing factor
Growth hormone-releasing hormone	Dopamine
Norepinephrine	Cholecystokinin
Anandamide	Leptin
γ-Aminobutyric acid	Glucagon-like peptide
Melanin-concentrating hormone	Thyroid-releasing hormone, Melanocyte-stimulating hormone, enterostatin, calcitonin, amylin, bombesin
Hypocretins/orexins	
Ghrelin	
Peptide YY	
Pancreatic polypeptide	Somatostatin, cytokines
	Melanocortin and agouti protein
	Pancreatic polypeptide

Adapted from Kalra SP, Dube MG, Pu S, et al. Interacting appetite-regulating pathways in the hypthalamic regulation of weight. *Endocr Rev* 1999;20(1):68–100.

been increased interest in the study of CNS 5-HT function and its general relationship to behavior (34). This research had produced an array of findings that have been among the most replicated in modern biologic psychiatry. Central to these studies is the finding that a low cerebrospinal fluid (CSF) concentration of 5-hydroxyindoleacetic acid (5-HIAA), a measure of CNS 5-HT activity, is correlated with impaired impulse control and with violence toward others and self. In all rearing conditions, the low 5-HIAA monkeys drink alcohol uncontrollably (34,35). Low 5-HIAA personality indices observed in human studies include chronic irritability, low-grade chronic somatic anxiety, dysphoria, violence (acting or lashing out), alcohol-related problems, and suicide attempts. Finally, the increased frequency of anger attacks among patients with eating disorders (36) are attributed to central serotonergic dysregulation that was previously associated with impulsive aggressive behavior (37). Patients with eating disorders exhibit several clinical features and biologic findings indicative of 5-HT dysregulation, including feeding abnormalities, depression, suicide, impulsivity, violence, anxiety, harm avoidance, obsessive-compulsive features, seasonality, and simultaneous dis-

turbances in neuroendocrine and neurochemical systems linked to 5-HT (38).

Neuropeptide Y

Neuropeptide Y (NPY) is a good place to start as a model for uncontrolled hyperphagia. NPY is one of the most abundant and widely distributed neuropeptides known. It is a member of the pancreatic polypeptide family but has a number of unique actions in the regulation of body weight by driving food intake. NPY is involved in the regulation of other hormones and neurotransmitters and appears involved in circadian rhythms. Studies indicate that 5-HT may play an antagonistic role with NPY in the regulation of feeding (39). 5-HT neurons innervate NPY-containing neurons in the arcuate nucleus. Central injections of 5-HT inhibit food intake through NPY as we might expect serotonin-specific reuptake inhibitors (SSRIs) to act. NPY infusions in the hypothalamus decrease 5-HT release. NPY is the most potent activator of feeding behavior yet discovered. Its levels seem to vary inversely with those of 5-HT. Administration of NPY into the hypothalamic PVN induces feeding in satiated animals and may selectively induce extraordinary carbohydrate intake. Administration of anti-NPY decreases spontaneous carbohydrate intake in animals. Chronic administration of NPY produces an obesity syndrome indistinguishable from naturally occurring obesity. NPY is a potent orexigenic compound and a viable model for driven overeating and obesity.

Neuroanatomic studies show that links exist between many of the neuropeptide systems, possibly indicating a feedback loop (40). NPY and endorphin relationships have been studied in animals. NPY administered intracerebroventricularly and into the PVN of the hypothalamus stimulates feeding and decreases brown adipose tissue thermogenesis. Although specific NPY antagonists are not yet being tested in humans, studies in non-human primates demonstrated that antagonist completely blocked the feeding response induced by NPY infused centrally. Additionally feeding induced by food deprivation was partially inhibited by a NPY antagonist (41).

Studies show that the opioid antagonist naloxone blocked NPY-induced feeding when both drugs were injected intracerebroventricularly. Peripheral naloxone blocked intracerebroventricular NPY-induced feeding and brown fat alterations. Fourth ventricular naloxone decreased PVN NPY-induced feeding and naltrexone given into the nucleus of the solitary tract blocked PVN NPY-induced alterations in feeding and brown fat. These data indicate that NPY–endorphin interactions in the PVN may act on feeding and the nucleus of the solitary tract (42). NPY has a number of known, and probably some unknown, receptors in brain and elsewhere. Which receptor is responsible for NPY effect on feeding and carbohydrate drive is unknown. It is also possible that neuropeptides reinforce existing macronutrient preference and simply increase the attachment for the preferred food, especially those with specific taste, smell, or texture. NPY and also galanin may induce eating in satiated animals and preferentially stimulate carbohydrate and fat intake, respectively, by this mechanism.

With the belief that NPY may induce eating, its role in the pathogenesis of bulimia and other eating disorders is under investigation. Bulimic patients have been found to have normal cerebrospinal fluid neuropeptide Y values. Kaye and associates found (43) that underweight anorexics had significantly elevated concentrations of cerebrospinal fluid NPY compared to healthy volunteers. CSF NPY levels appeared to return to normal with recovery, although anorexia nervosa (AN) with amenorrhea continued to have higher CSF NPY levels. However, elevated cerebrospinal fluid NPY levels appear to be an ineffective stimulant of feeding in underweight anorexics because they are notoriously resistant to eating and weight restoration. Alternatively, chronic elevation of NPY could be associated with a downregulation of the NPY receptors that modulate feeding in AN. Different trends were found upon investigation of plasma. When plasma NPY were measured, concentrations in AN patients were lower than in controls; patients with bulimia nervosa (BN) had significantly higher levels than either AN patients or controls (44,45).

d-Fenfluramine, a potent 5-HT agonist previously used in the treatment of obesity, blocks or attenuates NPY-induced or driven feeding in animals. Acute *d*-fenfluramine administration actually decreases NPY content in the hypothalamus, selectively in the paraventricular and arcuate nuclei. While the precise mechanism of fenfluramine's effects on eating is unknown, it does appear that it is an effect dependent on the presence of the medication and related to inducing a NPY store deficiency in the hypothalamus. These are very exciting and important studies because of the basic literature that supports a critical role for NPY. Studies of NPY microinjections into the hypothalamic PVN elicit a binge-type behavior similar to the binges of bulimic patients, even overriding states of satiety. NPY may be the brain's physiologic signal that means hunger and is the physiologic signal that drives feeding.

Neuroscientific progress allows certain patients with eating disorders to be categorized according to neuropeptide and treated accordingly. For example, testing patients for NPY or galanin abnormalities may identify important obesity subgroups, which may also explain clinical characteristics such as excessive fat eating. Leptin or other chemical abnormalities may also be defined. Although our body of knowledge in this area is expanding greatly, we still cannot diagnose or treat eating disorders via neurochemical markers. Neurotransmitter modulation of neuropeptides may also yield new treatments. 5-HT is demonstrated in animal and human studies to inhibit feeding and produce satiety. Administration of 5-HT agonists, including dexfenfluramine (46–48), sertraline (49), and fluoxetine (50,51) all result in weight loss and decreased food intake for as long as they are administered. New treatments for eating disorders may lead to novel approaches to cocaine and other addictions.

Peptide YY

Another key modulator of food intake is peptide YY (PYY), a neuropeptide cleaved from the larger molecule that includes NPY and pancreatic polypeptide. The substance is released in response to fatty nutrients and acts to inhibit gastric motility and gastric and insulin secretion (52,53). Although mainly found in the ileum and large intestine, lower doses have been reported in the mammalian central nervous system. Receptors have been located throughout the brain with higher density in the thalamic, limbic and hindbrain nuclei (54–56).

It is believed that PYY is an even more potent orexigen than NPY (57). PYY produces hyperphagia when injected into either of the cerebroventricles, the PVN, and the hippocampus, an extrahypothalamic site not usually associated with ingestive responses. Among all orexigenic peptides and neurotransmitters known, PYY is the most potent acute stimulator of food intake.

Clinically, PYY levels are significantly elevated in the CSF of 30-day–abstaining bulimia nervosa patients when compared either to healthy controls, to anorexia nervosa patients, or to their own CSF PYY levels shortly after binge eating and vomiting (58,59). CSF elevations of PYY may affect gastrointestinal levels of PYY to mobilize functions ameliorative to purging-induced injury. Some of these functions include delayed gastric emptying to optimize absorption of nutrients (60), maintenance of electrolyte balance (61), and protection of gastric mucosa (62). Agents that attenuate PYY-induced hyperphagia in rats such as opioid antagonists and serotonin reuptake inhibitors (63) ameliorate bulimic symptomatology (64,65). These facts argue for a role of PYY in bulimia nervosa. In contrast, patients with AN, whether underweight or recovered, had normal CSF PYY concentrations.

Assessment of CSF and plasma PYY in binge-eating disorder (BED) patients will clarify to what degree PYY is linked to long-lasting physiologic adaptations versus compensatory behaviors, since these behaviors are absent in BED patients (66).

Pancreatic Polypeptide

Pancreatic polypeptide (PP) is a 36-amino-acid peptide that belongs to a family including NPY and PYY. PP is produced in the endocrine type F cells located in the periphery of pancreatic islets and is released into the circulation after ingestion of food and exercise (67–71). PP released by food ingestion inhibits further food intake by modulating the rate of gastric emptying during the meal. On the other hand, central administration of PP elicits food intake and gastric emptying via NPY receptors. Therefore, PP actions on food intake may be, in part, attributable to gastric emptying. PP is an anorexigenic signal in the periphery and an orexigenic signal in the central nervous system (72,73).

A recent study in healthy volunteers investigated the effect of intravenous PP on appetite and energy expenditure. The data demonstrates that PP causes a sustained decrease in both appetite and food intake. As expected, appetite and energy intake decreased 2 hours after infusion. More importantly the inhibition of food intake was sustained, such that the 24-hour energy intake was significantly reduced. This data demonstrates that PP causes a sustained decrease in both appetite and food intake (74).

Ghrelin

Ghrelin is a neuropeptide, produced in the hypothalamus, which stimulates the release of growth hormone. Ghrelin is also an important regulator of food intake, being released from the stomach in response to fasting. Masamitsu and colleagues confirmed the belief when they demonstrated that intraventricular injections of ghrelin stimulated feeding in rats and increased body weight. Antighrelin immunoglobulins greatly suppressed feeding. Ghrelin also increases NPY gene expression and antagonized the effect of leptin-induced feeding reduction (75). In obese individuals, plasma ghrelin is low (76). Increased fasting plasma ghrelin levels (77) are reported in patients with anorexia nervosa (AN). Specifically, those with the binge–purge variety have a statistically higher level than their restricting counterparts (78). Bulimic patients who used vomiting as their purging method also appear to have higher ghrelin levels than their nonpurging peers. Leading hypotheses regarding these results include that vomiting may accelerate the release of ghrelin or damage the ghrelin-producing endocrine cells or influence circulating ghrelin levels via the vagal system (79). Ghrelin continues to play important roles in the understanding and treatment of eating disorders and obesity.

BEHAVIORAL SIMILARITIES

Addictions and eating disorders share many common clinical features. Some researchers suggest that classifying eating disorders as addictions based on phenomenologic analogy is an example of overgeneralization and selective reduction (80). However, it is clear that the commonalties between these disorders are not limited to behavioral observations but involve an array of still to be elucidated neurotransmitter abnormalities that converge in the centers of brain reward. Addiction has been defined as a disease characterized by the repetitive and destructive use of one or more mood-altering drugs that stems from a biologic vulnerability exposed or induced by environmental factors

(81). It is a maladaptive pattern of substance use leading to clinically significant impairment or distress with 3 or more of the following in the same 12-month period:

1. Tolerance.
2. Withdrawal.
3. The substance is often taken in larger amounts or over longer periods than was intended.
4. Persistent desire or unsuccessful efforts to cut down or control use.
5. A great deal of time is spent in activities necessary to obtain the substance, use the substance, or recover from its effects.
6. Important social, occupational, or recreational activities are given up or reduced because of substance abuse.
7. Continued substance use despite knowledge of having a persistent or recurrent physical or psychological problem that was likely to have been caused or exacerbated by the substance.

If current psychiatric diagnostic categories did not define addiction in terms of a psychoactive substance, would eating disorders qualify? Yes. The phenomenologic similarities between eating disorders and traditionally recognized substance abuse disorders are (a) a higher-than-average family history of alcohol or drug abuse; (b) cravings for food or a psychoactive substance; (c) cognitive dysfunction; (d) the use of food or psychoactive substances to relieve negative affect (e.g., anxiety and depression); (e) secretiveness about the problem behavior; (f) social isolation and maintenance of the problem behavior despite adverse consequences; (g) denial of the presence and severity of the disorder; (h) depression; and (i) experience of a transition where food or the psychoactive substance no longer relieves negative affect but creates the feelings they were originally used to allay. With the change away from considering tolerance and withdrawal as essential pieces of dependence, eating disorders share many of the most salient features of addictions (82). In the eating disorders currently classified in the *Diagnostic and Statistical Manual of Mental Disorders*, 4th ed., text revision (*DSM–IV–TR*), anorexia nervosa, bulimia nervosa, and binge-eating disorder, food is a substance used both repetitively and destructively by either its prolonged restriction or episodic overconsumption (66).

EATING DISORDERS

Eating disorders share the primary reward of feeding but differ in the paired stimuli. Feeding in this context is typically not a response that promotes survival, but rather serves to satisfy other paired stimuli. Various classifications of eating disorders abound in the literature. These classifications have established objective diagnostic criteria that are not correlated with neurotransmitter or other medical abnormality. The recent basic neurobiologic studies show a plethora of neurotransmitter systems are involved in the regulation of feeding, in mood, and in the pathogenesis of psychiatric and addictive disorders. While we have reported similarities between certain patients with eating disorders and those with addictive illness, others have argued for the inclusion of bulimia nervosa and anorexia nervosa into depressive illness or as an obsessive-compulsive spectrum disorder because of the many similarities between obsessive-compulsive disorder and eating disorders (83). They even further suggest that these disorders appear to be related to mood disorder, thus the obsessive-compulsive spectrum disorder family may be a subset of an affective disorder spectrum family (84).

Weight and food preoccupation are the primary symptoms in both anorexia nervosa and bulimia nervosa. Many patients demonstrate both anorexic and bulimic behaviors. Obese, especially morbidly obese, patients describe similar preoccupations. Anorexia nervosa appears in restricting and bulimic subtypes. Up to 50% of anorexia nervosa patients develop bulimic symptoms; significant numbers of patients who are initially bulimic develop anorexic symptoms, and restricting and bulimic subtypes may occasionally alternate in the same patient. The diagnostic process is confusing or confused.

Regardless of the diagnosis, the prevalence of *all* eating disorders appears to be increasing. Age- and gender-specific estimates suggest that approximately 0.5% to 1% of teenage females develop AN; up to 5% of older adolescent and young adult females develop BN. However, a recent population-based study by the Commonwealth Fund estimates that 25% of adolescents regularly engage in self-induced purging as a means of controlling their weight (85). Although there are no reliable population estimates for BED among children and adolescents, clinical experience with obesity in adults suggests that it is at least as common as the other conditions combined. The increase in prevalence rates over time for eating disorders is accounted for primarily by increases in the incidence of BN, increased media attention, improved detection, and less-stringent diagnostic criteria also probably contribute to the apparent "epidemic" of eating disorders.

Eating disorders are not distributed uniformly in the population. More than 90% of patients are female (86), more than 95% are white, and more than 75% are adolescents when they first develop their eating disorder. Most patients are from middle to upper socioeconomic status families, but patients can be of any gender, race, age, or social stratum. Recent studies suggest that the prevalence of eating disorders among minority females is much higher than previously suspected.

Currently, according to the Obesity Educational Initiative compiled by the National Lung, Heart and Blood Institutes, there are 97 million Americans who are overweight or obese. This is a dramatic increase since 1960. Over the last decade 54% of adults over the age of 20 years would now be classified as overweight or obese (87). This increase occurs despite personal trainers, home exercise equipment, and other fitness developments. The specific impact the binge-eating disorder has on this prevalence is not exactly known. However, it is diagnosable in more than 28% of patients who are seen in a weight-loss clinic. A better understanding of the disorder is needed to stop this epidemic.

Anorexia nervosa and bulimia nervosa are the two eating disorder syndromes recognized in the current *DSM–IV*, which was published in 1994 (66). Binge-eating disorder, while officially classified as an eating disorder not otherwise specified (NOS), is being considered for acceptance as a distinct diagnostic entity.

Anorexia Nervosa

Anorexia nervosa is a disease that has been documented back to at least the seventeenth century. While some experts suggest that there are no cases of anorexia nervosa, only starvation, in cultures without food abundance, it appears across the globe in various cultures. In fact, symptoms of anorexia were reported as early as the Middle Ages in female Christian saints (88). Anorexia nervosa is noted, however, to be more prevalent in industrialized societies where "one can never be too rich or too thin." It also occurs in non-Western cultures where weight concern is not apparent (89) and the expressed motivation for food restriction may be epigastric discomfort or distaste for food (66).

The diagnostic criteria for Anorexia nervosa are listed in the *DSM–IV* (66). The name anorexia is a misnomer because loss of appetite is actually rare. Anorexics tend to be obsessed with food, and may even hoard food and exercise for hours daily. They become socially isolated and depressed. Despite steady diminution in social and occupational functioning and the appearance of life-threatening physical disturbances, they will typically deny the severity of their symptoms and respond with disinterest and even resistance to treatment attempts (90). A cognitive distortion develops in which the anorexic's self-worth becomes inexplicably tied to her ability to achieve and maintain an emaciated state. Amenorrhea can appear before noticeable weight loss has occurred. Delayed sexual development in adolescents and poor sexual adjustment in adults is common (90).

Anorexics are classified into two subtypes. The restricting subtype limits their weight loss techniques to calorie restriction and excessive exercise. They tend to exhibit obsessive-compulsive behaviors (91), including, but not limited to, bizarre diet and exercise routines, and express diminished sexual interest. The binge-eating/purging subtype regularly engages in binge eating and purging. Purging methods include self-induced vomiting and the abuse of laxatives, diuretics, or enemas. The presence of binging and purging in anorexics is associated with impulsive behaviors, such as substance abuse, promiscuity, suicide attempts, self-mutilation, and stealing (91). Bulimic symptoms occur in 30% to 80% of anorexics (92) and subtypes can alternate in the same patient (91).

The incidence of anorexia nervosa has increased dramatically in the past 30 years (90). Eating disorders affect an estimated 5 million Americans every year (93). Females continue to comprise most of the cases, with only 5%–15% being male. Prevalence is 0.5% to 1% among late adolescents and adult females with subsyndromal cases even more common (85). The mean age of onset is 17 years and occurrence is rare in persons older than 40 years of age (90). Anorexia has an impressive mortality rate of 0.5% to 1% per observational year. Death is as a consequence of suicide in 30% to 50% of the cases, with the remaining morbidity secondary to medical complications (94). There is complete recovery in approximately 40% of anorexic patients. In another 20% of anorexic patients there is resolution of the eating disorder, but subsequent emergence of other significant psychiatric pathology, including schizophrenia, bipolar disorder, depression, personality disorders, and substance abuse.

Eating disorders, like classical addictions, can have quite tragic outcomes with a high degree of mortality. Anorexia nervosa mortality as estimated from (50) published studies in a recent meta-analysis is substantially greater than for female psychiatric outpatients, 200 times greater than the suicide rate in the general population at approximately 5.6% per decade (96).

The etiology of anorexia is unknown. Many psychosocial and psychodynamic theories have tried to explain its resurgence in modern times, but none define a mechanism for understanding the persistence of this unique symptom complex. The prelude to anorexia is exposure to severe food deprivation (90). This can occur both voluntarily to improve one's appearance or professional performance (e.g., ballet dancers, gymnasts, jockeys) (97) and involuntarily as a consequence of illness, severe stress, or involuntary starvation (90). But as Halmi asks, "What is unique about the individual who goes on to develop anorexia nervosa?" (90) This same question has been contemplated by addiction specialists for decades; that is, why are millions exposed to drugs such as alcohol and tobacco, but only smaller percentage become addicts? Exposure is the common risk factor, but a common neurobiologic process must be operant in all those who use a substance (food in case of anorexics) in a manner that is dangerous to their survival with little insight or regard for negative consequences.

Biologic explanations for the occurrence of this disease date back to the early 1950s when scientists found that lesions of the lateral hypothalamus lead to an avoidance of food in malnourished rats. More recent research indicates that the lateral hypothalamic area may be involved in the discrimination between food and nonfood through both visual and gustatory stimuli. This area also appears to mediate perception of reward and drive for food (98). A genetic association or common neurobiologic risk is evident from the high concordance of this disease between monozygotic twins (99). A definitive pathogenesis is unknown, although numerous investigations have identified reproducible abnormalities.

5-HT, DA, opioid peptides, and other food-relevant messengers are thought to have a critical role in the pathogenesis of anorexia nervosa. Many studies show that 5-HT activity parallels behavioral characteristics of anorexia nervosa, with the phenomenology of anorexia nervosa being related to serotonergic hyperactivity (100). These authors relate the disparity in gender prevalence to the greater hypophagic effect of serotonergic agents in female rats than in male rats (100,101). Human 5-HT levels have long been shown to diverge between the sexes. While men have been reported with anorexia nervosa, cases are extremely rare (102). Anorexia nervosa occurs before the onset of menses in approximately one-third of patients but is commonly followed by correlating amenorrhea and active disease state. Rather than thinking of the disease of some sort of rejection of adult sexuality, brain mechanisms common to luteinizing hormone rhythmicity and food reward may be particularly vulnerable in early adolescence. In all women, changes in levels of sex hormones during the normal menstrual cycle appear to affect 5-HT's influence on appetite. Furthermore, sexual repression frequently observed in anorexics mirrors the inhibition of female sexual behavior in other species by 5-HT (103).

Overall, 5-HT seems to be more potent as an appetite suppressant in women. It would be logical to believe that increased levels of 5-HT would be involved in the development of anorexia nervosa. Cocaine, which increases 5-HT and other essential brain messengers, produces anorexia in men and women who chronically self-administer cocaine. It also is associated with amenorrhea and delusions of well-being.

In actuality, however, the level of the major brain metabolite of 5-HT, 5-HIAA, appears to be reduced in the cerebral spinal fluid of anorexics rather than elevated (104). Following this observation, the serotonergic antidepressant fluoxetine has shown some favorable results in uncontrolled clinical trials with anorexics (105,106). To incorporate the observed efficacy of a serotonergic agent into the hyperserotonergic model it has been postulated that the chronic use of fluoxetine, through the downregulation of 5-HT receptors (107) results in a decrease in serotonergic hypersensitivity (108). Alternatively, fluoxetine's beneficial effect may be on obsessive-compulsive symptomatology (108). Certainly the SSRIs are not a cure for anorexia nervosa and are of limited value in supporting a 5-HT hypothesis. Another confounding finding is the modest response obtained with the antiserotonergic agent cyproheptadine (109).

Central DA dysfunctions have been suggested to be involved in the development and course of AN. Because dopamine is a physiologic inhibitor of hunger, a hypersecretion has been proposed to be responsible for anorexia and weight loss (110). Studies of central secretion of DA and its metabolites in AN are contradictory; with CSF concentrations of DA and its main metabolite homovanillic acid (HVA), having found to be normal (111), increased (112), or decreased (113–118) during disease active state.

Even with this suggested connection to dopamine, medications involving this neural system for the treatment of anorexia nervosa are limited. Few trials with older dopamine antagonists showed a possible trend for higher weight gain. While the data for chlorpromazine (Thorazine) showed statistical significance as compared to placebo, side effects were severe and frequent (119,120). Recent studies using the newer atypical antipsychotics that involve dopamine and serotonin receptors are in the initial stages, although results are promising (121–123).

Anorexia nervosa is also described by some as an "autoaddiction." The absence of food produces a state of strikingly bizarre well-being, which is supported by continued starvation. Marrazzi and Luby (124) proposed that, in an autoaddictive model, the disease might begin as a phobic fear arising from more general concerns about body image. Secondarily, the patient develops a ritualistic behavior revolving around dieting, exercise, and burning calories. Finally, chronicity leads to the condition of anorexia nervosa. They suggest that this psychobiologic process alters brain feeding mechanisms that gradually are recognized as a "normal" state, much like drug addicts of all types consume their drugs of choice to feel normal. In this sense, the disease state is a result of tolerance, dependence, and neuroadaptive mechanisms at a critical period in the developing organism's existence.

Central to this model is the role of opioids (124). It is during the initial period of dieting that opioids are released, reflected in increased CSF activity. This release of opioids affects the primitive dopaminergic reward system so as to reinforce the dieting behavior. The result is that the anorexic behavior of suppressing the drive for food is reinforced by the very signal which causes the drive to eat, namely increased opioid activity: opioids downregulate metabolism as an adaptation to starvation. Upregulation is seen with physical exercise. Confirming this theory, increased levels of endogenous opioids activity were discovered in the CSF of patients with anorexia nervosa (125). The results of this molecular change are the potentially tragic consequences of anorexia nervosa (126).

Bulimia Nervosa

Like adolescent alcohol and drug use, while many young men and women experiment with severe diets, starvation, fasting, and self-induced vomiting, few apparently lose control and become anorexic or bulimic. The diagnostic criteria for bulimia nervosa are listed in the *DSM–IV* (66). As initially described by Russell in 1979 (92), the defining behaviors in bulimia nervosa are episodes of binge eating combined with compensatory techniques to avoid gaining weight. Whether it is planned or spontaneous, the impulse to binge is perceived as irresistible by the bulimic. There is a subjective loss of control during the binge, with rapid consumption until the bulimic is uncomfortably, or even painfully, full. Because of significant shame engendered by this behavior, binge eating is typically done only in private and stopped if inadvertently discovered (92). After the binge-eating episode has run its course, the individual can be left with feelings of depression, guilt, or self-disgust.

The compensatory methods in bulimia are categorized as purging and nonpurging. Purging behaviors are self-induced vomiting and abuse of laxatives, diuretics, or enemas. Self-induced vomiting is practiced by 80% to 90% of patients. If fingers are used, scars and abrasions can often be found on the dorsum of the hand known as *Russell sign*. Other implements and, rarely, syrup of ipecac are used to induce vomiting, but most bulimics eventually learn how to vomit spontaneously. For some bulimics vomiting becomes a reinforcing goal in itself, occurring even after small meals. Laxatives, either alone or in combination with other purging methods, are employed by 38% to 75% of bulimic women (127). Bulimics practicing laxative abuse appear to exhibit greater psychiatric pathology, as reflected by an increased frequency of suicide attempts, self-injurious behaviors, and hospitalized depression (128), than do bulimics who use self-induced vomiting only. Nonpurging compensatory methods include fasting, excessive exercise, surreptitious use of thyroid hormone, and reduction of insulin dosage by diabetics to avoid metabolism of consumed food. Bulimics try to restrict caloric intake between binges and avoid foods that are binge triggers for them.

Bulimia nervosa is more common than anorexia nervosa, with prevalence among women of 1% to 3% (129,130). Only 10% to 15% of bulimics are men. Bulimia nervosa has traditionally been regarded as a disease afflicting middle to upper class white women (131), but recent reports suggest that its prevalence among ethnically diverse groups, although not as great, is significant (132). The age of onset ranges from 12 to 35 years of age, with a mean of 18 years of age (133). It is thought that bulimia nervosa tends to occur in overweight individuals during or following a dieting attempt and up to a third may be previous anorexics (90). The body weight of bulimics fluctuates but tends to remain in the normal range. There is an increased incidence of mood disorders, specifically dysthymia and major depression; the prevalence of borderline personality disorder in bulimics ranges from 25% to 48% (134). The reported incidence of drug abuse among bulimics is as high as 46% (135). Bulimia has a significant relapse rate (31%) within 2 years following treatment, but relapse after 6 months of symptom control is unusual

(136). Relapse occurs more often in patients who are vomiting than in those who are bingeing, but the significance of this fact is unknown.

As with classical addictions, eating disorders interfere with normal life patterns. Preoccupation with the substance in question, such as supermarket gazing and cooking for others, is common (99). Just as with other addictive substances, the over consumption of food or binging is frequently conducted at night or in secret, both historically and in current practice (137). Bulimics, like other addicts, appear to have a favorite "drug" of abuse, consuming proportionally more sweet, high-fat foods during larger meals (44). It is quite common to hear of a bulimic trigger in the same way an addict describes a drug cue that precipitates intense cravings and use. Bulimics describe external and internal cues such as seeing a pizza delivery truck or feeling depressed as triggering thoughts that they are fat or in need of a binge–purge episode. They describe rituals similar to drug-using rituals with similar foods and environments.

Bulimia nervosa, like anorexia nervosa, is characterized by abnormalities in the regulation of feeding. It has long been known to have a high comorbidity with substance abuse (138), particularly alcoholism (139). A review of 51 comorbidity studies conducted since 1977 found that greater comorbidity with substance abuse was present among bulimics than anorexics and among bulimic anorexics than restrictor (140). In a recent comorbidity study, 37% of 105 female patients with eating disorders met *DSM–III–R* criteria for either alcohol or drug dependence (141). The most commonly abused drugs were cannabis, cocaine, stimulants, and diet pills. Substance dependence was more common in patients with personality disorders. Thirty-one percent of the bulimic subgroups had cluster B personality disorders, with borderline personality disorder the most common, while none of the restrictor anorexics had a cluster B disorder. Restrictor anorexics were significantly less likely to be alcohol or drug dependent than the group as a whole. Similarly, in retrospective review of female psychiatric inpatient records from 1978 to 1990, the high incidence of alcohol abuse in the patients with eating disorders was accounted for by the subset of patients with borderline personality disorders. The occurrence of borderline personality disorders was significantly higher (11.4% vs. 2.9%) in patients with eating disorders than in others (142). While some findings are controversial it is clear that there is a very high incidence of alcohol abuse, drug abuse, or both among bulimic women.

Garfinkel and Garner (143) reported that 18.3% of their bulimics used alcohol at least weekly and 21.2% were frequent illicit drug users. Mitchell and coworkers (144) found that 34.4% of bulimics had a history of drug or alcohol problems and 23% had very serious alcohol abuse, with 17.7% having treatment for a chemical dependency. These data are consistent with the Yager et al. survey of 628 women with eating disorders (145) in which 38% reported

weekly alcohol use and 22.7% reported daily alcohol use. These authors also reported on a very high level of illicit drug use, with daily use in excess of 10% for marihuana alone. The authors reported, as have others, that the converse is also true and that eating disorders are very common among cocaine addicts, alcoholics, and other addicts in primary addiction treatment.

5-HT, dopamine, and opioids also seem to be important neurotransmitters involved in the pathogenesis of bulimia nervosa. Studies show low levels of 5-HT metabolite (5-HIAA) and low DA metabolite (HVA) in the CSF of bulimic patients when compared with normal controls. Low 5-HT and low DA in nAC and elsewhere is the critical chemical link to pathologic alcohol reward or preference (146). Decreased release of DA in the mesocorticolimbic system may affect taste preference of bulimic patients resulting in a decreased enjoyment of food. Bulimics' preference for high sucrose solutions may indicate that the impaired reward function could contribute to addictive cravings for food (147). Low 5-HT levels are also known to be associated with increased appetite, alcoholism, and impassivity.

Bulimic patients were found to exhibit higher pleasantness ratings for highly sweetened sucrose solution than controls or bulimics with a history of anorexia. These foods might produce a pathologic reward and attachment in the same way that alcohol produces excessive mesolimbic DA release in response to alcohol availability or use in alcohol preferring animals. Perceived deprivation of the normal level of hedonistic response to food could induce an addiction-like craving for food, culminating in a binge episode. Again, like alcohol, there is evidence that the hedonistic response to sweet taste involves both endogenous opioids (133) and central DA in the mesolimbic reward pathways. Interestingly, in addition to decreased CSF β-endorphin levels, bulimic patients with frequent binge episodes have lower CSF concentrations of the DA metabolite homovanillic acid (147). Decreased central DA appears to be a common feature of early drug abstinence and is related to dysphoria and craving as well as to depression. CSF β-endorphin levels in bulimic patients were found to be lower than in controls (148), which, interestingly, have been reported for alcoholic patients who have also responded to naltrexone (ReVia).

In the case of bulimia nervosa, the theory of 5-HT hypoactivity has been posited (44). According to this model, bulimics binge to improve their mood (i.e., self-medicate) by elevating brain 5-HT levels (44). Cocaine acutely elevates brain 5-HT and, while producing euphoria, inhibits appetite. High-carbohydrate, low-protein meals favor the transport of tryptophan into the CNS, which is the rate-limiting step in the synthesis of 5-HT (149). CSF 5-HIAA was found to be reduced in bulimic patients who binged at least twice a day (147), and in bulimic women, acute tryptophan depletion caused significant increased food intake, mood lability, irritability, and retarded affect over controls (150). Further support for serotonergic involvement is the seasonal variation in mood and eating symptoms among 10% to 45% of bulimic patients (151–154). Light therapy improved mood and eating behavior in a preliminary study with 17 bulimic patients (155). Light therapy may influence serotonergic pathways (156), as well as correct circadian rhythm disturbances (157,158). Serotoninergic theories appear to be the most relevant to bulimia, and a 5-HT subgroup may be quite important. Still, there are major problems with this theory. Problems with the 5-HT theory of bulimia nervosa are the observations that (a) binge meals do not generally contain a higher proportion of carbohydrates than do nonbinge meals (159) and (b) selective serotonergic antidepressants are no more efficacious than other antidepressant classes in the treatment of bulimia (108).

Knowing that 5-HT inhibits feeding, a number of studies have investigated the effect of antidepressants on bulimia. The SSRI fluoxetine (Prozac) is approved by the U.S. Food and Drug Administration for treatment of this disorder in adults. Symptoms that appeared to improve include binge/purge behavior and concerns regarding body weight (160). Patients treated with monoamine oxidase (MAO) inhibitors, which increase 5-HT, especially in high doses, report binge eating as a side effect of their treatment; however, it is not certain that this is a drug-driven effect and not a rebound from depressive illness. Studies of other medications that interact with the serotonin system, such as the serotonergic precursor L-tryptophan (161) and serotonergic agonist dexfenfluramine (162,163) were not impressive.

Scientists have tried to further understand the role opioids may have in the abnormal eating pattern seen in bulimia. Bulimic patients have been found to have low cerebrospinal fluid β-endorphin levels (164). Ingesting sweets has been correlated with increased opioid activity (165). Bulimics are known to binge on sweet, high-fat foods. Thus, abnormal endorphin levels may be related to bingeing behavior.

Research suggests (166) that opioid agonists increase and opioid antagonists decrease food intake. This information along with the noted rewarding aspects of feeding prompted studies investigating the effect of the opioid antagonist, naltrexone in both humans and animals. Open trials of high dosages of naltrexone have been reported to reduce binge frequency in bulimia (167–169). However, all but one (170) of the several double-blind, controlled trials using naltrexone showed no effects on binge frequency (171,172). The role of endogenous opioids in the pathogenesis and treatment of BN remains to be determined.

Binge-Eating Disorder

Obesity has many possible causes and may be divided into groups including hypothyroidism, diabetes mellitus, or binge-eating disorders. Binge-eating disorder is perhaps the most common, yet least studied, of the eating disorders (173). Binge-eating disorders, like drug addiction, are characterized by a pathologic attachment. Both include obsessive thoughts about food and compulsions to eat more food than most people would eat within similar periods of time and in similar circumstances. Like cocaine addiction or alcoholism, the binge eater cannot take or leave it—they "can't eat just one." The binge episodes generally cause the binge eater much distress, leaving them with feelings of guilt, disgust, and depression.

Research criteria for binge-eating disorder are listed in *DSM–IV* (66). Binge-eating disorder as defined is essentially bulimia nervosa in the absence of regular inappropriate compensatory behaviors, that has a duration of at least 6 months (174). A large multisite *DSM–IV* field trial with 2,727 subjects found a prevalence rate of 4.6% in a community sample and 28.7% among weight-loss program patients (175). The prevalence was significantly greater among women in the weight-loss patients (29.7% vs. 21.8%), yet the rate among men was substantial. As McElroy et al. note, "given that 34 million adults in the United States are overweight, even if only a small fraction of these individuals had binge-eating disorder, it would represent a large number of individuals" (84). By contrast, purging bulimia was found in only 0.5% of the community sample and 6.7% of the weight-loss patients.

Also in contrast to bulimia nervosa, binge-eating disorder appears to occur at least as often among ethnic minorities as among whites (176). Smith (132) suggests that such a finding should be anticipated because binge-eating disorder is more common in the obese (177) and obesity is more prevalent in minorities such as Native Americans, Hispanics, and African Americans. In some individuals, binge eating occurs prior to the development of obesity (178). Wurtman has previously described what she calls carbohydrate-craving obesity (179). In this disorder subjects preferentially consume carbohydrates at particular times during the day, typically in the early evening. Commonly these patients meet *DSM–IV* criteria for binge-eating disorder. Many of these patients give a strong family history for alcoholism and multiple previous attempts and failures in dieting, exercising, and surgeries.

Higher rates of depression, psychological distress, and impulsivity have been reported among those who binge than among obese subjects who do not (179). Preliminary studies did not consistently demonstrate an increased incidence of substance abuse or dependence in individuals with binge-eating disorder (180–183). In a study comparing men and women with BED, men appeared to have higher lifetime prevalence for alcohol dependence than the general population. However, the rate of substance abuse among their first-degree relatives was reported to be 49% (182), greater than the rate of 37% in the first-degree relatives of bulimics.

Sweet cravings occur with opiate addiction (185) and sweets can sometimes improve opiate withdrawal (186).

Drugs affecting the same neurotransmitter systems have been found to be efficacious in treating both eating disorders and the classical drug addictions. The serotonergic agent fenfluramine, in combination with the weak amphetamine phentermine (Adipex-P) that is currently being used in the treatment of obesity, has been reported to decrease craving and self-reported use in cocaine addicts (187). Naltrexone, which reduces the frequency of binge eating, reduces craving and relapse in alcoholics (188). A careful look at the neural events involved in pathologic drug attachment appears essential in links to pathologic eating.

Dopamine involvement in normal and pathologic food intake appears to be related to its role in reward and reinforcement. While no data is available specifically in the binge-eating disorder population, information is increasing about dopamine in obese patients. Imaging studies using positron emission tomography implicate low brain DA activity in obese individuals Specifically, it has been shown that the dopamine D2 receptor availability was decreased in obese individuals in proportion to their body mass index (189,190). It is believed that pathologic eating in obese individuals may serve to increase activation of this underactive system. It is important to note that low levels of dopamine D2 receptors have also been reported in individuals addicted to various types of drugs, including cocaine (191), alcohol (192), and opiates (193). This reinforces the central role of dopamine in addictive behavior, be it disordered eating or substance use.

Studies show that consumption of carbohydrates can selectively increase the levels of 5-HT in the brain (194). This process involves consumption of carbohydrates, which increases levels of tryptophan in the blood. Tryptophan is subsequently transported across the blood–brain barrier where it is converted to 5-HT. The studies show that consumption of carbohydrates is likely a specific response to decreased brain 5-HT. (Subjects with carbohydrate-craving obesity are thought to have lower 5-HT levels than control subjects.) Thus, carbohydrates are not necessarily consumed during times of food hunger, but instead are likely consumed to correct this deficit in 5-HT. Lowered brain 5-HT function may be caused by a calorie restricted, carbohydrate-limited, weight-loss regimen and result in negative mood changes leading to termination of the diet (195). These studies also show that the consumption is specific to carbohydrates: consumption of protein and fat does not increase. Consumption of carbohydrate-rich, protein-poor foods has been shown to result in an increased uptake of tryptophan and increased serotonergic synthesis and activity. Foods rich in protein inhibit this effect. Consumption of proteins may increase blood levels of tryptophan as well as other similar amino acids, but all compete for transport into the brain; thus there is no appreciable rise in brain tryptophan. Studies of 5-HT replacement also show decreases in the amounts of carbohydrate consumed, further indicating that increased carbohydrate consumption is in likely response to decreased

brain 5-HT (99). Extrapolating from this example, one can see how feeding in eating disorders is a result of the reward of feeding becoming paired with stimuli other than hunger. This results in an excess of feeding that bypasses or disrupts the normal mechanisms of appetite, hunger, and satiety control.

A recent small study using used single-photon emission computed tomography (SPECT) suggested that 5-HT transporter binding in the mid-brain is decreased in obese binge-eating women (196). Followup of treated patients with symptomatically recovered binge-eating disorder showed significantly increased 5-HT transporter binding, as compared to unchanged results in controls (197). These studies strongly support the role of serotonin and disordered eating.

It is known that medications that increase available 5-HT decrease carbohydrate consumption (198). The use of antidepressants to suppress binge eating in patients with BED is based on their demonstrated efficacy in bulimia nervosa. Serotonin reuptake inhibitors, used in high dosage, and tricyclic antidepressants yield substantially greater reduction in binge eating than placebo. Six-week trials of sertraline (Zoloft) (199), fluoxetine (200), and citalopram (Celexa) (201) for binge-eating disorder also show significant weight loss in treated patients. Long-term studies of these medications are needed to determine their long-term efficacy for both binge symptomatology and associated weight loss. It is noteworthy that nortriptyline (Pamelor), a tricyclic antidepressant, is efficacious for eliminating nicotine addiction (202).

Like the antidepressants, appetite suppressants such as phentermine and dexfenfluramine (which has been withdrawn from the market because of an association with heart valve disease) were found to produce short-term binge suppression with postdiscontinuation relapse (203–205). One open-label study using sibutramine (Meridia), a reuptake inhibitor of both serotonin and noradrenaline, showed significant loss of weight and improvement in binge episodes over a 12-week trial (206). Further studies are underway to determine the usefulness of this medication in the treatment of binge-eating disorder.

Several medications are in use for the treatment of substance abuse disorders, as well as eating disorders. As mentioned earlier, naltrexone has been investigated for its potential role in the treatment of cravings in anorexia, bulimia, and binge-eating disorder. Bupropion (Wellbutrin), is an antidepressant that is FDA approved for assisting in smoking cessation (207). A recent study showed its effectiveness in assisting weight loss in overweight and obese woman during an 8-week trial (208). These patients were not assessed for a binge pattern being a factor in their current weight.

Two studies (one case series and one open label) of topiramate (Topamax), an antiepileptic, for binge-eating disorder have been encouraging; both showed a significant reduction in binging and subsequently body weight in the majority of patients (209). Topiramate is an antiepileptic medication that facilitates γ-aminobutyric acid (GABA), leading to a decrease in extracellular release of dopamine in the midbrain (210). Studies for its use in binge-eating disorder have been encouraging. One case series and one open-label trial have both showed a significant reduction in bingeing, and subsequently of body weight, in the majority of patients (209). Recently, researchers have started to investigate the role of topiramate for the treatment of alcohol dependence. The initial randomized controlled study seems promising, with the study drug being more efficacious than placebo as an adjunct to standardized management (211). Multicenter trials are underway to further elucidate the role of this medication both in the treatment of eating disorders and substance addiction.

OTHER TREATMENT MODALITIES

We have examined the many similarities between substance addiction and eating disorders. As stated earlier, many of the same psychopharmacologic agents are used in the management of these syndromes. As important to treatment are the psychosocial and behavioral interventions frequently used. Group therapy is one of the most frequently used techniques in both substance abuse and eating disorder treatment programs. It allows communication of feelings, the sharing of frustrations, and offers the experience of closeness. It is a mechanism to provide strength for others who are struggling with control of substances or food. A 40-study meta-analysis with an average followup of 1 year suggests that group therapy for bulimia is moderately effective. Although commonly used as a component of their treatment, limited evidence is available for the use of group therapy in anorexia and binge-eating disorder patients.

Marital therapy and family therapy focuses on the maladaptive behaviors of the identified patient and on abnormal patterns of family interaction. It includes family members as active participants in the healing process. With their help, medication compliance and session attendance is ensured. Therapy focused on improving family dynamics and restructuring poor communication patterns. The goal being the establishment of a more supportive, appropriate environment for the person in recovery. Several well-designed research studies support the effectiveness of behavioral relationship therapy in improving the functioning of families and improving treatment outcomes for individuals with substance addiction (212), as well as anorexia nervosa (213).

Cognitive–behavioral therapy (CBT) attempts to alter the cognitive processes that lead to maladaptive behavior, intervene in the chain of events that lead to the disorder, and then promote and reinforce necessary skills and behaviors for achieving and maintaining remission. Research studies consistently demonstrate that such techniques improve self-control and social skills, thus helping to reduce drinking (American Psychiatric Association, 1995) (91). In eating-disorder patients, the aim is to help patients re-

think their eating and exercise habits and find other ways to cope with situations and feelings that induce binges. Many studies have found CBT to be successful in reducing the frequency of binge eating and self-induced vomiting, as well as in improving attitudes toward eating (214), in bulimic patients. As expected, this intervention is also being used to help control binge episodes in those with binge-eating disorder. Preliminary results are encouraging (215–217).

Self-help groups are defined as "a supportive, educational, usually change-oriented mutual aid group that addresses a single life problem or condition shared by all members" (217). Twelve-step groups such as Alcoholics Anonymous, Narcotics Anonymous, and Cocaine Anonymous are the backbone of many substance treatment efforts as well as a major form of continuing care. In 1990, *Twelve Steps of Overeaters Anonymous* was published, which has attempted to adapt the 12-step philosophy to the area of eating disorders (218). These fellowships help persons change old behavior patterns and maintain hope and determination to become and remain well.

IMPORTANCE OF DRUG STATE TO BEHAVIOR

Most current drugs of abuse have profound and important effects on eating and food preference. Alcoholics report appetite loss during intoxication and specific food cravings during abstinence. Nicotine dependence is associated with loss of weight and weight gain with abstinence. Marihuana induces eating and specific eating patterns descried as the "munchies." Cocaine and amphetamines are potent anorexics. Opiates appear to induce and opiate antagonists to decrease eating (Table 27.2). Drug abstinence states are referred to in terms of food. Hunger for drugs, the taste of drugs, and cravings are commonplace and can just as easily be heard on an eating disorder ward as an addiction service.

There have been numerous reports of comorbidity between eating disorders and substance abuse (33). Eating disorders run in addiction families and vice versa. Eating patterns change among alcoholics and other addicts depending on their drug status. Alcoholics in early abstinence report carbohydrate craving. NPY is a primary mediator of carbohydrate "drive" and norepinephrine is also a possible mediator, but DA is not. While norepinephrine and NPY drive carbohydrate cravings and intake, 5-HT

TABLE 27.2. *Effects of addictive drugs on eating*

Drug	Administration	Withdrawal
Nicotine	Decreases	Increases
Stimulant	Decreases	Increases
Marihuana	Increases	—
Opiate	Increases fat intake	—
Ethanol	Decreases by providing empty calories	Increases sugar, carbohydrate intake

is a primary inhibitor of carbohydrate intake. Although humans have well-developed and highly regulated drives for micronutrients in food, we appear to have poorly developed satiety. If we are deprived of a food or drink which we are accustomed to, the brain increases appetite for nutrients, appetites for specific foods, and/or alcohol ingestion, causing decreased perception of anxiety and stress. NPY appears to reduce anxiety, so carbohydrate or alcohol intake can actually increase self-perceptions of well-being. Another neuromodulator of eating, galanin, is also known to be a potent analgesic. This suggests that eating, especially eating fat, may reduce pain. Just putting a galanin antagonist in the hypothalamus of animals totally stops the eating of fat. Like opioids and other drugs, the more fat we eat, the more we want. The more eating of fat, the more galanin Liebowitz and her colleagues (35) find in the brain. In this way, she explains the "drive" for fat and a mechanism for fat craving. The resultant obesity occurs as a consequence of our poor fat satiety control. We eat carbohydrates generally in the morning; we eat fat between lunch and dinner. Alcoholics, in the early abstinence stage, report bingeing not only on fats but also on carbohydrates throughout the day.

Tobacco, alcohol, and other drug use starts and increases dramatically during adolescence. Fat intake rises dramatically at puberty. Appetite for ethanol also rises at puberty. Are the new appetites and drives that come along after puberty related? NPY stimulates intake of carbohydrate, galanin stimulates fat and some carbohydrate intake, and opiates stimulate fat and some protein intake after direct injection into the brain. Fluoxetine suppresses carbohydrate with no change in fat or protein. Opiate antagonists work in a different system and more generally stop fat intake. 5-HT works at special times in circadian and developmental stages, not at all times. Drug experimentation is a necessary precondition to abuse and addiction. Brain reward is essential in making the experimentation more likely to continue and in cementing the attachment necessary for dependence to occur. Dieting may be essential in the onset of anorexia nervosa, bulimia, and even obesity. In many cases, overeating is a paradoxical consequence of attempts at caloric restriction including dieting. Losing weight is the motivation behind diets and diets are rarely successful in achieving the desired effects. What diets may be doing is priming the neurotransmitter and neuromodulator systems to eat more and may be triggers for disinhibited eating.

CONCLUSION

The American media has expanded the country's interpretation of addictions and substance abuse. Pop culture has broadened its concept of addictions to encompass other self-destructive, yet seemingly compulsive, behaviors. These include "workaholics," gamblers, compulsive spenders, and food addicts, the self-confessed "foodaholics." Although this process may provoke a knee-jerk

rejection of commonalties, this chapter has addressed the issue of whether the eating disorders should legitimately be considered as forms of addiction. It appears that this tendency to consider every potentially harmful compulsive or repetitive behavior as an addiction is a major reason for not considering some eating disorders as addictive or autoaddictive disorders. Some believe that the conception of eating disorders as another form of addiction disorder is a "therapeutic dead end" (219). One concern raised is that the addiction-as-disease model is primarily an abstinence model and dieting and food avoidance are risk factors for eating disorders. It must be recognized, however, that with the evolution of our understanding of brain reward systems, the future addiction-as-disease model will include appropriate medication management for relapse prevention. It has also been proposed that patients with eating disorders embrace the suggestion that they have an addiction because then no self-responsibility is involved (82). However, it is clear that eating disorders are not a result of a lack of self-control. In addition to the neurotransmitter aberrations that have been described on SPECT imaging, bulimics exhibit low or negative changes in regional blood flow to the frontal lobe area (220). In answer to the initial question as to whether eating disorders should be classified as addictions, we propose that both disorders involve similar brain systems and result in similar behaviors and feeling states. Both are important diseases where loss of control and compulsive use are preeminent. Both are diverse groups of people with illnesses of unknown etiology, characterized by a chronic relapsing course without specific pathophysiology or treatment. Both involve the acquired pathologic attachment with the agent(s) of their ultimate compromise and possible destruction. Both may involve host or risk factors that predispose a person to extreme reward after consumption or use thereby making repetition more likely to occur. Both involve denial and reluctance to accept that they are in fact ill and in need of treatment. Both can result in early death. Both generally require early experimentation—one with drugs, the other with dieting. Both can be relapse triggers for each other. Drugs are used to decrease eating and eating is used to decrease drug taking. Both are used to accentuate the other. The similarities are numerous and striking. But as long as the diagnostic scheme is descriptive and not neurobiologic it will be difficult to identify which patients have one disorder and which have two disorders. Food is a powerful mood-altering substance that is repetitively and destructively used (or restricted) in eating disorders, and there is considerable experimental evidence of biologic vulnerability. Finally, categorizing eating disorders as addictions also has ramifications for prevention. Epidemiologic studies among high school students show that eating disorders are associated with alcohol use (221), and that even dieting in adolescents is related to alcohol and tobacco abuse (222). With our current appreciation of eating disorders as yet another form of dangerous addiction, it is time that educational efforts be targeted to the adolescent population to halt its current burgeoning growth in our society (223). It is time that individuals with eating disorders are not held "responsible" for a disease process any more than patients with diabetes or heart disease are held responsible. Hopefully this is true for other addicts. Experts worry whether such a discussion might lead to gambling or compulsive sexual behaviors being proposed for inclusion as addictions. However, as the well-known adage goes, if it looks like a duck, acts like a duck, and quacks like a duck, it must be a duck: patients with binge eating, obesity, anorexia, and bulimia have a chronic disorder characterized by loss of control, relapse, compulsivity, reprioritization, and continuation despite severe and adverse consequences. The *DSM–IV* eating disorder category naturally encompasses a diverse patient group. Some have a history

of anorexia nervosa without obesity, whereas others are restrictors, some purge, and still others have amenorrhea. Arguments have been made to consider eating disorders as personality disorders, obsessive-compulsive disease, and depression, and as an addictive disorder. Addiction treatment programs have alerted us to the high comorbidity of eating disorders in addiction patients, the high degree of eating disorders that appear to run in families, the common occurrence of eating binges or starvation as relapse triggers in newly abstinent patients, and patient reports of enhancing drugs' euphorigenic properties through starvation or purging. These observations support the importance of continued questioning and consideration to the hypothesis that eating disorders are related to tobacco, alcohol, and other addictive disorders.

REFERENCES

1. DuPont RL, Gold MS. Withdrawal and reward: implications for detoxification and relapse prevention. *Psychiatric Ann* 1995;25(11):663–668.
2. Gold MS. Clinical implications of the neurobiology of addiction. In: *ASAM Official Manual, Basic Science.* Bethesda: American Society of Addiction Medicine 1995;1(4):1–9.
3. Benveniste H, Huttmeir PC. Microdialysis theory and application. *Prog Neurobiol* 1990;35:195–215.
4. Church WH, Justice JB, Neill DB. Detecting behaviorally relevant changes in extracellular dopamine with microdialysis. *Brain Res* 1987;412:397–399.
5. Imperato A, Di Chiara G. Trans-striatal dialysis coupled to reverse-phase high-performance liquid chromatography with electrochemical detection: a new method for the study of the in vivo release of endogenous dopamine and metabolites. *J Neurosci* 1984;4:966–977.
6. Ungerstedt V, Hallstrom A. In vivo microdialysis. A new approach to the analysis of neurotransmitters in the brain. *Life Sci* 1987;41:861–864.
7. Fuxe K, Hokfelt T, Johansson O, et al. A. The origin of the dopamine nerve terminals in limbic and frontal cortex: evidence for mesocortico dopamine neurons. *Brain Res* 1974;82:349–355.
8. Hernandez L, Hoebel B. Feeding and hypothalamic stimulation increase dopamine turnover in the accumbens. *Physiol Behav* 1988;44:599–606.
9. Hernandez L, Hoebel BG. Feeding can enhance dopamine turnover in the prefrontal cortex. *Brain Res Bull* 1990; 24:975–979.
10. Mogenson GJ. Studies of the nucleus accumbens and its mesolimbic dopaminergic affects in relation to ingestive behaviors and reward. In:

Hoebel GB, Noving D, eds. *Neural basis of feeding and reward.* Brunswick, ME: Haer Institute, 1982:275–506.
11. Radhakishun FS, van Ree JM, Westerink BH, et al. Scheduled eating increases dopamine release in the nucleus accumbens of food-deprived rata as assessed with on-line brain dialysis. *Neurosci Lett* 1988;82:351–356.
12. Yoshida M, Yokoo H, Mizoguchi K, et al. Eating and drinking cause increased dopamine release in the nucleus accumbens and ventral tegmental area in the rat: measurement by *in vivo* microdialysis. *Neurosci Lett* 1992;139: 73–76.
13. Young AM, Joseph MN, Gray JA. Increased dopamine release in vivo in nucleus accumbens and caudate nucleus of the rat during drinking: a microdialysis study. *Neuroscience* 1992;48:871–876.
14. Miller NS, Gold MS. A hypothesis for a common neurochemical basis for alcohol and drug disorders. *Psychiatr Clin North Am* 1993;16:105–117.
15. Fantino M. Properties sensorielles des aliments et controle de la prise alimentaire. *Sci Alim* 1987;7:5–16.
16. Grill HJ, Berridge KC. Taste reactivity as a measure of the neural control of palatability. *Prog Psychobiol Physiol Psychol* 1985;11:1–61.
17. Louis-Sylvestre J, Giachetti I, Le Magnen J. Sensory vs. dietary factors in cafeteria-induced overweight. *Physiol Behav* 1984;32:901–905.
18. Rolls BJ. Palatability and food preference. In: Diaffi AL, et al., eds. *The body weight regulatory system: normal and disturbed mechanisms.* New York: Raven Press, 1981:271–278.
19. Sclafani A, Berner CN. Influence of diet palatability on the meal taking behavior of hypothalamic hyperphagic and nor-

mal rats. *Physiol Behav* 1976;16:355–363.
20. Gold MS. *Drugs of abuse: a comprehensive series for clinicians,* vol. IV. *Nicotine.* New York: Plenum, 1995.
21. Dackis CA, Gold MS. New concepts in cocaine addiction: the dopamine depletion hypothesis. *Neurosci Biobehav Rev* 1985;9(3):469–477.
22. Koob GF. Drugs of abuse: anatomy, pharmacology and function of reward pathways. *Trends Pharmacol Sci* 1992;13:177–184.
23. Gold MS. Neurobiology of addiction and recovery: the brain, the drive for the drug and the 12-step fellowship. *J Subst Abuse Treat* 1994;11(2):93–97.
23a. Lijun L, Gold MS. Human fMRI of Eating and Satiety in Eating Disorders and Obesity. *Psych Annals* 2003;33;127–132;87–90 .
23b. James GA, Gold MS, Liu Y. Interaction of Satiety and Reward Response to Food Stimulation. *J Add Dis* 2004;23:(3):23–39.
24. Gold MS. *Drugs of abuse: a comprehensive series for clinicians,* vol. III. *Cocaine.* New York: Plenum, 1993.
25. Kornetsky CR, et al. Intracranial self-stimulation thresholds: a model for the hedonic effects of drugs of abuse. *Arch Gen Psychiatry* 1979;36:289–292.
26. Gold MS, Miller NS. Seeking drugs/alcohol and avoiding withdrawal: the neuroanatomy of drive states and withdrawal. *Psych Ann* 1992;22(8): 430–435.
27. Jonas JM, Gold MS. Cocaine abuse and eating disorders. *Lancet* 1986; 1(8477):390.
28. Wise RA. The role of reward pathways in the development of drug dependence. *Pharmacol Ther* 1987;35:227–263.
29. Gold MS, Miller NS. A hypothesis for a common neurochemical basis for

alcohol and drug disorders. *Psychiatric Clin North Am* 1993;16(1):105–117.

30. Blundell JE. Appetite disturbances and the problems of overweight. *Drugs* 1990;39(Suppl 3):1–19.

31. Weingarten HP, Parkinson W. Ventromedial hypothalamic lesions eliminate acid secretion elicited by anticipated eating. *Appetite* 1988;10:205–219.

32. Kaschow J, Nemeroff CB. The neurobiology of neurotensin: focus on neurotensin-dopamine interactions. *Regul Pept* 1991;26:153–164.

33. Gold MS. Are eating disorders addictions? *Adv Biosci* 1993;90:455–463.

33a. Hodgkins CC, Cahill KS, Seraphine AE, Frost-Pineda K, Gold MS. Adolescent Drug Addiction Treatment and Weight Gain. *J Add Dis* 2004;23(3):55–66.

33b. Kleiner K, Jacobs WS, Lenz-Brunsman B, Perri MG, Frost-Pineda K, Gold MS. Body Mass Index and Alcohol Use. *J Add Dis* 2004;23(3):105–118.

34. Mehlman PT, Higley JD, Faucher I, et al. Correlation of SCF 5-HIAA concentration with sociality and the timing of emigration in free-ranging primates. *Am J Psychiatry* 1995;152:907–913.

35. University of Florida. *Facts about tobacco, alcohol, other drugs.* www.addictionandpsychiatry.com

36. Fava M, Rappe SM, West J, et al. Anger attacks in eating disorders. *Psychiatry Res* 1995;56:205–212.

37. Coccaro EF, Seiver LJ, Klar HM, et al. Serotonergic studies in patients with affective and personality disorders. *Arch Gen Psychiatry* 1989;46:587–599.

38. Brewerton TD. Toward a unified theory of serotonin dysregulation in eating and related disorders. *Psychoneuroendocrinology* 1995;20:561–590.

39. Pu S, Jain MR, Honath TL, et al. Interactions between Neuropeptide y and gamma-aminobutyric acid in stimulation of feeding: morphological and pharmacological analysis. *Endocrinology* 1999;140(2):933–940.

40. Guy J, Pelletier G, Boster D, et al. Serotonin innervation of neuropeptide-Y containing neurons in the rat arcuate nucleus. *Neurosci Let* 1988;85:9–13.

41. Larsen PJ, Tang-Christenson M, Stidsen CE, et al. Activation of central neuropeptide Y Y1 receptors potently stimulates food intake in male Rhesus monkeys. *J Clin Endocrinol Metab* 1999;84:3781–3791.

42. Kotz CM, Grace MK, Briggs J, et al. Effects of opioid antagonists naloxone and naltrexone on neuropeptide Y-induced feeding and brown fat thermogenesis in the rat. *J Clin Invest* 1995;96:163–170.

43. Kaye WH, Berrettini W, Gwirtsman H, et al. Altered cerebrospinal fluid neu-ropeptide Y and peptide YY immunoreactivity in anorexia and bulimia nervosa. *Arch Gen Psychiatry* 1990;147:548–556.

44. Kaye WH, Weltzin TE. Neurochemistry of bulimia nervosa. *J Clin Psychiatry* 1991;52[10 Suppl]:21–28.

45. Baranowska B. Plasma leptin, neuropeptide Y (NPY) and galanin concentrations in bulimia nervosa and in anorexia nervosa. *Neuroendocrinol Lett* 2001;22:356–358.

46. Sugrue MF. Neuropharmacology of drugs affecting food intake. *Pharmacol Ther* 1987;32:145–182.

47. McTavish D, Heel RC. Dexfenfluramine. A review of its pharmacological properties and therapeutic potential in obesity. *Drugs* 1992;43(5):713–733.

48. O'Conner HT, Richman RM, Steinbeck KS, et al. Dexfenfluramine treatment of obesity: a double-blind trial with post-trial follow-up. *Int J Obesity* 1995;19:181–189.

49. Nielson JA, Chapin DS, Johnson JL Jr, et al. Sertraline, a serotonin-uptake inhibitor, reduces food intake and body weight in lean rats and genetically obese mice. *Am J Clin Nutr* 1992;55:5s–8s.

50. Wise SD. Clinical studies with fluoxetine in obesity. *Am J Clin Nutr* 1992;55:181s–184s.

51. Spring S, Wurtman J, Wurtman R, et al. Efficacies of dexfenfluramine and fluoxetine in preventing weight after smoking cessation. *Am J Clin Nutr* 1995;62:1181–1187.

52. Bottcher G, Ekblad E, Ekman R, et al. Peptide YY: a neuropeptide in the gut: immunocytochemical and immunochemical evidence. *Neuroscience* 1993;55:281–290.

53. Pappas TN, Debas HT, Goto Y, et al. Peptide YY inhibits meal-stimulated pancreatic and gastric secretion. *Am J Physiol* 1985;248:G118–G123.

54. Dumont A, Fournier S, St. Pierre R. Quirion, autoradiographic distribution of [125I]Leu31, Pr034 PYY and [125I]PYY 3-36 binding sites in the rat brain evaluated with two newly developed y1 and y2 receptor radioligands. *Synapse* 1996;22:139–158.

55. Lynch DR, Walker MW, Miller RJ, et al. Neuropeptide Y receptor binding sites in rat brain: Differential autoradiographic localizations with 125I-peptide YY and 125I-neuropeptide Y imply receptor heterogeneity. *J Neurosci* 1989;9:2607–2619.

56. Yang H, Li WP, Reeve JR, et al. PYY-preferring receptor in the dorsal vagal complex and its involvement in PYY stimulation of gastric acid secretion in rats. *Br J Pharmacol* 1998;123:1549–1554.

57. Morley JE, Levine AS, Grace M, et al.

Peptide YY (PYY), a potent orexigenic agent. *Brain Res* 1985;341:200–203.

58. Berg BM, Croom J, Marcos Fernandez J, et al. Peptide YY administration decreases brain aluminum in the Ts65Dn Down Syndrome mouse model. *Growth Dev Aging* 2000;64:3–19.

59. Kaye WH, Berrettini W, Gwirtsman H, et al. Altered cerebrospinal fluid neuropeptide Y, and peptide YY immunoreactivity in anorexia and bulimia nervosa. *Arch Gen Psychiatry* 1990;47:548–556.

60. Taylor IL. Role of peptide YY in the endocrine control of digestion. *J Dairy Sci* 1993;76:2094–2101.

61. Playford RJ, Cox HM. Peptide YY, and neuropeptide Y two peptides intimately involved in electrolyte homeostasis. *Trends Pharmacol Sci* 1996;17:436–438.

62. Yang H, Kawakubo K, Tache Y. Intracisternal PYY increases gastric mucosal resistance: role of cholinergic, CGRP, and NO pathways. *Am J Physiol* 1999;227:G555–G562.

63. Hagan MM, Moss DE. Effect of naloxone and antidepressants on hyperphagia produced by peptide YY. *Pharmacol Biochem Behav* 1993;45:941–944.

64. Marrazzi MA, Wroblewski JM, Kinzie J, et al, High-dose naltrexone and liver function safety. *Am J Addict* 1997;6:21–29.

65. Walsh BT, Agras WS, Devlin MJ, et al. Fluoxetine for bulimia nervosa following poor response to psychotherapy. *Am J Psychiatry* 2000;157:1332–1334.

66. American Psychiatric Association. *Diagnostic and statistical manual of mental disorders, 4th ed.* Washington, DC: Author, 1994.

67. Adrian TE, Besterman HS, Cooke TJ, et al. Mechanism of pancreatic polypeptide release in man. *Lancet* 1997;I:161–163.

68. Inui A, Okita M, Miura M, et al. Plasma and cerebroventricular fluid levels of pancreatic polypeptide in the dog: effects of feeding, insulin-induced hypoglycemia, and physical exercise. *Endocrinology* 1993;132:1235–1239.

69. Kimmel JR, Hayden LJ, Pollock HG. Isolation and characterization of a new pancreatic polypeptide hormone. *J Biol Chem* 1975;50:9369–9376.

70. Sive AA, Vinik AI, van Tonder SV. Pancreatic polypeptide (PP) responses to oral and intravenous glucose in man. *Am J Gastroenterol* 1979;71:183–185.

71. Taylor IL, Impicciatore M, Carter DC, et al. Effect of atropine and vagotomy on pancreatic polypeptide response to a meal in dogs. *Am J Physiol* 1979;235:E443–E447.

72. Jia BQ, Taylor IL. Failure of pancreatic polypeptide release in

congenitally obese mice. *Gastroenterology* 1984;77:338–343.

73. Katsuura G, Asakawa A, Inul A. Roles of pancreatic polypeptide in regulation of food intake. *Peptide* 2002;23:323–329.

74. Batterham RL, Le Roux CW, Cohen MA, et al. Pancreatic polypeptide reduces appetite and food intake in humans. *J Clin Endocrinol Metab* 2003;88(8):3989–3992.

75. Nakazato M, Murakami N, Date Y, et al. A role for ghrelin in the central regulation of feeding. *Nature* 2002;409:194–198.

76. Lustig RH. The neuroendocrinology of obesity. *Endocrinol Metab Clin North Am* 2001;30:765–785.

77. Otto B, Cuntz U, Fruehauf E, et al. Weight gain decreases elevated plasma ghrelin concentrations of patients with anorexia nervosa. *Eur J Endocrinol* 2001;145(5):669–673.

78. Matsukura S, Nozoe S. Fasting plasma ghrelin levels in subtypes of anorexia nervosa. *Psychoneuroendocrinology* 2003;28(7):829–835.

79. Tanaka M, Naruo T, Nagai N, et al. Habitual binge/purge behavior influences circulating ghrelin levels in eating disorders. *J Psychiatr Res* 2003;37(1):17–22.

80. Vandereycken W. The addiction model in eating disorders: some critical remarks and selected bibliography. *Int J Eat Disord* 1990;9:95–101.

81. Gold MS. *The good news about drugs, alcohol.* New York: Villard Books, 1991.

82. Varner LM. Dual diagnosis. Patients with eating and substance-related disorders. *J Am Diet Assoc* 1995;95(2):224–225.

83. McElroy SL, Keck PE Jr, Phillips KA. Kleptomania, compulsive buying and binge-eating disorder. *J Clin Psychiatry* 1995;56[Suppl 4]:14–26.

84. McElroy SL, Phillips KA, Keck PE Jr. Obsessive compulsive spectrum disorder. *J Clin Psychiatry* 1994;55[Suppl]:33–51.

85. Schoen C, Davis K, Collins KS, et al. *The Commonwealth Fund survey of the health of adolescent girls.* New York: The Commonwealth Fund, 1997.

86. Kaplan AS, Garfinkel PR. General principles of outpatient treatment—eating disorders. In: Gabbard GO, ed. *Treatments of psychiatric disorders,* vol. 2. Washington, DC: American Psychiatric Press, 1995.

87. National Institute of Health. *Clinical guidelines on the identification, evaluation, and treatment of overweight and obesity in adults* 2004. www.nhlbi.nih.gov/guidelines/obesity/ob_gdlns.pdf

88. Bell RM. *Holy anorexia.* Chicago: University of Chicago Press, 1985.

89. Palmer RL. Weight concern should not be a necessary criterion for the eating disorders: a polemic. *Int J Eat Disord* 1993;14:459–466.

90. Halmi K. *Understanding eating disorders: anorexia nervosa, bulimia nervosa, and obesity.* Washington, DC: American Psychiatric Press, 1994.

91. American Psychiatric Association. *Practice guidelines for eating disorders.* Washington, DC: Author, 1993.

92. Russell G. Bulimia nervosa: an ominous variant of anorexia nervosa. *Psychol Med* 1979;9(3):429–448.

93. Becker AE, Grinspoon SK, Klibanski A, Heozoy DA. Eating disorders. *NEJM* 1999;340:1092–1098.

94. Herzog W, Rathner G, Vandereychken W. Long-term course of anorexia nervosa: a review of the literature. In: Herzig W, Deter HC, Vandereychken W, eds. *The course of eating disorders.* New York: Springer-Verlag, 1992:15–29.

95. Pirke KM, Pahy S, Schweiger V, et al. Metabolic and endocrine indices of starvation in bulimia: a comparison with anorexia nervosa. *Psychiatry Res* 1985;15:33–39.

96. Sullivan PF. Mortality in anorexia nervosa. *Am J Psychiatry* 1995;152:1073–1074.

97. Devlin B, Bacanu SA, Klump RL. Linkage analysis of anorexia nervosa incorporating behavioral covariates. *Hum Mol Gent* 2002;11(6):689–696.

98. Fukuda M, Ono T, Nishino H, Nakamura K. Neuronal responses in monkey lateral hypothalamus during operant feeding behavior. *Brain Res Bull* 1986;17:879–884.

99. Treasure J, Campbell I. The case for biology in the etiology of anorexia nervosa [editorial]. *Psychol Med* 1994;24:3–8.

100. Rowland NE. Effect of continuous infusions of dexfenfluramine on food intake, body weight and brain amines in rats. *Life Sci* 1986;39:2581–2586.

101. Haleem DJ. *Serotonergic functions in rat brain: sex-related differences and responses to stress [PhD thesis].* London: University of London, 1988.

102. Olivardia R, Pope HG Jr, Mangweth B, et al. Eating disorders in college men. *Am J Psychiatry* 1995;152(9):1279–1285.

103. Carter A, Davis ST. Biogenic amines, reproductive hormones and female sexual behavior. A review. *Behav Res* 1977;1:213–225.

104. Kaye WH, Ebert MH, Gwirtsman HE, et al. Differences in brain serotoner-

gic metabolism between nonbulimic and bulimic patients with anorexia nervosa. *Am J Psychiatry* 1984;141:1598–1601.

105. Gwirtsman HE, Guze BH, Yager J, et al. Fluoxetine treatment of anorexia nervosa: an open clinical trial. *J Clin Psychiatry* 1990;51:378–382.

106. Kaye WH, Weltzin TE, Hsu LKG, et al. An open trial of fluoxetine in patients with anorexia nervosa. *J Clin Psychiatry* 1991;52:464–471.

107. Beasley CM, Masica DN, Potvin JH. Fluoxetine. A review of receptor and functional effects and their clinical implications. *Psychopharmacol (Berl)* 1992;107:1–10.

108. Advokut C, Kutlesic V. Pharmacotherapy of the eating disorders: a commentary. *Neurosci Biobehav Rev* 1995;19:59–66.

109. Halmi KA, Eckert E, LaDu TJ, et al. Anorexia nervosa: treatment efficacy of cyproheptadine and amitriptyline. *Arch Gen Psychiatry* 1986;43:177–181.

110. Barry V, Klavans HL. On the role of dopamine in the pathophysiology of anorexia nervosa. *J Neural Transm* 1976;38:107–122.

111. Gerner RH, Cohen DJ, Fairbanks L, et al. CSF neurochemistry of women with anorexia nervosa and normal women. *Am J Psychiatry* 1984;141:1441–1444.

112. Bowers MB, Mariera CM, Greenfeld DG. Elevated plasma monoamine metabolites in eating disorders. *Psychiatry Res* 1994;52:11–16.

113. Gross HA, Lake CR, Ebert MH, et al. Catecholamine metabolism in primary anorexia nervosa. *J Clin Endocrinol Metab* 1979;49:805–809.

114. Riederer P, Toifl K, Boltzman L. Excretion of biogenic amine metabolites in anorexia nervosa and other diseases accompanied by severe weight loss. In: *III world congress of biological psychiatry.* Stochkolm: 1981(abstr).

115. Gillberg C. Low dopamine and serotonin in anorexia nervosa. *Am J Psychiatry* 1983;40:948–949.

116. Kaye WH. Neuropeptide abnormalities in anorexia nervosa. *Psych Res* 1996;62:65–74.

117. Kaye WH, Eber MH, Raleigh M, et al. Abnormalities in CNS monoamine metabolism in anorexia nervosa. *Arch Gen Psychiatry* 1984;41:350–355.

118. Ebert MH, Kaye WK, Gold PW. Neurotransmitter metabolism in anorexia nervosa. In: Pirke KM, Ploog D, eds. *The psychobiology of anorexia nervosa.* Berlin: Springer-Verlag, 1984:58–72.

119. Vandereycken W. Neuroleptics in short-term treatment of anorexia nervosa: a double-blind placebo controlled

study with sulpiride. *Br J Psychiatry* 1984;144:288–292.

120. Dally P, Sargant W. Treatment and outcome in anorexia nervosa. *BMJ* 1996;2:793–79.

121. La Via MC, Gray N, Kaye WH. Case reports of olanzapine treatment of anorexia nervosa. *Int J Eat Disord* 2000;27(3):363–366.

122. Newman-Toker J. Risperidone in anorexia nervosa. *J Am Acad Child Adolesc Psychiatry* 2000;39(8):941–942.

123. Powers PS, Santana CA, Bannon YS. Olanzapine in the treatment of anorexia nervosa: an open label trial. *Int J Eat Disord* 2002;32(2):146–154.

124. Marrazzi MA, Luby ED. An auto-addiction opioid model of chronic anorexia nervosa. *Int J Eat Disord* 1986;5(2):191–208.

125. Kaye WH, Pickar D, Naber D, et al. Cerebrospinal fluid opioid activity in anorexia nervosa. *Am J Psychiatry* 1982;139:643–165.

126. Marrazzi MA, Luby ED. Anorexia nervosa as an auto-addiction. *Ann N Y Acad Sci* 1989;575:545–547.

127. Bulik CM. Abuse of drugs associated with eating disorders. *J Subst Abuse* 1992;4:69–90.

128. Mitchell JE, Boutacoff LI, Hatsukami D, et al. Laxative abuse a variant of bulimia. *J Nerv Ment Dis* 1986;174:174–176.

129. Garfinkel PE, Lin E, Goening P, et al. Bulimia nervosa in a Canadian community sample: prevalence and comparison of subgroups. *Am J Psychiatry* 1995;152:1052–1058.

130. Kendler KS, Maculae C, Neil M, et al. The genetic epidemiology of bulimia nervosa. *Am J Psychiatry* 1991;148:1627–1637.

131. Striegel-Moore RH, Silberstein LR, Roudin J. Toward an understanding of risk of factors for bulimia. *Am Psychol* 1986;41:246–263.

132. Smith D. Binge eating in ethnic minority groups. *Addict Behav* 1995;20:695–703.

133. Drewnowski A. Metabolic determinants of binge eating. *Addict Behav* 1995;20:733–745.

134. Rossiter EM, Agras WS, Telch CF, et al. Cluster B personality characteristics predict outcome in the treatment of bulimia nervosa. *Int J Eat Disord* 1993;13:349–357.

135. Powers PS, Coovert DL, Brightwell DR, et al. Other psychiatric disorders among bulimic patients. *Compr Psychiatry* 1988;29:503–508.

136. Olmstead MP, Kaplan AS, Rockert W. Rate and prediction of relapse in bulimia nervosa. *Am J Psychiatry* 1994;151:738–743.

137. Parry-Jones WL, Parry-Jones B. Implications of historical evidence for the classification of eating disorders. *Br J Psychiatry* 1994;165:287–292.

138. Mitchell JE, Specker SM, de Zwaan M. Comorbidity and medical complications of bulimia nervosa. *J Clin Psychiatry* 1991;52[Suppl 10]:13–20.

139. Epik A, Arikan Z, Boratav C, et al. Bulimia in a male alcoholic: a symptom substitution in alcoholism. *Int J Eat Disord* 1995;17(2):201–204.

140. Holderness CC, Brooks P Gunn J, Warren MP. Co-morbidity of eating disorders and substance abuse. Review of the literature. *Int J Eat Disord* 1994;16:1–34.

141. Braun DL, Sunday SR, Halmi KA. Psychiatric co-morbidity in patients with eating disorders. *Psychol Med* 1994;24:859–867.

142. Koepp W, Schildbach S, Schmager C, et al. Borderline diagnosis and substance abuse in female patients with eating disorders. *Int J Eat Disord* 1993;14:107–110.

143. Garfinkel PE, Garner DM. *Anorexia nervosa: a multidimensional perspective.* New York: Brunner Mazel, 1982.

144. Mitchell JE, Hatsukami DK, Eckert ED, et al. Characteristics of 275 patients with bulimia. *Am J Psychiatry* 1985;142:482–485.

145. Yager J, Landsverk J, Edelstein CK, et al. A 20-month follow-up study of 628 women with eating disorders: II. Course of associated symptoms and related features. *Int J Eat Disord* 1988;7:503–513.

146. McBride WJ, Bodart B, Lumberg L, et al. Association between low contents of dopamine and serotonin in the nucleus accumbens and high alcohol preference. *Alcohol Clin Exp Res* 1995;19:1420–1422.

147. Jimerson DC, Lesem MD, Kaye WH, et al. Low serotonin and dopamine metabolite concentrations in cerebrospinal fluid from bulimic patients with frequent binge episodes. *Arch Gen Psychiatry* 1992;49:132–137.

148. Brewerton TD, Lydiard RB, Laraia MT, et al. CSF beta-endorphin and dynorphin in bulimia nervosa. *Am J Psychiatry* 1992;149:1086–1090.

149. Wallin MS, Rissanen AM. Food and mood: relationship between food, serotonin and affective disorders. *Acta Psychiatr Scand Suppl* 1994;377:36–40.

150. Weltzin TE, Fernstrom MH, Fernstrom JD, et al. Acute tryptophan depletion and increased food intake and irritability in bulimia nervosa. *Am J Psychiatry* 1995;152:1668–1671.

151. Fornari VM, Braun DL, Sunday SR, et al. Seasonal patterns in eating disorder subgroups. *Compr Psychiatry* 1994; 35:450–456.

152. Hardin TA, Wehr TA, Brewerton T, et al. Evaluation of seasonality in six clinical populations. *J Psychiatr Res* 1991;25:75–87.

153. Fornari WM, Sandberg DE, Lachenmeyer J, et al. Seasonal variations in bulimia nervosa. *Ann N Y Acad Sci* 1989;575:509–511.

154. Lam RW, Solyom L, Tompkins A. Seasonal mood symptoms in bulimia nervosa and seasonal affective disorder. *Compr Psychiatry* 1991;32:552–558.

155. Lam RW, Goldner EM, Solyom L, et al. A controlled study of light therapy for bulimia nervosa. *Am J Psychiatry* 1994;151:744–750.

156. Lewy AJ, Sack RL, Miller LS, et al. Antidepressant and circadian phase-shifting effects of light. *Science* 1987; 235:352–354.

157. Lewy AJ, Sack RL, Singer CM, et al. Winter depression and the phase-shift hypothesis for bright light's therapeutic effects: history, theory, and experimental evidence. *J Biol Rhythms* 1988;3:121–134.

158. Oren DA, Jacobsen FM, Wehr TA, et al. Predictors of response to phototherapy in seasonal affective disorder. *Biol Psychiatry* 1992;15:32(8):700–704.

159. Kales EF. Macronutrient analysis of binge eating in bulimia. *Physiol Behav* 1990;48:837–840.

160. Fluoxetine Bulimia Nervosa Collaborative Study Group. Fluoxetine in the treatment of bulimia nervosa: a multicenter, placebo-controlled trial. *Arch Gen Psychiatry* 1992;49:139–147.

161. Krahn D, Mitchell J. Use of L-tryptophan in treating bulimia. *Am J Psychiatry* 1985;142:1130.

162. Fahy TA, Eisler I, Russell GFM. A placebo-controlled trial of d-fenfluramine in bulimia nervosa. *Br J Psychiatry* 1993;162:597–603.

163. Russell GFM, Checkly SA, Feldman J, et al. A controlled trial of d-fenfluramine in bulimia nervosa. *Clin Neuropharmacol* 1988;11[Suppl 1]: S146–S159.

164. Brewerton TD, Lydiard RD, Laraia MT, et al. CSF beta-endorphin and dynorphin in bulimia nervosa. *Am J Psychiatry* 1992;149:1086–1090.

165. Fullerton DT, Getto CJ, Swift WF, et al. Sugar, opioids and binge eating. *Brain Res Bull* 1985;14:673–680.

166. Morley JE, Levine AS, Yim GK, et al. opioid modulation of appetite. *Neurosci Biobehav Rev* 1983;7:281–305.

167. Jonas JM, Gold MS. Naltrexone reverse bulimic symptoms. *Lancet* 1986;1:807.

168. Jonas JM, Gold MS. Treatment of antidepressant resistant bulimia with

naltrexone. *Int J Psychiatry Med* 1987; 16:305–309.

169. Jonas JM, Gold MS. The use of opiate antagonists in treating bulimia: a study of low dose versus high dose naltrexone. *Psychiatry Res* 1988;24:195–199.

170. Marrazzi MA, Bacon JP, Kinzie J, et al. Naltrexone use in the treatment of anorexia nervosa and bulimia nervosa. *Int Clin Psychopharmacol* 1995;10:163–172.

171. Agger SA, Schwalberg MD, Bigaouette JM, et al. Effect of a tricyclic antidepressant and opiate antagonist on binge eating behavior in normal weight bulimia and obese, binge-eating subjects. *Am J Clin Nutr* 1991;53:865–871.

172. Mitchell JE, Christenson G, Jennings J, et al. A placebo-controlled, double-blind crossover study of naltrexone hydrochloride in outpatients with normal weight bulimia. *J Clin Psychopharmacol* 1989;9:94–97.

173. Bruce B, Wilfley D. Binge eating among the overweight population: a serious and prevalent problem. *J Am Diet Assoc* 1996;96(1):58–61.

174. Marcus MD. Introduction—binge eating: clinical and research directions. *Addict Behav* 1995;20:691–693.

175. Spitzer RL, Yanovski S, Wadden T, et al. Binge eating disorder: its further validation in a multisite study. *Int J Eat Disord* 1993;13:137–153.

176. Bruce B, Agras WS. Binge eating disorder in females: a population-based investigation. *Int J Eat Disord* 1992; 12:365–373.

177. Mussell MP, Mitchell JE, Weller CL, et al. Onset of binge eating, dieting, obesity, and mood disorders among subjects seeking treatment for binge eating disorder. *Int J Eat Disord* 1995;14:395–401.

178. Wurtman JJ. Depression and weight gain: the serotonin connection. *J Affect Disord* 1993;29:183–192.

179. Mitchell JE, Mussell MP. Comorbidity and binge eating disorder. *Addict Behav* 1995;20:725–732.

180. Marcus MD, Wing RR, Ewing L, et al. M. Psychiatric disorders among obese binge eaters. *Int J Eat Disord* 1990;9:69–77.

181. Yanovski SZ, Nelson JE, Dubbert BK, et al. Association of binge eating disorder and psychiatric comorbidity in obese subjects. *Am J Psychiatry* 1993; 150:1472–1479.

182. Brody ML, Walsh T, Devlin MJ. Binge eating disorder: reliability and validity of a new diagnostic category. *J Consult Clin Psychol* 1994;62:381–386.

183. Specker S, deZwaan M, Raymond N, et al. Psychopathology in subgroups of obese women with and without binge eating disorder. *Compr Psychiatry* 1994;35:185–190.

184. Mitchell JE, Hatsukami D, Pyle R, et al. Bulimia with and without a family history of drug abuse. *Addict Behav* 1988;13:245–251.

185. Willenbring ML, Morley JE, Krahn DD, et al. Psychoneuroendocrine effects of methadone maintenance. *Psychoneuroendocrinology* 1989;14:371–391.

186. Moraia A, Fabre J, Chee E, et al. Diet and opiate addiction, a quantitative assessment of the diet of non-institutionalized opiate addicts. *Br J Addict* 1989;84:173–180.

187. Rothman RB, Gendron T, Hitzig P. Letter to the editor. *J Subst Abuse Treat* 1994;11:273–275.

188. Volpicelli JR, Alterman AI, Hayashida M, et al. Naltrexone in the treatment of alcohol dependence. *Arch Gen Psychiatry* 1992;49:876–880.

189. Wang GJ, Volkow ND, Fowler JS. The role of dopamine in motivation for food in humans: implications for obesity. *Expert Opin Ther Targets* 2002;6(5):601–609.

190. Wang GJ, Volkow ND, Logan J, et al. Brain dopamine and obesity. *Lancet* 2001;3;357(9253):354–357.

191. Volkow ND, Fowler JS, Wang G-J, et al. Decreased dopamine D2 receptor availability is associated with reduced frontal metabolism in cocaine abusers. *Synapse* 1993;14:169–177.

192. Hietala J, West C, Syvalahti E, et al. Striatal D2 dopamine receptor binding characteristics *in vivo* in patients with alcohol dependence. *Psychopharmacology (Berl)* 1996;116:285–290.

193. Wang G-J, Volkow ND, Fowler JS, et al. Dopamine D2 receptor availability in opiate-dependent subjects before and after naloxone-precipitated withdrawal. *Neuropsychopharmacology* 1997;16:174–182.

194. Fernstrom JD. Food-induced changes in brain serotonin synthesis: is there a relationship to appetite for specific macronutrients? *Appetite* 1987;8:163–182.

195. Walsh A, Oldman A, Franklin M, et al. Dieting decreases plasma tryptophan and increases the prolactin response to d-fenfluramine in women but not men. *J Affect Disord* 1995;33:89–97.

196. Kuikka JT, Tammela L, Karhunen L, et al. Reduced serotonin transporter binding in binge eating women. *Psychopharmacology (Berl)* 2001;155(3):310–314.

197. Tammela LI, Rissanen A, Kuikka JT, et al. Treatment improves serotonin transporter binding and reduces binge eating. *Psychopharmacology (Berl)* 2003;170(1):89–93.

198. Wurtman JJ, Wurtman RJ. Drugs that enhance central serotonergic transmission diminish elective carbohydrate consumption by rats. *Life Sci* 1979; 24:895–904.

199. McElroy SL, Casuto LS, Nelson EB, et al. Placebo-controlled trial of sertraline in the treatment of binge eating disorder. *Am J Psychiatry* 2000;157(6):1004–1006.

200. Arnold LM, McElroy SL, Hudson JI, et al. A placebo-controlled, randomized trial of fluoxetine in the treatment of binge-eating disorder. *J Clin Psychiatry* 2002;63(11):1028–1033.

201. McElroy SL, Hudson JI, Malhotra S, et al. Citalopram in the treatment of binge-eating disorder: a placebo-controlled trial. *J Clin Psychiatry* 2003; 64(7):807–813.

202. Hall SM, Reus VI, Munoz RF, et al. Nortriptyline and cognitive-behavioral therapy in the treatment of cigarette smoking. *Arch Gen Psychiatry* 1998;55(8):683–690.

203. Weintraub M, Hasday JD, Mushlin AI, et al. A double-blind clinical trial in weight control: use of fenfluramine and phentermine alone and in combination. *Arch Intern Med* 1984;144:1143–1148.

204. Weintraub M. Long-term weight control: the National Heart, Lung, and Blood Institute funded multimodal intervention study. *Clin Pharmacol Ther* 1992;51:581–646.

205. Stunkard A, Berkowitz R, Tanrikut C, et al. *d*-Fenfluramine treatment of binge eating disorder. *Am J Psychiatry* 1996;153:1455–1459.

206. Appolinario JC, Godoy-Matos A, Fontenelle LF, et al. An open-label trial of sibutramine in obese patients with binge-eating disorder. *J Clin Psychiatry* 2002;63(1):28–30.

207. Hurt RD, Sachs DP, Glover ED, et al. A comparison of sustained-release bupropion and placebo for smoking cessation. *N Engl J Med* 1997;337:1195–1202.

208. Gadde KM, Parker CB, Maner LG, et al. Bupropion for weight loss: an investigation of efficacy and tolerability in overweight and obese woman. *Obesity Res* 2001;9:544–551.

209. Shapira NA, Goldsmith TD, McElroy SL. Treatment of binge eating disorder with topiramate: a clinical case series. *J Clin Psychiatry* 2000;61:358–372.

210. Moghaddam B, Bolinao ML. Glutamatergic antagonists attenuate ability of dopamine uptake blockers to increase extracellular levels of dopamine: implications for tonic influence of

glutamate on dopamine release. *Synapse* 1994;18:337–342.

211. Johnson BA, Ait-Daoud N, Bowden CL, et al. Oral topiramate for treatment of alcohol dependence: a randomized controlled trial. *Lancet* 2003; 361(9370):1677–1685.

212. Landry 1996; Institute of Medicine 1990; American Psychiatric Association 1995.

213. Robin AL, Siegel PT, Moye AW, et al. A controlled comparison of family versus individual therapy for adolescents with anorexia nervosa. *J Am Acad Child Adoles Psychiatry* 1999;38: 1482–1489.

214. Fairburn CG, Marcus MD, Wilson GT. Cognitive-behavioral therapy for binge eating and bulimia nervosa: a comprehensive treatment manual. In: Fairburn CG, Wilson GT, eds. *Binge eating: nature, assessment and treatment.* New York: Guilford Press, 1993:361–404.

215. Chambless DL, Ollendick TH. Empirically supported psychological interventions: controversies and evidence. *Annu Rev Psychol* 2001;52:685–716.

216. Wilfley DE, Cohen LR. Psychological treatment of bulimia nervosa and binge eating disorder. *Psychopharmacol Bull* 1997;33:437–454.

217. Kurtz LF. *Self help and support groups: a handbook for practitioners.* Thousand Oaks, CA: Sage Publications, 1997.

218. *The Twelve-Steps of Overeaters Anonymous.* Los Angeles: Overeaters Anonymous, 1990.

219. Wilson GT. The addiction model of eating disorders: a critical analysis. *Adv Behav Res Ther* 1991;13:27–72.

220. Nazoe S, Naruo T, Yonekura R, et al. Comparison of regional cerebral blood flow in patients with eating disorders. *Brain Res Bull* 1995;36(3):251–255.

221. Watts WD, Ellis AM. Drug abuse and eating disorders: prevention implications. *J Drug Educ* 1992;22(3):223–240.

222. French SA, Story M, Duwnes B, et al. Frequent dieting among adolescents: psychosocial and health behavior correlates. *Am J Public Health* 1995;85:695–701.

223. Ash JB, Piazza E. Changing symptomatology in eating disorders. *Int J Eat Disord* 1995;18:27–38.

CHAPTER 28

Pathologic Gambling

SHEILA B. BLUME AND HERMANO TAVARES

Gambling in one form or another has been part of human behavior since prehistory. Records of games of chance and related artifacts have been discovered among the ruins of the ancient city of Babylon, dating from 3000 BC (1). Gambling is mentioned in both the Old and New Testaments and in the classical literature of many cultures. Private lotteries were common in Europe throughout the Middle Ages, and Elizabeth I of England chartered the first government-sponsored lottery in 1566. European settlers who came to North America employed lotteries as a means of raising funds in all of the original 13 colonies. The first great universities established in the New World also relied on lotteries to raise money (2).

Along with the human tendency to gamble have come gambling-related problems, including the loss of control of gambling behavior, commonly referred to as compulsive gambling. The Mahabahrata, for example, tells the story of how a fair and wise king is brought low by his only fault, his addiction to gambling. He gambles away his wealth, his kingdom, his brothers and himself (into slavery), and, finally, his wife. Famous compulsive gamblers in modern history have included a seventeenth century Venetian rabbi (3) and the Russian novelist Feodor Dostoyevsky. Dostoyevsky wrote a novel called *The Gambler* in 1866, during a period of catastrophic gambling losses, in an effort to preserve his financial integrity (4).

In a 1928 essay entitled *Dostoyevsky and Parricide* (5), Sigmund Freud discussed the writer's compulsive gambling and hypothesized its relationship to traumatic events in his life, particularly his father's death. Interestingly, Freud conceptualized Dostoyevsky's behavior as gambling for its own sake (rather than as a means to acquire money) and considered it an addiction. Several psychoanalysts studied and treated compulsive gamblers from the 1920s through the 1960s (6). However, there was relatively little interest in scientific research in the field of compulsive gambling or in the treatment of this disorder until the 1970s and 1980s. These decades saw an increased focus on gambling problems, which had several roots. The first treatment unit for compulsive gamblers was established by Dr. Robert Custer at the Brecksville, Ohio, Veterans Administration Hospital in 1971 (7). This unit adapted the treatment methods used in alcoholism rehabilitation to the treatment of gambling disorders, relying on group, individual, and family therapies and employing self-help fellowships, such as Gamblers Anonymous (GA) and Gam-Anon, as adjuncts to professional treatment. The model was found effective and subsequently adopted by other addiction treatment facilities throughout the United States. Articles in the popular press alluded to these treatment programs and to GA as a means of helping troubled gamblers. In addition, the 1980s and 1990s saw a worldwide trend toward governmental legalization of many types of gambling. Legislatures looked increasingly to state lotteries and taxes from legal gambling as revenue sources in an atmosphere of rising government expenses and citizen unwillingness to accept tax increases. The result was an explosive growth in the availability of a wide variety of games of chance to the general public. Also, the spread of computer use and growth of online wagering made gambling accessible to a larger audience in their own homes, and at all hours. The establishment of a virtual casino takes less than 1% of the capital needed to build a real one. Consequently, the next few years may witness an explosion of Internet gambling requiring governmental regulation, although it is not clear how best to assure the fairness of games and how to make game operators accountable (8). Recent surveys indicate that 80% to 90% of American adults gamble to some extent (9), a significantly greater proportion than those who use alcohol or other drugs.

TERMS AND DEFINITIONS

For the purpose of understanding gambling problems, it is important to define gambling narrowly rather than to use a broad definition. Gambling or wagering involves either playing a game for money or staking something of value (usually money) on an event influenced by chance (e.g., betting on whether a specific set of numbers will be picked in a lottery). To be important to the development of gambling problems, this wagering must be short-term, so that a feeling of excitement can be produced while awaiting the outcome. Thus, a long-term financial investment would not be considered gambling for this purpose, although chance may play a role in its gain or loss of value.

The term *gambling problems* is used as an umbrella term for a wide range of problems related to gambling activities, such as underage gambling, illegal gambling, and dishonest games, in addition to personal and family problems related to excessive gambling by an individual. *Problem gambler* is sometimes used to refer to a person whose gambling creates problems, whereas *compulsive gambler* or *pathologic gambler* applies specifically to an individual suffering from the disorder described in the American Psychiatric Association's *Diagnostic and Statistical Manual of Mental Disorders,* 4th ed. (*DSM–IV*), as "Pathological Gambling" (10).

Different varieties of currently popular gambling involve differing proportions of chance and skill. Playing chess for money involves significantly more skill than chance. Betting on horse races may involve considerable knowledge of the competitors and skill in handicapping, whereas playing the lottery or roulette relies entirely on chance. Forms of gambling also differ in the immediacy of their payoff. Casino games such as blackjack tend to be short-interval gambling, and slot machines offer an almost immediate payoff. However, little research has been devoted to the impact of different games on gamblers and most ideas about these differences are based on clinical experience.

DIAGNOSIS OF PATHOLOGIC GAMBLING

In the current edition, *DSM–IV* (10), the disorder is characterized as persistent and recurrent maladaptive gambling behavior, not better accounted for as a component of a manic episode. At least 5 of the following 10 criteria must be present for the diagnosis to be made:

1. "Is preoccupied with gambling (e.g., preoccupied with reliving past gambling experience, handicapping or planning the next venture, or thinking of ways to get money with which to gamble)." Preoccupation is sometimes extreme. Pathologic gamblers have been known to go to the racetrack on their wedding day. Pathologic sports bettors may follow several games simultaneously on two or three radios or television sets.

2. "Needs to gamble with increasing amounts of money in order to achieve the desired excitement." This phenomenon is comparable to the tolerance seen in substance dependence.

3. "Has repeated unsuccessful efforts to control, cut back, or stop gambling." This criterion refers to impaired control.

4. "Is restless or irritable when attempting to cut down or stop gambling." This describes the equivalent of a withdrawal state in substance dependence. Approximately 65% of GA members reported such withdrawal symptoms, which also included insomnia, headaches, upset stomach or diarrhea, anorexia, palpitations, weakness, shaking, sweating and breathing problems (11).

5. "Gambles as a way of escaping from problems or relieving a dysphoric mood (e.g., feelings of helplessness, guilt, anxiety, depression)." Female pathologic gamblers often describe such "escape" as a primary reason for gambling (12).

6. "After losing money gambling, often returns another day to get even ('chasing' one's losses)." Chasing is a common symptom of this disorder (13). It has no equivalent in alcohol or other drug addictions.

7. "Lies to family members, therapist, or others to conceal the extent of involvement with gambling."

8. "Has committed illegal acts such as forgery, fraud, theft, or embezzlement to finance gambling." Individuals who are normally honest and law-abiding often begin to appropriate other people's money when they develop pathologic gambling. They characteristically rationalize this activity as temporary borrowing, but their need for money eventually overpowers their moral standards. Pathologic gambling is closely associated with criminal activity, especially white-collar crime (14,15).

9. "Has jeopardized or lost a significant relationship, job, or educational or career opportunity because of gambling." Marital and other family relationships are usually the first to be affected as the gambler becomes preoccupied with gambling activity, although all relationships and activities are eventually damaged by the disease.

10. "Relies on others to provide money to relieve a desperate financial situation caused by gambling." This is generally known as a "bailout" and is often elicited from family or friends without revealing that the indebtedness is caused by gambling. If the donors of the

funds are aware of the gambling, they often insist on a promise that the pathologic gambler will give up or reduce this activity.

These criteria have much in common with the criteria for substance dependence and some authors consider pathologic gambling a behavioral addiction (16). Pathologic gambling is a progressive disease that often has its onset in adolescence, but may begin at any age. Its characteristics may differ with age and sex. Female pathologic gamblers show both a faster progression of the disease and higher comorbidity with anxiety and depression (17–19). They are less likely to commit crimes than males and report less indebtedness. Women also more often report gambling to escape from the psychological distress produced by a painful situation, for example, an abusive relationship or a husband who is often absent (12). Volberg (20) has pointed out the increasing availability of gambling machines, a form of gambling that particularly appeals to women, at supermarkets, Laundromats, and other places frequented by women. This increase in exposure may lead to an equalization of gambling problem rates between men and women in the near future. In spite of methodologic differences, studies conducted in North America in the early 1990s generally agreed that the male:female ratio for pathologic gambling was approximately 2:1 in most populations (21), but a general population study of U.S. adults published in 2001 found a male:female ratio close to 1:1 (22).

Epidemiologic and genetic data show that pathologic gambling runs in families and is highly associated with alcoholism, therefore, special attention should be paid to children of problem gamblers and problem drinkers when screening for pathologic gambling (22,23).

EPIDEMIOLOGY OF GAMBLING PROBLEMS

Prevalence Rates

In spite of varying methodologies, prevalence studies in the United States have reported rates between 1% and 2% for current pathologic gambling among adults, and an additional 2% to 4% for problem gamblers who do not meet criteria for pathologic gambling (24). To date, only four studies have investigated national samples (22,25–27). One of these is a meta-analysis of state and regional prevalence studies across North America. In its review of this topic, the National Research Council (28) stresses the experience of the states of Iowa, Minnesota, Texas, and Connecticut where repeated surveys demonstrated an increase in prevalence rates after the introduction of legal gambling. Reviewing the evidences one may fairly conclude that the greater the availability of gambling, the greater the prevalence of pathologic gambling.

At-Risk Populations

The picture of the "typical" pathologic gambler emerging from epidemiologic studies is a male subject, married with children, in his thirties, white, from a low socioeconomic stratum, and having a high school education. Nevertheless, more women are gambling now than in previous generations (18), and the proportion of nonmarried subjects (single, divorced, or separated) is higher among pathologic gamblers than in the general population, suggesting loneliness as an associated factor (26). Also, a number of studies have reported higher rates of pathologic gambling among ethnic minorities, including African Americans, Hispanics, Native Americans, and other populations (28). Little is known about the impact of social and cultural variables on gambling behavior. For instance, although low socioeconomic status is associated with pathologic gambling, it is not clear whether this may be cause or effect.

Age seems to play an important role in pathologic gambling. Today's youngsters are the first generation to be fully exposed to new societal rules in which gambling is not only accepted, but promoted by federal and state governments and entrepreneurs as a legitimate amusement and source of revenue (24). Studies conducted in the last 10 years in the United States and Canada show current prevalence rates up to almost 6% for current probable pathologic gambling among students in the sixth to twelfth grades, a rate almost six times higher than in the adult population (29,30). Studies point out the possibility of artificial inflation of prevalence rates by the use of instruments originally meant for screening in older subjects (31), but the higher frequency among adolescents and young adults has been so often replicated that it is a legitimate cause for public concern (28). On the other hand, while pathologic gambling is consistently reported as less frequent among older people, the population segment over the age of 65 years has had the greatest growth in gambling engagement in the last 20 years (26). The effect of this increase has not yet been fully investigated.

Prevalence rates for pathologic gambling are higher among patients in treatment for substance use disorders than in the general population. Studies conducted at addiction treatment sites report rates of pathologic gambling 4 to 10 times higher for substance abusers and dependents than for the general population (32). Two telephone surveys (22,33) and one household survey (34) have replicated the association between pathologic gambling and substance use disorders. The latter was a study conducted in St. Louis, Missouri, a site-specific investigation as part of the broader Epidemiological Catchment Area study. This study showed that the risk for alcohol abuse/dependence and nicotine dependence increased as the severity of gambling rose.

The prevalence of pathologic gambling among other psychiatric patients has also been studied. Lesieur and Blume (35) found a lifetime prevalence of 6.7% for probable pathologic gambling in a survey of 105 patients admitted to an acute adult psychiatric service for primary psychiatric problems. Another study reported a prevalence rate of pathologic gambling of 6% among patients presenting to primary care settings (36).

Reports on comorbidity show substance-related, anxiety and mood disorders as the main syndromes comorbid with pathologic gambling, but the temporal relationship between pathologic gambling and affective syndromes remains unclear (37). One epidemiologic study described anxiety and depression symptoms preceding gambling activity (34) suggesting that they could be potential catalysts for problem gambling.

High rates of pathologic gambling have been described among jail and prison inmates. Conversely, high comorbidity with antisocial personality disorder is also reported (27).

PHENOMENOLOGY OF PATHOLOGIC GAMBLING

Pathologic gambling is currently understood as a disease characterized by an addiction to what gamblers call "being in action" (38). This term describes an aroused state compared by some gamblers to the "high" experienced after using stimulants such as cocaine. A gambler is "in action" while awaiting the result of a significant wager. In some cases, a feeling of altered identity or dissociation is experienced (39). Both the "high" and the dissociated state afford a relief from dysphoric feelings such as boredom, anxiety, and depression. They allow a reduction in self-criticism, worry, and guilt, and permit the gambler to indulge in fantasies about the next "big win."

Pathophysiology

There are considerable gaps in our knowledge about how gambling impacts the brain. The research into gambling neurobiology started timidly in the late 1980s (40,41), but grew impressively throughout the 1990s. Different studies found altered regulation of monoamine neurotransmitters such as noradrenaline, serotonin, and dopamine, which, in turn, were related to the regulation of motivated behaviors and impulse control (42).

Blum has proposed that decreased dopamine activity on the mesocorticolimbic circuitry is related to addictions and addiction-like behaviors, the so-called reward deficiency syndrome (43). Genetic studies relate pathologic gambling to gene polymorphism at dopamine receptors, D1, D2, and D4 (44). Conversely, 3 studies reported 13 cases of pathologic gambling that started among Parkinson disease patients after the introduction of L-dopa therapy (45–47), noting that hyperactivity of dopamine circuitry could be responsible. The only study addressing the actual impact of gambling on neurotransmitters reported an increase of peripheral norepinephrine at the beginning of a winning streak and an increase of dopamine at the end of it (48).

A genetic alteration in norepinephrine receptors in pathologic gamblers has been reported (44), and elevated activity has been suggested by both peripheral and central measures of norepinephrine metabolites (41,42).

Both a decreased level of peripheral monoamine oxidase and genetic polymorphism for monoamine oxidase (MAO) types A and B among pathologic gamblers support the hypothesis that deregulated monoamine activity contributes to altered motivated behavior (49).

A functional magnetic resonance imaging (MRI) study of normal volunteers identified several brain sites involved in active gambling, for example, ventral tegmental area, orbitofrontal cortex, sublenticular extended amygdala, and the hypothalamus, identified by the authors as areas also involved in brain stimulation by cocaine infusion (50). A study of event-related potentials in the brain identified an electric activity generated by a medial-frontal region, probably related to the anterior cingulate cortex that reacted to monetary losses, that is, punishment (51). Overall, both studies show that gambling is a complex behavior that involves different parts of the brain depending upon a combination of previous expectancies (expected to win/expected to lose) and actual outcome.

Psychodynamics

Considerable attention has been devoted to the study of psychodynamic factors involved in pathologic gambling. Psychoanalysts stress the role of unconscious conflicts. Gambling enables the satisfaction of unacceptable erotic impulses, while providing masochistic punishment for the guilt caused by such satisfaction. Lately, the roles of narcissism and fantasies about power and control have also been explored (15). Behavioral psychologists point to the roles of classical and operant conditioning, and the self-reinforcement properties of gambling given its intermittent schedule of payout (52).

The possibility of predisposing personality features has been difficult to explore because of a lack of consensus about personality models. However, pathologic gamblers tend to score high on measures of impulsivity (53), and impulsivity assessed during mid-adolescence is related to problem gambling at late adolescence (54).

Course of the Disease

The progressive course of pathologic gambling is usually described in the three phases originally elucidated by Dr. Robert Custer, based on his experience at the Brecksville treatment unit. He described these as the winning, losing, and desperation phases (7). To this, Rosenthal has added the hopeless or "giving-up" phase (15). Because nearly all of Custer's patients were male, whereas about a third of probable pathologic gamblers identified in general population studies are female, it is not surprising that this progression of phases may not be characteristic of all gamblers. Women tend to start their gambling problems later than men, but they progress faster, coming to treatment at roughly the same age as men. This phenomenon, also described for alcohol dependence, has been called the *telescoping effect* (17–19).

Winning Phase

In some cases, the career of the pathologic gambler begins with a big win (equal to half the individual's annual earnings or more). Dostoyevsky describes such a progression in a character in *The Gambler,* with a rapid development of preoccupation, tolerance, and loss of control (4). For most gamblers, however, the winning phase reflects the time and effort they devote to gambling on skill-related forms of wagering such as horse race betting, playing the stock market, or playing cards. Winning induces a feeling of power, wealth, and omnipotence. As the gambler's involvement with gambling grows, the gambler depends increasingly on the "high" derived from being in action and less on other mechanisms of defense to deal with problems and to counteract negative emotional states. The gambler pulls away from intimate interpersonal relationships and derives a growing proportion of his or her self-esteem from both gambling skill and the feeling of being favored by God, Fate, or Lady Luck. Whereas others must work for a living, the gambler feels empowered to obtain money through magical means. Although pathologic gamblers both win and lose during this phase, they tend to recall and talk about their wins and deny, rationalize, or minimize their losses. For this reason, they are often unable to account for money claimed to be won. The winning phase is more characteristic of pathologic gamblers whom Lesieur describes as "action-seekers" as opposed to initial "escape-seekers" who begin their gambling involvement as a way to relieve situation-related dysphoria. In a study of female members of GA, more than half started as "escape-seekers" (12). Gambling for escape is also associated with the kinds of "hypnotic," "blackout," or dissociated status described by Jacobs (39).

Losing Phase

This phase often begins with the kind of unpredictable losing streak experienced by anyone who gambles. Sometimes it begins with a "bad beat" (an unexplained bizarre circumstance that turns an expected win into a loss) (55). For example, a horse approaching the finish line well in front of the pack suddenly drops dead, or a winning horse is disqualified because of a technicality irrelevant to the race itself. The experience of losing would be distressing for the ordinary gambler, but for the pathologic gambler it is experienced as a severe narcissistic blow, and may begin a pattern of "chasing" losses (13). This experience may be related to the phenomenon described by gamblers as "going on tilt" (an acute deterioration of play). In any case, the gambler now feels compelled to win back money the gambler has lost and begins to gamble less cautiously, thereby compounding losses. As losses mount, gambling becomes more urgent and also more solitary. Lying to cover losses, appropriating assets from family members, taking out loans, and continually searching for money

become prevalent activities. Interpersonal relationships are further strained. Family members find themselves isolated and confused by the gambler's behavior and the disappearance of family funds. Spouses sometimes suspect the gambler is having an affair. Even when they know about the gambling, spouses are usually unaware of the extent of the gambler's indebtedness.

Comorbidities, including affective disorders, may become more apparent during this phase (56), described by some patients and families as "like being on an emotional roller coaster." The gambler both wins and loses during this phase, but money won is only partially used to pay debts. Most of it is gambled.

During this phase the gambler may seek a bailout, promising to cut down or stop gambling in return. The bailout, however, is treated like a "big win," partly gambled, and accepted as further evidence of the gambler's omnipotence (15).

Desperation Phase

This phase may begin with the gambling away of funds from a bailout or some other grave disappointment. The gambler is now desperate. Immoral and/or illegal acts (e.g., fraud, embezzling, writing bad checks) become a necessity, as does the compensatory belief in a big win "just around the corner." Irritability, mood swings, isolation, escape fantasies, and suicidal ideation or attempts are common. Debts mount. Additional bailouts are sought. The gambler may be arrested and prosecuted.

Most members of GA who come for help reporting they have "hit bottom" do so in this phase. Surveys of GA members have reported severe depression in 72% and suicidal attempts in 17% to 24% (56).

Giving Up Phase

Pathologic gamblers who reach this phase no longer cling to the fantasy of "winning it all back." They gamble sloppily. Their goal is just to stay in action.

Comorbid psychiatric conditions have already been mentioned. Depression, bipolar disorder, and suicidal attempts are particularly common, as are substance use disorders (15). Physical conditions generally thought of as stress-related (e.g., hypertension, gastrointestinal problems, respiratory symptoms) are also common at all stages of the disease. Spouses of pathologic gamblers often suffer from a variety of physical and emotional disorders, and may experience several phases in their own reactions, as the disease develops. These have been described as denial (broken through in "cycles of discovery"), stress, and exhaustion (15). Studies of children of pathologic gamblers have found increased rates of such health-threatening behaviors as drinking, drug use, smoking, overeating, and gambling. These problems are especially evident in children of parents with comorbid conditions such as combined pathologic gambling and substance dependence (57,58).

PATHOLOGIC GAMBLING AND SUBSTANCE-USE DISORDERS: IDENTIFICATION IN CLINICAL POPULATIONS

Because of the high prevalence of pathologic gambling among persons suffering from substance use disorders, all such patients should be evaluated for gambling problems. The relationship between substance use and gambling is a complex one (32). The two activities are often combined. Alcoholic beverages are served in casinos and at sports events. Both licit and illicit gambling activities may be centered at bars, where illicit drugs are also sold. Substance dependence may develop simultaneously with pathologic gambling or may develop before or afterward. It is, therefore, important to assess risk in substance dependent patients who do not report current gambling problems. Patients with a history of intense interest in gambling before the onset of substance dependence, patients with a family history of pathologic gambling, and patients with a history of gambling problems in remission are at special risk. The altered psychological state experienced during gambling may lead to relapse in a newly abstinent substance-dependent patient. Alternatively, abstinence from alcohol and drugs may be sustained, but a "switch of addictions" experienced (59). The action of gambling is easily substituted for the substance-induced "high" in the patient's pattern of dependence, leading to a rapid development of pathologic gambling.

The South Oaks Gambling Screen (SOGS) (Figure 28.1) is available to screen clinical populations (60). It can be administered as a pencil-and-paper test or a clinical interview. It should be scored with the score sheet (Figure 28.2) because not all questions are counted in the total score. The first few questions, although not scored, give the evaluator a quick survey of the kinds and amounts of wagering done by the subject, and of family history. The amounts wagered must be evaluated relative to the subject's total disposable income. The family history is useful in judging risk. Question 12 is not scored, but acts as a lead-in to question 13. In addition, although questions 16 (j) and (k) are not scored, they provide valuable information to the rater. The maximum SOGS score is 20. Scores of 5 or more are indicative of probable pathologic gambling, while a score of between 1 and 4 may indicate some gambling problem. Note that the questions are written in a lifetime mode. Patients who score 5 or more should be evaluated using *DSM–IV* diagnostic criteria for pathologic gambling (10), either current or in remission.

The SOGS has been translated into many languages, including Spanish, Italian, German, Turkish, Japanese, Hebrew, and several Southeast Asian languages, and adapted to different cultures (61).

In addition to screening for pathologic gambling in chemically dependent populations, the SOGS is recommended for patients in mental health and general medical settings and in employee assistance programs (EAPs) (62). In a poll of 86 programs and EAP professionals, 64% reported having had experience with pathologic gamblers among their caseloads (63). Jail and prison populations should also be screened, because pathologic gamblers who complete their sentences are highly likely to resume criminal activity if their disease is untreated.

The SOGS has demonstrated both adequate specificity and reliability in clinical populations but may overestimate when it is used to measure the prevalence of pathologic gambling in general population surveys (64).

TREATMENT OF PATHOLOGIC GAMBLING

Current treatment for pathologic gambling is in many ways similar to the treatment of substance use disorders. Most of the treatment is delivered on an outpatient basis, with inpatient or residential care reserved for patients in a crisis of some kind, treatment failures, and patients with comorbid disorders (65).

Modalities employed include psychoeducation, individual and group therapies, and family involvement, either in conjoint family sessions or in separate individual or group therapy for "significant others." Family members can and should be referred for help whether or not the problem gambler accepts treatment (66).

Referrals to GA and Gam-Anon (a 12-step fellowship for family members) are often made and attendance is encouraged as an adjunct to treatment. GA was established in 1957, based on the 12 steps of Alcoholics Anonymous (AA), as adapted to the recovery of pathologic gamblers. GA has developed several specific strategies in dealing with the extreme financial indebtedness of new members and their initial difficulties in handling money (67).

Abstinence is the ultimate goal in most treatment programs, although reduction or control of gambling is sought in some programs, presumably for earlier-stage problem gamblers.

Initial Treatment

Patients may begin treatment for a variety of reasons. There is often an external motivation, for example, an arrest or threatened arrest, pressure from the family as a condition of providing a bailout, or job jeopardy. The patient may have been diagnosed through screening while in treatment for a psychiatric or substance use disorder, or there may be a crisis such as a suicide attempt or personal bankruptcy. Initial treatment attempts to prevent gambling from doing further harm. Many clinicians recommend limiting access to money, to credit, and to gambling venues and partners early in treatment (68). Such a strategy involves some loss of autonomy and patients may resist

Name_____ Date _____

1. Please indicate which of the following types of gambling you have done in your lifetime. For each type, mark one answer: "not at all," "less than once a week," or "once a week or more."

	not at all	less than once a week	once a week or more	
a.	_____	_____	_____	play cards for money
b.	_____	_____	_____	bet on horses, dogs or other animals (at OTB, the track or with a bookie)
c.	_____	_____	_____	bet on sports (parlay cards, with a bookie, or at Jai Alai)
d.	_____	_____	_____	played dice games (including craps, over and under or other dice games) for money
e.	_____	_____	_____	gambled in a casino (legal or otherwise)
f.	_____	_____	_____	played the numbers or bet on lotteries
g.	_____	_____	_____	played bingo for money
h.	_____	_____	_____	played the stock, options and/or commodities market
i.	_____	_____	_____	played slot machines, poker machines or other gambling machines
j.	_____	_____	_____	bowled, shot pool, played golf or some other game of skill for money
k.	_____	_____	_____	pull tabs or "paper" games other than lotteries
l.	_____	_____	_____	some form of gambling not listed above
				(please specify) _____

2. What is the largest amount of money you have ever gambled with on any one day?

_____ never have gambled   _____ more than $100 up to $1,000
_____ $1 or less   _____ more than $1,000 up to $10,000
_____ more than $1 up to $10   _____ more than $10,000
_____ more than $10 up to $100

3. Check which of the following people in your life has (or had) a gambling problem.

_____ father   _____ mother   _____ a brother or sister   _____ a grandparent
_____ my spouse or partner   _____ my child(ren)   _____ another relative
_____ a friend or someone else important in my life

4. When you gamble, how often do you go back another day to win back money you lost?

_____ never
_____ some of the time (less than half the time I lost)
_____ most of the time I lost
_____ every time I lost

5. Have you ever claimed to be winning money gambling but weren't really? In fact, you lost?

_____ never (or never gamble)
_____ yes, less than half the time I lost
_____ yes, most of the time

6. Do you feel you have ever had a problem with betting money or gambling?

_____ no
_____ yes, in the past but not now
_____ yes

7. Did you ever gamble more than you intend to? . . . . _____ yes _____ no

8. Have people criticized your betting or told you that you had a gambling problem, regardless of whether or not you thought it was true? . . . . _____ yes _____ no

9. Have you ever felt guilty about the way you gamble or what happens when you gamble?. . . . . _____ yes _____ no

10. Have you ever felt like you would like to stop betting money or gambling but didn't think you could? . . . . _____ yes _____ no

11. Have you ever hidden betting slips, lottery tickets, gambling money, I.O.U.s or other signs of betting or gambling from your spouse, children or other important people in your life? . . . . _____ yes _____ no

12. Have you ever argued with people you live with over how you handle money?. . . . . _____ yes _____ no

13. (If you answered yes to question 12): Have money arguments ever centered on your gambling? . . . . _____ yes _____ no

14. Have you ever borrowed from someone and not paid them back as a result of your gambling?. . . . . _____ yes _____ no

15. Have you ever lost time from work (or school) due to betting money or gambling? . . . . _____ yes _____ no

16. If you borrowed money to gamble or to pay gambling debts, who or where did you borrow from? (check "yes" or "no" for each)

	no	yes
a. from household money _____	( )	( )
b. from your spouse _____	( )	( )
c. from other relatives or in-laws _____	( )	( )
d. from banks, loan companies or credit unions_____	( )	( )
e. from credit cards_____	( )	( )
f. from loan sharks _____	( )	( )
g. you cashed in stocks, bonds or other securities _____	( )	( )
h. you sold personal or family property _____	( )	( )
i. you borrowed on your checking account (passed bad checks)_____	( )	( )
j. you have (had) a credit line with a bookie _____	( )	( )
k. you have (had) a credit line with a casino _____	( )	( )

FIG. 28.1. South Oaks Gambling Screen. Copyright 1992, South Oaks Foundation. Used with permission.

Scores on the SOGS itself are determined by adding up the number of questions which show an "at risk" response:

Questions 1, 2 & 3 not counted:

_____ Question 4 —most of the time I lost
or
every time I lost

_____ Question 5 —yes, less than half the time I lost
or
yes, most of the time

_____ Question 6 —yes, in the past but not now
or
yes

_____ Question 7 —yes

_____ Question 8 —yes

_____ Question 9 —yes

_____ Question 10 —yes

_____ Question 11 —yes

Question 12 not counted

_____ Question 13 —yes

_____ Question 14 —yes

_____ Question 15 —yes

_____ Question 16a—yes

_____ Question b—yes

_____ Question c—yes

_____ Question d—yes

_____ Question e—yes

_____ Question f—yes

_____ Question g—yes

_____ Question h—yes

_____ Question i—yes
questions 16j & k not counted

Total = _____ (there are 20 questions that are counted)

0 = no problem
1–4 = some problem
5 or more = probable pathological gambler

FIG. 28.2. South Oaks Gambling Screen score sheet. Copyright 1992, South Oaks Foundation. Used with permission.

the idea. Because noncompliance may lead to relapse and treatment dropout, motivational techniques can be useful (69). Initial treatment also involves educating the patient and family about the nature of the disease and its treatment, and dealing with concomitant psychiatric, physical, and social problems.

Various psychoactive medications have been tried in pathologic gamblers, including mood stabilizers, antidepressants, antipsychotics, and opiate receptor blockers. Double-blind trials have been limited to fluvoxamine (Luvox), paroxetine (Paxil), and naltrexone (ReVia) (70–72). One single-blind study found both lithium and valproate associated with improvement over a 14-week period (73). Further investigation is needed to clarify the effectiveness

and role of psychopharmacology. It is also important to note that a high initial placebo-response rate has been reported, up to 59% (70), so that extended studies are required.

Rehabilitation

Continued treatment includes exploring the role of gambling in patients' lives and helping them develop other healthier means to satisfy these needs. Understanding relapse triggers, learning relapse prevention techniques, and practicing stress management are helpful, as are measures to improve the interpersonal and social functioning of the patient. Family treatment is also critical to rehabilitation. In some patients long-term psychodynamic psychotherapy is required for stable recovery.

Few random controlled trials of treatment for pathologic gambling have been conducted, most of them employing cognitive–behavioral approaches (74). Cognitive therapy is based on the hypothesis that false assumptions regarding chance events and the laws of probability account for gambling attractiveness. The overestimation of one's skills, fantasies about being able to influence random events, and ideas that deny the independence of chance events (e.g., "odd numbers have come out so many times in a row, that now there will be an even number") feed into fantasies of restitution and the desire to resume gambling (75). Cognitive therapy asks that the patient keep a log of gambling thoughts, identify those pertaining to the distorted belief system, and challenge these misconceptions with more rational thoughts (76). Preliminary reports of progressive exposure to gambling machines coupled with response prevention has found this method potentially useful in diminishing cravings elicited by gambling cues (68).

Long-Term Followup

Pathologic gambling is a lifelong disorder. As with substance dependence, patients may relapse after years of abstinence. Therefore, long-term followup in GA is helpful, with the availability of professional assistance as needed in times of increased stress or risk of relapse. Likewise, long-term Gam-Anon involvement is helpful for family members. Unfortunately, Gamateen, a self-help, 12-step-based fellowship for adolescent children of pathologic gamblers, is not yet widely available.

The majority of published studies on treatment of pathologic gambling are case reports, uncontrolled trials, or open studies. However, the overall picture points to pathologic gambling as a treatable condition (77). Stinchfield and Winters (78) analyzed the outcome of four state-supported outpatient programs. The treatments combined varied techniques and a 12-step approach, which has been the standard for addiction treatment. Altogether 348 men and 220 women were treated between 1992 and 1995. Almost half of the sample (48%) showed significant improvement at 6-month followup. Twenty-eight percent had totally abstained and an additional 20% reported having gambled less than once a month. As the authors noted, these numbers are similar to the treatment efficacy observed for alcohol and drug treatment.

A 1985 study examined the cost-effectiveness of pathologic gambling treatment (79). The authors concluded that an overall benefit:cost ratio of 20:1 was realized to society.

PREVENTION OF PATHOLOGIC GAMBLING

In spite of the immense social and personal costs of pathologic gambling, there has been very little research or programmatic attention paid to the prevention of this disorder (80). Some attempts at prevention have been made through public education (e.g., posting signs in casinos) and the establishment of toll-free referral numbers. However, the shortage of treatment resources and the long waiting lists at many clinics hamper efforts to connect individuals and families in need with professional help.

A comprehensive prevention plan should address both education of those at risk for developing gambling problems, and lowering treatment barriers for those experiencing them already. Informative material for adolescents may be useful to address misconceptions about gambling (81),

but their utility in preventing pathologic gambling is still under investigation. A wider range of treatment options is needed to address different stages of illness (82). Shame, secrecy, and lonely attempts at financial recovery through gambling have been associated with treatment delay (83), and should be addressed in messages specifically targeting pathologic gamblers.

Another promising field of investigation is strategies to reduce the addictive potential of games (84). Cox and colleagues (85) report that betting at casinos and gambling machines, rather than buying lottery tickets, distinguishes problem from recreational gambling.

A more rapid onset of pathologic gambling among players of computerized games has been described. Because computer games are fast paced and allow immediate rebetting, they enable dysfunctional gambling (86). Furthermore, computer games reach a greater proportion of the population because they are not as associated with male culture as are more traditional games such as card games and horse racing (17,21).

Clearly, the growth of commercial gambling coupled with technologic advances set important challenges for the future. Enhanced societal support for research, prevention and treatment will be needed if we are to remedy the individual, family and community devastation produced by pathologic gambling.

REFERENCES

1. Fleming AM. *Something for nothing: a history of gambling.* New York: Delacorte Press, 1978. Cited by McGurrin MC, ed. *Pathological gambling: conceptual, diagnostic, and treatment issues.* Sarasota, FL: Professional Resource Press, 1992.
2. Clotfelter CT, Cook PJ. *Selling hope: state lotteries in America.* Cambridge, MA: Harvard University Press, 1989.
3. Hertzberg L. Leon Modena, Renaissance rabbi. 1571-1648. *Harv Mag* 1985(Sept-Oct):41–43.
4. Dostoyevsky F. *The gambler/ bobok/a nasty story.* New York: Penguin Books, 1966:7–16. Coulson J, translator.
5. Freud S. Dostoyevsky and parricide. In: *Collected Papers, vol. 5:* pp. 222–242. London: Hogarth Press, 1928.
6. Rosenthal RJ. The psychodynamics of pathological gambling: a review of the literature. In: Galski T, ed. *The handbook of pathological gambling.* Springfield, IL: Charles C Thomas, 1987.
7. Custer R, Milt H. *When luck runs out: help for compulsive gamblers and their families.* New York: Facts On File Publications, 1985.
8. Clarke R, Dempsey G. The feasibility of regulating gambling on the Internet. *Manage Decis Econ* 2001;22:125–132.
9. Volberg RA. Prevalence studies of prob-

lem gambling in the United States. *J Gambl Stud* 1996;12(2):111–128.
10. American Psychiatric Association. *Diagnostic and statistical manual of mental disorders,* 4th ed. Washington, DC: Author, 1994.
11. Rosenthal RJ, Lesieur HR. *Withdrawal symptoms and pathological gambling.* Paper presented at the International Conference on Gambling and Risk Taking. London, 1990.
12. Lesieur HR, Blume SB. When lady luck loses: women and compulsive gambling. In: Van Den Bergh N, ed. *Feminist perspectives on addictions.* New York: Springer-Verlag, 1991:181–197.
13. Lesieur HR. *The chase: career of the compulsive gambler.* Cambridge, MA: Schenkman, 1984.
14. Rosenthal RJ, Lorenz VC. The pathological gambler as criminal offender: comments on evaluation and treatment. *Clin Forens Psychiatry* 1992;15(3):647–660.
15. Lesieur HR, Rosenthal RJ. Pathological gambling: a review of the literature (prepared for the American Psychiatric Association Task Force on DSM-IV Committee on Disorders of Impulse Control Not Elsewhere Classified). *J Gambl Stud* 1991;7(1):5–39.
16. Holden C: "Behavioral" addictions: do they exist? *Science* 2001;294:980–982.

17. Tavares H, Zilberman M, Beites FJ, et al. Gender differences in gambling progression. *J Gambl Stud* 2001;17:151–159.
18. Potenza MN, Steinberg MA, McLaughlin SD, et al. Gender-related differences in the characteristics of problem gamblers using a gambling helpline. *Am J Psychiatry* 2001;158:1500–1505.
19. Martins SS, Lobo DSS, Tavares H, et al. Pathological gambling in women: a review. *Rev Hosp Clin Fac Med Sao Paulo* 2002;57:235–242.
20. Volberg RA. Has there been a "feminization" of gambling and problem gambling in the United States? *The Electronic Journal of Gambling Issues: eGambling,* Issue 8, 2002. Available at: http://www.camh.net/egambling.
21. Volberg RA. The prevalence and demographics of pathological gamblers: implications for public health. *Am J Public Health* 1994;84(2):237–241.
22. Welte J, Barnes G, Wieczorek W, et al. Alcohol and gambling pathology among U.S. adults: prevalence, demographic patterns and comorbidity. *J Stud Alcohol* 2001;62(5):706–712.
23. Slutske WS, Eisen S, True WR, et al. Common genetic vulnerability for pathological gambling and alcohol dependence in men. *Arch Gen Psychiatry* 2000;57(7):666–673.

24. Shaffer HJ, Korn DA. Gambling and related mental disorders: a public health analysis. *Annu Rev Public Health* 2002;23:171–212.

25. Kallick M, Suits D, Dielman T, et al. *A survey of American gambling attitudes and behavior.* Ann Arbor, MI: University of Michigan Press, 1979.

26. Gerstein D, Murphy S, Toce, et al. *Gambling impact and behavior study: final report to the National Gambling Impact Study Commission.* Chicago: National Opinion Research Center, 1999.

27. Shaffer HJ, Hall MN, Vander Bilt J. Estimating the prevalence of disordered gambling behavior in the United States and Canada: a research synthesis. *Am J Public Health* 1999;89(9):1369–1376.

28. National Research Council. *Pathological gambling: a critical review.* Washington, DC: National Academy Press, 1999.

29. Westphal JR, Rush JA, Stevens L, et al. Gambling behavior of Louisiana students in grades 6 through 12. *Psychiatr Serv* 2000;51(1):96–99.

30. Adlaf EM, Ialomiteanu A. Prevalence of problem gambling in adolescents: findings from the 1999 Ontario Student Drug Use Survey. *Can J Psychiatry* 2000;45(8):752–755.

31. Poulin C. An assessment of the validity and reliability of the SOGS-RA. *J Gambl Stud* 2002;18(1):67–93.

32. Spunt B, Dupont I, Lesieur H, et al. Pathological gambling and substance misuse: a review of the literature. *Subst Use Misuse* 1998;33(13):2535–2560.

33. Feigelman W, Wallisch LS, Lesieur HR. Problem gamblers, problem substance users, and dual-problem individuals: an epidemiological study. *Am J Public Health* 1998;88(3):467–470.

34. Cunningham-Williams RM, Cottler LB, Compton WM 3rd, et al. Taking chances: problem gamblers and mental health disorders—results from the St. Louis Epidemiologic Catchment Area Study. *Am J Public Health* 1998;88(7):1093–1096.

35. Lesieur HR, Blume SB. Characteristics of pathological gamblers identified among patients on a psychiatric admissions service. *Hosp Community Psychiatry* 1990;41(9):1009–1012.

36. Pasternak AV 4th, Fleming MF. Prevalence of gambling disorders in a primary care setting. *Arch Fam Med* 1999; 8(6):515–520.

37. Crockford DN, el-Guebaly N. Psychiatric comorbidity in pathological gambling: a critical review. *Can J Psychiatry* 1998;43(1):43–50.

38. Blume SB. Compulsive gambling and the medical model. *J Gambl Behav* 1988;3:237–247.

39. Jacobs DF. Evidence for a common dissociative-like reaction among addicts. *J Gambl Behav* 1988;4(1):27–37.

40. Roy A, Adinoff B, Roehrick L, et al. Pathological gambling: a psychobiological study. *Arch Gen Psychiatry* 1988;45:369–373.

41. Roy A, DeJong J, Linnoila M. Extraversion in pathological gamblers, correlates with indices of noradrenergic function. *Arch Gen Psychiatry* 1989;46: 679–681.

42. Potenza MN. The neurobiology of pathological gambling. *Semin Clin Neuropsychiatry* 2001;6(3):217–226.

43. Blum K, Braverman ER, Holder JM, et al. Reward deficiency syndrome: a biogenetic model for the diagnosis and treatment of impulsive, addictive, and compulsive behaviors. *J Psychoactive Drugs* 2000;32[Suppl i-iv]:1–112.

44. Comings DE, Gade-Andavolu R, Gonzalez N, et al. The additive effect of neurotransmitter genes in pathological gambling. *Clin Genet* 2001;60(2):107–116.

45. Molina JA, Sainz-Artiga MJ, Fraile A, et al. Pathologic gambling in Parkinson's disease: a behavioral manifestation of pharmacologic treatment? *Mov Disord* 2000;15(5):869–872.

46. Seedat S, Kesler S, Niehaus DJ, et al. Pathological gambling behaviour: emergence secondary to treatment of Parkinson's disease with dopaminergic agents. *Depress Anxiety* 2000;11(4):185–186.

47. Gschwandtner U, Aston J, Renaud S, et al. Pathologic gambling in patients with Parkinson's disease. *Clin Neuropharmacol* 2001;24(3):170–172.

48. Shinohara K, Yanagisawa A, Kagota Y, et al. Physiological changes in Pachinko players; beta-endorphin, catecholamines, immune system substances and heart rate. *Appl Hum Sci* 1999;18(2):37–42.

49. Ibanez A, de Castro IP, Fernandez-Piqueras J, et al. Pathological gambling and DNA polymorphic markers at MAO-A and MAO-B genes. *Mol Psychiatry* 2000;5(1):105–109.

50. Breiter HC, Aharon I, Kahneman D, et al. Functional imaging of neural responses to expectancy and experience of monetary gains and losses. *Neuron* 2000;30(2):619–639.

51. Gehring WJ, Willoughby AR. The medial frontal cortex and the rapid processing of monetary gains and losses. *Science* 2002;295(5563):2279–2282.

52. Petry NM, Roll JM. A behavioral approach to understanding and treating pathological gambling. *Semin Clin Neuropsychiatry* 2001;6(3):177–183.

53. Steel Z, Blaszczynski A. Impulsivity, personality disorders and pathological gambling severity. *Addiction* 1998; 93(6):895–905.

54. Vitaro F, Brendgen M, Ladouceur R, et al. Gambling, delinquency, and drug use during adolescence: mutual influences and common risk factors. *J Gambl Stud* 2001;17(3):171–190.

55. Rosecrance J. Attributions and the origins of problem gambling. *Sociol Q* 1986;27:463–477.

56. Linden RD. Pathological gambling and major affective disorder: preliminary findings. *J Clin Psychiatry* 1985;47:201–203.

57. Jacobs DF, Marston AR, Singer RD, et al. Children of problem gamblers. *J Gambl Behav* 1989;5(4):261–268.

58. Lesieur HR, Rothschild J. Children of Gamblers Anonymous members. *J Gambl Behav* 1989;5(4):269–281.

59. Blume SB. Pathological gambling and switching addictions: report of a case. *J Gambl Stud* 1994;10(1):87–96.

60. Lesieur HR, Blume SB. The South Oaks Gambling Screen (SOGS): a new instrument for the identification of pathological gamblers. *Am J Psychiatry* 1987;144(9):1184–1188.

61. Lesieur HR, Blume SB. Revising the South Oaks Gambling Screen in different settings. *J Gambl Behav* 1992;9(3):213–219.

62. Lesieur HR. Pathological gambling, work, and employee assistance. *J Empl Assist Professionals Assoc* 1992;1(1): 32–62.

63. Lesieur HR. Experience of employee assistance programs with pathological gamblers. *J Drug Issues* 1989;19(4):425–436.

64. Stinchfield R. Reliability, validity, and classification accuracy of the South Oaks Gambling Screen (SOGS). *Addict Behav* 2002;27(1):1–19.

65. Blume SB. Treatment for the addictions in a psychiatric setting. *Br J Addict* 1989;84:727–729.

66. Heineman M. *Losing your shirt.* Minneapolis: CompCare Publishers, 1992.

67. Gamblers Anonymous. *Sharing recovery through Gamblers Anonymous.* Los Angeles, CA: Author, 1984.

68. Echeburua E, Baez C, Fernandez-Montalvo J. Comparative effectiveness of three therapeutic modalities in the psychological treatment of pathological gambling: long-term outcome. *Behav Cogn Psychotherapy* 1996;24(1):51–72.

69. Hodgins DC, Currie SR, el-Guebaly N. Motivational enhancement and self-help treatments for problem gambling. *J Consult Clin Psychol* 2001;69(1):50–57.

70. Blanco C, Petkova E, Ibanez A, et al. A pilot placebo-controlled study of fluvoxamine for pathological gambling. *Ann Clin Psychiatry* 2002;14(1):9–15.

71. Kim SW, Grant JE, Adson DE, et al. A double-blind placebo-controlled study of the efficacy and safety of paroxetine in the treatment of pathological gambling. *J Clin Psychiatry* 2002;63(6):501–507.

72. Kim SW, Grant JE, Adson DE, et al. Double-blind naltrexone and placebo comparison study in the treatment of pathological gambling. *Biol Psychiatry* 2001;49(11):914–921.
73. Pallanti S, Quercioli L, Sood E, et al. Lithium and valproate treatment of pathological gambling: a randomized single-blind study. *J Clin Psychiatry* 2002;63(7):559–564.
74. Oakley-Browne MA, Adams P, Mobberley PM. Interventions for pathological gambling. *Cochrane Database Syst Rev* 2000;(2):CD001521.
75. Toneatto T. Cognitive psychopathology of problem gambling. *Subst Use Misuse* 1999;34(11):1593–1604.
76. Ladouceur R, Sylvain C, Boutin C, et al. Cognitive treatment of pathological gambling. *J Nerv Ment Dis* 2001;189(11):774–780.
77. Lopez Viets VC, Miller WR. Treatment approaches for pathological gamblers. *Clin Psychol Rev* 1997;17(7):689–702.
78. Stinchfield R, Winters KC. Outcome of Minnesota's gambling treatment programs. *J Gambl Stud* 2001;17(3):217–245.
79. Politzer RM, Morrow JS, Leavey SB. Report on the cost-benefit/effectiveness of treatment at the Johns Hopkins Center for Pathological Gambling. *J Gambl Behav* 1985;1:131–142.
80. *The need for a national policy on problem and pathological gambling in America.* New York: National Council on Problem Gambling, November 1, 1993.
81. Ferland F, Ladouceur R, Vitaro F. Prevention of problem gambling: modifying misconceptions and increasing knowledge. *J Gambl Stud* 2002;18(1):19–29.
82. Hodgins DC, el-Guebaly N. Natural and treatment-assisted recovery from gambling problems: a comparison of resolved active gamblers. *Addiction* 2000;95(5):777–789.
83. Tavares H, Martins SS, Zilberman ML, et al. Gamblers seeking treatment: why haven't they come earlier? *Addict Disord Treat* 2002;1(2):65–69.
84. Loba P, Stewart SH, Klein RM, et al. Manipulations of the features of standard video lottery terminal (VLT) games: effects in pathological and non-pathological gamblers. *J Gambl Stud* 2001;17(4):297–320.
85. Cox BJ, Kwong J, Michaud V, et al. Problem and probable pathological gambling: considerations from a community survey. *Can J Psychiatry* 2000;45(6):548–553.
86. Breen RB, Zimmerman M. Rapid onset of pathological gambling in machine gamblers. *J Gambl Stud* 2002;18(1):31–43.

CHAPTER 29

Addiction and Cults: Synthesizing a Model for Treating Ex-Members

RON BURKS

Fanaticism, an extreme devotion to a person or cause, seems to share many features with addiction. Schaef and Fassel (1) describe the "addictive organization" as both substance and setting for acting out using behaviors. The organization promises what substances promise: that answers, security, and a sense of worth are only found outside the self. Other observers of the cult phenomenon suspect certain combinations of behavior and belief on the part of the leader, combined with the inherent ability of groups to reinforce behavior change, is responsible for the unusual level of control over personal choice observed in some groups. Still other observers point to the contribution of family background and preexisting emotional problems as primary factors in the decision to involve oneself in a high-demand group. All successful addiction treatment requires knowledge. Helping patients recover from an experience in a cult is no exception.

The clinician's job is complicated by the word "cult" itself. It cannot be applied to a group without assuming a negative connotation. Here, the word is used to refer to a subculture that treats people as objects to be manipulated by the leader. Its ends are considered so noble that any means is justified in fulfilling them including deception or harming outsiders or even its own members if necessary. There are many harmful and dangerous groups where the results of membership are so well known that the clinician would not need this chapter to know how to proceed with treatment. The focus of this chapter is on groups that, although apparently benign, are of concern to the clinician because of persistent presenting problems of ex-members.

The incredible diversity of beliefs of groups that, under this rubric, might be called cults further complicates the clinician's job. By far the most familiar are those groups with some form of religious perspective. Cults may be strictly or loosely based on the Bible or on Indo-Asian religious tradition. But cults exist that have nothing to do with religion. Some cults form around certain political/ideological views, business/motivational concepts, and psychology/counseling/psychotherapy theories, including 12-Step groups (2–4).

Cults are a surprisingly large problem. Research indicates that from 2 to 20 million people are involved in cults at any given time (5–7). According to some estimates, cults, if they were a disease, would be the fourth most common malady affecting the American population. The tragedy of 9/11 illustrates the impact a cult can have to society.

The needs of patients still in a cultic environment differ from those who have left the cult. The focus of this chapter is on the care of patients who have left the cult and are suffering the aftereffects.

Involvement in a cult may be conceptualized in three ways, an addiction model, a social influence model, and an individual factor model. Each has its strengths and weaknesses as a foundation for choosing modality of treatment. A synthesis of the models follows the descriptions in the hope that treatment choices may be clarified and outcomes may be enhanced.

THE MODELS

Belonging as a Drug: The Addiction Model

Proponents of this model see involvement in a cult as a characteristic of the person who joins. People join cults because they feel a compulsive drive to connect with a person or group and panic at the thought of living without them. Ex-members feel there is no place to go and no way to end the discomfort. Cravings for the people and feelings experienced in the group can be overwhelming. After leaving or otherwise losing the group experience, the addict/member feels elation, liberation and a sense that he or she has accomplished something. Often there is no sense of mourning, a gradual acceptance and adjustment that is part of healing for the nonaddict. Hunger for attachment is at the basis of all addiction and there can be no better example than the promises of cults. Cults promise stable attachment in a context that is intense, and transcendent, even cosmic (8). Halperin focused on "addiction to a person" but his insights can be applied to members of cults.

Schaef and Fassel (1) asserted that no person or organization is addictive in itself but anything can become addictive when it becomes central to life. The cult becomes the central focus of life and the member becomes totally preoccupied with it, reducing touch with other aspects of life. Gradually the addict gives up what the addict knows, feels, and believes in favor of the teachings, experiences, and beliefs of the group. In exchange, cults promise the member recognition, approval, better social skills, and care. Membership is conditional on not being oneself or following one's own path. The member is taught to focus on what is required to stay in the group's good graces and that approval must be won by submitting to external control and by reducing awareness of the member's own needs.

The promised mission of the "addictive organization" or cult is usually so grandiose as to be unattainable, yet it is articulated in a way that makes it seem just possible enough given intense, focused effort. The promise of the mission is so compelling that members choose to overlook how the group actually works. The loftier the group's mission, the greater the divergence becomes between its stated mission and its actual day-to-day operation. Greater divergence requires greater denial, paving the way for greater grandiosity. Members cling to the lofty mission because it connects them to the group, giving them a sense of identity. Ironically, the member must seek identity through the group because the conditional acceptance practiced by the group has stripped them of their own. The daily grind seems purposeful, even joyful and apparently meaningful, but only if they become numb to the discrepancies and stay in the group.

Treatment, according to this model, involves facilitating a paradigm shift in the individual away from the need to feel in control. The cult member feels in control not by exercising control over others or even their own lives but through the predictability of life under the group's control. Like the alcoholic, the ex-member must eventually release patterns of dishonesty, let go of dualistic thinking patterns, and move toward flexibility, honesty, and multiple options. Dubrow-Eichel (9) observed that treatment of the adolescent ex-member of a cult resembled substance abuse counseling. Persons still in the mindset of the group resemble Prochaska's "precontemplative" stage with regard to therapy. He found ambivalence about counseling process itself, along with perceptual distortions. The problem, from the perspective of the adolescent still in the mindset of the group, was the lack of acceptance of them by significant others in their lives, because of their affiliation. The individual is suspicious of helpers and family even though they might have significant doubts about the group. The patient feels they are being manipulated by yet another system. The clinician must provide experiences that establish the patient as directing their own process of healing.

A judgmental attitude toward the ex-member/ recovering addict will lead to their becoming defensive, providing a way for them to avoid confronting the denial that perpetuated the addictive relationship to the group. From this perspective, the ex-member is not a bad or stupid person, but a sick person who needs to heal. The ex-member needs to establish a sense of core identity apart from the group and become aware of their needs and right to express them and work toward their fulfillment. Halperin suggests thought-stopping techniques such as one-line sayings, or aphorisms such as "guilt is not a good enough reason to stay," "the pain won't last forever," or "the intensity of withdrawal symptoms do not indicate the strength of the group but the strength of your addiction."

Surrender Without Informed Consent: The Social Influence Model

The social influence model shifts the focus of treatment from the internal dynamics of the ex-member to the aftereffects of the experience in the group. According to this model, the problems of ex-members do not arise from dynamics within the individual or the person's past life experience, but directly from abusive experiences perpetrated by the group. Questions of individual responsibility versus induced loyalty through social control make this model the most controversial of the three models. It is also the only perspective that has been tested empirically in a treatment context and shown helpful to patient recovery (7).

Tragedies such as Jonestown and Waco suggest that some members of cults do things they might not otherwise have done, had it not been for their involvement with the cult (10), even participate in murder (11). Singer and

Lalich suggest cults might have the ability to induce behavior that violates the members' basic values. Membership in some groups appears to inhibit clear thinking and thoughtful behavior.

Thought reform or "brainwashing," a specific set of procedures or conditions alleged to occur in cults is the centerpiece of most, but not all, of the variations of this perspective. Initially described by Robert Lifton (12) in his study of Korean prisoners of war, these procedures were found to make individuals exposed to them far more likely to be compliant with the demands of interrogators than those who were physically beaten or abused. Ten percent of those exposed to the procedures, an astonishingly high number given the times and the prevailing patriotism and intelligence of pilots and others, made public "confessions" to outrageous allegations. Many actually had temporary feelings that they had "done the right thing." Many others felt strongly that they should support their interrogators but did not because of a variety of factors.

In Chinese, thought reform is represented by the characters, *hsi,* to reform or cleanse and *nao,* thought or brain or mind. *Hsi nao,* "reform thought" could also be literally translated, "wash brain." American journalist, and some say intelligence agent, Edward Hunter made the connection and invented the English word "brainwashing" to describe the techniques used in the many "thought reform" camps scattered throughout China (13).

Lifton described eight interpersonal dynamics from his research with former prisoners after the Korean War and survivors of "thought reform" camps in China. In the introduction to the 1989 edition of his book, *Thought Reform and the Psychology of Totalism* (12), he expressed his agreement, from his own study of cults, that his dynamics could be applied to them. Individuals Lifton interviewed who had been subjected to these eight processes could be influenced to adopt new ways of looking at self or the world, enabling them to make rapid changes in convictions, values, attitudes, and behavior. Initially, Lifton may have seen thought reform as a process that required an atmosphere of physical coercion or deprivation. After his study of the rise of the Nazi party in Germany and of "doomsday cults," he made the connection between thought reform and fundamentalist, totalistic social systems. He saw in them the ability to "draw very ordinary people into murderous activities." The right context, the right recruiter with a message that, at least initially, is somewhat in line with the individual's interests at a transitional time in life, can make thought reform an extremely powerful psychological process. Lifton found thought reform effective when used in adversarial situations. One can only imagine how powerful it becomes when applied in a context of ostensible caring and support in a cult.

With few exceptions, thought reform is largely ineffective outside the totalist environment (14). After departure, ex-members are left with no clear explanation of how their beliefs, behavior, and attitudes could have been so radically manipulated. Successful thought reform environments do not seem manipulative. Members believe they are making informed choices. After leaving, isolation, alienation, and self-doubt are common.

Treatment, according to the social influence model, involves exposing the ex-member to large amounts of information about these dynamics and other principles of social influence. The thought reform environment is exposed as fraudulent. What appeared to be informed choice was really choosing among only group-sanctioned options. Ex-members gain an appreciation for the limitations of human perception and information processing that makes all humans susceptible to a thought reform program if it is imposed at the right time in life by the right recruiter promoting a cause or ideal already valued by the potential inductee. The uniqueness and alienation of the experience gives way to understanding and self-acceptance. The ex-member recovers by accepting that the limitations and idealism they share with all humans combined with being in the wrong place at the wrong time resulted in being controlled by the group. The patient is then free to cognitively restructure the experience without guilt or shame. As symptoms decrease and attitude toward self-acceptance increases, the ex-member is able to forward with life (7,10).

Born to Submit: The Individual Factor Model

The individual factor model assumes that if individuals experience harm while participating in a group, it is because of preexisting conditions in the individual, not to conditions in the group. The member's own biology and life experience are to blame for any ills experienced in a group or for joining a group that eventually turned out to be dangerous. The individual factor model shares some features with the addiction model.

New religious movements (NRMs), the term for cults preferred by proponents of this model, stimulate intellectual and behavioral diversity (15–18). Proponents of this model found members of NRMs used fewer substances and had fewer psychiatric symptoms, and long-term members were well adjusted, socially poised, independent, and exhibited flexible thinking (19–23). Latkin concluded that the NRM members he studied had strong opinions and would be hard to persuade, contradicting the assumption that those who join NRMs are gullible. Proponents of this model would deny that NRMs create an atmosphere that induces addiction, allowing that persons who have needs that lead them to become addicted might be attracted to an NRM.

Proponents of this model found that joining an NRM and ex-member maladjustment after leaving was a result of preexisting characteristics such as anxiety, unhappiness, egotism, depression, loneliness, rejection, sadness, meaninglessness, a lack of belonging, and an unhappy childhood (24–28).

These researchers suggest that NRM members have nothing but their parents, their pasts, their present vulnerability, or their preexisting psychopathology to blame for being recruited into a NRM, and their distress is, therefore, unrelated to their NRM experience.

Basic methodological problems were identified in these studies (29) long after their publication, raising peer review and other academic protocol concerns. The events surrounding the disaster at Jonestown and the many highly publicized events in the intervening decades, may seem to make this perspective moot. Sudden migrations of whole groups and mass suicides would seem to indicate that members of NRMs behave in ways that suggest a lack of critical thinking.

Nevertheless, the prior pathology model seems to have considerable influence over how ex-members are diagnosed and treated by the healthcare professions. A frequent complaint of ex-members presenting for treatment at Wellspring Retreat and Resource Center is that physicians who treat them are generally more interested in their families of origin and often express less interest in their more recent experience in a cult.

Treatment suggestions for this model may exist in the literature but were not found during this investigation. This perspective implies that ex-members of NRMs do not suffer harm from the NRM. It would follow, then, that treatment informed by the individual factor model focuses on empowering the patient to accept that their background and life experience is the cause of their distress. Membership in the group was a symptom, not a cause, of their present struggle. Ex-members who continue to focus on the conditions in the group are using their experience to escape their real problems. Recovery begins by taking responsibility for present feelings and attitudes. Telling "horror stories" of conditions in the group or otherwise focusing on it only delays recovery. The ex-member just made a mistake in judgment. Admitting the choice to be involved with the group was a lapse in good judgment allows patients to learn from their mistakes and move on with their lives. Of course, when groups inflict psychological harm or physical abuse on members or on society, whether NRM or old-time religion, those acts should be condemned (14).

Synthesis: Researching a Model as Complex as our Humanity

Each of these perspectives have their flaws and has something to offer in understanding those who seek medical care in the aftermath of a cult experience. The perspectives are so different that any real synthesis is likely to be artificial. Complicating the path to synthesis is the overwhelming complexity of the human brain. Ex-members are like snowflakes. Individual members of the same groups exposed to the same processes react differently. These are, after all, only models. No model can be expected to serve

perfectly in all applications. Still, successful medical treatment depends to a great extent on perspective. although each model has important philosophical shortcomings, each builds on the others toward a perspective that enhances treatment outcomes. In medicine, good treatment is based on good research.

A BRIEF REVIEW OF RESEARCH INTO TREATMENT OF EX-CULTISTS

Some investigators (26–28,30) found that the cult serves as a replacement family and when members leave they feel stress upon return to the family of origin. Maron (31), on the other hand, found that family background was not a likely factor in cult involvement.

Aronoff et al. (29) reviewed the literature and found the most common symptom reported by clinicians was dissociation. Dissociation for the ex-cultist is called *floating* in the literature (30,32,33), the experience of profound ambivalence toward the group, along with feelings of being in the milieu of the group, even years after leaving. Cognitive deficiencies, particularly difficulty making decisions and simplistic, black-and-white thinking were often reported (32,34). Depression (18,30) and anxiety were also commonly reported. Florid psychotic symptoms are less-frequently noted (34), although clinicians unfamiliar with cults sometimes mistake reports of bizarre conditions in groups as delusional thinking.

Singer and Offshe (34) identified areas they felt were common characteristics of ex-members of cults. Most ex-members Singer interviewed struggled with depression, loneliness, indecisiveness, slipping into altered states, trigger experiences, floating, subtle cognitive inefficiencies, fear of the cult, and the feeling of being in a "fish bowl," constantly watched by family and friends. Having to repeat explanations of why they joined and why they stayed gradually became agonizing for them. Ex-members often feel guilt over having brought difficulty into the family or over having recruited others into the group. To make matters worse, the ex-member now realizes that he or she was not part of an elite, historic, or cosmic company on a mission to save the world.

Conway and Siegelman (35) found seven symptoms—altered states, nightmares, inability to break mental rhythms of chanting, amnesia, suicidal/self-harm tendencies, hallucinations, and violent acting out among ex-members—they studied. Swartling and Swartling (36) found anxiety, guilt, emptiness, nightmares, difficulty concentrating, suicidal thoughts, and a loss of identity in ex-members of a Swedish group.

In 1992, Martin et al. (37) administered standard psychometric instruments to inpatients, all of whom had sought treatment at Wellspring Retreat and Resource Center, a facility that combined a bed-and-breakfast residential setting with a 2-week program of individual counseling and workshops. They found that those ex-members of cults who seek treatment after leaving the cult exhibit clinically significant symptoms. Six months after a 2-week intensive treatment program, they reported significant improvement. Martin et al. concluded that the changes in scores 6 months after treatment indicate that the admission scores did not indicate long-standing personality traits, but that the environment of the cult tends to "produce and/or exacerbate dependent-compulsive types."

Synthesis: Trauma and Cults

Synthesis is often achieved when another perspective illuminates the common elements in otherwise divergent ideas. The literature on the effects of trauma provides this perspective and draws the best from each model.

Trauma is an assault on the emotional and cognitive resources of the human organism by an overwhelming stressor. Psychologically, trauma occurs in situations where the individual's conception of a predictable world is shattered. This is where the study of cults and psychological trauma meet in the literature (38,39). Trauma is the result of specific biologic changes that occur in the brain in response to overwhelming stress. Interpersonal trauma is more insidious and more damaging that trauma from accidents and disasters. Trauma sustained in childhood is more difficult to recover from as an adult than trauma suffered as an adult. Trauma inflicted by a supposed caring relative or friend is more difficult to recover from than trauma inflicted by fires or floods. Cumulative trauma occurs when no single event can be characterized as trauma, but many small events, considered together, can have the same effect as overwhelming events. If the perpetrator succeeds in convincing the victim that it was the victim's fault the victim was abused, recovery is stymied (40).

When the source of the trauma is evident and the blame is correctly placed on the perpetrator, the victim is able to reconstruct a safe conception of the world and integrate the experience. When the source of the trauma is vague, victims tend to conclude they have only themselves to blame (40). Cults are successful at masking the harm they do to members usually by blaming some cosmic defect in the member for any ill effect. The individual factor model's contribution, namely that preexisting conditions in the member led to joining and staying, becomes a liability when twisted by the group.

Patients who have experienced periods of intense fear due to the group's emphasis on some form of unpredictable cataclysm or some perceived vulnerability to eternal harm may have been more traumatized than patients whose lives were threatened, or who witnessed an act of physical violence. Control in cults is often maintained using a threat of cosmic consequences that can only be predicted and neutralized through dedication to the group. The leader is then able to control the level of fear by mediating relief only to those who don't ask questions. The sad physical or emotional state of the patient in the clinician's office is proof to the group and, on some level, to the patient, that bad things happen to those who leave. Somewhere in their heart of hearts, the patient wonders if they should never have left.

When the patient in the examining room is considered from the perspective of having suffered psychological trauma, the resources of all three models are able to inform the attitude of the treatment professional to facilitate the patient's recovery. The social influence model tells the clinician that the patient has accepted traumatic experiences from the group because processes used by the group temporarily impaired the patient's judgment. The addiction model explains that the leader, in essence, the addict, has managed to induce a sense of codependence in the ex-member, leaving them with feelings of loss and anger at the same time. The individual factor model suggests that all of the trauma the patient might have experienced might not have been in the group, and that any preexisting conditions must be considered as part of a complete treatment plan.

The confused messages coming from the patient, cursing the group one minute and praising it the next, now have a context. Ambivalence toward the cause of suffering is a common occurrence in recovery from trauma, addiction, and betrayal (social influence model). The patient may alternately blame their family background, a previous failed relationship and the cult for their present suffering. Blending the perspectives of the models explains that all are the problem and all will have to be considered in treatment.

ESSENTIALS FOR TREATMENT

Ex-members of cults often have neglected basic medical and dental care for themselves and for their children. They may be resistant to routine or even necessary care, giving reasons that relate to the beliefs or their former group. Primary health care needs of ex-members of cults are as follows:

1. Ex-members often distrust medical professionals. They have not been well served by those who presented themselves as having special knowledge of their needs. They need an accepting but not condescending attitude from an informed clinician.
2. Ex-members of cults tend to underreport symptoms, having had plenty of practice in denying physical and emotional needs. This tendency can persist long after leaving the group, complicating psychiatric interventions. Answers to the same diagnostic questions may differ from one examination to the next.
3. Ex-members have often had bizarre experiences. Most reports of experiences that would otherwise be diagnosed as hallucinations or delusions are expected experiences in the group and, as such, must be viewed from a multicultural perspective.

4. Some cults are multinational. Ex-members may have lived in several countries in harsh or primitive conditions resulting in symptoms not usually seen the West.

5. Depending on the group, ex-members may have old injuries from physical abuse.

6. Some groups exercise control by strictly regulating sleep and food intake, and after leaving, suffer from forms of malnutrition or experience ongoing interruption of the sleep–wake cycle.

7. Ex-members may experience self-condemning thoughts that are highly resistant to cognitive interventions, even after they have renounced the beliefs of the group. Habitual patterns of thinking may need treatment informed by addiction recovery concepts. Note that some groups twist the 12-Steps to control their followers. Therapeutic or recovery language may be triggering to the ex-member/patient.

Triggers, ambivalence, mistrust of authority figures, inadequate reporting of symptoms, and the possibility of exotic diseases make ex-members of cults a complex but interesting population to treat.

Ex-members of cults need encouragement to counter habitual, self-condemning thought patterns, whether induced by the atmosphere of the group or as a consequence of prior developmental experiences. Understanding clinicians are able to provide an honestly noncritical atmosphere that serves to enhance the patient's ability to trust. Information about influence processes and how the ex-member has been affected, that is, the aftereffects of trauma, enable the ex-member to restart their critical thinking processes. The ex-member's facility to think clearly was impaired by the indoctrination process of the group and the denial that the ex-member has used to cope with the dissonance between the espoused goals of the group and its day-to-day reality. When the clinician provides an atmosphere of emotional safety by accepting and affirming the patient's feelings, the patient is enabled to process the trauma and move toward a life of their own choosing.

REFERENCES

1. Schaef AW, Fassel D. *The addictive organization.* San Francisco: Harper & Row, 1988.

2. Hochman J. Miracle, mystery, and authority: the triangle of cult indoctrination. *Psychiatric Ann* 1990;20:179–184, 187.

3. Singer MT, Temerlin MK, Langone MD. Psychotherapy cults. *Cultic Stud J* 1990;7:101–125.

4. Khantzian EJ. Alcoholics Anonymous—cult or corrective: a case study. *J Subst Abuse Treat* 1995;12:157–165.

5. Bird F, Reimer B. Participation rates in new religions and para-religious movements. *J Scientif Study Relig* 1982;12:1–14.

6. Zimbardo PG, Hartley CF. Cults go to high school: a theoretical and empirical analysis of the initial stage in the recruitment process. *Cultic Stud J* 1985;2:91–147.

7. Martin PR. Post-cult recovery: Assessment and rehabilitation. In: Langone MD, ed. *Recovery from cults: help for victims of psychological and spiritual abuse.* New York: WW Norton, 1993;203–231.

8. Halpern HM. *How to break your addiction to a person.* New York: Bantam, 1983.

9. Dubrow-Eichel SK. Saying goodbye to the guru: brief intermittent developmental therapy with a young adult in a high demand group. *J Coll Stud Psycother* 2001;16:153–170.

10. Singer MT, Lalich J. *Cults in our midst.* San Francisco: Jossey-Bass, 1994.

11. State of Ohio vs. Daniel D. Kraft, Jr. Case No. 90CR 012, in the Court of Common Pleas. Lake County, Ohio.

12. Lifton RJ. *Thought reform and the psychology of totalism.* Chapel Hill, NC: University of North Carolina Press, 1997.

13. Hassan S. *Combating cult mind control.* Rochester, VT: Park Street Press, 1988.

14. Melton JG, Introvigne M. *The brainwashing controversy: an anthology of essential documents, introduction, in center on studies of new religions* [online], 2002. Date of last access: January 16, 2003. Available at: www.cesnur.org/testi/melton.htm.

15. Alexander JW. Religious freedom at secular schools. *Cultic Stud J* 1983;2:318–320.

16. Anthony D, Robbins T. Law, social science and the "brainwashing" exception to the First Amendment. *Behav Sci Law* 1992;10:3–29.

17. Coleman, L. New religions and the myth of mind control. *Am J Orthopsychiatry* 1984;54:322–325.

18. Wright SA, Malony HN. Leaving cults: the dynamics of defection. *Contemp Psych* 1989;34:383–384.

19. Robbins T, Anthony D. Getting straight with Meher Baba: a study of drug rehabilitation, mysticism, and post-adolescent role conflict. *J Scientif Study Relig* 1972;11:122–140.

20. Galanter M, Buckley P. Evangelical religion and meditation: psychotherapeutic effects. *J Nerv Ment Dis* 1978;166:685–691.

21. Levine SV. Cults and mental health: clinical conclusions. *Can J Psychiatry* 1981;26:534–539.

22. Sundberg ND, Latkin CA, Littman RA, et al. Pitfalls and pratfalls in research on an experimental community: lessons in integrating theory and practice from the Rajneeshpuram Research Project. *J Comm Psychol* 1993;21:35–48.

23. Latkin, CA. Self-consciousness in members of a new religious movement: the Rajneeshees. *Journal of Social Psychology,* 1990;130:557–558.

24. Spero MH. Some pre- and post-treatment characteristics of cult devotees. *PerceptMotor Skills* 1984;58:749–750.

25. Levine SV, Salter NE. Youth and contemporary religious movements: psychosocial findings. *Can Psychiatric Assoc J* 1976;21:411–420.

26. Ash SM. Cult induced psychopathology, part 1: clinical picture. *Cultic Stud J* 1985;2:31–90.

27. Deutsch A, Miller MJ. A clinical study of four Unification Church members. *Am J Psychiatry* 1983;140:767–770.

28. Nicholi AM. A new dimension of youth culture. *Am J Psychiatry* 1974;131:396–401.

29. Aronoff J, Lynn SJ, Malinoski P. Are cultic environments harmful? *Clin Psychol Rev* 2000;1:91–111.

30. West LJ, Singer MT. Cults, quacks, and nonprofessional psychotherapies. In: Kaplan HI, Freedman AM, Shaddock BC, eds. *Comprehensive textbook of psychiatry,* Baltimore: Williams & Wilkins, 1980;3245–3258.

31. Maron N. Family environment as a

factor in vulnerability to cult involvement. *Cultic Stud J* 1988;5:23–43.

32. Goldberg L, Goldberg W. Group work with former cultists. *Social Work* 1982;27:163–170.

33. West LJ, Martin PR, Pseudo-identity and the treatment of personality change in victims of captivity and cults. In: Lynn SJ, Rhue JW, eds. *Dissociation: clinical and theoretical perspectives.* New York: Guilford Press, 1994:268–288.

34. Singer MT, Ofshe R. Thought reform programs and the production of psychiatric casualties. *Psychiatric Ann* 1990;20:188–193.

35. Conway F, Siegelman J. Information disease: have cults created a new mental illness? *Sci Dig* 1982;10:86–92.

36. Swartling G, Swartling PG, Psychiatric problems in ex-members of Word of Life. *Cultic Stud J* 1992;9:78–88.

37. Martin PR, Langone MD, Dole AA, et al. Post-cult symptoms as measured by the MCMI before and after residential treatment. *Cultic Stud J* 1992;9:219–249.

38. Herman J. *Trauma and recovery.* New York: Basic Books, 1992.

39. van der Kolk BA, The body keeps score: approaches to the psychobiology of post-traumatic stress disorder. In: van der Kolk BA, Mc Farlane AC, eds. *Traumatic stress: the effects of overwhelming experience on mind, body, and society.* New York: Guilford Press, 1996:214–241.

40. Lourie JB. Cumulative trauma: the nonproblem problem. *Transact Analysis J* 1996;26:276–283.

CHAPTER 30

Sexual Addiction: Nosology, Diagnosis, Etiology, and Treatment

AVIEL GOODMAN

NOSOLOGY

More than 100 years ago, Krafft-Ebbing described a condition in which a person's sexual appetite is abnormally increased

> to such an extent that it permeates all his thoughts and feelings, allowing of no other aims in life, tumultuously, and in a rut-like fashion demanding gratification without granting the possibility of moral and righteous counter-presentations, and resolving itself into an impulsive, insatiable succession of sexual enjoyments.... This pathological sexuality is a dreadful scourge for its victim, for he is in constant danger of violating the laws of the state and of morality, of losing his honor, his freedom, and even his life. (1, pp. 70–71)

Most clinicians agree that what Krafft-Ebbing described as pathologic sexuality does exist, in the form of paraphilias and syndromes of similarly driven nonparaphilic sexual behavior that causes either subjective distress or functional impairment. However, questions remain about whether this condition should be classified as an obsessive-compulsive disorder (2–8), as an impulse-control disorder (9,10), or as an addictive disorder (11–16). The focal point of these questions is how this syndrome of driven sexual behavior should be designated and classified in future editions of the American Psychiatric Association's *Diagnostic and Statistical Manual of Psychiatric Disorders (DSM)*. The influence of the *DSM* reaches far beyond clinical diagnosis to mental health research, third-party payments for treatment, legal decisions, societal morality, and public policy. Consequently, the significance of whether the second word in a disorder's name is compulsivity, impulsivity, or addiction is much more than just semantic. Moreover, sexual matters are heavily laden with strong emotions, and many of the sexual behaviors in which sufferers of this condition engage can cause serious psychological damage and social disruption. The strong feelings that tend to be associated with the sexual behaviors that characterize this condition often intensify the controversy that attends disagreements over the condition's designation. Because the issue of terminology not only is controversial but also has far-reaching implications for both theory and treatment, I believe that it is worth considering in detail.

Obsessive-Compulsive Disorder

Quadland (7) and Weissberg and Levay (8) advocated that this syndrome of driven sexual behavior be called "sexual compulsivity" and classified as an obsessive-compulsive disorder (OCD). They argued that the sexual behavior in this condition is compulsive, because it functions to reduce anxiety and other painful affects. The *Diagnostic and Statistical Manual of Psychiatric Disorders,* 4th ed. (*DSM-IV*) definition of compulsive behavior includes its function of reducing anxiety and other painful affects. However, it also specifies that the behavior does not produce pleasure or gratification (17). While reduction of anxiety or distress contributes to a person's motivation to engage in the sexual behavior that characterizes this disorder, pleasure or gratification also contributes, particularly in the early stages of the syndrome. Perhaps because they also provide gratification, these sexual behaviors are more often ego-syntonic (i.e., accepted by the subject as consistent with his or her sense of self) during their enactment than are compulsive behaviors. The *Diagnostic and Statistical Manual of Psychiatric Disorders,* 3rd ed. revised (*DSM–III–R*) explicitly clarified the relationship between compulsion and the sexual behavior syndrome that we are considering, as follows:

Some activities, such as eating (e.g., Eating Disorders), sexual behavior (e.g., Paraphilias), gambling (e.g., Pathological Gambling), or drinking (e.g., Alcohol Dependence or Abuse), when engaged in excessively may be referred to as "compulsive." However, the activities are not true compulsions because the person derives pleasure from the particular activity, and may wish to resist it only because of its secondary deleterious consequences. (18, p. 246)

Finally, evidence against classifying this condition as a compulsive disorder has emerged from studies that found it to differ from OCD in how it responds to antidepressant medication. The symptoms of OCD typically respond significantly more strongly to serotonin reuptake inhibitors (SRIs) and to clomipramine (Anafranil), than they do to nefazodone or to tricyclic antidepressants; and they respond particularly poorly to desipramine, which has little effect on serotonin activity. Studies by Kafka (19) and by Kruesi et al. (20) found that the behavioral symptoms of paraphilias and nonparaphilic sexual addictions responded similarly to both SRIs and tricyclic antidepressants, even when the tricyclic that was used was desipramine (Norpramin). More recently, Bradford and Gratzer (21) reported a case of paraphilia that responded to sertraline (Zoloft) but not to clomipramine (Anafranil), and Coleman et al. (22) reported significant remission of nonparaphilic "sexual obsessions and compulsions" with nefazodone (Serzone) treatment. These patterns of response to antidepressants resemble the response pattern that is typically observed in depression, but differs from the response pattern that is typically observed in OCD. The study by Kruesi's group also reported a placebo response rate of 17%, which is worthy of note because placebo response in adults with OCD is rare. Moreover, Stein et al. (23) found that the sexual symptoms of paraphilic and sexually addicted patients who were depressed improved when their emotional state improved, while those of paraphilic and sexually addicted patients who also had OCD often did not improve when their OCD improved. These research findings suggest that, while the condition that we are considering could be related to OCD, it is unlikely to be a form of OCD.

Both the definition of compulsion and the findings of the pharmacologic treatment studies suggest that calling this condition "sexual compulsivity" is inappropriate. The appropriate name would designate behavior that, like compulsive behavior, (a) feels driven, (b) entails harmful or unpleasant consequences, and (c) functions to reduce anxiety or other painful affects; and also that, unlike compulsive behavior, (d) functions to produce pleasure or gratification. I believe that *addiction* is the term that fits this description best. Drug addiction, for example, has the characteristics of feeling driven, entailing harmful consequences, and functioning both to relieve painful affects and to produce pleasure.

Impulse-Control Disorder

Barth and Kinder (9) argued that this syndrome of driven sexual behavior should be designated "sexual impulsivity" because it met the diagnostic criteria for atypical impulse control disorder in the then-current *Diagnostic and Statistical Manual of Psychiatric Disorders,* 3rd ed. (*DSM–III*). *DSM–IV* includes the following description of impulse-control disorders:

The essential feature of Impulse-Control Disorders is the failure to resist an impulse, drive, or temptation to perform an act that is harmful to the person or to others. For most of the disorders in this section, the individual feels an increasing sense of tension or arousal before committing the act and then experiences pleasure, gratification, or relief at the time of committing the act. (17, p. 609)

The DSM description of impulse-control disorder does seem to accurately characterize this condition. At the same time, it seems to characterize substance dependence equally well. If substance dependence, which is readily acknowledged to be an addictive disorder, is also an impulse-control disorder, then a condition that meets the diagnostic criteria for impulse-control disorder is not thereby precluded from being identified also as an addictive disorder.

Addictive Disorder

What then is the difference between impulse-control disorder and addictive disorder? This question can be answered only if a behaviorally nonspecific definition of addictive disorder is available. More to the point, the term *nonparaphilic sexual addiction,* which was listed in *DSM–III–R* as an example of a Sexual Disorder Not Otherwise Specified, was excluded from *DSM–IV* because there were "no scientific data to support a concept of sexual behavior that can be considered addictive" (24). However, because no definition of "addictive" or "addiction" was specified, we are left to wonder what reasoning could have led to the conclusion that scientific data did not support the concept of sexual addiction. Discussion of whether a syndrome should be classified as an addiction is difficult in the absence of a clear and meaningful definition of addiction.

The definition of addiction itself is a matter of controversy, and *DSM–IV* does not employ the term at all. However, we can begin to formulate a definition of addictive disorder by identifying the key features of drug addiction, the paradigm of addictive disorders.

To start, we now recognize that neither physiologic tolerance nor physical withdrawal is a key feature of drug addiction. Addictive use of some recreational drugs—hallucinogens, for example—is not typically associated with tolerance or withdrawal symptoms. Meanwhile, tolerance and withdrawal occur with therapeutic as well as addictive use of opiates, and can occur also with therapeutic use of other types of medication, such as decongestants and antidepressants. These processes reflect the natural adaptive responses of our bodies' cells to a changed chemical environment, regardless of whether the chemicals had been used addictively. Furthermore, psychological research has demonstrated that withdrawal in drug addiction is not simply an automatic physiologic response to decreased levels of exogenous chemicals, but is a complex process that is significantly shaped by learning (25–33). While tolerance and withdrawal symptoms can contribute to maintaining or increasing drug use, many investigators of the neurobiology of drug addiction (including Miller, Dackis, and Gold [34], Goldstein [35], and Jaffe [36]) agree with *DSM–IV* that "neither tolerance nor withdrawal is necessary or sufficient for a diagnosis of Substance Dependence" (p. 178). Current psychobiologic theories of drug addiction attribute considerably more significance to the effects of drugs on addicts' affect systems than to physical tolerance and withdrawal (37,38).

So, if tolerance and withdrawal symptoms are not the key features of drug addiction, what are? For us to identify a pattern of drug use as an addiction, what characteristics are both (a) necessary—that is, so essential that if one of them is absent, the pattern of drug use is not an addiction (whatever other characteristics may be present); and (b) sufficient—that is, so important that if all of them are present, the pattern of drug use is an addiction (whatever other characteristics may be absent)?

The characteristics that I believe are both necessary and sufficient for identifying a pattern of drug use as drug addiction are (a) recurrent failure to control the use of one or more drugs and (b) continuation of drug use despite significant harmful consequences. (What do I mean by "recurrent failure to control?" Not that addicted individuals invariably lose control when they use drugs, but that their predictions that they would remain in control of their drug use have repeatedly proved to be unreliable.) When I then adapt these necessary and sufficient characteristics from drug addiction to addiction in general by making them behaviorally nonspecific, what I come up with is the following: the key features of addiction are (a) recurrent failure to control the behavior and (b) continuation of the behavior despite significant harmful consequences. Readers who are familiar with 12-step programs might recognize a similarity between these two key features of addiction and the concepts of powerlessness and unmanageability.

If we combine these key features of addiction with our earlier recognition that addictive behavior resembles compulsive behavior in its capacity to reduce painful affects, but differs from compulsive behavior in its capacity to produce pleasure, then we have the makings of a definition of addiction. We can now define addiction as a condition in which a behavior that can function both to produce plea-

sure and to reduce painful affects is employed in a pattern that is characterized by two key features: (a) recurrent failure to control the behavior and (b) continuation of the behavior despite significant harmful consequences.

Some might argue that although such a definition of addiction might be convenient, it lacks the validity and reliability of the descriptive diagnostic criteria for disorders that are listed in *DSM–IV*. In response, we can offer a provisional *DSM*-type set of behaviorally nonspecific diagnostic criteria for addictive disorder (39–43):

Addictive Disorder
A maladaptive pattern of behavior, *leading to clinically significant impairment or distress,* as manifested by three (or more) of the following, occurring at any time in the same 12-month period:
(1) tolerance, as defined by either of the following:
　(a) a need for markedly increased amount or intensity of the behavior to achieve the desired effect
　(b) markedly diminished effect with continued involvement in the behavior at the same level of intensity
(2) withdrawal, as manifested by either of the following:
　(a) characteristic psychophysiologic withdrawal syndrome of physiologically described changes and/or psychologically described changes upon discontinuation of the behavior
　(b) the same (or a closely related) behavior is engaged in to relieve or avoid withdrawal symptoms
(3) the behavior is often engaged in over a longer period, in greater quantity, or at a higher level of intensity than was intended
(4) there is a persistent desire or unsuccessful efforts to cut down or control the behavior
(5) a great deal of time is spent in activities necessary to prepare for the behavior, to engage in the behavior, or to recover from its effects
(6) important social, occupational, or recreational activities are given up or reduced because of the behavior
(7) the behavior continues despite knowledge of having a persistent or recurrent physical or psychological problem that is likely to have been caused or exacerbated by the behavior

The origin of this set of diagnostic criteria need not be a mystery. It was derived from the *DSM–IV* criteria for substance dependence, the prototypal addiction, by replacing the specific terms *substance* and *substance use* with the nonspecific term *behavior,* and by replacing "characteristic withdrawal syndrome for the substance" with a general definition of withdrawal that is applicable to all categories of behavior. One of my reasons for formulating the diagnostic criteria for Addictive Disorder in this way was that they then could be readily recognized as being consistent with the currently accepted system. My objective was not necessarily to devise the best possible set of diagnostic criteria for Addictive Disorder (which, in any case, would need to be determined empirically), but to demonstrate that such diagnostic criteria could be formulated that were consistent with the form and content of the current *DSM*, that were expressed in the same descriptive language, and that were likely to be as reliable and valid as were the *DSM* diagnostic criteria for substance dependence.

We now can return to the question, What is the difference between impulse-control disorder and addictive disorder? Both kinds of disorder involve failure to control and harmful consequences. Both also involve pleasure or gratification. The major difference between impulse-control disorder and addictive disorder seems to be the relative importance of reducing painful affects. The definition of addictive disorder specifies that the behavior in question functions to reduce painful affects. The description of impulse-control disorder mentions tension and relief, but the context is drive, temptation, and arousal. Relief from the tension of an aroused drive is not the same as reduction of painful affects (such as anxiety or depressive affect). The latter process seems to be an important aspect of addictive disorders, but not of impulse-control disorders, as they are defined in *DSM–IV*.

We are now in a position to sketch a big-picture view of the relationship between impulse-control disorder, obsessive-compulsive disorder, and addictive disorder. All three types of disorder involve difficult-to-resist urges to engage in overt behaviors that entail harmful or unpleasant consequences. The primary function of impulsive behavior (as it is defined in *DSM–IV*) is to produce pleasure or gratification. In terms of learning theory, it is motivated primarily by positive reinforcement. Meanwhile, the primary function of compulsive behavior is to reduce anxiety or other painful affects. In terms of learning theory, it is motivated primarily by negative reinforcement. Finally, addictive behavior functions both to produce pleasure and to reduce painful affects. It is motivated by positive reinforcement and by negative reinforcement. Addictive behavior thus shares core characteristics with both impulsive behavior and compulsive behavior. These three classes of disorder can be subsumed under a superordinate class, which could be descriptively named "driven behavior spectrum disorders." In all three subclasses of this spectrum, an urge for some form of reinforcement (negative, positive, or both) in the short-term overrides consideration of longer-term consequences, both negative and positive.

Further support for grouping this syndrome of driven sexual behavior with the substance addictions is provided by their phenomenologic similarities. Orford (44) observed that patients' descriptions of their subjective experience of the sexual behavior syndrome were qualitatively similar to patients' descriptions of their experience of drug addiction. I have expanded on Orford's observation and noted a number of other characteristic features that are shared by sexual addiction and substance addiction (40–43). These include (a) characteristic course—the disorder typically begins in adolescence or early adulthood and follows a chronic course with remissions and exacerbations; (b) behavioral features—narrowing of behavioral repertoire, continuation of the behavior despite harmful consequences; (c) individuals' subjective experience of the condition—sense of craving, preoccupation, excitement during preparatory activity, mood-altering effects of the behavior, sense of loss of control; (d) progressive development of the condition—craving, loss of control, narrowing of behavioral repertoire, and harmfulness of consequences all tending to increase as the duration of the condition increases; (e) experience of tolerance—as the behavior is repeated, its potency to produce reinforcing effects tends to diminish; (f) experience of withdrawal phenomena—psychological and/or physical discomfort when the behavior is discontinued; (g) tendency to relapse—that is, to return to harmful patterns of behavior after a period of abstinence or control has been achieved; (h) propensity for behavioral substitution—when the behavioral symptoms of the disorder have come under control, tendency for addictive engagement in other behaviors to emerge or intensify; (i) relationship between the condition and other aspects of affected individuals' lives—for example, neglect of other areas of life as the behavior assumes priority; and (j) recurrent themes in the ways individuals with these conditions relate to others and to themselves—including low self-esteem, self-centeredness, denial, rationalization, and conflicts over dependency and control. Significantly, this syndrome of driven sexual behavior, like substance addiction, is characterized by the traditional hallmarks of addiction: experiences of craving, loss of control, tolerance, and withdrawal.

The foregoing discussion leads us to conclude that "sexual addiction" is the most appropriate designation for the pattern of sexual behavior that we are considering. We can also note, in passing, that the term "sexual addiction" is not a recent product of pop psychology, nor is it a creation of the 12-step movement. It was originally used by the psychiatrist Otto Fenichel in his classic text, *The Psychoanalytic Theory of Neurosis*, which was published in 1945 (45). To put this date into perspective, it was 7 years before the first psychiatric diagnostic and statistical manual, *DSM–I*, was published (1952), and more than three decades before the first 12-step groups for sex addicts were formed in the late 1970s. Even earlier, before the turn of the century, Sigmund Freud had identified masturbation as an addiction (46).

A variety of objections have been raised to the concept of sexual addiction. Some are based on an erroneous understanding of addiction, while others make points that are valid but true also of other psychiatric conditions. A few reflect the neonatal status of the sexual addiction field, and can be understood more as a call for action than as a criticism. I have addressed these objections in detail in other publications (40,42,47).

DIAGNOSIS AND EPIDEMIOLOGY

Diagnosis of Sexual Addiction

So, what is sexual addiction? The definition of a specific addictive disorder can be derived from the definition of addiction that we came up with in the "Nosology" section by replacing the phrase "a behavior that can function both to produce pleasure and to reduce painful affects" with the name of a behavior that can perform both of these functions. Accordingly, sexual addiction is defined as a condition in which some form of sexual behavior is employed in a pattern that is characterized by two key features: (a) recurrent failure to control the behavior, and (b) continuation of the behavior despite significant harmful consequences. In other words, sexual addiction is a condition in which some form of sexual behavior relates to and affects a person's life in such a manner as to accord with the definition of addiction.

A definition tells us what something is, and diagnostic criteria tell us how to recognize it when we see it, how to distinguish it from other things that may be similar ("diagnosis" derives from the Greek word *diagignoskein,* which means to distinguish). Diagnostic criteria are more formal and specific than is a definition, which makes them more preferable in some circumstances and less preferable in others. Diagnostic criteria for sexual addiction can be derived from the behaviorally nonspecific diagnostic criteria for addictive disorder that were proposed earlier, by replacing "behavior" with "sexual behavior," as follows:

Sexual Addiction
A maladaptive pattern of sexual behavior, *leading to clinically significant impairment or distress,* as manifested by three (or more) of the following, occurring at any time in the same 12-month period:
(1) tolerance, as defined by either of the following:
(a) a need for markedly increased amount or intensity of the sexual behavior to achieve the desired effect
(b) markedly diminished effect with continued involvement in the sexual behavior at the same level of intensity
(2) withdrawal, as manifested by either of the following:
(a) characteristic psychophysiologic withdrawal syndrome of physiologically described changes and/or psychologically described changes upon discontinuation of the sexual behavior
(b) the same (or a closely related) sexual behavior is engaged in to relieve or avoid withdrawal symptoms
(3) the sexual behavior is often engaged in over a longer period, in greater quantity, or at a higher level of intensity than was intended
(4) there is a persistent desire or unsuccessful efforts to cut down or control the sexual behavior
(5) a great deal of time is spent in activities necessary to prepare for the sexual behavior, to engage in the behavior, or to recover from its effects
(6) important social, occupational, or recreational activities are given up or reduced because of the sexual behavior

(7) the sexual behavior continues despite knowledge of having a persistent or recurrent physical or psychological problem that is likely to have been caused or exacerbated by the behavior

Significantly, no form of sexual behavior in itself constitutes sexual addiction. Whether a pattern of sexual behavior qualifies as sexual addiction is determined not by the type of behavior, its object, its frequency, or its social acceptability, but by how the behavior relates to and affects a person's life. Any sexual behavior has the potential to be engaged in addictively, but constitutes an addictive disorder only to the extent that it occurs in a pattern that meets the diagnostic criteria or accords with the definition. The key features that distinguish sexual addiction from other patterns of sexual behavior are (a) the person is not reliably able to control the sexual behavior; and (b) the sexual behavior has significant harmful consequences and continues nonetheless.

Differential Diagnosis

The hypersexual activity and paraphilic (i.e., perverse or unconventional) sexual behaviors that characterize sexual addiction can occur also as manifestations of underlying organic pathology, and occasionally are its earliest or most prominent symptoms. Paraphilic or hypersexual behavior can be a symptom of a brain lesion, particularly a lesion in the medial basal-frontal, diencephalic, or septal region. Anomalous sexual behavior can occur also in the context of a seizure disorder, especially in association with temporal lobe epilepsy (48–53). More broadly, any disorder that is associated with an impairment of cerebral functioning can weaken normal inhibitory controls and thereby allow the expression of sexual behaviors that ordinarily are suppressed. Hypersexual behavior can occur also as a side effect of medication, particularly antiparkinsonian agents. Finally, sexually aggressive behavior has been associated with elevated levels of testosterone (54,55). The differential diagnosis is usually facilitated by the presence of additional symptoms or circumstances that suggest the underlying etiology, although altered sexual behavior may be the earliest manifestation in some cases of brain pathology. Clues that invite an organic evaluation include onset in middle age or later; regression from previously normal sexuality; excessive aggression; report of auras or seizure-like symptoms prior to or during the sexual behavior; abnormal body habitus; and presence of soft neurologic signs. Also of value in determining whether a case of paraphilia or hypersexuality represents sexual addiction are the diagnostic criteria for sexual addiction. Patterns of paraphilic or hypersexual behavior that are not part of the sexual addiction syndrome generally are not characterized by tolerance, psychophysiologic withdrawal symptoms on discontinuation of the behavior (usually affective discomfort, irritability, or restlessness), and a persistent desire to cut down or control the behavior. The diagnostic criteria for sexual addiction are useful also in distinguishing sexual addiction from nonaddictive patterns of exploitative or aggressive sexual behavior that can occur with antisocial personality disorder.

Obsessions and compulsions with sexual content can occur in obsessive-compulsive disorder. Sexual obsessions are fairly common in OCD, and were reported in 32% of the patients in a large study. The content of these obsessions, however, consisted most often not of sexual fantasies, but of fears of acting on sexual impulses or fears of being a pervert (56,57). More generally, symptoms of sexual addiction differ from sexual obsessions and compulsions in that the former are associated with sexual arousal and sexual pleasure, while the latter typically are not (57,58).

A syndrome that meets the diagnostic criteria for sexual addiction can occur in the context of other psychiatric disorders, including manic-depressive conditions, schizophrenia, personality disorders, and substance dependence. When the diagnostic criteria for both sexual addiction and another psychiatric disorder are met, both diagnoses are warranted, regardless of whether sexual addiction might be secondary to the other psychiatric disorder. The diagnosis of sexual addiction is a descriptive designation of how a pattern of sexual behavior relates to and affects a person's life. It does not presume anything about how the pattern of sexual behavior developed, nor is it precluded by the presence of other conditions that may have influenced its development.

Prevalence

Carnes (12) reported that 3% to 6% of Americans suffer from sexual addiction, and Coleman (5) reported that approximately 5% of the population meet diagnostic criteria for "sexual compulsivity." Neither report indicated how the data were obtained. A literature review at the end of 2002 revealed no further data on the prevalence of sexual addiction.

Gender and Age Features

Approximately 80% of individuals who use sexual behavior addictively are male (59–61). Gender differences in prevalence are greater for paraphilias than for nonparaphilic sexual addictions. Within the nonparaphilic arena, males tend to focus more on physical sexual gratification, and thus more often engage addictively in masturbation, use of prostitutes, and impersonal sex. Females, meanwhile, tend to focus more on the emotional aspects of sexuality, and thus more often engage addictively in romantic relationships. Sexual addiction is usually a chronic disorder, with remissions and exacerbations. Addictive use of sexual behavior typically begins in the teens or early twenties, peaks between the ages of 20 and 40 years, and then gradually declines (61,62). Kafka and Prentky (62) char-

acterized the "modal subject" in a cohort that responded to an advertisement for evaluation and treatment of sexual addictions and compulsive sexual behaviors as a 34-year-old, white, married, Catholic college graduate earning a middle-class income.

Comorbidity and Familial Patterns

A review of comorbidity findings is prefaced by the observation that little research has actually been conducted specifically with individuals who use sexual behavior addictively. For a variety of reasons, most of the reviewed research studied paraphilic subjects and sex offenders. While the group of sex addicts overlaps with the group of sex offenders, and overlaps even more with the group of paraphilic subjects, these groups are not identical.

Researchers have noted significant comorbidity among different forms of sexual addiction: that is, individuals who engage addictively in one form of sexual behavior are likely also to engage addictively in other forms of sexual behavior. High frequencies of comorbidity have been observed not only within the category of paraphilic sexual addictions (20,63–66), but also between paraphilias and nonparaphilic sexual addictions (12,62,67). A variety of psychiatric disorders have been reported to be comorbid with sexual addiction at a rate that is higher than their prevalence in the general population. The strongest trend that the research reveals is significant comorbidity of sexual addiction with substance dependence and with other addictive disorders, including pathologic gambling, bulimia, and compulsive buying (4,20,59,61,68–76). Significant comorbidity between sexual addiction and mood disorders, anxiety disorders, attention deficit disorder, and personality disorders is indicated by the literature as well (19,20,65,66,69,75–80). The one family history study that has been published (71) found a significantly increased prevalence of sexual addiction and other addictive disorders (substance dependence, eating disorders, and pathologic gambling) in the parents of sex addict probands. Clearly, more research needs to be conducted in the areas of sexual addiction comorbidity and family history, particularly in light of the usefulness of such findings in understanding etiology and in formulating treatment plans.

ETIOLOGY

While all of us were genetically programmed to experience sexual activity as pleasurable, only 3% to 6% (or 5%) of us are sex addicts. Apparently, the pleasure that sexual activity produces is not the primary factor that determines whether or not sexual addiction develops. What then are the primary determining factors?

I have developed a theory of sexual addiction, but before I lay it out, I would like to provide an overview of other theories that have been proposed. On the one hand, I would like to give credit where credit is due. Most of what I offer are not new ideas but just new ways of putting together ideas that other people have already presented. On the other hand, I would like to sketch a frame of reference that indicates how my ideas are related to the field as a whole. Finally, my review mentions other investigators whose work some readers might wish to explore further, and I will be glad to have made the introductions.

In passing, I would like to mention that very little research or theory that addresses sexual addiction has been published. Most of the literature that could be relevant explicitly pertains not to sexual addiction but to paraphilias or perversions. Probably the chief reason for this unfortunate state of affairs is that sexual addiction was not until recently clearly defined in a way that made it suitable for scientific study, while paraphilias or perversions have an established history as psychiatric diagnoses. They also include a number of conditions that constitute serious law enforcement problems, and they thus attract the interest and resources that serious law enforcement problems attract. I am including theories of paraphilias or perversions in this discussion of sexual addiction, partly because at least some components of these theories may be applicable also to sexual addiction, and partly because limiting the discussion to theories that were developed specifically to account for sexual addiction would result in an unsatisfyingly brief and narrow discussion. Sexual addiction differs from paraphilia and perversion in that it can occur with behaviors that are socioculturally normal, and in its inclusion of impaired control as one of its defining characteristics. The group of all individuals with sexual addictions and the group of all individuals with paraphilias or perversions overlap, but are not identical. The sexual addiction group, but not the paraphilia and perversion groups, includes individuals who engage addictively only in socioculturally normal sexual behaviors. Meanwhile, unlike the sexual addiction group, the perversion group includes individuals whose unconventional sex lives do not entail harmful consequences, and both paraphilia and perversion groups include individuals who reliably remain in control of their sexual behavior.

Theories that could enhance our understanding of sexual addiction can be grouped into five general categories: biologic, sociocultural, cognitive-behavioral, psychoanalytic, and integrated.

Biologic Theories

Contemporary biologic approaches to understanding sexual addiction or paraphilias focus on the brain. Some earlier theories had attributed paraphilias to abnormalities of androgen metabolism, but recent reviews concluded that research results have provided little support for these theories (81–83). Brain-oriented approaches can be divided into two groups, one that emphasizes brain anatomy and another that emphasizes brain chemistry.

Brain Anatomy

Most studies of the relationship between hypersexual or paraphilic behavior and brain anatomy have focused on the temporal lobes. Temporal lobe epilepsy may be associated with changes in sexual behavior. Most often the results are loss of libido and impotence. However, in other cases, libido increases and, in some epileptic individuals, paraphilic or hypersexual behavior appears. The sexual behaviors that have been most frequently associated with epilepsy are fetishism and transvestism, although a wide range of sexual behavior anomalies have been reported (48–53,84). Several studies by groups of investigators led by Hendricks (85), Hucker (86,87), and Langevin (82,88,89) were consistent in their findings of right temporal lobe abnormalities in sexual sadists and left temporal lobe abnormalities in pedophiles. Flor-Henry's group (90,91) recorded electroencephalograms (EEGs) on 50 exhibitionists, and reported that the recordings showed altered left hemisphere function and disruption of interhemispheric EEG relationships. These findings are significant, but they are unlikely to have much relevance to sexual addiction. As I noted in the consideration of differential diagnosis, paraphilic or hypersexual behavior that results from demonstrable brain pathology is only rarely associated with tolerance (diminution of reinforcing effects as the behavior is repeated), psychophysiologic withdrawal symptoms on discontinuation of the behavior, or a persistent desire to cut down or control the behavior. Our understanding of the relationship between sexual addiction and brain pathology would benefit more from neurologic and neuropsychological research with subjects who met the diagnostic criteria for sexual addiction.

Brain Chemistry

The biologic approaches that emphasize brain chemistry consider sexual addiction to be part of a "spectrum" of disorders that share a number of clinically significant features, including demographic and clinical characteristics, comorbidity patterns, family history patterns, and response to pharmacologic treatments. Hollander and his colleagues (2,6,23) identified sexual addiction as part of what they called the obsessive-compulsive disorder spectrum. Meanwhile, two separate groups of investigators, one led by Kafka (62) and the other by McElroy (10), considered it to belong to what they called the affective disorders spectrum. Both of these approaches hypothesize that the primary neurobiologic abnormality that is associated with the disorders in its spectrum is a disturbance of the serotonin system. They have much in common, and obsessive-compulsive spectrum disorders could probably be understood to represent a subset of affective spectrum disorders, a relationship that was implied in the paper by McElroy's group and that does not seem to be contradicted in the reviewed papers by Hollander's group.

The spectrum disorder theories enhance our understanding of sexual addiction and its relationship to other psychiatric disorders. They also could be helpful in treatment situations, informing the selection of therapeutic modalities and alerting clinicians to the possibility that sex addicts could be suffering from one of these other conditions in addition to sexual addiction. However, they say little about what actually occurs in the brain of a sex addict, and even less about how sexual addiction differs neurobiologically from other disorders in its spectrum or about how sexual addiction develops.

Sociocultural Theories

As far as I know, no sociocultural theories have been developed specifically to account for sexual addiction. Most of the sociocultural theories have been concerned primarily with sexual aggression, while the sociocultural components of psychoanalytic theories have addressed either perversion or addiction in general.

In recent years, a number of publications have addressed the sociocultural contribution to the etiology of sexual aggression from a feminist perspective (reviewed in references 92 and 93). They describe the male-centered, power-oriented structure of our society; they identify relationships between sexual aggression and social attitudes toward women; and they criticize the social acceptance and the prevalence of sexual aggression in various forms. While these characteristics of our society are likely to be correlated with a significant prevalence of sexual aggression against women, such correlations do not necessarily indicate the nature of the relevant causal relationships. For example: Do these destructive characteristics of our society generate and shape sexual aggression against women? Does sexualized aggression toward women, in various forms, generate and shape these destructive characteristics of our society? Or does some third factor generate and shape both sexual aggression against women and these destructive characteristics of our society? The answer is likely to involve all of the above. Moreover, while almost all males in our society are exposed to much the same array of sociocultural messages, images, and attitudes, only a limited number of men engage in sexually aggressive behaviors. Sociocultural factors undoubtedly foster and shape the expression of sexually aggressive behavior. However, an adequate understanding of the development of sexual aggression in some, but not all, men in our sociocultural milieu requires that other, more specific factors be considered. Thus, as Marshall (94) concluded, theories that attribute sexually aggressive behavior to sociocultural messages, images, and attitudes are inadequate to account for the etiology of sexual aggression.

Psychoanalysis, in general, has been interested primarily in the meaning–providing functions of the sociocultural milieu, rather than in its possible causal functions. A number of psychoanalysts emphasize the importance of the sociocultural context in determining what constitutes a perversion or paraphilia, and what such behavior might mean to the individual who engages in it. Khan stated that "perversion-formations are much nearer to cultural artifacts than disease syndromes as such" (95, p. 555), and Goldberg observed that the sociocultural environment is relevant to the definition of perversion, "not so much as a standard, but rather as playing a particular role in the psyche of the individual" (96, p. 22). Approaching from another perspective, I have discussed the relationship between addiction in general and the technologic orientation of our society, which idealizes control and promotes a reliance on external, material things that we believe we can control as a means of solving our inner emotional and spiritual problems (97). These sociocultural hypotheses, isolated from the psychoanalytic formulations that constitute the bulk of these authors' theories, do not address why some individuals in our society develop clinically significant addictive disorders but most do not, even though virtually all are exposed to the same general set of sociocultural influences.

In short, while sociocultural factors are critical determinants of how sexuality is expressed and of how normal sexual behavior is defined, they are of limited utility in explaining sexual aggression, perversion, or addiction in general. Their utility in explaining sexual addiction is unlikely to be significantly greater. Nonetheless, sociocultural factors are worthy of attention and study. In addition to their defining and meaning-providing functions, they shape the etiologic pathway of sexual addiction (as they do the pathways of other psychiatric disorders), and they can function as a steady pressure toward relapse. Moreover, those who treat sexual addiction are exposed to the same sociocultural influences as are those who suffer from it. As Carnes observed, "all helping professionals struggle with two levels of pathology: the illness of the people who need help and the cultural pathology" (12, p. 50). We clinicians are no more capable than is anyone else of transcending our sociocultural context. But the more aware we are of how our sociocultural context influences our perceptions, our beliefs, and our feelings, the less likely are such contextual influences to undermine our therapeutic effectiveness.

Sexual Addiction and Childhood Sexual Abuse

The relationship between sexual addiction and childhood sexual abuse has been the focus of considerable attention (4,12,59,98–103). Carnes asked a group of men and women who used sexual behavior addictively, and a comparison group of men and women who did not, whether they had been sexually abused as children (12). He found that 39% of the 160 male sex addicts and 63% of the 24 female sex addicts reported having been sexually abused, as compared to 8% of 78 nonaddicted men and 20% of 98 nonaddicted women. Carnes and Delmonico reported that 78% of 290 persons in treatment for sexual addiction gave a history of childhood sexual abuse (59). Meanwhile, in a study by Black et al. (61) of 28 men and 8 women who responded to advertisements for persons with compulsive sexual behavior, only 31% reported that they had been sexually abused as children. And studies by Kafka and Prentky (62,72) of men in outpatient psychiatric treatment for sexual addiction yielded positive histories for childhood sexual abuse in 28% and 15% (respectively) of their subjects. The differences between these studies may have reflected differences in the kind of person who self-selected for one or the other pool of subjects, and differences between the research sites in the degree and kind of support that was felt to be provided for reporting childhood sexual abuse. In any case, the trend of the research seems to support the claim that childhood sexual abuse is more common in the histories of sex addicts than it is in the general population. In other words, sexual abuse during childhood and later development of sexual addiction seem to be positively correlated.

But what does that correlation mean? It could indicate that childhood sexual abuse predisposes to later development of sexual addiction. But it also could indicate that childhood sexual abuse generates a psychological imbalance that can lead to one or more of a whole host of psychiatric disorders, without any specific predilection for sexual addiction. Or, it could indicate that fathers who are sex addicts tend both to sexually abuse their children and to pass on to their children a genetically based predisposition to sexual addiction. Or, it could indicate that children in families that are seriously dysfunctional from any cause are at increased risk (compared to the general population) both to be sexual abused and later to become sex addicts.

A number of studies bear on the question of how specific a history of childhood sexual abuse is to sexual addiction. Two articles reviewed the literature on the proportion of convicted sexual abusers of children who were themselves sexually victimized during their childhood. Hanson and Slater (102) found that an average of approximately 28% of the offenders reported having been sexually victimized as children. This rate was higher than the base rate for community samples of nonoffending males (approximately 10%), but was similar to the rates that were found in populations of offenders whose offenses were nonsexual. Garland and Dougher (103) found that a history of childhood or adolescent sexual contact with adults did not differentiate sex offenders who victimized children (0 to 57%) from other sex offenders (8% to 57%) or from offenders whose offenses were nonsexual (10% to 47%). The authors concluded that the relationship between childhood sexual victimization and sexually abusing children as an adult did not appear to be specific, but rather seemed to be an unexceptional example of the general statement that many forms of childhood maltreatment can lead to many forms of behavioral and psychological problems in adult-

hood. (We can keep in mind that conclusions from studies of sex offenders may be of limited applicability to sexual addiction, yet remain open to whatever we can learn from these studies.)

Another body of research has documented the association between childhood sexual abuse and adult psychopathology (disordered psychological and behavioral functioning), most notably borderline personality disorder (104–108). While most of the patients who were the subjects of these studies were female, a study by Swett et al. (109) of 125 consecutive male psychiatric outpatients found that 48% reported histories of sexual abuse and/or physical abuse, and that a reported history of childhood abuse was correlated with more severe psychiatric symptoms and significantly higher mean scores on the global severity index of the Symptoms Checklist 90 Revised (SCL-90-R). The higher incidence of childhood sexual victimization in sex addicts than in the general population could thus reflect a high correlation between sexual addiction and borderline personality disorder or other serious psychopathology. Finally, a high correlation between childhood sexual abuse and sexual addiction, even if specific to sexual addiction, would not necessarily mean that sexual abuse was the critical factor in that disorder's etiology (origin). Sexual abuse of children is highly correlated with a disturbed family environment, and it could be a marker for other pathogenic factors within the family environment (a point that Paris and Zweig-Frank [110] made when they discussed the high incidence of childhood sexual abuse in patients with borderline personality disorder).

An association between childhood sexual abuse and sexual addiction makes intuitive sense, and the personal significance of sexual abuse in the histories of the sex addicts who report it is difficult to deny. I can add that in my experience, the frequency with which childhood sexual abuse is reported by sex addicts is considerably higher than the frequency with which it is reported by people with other psychiatric disorders. However, I do not know how representative the people I see in my practice are of sex addicts and sufferers of other psychiatric disorders in general. We are well advised to be cautious about the conclusions we draw from what we read and hear, and even from our own direct experience. The more important a subject is, the more it deserves our best critical thinking.

Cognitive–Behavioral Theories

A number of investigators have proposed psychological theories of sexual addiction, which they identify as cognitive–behavioral. These theories actually go beyond cognitive–behavioral psychology and incorporate elements of social learning, family systems, and psychodynamic approaches, as well as cognitive and behavioral theories.

Schwartz and Brasted (16) attributed the origin of "sexual impulsivity" to an irrational belief system that consists of poor self-image, unrealistic expectations of what life has to offer, anticipation of personal failure, and a general feeling of helplessness. They added that religious beliefs and social expectations also play roles in the development of the disorder, by burdening the individual with shame, guilt, and low self-esteem. Finally, they proposed that marital difficulties can lead to or exacerbate addictive sexual behavior.

The theory that was presented by Coleman (3,4) attributed the development of "compulsive sexual behavior" to two dynamics, one that predisposes an individual to compulsively use substances or behaviors as a means of alleviating emotional pain, and a second that leads individuals who are thus predisposed to select certain sexual behaviors as their preferred mode of pain alleviation. According to Coleman's theory, the basis of the predisposition is some type of intimacy dysfunction in an individual's family of origin, such as child abuse or neglect. In response to this trauma, the child develops a sense of shame, perceiving himself or herself to have been the cause of the abuse or neglect, and as a result experiences feelings of unworthiness and inadequacy. Shame and low self-esteem interfere with healthy interpersonal functioning, intimate relationships are dysfunctional or nonexistent, and loneliness compounds the individual's low self-esteem. Coleman identified these events and feelings as the origin of the compulsive predisposition:

> All of these events and feelings cause psychological pain for the client, and to alleviate this pain, the client begins to search for a "fix," or an agent that has analgesic qualities to it. For some, this agent is alcohol. For others, it could be drugs, certain sexual behaviors, particular foods, working patterns, gambling behaviors, and the like. All seem to cause physical and psychological changes which alleviate the pain and provide a temporary relief (3, p. 9; 4, pp. 196–197).

Coleman hypothesized that the specific dynamic that then leads predisposed individuals to use sexual behavior for their "fix" is a background of restrictive and conservative attitudes regarding sexuality. Coleman mentioned sexual abuse as one of the forms of child abuse or neglect that contribute to the general predisposition to compulsively depend on an external substance or behavior as a means of alleviating emotional pain, but he did not identify sexual abuse as a factor in the selection of sexual behavior as the specific means of alleviating pain.

Carnes (12) also distinguished between an individual's general addictive tendencies and the catalytic events and/or environments that interact with the addictive tendencies to precipitate a specific addictive problem. He represented the general addictive tendencies as a set of three core beliefs: (a) I am a bad, unworthy person; (b) no one would love me as I am; and (c) my needs will not be met if I have to depend on others. The faulty belief system that develops around these core beliefs then promotes the impaired thinking—denial, rationalization,

self-righteousness, and blame of others—that enables addictive behavior to flourish. Carnes attributed the development of addictive core beliefs to addicts' families of origin. He characterized these families as unbalanced along the dimensions of structure and intimacy, with structure being either chaotic or rigid and intimacy being either enmeshed or disengaged. As a result of this family pathology, many of the child's basic human needs remain unmet. The child, consequently, not only fails to develop healthy self-esteem, but also learns that other people are unreliable, that one can count only on oneself, and that to survive one must remain in control. What has been discussed so far applies to all forms of addiction. Sex addicts then develop a fourth core belief that distinguishes them from other addicts: (d) sex is my most important need. Carnes ascribed the development of this core belief to childhood experiences of being sexually abused, either overtly or covertly. He noted that "covert incest," in which parents are flirtatious, suggestive, or sexually titillating with their children, may be even more pathogenic than is overt incest. In addition to the distress and shame that are experienced by victims of overt incest, covert incest children are likely also to feel crazy, doubting that their sense of reality is reliable.

The theories that were presented by Schwartz and Brasted, Coleman, and Carnes are quite compatible with each other. While they vary in breadth and depth, none of the theories seems to be saying anything with which any of the others would seriously disagree. The most purely cognitive–behavioral of the three, Schwartz and Brasted's theory, focuses on a system of irrational beliefs that resemble those that Beck and others (111,112) described in cognitive theories of depression. Schwartz and Brasted offered no hypothesis about how the irrational belief system develops. Moreover, they did not consider what distinguishes those individuals with low self-esteem and depressing thoughts who become sexually impulsive from those who become depressed (and not sexually impulsive). These apparent shortcomings do not invalidate Schwartz and Brasted's theory, but rather suggest that it could be a cognitive–behavioral analogue of the biologic theory according to which sexual addiction is an affective spectrum disorder. Coleman identified two dynamics in the development of compulsive sexual behavior: one that predisposes an individual to compulsively use pleasure-producing substances or behaviors as means of alleviating emotional pain, and a second that leads predisposed individuals to select certain sexual behaviors as their preferred "fix." The idea of two dynamics, one of general predisposition and one of specific selection, seems to apply not only to sexual addiction but to all addictive disorders. Thus applied, I believe that it represents the most important concept in the entire body of theories about addiction. Coleman's description of the development of the first dynamic was clear, intuitively sound, and consistent with the more detailed psychoanalytic theories (which I discuss in the next section). His account of the second dynamic as being the result of restrictive and conservative attitudes regarding sexuality, however, seems to me to be insufficient. Sexually compulsive individuals come from a broad range of cultural backgrounds, and not every compulsively predisposed individual who grows up in a sexually restrictive or conservative subculture becomes sexually compulsive. Selection of sexual behavior by compulsively predisposed individuals, therefore, must be guided by factors that are more specific than are cultural attitudes about sexuality (as we noted in our earlier consideration of sociocultural theories). Carnes' account of sexual addiction synthesized cognitive–behavioral and family systems approaches to yield a theory that is both far-reaching and experience-near. His thoughts on the development of general addictive tendencies probably deserved more attention in the substance addiction field than they received. Interestingly, Carnes focused on the use of sexual behavior as a substitute means of gratifying unmet needs, while Coleman focused on its use as a means of alleviating emotional pain. As we considered earlier, gratification represents the primary function of impulsive behavior, while alleviation of emotional pain represents the primary function of compulsive behavior. And addiction involves both gratification and alleviation of emotional pain. Carnes and Coleman thus seemed to be emphasizing complementary aspects of addiction.

Psychoanalytic Theories

The psychoanalytic literature includes more material that pertains to sexual addiction than does the literature of all other areas of psychiatry and psychology combined. While some of it was written about driven heterosexual genital intercourse or pathologic hypersexuality—often referred to in colorful terms such as "Don Juanism" and "nymphomania"—most of it was written about perversions. Interestingly, although this literature spans a century and a variety of theoretical orientations, the themes around which it crystallizes have remained remarkably stable. The underlying processes that writers from different decades and orientations hypothesized to account for perversions not only are fairly consistent with each other; they also are fairly consistent with the underlying processes that were hypothesized to account for pathologic hypersexuality. For the remainder of this discussion, I lump pathologic hypersexuality in with the perversions, primarily for the sake of convenience, but also because pathologic hypersexuality can be regarded as a perversion-like use of heterosexual genital intercourse.

A review of this literature would dwarf the preceding chapters, so for now I content myself with summarizing it. In the process, I sacrifice depth and attention to differences among the various writers' contributions. (A comprehensive review of this literature can be found in my textbook, *Sexual Addiction: An Integrated Ap-

proach* [40].) Investigators whose work is incorporated into the summary include (in chronologic order): Freud (113,114), Payne (115), Fenichel (45), Gillespie (116), Bak (117,118), Greenacre (119,120), Khan (121–123), Glover (124), Hoffman (125), Kernberg (126,127), Hammer (99), Kohut (128), McDougall (129,130), Ovesey and Person (131), Chasseguet-Smirgel (132,133), Goldberg (134,135), Stolorow (136,137), Person and Ovesey (138), Stoller (139), Glasser (140,141), Rosen (142,143), Coen (144), Eber (145), Socarides (146), Hershey (147), Trop and Alexander (148), and Myers (149).

If we consider the work of these psychoanalytic investigators as a whole, the psychodynamic and etiologic factors in perversion and pathologic hypersexuality can be grouped in two categories: nonspecific factors that promote the development of addictive patterns in general, and specific factors that foster sexualization and thus promote the development of sexual addiction in particular.

The primary nonspecific factors have been described as (a) ego weakness—impaired self-regulatory and adaptational functioning; (b) unusually intense castration anxiety—anxiety about the vulnerability of one's body self; (c) a fantasy of "bisexuality" (being both male and female) and a general denial of limitations; (d) splitting—keeping incompatible experiences of self or others from being in awareness at the same time; (e) superego pathology—impairment in the mental functions that maintain values and standards; (f) impaired object relations—maladaptive influence on our thoughts, emotional states, and behavior of our self and object representations and the ways that we unconsciously manage them; (g) deficient psychic structuralization—ego or superego dysfunction of developmental origin; and (h) narcissistic pathology—disturbances in self-esteem, sense of self, and self-regulation. These factors are interrelated, often developing together and fostering one another's development. Psychoanalytic theories attribute their genesis to some combination of constitutional (genetic) factors and disturbances in the mother–child relationship. In general, they focus their energies on experiential relationship factors and have little to say about constitutional factors. Most of them consider the central experiential factor to be deficiencies and distortions in mothers' responsiveness to their children's needs during the first 2 or 3 years of their lives. These mothers do not consistently relate to their children as separate beings with needs and feelings of their own, but use their children as means of meeting their emotional needs and their narcissistic needs (i.e., needs having to do with their self-esteem or sense of self). Such impaired maternal responsiveness can disrupt the separation–individuation process, distort gender identity development, and generate high levels of aggression because of frustration of early needs. Moreover, it can interfere with internalization and thus result in deficient psychic structure, impaired self-regulatory functions, and an unstable or brittle sense of self.

However, we may have noticed that narcissistic pathology, ego weakness, superego pathology, impaired object relations, and deficient psychic structuralization, all are nonspecific terms. They are involved in just about any kind of disorder we can think of, so they don't tell us much beyond the potential relevance of the theoretical strand that a particular term represents. We can obtain some information that is more specific by looking at how the functions of perversion are understood from the perspectives of the three major strands of psychoanalytic theory: ego psychology (classical and contemporary), object relations theory, and self-psychology.

From the perspective of classical theory, perversion represents a compromise between sexual impulses (to discharge sexual tension and to establish a sexual object relationship) and ego defenses against castration anxiety. It functions also to compensate for inadequate oral gratification during infancy and to provide a feeling of security, because it reflects a level of development at which sexual satisfaction, oral gratification, and security are not yet well differentiated.

From the perspective of contemporary ego psychology, the primary function of perversion is to defend against, to relieve, or to master intolerable affects, such as depression, anhedonia, anxiety, guilt, loneliness, helplessness, and grief. Perverse sexual behavior can ward off dread by simulating a contradiction of the feared alienation, emptiness, inertia, and deadness. And, in a similar manner, it can function as a manic defense against threats of despair, ego disintegration, and personality dissolution and as a counterphobic defense against feelings of inadequacy, shame, humiliation, and narcissistic mortification. Perversion can provide a sense of mastery, power, and control, and thus it can function as a flight from and a denial of weakness and dependency. More specifically, perversion can serve as a means by which passively experienced traumatic intrapsychic states that threaten the pervert's ego are transformed into active, ego-directed mastery of objects in external reality. A significant aspect of this process of turning active into passive involves doing to others what has been done to oneself, and thereby actively making the object suffer what one once passively endured. This process can represent not only an interpersonal reversal of the traumatic experience of victimization, but also an intrapsychic reversal of the traumatic experience of being overwhelmed by painful affects.

From the perspective of object relations theory, perversion functions both (a) to express aggression toward the object and to affirm a separate identity, and (b) to preserve the object from being destroyed by the subject's aggression. One aspect of the aggression that perversion can express is revenge for childhood victimization, as we just noted. A wish for revenge can be inspired not only by active victimization, but also by early deprivation of needed oral and narcissistic supplies. In such cases, the revenge fantasy may involve "robbing" the frustrating oral mother

sexually of what she denied orally. A second aspect of the aggression that perversion can express relates to the separation–individuation process and the wish to affirm one's own separate identity. Aggression can operate in the service of identity affirmation (a) by defying the overbearing influence of the internal mothering figure; (b) by defining the boundaries of the self; and (c) by warding off the wish to depend on or to merge with the maternal imago. Meanwhile, perversion converts aggression and the urge to destroy into sadism and the urge to control, so it can function to preserve the object and those aspects of the self that are identified with the object. Beyond its specific functions in the context of aggression and identity, perversion also serves more broadly to fill in or to compensate for what is missing or damaged in the individual's internal object world that would regulate affects and provide a sense of wholeness.

From the perspective of self-psychology, perversion can function as a splint for an individual's self-esteem or sense of self or as an attempt to heal the self. Perverse sexual behavior can represent an expression of incorporative longings (a) to fill in missing narcissistic structure to regulate self-esteem; (b) to revive a sense of having a cohesive self; (c) to ward off self-depletion and self-fragmentation; and (d) to consolidate and stabilize a sense of self. In these cases, the perverse behavior or its object is being employed to substitute for self-regulatory intrapsychic structures that are missing or damaged because the caregiver functions that were needed for the internalization of these structures during the developmentally sensitive period were lacking. In two senses, perversion can also represent an attempt to heal the self. In one sense, perverse sexual behavior can function as an attempt to repair the sense of self. In a more profound sense, perverse sexual behavior can function as an attempt to achieve a "corrective emotional experience" through which the splits in the pervert's personality and representational world can be healed. The perverse sexual object and scenario then become containers for the individual's split-off parts, which the pervert tries to bring together and master by controlling the object or the scenario. Perversion thus can represent a reparative effort to restore missed opportunities for the integration of ego and self.

The functions of perversion provide us with more specific information, but still not enough to be satisfying. The psychoanalytic literature on alcoholism, drug addiction, bulimia, and pathologic gambling describes the development and dynamics of these other disorders in similar terms. Why might someone develop a perversion, rather than alcoholism or bulimia? The key factor seems to be sexualization. Sexualization is a use of sexual behavior and sexual fantasy in which their self-protective or self-preservative functions have greater urgency and significance in the person's motivational hierarchy than does sexual drive gratification. A tendency to rely on sexualization begins in childhood, often in early childhood, and when present in the context of the nonspecific factors that potentiate addictive disorders, it can tilt the balance toward perversion. Coen (144) proposed that sexualization most commonly develops in a child whose mother relies on sexualization to deal with her inner problems and brings it into her relationship with her child, overtly or covertly. According to Coen, the mother's relative neglect of the child's emotional needs combine with her seductive overstimulation of him to give sexual feelings an unusually significant role during his early development. He then draws on the predominantly available mode of relating with his mother to compensate for her relative unavailability and to stimulate her renewed interest in him. In effect, he identifies with his mother's sexualization so as to preserve his connection with her. Once this process has been set in motion, sexualization can readily become a preferred means of dealing with all sorts of painful or stressful feelings. It also can be additionally reinforced through its capacity to convert aggression into sadism, as I noted earlier.

Before we move on, let us consider the relationship between the cognitive–behavioral theories and the psychoanalytic theories. The two groups of theories turn out to be quite compatible with each other. For the most part, the cognitive–behavioral theories can be understood as simpler, less-detailed versions of the psychoanalytic theories, with four major differences. First, the cognitive–behavioral theories place greater emphasis on beliefs as etiologic factors, whereas the psychoanalytic theories place greater emphasis on affects and psychological functions. Second, the psychoanalytic theories focus on mother–child relationship as the nucleus of the etiologic matrix, and they explore in detail how it contributes to the development of psychopathology. Meanwhile, the cognitive–behavioral theories expand the etiologic matrix to include the entire family of origin and the sociocultural milieu, but they say little about the mother–child relationship or about specific pathogenic interactional patterns other than sexual abuse. In addition, the pathogenic interactions on which most of the psychoanalytic theories focus occur earlier in life than do those that the cognitive–behavioral theories typically discuss. Third, aggression and sadism are significant factors in the psychoanalytic theories, but cognitive–behavioral theories hardly mention either of them. Finally, the psychoanalytic theories emphasize overt sexual abuse less, and covert seduction and narcissistic exploitation more, than do the cognitive–behavioral theories.

Integrated Theories

The human being is both biologic and psychological, and the development of sexual addiction is likely to be most fully understood through a theory that integrates both biologic and psychological understandings. Prior to the 1990s, the theory of fetishism that was proposed by

Epstein (49) was the only coherent attempt to integrate biologic theory and psychological theory (in this case, psychoanalytic theory) to account for a condition similar to sexual addiction. Epstein identified the primary disturbance in fetishism as a state of increased organismic excitability or impaired organismic control, which he regarded as the product of cerebral pathophysiology. Epstein characterized the typical mother–child relationship of the fetishist in much the same way as did other psychoanalytic investigators of perversion. He added, however, that increased organismic excitability or dyscontrol would intensify the child's responses to disturbed maternal behavior, thereby exacerbating its pathogenic potential. According to Epstein's theory, fetishistic behavior represents a result of both the forces of excitability–dyscontrol and attempts to establish control by providing a focus toward which sexual and aggressive drives could be directed.

More recently, I proposed an integrated theory of sexual addiction that was based on a general theory of addictive disorders (39–41,43), which, in turn, was born through my attempt to make sense of patterns of comorbidity, family history relationships, and symptom substitution that I observed in the course of my work with alcoholics, drug addicts, bulimics, pathologic gamblers, compulsive buyers, and sex addicts. I also noticed that many of the characteristic features of alcoholism and drug addiction (those that I listed at the end of the "Nosology" section above) were shared also by bulimia, pathologic gambling, compulsive buying, and sexual addiction. What I observed led me to suspect that these conditions had something important in common. I then conducted an extensive review of the literature on these disorders, which revealed that these disorders are characterized by significant lifetime comorbidity, family history relationships, psychometric parallels, and neurobiologic similarities—similar neurochemical correlates of the behaviors that characterize each of these disorders, and similar responses of the disorders to pharmacotherapy. With such a wealth of research findings supporting the hypothesis that alcoholism, drug addiction, bulimia, pathologic gambling, compulsive buying, and sexual addiction have something important in common, I was ready to jump to the next step. Identifying each of these conditions as an addictive disorder (according to the criteria I discussed earlier), I hypothesized that all addictive disorders, whatever the types of behavior that characterize them, share an underlying psychobiologic process, which I called the *addictive process*. I suggested the addictive process be defined in two ways: a descriptive way and a subjective way. The descriptive definition of addictive process (i.e., what it looks like) is an enduring, inordinately strong tendency to engage in some form of pleasure-producing behavior in a pattern that is characterized by impaired control and continuation despite significant harmful consequences. Its subjective definition (i.e., what it feels like) is an enduring tendency to feel driven to use some form of pleasure-producing behavior as a consciously or unconsciously intended means of relieving painful affects and regulating one's sense of self. Thus, when we talk about addictive disorders as a group, what we are talking about is not a collection of distinct disorders, but an underlying process that can be expressed in one or more of various behavioral manifestations. Sexual addiction then can be succinctly characterized as an expression through sexual behavior of the addictive process.

The concept of the addictive process forms the cornerstone of my theory of addiction. Similar to the theories that were presented by Coleman (3,4) and Carnes (11,12), my theory identifies two sets of factors that shape the development of an addictive disorder: those that concern the underlying addictive process, and those that relate to the selection of a particular substance or behavior as the one that is preferred for addictive use. I begin by outlining a theory of the addictive process, and then I address the matter of behavior selection. Finally, I consider factors that may contribute to the selection of sexual behavior as an individual's "drug of choice."

When I introduced the addictive process, I referred to it as a psychobiologic process. What I mean when I say that the addictive process is psychobiologic is not that it represents an interaction between psychological and biologic, nor that it has psychological properties that emerge out of relationships within its biologic system. What I mean is something simpler, but perhaps initially more difficult to grasp: that the addictive process is both biologic and psychological. I am approaching it from the standpoint that biologic and psychological are not distinct forms of reality, but distinct ways of describing and understanding a unitary human reality (150,151). The addictive process is thus a unitary psychobiologic process that can be described and understood in either biologic or psychological terms. Accordingly, I present my understanding of the addictive process in two complementary formulations, a biologic (neurobiologic) formulation and a psychological (primary psychodynamic or psychoanalytic) formulation.

Biologic Formulation of the Addictive Process

In developing this formulation, I proceeded from my earlier conclusion that research findings sufficiently support the hypothesis that all addictive disorders, whatever behaviors they involve, share an underlying psychobiologic process. My intention was not to prove that the addictive process existed by explicating its neurobiology, but to stimulate further thought and to demonstrate that a neurobiologic theory of the addictive process was possible. After I had reviewed neurobiologic theories of alcoholism, drug addiction, bulimia, and pathologic gambling, I developed a biologic formulation of the addictive process on the foundation that was provided by the components of these theories that could fit together.

According to the formulation that I developed, the addictive process involves impaired affect regulation, aberrant function of the motivational–reward system, and impaired behavioral inhibition. Impaired affect regulation renders us chronically vulnerable to painful affects and emotional instability. In the context of impaired affect regulation, behaviors that are associated with escape from or avoidance of painful affects are more strongly reinforced (via negative reinforcement) than they otherwise would have been. Aberrant function of the motivational–reward system subjects us to unsatisfied states of irritable tension, emptiness, and restless anhedonia (incapacity to experience happiness or joy). In the context of aberrant motivational–reward function, behaviors that are associated with activation of the reward system are more strongly reinforced (via positive and negative reinforcement) than they otherwise would have been. Impaired behavioral inhibition increases the likelihood that an urge for some form of reinforcement (negative, positive, or both) in the short-term will override consideration of longer-term consequences, both negative and positive. When affect regulation is impaired and motivational–reward function is aberrant, impaired behavioral inhibition means that urges to engage in behaviors that are associated with both (a) escape from or avoidance of painful affects and (b) activation of the reward system, are extraordinarily difficult to resist, despite the harmful consequences that they might entail.

I hypothesized that impaired affect regulation, impaired behavioral inhibition, and aberrant function of the motivational–reward system are primarily associated with dysfunctions in the norepinephrine, serotonin, and dopamine systems (respectively, although probably not in a simple one-to-one fashion), and that dysfunction in the endogenous opioid system can contribute to all of these functional impairments. Activity of the norepinephrine system is associated with affect regulation and ability to manage emotional stress (152–154). Serotonin system activity is associated with emotional stabilization (155), behavioral inhibition (156,157), appetite modulation (158), sensory reactivity (159,160), and pain sensitivity (160,161). Dopamine is the principal neurotransmitter in the brain–reward system, and activity of dopaminergic pathways is associated also with behavioral activation, novelty seeking, and incentive functions (162–164). Endogenous opioids are involved in reward, hedonic tone (165), and analgesia. Significantly, they are involved in alleviation of psychosocial pain as well as somatic pain (166,167). They also have an ancillary role in appetitive, emotional, and behavioral regulation (168–172). I suggested that the addictive process may develop concurrently with a similar primary defect in each of these systems: low baseline activity of the neuromodulator, which is associated with supersensitivity of postsynaptic receptors in the cases of norepinephrine and dopamine, and perhaps also in the case of endogenous opioids. Dysfunction of the serotonergic system may be the most critical neurochemical correlate of the addictive process. Serotonin is released from all of the axonal varicosities (swellings) where it is concentrated, not only from those that make typical synaptic contacts (173,174). Such widespread release suggests that serotonin diffuses as a neurohumoral agent to reach relatively distant targets. The serotonergic system is, moreover, characterized by tonic activity, with serotonergic neurons firing at rates of about one spike per second (175). These findings suggest that the serotonergic system serves a widespread pacemaker or homeostatic regulatory function (176).

The neuroanatomic correlates of the addictive process, I hypothesized, may involve dysfunctions in two systems within the brain: one that is constituted by the orbitofrontal cortex, the septum, and the hippocampus; and one that includes the nucleus accumbens, the ventral tegmental area, and related structures. Dysfunction in the former system may be primarily associated with impaired affect regulation and impaired behavioral inhibition (177–181). Dysfunction in the latter system may be primarily associated with aberrant function of the motivational–reward system (182,183) and with dysregulation of the orbitofrontal cortex (178), which is the cortical component of the former system.

According to the hypothesized formulation, these impairments in neurochemical and neuroanatomic functioning develop out of the interaction between genetic propensities and deficiencies in the early caregiving environment. This interaction is particularly important in the developmental critical periods of the first years of life, during which the maturing brain is most sensitive to environmental influences and is dependent on particular qualities of environmental interchange for its healthy development (153,181,184–193). I proposed that the addictive process begins with genetically based temperamental tendencies and develops when parent–child interactions exacerbate the child's inherited vulnerability to developing addictive pathology.

Although this formulation brought us a step closer to understanding the neurobiology of the addictive process, it was a heuristic oversimplification. Each neuromodulator involves a diverse system of connections and receptors, and interactions among the neuromodulator systems are complex. Functional neuroanatomy also is more complex than my formulation can accommodate. Brain regions are interconnected by tangled networks through which they influence each other, and serious questions have been raised by neuroscientists about the extent to which functions can be meaningfully localized within the brain (177,194–196).

Psychological Formulation of the Addictive Process

In a manner analogous to how I developed the biologic formulation, I first reviewed psychoanalytic and learning theory-based theories of alcoholism, drug addiction, bulimia, pathologic gambling, and sexual addiction, and then I developed a psychological formulation of the addictive process on the foundation that was provided by core features that these theories shared (40,197).

The way of understanding the addictive process that I find most helpful is to see it as originating in an impairment of self-regulation. The self-regulation system is the internal psychobiologic system that regulates our subjective states and our behavior. The subjective states that are most affected when self-regulation is impaired are affects and sense of self. (Volition, sensory experience, and thought processes often also are affected, but less dramatically.) Impaired regulation of people's subjective states leads them to depend on external actions to regulate their affects and their sense of self, to the extent that potentially traumatic affects may be experienced not as emotions but as urges to act. Impaired behavioral regulation limits their capacity to resist urges to engage in actions that seem to promise, however illusory, to protect them from emotional trauma.

The self-regulation system is a complex system of functions that are interrelated both functionally and developmentally. It can be understood to consist of three primary components: affect regulation functions (the most basic and significant), self-care functions, and self-governance functions.

An affect is a complex emotional process that has subjective, physiological, behavioral, and interpersonal aspects. ("Affect" is similar in meaning to "emotional state" or "emotional event," but not to "feeling," which designates only the subjectively experienced aspect of an affect.) Hence, affect regulation functions are the psychobiologic functions that regulate our emotional processes. These functions include self-soothing, self-enlivening, keeping affects in balance, and tolerating affects without being overwhelmed.

Self-care functions consist primarily of self-protection and self-nurturing. Self-protection includes recognizing, assessing, warning ourselves of, and protecting ourselves from dangers. Self-nurturing includes recognizing, assessing, setting priorities among, and taking care of our needs. Self-care is a multiplex functional system that involves a variety of affective and cognitive processes, survival operations, reality testing, judgment, control, delay, synthesis, cause–consequence reasoning, and relatively stable self-governance functions. A critical component of self-care is the ability to use affects as signals or guides for appropriate action.

Self-governance functions include values, standards, self-esteem, self-punishment, and maintenance of a stable and cohesive sense of self. Self-governance thus subsumes (a) what psychoanalytic theory identifies as the superego, in its encouraging, approving, and rewarding aspects, as well as its prohibiting, condemning, and punishing aspects; (b) the ego ideal or self ideal—a fantasied representation of oneself that embodies all one's ideals; and (c) the processes that are involved in regulating one's sense of self.

The self-regulation system develops through the interaction between our genetic endowment and our relationships with our primary caregivers during the first years of life. In healthy development, our biologic maturation interacts with numerous occasions of our caregivers providing regulatory functions for us; and, through a process that has been called "internalization," we gradually become able to provide these functions for ourselves. However, various combinations of genetic and environmental factors can interfere with internalization and disrupt the development of the self-regulation system.

To the extent that people's affect regulation is impaired, their emotional states tend to be unstable, intense, and disorganizing. They are vulnerable to being traumatically overwhelmed by affects that intact individuals do not experience as potentially traumatic. Especially threatening are separation anxiety, claustrophobic anxiety (anxiety associated with the general idea of being closed in, trapped, or smothered), depressive affects, the "superego affects" of guilt and shame, and affects that are associated with narcissistic injury. ("Narcissistic" means having to do with a person's self-esteem or sense of self; it can refer also to psychological and behavioral operations that are performed, often unconsciously, in order to sustain or repair a person's self-esteem or sense of self.) But almost any intense affect, including excitement and love, can be experienced as threatening when affect regulation is impaired.

To the extent that people's self-care is impaired, they are deficient in their abilities to avoid danger, to protect themselves, and to take care of their needs. The dangers to which they expose themselves include physical, emotional, and narcissistic dangers. Similarly, the needs to which they do not adequately attend include physical, emotional, and narcissistic needs. As a result, they are particularly susceptible to getting hurt and to being chronically dissatisfied, on all three levels.

To the extent that people's self-governance is impaired, they lack a stable self-esteem, a consistent sense of self, and a clear sense of direction. They may have skewed or fragmented values, ideals, and sense of meaning. Their behavior tends to oscillate between extremes, and they may swing from actions that violate their values to actions that are self-injurious or that invite punishment from the environment.

When people's self-regulation is impaired, they tend to respond with overwhelmingly intense affects to events that most others seem to take in stride. They experience the risk of being thus affectively overwhelmed and losing their self-coherence as a threat to their survival, so they do what they can to avoid affective states that are potentially traumatic. Many seek desperately for something that can perform for them the self-regulatory functions that peo-

ple with intact self-regulation systems are able to do autonomously. Often, they develop fantasies (usually unconscious) that the solution for their self-regulatory problems lies in something outside their selves: a substance, a person, a nonhuman object, a bodily state, or an institution. Many of them learn to ward off traumatic affects and self-states by engaging in a rewarding activity, for example, eating, or taking a mood-altering substance into their bodies, or gambling, or engaging in some form of sexual behavior. They then tend to become dependent on this activity to provide self-regulatory functions that they have not been sufficiently able to provide for themselves. This sequence is an example of a process that is called externalization: acting as though a particular psychological function, which a person either has or (unconsciously) imagines, belongs to something external to his or her self. The addictive process involves the externalization of self-regulatory functions that addicts imagine (via unconscious fantasy), in a desperate attempt to compensate for the self-regulatory functions that are impaired. In the process, external or internal cues that are associated with intense affects or with loss of self-coherence can become conditioned to particular craving sensations, or can become discriminative stimuli for particular addictive-behavioral responses. As a result, these cues can trigger or can be experienced as urges to engage in the behavior. Because engaging in the behavior is an attempt to ward off traumatic affects and self-states that threaten their survival, their urges to engage in the behavior typically are so imperative that their patterns of engaging in it are likely to be characterized by impaired control and by relative imperviousness to the restraining influence of harmful consequences.

This, then, is the essence of the addictive process: (a) as a consequence of some combination of genetic and environmental factors, individuals' self-regulatory functions are impaired; (b) impaired self-regulation leaves them abnormally vulnerable to being overwhelmed by intense emotional states and by loss of self-coherence; and (c) in attempts to protect themselves from the danger of being thus overwhelmed, they externalize their self-regulatory fantasies onto nonself entities or processes over which they believe that they have control. When the behavior that results occurs in a pattern that is characterized by recurrent loss of control and by continuation of the behavior despite significant harmful consequences, they then can be characterized as "addicts," whatever the behaviors in which they addictively engage.

The "Drug of Choice" Question

Now that we have a general understanding of the addictive process, we can consider the "drug of choice" question: Given a sufficient degree of predisposition to develop addictive behavior patterns, as represented in the addictive process, what determines which behaviors are selected for addictive use? In other words, what leads a person to choose sex, rather than consuming alcohol or eating?

In general, the selection of a substance or a behavior for addictive use seems to depend both on factors of learning and on genetic factors. Three components of the learning process may be particularly influential: affect, expectancy, and exposure. The affect(s) from which an individual is most motivated to seek relief are those that he or she experiences as most painful or dangerous. The substance or experience that brings relief from such affects is thereby most strongly reinforced (via negative reinforcement). Meanwhile, learned expectations about how a substance or a behavior will alter one's affective state or sense of self are an integral part of the substance's or behavior's effects. The third component, exposure, can consist of either direct experience or modeling of another person who engages in the behavior. Exposure gives the contingencies of reinforcement a chance to operate.

The selection process is influenced also by genetic factors, especially those that affect the hedonic quality of specific experiences. Genetically based variation influences (a) the sensitivity of the reward system to different substances and behaviors, which determines their positive reinforcement value; (b) an individual's sensitivity to the immediate aversive consequences of a substance or a behavior, such as standing ataxia or flushing after ingestion of alcohol; and (c) the negatively reinforcing properties of a substance or a behavior (e.g., its capacity to attenuate physiologic responses to stress).

The addictive process is not separable from the addict's personality and character organization, except by theoretical abstraction, and neither is the addict's selection of a particular substance or behavior for addictive use. An addict's drug of choice or behavior of choice is typically an agent or action that is congruent with the addict's characteristic modes of adaptation: one that facilitates the addict's preexisting means of managing and integrating affective, behavioral, and cognitive responses. The selection of a particular substance or behavior is facilitated also by its capacity to enhance the individual's adaptation, by compensating for defects or weaknesses in the individual's adaptational system.

The development of a particular addictive disorder thus seems to have three components: (a) an individual is predisposed to depend on some form of pleasure-producing behavior to regulate his or her (dysregulated) affects and sense of self, by virtue of the addictive process; (b) the individual takes a mood-altering substance into his or her body, or engages in some other rewarding behavior; and (c) the effects of the substance or behavior (negatively reinforcing, positively reinforcing, and aversive) and the individual's expectations about its effects in the future combine to determine the likelihood that the individual will select that substance or behavior as his or her addictive "drug of choice." These effects and expectations are determined by both genetic and environmental factors. Meanwhile, the adaptive human organism, once having developed the capacity to use an external action as a means of regulating internal states, can shift among different behaviors (and substances) or combine them, according to the opportunities and limitations of the situation.

Selection of Sexual Behavior

The "drug of choice" theory suggests that sexual addiction develops in addictively predisposed individuals (i.e., predisposed by virtue of the addictive process) who experience some form of sexual stimulation and who learn to expect that sexual behavior not only will provide pleasure but also will relieve the affects that they experience as most painful or dangerous, through means that are congruent with their characteristic modes of adaptation. Childhood seems to be the developmentally sensitive period when sexual stimulation is most likely to result in dependence on sexual behavior for self-regulation, and the context of the sexual stimulation is critical. Children naturally explore their bodies with their hands and their physical surroundings with their bodies, so exposure to sexual sensations is virtually inevitable. Yet not all of us who are addictively predisposed become sex addicts. The kind of experience that leads to the development of sexual addiction in addictively predisposed individuals typically results from sexual seduction, which can be overt or covert. In addition to seduction, characteristics of the mother–child relationship that promote sexualization, including the mother's use of sexualization to protect herself from emotional pain, are likely also to contribute to a person's selection of some form of sexual behavior as his or her addictive "drug of choice."

The higher prevalence of sexual addiction in men than in women suggests that gender-related factors play a significant role in its development. A critical component seems to be the developmental crisis that little boys undergo when formation of their core gender identity is superimposed on the ongoing process of separation–individuation period. We all start out in a condition of primary identification with our primary caregivers, usually our mothers. Our subjective experience does not yet differentiate between ourselves and them. As little boys' core gender identity consolidates over the third year of their lives, the person with whom they identify shifts from mother to father. To identify with their fathers, boys have to dis-identify from their mothers, and this dis-identification can interact in complex ways with the ongoing separation–individuation process. In a sense, boys have to choose between a male identity and continuation of the early identification-based connection with their mother, whom they now recognize is female. The ensuing conflict between separation anxiety and vulnerability or castration anxiety is then superimposed on the basic conflict between wish for merger (with fear of separation or abandonment) and wish for individuation or mastery (with fear of being engulfed or controlled). If they are already having a hard time negotiating the separation–individuation process—for example, if important early maternal needs were not met and they are trying to postpone separation in the hope that those needs might still be met—the prospect of relinquishing the identification-based connection with their mother in favor of a male identity can seem unbearable. On the other hand, foregoing their male gender identity amounts to a castration at the level of the self, which can seem unbearable as well. Sexualization might emerge as a solution to this dilemma, a way of affirming male gender while denying separateness. For boys who go this route, narcissistic investment in their genital activity could become a substitute for a stable male gender identity, while their denial of separateness and the fantasies that sustain the denial become sexualized. In addition, the mother's narcissistic bond with a male child may be more sexually infiltrated than it is with a female child, and her tendency to sexualize may emerge more strongly or with a more genital tinge when the child is a boy. Open to speculation is how the development of sexual addiction in males compares to the development of bulimia in females. Interestingly, the percentage of sex addicts who are male, 80% (58–60), is similar to the percentage of bulimics who are female, 90% (17).

In short, if we were to sum up the etiology of sexual addiction in one brief equation, it would be: sexual addiction = the addictive process + sexualization.

TREATMENT

The modalities that have been employed in treating sexual addiction include medication, behavior modification, cognitive–behavioral therapy, therapeutic groups, couple or family therapy, and psychodynamic psychotherapy.

Medication

Two different kinds of pharmacologic treatment may be used in the treatment of sexual addiction, endocrinologic agents and affect-regulating agents. A number of other medications have side effects of decreased sex drive or erectile dysfunction and are, on occasion, used informally, often by patients on their own initiative and sometimes without informed medical direction, in attempts to reduce the symptoms of sexual addiction. These include antihypertensive agents, anticholinergics, antihistamines, disulfiram, antipsychotic medications, and hair growth stimulants. None of these have been studied for use in controlling sexual fantasies, urges, or behavior.

Endocrinologic Agents

Endocrinologic agents are used primarily to reduce the sex drive in paraphilic men. Those that are in use at this time include antiandrogenic agents and gonadotropin-releasing hormone (GnRH) agonists. Estrogens have been studied for use in controlling sexual behavior, but they were found to have too many undesirable effects to be worthy of consideration.

Medroxyprogesterone acetate (Depo-Provera) and cyproterone acetate are the antiandrogenic agents that are being used in the treatment of paraphilias. The latter is not currently available in the United States. A number of clinical studies demonstrate that medroxyprogesterone acetate can reduce sex drive, sexual thoughts, sexual behavior, and aggressiveness (198–208). Cyproterone acetate has been reported to decrease sexually driven aggression, and to reduce arousal responses to pedophilic and coercive sexual stimuli, but not to mutually consenting adult sex scenes (209–216). Administration of these agents is, however, frequently associated with unpleasant side effects, and serious side effects (including thrombophlebitis, pulmonary embolism, and hepatic dysfunction) occasionally occur. Noncompliance also is a significant problem, and one study (203) had a dropout rate of greater than 50%. Most reviewers agree that antiandrogenic agents do not by themselves constitute adequate treatment for paraphilias, but that they can be a valuable adjunct to behavior modification, group therapy, or individual psychotherapy with some patients, particularly during early stages of treatment (206,217,218).

Analogues of GnRH have been developed that have higher potency and longer duration of action than does naturally occurring GnRH. Initial administration of these agents raises serum testosterone by stimulating pituitary gonadotrope cells to increase production of luteinizing hormone (LH) and follicle-stimulating hormone (FSH), the former of which then stimulates testicular Leydig cells to synthesize more androgens. However, continuous administration of long-acting GnRH analogues produces downregulation of GnRH receptors on the pituitary gonadotropes, which leads to a decrease in secretion of LH and FSH, and a consequent decrease in the synthesis of testosterone. Four reports of uncontrolled open-label trials of GnRH agonists in the treatment of paraphilias and hypersexual disorders have been published (219–223). All demonstrated significant positive effects. In the largest study, Rösler and Witztum in Israel (221) reported studies in which 30 men with severe long-standing paraphilia were treated with the GnRH-agonist triptorelin pamoate (Trelstar). All 30 of the men had marked decreases in deviant sexual fantasies, desires, and behaviors. The main side effects were erectile dysfunction, hot flashes, and decrease in bone density. These results suggest that GnRH agonists could prove to be a more effective, safer, and less noxious alternative to the direct antiandrogenic agents. More study of this promising agent is warranted.

Although these medications do not change the direction of the paraphilic person's sexual interest, they decrease the intensity of his sexual drive, so he is more in control and less likely to act on his paraphilic interest. Their primary therapeutic function is to reduce sex drive to manageable levels in those individuals whose ability to control their behavioral impulses is so impaired as to put them at risk either to injure themselves or others, or to render them unresponsive to psychological interventions. Endocrinologic agents can lower the risk of problematic sexual behavior during the interval between the initiation of treatment and the consolidation of the changes that affect-regulating agents, behavior modification, group therapy, or psychotherapy can induce.

Affect-Regulating Agents

A number of reports have provided evidence for the efficacy of affect-regulating agents (primarily antidepressants) in the treatment of paraphilias, even in patients who are not suffering from a major affective disorder (224,225). Agents that have been found to be effective include fluoxetine (Prozac) (19,61,226–231), sertraline (Zoloft) (77,231), paroxetine (Paxil) (232), fluvoxamine (Luvox) (231), nefazodone (Serzone) (22), imipramine (Tofranil) (19,233), desipramine (Norpramin) (20), clomipramine (Anafranil) (20,234–237), lithium (19,238–240), buspirone (Zyban) (241), and electroconvulsive therapy (242). Kafka (19,78,243) and Prentky (62) treated nonparaphilic sexual addictions, as well as paraphilias, with affect-regulating agents, and found that both conditions responded favorably. Most of these studies reported a positive response rate in the range of 50% to 90%. While antidepressant medications, especially the serotonin reuptake inhibitors, can produce decreased libido as a side effect, a number of the studies noted that antidepressants reduced the drive for pathologic sexual behavior, but not the drive for healthy sexual behavior. Such a large number of positive findings is encouraging, but the confidence with which conclusions can be drawn from them is limited by the paucity of controlled studies.

Ward, the author of one of the earliest of these reports (240), explained his findings with the hypothesis that paraphilic behavior had been maintained by mood-dependent motives, and that pharmacologic treatment of the underlying mood disorder reduced the paraphilic behavior by alleviating the mood conditions that motivated it. A number of investigators have found that paraphilias respond to antidepressants in a pattern that closely resembles the response pattern of affective disorders (19–23). Both Kafka (19) and Stein and his colleagues (23) also observed that paraphilic patients with comorbid depression showed concurrent decrease in paraphilic behavior when depressive symptoms improved.

Shifting to consider issues of theory, the reviewed findings of pharmacologic treatment—that the symptoms of sexual addiction respond to medications in a pattern that resembles the response pattern of affective disorder symptoms—make sense when the biopsychological process that underlies sexual addiction (the addictive process) is understood to originate in impaired affect regulation, impaired behavioral inhibition, and aberrant function of the motivational–reward system. Addictive urges can then be recognized to represent both (a) expressions of dysregulated affect—a nonspecific tense or irritable dysphoria that is experienced consciously as an urge to do something, usually to engage in addictive behavior; and (b) conditioned stimuli for coping responses (responses to cope with dysregulated affect) that have been learned in the context of impaired behavioral inhibition and aberrant motivational–reward function. Interventions that enhance affect regulation and behavioral inhibition can thus be expected to diminish addictive craving and addictive behavior.

Behavior Modification

Behavioral methods have been employed in the treatment of paraphilias, but not in the treatment of nonparaphilic sexual addictions. They are oriented toward assisting individuals to reduce their erotic arousal to paraphilic subjects, or to shift the balance of erotic arousal potential from paraphilic to nonparaphilic interests. The primary forms of behavioral treatment for paraphilias are aversion conditioning, covert sensitization, masturbatory training, and imaginal desensitization.

Aversion Conditioning

In aversion conditioning, unwanted patterns of sexual behavior are linked repeatedly with unpleasant stimuli, most often electric shock or foul odors. This classical or pavlovian conditioning procedure is intended to transform stimulus features of the sexual behavior into conditioned stimuli or triggers for the aversive responses to the unpleasant stimuli. A number of uncontrolled studies found that aversion conditioning yielded positive results (244–253); only one found no significant effects (254). Another study found that the success of aversion conditioning depended on the availability of appropriate sexual outlets and the absence of severe nonsexual pathology (255).

Covert Sensitization

Covert sensitization was developed as an imaginary form of aversion conditioning, in which fantasies of paraphilic arousal are paired with fantasies of aversive events to promote a learned association between paraphilic themes and unpleasant feelings. In covert sensitization, patients are first led through a relaxation exercise, which enhances their receptiveness to vivid mental imagery and helps them to focus their attention on the imagery rather than on external events. They then are instructed to visualize themselves engaging in some aspect of their paraphilic behaviors, and they are encouraged to feel personally involved.

At that point, patients are told to imagine either an unpleasant event, such as nausea and vomiting, or an aversive consequence that could follow the behavior in reality, such as public humiliation or shame at being discovered by a superego figure (a parent or a clergyperson, for example). The aversive valence of the imagined noxious scene can be reinforced by the presentation of a nauseating odor. Studies have found covert sensitization to be effective in the treatment of exhibitionism and pedophilia (256–262). It neither inflicts physical discomfort nor requires expensive technology, and patients can be taught to self-administer the treatment. Consequently, many behavior therapists prefer to begin with covert sensitization, turning to aversion therapy only for patients who do not respond to covert sensitization.

Masturbatory Training

Masturbatory training attempts to shift paraphilic patients' arousal patterns in the conventional direction by controlling the fantasies or visual stimuli that they experience while masturbating. The two main forms of masturbatory training are satiation and fading. Satiation involves instructing male patients to masturbate to orgasm with conventional sexual stimuli or fantasies, and then to continue masturbating while visualizing their deviant objects. The idea is that masturbating after orgasm will extinguish erotic arousal to paraphilic fantasies. In the fading technique, paraphilic patients' fantasies are gradually shifted from deviant to conventional during periods of sexual arousal. Patients may be provided with visual stimuli on which to focus, such as photographic slides or computer graphics that automatically fade from one kind of scene to another; or they may be instructed to gradually alter the scenarios that they fantasize while masturbating. One study (263) of masturbatory satiation reported mild success, but other therapeutic modalities were provided at the same time and no posttreatment followup was mentioned.

Imaginal Desensitization

The technique of imaginal desensitization is based on the theory that, once an individual has developed a sequence of sexual activity that begins with a sexual thought or fantasy and ends with overt behavior, interruption of the sequence results in anxiety, which then motivates completion of the sequence. Imaginal desensitization uses the methods of systematic desensitization to diminish the anxiety that is aroused by interruption of that sequence. The procedure begins with the patient describing a scene in which he is stimulated to carry out the sexual activities for which he sought treatment. After relaxation is induced, the patient visualizes performing a sequence of behaviors that leads to noncompletion of the act. Relaxation is allowed to develop with each visualized behavior before the patient

proceeds to the next behavior in the sequence. The patient is thus trained to visualize not completing the sexual act, while remaining relaxed. One study reported imaginal desensitization to be more effective than covert sensitization (264).

Cognitive–Behavioral Therapies

Quadland (7), Schwartz and Brasted (16), and Carnes (11,12) described programs for treating sexual addiction that were predominantly cognitive–behavioral in their approach. In addition to their cognitive–behavioral orientation, the three programs shared a reliance on group therapy as their primary form of treatment.

Quadland (7) described a group therapy program for treating "compulsive sexual behavior." The program was intended to help group members both (1) to change their sexual behavior and (2) to recognize and understand the factors that drove their sexual behavior. Quadland identified two cognitive–behavioral techniques that the program employed: self-monitoring and contracting. In the self-monitoring component, participants kept journals of their sexual thoughts, feelings, and experiences. They then talked in group sessions about what they had entered in their journals. In the contracting component, participants made contracts with the group about changes that they wanted to make each week. Group sessions then usually began with a review of contracts from the previous week, and individuals shared their thoughts and feelings about their various successes and failures. Quadland noted the benefits of mutual support and of confrontation by peers of participants who seemed to be less than honest with themselves or with the group.

Schwartz and Brasted (16) presented a cognitive–behavioral treatment program that involved six stages. The first stage focused on stopping the undesired sexual behavior. Behavior modification techniques and/or pharmacotherapy were employed, as needed, to modify patients' sexual drives. The goal of the second stage, which the authors identified as the "admission" stage, was for the patient to accept the existence of a problem and to promise to keep no secrets from the therapist or from fellow group members. In the third stage, patients were taught anxiety reduction techniques, such as progressive relaxation, so they would no longer need to rely on sexual behavior to alleviate their anxiety. The fourth stage represented the core of Schwartz and Brasted's program. It consisted of cognitive therapy that was directed toward modifying the irrational beliefs that the authors hypothesized to underlie the sexual addiction. In the fifth stage, patients were trained in such skills as assertiveness and problem solving, to facilitate their adaptive social functioning. Finally, the sixth stage focused on resolving whatever residual problems the individual had in establishing a primary sexual relationship. This stage most often involved couple therapy with the pretreatment sexual partner.

The program for treating sexual addiction that was developed by Carnes (11,12) shared with Schwartz and Brasted's program an initial focus on stopping the addictive sexual behavior and a subsequent emphasis on altering the maladaptive core beliefs that were thought to underlie the patient's addictive system. It differed from the programs that were described by Quadland and by Schwartz and Brasted in several ways that reflected the more complete adoption by Carnes of the addiction model. Carnes developed a structured, intensive program that in many ways resembled a traditional chemical-dependency treatment program. A series of lectures and workshops were interwoven with group therapies and homework assignments. The program incorporated principles and methods from the 12-step approach, and participants were encouraged to regularly attend meetings of a 12-step fellowship for recovering sex addicts after they had completed the program. Carnes's program also directly involved members of sex addicts' families, who were invited to participate in special lectures and groups. Finally, Carnes's program was distinguished from the others by its inclusion of relapse prevention techniques. Participants were guided in compiling an inventory of their relapse risk factors, and then in preparing for what could be done before a "slip" (an episode of symptomatic behavior), during a slip, and after a slip had occurred. They learned to anticipate "triggers" that could precipitate a slip, and to devise a series of action steps that could serve to prevent a slip from occurring. Participants were then instructed to rehearse the slip-prevention steps so thoroughly that, when a potentially seductive situation occurred, they would be able to perform the steps automatically. Carnes added that an effective relapse-prevention plan must also build in rewards, so that the addict would not wind up feeling deprived.

Quadland (7) reported that participants in his program indicated a decrease in their frequency of compulsive sexual behavior at follow-up 6 months after treatment. No other studies have been published that specifically assessed the efficacy of cognitive–behavioral treatment for sexual addiction. In a review of treatment outcomes with sex offenders (a category that overlaps but is not identical with the category of sex addicts), Marshall and his colleagues (265) concluded that evaluations of comprehensive cognitive–behavioral programs were encouraging, at least for the treatment of child molesters and exhibitionists. However, they noted, the programs were not uniformly effective.

Therapeutic Groups

Many clinicians believe that group therapy and self-help groups are the most effective modalities for the treatment of individuals who use sexual behavior addictively. The types of therapeutic group that have been employed in treating sex addicts include cognitive–behavioral groups, psychodynamic psychotherapy groups, and support groups. Although group therapy can range from highly structured to relatively unstructured, most investigators have concluded that individuals who use sexual behavior addictively seem to do best in groups that are at least moderately structured. Mathis and Collins (266) and Truax (267) emphasized the importance of treating paraphilic patients in groups that consist of individuals with similar problems, where shared experiences and needs can help to dissolve rationalization, isolation, and denial. Ganzarain and Buchele (268) noted that, for many paraphilic patients, groupmates and the group peer culture become a surrogate benign superego. Group members often can more readily receive guidance, confrontation, and support from groupmates than from therapists or other individuals in their lives. Three studies reported positive results from psychodynamic group psychotherapy treatment of patients who suffered from perversions (268–270).

The most widespread and easy-to-access therapeutic groups for individuals who use sexual behavior addictively are the 12-step groups that are based on the model of Alcoholics Anonymous and adapted for sexual addiction. Since the 1970s, four 12-step fellowships of recovering sex addicts have developed: Sex Addicts Anonymous (SAA), Sex and Love Addicts Anonymous (SLAA), Sexaholics Anonymous (SA), and Sexual Compulsives Anonymous (SCA). The primary differences between the four fellowships are encapsulated in their definitions of sobriety. Sobriety in SAA is defined as no "out-of-bounds" sex. In consultation with their sponsors and fellow group members, sex addicts in SAA identify the sexual behaviors that are likely to lead to harmful consequences, and then define "boundaries" that exclude these behaviors (271). In SLAA, sobriety is similarly defined as no "bottom-line" sex: "Define your bottom-line behavior . . . any sexual or emotional act which, once engaged in, leads to loss of control over rate, frequency, or duration of its recurrence, resulting in worsening self-destructive consequences" (272, p. 4). Sobriety in SA is more strictly defined as no sexual activity other than with a spouse: "Any form of sex with one's self or with partners other than the spouse is progressively addictive and destructive" (273, p. 4). In SCA, members are encouraged to define sexual sobriety for themselves and to develop sexual recovery plans that are consistent with their own values (274). The differences between the 12-step fellowships may, however, be less important than the differences between individual groups. Because the fellowships lack formal leadership structures and internal controls, the characteristics of a particular group are determined primarily by the individuals who attend it.

Couple and Family Therapy

As I noted earlier, the sexual addiction treatment programs that were presented by Schwartz and Brasted (16) and by Carnes (11,12) both involved couple or family therapy. The inclusion of couple or family therapy in the treatment of sexual addiction is also recommended by psychiatric and psychoanalytic clinicians. Reid (217) and Gabbard (275) observed that marital therapy can elucidate pathogenic factors in the marital relationship, while Wise (276) emphasized that marital therapy can engage the spouse and the energy in the relationship as agents of therapeutic change. Both the cognitive–behaviorally oriented therapists and the psychodynamically oriented therapists, while noting that couple or family therapy can be important in the treatment of sexual addiction, accorded it a supplemental or adjunctive status.

Psychodynamic Psychotherapy

A number of psychoanalytically oriented clinicians have stated that intensive psychodynamic psychotherapy is the treatment of choice for paraphilias (275–278). Significantly, researchers who were not primarily oriented toward psychodynamic psychotherapy have observed that the beneficial effect of antidepressant medications in sexual addiction "may only be seen in combination with intensive psychotherapy" (22, p. 270), and that the success of behavioral treatments depends to a great extent on the relationship between the patient and the therapist and on how the issues that emerge in the context of this relationship are managed (279).

The primary focus of psychodynamic treatment is on patients' character pathology, rather than on their pathological behavior. Thus, as Rosen (278) noted, the more pronounced the accompanying personality disorder, the greater the need for psychodynamic therapy that emphasizes transference work. All of the investigators who recommended psychodynamic psychotherapy qualified their recommendations with statements to the effect that the general criteria of suitability for psychodynamic psychotherapy apply to sex addicts as well. One study (278) reported that 5 of 6 exhibitionists who were treated in individual psychodynamic psychotherapy for an average of 21 sessions lost all urges to expose themselves and had not relapsed at the 24-month follow-up. I discuss how psychodynamic psychotherapy works in treating the addictive process when I present my approach to integrated treatment.

Integrated Treatment

Many investigators have concluded that no single treatment is effective for all paraphilic patients, and that the best approach for most patients seems to be to provide individually tailored combinations of behavioral, psychosocial, psychodynamic, and pharmacological modalities (217,275,277,280–282). A number of clinicians have presented programs for treating sexual addiction that combine two or more therapeutic modalities. Interestingly, those multimodality programs that had a cognitive–behavioral core were usually described by their authors as "cognitive–

behavioral," while those multiple-modality programs that had a psychodynamic core were described as "integrated." Having reviewed a couple of the cognitive–behavioral programs (11,12,16), I now consider a couple of integrated programs.

Travin and Protter

Travin and Protter (283,284) were the first to introduce an integrated paradigm for the treatment of paraphilic disorders. They described their "bimodal approach" as a synthesis of cognitive–behavioral and focused psychodynamic treatment modalities, with which could be integrated other modalities, such as medication, family therapy, and longer-term psychodynamic psychotherapy. The cognitive–behavioral protocol that Travin and Protter recommended consists of (a) measures that enhance behavioral control, which include covert sensitization and/or masturbatory satiation, and (b) measures that address social–interpersonal deficits, which include stress management, assertiveness training, and social–communicative skills training. While relapse prevention was included among the self-control techniques that were identified in the authors' book (284), it was not further discussed in the book, and it was not mentioned at all in the initial paper by Protter and Travin (283) or in a more recent paper by Travin (285). Travin and Protter described the psychodynamic component of their approach as more active, more directive, and more focused on symptoms than is psychoanalytic psychotherapy. They directed attention to sexual fantasy both as a bridge that links the cognitive–behavioral and psychodynamic components, and as an organizing schema for treatment intervention. In the psychotherapy component of their approach, the therapist treats the patient's conscious fantasy productions and ritualized sexual behavior as symbolic transformations of the unconscious perverse fantasy that organizes the patient's sexual life. Travin and Protter noted that the way in which the various components of their treatment approach are implemented depends on a variety of factors that concern the patient, the severity of the disorder, and the treatment context. With patients who have little behavioral control and are at risk for victimizing others, covert sensitization and masturbatory satiation are initiated immediately, so as to promote the development of self-control. Until symptomatic control stabilizes, psychodynamic intervention assumes a secondary role. Such patients are likely also to require fairly comprehensive social rehabilitation. Meanwhile, the treatment of patients whose disorder is less severe and whose behavior is less likely to be harmful to others consists primarily of psychodynamic psychotherapy that addresses characterologic issues. Specific cognitive–behavioral interventions are then added, as they are needed. More recently, Travin (285) fine-tuned his bimodal approach in a few ways. He singled out Kohut's self-psychology as a particularly useful framework for the psychodynamic psychotherapy of patients with "compulsive sexual behaviors;" and he observed that, among the medications that are available, serotonergic agents seemed to be the most effective. Travin also identified group therapy as the primary means of treatment in his approach, noting that patients were seen individually as well when such treatment was deemed to be appropriate.

Goodman

Another integrated approach to treating sexual addiction was developed by me (14,39,46). It differs from the approach that was developed by Travin and Protter in three ways: (a) it follows Carnes (11,12) in including relapse prevention and in recognizing the usefulness of 12-step groups; (b) it emphasizes behavioral treatment less and pharmacologic treatment more than do Travin and Protter; and (c) its psychodynamic psychotherapy component is less focal and directive except when warranted by current circumstances, and hence it tends to address a broader range of characterologic issues more deeply (and consequently is of longer duration).

The understanding of addictive disorders that I presented earlier has a broad range of implications for treatment. But the principal implication is that treatment for an addictive disorder is most likely to be effective when it addresses both the addictive behavior and the underlying addictive process. My integrated approach addresses addictive sexual behavior through symptomatic behavior management, which consists primarily of relapse prevention and other cognitive–behavioral techniques. On occasion, symptomatic behavior management may also require behavioral therapy and/or antiandrogenic medication. The addictive process, meanwhile, can be addressed through psychodynamic psychotherapy, therapeutic groups, and psychiatric pharmacotherapy.

Relapse Prevention and Other Cognitive–Behavioral Techniques

Relapse prevention consists of three primary components: risk-management, urge-coping, and slip-handling. Relapse-prevention strategies help people who use sexual behavior addictively (a) to recognize factors and situations that are associated with an increased risk of acting out sexually, (b) to cope more effectively with sexual urges, (c) to recover rapidly from episodes of symptomatic behavior, and (d) to use such "slips" as opportunities to learn about how their recovery plans can be improved. Because many readers might not be familiar with relapse prevention, and it is good to know about even apart from the context of sexual addiction, I will say more about each of these four components.

Symptomatic behavior is more likely to occur under some conditions than others. *Risk management* teaches the person who uses sexual behavior addictively to be aware of factors that increase the likelihood of symptomatic sexual behavior, and to recognize these factors before they overwhelm his or her ability to cope with them. A detailed review of specific instances of acting out, with a focus on the thoughts, feelings, and circumstances that led up to the act, often can illuminate sequences of steps that culminate in episodes of symptomatic behavior, key features or patterns that different sequences share, and triggers that precipitate the sequences. Recognition of risk factors is facilitated also when the addict practices self-monitoring—for example, by keeping a daily journal of situations, times of day, moods, people, activities, and thoughts that are associated with urges to engage in symptomatic behavior. The earlier in the process leading up to symptomatic behavior that a person's healthy resources can be mobilized, the less likely is he or she to engage in symptomatic behavior. Consequently, a critical component of risk-management is identification of specific risk indicators—behaviors that occur early in the sequence that leads up to acting out and thus signals that such a sequence has already begun.

During the course of recovery from sexual addiction, urges to engage in symptomatic behavior are inevitable. *Urge-coping* skills are behavioral and cognitive skills that help people who use sexual behavior addictively to manage these urges without lapsing into symptomatic behavior. Behavioral skills are actions that can be put into practice. They include avoidance of identified risk factors, and specific protective responses that people can enact when they are exposed to a risk factor—for example, physically leaving the location, or engaging in an activity that precludes the next step toward sexually acting out, or contacting a peer and talking about the situation. Behavioral skills are most effective when planned in advance and rehearsed to the point where they become second nature, because the concentration that formulation and performance of an unfamiliar behavioral plan requires may not be available in the midst of a strong addictive urge. Cognitive skills are methods that people can employ to modify their own thoughts. They include (a) accepting urges to engage in symptomatic behavior as natural accompaniments of the recovery process; (b) recognizing that urges are not imperatives to act, but surface manifestations of affects—and that the affects are not in themselves lethal and will eventually subside; (c) reviewing the benefits of abstaining from symptomatic behavior and the potential negative consequences of engaging in that behavior; and (d) when fantasies of engaging in the behavior persist, prolonging the fantasies beyond the pleasurable experiences and imagining the harmful consequences that could ensue, especially those that entail shame, humiliation, or guilt. Particularly in the early phases of recovery, cognitive skills are most likely to be effective in practice when they have been verbally rehearsed with another person.

A discussion of slip-handling skills presupposes that slips can happen and thus seems to imply that slips can to some degree be tolerated. Such tolerance may make sense when the symptomatic behavior is visiting strip clubs or masturbating to pornography. But some sexual behaviors, such as pedophilia and rape, are so harmful to others that zero tolerance of the behavior is the only reasonable treatment stance. If a person who uses sexual behavior addictively is not reliably able to restrain himself from acting on urges to engage in such seriously harmful sexual behavior, then treatment should begin with behavior modification or endocrinologic pharmacotherapy or both, which would continue until such time as the patient is reliably able to restrain himself. If a sexually addicted person who is not reliably able to restrain himself from acting on urges to engage in seriously harmful sexual behavior does not accept a recommendation for behavior modification and/or antiandrogen pharmacotherapy, then a clinician would be well advised not to undertake the treatment of this person. The risks are considerable, and if the patient is not sufficiently motivated to cooperate with a recommendation of this type, then the likelihood of significant progress in treatment is too small to justify such risks. The discussion of slip-handling that follows thus applies only to the treatment of sexually addicted individuals whose sexual behaviors, while far from benign, are not so seriously harmful to others.

Slip-handling skills are developed to prevent progression to relapse after an episode of symptomatic sexual behavior, or a slip, has occurred. First, how do we distinguish between a slip and a relapse? I do not know whether any "official" version of the distinction exists, but I can offer one that I have found to be useful. I define a slip as an episode of symptomatic behavior (a) that has no significant harmful consequences; (b) that the addict terminates on his or her own initiative; and (c) that is immediately followed by a reinstitution of the recovery process, which includes talking about the episode with the person or persons who are significant sources of support in the addict's recovery. Meanwhile, I define a relapse as an episode or a series of episodes of symptomatic behavior that follows a period of abstinence from symptomatic behavior and that fits the definition of addiction—that is, characterized by loss of control and significant harmful consequences. Thus, the objectives of slip-handling skills are (a) to terminate an episode of symptomatic behavior before it can cause harmful consequences, and (b) to reinstitute the recovery process.

Even when motivation is genuine and therapeutic management is competent, slips can happen. However much an individual who has used sexual behavior addictively may consciously wish to abstain from the addictive behavior, a strong motivation to resume the behavior—which derives from the self-regulating functions that the behavior had served—persists unconsciously, if not at a conscious level. Some combination of emotional stress, narcissistic injury, weakening of internal behavioral controls, and gaps in the external support structure can converge momentar-

ily to shift the motivational balance in favor of resuming the behavior. If such a motivational shift happens to coincide with the availability of an opportunity to engage in the behavior, then a slip can occur. Like urge-coping skills, slip-handling skills consist of behavioral and cognitive skills. Behavioral skills are actions that limit the progression of symptomatic behavior and reinstitute recovery, such as communicating with the therapist, getting together with a supportive friend, and attending a 12-step meeting. Similar to the behavioral skills of urge-coping, those of slip-handling are most effective when they are planned in advance and rehearsed. Cognitive skills for handling slips involve reframing the slip, or reconceptualizing what it means to have engaged in symptomatic behavior. A slip or episode of symptomatic behavior is most usefully understood, not as a sign of failure or as the beginning of relapse, but as a signal that a change in the addict's self-management program is needed. It represents a combination of affect and opportunity for which he or she has not yet developed an appropriate coping strategy. A slip thus reframed becomes an opportunity to learn and to improve the therapeutic program. A problem-solving approach is ultimately more effective in containing slips and promoting recovery than is judgmental reproof or self-reproach. In the case of both behavioral and cognitive skills for slip-handling, the sooner after a slip that an intervention occurs, the greater the probability of preventing relapse.

Relapse prevention conceptualizes urges to engage in symptomatic sexual behavior as signals of disruptive affects that addicts need to develop healthier, more adaptive means to manage. In thus shifting the focus from controlling the behavior to understanding the affects, relapse prevention provides a natural bridge from behavior management to psychodynamic psychotherapy.

Cognitive–behavioral techniques other than relapse prevention have a variable role in the treatment of sexual addiction, depending on the addict's needs and limitations. They comprise directive or didactic procedures that focus not on the symptomatic sexual behavior itself, but on other aspects of a person's life that predispose to reliance on symptomatic behavior as a means of coping with painful affects and unmet needs. Applicable cognitive–behavioral techniques may be divided into two groups: skills training, which helps patients to learn thoughts and behaviors that will result in more effective management of their affects and meeting of their needs (e.g., anger management, assertiveness training), and lifestyle regeneration, which helps patients learn to achieve and maintain a healthy, balanced lifestyle.

Psychodynamic Psychotherapy

Psychodynamic psychotherapy is the core treatment for dysfunctions of the character or personality system. While behavioral and cognitive-behavioral therapy are the primary modalities for changing behavior and psychiatric pharmacotherapy is the primary modality for stabilizing affects, psychodynamic psychotherapy is the primary modality for healing the character. In so doing, it enhances addicts' self-regulation and fosters their capacity for meaningful interpersonal connections. Because it treats the addictive process, which is shared by all addictive disorders, the material that I discuss is not specific to sexual addiction but applies to all addictive disorders. The fabric of psychodynamic psychotherapy is woven from three strands: understanding, integration, and internalization.

Understanding is verbally mediated knowledge that the therapeutic process conveys or elicits, and it encompasses description, explanation, and articulation of meanings. It is a primarily cognitive process that is not specific to psychodynamic psychotherapy, and its domain overlaps that of cognitive–behavioral therapy. Both general and specific understanding are useful. The former concerns general information about the conditions from which people may be suffering, and it can be imparted either directly or by recommending something to read. For example, in my work with sex addicts and with others who use some kind of behavior addictively, I inform them about the addictive process and about how their addictive behavior represents an attempt to modulate dysregulated inner states. Such information provides a framework that can help people name their experiences and find order in them. Having words to describe inner states and processes gives our conscious mind a handle by which to apprehend them, and naming our inner realities provides perspective. The part of the mind that names, in so doing, steps back from the part of the mind that feels. Our emotional states and self-states thus no longer occupy the totality of our subjective psychic space, and we are much less likely to be overwhelmed by them. Our affects are signals that we send to ourselves, signals of something that an automatic process within us interprets as psychologically important. But when they become overwhelming, they feel like threats to our survival. Our survival instincts then drive us to ward off or shut down our affects, and we cannot benefit from their signal function. When we get perspective and become less overwhelmed, we can begin to experience our affects as signals, rather than as states of emergency, and we become more open to learning what they can teach us. Moreover, sex addicts in particular benefit from information that helps them realize that the condition that afflicts them is a recognized disorder that can be treated, not just a weakness of will. While this realization alleviates their self-blame for having the condition, it also indicates their responsibility for doing what they can to promote their recovery.

Specific understanding concerns the patient himself or herself, and what actually is going on or has gone on in his or her life. In the treatment of sexual addiction, it initially tracks the relationship between episodes of symptomatic sexual behavior or of urges to engage in such behavior, experiences preceding the episode or the urge that may have tapped into a vulnerable area and triggered affects that threatened to overwhelm the person, and specific vulnerabilities that were shaped by personal history and intensified beyond the range of ordinary manageability by impaired self-regulation. This process is similar to behavior analysis or chain analysis in cognitive–behavioral therapy, but with more emphasis on affects, on helping patients become aware of inner processes that previously had operated outside their awareness, and on discovering how the current complex of affect, thought, and behavior fits into the big picture of the person's life story. When we understand that addictive behaviors typically are patients' attempts to regulate their affective states, which threaten to overwhelm them because their built-in regulation systems are impaired, we see urges and acting out behavior in a new light. An urge to engage in symptomatic sexual behavior is not simply the first step in an experience of being out of control or a force that must be either resisted or submitted to. It is an indication that the coping system is trying to ward off a disruptive affect that is not being effectively managed. An urge is thus a signal of an affect that the person needs to manage in a healthier, more adaptive manner. Similarly, a slip or episode of symptomatic behavior is most usefully understood as a signal of a motivational factor, usually an anxiety, that has remained outside awareness or has not been adequately appreciated. Our focus shifts from behavior to affect, and affects then guide our explorations: What affects are emerging? What events triggered the affects? What core beliefs, inner conflicts, and personal history are involved?

Specific understanding is usually first directed toward urges and episodes of symptomatic behavior, initially focusing on external circumstances or events that may have triggered the affects that were experienced as urges to engage in the behavior. When patients begin psychotherapy, most are only minimally aware of the affects that intervene between the circumstances and their behavior. After all, one of the functions of addiction is to keep affects out of their awareness. The disturbing affects that threaten to overwhelm them may reach the surface of their awareness only as a vague restless discomfort, or they might experience them not as anything affective but only as urges to engage in the behavior. As patients move forward in therapy, they become increasingly able to be aware of their inner states. They come to recognize that behind the behaviors and urges are affects, they develop greater sensitivity to emotional stirrings or shifts in their emotional states, and they become more capable of differentiating among and naming their emotional experiences. The process of being aware also evolves, from a directed retrospective examination of the affective landscape at a particular time in the past to an ongoing undirected receptiveness to changes great and small in the current emotional climate. Concurrently, patients' angle of view widens from addictive behaviors and urges to other problematic behaviors (e.g., verbally flying off the handle, spending excessively, arriving late) and gradually to life in general, as it changes from a means of problem solving to a mode of living. A searchlight at night becomes a panorama at daybreak. The mode of living that is characterized by ongoing cultivation of inner awareness and active receptivity to one's subjective experience can be called mindfulness. Mindfulness emerges out of understanding, but its development usually depends also on integration, the second strand in the fabric of psychodynamic psychotherapy.

Integration refers to integration of the patient's personality or self, bringing its various aspects together as a coherent whole. The process of bringing together occurs through consciousness, and the critical step is patients' becoming consciously aware of what is going on in their minds: not only their beliefs and expectations, but also their affects, needs, wishes, fears, and inner conflicts. Conscious awareness is primarily a verbally mediated process, so becoming aware of what is going on in one's mind typically involves experiencing at the same time a mental or subjective process and its verbal description, and cognitively linking the description with the subjective experience. The mental processes that concern us most here are affects, needs, wishes, fears, inner conflicts, and patients' core beliefs about themselves and about other people.

People who use any kind of behavior addictively tend to be characterized by deficits in integration on several levels. Automatically, without conscious intent or awareness, they engage in a variety of mental processes that function to protect them from emotional trauma. Most of these self-protective processes can be understood as ways of keeping out of awareness material that patients unconsciously imagine would lead to overwhelming pain or to self-fragmentation if they were to become aware of it. Such material may include affects, needs, wishes, fears, inner conflicts, core beliefs, and the self-protective processes themselves. Ultimately, what patients are protecting themselves from most of the time are affects that they fear would overwhelm and psychologically destroy them. For example, when patients automatically push a need or wish out of their awareness, they do so usually not because the need or wish is dangerous in itself, but because past experiences of other people's responses to their expressing it have led them to associate it with potentially overwhelming feelings of disappointment and humiliation. Similarly, when patients automatically keep an inner conflict unconscious—for example, by allowing only one of its components into awareness at a time—they do so because it is fraught with unbearable anxiety, which, in turn, is because choosing one of the alternatives and giving up the other is associated with painful affects that could be traumatic, whichever alternative is chosen. Finally, the self-protective processes that are kept out of awareness are typically not themselves imbued with overwhelming affects. But if patients were aware that they were operating, they would be less likely to succeed in hiding the affect-laden material, so they, too, must be hidden from the inner view.

Integration concerns present experience. It entails becoming aware of affects, needs, wishes, fears, inner conflicts, core beliefs, and self-protective processes that are operating outside of awareness in the here and now. Nonetheless, memories of events that were associated with traumatic affects are important in the integration process, for three reasons. First, when patients are able to remember past experiences—when they can represent them verbally and thus be conscious of them—they then can process them with the conscious functions of their minds and can evaluate whether the responses that they learned in the past are suitable today. For example, at a time in patients' lives when they had few internal resources for dealing with intense affects and no one around to help them deal with their affects, they may have learned that closing their awareness to experiences associated with such affects was the only way to keep from being overwhelmed and traumatized. Since then, they have developed inner capacities to maintain their emotional balance, actions they can take to stabilize their affects or address the sources of their distress, and relationships with people who can help them. They now might be able to manage being aware of experiences and affects that in the past would have overwhelmed and traumatized them. Unfortunately, if they automatically avoid awareness of these experiences and affects, they do not get a chance to learn about the changes. So they are in a catch-22 kind of situation. If they wait to move forward until after the anxiety drops, they might not ever move forward. But when they remember the relevant past events and circumstances, their recognition of how past circumstances differ from present circumstances enables their conscious reasoning to override the anxiety and push them forward into experiences and affects that they otherwise automatically would avoid. While they feel the anxiety and accept it as real, they also recognize that the dangers it signals are not present but past, and that feeling the anxiety does not mean that they have to let it determine their decisions. They can make a conscious choice to "feel the fear and do it anyway." When they then act and directly experience that the anxiety's implicit prediction of doom does not come true, the anxiety loses some of its sting, and they become incrementally desensitized to the anxiety-evoking situation. The next round of learning then has less anxiety to overcome, and the learning process is accelerated. Without such conscious reasoning, they have to rely entirely on procedural learning and classical conditioning, unmediated by consciousness. Of course, this kind of reasoning does not require conscious memory of past events. It also can be based on theoretical knowledge, as it is in cognitive–behavioral therapy and in the "Understanding" component of psychodynamic psychotherapy. However, while the reasoning is the same, the process is different. Memories resemble theories in that they both consist of declarative knowledge. They differ from theories in that memories develop from and refer to specific experienced events, whereas theories develop from concepts and refer to abstract classes of events. Reasoning that is based on theoretical knowledge is often helpful. But reasoning that is based on experience, especially emotional experience, is significantly more effective and is less likely to be undermined by emotional factors that operate outside awareness.

At another level, remembering past experiences enables patients to address affective residues that have not been resolved. When the experiences and the associated affects are accessible to consciousness, they can use conscious thought to raise questions, recognize patterns, make connections, generate hypotheses, and solve problems. When unresolved affective residues are not available to conscious memory, their push toward resolution is restricted to nonverbal channels, that is, to physiology and behavior. Patterns of physiologic changes that are related to the original experiences, such as autonomic nervous system activity or muscular tension, may persist as "body memories" or predispose patients to psychosomatic illness. Patterns of behavior that are related to the original experiences, often representing attempts either to prevent them or to relive and rework them, may persist as driven enactments that undermine or thwart patients' consciously intended pursuits. These physiologic and behavioral patterns are not under conscious control, and they can be difficult to modify as long as unresolved affective residues of past experiences are restricted to nonverbal channels. However, when the past experiences and their associated affects are expressed in words as conscious memories and integrated into patients' personal narratives, the physiologic and behavioral patterns become more susceptible to modification and often dissipate on their own.

Finally, memories of events that were associated with traumatic affects do not exist in isolation. When patients shut out of their awareness past events and the related affects, they also in the process shut out the parts of their selves that experienced those events and affects. As vigorously as they automatically protect themselves from awareness of affects that seem to threaten to overwhelm them, so they protect themselves from awareness of parts of their selves that have been associated with those affects. Those parts of their selves then are hidden from their introspective eye, left behind by their psychological development, and omitted from their evolving sense of identity. By the same token, when patients recover memories of past events and consciously reexperience their associated affects, they initiate a process of reintegrating lost parts of their selves.

As was noted earlier, becoming consciously aware of what goes on in one's mind is the critical step in integration, and it typically involves experiencing a subjective mental process (an affect, need, wish, etc.) and its verbal description at the same time, and mentally linking the subjective experience with its description. Psychodynamic psychotherapy promotes integration by (a) providing an intimate interpersonal situation that tends to stir up affects, needs, wishes, fears, inner conflicts, core beliefs, and self-protective processes; (b) emphasizing verbal communication and meaning, with both patient and therapist working together to create verbal renditions of the patient's subjective experience; and (c) facilitating identification and working through of self-protective processes that interfere with the flow of experience or communication. It thus provides optimal conditions for patients to link their subjective experiences with the cocreated verbal descriptions of them, and thus to develop the self-awareness that leads to integration.

Because integration concerns present experience, psychotherapy tends to be most effective in promoting integration when it addresses issues as they arise in the here and now. In the psychotherapeutic situation, the most here-and-now issues are those that concern the relationship between the patient and the therapist. Hence, these issues often are the most productive issues to address. Early in life, people begin to develop inner models for how they perceive, experience, and respond to others, and also for how they perceive and experience themselves in relationships with others. These models are much more than verbal descriptions or audiovisual recordings. They encompass the somatic and behavioral residues (or representations) of the complex of affects, needs, wishes, fears, inner conflicts, core beliefs, and self-protective processes that were experienced in or developed in response to interactions with other people. Experiences with people during the first years of life have the most profound and enduring influence on the developing models, for two reasons that probably are related. Human beings are helpless at birth and during their early years they depend on their caregivers for their survival. Because what they learn about their caregivers and about how to respond to them is literally a matter of life or death, natural selection has favored those who learned quickly and held on tightly to what they learned. Meanwhile, human beings are born with central nervous systems that are only partially developed. Most of the remaining development occurs during the first 2 or 3 years of life and is shaped by interactions with the environment. And during the first years of human beings' lives, their environment consists primarily of their caregivers. The developmental plasticity of humans' central nervous systems enables them to be much more specifically adapted to their particular environments than the genetic code ever could do by itself. But it also means that the people who constitute a person's early environment have a profound and enduring influence on how the person's central nervous system functions.

People's inner models are of great value in their early relationships with their primary caregivers, on whom they depend for survival. Their models guide them to act in ways that increase the likelihood that their needs will be met, decrease the likelihood that they will experience affective–somatic pain, and in general enhance the chance that they will survive. As people's interpersonal world expands, their inner models continue to be adaptive to the extent that the people with whom they are now interacting are similar to those who were around when the models initially developed. If the differences are modest, they are able to get by. And if they persist long enough, the models often evolve to accommodate them. But sometimes the differences between people's models and the people in their current lives are so large or in such important areas that they cannot get by. And sometimes the models are not flexible enough to accommodate, particularly if they are suffused with anxiety about threats to survival. In those cases, people's inner models guide them to perceive, experience, and respond to significant others in ways that may cause them emotional distress and impair their social and occupational functioning. Often, this emotional distress and these functional impairments are what lead them to seek help.

In psychodynamic psychotherapy, the relationship between the patient and the therapist is both the stage on which the patient's inner models reveal themselves, and the medium through which the models can be changed. As patient and therapist spend time together, interacting at a level more intimate than ordinary discourse, the emotional significance of their relationship deepens and the patient's inner models become increasingly activated. The affects, needs, wishes, fears, inner conflicts, core beliefs, and self-protective processes that influence the patient's other significant relationships increasingly affect how the patient perceives, experiences, and responds to the therapist. The therapeutic relationship, however, differs from other close relationships in a crucial respect. The therapist does not react behaviorally to the content of the patient's words and actions the way he or she might if the patient's responses were taken personally and experienced as being only about who the therapist actually is. Instead, he or she takes the patient's responses as indications that the patient's inner models are active, and as opportunities for both patient and therapist to see how they operate. The therapeutic relationship then provides a safe environment in which both of them together can explore "in real-time" the meaning of the patient's responses in terms of the patient's affects, needs, wishes, fears, inner conflicts, core beliefs, and means of self-protection. This collaborative exploration gives words to the patient's subjective experience of these processes while they still are fresh, thus expanding the patient's awareness of them and promoting their integration into the patient's living narrative. Bringing together in consciousness the various disintegrated aspects of a person's psychic processes gradually heals the personality and enables it increasingly to function as an integrated whole. The net result is more conscious choice, more flexibility, and more freedom.

Internalization is the least-understood component of psychodynamic psychotherapy. As was noted earlier, it is the process whereby children gradually become able to provide for themselves the regulatory functions that had been provided for them by their caregivers. It occurs gradually over the course of numerous child–caregiver interactions in which the caregivers respond more or less appropriately to the children's needs for nurturing, soothing, and holding. The term *internalization* itself is a metaphor that can be translated most clearly as a combination of procedural learning and classical conditioning that interacts dialectically with genetically guided maturation. The capacity for developmental internalization of self-regulatory functions is greatest during early childhood, but it continues throughout life.

The function of internalization in psychodynamic psychotherapy derives from its role in the development of self-regulation. A primary means by which psychotherapy promotes the healing of impaired self-regulation is by providing new opportunities for patients to internalize self-regulatory functions that they did not adequately internalize during their childhood. Affect–regulation functions can develop through internalization of therapists' provision of a holding environment, their soothing and enlivening functions, and their treatment of affects as indications of internal states that deserve attention. (By "holding environment," I mean a place within the therapeutic relationship where patients can feel safe with affects that they by themselves are not able to tolerate. Therapists contribute to the creation of this place by being with patients' affects and not suppressing them, withdrawing, acting out, or being overwhelmed.) Self-care functions can develop through internalization of the therapist's nurturing and protective functions, accompanied by internalization of the message that the patient is valued as a person and is worth taking care of. Healthy self-governance functions can develop through internalization of the therapist's integrity, respectfulness, nonjudgmental acceptance, and general stabilizing function.

Psychodynamic psychotherapy is not the only context in which self-regulatory functions can be internalized. Internalization can occur in any significant relationship, and also in some group situations. What distinguishes psychotherapy is the depth of the relationship; the therapeutic frame of a dyadic relationship with a person who combines caregiving attributes and authority attributes; the therapist's ability to facilitate the patient's personality integration, and thus to minimize the extent to which the patient's projections distort the internalization process, and (as we have a right to expect) the therapist's level of psychological and emotional health.

In psychodynamic psychotherapy with sex addicts (and with addicts who specialize in other behaviors), internalization is facilitated by addicts' tendencies to experience their self-regulatory functions as being located in the external world, and to seek them there. This tendency is continuous with the addictive process itself. Paradoxically, the very process that determines addictive dependence on external behavior is thus an important facilitator of therapeutic internalization in psychotherapy.

Therapeutic Groups

Therapeutic groups can facilitate the development of abilities to make meaningful connections with others and to turn to people in times of need instead of turning to addictive behavior. Treatment in groups is particularly helpful for relapse prevention and for other cognitive–behavioral techniques. Therapeutic groups can provide a variety of beneficial processes, including support, commonality (the "I'm not the only one" experience), empathic bonding, group cohesiveness, and sense of belonging. They also can offer opportunities to learn interpersonal skills while receiving feedback, to develop social confidence, to learn vicariously by identifying with others in the group, and to help others. In therapeutic groups, the emotional energy of the interpersonal connection and consequent transference responses are typically weaker and more diffuse than they are in individual psychotherapy. One consequence of this difference is that character healing is more likely to occur in individual psychodynamic psychotherapy than it is in therapeutic groups, and closeness is likely to be less intense in therapeutic groups than in individual psychotherapy. As a result, groups can often be more rapidly effective than is individual therapy in supplementing members' impaired self-care and self-governance functions.

Unfortunately, treatment groups for sex addicts are typically feasible only in larger clinics or in association with treatment centers, hospitals, or other institutions. Independent practitioners are more likely to integrate relapse prevention and other cognitive–behavioral techniques into individual psychotherapy. Meanwhile, 12-step groups for individuals who use sexual behavior addictively are readily available across the United States and in other countries as well. Twelve-step groups can potentially provide all of the beneficial effects of therapeutic groups that I mentioned earlier. In addition, they offer membership at no charge for as long as a person wishes, round-the-clock support, and connection with a worldwide support network. They present a coherent framework for approaching addictive problems and life in general, including honesty with self and acceptance of limitations. In addition, 12-step groups offer (but do not impose) a nonjudgmental, nondogmatic spiritual foundation. The 12-step groups for sex addicts were briefly described earlier, in the "Therapeutic Groups" portion of the "Treatment" section.

Psychiatric Pharmacotherapy

Psychiatric pharmacotherapy is direct intervention to enhance emotional and behavioral self-regulation, as well as to treat other symptoms of comorbid psychiatric disorders. In sexual addiction, craving and urges to act out are expressions of dysregulated emotional states, and such urges are more likely to be acted out when behavioral regulation is impaired. Consequently, enhancement of affect regulation tends to diminish the frequency and intensity of addictive urges, whereas enhanced behavioral regula-

tion reduces the likelihood that urges will lead to acting out. As we noted earlier, a number of studies have indicated that antidepressant medications, particularly the serotonin reuptake inhibitors, can reduce the frequency of addictive sexual behavior and the intensity of urges to engage in addictive sexual behavior, even when the patient is not suffering from major depression. Kafka (243) reported anecdotally that augmentation of a serotonin reuptake inhibitor with bupropion or with a psychostimulant can further reduce sexual fantasies, urges, and behavior, particularly when concurrent depressive symptoms have not responded adequately to the SRI or when symptoms of attention deficit disorder are present. My clinical experience is consistent with Kafka's report. I also have found that divalproex (Depakote) or lamotrigine (Lamictal) can be helpful for sexual addiction symptoms that arise in the context of atypical manic-depressive conditions or "emotionally unstable character disorders," and that gabapentin (Neurontin) can alleviate accompanying irritability and feelings of being overwhelmed.

In nontechnical terms, the impairment of affect regulation that underlies addiction can be seen as an imbalance between the intensity of patients' affects, particularly their painful affects, and the capacity of their built-in coping systems. Painful affects, such as anxiety and dysphoria, are not in themselves bad. They are signals that we send to ourselves to call our attention to something that is important for our physical or psychological survival. Painful affects become a problem when their intensity overwhelms or threatens to overwhelm a person's coping system. The affects can then no longer be used as signals, but are experienced as extreme dangers that must be escaped or avoided. Often, patients will not consciously experience the painful affects, or even the threats of these affects, but will feel only a vague unease. Or they may be closed off to affects, and may experience only bodily states that they interpret as urges to engage in some kind of symptomatic behavior. People who have learned that certain self-initiated behaviors can quell such dangerous affects and prevent the system from being overwhelmed will experience strong urges to engage in these behaviors whenever such affects threaten. This process forms the core of addictive and compulsive patterns of behavior. Psychiatric medication works by restoring or reinforcing the brain chemistry that is associated with the built-in coping systems. While psychodynamic psychotherapy also can enhance the capacity of patients' coping systems, their accessibility to psychotherapy and to what it can offer may be limited when they are emotionally overwhelmed. To the extent that they shut down or shut out subjective experience because they unconsciously perceive that it threatens their psychological survival, their access to their inner lives will be compromised. Moreover, states of being overwhelmed can disorganize or disrupt cognitive functioning, so they not only are less aware of material that they can work with, they also are less able to work with the material of which they are aware. When psychiatric medication is effective in establishing a more stable balance between patients' affects and the capacity of their coping systems, the coping systems are less likely to be overwhelmed, and patients can better tolerate experiencing their painful affects as affects (rather than as states of emergency). Consequently, they will have more conscious access to their inner states, and their cognitive functions will be more organized and more free to operate. These developments provide them with more opportunity to work with their inner states in psychotherapy. Subsequent psychotherapeutic work can then help them to develop healthier, more adaptive ways of regulating and responding to their inner states, which may eventually enable them to manage without the psychiatric medication.

Treatment Organization and Course of Recovery

The specific functional impairments, needs, and inner resources that each of us brings to the treatment situation vary from person to person, and vary also within the same person, from one point during treatment to another. Treatment for sexual addiction is thus most likely to be effective when the treatment plan for each person is individually tailored and evolves as he or she progress through recovery. Recovery from sexual addiction is a developmental process that can be understood to proceed in four overlapping stages: stage I, initial behavior modulation; stage II, stabilization (of behavior and affect); stage III, character healing; and stage IV, self-renewal. Of course, this schema of stages is a heuristic device that oversimplifies the picture. Behavior, affect, character, and self are interrelated dimensions of a person that are together involved at all points in the developmental process. In general, the more concrete and directive treatment modalities (behavior modification, psychiatric pharmacotherapy, cognitive–behavioral therapy) tend to be more prominent during the earlier phases of recovery, while the more exploratory, interpersonal, and existential modalities (psychodynamic psychotherapy and spiritual regeneration [which I did not discuss here]) tend to be more prominent during the middle and later phases.

To date, no outcome studies have been published that evaluate the effectiveness of integrated treatment for sexual addiction. In fact, empirical research on almost every aspect of sexual addiction is sorely lacking: neurobiology, psychometrics, family history, diagnostic criteria (reliability, coverage, and predictive validity), and response to treatments. This deficit may have been a result of the unavailability, until recently, of clear and meaningful diagnostic criteria for sexual addiction. It may have been due also to a reluctance by many to consider sexual addiction as a fit subject for scientific study. My hope is that publications like this one will redress these conditions and stimulate the empirical research that this new field so desperately needs.

Prognosis

While the long-term response of sexual addiction to various types of treatment cannot at this time be reliably predicted, a number of factors have been identified that seem to influence the prognosis. These factors can be clustered in three groups: (a) illness factors (that tend to worsen the prognosis), which include early age of onset, high frequency of symptomatic sexual behavior, concomitant use of alcohol or other drugs, and absence of anxiety or guilt about the behavior; (b) recovery support factors (that tend to improve the prognosis), which include a stable job, a stable primary relationship, a supportive social network, and availability of appropriate sexual outlets; and (c) personality factors (that tend improve the prognosis), which include intelligence, creativity, self-observatory capacity, sense of humor, capacity to form interpersonal connections, and motivation for change—which is a function of people's ability to experience themselves as responsible, as well as their degree of subjective distress. Prognosis is influenced also by comorbidity with other psychiatric disorders, by the degree of associated character pathology, and by the kind of relationship that develops between the patient and the therapist (or whoever else is most involved in his or her treatment).

Significant recovery from sexual addiction, as from any other addictive disorder, requires a considerable period of time. Addiction interferes with normal development and corrodes interpersonal relationships. These problems remain after the addictive behavior has ceased, and only then can they begin to be addressed. Moreover, addiction is a chronic condition and, as we have seen, the core pathology in addiction is not readily separable from the affective and characterologic matrix from which it arises. However much they may have benefited from treatment, most addicts (of any behavioral type) will to some extent remain vulnerable to being overwhelmed by intense affects and loss of self-coherence in situations that would be neither traumatic nor disorganizing for individuals whose self-regulation systems are intact. And sex addicts are particularly likely to experience threats of being overwhelmed by these internal states as urges to engage in sexual behavior. Even after stable recovery has been achieved, ongoing maintenance activity may be required indefinitely to prevent relapse. Sexual addiction—like other addictive disorders, most psychiatric conditions, and the majority of diseases in medicine—is not an acute disease that effective treatment can cure, but a chronic disease that effective treatment can, with the patient's active collaboration, bring into and keep in remission. And the underlying pain is unlikely ever to disappear, though we can become better and better at accepting it, managing it, and living with it. As Albert Camus observed in *The Myth of Sisyphus* (286), "The important thing . . . is not to be cured, but to live with one's ailments."

REFERENCES

1. Krafft-Ebbing R. *Psychopathia sexualis* (1886). New York: Paperback Library 1965. Rebman FJ, translator.
2. Anthony DT, Hollander E. Sexual compulsions. In: Hollander E, ed. *Obsessive-compulsive related disorders.* Washington, DC: American Psychiatric Association 1993:139–150.
3. Coleman E. Sexual compulsion vs. sexual addition: The debate continues. *SIECUS Rep* 1986;7–11.
4. Coleman E. Sexual compulsivity: definition, etiology and treatment considerations. In: Coleman E, ed. *Chemical dependency and intimacy dysfunction.* New York: Haworth Press, 1987;189–204.
5. Coleman E. Is your patient suffering from compulsive sexual behavior? *Psychiatric Ann* 1992;22:320–325.
6. Hollander E. Introduction. In: Hollander E, ed. *Obsessive-compulsive related disorders.* Washington, DC: American Psychiatric Association 1993:1–16.
7. Quadland MC. Compulsive sexual behavior: definition of a problem and an approach to treatment. *J Sex Marital Ther* 1985;11:121–132.
8. Weissberg JH, Levay AN. Compulsive sexual behavior. *Med Aspects Hum Sex* 1986;20:127–128.
9. Barth RJ, Kinder BN. The mislabeling of sexual impulsivity. *J Sex Marital Ther* 1987;13:15–23.
10. McElroy SL, Hudson JI, Pope HG, et al. The *DSM–III–R* impulse control disorders not elsewhere classified: clinical characteristics and relationship to other psychiatric disorders. *Am J Psychiatry* 1992;149:318–327.
11. Carnes P. *Out of the shadows: understanding sexual addiction.* Minneapolis: CompCare, 1983.
12. Carnes P. *Contrary to love: helping the sexual addict.* Minneapolis: CompCare, 1989.
13. Goodman A. Sexual addiction: Designation and treatment. *J Sex Marital Ther* 1992;18:303–314.
14. Goodman A. Diagnosis and treatment of sexual addiction. *J Sex Marital Ther* 1993;19:225–251.
15. Marks I. Behavioural (non-chemical) addictions. *Br J Addict* 1990;85:1389–1394.
16. Schwartz MF, Brasted WS. Sexual addiction. *Med Aspects Hum Sex* 1985;19:103–107.
17. American Psychiatric Association. *Diagnostic and statistical manual of mental disorders,* 4th ed. *(DSM–IV).* Washington, DC: Author, 1994.
18. American Psychiatric Association. *Diagnostic and statistical manual of mental disorders,* 3rd ed., revised. *(DSM–III–R).* Washington, DC: Author, 1987.
19. Kafka MP. Successful antidepressant treatment of nonparaphilic sexual addictions and paraphilias in men. *J Clin Psychiatry* 1991;52:60–65.
20. Kruesi MJP, Fine S, Valladares L, et al. Paraphilias: a double-blind crossover comparison of clomipramine versus desipramine. *Arch Sex Behav* 1992;21:587–593.
21. Bradford JMW, Gratzer TG. A treatment for impulse control disorders and paraphilia: a case report. *Can J Psychiatry* 1995;40:4–5.
22. Coleman E, Gratzer T, Nesvacil L, et al. Nefazodone and the treatment of nonparaphilic compulsive sexual behavior: a retrospective study. *J Clin Psychiatry* 2000;6:282–284.
23. Stein DJ, Hollander E, Anthony DT, et al. Serotonergic medications for sexual obsessions, sexual addictions, and paraphilias. *J Clin Psychiatry* 1992;53:267–271.
24. Schmidt CW. Changes in terminology for sexual disorders in *DSM–IV. Psychiatric Med* 1992;10:247–255.
25. Wikler A. Some implications of conditioning theory for problems of drug abuse. *Behav Sci* 1971;16:92–97.
26. Ludwig AM, Wikler A. "Craving" and relapse to drink. *Q J Stud Alcohol* 1974;35:108–130.
27. O'Brien C. Experimental analysis of conditioning factors in human narcotic addiction. *Pharmacol Rev* 1975;27:533–543.
28. Leventhal H, Cleary PD. The smoking problem: a review of the research and theory in behavioral risk modification. *Psychol Bull* 1980;88:370–405.
29. Sideroff S, Jarvik ME. Conditioned responses to a videotape showing heroin-related stimuli. *Int J Addict* 1980;15:529–536.
30. Wikler A. A theory of opioid dependence. *NIDA Res Monogr* 1980;30:174–178.
31. Childress AR, McLellan AT, O'Brien CP. Abstinent opiate abusers exhibit conditioned craving, conditioned withdrawal, and reductions in both through extinction. *Br J Addict* 1986;81:701–706.
32. Sherman JE, Jorenby DE, Baker TB. Classical conditioning with alcohol: acquired preferences and aversions, tolerance, and urges/craving. In: Chaudron CD, Wilkinson DA, eds. *Theories on alcoholism.* Toronto: Addiction Research Foundation 1988:173–237.
33. Childress AR, Ehrman R, Rohsenow DJ, et al. Classically conditioned factors in drug dependence. In: Lowinson JH, Ruiz P, Millman RB, et al. *Substance abuse: a comprehensive textbook,* 2nd ed., Baltimore: Williams & Wilkins 1992:56–69.
34. Miller NS, Dackis CA, Gold MS. The relationship of addiction, tolerance, and dependence to alcohol and drugs: a neurochemical approach. *J Subst Abuse Treat* 1987;4:197–207.
35. Goldstein A. Introduction. In: Goldstein A, ed. *Molecular and cellular aspects of the drug addictions.* New York: Springer Verlag, 1989; XIII–XVIII.
36. Jaffe JH: Current concepts of addiction. In: O'Brien CP, Jaffe JH, eds. *Addictive states.* New York: Raven Press, 1992:1–21.
37. Cox WM, Klinger E. A motivational model of alcohol use. *J Abnorm Psychol* 1988;97:168–180.
38. Baker TB, Morse E, Sherman JE. The motivation to use drugs: a psychobiological analysis of urges. In: Rivers PC, ed. *Nebraska symposium on motivation,* vol. 34. *Alcohol and addictive behavior.* Lincoln, NE: University of Nebraska Press, 1987:257–323.
39. Goodman A. Addiction: definition and implications. *Br J Addict* 1990;85:1403–1408.
40. Goodman A. *Sexual addiction: an integrated approach.* Madison, CT: International Universities Press, 1998.
41. Goodman A. Addictive disorders: an integrated understanding. *Counselor* 2000;18:30–34.
42. Goodman A. What's in a name? Terminology for designating a syndrome of driven sexual behavior. *Sex Addict Compulsivity* 2001:8:191–214.
43. Goodman A. "Addictive disorders" as a diagnostic category. *Ital J Addict* 2003;38:39–46.
44. Orford J. Hypersexuality: implications for a theory of dependence. *Br J Addict* 1978;73:299–310.
45. Fenichel O. *The psychoanalytic theory of neurosis.* New York: Norton, 1945.
46. Freud S. Extracts from the Fleiss papers (Letter 79, dated Vienna, December 22, 1897). *Standard Edition (1892–1899),* vol. 1. London: Hogarth Press, 1966; 173–280.
47. Goodman A. Sexual addiction: diagnosis, etiology, and treatment. In: Lowenstein JH, Millman RB, Ruiz P, et al, eds. *Substance abuse: a comprehensive textbook,* 3rd ed. Baltimore: Williams & Wilkins 1997;340–354.
48. Blumer D. Changes in sexual behavior related to temporal lobe disorders in man. *J Sex Res* 1974;42:155–162.
49. Epstein AW. Fetishism: a study of its

psychopathology with particular reference to a proposed disorder in brain mechanism as an etiological factor. *J Nerv Ment Dis* 1960;130:107–119.

50. Epstein AW. Relationship of fetishism and transvestism to brain and particularly to temporal lobe dysfunction. *J Nerv Ment Dis* 1961;133:247–253.

51. Hoenig J, Kenna J. EEG abnormalities and transsexualism. *Br J Psychiatry* 1979;134:293–300.

52. Kolarsky A, Freund K, Machek J, et al. Male sexual deviation: association with early temporal lobe damage. *Arch Gen Psychiatry* 1967;17:735–743.

53. Mohan KJ, Salo MW, Nagaswami S. A case of limbic system dysfunction with hypersexuality and fugue state. *Dis Nerv Syst* 1975;36:621–624.

54. Raboch J, Cerna H, Zemek P. Sexual aggressivity and androgens. *Br J Psychiatry* 1987;151:398–400.

55. Seim HC. Evaluation of serum testosterone and luteinizing hormone levels in sex offenders. *Fam Pract Res J* 1988;7:175–180.

56. Abel G. Paraphilias. In: Kaplan HI, Sadock BJ, eds. *Comprehensive textbook of psychiatry*, 5th ed. Baltimore: Williams & Wilkins, 1989:1069–1085.

57. Rasmussen SA, Tsuang MT. Clinical characteristics and family history in DSM-III obsessive-compulsive disorder. *Am J Psychiatry* 1986;143:317–322.

58. Warwick HMC, Salkovskis PM. Unwanted erections in obsessive-compulsive disorder. *Br J Psychiatry* 1990;157:919–921.

59. Carnes PJ, Delmonico DL. Childhood abuse and multiple addictions: research findings in a sample of self-identified sexual addicts. *Sex Addict Compulsivity* 1996;3:258–268.

60. Schneider JP, Schneider BH. Couple recovery from sexual addiction/coaddiction: results of a survey of 88 marriages. *Sex Addict Compulsivity* 1996;3:111–226.

61. Black DW, Kehrberg LLD, Flumerfelt DL, et al. Characteristics of 36 subjects reporting compulsive sexual behavior. *Am J Psychiatry* 1997;154:243–249.

62. Kafka MP, Prentky R. Fluoxetine treatment of nonparaphilic sexual addictions and paraphilias in men. *J Clin Psychiatry* 1992;53:351–358.

63. Abel GC, Osborn C. The paraphilias: the extent and nature of sexually deviant and criminal behavior. *Psychiatric Clin North Am* 1992;15:675–687.

64. Rooth FG. Exhibitionism, sexual violence and paedophilia. *Br J Psychiatry* 1973;122:705–710.

65. Wilson GD, Gosselin C. personality characteristics of fetishists, transvestites, and sadomasochists. *Person Ind Diff* 1980;1:289–295.

66. Chalkley AJ, Powell GE. The clinical description of forty-eight cases of sexual fetishism. *Br J Psychiatry* 1983;142:292–295.

67. Breitner IE. Psychiatric problems of promiscuity. *South Med J* 1973;66:334–336.

68. Lesieur HR. Report on pathological gambling in New Jersey. In: *Report and Recommendations of the Governor's Advisory Commission on Gambling*. Trenton, NJ, Governor's Advisory Commission on Gambling, 1988;124.

69. Washton AM. Cocaine may trigger sexual compulsivity. *J Drug Alcohol Depend* 1989;13:8.

70. Steinberg MA. Sexual addiction and compulsive gambling. *Am J Prev Psychiatry Neurol* 1990;2:39–41.

71. Schneider JP, Schneider B. *Sex, lies, and forgiveness: couples speaking out on healing from sexual addiction*. Center City, MN: Hazelden Educational Materials, 1991.

72. Kafka MP, Prentky RA. Preliminary observations of *DSM–III–R* axis 1 comorbidity in men with paraphilias and paraphilia-related disorders. *J Clin Psychiatry* 1994;55:481–487.

73. McElroy SL, Keck PE Jr, Pope HG Jr, et al. Compulsive buying: a report of 20 cases. *J Clin Psychiatry* 1994;55:242–248.

74. Specker SM, Carlson GA, Christenson GA, et al. Impulse control disorder and attention deficit disorder in pathological gamblers. *Ann Clin Psychiatry* 1995;7:175–179.

75. Kafka MP, Prentky RA. Attention deficit hyperactivity disorder in males with paraphilias and paraphilia-related disorders: a comorbidity study. *J Clin Psychiatry* 1998;59:388–396.

76. Black DW. The epidemiology and phenomenology of compulsive sexual behavior. *CNS Spectr* 2000;5:26–35.

77. Irons RP, Schneider JP. Addictive sexual disorder. In: Miller N, ed. *Principles and practice of addictions in psychiatry* (sic). Philadelphia: WB Saunders, 1997:441–457.

78. Kafka MP. Sertraline pharmacotherapy for paraphilias and paraphilia-related disorders: An open trial. *Ann Clin Psychiatry* 1994;6:189–195.

79. Fagan PJ, Wise TN, Schmidt CW, et al. A comparison of five-factor personality dimensions in males with sexual dysfunction and males with paraphilia. *J Pers Assess* 1991;57:434–448.

80. Blair CD, Lanyon RI. Exhibitionism: etiology and treatment. *Psychol Bull* 1981;89:439–463.

81. Hucker SJ, Bain J. Androgenic hormones and sexual assault. In: Marshall WL, Laws DR, Barbaree HE, eds. *Handbook of sexual assault: issues, theories, and treatment of the offender*. New York: Plenum, 1990:94–102.

82. Langevin R, Ben-Aron MH, Coulthard R, et al. Sexual aggression: constructing a predictive equation: a controlled pilot study. In: Langevin R, ed. *Erotic preference, gender identity, and aggression in men: new research studies*. Hillsdale, NJ: Lawrence Erlbaum, 1985:39–76.

83. Marshall WL, Barbaree HE. An integrated theory of the etiology of sexual offending. In: Marshall WL, Laws DR, Barbaree HE, eds. *Handbook of sexual assault: issues, theories, and treatment of the offender*. New York: Plenum, 1990:209–229.

84. Purins J, Langevin R. Brain correlates of penile erection. In: Langevin R, ed. *Erotic preference, gender identity, and aggression in men: new research studies*. Hillsdale, NJ: Lawrence Erlbaum, 1985:113–133.

85. Hendricks SE, Fitzpatrick DF, Hartman K, et al. Brain structure and function in sexual molesters of children and adolescents. *J Clin Psychiatry* 1988;49:108–112.

86. Hucker S, Langevin R, Wortzman G, et al. Neuropsychological impairment in pedophiles. *Can J Behav Sci* 1986;18:440–448.

87. Hucker S, Langevin R, Wortzman G, et al. Cerebral damage and dysfunction in sexually aggressive men. *Ann Sex Res* 1988;1:33–47.

88. Langevin R. Sexual anomalies and the brain. In: Marshall WL, Laws DR, Barbaree HE, eds. *Handbook of sexual assault: issues, theories, and treatment of the offender*. New York: Plenum, 1990:103–113.

89. Langevin R, Bain J, Wortzman S, et al. Sexual sadism: brain, blood, and behavior. *Ann N Y Acad Sci* 1988;528:163–171.

90. Flor-Henry P, Koles ZL, Reddon JR, et al. Neuropsychological studies (EEG) of exhibitionism. In: Shagrasi MC, Josiassen RC, Roemer RA, eds. *Brain electrical potentials and psychopathology*. Amsterdam: Elsevier, 1986:279–306.

91. Flor Henry P, Lang R. Quantitative EEG analysis in genital exhibitionists. *Ann Sex Res* 1988;1:49–62.

92. Herman JL. Sexual offenders: a feminist perspective. In: Marshall WL, Laws DR, Barbaree HE, eds. *Handbook of sexual assault: issues, theories, and treatment of the offender*. New York: Plenum, 1990:177–193.

93. Stermac LE, Segal ZV, Gillis R. Social and cultural factors in sexual assault. In Marshall WL, Laws DR, Barbaree HE,

eds. *Handbook of sexual assault: issues, theories, and treatment of the offender.* New York: Plenum 1990:143–159.

94. Marshall WL. Intimacy, loneliness, and sexual offenders. *Behav Res Ther* 1989;27:491–503.

95. Khan MMR. Role of the "collated internal object" in perversion-formations. *Int J Psychoanal* 1969;50:555–565.

96. Goldberg A. *The problem of perversion: the view from self psychology.* New Haven: Yale University Press, 1995.

97. Goodman A. Addictive disorders: an integrated approach. Part two. An integrated treatment. *J Ministry Addict Recov* 1996;3:49–77.

98. McGuire RJ, Carlisle JM, Young BG. Sexual deviations as conditioned behaviour: a hypothesis. *Behav Res Ther* 1965;2:185–190.

99. Hammer EF. Symptoms of sexual deviation: dynamics and etiology. *Psychoanal Rev* 1968;55:5–27.

100. Anderson N, Coleman E. Childhood abuse and family sexual attitudes in sexually compulsive males: a comparison of three clinical groups. *Am J Prev Psychiatry Neurol* 1990;3:8–15.

101. Schwartz MF. Effective treatment for sex offenders. *Psychiatr Ann* 1992;22:315–319.

102. Hanson RK, Slater S. Sexual victimization in the history of sexual abusers: a review. *Ann Sex Res* 1988;1:485–499.

103. Garland RJ, Dougher MJ. The abused/abuser hypothesis of child sexual abuse: a critical review of theory and research. In: Feierman JR, ed. *Pedophilia: biosocial dimensions.* Springer-Verlag, 1990:488–509.

104. Herman JL, Perry JC, van der Kolk BA. Childhood trauma in borderline personality disorder. *Am J Psychiatry* 1989;146:490–495.

105. Zanarini MC, Gunderson JG, Marino MF, et al. Childhood experiences of borderline patients. *Compr Psychiatry* 1989;30:18–25.

106. Ogata SN, Silk KR, Goodrich S, et al. Childhood sexual and physical abuse in adult patients with borderline personality disorder. *Am J Psychiatry* 1990;147:1008–1013.

107. Links PS, van Reekum R. Childhood sexual abuse, parental impairment and the development of borderline personality disorder. *Can J Psychiatry* 1993;38:472–474.

108. Salzman JP, Salzman C, Wolfson AN, et al. Association between borderline personality structure and history of childhood abuse in adult volunteers. *Compr Psychiatry* 1993;34:254–257.

109. Swett C, Surrey J, Cohen C. Sexual and physical abuse histories and psychiatric symptoms among male psychiatric outpatients. *Am J Psychiatry* 1990;147:632–636.

110. Paris J, Zweig-Frank H. A critical review of the role of childhood sexual abuse in the etiology of borderline personality disorder. *Can J Psychiatry* 1992:37:125–128.

111. Beck AT. Depression: *Clinical, experimental and theoretical aspects.* New York: Harper & Row, 1967.

112. Beck AT, Rush AJ, Shaw BF, et al. *Cognitive therapy of depression.* New York: Guilford Press, 1979.

113. Freud S. Three essays on the theory of sexuality. In: Strachey J, ed. and translator. *The standard edition of the complete psychological works of Sigmund Freud,* vol. 7. London: Hogarth Press, 1905(1953):123–245.

114. Freud S. Fetishism. In: Strachey J, ed. and translator. *The standard edition of the complete psychological works of Sigmund Freud,* vol. 21. London: Hogarth Press, 1927(1953):149–157.

115. Payne SM. Some observations on the ego development of the fetishist. *Int J Psychoanal* 1939;20:161–170.

116. Gillespie WH. Notes on the analysis of sexual perversions. *Int J Psychoanal* 1952;3:397–402.

117. Bak RC. Fetishism. *J Am Psychoanal Assoc* 1953;1:285–298.

118. Bak RC: Aggression and perversion. In Lorand S, ed. *Perversions: psychodynamics and therapy.* London: Ortol, 1965:231–240.

119. Greenacre P. Further considerations regarding fetishism. *Psychoanal Stud Child* 1955;10:187–194.

120. Greenacre P. Fetishism. In: Rosen I, ed. *Sexual deviation,* 2nd ed. Oxford: Oxford University Press, 1979:79–108.

121. Khan MMR. The role of polymorph-perverse body-experiences and object-relations in ego-integration. *Br J Med Psychol* 1962;35:245–261.

122. Khan MMR. Role of the "collated internal object" in perversion-formations. *Int J Psychoanal* 1969;50:555–565.

123. Khan MMR. *Alienation in perversions.* London: Hogarth Press, 1979.

124. Glover E. Aggression and sado-masochism. In: Rosen I, ed. *Pathology and treatment of sexual deviation: a methodological approach.* London: Oxford University Press, 1964;146–162.

125. Hoffman M. Drug addiction and "hypersexuality": related modes of mastery. *Compr Psychiatry* 1964;5:262–270.

126. Kernberg OF. Borderline personality organization. *J Am Psychoanal Assoc* 1967;15:641–685.

127. Kernberg OF. *Aggression in personality disorders and perversions.* New Haven: Yale University Press, 1992.

128. Kohut H. *The analysis of the self: a systematic approach to the psychoanalytic treatment of narcissistic personality disorders.* New York: International Universities Press, 1971.

129. McDougall J. Primal scene and sexual perversion. *Int J Psychoanal* 1972;53:371–384.

130. McDougall J. Identifications, neoneeds and neosexualities. *Int J Psychoanal* 1986;67:19–31.

131. Ovesey L, Person E. Gender identity and sexual psychopathology in men: a psychodynamic analysis of homosexuality, transsexualism, and transvestism. *J Am Acad Psychoanal* 1973;1:53–72.

132. Chasseguet-Smirgel J. Perversion, idealization and sublimation. *Int J Psychoanal* 1974;55:349–357.

133. Chasseguet-Smirgel J. Loss of reality in perversions—with special reference to fetishism. *J Am Psychoanal Assoc* 1981;29:511–534.

134. Goldberg A. A fresh look at perverse behavior. *Int J Psychoanal* 1975;56:335–342.

135. Goldberg A. *The problem of perversion: the view from self psychology.* New Haven, CT: Yale University Press, 1995.

136. Stolorow RD. The narcissistic function of masochism (and sadism). *Int J Psychoanal* 1975;56:441–448.

137. Stolorow RD. Psychosexuality and the representational world. *Int J Psychoanal* 1979;60:39–45.

138. Person E, Ovesey L. Transvestism: new perspectives. *J Am Acad Psychoanal* 1978;6:301–323.

139. Stoller RJ. *Perversion: the erotic form of hatred.* New York: Pantheon, 1975.

140. Glasser M. Some aspects of the role of aggression in the perversions. In Rosen I, ed. *Sexual deviation,* 2nd ed. Oxford: Oxford University Press, 1979:278–305.

141. Glasser M. Identification and its vicissitudes as observed in the perversions. *Int J Psychoanal* 1986;67:9–17.

142. Rosen I. The general psychoanalytic theory of perversion: a critical review. In: Rosen I, ed. *Sexual deviation,* 2nd ed. Oxford: Oxford University Press, 1979:29–64.

143. Rosen I. Perversion as a regulator of self-esteem. In: Rosen I, ed. *Sexual deviation,* 2nd ed. Oxford: Oxford University Press, 1979:65–78.

144. Coen SJ. Sexualization as a predominant mode of defense. *J Am Psychoanal Assoc* 1981;29:893–920.

145. Eber M. Don Juanism: A disorder of the self. *Bull Menninger Clin* 1981;45:307–316.

146. Socarides CW. *The preoedipal origin and psychoanalytic therapy of sexual*

perversions. Madison, CT: International Universities Press, 1988.

147. Hershey DW. On a type of heterosexuality, and the fluidity of object relations. *J Am Psychoanal Assoc* 1989;37:147–171.

148. Trop JL, Alexander R. The concept of promiscuity: a self psychological perspective. In: Stern EM, ed. *Psychotherapy and the promiscuous patient.* New York: Haworth Press, 1992:39–49.

149. Myers W. Sexual addiction. In: Dowling S, ed. *The psychology and treatment of addictive behavior.* Madison, CT: International Universities Press, 1994; 115–130.

150. Goodman A. Organic unity theory: the mind-body problem revisited. *Am J Psychiatry* 1991;148:553–563.

151. Goodman A. Organic unity theory: An integrative mind-body theory for psychiatry. *Theoret Med* 1997;18:357–378.

152. Gold PW, Goodwin FK, Chrousos GP. Clinical and biochemical manifestations of depression: relation to the neurobiology of stress (first of two parts). *N Engl J Med* 1988;319:348–353.

153. Kraemer GW. Causes of changes in brain noradrenaline systems and later effects on responses to social stressors in rhesus monkeys: the cascade hypothesis. In: Porter R, Bock G, Clark S, eds. *Antidepressants and Receptor Function.* (CIBA Foundation Symposium 123) New York: Wiley, 1986;216–233.

154. Post RM. Transduction of psychosocial stress into the neurobiology of recurrent affective disorder. *Am J Psychiatry* 1992;149:999–1010.

155. Mandell AJ, Knapp S. Asymmetry and mood, emergent properties of serotonin regulation. *Arch Gen Psychiatry* 1979;36:909–916.

156. Coccaro EF, Siever LJ, Klar HM, et al. Serotonergic studies in patients with affective and personality disorders. *Arch Gen Psychiatry* 1989;46:587–599.

157. Stein DJ, Hollander E, Liebowitz MR. Neurobiology of impulsivity and the impulse control disorders. *J Neuropsychiatry Clin Neurosci* 1993;5:9–17.

158. Blundell JE. Serotonin and appetite. *Neuropharmacology* 1984;23:1537–1552.

159. Sheard MH, Aghajanian GK. Stimulation of midbrain raphe neurons: behavioral effects of serotonin release. *Life Sci* 1968;7:19–25.

160. Harvey JA, Yunger LM. Relationship between telencephalic content of serotonin and pain sensitivity. In: Barchas J, Usdin E, eds. *Serotonin and behavior.* New York: Academic Press, 1973:179–189.

161. Akil H, Liebeskind JC. Monoaminergic mechanisms of stimulation produced analgesia. *Brain Res* 1975;94:279–296.

162. Cloninger CR. Neurogenetic adaptive mechanisms in alcoholism. *Science* 1987;236:410–416.

163. Ramsey NF, Van Ree JM. Reward and abuse of opiates. *Pharmacol Toxicol* 1992;71:81–94.

164. Wise RA. The role of reward pathways in the development of drug dependence. *Pharmacol Ther* 1987;35:227–262.

165. Herz A, Shippenberg TS. Neurochemical aspects of addiction: opioids and other drugs of abuse. *Alc Clin Exp Res* 1989;24:1724–1729.

166. Panksepp J, Herman B, Conner R, et al. The biology of social attachments: opiates alleviate separation distress. *Biol Psychiatry* 1978;13:607–618.

167. Amir S, Brown ZW, Amit Z. The role of endorphins in stress: evidence and speculations. *Neurosci Biobehav Rev* 1980;4:77–86.

168. Baile CA, McLaughlin CL, Della-Fera MA. Role of cholecystokinin and opioid peptides in control of food intake. *Physiol Rev* 1986;66:172–234.

169. Morley JE, Levine AS. Pharmacology of eating behavior. *Ann Rev Pharmacol Toxicol* 1985;25:127–146.

170. Morley JE, Levine AS, Rowland NE. Stress-induced eating. *Life Sci* 1983;32:2169–2182.

171. Pfaus JG, Gorzalka BB. Opioids and sexual behavior. *Neurosci Biobehav Rev* 1987;11:1–34.

172. Graeff FG. Neuroanatomy and neurotransmitter regulation of defensive behaviors and related emotions in mammals. *Brazilian Journal of Medical and Biological Research* 1994;27:811–829.

173. Chan-Palay V. *Cerebellar dentate nucleus: organization, cytology and transmitters.* Berlin: Springer-Verlag, 1977.

174. Beaudet A, Descarries L. Quantitative data on serotonin nerve terminals in adult rat neocortex. *Brain Res* 1976;111:301–309.

175. Aghajanian GK, Wang RY. Physiology and pharmacology of central serotonergic neurons. In: Lipton MA, DiMascio A, Killam KF, eds. *Psychopharmacology: a generation of progress.* New York: Raven Press, 1978;171–183.

176. Smith BH, Sweet WH. Monoaminergic regulation of central nervous system function: I. Noradrenergic systems. *Neurosurgery* 1978;3:109–119.

177. Gorenstein EE, Newman JP. Disinhibitory psychopathology: a new perspective and a model for research. *Psychol Rev* 1980;87:301–315.

178. Modell JG, Mountz JM, Beresford TP. Basal ganglia/limbic striatal and thalamocortical involvement in craving and loss of control in alcoholism. *J Neuropsychiatry Clin Neurosci* 1990;2:123–144.

179. Tarter RE, Alterman AI, Edwards KL.

Vulnerability to alcoholism in males: A behavior-genetic perspective. *J Stud Alcohol* 1985;4:329–356.

180. Eyzaguirre C, Fidone SJ. *Physiology of the nervous system,* 2nd ed. Chicago: Year Book Medical, 1975.

181. Schore AN. *Affect regulation and the origin of the self: the neurobiology of emotional development.* Hillsdale, NJ: Lawrence Erlbaum, 1994.

182. Watson SJ, Trujillo KA, Herman JP, et al. Neuroanatomical and neurochemical substrates of drug-seeking behavior: overview and future directions. In: Goldstein A, ed. *Molecular and cellular aspects of the drug addictions.* New York: Springer-Verlag, 1989:29–91.

183. Louilot A, Taghzouti K, Simon H, et al. Limbic system, basal ganglia, and dopaminergic neurons: executive and regulatory neurons and their role in the organization of behavior. *Brain Behav Evol* 1989;33:157–161.

184. Kraemer GW. Effects of differences in early social experience on primate neurobiological-behavioral development. In Reite M, Field T, ed. *The psychobiology of attachment and separation.* New York: Academic Press, 1985:135–161.

185. Edelman GM. *Neural darwinism: the theory of neuronal group selection.* New York: Basic Books, 1987.

186. Greenough WT, Black J, Wallace C. Experience and brain development. *Child Dev* 1987;58:539–559.

187. Kraemer GW, Ebert MH, Schmidt DE, et al. A longitudinal study of the effects of different rearing environments on cerebrospinal fluid norepinephrine and biogenic amine metabolites in rhesus monkeys. *Neuropsychopharmacology* 1989;2:175–189.

188. Kraemer GW, Ebert MH, Schmidt DE, et al. Strangers in a strange land: a psychobiological study of infant monkeys before and after separation from real or inanimate mothers. *Child Dev* 1991;62:548–566.

189. Greenough WT, Black JE. Induction of brain structure by experience: substrates for cognitive development. In: Gunnar MR, Nelson CA, eds. *Minnesota symposium on child psychology,* vol. 24. *Developmental behavioral neuroscience.* Hillsdale, NJ: Lawrence Erlbaum, 1992:155–200.

190. Tucker DM. Developing emotions and cortical networks. In: Gunnar MR, Nelson CA, eds. *Minnesota symposium on child psychology,* vol. 24. *Developmental behavioral neuroscience.* Hillsdale, NJ: Lawrence Erlbaum, 1992:75–128.

191. Higley JD, Suomi SJ, Linnoila M. A nonhuman primate model of type II excessive alcohol consumption? Part 1. Low cerebrospinal fluid

5-hydroxyin-doleacetic acid concentrations and diminished social competence correlate with excessive alcohol consumption. *Alcohol Clin Exp Res* 1996;20:629–642.

192. Higley JD, Linnoila M. A nonhuman primate model of excessive alcohol intake. Personality and neurobiological parallels of type I- and type II-like alcoholism. *Recent Dev Alcohol* 1997;13:191–219.

193. Fahlke C, Lorenz JG, Long J, et al. Rearing experiences and stress-induced plasma cortisol as early risk factors for excessive alcohol consumption in nonhuman primates. *Alcohol Clin Exp Res* 2000;24:644–650.

194. Kiernan RJ. Localization of function: the mind-body problem revisited. *J Clin Neuropsychol* 1981;3:345–352.

195. Luria AR. *The working brain.* New York: Basic Books, 1973.

196. Miller L. "Narrow localizationism" in psychiatric nosology. *Psychol Med* 1986;16:729–734.

197. Goodman A: The addictive process: a psychoanalytic understanding. *J Am Acad Psychoanal* 1993;21:89–105.

198. Money J. Use of androgen depleting hormone in the treatment of male sex offenders. *J Sex Res* 1970;6:165–172.

199. Freund K. Therapeutic sex drive reduction. *Acta Psychiatr Scand* 1980;287[Suppl]:5–38.

200. Hermann WM, Beach RC. Pharmacotherapy for sexual offenders: review of the actions of antiandrogens with special references to their psychic effects. *Mod Probl Pharmacopsychiatry* 1980;15:182–194.

201. Gagne P. Treatment of sex offenders with medroxyprogesterone acetate. *Am J Psychiatry* 1981;138:644–646.

202. Berlin FS, Meinecke CF. Treatment of sex offenders with antiandrogenic medications: conceptualization, review of treatment modalities, and preliminary findings. *Am J Psychiatry* 1981;138:601–607.

203. Berlin FS. Sex offenders: a biomedical perspective and a status report on biomedical treatment. In: Greer JG, Sturat IR, eds. The sexual aggressor: current perspectives on treatment. New York: Van Nostrand Reinhold, 1983:83–123.

204. Cordoba OA, Chapel JL. Medroxyprogesterone acetate antiandrogen treatment of hypersexuality in a pedophiliac sex offender. *Am J Psychiatry* 1983;140:1036–1039.

205. Wincze JT, Bansai S, Malamud M. Effects of medroxyprogesterone acetate on subjective arousal, arousal through erotic stimulation, and nocturnal penile tumescence in male sexual offenders. *Arch Sex Behav* 1986;15:293–305.

206. Bradford JM. Organic treatment for the male sexual offender. *Ann N Y Acad Sci* 1988;528:193–202.

207. Bradford JMW. The antiandrogen and hormonal treatment of sexual offenders. In: Marshall WL, Laws DR, Barbaree HE, eds. *Handbook of sexual assault: issues, theories, and treatment of the offender.* New York: Plenum, 1990:297–310.

208. Maletzky BM. Somatic therapies. In: Maletzky BM, ed. *Treating the sexual offender.* Newbury Park, CA: Sage, 1991.

209. Laschet U. Antiandrogen in the treatment of sex offenders: mode of action and therapeutic outcome. In: Zubin J, Money J, eds. *Contemporary sexual behavior: critical issues in the 1970s.* Baltimore: Johns Hopkins University Press, 1973:311–319.

210. Bancroft J, Tennent G, Loucas K, et al. The control of deviant sexual behavior by drugs: behavioural changes following estrogens and anti-androgens. *Br J Psychiatry* 1974;125:310–315.

211. Laschet U, Laschet L. Antiandrogens in the treatment of sexual deviations in men. *J Steroid Biochem* 1975;6:821–826.

212. Murray MAF, Bancroft JHH, Anderson DC, et al. Endocrine changes in male sexual deviants after treatment with antiandrogens, oestrogens or tranquilizers. *J Endocrinol* 1975;67:179–188.

213. Cooper AJ. A placebo-controlled trial of antiandrogen cyproterone acetate in deviant hypersexuality. *Compr Psychiatry* 1981;22:458–465.

214. Gilby R, Wolf L, Goldberg B. Mentally retarded adolescent sex offenders: a survey and pilot study. *Can J Psychiatry* 1989;34:452–458.

215. Bradford JMW, Pawlak A. The effects of cyproterone acetate in the treatment of the paraphilias. *Arch Sex Behav* 1993;22:383–402.

216. Bradford JMW, Pawlak A. The effects of cyproterone acetate on the sexual arousal patterns of pedophiles. *Arch Sex Behav* 1993;22:629–641.

217. Reid WH. Sexual disorders. In: Reid WH. *The treatment of psychiatric disorders: revised for the DSM–III–R.* New York: Brunner/Mazel, 1989:273–295.

218. Marshall WL, Jones R, Ward T, et al. Treatment outcome with sexual offenders. *Clin Psychol Rev* 1991;11:465–485.

219. Thibaut F, Cordier B, Kuhn J-M. Effect of a long-lasting gonadotrophin hormone-releasing hormone agonist in six cases of severe male paraphilia. *Acta Psychiatr Scand* 1993;87:445–450.

220. Thibaut F, Cordier B, Kuhn J-M. Gonadotrophin releasing hormone agonist in cases of severe paraphilia: a lifetime

treatment? *Psychoneuroendocrinology* 1996;21:411–419.

221. Rösler A, Witztum E. Treatment of men with paraphilia with a long-acting analogue of gonadotropin-releasing hormone. *N Engl J Med* 1998;338:416–422.

222. Briken P, Nika E, Berner W. Treatment of paraphilia with luteinizing hormone-releasing hormone agonists. *J Sex Marital Ther* 2001;27:45–55.

223. Krueger RB, Kaplan MS. Depotleuprolide acetate for treatment of paraphilias: a report of twelve cases. *Arch Sex Behav* 2001;30:409–422.

224. Federoff JP. Serotonergic drug treatment of deviant sexual interests. *Ann Sex Res* 1993;6:105–121.

225. Greenberg DM, Bradford JMW. Treatment of the paraphilic disorders: a review of the role of selective serotonin reuptake inhibitors. *Sex Abuse* 1997;9:349–360.

226. Bianchi MD. Fluoxetine treatment of exhibitionism [Letter]. *Am J Psychiatry* 1990;147:1089–1090.

227. Jorgensen VT. Cross-dressing successfully treated with fluoxetine [Letter]. *N Y State J Med* 1990;90:566–567.

228. Emmanuel NP, Lydiard RB, Ballenger JC. Fluoxetine treatment of voyeurism [Letter]. *Am J Psychiatry* 1991;148:950.

229. Lorefice LS. Fluoxetine treatment of a fetish. *J Clin Psychiatry* 1991;52:41.

230. Perilstein RD, Lipper S, Friedman LJ. Three cases of paraphilias responsive to fluoxetine treatment. *J Clin Psychiatry* 1991;52:169–170.

231. Greenberg DM, Bradford JMW, Curry S, et al. A comparison of treatment of paraphilias with three serotonin reuptake inhibitors: a retrospective study. *Bull Am Acad Psychiatry Law* 1996;24:525–532.

232. Abouesh A, Clayton A. Compulsive voyeurism and exhibitionism: a clinical response to paroxetine. *Arch Sex Behav* 1999;28:23–30.

233. Snaith RP, Collins SA. Five exhibitionists and a method of treatment. *Br J Psychiatry* 1981;138:126–130.

234. Casals-Ariet C, Cullen K. Exhibitionism treated with clomipramine [Letter]. *Am J Psychiatry* 1993;150:1273–1274.

235. Clayton AH. Fetishism and clomipramine [Letter]. *Am J Psychiatry* 1993;150:4.

236. Torres AR, de Abreu Cerquiera AT. Exhibitionism treated with clomipramine [Letter]. *Am J Psychiatry* 1993;150:1274.

237. Wawrose FE, Sisto TM. Clomipramine and a case of exhibitionism [Letter]. *Am J Psychiatry* 1992;149:843.

238. Bartova D, Nahumek K, Svestke J. Pharmacological treatment of deviant

sexual behavior. *Activitas Nervosa Superior (Praha)* 1978;20:72–74.

239. Cesnik JA, Coleman E. Use of lithium carbonate in the treatment of autoerotic asphyxia. *Am J Psychother* 1989;63:277–286.

240. Ward NG. Successful lithium treatment of transvestism associated with manic-depression. *J Nerv Ment Dis* 1975;161:204–206.

241. Federoff JP. Buspirone hydrochloride in the treatment of transvestic fetishism. *J Clin Psychiatry* 1988;49:408–409.

242. Eyres A. Transvestism: Employment of somatic therapy with subsequent improvement. *Dis Nerv Syst* 1960;1:52–53.

243. Kafka M. Psychopharmacologic treatments for nonparaphilic compulsive sexual disorders. *CNS Spectr* 2000;1:49–59.

244. Marks IM, Rachman S, Gelder MG. Methods for assessment of aversion treatment in fetishism with masochism. *Behav Res Ther* 1965;3:253–258.

245. Marks IM, Gelder MG, Bancroft JHJ. Sexual deviants two years after electric aversion. *Br J Psychiatry* 1970;117:173–185.

246. Evans DR. Masturbatory fantasy and sexual deviation. *Behav Res Ther* 1968;6:17–19.

247. Evans DR. Subjective variables and treatment effects in aversion therapy. *Behav Res Ther* 1970;8:147–152.

248. Fookes BH. Some experience in the use of aversion therapy in male homosexuality, exhibitionism, and fetishism-transvestism. *Br J Psychiatry* 1969;115:339–341.

249. Abel GG, Lewis DJ, Clancy J. Aversion therapy applied to taped sequences of deviant sexual behavior in exhibitionism and other sexual deviations: A preliminary report. *J Behav Ther Exp Psychiatry* 1970;1:59–66.

250. Birk L, Huddleston W, Miller E, et al. Avoidance conditioning in homosexuality. *Arch Gen Psychiatry* 1971;25:314–323.

251. MacCulloch MJ, Williams C, Birtles CJ. The successful application of aversion therapy to an adolescent exhibitionist. *J Behav Ther Exp Psychiatry* 1971;2:61–66.

252. Wijesinghe B. Massed aversion treatment of sexual deviance. *J Behav Ther Exp Psychiatry* 1977;8:135–137.

253. Quinsey VL, Bergersen SG, Steinman CM. Changes in physiological and verbal responses of child molesters during aversion therapy. *Can J Behav Sci* 1976;8:202–212.

254. Feldman MP, MacCulloch MJ. The aversion therapy treatment of a heterogeneous group of five cases of sexual deviation. *Acta Psychiatr Scand* 1968;44:113–123.

255. Callahan EJ, Leitenberg H. Aversion therapy for sexual deviation: contingent shock and covert sensitization. *J Abnorm Psychol* 1973;81:60–73.

256. Maletzky BM. "Assisted" covert sensitization in the treatment of exhibitionism. *J Consult Clin Psychology* 1974;42:34–40.

257. Maletzky BM. Self-referred versus court-referred sexually deviant patients: success with assisted covert sensitization. *Behav Ther* 1980;11:306–314.

258. Brownell KD, Hayes SC, Barlow DH. Patterns of appropriate and deviant sexual arousal: the behavioral treatment of multiple sexual deviations. *J Consult Clin Psychology* 1977;45:1144–1155.

259. Hayes SC, Brownell KD, Barlow DH. The use of self-administered covert sensitization in the treatment of exhibitionism and sadism. *Behav Ther* 1978;9:283–289.

260. Alford GS, Webster JS, Sanders SH. Covert aversion of two interrelated sexual practices: obscene phone calling and exhibitionism. A single case analyis. *Behav The* 1980;11:15–25.

261. Lamontagne Y, Lesage A. Private exposure and covert sensitization in the treatment of exhibitionists. *J Behav Ther Exp Psychiatry* 1986;17:197–201.

262. Abel GG, Osborn C. Stopping sexual violence. *Psychiatr Ann* 1992;22:301–306.

263. Hunter JA, Goodwin DW. The clinical utility of satiation therapy with juvenile offenders: variations and efficacy. *Ann Sex Res* 1992;5:71–80.

264. McConaghy N, Armstrong MS, Blaszczynski A. Expectancy, covert sensitization and imaginal desensitization in compulsive sexuality. *Acta Psychiatr Scand* 1985;72:176–187.

265. Marshall WL, Barbaree HE. Outcome of comprehensive cognitive-behavioral treatment programs. In: Marshall WL, Laws DR, Barbaree HE, eds. *Handbook of sexual assault: issues, theories, and treatment of the offender.* New York: Plenum, 1990:363–385.

266. Mathis JL, Collins M. Mandatory group therapy for exhibitionists. *Am J Psychiatry* 1970;126:1162.

267. Truax RA. Discussion of Mathis and Collins [ref. 266]. *Am J Psychiatry* 1970;126:1166.

268. Ganzarain R, Buchele BJ. Incest perpetrators in group therapy: a psychodynamic perspective. *Bull Menninger Clin* 1990;54:295–310.

269. Rosen I. Exhibitionism, scopophilia and voyeurism. In: Rosen I, ed. *Pathology and treatment of sexual deviation: a methodological approach.* London: Oxford University Press, 1964:293–350.

270. Witzig JS. The group treatment of male exhibitionists. *Am J Psychiatry* 1968;125:179–185.

271. Anonymous. *Abstinence and boundaries in S.A.A.* [booklet]. Minneapolis: Sex Addicts Anonymous, 1986.

272. Anonymous. *Suggestions for newcomers* [pamphlet]. Boston: The Augustine Fellowship, Sex and Love Addicts Anonymous, 1986.

273. Anonymous. *Sexaholics anonymous.* Simi Valley, CA: SA Lit, 1989.

274. Anonymous. *SCA—a program of recovery* [booklet]. New York: SCA, 1989.

275. Gabbard G. Paraphilias and sexual dysfunctions. In: Gabbard G. *Psychodynamic psychiatry in clinical practice.* Washington, DC: American Psychiatric Press, 1994:327–357.

276. Wise TN. Fetishism and transvestism. In: Karasu TB, ed. *Treatment of psychiatric disorders: a task force of the American Psychiatric Association,* vol. 1. Washington, DC: American Psychiatric Press, 1989:633–646.

277. Wakeling A. A general psychiatric approach to sexual deviation. In: Rosen I, ed. *Sexual deviation,* 2nd ed. Oxford: Oxford University Press, 1979:1–28.

278. Rosen I. Exhibitionism, scopophilia and voyeurism. In: Rosen I, ed. *Sexual deviation,* 2nd ed. Oxford: Oxford University Press, 1979:139–194.

279. Meyer V, Gelder MG. Behaviour therapy and phobic disorders. *Br J Psychiatry* 1963;109:19–28.

280. Adson PR. Treatment of paraphilias and related disorders. *Psychiatr Ann* 1992;22:299–300.

281. Kilmann PR, Sabalis RF, Gearing ML, et al. The treatment of sexual paraphilias: a review of outcome research. *J Sex Res* 1982;18:193–252.

282. Schwartz MF. Effective treatment for sex offenders. *Psychiatr Ann* 1992;22:315–319.

283. Protter B, Travin S. Sexual fantasies in the treatment of paraphilic disorders: a bimodal approach. *Psychiatr Q* 1987;58:279–297.

284. Travin S, Protter B. *Sexual perversion: integrative treatment approaches for the clinician.* New York: Plenum Press, 1993.

285. Travin S. Compulsive sexual behaviors. *Psychiatric Clin North Am* 1995;18:155–169.

286. Camus A. The myth of Sisyphus. In: Camus A. *The Myth of Sisyphus and other essays* (1955; O'Brien J, translator). New York: Vintage, 1991:1–138.

CHAPTER 31

Internet/Computer Addiction

ZEBULON TAINTOR

This chapter discusses issues relating to computers and the Internet, both as the subjects and tools for addiction and as tools in the treatment of other addictions. Addiction related to computers and the Internet as the medium is rarely involved; more frequently, addiction is related to the messages carried by the medium, especially sex, games, gambling, crime, identity manipulation, and substances of abuse. However, the end user experiences both the medium and the message together, and there are aspects of each that work in synergy to promote use.

DEFINITIONS

Internet/computer addiction is defined as such a strong involvement with a machine or what can be displayed on it that the usual criteria for impairment through addiction are met. The concept is somewhat controversial (actually coined by Ivan Goldberg in 1995 as a joke [1]) in that some might complain that there are (a) no substances involved with this sort of addiction, thus no physiologic withdrawal, and (b) computer overuse is a symptom of diagnostic entities already included in standard classifications (2). However, the support group Dr. Goldberg set up (and many others since) attracted many people who described themselves as "computer addicted." The lay public understands the term and describes people who have it without other obvious diagnoses. The public sees a similarity to gambling and/or sex addiction, which, indeed, are related. The concept has been promoted in other mental health professions (3). It is evident that the usual addiction categories of use, abuse, dependency and addiction pertain to computer and Internet use. Initial attempts to define these categories by the amount of time spent on the computer have been abandoned for two reasons: (a) a general increase in time spent using computers, and (b) lack of measurable impairment related to time spent. Although computers preceded the Internet (which now is available without needing a computer) the terms *computer addiction* and *Internet addiction* are used interchangeably to cover the range of what is occurring. Dr. Goldberg's recommended *pathologic Internet use* is more exact, but hasn't caught on.

Use

Computers and the Internet are useful for communication, computation, and information. Of these, communication has become the most time intensive, with an estimated 40 million Americans spending at least 2 hours daily writing and receiving e-mail (4). The arrival of new technologies is likely to intensify communication and to blur some technologic boundaries. Instant messaging by computer has soared, with America Online (AOL) reporting that 195 million people use its service, generating more than 1.6 billion messages a day. Instant messaging is used extensively with handheld devices, which increasingly blend telephone and computer abilities with Internet access to offer images (5). Other figures show less change, for example, online sales, while increasing, are only 1.5% of total sales (6). Use figures are confusing as the boom-and-bust of dot coms was accompanied by wild exaggeration and pessimism. ComScore Media Matrix tracks web site usage as a way of attracting advertisers and setting rates. It revised its figures for the fourth quarter of 2002 upward to take into account web access from the workplace: there were 107.6 million unique (separate individual) visitors to its web site, followed by 100.6 million to Microsoft sites, 101.9 million to Yahoo sites, and so on (7). The reader will note the discrepancy (65%) between AOL's report of its instant messaging users and the ComScore web visitor estimate.

Perhaps the best estimates of computer usage come from George Lundberg, editor-in-chief of *Medscape*. Addressing the American Association for Technology in Psychiatry in May 2003, he suggested that in a population well exposed to computers educationally, at work, and at home, that one-third uses computers and the Internet often, one-third occasionally, and one-third rarely. Students of addiction will note some resonance with statistics of use by a population exposed to various drugs. Use and attitudes will be very much affected by the success or failure of efforts to control spam (unwanted flood of e-mail) and computer viruses and worms.

Abuse

Abuse is use plus problems. It is not necessarily time-consuming and therefore more related to the message than the medium. Impairment is measured in terms of the resulting problems. As with trying an unknown substance from a not necessarily trustworthy source, risk is underestimated, impulses should be controlled better, and there is a price for naiveté. Use of computers and the Internet require a level of literacy and education, although that requirement is decreasing as software has become more user-friendly. Education about computers typically does not touch on potential overuse. It should, although that may be no more protective than knowing the potential harmful effects of a frequently abused substance. Despite injunctions not to open an attachment unless one is expecting it, there are enough people eager for wicked screensavers that they will blithely open such attachments from strangers or friends (whose e-mail has been taken over by a virus) who would not be expected to send them such things. As noted in the drive against spam, there are enough gullible responders to messages offering to transfer millions to one's bank account, just as there are enough buyers of treatments for breast and penis enlargement to make sending such messages worthwhile. It takes only a few minutes to lose a substantial amount of money through online gambling or to become the victim of a credit card scam. The role of the medium is to make it possible to be robbed or otherwise exploited at any time of day or night without leaving the safety of one's own home. Abuse at the job, in the sense of use + trouble, can be more than just violating policies prohibiting access to certain web sites (e.g., pornography), but can include being found out spending excessive time on permitted but non job-related web sites, personal e-mails, playing solitaire or other games, etc. As access and key strokes can be tracked, the user can be found out and disciplined. "Cyberloafing" is estimated to cost 50 billion/year in lost productivity.

Criminals perpetrating cybercrime (viruses, credit card fraud, etc.) are also computer abusers, although they engender anger rather than sympathy, and the clinical attention they get is more usually a forensic psychiatric evaluation. Predators, sexual and otherwise, also fall into the category of abusers and combine their online work with meetings in person that can have disastrous results.

Dependency

More time is involved in dependency, and the pattern is the usual one seen by the addictionologist: an increasing amount of time is spent in the condition associated with the activity, increasingly the person's life is oriented around it, and relationships tend to grow or die away depending on the other person's attitude toward the activity and ability to add to it. Habituation and tolerance set in. Although computer and Internet use are not associated with an altered state of consciousness produced by an exogenous chemical substance, there is an altered state of consciousness from endogenous chemicals associated with the activity, for example, sexual arousal, gambling, and games. Computers lend themselves to identity falsification, which can bring its own sort of "high." While getting high on a substance can be a path to living out a fantasy, prolonged e-mail exchanges enable claiming an elaborating an identity far beyond what can be done in a chance encounter in a bar. Dependency is a need to be devoting considerable time to being at the computer, online or playing games.

Addiction

This term is reserved for severe dependency. The afflicted individual is described as unable to function without being at the computer for long periods of time and is severely impaired. While the absence of an exogenous chemical and accompanying enzymatic changes may preclude the use of the term addiction in the strictest sense, there is a withdrawal syndrome of nervousness, agitation, aggression, insomnia, and varying amounts of depression. The end of a life can be taken as a measure of severity, and there are documented cases of suicide and homicide after being denied use of a computer game, as well as playing to the point of death from exhaustion (8).

Clinicians are seeing patients with complaints in all the problematic categories above and major treatment facilities have developed special programs.

EPIDEMIOLOGY

This discussion does not include comorbidities, which may occur frequently. Recognition of psychopathology understandably lags Internet use, itself new. Technological changes, for example, use of cable and DSL lines, make both use and subsequent complications data into a moving target. Inevitably norms on rate of use are superseded shortly by reports of higher use.

Web searches show an enormous amount of interest. One carried out on August 27, 2003 (the date for all searches reported here) yielded the following number of hits on msn.search: computer addiction, 221,283; computer dependency, 106,798; computer abuse, 838,742.

There are no large-scale studies of psychopathology associated with computer and/or Internet use. To the extent that problems are recognized, such as sending spam, they are criminalized. Research funding is scant. Sources outside the industry have higher priorities. The computer industry, eager to encourage use, has minimized cybercrime (now estimated at "untold billions" [9]) along with hardware, software, and privacy problems, so it is unlikely to start research and/or educational campaigns on computer addiction. Among those interested, the general debate is on how much the Internet is an integrating force bringing society together versus a fragmenting force that isolates family members from one another and substitutes virtual relationships for real ones. Studies support both views. Morgan and Cotten found decreased depressive symptoms when college freshman were using the Internet for communication, but increased depression when playing games, shopping, or doing research (10). Young, whose 1997 presentation on Internet addiction lent new momentum to the concept, devised a 20-item questionnaire for Internet addiction. Items were based on the idea that it was an impulse control disorder (like pathologic gambling), but including some items designed to elicit behavior seen in alcoholics (11). In Korea, where more than 30% (50% by late 2002 [12]) of households have super high-speed Internet services (ADSL) and 69% of teenagers spend more than 2 hours daily playing computer games, use of Young's scale yielded (on a sample of 13,588 users of a major portal site) an addiction rate of 3.5%. Internet addicts tried to escape from reality, to access the Internet when stressed, and to show more dysfunctional behavior. They reported the highest degree of loneliness, depressed mood, and compulsivity compared to nonaddicts. "They seemed more vulnerable to interpersonal dangers than others, showing an unusually close feeling for strangers" (13).

The prime demographic variables affecting the epidemiology of computer/Internet addiction are age, education, and economic status. As with other addictions, men seem to be more at risk than women, in that two-thirds of Internet users are men, accounting for 77% of time online, but this difference may diminish (14).

Adolescence poses the same risk factors for this sort of addiction as for any other, enhanced by the fact that young people pick up technologic savvy very quickly and often are able to outmaneuver their parents. College students seem particularly vulnerable (15). Norms for computer and Internet use in the young are constantly shifting to greater use. This greater engagement (as contrasted to dependency) makes it likely that behavioral addiction may be mild and self-reports "classifying individuals as exhibiting pathologic computer use using checklists based upon adaptations of the *DSM* [American Psychiatric Association's *Diagnostic and Statistical Manual of Mental Disorders*] criteria for pathological gambling is likely to overestimate the number of people addicted to computing activities" (16). Young people are used to computers and the Internet in the way baby boomers grew up with television. The Internet is more interactive and thus reinforcing. The question to ask in assessing use and overuse is what is being reinforced.

While education and economic status generally are associated with lower risk for mental illness, they both presently work paradoxically to add to risk. One must be literate in computers and the Internet to use them effectively. Higher levels of education, to the degree they are associated with purposeful behavior, may diminish risk. However, one must be at least computer literate to use a computer well. Some knowledge of search engines is needed to find the right web sites. Economic factors strongly affect epidemiology. As of September 2001, 79% of the wealthiest families were using the Internet, as contrasted to 25% of the poorest, with use increasing more among the wealthiest (17). None of the phenomena described here can take place without money. One must be able to buy a computer, games, Internet service, and the like. Purveyors of the potentially addicting content are out to get more money from the users and pitch their content to varying tastes and economic status. As with addicting substances and other commercial enterprises, there are loss leaders, free come-ons, and subtle means of extracting money such as free registration. Economics also affect web content: There are some interests working hard (with varying success) to make sure some things are not for sale, such as wine across state lines, music, legal medications from other countries, unprescribed medications, some gambling, and unsolicited advertisements that constitute spam (which currently makes up to 50% of all e-mails). As a result, reported transactions in some areas represent only the tip of the iceberg.

SYMPTOMS OF INTERNET ADDICTION

There are various lists of symptoms (e.g., www.addictions.org/internet.htm), but they come down to excessive time on the Internet, feeling unhappy when off the Internet, and impaired role performance (relationships, work, etc.) as an apparent result of less time and interest being available. Other signs include, for example, preoccupation with the Internet when offline; inability to control amount of use; feeling restless and irritable when attempting to cut down use; using the Internet to escape from problems or to relieve a poor mood; lying to others about the extent of one's use; jeopardizing or risking the loss of a significant relationship, work, or opportunity because of the Internet (http://www.breining.edu/ce1301p1.pdf). As with most dependencies, impairment is often more obvious to others than to the potential patient, although self-reports include an awareness of compulsive use, using the Internet to escape negative feelings, time distortion, accelerated intimacy, and feeling uninhibited when on line.

Surveys on Internet users find 4% to 10% of users meet criteria for "Internet addiction," defined as having at least five of the following indicators: preoccupation with the Internet; increasing amount of time spent online; failure to cut back use with concomitant restlessness, moodiness, or depression; staying online longer than originally intended; running the risk of losing a job, relationship, or other opportunity because of Internet use; lying to conceal the extent of Internet use; and/or using the Internet to escape negative feelings. Subgroups include cybersex addiction (viewing pornography), cyber-relational addiction (online relationships become more important than those in one's physical world), gaming (gambling, stock trading, shopping, etc.), and information overload. There are web pages that offer a chance to evaluate one's Internet use as possibly pathologic and offer both education and online counseling, with some urging face-to-face counseling as a way of becoming less involved with the Internet (see www.netaddiction.com).

Case Examples

A wide range of psychopathology has been reported, including:

- A 21-year-old Washington State University student who played an online fantasy game for 36 hours straight, had a psychotic episode from lack of sleep, and ended up in a psychiatric unit.
- A 29-year-old in middle management who played an online game at work until he got fired and ended up living back home with his mother.
- A manager who was fired from two computer companies because he couldn't stop playing *Dungeons and Dragons* at work.
- A 16-year-old who became suicidal when his parents took away his modem. (18)

Internet Characteristics

Some factors promote overuse and addiction. The Internet is

- Always available, 24 hours a day, 7 days a week, lending itself to impulsive access and marathon sessions.
- Convenient, with no need to leave one's home or workplace (a surprising amount of downloads occur during work time).
- Inexpensive, with the only cost being to pay one's Internet service provider.
- Rewarding in that it is content rich, with a combination of web sites that are consistently present and calculated to please, some interactivity, and a continuous flow of new sites that offer novelty. Searches often show thousands of sites contain key words of interest. Most sites offer attractive and changing colors and sounds. Internet responses are getting faster and faster as speed of transmission increases.
- Controllable, with the user being able to go wherever desired without feeling threatened (especially as many users are oblivious or don't care about leaving a trail of sites accessed).
- Escapist, in that the sites of interest to the potentially addicted, offer a welcoming reality in which all sexual partners are attractive and willing, games are fascinating, bets seem likely to be won, and so on. It also offers a chance to escape one's own identity. One can be anonymous or misrepresent whatever characteristics one chooses. Women are said to be attracted to the Internet because they can act like men (19). Introverts often choose to become extroverts (20).
- Validating, in that one finds that which caters to one's interests and tastes, thus verifying that these are legitimate because there are other people who somehow share these interests and tastes.

What is not so obvious is the enormity of the number of interactions occurring constantly. Music downloading recently has centered around a site called KaZaA.com. It is usual to see that four million users are signed on at once. Yet many observers don't stop to think how many users might be signed on to get drugs of abuse via the Internet as a way of accounting for their widespread use, seeking instead to limit physician prescribing powers.

These features point to the power of the Internet/computer medium. What is available on the medium includes content related to abused substances, games and gambling, sex, chat groups, and information itself. There are all sorts of combinations: the number of sites mentioning "Cybersex" (862,000) has a variant in the 19,900 sites mentioning both "cybersex" and "casino."

Psychological risk factors for Internet/computer addiction involve a combination of susceptibility to the general issues above and to the specific content.

Substances

One can infer that the web and e-mail are used to set up sites for buying and selling illicit substances and that those so involved have developed codes to avoid detection. A study by the United Nations International Narcotics Control Board (21), issued February 20, 2002, described how such codes operate in chat rooms to keep wholesalers, retailers, and users in touch. Other web sites describe how to make or refine cocaine, heroin, and other substances at home. Although some of the information is patently false, other sites offer recipes that seem likely to produce good results. While buying codeine and heroin online yields few hits, there are 61 hits for ecstasy, of which more than half seem to promise delivery, often within a day. A search for buying marijuana online yields 520 hits, many of which promise delivery and offer seeds for growing at home. Although a search for buying methadone online was not very fruitful, it is stocked in many online pharmacies, so the paucity of hits may simply be its relative lack of profitability. A search for buying OxyContin online yielded 43 hits, with many sites offering the lowest prices and next day delivery. This represents a conservative estimate, because many other web sites offer OxyContin in a way calculated to avoid detection by search engines. Thus there is little change in a year from a 2002 *Time* magazine story (22) in which a reporter found prescription drug sales for OxyContin, methadone, codeine, testosterone, anabolic steroids, and other substances in a few hours and who concluded it is possible to order thousands of dollars of opiates online. OxyContin is described as causing 500 to 1,000 deaths a year, part of the rapidly increasing use of narcotics (an estimated 2 million recreational users in 2001) and devastating areas like Appalachia (that previously were protected by geographic isolation and relatively low returns from face-to-face marketing) has so severe a problem that regulations have been suggested to limit prescriptions (23). While the music industry sues to prevent file sharing (24), and drug companies and pharmacies work to prevent online purchases of inexpensive medications from Canada (25), such activities do not engender much law enforcement activity. Officials cite a lack of resources to deal with the 183 percent increase (from 1995 to 2002 in emergency room visits tied to prescription drug abuse, http://abcnews.go.com/sections/living/Business/csm_drugabuse_031006.html). Perhaps this is a measure of the economic interests at stake in the other activities. Online pharmacies promise prescriptions for Viagra, phendimetrazine, Soma, and other drugs, and offer a free online consultation before purchase to get somewhat around the issue of consultation. Many sites offer Xanax and other habit-forming drugs at "80% off of U.S. prices" and say that no prescription is necessary (although anyone signing up for membership in the plan must be at least 18 years old). Internet sales are cited as the prime source of counterfeit medicines (26).

Other substances available on the Internet are unregulated and may contain chemicals that are habit-forming and addictive. Spam offering herbal remedies for breast and/or penis enlargement are endemic. A new disease, such as severe acute respiratory syndrome (SARS), quickly engenders a host of unscientific and unproven remedies that nonetheless sell well enough that they are promoted (27). Civil litigation for deceptive marketing has not been used much, as the senders often cannot be found, have negligible assets to seize, and often are several steps ahead of the enforcers (28). A recent study of the major herbal remedies available on the Internet (29) noted the ease of availability of such substances as valerian, ginseng, kava kava, and St. John's wort, offered with misleading claims for efficacy in treating anxiety, stress, and depression that violate existing, but unenforced, regulations. Addiction has been described for the first three herbs. Many sites urge customers to try free samples of various substances.

Games

Electronic games have developed rapidly from their pinball arcade ancestors, with about 1,000 introduced yearly and annual sales of $10.3 billion in 2002 (up 10% from 2001). In 2003, approximately 33% of games carry warnings about sexual or violent content, compared with just 5% 3 years ago (30). A big seller is *Grand Theft Auto* in which the game link to drug abuse and sociopathy is clear as players roam the city delivering cocaine to crime bosses and soliciting favors from prostitutes (30). Games are also linked to gambling in that players pay to participate in games of "skill" (including Internet games) that are legal in all states but Arizona, Iowa, Louisiana, and Vermont and can win money. Amounts of skill and luck needed vary for each game; some are labeled "gambling" (see http://www.absolutefreebies.com/gaming/make_money_games.html).

There is a debate about the worth of video games (e.g., whether they promote visual observation skills [32] or that action games promote violence). Proponents claim that the roles and relationships developed in fantasy can help one overcome problems and otherwise improve real life. This may be true in some cases, although other players in a game may be motivated to act out their psychopathic urges so as to be less troubled by them in real life. Virtual reality has been reported to be useful in treating various psychiatric conditions, especially phobias (33). Games provide particularly rich visual rewards. Game players are mostly young (age <18 years = 37.9%; age 18 to 35 years = 39.5%; only 22.7% are age 36 years or older). Adolescents in various developed countries spend an average of 28 (Netherlands) to 65 (Israel) minutes a day playing games. The best-selling games are action (42.1%), sports (19.5%), and racing (16.6%) oriented. Players spend an increasing amount of time playing online (37%), often with other players (34). About one-third of Everquest players

surveyed spend more time at it than on their paying jobs. The common element of all games is fantasy. One is in a different, usually attractive (or there would be no sale) reality, often with different personal characteristics and usually greater powers. However, the debate about games should not be about their intrinsic worth any more than this chapter is about the worth of the Internet, but rather about the significance and consequences of excessive use. More time spent playing games is associated with a person's withdrawing into fantasy. There simply is less time to do anything else. Sometimes the fantasies are so strong that the role being played spills over into reality, as in the report of Koreans fighting in games on the Internet and later meeting to fight face to face (12). Multilayer online gaming took hold as of November 2002 with the Sims Family Online with 430,000 subscribers, 20 million copies sold, and users reporting spending up to 5 hours a night online (35).

Gambling

The Internet has greatly increased the volume of betting, which has made it possible for bookmakers to earn real money, but has also provided bettors with sites where they can get important information (e.g., The Rx.com, ESPN.com). Offshore betting is the rule, with immunity from prosecution for activities that are illegal in the United States. Enforcers are able to go after bank and credit card transactions and American bookmakers have to conceal their identities, lest they be arrested on returning to the United States (36). Although traditional gambling has adapted to the Internet with online casinos (with thousands of sites, ranked and rated on review sites), there are many new forms that blur the distinction between games and gambling. There are more ways of winning than money. However, money lost gaming on the Internet is a convenient measure of impairment (see Abuse, above) and a prime motivator for treatment for gambling. Overall, Internet casinos were reckoned to have had revenue of $4.2 billion in 2003 despite increasing enforcement (37), which probably will engender new evasive tactics. Although there are day traders who make a living at it, day traders often present with the usual symptoms of Internet addiction and have lost legally amounts of money similar to those lost illegally by typical Internet gamblers.

Sex

Sexual content on the Internet has been described as its most dependable and best moneymaker (38). It has many manifestations and uses, some therapeutic (39). It is estimated that there are 2 million sexually addicted Internet users, both in and out of recovery. One of 10 respondents to an MSNBC.com poll confessed to being an Internet sex addict, with most going online to escape their daily routines (40). There are three basic forms of delivery. First, are online exchanges of pornography in snapshot and video formats. This exchange may take place via e-mail, newsgroups, or home pages. The second is synchronous communication via chat groups or interactive home pages. The third is downloadable files, videotapes, or videodiscs that can be ordered online (www.ncsac.org/cybersex.htm). The Internet can also lead to meetings, some of which are predatory, with disastrous results (41–43). Men are thought to be more likely to view cyberporn, while women are more likely to engage in erotic chat. Hallmarks of this problem are using anonymous communication to engage in sexual fantasies typically not carried out in real life, hiding online interactions from one's partner, masturbating while online, and preferring cybersex as a primary form of sexual gratification. Risk factors include low self-esteem, social incompetence, distorted body image, untreated sexual dysfunction, and/or prior sexual addiction. Sex addicts often use the Internet as a way of avoiding expensive 900-lines, the fear of being seen in adult bookstores, or the fear of disease from prostitutes ("the only virus you can get is from a dirty laptop"). While cybersex is "safe," one sign of excess and potential problems is that 70% of all e-porn traffic occurs during the 9 AM to 5 PM workday (44). The market is highly differentiated, with a language of its own that caters to those who know what they're looking for, as can be seen from the following search results: pornography, 4,320,000 hits; pornography + Internet, 79,500 hits; orgasmic dysfunction, 23,900 hits; "erectile dysfunction," 312,000 hits; "sexual dysfunction," 271,000 hits; "sexual dysfunction" + Internet, 79,500 hits; "bondage and discipline," 313,000 hits; B&D, 175,000 hits; BDSM, 6,430,000 hits. Much of the sex available on the Internet is free, either as come-ons for pay sites or placed there by sex-style advocacy groups. Nonetheless, people choose to pay for perceived better thrills, just as they are willing to pay more for cars, watches, and other luxury goods.

Chat Groups

Also known as cyber-relational addiction, this problem entails overinvolvement in online relationships, which take up more time and become more important than real-life relationships with family and friends. In many instances, this leads to marital discord and instability. Identity issues may range from the blatant to the subtle. Role theorists argue that we have no "self" as such, just different masks we wear in response to various social situations. The Internet offers a new set of social situations to which people respond by grabbing for new masks. Because most communication is still just in words without other means of verification, people exercise wide and surprising choices, often with great verisimilitude, such as the 15-year-old who was ranked #1 for giving legal advice (45). Chat groups, even with supposedly nonsexual foci such as on the works of Jane Austen, often are pickup spots, and often are populated by the underaged (46). Many chat groups are blatantly sexual, as described by Nicholas Thompson: " . . . in almost all of them, users mainly flirt or talk about sex. The chat rooms aren't much more than a sprawling singles bar with sec-

tions for every sexual fetish known to humanity—and, it often seems, a few others that must have just been dreamed up" (47).

PREVENTION

The Internet poses special challenges to understanding the world of the addict and the "scene."

- *Size, scope, and volume of use:* The Internet is filled with words and pictures to which users relate specifically. Those who don't spend much time on the Internet (as inevitably is the case with those who are getting on with their real lives and work), typically underestimate the scale of activity involved and scoff at the notion that "millions" of people are doing this or that on the Internet.

- *Excessive use:* Typically the virtues of the Internet are cited to mask the issue of time spent and resulting impairment. For example, much is made of online help and the potential for e-therapy. A rough idea of the ratio of what is offered to possible sources of help online is the number of sites mentioning "Cybersex" (862,000) compared to those mentioning "cybersex addiction" (about 1,600). The Internet has many clear benefits, but they are not the problem.

- *Technology:* Prevention depends on appreciating the technology well enough to understand what computer/Internet addicts do, the effectiveness of efforts to prevent them from doing it, and what they will do next.

- *Ineffective laws, regulations, and enforcement:* Many things offered on the Internet are illegal. While enforcement lags and seems dispirited and desultory, the main problem may be that offenders can now move so fast that even determined (not yet available because of different approaches) enforcement may not be able to keep up with them. The few swindlers who have been prosecuted often have managed several more schemes since the one for which they are prosecuted. Most simply never are caught, staying several e-mail addresses ahead of detection (48).

- *Limiting access:* The simplest maneuver is to limit access to the computer, or to allow it only under observation (such as moving the computer from a bedroom to the living room). The government of Thailand tried a computer game curfew in the summer of 2003, from 10 PM to 6 AM, shutting down servers and Internet cafes (49). There are dozens of web site-blocking software packages (e.g., ChildWeb Guardian, Chaperon 2000, WiseChoice) to which one may subscribe for periodic updates. There are specific programs for particular problems, such as CyberPatrol, Netnanny, and Surfwatch, for sex addiction. The programs prevent access to unwanted or unexpected sites, depending on the presence of certain words or content. While some ingenious ways around the blocks have been devised, the net effect slows the flood to less than a trickle. During recovery from the addiction, other software programs that monitor Internet use without blocking sites can be used. For purchasing software, the games industry introduced a five-category rating system in 1994: EC = early childhood; E = for everyone over age 6 years; T = teens; M = for age 17 years and older; AO = adults only. Responding to criticisms, especially on "T" content, the system is now more detailed, specifying, for example, that violence is either "comic" or "fantasy." However, complaints continue. Those wishing to know much about a game may before allowing its use may have to sift through gamers' reviews on Amazon.com (34).

- *Community education:* Although the popular press has called attention to computer/Internet addiction, the effort should be sustained and involve the professional community more as a planned public mental health priority.

TREATMENT

Treatment for Internet/computer addiction is like treatment for any other addiction, involving professional involvement, use of medication to treat symptoms, and self-help. Twelve-step methods are frequently used. There are some special features described below.

Online

The Internet abounds in sites that provide education for patients, families, and significant others. There are online meetings, recovery discussion groups, and combinations of online help with face-to-face meetings. The term "computer addicts anonymous" elicits 10,051 hits. For sexual addiction the National Council on Sexual Addiction and Compulsivity maintains online resources (www.ncsac.org). In using the Internet to combat Internet addiction, clinicians must guard against dependency on the treatment. One study of a virtual reality online treatment program revealed a high rate of self-described Internet addiction (50).

Face-to-Face

Treatment for Internet/computer addiction is similar to treatment for other addictions as described elsewhere in this volume, so only a few considerations need be mentioned.

Medication

There are no special considerations regarding medication, although depression (51) is more closely associated with Internet overusage as 30% of self-reported computer addicts say they have come to depend on the Internet as an escape from negative feelings. Anxiety appears in those who feel that at least the technologic revolution, possibly the explosion of knowledge, and perhaps life in general,

are passing them by. Often the anxiety-prone are actually somewhat computer-phobic, and show reaction formation as they force themselves to use it. They keep looking for what they think they are missing. Usually they benefit more from reassurance that many productive people use the Internet sparingly than from medication. Because Internet overusage is associated with marathon sessions, it is important to restore a normal sleep–wake routine, in which medication may help. Internet/computer addicts who have psychotic symptoms as a result of sleep deprivation or a preference for virtual reality may be helped by antipsychotics.

Individual Psychotherapy

Sessions must explore the many different reasons the patient is involved with what is on the monitor instead of reality—both the attractions of the former and what problems exist in with the latter. As with all addictions, impairment may be more apparent to onlookers than to the patient and the usual rationalizations are harder to refute because the Internet has many positive sides. Most interesting and challenging is exploring the question of one's identity on the Internet as contrasted to real life, which is likely to be quite well differentiated. Using the list of reasons the Internet lends itself to overuse in taking a history points to directions to be taken in psychotherapy. Behavioral and cognitive approaches are likely to be as effective as in other addictions.

Group Psychotherapy

It is important to prevent sessions from turning technical, which both promotes Internet use and provides a vehicle for one-upmanship.

Self-Help Groups

These are best kept as much offline as possible because use of the Internet may still be reinforcing lack of engagement in real life. More data are needed on why some patients would choose (besides, e.g., convenience or cost) to get treatment online rather than face-to-face. One small study in Taiwan suggests such patients tend to be younger, better educated, first-time users of services and to have more anxiety disorders than patients seen in a real clinic (who tended to have more mood disorders) (52).

Reimbursement

Although there is no reimbursement or diagnostic code for Internet computer/addiction, services can be billed under the general diagnoses of impulse control and compulsive disorders. Because comorbidities abound, the other diagnos(es) may be billed while they and the computer/Internet addiction are being treated.

PROGNOSIS

The prognosis for any individual depends on the strength of the attraction of the virtual world versus the attraction of the real world. It also depends on ego strength, motivation, intelligence (especially abstracting ability), and other personal assets that can lead to getting in the real world whatever one is seeking in the virtual world, especially a preferred identity. As with other addictions, a support system and high-quality treatment are important determinants of outcome.

The prognosis for the diagnosis actually being accepted into the standard nomenclature depends in part on further research. Research in this area is not costly, although correlations with physiologic and chemical variables would help validation. There should be some urgency, because the cost of electronic devices continues to decrease while their capabilities increase, bandwidth increases, communication gets faster, and content becomes more stimulating and increasingly directed at the limbic system. Presently unanticipated future developments are likely.

REFERENCES

1. Mitchell P. Internet addiction: genuine diagnosis or not? *Lancet* 2000;355: 632.
2. Shaffer HJ, Hall MN, Vander Bilt J. "Computer addiction": a critical consideration. *Am J Orthopsychiatry* 2000;70(2):162–168.
3. Christensen MH, Orzack MH, Babington LM. Computer addiction. When monitor becomes control center. *J Psychosoc Nurs Ment Health Serv* 2001;39(3):40–7.
4. Clark D. New inventions are designed to solve problems of old ones. *Wall Street Journal* 2003;Feb 20:B7.
5. Quain JR. Instant messaging moves beyond chat to multimedia. *New York Times* 2003;May 15:G6.
6. Bloomberg News. Internet sales rise as share of all sales. *New York Times* 2003;Aug 25:C6.
7. Hansell S. Ratings agency says it erred in measuring web site use. *New York Times* 2003;Feb 24:C1.
8. Man dies after playing computer games non-stop. *Sidney Morning Herald* 2002;Oct 10.
9. Tedeschi B. E-commerce report. *New York Times* 2003;Jan 27:C4.
10. Morgan C, Cotten SR. The relationship between Internet activities and depressive symptoms. *Cyberpsychol Behav* 2003;6(2):133–142.
11. Young KS. Internet addiction: symptoms, evaluation, and treatment. In: Vande Creek L, Jackson T, eds. *Innovations in clinical practice: a source book, vol. 17.* Sarasota, FL: Professional Resource Press, 1999:19–31.
12. French H. Korea's real rage for virtual games. *New York Times* 2002;Oct 9:A8.
13. Whang LS, Lee S, Chang G. Internet over-users' psychological profiles: a behavior sampling analysis on Internet addiction. *Cyberpsychol Behav* 2003;6(2):143–150.
14. Morahan-Martin J. The gender gap in Internet use: why men use the Internet more than women—a literature review. *Cyberpsychol Behav* 1998;1(1):3–10.
15. Kandell JJ. Internet addiction on campus: the vulnerability of college students. *Cyberpsychol Behav* 1998;1(1):11–18.
16. Charlton JP. A factor-analytic investigation of computer "addiction" and engagement. *Br J Psychol* 2002;93[Pt 3]:329–344.
17. Guernsey L. A dissent on the digital divide. *New York Times* 2003;Sep 8:G4.
18. Walden A. The web can become a trap for heavy online users. *Poughkeepsie (NY) Journal* 2002;Feb 19:7A.
19. Grigoradis V. The casual sex revolution: how the Internet took the sting out of sleeping with strangers. *New York Magazine* 2003;Jan 13:17–20.
20. Amichai-Hamburger Y, Wainapel G, Fox S. "On the Internet no one knows I'm an introvert": extroversion, neuroticism, and Internet interaction. *Cyberpsychol Behav* 2002;5(2):125–128.
21. International Narcotics Control Board. Globalization and new technologies: challenges to drug law enforcement in the twenty-first century. In: *Report of the International Narcotics Control Board for 2001. Issued February 27, 2002.* New York: United Nations Publication Sales No. E. 02.XI.1. Available online at www.incb.org.
22. Reaves J. Clicking for a fix: drugs online. *Time* 2002;Feb 27.
23. Harris G. Drug panel rejects please to curb sales of a widely abused painkiller. *New York Times* 2003;Sep 11:C1.
24. Wingfield N, Smith E. The high cost of sharing. *Wall Street Journal* 2003; Sep 9:B1.
25. Heinzl M, Carlisle T. Canadian pharmacies vs. big drug makers. *Wall Street Journal* 2003;Aug 13:D4.
26. Abboud L, Mathews A, Tesriero H. Fakes in the medicine chest. *Wall Street Journal* 2003;Sep 22:B1.
27. Petersen M. The Internet is awash in ads for products promising cures or protection. *New York Times* 2003;Apr 14: A12.
28. Lee J. Spam: an escalating attack of the clones. *New York Times* 2002;Jun 27: G1.
29. Morris C, Avron J. Internet marketing of herbal products. *JAMA* 2003;290(11):1505–1509.
30. Pereira J. Games get more explicit—and so do warning labels. *Wall Street Journal* 2003;Sep 25:D1.
31. Clark D. Gamer offers form of instant replay to prevent cheating. *Wall Street Journal* 2003;Sep 24:D4.
32. Green CS, Bavelier D. Action video game modifies visual selective attention. *Nature* 2003;423:534–537.
33. Maltby N, Kirsch I, Makers M, et al. Virtual reality therapy for the treatment of fear of flying: a controlled investigation. *J Consult Clin Psychol* 2002;70:1112–1118.
34. Gluteal F. Overloaded? *Newsweek* 2002;November 25:E4–6.
35. Croal N. Sims family values. *Newsweek* 2002;Nov 25:45–54.
36. Berlind W. Bookies in exile. *New York Times Magazine* 2003;Aug 17:34–39.
37. Bulkeley W. Internet casinos lose allies, threatening winning streak. *Wall Street Journal* 2003;Nov 26:B1.
38. Schwartz J. From unseemly to lowbrow, the web's real money is in the gutter. *New York Times* 2002;Aug 26:C1.
39. Cooper A, Ed. *Sex and the Internet: a guidebook for clinicians.* New York: Brunner-Routledge, 2002.
40. Gill L. One in ten confesses to Internet sex addiction. *NewsFactor Network* 2001;Jul 20.
41. Gootman E. On stand, girl recalls week of captivity and rape on L. I. *New York Times* 2002;Nov 26:B5.
42. Cowan A. Inmate sought pen pals online after plea in Internet sex case. *New York Times* 2003;Jul 8:B5.
43. Morgan CJ. Travel plans foiled, sex crime averted. *The Village Times Herald (Stony Brook, NY)* 2003;Mar 13:1.
44. Corley D. Cybersex addiction as lethal as crack cocaine. *Paradigm* 2002;Winter:12–22.
45. Lewis M. Faking it. *New York Times Magazine* 2001;Jul 15:32–63.

46. Max DT. Mouse trapped. *New York Magazine* 2002;Feb 25:23–27, 78.
47. Thompson N. Sex in the digital city. *Washington Monthly* 2000; July–August.
48. Hitt J. Confessions of a spam king. *New York Times Magazine* 2003;Sep 28:48–51.
49. Pratchatt R. Virtually addicted. *Guardian Unlimited Online* 2003;July 12.
50. Bai YM, Lin CC, Chen JY. Internet addiction disorder among clients of a virtual clinic. *Psychiatr Serv* 2001;52(10):1397.
51. Young KS, Rogers RC. The relationship between depression and Internet addiction. *Cyberpsychol Behav* 1998;1(1):25–28.
52. Bai YM, Lin CC, Chen JY, et al. The characteristic differences between clients of virtual and real psychiatric clinics. *Am J Psychiatry* 2001;158:1160–1161.

CHAPTER 32

Collecting, Accumulation, and Hoarding: Acquisitions and Their Discontents

DAVID A. HALPERIN AND JANE GLICK

In a society increasingly driven by consumerism and impulse buying, it is not surprising that increasing interest is being paid to issues of consumption and accumulation (1). Indeed, the past two decades have seen the creation of a new sport (according to its participants), a new form of investment (according to its gurus), and a new form of postmodern esthetic (according to a cadre of academics). This new leisure-time activity, which has assumed an overdetermined status as every weekend its acolytes check the Yard Sales columns of newspapers across the country, is simply the accumulation of collectibles. Adherents' activities are hardly limited to the haphazard attendance at a Saturday morning flea market or their dropping over to a neighbor's garage sale there. Rather, the passionate acolyte pursues and accumulates collectibles spurred on by memorable finds displayed on the Antique Road Show, and educated by the numerous newspapers devoted to antiques/collectibles or the ubiquitous catalogs by the Kovels suggesting values and prices for such items. A *collectible* differs from an *antique* (a) by its relatively recent origin, and (b) because the collectible itself may not be an obviously attractive object. The desirability of a collectible—its "collectibility"—is often a matter initiated by popular consensus in which the object's eccentricity and potential for eliciting nostalgia is important. The esthetic value of the collectible may be validated only by using the complex tenets of postmodern deconstruction according to which the act of validating some objects over others is esthetically elitist circumvention or invalidation of more populist perspectives. Collectibles differ from antiques or other traditional objets d'art by their *mana*—the emotional quotient of an object—and are often significantly grounded in both the collector's childhood and the collectors' nostalgia for the world of their childhood. In this way, collectibles function as signifiers for a recently vanished past that the collector experienced as having offered great security and integrity—issues considered at length in Arthur Phillips' recent, highly praised novel, *Prague* (2). The possibility that some collectibles were created by talented artists, for example, the original Campbell's soup cans, and are esthetically successful pieces may add to their appeal, but it is not intrinsic to the collectors' interest.

This chapter examines the process by which individuals pursue the collection and accumulation of objects. The pursuit of the collectible is a multidimensional process. It deserves the interest of the mental health professional because individuals may pursue their grails to the extent of almost literally eating themselves out of house and home, leading to the transformation of their dwellings into profoundly nonfunctional environments. But, the transformation of the home is only one aspect of this process, because in the accumulation of objects individuals may grossly overextend themselves financially, and divert themselves from activities that are more creative. In this examination, however, it is important to recognize that collection, consumption, accumulation, and hoarding may reflect different psychopathologic issues within the individual, each of which deserves the respect and the attention of the mental health professional. Above all, it is important to appreciate that neither accumulation nor collection is necessarily pathologic—the collections and accumulations that have led to the creation of world-famous museums are clearly distinguishable from the piles of debris littering the hoarders' rooms which invoke the purely pathologic. Not every collector is driven by an unreasoning need to accumulate objects beyond rational desire, and collections may be the creation of individuals who are able to recognize the esthetic merit inherent in the most commonplace objects. Above all, a certain humility should be retained when criticizing the size or content of an individual's collection. After all, some of the most exquisite Tiffany Lamp Shades were destroyed during the 1930s for their lead, leaving extraordinary shards of stained glass to be swept into the street unrecognized and unappreciated. The mental health professional must distinguish from the passionate collector who buys a Tiffany lamp for its beauty and the grandiosity of the former patient who dealt in art nouveau and stated in his first session therapy that he personally resented anyone who possessed an attractive art nouveau object.

Acquisitive activities may be seen for some as comparable to binge eating in which recurrent episodes and physiologic impairment. Indeed, one collector/patient noted an almost narcotic-like effect when in the throes of a collecting frenzy until the preoccupation with acquisition subsided, and there was an increased awareness of a chronic and debilitating lumbosacral pain. For many collectors, concerns about a current acquisition enable them to temporarily suppress or dissociate other, more usual obsessive concerns (3). In dynamic terms, collecting, accumulation, and hoarding can be seen as overdetermined activities subject to a variety of interpretations (1). The possibility that collection/accumulation may be related to other forms of addiction is suggested by the intriguing conjunction of collection, accumulation, and creativity illustrated by Charcot and Freud (and in the world of fiction by Des Esseintes and the master of ratiocination, Sherlock Holmes) with the use of cocaine. The French diarist Edmond de Goncourt stated that the mature Doctor Charcot relied on a powerful narcotic potion of bromide, morphine, and codeine to "produce" such "exhilarating dream on a daily basis" (4). The relationship of collection and accumulation to substance abuse and its potential association with addictions of other types—its comorbidity—is highlighted in this chapter through an examination of clinical examples.

GENERAL CONSIDERATIONS ON COLLECTION, ACCUMULATION, AND HOARDING

Freud was a notable collector of antique statuary. John Gedo, in his *Art Alone Endures* (5), attributes Freud's being a "passionate" collector of antiquities to a multiplicity of causes, including Freud's ambivalent identification with the Jewish people. Gedo sees his collection as part of Freud's attempts at identification with his Germanic surround with its "commitment to classical ideals" acted out in the "struggle between Aryan Rome and Semitic Carthage, a conflict in which he identified with both sides." Thus, his antiquities played the role as transitional objects, allowing Freud to transcend his background in his drive to acquire a more cosmopolitan identification.

The acquisition of objects may be overdetermined. It can be fully understood only if intrapsychic, historical, social, and a wide variety of other external factors are considered. Individuals must be examined within their specific historical contexts. The acquisition of boatloads of art and antiquities by wealthy Englishmen or Americans was normative during their grand tours, or the collection of tulips during the Tulipmania that swept across Holland during the seventeenth century. Yet despite the appreciation of the context in which the "passionate" collector operates, it is important to note the presence of psychopathology.

Even so redoubtable and controversial a figure as Lord Elgin who collected the friezes on the Parthenon ostensibly guided by his interest in preserving art, and secondarily by his identification with the global cultural mission of the Empire, did so to the point of his financial destruction.

COLLECTORS AND THE RENOVATION NEXT DOOR

The problematic aspects of collection and accumulation may surface in less-exotic contexts. A recent article in the *New York Times* (6) describes Mr. and Mrs. XY renovating their apartment at great expense to accommodate Mr. XY's collection of stamps and Mrs. XY's collection of glass and porcelain. The article notes that "fortunately, Mr. XY is an architect, and so when he and his wife, bought an apartment, his first concern was finding and creating appropriate space for his collection of stamps and her collection of glass and porcelain." The article coyly notes that "collections by definition continue to grow" and that his stamp collection has increased exponentially during the course of their marriage—so much so that only a portion of his collection is housed in their home—the rest is housed in his office. Certain problematic issues have already surfaced because Mrs. XY sees her collection as far less invasive than his, even though it constitutes a few hundred pieces of ceramics, glass, and amber.... " And the writer comments that "it is a running theme as they give a tour of the apartment; who will get which space? When Mrs. XY showed off the very deep linen closet in the hallway, she said that it was roomy and that it could hold even some of his stamps. He [Mr. XY] seized the moment: 'Is this going to go into print? That I can have some of this space for my stamps?' He looked victorious; she looked resigned; they moved on" (6).

This vignette from the life of two affluent, upwardly mobile New Yorkers illustrates several significant issues relating to collecting and accumulation. Of primary importance, it illustrates the intensity of the collector's zeal. The XYs will be spending a large amount of money to accommodate their collections. The reader must presume that they are responsible, realistic individuals, capable of judging their financial commitments in their pursuit of creating storage space for their collections. But it is also possible that their zeal and vision outruns their financial capabilities, that their determination may lead to an unforeseen and unfortunate financial overcommitment. In the article, Mr. XY alludes to his dealing in stamps. One wishes him well. However, his reliance upon the possibility of his being able to sell his stamps—objects without intrinsic liquidity or value—may create financial difficulties. Does his seeing himself as a dealer as opposed to being a mere collector have some element of rationalization concealed within it? Many dealers in the arts and antiquities were collectors whose collections outgrew their space. But the step between one role and the other is not necessarily an easy one to take, especially when it entails selling the objects that one prizes, especially because the highest returns are often found in selling precisely those objects that one prizes for one's own collection! Moreover, hobbies/collections are creatures of a cultural climate, and as such the objects bought at considerable expense and assembled in a collection may *not* gain in value. There is a downside risk, which enthusiastic collectors may not appreciate in their zeal to amass a significant collection. Many blue chip collectibles, such as electric trains, are less appealing to younger collectors; the pool of train collectors is aging and diminishing. In this context, one author remembers his childhood in which every young male was a stamp collector and was aware of the older males who were engaged in the hobby, for example, President Franklin Delano Roosevelt and King George VI. More recently, he was disappointed when his own children showed little or no interest in his onetime hobby. Finally, the *New York Times* article refers to the possibility of familial conflict over space allotment for their respective collections: What happens when Mr. XY's collection outgrows storage in his office? This conflict over turf can express itself on many levels. It has the potential for creating serious disruption within a relationship over issues of finance, time allocation (e.g., collectors like to visit conventions), or the developing of resentment over a total commitment to the accumulation of objects. Yet, the XYs are collectors. Their accumulations are in precisely delimited areas, and may provide areas of healthy separation. Significant issues can arise, however, when individuals see no need limit to their acquisitions, as the following illustrates.

THE COLLECTOR IN CONTROL?

Tracey is a "self-regulating" collector. She has assembled a tasteful collection of twentieth century art which was recently exhibited in a prominent New York gallery. However, when questioned about her collection, she comments that "I never planned it; it just happened." She notes that she had always liked art and objects of beauty, but in addition to her pleasure in looking at art in museums and galleries, and she enjoyed the camaraderie she experienced with her dealer and fellow collectors on her "rounds." In college, she had decided that although she could never become a great artist, she could become a great art collector. The sublimatory aspect of being a great collector in lieu of being a great artist—that the great collector is often an "artiste manqué" (failed artist)—is frequently noted. But the pleasure in sublimation or provided on a social level gives only a partial explanation for the activity that occupies a great deal of the passionate collector's time and energy. A parallelism between the collector and the hunter has been noted as another significant factor in the development of the "committed" collector.

Olmstead (7) in his *Justifying Collecting—Metaphors and Functions*, notes that the hunting metaphor is often used "in the title of books about collecting, for example, *The Joys of Hunting Antiques* (Salter), *Treasure Hunting for All* (Fletcher), and *The Chase, The Capture: Collecting at the Metropolitan* (Hoving et al.)." As Dunford remarked: "People who don't get thrift shopping confuse the impulse with thrift. But thrift shopping for hobbyists has little to do with thrift and less to do with shopping in any conventional sense. It is a sport, much like bird-watching or fly-fishing. Over the years you develop skills that help to place you in the path of good and to seize it when it comes. The thrill comes directly after" (8). It is important to appreciate the addictive aspect of collecting/hunting. But Tracey notes that "I've gone through phases." She describes the satisfaction of being able to have things that were denied to her in the past as a motivating factor. However, following her parents' death within months of each other, she became depressed. As part of a moratorium on many aspects of her life, she stopped collecting (unlike Freud who began to collect after his father's death, perhaps because he felt liberated to pursue an expansion of his area of identification). Then, after about 2 years, she felt a renewed interest in life, including collecting. However, acquisition in and of itself became an ego dystonic activity. Pure possession did not seem to afford sufficient gratification. This changing attitude towards collection has enabled Tracey to impose some measure of self-regulation. Her modification of her behavior is a product of a number of factors including her increased sense of satiation, and her sense that the rapidly increasing price of art has made it increasingly difficult to find objects that she would prefer to those she has already acquired. At this point, "It stopped as rapidly as it started." Tracey considers herself "a controlled (self-regulated) addict." She acknowledges that she had an addiction for a time, but adds she now has the ability to "hold tight and stop." To maintain her sense of control, she imposes limits on herself such as frequenting only "safe" shows, that is, exhibitions at which the objects are either prohibitively expensive or not for sale. She compares her current attempts to maintain control as being comparable to her mother's attempts to limit her smoking addiction by not allowing herself (an observant Jew) to smoke on the Sabbath or to smoke only in a particular room of the house. Both Tracey and her mother control their addictions by the imposing compulsive controls, that is, two drinks per day no more no less, an approach that is often of initial benefit to the addict in recovery. However, such approaches do not deal with underlying aspects of an addiction, and often become less effective over time. Tracey comments that she would still like to find things that are "very special," but notes she does not feel driven while making her rounds. She is able to accept "just looking" in the same fashion that passing a bakery and merely inhaling the scent of pastries may satisfy a diabetic. Tracey has a sense of accomplishment over her self-control, but she is realistic enough to acknowledge that were she to move to a larger apartment. Tracey is a social collector; the rounds and the camaraderie of fellow collectors and dealers are important to her. But times change, consider the difficulties of the solitary "collector/addict" seated at a computer monitor seduced by the allure of the Internet, increasingly preoccupied with scoring a hit on eBay and operating without limits except those imposed by the fortuitous presence of a hectoring, nagging companion or spouse.

COLLECTION AS AN ESTHETIC ENTERPRISE

The formation of a collection is neither essentially nor primarily a pathologic enterprise. Tracey's collection does reflect her self-deprecating judgment on her artistic ability. But it is primarily an expression of her desire to possess objects of beauty. Comparably, the desire to collect objects of beauty underlies the collections of Clare and Eugene Thaw (9). Clare and Eugene Thaw have formed a number of museum-quality collections of widely disparate objects. Mr. Thaw describes his passionate collecting "as a combination of esthetic pleasure, the desire to possess the objects and the need to order the resulting accumulation." He "grants his collecting is a 'little bit obsessional'" but he considers it a rational endeavor nonetheless: "That's the way I get close to objects, and then, after I've owned them and learned about them, I don't need them anymore. They're with me and I can give them away." Thus museums have received his collections and as the recipients of his philanthropy have benefitted from his connoisseurship and expertise. For Mr. Thaw, ownership in its complex dimensions provides a motive underlying the formation of his collections. He shares with other collectors of great works of art a profound sense that certain works of art have a visual gravitas and a passionate intensity which remain with their owner after the actual object is donated. His serial formation of collections is a reflection that the esthetic bounty granted the passionate collector in one area exists in the art of superficially different areas, that there are esthetic rewards to be found among a multiplicity of cultures. The Thaws collect works of high esthetic merit from many sources. But collectors do not necessarily collect works of high art. Yet their collections become the focus of their passions and finances. The case of Ted M. presents these issues with his multiplicity of motivations and collections.

TED M. AND THE NEED TO BUY EVERYTHING

Ted M. is a successful architect. He entered treatment in his mid-thirties to resolve the complexities of his marital situation. He could not decide whether or not to leave his constricted, phobic wife for his current girlfriend. Soon after graduation from a prestigious school of architecture, he married his wife. He is the father of two children. Professionally, his work has been illustrated in a number of professional journals, although he feels he has not received adequate professional recognition. Within a few years after his marriage, Ted began entering into a series of long-term, tempestuous extramarital relationships. Characteristically, the relationships would begin explosively, rapidly turning into all-consuming relationships. He would respond explosively to any suggestions by his partners that they separate, or "at least cool things off," for example, throwing a computer monitor through a glass wall at his girlfriend Opal when she suggested establishing some boundaries. Despite his professed interest in resolving his marital situation, Ted remained unable to change his ambivalent relationship with his wife. He rationalized his passivity as reflecting his "kindness" and concern for his passive, phobic wife whom he was convinced could never survive his departure. Diagnostically, Ted was characterized as a borderline personality disorder with obsessive-compulsive features, particularly because of his (a) pattern of unstable and intense interpersonal relationships characterized by alternating between extremes of overidealization and devaluation; (b) impulsiveness in at least two areas that are potentially self-damaging, for example, spending and sex; (c) affective instability; (d) inappropriate intense anger or lack of control of anger; and (e) marked persistent identity disturbance manifested by uncertainty about self-image, sexual orientation, type of friends desired, and preferred values. Ted did not simply form friendships, he collected friends. For Ted, separation from a girlfriend like Opal was truly intolerable. Even after terminating the period of intense intimacy with a girlfriend, Ted would hire her as an employee at high salaries, often lending them large sums of money in the process. He kept an open box filled with money in his desk knowing that these employees or other "friends" would surreptitiously "borrow" from his petty cash. And he collected objects and clothing. If he found a shirt style he liked, he would impulsively buy the same shirt in every available color. His wardrobe became enormous. Yet he rarely, if ever, wore many of his clothes. Like Imelda Marcos, he could never throw any items of clothing away. His impulsive acquisition of clothing reflected his "chronic restiveness . . . an unrelenting need, even hunger for acquisitions . . . which derives from a memory of deprivation" (10). Nor were his acquisitions simply limited to friends or clothing. He collected other objects as well, developing a particular focus on elephants. He collected hundreds of objets d'art in the form of elephants. Unlike politicians for whom the elephant (or donkey) assumes a totemic value, his elephants reflected his being a "collector, not unlike the religious believer, [who] assigns power and value to these objects. . . . [in which] affection becomes attached to things, which . . . can become animated like the amulets and fetishes of preliterate humankind or the holy relics of the religionist" (11). On a more creative level, Ted assembled debris and found objects into sculptures of elephants (which he later exhibited in a gallery as the elephants of Ted M.). Eventually, his collection of clothing and objects became so large that he was forced to move into a larger apartment to accommodate his collections. This move precipitated a severe financial crisis because he felt obligated to extensively remodel his new apartment to make it consistent with his grandiose self-image of the architect as artist. He installed an expensive internal telephone complex ostensibly for business reasons to avoid missing "important" calls, but in reality his fear of being left out of the loop reflected a childhood filled with his profound sense of having been ignored or deprived of the attention he felt was his due. Borderline personality disorder is often characterized by identity disturbance. The formation of collections and the accumulation of objects may be an expression of ambivalence in core identity issues. Ted's identity disturbance manifested itself in the objects collected. He bought an enormous amount of clothing which was by the standards of the day often bizarre and inappropriately androgynous—clothing which he then often denigrated. Nor was clothing the only area in which his identity confusion expressed itself. Ted changed his professional name from a fairly standard Jewish name to one redolent of Anglophilia, doubtless assuming in the process another identity and collecting another history.

Therapeutic work with Ted focused around issues of identification in both sexual and vocational terms, and his inability to separate from individuals and objects, to enable Ted to develop other means of dealing with his separation anxiety than the blind accumulation of objects, allowing him in the process to separate from old relationships and old internal and external objects. Thus the ultimate goal of Ted's treatment was to allow him to form new relationships without being preoccupied with the loss of old ones, and in material terms, to allow him to selectively limit his purchases only to new objects that truly met his standards. In short, the goal of treatment was the transformation of Ted from being an accumulator to becoming a connoisseur. In this context, to transform Ted from being an individual who acquired objects only for the sake of accumulation to becoming the connoisseur who acquired only those objects that met his "carefully' defined esthetic standards reflecting his heightened artistic sensibility and leading him to "upgrade" his collection. During the course of treatment, Ted was able to make real distinctions within his collections and separate from many of his possessions. He was able to adopt other objects that were much more meaningful in personal and objective terms. Ted was enabled to face his temor vacuui, his fear of emptiness. Despite his professional success, Ted had always regarded his work as the product of his creative and esthetic subservience to his clients, unlike the work of "real artists." By supporting his adoption of a more personalized and esthetically consistent attitude toward his clients, he was able to enhance his sense of self-worth and achieve a measure of professional satisfaction. He felt a lessened need to accumulate and the store his "wardrobe." And he was ultimately able to form a lasting relationship with one partner.

ACCUMULATION AND COLLECTION: THE ACCUMULATOR AS ARTIST

Each possession you possess
Helps your spirits to soar
That's what's soothing about excess
Never settle for something less
Something's better than nothing, yes
But nothing's better than more
From "MORE," by Stephen Sondheim, 1990

Accumulation and collection exist on a spectrum. The XYs, Tracey, and the Thaws are collectors. Each of them have clearly defined areas and objects of desire. Above all, each appears to be in good control of their particular impulses to collect. All three collectors are contrasted with Ted who required psychotherapeutic intervention place limits on his impulsivity and his need to accumulate objects (and people). These individuals represent only relatively straightforward aspects of the accumulation–collection spectrum. More complex examples are provided by such well known artists as Joseph Cornell and Andy Warhol, and by a younger, lesser-known local artist, Renee G.

Renee G., a 30-year-old artist, has lived in the same apartment for 6 years. Recently, the character of the neighborhood started to change, and she was threatened by local denizens who threw rocks at her and fired a pistol. She luckily escaped without serious injury, but was clearly quite shaken by this experience. She states that she wants to live in a less-problematical neighborhood. She has entered treatment to enable her to move; however, a major difficulty that she will face should she choose to move will be disassembling her apartment. She has shown her therapist photographs and a videotape of her apartment, which is filled (the word is used advisedly) with an incredible assortment of objects. The walls of the apartment (which are not visible) are layered with an extraordinary assemblage of objects. The objects, themselves, include toys of every description, and a very wide variety of material referring to pop culture icons, particularly Elvis Presley. Renee is not unique in either her preoccupation with pop culture, or in her decorative style. She has layered her apartment to create an environment that appears to be a cross between The Old Curiosity Shop and a museum of pop culture. For example, a recent restaurant review of the Trailer Park Lounge and Grill is illustrated by a photo bearing a resemblance to Renee's apartment. Another recent article celebrates Billy Hibble, an Australian, characterized as a "pop culture vulture." The article mentions "an eye-popping assortment of rare collectibles from

Disney, Hanna-Barbera, and Warner Brothers, to name a few. A lot of the bounty that crowds Hibble's bedroom was won in the competitions he enters compulsively . . . " (12). Both Renee and Billy Hibble's homes are assemblages reflecting a comparable esthetic, summarized by standing the classic modernist phrase of "less is more" on its head and arriving at the postmodernist "less is a bore." Renee's esthetic is more than an assemblage of an overwhelming collection of pop culture icons. The objects collected present a challenge to prevailing establishment esthetic criteria. Renee and Billy Hibble's homes are statements that they will live in an environment that does not adhere to mainstream cultural criteria. Their esthetic reflects the free market at work—that if a million children and their parents buy and enjoy Disney toys or Hanna-Barbera dolls or visit Graceland as an act of cultural hommage, then attention must be paid to them and that disregarding these objects is to disregard a significant segment of society. Renee's formation of a hoard that layers every surface of her home is a conscious act of identification with the outsider as a cultural hero. There are other dimensions in this process of identification. Renee has rejected conventional sexual roles, which she regards as stereotypic. Her idealization of Elvis as an androgynous culture hero reflects her own sexual ambivalence and her own adoption of an androgynous sexual role. The objects she has accumulated also celebrate a cultural context strongly associated with a blue-collar social background (viz. Trailer Park Lounge) quite at odds with her parents' cultural tastes and values. She identifies the upper-middle-class style of her parents as being lean, wearing relatively tight-fitting clothing, and as adopting a minimalist decorative style with certifiable antiques. Thus Renee always wears baggy clothing, which loosely hangs from her hips—"home boy" style—cuts her hair in a "duckback" reminiscent of Elvis, and layers her walls with posters and objects that clash and clamor for attention. Renee can barely maneuver within her apartment; having visitors is difficult and finding any lost objects would certainly be problematical. The accumulation of these objects occupies her time and requires money. When questioned about her accumulation in view of her expressed desire to find an apartment in a more secure neighborhood and live in less-financially straitened circumstances, Renee emphasizes that she views her "collection" as investments! Renee, like many hoarders, regards her accumulations as money in the box (if not in the bank). Renee's accumulation is not simply the product of a "rational" financial decision, even if she rationalizes her accumulation in those terms.

The persistent decline of the stock market, the low rate of interest paid by conventional banks, and the high cost of real estate have led many to alternate forms of investment. Television programs such as the Antiques Road Show and publications such as Kovel's *Antique Guide* (to name just one) have heightened the appeal of the collectible as a form of investment. The creation of eBay and the In-

ternet have created a much greater degree of liquidity for antiques and collectibles lending a certain cachet to the accumulation of objects/collectibles as being reasonable alternatives to more traditional forms of investment. After all, eBay, itself, was created to enable its founder's girlfriend to readily dispose of her collection of Pez dispensers! In a sense, Renee is participating in a world where baseball cards are collected by the Metropolitan Museum of Art and auctioned off for extraordinary sums of money, and comic books may become valuable works of art. If Vietnam created a distrust of the political establishment, and the failure of "promised" medical miracles has lead to a burgeoning field of alternative medicine, it is not surprising that the collapse of the stock market and traditional forms of investment has led many people such as Renee to view their countercultural esthetic as presenting a financial refuge in uncertain times. In this context, the therapist can encourage patients, such as Renee, to recognize the unpredictable nature of fashion—that one decade's cultural icon is another decade's cultural bore—and dispose of their collection when a profitable opportunity presents itself. However, the therapist may meet with resistance. At times, Renee refers to her apartment as an example of installation art existing in the borderline between sculptural space and social commentary, rather than as an assemblage of hoarded objects preventing her from living comfortably in her apartment. Or, more grandiosely, she will compare her apartment to Francis Bacon's studio, which was moved lock, stock, dust, and debris to the National Museum in Ireland. Renee's apartment functions as a wry commentary on the often arbitrary assignment of esthetic worth or financial value to objects, but despite these esthetic precedents, her refusal to dispose of memorabilia, found objects, and pieces without inherent value reflects a pathologic inability either to dispose or discard. But Renee does not experience herself as a "pathologic accumulator" unable to discard useless objects. Her home functions as an esthetic expression and as a preserver of her sense of continuity and of her sense of individuality. She sees herself as having transformed the interior space of an apartment into a home with all its potentially accumulative connotations. She regards the interior space as a tabula rasa onto which she has imposed her unique esthetic sensibility, although she does acknowledge that her accumulation and hoarding have acted to the detriment of function and efficiency. And yet Renee presented herself as feeling like Freud, her apartment like his office dominated by a striking collection of objects and functioning as a museum from whose valences she drew inspiration.

The relationship between collection, accumulation, and art is multidetermined. Freud, himself, acknowledged that his maitre d'Charcot introduced into the clinical studies of psychopathology "the sensibility of the artist" and characterized Charcot's home as the "magic castle in which he lives. . . . in short a museum" (13). Charcot clearly saw a relationship between the act of collection and the act of creation: "The tension between reason and fantasy, order and disorder that shaped Charcot's artistic-medical persona was expressed in his personal practice of interior design. Charcot collaborated with his family to create a unified personal environment where historical materials were animated by private memories and "exteriorized dreams" (13). Likewise, Freud saw a relationship between collection and creation. Intriguingly, his first attempt at applied psychoanalysis, *Delusions and Dreams* in Jensen's *Gravida* (1907), examines the tension between an artist and his possession. Renee's collection of pop art objects and icons has appeared in her sculpture, film, and drawings. For her, as for Freud, her collection both grounds her sense of self and has become an expression of her individuality, for which she pays the price of immobility.

Certain issues are of particular importance for the therapist working with "pathologic" accumulators and hoarders. It is very important for the therapist to adopt a nonjudgmental stance, even given the reality that the patient's lifestyle revolves around the accumulation and hoarding of objects of dubious value which reflect a fixation on immature choices. Renee, like other accumulators/hoarders, brought to the treatment process her expectation that the therapist as a middle-class authority figure (like her parents) would object to her accumulations because of his middle-class esthetic views and values. Her expectations initially interfered with the formation of a therapeutic alliance, particularly because of her borderline pathology, which enabled her to focus (with exquisite sensitivity) onto any perceived judgmental stance by the therapist. However, the therapist who is working with an individual apparently functioning well below her capacity and who had chosen to identify with a cultural context where widespread drug abuse and other potentially dangerous behavior exists, must be alert to his own countertransference, which may lead him to be either overly protective or overly judgmental. The formation and maintenance of a therapeutic alliance with an immature, suspicious post adolescent is realistically very difficult. Yet, without the formation of this therapeutic alliance, the depressed, isolated postadolescent is left to his or her own dubious devices and rationalizations.

A dynamic issue that seemed to be particularly relevant in working with Renee, but which is present in other accumulators/hoarders, is that these are individuals with a poorly defined identity and identity diffusion. Thus, the objects accumulated are often those whose presence enables the accumulator to retain or more precisely define their identity. Renee's childhood, until the onset of puberty, was relatively conflict free, thus it is not surprising she collected objects reminiscent of a prepubertal toy shop, harking back to a period when issues of sexual identity and gender were significantly less problematic. Likewise, for Renee whose pervasive affect of depression was a product of her preoccupation with issues of separation and loss, her accumulations of childhood quasitransitional objects was helpful because it gave her home a gloss of permanence and of stasis without change. If one is fearful of growth and extremely fearful of illness, then growing older is experienced primarily as increasing one's exposure to greater losses. Thus, there is a certain inner logic to Renee's maintaining a household in which growth, illness, and aging appear to be permanently excluded. Enabling the accumulator to work on these dynamic issues may lead to lessening of the need to retain objects. Everyone (except for the most ascetic or minimalist) needs to retain objects from their past, objects symbolic of past experiences, of souvenirs and tokens from a life fully and pleasurably lived. But the accumulator retains objects not primarily for their "evidentiary" value but because they incorporate a mana that enables their possessor to retain a key for the door that opens to a happier and more fulfilling past (thus the fragments of walls have "auric" value by retaining the mana of the objects contained within the walls) (14). Identity issues arose when Renee chose to confront her parents by her dressing as a home boy and parading her identification with Elvis. Her parents responded to her venture in cultural diversity with a critical counterappraisal. Here, the therapist was able to help her by enabling her to appreciate how difficult it may be for people of her parents' generation to accept her tattoos, that if she chooses to maintain a relationship with them, some compromises might be helpful. Above all, the therapist must respect that for the accumulator, their accumulations are a form of personal archeology in which the accumulator discovers and preserves objects emblematic of their newfound identity, rather like the process of preservation in newly formed nations where each excavated object and each renamed coin provides a proof of continuity and a prophecy of permanence.

Renee is not unique among artists in her need to create an installation in which the passage of time is kept permanently at bay. Joseph Cornell is a widely esteemed artist whose art was grounded in similar ambitions. Cornell was able to transform found objects—the flotsam and jetsam of everyday life—into magical shadow boxes. He used collage-like techniques in the directing the individual towards an appreciation of the onward, irresistible rush of time. His is an art of nostalgia created out of the bits and pieces of everyday life (15), directed toward preserving an individual's sense of existing beyond time and its ravages. After all, great art does, in a profound sense, rescue the individual and their creations from the wrath of time.

HOARDING AND ENDSTAGE ACCUMULATION

Hoarding is more than a matter of the unregulated and impulsive accumulation of objects. It has been defined as "the acquisition of and failure to discard large numbers of possessions that appear to be useless or of limited value" (16).

It "spans a continuum from normal collecting to patho-logical self-neglect and can be associated with a number of disorders, most frequently organic mental disorders, psychotic disorders, obsessive-compulsive personality disorder, and obsessive-compulsive disorder (OCD)" (16). An intriguing example is presented in the life of D. D. Smalley, "a Houston eccentric (for whom) even a pencil stub was an object worth collecting." Lisa Germany (17) describes him as "a mapmaker, husband, and father living in the Hyde Park district of Houston whose 'seemingly limitless curiosity' allowed him to collect rows and rows of arrowheads and American Indian tools, mastodon teeth and a ribcage with an arrowhead caught betwixt its bones was treated exactly the same as a corset stay, an old spark coil, a shoe button hook, bullets from No Man's Land, a seed from a cucumber tree on the Texas Capitol grounds, a jar of soil from the Brazos River, and another jar of pencils so short that the eraser sits just above the point. And so on, totaling more that 1,500 similarly quirky irresistible ob-jects. It is as if Smalley had opened the bureau drawers of a generation and lifted out the fragments of lives lived, of moments enjoyed or (as with its collection of World War I bullets) simply endured." Smalley's innumerable collec-tions of objects are his hoards. He did not hoard materials and proceed to layer his home in the manner of Renee G. or Billy Hibble. Rather, he stored materials in his at-tic and shared them with children (who to judge from reports were enchanted with them). Smalley's need to hoard reflected his reluctance to leave the miniaturized world of childhood, where each object—no matter how small or functionally insignificant—retains a certain mana (rather like the tickets to a prized production of a play or the program to a football game played decades ago that suddenly materializes at the bottom of a pile of paper).

D. D. Smalley and Renee G. represent different points on the spectrum of accumulation and hoarding. For Renee, hoarding and the accumulation of objects is an end in it-self. Even if she documents her accumulation and regards it as an artistic-shaped environment, she isolates herself within it and has relatively little interest in reaching out to the wider society. Renee is not secretive about her accu-mulations, but her primary agenda is in the very personal way that these objects reflect her own attempts at iden-tification and rebellion. Renee uses her accumulations to confront the adult conforming mainstream world. In con-tradistinction, there seems to have been little interest in issues of identification or self-assertion as Smalley cre-ated his accumulations. Indeed, Smalley appears to have been comfortable in his role as father and husband, and in his vocation of mapmaker. In the creation of his collec-tions, there is no attempt to confront the mainstream world in terms of its values or as a reflection of a countercul-tural agenda. Rather, like other individuals who continue to own and expand the dollhouses of their childhood, or who continue to accumulate large collections of models,

the underlying basis of Smalley's collection would seem to reside primarily in his retaining objects in which reside a certain childhood magic. Like children fearful of growing older or preoccupied with losing the memory of signifi-cant events through the passage of time, Smalley collected a lifetime of objects and his collections kept his fear of loss at bay. His hoard has been preserved in the Small Museum of Houston where it still attracts and charms children.

ANDY WARHOL: THE HOARDER AS CREATOR OR AS ADDICT?

D. D. Smalley and Renee G. are accumulators/hoarders who have used their accumulations in a creative manner. However, the prize for hoarding in the possible service of creativity must go to Andy Warhol. Andy Warhol was/is an extraordinarily influential artist. He helped define art and fashion for an entire generation. He was also a collec-tor/accumulator/hoarder on a truly remarkable scale. His creative energy was unquestionable. Was his accumula-tive activity and hoarding just another facet of his creative process or is it more properly regarded as an addiction? Hellinger noted in *The Archives of the Andy Warhol Mu-seum* (18) that

> Warhol had filled his town house at 57 East 66th Street with a treasure trove of fine art, furnishings, objets d'art, and jewelry—all uncatalogued and much of it tucked into shopping bags and boxes stacked in rooms so full that the door could not be opened or closed.... [Only five rooms] out of the 27-room townhouse had [not] served as warehouse for the objects he acquired each day.... A team of appraisers labored for months, pro-ducing a six-volume auction catalog.... Warhol's lim-itless collecting interests ranged from "Canova (a great French sculptor) to cookie jars."... The auction re-sulted in the sale of a staggering amount of collectibles [and] established Warhol as an insatiable collector who was interested in everything and could part with nothing.

Was Andy Warhol a hoarder—a Collier brother with taste—or were his accumulations part and parcel of his creative process? Hellinger considers his accumulations to have been Warhol's "source material" (19). But when "letters from a Warhol Superstar are found in a cookie tin containing used batteries and a broken camera" it is difficult to see in this anything other than his inability to decrease his expanding hoard. Warhol also produced his "Time Capsules" in which he would dump seemingly un-related materials that were products of a certain period of creative activity. The Warhol Archives have chosen to pre-serve these "Time Capsules" in their original form because they reflect Warhol's perceptions of a particular period, from which Warhol then "selected and manipulated mass produced images of American pop culture—transforming the most poignant and at times horrific representations of our culture into fine art."

Andy Warhol's collection of objects was both an addiction and an artistic statement. He created a breach of the border between the antique and the "collectible" or, in other terms, high art and elitism versus kitsch and popular preference. In Warhol's sanctification of the collectible lies its emergence from under the shadow cast by the "genuine" antique. Warhol assisted in the recognition and heightened appreciation of the products of popular culture, a recognition celebrated every weekend across the country at flea markets and tag sales. In his refusal to accept the strictures dividing high art and its estheticism from kitsch with its acceptance of sentimentality and nostalgia, he provided an antidote to the anhedonic, almost puritanical strictures of modernism. Ironically, Warhol's hoards have provided sanction for collectibles which, unlike antiques (or Warhol's artistic creations), are objects considered worthy of attention precisely because of the feeling tone they elicit (hence cookie jars that are redolent of nurturing and comfort), without a formal consideration of their esthetic merit. Warhol presided with other "Pop" Artists over the transformation which eliminated "kulchur" as an object of derision and transformed it into the substance of blockbuster auctions within the august precincts of Sotheby's and Christie's. Warhol participated in the transfiguration of popular culture into the realm of high art. But when does the irresistible accumulation of collectibles become the pathologic expression of an addiction as opposed to being the expression of an esthetic passion?

Andy Warhol's need to acquire objects reflected his ideologic convictions and his restless intellectual curiosity. He (and his fellow archeologists of the "collectible") transformed "old junk into antiques." But, there was a darker side to his activities. Warhol's pathologic hoarding is reflected in the absence of any real attempt to organize his objects into a collection or provide any venue for others to appreciate them. Objects were piled in an addictive frenzy. Warhol, himself, was not addicted to drugs, but many of his collaborators, such as the talented painter Basquiat, were. Warhol's ambivalence towards Basquiat focused particularly around the issue of Basquiat's substance abuse. It may be that in a profound sense, Warhol's addictive accumulation of objects provided him with an area of transcendence that allowed him to avoid prolonged substance abuse. Others may not be so fortunate. Warhol despite his purchases became (and remained) a wealthy man. But for others, such as Ted and Renee, their constant purchases represented a flight from severe depressive affect into hypomanic behavior. And the accumulation of hoards by Ted and Renee were disruptive on a personal level. Their expenditures led to acquiring unnecessary objects but also significant personal debt. Indeed, a motive behind Ted's entry into psychiatric treatment was his family's concern for their financial future. When a patient discusses their accumulations as a form of "investment," they are reassuring the therapist and themselves that the accumulation of objects will provide secure and superior financial returns; it then becomes the therapist's responsibility to help that patient examine reality.

HERMANN GOERING: THE ADDICT AS HOARDER

The need to hoard vast amounts of property without any consideration of the human cost of its acquisition is a tragic aspect of human history. The human cost of the depredations by Hermann Goering are only one aspect of his need to accumulate and hoard art on an archetypal scale. His actions went beyond any civilized boundaries and deserve examination as representing an example of hoarding and accumulation by an individual with profoundly psychopathic traits and a significant history of narcotics addiction.

Hermann Goering has been characterized as the "most complex and many sided of all Nazi leaders, at once a figure of ridicule and of fear, a man of huge talents and of strange flaws.... He was also a drug addict, a glutton, a dandy, and the greediest and most insatiable of art collectors" (20). Goering presented the remarkable picture of an individual seemingly addicted to whatever object appeared to arrest his attention. While the florid, epicene figure of his later years is certainly an accurate portrayal, he also presents the complex union of a war hero (World War I), an apparently effective military leader (World War I) joined to a history of narcotics addiction and an addiction to art—activities he pursued while acquiring numerous extraordinarily gaudy uniforms, palaces, hunting lodges and economic control over much of Germany and German-occupied Europe. Ostensibly, Goering's addiction to morphine was the product of wounds he sustained during the Beer Hall Putsch in 1923. His addiction lasted for the next 2 to 3 years and was treated in a succession of Swedish sanitoria by enforced abstinence, that is, "cold turkey," followed by hospitalization.

His later desire to accumulate a vast art collection may have reflected some genuine appreciation of the objects themselves (but little connoisseurship as he was a major purchaser of fake Vermeers). Much of Goering's activity appears to have been the product of his ambivalent and competitive relationship with Hitler. Goering, himself, identified with the Italian condottiere and seemingly needed to establish himself as a type of Renaissance man. To establish himself as a twentieth century Maecenas, he planned to open his museum, Carin Halle, as the Hermann Goering Museum, in 1953, to celebrate his sixtieth birthday but characteristically (and no doubt wisely) later than Hitler's planned opening of his museum in Linz (scheduled for 1951) (21). The vast number of works of art acquired by Goering appears to reflect primarily art's traditional role as an icon of possession and conquest. But in addition, Goering would acquire and sell pieces of art in order to demonstrate his control of the men who were his underlings within the Nazi hierarchy and as an expression of his grandiosity. "Goering sold pictures to Gauleiters, as he told me with a childish smile, for many times what he had paid—adding, moreover, an extra something to the price for the glory of the painting having come 'from the famous Goering collection'" (21). His accumulative activity may be compared to Napoleon's if only to illustrate Marx' dictum that "when history repeats itself it does so the first time as tragedy, and the second time as farce." Comparisons are difficult, but consider other comparable rulers such as Saddam Hussein with his multitude of palaces or Stalin naming innumerable cities in the former Soviet Union in his honor. Fortunately, individuals such as Goering are rare. But it is important to consider Goering as an exemplar of the manner in which addictions to drugs, clothing, possessions, and fine art can be joined in an individual who, when placed in an unstructured setting, is tragically able to function in a very efficient manner.

HOARDING AS A CLINICAL PROBLEM

Hoarding and excessive accumulation do not usually present themselves in the grandiose terms of a Goering, or the esthetically complex conundrum presented by Andy Warhol. Rather, hoarding and excessive accumulation present themselves more prosaically in the clinical dilemmas faced by visiting nurses or families who attempt to provide adequate and appropriate care for clients/family members whose homes are dysfunctional because of the massive accumulations which interfere/prevent the appropriate use of housing and which prevent caretakers from gaining access to needy individuals (22–26). The classic picture presented is of an elderly (often but not necessarily) single individual whose home is filled with debris which prevents them from gaining ready access to rooms, prevent them from using the kitchen, and whose social life has decreased to the point of isolation because they are unable to invite friends to visit. These individuals often rationalize their accumulations by talking about being unable to throw materials away because they will be needed at some future time, and obsessively ruminate about their need to retain papers. The following is a typical example.

Mr. Q. portrays a scenario all too familiar to the health care practitioner serving the elderly, homebound population. These individuals may not consider their environments to be problematic and may continue in their lifestyle, despite obvious difficulties, until the loss of independence brings them into conflict with society's dictates. Mr. Q., a spirited 90-year-old Chinese gentleman, retired from a successful business. He had been widowed for several years, and was in the process of arranging for a third marriage, having lived alone in an apartment close

to his daughter's home. During his retirement years, he had continued to occupy himself as a writer and as an avid collector of Chinese calligraphy. Volumes of calligraphy filled bookcases in every room and blocked pathways in the halls of his apartment with 30 years' accumulation. He had been living precariously in his apartment, assisted by home nursing visits and several hours' of aide service per week, in addition to help from his daughter, whose time for him was extremely limited. When he came to the author's attention, he had already had multiple recent hospitalizations for pneumonia and minor injuries secondary to falls at home.

As Mr. Q.'s medical problems began to resolve, the question of how he could remain safely in his home became paramount. He had just received notice of acceptance into the Medicaid program, which would provide adequate hours of help, but the home care agency that had been providing service was unwilling to (and legally restricted from participating in a plan previously evaluated as unsafe) accept the case again, even with increased hours of help, unless Mr. Q. considerably reduced the clutter that had put him at risk.

Mr. Q. was more fortunate than many frail, elderly individuals in comparable situations, in that his daughter was willing to take responsibility for rearranging his living quarters, and worked closely with the home nursing agency in coordinating his ongoing care. The presence of a responsible family member and community agency willing to be flexible enabled Mr. Q. to remain in his home. However, individuals who are more physically and/or cognitively impaired, unable to obtain effective family intervention or who are otherwise isolated, are likely to come to the attention of a variety of health care, mental health, and welfare agencies. Moreover, their unwillingness to cooperate in their rehabilitation and/or their lack of response to pharmacologic intervention creates problems (26,27) that may require legal intervention with its concomitant loss of individual autonomy as agencies are forced to assume control. Clearly, this area of problematic behavior with its psychological and legal dimensions will only increase in importance in a society with an aging population. It deserves increased scrutiny now and in the future.

SUMMARY

Collection, accumulation, and hoarding are activities that are overdetermined and have characterized all societies since Maecenas and his colleagues transported Greek statues from Athens to Rome. The acquisition of objects may be viewed as a normative nonpathologic action, but it may also be viewed as an expression of an intrapsychic conflict in which the objects acquired allow the collector/accumulator to avoid a sense of loss or deprivation. For some individuals, it may reflect an addictive need to continually acquire and accumulate objects without regard to their merit or the individual's actual needs. For these individuals, the acquisition of objects is tied in a profound sense to a system in which "life is a game and he/she who dies with the most toys wins." For these individuals, the very acquisition of objects is seen both as a display of the inherent power/mana of the objects and as an attempt to incorporate the power resident in the objects themselves. On a less pathologic level, the accumulation of objects may be part of a creative process, in which the artist acquires objects as part of the exploration and transformation which accompanies the creative process. However, the process of accumulation and collection may share many characteristics of an addiction. In this case, the process of accumulation—the creation of a hoard—supersedes any attempt at differentiation or organization of the hoard. There is no simple means to differentiate between the addict's accumulation or the esthete's collection of objects. However, when the collection's growth appears to be fueled primarily by its own inner dynamic, the presence of severe pathology should become a matter of concern for the therapist. Timely intervention by the therapist with an exploration of the individual's need to acquire objects, as well as a consideration of the problems posed by the presence of severe borderline pathology and/or a bipolar disorder for which the aggressive accumulation may be a significant marker, may enable the addictive accumulator to avoid personal and financial ruin. Finally, consideration of hoarding as a significant problem within the elderly is raised. Grandiose and narcissistic leaders such as Goering are, fortunately, rare. Unfortunately, the frail, isolated elderly individuals trapped in labyrinths of their own devising are both too common and inaccessible to therapeutic intervention.

REFERENCES

1. Hartston HJ, Koran, LM. Impulsive behavior in a consumer culture. *Int J Psych Clin Pract* 6:65–68.
2. Phillips A. *Prague.* New York: Random House, 2002.
3. Kinsella S. *Confessions of a shopaholic.* New York: Dell/Random House, 2001.
4. Silverman DL. *Art nouveau in Fin-de-Siecle France: politics, psychology and style.* Berkeley, CA: University of California Press, 1989.
5. Gedo JE. *Art alone endures.* 1990.
6. River views plus space for a couple's collections. *New York Times* 2003 Jan 26;9:2.
7. Olmstead AD. Justifying collecting—metaphors and functions. *The Brimfield Antique Guide* 1996;Fall:9–10.
8. Treasures buried in plain sight. *New York Times* 2003 Feb 7;6:35.
9. A collector who can let go of his treasures. *New York Times* 2002 Nov 24;2:42.
10. Muensterberger W. *Collecting: an unruly passion-psychological perspectives.* Princeton, NJ: Harcourt Brace, 1994:3.
11. Muensterberger W. *Collecting: an unruly passion-psychological perspectives.* Princeton, NJ: Harcourt Brace, 1994:9–10.
12. Home design. *New York Times* 2002 Oct13:77.
13. Silverman, DL. Ibid. Letter of 01/20/1886 to Martha Bernays; E Freud, 1960,p. 102.
14. Magazine. *New York Times* 2003 Feb 16; magazine:36.
15. Gopnik A. Joseph Cornell's boxed nostalgia. *The New Yorker* 2003 Feb 17;184.
16. Damecour CL, Charron M. Hoarding: a symptom, not a syndrome. *J Clin Psychiarty* 1998;59:5.
17. Germany L. Home design. *New York Times* 2002 Oct 24:24–28.
18. Hellinger. *Archives of the Andy Warhol museum.* 1994:195.
19. Hellinger. *Archives of the Andy Warhol museum.* 1994:196.
20. Moseley L. *The Reichmarshall: a biography of Hermann Goering.* New York: Dell, 1974.
21. Moseley L. *The Reichmarshall: a biography of Hermann Goering.* New York: Dell, 1974:319.
22. Damecour CL, Charron M. Hoarding: a symptom, not a syndrome. *J Clin Psychiatry* 1998;59:267–272.
23. Frankenburg FR. Hoarding in anorexia nervosa. *Br J Med Psychiatry* 1984; 57:57–60.
24. Winsberg ME, Cassic KS, Koran LM. Hoarding in obsessive-compulsive disorder: a report of 20 cases. *J Clin Psychiatry* 1999;60(9):592–597.
25. Hwang JP, Tsai SJ, Yang CH, et al. Hoarding behavior in dementia. A preliminary report. *Am J Geriatr Psychiatry* 1998;6(4):285–289.
26. Steketee G, Frost RO, Kim HJ. Hoarding by elderly people. *Health Soc Work* 2001;26(3):176–184.

Evaluation and Early Treatment

CHAPTER 33

Diagnosis and Classification: *DSM–IV–TR* and ICD-10

JOHN CACCIOLA AND GEORGE E. WOODY

The *Diagnostic and Statistical Manual of Mental Disorders*, 4th ed. (*DSM–IV*) (1) is the diagnostic classification system developed by the American Psychiatric Association. Although the *DSM–IV* was updated and published as the *DSM–IV–TR* (*Text Revision*), the disorders and the diagnostic criteria did not change (2). The International Classification of Disease, Tenth Revision (ICD-10) (3) is the system used by the World Health Organization. The substance use disorders sections of previous iterations of each classification system differed significantly from each other, though many of the concepts they contained were similar. As a result, considerable efforts were made to make the current versions of these two systems as similar as possible and these efforts were mostly successful. ICD-10 actually has two versions: the clinical and the research. The clinical version is the manual that is used in clinical practice and is the main focus of this chapter, although the research version of ICD-10 is mentioned briefly in the discussion of course modifiers for dependence.

This chapter compares the sections of ICD-10 and *DSM–IV/–TR* that deal with substance-related disorders. Many details are only mentioned or described in very general terms so as to present an easily readable and memorable comparison of the two systems.

OVERVIEW

Psychiatric disorders attributable to abusable substances are of two general types: (a) disorders related to the pattern and/or consequences of substance use itself (i.e., dependence, abuse [in *DSM–IV/–TR*], and harmful use [in ICD-10]), and (b) disorders produced by the pharmacologic effects of the substances themselves (i.e., intoxication, withdrawal, and substance-induced mental disorders).

The edition preceding *DSM–IV/–TR, the Diagnostic and Statistical Manual of Mental Disorders,* 3rd ed., revised (*DSM–III–R*), organized these two general types of disorders into two areas, whereas ICD-10 placed them in one section. In *DSM–III–R*, the substance-induced disorders were found in a section entitled "Psychoactive Substance-Induced Organic Mental Disorders," whereas dependence and abuse were found in the "Psychoactive Substance Use Disorders" section. A major accomplishment of *DSM–IV* was to place all of these disorders into one section, "Substance Related Disorders," consisting of two parts: "Substance Use Disorders," which includes dependence and abuse, and "Substance-Induced Disorders," which includes intoxication, withdrawal, and substance-induced mental disorders. This major change in the organization of *DSM–IV*, and retained in the *DSM–IV–TR*, has made their overall organization much more similar to that of ICD-10. Nevertheless, there still exist substance-induced disorders that are not shared by the two classification systems, and criteria-level differences still exist between disorders that are shared by the two systems.

In each classification system, abusable substances or their general drug class are listed and criteria are provided so that any of the disorders attributable to that substance can be identified and numbered. For example, "Alcohol Withdrawal" in the *DSM–IV/–TR* is described and diagnostic criteria are summarized and coded as 291.8; "Amphetamine-Induced Mood Disorder" is identified and coded as 292.84; "Cocaine Dependence" is described and coded as 304.20; and so on. In general, the descriptive text for each of the diagnostic categories in *DSM–IV/–TR* is more detailed than that found in ICD-10.

Differences remain, however, the most prominent of which is found in the use of the terms "abuse" in *DSM–IV/–TR* and "harmful use" in ICD-10. Most importantly, each classification system is founded on the Edwards and Gross definition of the dependence syndrome (4,5), a concept that was originally developed from work with individuals having problems with alcohol but later expanded to all abusable substances.

DEPENDENCE AND ITS COURSE MODIFIERS, ABUSE, AND HARMFUL USE

Dependence

DSM–IV/–TR has seven criteria items for dependence and ICD-10 has six. In each classification system, three items are necessary to make a diagnosis of dependence. Specific items are ordered differently in each system; however, as Table 33.1 illustrates, their similarities are readily apparent when they are compared.

In *DSM–IV/–TR*, dependence is specified as being either with or without physiologic features. Dependence with physiologic features is present if there is evidence of tolerance or withdrawal (i.e., criterion items 1 or 2 are present). Dependence without physiologic features is present if three or more items are present but none of these are items 1 or 2. There is no comparable subtyping of dependence in ICD-10.

Both *DSM–IV/–TR* and ICD-10 include course modifiers for dependence. *DSM–IV* expanded the limited number of course modifiers that were present in *DSM–III–R*, again resulting in greater consistency between *DSM–IV/–TR* and ICD-10. The course modifiers for both classification systems apply only to dependence and not to abuse or harmful use.

DSM–IV/–TR

DSM–IV/–TR organizes its course modifiers in terms of stage of remission, agonist therapy, or being in a controlled environment.

Remission

A person is not classified as being in remission until that person has been free of all criteria items for dependence and all of the "A" items for abuse (to be described later in Table 33.2) for at least 1 month. The first 12 months following cessation of problems with the substance is a period of particularly high risk for relapse; thus it is given the special designation of "Early Remission." There are two categories:

- *Early Full Remission:* No criteria for dependence, and none of the "A" criteria for abuse, have been met for the last 1 to 12 months.
- *Early Partial Remission:* Full criteria for dependence or abuse have not been met for the last 1 to 12 months; however, one or two dependence, or one or more of

TABLE 33.1. *Comparison of DSM–IV and ICD-10 criteria items for dependence*

DSM–IV	ICD-10
Three or more of:	same
1) tolerance	iv) same
2) withdrawal	iii) same
3) the substance is often taken in larger amounts or over a longer period than was intended	ii) difficulties in controlling substance-taking behavior in terms of its onset, termination, or levels of use
4) any unsuccessful effort or a persistent desire to cut down or control substance use	no corresponding ICD category
5) a great deal of time is spent in activities necessary to obtain substance or recover from its effects	v) increased amounts of time necessary to obtain or take the substance or recover from its effects. Note: (v) item has two parts; this phrase represents one part
6) important social, occupational, or recreational activities given up or reduced because of substance use	v) progressive neglect of the alternative pleasures or interests. Note: (v) item has two parts; this phrase represents one part
7) continued substance use despite knowledge of having had a persistent or recurrent physical or psychological problems that are likely to be caused or exacerbated by the substance	vi) persisting with substance use despite evidence of overtly harmful problem consequences
no corresponding *DSM* category	i) a strong desire or sense of compulsion to take the substance

the "A" abuse criteria have been met, intermittently or continuously, during this period of Early Remission.

When 12 months of Early Remission have passed without relapse to dependence, the person is in "Sustained Remission." There are two categories:

- *Sustained Full Remission:* None of the criterion items for dependence and none of the criterion items for abuse have been present in the last 12 months.
- *Sustained Partial Remission:* Full criteria for dependence have not been met for a period of 12 months or longer. However, one or two dependence, or one or more of the "A" criteria for abuse have been met, either continuously or intermittently, during this period of Sustained Remission.

On Agonist Therapy

The person is on prescribed, supervised agonist medication related to the substance, and the criteria for dependence or abuse (other than tolerance or withdrawal) have not been met for the agonist medication in the last month.

This category also applies to persons being treated for dependence using an agonist/antagonist with prominent agonist properties.

In a Controlled Environment

No criteria for dependence or abuse are met but the person has been in an environment for 1 month or longer where controlled substances are highly restricted. Examples are closely supervised and substance-free jails, therapeutic communities, or locked hospital units. Occasionally, persons will be on agonist therapy while also in a controlled environment. In such cases, both course modifiers apply.

Just as the remission categories require a transitional month without satisfying any criteria for dependence or abuse, the 1-month period after cessation of agonist therapy or release from a controlled environment is a corresponding transition period. Thus, persons in this 1-month period are still considered dependent. They will move into an early remission category after being free of all criteria for dependence and of the "A" abuse criteria for 1 month.

ICD-10

The course modifiers for ICD are similar but not identical and are as follows:

- Currently abstinent
- Currently abstinent, but in a protected environment (e.g., hospital, therapeutic community, prison, etc.)
- Currently on a clinically supervised maintenance or replacement regime [controlled dependence] (e.g., with methadone, nicotine gum or nicotine patch)

- Currently abstinent, but receiving treatment with aversive or blocking drugs (e.g., naltrexone [Narcan] or disulfiram [Antabuse])
- Currently using the substance [active dependence]
- Continuous use
- Episodic use [dipsomania]

After publication of the ICD-10 clinical criteria, the ICD-10 research criteria were published. The section on course modifiers in the research criteria were made even more similar to those of *DSM–IV–TR* by adding three subcategories to "Currently abstinent," namely, "Early remission," "Partial remission," and "Full remission." Also, two subcategories were added to "Currently using the substance," "Without physical features" and "With physical features." The phrase "The course of the dependence may be further specified, if desired, as follows:" was added before the terms "Continuous use" and "Episodic use [dipsomania]." These changes to the ICD-10 research criteria set the stage for even more integration between the next iterations of the ICD and *DSM* criteria.

Abuse and Harmful Use

Although the current ICD and the *DSM* definitions of dependence are very similar, they differ sharply on the concepts of abuse and harmful use. In *DSM–IV/–TR*, abuse is defined in social terms, that is, problematic use in the absence of compulsive use, tolerance, and withdrawal. ICD has been reluctant to accept criteria items that are defined in terms of social impairment. However, ICD does recognize a nondependent type of substance use disorder. In ICD-10, this disorder is called "Harmful Use" and involves substance use that results in actual physical or mental damage.

This difference between *DSM* and ICD in the acceptability of social criteria for defining a disorder is primarily because ICD must be applicable to a wide range of cultures. Social mores differ so markedly between countries that it is difficult to develop socially defined criteria that can be applied across cultures. For example, any use of alcohol in a Moslem country can lead to major adverse social consequences, whereas Western societies have integrated alcohol use into their social fabric. The ICD-10 category of harmful use is one that can be applied cross-culturally, and is the closest that ICD comes to the *DSM* concept of abuse. However, harmful use is really a different construct because it is limited to use that causes actual physical or mental damage. Harmful use is in many ways a more restrictive category than abuse, and some persons having a *DSM–IV/–TR* abuse diagnosis do not meet criteria for harmful use. Table 33.2 is a summary comparison of Abuse and Harmful Use.

In addition to pointing out the major differences between *DSM–IV/–TR* and ICD-10 in this area, Table 33.2 summary also reflects a major change made to the

TABLE 33.2. *A comparison of abuse and harmful use*

DSM-IV	ICD-10
Abuse	**Harmful Use**
One or more of the following occurring over the same 12-month period:	Clear evidence that the substance use was responsible for (or substantially contributed to) physical or psychological harm, including impaired judgment or dysfunctional behavior.
1) recurrent substance use resulting in a failure to fulfill major role obligations at work, school, or home	
2) recurrent substance use in situations in which it is physically hazardous	
3) recurrent substance-related legal problems	
4) continued substance use despite having persistent or recurrent social or interpersonal problems caused or exacerbated by the effects of the substance	
Never met criteria for dependence	

definition of abuse. Unlike *DSM–III–R* and other earlier iterations of the *DSM*, *DSM–IV/–TR* clearly separate the criteria items for abuse from those for dependence. This change was done by attempting to identify only items that signify problematic or hazardous use as abuse and by leaving only items signifying compulsive use, tolerance, or withdrawal as dependence.

Four *DSM–IV* criteria items were developed for abuse. One (hazardous use) had been part of earlier definitions. Another (use resulting in failure to fulfill role obligations) was moved from a *DSM–III–R* dependence criterion item to abuse. The third and fourth items (recurrent substance-related legal problems; continued use despite having recurrent social or interpersonal problems) were split from one *DSM–III–R* dependence item and moved to abuse. Portions of that original item (recurrent substance-related medical or psychiatric problems) remained in a *DSM–IV* dependence item. Because diagnostic criteria did not change from *DSM–IV* to *DSM–IV–TR*, the operationalization of abuse is the same for both.

SUBSTANCE-INDUCED DISORDERS

As described above, intoxication, withdrawal, and the wide range of substance-induced mental disorders are included in a single section in both *DSM–IV/–TR* and ICD-10. *DSM–IV/–TR* provides a brief description of the clinical manifestations of intoxication and withdrawal for each substance; exceptions are those few substances that do not have an identified withdrawal syndrome, such as lysergic acid diethylamide (LSD). ICD-10 provides less detail about each substance but provides general criteria that allow for classification of intoxication or withdrawal according to specific substances.

DSM–IV/–TR also provides considerable detail for the substance-induced mental disorders. Table 33.3 identifies and summarizes the wide range of mental disorders that can be produced by substances.

Each of the mental disorders that are listed in Table 33.3 are referenced and coded in the text accompanying that

TABLE 33.3. *Diagnoses associated with class of substances*

Alcohol	X	X	X	X	I	W	P	P	I/W	I/W	I/W	I	I/W
Amphetamines	X	X	X	X	I				I	I/W	I	I	I/W
Caffeine			X								I		I
Cannabis	X	X	X		I				I		I		
Cocaine	X	X	X	X	I				I	I/W	I/W	I	I/W
Hallucinogens	X	X	X		I				Iª	I	I		
Inhalants	X	X	X		I		P		I	I	I		
Nicotine	X			X									
Opioids	X	X	X	X	I				I	I		I	I/W
Phencyclidine	X	X	X		I				I	I	I		
Sedatives, hypnotics, or anxiolytics	X	X	X	X	I	W	P	P	I/W				I/W
Polysubstance	X												
Other	X	X	X	X	I	W	P	P	I/W	I/W	I/W	I	I/W

ª Also "Hallucinogens Persisting Disorder (Flashbacks)."

Note: X, I, W, I/W, and P indicate that the category is recognized in *DSM–IV*. In addition, I indicates that the specifier "With Onset During Intoxication" may be noted for the category (except for "Intoxication Delirium"); W indicates that the specifier "With Onset During Withdrawal" may be noted for the category (except for "Withdrawal Delirium"); and I/W indicates that either "With Onset During Intoxication" or "With Onset During Withdrawal" may be noted for the category. P indicates that the disorder is persisting. Reproduced with permission from Frances A, Pincus HA, First MB, eds. Diagnostic and statistical manual of mental disorders, 4th ed. Washington, DC: American Psychiatric Association Press, 1994:177.

specific substance. They are also cross-referenced with the section of *DSM–IV/–TR* that deals with that type of disorder. For example, psychotic disorders attributable to alcohol intoxication or withdrawal are mentioned and coded in the text dealing with alcohol, and the reader is directed to the psychotic disorders section of *DSM–IV/–TR* for a more complete description of these disorders. ICD-10 provides a more general format that allows for classification of substance-induced mental disorders, but provides much less substance-specific detail than *DSM–IV/–TR*.

COMPARISONS OF DIFFERENCES IN SPECIFIC DIAGNOSTIC CATEGORIES

There are a few other important categories that are found in one system but not the other. For instance, *DSM–IV/–TR* has three categories that are not specified in ICD-10: "Polysubstance Dependence;" "Other (or Unknown) Substance-Related Disorders;" and "Phencyclidine (or Phencyclidine-Like)-Related Disorders." These categories would likely be classified under the ICD-10 heading of "Disorders Resulting from Multiple Drug Use and Use of Other Psychoactive Substances."

A number of substances have limited diagnostic possibilities in *DSM–IV/–TR* but have a wider range of ICD-10 diagnostic labels. For instance, caffeine is included in the stimulant section of ICD-10 and thus is open to a wide range of subcategories. In contrast, "Caffeine Intoxication," "Caffeine-Induced Anxiety Disorder," and "Caffeine-Induced Sleep Disorder" are the only categories available for this substance in *DSM–IV*. Similarly, *DSM–IV/–TR* has only two categories involving nicotine: dependence and withdrawal. ICD-10 has the same wide range of diagnostic categories for nicotine that is available for all other substances.

ICD-10 has a section (listed as a subsection of "Behavioural Syndromes Associated with Physiological Disturbances and Physical Factors") that is separate from the psychoactive substance use section and that is used for classifying abuse of non–dependence-producing substances. This includes problematic use of antidepressants, laxatives, steroids, and hormones. A comparable section in *DSM–IV/–TR* is found under "Other (or Unknown) Substance-Related Disorders."

SUMMARY

Many of the major differences between the *DSM* and ICD classification systems have been eliminated or considerably reduced by the devlopment of the *DSM–IV/–TR* and ICD-10. The most prominent remaining difference is in the concepts underlying abuse and harmful use. Less-prominent differences are found in the less-detailed descriptions of the various clinical syndromes in ICD-10 as compared to *DSM–IV/–TR*, and in ICD-10's ability to attach the entire range of substance-related diagnoses to any drug class, whereas *DSM–IV/–TR* provides more limits on the number of diagnostic possibilities. Generally, ICD-10 has more categories available for each substance than *DSM–IV/–TR*, but many of these categories are never used because they do not exist. An example is hallucinogen withdrawal—a possible category in ICD-10 that is not present in *DSM–IV/–TR*, but that is probably never used in ICD-10 because there is little evidence that it ever occurs.

Overall, there are many more similarities than differences, especially when one focuses on the specific categories described (with the exception of abuse and harmful use), and on the similarities in the ways dependence and its course modifiers are defined. It is hoped that future work will succeed in creating even more consistency between these two classification systems. A recent reveiw of the two systems by Rounaville discusses the remaining barriers to reconciling ICD and *DSM* in the future (6). He concludes, as suggested by this review, that reconcilliation may be most difficult for the abuse/harmful use disparity, perhaps less so for the substance-induced disorders, and most readily achieved for dependence.

REFERENCES

1. American Psychiatric Association. *Diagnostic and statistical manual of mental disorders,* 4th ed. (*DSM-IV*). Washington, DC: Author, 1994.
2. American Psychiatric Association. *Diagnostic and statistical manual of mental disorders,* 4th ed., text revision (*DSM-IV-TR*). Washington, DC: Author, 2000.
3. World Health Organization. *Tenth revision of the international classification of disease (ICD-10).* Geneva: World Health Organization, 1992.
4. Edwards G, Gross MM. Alcohol dependence: provisional description of a clinical syndrome. *Br J Med* 1976;1:1058–1061.
5. Edwards G. The alcohol dependence syndrome: a concept as stimulus to enquiry. *Br J Addict* 1986;81:171–183.
6. Rounsaville B. Experience with ICD-10/*DSM-IV* substance use disorders. *Psychopathology* 2002;35:82–88.

CHAPTER 34

Diagnostic Laboratory: Screening for Drug Abuse

KARL G. VEREBEY, GERARD MEENAN, AND BETTY J. BUCHAN

Alcohol and drug abuse are two major health care problems in America. This has prompted advancement in laboratory methods diagnosing substance abuse in psychiatric patients and suspected drug abusers. Physicians are more knowledgeable today than in the past about the nature of drug abuse, yet uncertainty remains in the use of the "diagnostic laboratory." The confusion surrounding drug abuse testing is a result of many variables. Each individual drug is unique, and detectability depends on the type of drug, size of the dose, frequency of use, the type of biologic specimen tested, differences in individual drug metabolism, sample collection time in relation to use, and sensitivity of the analytical method (1). All these variables make each test request an individual case, and there are no general rules for all drugs and all situations.

This chapter reviews testing of drugs of abuse from several perspectives. A brief history of drug testing is followed by a section on the reasons for testing. Described in detail are the available methodologies, testing strategies, and data interpretation methods.

HISTORY OF DRUG TESTING

The modern drug-abuse testing laboratory is a recent development. Initially, drug testing was exclusively part of the pathology services in which overdose or fatal toxicity cases were investigated for the causative agents. Very large sample volumes were processed with crude, nonspecific methodology. As drugs of abuse became a major social problem, overdose cases also became more common. Hospital laboratories were called upon to perform emergency toxicology procedures to identify drug classes or specific drugs.

Another branch of testing developed when identified drug abusers in treatment programs needed followup to objectively monitor abstinence from drugs. Such rehabilitation testing was performed in hospitals or private clinical laboratories that initially were not designed for drug testing.

Drug testing has increased rapidly over the last decade as a consequence of widespread employee testing by the federal government, the military, and private industry. This has influenced the rapid development of specific urine drug-testing laboratories.

Forensic drug testing is the newest to appear on the scene, forced upon the clinical laboratories by the legal profession. Positive results were sometimes questioned or flatly denied, and lawyers started to scrutinize every step of the testing process from collection to reporting of results. Forensic accountability was then required to protect the "due process rights" of clients. After losing court cases, clinical laboratories that performed legally sensitive testing began to reorganize. "Chain of custody" procedures were designed, and quality control and quality assurance procedures were implemented to promote reliability and reproducibility of test results. Drug-testing procedures and instrumentation became more sophisticated, more sensitive, and more specific. As a result, extremely small amounts of drugs can be determined reliably at the nanogram and picogram range, and gas chromatography-mass spectrometry (GC-MS) and gas chromatography-tandem mass spectrometry (GC-MS-MS) provides assurance of specific analyte identification (2).

RATIONALE FOR TESTING

Drug abuse is characterized by impulsive drug-seeking behavior with occasional breaks and almost certain relapses. A common feature of drug abusers is denial. Abusers lie to themselves and the forbidding outside world to protect their continued, obsessive addiction to drugs and/or alcohol. For this reason, physicians seldom are given voluntarily the diagnostically important information about addictive habits.

The drug choice and the abuse pattern are important parts of the medical history. The attending physician cannot properly design treatment when kept in the dark about the patient's addiction. Symptoms of physical and/or psychiatric illness may be simulated by the presence or absence of certain drugs. The dichotomy of symptoms associated with the presence or absence of a drug is best illustrated by the opioid class of drugs (3). While under the influence of an opioid, the addict experiences euphoric, anxiolytic sedation, mental clouding, sweating, and constipation. The common opioid withdrawal signs and symptoms appear characterized by pupillary mydriasis, agitation, anxiety, panic, muscle aches, gooseflesh, rhinorrhea, salivation, and diarrhea. Thus, the two different sets of symptoms belong to the abuse of the same drug, observed at times of opioid presence and at times of opioid absence.

In predisposed individuals, drugs can trigger behavior similar or identical to psychosis. For example, phencyclidine (PCP), lysergic acid diethylamide (LSD), amphetamines, or cocaine can cause toxic psychosis that is indistinguishable from paranoid schizophrenia. These drugs can produce model psychosis in anyone given an adequate dose. Drug-induced psychosis has a different prognosis and must be treated differently from psychosis related to endogenous organic, anatomic, or neurochemical disorders (4).

Treatment of drug abusers in therapy would be extremely handicapped if testing were not used. Therefore, comprehensive drug testing is important for making precise followup evaluations and selecting appropriate treatment (5). Thus the first good reason for laboratory drug testing is to provide objective identification of drug abusers and identify the substance abused.

Testing is also important after drug abusers are identified. Treatment strategies are intimately connected to frequent urinalyses to monitor recovering addicts. Negative results support the success of treatment, while positive results alert the physician to relapses. Objective testing, therefore, is a necessary component of modern treatment (5).

Drug-abuse testing may also be forensic in nature. Parole officers monitor ex-drug abusers after release from incarceration. A positive drug test may signal to law enforcement the parolee's involvement with drugs and may invalidate the parole.

More often than is seen in the general population, health professionals such as doctors, dentists, and nurses are afflicted with drug abuse problems. Once involvement with drugs is exposed, professional medical licenses are in danger of suspension. Rehabilitation of addicted health professionals is linked to drug testing as a condition of probation.

Professional athletes often abuse drugs. Teams and national or international sport associations may prohibit the use of performance-enhancing drugs (6). Staying drug-free is often a prerequisite for athletes to be allowed to compete. Laboratory testing of body fluids for drugs of abuse is the objective technique used to enforce these rules.

Finally, the conduct of business and the public's safety may be endangered by impaired or intoxicated employees. Bankers and stockbrokers who handle investors' money should not be influenced by psychoactive drugs, especially drugs that cause delusions and impulsive risk-taking behavior. Similarly, other drug-abusing professionals may endanger the public. Drug abuse has been identified among airline pilots, bus drivers, railroad engineers, and police officers. In all these examples, drug-abuse testing is advantageous to the drug abuser and the general public. The abuser gets early treatment and a chance for early rehabilitation, and the public is saved from drug-related wrongdoing.

A decrease in drug abuse as a result of testing has been demonstrated clearly in the military. Prior to the institution of testing in 1981, 48% of armed forces personnel used illegal drugs. Three years after testing began, fewer than 5% were using drugs (7). Although critics often attack testing as ineffective, drug use clearly decreases where effective drug testing exists.

TABLE 34.1. *Panel groups of abused drugs: tests performed by laboratories*

I: Required[a]	II: Commonly performed	III: Not commonly performed
Amphetamines	Barbiturates	LSD
Cannabinoids	Benzodiazepines	Fentanyl
Cocaine	Methadone	Psilocybin
Opioids	Propoxyphene	MDMA
Phencyclidine	Methaqualone	MDA
	Ethanol	Designer drugs

[a]Testing required for certification by the DHHS/SAMHSA National Laboratory Certification Program.

ABUSED DRUGS TESTED

Epidemiologic studies expose the types of drugs used, new trends, and frequency of drug abuse by different populations in specific geographic regions and countries. In effective drug-abuse testing, such information is used to help identify drug abusers. The testing of five drugs, selected by the Department of Health and Human Services Substance Abuse and Mental Health Services Administration (DHHS/SAMHSA), is required for accreditation by their National Laboratory Certification Program (NLCP) (Table 34.1). Panel I testing includes amphetamines, cannabinoids, cocaine, opioids, and phencyclidine. Panel II represents other commonly abused drugs, such as barbiturates, benzodiazepines, methaqualone, propoxyphene, methadone, and ethanol. Interestingly, some powerful hallucinogens seldom are tested routinely. They are listed in Panel III: LSD, methylenedioxyamphetamine (MDA), methylenedioxymethamphetamine (MDMA), psilocybin, and other designer drugs. These drugs are psychoactive in very low doses. Therefore, when they are diluted in total body water, detection is difficult or impossible unless large doses are taken or samples are collected immediately after drug use.

"Designer drugs" are structural congeners of common drugs of abuse. Often they are not yet regulated when sold and used. "Street chemists" are occasionally synthesizing new and often dangerous drugs. They will operate as long as abusers will try new drugs, and their trade remains profitable. The laboratory's role is to develop sensitive methods for the detection of designer drugs in the biofluids of users.

CLUB DRUGS OF ABUSE

Gamma hydroxybutyrate (GHB) is a central nervous system depressant. It is an endogenous substance in human and mammalian tissues at very low concentrations and thought to be a neurotransmitter. It had some clinical use as an anesthetic and hypnotic drug in the past, but now it is used only in research. Some of the pharmacologic effects are amnesia and hypotonia and, at large doses, sleep (8).

Use of this drug in date rapes are for its amnesia-producing effects. The perpetrator hopes that the victim will have no recollection of the sexual attack after the drug wears off. Detection of GHB is accomplished with analysis by gas chromatography (GC) and/or high-performance liquid chromatography (HPLC).

Another drug used in clubs and date rapes is flunitrazepam (Rohypnol) a member of the benzodiazepine family of drugs. Only available in Europe, however, it is also abused in the United States as a club drug. At low doses it causes sleepiness, and at larger doses, anesthesia. Detection, as for several other benzodiazepines, is performed by screening with an immunoassay and confirmation with GC-MS or HPLC (8).

Recently ketamine (Ketalar) or Special K appeared in clubs. It is chemically related to phencyclidine (PCP) or angel dust (8). Both of these drugs were used for rapidly acting dissociative anesthetics. However, in some individuals ketamine and PCP produce exit psychosis with paranoid ideation. For this reason ketamine currently is mainly used in veterinary medicine. Abuse of ketamine results in a diverse set of reactions depending on individual predispositions: numbness, loss of coordination, sense of invulnerability, muscle rigidity, aggressive/violent behavior, slurred speech, blank stare, and an exaggerated sense of strength. Recently, immunoassays were developed for ketamine screening. Positive results are confirmed by GC-MS or GC-MS–MS.

TESTS AVAILABLE

A number of different laboratory methods are available for drug screening. When the drug-abuse habit of the patient is unknown, physicians usually request a "comprehensive drug screen." Different laboratories have different definitions of the term *comprehensive drug testing*. The physician should be familiar with laboratory procedures and menus to ensure effective use of the drug testing laboratory.

Urine samples are most commonly sent for "routine drug screen." But oral fluid (saliva) testing is becoming more popular because of the ease of collection. Psychiatrists and other physicians assume that a comprehensive drug test detects all abused drugs. Thin-layer chromatography (TLC), mostly used in the past, is not sensitive enough to detect drugs such as marijuana, PCP, LSD, MDA, MDMA, mescaline, and fentanyl, among others. Thus, a negative drug screen may mean that the test cut-off is too high, the test menu doesn't contain the drug(s) of interest, or there is no evidence of high-dose and/or recent abuse of drugs commonly detected by the screening method used. Low-level abuse of drugs is not likely to be detected, therefore "false negatives" are very common for drug screens performed by TLC (9). More recently enzyme immunoassays (EIA) have replaced TLC as a

screening procedure. EIA, enzyme-linked immunoabsorbent assay (ELISA), and fluorescent polarization immunoassay (FPIA) are routinely used with biologic fluids screening such as urine, oral fluid, sweat, and hair.

If, for example, a physician suspects marihuana abuse, the physician must specifically request that a marijuana screen be performed by an immunoassay at the lowest available cut off. Currently, screening for prescription drugs and drugs of abuse is performed by EIA, such as the enzyme multiplied immunoassay test (EMIT), ELISA, radioimmunoassay (RIA), or FPIA, and a modern version of TLC, high-performance TLC (HPTLC), which has improved sensitivity over that of conventional TLC systems. In a very few laboratories, drug screening is performed by capillary gas-liquid chromatography (GLC). In a single GLC analysis more than 25 drugs can be identified. This system is advantageous when there is no clue to the identity of the abused substance; however, GLC, HPTLC, and GC-MS are time-consuming, labor-intensive, and usually expensive procedures. HPLC is similar to GLC in principle. It is usually less sensitive than GLC, but sample preparation is easier. The EIA, ELISA, and RIA tests are significantly less expensive and more practical than the more specific GC, HPTLC, and GC-MS methods. EIA procedures are easily adaptable for high-volume automated screening of drugs. In fact, most good laboratories offer a five- or ten-drug panel, with or without alcohol, performed by EIA.

ANALYTIC METHODOLOGIES

Alcohol Methods of Analysis

Alcohol abuse is a legal version of drug abuse in the United States and most parts of the world. The addictive chemical substance in all alcoholic beverages is ethanol or ethyl alcohol. Ethanol is present in beer (3% to 6%), wine (11% to 13%), and distilled beverages (22% to 60%). A 160-pound subject must ingest 4 to 5 drinks (12 oz beer, 4 oz wine, or 1 oz whiskey) in 1 hour to reach an ethanol level of 0.10 g/100 mL blood, or 100 mg/100 mL blood, which is the per se illegal limit to operate an automobile in most states, although many states have reduced this limit to 0.08 g%.

Ethanol is one of the few drugs for which blood levels can be correlated with levels of intoxication or impairment, although large individual variations do exist. Ethanol is analyzed by means of chemical assays and enzymatic and GLC methods (8). The most specific quantitative method for blood alcohol determination is GLC or "head space" analysis by GLC. Volatile substances such as ethanol are driven out of aqueous biofluids into the "head space" or air space of heated and sealed vials. Air samples are taken from the test tubes by an airtight syringe and injected into the gas chromatograph for separation and quantitation.

This method separates ethanol from other alcohols and other volatile substances.

If ethanol analysis is performed on breath by means of a breathalyzer, or on blood or urine by one of the chemical or enzymatic assays the results are reliable for general use. Some states allow breathalyzer results, as acceptable values, to determine legal impairment in driving accidents. In most forensic cases, however, results should be confirmed with a blood specimen using the GLC "head space" method. Alcoholism, like drug addiction, is hidden by denial. Therefore, when drug screening is requested, ethanol analysis should also be ordered. Ethanol measurement must be requested in addition to a drug screen because alcohol testing is not performed routinely by most laboratories. For clinical purposes, urine alcohol levels can be ordered. The conversion factor is 1.3 urine:blood ratio (8).

Thin-Layer Chromatography

TLC is a qualitative method and it is the least-sensitive analytic technique for most drugs. Visualization of the spots on TLC is achieved by illumination with ultraviolet or fluorescent lights, or by color reactions of the spots after spraying with chemical dyes. Identical molecules are expected to migrate to the same area and to give specific color reactions. Thus migration and color give TLC specificity not recognized in recent years with the advancement of more sophisticated techniques.

Radioimmunoassay Enzyme Immunoassay, and Enzyme-Linked Immunoabsorbent Assay

Figure 34.1 depicts the principle of immunoassays in drug detection. Antibodies are used to seek out specific drugs in biofluids. In samples containing one or more drugs, competition exists for available antibody-binding sites. The presence or absence of specific drugs is determined by the percent binding.

The specificity and sensitivity of the antibodies to a given drug differ depending on the particular drug assay and the assay manufacturer. Immunoassay can be very specific; however, compounds structurally similar to the drug of interest (i.e., metabolites or structural congeners) often cross-react. Interaction of the antibody with a drug plus its metabolites increases the sensitivity of the assay.

EIA, ELISA, and FPIA are commonly used for drug-abuse screening because no complicated extraction is required and the system lends itself to easy automation. EIA is more sensitive for most drugs and detects lower drug concentrations than TLC.

ELISA offers greater sensitivity than some other screening assays. The sensitivity and specificity of the ELISA assays provide valuable utility to the clinician. A variety of biologic samples are applicable to ELISA assays

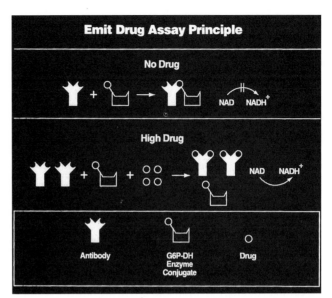

FIG. 34.1. The basic principle of enzyme immunoassay (EIA) reactivity as it relates to drug detection. Molecules with similar functional groups cross-react, hence immunoassays have less specificity than do chromatographic assays. EIA is the most popular screening procedure. G6P-DH = glucose-6-phosphate dehydrogenase; NAD = nicotinamide adenine dinucleotide; NADH = nicotinamide adenine dinucleotide (reduced form). (Reproduced with the permission of Syva Company, Inc.)

such as urine, serum/plasma/blood, and oral fluid or saliva. Depending on the concentration of drug expected in the specimen, sample size can be adjusted accordingly. ELISA assays are available for manual, semiautomated, and fully automated platforms. Analysis time varies between 1 and 2 hours. Cut-off levels and limits of detection (LOD) for saliva samples are very low compared to conventional immunoassays: amphetamines 50 ng/mL and 1 ng/mL, respectively; barbiturates 20 ng/mL and 1 ng/mL, respectively; Benzodiazepines 5 ng/mL and 2 ng/mL, respectively; cocaine 20 ng/mL and 1 ng/mL, respectively; methadone 5 ng/mL and 1 ng/mL, respectively; opiates 40 ng/mL and 0.25 ng/mL, respectively; PCP 10 ng/mL and 0.5 ng/mL, respectively; THC 4 ng/mL and 0.1 ng/mL. Also sample volumes are as low as 10 μL per analysis (10).

As seen above, allowing for detection of low levels of drug abuse, the levels of sensitivity or LOD are in the very low nanogram range (10).

The scientific literature supports oral fluid as an excellent alternative to urine and blood for the identification of drug abuse. Because oral fluid collection is convenient, noninvasive, fast, and observable, thus, sample adulteration is not likely to occur.

Several oral fluid sample collection devices are available. However, neat saliva collected in test tubes contained the highest concentrations of drugs when compared to oral fluid. On the other hand, spitting into a tube is not as acceptable to subjects as are the "lollipop" type collectors.

On-Site Screening Immunoassays

The increased prevalence of drug use has prompted the development of new drug-screening technology that produce results in as little as 10 minutes. Many situations require immediate testing and results for drugs of abuse. Hospital emergency departments have an immediate need for detecting drug overdoses. In addition, rapid results are useful for monitoring psychiatric patients, monitoring compliance within a drug rehabilitation program, and supervising parolees. Because these tests are designed to be performed on-site, they may be performed directly in front of the person being tested or, certainly, at the site of collection. This is particularly useful for preemployment screening, random or probable cause workplace testing, and for workplace accident-related injuries. It may also be important to conduct drug testing on-site in safety-oriented occupations, such as public transportation.

Visually interpreted competitive immunoassays that require no instrumentation have been developed in recent years. These kits are particularly effective because there is no calibration, maintenance or downtime required, and no special skills are needed to perform these tests. Most kits have built-in quality control zones in each panel, which ensures reagent integrity, and most have an extended shelf-life at room temperature.

There are currently a half dozen or more on-site kits on the market. Two kits use novel approaches. The Triage Panel for Drugs of Abuse plus Tricyclic Antidepressants (Biosite Diagnostics, Inc., San Diego, CA) is based on the use of Ascend Multiimmunoassay (AMIA) technology for simultaneous detection of multiple analytes in a sample. A urine sample is placed in the reaction cup in contact with lyophilized reagents and the reaction mixture is allowed to come to equilibrium for 10 minutes. The chemically labeled drugs (drug conjugate) compete with drugs that may be present in the urine for antibody binding sites. The reaction mixture is transferred to the solid-phase membrane in the detection area that contains various immobilized antibodies in discrete drug class-specific zones. After a washing step, the operator visually examines each zone for the presence of a red bar. The method incorporates preset threshold concentrations that are independent for each drug. The assay response is proportional to the concentration of the unbound drug conjugate so that no signal is observed at drug concentrations less than the threshold concentrations (11). A positive specimen produces a distinct red bar in the drug detection zone adjacent to the drug name. A negative specimen does not produce a colored bar.

Newer on-site screening analyzer is the PROFILE-II ER 9-panel for drugs of abuse (Medtox Diagnostics, Inc., Burlington, NC) (Figure 34.2). It is a one-step immunochromatographic test for the rapid, qualitative de-

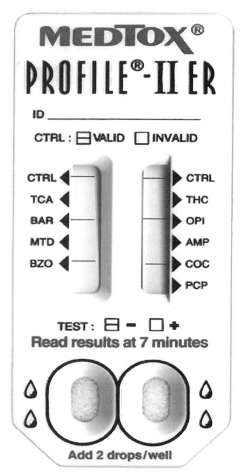

FIG. 34.2. The Medtox PROFILE-II ER hand-held point of care analyzer. (Reprinted with permission of Medtox Diagnostics, Inc. Burlington, NC).

tection of cannabinoids, cocaine, opiates, amphetamines, phencyclidine, tricyclic antidepressants, barbiturates, methadone, and benzodiazepines in human urine. A 10-panel configuration includes propoxyphene, methamphetamine and 3,4 methylenedioxymethamphetamine (MDMA). The test detects 11 drug classes at the following cutoff concentrations:

Cannabinoids (THC; 11-*nor*-9-carboxy-Δ9-THC), 50 ng/mL; opiates (OPI; morphine), 300 ng/mL; cocaine (COC; benzoylecgonine), 300 ng/mL; amphetamines (AMP; *d*-amphetamine), 1,000 ng/mL; phencyclidine (PCP), 25 ng/mL; tricyclic antidepressants (TCA; Desipramine), 300 ng/mL; barbiturates (BAR; phenobarbital), 200 ng/mL; methadone (MTD), 300 ng/mL; benzodiazepines (BZO; nordazepam), 300 ng/mL; propoxyphene (PPX; norpropoxyphene), 300 ng/mL; and methamphetamine–3,4 methylenedioxymethamphetamine (MAMP-MDMA), 1,000 to 1,500 ng/mL. PROFILE-II ER provides stat screening of selected target analytes. Two drops of urine are added to the sample well and the results are interpreted in 7 minutes. The PROFILE-II ER 9- or 10-panel test is a

1-step, competitive, membrane-based immunochromatographic assay. A single urine sample can be evaluated for the presence of each of the specified classes of drugs on two or three parallel strips in a single or dual device. Cannabinoids (THC), cocaine, opiates, amphetamines, and phencyclidine are assayed on one strip; tricyclic antidepressants, barbiturates, methadone, and benzodiazepines are assayed on the second strip; and propoxyphene and methamphetamine-MDMA are assayed on the third strip. When one or more drugs are present in a urine sample, they generate easily visible red lines at each of the labeled locations in the result window.

Another unique screening device is the OnTrak TesTcup Collection/Urinalysis Panel (Roche Diagnostic Systems, Inc., Somerville, NJ). The OnTrak TesTcup, shown in Figure 34.3, simultaneously tests for the presence of three drugs (with respective threshold/cut-off concentrations)—cocaine (COC) (300 ng/mL), tetrahydrocannabinol (THC) (50 ng/mL), and morphine (MOR) (300 ng/mL)—and has the capability for a total of five different drugs. OnTrak TesTcup assays are based on the principle of microparticle capture inhibition. The test relies on the competition between drug, which may be present in the urine being tested, and drug conjugate immobilized on a membrane in the test chamber. Urine is collected directly in the OnTrak TesTcup and therefore provides the advantage of eliminating transfer or direct contact with the sample. After closing the cap and moving it to the test position, the sample reservoir is filled by tilting the cup for 5 seconds. Urine proceeds down immunochromatographic strips by capillary action and reacts with antibody-coated microparticles and drug conjugate present on the membrane. In approximately 3 to 5 minutes, the Test Valid bars appear, a decal is removed from the detection window, and the results are interpreted as positive or negative. In the absence of drug, the antibody is free to interact with the drug conjugate, causing the formation of a blue band as a negative sign. When drug is present in the specimen, it binds to the antibody-coated microparticles and no blue band is formed. A positive sample causes the membrane to remain white (OnTrak TesTcup package insert, April 1995).

These on-site screening kits have demonstrated greater than 97% agreement with confirmatory tests such as GC-MS (11). However, it must be stressed that these kits provide only preliminary analytical test results, just like immunoassay tests run in a laboratory. A more specific alternate chemical method must be used to confirm positive screening results. GC-MS is the most specific confirmation method.

Gas Liquid Chromatography and Gas Chromatography-Mass Spectrometry

GLC is an analytic technique that separates molecules by migration as described for TLC. The TLC plate is replaced by lengths of glass or metal tubing called columns, which are packed or coated with stationary materials of variable polarity. Figure 34.4 is an example of a GLC tracing showing separation of drugs in a mixture. The extracted analyte is carried through the column to the detector by a steady flow of heated gas. The detector responds to the drugs and other molecules. This response is graphically recorded and quantified, and is proportional to the amount of substance present in the sample. Identical compounds travel through the column at the same speed because they have identical interaction with the stationary column packing. The time between injection and an observed response at the recorder is the retention time. Identical retention times of substances on two different polarity columns constitute strong evidence that the substances are identical.

Stronger evidence can be obtained by the use of GC-MS, which identifies substances by gas chromatography separation and mass spectrometry fragmentation patterns. Figure 34.5 shows a GC-MS separation and fragmentation pattern of cocaine and its major metabolite benzoylecgonine. The separation is shown at the bottom of the figure, while the fragmentation is shown in the top two panels. Cocaine has the fragments 82, 182, and 303, while benzoylecgonine has 82, 240, and 361.

Not all bonds in molecules are of equal strength. The weak bonds are more likely to break under stress. In the mass spectrometer detector, electron beam bombardment

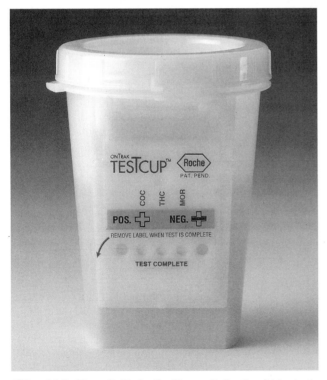

FIG. 34.3. The OnTrak TesTcup Collection/Urinalysis Panel. (Reprinted with permission of Roche Diagnostic Systems, Inc., Somerville, NJ.)

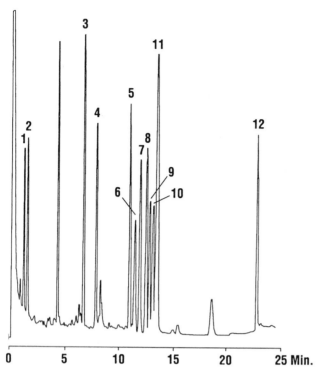

FIG. 34.4. Gas liquid chromatographic (GLC) tracing showing separation of a drug mixture. The abscissa is time in minutes, the ordinate is detector response. The different drugs are number coded on the tracing. The drugs are *1,* amphetamine; *2,* methamphetamine; *3,* meperidine; *4,* phencyclidine (PCP); *5,* methadone; *6,* amitriptyline; *7,* imipramine; *8,* cocaine; *9,* desipramine; *10,* pentazocine; *11,* codeine; and *12,* oxycodone. (Reprinted with permission of Alltech Associates, Inc., Deerfield, IL.)

of molecules breaks weak bonds. The exact mass and quantity of the molecular fragments or breakage products are measured by the mass detector. The breakage of molecules results in fragments unique for a drug. They occur in specific ratios to one another, thus the GC-MS method is often called "molecular fingerprinting." GC-MS is the most reliable, most definitive procedure in analytic chemistry for drug identification (12).

The fragmentation pattern of unknowns is checked against a computer library that lists the mass of drugs and related fragments. Matching a control's fragments and fragment ratios is considered absolute confirmation of a particular compound. The sensitivity of GLC for most drugs is in the nanogram range, but with special detectors some compounds can be measured at picogram levels. GLC and GC-MS can also be used quantitatively, which provides additional information helping to interpret a clinical syndrome or explain corroborating evidence in forensic cases. Tandem mass spectrometry (MS-MS) offers greater sensitivity than GC-MS. For example, LSD confirmation by GC-MS-MS is as low as 200 pg. As the screening method's sensitivity approaches the low nanogram range, confirmation often requires picogram-level sensitivity to confirm positive samples.

Technically, samples are introduced into MS-MS detectors from gas chromatographs, liquid chromatographs, or direct insertion probes. The choice depends on sample volatility and purity. Thus MS-MS provides a confirmation procedure for the ever-more-sensitive screening methods (e.g., ELISA) and use with very low drug concentrations such as is present in oral fluids, sweat, and hair analysis.

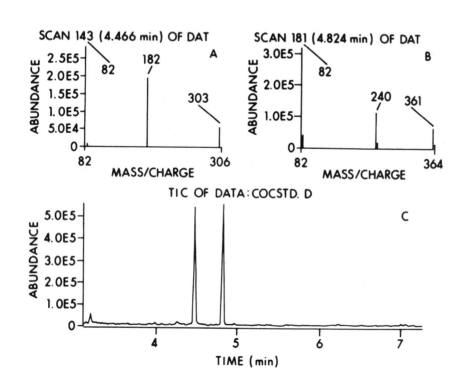

FIG. 34.5. Gas chromatography-mass spectrometry showing and the fragmentation pattern of cocaine (**A**) and benzoylecgonine (**B**). **C,** the chromatographic separation of cocaine (4 min, 28 sec) and benzoylecgonine (4 min, 51 sec). (Reproduced with the permission of Drs. R. W. Taylor, N. C. Jain, and the *Journal of Analytical Toxicology.*)

TABLE 34.2. *Performance characteristics of different assays for drugs of abuse*

Assay	Sensitivity	Specificity	Accuracy	Turn-around time	Cost ($)
On-site	Moderate-high	Moderate	Qualitative[a]	Minutes	4–25
EMIT; FPIA; RIA; KIMS	Moderate-high	Moderate	Low-high	1–4 hours	1–5
TLC	Low-high	High	Qualitative[a]	1–4 hours	1–4
GC	High	High	High	Days	5–20
GC-MS	High	High	High	Days	10–100

Abbreviation: EMIT-enzyme multiplied immunoassay technique; FPIA-fluorescent polarization immunoassay; GC-gas chromatography; GC-MS-gas chromatography-mass spectrometry; KIMS-kinetic interaction of microparticles in solution; RIA-radioimmunoassay; TLC-thin-layer chromatography.

[a]Results are generally expressed only in qualitative terms (i.e., positive/negative); consequently, accuracy may be difficult to assess.

From Cone EJ. New developments in biological measures of drug prevalence. *NIDA Res Monogr Ser* 1986;167:104–126.

HPLC is used especially for drugs that are not volatile or that cannot be made volatile by derivatization. These drugs are not amenable for analysis by GC-MS or GC. Examples of drugs or drug groups for which HPLC is the choice of analysis are the benzodiazepines, tricyclic antidepressants, and acetaminophen.

When a routine toxicology screen is ordered, the physician is often not aware that options are available for more specific screening and confirmation. Table 34.2 shows the performance characteristics of different types of assays for drugs of abuse.

CHOICE OF BODY FLUIDS AND TIME OF SAMPLE COLLECTION

Some drugs are metabolized extensively and are excreted very quickly, whereas others stay in the body for a long time (1). Thus success of detection depends not only on the time of sample collection after last use, but also on the drug used and whether the analysis is performed for the drug itself or for its metabolites. Table 34.3 illustrates the typical screening and confirmation cutoff concentrations, and the expected time scales of detectability for some commonly abused drugs.

When drug-abuse detection is the goal, the following questions should be asked: (a) How long does the suspected drug stay in the body, or, what is its biologic half-life? (b) How fast and how extensively is the drug biotransformed? Should one look for the drug itself or its metabolites? (c) Which body fluid is best for analysis, or, what is the major route of excretion? Intravenous use or smoking drugs of abuse provides nearly instantaneous absorption into the bloodstream and excretion of the drug and/or metabolites in urine occurs almost immediately. Inhalation (smoking or snorting) or oral use of drugs will result in slower absorption and excretion in urine may not be detected immediately after use.

Cocaine is rapidly biotransformed into benzoylecgonine and ecgonine methyl ester. Less than 10% unchanged

cocaine is excreted into the urine and is detectable only for 12 to 18 hours after use. What does this suggest to the clinician who wants to identify cocaine abusers? Because cocaine has a short half-life, unless use is suspected within hours or the patient is suspected to be under the influence of cocaine at the time of sample collection, the parent compound is unlikely to be found in detectable concentrations in either blood or urine (13). Plasma enzymes continue to metabolize cocaine even after blood is taken out of the body. Therefore, blood samples must be collected into tubes containing sodium fluoride to inactivate the enzymes. Benzoylecgonine is the major metabolite of cocaine; its half-life is about 6 hours and it is excreted in urine at levels totaling approximately 45% of the dose. Thus cocaine-abuse detection is best accomplished by collecting urine and analyzing it for benzoylecgonine.

Cocaine metabolism and disposition is contrasted with methaqualone, which is also very lipid-soluble but has a half-life of 20 to 60 hours as a consequence of slow biotransformation. Thus, either blood or urine tests are effective for many days to detect methaqualone itself. Methaqualone was detected for 21 days in urine after a single 300-mg oral dose and in blood for 7 days (14). Pharmacokinetic and drug excretion information are important to determine target chemicals (drug or metabolite) for detection. Many physicians prefer blood to urine for drug screening because blood levels constitute stronger evidence of recent use and are related more closely to brain levels and drug-related behavioral changes than are urine levels.

The collection of urine specimens must be supervised to ensure donor identity and to guarantee the integrity of the specimen. It is not unusual to receive someone else's urine or a highly diluted sample when collection is not supervised or screened by the laboratory for pH, specific gravity, and creatinine levels. As a rule, first morning urine samples are more concentrated, therefore, drugs are easier to detect than in more diluted samples. The decision

TABLE 34.3. *Typical screening and confirmation cut-off concentrations and detection times for drugs of abuse*

Drug	Screening cutoff concentrations (ng/mL)	Analyte tested in confirmation	Confirmation cutoff concentrations (ng/mL)	Urine detection time
Amphetamine	1,000	amphetamine	500	2–4 days
Barbiturates	200	amobarbital; secobarbital; other barbiturates	200	2–4 days for short acting; up to 30 days for long acting
Benzodiazepines	200	oxazepam; diazepam; other benzodiazepines	200	Up to 30 days
Cocaine	300	benzoylecgonine	150	1–3 days
Codeine	300	codeine	300	
		morphine	300	1–3 days
Heroin	300	morphine	300	1–3 days
		6-acetylmorphine	10	
Marijuana	100; 50; 20	tetrahydrocannabinol	15	1–3 days for casual use; up to 30 days for chronic use
Methadone	300	methadone	300	2–4 days
Methamphet-amine	1000	methamphetamine	500	2–4 days
		amphetamine	200	
Phencyclidine	25	phencyclidine	25	2–7 days for casual use; up to 30 days for chronic use

From Cone EJ. New developments in biological measures of drug prevalence. *NIDA Res Monogr* 1986;167:104–126.

to use blood or urine must be based on the information needed and the specific drug's pharmacokinetic and excretion data. Drug levels in urine are higher than in blood, therefore, urine is usually the biofluid of choice for drug detection.

INTERPRETATION OF RESULTS

Psychoactivity of most drugs lasts only a few hours, while urinalysis can detect some drugs and/or metabolites for days or even weeks (15). Thus, the presence of a drug (or metabolite) in urine is only an indication of prior exposure, not proof of intoxication or impairment at the time of sample collection. In some cases, quantitative data in blood or urine can corroborate observed behavior or action of a subject, especially when the levels are so high that it is impossible for the subject to be free of drug effects. Nevertheless, laboratory data and corroborating drug-induced behavior must be interpreted by experts in pharmacology and toxicology with experience in drug biotransformation and pharmacokinetics.

Drug analysis reports, either positive or negative, may raise questions about the absolute truth of the results. The usual questions are (a) What method was used? (b) Did the laboratory analyze for the drug only, the metabolite only, or both? (c) What is the "cut-off" value for the assay? and

(d) Was the sample time close enough to the suspected drug exposure?

False-negative results occur more easily than false-positive results, mainly because once a test is screened negative it is not tested further. Negative reports based on TLC alone are inconclusive because of a lack of sensitivity. Additionally, if the screening method is RIA or EIA, the cut-off may have been set too high, in which case, drugs present below the cut-off concentration are reported as negative. It is imperative for the physician to know the cut-off for each drug tested and, for diagnostic purposes, ask for any drug presence above the blank. Another possibility for false negatives is that the sample was taken too long after the last drug exposure. Whatever the case may be, if the suspicion of drug use is strong, the clinician must repeat testing and ask the laboratory for more sensitive drug-screening procedures.

In general, analytic methods have improved significantly in the past decades and the trend is toward further improvement (16). As technology advances, more drugs and chemicals will be analyzed in biofluids at the nanogram and picogram level. Advancement, however, does not mean that modern methodologies are infallible, nor that they replace clinical judgment. Theoretically and practically, technical or human error can influence testing results. A nationally certified laboratory, with a full spectrum of drug-abuse tests, enables the well-trained clinician to make drug-abuse diagnoses that were not possible in the past. With knowledge of the available analytic methods, one can scrutinize laboratory results with confidence as to their validity.

CLINICAL DRUG TESTING

Clinical drug testing has three components: emergency toxicology, rehabilitation toxicology, and diagnostic toxicology. Each has slightly different goals and requirements. Emergency toxicology requires quick analysis, responding to critical situations in overdose cases. Sometimes the clinical symptoms or the leftover drug is a sufficient clue to the laboratory for what drug to test, but most often the chemist must determine the toxic compound's identity. Thus, the emergency toxicology laboratory must be located near emergency services for speedy response and must use proved methods to provide quick answers. On-site, one-step, nontechnical kit screening is becoming more common. Instrumental immunoassays are also quick and practical, but as in all screening techniques, they give only "yes" or "no" results for each drug or drug class tested. If the target drug is not tested, no identification is possible, and tracking down the unknown one by one is a slow process. However, if there is a clue to drug identity, immunoassays provide quick answers. Confirmation of positive results is performed by an alternate scientific method and it is at the discretion of the physician to request confirmation.

In rehabilitation programs, drug testing is of foremost importance. Identified ex-drug abusers need to know that the therapist or the counselor knows objectively that they are in good standing or in danger of relapsing to drug use. In this situation, drug-abuse testing is a deterrent and an important component of the treatment process. However, from the laboratory's point of view, testing is significantly different from emergency toxicology. The test results may not be available for at least 24 hours, and large numbers of samples are analyzed in a batch for rehabilitation clinics. The laboratory usually performs a screening test recheck and/or confirms positives by means of an alternate scientific method. The choice of method depends on assay sensitivity, specificity, expense, and practicality. Instrumental immunoassay methods, such as EIA and ELISA are used most frequently for screening when large numbers of samples must be tested at a reasonable cost. An FDA-approved sweat patch aids rehabilitation drug testing. The patch placed on the skin is worn for several days and it detects drugs used during that period, thus use of short-acting drugs will also be detected (17).

Testing for diagnostic drugs of abuse is another important and slightly different area. Denial is typical of drug abusers. Astute physicians are now frequently testing their patients for drug abuse. A critical role of diagnostic testing is to prevent false negatives caused by poor timing of sample collection. Another essence of diagnostic testing is sensitivity. From the laboratory's perspective, the most sensitive methods and a large drug panel screening technique are most appropriate. Immunoassays and GLC techniques must be used for ultimate sensitivity.

FORENSIC DRUG TESTING

Forensic drug testing has three components: workplace testing, postmortem testing (medical examiner), and criminal justice (correctional and parole) testing.

Historically, forensic drug testing developed from clinical and pathologic testing. Laboratories had to implement numerous legally acceptable procedures, and testing also needed improvement. Certified laboratories must be able to prove that positive test results are accurate and reliable and that the tests performed were from the individual listed on the report. Weak links in external or internal chain-of-custody procedures or poor standards and/or quality control in the testing process provide sufficient ammunition to defense attorneys and expert witnesses to contradict the validity of positive results. For this reason the forensic drug-testing facility must be significantly more secure and better organized than that of a clinical drug-testing laboratory.

Workplace testing is performed on subjects at their place of employment. Many industries and governmental agencies mandate testing of individuals performing critical duties. These places of employment have strict drug policies in place, informing employees that drug abuse is not tolerated and that tests are performed to protect the public interest. The different types of tests performed are pre-employment, for cause, and random drug testing. Positive findings can result in loss of job or job opportunity. The consequences of workplace testing are very serious and often disputed. People's livelihoods depend on laboratory results; therefore, sufficient safeguards must be built into the system to provide assurance that the results are reliable. In forensic testing, the usual procedure is screening with a large-volume automated immunoassay analyzer (i.e., EIA, ELISA and FPIA) and confirmation of positives by GC-MS, LC-MS or MS-MS.

Other forms of forensic drug testing requiring "litigation documentation" are *medicolegal cases* and postmortem analysis of body fluids for the presence of drugs, alcohol, and poisons. Before workplace testing became common, even the medicolegal or postmortem toxicology testing was less stringent. As a result of the very strict rules and regulations governing workplace testing, more rigorous and complete chain-of-evidence documentation and more accurate methods are also required in medicolegal and postmortem testing.

Another example of drug testing is in *correctional cases* and testing in the prison system. A very large percentage of the prisoners' criminal activity is connected either with drug use or drug trafficking. It is not unusual to find that drug abuse continues in the prisons. Consequently, correctional facilities have adopted a drug-abuse testing policy in the prison system and also during parole. Although the consequences of testing are potentially punitive, testing of inmates in many states require only screening without confirmation of positive results.

TESTING DRUGS IN SALIVA, SWEAT, AND HAIR

Most drugs enter saliva by passive diffusion. The major advantages of saliva as a test specimen are that it is readily available, collection is noninvasive, the presence of parent drug is in higher abundance than its metabolites, and a high correlation of saliva drug concentration that can be compared with the free fraction of drug in blood (17). The pharmacologic activity of drugs are related to the free drug in blood. However, the use of saliva to predict blood concentrations is limited because of the possibility of contamination of saliva from drug use by oral, smoked, and intranasal routes. Cone (18) reported that marihuana smoking produced contamination of the oral cavity by THC. Even though saliva concentrations of THC were derived from contamination, they were highly correlated with plasma concentrations (17). Detectability of other drugs in saliva did correlate with the drug presence in blood. Thus, the shorter window of detectability of drugs in saliva, than in urine, can be used to detect recent drug use. This may be useful in testing automobile drivers involved in accidents. High salivary drug levels are more relevant to being under the influence than drug presence in urine. This is because drug excretion into urine may take days and by that time pharmacologic effects are no longer observed.

Sweat is approximately 99% water and is produced by the body as a heat-regulation mechanism. Because the amount of sweat produced is dependent on environmental temperatures, routine sweat collection is difficult because of a large variation in the rate of sweat production and the lack of adequate sweat-collection devices. However, cocaine, morphine, nicotine, amphetamine, ethanol, and other drugs have been identified in sweat (17). A recently developed "sweat patch" resembles an adhesive bandage and is applied to the skin for a period of several days to several weeks. Sweat is absorbed and concentrated on the cellulose pad, which is then removed from the skin and tested for drug content. Cone et al. (19) recently evaluated sweat testing for cocaine. Generally, there appeared to

be a dose–concentration relationship; however, there was wide intersubject variability, which is a disadvantage of this technology. Research in this testing technology is still developing and is indicating apparent advantages of the sweat patch, such as high subject acceptability of wearing the patch for drug monitoring and the ability to monitor drug intake for a period of several weeks with a single patch (17).

Testing for drugs in hair is an alternate method to the drug-abuse detection technology (20). Because of the very low concentrations of drugs incorporated in hair, very sensitive methodology must be used. Screening is performed by RIA with ultrasensitive antibodies, or by ELISA, with confirmation by GC-MS or MS-MS. Drug representatives from virtually all classes of abused drugs have been detected in hair (17). It remains unclear how drugs enter the hair, although the most likely entry routes involve (a) diffusion from blood into the hair follicle and hair cells with subsequent binding to hair cell components (Figure 34.6); (b) excretion in sweat, which bathes hair follicles and hair

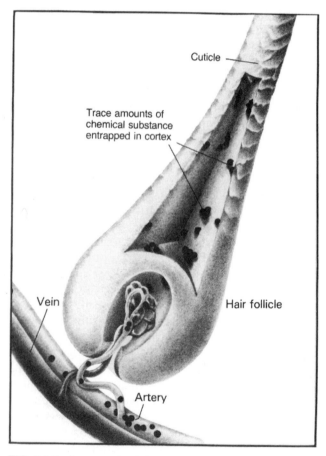

FIG. 34.6. A conceptual drawing of drug transfer from the blood to hair follicle and its subsequent encapsulation in the hair shaft. (Reproduced with the permission of Psychemedics, Inc., Santa Monica, CA.)

TABLE 34.4. *Comparative usefulness of urine, saliva, sweat, and hair as a biologic matrix for drug detection*

Biological matrix	Drug detection time	Major advantages	Major disadvantages	Primary use
Urine	2–4 days	Mature technology; on-site methods available; established cut-offs	Only detects recent use	Detection of recent drug use
Saliva	12–24 hours	Easily obtainable; samples "free" drug fraction; parent drug presence	Short detection time; oral drug contamination; collection methods influence pH and s/p ratios; only detects recent use; new technology	Linking positive drug test to behavior and performance impairment
Sweat	1–4 weeks	Cumulative measure of drug use	High potential for environmental contamination; new technology	Detection of recent drug use (days-weeks)
Hair	months	Long-term measure of drug use; similar sample can be recollected	High possibility for environmental contamination; new technology	Dectection of drug use in recent past (1–6 months)

From Cone EJ. New developments in biological measures of drug prevalence. *NIDA Res Monogr* 1986;167: 104–126.

strands; (c) excretion in oily secretions into the hair follicle and onto the skin surface; and (d) entry from the environment (17). Two controversial issues in hair drug testing are the environmental contamination of hair that may result in a false-positive test result and the interpretation of dose and time relationships. Although it has been generally assumed that the hair strand, when sectioned, provides a long-term time course of drug-abuse history, studies with labeled cocaine have not supported this interpretation. Henderson et al. (21) concluded that "... there is not, at present, the necessary scientific foundation for hair analysis to be used to determine either the time or amount of cocaine use." Cone, on the other hand, found good dose–response relationship and time profile of morphine and codeine in human beard (22). In spite of some controversial aspects of hair testing, this technique is being used on an increasingly broad scale in a variety of circumstances (23). This technology may be used to estimate the drug abuse habit of the patient who is in denial. Self-reported drug use over a period of several months can be compared to hair test results from a hair strand (about 3.9 cm long) representative of the same time period (17). It is expected that this type of comparison would be more effective than urine testing because urine provides a historical record of only 2 to 4 days under most circumstances (17). Because denial is a major problem with drug abusers, this technology is an invaluable tool in drug-abuse diagnosis and therapy. Table 34.4 illustrates the comparison of usefulness of urine, saliva, sweat, and hair as a biologic matrix for drug detection. Advantages and disadvantages of urine, saliva, hair and sweat are reviewed by Caplan and Goldberger (24) (Table 34.5).

ETHICAL CONSIDERATIONS

Legitimate need for drug-abuse testing in the clinical setting is indisputable. Denial makes identification of drug abuse difficult; therefore, testing is necessary both for identification of drug abusers and monitoring of treatment outcome. Drug testing in the workplace and in sports is more controversial because positive test results may be used in termination of long-time employees or refusal to hire new ones.

Private companies believe that it is their right to establish drug- and alcohol-free workplaces and sports arenas. The opposition believes that one is ill-advised to terminate individuals for a single positive test result, even when it is confirmed by forensically acceptable procedures. A testing program is reasonable when a chance for rehabilitation is offered. Probationary periods provide an opportunity to stop using drugs through treatment or self-help programs. Employee assistance programs, which refer employees to drug counseling, are available in larger companies and governmental organizations.

It is important that this new, powerful tool, drug testing, be used judiciously as a means of early detection, rehabilitation, and prevention. Test results must be interpreted only by individuals who understand drugs of abuse medically and pharmacologically. The federal

TABLE 34.5. *Summary of advantages and disadvantages of urine, oral fluid, hair, and sweat*

Specimen	Advantages	Disadvantages
Urine	Drugs and drug metabolites are highly concentrated Extensive scientific basis for testing methodology Performance testing is liberally practiced Results are frequently accepted in court Uniform testing criteria (e.g., cut-offs) established Easily tested by commercial screening methods	Period of detection 2–3 days No dose-concentration relationship Drug concentration influenced by the amount of water intake Susceptible to adulteration and substitution
Oral fluid	Useful in the detection of *recent drug use* Results may be related to *behavior/performance* Ready accessibility for collection Observed collection	Detection window may be shorter *Contamination following oral, smoked and intranasal* routes of drug administration *Collection volume may be device dependent* Performance testing under development
Hair	Detects *parent drugs and metabolites* Provides a longer estimate of time of drug use Detects parent drugs and metabolites (e.g., 6-acetylmorphine) Observed collection	Inability to detect recent drug use Potential hair color bias Possible environmental contamination for some drug classes Susceptible to adulteration by treatment prior to collection
Sweat	Ease of obtaining, storing and shipping specimens Second specimen can be obtained from original source Provides cumulative measure of drug exposure Ability to monitor drug intake for a period of days to weeks Detects parent drugs and metabolites (e.g., 6-acetylmorphine) Noninvasive specimen collection Collection device is relatively tamper-proof	Large variation in sweat production Specimen volume unknown Limited collection devices High intersubject variability Risk of accidental removal Risk of contamination during application/removal Cannot detect prior exposure Performance testing under development

From Caplan, YH, Goldberger BA. Alternative specimens for workplace drug testing. *J Anal Toxicol* 2001;25: 396–399.

government requires that in its drug-testing program the results go directly to medical review officers, who are supposed to be trained to interpret such reports. Improper testing or improper interpretation of drug testing data must be prevented.

CONCLUSION

As long as illegal drug use is prevalent in our society, drug-abuse testing will have an important clinical and forensic role. Testing in the clinical setting aids the physician who treats subjects with psychiatric signs and symptoms secondary to drug abuse, monitors treatment outcome, and handles serious overdose cases. Drug testing in the forensic setting will be used for workplace testing and monitoring of parolees convicted of drug-related charges.

Civil rights must be respected to protect the innocent. Names of subjects should be known only to the medical office where the sample is collected. Testing must follow strict security and chain-of-custody procedures to ensure anonymity and prevent sample mix-up during testing. Many progressive laboratories have instituted barcode labeling of samples and related documents to ensure confidentiality. Barcoding also improves accuracy of reporting and tracking of samples and records. This system ultimately prevents sample mix-up as a consequence of human error during accessioning and processing.

The reliability of testing procedures is also of foremost importance. Good laboratories institute internal open, blind, and external quality control systems to assure high quality of testing (2). Reliability depends on three major factors: well-qualified and well-trained laboratory personnel, state-of-the-art instrumentation, and logical organization of the testing laboratory.

Before issuing certification, governmental agencies require laboratories to adhere to strict standards in personnel qualifications, experience, quality control, quality assurance programs, chain of custody procedures, and multiple data review prior to reporting results.

Two nationally recognized agencies protect the rights of individual citizens by assuring proper procedures in forensic drug testing. DHHS/SAMHSA administers its National Laboratory Certification Program and the College of American Pathologists runs its Forensic Toxicology Inspection and Proficiency Program. In addition, numerous state and city regulatory agencies, such as the New York State Health Department, inspect and certify drug-testing laboratories. Good laboratories are easily identified by having current certificates of qualification issued by national and local regulatory agencies.

Drug-abuse testing has come a long way in terms of accuracy and reliability (16). Testing started in traditional "wet chemistry" laboratories, using huge sample volumes and crude methodologies of low sensitivity. Now autoanalyzers perform hundreds of tests on minute sample volumes, accurately measuring low-nanogram, and in some cases, picogram, amounts of drugs. The insecurity of physicians, counselors and forensic investigators about drug-abuse testing should not be a concern when using properly certified licensed laboratories.

REFERENCES

1. Verebey K, Martin D, Gold MS. Drug abuse: interpretation of laboratory tests. In: Hall W, ed. *Psychiatric medicine.* Washington, DC: U.S. Government Printing Office, 1982:155–167.
2. Blanke RV. Accuracy in urinalysis. *NIDA Res Monogr* 1986;73:43–53.
3. Jaffee JH. Drug Addiction and Drug Abuse. In: Gilman AS, Rall TW, Nies AS and Taylor P, eds. *The Pharmacological Basis of Therapeutics,* 8th ed. New York: Macmillan, 1990:522–535.
4. Gold MS, Verebey K, Dackis CA. Diagnosis of drug abuse: drug intoxication and withdrawal states. *Fair Oaks Hospital Psychiatry Letter* 1980;3(5):23–34.
5. Pottash ALC, Gold MS, Extein I, The use of the clinical laboratory. In: Sederer LI, ed. *Inpatient psychiatry: diagnosis and treatment.* Baltimore: Williams & Wilkins, 1982:205–221.
6. Wadler GI, Heinline B, *Drugs and athletes.* Philadelphia: FA Davis, 1989:195–210.
7. Willette E. Drug testing programs. *NIDA Res Monogr* 1986;73:5–12.
8. Baselt RC, Cravey RH, eds. *Disposition of toxic drugs and chemicals in man,* 5th ed. Foster City, CA: Chemical Toxicology Institute, 2000:360, 386.
9. Manno JE. Interpretation of urinaly-

sis results. *NIDA Res Monogr* 1986;73:54–61.
10. Immunoanalysis Corporation ELISA Kit Package Inserts, 2003 and *Mandatory Guidelines and Proposed Revisions to Mandatory Guidelines for Federal Workplace Drug Testing Programs; Notices. Federal Register* 4/13/2004; 69:19697.
11. Buechler KF, Moi S, Noar B, et al. Simultaneous detection of seven drugs of abuse by the Triage Panel for Drugs of Abuse. *Clin Chem* 1992;38:1678–1684.
12. Hawks RL. Analytical methodology. *NIDA Res Monogr* 1986;73:30–42.
13. Verebey K. Cocaine abuse detection by laboratory methods. In: Washton AM, Gold MS, eds. *Cocaine: a clinician's handbook.* New York: Guilford Press, 1987:214–228.
14. Kogan MJ, Jukofsky D, Verebey K, et al. Detection of methaqualone in human urine by radio immunoassay and gas-liquid chromatography after a therapeutic dose. *Clin Chem* 1987;24:1425–1427.
15. Dackis CA, Pottash ALC, Annitto W, et al. Persistence of urinary marijuana levels after supervised abstinence. *Am J Psychiatry* 1982;139:1196–1198.
16. Frings CS, Battaglia DJ, White RM. Status of drugs of abuse testing in urine un-

der blind conditions: an AACC study. *Clin Chem* 1989;35(5):891–944.
17. Cone EJ. New developments in biological measures of drug prevalence. *NIDA Res Monogr* 1986;167:104–126.
18. Cone EJ. Saliva testing for drugs of abuse. *Ann N Y Acad Sci* 1993;694:91–127.
19. Cone EJ, Hillsgrove MJ, Jenkins AJ, et al. Sweat testing for heroin, cocaine, and metabolites. *J Anal Toxicol* 1994;18(6):298–305.
20. Baumgarten WA, Hill VA, Blahd WH. Hair analysis for drugs of abuse. *J Forensic Sci* 1989;34(6):1433–1453.
21. Henderson GL, Harkey MR, Zhou C, et al. Incorporation of isotopically labeled cocaine and metabolites into human hair: 1- dose-response relationships. *J Anal Toxicol* 1996,20:1–12.
22. Cone EJ. Testing human hair for drugs of abuse. I. Individual dose and time profiles of morphine and codeine in plasma, saliva, urine, and beard compared to drug induced effects on pupils and behavior. *J Anal Toxicol* 1990;14:1–7.
23. Spiehler V. Hair analysis by immunological methods from the beginning to 2000. *Forensic Sci Int* 2000;107:249–259.
24. Caplan YH, Goldberger BA, Alternative specimens for workplace drug testing. *J Anal Toxicol* 2001;25:396–399.

Treatment Approaches

CHAPTER 35

Detoxification

GRACE CHANG AND THOMAS R. KOSTEN

Detoxification has been defined as the process of withdrawing an individual from a specific psychoactive substance in a safe and effective manner (1). Withdrawal is recognized for the following groups of substances: alcohol, amphetamines and related substances, cocaine, nicotine, opioids, sedatives, hypnotics, and anxiolytics. With signs and symptoms of withdrawal generally being the opposite of those observed in intoxication with the substance, three diagnostic criteria have been established for substance withdrawal: (a) development of a substance specific syndrome as a consequence of cessation of (or reduction in) substance use that has been heavy and prolonged; (b) the substance-specific syndrome causes clinically significant distress or impairment in social, occupational, or other important areas of functioning; and (c) the symptoms are not a result of a general medical condition and are not better accounted for by another medical or mental disorder (2).

Detoxification may take place in either inpatient or outpatient settings. Detoxification, or the achievement of substance-free state, is but the beginning of substance-abuse treatment and sustained abstinence from alcohol and drugs. This chapter describes the detoxification process for all of the major substances of abuse and dependence, except for nicotine. Current research on the status of marijuana withdrawal is included.

ALCOHOL WITHDRAWAL

Diagnostic Criteria

The essential feature of alcohol withdrawal is the presence of a characteristic withdrawal syndrome that results after the cessation of (or reduction in) heavy drinking and prolonged alcohol use. According to the *Diagnostic and Statistical Manual of Mental Disorders,* 4th ed., text revision (*DSM–IV–TR*) criteria, the withdrawal syndrome includes at least two of the following symptoms developing within several hours to a few days after the decline in blood alcohol concentration:

1. Autonomic hyperactivity (e.g., pulse rate >100 beats per minute)
2. Increased hand tremor
3. Insomnia
4. Nausea or vomiting
5. Transient visual, tactile, or auditory hallucinations or illusions
6. Psychomotor agitation
7. Anxiety
8. Grand mal seizures (2)

The *DSM–IV–TR* diagnostic criteria also require that these symptoms cause clinically significant distress or impairment in social, occupational, or other important areas of functioning. Moreover, these symptoms are not caused by another medical condition or mental disorder. Perceptual disturbances, such as auditory, visual, or tactile illusions in the absence of delirium, may accompany the withdrawal syndrome. Differential diagnoses include withdrawal from anxiolytics or sedative-hypnotics and generalized anxiety disorder (2).

The milder symptoms appear within hours of cessation or reduction of alcohol consumption and remit over several days to a week. Seizures usually appear within 24 to 48 hours of alcohol withdrawal and are either single or as a series. Approximately 30% of those who experience seizures will experience delirium tremens (DTs). Delirium tremens typically manifest 48 to 72 hours after alcohol withdrawal. (3,4). A model for predicting alcohol withdrawal delirium, based on a sample of 334 alcohol-dependent patients, has been developed. The five risk

TABLE 35.1. *CIWA-Ar categories and range of scores*

Agitation	0–7	Examples:	0 = normal activity
			7 = constantly thrashes about
Anxiety	0–7		0 = no anxiety, at ease
			7 = acute panic states
Auditory disturbances	0–7		0 = not present
			7 = continuous hallucinations
Clouding of sensorium	0–4		0 = oriented, can do serial additions
			4 = disoriented for place and/or person
Headache	0–7		0 = not present
			7 = extremely severe
Nausea/vomiting	0–7		0 = no nausea, no vomiting
			7 = constant nausea, frequent dry heaves and vomiting
Paroxysmal sweats	0–7		0 = no sweat visible
			7 = drenching sweats
Tactile disturbances	0–7		0 = none
			7 = continuous hallucinations
Tremor	0–7		0 = no tremor
			7 = severe, even with arms not extended
Visual disturbances	0–7		0 = not present
			7 = continuous hallucinations

factors significantly correlated with alcohol withdrawal delirium are current infectious disease, tachycardia defined as a heart rate in excess of 120 beats per minute at admission; signs of withdrawal accompanied by an alcohol concentration greater than 1 g/L of body fluid: history of epileptic seizures; and history of delirious episodes (5). A history of multiple previous detoxifications is associated with more severe alcohol withdrawal symptoms (6).

Measurement

The use of a rating scale to quantify the alcohol withdrawal syndrome provides valuable clinical information. The ideal scale would aid in the diagnosis of the withdrawal syndrome, indicate when drug therapy is required, alert staff to the development of serious withdrawal symptoms requiring more intensive medical input, and reveal when medication can be discontinued and the patient discharged (7). The Clinical Institute Withdrawal Assessment scale–alcohol (CIWA-A) and an abbreviated version, the CIWA-A Revised (CIWA-Ar), are among the best known and studied. The CIWA-Ar is not copyrighted and may be used freely.

The CIWA-Ar measures ten symptom categories, with a range of scores in each. The total maximum score is 67. Scores of less than 8 to 10 indicate minimal to mild withdrawal. Moderate withdrawal (marked autonomic arousal) results in scores of 8 to 15. Severe withdrawal results in scores of 15 or more. High CIWA-Ar scores are predictive of seizures and delirium (8).

Pharmacology

Alcohol affects endogenous opiates and several neurotransmitter systems in the brain, including γ-aminobutyric acid (GABA), glutamate, and dopamine. The central ner-

vous system adapts to the overall inhibitory effects of long-term alcohol exposures on inhibitory GABA$_A$-type and excitatory N-methyl-D-aspartate (NMDA)-type glutamate receptor transmission by adjustments in receptor number and function. In the absence of alcohol, the adaptations result in greater central nervous systems excitability (9–11).

Pharmacologic management of alcohol withdrawal has been attempted with medications ranging from benzodiazepines, anticonvulsants, barbiturates, and neuroleptics to sympatholytics, and even to alcohol itself. Comprehensive reviews of treatment options have all come to the same conclusion—benzodiazepines are the preferred pharmacologic agents for the treatment of alcohol withdrawal. Benzodiazepines alone reduce withdrawal severity, reduce the incidence of delirium, and reduce seizures (9,12–17).

All benzodiazepines appear to be equally efficacious in the treatment of alcohol withdrawal. Some clinical considerations may be of assistance in selection. For example, short-acting benzodiazepines may have a lower risk of oversedation. Long-acting agents may be more effective in preventing withdrawal seizures and can contribute to a smoother withdrawal with fewer rebound symptoms. Other benzodiazepines may have a higher liability for abuse, such as those with rapid onset of action. The main disadvantage of the benzodiazepines is the risk of subsequent dependency, but that risk should be avoided if their use is confirmed to the withdrawal period (6,12).

Other Treatment Options

Anticonvulsants may be an alternative to benzodiazepines in the treatment of alcohol withdrawal. Advantages are threefold: they do not interact with alcohol, they lack abuse liability, and they ameliorate psychiatric symptoms (18). However, disadvantages of anticonvulsants include their gastrointestinal and other side effects, rare cytopenias, and unproven efficacy in preventing seizures and treating delirium tremens (19).

Carbamazepine was found to be superior to placebo and equal in efficacy to barbital and oxazepam for patients with mild to moderate withdrawal in several studies (20–22). Moreover, it had no significant hematologic or hepatic toxic effects when used in 7-day protocols for alcohol withdrawal, and it reduced psychiatric distress and hastened the return to work more than oxazepam (23). When compared in a 5-day protocol using lorazepam, carbamazepine treated subjects had fewer withdrawal symptoms and less relapse to alcohol use (24). However, dizziness, vomiting, and nausea were common side effects, particularly at the initial 800-mg dose. Carbamazepine prevents alcohol withdrawal seizures in animal studies, but human data are limited, and it has not been evaluated for treating delirium tremens (25).

Valproate may also reduce symptoms of alcohol withdrawal, based on several open-label studies, as well as two controlled studies. About 2,500 subjects have been enrolled in predominantly open-label studies of valproate, but seizure rates are not reported. Two double-blind, randomized studies treated patients for 4 to 7 days on 500 to 1,200 mg of valproate and found fewer seizures, less dropout, less-severe withdrawal, and less use of oxazepam than in patients on placebo or carbamazepine (26).

Adjuvant Treatments

Except as adjuvant treatments most other agents have poor justification as sole medications during alcohol withdrawal. The phenothiazines and haloperidol reduce signs and symptoms of withdrawal, but are significantly less effective than benzodiazepines in preventing delirium (risk difference: 6.6 cases per 100 patients) and seizures (risk difference: 12.4 seizures per 100 patients treated) (P <0.01 for each) (27). β-Adrenergic antagonists and clonidine reduce autonomic manifestations of withdrawal, but have no known anticonvulsant activity (28,29). Symptoms of early withdrawal or impending delirium may be masked by propranolol (30). Centrally acting α-adrenergic agonists, such as clonidine, ameliorate symptoms in patients with mild to moderate withdrawal, but the reduction of delirium or seizures is unlikely (31). These adrenergic agents may be used in conjunction with benzodiazepines for patients with certain coexisting conditions, such as coronary artery disease.

Although neither thiamine nor magnesium will reduce delirium or seizures, each might also be administered as part of the pharmacologic management of alcohol withdrawal (9,13,32). Individuals with alcohol dependence are frequently deficient of both thiamine and magnesium.

Administration of thiamine will prevent Wernicke-Korsakoff syndrome, which includes acute encephalopathy characterized by ataxia, dysarthric, and oculomotor paralysis, and then psychological symptoms, with anterograde amnesia, confabulation, and some degree of retrograde amnesia. A parenteral dose of thiamine, 100 mg, is given initially and then followed by 50 to 100 mg daily by mouth, for 7 days.

Supplementation with magnesium has also been recommended, particularly for elderly patients (32). Serum magnesium levels are generally unhelpful when trying to decide if magnesium replacement is needed. Magnesium, 2 to 4 mEq/kg intravenously on day 1, and then 0.5 to mEq/kg orally or intravenously on days 2, 3, and 4, is safe in the absence of renal impairment. Patients with hypomagnesemia are at risk for cardiac dysrhythmias and other nonspecific signs and symptoms such as weakness, tremor, and hyperactive reflexes. In contrast to the administration of thiamine, for which there is consensus, routine administration of magnesium is not uniformly endorsed (13).

Treatment Regimens

There are three treatment regimens for the management of alcohol withdrawal using benzodiazepines. The regimens are fixed dose, front loading, and symptom triggered.

The fixed-dose method relies on the administration of benzodiazepines at predetermined intervals and doses. An example is chlordiazepoxide, 50 to 100 mg given every 6 hours for the first 24 hours, then 25 to 50 mg every 6 hours for the next 2 days. Additional medication is given if needed. This approach may be particularly suitable for patients with a history of delirium tremens or a history of seizures. Pregnant women or people with acute medical or surgical illness might also be appropriate candidates (13).

The front-loading method relies on high doses of medication given early in the course of withdrawal. An example is 20 mg of diazepam given every 2 hours until there is resolution of withdrawal symptoms. Usually, three doses are required, but at least one dose should be given if an asymptomatic patient has a history of seizures or an acute medical illness. The use of long-acting benzodiazepines provides a self-tapering effect. This method is more labor-intensive at the outset of treatment, but requires less medication and time than the fixed-dosed approach (9).

The symptom-triggered method gives each patient an individualized treatment regimen that studies have demonstrated to result in less medication and more rapid withdrawal treatment (33–35). An example is the administration of 25 to 100 mg of chlordiazepoxide hourly whenever the patient is symptomatic and has a CIWA-Ar score greater than or equal to 8.

Treatment of Seizures and Delirium Tremens

Uncomplicated alcohol withdrawal seizures do not require the long-term use of antiepileptics. The generalized seizures typically resolve spontaneously and are usually single. Severe or repeated seizures can be treated with intravenous diazepam 5 to 10 mg. The development of delirium tremens requires the constant observation offered in a hospital, as well as active treatment to achieve stabilization. Intravenous diazepam is the most effective and safest treatment regimen for delirium tremens (9).

ANXIOLYTIC, SEDATIVE, OR HYPNOTIC WITHDRAWAL

Diagnostic Criteria

Commonly abused substances in this class include benzodiazepines. The characteristic withdrawal syndrome is precipitated by a marked decrease or cessation of intake after several weeks or more of regular use. According to the *DSM–IV–TR* criteria, at least two or more of the following symptoms are manifest:

1. Autonomic hyperactivity (e.g., sweating)
2. Increased hand tremor
3. Insomnia
4. Nausea or vomiting
5. Transient visual, tactile, or auditory hallucinations or illusions
6. Psychomotor agitation
7. Anxiety
8. Grand mal seizures (2)

Withdrawal from anxiolytics, sedatives, or hypnotics produces a syndrome similar to that associated with alcohol withdrawal. Perceptual disturbances should be specified if the transient visual, tactile, or auditory hallucinations occur in the absence of delirium. Twenty percent to 30% of individuals undergoing untreated withdrawal will experience grand mal seizures (2).

The half-life of the substance will generally predict the time course of withdrawal. Substances with a half-life of 10 hours or less will produce withdrawal symptoms 6 to 8 hours after decreasing blood levels. The symptoms will then peak by the next day and improve by the fourth or fifth day. Withdrawal may persist until the second week, and subside by the third or fourth week. Chances for a severe withdrawal are increased if the substance has been used at high doses (more than 40 mg of diazepam daily) for a long time (2).

Measurement

The CIWA-Ar has been adapted for benzodiazepine withdrawal assessment (36).

Pharmacology

Benzodiazepines cause an increase of gamma aminobutyric acid inhibitory impulses in the central nervous system (37). The benzodiazepine antagonist flumazenil selectively blocks the central effects of benzodiazepines by competitive interaction at the benzodiazepine receptors (38).

Treatment

Predictors of withdrawal severity from benzodiazepines include both pharmacologic and clinical variables. Pharmacologic variables that increase the risk of severity are higher daily dose of benzodiazepine, shorter benzodiazepine half-life, longer duration of benzodiazepine therapy, and a rapid taper, particularly in the last half. Clinical variables that increase the severity of withdrawal include diagnosis of panic, higher pretaper levels of anxiety or depression, higher levels of psychopathology, and concomitant abuse or dependence of alcohol and/or other substances (39,40).

If the amount of anxiolytic or sedative–hypnotic is known, and there are no additional complicating factors, it may be possible to offer a medically supervised outpatient taper over the course of 4 or more weeks. This may be most effective for low-dose withdrawal, where patients have exceeded recommended doses on a daily basis for more than 1 month. High-dose withdrawal is considered for patients who have been using more than the equivalent of 40 mg of diazepam daily for 8 months. In this case, the patient is tolerance tested with diazepam, and if dependent, tapered off medications at the rate of 10% per day in a medically supervised setting (41). Where patients have significant levels of anxiety or depression prior to initiation of a benzodiazepine taper, other pharmacologic or therapeutic measures should be undertaken while the patient continues to take his or her established benzodiazepine dose. Once levels of psychopathology are reduced, then the taper may begin. Reduced levels of benzodiazepine may be maintained for several months before the final taper is attempted (39,42).

If the dose of a sedative–hypnotic is not known, or if the patient may be using several simultaneously, one strategy may be to offer a pentobarbital challenge test, estimate phenobarbital equivalences for drugs of abuse, and then begin a phenobarbital taper (43). The details of the pentobarbital challenge test have been widely described and can be summarized as follows. An awake patient is given 200 mg of pentobarbital by mouth and carefully observed. If the patient falls asleep, it is most likely that the patient is not dependent on sedative–hypnotics and the diagnosis revised. If the patient appears intoxicated (with nystagmus, ataxia, dysarthria), then the patient's 6-hour pentobarbital requirement is between 100 and 200 mg. If the patient does not appear to be intoxicated, then a 100-mg pentobarbital challenge can be administered every 2 hours until intoxication is achieved or 500 to 600 mg of pentobarbital are administered. The total pentobarbital dose is calculated and then converted to phenobarbital (100 mg pentobarbital = 30 mg phenobarbital). The patient is then stabilized with a standing dose of phenobarbital for 48 hours, after which point the daily dose is decreased by 30 mg, until detoxification is achieved.

COCAINE AND AMPHETAMINE WITHDRAWAL

Diagnostic Criteria

The withdrawal syndrome for both cocaine and amphetamine withdrawal is characterized by the development of dysphoric mood and at least two of the following, according to *DSM–IV–TR* criteria:

1. Fatigue
2. Vivid, unpleasant dreams
3. Insomnia or hypersomnia
4. Increased appetite
5. Psychomotor agitation or retardation (2)

These developments follow a few hours to a few days after the cessation of or reduction in amphetamine or cocaine use that has been heavy and prolonged. Moreover, these symptoms cause significant distress or impairment in social, occupational, or other important areas of functioning. These symptoms cannot be attributable to another general medical or mental disorder (2).

An episode of intense, high-dose use of amphetamines or cocaine can be followed by a period of acute withdrawal. The individual may experience intense and unpleasant feelings of lassitude and depression, and may need several days of rest and recuperation. Some may experience suicidal ideation or behavior, which would warrant close observation (43).

Measurement

The Cocaine Selective Severity Assessment is a measure of cocaine abstinence signs and symptoms. It is an 18-item clinician administered instrument that includes the symptoms most often associated with early cocaine abstinence, including depression, fatigue, anhedonia, anxiety, irritability, and sleep disturbance, rated on a scale of 0 to 7, with a maximum total score of 112. The instrument appears to be helpful in predicting early treatment failure (44,45).

Pharmacology

Neural circuits of dopamine-containing and dopamine-receptive neurons are altered functionally after repeated intermittent administration of cocaine and its withdrawal in animal models. The neuroadaptive changes are important because they may relate to addictive or withdrawal states associated with cocaine abuse and suggest targets for the development of medications to treat cocaine dependence (46,47).

Treatment

The symptoms associated with withdrawal from central nervous system (CNS) stimulants are usually transient. Inpatient studies of the acute symptoms of abstinence from cocaine suggest that they are minimal, and not clinically significant (48–50). However, ambulatory treatment may be associated with more severe symptoms for any number of reasons, including the psychosocial stressors of everyday life, cocaine availability, and triggers for craving (42,43,51,52). A prior history of depression might be related to whether or not a cocaine abuser reports withdrawal symptoms (53). Indeed, suicidal ideation, intent, or plan in the context of CNS stimulant withdrawal should warrant careful evaluation and observation.

Several new approaches to the management of severe cocaine withdrawal have been studied. Amantadine (Symmetrel), an indirect dopamine agonist, might be able to stimulate the release of dopamine and therefore offer particular relief to those with severe cocaine withdrawal symptoms (54). Propanolol (Inderal), a β-blocker, may have some utility for the treatment of the symptoms of autonomic arousal associated with early cocaine abstinence (55). Disulfiram (Antabuse), which acts centrally by inhibiting dopamine β-hydroxylase, leading to an excess of dopamine and decreased synthesis of norepinephrine, may blunt cocaine craving, resulting in a decreased desire to use cocaine (56).

OPIATE WITHDRAWAL

Diagnostic Criteria

Commonly abused opioids include heroin, hydromorphone hydrochloride, oxycodone, propoxyphene, meperidine, opium, and codeine. The characteristic withdrawal syndrome can be precipitated by either cessation or reduction of opiate use that has been heavy or prolonged or the administration of an opiate antagonist such as naloxone (Narcan) after a period of opiate use. According to the *DSM–IV–TR* criteria, three or more of the following, developing minutes to several days after last use or administration of the antagonist, are required:

1. Dysphoric mood
2. Nausea or vomiting
3. Muscle aches
4. Lacrimation or rhinorrhea
5. Pupillary dilation, piloerection, or sweating
6. Diarrhea
7. Yawning
8. Fever
9. Insomnia (2)

These symptoms cause clinically significant distress or impairment in social, occupational, or other important areas of functioning. The symptoms cannot be attributable to another medical condition or mental disorder (2).

The onset of these withdrawal symptoms depends on the amount and type of opiate abused. Withdrawal from heroin, which has a short half-life, begins 4 to 8 hours after last use, peaks within 24 to 48 hours, and may persist for as long as 2 weeks. Withdrawal from methadone does not begin until 24 to 36 hours after last use, and may go on for several weeks. As uncomfortable as opiate withdrawal may seem, it differs from alcohol or anxiolytic withdrawal because serious complications such as seizures or delirium tremens do not typically occur (57).

Measurement

A measure of opiate withdrawal distress may helpful for both clinical and theoretical reasons. The opiate withdrawal scale (OWS) is a 32-item measure of withdrawal signs and symptoms that has been shortened to a 10-item version (58). The short opiate withdrawal scale (SOWS) asks patients to rate ten items (e.g., feeling sick) on a Likert scale ranging from none to severe (59). A more recent version is the clinical opiate withdrawal scale (COWS), which consists of 11 items rated by a clinician. An estimate of mild (score: 5 to 12), moderate (score: 13 to 24), moderately severe (score: 25 to 36), and severe (score: >36) withdrawal is thus generated (60).

Pharmacology

Repeated administration of opioids that activate the μ opioid receptor results in tolerance and dependence. Reduction or cessation of opiate use results in the characteristic, spontaneous withdrawal syndrome. Withdrawal may also be precipitated by the administration of an opiate antagonist such as naltrexone (ReVia) or naloxone. The duration of the precipitated withdrawal will depend on the half-life of the antagonist.

Treatment

No clear guidelines to assist with the choice between detoxification and opioid-agonist therapy exists for the opiate-dependent patient. There are advantages and disadvantages to either approach. Specific state and federal regulations govern admission criteria for methadone and levo-alpha-acetylmethadol (LAAM) maintenance. These criteria include a documented history of some period of opiate addiction, 1 year of addiction prior to admission, and evidence of current narcotic dependence (61). Treatment selection should be guided by good clinical judgment informed by patient participation in treatment planning and local regulations.

There are four major categories of opiate detoxification options: (a) detoxification using opiate agonists, (b) detoxification using nonopioid medications, (c) rapid and ultrarapid detoxification, and (d) opioid detoxification in physician offices. Detoxification may be precipitated by a naloxone challenge test to establish actual physical dependence on the opiate.

The general principle of detoxification using opiate agonists is to substitute the opiate being abused with one that will be tapered under medical supervision. Methadone is the most commonly used opiate substitute for this pur-

pose. Buprenorphine (Buprenex), is a partial opiate agonist approved by the FDA in October 2002 for use in detoxification (62). The total amount of opiate used by an individual in a 24-hour period is estimated and the physical findings of withdrawal are observed. The patient is given an initial dose of methadone, 15 to 30 mg p.o. Additional medication can be given on the basis of physical findings consistent with withdrawal. Once the correct daily dose is established, the rate of tapering reflects the planned rate of detoxification (e.g., 5% to 10% per day).

In addition to short-term detoxification, long-term (up to 180 days) detoxification was approved in 1989 as a treatment option for opioid-dependent patients who are ineligible for methadone maintenance or who do not want it (63). A comparison of retention, illicit drug use, and illicit human immunodeficiency virus (HIV) risk behaviors in 179 subjects satisfying *Diagnostic and Statistical Manual of Mental Disorders,* 3rd ed., Revised (*DSM–III–R*) criteria for opiate dependence randomized to receive either methadone maintenance or 180-day psychosocially enriched detoxification found that those in the methadone maintenance group had superior results (64). Additional outcome data for long-term detoxification are needed.

LAAM is associated with potential cardiovascular complications. Patients maintained on LAAM may experience symptomatic arrhythmia with prolongation of the QT interval. Thus LAAM is contraindicated in patients with known or suspected QT prolongation, and may be best reserved for appropriate patients who have failed with methadone treatment. (65).

Detoxification with nonopioid medications is also a possibility. Clonidine (Catapres), an α_2-agonist, has been the best studied. The rationale for the use of clonidine is to diminish norepinephrine activity associated with opiate withdrawal. The patient is given up to 1.2 mg in divided doses over a 24-hour period, with careful monitoring of blood pressure. The peak clonidine dose is given on day 3 for detoxification from heroin, and on day 5 for detoxification from methadone. The peak dose is then tapered down over 4 to 7 days by 0.2 to 0.1 mg per day. Variations of clonidine detoxification include combining it with an opioid antagonist or using a transdermal patch.

Rapid and ultrarapid detoxification have been proposed to shorten the time necessary for withdrawal (66). Rapid detoxification begins by precipitating withdrawal through the administration of an opioid antagonist such as naloxone or naltrexone, followed by naltrexone maintenance and adjuvant medications such as antiemetics, analgesics, sedative–hypnotics, or buprenorphine for withdrawal symptoms. In ultrarapid opioid detoxification, patients undergo opioid-antagonist–precipitated withdrawal while under general anesthesia or heavy sedation (67). The efficacy of the rapid and ultrarapid techniques needs to be compared with more traditional approaches in randomized trials. The high costs and anesthesia risks of ultrarapid detoxification warrant careful consideration, because detoxification is the not the end of treatment.

The Drug Addiction Treatment Act of 2000 (21 USC §823(g)) allows qualified physicians to use buprenorphine products for office based treatment for detoxification or maintenance. Prior to the initiation of office-based treatment, the secretary of Health and Human Services requires notification. Physicians are qualified to offer office-based opiate treatment if they have subspecialty board certification in addiction psychiatry from the American Board of Medical Specialties, addiction certification from the American Society of Addiction Medicine, or completion of not less than 8 hours of training for the treatment and management of dependent patients provided by an approved organization (e.g., American Academy of Addiction Psychiatry). Careful selection of appropriate patients for office-based detoxification is essential. The *Field Review Draft of Buprenorphine Clinical Practice Guidelines* suggest that individuals with comorbid dependence on high doses of alcohol, benzodiazepines, or other central nervous systems depressants; significant psychiatric comorbidity; active or chronic suicidal or homicidal ideation or attempts; multiple previous treatments and relapses; and previous nonresponse to buprenorphine are not optimal candidates for office-based treatment (68).

The patient must be in early withdrawal before buprenorphine is administered. In the case of a patient dependent on short-acting opioids, 12 to 24 hours should lapse since the last opioid use. Patients dependent on longer-acting opioids must also be in withdrawal prior to initiation of buprenorphine. In the case of methadone dependence, the last dose should be 40 mg or less of methadone, 24 hours ago. For LAAM, the last dose should be 40 mg or less, 48 hours ago. The patient is given up to 8 mg of buprenorphine with 2 mg naloxone on the first induction day, after an initial dose followed by at least 2 hours of observation for withdrawal symptoms. The patient should be stabilized on an appropriate dose for 48 hours. If there is a compelling reason for a rapid taper, then buprenorphine can be reduced over the course of 3 to 6 days and then discontinued. If a rapid taper is not necessary, the patient can be stabilized on buprenorphine/naloxone for at least 1 week, after which a taper from the combination therapy over the course of 2 weeks should be initiated. If no withdrawal symptoms emerge, then the taper can continue until the medication is discontinued. If withdrawal symptoms are evident, divided daily doses of the medication can be tried until the medication is discontinued. Patients maintained on buprenorphine are likely to have doses as high as 24 to 32 mg each day and probably should have these doses tapered over several weeks to maximize successful achievement of abstinence.

MARIJUANA AND HALLUCINOGEN WITHDRAWAL

A withdrawal syndrome specific to marijuana and hallucinogens is not formally recognized. Of the limited research available, most has focused on marijuana, which is not commonly perceived to result in a physical withdrawal syndrome when regular use is stopped (69). A possible explanation is the long half-life of *cannabis,* which would allow for a "self-tapering" drug effect.

The development of a specific cannabinoid antagonist, SR141716A, however, has advanced the notion that there is a physiologic basis for *cannabis* dependence. This antagonist has been tested in both animal and human subjects. Rats treated daily with the potent synthetic cannabinoid HU-210 for 2 weeks were then given antagonist SR141716A. The induced withdrawal was accompanied by a marked elevation in extracellular corticotropin-releasing factor concentration and a distinct pattern of Fos activation in the central nucleus of the amygdala, supporting the possibility that long-term cannabinoid administration alters corticotropin-releasing factor function in a manner similar to that observed with other drugs of abuse, and also induces neuroadaptive processes (70).

Other studies of controlled marijuana administration to known marijuana users have described abstinence symptoms. For example, subject reports of anxiety, irritability, stomach pain, and objectively decreased food intake compared to baseline have followed abstinence from marijuana and THC (71–73). Others have described signs and symptoms of *cannabis* withdrawal as including restlessness, dysphoria, insomnia, muscle tremor, increased reflexes, and autonomic effects (74–77).

To date, unequivocal support for a marijuana withdrawal syndrome is elusive. More rigorous studies, which include control groups, comparable substance administration, and symptom severity measurement, are needed, particularly in light of the prevalence of marijuana use.

SUMMARY

Detoxification can take place in either inpatient or outpatient settings. An accurate and competent clinical assessment is essential when detoxification and subsequent treatment plans are formulated, particularly as some patients are dependent on more than one substance. The most appropriate setting for treatment will be determined by clinical judgment, treatment availability, and patient cooperation. Detoxification is but the first step to sustained abstinence.

REFERENCES

1. Mee-Lee D, ed. *ASAM PPC-2R, ASAM patient placement criteria for the treatment of substance-related disorders.* Chevy Chase, MD: American Society of Addiction Medicine, 2001.

2. American Psychiatric Association. *Diagnostic and Statistical Manual of Mental Disorders,* 4th edi., text revision. Washington, DC: Author, 2000:191–296.

3. Williams D, McBride A. The drug treatment of alcohol withdrawal symptoms: a systematic review. *Alcohol Alcohol* 1998;33:103–115.

4. Foy A, Kay J, Taylor A. The course of

alcohol withdrawal in a general hospital. *QJM* 1997;90:253–261.

5. Palmstierna T. A model for predicting alcohol withdrawal delirium. *Psychiatr Serv* 2001;52:820–823.

6. Malcolm R, Roberts JS, Wang W, et al. Multiple previous detoxifications are associated with less responsive treatment and heavier drinking during an index outpatient detoxification. *Alcohol* 2000;22:159–164.

7. Williams D, Lewis J, McBride A. A comparison of rating scales for the alcohol-withdrawal syndrome. *Alcohol Alcohol* 2001;36:104–108.

8. Sullivan JT, Sykora K, Schneiderman J, et al. Assessment of alcohol withdrawal. The revised clinical institute withdrawal assessment for alcohol scale (CIWA-Ar) *Br J Addict* 1989;84:1353–1357.

9. Saitz R, O'Malley SS. Pharmacotherapies for alcohol abuse, withdrawal and treatment. *Med Clin North Am* 1997;81:881–907.

10. Heinz A, Ragan P, Jones DW, et al. Reduced central serotonin transporters in alcoholism. *Am J Psychiatry* 1998;155:1544–1549.

11. Davis KM, Wu JY. Role of glutaminergic and GABAergic systems in alcoholism. *J Biomed Sci* 2000;8:7–19.

12. Shaw GK. Detoxification: the use of benzodiazepines. *Alcohol Alcohol* 1995;30:765–770.

13. Mayo-Smith MF. Pharmacological management of alcohol withdrawal: a meta-analysis and evidence-based practice guideline. *JAMA* 1997;278:144–151.

14. Lejoyeux M, Solomon J, Ades J. Benzodiazepine treatment for alcohol-dependent patients. *Alcohol Alcohol* 1998;33:563–575.

15. Williams D, McBride AJ. The drug treatment of alcohol withdrawal symptoms: a systematic review. *Alcohol Alcohol* 1998;33:103–115.

16. O'Connor PG, Schottenfeld RS. Medical progress: patients with alcohol problems. *N Engl J Med* 1998;338:592–602.

17. Holbrook A, Crowterh R, Lotter A, et al. Meta-analysis of acute alcohol withdrawal. *CMAJ* 1999;160:649–655.

18. Myrick H, Brady KT, Malcolm R. New developments in the pharmacotherapy of alcohol dependence. *Am J Addict* 2001;10S:3–15.

19. Pages KP, Ries RK. Use of anticonvulsants in benzodiazepine withdrawal. *Am J Addict* 1998;7:198–204.

20. Malcolm R, Myrick H, Roberts J, et al. The effects of carbamazepine and lorazepam on single vs multiple previous withdrawal in an outpatient randomized trial. *J Gen Intern Med* 2002;17:349–355.

21. Bjorkquist SE, Isohanni M, Makella R, et al. Ambulant treatment of alco-hol withdrawal symptoms with carba-mazepine: a formal multicentre double-blind comparison with placebo. *Acta Psychiatr Scand* 1976;53:333–342.

22. Malcolm R, Ballenger JC, Sturgis ET, et al. Double-blind controlled trial comparing carbamazepine to oxazepam treatment of alcohol withdrawal. *Am J Psychiatry* 1989;146:617–621.

23. Stuppaeck CH, Pycha R, Miller C, et al. Carbamazepine versus oxazepam in the treatment of alcohol withdrawal: a double-blind study. *Alcohol Alcohol* 1992;27:153–158.

24. Malcolm R, Myrick H, Brady KT, et al. Update on anticonvulsants for the treatment of alcohol withdrawal. *Am J Addict* 2001;10:16–23.

25. Chu N. Carbamazepine: prevention of alcohol withdrawal seizures. *Neurology* 1979;29:1397–1401.

26. Reoux JP, Saxon AJ, Malte CA, et al. Divalproex sodium in alcohol withdrawal: a randomized double-blind placebo-controlled clinical trial. *Alcohol Clin Exp Res* 2001;25:1324–1329.

27. Palestine ML, Alatorre E. Control of acute alcoholic withdrawal symptoms: a comparative study of haloperidol and chlordiazepoxide. *Curr Ther Res Clin Exp* 1976;20:289–299.

28. Horwitz RI, Gottlieb LD, Kraus ML. The efficacy of atenolol in the outpatient management of the alcohol withdrawal syndrome: results of a randomized clinical trial. *Arch Intern Med* 1989;149:1089–1093.

29. Worner TM. Propranolol versus diazepam in the management of the alcohol withdrawal syndrome: double-blind controlled trial. *Am J Drug Alcohol Abuse* 1994;20:115–124.

30. Zilm DH, Jacob MS, MacLeod SM, et al. Propranolol and chlordiazepoxide effects on cardiac arrhythmias during alcohol withdrawal. *Alcohol Clin Exp Res* 1980;4:400–405.

31. Robinson BJ, Robinson GM, Maling TJ, et al. Is clonidine useful in the treatment of alcohol withdrawal? *Alcohol Clin Exp Res* 1989;13:95–98.

32. Kraemer KL, Conigliaro J, Saitz R. Managing alcohol withdrawal in the elderly. *Drugs Aging* 1999;14:409–425.

33. Daeppen JB, Gache P, Landry U, et al. Symptom-triggered vs. fixed-schedule doses of benzodiazepine for alcohol withdrawal: a randomized treatment trial. *Arch Intern Med* 2002;162:1117–1121.

34. Saitz R, Mayo-Smith MF, Roberts MS, et al. Individualized treatment for alcohol withdrawal: a randomized double-blind controlled trial. *JAMA* 1994;272:519–523.

35. Wartenberg AA, Nirenberg TD, Leipman MR, et al. Detoxification of al-coholics: improving care by symptom-triggered sedation. *Alcohol Clin Exp Res* 1990;14:71–75.

36. *ASAM PPC-2R.* Chevy Chase, MD: American Society of Addiction Medicine 2001:355.

37. Moller HJ. Effectiveness and safety of benzodiazepines. *J Clin Psychopharmacol* 1999;19:2S–11S.

38. Mintzer MZ, Stoller KB, Griffiths RR. A controlled study of flumazenil-precipitated withdrawal in chronic low-dose benzodiazepine users. *Psychopharmacology (Berl)* 1999;147:200–209.

39. Rickels K, DeMartinis N, Ryan M, et al. Pharmacologic strategies for discontinuing benzodiazepine treatment. *J Clin Psychopharmacol* 1999;196:12s–16s.

40. O'Connor K, Belanger L, Marchand A, et al. Psychological distress and adaptational problems. *Addict Behav* 1999;24:537–531.

41. Alexander B, Perry PJ. Detoxification from benzodiazepines: schedules and strategies. *J Subst Abuse Treat* 1991;8:9–17.

42. Spiegel DA. Psychological strategies for discontinuing benzodiazepine treatment. *J Clin Psychopharmacol* 1999;19:17s–22s.

43. Weiss RD, Greenfield SF, Mirin SM. Intoxication and withdrawal syndromes. In: Hyman SE, Tesar GE, eds. *Manual of psychiatric emergencies,* 3rd ed. Boston: Little, Brown, 1994:279–293.

44. Kampman KM, Volpicelli JR, McGinnis DE, et al. Reliability and validity of the cocaine selective severity assessment. *Addict Behav* 1998;23:449–461.

45. Mulvaney FD, Alterman AI, Boardman CR, et al. Cocaine abstinence symptomatology and treatment attrition. *J Subst Abuse Treat* 1999;16:129–135.

46. Pilotte NS. Neurochemistry of cocaine withdrawal. *Curr Opin Neurol* 1997;10:534–538.

47. Cadet JL, Bolla KI. Chronic cocaine use as a neuropsychiatric syndrome: a model for debate. *Synapse* 1996;22:28–34.

48. Dudish-Poulsen S, Hatsukami DK. Acute abstinence effects following smoked cocaine administration in humans. *Exp Clin Psychopharmacol* 2000;8:472–482.

49. Satel SL, Price LH, Palumbo JM, et al. Clinical phenomenology and neurobiology of cocaine abstinence: a prospective inpatient study. *Am J Psychiatry* 1991;148:1712–1716.

50. Weddington WW, Brown BS, Haertzen CA, et al. Changes in mood, craving, and sleep during short-term abstinence reported by male cocaine addicts. *Arch Gen Psychiatry* 1990;47:861–868.

51. Ehrman RN, Robbins SJ, Childress AR, et al. Conditioned responses to cocaine-related stimuli in cocaine abuse

patients. *Psychopharmacology (Berl)* 1992;107:523–529.

52. Franken IH, Droon LY, Hendricks VM. Influence of individual differences in craving and obsessive cocaine thoughts on attentional processes in cocaine abuse patients. *Addict Behav* 2000;25:99–102.

53. Helmus TC, Downey KK, Wang LM, et al. The relationship between self-reported cocaine withdrawal symptoms and history of depression. *Addict Behav* 2001;26:461–467.

54. Kampman KM, Volpicelli JR, Alterman AI, et al. Amantadine in the treatment of cocaine-dependent patients with severe withdrawal symptoms. *Am J Psychiatry* 2000;157:2052–2054.

55. Kampman KM, Volpicelli JR, Mulvaney F, et al. Effectiveness of propanolol for cocaine dependence treatment may depend on cocaine withdrawal symptom severity. *Drug Alcohol Depend* 2001;63:69–78.

56. Petrakis IL, Carroll KM, Nich C, et al. Disulfiram treatment for cocaine dependence in methadone-maintained opioid addicts. *Addiction* 2000;95:219–228.

57. O'Connor PG, Fiellin DA. Pharmacologic treatment of heroin-dependent patients. *Ann Intern Med* 2000;133:40–54.

58. Bradley BP, Gossop M, Phillips GT, et al. The development of an opiate withdrawal scale. *Br J Addict* 1987;82:1139–1142.

59. Gossop M. The development of a short opiate withdrawal scale. *Addict Behav* 1990;15:487–490.

60. American Society of Addiction Medicine. *State of the art conference syllabus.* Washington, DC: Author: November 2001.

61. McCann MJ, Rawson RA, Obert JL, et al. *Treatment of opiate addiction with methadone.* Rockville, MD: U.S. Department of Health and Human Services, 1994.

62. Barnett PG, Rodgers JH, Bloch DA. A meta-analysis comparing buprenorphine to methadone for treatment of opiate dependence. *Addiction* 2001;96:683–690.

63. 54 Fed Reg 8954 (1989) Vol: 54 (codified at CFR §291).

64. Sees KL, Delucchi KL, Masson C, et al. Methadone maintenance vs. 180-day psychosocially enriched detoxification for treatment of opioid dependence: a randomized controlled trial. *JAMA* 2000;283:1303–1310.

65. Food and Drug Administration. *OR-LAMM.* In: Index of safety-related drug labeling change summaries approved by FDA center for drug evaluation and research (CDER) 2001. Medwatch. www.fda.gov/medwatch/SAFETY/2003/safety03.htm

66. O'Connor PG, Kosten TR. Rapid and ultrarapid opioid detoxification techniques. *JAMA* 1998;279:229–234.

67. Kienbaum P, Scherbaum N, Thurauf N, et al. Acute detoxification of opioid-addicted patients with naloxone during propofol or methohexital anesthesia: a comparison of withdrawal symptoms, neuroendocrine, metabolic, and cardiovascular patterns. *Crit Care Med* 2000;28:969–976.

68. McNichols L, Howell EF. *Buprenorphine clinical practice guidelines. Field review draft.* SAMSA, CSAT Office of Pharmacologic and Alternative Therapies, Columbia, MD, November 2000.

69. Smith NT. A review of the published literature into *cannabis* withdrawal symptoms in human users. *Addiction* 2002;97:621–632.

70. DeFonseca FR, Carrera MRA, Navarro M, et al. Activation of corticotropin-releasing factor in the limbic system during cannabinoid withdrawal. *Science* 1997;276:2050–2054.

71. Haney M, Ward AS, Comer SD, et al. Abstinence syndrome following oral THC administration to humans. *Psychopharmacology (Berl)* 1999;141:385–394.

72. Haney M, Ward AS, Comer SD, et al. Abstinence symptoms following smoked marijuana in humans. *Psychopharmacology (Berl)* 1999;141:395–404.

73. Haney M, Ward AS, Comer SD, et al. Bupropion SR worsens mood during marijuana withdrawal in humans. *Psychopharmacology (Berl)* 2001;143:171–179.

74. Mendelson JH, Mello NK, Lex BW, et al. Marijuana withdrawal syndrome in a woman. *Am J Psychiatry* 1984;141:1289–1290.

75. Andrews JS. Psychiatric effects of cannabis. *Br J Psychiatry* 2001;178:116–122.

76. Wiesbeck GA, Schuckit MA, Kalmijn JA, et al. An evaluation of the history of a marijuana withdrawal syndrome in a large population. *Addiction* 1996;91:1469–1478.

77. Crowley TJ, Macdonald MJ, Whitmore DA, et al. *Cannabis* dependence, withdrawal, and reinforcing effects among adolescents with conduct symptoms and substance use disorders. *Drug Alcohol Depend* 1998;50:27–37.

CHAPTER 36
Alcoholics Anonymous

EDGAR P. NACE

For more than six decades Alcoholics Anonymous (AA) has influenced, guided, and shaped the treatment of alcoholism. It would be difficult today to find a substance abuse treatment program that does not espouse the principles of AA. The appeal of AA's Twelve Steps program has been extended to other disorders, including drug addiction (Narcotics Anonymous), eating disorders (Overeaters Anonymous), and gambling (Gamblers Anonymous).

From an inauspicious founding by two chronic alcoholics, AA has grown in numbers and scope to reach around the world. Men and women whose lives have been touched, even saved, by the program's deceptively simple Twelve Steps offer fervent testimony to AA's efficacy. This chapter highlights some of the history, growth, and dynamics of AA. A more in-depth understanding can be acquired through reading the "Big Book," *Alcoholics Anonymous* (1), *Twelve Steps and Twelve Traditions* (2), Kurtz's *Not-God: A History of Alcoholics Anonymous* (3), and Bean's series of articles (4).

WHAT IS AA?

AA is a fellowship, that is, a "mutual association of persons on equal and friendly terms; a mutual sharing, as of experience, activity, or interest" (5). AA is open to all men and women who want to do something about their drinking problems. Interestingly, members need not consider themselves alcoholics or seek abstinence. AA is nonprofessional, self-supporting, nondenominational, apolitical, and multiracial. There are no age or education requirements (6).

At the start of an AA meeting the "AA preamble" is usually read. The preamble is a concise description of AA (7):

> Alcoholics Anonymous is a fellowship of men and women who share their experience, strength, and hope with each other that they may solve their common problem and help others to recover from alcoholism. The only requirement for membership is a desire to stop drinking. There are no dues or fees for AA membership; we are self-supporting through our own contributions. AA is not allied with any sect, denomination, politics, organization, or institution; does not wish to engage in any controversy, neither endorses nor proposes any causes. Our primary purpose is to stay sober and help other alcoholics to achieve sobriety.

The Program of AA

The program of AA consists of studying and following the "Twelve Steps" of AA (Table 36.1). In addition, AA groups are careful to adhere to the "Twelve Traditions" of AA (Table 36.2). The Twelve Steps offer the alcoholic a sober way of life. This program is presented and discussed in AA meetings. Meetings may be "open" or "closed." Closed meetings are for AA members only or prospective AA members, whereas open meetings are for nonalcoholics as well. AA meetings usually last 1 hour and are preceded and followed by informal socializing. There are different types of meetings: In speaker meetings, AA members tell their "stories." They describe their experiences with alcohol and their recovery—what it was like, what happened, and what it is like now. In discussion meetings, an AA member briefly describes some of the member's experiences and then leads a discussion on a topic related to recovery. Step meetings usually are closed meetings and consist of a discussion of the meaning and ramifications of one of the Twelve Steps.

AA groups are autonomous. Some groups provide proof of attendance that may be required by a court or probation office, whereas other groups choose not to sign court slips.

Sponsorship is an essential function of AA. Each person who joins AA is encouraged to obtain a sponsor, that is, another AA member willing to offer person-to-person guidance in working the AA program. A sponsor typically is a person who has a substantial period of sobriety and who has studied and worked the Twelve Steps. The sponsorship relationship is informal, and the styles of sponsorship vary greatly. The neophyte to AA need not hesitate to ask another member to be a sponsor for fear of being a burden. Members who become sponsors do so, in part, because it helps them in recovery as well—"you keep it [sobriety] by giving it away."

TABLE 36.1. *The Twelve Steps of Alcoholics Anonymous*

1. We admitted we were powerless over alcohol and that our lives had become unmanageable.
2. Came to believe that a Power greater than ourselves could restore us to sanity.
3. Made a decision to turn our will and our lives over to the care of God as we understood Him.
4. Made a searching and fearless moral inventory of ourselves.
5. Admitted to God, to ourselves, and to another human being the exact nature of our wrongs.
6. Were entirely ready to have God remove all these defects of character.
7. Humbly asked Him to remove our shortcomings.
8. Made a list of all persons we had harmed, and became willing to make amends to them all.
9. Made direct amends to such people wherever possible, except when to do so would injure them or others.
10. Continued to take personal inventory and when we were wrong promptly admitted it.
11. Sought through prayer and meditation to improve our conscious contact with God as we understood Him, praying only for knowledge of His will for us and the power to carry that out.
12. Having had a spiritual awakening as the result of these steps, we tried to carry this message to alcoholics, and to practice these principles in all our affairs.

The Twelve Steps and Twelve Traditions are reprinted with permission of Alcoholics Anonymous World Services, Inc. Permission to reprint this material does not mean that AA has reviewed or approved the contents of this publication, nor that AA agrees with the views expressed herein. AA is a program of recovery from alcoholism. Use of the Twelve Steps and Twelve Traditions in connection with programs and activities which are patterned after AA but which address other problems does not imply otherwise.

That AA is a fellowship distinguishes it from professional treatment or programs. Alcoholism provides a bond between one AA member and another. In contrast, professional relationships establish a boundary between doctor and patient or therapist and client. The clinician, when confronted with an alcoholic patient, uses the diagnosis of alcoholism to erect a boundary from which role relationships are carefully defined. From the structure of the professional relationship the clinician applies his or her skills and technologies. There is no mutual sharing of experience or any pretense of equality in the relationship. According to Bean, the nonalcoholic professional often seems unattainably happy to the alcoholic, and the professional may "reinforce the picture of himself [or herself] as superior, powerful, and omniscient. The moral culpability of the alcoholic and the moral superiority of the helper, even though unstated, are always clearly understood" (4, p. 32).

TABLE 36.2. *The Twelve Traditions of Alcoholics Anonymous*

1. Our common welfare should come first; personal recovery depends upon AA unity.
2. For our group purpose there is but one ultimate authority—a loving God as He may express Himself in our group conscience. Our leaders are but trusted servants; they do not govern.
3. The only requirement for AA membership is a desire to stop drinking.
4. Each group should be autonomous except in matters affecting other groups or AA as a whole.
5. Each group has but one primary purpose—to carry its message to the alcoholic who still suffers.
6. An AA group ought never endorse, finance, or lend the AA name to any related facility or outside enterprise, lest problems of money, property, and prestige divert us from our primary purpose.
7. Every AA group ought to be fully self-supporting, declining outside contributions.
8. Alcoholics Anonymous should remain forever nonprofessional, but our service centers may employ special workers.
9. AA, as such, ought never be organized; but we may create service boards or committees directly responsible to those they serve.
10. Alcoholics Anonymous has no opinion on outside issues; hence the AA name ought never be drawn into public controversy.
11. Our public relations policy is based on attraction rather than promotion; we need always maintain personal anonymity at the level of press, radio, and films.
12. Anonymity is the spiritual foundation of all our Traditions, ever reminding us to place principles before personalities.

What AA Promises

Working the Twelve Steps and adhering to the Twelve Principles leads to possibilities contained in the Twelve Promises:

1. We are going to know a new freedom and a new happiness.
2. We will not regret the past nor wish to shut the door on it.
3. We will comprehend the word serenity.
4. We will know peace.
5. No matter how far down the scale we have gone, we will see how our experience can benefit others.
6. That feeling of uselessness and self-pity will disappear.
7. We will lose interest in selfish things and gain interest in our fellows.
8. Self-seeking will slip away.
9. Our whole attitude and outlook on life will change.
10. Fear of people and economic insecurity will leave us.
11. We will intuitively know how to handle situations which used to baffle us.
12. We will suddenly realize that God is doing for us what we could not do for ourselves. (1, pp. 83–84)

The "Big Book" (*Alcoholics Anonymous*) goes on to say: "Are these extravagant promises? We think not. They are being fulfilled among us—sometimes quickly, sometimes slowly. They will always materialize if we work for them" (1, p. 84).

What AA Does Not Do

Part of appreciating the role of AA in the recovery of alcoholics is understanding what AA does not do. From such an understanding, we will be better prepared to focus on what it does do. The list below was obtained from AA literature (6). AA does not:

1. Furnish initial motivation for alcoholics to recover
2. Solicit members
3. Engage in or sponsor research
4. Keep attendance records or case histories
5. Join "councils" of social agencies
6. Follow up or try to control its members
7. Make medical or psychological diagnoses or prognoses
8. Provide drying-out or nursing services, hospitalization, drugs, or any medical or psychiatric treatment
9. Offer religious services
10. Engage in education about alcohol
11. Provide housing, food, clothing, jobs, money, or any other welfare or social services
12. Provide domestic or vocational counseling
13. Accept any money for its services, or any contributions from non-AA sources
14. Provide letters of reference to parole boards, lawyers, court officials

THE GROWTH OF AA

The birth date of AA is given as June 10, 1935. On this date Dr. Bob Smith, the Akron surgeon who cofounded AA with Bill Wilson, had his last drink. The official founding of AA was established with that event. Two and one-half years later, "Dr. Bob" and "Bill W." estimated that as a result of their combined efforts in both Akron and New York City, there were nearly 40 sober recovering alcoholics. The cofounders knew they were onto something (one alcoholic talking to another) and continued the struggle of carrying their hope, strength, and experience to other alcoholics. Most of those they contacted, however, were not maintaining sobriety nor had any interest in their ideas (3). But by the end of 4 years, membership was estimated to be about 100, and by the end of 1941, 8,000 members could be counted. By 1968, 170,000 members were estimated (8). In spite of early periods of discouragement, the growth of AA has been phenomenal and continues today, exceeding 1 million members worldwide.

Anonymous surveys of AA have been conducted every 3 years since 1968 by the AA General Services Office. The 2001 survey (available from AA World Services) determined that there are more than 97,000 AA groups worldwide (9).

COMPOSITION OF AA

Approximately 7,500 members in the United States and Canada were surveyed in 2001. The average age of an AA member is 46 years; 75% of members are between the ages of 31 and 60 years. Women make up 33% of the membership and whites make up 88% of the membership; 37% of members are married, 31% single, and 24% divorced. The average AA member has 7 years sobriety and attends two AA meetings per week (9).

An interesting trend is the percentage of AA members reporting addiction to drugs. In 1977, 18% reported drug addiction, but by 1989, 46% were reporting a history of drug addiction. Women and younger people in AA were more likely to report a history of drug addiction.

THE ORIGINS OF AA

The origins of AA arise from the experience and insight of Bill Wilson ("Bill W."). The sequence of events and the major influences affecting him were described by Ernest Kurtz (3).

Kurtz described four founding moments of AA. Carl Jung played a role in the first founding moment through his extended and frustrating treatment of an American businessman. Jung eventually advised this man (Roland H.) that medicine and psychiatry had no more to offer. Only a spiritual change or awakening, however unlikely, could be expected to release the continuing compulsion to drink. Roland H. proceeded to join the Oxford Group, a popular nondenominational religious group that sought to recapture the essence of first century Christianity and was interested in alcoholics. Roland H.'s successful conversion and abstinence constituted the first founding moment.

Roland H.'s experience was shared with an old friend and alcoholic, Edwin T. ("Ebby"). He, too, found the evangelical efforts of the Oxford Group sufficient to release him from further drinking (at least, temporarily). Ebby, a friend of Bill Wilson, called on Bill in November 1934. Wilson was at his home in New York City drinking. Ebby refused a drink, stating, "I don't need it anymore. I've got religion" (3, p. 7), and described his recent success in giving up alcohol. This conversation (between Bill and Ebby) was the second founding moment. In spite of Bill's disdain for his friend's newfound "religion," he couldn't shake the image of his friend—sober and confident. Bill was influenced through his conversation with Ebby to try again. Bill had himself admitted to the Charles B. Towns Hospital under the care of a psychiatrist, Dr. William Silkworth.

During this hospitalization Bill became increasingly depressed. Concomitant with his worsening condition there occurred one of those inexplicable events that one describes as a spiritual experience. Wilson experienced "ecstasy." He couldn't describe it, and he feared that it indicated brain damage. Dr. Silkworth reassured him concerning the latter, and Bill began to read James's *Varieties of Religious Experience* (10) in an effort to understand what had happened to him. The spiritual experience, the influence of James's writings, and the recognition of the utter hopelessness of his drinking were the third founding moment.

Bill then imagined that conversations between one alcoholic and another, such as his with Ebby, could lead to a "chain reaction" among alcoholics. Months later, in May 1935, an opportunity occurred in Akron, where Bill, a stockbroker, was on a business trip. A deal had fallen through, and Bill felt a mounting urge to drink. It was late Saturday afternoon, the day before Mother's Day. He consulted a church directory, reached an Oxford Group minister, and ultimately was referred to a woman who was receptive to his need to talk to another alcoholic. Mrs. Henrietta Sieberling arranged for Bill to come to her house and meet with Dr. Bob Smith, a deteriorating alcoholic surgeon. Dr. Smith was reluctant to accept this invitation but went with his wife to meet Bill W. Their historic meeting, the fourth founding moment, is described as follows (3, p. 29):

> ... here was someone who did understand, or perhaps at least could. This stranger from New York didn't ask questions and didn't preach; he offered no "you musts" or even "let's us's." He had simply told the dreary but fascinating facts about himself, about his own drinking. And now, as Wilson moved to stand up to end the conversation, he was actually thanking Dr. Smith for listening. "I called Henrietta because I needed another alcoholic. I needed you, Bob, probably a lot more than you'll ever need me. So, thanks a lot for hearing me out. I know now that I'm not going to take a drink, and I'm grateful to you." While he had been listening to Bill's story, Bob had occasionally nodded his head, muttering "Yes, that's like me, that's just like me." Now he could bear the strain no longer. He'd listened to Bill's story, and now, by God, this "rum hound from New York" was going to listen to him. For the first time in his life, Dr. Bob Smith began to open his heart.

Bill Wilson and Bob Smith became the cofounders of AA. Wilson went on to develop the fellowship of AA and to provide a remarkable chapter in the social history of twentieth century America. Bill W. learned to weave a careful course between religious dogma, on the one hand, and a humanistic liberal psychology on the other. The AA program was successful in incorporating the concepts of "surrender," "powerlessness," and appeal to a "Higher Power." These elements reflect its roots in the evangelical Christianity of the Oxford Group. Yet Bill W. avoided the Oxford Group's focus on attaining "Four Absolutes": absolute honesty, absolute purity, absolute unselfishness, and absolute love (3). He was aware of the psychological vulnerability of the alcoholic to strive for "absolutes," and, when the mark is missed, to indulge in self-castigation, self-hatred, and, finally, drunkenness.

The AA Fellowship evolved a system and a way of life reflected in the Twelve Steps and Twelve Traditions. The Traditions of AA are less familiar to most clinicians (see Table 36.2) than the Steps. Even a cursory reading of the Traditions conveys these three principles:

1. The singleness of purpose of AA
   - "The only requirement for AA membership is a desire to stop drinking" (Tradition 3)
   - "... primary purpose—to carry its message to the alcoholic who still suffers" (Tradition 5)
2. The avoidance of personal power and influence
   - "... there is but one ultimate authority—a loving God...." (Tradition 2)
   - "... each group should be autonomous...." (Tradition 4)
   - "An AA group ought never endorse, finance, or lend the AA name to any related facility or outside enterprise...." (Tradition 6)
   - "AA, as such, ought never be organized...." (Tradition 9)
3. The need for humility
   - "Our common welfare should come first...." (Tradition 1)
   - "Alcoholic Anonymous should remain forever nonprofessional" (Tradition 7)
   - "Alcoholics Anonymous has no opinion on outside issues...." (Tradition 10)
   - "Our public relations policy is based on attraction rather than promotion...." (Tradition 11)
   - "... place principles before personalities" (Tradition 12)

The AA program counters pathologic narcissism by assisting the alcoholic to be "not-God," to accept limitations, and to serve others. Furthermore, the AA program provides a means for overcoming guilt, for example, by taking a personal inventory (Step 4) and making amends (Step 9) without triggering harsh superego responses. Although the origins of AA are rooted in the sacred and the religious, it has widened its appeal by cloaking the program in spiritual and secular garb.

AFFILIATION WITH ALCOHOLICS ANONYMOUS

The 2001 AA General Services Office survey (9) reports that of the factors most responsible for coming to AA, 32% of newcomers were referred by treatment facilities. Thirty-three percent were attracted to AA by an AA member and 33% reported being self-motivated.

Gradually, AA is receiving greater emphasis from physicians. Historically, things got off to a slow start with doctors. The first edition of *Alcoholics Anonymous* was published in 1939 (1). AA members were enthusiastic about reaching out to the medical community and sent 20,000 announcements of the "Big Book." Only two orders for *Alcoholics Anonymous* were received (11). Since then, of course, physicians have become much more aware of AA; one study from Great Britain reports that 65% of general practitioners believed that AA had something to offer beyond what could be obtained through medical efforts (12). The 2001 General Services Survey (9) reports that 38% of members were referred to AA by a health care professional and that 73% of member's doctors know they are in AA.

Once someone gets to AA, what are the chances that person will stay? Figures from AA General Services Office surveys indicate that only 50% of those who come to AA remain more than 3 months. In a review of AA affiliation (13), approximately 20% of problem drinkers referred to AA were found to attend regularly. In a 4-year followup of alcoholism treatment (14), 27% of those who had ever gone to AA reported attendance at AA the month prior to followup, and of those who reported attending AA regularly, 39% had attended a meeting during the month prior to followup. In a review of the literature (14), dropout rates from AA varied from 68% before 10 meetings were attended to 88% by 1 year after discharge. A recent followup study of an outpatient program found that a majority of patients were attending AA 6 months after discharge (15). The latter study plus data from the 2001 AA Survey (9) indicate an emerging trend; that is counseling or other related treatments are influencing AA affiliation as 74% of AA members who received treatment report that it played an important part in their going to AA.

The "dropout" problem raises the question of who is likely to make a stable affiliation with AA. Early research on this problem (4,13,16) suggests that those who join AA are middle class, guilt ridden, sociable, cognitively rigid, and socially stable. They also are more likely to be chronic alcoholics or loss-of-control drinkers and to have more alcohol-related problems. A comprehensive recent review (14) of the affiliation process fails to support earlier findings. Emrick (14) compared variables used to distinguish between stable and unstable affiliations and found that 64% bear no relationship, 29% show a positive relationship favoring AA affiliation, and only 7% bear a negative relationship to AA affiliation. This leads to the conclusion that most alcoholics have the possibility of making an affiliation with AA. Only those whose goal is not to abstain from alcohol would be seen as exceptions. Demographic variables such as education, employment, socioeconomic status of the alcoholic or of the parents, social stability, religion, and measures of social competence are unrelated to the affiliation process. Age favors, although not consistently, older alcoholics' making a positive affiliation. Marital status (married) and gender (male) also show some positive relationship to affiliation. Alcoholism variables bear little relationship to making a positive affiliation. For example, loss of control, quantity drunk daily, age at first drink, degree of physiologic dependence, and drinking style bear no consistent relationship to affiliation. On the other hand, a recent study (17) of drug abusers found that frequent attenders of Narcotics Anonymous (NA) or AA were likely to have had more severe histories of drug abuse and more criminal activity.

Currently, it is best to accept as unpredictable who will affiliate with AA, which again emphasizes the importance of recommending AA to all possible members.

ALCOHOLICS ANONYMOUS OUTCOME

Many efforts have been made to assess the effectiveness of AA attendance. Measurement of "outcome" typically is limited to abstinence or lack of abstinence from alcohol. In studies of AA from the 1940s to the early 1970s (18), sampling difficulties and other methodological problems were immense. Nevertheless, the findings indicated that thousands of AA members had achieved sobriety through AA. In a study of 393 AA members conducted by an AA member, it was determined that 70% who stayed sober for 1 year would be sober at 2 years, and that 90% of those sober at 2 years would be sober at 3 years (15). In two early studies of AA, sobriety of more than 2 years' duration was found in 46% of those sampled (19,20).

A review of survey studies (14) found that 35% to 40% of respondents reported abstinence of less than 1 year, with 26% to 40% reporting abstinence of 1 to 5 years, and 20% to 30% having been sober 5 or more years. Overall, 47% to 62% of active AA members had at least 1 year of continuous sobriety.

The 1989 AA General Services Office survey consisting of 9,994 responses from a mailing of 12,000 reported an average sobriety length of 50 months. This figure was somewhat lower than the 52-month average in the 1986 survey, but higher than the 45-month average reported in 1983. The 2001 survey (9) reported the average sobriety of members to be 84 months, with 18% sober more than 5 years and 30% sober less than 1 year.

AA involvement correlates favorably with a variety of outcome measures. Those patients who attend AA before, during, or after a treatment experience have a more favorable outcome in regard to drinking (14). In the few studies available that assess the outcome on other variables, AA involvement is associated with a more stable social adjustment, more active religious life, internal locus of control, and better employment adjustment (14). Increased ethical concern for others, an increased sense of well-being, and increasing dependence on a Higher Power with less dependence on others also have been described (21). Finally, there is a positive relationship between outcome and extent of AA participation (14). Outcome is more favorable for those who attend more than one meeting per week and for those who have a sponsor, sponsor others, lead meetings, and work Steps Six through Twelve after completing a treatment program. Taking Step Four or Five is not consistently related to outcome, nor is telling one's story or doing Twelve Step work.

THE DYNAMICS OF ALCOHOLICS ANONYMOUS

The reasons for AA's effectiveness may be as varied as the individuals involved. At the most basic level, the program works because one follows the Twelve Steps. It may be that these deceptively simple steps provide a concrete, tangible course of action; they may trigger cognitive processes previously unformed, unfocused, or abandoned; and they may encapsulate powerful dynamics capable of having an impact on craving, conditioning, and character. The AA program revolves around the Twelve Steps, and most members would offer the common-sense explanation that working the steps keeps them sober. This sentiment is reflected in the "Big Book's" chapter on how it works: "Rarely have we seen a person fail who has thoroughly followed our path" (1).

GROUP PROCESS

The utility of the slogan "keep it simple" is well-known to AA members, but need not deter further inquiry into the process or dynamics of AA's effectiveness. Any effort to understand the efficacy of AA must take into account the ubiquitous group process that is operating. The elements of group therapy as enumerated by Yalom (22) are apparent:

1. *Hope* is provided by associating with other alcoholics who are not drinking and who apparently are happy, satisfied, or, indeed, grateful not to be drinking. In other words, change is possible.
2. *Universality* is formed through sharing stories and experiences involving alcohol. The newcomer is struck by the value of his or her experience as AA members identify with it and express thanks and gratitude to the

newcomer for sharing the story. Instead of feeling condemned, the newcomer feels bonded to these other alcoholics by virtue of his or her experience.

3. *Information* is provided informally through conversations, through literature published by AA, and through the topics and content of the meetings themselves.

4. *Imitation* is a very prominent aspect of the group process. Phrases are repeated and rituals followed.

5. *Learning* occurs at multiple levels and includes how sober alcoholics view their disease, how they relate to others, and what they do to stay sober. The member also learns that the problem is alcohol (not a spouse, or job, or a lack of willpower). It is learned that one has a disease and that alcoholism is cunning, powerful, and baffling.

6. *Catharsis* can occur. The opportunity is provided (but not demanded) through discussion, speaker, and Step study meetings. Again, one's experiences are appreciated and not subjected to condemnation or judgment.

7. *Cohesiveness* follows from the ability to identify, usually quickly, with the viewpoints and experiences of fellow members. Cohesiveness is also facilitated by participating in the informal socializing characteristic of AA meetings. One feels at home by helping to make coffee, set up chairs, and eventually greet newcomers.

The beneficial aspects of group process may be found in many settings, for example, group therapy, religious groups, and organizational activities. The dynamics operative in coherent group settings as described by Yalom (22) cannot fully account for the impact of AA on alcoholics. If group process variables were the key to the transformation from inebriety to sobriety, substantial progress in arresting alcoholism could have been expected before the establishment of the AA program. Equal success might have been expected from a variety of group approaches. This has not been the case. It is necessary to look further. This chapter describes several formulations of AA effectiveness. These formulations, or explanations of the efficacy of AA, are superordinate to the group process variables described above, are not mutually exclusive, and are not necessarily contradictory.

EGO FUNCTIONS

Mack (23) introduces the concept of "self-governance," which refers to an aspect of the ego (or self) concerned with choosing, deciding, and directing the personality. Self-governance, according to Mack, encompasses a group of functions in the ego system and provides the individual with a sense of being and a sense of power to be in charge of oneself. Self-governance differs somewhat from the concept of autonomous and executive functions of the ego in that it acknowledges the interdependence among the ego and other individuals and groups. The concept of self-governance allows a sharing of control with others, and, indeed, indicates that survival and sense of personal value require interdependent participation in social structures.

The success of AA, according to Mack, is "due to its intuitive and subtle grasp of the complex psychosocial and biological nature of self-governance, not only for the control of problem drinking but in a far more general sense" (20, p. 134). The alcoholic has lost control over alcohol, and alcohol is making life unmanageable. AA recognizes the powerlessness of the individual in the face of the drive to drink and provides a counterforce to the drive to drink through caring, supportive interaction with others. The social aspects of group process operating in AA strengthen the individual's capacity for self-governance by "borrowing" such capacity from fellowship with AA members, the group process, and the acceptance of a Higher Power. In simplest terms, the alcoholic learns to substitute people for alcohol.

Khantzian and Mack (24) further implicate ego functions in the etiology of and recovery from alcoholism. They view the alcoholic as not necessarily suffering from structural defects in the ego (as is more commonly noted in drug addicts) but rather see certain ego functions as being poorly developed. One such ego disability commonly observed in alcoholics and other addicts is a diminished capacity to recognize, regulate, and tolerate affect. Feelings may seem unmanageable and, therefore, threatening. The ability to describe how one feels may be lacking. The individual who feels overwhelmed, confused, or intolerably uncomfortable with affect is subject to develop counterdependent personality traits or other exaggerated character traits that serve as an affect defense (25). Such defenses constitute, in part, the defects of character that the AA Step Program seeks to remove. Thus AA, through the working of the Steps (see Steps 6, 7, and 10), challenges the past faulty coping strategies of the alcoholic through its recognition that failure to do so will lead back to drinking.

Another ego function that may be deficient in substance-abusing individuals is that of "self-care." This capacity is part of the larger function of self-governance and involves reality testing, judgment, anticipation of consequences, and impulse control. AA may strengthen the self-care capacity of the individual by offering self-soothing slogans ("Easy does it"; "One day at a time"; "Live and let live") and by providing a caring milieu the alcoholic gradually identifies with, internalizes, and uses to modulate his or her behavior.

PATHOLOGIC NARCISSISM

In addition to the specific ego dysfunctions mentioned earlier, Khantzian and Mack (24) emphasize the importance of pathologic narcissism in substance abusers. Strands of pathologic narcissism that may be observed in alcoholics and other addicts include the belief that they can take care of problems themselves, that they are self-sufficient, and that they are able to retain the necessary control over alcohol as well as other areas of their lives. Further, alcohol induces a feeling of personal power and adequacy (26). The person vulnerable to alcoholism or drug addiction may enter adult life wounded by empathic failures in being parented and therefore may retain archaic narcissistic tendencies such as grandiosity (including self-sufficiency), an overvaluation or devaluation of others, and a reliance on external supplies and sources to feel complete (27). An adult burdened by these narcissistic themes is doomed to continuous disappointment in self and others. Depression, anxiety, guilt, and shame can be expected. It is a short step to the discovery of relief from such emotional pain through alcohol. In addition, alcohol's pharmacologic restoration of a feeling of personal power (26) reinforces the original pathologic narcissism (28). As Mack (23) points out, AA tradition recognized the artificial inflation of the self in alcoholism and the chance of stimulating "power drives" in authoritarian systems. Thus, the AA traditions (see Traditions 1, 2, 6, 9, 10, and 11) de-emphasize and discourage prestige, status, and power. A focus is kept on Tradition 5. At a very practical level, AA groups do not let money from their collections accumulate lest ambitious members covet a special project. The emphasis in Tradition 2 is to serve, not govern. The Traditions of AA, therefore, serve to curb and discourage expressions of unhealthy narcissism.

Even more cogent to the theme of narcissism are the Twelve Steps. The First Step, acknowledging powerlessness and loss of control, is the sine qua non of recovery. Without the recognition and acceptance of one's loss of control, recovery remains postponed. Brown (29) places particular emphasis on the alcoholic's need to accept loss of control (that is, accept Steps 1 and 2), for such acceptance is considered the nucleus of one's identity as an alcoholic from which the stages of recovery may unfold. A reading of the Steps makes clear how they offer a healthy alternative to pathologic expressions of personality, whether the latter are premorbid or secondary to chronic intoxication. Humility, powerlessness, consideration of others, the need for self-examination, and service are clearly put forth, not as abstract ideals, but as tools to ward off a return to the insanity of alcoholism.

The narcissistic problems just described were recognized earlier by Tiebout (30). He points out that defiance and grandiosity stand in the way of the alcoholic's "surrender" and result in fleeting states of compliance but not a deep acceptance of defeat at the hands of alcohol.

The problem of retained pathologic narcissistic traits is more central to the recovery process than are the ego functions described by Khantzian and Mack (24). This assertion is based on the unlikelihood of achieving a mature capacity for self-governance in the face of grandiosity, self-sufficiency, and a devaluing of others. Such narcissistic defenses shut out the social field from which mature self-governance may grow. Narcissistic pathology necessarily results in a diminished capacity for self-governance. Thus the modification of narcissistic traits, as facilitated by the caring confrontation of AA, opens the door to an improvement in other areas of ego development.

AN EMPATHIC UNDERSTANDING OF THE ALCOHOLIC

In a series of classic papers, Bean provides a second description of the mechanisms of AA's effectiveness, integrating its phenomenologic and psychodynamic aspects: AA has "accomplished a shift from a society-centered view of alcoholism to an abuser-centered one" (4, p. 6). For the bereft or discouraged alcoholic, this shift is a startling, powerful encounter. AA provides the alcoholic with a protected environment. After years of feeling debased and worthless, the alcoholic is offered an environment free from the conventional view of drunken behavior. The alcoholic discovers that his or her experience is of value and even interesting to others. Furthermore, the alcoholic's experiences may be useful to someone else, and others thank him or her for sharing it. As Bean explains, "This idea, that a person's experience is of value, is gratifying to anyone and is especially heady stuff to the chronically self-deprecating alcoholic" (4, p. 10).

Along with the shift in how alcoholism is viewed, AA provides a shift in what is expected of the alcoholic. First, the alcoholic is not asked to admit that he or she is an alcoholic. AA simply asks that one have a sincere desire to stop drinking. There is no effort to point out the error of one's ways or the evils of drink. In fact, the attraction of alcohol and the pleasure of alcohol are openly acknowledged but linked with the statement that "we couldn't handle it." The alcoholic who comes to AA is not asked to change, only to listen, identify, and keep coming back. The style of interpersonal contact is nonthreatening. Last names are not given, attendance is not taken, the setting is casual, and humor and friendliness abound. Nevertheless, the meeting is serious. Each member conveys that there is a lot to lose, regardless of how much has actually been lost, but also that there is much to gain—sobriety. Sobriety is the focus, and remains so, unvaryingly. Not drinking is the coin of the realm. Relapses or "slips" do not represent a failure on the part of the alcoholic or of AA. Rather, slips are further demonstration of the power of alcohol and, therefore, the necessity of AA as a counterforce.

Bean (4) emphasizes the regressive effect of alcohol on the alcoholic's personality functioning. The regression results from the toxic disinhibiting effect of alcohol on the brain, the stress of losing control, and the impact of opprobrium, failure, and stigma. AA is seen by Bean to facilitate surrendering immature defenses for mature defenses. Denial is relinquished partly as a result of the crisis that usually brings the alcoholic to AA in the first place, but also because the alcoholic is offered hope that there is a way out. The alcoholic is not expected to appreciate fully the consequences of his or her behavior. This would be overwhelming. The only expectation is to stop drinking one day at a time. Repression, therefore, replaces denial, according to Bean. Reaction formation and undoing are manifested in the change from love of drinking to love of sobriety.

The central point in Bean's explication of psychodynamic change through AA is that the drinking alcoholic is accepted as he or she presents (4). One is permitted to express oneself as he or she is rather than as others may wish him or her to be. The alcoholic in AA may continue unchanged in character and so is granted the opportunity to put his or her energy into abstinence. Not drinking allows the brain to heal and nurtures confidence, hope, and the gradual restoration of self-esteem. Not drinking and following the AA way promote maturity, that is, a shift from primitive defenses to higher-order defenses (26).

As the alcoholic advances in recovery, self-esteem is protected by abstinence but threatened by remorse over the past. According to Bean, AA techniques to handle this aspect of recovery are

1. The decision not to drink—repent and reform to build upon the wreckage of the past
2. Place blame on the illness, not the alcoholic
3. Avoid censure
4. Reward good behavior—this is done by dispensing 30-day, 60-day, 90-day, or 1-year "chips" as milestones in sobriety are achieved
5. Allow expression of low self-esteem in nondestructive ways rather than by drinking

AA does not ask the alcoholic to get a job, be a better family member, or become more responsible. Sobriety is the goal from which other desirable efforts may emerge. The "depressurization" techniques of AA ("one day at a time," "keep it simple," etc.) and the social dimension—sharing "experiences, strength, and hope"—are, from Bean's perspective, critical components of the AA experience.

ACCEPTING LIMITATIONS

The writings of Kurtz provide not only a definitive history of AA but also critical insights into AA's effectiveness (3,31). The core dynamic of AA therapy, according to Kurtz, is "the shared honesty of mutual vulnerability openly acknowledged . . . " (31, p. 30).

An essential insight of AA for the alcoholic is its recognition and acceptance that one is "not-God" (3). With this term Kurtz is referring to the necessity for the alcoholic to accept personal limitation. The First Step of AA communicates to the alcoholic: "We admitted we were powerless over alcohol and that our lives had become unmanage-

able." The acceptance of personal limitation—a condition of existence for all—is a life or death matter for the alcoholic. AA, in teaching that the first drink gets the alcoholic drunk, implies that the alcoholic does not have a drinking limit, the alcoholic is limited (31). To experience limitation is tantamount to experiencing shame. As painful as the shame is, it is an affect pivotal to recovery. Acceptance of shame distinguishes the alcoholic who, in Tiebout's (30) terms, complies rather than surrenders. Compliance is motivated by guilt, is superficial, and ultimately is useless to extended recovery. Surrender involves recognition of powerlessness (and the affect associated with feeling limited or of having fallen short). Through surrender the alcoholic becomes open to the healing forces within AA. Kurtz (31) considers that Steps 2, 6, 7, and 10 influence the experience of shame in the alcoholic. The AA program treats shame by enabling the alcoholic to accept his or her need for others, by promoting the acceptance of others as they are ("live and let live"), and by valuing and reinforcing traits of honesty, sharing, and caring.

SPIRITUAL DIMENSION

Earlier it was noted that the effectiveness of AA could not be explained fully by the variables operating within group dynamics. Other mechanisms or explanations have been reviewed in the effort to understand better the dynamics of AA. Among these explanations are AA's impact on ego functions and pathologic narcissism (23,24), AA's understanding of the alcoholic and alcoholism from the viewpoint of the alcoholic (4), AA's confrontation of the powerlessness and loss of control of the alcoholic (29), and AA's ability to shift the alcoholic from self-centeredness to self-acceptance (31). These analyses of AA's effectiveness (like examination of group process variables) contribute to our understanding of the AA program but are incomplete in their capture of the AA process. The dimension of spirituality must be introduced and considered in the equation of our understanding.

At the beginning of this chapter it was suggested that working the Twelve Steps is what makes AA effective. This simple explanation may disguise the impact of spirituality on the recovery process. Spirituality rarely is part of the lexicon of the mental health professional but is a dimension of the AA program understood by those who work and live the Twelve Steps. The spirituality of the AA program is distinct from religious dogma and may be understood as a series of overlapping themes (32). The first theme is release. Release refers to the "chains being broken"—freedom from the compulsion to drink. The experience of release is a powerful and welcome event for the alcoholic and seems to occur naturally or to be given rather than achieved.

A second theme of spirituality is gratitude. Gratitude may flow from the feeling of release and includes an awareness of what we have—for example, the gift of life. According to Kurtz, the words "think" and "thank" share a common derivation (32). Thinking leads to remembrance (e.g., as the AA speaker tells his or her story), and from remembrance an attitude of thankfulness (gratitude) may be experienced—gratitude, for example, that one is now sober.

The third theme is humility. Humility conveys the attitude that it is acceptable to be limited, to be simply human. The alcoholic's awareness of powerlessness over alcohol engenders humility.

Finally, a fourth theme or component to spirituality is tolerance. A tolerance of differences and limitations fosters the serenity often experienced by AA members.

These themes of spirituality are very similar to the healing process in mystical traditions as described by Deikman (33). According to Deikman, the process of attaining higher psychological development involves renunciation, humility, and sincerity. Renunciation refers to an attitude, that is, a giving up of the attachment to the things of the world. The alcoholic's giving up alcohol would demonstrate renunciation. Humility, according to Deikman, is "the possibility that someone else can teach you something you do not already know, especially about yourself" (33, p. 81), and sincerity simply refers to honesty of intention. It is apparent that the alcoholic working the Twelve Steps (see Table 36.1) is involving himself or herself in the processes of renunciation, humility, and sincerity.

More recently, Emmonds (34) empirically demonstrated that goals, especially goals of spiritual striving and goals with religious significance, seem to promote personality integration and assist in resolving the pernicious effect of conflict on mental and physical health. AA provides goals for the alcoholic; not only the goal and "promises" of sobriety, but the goals of understanding, embracing, and following the 12 Steps.

In addition to the spiritual themes mentioned earlier, an additional healing dynamic may be significant: forgiveness. The seeking of forgiveness is implied, not directly expressed, in the Twelve Steps. For example, Steps 6 and 7 (see Table 36.1) ask God to remove defects of character and remove shortcomings. The behavior of AA members toward newcomers (welcoming, accepting, friendly, caring) communicates forgiveness. Forgiveness is neither asked for nor offered at AA. The word itself may or may not be heard at AA meetings, but its meaning pervades the transactions of the meetings. For example, Bean writes (4, p. 10):

> Alcoholics know how deeply and painfully ashamed and guilty other alcoholics are about their drinking, how they lie and minimize it, and how this reinforces their sense of worthlessness. The discovery that others have committed what they thought was their own

uniquely unforgivable crime brings longed-for solace. Speakers repeatedly report their sense of relief when they first come to AA. They had no further need for dissembling and fear. Here they were among their own kind and were accepted.

Forgiveness may be a precondition for the dynamic forces described in this chapter to be operative. For example, forgiveness precedes hope. Hope is necessarily very tenuous for a newcomer to AA and requires a future orientation, an orientation minimized by AA's emphasis on "one day at a time." Forgiveness is experienced in a moment and may be the foundation for a growing sense of hope. Abandoning narcissistic defenses, strengthening the capacity for self-governance, and accepting "powerlessness" over alcohol all may be contingent on feeling forgiven or feeling capable of being forgiven. To be forgiven, to feel forgiven implies being accepted, a common description of the AA experience. The experience of shame (31) as a pivotal affect and the treatment of shame in AA may become possible only if preceded by a sense of being forgiven.

The concepts of spirituality, including forgiveness, are put forth only as one further effort to explain the impact and mechanisms of the AA program. Perhaps that which is effective in the AA program varies considerably from member to member. An AA member may have limited awareness of (and equally little interest in) the dynamic forces accounting for AA's effectiveness. But, possibly, for some, the program may be a secular expression of the Christian concept of grace—an unmerited gift from God.

LIMITATIONS OF ALCOHOLICS ANONYMOUS

AA is predominantly a white, middle-class organization consisting of middle-aged married males (4). This broad demographic characterization of AA does not indicate a limitation of the AA program itself but may impose some barriers for those out of the mainstream. AA does attract a young population. Eleven percent of members are 30 years of age or younger (9). The percentage of women is 33% (9). Adoption of the AA program by minorities has been slower to occur. Yet, most urban areas have several meetings with a predominantly African American or Hispanic population. African American affiliation with AA is growing stronger and may exceed white affiliation on some variables (35).

Psychiatric comorbidity may impede AA affiliation for some alcoholics. Personality disorders of the schizoid, avoidant, or paranoid type may not adapt well to the interaction and emotionality of AA meetings. At times, a patient on medications is thrown into conflict by AA members who may advise against the use of any drugs. AA as an organization does not hold opinions on psychotropic medications, but occasionally an AA member may inappropriately influence a fellow member who requires specific psychiatric treatment. An alcoholic persuaded to discontinue lithium or neuroleptics may relapse into psychosis, at great personal expense. As more alcoholics are reaching AA through rehabilitation programs, AA's familiarity with and understanding of individual needs may be increased, and the AA member under psychiatric treatment will be less likely to experience conflict and inappropriate advice. However, in one study (36), 29% of AA members reported feeling pressure to stop medication, but 89% of these continued their medications. Only 17% of 277 surveyed AA members believed that medications, for example, naltrexone (ReVia), should not be used.

Should AA be recommended only for certain alcoholics? There is no empirical base from which such a decision-making process could follow. AA generally seems to accommodate a wide variety of personalities and backgrounds. On a case-by-case basis, social or psychodynamic factors may deter the efficacy of AA use, but that can be ascertained on an individual basis only, not by currently available data. The question of whether some alcoholics are suited for AA and others not is seen by Brown less as an empirical question and more as reflecting a misunderstanding of or bias toward AA (26, p. 187):

> The position that AA is for some and not for others widens the gap between professionals and AA members. Patients and therapists alike tend to believe that being able to stay sober without the use of AA is superior to using it. Patients and therapists may both believe that AA is not for bright, capable people who can make use of a therapist.

Brown recommends that anyone concerned about drinking be referred to AA.

Apart from the issue of whether every alcoholic should be referred to AA, there are specific limitations to the AA method. These were summarized by Bean (4) and include AA's being rigid, superficial, regressive, inspirational, fanatical, stigmatizing, and focusing only on alcohol. The rigidity is more likely to lie in individual members than the AA program itself. Questioning and intellectualizing are discouraged, but this seems more a means to hold back the ever-present threat of denial than a commitment to absolute dogma. The criticism of superficiality is appropriate if one's goals are to unravel the complex etiologies of alcoholism or to understand the dynamics of behavior change. AA chooses to put its energy into abstaining from drinking and into simultaneously providing and tolerating a system that fosters dependency (hence the criticism of being regressive). AA certainly is inspirational rather than reflective, but again, the alcoholic early in recovery cannot be expected to obtain or use

insight. Morale is of critical concern, and the emotional pitch of AA strikes a respondent chord in the demoralized. Unfortunately, fanaticism or zealotry may form part of the operation of AA loyalty. Such members are repellent to some newcomers, who may feel that their emotional needs are not understood or validated. Some charismatic AA members convert many alcoholics but alienate others, including the professionals to whom they relate in a condescending manner. Is there a stigma about attending AA? If there is, it is less than in past years, because acclaim for AA is easily found in popular literature and the media. At the least, any stigma attached to the AA program would be substantially less than that of chronic drunkenness.

To conclude, AA, like all other therapies for alcoholism, is limited. Considering our current state of knowledge, the clinician is obligated to become conversant with the purpose, principles, and utility of the AA program. By gaining an understanding of the Twelve Steps program, the clinician will be prepared to motivate and advocate AA to his or her alcoholic patients. This understanding is gained best by attending AA meetings, discussing AA with experienced members, and reading widely, including the AA literature as well as professional writings on AA. From this effort the physician can inform each patient appropriately of the advantages of AA as well as any potential drawbacks he or she may encounter.

THE MENTAL HEALTH PROFESSIONS AND ALCOHOLICS ANONYMOUS

The clinician would be remiss to overlook, ignore, or disparage the value of AA for any patient with a substance use disorder. Familiarity with AA can be obtained by attending open AA meetings, developing friendly relationships with AA members, and insisting that one's patients meet with AA members for an initial, informed introduction to AA. Such efforts can facilitate an alliance with the AA community and foster the development of mutual respect.

Such grassroots efforts, however, do not dispel conceptual differences between AA and the treatments offered by the mental health field. Table 36.3 outlines potential differences, and, for the sake of comparison, presents these differences in extreme form. A modulation of the differences is suggested.

Chappel (37) effectively integrates working the Twelve Steps with the process of psychotherapeutic change. For example, Step One requires self-examination and honesty and is critical to overcoming the defense of denial; Step Three is, in part, a process of "letting go" and ridding oneself of obsessive tendencies; and Step Four promotes the development of an observing ego as one confronts issues of guilt and shame. If one conscientiously applies the Twelve Steps to one's life an openness to new experiences will be gained, the courage to attempt personal change

TABLE 36.3. *Modulation of differences between AA and psychiatry*

Subject	AA	Psychiatry	Modulation
Cause of drinking	One drinks because one is an alcoholic. Therapy can lead to intellectualization and denial.	One needs to understand the dynamics that influence behavior in order for change to be lasting.	Initially, the emphasis is put on cessation of drinking; later, an understanding of one's emotional pain or vulnerabilities.
Recovery	Simple—just follow the program.	Lengthy therapeutic quest.	Explore with the alcoholic resistances to AA, and/or why he or she can't avoid people, places, or things that facilitate drinking.
AA	A divine gift. It saved my life.	It's rigid.	It's both. Early in treatment the alcoholic needs a concise, rigid formula to contain drinking impulses and to counter despair.
Controlled drinking	A myth that kills.	Sometimes it seems possible.	Controlled drinking is a very unlikely outcome for the large majority of alcoholics. Mildly dependent, early-stage alcoholics sometimes reverse loss of control.
Medication	It's bad.	Good—corrects biochemical defects.	Medication may be essential during detoxification and in cases of psychiatric comorbidity.
Psychopathology	Alcoholics are normal once they stop drinking.	All alcoholics have specific conflicts that predate their alcoholism.	Psychopathology often predates the alcoholism but many times is the result of drinking. Sobriety leads to improvement in either case, but additional treatment is often useful.
Treatment	The Twelve Steps	Medical and psychological.	The two are not contradictory but can be used effectively by most alcoholics, with one receiving more emphasis at certain times.
Basis of treatment	Personal experience of others.	Scientifically based and empirically validated procedures.	Divergent sources of understanding enable the experience of many to make an impact on a complex disease.

will be acquired, and a greater acceptance of oneself and others can be expected (37).

CONCLUSION

This chapter outlines the origins of AA and describes its growth and basic situations. AA works. How well and for whom remain unsatisfactorily researched.

Particular emphasis is placed on reviewing the dynamics of AA. Just as group process variables seem to have only partial explanatory power, the same may be said of sophisticated psychodynamic formulations. The underacknowledged, understudied area of spirituality bears serious consideration by the clinician. The theme of spirituality and the homilies expressed in AA slogans may someday catalyze an understanding of behavior change.

REFERENCES

1. Alcoholics Anonymous. *Alcoholics Anonymous,* 2nd ed. New York: AA World Services, 1955.
2. Alcoholics Anonymous. *Twelve steps, twelve traditions.* New York: AA World Services, 1978.
3. Kurtz E. *Not-God: a history of Alcoholics Anonymous.* Center City, MN: Hazelden, 1979.
4. Bean MH. Alcoholics Anonymous: AA. *Psychiatr Ann* 1975;5(2):3–64.
5. *Webster's new twentieth century dictionary of the English language, unabridged,* 2nd ed. New York: William Collins Publishers, 1980.
6. Alcoholics Anonymous. *Information on Alcoholics Anonymous.* New York: AA World Services, 1988.
7. Alcoholics Anonymous. *Grapevine.* New York: The AA Grapevine, 1992.
8. Alcoholics Anonymous. *About AA: a newsletter for professional men and women.* Fall, 1984.
9. Alcoholics Anonymous 2001 Membership Survey, AA World Services. Grand Central Station, Box 459 New York, NY 10163.
10. James W. *The varieties of religious experience.* New York: Mentor, 1958.
11. Thomsen R. *Bill W.* New York: Harper and Row, 1975.
12. Henry S, Robinson D. Understanding Alcoholics Anonymous. *Lancet* 1978;2: 372–375.
13. Ogborne AC, Glaser FB. Characteristics of affiliates of Alcoholics Anonymous. *J Stud Alcohol* 1981;42(7):661–675.
14. Emrick C. Alcoholics Anonymous: affiliation processes and effectiveness as treatment. *Alcohol* 1987;11:416–423.
15. Thomassen L. AA utilization after introduction to treatment. *Subst Use Misuse* 2002;37(2):239–253.
16. Boscarino J. Factors related to "stable" and "unstable" affiliation with Alcoholics Anonymous. *Int J Addict* 1980; 15(6):839–848.
17. Brown BS, O'Grady KE, Farrell EV, et al. Factors associated with frequency of 12-step attendance by drug abuse clients. *Am J Drug Alcohol Abuse* 2001;27(1):147–160.
18. Leach B, Norris JL. Factors in the development of Alcoholics Anonymous (AA). In: Kissin B, Begleiter H, eds. *The biology of alcoholism: treatment and rehabilitation of the chronic alcoholic.* New York: Plenum Press, 1977;5:441–543.
19. Bailey MB, Leach B. *Alcoholics Anonymous: pathway to recovery: a study of 1058 members of the AA fellowship in New York City.* New York: National Council on Alcoholism, 1965.
20. Edwards G, Hensman C, Haukes A, et al. Alcoholics Anonymous: the anatomy of a self-help group. *Soc Psychiatry* 1967;1:195.
21. Eckhardt W. Alcoholic values and Alcoholics Anonymous. *Q J Stud Alcohol* 1967;28:277–288.
22. Yalom ID. *The theory and practice of group psychotherapy,* 2nd ed. New York: Basic Books, 1975.
23. Mack JE. Alcoholism, AA, the governance of the self. In: Bean MH, Zinberg NE, eds. *Dynamic approaches to the understanding and treatment of alcoholism.* New York: The Free Press, 1981, pp 128–162.
24. Khantzian EJ, Mack JE. Alcoholics Anonymous and contemporary psychodynamic theory. In: Galanter M, ed. *Recent developments in alcoholism.* New York: Plenum Press, 1989, pp 67–89.
25. Wurmser L. Psychoanalytic considerations of the etiology of compulsive drug use. *J Am Psychoanal Assoc* 1974;22: 820–843.
26. McClelland DC, Davis WN, Kelin R, et al. *The drinking man.* New York: The Free Press, 1972.
27. Kohut H. *The restoration of the self.* New York: International Universities Press, 1977.
28. Nace EP. *The treatment of alcoholism.* New York: Brunner/Mazel, 1987.
29. Brown S. *Treating, the alcoholic: a developmental model of recovery.* New York: John Wiley, 1985.
30. Tiebout HM. Surrender versus compliance in therapy. *Q J Stud Alcohol* 1953;14:58–68.
31. Kurtz E. *Shame and guilt: characteristics of the dependency cycle.* Center City, MN: Hazelden Foundation, 1981.
32. Kurtz E. *Alcoholics Anonymous and spirituality.* Workshop presented by Green Oaks Psychiatric Hospital, Dallas, TX, June 9, 1989.
33. Deikman AJ. *The observing self—mysticism and psychotherapy.* Boston: Beacon Press, 1982.
34. Emmonds RA. *The psychology of ultimate concerns: motivation and spirituality in personality.* New York: The Guilford Press, 1999.
35. Kastutas LA, Weisner, C, Lee M, et al. Alcoholics Anonymous affiliation at treatment intakes among white and black Americans. *J Stud Alcohol* 1999;60(6):810–816.
36. Rychtarik RG, Connors GJ, Dermen RH, Stasiewicz PR. Alcoholics Anonymous and the use of medications to prevent relapse; an anonymous survey of member attitudes. J Stud Alochol 2000 Jan;61(1):134–8.
37. Chappel JN. Teaching, learning recovery. Substance abuse. *AMERSA* 1995;16(3):141–153.

CHAPTER 37

Alternative Support Groups

ARTHUR T. HORVATH

This chapter overviews five support groups for addictive behavior. These groups are in many aspects fundamentally different from and hence alternatives to 12-step groups such as Alcoholics Anonymous (AA; which is discussed in Chapter 36). These groups, in order of longevity, are Women for Sobriety (WFS), Secular Organizations for Sobriety/Save Our Selves (SOS), Moderation Management (MM), SMART (Self-Management and Recovery Training) Recovery (SMART), and LifeRing Secular Recovery (LSR). They appear to comprise, as of 2004, the complete list of widely available secular addiction support groups. This chapter is oriented toward providing information that would help professionals and their patients identify whether alternatives in general, and which alternative in particular, might be helpful for a particular patient.

Rational Recovery (RR) is not covered. As of January 1, 2000, RR no longer offers support groups, because it now views support groups as a serious impediment to quitting an addiction (1). Also not covered are groups that have a religious orientation (e.g., Overcomers Outreach, Overcomers in Christ, the Calix Society), and Men for Sobriety (MFS), which as of the publication date offered only three meetings, all in Canada.

These alternatives are relatively young and unknown. AA began in 1935. The oldest of the alternatives, WFS, began in 1976. Despite the continued predominance of 12-step groups in the United States, the alternatives appear to be gaining recognition. Where available, they have become options for professionals and their patients to consider in treatment planning.

The history, program (including primary publications and intended membership), meeting format, and organizational aspects of each alternative is discussed. A review of the limited empirical findings is also presented. Contact information for each group is included at the end of the chapter.

These alternatives have significant similarities with 12-step groups. All are without substantial empirical support of effectiveness. All offer 60-to 90-minute meetings at no charge, but request donations. All are essentially self-supporting, primarily through member donations and the sale of recovery materials (including newsletters, books, workbooks, audio- and videotapes, and software, some of which may be produced by lay individuals or professionals not directly affiliated with the organization). All have an extensive Internet presence, including online meetings, listserves, message boards, or chat rooms. All (except MM) are abstinence-oriented. All (except SMART and LSR) were founded by one or two individuals who had a vision about recovery from addictive behavior. All are nonprofit corporations.

The programmatic and organizational differences between these alternatives and 12-step groups are substantial and numerous. None emphasize reliance on a "higher power" for recovery. On the other hand, none are opposed to religious or spiritual beliefs in their members. None offer formal sponsorship of new members by experienced members. All are supportive, both in principle and in practice, of appropriate professional treatment for addictive behavior. None expect members to attend for life, but rather to attend for as long as (or whenever) it is helpful. Typical attendance during the period of active involvement is one to three meetings per week, but there are few guidelines about frequency of attendance (versus AA's "90 meetings in 90 days"). All apparently appeal primarily to higher-functioning individuals (although this may be an artifact of the effort often required to locate these alternatives). All are accepting, both in principle and in practice, of individuals with neurotic (but not necessarily psychotic) comorbidity, and all encourage professional treatment of these conditions. All are flexible in the application of their program principles to the individual case. All are supportive of 12-step groups for individuals who benefit from them. All suggest that some individuals may be impeded in their recovery by 12-step groups, or benefit more from alternative groups, or both. All are

small (in comparison to AA's more than approximately 100,000 meetings worldwide). All operate on very limited budgets.

The differences with respect to meetings and meeting leaders are also substantial and numerous. All groups typically devote major portions of their meetings to discussion ("crosstalk"). None have speaker meetings (although their leaders may give separate public presentations). All have, or prefer to have, small meetings (approximately 6 to 12 members), to allow ample opportunity for individual participation. All have meeting formats, but tolerate (or even encourage) significant variation based on local custom or preference. None have extensive meeting rituals. All are led by a facilitator who guides the discussion. The facilitator is typically a peer, and a member of the group's recovery program (but a significant minority of facilitators in some alternatives are behavioral health professionals). Because of the responsibility involved in being a facilitator, all appear to experience difficulty finding facilitators. Because of the lack of a lifetime membership requirement, all experience difficulty retaining facilitators. All aspire to international availability, as qualified facilitators can be identified.

The five alternatives differ from one another primarily on their view of addiction as a disease. WFS takes a disease approach. SOS and LSR leave this issue up to the individual, but emphasize physiologic aspects of addiction more than psychological ones. Both MM and SMART view addictive behavior as a learned maladaptive behavior, not a disease.

Contact information is also provided for the American Self-Help Clearinghouse, which maintains a database of nationally available support groups, many of them for addictive behavior. Specialized support groups with a 12-step or similar orientation are available for various faiths, occupations, and addictive behaviors (2).

Several issues pertinent to alternative support groups can be identified but are not explored here. Serious ethical and legal issues may arise when an individual, for considered and responsible reasons, chooses to pursue an alternative approach to recovery, but a treatment provider or third party insists on 12-step-oriented treatment. A number of appeals court decisions have held that government-required 12-step attendance violates the establishment clause of the U.S. Constitution's First Amendment (3). The conditions that have allowed the alternatives to emerge may facilitate the emergence of others. The alternatives may increase the number of individuals involved in recovery, or they may draw their participants only from those who otherwise would have attended 12-step groups.

WOMEN FOR SOBRIETY

History

Women for Sobriety (WFS) was founded in 1976 by Jean Kirkpatrick, PhD, to address the unique problems of women alcoholics. She suggested that these problems include self-value, self-worth, guilt, and humiliation. Kirkpatrick's own experience was that AA was only partially helpful to her as a woman alcoholic.

Despite professional treatment and AA attendance, Kirkpatrick had a 30-year drinking history, including hospital and mental hospital admissions, hit-and-run accidents (during blackouts), and jail time. She had recurring episodes of depression and attempted suicide several times. She nevertheless managed to earn a doctorate in sociology from the University of Pennsylvania by age 50 years. She died in June 2000, at the age of 77 years.

Kirkpatrick's AA experience was one that she believes is typical for women. The recounting of the harm caused by drinking seemed to be good for men in AA and reminded them of their reasons not to relapse. For her, however, recounting painful and often humiliating past drinking experiences seemed to make even more difficult the task of accepting herself and gaining mastery of her life. Additionally, AA did not address how societal views of women (versus men) alcoholics posed additional challenges for recovering women.

Program

WFS has two primary publications (4,5). The WFS newsletter is *Sobering Thoughts*. WFS is intended for women alcoholics (including those who also have prescription medication problems). Kirkpatrick has suggested that for some women, AA may be more effective at achieving initial sobriety, because initially a woman may be overwhelmed by the complexity of the WFS program. After several months of abstinence, however, most women are believed to be ready to appreciate the idea that women need a different approach to recovery.

Kirkpatrick was ultimately able to stop drinking in her early fifties by relying on the philosophies of the Unity Church, Emerson, and Thoreau. Several years after achieving sobriety she formulated the principles of WFS, based in part on these philosophies. She also included in WFS cognitive–behavioral change techniques, and an emphasis on health promotion and peer support.

WFS views alcoholism as a physical disease that a woman can grow beyond by learning new self-enhancing behavior via:

1. Positive reinforcement (approval and encouragement),
2. Cognitive strategies (positive thinking),
3. Letting the body help (relaxation techniques, meditation, diet, and physical exercise), and
4. Dynamic group involvement (6).

Table 37.1 presents the WFS "New Life" Acceptance Program.

TABLE 37.1. *The WFS "New Life" acceptance program*

Level I: Accepting alcoholism as a physical disease.
 "I have a life-threatening (drinking) problem that once had me." (#1)
Level II: Discarding negative thoughts, putting guilt behind, and practicing new ways of viewing and solving problems.
 "Negative thoughts destroy only myself." (#2)
 "Problems bother me only to the degree I permit them to." (#4)
 "The past is gone forever." (#9)
Level III: Creating and practicing a new self-image.
 "I am what I think." (#5)
 "I am a competent woman and have much to give life." (#12)
Level IV: Using new attitudes to enforce new behavior patterns.
 "Happiness is a habit I will develop." (#3)
 "Life can be ordinary or it can be great." (#6)
 "Enthusiasm is my daily exercise." (#11)
Level V: Improving relationships as a result of our feelings about self.
 "Love can change the course of my world." (#7)
 "All love given returns." (#10)
Level VI: Recognizing life's priorities: emotional and spiritual growth, self-responsibility.
 "The fundamental object of life is emotional and spiritual growth." (#8)
 "I am responsible for myself and my actions." (#13)

From Kirkpatrick J. *WFS "new life" acceptance program* [brochure]. Quakertown, PA: Women for Sobriety, 1993, with permission. Copyright Jean Kirkpatrick, 1993.

Meeting Format

WFS meetings are lead by a Certified Moderator. Certification is based on having at least 1 year of continuous sobriety, reading *Turnabout* (4), subscribing to the WFS newsletter, and passing a written test about WFS principles and their application in meetings. WFS instituted certification to assure that moderators with a history of AA attendance understood the differences between WFS and AA principles and meeting formats.

Meetings are open to all women alcoholics. Newcomers are given a packet of introductory information. Meetings begin with a reading of the Statement of Purpose, followed by introductions ("Hello, my name is Jean, and I'm a competent woman"). Most of the meeting is devoted to discussion of member's concerns, and how the 13 Statements (see Table 37.1) can be applied to them. Following discussion each member is asked to describe something positive she has accomplished in the past week.

The meeting closes with the members standing, holding hands, and saying: "We are capable and competent, caring and compassionate, always willing to help another, bonded together in overcoming our addictions."

Organizational Aspects

As of 2004, WFS reports approximately 100 face-to-face meetings in the United States, and 50 meetings in other countries (primarily Canada, Australia, New Zealand, Ireland, and Finland), plus online meetings. The Board of Directors is composed of professional women who have recovered through WFS and who lead groups. In Australia and New Zealand, WFS receives some government funding.

Empirical Findings

Kaskutas (7–10) collected responses from 579 women who attended WFS only, or both WFS and AA. These responses support the suggestion that women may need a different approach to recovery. Women who attended only WFS reported that they did not feel that they fit in at AA, that AA was too negative, that they disliked the "drunk-alogues" and the focus on the past, and that AA is better suited to men's needs than to women's needs. Women attended WFS for support and nurturance, for a safe environment, for discussion about women's issues, and for the emphasis on positives and self-esteem. Attending WFS for 1 year was associated with an increase in self-esteem. For women who attended both WFS and AA, insurance against relapse and AA's availability were frequently cited reasons to attend AA. Respondents were primarily white, educated, middle aged, and middle or upper class. Most had also participated in individual psychotherapy.

SECULAR ORGANIZATIONS FOR SOBRIETY/SAVE OUR SELVES

History

Secular Organizations for Sobriety/Save Our Selves (SOS) was established in 1985 by Jim Christopher, in Hollywood, CA. Christopher had been sober since 1978, initially using AA. He separated from AA early in his recovery, because he wanted an approach that was based on personal responsibility rather than reliance on a higher power. In 1985, he wrote "Sobriety without Superstition" for *Free Inquiry,* a leading U.S. secular humanist journal. Because of the strong positive response to the article he founded SOS.

Program

SOS has two primary publications (11,12), and publishes the *SOS International Newsletter.* Originally intended for alcoholics, SOS has been extended to the full range of addictive behavior, both substance and activity addictions, and in some cases to family members as well. SOS is for individuals who desire recovery but are uncomfortable with the spiritual content of 12-step groups and would pre-

fer a personal responsibility approach. Specialized groups for family members, youth, or youth in dysfunctional families are also allowed. The only requirements of an SOS meeting are that it be secular and promote total abstinence.

SOS views the cycle of addiction as having three elements: physiologic need for the substance, the learned habit of using and all the associations to using, and the denial of both the need and the habit. Over time the addiction becomes the highest priority, and it begins to destroy the rest of life. However, the cycle of addiction can be replaced by the cycle of sobriety: acknowledgement of the addiction, acceptance of the disease or habit, and making sobriety highest priority in life (the "Sobriety Priority"). The Sobriety Priority is a cognitive strategy to be applied daily, to weaken associations to using, and to allow new associations to develop. SOS accepts that participants may use a wide variety of techniques or approaches in recovery. SOS emphasizes that it concerns itself only with helping participants accomplish the Sobriety Priority, and not with transforming the rest of life. With sobriety secured, participants are in a much better position to grow as individuals, but this remains a personal matter. Table 37.2 reproduces the Suggested Guidelines for Sobriety, and the General Principles of SOS.

Meeting Format

The suggested meeting format includes an opening statement summarizing the purpose of the meeting, announcements (e.g., the availability of new literature), anniversaries (of sobriety), the reading of the Guidelines for Sobriety, and introductions of all present. The meeting proper is next ("This meeting is now open. We ask that you try to keep your sharing to a reasonable length of time so that everyone can participate."). The closing includes passing the hat, and a ritual ("Let's close by giving ourselves a hand for being here to support and celebrate each other's sobriety.").

The members of each SOS group are allowed to create a meeting structure that meets their needs. Most SOS meetings have an active exchange of information, experiences, and ideas.

Organizational Aspects

As of 2004, the SOS International Clearinghouse reports that there are approximately 500 SOS meetings, and an additional 250 that are held in correctional facilities, plus online meetings. SOS maintains a database of approximately 20,000 individuals, 500 meetings in the United States and abroad, and over 250 prisoner inmate meetings. In addition to the United States, meetings are also available in 36 other countries countries. SOS is also allied with secular recovery groups in Italy and Poland. SOS is a subcommittee of the Council for

TABLE 37.2. *Suggested guidelines for sobriety, and general principles of SOS*

Suggested Guidelines for Sobriety
1. To break the cycle of denial and achieve sobriety, we first acknowledge that we are alcoholics or addicts.
2. We reaffirm this truth daily and accept without reservation the fact that, as clean and sober individuals, we can not and do not drink or use, no matter what.
3. Since drinking or using is not an option for us, we take whatever steps are necessary to continue our Sobriety Priority lifelong.
4. A quality of life—"the good life"—can be achieved. However, life is also filled with uncertainties. Therefore, we do not drink or use regardless of feelings, circumstances, or conflicts.
5. We share in confidence with each other our thoughts and feelings as sober, clean individuals.
6. Sobriety is our Priority, and we are each responsible for our lives and our sobriety.

General Principles of SOS
1. All those who sincerely seek sobriety are welcome as members in any SOS Group.
2. SOS is not a spin-off of any religious or secular group. There is no hidden agenda, as SOS is concerned with achieving and maintaining sobriety (abstinence).
3. SOS seeks only to promote sobriety amongst those who suffer from addictions. As a group, SOS has no opinion on outside matters and does not wish to become entangled in outside controversy.
4. Although sobriety is an individual responsibility, life does not have to be faced alone. The support of other alcoholics and addicts is a vital adjunct to recovery. In SOS, members share experiences, insights, information, strength, and encouragement in friendly, honest, anonymous, and supportive group meetings.
5. To avoid unnecessary entanglements, each SOS group is self-supporting through contributions from its members and refuses outside support.
6. Sobriety is the number one priority in a recovering person's life. As such, he or she must abstain from all drugs or alcohol.
7. Honest, clear, and direct communication of feelings, thoughts, and knowledge aids in recovery and in choosing nondestructive, nondelusional, and rational approaches to living sober and rewarding lives.
8. As knowledge of addiction might cause a person harm or embarrassment in the outside world, SOS guards the anonymity of its membership and the contents of its discussions from those not within the group.
9. SOS encourages the scientific study of addiction in all its aspects. SOS does not limit its outlook to one area of knowledge or theory of addiction.

Reprinted by permission, SOS International Clearinghouse.

Secular Humanism, a nonprofit corporation. Executive director Christopher autonomously administers the SOS International Clearinghouse. An International Advisory Board consists of a diverse group of community leaders, academics and professionals.

Empirical Findings

London et al. (13) found that SOS members were predominantly white, educated, and nontheistic. Most had negative experiences with AA. Conors and Dermen (14) found similar demographics, but less negative experience with AA. Both surveys found that SOS involvement was associated with sobriety.

MODERATION MANAGEMENT

History

Moderation Management (MM) was founded in 1993 by Audrey Kishline to support individuals who desire to moderate their alcohol consumption. Her own experience had been that it was difficult to obtain support for this goal.

During her twenties, Kishline's drinking increased to the level of a moderate problem. She eventually sought treatment. Ultimately, this treatment included two inpatient stays, an aftercare program, and consultation with at least 30 alcoholism treatment professionals, all of whom diagnosed her as "alcoholic." She also attended AA regularly for several years, attending hundreds of meetings. Her initial reaction to treatment was that her drinking became more severe. She suggested that at least in part this increase was a self-fulfilling prophecy based on what she had learned about alcoholism as a disease over which she was powerless. She also suggested that over several years she gradually matured out of her drinking problem, as she became more involved in the responsibilities and activities of life (e.g., marriage, children, homemaking, college courses, hobbies, and friends). As this maturing occurred, her beliefs about herself also evolved. Rather than believing herself to have a disease, she chose to abstain because of the kind of life she wanted to lead.

Several years prior to writing her 1994 book (15), Kishline chose to return to moderate drinking. She asserted that she was misdiagnosed initially, and that moderation of her alcohol consumption had been overlooked as an option for her. She founded MM in the hope that the moderation option would not be overlooked for others in similar situations.

Kishline had a drunk driving crash in spring 2000, in which she killed two passengers in an oncoming car (16). Moderation Management issued a statement regarding the significance of the event (17). A fact left out of many media reports was that at the time of the crash Kishline had stopped attending MM and had been attending AA for about 2 months. It would not appear to be reasonable to blame either AA or MM for her behavior.

Program

MM originally had one primary publication (15), and has now switched to another (18). MM also has a suggested reading list. MM is intended for individuals who fit the description "problem drinker" rather than "alcoholic." There are two fundamental requirements for membership: a willingness to accept responsibility for one's own behavior and a desire to moderate drinking. MM is not aimed at individuals who have experienced significant withdrawal symptoms from alcohol, who have medical conditions exacerbated by alcohol (e.g., heart disease, diabetes, gastrointestinal problems, etc.), or who are experiencing other relevant conditions including pregnancy or desired pregnancy, a behavioral health disorder, being on medications that interact negatively with alcohol, or being in personal crisis. Lastly, MM is not designed for individuals who are already abstaining successfully after a history of severe dependence.

MM also recommends that prospective members complete the Short Alcohol Dependence Data Questionnaire (SADD) (19), which is reproduced on the group's Web site. On this test scores from 1 to 9 suggest low dependence on alcohol, 10 to 19 medium dependence, and 20 or higher (maximum score 45) high dependence. Those who score below 16 are considered good candidates for MM. Those who score between 16 and 19 are encouraged to obtain professional assessment before attending a moderation program. Those who score 20 and above are encouraged to pursue abstinence. Even individuals with low scores are not discouraged from pursuing abstinence, but are offered the alternative of MM.

MM hopes to reach problem drinkers early in their problem drinking career by offering an approach that appeals to common sense and does not require excessive effort (relative to the intensity of the problem). MM is therefore partly a prevention program. If an individual is not successful following MM's moderation guidelines, the individual is encouraged to pursue abstinence.

MM views drinking problems as arising from bad habits, rather than being the manifestations of a disease. MM is based on empirically supported cognitive-behavioral moderation training (18). Table 37.3 reprints the Nine Steps of MM. MM suggests that 6 to 18 months of once-weekly attendance is usually needed for successful completion of its program.

MM understands moderate drinking to be (for men) no more than 4 standard drinks per day, no more than 4 drinking days per week, and no more than 14 standard drinks per week. A standard drink is the amount of alcohol in a 12-ounce bottle of beer, a 5-ounce glass of wine, or a 1.5-ounce shot of liquor, all of which, because of differing concentrations, have approximately equal amounts of pure alcohol. For women, moderate drinking is understood to be no more than 3 standard drinks per day, no more than 4 drinking days per week, and no more than 9 standard drinks per week. Both sexes are encouraged not to drink

TABLE 37.3. *The nine steps of moderation management*

1. Attend meetings and learn about the program of Moderation Management.
2. Abstain from alcoholic beverages for 30 days and complete steps three through six at this time.
3. Examine how drinking has affected your life.
4. Write down your priorities.
5. Take a look at how much, how often, and under what circumstances you used to drink.
6. Learn the MM guidelines and limits for moderate drinking.
7. Set moderate drinking limits and start weekly "small steps" toward positive lifestyle changes.
8. Review your progress at meetings and update your goals.
9. After achieving your goal of moderation, attend MM meetings any time you feel the need for support, or would like to help newcomers.

From Kishline A. *Moderate drinking: the Moderation Management Guide for people who want to reduce their drinking.* New York: Crown, 1995, with permission. Copyright Audrey Kishline, 1994.

and drive, or to drink in situations where the drinker or others might be endangered.

Meeting Format

Meetings are led by a moderator, and begin with the reading of an opening statement describing the purpose of MM, followed by a reading of the Nine Steps (see Table 37.3) and ground rules for members. Visitors (the meetings are open) and newcomers are invited to introduce themselves. Anyone who recently completed the recommended initial 30 days of abstinence is acknowledged.

The first working section of the meeting is devoted to giving every member the opportunity to update the group on the member's activities since the member's last meeting. Feedback by others may be offered. The next working section is general discussion. If no one has a topic to discuss, the moderator suggests one, which would typically be one of the ideas or techniques covered in the MM book. The meeting ends with the reading of a closing statement.

Organizational Aspects

As of 2004, the MM web site reports 15 meetings in 11 states, and a comparable number of online meetings. The board of directors is composed primarily of addictive behavior professionals and writers. MM seeks inquiries from behavioral health professionals, who are welcome to function as meeting moderators.

Empirical Findings

Humphreys and Klaw (20) found that MM attracts women and younger adults, most of whom were nondependent drinkers. However a significant minority of respondents had multiple alcohol-dependence symptoms. Klaw and Humphreys (21) also analyzed life story themes of MM members, most of whom were white, educated, and middle class. The themes were more consistent with MM's emphasis on self-control and choice than with a powerlessness approach.

SMART RECOVERY

History

SMART (Self-Management and Recovery Training) incorporated as a nonprofit organization in 1992 under the name Rational Recovery Self-Help Network. The organization entered into an agreement with Jack Trimpey, the founder and owner of Rational Recovery Systems, to use the name Rational Recovery and to operate Rational Recovery support groups. The board of directors, of which Trimpey was a member, had evolved from an informal group of advisors, mostly mental health professionals, that Trimpey had assembled for an initial meeting in 1991. Trimpey took the leading role in establishing and incorporating the organization.

Beginning about 1993 there was increasing disagreement between Trimpey and the organization about how the organization would be managed, and the nature of its program. These developments culminated in 1994 with the mutual agreement between Trimpey and the organization to separate. This separation was accomplished by changing the organization's name. The separation and related issues have been described in a series of articles (22–26). Individual support groups made their own decisions about which affiliation to maintain. As of 2000, Rational Recovery groups have ceased altogether.

Program

SMART has two primary publications (27,28) and a recommended reading list. The SMART newsletter is *SMART Recovery: News and View*. There is a specialized application for SMART in correctional facilities, the InsideOut program (29), which was developed on a grant from the National Institute on Drug Abuse. The InsideOut program includes a facilitator manual and videotape, participant workbook, and male and female participant videotapes. SMART is intended for individuals who desire to abstain from any addictive behavior (substance or activity), or who are considering abstinence. SMART assumes that there are degrees of addictive behavior, and that all individuals to some degree experience it. Individuals for whom the negative consequences of addictive behavior have become considerable are the ones likely to be considering or desiring abstinence.

The SMART program is consistent with a cognitive–behavioral perspective, and views addictive behavior as a complex maladaptive behavior. Table 37.4 reprints the SMART Purposes and Methods statement.

TABLE 37.4. *S.M.A.R.T recovery purposes and methods*

1. We help individuals gain independence from addictive behavior.
2. We teach how to
   Enhance and maintain motivation to abstain
   Cope with urges
   Manage thoughts, feelings and behavior
   Balance momentary and enduring satisfactions
3. Our efforts are based on scientific knowledge, and evolve as scientific knowledge evolves.
4. Individuals who have gained independence from addictive behavior are invited to stay involved with us, to enhance their gains and help others.

From S.M.A.R.T Recovery. S.M.A.R.T Recovery purposes and methods [brochure]. Beachwood, OH with permission. Copyright S.M.A.R.T Recovery, 1996.

There are four primary goals for an individual in the SMART program: motivational maintenance and enhancement, effective urge coping, rational thinking (leading to effective emotional and behavioral management), and lifestyle balance. In service of these goals, many cognitive–behavioral and other psychological techniques are taught. With respect to changing addictive behavior itself, the program draws from established references of the cognitive–behavioral approach (e.g., reference 30). Self-help literature on addictive behavior (e.g., references 31 to 34), as well as cognitive–behavioral self-help literature on a broad range of topics, including mood management, assertiveness training, relationships, effective communication, and stress management, is also recommended (35), and techniques derived from this literature are incorporated into the SMART program. Consistent with SMART's previous affiliation with Rational Recovery, as well as its cognitive–behavioral orientation, REBT techniques and terms (36,37) are a prominent aspect of the SMART program.

SMART does not employ "steps," or have a suggested sequence for change. It is assumed that each of the four primary goals will be important for most members, but the relative importance at different times, and the degree to which applicable ideas and techniques will need to be employed, is left to the individual. SMART suggests that there are as many routes to gaining independence from addictive behavior as there are individuals.

Although SMART limits its discussions to how to achieve abstinence, individuals unsure about adopting this goal are also encouraged to attend. SMART has a broad definition of abstinence, in part because individuals with any addictive behavior are invited to attend (e.g., abstinence from over involvement with food or sex, versus abstinence from all involvement, would be acceptable). SMART also encourages individuals unwilling to make a lifetime commitment to abstinence to consider a trial of abstinence.

Meeting Format

Meetings are open unless closed by local custom. Meetings begin with an opening statement by the Coordinator. The statement describes the four primary goals of the SMART program, and outlines the meeting to follow. Members check in and establish an agenda for who will be the primary focuses of the discussion. The major portion of the meeting follows, consisting of discussion guided by the Coordinator on the four primary goals of the SMART program, as they apply to the individual situations discussed. One of the principal approaches is to consider "activating events" volunteered by the members. Activating events can include urges, life circumstance changes, thoughts, social interactions, or other experiences that lead or potentially lead to undesired emotions or behavior, including addictive behavior. Activating events are typically analyzed using Ellis' ABCDE method (36,37). The Disputation step, in which irrational ideas are disputed, can draw upon the entire range of scientific knowledge about addictive behavior. The formal meeting concludes with a check out, possibly to include each member proposing a personal homework project, which would put into action the ideas or techniques from the meeting that have been significant for the member.

Organizational Aspects

As of 2004, SMART reports more than 250 face-to-face meetings, plus online meetings. The meetings are in most states and a few (mostly European) countries. More than 80 meetings are in correctional facilities. There are two part-time paid staff. The board of directors is composed primarily of addictive behavior professionals. An international advisory council is composed of leaders in the fields of addictive behavior treatment and research. SMART meeting Coordinators have the opportunity to consult with a Professional Advisor, who typically is a behavioral health professional. Depending on local circumstances and traditions, either the Professional Advisor or the Coordinator handles administrative matters at the local level. Often a Professional Advisor consults with more than one Coordinator. SMART seeks inquiries from behavioral health professionals who may be interested in serving as Professional Advisors.

Empirical Findings

Two studies (38,39) found that participants in SMART Recovery have a significantly higher level of internal locus of control than do AA members. Penn (40) found comparable outcomes for participants in a 12-step or SMART-oriented day-treatment program for the addicted mentally ill. Studies of Rational Recovery have some relevance and are reviewed in the previous edition (41).

LIFERING SECULAR RECOVERY

History

LifeRing Secular Recovery (LSR) began as the Northern California set of SOS meetings. In 1999, the final ruling of a federal lawsuit prohibited SOS from using that name in Northern California. Representatives of the Northern California meetings, meeting on May 23, 1999, adopted the name LifeRing Secular Recovery. During 2000, LSR emerged as an organization independent of SOS. A constitutional congress ratified bylaws on February 17, 2001. Some former SOS meetings from outside of Northern California are now affiliated with LSR.

Program

LSR has one primary publication (42) and additional suggested publications and a newsletter in development. The LSR program appears to be similar to the SOS program. After SMART and Rational Recovery separated, their programs became substantially different. It remains to be seen whether this also happens for LSR and SOS. LSR describes its fundamental principles as the "Three-S" Philosophy: Sobriety, Secularity, and Self-Help.

Meeting Format

The meeting format is also similar to SOS. Table 37.5 reprints the suggested Opening Statement for meetings. Meeting leaders are termed Conveners.

Organizational Aspects

As of 2004, LSR reports approximately 75 face-to-face meetings in 20 states and Canada, plus online meetings and about 12 listserves. LSR appears to be the most democratically operated alternative support group. Although LSR and SOS are programmatically similar, they are organizationally dissimilar. While LSR's central organization is more highly structured, SOS meetings operate with a greater degree of autonomy from the national organization provided they preserve the SOS doctrines of secularity and abstinence. It is conceivable that over time the differences in organizational environment will have an impact on LSR's program. Each active LSR meeting selects a delegate to the annual congress, which in turn elects a seven-member board of directors. Directors are required to be in recovery and have 2 years of sobriety. They are deemed to have resigned if they relapse.

Empirical Findings

There are no empirical studies of LSR.

TABLE 37.5. *LSR opening statement for meetings*

This is a regular open meeting of LifeRing Secular Recovery (LSR). LifeRing Secular Recovery is a self-help support group for all people who want to get and stay clean and sober. We feel that in order to remain in recovery, we have to make sobriety the top priority in our lives. By sobriety, we mean complete abstinence from alcohol and other addictive drugs. Out of respect for people of all faiths and none, we conduct our meetings in a secular way. We rely in our recovery work on our own efforts and on the help of our support systems. Everything that we share at this meeting is completely confidential. If you are under the influence of alcohol or drugs now, we ask that you maintain silence at this meeting. You may speak with members afterward. The meeting format is flexible. We generally begin by checking in and talking about our past week and our coming week in recovery. Please respect the right of others to speak by limiting your speaking time if necessary. If this is your first time at this meeting, you are welcome. Please introduce yourself by your first name and state your reason for coming. Thank you.

Reprinted by permission of LifeRing Secular Recovery.

CHOOSING AN ALTERNATIVE SUPPORT GROUP

If an individual has no experience with addictive behavior support groups, sampling all that are available would seem most sensible. If an individual has no strong preferences, 12-step groups would seem more desirable than the alternatives simply because of their availability and size (which increase the likelihood that suitable models of success would be identified). If alternatives are preferred, and more than one is reasonably proximate and not inappropriate for one's gender (WFS) or goal (MM), on what basis might one be selected over another? Although the information provided here may be helpful, probably the best test of compatibility is the individual's reaction to each available meeting. Because the quality of these meetings is quite dependent on the style and ability of the facilitator, it seems likely that the group environment the facilitator engenders may be a larger factor in the desirability of an individual meeting than the organization's official program or meeting format. Consequently, where more than one alternative is available, it should not be unexpected that an individual might attend selected meetings of each. Just as there is presumably a high degree of variability in the helpfulness of 12-step sponsors, there is presumably a high degree of variability in the helpfulness of the individual meetings of alternative support groups.

Excellent advice has been offered on how to integrate mental health treatment with 12-step attendance (43). This advice is needed because of the apparent contradictions between these two perspectives. There appear to be far fewer of such contradictions for the individual attending an alternative. On the other hand, contradictions are likely to arise if the individual attending an alternative is also attending 12-step-oriented addictive behavior treatment.

If no suitable group is available, an option for the motivated individual, depending on the desired affiliation, would be to start one's own group. Given that teaching a subject is often the best way to learn it, this option has much to recommend it. The objection that those in early recovery should be guided by those in long-term recovery overlooks the fact that recoveries without this guidance occur routinely (44). If attending or starting a group is not an option, the literature of one or more of these alternatives may by itself be helpful. All the alternatives have extensive Internet services, which may be of benefit to those who can access them. When there are not enough weekly meetings in a given locality to provide the level of support an individual desires, the literature and clinical experience suggest that some individuals may benefit from also attending 12-step groups (despite the programmatic contradictions).

Further research may provide guidance regarding matching individuals to addictive behavior support groups. However, the ultimate justification of a support group could not be established by an efficacy study. Millions have attended 12-step groups although there is little solid evidence of their efficacy. Support groups exist because recovering individuals choose to attend them.

A fundamental question regarding alternative support groups will likely be pertinent for some years. Will enough individuals attend them so that one or more come to exist as equal members of the recovery community, and not merely as "alternatives?"

CONTACT INFORMATION

Women for Sobriety (WFS)
  PO Box 618
  Quakertown, PA 18951–0618
  215-536-8026 (voice)
  215-538-9026 (fax)
  NewLife@nni.com
  www.womenforsobriety.org
Secular Organizations for Sobriety/Save Our Selves (SOS)
  4773 Hollywood Blvd
  Hollywood, CA 90027
  323-666-4295 (voice)
  323-666-4271 (fax)
  sos@cfiwest.org
  www.sossobriety.org
Moderation Management (MM)
  c/o HRC
  22 W 27th Street
  New York, NY 10001
  212-871-0974 (voice)

212-213-6582 (fax)
mm@moderation.org
www.moderation.org
SMART Recovery (SMART)
  7537 Mentor Avenue, Suite 306
  Mentor, Ohio 44060
  440-951-5357 (voice)
  440-951-5358 (fax)
  SRMai11@aol.com
  www.smartrecovery.org
LifeRing Secular Recovery (LSR)
LifeRing Service Center
  1440 Broadway, Suite 312
  Oakland, CA 94612-2029
  510-763-0779 (voice)
  510-763-1513 (fax)
  service@lifering.org
  www.unhooked.com

American Self-Help Clearinghouse
  St. Clare's Health System
  100 East Hanover Avenue, Suite 202
  Cedar Knolls, NJ 07927-2020
  Group Information: 973-326-6789 (from out of state)
  800-367-6274 (from within New Jersey)
  973-326-9467 (fax)

ACKNOWLEDGMENTS

The author gratefully acknowledges the assistance of Jim Christopher, Martin Nicolaus, Lois Trimpey, Jodi Dayton, and Becky Fenner. Assistance with the previous edition came from Jean Kirkpatrick, Beatrice (Cookie) Scott, Lois Trimpey, Audrey Kishline, Philip Tate, Michler Bishop, Rob Sarmiento, Randy Cicen, Jim Christopher, Vince Fox, Barbara McCrady, and Kris Figueroa. Nevertheless, all opinions and any errors are attributable solely to the author.

REFERENCES

1. www.rational.org. Last accessed April 10, 2004.
2. American Self-Help Clearinghouse. *The self-help source book,* 7th ed. Cedar Knolls, NJ: Author, 2002.
3. Apanovitch DP. Religion and rehabilitation: the requisition of God by the state. Available at: www.law.duke.edu/shell/cite.pl?47+Duke+L.+J.+785. Last accessed April 10, 2004.
4. Kirkpatrick J. *Turnabout. New help for the woman alcoholic.* New York: Bantam Books, 1990.
5. Kirkpatrick J. *Goodbye hangovers, hello life: self-help for women.* New York: Ballantine Books, 1986.
6. Women for Sobriety. *Women and addictions: a way to recovery* [brochure]. Quakertown, PA: Author, undated.
7. Kaskutas LA. What do women get out of self-help? Their reasons for attending Women for Sobriety and Alcoholics Anonymous. *J Subst Abuse Treat* 1994;11:185–195.
8. Kaskutas LA. Predictors of self esteem among members of Women for Sobriety. *Addict Res* 1996;4(3):273–281.
9. Kaskutas LA. Pathways to self-help among Women for Sobriety. *Am J Drug Alcohol Abuse* 1996;22(2):259–280.
10. Kaskutas LA. A road less traveled: choosing the "Women for Sobriety" program. *J Drug Issues* 1996;26(1):77–94.
11. Christopher J. *How to stay sober. Recovery without religion.* Buffalo, NY: Prometheus Books, 1988.
12. Christopher J. *Unhooked. Staying sober and drug free.* Buffalo, NY: Pometheus Books, 1989.
13. London WM, Courchaine KE, Yoho DL. Recovery experiences of SOS members. Preliminary findings. In: Christopher J, ed. *SOS sobriety: the proven alternative to 12-step programs.* Buffalo, NY: Prometheus Books, 1992:45–59.
14. Conors G, Derman K. Characteristics of participants in Secular Organizations for Sobriety (SOS). *Am J Drug Alcohol Abuse* 1996;22(2):281–295.
15. Kishline A. *Moderate drinking: the Moderation Management Guide for people who want to reduce their drinking.* New York: Crown, 1996.
16. www.moderation.org/media.html. Last accessed April 10, 2004.
17. The tragedy of Audrey Kishline and the future of moderation management. Available at www.moderation.org/Mmboard.htm. Last accessed April 10, 2004.
18. Rotgers F, Kern MF, Hoeltzel R. *Responsible drinking: a Moderation Management approach for problem drinkers.* Oakland, CA: New Harbinger, 2002.
19. Raistrick D, Dunbar G, Davidson R. Development of a questionnaire to measure alcohol dependence. *Br J Addict* 1983;78:89–95.
20. Humphreys K, Klaw E. Can targeting nondependent problem drinkers and providing Internet-based services expand access to assistance for alcohol problems? A study of the Moderation Management self-help/mutual aid organization. *J Stud Alcohol* 2001;62(4):528–532.
21. Klaw E, Humphreys K. Life stories of Moderation Management mutual help group members. *Contemp Drug Probl* 2000;27(4):779–803.
22. Trimpey J. Rational Recovery update. *Addict Newslett* [Newsletter of the American Psychological Association Division on Addictions] 1995;2:4, 14–15.
23. Bishop FM, Tate P, Horvath AT, et al. SMART Recovery/Rational Recovery update. *Addict Newslett* [Newsletter of the American Psychological Association Division on Addictions] 1995;2:4, 12–13.
24. McCrady BS. Don Cahalan was right–the alcohol field does act like a "Ship of Fools": commentaries on "SMART Recovery/Rational Recovery update" and "Rational Recovery update." *Addict Newslett* [Newsletter of the American Psychological Association Division on Addictions] 1995;2:5, 16–17.
25. Trimpey J. Ship of fools or riverboat casino? Response to Barbara McCrady. *Addict Newslett* [Newsletter of the American Psychological Association Division of Addictions] 1995;3:6, 23–24.
26. Bishop M. SMART Recovery. Response to Barbara McCrady. *Addict Newslett* [Newsletter of the American Psychological Association Division of Addictions] 1995;3:7–8.
27. SMART Recovery. *Member's manual.* Mentor, OH: Author, 1996.
28. SMART Recovery. *Coordinator's manual.* Mentor, OH: Author, 1996.
29. Inflexxion. *InsideOut: A SMART Recovery correctional program.* Newton, MA: Author, 2002.
30. Hester RK, Miller WR, eds. *Handbook of alcoholism treatment approaches: effective alternatives.* Boston: Allyn & Bacon, 2002.
31. Trimpey J. *The small book.* New York: Delacorte Press, 1992
32. Ellis A, Velten E. *When AA doesn't work for you: rational steps to quitting alcohol.* Fort Lee, NJ: Barricade, 1992.
33. Prochaska JO, Norcross JC, DiClemente CC. *Changing for good: the revolutionary program that explains the six stages*

of change and teaches you how to free yourself from bad habits. New York: William Morrow, 1994.

34. Horvath AT. *Sex, drugs, gambling and chocolate: a workbook for overcoming addictions.* San Luis Obispo, CA: Impact, 1999.

35. Norcross JC, Santrock JW, Campbell LF, et al. *Authoritative guide to self-help resources in mental health.* New York: Guilford Press, 2000.

36. Ellis A, Harper RA. *A new guide to rational living.* Englewood Cliffs, NJ: Prentice-Hall, 1975.

37. Ellis A, McInerney JF, DiGiuseppe R, et al. *Rational-emotive therapy with alcoholics and substance abusers.* Elmsford, NY: Pergamon Press, 1989.

38. Li EC, Feifer C, Strohm M. A pilot study: locus of control and spiritual beliefs in Alcoholics Anonymous and SMART Recovery. *Addict Behav* 2000;25(4):633–640.

39. Bogdonoff DA. *Resilience as a predictor of abstinence in the recovery from alcohol dependence.* San Diego: California School of Professional Psychology at Alliant University; 2002:160

40. Penn PE, Brooks AJ. Five years, Twelve Steps, and REBT in the treatment of dual diagnosis. *J Rational-Emotive Cognitive-Behavior Ther* 2000;18 (4):197–208.

41. Horvath AT. Alternative support groups. In: Lowinson JH, Ruiz P, Millman RB, et al., eds. *Substance abuse: a com-*prehensive textbook, 3rd ed. Baltimore: Williams & Wilkins, 1997:390–396.

42. Nicolaus M. *Recovery by choice: living and enjoying life free of alcohol and drugs.* Oakland, CA: LifeRing, 2001.

43. McCrady B, Horvath AT, Delaney SI. Self-help groups. In: Hester RK, Miller WR, eds. *Handbook of alcoholism treatment approaches: effective alternatives,* 3rd ed. Boston: Allyn & Bacon, 2002:165–187.

44. Sobell LC, Cunningham JA, Sobell MB. Recovery from alcohol problems with and without treatment: prevalence in two population surveys. *Am J Public Health* 1996;86:966–972.

CHAPTER 38

The Therapeutic Community

WILLIAM B. O'BRIEN
AND FERNANDO B. PERFAS

In the changing global landscape of drug abuse and varied socioeconomic conditions in different parts of the world, the Therapeutic Community (TC) provides an effective response to the scourge of drug abuse. The amphetamine epidemic in Asia has forced both governmental and nongovernmental drug programs to innovate, often using the TC approach as a treatment platform for both residential and outpatient programs. To the swollen prisons of developing countries in the world, where drug offenders of various ages comprise more than half of the prison population, the prison TC is making its most important contributions. While providing not only an effective rehabilitative approach, it serves to humanize the treatment of inmates as well.

The TC, which traces its origin to the late 1950s as a homespun approach to the problem of heroin addiction in the United States, has now grown into a worldwide movement under the banner of the World Federation of Therapeutic Communities (WFTC) (1). It has affiliates in six regional federations in North America, Latin America, Europe, Central and Eastern Europe, Asia, and Australasia. The TC treatment philosophy with its approach to the problem of addiction has taken its roots in diverse cultural and socioeconomic settings, spawning a global network of TCs uniquely adapted to local conditions.

The TC, as a treatment framework, has such wide appeal because it draws from universally practiced social and spiritual values that form part of its community standards and behavior norms. In fact, many of the TC approaches to behavior and psychological change not only result in improvements in psychosocial functioning of the ex-addict, but also promote a prosocial lifestyle. Furthermore, the treatment experience in the TC often results to an increase in self-awareness and a sense of responsibility for oneself and for the welfare of others. Its vigorous method of shaping attitudes and behaviors, as important determinants of sobriety and a safe lifestyle, offers a meaningful approach for influencing both high-risk and drug-using behaviors (2).

As a treatment philosophy that emphasizes the empowerment of the person, the importance of positive social or community support, and the value of teamwork, the TC has been successfully used as a model to organize a community-based drug treatment program. Daytop's contribution to a United Nations International Drug Control Program (UNDCP)-sponsored community-based project in Vietnam is a testimony to the versatility of the TC treatment methods (3,4).

To determine how responsive the TC is to the needs of its clientele and to assess its efficacy in treating clients with various needs and backgrounds, new research has focused on developing tools to measure the treatment processes of the TC (5). Various outcome studies have been conducted to investigate the efficacy of the TC for funding purposes and accountability (6). For program developers and clinicians who are seeking to improve the delivery of services and to identify factors that contribute to successful outcome, studies that look into therapeutic processes are equally important. Research on best treatment practices (7) was conducted to identify treatment aspects that contribute to program effectiveness.

THE WORLDWIDE GROWTH OF THE TC

Most of Europe traces the development of the present-day European TCs to two major influences. First is the democratic TC that evolved from the innovations in social psychiatry for the treatment of mentally ill patients. Second is the influx of ideas that originated from the concept-based TC pioneered by Synanon in California to treat narcotic addicts (1,8). The politics of social and health service delivery in Western Europe exerted tremendous influences on how the concept-based TC was adapted in an environment that is historically tolerant to drug maintenance. The medical profession played an important role in dispensing or regulating drug maintenance. Traditionally, Western Europe is more inclined to the more liberal democratic TC in contrast with the hierarchical model of the largely American concept-based TC (1). While the European TC developed along these two lines of kindred, but distinct, treatment philosophies, the Asian, and to a similar extent the Latin American TCs, adopted the concept-based TC as practiced currently in Daytop and in most of North America. The first TC in Asia, established in 1971 by DARE Foundation of the Philippines, was patterned after the Daytop model. The same TC model was later transported to Malaysia in 1974, and to Thailand in 1979. These initial isolated outgrowths of the TC led to the establishments of TCs in Singapore, Indonesia, Vietnam, China, Hong Kong, Pakistan, India, Sri Lanka, Nepal, the Maldives, and, recently, South Korea. Today, most, if not all, of the Asian TC programs in private or community-based treatment settings, prisons, juvenile detention homes, and parole and probation programs are established along the traditional concept-based TC that was pioneered by Synanon and later adopted by the second-generation TCs such as Daytop Village and Phoenix House.

Similar developments of the TC occurred in several countries in Latin America. Countries such as Colombia and Argentina received training assistance in the past from the Italian TC program, *Centro Italiano di Solidarieta* (CEIS) (1) but had also engaged actively in developing their TCs along the Daytop model. The CEIS TC program had been largely influenced in the beginning by Daytop, which provided staff trainers to develop the Italian TC in the 1980s. In recent years, Daytop, through grants from the Bureau for International Narcotics and Law Enforcement Affairs (INL) of the U.S. Department of State, has been able to assist in developing the TC as part of the drug demand reduction programs in Peru, Ecuador, Brazil, Argentina, and in most parts of Asia, as well as in some parts of Eastern Europe.

THE TC IN PRISONS

The cycle of drug use and crime has resulted in a worldwide trend of overpopulation in prisons. The overrepresentation of substance abusers among prisoners and parolees prompted the California legislature to appropriate $94 million since 1995 for the expansion of TC prison-based substance-abuse programs (9). Of the total inmates in California's 33 prisons, 28% were incarcerated for drug-related offenses and another 21% were incarcerated for property offenses, which are generally related to drug use (10). In 1999, the California Department of Corrections (CDC) (11) reported that 67% of the individuals entering the state's prison system were parole violators, with 55.5% of them charged with drug-related offenses. The rest of the major U.S. state prisons follow a similar trend in their prisoners' profile.

In England and Wales, there has been a significant rise in recent years in the proportion of offenders in the criminal justice system who are drug abusers, while treatment services offered to them have been inadequate (12). It was found that 11% of male and 23% of female prisoners were drug dependent prior to their incarceration in 1989. In a frank look into incidents of drug misuse in English prisons, the prison service, in 1995, acknowledged pronounced drug misuse in prisons and drafted the strategy document, "Drug Misuse in Prison" (13). This document provided the framework for reducing the supply of drugs in prison and in reducing drug demand by establishing several pilot, prison-based TCs in 19 prisons in England and Wales (12).

In the last 5 years, there have been bold efforts to bring the TC to the prisons in Peru and Ecuador, and to the facilities for juvenile offenders in Brazil. Some of these efforts were truly heroic given the substandard prison conditions and the absence of resources available for any meaningful drug treatment for drug-addicted prisoners in these countries. In Ecuador, a prison psychiatrist and his assistant psychologist were so moved after completing a TC training that they struck a deal with the prison authorities in the city of Quito to take over a psychiatric unit. They negotiated that they be allowed to start a prison TC pilot program for drug offenders while at the same time providing psychiatric services for mentally ill prisoners (14).

It is, however, in Asian prisons that the proliferation of the TC outside of the United States is happening dramatically.

DRUG ABUSE AND THE PRISON SITUATION IN ASIA

In Asia, the incidence of drug-related offenses among convicted prisoners is no different and perhaps, even worse. The Thai Department of Corrections (15) reports that there are 137 prisons and correctional institutions across the country with an approximate capacity of 90,000 inmates. As of December 2001, the total Thai prison population was 249,363, almost three times actual capacity. The drug offenders comprise a staggering 63.24% of the total prison population (15). The overcrowding of prisons was the direct result of the imposition of severe penalties for drug offenses in response to the raging amphetamine epidemic in Thailand and the rest of Asia as well as the increase in crimes spawned by drug abuse.

The picture of the drug and prison situation in the Philippines is similar. Overcrowding is the norm in all the national prisons and jails operated by the Bureau of

Corrections (BUCOR) and the Bureau of Jail Management and Penology (BJMP) (16,17). In the medium security prison of the National Penitentiary in Manila, 37.67% of inmates were convicted of drug-related offenses, and 38.12% of 648 inmates who had undergone diagnostics and assessment were found to have a history of drug abuse (16). It is estimated that between 50% and 60% of all inmates in provincial, municipal, or city jails are facing drug-related charges (17).

Malaysia with 17 million people had 127,000 registered heroin addicts in 1991 and possibly 250,000 by 1998. In 2000, one estimate puts the number of drug addicts to be 300,000, which does not account for the young people who are abusing amphetamine-type substances. These figures translate into a mushrooming in the number of inmates convicted for drug related-offenses, a fact observed in the statistics of drug offenders referred to the government-operated drug rehabilitation centers or boot camps (18).

The use of illegal drugs and crime go hand in hand. In far too many cases in Bangladesh, drug users will literally do anything to obtain drugs. During the last few years, because of an increase incidence of drug abuse, there has been a significant rise in crime rate (19). In Peshawar (20), located in northwestern frontier of Pakistan, where drug incidence is alarmingly critical, records show that 44% of prison inmates are charged with drug-related offenses.

Against this backdrop, the prison-based TC, applying the U.S. concept-based model, offered a much-needed treatment technology to stem the rising tide of drug abuse among prison inmates in Asia. What began in the prisons of Thailand and Malaysia in 1992 is now unfolding in the Philippines (21) and Singapore (22), with TCs operating to serve criminal justice clients both in prisons and in the community. The successful adaptation of the TC for criminal justice clients in the aforementioned countries have prompted prison agencies in Indonesia, Sri Lanka, Nepal, the Maldives, Bangladesh, and Pakistan to express their interest in developing their own prison-based TCs.

IMPLEMENTATION AND OPERATIONAL ISSUES IN PRISON-BASED TC

The implementation and development of the prison-based TC are often both exciting and frustrating to the TC professionals: exciting because it presents a radical opportunity to use the TC in a different setting that is full of new challenges; frustrating because the world of "corrections" with its massive institutions and traditional doctrines clash with the optimistic and humanistic culture of the TC. One is steeped in a largely retributive philosophy with heavy emphasis on security and total control of its inmates. The other is focused on providing treatment for its "residents" and the provision of services that allow the processes of change to take place. Two contrasting cultures require reconciliation of their differences in order to work toward a common goal, yet not willing to give up an inch of what they hold as their primary functions. These realities expe-

rienced by the pioneers of the prison-based TC initiatives in the United States are the very same hurdles and challenges encountered by the innovators of the TC within the prison systems of Asia. Adaptive changes have since been made by both the prison authorities and the treatment staff to establish viable TCs within the prison system. The constraints that the prison system and its special population of prisoners impose on the TC implementers might look daunting but it should not deter anyone willing to try (13).

The experiences and observations of prison-based TCs, such as Project REFORM in New York, were instructive as they declared that (a) prison-based treatment efforts were most likely to be effective when carried out jointly between correctional and treatment staff (TC trained staff), (b) the primary focus of these programs must be the reduction of criminal recidivism, (c) successful in-prison TCs must include a seamless continuum of care for graduates paroled in the community, and (d) evaluation outcomes must include objective measures such as urine monitoring, infractions, and official arrest records (23).

The following are common systemic and treatment issues encountered in prison-based TCs (9,24):

1. Collaboration and communication between the prison administration and prison-treatment personnel are often hampered by the contrasting ideologies of the correctional and treatment system. While the treatment system views drug abuse as a chronic treatable disorder, the correctional system views drug abuse as a crime while the prescription for controlling it is through punishment and incarceration. The former sees its primary function as the provider of treatment to reduce drug abuse and improve the physical and mental health of the person; whereas, the latter focuses on the crime that is committed and the sanctions to punish the offender and prevent him from committing further criminal activity.

2. Departments of corrections, by and large, are bureaucratic organizations that require strict adherence to the policy and procedure manual as standard operating procedure for its personnel. This fact, coupled with the underlying philosophies and objectives of the correctional system supports and reinforces a firmly established culture that puts emphasis on safety, security, and strict adherence to established policies and procedures. Reassignments of officers trained to operate the TC to other sections of the prison occur for this reason. Generally, such an organizational culture is intolerant of any other system that has different philosophies and objectives. However, for a treatment program to be able to operate effectively inside the prison, there must be a significant integration between these two systems.

3. The continued availability of sufficient resources properly directed to maintaining adequate treatment facilities and quality services is essential to ensuring treatment effectiveness. This includes the training and hiring of adequately trained drug treatment staff.

4. For prison-based TCs that use prison officers as TC personnel, assignment to the TC project could be perceived as a slower tract for career advancement, especially if the project is not given its due priority.
5. The TC is an intensive form of substance-abuse treatment that costs money to deliver. In addition, not every substance-abusing offender needs the TC treatment modality. This requires us to be judicious in identifying substance-abusing offenders whose treatment needs match the TC admission criteria.
6. The TC requires the full immersion of the members into the community environment and its culture in a seamless 24-hour structure. However, because of some conflicting programming priorities, the members may be required by prison authorities to spend several hours in profit-inducing cottage industries to meet business demands.
7. There is a high-rate of comorbidity among substance-abusing prisoners that requires prison-based TCs to have a well-established assessment and diagnostics procedure to assess residents' clinical needs and determine those who are appropriate for the TC.

THE TRANSFER OF TC TECHNOLOGY TO OTHER CULTURES AND THE ROLE OF TRAINING

The TC Philosophy and Culture

The TC has been defined as a treatment environment wherein members, who suffer from addiction or companion problems, consent to live together in an organized and structured setting that would facilitate the process of change and the acquisition of a lifestyle free from any form of substance abuse. It is a microcosmic representation of the larger society, where everyone fulfills distinctive roles and lives by established community norms that facilitate the resident's reintegration into the larger society. In short, it is helping oneself while helping others in the therapeutic process. Each resident takes responsibility for achieving personal growth, acquiring prosocial values, nurturing a meaningful and responsible life, and protecting the integrity of the community (25).

The TC could vary in several ways as it adapts itself to different conditions. There are, nevertheless, fundamental principles or elements that must be maintained. The most important of these is the philosophy and its belief system. The TC believes in the inherent goodness of the individual, in the individual's capacity to change, in helping others to help themselves, in a power greater than oneself, and in human values. The philosophy and the beliefs pervade the community and serve as reminder for the members as to the purpose for living as a community.

The Elements of the TC

Defining the essential elements of the TC is a crucial first step in conducting training and adapting the TC to other cultures. TC program fidelity represents an imperative in training staff and establishing the TC in a different culture. Personal backgrounds, cultural conditioning, and professional training determine how we interpret the TC treatment philosophy, assign importance to the different aspects of the TC, and select elements that we prefer to adopt. For this reason, there should be a certain consensus on the most basic elements present in a TC to fulfill its functions and operate as a treatment community. Different TC experts will attach varying degrees of importance to assorted aspects of the TC as constituting its essential elements. The following list of core elements of the TC is by no means exhaustive:

1. The philosophy, unwritten philosophy, and belief system of the TC.
2. A setting or environment dedicated for the purpose of the TC.
3. An effective method to shape and manage behavior.
4. A proven method to facilitate psychological change and spiritual healing.
5. Activities that increase self-competence and self-reliance.
6. A system that provides a daily structure with clearly defined member roles within the community.
7. A system of rewards and sanctions.
8. Reliance on self-help as a mode of treatment and the use of community as a social learning environment for healing and personal growth.
9. Peers and staff as role models.
10. A set of community norms, codes of conduct, and a value system that operationalizes the TC philosophy, unwritten philosophy, and belief system.
11. The use of public sharing in interpersonal communication.
12. A treatment process organized by stages designed to prepare the members for social reintegration.
13. A treatment curriculum that teaches the members the elements, processes, and methods of the TC as well as the maintenance of sobriety, health, and safe lifestyle.

Training the TC Staff

How must we train a potential TC worker? What skills must one acquire to work successfully in the TC environment? What personal attributes must one possess to be an effective staff member? There is no guaranteed training guide to meet all the requirements and there are no fool-proof tests that predict how one does as a TC staff member. One thing is certain: paraprofessionals and professionals are often attracted to working in the TC, not for the financial rewards it offers, because of its "meaning" and the intangible feeling of self-fulfillment it promises, whether to fill a personal void, work on unresolved issues or live out a meaningful career. A certain level of personal confrontation and accountability in this area are necessary if only to have some clarity on motivation and awareness of potential pitfalls as one interacts with others in the TC. Tragedy sometimes occurs from the inability of a staff member to be fully aware of his or her own needs or personal boundaries and the client's needs. Thus, the staff member proceeds to make decisions that satisfy more his or her needs than the client's.

Staff should be trained to be effective facilitators of the TC; not as the primary source of healing. To fulfill this function, staff must focus on three different levels of operation: (a) the community level, (b) the individual resident's level, and (c) the internal level of emotions and feelings (26).

The fundamental principle in the concept-based TC is that the community itself is the most effective means of providing treatment (2). To carry this out, the TC has its work ethic, various group encounters, and its own structure and hierarchy. Operating on this level, it is the main function of staff to determine how the community is functioning as a healing environment. Staff empower the residents in the hierarchy to develop the therapeutic standards of the community and are expected to use the community structure when dealing with individual residents (26).

Focusing on the "individual resident's level," staff work through the senior resident hierarchy and maintain some distance from the younger members of the community. However, staff need to be fully aware of all the members and must keep track of how they are responding to the environment and the kinds of problems that they encounter or create in the community.

Staff must have a good grip on their own feelings and should have a healthy self-awareness of their own internal processes. They should know when to get appropriate help from other staff to maintain their own personal boundaries. Working in the TC involves an intimate process of working with individual issues that trigger, at times, his inner and external conflicts requiring the resolution of those conflicts. The emotional challenge to staff to confront their own feelings and vulnerabilities is always present and tied to their ability to assist the residents in dealing with their own personal vulnerabilities.

Training the staff on the mechanics of the TC and attending to their own emotional issues may fall short in promoting healthy functioning among the TC staff. Formal and informal supervision by seasoned and trained supervisors must be always available and an essential part of the professional development program for all staff. The highly experiential nature of learning the TC dynamics and appropriate applications of the TC treatment tools require time and proper guidance for neophyte staff by highly experienced leaders. It will take 2 years approximately before a new staff member will be able to grasp the TC processes and integrate with the TC (26). However, for some staff, this process could prove very stressful, depending on personal and professional issues that the person brings to their work in the TC. Burnout is common and rapid staff turnover could leave the TC always in need of adequately trained staff.

THE DAYTOP INTERNATIONAL TRAINING PROGRAM

For more than two decades, Daytop has been host to hundreds of foreign visitors ranging from graduate students to all types of professionals and government officials. A particular group of visitors has sought more than just a quick study tour of the Daytop facilities but is interested in learning the TC by undergoing an intensive training on its methods. This group is comprised of government and private agencies whose primary purpose for coming to Daytop is to learn and to be able to adapt this treatment model to various treatment settings and clientele (juvenile, prison, psychiatric populations, etc.) (27).

The diverse group of professionals and paraprofessionals who come for this training spend between a month to a year in a carefully designed training curriculum that involves extended period of immersion in the TC environment. They experience a supervised residential program as TC residents among the regular clients in various Daytop facilities. They go through an accelerated process, rising through the ranks in the TC hierarchy in a highly experiential training experience.

The Daytop on-site training model, coupled with the Daytop International overseas training and consulting activities, is responsible for the successful transfer of the TC technology to different countries with diverse cultures. Even in non-English–speaking countries such as Thailand, China, Vietnam, South Korea, Peru, Colombia, Brazil, Bosnia Herzegovina, and Romania, the TC was adapted and developed through this process. The didactic and experiential approaches of the Daytop on-site training in the United States have helped assure program fidelity in the process of adapting the TC to various cultural settings.

THE CHANGE PROCESS IN THE TC AND THE ROLE OF SPIRITUALITY

What makes a TC therapeutic lies in how the community is constituted. The term "community" in therapeutic community is qualitatively different from the ordinary village, neighborhood, or housing complex. They might be structurally similar but they have different goals and espouse divergent ideologies. Affiliation with the TC requires a commitment to its philosophy and a willingness to live by a code of conduct that actualizes the ideals agreed upon by the members of the community. The philosophy and the ideals of the community are statements of what constitute to be the "good life" or "right living" (2) that each member aspires to achieve through mutual help and a willingness to learn from others. Implicit in TC participation is the recognition of one's limitations or personal flaws that can be overcome through genuine mutual feedback in a social learning relationship.

Driven by a collective purpose, the community develops its structure for organizing daily life and the sustenance of the system dedicated to serving the needs of the individual members and the community as a whole. Norms and rituals are evolved that embody the ideals and philosophy of the community. Community rituals to deal with transgressions of the norms and a method of redemption, by expressing remorse and offering restitution, both for sins of omission and commission, are developed. In the context of an Islamic TC, how sin, shame, and guilt are to be dealt with are central issues. By taking drugs, the individual has broken the laws of his society and religion, rejected common moral values, and betrayed his family and loved ones. This leaves the individual with strong feelings of shame and guilt, constantly haunting the person and making the person vulnerable to negative influences (28).

The social nature of humans and their development that is dependent on the reciprocal interactions of their personal traits, their behavior, and their social environment make the TC an appropriate setting for personal growth or change. A person's imitative tendency predisposes that person to learn through "role modeling," and an individual's need for social affiliation and affirmation drives the individual to conform to social norms (29). A person tends to represent his perception of reality and ideas in symbols and rituals. Rituals are used as symbolic vehicles for psychological and behavioral transformations.

The use of the community as a means for personal or spiritual transformation is not new. It is found in many cultures and practiced by many religions, from the "ashrams" of the Hindus to the sacred monasteries of the Buddhists and Christians. They share the common characteristic of a life in "community." Communal living requires a paradigm-shift in one's personal identity and locus of identification where one's ego is subsumed to the higher power for which the community is dedicated to serve. This lifestyle is designed to overcome the natural selfishness of people, which also breeds division and conflict. Compassion and real love, as expressions of spirituality, will not be possible if one fails to sublimate and transcend selfishness. In this community, "responsible love" for one another is an important covenant. This is the way of the spiritual life.

To this ideal community and the healing potential it promises to the "lost" soul of troubled individuals, the TC does trace part of its beginnings. When a person suffers from social or mental maladies, that person finds healing not in isolation but in communion with another human being. This is why therapy heals. Using the contact between two people or a group of people, it brings to bear the social context to alter thinking, feeling, and behavior.

Perhaps the very nature of addiction, with its encompassing impact on the total person, requires a global change to overcome it. The change process must go beyond the person's behavior and must include the person's outlook on life and living (30,31). The 12-step program with its roots in Christian traditions and the various forms and permutations of the TC attest to the spiritual qualities involved in personal change. The healing process from addiction, therefore, requires a paradigm-shift in the realms of values and lifestyle that finds itself at the heart of the treatment experience in the TC.

THE APPLICATION OF THE THERAPEUTIC COMMUNITY TO COMMUNITY-BASED PROGRAMS

The UNDCP has promoted the community-based program as the treatment model for developing countries. The model is based on the partnership of the local community and a group of experts in community development projects with the overall goal of reducing drug demand through a locally organized drug treatment and prevention initiative. The experts generally provide the organizational impetus to the project. They guide and empower the local organization to solve various social, economic, health and security problems often tied to the supply and demand for drugs. The approach involves using grassroots and indigenous organized efforts, with little help from the national government to solve community problems, such as drug abuse and other drug-related health or social problems (32).

The community-based program is a treatment approach designed to help the drug-addicted persons with the least disruption of their life and obtain treatment services that are located in the immediate community. This approach to drug treatment is characterized by a high degree of participation in project planning and implementation by the members of the community. It empowers local people to initiate action on their own; thereby, influencing the process and outcome of their activities (32).

EVALUATING TREATMENT OUTCOME

For the first time, the TC method was successfully used in Vietnam as a treatment framework that blended traditional community-based and residential-based drug programs. The project was conducted under the auspices of UNDCP and the government of Vietnam while Daytop International provided the technical expertise (3,4).

Evaluation research serves the important purpose of (a) determining if clients have made improvement, and (b) whether the improvement is truly the result of treatment (6). Of particular interest to funding agencies and treatment providers about outcome evaluations is to discover if the program is effective enough to justify putting resources there and to determine what aspects of the program work and where changes are needed for improvement (6).

Some studies focused on determining what variables are predictive of client successful treatment. For example, early studies of the TC (33) found that dynamic variables (e.g., type of treatment, length of treatment, and psychological profile) are more predictive of treatment outcome than static variables (e.g., race, gender, religion, education).

Most studies of TC treatment outcome are comprised of posttreatment outcome and psychological studies of in-treatment changes (6). Posttreatment studies usually classify the subjects into different groups (e.g., graduates and dropouts, or convicted and nonconvicted clients, or adolescent and adult drug users), comparing them based on a set of outcome measures (e.g., relapse rate, productivity or employment, criminality, or reconviction rates). Most of these studies found that retention is the most significant predictor of positive treatment outcome (6). However, a study of 255 ex-residents of Odyssey House in Australia (reference 34, cited in reference 6) found that instead of the length of time spent in treatment as critical to outcome, the amount of progress made in that time is a better predictor. Those residents who made faster progress did better than those who stayed the same amount of time but made slower progress in treatment.

Some studies compared the clients' psychological functioning and level of social skills at the onset and end of treatment using standard psychological tests and clinical progress reports (33,35). Recently, a retrospective study of 2,881 residents who were treated at Thanyarak TC in Thailand found that residents who relapsed are more likely to experience neurotic symptoms and reflect more introverted personalities, whereas those who remain absti-

nent have more extroverted personalities (36). Moreover, relapse cases are likely to exhibit labile mood strains and feel emotionally vulnerable. A retrospective study of residents in a Daytop TC for adolescent males (37) found that there were significant improvements in educational performance, family/social problems, mental health and medical status within 6 months of treatment. However, prior to discharge most of the subjects exhibited marked increase in perceived medical problems and psychological distress, which indicate possible anticipatory anxiety prior to discharge from treatment.

Some research studies have investigated particular aspects of the TC in an attempt to determine how and why it works. A study using 345 adult residents of Daytop Village investigated the validity and reliability of a theory-based set of instruments designed to measure and understand the change process of the resident in the TC. Based on the view of addiction as a disorder of the whole person, the instruments were designed to evaluate the developmental, socialization, and psychological changes in the resident as a result of treatment in TC (5).

Best practice studies using qualitative and quantitative methods have investigated drug treatment programs in Latin America, Europe, and Asia (7) in a bid to identify promising practices related to the programs studied.

REFERENCES

1. Kooyman M. The history of therapeutic communities: a view from Europe. In: Rawlings B, Yates R, eds. *Therapeutic communities for the treatment of drug users*. London: Jessica Kingsley Publishers, 2001, pp. 59–78.
2. De Leon G. *The therapeutic community: theory, model, and method*. New York: Springer Publishing, 2000.
3. Perfas F. *Drug situation analysis and training in community-based treatment and rehabilitation. Report*. Hanoi, Vietnam: United Nations International Drug Control Program, 2000.
4. United Nations International Drug Control Programme (UNDCP). *Drug situation analysis. Report at the National Forum on Community-based Program*. Hanoi, Vietnam, 2000.
5. Kressel D, De Leon G, Palij M, et al. Measuring client clinical progress in therapeutic community treatment: client assessment inventory, client assessment summary, and staff assessment summary. *J Subst Abuse Prev* 2000;19:267–272.
6. Rawlings B. Evaluative research in therapeutic communities. In: Rawlings B, Yates R, eds. *Therapeutic communities for the treatment of drug users*. London: Jessica Kingsley Publishers, 2001, pp. 209–223.
7. Landis R, Kaplan L, Nemes S, et al. *A study of promising treatment practices in Latin America, Europe, and

Asia*. Paper presented at the 5th Asian Federation of Therapeutic Communities Conference. Bangkok, Thailand, August 2002.
8. Raimo S. Democratic and concept-based therapeutic communities and the development of community therapy. In: Rawlings B, Yates R, eds. *Therapeutic communities for the treatment of drug users*. London: Jessica Kingsley Publishers, 2001, pp. 43–56.
9. Burdon WM, Farabee D, Prendergast ML, et al. *Evaluating prison-based therapeutic community substance abuse programs: the California initiative*. Paper presented at the 21st World Conference of the World Federation of Therapeutic Communities, Melbourne, Australia, February 2002.
10. Lowe L. *A profile of the young adult offender in California prisons as of December 31, 1989–1994 (prepared for the Substance Abuse Research Consortium, Spring 1995)*. Sacramento: Office of Substance Abuse Programs, California Department of Corrections, 1995.
11. California Department of Corrections. California Prisoners and Parolees-preliminary. 2000. Available at: http://www.cdc.state.ca.us/reports/offenders.htm.
12. Mason P, Mason D, Brooks N. Therapeutic communities for drug-misusing offenders in prison. In: Rawlings B, Yates

R, eds. *Therapeutic communities for the treatment of drug users*. London: Jessica Kingsley Publishers, 2001, pp. 163–177.
13. *Drug misuse in prison. Prison Service Strategy Document*. London: HMSO, 1995.
14. Daytop International. *Training report for Ecuador*. New York: Author, 2000.
15. Chisawang N. *Therapeutic community for drug-addicted inmates in the Department of Corrections, Thailand*. Paper presented at the 21st World Conference of the World Federation of Therapeutic Communities, Melbourne, Australia, February 2002.
16. Patac E. *Establishment of a therapeutic community center: the first in Philippine national prisons*. Paper presented at the 5th Asian Federation of Therapeutic Communities Conference. Bangkok, Thailand, August 2002.
17. Lim I. *Adaptation of therapeutic community concept for special population in Asia: Therapeutic community in the Philippine jail setting*. Paper presented at the 5th Asian Federation of Therapeutic Communities Conference. Bangkok, Thailand, August 2002.
18. Rajenthiran SP. *The TC within the correctional setting: Persada's experience*. Paper presented at the 5th Asian Federation of Therapeutic Communities Conference. Bangkok, Thailand, August 2002.

19. Huq ME. *Drug menace: Bangladesh-global perspective.* Paper presented at the Seminar on Anti-Drug of Asian Countries of International Police, Beijing, China, 1989.

20. United Nations Office for Drug Control and Crime Prevention. *Drug abuse in Pakistan: results from the year 2000 national assessment study.* Pakistan: 2002.

21. Bacolod G. *Drug abuse treatment in Philippine correctional facilities: community-based program.* Paper presented at the 5th Asian Federation of Therapeutic Communities Conference. Bangkok, Thailand, 2002.

22. Salim I. *Reentry and aftercare program: Pertapis, Singapore.* Paper presented at the 5th Asian Federation of Therapeutic Communities Conference. Bangkok, Thailand, 2002.

23. Wexler HK, Blackmore J, Lipton DS. Three-year re-incarceration outcomes for Amity in-prison therapeutic community and aftercare in California. *Prison J* 1991;79(3):312–336.

24. Hooper RM, Lockwood D, Inciardi JA. Treatment techniques in corrections-based therapeutic communities. *Prison J* 1993;73(3&4):290–306.

25. Ottenberg D, Broekaert E, Kooyman M. What cannot be changed in a therapeutic community? In: Broekaert E, Van Hove G, eds. *Special education Ghent 2: therapeutic communities.* Ghent: vzw OOBC, 1993.

26. Woodhams A. The staff member in the therapeutic community. In: Rawlings B, Yates R, eds. *Therapeutic communities for the treatment of drug users.* London: Jessica Kingsley Publishers, 2001, pp 123–137.

27. Daytop International. *A guide to Daytop International.* New York: Author, 1999.

28. Yunus P. (*Spiritual program within the therapeutic community.* Paper presented at the 5th Asian Federation of Therapeutic Communities Conference. Bangkok, Thailand, August 2002.

29. Miller PH. *Theories of developmental psychology.* New York: W H. Freeman, 1989.

30. Koe G. *Spirituality and its role in the healing process.* Paper presented at the 21st World Conference of the World Federation of Therapeutic Communities, Melbourne, Australia, February 2002.

31. Johnson B. A developmental model of addiction and its relationship to the twelve-step program of Alcoholics Anonymous. *J Subst Abuse Prev* 1993;10:23–34.

32. Economic and Social Council of Asia and the Pacific. *Community-based drug demand reduction and HIV/AIDS prevention: a manual for planners, practitioners, trainers, and evaluators.* New York: United Nations, 1995.

33. De Leon G.. *The therapeutic community: study of effectiveness.* DHHS Publication No. (ADM) 84-1286. Washington, DC: U.S. Government Printing Office, 1984.

34. Toumbourou JW, Hamilton M, Fallon B. Treatment level, progress and time spent in treatment in the prediction of outcomes following drug-free therapeutic community treatment. *Addiction* 1998;93(7):1051–1064.

35. Kennard D. *An introduction to therapeutic communities.* London: Jessica Kingsley Publishers, 1998.

36. Virachai V, Punjawatnun J, Perfas FB. *The results of drug dependence treatment by therapeutic community for Thais in Thanyarak Hospital.* Paper presented at the 5th Asian Federation of Therapeutic Communities Conference. Bangkok, Thailand, 2002.

37. Solkhah R, Bunt GC, Schulman MN. *Adolescent treatment interventions and outcomes in the therapeutic community (TC).* Paper presented at the 21st World Conference of the World Federation of Therapeutic Communities, Melbourne, Australia, 2002.

CHAPTER 39

Methadone Maintenance

JOYCE H. LOWINSON, IRA MARION,
HERMAN JOSEPH, JOHN LANGROD,
EDWIN A. SALSITZ, J. THOMAS PAYTE, AND
VINCENT P. DOLE

This chapter reviews the historical perspectives leading to the development of methadone maintenance treatment (MMT), clinical procedures, and summaries of studies and evaluations regarding its effectiveness. Under the leadership of Dr. Vincent P. Dole, a metabolic scientist, and Dr. Marie E. Nyswander, a psychiatrist specializing in the treatment of heroin addiction, the development of methadone maintenance at The Rockefeller University in 1964 and 1965 ushered in the modern era of medical treatment and neurobiologic research for the treatment of opioid dependency. In 2002, approximately 215,600 patients were enrolled in 1,080 methadone treatment centers throughout the United States (1). By 2004, 47 countries had established methadone maintenance programs, treating about 500,000 patients worldwide (2).

HISTORICAL PERSPECTIVE

The Harrison Act, a revenue law passed to honor the United States' international commitment to the 1912 Hague Convention to control narcotics, made the sale or transfer of all narcotic drugs a matter of record and subject to taxes and fees. At that time, many patent and prescription medications contained "narcotic" drugs, including cocaine, heroin, and morphine, and addiction was not uncommon (3). Physicians, faced with persons addicted to narcotic drugs, prescribed them. However, the United States Treasury Department viewed addiction as a criminal and moral problem, rather than a medical concern. The Harrison Act was used as the legal basis to systematically prosecute these physicians, known as the "Doctor Cases" (see Chapter 1, "Historical Perspectives"). Most significant among these cases was *Linder vs. the United States*, because it established that physicians could provide "good faith" treatment for addicts (4). Despite this favorable decision, physicians continued to be harassed and increasingly often refused to treat narcotic addicts.

By 1918, clinics dispensing morphine and other drugs were established in 14 cities in an effort either to maintain or withdraw addicts from addictive drugs. The two most famous of these clinics were in New York City and Shreveport, Louisiana. By 1923, however, the active campaign by the United States government ended this form of clinical intervention until methadone maintenance treatment research began in the mid-1960s (5).

Once the United States narcotics clinics were closed, treatment for addiction became largely unavailable until 1935, when the United States Public Health Service opened a hospital for this purpose in Lexington, Kentucky. This facility and another in Fort Worth, Texas, which opened in 1938, operated much like a prison, treating both involuntary criminal and volunteer addicts. They remained the only two public facilities treating addiction until the mid-1950s, when Riverside Hospital opened in New York City. Treatment consisted of detoxification with a goal of abstinence. However, a followup study of patients discharged from Riverside showed that more than 90% relapsed to heroin use (6).

The first renewed attempt of organized medicine to advocate treatment and medical research for narcotics addiction came in 1955 when the New York Academy of Medicine strongly objected to federal regulations that "prohibited physicians from prescribing a narcotic drug to keep comfortable a confirmed addict who refuses withdrawal, but who might, under regulated dosage, lead a useful life and later might agree to withdrawal" (7). The Academy report observed that the early morphine maintenance clinics opened after World War I were closed in 1923, not because they had failed, but because their goals were not in accordance with the prevailing philosophy of a punitive approach to the so-called criminal problem. This report led to a renewed debate on narcotic maintenance at a time when the number of young heroin addicts in urban ghettos was increasing and concern over rising overdose deaths and drug-related crime was escalating. As a result, a position paper was generated by the Joint Committee of the American Bar Association and the American Medical Association in 1959, calling for a softening of penalties and the establishment of an experimental outpatient clinic for the treatment of drug addicts (8).

In 1962, the Medical Society of the County of New York recognized the need for systematic clinical investigation of medical maintenance treatment programs and ruled that "physicians who participate in a properly controlled and supervised clinical research project for addicts on a noninstitutional basis would be deemed to be practicing ethical medicine" (8). By 1963, the available treatment for narcotics addicts in New York City, where half of the nation's addicts lived, consisted of detoxification in Manhattan General Hospital and Metropolitan Hospital. Also that year, New York's first therapeutic community (Daytop Lodge) opened on Staten Island under the leadership of Monseigneur William O'Brien.

With the medical and legal professions calling for a reevaluation of American narcotics policies, the climate became more favorable for a maintenance approach to treating addiction in outpatient clinics. In 1963, the New York Academy of Medicine recommended again that clinics be established in affiliation with hospitals to dispense narcotics to addicts. The same year, President Kennedy's Advisory Committee on Narcotics and Drug Abuse made similar recommendations (8). By the early 1960s, heroin-related mortality became the leading cause of death for young adults between the ages of 15 and 35 years. Serum hepatitis cases related to injection of narcotics with contaminated needles were increasing markedly. A record number of addicts was being arrested for drug-related crimes (possession, sale of narcotics, property crimes) and jails were overcrowded (9). Drug-free approaches were unable to impact on the post-World War II heroin epidemic on a cost-effective basis, and a public health medical intervention was needed.

In 1962, in response to the growing concern over the spread of heroin addiction, the New York City Health Research Council, viewing narcotic addiction as a public health emergency, recommended research in this area. Dr. Vincent Dole, of The Rockefeller University, an expert in metabolic research and Dr. Marie Nyswander, a psychiatrist with extensive experience in narcotic addiction, undertook this endeavor. As a result of her experiences at the U.S. Public Health Hospital in Lexington, Kentucky, at the Musicians Clinic, and in her private psychoanalytic practice in New York City, Dr. Nyswander became convinced that traditional psychiatric approaches alone could not help addicts to discontinue their use of narcotics (10). Recognizing that relapse in most cases was related to persistent or recurring narcotic craving, Dole and Nyswander hypothesized that the relief of this craving constituted a critical first step to transform intractable addicts into patients leading normal lives.

To test their theory, they admitted to the hospital at The Rockefeller Institute (now known as The Rockefeller University) six heroin addicts, between 20 and 40 years old with minimum addiction histories of at least 5 years, and at least two prior failures in treatment. All had histories of criminal activity related to their addictions to heroin. An initial attempt to stabilize them on short-acting narcotics such as morphine proved problematic because the patients required multiple daily injections and were preoccupied with their scheduling, as well as experiencing mood-altering effects ("highs and lows," as well as experiencing withdrawal). In contrast, methadone, a long-acting narcotic, could be administered orally once daily in doses greater than 80 mg. As a result, the sharp mood swings and withdrawal symptoms of short-acting narcotics were eliminated, and patients could function normally. A daily maintenance dose of 80 to 120 mg produced a pharmacologic cross-tolerance, or "blockade," so that patients would not feel any narcotic or euphoric effects if they were to self-administer a normal dose of a short-acting narcotic (e.g., 25 mg of heroin). Finally, methadone appeared to be safe and nontoxic, with only minimal side effects (11).

With the support of Dr. Ray Trussell, the New York City Commissioner of Hospitals, an expanded pilot program with 120 patients was conducted at Manhattan General Hospital, which later became affiliated with the Beth Israel Medical Center (12). In 1967, 107 patients remained in treatment, of whom 71% were employed in steady jobs, attending school, or both. Dole and Nyswander stated: "To date we have seen no indication to remove the blockade from any patient in the treatment program since all of them are still in the process of rehabilitation and no patient has been limited by intolerance of the medication" (11). The Columbia University School of Public Health was enlisted to conduct an independent evaluation of the project under the leadership of Dr. Frances Rowe Gearing as committee chair. These evaluations continued for the first 10 years of methadone maintenance treatment and yielded the following positive outcomes: (a) a decrease in antisocial behavior measured by arrest and/or incarceration; (b) an increase in social productivity measured by employment and/or schooling, homemaker, or vocational training; (c) clinical impression of relief of heroin craving confirmed by negative urine specimens after stabilization on methadone; and (d) a recognition of, and willingness by motivated patients to accept help for, psychiatric and other problems, including those related to excessive use of alcohol or other drugs.

Based on these evaluations, further expansion of the program was recommended (13). As a result methadone maintenance treatment programs were opened in many urban areas throughout the United States. Reports of their success were published in the medical literature. Annual methadone conferences were held, giving an opportunity for in-depth discussion of this new treatment. Some of the programs followed the Dole-Nyswander protocols (11,14). Others used methadone medication but developed programs with divergent goals and objectives including abstinence, low-dose therapy, and combinations of residential, outpatient, mental health, and other modalities (15,16).

By 1969 there were 2,000 patients enrolled in methadone maintenance programs in New York City alone, and 10,000 applicants were awaiting admission. The New York Academy of Medicine termed the situation a crisis. Although they recognized that treatment of heroin addiction with methadone, a long-acting narcotic, might be a lifelong affair, they felt that "no other regimen currently available offers as much to the chronic addict" (17). New York State legislators responded by appropriating $10 million for the establishment of additional methadone maintenance programs. In 1970, the Bureau of Narcotics and Dangerous Drugs, in a joint statement with the United States Food and Drug Administration (FDA), approved the use of methadone as an investigational drug for "experimental" maintenance programs and interdicted

further research except in accordance with guidelines to be promulgated by regulations. Other established uses of methadone were adversely impacted when it was removed from retail pharmacies and made available only through hospital pharmacies subject to specific restrictions. Emphasis continued to focus on eventual abstinence. In 1971, Dr. Jerome Jaffe, appointed to direct the White House Special Action Office for Drug Abuse Prevention, played a major role in stemming the rise of heroin addiction in the United States by expanding methadone treatment nationwide.

In 1972, the FDA approved the use of methadone hydrochloride for the treatment of narcotic addiction (18). Subsequently, other medications have been approved by the FDA to treat addiction. In 1985, naltrexone hydrochloride (ReVia) received the same approval but is of limited use because it is an antagonist, does not effectively relieve craving and is rejected by large segments of the patient population. In 1993, LAAM (levo-alpha-acetylmethadol) a longer-acting methadone analogue was approved. However, it was found to be associated with torsade de pointes in Europe, was subsequently banned in Europe, and is no longer manufactured in the United States. In 2002, buprenorphine (Buprenex), a partial agonist, was approved for use in United States in office-based practices and is now a used for opioid withdrawal as well as maintenance treatment (see Chapter 40). At present, methadone is the major modality worldwide for the treatment of opioid dependency. It has been researched thoroughly and evaluated extensively for four decades (19). Methadone treatment also has relevance to the prevention and treatment of the human immunodeficiency virus (HIV) and hepatitis C by curtailing intravenous drug use (19).

Despite the resistance of some segments of the treatment community, who do not accept agonist maintenance therapy for ideological and funding reasons, methadone has become the most accepted and cost-effective public health approach to the treatment of opioid addiction throughout the world. Unfortunately, the Dole-Nyswander models are not universally applied. This has resulted in methadone programs of less-than-optimal quality (20). It is, therefore, critical to educate the treatment community regarding best practices. Despite the need for further education and quality assurance, methadone maintenance treatment in general has remained an important intervention for the disenfranchised, population at risk for HIV and hepatitis C, as well as for sexually transmitted diseases (STDs) and tuberculosis. Despite its cost-effectiveness, waiting lists continue to exist because of inadequate funding, and a lack of political and community support.

USE OF METHADONE AS A MEDICATION

Methadone is a synthetic narcotic analgesic compound developed in Germany just prior to World War II (21). It was patented in 1941 but was not used since German physicians did not know how to safely prescribe it. After the war methadone was studied at the U.S. Public Health Hospital in Lexington, Kentucky, and was found to have effects similar to those of morphine but longer in duration. These initial studies led to the use of methadone for analgesia and for withdrawal from heroin. Although methadone continues to be used for these purposes, its unique pharmacologic properties can be used for maintenance (22,23).

As a maintenance medication, methadone has distinct advantages. When administered in adequate oral doses, a single dose in a stabilized patient lasts between 24 and 36 hours without creating euphoria, sedation, or analgesia. Therefore, the patient can function normally and can perform any mental or physical tasks without impairment. Patients continue to experience normal physical pain and emotional reactions. Most importantly, methadone relieves the persistent narcotic craving or hunger that is believed to be the major reason for relapse. According to Dr. Dole, this narcotic craving has a metabolic component. He summarizes the relationships among craving, addiction, and methadone treatment as follows:

> A modern theory of narcotic addiction is that the compulsive (and quite specific) craving for narcotic drugs is a symptom of deficiency in function of the natural opiate-like substances in the brain. To be sure, sociological and psychological forces enter into the making of an addict, but these factors determine exposure—whether or not addictive drugs are available in the environment and whether a person chooses to experiment with them. In any person with repeated exposure to a narcotic drug, the brain adapts and becomes pharmacologically dependent on a continuing input. In some susceptible persons—fortunately a minority of the population—the adaptation becomes fixed and with repeated use a regular input of narcotic becomes a necessity. The experimenter has become an addict. From this perspective methadone maintenance is replacement treatment, compensating for impairment in function of natural opiate-like substances. (24)

Stimmel and Kreek (25) report that chronic abuse of short-acting opioids profoundly alters stress responsivity including hyporesponsivity to stressors during cycles of heroin addiction, hyperresponsivity during periods of abstinence, and normalization during methadone maintenance treatment. These states are reflected in physiologic changes of the hypothalamic–pituitary–adrenal axis, which is normalized in long-term methadone-maintained patients. Recent studies also indicate that a genetic vulnerability to addiction may exist and early environmental factors may increase vulnerability (26). Furthermore imaging studies suggest that neurobiologic abnormalities in the brain caused by addiction to narcotics can persist and that the brains of methadone-maintained patients are closer to normal controls than to abstinent addicts (27).

Narcotic cross-tolerance, or "blockade," is another important property of the medication. In sufficient doses, methadone "blocks" the narcotic effects of normal street doses of short-acting narcotics such as heroin and can lessen the likelihood of self-administered drug overdose. Because tolerance to methadone remains steady, patients can be maintained indefinitely (e.g., in some cases more than 20 years) on the same dose.

Finally, methadone is a medically safe treatment medication, with minimal side effects (15,16,28). Much has been said about the importance of appropriate and adequate dosages of methadone. Since its early development, many practitioners have deviated from the original Dole-Nyswander protocol with the desire to conduct research to determine the most effective approach to treatment and detoxification. However, others, because of preconceived notions that abstinence was an achievable goal for the majority of addicts, that lower doses were less toxic, and that less diversion would occur, believed in administration of low-dose methadone. They also assumed, incorrectly, that it would be easier to withdraw patients from low doses of methadone. Patients, themselves, continued to resist adequate dosages based on mythologies that methadone "rots the bones," decreases libido, and is more difficult to "kick" than heroin (29,30).

Nevertheless, scientific evidence is now available to support the use of the original dosage protocol and that lower doses (less than 60 mg) are appropriate for only a limited number of patients. A series of large-scale studies has emerged showing that patients maintained on doses of 60 mg per day or more had better treatment outcomes than those maintained on lower doses. Hartel reports data based on 2,400 patients enrolled over a 15-year period. She observed that those patients maintained on a daily dose of 60 mg or more had longer retention in treatment, less use of heroin and other drugs, including cocaine, and a lower incidence of HIV infection and acquired immunodeficiency syndrome (AIDS). The effectiveness of methadone was even greater for patients on a 70-mg dose and was still more pronounced for patients on 80 mg per day or more (31–33). Ball and Ross (19) reported on a 3-year study of six methadone programs in three northeastern cities. They showed that patients reduced their use of intravenous heroin by 71% when compared with the preadmission level. Most importantly, this study revealed that opiate use was directly related to methadone dose levels. In patients on doses above 70 mg per day, no heroin use was detected, whereas those patients on doses below 46 mg per day were 5.16 times more likely to use heroin than were those receiving higher doses (19). Similar results were found by Caplehorn and Bell (34), who found that patients in Australia on higher doses remained in treatment longer. Finally, in a review of 24 methadone treatment programs, the United States General Accounting Office (20) concluded that "sixty milligrams of methadone is the lowest effective dose to stop heroin use and low dose maintenance (20 to 40 milligrams) is inappropriate."

Kreek (28,35) used blood plasma levels to establish optimal methadone doses and stated that whatever method is used, methadone dosages should never be used for social rewards or punishment because this is mostly a physiologic issue (28,35). Also, all doses must be determined individually, because of differences in metabolism, body weight, length and amount of heroin use, its purity, and, most importantly, maintenance of appropriate methadone blood levels throughout the 24-hour period.

These studies confirm that dosages below 60 mg appear inadequate for most patients. This is especially important at the beginning of treatment, when patients may experiment with heroin to test the effectiveness of the medication. Inadequate doses will reinforce the euphoric effects of heroin, thus making it more difficult to extinguish its use. Therefore, low doses of methadone are generally inappropriate.

CLINICAL APPLICATIONS: METHADONE MAINTENANCE PHARMACOTHERAPY

Goals for pharmacotherapy for addiction are to prevent or reduce withdrawal symptoms, drug craving, and relapse, and to restore to normalcy and physiologic functions disrupted by drug abuse (36).

For ease of discussion methadone dosing can be divided into simple phases as described in Table 39.1. Elsewhere in this chapter there is a separate discussion of methadone treatment phases looking at treatment in a broader context. The benefits of adequate individualized methadone dosing are well documented, as are the problems associated with inadequate dosing levels (19,34,37,38). This section focuses on how to ensure adequate dosing rather than why.

TABLE 39.2. *Initial dose*

Degree of tolerance	Dose range
Nontolerant	10 mg +/−5
Unknown tolerance	20 mg +/−5
Known tolerance	20–40 mg

Reproduced with permission from Payte JT. *Adequate dose lecture series.* Paper presented at the Albert Einstein College of Medicine, Division of Substance Abuse, New York, November 26, 1996.

Terms such as "high dose" and "low dose" are set aside to encourage the concept of individually determined adequate dose.

The initial dose of methadone is most commonly given at a time when the patient is having both signs and symptoms of opioid withdrawal. The immediate purpose is to relieve the withdrawal that is present and also to establish a dose reference point on which future dose adjustments can be made. Table 39.2 summarizes initial dose.

Michael Gossop and colleagues reported experiences that fail to support the accepted view that dose is the major determinant of withdrawal severity (39). Clinical experience of three of the authors (JHL, JTP, VPD) supports this observation. Patients present in varying stages of withdrawal. The presence or appearance of more severe withdrawal does not necessarily mean a high level of physical dependence or tolerance, or a higher initial or maintenance dose of methadone.

As indicated in Table 39.1 the purpose of the early induction is to bring the methadone dose to approximate the established opioid tolerance in a prompt but safe manner. To enable the patient to abstain from heroin or other opioids it is essential to relieve the withdrawal and to reduce

TABLE 39.1. *Principles of methadone dosing*

Phase	Purpose	Range in Mg/Comments
Initial Dose	Relieve abstinence symptoms	20–40 mg
Early Induction	Reach established tolerance level	Plus or minus 5–10 mg q 3–24 h
Late Induction	Establish *adequate* dose (desired effects)	Plus or minus 5–10 mg q 5–10 days
Maintenance/ Stabilization	Maintain desired effects (steady-state occupation of opiate receptors)	Ideally 60–120 mg, may be more than 120 mg or less than 60 mg
Maintenance to Abstinence	Medically supervised withdrawal	As Individually tolerated, up to 10% reduction q 5–10 days
Medical Maintenance	Indefinite maintenance of rehabilitated patient in a medical setting	Adequate dose with 2–4 weeks' medication at a time

Reproduced with permission from Payte JT, Khurl ET. Principles of methadone dose determination. In: State methadone treatment guidelines. Rockville, MD: Center for Substance Abuse Treatment, Treatment Improvement Protocol Series 1993;1:47–58.

the craving or drug hunger. If this process is too slow, the patient may continue to use heroin or other unprescribed narcotics; if the process is too fast, some degree of intoxification or overdose may result. Induction overdoses can result from exaggeration of tolerance and dependence by the newly admitted patient, overestimation on the part of the clinician, and the failure to consider basic steady-state pharmacology. Because the pharmacology of methadone differs from that of other opioids, the initial dose on the first day should be in the range of 20 to 40 mg, but not more than 40 mg.

Methadone has a half-life of 24 to 36 hours. Twenty-four hours after the initial dose is administered about half remains to which the second dose is added. The result is a significant increase in mean methadone levels with no increase in dose. This accumulation process continues until steady-state is achieved at some 4 to 5 half-lives or days The important clinical lesson is that the effect of the medication will increase in the absence of a dose increase, and that relief of withdrawal may require more time before the dose is increased. Both the clinician and the patient should be alert to any sedation on day one or two as subsequent days may result in overmedication.

The peak serum plasma levels occur between 2 and 4 hours after oral administration of methadone. During early induction when signs and symptoms of withdrawal, persist it is prudent to wait at least 3 hours before additional doses of 5 to 10 mg are provided (40,41).

Once the initial relief of withdrawal has been achieved, a more gradual dose adjustment may be indicated to establish an adequate maintenance dose to ensure realization of the goals listed earlier. An example would be the patient who has an initial elimination of withdrawal and craving at 50 mg per day but who is exposed to opportunistic heroin use, suggesting the need to establish a "blockade" level of cross-tolerance, usually requiring doses of 80 mg or more. In other situations, the late induction may involve a gradual reduction to find the lowest effective dose.

Once the stabilization dose is achieved, its indefinite administration should ensure continued maintenance of the desired effects. This stability is presumed to result from a steady-state occupation of the appropriate opiate receptors. Most patients may remain on a stable dose for decades while others, at times, may require some adjustment either an increase or decrease of the dose. However, both patients and clinicians should avoid the tendency to lower the dose simply because the patient is stable and doing well.

Maintenance to Abstinence

Medically supervised withdrawal should be attempted only when desired by the rehabilitated patient with adequate supervision and support. Staff should carefully explore the motivation for withdrawal. In many cases the motivation is based on external pressures, such as family and friends or regulatory or program policies that result in continued disruption of any efforts to achieve a normal, stable lifestyle. In consideration of the high rate of relapse to intravenous drug use and its concomitant medical and social risks, patients who have withdrawn or who are withdrawing should be carefully monitored in a clinical setting. In the event of relapse or impending relapse, appropriate intervention should be initiated, including rapid resumption of maintenance pharmacotherapy (42). Magura and Rosenblum, in a comprehensive review of numerous studies completed throughout the world over a 30-year period, demonstrated the risks of withdrawal from methadone maintenance, even under optimal conditions. A common finding was a high rate of relapse, arrests, and death after withdrawal (43).

The method of withdrawal usually involves a gradual reduction in dose over time. The schedule must be carefully individualized. Many patients will tolerate up to a 10% reduction in current dose at intervals of 5 to 10 days. (See Chapter 35, "Detoxification," for a discussion of detoxification.)

Use of Plasma Levels of Methadone

In recent years, reliable determination of methadone levels have become more available and affordable (44). Adequate dosing can be based on clinical findings in the majority of the cases. Blood levels may be considered in the following situations:

- To clarify a clinical picture that does not correspond to the dose of methadone
- To confirm suspected drug interactions (Table 39.3)
- To ensure adequacy of a given dose
- To document or justify the need for a particular dose or schedule
- To determine the need for and the effectiveness of split dose practices

Plasma levels of 150 to 200 ng/mL are adequate to prevent most craving and withdrawal (45,46). Adequate cross-tolerance or "blockade" is achieved at plasma levels at or above 400 ng/mL (47). The rate of change in plasma blood levels is critical and can be determined by calculating a peak-to-trough ratio. Ideally, this ratio is two or less. Higher ratios indicate rapid metabolism and the possible need for a split-dose twice per day. Split-dose induction is facilitated by giving the full customary dose on day 1 followed in about 12 hours with one-half the anticipated total daily dose. This "half-dose" is then continued twice daily.

Tolerance to the narcotic properties of methadone (sedation, analgesia) develops within a period of about 4 to 6 weeks. However, tolerance to the autonomic effects, most commonly constipation, libido, and sweating, develops at slower rates. Therefore, it is important to monitor the

TABLE 39.3. *Common methadone-drug interactions*

Drug	Mechanism	Effects/remarks	Reference
Rifampin	Induction CYP-450 enzyme activity	Withdrawal Symptoms	49
Phenytoin	Induction CYP-450 enzyme activity	Withdrawal Symptoms	85
Ethyl Alcohol	Induction CYP-450 enzyme activity	Acute and chronic effects may differ	16, 51
Barbiturates	Induction CYP-450 enzyme activity	Acute and chronic effects may differ	86
Carbomozepine	Induction CYP-450 enzyme activity	Acute and chronic effects may differ	87
Oploid Agonist/ Antagonists	Oploid displaced from receptor sites	Withdrawal, usually Inadvertent	41, 88

Reproduced with permission from Payte JT. Khuri ET. Principles of methadone dose determination. In: *State methadone treatment guidelines.* Rockville, MD: Center for Substance Abuse Treatment, Treatment Improvement Protocol Series 1993;1:47–58.

stabilization process carefully to minimize narcotic effects and withdrawal symptoms (15,48). Kreek has demonstrated that methadone prescribed in high doses up to 150 mg/day on a long-term basis has no toxic effects and minimal side effects for adult patients maintained in treatment for up to 14 years and for adolescent patients treated for up to 5 years (49–51).

At admission all patients are given a complete physical examination, including blood work, urinalysis, as well as screening for infectious diseases including purified protein derivative (PPD) for tuberculosis and serology. HIV testing should not be and is not given at admission because of the extensive orientation regarding this matter. Testing is voluntary and is completed after orientation subsequent to treatment entry.

Medical conditions identified among methadone patients include worsening of illnesses that existed prior to or while in treatment. Included are chronic hypertension, dental complications, diabetes, alcoholism, multiple substance abuse, HIV/AIDS, hepatitis C, chronic liver disease and cirrhosis, alcoholism, asthma, tuberculosis, STDs, endocarditis, and psychiatric disorders, and as well as other diseases associated with aging. However, following entry into treatment, health status usually improves with access to medical care, elimination of injections with contaminated needles, and improved quality of life. See (Gourevitch's Chapter 54).

As noted previously, the major side effects during methadone maintenance treatment occur during the initial stabilization process. Although these effects are minor and usually subside over time, they can also be reduced or eliminated by an appropriate dose adjustment. In addition to constipation and sweating, the following have been ascribed to methadone such as transient skin rash, weight gain, and water retention. Some patients

have reported changes in libido. Where there is a reduction in libido, Viagra (sildenafil citrate) is being prescribed to males. Most females who experienced amenorrhea while addicted to heroin report a return of menses when stabilized on methadone. However, some female patients complain about irregular menses or continued amenorrhea. To address the issues of side effects, appropriate medications may be prescribed, as well as providing counseling, education about methadone, family planning, nutritional guidance, and the prescribing of birth control medications and/or diaphragms for those who request it. Condoms are also distributed in clinics and orientation related to their use is provided. However, some of these side effects may be complications of coexisting alcoholism, multiple substance abuse, smoking, advanced age, other medical conditions, diet, and lifestyle (52).

Methadone maintenance, itself, does not impair the normal functioning of patients. Psychomotor performance tests that measure skills such as reaction time, driving ability, intelligence, attention span, and other important abilities were administered to methadone patients, volunteers, and normal college students with no drug history. The performance of methadone patients did not differ from those of normal volunteers or college students. Studies of patients' driving records in both Texas and New York found that the driving records of methadone patients did not differ significantly from those of the driving population at large (53). On the Wechsler Adult Intelligence Scale, the mean intelligence quotient (IQ) of methadone patients at the time of entry into treatment was slightly higher than that of the general population. Ten years later, the same patients showed even higher scores, possibly as a consequence of improved quality of life. Based on these studies, it can be concluded that methadone maintenance does not impair normal functioning or intellectual capacity (54–58).

METHADONE PROGRAMS

Methadone maintenance programs are controlled and regulated by federal and state agencies to an extent not found in any other form of medical treatment. In many states, the original Dole-Nyswander protocol has been altered to make abstinence the priority. In 1972, to establish minimal standards and quality, the FDA promulgated regulations governing the use of methadone; the Drug Enforcement Administration (DEA) was established to oversee the security and dispensing of the medication. In 2000, new federal regulations went into effect. The role of the DEA remains, but the FDA no longer is involved with the regulation of methadone. The Center for Substance Abuse Treatment (CSAT) has assumed the oversight of methadone and management of the accreditation process on the federal level. States have the right, and often exercise it, to make their licensing criteria more stringent than the federal regulations. They cannot, however, loosen the criteria beyond those permitted on a federal level. These minimum standards regulate admissions, staffing patterns, record keeping, treatment planning, service provision, storage, facility standards, frequency of visits and of urine testing, and dose limitations. Six states totally interdict the practice of methadone maintenance. Some states place a ceiling on the maximum dose, making it impossible to produce a narcotic blockade or to remove narcotic craving. Some prohibit take-home medication, and others place a limit on time in treatment before a patient must be withdrawn from methadone. Such restrictions present physicians with serious dilemmas. Instead of being able to rely on their professional judgment and clinical experience, they are often forced to make medical decisions independent of the needs of the patients. The effectiveness of methadone treatment can be reduced as a consequence of these factors. Also, some individual programs may exceed CSAT guidelines and state regulations, compromising effective treatment even further.

For admission to methadone treatment, federal standards mandate a minimum of 1 year of addiction to opiates as well as current evidence of addiction, although they allow for exceptions such as pregnancy or recent discharge from a chronic care institution or prison. The minimum age for admission is 18 years (younger than 18 years with parental or legal guardian consent). Applicants younger than age 18 years must have at least two prior documented treatment episodes, either short-term detoxification or drug-free treatment, before they can be considered for methadone maintenance. Pregnant women are routinely accepted for methadone treatment and can now be admitted without a 1-year addiction history because it is recognized that methadone maintenance treatment greatly improves the pregnancy outcome for the woman and her unborn child (see Chapter 53, "Maternal and Neonatal Effects of Alcohol and Drugs"). Applicants with major medical conditions such as AIDS are eligible and should be routinely accepted for methadone treatment (59).

In the United States, methadone treatment has evolved into three phases (not to be confused with the "dosing" phases previously discussed) during the past two decades. The first phase consists of a stabilization period that can last for about 3 months, during which patients adjust to the medication, receive their first annual physical examination, and are oriented to program regulations, expectations, routines, and services offered. Treatment planning begins with a thorough psychosocial history and assessment. Emergency situations and entitlements are addressed. Referrals are made to appropriate medical and social service agencies. New patients must report to the program daily (6 or 7 days per week) during this initial period. During the second phase, the treatment plan is reviewed and revised if necessary. This often involves implementing vocational goals such as job training or employment and providing ongoing medical and mental health treatment. For patients with serious medical problems such as HIV/AIDS, hepatitis C, or tuberculosis, or those with serious alcohol or multiple-drug problems, this phase of treatment can be extended as long as necessary. Many patients profit relatively quickly from the relevant services that are provided and are able to improve family relationships, find employment, attend school, and function productively. During this phase, patients may receive take-home medication, depending on their progress and adjustment to treatment. The third and final phase of treatment consists of continued methadone maintenance, but a minimum of other services. These patients most often are employed and no longer require the intensive services provided in other phases but still require ongoing methadone maintenance. They continue to submit urine specimens for drug screening and ingest a dose of methadone under observation of a nurse, and they can consult with program staff if necessary. Many patients visit only once a week at this time. However, a limited number of experimental projects are currently operating that allow patients to visit even less frequently. These projects should be expanded for addicts seeking help.

The modern urban methadone treatment program is a full-scale medical and human service agency attempting to address major social and medical problems using a variety of techniques. A study at the Veterans Administration Medical Center in Philadelphia showed that minimal or low-threshold treatment did not significantly reduce illicit drug use. Therefore, skilled counseling, an adequate dose, and case management are essential components of an effective program (60).

During the past decade, patient characteristics have changed markedly as a consequence of HIV/AIDS, increases in hepatitis C infection among intravenous drug abusers, the epidemic of cocaine and crack, and homelessness (see Chapter 72, "The Homeless"). These problems and their sequelae require methadone providers to create and enhance services to meet these needs. These programs require expanded and more sophisticated physical facilities for an expanding population, better trained staff, and greater funding. However, public funding has not kept pace with program needs, and a pervasive downsizing and reform agendas in welfare and Medicaid managed care at the time of this writing do not allow for much hope in this area (for more information, see Chapter 86, "Treatment for Alcohol and Drug Dependence: History, Workforce, Organization, Financing, and Emerging Policies"). However, providing primary care to substance abusers treated in methadone maintenance clinics could reduce the demand placed on emergency rooms and the need for hospitalization, reducing the overall cost of their care.

Methadone maintenance treatment programs can be established in a variety of health care and social service settings. Whether located in a hospital, a primary care clinic, or a social service agency, methadone programs should be organized and managed to ensure optimal outcomes for patients in an environment conducive to health, safety, and good treatment.

In organizing and operating a program, concerns about how space is allocated and used can be critical to operations. Clinics operating in cramped or inadequate quarters cannot provide the kind of care or privacy needed for physical examinations or effective counseling and casework.

A quality program should have clear, cogent, consistent, and humanistic policies and procedures that are known and understood by both patients and staff. There should be a multidisciplinary approach that is flexible in order to provide individualized treatment planning and implementation based on assessed patient needs (61,62).

A well-organized methadone maintenance treatment program must have enough space to allow staff to function in a professional manner consistent with good medical and mental health standards. Most states require programs to meet some degree of facility standards, and the federal government requires that facilities receiving federal funds provide unrestricted access for disabled persons. Over and above the minimum federal and state standards, programs should provide a clean, safe, and attractive environment that is friendly, cheerful, and accommodating. Although it is difficult to estimate the optimal size of an adequate program, between 15 and 20 square feet for each patient in treatment should be allotted, based on a patient census of 300.

Each clinic should be organized around the services it provides, and services should flow into each other easily. There must be a methadone dispensing area that is easily accessible to the patients it will serve. Ideally, a nurses' station or dispensing area is constructed adjacent to a comfortable patient waiting area. The nurses' station should be well lighted and should allow for easy communication between nurse or dispenser and patient, as this interaction is the most frequent contact the patient has with staff. It allows the nurse to assess the patient and note any changes in appearance and demeanor, as well as to ensure that the patient ingests his or her medication. Generally, the medication is stored in a safe equipped for this purpose (the DEA currently requires a General Services Administration Class 5 safe within or adjacent to the nurses' station).

With the current concern about hepatitis C, HIV infection, and other health issues, the waiting room can be used to impart information about the program and its services, hepatitis C and HIV education, prenatal care, and parenting skills as well as other important information. Through the creative use of videotapes that can run continuously while patients are waiting, a clinic can impart important information to its patients. Because patients often bring young children with them to the clinic, the area should be safe for young children and out of sight of the actual dispensing area.

The medical suite should be organized to ensure privacy and encourage patients to meet with the physician and other medical staff. The examination room must be well equipped and comfortable and there should be an adjacent office for staff to consult with patients. This area, as well as the entire clinic, should be equipped with adequate air exchange to prevent, as much as possible, airborne infections. Ultraviolet lighting and high-efficiency particulate air (HEPA) filtration systems can also be helpful. Patient records should be stored in a secure area but should be easily accessible to those who must use them frequently. Programs should also provide offices for individual staff members, rooms to hold patient groups and staff meetings, and a staff lounge.

The space should encourage patient and staff interaction, ensure privacy, and provide access to the services the program provides. This can best be accomplished by eliminating barriers between the patient and staff areas and by establishing an effective communications system that allows staff to communicate freely with each other whenever necessary.

Appropriate bathrooms are crucial, as programs must collect urine specimens from patients to clinically monitor whether patients continue to take methadone and do not misuse other drugs. The bathrooms should also be clean and neat and allow for privacy. Some clinics turn off the hot water in patient bathrooms to prevent the warming of urine specimens brought from elsewhere. The bathrooms should also be located where staff can monitor use.

Clinics should be decorated in a friendly and inviting style to prevent a drab and institutional look. Bulletin boards should be hung in the waiting area and elsewhere to provide current information to patients.

Where space and funding allows, programs can experiment with recreation areas, classrooms, skills training (such as typing or word processing), or other methods to prevent patients from congregating directly outside the clinic or in the neighboring community.

Programs with clear, cogent policies, procedures, goals, and objectives that are familiar to both staff and patients and consistent with state of the art knowledge will provide the best outcomes. Programs must be operated with flexibility and understanding of patient behavior, but with clear rules against violence or threats of violence. Patients must see the clinic site as distinct from the hostile environments where they formerly used heroin and understand that different rules apply inside the clinic. However, the methods used to communicate these basics and the program's policies and procedures often can facilitate making the distinction. Patients must always be treated with compassion, dignity, and respect.

The dispensing of methadone is an important aspect of the treatment process, and the relationship between the patient and the nurse is very important. Program directors should endeavor to make this a therapeutic process. Therefore, the collection of clinic fees, urine specimens, or other clinic matters should be handled apart from the dispensing process to allow patients to view the dispensing of methadone in a therapeutic manner.

Because patient motivation is high upon entry into treatment, it is important that the entire treatment team engage the patient early. The medical history, physical examination, laboratory tests, psychosocial history, and medical, mental health, and social assessments should be accomplished during the first weeks of treatment. Most important in this process is staff–patient contact and the initial orientation. The initial physician–patient contact gives the doctor an opportunity to establish a relationship of trust, to explain the effectiveness and pharmacology of methadone, and to treat acute medical problems. Patients must learn to respect methadone as a legitimate medication and not regard it as a substitute "street drug." Patients should be educated to dispel destructive myths and misunderstandings about methadone, understand how it is used, its effects and its side effects, how the maintenance dose will be achieved, how to request a dosage change, and how to store methadone safely, if take-home doses are dispensed. They also should be educated about the nature of addiction and the need for long-term treatment. Patients must understand how the program functions and be introduced to the program staff. The patient should participate in the development of an individualized treatment plan and clearly understand the goals and objectives the program has for his or her treatment and what the program expects. Most treatment plans are based on a triage concept, dealing with critical needs first. Housing, financial assistance, health care, and pending court cases are of primary importance. Later, vocational and educational goals can be pursued. Patients should know the services to which they entitled, what services are provided at the program and, if necessary, by referral to cooperating agencies.

Despite the poor prognosis indicated in early studies of methadone to abstinence (37,63), many patients who do well in treatment request to withdraw from methadone after a successful period of maintenance. Programs must advise patients of the risks and benefits of tapering the dose and provide service and support for those who elect to undergo withdrawal. Service should continue after zero dose is achieved and should involve individual, family, and group treatment. Because craving may invariably return, the patient should be provided with tools and support in this area, including possible return to maintenance treatment without delay, if this becomes necessary.

Some methadone treatment programs have taken advantage of the fact that patients visit regularly and remain in treatment to offer needed services that are usually difficult to obtain. This model, "one-stop shopping," provides HIV/hepatitis C-related services, services for children and families, services for pregnant and postpartum women (see Chapters 53 "Children of Substance Abusing Parents" and 61 "Maternal and Neonatal Effect of Alcohol and Drugs"), vocational and educational services, primary medical care, mental health services, and an array of substance abuse treatment services to deal with those who continue to abuse drugs and/or alcohol. Counseling and casework, relapse prevention techniques, 12-step groups, and other services are offered to patients with these problems.

A methadone maintenance treatment program is a complex system of health care and social services. Health concerns require a sanitary environment. Medical and psychiatric care, nursing, counseling, casework, finance, public and community relations, pharmacy, administration, medical records management, clerical, housekeeping, security, communications systems, safety, biohazard disposal all play a role in a successful and well-run program.

METHADONE TREATMENT HIV/AIDS AND HEPATITIS C

Several studies have confirmed that continuous methadone treatment is associated with a reduced risk of contracting HIV and may prevent infection of those patients not yet exposed to the virus. Infection rates among intravenous drug abusers in New York are estimated at 50%. Yet, studies in New York and Sweden examined patients in continuous treatment during the years when HIV exposure increased markedly (1983 was the pivotal year when HIV infection rates soared in both New York and Sweden). Infection rates for these groups of patients were extremely low (3% in Sweden; less than 10% in New York) compared with those for newly admitted patients and active addicts, leading investigators in these locations to conclude that continuous methadone treatment was associated with reduced risk of contracting HIV (31,64). A study of 58 long-term socially rehabilitated patients showed that all were seronegative for HIV. These patients were enrolled in treatment for more than 16 years and were maintained on a median dose of 60 mg per day (range: 5 to 100 mg per day). Prior to entry into treatment, these patients had used heroin by injection for an average of 10.3 years and engaged in high-risk behavior for contracting HIV, including sharing needles and "works," using "shooting galleries," and having unprotected sexual contacts. Successful methadone treatment was the major factor associated with the absence of HIV infection (65). Because of the high prevalence of infectious diseases (e.g., HIV/AIDS, hepatitis, tuberculosis) among methadone patients, many programs have developed research and service delivery systems to deal with the high numbers of infected patients. Staff with special training in HIV spectrum disease provide risk reduction education, distribute condoms, and assist with referrals to infectious disease clinics (see Chapter 58 "Medical Aspects of HIV Infection and Its Treatment in Injection Drug Users"). An increase in tuberculosis, especially treatment-resistant tuberculosis, among this group has resulted in tuberculosis case management projects including direct observation therapy (DOT), the provision of medications for prophylaxis and treatment (66,67). Some hospitals have developed specific methadone programs for HIV infection. At Montefiore Medical Center in the Bronx, research into the natural history of HIV disease among intravenous drug abusers has been ongoing.

Hepatitis C is now the most prevalent infectious disease among MMT patients with histories of intravenous drug use. The infection is usually acquired during the first year of injection. Therefore, it is estimated that the prevalence of hepatitis C among former injectors who are now in treatment is between 64% and 88% depending on the geographic location. Many clinics provide diagnostic services. However, patients are mostly referred to specialized services for ongoing treatment if the clinic is unable to provide it. In the 1980s AIDS was the major cause of death among methadone patients. However, by the late 1990s the death rate from AIDS stabilized and the death rate from hepatitis C had increased; eventually the death rate from hepatitis C may supersede that from AIDS (68).

EFFICACY OF METHADONE MAINTENANCE TREATMENT

Despite the differences in goals and policies among programs, methadone maintenance treatment has yielded consistently positive evaluations since it was implemented in 1964. To fully understand methadone treatment, the program goals "... to reduce illicit drug consumption and other criminal behavior and secondarily to improve productive social behavior and psychological well being" must be considered (69). As stated previously, when appropriate doses are provided, heroin use is markedly decreased or eliminated in most patients (70).

Alcohol and cocaine (crack and cocaine hydrochloride) have been and continue to be major substances of abuse among methadone maintenance patients. Alcohol in particular has been a major cause of death since the program's inception (71). With this increase in use, programs have begun investigating 12-step models, self-help programs, cognitive–behavioral therapy, relapse prevention, and harm reduction, as well as other pharmacotherapies and other modalities to address these serious problems.

In its review of methadone treatment programs, the General Accounting Office reported that in 1989, 14% of the patients in the programs surveyed had problems with cocaine or crack. In 8 of the programs, up to 40% of the patients used the drug, while in 16 programs, cocaine was used by 0% to 15% of the patients (20). In 2003, the New York State Office of Alcoholism and Substance Abuse reported that 35% of 16,179 patients reported cocaine or crack as a secondary substance of abuse upon admission to the program. This high prevalence of self-reported cocaine or crack abuse has led policy makers to criticize methadone maintenance treatment for failing to reduce these numbers. Yet studies suggest that the level of cocaine use decreases from time of admission. In the 1990s, Magura reported a decrease in cocaine use from 84% at admission to 66% after 6 months in treatment (72) in a population with an exceptionally high prevalence of cocaine use; Hartel et al. (32) report that prevalence of cocaine use is lower for those patients receiving more than 70 mg per day of methadone (35).

Prior to the increase in cocaine use and HIV infection, alcohol and the medical complications of alcoholism were the most serious problem found among methadone patients, affecting approximately 20% to 25% of the patients (71,73). Before 1986, medical conditions related to alcoholism were the major cause of mortality in methadone maintenance treatment. Studies also suggest that when patients leave methadone treatment, their drinking behavior increases, possibly to obtain relief from symptoms of narcotic craving without relapsing to the use of heroin. However, many patients used alcohol in conjunction with heroin prior to entering treatment (71). Also, because patients with alcohol and other drug problems were routinely admitted into methadone treatment, these problems had program implications and decreased positive treatment response.

Many studies have documented a substantial reduction in criminal behavior from pretreatment levels. Like most other treatment variables, reduction in criminal behavior increases with length of time in treatment. These trends have been consistent throughout the more than two decades of methadone treatment and in a variety of settings. In Hong Kong, after methadone was introduced in 1976, there was an 85% reduction in the number of heroin addicts sent to prisons during a 4-year period (74). In the study conducted in three northeastern cities, Ball and Ross (19) reported a 79% decrease in the number of crimes committed by patients during their first 6 months of treatment. The improvement in patients' behavior while in methadone treatment can be reflected in citywide statistics. From 1970 to 1973 the number of patients in methadone treatment in New York City increased by 20,000 to 34,000 patients. Reductions in citywide drug-related arrests, new cases of hepatitis, and drug-related mortality were reported.

Socially productive behavior as measured by employment, schooling, or homemaking also improves with length of time in treatment. During the first 15 years of methadone treatment in New York, employment rates were just below 60%. During the 1980s, when the employment market changed, cocaine and crack use increased, and homelessness and HIV infection rates increased, while social productivity and employment levels in New York declined to less than 40% in 1990 (75). A study of employed methadone patients in New York showed that they held positions across the spectrum of the job market, including lawyer, architect, musician, film producer, housewife, chef, construction worker, social worker, secretary, laborer, drivers, and doorman. There was no relationship between the nature of employment and dose or number of treatment episodes. Many of these successful patients had attempted to become abstinent, relapsed, and subsequently returned to methadone treatment to maintain their employment. For the majority of inner-city patients, lack of education, job skills, and child care, as well as unemployment and poverty, continue to have an adverse impact on socially productive behavior and treatment response.

Recent research has concluded that program characteristics are the critical factor in successful outcomes. In their study, Ball and Ross (19) opened what they call the "black box" of treatment, indicating that the major factor in outcome is the length of time in treatment. Factors that influence longer retention are adequate dose, well-trained staff, trusting and confidential relationships between the patients and program staff, clear policies and procedures, low staff turnover and high morale, flexible take-home policies, and other pertinent program characteristics. Although many clinicians consider abstinence as a critical treatment goal, it is problematic and difficult to attain for most patients. There is a high degree of consistency in the results of studies of patients who leave treatment. The majority of discharged patients revert to use of heroin, other illicit narcotics, and/or alcohol. Ball and Ross (19) found that 82% of the patients had relapsed to intravenous drug use after having been out of treatment for 10 months or more, with almost half (45.5%) relapsing after having been out of treatment for 1 to 3 months. Dole and Joseph (76) found that relapse occurred independently of patient variables such as ethnicity, gender, or education level. Older patients may substitute heavy alcohol use for heroin, and favorable outcome is associated with shorter duration of heroin use, longer duration of treatment, employment, and an absence of behavioral problems while in treatment. Withdrawal from treatment may have fatal consequences. Appel, Joseph, and Richman found that the death rate for discharged persons was more than twice those of patients still in treatment. The major difference in the causes of death between treatment and posttreatment is the sharp increase in narcotics-related deaths after leaving treatment. No evidence was found of narcotics-related deaths among properly stabilized patients during methadone treatment (68). However, this study was completed prior to the advent of the HIV epidemic. By 1986, AIDS had become the major cause of death among methadone patients in New York City programs (68).

Methadone maintenance treatment is cost-effective and beneficial to society. Rufener and colleagues (77) studied the cost effectiveness of methadone maintenance and other treatment modalities and yielded a benefit:cost ratio of 4.4:1. The most comprehensive examination of economic benefits and costs was performed on data from the Treatment Outcome Prospective Study (TOPS) (78). After examining the average cost of a treatment day, detailed measurements of rates of criminal activities, and the costs to society of various crimes, the study yielded a final benefit:cost ratio of 4:1. Using any of the studies, it is clear that methadone maintenance pays for itself on the first day it is delivered and that posttreatment effects are an economic bonus. These benefits accrue not only to the patient but to society in general.

SPECIAL ISSUES AND NEW TREATMENT APPROACHES

The current methadone maintenance system faces many problems in the United States. Numerous programs are publicly funded and have been subject to stigma, apathy, hostility, decreased funding, deteriorating physical facilities, high staff turnover, and community opposition to the opening and/or continued operation of clinics. Programs are now addressing many critical issues: loitering, diversion, and community concerns A particular problem is the lack of readily accessible treatment to people residing in suburban/rural areas as well as in cities where public transportation does not exist or is inadequate. Vans and pharmacies for dispensing are now being considered.

Funding, always problematic, needs to be secured for physical facilities as well as for ongoing operations. Programs have developed strategies to secure additional funding from agencies that did not traditionally fund drug treatment, such as HIV/AIDS service systems and social services agencies. New models of treatment and services are being developed and piloted to supplement existing program models. Service providers and funding and regulatory agencies must work cooperatively to improve treatment and seek solutions to existing problems. Provider coalitions on a state, national, and international basis can provide a forum for this to occur. Broad-based conferences can also serve to discuss, debate, and resolve concerns while serving as vehicles for the transfer of technology from researchers to clinicians.

To enhance the traditional outpatient methadone clinic, changing patient needs dictate that new and innovative approaches be piloted. Since the 1980s, several such efforts have been implemented. Some were developed specifically in response to HIV spectrum disease, as well as to hepatitis C and the mentally ill, chemically dependent patient, whereas others sought to provide innovative ways to expand or enhance programs.

To address homelessness and/or abuse of cocaine and other drugs, Short Stay, a residential short-stay methadone treatment program, was developed by the Lower East Side Service Center in New York for patients who were not functioning well (e.g., because of mental illness and substance abuse). Other residential programs, such as Samaritan and Promesa, provide methadone but they require tapering the dose over a 6-month period. Short Stay provides methadone maintenance and residential treatment while endeavoring to resolve the difficulties that interfered with adjustment to outpatient treatment. The program is usually 3 to 6 months in duration and the patient is returned to the patient's outpatient clinic after completion. Methadone dose is maintained throughout the program. Within the past 3 years, Project Renewal, a program that deals with issues of homelessness in New York City, developed a methadone residence within the New York Cityshelter system. Methadone patients are provided psychosocial services including assistance in finding housing. Although patients at this time receive methadone in designated outpatient clinics, a special shelter methadone-dispensing program is being planned for the homeless.

In New York City's Rikers Island Correctional Facility, the Key Extended Entry Program (KEEP) offers methadone maintenance treatment to narcotic-addicted inmates who request treatment upon incarceration. Eligible inmates are those with sentences of no more than 1 year who meet admission criteria. They are maintained while in jail and are referred to a community clinic where they are guaranteed continued treatment. Arrested methadone patients who meet KEEP criteria are maintained on methadone at their regular clinic dose and returned to their clinics upon release. This program involves the cooperation of the New York City Department of Corrections, the prison health services, and a network of community-based methadone treatment providers (79).

Methadone Medical Maintenance

Methadone medical maintenance (MMM) is the integration of socially rehabilitated methadone patients into general medical practice. They are not isolated in special clinics, as are regular maintenance and aftercare patients, but are treated by internists or other primary care physicians in a private practice setting, indistinguishable from other patients. This program was started in 1983 at The Rockefeller University by Drs. Dole, Nyswander, and Kreek. In 1985, 25 of their stable long-term methadone patients were transferred into the general medical practices of Drs. David Novick and Edwin A. Salsitz at Beth Israel Medical Center (80,81). As of July 2004 approximately 225 patients are enrolled in this ongoing project. However, in New York State, six other programs were developed based on the Beth Israel model, treating a total of approximately 400 patients. Two models have been to modified by allowing for dispensing of methadone in a commercial pharmacy and in a community primary care setting.

All patients have to meet the following criteria: 3 consecutive years of methadone treatment with employment or other socially productive activities, as well as absence of criminality, drug or alcohol abuse, and resources to store the medication safely. Patients with psychological and/or medical conditions should be in treatment for either with the medical maintenance physician or an appropriate specialist.

Patients are seen monthly or, if indicated, more frequently, if problems should arise. At the time of the office visit a urine toxicology is obtained, a 28-day or an appropriate supply of methadone diskets or tablets is dispensed, a dose of methadone is taken under observation by the physician, medical problems are treated and addressed, and other problems or issues are discussed. Most patients return every 28 days, or more frequently if problems should arise that need attention. Fees are collected at the time of the office visit. In the pharmacy project, the physician collects the urine and delivers the methadone order to the pharmacy either electronically or in person. The physician meets with the pharmacist once per month but remains in contact if changes in prescriptions are needed. The patient receives the methadone without observed ingestion but is subject to random call backs for counting of methadone tablets to assure quality control. Street ethnography observations by the New York State Office of Alcoholism and Substance Abuse Services have been made periodically to determine if methadone tablets are being diverted. After 1 year of operation the pharmacy unit has functioned without incident or division of tablets in the neighborhood. Call backs have shown that patients have managed their methadone supply as directed and prescribed by the physician.

The fee for MMM includes the office visit, the urinalysis, an annual physical, and the methadone. However, in the pharmacy program, the patient pays the pharmacy for the methadone.

MMM is the essential "next phase" of methadone treatment for socially rehabilitated patients. The methadone clinic system, with its controls, prevents some patients from developing their full potentials. These controls may be appropriate at the beginning of treatment but they become obstacles to further rehabilitating experiences, such as business opportunities, job-related and personnel travel, confidentiality issues, or the need to quickly change an appointment.

Furthermore, the MMM patient is removed from the clinic environment, away from patients who may present social and/or medical polydrug abuse and behavioral problems, into an office-based practice where these problems are no longer an issue. MMM physicians report that the personality profiles of MMM patients do not appear to be different than patients with other chronic medical conditions (26).

A 15-year followup study of 158 patients (81) showed that 83.5% of the patients had been compliant with the rules and regulations of the program. The projected median retention time for this group of patients was 13.8 years. Noncompliant patients (16.5%) were referred back to their clinics for failure to report as directed and abuse of cocaine/crack. Approximately 8% were able to successfully withdraw from methadone. Forty percent of the 20 deaths in MMM were caused by smoking-related medical conditions (8), the leading cause of death in this group. Other causes of death included hepatitis C (4), AIDS (3), cancer (1), brain aneurysm (1), meningitis (1) complications of morbid obesity (1) and homicide (1). Twelve compliant patients (8.2%) electively withdrew from methadone in good standing, and one compliant patient voluntarily returned to the clinic. Other factors were noted: A higher proportion of compliant patients were either married or lived in stable relationships than did noncompliant patients (68% vs. 46%, $p < 0.03$). A higher proportion of compliant patients had two or more admissions to convention methadone programs prior to being admitted to MMM (36% vs. 12%, $p < 0.002$). This may imply that compliant patients were committed to long-term methadone treatment since they had relapsed during previous episodes of methadone treatment. Noncompliant patients had significantly shorter periods of treatment in the traditional methadone clinics than did compliant patients prior to entrance into MMM (12.5 years vs. 15.8 years, $p < 0.02$). However, the patients who were able to successfully withdraw from methadone had an average of 17.7 years of methadone treatment in traditional clinics and MMM. Although not statistically significant, a clinical trend that was identified and should be investigated further is that those who were able to withdraw from methadone successfully had shorter histories of heroin use than other compliant patients (5.8 [standard deviation (SD) 3.6] years vs. 9.3 [SD 10.3] years). In 1988, the first 58 MMM patients were tested for HIV. All were HIV-negative, and none seroconverted. Prior to entry into methadone treatment, these patients had injected heroin daily, and approximately 90% had contracted hepatitis from use of contaminated needles. Successful adjustment in methadone treatment therefore appears to have had a protective effect HIV because these patients stopped use of heroin by injection after entering methadone treatment and did not contract HIV (26).

A survey of 80 medical maintenance patients treated by Dr. Edwin A Salsitz, director of the Beth Israel Medical Center, revealed 55% of patients had an undergraduate or graduate degree (26). Average family income was $62,000 (range: $12,000 to $400,000), mean duration of methadone treatment was 22 years (range: 8 to 30 years), and mean dose was 60 mg (range: 5 to 100 mg). There was no correlation between dose level, job description, or income level.

MMM is a proven method of methadone treatment. Physicians must be properly trained and not harbor the many and pervasive methadone myths. They must be flexible and sensitive to the patients' needs for confidentiality and changes of appointments. When referrals are made, contact must be made by the MMM physician with the consulting physician, or dentist to dispel misinformation and educate them about methadone treatment, possible drug interactions and to insure that patients receive proper pain management. MMM and office based prescribing of methadone has been established in New York, Oregon, Maryland, New Mexico, and California.

Stigma

Despite the years of favorable evaluations and research studies, methadone programs, their patients, and their staff are stigmatized by the general public, elected officials, treatment providers, the health care profession, social service agencies, the criminal justice system, and some outreach and harm-reduction programs. Methadone is misunderstood and misperceived as just "substituting one addiction for another." This is reflected in the lack of funding, the rejection of methadone maintenance as viable treatment and recovery, the undertreatment or no treatment of pain if patients are hospitalized for surgery or other painful procedures or medical conditions, and the inability to establish new programs because of community opposition. The stigma is pervasive and can carry over into everyday life and the relationships that patients have with their families, friends, employers, health care providers, and others. Patients may not tell spouses, other members of their families, or physicians and nurses who treat them that they are enrolled in methadone treatment. Entering into MMM may help to reduce the tensions and anxiety associated with the social stigma directed to methadone treatment because the patients' movements and confidentiality are less compromised. However, the social stigma still exists and affects the self-esteem of patients. Salsitz (26) reports that the stigma directed to methadone treatment is the most powerful destructive social force that patients face. Clinicians, both in the clinics and MMM, must support and educate patients and their families about the nature of addictive disease and the role of methadone as an effective medication that may be necessary for the duration of a patient's life. However, agencies that fund methadone programs and the programs themselves must undertake educational campaigns targeted to the general public, health professionals, the criminal justice system, and elected officials to dispel misunderstandings about methadone and to emphasize its important role in public health and the treatment of narcotic addiction (82).

Treatment Issues: Access, Expansion and Retention

Several models have been proposed and developed to address these issues. At the Albert Einstein College of Medicine in the Bronx, two such models are now being developed. One will attempt to provide culturally sensitive, family-centered treatment. The other model involves "front-loading" services to newly admitted patients, in an effort to mobilize intensive resources at the time of greatest need and to integrate the patient more fully into the treatment system. These models are examples of ways to enhance or expand treatment to meet current needs and to improve retention in treatment.

At present, methadone treatment programs in the United States treat approximately 15% to 20% of narcotics addicts at any given time The human and financial cost to society of more than 500,000 untreated narcotics addicts is a major public health problem. Mobile vans have been used in the Netherlands and in Boston to reach addicts where it has not been possible to establish permanent clinic sites. Such a strategy could be used to introduce treatment to shelters and other social service agencies directly serving addicted people. Pilot projects have been developed in California and New Mexico to expand the intake of untreated heroin addicts into treatment by using vans as clinics and dispensing units as well as community pharmacies working with private physicians to dispense methadone and become part of the treatment process.

Outreach and harm reduction workers themselves may harbor biases against methadone treatment and therefore, may not refer untreated addicts to treatment. Heroin addicts also harbor unfounded biases and myths about methadone treatment (e.g., rots the bones) and object to the regulations. Many do not have the necessary identification for entrance into treatment and benefits. Rosenblum, Magura, and Joseph reported that untreated addicts are ambivalent about methadone treatment because of misunderstandings about methadone and its use as a medication to treat addiction (30). These views and beliefs have adversely impacted on their decisions to enter and remain in treatment. Appel showed that in New York City, only 5% of untreated street addicts who are known to outreach services have entered treatment because of lack of identification for insurance, waiting lists, attitudes of treatment staff, police insensitivity, lack of housing, and child care issues (83).

A recent study by Goldstein et al. (83a) followed up 175 patients in East Harlem who had dropped out of methadone maintenance treatment. To participate, patients had to be 18 years of age or older, and had to have dropped out of treatment within the past 12 months. Participants were recruited through word of mouth and by seeking out those who had dropped out of treatment. The outreach workers who did the recruiting were familiar with the neighborhood. The patients were placed in one of three treatment conditions: (a) attending cognitive behavioral therapy sessions; (b) receiving only limited cognitive behavioral therapy; or (c) no intervention. All patients, if interested, were referred to methadone maintenance programs. In the cognitive–behavioral therapy group, 72% of patients returned to treatment. Among those who received limited therapy, 53% returned to treatment. In the no intervention group, 50% returned. The data were significant to the 0.005 level. This study suggests that patients who drop out of treatment will return to treatment provided they are followed up and given services, and that granting funding to individual methadone programs or a consortium of programs to employ outreach workers for this purpose would be beneficial. Such intervention would be cost-effective in terms of decreasing costs of criminal activity, incarceration, and the spread of communicable diseases such as HIV and hepatitis. Followup has been sorely lacking in this area, primarily because of funding. If meaningful expansion of treatment to be accomplished, efforts to overcome community concerns and opposition to the location of new clinics must be addressed. Community and political leaders must be educated to understand the public health value of expanded methadone treatment.

Methadone maintenance, as a chronic condition of long duration, does not fit in easily with recent changes in federal benefits. As a result, some states have "carved out" methadone treatment, while others have ignored or incorporated it into their managed care plans. These changes represent an additional challenge to providers to improve and expand treatment.

DIVERSION AND MORTALITY

On February 6, 2004, the Substance Abuse and Mental Health Services Administration (SAMHSA) reported at the Sixth International Pain and Chemical Dependency Conference in New York City, that the major source of methadone found in deaths where methadone is cited in autopsy reports across the United States is from sources outside the clinic system. The majority of deaths where methadone was identified at autopsy were polydrug abuse deaths involving other psychoactive substances. Although data remain incomplete, a National Assessment meeting attended in May 2003 "by state and federal experts including researchers, epidemiologists, medical examiners, coroners, pain management specialists, addiction medicine specialists, and others" recommended "creation of case definitions that would make a distinction between deaths caused by methadone and deaths in which methadone is a contributing factor or merely present." The panel noted that increasing numbers of prescriptions by physicians for methadone to treat pain "are paralleling the increase in prescriptions for oxycodone, hydrocodone, and morphine, as physicians prescribe to meliorate chronic pain." Therefore, the panel recommends the inclusion in health care curricula of information about the "diagnosis and treatment of addiction and appropriate pharmacotherapies for pain."

The panel is of the opinion that reports of methadone mentions in deaths "involve one of three scenarios:

- Illicitly obtained methadone used in excessive or repetitive doses in an attempt to achieve euphoric effects;
- Methadone, either licitly or illicitly obtained, used in combination with other prescription medication such as benzodiazepines (antianxiety medication), alcohol or other opioids;
- Or an accumulation of methadone to harmful serum levels in the first days of treatment for addiction or pain, before tolerance is developed."

Dr. H. Westley Clark, Director of the Center for Substance Abuse Treatment stated that "Methadone continues to be a safe, effective treatment for addiction to heroin or prescription pain killers. While deaths involving methadone increased, experiences in several states show that addiction treatment programs are not the culprits." (84)

SUMMARY AND CONCLUSION

When the Dole-Nyswander protocol and philosophy (11,14) are followed, methadone maintenance has proven to be a highly effective treatment and has been recognized throughout the world, as well the by National Institutes of Health and the Institute of Medicine. However, since the early years of methadone maintenance, many new social and health problems have emerged. These have had an adverse effect on methadone patients and the programs that treat them. HIV/AIDS, hepatitis C, problems of an aging patient population, homelessness, chronic unemployment, and destitution have placed methadone programs in the position of assuming ever-wider responsibilities (see Chapter 72 "The Homeless").

The frequency of clinic attendance by patients give programs the opportunity and the responsibility to provide the medical and social care that a chronic, debilitating and potentially terminal illness requires. Some programs are now moving in the direction of providing primary care with expanded social services for their patients in addition to methadone treatment. Patients are also educated about the transmission of infectious diseases and are either treated on site or referred to other facilities. Therefore, a quality methadone maintenance treatment program is one that continuously evaluates and assesses the changing needs of its patients and seeks to meet them to the best of its ability. The recession and economic volatility, including cuts in benefits beginning in the late 1990s, have made it mandatory for programs to seek new and creative funding. As the public currently demands programs that are cost-effective, it is important that programs develop the capability to evaluate and document their productivity and the improved status of their patients.

In conclusion, notwithstanding all of the social and medical challenges that methadone treatment has faced over the past 40 years, The Rockefeller University, in 2001, included methadone maintenance as 1 of 10 outstanding achievements developed at the university during its first century.

REFERENCES

1. Substance Abuse and Mental Health Services Administration (SAMHSA) Office of Applied Studies. *National survey of substance abuse treatment services (N-SSATS) data on substance abuse treatment facilities, DASIS Series: S-19.* DHHS publication no. (SMA) 03-3777. Rockville, MD: Substance Abuse and Mental Health Services Administration, 2002.
2. International Center for the Advancement of Addiction Treatment web site at: www.OpiateAddictionRx.info. Last accessed April 10, 2004.
3. Courtwright DT. *Dark paradise: opiate addiction in America before 1940.* Cambridge, MA: Harvard University Press, 1982.
4. Gewirtz PD. Notes and comments: methadone maintenance for heroin addicts. *Yale Law J* 1969;78:1175–1211.
5. Courtwright DT, Joseph H, Des Jarlais D. *Addicts who survived: an oral history of narcotic use in America, 1923–1965.* Knoxville: University of Tennessee Press, 1989.
6. Alksne H, Trussel RE, Elinson J, et al. *A follow-up study of treated adolescent narcotics users* [Mimeographed report]. New York: Columbia University School of Public Health and Administrative Medicine, 1959.
7. Report on drug addiction by the NY Academy of Medicine Committee on Public Health Subcommittee on Drug Addiction. *Bull NY Acad Med* August 1955;31(8):592–607.
8. Brecher EM. *Licit and illicit drugs: Consumers Union report on narcotics, stimulants, depressants, inhalants, hallucinogens, and marijuana.* Boston: Little Brown and Company, 1972.
9. Joseph H, Dole VP. Methadone patients on probation and parole. *Fed Prob* 1970 (June):42–48.
10. Nyswander ME. *The drug addict as a patient.* New York: Grune & Stratton, 1956.
11. Dole VP, Nyswander ME, Kreek MJ. Narcotic blockade. *Arch Intern Med* 1966;118:304–309.
12. Lowinson JH. The methadone maintenance research program. In: *Rehabilitating the narcotic addict.* Report of Institute on New Developments in the Rehabilitation of the Narcotic Addict, Fort Worth, TX, February 16-18, 1966. Sponsored jointly by the Division of Hospitals of the United States Public Health Service, Vocational Rehabilitation Administration, and Texas Christian University. Washington, DC: U.S. Government Printing Office, 1967:271–284.
13. Gearing FR, Schweitzer MD. An epidemiological evaluation of long-term methadone maintenance treatment for

heroin addiction. *Am J Epidemiol* 1974;100:101–112.

14. Dole VP, Nyswander ME. A medical treatment for diacetyl-morphine (heroin) addiction. *JAMA* 1965;193:646.

15. Goldstein A. Blind dosage comparisons and other studies in a large methadone program. *J Psychedelic Drugs* 1971; 4:177–181.

16. Jaffe JH. Further experience with methadone in the treatment of narcotic users. *Int J Addict* 1970;5:375–389.

17. New York Academy of Science, Committee on Public Health. Methadone management of heroin addiction. *Bull N Y Acad Med* 1990;46:391.

18. *Fed Reg* for methadone treatment 1972; 37:16790.

19. Ball JC, Ross A. *The effectiveness of methadone maintenance treatment.* New York: Springer-Verlag, 1991.

20. U.S. General Accounting Office. *Methadone maintenance: some treatment programs are not effective. Greater federal oversight needed.* Publication no. GAO/HRD-90-104, 1990. Washington, DC: U.S. Government Printing Office, 1990.

21. Goldstein A, Aronow L, Kalman S. *Principles of drug action: the clinical basis of pharmacology,* 2nd ed. New York: John Wiley, 1974.

22. Isbell H. Methods and results of studying experimental human addiction to the newer synthetic analgesics. *Ann N Y Acad Sci* 1948;51:108.

23. Isbell H, Vogel V. The addiction liability of methadone (Amidone, Dolophine, 10820) and its use in the treatment of the morphine abstinence syndrome. *Am J Psychiatry* 1949;105:909.

24. Dole VP. Methadone maintenance: optimizing dosage by estimating plasma level [Editorial]. *J Addict Dis* 1991;13(1):1–4.

25. Stimmel B, Kreek MJ. Neurobiology of addictive behaviors and its relationship to methadone maintenance. *Mt Sinai J Med* 2000;67(5&6):375–380. Available at: www.mssm.edu/msjournal.

26. Salsitz EA, Joseph H, Frank B, et al. Methadone medical maintenance: treating chronic opioid dependence in private medical practice—a summary report. *Mt Sinai J Med* 2000;67(5&6):388–397. Available at: www.mssm.edu/msjournal.

27. Galynker EE, Watras-Ganz S, Miner C, et al. Cerebral metabolism in opiate-dependent subjects: effects of methadone maintenance. *Mt Sinai J Med* 2000;67(5&6):381–387. Available at: www.mssm.edu/msjournal.

28. Kreek MJ. Plasma and urine levels of methadone. *N Y State J Med* 1973;73:2773–2777.

29. Goldsmith DS, Hunt DE, Lipton DS, et al. Methadone folklore: beliefs about side effects and their impact on treatment. *Hum Organ* 1984;43(4):330–340.

30. Rosenblum AR, Magura S, Joseph H. Ambivalence towards methadone treatment among intravenous drug users. *J Psychoactive Drugs* 1991;23(1):21–27.

31. Hartel D, Selwyn PA, Schoenbaum EE, et al. *Methadone maintenance treatment and reduced risk of AIDS and AIDS-specific mortality in intravenous drug users* [Abstract 8526]. Paper presented at the Fourth International Conference on AIDS, Stockholm, Sweden, June, 1988.

32. Hartel D, Schoenbaum EE, Selwyn PA, et al. *Temporal patterns of cocaine use and AIDS in intravenous drug users in methadone maintenance* [Abstract]. Paper presented at the Fifth International Conference on AIDS, Montreal, Canada, June, 1989.

33. Hartel D. Cocaine use, inadequate methadone dose increase risk of AIDS for IV drug users in treatment. *NIDA Notes* 1989/1990; 5(1).

34. Caplehorn JRM, Bell J. Methadone dosage and retention of patients in maintenance treatment. *Med J Aust* 1991;154:195–199.

35. Kreek MJ. *Methadone maintenance for harm reduction.* Paper presented at the International Symposium on Addiction and AIDS, Vienna, Austria, February, 1991.

36. Kreek MJ. Rationale for maintenance pharmacotherapy of opiate dependence. In: O'Brien CP, Jaffe JH, eds. *Addictive states. Research publications: Association for Research in Nervous and Mental Disease.* New York: Raven Press, 1992;70:210.

37. Cooper JR. Ineffective use of psychoactive drugs—methadone treatment is no exception. *JAMA* 1992;267(2):281–282.

38. D'Aunno T, Vaughn TE. Variations in methadone treatment practices result from a national study. *JAMA* 1992;267(2):253–258.

39. Gossop M, Bradley B, Phillips GT. An investigation of withdrawal symptoms shown by opiate addicts during and subsequent to a 21-day in-patient methadone detoxification procedure. *Addict Behav* 1987;12:1–6.

40. Institute of Medicine. Treatment standards and optimal treatment. In: Rettig RA, Yarmolinsky A, eds. *Federal regulation of methadone treatment.* Washington, DC: National Academy Press, 1995:185–216.

41. Payte JT, Khuri ET. Principles of methadone dose determination. In: *State methadone treatment guidelines.* Center for Substance Abuse Treatment, Treatment Improvement Protocol Series 1991;1:47–58.

42. American Society of Addiction Medicine (ASAM). *American Society of Ad-*

diction Medicine policy statement on methadone treatment. Washington, DC: Author, 1991.

43. Magura S, Rosenblum A. Leaving methadone treatment: lessons learned, lessons forgotten, lessons ignored. *Mt Sinai J Med* 2001;68(1):62–74.

44. Borg L, Ho A, Peters JE, et al. Availability of reliable serum methadone determination for management of symptomatic patients. *J Addict Dis* 1995;14(3):83–96.

45. Dole VP. Implications of methadone maintenance for theories of narcotic addiction. *JAMA* 1988;260:3025–3029.

46. Loimer N, Schmid R. The use of plasma levels to optimize methadone maintenance treatment. *Drug Alcohol Depend* 1992;30(3):241.

47. Loimer N, Schmid R, Grunberger J, et al. Psychophysiological reactions in methadone maintenance patients do not correlate with methadone plasma levels. *Psychopharmacology (Berl)* 1991;103(4):538.

48. Gotsis CA. Personal communication, 1991.

49. Kreek MJ. Drug interactions with methadone. *Ann N Y Acad Sci* 1976;281: 350–371.

50. Kreek MJ. Medical complications in methadone patients. *Ann N Y Acad Sci* 1978;311:29,110–134.

51. Kreek MJ. Opiate-ethanol interactions: implications for the biological basis of treatment of combined addictive diseases. *NIDA Res Monogr* 1987;81:428–439.

52. Langrod J, Lowinson J, Ruiz P. Methadone treatment and physical complaints: a clinical analysis. *Int J Addict* 1981;16(5):947–952.

53. Babst DV, Newman S, Gordon NB, et al. *Driving records of methadone maintained patients in New York State.* New York State OASAS and the Rockefeller University. 1973, New York City.

54. Appel PW, Gordon NB. Digit-symbol performance in methadone-treated ex-heroin addicts. *Am J Psychiatry* 1976;133:1337–1340.

55. Blumberg RD, Pruesser DF. *Drug abuse and driving performance. Final report.* Control DOT-HS-009–1–184. Washington, DC: U.S. Department of Transportation, 1972.

56. Gordon NB. Influence of narcotic drugs on highway safety. *Accid Anal Prev* 1976;8:3–7.

57. Gordon NB, Lipset JS. *Intellectual and functional status of methadone patients after nearly ten years of treatment. Internal report.* The Rockefeller University and New York State Office of Drug Abuse Services. Presented at the 85th annual convention of the American Psychological Association, Washington, DC, September 5, 1976.

58. Moskowitz H, Sharma S. *Skills performance in methadone patients and ex-addicts*. Paper presented at the annual meeting of the American Psychological Association, New York City, September 5, 1979.

59. Novick DM, Joseph H, Croxson TS, et al. Absence of antibody to human immunodeficiency virus in long-term, socially rehabilitated methadone maintenance patients. *Arch Intern Med* 1990;150:97–99.

60. McLellan AT, Woody GE, Luborsky L, Goehl L. Is the counselor an "active ingredient" in substance abuse rehabilitation? An examination of treatment success among four counselors. *J Nerv Ment Dis* 1988;176:423–430.

61. Lowinson JH. Commonly asked clinical questions about methadone maintenance. *Int J Addict* 1977;12:821.

62. Lowinson JH, Millman RB. Clinical aspects of methadone maintenance treatment. In: Dupont R, Goldstein A, O'Donnell J, eds. *Handbook on drug abuse*. Washington, DC: National Institute on Drug Abuse, 1979:49–56.

63. Lowinson JH. Methadone maintenance in perspective. In: Lowinson JH, Ruiz P, eds. *Substance abuse: clinical problems and perspectives*. Baltimore: Williams & Wilkins, 1981:344–354.

64. Blix O, Gronbladh L. AIDS and IV heroin addicts: the preventive effect of methadone maintenance in Sweden. In: *Programs and abstracts of the Fourth International Conference on AIDS, June 12–16, 1988, Stockholm, Sweden*.

65. Novick DM, Ochshorn M, Ghail V, et al. Natural killer activity and lymphocyte subsets in parenteral heroin abusers and long term methadone maintenance patients. *J Pharmacol Exp Ther* 1989;250:606–610.

66. Division of Substance Abuse of the Albert Einstein College of Medicine of Yeshiva University, New York City. *Annual report*. 1989.

67. Joseph H, Springer E. Methadone maintenance treatment and the AIDS epidemic. In: Platt JJ, Kaplan CD, McKim PJ, eds. *The effectiveness of drug abuse treatment: Dutch and American perspectives*. Malabar, FL: Robert E. Krieger, 1990:261–274.

68. Appel PW, Joseph H, Richamn B. Causes and rates of death among methadone maintenance patients before and after the onset of the HIV/AIDS epidemic. *Mt Sinai J Med* 2000;57(5&6):444–451. Available at: www.mssm.edu/msjournal.

69. Committee for the Substance Abuse Coverage Study, Division of Health Care Services, Institute of Medicine. The effectiveness of treatment. In: Gerstein DR, Harwood HJ, eds. *Treating drug problems*. Washington, DC: National Academy Press, 1990;1:132–199.

70. Joseph H, Stancliff S, Langrod J. Methadone maintenance treatment: a review of historical and clinical issues. *Mt Sinai J Med* 2000;67(5&6):347–364.

71. Joseph H, Appel P. Alcoholism and methadone treatment: consequences for the patient and the program. *Am J Drug Alcohol Issues* 1985;11(1&2):37–53.

72. Magura S, Siddiqi Q, Freeman R, et al. *Changes in cocaine use after entry to methadone treatment* [Mimeographed report]. New York: Narcotic and Drug Research, 1991.

73. Bickel WK, Marion I, Lowinson J. The treatment of alcoholic methadone patients: a review. *J Subst Abuse Treat* 1987;4:15–19.

74. Joseph H. The criminal justice system and opiate addiction: a historical perspective. *NIDA Res Monogr* 1988;86:106–125.

75. Armstrong G. *Methadone programs: a snapshot*. Report prepared for the New York State Office of Alcoholism and Substance Abuse Services (OASAS), 1990, New York City.

76. Dole VP, Joseph H. Long-term outcome of patients treated with methadone maintenance. *Ann N Y Acad Sci* 1978;311:181–189.

77. Rufener BL, Rachal JV, Cruze AM. *Management effectiveness measures for NIDA drug abuse treatment programs. Cost benefit analysis*. DHEW publication no. (ADM) 77–423. Rockville, MD: National Institute on Drug Abuse, 1977.

78. Harwood HJ, Hubbard RL, Collins JJ, et al. The costs of crime and the benefits of drug abuse treatment: a cost-benefit analysis using TOPS data. *NIDA Res Monogr* 1988;86:209–235.

79. Tomasino V, Swanson AJ, Nolan J, et al. The Key Extended Entry Program (KEEP): a methadone treatment program for opiate-dependent inmates. *Mt Sinai J Med* 2001;68(1):14–20.

80. Novick DM, Pascarelli EF, Joseph H, et al. Methadone maintenance patients in general medical practice: a preliminary report. *JAMA* 1988;259:3299–3302.

81. Novick DM, Joseph H, Salsitz EA, et al. Outcomes of treatment of socially rehabilitated methadone maintenance patients in physicians' offices (medical maintenance): follow-up at three and a half to nine and a fourth years. *J Gen Intern Med* 1994;9(3):127–130.

82. Joseph H. *Methadone Medical Maintenance: the further concealment of a stigmatized condition* [Dissertation]. New York: Library of the Graduate Center of the City University of New York, 1995.

83. *Bureaucracy and insurance issues contributing to low enrollment in treatment among New York City's injection drug users* [News release]. Available at: www.saprp.org/MediaResources/NewsReleases/Appe1040104.htm. Last accessed April 10, 2004.

83a. Goldstein MF, Deren S, Kang SY, et al. Evaluation of an alternative program for MMTP drop-outs: impact on treatment re-entry. *Drug Alcohol Depend* 2002;66(2):181–187.

84. SAMHSA. Methadone deaths not linked to misuse of methadone from treatment centers [News release]. Available at: www.samhsa,gov/news/newsreleases/040206nr_deaths.htm. (Last accessed July, 2004.)

85. Tong TG, Pond SM, Kreek MJ, et al. Phenytoin-induced methadone withdrawal. *Ann Intern Med* 1981;94(3):349–351.

86. Liu SJ, Wang RI. Case report of barbiturate- induced enhancement of methadone metabolism and withdrawal syndrome. *Am J Psychiatry* 1988;141:1287–1288.

87. Kuhn KL, Halikas JA, Kemp KD. Carbamazepine treatment of cocaine dependence in methadone maintenance patients with dual opiate-cocaine addiction. *NIDA Res Monogr* 1989;95:316–317.

88. Zweben JE, Payte JT. Methadone maintenance in the treatment of opioid dependence: a current perspective. *West J Med* 1990;152(5):588–599.

SUGGESTED READINGS

Cushman P. Ten years of methadone maintenance treatment: some clinical observations. *Am J Drug Alcohol Abuse* 1977;4:543–553.

Fed Reg[FES10] 1970;35:9013.

Fed Reg 21 CFR, part 21. Washington, DC: Food and Drug Administration, March 2, 1989.

Joseph H, ed. *Methadone symposium. Mt Sinai J Med* 2000;67(5&6 and 2001;68(1). Available at: www.mssm.edu/msjournal.

Kreek MJ. Presentation at 1988 meeting of the Committee on Problems of Drug Dependence. *NIDA Notes* 1988(Fall):12, 25.

Stimmel B, Goldberg J, Rotkopf E. Ability to remain abstinent after methadone maintenance detoxification. A six-year study. *JAMA* 1977;237:1216–1220.

CHAPTER 40

Buprenorphine for the Treatment of Opioid Addiction

PAUL J. FUDALA AND CHARLES P. O'BRIEN

There are a number of effective pharmacotherapies currently available for the treatment of opioid addiction and they are discussed in other chapters of this volume. They include opioid agonists (e.g., methadone, levo-alpha-acetylmethadol), an opioid antagonist (naltrexone), and centrally acting α-adrenergic agonists (clonidine, lofexidine). Recently, however, another medication that is changing the direction of addiction treatment has been made available, and it may represent the most important advance in addiction medicine since the introduction of methadone substitution pharmacotherapy approximately 40 years ago. That medication is buprenorphine. It has a unique pharmacologic profile and, in the United States (as it has been in other countries since its introduction), it will be made available to patients in a manner unlike previous maintenance medications such as methadone or LAAM.

OVERVIEW OF PHARMACODYNAMICS, PHARMACOLOGY, AND PHARMACOKINETICS

Buprenorphine, a derivative of the morphine alkaloid thebaine (1), has been available in numerous countries as an analgesic for parenteral and sublingual administration since the 1970s, and a parenteral dosage form has been available in the United States since the early 1980s. As an analgesic, buprenorphine is approximately 25 to 50 times more potent than morphine (2–4). Typically, 0.3 mg of buprenorphine is considered to produce analgesia approximately equivalent to 10 mg of morphine when both medications are given parenterally.

Unlike methadone and LAAM, which can be characterized as full μ-opioid agonists, buprenorphine may be described as a partial agonist (5). That is, buprenorphine produces submaximal effects relative to those produced by full μ-opioid agonists when a maximally effective dose of buprenorphine is given. While this description does not detail the molecular mechanisms involved in the drug's actions, it does provide a basis for understanding the potential utility and limitations of using buprenorphine as an opioid-addiction treatment medica-

tion. Although buprenorphine has a high affinity for the μ-opioid receptor, it also has a low intrinsic activity (6,7). This high affinity makes buprenorphine extremely difficult to displace from the receptor by opioid antagonists; the clinical implications of this is discussed later in the Safety section of this chapter. Furthermore, buprenorphine dissociates very slowly from the receptor and it is very lipophilic (8,9), both factors contributing to the relatively long duration of activity of buprenorphine. Buprenorphine also binds with high affinity to the κ-opioid receptor but functions there as an antagonist (10–12). Buprenorphine binding at other receptor types has also been demonstrated (7,13), but it is its activity at the μ and κ receptors that is associated with its unique and often complex pharmacologic profile.

Buprenorphine has poor oral bioavailability (14), less than 10% compared to that when given intravenously. This is secondary to extensive gastrointestinal and hepatic metabolism (15). The primary metabolite of buprenorphine is norbuprenorphine, which, being a more polar compound, is associated with less penetration into the central nervous system (16). Buprenorphine and norbuprenorphine also form glucuronide conjugates. Given the low oral bioavailability of buprenorphine, and a concern that a parenteral dosage form should not be used for the treatment of opioid addicts (so as not to reinforce injection-associated behaviors), the sublingual route of administration has generally been considered to be the most appropriate for opioid-addiction treatment.

Initially, in many clinical studies assessing the safety and efficacy of buprenorphine, a sublingual solution was used. This solution was commonly formulated to contain 30% or 40% ethanol secondary to buprenorphine's poor solubility in a totally aqueous medium. The bioavailability of this solution typically has been reported to be between 30% and 50% (17–19). However, there are many factors that could make a hydroalcoholic solution impractical for general use. These include concerns regarding storage requirements and ease (or lack thereof) of dispensing, as well as potential diversion and illicit use.

To obviate these concerns, two sublingual buprenorphine tablet formulations were developed—one containing only buprenorphine and one containing a combination of buprenorphine and naloxone in a 4:1 ratio (to reduce its potential for diversion and illicit use). The bioavailability of the buprenorphine tablet has been reported to be approximately 50% to 65% (20,21) compared to the sublingual solution. Naloxone itself has poor sublingual bioavailability (22). Thus, when taken sublingually as directed, naloxone will not interfere with the therapeutic effects of buprenorphine. However, when taken parenterally by opioid-dependent individuals, the naloxone component may be expected to produce signs and symptoms characteristic of opioid withdrawal.

DEVELOPMENT OF BUPRENORPHINE AS A TREATMENT FOR OPIOID ADDICTION

The results of a clinical study published in 1978 by Jasinski and his coworkers (23) fostered interest in, and suggested the utility of, buprenorphine for the treatment of opioid addiction. Subsequent studies generally confirmed the initial observations regarding the potential effectiveness of buprenorphine by providing evidence for its patient acceptability, ability to substitute for and block the effects of other opioids, safety, and its utility in maintaining individuals in treatment.

Findings from a number of studies indicate that buprenorphine can substitute for other opioids and decrease illicit opioid use. In one of the first clinical pharmacology investigations, Mello and her colleagues (24) reported the results from an inpatient study in which individuals maintained on placebo or buprenorphine could make operant responses to earn money or receive intravenous heroin; those receiving buprenorphine took significantly less heroin. Over the next 20 years, numerous clinical laboratory and treatment–research studies, conducted in a variety of settings over varying periods of time and using various schedules of buprenorphine administration, provided evidence that buprenorphine can be used effectively and safely as an opioid-substitution pharmacotherapy (for reviews see references 25 to 32).

Demonstration of the efficacy and safety of buprenorphine for opioid-addiction treatment comes from three basic types of clinical trials: (a) comparisons of buprenorphine to other opioid agonists used for treatment (methadone and LAAM), (b) comparisons of buprenorphine to placebo, and (c) studies providing buprenorphine dose–response data. It must be pointed out that most of the trials were conducted using a sublingual liquid formulation of buprenorphine, not the sublingual tablet formulation of buprenorphine (or buprenorphine-naloxone) that is currently approved for use. Nonetheless, without reviewing in detail each of the trials, certain general observations can be discussed.

It is likely that the maximum agonist effects from higher therapeutic dosages of buprenorphine (approximately 8 mg per day of the sublingual liquid or 16 mg per day of the sublingual tablet) is likely to be comparable to methadone dosages no higher than about 60 mg per day (33–38). As a partial agonist, the effects of buprenorphine are dose-dependent within a limited range, above which increasing doses to not produce corresponding increases in effect. Thus patients who have been maintained on higher dosages of methadone (or corresponding dosages of LAAM) may not be good candidates for buprenorphine treatment. Buprenorphine, however, was not developed to replace methadone and LAAM, but rather to provide a treatment alternative for patients and clinicians who could not or would not consider treatment with one of the other available therapies. Furthermore, the same μ-opioid, partial-agonist profile that provides a ceiling to the therapeutic effects of buprenorphine also provides for a greater safety margin for buprenorphine as discussed later in the Safety section of this chapter.

Patients initiating treatment may be inducted onto therapy using either buprenorphine or the buprenorphine-naloxone combination. Consideration should be given to the type of opioid the patient has been abusing (e.g., heroin, morphine, methadone), the time since the patient last used opioids, and the current level of the patient's opioid addiction. Generally, the induction process will be easier in patients using shorter-acting (e.g., heroin) than in those using longer-acting (e.g., methadone, LAAM) opioids; patients experiencing mild withdrawal symptoms will be easier to induct than those who aren't and who have recently (i.e., within the last 4 to 6 hours) used other opioids; and patients with lower levels of addiction will be easier to induct than those with higher levels. Initial doses of buprenorphine will typically range from 4 to 8 mg per day (i.e., 4/1 to 8/2 mg per day of the buprenorphine-naloxone combination). Administering the first day's dosage as two or three individual doses may also be useful. Dosages on subsequent days are then gradually increased to the desired level. For patients transferring to buprenorphine therapy who have been actively maintained on methadone or LAAM, lowering the dose of that medication to the equivalent of no more than 30 to 40 mg per day of methadone will also facilitate a smooth transition onto buprenorphine. For individuals maintained on higher doses of methadone, the use of adjunct medications (e.g., clonidine, oxazepam) while rapidly reducing the daily methadone dosage (39), or administering the first dose of buprenorphine more than 24 hours following the last methadone dose (40), may be useful.

Although buprenorphine has been used effectively to substitute for other opioids and to suppress the development of opioid withdrawal signs and symptoms, its partial agonist properties are also responsible for its potential to precipitate an opioid withdrawal syndrome under certain conditions. This precipitated withdrawal phenomenon has been observed or suggested by both preclinical (2,3,41–43) and clinical studies (44,45). It may not always be clear in clinical situations, however, whether withdrawal symptomatology is a result of an insufficient or excessive dosage of buprenorphine being administered. Furthermore, for patients being maintained on high dosages of methadone or LAAM, or addicts using large amounts of heroin or other opioids, there may not be a dosage of buprenorphine that will fully substitute for the other opioid drug. The administration of buprenorphine to these individuals may result in the production of significant opioid withdrawal effects.

Of particular interest with respect to substitution therapy with buprenorphine has been its long duration of action. It was reported in some of the initial studies that at sufficient doses, buprenorphine could be effectively administered once daily (46–48). Those findings were subsequently supported by results from numerous clinical trials. Later studies indicated that alternate-day, or even less-frequent dosing was possible (49–64). However, given the permissibility of buprenorphine take-home dosing (discussed in "Office-Based Treatment with Buphrenorphine and Buprenorphine-naloxone" section), the desirability or necessity for less than once-daily dosing is likely to be minimal.

POTENTIAL FOR ABUSE

It is obvious that a medication must be acceptable to the targeted treatment population if it is to be effective, and studies assessing the utility of buprenorphine as a treatment agent for opioid addiction have provided evidence of its acceptability. Subjects have reported "liking" buprenorphine and have reported opioid-like effects following its administration (24,46,47,65,66). These "positive" subjective effects may be important for initiating and maintaining individuals on buprenorphine.

However, as is true for methadone and LAAM, buprenorphine should be considered to have a potential for abuse. In various drug-discrimination paradigms, buprenorphine has been discriminated by human subjects to be one of various opioid agonists or agonist–antagonists (67–70). In a controlled clinical trial (71), intravenously administered buprenorphine was associated with positive subjective effects in individuals not dependent on opioids and, in another (72), buprenorphine was self-administered by individuals who were not opioid-dependent. The former also indicated that the effects of buprenorphine were not consistently dose-related, consonant with buprenorphine's partial agonist profile. Results from other studies (45,73,74) that assessed the effects of buprenorphine in methadone-maintained patients suggest that buprenorphine would have a limited potential for abuse in these individuals, and that the time of buprenorphine administration relative to that of the last methadone dose may be an important determinant of buprenorphine's subjective effects.

As mentioned previously, the combining of naloxone with buprenorphine is expected to reduce the abuse liability of buprenorphine used clinically. Support for this assertion has been obtained from studies (22,73,75–81) using various ratios of buprenorphine to naloxone (e.g., 2:1, 4:1, and 8:1), various subject populations (e.g., non-dependent, methadone-maintained, morphine-stabilized), and various routes of buprenorphine-naloxone administration (e.g., sublingual, intramuscular). Furthermore, a number of studies provide evidence that the naloxone component will not interfere with the therapeutic effectiveness of buprenorphine (82–84).

Since 1983 (85), reports of buprenorphine abuse have come from various countries (86–99), although its relative availability and the availability of licit and illicit alternatives needs to be taken into account when interpreting these reports. Thus, buprenorphine abuse has often been associated with a lower cost and more ready availability than other opioid alternatives.

SAFETY

The use of buprenorphine has not been associated with an adverse effect profile that would appear to limit its utility as an opioid-addiction pharmacotherapy. Adverse effects reported following the administration of buprenorphine for opioid addiction treatment have included primarily sedation, drowsiness, and constipation, and other effects typical of μ-opioid agonists in general (71,100–102). Tolerance to these effects can be expected to develop during continued buprenorphine therapy. The safety of buprenorphine is, like its pharmacodynamic profile, related to its partial agonist properties. In particular, the potential for severe drug-induced respiratory depression, a concern for medications such as methadone and LAAM, as well as drugs primarily used illicitly, such as heroin, does not appear to be a relevant concern for buprenorphine. Even 32 mg of buprenorphine administered sublingually (approximately 70 times higher, corrected for differences in bioavailability, than a 0.3-mg analgesic dose given intramuscularly) produced only marginal effects on respiratory function in individuals not dependent on opioids (49), and 12 mg given intravenously (also in individuals who were not opioid-addicted) was shown to have a high margin of safety (103).

The high affinity of buprenorphine for the μ-opioid receptor would also render usual therapeutic doses of naloxone or nalmefene ineffective in the management of respiratory depression secondary to that which might be seen following an overdose of buprenorphine; doses of naloxone ranging from 10 to 35 mg per 70 kg could be required (104,105). Furthermore, buprenorphine has a longer duration of action and greater μ-opioid receptor affinity than either naloxone or nalmefene, such that mechanical support of respiration could be required in an overdose situation (106).

Deaths have been reported when buprenorphine has been combined with other drugs, particularly central nervous system depressants such as benzodiazepines (107–110). These reports come from France, where buprenorphine was approved for use in 1996 and where more patients have received buprenorphine therapy than have in any other country. In these cases, buprenorphine tablets typically have been pulverized and then administered intravenously.

Buprenorphine is widely available in France with minimal regulatory constraints upon its use (111–113).

However, even with fewer restrictions placed on buprenorphine compared to methadone treatment, buprenorphine appears to be a safe alternative to methadone. From 1994 to 1998, there were an estimated 1.4 times more buprenorphine-related deaths than methadone-related deaths in France (107). However, for each of those years (except for 1994 when no deaths were reported), the calculated death rate was always *higher* (ranging from 3.5 to 30 times higher) for methadone than for buprenorphine. Considering 1998, for example, the latest year for which data were available, buprenorphine was associated with slightly more than three times the number of deaths (13 compared to 4 for methadone), but there were more than 10 times as many patients receiving buprenorphine (55,000) compared to methadone (5,360).

In addition to the obvious drug interactions that may occur when buprenorphine is combined with central nervous system depressants, other potential interactions may occur with medications that either induce or inhibit cytochrome P450 3A4, which catalyzes the dealkylation of buprenorphine to norbuprenorphine (15,114). Because patients receiving buprenorphine may also be human immunodeficiency virus (HIV)-positive, potential interactions of buprenorphine with anti-HIV medications is a concern. Although a recent *in vitro* study indicated that ritonavir (Norvir), saquinavir (Fortovase), and indinavir (Crixivan) (all HIV protease inhibitors) competitively inhibited the metabolism of buprenorphine (115), another study did not indicate that buprenorphine influenced viral load in patients receiving highly active antiretroviral therapy (116).

OFFICE-BASED TREATMENT WITH BUPRENORPHINE AND BUPRENORPHINE-NALOXONE

Since methadone substitution therapy was developed in the 1960s by Dole and Nyswander (117), methadone has become the prototypical pharmacotherapy for opioid addiction treatment. LAAM, also a μ-opioid agonist, is pharmacologically similar to methadone but is administered on an alternate-day or three-times-weekly schedule, rather than daily (118). In the United States, both medications are Schedule II substances under the Controlled Substances Act and can only be used in a strictly regulated environment. Thus the medications are taken under direct observation or with limited privileges for take-home dosing. Regulations also govern treatment eligibility criteria, administrative oversight, requirements for mandatory urine testing of participants, and how the medications are to be stored and secured.

Unfortunately, while born from concerns related to the possible diversion and illicit use of the treatment medications, the regulations governing methadone and LAAM treatment also serve as barriers to treatment for certain individuals. Some individuals will not qualify for treatment because they do not meet regulatory criteria. Others may not live within a reasonable proximity to a "methadone clinic." Others who could qualify for treatment do not present themselves for it secondary to real or perceived fears regarding the medications themselves. Still others have attempted treatment and failed, sometimes on multiple occasions.

From the standpoint of many clinicians and patients, both regulatory reform and enhanced treatment options were necessary. Some regulatory reform regarding the existing federal regulations covering the use of methadone and LAAM has recently been adopted (119). An important part of this reform was a liberalization of the take-home dosing policies for methadone, and an allowing of take-home dosing for LAAM. More dramatic, however, was federal legislation that can literally mainstream addiction treatment and may substantially increase the availability and accessibility of opioid-addiction treatment.

In October, 2000, Public Law 106-310, the Children's Health Act of 2000, became effective. A part of that law, the Drug Addiction Treatment Act of 2000 (DATA), allows qualified physicians to prescribe medications in Schedule III, IV, or V as part of office-based maintenance or detoxification treatment for opioid addiction. Physicians must also have the capacity to refer patients for counseling and other appropriate ancillary services, and no more than 30 patients may be treated by an individual physician at any one time. Furthermore, individual states may not preclude clinicians from prescribing or dispensing these medications unless a particular state specifically enacts a law prohibiting such activity.

Both buprenorphine and the buprenorphine-naloxone combination are currently in Schedule III, and thus may be used for opioid-addiction treatment under DATA. Recent clinical trials of buprenorphine and buprenorphine-naloxone sublingual tablets in an office-based setting have shown buprenorphine to be effective and safe in the study paradigms (82–84). In a smaller study, buprenorphine given as a sublingual solution also was associated with more favorable outcomes in an office-based than in a clinic-based treatment environment (120). There are numerous potential advantages regarding the use of office-based addiction treatment including expansion of treatment availability, better matching of treatment services to individual needs, minimizing the stigma that often accompanies drug addition and its treatment, and limiting patients' contact with other drug-addicted and substance-abusing individuals (121,122).

CONCLUSIONS

Buprenorphine is a safe and effective treatment for opioid addiction. Its partial agonist character makes it a potentially safer medication than methadone or LAAM, particularly with regards to drug-induced respiratory depression. The combination product containing buprenorphine and naloxone is expected to decrease the abuse liability of buprenorphine yet provide comparable efficacy. Importantly, buprenorphine and buprenorphine-naloxone may be used for addiction treatment in office-based settings, thereby likely increasing the availability and accessibility of opioid-addiction treatment.

REFERENCES

1. Heel RC, Brogden RN, Speight TM, et al. Buprenorphine: a review of its pharmacological properties and therapeutic efficacy. *Drugs* 1979;17:81–110.
2. Cowan A, Doxey JC, Harry EJ. The animal pharmacology of buprenorphine, an oripavine analgesic agent. *Br J Pharmacol* 1977;60:547–554.
3. Cowan A, Lewis JW, Macfarlane IR. Agonist and antagonist properties of buprenorphine, a new antinociceptive agent. *Br J Pharmacol* 1977;60:537–545.
4. Houde RW. Analgesic effectiveness of the narcotic agonist-antagonists. *Br J Cin Pharmacol* 1979;7:297S–308S.
5. Martin WR, Eades CG, Thompson JA, et al. The effects of morphine- and nalorphine-like drugs in the nondependent and morphine-dependent chronic spinal dog. *J Pharmacol Exp Ther* 1976;197:517–532.
6. Villiger JW, Taylor KM. Buprenorphine: high-affinity binding to dorsal spinal cord. *J Neurochem* 1982;38:1771–1773.
7. Villiger JW, Taylor KM. Buprenorphine: characteristics of binding sites in the rat central nervous system. *Life Sci* 1981;29:2699–2708.
8. Tallarida RJ, Cowan A. The affinity of morphine for its pharmacologic receptor *in vivo*. *J Pharmacol Exp Ther* 1982;222:198–201.
9. Boas RA, Villiger JW. Clinical actions of fentanyl and buprenorphine. The significance of receptor binding. *Br J Anaesth* 1985;57:192–196.
10. Leander JD. Buprenorphine is a potent kappa-opioid receptor antagonist in pigeons and mice. *Eur J Pharmacol* 1988;151:457–461.
11. Leander JD. Buprenorphine has potent kappa opioid receptor antagonist activity. *Neuropharmacology* 1987;26:1445–1447.
12. Richards ML, Sadee W. In vivo opiate receptor binding of oripavines to mu, delta and kappa sites in rat brain as determined by an *ex vivo* labeling method. *Eur J Pharmacol* 1985;114:343–353.
13. Bloms-Funke P, Gillen C, Schuettler AJ, et al. Agonistic effects of the opioid buprenorphine on the nociceptin/OFQ receptor. *Peptides* 2000;21:1141–1146.
14. Jasinski DR, Haertzen CA, Henningfield JE, et al. Progress report of the NIDA Addiction Research Center. *NIDA Res Monogr* 1982;41:45–52.
15. Iribarne C, Picart D, Dreano Y, et al. Involvement of cytochrome P450 3A4 in N-dealkylation of buprenorphine in human liver microsomes. *Life Sci* 1997;60:1953–1964.
16. Ohtani M, Kotaki H, Nishitateno K, et al. Kinetics of respiratory depression in rats induced by buprenorphine and its metabolite, norbuprenorphine. *J Pharmacol Exp Ther* 1997;281:428–433.
17. Everhart ET, Cheung P, Shwonek P, et al. Subnanogram-concentration measurement of buprenorphine in human plasma by electron-capture capillary gas chromatography: application to pharmacokinetics of sublingual buprenorphine. *Clin Chem* 1997;43:2292–2302.
18. Mendelson J, Upton RA, Everhart ET, et al. Bioavailability of sublingual buprenorphine. *J Clin Pharmacol* 1997;37:31–37.
19. Kuhlman JJ Jr, Lalani S, Magluilo J Jr, et al. Human pharmacokinetics of intravenous, sublingual, and buccal buprenorphine. *J Anal Toxicol* 1996;20:369–378.
20. Nath RP, Upton RA, Everhart ET, et al. Buprenorphine pharmacokinetics: relative bioavailability of sublingual tablet and liquid formulations. *J Clin Pharmacol* 1999;39:619–623.
21. Schuh KJ, Johanson CE. Pharmacokinetic comparison of the buprenorphine sublingual liquid and tablet. *Drug Alcohol Depend* 1999;56:55–60.
22. Harris DS, Jones RT, Welm S, et al. Buprenorphine and naloxone coadministration in opiate-dependent patients stabilized on sublingual buprenorphine. *Drug Alcohol Depend* 2000;61:85–94.
23. Jasinski DR, Pevnick JS, Griffith JD. Human pharmacology and abuse potential of the analgesic buprenorphine: a potential agent for treating narcotic addiction. *Arch Gen Psychiatry* 1978;35:501–516.
24. Mello NK, Mendelson JH, Kuehnle JC. Buprenorphine effects on human heroin self-administration: an operant analysis. *J Pharmacol Exp Ther* 1982;223:30–39.
25. Mello NK, Mendelson JH, Lukas SE, et al. Buprenorphine treatment of opiate and cocaine abuse: clinical and preclinical studies. *Harv Rev Psychiatry* 1993;1:168–183.
26. Johnson RE, Fudala PJ. Development of buprenorphine for the treatment of opioid dependence. *NIDA Res Monogr* 1992;121:120–141.
27. Fudala PJ, Johnson RE. Clinical efficacy studies of buprenorphine for the treatment of opiate dependence. In: Cowan A, Lewis JW, eds. Buprenorphine: combatting drug abuse with a unique opioid. New York: Wiley-Liss, 1995:213–239.
28. Bickel WK, Amass L. Buprenorphine treatment of opioid dependence: a review. *Exp Clin Psychopharmacol* 1995;3:477–489.
29. Raisch DW, Fye CL, Boardman KD, et al. Opioid dependence treatment, including buprenorphine/naloxone. *Ann Pharmacother* 2002;36:312–321.
30. Johnson RE, McCagh JC. Buprenorphine and naloxone for heroin dependence. *Curr Psychiatry Rep* 2000;2:519–526.
31. Kreek MJ. Methadone-related opioid agonist pharmacotherapy for heroin addiction. History, recent molecular and neurochemical research and future in mainstream medicine. *Ann N Y Acad Sci* 2000;909:186–216.
32. Ling W, Rawson RA, Compton MA. Substitution pharmacotherapies for opioid addiction: from methadone to LAAM and buprenorphine. *J Psychoactive Drugs* 1994;26:119–128.
33. Johnson RE, Jaffe JH, Fudala PJ. A controlled trial of buprenorphine treatment for opioid dependence. *JAMA* 1992;267:2750–2755.
34. Strain EC, Stitzer ML, Liebson IA, et al. Comparison of buprenorphine and methadone in the treatment of opioid dependence. *Am J Psychiatry* 1994;151:1025–1030.
35. Schottenfeld RS, Pakes JR, Oliveto A, et al. Buprenorphine vs methadone maintenance treatment for concurrent opioid dependence and cocaine abuse. *Arch Gen Psychiatry* 1997;54:713–720.
36. Uehlinger C, Deglon J, Livoti S, et al. Comparison of buprenorphine and methadone in the treatment of opioid dependence. Swiss multicentre study. *Eur Addict Res* 1998;4:13–18.
37. Pani PP, Maremmani I, Pirastu R, et al.

Buprenorphine: a controlled clinical trial in the treatment of opioid dependence. *Drug Alcohol Depend* 2000;60:39–50.

38. Petitjean S, Stohler R, Deglon JJ, et al. Double-blind randomized trial of buprenorphine and methadone in opiate dependence. *Drug Alcohol Depend* 2001;62:97–104.

39. Levin FR, Fischman MW, Connerney I, et al. A protocol to switch high-dose, methadone-maintained subjects to buprenorphine. *Am J Addict* 1997;6:105–116.

40. Bouchez J, Beauverie P, Touzeau D. Substitution with buprenorphine in methadone- and morphine sulfate-dependent patients. Preliminary results. *Eur Addict Res* 1998;4:8–12.

41. Aceto MD. Characterization of prototypical opioid antagonists, agonist-antagonists, and agonists in the morphine-dependent rhesus monkey. *Neuropeptides* 1984;5:15–18.

42. Dum JE, Herz A. *In vivo* receptor binding of the opiate partial agonist, buprenorphine, correlated with its agonistic and antagonistic actions. *Br J Pharmacol* 1981;74:627–633.

43. Fukase H, Fukuzaki K, Koja T, et al. Effects of morphine, naloxone, buprenorphine, butorphanol, haloperidol and imipramine on morphine withdrawal signs in cynomolgus monkeys. *Psychopharmacology (Berl)* 1994;116:396–400.

44. Kosten TR, Kleber HD. Buprenorphine detoxification from opioid dependence: a pilot study. *Life Sci* 1988;42:635–641.

45. Walsh SL, June HL, Schuh KJ, et al. Effects of buprenorphine and methadone in methadone-maintained subjects. *Psychopharmacology (Berl)* 1995;119:268–276.

46. Bickel WK, Stitzer ML, Bigelow GE, et al. A clinical trial of buprenorphine: comparison with methadone in the detoxification of heroin addicts. *Clin Pharmacol Ther* 1988;43:72–78.

47. Fudala PJ, Jaffe JH, Dax EM, et al. Use of buprenorphine in the treatment of opioid addiction. II. Physiologic and behavioral effects of daily and alternate-day administration and abrupt withdrawal. *Clin Pharmacol Ther* 1990;47:525–534.

48. Bickel WK, Stitzer ML, Bigelow GE, et al. Buprenorphine: dose-related blockade of opioid challenge effects in opioid dependent humans. *J Pharmacol Exp Ther* 1988;247:47–53.

49. Walsh SL, Preston KL, Stitzer ML, et al. Clinical pharmacology of buprenorphine: ceiling effects at high doses. *Clin Pharmacol Ther* 1994;55:569–580.

50. Chawarski MC, Schottenfeld RS, O'Connor PG, et al. Plasma concentrations of buprenorphine 24 to 72 hours after dosing. *Drug Alcohol Depend* 1999;55:157–163.

51. Amass L, Bickel WK, Crean JP, et al. Alternate-day buprenorphine dosing is preferred to daily dosing by opioid-dependent humans. *Psychopharmacology (Berl)* 1998;136:217–225.

52. Amass L, Bickel WK, Higgins ST, et al. Alternate-day dosing during buprenorphine treatment of opioid dependence. *Life Sci* 1994;54:1215–1228.

53. Amass L, Kamien JB, Mikulich SK. Efficacy of daily and alternate-day dosing regimens with the combination buprenorphine-naloxone tablet. *Drug Alcohol Depend* 2000;58:143–152.

54. Amass L, Kamien JB, Mikulich SK. Thrice-weekly supervised dosing with the combination buprenorphine-naloxone tablet is preferred to daily supervised dosing by opioid-dependent humans. *Drug Alcohol Depend* 2001;61:173–181.

55. Petry NM, Bickel WK, Badger GJ. A comparison of four buprenorphine dosing regimens in the treatment of opioid dependence. *Clin Pharmacol Ther* 1999;66:306–314.

56. Petry NM, Bickel WK, Badger GJ. A comparison of four buprenorphine dosing regimens using open-dosing procedures: is twice-weekly dosing possible? *Addiction* 2000;95:1069–1077.

57. Petry NM, Bickel WK, Badger GJ. Examining the limits of the buprenorphine interdosing interval: daily, every-third-day and every-fifth-day dosing regimens. *Addiction* 2001;96:823–834.

58. Johnson RE, Eissenberg T, Stitzer ML, et al. Buprenorphine treatment of opioid dependence: clinical trial of daily versus alternate-day dosing. *Drug Alcohol Depend* 1995;40:27–35.

59. Bickel WK, Amass L, Crean JP, et al. Buprenorphine dosing every 1, 2, or 3 days in opioid-dependent patients. *Psychopharmacology (Berl)* 1999;146:111–118.

60. O'Connor PG, Oliveto AH, Shi JM, et al. A pilot study of primary-care-based buprenorphine maintenance for heroin dependence. *Am J Drug Alcohol Abuse* 1996;22:523–531.

61. O'Connor PG, Oliveto AH, Shi JM, et al. A randomized trial of buprenorphine maintenance for heroin dependence in a primary care clinic for substance users versus a methadone clinic. *Am J Med* 1998;105:100–105.

62. Schottenfeld RS, Pakes J, O'Connor P, et al. Thrice-weekly versus daily buprenorphine maintenance. *Biol Psychiatry* 2000;47:1072–1079.

63. Perez de los Cobos J, Martin S, Etcheberrigaray A, et al. A controlled trial of daily versus thrice-weekly buprenorphine administration for the treatment of opioid dependence. *Drug Alcohol Depend* 2000;59:223–233.

64. Johnson RE, Chutuape MA, Strain EC, et al. A comparison of levomethadyl acetate, buprenorphine, and methadone for opioid dependence. *N Engl J Med* 2000;343:1290–1297.

65. Mello NK, Mendelson JH. Buprenorphine suppresses heroin use by heroin addicts. *Science* 1980;207:657–659.

66. Johnson RE, Cone EJ, Henningfield JE, et al. Use of buprenorphine in the treatment of opiate addiction. I. Physiologic and behavioral effects during a rapid dose induction. *Clin Pharmacol Ther* 1989;46:335–343.

67. Preston KL, Bigelow GE. Drug discrimination assessment of agonist-antagonist opioids in humans: a three-choice saline-hydromorphone-butorphanol procedure. *J Pharmacol Exp Ther* 1994;271:48–60.

68. Preston K, Bigelow G, Bickel W, et al. Drug discrimination in human post-addicts: agonist/antagonist opioids. *NIDA Res Monogr* 1988;81:209–215.

69. Preston KL, Liebson IA, Bigelow GE. Discrimination of agonist-antagonist opioids in humans trained on a two-choice saline-hydromorphone discrimination. *J Pharmacol Exp Ther* 1992;261:62–71.

70. Jones HE, Bigelow GE, Preston KL. Assessment of opioid partial agonist activity with a three-choice hydromorphone dose-discrimination procedure. *J Pharmacol Exp Ther* 1999;289:1350–1361.

71. Pickworth WB, Johnson RE, Holicky BA, et al. Subjective and physiologic effects of intravenous buprenorphine in humans. *Clin Pharmacol Ther* 1993;53:570–576.

72. Comer SD, Collins ED, Fischman MW. Intravenous buprenorphine self-administration by detoxified heroin abusers. *J Pharmacol Exp Ther* 2002;301:266–276.

73. Strain EC, Preston KL, Liebson IA, et al. Acute effects of buprenorphine, hydromorphone and naloxone in methadone-maintained volunteers. *J Pharmacol Exp Ther* 1992;261:985–993.

74. Strain EC, Preston KL, Liebson IA, et al. Buprenorphine effects in methadone-maintained volunteers: effects at two hours after methadone. *J Pharmacol Exp Ther* 1995;272:628–638.

75. Fudala PJ, Yu E, Macfadden W, et al. Effects of buprenorphine and naloxone in morphine-stabilized opioid addicts. *Drug Alcohol Depend* 1998;50:1–8.

76. Mendelson J, Jones RT, Fernandez I, et al. Buprenorphine and naloxone interactions in opiate-dependent volunteers. *Clin Pharmacol Ther* 1996; 60:105–114.

77. Mendelson J, Jones RT, Welm S, et al. Buprenorphine and naloxone combinations: the effects of three dose ratios in morphine-stabilized, opiate-dependent volunteers. *Psychopharmacology (Berl)* 1999;141:37–46.

78. Mendelson J, Jones RT, Welm S, et al. Buprenorphine and naloxone interactions in methadone maintenance patients. *Biol Psychiatry* 1997;41:1095–1101.

79. Preston KL, Bigelow GE, Liebson IA. Buprenorphine and naloxone alone and in combination in opioid-dependent humans. *Psychopharmacology (Berl)* 1988;94:484–490.

80. Strain EC, Stoller K, Walsh SL, et al. Effects of buprenorphine versus buprenorphine/naloxone tablets in non-dependent opioid abusers. *Psychopharmacology (Berl)* 2000;148: 374–383.

81. Weinhold LL, Preston KL, Farre M, et al. Buprenorphine alone and in combination with naloxone in non-dependent humans. *Drug Alcohol Depend* 1992;30:263–274.

82. Casadonte P, Walsh R, Vocci F, et al. Treatment of opiate dependence with buprenorphine/naloxone in a solo private psychiatry office. *Drug Alcohol Depend* 2001;63:S26.

83. Fudala PJ. United States multisite evaluations of office-based buprenorphine treatment. *NIDA Res Monogr* 2002;182:31–32.

84. Fudala PJ, Bridge TP, Herbert S, et al. A multisite efficacy evaluation of a buprenorphine/naloxone product for opiate dependence treatment. *NIDA Res Monogr* 1998;179:105.

85. Harper I. Temgesic abuse. *N Z Med J* 1983;96:777.

86. Quigley AJ, Bredemeyer DE, Seow SS. A case of buprenorphine abuse. *Med J Aust* 1984;140:425–426.

87. Strang J. Abuse of buprenorphine. *Lancet* 1985;2:725.

88. Rainey HB. Abuse of buprenorphine. *N Z Med J* 1986;99:72.

89. O'Connor JJ, Moloney E, Travers R, et al. Buprenorphine abuse among opiate addicts. *Br J Addict* 1988;83:1085–1087.

90. Sakol MS, Stark C, Sykes R. Buprenorphine and temazepam abuse by drug takers in Glasgow—an increase. *Br J Addict* 1989;84:439–441.

91. Hammersley R, Lavelle T, Forsyth A. Buprenorphine and temazepam—abuse. *Br J Addict* 1990;85:301–303.

92. Chowdhury AN, Chowdhury S. Buprenorphine abuse: report from India. *Br J Addict* 1990;85:1349–1350.

93. Strang J. Abuse of buprenorphine (Temgesic) by snorting. *BMJ* 1991;302:969.

94. Stewart MJ. Effect of scheduling of buprenorphine (Temgesic) on drug abuse patterns in Glasgow. *BMJ* 1991; 302:969.

95. Lavelle TL, Hammersley R, Forsyth A. The use of buprenorphine and temazepam by drug injectors. *J Addict Dis* 1991;10:5–14.

96. Frischer M. Estimated prevalence of injecting drug use in Glasgow. *Br J Addict* 1992;87:235–243.

97. Singh RA, Mattoo SK, Malhotra A, et al. Cases of buprenorphine abuse in India. *Acta Psychiatr Scand* 1992; 86:46–48.

98. Robinson GM, Dukes PD, Robinson BJ, et al. The misuse of buprenorphine and a buprenorphine-naloxone combination in Wellington, New Zealand. *Drug Alcohol Depend* 1993;33:81–86.

99. Baumevieille M, Haramburu F, Begaud B. Abuse of prescription medicines in southwestern France. *Ann Pharmacother* 1997;31:847–850.

100. Lange WR, Fudala PJ, Dax EM, et al. Safety and side-effects of buprenorphine in the clinical management of heroin addiction. *Drug Alcohol Depend* 1990;26:19–28.

101. Ling W, Charuvastra C, Collins JF, et al. Buprenorphine maintenance treatment of opiate dependence: a multicenter, randomized clinical trial. *Addiction* 1998;93:475–486.

102. Ling W, Wesson DR, Charuvastra C, et al. A controlled trial comparing buprenorphine and methadone maintenance in opioid dependence. *Arch Gen Psychiatry* 1996;53:401–407.

103. Umbricht A, Huestis MA, Cone EJ, et al. Safety of buprenorphine: Ceiling for cardio-respiratory effects at high IV doses. *NIDA Res Monogr* 1998; 179:225.

104. Kosten TR, Krystal JH, Charney DS, et al. Opioid antagonist challenges in buprenorphine maintained patients. *Drug Alcohol Depend* 1990;25:73–78.

105. Eissenberg T, Greenwald MK, Johnson RE, et al. Buprenorphine's physical dependence potential: antagonist-precipitated withdrawal in humans. *J Pharmacol Exp Ther* 1996;276:449–459.

106. Reckitt Benckiser Pharmaceuticals Inc. *Suboxone and Subutex product labeling.* Richmond, VA 2002.

107. Auriacombe M, Franques P, Tignol J. Deaths attributable to methadone vs buprenorphine in France. *JAMA* 2001; 285:45.

108. Kintz P. Deaths involving buprenorphine: a compendium of French cases. *Forens Sci Int* 2001;121:65–69.

109. Tracqui A, Kintz P, Ludes B. Buprenorphine-related deaths among drug addicts in France: a report on 20 fatalities. *J Anal Toxicol* 1998;22:430–434.

110. Tracqui A, Tournoud C, Flesch F, et al. [Acute poisoning during substitution therapy based on high-dosage buprenorphine. 29 clinical cases-20 fatal cases]. *Presse Med* 1998;27:557–561.

111. Thirion X, Barrau K, Micallef J, et al. [Maintenance treatment for opioid dependence in care centers: the OPPIDUM program of the Evaluation and Information Centers for Drug Addiction]. *Ann Med Interne (Paris)* 2000;151:A10–A17.

112. Thirion X, Lapierre V, Micallef J, et al. Buprenorphine prescription by general practitioners in a French region. *Drug Alcohol Depend* 2002;65:197–204.

113. Thirion X, Micallef J, Barrau K, et al. Recent evolution in opiate dependence in France during generalisation of maintenance treatments. *Drug Alcohol Depend* 2001;61:281–285.

114. Kobayashi K, Yamamoto T, Chiba K, et al. Human buprenorphine N-dealkylation is catalyzed by cytochrome P450 3A4. *Drug Metab Dispos* 1998;26:818–821.

115. Iribarne C, Berthou F, Carlhant D, et al. Inhibition of methadone and buprenorphine N-dealkylations by three HIV-1 protease inhibitors. *Drug Metab Dispos* 1998;26:257–260.

116. Carrieri MP, Vlahov D, Dellamonica P, et al. Use of buprenorphine in HIV-infected injection drug users: negligible impact on virologic response to HAART. The Manif-2000 Study Group. *Drug Alcohol Depend* 2000;60:51–54.

117. Dole VP, Nyswander M. Successful treatment of 750 criminal addicts. *JAMA* 1968;26:2708–2710.

118. Fudala PJ. LAAM - Pharmacology and pharmacokinetics, development history, and therapeutic considerations. *Subst Abuse* 1996;17:127–132.

119. 42 CFR 8.12. *Federal opioid treatment standards: Public Health Service,* 2001.

120. Fiellin DA, Pantalon MV, Pakes J, et al. Treatment of heroin dependence with buprenorphine in primary care. *Am J Drug Alcohol Abuse* 2002;28:231–241.

121. Fiellin DA, O'Connor PG. Office-based treatment of opioid-dependent patients. *N Engl J Med* 2002;347:817–823.

122. Fiellin DA, Rosenheck RA, Kosten TR. Office-based treatment for opioid dependence: reaching new patient populations. *Am J Psychiatry* 2001;158:1200–1204.

CHAPTER 41

Alternative Pharmacotherapies for Opioid Addiction

PAUL J. FUDALA, ROBERT A. GREENSTEIN, AND CHARLES P. O'BRIEN

The development of methadone maintenance by Dole and Nyswander in the mid-1960s (1) ushered in the modern era of pharmacologic treatment for opioid dependence. Previously, except for a brief period of legalized opioid maintenance in several United States cities in the early 1900s, abrupt discontinuation of opioids or substitution of decreasing doses of methadone or shorter-acting legally prescribed opioids for patients' drugs of choice were used to detoxify opioid addicts. However, detoxification alone is a generally unsuccessful treatment for opioid dependence because relapse occurs shortly after the patient leaves the hospital (2).

Detoxification followed by incarceration or inpatient or outpatient treatment has a somewhat better outcome but is highly influenced by patient selection and by availability of drugs in the community. Opioid substitution using methadone or levo-alpha-acetylmethadol (LAAM), with or without adjunctive therapy such as counseling or vocational rehabilitation, enables many patients to reduce or stop use of illicit opioids and to stabilize their lives. Nonetheless, methadone-maintained patients also have a high rate of relapse following discontinuation of the medication. Hence, many addicts require recurrent or extended courses of treatment.

Although social and physiologic factors are involved in the vulnerability to relapse, including lability of mood and stress intolerance associated with the protracted abstinence syndrome (3), drug-related stimuli alone may elicit conditioned withdrawal effects in the absence of pharmacologically induced changes (4). Hence, addicts may experience physical symptoms similar to those related to the withdrawal of opioids when they are exposed to environmental cues or settings previously associated with drug use. Addicts may be more vulnerable to conditioned withdrawal effects during the period of autonomic instability known as protracted withdrawal, and they may resume drug use to relieve these symptoms. Methadone or LAAM maintenance reduces craving for opioids (5) but may prolong physical dependence.

Psychopharmacologists have searched for nonaddicting analgesics and treatments for opioid dependence for decades. Although methadone maintenance has helped thousands of opioid addicts in the United States during the past 40 years, there remain considerable philosophical objections to its use. This has given added impetus to the development of alternative pharmacologic treatments that would not prolong physical dependence on opioids, thus enabling addicts to recover without months or years of treatment with methadone, and without the high rate of relapse that follows most drug-free treatments for substance dependence. This effort has led to the development of new therapeutic options for those patients who prefer a nonmethadone treatment or who respond less well to methadone.

Many addicts begin experimenting with or abusing drugs in adolescence and progress over a period of months or years to dependence. As dependence continues, addicts spend more of their time and energy securing drugs, which leads to disruption of interpersonal and family relationships, and diminished educational and vocational achievement. This results in increasing antisocial behavior and criminality, and high emotional and economic costs for sustaining dependence. Nonetheless, even individuals professing a strong desire to interrupt the addiction cycle are often ambivalent about achieving abstinence. Most have not learned to manage stress without opioids and look to drugs for immediate symptom relief. For any treatment, whether pharmacologically based or not, to produce significant benefit, the natural course of the opioid dependence process, the presence of concurrent psychiatric illness, and the abuse of other drugs or alcohol must be recognized and addressed. Additionally, treatment goals themselves may vary. For example, if a patient is early in the course of addiction or an older patient near the end of an addiction cycle, then total abstinence may be a realistic goal. Conversely, if a patient is in the throes of his or her addiction, a decrease in the amount and/or frequency of illicit drug abuse may be a more attainable and realistic goal than immediate abstinence.

Experience has taught us that interrupting the powerfully reinforcing effects of opioids and drug-seeking behavior requires a concerted effort by therapists, patients, and their families to permanently overcome addiction. This is particularly true once an addiction is established as a chronic condition, when most patients will require multiple interventions. During the past three decades, much research has focused on three classes of treatment medications: nonopioids that alleviate withdrawal symptomatology; opioid agonists other than methadone; and opioid antagonists, partial agonists, and mixed agonists/antagonists that can block or competitively inhibit opioids at their receptors. This chapter reviews the literature on alternative pharmacotherapies to methadone and discusses strategies for developing more effective treatments for opioid dependence.

NONOPIOID TREATMENT ALTERNATIVES: CLONIDINE AND LOFEXIDINE

The acute opioid withdrawal syndrome is a time-limited phenomenon, generally of brief duration. Following the abrupt termination of short-acting opioids such as heroin, morphine, or hydromorphone, withdrawal signs and symptoms usually subside by the second or third opioid-free day. Although uncomfortable for the addict, the opioid withdrawal syndrome, in contrast to the syndrome associated with the withdrawal of other drugs such as benzodiazepines and alcohol, does not pose a medical risk to the individual. Thus, there is a particular appeal for treating this syndrome symptomatically, especially with medications that do not themselves produce physical dependence. It should be recognized, however, that detoxification from opioids is only one of the initial steps in the process of rehabilitating opioid-addicted individuals if complete and permanent abstinence is the treatment goal.

Clonidine is an α_2-adrenergic agonist indicated for the treatment of hypertension (6) and has also been used to treat autism (7–9), attention-deficit hyperactivity disorder (10,11), and various types of pain (12). Clonidine is useful in the medical detoxification of patients from methadone (13–15), as well as from commonly abused opioids such as heroin (16,17), morphine (18), propoxyphene (19), and meperidine (20). In particular, it has been shown to be useful in preparing individuals for stabilization onto the opioid antagonist naltrexone (21–24). Clonidine has also been reported to be useful in decreasing withdrawal signs and symptoms associated with the cessation of alcohol (25–27) and tobacco (28–31) use.

The capacity of clonidine to ameliorate withdrawal-associated effects (e.g., lacrimation and rhinorrhea) is linked to its modulation of noradrenergic hyperactivity in the locus ceruleus (32–34). Additionally, clonidine may affect central serotonergic (35,36), cholinergic (37,38), and purinergic systems (37–41). It seems to be most effective in suppressing certain opioid withdrawal signs and symptoms, such as restlessness and diaphoresis. However, clonidine is not well accepted by addicts because it does not produce morphine-like subjective effects or relieve certain types of withdrawal distress, such as anxiety (18). Sedation and hypotension also limit its utility. No fixed-dosing guidelines are currently available and dosages are generally individualized to each patient based on therapeutic response and side-effect limitations.

Interestingly, clonidine abuse by users of illicit opioids and other drugs has been reported since the early 1980s (42). This abuse may be secondary to a desire to obtain various drug-related effects, such as sedation, euphoria, or hallucinations (42–44). Clonidine may also be used to prolong and enhance the effects of heroin or other opioids (45–47).

Secondary to an effort to identify an agent with less sedating and hypotensive effects than clonidine, a number of other α_2-adrenergic agonists have been evaluated for their ability to moderate the opioid-withdrawal syndrome. Of these, lofexidine, a clonidine analogue licensed in the United Kingdom for opioid detoxification treatment, has been the subject of much clinical evaluation. Although lofexidine has not been as extensively studied as clonidine in the United States, it has enjoyed widespread usage in the United Kingdom (48). Lofexidine is suggested to be used for a period of 7 to 10 days at dosages ranging from 0.4 to 2.4 mg per day (49).

Studies conducted in the early 1980s provided initial data indicating that lofexidine could be effective in suppressing some of the signs and symptoms of opioid withdrawal (50–55). More recent trials have provided further evidence for the efficacy of lofexidine. These trials included both open-label and double-blind evaluations, using both inpatient and outpatient populations.

When compared to methadone for the treatment of opioid withdrawal in polydrug-abusing opioid addicts, lofexidine treatment was associated with more severe symptomatology at various time points on and before the tenth (last) day of treatment, but both groups were observed to have a similar course of symptom decline thereafter (56). Both groups also showed similar rates of detoxification treatment completion. In a subsequent open-label study by the same research group (57), the authors found that a 5-day lofexidine treatment regimen may attenuate opioid withdrawal symptoms more rapidly than a 10-day lofexidine- or methadone-treatment schedule without exacerbating hypotensive side-effects.

When lofexidine was compared to clonidine, both treatments were generally found to produce similar therapeutic effects, but lofexidine typically was better tolerated. When lofexidine was compared to clonidine in an outpatient, double-blind trial, both medications produced positive treatment outcomes, but clonidine was associated with more hypotensive effects and more required home visits by medical staff (58). In a double-blind, inpatient study, lofexidine and clonidine were reported to be equally effective in treating the withdrawal syndrome. Clonidine, however, was associated with more hypotension and better treatment retention than was noted for lofexidine (59). In another double-blind, inpatient study using methadone-stabilized opioid addicts, both lofexidine and clonidine produced a similar suppression of withdrawal symptoms, but lofexidine was associated with less hypotension and fewer adverse events (60).

Additional studies using diverse paradigms have also supported the therapeutic effectiveness of lofexidine. For example, a naltrexone-lofexidine combination was associated with a more rapid resolution of the opioid withdrawal syndrome than was a 7-day lofexidine-only treatment schedule, without substantial increases in withdrawal symptoms or hypotensive side-effects (61). When used in a 3-day opioid detoxification procedure with adjunct medications (oxazepam, baclofen, ketoprofen, naloxone, and naltrexone), lofexidine-treated individuals showed significantly lower levels of withdrawal symptoms and fewer mood problems, as well as less sedation and hypotension (62). In an inpatient evaluation of a high-dose, 3-day regimen of buprenorphine compared to a standard 5-day course of clonidine, buprenorphine was found to provide for more effective early relief of withdrawal symptoms (63). Similarly, when lofexidine was compared to buprenorphine in an open-label study, patients receiving buprenorphine reportedly had less-severe withdrawal symptoms and were more likely to complete detoxification treatment (64).

Few data relevant to the potential effectiveness of other α_2 adrenergic agonists, guanabenz (65–67) and guanfacine (68–71) are available, with some indication that guanfacine may be more effective than clonidine (72). One study (73), however, indicated that guanfacine was unable to effectively control methadone-associated withdrawal symptoms.

LAAM: AN OPIOID AGONIST ALTERNATIVE TO METHADONE

LAAM is a derivative of methadone, and like methadone, is a synthetic μ-opioid agonist. LAAM was approved in the United States for the management of opioid dependence in 1993 (74). It was initially developed in the late 1940s by chemists in Germany seeking an analgesic substitute for morphine. Subsequent studies indicated that LAAM would be unsuitable for the treatment of acute pain given its slow onset of effect and extended duration of action (75,76). However, the data are mixed concerning the onset of effect of LAAM. Initial studies indicated that LAAM given orally produced a more rapid onset of effect than when it was given intravenously or subcutaneously (77,78), although recent data (79) suggests that LAAM produces effects of immediate onset when administered parenterally. While it was noted early in LAAM's development that LAAM could alleviate the signs and symptoms of opioid withdrawal following the termination of morphine administration, it was also observed that giving LAAM on a daily basis could lead to signs indicative of opioid toxicity, such as severe nausea and vomiting and respiratory depression.

The use of methadone to treat opioid-dependent individuals, which began in the mid-1960s, provided a new and important therapeutic option for managing opioid addiction. Methadone, which has a plasma half-life of about 30 hours (80–82), requires administration on a daily basis to be optimally effective. There were concerns related to the potential diversion of this medication to illicit channels when it was dispensed to patients for consumption outside of the clinic environment. The opioid effects produced by LAAM and its active metabolites, along with the potential for administering the parent drug on alternate days or on a three-times-weekly schedule (thus eliminating the

need for "take-home" doses), fostered interest in its potential use as an alternative to methadone. LAAM had already been shown to produce effects that were qualitatively similar to morphine and methadone. Also, LAAM is converted to two pharmacologically active compounds by N-demethylation (nor-LAAM and dinor-LAAM) in addition to inactive compounds (83–85). The long half-lives of the nor-LAAM and dinor-LAAM metabolites, 48 and 96 hours, respectively, contribute to the extended duration of activity of LAAM (79,86).

Numerous studies (87) provide evidence for the effectiveness of LAAM as an opioid-dependence treatment agent. Most of these investigations compared LAAM to methadone, because the latter is considered the standard for opioid-addiction treatment. Outcome measures most often assessed in these studies include the amount of time individuals remained in treatment, patients' illicit use of opioids and other drugs during the course of treatment, various elements related to individuals' social functioning (such as employment history and interactions with legal system), and general medical and psychiatric parameters, including adverse events potentially related to the treatment medication.

Three phase III, multicenter clinical studies were considered pivotal with respect to the approval of LAAM by the Food and Drug Administration (FDA). Two of these (88,89) were conducted in the 1970s and involved 25 clinical sites and approximately 1,100 individuals, of which 470 received LAAM. The first study (88) used a randomized, double-blind, parallel-group design and compared one targeted dosage regimen of LAAM (80 mg given on Mondays, Wednesdays, and Fridays) to two regimens of methadone (50 or 100 mg daily). Overall, the group that received LAAM was associated with results similar to the one given methadone 100 mg with respect to safety assessments and various measures of efficacy. The second study (89) was open-label in design and used dosages of methadone and LAAM that were titrated by the site investigators to the clinical response of the study participants. The primary purpose of this study was to gain additional clinical experience with LAAM, with particular emphasis on accumulating safety data. Again, few differences were noted between LAAM-treated and methadone-treated groups with respect to measures of efficacy and safety.

The third pivotal trial (90) was the final one conducted prior to the approval of the medication by the FDA. Its primary purpose was to assess the adequacy of the prototype product labeling and treatment regulations which had been developed to guide clinicians in the use of LAAM as an opioid-dependence treatment. The study was also conducted to generate additional safety data regarding LAAM. Six-hundred twenty-three individuals who had been using opioids illicitly or receiving methadone in a dependence-treatment program received LAAM during the course of the 52-week, 26-site study. In contrast to previous trials of LAAM safety and efficacy that generally excluded women, the subject population of this study was 33% female. Additionally, issues related to the human immunodeficiency virus and the use of "crack" cocaine, which were not relevant to earlier evaluations, were considered in this study. Data from this trial confirmed previous observations regarding the general safety of LAAM in a "current" population of opioid-dependent individuals.

Because LAAM may be administered on alternate days or three times weekly, it may provide advantages over methadone for some patients (86,91). Some individuals, because of the distance of their place of residence or employment from the treatment program, may find it difficult to receive their methadone doses on a daily basis. Take-home doses of methadone may provide an alternative; however, methadone is sometimes diverted for illicit sale and street use. The use of LAAM eliminates the need for a schedule of daily medication administration; additionally, take-home doses of LAAM are now permitted by current federal regulations.

As with the use of any opioid-dependence treatment medication, patients must be carefully evaluated prior to the initiation of therapy. Close monitoring is especially important during the first few weeks following the beginning of LAAM therapy while a pharmacokinetic steady state is being attained. Although alcohol and illicit drug use should be discouraged throughout the entire course of treatment, this is especially important during the first few weeks of LAAM therapy when the potential for cumulative toxicity with other agents may be particularly difficult to predict. Additionally, because of the nature of LAAM's metabolism, microsomal enzyme inducers such as phenobarbital and rifampin, and inhibitors such as cimetidine or ketoconazole, may have variable effects on the apparent activity or duration of action of LAAM. LAAM, unlike methadone, however, does not significantly affect the pharmacokinetics of the reverse transcriptase inhibitor zidovudine (92).

A number of factors have served to limit the widespread use of LAAM, including regulatory issues, clinic–staff resistance, and the reluctance by practitioners to consider LAAM as a viable alternative to methadone (93). Most recently, however, LAAM was associated with serious cardiac adverse events, including *torsade de pointes* (94). LAAM is no longer indicated as a first-line addiction treatment agent, and should never be used with drugs that may prolong the QT interval, but it should be reserved for individuals who fail to show an adequate response to other treatments (95).

OPIOID ANTAGONISTS

Antagonists help addicts to avoid relapse by occupying opioid receptor sites and blocking the effects of agonists at the cellular level (96). Relatively pure opioid antago-

nists, such as naltrexone, are not in themselves addicting and do not have the pharmacologically reinforcing effects of agonists. However, if an individual stabilized on naltrexone administers an opioid agonist, the effects of that drug are effectively blocked. Partial agonists such as buprenorphine may block or enhance the effects of other opioids and may have an abuse potential of their own.

Among the opioid antagonists, naltrexone has emerged as the most extensively studied agent. Despite its relatively pure antagonist activity and minimal side effects, naltrexone has not been widely accepted by addicts. This may be a result of several factors, including the risk of precipitating a withdrawal syndrome during naltrexone induction and the absence of reinforcing opioid effects, such as feelings of well-being and euphoria. Many addicts stop taking naltrexone before they have learned new, nonopioid methods for controlling anxiety or depression, or before they can recognize cues that can trigger withdrawal symptoms and the urge to use illicit drugs.

Pharmacology of Opioid Antagonists

Opioid antagonists are substances that bind to opioid receptors but do not produce morphine-like effects. They compete at the receptors with both exogenous (e.g., morphine) and endogenous (e.g., endorphins) opioid agonists. When an antagonist is given in sufficient quantities, drugs such as heroin are prevented from interacting with their receptors. Opioid antagonists with high receptor affinity also displace agonists from receptor sites, reversing agonist effects. This is the basis for using naloxone to treat opioid overdoses. Antagonists also may be used to assess physical dependence, because they precipitate a withdrawal syndrome in chronic opioid users (97–101). Failure to respond to an opioid antagonist can be regarded as evidence against current physical dependence on opioids.

There are at least three types of opioid receptors referred to as μ, κ, and δ, with different opioids and opioid antagonists having varying affinities for each (102,103). The first clinically useful antagonist was nalorphine, which reduced morphine effects, but also produced some direct or agonist effects (104,105). Because of its potential for increasing rather than decreasing respiratory depression, nalorphine has been replaced by naloxone, which has no agonist effects over a reasonable range of doses and is, therefore, considered to be a "pure" μ-opioid antagonist (106). Such an antagonist would be preferable for preventing readdiction, because it blocks opioid effects without producing direct effects of its own. While opioid antagonists could potentially interfere with normal central pain inhibitory systems, consistent experimental evidence of this effect in human subjects has not been produced.

Naloxone has limited utility as a maintenance agent because it is poorly absorbed and has a duration of only a few hours following oral administration (107,108). Naltrexone, an analogue of naloxone synthesized in 1963, also has a high affinity for opioid receptor (109). It is well-absorbed in the gastrointestinal tract and has antagonist activity for up to 72 hours after oral ingestion (110). Weak opioid agonist activity has been reported for naltrexone (111), but this has not been shown to be clinically significant. Volavka and colleagues (112) reported acute rises in adrenocorticotropic hormone and cortisol after naloxone injections, and Mendelson and coworkers (113) reported increases in luteinizing hormone and little alteration in testosterone levels after acute oral ingestion of naltrexone. They also noted affective changes in normal volunteers who ingested 50 mg of naltrexone on a single occasion (114). Some individuals reported penile erections. Dysphoria was also reported in that study and in others (115,116). A subsequent investigation (117) did not indicate significant alterations in mood in nonaddicted, healthy individuals given 100 mg of naltrexone twice daily.

Formerly opioid-dependent patients have been maintained on effective blocking doses of naltrexone for up to 20 years, and large-scale, short-term studies that included several thousand patients failed to show evidence of naltrexone toxicity or significant laboratory abnormalities (118–120).

Results from liver function tests in particular were a matter of concern because of the high frequency of hepatitis among addicts. A study of nonaddict groups treated with high doses of naltrexone showed dose-related increases in transaminase levels that were reversible when the medication was stopped. The individuals in that study received naltrexone 300 mg per day, or about six times the therapeutic dose in opioid-dependence treatment (121). Subsequently, however, Marrazzi and coworkers (118) measured liver function in response to high doses of naltrexone (up to 400 mg per day) in an eating disorders study, and found no adverse clinical or laboratory changes in liver function.

Because medication compliance with the oral preparation of naltrexone has been low, the safety and effectiveness of a depot formulation of naltrexone is currently under study. Comer and colleagues (122) found that low-dose (192 mg) and high-dose (384 mg) depot naltrexone antagonized heroin-induced subjective ratings for 3 and 5 weeks, respectively. Other than initial discomfort associated with injection of the depot formulation, there were no adverse effects, suggesting that depot naltrexone may provide safe, effective, and long-lasting opioid antagonism. Additional studies are required before depot naltrexone is approved for general clinical use.

Clinical Studies of Naltrexone

While the plasma half-life of naltrexone (following oral administration) ranges from about 4 to 10 hours and that of its active metabolite, 6β-naltrexol, from approximately 10 to 12 hours (111,123–125), the duration of naltrexone's opioid receptor blockade is much longer. A single 50-mg dose produces 80% inhibition of binding of the ^{11}C-labeled μ ligand, carfentanil, to brain receptors at 72 hours (126). The first human studies showing the potential of naltrexone blockade for treating opioid abuse were conducted in the early 1970s. Martin and coworkers (127) found that 30 to 50 mg of naltrexone administered orally blocked subjective effects of morphine for up to 24 hours. A carefully conducted double-blind study of naltrexone-opioid interactions in human subjects (128) subsequently demonstrated that 150 to 200 mg of naltrexone attenuated heroin or hydromorphone effects for 72 hours, although some patients did report a "rush" or brief high after administration of the agonist.

Recently detoxified patients, particularly those discontinuing methadone maintenance, need to be opioid-free for at least 7 to 14 days to avoid precipitation of a withdrawal syndrome following the first dose of naltrexone (129,130). As an added precaution, it is advised that an intravenous or subcutaneous challenge of 0.4 to 0.8 mg naloxone be given prior to administration of naltrexone to ensure that withdrawal signs and symptoms are not produced (99,101,131). If the challenge is negative, patients are usually asymptomatic during naltrexone induction. If positive (i.e., there is the production of a short episode of yawning, abdominal cramps, irritability, anxiety, chills, and related signs and symptoms), the first naltrexone dose given shortly thereafter is also likely to precipitate a withdrawal syndrome, but of longer duration. After a negative naloxone challenge, patients are given graduated doses of naltrexone, beginning with a 25 mg test dose, followed by 50, 75, and 100 mg on subsequent days. Most patients who tolerate 100 mg without side effects can be maintained on 100 mg of naltrexone on Mondays and Wednesdays and given 150 mg on Fridays.

Patients involved in meaningful relationships, employed full-time, or attending school and living with family members are most likely to benefit from naltrexone treatment (132). Nonetheless, naltrexone treatment has a very high, early dropout rate. Only 20% to 30% of street heroin addicts successfully complete opioid detoxification, "pass" a naloxone challenge test, and begin naltrexone treatment; 40% of them may leave treatment before completing the first month. Only 10% to 20% take naltrexone for 6 months or longer, although addicted professionals (133) and former prisoners on probation (134) have significantly higher rates of accepting naltrexone and remaining in treatment. In one report acknowledging the difficulty in recruiting inner-city patients (135), only 15 of 300 (5%) offered naltrexone agreed to take it, and only three continued on naltrexone for more than 2 months.

Up to 20% of naltrexone patients have more than one treatment episode (136). During treatment, about a third of the patients will test naltrexone's blockade at least once, although most urine samples collected during treatment are negative for opioids. If patients have a pattern of missing naltrexone doses and using opioids, they soon discontinue naltrexone and relapse to opioid use. No evidence indicates that patients switch to nonopioid drugs while maintained on naltrexone, but those with histories of cocaine or other drug abuse may continue to use other substances. Followup of naltrexone-treated patients indicates that 30% to 40% are opioid-free for 6 months after terminating treatment (137). However, results depend on the population studied and the length of time patients have remained on naltrexone.

Naltrexone has no reinforcing properties of its own and is perceived as a subjectively neutral drug that prevents addicts from getting "high." Because most patients are ambivalent about stopping drug use and miss the reinforcing effects of opioids, many choose very early on to discontinue naltrexone or switch to methadone maintenance. Behavioral therapies using contingency management and reinforcers such as money or vouchers as a reward for opioid negative urine samples or continued treatment have been used with some success to induce patients to remain longer on naltrexone, although monetary rewards have obvious practical limitations (138–141).

PATIENTS SUITED FOR TREATMENT WITH OPIOID ANTAGONISTS

The best results with naltrexone have been reported in the treatment of health care professionals. Washton and coworkers (133) found, in a study of physicians, that 74% completed at least 6 months of treatment with naltrexone and were opioid-free and practicing medicine at 1-year followup. Ling and Wesson (142) found that 78% of health care professionals treated for an average of 8 months were rated as "much" or "moderately" improved at followup. Both studies involved comprehensive treatment, including medical evaluation, detoxification, psychiatric and family evaluation, and individual and family therapy (as well as confirmation of naltrexone ingestion). Roth and colleagues (143) conducted a program for professionals that included naltrexone administration for the first several months, followed by continued group therapy without naltrexone. Mean duration of naltrexone ingestion was 8 months, and mean duration in the program was 1.9 years. Of patients referred to the program, 94% had long-term abstinence and 66% worked in their profession during treatment.

Tennant and colleagues (144) described a group of suburban practitioners in southern California who treated opioid addicts from a wide range of socioeconomic groups. The majority of their patients were employed and expressed a desire for abstinence-oriented treatment. The program was conducted on an outpatient basis beginning with detoxification and a naloxone challenge. In addition

to naltrexone administered three times weekly, patients received counseling and drug and alcohol testing using breath and urine tests. Patients paid a fee if treatment was not covered by insurance. Although individuals were treated for a mean of 51 days (with an upper limit of up to 635 days), the majority were short-term patients, with only 17% remaining on naltrexone more than 90 days. Only 1% to 3% of tests for illicit drug and alcohol use were positive.

Washton and colleagues (133) treated a group of business executives addicted for at least 2 years to heroin, methadone, or prescription opioids. Most were white males, about 30 years of age, with an average income of more than $40,000 per year. This group was under external pressure to accept treatment, and almost half were in jeopardy of losing their jobs or suffering legal consequences. The program was oriented toward abstinence and began with 4 to 10 weeks of inpatient treatment, during which detoxification and induction onto naltrexone were accomplished. Individual psychotherapy and self-help groups were used. The posthospital phase was emphasized, and all patients signed a contract for aftercare treatment. All patients in the study completed naltrexone induction, and 61% remained on naltrexone for at least 6 months with no missed clinic visits or positive urine drug screens. Twenty-eight percent took naltrexone for less than 6 months, but remained in the program with drug-free urine samples following naltrexone cessation. Of the entire group, 64% were opioid-free at 12- to 18-month followup.

Relapse to drug use and crime after release from prison is common for individuals with drug-related convictions. In efforts to reduce recidivism, naltrexone was studied in former opioid-dependent probationers and parolees. In one study (134), former addict inmates who volunteered for a work-release program and who were using naltrexone were monitored for illicit drug use by random urine drug screening. Participants were offered additional treatment after their sentences were served. Success rates of former addicts in the work-release program were equal to those of inmates without drug histories. After completing the program, naltrexone-treated individuals had fewer drug arrests than did opioid abusers who did not receive naltrexone treatment. In another study, Cornish and coworkers (145) reported on federal probationers and parolees with a history of opioid addiction who volunteered for a 6-month, randomized controlled study of naltrexone and brief counseling, which was compared to counseling alone. More than 50% of subjects in the naltrexone-plus-counseling group remained in treatment for 6 months, as opposed to 33% of subjects who received only counseling. Opioid use was significantly lower in the naltrexone group, and fewer naltrexone-treated subjects (26% compared to 56% for the nonnaltrexone treated) had their probation status revoked with a subsequent return to prison during the 6-month period.

NALTREXONE AS PART OF A COMPREHENSIVE DRUG TREATMENT PROGRAM

Naltrexone treatment retention is enhanced by the presence of family support and supportive or behavioral therapy (146). Licensed physicians in private offices or clinic settings may prescribe naltrexone, but it is recommended that it be used by clinicians knowledgeable about substance abuse. Baseline laboratory tests should include liver function studies, and monthly testing should occur during the first 3 months, and at intervals of 3 to 6 months thereafter. It is recommended that opioid addicts in hepatic failure not be treated with naltrexone, although those with minor liver function abnormalities may receive treatment. After medical and psychosocial assessment, patients physically dependent on opioid agonists must undergo detoxification and a naloxone challenge as discussed in "Pharmacology of Opioid Antagonists."

In 1991, Loimer and colleagues (147) reported a procedure using intravenous midazolam and naloxone to shorten the transition time from methadone to naltrexone maintenance, enabling patients to receive therapeutic doses of naltrexone within hours of beginning this rapid detoxification procedure. Highly motivated patients were willing to tolerate opioid withdrawal in order to return quickly to their jobs or to a more normal lifestyle. Subsequent studies of rapid detoxification have been conducted with clonidine, lofexidine, buprenorphine and naloxone; ultrarapid detoxification with naloxone or naltrexone under anesthesia has also been used (148–158). These studies produced mixed results, with some describing uncomplicated naltrexone induction and reasonable retention and outcome, while others reported complicated induction, with vomiting and aspiration occurring under anesthesia, moderately severe withdrawal discomfort, and early dropout.

Scherbaum and colleagues (159) found that patients undergoing ultrarapid detoxification with anesthesia and naloxone experienced mid-level withdrawal symptoms for several days. Nonetheless, 75% of them went on to the next stage of treatment. Because of risks inherent in general anesthesia and the cost of the procedure, the authors recommended that ultrarapid detoxification under anesthesia be restricted to patients addicted to opioids only or in situations where other detoxification strategies are unsuitable. Lawental (160) found, in a nonrandomized pilot study, that ultrarapid detoxification may be less effective and more expensive than traditional 30-day inpatient opioid detoxification in achieving long-term abstinence.

Several authors have warned of potential complications of ultrarapid detoxification. Elman and coworkers (161) studied acute and prolonged effects of ultrarapid detoxification on cardiopulmonary physiology, stress hormones, and clinical outcomes in seven patients inducted onto naltrexone. They found no significant changes in cardiac and pulmonary physiology during the anesthesia phase of ultrarapid detoxification, but plasma adrenocorticotropic hormone (ACTH) and cortisol increased 15- and 13-fold, respectively. During the postanesthesia phase, patients experienced marked withdrawal and tachypnea, and one developed respiratory distress. Withdrawal scores were significantly elevated for 3 weeks following induction, but opioid cravings were reduced. Because of the effects on breathing and stress hormones, the authors recommended further research on ultrarapid detoxification safety and efficacy, and that it be conducted only by experienced anesthesiologists. Hamilton and colleagues (162) described six cases in which patients undergoing a ultrarapid detoxification procedure with subcutaneous naltrexone pellets developed life-threatening complications, including pulmonary edema, prolonged withdrawal, drug toxicity, withdrawal from benzodiazepine and alcohol coaddiction, aspiration pneumonia, and death. It should be noted that the formulation of the pellets used in these patients was *not* the same as the depot formulation currently undergoing phase II evaluation according to FDA procedures for naltrexone maintenance.

Following naltrexone induction, compliance with naltrexone ingestion should be verified in the office or clinic, or by significant people in the patient's life. When treatment is progressing well, as determined by treatment engagement, job performance and absence of illicit drug use confirmed by urinalysis, naltrexone dosing may be reduced to twice weekly. Once patients are stabilized, naltrexone maintenance is associated with few side effects, although nausea, abdominal pain or headache, and mild increases in blood pressure have been noted (127,136). Years of chronic opioid use potentially alter endocrine responses, libido, mood, and pain threshold, so patients may experience rebound effects when opioids are discontinued. Such effects appear to be milder in naltrexone-maintained individuals than in those experiencing the naturally occurring lability of prolonged opioid abstinence without naltrexone. Some individuals taking naltrexone report an increased sex drive (163), a finding observed in rodents (164) and also seen after patients discontinue methadone and other opioids (165). Although variable effects on appetite following the administration of naltrexone have been reported, decreases appear to predominate (166–168). Long-term opioid-receptor blockade by naltrexone does not appear to lead to alteration in mood, and increases in depression have infrequently been encountered.

NALMEFENE: A LONG-ACTING OPIOID ANTAGONIST

Nalmefene is an opioid antagonist that has been approved for use in the management of opioid overdose and for the reversal of opioid drug effects. It is an orally active analogue of naltrexone (169) with a terminal phase plasma half-life of approximately 8 to 9 hours (170). This is in contrast to the poor oral bioavailability and approximately 1- to 2-hour half life of naloxone (171,172).

Numerous clinical pharmacology and efficacy studies have assessed the antagonist properties of nalmefene in human subjects. A single oral dose of nalmefene 50 mg administered to healthy volunteers blocks for 48 to 72 hours the respiratory depression, analgesia, and subjective effects (e.g., drowsiness, nausea, itching) secondary to intravenously administered fentanyl, 2 μg/kg (173). A subsequent study confirmed the ability of nalmefene to antagonize respiratory depression induced by multiple fentanyl challenges (174). In the only study to assess dose effects and duration of opioid blockade in opioid abusers administered oral nalmefene (175), both the 50- and 100-mg doses blocked various physiologic (e.g., pupillary constriction) and subjective (e.g., morphine-induced euphoria) effects produced by 10 and 20 mg of morphine given intravenously. Nalmefene did not produce noticeable physiologic or subjective effects either alone or in combination with morphine.

Results also indicated that intravenous nalmefene (0.4 mg per 70 kg body weight) was comparable to a four times greater dose of naloxone in reversing morphine-induced respiratory depression, and that nalmefene had a longer duration of action (176). In contrast, it was later reported that nalmefene and naloxone were equipotent in reversing fentanyl-induced respiratory depression following a single, intravenous dose of the antagonist (177). Other studies have shown nalmefene to be more effective or potent in reversing opioid-induced respiratory sedation (178) and to be effective in the emergency management of opioid overdosage (179,180).

Nalmefene has generally been reported to be well-tolerated in healthy volunteers. In one study, lightheadedness was the most commonly reported subjective effect following the administration of both single oral nalmefene doses of 50 to 300 mg, and 20-mg doses given twice daily for 7 days (181). Similarly, the parenteral administration of nalmefene in doses up to 24 mg was also well tolerated, with lightheadedness, dizziness, and mental fatigue being reported. In a study using individuals with a history of opioid abuse, a somewhat different effect profile was reported when nalmefene in single oral doses up to 100 mg was compared to morphine and placebo (182). Side effects reported only after nalmefene administration included agitation and irritability, muscle tension, abdominal cramps, and a "hungover feeling." Drowsiness or sleepiness was the most common effect reported following each of the treatments. These effects did not appear to be dose related and nalmefene did not produce typical morphine-like effects.

Nalmefene, like naltrexone, apparently does not produce morphine-like subjective effects that could be considered desirable by opioid-dependent or abusing individuals (175). Additionally, as noted previously, nalmefene may produce effects that could limit its use in the abstinence treatment of individuals previously dependent on opioids. However, naltrexone, which has some utility in the maintenance treatment of certain patient populations, has also been reported to produce dysphoria, depressed mood, and other untoward effects in individuals not currently dependent on opioids (115,183). The successful use of nalmefene, like naltrexone, as an adjunctive treatment for the maintenance of opioid abstinence will probably require highly motivated patients.

CURRENT STATUS OF ANTAGONIST TREATMENT

Naltrexone treatment currently is limited to a relatively small number of patients, primarily because of low interest by most opioid-dependent individuals, difficulties associated with naltrexone induction, and high early treatment dropout rates. Kirchmayer and colleagues (184) systematically reviewed controlled clinical trials and concluded that there was insufficient evidence to justify naltrexone use in the maintenance of addicts, except to decrease the probability of reincarceration of prisoners treated with combined naltrexone and behavioral therapy. Nonetheless, selected patients, particularly health care professionals and others with strong social and family support and good jobs, have benefited greatly from naltrexone, and have used even relatively short treatment episodes as a stepping stone toward opioid abstinence. Depot naltrexone may produce better long-term treatment compliance, but problems in recruiting and successfully inducting patients into treatment must be overcome before this type of naltrexone therapy becomes widely accepted. Because opioid dependence is a chronic relapsing disorder, no single treatment may result in long-term abstinence, but a cumulative effect produced by multiple treatments with naltrexone and other modalities may be required.

SUMMARY

Various types of pharmacotherapies with different modes of action have been used and continue to be evaluated as treatments for opioid addiction. Because no single medication is appropriate for every individual, it is important that clinicians have a variety of therapeutic agents available to them. Additionally, pharmacotherapy is not a treatment end in itself; other adjuncts to successful treatment may include psychotherapy, social rehabilitation, vocational training, and others. Intraindividual treatment may also change over time as patients cycle through periods of abstinence and drug use. Rational medication therapy begins with an understanding of not only the disease state generally, but also of the specific dynamics of the addiction process that affect the overall success of treatment.

REFERENCES

1. Dole VP, Nyswander M. A medical treatment for diacetylmorphine (heroin) addiction. A clinical trial with methadone hydrochloride. *JAMA* 1965;193:80–84.
2. Kreek MJ. Multiple drug abuse patterns and medical consequences. In: Meltzer HY, ed. *Psychopharmacology: the third generation of progress.* New York: Raven Press; 1987:1597–1604.
3. Martin WR, Jasinski DR. Physical parameters of morphine dependence in man: tolerance, early abstinence, protracted abstinence. *J Psychiatr Res* 1969;7:9–17.
4. Wikler A. Dynamics of drug dependence: implication of a conditioning theory for research and treatment. *Arch Gen Psychiatry* 1973;28:611–616.
5. Childress AR, McLellan AT, O'Brien CP. Abstinent opiate abusers exhibit conditioned craving, conditioned withdrawal and reductions in both through extinction. *Br J Addict* 1986;81:655–660.
6. van Zwieten PA. Centrally acting antihypertensive drugs. Present and future. *Clin Exp Hypertens* 1999;21:859–873.
7. Koshes RJ, Rock NL. Use of clonidine for behavioral control in an adult patient with autism. *Am J Psychiatry* 1994;151:1714.
8. Jaselskis CA, Cook EH Jr, Fletcher KE, et al. Clonidine treatment of hyperactive and impulsive children with autistic disorder. *J Clin Psychopharmacol* 1992;12:322–327.
9. Fankhauser MP, Karumanchi VC, German ML, et al. A double-blind, placebo-controlled study of the efficacy of transdermal clonidine in autism. *J Clin Psychiatry* 1992;53:77–82.
10. Connor DF, Fletcher KE, Swanson JM. A meta-analysis of clonidine for symptoms of attention-deficit hyperactivity disorder. *J Am Acad Child Adolesc Psychiatry* 1999;38:1551–1559.
11. Silver LB. Alternative (nonstimulant) medications in the treatment of attention-deficit/hyperactivity disorder in children. *Pediatr Clin North Am* 1999;46:965–975.
12. Quan DB, Wandres DL, Schroeder DJ. Clonidine in pain management. *Ann Pharmacother* 1993;27:313–315.
13. Gold MS, Pottash AL, Extein I, et al. Clonidine in acute opiate withdrawal. *N Engl J Med* 1980;302:1421–1422.
14. Kleber HD, Gold MS, Riordan CE. The use of clonidine in detoxification from opiates. *Bull Narc* 1980;32:1–10.
15. Washton AM, Resnick RB. Clonidine for opiate detoxification: outpatient clinical trials. *Am J Psychiatry* 1980;137:1121–1122.
16. Spencer L, Gregory M. Clonidine transdermal patches for use in outpatient opiate withdrawal. *Journal of Substance Abuse Treatment.* 1989;6:113–117.
17. Cuthill JD, Beroniade V, Salvatori VA, et al. Evaluation of clonidine suppression of opiate withdrawal reactions: a multidisciplinary approach. *Can J Psychiatry* 1990;35:377–382.
18. Jasinski DR, Johnson RE, Kocher TR. Clonidine in morphine withdrawal. Differential effects on signs and symptoms. *Arch Gen Psychiatry* 1985;42:1063–1066.
19. Johnson DA, Bohan ME. Propoxyphene withdrawal with clonidine. *Am J Psychiatry* 1983;140:1217–1218.
20. Haggerty JJ, Jr., Slatkoff S. Clonidine therapy and meperidine withdrawal. *Am J Psychiatry* 1981;138:698.
21. Charney DS, Riordan CE, Kleber HD, et al. Clonidine and naltrexone. A safe, effective, and rapid treatment of abrupt withdrawal from methadone therapy. *Arch Gen Psychiatry* 1982;39:1327–1332.
22. Charney DS, Heninger GR, Kleber HD. The combined use of clonidine and naltrexone as a rapid, safe, and effective treatment of abrupt withdrawal from methadone. *Am J Psychiatry* 1986;143:831–837.
23. Kleber HD, Topazian M, Gaspari J, et al. Clonidine and naltrexone in the outpatient treatment of heroin withdrawal. *Am J Drug Alcohol Abuse* 1987;13:1–17.
24. Vining E, Kosten TR, Kleber HD. Clinical utility of rapid clonidine-naltrexone detoxification for opioid abusers. *Br J Addict* 1988;83:567–575.
25. Bjorkqvist SE. Clonidine in alcohol withdrawal. *Acta Psychiatr Scand* 1975;52:256–263.
26. Bjorkqvist SE. Clonidine therapy for alcohol withdrawal. *Acta Psychiatr Scand Suppl* 1986;327:114–120.
27. Wilkins AJ, Jenkins WJ, Steiner JA. Efficacy of clonidine in treatment of alcohol withdrawal state. *Psychopharmacology (Berl)* 1983;81:78–80.
28. Glassman AH, Covey LS, Dalack GW, et al. Smoking cessation, clonidine, and vulnerability to nicotine among dependent smokers. *Clin Pharmacol Ther* 1993;54:670–679.
29. Glassman AH, Jackson WK, Walsh BT, et al. Cigarette craving, smoking withdrawal, and clonidine. *Science* 1984;226:864–866.
30. Glassman AH, Stetner F, Walsh BT, et al. Heavy smokers, smoking cessation, and clonidine. Results of a double-blind, randomized trial. *JAMA* 1988;259:2863–2866.
31. Ornish SA, Zisook S, McAdams LA. Effects of transdermal clonidine treatment on withdrawal symptoms associated with smoking cessation. A randomized, controlled trial. *Arch Intern Med* 1988;148:2027–2031.
32. Aghajanian GK. Tolerance of locus coeruleus neurones to morphine and suppression of withdrawal response by clonidine. *Nature* 1978;276:186–188.
33. Crawley JN, Laverty R, Roth RH. Clonidine reversal of increased norepinephrine metabolite levels during morphine withdrawal. *Eur J Pharmacol* 1979;57:247–250.
34. Roth RH, Elsworth JD, Redmond DE Jr. Clonidine suppression of noradrenergic hyperactivity during morphine withdrawal by clonidine: biochemical studies in rodents and primates. *J Clin Psychiatry* 1982;43:42–46.
35. Redrobe JP, Bourin M. Clonidine potentiates the effects of 5-HT$_{1A}$, 5-HT$_{1B}$ and 5-HT$_{2A/2C}$ antagonists and 8-OH-DPAT in the mouse forced swimming test. *Eur Neuropsychopharmacol* 1998;8:169–173.
36. Lin MT, Su CF. Spinal 5-HT pathways and the antinociception induced by intramedullary clonidine in rats. *Naunyn Schmiedebergs Arch Pharmacol* 1992;346:333–338.
37. Buccafusco JJ. Mechanism of the clonidine-induced protection against acetylcholinesterase inhibitor toxicity. *J Pharmacol Exp Ther* 1982;222:595–599.
38. Buccafusco JJ, Spector S. Influence of clonidine on experimental hypertension induced by cholinergic stimulation. *Experientia* 1980;36:671–673.
39. Katsuragi T, Su C. Facilitation by clonidine of purine release induced by high KCl from the rabbit pulmonary artery. *Br J Pharmacol* 1981;74:709–713.
40. Katsuragi T, Ushijima I, Furukawa T. The clonidine-induced self-injurious behavior of mice involves purinergic mechanisms. *Pharmacol Biochem Behav* 1984;20:943–946.
41. Katsuragi T, Kuratomi L, Furukawa T. Clonidine-evoked selective P1-purinoceptor antagonism of contraction of guinea-pig urinary bladder. *Eur J Pharmacol* 1986;121:119–122.
42. Schaut J, Schnoll SH. Four cases of clonidine abuse. *Am J Psychiatry* 1983;140:1625–1627.
43. Beuger M, Tommasello A, Schwartz R, et al. Clonidine use and abuse among methadone program applicants and patients. *J Subst Abuse Treat* 1998;15:589–593.
44. Brown MJ, Salmon D, Rendell M.

Clonidine hallucinations. *Ann Intern Med* 1980;93:456–457.

45. Dennison SJ. Clonidine abuse among opiate addicts. *Psychiatr Q* 2001;72:191–195.

46. Sharma A, Newton W. Clonidine as a drug of abuse. *J Am Bd Fam Pract* 1995;8:136–138.

47. Dy EC, Yates WR. Atypical drug abuse: a case report involving clonidine. *Am Fam Physician* 1996;54:1035–1038.

48. Strang J, Bearn J, Gossop M. Lofexidine for opiate detoxification: review of recent randomised and open controlled trials. *Am J Addict* 1999;8:337–348.

49. *Britlofex data sheet*. Redhill, Surrey, UK: Britannia Pharmaceuticals, January, 1996.

50. Gold MS, Pottash AC, Sweeney DR, et al. Opiate detoxification with lofexidine. *Drug Alcohol Depend* 1981;8:307–315.

51. Gold MS, Pottash AC, Sweeney DR, et al. Lofexidine blocks acute opiate withdrawal. *NIDA Res Monogr* 1982;41:264–268.

52. Washton AM, Resnick RB. Clonidine in opiate withdrawal: review and appraisal of clinical findings. *Pharmacotherapy* 1981;1:140–146.

53. Washton AM, Resnick RB. Lofexidine in abrupt methadone withdrawal. *Psychopharmacol Bull* 1982;18:220–221.

54. Washton AM, Resnick RB, Perzel JF, et al. Opiate detoxification using lofexidine. *NIDA Res Monogr* 1982;41:261–263.

55. Washton AM, Resnick RB, Geyer G. Opiate withdrawal using lofexidine, a clonidine analogue with fewer side effects. *J Clin Psychiatry* 1983;44:335–337.

56. Bearn J, Gossop M, Strang J. Randomised double-blind comparison of lofexidine and methadone in the inpatient treatment of opiate withdrawal. *Drug Alcohol Depend* 1996;43:87–91.

57. Bearn J, Gossop M, Strang J. Accelerated lofexidine treatment regimen compared with conventional lofexidine and methadone treatment for in-patient opiate detoxification. *Drug Alcohol Depend* 1998;50:227–232.

58. Carnwath T, Hardman J. Randomised double-blind comparison of lofexidine and clonidine in the out-patient treatment of opiate withdrawal. *Drug Alcohol Depend* 1998;50:251–254.

59. Lin SK, Strang J, Su LW, et al. Double-blind randomised controlled trial of lofexidine versus clonidine in the treatment of heroin withdrawal. *Drug Alcohol Depend* 1997;48:127–133.

60. Kahn A, Mumford JP, Rogers GA, et al. Double-blind study of lofexidine and clonidine in the detoxification of opiate addicts in hospital. *Drug Alcohol Depend* 1997;44:57–61.

61. Buntwal N, Bearn J, Gossop M, et al. Naltrexone and lofexidine combination treatment compared with conventional lofexidine treatment for in-patient opiate detoxification. *Drug Alcohol Depend* 2000;59:183–188.

62. Gerra G, Zaimovic A, Giusti F, et al. Lofexidine versus clonidine in rapid opiate detoxification. *J Subst Abuse Treat* 2001;21:11–17.

63. Cheskin LJ, Fudala PJ, Johnson RE. A controlled comparison of buprenorphine and clonidine for acute detoxification from opioids. *Drug Alcohol Depend* 1994;36:115–121.

64. White R, Alcorn R, Feinmann C. Two methods of community detoxification from opiates: an open-label comparison of lofexidine and buprenorphine. *Drug Alcohol Depend* 2001;65:77–83.

65. Levadi DI. Use of guanabenz in methadone withdrawal. *Am J Psychiatry* 1985;142:1128–1129.

66. Mulry JT. Guanabenz therapy for opiate withdrawal. *Clin PharmDrug Intell Clin Pharm* 1985;19:32–33.

67. Tennant FS, Jr., Rawson RA. Guanabenz acetate: a new, long-acting alpha-two adrenergic agonist for opioid withdrawal. *NIDA Res Monogr* 1984;49:338–343.

68. Rubio G, Alguacil LF, Alamo C, et al. Cardiovascular parameters of heroin-withdrawn addicts treated with guanfacine. *Methods Find Exp Clin Pharmacol* 1997;19:189–192.

69. San L, Cami J, Peri JM, et al. Success and failure at inpatient heroin detoxification. *Br J Addict* 1989;84:81–87.

70. Schubert H, Fleischhacker WW, Meise U, et al. Preliminary results of guanfacine treatment of acute opiate withdrawal. *Am J Psychiatry* 1984;141:1271–1273.

71. Soler Insa PA, Bedate Villar J, Theohar C, et al. Treatment of heroin withdrawal with guanfacine: an open clinical investigation. *Can J Psychiatry* 1987;32:679–682.

72. San L, Cami J, Peri JM, et al. Efficacy of clonidine, guanfacine and methadone in the rapid detoxification of heroin addicts: a controlled clinical trial. *Br J Addict* 1990;85:141–147.

73. San L, Fernandez T, Cami J, et al. Efficacy of methadone versus methadone and guanfacine in the detoxification of heroin-addicted patients. *J Subst Abuse Treat* 1994;11:463–469.

74. Nightingale SL. Levomethadyl approved for the treatment of opiate dependence. *JAMA* 1993;270:1290.

75. Keats AS, Beecher HK. Analgesic activity and toxic effects of acetyl-methadol isomers in man. *J Pharmacol Exp Ther* 1952;105:210–215.

76. David NA, Semler HJ, Burgner PR. Control of chronic pain by dl-alpha-acetylmethadol. *JAMA* 1956;161:599–603.

77. Fraser HF, Isbell H. Actions and addiction liabilities of alpha-acetyl-methadols in man. *J Pharmacol Exp Ther* 1952;105:458–465.

78. Isbell H, Fraser HF. Addictive properties of methadone derivatives. *J Pharmacol Exp Ther* 1954;13:369.

79. Walsh SL, Johnson RE, Cone EJ, et al. Intravenous and oral 1-alpha-acetylmethadol: pharmacodynamics and pharmacokinetics in humans. *J Pharmacol Exp Ther* 1998;285:71–82.

80. Inturrisi CE, Verebely K. The levels of methadone in the plasma in methadone maintenance. *Clin Pharmacol Ther* 1972;13:633–637.

81. Sawe J. High dose morphine and methadone in cancer patients. Clinical pharmacokinetic considerations for oral treatment. *Clin Pharmacokinet* 1986;11:87–106.

82. Inturrisi CE, Colburn WA, Kaiko RF, et al. Pharmacokinetics and pharmacodynamics of methadone in patients with chronic pain. *Clin Pharmacol Ther* 1987;41:392–401.

83. Leimbach DG, Eddy NB. Synthetic analgesics. III. Methadols, isomethadols and their acyl derivatives. *J Pharmacol Exp Ther* 1954;110:135–147.

84. McMahon RE, Calp HW, Marshal FJ. The metabolism of alpha-*dl*-acetyl methadol in the rat: the identification of a probable active metabolite. *J Pharmacol Exp Ther* 1965;149:436–445.

85. Moody DE, Alburges ME, Parker RJ, et al. The involvement of cytochrome P450 3A in the N-demethylation of 1-alpha-acetylmethadol (LAAM), nor-LAAM and methadone. *Drug Metabl Dispos* 1997;25:1347–1353.

86. Fudala PJ. LAAM—pharmacology and pharmacokinetics, development history, and therapeutic considerations. *Subst Abuse* 1996;17:127–132.

87. Jaffe JH, Schuster CR, Smith BB, et al. Comparison of acetylmethadol and methadone in the treatment of long-term heroin users. A pilot study. *JAMA* 1970;211:1834–1836.

88. Ling W, Charuvastra C, Kaim SC, et al. Methadyl acetate and methadone as maintenance treatments for heroin addicts. A veterans administration cooperative study. *Arch Gen Psychiatry* 1976;33:709–720.

89. Ling W, Klett CJ, Gillis RD. A cooperative clinical study of methadyl acetate. I. Three-times-a-week regimen. *Arch Gen Psychiatry* 1978;35:345–353.

90. Fudala PJ, Vocci F, Montgomery A, et al. Levomethadyl acetate (LAAM) for the treatment of opioid dependence: a multisite, open-label study of LAAM safety and an evaluation of the product labeling and treatment regulations. *J Maint Addict* 1997;1:9–39.

91. Finn P, Wilcock K. Levo-Alpha Acetyl Methadol (LAAM). Its advantages and drawbacks. *J Subst Abuse Treat* 1997;14:559–564.

92. McCance-Katz EF, Rainey PM, Friedland G, et al. Effect of opioid dependence pharmacotherapies on zidovudine disposition. *Am J Addict* 2001;10:296–307.

93. Rawson RA, Hasson AL, Huber AM, et al. A 3-year progress report on the implementation of LAAM in the United States. *Addiction.* 1998;93:533–540.

94. Deamer RL, Wilson DR, Clark DS, et al. Torsades de pointes associated with high-dose levomethadyl acetate (ORLAAM). *J Addict Dis* 2001;20:7–14.

95. Schwetz BA. From the Food and Drug Administration. *JAMA* 2001;285:2705.

96. O'Brien C, Greenstein R, Ternes J, et al. Clinical pharmacology of narcotic antagonists. *Ann N Y Acad Sci* 1978;311:232–233=240.

97. Blachly PH. Naloxone for diagnosis in methadone programs. *JAMA* 1973;224:334–335.

98. Fudala PJ, Berkow L, Fralich J, et al. Use of naloxone in the assessment of opiate dependence. *Life Sci* 1991;49:1809–1814.

99. Zilm DH, Sellers EM. The quantitative assessment of physical dependence on opiates. *Drug Alcohol Depend* 1978;3:419–428.

100. Peachey JE, Lei H. Assessment of opioid dependence with naloxone. *Br J Addict* 1988;83:193–201.

101. Judson BA, Himmelberger DU, Goldstein A. The naloxone test for opiate dependence. *Clin Pharmacol Ther* 1980;27:492–501.

102. Martin WR. Opiate antagonists. *Pharmacol Rev* 1967;19:463–521.

103. Gilbert PE, Martin WR. The effects of morphine and nalorphine-like drugs in the nondependent and morphine-dependent and cyclazocine-dependent chronic spinal dog. *J Pharmacol Exp Ther* 1976;198:66–82.

104. Jasinski DR. Human pharmacology of narcotic antagonists. *Br J Pharmacol* 1979;7:287S–290S.

105. Fraser HR. Human pharmacology and clinical uses of nalorphine (N-Allylnormorphine). *Med Clin North Am* 1957;23:1–11.

106. Jasinski DR, Martin WR, Haertzen CA. The human pharmacology and abuse potential of n-allylnoroxymorphine

107. Fishman J, Roffwarg H, Hellman L. Disposition of naloxone in normal and narcotic dependent men. *J Pharmacol Exp Ther* 1973;187:575–580.

108. Heilman RD, Hahn EF, Fishman J. Narcotic antagonists. 4. Cabon-6 derivatives of N-substituted noroxymorphones as narcotic antagonists. *J Med Chem* 1975;18:259–262.

109. Archer S, Michne WF. Recent progress in research on narcotic antagonists. *Prog Drug Res* 1976;20:45–100.

110. Resnick RB, Freedman AM, Thomas M. Studies of EN-1639A (naltrexone): a new narcotic antagonist. *Am J Psychiatry* 1974;131:646–650.

111. Verebey K, Volavka J, Mule SJ, et al. Naltrexone: disposition, metabolism and effects after acute chronic dosing. *Clin Pharmacol Ther* 1976;20:315–328.

112. Volavka J, Cho D, Mallya A, et al. Naloxone increases ACTH and cortisol in man. *N Engl J Med* 1979;300:1056.

113. Mendelson JH, Ellingboe J, Keuhnle JC, et al. Heroin and naltrexone effects on pituitary-gonadal hormones in man: interaction of steroid feedback effects, tolerance and supersensitivity. *J Pharmacol Exp Ther* 1980;214:503–506.

114. Mendelson JH, Ellingboe J, Keuhnle JC, et al. Effects of naltrexone on mood and neuroendocrine function in normal adult males. *Psychoneuroendocrinol* 1978;3:231–236.

115. Crowley TJ, Wagner JE, Zerbe G, et al. Naltrexone-induced dysphoria in former opioid addicts. *Am J Psychiatry* 1985;142:1081–1085.

116. Hollister L, Johnson K, Boukhabza D, et al. Aversive effects of naltrexone in subjects not dependent on opiates. *Drug Alcohol Depend* 1981;8:37–41.

117. Malcolm R, O'Neil PM, Von JM, et al. Naltrexone and dysphoria: a double-blind placebo controlled trial. *Biol Psychiatry* 1987;22:710–716.

118. Marrazzi MA, Wroblewski JM, Kinzie J, et al. High-dose naltrexone and liver function safety. *Am J Addict* 1997;6:21–29.

119. National Research Council Committee. Clinical evaluation of naltrexone treatment of opiate-dependent individuals. *Arch Gen Psychiatry* 1978;35:335–340.

120. Croop RS, Faulkner EB, Labriola DF. The safety profile of naltrexone in the treatment of alcoholism. Results from a multicenter usage study. The Naltrexone Usage Group. *Arch Gen Psychiatry* 1997;54:1130–1135.

121. Maggio CA, Presta E, Bracco EF, et al. Naltrexone and human eating behavior: a dose-ranging inpatient trial in moderately obese men. *Brain Res Bull* 1985;14:657–661.

122. Comer SD, Collins ED, Kleber HD, et al. Depot naltrexone: long-lasting antagonism of the effects of heroin in humans. *Psychopharmacology (Berl)* 2002;159:351–360.

123. Wall ME, Brine DR, Perez-Reyes M. Metabolism and disposition of naltrexone in man after oral and intravenous administration. *Drug Metab Dispos* 1981;9:369–375.

124. Meyer MC, Straughn AB, Lo MW, et al. Bioequivalence, dose-proportionality, and pharmacokinetics of naltrexone after oral administration. *J Clin Psychiatry* 1984;45:15–19.

125. Crabtree BL. Rieview of naltrexone, a long-acting antagonist. *Clin Pharm* 1984;3:273–280.

126. Lee MC, Wagner HN, Tanada S, et al. Duration of occupancy of opiate receptors by naltrexone. *J Nucl Med* 1973;29:1207–1211.

127. Martin WR, Jasinski D, Mansky P. Naltrexone. An antagonist for the treatment of heroin dependence. *Arch Gen Psychiatry* 1973;28:784–791.

128. O'Brien CP, Greenstein R, Mintz J, et al. Clinical experience with naltrexone. *Am J Drug Alcohol Abuse* 1975;2:365–377.

129. Bradford H, Kaim, S. *National Institute on Drug Abuse studies evaluating the safety of the narcotic antagonist naltrexone.* Washington, DC: Biometric Research Institute, 1977.

130. Hollister L. Clinical evaluation of naltrexone treatment of opiate-dependent individuals. Report of the National Research Council Committee on Clinical Evaluation of Narcotic Antagonists. *Arch Gen Psychiatry* 1978;35:335–344.

131. Wang RIH, Wiesen RL, Lamid S, et al. Rating the presence and severity of opiate dependence. *Clin Pharmacol Ther* 1974;16:653–658.

132. Resnick R, Schuyten-Resnick E, Washton AM. Narcotic antagonists in the treatment of opioid dependence: Review and commentary. *Compr Psychiatry* 1979;20:116–125.

133. Washton AM, Pottash AC, Gold MS. Naltrexone in addicted business executives ans physicians. *J Clin Psychiatry* 1984;45:39–41.

134. Brahen LS, Henderson RK, Capone T, et al. Naltrexone treatment in a jail work-release program. *J Clin Psychiatry* 1989;45:49–52.

135. Fram DH, Marmo J, Hoden R. Naltrexone treatment - The problem of patient acceptance. *J Subst Abuse Treat* 1989;6:119–122.

136. Greensein RA, Arndt IC, McLellan AT, et al. Naltrexone: a clinical perspective. *J Clin Psychiatry* 1984;45:25–28.

137. Resnick RB, Washton AM, Thomas MA, et al. Natrexone in the treatment of

opiate dependence. *NIDA Res Monogr* 1978;19:321–332.

138. Grabowski J, O'Brien CP, Greenstein RA, et al. Effects of contingent payment on compliance with a naltrexone regimen. *Am J Drug Alcohol Abuse* 1979;6:355–365.

139. Carroll KM, Ball SA, Nich C, et al. Targeting behavioral therapies to enhance naltrexone treatment of opioid dependence: efficacy of contingency management and significant other involvement. *Arch Gen Psychiatry* 2001;58:755–761.

140. Church SH, Rothenberg JL, Sullivan MA, et al. Concurrent substance use and outcome in combined behavioral and naltrexone therapy for opiate dependence. *Am J Drug Alcohol Abuse* 2001;27:441–452.

141. Preston KL, Silverman K, Umbricht A, et al. Improvement in naltrexone treatment compliance with contingency management. *Drug Alcohol Depend* 1999;54:127–135.

142. Ling W, Wesson DR. Naltrexone treatment for addicted health-care professionals: a collaborative private practice experience. *J Clin Psychiatry* 1984;45:46–48.

143. Roth A, Hogan I, Farren C. Naltrexone plus group therapy for the treatment of opiate abusing health-care professionals. *J Subst Abuse Treat* 1997;14:19–22.

144. Tennant FSJ, Rawson RA, Cohen AJ, et al. Clinical experiences with naltrexone in suburban opioid addicts. *J Clin Psychiatry* 1984;45:42–45.

145. Cornish JW, Metzger D, Woody GE, et al. Naltrexone pharmacotherapy for opioid dependent federal probationers. *J Subst Abuse Treat* 1997;14:529–534.

146. Gonzalez JP, Brogden RN. Naltrexone, a review of its pharmacodynamic and pharmacokinetic properties and therapeutic efficacy in the management of opioid dependence. *Drugs* 1988;35:192–213.

147. Loimer N, Lenz K, Schmid R, et al. Technique for greatly shortening the transition from methadone to naltrexone maintenance of patients addicted to opiates. *Am J Psychiatry* 1991;148:933–935.

148. McGregor C, Ali R, White JM, et al. A comparison of antagonist-precipitated withdrawal under standard inpatient withdrawal as a precursor to maintenance treatment in heroin users: outcomes at 6 and 12 months. *Drug Alcohol Depend* 2002;68:5–14.

149. Seoane A, Carrasco G, Cabre L, et al. Efficacy and safety of two new methods of rapid intravenous detoxification in heroin addicts previously treated without success. *Br J Psychiatry* 1997;171:340–345.

150. O'Connor PG, Kosten TR. Rapid and ultrarapid opioid detoxification techniques. *JAMA* 1998;279:229–234.

151. Albanese AP, Gevirtz D, Oppenheim B, et al. Outcome and six-month follow up of patients after ultra rapid opiate detoxification (UROD). *J Addict Dis* 2000;19:11–28.

152. Cucchia AT, Monnat M, Spagnoli JH, et al. Ultra-rapid opiate detoxification using deep sedation with oral midazolam: short- and long-term results. *Drug Alcohol Depend* 1998;52:243–250.

153. Umbricht A, Montoya ID, Hoover DR, et al. Naltrexone shortened opioid detoxification with buprenorphine. *Drug Alcohol Depend* 1999;56:181–190.

154. Bruntwal N, Bearn J, Gossop M, et al. Naltrexone and lofexidine combination treatment compared with conventional lofexidine treatment for in-patient opiate detoxification. *Drug Alcohol Depend* 2000;59:183–188.

155. Gold CG, Cullen DJ, Gonzales S, et al. Rapid opioid detoxification during general anesthesia: a review of 20 patients. *Anesthesiology* 1999;91:1639–1647.

156. Gerra G, Zaimovic A, Giusti F, et al. Lofexidine versus clonidine in rapid opiate detoxification. *J Subst Abuse Treat* 2001;21:11–17.

157. Pozzi G, Conte G, De Risio S. Combined use of trazodone-naltrexone verus clonidine-naltrexone in rapid withdrawal from methadone treatment. A comparative inpatient study. *Drug Alcohol Depend* 2000;59:287–294.

158. Bartter T, Gooberman LL. Rapid opiate detoxification. *Am J Drug Alcohol Abuse* 1996;2:489–495.

159. Scherbaum N, Klein S, Kaube H, et al. Alternative strategies of opiate detoxification: evaluation of the so-called ultrarapid detoxification. *Pharmacopsychiatry* 1998;31:205–209.

160. Lawental E. Ultra rapid opiate detoxification as compared to 30-day inpatient detoxification program—a retrospective follow-up study. *J Subst Abuse Treat* 2000;11:173–181.

161. Elman I, D'Ambra MN, Krause S, et al. Ultrarapid opioid detoxification: effects on cardiopulmonary physiology, stress hormones and clinical outcomes. *Drug Alcohol Depend* 2001;61:163–172.

162. Hamilton RJ, Olmedo RE, Shah S, et al. Complications of ultrarapid opioid detoxification with subcutaneous naltrexone pellets. *Acad Emerg Med* 2002;9:63–68.

163. Sathe RS, Komisaruk BR, Ladas AK, et al. Naltrexone-induced augmentation of sexual response in men. *Arch Med Res* 2001;32:221–226.

164. Christian MS. Reproductive toxicity and teratology evaluations of naltrexone. *J Clin Psychiatry* 1984;45:7–10.

165. Mirin SM, Meyer RE, Mendelson JH, et al. Opiate use and sexual function. *Am J Psychiatry* 1980;137:909–915.

166. Spiegel TA, Stunkard AJ, Shrager EE, et al. Effect of naltrexone on food intake, hunger, and satiety in obese men. *Physiol Behav* 1987;40:135–141.

167. Yeomans MR, Gray RW. Effects of naltrexone on food intake and changes in subjective appetite during eating: evidence for opioid involvement in the appetizer effect. *Physiol Behav* 1997;62:15–21.

168. de Zwaan M, Mitchell JE. Opiate antagonists and eating behavior in humans: a review. *J Clin Pharmacol* 1992;32:1060–1072.

169. Hahn EF, Fishman J, Heilman RD. Narcotic antagonists. 4. Carbon-6 derivatives of N-substituted noroxymorphones as narcotic antagonists. *J Med Chem* 1975;18:259–262.

170. Dixon R, Howes J, Gentile J, et al. Nalmefene: intravenous safety and kinetics of a new opioid antagonist. *Clin Pharmacol Ther* 1986;39:49–53.

171. Ngai SH, Berkowitz BA, Yang JC, et al. Pharmacokinetics of naloxone in rats and man: basis for its potency and short duration of action. *Anesthesiology* 1976;44:398–401.

172. Aitkenhead AR, Derbyshire DR, Pinnock CA, et al. Pharmacokinetics of intravenous naloxone in health volunteers. *Anesthesiology* 1984;40:537–542.

173. Gal TJ, DiFazio CA, Dixon R. Prolonged blockade of opioid effect with oral nalmefene. *Clin Pharmacol Ther* 1986;40:537–542.

174. Moore LR, Bikhazi GB, Tuttle RR, et al. Antagonism of fentanyl-induced respiratory depression with nalmefene. *Methods Find Exp Clin Pharmacol* 1990;12:29–35.

175. Jones HE, Johnson RE, Fudala PJ, et al. Nalmefene: blockade of intravenous morphine challenge effects in opioid-abusing humans. *Drug Alcohol Depend* 2000;60:29–37.

176. Konieczko KM, Jones JG, Barrowcliffe MP, et al. Antagonism of morphine-induced respiratory depression with nalmefene. *Br J Anaesth* 1988;61:318–323.

177. Glass PS, Jhaveri RM, Smith LR. Comparison of potency and duration of action of nalmefene and naloxone. *Anesth Analg* 1994;78:536–541.

178. Barsan WG, Seger D, Danzl DF, et al. Duration of antagonistic effects of nalmefene and naloxone in

opiate-induced sedation for emergency department procedures. *Am J Emerg Med* 1989;7:155–161.

179. Kaplan JL, Marx JA. Effectiveness and safety of intravenous nalmefene for emergency department patients with suspected narcotic overdose: a pilot study. *Ann Emerg Med* 1993;22:187–190.

180. Kaplan JL, Marx JA, Calabro JJ, et al. Double-blind, randomized study of nalmefene and naloxone in emergency department patients with suspected narcotic overdose. *Ann Emerg Med* 1999;34:42–50.

181. Dixon R, Gentile J, Hsu HB, et al. Nalmefene: safety and kinetics after single and multiple oral doses of a new opioid antagonist. *J Clin Pharmacol* 1987;27:233–239.

182. Fudala PJ, Heishman SJ, Henningfield JE, et al. Human pharmacology and abuse potential of nalmefene. *Clin Pharmacol Ther* 1991;49:300–306.

183. Hollister LE, Johnson K, Boukhabza D, et al. Aversive effects of naltrexone in subjects not dependent on opiates. *Drug Alcohol Depend* 1981;8:37–41.

184. Kirchmayer U, Davoli M, Verster AD, et al. A systematic review on the efficacy of naltrexone maintenance for opioid dependence. *Addiction* 2002;97:1241–1249.

CHAPTER 42

Individual Psychotherapy

BRUCE J. ROUNSAVILLE, KATHLEEN M. CARROLL, AND SUDIE BACK

This chapter focuses on those aspects of individual therapy that are unique to the one-to-one format of treatment delivery. The chapter presents guidelines on individual therapy that are applicable to those dependent on alcohol as well as other drugs. The chapter emphasizes a review of research findings relative to illicit drugs because the extensive literature on psychosocial treatments for alcoholics has been reviewed elsewhere (1–4).

The history of individual psychotherapy for addictive disorders has been one of importation of methods first developed to treat other conditions. Thus, when psychoanalytic and psychodynamic therapies were the predominant modality for treating most mental disorders, published descriptions of the dynamics of substance abuse or of therapeutic strategies arose from using this established general modality to treat the special population of individuals with addictive disorders (5). Similarly, with the development of behavioral techniques, client-centered therapies, and cognitive–behavioral treatments, earlier descriptions based on other types of patients were followed by discussions of the special modifications needed to treat addictive disorders.

Psychosocial treatment approaches that have originated with treating addictive disorders, such as Alcoholics Anonymous (AA) and therapeutic communities, have emphasized large and small group treatment settings. Although always present as a treatment option, individual psychotherapy has not been the predominant treatment modality for drug abusers since the 1960s, when inpatient 12-step–informed milieu therapy, group treatments, methadone maintenance, and therapeutic community approaches came to be the fixtures of addictive disorder treatment programs.

In fact, these newer modalities derived their popularity from the failures of dynamically informed ambulatory individual psychotherapy when it was used as the sole treatment for addictive disorders. There are several reasons why this approach was poorly suited to the needs of addicts when it was offered as the sole ambulatory treatment.

First, the lack of emphasis on symptom control and the lack of structure in the therapist's typical stance allowed the patient's continued drug or alcohol use to undermine the treatment. Therapists did not develop methods for addressing patient's needs for coping skills because this removal of symptoms was seen as palliative and likely to result in symptom substitution. As a result, substance use often continued unabated while the treatment focused on underlying dynamics. The major strategy that is now common to all currently practiced psychotherapies for addictive disorders is to place primary emphasis on controlling or reducing drug use, while pursuing other goals only after such use has been at least partly controlled. This means that either (a) the individual therapist uses techniques designed to help the patient stop alcohol or drug use as a central part of the treatment, or (b) the therapy is practiced in the context of a comprehensive treatment program in which other aspects of the treatment curtail the patient's use of alcohol or other drugs (e.g., pharmacotherapy or residential treatment).

A second major misfit between individual dynamic therapy and addictive disorders is its anxiety-arousing nature coupled with the lack of structure provided by the neutral therapist. Because addicts frequently react to increased anxiety or other dysphoric affects by resuming substance use, it is important to introduce anxiety-arousing aspects of treatment only after a strong therapeutic alliance has been developed or within the context of other supportive structures (e.g., an inpatient unit, a strong social support network, or methadone maintenance) that guard against relapse to substance use when the patient experiences heightened anxiety and dysphoria in the context of therapeutic exploration.

Individual psychotherapy has become a resurgent approach since the 1980s, as the limitations of other modalities became apparent (e.g., methadone maintenance without ancillary services) (6,7), and necessary modifications in technique were made to address the factors underlying earlier failures. A major development in recent years is the growing list of individual psychotherapies for addictive disorders that have demonstrated efficacy in rigorously conducted randomized clinical trials (8–10).

Two key research developments have encouraged renewed interest in individual psychotherapies. The first development was the publication of results of Project MATCH (Matching Alcoholism Treatments to Client Heterogeneity), a landmark multisite clinical trial in which 3 months of treatment with one of three individual psychotherapies—motivational enhancement treatment (MET) (11), 12-step facilitation (TSF) (12), and cognitive–behavioral therapy (CBT) (13)—was followed by marked and sustained reductions in alcohol consumption (14,15). To illustrate, in all three treatments, patients, on average, who entered treatment drinking more than 80% of days, rapidly reduced their consumption to less than 15% of days, and kept those levels down at followup visits over 3 years.

The second development was the growing evidence for the efficacy of brief psychotherapies (2,4,16,17). This approach includes brief advice to nondependent, heavy substance users in medical settings (18,19). There also was mounting evidence for the efficacy of four or fewer sessions of MET, one of the three treatments included in Project MATCH.

To encourage more widespread use of efficacious treatments, the National Institute on Drug Abuse (NIDA), the National Institute on Alcohol Abuse and Alcoholism, and the Center for Substance Abuse Treatment disseminated training manuals for many of these treatments, either through the Internet from their Web sites (www.nida.nih.gov *or* www.niaaa.nih.gov) or in a printed format that can be ordered through the National Clearinghouse on Alcohol and Drug Abuse Information (PO Box 2345, Rockville, MD 20847).

WHEN IS PSYCHOTHERAPY INDICATED?

Some form of behavioral therapy should be considered as a treatment option for all patients who seek help for a substance use disorder. Treatment seekers represent only approximately 20% of community members who meet the criteria for current substance use disorders (20), and they are likely to represent the more severe end of the spectrum, as most of those who seek treatment do so only after numerous unsuccessful attempts to stop or reduce drug use on their own (21). The alternatives to psychotherapy are either pharmacologic or structural (as through sequestration from access to drugs and alcohol in a residential setting), and both treatments have limited effectiveness if not combined with psychotherapy or counseling. Removal from the substance-using setting is a useful and, sometimes, necessary part of treatment, but it seldom is sufficient in itself, as demonstrated by the high relapse rates typically

seen from residential detoxification programs or incarceration during the year after the patient's return to his or her community (22,23).

PSYCHOTHERAPY AND PHARMACOTHERAPY

The most powerful and commonly used pharmacologic approaches to drug abuse are maintenance on an agonist that has an action similar to that of the abused drug (e.g., methadone for opioid addicts or nicotine gum for cigarette smokers), use of an antagonist that blocks the effect of the abused drug (e.g., naltrexone [ReVia] for opioid addicts), the use of an aversive agent that provides a powerful negative reinforcement if the drug is used (e.g., disulfiram [Antabuse] for alcoholics), or the use of agents that reduce the desire to use the substance (e.g., naltrexone and acamprosate for alcoholics). Although all of these agents are widely used, they seldom are employed without adjunctive psychotherapy, because, for example, naltrexone maintenance alone for opioid dependence is plagued by high rates of premature dropout (24,25), and disulfiram use without adjunctive psychotherapy is not superior to placebo (26–28).

In particular, the large body of literature on the effectiveness of methadone maintenance points to the success of methadone maintenance in retaining opioid addicts in treatment and reducing their illicit opioid use and illegal activity (7). However, there is a great deal of variability in success rates across different methadone maintenance programs, which is at least partially a result of wide variations in the provision and quality of psychosocial services (7).

The shortcomings of even powerful pharmacotherapies delivered without psychotherapy were convincingly demonstrated by McLellan and colleagues at the Philadelphia Veterans Affairs Medical Center (29). In a 24-week trial, 92 opioid addicts were randomly assigned to receive either (a) methadone maintenance alone, without psychosocial services; (b) methadone maintenance with standard psychosocial services, which included regular individual meetings with a counselor; and (c) enhanced methadone maintenance, which included regular counseling plus access to on-site psychiatric, medical, employment, and family therapy. In terms of drug use and psychosocial outcomes, the best outcomes were seen in the enhanced methadone maintenance condition, with intermediate outcomes for the standard methadone services condition, and poorest outcomes for the methadone alone condition. Although a few patients did reasonably well in the methadone alone condition, 69% had to be transferred out of that condition within 3 months of initiation of the study inception because their substance use did not improve or even worsened or because they experienced significant medical or psychiatric problems that required a more intensive level of care.

The results of this study suggest that although methadone maintenance alone can be sufficient for a small subgroup of patients, the majority will not benefit from a purely pharmacologic approach, and the best outcomes are associated with higher levels of psychosocial treatments. Even when the principal treatment is seen as pharmacologic, psychotherapeutic interventions are needed to complement the pharmacotherapy by (a) enhancing the motivation to stop substance use by taking the prescribed medications, (b) providing guidance for the use of prescribed medications and management of side effects, (c) maintaining motivation to continue taking the prescribed medications after the patient achieves an initial period of abstinence, (d) providing relationship elements to prevent premature termination, and (e) helping the patient to develop the skills to adjust to a life without drug and alcohol use.

The elements that psychotherapy can offer to complement pharmacologic approaches are likely to be needed even if "perfect" pharmacotherapies become available. This is because the effectiveness of even the most powerful pharmacotherapies is limited by patients' willingness to comply with them, and the strategies found to enhance compliance with pharmacotherapies (monitoring, support, encouragement, education) are inherently psychosocial. Moreover, the provision of a clearly articulated and consistently delivered psychosocial treatment in the context of a primarily pharmacologic treatment is an important strategy for reducing noncompliance and attrition, thereby enhancing outcomes in clinical research and clinical treatment (30).

Moreover, the importance of psychotherapy and psychosocial treatments is reinforced by recognition that the repertoire of pharmacotherapies available for treatment of drug addicts is limited to a handful, with the most effective agents limited in their utility to treatment of opioid dependence (31–34) and alcohol dependence (26,35–38). Effective pharmacotherapies for dependence on cocaine, marijuana, hallucinogens, sedative–hypnotics, and stimulants have not yet been developed, and behavioral therapies remain the principal approaches for the treatment of these classes of drugs (32,39).

Although the foregoing has emphasized the need for psychotherapy to enhance the effectiveness of pharmacotherapy, this section would not be complete without considering the role of pharmacotherapy to enhance the efficacy of psychotherapy. These two treatments have different mechanisms of action and targeted effects that can counteract the weaknesses of either treatment alone. Psychotherapies effect change by psychological means in psychosocial aspects of drug abuse, such as motivation, coping skills, dysfunctional thoughts, or social relationships. Their weaknesses include limited effects on the physiologic aspects of drug use or withdrawal. Also, the effects of behavioral treatments tend to be delayed, requiring practice, repeated sessions, and a "working through" process.

In contrast, the relative strengths of pharmacologic treatments are their rapid actions in reducing immediate or protracted withdrawal symptoms, drug craving, and/or the rewarding effects of continued drug use. In effect, pharmacotherapies for drug dependence reduce the patients' immediate access to and preoccupation with drugs, freeing the patient to address other concerns such as long-term goals or interpersonal relationships.

Dropout from psychotherapy is reduced because drug urges and relapse are mitigated by the effects of the medication. Greater duration of abstinence can further enhance the effects of psychotherapy because substance-related effects on attention and mental acuity are prevented, maximizing new learning that therapy can induce. Because of the complementary actions of psychotherapies and pharmacotherapies, combined treatment has a number of potential advantages. As reviewed later under "Efficacy Research," research evidence on combined treatment is sparse but generally supportive of this approach. Although factors such as cost and patient acceptance can limit use of combined approaches, it is important to note that no studies have shown that combined treatments are less than effective with either psychotherapy or pharmacotherapy alone.

Individual Versus Group Therapy

If psychotherapy is necessary for at least a substantial number of treatment-seeking drug addicts, when is individual therapy a better choice than other modalities such as family therapy or group therapy? Because group therapy has become the modal format for psychotherapy of drug addicts, evaluation of the role of individual therapy should take the strengths and weaknesses of group therapy as its starting point.

A central advantage of group over individual psychotherapy is economy, which is a major consideration in an era of generally skyrocketing health care costs and increasingly curtailed third-party payments for the treatment of addictive disorders. Groups typically have a minimum of six members and a maximum of two therapists, yielding at least a threefold increase in the number of patients treated per therapist hour. Although the efficacy of group versus individual therapy has only rarely been systematically studied with drug addicts, no evidence is available from other populations that individual psychotherapy yields superior benefits (40).

In addition to the general concept that group therapy can be just as effective as, but less expensive than, individual therapy (41), there are aspects of group therapy that can be argued to make this modality more effective than individual treatment of drug addicts. For example, given the social stigma attached to having lost control of substance use, the presence of other group members who acknowledge having similar problems can provide comfort. Related to this aspect, other group members who are farther along in their recovery from addiction can act as models to illustrate that attempting to stop drug and alcohol use is not a futile effort. These more experienced group members can offer a wide variety of coping strategies that go beyond the repertoire known even by the most skilled individual therapist. Moreover, group members frequently can act as "buddies" who offer continued support outside of the group sessions in a way that most professional therapists do not.

Finally, the "public" nature of group therapy, with its attendant aspects of confession and forgiveness, coupled with the pressure to publicly confess future slips and transgressions, provides a powerful incentive to avoid relapse. The ability to publicly declare the number of days sober, coupled with the fear of having to publicly admit to "falling off the wagon," are strong forces that push an addict toward recovery. This public affirmation or shaming can be all the more crucial in combating a disorder that is characterized by a failure of internalized mechanisms of control. Drug addicts have been characterized as having poorly functioning internal self-control mechanisms (42,43), and the group process—with many eyes watching—provides a robust source of external control. Moreover, because the group is composed of recovering addicts, members may be better able to detect each other's attempts to conceal relapse or early warning signals for relapse than would an individual therapist who may not have personal experience with an addictive disorder.

Given these strengths of group therapy, what are the advantages of individual therapy that can justify its greater expense? First, a key advantage of individual therapy is that it provides privacy. Although self-help groups such as Alcoholics Anonymous (AA) attempt to protect the confidentiality of group members by asking for first names only, and routine group therapy procedures involve instructions to members to keep identities of individuals and the contents of sessions confidential, participation in group therapy always risks a breach in confidentiality, especially in small communities. Although publicly admitting to one's need for help can be a key element of the recovery process, it is a step that is very difficult to take, particularly when the problems associated with substance use have not yet become severe. Public knowledge of drug and alcohol use still can ruin careers and reputations.

Second, the individualized pace of individual therapy allows the therapist more flexibility to address the patient's problems as they arise, whereas group therapy can be out of sync with some members while suiting the needs of the majority. This situation is particularly an issue for open groups that add new members throughout the life of the group, necessitating repetition of many therapeutic elements so as to acquaint new members with the group's history and to address the needs of individuals who have just begun treatment.

Third, from the patient's point of view, individual therapy allows a much higher percentage of therapy time to concentrate on issues that are uniquely relevant to that individual. Members of therapy groups usually have the experience of spending many hours discussing issues that are not problems for them, and the individual tailoring of therapy sessions to fit particular needs ultimately can be more efficient.

Fourth, logistical issues make individual therapy more practical in many settings. Given the decentralization of much mental health service delivery, individual therapy is most feasible for many mental health professionals or medical practitioners who do not have a caseload of addicts large enough to conduct group treatment. If group therapy is to be started with a new group, it can be many weeks before enough members are screened to be entered into a new group, resulting in patients' discouragement and high dropout rates while awaiting the onset of treatment. If group therapy involves addition to an ongoing group, this situation can present formidable obstacles to joining. Also, unless group therapy is offered in the context of a large clinic or practice with many ongoing groups, scheduling can be very difficult for those patients whose employer is not apprised of the need for treatment.

Fifth, the process and structure of individual therapy can confer unique advantages in dealing with some kinds of problems presented by patients. For example, individual therapy can be more conducive to the development of a deepening relationship between the patient and therapist over time, which can allow exploration of relationship elements not possible in group therapy. Alternatively, patients with particular personality disorders, such as borderline or schizoid patients, may be unable to get involved with other group members, as can patients who are so shy that they cannot bring themselves to attend group sessions.

SPECIALIZED KNOWLEDGE NECESSARY FOR THERAPY WITH ADDICTS

This section bases its recommendations on the supposition that most individual psychotherapists who attempt to work with addicts obtained their first psychotherapy experience and training with other groups of patients, such as those typically seen at inpatient or outpatient general psychiatric clinics. This supposition is based on the status of addiction treatment as a subspecialty placement within training programs for the major professions that practice psychotherapy, including psychologists, psychiatrists, and social workers. Thus, to treat addicts, the task for the typical psychotherapist is to acquire necessary new knowledge and modify already learned skills.

Pharmacology, Use Patterns, Consequences, and Course of Addiction

The principal areas of knowledge to be mastered by the beginning therapist are pharmacology, use patterns, consequences, and course of addiction for the major types of abused substances. For therapy to be effective, it is useful not only to obtain the textbook knowledge about frequently abused drugs, but also to become familiar with street knowledge about drugs (e.g., slang names, favored routes of administration, prices, and availability) and the clinical presentation of individuals when they are intoxicated or experiencing withdrawal from the various abused drugs. This knowledge has many important uses in the course of individual therapy.

First, it fosters a therapeutic alliance by allowing the therapist to convey an understanding of the addict's problems and the world in which the addict lives. This issue is especially important when the therapist is from a different racial or social background from the patient. In engaging the patient in treatment, it is important to emphasize that the patient's primary presenting complaint is likely to be substance abuse, even if many other issues also are amenable to psychotherapeutic interventions. Hence, if the therapist is not comfortable and familiar with the nuances of problematic drug and alcohol use, it can be difficult to forge an initial working alliance. Moreover, by knowing the natural history of addiction and the course of drug and alcohol effects, the clinician can be guided in helping the patient anticipate problems that will arise in the course of initiating abstinence. For example, knowing the typical type and duration of withdrawal symptoms can help the addict recognize their transient nature and develop a plan for successfully completing an ambulatory detoxification.

Second, knowledge of drug actions and withdrawal states is crucial for diagnosing comorbid psychopathology and for helping the addict to understand and manage dysphoric affects. It has been observed in clinical situations and demonstrated in laboratory conditions (44–46) that most abused drugs are capable of producing constellations of symptoms that mimic psychiatric syndromes, such as depression, mania, anxiety disorders, or paranoia. Many of these symptomatic states are completely substance-induced and resolve spontaneously when such use is stopped. It often is the therapist's job to determine whether or not presenting symptoms are part of an enduring, underlying psychiatric condition or a transient, drug-induced state. If the former, then simultaneous treatment of the psychiatric disorder is appropriate; if the latter, reassurance and encouragement to maintain abstinence usually are the better course.

This need to distinguish transient substance-induced affects from enduring attitudes and traits also is an important psychotherapy task. Affective states are linked closely with cognitive distortions, as Beck and colleagues (47) demonstrated in their delineation of the cognitive distortions associated with depression. While experiencing depressive symptoms, a patient is likely to have a profoundly different view of himself or herself, the future, the satisfactions available in life, and his or her important interpersonal relationships. These views are likely to change radically with remission of depressive symptoms, even if the remission of symptoms is induced by pharmacotherapy and not by psychotherapy or actual improvement in life circumstances (48,49). Because of this tendency for substance-related affective states to greatly color the patient's view of self and world, it is important for the therapist to be able to recognize these states so that the associated distorted thoughts can be recognized as such rather than being taken at face value. Moreover, it is important that the patient also be taught to distinguish between sober and substance-affected conditions and to recognize when, in the colloquial phrase, it is "the alcohol talking" and not the person's more enduring sentiments.

Third, learning about drug and alcohol effects is important in detecting when patients have relapsed or come to sessions intoxicated. It is very rarely useful to conduct psychotherapy sessions when the patient is intoxicated and, when this happens, the session should be rescheduled for a time when the patient can participate while sober. For alcoholics, noticing the smell of alcohol or using a Breathalyzer is a useful technique for detecting intoxication. A number of inexpensive and rapid urine tests are commercially available that can be used in the office to detect recent drug use. Samples also can be sent to commercial laboratories for verification. The clinician then must rely on his or her own clinical skills to determine whether or not the patient is drug free and able to participate fully in the psychotherapy.

Other Treatment and Self-Help Group Philosophies and Techniques

A second area of knowledge to be mastered by the psychotherapist is an overview of treatment philosophies and techniques for the range of treatments and self-help groups that are available to substance-using patients. As noted earlier, the early experience of attempting individual psychotherapy as the sole treatment of the more severe types of drug addiction was marked by failure and early dropout. Hence, for many addicts, individual psychotherapy is best conceived as a component of a multifaceted program of treatment to help the patient overcome a chronic, relapsing condition. In fact, one function of individual psychotherapy can be to help the patient choose which additional therapies to employ in the patient's attempt to stop using alcohol or other drugs. Thus, even when the therapist is a solo practitioner, the therapist should know when detoxification is necessary, when inpatient treatment is appropriate, and what pharmacotherapies are available.

Another major function of knowing about the major alternative treatment modalities for addicts is to be alert to the possibility that different treatments can provide contradictory recommendations that may confuse the patient or foster the patient's attempts to sabotage treatment. Unlike a practitioner whose treatment is likely to be sufficient in itself, the individual psychotherapist does not have the option of simply instructing the patient to curtail other treatments or participation in self-help groups while individual treatment is taking place. Rather, it is vital that the therapist attempt to adjust his or her own work to bring the psychotherapy into accord with other treatments.

A commonly occurring set of conflicts arises between the treatment goals and methods employed by professional therapists and those of 12-step self-help movements such as AA, Cocaine Anonymous (CA), and Narcotics Anonymous (NA). For example, the recovery goal for many who use a 12-step approach is a life of complete abstinence from psychotropic medications. This approach may conflict with professional advice when the therapist recommends use of psychopharmacologic treatments for co-occurring psychiatric disorders such as depression, mania, or anxiety. Although the 12-step literature supports use of appropriately prescribed medications of all kinds, many individual members draw the line at prescribed psychotropic medications. In the face of disapproval from fellow members, patients may prematurely discontinue psychotropic medications and experience relapse of psychological symptoms, with consequent return to substance use.

To avoid this situation, it is important for the therapist who recommends or prescribes psychotropic medications to warn the patient about the apparent contradiction between the 12-step admonition to lead a drug-free life and the clinician's use of prescribed psychotropic medications. One way to approach this issue is to describe the psychiatric condition for which the medications are prescribed as a disease separate from the addictive disorder and to impress on the patient that medications are as necessary for the treatment of this separate condition as insulin would be for diabetes. The fact that the medications are intended to affect brain functioning and attendant mental symptoms, while insulin affects other parts of the body, is less important than the concept that two diseases are present and not one.

A second common area of conflict between some forms of psychotherapy and the 12-step philosophy is the role played by family members. The Al-Anon approach tends to suggest that family members get out of the business of attempting to control the addict's use of drugs and alcohol. Separate meetings are held for family members and addicts. In contrast, many therapists encourage involvement of family members in dealing with family dynamics that can foster substance use and/or in acting as adjunctive therapists (50). As with the use of psychotropic medications, the major way to prevent a patient's confusion is to anticipate the areas of contradictory advice and to provide a convincing rationale for the therapist's recommendations. In doing so, it is advisable to acknowledge that different strategies appear to work for different individuals and that alternative approaches may be employed sequentially if the initial plan fails.

COMMON ISSUES AND STRATEGIES

This section reviews issues that must be addressed, if not emphasized, for individual psychotherapy to be effective. As noted in reviewing the difficulties encountered by early psychodynamic practitioners, the central modification that is required of psychotherapists is to be aware that the patient being treated is an addict. Hence, even when attempting to explore other issues in depth, the therapist should (a) devote at least a small part of every session to monitoring the patient's most recent successes and failures in controlling or curtailing substance use and (b) be willing to interrupt other work to address slips and relapses as they occur.

Implicit in the need to remain focused on the patient's substance use is the recognition that psychotherapy with these patients entails a more active therapist stance than does treatment of patients with other psychiatric disorders, such as depression or anxiety. This need is related to the fact that the principal symptom of substance abuse—compulsive use—is at least initially gratifying, whereas it is the long-term consequences of substance use that induce pain and the desire to stop. In contrast, the principal symptoms of depression or anxiety disorders are inherently painful and alien. Because of this key difference, psychotherapy with addicts typically requires both empathy and structured limit-setting, whereas the need for limit-setting is less marked in psychotherapy with depressed or anxious patients.

Beyond these key elements, this section also elaborates on the following set of psychotherapy tasks: enhancing motivation to stop drug use, teaching coping skills, changing reinforcement contingencies, fostering management of painful affects, improving interpersonal functioning, and enhancing social supports. Although different schools of thought about therapeutic action and behavior change can vary in the degree to which emphasis is placed on the various tasks, some attention to each area is likely to be part of any successful treatment.

Enhancing Motivation

Addicts often enter treatment not with the goal to stop, but rather to return to the days when drug and alcohol use was enjoyable (51). The natural history of substance abuse (21,22,52,53) typically is characterized by an initial period of episodic use lasting months to years in which substance-related consequences are minimal and use is perceived as beneficial. Even at the time of treatment-seeking, which usually occurs only after substance-related problems have become severe, patients usually can identify many ways in which they want or feel the need for drugs or alcohol and have difficulty developing a clear picture of what life without these substances might be like. To be able to achieve and maintain abstinence or controlled use, such patients need a clear conception of their treatment goals.

Several investigators (54,55) have postulated stages in the development of addicts' thinking about stopping use, beginning with precontemplation, moving through contemplation, and culminating with determination as the ideal cognitive set with which to derive the greatest benefit from treatment.

Regardless of the treatment type, an early task for psychotherapists is to gauge the patient's level of motivation to stop his or her substance use by exploring the patient's treatment goals. In this task, it is important to challenge overly quick or glib assertions that the patient's goal is to stop using the substance altogether. One way to approach the patient's likely ambivalence is to attempt an exploration of the patient's perceived benefits from use of alcohol or drugs, or the patient's perceived need for them. To obtain a clear report of the patient's positive attitudes toward substance use, it may be necessary to elicit details of the patient's early involvement with drugs and alcohol. After the therapist has obtained a clear picture of the patient's perceived needs and desires, it is important to counter these perceptions by exploring the advantages of a drug-free life.

As noted earlier, although virtually all types of psychotherapy for addiction addresses the issue of motivation and goal-setting to some extent, motivational therapy or interviewing (56) makes this the sole initial focus of treatment. Motivational approaches, which usually are quite brief (e.g., two to four sessions) are based on principles of motivational psychology and are designed to produce rapid, internally motivated change by seeking to maximize patients' motivational resources and commitment to abstinence. Active ingredients of these approaches are hypothesized to include objective feedback of personal risk or impairment, emphasis on personal responsibility for change, clear advice to change, a menu of alternative change options, therapist empathy, and facilitation of patient self-efficacy (11,57). Motivational approaches have substantial empirical evidence supporting their effectiveness with alcoholics (2,4,17), but have comparatively recently been evaluated for drug-abusing populations (58–61).

One major controversy in this area is whether controlled use can be an acceptable alternative treatment goal to abstinence from all psychoactive drugs. Many, if not most, patients enter treatment with a goal of controlled use, especially of alcohol (62), and failure to address the patient's presenting goal may result in failure to engage the patient. At the heart of the issue is whether or not drug abuse is seen as a categorical disease, for which the only treatment is abstinence, or as a set of habitual dysfunctional behaviors that are aligned along a continuum of severity (63,64). For illicit drugs of abuse (such as cocaine or heroin), it is unwise for a clinician to take a position that advocates any continued use, because such a stance allies the therapist with illegal and antisocial behavior. Even advocates of controlled use as an acceptable treatment goal usually acknowledge that patients with more severe de-

pendence should seek an abstinence goal. In practice, the therapist cannot force the patient to seek any goal that the patient does not choose. The process of arriving at an appropriate treatment goal frequently involves allowing the patient to make several failed attempts to achieve a goal of controlled use. This initial process may be necessary to convince the patient that a goal of abstinence is more appropriate.

Teaching Coping Skills

The most enduring challenge in treating addicts is to help the patient avoid relapse after achieving an initial period of abstinence (65). A general tactic for avoiding relapse is to identify specific circumstances that increase an individual's likelihood of resuming substance use and to help the patient anticipate and practice strategies (e.g., refusal skills, recognizing and avoiding cues for craving) for coping with these high-risk situations. Approaches that emphasize the development of coping skills include CBT (13,65–67), in which a systematic effort is made to identify high-risk situations and master alternative behaviors, as well as coping skills intended to help the patient avoid drug use when these situations arise. A postulate of this approach is that proficiency in coping skills that are generalizable to a variety of problem areas will help foster durable change. Evidence is emerging that points to the durability and in some cases the delayed emergence of effects of coping skills treatments (68–72). For other approaches, enumeration of risky situations and development of coping skills is less structured (73,74) and embedded in a more general exploration of patients' wishes and fears.

Changing Reinforcement Contingencies

Edwards and colleagues (64,75) have noted that a key element of deepening dependence on alcohol or other drugs is the rise of substance-related behavior to the top of an individual's list of priorities. As dependence deepens, it can take precedence over concerns about work, family, friends, possessions, and health. As compulsive use becomes a part of every day, previously valued relationships or activities may be given up, so that the rewards available in daily life are narrowed progressively to those derived from use of the substance. When such use is ended, its absence may leave the patient with a need to fill the time that had been spent using drugs or alcohol and to find rewards to substitute for those derived from their use.

The ease with which the patient can rearrange priorities is related to the level of achievement before the patient became involved with alcohol or drugs and the degree to which substance use destroyed or replaced valued relationships, jobs, or hobbies. Because the typical course of illicit drug use entails initiation of compulsive use between the ages of 12 and 25 years (76,77), many patients come to treatment without having achieved satisfactory adult relationships or vocational skills. In such cases, achieving a drug- and alcohol-free life may require a lengthy process of vocational rehabilitation and development of meaningful relationships. Individual psychotherapy can contribute importantly to this process by helping maintain the patient's motivation throughout the recovery process and by helping the patient to explore factors that have interfered with achievement of rewarding ties to others. An example of an approach that actively changes reinforcement contingencies is the one developed by Higgins and colleagues (78,79), which incorporates positive incentives for abstinence into a community reinforcement approach (80).

Fostering Management of Painful Affects

Marlatt and Gordon (81) demonstrated that dysphoric affects are the most commonly cited precipitant for relapse, and many psychodynamic clinicians (42,43) have suggested that failure of affect regulation is a central dynamic underlying the development of compulsive alcohol or drug use. Moreover, surveys of psychiatric disorders in treatment-seeking and community populations concur in demonstrating high rates of depressive disorders among drug users (82–85).

A key element in developing ways to handle powerful dysphoric affects is learning to recognize and identify the probable cause of such feelings. The difficulty in differentiating among negative emotional states has been identified as a common characteristic among addicts (42,43). To foster the development of mastery over dysphoric affects, most psychotherapies include techniques for eliciting strong affects within a protected therapeutic setting and then enhancing the patient's ability to identify, tolerate, and respond appropriately to them. Given the demonstrated efficacy of pharmacologic treatments for affective and anxiety disorders and the high rates of these disorders seen in treatment-seeking populations, the individual psychotherapist should be alert to the possibility that a patient may benefit from combined treatment with psychotherapy and medications.

Moreover, as evidence points to the difficulty many patients face in articulating strong affect (86), which can have an effect of treatment response (87), clinicians should be alert to the need to assess and address difficulties in expression of affect and cognition when working with addicts in psychotherapy.

Improving Interpersonal Functioning and Enhancing Social Supports

A consistent finding in the literature on relapse is the protective influence of an adequate network of social supports (88,89). Gratifying friendships and intimate relationships provide a powerful source of rewards to replace those obtained from drug and alcohol use, and the threat of losing those relationships can furnish a strong incentive to maintain abstinence. Typical issues presented by addicts are the loss of or damage to valued relationships that occurred when alcohol or drug use became the individual's principal priority, failure to have achieved satisfactory relationships even before having initiated substance use, and inability to identify friends or intimates who are not, themselves, engaged in substance abuse. For some types of psychotherapy (such as interpersonal therapy and supportive-expressive treatment), working on relationship issues is the central focus of the work, while for others this aspect is implied in other therapeutic activities such as identifying risky and protective interpersonal situations (65).

A major potential limitation of individual psychotherapy as the sole treatment for alcohol or drug dependence is its failure to provide adequate social supports to patients who lack a supportive social network of friends who are not engaged in substance abuse. Individual psychotherapy can fill only one to several hours per week of a patient's time.

Again, although most approaches address these issues to some degree in the course of treatment, approaches that emphasize the development of a strong relationship with persons who are not substance users are traditional counseling, 12-step facilitation (12), and other approaches that underline the importance of involvement in self-help groups. Self-help groups offer a fully developed social network of welcoming individuals who are understanding and committed to leading a substance-free life. Moreover, in most urban and suburban settings, self-help meetings are held daily or several times a week, and a sponsor system is available to provide the recovering person with individual guidance and support on a 24-hour basis, if needed. For psychotherapists who working with addicts, encouraging patients to become involved in self-help groups can provide a powerful source of social support that protects the patient from relapse while the work of therapy progresses.

EFFICACY RESEARCH

Early efforts to engage and treat drug users with dynamically oriented individual psychotherapy as the sole treatment were marked by failure. These failures led researchers to focus increasingly on the evaluation of psychotherapy as a treatment for addiction in terms of the context in which individual psychotherapy is delivered most effectively, as well as the types of patients most likely to benefit from individual psychotherapy. Hence, the following section reviews empiric evidence for the effectiveness of individual psychotherapy by substance of abuse and treatment setting. The section reviews findings from the growing number of studies that have used rigorous methodologies associated with the technology model of psychotherapy research

(90,91). Akin to specification of the formulation and dosage of medications in pharmacotherapy trials, this approach has generated methods for specifying the techniques to be evaluated, for training therapists to use these techniques consistently, and for monitoring the dose and delivery of these techniques over the course of clinical trials. These methodological features include random assignment to treatment conditions, specification of treatments in manuals, selection of well-trained therapists committed to the type of approach they conduct in the trial, extensive training of therapists, ongoing monitoring of therapy implementation, multidimensional ratings of outcome by independent evaluators blind to the study treatment received by the patient, and adequate sample sizes.

In this review, we have focused on studies of opiate and cocaine addicts because the more extensive literature on psychosocial treatments of alcohol has received detailed review elsewhere (2,3).

Individual Psychotherapy for Opioid Dependence

Opioid Agonist Therapy

Only a few studies have evaluated the efficacy of formal psychotherapy to enhance outcomes with agonist treatments. The landmark study in this area was done by Woody and colleagues (92) and was also replicated in community settings (93). Although the original study is now nearly 20 years old, it is reviewed here because it remains an impressive demonstration of the benefits and role of psychotherapy in the context of methadone maintenance. In the study, 110 opiate addicts entering a methadone maintenance program were randomly assigned to one of three treatments: drug counseling alone, drug counseling plus supportive-expressive psychotherapy (SE), which is a short-term dynamic approach, or drug counseling plus cognitive psychotherapy, a structured cognitive approach. After a 6-month course of treatment, although the SE and cognitive psychotherapy groups did not differ significantly from each other on most measures of outcome, subjects who received either form of professional psychotherapy evidenced greater improvement in more outcome domains than did the subjects who received drug counseling alone (92). Moreover, gains made by the subjects who received professional psychotherapy were sustained over a 12-month followup period, whereas subjects who received drug counseling alone evidenced some attrition of gains (94). The study also demonstrated differential responses to psychotherapy as a function of patient characteristics, which can point to the best use of psychotherapy (relative to drug counseling) when resources are scarce: although methadone-maintained opiate addicts with lower levels of psychopathology tended to improve regardless of whether they received professional psychotherapy or drug counseling, those with higher levels of

psychopathology tended to improve only if they received psychotherapy.

Contingency Management

Several studies have evaluated the use of contingency management to reduce the use of illicit drugs in addicts who are maintained on methadone. In these studies, a reinforcer (reward) is provided to patients who demonstrate specified target behaviors such as providing drug-free urine specimens, accomplishing specific treatment goals, or attending treatment sessions. For example, offering methadone take-home privileges contingent on reduced drug use is an approach that capitalizes on an inexpensive reinforcer that is potentially available in all methadone maintenance programs. Stitzer and colleagues (95–97) have done extensive work in evaluating methadone take-home privileges as a reward for decreased illicit drug use. In a series of well-controlled trials, these researchers demonstrated (a) the relative benefits of positive (e.g., rewarding desired behaviors such as abstinence) compared with negative (e.g., punishing undesired behaviors such as continued drug use through discharges or dose reductions) contingencies (97), (b) the attractiveness of take-home privileges over other incentives available within methadone maintenance clinics (95), and (c) the relative effectiveness of rewarding drug-free urine specimens compared with other target behaviors (98).

Silverman and colleagues (99,100), drawing on the compelling work of Higgins and colleagues (described under "Individual Psychotherapy for Cocaine Dependence"), evaluated a voucher-based contingency management system to address concurrent illicit drug use (typically cocaine) among methadone-maintained opioid addicts. In this approach, urine specimens are required three times a week to systematically detect all episodes of drug use. Abstinence, verified through drug-free urine screens, is reinforced through a voucher system in which patients receive points redeemable for items consistent with a drug-free lifestyle that are intended to help the patient develop alternate reinforcers to drug use (e.g., movie tickets and sporting goods). In a very elegant series of studies, Silverman and colleagues (99,100) demonstrated the efficacy of this approach in reducing illicit opioid and cocaine use and producing a number of treatment benefits in this very difficult population.

Behavioral Therapies

Opioid-antagonist treatment (naltrexone) offers many advantages over methadone maintenance, including the fact that it is nonaddicting and can be prescribed without concerns about diversion, has a benign side effect profile, and can be less costly in terms of demands on professional time and of patient time than the daily or near-daily clinic visits required for methadone maintenance (101). Most important are the behavioral aspects of treatment, as unreinforced opiate use allows extinction of relationships between cues and drug use. Although naltrexone treatment is likely to be attractive only to a minority of opioid addicts (34), naltrexone's unique properties make it an important alternative to methadone maintenance and other agonist approaches.

However, naltrexone has not, despite its many advantages, fulfilled its promise. Naltrexone treatment programs remain comparatively rare and underused as compared to methadone maintenance programs (101). This situation is largely a result of problems with retention, particularly during the induction phase, when an average of 40% of patients drop out during the first month of treatment and 60% drop out by 3 months (34). In the 1970s, several preliminary evaluations of behavioral interventions used to address naltrexone's weaknesses, including providing incentives for compliance with naltrexone (102,103) and the addition of family therapy to naltrexone treatment (104), suggested the promise of these strategies. However, the interventions were not widely adopted, compliance remained a major problem, and naltrexone treatment and research dropped off considerably until the past few years, when the need for alternatives to methadone maintenance stimulated a modest revival of interest in naltrexone.

Some of the most recent promising data about strategies to enhance retention and outcome in naltrexone treatment has come from investigations of contingency management approaches. Preston and colleagues (105) found improved retention and naltrexone compliance with an approach that provided vouchers for naltrexone compliance, as compared with standard naltrexone treatment that did not provide vouchers. Carroll and colleagues (106,107) found that reinforcement of naltrexone compliance and drug-free urine specimens, alone or in combination with family involvement in treatment, improved retention and reduced drug use among recently detoxified opioid-dependent individuals.

Individual Psychotherapy for Cocaine Dependence

Compared with the results of trials evaluating pharmacologic treatment of cocaine dependence, evaluations of behavioral therapies—particularly contingency management, CBT, and manualized disease-model approaches—are much more promising (8,108). Because of the lack of an effective pharmacologic platform for cocaine dependence (analogous to methadone maintenance for the treatment of opioid dependence), behavioral therapies for cocaine-dependent individuals have had to focus on key outcomes such as retention and the inception and maintenance of abstinence, rather than placing initial emphasis on secondary psychosocial problems (e.g., family, psychological, legal problems). Major findings from randomized controlled trials evaluating each of these treat-

ments for adult cocaine dependent groups are summarized here.

Contingency Management

Perhaps the most exciting findings pertaining to the effectiveness of behavioral treatments for cocaine dependence have been the reports by Higgins and colleagues (78,109–111) on the use of behavioral incentives for abstinence, as described earlier. The strategy of Higgins has four organizing features that are grounded in principles of behavioral pharmacology: (a) drug use and abstinence must be swiftly and accurately detected, (b) abstinence is positively reinforced, (c) drug use results in loss of reinforcement, and (d) emphasis is placed on the development of reinforcers to compete with drug use (79). In this approach, urine specimens are required three times weekly to systematically detect all episodes of drug use. Abstinence, verified through drug-free urine screens, is reinforced through a voucher system in which patients receive points redeemable for items consistent with a drug-free lifestyle (such as movie tickets and sporting goods).

In a series of well-controlled clinical trials, Higgins demonstrated high acceptance, retention, and rates of abstinence for patients receiving this approach, as compared with standard counseling oriented toward 12-step programs (78,109). Rates of abstinence do not decline substantially when less valuable incentives are substituted for the voucher system (109). The value of the voucher system itself, as opposed to other program elements, in producing good outcomes was demonstrated by comparing the behavioral system with and without the vouchers (112). Although the strong effects of this treatment declined somewhat after the contingencies were terminated, the voucher system has durable effects (110). Moreover, the efficacy of a variety of contingency management procedures (including vouchers, direct payments, and free housing) have been replicated in other settings and samples, including cocaine-dependent individuals within methadone maintenance (99,100), homeless addicts (113), freebase cocaine users (114), and pregnant drug users (115).

These findings are of great importance because contingency management procedures are potentially applicable to a wide range of target behaviors and problems, including treatment retention and compliance with pharmacotherapy (such as retroviral therapies for individuals with human immunodeficiency virus [HIV]). For example, Iguchi and colleagues (98) showed that contingency management can be used effectively to reinforce desired treatment goals (e.g., looking for a job) in addition to abstinence.

Nevertheless, despite the very compelling evidence of the effectiveness of these procedures in promoting retention in treatment and reducing cocaine use, the procedures rarely are used in clinical treatment programs. One major impediment to broader use is the expense associated with the voucher program; average earnings for patients are about $600 (78,112,116). Recently developed low-cost contingency-management procedures may be a way to bring these effective approaches into general clinical use. In a recently completed study, Petry and colleagues (117,118) demonstrated that a variable ratio schedule of reinforcement that provides access to large reinforcers (but at low probabilities) is effective in retaining subjects in treatment and reducing substance use. Rather than earning vouchers, subjects earn the chance to draw from a bowl and win prizes of varying magnitudes. The prizes range from small $1 prizes (bus tokens, McDonald's coupons) to large $20 prizes (portable radios, watches, and phone cards), to jumbo $100 prizes (e.g., small televisions). This system is far less expensive than the standard voucher system, because only a proportion of behaviors are reinforced with a prize. In a study of 42 alcohol-dependent veterans who were randomly assigned to standard treatment or standard treatment plus contingency management, 84% of the contingency-management subjects were retained in treatment throughout an 8-week period, compared with 22% of standard treatment subjects. By the end of the treatment period, 69% of those receiving contingency-management treatment had not experienced a relapse to alcohol use, but only 39% of those receiving standard treatment were abstinent (118), with similar findings among cocaine abusers (117).

Cognitive–Behavioral Therapies

Another behavioral approach that is effective in treating cocaine abusers is CBT. This approach is based on social learning theories on the acquisition and maintenance of substance use disorders (119). Its goal is to foster abstinence by helping the patient master an individualized set of coping strategies as an effective alternative to substance use. Typical skills include fostering the patient's resolve to stop using cocaine and other substances by exploring positive and negative consequences of continued use, functional analysis of substance use (that is, understanding substance use in relationship to its antecedents and consequences), development of strategies for coping with cocaine craving, identification of seemingly irrelevant decisions that could culminate in high-risk situations, preparation for emergencies and coping with a relapse to substance use, and identifying and confronting thoughts about substance use.

A number of randomized clinical trials among several diverse cocaine-dependent populations have demonstrated that (a) compared with other commonly used psychotherapies for cocaine dependence, CBT appears to be particularly more effective with more severe cocaine users or those with comorbid disorders (120–125); (b) CBT is sig-

nificantly more effective than less-intensive approaches that have been evaluated as control conditions (126,127); and (c) CBT is as or more effective than manualized disease-model approaches (124,126). Moreover, CBT appears to be a particularly durable approach, with patients continuing to reduce their cocaine use even after they leave treatment (68,69,71,72).

Manualized Disease-Model Approaches

Until very recently, treatment approaches based on disease models were widely practiced in the United States, but virtually no well-controlled randomized clinical trials had evaluated their efficacy alone or in comparison with other treatments. Thus, another important finding emerging from randomized clinical trials that has great significance for the treatment community is the effectiveness of manualized disease-model approaches. One such approach is TSF (12), a manual guided, individual approach that is intended to be similar to widely used approaches that emphasize principles associated with disease models of addiction and has been adapted for use with cocaine-dependent individuals (126). Although this treatment has no official relationship with AA or CA, its content is intended to be consistent with the Twelve Steps of AA, with primary emphasis given to Steps 1 through 5 and the concepts of acceptance (e.g., to help the patient accept that the patient has the illness, or disease, of addiction) and surrender (e.g., to help the patient acknowledge that there is hope for sobriety through accepting the need for help from others and a "Higher Power"). In addition to abstinence from all psychoactive substances, a major goal of the treatment is to foster active participation in self-help groups. Patients are actively encouraged to attend AA or CA meetings, become involved in traditional fellowship activities, and maintain journals of their self-help group attendance and participation.

In a comparison of TSF, CBT, and clinical management (a supportive approach in which patients received comparable empathy, support, and other "common elements" of psychotherapy but none of the unique "active ingredients" of TSF or CBT) for alcoholic cocaine-dependent individuals, TSF was found to be significantly more effective than clinical management and was comparable to CBT in reducing cocaine use (126). In addition, a 1-year followup suggested that gains from treatment were maintained for subjects who received TSF or CBT, who reported continuing to reduce their cocaine use throughout the followup period, compared with subjects who received clinical management. Moreover, there was a strong relationship between the attainment of significant periods of abstinence during treatment and abstinence during followup, which emphasizes that the inception of abstinence, even for comparatively brief periods, is an important goal of treatment (69,110).

More recently, the NIDA Collaborative Cocaine Treatment Study, a multisite, randomized trial of psychotherapeutic treatments for cocaine dependence (128,129), suggested the effectiveness of a similar approach: individual drug counseling (130). In that study, 487 cocaine-dependent participants in 4 sites were randomly assigned to 1 of 4 manual-guided treatment conditions: (a) cognitive therapy (131) plus group drug counseling; (b) SE therapy, a short-term psychodynamically oriented approach (73) plus group drug counseling; (c) individual drug counseling plus group drug counseling; or (d) group drug counseling alone. The treatments offered were intensive (36 individual and 24 group sessions over 24 weeks, for a total of 60 sessions) and were met with comparatively poor retention, with patients on average completing less than half the sessions offered, with higher rates of retention for subjects assigned to cognitive therapy or SE therapy (128). On the whole, outcomes were good, with all groups significantly reducing their cocaine use from baseline; however, the best cocaine outcomes were seen for subjects who received individual drug counseling (a related point is that this study suggests that psychodynamic and cognitive approaches, which rarely have been studied with this population, may not be optimal initial approaches for general populations of cocaine users) (132).

Considered together with the findings of Project MATCH (14,133), TSF was found to be comparable to CBT and MET in reducing alcohol use among 1,726 alcohol-dependent individuals. The findings from these studies offer compelling support for the efficacy of manual-guided disease-model approaches. This finding has important clinical implications because these approaches are similar to the dominant model applied in most community treatment programs (134) and thus can be more easily mastered by "real-world" clinicians than can approaches such as contingency management or CBT—treatments whose theoretical underpinnings may not be perceived highly compatible with disease-model approaches (although such incompatibility has yet to be demonstrated) (135).

Moreover, it is critical to recognize that the evidence supporting disease-model approaches has emerged from well-conducted clinical trials in which therapists were selected on the basis of their expertise in this approach and were trained and closely supervised so as to foster high levels of adherence and competence in delivering the treatments, and it remains to be seen whether these approaches will be as effective when applied under less-than-ideal conditions. Likewise, these professional, individual approaches should be distinguished from merely referring patients to self-help meetings. It is noteworthy that a large randomized trial that directly compared referral to self-help with professional treatments found poorer outcomes with high rates of treatment use for the patients referred to self-help compared with inpatient treatment (136).

Individual Psychotherapy for Marijuana Dependence

Although marijuana is the most commonly used illicit substance, treatment of marijuana abuse and dependence is a comparatively understudied area to date, in part because comparatively few individuals present for treatment with a primary complaint of marijuana abuse or dependence. Currently, no effective pharmacotherapies for marijuana dependence exist, and only a few controlled trials of behavioral approaches have been completed. Stephens and colleagues (137,138) compared a delayed-treatment control group with a two-session motivational approach and to an intensive (14-session) relapse prevention approach, and found better marijuana outcomes for the two active treatments than with the delayed-treatment control group, but found no significant differences between the brief and the more intensive treatment. More recently, a replication and extension of that study, involving a multisite trial of 450 marijuana-dependent patients, compared 3 approaches: (a) a delayed treatment control, (b) a 2-session motivational approach, and (c) a 9-session combined motivational/coping skills approach. Results suggested that both active treatments were associated with significantly greater reductions in marijuana use than the delayed treatment control through a 9-month followup period (139). Moreover, the nine-session intervention was significantly more effective than the two-session intervention, and this effect also was sustained through the 9-month followup period. Budney and colleagues have extended the application of contingency management to marijuana users, and recently reported that adding voucher-based incentives to coping skills and motivational enhancement improves outcomes during treatment for marijuana dependence (140).

CONCLUSIONS

The empirical evidence reviewed here and the literature on behavioral treatments of alcoholism reviewed elsewhere (2,3) suggest the following:

- To date, most studies suggest that individual psychotherapy is superior to control conditions as a treatment for patients with substance use disorders. This finding is consistent with the bulk of findings from psychotherapy efficacy research in areas other than substance use, which suggests that the effects of many psychotherapies are clinically and statistically significant and are superior to no treatment and placebo conditions.
- No particular type of individual psychotherapy was found to be consistently superior as a treatment for substance use disorders.
- The effects of even comparatively brief psychotherapies appear to be durable among patients with substance use disorders.

Ongoing Development of Innovative Behavioral Therapies

Our review of rigorously conducted efficacy research on psychotherapies for substance use disorders provides support for the use of a number of innovative approaches: SE treatment for methadone-maintained opioid addicts, CBT for cocaine and marijuana dependence, and contingency management for a wide range of substance use disorders.

This growing list of empirically validated treatments is attributable, in part, to the behavioral therapies initiative begun in the early 1990s by NIDA (141). That initiative was begun to encourage development and testing of new and improved psychotherapies for drug addicts. Although strong evidence suggests that addiction treatment works, the field needs better methods, as too few addicts enter treatment, complete treatment, and achieve lasting improvement. Novel treatment ideas can come from any source, but widespread adoption of new methods should be reserved for those treatments with proven efficacy.

The behavioral therapies initiative was instituted to promote the process of moving new treatments from the stage in which they represent "good ideas" to one in which they are shown to be effective, are fully specified in training manuals, and are ready for use in community programs. This process is guided by a new stage model of behavioral therapies research (142), demarcating three divisions in a rigorous scientific process that leads from initial innovation through efficacy research to effectiveness research. Stage I consists of pilot/feasibility testing, manual writing, training program development, and adherence/competence measure development for new and untested treatments. Stage II initially consists of randomized clinical trials (RCTs) to evaluate efficacy of manualized and pilot-tested treatments that have shown promise or efficacy in earlier studies. Stage II research also can address mechanisms of action or effective components of treatment for approaches with evidence of efficacy derived from RCTs. Stage III consists of studies to evaluate transportability of treatments whose efficacy has been demonstrated in at least two RCTs (143,144). Key stage III research issues revolve around (a) generalizability (i.e., will this treatment maintain effectiveness with different practitioners, patients, and settings?), (b) implementation issues (i.e., what kinds of training by what kinds of trainers are necessary to train what kinds of clinicians to learn a new technique?), (c) cost-effectiveness issues (i.e., compared with the costs of learning and implementing this treatment, what are the savings, particularly in comparison to existing methods?), and (d) consumer/marketing issues (i.e., how acceptable is a new treatment to clinicians, patients, and payers outside of research settings?).

The stage model was developed in an attempt to bridge the gap (145) between research and practice in the treatment of addiction. Although psychotherapies are widely practiced, the types of treatments most widely used have not been shown to be effective in RCTs. Conversely, comparatively few practitioners use the empirically validated treatments listed above. This gap is attributable, in part, to bottlenecks at stage I and stage III.

At the front end, creative clinicians have proffered many new treatments, but few of the originators have had an opportunity to prove their efficacy of their treatments in clinical trials. As a result, many promising, potentially effective treatments have been ignored. By following guidelines for stage I research (142), clinicians can move their treatments to a stage at which efficacy testing can take place.

Another bottleneck occurs after a treatment is shown to be efficacious in rigorous clinical trials, but before community programs are ready to adopt the new treatments. The role of stage III research is to answer important questions about a new treatment's effectiveness and cost-effectiveness in real-world settings. In addition to articulating the stage model, NIDA has taken a major role in stage III research by developing the National Drug Abuse Treatment Clinical Trials Network (CTN). The CTN is a network of academically based regional research and training centers that are linked in partnership with clinical treatment programs to provide the infrastructure for large-scale trials to evaluate the effectiveness of promising pharmacologic and/or behavioral treatments in representative community settings. NIDA's CTN plays a unique role for behavioral treatments. Unlike medication treatments that are distributed for profit by commercial pharmaceutical manufacturers, behavioral treatments have no organizational resources or advocates to promote their dissemination into community practice.

From the preceding summary, it is clear that the empirical literature offers only the most general sort of guidance about the choice of which individual psychotherapy is likely to be useful for a particular patient and when in the course of treatment it should be offered. Hence, the following recommendations are made on the basis of clinical experience rather than research evidence. With this *caveat*, it is suggested that individual psychotherapy may have the following uses: (a) as an initial treatment or an introduction into treatment, (b) to treat patients with low levels of substance dependence, (c) to treat patients who failed in other modalities, (d) to complement other ongoing treatment modalities for selected patients, and (e) to help the patient solidify gains after achievement of stable abstinence (146).

Psychotherapy as Initial Treatment

As noted previously, a key advantage of individual therapy is the privacy and confidentiality it affords. This aspect can make individual therapy or counseling an ideal setting in which to clarify the treatment needs of patients who are in the early stages (i.e., contemplation, precontemplation) of thinking about changing their patterns of substance use (55). Notably, the growing evidence for the efficacy of brief (two to four sessions) motivational interviewing approaches suggests that this can be sufficient for certain patients (147). For individuals with severe dependence who deny the seriousness of their involvement, a course of individual therapy in which the patient is guided to a clear recognition of the problem can be an essential first step toward more intensive approaches such as residential treatment or methadone maintenance. An important part of this process may involve allowing the patient to fail one or more times at strategies that have a low probability of success, such as attempting to cut down on substance use without stopping or attempting outpatient detoxification.

A general principle underlying this process is the successive use of treatments that involve greater expense and/or patient involvement only after less-intensive approaches have failed. Hence, brief individual treatment may be sufficient alone or may serve a cost-effective triage function.

Psychotherapy for Patients with Mild to Moderately Severe Substance Dependence

Although less studied with nonalcoholic drug abusers, the drug-dependence syndrome concept (75) has received considerable attention in the study of alcoholism. This concept, first described by Edwards and Gross (64), suggests that drug dependence is best understood as a constellation of cognitions, behaviors, and physical symptoms that underlie a pattern of progressively diminished control over drug use. This dependence syndrome is conceived to be aligned along a continuum of severity, with higher levels of severity associated with poorer prognosis and the need for more intensive treatment, and lower levels of severity requiring less intensive interventions. The dependence syndrome construct has generated a large empiric literature, suggesting its validity with alcoholics (63). Moreover, several scales have been developed for gauging the severity of alcohol dependence (148). Generally, measures of quantity and frequency of alcohol use show a high correlation with dependence severity, and similar quantity/frequency indices for other drugs of abuse can be an adequate gauge of dependence severity. Evidence from studies of individuals who are mildly to moderately dependent on alcohol indicates that a brief course of psychotherapy is sufficient for many to achieve substantial reductions in, or abstinence from, drinking (2,4,16,17). Although these findings have yet to be replicated with other types of substance use disorders, they are likely to be generalizable.

Psychotherapy for Patients Who Failed in Other Therapies

Although numerous predictors of outcomes for addiction treatment have been identified (149), only a few are robust and still fewer have been evaluated in terms of the issue of matching patients to treatments (150). As a result, the choice of treatment often involves a degree of trial and error. Each type of treatment has its strengths and weaknesses, which can result in a better or worse "fit" for a particular patient. For example, individual therapy is more expensive but more private than group therapy, more enduring and less disruptive to normal routine than residential treatment, and less troubled by side effects and medical contraindications than pharmacotherapies. Each of these advantages may be crucial to a patient who has responded poorly to other therapeutic approaches.

Psychotherapy as Ancillary Treatment

In considering psychotherapy as part of an ongoing comprehensive program of treatment, it is useful to distinguish between treatment of opioid addicts and alcoholics, for which powerful pharmacologic approaches are available, and treatment of other drugs of abuse, for which strong alternatives to behavioral approaches are not yet available (32,39). For alcoholics, naltrexone, acamprosate, and disulfiram have strong potential for improving treatment outcome and reducing relapse rates. However, the effectiveness of disulfiram in the absence of a strong psychosocial treatment was no greater than placebo (26), and most studies demonstrating the efficacy of naltrexone and acamprosate have been done in the context of a comparatively intense psychosocial intervention (35,37,38,70,151,152). For opioid-dependent patients, the modal treatment approach remains methadone maintenance, which is used with the majority of those in treatment, whereas an alternative pharmacotherapy, naltrexone, can be highly potent for the minority who choose this approach. Because of their powerful and specific pharmacologic effects, either to satisfy the need for opioids or to prevent illicit opioids from yielding their desired effect, these agents—provided that they are delivered with at least minimal counseling—can be sufficient for many opioid addicts (29). The choice of those who might benefit from additional individual psychotherapy may be guided by the unique but robust empiric findings of Woody and colleagues (153a,154a) and McLellan (153,154) which suggest that psychotherapy is most likely to be of benefit to those opioid addicts with higher levels of psychiatric symptoms. Because the benefits of psychotherapy can be maximized when instituted relatively soon after the patient enters treatment, assessment instruments such as the Addiction Severity Index (155) can be used to quickly identify those with psychopathology or depression, alerting staff to the need to refer the client for psychotherapy.

For nonopioid drugs of abuse, an active search for effective pharmacotherapies currently is under way. In the interim, the mainstay of treatment for such patients remains some form of psychosocial treatment offered in a group, family, residential, or individual setting. For cocaine use, forms of treatment that currently have the strongest levels of empirical support for general groups of cocaine users include contingency management and cognitive behavioral therapy. However, there is as yet no strong empirical evidence as to the optimal duration of treatment, nor are there clear guidelines for matching patients to treatment.

For other types of drug abuse, in the absence of empirically validated guidelines, the choice of individual psychotherapy can be based on such factors as expense, logistical considerations, patient preference, or the clinical fit between the patient's presenting picture and the treatment modality (e.g., family therapy is ruled out for those without families).

Psychotherapy After Achievement of Sustained Abstinence

An individual who experiences frequent relapses or who is only tenuously holding onto abstinence can be a poor candidate for certain types of psychotherapy, particularly those that involve bringing into focus painful and anxiety-provoking clinical material as an inevitable part of helping the patient to master his or her dysphoric affects or avoid recurrent failures in establishing enduring intimate relationships. In fact, some arousal of anxiety or frustration may occur with most types of psychotherapy, even those that are conceived as being primarily supportive. Because of this situation, individual psychotherapy may be effective for many individuals only after they have achieved abstinence through some other treatment approach, such as residential treatment, methadone maintenance, or group therapy. Given the vulnerability of these patients to relapse (which can extend over a lifetime), and the frequency with which dysphoric affects or interpersonal conflict are noted as precipitants of relapse (81), individual psychotherapy may be particularly indicated for those whose psychopathology or disturbed interpersonal functioning is found to endure after the achievement of abstinence. Given findings pointing to the delayed emergence of effects of individual psychotherapy for both cocaine and opioid users, psychotherapy aimed at these enduring issues can be helpful not only for such problems independent of their relationship to drug use, but also as a form of insurance against the likelihood that these continuing problems eventually will lead to relapse.

REFERENCES

1. Miller WR, Heather N. *Treating addictive behaviors,* 2nd ed. New York: Plenum, 1998.
2. Miller WR, Wilbourne PL. Mesa Grande: a methodological analysis of clinical trials of treatments for alcohol use disorders. *Addiction* 2002;97:265–277.
3. Institute of Medicine. *Broadening the base of treatment for alcohol problems.* Washington, DC: National Academy Press, 1990.
4. Babor TF. Avoiding the horrid and beastly sin of drunkenness: does dissuasion make a difference? *J Consult Clin Psychol* 1994;62:1127–1140.
5. Blatt SJ, McDonald C, Sugarman A, et al. Psychodynamic theories of opiate addiction: new directions for research. *Clin Psychol Rev* 1984;4:159–189.
6. Dole VP, Nyswander ME, Warner A. Methadone maintenance treatment: a ten-year perspective. *JAMA* 1976;235:2117–2119.
7. Ball JC, Ross A. *The effectiveness of methadone maintenance treatment.* New York: Springer-Verlag, 1991.
8. DeRubeis RJ, Crits-Christoph P. Empirically supported individual and group psychological treatments for adult mental disorders. *J Consult Clin Psychol* 1998;66:37–52.
9. Leshner AI. Science-based views of drug addiction and its treatment. *JAMA* 1999;282:1314–1316.
10. McLellan AT, McKay JR. The treatment of addiction: what can research offer practice? In: Lamb S, Greenlick MR, McCarty D, eds. *Bridging the gap between practice and research: forging partnerships with community based drug and alcohol treatment.* Washington, DC: National Academy Press, 1998:147–185.
11. Miller WR, Zweben A, DiClemente CC, et al. *Motivational enhancement therapy manual: a clinical research guide for therapists treating individuals with alcohol abuse and dependence.* Rockville, MD: NIAAA, 1992.
12. Nowinski J, Baker S, Carroll KM. *Twelve-step facilitation therapy manual: a clinical research guide for therapists treating individuals with alcohol abuse and dependence.* Rockville, MD: NIAAA, 1992.
13. Kadden R, Carroll KM, Donovan D, et al. *Cognitive-behavioral coping skills therapy manual: a clinical research guide for therapists treating individuals with alcohol abuse and dependence.* Rockville, MD: NIAAA, 1992.
14. Project MATCH Research Group. Matching alcohol treatments to client heterogeneity: project MATCH posttreatment drinking outcomes. *J Stud Alcohol* 1997;58:7–29.
15. Project MATCH Research Group. Matching alcoholism treatments to client heterogeneity: project MATCH three-year drinking outcomes. *Alcohol Clin Exp Res* 1998;22:1300–1311.
16. Bien TH, Miller WR, Tonigan JS. Brief interventions for alcohol problems: a review. *Addiction* 1993;88:315–335.
17. Wilk AI, Jensen NM, Havighurst TC. Meta-analysis of randomized controlled trials addressing brief interventions in heavy alcohol drinkers. *J Gen Intern Med* 1997;12:274–283.
18. Babor TF, Grant M, Acuda W, et al. A randomized clinical trial of brief interventions in primary care: summary of a WHO project. *Addiction* 1994;89:657–660.
19. WHO Brief Intervention Study Group. A randomized cross-national clinical trial of brief interventions with heavy drinkers. *Am J Public Health* 1996;86:948–955.
20. Norquist G, Regier DA. The epidemiology of psychiatric disorders and the de facto mental health care system. *Ann Rev Med* 1996;47:473–479.
21. Robins LN. Addicts' careers. In: Dupont RI, Goldstein A, O Donnell J, et al., eds. *Handbook on drug abuse.* Rockville, MD: NIDA, 1979:17–31.
22. Valliant GE. Twelve-year follow-up of New York addicts. *Am J Psychiatry* 1966;122:727–737.
23. Simpson DD, Joe GW, Bracy SA. Six-year follow-up of opioid addicts after admission to treatment. *Arch Gen Psychiatry* 1982;39:1318–1326.
24. Kosten TR, Rounsaville BJ, Kleber HD. A 2.5- year follow-up of depression, life events, and treatment effects on

abstinence among opioid addicts. *Arch Gen Psychiatry* 1986;43:733–738.

25. Kleber HD, Kosten TR. Naltrexone induction: psychologic and pharmacologic strategies. *J Clin Psychiatry* 1984;45:29.

26. Fuller RK, Branchey L, Brightwell DR, et al. Disulfiram treatment of alcoholism: a Veterans Administration cooperative study. *JAMA* 1986;256:1449–1455.

27. Ling W, Weiss DG, Charuvastra VC, et al. Use of disulfiram for alcoholics in methadone maintenance programs: a Veterans Administration Cooperative Study. *Arch Gen Psychiatry* 1983;40:851–854.

28. Chick J, Gough K, Falkowski W, et al Disulfiram treatment of alcoholism. *Br J Psychiatry* 1992;161:84–89.

29. McLellan AT, Arndt IO, Metzger D, et al. The effects of psychosocial services in substance abuse treatment. *JAMA* 1993;269:1953–1959.

30. Carroll KM. Manual guided psychosocial treatment: a new virtual requirement for pharmacotherapy trials? *Arch Gen Psychiatry* 1997;54:923–928.

31. Senay E. Methadone maintenance. In: Karasu TB, ed. *Treatments of psychiatric disorders.* Washington, DC: American Psychiatric Association Press, 1989:1341–1358.

32. O'Brien CP. A range of research-based pharmacotherapies for addiction. *Science* 1997;278:66–70.

33. Lowinson JH, Marion IJ, Joseph H, et al. Methadone maintenance. In: Lowinson JH, Ruiz P, Millman RB, eds. *Substance abuse: a comprehensive textbook,* 2nd ed. Baltimore: Williams & Wilkins, 1992:550–561.

34. Greenstein RA, Fudala PJ, O'Brien CP. Alternative pharmacotherapies for opiate addiction. In: Lowinson JH, Ruiz P, Millman RB, et al., eds. *Substance abuse: a comprehensive textbook,* 3rd ed. Baltimore: Williams & Wilkins, 1997:415–425.

35. Volpicelli JR, Alterman AI, Hayashida M, et al. Naltrexone in the treatment of alcohol dependence. *Arch Gen Psychiatry* 1992;49:876–880.

36. O'Malley SS, Jaffe AJ, Chang G, et al. Naltrexone and coping skills therapy for alcohol dependence: a controlled study. *Arch Gen Psychiatry* 1992;49:881–887.

37. Whitworth AB, Fischer F, Lesch OM. Comparison of acamprosate and placebo in long-term treatment of alcohol dependence. *Lancet* 1996;347:1438–1442.

38. Sass H, Soyka M, Mann K, et al. Relapse prevention by acamprosate. *Arch Gen Psychiatry* 1996;53:673–680.

39. Kosten TR, McCance Katz EF. New pharmacotherapies. In Oldham JM, Riba MB, eds. *American Psychiatric Press Review of Psychiatry, vol. 14.* Washington, DC: American Psychiatric Press, 1995:105–126.

40. Smith M, Glass C, Miller T. *The benefits of psychotherapy.* Baltimore: Johns Hopkins Press, 1980.

41. Marques AC, Formigoni ML. Comparison of individual and group cognitive behavioral therapy for alcohol and/or drug dependent patients. *Addiction* 2001;96:835–846.

42. Khantzian EJ. The self-medication hypothesis of addictive disorders: focus on heroin and cocaine. *Am J Psychiatry* 1985;142:1259–1264.

43. Wurmser L. *The hidden dimension: psychopathology of compulsive drug use.* New York: Jason Aronson, 1979.

44. Mendelson JH, Mello NK. Experimental analysis of drinking behavior in chronic alcoholics. *Ann N Y Acad Sci* 1966;133:828–845.

45. Mirin SR, Meyer RE, McNamme B. Psychopathology and mood duration in heroin use: acute and chronic effects. *Arch Gen Psychiatry* 1980;33:1503–1508.

46. Gawin FH, Ellinwood EH. Stimulants: actions, abuse, and treatment. *N Engl J Med* 1988;318:1173–1183.

47. Beck AT, Rush AJ, Shaw BF, et al. *Cognitive therapy of depression.* New York: Guilford Press, 1979.

48. Raimo EB, Schuckit MA. Alcohol dependence and mood disorders. *Addict Behav* 1998;23:933–946.

49. Schuckit MA, Smith TL, Danko GP, et al. Five-year clinical course associated with *DSM–IV* alcohol abuse or dependence in a large group of men and women. *Am J Psychiatry* 2001;158:1084–1090.

50. Stanton MD, Shadish WR. Outcome, attrition, and family-couples treatment for drug abuse: a meta-analysis and review of the controlled, comparative studies. *Psychol Bull* 1997;122:170–191.

51. Cummings N. Turning bread into stones: our modern anti-miracle. *Am Psychologist* 1979;34:1119–1129.

52. Valliant GE. A long-term follow-up of male alcohol abuse. *Arch Gen Psychiatry* 1996;53:243–249.

53. Hser Y, Hoffman V, Grella CE, et al. A 33-year follow-up of narcotics addicts. *Arch Gen Psychiatry* 2001;58:503–508.

54. Prochaska JO, DiClemente CC. Transtheoretical therapy: toward a more integrative model of change. *Psychother Theory Res Pract* 1982;19:276–288.

55. Prochaska JO, DiClemente CC, Norcross JC. In search of how people change: applications to addictive behaviors. *Am Psychologist* 1992;47:1102–1114.

56. Miller WR, Rollnick S. *Motivational interviewing: preparing people for change,* 2nd ed. New York: Guilford Press, 2002.

57. Miller WR. Rediscovering fire: small interventions, large effects. *Psychol Addict Behav* 2000;14:6–18.

58. Saunders B, Wilkinson C, Philips M. The impact of a brief motivational intervention with opiate users attending a methadone programme. *Addiction* 1995;90:415–424.

59. Carroll KM, Libby B, Sheehan J, et al. Motivational interviewing to enhance treatment initiation in substance abusers: an effectiveness study. *Am J Addict* 2001;10:335–339.

60. Swanson AJ, Pantalon MV, Cohen KR. Motivational interviewing and treatment adherence among psychiatric and dually diagnosed patients. *J Nerv Ment Dis* 1999;187:630–635.

61. Stotts AL, Schmitz JM, Rhoades HM, et al. Motivational interviewing with cocaine-dependent patients: a pilot study. *J Consult Clin Psychol* 2001;69:858–862.

62. Sanchez-Craig M, Wilkinson DA. Treating problem drinkers who are not severely dependent on alcohol. *Drugs Soc* 1986;1:39–67.

63. Edwards G. The alcohol dependence syndrome: a concept as stimulus to enquiry. *Br J Addict* 1986;81:171–183.

64. Edwards G, Gross MM. Alcohol dependence: Provisional description of a clinical syndrome. *Br Med J* 1976;1:1058–1061.

65. Marlatt GA, Gordon JR. *Relapse prevention: maintenance strategies in the treatment of addictive behaviors.* New York: Guilford Press, 1985.

66. Monti PM, Rohsenow DJ, Abrams DB, et al. *Treating alcohol dependence: a coping skills training guide in the treatment of alcoholism.* New York: Guilford Press, 1989.

67. Carroll KM. *A cognitive-behavioral approach: treating cocaine addiction.* Rockville, MD: NIDA, 1998.

68. Carroll KM, Rounsaville BJ, Nich C, et al. One year follow-up of psychotherapy and pharmacotherapy for cocaine dependence: delayed emergence of psychotherapy effects. *Arch Gen Psychiatry* 1994;51:989–997.

69. Carroll KM, Nich C, Ball SA, et al. One year follow-up of disulfiram and psychotherapy for cocaine-alcohol abusers: sustained effects of treatment. *Addiction* 2000;95:1335–1349.

70. O'Malley SS, Jaffe AJ, Chang G, et al. Six month follow-up of naltrexone and psychotherapy for alcohol dependence. *Arch Gen Psychiatry* 1996;53:217–224.

71. McKay JR, Alterman AI, Cacciola JS, et al. Continuing care for cocaine

dependence: comprehensive 2-year outcomes. J Consult Clin Psychol 1999; 63:70–78.

72. Rawson RA, Huber A, McCann MJ, et al. A comparison of contingency management and cognitive-behavioral approaches during methadone maintenance for cocaine dependence. *Arch Gen Psychiatry* 2002;59:817–824.

73. Luborsky L. *Principles of psychoanalytic psychotherapy: a manual for supportive-expressive treatment.* New York: Basic Books, 1984.

74. Rounsaville BJ, Gawin FH, Kleber HD. Interpersonal psychotherapy adapted for ambulatory cocaine abusers. *Am J Drug Alcohol Abuse* 1985;11:171–191.

75. Edwards G, Arif A, Hodgson R. Nomenclature and classification of drug and alcohol related problems. *Bull WHO* 1981;59:225–242.

76. Kandel DB, Yamaguchi K, Chen K. Stages of progression in drug involvement from adolescence to adulthood. *J Stud Alcohol* 1992;53:447–457.

77. Kandel D, Faust R. Sequence and stages in patterns of adolescent drug use. *Arch Gen Psychiatry* 1975;32:923–932.

78. Higgins ST, Delany DD, Budney AJ, et al. A behavioral approach to achieving initial cocaine abstinence. *Am J Psychiatry* 1991;148:1218–1224.

79. Budney AJ, Higgins ST. *A community reinforcement plus vouchers approach: treating cocaine addiction.* Rockville, MD: NIDA, 1998.

80. Azrin NH. Improvements in the community-reinforcement approach to alcoholism. *Behav Res Ther* 1976;14:339–348.

81. Marlatt GA, Gordon GR. Determinants of relapse: implications for the maintenance of behavior change. In: Davidson PO, Davidson SM, eds. *Behavioral medicine: changing health lifestyles.* New York: Brunner/Mazel, 1980:410–452.

82. Regier DA, Farmer ME, Rae DS, et al. Comorbidity of mental disorders with alcohol and other drug abuse. Results from the Epidemiologic Catchment Area (ECA) study. *JAMA* 1990;264:2511–2518.

83. Rounsaville BJ, Weissman MM, Kleber HD, et al. Heterogeneity of psychiatric diagnosis in treated opiate addicts. *Arch Gen Psychiatry* 1982;39:161–166.

84. Rounsaville BJ, Anton SF, Carroll KM, et al. Psychiatric diagnosis of treatment seeking cocaine abusers. *Arch Gen Psychiatry* 1991;48:43–51.

85. Khantzian EJ, Treece C. *DSM-III* psychiatric diagnosis of narcotic addicts. *Arch Gen Psychiatry* 1985;42:1067–1071.

86. Keller DS, Carroll KM, Nich C, et al. Differential treatment response in alexithymic cocaine abusers: findings from a randomized clinical trial of psychotherapy and pharmacotherapy. *Am J Addict* 1995;4:234–244.

87. Taylor GJ, Parker JD, Babgby RM. A preliminary investigation of alexithymia in men with psychoactive substance dependence. *Am J Psychiatry* 1990;147:1228–1230.

88. Longabaugh R, Beattie M, Noel R, et al. The effect of social support on treatment outcome. *J Stud Alcohol* 1993;54:465–478.

89. Galanter M. *Network therapy for alcohol and drug abuse: a new approach in practice.* New York: Basic Books, 1993.

90. Waskow IE. Specification of the technique variable in the NIMH Treatment of Depression Collaborative Research Program. In: Williams JBW, Spitzer RL, eds. *Psychotherapy research: where are we and where should we go?* New York: Guilford Press, 1984.

91. Carroll KM, Rounsaville BJ. Can a technology model be applied to psychotherapy research in cocaine abuse treatment? In: Onken LS, Blaine JD, eds. *Psychotherapy and counseling in the treatment of drug abuse.* Rockville, MD: NIDA, 1991:91–104.

92. Woody GE, Luborsky L, McLellan AT, et al. Psychotherapy for opiate addicts: does it help? *Arch Gen Psychiatry* 1983;40:639–645.

93. Woody GE, McLellan AT, Luborsky L, et al. Psychotherapy in community methadone programs: a validation study. *Am J Psychiatry* 1995;152:1302–1308.

94. Woody GE, McLellan AT, Luborsky L, et al. Twelve-month follow-up of psychotherapy for opiate dependence. *Am J Psychiatry* 1987;144:590–596.

95. Stitzer ML, Bigelow GE. Contingency management in a methadone maintenance program: availability of reinforcers. *Int J Addict* 1978;13:737–746.

96. Stitzer ML, Iguchi MY, Felch LJ. Contingent take-home incentives: effects on drug use of methadone maintenance patients. *J Consult Clin Psychol* 1992;60:927–934.

97. Stitzer ML, Bickel WK, Bigelow GE, et al. Effect of methadone dose contingencies on urinalysis test results of polydrug abusing methadone maintenance patients. *Drug Alcohol Depend* 1986;18:341–348.

98. Iguchi MY, Lamb RJ, Belding MA, et al. Contingent reinforcement of group participation versus abstinence in a methadone maintenance program. *Exp Clin Psychopharmacol* 1996;4:1–7.

99. Silverman K, Higgins ST, Brooner RK, et al. Sustained cocaine abstinence in methadone maintenance patients through voucher-based reinforcement therapy. *Arch Gen Psychiatry* 1996;53:409–415.

100. Silverman K, Wong CJ, Umbricht-Schneiter A, et al. Broad beneficial effects of cocaine abstinence reinforcement among methadone patients. *J Consult Clin Psychol* 1998;66:811–824.

101. Rounsaville BJ. Can psychotherapy rescue naltrexone treatment of opioid addiction? In: Onken LS, Blaine JD, eds. *Potentiating the efficacy of medications: integrating psychosocial therapies with pharmacotherapies in the treatment of drug dependence.* Rockville, MD: NIDA, 1995:37–52.

102. Grabowski J, O'Brien CP, Greenstein RA, et al. Effects of contingent payments on compliance with a naltrexone regimen. *Am J Drug Alcohol Abuse* 1979;6:355–365.

103. Meyer RE, Mirin SM, Altman JL, et al. A behavioral paradigm for the evaluation of narcotic antagonists. *Arch Gen Psychiatry* 1976;33:371–377.

104. Anton RF, Hogan I, Jalali B, et al. Multiple family therapy and naltrexone in the treatment of opioid dependence. *Drug Alcohol Depend* 1981;8:157–168.

105. Preston KL, Silverman K, Umbricht A, et al. Improvement in naltrexone treatment compliance with contingency management. *Drug Alcohol Depend* 1999;54:127–135.

106. Carroll KM, Ball SA, Nich C, et al. Targeting behavioral therapies to enhance naltrexone treatment of opioid dependence: efficacy of contingency management and significant other involvement. *Arch Gen Psychiatry* 2001;58:755–761.

107. Carroll KM, Sinha R, Nich C, et al. Contingency management to enhance naltrexone treatment of opioid dependence: a randomized clinical trial of reinforcement magnitude. *Exp Clin Psychopharmacol* 2002;10:54–63.

108. Van Horn DH, Frank AF. Psychotherapy for cocaine addiction. *Psychol Addict Behav* 1998;12:47–61.

109. Higgins ST, Budney AJ, Bickel WK, et al. Achieving cocaine abstinence with a behavioral approach. *Am J Psychiatry* 1993;150:763–769.

110. Higgins ST, Wong CJ, Badger GJ, et al. Contingent reinforcement increases cocaine abstinence during outpatient treatment and one year follow-up. *J Consult Clin Psychol* 2000;68:64–72.

111. Petry NM. A comprehensive guide to the application of contingency management procedures in clinical settings. *Drug Alcohol Depend* 2000;58:9–25.

112. Higgins ST, Budney AJ, Bickel WK, et al. Incentives improve outcome in outpatient behavioral treatment of cocaine

dependence. *Arch Gen Psychiatry* 1994;51:568–576.

113. Milby JB, Schumacher JE, Raczynski JM, et al. Sufficient conditions for effective treatment of substance abusing homeless persons. *Drug Alcohol Depend* 1996;43:39–47.

114. Kirby KC, Marlowe DB, Festinger DS, et al. Schedule of voucher delivery influences initiation of cocaine abstinence. *J Consult Clin Psychol* 1998;66:761–767.

115. Svikis DS, Haug NA, Stitzer ML. Attendance incentives for outpatient treatment: effects in methadone- and nonmethadone-maintained pregnant drug-dependent women. *Drug Alcohol Depend* 1997;25:33–41.

116. Higgins ST, Silverman K. *Motivating behavior change among illicit-drug abusers.* Washington, DC: American Psychological Association, 1999.

117. Petry NM, Martin B. Low-cost contingency management for treating cocaine- and opioid-abusing methadone patients. *J Consult Clin Psychol* 2002;70:398–405.

118. Petry NM, Martin B, Cooney JL, et al. Give them prizes and they will come: contingency management treatment of alcohol dependence. *J Consult Clin Psychol* 2000;68:250–257.

119. Carroll KM. Behavioral and cognitive behavioral treatments. In: McCrady BS, Epstein EE, eds. *Addictions: a comprehensive guidebook.* New York: Oxford University Press, 1999:250–267.

120. Carroll KM, Rounsaville BJ, Gawin FH. A comparative trial of psychotherapies for ambulatory cocaine abusers: relapse prevention and interpersonal psychotherapy. *Am J Drug Alcohol Abuse* 1991;17:229–247.

121. Carroll KM, Rounsaville BJ, Gordon LT, et al. Psychotherapy and pharmacotherapy for ambulatory cocaine abusers. *Arch Gen Psychiatry* 1994;51:177–197.

122. Carroll KM, Nich C, Rounsaville BJ. Differential symptom reduction in depressed cocaine abusers treated with psychotherapy and pharmacotherapy. *J Nerv Ment Dis* 1995;183:251–259.

123. McKay JR, Alterman AI, Cacciola JS, et al. Group counseling versus individualized relapse prevention aftercare following intensive outpatient treatment for cocaine dependence. *J Consult Clin Psychol* 1997;65:778–788.

124. Maude-Griffin PM, Hohenstein JM, Humfleet GL, et al. Superior efficacy of cognitive-behavioral therapy for crack cocaine abusers: main and matching effects. *J Consult Clin Psychol* 1998;66:832–837.

125. Rosenblum A, Magura S, Palij M, et al. Enhanced treatment outcomes for cocaine-using methadone patients. *Drug Alcohol Depend* 1999;54:207–218.

126. Carroll KM, Nich C, Ball SA, et al. Treatment of cocaine and alcohol dependence with psychotherapy and disulfiram. *Addiction* 1998;93:713–728.

127. Monti PM, Rohsenow DJ, Michalec E, et al. Brief coping skills treatment for cocaine abuse: substance abuse outcomes at three months. *Addiction* 1997;92:1717–1728.

128. Crits-Christoph P, Siqueland L, Blaine JD, et al. Psychosocial treatments for cocaine dependence: results of the National Institute on Drug Abuse Collaborative Cocaine Study. *Arch Gen Psychiatry* 1999;56:495–502.

129. Crits-Christoph P, Siqueland L, McCalmont E, et al. Impact of psychosocial treatments on associated problems of cocaine-dependent patients. *J Consult Clin Psychol* 2001;69:825–830.

130. Mercer DE, Woody GE. *An individual drug counseling approach to treat cocaine addiction: the Collaborative Cocaine Treatment Study model.* Rockville, MD: NIDA, 1999.

131. Beck AT, Wright FD, Newman CF, et al. *Cognitive therapy of substance abuse.* New York: Guilford Press, 1993.

132. Carroll KM. Old psychotherapies for cocaine dependence . . . revisited. *Arch Gen Psychiatry* 1999;56:505–506.

133. Project MATCH Research Group. Matching alcoholism treatments to client heterogeneity: treatment main effects and matching effects on drinking during treatment. *J Stud Alcohol* 1998;59:631–639.

134. Horgan CM, Levine HJ. The substance abuse treatment system: what does it look like and whom does it serve? In: Lamb S, Greenlick MR, McCarty D, eds. *Bridging the gap between practice and research: forging partnerships with community-based drug and alcohol treatment.* Washington, DC: National Academy Press, 1999:186–197.

135. Morgenstern J, Morgan TJ, McCrady BS, et al. Manual-guided cognitive behavioral therapy training: a promising method for disseminating empirically supported substance abuse treatments to the practice community. *Psychol Addict Behav* 2001;15:83–88.

136. Walsh DC, Hingson RW, Merrigan DM, et al. A randomized trial of treatment options for alcohol-abusing worker. *N Engl J Med* 1991;325:775–782.

137. Stephens R, Roffman RA, Simpson EE. Treating adult marijuana dependence: a test of the relapse prevention model. *J Consult Clin Psychol* 1994;62:92–99.

138. Stephens R, Roffman RA, Curtin L. Comparison of extended versus brief treatments for marijuana use. *J Consult Clin Psychol* 2000;68:898–908.

139. MTP Research Group. Treating cannabis dependence: findings from a multisite study. 2004;72(3):455–465.

140. Budney AJ, Higgins ST, Radonovich KJ, et al. Adding voucher-based incentives to coping skills and motivational enhancement improves outcomes during treatment for marijuana dependence. *J Consult Clin Psychol* 2000;68:1051–1061.

141. Onken LS, Blaine JD, Battjes R. Behavioral therapy research: a conceptualization of a process. In: Hennegler SW, Amentos R, eds. *Innovative approaches for difficult-to-treat populations.* Washington, DC: American Psychiatric Press, 1997:477–485.

142. Rounsaville BJ, Carroll KM, Onken LS. A stage model of behavioral therapies research: getting started and moving on from stage I. *Clin Psychol Sci Pract* 2001;8:133–142.

143. Carroll KM, Rounsaville BJ. Bridging the gap between research and practice in substance abuse treatment: a hybrid model linking efficacy and effectiveness research. Psychiatric Services 2003;54(3):333–339.

144. Carroll KM, Nuro KF. One size can't fit all: a stage model for psychotherapy manual development. *Clin Psychol Sci Pract* 2002;9:396–406.

145. Institute of Medicine. *Bridging the gap between practice and research: forging partnerships with community-based drug and alcohol treatment.* Washington, DC: National Academy Press, 1998.

146. Rounsaville BJ, Kleber HD. Psychotherapy/counseling for opiate addicts: strategies for use in different treatment settings. *Int J Addict* 1985;20:869–896.

147. Miller WR, Brown JM, Simpson TL, et al. What works? A methodological analysis of the alcohol treatment literature. In: Hester RK, Miller WR, eds. *Handbook of alcoholism treatment approaches: effective alternatives.* Boston, MA: Allyn & Bacon, 1995:12–44.

148. Sobell LC, Toneatto T, Sobell MC. Behavioral assessment and treatment planning for alcohol, tobacco, and other drug problems: current status with an emphasis on clinical applications. *Behav Ther* 1994;25:533–580.

149. McLellan AT, Alterman AI, Metzger DS, et al. Similarity of outcome predictors across opiate, cocaine, and alcohol treatments: role of treatment services. *J Consult Clin Psychol* 1994;62:1141–1158.

150. McLellan AT, Luborsky L, Woody GE, et al. Predicting response to alcohol and drug treatments: role of psychiatric severity. *Arch Gen Psychiatry* 1983;40:620–625.

151. Krystal JH, Cramer JA, Krol WF, et al. Naltrexone in the treatment of alcohol dependence. *N Engl J Med* 2001;345:1734–1739.

152. Anton RF, Moak DH, Waid LR, et al. Naltrexone and cognitive-behavioral therapy for the treatment of outpatient alcoholics: results of a placebo-controlled trial. *Am J Psychiatry* 1999;156:1758–1764.

153. McLellan AT, O'Brien CP, Kron R, et al. Matching substance abuse patients to appropriate treatments: a conceptual and methodological approach. *Drug Alcohol Depend* 1980;5:189–195.

153a.Woody GE, McLellan AT, Luborsky L, O'Brien CP. Sociopathy and psychotherapy outcome. *Arch Gen Psychiatry* 1985;42:1081–1086.

154. McLellan AT, Grissom GR, Zanis D, et al. Problem-service "matching" in addiction treatment: a prospective study in four programs. *Arch Gen Psychiatry* 1997;54:730–735.

154a.Woody GE, McLellan AT, Luborsky L, et al. Severity of psychiatric symptoms as a prediction of benefits from psychotherapy: The Veterans Administration-Penn study. *Am J Psychiat* 1984.

155. McLellan AT, Luborsky L, Woody GE, et al. An improved diagnostic evaluation instrument for substance abuse patients: the Addiction Severity Index. *J Nerv Ment Dis* 1980;168:26–33.

CHAPTER 43

Group Therapy with Outpatients

ARNOLD M. WASHTON

This chapter discusses practical considerations involved in providing group therapy for addiction in outpatient treatment settings. Group therapy has evolved over the years as the treatment modality of first choice for chemical dependency. It has been the primary form of treatment in structured inpatient and outpatient addiction programs for decades. As managed care has moved treatment increasingly from inpatient to outpatient settings, use of outpatient group therapy has risen steadily. A growing trend in recent years is the proliferation of addiction treatment services into office-based practice (1,2). Addiction specialists from a variety of professional disciplines (e.g., psychologists, psychiatrists, clinical social workers, professional counselors) have been adding substance abuse services, including group therapy in some cases, to the array of mental health services they already provide in office practice.

Although group therapy is the focus of this chapter, it is not touted here as the most effective treatment for everyone with an addiction problem. Addiction specialists generally agree that a combination of different approaches works best in most cases and that matching treatment interventions to specific patient needs is the most effective way to produce successful clinical outcomes. Given that this is only one chapter in a comprehensive textbook that covers a wide range of therapeutic approaches and treatment orientations, the material presented here focuses on practical rather than theoretical aspects of delivering treatment in a group format. The material in this chapter is applicable to all types of chemical dependencies, recognizing that treatment must address the addictive disorder regardless of the patient's substance(s) of choice. It is also applicable to all types of outpatient settings, including intensive outpatient programs, halfway houses, day hospital programs, and office-based practices.

ADVANTAGES OF GROUP THERAPY

Group therapy provides a unique mixture of therapeutic ingredients not available in any other single format of treatment delivery (3–5). Groups provide patients with opportunities for (a) mutual identification and reduced feelings of isolation and shame; (b) peer acceptance, support, and role modeling; (c) therapeutic confrontation and realistic feedback; (d) peer pressure, social support, structure, and accountability for making positive changes; (e) acquisition of new coping skills; (f) exchange of factual information; and, (f) instillation of optimism and hope. The gathering together of people who share a common problem often creates a common bond between them, stemming from a sense of belonging and an expectation of being intuitively understood. This is critically important in counteracting the intense feelings of isolation, shame, and guilt typically associated with chemical dependency. The social stigma of addiction and the humiliation of having lost control over one's behavior makes rapid acceptance into a peer group all the more important for newcomers. The group instills hope by giving the person a chance to make contact with others who are getting better and by instantly supplying the individual with a positive support network committed to the pursuit of healthy, shared ideals. Groups provide a broad power base for positive reinforcement (approval) of adaptive behaviors and negative reinforcement (disapproval) of maladaptive behaviors. Because groups typically place high value on self-disclosure, active participation, compliance with group norms (e.g., abstinence, punctuality, attendance, honesty), a spirit of cooperation among group members, and facing rather than avoiding problems, it is difficult for resistant or noninteractive patients to "hide out" in small groups because every member is subjected regularly to the scrutiny of the group. Groups are also an excellent way to facilitate treatment retention and compliance as a by-product of bonding between members.

In addition to clinical benefits, group therapy also has economic advantages over other forms of treatment. As compared with individual therapy, groups are more cost-effective. Groups typically have no more than 8 to 10 members and one or two group leaders. The length of each group session is usually 1 to 2 hours. Accordingly, groups allow both programs and practitioners to treat larger numbers of patients than would be the case if individual sessions were the only option. Also, because group session fees are usually a fraction of those for individual therapy, groups allow addiction treatment to be more accessible to those who otherwise could not afford it.

Another unique benefit of group therapy is that it serves as an excellent training ground for student therapists who can be brought in as coleaders to observe and role model the clinical skills of an experienced group leader. Last, but certainly not least among its advantages, is that from a therapist's standpoint, delivering treatment in a group format is professionally stimulating and rewarding. Addiction recovery groups provide a continuous source of personal and professional growth even for the most seasoned clinician.

LIMITATIONS OF GROUP THERAPY

Given the many benefits of group therapy, what are some of its limitations and when might individual therapy be preferable? First, unlike individual therapy where patients enjoy total privacy and confidentiality, group therapy inevitably requires patients to disclose their identity and personal problems to strangers. This can be a problem especially for patients who live in small communities where the chances of encountering people who might know them can be substantial. While maintaining strict confidentiality regarding group members' identities and the content of sessions is a cardinal rule of group therapy, there is no way to control what group members might say or do outside of group sessions. Despite increasing public enlightenment about addiction as a widespread disorder affecting people from all walks of life, unwanted disclosure of information about an individual's alcohol/drug problem still holds the potential to damage careers, reputations, and relationships.

A second limitation of group therapy is that the content and pace of the treatment is determined by the group as a whole and not by the needs of any one individual. Inevitably there will be times when group therapy is out of step with the needs of some members while focusing on the needs of others. This limitation is most evident in open membership groups where new members are admitted throughout the life of the group when others leave. Each time newcomers enter the group, the continuity of treatment is interrupted as attention shifts back to beginner issues. By contrast, individual therapy allows the therapist to address patient's issues as they arise and to spend as much time or as many sessions as necessary to deal with these issues.

A third limitation of groups is that typically only a small portion of the therapy time is devoted to the needs of any one individual. This is offset to some extent by the benefits that patients derive indirectly from participating in group discussions focusing on other members' issues. Nonetheless, individual therapy devotes 100% of the therapy time to the needs of one person, which may be more effective for at least some patients in producing therapeutic benefit.

A fourth limitation is that there are practical obstacles to delivering group therapy in certain treatment settings. For example, office practitioners typically do not have an adequate caseload or referral volume of chemically dependent patients needed to both initiate and maintain ongoing recovery groups. It may take the therapist several weeks or longer to gather together enough patients to start a group. While waiting for the group to begin, some patients may change their mind about entering the group, others may enter group therapy elsewhere, and still others may relapse. Even after the group gets started, the therapist may not have an adequate referral volume of newcomers to maintain adequate group census as some patients inevitably leave the group because of treatment completion or premature dropout. Another practical limitation is that group meeting times are generally inflexible. Groups typically meet one or more times per week on the same days and at the same times of the day every week. Unless there are enough patients to maintain several groups that run at different times of the day or evening (an unlikely occurrence for most private practitioners or small treatment programs) many patients who want and need group therapy will be unable to attend because of scheduling conflicts.

A fifth limitation is that group therapy is neither suitable nor appropriate for all chemically dependent patients. While many, if not most, patients can benefit from group therapy and prefer it to other forms of treatment, others are simply not good candidates for group treatment. Patients with severe borderline personality disorders often find the intense interpersonal interaction and scrutiny in group sessions intolerably stressful. Similarly, patients who are avoidant, shy, or schizoid may be unable to participate actively in group discussions or form meaningful connections with other group members. Apart from psychiatric impairment, some patients simply have no desire or willingness to be in group therapy for whatever reasons and flatly refuse to participate, preferring individual therapy instead. Although further exploration of this unreceptive stance may help to allay certain commonly held fears and misconceptions about group therapy (e.g., expectations of harsh confrontation by peers), some patients remain adamant about not wanting group therapy and it is important for therapists to respect their wishes.

GROUP THERAPY VERSUS SELF-HELP GROUPS

Group therapy and self-help groups such as Alcoholics Anonymous (AA) are not good substitutes for one another.

Each provides a unique form of help and, ideally, they should be seen as synergistic rather than competing activities (5). Self-help groups are invaluable, but the in-depth attention given to psychological and personal issues that takes place in professionally led recovery groups is simply not available in self-help meetings. Moreover, in group therapy sessions members are strongly encouraged to give objective feedback to one another whereas in self-help meetings giving feedback (known as "crosstalk") is strictly prohibited. These are not criticisms of self-help groups, which contain their own unique blend of therapeutic forces, but fundamental differences between these two very different forms of help for people struggling with chemical dependency. Unlike group therapy, self-help meetings are characterized by peer rather than professional leadership, an absence of screening or exclusion criteria, unlimited size of membership, widespread availability of different types of self-help meetings at various times during the day and night especially in highly populated areas, and no time limits on the length of participation which may extend over a participant's lifetime.

GROUPS FOR DIFFERENT STAGES OF RECOVERY

Phase-Specific Groups

The types of therapeutic interventions that work best in the treatment of addiction often depend on what phase of recovery or stage of change the person is in (6). Chemically dependent patients progress through a series of phases as they move from active use toward sustained abstinence and recovery. Accordingly, many treatment programs offer phase-specific groups that focus on the tasks and goals most relevant to each stage. This may include motivation enhancement or pretreatment induction groups for those who need preparatory work before making an abstinence commitment or entering a formal treatment program; early abstinence groups for those in the process of stopping their alcohol/drug use; and, relapse prevention or continuing care groups for those in the middle and later stages of recovery (7). This stratification offers a number of clinical advantages: (a) it focuses the therapeutic work on the specific problems, tasks, and goals relevant to each phase; (b) it provides predefined progress markers that give clients a sense of personal accomplishment as they complete one phase and move on to the next; (c) it makes it is easier for individuals to identify and relate to the content material being addressed within each stage and to bond with others who are dealing with similar issues; and (d) it facilitates patient placement into a group best suited to meet patients' needs at each point in the recovery process. The rationale for stratification is based on the assumption that matching treatment interventions to meet the specific needs of patients as they progress through different stages of recovery is likely to enhance clinical outcomes. There is a natural progression from an initial focus on stopping

all substance use, to securing abstinence, to preventing relapse, and eventually to addressing a variety of psychological issues. The dividing lines between different stages are somewhat arbitrary and the duration of each stage varies from person to person because patients move through them at different rates.

Mixed-Phase Groups

Despite the numerous advantages of phase-specific groups, there are also drawbacks. One significant disadvantage is the disruption caused by members leaving a group in which they have bonded with others and shared intimate details of their personal lives. Another limitation is that private practitioners or small treatment programs may not have sufficient caseloads or manpower to reliably maintain different groups for patients in each phase of treatment and thus mixed-phase groups may be the only feasible alternative. In a mixed-phase model, participants stay in a group as long as needed to achieve their treatment goals and/or as long as their participation in group remains productive. People in recovery move through the process at such different rates that it is not possible to specify in advance how long it will take for a given group member to reach these points. As compared to phase-specific groups, mixed groups contain a broader array of patients at different phases of recovery: some in the beginning phases of recovery, others farther along in the process, and still others somewhere in between. All have an opportunity to interact with one another in a group setting and derive mutual benefits from doing so. A potential drawback, however, is that inevitably there will be times when the group membership becomes skewed as, for example, when a majority of members is in the early phases of recovery. When this happens the smaller number of advanced members may become disenchanted or bored with the types of issues that consume the group's time.

Early Recovery Groups

Early recovery groups focus on issues most relevant to the beginning stages of treatment: helping members to establish initial abstinence, to stabilize their overall functioning, to acknowledge and accept their addiction problem, to work through their initial ambivalence and reluctance about giving up alcohol/drug use, to establish a social support network, to become bonded to other members and integrated into the group, to overcome early relapses and other setbacks without dropping out, to deal effectively with both immediate and delayed consequences of their addiction, and to begin the process of identifying and changing some of the dysfunctional self-defeating cognitions, emotions, and behaviors that perpetuate their addiction. This is an ideal wish list and certainly not all members will achieve all of these goals during their tenure in the group. In the absence of strict economic constraints on length of stay, tenure in the group varies according to how quickly patients progress toward achieving their goals, ranging usually from several months to as much as a year, if circumstances permit.

Newcomers struggling to establish or maintain initial abstinence usually need specific guidance from other group members on fundamental issues such as (a) discarding all drug supplies and paraphernalia; (b) avoiding contact with dealers, users, parties, bars, and other high-risk situations; (c) learning how to recognize self-sabotaging behaviors and other "setups" for drug/alcohol use; and (d) learning how to manage urges and cravings. Once initial abstinence is established, the focus predictably shifts to stabilization of the individual's functioning. Often, a profound sense of disappointment emerges in the newly abstinent patient soon after the patient realizes that life is still fraught with problems despite having given up alcohol/drugs. This realization may lead the patient to seriously question whether the struggle of staying abstinent is really worthwhile, especially if and when delayed consequences of prior substance use such as financial, legal, and relationship problems begin to surface while the patient is actually doing well. Support and advice from established group members who have "been there" can be extremely helpful at this point to counteract the newcomer's tendency to impulsively self-medicate their resentment, anxiety, and fear.

The issues discussed in early recovery groups are largely patient-driven so that members' problems, crises, and issues can be effectively dealt with as they arise. The leader often plays a very active, and at times directive, role in guiding the group discussion by keeping it focused on relevant issues, encouraging participation of all members, and insuring that members provide helpful therapeutic feedback to one another without lecturing, advice-giving, hostile confrontation, and other unhelpful behaviors (8). At times, the group leader may suggest that a certain topic or issue be addressed in the group based on important themes that have emerged in recent group sessions. Where appropriate, the leader may take a portion of the session to review group rules or guidelines such as those regarding how group members can give good feedback to one another, especially when there is an influx of new members. In early recovery groups, members are actively encouraged to maintain contact with one another outside the group. This stands in marked contrast to traditional (psychodynamic) group psychotherapy where outside contact between group members is viewed as undesirable "contamination" that must be avoided.

Relapse Prevention and Continuing Care Groups

The essential tasks and goals of this phase are to strengthen the commitment to abstinence, work through residual ambivalence about giving up alcohol and drugs, and both learn and practice relapse prevention strategies including identification of relapse warning signs, as well

as behavioral coping and affect-management skills as alternatives to self-medication with alcohol/drugs. Although relapse prevention is the primary focus of this phase, the group does not focus exclusively on substance use but on a wider range of issues in greater depth. These issues may include the recovery tasks of repairing damaged relationships, forming new ones, working toward resolving the lingering impact of developmental and trauma issues, enhancing self-esteem, and creating a reasonably satisfying lifestyle that is free of alcohol and other drugs. Relapses that occur after abstinence has been firmly established and practiced for at least several months are frequently caused not so much by environmental triggers (which is more typical during the early phases) as by failure of the patient to cope adequately with negative emotions generated by interpersonal conflicts and other types of life problems and stressors. Research on the relapse process indicates that the most common precipitants of relapse are negative mood states, interpersonal conflict, and social pressures to use alcohol/drugs (9). Among the many topics addressed in this phase of treatment are how to identify negative feelings; how to manage anger; how to avoid impulsive decision-making; how to relax and have fun without drugs; how to give and receive constructive criticism; how to be assertive without being aggressive; and how to deal with problems in interpersonal relationships.

In addition to providing coping skills training, it is equally important to sensitize patients to relapse warning signs so that appropriate measures can be taken to "short-circuit" what is often a progressive backsliding in attitudes and behaviors. Explaining the relapse dynamic (9) as a progressive identifiable process that is set in motion long before returning to substance use empowers group members to interrupt what otherwise might be an insidious slide toward relapse, which they are unable to recognize while it is happening. Moreover, group members must be alerted to the possibility that flare-ups can occur many months (or even years) after stopping alcohol and drug use.

The relapse prevention group should also address psychological issues that go beyond the basic cognitive and behavioral factors that promote relapse. This involves exploring in detail the inner emotional life of each group member and interpersonal problems that repeatedly give rise to the compulsive desire to "self-medicate" (10). Patients with long, destructive histories of substance use often lack the ability to identify, manage, tolerate, and appropriately express feelings. The ultimate goal here is not merely the acquisition of self-knowledge and insight, but fundamental change in the individual's characteristically maladaptive patterns of thinking, feeling, behaving, and interacting. For example, learning how to tolerate unpleasant feelings instead of impulsively obliterating them with chemicals is an essential part of group treatment at this stage. At an appropriate time the group should also address members' long-standing, deep-seated problems that may stem from parental alcoholism, physical/sexual abuse, or other developmental and life traumas. Coordination between individual and group therapy is especially vital here. Moreover, whenever such sensitive highly charged issues are being discussed, the group leader must be especially mindful of the possibility that group members may be at increased risk of relapse. Even when in-depth exploration of difficult issues appears to be well-tolerated, patients should always be alerted to the possibility of relapse as an attempt to avoid painful material.

PRACTICAL CONSIDERATIONS IN SETTING UP GROUPS

Group Size and Member Selection

Optimal group size is usually 8 to 10 members and optimal length of group sessions is usually 90 to 120 minutes. When groups are longer than 2 hours and/or exceed 10 members, often it becomes difficult to for the discussion to remain focused and for everyone to remain sufficiently involved. In a large group, the more vocal members tend to dominate the discussion while the more passive members sit quietly as spectators content that the action is not focusing on them.

There is no reliable formula for choosing the optimal mixture of candidates for group membership. As a general rule, however, the composition of a group should be neither too heterogeneous nor too homogeneous. Groups function best when there is a reasonable degree of diversity among members in terms of age, gender, race, socioeconomic status, educational level, and other relevant variables. Diversity of membership enhances the richness of the group experience, but too much diversity can make it more difficult for patients to adequately identify and bond with one another. Ideally, newcomers should be placed in groups where they have an opportunity to identify readily with at least one or two other members. Single "outliers" (4) who are different from all other group members in an important respect (e.g., one woman among all men, one gay person among all heterosexuals, one seriously impaired patient among all highly functional people) are likely to feel out of place and to drop out prematurely. In addition to differing demographics, wherever possible there should be diversity among group members with regard to substances of choice. Group membership should not be based on the patients' primary drug of choice because it is the addictive disorder not the drug that is the focus of treatment. While patients with different types of chemical dependencies can be treated effectively in the same groups, it is nonetheless essential to address problems uniquely associated with different types of substances such as sexual acting-out behaviors in cocaine-dependent males (11); lingering withdrawal symptoms of depression and insomnia in recently detoxified opioid addicts; and residual cognitive impairments in newly sober alcoholics. It is therapeutic for patients to realize that

different types of substances can all lead to the same disorder and that the types of changes required to recover successfully are the same regardless of a person's substance(s) of choice.

Open Versus Closed Membership

The choice of open versus closed membership is often decided on purely practical grounds. Open membership groups allow new members to enter as others leave, whereas closed membership groups do not. While it may be ideal for all members of a group to start and finish at the same time, in actual practice this rarely happens. In addition to the difficulty of assembling an entire cohort of patients to start group therapy all at the same time, some patients inevitably will leave the group before completing treatment no matter what measures are taken to prevent this from occurring. Thus in nearly all addiction treatment settings open group membership is the norm.

In open groups, the dynamics of the group change significantly whenever new members arrive. Usually, a certain degree of initial discomfort and readjustment are created by the entry of new members, but with proper management by the group leader the potential benefits of adding new members usually outweigh the drawbacks (8). New members add new points of view, new problems, new ideas, and a new set of life experiences, all of which can broaden the scope and effectiveness of the group experience for its members (3). Because newcomers are typically at an earlier stage of recovery than established members, they often stimulate anxiety and even overt expressions of discomfort in established members by reminding them of their own painful struggles to stop using and accept the reality that they had lost control. More advanced members experience a renewed sense of accomplishment when exposed to those who are just starting out. Additionally, newcomers give the more advanced members a chance to express altruism by taking a fledgling "under their wing" and helping him or her to assimilate into the group. Certainly, from the standpoint of the newcomer, having immediate access to a ready-made group of recovering peers who are eager to share knowledge and lend emotional support is decidedly positive.

Urine Drug Testing

Urine drug testing is a valuable treatment tool that should be a standard feature of group therapy in outpatient settings. Drug testing helps to establish and maintain the integrity of the treatment environment by establishing behavioral accountability for substance use. It also serves as an objective marker of clinical progress and as a tool that helps patients resist their impulses to use or deny that use has actually occurred. Most patients respond positively to the introduction of urine testing because they intuitively recognize its therapeutic value. Not having secrets about using can prevent a patient who is struggling to maintain abstinence from devaluing the treatment. And with urine monitoring, family members and employers can breathe a little easier and be more supportive of the patient's recovery when they no longer feel the need to vigilantly scrutinize his or her behavior for possible signs of intoxication. (Because alcohol cannot be reliably detected in urine by most testing methods, a breath or saliva test is typically used instead.)

There are several ways to maximize the accuracy and clinical value of urine testing. (a) Steps must be taken to prevent and deter falsification of urine samples. Given that it is not at all feasible for therapists to directly observe patients voiding urine into a specimen cup, other methods must be used to insure the integrity of the sample. One way is to use on-site drug testing kits that yield instant results along with instant readings of urine temperature, pH, and specific gravity to detect adulteration of the sample. (These kits can be purchased from suppliers found on the internet by searching for "drug tests.") (b) Urine samples should be taken frequently enough, generally at least every 3 to 4 days, to remain within the detection limits of most tests. (c) Each sample should be tested for the most commonly abused drugs- cocaine, amphetamines, opioids, marijuana, benzodiazepines, and barbiturates and for whatever other substances the patient may have been using prior to entering treatment. (d) Wherever possible, drug testing should be done throughout the entire duration of treatment.

GROUP MANAGEMENT CONSIDERATIONS

Leadership Roles and Responsibilities

Among the group leaders' most important functions are (a) to establish and enforce group rules in a caring, consistent, nonpunitive manner to protect the group's integrity and progress; (b) to screen, prepare, and orient potential group members to ensure suitability and proper placement in the group; (c) to keep group discussions focused on important issues and to do so in ways that try to maximize the therapeutic benefit of these discussions for all members; (d) to emphasize, promote, and maintain group cohesiveness and reduce feelings of alienation, wherever possible; (e) to create and maintain a caring, nonjudgmental, therapeutic climate in the group that both counteracts self-defeating attitudes and promotes self-awareness, expression of feelings, honest self-disclosure, adaptive alternatives to drug use; (f) to handle problem members who are disruptive to the group in a timely and consistent manner to protect the membership and integrity of the group; and (g) to educate patients about selected aspects of drug use, addiction, and recovery.

Effective group leadership demands that the leader adopt a certain posture in the group that differs significantly from that of traditional psychotherapy groups, particularly in the early stages of recovery. In traditional groups, the therapist gently guides and focuses the attention of group members on matters pertaining to group process, group dynamics, and the complicated interpersonal interaction among group members. With the exception of carefully timed comments, the therapist may remain passive, quiet, and nondirective in the customary mode of psychodynamic psychotherapy. By contrast, in early abstinence groups the therapist must work actively to keep the group focused on concrete here-and-now issues that pertain directly to addiction-related issues. The therapist plays a very active and directive leadership role that includes questioning, confronting, advising, and educating group members on relevant issues. The therapist keeps the group task-oriented and reality-based, and serves as the major catalyst for group discussion. Addressing substance-related issues is always the number one priority of the group, and the therapist must be sure always to keep the group focused on this task.

It is not the group leader's role to direct the group per se, but rather to facilitate a process whereby members learn how to interact with one another in an increasingly open, honest, empathetic manner that promotes positive changes in attitude and behavior (12). When the group is working properly the leader functions as a group manager staying in the background while the group takes full responsibility for the therapeutic work. When the group is not working properly the leader is doing a lot of talking and/or spending a lot of time exhorting members to participate in the group discussion. This requires deliberate and persistent intervention by the group leader to return maximum responsibility for what goes on in the group to the group, consistent with the psychotherapeutic principle of analyzing resistance before dealing with content (12). It is much more important to help group members recognize their passivity than it is to try to drag them into doing the therapeutic work. As compared to early recovery groups, where the group leader plays a much more active role, latter stage groups should be helped to focus increasingly on group process and become reliably self-correcting when the discussion strays off track or becomes unproductive.

Preparing New Members for Group Entry

Preparing new patients for group entry involves not only orienting them to group rules (Table 43.1), but also establishing realistic goals and expectations. Before admitting new patients, the group leader should meet individually with the prospective newcomer for at least one or two sessions to assess motivation, clarify myths and misconceptions about group therapy, and address resistances to group participation. Patients should also be informed about how the group works, how to give useful feedback, and how to refrain from unhelpful group behaviors (8). Before newcomers attend a first group meeting they should agree in writing to adhere to the group rules. They also must be

TABLE 43.1. *Group rules*

1. You are expected to come to group sessions not under the influence of any mood-altering chemicals whatsoever.

2. You are expected to abstain from the use of alcohol and all other mood-altering chemicals during your participation in the group. In the event of relapse, you must notify the group leader before attending the next session and you must bring up the relapse for discussion at the *beginning* of that next session. Relapse will be viewed as a potential learning experience, but you will not be able to continue in the group if you are unable to regain and sustain abstinence.

3. You agree to attend all scheduled sessions and arrive on time reliably. This may require you to rearrange other obligations and perhaps even postpone vacations and out-of-town trips while participating in the group.

4. You agree to preserve the anonymity and confidentiality of all group members. You must not divulge the identity of any group member or the content of any group discussions to persons outside the group.

5. You agree to remain in the group until you have completed treatment as agreed upon in your original treatment plan . . . . If you have an impulse or desire to leave the group prematurely, you will raise and process this issue in the group before taking any action to leave . . . .

6. You agree to refrain throughout your participation in the program from becoming involving romantically, sexually, financially, or professionally with other group members.

7. You will be terminated from the program immediately if you offer drugs/alcohol to any other group member or use alcohol/drugs together with another group member.

8. You agree to have your telephone number(s) added to the contact list distributed to all group members.

9. You agree to give a urine sample whenever the group leader may request it.

10. You agree to raise for discussion in the group any issue that threatens your own or another member's recovery. You will not keep secrets regarding another member's alcohol or drug use or other destructive behaviors.

notified that violation of any of these rules is potential grounds for termination from the group. One useful way to enhance the induction of newcomer into the group is to arrange an orientation meeting between the newcomer and a more advanced group member.

A vital prerequisite for entering an early recovery group is for prospective new members to achieve at least 1 to 2 weeks of continuous abstinence from all psychoactive substances just prior to attending their first group session.

This is important because it provides the time that may be needed to recover from the acute aftereffects of recent alcohol/drug use, and just as importantly, concretizes the patient's motivation and ability to comply with the group requirement of total abstinence.

Introducing Newcomers into the Group

It is essential to introduce newcomers into the group in a manner that fosters mutual identification and bonding with existing members. The following techniques can be used for introducing new members to the group at their first session. First, ask each group members to give a 2- to 3-minute synopsis of how and why they came to the group, including a brief overview of their addiction/treatment history, what issues they have been working on in the group, and what role group therapy has played thus far in their recovery. Second, ask the newcomer to describe the circumstances surrounding his or her entry into the group; a brief overview of his or her addiction and treatment history including any prior group therapy and/or experience with self-help programs; and what he or she expects to get out of being in the group. Third, encourage group members to offer feedback to the newcomer based on what they heard thus far and where possible to identify with selected aspects of the newcomer's experiences.

Because outpatient group therapy can be effective only if patients actually show up, integrating newcomers into the group quickly is absolutely critical. This process can be facilitated by asking one or more established group members to maintain daily contact with the newcomer outside the group, including accompanying him or her to local self-help meetings. Newcomers must be helped to see as quickly as possible that their punctual attendance at all group sessions is essential to their recovery and to healthy functioning of the group. When patients miss a group session, it is critical that group members and the group leader call to express concern and communicate that the patient's presence definitely was missed. One such phone call may go a long way toward preventing precipitous dropout in a newcomer who assumes, incorrectly, that "no one really cares."

Managing Peer Confrontation and Feedback

Peer confrontation by fellow group members can be extremely effective in helping others achieve a more realistic assessment of their maladaptive attitudes and behaviors. But heavy-handed, excessive, and poorly timed confrontation can be countertherapeutic and even damaging. Some patients enter groups with the mistaken idea that humiliation and aggressive confrontation are acceptable ways to force resistant members of the group to face reality. Sometimes harsh confrontations are rationalized as attempts to be "truly honest" with members who violate group expectations and norms. Group members typically have less tolerance for negative attitudes and obfuscations than do group leaders, especially when these attitudes are reminiscent of their own. Likely targets for attack are members who relapse repeatedly, those who remain defiant, superficial, or insincere, and those who minimize their problem and fail to affiliate genuinely with other members. The group leader must never allow unpopular, frustrating, resistant, or severely troubled group members to be verbally scapegoated and bludgeoned by their peers, even when the content of what is being said is entirely accurate. Harsh or excessive confrontation must not be used as a means to push unpopular or troubled members out of the group and discourage them from coming back.

It is often the style rather than content of peer confrontation that determines its impact on the designated group member. The main goal of confrontation is to make the person more receptive to change without eliciting defensiveness or destructive acting-out behavior. Presenting group members with specific guidelines for therapeutic confrontation can be extremely helpful (8).

Managing Common Problems

The most common problems that arise in group therapy include the following: chronic lateness and absenteeism, hostility and other disruptive behaviors, lack of active participation, superficial presentations, proselytizing and hiding behind AA, and playing cotherapist. Because of space limitations, these problems are touched on only briefly here. More in-depth discussion of these issues can be found elsewhere (4,8,12,13).

Lateness and Absenteeism

An atmosphere of consistency and predictability is essential for group therapy to be effective. Because most patients have histories of irresponsible behavior during active addiction, when this type of behavior arises in the group it should not be ignored. A pattern of repeated lateness and/or absenteeism adversely affects group morale and cohesion. It is almost always a sign of ambivalence about being in the group and should be addressed as such.

Hostility and Other Disruptive Behaviors

Sometimes the content of what is said in group is less important than the way it is said. The group leader must attend continuously to the affect, body language, voice intonation, and overall communication style of group members. Some members are chronically antagonistic, argumentative, and sarcastic. They repeatedly devalue the group, complain about how poorly it is run, point out minor inconsistencies, and reject advice or suggestions offered by other group members or the group leader. The group leader must not allow these types of negative behaviors to go by unnoticed and unaddressed. An appropriate intervention by the group leader might be: "I wonder if anyone else is experiencing Tom's remarks as hostile and devaluing? Can someone offer him feedback about how he's coming across and how it is affecting the atmosphere in the group?" The group leader should guide the ensuing discussion to make sure that group members do not use this as an opportunity to assault and demean the problem group member for "bad" behavior, but rather help him to see the self-defeating nature of his actions as well as the negative impact of his behavior on the entire group.

Silence and Lack of Participation

Some group members sit quietly on the sidelines as observers of the group discussion glad to have the focus of attention not be on them. Silent members may secretly harbor intense feelings of ambivalence, resentment, and annoyance about being in treatment, and doubting whether they need to be in the group or if it is useful for them. Some members are just shy and need gentle coaxing and encouragement from the group to open up. An example of how to address a silent group member is as follows: "I've noticed that Dale has not participated at all during the past two or three group sessions. Maybe the group can try to find out what's holding her back and perhaps encourage or make it easier for her to join in the discussion?"

Superficial Presentations

Terse or superficial presentations that focus on facts rather than feelings and reveal little or nothing about the presenter is another form of resistance to the group's therapeutic work. In these situations, the group leader can intervene by saying something like, "I've noticed that when Jason talks about himself his statements are very brief and factual. They tell us very little about what's on his mind or what he is actually feeling. I'm wondering if others share my observations and concerns?" Similarly, some group members present lengthy stories recounting external events and circumstances full of irrelevant details and devoid of emotional content. This is often indicative of a member who is just going through the motions of being in treatment to satisfy a spouse, employer, or mandate. The group leader might intervene by saying, "Jeff, you've just given the group a very long and detailed account of the events of last week, but we heard very little about how you were feeling these past few days on the heels of your recent relapse. I'm wondering if other group members are getting the type of information from you that they would need to give you meaningful feedback. I notice that some group members look bored and uninterested. How are you all feeling right now?"

Proselytizing and Hiding Behind Alcoholics Anonymous

This is a one of the most difficult problems to address in group therapy for addiction (4). In almost every recovery group there are likely to be some members solidly linked into AA or other 12-step programs who insist with absolute conviction that AA is the one and only pathway to successful recovery. They are frequently intolerant of others in the group who do not embrace AA and take it as their mission to proselytize the benefits of AA in the hopes of converting nonbelievers. Additionally, they may complain that there is not enough "recovery talk" in the group and that the format of group sessions does not sufficiently parallel that of an AA meeting. These patients will often polarize the group into opposing factions: those who embrace AA enthusiastically and wholeheartedly versus those who are more tempered in their posture toward AA or reject it completely. If this polarization is not addressed, it ultimately will destroy group cohesion, create an unsafe climate in the group, divert valuable attention from other important issues, and stall the group's therapeutic work. (It is important for group leaders to acknowledge that although AA can be extremely helpful to people struggling with addiction, many are not receptive to it at first and should be coaxed not coerced into giving AA a try. Moreover, no single method of recovery is best for everyone with an addiction problem.) A potentially helpful intervention may include something like, "Well group, we could probably debate the pros and cons of AA here for group many sessions and still not reach agreement among everyone in the room. I think it would be more useful to talk about how group members feel that there is a serious split among you on this issue and how it is affecting what we do here in the group."

Playing Cotherapist

Some group members play the role of therapist's helper which serves (unconsciously) as a diversion or smoke-screen for dealing with their own issues. They often perform certain of the group leader's functions such as keeping the group discussion on track, confronting other members on inappropriate behaviors, and reinforcing group norms. Because their input is often very helpful to the group it is easy for other members and sometimes the group leader to overlook the fact that the self-appointed "cotherapist" spends so much time being a helper that the cotherapist fails to address his or her own issues. An appropriate intervention might include a statement like, "Robert, you've been extremely helpful to other group members and it's very clear that everyone here values your input. But I'm wondering if the group can take some time to get to know you a little better and try to help you identify what you want to work on here."

Responding to Relapses

When group members report that they have used alcohol/drugs since the last session, the group must give top priority to addressing this issue. In doing so, the group leader should portray a leadership style that models clear, consistent, and nonpunitive behavior. The group leader's task is to help the group use the discussion of member's relapse as an opportunity to learn something useful. Suggested guidelines for dealing with a relapsed group member are as follows: (a) Ask the patient to give the group a detailed account of the sequence of feelings, events, and circumstances that led up to the relapse. (b) Invite others to ask the patient about early warning signs, self-sabotage, and other factors that may have preceded the actual substance use. (c) Ask others to share any suggestions or feedback they can offer the patient about the relapse and how to prevent it from happening again. Also ask them to share their feelings about the relapse, reminding them to avoid any tendency they may have to scapegoat the patient or to act out feelings of anger and frustration with negative comments. (d) With the patient's active participation, ask the group to develop a list of suggested strategies and behavioral changes to guard against the possibility of further substance use.

Although most group members respond supportively to a fellow member's relapse there is an unspecified limit as to how often relapsing members can expect this type of supportive response. When a group member who is having trouble remaining abstinent shows little evidence of using previous suggestions about how to prevent further relapses, other members frequently become intolerant and feel that the person may be jeopardizing the integrity of the group. Peer confrontation can become very intense when dealing with relapse issues and the group leader must guard vigilantly against the group's tendency to scapegoat or ostracize the relapsed member.

FINAL COMMENT

This chapter discusses practical considerations involved in providing group therapy for addiction in outpatient treatment settings. Because it is both clinically effective and cost-effective, group therapy has become the treatment of choice for addiction. Stage-specific groups that address the changing needs of patients as they move through different phases of recovery can be particularly effective. Nonetheless, group therapy is not the best or only treatment option for everyone with an addiction problem. Group therapy not should be used as a stand-alone treatment, but as one component of a more comprehensive treatment approach. Group therapists face many challenging tasks including deciding which patients to bring together in a group, keeping group discussions focused and on track, and handling various types of clinical and behavior problems that arise during group sessions. In addition to its therapeutic benefits for patients, groups provide a valuable source of personal and professional growth even for the most seasoned clinician.

REFERENCES

1. Washton AM, Zweben JE. *Treating substance use disorders in office-based practice: a psychotherapist's guide.* New York: Guilford Press, in press.
2. Washton AM, ed. *Psychotherapy and substance abuse: a practitioner's handbook.* New York: Guilford Press, 1995.
3. Yalom I. *The theory and practice of group psychotherapy.* New York: Basic Books, 1995.
4. Vannicelli M. *Removing the roadblocks: group psychotherapy with substance abusers and family members.* New York: Guilford Press, 1992.
5. Spitz HI, Brook DW. *The group therapy of substance abuse.* New York: Haworth Medical Press, 2002.
6. Prochaska JO, DiClemente CC, Norcross JC. In search of how people change: applications to addictive behaviors. *Am Psychol* 1992;47:1102–1114.
7. Washton AM. Outpatient groups at different stages of substance abuse treatment: preparation, initial abstinence, and relapse prevention. In: Brook DW, Spitz HI, eds. *The group therapy of substance abuse.* New York: Haworth Medical Press, 2002:99–119.
8. Washton AM. Group therapy: a clinician's guide to doing what works. In: Coombs RH, ed. *Addiction recovery tools: a practical handbook.* Thousand Oaks, CA: Sage Publications, 2001:239–256.
9. Marlatt GA, Gordon J. *Relapse prevention: preparing people to change addictive behaviors.* New York: Guilford Press, 1985.
10. Khantzian EJ, Halliday KS, McAuliffe WE. *Addiction and the vulnerable self: modified dynamic group therapy for substance abusers.* New York: Guilford Press, 1990.
11. Washton AM. *Cocaine addiction: treatment, recovery, and relapse prevention.* New York: Guilford Press, 1989.
12. Edelwich J, Brodsky A. *Group counseling for the resistant client: a practical guide to group process.* New York: Lexington, 1992.
13. Elder IR. *Conducting group therapy with addicts.* Brandenton, FL: Human Services Institute, 1990.

CHAPTER 44

Family/Couples Approaches to Treatment Engagement and Therapy

M. DUNCAN STANTON AND
ANTHONY W. HEATH

For many years, substance abusers, especially drug addicts, were viewed as "loners" as people who were cut off from primary relationships and living a kind of "alley cat" existence. It was not until researchers began inquiring about addicts' living arrangements and familial contacts that the picture began to shift. The realization began to emerge that most substance abusers are closely tied to their families or the people who raised them.

It should be noted that this is not a strictly North American phenomenon. Reports from other countries have arrived at the following percentages of drug addicts who reside with their parents: England, 50% (two-study mean); Greece, 84%; Italy, 80%; Puerto Rico, 67%; Thailand, 80% (78; V. Pomini [Athens, Greece], personal communication, July 25, 2000).

In general, the findings are that 60% to 80% of adult drug abusers either live with their parent(s), or are in regular contact (e.g., four to seven times per week) with at least one parental figure, while 75% to 95% are reported to be in at least weekly contact with one or both parents. Thirty of 32 reports, across 7 countries, attest to the prevalence of

such patterns (71,72,78). Furthermore, normative studies indicate that the living-with-parent(s) rates for U.S. drug-dependent people are dramatically higher (i.e., an average of five times greater) than the rates for same-age adults in the general population (12,22,64,83).

Questions of family-of-origin contact have received very little attention in regard to alcohol-dependent individuals. This, despite what the first author has observed during 35 years of treating alcoholics: A male drinker's wife typically voices a complaint something like, "I don't see him during weeknights because he's in the bars, and I don't see him during the weekend because he's over at his mother's putting up storm windows or something." In other words, present-day perception of this issue among professionals and researchers is analogous to that which existed in the drug abuse field 35 years ago: nobody asked, so nobody knew. One study, conducted by the first author and colleagues (75), examined 111 consecutive admissions (ages 20 to 59 years, mean = 36.2 years; 44% female) in three different alcoholism programs in two cities; all were diagnosed alcohol dependent. Seventy-one percent of the subjects reported being in touch with one or both parents at least two to three times per month, while for 56% the contact was at least weekly. When the analysis was limited to those who had at least one living parent (i.e., 82.2% of the sample), the frequency of contact percentages rose to 87% and 68%, respectively. In addition, a study by Abtin (1) comparing 200 alcohol-dependent adults with 251 non–alcohol-dependent adults from the same community (total sample age range: 18 to 68 years, mean = 39.6 years; 55% female) found the living-with-mother rate for the alcohol-dependent group, at 19.9%, to be (a) twice as high as the 8.1% obtained for the community sample, and (b) five times the national rates of 4.2% for 35- to 54-year-old adults, and 3.8% for all adults (12,64). Abtin's comparative rates for seeing mother at least three to five times a week were 34.9% for the addicted group versus 21.1% for the community group. These two studies reveal parental contact/coresidence patterns similar to those observed with drug abusers, although at slightly lower levels, possibly because they represent a somewhat older age group. They are, as well, significantly higher than the levels observed in the overall adult population.

Of course, living with or regularly contacting parents is not in and of itself pathognomonic; such practices are the rule in some ethnic groups. We emphasize such patterns of connectedness here because (a) they are often overlooked by treatment programs and (b) they underscore that family members are important to substance abusers, and substance abusers are important to their families. Furthermore, as discussed in the section on treatment/self-help engagement, family members can be a tremendous resource toward getting reluctant substance abusers to seek help (72).

SOME RELEVANT FAMILY DYNAMICS

There is an extensive body of literature, covered by a number of reviews (e.g., 4–7,32,44,63,78,79), on the family and marital/couples aspects of substance abuse. While most of this literature lies beyond the scope of the present chapter, much of it independently corroborates the family contact studies noted above. Some highlights are presented below.

Deaths, Losses, and Disruptions

A number of researchers have documented that both the initial onset of, and subsequent relapses in, substance abuse are commonly tied to unexpected and/or disruptive losses—such as a sudden death, forced immigration, even an undesired retirement—within a substance abuser's family-of-origin and extended family (e.g., 3,9,17,30,33,34,37,53,62). Extending the well-established finding with children that events occurring with parents are more likely to predict child symptoms than are the child's own life events (such as moving to a new school), Duncan (14) found that (a) a family stress event preceded an adolescent's initiation of drug abuse in 94% of cases, and (b) there was an average of 3.5 family stress events—particularly major family losses such as a death, or disruption (e.g., onset of a life-threatening illness in a parent, a parent getting laid off)—in the year prior to onset. Furthermore, a Chicago study with opiate addicts found that the initial onset of drug abuse, as well as subsequent overdoses, were precipitated 80% of the time by such major family losses or disruptions (54).

In another example, a recent study reviewed the literature on early deaths/losses and subsequent addiction, and presented data on such questions, with 592 adult, out-of-

treatment, intravenous drug users (3). It found that the regularity with which these participants injected heroin and engaged in other human immunodeficiency virus (HIV)-related risks (e.g., needle sharing, unprotected sex) was significantly correlated ($p < 0.001$) with both (a) the number of their close family members who had died suddenly when the respondents were age 15 years or younger, and (b) the extent to which they and their families had effectively mourned those losses (e.g., very little manifestation of mourning of someone "close" to a participant was regarded as "inadequate" mourning). The canonical correlations between risk-taking and measures of inappropriate or inadequate mourning were 0.55 for the total sample and 0.70 for the subsample who experienced early and sudden family deaths. Findings from this and other studies (9,26,70) are consistent with Reilly's (61) conclusion that the addicted person often serves as a "revenant," or "replacement," for a deceased loved one. The addict is thus held onto in an enmeshed, overattached way as a means of retaining—or perhaps even symbolically "bringing back"—the lost family member. This is undoubtedly a factor in the aforementioned high levels at which most substance abusers maintain contact with their families of origin.

Other Patterns and Dynamics

While genetics can play a role in many cases, a number of other family factors can also have direct bearing on the genesis and remediation of addiction. For instance: (a) parental modeling of drug and alcohol taking is important (4,23); (b) the substance abuse may help to maintain family homeostasis, or even serve as a means for getting the drug abuser's parents into treatment (32,78); and (c) family members can engage in "enabling" behaviors that perpetuate the substance abuse of a member (10,43).

A particularly cogent process is the "family addiction cycle" (32,78). A cyclical, homeostatic pattern has been described with families of addicts in which, when the addict improves in some way, the parents begin to fight and to separate emotionally from each other. When the addict "fails," such as by taking drugs or losing a job, the parents shift attention from their couple problem and address the addict's problem. Thus the family becomes, in a sense, "unified." In this way, the addict's behavior serves a purpose of keeping the family together, at least temporarily. Furthermore, from this viewpoint the chemical taking is simply one event within an interpersonal sequence of behavior. It is not an independent phenomenon occurring in a vacuum, but a response to a series of others' behaviors that precede (and succeed) it. That is the reason for the term *family* addiction cycle. Professionals who are not attuned to these kinds of sequences taking place in a client's life put themselves at a disadvantage. They run the risk of being constantly mystified by onset and cessation of chemical taking.

Implications for Prevention

Family dynamics and patterns have also emerged as important in the prevention of substance abuse (25). Of the six protective factors identified by the United States National Institute on Drug Abuse (NIDA) as key to prevention of drug abuse, four (such as strong and positive parental bonds, parental monitoring, clear and consistently enforced rules of conduct) are family-related, as are four of the eight most important risk factors (e.g., chaotic home environment, ineffective parenting) (8). Further, of the ten evidence-based drug-abuse prevention programs endorsed by NIDA, seven involve parents/family, four very strongly so (67). As an example, parent–family interventions in the "Project Family" randomized prevention trial have been shown to hold up over a 4-year period (69). And, regarding alcohol, working with parents reduces drinking and related consequences in college students (82).

FAMILY/COUPLES/NETWORK APPROACHES TO GETTING SUBSTANCE ABUSERS TO ENGAGE IN TREATMENT/SELF-HELP

A major concern in the addiction field is that, in any given year, 90% to 95% of drug- and/or alcohol-dependent persons do not get into either treatment or self-help groups (35,60,68). This disturbing finding underscores the need to find new and better ways to get help for these individuals. Family members and significant others can be major sources of energy, competence, and motivation for addressing this problem.

At least 11 approaches have been developed, 10 of which have been examined in at least 19 outcome studies involving 1,501 cases, regarding the means for helping family members or significant others get a reluctant substance-abusing person to enroll in treatment or to begin attending a self-help group such as Alcoholics Anonymous or Cocaine Anonymous. While the last few years have seen reviews of various subsets of this research literature (e.g., 51,57,59,63,71), the first author recently published, in the *Journal of Marital and Family Therapy,* an overview of the complete body of engagement outcome studies (72). We present here some of the major conclusions and clinical recommendations from that review.

All of the approaches start with what has been termed a "concerned other" person or a "concerned significant other" that is, the person who contacts a treatment program to get help for a substance abuser. The concerned other might be a family member or relative, a spouse/partner, a friend, a member of the clergy, or anyone else who is motivated and connected enough to have some influence on the substance abuser.

The various approaches fall into two general categories: dual-purpose approaches and engagement-primary approaches. Dual-purpose methods tend to work with one person, most commonly a spouse/partner or an immediate family member such as a parent. The term "dual" refers to the two goals subscribed to by the approach. The first goal is to get the substance abuser engaged in treatment or self-help. The second goal is to help the concerned other to cope more effectively with both the substance abuser and (through counseling and educational material) the patterns that attend the addictive process itself, for example, to cease enabling, nagging, or escalating to the extreme. In this way, the approach resembles a form of personal counseling for the concerned other. Hence, the number of sessions conducted with the concerned other can range from 6 to 36 over a period of 3 to 6 months, depending on the particular model applied (the exception being Cooperative Counseling, which involves 1 to 6 sessions).

Engagement-primary approaches are pitched almost wholly toward the task of getting the substance abuser to enter treatment or self-help; they don't include an additional counseling component per se. The earliest and best known of these approaches is the Johnson Institute's "Intervention" (31), although at least four other engagement-primary approaches have been subsequently developed.

Overall Engagement Rates and Time-Period Comparisons

Some of the general findings and conclusions from Stanton's (72) review, particularly regarding the intent-to-treat rates/proportions of substance abuser who were engaged within 6 months from concerned other intake, are as follows:

1. As might be expected, later (1995-on) studies tended to achieve higher engagement rates (overall mean = 69%) than earlier (1983–1990) studies (52%), partly because the former had the advantage of being able to build on and refine the work of their predecessors.
2. As a group, the engagement experimental conditions performed significantly better (65%) than both wait-list controls (6%) and self-help conditions (17%). Experimental conditions in later studies also outperformed "engagement-as-usual" comparison groups (69% vs. 52%), whereas those in earlier studies obtained an identical rate of 52%.
3. The overall engagement rate with adolescents was 83%, which differed significantly from the overall rate of 59% for adults. However, this is confounded by substance of abuse, in that all the adolescent studies were with drug abusers, whereas there were no studies with adolescent alcohol abusers. A comparison between adolescent and adult drug abusers yielded figures, respectively, of 83% and 78%, and those rates did not differ significantly.
4. Following from the above, the aforementioned 78% rate for adult drug abusers, all of which were from later studies, was significantly higher than the 49% rate for later study alcohol abusers, implying that higher rates can be expected with the former group. However, this difference may be confounded by age, because the

alcohol abuser sample appeared (based on incomplete data) to be older.

Comparison of Dual-Purpose and Engagement-Primary Approaches

The two groups did not differ significantly, overall, in the design quality of their studies. Nor did dual-purpose and engagement-primary approaches differ significantly in their overall engagement rates with adult problems drinkers, that is, 40% versus 45% (identical 49% rates for later studies). However, among the six experimental conditions (within five studies) with adult drug abusers the engagement-primary approach attained a significantly higher engagement rate than did the dual-purpose approach (88% vs. 69%).

Note was also made of the fact that, although the additional counseling provided by dual-purpose approaches appears, in and of itself, to be of clear value to the concerned others who participate in it, such a requirement is not indicated for a certain proportion of concerned others. For some sorts of concerned others who may call in to get help for a substance abuser (e.g., employers, work associates, friends, clergy, second-degree relatives), the quasi-personal counseling component may not be appropriate. Additionally, others who do seem appropriate may still refuse such an option, especially if, or because, it requires a significant number of individual sessions.

Other Conclusions

Additional conclusions emerging from Stanton's (72) review were the following:

1. The four groups of investigators who examined them determined that heavily confrontational approaches, such as the traditional form of the Johnson Intervention (31), are not indicated in most cases, particularly because the majority (70% to 100%) of concerned others to whom they are offered refuse to carry them out due to the stressful nature of the confrontation, the secretiveness involved, and the potential damage to the relationship. While in recent years several less-aggressive versions of intervention have been developed, none of them have been examined in engagement outcome studies.
2. Involving parents, not only with adolescents but also with adults, appears to increase the likelihood of substance abuser engagement.
3. Involving greater numbers of significant others in the endeavor may produce better engagement results for less professional effort.

Clinical Options

In light of the above, thinking clinicians are likely to ask, "What are the 'better edge,' manual-guided options if one

wants to get an substance abuser into treatment or self-help?" Based on the existent studies in this still-evolving field, below are the first author's (72) recommendations for engaging seven particular clinical subgroups. This is not meant to imply, incidentally, that approaches not mentioned here have no value, but rather that the research evidence indicates that those listed appear, generally, to be more likely to succeed.

Dual-Purpose Preferred Options

If the intent is to help the concerned other both to participate in counseling to better cope with the substance abuser (and perhaps to benefit personally), as well as to get the substance abuser to enter treatment or self-help, the following are recommended:

- Adults with Substance Use Disorder (Drug Abuse)

  The Community Reinforcement and Family Training (CRAFT) approach, with its rigorous research underpinnings, is clearly the best option here. CRAFT is a behaviorally oriented, problem-focused, skill-based approach using role-play techniques, and involves, in its latest version, an average of 10 to 12 sessions. The overall mean engagement rate for drug abusers across three experimental conditions in two studies was 71%, with some indication that engagement may be additionally improved by providing the concerned other with group aftercare sessions (47,48).

  A credible second choice to CRAFT is another behaviorally based method known as Community Reinforcement Training (CRT). A nonconfrontational approach averaging 12 to 13 sessions over an 8 to 9 week period, CRT provides motivational training, encourages independence from the substance abuser, and provides training in contingency management. It attained an engagement rate of 64% (56% of those randomized) with adult drug abusers (36).

- Adults with Alcohol Use Disorder

  Based on its high-quality outcome research, CRAFT is the first choice here, too. A study with adult problem drinkers, in which concerned other person's attended an average of 10 to 11 sessions, achieved a 64% engagement rate (51).

Engagement-Primary Preferred Options

If engagement of substance abusers in treatment/self-help is, in and of itself, the clinical or programmatic goal, the recommendations are as follows:

- Adolescents with Substance Use Disorder (Drug Abuse)

  The (CRT-influenced) Intensive Parent and Youth Attendance Intervention appears to be the most cost-efficient mode, especially if engagement of the youth, per se, is the goal. In particular, its cost-effectiveness, that is, its high rate of return for only 2 hours of professional effort, sets it apart. It involves a standardized handling of the first call, the setting of a parent plus youth intake appointment within 2 to 7 days, and preparatory calls to both parent and adolescent 2 to 3 days prior to the appointment. Donahue et al. (13) obtained an 89% success rate with this method, which was a marked improvement over the typical appointment procedure rate of 45%.

- Adolescents with Substance Use Disorder (Drug Abuse) and Their Families

Adding family engagement to the agenda evokes the Strategic Structural Systems Engagement (SSSE) option. One of the two best-researched methods, SSSE, in particular, is effective with Hispanic families. The procedure is to use from (on average) 2.5 to 5.3 "contacts" (phone calls, home visits, office sessions) with the concerned other and resistant family members (including, of course, the substance abuser) in applying techniques such as "joining" and family "restructuring" in an effort to overcome the family's resistance to engagement. Its success rate across two experimental conditions with youthful drug abusers was 87% (65,81).

- Adults with Either Substance Use (Drug Abuse) or Alcohol Use Disorder

An approach called A Relational Intervention Sequence for Engagement (ARISE) is the most cost-effective choice here. It combines rapid results and a relatively low demand on staff time (an average of 1.5 total hours per case) to attain high rates with both categories of disorder. Primarily developed by Garrett (19–21), the approach involves up to three stepped stages: (a) starting with the concerned other's first call (which is pivotal, and involves the message, "You can't do this alone"), (b) holding one or (if necessary) more sessions with significant others (to which the substance abuser is also invited), and (c) culminating in a modified, less-confrontational Johnson Intervention for the small proportion (2% to 3%) of cases that require it. Outcome results yielded an 87% rate with adult drug abusers, and a 77% rate with adult alcohol abusers (40). Of those who engaged, most (76%) did so within 2 weeks from the first call.

- Mothers with Substance Use Disorder (Drug Abuse)

The Engaging Moms approach, with its uniquely tailored protocol, has carved out a distinctive niche in the engagement of women under such circumstances, that is, in which either a mother or her infant tested positive for cocaine. An integrative approach, using techniques from several family and women's treatment models, it entails an average of 15 family, individual, and case management contacts (not necessarily "sessions"), averaging

about 7 to 8 total hours, over an 8-week period (11). The approach obtained an 88% treatment engagement rate with such women.

FAMILY/COUPLES TREATMENT CONSIDERATIONS

About Family/Couples Treatment

Fundamentally, family therapy is a way of thinking about human problems that suggests certain actions for their alleviation, rather than a modality of treatment per se. The term *systems therapy* actually is preferred by many family therapists, but most agree that it is too late to change the tag. Indeed, it is the systemic (relational, interactional) manner of their thought and interventions that defines the approach, not the attention to the social unit called a "family." Family therapists work with families because the family is one of the systems in which human problems can be most easily understood, and because families often provide a significant resource for solving problems. Furthermore, the term *family therapist* applies to *all* professionals who "think family" in their clinical work, including psychiatrists, psychologists, social workers, counselors, nurses, and clergy, as well as, of course, professional marriage and family therapists. Indeed, family and marital/couples therapy traces its beginnings to pioneers in all of these various fields.

Treating Families with a Substance Abuse Problem

The case can be made that family/couples therapy is appropriate and helpful throughout the process of recovery. This includes, in addition to the substance abuser engagement effort described above, both outpatient and residential treatment contexts. All are fitting settings for the family and its members to learn new ways to continue their lives without chemicals of abuse.

Taking this point further, the converse is also true: A lack of family-oriented services in substance abuse treatment can have calamitous consequences. As Liepman et al. (43) stated in the conclusion to their review of the research on treatment of children of alcoholics, "Without family therapy, most families would suffer serious 'side effects' if the alcoholic were to stop drinking" (p. 53). In fact, without concurrent treatment for nonabusing members, families have been known (in order to preserve the familiar and perhaps avoid the illumination of other problems) to attempt to sabotage treatment efforts, when those efforts begin to succeed. Examples of this are commonly reported in the literature; they range from a spouse slipping beer to a recovering alcoholic, to the parents who refuse to work together in maintaining rules for their out-of-control adolescent. Contrast that with a community reinforcement approach study by Higgins et al. (29) that found that the best predictor of achieving cocaine abstinence in treatment was whether a case involved participation by a significant other—involvement increased the odds of success by a factor of 19.3. Indeed, recognition of such variables led Craig, in an overview of trends in the substance abuse field, to conclude that, "The need to address family issues in a comprehensive treatment program is now widely recognized in drug abuse treatment" (10, p. 185).

Sometimes it is difficult to convene the whole family of an substance abuser for therapy (65,71,78). Fathers of substance-abusing young people, in particular, often appear threatened by treatment and defensive about their contributions to the problem. Because many have drinking problems themselves, they may also fear discovery, being blamed for the problem, or that their own addiction will be challenged.

Recognizing such hesitancies, family therapists try to recruit families into therapy. Sometimes they ask other family members to help with recruiting, but they are cognizant that this approach may not be sufficient. Thus they extend personal invitations to the reluctant members. In less seriously disturbed families, one telephone call may enable a therapist to reassure family members that their contributions are important to the solution of the substance abuse. In more disturbed families, it may be necessary to meet family members on "neutral turf" (such as at a restaurant), or to write multiple letters, or even to pay family members for participation in treatment (77,78). There are many standardized and creative techniques for involving families of drug or alcohol abusers in treatment (38,78).

Involving Parents in Decisions

Parents should be involved in all decisions about treatment when a substance abuser is an adolescent or a young adult. This includes decisions about hospitalization, medication, and drug tests. Family therapists make the parents part of the treatment team because it helps to get the couple working together and because the responsibility for the resolution of the problem is correctly theirs. When the parents of a young abuser are divorced or unmarried, the same holds true; adult caretakers must be encouraged to work together to help their children.

Detoxification at Home

Physical dependence on alcohol or other drugs must, of course, be assessed and managed early in treatment. When dependence exists, the client may be hospitalized for detoxification, especially if the dependence is on sedative hypnotics such as alcohol or barbiturates. However, for some other substances, and given medical backup, the family may attempt, following certain procedures, to conduct the detoxification at home (66,78). In fact, home detoxification appears to be a cost-effective option in many cases, with savings of 70% to 85% of the cost of hospitalization (74,76).

Dealing with Intergenerational Losses and Patterns

Stemming from the earlier discussion regarding how major losses within an substance abuser's extended family can lead to unresolved mourning (3,9,26,70), or to the family's otherwise getting "stuck" in an intergenerational pattern of addiction, Landau and Stanton (39,73) developed a conceptual model of how such patterns develop within a family. Using a genogram covering at least four generations, the method starts by asking, "When, in this family's history, was the family so stressed that it had to change its relational patterns or organization and develop a drinking or drug problem?" That information is then used therapeutically, taking the family back to the point of loss and symbolically "going through" it again from a present-day vantage point. This joins the poles of past, present, and future—spanning the family's generations. The process also depathologizes those members from the past who had problems, and reinstates them, instead, as people who may have been pained and besieged. By granting the forebears their honorable place, honor is also bestowed on the living, their descendants. Such uncovering and rebuilding gives the family members the kind of information that can free them up to make a choice: whether to keep, revise, or replace the scripts—the intergenerational instructions—that have been carried down. In other words, it helps them acquire flexibility in coming to grips with the question as to whether, and how, to move on in life. In experience with several thousand cases, as well as more systematic qualitative study with more than 200 clinical and nonclinical families, the method shows great promise in bringing about long-term change in the intergenerational family addiction pattern.

An Integrative View

More than two dozen books have been written specifically about family/couples therapy with substance abusers. Similarly, many different modalities of family treatment have been described, including marital/couples therapy; group therapy for parents or relatives; concurrent parent and index patient therapy; therapy with individual families, both inpatient and outpatient; sibling-oriented therapy; multiple-family therapy; social network therapy (including friends, neighbors, other therapists, social agents and, often, systems external to the family); and family therapy with one person. To bring greater coherence to this multifaceted and expanding field, we have set forth an integrative model of the stages of family/couples therapy with substance abusers (27). The model synthesizes the relevant literature for both alcohol- and drug-dependent adults, as well as for substance-abusing adolescents. It emphasizes the consensus among the various authors in the field, and offers a rich collection of the clear and specific family therapy methods they have developed. The interested reader is referred to that publication for the principles it delineates and the literature it covers.

OUTCOME RESEARCH

Subsequent to the comprehensive reviews of the outcome studies of family/couples treatment for alcoholism by Edwards and Steinglass (15) and McCrady (46), and for drug abuse by Liddle and Dakof (41), at least 16 additional reviews have emerged pertaining to that literature. Four of these more recent reviews dealt specifically with adult alcohol studies (7,56–58), and five specifically with drug abuse, three of which cover adolescents (6,59,84) and the remaining two cover both adolescents and adults (63,74). Seven other reviews encompassed research on both alcohol and drugs: two regarding adults (16,55), three pertaining to adolescents (85–87), and two including both adult and adolescent studies (49,50). In line with the growing emphasis on evidence-based treatments for mental health and addictive disorders, most of the studies which were reviewed, and nearly all of the more recent studies, have been randomized clinical trials (RCTs). Because RCTs generally provide the proof-in-the-pudding in regard to questions of efficacy and effectiveness, this section is essentially confined to studies that incorporated an RCT design. Furthermore, it will not be our purpose here to go over the ground already covered by these reviewers, such as summarizing studies they have already presented. Rather, where indicated, we will highlight some of their major conclusions, as well as briefly describe a few studies which have come to light since their reviews.

Alcohol

Regarding family/couples treatment for adult drinking problems, O'Farrell and Fals-Stewart (56) found that the number of relevant RCTs had increased measurably since Edwards and Steinglass' 1995 meta-analysis (15). Consequently, they calculated effect sizes for five outcome variables (e.g., alcohol use, treatment attendance, couple/family adjustment). Of most relevance here was their drinking outcome finding across the 16 family/couples RCTs that examined it, as they obtained a highly significant effect size in favor of family involved treatment relative to individually based treatment or wait-list control conditions (median effect size = 0.30, p <0.00001). More specifically, they found the strongest evidence (8 of 10 studies) for couples approaches, particularly behavioral couples therapy, in comparison to the other conditions. The evidence for family systems approaches, which had grown to seven RCTs from 1 in 1989 (46), was generally positive, but more mixed: 3 of 4 comparisons with other conditions favored family systems therapy, whereas 1 of 4 comparisons with other family approaches favored the family systems approach (the other 3 yielding equivalent results). These findings were reinforced in a sub-

sequent review, by the same authors, of 29 RCTs and 2 sequential assignment studies (58). Furthermore, Miller et al. (50), in their summary of the efficacy of specific family/couples approaches to alcohol abuse, provided additional confirmation in their conclusions that, regarding adults, effectiveness is (a) now established for behavioral couples approaches, and (b) probable for psychodynamic/eclectic conjoint couples groups.

In contrast to the burgeoning research with adult alcohol abusers, it is rather surprising that, whereas at least 19 RCTs have emerged exploring family oriented treatments with drug-abusing adolescents (see Drug Abuse, below), there is a dearth of such studies with adolescents whose primary substance of abuse is alcohol, even though alcohol has persisted for decades as the number one chemical abused by youth (52). The single such RCT we were able to find was conducted in Sweden by Hansson (24) with 89 youths (10% female) who were apprehended by the police. Alcohol was a problem for 75%, the rest having drug-abuse problems. Two conditions were compared: treatment-as-usual counseling (TAU), and functional family therapy (FFT) (2). In a 1-year followup, 65% of the TAU cases had relapsed versus 33% of the FFT cases (Fisher's Exact Test p <0.003), while at 2-year followup the rates, respectively, were 82% and 41% (p <0.00008). In addition, 53% of the TAU cases dropped out before completing treatment, whereas none of the FFT cases did so.

Drug Abuse

In terms of the effectiveness of family/couples treatment for drug abuse, in 1997 Stanton and Shadish (74) performed a review and meta-analysis across 15 RCT outcome studies, 6 with adults and 9 with adolescents. Some of the major conclusions from that review were as follows:

1. Overall, the studies' design quality was rated very good.
2. Compared to the nonfamily modalities of individual counseling/therapy, group therapy, and treatment-as-usual, family/couples therapy showed superior results, with significant (p <0.01) effect sizes of 0.55, 0.51, and 0.38, respectively. This was not meant to imply that the nonfamily approaches are ineffective, for most of them are effective, but rather that either (a) their results can be improved by the addition of family/couples therapy—such as to methadone maintenance, or (b) family/couples therapy presents a more effective and/or cost-effective alternative.
3. Comparisons between family therapy and other forms of family intervention gave an edge to family therapy over family psychoeducation (effect size = 0.66), but equivalent effects for relatives' groups.
4. These findings hold for both adolescent and adult drug abusers.

5. Comparisons between different "schools" of family therapy are inconclusive. One reason is that many of these schools have not been involved in outcome research with this population. A second reason is that most of the approaches that have been tested share many commonalities with each other, so that differences among them in effectiveness, if such differences exist, are difficult to tease out.

6. Compared with other studies and approaches to psychotherapy with drug abusers, family therapy conditions have attained relatively high rates of engagement and retention in treatment.

7. Differences between different treatment conditions as to their early dropout rates pose a potential problem. All too commonly, such dropouts have been excluded from outcome analyses. When, as part of the meta-analytic review, dropouts were reintroduced into the data analysis as treatment failures, it became apparent that family treatment, which was likely to have fewer dropouts, had, in the original analyses, been modestly penalized relative to other modalities.

Subsequent to that meta-analysis, the number of family/couples treatment RCTs for drug abuse has more than doubled, to at least 32. Seven of the newer studies have been with adults, and 10 with adolescents. Sixteen of the 17 are confirmatory of the Stanton and Shadish (74) conclusions given above. Most of these newer studies are incorporated within the 12 drug-abuse reviews cited earlier.

Adults

Not covered in those 12 reviews are, in addition, the following recent RCTs of family/couples treatment for adult drug abusers:

- In a study with 58 patients receiving short-term buprenorphine (Buprenex) maintenance, Galanter et al. (18) compared buprenorphine augmented by network therapy sessions (averaging 2.3 members) in 24 cases, to 34 cases in which buprenorphine was augmented by medical management sessions of equal duration. During an 18-week treatment period, significantly more of the network therapy patients' twice-weekly urine tests were opiate free, that is, 64.6%, compared to 43.2% of those from the medical management patients (t = 55.2, p <0.03).
- McCollum et al. (45) compared 122 female drug abusers (a minority of whom also abused alcohol) across three conditions: (a) 12 weeks of outpatient TAU; (b) TAU accompanied by 12 sessions of systemic couple therapy (SCT), an integrative method that incorporated both couple and intergenerational family concepts, and which also conjointly included the woman's partner/spouse; (c) TAU accompanied by 12 sessions of systemic individual therapy (SIT) which used SCT methods

and concepts, but without the partner being present. Although no differences emerged in alcohol use, all three conditions demonstrated marked reductions in drug use between pretest and 3 months posttest. However, the TAU group showed a significant return to drug abuse after 3 months, while the two couples' conditions maintained their gains at 6 and 12 months.

- A United Kingdom (London) study by Yandoli at al. (88) involved 119 male and female opioid-dependent patients within a methadone program. Three conditions were compared: (a) A nonnegotiable methadone reduction regimen accompanied by structural/strategic family therapy (78), which, with the 80% of cases who were living with a partner, involved mainly couples work (although other family members were invited to some sessions and, "conceptually, the family as a whole was always part of the therapists' consideration" (88, p. 407); (b) standard clinic treatment, an open-ended modality that included counseling, but with a more flexible methadone reduction regimen; (c) "low contact" treatment involving up to 12 monthly sessions plus the nonnegotiable methadone-reduction regimen. Results indicated that, in terms of abstinence from illegal drugs, "overall there was a consistent pattern for family therapy to produce better results at both 6 and 12 months" following intake than the other two conditions (88, p. 412). In addition, although the standard treatment condition included more sessions (18.1) than did family therapy (10.1) and low-contact treatment (8.9), its illegal drug abstinence outcomes were significantly worse than those for the other 2 conditions.

Adolescents

A recent, comprehensive review by Rowe and Liddle (63) provides additional documentation, including data on cost-effectiveness, reinforcing the validity of the seven aforementioned conclusions as they pertain to adolescents. Furthermore, Williams and Chang (86), in their overview of treatments for adolescent substance abusers, concluded both that "outpatient family therapy appears superior to other forms of outpatient treatment" (p. 138), and that it should be a component of any treatment program for such youth.

Specific Approaches

In terms of particular models of family/couples treatment for drug abuse, Miller et al. (50) concluded that effectiveness is (a) established for integrative structural-strategic models (e.g., references 78, 80, and 88), and (b) probable for multisystemic family therapy (28). Using their criteria for "established" (four or more quality studies, or one quality study replicated by another researcher), and based on subsequent research, we would add three other approaches to the list of family/couples approaches with established effectiveness for these sorts of disorders. They are, for adolescents, multidimensional family therapy (42) and functional family therapy (2), and, for adults, behavioral couples therapy (16). In fact, regarding the last, Fals-Stewart et al. (16) make the case that behavioral couples therapy, which has been examined in at least five RCTs (with several more currently underway), is a strong, and relatively inexpensive, option for application with adult drug abusers of either sex, as well as in conjunction with both methadone and naltrexone (ReVia) regimens.

So, overall, Stanton and Shadish's (74) seven conclusions appear to have been upheld by the reviews and studies that have subsequently emerged. In other words, evidence continues to accumulate that family and couples treatments for substance abuse are both efficacious and cost-effective.

REFERENCES

1. Abtin A. Frequency of contact with family of origin in individuals with alcohol dependence [Doctoral dissertation, Spalding University, 2001]. *Dissertation Abstracts Int* 2001;61(11B):6123.
2. Alexander JF, Parsons BV. *Functional family therapy.* Monterey, CA: Brooks/Cole, 1982.
3. Bowser BP, Word CO, Stanton MD, et al. Death in the family and HIV risk-taking among intravenous drug users. *Fam Process* 2003;42:291–304.
4. Brook JS, Brook DW, Arencibia-Mireles O, et al. Risk factors for adolescent marijuana use across cultures and time. *J Genet Psychology* 2001;162(3):357–374.
5. Brown S, Lewis V. *The alcoholic family in recovery: a developmental model.* New York: Guilford Press, 1999.
6. Carr A. Evidenced-based practice in family therapy and systemic consultation: I. Child-focused problems. *J Fam Ther* 2000;22:29–60.
7. Carr A. Evidenced-based practice in family therapy and systemic consultation: II. Adult-focused problems. *J Fam Ther* 2000;22:273–295.
8. Cire B. NIDA conference reviews advances in prevention science, announces new national research initiative. *NIDA Notes* 2002;16(6):1,5–7.
9. Coleman S, Kaplan J, Downing R. Life cycle and loss: the spiritual vacuum of heroin addiction. *Fam Process* 1986;25(1):5–23.
10. Craig RJ. Contemporary trends in substance abuse. *Pro Psychol Res Pract* 1993;24:182–189.
11. Dakof GA, Quille TJ, Tejeda MJ, et al. Enrolling and retaining mothers of substance-exposed infants in drug abuse treatment. *J Consult Clin Psychol* 2003;71(4):764–772.
12. Davis JA, Smith TW. *General social surveys, 1972–99: cumulative codebook.* Chicago: National Opinion Research Center. Retrieved (1994 cohort) May 17, 2000, from http://www.icpsr.umich.edu/gs99/codebook/mavisit.htm.
13. Donahue B, Azrin NH, Lawson H, et al. Improving initial session attendance of substance abusing and conduct disordered adolescents: a controlled study. *J Child Adolesc Subst Abuse* 1998;8(1):1–13.
14. Duncan DF. Family stress and the initiation of adolescent drug abuse: a retrospective study. *Correct Soc Psychiatry* 1978;24(3):111–114.
15. Edwards M, Steinglass P. Family therapy treatment outcomes for alcoholism. *J Marital Fam Ther* 1995;21:475–509.
16. Fals-Stewart W, O'Farrell T, Birchler GR, et al. Behavioral couples therapy for alcoholism and drug abuse: where we've been, where we are, and where we're going. *J Cognit Psychother* (in press).
17. Frone MR, Cooper ML, Russell M. Stressful life events, gender, and substance use: an application of tobit regression. *Psychol Addict Behav* 1994;8(2):59–69.
18. Galanter M, Dermatis H, Resnick R, et al. *Short-term buprenorphine maintenance: a comparison of the relative efficacy of network therapy and medication management* [Unpublished manuscript]. New York: New York University School of Medicine, 2003.
19. Garrett J, Landau J, Shea R, et al. The ARISE Intervention: using family and networks links to engage addicted persons in treatment. *J Subst Abuse Treat* 1998;15(2):333–343.
20. Garrett J, Landau-Stanton J, Stanton MD, et al. ARISE: a method for engaging reluctant alcohol- and drug-dependent individuals in treatment. *J Subst Abuse Treat* 1997;14(3):235–248.
21. Garrett J, Stanton MD, Landau J, et al. The "concerned other" call: using family links and networks to overcome resistance to addiction treatment. *Subst Use Misuse* 1999;34:363–382.
22. Goldscheider F. Recent changes in U.S. young adult living arrangements in comparative perspective. *J Fam Issues* 1997;18(6):708–724.
23. Gorsuch RL, Butler MC. Initial drug abuse: a review of predisposing social psychological factors. *Psychol Bull* 1976;83(1):120–137.
24. Hansson K. *The Swedish model of functional family therapy: results and reflections from four replications.* Plenary address at the Eighth International Conference on Treatment of Addictive Behaviors, Sante Fe, New Mexico, January 1998.
25. Hawkins JD, Catalano RF, Miller JY. Risk and protective factors for alcohol and other drug problems in adolescence and early adulthood: implications for substance abuse prevention. *Psychol Bull* 1992;112:64–105.
26. Heard D. Death as a motivator: using crisis induction to break through the denial system. In: Stanton MD, Todd TC, and Associates. *The family therapy of drug abuse and addiction.* New York: Guilford Press, 1982:203–234.
27. Heath AW, Stanton MD. Family-based treatment: stages and outcomes. In: Frances RJ, Miller SI, Mack A, eds. *Clinical textbook of addictive disorders,* 3rd ed. New York: Guilford Publications, 2004: in press.
28. Henggeler SW, Borduin CM. *Family therapy and beyond: a multisystemic approach to treating the behavior problems of children and adolescents.* Pacific Grove, CA: Brooks/Cole, 1990.
29. Higgins, ST, Budney AJ, Bickel WK, et al. Participation of significant others in outpatient behavioral treatment predicts greater cocaine abstinence. *Am J Drug Alcohol Abuse* 1994;20(1):47–56.
30. Hope S, Power C, Rodgers B. The relationship between parental separation in childhood and problem drinking in adulthood. *Addiction* 1998;93:505–514.
31. Johnson VE. *Intervention: how to help someone who doesn't want help.* Minneapolis, MN: Johnson Institute Books, 1986.
32. Kaufman E. Family systems and family therapy of substance abuse: an overview of two decades of research and clinical experience. *Int J Addict* 1985;20(6&7):897–916.
33. Kendler KS, Neale MC, Prescott CA, et al. Childhood parental loss and

alcoholism in women: a causal analysis using a twin-family design. *Psychol Med* 1996;26:79–95.

34. Kessler RC, Davis CG, Kendler KS. Childhood adversity and adult psychiatric disorder in the US National Comorbidity Survey. *Psychol Med* 1997;27:1101–1119.

35. Kessler RC, McGonagle KA, Zhao S, et al. Lifetime and 12-month prevalence of *DSM-III-R* psychiatric disorders in the United States: results from the National Comorbidity Survey. *Arch Gen Psychiatry* 1994;51:8–19.

36. Kirby KC, Marlowe DB, Festinger DS, et al. Community reinforcement training for family and significant others of drug abusers: a unilateral intervention to increase treatment entry of drug users. *Drug Alcohol Depend* 1999;56:85–96.

37. Krueger DW. Stressful life events and the return to heroin use. *J Hum Stress* 1981;7(2):3–8.

38. Landau J, Garrett J, Shea RR, et al. Strength in numbers: the ARISE method for mobilizing family and network to engage substance abusers in treatment. *Am J Drug Alcohol Abuse* 2000;26(3):379–398.

39. Landau J, Stanton MD. A model for alcoholism and addiction within the family: I. Intergenerational genesis and the "when did it start?" question. [*Manuscript submitted for publication.*]

40. Landau J, Stanton MD, Brinkman-Sull D, et al. Outcomes with the ARISE approach to engaging reluctant drug- and alcohol-dependent individuals in treatment. *Am J Drug Alcohol Abuse* 2004; 30(4): *in press*.

41. Liddle HA, Dakof GA. Efficacy of family therapy for drug abuse. *J Marital Fam Ther* 1995;21:511–543.

42. Liddle HA, Hogue A. Multidimensional family therapy for adolescent substance abuse. In: Wagner EF, Waldron HB, eds. *Innovations in adolescent substance abuse interventions.* New York: Pergamon/Elsevier Science, 2001:229–261.

43. Liepman MR, White W, Nirenberg TD. Children of alcoholic families. In: Lewis D, Williams C, eds. *Providing care for children of alcoholics: clinical and research perspectives.* Pompano Beach, FL: Health Communications, 1986:39–64.

44. Mackenson G, Cottone RR. Family structural issues and chemical dependency: a review of the literature from 1985 to 1991. *Am J Fam Ther* 1992;20(3):227–241.

45. McCollum EE, Lewis RA, Nelson TS, et al. Couple treatment for drug abusing women: effects on drug use and need for treatment. *J Couple Relationship Ther* 2003;2(4):1–18.

46. McCrady BS. Outcomes of family-involved alcoholism treatment. In: Galanter M, ed. *Recent developments in alcoholism, vol. 7: treatment research.* New York: Plenum Press, 1989:165–182.

47. Meyers RJ, Miller WR, Hill DE, et al. Community reinforcement and family training (CRAFT): engaging unmotivated drug users in treatment. *J Subst Abuse* 1999;10(3):291–308.

48. Meyers RJ, Miller WR, Smith JE, et al. A randomized trial of two methods for engaging treatment-refusing drug users through concerned significant others. *J Consult Clin Psychol* 2002;70(5):1182–1185.

49. Meyers RJ, Smith JE, Lash DN. The community reinforcement approach. In: Galanter M, ed. *Recent developments in alcoholism, vol. 16: research on alcoholism treatment.* New York: Kluwer Academic/Plenum Publishers, 2003:183–195.

50. Miller RB, Johnson LN, Sandberg JG, et al. An addendum to the 1997 outcome research chart. *Am J Fam Ther* 2000;28:347–354.

51. Miller WR, Meyers RJ, Tonigan JS. Engaging the unmotivated in treatment for alcohol problems: a comparison of three intervention strategies. *J Consult Clin Psychol* 1999;67(5):688–697.

52. Morrison SF, Rogers PD, Thomas MH. Alcohol and adolescents. *Pediatr Clinic North Am* 1995;42(2):371–387.

53. Newcomb MD, Huba GJ, Bentler PM. Life change events among adolescents: an empirical consideration of some methodological issues. *J Nerv Ment Dis* 1986;174(5):280–289.

54. Noone RJ. Drug abuse behavior in relation to change in the family structure. In: McCullough PG, Carolin JC, eds. *Pittsburgh Family Systems Symposia: collection of papers.* Pittsburgh, PA: Western Psychiatric Institute and Clinic, 1979-1980:174–186.

55. O'Farrell TJ, Fals-Stewart W. Behavioral couples treatment for alcoholism and drug abuse. *J Subst Abuse Treat* 2000;18:51–54.

56. O'Farrell TJ, Fals-Stewart W. Family-involved alcoholism treatment: an update. In: Galanter M, ed. *Recent developments in alcoholism, vol. 15: services research in the era of managed care.* New York: Plenum Press 2001:329–356.

57. O'Farrell TJ, Fals-Stewart W. Marital and family therapy. In: Hester R, Miller WR, eds. *Handbook of alcoholism treatment approaches,* 3rd ed. Boston: Allyn & Bacon, 2002:188–212.

58. O'Farrell TJ, Fals-Stewart W. Alcohol abuse. *J Marital Fam Ther* 2003; 29(1):121–146.

59. Ozechowski TJ, Liddle HA. Family-based therapy for adolescent drug abuse: knowns and unknowns. *Clin Child Fam Psychol Rev* 2000;3(4):269–298.

60. Regier DA, Narrow WE, Rae DS, et al. The de facto U. S. mental and addictive disorders service system. *Arch Gen Psychiatry* 1993;50:84–94.

61. Reilly D. Family factors in the etiology and treatment of youthful drug abuse. *Fam Ther* 1976;2:149–171.

62. Rosenbaum M, Richman J. Family dynamics and drug overdoses. *Suicide Life Threat Behav* 1972;2:19–25.

63. Rowe CL, Liddle HA. Substance abuse. *J Marital Fam Ther* 2003;29(1):97–120.

64. Russell C. *The baby boom: Americans aged 35-54,* 2nd ed. Ithaca, New York: New Strategist Publications, 1999.

65. Santisteban DA, Szapocznik J, Perez-Vidal A, et al. Efficacy of intervention for engaging youth and families into treatment and some variables that may contribute to differential effectiveness. *J Fam Psychol* 1996;10(1):35–44.

66. Scott S, Van Deusen J. Detoxification at home: a family approach. In: Stanton MD, Todd TC, and Associates. *The family therapy of drug abuse and addiction.* New York: Guilford Press, 1982:310–334.

67. Sloboda Z, David SL. *Preventing drug use among children and adolescents: a research-based guide.* NIH Pub. No. 97-4212. Rockville, MD: National Institute on Drug Abuse, 1997.

68. Sobell LC, Cunningham JA, Sobell MB. Recovery from alcohol problems with and without treatment: prevalence in two population surveys. *Am J Pub Health* 1996;86:966–972.

69. Spoth RL, Redmond C, Shin C. Randomized trial of brief family interventions for general populations: adolescent substance use outcomes 4 years following baseline. *J Consult Clin Psychol* 2001;69(4):627–642.

70. Stanton MD. The addict as savior: heroin, death and the family. *Fam Process* 1977;16:191–197.

71. Stanton MD. The role of family and significant others in the engagement and retention of drug-dependent individuals. *NIDA Res Monogr* 1997;165:157–180.

72. Stanton MD. Getting reluctant substance abusers to engage in treatment/self-help: a review of outcomes and clinical options. *J Marital Fam Ther* 2004;30(1):165–182.

73. Stanton MD, Landau J. A model for alcoholism and addiction within the family: II. Intergenerational transmission, maintenance of the symptom, and therapeutic

implications. [*Manuscript submitted for publication.*]

74. Stanton MD, Shadish WR. Outcome, attrition and family/couples treatment for drug abuse: a meta-analysis and review of the controlled, comparative studies. *Psychol Bull* 1997;122(2):170–191.

75. Stanton MD, Shea R, Garrett J. *Family-of-origin contacts of alcoholics: an overlooked phenomenon* [Unpublished manuscript]. Rochester, NY: University of Rochester Medical Center, 1997.

76. Stanton MD, Steier F, Cook L, et al. *Narcotic detoxification in a family and home context: updated summary of final report results—1997.* (Grant No. R01 DA03097). Rockville, MD: National Institute on Drug Abuse, Treatment Research Branch, 1997.

77. Stanton MD, Steier F, Todd TC. Paying families for attending sessions: counteracting the dropout problem. *J Marital Fam Ther* 1982;8:371–373.

78. Stanton MD, Todd TC, and Associates. *The family therapy of drug abuse and addiction.* New York: Guilford Press, 1982.

79. Steinglass P, Bennett L, Wolin S, et al. *The alcoholic family.* New York: Basic Books, 1987.

80. Szapocznik J, Kurtines WM. *Breakthroughs in family therapy with drug abusing and problem youth.* New York: Springer Publishing, 1989.

81. Szapocznik J, Perez-Vidal A, Brickman AL, et al. Engaging adolescent drug abusers and their families in treatment: a strategic structural-systems approach. *J Consult Clin Psychol* 1988;56(4):552–557.

82. Turrisi R, Jaccard J, Taki R, et al. Examination of the short-term efficacy of a parent intervention to reduce college student drinking tendencies. *Psychol Addict Behav* 2001;15(4):366–372.

83. U.S. Bureau of the Census. *Marital status and living arrangements (current population reports, series P-20–514).* Washington, DC: U.S. Government Printing Office, 1998 (March).

84. Waldron HB. Adolescent substance abuse and family therapy outcome: a review of randomized trials. In: Ollendick TH, Prinz RJ, eds. *Advances in clinical child psychology.* New York: Plenum Press, 1997;19:199–234.

85. Weinberg NZ, Rahdert E, Colliver JD, et al. Adolescent substance abuse: a review of the past 10 years. *J Am Acad Child Adolesc Psychiatry* 1998;37:252–261.

86. Williams RJ, Chang SY. A comprehensive and comparative review of adolescent substance abuse treatment outcome. *Clin Psychol Sci Pract* 2000;7(2):138–166.

87. Winters KC, Latimer WL, Stinchfield RD. Adolescent treatment for alcohol and other drug abuse. In: Ott PJ, Tarter RE, Ammerman RT, eds. *Sourcebook on substance abuse: etiology, epidemiology, assessment, and treatment.* New York: Allyn & Bacon, 1999:350–361.

88. Yandoli D, Eisler I, Robbins C, et al. A comparative study of family therapy in the treatment of opiate users in a London drug clinic. *J Fam Ther* 2002;24(2):402–422.

CHAPTER 45

The Role of Coercion in Drug Treatment

SALLY L. SATEL AND DAVID J. FARABEE

To judge by the character of the present debate over national drug control policy, an observer would never guess how completely the participants agree about some very important things. The debate is dominated by its extremes, opposing camps that deride each other's arguments. On one side, the "drug warriors," as their critics label them, want to stamp out drug use altogether: They advance strict controls on drug production and harsh punishments for trafficking. At the other end of the continuum, drug legalizers condemn the abolitionist strategy as costly, punitive, and unrealistic, promoting in its place a regime of relaxed controls plus regulation for some or all drugs.

Yet all assent to two crucial points. First, many drug addicts need drug treatment if they are to lead productive and satisfying lives. Second, the more treatment available to each of these addicts, the better. The White House's Office of National Drug Control Policy estimates that the nation's present treatment capacity can accommodate only half the country's 3.5 million addicts, (1) and there is need to narrow the gap.

WHY COERCION?

These agreed-on propositions have not been acknowledged for what they are: starting points from which to work toward a policy consensus. The reason for this avoidance is a large, uncomfortable fact. Even if we close the so-called treatment gap, the most promising way—perhaps the only way—to put enough addicts into treatment for long enough to make a difference entails a considerable measure of coercion. This is a proposition massively supported by the empirical data on drug treatment programs, yet it runs counter to some of today's most powerful political and cultural currents.

Data consistently show that treatment, when completed, is quite effective. Indeed, during even brief exposures to treatment, almost all addicts will use fewer drugs and commit less crime than they otherwise would, which means that almost any treatment produces benefits in excess of its cost (2). But most addicts, given a choice, will not enter a treatment program at all. Those addicts who do enter a program rarely complete it. About half drop out in the first 3 months, and 80% to 90% have left by the end of the first year. Among such dropouts, relapse within a year is the rule.

In short, if treatment is to fulfill its considerable promise as a key component of drug control policy, whether strict or permissive, addicts not only must enter treatment but must stay the course and "graduate." And if they are to do so, most will need some incentives that can properly be considered coercion.

In the context of treatment, the term *coercion*—used more or less interchangeably with "compulsory treatment," "mandated treatment," "involuntary treatment," "legal pressure into treatment," and "criminal justice referral to treatment" (3)—refers to an array of strategies that shape behavior by responding to specific actions with external pressure and predictable consequences. Terminology in this area is important: What may appear to be academic hairsplitting is actually one of the primary drawbacks of the coerced treatment literature. While some of these terms likely refer to similar actions (e.g., "mandated" and "compulsory"), the presence of a legal mandate to participate in treatment tells us nothing about whether the mandated client wanted treatment in the first place. In a study of parolees referred to outpatient psychiatric treatment, Farabee, Shen, and Sanchez found that coerced patients were not necessarily unwilling patients, and the discrepancy was substantial: More than three-quarters of the patients in their study who reported *no control* over their admission to the clinic (i.e., high coercion) acknowledged that they needed psychiatric treatment. (4) The use of the "criminal justice net" to facilitate, rather than coerce, treatment admission is widely acknowledged, but such distinctions remain scarce in the research literature. Coercive drug-treatment strategies are already common. Both the criminal justice system and the workplace, for example, have proved to be excellent venues for identifying individuals with drug problems and then exerting leverage, from risk of jail to threat of job loss, to provide powerful incentives to start and stay in treatment.

Moreover, evidence shows that addicts who get treatment through court order or employer mandates benefit as much as, and sometimes more than, their counterparts who enter treatment voluntarily.

This chapter presents the case for employing coercion to increase the efficacy of treatment for drug addicts. With the aid of coercion, substance abusers can be rescued earlier in their "careers" of abuse, at a time when intervention can produce greater lifetime benefits. With coercion, more substance abusers will enter treatment than would enroll voluntarily, and those who enroll will enjoy an increased likelihood of success.

The argument begins by recounting the story of early formal efforts to rehabilitate drug addicts and by drawing the lessons of those efforts. It proceeds to explore modern approaches to coercive treatment and to examine the effectiveness of those approaches. It then presents the sources of current resistance to coercive strategies and, finally, suggests ways to integrate the theory and practice of coercive treatment into current policy.

The aim of the examination is to make the case that unless we acknowledge the necessity for coercive strategies, we will lose the best chance we have for treating addicts in ways that will significantly improve the quality of their lives and that of the society they inhabit.

A BRIEF HISTORY OF COERCION IN DRUG TREATMENT

America had a perceived drug problem for some 50 years before coercive strategies arose in response to the problem.

The Rise of Coercive Treatment

The first wave of cocaine, heroin, and morphine addicts was inadvertently created from the 1880s to the early 1900s, originally by well-meaning physicians, later by hawkers of patent remedies. Most of the resulting "medical addicts," as they were called, were genteel women, personified by the heroin-addicted mother Mary Tyrone in Eugene O'Neill's *Long Day's Journey into Night*. They did not evoke moral censure.

Very different were the addicts who emerged over the first two decades of the twentieth century. These were poor male "pleasure" addicts, harshly condemned as a social menace (5). In response, the Treasury Department, in 1919, cracked down on physicians who prescribed cocaine, heroin, and morphine. States imposed and enforced criminal penalties for use. Officials in big cities, fearing that the hundreds of male addicts thus deprived of their prescriptions would turn in desperation to violent crime, established opiate clinics to dispense morphine and heroin. By 1920, some 40 such clinics had been established.

Some of the clinics were worse than ineffective. The most notorious, like the Worth Street Clinic in New York City, were corrupted by their patients' diversion of drugs. The clinics presented the spectacle of bedraggled dope fiends, as the patients were portrayed, loitering around the neighborhood.

The best-run of these facilities, like those in New Haven, Connecticut, Los Angeles, California, and Shreveport, Louisiana, did reduce drug-related crime and illicit trafficking, but they were still unable to point to addicts whom the clinics had cured of their addiction (6). The Shreveport clinic, however, did keep a close eye on its 198 patients. It maintained meticulous records and required that its addicts hold down jobs and keep up their physical appearance or be cut off from the clinic. This requirement, historian Jill Jonnes notes, "probably weeded out most of the 'sporting' addicts and other unsavory types who so frustrated the New York doctors" (7).

In time, the federal government extended its policy of total drug abstinence to the clinics, which had all closed their doors by 1925. By then all the medical staffs had been threatened with indictment by federal authorities. With the end of this short-lived clinical era, treatment for opiate dependence was largely unavailable between the early 1920s and the end of World War II. Although relatively few new addicts were created during this period, those who had become afflicted in the early 1900s tended to remain opiate-dependent. In particular, a growing population of aging addicts came to inhabit federal prisons, to which addicts convicted of selling or possessing drugs were routinely sent.

Narcotics Farms

As early as 1919, when governments began reining in physicians prescribing the use of opiates, the Narcotics Unit of the Treasury Department urged Congress to set up a series of federal narcotics farms where users could be confined and treated (8). It wasn't until 1935, however, in response to the problem of aging addicts, that the U.S. Public Health Service opened a facility in Lexington, Kentucky. Three years later another federal farm was established in Fort Worth, Texas. These facilities received both criminal violators and addicts who enrolled in treatment voluntarily.

The Lexington facility was a hospital-prison-sanitarium in which medical and moral approaches to treatment converged. It was located, as Jonnes has described it,

> on 1,100 acres of rolling bluegrass... an Art Deco campus-like affair with barred windows. In its early years, Lexington was literally a working farm operated by patient-inmates with chicken hatcheries, slaughter houses, four large dairy barns, a green house, and a utility barn. When not farming, inmates could work in sewing, printing, or woodworking shops (9).

The facilities did not, however, succeed in providing a wholesome and salutary rural respite. According to Jonnes, the "effect of going to KY [as patient-inmates called the Lexington farm] for most addicts was to expand their network of addict pals." The doctors were dedicated but frustrated, often noting that their patients would likely relapse upon returning to the inner cities from which they came.

The data confirmed the doctors' impressions. According to a report by the U.S. comptroller general, approximately 70% of the hospital's voluntary patients signed out against medical advice before completing the 6- to 12-month treatment program; and within a few years, 90% had relapsed (10). Most who remained in treatment did so under legal pressure from a court.

Poor communication between treatment and criminal justice organizations inevitably diminishes the provider's ability to enact immediate sanctions for nonattendance or noncompliance. A notable example of this problem was observed in the administration of the narcotics farms in Lexington, Kentucky, and Fort Worth, Texas. A commonly cited problem with these programs was the providers' lack of autonomy and their inability to communicate efficiently with the court system. In fact, any movement or status change of an addict in these programs required court approval, which, in turn, required that the addict be transported to and from the federal court for the case to be presented (Anglin & Hser, 1991). Despite some positive findings for these programs, the cumbersome administrative structure and poor linkages between the treatment providers and the court system led to their eventual closure in 1972.

Although the farms are generally considered to have been failures, they did generate useful clinical information. Most important, several followup studies of the participants indicated that addicts who after treatment were supervised under legal coercion had better outcomes than those not so supervised. A followup of more than 4,000 addicts 6 months after discharge from treatment found that those on probation or parole were more than twice as likely to remain abstinent as were voluntary patients, probably because the former had compulsory posthospital supervision (11). A longer-term followup of the same population confirmed the critical role of posthospital surveillance: it found that of those serving more than 12 months of parole, 67% remained drug-free a year after discharge, while the figure for voluntary patients was only 4% (12).

The data showed, in sum, that some kind of postdischarge supervision was needed. The information also yielded the lessons that (a) a 6- to 12-month treatment stay was too brief; (b) the need was for intensive vocational services rather than for psychological services aimed at personality change; and (c) the threat of reinstitutionalization had to have teeth.

Therapeutic Communities

After World War II, organized crime was able to reactivate the old heroin trafficking routes disrupted by the war, and inner-city physicians began to encounter the next generation of heroin addicts. As a result, the 1950s saw a resurgence of interest in the treatment of addiction, particularly, the emergence of the notion of the self-regulating therapeutic community (TC). This concept was enthusiastically welcomed by clinicians and policymakers alike, who were heartened by early TC success stories and demoralized by the gloomy results of previous treatment efforts.

The idea of a therapeutic community was exemplified by Synanon, a residential facility established by former alcoholic Charles Dederich in Santa Monica, California, to treat both alcohol and heroin addicts. Synanon was followed by the establishment in New York City of Daytop Village and, in 1967, of Phoenix House. The latter, a residential center on the Upper West Side, was founded by psychiatrist Mitchell Rosenthal. It was inspired by the efforts of six former addicts who enlisted Dr. Rosenthal's help in their commitment to keep themselves clean.

Modern therapeutic communities immerse patients in a comprehensive 18- to 24-month treatment regimen built around the philosophy that the addict's primary problem is not the drug he abuses but the addict himself. Although psychiatric orthodoxy holds that addiction is a discrete, self-contained "disease," the therapeutic community's approach recognizes drug abuse as a symptom of a deeper personal disturbance. The strategy for rehabilitation is to transform the destructive patterns of feeling, thinking, and acting that predispose a person to use drugs.

In this effort, the primary "therapist" is the community itself—not only peers but also staff members, some of whom are graduates of a program themselves and can serve as role models. The dynamic is mutual self-help; residents continually reinforce, for each other, the expectations and rules of the community. For meeting community expectations, residents win rewards such as privileges, like weekend passes, or increasing responsibility, culminating in leadership roles. If a resident defies the rules, the resident loses privileges and must perform the least-desirable chores. All residents must work, so that they learn to accept authority and supervision, which is vital to their future success in the workforce.

Researcher George DeLeon identified three stages in a resident's attitude toward such communities (13):

1. *Compliance:* adherence to rules simply to avoid negative consequences such as disciplinary action, discharge from the program, or reincarceration.
2. *Conformity:* adherence to the recovery community's norms to avoid loss of approval or disaffiliation.
3. *Commitment:* development of a personal determination to change destructive attitudes and behaviors.

Those who negotiate the commitment stage have excellent outcomes. DeLeon, in a long-term followup study of addicts admitted to Phoenix House, found that after 5 to 7 years, 90% of those who had graduated were employed and crime-free, and 70% were drug-free (14).

But the graduates constituted only 20% of DeLeon's sample. Generally, half of voluntarily committed patients leave therapeutic communities prematurely within the first ninety days, the threshold at which most individuals form an independent commitment to a treatment program. Perhaps 1 in 5 to 10 fully completes a program (15).

These dropout rates are not hard to understand. In the early months of a program, residents of a therapeutic community often rebel against the rigid structure, loss of status they enjoyed on the street, and deprivation of getting high. Ambivalence about relinquishing drugs is a powerful psychological force pulling patients back to the street. Even patients with strong motivation experience flagging resolve, momentary disillusionment, or intense cravings. If a patient succumbs to these pressures and leaves treatment prematurely, the patient may have gained some benefit from even the brief exposure to treatment but is at high risk for relapse into drug use and crime.

DeLeon therefore sees legal pressure as the initial force that can literally get patients through the door into treatment and keep them there until they internalize the values and goals of recovery. Coercion alone cannot do the job: one researcher observed that "if contact with therapy does not bring its own rewards, the potency of coercion will decline precipitously, and could ultimately work against

treatment goals" (16). But the threat of consequences like incarceration, the loss of a job, or some other aversive event can sustain an ambivalent or flatly resistant patient during the early months of treatment until those rewards—newly learned skills, a transformed self-concept, social maturation, and optimism about the future—ultimately inspire the patient to change.

Thus it is of interest that in DeLeon's Phoenix House sample, it did not matter statistically to a patient's chances of "graduating" whether the patient had enrolled voluntarily or been mandated to treatment (17). This similarity did not mean, in DeLeon's view, that compelled treatment made no difference; it was just the opposite. The compelled patients began with worse prognoses, because of their legal involvement and their higher incidence of antisocial personality disorder and low motivation (18) Counteracting these disadvantages, however, was the fact that individuals who had court cases pending or had been legally referred to the community spent, on average, more days in treatment than did voluntary patients (19). The relatively bad prognosis was made up for by more treatment days. "Retention in treatment," DeLeon therefore concluded, "is the best predictor of outcome, and legal referral is a consistent predictor of retention."

There are not many studies of the relationship between compelled treatment and methadone therapy because, although methadone is one of the best-studied antiaddiction therapies to date, few patients are legally mandated to maintenance treatment. The major source of compelled treatment, the criminal justice system, prefers rehabilitation that aims for total abstinence rather than substitution of one dependence-producing agent for another.

More than 20 years ago, however, M. Douglas Anglin of the University of California, Los Angeles, conducted an important study to determine whether addicts coerced into drug treatment differed from voluntary patients in their responses to treatment (20). Anglin categorized some 600 methadone-maintenance patients according to whether they were subject to high, moderate, or low levels of coercion. The 19% in the high-level category were under official legal supervision, including required urine testing, and perceived their entry into treatment as motivated primarily by the legal system. Another 19%, moderately coerced, were under active legal supervision and either were submitting to urine tests or perceived coercion as the reason for their entry into treatment. Finally, 62% of the sample, under a low level of coercion, were not under legal supervision and not subject to monitoring via probation or parole. The majority of these reported feeling no legal pressure, even as minor as a fear of arrest, impelling them toward treatment.

When Anglin compared the three groups, he found that all of them showed substantial improvement when measured on narcotics use, crime, and social functioning. Once again, compelling patients to accept treatment did not bar clinical progress; given the relatively poor prognoses of those involved, it probably aided such progress.

The same lesson emerged from a more recent experience with methadone treatment at the Southeast Baltimore Drug Treatment program. A research team led by psychologist Michael Kidorf of Johns Hopkins University noted that unemployment was a common problem among inner-city drug users and lamented that "standard drug abuse treatment services appear to have only small effects on employment" (21). In response, the Baltimore clinic, like its predecessor clinic in Shreveport some 70 years earlier, instituted the once-again-innovative requirement that its methadone patients be employed for at least 20 hours a week in order to receive methadone and related services. Patients were given 2 months to find employment or to enroll in job training or community service programs. If they did not, they received 5 weeks of intensive counseling. Those who did not obtain employment after counseling were tapered off methadone.

Because these patients had been enrolled in the same clinic before the requirement went into effect, their performance prior to the new rule could be compared with the same population's performance afterward. Before the requirement, despite enhanced counseling with vocational training, none had managed to secure either paying or volunteer employment. Two months after the imposition of the requirement, however, 75% of the sample had secured and maintained verified paid employment, volunteer work, or education.

Civil Commitment

Compelled treatment showed its potential in the California Civil Addict program, created in 1961 as the first-implemented statewide civil commitment program in the country. Serving mostly heroin addicts, the program flourished during the 1960s (22). The California Department of Corrections ran the program, providing high-quality treatment by specifically recruited and specially trained corrections personnel.

During the program's most active years, its protocol included an average of 18 months of inpatient treatment out of a total commitment period of 7 years. After 18 to 24 months in residential treatment, patients spent up to 5 years being closely supervised by specially trained parole officers with small caseloads, who monitored patients closely and administered weekly urine toxicology tests. For any narcotics use violation discovered by these tests, the officers had authority to take action—including returning patients for treatment to the institutions from which they had been discharged.

This program became the venue for an unfortunate natural experiment. During the program's first 2 years, judges and other officials unfamiliar with its procedures mistakenly released about half of the committed population after only minimal exposure to the inpatient part of the program. Anglin's research team took advantage of this circumstance, selecting a sample of individuals who had participated in the program's inpatient treatment for a sustained length of time and comparing it with a matched sample of individuals who had been erroneously released. The team compared the two groups on their self-reported percentages of time spent on drug use and criminal activity, then verified the data through arrest records and urine specimens taken at followup interviews.

By 1 year after the premature release of half the study population, the two groups had sharply diverged. Individuals who had been prematurely released were more than twice as likely to use narcotics as those who had completed 18 months as inpatients. During the subsequent years of outpatient supervision, narcotics use declined for both groups; but the decline for those who had been kept as inpatients averaged 22%, while the figure for the discharged group was only 7%.

Criminal activity followed a similar pattern. Before commitment, both groups had devoted approximately 60% of their time to such activity. A year after one group had been prematurely discharged, the figure for the treated group was 20%, while the figure for the discharged group was 48%. At the end of 7 years, criminal activity among the treated group had undergone a further reduction of 19%, but the reduction figure for the discharged group was only 7%.

New York followed California's model, with a crucial and deleterious difference. Prompted by California's success, New York began its own civil commitment program in 1966. New York had the advantage of that year's federal Narcotic Addict Rehabilitation Act, which aimed to link criminal justice agencies to community-based treatment programs. The act provided for compulsory treatment for addicts charged with certain nonviolent federal crimes; for treatment instead of sentencing for those convicted of such crimes; and for voluntary commitment of drug users not involved in criminal proceedings. The act also began what was to become, in the 1970s, massive federal funding of treatment programs.

But New York—unlike California, which mandated addicts to rehabilitation—allowed addicts to choose between treatment and incarceration. Those who chose the former were treated in residential settings developed during those years by the state Narcotics Addiction Control Commission, but this phase of treatment lasted only about 9 months. Inpatient treatment was followed by parole-like supervision for another 2 to 4 years. Unfortunately, supervision was loose, and a high percentage of patients went absent without leave. Governor Nelson Rockefeller was, not surprisingly, discouraged. "Let's be frank," he said in his 1973 address to the legislature, "we have achieved very little permanent rehabilitation, we have found no cure" (23).

In contrast, the civil addict program in California still exists, but operates at about half its capacity from the late

1960s (from nearly 3,000 in 1968 to about 1,600 in 2002), in spite of California's felon population having grown from approximately 20,000 to 160,000 over this same period.

MODERN EVALUATIONS OF THE EFFECTIVENESS OF COMPELLED TREATMENT

National Outcome Studies

The first evaluation of this network of community-based programs began in 1968, when the National Institute of Mental Health funded a proposal by Saul B. Selis, director of the Institute of Behavioral Research at Texas Christian University, for the Drug Abuse Reporting Project (DARP). Data collection began in 1969 and lasted 4 years, following about 44,000 patients enrolled in 52 federally funded programs. The project followed subgroups for 5 and 12 years following discharge from treatment.

In 1974, the Institute transferred control of the project to the newly created National Institute on Drug Abuse (NIDA). NIDA subsequently funded two more large studies: the Treatment Outcome Prospective Study (TOPS), which followed 12,000 patients who entered treatment between 1979 and 1981, and the Drug Abuse Treatment Outcome Study (DATOS), which followed 11,000 patients who entered between 1991 and 1993. More recently, another federal agency, the Center for Substance Abuse Treatment, undertook the National Treatment Improvement and Evaluation Study of 4,400 patients who entered the project between 1993 and 1995. Together these studies assessed roughly 70,000 patients, of whom 40% to 50% were court-referred or otherwise mandated to residential and outpatient treatment programs (24).

Two major findings emerged from these huge evaluations. The first was that the length of time a patient spent in treatment was a reliable predictor of the patient's posttreatment performance. Beyond a 90-day threshold, treatment outcomes improved in direct relationship to the length of time spent in treatment, with 1 year generally found to be the minimum effective duration of treatment (25).

The second major finding was that coerced patients tended to stay longer. (On this second point, DARP was an exception, finding no correlation between criminal justice status and either time spent in treatment or improvement. One can say only that DARPs compelled patients stayed as long as, and did no worse than, voluntary patients.)

To evaluate these findings, it is important to know whether addicts who entered treatment under legal coercion were meaningfully different from other patients. The findings from these studies are mixed. Some show that legally coerced addicts had a relatively unfavorable preadmission profile—more crime and gang involvement, more drug use, worse employment records than had their noncoerced counterparts. Other studies detected little difference

other than the particular offense that triggered the mandate to treatment (26). The primary difference between these groups, as might be expected, lies in their motivation. Farabee, Nelson, and Spence compared psychosocial profiles of voluntary and criminal justice-referred substance abuse clients in community-based treatment. The rationale for the study arose from the observation that voluntary and involuntary clients were receiving identical treatment despite the possibility that the treatment needs of these groups differ. Between-group comparisons indicated that these two groups were almost identical in terms of standard psychological features (e.g., depression, hostility, anxiety, childhood problems). However, these groups differed significantly on the three motivation indices, with involuntary clients scoring lower on recognition of their drug problems, desire for help, and readiness for treatment (27).

In the DARP study, the baseline characteristics of voluntary and legally referred patients were similar. Because the subjects were relatively homogeneous on these dimensions—being primarily young, male, inner-city "street addicts," more than 80% with at least one previous arrest, and more than half previously incarcerated—the authors speculate that legal status was unlikely to have been a very discriminating variable.

The TOPS study, by contrast, discovered some differences. True, legally mandated and voluntary patients alike had similar drug use patterns, comparable previous criminal justice involvement, and equivalent numbers of prior treatment episodes, but the legally mandated patients were younger than their voluntary counterparts and more likely to be male. When researchers looked specifically at patients who reported that the criminal justice system was the primary source of their referral to treatment, they found that these legal referrals not only were younger but also used mainly alcohol and marijuana rather than "harder" drugs. The authors speculate that the legally mandated patients were "caught" earlier in their careers, or that they were incarcerated too recently to have reestablished their habits, or both.

Although the studies do not present a consistent picture of pretreatment characteristics of legally mandated patients, they do make it reasonable to conclude that even legally coerced addicts having relatively unfavorable prognoses can benefit from treatment as much as voluntary patients can, because the latter often remain in treatment for a shorter period (28).

A 1990 report from the Institute of Medicine summarized that "contrary to earlier fears among clinicians, criminal justice pressure does not seem to vitiate treatment effectiveness, and it probably improves retention" (29). Thus, while there is conflicting evidence on whether a legal mandate brings individuals into treatment earlier, coercion can almost surely be credited with derailing many an addiction career once individuals have been brought into treatment (30).

Of special significance, in light of the importance of length of treatment, is that all four national outcome studies showed high rates of attrition among patients, with half dropping out inside of 90 days. For these early dropouts, the benefits of treatment disappeared within the year. With substantial, durable change rarely occurring in less than a year or two of treatment, the high dropout rate makes retaining patients in treatment a pressing challenge.

Some researchers have hypothesized that the key to retention is to match each individual patient with the proper type of treatment. Although in principle such matching makes clinical and economic sense, there is surprisingly little tested information about such attempts. Two prospective studies by A. Thomas McLellan of the University of Pennsylvania suggest that tailoring patient care can indeed make a difference (31). McLellan assigned patients to programs according to particular psychiatric, medical, or family needs and found better outcomes for these patients than for those without such treatment. DATOS similarly found that even severely drug-dependent patients were more likely to be abstinent at their 1-year followup if they had received support services targeted to specific needs.

But these findings are not uniform. The American Society for Addiction Medicine has developed widely used criteria for placing patients in specific treatment modalities; the few studies assessing the validity of these criteria, however, have not found an effect on outcomes (32).

Thus far it appears that "patient matching," although it may be one means of assigning patients to treatment, is no substitute for length of treatment. It is length of exposure to treatment that powerfully predicts patient success, no matter what the treatment setting. The federal Center for Substance Abuse Treatment, in a recent study examining the relationship between these two variables, compared one sample of addicts who had 10 months of residential care followed by 2 months of outpatient care with another sample who had 6 months of residential care followed by another 6 months of outpatient care. Regardless of the treatment scheme to which patients were assigned, those who completed the entire 12-month treatment period had the best outcomes. And those most likely to complete the course of treatment were patients under probation, parole, or pretrial supervision (33).

But the utility of legal pressure alone cannot replace the programs' role in engaging clients in the treatment process. A recent study using a national sample of clients admitted to long-term residential drug treatment programs found high retention levels among clients who expressed high treatment readiness, as well as among those who were admitted under legal pressure, but only treatment readiness significantly predicted whether the clients ultimately engaged in treatment (34).

Project MATCH (Matching Alcoholism Treatments to Client Heterogeneity) represents another attempt to identify the most appropriate treatment based on the specific needs and characteristics of patients. In this study, 1,700 patients with alcohol problems were randomly assigned to 12-step, cognitive–behavioral coping skills, or motivational enhancement therapy and followed for 1 year after completing a 12-week program. The project achieved fairly positive outcomes overall, but the hypothesized differences by treatment condition—and the interaction of these treatment programs with 10 selected patient characteristics—were not supported. Thus, there remains a common perception that, although matching clients to treatment makes intuitive sense, the key ingredients to client-treatment matching have yet to be empirically established (35).

Treatment Alternatives to Street Crime

Treatment alternatives to street crime (TASC), established as a federal program in 1972 as one of the first initiatives of the Nixon administration's war on drugs, was moderately successful in cutting the number of street crimes committed by addicts. TASC was meant to serve as a bridge between the criminal justice and the treatment systems. It functioned as a diversion program for drug abusers, diverting them from jail or prison by identifying nonviolent addicted criminals and referring them to treatment in the community. TASC assigned arrestees to case managers who were to get them into treatment and send progress reports back to the courts. The program, now supported primarily by state and local governments, subsequently expanded to supervising probationers and to postsentencing disposition.

TASC has been the subject of a number of evaluations. Most are positive; others are partly so. In one such study, the TOPS project compared a subgroup of TASC-referred patients with a group of voluntary, unmonitored patients involved in the criminal justice system (36). Comparing patients' drug use 1 year before treatment with their drug use after the first 3 to 6 months of treatment, the TOPS researchers found that the TASC patients' use had declined by 81%; the comparable figure for the control group was 74%. Predatory illegal acts had declined by 96% for the TASC group, but only by 71% for the control group.

The Education and Assistance Corporation analyzed results from the Brooklyn, New York, TASC program (37). Of 173 felons placed in treatment in 1992, 71% remained in the program for at least 2 years. At 29 months after completion of the program, the group's rearrest rate was 9%. This was much lower than either the 25% rearrest rate among offenders from a control program or the 28% rearrest rate among the general inmate population in New York State correctional facilities.

In Texas, a study found that 7% of TASC-referred offenders were incarcerated during an 18-month observation period, compared with 28% of offenders who did not enter treatment or who stayed fewer than 3 months (38).

Finally, researchers at UCLA and at the RAND Corporation studied five regional sites and compared TASC offenders mandated to treatment or to surveillance, including urine testing and case management, with a control group of offenders who received standard probation with little supervision (39). The TASC and control groups were similar on most demographic, drug, and criminal record variables. At 6 months after patients' entry into the study, the researchers measured police-confirmed new arrests and technical violations, along with unverified self-reports of drug use.

The findings varied across the sites. In three places, TASC patients showed greater reductions in all three outcomes. In some places there was no difference in one or another outcome. At two sites, Birmingham, Alabama, and Portland, Oregon, the researchers actually found more criminal involvement and technical violations among TASC patients—but the authors attributed this phenomenon to the fact that the TASC offenders were being watched more closely and were thus more likely to get caught. (The authors also thought that the figures on self-reported drug use among TASC patients might be artificially low because heavily monitored groups might be more likely to minimize their reporting of punishable behavior.)

This evaluation also identified a common problem with the use of coercion, namely, that its overuse can lead to poorer overall outcomes. In their evaluation, Anglin et al. found that TASC referrals with the lowest problem severity demonstrated the least improvement overall. In contrast, substance abuse treatment appeared to have more favorable effects on "hard core" TASC referrals, as defined by baseline drug use prior to TASC involvement (40). These findings suggest that coercion should not become a uniform response to all drug-involved offenders, but should be reserved for those with the highest criminal and drug use severity.

Coercion of Criminals

An estimated 60% of the cocaine and heroin used in the United States is consumed by the 5 million Americans who are supervised by or incarcerated within the criminal justice system. Moreover, offenders who abuse drugs are more likely than nonabusing offenders to return to crime following release from incarceration (41). Therefore there is considerable potential within the criminal justice system for reducing drug abuse and related crime by mandated treatment. Evidence indicates that diversionary and in-prison treatment programs, although currently available only to some 15% of offenders, have a benefit beyond the crime-reducing effects of incarceration or probation as usual (42). Results from several categories of criminal commitment show that treated offenders have lower rates of recidivism. Although these studies do not always directly measure posttreatment drug use, crime it-

self can reasonably be used as indirect evidence of drug involvement, because the two activities are so highly correlated. Conversely, declines in drug use are accompanied by declines in crime, particularly income-generating crime (43).

Drug Courts

One major category of coerced treatment of criminals occurs in drug courts, which offer nonviolent offenders, usually recidivists, the prospect of dismissed charges if they plead guilty and agree to be diverted to a heavily monitored drug treatment and testing program overseen by a judge. Although in the TASC model judges do not have direct contact with treatment personnel, a drug court is a hub from which services such as treatment, case management, and vocational training radiate (44).

Drug courts originated in southern Florida in the late 1980s, when the area was hit hard by cocaine-related arrests that flooded courtrooms and overwhelmed jails. Addicts out on probation were quickly rearrested for new drug-related crimes, and the revolving door to the justice system seemed to be spinning out of control. Drug courts promised a way to break the cycle by "reserving" jail and prison beds for dangerous offenders while sending criminally involved addicts to treatment. The first one opened in Miami in 1989.

Enthusiasm about drug courts has spawned a drug court movement. As of January 2003, according to the National Association of Drug Court Professionals, there are nearly 1,000 drug courts in operation (up from about 20 in 1994), and another 473 being planned (45). Currently, every state has at least one drug court in operation. California, where nearly a quarter of all state prisoners are incarcerated because of a drug offense, has more than 70.

Although the accumulated evidence of drug courts' effectiveness has yet to reach a critical threshold because only a handful of independently evaluated studies have been performed, the early data look promising. More than 70% of drug court participants have been incarcerated at least once previously, almost three times more than have been in drug treatment (46); thus for many offenders, drug court is the route of entry into rehabilitation. In almost all drug courts, retention in court-ordered drug treatment is consistently several times greater than it is in voluntary treatment (47).

A General Accounting Office (GAO) report found that the average retention rate of drug court programs was a highly respectable 71%. Even the lowest retention rate that the GAO found in a drug court, 31%, exceeds the average 1-year retention rate of some 15% for noncriminal addicts in public-sector treatment programs (48). This comparison is all the more impressive in light of the fact that the criminally involved addict is generally considered the hardest to treat in conventional settings. The GAO report also found, like other studies, that the longer a participant stayed in drug court treatment, the better the participant fared.

A survey by the Drug Court Clearinghouse at American University found similar patterns. Survey results first emphasized the element of coercion in drug court participation. Although 80% of offenders who were offered the drug court option chose to take it, many saw it simply as an expeditious way to get their charges dropped. Indeed, some actually said they planned to return to drugs after they "went through the motions" in the program (49).

Yet the survey also found that drug courts operational for 18 months or more reported completion rates of 48%. Rearrest rates, primarily for drug crimes, varied according to graduates' characteristics and degree of social dysfunction, but they averaged just 4% at 1 year after graduation. Even among those who failed to finish the program, rearrest rates 1 year after enrollment ranged from 5% to 28%. By contrast, the Bureau of Justice Statistics reports a 26% to 40% rearrest rate for individuals convicted of drug possession who are traditionally adjudicated (50).

Evaluations of particular drug courts also show good results. The Portland, Oregon, drug court was evaluated in 1998 by the State Justice Institute, which made careful efforts to match drug court participants with other arrestees having similar demographic characteristics and criminal histories who had either refused drug court or were ineligible for administrative reasons. Two years after adjudication, drug court program participants had 61% fewer arrests than had offenders who were eligible but did not participate. Drug court graduates performed best, with 76% fewer arrests 2 years later. The longer the retention, the better the outcomes: those who stayed for less than one-third of the program duration had three times as many arrests as had those who graduated, and twice as many as those who completed at least one-third (51).

The Maricopa, Arizona, drug court was the subject of a 1996 evaluation by the RAND Corporation, which found that among a sample randomly assigned to the drug court, rates of rearrest for any crime were significantly lower than for those randomly assigned to probation alone (52). These findings were similar to those obtained in a randomized study of addicts in Baltimore who were assigned to drug court or "treatment as usual." During the 12 months following randomization, 48% of the drug court clients had been rearrested, compared to 64% of the controls. For serious offenses, the difference between groups was even greater, with 32% of drug court clients being rearrested for a serious crime versus 57% of the controls (53).

A recent review of the Broward County, Florida, drug court found that drug court graduates were half as likely to be rearrested for a felony, and one-third as likely to be rearrested for a drug felony, as demographically similar offenders who were eligible for drug court but had instead chosen and completed probation (54).

An independent evaluation found the Dade County, Florida, drug court superior to "disposition as usual" (55).

Between June 1989 and March 1993, the Dade County program enrolled 4,500 defendants, 20% of all arrestees in the county who were charged with drug-related offenses. During that same period, 60% of the enrollees graduated or remained in the program. A year after graduation, only 11% were rearrested in Dade County on any criminal charge. By contrast, the rearrest rate was some 60% for a matched sample of drug offenders in 1987, 2 years before institution of the drug court. Furthermore, the time that elapsed between graduation and first reoffense was two to three times longer in the drug court group than in the nondrug court group.

In the most mixed evaluation of results in a drug court, the Urban Institute found that participants randomly assigned to the District of Columbia drug court from 1993 to 1995 were twice as likely to be drug free in the month before sentencing than were those assigned to probation as usual; the figures were 27% versus 12% (56). Six months after sentencing, however, rearrest rates for any crime averaged 4% for the treatment track versus 6% for the control track, not a statistically significant difference.

More than 100 evaluations of drug courts have found their way into the literature. Reviews of these evaluations by the Government Accounting Office (57) and Steve Belenko (58,59) mirror those of the studies discussed above. Specifically, drug courts appear to foster closer supervision and accountability than traditional treatment diversion approaches. Consequently, offenders under drug court supervision tend to be more likely to enter and remain in treatment. Moreover, drug courts are associated with lower levels of drug use and crime over the course of the treatment period, relative to similar offenders who are not under drug court supervision. However, the majority of these evaluations emphasize during-treatment measures, rather than long-term outcomes. Furthermore, many of these programs were evaluated while they were still quite new. For these reasons, the GAO (57) researchers recommended that these aggregate findings, while positive, should be interpreted with caution.

As this body of literature expands, however, so does our knowledge base concerning how individual client characteristics interact with levels of judicial supervision. One recent study, for example, examined the relationship between antisocial personality disorder (ASPD) and "dosage" of judicial control (60). Specifically, drug court clients were randomly assigned to see the judge every 2 weeks or on an as-needed basis. Overall, the biweekly and as-needed groups showed similar patterns of drug use and treatment completion rates, but when ASPD was taken into consideration, a different pattern emerged. Specifically, drug court clients who were classified as having ASPD had better completion rates and drug use outcomes when they were required to see a judge on a regular basis. Moreover, for the non-ASPD clients, the as-needed condition produced superior results. These findings suggest that the levels of coercion and judicial supervision should be increased for drug offenders with ASPD and actually *decreased* for those without ASPD.

Prison-Based Programs

Approximately 70% of all state prison inmates are in need of substance abuse treatment (61). Based on a national survey of inmates in 1997, only 1 in 8 state inmates were treated for substance abuse. Moreover, the reported levels of drug treatment in prison declined since a similar survey was conducted in 1991 (62).

Approximately 12% of prisons have intensive treatment programs based on therapeutic community principles (63), lasting from 6 to 15 months and open to nonviolent offenders who are within 18 months of eligibility for work release or parole. Within the prison, these offenders are segregated from the rest of the inmate population, in order to maintain the integrity of the program and to protect participants from other prisoners.

In a comprehensive review of the prison-based programs of the 1970s and 1980s, Falkin and coauthors concluded that in-prison therapeutic communities are effective (64). Examining programs such as New York's Stay'n Out (which they praised as a national model), Oregon's Cornerstone Program, and others, the authors found that the treatment experience, optimally sustained for 9 to 12 months, was strongly correlated with successful subsequent parole. For example, violations of parole occurred among 50% of the offenders who stayed for less than 3 months in Stay'n Out; among 39% of those who stayed longer than 3 months; and among only 15% of those who completed the program. Reincarceration rates within 3 years of release from prison were significantly lower for Stay'n Out participants, no matter how long they participated, than for matched offenders who had expressed interest in being treated but did not meet technical eligibility requirements.

Similarly, Cornerstone graduates had a 36% reincarceration rate over a 3-year followup period, while the figure was 63% for parolees-as-usual. The graduates' relative success occurred despite the fact that they had begun with more severe criminal and substance abuse histories than had the comparison group.

More recently, 3-year outcomes of several of the most prominent prison-based therapeutic communities were published in a special issue of *The Prison Journal* (65). These evaluations provide continued support for the overall effectiveness of the therapeutic community approach in correctional settings. However, the effects of prison treatment-only did not tend to be sustained over the full 3-year postrelease period unless the program graduates had continued treatment in the community.

Coerced treatment in prison settings is often justified on the grounds of the previous research summarized earlier indicating that coerced clients do as well or better than voluntary clients. However, these prior studies are based on community treatment samples where, typically, drug users are required to enter treatment as a condition of probation or parole. But most of the incentives (e.g., expunged records, diversion from prison) and consequences (e.g., revocation of probation or parole) offered to offenders in the community are not available in prison settings. Given the option to go to treatment *or* go to prison is clearly not the same as being required to go to treatment *and stay* in prison. Hence, it is possible that the apparent effectiveness of coercion demonstrated with community-based offender samples may not apply to incarcerated offenders. In fact, in a recent evaluation of a large prison-based therapeutic community in California, Farabee, Prendergast, and Cartier (2002) found that inmates who were coerced into treatment had significantly higher recidivism rates than those who expressed a desire for—and received—treatment. Overall, the best outcomes were for inmates whose desire for treatment was concordant with whether or not they received it.

Work Release

In 1987, the Delaware Department of Corrections established the Crest program, the first therapeutic community work-release center in the United States (66). Offenders who had been released from prison after participating in the Key program, a prison-based therapeutic community for drug-involved offenders at a maximum security prison, entered the Crest Center for 3 months of on-site treatment, 3 months of additional treatment, and job training, also within a therapeutic community.

Led by the center's director, James Inciardi, researchers from the University of Delaware's Center for Drug and Alcohol Studies compared four groups of mostly male participants: Key participants who did not go on to Crest; Crest participants who had not gone through the Key program; Key and Crest combined; and a control group that had first been incarcerated without treatment, then had gone on to conventional work release. The Key and Key-Crest groups had begun with higher levels of drug abuse and longer criminal histories. The Key-only group was older and less likely to be white.

The study found that the longer a participant's tenure in treatment was and the closer to time of release the treatment was received, the better the postrelease outcome. In sum, the therapeutic element of the prison–parole combination appears to reside more heavily in the parole phase than in the incarceration.

At an early followup, in-prison treatment was found to be somewhat more beneficial than no treatment. By 18 months, however, there was no significant difference between the Key and control groups in rearrest rates and urinalysis-confirmed drug use. By contrast, at 18 months Crest-only participants maintained an advantage over the control group. In addition, at the 6-month followup, the Crest group was as successful as the Key-Crest group;

but by 18 months, the Key-Crest group was superior, with 77% being arrest-free and 47% being drug-free among Key-Crest participants, while the figures were only 57% arrest-free and 31% drug-free among the Crest group.

The Key-Crest combination outranked all the others, with nearly half the individuals being drug-free at 18 months, a figure three times higher than that of the control group, while Crest-only participants had an intermediate likelihood of being drug-free.

Diversion from Prison

In 1990, the office of the Kings County (Brooklyn, NY) District Attorney developed the Drug Treatment Alternative to Prison (DTAP) program in response to the increasing pressure of drug-related commitments on the state prison system. (By the mid-1990s, drug offenders would constitute nearly one-half of admissions to state prisons.) The program diverts nonviolent drug felons to long-term, community-based residential drug treatment at about two-thirds the cost of incarceration. Like drug court, the program offers dismissal of charges in return for an offender's completing treatment under close judicial supervision. Also like drug court, DTAP may be chosen by offenders for reasons having little to do with a desire to become drug-free. For some, the program is a way to avoid incarceration; for others, it promises an expunged criminal record.

The Vera Institute of Justice in New York City conducted an independent evaluation of DTAP (67). Vera found that participants began with more severe pretreatment deficits—in education, employment, and legal involvement—than those of offenders placed in other diversion programs. Yet DTAP's total retention rate at 1 year was 64%, two to four times higher than that of residential programs in general. At 1 year, 11% of DTAP participants had been rearrested, half for drug offenses; by comparison, drug offenders sent to prison are more than twice as likely to be rearrested within a year of release, with more than half those arrests being drug-related. Fewer than 5% of ex-prisoners are rearrested while in treatment, but dropouts have high rates of reoffense, ranging from 80% to 92%, with an average time before return to custody of only 1 week.

A more recent study of the DTAP confirmed that clients with high perceived coercion remained in treatment for a longer period of time than those with low perceived coercion (68). But Douglas Young's research went beyond the usual categories of "coerced" and "voluntary" and explored the specific qualities of coercion that appeared to drive this effect. Interestingly, Young found that close monitoring and severe penalties were not as predictive of treatment retention as providing information to clients about treatment, describing the contingencies of treatment participation, and convincing the clients that the contingencies will be strictly enforced. As stated earlier in this

chapter, the majority of coerced treatment studies have relied on imprecise measures (e.g., whether or not a client was referred to treatment by a criminal justice agency) to assess the impact of coercion. This study represents a important advance in this line of research by attempting to identify the "active ingredients" of coerced treatment approaches.

In a review of 170 English-language articles (published since 1988) concerning compulsory substance abuse treatment, Wild, Roberts, and Cooper described study methods and identified points of consensus in the literature. Only about half of these articles were empirical studies, and only 18 of these were identified as effectiveness studies. Of this subsample, the most popular outcome measured was treatment retention, accounting for 56% of the studies; only one-third of the studies (6 of 18) examined criminal behaviors between coerced and noncoerced subjects. The authors reported mixed findings, often varying by the type of outcome measured. For example, 80% of the studies examining referral patterns showed a positive effect for compulsory treatment; regarding retention, compulsory treatment was superior in 55% of the studies; 33% of the studies showed lower recidivism for coerced clients (half of the studies showed no difference); and 25% of the studies examining drug use showed superior results for compulsory clients, while 75% showed no difference (69). In short, most of the studies emphasizing treatment referral and participation showed positive effects of compulsory treatment, while most of the studies focused on drug use and criminal behavior showed no differences. These trends provide further support for the claim that coerced clients do as well or better than noncoerced clients, but they also point to the complexity of the issue. Superior referral rates and retention do not always translate into superior long-term outcomes. In addition, as we have already described, compulsory treatment and coercion are not always synonymous. Gaining a better understanding of the *effectiveness* of *coerced* treatment will depend on how precisely these two variables are measured in the future.

RESISTANCE TO COERCION

Coercive strategies for drug treatment range from the least intrusive, that is, social contracting, in which individuals are simply given incentives to behave in certain ways, to the most restrictive, such as forced treatment and confinement, in the face of life-threatening behavior. No matter where on this continuum a particular coercive strategy lies, however, it has met with significant resistance.

One source of this resistance is the healthy reluctance we all feel to curtail anyone's personal autonomy. Political scientist James Q. Wilson has observed that this reluctance sometimes leads us to insist on the same freedom for others that we want for ourselves, even when the others in question have great difficulty in making use of such freedom.

Many clinicians voice another objection to coercive strategies: they believe, mistakenly, that a patient must desire drug treatment in order to benefit from it.

A third source of resistance is the current "medicalization" of addiction, the most recent round in the century-long debate over whether drug abuse should be treated on the medical model or the moral model (70). Thus the National Institute on Drug Abuse of the National Institutes of Health now dubs addiction a "chronic and relapsing brain disease," as part of the institute's attempt to define addiction as simply another long-term medical condition like asthma or high blood pressure. This view, instead of challenging the inevitability of relapse by holding patients accountable for their choices, suggests the need for biologic remedies for addiction. It also discounts the therapeutic potential of the coercion that the criminal justice system can exercise (71).

Contrary to what this medicalized view would predict, however, the compulsion to take drugs does not necessarily dominate an addict's minute-to-minute or even day-to-day existence. The temporal architecture of the addict's routine reveals that the addict is capable of reflection and purposeful behavior for some, perhaps a good deal, of the time. During the course of a heroin addict's day, for example, the addict may feel calm and with lucid thoughts as long as the addict is confident of access to drugs and is using them in dosages adequate to prevent withdrawal but not large enough to be sedating. Likewise, there are periods in a cocaine addict's week when the addict is neither engaged in a binge nor wracked with intense craving for the drug. At these moments, the addict is not a victim controlled by brain disease. The addict might even choose to change his or her behavior, depending on what the addict thinks is at stake (72).

This potential for self-control permits society to entertain and enforce expectations for addicts that would never be possible for someone who had, say, a brain tumor. Making such demands is of course no guarantee that they will be met. But confidence in the legitimacy of such demands would encourage a range of policy and therapeutic options, using consequences and coercion, that are incompatible with the idea of an exclusively no-fault brain disease.

A final source of resistance to coercion in this therapeutic age is the belief that self-improvement is more successful and admirable when undertaken for one's self and one's self alone, not for anyone else or for the larger good. In this view, betterment achieved as a result of intrinsic motivation is more durable, and even more worthy, than is personal gain that is externally compelled.

But as we know, addicts are notoriously poor self-disciplinarians. They are also extremely ambivalent about giving up drugs, in spite of all the damage that drugs have caused them. Addicts' problems of self-governance demand that a rehabilitative regime for them include limit-setting, consistency, and sometimes physical containment.

Civil Commitment

Perhaps the greatest controversy about coercive strategies has arisen over the issue of civil commitment. When an addict has sustained significant temporary brain damage from compulsive drug taking, this ultimate intrusion is warranted (73). Such time-limited, often life-saving suspension of autonomy allows for urgent medical attention to suicidal impulses, severe depression, or psychosis.

More than half the states now have statutes that allow judges to commit an addicted person to treatment without the addict's consent in much the same way that they can mandate a gravely disabled mentally ill person to undergo treatment in a psychiatric hospital (74). The process is appropriate for addicted individuals considered incompetent to attend to their own welfare and safety; the standard for this form of coercion is helplessness, not necessarily dangerousness to society.

As early as 1870, the American Association for the Cure of Inebriety tried to persuade states to create institutions in which doctors could treat and confine alcoholics and drug "habitués" rather than send them to jail. In the 1930s, narcotics farms were able, in a similar way, to accommodate some so-called civil addicts whose severe addiction made them dysfunctional but who were not involved in crime.

As we have seen, California and New York used civil commitment extensively in the 1960s and 1970s. Unsurprisingly, the constitutionality of the process has been challenged; but the Supreme Court has upheld the process. Since then, the California Supreme Court and the New York State Court of Appeals have also upheld civil commitment, reasoning that life-threatening developments—the college student so heavily addicted to cocaine that the student drops out of school to work as a prostitute in a crack house, or the homeless addict who refuses to see a doctor for a gangrenous foot—can justify the intrusion into personal autonomy (75).

Nevertheless, civil commitment of addicts now occurs only occasionally, usually when a desperate loved one or concerned physician brings an addicted individual to the attention of a judge.

CONCLUSION

Coercion has been applied in the service of rehabilitating addicts for more than 70 years. The experience has yielded a powerful clinical lesson: Addicts need not be internally motivated at the outset of treatment to benefit from it. Indeed, addicts who are legally pressured into treatment may outperform voluntary patients, because they are likely to stay in treatment longer and are more likely to graduate. Without formal coercive mechanisms, the treatment system would not attract many of the most dysfunctional addicts, and surely could not retain them.

But although official bodies—especially criminal justice organizations—are accustomed to wielding such leverage, they do not do so systematically enough to yield maximum benefit (76). Some judges will forgo referral to treatment altogether if they perceive an offender not to be motivated toward rehabilitation (77). Other judges express disappointment with the laxity of supervision addicts receive in treatment, citing failure to follow up with the court, verify patient participation, and perform drug testing—the very surveillance mechanisms that are necessary to retain unmotivated addicts.

Ironically, it appears that among current programs, with their various mixtures of treatment and coercion, the treatment component has relatively less clout than other forces have in shaping addicts' behavior. That is why examples of combining treatment with external monitoring, as in employee assistance programs and drug courts, are so encouraging. If more institutions, including public housing or even disability programs, adopted principles of contingency management, individuals would be likely to remain in treatment longer and enjoy greater improvement. Such behavioral gains would serve both addicts and the communities whose resources they strain.

A coordinated effort by social service agencies to track and monitor drug use and to enforce consequences for that use will be costly in the short run. In addition, it will require the creation of a certain amount of new bureaucracy. Those facts make coercive strategies unattractive even to those who are sympathetic to the need for aggressive intervention. It remains true, however, that as a clinical strategy, coercion is solidly promising. What is more, increasing our capacity to leverage addicts into treatment will be important whether we maintain our present policy of drug prohibition, decide on a policy of outright legalization, or choose anything in between, because any one of these policies will depend on drug treatment to rehabilitate addicts.

Addiction impairs participation in a free society. It interferes with the ability to ensure one's own welfare, respect the safety of others, and discharge responsibilities as a parent, spouse, worker, neighbor, or citizen. Addiction is a behavioral condition for which the prescription of choice is the imposition of reliable consequences and rewards, often combined with coercion that keeps the addicted individual from fleeing treatment. To say this, is not punitive; it is clinically sound and empirically justified.

Every day, all people respond to contingencies, incentives, and consequences. If we do not work, we do not get paid. If rent is not paid, we are evicted. If children are mistreated, they can be taken away. Meeting obligations in these circumstances is not the antithesis of freedom but a prerequisite to it. No less is this true of individuals with drug problems, although it is our job to structure the contingencies before them in creative ways to help them regain their freedom.

REFERENCES

1. The Office of National Drug Control Policy (ONDCP), Executive Office of the President, defines treatment gap as the difference between the number of people needing treatment and the number receiving it. Based on data from the National Household Survey on Drug Abuse, the gap in 1994 was 1.7 million people: an estimated 3,553,000 needed treatment and 1,847,000 received it. Information from the Uniform Crime Report and the Uniform Facility Data Set are also used to calculate the gap. (From personal communication with Janie B. Dargan, Office of Planning, Budget, and Research, May 29, 1998.) Typically, 6 to 8 years elapse between initiation of problem use and first treatment, according to the Drug Abuse Treatment Outcome Study (DATOS). (See *Psychology of Addictive Behaviors,* entire December 1997 issue, vol. 11.) The shorter the period of dysfunction, the better the chance of regaining social and personal competence.
2. Langenbucher J, McCrady BS, Brick J, et al. *Socioeconomic evaluations of addictions treatment.* Washington, DC: White House Printing Office, 1993.
3. Definitional and methodological issues abound. The term *coerced treatment* has been used interchangeably with compulsory treatment, mandated treatment, involuntary treatment, legal pressure into treatment, and criminal justice referral to treatment. See Anglin MD, Prendergast ML, Farabee D. *The effectiveness of coerced treatment for drug abusing offenders.* Presented at the Office of National Drug Control Policy's Conference of Scholars and Policy Makers, Washington, DC, March 25, 1998. (Paper available on ONDCP web site at: www.whitehousedrugpolicy.gov.) Researcher George DeLeon considered separately the often interchangeable terms legal status, legal referral, and legal pressure. Legal status, he noted, means any form of legal involvement, including being arrested, in jail, awaiting trial, or out on bail. Legal referral indicates any one of a variety of criminal justice procedures that direct addicts to a treatment alternative, such as pretrial rehabilitation services, parole, probation, or sentencing stipulations. Legal pressure, however, refers to the individual's perception of the forces impinging on him. In one analysis, it appeared that retention depended more on the mere presence of criminal justice pressure than on its level of intensity. (See Hiller ML, Knight K, Broome KM, et al. Legal pressure and treatment retention in a national sample of long-term residential program, Crim Just Behav 1998;25:463–481.)

Differences in the personal meaning of coercion have prompted evaluators to consider a more subtle analysis of "treatment under pressure." After all, not every formally coerced addict is a resistant one. Indeed, approximately 50% of inmates surveyed in a Texas prison said they would be willing to participate in treatment, even if it meant remaining incarcerated for 3 additional months. See Farabee D. *Substance abuse among male inmates entering the Texas Department of Criminal Justice-Institutional Division.* Austin, TX: Texas Commission on Alcohol and Drug Abuse, 1993. Yet 25% to 35% of incarcerated offenders still refuse the option of treatment and prefer jail time, dispelling the popular belief that drug treatment "coddles" addicts. See MacKenzie DL, Sourya C. *Multisite evaluation of shock incarceration.* Washington, DC: National Institute of Mental Health, 1994; Petersilia J, Turner S. *Evaluating intensive supervision probation/parole: results of a nationwide experiment.* Washington, DC: National Institute of Justice, 1993; Taxman F. *Report to ONDCP:. reducing recidivism through a seamless system of care: components of effective treatment, supervision* and transition services in the community. February 20, 1998. According to criminologist Faye Taxman at the University of Maryland, author of the February 20, 1998, report, some defense attorneys consider treatment programs "a risk for their clients because failure to comply may result in more incarceration time [than otherwise imposed]."

But what about addict-offenders who are not given the option of refusing treatment? Douglas Young and colleagues at the Vera Institute for Justice explored this question. They devised a construct called Perceived Legal Pressure (PLP) and applied the measure to a modest-sized group of drug felons in mandatory residential treatment. The PLP index measured respondents' views that (a) conditions of the treatment mandate would be enforced, (b) their behavior would be closely monitored, and (c) the consequences for failing treatment would be severe. After controlling for other clinical characteristics, the researchers found that retention correlated with the perception that monitors were vigilant and that absconding from the program agents would result in certain and immediate apprehension. Notably, the perceived aversion to prison was only marginally associated with higher retention. (See Young D, Dynia P, Belenko S. *How compelling is coerced treatment: a study of different mandated approaches?* Presented at the annual meeting of the American Society of Criminology, Chicago, November 22, 1996.)

4. Farabee D, Shen H, Sanchez S. Perceived coercion and treatment need among mentally ill parolees. *Crim Just Behav* 2002;29(1):76–86.
5. Jonnes J. *Hep-cats, narcs, and pipe dreams: a history of America's romance with illegal drugs.* New York: Scribner, 1996.
6. Musto DF. *The American disease: origins of narcotic control,* 2nd ed. New York: Oxford University Press, 1987; also White WL. *Slaying the dragon: the history of addiction treatment and recovery in America.* Bloomington, IL: Chestnut Health Services/Lighthouse Institute, 1998.
7. Jonnes J. *Hep-cats, narcs, and pipe dreams: a history of America's romance with illegal drugs.* New York: Scribner, 1996:55.
8. Inciardi JA. Some considerations on the clinical efficacy of compulsory treatment: reviewing the New York experience. *NIDA Res Monogr* 1988;86:126–138.
9. Jonnes J. *Hep-cats, narcs, and pipe dreams: a history of America's romance with illegal drugs.* New York: Scribner, 1996:111–112.
10. U.S. Comptroller General. *Limited use of federal programs to commit narcotics addicts for treatment and rehabilitation.* September 20, 1971.
11. Pescor MJ. *Public Health Rep* 1943; [Suppl]:170, follow-up study of treated narcotics addicts. For more discussion, see Leukefeld CG, Tims FM, eds., *Compulsory treatment of drug abuse: research and clinical practice.* Washington, DC: U.S. Government Printing Office, 1988.
12. Vaillant GE. The role of compulsory supervision in the treatment of addiction. *Fed Prob* 1966;30:53–59.
13. De Leon G. Legal pressure in therapeutic communities. In: Leukefeld CG, Tims FM, eds., *Compulsory treatment of drug abuse: research and clinical practice.* Washington, DC: U.S. Government Printing Office, 1988. Although he has studied this process most extensively among patients treated in residential programs—self-contained, live-in "therapeutic communities" lasting 1 to 2 years—De Leon's scheme likely operates in any compulsory treatment setting. De Leon G, Melnick G, Kressel D. Motivation and readiness for therapeutic community treatment among cocaine and other drug abusers. *Am J Drug Alcohol Abuse* 1997;23:169–189.

What can we expect from treatment? The major studies show that patient drug use and criminal activity are markedly reduced during treatment itself. Upon completion, between one-third and one-half of patients are able to remain abstinent from their "drug of choice" 1 year later. (See Prendergast ML, Hser YI, Chen J, et al. *Drug treatment need among offender populations.* Paper presented at the 44th annual meeting of the American Society of Criminology, New Orleans, Louisiana, November 4–7, 1992.) Because few patients complete programs, however, enduring abstinence is a rare result of treatment. Nevertheless, considerable reductions in drug use and crime are consistently demonstrated.

In the Drug Abuse Reporting Project (DARP), daily use of heroin was down by an average of 60% 1 year after treatment, irrespective of modality, ranging from 64% among methadone patients to 56% among outpatient clinic patients. Employment increased two- to threefold at 1 year, and incarceration declined by one-half to two-thirds, relative to pretreatment levels. Within the subset of patients followed for 12 years, 63% had been drug-free for 3 years. This is almost twice the rate of developmental "maturing out" (or, retirement from a lifelong career of addiction) that one expects to see among a cohort of aging heroin users. Unless a patient stayed beyond a threshold treatment stay of 3 months, however, the patient's status 1 year after treatment would be unchanged from pretreatment levels.

Among Treatment Outcome Prospective Study (TOPS) patients, daily cocaine and heroin rates were down by about half at 1 year after treatment, as long as the length of stay exceeded 3 months. But the most impressive reductions were seen among those who stayed at least 1 year. Patients who remained for at least 3 months dropped at-least-weekly use of cocaine by one-third to two-thirds by the fifth year. Regular heroin use declined between 50% and 75% by the fifth year. Predatory crime declined by one-third to one-half, while employment doubled among those in outpatient and residential programs; it declined for those on methadone. Unfortunately, however, use of alcohol and marijuana increased. Similarly, DATOS patients at 1-year followup cut both weekly and daily usage of cocaine and heroin by one-half, if they stayed for at least 3 to 6 months.

14. De G Leon, Wexler HK, Jainchill N. The therapeutic community: success and improvement rates five years after treatment. *Int J Addict* 1982;17(4):703–747.
15. Leukefeld CG, Tims FM, eds., *Compulsory treatment of drug abuse: research and clinical practice.* Washington, DC: U.S. Government Printing Office, 1988. See also Anglin MD, Hser Y. Legal coercion and drug abuse treatment: research findings and social policy implications. In: Inciardi JA, ed. *Handbook of drug control in the United States.* New York: Greenwood Press, 1990; and Hiller ML, Knight K, Broome KM, et al. Legal pressure and treatment retention in a national sample of long-term residential program, *Crim Just Behav* 1998;25:463–481. A recent analysis from a large treatment sample (DATOS) suggests that retention may depend more on the mere presence of the criminal justice pressure than on the level of its intensity and the risk of incarceration; see Anglin MD, Prendergast ML, Farabee D. *The effectiveness of coerced treatment for drug abusing offenders.* Presented at the Office of National Drug Control Policy's Conference of Scholars and Policy Makers, Washington, DC, March 25, 1998. (This paper is available at the ONDCP web site: www.whitehousedrugpolicy.gov.) In the paper, Douglas Anglin and colleagues at the Drug Abuse Research Center at UCLA explicitly took differing terminology into account in their review of studies of coerced treatment. They concluded that "legally referred clients do as well or better than voluntary clients in and after treatment . . . and [because] controlling drug abuse and addiction benefits

society as a whole, the criminal justice system should bring drug-abusing offenders into treatment as a safeguard and [so] promote the interests and well-being of the community." See also Marlowe DB, Glass DJ, Merikle EP, et al. Efficacy of coercion in substance abuse treatment. In: Tims F, Leukefeld C, Platt JJ, eds. *Relapse and recovery in the addictions.* New Haven, CT: Yale University Press, 2001:_____, and Langenbucher J, McCrady BS, Brick J, et al. *Socioeconomic evaluations of addictions treatment.* Washington, DC: White House Printing Office, 1993.

16. Marlowe DB, Kirby KC, Bonieskie LM, et al. Assessment of coercive and noncoercive pressures to enter drug abuse treatment. *Drug Alcohol Depend* 1996;42:77–84. See also Marlowe DB, Glass DJ, Merikle EP, et al. Efficacy of coercion in substance abuse treatment. In: Tims F, Leukefeld C, Platt JJ, eds. *Relapse and recovery in the addictions.* New Haven, CT: Yale University Press, 2001:308–327.

17. De G Leon, Wexler HK, Jainchill N. The therapeutic community: success and improvement rates five years after treatment. *Int J Addict* 1982;17(4):703–747.

18. Leukefeld CG, Tims FM, eds., *Compulsory treatment of drug abuse: research and clinical practice.* Washington, DC: U.S. Government Printing Office, 1988. According to Drug Abuse Treatment Outcome Study, patients most likely to stay in treatment are those with high motivation; legal pressure; no prior trouble with the law; psychological counseling while in treatment; and lack of other psychological problems, especially antisocial personality disorder.

19. De Leon G. Legal pressure in therapeutic communities. In: Leukefeld CG, Tims FM, eds., *Compulsory treatment of drug abuse: research and clinical practice.* Washington, DC: U.S. Government Printing Office, 1988.

20. Anglin MD. The efficacy of civil commitment in treating narcotic addiction. In: Leukefeld CG, Tims FM, eds., *Compulsory treatment of drug abuse: research and clinical practice.* Washington, DC: U.S. Government Printing Office, 1988; Anglin MD. Efficacy of civil commitment in treating narcotics addiction. *J Drug Issues* 1988;18:527–545.

21. Kidorf M, Hollander JR, King VL, et al. Increasing employment of opioid dependent outpatients: an intensive behavioral intervention. *Drug Alcohol Depend* 1998;50:73–80.

22. McGlothlin WH, Anglin MD, Wilson BD. *An evaluation of the California Civil Addict Program.* DHEW pub. no. (ADM) 78–558. Washington, DC: National Insti-

tute on Drug Abuse, 1977. According to Anglin, the California Civil Addict Program (CAP) program changed dramatically after the advent of determinant sentencing in California in the 1970s. After determinant sentencing, it was possible for the required stay in CAP to be longer than the incarceration period, a condition that mitigated against the offender choosing treatment. Treatment at the main incustody facility, the California Rehabilitation Center in Corona, now consists primarily of drug education efforts. Currently, the state legislature is considering a bill to revitalize the CAP and return the services provided to a level reminiscent of its initial decade. (Personal communication, July 1, 1998.)

23. Annual address, Message to the legislature. State of New York, January 3, 1973.

24. Simpson, Sells. Effectiveness of treatment for drug abuse; Hubbard et al. *Drug abuse treatment;* Simpson, Curry. Special issue: drug abuse outcome study; Center for Substance and Abuse Treatment, *One year later.*

25. De Leon G. Legal pressure in therapeutic communities. In: Leukefeld CG, Tims FM, eds., *Compulsory treatment of drug abuse: research and clinical practice.* Washington, DC: U.S. Government Printing Office, 1988; De Leon G, Melnick G, Kressel D. Motivation and readiness for therapeutic community treatment among cocaine and other drug abusers. *Am J Drug Alcohol Abuse* 1997;23:169–189. Attrition rates in the major studies were high. Among DARP patients, 13% completed outpatient treatment, 20% completed therapeutic community (TC) treatment, and 28% completed methadone maintenance. These high dropout rates were associated with a pattern of readmission to the same or another clinic within a few years. During the 12-year followup period, for example, the average addict in outpatient treatment had 3.4 more treatment admissions; one in a TC had 4.6 more admissions, and one in methadone maintenance had 5.1 more treatment admissions.

Attrition in TOPS and DATOS was also considerable. In TOPS, 8% finished a year in outpatient, 12% a year in a TC, and 33% a year in methadone treatment. Among DATOS patients, approximately 5% finished 1 year in outpatient, 8% in a TC, and 44% in methadone treatment. A number of factors likely account for what appears to be a trend toward declining retention; they include the shrinking of adjunct social services provided by the clinic and a higher proportion of cocaine abusers in later studies, and thus fewer patients in all who could benefit from the stabilizing effect of methadone.

The proportion of young patients and multiple-drug abusers—features associated with poorer prognoses—has also increased. In addition, a higher proportion of women in the later studies may also contribute to the attrition trend. Women's notorious skittishness as patients in residential programs is generally attributed to the competing demands of childcare and the distractions of what is often a chaotic family scene. Newer residential programs, therefore, try to accommodate one or more of their children as well. See also Simpson DS, Joe GW, Brown BS. Treatment retention and follow-up outcomes in the drug abuse treatment outcome study. *Psychol Addict Behav* 1997;11:294–307; Maxwell JC. Substance abuse trends in Texas, December 1995. In: *TCADA research briefs.* Austin, TX: Texas Commission on Drug and Alcohol Abuse, 1996; Price RH, D'Aunno T. *NIDA III respondent report drug abuse treatment system survey: a national study of the outpatient drug-free and methadone treatment systems, 1988–1990 results.* Ann Arbor, MI: University of Michigan Institute for Social Research, 1992. Also see Anglin MD, Hser Y. Treatment of drug abuse. In: Tonry M, Wilson JQ, eds. Drugs and crime. Chicago: University of Chicago Press, 1990.

26. Dr. David F. Duncan (Brown University, Department of Psychiatry) presented data at the 1997 annual meeting of the Drug Policy Foundation on drug abusers mandated to treatment in Rhode Island. He had found that this group was significantly more likely to designate marijuana as their problem drug, and he expressed concern that these individuals were occupying treatment slots that should more properly go to people addicted to heroin or cocaine, who were on waiting lists for treatment. As of this writing, DATOS researchers are still looking at pretreatment characteristics and outcome by voluntary versus involuntary status. See McGlothlin WH. Criminal justice clients. In DuPont, Goldstein, O'Donnell, *Handbook of drug abuse.*

27. Farabee D, Nelson R, Spence R. Psychosocial profiles of criminal justice- and non-criminal justice-referred clients in treatment. *Crim Just Behav* 1993;20: 336–346.

28. McGlothlin WH. Criminal justice clients. In DuPont, Goldstein, O'Donnell, *Handbook of drug abuse.*

29. Gerstein DR, Harwood HJ, eds. *Treating drug problems,* vol. 1. Washington, DC: Institute of Medicine, National Academy Press, 1990.

30. Collins JJ, Allison M. Legal coercion and retention in drug abuse treatment. *Hosp*

Community Psychiatry 1983;34:1145–1149; Anglin MD, Hser Y. Treatment of drug abuse. In: Tonry M, Wilson JQ, eds. *Drugs and crime*. Chicago: University of Chicago Press, 1990.

31. McLellan AT, Arndt IO, Metzger DS, et al. The effects of psychosocial services in substance abuse treatment. *JAMA* 1993;269(15):1953–1959; McLellan AT, Grissom GR, Zanis D et al. Problem-service "matching" in addiction treatment: a prospective study in four programs. *Arch Gen Psychiatry* 1997;54(8):730–735; Hser Y. A referral system that matches drug users to treatment programs: existing research and relevant issues. *J Drug Issues* 1995;25(1):209–24.

    Indeed, duration of treatment may be more important, and is certainly no less important, than the particular modality. It's true that patients tend to sort themselves out, but with the most severely addicted finding their way into residential treatment, the ratio of outpatient to residential slots is so high that outpatient facilities inevitably serve a rather heterogeneous population. This population includes a sizable percentage of heavily addicted and criminally involved individuals. There is considerable similarity between patient outcomes across modalities.

32. McKay JR, McLellan AT, Alterman AI. An evaluation of the Cleveland criteria for inpatient substance abuse treatment. *Am J Psychiatry* 1992;149:1212–1218.

33. Nemes S, Wish E, Messina N. *The District of Columbia treatment initiative*. College Park, MD: Center for Substance Abuse Research, University of Maryland, 1998.

34. Knight K, Hiller ML, Broome KM, et al. Legal pressure, treatment readiness, and engagement in long-term residential programs. *J Offend Rehabil* 2000;31:101–115.

35. Finney JW. Some treatment implications of project MATCH. *Addiction* 1999;94:42–45.

36. Collins JJ, Allison M. Legal coercion and retention in drug abuse treatment. *Hosp Community Psychiatry* 1983;34:1145–1149.

37. Education and Assistance Corporation. Brooklyn TASC predicate program: a program briefing. Carle Place, New York: Education and Assistance Corporation, Criminal Justice Division, 1995.

38. Criminal Justice Policy Council. *Treatment alternatives to incarceration program: an analysis of retention and treatment and outcome evaluation*. Austin, TX: Criminal Justice Policy Council, 1995.

39. Anglin MD, Longshore D, Turner S, et al. *Studies of the functioning and effective-*
    ness of treatment alternatives to street crime. Final report. Los Angeles: UCLA Drug Research Center, 1996.

40. Anglin MD, Longshore D, Turner S, et al. *Studies of the functioning and effectiveness of treatment alternatives to street crime (TASC) programs.* Los Angeles: UCLA Drug Abuse Research Center, 1996.

41. Taxman FS. *Reducing recidivism through a seamless system of care: components of effective treatment, supervision, and transition services in the community.* College Park, MD: 1998 (paper prepared for the Office of National Drug Control Policy Conference on Treatment and the Criminal Justice System, February 20, 1998). *Felony defendants in large urban counties in 1992.* Bureau of Justice Statistics (NCJ-148826). 1995.

42. National Center on Addiction and Substance Abuse at Columbia University. *Behind bars: substance abuse and America's prison population.* New York: 1998:127; Harlow CW. *Profile of jail inmates, 1996.* Bureau of Justice Statistics (NCJ-164620), 1998; Prisoners in 1996. *Bur Just Stat Bull* 1997; June.

    An arrestee who participated in Drug Use Forecasting in 1990 was considered to be probably in need of drug treatment if the arrestee tested positive for one of the drugs and met one of the following conditions: (a) reported frequent use of the drug (at least 10 times in the past month); (b) reported being dependent on the drug at some time in the past; (c) reported being currently in treatment; or (d) reported being in need of treatment. According to this definition, the percentage of arrestees who were probably in need of treatment was 45% of those who tested positive for cocaine, 59% of those who tested positive for opiates, 10% of those who tested positive for amphetamines, and 77% of those who tested positive for cocaine, opiates, or amphetamines and who reported injection drug use. From Prendergast ML, Hser YI, Chen J, et al. *Drug treatment need among offender populations.* Paper presented at the 44th annual meeting of the American Society of Criminology, New Orleans, Louisiana, November 4–7, 1992.

43. Speckart GR, Anglin MD. Narcotics and crime: a causal modeling approach. *J Quant Criminol* 1986;2:3–28; Nurco DN, Kinlock TW, Hanlon TE. The drugs–crime connection. In: Inciardi JA, ed. *Handbook of drug control in the United States.* Westport, CT: Greenwood Press, 1990:71–90; Chaiken MR. Crime rates and substance abuse among types of offenders. In: Johnson BD, Wish E, eds. *Crime rates among drug-abusing of-*
    fenders: final report to the national institute of justice. New York: Narcotic and Drug Research, 1986. For a detailed discussion of the history and effectiveness of TASC, see Anglin MD, Longshore D, Turner S, et al. *Studies of the functioning and effectiveness of treatment alternatives to street crime (TASC) programs.* Los Angeles: UCLA Drug Abuse Research Center, 1996. Also see Taxman FS. *Reducing recidivism through a seamless system of care: components of effective treatment, supervision, and transition services in the community.* College Park, MD: 1998 (paper prepared for the Office of National Drug Control Policy Conference on Treatment and the Criminal Justice System, February 20, 1998).

44. "The arrangement of the judge at the center of the operation reflects the growing desire of judges to have more control," says Judge Jeffrey Tauber, president and founder of the National Association of Drug Court Professionals. This may be one reason why TASC programs have declined, while drug courts have expanded. (From personal communication, August 1997.)

45. Office of Justice Programs Drug Court Clearinghouse at American University, January 17, 2003.

46. Belenko S. Research on drug courts. *Natl Drug Court Instit Rev* 1998;1(1):1–44.

47. Experimental designs are difficult to implement. Researchers associated with the Brooklyn Treatment Court in New York are comparing its participants with matched offenders from neighboring areas who do not have access to drug court but who would choose that option if it were available. This avoids introducing the confounding variable of motivation, a problem intrinsic to studies that compare individuals who choose drug court with those who actively reject it. But perhaps the most clinically informative comparison, which has yet to be conducted, would include drug court participants with matched patients who were court-referred to the same treatment program. This would help tease apart the combined effects of sanctions and heavy judicial supervision from the influence of treatment.

48. U.S. General Accounting Office. *Drug courts: overview of growth, characteristics and results.* Washington, DC: Author, 1997.

49. Cooper CA, Bartlett SR, Shaw MA, et al. *Drug courts: 1997 overview of operational characteristics and implementation issues,* vol. 1. Washington, DC: Office of Justice Programs Drug Court Clearinghouse and Technical Assistance Project, American University, May 1997; Satel S. Do drug courts really work? *City J* 1998;Summer:81–87.

50. Bureau of Justice Statistics Special Report. *Recidivism of felons on probation, 1986–1989.* Washington, DC: U.S. Department of Justice, Office of Justice Programs, 1992.

51. Finigan M. *An outcome program evaluation of the Multnomah County S.T.O.P. drug diversion program.* Prepared by the State Justice Institute of Alexandria, Virginia, for the Multnomah County, Oregon, Department of Corrections, January 6, 1998.

52. Deschenes EP, Turner S, Greenwood PW, et al. *An experimental evaluation of drug testing and treatment interventions for probationers in Maricopa County, Arizona.* Prepared for the National Institute of Justice by RAND Corporation, July 1996.

53. Gottfredson DC, Exum ML. The Baltimore city drug treatment court: one-year results from a randomized study. *J Res Crime Delinquency* 2002;39(3):337–356.

54. Terry WC III. Broward County's dedicated drug treatment court: from post-adjudication to diversion. In: Terry WC III, ed. *Judicial change and drug treatment courts: case studies in innovation.* Beverly Hills, CA: Sage, 1998.

55. Goldkamp JS, Weiland D. *Assessing the impact of Dade County's felony drug court: final report to the National Institute of Justice.* Philadelphia: Criminal and Justice Research Institute, 1993.

56. Harrell A, Cavanaugh S. *Preliminary results from the evaluation of the D.C. Superior Court drug intervention program for drug felony defendants.* Washington, DC: Urban Institute, 1997.

57. General Accounting Office. *Drug courts: overview of growth characteristics, and results.* Washington, DC: Author, 1997.

58. Belenko S. Research on drug courts: a critical review. *Natl Drug Court Instit Rev* 1999;2(2):1–58.

59. Belenko S. Drug courts. In: Leukefeld CG, Tims F, Farabee D, eds. *Treatment of drug offenders: policies and issues.* New York: Springer, 2002:301–318.

60. Festinger DS, Marlowe DB, Lee PA, et al. Status hearings in drug court: when more is less and less is more. *Drug Alcohol Depend* 2002;68:151–157.

61. Office of Justice Programs. *OJP drugs and crime and CASA behind bars 1998,* appendix D; Working group, Department of Justice, *A report to the assistant attorney general, January 1996.*

62. Bureau of Justice Statistics. *Substance abuse and treatment, state and federal prisoners, 1997.* Washington, DC: U.S. Department of Justice, 1999.

63. Douglas S. Lipton, National Drug Research Institute, New York City; personal communication, July 6, 1998.

64. Falkin GP, Wexler HK, Lipton DS. Drug treatment in state prisons. In: Gerstein DR, Harwood HJ, eds. *Treating drug problems,* vol. 2. Washington, DC: National Academy Press, Institute of Medicine, 1990.

65. Simpson DD, Wexler HK, Inciardi JA, eds. Drug treatment outcomes for correctional settings, part 1. *Prison J* 79(3).

66. Inciardi JA, Martin SS, Butzin CA, et al. An effective model of prison-based treatment for drug-involved offenders. *J Drug Issues* 1997;27(2):261–278. The effectiveness of drug treatment in jails is less well characterized.

67. Young D. *Bridging drug treatment and criminal justice.* New York: Vera Institute of Justice, 1996.

68. Young D. Impacts of perceived legal pressure on retention in drug treatment. *Crim Just Behav* 2002;29(1):27–55.

69. Wild TC, Roberts AB, Cooper EL. Compulsory substance abuse treatment: an overview of recent findings and issues. *Eur Addict Res* 2002;8:84–93.

70. Gerstein DR, Harwood HJ, eds. *Treating drug problems,* vol. 1. Washington, DC: Institute of Medicine, National Academy Press, 1990.

71. Sullum J. Drug test. *Reason Magazine* 1998;Mar:22–31; Leshner AI. Addiction is a brain disease, and it matters. *Science* 1997;278:45; Consensus Statement, Physician Leadership on National Drug Policy, July 9, 1997. See also Medical news and perspective. *JAMA* 1997;278(5):378; Moyers B. *Addiction: close to home.* Public Broadcasting Service, March 29–31, 1998.

72. Psychologist Gene M. Heyman of Harvard University points to epidemiologic data to show that relapse is not universal among addicts. The large Epidemiologic Catchment Area (ECA) study, funded by the National Institute of Mental Health, shows that in the general population, remission rates are the norm, not the exception. According to ECA criteria for remission—defined as no symptoms for the year just prior to the interview—59% of roughly 1,300 respondents who met lifetime criteria were free of drug problems. The average duration of remission was 2.7 years and the mean duration of illness was 6.1 years, with most cases (75th percentile) lasting no more than 8 years. Furthermore, the addicts most likely to serve as subjects in treatment-outcome studies—treatment seekers—form a subgroup of the general addict population that is most prone to relapse. While roughly only one-third of drug abusers seek treatment, more than 60% of them are diagnosed with additional psychiatric disorders, according to the National Co-Morbidity Study. Among abusers who have not sought treatment, however, approximately 29% have additional psychiatric diagnoses, a proportion not much different from the prevalence of psychiatric illness in the general population. Also see Satel S. The fallacies of no-fault addiction. *Public Interest* 1999;Winter: .

73. For a discussion of the possible negative consequences of coercion, see Schottenfeld RS. Involuntary treatment of substance abuse disorders—impediments to success. *Psychiatry* 1989;52:1640–1676. Civil commitment and diversion programs are expensive to implement effectively. (Personal communication from Jerome Jaffe, MD, former director of the Special Action Office for Drug Abuse Prevention under President Nixon.) J. J. Platt concluded that such programs are typically effective only if the heroin abuser is placed on long-term probation or parole (5 to 10 years), with close supervision, regular urine testing, and a realistic threat of reincarceration for serious instances of relapse. Platt JJ. *Heroin addiction: theory, research and treatment,* vol. 2. *The addict, the treatment process, and social control.* Malabar, FL: Krieger, 1995.

74. Galon PA, Liebelt RA. Involuntary treatment of substance abuse disorders. In: Munetz MR, ed. *Can mandatory treatment be therapeutic?* New Directions for Mental Health Services, no. 75. San Francisco: Jossey-Bass, Fall 1997.

75. This was the type of rationale described by psychologist Barbara Lex at McLean Hospital in Boston, who examined data for 500 women civilly committed to treatment in Massachusetts in 1995. Except for the severity of the condition precipitating commitment, these women were demographically similar to a comparison set of women who were voluntarily admitted. The committed group stayed in treatment an average of four times longer. Lex BW. *Women civilly committed to substance abuse treatments in Massachusetts.* Data presented at the American Society of Addiction Medicine, 29th annual meeting, New Orleans, Louisiana, 1998.

76. Taxman and Byrne, "Locating absconders"; Langan and Cunliffe, "Recidivism of felons on probation."

77. Belenko S, Nikerson G, Rubinstein T. *Crack and the New York courts: a study of judicial responses and attitudes.* New York: New York City Criminal Justice Agency, 1990. This study examined perceptions affecting judges' decisions regarding the adjudication of crack and powdered cocaine offenders. Most of them believed that only motivated defendants would benefit from treatment.

CHAPTER 46

Treatment in Prisons and Jails

ROGER H. PETERS, CHARLES O. MATTHEWS, AND JOEL A. DVOSKIN

To understand the context in which correctional substance abuse treatment services are provided, it is important to highlight several key differences between jails and prisons. Prisons are distinct from jails in that they only house inmates who are sentenced for more than 1 year of incarceration, and who have generally committed serious and/or more frequent offenses in comparison to jail inmates. Inmates confined in jails are either sentenced for a period of less than 1 year, or are unsentenced and awaiting trial or sentencing. Prison systems are typically much larger than jails, and sometimes feature separate institutions for inmates of differing security levels, or for inmates who need treatment for their mental health or substance abuse problems. Jails are typically operated by municipalities or counties, whereas prisons are operated by state or federal governments. Both jail and prison systems vary widely in the amount and type of resources that are allocated for substance abuse treatment.

Jail and prison populations in the United States have increased dramatically during the last several decades, in large part as a result of the arrest and incarceration of drug offenders. There are currently 1.3 million adult offenders incarcerated in state and federal prisons, and 631,000 adult offenders incarcerated in jails (1). This represents a 415% increase in prison populations and a 340% increase in jail populations since 1980. There are now more than 250,000 drug offenders in state prisons, up from 19,000 in 1980, and approximately 3% of all U.S. citizens are under some type of correctional supervision (2). Several factors have contributed to the growing correctional populations, including new sentencing laws and policies (e.g., laws establishing mandatory minimum sentences) adopted in the 1980s and 1990s, abolition of parole in many jurisdictions, and law enforcement practices that have focused on street-level drug users and sellers.

The costs associated with expanding jails and prison systems are enormous. The average cost for incarcerating a jail or prison inmate ranges from $20,000 to $23,000 per year (3). Approximately $40 billion was spent on U.S. prisons and jails in 2000, including $24 billion to incarcerate nonviolent offenders, many of whom are drug offenders. An estimated 77% of correctional costs are linked to substance abuse, representing approximately 10 times the amount that states spend on substance abuse treat-

ment, prevention, and research (4). In response to the high cost of incarcerating drug offenders, states have begun to revise sentencing statutes to provide early release and reduced sanctions for drug offenders (5). Ballot initiatives passed in a number of states authorize participation in substance abuse treatment in lieu of incarceration for nonviolent drug offenders. Proposition 36 in California was one of the first such initiatives, and allocates $60 to $120 million per year to fund treatment services, vocational training, family counseling, literacy training, and probation supervision and court monitoring. According to analyses conducted by the California Legislature, Proposition 36 would result in the need for 11,000 fewer prison beds, and would result in an annual savings of $200 to $250 million (6).

TREATMENT NEEDS IN JAILS AND PRISONS

With the closing of state mental hospitals, reductions in public treatment services, and the narrowing scope of private insurance coverage, jails and prisons have increasingly served as "public health outposts" and human service providers of "last resort" (7). In recent years, an increasingly greater proportion of jail and prison inmates are homeless, mentally ill, and have substance use disorders and other chronic health problems (8). For example, between 6% and 12% of jail inmates have a severe mental disorder (9–11), and approximately 10% of jail and prison inmates report mental health problems or a history of residential mental health treatment (12). Jails and prisons have had to adapt new types of services for the growing numbers of inmates with specialized health care needs, including those with human immunodeficiency virus (HIV)/acquired immunodeficiency syndrome (AIDS) and those with co-occurring mental health and substance use disorders (13). Many offenders have not previously received adequate dental, mental health, substance abuse, or other health care services, and arrive at jails or prisons with preexisting conditions and a range of acute care needs. A significant proportion of these individuals do not have established relationships with community substance abuse or health care programs (7).

Well over half of jail and prison inmates have significant substance abuse problems, and need treatment services (14,15). Within jails, 66% of adult arrestees in metropolitan jails test positive for drugs, and 70% of inmates are either arrested for a drug offense or report using drugs on a regular basis (16,17). The lifetime prevalence rates of substance abuse or dependence disorders among prisoners is 74%, including 46% for drug dependence and 37% for alcohol dependence (18). These rates are markedly higher than in the general population (19). In recognition of the significant need for substance abuse treatment in jails and prisons and the lengthy amount of time that is often available to provide services in these settings, incarceration is seen by many as an important opportunity to capitalize on periods of emotional crisis and to promote major lifestyle change (20).

In recent years there has been an emerging gap between the need for substance abuse treatment services in jails and prisons and the scope of services provided (15,20–24). Less than 6% of state and federal prison budgets are currently spent on substance abuse treatment (25), and only 10% to 12% of prison inmates receive any form of substance abuse treatment (12,26). The "war on drugs" has not apparently been waged in correctional settings, as the rate of inmate participation in treatment declined from 25% to 10% between 1991 and 1997 (12). A recent national survey of correctional and detention facilities determined that only 56% of state prisons, and 33% of jails provided any type of substance abuse treatment services (27,28). Only 21% of treatment services in jails, and 31% in state prisons are provided in treatment units that are isolated from the general inmate population. Moreover, many jail and prison treatment programs are not comprehensive in scope, and rely on peer or inmate "counselors" to provide Alcoholics Anonymous (AA) and Narcotics Anonymous (NA) groups. Similarly, the staff:inmate ratio is quite low in correctional treatment programs, averaging 1:25 in state prisons (27,28).

Several national surveys confirm the need for more extensive substance abuse treatment services in jails and prisons. A survey conducted by the American Jail Association (29) found that only 28% of jails reported substance abuse treatment services. Among jails reporting treatment services, only 18% featured paid staff, and only 7% had a comprehensive level of services. Few jails were found to provide transition or reentry services. Surveys conducted by the U.S. Department of Justice in 1997 and 1998 found that 43% of jails and 56% of state prisons reported substance abuse treatment programs (1,16). Among the jails surveyed, 64% reported self-help programs (e.g., AA, NA), 30% provided drug-education services, and only 12% provided a combination of treatment, self-help groups, and drug-education programs. A striking finding of the survey was that only 4% of jail inmates received any type of treatment services during their current incarceration, and less than 2% received counseling services.

HISTORICAL TRENDS IN CORRECTIONAL TREATMENT SERVICES

Correctional substance abuse treatment services have been influenced by a cyclical pattern of political support for either punishment or rehabilitation of offenders (30). County and state fiscal problems, including recent revenue shortfalls, have also led to significant reductions in jail and prison substance abuse treatment services. Correctional treatment programs were first offered in the late 1920s, when the U.S. Congress established hospital-based programs for those with opiate addiction, although relatively few programs were developed in jails and prisons before the 1960s. During the 1960s, several states enacted civil commitment statutes that required substance abuse treatment in secure settings. The Narcotic Addict Rehabilitation Act (NARA) passed by Congress in 1966 required in-prison treatment of narcotic addicts who were convicted of federal crimes. The emerging NARA-supported treatment services were essentially residential hospital programs that were situated in prisons.

A number of correctional therapeutic community (TC) programs were implemented in the 1970s, but it wasn't until a decade later that TC programs received widespread support through federal initiatives such as Project REFORM and Project RECOVERY (31–33). These initiatives led to implementation of TCs in a number of state correctional systems, and supported a variety of training and technical support services. Since this time, the Residential Substance Abuse Treatment (RSAT) formula grant program funded by the U.S. Department of Justice has supported a wide range of treatment programs in state prisons and in local correctional and detention facilities. Additional prevention and treatment services have been funded through block grants provided by the Department of Justice.

The scope and quality of prison-based treatment services in the United States has varied considerably over the last several decades. Until recently, several of the most highly populated states (e.g., California) maintained only a few prison-based substance abuse treatment programs, whereas several smaller states (e.g., Oregon) developed an extensive array of in-prison and postrelease services. Perhaps the most comprehensive set of treatment services is provided by the Federal Bureau of Prisons (34). Several other countries, such as Canada, Denmark, and Germany, have developed a range of substance abuse treatment and harm reduction programs in correctional settings that are broader in scope and application than many of the correctional programs in the United States (35,36). In Canada, for example, correctional treatment programs focus not only on substance abuse, but also include cognitive–behavioral interventions, problem solving, and other psychosocial skills that are relevant to the broader inmate population.

THE CORRECTIONAL TREATMENT ENVIRONMENT

Several unique environmental elements of jails and prisons affect the ability to provide substance abuse treatment services (21). Jails house a large number of unsentenced inmates for short periods of time, many of whom may be released from incarceration with little advance warning. These individuals may be reluctant to disclose information that could adversely influence their pending case, and may be less interested in treatment than their judicial disposition. Jail and prison schedules are very regimented, and include large blocks of time when inmates are involved in structured work or educational activities, or are locked in their cells for "count." Because of the large volume of staff and inmate movement, and because of architectural constraints, jails and prisons are often very noisy and lack privacy and dedicated space for treatment activities. In recent years, several treatment-oriented prisons have been built that provide better accommodation for group space, staff offices, and privacy in treatment settings. Work activities in jails and prisons often compete with treatment. For example, in many prisons, inmates may receive early release for employment but not for involvement in substance abuse treatment.

Correctional systems have as their primary focus the control and security of inmates, and have not traditionally provided significant attention to the substance abuse needs of incarcerated offenders. Conflicts often arise within jails and prisons between treatment and security staff, who may have different perspectives regarding the importance of treatment and methods for dealing with inmate infractions, "critical incidents," and contraband. Although basic correctional mental health treatment services are mandated by the courts, there are fewer requirements for substance abuse treatment services. Similarly, while mental health disorders are widely viewed as having biologic and medical origins, substance abuse disorders are misunderstood by many as reflecting "moral weakness," and as intractable to treatment. As a result, jail and prisons systems vary widely in the scope and quality of substance abuse treatment services provided.

In times of budget shortfalls, cutbacks, and spiraling correctional costs, substance abuse services are often eliminated or scaled down, and are seen as dispensable relative to other health and security services. At the same time, many correctional systems have begun to experiment with privatized, or partially privatized health care services as a way of limiting liability and containing costs. However, unless substance abuse treatment services are specifically listed as deliverables in these contracts, it is unlikely that the private provider would offer these services.

STANDARDS FOR SUBSTANCE ABUSE TREATMENT IN PRISONS AND JAILS

Legal Standards

Although the courts have consistently rejected a general constitutional right to substance abuse rehabilitation or treatment in correctional facilities (37), case law indicates that inmates do have limited rights to substance abuse treatment in prisons and jails (15,38). If conditions in a correctional facility demonstrate "deliberate indifference" to inmates' serious medical needs (serious medical needs are defined as those diagnosed by a physician as requiring treatment or those that are so obvious that a layperson would easily recognize the necessity for

medical attention [see *Pace v. Fauver* (39)]), then substance abuse treatment might be court-ordered to be made available as part of the remedy. For instance in *Palmigiano v. Garrahy* (40), the court found that conditions in a Rhode Island prison were below constitutional standards and linked the prison's failure to identify inmates with substance dependence problems to increased prison drug trafficking, increased risk of suicide, and overall deterioration of prison conditions. Consequently, the prison was ordered by the court to implement substance abuse treatment services that met minimal professional organization and federal agency standards, including those that address the medical needs associated with substance abuse withdrawal.

While there is a limited legal mandate for substance abuse treatment services in jails and prisons, inmates' rights to medical treatment for withdrawal (i.e., detoxification) and other serious medical problems associated with substance abuse have consistently been upheld (15,38,41–43). Thus, when an inmate enters the correctional system while on methadone maintenance for heroin addiction, the courts have required medical management of methadone withdrawal, but have not required continuance on methadone (38). Partly as a result of the need to identify and treat potentially life-threatening consequences of substance dependence, including withdrawal, screening for substance abuse in prisons and jails appears to have a stronger legal basis than does substance abuse treatment (39,44–46).

Several lawsuits have also supported the need for correctional personnel in jails and prisons to be adequately trained to distinguish between intoxication from substance abuse and serious medical illnesses, which can mimic symptoms of intoxication (47). For instance, in *Ferguson v. Perry* (48), an individual was arrested for suspicion of drunk driving, placed in jail, and was mistakenly thought to be highly intoxicated. As a result, diagnosis and treatment of a cerebral hemorrhage was delayed, which contributed to his death three days later. In a similar case (49), an individual was arrested for public drunkenness and was placed in jail overnight for observation. The next day he was still unconscious, was hospitalized, and died of encephalitis several days later. In both of these cases the defendants (jail systems) were found liable, demonstrating the importance of adequate screening, examination, and close observation of inmates who appear to be intoxicated, in order to rule out serious health problems (47).

Legal cases in which correctional health care personnel have been found guilty of malpractice and/or negligence for *denial* of medical care include the following categories: "(a) denial of treatment for known and serious medical conditions, (b) denial of medical care to physically disabled prisoners, (c) denial of care from failure to diagnose health problems, and (d) denial, to prisoners, of access to their prison medical records" (47). Legal cases in which correctional health care personnel have been found guilty of malpractice and/or negligence for *delay* of medical care include the following: "(a) delay in diagnosis of life-threatening illnesses, (b) delay in treatment that results in hospitalization, and (c) delay in administering appropriate medications" (47). These findings from case law underscore the importance of attending to the serious medical consequences of substance abuse, including prompt medical screening to rule out other serious diseases when inmates appear intoxicated, and to address the risk of medical complications related to overdose or withdrawal.

Several new court decisions (50,51) have defined Alcoholics Anonymous (AA) and Narcotics Anonymous (NA) as religious-based activities (15). Thus, jails and prisons that coerce inmate participation in AA or NA (e.g., with institutional privileges and/or desirable security classifications) violate the First Amendment of the U.S. Constitution, which prohibits government-sponsored religious activities. Legal liability can be avoided by either removing coercive requirements to participate in such programs, or by providing nonreligious treatment alternatives (15,38).

Professional Standards

A number of professional standards have been developed to guide the implementation of correctional substance abuse treatment services (15,38,52). Standards developed by the National Commission on Correctional Health Care (NCCHC) and by the American Correctional Association (ACA) are among the most comprehensive and are generally more explicit and demanding than the legal standards described in the previous section. The following substance abuse services are listed as "essential" by the NCCHC (53–55) for both jails and prisons:

- Management of intoxication and withdrawal, including medical supervision, use of written policies and procedures, and provisions for transferring inmates experiencing severe overdose or withdrawal to a licensed acute care facility.
- A comprehensive health assessment (including substance abuse history) conducted within 7 days after arrival in prison or within 14 days after arrival in jail.
- A mental health evaluation conducted within 14 days of arrival in jail or prison, including an evaluation of substance abuse history (these services are listed as "essential" for prisons and as "important" for jails).

The NCCHC lists the following correctional services as "important" under its "Standards for Inmates with Alcohol or Other Drug Problems" for both jails and prisons (53–55):

- Written policies and actual practice to identify, assess, and manage inmates with substance abuse problems.
- Opportunities for counseling provided to all inmates with histories of substance abuse problems.

- Accreditation of counselors who provide substance abuse treatment services.
- Use of existing community resources, including referral to specified community resources on release.

Although similar to the standards developed by the NCCHC, the ACA's standards for jail and prison substance abuse treatment (56–58) give more detail regarding appropriate programmatic elements (15). The ACA's standards also call for mandatory substance abuse screening of inmates during the initial health examination, and offer the following additional recommendations regarding the use of standardized procedures for substance abuse screening and assessment:

- Inclusion of a standardized battery of instruments.
- Screening and sorting procedures, including clinical assessment and reassessment.
- Assessment and referral for substance abuse program assignment that is appropriate to the needs of individual inmates, including a standardized "needs assessment" administered to investigate the inmate's substance abuse history and identification of problem areas.
- Drug testing and monitoring.
- Routine diagnostic assessment.

ACA's guidelines for substance abuse treatment in jails and prisons (56–58) include the following:

- Development of individualized treatment objectives and goals by a multidisciplinary treatment team.
- Addressing counseling and drug education needs.
- Medical exams to determine health needs and/or observational requirements.
- Development of an aftercare discharge plan with the inmate's involvement.
- Use of staff who are trained in substance abuse treatment to design and supervise the program.
- Written treatment philosophy with goals and measurable objectives.
- Inclusion of recovered alcoholics/addicts as employees or volunteers, with appropriate training.
- Inclusion of self-help groups as adjuncts to treatment.
- Efforts to motivate addicts to receive treatment through incentives such as housing and clothing preference.
- Provision of a range of treatment services.
- Culturally sensitive treatment approaches.
- Prerelease relapse prevention education including risk management.
- Prerelease and transitional services, including coordination with community programs to ensure continuity of supervision and treatment.

Practice Guidelines

In addition to legal and professional standards for substance abuse treatment in correctional settings, practice guidelines have been established by the American

Psychiatric Association (APA) (59) that provide detailed recommendations related to clinical treatment for alcohol, cocaine, and opioid use disorders. Although these do not specifically address issues unique to correctional settings, they provide more comprehensive practice guidelines than the standards outlined above by the NCCHC and the ACA. APA's guidelines (59) give an overview of treatment principles and alternative treatments for these disorders, as well as recommendations regarding assessment, psychiatric management, pharmacology, psychosocial treatments, treatment planning and treatment settings, and legal/confidentiality issues.

A more recent set of guidelines (60) focuses on psychiatric services in jails and prisons, and includes brief but useful sections on treatment of substance-involved offenders, including those with co-occurring mental and substance use disorders. These guidelines note that, in jails, acute conditions can be present at the time of detainment, including intoxication and/or mental disorders. These conditions, along with the stress of arrest and confinement, increase the risks of suicidal and violent behavior, underscoring the need for adequate and timely screening and assessment procedures for both mental health and substance use disorders. For example, substance intoxication noted during mental health screening should immediately trigger screening for depressed mood and/or suicide potential. This is particularly important because most suicides in jail settings occur within 24 to 48 hours after admission, and are often carried out by inmates who are intoxicated or experiencing substance withdrawal. Psychiatrists should be involved in ensuring that screening for the above issues is adequate.

APA also calls for the integration of substance abuse services with mental health services in correctional settings, and notes that co-occurring disorders are often undetected in correctional settings because of inadequate screening and assessment procedures. Nondetection of one co-occurring disorder can lead to exacerbation of symptoms in the other type of disorder and increase the risk of suicide, recurrence of psychiatric symptoms, substance use relapse, and criminal recidivism. Thus, detection of one type of disorder should immediately trigger screening for the other type of disorder, and necessitates sharing and coordination of information across security and treatment staff and throughout the system. Treatment of co-occurring disorders must be comprehensive, integrated, and individualized, with adequate followup in the community.

SCREENING AND ASSESSMENT IN CORRECTIONAL SETTINGS

Screening and assessment procedures are an important part of any substance abuse treatment system in jails and prisons. Accurate screening and assessment can allow offenders to be routed efficiently into an appropriate level of treatment, while screening out those who do not need

such treatment. Screening and assessment are particularly important in criminal justice populations, which have high prevalence rates of substance abuse and other co-occurring disorders. Without adequate screening and assessment, offenders are likely to be released to the community with their substance use and co-occurring disorders untreated, leading to a high likelihood of criminal recidivism and substance relapse. Although there are currently no comprehensive national standards for substance abuse screening and assessment in jails and prisons, there are several important publications that offer useful guidelines (21,61–63).

Screening typically refers to use of brief measures that rapidly identify offenders with a potential need for substance abuse treatment, and thus informs determinations about eligibility for services. Screening also informs decisions regarding referral for more comprehensive assessment. Assessment typically requires more training than screening, and often includes a comprehensive battery of instruments and completion of a psychosocial interview to determine suitability for placement in available levels of treatment (21).

Key domains to be addressed during screening and assessment in correctional settings include the following (21):

- Substance use history, including current patterns of use, treatment history, and acute symptoms, including the need for detoxification
- Criminal history
- Personality traits related to criminality (e.g., features of psychopathy)
- Mental health issues, including suicide potential, acute symptoms, prescribed psychiatric medications, and treatment history
- History of abuse or trauma as a victim or perpetrator
- Motivation and readiness for treatment
- Physical health, including pregnancy status, acute conditions, and presence of infectious disease (especially sexually transmitted diseases, HIV/AIDS, hepatitis, and tuberculosis)
- Education and literacy
- Physical disabilities
- Housing issues
- Relationships with family members, significant others, and dependents

Motivation and readiness for treatment is useful to examine to match offenders to an appropriate level and intensity of treatment, and to provide specific interventions to address motivational issues (64). Nonconfrontational motivational interviewing techniques (65) are discussed later in this chapter in the section "Substance Abuse Treatment Approaches in Corrections," and can be used during assessment interviews to promote inmate motivation and engagement in treatment. Screening instruments that can be used to identify offenders' motivation and readiness for treatment include the University of Rhode Island Change Assessment Scale (66,67), the Stages of Change Readiness and Treatment Eagerness Scale (68), and the Circumstances, Motivation, Readiness, and Suitability Scale (69).

Offenders, as well as substance abusers in general, may be more likely than other populations to attempt to conceal or distort information obtained from self-report screening and assessment measures (70–73). Malingering in prison settings has been found to range from 15% (74) to 46% (75). In pretrial jail settings, malingering has been found to range from 8% (76) to 37% (77). Rogers' (71) review of the malingering literature found a range of 15% to 17% in forensic settings. Internal factors that might contribute to inaccurate self-report include antisocial, psychopathic, paranoid, or manipulative traits, "denial" as part of the patient's substance use disorder, a lack of readiness to participate in treatment, and poor memory as a result of a higher likelihood of neurologic problems associated with substance use disorders and/or head trauma (70,78).

External factors contributing to offender motivation to report inaccurately include malingering substance use problems to obtain treatment for nonclinical reasons. For example, inmates may inaccurately report a substance abuse history in an attempt to obtain reduced sentences, favorable housing arrangements, or institutional privileges (70). On the other hand, some inmates will exaggerate symptoms of real distress, because they believe that a high level of severity is required to obtain services. Additionally, inmates may attempt to conceal substance abuse because of the fear of legal consequences (i.e., adjudication and sentencing). Staff who provide screening and assessment in jails and prisons should be familiar with the potential reasons and motivations for inaccurate reporting of information.

The accuracy of self-report information can be enhanced through the use of effective screening and assessment measures. Several measures are more effective than others in classifying offenders who are suitable for treatment (63). These include the combined Addiction Severity Index (ASI)–Drug Use Section (79) and the Alcohol Dependence Scale (80), the Simple Screening Instrument (SSI) (81), and the Texas Christian University Drug Screen (TCUDS) (82). The 16-item SSI was developed by a panel of national experts who selected items from existing validated substance abuse screening instruments. The SSI is most useful when the purpose of screening is to maximize identification of inmates who have substance use disorders (e.g., during initial screening for treatment eligibility). The TCUDS is a 19-item instrument that was developed through funding from the National Institute of Drug Abuse, and is most useful when the purpose of screening is to maximize identification of inmates who do *not* require substance abuse treatment. The SSI and the TCUDS are quick and easy to administer and score, can be completed in either a paper-and-pencil or interview form, and are available in the public domain. Both measures outper-

formed the Substance Abuse Subtle Screening Inventory (SASSI)-2 (83) and a range of other screening instruments in identifying substance use disorders among incarcerated offenders (63).

The accuracy of screening and assessment can be further improved by obtaining collateral information from friends, associates, or family members of offenders, and from review of medical and other correctional records (e.g., to assess the inmate's history of drug screens in institutional and community settings). Some screening and assessment measures also include scales to measure malingering, as well as defensive, random, and/or inconsistent responding. Two such measures that have been validated for correctional populations include the Minnesota Multiphasic Personality Inventory-2 (84) and the Structured Interview of Reported Symptoms (85).

SUBSTANCE ABUSE TREATMENT APPROACHES IN CORRECTIONS

Motivational Interviewing

Motivational interviewing (MI; also referred to as motivational enhancement therapy [MET]) is a counseling approach designed to increase client motivation and readiness to change, (65,86) and is based in part upon the Transtheoretical Model of Stages of Change (64). MI is designed to help move clients from earlier stages (i.e., precontemplation and contemplation) to later stages of change (i.e., preparation and action) by increasing their motivation, commitment, and readiness for change. MI has a strong research base to support its effectiveness in community treatment, and has also been adapted successfully with criminal justice populations (87). Many offenders with substance use disorders are initially coerced into treatment by the court or correctional system, and may have little internal motivation to stop their addictive behaviors. MI encourages exploration and resolution of ambivalence about behavioral change, which is particularly useful in work with substance-involved offenders, who have high initial resistance to change (87). Thus, MI is useful to assist inmates in developing readiness and commitment to make lifestyle changes.

Cognitive Skills Training and Criminal Thinking

Cognitive skills interventions such as rational emotive–behavioral therapy (88) have emerged as significant treatments for a range of psychosocial disorders. These approaches recognize that behavioral problems are often rooted in distorted thought processes, such as rationalizations to engage in criminal or addictive behavior. Cognitive skills interventions provide self-monitoring skills to identify maladaptive thoughts and learn how to replace or restructure them. These interventions have been successfully adapted for use with substance-abusing offenders (89). For example, treatment activities have focused on modifying long-standing criminal thinking patterns and values that are closely linked with substance-abuse problems.

Criminal thinking problems are characterized by denial, minimization, externalization of blame, and self-centeredness—distortions that are similar to those used by substance abusers. For example, offenders may attribute their criminal behavior solely to their substance abuse disorder, to which the individual has fallen "victim" (90). Specific treatment strategies include self-assessment exercises, regular self-monitoring through completion of "thinking logs," and identification of different types of criminal thought patterns.

Relapse Prevention

The relapse prevention model (91) was developed to help prevent substance abusers who have become abstinent from returning to full-blown use. Because many substance-abusing offenders have a history of multiple prior relapses and unsuccessful attempts to maintain abstinence, relapse prevention is an important component of treatment in criminal justice settings, and has been implemented effectively in such settings (92). For many substance-involved offenders, incarceration may provide one of the first opportunities to experience an extended period of abstinence. Despite having relapsed frequently in the past, offenders are not typically aware of how the relapse process occurs and typically have few strategies for dealing with their high-risk situations for relapse.

Relapse prevention techniques combine elements of cognitive therapies, behavioral skill training, and lifestyle change to assist offenders in developing effective coping skills to maintain abstinence. Self-management strategies are developed, such as self-assessment of prior relapse episodes and learning ways to counteract relapse antecedents (e.g., negative emotions, drug cravings, social pressure to use), including learning drug-refusal skills. Prior to release, it is important to help offenders develop a relapse prevention plan that may include emergency coping skills used to deal with unexpected high-risk situations, strategies for avoiding high-risk situations (including neighborhoods and persons associated with the offender's prior substance abuse), and peer supports such as 12-step groups and sponsors. Relapse prevention plans may also address issues related to living arrangements (e.g., living with known substance abusers), employment, methods to cope with stress, warning signs for relapse, managing cravings and urges to use, and time management to maintain lifestyle balance.

Co-occurring Mental Health and Substance Abuse Disorders

An estimated 3% to 11% of jail and prison inmates have co-occurring substance use and major mental disorders (9,10,93–95). Incarcerated offenders with co-occurring disorders have more pronounced psychosocial problems than do other offenders in areas of employment, social skills and social supports, cognitive functioning, and adjustment to incarceration (13). Because of the absence of community services for persons with severe and persistent mental illness, and as a result of fragmented mental health and substance abuse service systems, many offenders with co-occurring disorders repeatedly cycle through the criminal justice system (96).

Co-occurring disorders frequently are undetected in jails and prisons (60). The resulting lack of treatment for one or both disorders contributes to poor treatment outcomes (97), which are often misattributed to client resistance, lack of motivation, or to staff or programmatic factors.

The American Psychiatric Association (60) has outlined the following treatment strategies for effective treatment of co-occurring disorders in criminal justice settings:

- Treatment should be integrated and focus concurrently on both substance use and mental disorders.
- Both types of disorders must be considered "primary," and treatment activities should provide greater understanding of how the disorders interact.
- Comprehensive assessment should lead to development of an individualized treatment plan, which should include input from the inmate and family members if available, and should address specific psychosocial problems and skill deficiencies.
- Intensity, length, and types of services should also be tailored to the specific correctional setting.
- Prescribed medications should be administered with caution, due to their potential interaction with substance use. If possible, inmates who have not previously been prescribed psychiatric medications should be provided a reasonable period of detoxification prior to beginning a trial on medication, unless psychotic or suicidal symptoms are present.
- Treatment must be extended into the community, with special attention to discharge/aftercare planning, and should include ways to address ongoing treatment needs, housing and employment needs, reconnection with the family, and development of support networks, including self-help groups.

In the last several years, a number of treatment programs for co-occurring disorders have been developed in state prisons and in the Federal Bureau of Prisons (13). Typically, such programs provide structured, intensive treatment activities in several phases, with gradually less-intensive services provided over time. Phases of treatment often include an orientation phase focused on motivation and engagement in treatment. This is followed by a more intensive treatment phase, with a final phase focused on relapse prevention, discharge planning, and transition services. In-prison co-occurring disorders treatment programs often consist of therapeutic communities that are modified to provide a longer period of treatment, a focus on psychoeducational and skill-building approaches, shorter duration of individual and group treatment sessions, and smaller staff caseloads (13). Such programs are less confrontative and provide more individual counseling and support in comparison to traditional correctional treatment programs (98,99).

Several programs have also been developed in recent years to divert inmates with co-occurring disorders from jail (96). Prebooking jail diversion programs provide coordination between law enforcement and community mental health and substance abuse treatment agencies and often include mobile crisis response teams that intervene in emergency situations when requested by law enforcement. Postbooking jail diversion programs involve arrangements between courts, defenders and prosecutors, probation agencies, and community mental health/substance abuse treatment agencies to identify and refer offenders who are eligible for community treatment as a condition of their sentence. Postbooking diversion programs help to identify eligible cases, and to negotiate with prosecutors and defense counsel regarding treatment alternatives to incarceration. Common elements of postbooking diversion programs include (a) screening and assessment of mental and substance use disorders, (b) counseling, (c) discharge planning, (d) "boundary spanning" staff who link the mental health, substance abuse, and criminal justice systems, (e) referral to community treatment, and (f) postrelease monitoring in the community (100).

Therapeutic Communities

The therapeutic community approach was developed more than 30 years ago as a long-term residential treatment for individuals with chronic and severe drug problems. The TC is based on development of a peer recovery community that promotes behavior change through a variety of social learning experiences (101). There is considerable research to support the effectiveness of TCs in reducing substance abuse and crime, and many TCs have been implemented effectively in prison settings (102). Although TCs vary widely in size and client demographics, they feature lengthy involvement in treatment, and have a similar programmatic structure, staffing pattern, theoretical perspective, and daily treatment regimen (102).

Within TC programs, substance abuse is viewed as a disorder of the whole person, which affects all areas of functioning. TCs focus on development of basic skills (e.g., social skills) that may have never been fully learned (102), and recovery is seen as involving major changes in lifestyle, behavior, and identity. While offenders usually enter TCs under coercion from the criminal justice system, these programs attempt to instill internal commitment to recovery through peer and staff feedback, and through other self-help and social learning experiences.

CORRECTIONAL SUBSTANCE ABUSE TREATMENT PROGRAMS

Over the past 25 years, a wide range of substance abuse treatment programs have been developed for correctional settings. Such programs are typically more comprehensive in prisons than in jails, as prisons often have more resources, provide longer periods of confinement, and offer a broader range of institutional settings than jails. Although numerous treatment program descriptions are available in the literature for both jails (15,45,103) and prisons (33,52,104–107), several of the more comprehensive treatment systems are reviewed in the following section.

Federal Bureau of Prisons

The Federal Bureau of Prisons (BOP) has a long history of providing substance abuse treatment (34). The BOP substance abuse treatment services employ a biopsychosocial approach, which focuses on modification of values, attitudes, and cognitive patterns associated with criminal behavior and substance abuse. Substance abuse treatment is provided at different levels of intensity, followed by postrelease transitional services in the community. To be eligible for residential treatment, inmates must volunteer and have a *Diagnostic and Statistical Manual of Mental Disorders,* 4th ed. (*DSM–IV*) diagnosis of substance dependence or abuse. Participants are housed in units that are isolated from the general prison population. Treatment services are provided for up to 10 months and include at least 500 hours of substance abuse treatment. Services provided include individual and group therapy, as well as psychoeducational approaches to help inmates develop positive coping skills and interpersonal skills, and cognitive restructuring techniques such as rational behavior therapy (RBT). Inmates enrolled in nonresidential treatment services are not separated from the general prison population. Services include individualized assessment and treatment planning, as well as individual and group therapy that addresses relapse prevention and restructuring of cognitive errors associated with criminal behavior and substance abuse.

Florida Department of Corrections

The Florida Department of Corrections (FDC) has provided prison-based substance abuse program services since the 1970s (15,108,109), which are located in major correctional institutions, as well as work and forestry camps, work-release centers, and road prisons (110). Long-term residential TCs are housed in isolated treatment units and provide 9 to 12 months of services. TC participants are encouraged to earn better jobs, greater privileges, and higher status through adhering to community rules and values, full participation in treatment activities, and commitment to recovery goals. Through multiple opportunities to learn from the consequences of their behaviors, these highly structured TCs help inmates to develop personal accountability and responsibility, self-discipline, and consistency. Structured TC activities are provided 7 days per week for a minimum of 60 hours weekly. Several TCs have also been designed for inmates who have co-occurring mental health and substance use disorders. These programs range in duration from 8 to 12 months, and include specialized psychoeducational skills groups, psychiatric medication and consultation services, group and individual counseling, relapse prevention, and transition services.

Intensive outpatient services are also provided by the FDC over a period of 4 to 6 months. At least 12 hours of program activities are provided weekly for a minimum of 4 days per week. In addition, nonintensive outpatient and reentry/transitional services are available and are intended primarily for inmates who were not released from custody after completion of the intensive outpatient or residential programs.

Oregon Department of Corrections

The Oregon Department of Corrections (ODC) has developed a linked, computerized tracking system to ensure that inmates are matched to services that meet their needs (15). Three TCs provide services for inmates with severe substance use disorders and extensive criminal histories. Inmates are admitted to these programs during the last 9 to 12 months of their incarceration, so that they may transition directly from treatment to the community. These TCs have small staff caseloads and provide approximately 30 hours of services per week. One TC provides specialized treatment for sex offenders with substance abuse disorders, while the other two are designed for inmates with severe substance use disorders, high levels of criminality, and moderately severe co-occurring mental disorders.

Two additional TCs have been modified to meet the needs of inmates with co-occurring mental disorders. These programs use a slower pace of treatment and provide fewer hours of core services per week (12 to 15 hours) than the other TCs. The ODC also operates three prerelease day treatment programs that are available to inmates during the last 6 to 7 months of their sentence. These programs provide 12 to 15 weekly hours of treatment services, and feature a bilingual, bicultural Spanish-English program that admits primarily Spanish-speaking inmates. To increase the likelihood of inmate involvement in aftercare services, these programs also facilitate "in-reach" linkage services with substance abuse treatment staff in the community, who establish contact with inmates prior to release.

CORRECTIONAL TREATMENT OUTCOME RESEARCH

A large number of prison and jail treatment outcome studies have been conducted and are summarized in several recent reviews (15,22,24,111). These studies provide strong evidence for the effectiveness of prison-based TCs (112–118) and other intensive prison-based treatment programs (119,120) in reducing relapse and recidivism. A recent meta-analysis of the correctional treatment literature also indicates the effectiveness of long-term prison-based TCs in reducing criminal recidivism (111). The meta-analysis found that approaches such as cognitive–behavioral therapies, methadone maintenance, and 12-step programs are promising approaches, but require additional research to establish their effectiveness in correctional settings. The study did not support the effectiveness of boot camps and "drug-focused group-counseling" programs. One recent study indicated that offenders diagnosed with antisocial personality disorder had positive outcomes similar to those of other offenders, following enrollment in community-based TC programs (121,122).

Compared to the relatively large body of outcome research evaluating prison substance abuse treatment programs, far fewer studies have focused on jail-based treatment programs. An inherent difficulty in conducting research in jails is that treatment programs are typically much shorter than those in prisons, which limits the type of services and program models that can be examined. Furthermore, many inmates released from prison are subsequently followed on parole, while people are released from jails to a wide array of settings and systems (e.g., state prison, probation), and many are lost to further contact. Nevertheless, a number of studies provide consistent evidence for the effectiveness of jail substance abuse treatment programs in reducing substance use relapse and criminal recidivism, and in extending the length of time that participants remain arrest-free in the community (103,123–130).

Research indicates that involvement in postrelease community treatment services improves the likelihood of positive outcomes for both prison and jail treatment participants (112–114,116,131–133). Additionally, longer treatment duration appears to improve outcomes for participants in both prison (134,135) and jail programs (103,127,136,137). The optimal length of treatment may be somewhat shorter in jails (1.5 to 5 months) (127,137) than in prisons (9 to 12 months) (135), although more research is needed in this area.

The cost-effectiveness of intensive prison TC programs was demonstrated in a recent study, (138), although only when postrelease aftercare treatment was provided. Intensive TC services were also found to be the most cost-effective for offenders who are at high risk of criminal recidivism. Jail treatment programs have also been found to yield considerable cost savings related to reductions in criminal recidivism and reincarceration. Annual savings are estimated at $156,000 to $1.4 million per program (125,139). Because there are numerous potential outcome variables to examine, treatment efficacy research is challenging, and it is hazardous to recommend programs solely on the basis of cost effectiveness. Nevertheless, the consistently positive findings from the correctional outcome literature indicate that these programs are a wise investment, and reflect sound public policy.

IMPLEMENTATION OF PRISON AND JAIL TREATMENT SERVICES

There are numerous challenges in implementing correctional substance abuse treatment services in correctional settings (15,140). Some correctional and treatment staff view substance abuse as a "moral weakness" rather than a biobehavioral problem that is amenable to treatment. As such, substance abuse treatment is seen by these staff as ineffective or merely delaying inmates' inevitable return to drugs and crime. Rationalization of criminal behavior is also a key component of ingrained criminal value systems (89,90), and treatment participants are often suspected of using their prior substance abuse experiences to rationalize and minimize the importance of criminal behavior. In reality, intensive substance abuse treatment programs in jails and prison can effectively identify and change patterns of criminal thinking and behaviors, and in this capacity are similar to long-term residential treatment programs in the community.

Program Funding and Administrative Support

Only limited funding and staff support are provided to many substance abuse programs in jails and prisons. For example, a national survey found that volunteer staff outnumbered salaried staff by a 2:1 ratio within jail treatment programs (29). Treatment in many correctional settings consists primarily of 12-step programs (e.g., AA or NA groups) or other peer support and peer-directed activities (52). In many other settings, programs that previously had adequate funding to support comprehensive treatment have been stripped of funding as a consequence of budget cutbacks or lack of administrative support (15). Administrative support may be compromised through transfer or retirement of facility administrators (e.g., prison wardens or superintendents), or through changes in political leadership at the state or local level. In many jails and prisons, professional advancement of correctional staff is contingent on their routine transfer to different units within the facility or to other institutions (141). Although this practice provides exposure to a range of different institutional settings, it can also undermine the stability and support for treatment programs. In attempts to overcome this problem, several treatment programs have worked closely with correctional administrators to develop a new professional "tier" for correctional officers that allows for specialized training and permanent assignment to substance abuse treatment units (141).

Structural Challenges

Recruitment of professional staff with training and experience in substance abuse treatment is often difficult in correctional settings. Correctional facilities are often sited in rural, remote areas that are underserved by health care professionals, and that are far from educational institutions. Some correctional systems provide substance abuse treatment services through contract providers, who are sometimes better able to recruit staff to these remote locations. Because of their location and undesirable working conditions, staff turnover is a frequent problem in many prison systems and jails. Research indicates that this turnover reduces the stability and effectiveness of correctional treatment programs, particularly when this occurs among experienced staff and in more recently established programs (141,142). Staff burnout and morale can also be problematic in correctional settings (21).

An isolated housing unit is vitally important for delivering effective substance abuse services in jails and prisons (143). Treatment gains established by program participants are sometimes undermined by inmates who are not enrolled in treatment, and treatment participants who are not separated from the general inmate population are subject to the corrosive effects of their attitudes, values, and behaviors (21). Participants in correctional treatment are sometimes ostracized by "general population" inmates, and under these conditions, it is quite difficult to establish a cohesive therapeutic environment. Effective correctional treatment programs typically include living quarters, dining area, and recreational activities that are isolated from the general correctional population (13,15).

One general disadvantage to providing treatment in correctional institutions is that inmates are not exposed to the same environment (e.g., stressors, high-risk situations) as they are when they return to the community. Although it is difficult to realistically simulate some situations in jails and prisons, drug-coping skills can be taught and rehearsed. Therapeutic communities in correctional settings also provide an important opportunity for extensive peer and staff feedback related to ingrained patterns of "criminal thinking" and antisocial behavior.

Most jails and prisons were not designed architecturally to address the specific needs of substance abuse treatment services (21). As a result, many treatment programs must share meeting rooms with educational and other correctional services. Program space is often not "soundproof," and staff offices and meeting rooms are often located outside the main housing unit. Treatment services must fit within the regimented schedule of the institution, including daily "counts," in which all inmates are required to return to their cells. In many cases, inmates may select or be assigned to other programs (e.g., vocational and educational services, work assignments) that compete directly with substance abuse treatment, despite clear evidence of an inmate's substance abuse problems. Incentives such as wages or early release that are provided for involvement in institutional employment are often unavailable for participants in substance abuse treatment.

Transition to the Community

One of the most significant obstacles to effective substance abuse treatment services in correctional settings is the absence of coordinated aftercare and transition services in the community (15,52,144). A national survey of jail treatment programs found that only 44% of programs offered these services upon release (29). Similarly, few prisons provide comprehensive discharge planning and transition services. Although jails and prisons appropriately view their primary mission as ensuring inmate security within the institution, substance-involved offenders are very likely to relapse and return to the justice system if they don't receive ongoing treatment in the community (92,116). The most effective correctional treatment programs are those that combine treatment in the institution with treatment for at least 3 months following release to the community (115,116,132).

A related issue is that many inmates are released to the community with no further criminal justice supervision (e.g., probation or parole), and are unlikely to enter and remain in treatment under these conditions. One solution is to provide early release from correctional facilities with treatment involvement required as a condition of probation or parole supervision. Case management services can provide an important bridge to assist in successful reintegration of offenders to the community (21). These services are often initiated while the inmate is still in jail or prison, with community treatment staff and/or case managers visiting the institution to begin planning for involvement in ongoing treatment, peer support programs, transitional housing, vocational and educational services, and continuation of medications and other health care needs (144). A recent initiative funded by the U.S. Department of Justice is designed to develop reentry partnerships to assist drug-involved offenders in the transition to the community (145). These partnerships will establish links between correctional institutions, courts, community treatment agencies, community supervision services, law enforcement, other faith-based and neighborhood organizations, and other ancillary services.

Maintaining Professional Boundaries

Providing substance abuse services in jails and prisons requires that treatment staff maintain the trust of both inmates and correctional staff and administrators (143,146), which can be challenging at times to achieve. Inmate participants in treatment tend to value the advice of staff who have experienced addiction and recovery, and who are willing to talk about these experiences. In contrast, correctional staff frequently express mistrust of former addicts, and are trained not to discuss their own problems, including those related to alcohol and drug abuse. This practice stems in part from the need for correctional staff members to maintain emotional distance between themselves and inmates, so as to ensure objectivity and fairness in dealing with inmates. Taken to the extreme, the need to maintain distance from inmates can lead to coldness, disrespect, and tension between staff and inmates. For treatment staff working in jails and prisons, it is important to assist correctional staff to see addicts as human beings deserving of respect and even empathy. On the other hand, inmates must never doubt that clinicians are corrections employees, and will carry out their responsibilities despite their respect for the inmates they treat.

Inmates sometimes attempt to gain the allegiance of treatment staff (147), or to compromise or manipulate treatment staff (148,149). For example, inmates may offer a secret on the condition that it not be repeated to others. If the secret is one that would legally require a report (e.g., planned escape, child abuse) the staff must decide between breaking a promise and breaking the law. When an inmate offers to trade information for an absolute promise of confidentiality, the answer should always be "no." Basic guidelines for correctional treatment staff include avoiding lying, avoiding promises that can't be kept, and ensuring the confidentiality of selected information (147).

Relationships Between Security and Treatment

Conflicts inevitably arise in jails and prisons between security and treatment staff, as a result of different perspectives on institutional safety, rehabilitation, sanctions, and the purpose of incarceration (141,147,149,150). It is important for staff working in jails and prisons to understand and appreciate these different professional cultures, values, and missions (151). Unfortunately, security has somehow become synonymous with punishment, and the misuse of this word is unfortunate. Security should mean safety for everyone who lives in, works at, or visits a jail or prison.

Experienced and competent correctional leaders know that correctional facilities are safest when the inmates are productively engaged, and therefore support treatment services. By the same token, experienced clinicians know that little learning or growth takes place unless the inmates are safe, and that institutional safety is the job of all paid staff within the correctional institution. By contributing to the institution's security, treatment staff are not betraying their clients, but are actually providing more effective services (21). When a jail or prison is not secure (i.e., unsafe), the most likely victims of violence are other inmates.

In addition to their traditional security obligations, correctional staff can make important contributions to treatment programs. Correctional staff have more frequent daily contact with inmates than treatment staff, and can provide valuable insights related to treatment planning, as well as information regarding inmate attitudes, functioning, and participation in community activities (150). In some facilities, correctional officers help to lead skills training groups, and are involved in community meetings, treatment planning, and discharge planning activities (147,152).

When conflicts arise with correctional officers or correctional administrators, treatment staff should avoid the temptation to view one side as "right" or "wrong (21,150). Treatment staff should recognize that their perspective is different than that of correctional staff, and that the objective of implementing treatment services is not to overcome the legitimate need of correctional administrators to preserve the security of the institution, but to find creative ways to meet inmates' needs in ways that contribute to the welfare and safety of the facility (150,153). By taking such a stance, treatment staff will quickly begin to be viewed as important institutional assets by administrators and correctional officers. In fact, treatment coordinators often become an integral part of the leadership team of correctional institutions (153). In contrast, treatment staff who view their role as one of protecting inmates from the institution and its custody staff will soon become marginalized and ineffective.

The best course of action in resolving conflict between treatment and custody staff is often some type of compromise between the two positions (21). Before any negotiation can occur, the respective sides must understand each other's legitimate concerns. This process will often lead to a third course of action that is seen as appropriate by both security and clinical staff, especially when it is clear that both groups share a commitment to safety within the institution. When forced to choose between the interests of treatment and security, correctional administrators will necessarily opt for enhanced security. Fortunately, most treatment programs are designed to support, rather than to compete with the goals of institutional security, and are recognized as among the safest, cleanest, and quietest units within jails and prisons (20). Effective correctional administrators are typically strong advocates for substance abuse treatment and other related inmate programs, because these services help to create a safer institution (150,154).

Some jail and prison treatment programs have found that use of joint coordinators from both treatment and corrections systems promotes more effective implementation of services (143). Joint coordinators can serve as an effective "bridge" between staff from both systems, and are engaged in program planning, debriefing critical incidents, training, and program modification. Cross-training activities involving substance abuse treatment, corrections, and mental health and other health care staff are quite useful in developing shared values and commitment to support correctional treatment programs (78,150, 155).

CONCLUSION

Prison and jail populations have grown tremendously over the past two decades as a result of an influx of drug-involved offenders to the criminal justice system. Well over half of jail and prison inmates have significant substance-abuse problems, although most have never participated in a comprehensive treatment program. Incarceration provides a significant opportunity to initiate treatment services for those with severe alcohol and drug problems. However, the treatment capacity in jails and prisons has not kept pace with the rising number of drug-involved inmates. In fact, our nation's correctional systems are now treating only a small fraction of inmates who need these services.

Many existing correctional treatment programs are limited to self-help and peer support activities (e.g., AA and NA groups), and are inadequate to address the pronounced behavioral, emotional, and psychiatric problems that are common among this population, and often do not provide key skills (e.g., employment, problem-solving, relapse prevention, interpersonal/social) that are necessary to make lifestyle changes and to maintain sobriety in the community. Although evidence-based substance abuse treatment techniques are available for female inmates and inmates with co-occurring mental disorders, few specialized programs in jails and prisons have been developed for these populations. Moreover, few services are available in most correctional systems to assist drug-involved inmates in making the difficult transition back to the community, and to ensure that offenders are enrolled in ongoing services once they are released from custody.

Several existing program models in prisons and jails feature a comprehensive treatment approach and a continuum of services from the correctional institution to the community. Convergent research findings during the past decade indicate that jail and prison treatment of sufficient intensity and duration (e.g., TC programs) can effectively reduce criminal recidivism and substance abuse in the community. An important corollary to these findings is that involvement in community treatment following participation in jail or prison is critical in ensuring the long-term maintenance of positive outcomes related to recidivism and substance abuse. Preliminary evidence suggests that jail and prison treatment programs are cost effective and pay significant dividends to society.

Further research is needed to examine alternatives to traditional TC treatment programs in jails and prisons, including those that are of high intensity, but moderate duration (i.e., 4 to 6 months). Research is also needed to identify methods of matching offenders with the appropriate type, duration, and intensity of treatment to maximize the clinical and financial benefits. Additional work is also needed to examine outcomes of specialized programs designed for "high-risk" inmates, such as those with co-occurring mental disorders. Several new reentry programs were recently funded by the U.S. Department of Justice that will help to determine the effectiveness of specialized case management services and other links to community treatment. Several reentry drug courts are also being implemented in sites around the country, and offer the promise of better coordination and monitoring of the transition process.

This chapter highlights the overwhelming need for substance abuse treatment services in correctional settings; the shortfall of services provided compared to need is almost impossible to exaggerate. Furthermore, while the failure to provide substance abuse treatment services may save money in the short-term, in the long-term it is a wasteful and ineffective public policy. Because correctional substance abuse treatment services are not required by existing case law, they have not been implemented to the same degree as mental health or other program services. However, it is of paramount importance that substance abuse treatment be made a top priority in our institutions and in our communities. To ignore this unmet need will only guarantee communities that are less safe and more wasteful of public resources and human lives.

REFERENCES

1. Bureau of Justice Statistics. US. Department of Justice, BJS home page, and social statistics briefing room: corrections facts at a glance, 2002. Available at: http://www.ojp.usdoj.gov/bjs/glance/corrtyp.htm.

2. Bureau of Justice Statistics. *National corrections population reaches new high: grows by 117,400 during 2000 to total 6.5 million adults.* Washington, DC: U.S. Department of Justice, 2001.

3. Office of National Drug Control Policy Drug Treatment in the Criminal Justice System. *Drug policy information clearinghouse: fact sheet.* Washington, DC: U.S. Department of Justice, 2001.

4. National Center on Addiction and Substance Abuse. *Shoveling up: the impact of substance abuse on state budgets.* New York: Columbia University, 2001.

5. Turner NR, Wilhelm DF. Are the politics of criminal justice changing? *Corrections Today* 2002;Dec:74–76.

6. California Legislative Analyst's Office. *Proposition 36*, 2000. Available at: http://www.lao.ca.gov/initiatives/2000/36_11_2000.html.

7. Wallenstein AM. Intake and release in evolving jail practice. In: Carlson PM, Garrett JS, eds. *Prison and jail administration: practice and theory.* Gaithersburg, MD: Aspen Publishers, 1999:49–58.

8. Council of State Governments Criminal Justice/Mental Health Consensus Project. Lexington, KY: 2002.

9. Abram KM, Teplin LA. Co-occurring disorders among mentally ill jail detainees: implications for public policy. *Am Psychol* 1991;46:1036–1045.

10. Teplin LA. The prevalence of severe mental disorder among urban male detainees: comparison with the epidemiologic catchment area program. *Am J Public Health* 1990;80(6):663–669.

11. Teplin LA. The prevalence of severe mental disorder among male urban jail detainees. *Am J Public Health* 1990;80:663–669.

12. Bureau of Justice Statistics. *Mental health and treatment of inmates and probationers. Special report.* Washington, DC: U.S. Department of Justice, 1999.

13. Edens JF, Peters RH, Hills HA. Treating prison inmates with co-occurring disorders: an integrative review of existing programs. *Behav Soc Sci Law* 1997;15:439–457.

14. Belenko S, Peugh J, Califano JA, et al. *Behind bars: substance abuse and America's prison population.* New York: Center on Addiction and Substance Abuse, Columbia University, 1998.

15. Peters RH, Matthews CO. Substance abuse treatment programs in prisons and jails. In: Fagan T, Ax R, eds. *Correctional mental health handbook.* Laurel, MD: Sage Publications, 2002:73–99.

16. Bureau of Justice Statistics. *Special report: drug use, testing, and treatment in jails.* Washington, DC: U.S. Department of Justice, 2000.

17. National Institute of Justice. *1999 Annual report on drug use among adult and juvenile arrestees. Arrestee Drug Abuse Monitoring Program.* Washington, DC: U.S. Department of Justice, 2000.

18. Peters RH, Greenbaum PE, Edens, JF, et al. Prevalence of *DSM-IV* substance abuse and dependence disorders among prison inmates. *Am J Drug Alcohol Abuse* 1998;24(4):573–587.

19. Robins LN, Regier DA. *Psychiatric disorders in America: the Epidemiologic Catchment Area Study.* New York: Free Press, 1991.

20. Lipton DS. The correctional opportunity: pathways to drug treatment for offenders. *J Drug Issues* 1994;24(2):331–348.

21. Center for Substance Abuse Treatment. Substance abuse treatment for adults in the criminal justice system. In: Peters RH, Wexler HK, eds. *Treatment improvement protocol (TIP).* Rockville, MD: Substance Abuse and Mental Health Services Administration, in press.

22. Peters RH, Matthews CO. Jail treatment for drug abusers. In: Leukefeld CG, Tims FM, Farabee D, eds. *Treatment of drug offenders: policies and issues.* New York: Springer Publishing, 2002:186–203.

23. Belenko S, Peugh J. Fighting crime by treating substance abuse. *Issues Sci Technol* 1998;Fall:53–60.

24. Lurigio AJ. Drug treatment availability and effectiveness: studies of the general and criminal justice populations. *Crim Just Behav* 2000;27(4):495–528.

25. Belenko S. *Behind bars: substance abuse and America's prison population.* New York: National Center on Addiction and Substance Abuse, Columbia University, 1998.

26. Simpson DD, Knight K, Pevoto C. *Research summary: focus on drug*

treatment in criminal justice settings. Ft. Worth, TX: Institute of Behavioral Research, Texas Christian University, 1996.

27. Substance Abuse and Mental Health Services Administration. *Substance abuse treatment in adult and juvenile correctional facilities: findings from the uniform facility data set 1997 survey of correctional facilities.* Rockville, MD: Author, 2000.

28. Substance Abuse and Mental Health Services Administration. *Substance abuse services and staffing in adult correctional facilities. The Drug and Alcohol Services Information System.* Rockville, MD: Author, 2002. Also available at: http://www.samhsa.gov/oas/2k2/justice/justice.htm.

29. Peters RH, May RL, Kearns WD. Drug treatment in jails: results of a nationwide survey. *J Crim Just* 1992;20(4):283–295.

30. Field GD. Historical trends of drug treatment in the criminal justice system. In: Leukefeld, CG, Tims FM, Farabee D, eds. *Treatment of drug offenders: policies and issues.* New York: Springer Publishing, 2002:9–21.

31. Deitch DA, Carleton S, Koutsenok IB, et al. Therapeutic community treatment in prisons. In: Leukefeld CG, Tims FM, Farabee D, eds. *Treatment of drug offenders: policies and issues.* New York: Springer Publishing, 2002:127–137.

32. Lipton DS. Prison-based therapeutic communities: their success with drug abusing offenders. *Natl Inst Just J* 1996:12–20.

33. Wexler HK, Lipton DS. From reform to recovery: advances in prison drug treatment. In: Inciardi J, ed. *Drug treatment and criminal justice.* Newbury Park, CA: Sage, 1993:209–227.

34. Weinman BA, Dignam JT. Drug-abuse treatment programs in the Federal Bureau of Prisons: past, present, and future directions. In: Leukefeld CG, Tims FM, Farabee D, eds. *Treatment of drug offenders: policies and issues.* New York: Springer Publishing, 2002:91–104.

35. Jacob J, Stover H. Drug use, drug control and drug services in German prisons: contradiction, insufficiencies and innovative approaches. In: Shewan D, Davies J, eds. *Drugs and prisons.* London: Harwood Academic Publishers, 2000:57–88.

36. Lightfoot LO. Treating substance abuse and dependence in offenders: a review of methods and outcomes. In: Latessa E, ed. *Strategic solutions: the International Community Corrections Association examines substance abuse.* Lanham, MD: American Correctional Association, 1999:43–80.

37. *Marshall v. United States,* 414 U.S. 417 (1974).

38. Cohen F. *The mentally disordered inmate and the law.* Kingston, NJ: Civic Research Institute, 1998.

39. *Pace v. Fauver,* 479 F. Supp. 456 (D.N.J. 1979).

40. *Palmigiano v. Garrahy,* 443 F. Supp. 956 (D.R.I. 1977).

41. *Pedraza v. Meyer,* 919 F.2d 317–319 (5th Cir. 1990).

42. *United States ex rel. Walker v. Fayette County, Pa.,* 599 F.2d 573, 575,576 (3d Cir. 1979).

43. *Wayne County Jail Inmates v. Lucas,* 216 N.W.2d 910 (Mich. 1974).

44. *Alberti v. Sheriff of Harris County, Texas,* 406 F. Supp. 649 (S.D. Tex. 1975).

45. Peters RH. Drug treatment in jails and detention settings. In: Inciardi J, ed. *Drug treatment and criminal justice.* Newbury Park, CA: Sage, 1993:44–80.

46. *Ruiz v. Estelle,* 503 F. Supp. 1265 (S.D. Tex. 1980).

47. Vaughn MS. Penal harm medicine: State tort remedies for delaying and denying healthcare to prisoners. *Crime Law Soc Change* 1999;31:273–302.

48. *Ferguson v. Perry,* 593 So.2d 273 (Fla. App. 5th Dist. 1992).

49. *Hart v. County of Orange,* 62 Cal. Rptr. 73 (Cal. App. 4th Dist. 1967).

50. *Griffin v. Coughlin,* 673 N.E. 2d 98 (N.Y. 1996).

51. *Kerr v. Farrey,* 95 F.3d 472 (7th Cir. 1996).

52. Peters RH, Steinberg ML. Substance abuse treatment services in U.S. prisons. In: Shewan D, Davies J, eds. *Drugs and prisons.* London: Harwood Academic, 2000:89–116.

53. National Commission on Correctional Health Care. *Standards for health services in jails.* Chicago: Author, 1996.

54. National Commission on Correctional Health Care. *Standards for health services in prisons.* Chicago: Author, 1997.

55. National Commission on Correctional Health Care. *Correctional mental health care: standards and guidelines for delivering services.* Chicago: Author, 1999.

56. American Correctional Association. *Standards for adult local detention facilities,* 3rd ed. Lanham, MD: Author, 1991.

57. American Correctional Association. *Standards supplement.* Lanham, MD: Author, 2002.

58. American Correctional Association. *Standards for adult correctional institutions,* 4th ed. Lanham, MD: Author, 2003.

59. American Psychiatric Association. *Practice guidelines.* Washington, DC: Author, 1996.

60. American Psychiatric Association. *Psychiatric services in jails and prisons: a task force report of the American Psychiatric Association,* 2nd ed. Washington, DC: Author, 2000.

61. Knight K, Simpson DD, Hiller M. Screening and referral for substance abuse treatment in the criminal justice system. In: Leukefeld CG, Tims, FM, Farabee DF, eds. *Clinical and policy responses to drug offenders.* New York: Springer Publishing, 2002:259–272.

62. Peters RH, Bartoi MG. *Screening and assessment of co-occurring disorders in the justice system.* Delmar, NY: National Gains Center, 1997.

63. Peters RH, Greenbaum PE, Steinberg ML, et al. Effectiveness of screening instruments in detecting substance use disorders among prisoners. *J Subst Abuse Treat* 2000;18:349–358.

64. Prochaska JO, DiClemente CC, Norcross JC. In search of how people change: Applications to addictive behaviors. *Am Psychol* 1992;47:1102–1114.

65. Miller WR, Rollnick S. *Motivational interviewing: preparing people for change,* 2nd ed. New York: Guilford Press, 2002.

66. McConnaughy EA, Prochaska JO, Velicer WF. Stages of change in psychotherapy: measurement and sample profiles. *Psychother Theory Res Pract* 1983;20:368–375.

67. DiClemente CC, Hughes SO. Stages of change profiles in outpatient alcoholism treatment. *J Subst Abuse* 1990;2:217–235.

68. Peters RH, Greenbaum PE. *Texas Department of Criminal Justice/Center for Substance Abuse Treatment prison substance abuse screening project.* Milford, MA: Civigenics, 1996.

69. DeLeon G, Jainchill N. Circumstance, motivation, readiness, and suitability as correlates of treatment tenure. *J Psychoactive Drugs* 1986;18:203–208.

70. Clements CB, McLearen AM. Research-based practice in corrections: a selective review. In: Fagan T, Ax R, eds. *Correctional mental health handbook.* Thousand Oaks, CA: Sage, 2003.

71. Rogers R. *Clinical assessment of malingering and deception,* 2nd ed. New York: Guilford Press, 1997.

72. Sierles FS. Correlates of malingering. *Behav Sci Law* 1984;2:113–118.

73. Wilson DJ. *Drug use, testing, and treatment in jails.* Bureau of Justice Statistics special report, NCJ Publication No. 179999. Washington, DC: National Criminal Justice Reference Service, 2000.

74. Haskett J. *Tehachapi malingering*

scale: research revision No. 5 manual. Modesto, CA: Logocraft, 1995.

75. Walters GD, White TW, Green RL. Use of the MMPI to identify malingering and exaggeration of psychiatric symptomatology in male prison inmates. *J Consult Clin Psychol* 1988;56:111–117.

76. Cornell DG, Hawk GL. Clinical presentation of malingerers diagnosed by experienced forensic psychologists. *Law Hum Behav* 1989;13:374–383.

77. Wasyliw OE, Grossman LS, Haywood T, et al. The detection of malingering in criminal forensic groups: MMPI validity scales. *J Personal Assess* 1988;52(2):321–333.

78. American Psychiatric Association. *Diagnostic and statistical manual of mental disorders,* 4th ed. (*DSM-IV*). Washington, DC: Author, 1994.

79. McLellan AT, Kushner H, Metzger D, et al. The fifth edition of the addiction severity index. *J Subst Abuse Treat* 1992;9:199–213.

80. Skinner H, Horn JL. *Alcohol dependence scale: user's guide.* Toronto: Addiction Research Foundation, 1984.

81. Center for Substance Abuse Treatment. *Simple screening instruments for outreach for alcohol and other drug abuse and infectious diseases. Treatment improvement protocol (TIP) series, #11.* Rockville, MD: U.S. Department of Health and Human Services, 1994.

82. Simpson DD, Knight K, Broome KM. *TCU/CJ forms manual: drug dependence screen and initial assessment.* Fort Worth, TX: Texas Christian University, Institute of Behavioral Research. TCU Drug Screen available online at www.ibr.tcu.edu or call 817—257—7226, 1997.

83. Miller GA. *The substance abuse subtle screening inventory (SASSI) manual.* Bloomington, IN: SASSI Institute, 1985.

84. Megargee EI. Using the MMPI-based classification system with the MMPI-2's of male prison inmates. *Psychol Assess* 1994;6:337–344.

85. Rogers R, Bagby RM, Dickens SE. *Structured interview of reported symptoms: professional manual.* Odessa, FL. Psychological Assessment Resources, 1992.

86. Miller W, Rollnick S. *Motivational interviewing: preparing people to change addictive behavior.* New York: Guilford Press, 1991.

87. Ginsburg J, Mann R, Rotgers F, et al. Motivational interviewing with criminal justice populations. In: Miller W, Rollnick S, eds. *Motivational interviewing: preparing people for change,* 2nd ed. New York: Guilford Press, 2002.

88. Ellis A, MacLaren C. *Rational emotive behavior therapy: a therapist's guide.* Atascadero, CA: Impact Publishers, 1998.

89. Wanberg KW, Milkman HB. *Criminal conduct and substance abuse treatment.* Thousand Oaks, CA: Sage Publications, 1998.

90. Yochelson S, Samenow SE. *The criminal personality. Volume III: the drug user.* Jason Aronson, Northvale, New Jersey, 1986.

91. Marlatt GA, Gordon JR. *Relapse prevention.* New York: Guilford Press, 1985.

92. Gorski TT, Kelly JM, Havens L, et al., eds. *Relapse prevention and the substance-abusing criminal offender: an executive briefing.* Rockville, MD: Center for Substance Abuse Treatment, 1994.

93. National GAINS Center. *The prevalence of co-occurring mental and substance abuse disorders in the criminal justice system. Just the Facts.* Delmar, NY: 1997.

94. Peters RH, Hills HA. Inmates with co-occurring substance abuse and mental health disorders. In: Steadman H J, Cocozza JJ, eds. *Providing services for offenders with mental illness and related disorders in prisons.* Washington, DC: National Coalition for the Mentally Ill in the Criminal Justice System, 1993: 159–212.

95. Teplin LA, Abram KM, McClelland GM. Prevalence of psychiatric disorders among incarcerated women: I. Pretrial jail detainees. *Arch Gen Psychiatry* 1996;53:505–512.

96. National GAINS Center. *Jail diversion: knowledge development and application program.* Rockville, MD: Substance Abuse and Mental Health Services Administration, 1998.

97. Drake RE, Alterman AI, Rosenberg SR. Detection of substance use disorders in severely mentally ill patients. *Commun Ment Health* 1993;29:175–192.

98. McLaughlin P, Pepper P. Modifying the therapeutic community for the mentally ill substance abuser. *New Direct Ment Health Serv* 1991;50:85–93.

99. Sacks S, Sacks J. *Recent advances in theory, prevention, and research for dual disorder.* Paper presented at the Middle Eastern Institute on Drug Abuse, Jerusalem, 1995.

100. Conly C. Coordinating community services for mentally ill offenders: Maryland's community criminal justice treatment program. *Am Jails* 1999;Mar-Apr:9–16, 99–114.

101. DeLeon G. Therapeutic communities for addictions: theoretical framework. *Int J Addict* 1995;30:1603–1645.

102. De Leon G. Therapeutic communities. In: Galanter M, Kleber HD, eds. *2nd ed.* Washington, DC: American Psychiatric Association, 1999.

103. Tunis S, Austin J, Morris M, et al. *Evaluation of drug treatment in local corrections.* Washington, DC: National Institute of Justice, 1996.

104. Early KE. *Drug treatment behind bars: prison-based strategies for change.* Westport, CT: Praeger, 1996.

105. Inciardi JA. *Drug treatment and criminal justice.* Newbury Park, CA: Sage, 1993.

106. Leukefeld CG, Tims FM. *Drug treatment in prisons and jails.* Rockville, MD: National Institute on Drug Abuse, 1992.

107. Wellisch J, Prendergast ML, Anglin MD. *Drug-abusing women offenders: results of a national survey. Research in brief.* Washington, DC: National Institute of Justice, 1994:1–19.

108. Chaiken M. *In-prison programs for drug-involved offenders.* Washington, DC: U.S. Department of Justice, 1989.

109. Florida Department of Corrections. Substance Abuse Program Services Office: Comprehensive report. Tallahassee: Author, 1995.

110. Florida Department of Corrections. Community corrections and institutional substance abuse program services. Tallahassee: Author, 2000.

111. Pearson FS, Lipton DS. A meta-analytic review of the effectiveness of corrections-based treatments for drug abuse. The Prison Journal 1999;79:384–410.

112. Butzin C, Martin S, Inciardi J. Evaluating component effects of a prison-based treatment continuum. Journal of substance abuse treatment 2001;22:63–69.

113. Inciardi J, Martin S, Butzin C, Hooper R, Harrison L. An effective model of prison-based treatment for drug-involved offenders. *J Drug Issues* 1997;27:261–278.

114. Knight K, Simpson D, Chatham L, et al. An assessment of prison-based drug treatment: Texas's in-prison therapeutic community program. *J Offend Rehabil* 1997;24:75–100.

115. Knight K, Simpson DD, Hiller ML. Three-year reincarceration outcomes for in-prison therapeutic community treatment in Texas. *Prison J* 1999;79(3):337–351.

116. Martin S, Butzin C, Saum C, et al. Three-year outcomes of therapeutic community treatment for drug-involved offenders in Delaware: from prison to work release to aftercare. *Prison J* 1999;79:294–320.

117. Wexler H, Melnick G, Lowe L, et al. Three-year reincarceration outcomes for amity in-prison therapeutic

community and aftercare in California. *Prison J* 1999;79:321–336.

118. Wexler HK, Melnick G, Lowe L, et al. Three-year reincarceration outcomes for amity in-prison therapeutic community and aftercare in California. *Prison J* 1999;79(3):321–336.

119. Pelissier B, Rhodes W, Saylor W, et al. *TRIAD drug treatment evaluation project: final report of three-year outcomes—part 1.* Washington, DC: Federal Bureau of Prisons, Office of Research and Evaluation, 2000.

120. Pelissier B, Wallace S, O'Neil J, et al. Federal prison residential drug treatment reduces substance use and arrests after release. *Am J Drug Alcohol Abuse* 2001;27:315–337.

121. Messina N, Wish E, Nemes S. Therapeutic community treatment for substance abusers with antisocial personality disorder. *J Subst Abuse Treat* 1999;17:121–128.

122. Messina N, Wish E, Hoffman J, et al. Antisocial personality disorder and TC treatment outcomes. *Am J Drug Alcohol Abuse* 2002;28:197–212.

123. Barron N, Finnigan M. *Self-report and system-report of arrests for alcohol/drug clients in the Target City context of assessment and referral to alcohol and drug treatment [Ministudy].* Portland, OR: Multnomah County, Portland Target City Project, 1999.

124. Finigan M, Barron N, Carey S. Effectively assessing and preparing inmates for community substance abuse treatment: the Portland target cities project in-jail intervention. In: Stephens R, Scott C, Muck R, eds. *Clinical assessment and substance abuse treatment: the target cities experience.* Albany, New York: SUNY Press (*in press*).

125. Hughey R, Klemke LW. Evaluation of a jail-based substance abuse treatment program. *Fed Probation* 1996;60(4):40–44.

126. Peters RH, Kearns WD, Murrin MR, et al. Examining the effectiveness of in-jail substance abuse treatment. *J Offend Rehabil* 1993;19(3/4):1–39.

127. Santiago L, Beauford J, Campt D, et al. *SISTER project final evaluation report: Sisters in Sober Treatment Empowered in Recovery, San Francisco County Sheriff's Office Department.* San Francisco: University of California, San Francisco, Clearinghouse for Drug-Exposed Children, 1996.

128. Taxman FS, Spinner DL. *The jail addiction services (JAS) project in Montgomery County, Maryland: overview of results from a 24-month follow-up study.* College Park, MD: University of Maryland, 1996.

129. Tucker TC. *Outcome evaluation of the Detroit target cities jail based substance abuse treatment program.* Detroit, MI: Wayne County Department of Community Justice, 1998.

130. Windell P, Barron N. Treatment preparation in the context of system coordination serves inmates well. *J Psychoactive Drugs* 2002;34:59–67.

131. Hiller M, Knight K, Simpson D. Prison-based substance abuse treatment, residential aftercare, and recidivism. *Addiction* 1999;94:833–842.

132. Wexler HK, Melnick G, Lowe L, et al. Three-year reincarceration outcomes for amity in-prison therapeutic community and aftercare in California. *Prison J* 1999;79(3):321–336.

133. Porporino F, Robinson D, Millson B, et al. An outcome evaluation of prison-based treatment programming for substance users. *Subst Use Misuse* 2002;37:1047–1077.

134. Siegal H, Wang J, Carlson R, et al. Ohio's prison-based therapeutic community treatment programs for substance abusers: preliminary analysis of re-arrest data. *J Offend Rehabil* 1999;28:33–48.

135. Wexler HK, Falkin GP, Lipton DS. Outcome evaluation of a prison therapeutic community for substance abuse treatment. *Crim Just Behav* 1990;17:71–92.

136. Swartz JA, Lurigio AJ. Final thoughts on IMPACT: a federally funded, jail-based, drug-user-treatment program. *Subst Use Misuse* 1999;34:887–906.

137. Swartz JA, Lurigio AJ, Slomka SA. The impact of IMPACT: an assessment of the effectiveness of a jail-based treatment program. *Crime Delinquency* 1996;42:553–573.

138. Griffith J, Hiller M, Knight K, et al. A cost-effectiveness analysis of in-prison therapeutic community treatment and risk classification. *Prison J* 1999;79:352–368.

139. Center for Substance Abuse Research. Washington county explores a structure for success. *CESAR Rep* 1992;2(2):1, 5.

140. Leukefeld CG, Tims FM, Farabee D, eds. *Treatment of drug offenders: policies and issues.* New York: Springer Publishing, 2002.

141. Farabee D, Prendergast M, Cartier J, et al. Barriers to implementing effective correctional drug treatment programs. *Prison J* 1999;79(2):150–162.

142. Petersilia J. Conditions that permit intensive supervision programs to survive. *Crime Delinquency* 1990;36(1):126–145.

143. Center for Substance Abuse Treatment. *Critical elements in developing effective jail-based drug treatment programming.* Rockville, MD: Substance Abuse and Mental Health Service Administration, 1996.

144. Center for Substance Abuse Treatment. *Continuity of offender treatment for substance use disorders from institution to community. Treatment improvement protocol (TIP) series #30.* Rockville, MD: 1998.

145. Travis J, Solomon AL, Waul M. *From prison to home: the dimensions and consequences of prisoner reentry.* Washington, DC: The Urban Institute, Justice Policy Center, 2001.

146. Wellisch J, Anglin MD, Prendergast ML. Treatment strategies for drug-abusing women offenders. In: Inciardi J, ed. *Drug treatment and criminal justice.* Newbury Park: Sage, 1993:5–29.

147. Metzner JL. An introduction to correctional psychiatry: part III. *J Am Acad Psychiatry Law* 1998;26 (1):107–115.

148. Allen B, Bosta D. *Games criminals play: how you can profit by knowing them.* Sacramento, CA: Rae John Publishers, 1981.

149. Robey A. Analysis and commentary: stone walls do not a prison psychiatrist make. *J Am Acad Psychiatry Law* 1998;26(1):101–105.

150. Appelbaum KL, Hickey JM, Packer I. The role of correctional officers in multidisciplinary mental health care in prisons. *Psychiatr Servi* 2001;52(10):1343–1347.

151. Faiver KL. Organizational issues: corrections and health care: working together. In: Faiver KL, ed. *Health care management issues in corrections.* Lanham, MD: American Correctional Association, 1998.

152. Condelli WS, Dvoskin JA, Holanchock H. Intermediate care programs for inmates with psychiatric disorders. *Bull Am Acad Psychiatry Law* 1994;22:63–70.

153. Bush CD, Hecht FR, LaBarbara M, et al. *Drug treatment in the jail setting: national demonstration program.* Washington, DC: Bureau of Justice Assistance, 1993.

154. Steadman HJ, McCarty DW, Morrissey JP. Scope and frequency of conflict between mental health and correctional staffs. In: *The mentally ill in jail: planning for essential services.* New York: Guilford Press, 1989.

155. Griffin PA, Hills H, Peters RH. Mental illness and substance abuse in offenders: overcoming barriers to successful collaboration between substance abuse, mental health, and criminal justice staff. In: *Criminal justice-substance abuse cross-training: working together for change.* Rockville, MD: Center for Substance Abuse Treatment, 1996.

CHAPTER 47

Cognitive and Behavioral Therapies

LISA M. NAJAVITS AND BRUCE S. LIESE,
AND MELANIE S. HARNED

Psychotherapies that focus primarily on individuals' thoughts and behaviors are generally known as cognitive–behavioral therapies (CBTs). There have been many different CBT approaches; some have attended mostly to cognitive processes, some have attended mostly to behavioral processes, and others have been equally attentive to both. CBT is typically active, structured, directive, focused, and present-oriented. Dobson and Block (1) reviewed the historical and philosophical bases of CBT. They credit Ellis (2) and Beck (3) with introducing the first CBT (rational emotive therapy and cognitive therapy, respectively), and they cite other important early contributors (4–11).

Early applications of CBT were to depression (12), anxiety (13), and various other problems, including anger, stress, somatic disorders, sexual dysfunction, and pain (14,15). More recently, CBT has been applied to such complex problems as personality disorders (16–18), schizophrenia (19,20), crisis intervention (21,22), and suicidal behavior (23). Consistent with this focus on more complex problems, CBT has increasingly been applied to substance abuse (24–31). Two major multisite, randomized, controlled studies of substance abuse included CBT as main treatment conditions (32,33). This chapter reviews three theories of CBT for substance abuse, discusses principles of treatment, and describes techniques.

COGNITIVE–BEHAVIORAL THEORIES OF SUBSTANCE ABUSE

The application of cognitive–behavioral theory to substance abuse is relatively recent. For most of the twentieth century until the mid-1980s, the field of psychotherapy largely ignored substance abuse, viewing it as a superficial symptom of more important underlying problems (34). As substance abuse became more widely recognized, interest in developing effective treatments increased.

This section describes three major cognitive–behavioral theories of substance abuse: *relapse prevention*, *cognitive therapy*, and *behavioral learning theory*. These theories provide the conceptual foundation for treatment strategies discussed later in the chapter. All of these theories make the following assumptions:

1. Substance abuse is mediated by complex cognitive and behavioral processes.

2. Substance abuse and associated cognitive–behavioral processes are, to a large extent, learned.
3. Substance abuse and associated cognitive–behavioral processes can be modified, particularly by means of CBT.
4. A major goal of CBT for substance abuse is to teach coping skills to resist substance use and to reduce the problems associated with substance abuse.
5. CBT requires comprehensive case conceptualization that serves as the basis for selecting specific CBT techniques.
6. To be effective, CBT must be provided in the context of warm, supportive, collaborative therapeutic relationships.

Relapse Prevention

Most CBT is derived at least in part from the work of Marlatt and Gordon (27). Their relapse prevention model is important for several reasons: it was the first major CBT approach to substance abuse; it provides practical, flexible interventions that can be applied by a wide range of clinicians; it can be used adjunctively with other treatments; and, it provides a straightforward conceptual model for understanding substance abuse. Their sensitive descriptions of substance abusers' subjective experiences, as well as their clear articulation of a theoretical model and specific interventions, have contributed to making Marlatt and Gordon's text the seminal CBT work on substance abuse (35,36). Some popular relapse prevention techniques include the identification and avoidance of high-risk situations, exploration of the decision chain leading to drug use, lifestyle modification (e.g., choosing friends who do not use), and learning from "slips" to prevent future relapses. Originally developed for substance abuse, relapse prevention has since been adapted for a variety of psychological problems (37,38).

According to Marlatt and Gordon (27), the potential for relapse begins with a high-risk situation, defined as any circumstance "that poses a threat to the individual's sense of control and increases the risk of potential relapse" (39, p. 37). The most common high-risk situations are negative emotional states, interpersonal conflicts, and social pressure (40). Individuals with effective coping responses (e.g., substance refusal skills) are most likely to develop self-efficacious beliefs (i.e., self-confidence) about their abilities to refrain from substance use. Self-efficacy, in turn, decreases their probability of relapse. In contrast, individuals without effective coping responses have decreased self-efficacy regarding their abilities to resist substance use. They are more likely to expect positive effects from initial substance use. Decreased self-efficacy and positive outcome expectancies lead to initial substance use (i.e., a "slip"), which may lead to the abstinence violation effect (AVE). The AVE is the often-seen cognitive phenomenon in which a single slip becomes the basis of a full-blown relapse ("I've had one drink, so I might as well give up on recovery altogether").

Cognitive Therapy of Substance Abuse

Cognitive therapy of substance abuse (24,41–44) is based on the same basic principles as cognitive therapy for other problems, such as depression (12), anxiety (13), and personality disorders (16). In cognitive therapy of substance abuse, the focus is on the complex behaviors that derive from substance-related beliefs, automatic thoughts, and facilitating beliefs. Complex behaviors involve the consumption of substances as well as actions to avoid the negative consequences of substance abuse (e.g., lying about drinking to avoid conflicts with a spouse). Substance-related beliefs involve positive ("anticipatory") beliefs about the effects of substance use (e.g., "Nothing feels as great as getting stoned!"), as well as negative ("relief-oriented") beliefs about the effects of refraining from substance use (e.g., "If I quit now, I'll get the shakes"). Automatic thoughts are brief ideas that spontaneously flash across a person's mind. Some automatic thoughts manifest themselves as sharp visual images, like frozen frames from a movie, such as the image of an ice-cold beer on a hot summer's day. Facilitating beliefs involve permission to use despite prior commitments to stop using (e.g., "I'll just have one drink").

"Triggers" are an important concept in cognitive therapy for substance abuse and other models such as relapse prevention. From the cognitive therapy perspective, substance use is initiated by activating stimuli ("high-risk situations"). Activating stimuli can be either internal or external. Internal cues may include negative feelings (e.g., anxiety, boredom), positive feelings (e.g., joy, excitement), memories (e.g., flashbacks of being abused), and physiologic sensations (e.g., cravings, pain). External cues include interpersonal conflicts, sights and sounds (e.g., seeing a wine advertisement), other substance users, problems at school or work, and celebration times such as parties and holidays.

In response to internal and external cues, people use psychoactive substances because they believe they will either increase positive feelings (pleasure), or they will alleviate negative feelings (pain). These anticipatory and relief-oriented beliefs lead to automatic thoughts and images (e.g., "I need a drink," "I want a hit"), that result in craving for the substance. Following these cravings, individuals may give themselves permission to use (e.g., "I'll quit soon," "Just one is okay"). Permissive beliefs lead to action plans, which eventually lead to continued use or relapse.

Although the focus in cognitive therapy is primarily in the present, the past may help explain the development of substance abuse problems and may be highly relevant for treatment. Liese and Franz (43), for example, have proposed a model that focuses on difficult or traumatic early life experiences. Such experiences contribute to basic beliefs about their own unlovability and inadequacy, which, in turn, increase the likelihood of experimentation with substances.

Behavioral Learning Theories of Substance Abuse

Behavioral theories contend that human behavior is learned and shaped via complex contingencies (45,46). Thus, behavioral theories of substance use are based on the assumption that the primary goal of treatment is to help patients unlearn old, ineffective behaviors and learn more adaptive ones (31,47). These theories suggest several ways that learning to use substances may occur.

Social learning theory (45) emphasizes the importance of modeling; that is, learning occurs by observing other people's behavior and its consequences. In terms of substance use, modeling can occur indirectly through cultural norms and prescriptions (e.g., media depictions of substance use) as well as directly through family and peer socialization (e.g., children observing their parents using alcohol to cope with problems). Such modeled behaviors get translated into attitudes, expectancies, and beliefs about substance use (e.g., the belief that alcohol enhances social interactions) (47). Given the vicarious nature of social learning, much learning about substance use can take place before an individual ever consumes any substances, such as in childhood.

A second way that learning may occur is through operant conditioning (46). Operant learning takes place when a behavior serves an instrumental function and, as a result, is reinforced by its consequences. A positive reinforcer strengthens any behavior that produces it, whereas a negative reinforcer strengthens any behavior that reduces or terminates it (46). The use of substances is established and maintained by both positive and negative reinforcers. Positive reinforcement occurs when substance use is rewarded by, for example, increasing social confidence, enhancing positive affect, and facilitating entry into social groups of substance-using peers. Conversely, substance use is negatively reinforced when it allows escape from aversive stimuli such as negative affect or the physiologic symptoms of withdrawal. The positive and negative reinforcers of substance use vary widely among individuals and it is important for clinicians to assess the specific reasons that any given person uses substances (31).

A third form of learning is classical conditioning. The first type of learning to be studied within the behaviorist tradition, classical conditioning was originally researched by Pavlov in the 1920s. In Pavlov's experiments with dogs, he found that repeated pairings of a conditioned stimulus (i.e., a bell ringing) with an unconditioned stimulus (i.e., food) would eventually cause the unconditioned response (i.e., salivating) to occur at the presentation of the conditioned stimulus. When applied to substance use, classical conditioning suggests that substance use may become paired with a variety of stimuli that reliably precede consumption of substances (e.g., drug paraphernalia, sights and smells associated with substance use, people, places, times of day, and negative emotions). Eventually, exposure to these stimuli may come to elicit a variety of substance-related conditioned responses such as intense cravings, physiologic changes (e.g., increased heart rate), and substance-related thoughts (31,48).

BASIC PRINCIPLES

Regardless of specific therapeutic techniques, certain principles are important to all CBT substance abuse treatments. These principles include case conceptualization, collaboration, psychoeducation, structure, attending to the multiple needs of patients, and monitoring substance use.

Case Conceptualization

Substance abuse patients comprise an extremely heterogeneous group. Some have no coexisting psychiatric problems while others have one or more psychiatric syndromes such as depression or panic disorder. Some are highly motivated to change while others deny that they have serious problems. Some have major coexisting life problems, such as acquired immunodeficiency syndrome (AIDS) or homelessness, while others are stable and high-functioning.

Case conceptualization involves the assessment of patients' backgrounds, presenting problems, psychiatric diagnoses, developmental profiles, and cognitive–behavioral profiles (24,41,43). Furthermore, the case conceptualization should include information about the unique variables responsible for the development and maintenance of substance use for the individual. This case formulation process may be facilitated by the use of standardized assessment instruments. For a guide to substance abuse assessment, see the recent chapter by Najavits (49), which provides a variety of Internet links to substance abuse measures that can be directly downloaded, as well as other resources. Additionally, several methods for organizing information about the chain of cognitive and behavioral events surrounding substance use have been developed, including conducting functional analyses of substance use behavior (31) and using the cognitive case conceptualization diagram created by Beck (50).

The therapist's selection and timing of therapeutic techniques should follow directly from the case conceptualization. For example, after conducting a functional analysis of an individual's substance use, treatment planning can focus on the specific skills necessary to intervene in the unique chain of events that lead to substance use for that individual (51). This approach reflects the CBT emphasis on adapting treatment to individuals, rather than expecting individuals to adapt to treatment. Other ways to individualize treatment include structuring sessions to include time for patient-driven material, repeating topics if patients have difficulty understanding a concept, and offering examples provided by the patient when presenting a new skill or topic (31).

The case conceptualization would be incomplete without an assessment of motivation to change. Prochaska, DiClemente, and Norcross (52,53) developed a system for assessing individuals' readiness to change. Substance abusers who believe that they have no problems are considered to be in the precontemplation stage. Those who believe that they may have problems are in the contemplation stage. Those taking steps to get ready for change are in the preparation stage. Those who have changed for at least 24 hours are in the action stage. And those who have endured change for at least 6 months are in the maintenance stage.

Research on the stages of change model has consistently shown evidence of a relationship between readiness to change and treatment outcome (52). Hence, CBT therapists are encouraged to carefully assess individuals' thoughts and behaviors regarding change and choose interventions accordingly. For example, precontemplators are unlikely to benefit from interventions that are heavy-handed and focus on specific methods of changing. Instead, precontemplators are likely to positively respond to discussions in which they are listened to empathetically and encouraged to discuss ambivalence.

Collaboration

CBT for substance abuse is highly collaborative, supportive, and empathetic (24,41–44,54–56). Collaboration is important because it creates a trusting atmosphere that supports the difficult work of changing addictive behaviors. In addition, substance abuse patients have notoriously high treatment dropout rates (57) and general therapeutic strategies aimed at cultivating rapport, collaboration, and alliance can help to maximize retention. Substance abusers tend to evoke more negative responses in therapists than many other patient populations (58,59). Some therapists feel frustrated, angry, or helpless because they are unable to stop patients from substance use. Many find that they cannot compete with substances that provide more intense and immediate effects than therapy. Some therapists feel frustrated because they cannot relate to the chronically impaired lives of such patients.

Cognitive–behavioral therapists are strongly encouraged to directly confront their thoughts about patients who abuse substances (42,43). For example, rather than thinking, "This drug addict will never change," therapists are taught to think, "If I am patient, this person may eventually make some important changes." Therapists are also encouraged to use effective communication skills with patients. For example, they are discouraged from lecturing and cajoling patients; instead, active listening and role playing are recommended. When patients want to discuss non–substance-related problems, therapists are encouraged to spend appropriate time discussing, rather than minimizing, these problems. Therapists are encouraged to regularly elicit feedback about patients' responses to therapy by asking such questions as, "What was most and least helpful about our talk today?" and "How will you implement what we've talked about?"

Psychoeducation

CBT usually incorporates significant psychoeducational efforts, particularly early in treatment. The complexity of biologic, behavioral, cognitive, and spiritual problems associated with substance abuse requires that CBT therapists be well informed about these areas. Psychoeducation is a delicate process. Just as individuals vary in their readiness to change, they also vary in their readiness for educational interventions. Both timing and style of delivery determine the value of psychoeducational presentations. Rather than randomly lecturing patients, CBT therapists elicit knowledge from patients in areas relevant to their circumstances and needs. Therapists offer opportunities for patients to learn more by means of brief lectures, written materials, videotapes, or workbooks on a variety of topics. Long lectures are inappropriate. ("too long" is defined as the point at which patients become bored or distracted). Areas for education might include the physiologic effects of particular substances, high-risk behaviors, the impact of substance use on the family, dual diagnosis, and psychological models for understanding substance abuse. Information in these areas may be found in CBT manuals, or free from resources such as the National Clearinghouse for Alcohol and Drug Information (800-729-6686).

Structure

Most CBT is quite structured. In cognitive therapy of substance abuse (24,41,43), for example, the structure includes setting the agenda, checking the patient's mood, bridging from the last visit (including a review of substance use, urges, cravings, and upcoming triggers), discussion of problems (including potential coping strategies and skill-building activities), frequent summaries, the assignment and review of homework, and feedback from the patient about the session. In the Seeking Safety model of CBT for the dual diagnosis of substance abuse and posttraumatic stress disorder (PTSD) (56,60), the structure includes a check-in, a brief inspiring quotation to emotionally engage patients, distribution of handouts to help instill new learning, and a check-out to end the session on a positive note (e.g., "Name one thing you got out of today's session") (56,60).

Attention to the Multiple Needs of Patients

CBTs for substance abuse recognize that patients typically suffer from serious life problems, including health,

legal, employment, family, and housing problems. In some cases, these are the result of substance use (e.g., a heroin abuser who has contracted human immunodeficiency virus [HIV] by sharing needles). In other cases, these life problems may have led to substance abuse (e.g., a teenage girl who uses alcohol to cope with childhood sexual abuse). Actively addressing these real-life issues is a necessary component of CBT.

There are numerous opportunities for CBT therapists to provide case management services. For example, they might refer patients for specialized assistance (e.g., medical, legal, family, or vocational counseling), give patients listings of sober houses, help patients fill out welfare forms, provide referrals to and basic information about self-help groups (e.g., Alcoholics Anonymous or other 12-step programs), review newspaper job listings during sessions, monitor patients' important visits to their physicians, help patients complete domestic abuse restraining orders, or call detoxification hospital units to determine whether beds are available. Thus, therapists must be familiar with community resources, including legal services, detoxification centers, HIV testing sites, and self-help groups.

In addition to general life problems, many substance-using patients have one or more comorbid psychiatric disorders that must be actively addressed, such as depression, personality disorders, and anxiety disorders (61). Such comorbidity presents significant treatment challenges; because these disorders are intricately bound to substance abuse in complex cyclical patterns and abstinence from substances may either decrease or increase psychological symptoms. The etiologies of dual diagnoses are typically multifactorial. While psychiatric disorders might lead some people to "self-medicate," resulting in alcohol or drug problems, substance abuse might lead others to develop psychiatric problems (e.g., cocaine addicts who develop secondary panic disorder). Comorbid disorders are known to affect treatment outcome, as seen in a classic study by Woody and colleagues (62), in which psychiatric severity predicted differential response to psychotherapy, including CBT.

In treating dually diagnosed patients, the most important step is the initial assessment and monitoring of symptoms throughout treatment. It is important to understand the relationship between psychiatric symptoms and drug use, cravings, and withdrawal (63). Following initial assessment, patients with coping skills deficits are taught new skills for managing their lives. While previously many patients were told to first become abstinent before comorbid disorders could be addressed (e.g., "First get clean, and then we'll talk about your depression"), most CBT models support integrated treatment (i.e., simultaneously addressing multiple disorders). Several CBT dual-diagnosis treatments have been developed and empirically evaluated for PTSD (60), personality disorders (64–67), bipolar disorder (68–70), and schizophrenia (71–74). When clinicians cannot directly provide dual diagnosis treatment, referral to adjunctive treatments is recommended.

Monitoring Substance Use

CBT therapists actively monitor the types, quantities, and routes of recent substance use at each treatment session. There are various methods for monitoring substance use (49). While self-report is the most common, urine and breathalyzer tests provide more objective data. Some forms of urine and breathalyzer testing are relatively easy to implement and some insurance companies will pay for this type of monitoring. One of the most commonly used self-report instruments for monitoring substance use is the Timeline Followback (TLFB) (75). Originally developed for alcohol use, the TLFB facilitates patients' recall of their substance use patterns over specified periods of time. This method has demonstrated reliability, especially when memory aids are used to facilitate recollection of substance use (75). Another method for assessing substance use is the widely used Addiction Severity Index (76). A common screening tool is Ewing and Rooss' four-question alcohol screening tool the CAGE (cut down [on drinking], annoyance, guilt [about drinking], [need for] eyeopener) (77). These instruments can be augmented with information from family members, probation officers, or other persons who have knowledge of patients' substance use. Regardless of the method chosen, asking patients about substance use at each session is an essential component of CBT and the accuracy of self-reports is enhanced when confidentiality is assured (49).

SPECIFIC TREATMENTS AND TECHNIQUES

CBT for substance abuse comprises a wide range of specific treatments and techniques that focus on general substance use disorders (24,27,78–81) as well as specific substances of abuse (26,29–31,82–88). Despite their diversity, there are several strategies common to most CBT approaches to substance abuse. These strategies include conducting functional analyses and providing training in coping skills to better manage the identified antecedents and consequences of substance use. Examples of these strategies are briefly described in this section.

Functional Analysis of Substance Use

Virtually all CBT attempts to identify the chain of cognitive, behavioral, and emotional events that precede and follow incidents of substance use. This process, referred to as *functional analysis* (or chain analysis), is defined as "the identification of important, controllable, causal functional relationships applicable to a specified set of target behaviors for an individual client" (89, p. 654). The goal of functional analysis is to understand the variables that

are controlling the target behavior (i.e., substance use) and to use this information to provide a focus for coping skills training.

Accordingly, the initial step is to conduct a functional analysis to help the patient recognize what factors tend to trigger and reinforce episodes of substance use, and to determine what skills they will need to learn to intervene in this process (31,51). This chain of events is composed of exposure to triggers for substance use, responses to these triggers, acquisition and actual use of the substance, and the positive and negative consequences of use (51). An important assumption of CBT is that patients can learn to alter this chain of events by managing these triggers and reinforcers (and thereby managing their substance use) after learning how they operate in their lives.

Functional analysis requires a careful assessment of the circumstances surrounding episodes of substance use and is often addressed through open-ended exploration of patients' substance abuse history (e.g., determinants of substance use, patterns of substance use, common thoughts and feelings associated with urges to use, reasons for using substances) (31). Standardized assessment instruments may also be useful in this process, such as the Inventory of Drinking Situations (90).

Coping Skills for Managing the Antecedents of Substance Use

Once antecedents of substance use have been identified via functional analysis, coping skills are taught to better manage these triggers in an effort to break their connection to substance use. A number of different types of antecedents may be involved in triggering substance use, including social, environmental, emotional, cognitive, and physical factors (31,51). Examples of CBT strategies for addressing these types of antecedents are briefly described.

Social Antecedents

Social antecedents for substance use include any social situations or interactions the patient may encounter in which they are at increased risk for substance use. Many substance users consume substances in social contexts and thus have developed networks of family, friends, dating partners, and coworkers with whom they have used substances in the past. These people may trigger urges to use directly by pressuring the individual to engage in substance use or indirectly by their conditioned association with substance use. Social triggers may also include attending social events such as parties or celebrations at which people are using substances.

Lifestyle Changes

One strategy for coping with social antecedents is to make lifestyle changes that help patients avoid exposure to social situations that trigger substance use. Lifestyle changes may range from informal discussions of lifestyle options to formal planning of, and participation in activities together (87). Other techniques include contracting to engage in new activities that are incompatible with substance use (e.g., exercise, meditation), referring patients to external resources to develop alternative pursuits (e.g., helping patients sign up for volunteer work), and identifying healthy activities.

Enhancing Social Support

Another strategy is to encourage the development of social support networks that are supportive of abstinence. Often patients' social networks include many people who use substances and, thus, may trigger urges to drink or use drugs. Strategies include minimizing contact with people who use substances, and developing a new social support network that is supportive of abstinence (93). In network therapy (79), for example, family or close friends are invited to attend sessions with patients and actively become involved in treatment contracting. In other treatments, such as cognitive therapy (24), family sessions are provided to enable family members to learn about the treatment and support patients' efforts.

Refusal Skills

Virtually all CBT includes training in substance-refusal skills to help patients cope with social pressure to use substances. Techniques include role playing to practice refusing offers of substances; educating patients about passive, aggressive, and assertive communication styles; anticipating consequences of refusal; and paying attention to body language and nonverbal cues.

Environmental Antecedents

Environmental antecedents to substance use include any external cues that are associated with substance use for an individual and increase urges to use. These include substance-related cues (e.g., advertisements for alcohol, the smell of alcohol) and general cues that have come to be associated with substance use through classical conditioning (e.g., money, times of day).

Cue Exposure

Drawing from classical conditioning theory, cue exposure treatment (CET) seeks to diminish conditioned responses to substance use cues by repeatedly exposing patients to these cues in the absence of actual substance use (91,92). CET involves repeated exposure to the environmental cues associated with substance use (e.g., drug-related paraphernalia, photographs of high-risk locations, and depictions of actual drug use), with the goal of decreasing respon-

sivity (e.g., cravings, substance-related thoughts) to these stimuli (51).

Decision-Making Skills

One strategy for managing environmental triggers of substance use is to train patients in decision-making skills that help them to decrease exposure to these stimuli. Relapse prevention models of substance use focus on the decision chain leading to drug use, including identifying "seemingly irrelevant decisions" that increase the risk of relapse (27), such as, "I can get a job as a bartender." Training in decision-making skills can help patients to interrupt these decision chains before substance use occurs. Strategies include identifying examples of poor decisions (e.g., keeping substances in the house), recognizing associations between decisions and exposure to high-risk situations, challenging cognitive distortions that encourage risky decisions, and practicing safe decision-making (31).

Emotional Antecedents

Negative emotions such as anger and anxiety can be a common trigger of relapse, and substance use often functions as a way to decrease or avoid these aversive emotional states. Conversely, positive affect (e.g., joy, excitement) can also trigger substance use, as it can remind patients of enjoyable times with others and pleasurable emotions they have experienced when using substances. CBT strategies for coping with emotional triggers focus on how to regulate and tolerate emotional states to decrease the risk of substance abuse.

Change Strategies

CBT for substance abuse includes many emotion regulation strategies that are focused on changing negative affect. Cognitive strategies include challenging distorted thoughts that fuel negative affect, completing daily thought records, and using positive coping statements (e.g., "I can handle these feelings without using"). Behavioral strategies include activities to decrease the intensity of negative affect such as distraction, engaging in pleasurable activities, self-soothing, acting opposite of emotions, and relaxation strategies.

Acceptance Strategies

In contrast to techniques aimed at changing negative affect, acceptance strategies focus on increasing tolerance for negative emotional states, decreasing emotional avoidance, and encouraging acceptance of emotional experiences (18,93,94). One common technique is mindfulness meditation. Mindfulness is a cognitive strategy that focuses attention on emotions by observing them in an objective, nonjudgmental way, rather than avoiding or suppressing them. The goal of mindfulness is to alter one's relationship to negative affect rather than to change or eliminate the emotion itself, and has been referred to as taking a "decentered perspective" or "cognitive distancing" (93–95). In substance abuse treatment, mindfulness is hypothesized to prevent relapse by increasing conscious awareness of automatic emotional (and cognitive) responses to substance use triggers (94). Mindfulness may serve as a form of covert exposure to emotions, thereby decreasing the need for patients to engage in substance use as a way to avoid aversive emotions (94).

Cognitive Antecedents

Cognitive antecedents of include drug-related beliefs (e.g., "Using drugs improves my mood"), automatic thoughts (e.g., "Smoke!"), and facilitating beliefs (e.g., "I can handle just one hit") that increase the risk of use or relapse. These cognitions often derive from core beliefs about the self (e.g., "I'm vulnerable") and resulting rules that a person has developed for survival (e.g., "If I let myself feel my emotions, I'll fall apart").

Modifying Automatic Thoughts and Drug-Related Beliefs

An initial step in cognitive therapy for substance use is to help patients identify their automatic thoughts and drug-related beliefs and to recognize that they may not be completely accurate (96). Patients are taught to identify logical errors in their thinking that may trigger substance use (e.g., ignoring evidence that substance use is becoming problematic, exaggerating their ability to quit, overemphasizing the positive aspects of substance use, devaluing non–substance-using friends and activities, and believing that life without substance use is boring) (97). A variety of cognitive restructuring techniques can be used to modify distorted automatic thoughts and drug-related beliefs, including examining the evidence, considering the alternatives, keeping daily thought records, using a cognitive continuum, surveying others, and the double-standard technique. In addition, patients can create flash cards on which they write their common automatic thoughts and effective challenges to them. Patients can refer to the flash cards when confronted with high-risk situations that trigger these cognitions.

Modifying Conditional Assumptions and Core Beliefs

A later step in cognitive therapy for substance use is to identify and modify patients' conditional assumptions and core beliefs that are fueling negative automatic thoughts (96). A variety of techniques are available for identifying core beliefs, including the downward arrow technique, looking for central themes in patients'

automatic thoughts, recognizing core beliefs that are expressed as automatic thoughts, Socratic questioning, and the what-if method. Once patients' core beliefs have been identified, strategies for modifying these beliefs include examining advantages and disadvantages, historical tests, keeping a daily log of evidence that supports and contradicts the core belief, and conducting behavioral experiments to test the conditional assumptions associated with core beliefs.

Physical Antecedents

Physical antecedents to substance use typically involve cravings and withdrawal symptoms. In addition, individuals may use substances to cope with other types of physical symptoms that may be unrelated to cravings or withdrawal (e.g., headaches, fatigue, nausea).

Distraction

Perhaps the most common technique for managing cravings is distraction. This involves engaging in activities that distract attention from the craving experience (e.g., physical exercise, talking with someone, snapping a rubber band on their wrist, relaxation strategies). Another version is thought-stopping wherein patients silently say "stop!" when experiencing cravings. Patients can create a coping card containing a list of distraction techniques to help them manage future cravings.

Urge Surfing

Similar to mindfulness techniques for coping with negative affect, urge surfing (going with the craving) involves letting cravings occur, peak, and pass without either fighting them or giving in to them (31). Urge surfing is done by focusing attention on the experience of craving and describing the physical sensations, feelings, and thoughts associated with it in an objective way (31). Urge surfing aids in increasing acceptance of craving as a time-limited, normal experience that patients can manage without using substances.

Focus on Consequences

Patients often overemphasize the positive aspects of substance use and ignore the negative consequences. Conversely, patients tend to minimize the benefits of abstinence and focus only on its disadvantages. One strategy for correcting these errors is to conduct an advantages–disadvantages analysis to identify the pros and cons of abstinence and continued use. Another strategy involves recalling the negative consequences of past substance use in order to make the disadvantages of giving in to the craving more salient. This can be done by having patients carry a reminder card that lists past negative effects of their substance use and having them review this card whenever cravings occur (51).

Coping Skills for Managing the Contingencies of Substance Use

In addition to providing training in coping skills for managing the antecedents of substance use, CBT also attempts to help patients manage the contingencies (i.e., positive and negative reinforcers) of their substance use. Examples of strategies for managing contingencies are briefly described here.

Contingency Management

Using principles of operant conditioning, contingency management techniques implement reinforcement to strengthen the incentive to become abstinent and weaken the incentive to continue using substances. Such reinforcement can be either positive (i.e., rewarding patients for abstinence) or negative (i.e., withdrawal of rewards for substance use). Less frequently, treatments have investigated the use of punishment in decreasing substance use (e.g., inducing nausea).

Some treatments (e.g., voucher-based incentive programs) use positive reinforcement as the central mechanism of treatment (98,99). Formal systems of are devised to motivate behavior change, such as paying patients for clean urines with increasing rates of pay for longer periods of abstinence (e.g., $1.50 for the first urine; $3.00 for the third). In some programs, patients are provided with vouchers that can be redeemed for items that could support substance-free activities and lifestyles (e.g., sports equipment and movie passes).

Another version of contingency management is the community reinforcement (80,81). This is designed to have patients participate in a social community that is highly reinforcing of abstinence. It involves providing patients with numerous services (e.g., individual and couples counseling, vocational counseling, a social club, recreational skills training) that reinforce abstinence in many areas of patients' lives.

Substituting Alternative Behaviors

Another behavioral strategy for addressing the reinforcers of substance use is to substitute the use of substances with functionally equivalent and more adaptive behaviors. It involves identifying both the positive and negative contingencies of substance use and finding less destructive behaviors that could serve the same function. For example, if substance use decreases negative affect, it could be substituted with emotion regulation strategies (e.g., distraction, self-soothing). If substance use serves a relaxation purpose, functionally equivalent alternative behaviors might include relaxation or meditation.

SUMMARY AND CONCLUSIONS

Over the past decade, numerous CBT approaches to substance abuse have been developed. These structured, focused, collaborative approaches have been based on the assumption that substance abuse is mediated by complex cognitive-behavioral processes. In this chapter, an overview of cognitive-behavioral substance abuse theories and techniques has been presented. According to Rotgers, these approaches "have been among the most productive of the last quarter century with respect to the advancement of empirically validated knowledge of the origins and treatment of . . . substance use disorders" (100, p. 198).

Liese and Franz (43) have described 10 lessons learned from applying cognitive therapy to substance abuse. Specifically, cognitive-behavioral therapists should (a) be knowledgeable about a wide variety of psychoactive drugs, addictive behaviors, and traditional treatment modalities; (b) communicate and collaborate with other addiction treatment personnel; (c) understand and address the role of substances in mood regulation; (d) conceptualize and treat coexisting psychopathology; (e) explore the development of all patients' substance abuse problems; (f) address therapeutic relationship issues; (g) confront patients appropriately and effectively; (h) stay focused in sessions; (i) use techniques appropriately and sparingly; and (j) never give up on addicted patients. Many more lessons will likely be learned as CBT continues to be applied to substance abuse.

REFERENCES

1. Dobson KS, Block L. Historical and philosophical bases of the cognitive–behavioral therapies. In: Dobson KS, ed. *Handbook of cognitive–behavioral therapies.* New York: Guilford Press, 1988:3–38.
2. Ellis A. *Reason and emotion in psychotherapy.* Secaucus, NJ: Citadel Press, 1962.
3. Beck AT. Thinking and depression: 1. Idiosyncratic content and cognitive distortions. *Arch Gen Psychiatry* 1963;9:36–46.
4. D'Zurilla TJ, Goldfried MR. Problem-solving and behavior modification. *J Abnorm Psychol* 1971;78:107–126.
5. Goldfried MR, Decenteceo ET, Weinberg L. Systematic rational restructuring as a self-control technique. *Behav Ther* 1974;5:247–254.
6. Guidano VF, Liotti G. *Cognitive processes and emotional disorders: a structural approach to psychotherapy.* New York: Guilford Press, 1983.
7. Mahoney MJ. *Cognition and behavior modification.* Cambridge, MA: Ballinger, 1974.
8. Maultsby MC. *Rational behavior therapy.* Englewood Cliffs, NJ: Prentice-Hall, 1984.
9. Meichenbaum DH. *Cognitive behavior modification.* New York: Plenum, 1977.
10. Rehm L. A self-control model of depression. *Behav Ther* 1977;8:787–804.
11. Spivack G, Platt JJ, Shure MB. *The problem-solving approach to adjustment.* San Francisco: Jossey-Bass, 1976.

12. Beck AT, Rush AJ, Shaw BF, et al. *Cognitive therapy of depression.* New York: Guilford Press, 1979.

13. Beck AT, Emery G, Greenberg RL. *Anxiety disorders and phobias: a cognitive perspective.* New York: Basic Books, 1985.

14. Foreyt JP, Rathjen DP, eds. *Cognitive behavior therapy: research and application.* New York: Plenum, 1978.

15. Kendall PC, Hollon SD, eds. *Cognitive-behavioral interventions: theory, research, and procedures.* New York: Academic Press, 1979.

16. Beck AT, Freeman A, et al. *Cognitive therapy of personality disorders.* New York: Guilford Press, 1990.

17. Layden MA, Newman CF, Freeman A, et al. *Cognitive therapy of borderline personality disorder.* Boston: Allyn & Bacon, 1993.

18. Linehan MM. Cognitive-behavioral treatment of borderline personality disorder. New York: Guilford Press, 1993.

19. Kingdon DG, Turkington D. *Cognitive-behavioral therapy of schizophrenia.* New York: Guilford Press, 1994.

20. Perris C. *Cognitive therapy with schizophrenic patients.* New York: Guilford Press, 1989.

21. Dattilio FM, Freeman A, eds. *Cognitive–behavioral strategies in crisis intervention.* New York: Guilford Press, 1994.

22. Roberts AR, ed. *Crisis intervention and time-limited cognitive treatment.* Thousand Oaks, CA: Sage, 1995.

23. Freeman A, Reinecke MA. *Cognitive therapy of suicidal behavior: a manual for treatment.* New York: Springer, 1993.

24. Beck AT, Wright FD, Newman CF, et al. *Cognitive therapy of substance abuse.* New York: Guilford Press, 1993.

25. Ellis A, Velten E. *Rational steps to quitting alcohol.* Fort Lee, NJ: Barricade Books, 1992.

26. Kadden R, Carroll K, Donovan D, et al. *Cognitive–behavioral coping skills therapy manual: a clinical research guide for therapists treating individuals with alcohol abuse and dependence. NIAAA Project MATCH Monograph Series,* vol. 3. Washington, DC: U.S. Department of Health and Human Services, 1995.

27. Marlatt GA, Gordon JR. *Relapse prevention: maintenance strategies in the treatment of addictive behavior.* New York: Guilford Press, 1985.

28. Miller WR, Munoz RF. *How to control your drinking.* Englewood Cliffs, NJ: Prentice-Hall, 1976.

29. Monti PM, Abrams DB, Kadden RM, et al. *Treating alcohol dependence: a coping skills training guide.* New York: Guilford Press, 1989.

30. Sobell MB, Sobell LC. *Problem drinkers: guided self-change treatment.* New York: Guilford Press, 1993.

31. Carroll KM. *A cognitive-behavioral approach: treating cocaine addiction.* NIH Pub No 98–4308. Rockville, MD: U.S. Department of Health and Human Services, 1998.

32. Project MATCH Research Group. 1993 Project MATCH: rationale and methods for a multisite clinical trial matching patients to alcoholism treatment. *Alcohol Clin Exp Res* 1993;17:1130–1145.

33. Crits-Christoph P, Siqueland L, Blaine J, et al. The NIDA Collaborative Cocaine Treatment Study: rationale and methods. *Arch Gen Psychiatry* 1997;54:721–726.

34. Najavits LM, Weiss RD. The role of psychotherapy in the treatment of substance use disorders. *Harv Rev Psychiatry* 1994;2:84–96.

35. Rawson RA, Obert JL, McCann MJ, et al. Relapse prevention models for substance abuse treatment. *Psychotherapy* 1993;30:284–298.

36. Rawson RA, Obert JL, McCann MJ, et al. Relapse prevention strategies in outpatient substance abuse treatment. *Psychol Addict Behav* 1993;7:85–95.

37. Brownell KD, Marlatt GA, Lichtenstein E, et al. Understanding and preventing relapse. *Am Psychol* 1986;41:765–782.

38. Wilson PH. *Principles and practice of relapse prevention.* New York: Guilford Press, 1992.

39. Marlatt GA. Relapse prevention: theoretical rationale and overview of the model. In: Marlatt GA, Gordon JR, eds. *Relapse prevention: maintenance strategies in the treatment of addictive behavior.* New York: Guilford Press, 1985:3–70.

40. Cummings C, Gordon JR, Marlatt GA. Relapse. Prevention and prediction. In: Miller WR, ed. *The addictive behaviors: treatment of alcoholism, drug abuse, smoking, and obesity.* Oxford, England: Pergamon Press, 1980:291–321.

41. Liese BS. Brief therapy, crisis intervention, and the cognitive therapy of substance abuse. *Crisis Interv Time Limit Treat* 1994;1:11–29.

42. Liese BS, Beck AT. Back to basics: fundamental cognitive therapy skills for keeping drug-dependent individuals in treatment. *NIDA Res Monogr* 1997;207–237.

43. Liese BS, Franz RA. Treating substance use disorders with cognitive therapy: lessons learned and implications for the future. In: Salkovskis P, ed. *Frontiers of cognitive therapy.* New York: Guilford Press, 1996:470–508.

44. Wright FD, Beck AT, Newman CF, et al. Cognitive therapy of substance abuse: theoretical rationale. *NIDA Res Monogr* 1992;137:123–146.

45. Bandura A. *Social learning theory.* Englewood Cliffs, NJ: Prentice-Hall, 1977.

46. Skinner BF. *About behaviorism.* New York: Vintage Books, 1974.

47. Abrams DB, Niaura RS. Social learning theory. In: Blane HT, Leonard KE, eds. *Psychological theories of drinking and alcoholism.* New York: Guilford Press, 1987:131–178.

48. Ruzek JI, Polusny MA, Abueg FR. Assessment and treatment of concurrent posttraumatic stress disorder and substance abuse. In: Follette VM, Ruzek JI, Abueg FR, eds. *Cognitive–behavioral therapies for trauma.* New York: Guilford Press, 1998:226–255.

49. Najavits LM. Assessment of trauma, PTSD and substance abuse: a practical guide. In: Wilson JP, Keane TW, eds. *Assessment of psychological trauma and PTSD.* New York: Guilford Press (2004).

50. Beck JS. *Cognitive therapy: basics and beyond.* New York: Guilford Press, 1995.

51. Kadden RM. Cognitive behavior therapy. In: Ott, PJ, Tarter, RE, Ammerman, RT, eds. *Sourcebook on substance abuse: etiology, epidemiology, assessment, and treatment.* Boston: Allyn & Bacon, 1999:272–283.

52. Prochaska JO, DiClemente CC, Norcross JC. In search of how people change: applications to addictive behaviors. *Am Psychol* 1992;47:1102–1114.

53. Prochaska JO, Norcross JC, DiClemente CC. *Changing for good.* New York: William Morrow, 1994.

54. Miller WR, Rollnick S. *Motivational interviewing: preparing people to change addictive behavior.* New York: Guilford Press, 1991.

55. Najavits LM, Weiss RD. Variations in therapist effectiveness in the treatment of patients with substance use disorders: an empirical review. *Addiction* 1994;89:679–688.

56. Najavits LM. Seeking Safety: a new psychotherapy for PTSD and substance abuse. In: Ouimette P, Brown PJ, eds. *Trauma and substance abuse: causes, consequences and comorbid conditions.* Washington, DC: American Psychological Association, 2002;147–170.

57. Crits-Christoph P, Siqueland L. Psychosocial treatment for drug abuse: selected review and recommendations for national health care. *Arch Gen Psychiatry* 1996;53:749–756.

58. Imhof J. Countertransference issues in alcoholism and drug addiction. *Psychiatr Ann* 1991;21:292–306.

59. Najavits LM, Griffin ML, Luborsky L,

et al. Therapists' emotional reactions to substance abusers: a new questionnaire and initial findings. *Psychotherapy* 1995;32:669–677.

60. Najavits LM. *Seeking safety: a treatment manual for PTSD and substance abuse.* New York: Guilford Press, 2002.

61. Regier DA, Farmer ME, Rae DS, et al. Comorbidity of mental disorders with alcohol an other drug abuse: results from the Epidemiological Catchment Area (ECA) study. *JAMA* 1990;264:2511–2518.

62. Woody GE, Luborsky LL, McLellan AT, et al. Psychotherapy for opiate addicts: does it help? *Arch Gen Psychiatry* 1983;40:639–645.

63. Mirin SM, Weiss RD. Substance abuse and mental illness. In: Frances RJ, Miller SI, eds. *Clinical textbook of addictive disorders.* New York: Guilford Press, 1991:271–298.

64. Linehan MM, Dimeff LA, Reynolds SK, et al. Dialectical behavior therapy versus comprehensive validation therapy plus 12-step for the treatment of opioid dependent women meeting criteria for borderline personality disorder. *Drug Alcohol Depend* 2002;67:13–26.

65. van den Bosch LMC, Verheul R, Schippers GM, et al. Dialectical behavior therapy of borderline patients with and without substance use problems: implementation and long-term effects. *Addict Behav* 2002;27:911–923.

66. Linehan MM, Dimeff LA. *Dialectical behavioral therapy manual of treatment interventions for drug abusers with borderline personality disorder.* Seattle: University of Washington, 1997.

67. Ball SA. Manualized treatment for substance abusers with personality disorders: dual-focus schema therapy. *Addict Behav* 1998;23:883–891.

68. Weiss RD, Greenfield SF, Najavits LM. Integrating psychological and pharmacological treatment of dually diagnosed patients. *NIDA Res Monogr* 1995;150:110–128.

69. Weiss RD, Najavits LM, Greenfield SF. A relapse prevention group for patients with bipolar disorder and substance use disorders. *J Subst Abuse Treat* 1999;16:47–54.

70. Weiss RD, Griffin ML, Greenfield SF, et al. Group therapy for patients with bipolar disorder and substance dependence: results of a pilot study. *J Clin Psychiatry* 2000;61:361–367.

71. Ziedonis D, Fisher W. *Motivation-based assessment and treatment of substance abuse in patients with schizophrenia. Directions in psychiatry 16.* New York: Hartherleigh Co., 1996.

72. Roberts L, Shaner A, Eckman T. *Overcoming addictions: skills training for people with schizophrenia.* Norton Professional Books, New York, 1999.

73. Bennett ME, Bellack AS, Gearon JS. Treating substance abuse in schizophrenia: an initial report. *J Subst Abuse Treat* 2001;20:163–175.

74. Bellack AS, DiClemente CC. Treating substance abuse among patients with schizophrenia. *Psychiatr Serv* 1999;50:75–80.

75. Sobell LC, Sobell MB. Timeline Followback: a technique for assessing self-reported alcohol consumption. In: Litten RZ, Allen J, eds. *Measuring alcohol consumption: psychosocial and biological methods.* Totowa, NJ: Humana Press, 1992:41–72.

76. McLellan T, Kushner H, Metzger D, et al. The fifth edition of the Addiction Severity Index. *J Subst Abuse Treat* 1992;9:199–213.

77. Ewing JA. Detecting alcoholism: The CAGE questionnaire. *JAMA* 1984;252:1905–1907.

78. Childress A, Ehrman R, McLellan A, et al. Update on behavioral treatments for substance abuse. *NIDA Res Monogr* 1988;90:183–192.

79. Galanter M. Network therapy for addiction: a model for office practice. *Am J Psychiatry* 1993;150:28–36.

80. Meyers, RJ, Miller, WR, eds. *A community reinforcement approach to addiction treatment.* New York: Cambridge University Press, 2001.

81. Smith JE, Meyers RJ, Miller WR. The community reinforcement approach to the treatment of substance use disorders. *Am J Addict* 2001;10:51–59.

82. Carroll KM, Rounsaville BJ, Keller DS. Relapse prevention strategies for the treatment of cocaine abuse. *Am J Drug Alcohol Abuse* 1991;17:249–265.

83. Rawson RA, Obert JL, McCann MJ, et al. *The neurobehavioral treatment manual: a therapist manual for outpatient cocaine addiction treatment.* Beverly Hills, CA: Matrix Center, 1989.

84. Wallace BC. *Crack cocaine.* New York: Brunner/Mazel, 1991.

85. Washton AM. *Cocaine addiction: treatment, recovery, and relapse prevention.* New York: WW Norton, 1989.

86. Roffman RA, Stephens RS, Simpson EE, et al. Treatment of marijuana dependencies: preliminary results. *J Psychoactive Drugs* 1990;22:129–137.

87. McAuliffe WE, Ch'ien JMN. Recovery training and self-help: a relapse prevention program for treated opiate addicts. *J Subst Abuse Treat* 1986;3:9–20.

88. Annis HM. A relapse prevention model for the treatment of alcoholics. In: Miller WR, Heather N, eds. *Treating addictive behaviors: process of change.* New York: Plenum, 1986:407–433.

89. Haynes SN, O'Brien WH. Functional analysis in behavior therapy. *Clin Psychol Rev* 1990;10:649–668.

90. Annis HM, Graham JM, Davis CS. *Inventory of Drinking Situations (IDS): users guide.* Toronto: Addiction Research Foundation, 1987.

91. Rohsenow DJ, Monti PM, Rubonis AV, et al. Cue exposure with coping skills training and communication skills training for alcohol dependence: 6- and 12-month outcomes. *Addiction* 2001;96:1161–1174.

92. Conklin CA, Tiffany ST. Applying extinction research and theory to cue-exposure addiction treatments. *Addiction* 2002;97:155–167.

93. Hayes SC, Strosahl KD, Wilson KG. *Acceptance and commitment therapy: an experiential approach to behavior change.* New York: Guilford Press, 1999.

94. Breslin FC, Zack M, McMain S. An information-processing analysis of mindfulness: implications for relapse prevention in the treatment of substance abuse. *Clin Psychol Sci Prac* 2002;9:275–299.

95. Teasdale JD, Seagal ZV, Williams JMG. How does cognitive therapy prevent depressive relapse and why should attentional control (mindfulness) training help? *Behav Res Ther* 1995;33:25–39.

96. Beck JS, Liese BS. Cognitive therapy. In: Frances RJ, Miller SI, eds. *Clinical textbook of addictive disorders,* 2nd ed. New York: Guilford Press, 1998;547–573.

97. Thase ME. Cognitive–behavioral therapy for substance abuse disorders. In: Dickstein LJ, Riba MB, Oldham JM, eds. *American Psychiatric Press review of psychiatry,* vol. 16. Washington, DC: American Psychiatric Press, 1997.

98. Higgins ST, Budney AJ, Bickel WK, et al. Incentives improve outcome in outpatient behavioral treatment of cocaine dependence. *Arch Gen Psychiatry* 1994;51:568–576.

99. Messina N, Farabee D, Rawson R. Treatment responsivity of cocaine-dependent patients with antisocial personality disorder to cognitive-behavioral and contingency management interventions. *J Consult Clin Psychology* 2003;71:320–329.

100. Rotgers F. Behavioral theory of substance abuse treatment: bringing science to bear on practice. In: Rotgers F, Keller DS, Morganstern J, eds. *Treating substance abuse: theory and technique.* New York: Guilford Press, 1996:174–201.

CHAPTER 48
Network Therapy

MARC GALANTER

There is a need for innovative techniques to enhance the effectiveness of psychotherapy with abusers of alcohol and other drugs in the office treatment setting in individual practice. Augmentation of treatment by group and family therapy in the multimodality clinic setting has led to considerably more success (1,2), and in the clinic, these therapies may be supplemented by a variety of social rehabilitation techniques. Groups such as Alcoholics Anonymous (AA) also offer invaluable adjunctive support. Nonetheless, a model for enhancing therapeutic intervention in the context of insight-oriented individual therapy would be of considerable value, given the potential role of the individual practitioner as primary therapist for many patients with addictive problems.

A LEARNING THEORY APPROACH

Classical Conditioning of Addiction Stimuli

An important explanatory model of drug dependence was elaborated by Wikler (3) based on his clinical investigations. In an attempt to explain the spontaneous appearance of drug craving in the absence of physiologic withdrawal, Wikler looked to certain stimuli that may have been conditioned to evoke withdrawal phenomena. He pointed out that addictive drugs produce counteradaptive responses in the central nervous system (CNS) at the same time that their direct pharmacologic effects are felt, and that these are reflected in certain physiologic events. With alcohol, for example, electroencephalogram (EEG)-evoked response changes characteristic of withdrawal may be observed in the initial phases of intoxication under certain circumstances (4). With opiates, administration of a narcotic antagonist to an addict who is "high" will precipitate a withdrawal reaction, which may be said to have been present in a latent form. Such responses are overridden by the direct effect of the drug and generally are observed only after the cessation of a prolonged period of administration, when they are perceived as physiologic withdrawal feelings or craving.

Hence, the drug euphoria inevitably is followed by the counteradaptive responses that occur on a physiologic level, shortly after the initial drug administration. The pairing of this administration with stimuli from the environment or with internal subjective stimuli in a consistent manner causes these stimuli to elicit the central counteradaptive response in the absence of prior drug administration. Wikler primarily discussed conditioning

or a psychophysiologic response. With regard to the issues presented here, however, it should be pointed out that the conditioned stimulus of the drug or the affective state may lead directly to the behavioral response before the addict consciously experiences withdrawal feelings. The addict may therefore automatically act to seek out drugs by virtue of this conditioning upon entry into the addict's old neighborhood, or upon experiencing anxiety or depression, all of which may have become conditioned stimuli. O'Brien and associates (5) have demonstrated the conditioning of addicts of opiate withdrawal responses to neutral stimuli, such as sound and odor. This conditioning, produced in a laboratory setting, provided experimental corroboration of Wikler's hypothesis. Ludwig and associates (6) demonstrated the direct behavioral correlates of such conditioned stimuli in relation to alcohol administration. They found that, for the alcoholic, the alcohol dose itself might serve as a conditioned stimulus for enhancing craving, as could the appropriate drinking context.

The following example illustrates the precipitation of drug-seeking by a stimulus previously conditioned through its association with drug-taking behavior. Two conditioned stimuli—a subjective anxiety state and the visual cue of the bottle—both combined to precipitate a relapse into drug-seeking behavior without intermediate steps of deliberation, and without the intervening sensation of craving.

> A 41-year-old recovered alcoholic had been abstinent for 6 years. She was a regular, if infrequent, attender at AA meetings and had no interest in resuming drinking. One day, her 10-year-old daughter had not returned home from school. The daughter was sufficiently late so that the mother called the homes of her daughter's friends and then the police to find out whether there had been any reports of her whereabouts. The mother was sitting in her living room near the telephone awaiting a possible call and was quite anxious. At one point, she glanced over at a liquor cabinet and her attention was caught by a bottle of gin, which had been her preferred alcoholic beverage before achieving sobriety. The liquor cabinet was placed in the open because of her confidence and that of her family in the reliability of her maintaining abstinence. Without thinking, she went over to the bottle and poured a drink. This information was obtained from her in an interview by a detoxification service, some 6 months later; her drinking had increased to the point that she required hospital admission. The particular incident had been forgotten and was elicited only after a lengthy guided interview.

It should be noted that the initial dose of alcohol described here itself served as a conditioned stimulus for further alcohol seeking. As noted already, the enhancement of craving by an initial alcohol dose has been demonstrated in an experimental context. It is by this mechanism that a small amount of the addictive agent has been observed to precipitate "loss of control," i.e., unmoderated alcohol or drug use.

Learning Theory and the Treatment of Addiction

Mello (7) describes systematic research on behavioral variables during intoxication by studying ethanol self-administration among alcoholics. With colleagues, she investigated effects of a number of variables, including altering the amount of effort necessary to obtain ethanol. Nathan and colleagues (8) have undertaken the use of within-subject experimental manipulations to study psychological factors such as socialization versus isolation and affective state. Such studies gradually have led to a better understanding of the possibility for manipulating an alcoholic's drinking patterns. Further elaboration has been undertaken by behavioral researchers for the therapy of alcoholism (9).

This experimental work is cited to illustrate a perspective for defining and modifying drinking behavior. Certain conditioned drinking behaviors may be extinguished if the appropriate extinguishing stimulus is interposed in a systematic way. This may be done by using noxious stimuli or by reinforcing constructive behavior patterns.

Cognitive Labeling

The question may then be raised as to what would serve as a minimally noxious aversive stimulus that would be both specific for the conditioned stimulus and unlikely to be generalized, thereby yielding a maximal positive learning experience. To answer this, we may look at Wikler's initial conception of the implications of this conditioning theory. He pointed out (10) that the user would become entangled in an interlocking web of self-perpetuating reinforcers, which perhaps explain the persistence of drug abuse, despite disastrous consequences for the user, and the user's imperviousness to psychotherapy that does not take such conditioning factors into account because neither the user nor the therapist is aware of their existence.

In addition, Ludwig et al. point out that the conditioned stimuli can be cognitively labeled so as to manipulate their role in precipitating craving and drug-seeking behavior (6). That is to say, by tagging the stimulus with some perceived label, the effect of the stimulus itself can be manipulated.

Because of the unconscious nature of the conditioned response of drug-seeking, the patient's attempt to alter the course of the stimulus–response sequence is generally not viable, even with the aid of a therapist. Neither party is aware that a conditioned sequence is taking place. However, sufficient exploration may reveal the relevant stimuli and their ultimate effect through conditioned sequences of drug-seeking behavior. By means of guided recall in a psychotherapeutic context, the alcoholic or addict can become aware of the sequence of action of conditioned

stimuli. The user can then label those stimuli. The therapeutic maneuver consists of applying an aversive stimulus to conditioned responses that are to be extinguished.

At this point, the patient's own distress at the course of the addictive process, generated by the patient's own motivation for escaping the addictive pattern, may be mobilized. This motivational distress then serves as the aversive stimulus. The implicit assumption behind this therapeutic approach is that the patient in question wants to alter his or her pattern of drug use and that the recognition of a particular stimulus as a conditioned component of addiction will allow the patient, in effect, to initiate the extinction process. If a patient is committed to achieving abstinence from an addictive drug such as alcohol or cocaine but is in jeopardy of occasional slips, cognitive labeling can facilitate consolidation of an abstinent adaptation. Such an approach is less valuable in the context of (a) inadequate motivation for abstinence, (b) fragile social supports, or (c) compulsive substance abuse unmanageable by the patient in the patient's usual social settings. Hospitalization or replacement therapy (e.g., methadone) may be necessary here, because ambulatory stabilization through psychotherapeutic support is often not feasible. Under any circumstances, cognitive labeling is an adjunct to psychotherapy and not a replacement for group supports such as AA, family counseling, or outpatient therapeutic community programs, where applicable. The following clinical examples may be helpful in illustrating this approach.

A 30-year-old amphetamine addict had been taking pills on binges for 10 years, with very few periods of abstinence longer than a few weeks. Early in the process of insight treatment, the various cues and behavior patterns associated with the initiation of binges were explored. After a 1-month period of abstinence the patient was encouraged to recall the particulars surrounding a relapse into drug taking that had occurred 3 days before. The drug taking began after a disappointment concerning her boyfriend. She reported going to a physician who supplied pills to abusers (under the nominal excuse of dieting) the day after her disappointment. She related a lengthy tale of going through the entire acquisition procedure, obtaining the pills, and ultimately taking them after a series of evasive arrangements to avoid her roommate's attention. When specifically asked, she said that all this occurred without her specific awareness of an intent to take the pills. Only after working on the guided recall was it clear to her that her actions were undertaken so as to assure that she could ingest the pills that day. The trip to the physician had been rationalized by saying it would make her feel more comfortable to have pills "in the house." By repeatedly examining such behaviors, she could ascertain each sequential stimulus that triggered an ensuing one. This allowed her to label these events and the feelings associated with them. After 9 months of such treatment she was able to terminate the episodes of amphetamine binging and remain abstinent over the course of psychotherapy for an ensuing 2 years.

Emphasis was placed on bringing into awareness each behavior from the initial conditioned stimulus to the final addictive act. Behaviors were labeled according to associated feelings and their role in the sequence.

Adjunctive support, such as disulfiram (Antabuse) treatment and/or AA, is indicated for someone who is truly alcohol dependent. At such times, cognitive labeling may also play a role in the therapy.

A 40-year-old writer-publicist had been drinking heavily since his late teens, at least a pint daily for the past 10 years. He was referred to consultation by his child's therapist. This and a recent work-related crisis led him to appreciate the extensive damage caused by his drinking. He agreed to seek abstinence and to take disulfiram, but refused to attend AA. Although drinking presented a problem during only one subsequent episode, conditioned drinking cues emerged as an issue in therapy. These were illustrated by three contexts previously associated with drinking in which the patient experienced malaise and restlessness. All three were examined in depth in terms of the drinking antecedents as well as the patient's contemporaneous feelings. This allowed him to understand his malaise and consciously mobilize himself to deal with the craving he felt in these situations. The first setting was when he stayed up late at night, as was his habit, to do his writing; he had regularly drunk heavily at these times to allay anxiety aroused by his conflicts over his creative work. Second, he suffered from a mild phobia of airplane flights and would drink heavily before flying. Third, before major speeches out-of-town, he would spend the evening in a bar, sometimes to the point of affecting his ability to present his material the next day. Addressing the symptoms experienced at these times served as a basis for understanding the patient's conflicts and helped to bolster his commitment to abstinence.

Altogether, these examples illustrate enhanced means for approaching psychotherapy with the alcohol and drug abuser. They may provide the therapist with another tool to assist the patient at a time when more traditional therapeutic maneuvers may be less successful.

THE NETWORK THERAPY TECHNIQUE

This approach can be useful in addressing a broad range of addicted patients characterized by the following clinical hallmarks of addictive illness. When they initiate consumption of their addictive agent, be it alcohol, cocaine, opiates, or depressant drugs, they frequently cannot limit that consumption to a reasonable and predictable level; this phenomenon has been termed *loss of control* by clinicians who treat persons dependent on alcohol or drugs (11). Second, they have consistently demonstrated relapse to the agent of abuse; that is, they have attempted to stop

using the drug for varying periods of time but have returned to it, despite a specific intent to avoid it.

This treatment approach is not necessary for those abusers who can, in fact, learn to set limits on their use of alcohol or drugs; their abuse may be treated as a behavioral symptom in a more traditional psychotherapeutic fashion. Nor is it directed at those patients for whom the addictive pattern is most unmanageable, such as addicted people with unusual destabilizing circumstances such as homelessness, severe character pathology, or psychosis. These patients may need special supportive care such as inpatient detoxification or long-term residential treatment.

Key Elements

Three key elements are introduced into the network therapy technique. The first is a cognitive behavioral approach to relapse prevention, independently reported to be valuable in addiction treatment (12). Emphasis in this approach is placed on triggers to relapse and behavioral techniques for avoiding them, in preference to exploring underlying psychodynamic issues.

Second, support of the patient's natural social network is engaged in treatment. Peer support in AA has long been shown to be an effective vehicle for promoting abstinence, and the idea of the therapist's intervening with family and friends in starting treatment was employed in one of the early ambulatory techniques specific to addiction (13). The involvement of spouses (14) has since been shown to be effective in enhancing the outcome of professional therapy.

Third, the orchestration of resources to provide community reinforcement suggests a more robust treatment intervention by providing a support for drug-free rehabilitation (15). In this relation, Khantzian points to the "primary care therapist" as one who functions in direct coordinating and monitoring roles in order to combine psychotherapeutic and self-help elements (16). It is this overall management role over circumstances outside as well as inside the office session which is presented to trainees, in order to maximize the effectiveness of the intervention.

Initial Encounter: Starting a Social Network

The patient should be asked to bring his or her spouse or a close friend to the first session. Alcoholic patients often dislike certain things they hear when they first come for treatment and may deny or rationalize, even if they have voluntarily sought help. Because of their denial of the problem, a significant other is essential to both history taking and to implementing a viable treatment plan. A close relative or spouse can often cut through the denial in a way that an unfamiliar therapist cannot and can therefore be invaluable in setting a standard of realism in dealing with the addiction.

Some patients make clear that they wish to come to the initial session on their own. This is often associated with their desire to preserve the option of continued substance abuse and is born out of the fear that an alliance will be established independent of them to prevent this. Although a delay may be tolerated for a session or two, it should be stated unambiguously at the outset that effective treatment can be undertaken only on the basis of a therapeutic alliance built around the addiction issue that includes the support of significant others and that it is expected that a network of close friends and/or relatives will be brought in within a session or two at the most.

The weight of clinical experience supports the view that abstinence is the most practical goal to propose to the addicted person for his or her rehabilitation (17,18), although as Pattison has pointed out (19), patients may sometimes achieve an outcome of limited drinking. For abstinence to be expected, however, the therapist should assure the provision of necessary social supports for the patient. Let us consider how a long-term support network is initiated for this purpose, beginning with availability of the therapist, significant others, and a self-help group.

In the first place, the therapist should be available for consultation on the phone and should indicate to the patient that the therapist wants to be called if problems arise. This makes the therapist's commitment clear and sets the tone for a "team effort." It begins to undercut one reason for relapse, the patient's sense of being on the patient's own if unable to manage the situation. The astute therapist, however, will assure that he or she does not spend excessive time on the telephone or in emergency sessions. The patient will therefore develop a support network that can handle the majority of problems involved in day-to-day assistance. This generally will leave the therapist to respond only to occasional questions of interpreting the terms of the understanding among himself or herself, the patient, and support network members. If there is a question about the ability of the patient and network to manage the period between the initial sessions, the first few scheduled sessions may be arranged at intervals of only 1 to 3 days. In any case, frequent appointments should be scheduled at the outset if a pharmacologic detoxification with benzodiazepines is indicated, so that the patient need never manage more than a few days' medication at a time.

What is most essential, however, is that the network be forged into a working group to provide necessary support for the patient between the initial sessions. Membership ranges from one to several persons close to the patient. Larger networks have been used by Speck (20) in treating schizophrenic patients. Contacts between network members at this stage typically include telephone calls (at the therapist's or patient's initiative), dinner arrangements, and social encounters and should be preplanned to a fair extent during the joint session. These encounters are most often undertaken at the time when alcohol or drug use is

likely to occur. In planning together, however, it should be made clear to network members that relatively little unusual effort will be required for the long term, and that after the patient is stabilized, their participation will amount to little more than attendance at infrequent meetings with the patient and therapist. This is reassuring to those network members who are unable to make a major time commitment to the patient as well as to those patients who do not want to be placed in a dependent position.

Defining the Network's Membership

Once the patient has come for an appointment, establishing a network is a task undertaken with active collaboration of patient and therapist. The two, aided by those parties who join the network initially, must search for the right balance of members. The therapist must carefully promote the choice of appropriate network members, however, just as the platoon leader selects those who will go into combat. The network will be crucial in determining the balance of the therapy. This process is not without problems, and the therapist must think in a strategic fashion of the interactions that may take place among network members. The following case illustrates the nature of their task.

A 25-year-old graduate student had been abusing cocaine since high school, in part drawing from funds from his affluent family, who lived in a remote city. At two points in the process of establishing his support network, the reactions of his live-in girlfriend, who worked with us from the outset, were particularly important. Both he and she agreed to bring in his 19-year-old sister, a freshman at a nearby college. He then mentioned a "friend" of his, apparently a woman whom he had apparently found attractive, even though there was no history of an overt romantic involvement. The expression on his girlfriend's face suggested that she did not like this idea, although she offered no rationale for excluding this potential rival. However, the idea of having to rely for assistance solely on two women who might see each other as competitors was unappealing. I therefore finessed the idea of the "friend," and we moved on to evaluating the patient's uncle, whom he initially preferred to exclude, despite the fact that his girlfriend thought him appropriate. It later turned out (as I had expected) that the uncle was perceived as a potentially disapproving representative of the parental generation. I encouraged the patient to accept the uncle as a network member nonetheless, so as to round out the range of relationships within the group, and did spell out my rationale for his inclusion. The uncle did turn out to be caring and supportive, particularly after he was helped to understand the nature of the addictive process.

Defining the Network's Task

As conceived here, the therapist's relationship to the network is like that of a task-oriented team leader, rather than that of a family therapist oriented toward insight. The network is established to implement a straightforward task, that of aiding the therapist in sustaining the patient's abstinence. It must be directed with the same clarity of purpose that a task force is directed in any effective organization. Competing and alternative goals must be suppressed, or at least prevented from interfering with the primary task.

Unlike family members involved in traditional family therapy, network members are not led to expect symptom relief for themselves or self-realization. This prevents the development of competing goals for the network's meetings. It also assures the members protection from having their own motives scrutinized and thereby supports their continuing involvement without the threat of an assault on their psychological defenses. Because network members have—kindly—volunteered to participate, their motives must not be impugned. Their constructive behavior should be commended. It is useful to acknowledge appreciation for the contribution they are making to the therapy. There is always a counterproductive tendency on their part to minimize the value of their contribution.

The network must, therefore, be structured as an effective working group with high morale. This is not always easy:

A 45-year-old single woman served as an executive in a large family held business—except when her alcohol problem led her into protracted binges. Her father, brother, and sister were prepared to banish her from the business but decided first to seek consultation. Because they had initiated the contact, they were included in the initial network and indeed were very helpful in stabilizing the patient. Unfortunately, however, the father was a domineering figure who intruded in all aspects of the business, evoking angry outbursts from his children. The children typically reacted with petulance, provoking him in return. The situation came to a head when both of the patient's siblings angrily petitioned me to exclude the father from the network, 2 months into the treatment. This presented a problem because the father's control over the business made his involvement important to securing the patient's compliance. The patient's relapse was still a real possibility. This potentially coercive role, however, was an issue that the group could not easily deal with. I decided to support the father's membership in the group, pointing out the constructive role he had played in getting the therapy started. It seemed necessary to support the earnestness of his concern for his daughter, rather than the children's dismay at their father's (very real) obstinacy. It was clear to me that the father could not deal with a situation in which he was not accorded sufficient respect and that there was no real place in this network for addressing the father's character pathology directly. The hubbub did, in fact, quiet down with time. The children became less provocative themselves, as the group responded to my pleas for civil behavior.

The Use of Alcoholics Anonymous

Use of self-help modalities is desirable whenever possible. For the alcoholic, certainly, participation in AA is strongly encouraged. Groups such as Narcotics Anonymous, Pills Anonymous, and Cocaine Anonymous are modeled after AA and play a similarly useful role for drug abusers. One approach is to tell the patient that he or she is expected to attend at least two AA meetings a week for at least 1 month so as to become familiar with the program. If after a month the patient is quite reluctant to continue, and other aspects of the treatment are going well, the patient's nonparticipation may have to be accepted.

Some patients are more easily convinced to attend AA meetings; others may be less compliant. The therapist should mobilize the support network as appropriate, so as to continue pressure for the patient's involvement with AA for a reasonable trial. It may take a considerable period of time, but ultimately a patient may experience something of a conversion, wherein the patient adopts the group ethos and expresses a deep commitment to abstinence, a measure of commitment rarely observed in patients who undergo psychotherapy alone. When this occurs, the therapist may assume a more passive role in monitoring the patient's abstinence and keep an eye on the patient's ongoing involvement in AA.

Use of Pharmacotherapy in the Network Format

For the alcoholic, disulfiram may be of marginal use in assuring abstinence when used in a traditional counseling context (21) but becomes much more valuable when carefully integrated into work with the patient and network, particularly when the drug is taken under observation. It is a good idea to use the initial telephone contact to engage the patient's agreement to abstain from alcohol for the day immediately prior to the first session. The therapist then has the option of prescribing or administering disulfiram at that time. For a patient who is earnest about seeking assistance for alcoholism, this is often not difficult, if some time is spent on the phone making plans to avoid a drinking context during that period. If it is not feasible to undertake this on the phone, it may be addressed in the first session. Such planning with the patient almost always involves organizing time with significant others and therefore serves as a basis for developing the patient's support network.

The administration of disulfiram under observation is a treatment option that is easily adapted to work with social networks. A patient who takes disulfiram cannot drink; a patient who agrees to be observed by a responsible party while taking disulfiram will not miss his or her dose without the observer's knowing. This may take a measure of persuasion and, above all, the therapist's commitment that such an approach can be reasonable and helpful.

Disulfiram typically is initiated with a dose of 500 mg, and then reduced to 250 mg daily. It is taken every morning, when the urge to drink is generally least. Particulars of administration in the context of treatment should be reviewed (22).

As noted previously, individual therapists traditionally have seen the abuser as a patient with poor prognosis. This is largely because in the context of traditional psychotherapy, there are no behavioral controls to prevent the recurrence of drug use, and resources are not available for behavioral intervention if a recurrence takes place—which it usually does. A system of impediments to the emergence of relapse, resting heavily on the actual or symbolic role of the network, must therefore be established. The therapist must have assistance in addressing any minor episode of drinking so that this ever-present problem does not lead to an unmanageable relapse or an unsuccessful termination of therapy.

How can the support network be used to deal with recurrences of drug use, when in fact the patient's prior association with these same persons did not prevent him or her from using alcohol or drugs? The following example illustrates how this may be done when social resources are limited. In this case, a specific format was defined with the network to monitor a patient's compliance with a disulfiram regimen:

A 33-year-old public relations executive had moved to New York from a remote city 3 years before coming to treatment. She had no long-standing close relationships in the city, a circumstance not uncommon for a single alcoholic in a setting removed from her origins. She presented with a 10-year history of heavy drinking that had increased in severity since her arrival, no doubt associated with her social isolation. Although she consumed a bottle of wine each night and additional hard liquor, she was able to get to work regularly. Six months before the outset of treatment, she attended AA meetings for 2 weeks and had been abstinent during that time. She had then relapsed, though, and became disillusioned about the possibility of maintaining abstinence. At the outset of treatment, it was necessary to reassure her that prior relapse was in large part a function of not having established sufficient outside supports (including more sound relationships within AA) and of having seen herself as failed after only one slip. However, there was basis for real concern as to whether she would do any better now, if the same formula was reinstituted in the absence of sufficient, reliable supports, which she did not seem to have. Together we came up with the idea of bringing in an old friend whom she saw occasionally and whom she felt she could trust. We made the following arrangement with her friend. The patient came to sessions twice a week. She would see her friend once each weekend. On each of these thrice-weekly occasions, she would be observed taking disulfiram, so that even if she missed a daily dose in between, it would not be possible for her to resume drinking on a regular basis, undetected. The interpersonal support inherent in this arrangement, bolstered by conjoint meetings with her and her friend,

also allowed her to return to AA with a sense of confidence in her ability to maintain abstinence.

The following case history illustrates the implementation of a regimen designed to secure the use of pharmacotherapy in an unstable patient with better access to a social network.

A 24-year-old college dropout, involved in the arts, came for treatment after she had been using heroin intranasally daily, and drinking heavily for 7 days. This was a relapse to her previous long-standing pattern of drug dependence, as she had been hospitalized twice for heroin addiction in the previous 2 years. Her last hospitalization, 6 months before, had been followed by episodic heroin insufflation and bouts of heavy drinking. Her polysubstance abuse as well as her promiscuity and rebellious behavior dated back to her early teens. One month prior to presenting, while living in a rural area, she had been abducted by a man whom she had befriended at an AA meeting, and managed to escape after being held captive in a motel for a week. She was now living alternately with a friend in the city where she presented for treatment, and with her parents who lived 200 miles away; she commuted by train. She had not admitted to her parents that she had relapsed to heroin use. As the patient's history unfolded in her first session, it was clear that she had a long history of major problems of social and residential instability, as well as clear evidences of poor judgment since her hospitalization. Nonetheless, she wanted to escape from her self-destructiveness and her pattern of drug use.

The preliminary structure of a network was established in the second session with her and with the friend with whom she was staying some of the time. The patient, however, acknowledged she was still using heroin intermittently in this session. In the third session, her parents were added, having them participate via speakerphone. This arrangement allowed for simultaneous planning along with the parties with whom her current life was rooted. Given her previous exposure to addiction treatment and AA, she was willing to accept a concrete plan for achieving abstinence from both alcohol and heroin as an appropriate course of action. She agreed to undergo detoxification from heroin while staying in her parents' home with the aid of clonidine (Catapres), and to then continue with naltrexone (ReVia) and disulfiram treatment. The former was for opiate blockade and for alcohol craving, and the latter was for securing alcohol abstinence. These medications were to be taken under observation, using the format developed within the network therapy regimen as described below.

The patient was initially concerned that her parents would be upset if she told them that she had relapsed to heroin use after her last hospitalization. The therapist pointed out that it was important for them to be told in order for them to serve as properly informed members of the network. It was agreed in an individual session that this need not be done until the patient's abstinence was stabilized over 2 weeks of use of the medications. The patient's concern was discussed in light of the judgmental and highly critical attitude of her mother, which had been influential over the course of the patient's adolescence, and had contributed greatly to her rebellious use of drugs. On a few occasions during the initial weeks, the mother became angry when the patient, while staying at home, had not attended AA meetings as planned.

It was therefore important for the sake of the network's stability to make clear that the principal role of network members is to participate with the patient and therapist in discussing opportunities for abstinence and stabilization, and not to scrutinize all aspects of the patient's behavior. Problems in compliance with the regimen of medication observation or AA meetings are discussed in network and individual sessions, and not policed by network members. Thus, if the patient misses a pill, the therapist was to be called and the patient not confronted. This removes network members from the role of independent enforcers, although their perspective and assistance may be solicited by mutual agreement with the patient. In this way, it is the implicit social pressure from members of the network for compliance that is most directed at stabilizing of the treatment. Two more of the patient's friends were added to the network after the initial month of stabilization. This helped dilute the role of her parents in the network, and added additional practical resources, perspective, and support for recovery. The patient herself continued to take the medications under the observation of either her father or her friend, depending on where she was residing.

This patient's circumstances illustrate the value of drawing supportive figures into the treatment early on, and using this network resource in combination with the observation of ingestion of a blocking agent or an antidipsotropic. (Both were used in this case.) The fact that the patient was taking these two medications on any given day undercut her craving and left her prepared to be compliant with the medication regimen the next day, as well as with the overall treatment plan. In practice, patients experience less craving when such medications are integrated into the treatment regimen, because they know that opiates or alcohol, respectively, are not available to them for the next few days after ingestion of the medication.

Format for Medication Observation by the Network

1. Take the medication every morning in front of a network member.
2. Take the pill so that that person can observe you swallowing them.
3. Have the observer write down the time of day the pills were taken on a list prepared by the therapist.
4. The observer brings the list in to the therapist's office at each network session.
5. The observer leaves a message on the therapist's answering machine on any day in which the patient had not taken the pills in a way that ingestion was not clearly observed.

Meeting Arrangements

At the outset of therapy, it is important to see the patient with the group on a weekly basis for at least the first month. Unstable circumstances demand more frequent contacts with the network. Sessions can be tapered off to biweekly and then to monthly intervals after a time.

To sustain the continuing commitment of the group, particularly that between the therapist and the network members, network sessions should be held every 3 months or so for the duration of the individual therapy. Once the patient has stabilized, the meetings tend less to address day-to-day issues. They may begin with the patient's recounting of the drug situation. Reflections on the patient's progress and goals, or sometimes on relations among the network members, then may be discussed. In any case, it is essential that network members contact the therapist if they are concerned about the patient's possible use of alcohol or drugs, and that the therapist contact the network members if the therapist becomes concerned about a potential relapse.

Adapting Individual Therapy to the Network Treatment

As noted previously, network sessions are scheduled on a weekly basis at the outset of treatment. This is likely to compromise the number of individual contacts. Indeed, if sessions are held once a week, the patient may not be seen individually for a period of time. The patient may perceive this as a deprivation unless the individual therapy is presented as an opportunity for further growth predicated on achieving stable abstinence assured through work with the network.

When the individual therapy does begin, the traditional objectives of therapy must be arranged so as to accommodate the goals of the substance abuse treatment. For insight-oriented therapy, clarification of unconscious motivations is a primary objective; for supportive therapy, the bolstering of established constructive defenses is primary. In the therapeutic context that is described here, however, the following objectives are given precedence.

Of first importance is the need to address exposure to substances of abuse or exposure to cues that might precipitate alcohol or drug use (23). Both patient and therapist should be sensitive to this matter and explore these situations as they arise. Second, a stable social context in an appropriate social environment—one conducive to abstinence with minimal disruption of life circumstances—should be supported. Considerations of minor disruptions in place of residence, friends, or job need not be a primary issue for the patient with character disorder or neurosis, but they cannot go untended here. For a considerable period of time, the substance abuser is highly vulnerable to exacerbations of the addictive illness and in some respects must be viewed with the considerable caution with which one treats the recently compensated psychotic.

Finally, after these priorities have been attended to, psychological conflicts that the patient must resolve, relative to his or her own growth, are considered. As the therapy continues, these come to assume a more prominent role. In the earlier phases, they are likely to reflect directly issues associated with previous drug use. Later, however, as the issue of addiction becomes less compelling from day to day, the context of the treatment increasingly will come to resemble the traditional psychotherapeutic context. Given the optimism generated by an initial victory over the addictive process, the patient will be in an excellent position to move forward in therapy with a positive view of his or her future.

RESEARCH ON NETWORK THERAPY

Network therapy is included under the American Psychiatric Association (APA) *Practice Guidelines* (24) for substance use disorders as an approach to facilitating adherence to a treatment plan, and to date, four studies have demonstrated its effectiveness in treatment and training. Each addressed the technique's validation from a different perspective: a trial in office management; studies of its effectiveness in the training of psychiatric residents and of counselors who work with cocaine-addicted persons; and an evaluation of acceptance of the network approach in an Internet technology transfer course.

An Office-Based Clinical Trial

A chart review was conducted on a series of 60 substance-dependent patients, with followup appointments scheduled through the period of treatment and up to 1 year thereafter (25). For 27 patients, the primary drug of dependence was alcohol; for 23, it was cocaine; for 6, it was opiates; for 3, it was marijuana; and for 1, it was nicotine. In all but eight of the patients, networks were fully established. Of the 60 patients, 46 experienced full improvement (i.e., abstinence for at least 6 months) or major improvement (i.e., a marked decline in drug use to nonproblematic levels). The study demonstrated the viability of establishing networks and applying them in the practitioner's treatment setting. It also served as a basis for the ensuing developmental research supported by the National Institute on Drug Abuse.

Treatment by Psychiatry Residents

We developed and implemented a network therapy training sequence in the New York University psychiatric residency program and then evaluated the clinical outcome of a group of cocaine-dependent patients treated by the residents. The psychiatric residency was chosen because of the growing importance of clinical training in the management of addiction in outpatient care in residency programs, in line with the standards set for specialty certification.

A training manual was prepared on the network technique, defining the specifics of the treatment in a manner allowing for uniformity in practice. It was developed for use as a training tool and then as a guide for the residents during the treatment phase. Network therapy tape segments drawn from a library of 130 videotaped sessions were used to illustrate typical therapy situations. A network therapy rating scale was developed to assess the technique's application, with items emphasizing key aspects of treatment (26). The scale was evaluated for its reliability in distinguishing between two contrasting addiction therapies, network therapy and systemic family therapy, both presented to faculty and residents on videotape. The internal consistency of responses for each of the techniques was high for both the faculty and the resident samples, and both groups consistently distinguished the two modalities. The scale was then used by clinical supervisors as a didactic aid for training and to monitor therapist adherence to the study treatment manual.

We trained third-year psychiatry residents to apply the network therapy approach, with an emphasis placed on distinctions in technique between the treatment of addiction and of other major mental illness or personality disorder. The residents then worked with a sample of 47 cocaine-addicted patients. Once treatment was initiated, 77% of the subjects did establish a network, that is, bring in at least one member for a network session. In fact, 1.47 collaterals on average attended any given network session, across all the subjects and sessions. This is notable, because compliance after initial screening was not necessarily assured. Almost all of those who completed a 24-week regimen (15 of 17) produced urines negative for cocaine in their last 3 toxicologies. On the other hand, only a minority of those who attended the first week but who did not complete the sequence (4 of 18) met this outcome criterion (27). The residents, inexperienced in drug treatment, achieved results similar to those reported for experienced professionals (28–30). These comparisons supported the feasibility of successful training of psychiatry residents naive to addiction treatment and the efficacy of the treatment in their hands.

Treatment by Addiction Counselors

This study was conducted in a community-based addictions treatment clinic, and the network therapy training sequence was essentially the same as the one applied to the psychiatry residents (31). A cohort of 10 cocaine-dependent patients received treatment at the community program with a format that included network therapy, along with the clinic's usual package of modalities, and an additional 20 cocaine-dependent patients received treatment as usual and served as control subjects. The network therapy was found to enhance the outcome of the experimental patients. Of 107 urinalyses conducted on the network therapy patients, 88% were negative, but only 66% of the 82 urine samples from the control subjects were negative, a significantly lower proportion. The mean retention in treatment was 13.9 weeks for the network patients, reflecting a trend toward greater retention than the 10.7 weeks for control subjects.

The results of this study supported the feasibility of transferring the network technology into community-based settings with the potential for enhancing outcomes. Addiction counselors working in a typical outpatient rehabilitation setting were able to learn and then incorporate network therapy into their largely 12-step–oriented treatment regimens without undue difficulty and with improved outcome.

Use of the Internet

We studied ways in which psychiatrists and other professionals could be offered training by a distance-learning method using the Internet, a medium that offers the advantage of not being fixed in either time or location. An advertisement was placed in *Psychiatric News*, the newspaper of the American Psychiatric Association, offering an Internet course combining network therapy with the use of naltrexone for the treatment of alcoholism.

The sequence of material presented on the Internet was divided into three didactic "sessions," followed by a set of questions, with a hypertext link to download relevant references and a certificate of completion. The course took about 2 hours for the student to complete. Our assessment was based on 679 sequential counts, representing 240 unique respondents who went beyond the introductory web page (32). Of these respondents, 154 were psychiatrists, who responded positively to the course. A majority responded "a good deal" or "very much" (a score of 3 or 4 on a 4-point scale) to the following statements: "It helped me understand the management of alcoholism treatment" (56%); "It helped me learn to use family or friends in network treatment for alcoholism" (75%); and "It improved my ability to use naltrexone in treating alcoholism" (64%). The four studies described in this section support the use of network therapy as an effective treatment for addictive disorders. They are especially encouraging given the relative ease with which different types of clinicians were engaged and trained in the network approach. Because the approach combines a number of well-established clinical techniques that can be adapted to delivery in typical clinical settings, it is apparently suitable for use by general clinicians and addiction specialists.

PRINCIPLES OF NETWORK TREATMENT
Start a Network as Soon as Possible

1. It is important to see the alcohol or drug abuser promptly, because the window of opportunity for openness to treatment is generally brief. A week's delay can result in a person's reverting back to drunkenness or losing motivation.
2. If the person is married, engage the spouse early on, preferably at the time of the first phone call. Point out that addiction is a family problem. For most drugs, you can enlist the spouse in assuring that the patient arrives at your office with a day's sobriety.
3. In the initial interview, frame the exchange so that a good case is built for the grave consequences of the patient's addiction, and do this before the patient can introduce his or her system of denial. That way you are not putting the spouse or other network members in the awkward position of having to contradict a close relation.
4. Then make clear that the patient needs to be abstinent, starting now. (A tapered detoxification may be necessary sometimes, as with depressant pills.)
5. When seeing an alcoholic patient for the first time, start the patient on disulfiram treatment as soon as possible, in the office if you can. Have the patient continue taking disulfiram under observation of a network member.
6. Start arranging for a network to be assembled at the first session, generally involving a number of the patient's family or close friends.
7. From the very first meeting you should consider how to ensure sobriety till the next meeting, and plan that with the network. Initially, their immediate company, a plan for daily AA attendance, and planned activities may all be necessary.

Manage the Network with Care

1. Include people who are close to the patient, have a long-standing relationship with the patient, and are trusted. Avoid members with substance problems, because they will let you down when you need their unbiased support. Avoid superiors and subordinates at work, because they have an overriding relationship with the patient independent of friendship.
2. Get a balanced group. Avoid a network composed solely of the parental generation, or of younger people, or of people of the opposite sex. Sometimes a nascent network selects itself for a consultation if the patient is reluctant to address his or her own problem. Such a group will later supportively engage the patient in the network, with your careful guidance.
3. Make sure that the mood of meetings is trusting and free of recrimination. Avoid letting the patient or the network members feel guilty or angry in meetings.

Explain issues of conflict in terms of the problems presented by addiction; do not get into personality conflicts.

4. The tone should be directive. That is to say, give explicit instructions to support and ensure abstinence. A feeling of teamwork should be promoted, with no psychologizing or impugning members' motives.

5. Meet as frequently as necessary to ensure abstinence, perhaps once a week for a month, every other week for the next few months, and every month or two by the end of a year.

6. The network should have no agenda other than to support the patient's abstinence. But as abstinence is stabilized, the network can help the patient plan for a new drug-free adaptation. It is not there to work on family relations or help other members with their problems, although it may do this indirectly.

Keep the Network's Agenda Focused

1. Maintaining abstinence. The patient and the network members should report at the outset of each session any exposure of the patient to alcohol and drugs. The patient and network members should be instructed on the nature of relapse and plan with the therapist how to sustain abstinence. Cues to conditioned drug-seeking should be examined.

2. Supporting the network's integrity. Everyone has a role in this. The patient is expected to make sure that network members keep their meeting appointments and stay involved with the treatment. The therapist sets meeting times and summons the network for any emergency, such as relapse; the therapist does whatever is necessary to secure stability of the membership if the patient is having trouble doing so. Network members'

responsibility is to attend network sessions, although they may be asked to undertake other supportive activity with the patient.

3. Securing future behavior. The therapist should combine any and all modalities necessary to ensure the patient's stability, such as a stable, drug-free residence; the avoidance of substance abusing friends; attendance at 12-step meetings; medications such as disulfiram or blocking agents; observed urinalysis; and ancillary psychiatric care. Written agreements may be handy, such as a mutually acceptable contingency contract with penalties for violation of understandings.

Make Use of Alcoholics Anonymous and Other Self-Help Groups

1. Patients should be expected to go to meetings of AA or related groups at least two to three times, with followup discussion in therapy.

2. If patients have reservations about these meetings, try to help them understand how to deal with those reservations. Issues such as social anxiety should be explored if they make a patient reluctant to participate. Generally, resistance to AA can be related to other areas of inhibition in a person's life, as well as to the denial of addiction.

3. As with other spiritual involvements, do not probe the patients' motivation or commitment to AA once engaged. Allow them to work out things on their own, but be prepared to listen.

ACKNOWLEDGMENTS

This chapter was adapted in part from articles previously published by the author (33–36).

REFERENCES

1. Institute of Medicine. *Broadening the base of treatment for alcohol problems.* Washington, DC: National Academy Press, 1990.
2. Galanter M, Castaneda R. Alcoholism and substance abuse: psychotherapy. In: Bellack AS, Hersen M, eds. *Comparative handbook of treatment for adult disorders.* New York: John Wiley, 1990:463–478.
3. Wikler A. Dynamics of drug dependence. *Arch Gen Psychiatry* 1973;28:611–616.
4. Begleiter H, Porjesz B. Persistence of a subacute withdrawal syndrome following chronic ethanol intake. *Drug Alcohol Depend* 1979;4:353–357.
5. O'Brien CP, Testa T, O'Brien TJ, et al. Conditioned narcotic withdrawal in humans. *Science* 1977;195:1000–1002.
6. Ludwig AM, Wikler A, Stark LM. The

first drink. *Arch Gen Psychiatry* 1974;30:539–547.
7. Mello NK. Behavioral studies of alcoholism. In: Kissin B, Begleiter H, eds. *The biology of alcoholism.* New York: Plenum, 1972;2:219–292.
8. Nathan P, Titler N, Lowison L, et al. Behavioral analysis of chronic alcoholism. *Arch Gen Psychiatry* 1970;22:419–430.
9. Miller WE, Heather N, eds. *Treating addictive behaviors.* New York: Plenum, 1986.
10. Wikler A. Some implications of conditioning theory for problems of drug abuse. *Behav Sci* 1971;16:92–97.
11. Jellinek EM. *The disease concept of alcoholism.* New Haven, CT: Hillhouse, 1963.
12. Marlatt GA, Gordon J. *Relapse prevention: maintenance strategies in the treat-

ment of addictive behaviors.* New York: Guilford Press, 1985.
13. Johnson VE. *Intervention: how to help someone who doesn't want help.* Minneapolis: Johnson Institute, 1986.
14. McCrady BS, Stout R, Noel N, et al. Effectiveness of three types of spouse-involved behavioral alcoholism treatment. *Br J Addict* 1991;86:1415–1424.
15. Azrin NH, Sisson RW, Meyers R. Alcoholism treatment by disulfiram and community reinforcement therapy. *J Behav Ther Psychiatry* 1982;13:105–112.
16. Khantzian EJ. The primary care therapist and patient needs in substance abuse treatment. *Am J Drug Alcohol Abuse* 1988;14(2):159–167.
17. Helzer JE, Robins LN, Taylor JR, et al. The extent of long-term drinking among alcoholics discharged from

medical and psychiatric facilities. *N Engl J Med* 1985;312:1678–1682.

18. Gitlow SE, Peyser HS, eds. *Alcoholism: a practical treatment guide.* New York: Grune & Stratton, 1980.

19. Pattison EM. Non-abstinent drinking goals in the treatment of alcoholism: a clinical typology. *Arch Gen Psychiatry* 1976;33:923–930.

20. Speck R. Psychotherapy of the social network of a schizophrenic family. Fam Process 1967;6:208.

21. Fuller R, Branchey L, Brightwell DR, et al. Disulfiram treatment of alcoholism. A Veterans Administration cooperative study. *JAMA* 1986;256:1449–1455.

22. Gallant DM. *Alcoholism: a guide to programs, intervention and treatment.* New York: Norton, 1987.

23. Galanter M. Network therapy for addiction: a model for office practice. *Am J Psychiatry* 1993;150:28–36.

24. American Psychiatric Association. Practice guidelines for the treatment of patients with substance use disorders: al-

cohol, cocaine, opioids. *Am J Psychiatry* 1995[Supple]:152.

25. Galanter M. Network therapy for substance abuse: a clinical trial. *Psychotherapy* 1993;30:251–258.

26. Keller D, Galanter M, Weinberg S. Validation of a scale for network therapy: a technique for systematic use of peer and family support in addiction treatment. *Am J Drug Alcohol Abuse* 1997;23:115–127.

27. Galanter M, Dermatis H, Keller D, et al. Network therapy for cocaine abuse: use of family and peer supports. *Am J Addict* 2002;11:161–166.

28. Carroll KM, Rounsaville BJ, Gordon LT, et al. Psychotherapy and pharmacotherapy for ambulatory cocaine abusers. *Arch Gen Psychiatry* 1994;51:177–187.

29. Higgins ST, Budney AJ, Bickel WK, et al. Achieving cocaine abstinence with a behavioral approach. *Am J Psychiatry* 1993;150:763–769.

30. Shoptaw S, Rawson RA, McCann MJ, et al. The matrix model of outpatient stimulant abuse treatment: evidence of

efficacy. *J Addict Dis* 1994;13:129–141.

31. Keller D, Galanter M, Dermatis H. Technology transfer of network therapy to community-based addiction counselors. *J Subst Abuse Treat* 1999;16:183–189.

32. Galanter M, Keller DS, Dermatis H. Using the Internet for clinical training: a course on network therapy. *Psychiatr Serv* 1997;48:999. Available at: http://mednyu/substanceabuse/course.

33. Galanter M. Psychotherapy for alcohol and drug abuse: an approach based on learning theory. *J Psychiatr Treat Eval* 1983;5:551–556.

34. Galanter M. *Network therapy for alcohol and drug abuse: a new approach in practice.* New York: Basic Books, 1993.

35. Galanter M. Social network therapy for cocaine dependence. *Adv Alcohol Subst Abuse* 1987;6:159–175.

36. Galanter M. Management of the alcoholic in psychiatric practice. *Psychiatr Ann* 1989;19:226–270.

CHAPTER 49

Acupuncture

JI-SHENG HAN, ALAN I. TRACHTENBERG, AND JOYCE H. LOWINSON

Acupuncture (derived from the word *acus*, meaning a sharp point, and *punctura*, meaning to pierce), is defined as "stimulation, primarily by the use of solid needles, of traditionally and clinically defined points on or beneath the skin, in an organized fashion for therapeutic and/or preventive purposes" (1). The original acupuncture points (or *acupoints*) are superficial anatomic loci described in traditional Asian texts. The skin directly over these points is generally lower in transdermal electrical resistance than the skin surrounding them. There is considerable overlap between these traditional acupoints and locations defined in modern physical medicine such as "trigger points," "motor points," or "osteopathic lesions." Acupuncture points are often palpable as either mild depressions or small, and sometimes tender, subcutaneous nodules. In traditional Asian medicine, these points are stimulated either by puncture and manipulation with solid needles or by local heating. Heating is generally accomplished by the burning of dried, powdered *Artemisia vulgaris* (moxa), referred to as *moxibustion*. This moxa is either held just above the acupoint by the acupuncturist (indirect moxibustion), attached to a needle penetrating the point, or applied directly to the skin (direct moxibustion). In modern times, new methods of stimulating the acupoints include applications of electric current to needles in the points (electroacupuncture) or skin electrodes over the points, injections into the points, laser-light directed onto the points, or finger-pressure massage of selected points, called *acupressure*. In addition, many new points and whole new "microsystems" of points have been described on specific body parts on which an entire homunculus is represented, leading to, for instance, scalp acupuncture, hand acupuncture, and (of particular interest for addiction treatment) ear acupuncture, also known as auricular acupuncture.

Although acupuncture and related acupoint therapies are most commonly known for their analgesic effects, their medical applications are by no means limited to pain treatment. After a careful literature and clinical survey, the World Health Organization (WHO) listed 42 medical problems that are were considered suitable for acupuncture treatment, including the treatment of drug abuse. A smaller group of definite or possible indications for acupuncture were recommended by an National Institutes of Health (NIH) Consensus Panel in 1997 as follows: "Promising results have emerged, for example, showing efficacy of acupuncture in adult postoperative and chemotherapy nausea and vomiting and in postoperative dental pain. There are other *situations such as addiction,* stroke rehabilitation, headache, menstrual cramps, tennis elbow, fibromyalgia, myofacial pain, osteoarthritis, low back pain, carpal tunnel syndrome, and asthma *where acupuncture may be useful as an adjunct treatment or an acceptable alternative or be included in a comprehensive management program*" (2). Although a consensus on the clinical efficacy of acupuncture for the treatment of addictions has not yet been achieved in the United States, it has been amply demonstrated that acupuncture is an addiction treatment service now being sought by many potential patients (3). Thus, as with many low-cost alternative-healing practices, acupuncture may serve an important role in social marketing of the entire treatment package, enhancing use and compliance. This is an important potential benefit that is additional to any specific physiologic effect(s) of acupoint stimulation, which is documented in the rest of this chapter.

CLINICAL OBSERVATION

The application of acupuncture in the treatment of opioid addiction originated from a serendipitous observation made by Dr. H. L. Wen in Hong Kong in 1972. The following is a brief description quoted from Dr. Wen's report on this case:

> In early November 1972, a 50-year-old man was admitted to the Neurosurgical Unit of the Kwong Wah Hospital, Tung Wah Group of Hospitals, Kowlong, in Hong Kong, because of brain concussion. He was a known opium addict of 5 years' duration. While in the ward, he was given tincture of opium to relieve his withdrawal syndrome. After the cerebral concussion had improved, the patient was asked whether he would agree to cingulotomy to relieve his drug abuse problem. He agreed. He was scheduled for surgery on the 9th of November 1972. During the operation for surgery, instead of local anesthesia being injected under the scalp (where the incision was to be made), acupuncture anesthesia (analgesia) was used.
>
> Four needles were inserted into the right hand (IL-4 and SI-3) and in the arm (EH-4 and TB-9), and another two needles were inserted into the right ear (brainstem and Shenmen). Stimulation with an electrical stimulator was carried out for half an hour. At that time, our interest was in discovering whether the patient obtained analgesia in the scalp prior to surgery. During stimulation, 15 to 30 minutes later, the patient voluntarily stated that his withdrawal syndrome had completely cleared up. We examined him and found that he was free of withdrawal syndrome. Operation was canceled and the patient returned to the ward with advice to the nursing staff that doctor should be informed if the patient showed withdrawal symptoms again. At 9:00 P.M. I [HKW] was informed that the patient had another withdrawal syndrome. Again, acupuncture and electrical stimulation was carried out in a similar manner, the withdrawal symptoms again disappeared. The next day, we saw two other patients in the orthopedic wards who were both opium abusers. When we explained how we wanted to treat their withdrawal symptoms, both agreed to the procedure. Both responded well to the half hour of acupuncture and electrical stimulation and their withdrawal symptoms stopped.

After the above observation, Dr. Wen and his colleague, Dr. Cheung, at the Kwong Wah Hospital, subsequently reported that, in a study of 40 heroin and opium addicts, acupuncture combined with electrical stimulation was effective in relieving the symptoms of narcotic withdrawal (4).

This method was later adopted in many clinical settings in Western countries, including at Lincoln Hospital in New York City. However, as time and experience accumulated, the body acupuncture points originally used by Wen and Cheung on the arm and hand were gradually omitted, retaining only the ear points for acupuncture in drug abuse treatment (5) and doing without additional electrical stimulation. The protocol developed at Lincoln Hospital by Dr. Michael Smith and his colleagues was subsequently promulgated by the National Acupuncture Detoxification Association (NADA) on a national basis, with formalized training and standards for the application of ear acupuncture in a group setting without the use of electricity. This has been the predominant approach studied by clinical trials and practiced in the United States since then, and is described in more detail later in the Clinical Trials section.

IMPLICATION FROM ANIMAL EXPERIMENTS

The use of acupuncture as a method of anesthesia and/or analgesia for surgery in the People's Republic of China in the late 1950s raised a great deal of interest among the public and the biomedical community. This led to exploration of the biologic mechanisms underlying the actions of acupuncture. Starting in 1965, the Department of Public Health of the Chinese government sponsored extensive research in this area. The discovery of morphine-like substances (endorphins) in the mammalian brain (6) in 1975 had a great impact on modern concepts of pain and analgesia. It was soon clear that acupuncture (manual needling)-induced analgesia can be blocked by the opioid antagonist naloxone (Narcan), suggesting the involvement of endogenous opioid substances in acupuncture analgesia (7). In animal experiments, manual acupuncture or acupuncture combined with electrical stimulation (electroacupuncture) was shown to accelerate the production and release of endorphins which could then interact with various opioid receptors to relieve or prevent pain (8). It was further clarified that endorphins are a group of peptides possessing a variety of specific characteristics. Among those peptides, β-endorphin and enkephalin are primarily agonists of the μ and δ opioid receptors, whereas dynorphin is the agonist for the κ opioid receptors (9). Interestingly, electrical stimulation of different frequencies can specifically induce the release of different endorphins. For example, low-frequency (2 to 4 Hz) electroacupuncture stimulates release of the enkephalins that interact with μ and δ opioid receptors, whereas high-frequency (100 Hz) electroacupuncture can stimulate the release of dynorphin to interact with κ opioid receptors (10). These findings provided a biochemical explanation for traditional practice and suggested that the usefulness of acupuncture might be much broader than pain control.

China had suffered seriously from problems of opiate addiction in the 1800s and early 1900s. This problem was minimized from 1949 to 1951 because of the complete closure of overseas trade involving opioids. However, concurrent with the implementation of the "open door policy" of the 1980s, large amounts of opiates began to be smuggled into border areas and increasing problems were seen with opiates and heroin addiction. In that period, the number of persons abusing or addicted to heroin was estimated to be increasing as much as 10% to 40% per year. Accompanying this, hand in hand with heroin injection, was the problem of human immunodeficiency virus (HIV) infection and acquired immunodeficiency syndrome (AIDS). It was natural to think that if acupuncture can release endogenous opioids in the brain to ease pain, why not make use of it to relieve withdrawal symptoms? This idea was initially tested in morphine-dependent rats. The withdrawal symptoms were significantly reduced by high-frequency (100 Hz) electroacupuncture administered at the hind limbs. This effect was found to be much greater than that induced by low-frequency (2 Hz) stimulation (11). Encouraged by the experimental results, electroacupuncture was applied clinically to heroin-addicted patients to see if it suppressed withdrawal symptoms. The results here were also promising. However, it was soon found that it was not always feasible for patients to attend the clinic to obtain professional treatment one or more times a day, and, as a result, patients often missed many of the recommended number of sessions of acupuncture, with adverse consequences for therapeutic results. Technology for self-administration of the stimulation was developed to see whether it would be possible for patients to treat themselves as many times per day as they might desire, by using electrical acupoint stimulation without a needle, as part of the treatment program for their addiction.

Experimental findings obtained in the rat model had showed that electrical stimulation applied to the surface of the skin could produce analgesic effects similar to that produced by electroacupuncture, as long as the stimulator provided a controlled current (to correct for varying skin resistance in the absence of a penetrating needle electrode) (12). Satisfactory subjective results were obtained for the treatment of heroin withdrawal in humans using the same method of electrical acupoint stimulation via skin electrodes (13). Later it was found that this device was also useful in suppressing the conditioned place preference (CPP) to morphine in the rat (14). This is an animal model

of craving for drugs of abuse. Subsequent human studies revealed that this form of stimulation could also inhibit the craving for heroin in addiction patients (see below).

Data are presented in the following sections on the role of acupuncture and related techniques in treating both withdrawal from, and craving for, drugs of abuse, especially cocaine and possibly heroin, as well as other substances of abuse, such as alcohol. Results obtained in animal experiments are presented as a method of exploring acupuncture's potential mechanisms of action.

ACUPUNCTURE AND RELATED TECHNIQUES

Manual Needling

As discussed in the previous paragraphs, classical acupuncture involves the piercing of the skin by a sharp metallic needle and manipulation by up-and-down and twisting or twirling movements. The traditional purpose of these movements is supposedly to stimulate the underlying anatomic conceptual structures described as meridians or channels (*jing*) and their branches (*luo*). The meridians may represent networks of connective tissue and nerves or may be merely allegorical and/or functional entities that serve as mnemonic aides to point locations. The correct placement of the needle at the acupoint and the optimal manipulation are generally characterized by feedback from the patient concerning a subjective feeling called *de-qi*. This sensation, reported by patients to include heaviness, soreness, numbness, and sense of swelling, occasionally also involves the trembling of the local muscle. In the meantime, the operator of the needle (the acupuncturist) often has a feeling resembling that experienced during fishing when a fish is nibbling at or swallowing the bait. This is likely the result of the rhythmic contraction of muscle fibers surrounding the needle. With this approach, the tip of the needle is felt to go deep into the tissue and believed to stimulate the structures to induce maximal *de-qi*, experienced by both patient and acupuncturist. The shortcoming of this method, especially for research purposes, is that it is empirical and subjective in nature, difficult to describe precisely, and by no means easy to replicate by others. According to the traditional acupuncturist, it takes years to really master the particular modes of manual stimulation.

Electroacupuncture

It has been made clear that the analgesic effect induced by acupuncture can be completely blocked by a local procaine injection deep into the acupoint, but not by its subcutaneous injection, suggesting that the signal of acupuncture originates mainly from nervous tissues (or tissues susceptible to procaine blockade) located in deep structures rather than in the superficial layer of the skin (15). Using single nerve fiber recording technique to record the afferent impulses of the nerve innervating the site of stimulation, it was found that the nerve fibers responsible for transmission of acupuncture signals belong to the group II (Aβ) fibers (16). Strong twisting and up-and-down movements of the needle produces a firing as high as 50 to 80, but no more than 100, spikes per second. Because the analgesic effect induced by manual needling can be totally abolished by local nerve blockade (15) or nerve transection, a neural mechanism is strongly implicated. It is thus rational to use electrical stimulation administered via the metallic needles in lieu of its mechanical movement. This has been called *electroacupuncture*. The advantage of the electroacupuncture is that the frequency, amplitude, and pulse width of the electrical stimulation can be determined precisely and objectively. Consequently, it can be replicated by other acupuncturists or experimenters without difficulty. Moreover, the procedure of inserting the needle at a precise skin location, as well as changing the direction and the depth of the needle to an optimal status, can still be performed by an experienced acupuncturist to achieve a maximal *de-qi* for confirmation of placement. It is only at the end of the placement procedure that the needles are connected to the electrical stimulator in place of further manual stimulation. This is exactly the procedure described by Dr. Wen in his first report, that is, "acupuncture and electrical stimulation" (4). Having said that, it should be mentioned that because electroacupuncture should optimally be given daily, or even on an as-needed basis, several times per day in the period of detoxification, which may be difficult for outpatients who are at a distance away from the clinic. A procedure that can be operated by the patient at home under the supervision of the physician might be a desirable alternative to daily treatment in the clinic or inpatient care.

In addition, because drug-addiction patients, especially those using injection routes of administration, have a high incidence of blood-borne viral infections, it may be more convenient for invasive procedures to be replaced by non-invasive methods that do not produce sharp biohazardous waste.

Han's Acupoint Nerve Stimulator

An alternative to use of the electroacupuncture (insertion of a needle through the skin to deliver electrical stimulation for the underlying tissue) is to use a transcutaneous route of electrical administration. However, because the skin has a very high impedance, which is more than 10 times that of the muscle tissue, it is necessary to use a constant current output device to assure an regular level of stimulation without being affected by the degree of moisture of the skin surface or the change of blood flow rate within the skin. Because the tip of the needle goes several millimeters or even centimeters below the skin, the placement of the skin electrodes should ensure the maximal stimulation of the deep structures underlying the acupoint. For example, to stimulate the Hegu point (coded as

Large Intestine 4 [LI-4]) located in the thenar muscle of the hand, the correct placement of the skin electrodes should be one on the dorsal side and the other on the palm side of the point, so that the current is forced to pass through the thenar muscle with little deviation.

Regarding the frequency of stimulation, it is commonly accepted that conventional transcutaneous electric nerve stimulation (TENS) is based on the gate-control theory (17) that high-frequency (e.g., 100 Hz) low-intensity stimulation is preferable to activate the large-caliber nerve fibers in order to suppress the pain mediated by the unmyelinated small-caliber fibers. On the other hand, "acupuncture-like" stimulation is characterized by low-frequency (e.g., 2 Hz), high-intensity stimulation. The current approach attempts to combine TENS-like and acupuncture-like stimulation to create what is hoped to be an optimal mode of stimulation to maximize the release of both classes of endorphins. A device that possesses these features was designed and named Han's Acupoint Nerve Stimulator (HANS), and used in a series of animal and clinical experiments, the details of which follow.

OPIOID DETOXIFICATION

Experimental Studies

Systemic studies reveal that the mechanism of acupuncture analgesia is attributed mainly to the increased release of endogenous opioid peptides in the central nervous system (CNS) (8). A rational extrapolation is that the activation of endogenous opioid systems by acupuncture should be useful to ease opiate withdrawal symptoms.

It has been reported that transauricular electrostimulation suppressed the naloxone-induced morphine withdrawal syndrome in mice (18) and in rats (19). Auriacombe et al. (20) demonstrated that TENS with an intermittent high-frequency current effectively attenuated the abstinence syndrome of the rat after abrupt cessation of morphine administration. The mechanisms of action remained obscure. Based on our previous findings that low-frequency electroacupuncture (e.g., 2 Hz) accelerated the release of β-endorphin and enkephalin in the CNS, whereas high-frequency electroacupuncture (e.g., 100 Hz) accelerated the release of dynorphin (10,21) in the spinal cord, we tested the effect of electroacupuncture in a naloxone-precipitated morphine withdrawal model of the rat. The original perspective was that 2 Hz would be more effective than 100 Hz in suppressing withdrawal syndrome, if the effect of electroacupuncture is to accelerate the release of morphine-like opioid peptides (enkephalin and endorphin) to replace morphine, thus ameliorating abstinence syndrome. To our surprise, the results showed that 2-Hz electroacupuncture was only marginally effective in reducing withdrawal in 2 of 5 signs, whereas 100 Hz electroacupuncture produced a dramatic suppression of all 5 withdrawal signs. In other words, 100-Hz electroacupuncture was far more effective than 2-Hz electroacupuncture in suppressing withdrawal syndrome (11).

This outcome can be explained in three ways. First, the experimental design was that naloxone was given immediately after the electroacupuncture, therefore the effect of electroacupuncture itself may be partially blocked by naloxone. One may expect that if 2-Hz electroacupuncture is used to treat spontaneous withdrawal rather than naloxone-precipitated withdrawal, the therapeutic effect might be more prominent. This was verified in the human studies cited in the Human Observations section. Second, compared with 2 Hz, the effect of 100-Hz electroacupuncture is less likely to be affected by naloxone at this dose, because 100-Hz electroacupuncture effect is mediated by dynorphin, which is a κ opioid agonist and is relatively resistant to naloxone blockade ($ID_{50} = 10$ mg/kg) (22). Third, dynorphin suppresses the withdrawal syndrome in heroin-dependent humans (23) and in morphine-dependent monkeys (24), and the site of action is in the spinal cord (25).

To explore the possible involvement of dynorphin and κ opioid receptor in the effect of 100-Hz electroacupuncture for modulating withdrawal syndrome in rats, Cui et al. (26) used rats made dependent on morphine. These rats were then given spinal intrathecal administration of a κ opioid receptor agonist U-50488 or its antagonist nor-binaltorphimine dihydrochloride (nor-BNI). Naloxone (0.5 mg/kg) was then administered to precipitate withdrawal syndrome. U-50488 produced a dose-dependent suppression, whereas nor-BNI elicited a dose-dependent augmentation of naloxone-precipitated withdrawal. The latter result implies that an endogenous κ agonist, most probably dynorphin, exerts a tonic suppressive effect on morphine withdrawal syndrome at the spinal level.

Withdrawal syndromes have multiple manifestations. One of the cardiovascular manifestations of the withdrawal syndrome is an increase in heart rate. In a mouse model of morphine dependence induced by multiple injections of increasing doses of morphine for 8 days, the heart rate and blood pressure were measured by tail cuff method (27,28). Morphine abstinence resulted in a 20% increase of the heart rate without affecting the blood pressure. Electroacupuncture of 100 Hz or 15 Hz was very effective in bringing down the heart rate to approach normal level; 2 Hz produced only a mild effect.

An intriguing finding was that the therapeutic effect of electroacupuncture was achieved only when the stimulation intensity was kept at a low level (1 mA). The effect of electroacupuncture disappeared when the intensity was increased to 2 to 3 mA. This is probably a result of the stressful effect produced in mice by high-intensity stimulation that activates the sympathetic system, thus antagonizing the calming effect of electroacupuncture. Subsequent studies revealed that the intensity tolerated by the mouse is indeed smaller than that for the rat. For example, to induce an analgesic effect, the optimal intensity is

0.5 to 1.5 mA for mice (29), in contrast to 1 to 3 mA for rats (30).

To summarize, for the purpose of opioid detoxification in rats and mice, it is preferable to use electroacupuncture of higher frequency and lower intensity, which may have some implication for its application in humans.

Human Observations

To observe the effect of HANS on the withdrawal syndromes in heroin addiction, HANS was used once a day for 30 minutes for a period of 10 days in a drug-addiction treatment center (13). Aside from the subjective answer to a standard questionnaire, two objective parameters were measured, that is, heart rate and body weight.

Single Treatment

To observe the immediate effect of HANS on the heart rate of patients in withdrawal from heroin, the two pairs of output leads of the HANS were connected to four acupoints in the upper extremities. One pair of skin electrodes was placed on the Hegu point (LI-4, at the dorsum of the hand on the thenar eminence) and the other at the palmar side on Laogon (P-8, opposite to LI-4), to complete an electric circuit. Another pair of electrodes were placed on Neiguan (P-6, located at the palmar side of the forearm, 2 inches proximal to the palmar groove, between the tendons of the palmaris longus and flexor carpi radialis) and Waiguan (TE-5, on the dorsal surface of the forearm opposite the P-6) point, to complete a circuit. A "dense-and-disperse" mode of stimulation was administered, in which 2-Hz stimulation alternated automatically with 100-Hz stimulation, each lasting for 3 seconds. This mode of stimulation releases all four kinds of opioid peptides in the central nervous system (CNS) (10), hopefully producing a maximal opioidergic effect. The control group received the same treatment of placing the skin electrodes on site, except that the electrodes were disconnected from the electronic circuitry. The average heart rate of the patients in opioid withdrawal was 109 beats per minute before treatment. The dense-and-disperse mode stimulation for 30 minutes reduced the heart rate in a significant extent, as shown in Figure 49.1. Suppression of the tachycardia occurred within the first 5 to 10 minutes. Heart rate continued to fall through the 20th minute, and leveled at 90 beats per minute for the last 10 minutes. This change is statistically significant, although the effect is short lasting. The full effect remained for only 20 minutes after the stimulation; thereafter, heart rate began returning to its original level (31).

Multiple Treatments

To observe the cumulative effect of multiple daily treatments with HANS, 117 heroin-addiction patients were

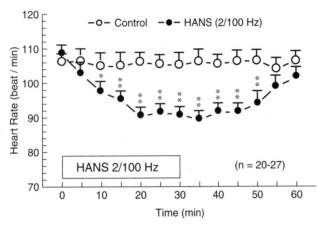

FIG. 49.1. Effect of 2/100 Hz electrical stimulation (HANS) on the heart rate of heroin addicts during episodes of withdrawal. *, ** represent $p < 0.05$ and $p < 0.01$ respectively, compared with the control (Mock HANS) group. (From Wu LZ, Cui CL, Han JS. Effect of Han's acupoint nerve stimulator (HANS) on the heart rate of 75 inpatients during heroin withdrawal. *Chin J Pain Med* 1996;2:98–102, with permission.)

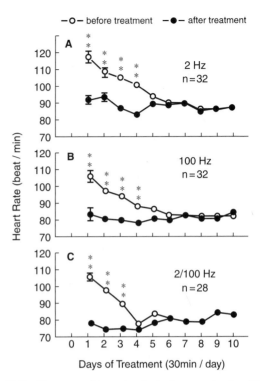

FIG. 49.2. Change of heart rate before and after HANS treatment once a day for 10 days. ** $p < 0.01$ compared with the after-treatment value. (Modified from Wu LZ, Cui CL, Han JS. Han's acupoint nerve stimulator for the treatment of opiate withdrawal syndrome. *Chin J Pain Med* 1995;1:30–35, with permission.)

randomly divided into 4 groups. Three groups received HANS of 2 Hz (constant frequency), 100 Hz (constant frequency), or 2/100 Hz (2 Hz alternating with 100 Hz, or "dense-and-disperse mode") respectively. The control group received mock stimulation, where the skin electrodes were placed on site and connected to the stimulator with blinking signals, yet the electric circuitry was disconnected. The treatment was for 30 minutes a day and was given for 10 consecutive days. Heart rate was measured with an electrocardiogram before and immediately after the HANS stimulation. Figure 49.2 shows the results. Taking the 2-Hz group as an example, in the first day of observation, the heart rate averaged 110 beats per minute, which dropped to 90 beats per minute immediately after the HANS treatment ($p < 0.01$). In the second day, the heart rate averaged 102 beats per minute, and then dropped to 91 beats per minute after the treatment ($p < 0.01$). This trend continued for days 3 and 4. On day 5, no significant difference was found in heart rate before and after the treatment (91 beats per minute vs. 89 beats per minute), suggesting that the heart rate had returned to "normal" range (13).

Comparing the effects among the three HANS groups, the 100-Hz group produced a slightly better result than that of 2 Hz. In the 2/100-Hz group, the after-HANS heart rate reached an even lower level (72 beats per minute). Additionally, the heart rate of the 2/100-Hz group returned to "normal" range on day 4, 1 day earlier than the fixed frequency groups (day 5). In the control group (n = 30) receiving mock HANS, heart rate did not come down to a level of 100 beats per minute until 8 days after the treatment. The results suggest that repeated daily electroacupuncture treatment is effective in reducing the tachycardia of heroin withdrawal, with an effective order of dense-and-disperse > 100Hz > 2 Hz.

Another objective parameter for measuring the severity of heroin withdrawal is body weight. The heroin addicted subjects recruited in this study were aged 17–35, their average body weight was only 49–51 kg. In the control group receiving mock HANS, body weight showed a reduction of 1 kg at the end of the first week, probably due to the presence of withdrawal distress. In the HANS treated groups, a significant increase of body weight developed after 4 days of treatment, and continued to increase thereafter. A net increase of 5 kg was recorded in the HANS groups compared with the control group at the end of 10 day observation period. This increase of body weight (approximately 10%) is apparently due to the reduction of the withdrawal syndrome and an increase of food and water intake in the HANS-treated groups. It is interesting to find that while the dense-and-disperse mode is significantly better than the fixed frequency groups in ameliorating the tachycardia, no significant difference was observed among the three HANS groups in terms of body weight changes, suggesting that the mechanisms of action underlying heart rate- and body weight-modulation may not be identical (13).

In clinical practice with Chinese inpatients, opiate withdrawal symptoms have been significantly reduced, but not totally abolished by the HANS treatment, especially in those who had a history of heroin abuse for more than 5 years. To obtain a quantitative estimate of the effect of HANS, the following protocol was established (32): (a) HANS was used several times a days, with a maximum of four times a day on days 1 and 2, then two to three times a day on days 3 to 7, and twice a day on days 8 to 14. (b) A four-channel HANS device was used instead of two-channel device. The acupoints used were Hegu/Laogong for left (or right) hand, Neiguan/Waiguang for right (or left) arm, and Xingjian/Sanyinjiao (LV-2/SP-6) for left leg, as well as for right leg. (c) The intensity of stimulation was 5 to 7 mA for the first day (5 to 6 mA being the threshold value [T]), 1.5 to 2.0 T for the second day, and 2.5 to 3.0 T for the third day and thereafter. (d) Buprenorphine (Buprenex) i.m. was used as a supplement to HANS when the patient experienced a certain degree of withdrawal distress. Patients were allowed to ask for buprenorphine as much as they liked, and medication was administered on request. The purpose of this arrangement was to maintain a comfortable detoxification procedure with minimal withdrawal discomfort. In a study to quantify the role of HANS in a combined HANS/buprenorphine treatment, 28 heroin addiction patients were randomly divided into 2 groups, receiving buprenorphine only, or HANS plus buprenorphine. The results are shown in Figure 49.3A. In the buprenorphine-only group, the total dose requested in 14 days averaged 12.91 ± 1.34 mg (X ± SEM [standard error of mean]), whereas the total dosage requested by the HANS-plus-buprenorphine group averaged only 1.01 ± 0.09 mg, which was consumed only in the first 5 days. In other words, the total amount of buprenorphine used in the HANS group was only 7.8% of that needed in the pure buprenorphine group. This can be taken as a quantitative estimate of the effect of HANS for opioid detoxification. Compared with the relatively mild and short-lasting therapeutic effect observed in the first day treatment (see Fig. 49.1), the marked symptomatic improvement of the 14-day multiple treatment regime (Fig. 49.3) is apparently a result of an accumulation of the therapeutic effect produced by repetitive treatments. These results of short-term withdrawal are described primarily to illustrate the physiologic effects of the acupoint stimulation. Because short-term withdrawal does not have significant effects on the long-term course of addiction, these results are not described as a measure of true clinical or therapeutic benefits.

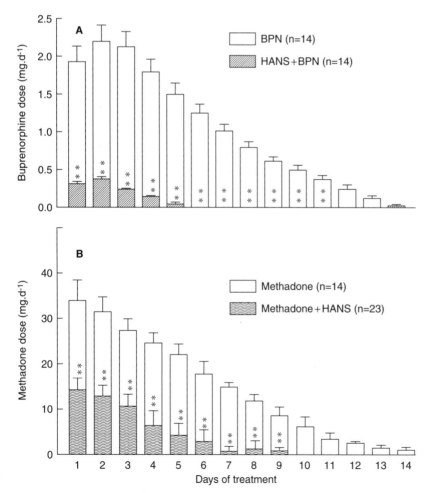

FIG. 49.3. Influence of 2/100Hz electric stimulation (HANS) on the requirement of buprenorphine (BPN) (**A**) or methadone (**B**) for heroin detoxification. ** $P<0.01$ compared with the corresponding control group. (Modified from Wu LZ, Cui CL, Han JS. Treatment on heroin addicts by 4-channel Han's Acupoint Nerve Stimulator (HANS). *J Beijing Med Univ* 1999;31:239–242, and Wu LZ, Cui CL, Han JS. Reduction of methadone dosage and relief of depression and anxiety by 2/100 Hz TENS for heroin detoxification. *Chin J Drug Depend* 2001;10:124–126, respectively, with permission.)

Similar observations were made in another group of heroin-addicted subjects using a methadone reduction protocol as control group and HANS (2/100 Hz) plus methadone as the experimental group (33). Figure 49.3B depicts the results. The total dose of methadone used in the control group averaged 202 ± 15 mg (X $\pm$ SEM), whereas in the HANS-plus-methadone group the total dose of methadone was only 50.5 ± 8.2 mg, showing a reduction of 75% (p<0.001).

A bonus effect of HANS treatment is on the injection mark syndrome (32). At the end of the 14-day detoxification period, the injection marks on the skin were significantly reduced in the HANS-plus-buprenorphine group as compared with the buprenorphine-only group. Among the five indicators, such as the venous collapse, fibrotic thickening of the venous wall, thrombosis, bluish streak, and scarred mainliners, the first two indicators showed the most striking difference. Although a minor finding, the disappearance of the injection marks made the patients very happy, because was a symbol indicating the beginning of a new and normal life. The mechanisms underlying these structural changes remain unclear. A plausible hypothesis is that an improvement of the microcirculation as a result of the decrease of the peripheral sympathetic tone is responsible for the facilitation of tissue repair as well as the production of the "warm feeling" (13) experienced by the patient during the HANS treatment.

Peking University Clinical Bases Treatment Protocol

The following protocol is based on the clinical practice evolved over the past 10 years at Peking University Drug Abuse Treatment Clinical Bases (PUCB):

1. Patients with drug addiction are admitted for inpatient treatment once their status has been verified by physical examination and urine toxicology and informed consent is obtained.
2. No drug whatsoever, including narcotics and nonnarcotics, can be brought into the PUCB from the outside.
3. The principle of electrically stimulated acupoint treatment (to make full use of the resources existing in the central nervous system to counter the pathophysiologic changes produced by drug abuse) is explained to the patient. Although this is a nonpharmacologic treatment, enough pharmacologic supplements will be available, if needed, to avoid any excessive withdrawal symptoms.
4. HANS is immediately administered to the patient upon admission. A four-channel device is used, with the four electrical leads connected to four pairs of skin electrodes placed at four pairs of acupoints: Hegu and Laogong on the left (or right) hand; Neiguan and Waiguan on the right (or left) arm; and Xingjian (LV-2) and Sanyinjiao (Sp-6) on the left and the right legs.

5. Unless otherwise stated, the frequency is put at the dense-and-disperse mode, that is, 2 Hz alternating with 100 Hz at 3-second intervals. The pulse width changed automatically with the frequency, that is, 0.2 ms pulse width for 100-Hz stimulation and 0.6 ms for the 2-Hz stimulation.
6. The intensity of the electric stimulation is determined according to the sensitivity of the subject to the stimulation. In the first treatment when the patient is not familiar with the electrical stimulation, a threshold (T) intensity (5 to 6 mA) is preferable. When patients become familiar with the stimulation, they usually prefer to have higher intensity in order to strengthen the relief experienced from withdrawal symptoms. The stimulation intensity can then be increased to twice threshold (2T or 10 to 12 mA), or even greater, so long as the patient feels comfortable. Rhythmic contraction of the local muscle is often observed. One treatment session lasts for 30 minutes. The electric output is automatically cut off at the end of that period.
7. HANS treatment is given for no more than four times a day in days 1 and 2 of drug abstinence. Thereafter it is administered three times a day for the first week, and then twice a day for the second week. Irrespective of how many times a day HANS treatment is given, a session before going to bed is always administered with the intention of ensuring a good night's sleep.
8. Buprenorphine (32) or methadone (33) can be used as supplement when the patient feels excessive degrees of withdrawal distress. The dose for the first 2 days is 30 to 40 mg for methadone or 2 to 3 mg for buprenorphine. It should then be gradually reduced according to the individual's requirements. Opioid supplementation usually lasts for 2 to 7 days. Compared with the purely pharmacologic regimen, the HANS-treated patients report an easier time in becoming drug free.
9. Patients that are coaddicted to sedatives or other drugs of abuse often ask for the relevant drugs. These requests are usually not fulfilled. The standard treatment regime usually takes care of all the related symptoms (see "Lincoln Hospital Protocol" below).
10. Close contact between doctor and patient and communication between patients are highly encouraged.
11. Detoxification is usually completed in 14 days. However, the patient is welcome to stay longer in the treatment center for consolidation of the therapeutic effect. In that case, HANS can be given once or twice a day for another 2 weeks.

Lincoln Hospital Protocol

Acupuncture treatment for drug and alcohol problems was originally introduced in 1974 at Lincoln Hospital (LH), a city-owned facility in the South Bronx of New York

City for the treatment of drug and alcohol problems. The Substance Abuse Division at LH is a state-licensed treatment program that has provided more than 500,000 acupuncture treatments in the past 20 years. Initially, in 1974, LH used Dr. H. L. Wen's method, applying electrical stimulation to the lung point in the ear. At that time acupuncture was used as an adjunctive treatment for prolonged withdrawal symptoms after a 10-day detoxification cycle. Subsequently twice daily acupuncture was used concurrently with tapering methadone doses. Reduction in opiate withdrawal symptoms and higher retention rates were reported (34).

It was serendipitously discovered that electrical stimulation was not necessary to produce symptomatic relief. Instead, simple manual needling was found to produce a more prolonged effect. Patients using acupuncture only one time a day still experienced a suppression of their withdrawal symptoms. Gradually the acupuncture protocol was expanded by adding the "Shen Men" (spirit gate), an ear point that is well known for producing relaxation. Other points were tried on the basis of lower skin resistance, pain sensitivity, and clinical indications during a several-year developmental process. Dr. Smith of LH added the "sympathetic," "kidney," and "liver" points to create a basic five-point formula. Over time, patients receiving ear needling reported continuing benefits from use of this protocol and were allowed to continue to attend LH for acupuncture on a "drop-in" basis, often continuing to attend several times per week for months or even years. Patients received frequent (on-site) urine testing for drugs, and were given their results in an immediate and nonjudgmental fashion. Although they came to LH for acupuncture, patients often took advantage of a variety of treatment services that were available there. Over time, although still called "acu-detox," the program included as-needed "aftercare" to such a large degree that that it came to resemble more of an ongoing or maintenance program than a detoxification program. This was seen as a good thing, because results in the literature were making it clearer that length of stay in any modality of treatment was a key predictor of better outcomes (35).

The standard formula seemed to be equally helpful for different drugs of abuse and at different stages of treatment (36). Patients responded better when acupuncture treatment was administered quickly without a self-conscious, diagnostic prelude. A group setting enhanced the acupuncture effect. A group size of fewer than six members seemed to diminish symptom relief and retention significantly. Patients receiving acupuncture in an individual setting were often self-conscious and easily distracted. These problems are more evident in the management of new patients. In general acupuncture treatment, sessions usually last for 20 to 25 minutes. Because chemical dependency patients seemed more resistant and dysfunctional, their length of treatment session in the acupuncture group setting was prolonged to 40 to 45 minutes, for a fuller effect to be reported.

The atmosphere of the treatment room should be adjusted to fit varying clinical circumstances. Programs with a significant number of new intakes or socially isolated patients should use a well-lighted room and allow a moderate amount of conversation to minimize alienation and encourage social bonding. On the other hand, programs with relatively fixed clientele who relate to each other frequently in other group settings should dim the lights and not allow any conversation to minimize distracting cross talk. Background music is often used in the latter circumstance. Dr. Smith developed an herbal formula known as "sleep mix," which can be used for the treatment of conventional stress and insomnia, as well as for providing an adjunctive support in addiction treatment settings. Although acupuncture was originally seen as a potential alternative to methadone maintenance, it has never shown comparable long-term efficacy against heroin addiction and is now seen as a potential adjunctive to opioid maintenance, perhaps assisting with cocaine or stimulant problems in methadone patients, or in other settings, to facilitate psychosocial treatment for addictions which do not have pharmacologic therapeutics available. While various numbers and combinations of ear points have been used, an important and interesting commonality to all of them is that the points reported as "active" and useful by clinical observation have all been located within the concha of the ear, which has the unique anatomic distinction of being the only exterior skin surface with sensory innervation from the vagus nerve. Auricular points are also notable in being the most well documented of the acupuncture microsystems, with some correspondences documented between the parts of the auricular homunculi and the anatomic areas or functions they are claimed to represent (37–39). The LH protocol was codified by NADA, which established training standards (including an emphasis on the clean-needle technique) for "acu-detox technicians" who, depending on specific state regulations, were sometimes addiction counselors without other acupuncture training. This model became especially popular in the drug court setting, where, paradoxically, methadone (a lifesaving treatment with well-established efficacy), is often seen as controversial, whereas acupuncture is accepted as very much a standard treatment. Some of the earliest U.S. trials came from an early drug court setting in Dade County, Florida, where acupuncture seemed to facilitate compliance with a drug-free treatment program (40). The same LH/NADA ear acupuncture protocol was adopted by a number of "detox" programs in the Boston area, where fewer subsequent detoxification readmissions where required by patients who attended programs incorporating acupuncture (41). This result held, suggesting that the risk of relapse was lower in patients with access to acupuncture, even when statistical adjustments were made between groups for clinical severity and other risk factors for relapse.

PREVENTION OF RELAPSE TO OPIOID ABUSE

Drug addiction is a chronic and recurrent condition. A high rate of relapse after prolonged drug-free periods characterizes the behavior of experienced abusers of heroin and other addictive drugs. Compared with physical dependence and withdrawal syndromes, addiction and relapse to opioids is an issue more difficult to deal with. It is typical that once addicted to heroin, the craving for heroin lasts a lifetime. It is the protracted patient's withdrawal syndromes (negative reinforcement) and the craving for drugs (positive reinforcement) that are the behavioral engines driving the patient to drug relapse. According to statistics from different sources, the relapse rate is no less than 95% and can be as high as 99%. If one confesses that for most patients craving will last their whole life, then long-acting opioid (methadone, levo-alpha-acetylmethadol [LAAM], or buprenorphine) maintenance is the principal choice to prevent relapse to heroin for most patients. Alternately, for some patients, especially those with strong resources for social support (or actual environmental control), one may try to find other ways to substantially reduce craving so that the occasional patient may become drug free for the rest of the patient's life. A radical change in the environment is often one of the most successful contributors to such efforts. The following sections explore whether acupuncture helps to reduce craving and postpone or prevent the relapse.

Experimental Studies in the Rat

There are several animal models (42) that can be used to study the problem of craving and relapse to drugs of abuse (the central issue in addictive disorders). Conditioned place preference (CPP) is one of the frequently used models (43). In a two-chamber or three-chamber experimental apparatus, the drug (unconditioned stimulus) is injected in the animal in one of the chambers. Thus it becomes associated with the environmental stimuli unique to that chamber (color of the surroundings, texture of the floor, etc.). After repeated training, the rat will choose to stay longer on the drug-associated side than in a chamber associated with normal saline injection or no injection. The ratio between the time spent in the drug-associated side and the saline-associated side can be taken as an index for the degree of craving. The CPP model is regarded as a relatively pure measure of addiction (as opposed to physical dependence) because the preference for the drug-associated compartment can be demonstrated when the animal is in the undrugged condition and free of withdrawal symptoms. Using this model, experiments were conducted to test whether acupuncture suppresses the expression of the CPP.

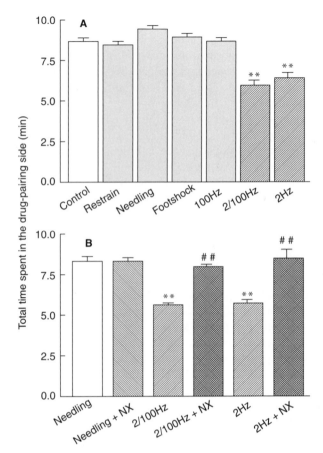

FIG. 49.4. A: Effect of electroacupuncture on 4 mg/kg morphine-induced CPP (n = 11–12). ** $P<0.01$, compared with the four control groups as well as the group treated with 100Hz stimulation. **B:** Naloxone blockade of the inhibitory effect of electroacupuncture on morphine-induced CPP (n = 9–10). ** $P<0.01$, compared with needling control group. ## $P<0.01$, compared with their corresponding naloxone treated group. (Modified from Wang B, Luo F, Xia YQ, et al. Peripheral electric stimulation inhibits morphine-induced place preference in rats. *Neuroreport* 2000;11:1017–1020, with permission.)

Wang et al. (14) (Fig. 49.4) were among the first to explore the effect of electroacupuncture on morphine CPP in the rat. A two-chamber apparatus was used. CPP was established by morphine injection at 4 mg/kg dose and the rats were trained for 10 days. The rats were then given electroacupuncture at 2 Hz, 100 Hz, or 2/100 Hz (dense-and-disperse mode) for 30 minutes, with intensity increasing stepwise from 1 mA to 2 mA to 3 mA within 30 minutes. Twelve hours after the end of electroacupuncture session, when the rats completely recovered from the manipulation of electroacupuncture procedure, they were put into the testing phase of CPP. CPP was significantly suppressed by electroacupuncture of 2 Hz and 2/100 Hz, but not of 100 Hz. Because the procedure of electroacupuncture consists of keeping the rat in the holder, the insertion of the stainless steel needles into the hind leg points (Zusanli and Sanyinjiao at both hind legs) and the administration of electrical stimulation, three control groups of rats received one of the following: (a) restraining in the holder for 30 minutes, (b) holder restraining plus needle insertion without electrical stimulation, or (c) intermittent electrical stimulation on the feet (foot shock). None of the three control groups showed any suppression of the CPP. Interestingly, electroacupuncture of 100 Hz was without effect, although the manipulation was exactly the same as for the 2-Hz group except for the difference in stimulation frequency. The results suggest that it is the low-frequency component of the electroacupuncture that suppressed the morphine CPP. Because the effect of electroacupuncture can be completely reversed by the opioid receptor antagonist naloxone at a small dose of 1 mg/kg, which is sufficient to block the opioid μ and δ, but not the κ, receptors, it seems evident that the effect of electroacupuncture is mediated by endogenously released μ- and δ-opioid agonists, most likely endorphins and enkephalins, to ease "craving" for exogenous opioids (in this case, the morphine). Another issue deserving attention is that the effect of electroacupuncture can still be revealed 12 hours after the episode of electroacupuncture, suggesting that this effect lasts longer than acupuncture-induced analgesia (which usually disappears within 60 minutes after the end of stimulation). Thus, a sensitization of the endogenous opioid circuits might be implied, which would readily release more opioids after electroacupuncture stimulation, resulting in a relatively long-lasting effect.

In practical life, craving and relapse can be easily induced by stress or by a very small dose of opioids. This phenomenon can be reproduced in animals using the CPP model. Wang et al. (44) reported that morphine-induced CPP disappeared after a 9-day extinction period. The extinguished CPP could be easily reinstated by foot shock stress, or by a small dose of morphine or amphetamine. Again, the reinstated CPP could be reversed by 2-Hz or 2/100-Hz electroacupuncture in a naloxone-preventable manner (45). It is worth mentioning that while both drug priming and foot shock stress can reactivate morphine CPP, the underlying mechanisms may be different. The drug-priming-induced reactivation can be totally blocked by the destruction of the mesolimbic dopamine system, including the ventral tegmental area (VTA) and the shell part of the nucleus accumbens, while the foot-shock-induced reactivation of CPP depends on the integrity of the central nucleus of the amygdala (46). Consequently, the mechanisms of electroacupuncture suppression of morphine CPP may involve a variety of neural pathways.

For simplicity and clarity of analysis, previous studies observed only the effects produced by a single session of electroacupuncture. However, in clinical practice, acupuncture or HANS is delivered daily in consecutive days or even several times a day. To mimic the clinical situation, animal experiments were designed using (a) electroacupuncture once a day for 3 consecutive days, (b) a

50% lower current intensity, and (c) a three-chamber device instead of a two-chamber device. The results showed that not only 2-Hz electroacupuncture, but also 100-Hz electroacupuncture is effective in suppressing morphine CPP (47). It seems plausible that by optimizing the parameters of electroacupuncture, its utility for the suppression of craving might be further improved.

Effect of HANS on Opiate Craving in Humans

To obtain a quantitative estimate of possible suppression of craving in response to acupuncture or related techniques, we used a visual analogue scale (VAS) to represent the degree of craving in a group of heroin-addicted patients who had completed the process of detoxification more than 1 month previously. A scale of 10 (10 cm in length) was used in the standard VAS, with VAS = 0 as having absolutely no craving and VAS = 10 as having the most severe craving imaginable. The experimenter can read the scale to the precision of 0.1 unit. The results from subjects with an initial VAS score of less than 2.0 were discarded. A total of 117 subjects were recruited, and were randomly and evenly assigned into 4 groups. Three groups received HANS treatment, each with a different frequency, 2 Hz, 100 Hz, or 2/100 Hz. Self-sticking skin electrodes were placed on four acupoints: Hegu and Laogong (palmar side of the Hegu point) in the left (or right) hand to complete a circuit, and Neiguan and Weiguan in the right (or left) arm to complete a circuit. The intensity was increased from the threshold level of the first day by two or three threshold values in the following days. The fourth group was processed as in the previous groups except that the intensity was minimal (15 Hz, threshold stimulation for 3 minutes, and then switched to 1 mA thereafter) to serve as a mock HANS control. There was a very slow decline of the VAS in the mock HANS control group. A dramatic decline of the degree of craving was observed in the groups receiving 2-Hz and 2/100-Hz electric stimulation, but not in the group receiving 100-Hz stimulation. In summary, the results observed in humans coincided with the findings obtained in the rat: low-frequency HANS is more effective than high-frequency HANS at reducing the craving for opiates (45) (Fig. 49.5). Interestingly, low-frequency electroacupuncture results in neural input to the CNS more like that of traditional acupuncture than does high-frequency electroacupuncture.

Drug Free for 1 Year as a Standard for Successful Prevention of Relapse

Heroin addiction is characterized by a high rate of relapse even after a long abstinence (for patients not in opioid-maintenance therapy). While the relapse rate after 3 months of being drug free is usually more than 50%, the relapse rate in 6 months can be as high as 95% to 99%. The hedonic concept holds that the fear of withdrawal

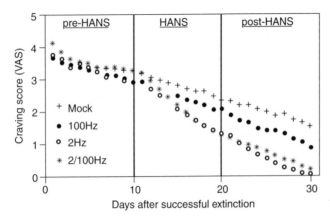

FIG. 49.5. Effect of Han's Acupoint Nerve Stimulation (HANS) on craving scores in heroin addicts (n = 29 to 30 in each group). HANS of 2 Hz and 2/100 Hz accelerated the decay of craving scores during the 10-day treatment period. (Modified from Wang B, Zhang BG, Yang C, et al. The suppressive effect of peripheral electric stimulation of different frequencies on the degree of craving in heroin addicts. *J Peking Univ (Health Sci)* 2003;35:(*in press*), with permission.)

symptoms and the craving for extreme pleasure constitute the two-wheel drive for relapse to drug-taking. Without taking special measures, the chance of complete drug abstinence for a period of 1 year is minimal. Consequently, we accept 1 year as a criterion of successful prevention of relapse. At least five factors determine the chance for success: (a) strong personal desire and determination to be rid of the drug; (b) warm and strong support from the family; (c) understanding from social relations; (d) having a job, even a part time job; and (e) having continuous care from the treatment center, including pharmacologic and non-pharmacologic and psychological interventions. Because methadone treatment has not been generally available in China, and based on the findings shown in the previous study concerning the effect of HANS on opiate craving, we encouraged the detoxified-addiction patients to take with them 1 unit of portable HANS when they are discharged from the detoxification center to ameliorate the protracted withdrawal syndrome and to suppress the craving induced by environmental cues. It is strongly recommended to the patient to have at least one session (30 minutes) before going to bed to facilitate sleep. It is also suggested that they use the device anytime there is a strong drug cue or a significant craving. The anticraving effect is usually reported to appear within 20 minutes.

Although there is a whole host of factors affecting the success of HANS in the prevention of relapse over 1 year, the most important one seems to be the effectiveness of the treatment system in taking care of the overall medical and psychological needs of the patient. In south China's Hainan province, a local rehabilitation center under the auspices of the Peking University Neuroscience Research Institute was established. The staff make friends and keep in close contact with all the drug-addiction patients discharged from the detoxification center. These patients can get HANS treatment from the rehabilitation center for free and ad lib. As an alternative, they can buy a unit of the device at an affordable cost and apply HANS at home under the staff's continuing supervision. A followup study was conducted on a group of 56 patients who used HANS at home. Using monthly urine test as criterion, the relapse rates at third, sixth, ninth, and twelfth months were 50.0%, 71.4%, 80.4%, and 83.9%, respectively. Those showing negative urine tests for 12 or 24 consecutive months were given a naloxone test (0.4 mg subcutaneously × 2 at 15-minute intervals) to further confirm their heroin-free status. Compared with the 97% relapse rate at 6 months and more than 99% relapse rate at 1 year in the majority of reports on heroin addiction (without methadone maintenance), an 83.9% relapse rate (16% success rate) at 1 year is encouraging. Similar studies were performed in treatment centers located in south China's Guangdong province. In Shanghai and in Tianjin, the 1-year success rate was between 2% and 10%, depending on the degree of followup medical care offered to the patients.

COCAINE ABUSE

Cocaine addiction is one of the most important challenges for acupuncture treatment of substance abuse for two reasons. First, the incidence of cocaine addiction has surpassed that of heroin in the whole world (13.4 vs. 9.2 million [48]). Second, there is no effective pharmacologic treatment available for cocaine addiction.

Compared with heroin addiction, cocaine addiction shows much less withdrawal syndrome on abstinence, yet more prominent and longer-lasting craving, serving as one of the most important cues leading to its relapse. Therefore the most important issue is whether acupuncture can have an effect in treatment on the prevention of cocaine craving. Data obtained from animal experiments is discussed first, followed by a discussion of the clinical trials.

Experimental Studies

In the last three decades, the self-administration technique has commonly been used to assess the degree of psychic dependence to cocaine in rats, that is, to mimic the degree of craving in humans. In recent years, CPP has also been used for this purpose. Drug-induced CPP is thought to mimic the cue-elicited conditioning that motivates drug-seeking behavior. The establishment of cocaine-induced CPP depends on the dose and route of administration, as well as the number of conditioning sessions used. Using an 8-day conditioning paradigm and the dose of cocaine at 1 mg/kg (intraperitoneally) and higher, Ren et al. (49) studied the expression of cocaine-induced CPP in rats, which maintained as long as 4 weeks at weekly checking, or 13 days at daily checking schedule. High-frequency electroacupuncture (100 Hz) applied at hind leg points for 30 minutes was found to significantly reduce the CPP, whereas low-frequency (2 Hz) electroacupuncture was without effect (Fig. 49.6A). The procedure of electroacupuncture might involve at least three stress factors: restraining, needling, and electric shocking. These possibilities have individually been ruled out by control studies. The results suggest that it is the specific parameter of electroacupuncture rather than a nonspecific stressful condition that played an important role in modulating cocaine CPP.

Electroacupuncture of identified frequencies mobilizes different kinds of endogenous opioid peptides. The attenuation of cocaine CPP by 100-Hz electroacupuncture may involve a κ-opioid mechanism. Indeed, the effect of 100 Hz can be blocked by the opioid antagonist naloxone only at a high dose of 10 mg/kg. This dose is sufficient to antagonize all three subtypes of opioid receptors, including κ. On the other hand, the lower doses (1 and 5 mg/kg) that are only able to inactivate μ- and δ-opioid receptors could not block the effect of electroacupuncture (Fig. 49.6B).

It is worth noting that (a) the effect of electroacupuncture can be detected 10 to 24 hours, but not 5 hours, after the termination of electroacupuncture, suggesting that this could be an effect involving a cascade of reactions, probably through transcriptional regulation. (b) Naloxone injected 20 minutes prior to electroacupuncture can block the effect of electroacupuncture as detected 24 hours post-electroacupuncture, suggesting that the role of naloxone is to block the initiation of the electroacupuncture effect. (c) The effect of electroacupuncture on suppressing cocaine CPP can be blocked by a specific κ opioid receptor antagonist administered into the nucleus accumbens, but not into the amygdala, suggesting that nucleus accumbens is one of the sites of action for endogenous opioid peptide, most probably dynorphin, to suppress cocaine CPP. (d) Injection of κ receptor agonist into the nucleus accumbens suppresses CPP in a dose-dependent manner (50). Together this suggests that cocaine-induced CPP can be suppressed by electroacupuncture in a frequency-dependent manner, being effective at 100 Hz, but not at 2 Hz. The effect of 100 Hz electroacupuncture can be reversed by naloxone at 10 mg/kg but not with lower doses, suggesting the involvement of a κ-opioid mechanism in mediating electroacupuncture effect. This was verified using highly specific κ agonist and antagonist, and the site of action was targeted to the nucleus accumbens. These results may suggest a role for 100-Hz electroacupuncture or HANS to reduce cocaine craving and to prevent

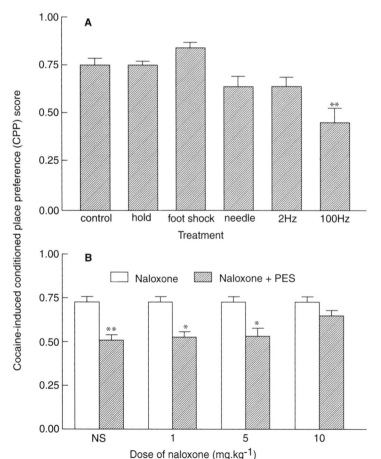

FIG. 49.6. A: Effect of electroacupuncture of different frequencies on CPP expression induced by 5 mg/kg of cocaine B: Naloxone reversal of the CPP-attenuating effect of 100 Hz electroacupuncture. (Modified from Ren YH, Wang B, Luo F, et al. Peripheral electric stimulation attenuates the expression of cocaine-induced place preference in rats. *Brain Res* 2002;957:129–135, with permission.)

relapse. Clinical trials of this approach are certainly indicated.

Clinical Trials

Ear acupuncture is often used for the treatment of cocaine addiction in the United States, using the same four to five ear points bilaterally originally developed at Lincoln Hospital for use against opioid addiction and promulgated by NADA for general use in addiction programs. In a series of 226 cases of users of cocaine or crack cocaine who had more than 20 visits to the Lincoln Hospital treatment center, 149 (65%) had more than 80% negative urine tests during the entire treatment involvement. Of the remaining patients, 39 (17%) had at least 80% negative urine test during the 2 weeks prior to data collection. While there is no control group, the success rate by itself was felt to be quite encouraging (36). The Yale group (51) studied 32 cocaine-dependent, methadone-maintained patients who received an 8-week course of auricular acupuncture for the treatment of cocaine dependence. Fifty percent completed treatment; 88% of study completers attained abstinence, defined as providing cocaine-free urine samples for the last 2 weeks of the study, yielding an overall abstinence rate of 44%. Post hoc comparisons to pharmacotherapy with desipramine (Norpramin), amantadine (Symmetrel) and placebo revealed a higher abstinence rate for acupuncture (44%) than for amantadine (15%) or placebo (13%), but not significantly higher than for desipramine (26%). Avants et al. (52) obtained similar results in a moderately sized randomized (n = 82) trial. Longitudinal analysis of the urine data for the intent-to-treat sample showed that patients assigned to acupuncture were significantly more likely to provide cocaine-negative urine samples relative to both the relaxation control (odds ratio: 3.41) and the needle-insertion control (odds ratio: 2.40). These findings suggested that acupuncture was effective for the treatment of cocaine dependence under the conditions at the site under study.

Encouraged by the aforementioned results, a randomized, controlled, single-blind, multisite large-scale clinical trial was conducted from 1996 to 1999. The results were published in the *Journal of the American Medical Association* in 2002 (53). This study included 620 cocaine-dependent adult patients, 420 of whom used cocaine only and 208 of whom used both cocaine and opiates and were receiving methadone maintenance. Patients were randomly assigned to receive auricular acupuncture (four needles schedule), a needle-insertion control (four needles inserted into the helix of the ear), or a relaxation control. Treatments were offered five times weekly for 8 weeks. Main outcome measures were cocaine use during treatment and at the 3- and 6-month followup based on urine toxicology screen and retention in treatment. Analysis of urine samples showed a significant overall reduction in cocaine use but no differences by treatment condition,

nor any difference in the rate of treatment retention. The conclusion is that within the clinical context of this study, acupuncture was not more effective than a needle insertion or relaxation control in reducing cocaine use. The authors concluded that the results do not support the use of acupuncture as a stand-alone treatment for cocaine addiction, yet it may play an ancillary role for the treatment of cocaine addiction. This conclusion is apparently in contrast to that derived from the animal experiments, as well as results from the preceding pilot study. Consideration of important differences between the conditions under which acupuncture demonstrated efficacy in the pilot and then failed to do so in the larger study leads to implications for the clinical conditions under which acupuncture may be most useful. Because of changes in available resources, it seems that the psychosocial and rehabilitative services made available for patients during the second study was fairly minimal, while in the first, the services had been considerable (54). Also, of particular methodologic importance, patients in the first trial were not paid, and those in the second were. This is, of course, quite different from the situation found in clinical practice. Although paying subjects is a common practice in clinical research, it could obviously create inferential problems when studying a therapy who's major effects may interact with or actually depend on patient motivation, especially when outcomes are so dependent on patient behavior. If acupuncture's major benefit lies in motivating patients to keep returning to the clinic, then paying subjects to participate in and complete the study could have easily eliminated most of the study's potential for showing such a difference between the groups.

Finally, in the planning of future large trials of acupoint therapy for cocaine addiction, attention should also be directed to the results obtained in rat experiments showing that 100-Hz, rather than 2-Hz, stimulation can suppress the cocaine-induced CPP. Recalling that this high-frequency, dynorphinergic (primarily κ-receptor activating) stimulation is quite different from the more closely related low-frequency or manual (primarily μ- and δ-receptor activating) stimulation, it may be important to include 100-Hz electroacupuncture (and possibly body electroacupuncture or HANS) stimulation in future American trials of acupoint therapy for the treatment of cocaine addiction.

ALCOHOLISM

Acupuncture was considered quite promising for the treatment of alcohol addiction in the 1980s. Two consecutive papers were published providing clearly positive results in this regard (55,56). The orthodox ear points suggested in the LH/NADA protocol were used, and points 3 to 5 mm apart were used as nonspecific points for control. The subject size was 54 and 80, respectively, and the observation period was 6 months. The results obtained were in favor of acupuncture treatment, as manifested in the reduced need for alcohol, fewer drinking episodes, fewer subsequent admissions requiring detoxification, less desire to drink, and more people to complete the acupuncture program. However, this result could not be replicated by Worner et al. (57) in the United States (56 cases) or by Sapir-Weise et al. (58) in Sweden (72 cases). In a recent randomized, placebo-controlled study of auricular acupuncture, Bullock et al. (59) conducted a large-scale clinical trial that included 503 cases. The unique feature of the design of the study for the patient grouping was that, aside from the "specific" ear acupuncture group, "nonspecific" ear acupuncture group, and the conventional treatment group, a fourth group was set using symptom-based acupuncture where the acupuncturists were not constrained to the four ear points stipulated in the other acupuncture treatment group, and point prescription could be changed on a day-to-day basis according to the patients' discomfort. The patients were given six treatments per week for as long as 3 weeks to maximize the therapeutic effects. The outcome, however, was quite different from the original hypothesis. All four groups showed a significant improvement. There were few differences associated with treatment assignment, and there were no treatment differences on alcohol use measures, although 49% of subjects reported that acupuncture reduced their desire for alcohol. These authors concluded that ear acupuncture did not make a significant contribution over and above that achieved by conventional treatment alone in the reduction of alcohol use.

Lots of data show that the euphoric effect of alcohol is mediated by endogenous opioid peptides (60) and the opioid antagonist naltrexone has been used to assist cognitive–behavioral therapy for alcoholics (61). Therefore, modulation of the endogenous opioid system should be considered as one of the approaches for the treatment of alcohol craving and reward in alcoholic patients. Yoshimoto et al. (62) reported that rats subject to repeated restriction stress consume more alcohol than the control animals. Electroacupuncture at hind limb points zusanli (ST-36) significantly reduced the alcohol-seeking behavior, whereas the lumbar point Shenshu (BL-23) was not effective. The effect of electroacupuncture stimulation at ST-36 was accompanied by an increase in dopamine level in the striatum, compared with that produced by electroacupuncture at BL-23. These findings provide new information for understanding alcohol-drinking behavior and for treating human alcoholics.

TECHNICAL COMMENTS ON USING ACUPUNCTURE IN THE TREATMENT OF ADDICTION

Because of the conflicting opinions regarding the efficacy of acupuncture for the treatment of substance abuse, the National Institute on Drug Abuse (NIDA) sponsored a technical review on October 23, 1991, to discuss this issue in an attempt to propose directions for future studies. A summary of the report was published in the *Journal of Substance Abuse Treatment* in 1993 (5). The review pointed out four major problems that required a solution: the nonstandard terminology used to describe it, the wide range of procedures that have been called acupuncture, the lack of a clear mechanism to explain the purported benefits of acupuncture treatment, and the lack of systematic clinical research in this area. Ten years have passed since the publication of the report. In that time, terminology has become somewhat more standardized, but not completely and clinical trials have begun to focus on a limited number of procedures, guided more by popularity than any particularly rational or planned approach. Perhaps the furthest progress has been made in the area of acupuncture's mechanisms. With a new wealth of neurochemical data and neuroanatomic imaging, it is no longer essential to postulate traditional paradigms such as yin and yang in order to approach the topic of acupuncture. However, the millennia of clinical experience encoded in the allegorical imagery of elements and meridians and functional concepts, such as the triple burner, may still have much to offer on the empiric clinical level. It may be useful to admit that we will never see the superego or id on an x-ray or under the microscope, or measure either on a meter or a blood test, and the same may be true for chi. Most of the important problems seem to remain, although many issues have become clearer than before for both research and practice.

Ear Acupuncture Versus Body Acupuncture

From an historical point of view, the 14 meridians or channels considered by ancient Chinese physicians as the linkage for acupuncture points, serving as the channel for the flow of "Qi", are distributed over the body rather than on the ear. Dr. H. L. Wen of the Kwong Wah Hospital of Hong Kong, the pioneer of the acupuncture treatment for drug addiction, used four needles in the hand and arm, plus two needles in the ear (4). These needles were manipulated to induce *de-qi* sensation and then connected to an electronic stimulator for further stimulation lasting for 30 minutes. In states that require fully licensed acupuncturists or physicians to administer ear needling to begin with, these operators may wish to consider the addition of body points or even additional treatment for other symptoms or complaints while the patient is being treated, concurrently with the NADA ear protocol. In states that have created the category of mid-level "acu-detox technicians" allowed only to administer the ear protocol, this would not be possible unless the fully licensed practitioner were called in. While training or certification to pierce the skin is not required for the use of a TENS or HANS device, a knowledge of the location of the relevant points is still required, as is the ability to communicate the finding of these points for patients who will be self-administering electrical acupoint stimulation. Whichever methods of point stimulation are chosen, it is vital to keep in mind that engagement of the patient with an adequate program and frequently recurring visits by the patient are just as, if not more, important than the acupoint stimulation itself. While clinical trial data are still somewhat equivocal on acupuncture and are not yet helpful in selecting one modality or protocol over another, it is still clear that increasing the length and frequency of clinical engagement with an otherwise adequate treatment program will improve the long-term outcome of patients being treated for addictive disorders. To the degree that acupuncture or other safe and low-cost alternative therapies will accomplish this, their benefits in incremental use and compliance may be enough to make them worthwhile for programs that wish to take advantage of current positive public perceptions. Having said this, such programs should feel obligated to follow the results of new research as it emerges. An upcoming Treatment Improvement Protocol (TIP) from the Center for Substance Abuse Treatment will include the clinical trial data to date, and current plans include the dissemination of further new trial data, especially U.S. trials, as they emerge.

Needle Staying Versus Manual Needling

According to traditional acupuncture practice, a needle inserted into the acupoint can be further processed in at least different three ways: (a) left *in situ* undisturbed for a period of time, which is defined as "needle staying;" (b) manually twisted to obtain maximal *de-qi* sensation; or (c) heated at the shaft of the needle to intensify the therapeutic effect. It is clear that needle staying is the most modest of the three procedures. Moreover, the efficacy of needle staying depends on the site of needle insertion. The ear comprises skin that is covering cartilage, which is quite sensitive to mechanical stimulation and may produce continuous input during the staying of the needle. The situation will be dramatically different if the needle is inserted into soft tissues. In our pilot experiment performed in human volunteers, it was evident that merely leaving the needle in the Hegu (LI-4) point for 30 minutes in the control group produced little change in the pain threshold of the skin (15). When a needle is inserted in most body points, to induce a marked elevation of the pain threshold one has to twist or otherwise stimulate it. Early in 1973, a research group at Jiangsu College of New Medicine in Nanjin, China, showed that insertion of a needle in the ear point Shenmen (single point) with manipulation for 60 minutes produced a gradual increase of the pain threshold of the skin over the body (chest and abdomen) as measured by the potassium iontophoresis method. It reached a plateau in 30 minutes and remained there for the duration of the study. The pain threshold went down when the needle was left *in situ* unmanipulated, and went up again when the needle was manipulated for another 50 minutes (Fig. 49.7). The results suggest that manipulation of the needle

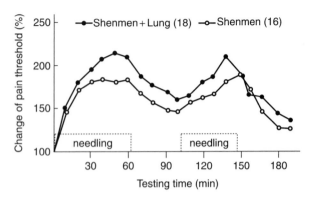

FIG. 49.7. Influence of manual needling at ear acupoint Shenmen (n = 16) or Shenmen plus lung (n = 18) on pain threshold of the skin over the chest and abdomen in humans. (Modified from Research Group of Ear Acupuncture, Jiangsu College of New Medicine. The effect of ear acupuncture on the pain threshold of the skin at thoracic and abdominal region. In: *Theoretical study on acupuncture anesthesia.* Shanghai People's Press, Shanghai, China 1973:27–32, with permission.)

produces much stronger physiologic effects than does needle staying, at least when pain modulation is measured (63).

Acupuncture and Electroacupuncture Versus Transcutaneous Electric Stimulation

A series of studies showed that the manipulation of the needle triggers a train of nerve impulses transmitted along the afferent nerve fibers to the CNS. The physiologic effects produced by acupuncture (e.g., the antinociceptive effect) can be readily blocked by the injection of local anesthetics deep into the point (15), or along the nerve trunk. If nerve activation accounts for the transmission of the acupuncture signals, then similar effects should be induced whether similar nerve impulses are generated by manipulation of a needle, or directly by electrical impulses through the needles inserted into the point, or even by electrodes on the surface of the skin over the point, that force a current to pass through the same underlying tissue and produce a feeling of *de-qi*. In an experiment performed in the rat, the analgesic effects induced by electroacupuncture (via needles) and by transcutaneous stimulation (via skin electrodes) were compared. No significant difference was found between the two approaches in the efficacy of inducing an analgesic effect (12). It is interesting to note that a similar mechanism seems to underlie the two analgesic effects. Thus, no matter the electrical stimulation is delivered via needles or skin electrodes, opioid antagonist naloxone at 2 mg/kg dose produced a complete reversal of 2-Hz stimulation-produced analgesia, a partial reversal of 15-Hz stimulation-induced analgesia, and no reversal on 100-Hz stimulation-produced analgesia (12). In a human study, the analgesic effect induced by manual needling was compared to that induced by transcutaneous electric stimulation at the Hegu (LI-4) point. The results indicated that they are essentially the same, if not identical (64). It should also be mentioned that this and other clear evidence of neuronal mediation of the analgesic effects of acupuncture, while not necessarily excluding the meridian model or the existence of chi, certainly demonstrates that this model (or allegory) of meridians and chi is not required for an explanation of acupuncture's effects.

In the past, blood-borne virus and anecdotal reports of bacterial infections have been associated with acupuncture (65). Woo et al. recently reported four cases encountered with acupuncture in a 2-year period with relatively alcohol-resistant mycobacteria infection at acupuncture-point-specific locations (66). The risk of acupuncture-mediated infection is minimized by strict adherence to the instructions for single use only, which are included in the packaging of all FDA-approved acupuncture needles. For those still concerned, use of skin electrodes rather than needles will reduce this risk from minimal to zero.

Opioid- Versus Nonopioid Mechanisms

The mechanism of acupuncture or electroacupuncture relies, at least partly, on the frequency-dependent release of opioid peptides in the CNS (67). For example, high-frequency (100 Hz) stimulation is more efficacious than low-frequency (2 Hz) stimulation in reducing opiate withdrawal syndrome through activation of the dynorphin system mediated by the κ-opioid receptors, whereas the low-frequency stimulation is more efficacious than high-frequency stimulation in reducing opiate craving by the activation of endorphin/enkephalin system mediated by μ- and d-opioid receptors. In contrast to opiate addiction, effects on cocaine addiction may work through a slightly different mechanism, such that the CPP for cocaine in the rat, a rodent model of cocaine craving, can be suppressed only by 100-Hz, but not 2-Hz, stimulation (49).

Aside from the opioid systems, electroacupuncture also activates nonopioid systems of the brain, including the norepinephrine system (68) and the serotonin (5-HT) system (69) of the CNS. Activation of these monoaminergic pathways may also help to ameliorate the withdrawal syndrome, although it has not been elucidated whether there is also a frequency dependence in this context.

How Frequently Should Acupuncture Be Used for the Treatment of Drug Abuse?

In an inpatient setting, it is clear that both electroacupuncture and HANS works to suppress opiate-withdrawal syndrome even if it is administered only once (for 30 minutes) a day (13). However, for the best results, it is recommended to use it three to four times a day for the first 5 days, followed by a reduction to twice a day for another 5 days,

and then once a day for the rest of the time for a total of 2 weeks. Too frequent an application results in the decrease of the therapeutic effect because of the development of tolerance (70). For the treatment of protracted withdrawal syndromes in the period of rehabilitation, once or twice a day is sufficient. The session applied immediately before sleep is critical for the treatment schedule, because this will facilitate a good sleep (13). It is noticeable that in the rat experiment, the effect of electroacupuncture in suppressing CPP induced by morphine or cocaine bears with a long latency of 10 hours and a long aftereffect of at least 24 hours (14,49). This may serve as a mechanism for the cumulative effect observed in the treatment of drug abuse with acupuncture.

Design Considerations

Acupuncture, as a procedure (or group of related procedures), is far more difficult to subject to a traditional double-blind clinical trial than is a drug. In this respect, clinical trials of acupuncture should be compared with trials for different types of psychotherapy or for surgical procedures, rather than drug trials. Considerable methodologic progress has been made in recent years, that will make better randomized trials possible and should help answer the many questions yet unanswered about acupuncture's efficacy.

Mock Needle

To design a study where mock acupuncture is administered is by no means an easy task, because needling by itself will produce a vague sensation. In fact no one can tell how far from an acupoint would needling become ineffective. So the determination of a "sham point" has no scientific basis. The invention of a mock needle seems to provide a solution to this question. The design of the mock needle is such that the needle looks like penetrating the skin, but it actually withdraws into a hollow space, leaving a touch sensation on the skin to mimic the *de-qi* sensation (71). This is a single-blind design, because the acupuncturist knows the difference between the conventional needle and the mock needle.

Frequency Specificity Design

Another design involves insertion of the needle to the real acupoint, but electrical stimulation at two different frequencies is used, which might induce a qualitatively different result. For example, it happens that 2 Hz and 2/100 Hz stimulations are effective in producing a suppression of the opiate craving, whereas 100-Hz stimulation is ineffective (see Fig. 49.5). In contrast, cocaine-induced CPP can be suppressed by 100-Hz, but not 2-Hz, electroacupuncture (49).

Intensity Specificity Design

To use electroacupuncture or TENS at different intensities is another choice. For example, using a constant current device, the threshold intensity for a 4×4-cm skin pad is 5 to 6 mA for most subjects. A desirable intensity is two times threshold, that is, 10 to 12 mA. By using the two different levels of intensity it can be expected that the higher intensity group would produce a more prominent effect, and that relapse would occur more often in the lower intensity group.

Outcome Measure

Urinalysis is an objective and essential measure. Three times per week during the detoxification period and once or twice a month during the rehabilitation period are reasonable design. It should be continued for as long as 1 year to obtain a 1-year abstinence record.

PSYCHOSOCIAL PERSPECTIVES

Dr. Michael Smith made an important statement (36) when he wrote that "it is essential to understand acupuncture's psychological and social mechanisms of action to use this modality effectively. Acupuncture has an impact on the patient's thoughts and feelings that is different from conventional pharmacological treatments."

Seeking Help from Outside or from Within

Conventional treatment efforts tend to focus on assessment of past activities and planning for the future. However, the past leaves nothing to the addicts but pain. As for the future, they feel hopeless because they lose confidence to themselves. What is important to them is the present: Can you solve my problem without my taking drugs? Acupuncture allows treatment staff to respond to one of the patient's immediate needs without using addictive drugs. That is, to meet the patient in present-time reality, validating their needs and providing substantial relief. The nonverbal, present-time aspects of the treatment make it easy to respond to a patient in whatever stage of crisis or denial that may exist. Additionally, and unlike talk therapy, acupuncture will not challenge the patient cognitively or emotionally. Acupuncture provides a way for patients to feel they are being helped by a health professional without being threatened or confronted. Having acupuncture in a group setting, and seeing fellow patients being similarly helped, may reinforce this message. This and other nonverbal interactions in the group acupuncture setting may be responsible for the observation from Lincoln Hospital that patients respond much better to acupuncture in the group setting.

One difference between pharmacologic treatment and acupuncture treatment is that the former relies more on external help whereas the latter builds up one's self-confidence. Addicts may well feel hopeless about their future, even for those who really want to quit drugs. They perceive themselves as being unable to change from within: "once an addict, always an addict." They seek external help to provide hospitalization and medication. The help can be pills or injections. Taking medications, for example, methadone or buprenorphine, may help to relieve their withdrawal syndrome, but does not improve their confidence, because they know that they will rely on the medication just as they relied on their drug of abuse. In contrast, acupuncture can be explained to reprogram their brain function, and thereby restore their ability to live a normal life. It is the patient's common feeling that after the first treatment, they often have a very good sleep that night, which has not been experienced for a very long period of time. The confidence and loyalty for this nonpharmacologic treatment becomes increasingly evident, and the compliance to acupuncture is built up quickly. Once a comfortable day-to-day support is established, we can approach past and future issues with a better alliance with the patient.

Group Setting or Single Treatment

According to Dr. Smith, a group setting may be more suitable for addiction patients to interact with others as compared to one-to-one conversation between the doctor and the patient. "We describe acupuncture as a foundation for psychosocial rehabilitation," stated Dr. Smith. In their practice, acupuncture for substance abuse is provided in a group setting, with a group being no fewer than six patients. "This encouraging and balancing group experience becomes a critically important basis for the entire process of substance abuse treatment."

Unexpected Physiologic Changes that Help to Build Psychological Confidence

In the treatment of opiate addiction, two unexpected changes in the body function help the patient to build their confidence. One is the disappearance of injection marks and the other is the recovery of the depressed sexual function. In an incidental case, the patient treated with HANS supplemented with a small dose of buprenorphine reported that his injection marks in the forearm disappeared and the veins reappeared at the end of the 14-day detoxification period. That was recognized as a strong indication that his body function was quickly recovering. A careful study was designed to record the injection marks as coded by the existence of fibrotic thickening of the blood vessel wall, thrombosis, bluish streak, scared mainliners, and venous collapse. Statistical analysis revealed that these changes were significantly less frequently revealed in the control group using only buprenorphine for detoxification (32). Another observation was on the sexual function as revealed by standard questionnaire. The sexual function of the 32 male patients was seriously depressed at their enrollment to the treatment center, and was markedly recovered (to 80% of the normal level) at the end of 1 month of treatment with HANS supplemented with small amount of buprenorphine, but not in the group using the full dose of buprenorphine (it remained at a level equivalent to 20% to 25% of the normal level of sexual function) (72). These changes provided the patient with positive psychological impact and confidence, and would certainly be helpful in the establishment of a normal life, thus delaying the occurrence of the relapse to drugs.

The friendship established between the patient and the staff in residential treatment can, and should be continued when the patients are discharged from the treatment center. The transfer from the treatment center to the home is a very critical period, especially for persons leaving prison. They are confronted with a bleak uncaring world. Their own feelings of inadequacy frequently become so overwhelming that a return to prior drug use may occur within hours of release. It is in this sense that family help, social caring, and medical instruction should be intimately organized from the first day of returning home, and acupuncture provides a unique chance to let the patient feel that there is something to rely on.

Acupuncture is an emerging treatment for drug abuse. This new approach is different from that of pharmacologic treatment. From a technical point of view, there is plenty of room for improvement and definitive evidence of efficacy remains to be shown. Many patients and providers remain convinced that it has something to add to the treatment package. The complicated network underlying drug abuse can be unraveled only through combined physiologic, neurobiologic, and psychological endeavors, and acupuncture can play a role at least as one of the tools in a comprehensive approach.

REFERENCES

1. Klein LJ, Trachtenberg AI, compilers. *Acupuncture [bibliography online].* Bethesda, MD: National Library of Medicine, 1997. (Current bibliographies in medicine; no. 97-6); 2,302 citations from January 1970 through October 1997. Available at: http://www.nlm.nih.gov/pubs/resources.html.
2. NIH Consensus Conference. Acupuncture. *JAMA* 1998;280:1518–1524.
3. CSAT. *Treatment improvement protocol (TIP) on the incorporation of acupuncture in addiction treatment programs.* 2004 (in press).
4. Wen HL, Cheung SYC. Treatment of drug addiction by acupuncture and electrical stimulation. *Asian J Med* 1973;9:138–141.
5. McLellan AT, Grossman DS, Blaine JD, et al. Acupuncture treatment for drug abuse: a technical review. *J Subst Abuse Treat* 1993;10:569–576.
6. Hughes J, Smith TW, Kosteritz HW, et al. Identification of two related pentapeptides from the brain with potent opiate agonist activity. *Nature* 1975;258:577–579.
7. Mayer DJ, Price DD, Rafii A. Antagonisms of acupuncture analgesia in man by the narcotic antagonist naloxone. *Brain Res* 1977;121:368–372.
8. Han JS, Terenius L. Neurochemical basis of acupuncture analgesia. *Annu Rev Pharmacol Toxicol* 1982;22:193–220.
9. Herz A, ed. *Handbook of experimental pharmacology,* vol. 104/I: *opioids I.* Berlin: Springer-Verlag, 1993.
10. Han JS, Wang Q. Mobilization of specific neuropeptides by peripheral stimulation of different frequencies. *News Physiol Sci* 1992;7:176–180.
11. Han JS, Zhang RL. Suppression of morphine abstinence syndrome by body electroacupuncture of different frequencies in rats. *Drug Alcohol Depend* 1993;31:169–175.
12. Wang Q, Mao LM, Han JS. Comparison of the antinociceptive effects induced by electroacupuncture and transcutaneous electrical nerve stimulation in the rat. *Int J Neurosci* 1992;65:117–129.
13. Wu LZ, Cui CL, Han JS. Han's acupoint nerve stimulator for the treatment of opiate withdrawal syndrome. *Chin J Pain Med* 1995;1:30–35.
14. Wang B, Luo F, Xia YQ, et al. Peripheral electric stimulation inhibits morphine-induced place preference in rats. *Neuroreport* 2000;11:1017–1020.
15. Research Group of Acupuncture Anesthesia, Peking Medical College. Effect of acupuncture on pain threshold of human skin. *Chin Med J* 1973;(3):151–157.
16. Lu GW. Characteristics of afferent fiber innervations on acupuncture point Zusanli. *Am J Physiol* 1983;245:R606–R612.
17. Melzack R, Wall PD. Pain mechanisms: a new theory. *Science* 1965;130:971–979.
18. Choy YM, Tso WW, Fung KP, et al. Suppression of narcotic withdrawals and plasma ACTH by auricular electroacupuncture. *Biochem Biophys Res Commun* 1978;82:305–309.
19. Ng LKY, Douthitt TC, Thoa NB, et al. Modification of morphine withdrawal syndrome in rats following transauricular electrostimulation: an experimental paradigm for auricular electroacupuncture. *Biol Psychiatry* 1975;10:575–580.
20. Auricombe M, Tignol J, Moal ML, et al. Transcutaneous electrical stimulation with Limoge current potentiates morphine analgesia and attenuates opiate abstinence syndrome. *Biol Psychiatry* 1990;28:650–656.
21. Han JS, Chen XH, Sun SL, et al. Effect of low- and high-frequency TENS on met-enkephalin-Arg-Phe and dynorphin A immunoreactivity in human lumbar CSF. *Pain* 1991;47:295–298.
22. Han JS, Xie GX, Goldstein A. Analgesia induced by intrathecal injection of dynorphin B in the rat. *Life Sci* 1984;34:1573–1579.
23. Wen HL, Ho WKK. Suppression of withdrawal symptoms by dynorphin in heroin addicts. *Eur J Phamacol* 1982;82:183–186.
24. Aceto MD, Dewey WL, Chang JK, et al. Dynorphin (1–13): effect on non-tolerant and morphine-dependent rhesus monkeys. *Eur J Pharmacol* 1982;83:139–142.
25. Green PG, Lee NM. Dynorphin (1–13) attenuates withdrawal in morphine-dependent rats: effect of route of administration. *Eur J Pharmacol* 1998;145:267–272.
26. Cui CL, Wu LZ, Han JS. Spinal kappa-opioid system plays an important role in suppressing morphine withdrawal syndrome in the rat. *Neurosci Lett* 2000;295:42–48.
27. Yu YG, Cui CL, Yu JR, et al. 100 Hz electroacupuncture amelioration of tachycardia of morphine withdrawal rats is mediated by kappa-opioid receptor in central nervous system. *J Beijing Med Univ* 1999;31:1–4.
28. Yu YG, Cui CL, Yu JR, et al. Tachycardia ameliorated by electroacupuncture in

morphine withdrawal rats. *Chin J Integr Trad West Med* 2000;20:353–355.

29. Huang C, Wang Y, Han JS, et al. Characteristics of electroacupuncture-induced analgesia in different strains of mice. *Brain Res* 2002;945:20–25.

30. Chen XH, Han JS. All three types of opioid receptors are important for 2/15 Hz electroacupuncture analgesia. *Eur J Pharmacol* 1992;211:203–210.

31. Wu LZ, Cui CL, Han JS. Effect of Han's acupoint nerve stimulator (HANS) on the heart rate of 75 inpatients during heroin withdrawal. *Chin J Pain Med* 1996;2:98–102.

32. Wu LZ, Cui CL, Han JS. Treatment on heroin addicts by 4-channel Han's Acupoint Nerve Stimulator (HANS). *J Beijing Med Univ* 1999;31:239–242.

33. Wu LZ, Cui CL, Han JS. Reduction of methadone dosage and relief of depression and anxiety by 2/100 Hz TENS for heroin detoxification. *Chin J Drug Depend* 2001;10:124–126.

34. Smith MO, Khan I. An acupuncture program for the treatment of drug addicted persons. *Bull Narc* 1988;40:35–41.

35. Simpson DD, Brown BS. Treatment retention and follow-up outcomes in the Drug Abuse Treatment Outcome Study (DATOS). *Psychol Addict Behav* 1998;11(4):294–307.

36. Smith MO, Brewington V, Culliton PD, et al. Acupuncture. In: Lowinson JH, Ruiz P, Millman RB, et al., eds. *Substance abuse, a comprehensive textbook,* 3rd edi. Baltimore: Williams & Wilkins, 1997:484–492.

37. Oleson T, Kroening R, Bresler D. An experimental evaluation of auricular diagnosis: the somatotopic mapping of musculoskeletal pain at ear acupuncture points. *Pain* 1980;8:217–229.

38. Alimi D, Geissmann A, Gardeur D. Auricular acupuncture stimulation measured on functional magnetic resonance imaging. *Med Acupunct* 2002;13:18–21.

39. Asamoto S, Takeshige C. Activation of the satiety center by auricular acupuncture point stimulation. *Brain Res Bull* 1992;29:157–164.

40. Konefal J, Duncan R, Clemence C. The impact of the addition of an acupuncture treatment program to an existing Metro-Dade County outpatient substance abuse treatment facility. *J Addict Dis* 1994;13(3):71–99.

41. Shwartz M, Saitz R, Mulvey K, et al. The value of acupuncture detoxification programs in a substance abuse treatment system. *J Subst Abuse Treat* 1999;17(4):305–312.

42. Markou A, Weiss F, Gold LH, et al. Animal models of drug craving. *Psychopharmacology (Berl)* 1993;163:182.

43. Bardo MT, Bevins RA. Conditioned place preference: what does it add to our preclinical understanding of drug reward? *Psychopharmacology (Berl)* 2000;153(1):31–43.

44. Wang B, Luo F, Xia YQ, et al. Stress or drug priming induces reinstatement of extinguished conditioned place preference. *Neuroreport* 2000;11:1017–1020.

45. Wang B, Zhang BG, Yang C, et al. The suppressive effect of peripheral electric stimulation of different frequencies on the degree of craving in heroin addicts. *J Peking Univ (Health Sci)* 2003;35:(in press).

46. Wang B, Luo F, Ge XC, et al. Effects of lesions of various brain areas on drug priming or foot-shock induced reactivation of extinguished conditioned place preference. *Brain Res* 2002;950:1–9.

47. Shi et al, 2003, to be published

48. WHO report 1988–2001.

49. Ren YH, Wang B, Luo F, et al. Peripheral electric stimulation attenuates the expression of cocaine-induced place preference in rats. *Brain Res* 2002;957:129–135.

50. Ren et al. to be published.

51. Margolin A, Avants KS, Chang P, et al. Acupuncture for the treatment of cocaine dependence in methadone-maintained patients. *Am J Addict* 1993;2:194–201.

52. Avants SK, Margolin A, Holford TR, et al. A randomized controlled trial of auricular acupuncture for cocaine dependence. *Arch Intern Med* 2000;160:2305–2312.

53. Margolin A, Kleber HD, Avants SK, et al. Acupuncture for the treatment of cocaine addiction. *JAMA* 2002;287:55–63.

54. Margolin A, Avants SK, Holford TR. Interpreting conflicting findings from clinical trials of auricular acupuncture for cocaine addiction: does treatment context influence outcome? *J Altern Complement Med* 2002;8(2):111–121.

55. Bullock ML, Umen AJ, Culliton PD, et al. Acupuncture treatment of alcoholic recidivism: a pilot study. *Alcohol Clin Exp Res* 1987;11:292–295.

56. Bullock ML, Culliton PD, Olander RT. Controlled trial of acupuncture for severe recidivist alcoholism. *Lancet* 1989;1:1435–1439.

57. Worner TM, Zeller B, Schwarz H, et al. Acupuncture fails to improve treatment outcome in alcoholics. *Drug Alcohol Depend* 1992;30:169–173.

58. Sapir-Weise R, Berglund M, Frank A, et al. Acupuncture in alcoholism treatment: a randomized out-patient study. *Alcohol Alcohol* 1999;34:629–635.

59. Bullock ML, Kiresuk TJ, Sherman RE, et al. A large randomized placebo-controlled study of auricular acupuncture for alcohol dependence. *J Subst Abuse Treat* 2002;22:71–77.

60. Olive MF, Koenig HN, Nannini MA, et al. Stimulation of endorphin neurotransmission in the nucleus accumbens by ethanol, cocaine, and amphetamine. *J Neurosci* 2001;21:RC184:1–5.

61. Anton RF, Moak FH, Waid LR, et al. Naltrexone and cognitive–behavioral therapy for the treatment of out patient alcoholics: results of a placebo–controlled trial. *Am J Psychiatry* 1999;156:1758–1764.

62. Yoshimoto K, Kato B, Sakai K, et al. Electroacupuncture stimulation suppresses the increase in alcohol-drinking behavior in restricted rats. *Alcohol Clin Exp Res* 2001;25:63S–68S.

63. Research Group of Ear Acupuncture, Jiangsu College of New Medicine. The effect of ear acupuncture on the pain threshold of the skin at thoracic and abdominal region. In: *Theoretical study on acupuncture anesthesia.* Shanghai People's Press, Shanghai, China 1973:27–32.

64. Research Group of Acupuncture Anesthesia, Beijing Medical College. Comparison between the analgesia induced by acupuncture or transcutaneous electric stimulation. In: *Theoretical study on acupuncture anesthesia.* Shanghai People's Press, Shanghai, China 1973:12–18.

65. Hoffman P. Skin infection and acupuncture. *Acupunct Med* 2001;19:112–116.

66. Woo PC, Leung KW, Wong SS, et al. Relatively alcohol-resistant mycobacteria are emerging pathogens in patients receiving acupuncture treatment. *J Clin Microbiol* 2002;40:1219–1224.

67. Han JS. Acupuncture: neuropeptide release produced by electrical stimulation of different frequencies. *Trends Neurosci* 2003;26:17–22.

68. Han JS, Ren MF, Tang J, et al. The role of central catecholamine in acupuncture analgesia. *Chin Med J (Engl)* 1979;92:793–800.

69. Han JS, Chou BH, Lu CC, et al. The role of 5-hydroxytryptamine in acupuncture analgesia. *Scientia Sinica* 1979;22:91–104.

70. Han JS, Li SJ, Tang J. Tolerance to acupuncture and cross tolerance to morphine. *Neuropharmacology* 1981;20:593–596.

71. Streitberger K, Kleinhenz J. Introducing a placebo needle into acupuncture research. *Lancet* 1998;352:364–365.

72. Wu LZ, Cui CL, Han JS. Effect of 2/100 Hz transcutaneous electric nerve stimulation on sexual dysfunction and serum sex hormone of heroin addicts. *Chin J Integ Tradit Med West Med* 2000;20:15–18.

CHAPTER 50
Faith-Based Approaches

JOHN G. LANGROD, JOHN MUFFLER,
JAMES ABEL, JAMES T. RICHARDSON,
EUGENIA CURET, HERMAN JOSEPH,
AND PEDRO RUIZ

Unlike other established approaches to treating substance abuse, both conventional and unconventional, religiously oriented programs are not adequately covered in the professional literature (1–3). This chapter examines these approaches in relation to their significance in aiding recovery, maintaining sobriety, and encouraging social reintegration. Their negative consequences are also reviewed, although this concern is dealt with in depth by Burks in his chapter. There appears to be an underestimation of the role of religious treatment modalities on the part of some "secular" professionals and an equal lack of recognition of "secular" approaches by religiously oriented practitioners. The dichotomy is further exacerbated by divisions within the religious community itself over theological grounding and methodological considerations in providing care for substance abusers. The increasing visibility of "ethnic" or "folk" religious practices, such as Santeria and Espiritismo, coupled with the growing awareness of, and, in some quarters, uneasiness with the emergence of new religious movements (NRMs) has added to the confusion.

Clearly, not all substance abusers can be reached, much less successfully treated, by way of religiously oriented programs. Nevertheless, faith-based approaches merit serious consideration, because for some individuals with a high degree of religious motivation they have produced positive results, comparable to those of other treatment modalities. For those persons, it is often the treatment of choice (1,4–6). This chapter focuses on one much neglected element of that context: the religious milieu and the relative importance of religiously oriented programs for some persons searching relief from their addictions. Twelve-step programs such as Alcoholics Anonymous (AA), which are also considered spiritually oriented, are discussed in Chapter 36.

Religion's major effort must be placed in the service of reversing technologic society's seeming tendency to trivialize human existence, while assisting humankind's search for meaning and purpose. Religious traditions remind us that the individual is quite willing to endure sacrifice, discipline, and moral and spiritual exaltation in the search for a commitment to freedom and dignity. We also are reminded that, in the name of human freedom and dignity, we are accountable for our choices and actions and, as such, people are capable of forgiving and being forgiven, of starting anew (7).

VARIETIES OF RELIGIOUS EXPERIENCE

The term *mainline church* generally refers to the members of the major Protestant denominations that were formed as a result of the Reformation in the sixteenth and seventeenth centuries. The Episcopalian, Lutheran, Presbyterian, Methodist, United Church of Christ, Unitarian, Universalist, and Reformed churches are examples of mainline denominations. For a variety of historical reasons, today such churches tend to have less literal interpretations of Scripture, more progressive theologies and social agendas, and an appreciation of modern science and biblical scholarship. To the degree that contemporary Catholicism shares these characteristics, without compromising its particular theological history and ecclesiology, it can also be considered as mainline; however, there exist evangelical and or charismatic elements within many of these churches. Their presence reflects the same theological tensions within the denominations that exist between the mainline and evangelical/charismatic churches. The term *evangelical,* derived from the Greek word meaning "gospel," has become the common designation for the revival movements that swept throughout Europe and the Americas during the eighteenth and nineteenth centuries. Proclamation of Christ's saving work through His death on the cross and the absolute necessity of personally trusting in Christ for eternal salvation constitute the pivotal beliefs (8). Evangelicals generally believe that a spiritual rebirth, a "born again" experience during which the individual acknowledges personal sinfulness and Christ's atonement, is required in order to be saved. When faced with the challenge of Darwin and more sophisticated forms of biblical critical scholarship, evangelicals, who already embraced a literal interpretation of the Bible, began to emphasize its inerrant nature (9).

Evangelicalism today cuts across denominational identity and includes any Christian willing to affirm these traditional tenets of faith: (a) the real historical character of God's saving work as recorded in the Bible; (b) salvation to eternal life based solely on the redemptive work of Christ; (c) the importance of a spiritually transformed life; (d) the centrality of evangelism and mission in the life of the church; and (e) the Reformation doctrine of the final authority of Scripture. Thus evangelicalism includes an amazingly diverse membership consisting of Holiness churches; Pentecostals; traditional Methodists; the various Baptist Conventions; elements of Presbyterian, Episcopalian, Reformed, and Lutheran churches; Anabaptists such as Mennonites; as well as Hispanic and African American churches. Within all of these traditions, recent surveys suggest that nearly 50 million Americans identify themselves as evangelical Christians (8–10).

Pentecostals comprise another segment of the evangelical community. Growing out of the holiness movement of the nineteenth century and the emotion-laden Pentecostal revivals of the early twentieth century, Pentecostals take their name from this latter ecstatic religious phenomenon. In addition to the tenets of faith described above, Pentecostals believe that the gifts of the Holy Spirit bestowed on the church of the apostles, as recounted by Luke in the New Testament's Acts of the Apostles, are available to modern-day believers. They insist that a spiritual experience of baptism, a "filling by the Holy Spirit," constitutes the mark of the truly authentic Christian. The "gifts of the Spirit" include speaking in tongues and interpreting the message thus presented, the ability to discern the needs and spiritual condition of the brothers and sisters, and divine healing. Holiness in one's personal life is stressed. Secular activities such as social dancing, smoking, and social drinking are discouraged. Worship is characterized by singing, clapping, and the spontaneous participation of the congregation. "Fellowship" among members, both within and away from church, is highly valued and highly evident in Pentecostal churches. The Church of God in Christ and the Assemblies of God are two of the more familiar Pentecostal denominations (6,9).

Charismatics form still another branch of the conservative evangelical family tree. Closely related to the Pentecostals in theology and style of worship, they also emphasize the availability of the gifts of the Holy Spirit. Charismatics generally are even more dramatic, demonstrative, and emotive in worship and spirituality. The term *Charismatic*, however, usually refers to those Christians who are not affiliated with the traditional Pentecostal denominations. Cutting across all the major denominations, Charismatic Christians are especially well-represented within the ranks of the more liturgical denominations, such as the Catholic and Episcopalian churches (8,9).

Although church attendance reportedly is declining in modern, industrialized societies, this is not true in the United States. Growth in this country has been especially noticeable among the Evangelical, Pentecostal, and Charismatic churches, as well as in the emergent NRMs. Although this growth is experienced across class and socioeconomic boundaries, these three churches' expressions of Christianity are especially well-represented among disadvantaged and low-income people. In cities, particularly, large numbers of Hispanic and African American Christians are active members of Pentecostal and Charismatic churches (8,10).

RELIGION AND REHABILITATION

A study of Hispanic Americans, largely Chicanos, in San Antonio by Desmond and Maddux (4) suggests that Pentecostal-type programs may prove effective in treating chronic opioid dependence. Research conducted by Larson et al. (3), using data from the Epidemiologic Catchment Area Program of the National Institute of Mental Health, found surprisingly positive results for frequent use of religious providers by persons with alcohol and drug-abuse disorders classified in the American Psychiatric As-

sociation's *Diagnostic and Statistical Manual of Mental Disorders*.

We now turn to a closer examination of religion and rehabilitation. The following sections summarize mainline and Evangelical/Pentecostal Christian involvement with those seeking relief from their addictions, followed by an analysis of Teen Challenge, Espiritismo, and the New Religious Movements.

Mainline Christianity

Most of the early church-related programs were Protestant. Although they stressed religious values and the importance of faith in a God who delivers people from their afflictions, these mainline churches tended to adopt a more secular professional approach to treatment. In essence, they became ecclesiastical social service delivery systems. Religious belief provided the basis and framework for the involvement of these churches, though this was not necessarily emphasized when treating the individual (11).

The current religious situation is quite a bit different. The Catholic Church, Islam, and Judaism have become increasingly involved in providing treatment and rehabilitation services to substance abusers since the late 1960s. Protestant, Catholic, and Jewish efforts have been institutionalized and coordinated through organizations such as Catholic Charities, Lutheran Social Services, and Federation of Jewish Philanthropies based primarily in hospitals and other community satellite centers. For the most part, the participation of local congregations is confined to providing sponsorship and meeting space in church or temple facilities for Alcoholics and/or Narcotics Anonymous groups. Some congregations offer a broader range of social services and referrals in conjunction with ministries to the homeless. Others have joined forces with neighboring churches and formally incorporated themselves into community not-for-profit organizations, such as Harlem Churches for Community Improvement in New York City, and Newark Fighting Back in Newark, New Jersey (11). Islamic groups, particularly the Nation of Islam, have reached out to addicts in the urban ghettos.

Evangelical and Pentecostal Approaches

The Evangelical and Pentecostal churches travel a different road. Programs such as Teen Challenge use religious conversion as the primary step to begin to combat addiction, they believe that there is no other effective way to overcome heroin or cocaine addiction, alcoholism, and other "deviant" behaviors. It is essential, according to their beliefs, that the troubled person, having sinned, be "born again" by accepting Jesus Christ as one's "personal savior." Ideally, the born-again person will then exhibit a life and personality change that is consistent with scriptural values and behaviors. Ultimately, the converted sinner is brought into the church as a brother or sister in a strong fellowship characterized by love and concern.

Those who come seeking "treatment" are taught to pray and to depend on God's assistance with all their personal problems, including addiction. Ideally, they are entirely freed from the mistakes of their former life, and the desire to continue the old, sinful ways will also fade with the passage of time and spiritual growth. Their interests become largely spiritual rather than "worldly." As the individual relates to a larger reality outside of oneself, the world view and value system becomes much less egocentric. Clearly, for Evangelical and Pentecostal Christians, faith is both the starting and end point of recovery. It is the healing power of Jesus Christ, in the Church, and not the intervention of behavioral science that brings about and maintains the individual's rehabilitation.

Teen Challenge

Teen Challenge is one of the oldest drug-free religious residential programs for drug abusers. Describing itself as a Christ-centered organization, it is a ministry for people who have "life-controlling problems and are without the necessary resources and opportunities to live productively" (12). Teen Challenge sees its mission as "helping people become mentally sound, emotionally balanced, socially adjusted, physically well, and spiritually alive," a haven for youth trapped in a world defined by drug and alcohol dependence and immorality. Founded in 1961 by the Rev. David Wilkerson, a minister in the Assemblies of God, the original program was located in the Williamsburg section of Brooklyn, New York.

Having spent 3 years in the slums of East Harlem, David Wilkerson judged narcotics addiction to be the greatest challenge facing the people of that community. He sensed that a reality more powerful, attractive, and rewarding than the needle was needed. He believed that this new reality could be brought about only by religious conversion. Most young people who came to the Teen Challenge Center were addicts seeking help. In 1964, Rev. Don Wilkerson, David's brother, assumed the directorship of the Center, presiding over its transition to an induction and detoxification center. The group also established a Training Center on a 200-acre farm in Rehrersburg, Pennsylvania, far away from the "temptations of the city."

As described above, Teen Challenge grew rapidly during the intervening years. Prizing independence, the program did not accept government funding or assistance. However, residents sign over their welfare checks and food stamps to the program. Teen Challenge has also expressed an interest in participating in accessing funding through President Bush's faith-based initiative. Teen Challenge induction centers now exist in most large cities. Referrals and financial contributions come through a vast network of individuals, churches, and other religious organizations. Today, there is a Teen Challenge Induction Center in most large cities in the United States, Canada, Puerto Rico, Europe, and Australia. Each local program remains autonomous and is only loosely affiliated with the others.

Teen Challenge accepts anyone who has been using drugs and is willing to abide by its rules and practices. However, the program was not prepared to provide services to the "mentally ill." It serves both adolescents and adults of all races and ethnic groups. The racial and ethnic makeup of the program generally reflects its locale. In New York, for example, most participants are Hispanic. This may reflect, in part, Rev. Wilkerson's original involvement with Puerto Rican gang members. Two-thirds of the group come from low-income ghetto backgrounds, while the remainder are middle class. There are facilities for both males and females. The majority of the residents, however, are male (6,12,13).

According to Teen Challenge philosophy, individuals using drugs cannot be helped until they "hit rock bottom." They must admit to having a problem and actively seek help (6,12,13). The Teen Challenge induction centers are crisis centers, accepting people from the streets for immediate help or counseling 24 hours a day. If the individual wishes to enter the residential program, he or she goes through an intake interview to determine whether the program is suitable.

From a research perspective, many of the participants select themselves into the program. Sometimes, however, candidates are referred by a judge, probation officer, minister, or counselor, whereas others find their way through street evangelization efforts or at the urging of relatives and recovering addict friends who are already in the program (12).

Four major outcome studies have been completed on Teen Challenge: see Calof (13), an internal evaluation reported by Langrod et al. (6), Glasscote et al. (14), and Hess (15).

Catherine B. Hess, MD, MPH, was formerly Assistant Commissioner of Health for New York City, and served as special consultant to Teen Challenge. Her 7-year followup study was on 366 selected individuals who entered the program in Brooklyn in 1968. At the time of the evaluation, 56% of all the participants reported being employed (15). Hess reports the Teen Challenge graduation rate at 18.3%, which is somewhat higher than the 15% reported by Smart (16) in a review of outcome studies of drug-free therapeutic communities. These data also appear consistent with subsequent findings by Anglin and Hser (17), DeLeon (18,19), DeLeon and Rosenthal (20), and Falkin (21). In terms of continued drug use, 24% of the population for which this information was available reported never using narcotics after leaving Teen Challenge. Seventy-six percent relapsed. Five percent of this group were drug-free at the time of followup, having been treated in other programs or having detoxified on their own.

Mayhew reports similar results and notes that of those who complete Teen Challenge's program a high proportion remains drug free and faith-based treatment costs less than "traditional" approaches (12).

Teen Challenge has been successful in reorienting the lives of some drug users. Future research should focus upon cost effectiveness, success rates compared with those of traditional secular approaches and an analysis of who would appear to benefit from this type of treatment (12).

Espiritismo

Espiritismo, often referred to as spiritism, is a belief system among Puerto Rican and other Hispanic cultures that transcends both socioeconomic status and national borders. At its core lies the assumption that spirits are able to influence and affect the lives of people existing here, in the material and tangible world. Spiritists believe that spirits have the ability to make people physically and mentally ill, including by using drugs and other substances of abuse, as well as have the power to cure them (22).

It is estimated that as many as 80% of Puerto Ricans believe in spiritism to some degree. Curet and Langrod (23) noted that 65% of their Puerto Rican substance-abuse patients reported utilizing Espiritismo as a support system at some point during their lives. Only one study has examined Espiritismo and alcohol abuse. Many Western mental health practitioners, however, tend to view such alternative healing systems as maladaptive or even pathologic. Thus, this animosity (both real and perceived) toward a strongly held cultural belief system acts as a deterrent, discouraging the individual from seeking modern medical and mental health assistance (23,24). Pentecostals and other fundamentalists are also hostile to Espiritismo, because they consider it to be the practice of "necromancy," which is biblically prohibited.

Espiritismo, in addition to its comforting familiarity, possesses other attractive qualities lacking in the everyday practice of modern health care. The atmosphere in which the medium, that is, folk healer, works is one of warmth and relaxation rather than cold, sterile efficiency. Patients usually do not have to wait endlessly for their names to be called. The medium is concerned not only with the entire person, but with the patient's entire family, living and dead as well as other social networks. Family and friends frequently are present to lend support. They are not seen as intruders who are "getting in the way" (22).

Perhaps the most significant reason many people seek out folk healing of any type is that it taps into one's reservoir of faith, and that faith, whether in a spirit, God, or oneself, can heal. It is within this latter context that Espiritismo has proven to be an effective support system in substance abuse treatment programs, as well as in other areas. This practice, of course, has been subject to abuse and must be used with caution, and in accordance with the patient's religious belief system. The clinician must be culturally competent, thoroughly conversant with Espiritista principles, as well as with the parallel, psychological dynamics, and the culture as a whole. The following case studies illustrate how Espiritismo has assisted patients receiving methadone maintenance treatment (23).

Case 1

S. G. is a 26-year-old woman of Puerto Rican descent who was doing well in treatment. However, upon learning that her husband was murdered in prison she developed what appeared to be a reactive depression. She started missing appointments or coming late to her clinic. She was disheveled and did not want to leave the house. She complained of an impulse to jump under a subway train or throw herself out the window. Further inquiry revealed that the suicidal ideation was in response to her belief that her deceased husband wanted her to join him in the spirit world. The clinician, knowledgeable about her belief system, asked whether and where she lit a candle in his honor. She said she lit it at home. The clinician knew that, according to Espiritista principles, a newly departed or "immature" spirit had difficulty in separating from the material plane and that lighting a candle would attract the spirit to the home. The clinician interpreted this to the patient. He suggested that if she wanted to honor her husband's memory, she could light a candle at the local church and, at the same time, become involved with a responsible Espiritista center with which the clinician was acquainted. This strategy had a twofold purpose. One was to mobilize the patient to get her out of the house and engage in constructive activity. The second was to therapeutically help the patient work out her grief process within the context of her belief system, in a safe manner designed to prevent any suicidal ideation or attempt. The patient did become more constructively engaged. The depression eventually remitted, and she responded positively to treatment once again.

Case 2

R. L. is a 31-year-old Puerto Rican woman and practitioner of Espiritismo who was diagnosed with schizophrenia. As previously noted, culturally competent clinicians understand that Espiritista doctrine differentiates illnesses and other problems to be of either "material" or "spiritual" causation, or a combination of both. This patient ceased taking her newly prescribed neuroleptic medication because voices were telling her that she was being poisoned. The clinician, in collaboration with the Espiritista, convinced this patient that the voices telling her not to take the medication were trying to create material problems for her by not permitting her illness to be treated. Accepting this interpretation, the patient resumed taking her medication. She averted a complete decompensation and possible rehospitalization.

The above cases demonstrate that a collaborative effort can exist between responsible clinicians, who represent the "material" world, and trained Espiritistas, who are able to distinguish spiritual causation from the material. If this collaboration had not existed in the cases cited above, these patients' belief systems might have been labeled as pathologic, and the patients would have been lost to treatment, with possibly tragic consequences.

Similarly, the Pentecostal faith has been used as a support system in one large methadone-maintenance program. A number of patients who subscribed to this belief found themselves rejected from churches because they were enrolled in methadone treatment. However, one counselor who was also a minister rehabilitated in a drug-free religious program presented methadone "as a gift from God like insulin for the diabetic" to those people who expressed guilt about receiving methadone. He was also able to locate a church which would be accepting of these persons and where methadone treatment was not an issue (6), thus allowing these patients to receive the best of both worlds.

Some of the possible positive clinical aspects and dynamics of faith-based substance abuse treatment can be summarized as the follows:

- Guilt is removed when the addict is "saved," because internalized guilt often causes the individual to continue to self-medicate with illicit or harmful substances.
- The fragmented, dysfunctional family background is replaced by a strongly knitted, cohesive, religious family providing spiritual and emotional support, as well as material/concrete assistance with the necessities of everyday life. The terms "brother" and "sister" illustrate the concept of this newly acquired family.
- Provision of an external organized structure which is internalized in terms of "bad" and "good," or "evil" and "God/Jesus-like" behaviors.
- Forgiveness is central to acceptance by an ideologic father figure "God/Jesus," hence the addict is once again valued as a worthy human being who was "lost" and now is "found, or born again," thus enhancing the addict's self-concept or self-worth.
- The addict—repented, accepted, and forgiven—uses his or her past life (addiction and sin) to "teach" others, which further enhances and reinforces the addict's self-concept, ego, and superego by becoming a role model.
- Contrary to the traditional and still existing therapeutic community approach of a devaluation of the self through harsh confrontation, the addict experiences validation of his or her life as worthy of God/Christ. However, in highly legalistic and abusive religious groups, the individual may also feel and be devalued..
- The support of the religious family continues after the addict finishes treatment and life is centered around the church and his "brothers" and "sisters."

Nonetheless, precautions must be taken when funding faith-based programs. Patients or clients entering such programs may be subjected primarily to the ideologic teachings of the faith-based program, both politically and theologically and not receive services or medications that have demonstrated their efficacy. Governmental agencies that fund faith-based programs must not only be evenhanded in their approach, but must also evaluate the teachings of such programs, their past histories, and mission to preclude the funding of fraudulent programs that have the potential to harm participants through brainwashing techniques and by not providing effective treatment. Also, because many faith-based programs will be entering drug treatment initiatives for the first time in their histories, outcome evaluation research must be undertaken to determine their strengths, weaknesses, cost-effectiveness, and appropriateness in treating substance abusers.

New Religious Movements

Since the inception of NRMs about three decades ago, there has existed controversy about the relationship between NRMs and drugs. Initially, it seemed to many that drugs and new religions were inextricably intertwined and that those involved in new religions were also often involved in drug use. We now know that such a view is overly simplistic, but the apparent co-occurrence of religious experimentation and drug use made such assumptions about the relationship easy to make (25–27).

We also now know that both drug use and religious experimentation are anathema to some people (including some professionals), which contributes to a misunderstanding about the relationship of drug use and religious experimentation among America's youth. Some commentators fail to fully differentiate between these two types of countercultural behavior patterns and, instead, may lump them together for purposes of treatment and public policy development (28,29). Although religious interventions may be beneficial to some, others have been harmed and require assistance. Abusive religion as an addictive phenomenon and its treatment is extensively discussed by Burks in Chapter ____.

Considerable research relevant to explaining the relationship between participation in new religions and drug use has now become available. Much of this research is based on personality assessment of participants and the effects of participation on psychological well-being (25–27), as well as discussion of specific therapeutic effects of participation in NRMs (25–27,30). This brief section cannot summarize all of that work but will trace some themes that have emerged from existing research.. Specifically, it focuses on the relationship of prevalence and incidence of drug abuse and participation in NRMs.

Prevalence of Heavy Prior Drug Use

One major theme derived from early research on NRMs was that many of those participating had previously been involved extensively in the drug subculture. The same applies to Pentecostals and Espiritistas, as well as to believers in other faiths.

This phenomenon is described by Downton (31) in relation to the Divine Light Mission, with presentation of case studies which illustrate this point. Nordquist (32) presents similar findings regarding Ananda Cooperative Village in

Grass Valley, California. Heavy drug-use histories among participants were found there, with 68% of his respondents admitting to using drugs prior to joining and 63% of those saying the use was "often." Johnson's study of the Hare Krishna in California, as well as other work about this group, also indicated heavy prior drug involvement among participants (33,34). Similarly, Richardson et al. in their research on a major Jesus movement organization (35,36) found that 90% of members had used drugs, with 72% of those admitting to the use of hard drugs and 75% saying that they had used drugs "all the time" (42%) or "fairly often" (33%).

Thus, any claim of an association or causal relationship between drug use and NRM participation is subject to question, because it cannot be clearly demonstrated that the relationship is not an artifact of both increased drug use and interest in new forms of religion among certain demographic categories arising from common social contextual factors.

Wuthnow (10,37,38) presents data suggestive of what type of individual is attracted to which type of NRM. He classifies NRMs into one of three categories—"countercultural," "personal growth," and "neo-Christian"—and compares the values of those individuals from the sample who are attracted to each of the group types on a number of issues, including a few measures of drug-related values and experiences. He found that those attracted to "countercultural" groups (such as Transcendental Meditation, Yoga, Zen, Hare Krishna, and Satanism) do, at least for this sample, have a higher propensity toward having the experience of being "high" on drugs and favoring the legalization of marihuana than those attracted to either "personal-growth" groups (est, Scientology, Synanon) or "neo-Christian" groups (Christian World Liberation Front, Children of God, Jews for Jesus, and Campus Crusade for Christ). "Personal-growth" group participants also usually ranked higher than "neo-Christian" group participants on these two measures. There was a fairly consistent pattern on the drug-related questions among this sample, suggesting that at least some of the more radical religious groups might be more attractive to those who had been most actively involved with drugs. Other studies show a marked relationship between earlier history of drug use and involvement in Eastern-oriented religions (39–41). These studies, however, were not controlled, simply comparing participants and nonparticipants on the matter of drug use and values. Thus care must be taken in making claims about the basic relationship between type and extent of NRM participation and drug use history.

NRMs as Halfway Houses: An Alternative Perspective

New religions, including some of the most controversial, have been reported to relieve psychiatric symptoms psychological distress, and drug dependence. On the other hand, there exist numerous reports of damage caused by participation in NRMs, suggesting that they "brainwash" people into joining, "destroy families," and create severe psychological and psychiatric problems (16,27–29,42). One counterargument that has been made, for example, is that NRMs do perform, for some persons, a "halfway house" function. Sociologist Tom Robbins and psychologist Dick Anthony describe this phenomenon among participants of Meher Baba groups (43). They show that at least some NRMs assisted in the reintegration of a number of young persons into "mainstream" society. Richardson et al. also presented supporting data in this regard. They maintain that NRMs reintegrate participants into a more normal existence, while at the same time teaching necessary skills for survival in ordinary society (43,44).

Another perspective on the reintegration hypothesis was offered by Kilbourne and Richardson (45) who presented a social-psychological model of healing based on similarities between communal new religions' practices and therapy situations. It was assumed that many participants chose to participate in either modality, seeking to be healed of drug addiction or other problems. They noted that numerous religious groups as well as many therapies involve common roles of healer (doctor) and healee (patient), and an underlying "deep structure" focused on healing. In her analysis of religion and healing, McGuire (46) suggested a similar idea that much of the interest in NRMs and alternative therapies derives from a deep desire to be healed. Psychiatrist Marc Galanter, as a result of doing several important studies of the effects of participation in controversial NRMs (47–49), posits a "relief effect" brought on by participation, in attempting to explain what it is about NRMs that causes such dramatic change in some individuals, including the relief of psychiatric symptoms and dependencies on drugs and alcohol (30).

It appears that some NRMs may serve a "halfway house" function for certain participants (16). This role was needed by those young people who were so disconnected from society that they were unable to access the usual modes of social support. Others counter that NRM participants are simply exchanging one form of dependency (drugs) for another (religion) (50–52) when they decide to embrace an NRM. Although there is some truth to this assertion, society in general would tend to agree that "nonpathologic" religious affiliation is usually more acceptable than drug addiction, provided that the religious affiliation does not harm its members.

NRMs as a Support Community

Many who join NRMs do so because their usual social supports are unavailable, either because they have left them voluntarily or because some external agent has alienated those relationships (53,54). Individuals may be seeking a surrogate family or simply need food and shelter. Thus we saw in the 1960s and 1970s a move toward "communalization of religious experience" for many youth as they explored alternatives to a normal lifestyle, for short periods of time (55).

Religious communal organizations assisted numbers of young people who were at least temporarily dislocated from their usual social moorings. This communal experience would appear to be most useful for those participants who desire to change their lifestyles. These groups typically share a belief system and an ethic built on its religious ideology, and their members support each other in the acting out of these newly acquired beliefs and values. Behavior deemed deviant and negatively sanctioned in previous reference groups may be accepted and encouraged in the new environment of a religious group (56). As Galanter (30) notes, the relief effect comes from participation in a human group that is accepting and personal. Participants are often helped with their problems, including drug dependence.

One major reason for contributing to positive response and outcome is self-selection. There is no denying that considerable self-selection occurs by those who enter a program, either because they are under social pressure or because they genuinely want to change their lives. Research demonstrates that treatment for any dependency is more successful if the person wants to change and acts in a manner to fulfill that goal. Many participants in NRMs and other faith-based programs act in a manner designed to change themselves. The key to NRMs and other modalities success at drug rehabilitation is the volition being exercised by those desiring to use the groups as vehicles of change (53,57,58).

NRM groups, as well as other religiously oriented programs, are not for everyone. This is evidenced by their extremely high attrition rates and small size. Many people who experiment with these groups as possible personal vehicles for change reject them for a variety of reasons. For some, the often quite rigorous and lengthy resocialization methods are simply too difficult to accept. Others find the belief system too strange to accept as a center for one's life. Still others may be repulsed by the actions teachings or practices of some groups their leaders or members, which they regard as abusive, unethical, hypocritical, or illegal (39,59).

Some who leave NRMs or other modalities voluntarily after a relatively short period of time, have used the experience to get themselves "straightened out" and reoriented. They "move back" to more normal types of existence, establishing families, obtaining and holding jobs, and/or returning to school. For some individuals, the NRM or Teen Challenge has provided a valuable halfway house function. In assisting participants to avoid the abuse of drugs or other problematic behaviors, participants have been afforded an opportunity to recoup and regroup. The community at large benefits from the groups' capacity to act as a vehicle for reintegration, by reinserting individuals into society after having assisted them. Nevertheless,

as previously noted, other participants fall victim to abuse in some of these religions or groups.

Final Thoughts Regarding NRM Approaches

This analysis of participation in NRMs requires some qualification and explication. It must be acknowledged that much negative attention has been focused on some NRMs, often referred to as "cults" in the media, as well as by many in positions of authority. The issues involved are complex. However, there exists a body of research, published in books and academic journals by psychologists, psychiatrists, and sociologists, that include data supporting the view that some NRMs and religious approaches serve a valuable role for stopping substance abuse of various kinds. It is important to identify and better understand the essential characteristics of those groups that are critical to producing positive outcomes in this area, but without harming their participants.

A few caveats are also in order. Obviously, participation in NRMs is not for everyone. Most who do participate apparently agree with that assertion, as evidenced by the high attrition rates from those organizations. Many people who try out NRMs as vehicles of personal growth do not find them acceptable and simply leave. Anthony et al. noted that not all "spiritual choices" are equal (60). Some NRMs may not foster personal growth and do not seek to be vehicles of personal change for their participants. Tragedies like those involving the People's Temple, the Branch Davidians, Heaven's Gate, and Aum Shirikyo do occur. Participation in traditional NRMs has not been a positive experience for all involved (59). Clearly one size does not fit all, and careful scrutiny must take place to establish that participants are helped and not harmed.

RECENT FAITH-BASED INITIATIVES

On January 29, 2001, President George W. Bush established the White House Office of Faith-Based and Community Initiatives by an Executive Order (61). The purpose of this office was to provide federal support for religiously based social services including substance abuse treatment and prevention. In the area of substance abuse, the president asked Congress to allocate $200 million to provide vouchers for persons seeking faith-based treatment. Similar initiatives have been proposed or are being funded in various states.

The University of Nebraska received a $3 million federal grant to develop faith-based behavioral health interventions for that state (62). On December 24, 2003, Governor Jeb Bush of Florida announced the opening of a "faith-based" prison. He noted that participation would be voluntary, as is said to be the case in relation to all federally funded faith-based substance abuse treatment. On December 8, 2003, Americans United for Separation of Church and State (63) expressed concern that there are coercive elements to these proposals because acceptance of religion is socially approved and rejection of faith-based substance abuse treatment or prisons could be viewed in a negative light and result in possible reprisals. Although secular options, such as Save Our Selves (SOS), SMART Recovery, Women for Sobriety, and Life Ring Secular Recovery, must be made available, this may not always be feasible because of waiting lists or a paucity of such programs in certain geographical areas. This is in addition to the possible reluctance of government to fund or assist such programs under the faith-based initiatives.

A related concern is that the government may fund only those religiously based programs that are in sympathy with its philosophy, political and theological, as well as its goals and objectives. A concrete example, in terms of the current administration, is preferential funding and/or support for fundamentalist-type programs, to the exclusion of others. Another area that is a cause for concern relates to qualifications of personnel working in the faith-based programs, as opposed to secular programs, regarding the employing of professional staff. In relation to equity in funding, James Towey, the current director of the White House Office of Faith-Based and Community Initiatives, noted that funding of programs sponsored by groups such as WICCA, a neopagan earth-centered religion, would not be acceptable. Programs that engage in punitive practices such as "brainwashing" or corporal punishment and that are spiritually abusive might also be funded if clear guidelines are not developed. In terms of personnel, staff of some faith-based programs are expected to be of the same religious faith as, or at a minimum subscribe to the principles of, the religious organization for which they are working. Religiously based programs are governmentally protected when engaging in these practices. This has been documented in a position paper issued by the White House Office of Faith-Based and Community Initiatives (64). A recent *New York Times* article notes that The Salvation Army is now requiring that employees reaffirm their religious faith or adherence to their principles (65). Because The Salvation Army receives substantial amounts of governmental funds, such a requirement may be in violation of fair employment practices. These issues are being litigated and conflicting decisions have been rendered in different jurisdictions. New York State, for example, in response to a decision of the U.S. Court of Appeals for the Second Circuit is now requiring that treatment providers who receive funding or accreditation must not coerce individuals into attending Alcoholics Anonymous, a spiritually based program. Opportunities have to be provided for those persons to attend alternate secular treatment. However, secular alternatives may not be readily available. However, this policy of the New York State Office of Alcoholism and Substance Abuse Services is an equitable resolution in response to the court's decision (66). Another concern is that funding may be diverted from existing, well-functioning, accredited secular programs to untried faith-based alternatives, whose staff or facilities may not be obliged to meet accreditation standards.

This issue is a complex one that is colored by the ideology of whomever is dispensing governmental funds.

CONCLUSION

Synthesizing the extensive sociocultural analyses of Hoge and Roozen (67,68), it can be suggested that a dichotomy exists in contemporary American culture. This dichotomy may be best expressed as a difference between the religious and the secular. It would seem that a sense of meaning and purpose that grounds the lives of individual persons could be derived from one or the other or from some combination of these seemingly differing world views.

Religiously oriented treatment is not suitable for everyone. For those persons who can accept the creeds, rituals, and commitments required of such programs, there seem to be advantages. The idea of being "born again" can be quite liberating for some, because the recovering addict would be provided with a "clean slate" and a "clean life." Then the central life interest no longer revolves around drugs. Within a new reference group, the recovering drug user is surrounded by significant others who can in some respects serve as role models for behavior appropriate to the drug user's new social identity. The person is now guided by newly acquired values and normative expectations that are constantly reinforced through membership in a religious community.

Another core religious belief is conversion. Conversion has its root meaning in the Greek word *metanoia*, literally, "to turn over." More idiomatically, it conveys the image of having a change of heart or turning over a new leaf. The fundamentalist community's idea of conversion does share with that of the secular community the reality that one must first accept drug use as life destroying, and then choose to discard it in favor of behavior that is life building, before rehabilitation can begin.

Clinicians providing services within ethnic communities need to be culturally attuned to their clients; particularly to the significance of faith and religious expression among Hispanic and other cultures. Neglect or derision of traditions that do not derive from Western constructs of science frequently result in the individuals' being lost to treatment, even among those acknowledging the need for both "professional" intervention and "spiritual" healing.

From the discussion presented in this chapter, one may conclude that religious commitment and religiously oriented treatment programs can be significant factors that merit consideration and inclusion when planning a mix of appropriate treatment alternatives. There remains a great need for additional rigorous research examining the significance of religious commitment and affiliation, experienced within mainline, fundamentalist, ethnic, and NRM communities, in treatment readiness and outcomes. Researchers also need to reduce emphasis on seeking predictive indicators of delinquency and deviance, steering the analysis toward issues of social reintegration, potentiating recovery, and maintaining sobriety, particularly in the posttreatment milieu. Finally, religious practitioners and researchers can and should begin to work collaboratively with their secular professional mental health counterparts. At the very least, serious and open communication needs to be attempted. On the other hand, taxpayer funding of sectarian programs raises serious questions regarding the separation of church and state, as well as se-

rious concern that such funding may interfere with the autonomy of religiously based institutions and generally discriminate against the funding of effective programs that may not be politically acceptable at a given time.

Note

This chapter presents the individual points of view of its authors and in no way represents the views of the agencies with which they are affiliated.

REFERENCES

1. Gorsuch R. Religious aspects of substance abuse and recovery. *J Soc Issues* 1995;51(2):65–83.
2. Larson D, Hohmann A, Kessler L, et al. The couch and the cloth: the need for linkage. *Hosp Community Psychiatry* 1988;39(10):1064–1069.
3. Larson D, Pattison M, Blazer D, et al. Systematic analysis of research on religious variables in four major psychiatric journals. *Am J Psychiatry* 1986; 143(3):329–334.
4. Desmond D, Maddux J. Religious programs and careers of chronic heroin users. *Am J Drug Alcohol Abuse* 1981;8(1):71–83.
5. Hathaway W, Pargament K. Intrinsic religiousness, religious coping, and psychosocial competence: a covariance structure analysis. *J Sci Stud Religion* 1990;20(4):423–441.
6. Langrod J, Joseph H, Valdes K. The role of religion in the treatment of opiate addictions. In: Brill L, Lieberman L, eds. *Major modalities in the treatment of drug abuse.* New York: Behavioral Publications, 1972.
7. Heschel AJ. The abiding challenge of religion. *Center Mag* 1958;March/ April:43–51 (reprinted 1973).
8. Marsden GM. *Understanding fundamentalism and evangelicalism.* Grand Rapids, MI: William B. Eerdmans Publishing, 1991.
9. Balmer R. *Mine eyes have seen the glory: a journey into the evangelical subculture in America.* New York: Oxford University Press, 1989.
10. Wuthnow R. *The struggle for America's soul: evangelicals, liberals, and secularism.* Grand Rapids, MI: William B Eerdmans Publishing, 1989.
11. Muffler J. *Church lady meets wolfman: towards a paradigm of salvation, stigmatization, and the urban church's involvement with drug abusers and people with AIDS.* New York: Society for the Study of Social Problems, 1995.
12. Available at www.teenchallenge.com. Last accessed: May 11, 2004.
13. Calof J. *A study of four voluntary treatment and rehabilitation programs for New York City's narcotic addicts.* New York: Community Service Society of New York, 1967.
14. Glasscote R, Sussex J, Jaffe J, et al. *The treatment of drug abuse: programs, problems, prospects.* Washington, DC: Joint Information Service of the American Psychiatric Association and the National Association for Mental Health, 1972.
15. Hess CB. A seven year follow-up study of 186 males in a religious therapeutic community. In: Schecter A, Alksne H, Kaufman E, eds. *Critical concerns in the field of drug abuse.* New York: Marcel Dekker, 1977.
16. Smart R. Outcome studies of therapeutic community and halfway house treatment for addicts. *Int J Addict* 1976; 11:143.
17. Anglin MD, Hser YI. Treatment of drug abuse. In: Tonry M, Wilson JQ, eds. *Drugs and crime.* Chicago: University of Chicago Press, 1990.
18. DeLeon G. The therapeutic community: status and evolution. *Int J Addict* 1985;20:823–844.
19. DeLeon G. *The therapeutic community: study of effectiveness.* Treatment research monograph series (ADM) 84–1286. Washington, DC: National Institute on Drug Abuse, 1984.
20. DeLeon G, Rosenthal MS. Treatment in residential therapeutic communities. In: Karasu TB, ed. *Treatment of psychiatric disorders,* vol. II. New York: American Psychiatric Press, 1989.
21. Falkin GP. *Policy development report on residential drug treatment programs. Report to the New York State Division of Substance Abuse Services 1991.* Albany, NY: mimeographed report, 1991.
22. Ruiz P, Langrod J. Cultural issues in the mental health of Hispanics in the United States. *Am J Soc Psychiatry* 1982;2(2)35–38.
23. Curet E, Langrod J. *Espiritismo as a support system in substance abuse treatment.* New York: mimeographed report, 1997.
24. Garrison V. Support systems of schizophrenic and nonschizophrenic Puerto Rican migrant women in New York City. *Schizophr Bull* 1978;4:561.
25. Richardson J. Clinical and personality assessment of participants in new religions. *Int J Psychol Religion* 1996;5(3):145–170.
26. Richardson J. Psychological and psychiatric studies of new religions. In: Brown LB, ed. *Advances in the psychology of religion.* New York: Pergamon Press, 1985.
27. Richardson J. Two steps forward, one back: psychiatry, psychology, and the new religions. *Int J Psychol Religion* 1996;5(3):181–186.
28. Clark J. Problems in referral of cult members. *J Natl Assoc Private Psychiatr Hosp* 1978;9:19–21.
29. Singer M. Therapy with ex-cult members. *J Natl Assoc Private Psychiatr Hosp* 1978;9:14–18.
30. Galanter M. The "relief effect": a sociobiological model for neurotic distress and large-group therapy. *Am J Psychiatry* 1978;135:588–591.
31. Downton JV. *Sacred journeys: conversion of young Americans to Divine Light Mission.* New York: Columbia University Press, 1979.
32. Nordquist T. *Ananda Cooperative Village. A study in the beliefs, values, and attitudes of a New Age religious community.* Uppsala: Borgstroms Tryckeri AB, 1978.
33. Johnson G. The Hare Krishna in San Francisco. In: Glock C, Bellah R, eds. *The new religious consciousness.* Berkeley, CA: University of California Press, 1976.
34. Rochford B. *Hare Krishna in America.* New Brunswick, NJ: Rutgers University Press, 1985.
35. Richardson J, Davis R. Experiential fundamentalism: revisions of orthodoxy in the Jesus Movement. *J Am Acad Religion* 1983;LI(3):397–425.
36. Richardson J, Stewart M, Simmonds R. *Organized miracles: a study of a contemporary, youth, communal,*

fundamentalist organization. New Brunswick, NJ: Transaction Books, 1979.

37. Wuthnow R. *The consciousness reformation.* Berkeley, CA: University of California Press, 1976.

38. Wuthnow R. The new religions in social context. In: Glock C, Bellah R, eds. *The new religious consciousness.* Berkeley, CA: University of California Press, 1976.

39. Deutsch A. Psychiatric perspectives on an Eastern-style cult. In: Halperin D, ed. *Psychodynamic perspectives on religion, sect, and cult.* Boston: John Wright, 1983.

40. Kilbourne B, Richardson J. Psychotherapy and new religion in a pluralistic society. *Am Psychol* 1984;39(3):237–251.

41. Needleman J. *The new religions.* Garden City, NY: Doubleday, 1970.

42. Robbins T, Anthony D. Deprogramming, brainwashing, and the medicalization of deviant religious groups. *Soc Probl* 1982;29:283–297.

43. Robbins T, Anthony D. Getting straight with Meher Baba: a study of drug rehabilitation, mysticism, and post-adolescent role conflict. *J Sci Study Religion* 1972;11(2):122–140.

44. Robbins T, Anthony D, Curtis T. Youth culture religious movements: evaluating the integrative hypothesis. *Sociol Q* 1975;16(1):48–64.

45. Kilbourne B, Richardson J. A social psychological analysis of healing. *J Integr Eclec Psychother* 1988;7(1):20–34.

46. McGuire M. Religion, healing. In: Hammond P, ed. *The sacred in a secular age.* Berkeley, CA: University of California Press, 1985.

47. Galanter M. *Cults. Faith, healing, and coercion.* New York: Oxford University Press, 1989.

48. Galanter M, Buckley P. Evangelical religion and meditation: psychotherapeutic effects. *J Nerv Ment Dis* 1978; 166:685–691.

49. Galanter M, Rabkin R, Rabkin F. The "Moonies": a psychological study of conversion and membership in a contemporary religious sect. *Am J Psychiatry* 1979;136:165–169.

50. Gerlach L. Pentecostalism. Revolution or counter-revolution? In: Zaretsky I, Leone M, eds. *Religious movements in contemporary America.* Princeton, NJ: Princeton University Press, 1984.

51. Rebhan J. The drug rehabilitation program: cults in formation? In: Halperin D, ed. *Psychodynamic perspectives on religion, sect, and cult.* Boston: John Wright, 1983.

52. Simmonds R. Conversion or addiction: consequences of joining a Jesus Movement group. In: Richardson J, ed. *Conversion careers: in and out of the new religions.* Beverly Hills, CA: Sage, 1980.

53. Kilbourne B. Equity or exploitation: the case of the Unification Church. *Rev Religious Res* 1986;28:143–150.

54. Kilbourne B, Richardson J. Cults versus families: a case of misattribution of cause? *Marriage Fam Rev* 1981;4:81–100.

55. Kilbourne B, Richardson J. Communalization of religious experience in contemporary religious groups. *J Community Psychol* 1986;14:206–213.

56. Stark R. Psychopathology and religious commitment. *Rev Religious Res* 1971;12:165–176.

57. Richardson J. The active versus passive convert: paradigm conflict in conversion/recruitment research. *J Sci Study Religion* 1985;24:163–179.

58. Straus R. Religious conversion as a per-

sonal and collective accomplishment. *Sociol Anal* 1979;40:158–165.

59. Balch R. Money and power in utopia. In: Richardson J, ed. *Money and power in the new religions.* Lewiston, NY: Edwin Mellen Press, 1988.

60. Anthony D, Ecker B, Wilber K. *Spiritual choices: the problem of recognizing authentic paths to inner transformation.* New York: Paragon, 1987.

61. Available at www.whitehouse.gov/ news/releases/2001/01/20010129-2.html. Last accessed May 11, 2004.

62. *State officials waiting to see Bush's faith-based drug, alcohol treatment plan.* Available at: http://theindependent.com/stories/013003/new_drugtreatment30.shtml. Last accessed May 11, 2004.

63. *Americans United criticizes plan to create "faith-based" prison in Florida.* Monday December 8, 2003. Available at: www.au.org/site/News2?page=NewsArticle&id=5017&abbr=pr&security=1002&news_iv_ctrl=1349. Last accessed May 11, 2004.

64. Available at: www.whitehouse.gov/ government/fbci/booklet.pdf. Last accessed May 11, 2004.

65. Wakin DJ. Suit claims group's staff is pressured on religion. *New York Times* 25 Feb 2004:B6 (col 6).

66. *Impact of recent federal court decision concerning Alcoholics Anonymous on government funded providers.* Available at: www.oasas.state.ny.us/mis/bulletins/lsb2002–05.htm. Last accessed May 11, 2004.

67. Hoge DR. *Division in the Protestant house: the basic reasons behind intrachurch conflicts.* Philadelphia: Westminster Press, 1976.

68. Hoge D, Roozen D. *Understanding church growth and decline.* New York: Pilgrim Press, 1980.

CHAPTER 51
Relapse Prevention

DENNIS C. DALEY AND G. ALAN MARLATT

Substance use disorders (SUDs) represent a serious public health problem in the United States. They are associated with many serious medical, psychiatric, family, occupational, legal, financial, and spiritual problems. SUDs not only cause impairment and suffering on the part of the affected individual, but they also create a significant burden for the family and society (18–20,36,37,81,83). For many clients, SUDs are chronic conditions that must be managed over the course of time. Similar to other chronic or recurrent medical or psychiatric disorders, relapse is a common problem among clients with a SUD (72). While many clients evidence significant benefits from treatment, lapses and relapses often occur (31,70). A challenge for any clinician treating clients with SUDs is to understand relapse and to integrate strategies to prevent relapse or reduce relapse risk.

This chapter provides an overview of relapse and relapse prevention. We define recovery and relapse, and review treatment outcome studies, causes of relapse, clinical models of relapse prevention, and empirical studies of relapse prevention approaches. We then integrate the relapse prevention literature by discussing 12 cognitive and behavioral strategies that clinicians can use with clients with any type of SUD, including those with co-occurring psychiatric disorders. These strategies can be used in individual, family or group therapy, and incorporated into structured groups in rehabilitation programs. By reducing the frequency or severity of relapses, the clinician helps the client improve the client's quality of life. This can also provide benefits to the family and society.

OVERVIEW OF RECOVERY AND RELAPSE

Recovery

Recovery from a substance use disorder is the process of initiating abstinence from alcohol or other drug use, as well as making intrapersonal and interpersonal changes to maintain this change over time. Specific changes vary among people with substance use disorders and occur in any of the following areas of functioning: physical, psychological, behavioral, interpersonal, family, social, spiritual, and financial (29,30,36). It is generally accepted that recovery tasks are contingent on the stage or phase of recovery the individual is in (12). Recovery is mediated by the severity and degree of damage caused by the substance use disorder, the presence of a comorbid psychiatric or medical illness, and the individual's perception, motivation, gender, ethnic background, and support system. Although some individuals may achieve full recovery, others achieve a partial recovery. The latter may experience multiple relapses over time.

Recovering from a substance use disorder involves gaining information, increasing self-awareness, developing skills for sober living, and following a program of change. The program of change may involve professional treatment, participation in self-help programs (Alcoholics Anonymous [AA], Narcotics Anonymous [NA], Cocaine Anonymous [CA], Rational Recovery, SMART Recovery, Men or Women for Sobriety, or Dual Recovery Anonymous) and self-management approaches. In the earlier phases of recovery, the individual typically relies more on external support and help from professionals, sponsors, or other members of support groups. As recovery progresses, more reliance is placed on oneself to handle problems and the challenges of living a sober lifestyle. The information and skills learned as part of relapse prevention offer an excellent mechanism to prepare for the maintenance phase of recovery.

Lapse and Relapse

The term *lapse* refers to the initial episode of alcohol or other drug use following a period of abstinence, whereas the term *relapse* refers to failure to maintain behavior change over time (70). Relapse can be viewed not only as the event of resumption of a pattern of substance abuse or dependency, but also as a process in which indicators or warning signs appear prior to the individual's actual substance use (29,82).

A lapse may end quickly or lead to a relapse of varying proportions. Shiffman (99), for example, reported that 63% of lapsers who called his Stay-Quit line were smoking 2 weeks later; only 37% were able to stop their lapses. The effects of the initial lapse are mediated by the person's affective and cognitive reactions. A full-blown relapse is more likely with the individual who has a strong perception of violating the abstinence rule (66). Although some individuals experience a full-blown relapse and return to pretreatment levels of substance abuse, others use alcohol and drugs problematically, but do not return to previous levels of abuse or dependence and suffer less-harmful effects as a result. Relapsers vary in the quantity and frequency of substance use as well as the medical and psychosocial sequelae that accompany a relapse.

TREATMENT OUTCOME STUDIES

Numerous reviews of the treatment outcome literature, as well as studies of specific clinical populations receiving treatment, document variable rates of relapse among alcoholics, smokers, and drug abusers. Despite the high relapse rates reported in some studies, treatment has a positive effect on multiple domains of functioning for treated alcoholics and drug-dependent individuals. Outcome is best viewed by considering multiple domains: substance use, social, family, and psychological functioning. Substance use disorders are not unlike other chronic or recurrent medical or psychiatric conditions in that recovery is not a linear process and relapses do occur, yet significant improvements are often made.

Miller and Hester reviewed more than 500 alcoholism outcome studies and reported that more than 75% of subjects relapsed within 1 year of treatment (77). In another analysis of the alcohol treatment outcome literature, Miller and colleagues reported that there was a "significant" treatment effect on at least one alcohol measure for at least one followup point for 146 of 211 studies (78, p. 17). Results of Project MATCH (Matching Alcoholism Treatments to Client Heterogeneity), a large-scale multisite, randomized clinical trial of three manual-driven treatments, showed significant reductions in days of alcohol use and drinks per day at both the 1- and 3-year followup periods (93).

McLellan and colleagues reviewed more than 100 clinical trials of drug abuse treatment and found that most clients show favorable outcomes at the 1-year followup period: 40% to 60% are continuously abstinent and 15% to 30% are not using addictively (72). Catalano and colleagues reviewed studies of relapse rates and found relapse rates ranging from 25% to 97% for opioid addiction and from 75% to 80% for tobacco dependence within 1 year of treatment (17). Relapse rates were lowest among opiate addicts who graduated from a therapeutic community in which they resided for a minimum of 18 to 24 months. Hoffmann and Harrison (54) followed 1,957 adult clients with alcohol and/or drug problems who were treated in five different treatment centers in the St. Paul, Minnesota, area. They reported that approximately 50% of clients were abstinent for the entire 2-year period. The Comprehensive Assessment and Treatment Outcome Research (CATOR) group, an independent evaluation service for the substance abuse field, followed 8,087 patients from 38 inpatient programs and 1,663 patients from 19 different programs for 1 year (55). Sobriety rates at 1 year were 60% for inpatient and 68% for outpatient subjects successfully contacted at 6 and 12 months. Even when these rates are adjusted and assume a 70% relapse rate for missing cases, sobriety rates at 1 year are 44% and 52% for the inpatient and outpatient cohorts. Numerous reports by the National Institute on Drug Abuse, the National Institute on Alcohol Abuse and Alcoholism, and the Center for Substance Abuse Treatments document the following positive outcomes for treatment of alcohol and drug abuse: cessation or reduction of substance use; decreases in posttreatment medical care and medical costs; decreases in work problems including absenteeism and working under the influence; decreases in traffic violations and other arrests; and improvement in psychological, social, and family functioning (18–20,81,83,84).

Individuals who relapse do not always return to pretreatment levels of substance use. The actual quantity and frequency of use may vary dramatically. A cocaine or heroin addict who injected large quantities of drugs on a daily basis for years may return to substance use after treatment. Yet this individual may not return to daily use, and the quantity of drugs used may be significantly less than the pretreatment level. Because drug and alcohol use is only one outcome measure, an individual may show improvement in other areas of life functioning despite an actual lapse or relapse to substance use.

RELAPSE PRECIPITANTS

Research by Marlatt and colleagues led to classifying relapse for alcoholics, smokers, heroin addicts, gamblers, and overeaters in two broad categories, intrapersonal and interpersonal determinants (70). This classification scheme has been found useful in other countries (97). Intrapersonal determinants contributing to relapse include negative emotional states, negative physical states, positive emotional states, testing of personal control, and urges and temptations. According to this research, the category that most frequently affected relapse of alcoholics, smokers, and heroin addicts was negative emotional states. Thirty-eight percent of alcoholics, 37% of smokers, and 19% of heroin addicts relapsed in response to a negative affective state that they were unable to manage effectively.

Interpersonal precipitants of relapse include relationship conflict, social pressure to use substances, and positive emotional states associated with some type of interaction with others (53,66,98,106). Social pressure to use drugs was identified by 36% of heroin addicts, 32% of smokers, and 18% of alcoholics as contributing to their relapses (68).

Catalano et al. (17) published an extensive review of rates and determinants of relapse. They investigated the strength of evidence for factors associated with relapse to alcohol, tobacco, and opiate use according to pretreatment, treatment, and posttreatment variables. For opiate addicts, the variables most strongly associated with relapse were degree of impairment caused by drug use, psychiatric impairment, length and modality of treatment, involvement in crime, lack of family and peer support, negative emotional states, and skill deficits. For alcoholics, the factors strongly associated with relapse were lack of family or peer support, negative emotional states, skill deficits, and negative life events. For smokers, the variables most strongly associated with relapse were negative emotional states and problems in family or peer relationships. Many other pretreatment, treatment, and posttreatment factors either had "some" association with relapse or were found to have an equivocal effect on outcome.

A review of the literature by Daley has led to a modification of Marlatt's categories of relapse precipitants (30–32). Relapse can be understood as resulting from an interaction of client-, family-, social-, and treatment-related factors (9,25,58,60,75,76,98,106,109). These include affective variables (e.g., negative or positive mood states), behavioral variables (e.g., coping skills or social skill deficits; impulsivity), cognitive variables (e.g., attitudes toward recovery, self-perception of ability to cope with high-risk situations, and level of cognitive functioning), environmental and interpersonal variables (e.g., lack of social or family stability, social pressures to use substances, lack of productive work or school roles, and lack of involvement in leisure or recreational interests), physiologic variables (e.g., cravings, protracted withdrawal symptoms, chronic illness or physical pain, or response to medications used for medical or psychiatric disorders), psychiatric variables (e.g., presence of a comorbid psychiatric illness, sexual trauma, a higher global rating of psychiatric severity), spiritual variables (e.g., excessive guilt and shame, feelings of emptiness, a sense that life lacks meaning), and treatment-related variables (e.g., negative attitudes of caregivers; inadequate aftercare services following rehabilitation programs; lack of integrated services for dual diagnosis clients).

OVERVIEW OF RELAPSE PREVENTION

Relapse prevention emerged as a way of helping the individual with a substance use disorder maintain change over time. Factors associated with achieving initial change (i.e., abstinence) differ from those associated with the maintenance of change over time (65). Relapse prevention generally refers to two types of treatment strategies. First, relapse prevention may be incorporated in any treatment aimed at helping an individual with a substance use problem maintain abstinence once substances are stopped. In a general sense, psychosocial treatments such as individual drug counseling, group drug counseling, 12-step facilitation therapy, cognitive–behavioral therapy, contingency management, and the MATRIX model, and pharmacologic treatments such as Trexan (Trexan for opiate addicts and ReVia for alcoholics), naltrexone (ReVia), or disulfiram (Antabuse), all aim to help the client remain substance free and prevent relapse or reduce relapse risk (81,84,94). Second, specific coping skills-oriented treatments incorporating the major tenets and interventions discussed in the section below may comprise a specific program referred to as relapse prevention (relapse prevention). While relapse prevention may be offered as a stand-alone program, it often is incorporated into a rehabilitation program in which relapse prevention is one component of the overall program. The focus of relapse prevention is to reduce the relapse risk by addressing potential precipitants of relapse and high-risk factors associated with addictive disorders.

A variety of models of relapse prevention are described in the literature. The more common approaches include (a) Marlatt and Gordon's cognitive–behavioral approach, which has been adapted for other clinical populations such as sex offenders, overeaters, and individuals with problems controlling sexual behaviors; (b) Annis' cognitive–behavioral approach, which incorporates concepts of Marlatt's model with Bandura's self-efficacy theory; (c) Daley's psychoeducational approach; (d) Gorski's neurologic impairment model; and (e) Zackon, McAuliffe, and Ch'ien's addict aftercare model. A more complete description of these and other relapse prevention models is available elsewhere (8,23,30,32,44,70,95,104,105,110,114).

Many inpatient, partial hospital and outpatient treatment programs have incorporated various aspects of these relapse prevention approaches. Some programs offer specific "relapse tracks" that are geared specifically for clients who have relapsed following a period of sustained recovery. The focus of these programs is primarily on problems and issues associated with relapse (32). Despite their differences, these relapse prevention approaches have many components in common. They focus on the need for individuals with a substance use disorder to develop new coping skills for handling high-risk situations and relapse warning signs; to make lifestyle changes to decrease the need for alcohol, drugs, or tobacco; to increase healthy activities; to prepare for interrupting lapses so that they do not end in a full-blown relapse; and to prepare for managing relapses so that adverse consequences may be minimized. All relapse prevention approaches emphasize the need to have a broad repertoire of behavioral, cognitive, and interpersonal coping strategies to help prevent a relapse. Most

are time-limited or brief, making them more feasible in the current climate of managed care.

Empirical Studies of Relapse Prevention

There is evidence that relapse prevention does help to improve recovery and reduce relapse rates (6–8,14,15,56). Carroll (14) reviewed 24 randomized controlled trials on the effectiveness of relapse prevention among smokers (12 studies), alcohol abusers (6 studies), marihuana abusers (1 study), cocaine abusers (3 studies), the opiate addicted (1 study), and other drug abusers (1 study). Carroll reported that the strongest evidence for efficacy of relapse prevention is with smokers and concluded that "there is good evidence for relapse prevention approaches compared with no-treatment controls... [and that] outcomes where relapse prevention may hold greater promise include reducing severity of relapses when they occur, durability of effects after cessation, and patient-treatment matching" (14, p. 53). Clients with higher levels of impairment along dimensions such as psychiatric severity and addiction severity appear to benefit most from relapse prevention when compared to those with less-severe levels of impairment. Thus, relapse prevention may be especially helpful for dual diagnosis clients.

A meta-analysis of 26 clinical trials by Irvin and colleagues involving 9,504 participants supports the efficacy of Marlatt and Gordon's relapse prevention model (56). This analysis found the strongest treatment effects for relapse prevention with clients who had problems with alcohol and polysubstance use.

Carroll and colleagues (15) conducted a study of outpatient cocaine abusers in which they compared relapse prevention to interpersonal psychotherapy (IPT). Relapse prevention was more effective than IPT for patients with more severe cocaine problems and, to some extent, for those with higher psychiatric severity. In another study of outpatient cocaine abusers, Carroll and colleagues (16) compared the outcomes of 12 weeks of treatment in which patients were randomized to psychotherapy (cognitive–behavioral relapse prevention or an operationalized clinical management condition) and pharmacotherapy (desipramine hydrochloride or placebo). Patients were followed for 1 year and the research team found a significant psychotherapy-by-time effect, indicating a delayed improved response to treatment for patients who received relapse prevention.

In a study of 60 men with problem drinking, subjects receiving a relapse program returned to problematic alcohol use at a rate four to seven times less rapidly than subjects in a discussion control group (98). A study of inpatient alcoholic veterans found that results consistently favored clients receiving relapse prevention over those receiving a discussion group (21). Clients in the relapse prevention group drank less, had fewer episodes of intoxication, experienced less-severe lapses for shorter periods of time, and stopped drinking significantly sooner after a relapse compared to clients in the discussion group. Another study of alcoholics receiving inpatient treatment, found that there was greater treatment adherence and satisfaction, reduced lengths of inpatient treatment, and fewer alcohol-related arrests among clients receiving relapse prevention compared to clients receiving other treatment modalities (60). A study of hospitalized male alcoholics found that clients receiving relapse prevention compared to interpersonal process therapy drank on fewer days, drank less alcohol, completed more aftercare, and had a slightly higher rate of continuous abstinence at 6-month follow-up (57).

Other studies have demonstrated relapse prevention to be effective in reducing substance abuse but not more effective than a comparison condition. For example, Stephens et al. (103) randomly assigned 161 men and 51 women seeking help for marihuana dependence to a relapse prevention or social support discussion intervention. Twelve-month posttreatment data indicate substantial reductions in frequency of marihuana use and associated problems but no significant differences between these two interventions on measures of days of use, related problems, or abstinence rates. A study by Wells and colleagues (112) of outpatient cocaine abusers comparing relapse prevention and 12-step counseling found that subjects in both treatment conditions reduced their use of cocaine, marihuana, and alcohol use at 6 months posttreatment. However, subjects in the 12-step counseling condition showed greater improvement in alcohol use when compared to those receiving relapse prevention at the 6-month followup period.

Several studies have included spouses in the relapse prevention intervention (71). A study of the first relapse episodes and reasons for terminating relapses of men with alcoholism who were treated with their spouses found that the relapses of clients receiving relapse prevention in addition to behavioral marital therapy were shorter than those of clients not receiving the relapse prevention (64). In a study of married alcoholics, O'Farrell (88) found that in couples assessed to be "high distress," abstinence rates were highest for those who received behavioral marital therapy in combination with relapse prevention. Alcoholics who received relapse prevention after completing behavioral marital therapy had more days of abstinence, fewer days drinking, and improved marriages than did those who received only behavioral marital therapy (89).

There are limitations to studies on relapse prevention. First, some studies have used relapse prevention as the single treatment intervention for cessation of drinking rather than for maintenance of change once drinking was stopped. Second, studies usually do not differentiate between subjects who are motivated to change substance use behavior and those who have little or no motivation to change. Third, in some studies, sample sizes are small and there is not enough power to detect statistical differences between experimental and control conditions. Fourth, studies do not always use random assignment or

operationalize the therapy being compared against relapse prevention, making it difficult to determine what factors contribute to treatment effects. And last, the followup period is often short-term (6 months or less). Despite these limitations, however, there is empirical evidence that relapse prevention strategies enhance the recovery of individuals with substance use disorders.

COGNITIVE AND BEHAVIORAL INTERVENTIONS

This section discusses practical relapse prevention interventions that can be used in multiple treatment contexts. These interventions reflect the approaches of numerous clinicians and researchers who have developed specific models of relapse prevention and/or written client-oriented relapse prevention recovery materials and the authors' experience with alcoholics and drugs addicts, including clients with comorbid psychiatric conditions. The interventions discussed herein include cognitive and behavioral ones. Whereas some of these interventions can be used by the client as part of a self-management recovery program, other interventions involve eliciting support or help from family or significant others. The literature emphasizes individualizing relapse prevention strategies, taking into account the client's level of motivation, severity of substance use, gender, ego functioning, and sociocultural environment.

The use of experiential learning (e.g., role playing, fantasy, behavioral rehearsal, monodramas, psychodrama, bibliotherapy, use of workbooks, interactive videos, and homework assignments) is recommended to make learning an active experience for the client. Such techniques enhance self-awareness, decrease defensiveness, and encourage behavioral change (31). In treatment groups, action techniques provide numerous opportunities for the clinician to elicit feedback and support for individual clients, identify common themes and issues related to relapse prevention, and practice specific interpersonal skills.

The use of a daily inventory is also recommended (50,93). A daily inventory aims to get clients to continuously monitor their lives so as to identify relapse risk factors, relapse warning signs, or significant life problems that could contribute to a relapse.

Interventions to Reduce Relapse Risk

Help Clients Identify Their High-Risk Relapse Factors and Develop Strategies to Deal With Them

The need to recognize the risk of relapse and high-risk factors is an essential component of relapse prevention. High-risk factors, or critical incidents, typically are those situations in which clients used alcohol or other drugs prior to treatment. High-risk factors usually involve intrapersonal and interpersonal situations (5,66). Because the availability of coping skills is a protective factor reducing relapse risk the clinician should assess coping skills and help the client develop new ones as needed (22).

Numerous clinical aids have been developed by researchers and clinicians to help clients identify and prioritize their individual high-risk situations and develop coping strategies to aid in their recovery. These include Annis' *Inventory of Drinking Situations* (3) and *Inventory of Drug-Taking Situations* (4); Daley's *Identifying High Risk Situations* inventory (29); Zackon, McAuliffe, and Ch'ien's *Your Dangerous Situations* worksheet (114); Gorski's *High-Risk Situation List* and *High-Risk Situations Worksheet* (50); Washton's *Staying Off Cocaine* workbook (111); and Daley and Marlatt's *High Risk Situations Worksheet* (36).

For some clients, identifying high-risk factors and developing new coping strategies for each are inadequate, because they may identify large numbers of risk factors. Such clients need help in taking a more global approach to recovery and may need to learn specific problem-solving skills. Marlatt (67,69), for example, suggests that in addition to teaching clients "specific" relapse prevention skills to deal with high-risk factors, the clinician should also use "global" approaches such as skill training strategies (e.g., behavioral rehearsal, covert modeling, assertiveness training), cognitive reframing (e.g., coping imagery, reframing reactions to lapse or relapse), and lifestyle interventions (e.g., meditation, exercise, relaxation). Numerous behavioral, skill training, and stress management approaches increase the effectiveness of treatment (see, e.g., references 1, 16, 21, 59, and 80). Figure 51.1 summarizes one paradigm for conceptualizing high-risk factors.

Help Clients Understand Relapse as a Process and as an Event

Clients are better prepared for the challenges of recovery if they are cognizant of the fact that relapse occurs within a context and that clues or warning signs typically precede an actual lapse or relapse to substance use. Although a relapse may be the result of an impulsive act on the part of the recovering individual, more often than not, attitudinal, emotional, cognitive, and/or behavioral changes usually manifest themselves prior to the actual ingestion of substances (29,74). An individual's clues or warning signs can be conceptualized as links in a relapse chain (13,36,70). Many relapsers reported to the authors that their warning signs appeared days, weeks, or even longer before they used substances (Fig. 51.2).

Clients in treatment for the first time can benefit from reviewing common relapse warning signs identified by others in recovery. The authors have found it helpful to have relapsers review their experiences in great detail so that they can learn the connections among thoughts, feelings, events or situations, and relapse to substance use. An evaluation of one of the authors' psychoeducational model of relapse prevention and a workbook used in conjunction with this program by 511 clients found that "Understanding the Relapse Process" was the topic rated as the most useful topic (31).

Help Clients Understand and Deal with Alcohol or Drug Cues as Well as Cravings

There is a growing body of research suggesting that alcoholics', drug addicts', and smokers' desire or craving for

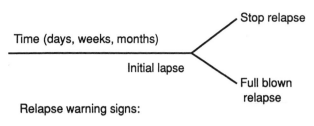

FIG. 51.2. Relapse process

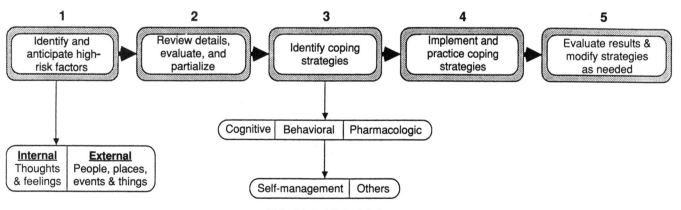

FIG. 51.1. High-risk factors

alcohol or other drugs can be triggered by exposure to environmental cues associated with prior use (73,82,85,107). Cues such as the sight or smell of the substance of abuse may trigger cravings that become evident in cognitive (e.g., increased thoughts of using) and physiologic (e.g., anxiety) changes.

The advice given in AA, NA, and CA for alcoholics and addicts to "avoid people, places, and things" associated with their substance abuse was developed as a way of minimizing exposure to cues that trigger cravings that can be so overwhelming that they contribute to a relapse. A practical suggestion is to encourage clients to remove from their homes substances as well as paraphernalia (pipes, mirrors, needles, etc.) used for taking drugs. This may be more difficult for smokers, however, because most relapse crises occur in association with food or alcohol consumption (100).

Cue exposure treatment is one method used to help reduce the intensity of the client's reactions to cues (82,86,102). This treatment involves exposing the client to specific cues associated with substance use. Cue exposure also involves teaching or enhancing coping skills (e.g., systematic relaxation, behavioral alternatives, visual imagery, and cognitive interventions) to improve the client's confidence in his or her ability to resist the desire to use.

Because it is impossible for clients to avoid all cues that are associated with substance use, the clinician can teach the client a variety of practical techniques to manage cravings (29,49,61,68,100,111). Clients should learn information about cues and how they trigger cravings

for alcohol or other drugs. Monitoring and recording cravings, associated thoughts, and outcomes can help clients become more vigilant and prepared to cope with them. Helpful cognitive interventions for managing cravings include changing thoughts about the craving or desire to use, challenging euphoric recall, talking oneself through the craving, thinking beyond the high by identifying negative consequences of using (immediate and delayed) and positive benefits of not using, using AA/NA/CA recovery slogans and delaying the decision to use. Behavioral interventions include avoiding, leaving, or changing situations that trigger or worsen a craving, redirecting activities or getting involved in pleasant activities, getting help or support from others by admitting and talking about cravings and hearing how others have survived them, attending self-help support group meetings, or taking medications such as disulfiram or naltrexone (for alcoholics). Shiffman and colleagues (100) recommend that ex-smokers carry a menu card that lists various ways to cope with a craving to smoke, a strategy that can also address alcohol or other drug cravings. Figure 51.3 represents a paradigm that the authors have found useful when helping clients understand and manage cravings.

Help Clients Understand and Deal with Social Pressures to Use Substances

Direct and indirect social pressures often lead to increased thoughts and desires to use substances, as well as anxiety regarding one's ability to refuse offers to drink alcohol or

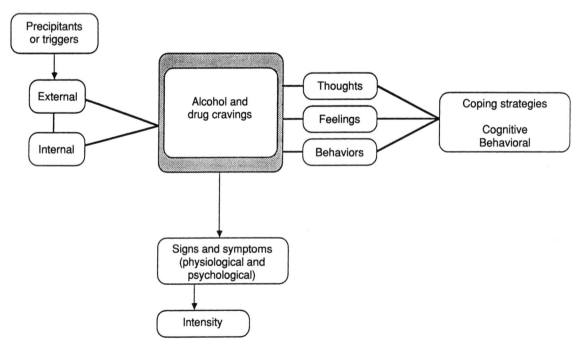

FIG. 51.3. Cravings

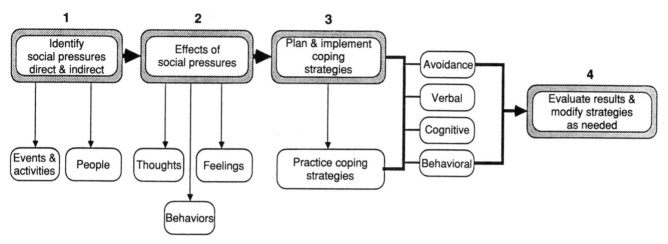

FIG. 51.4. Social pressures

use other drugs. Figure 51.4 outlines one method of helping clients understand and deal with social pressures. The first step is to identify high-risk relationships (e.g., living with or dating an active drug abuser or alcoholic) and situations or events in which the client may be exposed to or offered substances (e.g., social gatherings where people smoke cigarettes or drink alcohol). The next step is to assess the effects of these social pressures on the thoughts, feelings, and behaviors of the client. Planning, practicing, and implementing coping strategies is the next step. These coping strategies include avoidance and the use of verbal, cognitive, or behavioral skills. Using role playing to rehearse ways to refuse offers of drug or alcohol is one very practical and easy-to-use intervention. The final step of this process involves teaching the client to evaluate the results of a given coping strategy and to modify it as needed.

Pressures to use alcohol or other drugs may result from relationships with active drug users or alcoholics. The client needs to assess his or her social network and learn ways to limit or end relationships that represent a high risk for relapse (114).

Help Clients Develop and Enhance a Supportive Social Network

Several authors have addressed relapse prevention from a broader perspective that involves the family or significant others (27, 37, 50). McGrady (70) has modified Marlatt's cognitive-behavioral model of relapse prevention and applied it to couples in recovery. Gorski's model of relapse prevention (50) places strong emphasis on the need for relapse-prone people to involve significant individuals in their lives in a relapse prevention network. O'Farrell and colleagues (88,89) developed a relapse prevention protocol for use in combination with behavioral marital therapy. Maisto and colleagues (64) found that alcoholics who were treated with their spouses with relapse prevention in addi-

tion to marital therapy had shorter and less-severe relapses than clients not receiving relapse prevention.

Numerous studies have substantiated a positive correlation between abstinence from alcohol, drugs, and tobacco and the presence of family and social supports. Families are more likely to support recovery if they are involved in the process and have an opportunity to heal from the emotional pain they experienced. This is more likely to occur if the member with the substance use disorder understands the impact of substance abuse on the family and makes amends for some of the adverse effects on the family.

Involvement of immediate families or significant others in the recovery process provides them with an opportunity to deal with the impact of substance use on their lives as well as their own issues (e.g., enabling behaviors, preoccupation, feelings of anger, shame, and guilt) (37). Families are then in a much better position to support the recovering member. The authors have seen family members sabotage the recovery of the addicted member in a multiplicity of overt and covert ways. Such behavior usually is an indication that they have not had an opportunity to deal with their own issues or heal from their emotional pain.

Clients can be encouraged to get involved in AA, NA, or other support groups. Sponsors, other recovery and personal friends, and employers may become part of an individual's relapse prevention network (9,91). Clients generally should not try to recover in isolation, particularly during the early stages of recovery.

Following are some suggested steps for helping clients develop a relapse prevention network. First, the client needs to identify whom to involve in or exclude from this network. Others who abuse substances, harbor extremely strong negative feelings toward the recovering person, or generally are not supportive of recovery usually should be excluded.

The client should then determine how and when to ask for support or help. Behavioral rehearsal can help the client practice ways to make specific requests for support. Rehearsal also helps increase confidence as well as clarify thoughts and feelings regarding reaching out for help. Many clients, for example, feel guilty or shameful and question whether or not they deserve support from others. Yet others have such strong pride that the thought of asking others for support is very difficult to accept. Rehearsal may also clarify the client's ambivalence regarding ongoing recovery, and it helps better understand how the person being asked for support may respond. This prepares the client for dealing with potential negative responses from others. Clients should be advised to emphasize that recovery is ultimately their responsibility.

An action plan can then be devised, practiced, implemented, and modified as needed. Some clients find it helpful to put their action plan in writing so that all of those involved have a specific document to refer to. The action plan can address the following issues: how to communicate about and deal with relapse warning signs and high-risk situations; how to interrupt a lapse; how to intervene if a relapse occurs; and the importance of exploring all the details of a lapse or relapse after the client is stable so that it can be used as a learning experience. Having a plan can make both the recovering person and family feel more in control even if faced with the possibility of an actual relapse. Additionally, it helps everyone take a proactive approach to recovery rather than sit back passively and wait for problems to occur. The authors' clinical experience has been that clients and families who are involved in such discussions are much more likely to intervene earlier in the relapse process than those not involved in these discussions.

Help Clients Develop Methods of Coping with Negative Emotional States

Negative affective states are associated with relapse across a range of addictions (70). Several investigators reported that depression and anxiety were major factors in a substantial number of relapses (52,63,92). Zackon (113) believes that addicts frequently relapse as a result of joylessness in their lives. Shiffman and colleagues (100) found that coping responses for high-risk situations were less effective for smokers who were depressed. Other negative affective states associated with relapse include anger, anxiety, and boredom. The acronym HALT used in AA and NA (which stands for, "don't get too hungry, angry, lonely, or tired") speaks to the importance of the recovering alcoholic's or drug addict's not allowing himself or herself to get too angry or lonely (2). These two emotional states are seen as high-risk factors for many.

Helping clients improve their ability to identify and manage their emotions is a helpful treatment strategy

(26,28). Interventions for helping clients develop appropriate coping skills for managing negative emotional states vary, depending on the sources, manifestation, and consequences of these emotions. For example, strategies for dealing with depression that accompanies the realization that addiction caused havoc in one's life may vary from those for dealing with depression that is part of a bipolar or major depressive illness that becomes manifest after the client is substance-free and creates significant personal distress.

Interventions to help the client who occasionally gets angry and seeks solace in drugs, tobacco, or alcohol vary from those needed to help the client who is chronically angry at self and others. The former may need help in expressing anger appropriately rather than in suppressing it. The chronically angry individual, on the other hand, may need to learn how not to express anger, since it is often expressed impulsively and inappropriately and often is not even justified. With this type of individual, cognitive techniques that teach the individual to challenge and change angry thoughts that are not justified are helpful. The chronically angry person may also benefit from seeing his or her angry disposition as a "character defect." Psychotherapy and/or use of the 12-step program of AA and NA are appropriate interventions to help modify such an ingrained character trait.

Interventions for clients who report feelings of chronic boredom, emptiness, or joylessness similarly depend on the specific nature of the emotional state. The client may need help in learning how to use free time or how to have fun without chemicals. Or, the client may need help in developing new values and new relationships or in finding new activities that provide a sense of meaning in one's life. Many clients need to alter their beliefs regarding fun, excitement, and what is important in life. The authors have encountered many cocaine addicts who reported that being drug-free was boring compared with the high provided by the drug or behaviors associated with getting the drug or "living on the edge." In such a case, the client needs to change not only behaviors but also beliefs and attitudes.

Assess Clients for Psychiatric Disorders and Facilitate Treatment If Needed

Numerous studies of community samples, psychiatric treatment populations, and substance abuse treatment populations evidence high rates of dual diagnoses (substance use plus psychiatric disorder) (38). Dual-diagnosis clients are at higher risk for substance use relapse than those with only a substance use diagnosis resulting from the effect of psychiatric symptomology on motivation, judgment, and functioning. In addition, dual-diagnosis clients who resume substance use frequently fail to adhere to psychiatric treatment and comply poorly with pharmacotherapy, psychotherapy, and/or self-help program attendance (41).

In a quality assurance/improvement study conducted by one of the authors of 25 substance abusers with mood disorders and 25 substance abusers with schizophrenia who were rehospitalized as a result of significant worsening of psychiatric condition, it was found that alcohol and drug abuse relapse played a significant role in 60% of these psychiatric relapses. In a study comparing psychiatric patients with (n = 127) and without (n = 102) substance abuse comorbidity, one of the authors found that the patients with co-occurring disorders were significantly more likely to relapse and be hospitalized (115).

Relapse prevention strategies can be adapted and tailored to the specific problems and symptoms of the client's psychiatric disorder. Monitoring target moods or behaviors, participating in pleasant activities, developing routine and structure in daily life, learning to cope with persistent psychiatric symptoms associated with chronic or recurrent forms of psychiatric illness, and identifying early warning signs of psychiatric relapse and developing appropriate coping strategies are helpful interventions for dual diagnosis clients (34,35,39).

Negative mood states that are part of an affective disorder (major depression, bipolar disease, etc.) or anxiety disorder (phobia, panic, etc.) may require pharmacotherapy in addition to psychotherapy and involvement in self-help programs. Clients on medications for these or other psychiatric disorders may also benefit from developing strategies for dealing with well-meaning members of self-help programs who encourage them to stop their medications because it is perceived as detrimental to recovery from their substance use disorder.

For Clients Completing Residential or Hospital-Based Treatment, Facilitate the Transition to Followup Outpatient or Aftercare Treatment

Many clients make significant gains in structured, hospital-based or residential substance abuse treatment programs only to have these negated as a consequence of failure to adhere to ongoing outpatient or aftercare treatment (40,43). Interventions used to enhance treatment entry and adherence that lower the risk of relapse include the provision of a single session of motivational therapy prior to discharge from inpatient treatment, the use of telephone or mail reminders of initial treatment appointments, integrating motivational interventions in early recovery, and providing reinforcers for appropriate participation in treatment activities or for providing drug-free urines (41,42,62,79). Studies of patients with schizophrenia and a substance use disorder (104) or patients with mood and substance use disorders (40) show that providing a single motivational therapy session prior to hospital discharge leads to a nearly twofold increase in the show rate for the initial outpatient appointment. Clients who show for their initial appointment and successfully "enter" outpatient treatment have a reduced risk of treatment dropout and subsequent psychiatric and/or substance use relapse.

Help Clients Learn Methods to Cope with Cognitive Distortions

Cognitive distortions or errors in thinking are associated with a wide range of mental health and substance use disorders (10,11,45). These distortions have also been implicated in relapse to substance use as well (30,68). Twelve-step programs refer to cognitive distortions as "stinking thinking" and suggest that recovering individuals need to alter their thinking if they are to remain alcohol- and drug-free.

Teaching clients to identify their cognitive errors (e.g., black-and-white thinking, "awfulizing," overgeneralizing, selective abstraction, catastrophizing, or jumping to conclusions) and evaluate how these affect the relapse process is often very helpful. Clients can then be taught to use counterthoughts to challenge their faulty beliefs or specific negative thoughts. The authors provide clients with a sample worksheet to help them learn to change and challenge relapse thoughts. This worksheet has three directives: (a) list the relapse-related thought; (b) state what's wrong with it; and (c) create new statements. A list of seven specific thoughts commonly associated with relapse is used to prompt clients in completing this therapeutic task. These examples include, "relapse can't happen to me"; "I'll never use alcohol or drugs again"; "I can control my use of alcohol or other drugs"; "a few drinks, tokes, pills, lines won't hurt"; "recovery isn't happening fast enough"; "I need alcohol or other drugs to have fun"; and "my problem is cured." Clients seldom have difficulty coming up with additional examples of specific thoughts that can contribute to a relapse.

Many of the AA and NA slogans were devised to help alcoholics and drug addicts alter their thinking and survive desires to use substances. Slogans such as "this, too, will pass," "let go and let God," and "one day at a time" often help the chemically dependent individual work through thoughts of using.

Help Clients Work Toward a Balanced Lifestyle

In addition to identifying and managing high-risk relapse factors, recovering individuals often need to make more global changes to restore or achieve a balance in their lifestyle (69,110). Development of a healthy lifestyle is seen as important in reducing stress that makes one more vulnerable to relapse.

The client's lifestyle can be assessed by evaluating patterns of daily activities, sources of stress, stressful life events, daily hassles and uplifts, balance between wants (activities engaged in for pleasure or self-fulfillment) and shoulds (external demands), health and exercise patterns, relaxation patterns, interpersonal activities, and religious beliefs (69). Helping clients develop positive habits or substitute indulgences (e.g., jogging, meditation, relaxation, exercise, hobbies, or creative tasks) for substance abuse can help to balance their lifestyle (47,87).

Consider the Use of a Pharmacologic Intervention as an Adjunct to Psychosocial Treatment

Because some clients benefit from pharmacological interventions to attenuate or reduce cravings for alcohol or other drugs, enhance motivation to stay sober, and increase confidence in their ability to resist relapse, a therapist should consider using a pharmacologic intervention as an adjunct to psychosocial treatment (7,48,81,84,101,108). Naltrexone, for example, is helpful for some alcoholics (46,96). Volpicelli and colleagues' study (108) of 70 male alcohol-dependent clients participating in a 12-week, double-blind, placebo-controlled trial of naltrexone found that 23% of subjects taking naltrexone met criteria for relapse compared with 54% of placebo-treatment subjects. The primary effect of naltrexone was that subjects were much less likely to continue drinking following the initial use of alcohol compared to control subjects. In a study of naltrexone combined with coping skills and/or relapse prevention training (N+RP) or supportive therapy (N+ST), O'Malley and colleagues (90) found that N+RP subjects who returned to drinking were less likely to experience a relapse to heavy drinking than were N+ST subjects.

As we mentioned in the previous discussion on dual-diagnosis, treatment of psychiatric symptoms with appropriate medications has important implications for recovery (24,38). Kranzler and colleagues (62) conducted a randomized, 12-week, placebo-controlled trial of buspirone (Zyban) in 61 anxious alcoholics who also received weekly relapse prevention therapy. Clients receiving buspirone showed greater retention in treatment at 12 weeks, reduced anxiety, a slower return to heavy alcohol use, and fewer drinking days than did those clients receiving placebo. In a randomized, controlled, double-blind clinical trial of 100 alcoholic patients, Gottlieb and colleagues (51) found that, among the 57 high-risk patients reporting cravings for alcohol at baseline, relapse rates were 90% for patients receiving placebo compared with 65% for those receiving atenolol, a β-adrenergic blocker. This study also found that poor levels of treatment adherence were strongly associated with adverse outcomes.

Help Clients Develop a Plan to Manage a Lapse or Relapse

The outcome literature shows that most alcoholics, smokers, and drug addicts lapse or relapse at one time or another. Therefore, it is highly recommended that clients have an emergency plan to follow if they lapse, so that a full-blown relapse can be avoided. If a full-blown relapse occurs, however, the client needs to have strategies to stop it. The specific intervention strategies should be based on the severity of the client's lapse or relapse, coping mechanisms, and prior history of relapse.

Helpful interventions include getting clients to use self-talk or behavioral procedures to stop a lapse or relapse, asking family, AA/NA/SA sponsors, friends, or professionals for help, carrying an emergency card with names and phone numbers of others who can be called on for support, or carrying a reminder card that gives specific instructions on what to do if a lapse or relapse occurs (29,68). Marlatt recommends developing a relapse contract with clients that outlines specific steps to take in the event of a future relapse. The aim of this contract is to formalize or reinforce the client's commitment to change.

Analyzing lapses or relapses is a valuable process that can aid ongoing recovery. This helps to reframe a "failure" as a "learning" experience and can help the individual prepare for future high-risk situations.

CONCLUSION

A variety of relapse prevention clinical treatment models and specialized programs have been developed for clients with alcohol, tobacco, or other drug problems. Many of the cognitive and behavioral interventions described in these relapse prevention approaches can be adapted for use with clients who have additional problems, such as other compulsive disorders, impulse control disorders, or comorbid psychiatric illnesses. Relapse prevention interventions aim to help clients maintain change over time and address the most common issues and problems raising vulnerability to relapse. Studies indicate that relapse prevention has efficacy in reducing both relapse rates and the severity of lapses or relapses. Relapse prevention strategies can be used throughout the continuum of care in primary rehabilitation programs, dual-diagnosis hospital programs, residential programs, halfway houses, or therapeutic community programs, as well as in partial hospital, outpatient, and aftercare programs. In addition, family members can be included in educational and therapy sessions and involved in the development of relapse prevention plans for members with substance use disorders.

Many of the relapse prevention approaches described in the literature can be considered short-term or brief treatments and can be provided in individual or group sessions, making them attractive and cost effective. Most clinical models of relapse prevention are supported by user-friendly, interactive recovery materials such as books, workbooks, videos, and audio tapes. These supplemental materials provide additional information and support to clients who can learn to use self-management techniques of relapse prevention on their own, following completion of formal treatment.

REFERENCES

1. Abrams D, Niaura R, Carey K, et al. Understanding relapse and recovery in alcohol abuse. *Ann Behav Med* 1986;8(2-3):27–32.
2. *Alcoholics Anonymous (Big Book),* 3rd ed. New York: AA World Services, 1976.
3. Annis H. *Inventory of drinking situations.* Toronto: Addiction Research Foundation, 1982.
4. Annis H. *Inventory of drug-taking situations.* Toronto: Addiction Research Foundation, 1985.
5. Annis H. A relapse prevention model for treatment of alcoholics. In: Miller W, Heather N, eds. *Treating addictive behaviors: process of change.* New York: Plenum, 1986.
6. Annis H. *Effective treatment for drug and alcohol problems: what do we know?* Paper presented at the annual meeting of the Institute of Medicine, National Academy of Sciences, Washington, DC, 1987.
7. Annis H. A cognitive-social learning approach to relapse: pharmacotherapy and relapse prevention counseling. *Alcohol Alcohol* 1991;[Suppl 1]:527–530.
8. Annis H, Davis C. Relapse prevention training. A cognitive–behavioral approach based on self-efficacy theory. *J Chem Depend Treat* 1989;2:2,81–104.
9. Barber JG, Crisp BR. Social support and prevention of relapse following treatment for alcohol abuse. *Res Soc Work Pract* 1995;5(3):283–296.
10. Beck A. *Cognitive therapy and the emotional disorders.* New York: New American Library, 1976.
11. Beck A, Wright F, Liese B. *Cognitive therapy of substance abuse.* New York: Guilford Press, 1994.
12. Brown S. *Treating the alcoholic: a developmental model of recovery,* 2nd ed. New York: John Wiley, 1995.
13. Brownell K, Rodin J. *The weight maintenance survival guide.* Dallas, TX: LEARN Education Center, 1990.
14. Carroll KM. Relapse prevention as a psychosocial treatment: a review of controlled clinical trials. *Exp Clin Psychopharmacol* 1996;4(1):46–54.
15. Carroll KM, Rounsaville BJ, Gawin FH. A comparative trial of psychotherapies for ambulatory cocaine abusers: relapse prevention and interpersonal psychotherapy. *Am J Drug Alcohol Abuse* 1991;17(3):229–247.
16. Carroll KM, Rounsaville BJ, Nich C, et al. One-year follow-up of psychotherapy and pharmacotherapy for cocaine dependence. Delayed emergence of psychotherapy effects. *Arch Gen Psychiatry* 1994;51(12):989–997.
17. Catalano R, Howard M, Hawkins J, et al. Relapse in the addictions: rates, determinants, and promising prevention strategies. In: *1988 Surgeon General's report on health consequences of smoking.* Washington, DC: U.S. Government Printing Office, 1988.
18. Center for Substance Abuse Treatment (CSAT). Treatment succeeds in fighting crime. In: *Substance abuse in brief.* Rockville, MD: Substance Abuse and Mental Health Services Administration, December 1999.
19. Center for Substance Abuse Treatment (CSAT). Substance abuse treatment reduces family dysfunction, improves productivity. In: *Substance abuse in brief.* Rockville, MD: Substance Abuse and Mental Health Services Administration, April 2000.
20. Center for Substance Abuse Treatment (CSAT). Treatment cuts medical costs. In: *Substance abuse in brief.* Rockville, MD: Substance Abuse and Mental Health Services Administration, May 2000.
21. Chaney E, O'Leary M. Skill training with alcoholics. *J Consult Clin Psychol* 1978;46(5):1092–1104.
22. Connors GJ, Longabaugh R, Miller WR. Looking forward and back to relapse: implications for research and practice. *Addiction* 1996;[Suppl 91]:191–196.
23. Connors GJ, Maisto SA, Donovan DM. Conceptualizations of relapse: a summary of psychological and psychobiological models. *Addiction* 1996;[Suppl 91]:S5–S13.
24. Cornelius JR, Salloum IM, Ehler JG, et al. Fluoxetine in depressed alcoholics: a double-blind placebo-controlled trial. *Arch Gen Psychiatry* 1997;54:700–705.
25. Cuffel BJ, Chase P. Remission and relapse of substance use disorders in schizophrenia: results from a one-year prospective study. *J Nerv Ment Dis* 1994;182(6):342–348.
26. Daley D. *Coping with feelings workbook,* 2nd ed. Holmes Beach, FL: Learning Publications, 2001.
27. Daley D. *Improving communications and relationships workbook,* 2nd ed. Holmes Beach, FL: Learning Publications, 2003.
28. Daley D. *Managing anger workbook,* 2nd ed. Holmes Beach, FL: Learning Publications, 2001.
29. Daley D. *Relapse prevention workbook for recovering alcoholics and drug-dependent persons,* 3rd ed. Holmes Beach, FL: Learning Publications, 2000.
30. Daley D. *Relapse prevention: treatment alternatives and counseling aids.* Bradenton, FL: Human Services Institute, 1988.
31. Daley D. Five perspectives on relapse in chemical dependency. *J Chem Depend Treat* 1989;2:2,3–26.
32. Daley D, ed. *Relapse. Conceptual, research and clinical perspectives.* New York: Haworth, 1989.
33. Daley D. *Surviving addiction workbook,* 2nd ed. Holmes Beach, FL: Learning Publications, 1999.
34. Daley D. *Preventing relapse,* 2nd ed. Center City, MN: Hazelden, 2003.
35. Daley D, Lis J. Relapse prevention: intervention strategies for mental health clients with comorbid addictive disorders. In: Washton A, ed. *Psychotherapy and substance abuse: a practitioner's handbook.* New York: Guilford Press, 1995:243–263.
36. Daley D, Marlatt GA. *Managing your alcohol or drug problem.* San Antonio, TX: Psychological Corporation, 1997.
37. Daley D, Miller J. *Addiction in your family: helping yourself and your loved ones.* Holmes Beach, FL: Learning Publications, 2001.
38. Daley D, Moss HB. *Dual disorders: counseling clients with chemical dependency and mental illness,* 3rd ed. Center City, MN: Hazelden, 2002.
39. Daley D, Roth L. *When symptoms return: a guide to relapse in psychiatric illness,* 2nd ed. Holmes Beach, FL: Learning Publications, 2001.
40. Daley D, Zuckoff A. Improving compliance with the initial outpatient session among discharged inpatient dual diagnosis clients. *Social Work* 1998;43(5):470–473.
41. Daley D, Zuckoff A. *Improving treatment compliance: counseling and system strategies for substance use and dual disorders.* Center City, MN: Hazelden, 1999.
42. Daley D, Salloum IM, Zuckoff A, et al. Increasing treatment compliance among outpatients with depression and cocaine dependence: results of a pilot study. *Am J Psychiatry* 1998;155:1611–1613.
43. deLeon G. Aftercare in therapeutic communities. Special issue: relapse prevention in substance misuse. *Int J Addict* 1990—1991;25(9A-10A):1225–1237.
44. Donovan D, Chaney E. Alcoholic relapse prevention and intervention: models and methods. In: Marlatt GA, Gordon J, eds. *Relapse prevention: maintenance strategies in the treatment of addictive behaviors.* New York: Guilford Press, 1985:351–416.
45. Ellis A, McInerney J, DiGiuseppe R, et al. *Rational-emotive therapy with*

alcoholics and substance abusers. New York: Pergamon Press, 1988.

46. Garbutt JC, West SL, Carey TS, et al. Pharmacological treatment of alcohol dependence: a review of evidence. *JAMA* 1999;281(14):1318–1325.

47. Gelderloos P, Walton KG, Orme-Johnson DW, et al. Effectiveness of the transcendental meditation program in preventing and treating substance misuse: a review. *Int J Addict* 1991;26(3):293–325.

48. Gorelick DA. Overview of pharmacologic treatment approaches for alcohol and other drug addiction. Intoxication, withdrawal, and relapse prevention. *Psychiatr Clin North Am* 1993;16(1): 141–156.

49. Gorski T. *Managing cocaine craving.* Center City, MN: Hazelden, 1990.

50. Gorski T, Miller M. *Staying sober workbook.* Independence, MO: Independence Press, 1988.

51. Gottlieb LD, Horwitz RI, Kraus ML, et al. Randomized controlled trial in alcohol relapse prevention: role of atenolol, alcohol craving, and treatment adherence. *J Subst Abuse Treat* 1994;11(3):253–258.

52. Hatsukami D, Pickins R, Svikis D. Post-treatment depressive symptoms and relapse to drug use in different age groups of an alcohol and other drug abuse population. *Drug Alcohol Depend* 1981;8(4):271–277.

53. Havassy BE, Hall SM, Wasserman DA. Social support and relapse: commonalities among alcoholics, opiate users, and cigarette smokers. *Addict Behav* 1991;16(5):235–246.

54. Hoffmann N, Harrison P. *CATOR 1986 report: findings two years after treatment.* St Paul, MN: CATOR, 1986.

55. Hoffmann NG, Miller NS. Treatment outcomes for abstinence-based programs. *Psychiatr Ann* 1992;22(8):402–408.

56. Irvin JE, Bowers CA, Dunn ME, et al. Efficacy of relapse prevention: a meta-analytic review. *J Consult Clin Psychol* 1999;67(4):563–570.

57. Ito JR, Donovan DM, Hall JJ. Relapse prevention and alcohol aftercare: effects on drinking outcome, change process, and aftercare attendance. *Br J Addict* 1988;83:171–181.

58. Johnson E, Herringer LG. A note on the utilization of common support activities and relapse following substance abuse treatment. *J Psychol* 1993;127(1):73–77.

59. Kadden RM, Mauriello IJ. Enhancing participation in substance abuse treatment using an incentive system. *J Subst Abuse Treat* 1991;8:133–144.

60. Koski-Jannes A. *Alcohol addiction and self-regulation: a controlled trial of re-lapse prevention program for Finnish inpatient alcoholics.* Finland: Finnish Foundation for Alcohol Studies, 1992.

61. Kosten TR. Can cocaine craving be a medication development outcome? Drug craving and relapse in opioid and cocaine dependence. *Am J Addict* 1992;1(3):230–239.

62. Kranzler HR, Burleson JA, Del Boca FK, et al. Buspirone treatment of anxious alcoholics. A placebo-controlled trial. *Arch Gen Psychiatry* 1994;51(9):720–731.

63. LaBounty LP, Hatsukami D, Morgan SF, et al. Relapse among alcoholics with phobic and panic symptoms. *Addict Behav* 1992;17(1):9–15.

64. Maisto SA, McKay JR, O'Farrell TJ. Relapse precipitants and behavioral marital therapy. *Addict Behav* 1995;20(3):383–393.

65. Marlatt GA. Relapse prevention: theoretical rationale and overview of the model. In: Marlatt GA, Gordon J, eds. *Relapse prevention: a self-control strategy in the maintenance of behavior change.* New York: Guilford Press, 1985:3–70.

66. Marlatt GA. Situational determinants of relapse and skill-training interventions. In: Marlatt GA, Gordon J, eds. *Relapse prevention: a self-control strategy for the maintenance of behavior change.* New York: Guilford Press, 1985:71–127.

67. Marlatt GA. Cognitive factors in the relapse process. In: Marlatt GA, Gordon J, eds. *Relapse prevention: a self-control strategy for the maintenance of behavior change.* New York: Guilford Press, 1985:128–200.

68. Marlatt GA. Cognitive assessment and intervention procedures for relapse prevention. In: Marlatt GA, Gordon J, eds. *Relapse prevention: a self-control strategy for the maintenance of behavior change.* New York: Guilford Press, 1985:201–279.

69. Marlatt GA. Lifestyle modification. In: Marlatt GA, Gordon J, eds. *Relapse prevention: a self-control strategy for the maintenance of behavior change.* New York: Guilford Press, 1985:280–350.

70. Marlatt GA, Gordon J, eds. *Relapse prevention: a self-control strategy for the maintenance of behavior change.* New York: Guilford Press, 1985.

71. McGrady B. Extending relapse prevention to couples. *Addict Behav* 1989;14:69–74.

72. McLellan A, Lewis DC, O'Brien CP, et al. Drug dependence, a chronic mental illness: implications for treatment, insurance, and outcomes evaluation. *JAMA* 2000;284(13):1689–1695.

73. McKay JR. Studies of factors of relapse to alcohol, drug, and nicotine use: a crit-ical review of methodologies and findings. *J Stud Alcohol* 1999;60:566–576.

74. McKay JR, Rutherford MJ, Alterman AI, et al. An examination of the cocaine relapse process. *Drug Alcohol Depend* 1995;38(1):35–43.

75. Miller L. Predicting relapse and recovery in alcoholism and addiction: neuropsychology, personality, and cognitive style. *J Subst Abuse Treat* 1991;8(4):277–291.

76. Miller NS, Gold MS. Dissociation of "conscious desire" (craving) from and relapse in alcohol and cocaine dependence. *Ann Clin Psychiatry* 1994;6(2):99–106.

77. Miller W, Hester R. Treating the problem drinker: modern approaches. In: *The addictive behaviors: treatment of alcoholism, drug abuse, smoking and obesity.* New York: Pergamon Press, 1980.

78. Miller WR, Brown JM, Simpson TL, et al. What works? A methodological analysis of the alcohol treatment outcome literature. In: Hester R, Miller W, eds. *Handbook of alcoholism treatment approaches,* 2nd ed. Boston: Allyn & Bacon, 1995:12–44.

79. Miller WR, Rollnick S. *Motivational interviewing: preparing people to change addictive behavior,* 2nd ed. New York: Guilford Press, 2002.

80. Monti P, Adams D, Kadden R, et al. *Treating alcohol dependence.* New York: Guilford Press, 1989.

81. National Institute on Alcohol Abuse and Alcoholism (NIAAA). Highlights from the 10th special report to Congress. *Alcohol Res Health* 2000;24(1).

82. National Institute on Drug Abuse (NIDA). *Cue extinction techniques: NIDA technology transfer package.* Rockville, MD: National Institutes of Health, 1993.

83. National Institute on Drug Abuse (NIDA). Study sheds new light on the state of drug abuse treatment nationwide. *NIDA Notes* 1997;12(5):1–8.

84. National Institute on Drug Abuse (NIDA). *Principles of drug addiction treatment: a research-based guide.* Rockville, MD: National Institutes of Health, 1999.

85. O'Brien CP, Childress AR, Ehrman R, et al. Conditioning factors in drug abuse: can they explain compulsion? *Psychopharmacology (Berl)* 1998;12:15–22.

86. O'Brien CP, Childress AR, McLellan T, et al. Integrating systematic cue exposure with standard treatment in recovering drug-dependent patients. *Addict Behav* 1990;15(4):355–365.

87. O'Connell DF. The use of transcendental meditation in relapse

prevention counseling. *Alcohol Treat Q* 1991;8(1):53–68.

88. O'Farrell TJ. Couples relapse prevention sessions after a behavioral marital therapy couples group program. In: O Farrell TJ, ed. *Treating alcohol problems: marital and family interventions.* New York: Guilford Press, 1993:305–326.

89. O'Farrell TJ, Choquette KA, Cutter HS, et al. Behavioral martial therapy with and without additional couples relapse prevention sessions for alcoholics and their wives. *J Stud Alcohol* 1993;54(6):652–666.

90. O'Malley SS, Jaffe AJ, Chang G, et al. Naltrexone and coping skills therapy for alcohol dependence. *Arch Gen Psychiatry* 1992;49:881–887.

91. Peters RH, Witty TE, O'Brien JK. The importance of the work family with structured work and relapse prevention. *J Appl Rehabil Counsel* 1993;24(3):3–5.

92. Pickens R, Hatsukami D, Spicer J, et al. Relapse by alcohol abusers. *Alcohol Clin Exp Res* 1985;9(3):244–247.

93. Project MATCH. Matching alcoholism treatments to client heterogeneity: Project MATCH three-year drinking outcomes. *Alcoholism Clin Exp Res* 1998;22(6):1300–1311.

94. Rawson RA, Obert JL, McCann MJ, et al. Relapse prevention models for substance abuse treatment. Special issue: psychotherapy for the addictions. *Psychotherapy* 1993;30(2):284–298.

95. Rawson RA, Obert JL, McCann MJ, et al. Relapse prevention strategies in outpatient substance abuse treatment. Special series: psychosocial treatment of the addictions. *Psychol Addict Behav* 1993;7(2):85–95.

96. Salloum IM, Cornelius JR, Thase ME, et al. Naltrexone utility in depressed alcoholics. *Psychopharmacol Bull* 1998;34(1):111–115.

97. Sandahl C. Determinants of relapse among alcoholics: a cross-cultural replication study. *Int J Addict* 1984; 19(8):833–848.

98. Saunders B, Allsop S. Alcohol problems and relapse: can the clinic combat the community? *J Community Appl Soc Psychol* 1991;1(3):213–221.

99. Shiffman S. Relapse following smoking cessation: a situational analysis. *J Consult Clin Psychol* 1982;50:71–86.

100. Shiffman S, Read L, Maltese J, et al. Preventing relapse in ex-smokers: a self-management approach. In: Marlatt GA, Gordon J, eds. *Relapse prevention: a self-control strategy for the maintenance of behavior change.* New York: Guilford Press, 1985:472–520.

101. Smith JW, Frawley PJ. Treatment outcome of 600 chemically dependent patients treated in a multimodal inpatient program including aversion therapy and pentothal interviews. *J Subst Abuse Treat* 1993;10(4):359–369.

102. Staiger PK, Greeley JD, Wallace SD. Alcohol exposure therapy: generalization and changes in responsivity. *Drug Alcohol Depend* 1999;57(1):29–40.

103. Stephens RS, Roffman RA, Simpson EE. Treatment adult marijuana dependence: a test of the relapse prevention model. *J Consult Clin Psychol* 1994;62(1):92–99.

104. Swanson AJ, Pantalon MV, Cohen KR. Motivational interviewing and treatment adherence among psychiatric and dually diagnoses patients. *J Nerv Ment Dis* 1999;187(9):630–635.

105. Tims F, Leukefeld C, eds. Relapse and recovery in drug abuse. *NIDA Res Monogr* 1987;72.

106. Tucker JA, Vuchinich RE, Gladsjo JA. Environmental influences on relapse in substance use disorders. Special issues: environmental factors in substance misuse and its treatment. *Int J Addict* 1990-91;25(7A-8A):1017–1050.

107. Volkow ND, Fowler JS. Addiction, a disease of compulsion and drive: involvement of the orbitofrontal cortex. *Cereb Cortex* 2000;10:318–325.

108. Volpicelli JR, Alterman AI, Hayashida M, et al. Naltrexone in the treatment of alcohol dependence. *Arch Gen Psychiatry* 1992;49:876–880.

109. Wadsworth R, Spampneto AM, Halbrook BM. The role of sexual trauma in the treatment of chemically dependent women: addressing the relapse issue. *J Counsel Dev* 1995;73(4):401–406.

110. Wanigaratne S. *Relapse prevention for addictive behaviors.* London: Blackwell Scientific Publications, 1990.

111. Washton A. *Staying off cocaine: cravings, other drugs and slips.* Center City, MN: Hazelden, 1990.

112. Wells EA, Peterson PL, Gainey RR, et al. Outpatient treatment for cocaine abuse: a controlled comparison of relapse prevention and twelve-step approaches. *Am J Drug Alcohol Abuse* 1994;20(1):1–17.

113. Zackon F. Relapse, "re-joyment" observations and reflections. *J Chem Depend Treat* 1989;2(2):67–80.

114. Zackon F, McAuliffe W, Ch'ien J. *Addict aftercare: recovery training and self-help.* Rockville, MD: NIDA, 1992.

115. Zuckoff A, Daley DC. Engagement and adherence issues in treating persons with non-psychosis dual disorders. *Psychiatr Rehabil Skills* 2001;5(1):131–162.

SUGGESTED CLIENT EDUCATIONAL VIDEOTAPES

Living sober series 1, 2, and 3. Skokie, IL: Gerald T Rogers Production (800-227-9100) 1994, 1995, and 1996. These interactive videos focus on the most common relapse issues such as resisting social pressures, coping with cravings, managing feelings, dealing with family and interpersonal conflict, building a recovery network and sponsorship, coping with relapse warning signs, improving relations and support systems, improving motivation and improving adherence to treatment.

Staying Sober, Keeping Straight: Gerald T. Rogers Productions (800-227-9100). This includes three stories, which illustrate relapse warning signs, high-risk situations and positive coping strategies.

Relapse Prevention: National Institute on Drug Abuse, 1994. This provides an overview of relapse factors and RP strategies.

CHAPTER 52

Evaluation and Outcome of Treatment

ROBERT L. HUBBARD

Various treatments for both alcohol and drug abuse have been available since the turn of the century. However, only in the late 1960s and early 1970s did both alcohol and drug abuse treatment become major parts of the public health system in the United States. Much of what we know about treatment and current clinical approaches to treatment was developed during these years. In the early 1990s, a number of studies were initiated to update and expand this knowledge base. This knowledge will be especially important in shaping treatment in the rapidly changing cost containment environment which emerged in the late 1990s, and should inform the continuing efforts to identify science-based effective and efficient practices.

The alcohol treatment system emerged in the late 1960s in an effort to establish community-based alcohol treatment centers throughout many parts of the United States. Combined with this public approach was the proliferation of proprietary inpatient programs based on the "Minnesota model" treatment protocol (1,2). These short-term inpatient regimens helped guide alcohol abusers through the first phases of the Twelve Steps of the Alcoholics Anonymous recovery process. Treatment for drug abuse, particularly cocaine, began to be provided in these chemical-dependency programs originally designed for alcoholism. With increasing concerns about costs, the length of inpatient stays has been dramatically reduced and the chemical dependency model shifted largely to outpatient environments.

The rapid escalation of heroin addiction in communities in the late 1960s, coupled with the high rates of addiction among returning Vietnam veterans, led to the establishment of a national system of drug abuse treatment programs to deal with the increasing rates of addiction and associated crime (3). Since these early years there have been far-reaching changes in the drug abuse treatment system. The three major "modalities," or types of treatment, developed and under public funding in the United States have been the outpatient methadone clinics, therapeutic communities, and outpatient drug-free programs. Outpatient methadone programs treat opioid abusers, most of whom use heroin intravenously. After stabilization with medically prescribed doses of methadone, clients receive a variety of counseling and other services to help them resume productive lives. Therapeutic communities use group counseling with all types of drug abusers over long stays in a 24-hour community environment. Outpatient

drug-free programs tend to be oriented toward nonopioid users, emphasizing counseling, often in community mental health center settings. Among these modalities, there are great variations in program size, setting, organization, philosophy, structure, therapeutic approach, services, and funding. Although existing in their original form, the three traditional modalities have faced a rapidly changing environment and reduced resources.

A rich database, including three national multiprogram studies, was developed to describe the effectiveness of these modalities and approaches. In addition, a number of studies of individual programs using quasi-experimental and clinical trial designs have been conducted. The overwhelming weight of the evidence from these studies and carefully designed epidemiologic outcome studies is that treatment contributes significantly to change in client behavior during and after treatment. Many of these data were summarized in major literature reviews and deliberation of expert panels at the Institute of Medicine (IOM) (4–6). These major reviews have concluded that treatment is effective. A more limited number of studies indicate that the benefits of these changes considerably outweigh the costs of the treatment. Because of the lack of studies of elements of treatment or of alternative strategies for reducing demand and supply, the comparative cost effectiveness of different treatment components or treatment versus prevention or enforcement is not known. The need for such studies has become even more important as concern has risen over containing health care costs during the 1990s.

Questions continue to be raised about the overall effectiveness of treatment, the comparative effects of different treatment approaches, and the benefits of particular components of treatment. Despite the wealth of data, these questions are valid. Extensive, systematic research has not yet focused on the many components of treatment in typical programs in community settings. Furthermore, the treatment system and the client population have changed since the late 1970s. Very limited information exists for the programs and approaches in operation during the 1980s. Major new research and data collection efforts are only beginning for the treatment system into the next century. These efforts must not only confirm or revise previous findings but also anticipate questions that will emerge in a rapidly changing environment.

The treatment system in the United States in the 2000s includes a broader array of public and private program types. The proportion of privately funded alcohol and drug abuse treatment programs increased during the 1980s, but by 1987 utilization rates in many areas were only 50% of capacity (5). Drug abuse treatment is now delivered in a wider variety of settings, including chemical dependency programs (formerly exclusive alcohol treatment programs) and community mental health centers, as well as treatment programs designed primarily for alcohol. The administration of the public treatment system has shifted from the federal government to states under the Omnibus Budget

Reconciliation Act of 1981 and entered an era of managed care in the 1990s. The distinction between publicly funded and private treatment is blurred. The treatment of many clients in the traditional public treatment modalities is not fully supported by public funds. Clients pay for all or part of treatment through third-party reimbursements or their own resources, and costs are closely monitored by managed care organizations. In recognition of the paucity of up-to-date information, major new research and demonstration efforts were launched for the 1990s, including two new multisite evaluation studies, a large-scale clinical trial of matching for alcohol treatment, and the establishment of a clinical trial network as a platform to test the effectiveness of science-based intervention. While we await updated effectiveness and benefit:cost studies, and more detailed studies of treatment components and targeted interventions, we can have confidence that treatment is an effective and cost-effective strategy. However, more fundamental questions need to be addressed in analysis of treatment.

Although various treatments have been shown to have an aggregate effect and a favorable benefit:cost ratio, many factors limit the effectiveness of treatment. Many drug abusers do not enter treatment. Many do not stay a sufficient time to receive the full benefits of treatment. Services to deal with increasingly complex problems of clients need to be expanded in quantity and enhanced in quality. Even after extensive treatment experience, many clients relapse and renew their treatment careers. It is also critical to determine whether the positive outcomes of previous studies can be confirmed during periods of reduced resources and cost containment. Previous studies show that the full potential of treatment is not being realized. Questioning the aggregate effectiveness diverts research from a more fundamental issue of how to improve the many types of treatment currently available to clients with diverse backgrounds and impairments. The basic question facing us is how to maximize the return on each hour and dollar of resources invested in treatment.

This chapter first reviews and updates major findings on treatment effectiveness. Second, it outlines two major issues, client differences and treatment variations, which require extensive conceptual and empiric examination particularly when the environment is rapidly changing. The chapter broadens the reader's understanding of clients and treatment and their potential contribution to a more comprehensive investigation of the effectiveness of treatment. A broader perspective on client differences includes consideration of impairments and functioning of clients across multiple domains, exposure to many types and durations of programs during a treatment career, and dynamic, complex patterns of drug abuse. The development of a model of treatment structure and process components needs to include multilevel consideration of program structure, client–counselor interaction, and the process of service delivery and client change, as well as the health

and social system in which treatment is funded and delivered. In-depth investigation of these issues should build upon existing research to provide a more complete understanding of effectiveness of treatment and the factors that contribute to it. This chapter focuses primarily on prospective epidemiologic multiprogram studies, which provide the breadth of information necessary to identify the nature and range of client and treatment variables and their relative contribution to treatment outcomes.

EFFECTIVENESS

The effectiveness of both alcohol and drug abuse treatment has been continually questioned. One reason why is the difficulty of conducting broad-based epidemiologic outcome studies or controlled clinical trials of sufficient scope to answer the central questions about treatment. Prior to 1990, only one national study of alcohol treatment and two of drug abuse treatment had been mounted successfully in the previous 30 years. Clinical trials based on unblinded random assignment have often failed because of the limited compliance (7) and retention (8) for sufficiently long periods of time to demonstrate the efficacy of any particular treatment approach. Despite these limitations, IOM panels (5,9) and individual reviewers (4,6,10,11) have concluded that treatment does have positive effects. Since 1990, two major national epidemiologic outcome studies on drug abuse treatment and one clinical trial of alcohol treatment have been launched. The analysis of data bases from these studies are published in early stages. Where applicable, early results are included to broaden the base of knowledge presented in this chapter. Epidemiologic outcome studies do indicate positive effects. The major clinical epidemiologic study of alcohol treatment was conducted in the early 1970s, with a sample of 593 clients followed 18 and 48 months after treatment (12,13). After 4 years, 21% were abstinent for at least 1 year before the followup. A positive correlation was reported between those clients receiving five or more outpatient visits and those with more than 7 days' of inpatient visits. Using a cost-offset framework in an analysis of health insurance data, Holder and Blose (14) attributed substantial savings to alcohol treatment in health care costs. Other followup studies of proprietary programs reviewed in 1989 by the IOM Committee to Identify Research Effectiveness in the Prevention and Treatment of Alcohol-Related Problems (15) found abstinence rates between 40% and 60% in the first year after treatment. Similar results were found in studies of state programs (16) and private programs (17). Because of the often low rates of response to followup, the method of obtaining reports, and imprecise measurement of treatment process, including continuing care and other methodological considerations, these rates of abstinence likely exaggerate the positive effects of treatment.

In contrast to these findings and those for drug abuse treatment reported later in this section, the IOM committee found little evidence supporting longer-term treatment for alcohol abuse. Reviews (18–20) and a series of random assignment studies have found that neither length of treatment nor intensity (inpatient versus outpatient) influenced outcome. In such unblinded research, however, the levels of severity of client problems likely interact with selection bias from compliance and attrition to confound the interpretation of results. Furthermore, most alcohol treatment protocols tested, typically less than 3 months, may not be of sufficient duration or intensity to produce demonstrable effects. Controlled studies of alcohol treatment may need to focus more on comparison of different continuums of care to examine how inpatient and outpatient programs can contribute to long-term compliance with aftercare and relapse prevention. A major multisite clinical trial was initiated in 1989 to examine patient matching hypotheses for 952 alcohol-dependent clients in outpatient settings, and for 774 patients receiving aftercare following inpatient treatment (21). The findings were summarized as "results showed sustained improvement in drinking frequency and severity from pretreatment to 1 year posttreatment with little difference across treatments for both groups" (22). The changes in behavior were sustained for more than 3 years for the 952 outpatient clients (23).

A series of studies of drug abuse treatment conducted primarily over the past two decades has demonstrated the effectiveness of the publicly funded methadone maintenance and therapeutic community approaches (24,25). Use of most drugs declines during and after treatment (26–30). Criminal activity is reduced among program clients, particularly during treatment (31–34).

To conclusively demonstrate effectiveness, results must be replicated across different client populations and diverse programs. Three multisite national prospective studies have been undertaken to demonstrate effectiveness and to consider the multiple factors that contribute to treatment outcome. Beginning with the Drug Abuse Reporting Program (DARP) admission cohorts in 1969–1973, followed by the Treatment Outcome Prospective Study (TOPS) cohorts in 1979–1981, and continuing with the Drug Abuse Treatment Outcome Study (DATOS) of adult cohorts in 1991–1993, and adolescent cohorts in 1993–1995, each of the studies has built upon its predecessor. Fundamental to such studies is the most comprehensive assessment of clients and treatments feasible across multiple programs and large client samples. Applying the advances in instrument design, improvement in interviewer training, and enhancement of conceptual models of client characteristics and treatment, the DATOS research contained comprehensive client and treatment measurement in a sample of 99 programs for an estimated 10,000 adult clients. The complementary study in a sample of 37 programs for 3,400 adolescent clients adapted and applied the DATOS research framework to focus on the issues critical for the young drug abusers early in their treatment

careers (35). Until DATOS findings became available, much of our current knowledge about effectiveness of the broad range of community-based program clients, treatments, and their relationship to outcomes was based on TOPS and a limited number of other individual program studies.

The previous clinical epidemiologic study of drug abuse treatment, TOPS, assessed client characteristics, treatment, and outcomes for 10,000 clients (36) in 40 methadone, residential, and outpatient drug-free programs. Although less comprehensive than DATOS, TOPS has resulted in a substantial body of important knowledge about drug abuse treatment and treatment effectiveness. Major findings from TOPS are reported in the book-length manuscript (37) that considers the substantive findings of TOPS within an explicit policy and clinical context. These findings were updated and replicated with those in the DATOS studies.

Characteristics of Clients in Different Types of Treatment

The client populations of outpatient methadone, residential, and outpatient drug-free programs participating in TOPS in 1979–1981 had many common features, but differed on many sociodemographic and background characteristics (38). Although high percentages of the clients in each modality had similar characteristics (i.e., young adult males were the predominant type of client), large numbers of clients in each modality also had special needs. Thirty percent of clients, for example, were women, 25% of residential and outpatient drug-free clients were younger than 21 years of age, and large numbers were members of racial and ethnic minorities. Similar ethnic differences were found in DATOS programs in 1991–1993, but clients were older and more likely to be female (37). These special populations suggest the need for targeted treatment services to provide effective treatment and to retain such groups in treatment for a significant length of time.

The analyses briefly described in the following paragraphs emphasize the need to consider client characteristics carefully, especially drug-use patterns, extent of impairment, and experience with treatment and criminal justice systems, in the assessment of outcomes across modalities and in studies examining matching of clients to treatment. What type of treatment works best for a particular kind of client is still an unanswered question. The range of modalities and types of programs available may be part of the reason for the success of drug abuse treatment. The opportunity for a client or a referral source to choose may lead to an appropriate match of client and type of treatment. The high rates of self-referrals to methadone and criminal justice referrals to residential and outpatient drug-free treatment (3 in 10 in TOPS and 4 in 10 in DATOS) suggest differences in client motivations for seeking treatment and, consequently, differences in retention, services received, and outcomes (39).

Drug Use Patterns

Drug use by treatment clients frequently is described in terms of the major drug of abuse upon entering treatment. However, the exclusive use of the traditional primary drug of abuse diagnosis or a focus on a particular drug such as heroin or cocaine obscures the extensive nature of abuse of multiple drugs by clients entering treatment in 1979–1981 (39). Some index or typology is needed to better describe and categorize the complex patterns of use by clients. These patterns need to capture lifetime pretreatment and posttreatment use.

One approach developed for clients entering the TOPS programs was a hierarchical seven-category drug-use pattern summarizing the nature of drug use. The patterns are heroin/other narcotics, heroin, other narcotics, multiple nonnarcotics, single nonnarcotics, alcohol/marihuana, and minimal drug use. The categories were based on an extensive examination of the patterns of use of 20 drugs (including alcohol) combining statistical cluster analysis and clinical judgment. The procedures used to develop various typologic and quantitative measures of overall severity of drug use are described in Hubbard et al. (40) and Bray et al. (41).

The drug-abuse pattern index used for TOPS reveals the differential concentration of types of drug abusers across the major modalities. Methadone clients were primarily (52%) traditional heroin users who used only cocaine, marihuana, and alcohol in addition to heroin. However, 1 in 5 methadone clients used heroin and other narcotics, as well as a variety of nonnarcotic drugs. The remaining quarter of methadone clients were classified as former daily users who had histories of regular use but did not use heroin weekly or daily in the year before treatment. Residential clients were distributed more evenly among the patterns, and the majority of outpatient drug-free clients were alcohol and/or marihuana users (36%) or single nonnarcotics users (22%).

The seven-category drug-use pattern captures the complex multiple patterns of drug use of clients entering drug-abuse treatment in TOPS and may be used as one indicator of multiple drug use. However, this index needs to be reevaluated as a descriptor of drug-abuse patterns, particularly in light of the increased use of cocaine in the 1980s. One advantage of the hierarchical typologic approach is its flexibility for emphasizing the importance of specific drugs. For example, the seven-category pattern emphasizes heroin use because of its prominence in the 1970s. For the 1990s, in DATOS, cocaine was used to create an alternate hierarchical typology. Two thirds of long-term residential and 40% of methadone and outpatient drug-free program participants used cocaine at least once a week. Generally, this cocaine use was combined with marihuana

or alcohol. Use of other nonnarcotic drugs was much lower in 1991–1993 than in 1979–1981 (37). Lifetime patterns of drug dependence in addition to current use patterns were related to poorer outcomes (42).

Impairment

A critical issue in evaluation of effectiveness of treatment is the severity of impairment of clients. Work with the Addiction Severity Index (ASI) and assessment of the extent of alcohol and other drug-dependent and psychiatric comorbidities of clients suggest different expectations for clients with more- or less-severe impairments. Although more limited in-depth and clinical expertise is available in multiprogram studies than in clinically based research studies, the former have included some key indicators of impairment. The TOPS data set was one of nine data sets used by a consortium of researchers (43) to examine the drug-dependence syndrome (DDS) concept (44). The goals were to determine the DDS patterning in clinic samples of opioid- and alcohol-dependent persons, the generalizability of DDS to diverse cultural settings, the relation of DDS to certain antecedent and concurrent mediating variables, and the value of DDS as a predictor of treatment outcome. The results indicated that (a) almost all of the provisional DDS elements can be measured reliably in samples of alcoholics and opioid users (45–47); (b) summary measures of alcohol dependence before treatment predict reinstatement of alcohol dependence among relapsed alcoholics following a period of posttreatment abstinence (43); and (c) summary measures of drug dependence do not consistently predict reinstatement among opioid users (43).

Psychiatric impairment was a major interest at the inception of TOPS in 1975, but assessment instruments appropriate for use in multiprogram studies were not available when the TOPS instruments were designed. However, a brief hierarchy of indicators of depression was included to provide basic data on depressive and suicidal symptoms (48). Depression indicators were reported very commonly by clients entering drug-abuse treatment programs (49,50). Overall, approximately 60% of TOPS clients reported at least one item of a three-item scale at intake; nearly 75% of women younger than 21 years of age reported one or more depression indicators. A history of mental health treatment was predictive of depressive symptoms; however, prior drug-abuse treatment was unrelated to signs of depression. Clients who used multiple nonnarcotics weekly or daily were more likely to report signs of depression than were clients in other drug-abuse categories.

The residential clients were significantly more likely to report multiple use of drugs, more drug-related problems, suicidal thoughts and attempts, heavy drinking, predatory crimes, and less full-time employment than were methadone clients with similar backgrounds and demographic characteristics. Outpatient drug-free clients were more likely than similar methadone clients to report drug-related problems, suicidal thoughts or attempts, predatory crimes, and heavy drinking, but were less likely than comparable residential clients to use multiple drugs. Those results demonstrate that each modality does serve very different and important segments of the drug-abusing population. In DATOS, prevalence rates of the American Psychiatric Association's *Diagnostic and Statistical Manual of Mental Disorders,* 3rd ed., revised (*DSM–III–R*) antisocial personality and other comorbid disorders could be assessed with modules for substance dependence and for antisocial personality, depressive, and anxiety disorders from the Composite International Diagnostic Interview and the Diagnostic Interview Schedule (51). Prevalence rates were 39.3% antisocial personality and 13.9% lifetime Axis I disorders. These rates differed by drug-use pattern, age, gender, and race/ethnicity. Clients dependent on heroin, cocaine, and alcohol had higher rates of disorders than did clients dependent on only a single drug or on alcohol. For adolescents, psychiatric diagnoses were measured using modules from the Diagnostic Interview Schedule for Children. Among adolescents in DATOS, conduct disorder was the most common diagnosis (57%). While a third of adolescents reported suicidal thoughts or attempts, depression was diagnosed for less than 10% of the sample (52). Comorbid adolescents had a likelihood of poorer posttreatment outcomes (53).

Treatment Experience and Criminal Justice Involvement

Detailed data on number of admissions and on weeks of treatment obtained in TOPS (54) and DATOS (55) were used to describe the drug-abuse treatment career and to model the effects of the career on treatment outcomes. Drug-abuse treatment is a recurrent phenomenon in the lives of drug abusers. Other results indicate that the duration of regular drug use and the number of prior treatment episodes are important indicators of the effectiveness of any single treatment episode; those with lengthy drug abuse or drug treatment histories have poorer prognoses. On average, clients began regular drug use at age 16 years and entered drug-abuse treatment for the first time at age 24 years. They averaged five treatment admissions and 70 weeks in treatment during their treatment careers. Most have been in several modalities, implying changes during the life span in the nature and severity of drug abuse. About 1 in 5 had also been in alcohol treatment, and 1 in 4 in mental health treatment during their lives. Approximately 40% returned to treatment in the year after the TOPS episode. The time between treatment episodes averaged about 13 weeks. There was considerably more diversity in treatment histories in the DATOS sample and the average age of first admission was later (age 30 years) (55). A comparison of clients not previously admitted with treatment experi-

enced clients showed more problems and poorer outcomes (56). Basic analyses of the contributions of numbers of admissions or total weeks in treatment need to be developed further to investigate the effects of treatment experience. More refined assessment and analysis of patterns of treatment history should help determine the effects of treatment career on outcomes.

The results of the analyses of the treatment–criminal justice system link (57,58) support the basic belief that criminal justice clients do as well as or better than other clients in drug abuse treatment. Treatment Alternatives to Street Crimes (TASC) programs and other formal or informal criminal justice system mechanisms appear to refer individuals who had not been treated previously and many who were not yet heavily involved in drug use. Criminal justice system involvement also helps retain clients in treatment. The estimated 6 to 7 additional weeks of retention for TASC referrals provided programs with considerably more time for rehabilitation efforts (59). For adolescents in DATOS criminal justice supervised clients were more likely to have improved outcomes (60). There also seemed to be more substantial changes in behavior during treatment for criminal justice clients.

One major finding in both TOPS and DATOS research is that few clients referred from the criminal justice system entered outpatient methadone programs (37,57). The reasons for the low numbers in methadone programs need to be explored. There appear to be many heroin addicts in the criminal justice system who could benefit from methadone treatment to reduce their criminal behavior. A second finding is that criminal justice system clients in outpatient drug-free programs received fewer services than did other clients in the same program. Although criminal justice system clients reported fewer drug-related problems than did clients with no legal involvement, they still reported a wide array of problems. The reasons for differential services were unclear.

Treatment Programs

Drug-abuse treatment programs vary in the nature and intensity of treatment services provided, types of therapists and therapies provided, average length of stay, and inclusion of aftercare (61). The limited detailed research on the treatment process (62–64) suggests that the nature and intensity of treatment services are important determinants of treatment outcome. A description of variation in the nature of treatment across treatment settings can provide useful information about current drug-abuse treatment. In addition, information about aspects of the course of treatment, together with information about treatment outcomes, can help identify the most effective types of treatment. A particular concern is how the treatment received in traditional treatment modalities compares with the treatments in new chemical-dependency programs that treat drug abuse as well as alcohol abuse.

The study of the treatment process (62) in TOPS programs focused on the structure, nature, duration, and intensity of drug-abuse treatment. Descriptions of aspects of the treatment process were developed from client self-reports of treatment service needs, services received, and satisfaction, combined with abstractions of clinical/medical records and descriptions of programs by counselors and directors. The characteristics of TOPS clinics were compared with those in the National Drug and Alcohol Treatment Utilization Survey. TOPS clinics were found to be larger and more urban than the national norms for each modality. In 1980, the outpatient methadone and outpatient drug-free treatment programs had budgets per client of approximately $2,000 per year. Therapeutic communities had an average expenditure of $6,135 per bed. TOPS clinics appeared to reflect the continued national trend toward employing fewer ex-addicts and more counselors with advanced degrees (master's degrees and above). The overall philosophy of the clinic directors was that abstinence was an appropriate goal.

The number of services (medical, psychological, family, legal, educational, vocational, and financial) available during the years 1979–1981 varied. Fewer services appeared to be available in the later years of the study. The proportion of clients receiving family, educational, and vocational services decreased noticeably in residential treatment programs during the 3-year period. During this same period, client demand for services increased. However, similar proportions of treatment clients continued to receive services during the study period. Fewer received aftercare services in 1981 than in 1979. In outpatient drug-free program clinical/medical records, mention of aftercare services decreased from 26% in 1979 to 5% in 1981.

Findings from DATOS document a further decline in the resources available for drug-abuse treatment and the services being provided to clients in community-based drug-abuse treatment programs (65). In DATOS, the estimated annual costs of a year of outpatient treatment were $3,285 and for long-term residential treatment, $26,280. These costs in 1980 dollars show a decline in resources (66). A marked decrease over the intervening decade in the number and variety of services to clients was also reported. There was also a large increase in self-reported unmet service needs in both DATOS adult and adolescent samples (67). Clients reported having received at least some sessions of drug abuse counseling during treatment and the level of satisfaction with treatment and services was generally high across modalities, although drug-abuse counseling alone did not address their wider ranging service needs. An analysis of service clusters in adolescent programs indicated very different approaches to treatment. However, none of the clusters provided the full array of comprehensive services needed by adolescents (68). Methadone had the lowest level of drug abuse counseling and services/programs among the four modalities studied.

Programs in TOPS appeared to focus on the client's primary drug of abuse rather than addressing the client's multiple-drug use, drug-related problems, and social and economic functioning. Programs in DATOS having considerably fewer resources provided an even more restricted range of services. For heroin abusers, low-dose methadone (69% of admissions initially were treated with less than 30 mg oral methadone daily) was the most common pattern of methadone treatment in the programs participating in TOPS. Forty percent of clients in methadone treatment for at least 3 months received 30 mg of methadone or less daily; 26% received more than 50 mg. In DATOS, all participating programs reported higher methadone doses. Take-home privileges were common, but policies determining the qualification for the privilege and the number of doses varied greatly among the methadone treatment programs (69).

Treatment Outcomes

Many studies demonstrate that community-based methadone, residential, and outpatient drug-free treatment helped reduce the drug dependence of clients entering treatment in the early 1970s (70–72).

In TOPS, multiple measures of treatment outcome have been necessary to describe changes in the client's ability to function in society after treatment. The duration of abstinence, the predictors of relapse, the nature of posttreatment drug-use patterns, the reinstatement of dependence, and treatment reentry are central indicators of the impact of treatment. Severity of medical, social, and psychological problems directly related to drug use, as well as other indicators of functioning, such as alcohol use, employment, family stability, health, and psychological well-being, are also important evaluation measures considered. Extensive descriptive and multivariate analyses of posttreatment drug use indicators (73), depression (49), and criminal behavior (61) were conducted using the TOPS and DATOS data. In general, clients remaining in treatment for at least 3 months have more positive posttreatment outcomes (74), but the major changes in behavior are seen only for those who stay in treatment for more than 12 months (38). These findings were replicated in other national studies, such as the National Treatment Improvement Evaluation Study (NTIES) conducted from 1993 to 1995 with a sample of 6,593 clients in 78 treatment units (75), as well as studies in individual states, such as California (76). Combined with results from other research, the findings described in this section provide comprehensive and convincing evidence that long-term treatment is effective. Several studies, however, including experiments with random assignment (77) and evaluation of abrupt closures of methadone programs (78), provide evidence that the programs do produce effects independent of client motivation to remain in treatment. Furthermore, the multivariate analyses and the research design used in the author's study carefully considered alternative assumptions about measurement validity and took into account potential indicators of client motivation, including previous treatment and reasons for entering treatment (37).

Analyses of the TOPS data show that the posttreatment rate of daily heroin, cocaine, and psychotherapeutic drug use of clients who spent at least 3 months in treatment was half the pretreatment rate. The posttreatment rates of weekly or more frequent use for clients who stayed in treatment for at least 3 months were 10% to 15% lower than the rates for short-term clients. Despite these major reductions in rates of use, many clients in each modality reported posttreatment use of at least one drug other than marihuana or alcohol: 40% of methadone, 30% of residential, and 20% of outpatient drug-free clients who stayed in treatment for at least 3 months reported weekly or daily use after treatment. Multivariate log linear regression analyses were conducted to investigate the effects of client characteristics and treatment factors on treatment outcomes (73). Demographic factors (sex, age, race), treatment history, source of referral, and pretreatment drug-use patterns were included as control variables. Three regression analyses (one for each modality) were used to describe the effect of different categories of time in treatment on the odds of being a weekly or more frequent drug user during the year after treatment. The results showed that time spent in treatment was among the most important predictors of most treatment outcomes. Stays of 1 year or more in residential or methadone treatment, or continuing methadone maintenance, produced significant decreases in the odds of using heroin in the followup period.

TOPS clients also reported a substantial decrease in depression indicators during the years after treatment (49,50). Multivariate analysis using the logistic regression procedure revealed that, aside from pretreatment depression indicators, very few factors were significant predictors of posttreatment suicidal thoughts or attempts.

Analyses of the effects of treatment on criminal behavior have focused on reduction in predatory crime and costs associated with crime. Although treatment itself reduces predatory crime (37), those referred by the criminal justice system do not show a greater reduction in predatory illegal acts after treatment than do those who were not involved with the criminal justice system (57). The assessment of the benefit:cost ratio indicates that substantial benefits in reduction of crime-related costs are obtained regardless of the measures used or the time period for which benefits are calculated (79).

DATOS also collected 1-year followup outcomes for 2,966 clients in outpatient methadone, long-term residential, outpatient drug-free, and short-term inpatient programs in 1991–1993. Long-term residential, short-term inpatient, and outpatient drug-free clients reported 50% less weekly or daily cocaine use in the followup year than in the preadmission year. Reductions were greater (p < .01) for clients treated for 3 months or more. Clients still in the outpatient methadone program reported less weekly or daily heroin use than clients who left the outpatient methadone program. Multivariate analysis confirmed that 6 months or more in the outpatient drug-free and long-term residential programs and enrollment in the outpatient methadone program were associated with the reductions. Reductions of 50% in illegal activity and 10% increases in full-time employment for long-term residential program clients were related (p < .01) to treatment stays of 6 months or longer. The results replicated findings from TOPS for heroin use in the outpatient methadone program, and illegal activity and employment for the long-term residential program, but not for illegal activity in the outpatient methadone and outpatient drug-free programs (80).

A separate analysis of 1,605 cocaine-dependent patients found that 23.5% reported weekly cocaine use in the year following treatment, compared to 73.1% in the year before admission. Higher severity of patient problems at program intake and shorter stays in treatment (<90 days) were related to higher cocaine relapse rates (81).

A stratified followup sample including 1,393 of the same individuals in the 1-year followup sample was followed for 5 years. Reductions in prevalence of cocaine use in the year after treatment (compared to the preadmission year) by patients were associated with longer treatment durations (particularly 6 months or more in the long-term residential and outpatient drug-free programs). In addition, reductions in illegal activity and increases in full-time employment were related to treatment stays of 6 months or longer for patients in the long-term residential program. The DATOS results from the 1-year and 5-year posttreatment followup combined suggest the stability of outcomes of substance-abuse treatment (82).

Similar analyses were conducted for the 708 subjects who met *DSM–III–R* criteria for cocaine dependence when admitted in 1991–1993. Self-reported cocaine use showed high overall agreement with urine (79% agreement) and hair (80% agreement) toxicology analyses. Weekly cocaine use was reported by 25% of the sample in the fifth year of followup, slightly higher than the 21% for the first year after treatment. Illegal activity declined from 40% before intake to 25% in year 5 (up slightly from 16% in year 1) (83).

For adolescent clients, significant before-to-after treatment reductions were found in weekly or more frequent marihuana use, heavy drinking, use of other illicit drugs, criminal activities, and arrests. Better psychological adjustment in terms of reduced suicidal thoughts and hostility and increased self-esteem, better school attendance, and average or better-than-average grades after treatment (as compared with the year before) were also reported. As with adults, longer time in treatment (greater than 90 days in long-term residential and outpatient drug-free programs, and 21 days in short-term inpatient programs) was significantly related to lower drug use and lower arrest rates following treatment (84).

Conceptual models (85) and recent empiric findings (71,86) stress the key role of posttreatment experiences in long-term recovery. Procedures for reducing relapse (87) and standard aftercare protocols have been developed for alcohol treatment (21,45). DARP (71) analyses reveal that the positive effect of longer retention in a particular program diminishes over time. Treatment, employment, and other behaviors co-occurring with outcomes during a given year are hypothesized to be more important factors than prior treatment.

Benefit:Cost Studies and Cost-Effectiveness

Benefit:cost studies of drug-abuse treatment are needed to meet the increasing concerns about cost containment in both the public and private sectors. Most current benefit:cost studies are limited to the cost-effectiveness of alcohol-abuse treatment and merely calculate the difference between treatment costs and the savings in health care expenditures following treatment (14,88). To date, no study has rigorously assessed all economic benefits from drug-abuse treatment. The assessment of the crime reduction effects of drug-abuse treatment by Harwood and colleagues (79) is the first step in building a benefit:cost framework. That assessment used information on the societal costs of crime and drug treatment to estimate the economic benefits of drug-abuse treatment.

The economic costs imposed by drug abusers' criminal activities before, during, and after admission to residential, outpatient methadone, and outpatient drug-free programs were calculated in a secondary analysis of TOPS data. Using the framework from the Harwood social cost study (79), values were calculated for costs to victims, costs to the criminal justice system, and criminal career/productivity losses. Two alternative summary cost measures were defined: economic costs to society and economic costs to law-abiding citizens. The analysis demonstrated that drug-abuse treatment significantly reduced the economic costs associated with criminal activity of drug abusers, and treatment produced a positive benefit:cost ratio within the first year after completing treatment, regardless of the cost measures employed. A replication of this method in a study of California programs in 1992 indicated an overall return of $7 for each dollar invested, and savings of $1.5 billion, mostly as a consequence of crime reduction (76). Using DATOS data for adult clients dependent on cocaine, the positive benefit:cost ratios for crime costs alone were replicated in outpatient drug-free and long-term residential programs (66).

QUESTIONS

New research must build upon and expand the knowledge generated by previous research on treatment effectiveness and ongoing clinic-based research programs. We need to expand our substantive knowledge about drug-abuse treat-

ment effectiveness and refine theory about treatment itself, as well as about recovery and relapse. National prospective studies, such as the DARP study conducted on clients entering treatment during the late 1960s and early 1970s (29,70) and the TOPS studies conducted with clients entering drug-abuse treatment between 1979 and 1981 (38,39), provide rich databases that have been used to answer many of the basic questions about treatment effectiveness. These answers guided subsequent research, such as DATOS and NTIES. This also set the stage and framework for multisite effectiveness trials such as the National Institute on Drug Abuse's (NIDA) Clinical Trial Network.

Several events, however, necessitate broader perspectives in studies of drug-abuse treatment and treatment effectiveness. Major changes occurred in the nation's drug-abusing population and treatment system in the 1980s and 1990s, and continue to occur into the new century. New research questions have arisen because of these changes and because of the lessons learned from prior research. The prior research, however, has several inherent limitations. Finally, the acquired immune deficiency syndrome (AIDS) crisis has intensified interest in drug-abuse treatment as a strategy to reduce exposure to the cause of AIDS, the human immunodeficiency virus (HIV). It is therefore necessary to update information to reexamine what we have learned about treatment effectiveness and to augment the types of available data to examine new issues about the nature, effectiveness, and costs of current treatment approaches.

Changes in Treatment Clients and the Treatment System

Although many attempts have been made to control drug abuse during the past century, the problem has persisted and the nature and extent of abuse has changed dramatically during the past decade. Opioid dependence has persisted for the past century (3,89–92) and accounted for two-thirds of the estimated $60 billion social cost of drug abuse in 1980 (93). Extensive use of multiple drugs by young adults in the general population (94), as well as by drug abusers entering treatment (40), was common in the 1980s. By 1980, many of those for whom heroin was the primary drug of abuse were using a greater variety of drugs (40,95). Data from the National Household Survey on Drug Abuse show that the proportion of young adults (18 to 25 years of age) who had used marihuana increased from 48% in 1972 to 64% in 1982. Cocaine use tripled, and nonmedical use of stimulants, sedatives, and tranquilizers doubled (96). However, by 1985, the percentage of young adults who had used marihuana had decreased slightly, to 60%, and the prevalence of cocaine use was 25% (97). Clients entering treatment in the new century likely will reflect the trend in multiple-drug use in the general population, and will have a greater variety of problems and comorbidities (39,74,98), particularly psychiatric (99), than did drug-abuse clients in the 1970s and the 1990s.

The TOPS and DATOS data confirmed the impression that drug use patterns and problems of clients coming into community-based drug abuse treatment changed dramatically during the 1970s (39) and the 1990s (37). The TOPS clients entering treatment between 1979 and 1981 were much more likely to use multiple drugs than were DARP clients entering treatment between 1969 and 1973. Whereas the drug-use pattern of about half of DARP methadone clients was described as "daily opioid use only," only 1 in 5 TOPS methadone clients reported this use pattern. Daily opioid use was much more common for DARP residential (63%) and outpatient drug-free (35%) clients than for TOPS residential (30%) and outpatient drug-free (10%) clients. In TOPS, use of nonopioids was reported much more frequently in all modalities than in DARP and was the modal pattern for residential and outpatient drug-free clients. In DATOS, cocaine became the primary drug of interest.

The far-reaching changes in the drug-abuse treatment system since studies of the DARP and TOPS admission cohorts require reconsideration of these studies. The DARP and TOPS samples were composed primarily of publicly funded outpatient methadone, residential, and outpatient drug-free programs. Privately funded drug-abuse programs increased (99) during the 1980s, and decreased in the 1990s, in part because concerns about costs and the introduction of managed care and cost containment were not included in DARP or TOPS. The role of state funding and oversight has not been reexamined (100). The distinction between publicly funded (state or local) and private (self-pay or insurance) treatment has become blurred. The treatment of many clients in traditional "public" treatment modalities is not supported by public funds. Fee-for-service is now more common (101), and long waiting lists for publicly funded treatment slots are reported in many areas.

Based on an assessment of the outpatient treatment system, some researchers hypothesize that changes in the drug-abuse treatment environment will affect the way services are delivered and ultimately may influence treatment efficiency and effectiveness (102,103). With the increase in concern about cost containment there is greater concern for the cost-effectiveness of publicly delivered services. Cost issues were raised when Diagnostic Related Group costs for an episode of alcohol- and drug-abuse treatment were proposed in the Medicare system. It is assumed that the example set by Medicare may be followed by other public programs and private insurance companies. Although longer stays are related to more successful outcomes (26,38,70), cost constraints and public and client preference for short-term chemical dependency and methadone detoxification programs may pressure traditional programs to consider shorter treatment and more effective aftercare and relapse prevention efforts in place

of long-term retention (87). These changes in the drug-abuse treatment population and in treatment itself suggest that existing information may no longer be adequate to describe treatment. Although the three major modalities remain, treatment is now provided in a broader range of settings to a more diverse clientele. DATOS will provide important new information about the nature of drug abuse, the treatment system, and treatment effectiveness.

New Research Questions

Knowledge is cumulative and new questions continue to be asked about drug treatment effectiveness. These include questions about the role of psychiatric severity and depression in treatment outcomes; the effectiveness of the components of drug-abuse treatment such as psychological services, family therapy, and aftercare; the process of client change during and after treatment; the role of posttreatment experiences in relapse and recovery; how clients and programs can best be matched to improve the effectiveness of treatment; the predictive role of drug-use histories and dependence; and the chronicity of drug-treatment episodes in the effectiveness of specific treatment episodes. Furthermore, as discussed more fully later, the potential effect of drug-abuse treatment on the AIDS epidemic continues to receive increased attention. These questions continue to require investigation over a broad array of program types and across multiple sites.

Although the overall effectiveness of the major modalities has been examined in a number of studies, including DARP, TOPS, DATOS, and NTIES, the effectiveness of certain components of treatment—such as counseling and other types of services or of aftercare—has not been examined in detail. In recent years the perception of the need to evaluate the impact of treatment components has grown, but the complexity of the client process of change and the treatment factors involved pose many great challenges. Several studies have examined the role of relapse prevention and aftercare services in treatment outcome (87,104), cognitive factors have received more attention in research in therapeutic communities (105,106), and the TOPS/DATOS researchers have investigated the role of the number and intensity of treatment services in treatment outcomes (61). The TOPS research, for instance, suggests that more positive treatment outcomes result from more intense services and that service intensity may compensate for the trend toward shorter stays in treatment. Detailed analysis in DATOS, however, identified posttreatment self-help group participation as a major correlate of outcomes (107).

Coupled with these concerns about what occurs during treatment is a greater recognition that posttreatment experiences, such as social support and life events, can also significantly influence treatment outcomes. Conceptual models (85) and recent empiric findings (22,23,82,83,75,108) stress the role of posttreatment experiences in long-term recovery. As with treatment components, however, the study of the impact of posttreatment factors has received little attention because of the complexity of the issues involved. Posttreatment experiences, such as social support and life events, need to be developed and evaluated based on models of posttreatment recovery and relapse.

Research literature has found that some types of treatment are more effective for some types of client than for other types (109,110), and that problem severity may require attention to matching of clients and therapists (111). Yet, the major research on matching failed to detect any interaction effect, perhaps because of the complex statistical and methodological issues involved (22,23). However, several authors have developed models of client–treatment matching and reviewed the conceptual and methodological issues (109,112). The careful measurement of both clients and treatments should provide data that better inform researchers and clinicians about key factors to consider in controlled clinical studies such as Project MATCH (Matching Alcoholism Treatments to Client Heterogeneity) (21) and the ongoing Clinical Trial Network (113).

Potential of Drug Abuse Treatment in the AIDS Epidemic

Because of the central role of intravenous drug use in the spread of HIV infection, drug-abuse treatment has been mentioned increasingly as an effective strategy. Drug-abuse treatment not only can reduce intravenous drug use but, through its impact on reducing the number of drug users per se, it can reduce the transmission of HIV that is facilitated by the weakened immune systems of drug abusers (10,73). Furthermore, the treatment program provides a most appropriate site for educational messages on the prevention of HIV transmission. The National Commission on AIDS recommended doubling treatment capacity (114). Yet, few data are available to suggest where and how these resources can be directed most effectively. Reports of intravenous cocaine use by large numbers of abusers without a history of heroin use are a new and troubling phenomenon. Traditional publicly funded programs for intravenous drug abusers did not reduce cocaine use effectively (73). Treatment effectiveness for individuals entering programs because they fear AIDS or greater criminal sanctions (115) should continue to be carefully examined. The results of DATOS show that risk behaviors are reduced after treatment for both adolescents (116) and adults (117), but an association with treatment retention was not clear.

Broadened Economic Perspectives

The major types of publicly funded drug-abuse treatment are effective, and positive benefit:cost ratios are obtained for outpatient methadone, long-term residential, and outpatient drug-free modalities. Such results justify the overall investment in treatment, but provide little insight into ways to improve effectiveness and increase benefit:cost ratios.

If the investment in treatment is to produce a maximum return and guide payment justification for longer or more intense services, multiple approaches and improvements must be considered in resource allocation. Broader recruitment, more comprehensive assessment, improved services, matching of clients with services, increased retention, and an expanded continuum of care must be considered in terms of their contribution to outcomes. New frameworks need to include consideration of several factors:

1. Stage in the treatment career of clients
2. Components of treatment structure and process
3. Typology of client impairment
4. Complex patterns of alcohol and drug abuse

Such disaggregation of the entity of "treatment" and its appropriate application to clients of different types is essential. The specific elements and client–treatment matches can then be allocated costs and benefits, which should suggest ways to invest prudently new monies for demand reduction.

CLINICAL IMPLICATIONS OF CLIENT DIFFERENCES

Detailed consideration has begun to be given to how elements such as client characteristics and specific aspects of treatment affect treatment success (118) and to how client characteristics may interact with treatment type to affect treatment success (112,119). Client characteristics are important because they define treatment populations across treatment types and can contribute to differential treatment effectiveness. Description of pretreatment behaviors provides the baseline against which treatment effectiveness may be assessed. Treatment needs and prospects for successful outcomes differ by basic demographic characteristics such as gender (120), age (121,122), and ethnicity (123,124). Many aspects of a client's past and current treatment experience, such as prior treatment (38,54,108), the source of referral (57–59), method of paying for treatment (101), and sensitivity to client needs (125–127), could influence the course and outcome of a particular treatment episode. Thus, assessment of the nature of client characteristics is essential for accounting for the level of effectiveness of drug abuse treatment for any particular client. Different types of clients benefit differentially from the treatment experience. Differences in the types of clients entering a particular type of treatment program are also critical to the design, implementation, and outcome of the regimen. The major types of programs have been explicitly and implicitly designed to deal with specific types of drug abusers. Outpatient methadone programs admit only clients with documented histories of opioid addiction. Although residential and outpatient drug-free programs also serve opioid addicts, the use patterns of their clientele are more diverse (39). The broad-based orientation of residential treatment programs (128) attracts clients with a wide range of drug-use patterns, often coupled with psychological disturbance and social dysfunction. Consequently, knowledge about the nature of client populations across modalities, including client characteristics, psychiatric severity, and social and economic functioning, is essential for planning purposes.

Impairment

Indicators of both drug use patterns and impairment levels across an array of areas of function must be developed. The various components of each concept (i.e., types of drugs or types of impairment) must be considered as well as overall summary measures. For such complex concepts, both qualitative and typologic indices will be useful.

A major issue that emerged during the 1980s concerns the impact of impairment, particularly psychopathology, on treatment outcomes. Although the DARP study concluded that there were few differences in overall treatment outcomes for opioid abusers across treatment modalities, more recent work by McLellan and his colleagues suggests that psychological problems significantly detract from the treatment process (129,130). Jaffe (99) argues that opioid abusers with severe psychological problems do poorly in the confrontational context of a therapeutic community but may function better in a methadone program. On the other hand, Woody et al. (131) found that methadone clients with antisocial personality and depression showed substantial improvement on multiple outcomes. A similar finding was reported for adolescents (132). Data to examine this issue are largely unavailable outside programs closely linked with clinical research centers. The DATOS analysis of outcomes for cocaine abusers also found that severity of problems was related to posttreatment cocaine abuse (81).

Serious depression can affect the course of treatment and jeopardize successful outcomes (133,134). The prevalence and course of depressive symptoms among clients in drug-abuse treatment is, therefore, a topic of major concern among analysts of treatment effectiveness (26,49,50,135,136), and treatment requires more careful attention to the multiple problems of clients, particularly psychiatric severity (99).

Drug-Use Patterns

The TOPS and DATOS results (40,41,137) indicate that programs and researchers should move beyond the traditional diagnosis of primary drug of abuse or single-drug use to consider patterns of multiple-drug use. Using only basic single-drug measures obscures the extensive nature of multiple abuse, and may lead to similar treatments for clients with very different abuse patterns. In addition to

a primary diagnosis of drug use, many clients entering drug-abuse treatment programs appear to need treatment for alcohol abuse as well. Thus, problems related to alcohol abuse must also be assessed and treated. Programs also should consider how the general treatment regimen will affect multiple drug and alcohol use (138,139). Separate intensive therapies focusing on cocaine, marihuana, and alcohol use for clients with multiple-drug-use patterns may be needed to supplement the basic treatment regimen for the primary drug of abuse. Even in the treatment of primary heroin or cocaine users, the abuse of other drugs, especially marihuana and alcohol, should be assessed and treated. To plan for appropriate treatment, multiple-drug-use patterns and use of particular types of drugs within these multiple-drug-use patterns must be considered.

Treatment Experience

The recognition that drug-abuse treatment admissions—as with drug-abuse episodes—recur, and that improvement may be incremental through a number of treatment episodes (54,108,140,141), argues for closer consideration of the role in treatment outcomes of the client's treatment history. That is, is the client entering treatment for the first time, following a brief period of addiction, or has the client had multiple episodes of treatment? Research from the TOPS and DATOS shows that drug-abuse treatment clients are, in general, repeat clients; more than 40% of clients entering treatment had prior treatment experiences, and more than 30% reentered treatment in the year after leaving the TOPS program. Other analyses of the TOPS and DATOS data (38,142) found that treatment outcomes are related to treatment history; those with no or few prior treatment episodes had more positive treatment outcomes than did those with many such episodes. The integration of this life history perspective with measures of motivation and readiness for treatment (105) can suggest ways to enhance retention, particularly during the key first weeks of treatment. The role of a particular treatment episode in the treatment career or recovery process must be identified. Thus, such an episode need not be an isolated event but part of a continuum of care.

Multidimensional Client Assessment

A variety of serious medical and mental health problems, serious family disruption, and employment problems are closely associated with drug and alcohol abuse, and the severity of these problems also varies across modalities. These "addiction-related" problems are theoretically and clinically important (130). It is generally agreed that assisting clients to cope with these problems should be a major goal of treatment and that, to be successful, treatment must be oriented to a variety of client needs and provide services to meet those needs effectively. Analyses of the TOPS and DATOS data described previously indicate that clients entering each of the modalities had very different patterns of drug-related problems (39,74). There are two basic approaches to assessing problems. The nosologic approach is designed to categorize individuals as to the presence or absence of specific disorders—for example, using standard diagnostic criteria, such as those of the American Psychiatric Association's *Diagnostic and Statistical Manual of Mental Disorders*. The other type of assessment approach is dimensional, rather than categoric. This approach focuses more on symptom severity and the relative importance of different types of problems. For efficiency and cost-effectiveness, the nosologic and dimensional approaches could be combined by using a dimensional instrument as a screening scale to choose individuals for a followup interview by a clinician using an instrument with a nosologic approach.

In addition to psychiatric impairment, various other aspects of impairment that each can have a major influence on the response to treatment and on subsequent outcomes must be considered. Treatment history, criminal involvement, drug dependence, drug-related problems, health status, and employment all must be considered as elements of impairment and can also be considered as descriptors of client types.

The nature and extent of the multiple problems can have important implications for service needs for clients and potential outcomes. McLellan and colleagues developed the ASI for use in a clinical setting to evaluate the severity of problems in seven areas: drug abuse, alcohol abuse, medical, employment/support, family/social, legal, and psychological (130).

The psychological problems or psychiatric subscale of the ASI was found to be the best predictor of treatment outcome across all types of programs, and the appropriate matching of substance abusers with inpatient and outpatient programs was suggested (143). The TOPS interviews designed for field surveys collect similar data on most of the ASI problem areas. As in the ASI studies (130), analyses of the TOPS data indicate that the multiple problems reported by clients are not related.

The results from both TOPS and DATOS suggest that a quantitative composite measure of severity does not effectively summarize the nature and extent of multiple problems. A typology (81) may be a more appropriate and clinically useful method of describing and summarizing multiple problems. These results show that there are many combinations of problems among drug abusers. Multiple problems are most common among residential clients. It should also be noted that within each category of the typology, alcohol abuse accompanies drug abuse for 20% to 40% of the clients.

CLINICAL IMPLICATIONS OF TREATMENT STRUCTURE AND PROCESS

Program administrators, researchers, and policymakers are in general agreement that community-based drug-

abuse treatment "has been instrumental in the rehabilitation of significant numbers of drug-dependent individuals" (24). There is no question that treatment works, but little is known about how and why treatment works. In general, treatment outcomes are not linked with the nature of treatment that clients receive (28). Variables in the diverse approaches that comprise drug-abuse treatment must be better specified and their role in producing positive treatment outcomes better understood for methadone (118,144), residential (128,145), and outpatient treatment (146).

Treatment as currently rendered is a complex, multifaceted process delivered in a variety of contexts and environments to clients undergoing behavioral and cognitive changes at different rates. Thus, general descriptive information alone is insufficient to examine specific hypotheses regarding the nature of the drug-abuse treatment process.

Developing a typology of drug-abuse treatment program structure or descriptions of approaches assumes that there is an agreed-upon definition of treatment, that the dimensions of treatment are identified, and that there is a fair degree of consistency within treatment types. However, there is no consensus on what constitutes nonmedical psychological, mental health, alcohol, or drug "treatments." Similarly, the treatment process is poorly defined. It is useful, however, to regard treatment as a specific set of procedures, approaches, therapies, or services that are designed to achieve certain goals. Treatment process that can be thought of as the steps or the dynamic movement from addiction to recovery is also poorly defined. In the context of drug abuse, this process typically involves changes in one or more areas of a client's life. Simpson and his colleagues developed a treatment engagement model (147) and applied it to DATOS. Motivation was related to participation in treatment for adults and adolescents (148,149). More severe problems, such as hostility in adults and legal involvement for adolescents, interfered with the engagement process (150).

Approach to Assessing Structure and Process

Research from DARP, TOPS, and DATOS provides guidance for future consideration of treatment structure and process. One of the most comprehensive attempts to explore the issue of the interactive relationship of client and program typologies was initiated in the DARP studies. The early development of a treatment typology was based on client bimonthly status reports and program site visits (151). With this approach, it was possible to classify clients' treatment according to the services they received during the "majority" of each period covered by the status report. A second phase of the classification took into account "treatment objectives and rationales, program structure, staffing, and other program aspects within or between treatment categories" (152) that were assumed to be correlated with treatment outcome.

In TOPS, researchers described the overall structure and functioning of the major modalities based on director and counselor surveys (61) and examined the type and number of services received at the client level based on record abstractions and client self-reports. Although the treatment process was not fully elaborated, TOPS examined the relationship among treatment outcomes and treatment services, client characteristics, and the duration of treatment.

Client–Counselor/Service Interaction

Although the DARP, TOPS, and DATOS treatment process studies showed that it is possible to assess the main elements of treatment, drug-abuse treatment has a complex, multifaceted structure, and a dynamic process. To identify and quantify types of services or counseling, the client–counselor/staff interaction must be considered. Both within and across counseling sessions, many services may be provided, none necessarily as an independently structured service. Thus, any quantitative analysis may not be able to capture fully the complete dynamics of treatment. Encouraging findings on the relationship of the psychotherapy process to outcome (153) indicate that some of the key components and processes of drug-abuse treatment can be described. Recent findings on counselor effects by McLellan et al. (62) are further confirmation that research can lead to better understanding of why some types of programs work or some types of clients succeed.

A second general point underscores the importance of systematic evaluation of program, client, and therapist interaction variables. For example, researchers and policymakers often appear to assume that the different types of modalities or environments could serve the total population of individuals with drug-abuse problems equally well (8).

Finding variation among modalities and among clinics of different programs within modalities was not surprising. However, contrary to most expectations, in TOPS (38,61,69) extensive variation was found not only among clinics, but even within units of the same treatment program. This implies that, despite policies and plans at a general administrative level, distinctiveness of the counseling and services within clinics must be taken into account.

PSYCHOTHERAPY PROCESS RESEARCH

Although the modalities of psychotherapy are better defined than those of drug-abuse treatment, the general approach to the study of psychotherapy process can help guide the current research. The research in psychotherapy also has a longer history. Kiesler (154) summarized some of the early work in process research. Greenberg and Pinsof (155) build upon this conceptual and methodological base to develop a more comprehensive assessment of psychotherapeutic process. They cite major emerging trends that will help advance the field:

1. Integration of process and outcome studies
2. Theory of process
3. Involvement of clients
4. Analysis of context, patterns, and change
5. Quality instrumentation to measure process

They believe that the study of treatment process should emphasize a system in addition to an individual perspective. They define process research as the study of interaction between the client and therapist in order to identify the factors contributing to change within and outside of the system.

In addition to conceptual and theoretical advances, new analysis approaches have been recommended that assess the counseling sequence and pattern process (156). These approaches (157) must be consistent with the general model of events listing analysis that has received increased attention in the sociologic literature. The analysis plan for the treatment process study includes consideration of these techniques to link process with outcome. Orlinsky and Howard (153) review a range of variables that must be considered in the assessment of the process and outcome in psychotherapy and a conceptual framework for their interaction. These variables and models can be adapted for drug abuse treatment.

A Conceptual Model for Treatment Process and Structure

A number of researchers have examined elements of drug-abuse treatment and the treatment process at the aggregate program level (151,152,158,159). D'Aunno and Price (103) examined the organizational environment of drug-abuse treatment but include no client-level data on the treatment process. Magura (160) assessed participative decision making by clients in methadone clinics and its effects on process and outcomes. DeLeon (145) outlined the levels of the therapeutic approach as structure, elements, and process. Holland (27,64) included organizational, client, and process variables as predictors of planned duration. Allison et al. (61) focused on service for clients in the programs. Aiken, Losciuto, and colleagues (161) concentrated on the counselor characteristics and the progress of clients in terms of behavioral change, as have McLellan et al. (62). Biase and colleagues (106,162) focus more on the progress of the client through treatment in terms of cognitive development of self-concept. Joe et al. (163,164) conducted secondary analysis of TOPS to examine the process of services received and behaviors during treatment, as did Etheridge et al. (107).

None of these studies fully integrated the many elements of treatment structure and treatment process. A framework is proposed in Figure 52.1, drawn in part from psychotherapy models. This framework suggests that three levels of

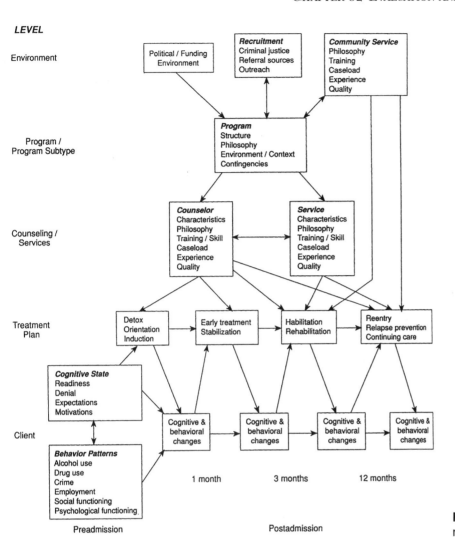

FIG. 52.1. Conceptual model of treatment process.

variables and the factors influencing each level must be considered (165):

1. The program (the administrative structures, policies and procedures, staff:client ratios, staff training, and other objective, clearly identifiable characteristics of the program environment)
2. The counseling and services (availability, nature, and quality)
3. The client (receipt of service and satisfaction with perceived need for services)

At the client level, it is also suggested that the process of individual change during the course of treatment be considered. This dynamic element of treatment process has often been neglected. At the counseling and service level, one should be more interested in functional aspects of different program components, including the more objective features, such as years of training and experience, as well as personal qualities, such as warmth, sensitivity, and empathy. Most programs implicitly or explicitly plan progression through treatment, either as a 12-step model,

a methadone-to-abstinence or methadone-to-maintenance regimen, or stages in a therapeutic community. Research has seldom, if ever, examined the nature and rate of this progression as either a dependent or predictor variable. The indicators of progression can include elements such as:

1. Readiness to progress
2. Relapse potential
3. Behavioral level or pattern of change (i.e., improvement or worsening)
4. Cognitive change (i.e., overcoming denial, commitment to recovery)
5. Changes in social functioning
6. Changes in psychological functioning

A major limitation of past drug-abuse treatment research is a failure to fully examine changes in attitudes, motivation, knowledge, and skills associated with participation in treatment. These alterations include changes in beliefs, attitudes, and knowledge about dependence and recovery, as well as behavioral changes during treatment

(166–168). The application of psychological learning theory to the study of relapse (169) has led to the development of specific treatment techniques designed to prevent relapse and to minimize the effects of brief lapses (170,171). Studies of coping strategies in response to stressful life events and to high-risk situations during the crucial transitional period after the termination of treatment have provided a scientific basis for these new approaches. To fully understand the treatment process, and to link the process with outcome after treatment, we must understand the external factors contributing to client change, as well as to the program and service/counseling-level components.

SUMMARY

During the 1990s outcome and effectiveness of drug-abuse treatment programs continued to be major public concerns. A variety of individual clinical studies, multiprogram evaluations, and research reviews substantiate the effectiveness of drug-abuse treatment in reducing drug use and improving functioning. Further analyses demonstrate that the benefits derived from drug-abuse treatment considerably outweigh the cost of the treatment. Despite these positive conclusions, treatment can and should be improved. Furthermore, effectiveness studies of individual programs and services are required to justify costs.

To identify the areas in which treatment should be supported and can be improved, new conceptual models and empiric studies are needed that focus on client and treatment. By augmenting our understanding of the various domains of client impairment and functioning, the patterns of multiple-drug abuse, and the diverse experiences with treatment and criminal justice systems, it should be possible to develop better treatment plans and services. By increasing our knowledge of treatment structure and process, including program organization and operation, engagement in the recovery process, client–counselor/service interaction, and the dynamics of service delivery and client change, more appropriate and effective treatment programs and components can be designed and implemented.

A new generation of treatment research is being developed for the next century that builds on prior multiprogram and clinically based research. These studies are focusing on improved assessment of clients and more refined measures of treatment. The results of this research should provide the foundation of knowledge to help improve drug abuse treatment into the next decade. This research conducted over three decades of the 1900s can identify the findings that remain constant despite rapidly changing environments. The studies can also identify the ways environment changes may affect outcomes and provide a framework for future research to improve treatment.

REFERENCES

1. Laundergan JC. *Easy does it: alcoholism treatment outcomes: Hazelden and the Minnesota model.* Duluth, MN: Hazelden Foundation, 1982.
2. Cook CCH. The Minnesota model in the management of drug and alcohol dependency: miracle, method, or myth? Part I. The philosophy and the programme. *Br J Addict* 1988;83:625–634.
3. Jaffe JH. The swinging pendulum: the treatment of drug users in America. In: DuPont RL, Goldstein A, O'Donnell J, eds. *Handbook on drug use.* Washington, DC: U.S. Government Printing Office, 1979:3–16.
4. Anglin MD, Hser Y. Treatment of drug abuse. In: Tonry M, Wilson JQ, eds. *Drugs and crime.* Chicago: University of Chicago Press, 1990:393–460.
5. Gerstein DR, Harwood HJ, eds. *Treating drug problems.* Washington, DC: National Academy Press, 1990.
6. Sisk JE, Hatziandren EJ, Hughes R. *The effectiveness of drug abuse treatment: implication for controlling AIDS/HIV infection.* Washington DC: Office of Technology Assessment, 1990.
7. Fuller RK, Branchey L, Brightwell DR, et al. Disulfiram treatment of alcoholism. *JAMA* 1986;245:1449–1455.
8. Bale RN, Van Stone WW, Kuldau JM, et al. Therapeutic communities vs. methadone maintenance. *Arch Gen Psychiatry* 1980;37:179–193.
9. Committee for the Study and Treatment and Rehabilitation Services for Alcoholism and Alcohol Abuse. *Broadening the base of treatment for alcohol problems.* Washington, DC: National Academy of Science, 1990.
10. Hubbard RL, Des Jarlais DC. Alcohol and drug abuse. In: Holland EE, Petels R, Knox G, eds. *Oxford textbook of public health,* vol. 3, 2nd ed. London: Oxford University Press, 1991.
11. Landry MJ. *Overview of addiction treatment effectiveness.* Rockville, MD: Substance Abuse and Mental Health Administration, 1996.
12. Armor DJ, Polich JM, Stambul HB. *Alcoholism and treatment.* New York: Wiley, 1978.
13. Polich JM, Armor DJ, Braiker HB. *The course of alcoholism: four years after treatment.* New York: Wiley, 1981.
14. Holder HD, Blose JO. Alcoholism treatment and total health care utilization and costs: a four-year longitudinal analysis of federal employees. *JAMA* 1986;256:1456–1460.
15. Institute of Medicine, Committee to Identify Research Effectiveness in the Prevention and Treatment of Alcohol Related Problems. *Prevention and treatment of alcohol problems.* Washington, DC: National Academy Press, 1989.
16. Hubbard RL, Anderson J. *A followup study of individuals receiving alcoholism treatment.* Research Triangle Park, NC: Research Triangle Institute, 1988.
17. Hoffmann N, Harrison P. *A 2-year followup of inpatient outpatient treatment.* St. Paul, MN: Chemical Abuse Treatment Outcome Registry, 1987.
18. Saxe L, Dougherty D, Esty K, et al. *Health technology case study 22: the effectiveness and costs of alcoholism treatment.* Washington, DC: Office of Technology Assessment, 1983.
19. Annis HM. Is inpatient rehabilitation of the alcoholic cost effective? Con position. *Adv Alcohol Subst Abuse* 1986;5:175–190.
20. Miller WR, Hester RK. Inpatient alcoholism treatment: who benefits? *Am Psychol* 1986;41:794–805.
21. Project MATCH Research Group. Project MATCH: rationale and methods

for a multisite clinical trial matching patients to alcoholism treatment. *Alcohol Clin Exp Res* 1993;17:1130–1145.

22. Project MATCH Research Group. Matching alcoholism treatments to client heterogeneity: Project MATCH posttreatment drinking outcomes. *J Stud Alcohol* 1997;58:7–29.

23. Project MATCH Research Group. Matching alcoholism treatments to client heterogeneity: Project MATCH three-year drinking outcomes. *Alcohol Clin Exp Res* 1998;22:1300–1311.

24. Tims FM. *Effectiveness of drug abuse treatment programs. Treatment research report.* DHHS publication no. (ADM) 84–1143. Rockville, MD: National Institute on Drug Abuse, 1981.

25. Tims FM, Ludford JP, eds. *Drug abuse treatment evaluation: strategies, progress, and prospects.* DHHS publication no. (ADM) 88–1329. Research monograph series 51. Rockville, MD: National Institute on Drug Abuse, 1984.

26. DeLeon G. *The therapeutic community: study of effectiveness.* DHHS publication no. (ADM) 84–1286. Rockville, MD: National Institute on Drug Abuse, 1984.

27. Holland S. *Residential drug-free programs for substance abusers: the effect of planned duration on treatment.* Chicago: Gateway Houses, 1982.

28. Sells SB. Treatment effectiveness. In: DuPont RL, Goldstein A, O'Donnell J, eds. *Handbook on drug use.* Washington, DC: U.S. Government Printing Office, 1979:105–118.

29. Sells SB, Simpson D. *The effectiveness of drug abuse treatment,* vols. 1–5. Cambridge, MA: Ballinger Publishing, 1976.

30. Smart RG. Outcome studies of therapeutic community and halfway house treatment for addicts. *Int J Addict* 1976;11:143–159.

31. Dole VP, Joseph H. Long-term outcome of patients treated with methadone maintenance. *Ann N Y Acad Sci* 1978;311:181–189.

32. Gorsuch RL, Abbamonte M, Sells SB. Evaluation of treatments for drug users in the DARP: 1971–1972 admissions. In: Sells SB, Simpson DD, eds. *The effectiveness of drug abuse treatment: evaluation of treatment outcomes for the 1971–1972 admission cohort.* Cambridge, MA: Ballinger Publishing, 1976;4:210–251.

33. Nash G. An analysis of twelve studies of the impact of drug abuse treatment upon criminality. In: *Drug use and crime: report of the panel on use and criminal behavior* [appendix]. Research Triangle Park, NC: Research Triangle Institute, 1976.

34. McGlothlin WH, Anglin MD. Long-term follow-up of clients of high- and low-dose methadone programs. *Arch Gen Psychiatry* 1981;38:1055–1063.

35. Kristiansen PL, Hubbard RL. Methodological overview and research design for adolescents in the Drug Abuse Treatment Outcome Studies. *J Adolesc Res* 2001;16:545–562.

36. Flynn PM, Craddock SG, Hubbard RL, et al. Methodological overview and research design for the Drug Abuse Treatment Outcome Study (DATOS). *Psychol Addict Behav* 1997;11:230–243.

37. Craddock SG, Rounds-Bryant JL, Flynn PM, et al. Characteristics and pretreatment behaviors of clients entering drug abuse treatment 1969 to 1993. *Am J Drug Abuse* 1997;23:43–59.

38. Hubbard RL, Marsden ME, Rachal JV, et al. *Drug abuse treatment: a national study of effectiveness.* Chapel Hill, NC: University of North Carolina Press, 1989.

39. Hubbard RL, Cavanaugh ER, Craddock SG, et al. *Drug abuse treatment client characteristics and pretreatment behavior: Treatment Outcome Prospective Study (TOPS), 1979–1981.* Rockville, MD: National Institute on Drug Abuse, 1986.

40. Hubbard RL, Bray RM, Craddock SG. Issues in the assessment of multiple drug use among drug treatment clients. *NIDA Res Monogr* 1986;68:15–40.

41. Bray RM, Schlenger WE, Craddock SG, et al. *Approaches to the assessment of drug use in the Treatment Outcome Prospective Study.* Report no. RTI/1901,01–05S. Research Triangle Park, NC: Research Triangle Institute, 1982.

42. Hser YI, Anglin MD, Fletcher BW. Comparative treatment effectiveness: effects of program modality and client drug dependence history on drug use reduction. *J Subst Abuse Treat* 1998;15:513–523.

43. Babor T, Cooney N, Hubbard R, et al. The syndrome concept of alcohol and drug dependence: results of the secondary analysis project. *NIDA Res Monogr* 1988;81:33–39.

44. Edwards G, Arif A, Hodgson R. Nomenclature and classification of drug- and alcohol-related problems: a WHO memorandum. *Bull World Health Organ* 1981;59:225–242.

45. Babor TF, Cooney NL, Lauerman RJ. The drug dependence syndrome concept as a psychological theory of relapse behavior: an empirical evaluation. *Br J Addict* 1987;82:393–405.

46. Kosten TR, Rounsaville BJ, Babor T, et al. Substance use disorders in *DSM–III–R:* the dependence syndrome across different psychoactive substances. *Br J Psychiatry* 1987;151:834–843.

47. Skinner HA, Goldberg AE. Evidence for a drug dependence syndrome among narcotic users. *Br J Addict* 1987;81:479–484.

48. Allison M, Hubbard RL, Ginzburg HM, et al. Validation of a three-item measure of depressive and suicidal symptoms. *Hosp Community Psychiatry* 1986;37:738–740.

49. Allison M, Hubbard RL, Ginzburg HM. *Indicators of suicide and depression among drug abusers. Research monograph 68.* DHHS publication no. (ADM) 85–1411. Rockville, MD: National Institute on Drug Abuse, 1985.

50. Magruder-Habib K, Hubbard RL, Ginzburg HM. Effects of drug abuse treatment on symptoms of depression and suicide. *Int J Addict* 1992;27:1036–1065.

51. Flynn PM, Craddock SG, Luckey JW, et al. Comorbidity of antisocial and mood disorders among psychoactive substance-dependent treatment clients. *J Personal Disord* 1996;10:56–67.

52. Rounds-Bryant JL, Kristiansen PL, Fairbank JA, et al. Substance use, mental disorders, abuse, and crime: gender comparisons among a national sample of adolescent drug treatment clients. *J Child Adolesc Subst Abuse* 1998;7:19–34.

53. Grella CE, Hser YI, Joshi V, et al. Drug treatment outcomes for adolescents with comorbid mental and substance use disorders. *J Nerv Ment Dis* 2001;189:384–392.

54. Marsden ME, Hubbard RL, Bailey SL. *Treatment histories of drug abusers.* Research Triangle Park, NC: Research Triangle Institute, 1988.

55. Anglin MD, Hser YI, Grella CE. Drug addiction and treatment careers among clients in the Drug Abuse Treatment Outcome Study (DATOS). *Psychol Addict Behav* 1997;11:308–323.

56. Hser Y, Grella CE, Hsieh S, et al. Prior treatment experience related to process and outcomes in DATOS. *Drug Alcohol Depend* 1999;57:137–150.

57. Hubbard RL, Collins JJ, Rachal JV, et al. The criminal justice client in drug abuse treatment. *NIDA Res Monogr* 1988;86:57–80.

58. Hubbard RL, Craddock SG, Anderson J. Replicated effects of criminal justice involvement on retention and outcomes. Fairfax, VA: Caliber Associates, 2002.

59. Collins JJ, Allison M. Legal coercion and retention in drug abuse treatment. *Hosp Community Psychiatry* 1983;34:1145–1149.

60. Farabee D, Shen H, Hser YI, et al. The effect of drug treatment on criminal behavior among adolescents in DATOS-A. *J Adolesc Res* 2001;16:679–696.

61. Allison M, Hubbard RL, Rachal JV. *Treatment process in methadone, residential, and outpatient drug-free abuse treatment programs.* Rockville, MD: National Institute on Drug Abuse, 1985.

62. McLellan AT, Woody GE, Luborsky L, et al. Is the counselor an "active ingredient" in substance abuse rehabilitation? An examination of treatment success among four counselors. *J Nerv Ment Dis* 1988;176:423–430.

63. Allison M, Hubbard RL. Drug abuse treatment process: a review of the literature. *Int J Addict* 1985;20:1321–1345.

64. Holland S. Measuring process in drug abuse treatment research. In: DeLeon G, Ziegenfuss JT, eds. *Therapeutic communities for addictions: readings in theory, research and practice.* Springfield, IL: Charles C Thomas, 1986;169–181.

65. Etheridge RM, Craddock SG, Dunteman GH, et al. Treatment services in two national studies of community-based drug abuse treatment programs. *J Subst Abuse Treat* 1995;7:9–26.

66. Flynn PM, Kristiansen PL, Porto JV, et al. Costs and benefits of treatment for cocaine addiction in DATOS. *Drug Alcohol Depend* 1999;57:167–174.

67. Etheridge RM, Smith JC, Rounds-Bryant JL, et al. Drug abuse treatment and comprehensive services for adolescents. *J Adolesc Res* 2001;16:563–589.

68. Delany PJ, Broome KM, Flynn PM, et al. Treatment service patterns and organizational structures: An analysis of programs in DATOS-A. *J Adolesc Res* 2001;16:590–607.

69. Hubbard RL, Allison M, Bray RM, et al. An overview of client characteristics, treatment services, and during treatment outcomes for outpatient methadone clinics in the Treatment Outcome Prospective Study (TOPS). In: Cooper JR, Altman F, Brown BS, et al, eds. *Research on the treatment of narcotic addiction: state of the art. Treatment research monograph series.* DHHS publication no. (ADM) 83–1281. Rockville, MD: National Institute on Drug Abuse, 1983:714–751.

70. Simpson DD, Sells SB. *Evaluation of drug abuse treatment effectiveness: summary of the DARP followup research.* Rockville, MD: National Institute on Drug Abuse, 1982.

71. Simpson DD, Savage LJ, Sells SB. *Evaluation of outcomes in the first year after drug abuse treatment: a replication study based on 1972–73 DARP admissions.* IBR report no. 80–8. Fort Worth: Texas Christian University, 1980.

72. Burt Associates. *Drug treatment in New York City and Washington, DC: followup studies.* Rockville, MD: National Institute on Drug Abuse, 1977.

73. Hubbard RL, Marsden ME, Cavanaugh ER, et al. Role of drug abuse treatment in limiting the spread of AIDS. *Rev Infect Dis* 1988;10:377–384.

74. Hubbard RL, Rachal JV, Craddock SG, et al. Treatment Outcome Prospective Study (TOPS): client characteristics and behaviors before, during, and after treatment. *NIDA Res Monogr* 1984;51:42–68.

75. Center for Substance Abuse Treatment. *The persistent effects of substance abuse treatment—one year later.* Rockville, MD: Center for Substance Abuse Treatment, 1996.

76. Gerstein DR, Johnson RA, Harwood HJ, et al. *Evaluating recovery services: The California drug and alcohol treatment assessment.* Sacramento: California Department of Alcohol and Drug Programs, 1994.

77. Newman RG, Whitehill WB. Double-blind comparison of methadone and placebo maintenance treatments of narcotic addicts in Hong Kong. *Lancet* 1979;8:485–489.

78. McGlothlin WH, Anglin MD. Long-term follow-up of clients of high- and low-dose methadone programs. *Arch Gen Psychiatry* 1981;38:1055–1063.

79. Harwood HJ, Hubbard RL, Collins JJ, et al. The costs of crime and the benefits of drug abuse treatment: a cost-benefit analysis using TOPS data. *NIDA Res Monogr* 1988;86:209–235.

80. Hubbard RL, Craddock SG, Flynn PM, et al. Overview of 1-year follow-up outcomes in the Drug Abuse Treatment Outcome Study (DATOS). *Psychol Addict Behav* 1997;11:261–278.

81. Simpson DD, Joe GW, Fletcher BW, et al. A national evaluation of treatment outcomes for cocaine dependence. *Arch Gen Psychiatry* 1999;56:507–514.

82. Hubbard RL, Craddock SG, Anderson J. Overview of 5-year followup outcomes in the drug abuse treatment outcome studies (DATOS). *J Subst Abuse Treat* 2003;25:125–134.

83. Simpson DD, Joe GW, Broome KM. A national 5-year follow-up of treatment outcomes for cocaine dependence. *Arch Gen Psychiatry* 2002;59:538–544.

84. Hser YI, Grella CE, Hubbard RL, et al. An evaluation of drug treatments for adolescents in 4 U.S. cities. *Arch Gen Psychiatry* 2001;58:689–695.

85. Cronkite RC, Moos RH. Determinants of the posttreatment functioning of alcoholic patients: a conceptual framework. *J Consult Clin Psychol* 1980;48:305–316.

86. Moos RH, Finney JW. The expanding scope of alcoholism treatment evaluation. *Am Psychol* 1983;38:1036–1044.

87. Tims FM, Leukefeld CG, eds. *Relapse and recovery in drug abuse.* DHHS publication no. (ADM) 86–1473. Research monograph series 72. Rockville, MD: National Institute on Drug Abuse, 1986.

88. Jones KR, Vischi TR. Impact of alcohol, drug abuse, and mental health treatment on medical care utilization. *Med Care* 1979;79:1–82.

89. Musto DF. *The American disease.* New Haven: Yale University Press, 1973.

90. Musto DF. *The American disease. Expanded ed.* New York: Oxford University Press, 1988.

91. Courtwright DT. *Dark paradise: opiate addiction in America before 1940.* Cambridge, MA: Harvard University Press, 1982.

92. Jaffe JH. Footnotes in the evolution of the American national response: some little known aspects of the first American strategy for drug abuse and drug traffic prevention [the Inaugural Thomas Okey Memorial Lecture]. *Br J Addict* 1987;82:587–600.

93. Harwood HJ, Napolitano DM, Kristiansen PL, et al. *Economic costs to society of alcohol and drug abuse and mental illness: 1980.* Report no. RTI/2734/00–01FR. Research Triangle Park, NC: Research Triangle Institute, 1984.

94. Clayton RR. Cocaine use in the United States: in a blizzard or just being snowed? *NIDA Res Monogr* 1985;61:8–34.

95. Des Jarlais DC. "Free" needles for intravenous drug users at risk for AIDS: current developments in New York City [Letter]. *N Engl J Med* 1985;313:1476.

96. Miller JD, Cisin IH, Gardner-Keaton H, et al. *National Household Survey on Drug Abuse: main findings 1982.* Rockville, MD: National Institute on Drug Abuse, 1983.

97. National Institute on Drug Abuse. *National Household Survey on Drug Abuse: main findings 1985.* Rockville, MD: National Institute on Drug Abuse, 1987.

98. National Institute on Drug Abuse. *Demographic characteristics and patterns of drug use of clients admitted to drug abuse treatment programs in selected states.* Rockville, MD: U.S. Government Printing Office, 1988.

99. Jaffe JH. Evaluating drug abuse treatment: a comment on the state of the art. *NIDA Res Monogr* 1984;51:13–28.

100. Tims FM. Introduction. *NIDA Res Monogr* 1984;51:9–12.

101. Rosenbaum M, Murphy S, Beck J. Money for methadone: preliminary findings from a study of Alameda County's new maintenance policy. *J Psychoactive Drugs* 1987;19:13–19.

102. Price RH, Burke AC, D'Aunno T, et al. Outpatient drug abuse treatment services, 1988: results of a national survey. *NIDA Res Monogr* 1991;106:63–92.

103. D'Aunno T, Price RH. Organizational adaptation to changing environments: community mental health and drug abuse services. *Am Behav Sci* 1985;28:669–683.

104. Marlatt GA, Gordon JR. *Relapse prevention: maintenance strategies in addictive behavior change.* New York: Guilford Press, 1984.

105. DeLeon G, Jainchill N. Circumstance, motivation, readiness, and suitability as correlates of treatment tenure. *J Psychoactive Drugs* 1986;18:203–208.

106. Biase DV, Sullivan AP, Wheeler B. Daytop Miniversity—phase 2—college training in a therapeutic community: development of self concept among drug free addict/abusers. In: DeLeon G, Ziegenfuss JT, eds. *Therapeutic communities for addictions: readings in theory, research and practice.* Springfield, IL: Charles C Thomas, 1986;121–130.

107. Etheridge RM, Craddock SG, Hubbard RL, et al. The relationship of counseling and self-help participation to patient outcomes in DATOS. *Drug Alcohol Depend* 1999;57:99–112.

108. Simpson DD, Sells SB, eds. *Opioid addiction and treatment: a 12-year followup.* Malabar, FL: Krieger Publishing, 1990.

109. Glaser FB. Anybody got a match? Treatment research and the matching hypothesis. In: Edwards G, Grant M, eds. *Alcoholism treatment in transition.* Baltimore: University Park Press, 1980:178–196.

110. McLellan AT, Luborsky L, Woody GE, et al. Predicting response to alcohol and drug abuse treatments. *Arch Gen Psychiatry* 1983;40:620–625.

111. Rounsaville BJ. Clinical assessment of drug abusers. In Kleber HD, ed. Treatment of substance use disorders (nonalcohol). Washington, DC: American Psychiatric Association Press, 1989; 11:1183–1191.

112. Finney JW, Moos RH. Matching patients with treatments: conceptual and methodological issues. *J Stud Alcohol* 1986;47:122–134.

113. National Institute on Drug Abuse. *National drug abuse treatment clinical trials network.* Washington, DC: National Institutes of Health, U.S. Department of Health and Human Services 2002.

114. Presidential Commission on the Human Immunodeficiency virus epidemic. Washington, DC: U.S. Government Printing Office, 1988.

115. Leukefeld CG, Tims FM. An introduction to compulsory treatment for drug abuse: clinical practice and research. *NIDA Res Monogr* 1988;86:1–7.

116. Joshi V, Hser YI, Grella CE, et al. Sex-related HIV risk reduction behavior among adolescents in DATOS-A. *J Adolesc Res* 2001;16:642–660.

117. National Institute on Drug Abuse. *Principles of HIV prevention in drug-using populations.* No.02-4733. Washington, DC: National Institutes of Health, U.S. Department of Health and Human Services, 2002.

118. Meyer R. Introduction: factors affecting the outcome of methadone treatment. In: Cooper JR, Altman F, Brown BS, et al, eds. *Research on the treatment of narcotic addiction: state of the art.* DHHS publication no. (ADM) 83–1281. Rockville, MD: U.S. Government Printing Office, 1983:495–499.

119. Skinner HA. Profiles of treatment-seeking populations. In: Edwards G, Grant M, eds. *Alcohol treatment in transition.* Baltimore: University Park Press, 1981.

120. Beschner G, Thompson P. *Women and drug abuse treatment: needs and services.* DHHS publication no. (ADM) 81–1057. Washington, DC: U.S. Government Printing Office, 1981.

121. Finnegan LP. Women in treatment. In: DuPont RL, Goldstein A, O'Donnell J, eds. *Handbook on drug abuse.* Washington, DC: U.S. Government Printing Office, 1979:121–131.

122. Friedman AS, Beschner GM, eds. *Treatment services for adolescent substance abusers.* DHHS publication no. (ADM) 85–1342. Rockville, MD: National Institute on Drug Abuse, 1985.

123. Austin GA, Johnson BD, Carroll EE, et al, eds. *Drugs and minorities.* DHEW publication no. (ADM) 78–507. Research issues 21. Rockville, MD: National Institute on Drug Abuse, 1977.

124. Espada F. The drug abuse industry and the "minority" communities: time for change. In: Dupont RL, Goldstein A, O'Donnell J, eds. *Handbook on drug abuse.* Washington, DC: U.S. Government Printing Office, 1979:293–300.

125. Rosenbaum M, Murphy S. Not the picture of health: women on methadone. *J Psychoactive Drugs* 1987;19:217–226.

126. Reed BG. Developing women-sensitive drug dependence treatment services: why so difficult? *J Psychoactive Drugs* 1987;19:151–164.

127. Anglin MD, Hser Y, Booth MW. Sex differences in addict careers: treatment. *Am J Drug Alcohol Abuse* 1987;13:253–280.

128. DeLeon G, Rosenthal MS. Therapeutic communities. In: DuPont RL, Goldstein A, O'Donnell J, eds. *Handbook on drug abuse.* Washington, DC: U.S. Government Printing Office, 1979:39–47.

129. McLellan AT, Childress AR, Griffith J, et al. The psychiatrically severe drug abuse patient: methadone maintenance or therapeutic community? *Am J Drug Alcohol Abuse* 1984;10:77–95.

130. McLellan AT, Luborsky L, Cacciola J, et al. *Guide to the Addiction Severity Index: background, administration, and field testing results.* DHHS publication no. (ADM) 85–1419. Rockville, MD: National Institute on Drug Abuse, 1985.

131. Woody GE, McLellan AT, Luborsky L, et al. Sociopathy and psychotherapy outcome. *Arch Gen Psychiatry* 1985;42:1081–1086.

132. Friedman AS, Glickman NW. Effects of psychiatric symptomatology on treatment outcome for adolescent male drug abusers. *J Nerv Ment Dis* 1987;175:1–6.

133. Dorus W, Senay EC. Depression, demographic dimensions, and drug abuse. *Am J Psychiatry* 1980;137:699–704.

134. Woody GE, Blaine J. Depression in narcotic addicts: quite possibly more than a chance association. In: DuPont RL, Goldstein A, O'Donnell J, eds. *Handbook on drug abuse.* Washington, DC: U.S. Government Printing Office, 1979:277–285.

135. DeLeon G. Phoenix House: psychopathological signs among male and female drug-free residents. *Addict Dis* 1974;1:135–151.

136. Weissman MM, Slobetz F, Prusoff B, et al. Clinical depression among narcotic addicts maintained on methadone in the community. *Am J Psychiatry* 1976;133:1434–1438.

137. Craddock SG, Bray RM, Hubbard RL. *Drug use before and during drug abuse treatment: 1979–1981 TOPS admission cohorts.* Rockville, MD: National Institute on Drug Abuse, 1985.

138. Hubbard RL, Marsden ME. Relapse to use of heroin, cocaine, and other drugs in the first year after treatment. *NIDA Res Monogr* 1986;72:157–166.

139. Hubbard RL. Treating combined alcohol and drug abuse in community-based programs. In: Galanter M, ed. *Recent developments in alcoholism.* New York: Plenum Press, 1990;8:273–283.

140. McLellan AT, Druley KA. A comparative study of response to treatment in court-referred and voluntary drug patients [Brief reports]. *Hosp Community Psychiatry* 1977;28:241–245.

141. Senay EC, Dorus W, Showalter C. Methadone detoxification: self versus physician regulation. *Am J Drug Alcohol Abuse* 1984;10:361–374.

142. Grella CE, Hser YI, Joshi V, et al. Patient histories, retention, and outcome models for younger and older

adults in DATOS. *Drug Alcohol Depend* 1999;57:151–166.

143. McLellan AT, Woody GE, Luborsky L, et al. Increased effectiveness of substance abuse treatment: a prospective study of patient-treatment "matching." *J Nerv Ment Dis* 1983;171:597–605.

144. Lowinson JH, Millman RB. Clinical aspects of methadone maintenance treatment. In: DuPont RL, Goldstein A, O'Donnell J, eds. *Handbook on drug abuse.* Washington, DC: U.S. Government Printing Office, 1979: 49–56.

145. DeLeon G. The therapeutic community for substance abuse: perspective and approach. In: DeLeon G, Ziegenfuss JT, eds. *Therapeutic communities for addictions: readings in theory, research and practice.* Springfield, IL: Charles C Thomas, 1986;185–189.

146. Kleber HD, Slobetz F. Outpatient drug-free treatment. In: DuPont RL, Goldstein A, O'Donnell J, eds. *Handbook on drug abuse.* Washington, DC: U.S. Government Printing Office, 1979:31–38.

147. Simpson DD, Joe GW, Rowan-Szal GA, et al. Drug abuse treatment process components that improve treatment. *J Subst Abuse Treat* 1997;14:565–572.

148. Joe GW, Simpson DD, Broome KM. Retention and patient engagement models for different treatment modalities in DATOS. *Drug Alcohol Depend* 1999;57:113–125.

149. Broome KM, Simpson DD, Joe GW. Patient and program attributes related to treatment process indicators in DATOS. *Drug Alcohol Depend* 1999;57:127–135.

150. Broome KM, Joe GW, Simpson DD. Engagement models for adolescents in DATOS-A. *J Adolesc Res* 2001;16:608–623.

151. Watson DD, Simpson DD, Spiegel DK. Development of a treatment typology for drug use in the DARP: 1969–1971 admissions. In: Sells SB, ed. *The effectiveness of drug abuse treatment: research on patients, treatments and outcomes,* vol. 2. Cambridge, MA: Ballinger Publishing, 1974;253–308.

152. Cole SG, James LR. A revised treatment typology based on the DARP. *Am J Drug Alcohol Abuse* 1974;2:37–49.

153. Orlinsky DE, Howard KI. Process and outcome in psychotherapy. In: Garfield SL, Bergin AE, eds. *Handbook of psychotherapy and behavior change.* New York: Wiley, 1986.

154. Kiesler DJ. *The process of psychotherapy.* Chicago: Aldine, 1983.

155. Greenberg LS, Pinsof WM, eds. *The psychotherapeutic process: a research handbook.* New York: Guilford Press, 1986.

156. Lichtenberg JW, Heck EJ. Analysis of sequence and pattern in process research. *J Counsel Psychol* 1986;33: 170–181.

157. Highlen PS. Analyzing patterns and sequence in counseling: reactions of a counseling process researcher. *J Counsel Psychol* 1986;33:186–189.

158. Ball JC. A schema for evaluating methadone maintenance programs. In: Harris LS, ed. *Problems of drug dependence 1989: proceedings of the 51st annual scientific meeting: the Committee on Problems of Drug Dependence, Inc.* Research monograph series 95. Washington, DC: U.S. Government Printing Office, 1990:74–77.

159. Ball JC, Lange R, Myers P, et al. Reducing the risk of AIDS through methadone maintenance treatment. *J Health Soc Behav* 1988;29:214–226.

160. Magura S, Goldsmith DS, Casriel C, et al. Patient-staff governance in methadone maintenance treatment: a study in participative decision making. *Int J Addict* 1988;23:253–278.

161. Aiken LS, LoSciuto LA, Ausetts MA, et al. Paraprofessional versus professional drug counselors: the progress of clients in treatment. *Int J Addict* 1984;19:383–401.

162. Wheeler BL, Biase DV, Sullivan AP. Changes in self-concept during therapeutic community treatment: a comparison of male and female drug abusers. *J Drug Educ* 1986;16:191–196.

163. Joe GW, Simpson DD, Hubbard RL. Treatment predictors of time in methadone maintenance. *J Subst Abuse Treat* 1991;3:73–84.

164. Joe GW, Simpson DD, Hubbard RL. Unmet service needs in methadone treatment. *Int J Addict* 1991;26:1–22.

165. Etheridge RM, Hubbard RL. Conceptualizing and assessing treatment structure and process in community-based drug dependency treatment programs. *Subst Use Misuse* 2000;35:1757–1795

166. Havassy BE, Tschann JM. Client initiative, inertia, and demographics: more powerful than treatment interventions in methadone maintenance. *Int J Addict* 1983;18:617–631.

167. Hunt DE, Lipton DS, Goldsmith DS, et al. Problems in methadone treatment: the influence of reference groups. *NIDA Res Monogr* 1984;46:8–22.

168. McCrady B, Sher K. Treatment variables. *NIDA Res Monogr* 1985;15:48–62.

169. Marlatt GA, George WH. Relapse prevention: introduction and overview of the model. *Br J Addict* 1984;79:261–274.

170. Sorensen JL, Acampora A, Trier M, et al. From maintenance to abstinence in a therapeutic community: follow-up outcomes. *J Psychoactive Drugs* 1987;19:345–351.

171. McAuliffe WE, Ch'ien JMN. Recovery training and self-help: a relapse-prevention program for treated opiate addicts. *J Subst Abuse Treat* 1986;3: 9–20.

Management of Associated Medical Conditions

CHAPTER 53

Maternal and Neonatal Effects of Alcohol and Drugs

LORETTA P. FINNEGAN AND
STEPHEN R. KANDALL

Despite the acknowledgment that the use of licit and illicit substances by women in our country is increasing, the exact magnitude of the problem has always been difficult to determine. It has not been widely publicized that, historically, women made up as many as two-thirds of America's opiate addicts and a significant percentage of users of cocaine, sedatives, and marijuana between 1850 and 1900 (1). Although the percentage of females in the addict population fell to approximately 20% during the Classic Era of drug repression (1914–1950s), it is now estimated that women represent about one-third of the drug abusers in the United States. This number would certainly be significantly higher if addiction to legal prescription medications were included, because women are overrepresented in that group of drug-dependent patients. Although "crack" cocaine use has recently declined from its peak in the late 1980s, the use of other "old" drugs such as heroin, now smoked as well as injected, and newer drugs such as methamphetamine and oxycodone hydrochloride (OxyContin) has increased.

Although their numbers are not exactly known, the fact that many drug-using women are of childbearing age translates into a large number of infants being born following intrauterine drug exposure. The use of questionable epidemiologic methodologies was highlighted by Dicker and Leighton (2), who found a huge disparity in "official" estimates of drug-exposed newborns born between 1979 and 1987, ranging from a low of about 13,000 to a high of about 700,000. In the late 1980s, Chasnoff (3) surveyed 36 hospitals throughout the United States and found an overall incidence of substance abuse in pregnancy, excluding alcohol, to be 11%, with an interhospital range of 0.4% to 27%. In their 1989 Pinellas County, Florida study, Chasnoff et al. (4) found that approximately 15% of the 715 urines screened during pregnancy were positive for illicit substances, including alcohol (1%). That study found similar rates of drug usage between "public" and "private" patients, and between black and white women. Combining 27 reports published in the 1980s with existing National Institute on Drug Abuse (NIDA) data, Gomby and Shiono (5) estimated that approximately 2% to 3% of babies (75,000/per year) may have been exposed to opiates during the intrauterine period, compared to 4.5% of babies (158,000/per year) exposed to cocaine and 17% (611,000 per year) to marihuana, all far less than the 73% (2.6 million per year) with possible exposure to alcohol.

The most comprehensive study of perinatal drug epidemiology was conducted between late 1992 and mid-1993 by the National Institute on Drug Abuse. Generating a probability sample of 2,613 women in 52 metropolitan and nonmetropolitan hospitals, the National Pregnancy and Health Survey (6) estimated that 5.5%, or 222,000 of the 4 million women who give birth annually, used some illicit drug during their pregnancy. Highest estimates were found for marijuana (119,000; 2.9%), followed by amphetamines, sedatives, tranquilizers, and analgesics in a nonmedical context (61,000; 1.5%), cocaine (45,000; 1.1%), and smaller numbers for methamphetamine, heroin, methadone, hallucinogens, and inhalants. Those numbers were all considerably less, however, than the numbers for alcohol use (757,000; 18.8%) and cigarette use (820,000; 20.4%) during pregnancy. The survey also found that estimated rates of drug use were higher for African American women (11.3%) than for either Hispanic (4.5%) or white women (4.4%).

During the decade of the 1990s, therefore, large numbers of pregnant drug-dependent women presented themselves to medical facilities, some to receive ongoing prenatal care but others only to deliver their babies without the benefit of prenatal attention. Unfortunately, the threat of confrontations with legal and child protection authorities, often with punitive outcomes, as well as the general unavailability of women-oriented treatment programs, has kept many drug-dependent women from seeking general medical and prenatal care. Failure of such women to receive comprehensive health care during pregnancy is a known cause of increased morbidity and mortality in both the mother and her infant.

This chapter reviews the past and current literature, as well as the experiences of the authors, with regard to the sociomedical characteristics of pregnant drug-dependent women. In addition, the effects of substances of abuse on the pregnant woman, the fetus, and the newborn on immediate and long-term morbidity and mortality, and recommendations for management of both the mother and her infant are presented. Readers may refer to the 1993–1994 Treatment Improvement Protocols (7,8) pertaining to pregnant substance-abusing women and drug-exposed infants as well as Center for Substance Abuse Treatment's (CSAT) 1994 publication (9), which describes treatment approaches for women who abuse alcohol and other drugs.

Other useful, more targeted monographs include the NIDA monographs (10–12). Throughout this discussion, because of the high incidence of polysubstance use, it is essential to remember the inherent difficulties involved in ascribing a specific perinatal effect to one specific substance. This chapter deals first with opiates (primarily heroin and methadone) and then stimulants (primarily cocaine and amphetamines). In addition, some brief comments about perinatal effects of alcohol are offered.

SOCIAL AND MEDICAL CHARACTERISTICS OF THE PREGNANT DRUG-DEPENDENT WOMAN THAT INFLUENCE THE INTRAUTERINE MILIEU

The lives of many drug-dependent women are chaotic and subject to influences that adversely affect their physical and psychosocial health and well-being (13). Because of preexisting conditions and ongoing active drug use, the drug-dependent woman frequently suffers from chronic anxiety and depression. Lacking self-confidence and hope for the future, these women often have interpersonal heterosexual difficulties and become victims of abuse and battering. Finnegan et al. (14) found that 83% of addicted women coming into treatment were raised in households marked by parental chemical abuse; 67% of those women had been sexually assaulted, 60% had been physically assaulted, and almost all of the women wished that they were someone else as they were growing up. Chavkin and coworkers (15) similarly found that almost 60% of drug-dependent women in New York City had been homeless within the past 2 years, half had experienced at least one forced sexual encounter, and two-thirds gave histories of drug or alcohol abuse in their upbringing. These serious social stresses and the need to engage in prostitution or other crimes to support a drug habit may overwhelm coping mechanisms and lead to involvement with the criminal justice system. In 1990, for example, the National Institute on Justice (16) found that almost two-thirds of arrested women were illicit drug users. Placed in the context of these serious and often crippling problems, the treatment and possible resolution of the superimposed addiction are usually complicated and require skill, understanding, compassion, and patience. Addiction is a chronic, progressive, relapsing disease, and one cannot expect a smooth and rapid recovery. It should not be surprising, therefore, that the lifestyle of the pregnant user of illegal drugs has a profound influence upon her psychological, social, and physiologic well-being.

It is well known that medical complications compromise many drug-involved pregnancies (Table 53.1). Sexually transmitted diseases have played an increasingly important role in this spectrum of diseases. Of most concern is that human immunodeficiency virus (HIV) disease is significantly linked to drug use. The practices of sharing contaminated needles to inject drugs, engaging in prostitution to buy drugs, or conducting direct sex-for-drugs transactions associated with "crack" smoking, have all contributed to this serious international health crisis. Addressing perinatal transmission, the landmark AIDS

TABLE 53.1. *Medical complications encountered in pregnant intravenous addicts*

Anemia
Bacteremia, septicemia
Cardiac disease, especially endocarditis
Cellulitis
Poor dental hygiene
Edema
Hepatitis, acute and chronic
Human immunodeficiency virus (HIV infection)
Hypertension
Phlebitis
Pneumonia
Sexually transmitted diseases
Tetanus
Tuberculosis
Urinary tract infections—cystitis, urethritis, pyelonephritis

Clinical Trials Group (ACTG) 076 study (17) showed that administration of zidovudine (AZT) to a woman beginning at 14 to 34 weeks of pregnancy and to the infant for 6 weeks after birth reduced the risk of perinatal HIV transmission by about two-thirds from the previous percentages of 25% to 30% if the woman is untreated. Newer recommendations call for treatment of HIV-infected women with HIV ribonucleic acid (RNA) >1000 copies/mL with a combination of highly active antiretroviral therapy (HAART) regimens, including AZT. The use of AZT alone is recommended with RNA copies <1000/mL. In all cases, AZT should be given to the woman during labor and continued for 6 weeks in the newborn infant. Aggressive HAART regimens appear to reduce the perinatal HIV transmission rate to <2%. In addition to acquired immunodeficiency syndrome (AIDS) prevention counseling, retention of women in prenatal care provides the matrix in which concrete, effective medical services can be offered to pregnant substance-abusing women or women involved in close relationships with addicted men.

The drug-dependent pregnant woman may develop a range of nutritional deficiencies either as a result of preoccupation with drug seeking at the expense of food intake, inhibition of the central mechanism that controls appetite and hunger, or toxic interference with the absorption or utilization of ingested nutrients. Abnormalities of nutrient absorption are common in drug addicts because of the high incidence of lesions of the intestine, liver, and pancreas. Iron and folic acid deficiencies, as well as peripheral neuritis as a consequence of thiamine, vitamin B_6, pantothenic acid, or nicotinic acid depletion, may occur. Hypoglycemia, vitamin B_6 deficiency, thiamine depletion, or magnesium deficiency may cause seizures in both alcoholics and drug addicts. Consequently, intensive dietary therapy is desirable in drug and alcohol addiction, and parenteral therapy may be necessary to correct fluid, mineral, and vitamin deficits in acutely ill patients.

Chronic heroin addicts have been said to show frequent endocrine aberrations, including amenorrhea, anovulation, and infertility, possibly through depression of adrenocorticotropic hormone (ACTH) release and adrenal function, as well as ovulation. The women themselves believe that amenorrhea and infertility always occur when they are using substantial amounts of heroin. Wallach et al. (18), however, found that women maintained on methadone have regular menstruation, ovulation, and apparently normal pregnancies. Other investigators also support the use of methadone to normalize the mother's endocrinologic status and to promote more normal pregnancies (19–25). When it occurs, severe dysmenorrhea is most likely caused by pelvic inflammatory disease.

In addition to these many potential medical problems, the lifestyle of the addict is also detrimental to herself and to society. Because most of her day is consumed by the two activities of either obtaining drugs or using drugs, she spends most of her time unable to function in the usual activities of daily living. The opiate addict has intermittent periods of normal alertness and well-being, but for most of the day she is either "high" or "sick." The "high," or euphoric state, keeps her sedated or tranquilized, absorbed in herself, and incapable of fulfilling familial responsibility. The "sick" stage, or the periods during which she is going through abstinence symptoms, generally is characterized by craving for narcotics accompanied by malaise, nausea, lacrimation, perspiration, tremors, vomiting, diarrhea, and cramps. The cocaine user may go on "binges" of drug use, resulting in lack of sleep, poor nutrition, and potentially acute life-threatening complications such as hypertensive crises, cerebrovascular accidents, and seizures.

Because of her lifestyle and because she may fear calling attention to her drug habit, the pregnant addict often does not seek prenatal care. The physician or nurse should be able to determine that the woman is drug-addicted by taking a thorough history and conducting a careful physical examination. Prenatal care, either in a hospital setting or in a private physician's office, may be sporadic and inconsistent, or even totally lacking. A history of sexually transmitted diseases may be obtained. Tattoos or self-scarring of the body to disguise needle marks may be evident. As a consequence of diminished pain perception when smoking while "high," burns of the fingertips and cigarette burns of the clothes may be found. The use of poorly cleaned needles or shared needles predisposes these women to serum hepatitis evidenced by jaundiced skin or sclera.

Additional history taking may reveal that the woman has several other children who are currently not living with her but instead with a relative or in placement. Housing situations frequently are chaotic, and plans for the impending birth of the child often have not been considered. Many drug-dependent women are innately intelligent, but a review of their formal education histories shows that many do not complete high school. In a Philadelphia

TABLE 53.2. *Obstetric complications associated with heroin addiction*

Abortion (spontaneous early loss)
Amnionitis
Intrauterine death (late)
Intrauterine growth retardation
Placental insufficiency
Postpartum hemorrhage
Preeclampsia, eclampsia
Premature labor
Premature rupture of membranes
Septic thrombophlebitis

Adapted from Finnegan LP, ed. *Drug dependence in pregnancy: clinical management of mother and child. A manual for medical professionals and paraprofessionals prepared for the National Institute on Drug Abuse, Services Research Branch, Rockville, MD.* Washington, DC: Government Printing Office, 1978.

series at a treatment program called Family Center, the average level of high school achievement was the 11th grade (26). Chavkin et al. (15) also found that the average number of educational years among their female addicts was 11.5.

Drug dependence in the pregnant woman is not only detrimental to her own physical condition, but also potentially dangerous to that of the fetus and eventually to the newborn infant. Table 53.2 lists the obstetric complications associated with heroin addiction. Most of these pregnancy-related problems can be diagnosed and treated antenatally, reinforcing the importance of enlisting and retaining drug-dependent women in prenatal care throughout the pregnancy (7).

NORMALIZING THE INTRAUTERINE MİLIEU

Because pregnant drug-abusing women are afflicted with numerous and potentially overwhelming problems, most experts advocate the provision of a comprehensive approach that will specifically meet the various needs of these women (7,9). It should be acknowledged, however, that some women might find this approach overwhelming and thus prefer a more targeted strategy aimed at solving specific lifestyle problems.

The primary focus of a program of comprehensive care for the pregnant drug abuser should be addiction treatment in a setting in which medical and obstetric care, psychosocial counseling, and long-term planning for the mother and her newborn infant are also provided. The underlying assumptions regarding drug treatment during pregnancy have changed, however, over the past 25 years. In 1972, the American Medical Association's Council on Mental Health and the Committee on Alcoholism and Drug Dependence recommended that a pregnant drug-dependent woman should undergo withdrawal prior to delivery. If there was insufficient time to accomplish withdrawal before delivery, the woman could be maintained on opiates during labor and then withdrawn after the delivery process (27). Current recommendations acknowledge that achieving the drug-free state is probably impossible for the large majority of opiate-addicted women. Most experts now advocate methadone maintenance as a way to reduce illegal drug use, remove the woman from a drug-seeking environment, prevent fluctuations of drug levels throughout the day, improve maternal nutrition, increase the likelihood of prenatal care, enhance the woman's ability to prepare for the birth of her baby, reduce obstetric complications, and offer the pregnant heroin addict an opportunity to restructure her life with a goal to continued stabilization after pregnancy (7). Although methadone maintenance as a treatment modality in and of itself has been extremely beneficial in the treatment of addiction during pregnancy, investigators stress that provision of psychosocial support in a structured treatment setting is extremely important (19,21,28).

Although methadone maintenance during pregnancy is clearly the treatment of choice, a small number of highly motivated women or those facing logistical or geographic barriers to methadone maintenance may be candidates for medical withdrawal during pregnancy. The CSAT Consensus Panel recommended that undertaking a medical withdrawal regimen could be most safely accomplished during the second trimester with careful monitoring of fetal welfare by perinatal experts (7). The panel advised that opiate withdrawal could be best accomplished through stabilization with methadone followed by gradual reduction of the methadone dosage by 2 to 2.5 mg every 7 to 10 days. Although medical withdrawal is not usually recommended during pregnancy, a pilot program conducted at Beth Israel Medical Center in New York between 1993 and 1995 showed that a multidisciplinary effort that included obstetrical and neonatal consultation, substance abuse treatment and counseling, and a women's support group offered a feasible and safe approach to medical withdrawal during pregnancy. If treatment staff and the woman agree to embark on this approach, careful monitoring of the fetus and woman are essential by expert staff in an appropriate clinical setting.

During the past 30 years, substantial experience with methadone maintenance during pregnancy has been accumulated. In 1972, Statzer and Wardell (29) developed a specialized program of prenatal care for the high-risk mother at the Hutzel Hospital in Detroit. In addition to receiving regular prenatal care, patients were seen by a nutritionist, social worker, public health nurse, and staff with specialized training in the psychological needs of the heroin user. From that program's experience, Strauss et al. (25) concluded that low-dose methadone maintenance in conjunction with comprehensive prenatal care reduced obstetric risk to a level comparable to that of nonaddicted women of similar socioeconomic circumstances.

At Beth Israel Medical Center in New York City, Blinick et al. (30,31) found that methadone maintenance eliminated maternal mortality and reduced complication rates of pregnancy and fetal wastage in 105 women. Although one-third of the infants were low birth weight, no serious effects attributable to methadone in the neonatal period were reported; followup of a small number of the infants revealed normal growth and development. Harper et al. (28) organized the Family and Maternity Care Program for pregnant addicts, their spouses, and their newborn infants at the State University of New York Downstate Medical Center in Brooklyn. Low-dose methadone maintenance coupled with intense psychosocial support appeared to alleviate many of the common problems associated with addiction in pregnancy. Although one would not expect that this regimen would prevent withdrawal in the newborn infant, symptomology was not associated with an increase in mortality or prolonged morbidity.

Kandall et al. (23), working in conjunction with the Bronx State Methadone Program, studied 230 infants born to drug-dependent women and 33 infants born to ex-addicts between 1971 and 1974. Compared with heroin use, methadone maintenance was associated with more consistent prenatal care, more normal fetal growth, and reduced fetal mortality. In this program, neonatal withdrawal from methadone seemed to be more severe than that from heroin, but severity of the withdrawal did not correlate with late pregnancy maternal methadone dosage. In New York City as a whole, Newman (32) reported an extraordinarily high retention rate (95%) in the city's methadone treatment programs after delivery.

In Philadelphia, Connaughton and Finnegan (19) developed Family Center, a comprehensive approach that has been used over several decades to care for more than 2,500 pregnant, addicted women. Combining methadone maintenance with consultations with obstetricians, medical consultants, psychiatric social workers, public health nurses, community workers, and psychiatrists, management of addiction was individualized to the patient's needs. Although most patients chose methadone maintenance, some patients became drug-free, whereas others were placed on a regimen of methadone withdrawal, if deemed medically safe. Those patients who are to be methadone-maintained are hospitalized and started on 10 mg of methadone daily, and the dose is titrated upward to prevent withdrawal symptomatology. Depending on the length of the woman's addiction, the duration of time in methadone treatment, the concomitant use of other drugs, and her own metabolic state, homeostasis was usually achieved with doses from 35 to 80 mg daily. Many women, however, require higher doses of methadone for stabilization. Family Center's multidisciplinary approach, combining outreach services with individual and interpersonal interventions to comprehensively address biologic/physiologic issues, psychological/behavioral/cognitive function, sociocultural/demographic issues, mother–infant interaction, and early childhood development, has significantly reduced the maternal and infant morbidity that previously have been associated with pregnancies complicated by opiate addiction.

METHADONE MAINTENANCE

Although methadone therapy has been used during pregnancy for about 30 years, no randomized trials comparing dosing regimens have been published on which to base specific therapeutic recommendations. In general, clinicians have tended to use dosages that are individually determined and will keep the woman and fetus subjectively comfortable physiologically, as well as stable. Although the health and comfort of the pregnant substance-using woman remain paramount considerations, higher dosages of methadone (50 to 150 mg/day) early in pregnancy have been reported to be associated with more normal fetal growth (33). Data on the relationship between maternal methadone doses, especially late in pregnancy, and

subsequent severity of neonatal abstinence are contradictory (see pages 814–816).

Plasma methadone levels during pregnancy show marked intrapatient and interpatient variability and usually are somewhat lower than those prior to pregnancy (34). This decrease can be explained by an increased fluid space, a large tissue reservoir (35), and altered drug metabolism by the placenta and fetus. These data suggest that pregnant women may need increasing methadone doses during gestation and that lowering the dosage in an attempt to minimize complications of the therapy would be medically inappropriate. Treatment with other drugs, such as tranquilizers, are strictly avoided unless the patient is addicted to these medications. In case of such addiction, the patient should be transferred to a special detoxification ward where she can be safely weaned from drugs potentially more dangerous than opiates.

Regardless of the dosing regimen, every woman should receive a detailed health history, comprehensive physical examination, and a family psychosocial, medical, and substance-using history (the father's history is also important) (7). An initial laboratory evaluation includes drug screening and blood work (blood group, Rh factor and antibody screen; rubella immune status; serologic test for syphilis; hepatitis B surface antigen screen; complete blood count; baseline liver function tests; baseline renal function tests). Other indicated tests include cervical cytology, cervical culture for gonorrhea, and chlamydia screen; hemoglobin electrophoresis, as indicated; tuberculin testing; and baseline sonogram. Optional studies such as human T-lymphotropic virus (HTLV)-1 testing, diabetic screening, maternal serum alpha-fetoprotein, and TORCH (toxoplasmosis, other infections, rubella, cytomegalovirus, and herpes simplex) studies, may also be considered. HIV education and counseling are essential, and maternal testing should be strongly advised as part of a campaign to achieve universal voluntary testing. The patient should meet with professionals involved in the program, including the obstetrician, neonatologist, public health nurse, community worker, and social worker, all of whom may be interacting with the patient during her hospital stay.

During labor, the patient is generally managed like any other parturient. Physicians in charge of the labor floor should be made aware of her drug use, and an effort made to start conduction anesthesia as early as possible to avoid the use of narcotic analgesics. The last dose of methadone is recorded, and, if necessary, methadone is given to the patient for analgesia and prevention of withdrawal symptoms. Because administration of naloxone (Narcan) or any other narcotic antagonist to an opiate-dependent woman in labor may result in stillbirth from fetal withdrawal, as well as more severe neonatal symptomatology immediately after birth, its use is contraindicated except as a last resort to reverse severe narcotic overdose.

IMPACT OF MATERNAL NARCOTIC USE ON FETAL WELFARE

Because of the obvious lack of quality control seen in street narcotics, the pregnant woman frequently may experience repeated episodes of withdrawal and overdose. Maternal narcotic withdrawal is associated with the occurrence of stillbirth (20,36). Severe maternal withdrawal is associated with increased muscular activity, metabolic rate, and oxygen consumption. At the same time, fetal activity also increases, and the increased oxygen needs of the fetus may not be met if labor contractions coincide with abstinence symptoms in the mother. As the pregnancy proceeds, the fetal metabolic rate and oxygen consumption increase; therefore, a pregnant woman undergoing severe abstinence symptoms during the latter part of pregnancy would be less likely to supply the withdrawing fetus with the oxygen it needs than would an addict in the first trimester of pregnancy (36).

Fetal Growth

Abundant animal laboratory evidence suggests that heroin directly causes fetal growth retardation; this observation is well supported by human data (21,32,37–39). Although earlier reports did not differentiate between premature infants and term infants who were small for gestational age, it is now evident that many of these low-birth-weight infants were, in fact, small for gestational age. Naeye (40) found that infants born to heroin addicts were, as a group, growth-retarded, with all of their organs affected. Naeye observed that the small size of many of these organs in infants exposed to heroin was mainly a result of a subnormal number of cells; this finding could not be explained by maternal undernutrition. Nearly 60% of the mothers or their newborn infants, most of whom delivered prematurely, showed evidence of acute infection. The placentas of the heroin-exposed infants commonly revealed meconium histiocytosis, suggesting that episodes of distress had occurred during fetal life.

In an analysis of 338 neonates, Kandall et al. (33) found that the mean birth weight of infants born to mothers using heroin during the pregnancy was 2,490 g, an effect primarily caused by intrauterine growth retardation. Low mean birth weight was also seen both in infants born to mothers who had used heroin only prior to this pregnancy (2,615 g) and to mothers who had used both heroin and methadone during the pregnancy (2,535 g). Infants born to mothers on methadone maintenance during the pregnancy, however, had significantly higher mean birth weights (2,961 g), although they remained lower than those of the control group (3,176 g). A highly linear significant relationship accounting for 27% of the variance was observed between maternal methadone dosage in the first trimester and birth weight. This study thus suggested that methadone administration to opiate-addicted mothers could promote fetal growth in a dose-related fashion.

In a subsequent study of 150 drug-exposed mother–infant pairs and 150 controls, Doberczak et al. (41) found that the mean birth weight of the drug-dependent infants was 2,800 g, significantly less than the 3,248-g mean birth weight of the controls. Low birth weight was primarily a consequence of intrauterine growth retardation (20% in drug-exposed group vs. 4% in controls); mean gestational age did not differ between the two groups. In addition, mean head circumference of the drug-exposed group was 32.6 cm, significantly less than the 33.8-cm mean head circumference of controls. This study thus documented a pattern of symmetric or proportional growth retardation in a large series of drug-exposed infants.

Various other parameters, including prostaglandin levels, corticosteroid production, estriol excretion, heat-stable alkaline phosphatase enzyme levels, liver function studies, serum immunoglobulin (Ig) M levels, and lecithin/sphingomyelin ratios in amniotic fluid have been used as research tools to assess fetal welfare; none are clinically employed on a widespread basis. Amniotic fluid lecithin:sphingomyelin (L:S) ratios as a marker of fetal lung maturity were found to be greater than that found in controls in ten narcotic-addicted pregnancies (42). This finding may correlate with animal studies by Roloff et al. (43) and Taeusch et al. (44) that demonstrated accelerated lung maturation in narcotic-exposed fetuses, as well as with a reduction in prematurity-related lung disease clinically observed by Glass et al. (45).

Laboratory and animal studies show that narcotics may have an inhibitory effect on enzymes of oxidative metabolism and oxygen-carrying cytochromes. Narcotics also alter fetal–placental perfusion by constricting the umbilical vessels and decreasing fetal brain oxygenation. These metabolic side effects may cause a decrease in oxygen availability to and utilization by the fetus, resulting in fetal hypoxia or acidosis. Chang et al. (46) reported that nalorphine, pethidine, morphine, and heroin each caused a decrease in pH and an increase in the pressure of carbon dioxide (PCO_2) in the maternal blood, and an independent decrease in pH and base excess in the fetal scalp blood. This was thought to be caused by the respiratory depressant effect of the drugs, supporting the suggestion that narcotic agents may have subtle adverse metabolic effects on the fetus.

Archie et al. (47) found a significant decrease in fetal movements and cardiac accelerations on nonstress testing following administration of a methadone dose (mean dose: 26 mg) to 30 women at a mean time of 34 weeks gestation. Richardson et al. (48), in a study of six methadone-maintained patients at between 28 and 40 weeks gestation, found that fetal breathing movements were decreased both before and after maternal methadone administration compared to controls; fetal respiratory responses were also blunted after administration of 5% carbon dioxide to the mothers. The authors suggested that this blunted response could be predictive of subsequent respiratory regulatory abnormalities such as sudden infant death syndrome (SIDS). Wittman et al. (49) found that a single dose of methadone averaging 40 mg (range: 30 to 75 mg) significantly reduced fetal activity and respiratory activity and increased periods of inactivity 1 hour after administration of the medication. Split-dosing every 12 hours, however, was associated with an insignificant change in parameters monitored. These studies suggest that certain women might benefit from split-dosing of daily methadone in achieving more optimal fetal stability.

Little information is available regarding the intrapartum course of opiate-using women. Silver et al. (50) reported that the duration of the first, second, and third stages of labor was similar in 112 drug-dependent women and 224 controls. The rate of cesarean sections and complications of labor also did not differ between the groups. Drug-dependent women, however, received more analgesia and anesthesia, specifically epidural anesthesia, which the authors speculated might have reduced perineal sensation and maternal bearing down, accounting for an increase in forceps deliveries.

Transition from intrauterine to extrauterine life usually proceeds smoothly in the opiate-exposed infant. As a measure of this transition, Apgar scores are usually normal. Kandall et al. (23) reported that meconium staining is seen more commonly in the setting of maternal heroin abuse than with methadone maintenance, reflecting the more stable intrauterine milieu in the latter. Airway toilet and mechanical aspiration of meconium and secretions from the infant's airway should be carried out with equipment that protects the resuscitator's mouth from blood and secretions. Universal precautions for handling of all newborn infants should be stressed in this population because of the increased risk of hepatitis B and HIV transmission.

Early studies found that heroin-exposed and methadone-exposed infants showed an increased incidence of chromosomal aberrations (51,52) and abnormal palmar creases (53). Based on such studies, concern was raised that drug abuse could produce irreversible fetal chromosome damage. Considering the many high-risk variables frequently associated with drug-involved pregnancies, and most notably in the absence of any specific teratology in drug-exposed infants, it has thus far been impossible to link either methadone or heroin with clinically evident genetic damage.

ACUTE MORBIDITY AND MORTALITY IN THE INFANT BORN TO THE NARCOTIC-DEPENDENT WOMAN

Many of the medical complications seen in the neonates of heroin-dependent women are secondary to low birth weight and prematurity. Therefore, in addition to the neonatal abstinence syndrome, conditions such as asphyxia

neonatorum, intracranial hemorrhage, nutritional deprivation, hypoglycemia, hypocalcemia, septicemia, and hyperbilirubinemia should be anticipated in opiate-exposed low-birth-weight babies. Because infants born to women who receive methadone maintenance are more apt to have higher birth weights and a decreased incidence of premature birth, medical complications in that group of infants generally reflect: (a) the amount of prenatal care that the mother has received; (b) whether she has suffered particular obstetric or medical complications, such as hypertension or toxemia of pregnancy, placental accidents, or infection; and, most importantly, (c) multiple-drug use that may produce an unstable intrauterine milieu complicated by withdrawal and overdose.

At Family Center in Philadelphia (20), morbidity in infants born to drug-dependent women was dependent upon the amount of prenatal care as well as the kind of maternal drug intake (heroin vs. methadone). More than 75% of infants born to heroin addicts without prenatal care, as well as those born to methadone-maintained women with suboptimal prenatal care, suffered neonatal morbidity. This morbidity was somewhat decreased in infants born to methadone-maintained women who had received adequate prenatal care. Mean duration of hospitalization was 17 days for infants of methadone-maintained mothers and 27 days for infants of heroin-addicted mothers.

Also at Family Center in Philadelphia, data on 278 infants born to drug-dependent women and 1,586 control infants from the general population delivering at the municipal hospital revealed an increased incidence of low birth weight and neonatal mortality in the infants of drug-dependent women (54). A study of infants born to heroin- and methadone-dependent mothers (the latter a stratified group of women having inadequate and adequate prenatal care), revealed an overall mortality incidence of 5.4% compared to 1.6% in controls. In low-birth-weight infants, mortality in the drug-dependent population reached 13.3%, compared with 10% in the controls. Within the methadone-dependent group, better outcomes were achieved with adequate prenatal care. Overall mortality in the methadone/inadequate care group was 10%, compared with 3% in the methadone/adequate prenatal care group and 4.8% in the heroin-dependent group. The same trend was found in the mortality rates seen in the low-birth-weight infants. These data confirmed that comprehensive care for pregnant drug-dependent women significantly reduced the morbidity and mortality in both the mother and the infant.

Detailed neuropathologic studies were performed following death of ten of the infants in the previous study (55). Eight categories of lesions were found, three of which were thought to bear some specific relationship to maternal drug dependence. These lesions included gliosis (5), foci of old infarction (4), and developmental retardation of the brain (3). In addition, minor microscopic brain malformations were found in three cases. Other lesions identified included those common to high-risk neonates: germinal plate hemorrhage (7), acute brain necrosis with and without hemorrhage (5), germinal plate cysts (4), and focal subarachnoid hemorrhages (3). Although the majority of the findings may be caused by nonspecific secondary gestational complications, these neuropathologic findings tentatively suggest primary and specific effects of addictive drugs with concomitant anoxic episodes on the developing nervous system.

NEONATAL NARCOTIC ABSTINENCE SYNDROME

Description of Symptomatology

During the 1950s and 1960s, numerous reports in the medical literature described the symptoms of heroin abstinence in the newborn (56–60). Since then an increasing number of reports have described the neonatal abstinence syndrome caused by combinations of heroin and methadone dependence exposure during pregnancy (23,61–66).

Clear delineation of narcotic-related abstinence has been made more difficult by the recognition that a number of nonnarcotic drugs are capable of causing fetal dependence and subsequent neonatal abstinence (Table 53.3). In addition to the barbiturates (67,68), certain sedatives, minor tranquilizers, and stimulants have been incriminated, including bromide, chlordiazepoxide (Librium), diazepam (Valium), diphenhydramine hydrochloride (Benadryl), ethchlorvynol (Placidyl), glutethimide (Doriden), hydroxyzine hydrochloride (Atarax), desipramine (Pertofrane), pentazocine (Talwin), and propoxyphene hydrochloride (Darvon) (69–82).

Alcohol (83,84) has also been reported to produce neonatal withdrawal symptomatology. A study of 60 drug-dependent infants randomly chosen from 275 consecutive births in the Philadelphia comprehensive care methadone maintenance program between 1975 and 1979 indicated

TABLE 53.3. *Pharmacologic agents that may cause abstinence symptoms in the neonate*

Alcohol
Barbiturates
Bromides
Chlordiazepoxide (Librium)
Diazepam (Valium)
Diphenhydramine hydrochloride (Benadryl)
Ethchlorvynol (Placidyl)
Glutethimide (Doriden)
Hydroxyzine hydrochloride (Atarax)
Desipramine (Pertofran)
Opioids: opium, meperidine, methadone, morphine, oxycodone hydrochloride
Pentazocine (Talwin)
Propoxyphene hydrochloride (Darvon)

TABLE 53.4. *Abstinence symptoms in the neonatal period: frequency seen in 138 newborns at family center program in Philadelphia*

Symptoms	Frequency (%)
Tremors	
Mild/disturbed	96
Mild/undisturbed	95
Marked/disturbed	77
Marked/undisturbed	67
High-pitched cry	95
Continuous high-pitched cry	54
Sneezing	83
Increased muscle tone	82
Frantic sucking of fists	79
Regurgitation	74
Sleeps <3 hours after feeding	65
Sleeps <2 hours after feeding	66
Sleeps <1 hour after feeding	58
Respiratory rate >60 breaths per minute	66
Poor feeding	65
Hyperactive Moro reflex	62
Loose stools	51
Sweating	49
Excoriation	43
Mottling	33
Nasal stuffiness	33
Frequent yawning	30
Fever less than 101°F	29
Respiratory rate >60 breaths per minute, retractions	28
Markedly hyperactive Moro reflex	15
Projectile vomiting	12
Watery stools	12
Fever higher than 101°F	3
Dehydration	1
Generalized convulsions	1

that changing patterns of polydrug abuse markedly increased the duration of pharmacotherapy needed for control of neonatal abstinence associated with maternal methadone administration (85).

Neonatal narcotic abstinence syndrome is described as a generalized disorder characterized by signs and symptoms of central nervous system hyperirritability, gastrointestinal dysfunction, respiratory distress, and autonomic symptoms that include yawning, sneezing, mottling, and fever (Table 53.4).

Central Nervous System

Opiate-exposed infants tend initially to develop mild high-frequency, low-amplitude tremors that progress in severity if untreated. High-pitched cry, increased muscle tone, irritability, increased deep tendon reflexes, and an exaggerated Moro reflex are all characteristic of neonatal abstinence. These infants show an exaggerated rooting reflex and a voracious appetite manifested as sucking of fists or thumbs, yet when feedings are administered the infants may have extreme difficulty because of an ineffectual sucking reflex and incoordination of the suck–swallow mechanism. Feeding may be so impaired that formula may have to be "milked" into the infant. Kron et al. (86) found that both heroin-exposed and methadone-exposed infants have reduced sucking rates and pressures, disordered sucking organization, and a reduction in amounts of nutrients consumed. Two early studies in small numbers of heroin-exposed infants reported alterations in rapid eye movement (REM) sleep (87,88). Pasto et al. (89) studied serial cerebral sonographic characteristics of methadone-exposed infants at birth, 1 month, and 6 months of age. Methadone-exposed infants showed significantly increased incidences of slit-like ventricles at all three examinations. Although the pathophysiology of this abnormality is not clear, neither cerebral edema nor increased intracranial pressure could be demonstrated.

Seizures may occur as the most dramatic drug-associated central nervous system abnormality. Reported incidences of seizures vary among published series, perhaps because these seizures may be subtle. In addition, recommended treatment for neonatal abstinence often calls for tightly swaddling the infant in a darkened room, exactly those conditions that could lead to failure to note seizure movements. Zelson et al. (39,66) found that seizures were seen more frequently in infants of methadone-dependent mothers compared to heroin-exposed infants. Finnegan (90) found that 1% of infants who had withdrawn from heroin and/or methadone had evidenced generalized seizures. Davis et al. (91) observed myoclonic jerks in 7 of 49 methadone-exposed babies and tonic–clonic seizures in 5 others; myoclonic jerks were seen in 2 of 21 heroin-exposed infants and tonic–clonic seizures in 1 additional infant.

The most extensive report on abstinence-associated seizures was published by Herzlinger et al. (92). Among 302 neonates passively exposed to narcotics during pregnancy, 18 (5.9%) had seizures that were attributed to withdrawal. Of these 18 infants, 10 were among the 127 infants (7.8%) exposed to methadone, 4 were among the 78 (5.1%) exposed to methadone and heroin, and 3 were among the 14 (21.4%) exposed to "other" drugs taken during pregnancy. There was no apparent relationship between maternal methadone dose (10 to 100 mg/day) and frequency or severity of seizures, and no correlations were found between seizures and birth weight, gestational age, occurrence of other withdrawal symptoms, day of onset of withdrawal symptoms, or the need for specific pharmacologic treatment. All infants with seizures manifested other withdrawal symptoms prior to the initial seizure. Only 2 of 48 infants initially treated for withdrawal with paregoric subsequently developed seizures, compared with 5 of the 12 infants initially treated with diazepam. Seizures occurred at a mean age of 10 days, with a range of 3 to 34 days. Generalized motor seizures or rhythmic myoclonic jerks, each of which occurred in seven infants, were the principal seizure manifestations. In 18 infants, however, seizure manifestations were complex, and 3 of the 18 had refractory seizure activity. Paregoric was more effective than diazepam in controlling both initial and subsequent seizure episodes. Six electroencephalograms (EEGs) were normal after clinical seizures had ceased. Although some reports indicate uncertainty with regard to the mechanism of neonatal myoclonic jerks in the neonatal abstinence syndrome (28,93,94), the report by Herzlinger et al. suggests that such movements are true seizures.

In a subsequent study, Kandall et al. (95) studied 153 infants born following intrauterine opiate exposure. Twelve (7.8%) of those 153 infants demonstrated neonatal seizures that could not be otherwise explained. Seizures were unrelated to maternal age, parity, last methadone dosage, length of drug use, degree of polydrug use, gender, gestational age, 1-minute Apgar score, time of initial treatment, or severity of abstinence. However, the seizure group did have lower 5-minute Apgar scores, suggesting that mild asphyxia may potentiate abstinence-associated seizures. Mean time of seizure onset was 9.7 days, with a range of 5 to 26 days. Noteworthy was the observation that none of the 49 infants treated with paregoric developed seizures, while 7 of the 62 phenobarbital-treated infants developed seizures. The authors postulated that phenobarbital dosages used to control abstinence (see page 819) were inadequate to provide antiseizure prophylaxis in the face of enhanced methadone clearance induced by phenobarbital.

The only followup of infants with abstinence-associated seizures was published by Doberczak et al. (96). Despite abnormal neurologic examinations in 8 of 12 infants early in life, all neurologic examinations and EEG tracings normalized during the first year of life. Infant assessment remained normal during the first year of life and did not differ from either passively addicted infants without seizures or from published norms. This short-term favorable prognosis suggests that the pathophysiologic mechanism of these seizures differs from that associated with more ominous types of neonatal seizures.

Gastrointestinal

Regurgitation, projectile vomiting, and loose stools may be seen in the course of neonatal abstinence. Dehydration as a consequence of poor intake, coupled with increased losses from the gastrointestinal tract, may cause excessive weight loss, electrolyte imbalance, shock, coma, and death. Weinberger et al. (97) found that drug-exposed newborns who developed mild abstinence not requiring specific pharmacotherapy lost an average of only 4% of birth weight, reached a weight nadir on day 3, and regained birth weight by day 7 of life. Newborns displaying more severe abstinence lost more weight and did not regain birth weight until an average of 2 weeks of age. These data suggest that timely and appropriate pharmacologic control of abstinence, as well as provision of extra fluids and calories to offset both clinically apparent and insensible losses, are important in the management of neonatal abstinence.

Respiratory

The opiate abstinence syndrome may include excessive secretions, nasal stuffiness, sometimes accompanied by retractions, intermittent cyanosis, and apnea (98). Severe respiratory distress occurs most often when the infant regurgitates, aspirates, and develops aspiration pneumonia. Infants with acute heroin withdrawal show increased respiratory rates, leading to hypocapnia and an increase in blood pH during the first week of life (99). As noted previously, the incidence of idiopathic respiratory distress syndrome is decreased in heroin-exposed infants, either as a result of chronic intrauterine stress or of accelerated heroin-mediated maturation of lung function, or perhaps both. Newborn infants have decreased levels of 2,3-diphosphoglycerate (DPG) and, therefore, cannot unload oxygen effectively at the tissue level. In one study (100), mean values of the oxygen half-saturation pressure of hemoglobin (P-50) in the cord blood and total 2,3-DPG in red blood cells were increased in the opiate-addicted infants when compared with normal controls.

Autonomic Nervous System

Behrendt and Green (101) found that 8 of 20 low-birth-weight infants of heroin-addicted mothers had spontaneous generalized sweating compared to only 2 of 108 healthy low-birth-weight babies. In addition, the pharmacologic threshold for sweating was decreased in the drug-exposed infants. Other autonomic nervous system signs seen during abstinence include hyperpyrexia and lacrimation, both of which increase water loss.

Other Effects

Nathenson et al. (102) found a lack of significant jaundice among infants of heroin-addicted mothers. Further investigation demonstrated increased bilirubin glucuronide transferase activity in morphine-addicted mice and an electron microscopic increase in the smooth endoplasmic reticulum of their liver cells. The significance of increased hepatic bilirubin glucuronide transferase activity by opiates may extend beyond the metabolism of bilirubin to enhanced excretion of other biologic substances requiring glucuronidation or to induction of other enzyme systems within and beyond the liver.

Burstein et al. (103) found a significant thrombocytosis in 33 prospectively studied methadone-exposed infants. Platelet counts rose during the second week of life, peaked at about 10 weeks of life, and returned to normal slowly during the next 8 months. Platelet levels exceeding 1,000,000/mm^3 were found in seven infants. Fifteen of the studied patients had increased circulating platelet aggregates. Despite this abnormal platelet pattern, other hematologic parameters, including hemoglobin concentration and white cell count, were normal.

Jhaveri et al. (104), in a study of 14 methadone-exposed infants, found increased levels of T_3 (triiodothyronine) on days 2 and 7, and increased levels of T_4 (thyroxine) on days 2, 3, and 7, when compared to control infants. Although maternal drug-taking was not limited to methadone and despite a range of gestational ages in the infants, the authors speculated that this biochemical evidence of hyperthyroidism was related either to altered autonomic function or increased metabolic activity associated with neonatal withdrawal.

Determinants and Patterns of Neonatal Abstinence

Confirmation of fetal drug exposure has classically been documented through urine toxicologic assay. These assays have been performed first with a screening method such as immunoassay, and then confirmed with a more specific testing procedure such as gas chromatography-mass spectroscopy. Confirmation is considered an essential part of drug testing because of the legal and social service implications of a positive test. It should be recognized, however, that the criteria for obtaining a urine toxicology and the actions that flow from a positive result vary widely from state to state and even within the same state.

There is increasing interest in the use of meconium for toxicologic testing. Throughout gestation, drugs are metabolized by the fetal liver and excreted into the urine or bile. Because the fetus does not usually pass stool *in utero*, meconium, containing its drug metabolites, represents a waste product that accumulates throughout the gestation. Meconium testing therefore represents a much wider window of drug exposure than does urine testing. Ostrea et al. (105) showed, in both human and animal studies, that meconium represented an excellent source from which metabolites of illicit drugs could be retrieved. In a subsequent study of more than 3,000 neonates at Hutzel Hospital in Detroit, Ostrea et al. (106) found that meconium drug testing yielded almost twice the number of positive drug tests than urine testing, and four times that found by maternal self-report.

Not all infants born to drug-dependent mothers show withdrawal symptomatology. Several investigators report that between 60% and 90% of infants show symptoms (23,39,53,56,58). Because the biochemical and physiologic processes governing withdrawal are still poorly understood, and because polydrug abuse, erratic drug taking, and vague and inaccurate maternal histories complicate accurate data gathering, it is not surprising to find differing descriptions and experiences in reports from different centers.

Time of onset of abstinence symptoms varies. Once the infant is delivered, serum and tissue levels of the drug or drugs used by the mother begin to fall. The newborn infant continues to metabolize and excrete the drug, and signs of abstinence occur when critically low tissue levels have been reached. Rosen and Pippenger (107) could not demonstrate a relationship between maternal methadone dosage and neonatal abstinence, but found that abstinence was most closely correlated with the rate of excretion of methadone by the drug-exposed neonate. The authors found that plasma levels of 0.06 μg/mL protected the infant from abstinence; levels falling below that point were associated with the onset of abstinence. Recovery from the abstinence syndrome is gradual and occurs as the infant's metabolism adjusts to the absence of the dependence-producing agent.

Immediately after birth, if the mother has continued her drug use, most passively dependent infants, whether born to heroin-addicted or methadone-dependent women, seem physically and behaviorally normal. Heroin is not stored by the fetus to any appreciable extent; if the mother has been on heroin alone, the majority (80%) of infants will develop clinical signs of withdrawal between 4 and 24 hours of age. Methadone, however, is stored by the fetus, primarily in the lung, liver, and spleen (34,35). If the mother has been on methadone alone, the baby's symptoms usually appear within the first 24 to 72 hours but may appear somewhat later. Several methadone-exposed babies have had their onset of major withdrawal after the first or second week of life (108).

The type and amount of drug or drugs used by the mother, timing of her dose before delivery, and the presence or absence of intrinsic disease in the infant which, may affect drug metabolism and excretion, may all play a role in determining the time of onset in the individual infant. Withdrawal may be mild and transient, delayed in onset, have a stepwise increase in severity, be intermittently present, or have a biphasic course that includes acute neonatal withdrawal followed by improvement and then an exacerbation of acute withdrawal.

In an early study, Blinick (109) reported mild to moderate withdrawal symptoms in 9 of 19 infants exposed to methadone; none of the infants developed severe symptoms. Rajegowda et al. (110) found a higher incidence and more prolonged duration of withdrawal symptoms in methadone-exposed infants than in those exposed to heroin. However, mothers in Rajegowda's study were on higher doses of methadone (80 to 160 mg/day) than were Blinick's patients (60 to 120 mg/day). Zelson et al. (39) found an increase in severity of withdrawal and a higher number of seizures among 34 infants born to mothers who had used methadone alone or in combination with heroin, than in 24 infants born to mothers who used heroin only. Davis et al. (111) found that 80% of infants born to women maintained on low doses of methadone (mean: 45 mg/day) had evidence of withdrawal, but fewer than one-third of the 80% showed signs that were severe enough to require therapy.

In a study of 196 drug-exposed infants at Hutzel Hospital in Detroit, Ostrea et al. (63) found that the severity of neonatal withdrawal did not correlate with the infant's gestational age, sex, race, or Apgar score, with maternal age, parity, or duration of heroin intake, or with the level of morphine measured in the infant's urine or blood. Reduction in the amount of illumination and noise in a study nursery also did not lower the incidence of severe withdrawal in the infants. A significant correlation between the severity of withdrawal in the infant and the maternal methadone dose prompted the recommendation that mothers on methadone treatment should be put on a low dose of drug (less than 20 mg/day) as soon as it is safely possible. Similar conclusions were reached by Madden et al. (112), who suggested a reduction of methadone to less than 20 mg daily in late pregnancy. A study at Philadelphia General Hospital (20) involving 260 pregnant addicts treated with methadone and street addicts on heroin showed a reduced incidence of severe withdrawal (12.5%) associated with low-dose methadone, compared with 25% among infants of mothers on heroin only.

In contrast to these reports, a pilot study in Philadelphia showed that dose does not correlate with severity of neonatal abstinence. Although the effects of methadone maintenance during pregnancy have been well investigated, the dosage range of methadone for pregnant women remains a topic of clinical debate. Clinicians either have followed regimens that recommend a low dose of 20 mg daily of methadone or a more flexible one where the most "effective" dose is given. The latter may be associated with an increased dose in the last trimester.

Very little information exists regarding doses of greater than 80 mg throughout the pregnancy. In Philadelphia, Kaltenbach and others studied women who received methadone in a dosage of greater than 80 mg and women who received 80 mg or less. The mean dose for the first group was 81 mg and for the second, it was 52 mg throughout pregnancy. No significant differences were found between the groups on birth weight, length, head circumference, and severity of withdrawal. Overall, women who received 80 mg or more were more successful in reducing their drug use during pregnancy as indicated by the percentage of urine drug screens that were positive only for methadone. However, length of time in methadone maintenance treatment, history of other drug use, and maintenance dose prior to pregnancy are factors that first must be taken into account in evaluating methadone dose during pregnancy (113).

Doberczak et al. (114) reported that more term infants (145 of 178) required treatment for abstinence than did the preterm infants (20 of 34) and that abstinence severity correlated with gestational age; less-mature infants showed lesser abstinence. The authors postulated that this reduced severity of abstinence could be a result of either

(a) developmental immaturity of the preterm nervous system, (b) reduced total drug exposure in shortened gestations, or (c) insensitivity of the testing instrument to gestational age and neurologic development of neonates.

A number of studies attempted to correlate drug levels in various body fluids to neonatal outcome. Blinick et al. (115) could not establish a simple relationship between the concentration of methadone in maternal plasma and urine of pregnant women on methadone to levels of amniotic fluid, cord blood, fetal urine, and breast milk, or to the intensity of the neonatal withdrawal syndrome. Harper et al. (22) found that the severity of neonatal abstinence correlated positively with the total amount of methadone ingested by the mother during the last 12 weeks of pregnancy, the maternal dose of methadone at the time of delivery, and the intrapartum maternal serum methadone level, suggesting that a strategy of reducing the methadone dose during pregnancy might constitute optimal management. Doberczak et al. (116) found an association between maternal methadone dosage at delivery and maternal plasma methadone level drawn 16 hours after delivery; the latter correlated significantly with the neonatal plasma methadone level on day 1 of life. The authors also found that severity of neonatal abstinence correlated with the rate of decline of neonatal plasma methadone level from day 1 to day 4. These data support those of Rosen and Pippenger in suggesting that the rate of disposition of methadone from tissue or plasma influences the onset and severity of neonatal abstinence.

Because of the variable severity of the withdrawal, the duration of symptoms may last anywhere from 6 days to 8 weeks. Although the infants are discharged from the hospital after drug therapy is stopped, their symptoms of irritability may persist for more than 3 or 4 months (117). Although unrecognized, untreated, prolonged abstinence carries a risk of death, earlier detection of the maternal drug use, more accurate laboratory diagnosis, and prompt treatment of the infant have essentially eliminated the mortality attributed to acute neonatal abstinence.

Behavioral Studies in the Neonatal Period

Many animal studies have demonstrated developmental, neuroendocrine, and behavioral effects of opiate exposure in young offspring. These effects include, among many others, an impaired ability to learn a condition suppression response (118), differences in reflex development (119), and altered response to stress (120).

In human neonates, the Brazelton Neonatal Assessment Scale has been used extensively to evaluate newborn behavior. This instrument assesses habituation to stimuli such as a light or bell sound, responsivity to animate and inanimate stimuli (face, voice, bell, rattle), state (sleep to alertness to crying) and the requirements of state change (such as irritability and consolability), and neurologic and motor development. Soule et al. (121) compared

19 methadone-exposed babies who had received no pharmacologic treatment prior to the first examination with 41 babies who were subjects of an unrelated developmental study. Group differences in scores on the Brazelton Scale at 48 and 72 hours of age indicated that methadone-exposed babies were restless, tended to be in a neurologically irritable condition, cried more often, and were state-labile. The infants were also more tremulous and hypertonic, and manifested less motor maturity than did the control group. In addition, although quite available and responsive auditorily, the methadone-exposed subjects responded poorly to visual stimuli.

Strauss et al. (122) also found that addicted infants were less able to be maintained in an alert state and less able to orient to auditory and visual stimuli, signs that were most pronounced at 48 hours of age. Despite increased irritability, drug-exposed infants were as capable of self-quieting and responding to soothing intervention as normal neonates. These findings have substantial implications for caregivers' perceptions of infants and thus may have long-term impact on the development of infant-caregiver interaction patterns. These implications have been further developed by Kaltenbach and Finnegan (123), who found that infants born to methadone-maintained women showed deficiencies in their attention and social responsiveness during the first few days of life; these abnormalities persisted during the infants' course of abstinence and treatment. Fitzgerald et al. (124) found that the interaction of drug-dependent mothers and their infants showed abnormalities on measures of social engagement; this dyadic interaction was explained by less maternal positive affect and attachment, as well as infant behavior impeding social involvement. Many of these interactive abnormalities normalized by 4 months of age, but the need for "parenting training" was underscored by these findings.

Lodge et al. (125) noted that infants born to mothers on varying doses of methadone showed withdrawal-associated heightened auditory responsiveness and orientation, lowered overall alertness, and poor attentiveness to a visual stimulus compared to controls. Electroencephalographic recordings revealed high-frequency dyssynchronous activity suggestive of central nervous system irritability, as well as low arousal responses to visual stimulation.

Drug-exposed infants show an uncoordinated and ineffectual sucking reflex as a major manifestation of abstinence. Kron et al. (86) measured the rate, pressure, and organization of sucking, as well as nutrient consumption in drug-exposed neonates. Sucking rates and pressure parameters were felt to be most sensitive in distinguishing between the control and the drug-exposed populations. Paregoric-treated infants tended to suck more vigorously than infants treated with sedatives such as phenobarbital and were even superior to those who received no therapy at all. Diazepam-treated infants were found to show depressed feeding behavior. These studies provide support for a pharmacotherapeutic approach to the treatment of neonatal abstinence.

Most recently a neurodevelopmental followup battery of tests was developed to assess substance-exposed infants as part of a multicenter prospective study in the National Institute of Child Health and Human Development (NICHD) Neonatal Research Network in conjunction with NIDA. This battery, called the Neonatal Network Neurobehavioral Scale (NNNS), developed by Lester, Tronick, Mayes and Zuckerman, is being used to assess developmental constructs at eight time-points from 1 to 36 months of age (126).

Assessment and Management of Neonatal Abstinence

It is important to stress that unrecognized and untreated neonatal opiate abstinence may result in death as a consequence of factors such as excess fluid losses, hyperpyrexia, seizures, respiratory instability, aspiration, and apnea. With proper management, the neonate's prognosis for recovery from the acute phase of abstinence should be excellent. It should also be stressed that because of the nonspecific nature of signs of neonatal abstinence, other potentially serious illnesses such as bacterial sepsis and/or meningitis, intracranial hemorrhage, and metabolic disorders such as hypoglycemia, hyponatremia, or hypernatremia, which may mimic abstinence, should also be considered in symptomatic opiate-exposed newborns.

Because not all infants born to drug-dependent women develop abstinence, prophylactic drug therapy is not recommended. The asymptomatic narcotic-exposed infant should be observed in the hospital for at least 4 days. Even if the infant is still symptom-free and evaluation of the home and mothering capability has been adequate to permit discharge, observation at close intervals must be continued. A disrupted social situation or polydrug abuse may mandate a longer period of observation in the hospital. In any case, a home visit or return appointment should be made within a few days after discharge and the mother alerted to the possibility of late onset of withdrawal signs (108) that might necessitate readmission.

When signs of abstinence do appear, simple nonspecific measures should be instituted. An individualized treatment program using supportive techniques may ameliorate the abstinence in opiate-exposed babies. These techniques include reducing noxious environmental stimuli, positioning which encourages flexion rather than extension, and individualized handling procedures based on the infant's level of tolerance. Gentle swaddling should be used to reinforce flexion and infant comfort. Demand feeding, sometimes as frequently as every two hours, has been found to reduce irritability.

Indications for specific pharmacotherapy, dosage schedules, and duration of treatment courses have varied widely. Some of this variation is undoubtedly a result

of observer difference in judging severity of symptoms. To improve the objectivity of these judgments, the use of a neonatal abstinence scoring system is strongly recommended. Although other scales have been proposed (127,128), the Finnegan's 21-symptom rating scale is most widely used as a research tool and treatment guide (Table 53.5). All infants born to drug-dependent mothers are assessed for withdrawal symptomatology by using this dynamic scoring scale at 2-hour intervals for the first 48 hours of life, then every 4 hours thereafter. If at any point the infant's score is 8 or greater (regardless of age), every 2-hour scoring is initiated and continued for 24 hours from the last total score of 8 or greater. If the 2-hour scores continue to be 7 or less for 24 hours, then 4-hour scoring intervals are resumed. Pharmacologic intervention is begun when the total abstinence score is 8 or greater for three consecutive scorings, or when the average of any three consecutive scores is 8 or greater. The total abstinence score also dictates the dosage of the pharmacotherapeutic agent (i.e., the dosage is titrated against the total abstinence score). The specific details of the use of the scoring system have been reported elsewhere (90,129).

Both a replacement opiate such as paregoric (camphorated tincture of opium) or a nonspecific central nervous system depressant such as phenobarbital (in cases complicated by polydrug use) appear to be effective in treating neonatal opiate abstinence (8). Generally, dosages of medication must be regulated so that the infant's symptoms are minimized without excessive sedation. Paregoric treatment begins with an oral dosage of 0.2 mL every 3 hours. If symptoms are not controlled based on the severity scale, dosages are increased by 0.05 mL to a maximum of 0.4 mL every 3 hours. The stabilizing dosage is maintained for 5 days, following which the dosage is slowly reduced by 0.05 mL every other day, maintaining a dosing regimen of every 3 hours.

Despite its record of efficacy and safety, recent concerns have been raised about the safety of other ingredients found in paregoric (130). The Committee on Drugs of the American Academy of Pediatrics cautioned that paregoric contains the isoquinoline derivatives noscapine and papaverine, which are antispasmodics. Paregoric also contains camphor, a potentially dangerous central nervous system stimulant (131), which is lipid-soluble and requires glucuronidation for excretion. In addition, paregoric also contains alcohol, anise oil, and glycerin. Finally, paregoric contains 4 mg/mL of benzoic acid, which may compete for bilirubin binding sites. Its oxidative product, benzyl alcohol, has been reported to cause a syndrome of severe acidosis, central nervous system depression, hypotension, renal failure, seizures, and death in small premature infants who receive large doses of benzyl alcohol (132).

Because of these concerns, the Committee on Drugs of the American Academy of Pediatrics recommends tincture of opium as the treatment of choice for neonatal opioid abstinence (130). The committee's recommendation

TABLE 53.5. *Neonatal abstinence scoring system*

System	Signs and symptoms	Score	AM	PM	Comments
Central Nervous System Disturbances	Excessive high-pitched (or other) cry	2			Daily Weight
	Continuous high-pitched (or other) cry	3			
	Sleeps <1 hour after feeding	3			
	Sleeps <2 hours after feeding	2			
	Sleeps <3 hours after feeding	1			
	Hyperactive Moro reflex	2			
	Markedly hyperactive Moro reflex	3			
	Mild tremors disturbed	1			
	Moderate-severe tremors disturbed	2			
	Mild tremors undisturbed	3			
	Moderate-severe tremors undisturbed	4			
	Increased muscle tone	2			
	Excoriation (specific area)	1			
	Myoclonic jerks	3			
	Generalized convulsions	5			
Metabolic Vasomotor Respiratory Disturbances	Sweating	1			
	Fever <101° (99–100.8°F or 37.2–38.2°C)	1			
	Fever >101° (38.4°C and higher)	2			
	Frequent yawning (>3–4 times/interval)	1			
	Mottling	1			
	Nasal stuffiness	1			
	Sneezing (>3–4 times/interval)	1			
	Nasal flaring	2			
	Respiratory rate >60/minute	1			
	Respiratory rate >60/minute with retractions	2			
Gastrointestinal Disturbances	Excessive sucking	1			
	Poor feeding	2			
	Regurgitation	2			
	Projectile vomiting	3			
	Loose stools	2			
	Watery stools	3			
	Total Score				
	Initials of scorer				

From Finnegan LP. Neonatal abstinence syndrome: assessment and pharmacotherapy. In: Rubaltelli FF, Granati B, eds. *Neonatal therapy: an update.* New York: Elsevier Science, 1986:136.

calls for the use of a 25-fold dilution of tincture of opium, which results in an equivalent concentration of morphine as in paregoric. Dosage regimens can therefore be used in the same way as paregoric, using one of the above regimens. Using one of the severity scoring systems, tincture of opium dosages may be tapered in the same way as with paregoric.

Although opiate abstinence is best treated with another opiate medication, polydrug abuse in which nonopiate use is suspected or confirmed is probably better treated by taking advantage of the wider therapeutic spectrum of phenobarbital (8,133). After a loading dose of 5 mg/kg of phenobarbital intramuscularly or intravenously, a maintenance dose of between 3 and 5 mg/kg per day should be started. Using the severity scale, phenobarbital dosages can be increased by 1 mg/kg to a stabilizing dosage that generally should not exceed 10 mg/kg per day. Others have recommended much higher loading dosages (22), but use of higher dosing carries the risk of excessive sedation and poor infant feeding.

Few controlled studies exist comparing the efficacy of these two therapies. Kandall et al. (95) found that control of abstinence appeared equally effective in 49 infants treated with paregoric and 62 infants treated with phenobarbital; however, seizures developed only in the phenobarbital-treated group. The superiority of higher-dosage paregoric over phenobarbital treatment was also demonstrated by Finnegan and Ehrlich (134) in a study of 300 neonates. In that study, paregoric-treated infants were brought under therapeutic control more rapidly and required a shorter treatment period than phenobarbital-treated infants. The use of other agents such as chlorpromazine or diazepam to treat neonatal opiate abstinence should be discouraged. In addition, methadone has been used very infrequently because its pharmacology in the human neonate has not been studied adequately.

LATER SEQUELAE OF INTRAUTERINE OPIATE EXPOSURE

Delayed Presentation of Abstinence

Late presentation of neonatal abstinence symptoms in newborns was reported by Kandall and Gartner (108). Significant symptoms, primarily irritability and tremulousness, first occurred in seven infants between 2 and 4 weeks of age. Seizures occurred in three infants, while a fourth infant showed progression of symptoms and died at 3 weeks of age. The delayed onset of symptoms may be explained by the accumulation of methadone in the lung, liver, kidney, and spleen, its gradual accumulation, and its subsequent slow excretion (34,35).

Sudden Infant Death Syndrome

Sudden infant death syndrome (SIDS) is defined as the sudden and unexpected death of an infant between 1 week and 1 year of age, whose death remains unexplained after a complete autopsy examination, full history, and death site investigation. Compared with an incidence of approximately 1 per 1,000 live births in the general population, opiate-exposed infants appear to have an increased risk of SIDS. Anecdotal and small population studies (93,135–139) have all found increased rates of SIDS in opiate-exposed infants.

The first large population study linking SIDS to maternal drug use was published by Ward et al. (140). Using a Los Angeles County, California, database from 1986 and 1987, the authors found an unadjusted SIDS rate of 8.87 per 1,000 live births, with the highest rate seen with maternal opiate use. The most extensive study was published by Kandall et al. (141), who studied SIDS rates in 1.21 million live births in New York City from 1979 to 1989. The authors identified 90 SIDS deaths among 16,409 drug-exposed infants (5.48 per 1,000 live births), about 4 times the rate in the general population. Maternal opiate use increased the risk of SIDS about sixfold; after control for high-risk variables including race/ethnicity, young maternal age, parity, maternal smoking, and low birth weight, the risk of SIDS was still three times that of the general population. Although the etiology of SIDS in either the general population or drug-exposed infants is not well understood, Olsen and Lees (142) and Richardson et al. (48) suggest that the mechanism in methadone-exposed infants lies in a reduced ventilatory arousal response to hypercapnia. The same mechanism is postulated in relation to cocaine exposure (see page 827). Kandall and Gaines (143) published an extensive review of maternal drug use and subsequent SIDS.

LONG-TERM OUTCOME OF CHILDREN EXPOSED *IN UTERO* TO NARCOTIC AGENTS

Once in-hospital pharmacologic and supportive therapy is discontinued, a paramount concern becomes appropriate discharge planning that will assure the infant's optimal growth and development. Because there is no standard method by which the disposition of these infants is decided, some infants may be discharged home with their mothers, some may be placed with relatives, and others may be placed in custody of a state agency or voluntarily released by the mother to private agencies for temporary or permanent placement. This last option may not be practical in cities where social services and courts are already understaffed and overworked. Appropriate foster care is expensive and hard to find. Pediatricians generally believe that the mother–infant association should not be dissolved except when clearly indicated. Aside from intensive drug rehabilitation and medical treatment, drug-dependent women need extensive educational and job training so that they will become productive citizens and loving mothers who will positively influence the development and socialization of their children. Supportive outpatient care or residential treatment may help to eliminate many of the medical and social problems experienced by drug-dependent women and their children.

At Family Center of Thomas Jefferson University in Philadelphia, mothers in recovery are given their infants when they are ready for discharge unless a team consisting of a nursery nurse, pediatrician, psychiatric social worker, obstetrician, and public health nurse find that the mother cannot care for her infant adequately with the supportive services available to her. With strong support from this team providing intensive psychosocial services during her pregnancy and immediately after delivery, the woman is usually prepared to cope more realistically with motherhood. However, if the team believes that she neither wishes nor is able to assume this responsibility, arrangements are made for temporary foster placement or for a relative to accept the major care duties.

Despite the fact that a drug-exposed newborn may be free of physical, behavioral, or neurologic deficits at the time of birth, one cannot assume that no adverse effect has occurred. It is generally accepted that the effects of pharmacologic agents may not become apparent for many months or years. Although heroin abuse during pregnancy has been recognized for more than 40 years and methadone treatment has been employed for more than 30 years, followup studies of opiate-exposed infants are notably fragmentary. Among the issues encountered in long-term followup assessment of this population are an inability to fully document a mother's drug intake, the difficulty in differentiating a drug's organic effects from high-risk obstetric and neonatal variables, problems in maintaining a cohort of infants for study, and the need to isolate a specific drug effect from the profound impact of parenting and the home environment. A number of long-term followup studies in opiate-exposed children commenced in the mid- to late-1970s, but with the onset of the cocaine epidemic in the mid-1980s, most of these studies were terminated. The following describes the early followup studies in opiate-exposed children.

In 1973, Wilson et al. (117) reported on the growth and development of 30 heroin-exposed infants who were observed from 3 to 34 months. Eighty percent had shown signs of neonatal withdrawal, and 60% continued to have subacute withdrawal signs for 3 to 6 months. Behavioral disturbances, predominantly hyperactivity, brief attention span, and temper outbursts were identified in 7 of 14 infants observed for 1 year or longer; 2 had neurologic abnormalities. These disturbances seemed to be unrelated to subsequent environmental factors. Despite behavioral abnormalities, infants performed at age-appropriate levels on Gesell adaptive and motor testing. In 1979, Wilson et al. (144) compared 3- to 6-year outcomes of 20 heroin-exposed infants to 55 infants at "high-risk" for suboptimal neurobehavioral outcomes for other reasons. Although overall testing of the heroin-exposed children fell within the normal range, those infants displayed significant deficits in behavioral adjustment, in perceptual measures, and specific subtests related to the process of organization, requiring attention, concentration, short-term memory, and the internal manipulation of symbols. Wilson et al. (145) found that at 1 year of age, methadone-exposed infants showed excessive crying and delay in establishing quiet sleep patterns, and showed deficits in fine motor coordination and attention despite testing within the normal range on Bayley mental scores.

Ramer and Lodge (146) studied 35 infants who were born to 32 mothers registered in a San Francisco city-operated methadone-maintenance treatment program. Sixty percent of the infants demonstrated mild or no symptoms, and 40% developed moderate or severe symptoms of withdrawal. The infants whose symptoms were most severe were born to mothers who had documented histories of polydrug abuse. Although many infants were slow to gain weight in the neonatal period, thereafter growth and development remained generally within the normal range. Bayley Scales of Infant Mental and Motor Development revealed that the older infants (up to 3 years of age) showed age-appropriate development in the area of vocalization and language, but performance on perceptual motor tasks was somewhat less adequate.

In 1976, Strauss et al. (147) evaluated 60 infants born to narcotic-addicted women enrolled in the Hutzel Hospital's perinatal methadone treatment program and 53 control infants. Psychological development of a subset of the addicted infants (n = 25), using the Bayley Scales of Infant Development at 3, 6, and 12 months of age, fell within the normal range, but psychomotor development scores of

these children declined from 119 to 103 through the first year.

In 1979, Strauss and colleagues (148) evaluated 5-year-old children from their original cohort reported in 1976. The children were from Strauss' original sample of newborns but not necessarily the children studied at 3, 6, and 12 months of age. The investigators had not contacted the previously studied children in 4 years. Children in the drug-exposed group were born to methadone-treated heroin-addicted women who had participated in the Methadone Maintenance Obstetric Care Program. No maternal drug use information was provided. Children were assessed with the McCarthy Scales of Children's Abilities and a 15-minute videotape of behavior in the waiting room. No differences were found between 33 methadone-exposed children and 30 non–drug-exposed comparison children on the McCarthy General Cognitive Index or any of the subscales. Scores for both groups were well below the standardization means at 86.8 for the narcotic-exposed children and 86.2 for controls. Videotapes of waiting room behavior were coded for children's playing and talking, interaction with caregiver and other children, wandering, for the mother's playing with the child, positive/negative responses, and initiation of interaction and reprimands. During this observation, no differences were found in the children's or mother's responses between the two groups. The drug-exposed children were found to be more active, energetic, and immature, and displayed more task-irrelevant activity during the structured testing situation.

In 1985, Lifschitz and colleagues (149) evaluated 92 children between the ages of 3 and 6 years who were drawn from a previous sample studied in 1981. The study sample was composed of 26 methadone-exposed, 25 heroin-exposed, and 41 drug-free comparison children. The methadone-exposed infants were born to women enrolled in a treatment program, whereas the heroin-exposed infants were born to women who were not in a treatment program. Methadone-maintained women (95%) continued to use illicit and/or prescription psychoactive agents. The McCarthy Scales of Children's Abilities was used to assess cognitive development of the sample. Physical and psychological characteristics of the child's home were measured by the HOME (Home Observation of Measurement of the Environment) Inventory (150). Performance on the McCarthy Scales was comparable for all of the groups. Despite overall testing which fell within the normal range, heroin- and methadone-exposed infants were overrepresented in the group of infants showing low-average and mildly retarded intellectual performance at 3 to 6 years of age. Although the degree of maternal opiate use was not a factor in predicting cognitive performance, amount of prenatal care, prenatal risk, and the HOME scores were.

Rosen and Johnson (151) reported followup to 18 months of age of 45 methadone-exposed infants and 25 comparison infants. The drug-exposed group displayed both hypertonia and hypotonia, as well as delays in sitting, transfer ability, fine motor coordination, and language acquisition. Although both study and control infants scored within the normal range on the Bayley Mental Developmental Index (MDI) and Physical Development Index (PDI) scales, scores for methadone-exposed infants were lower; differences were statistically significant at both 12- and 18-month examinations.

In a later study, Rosen and Johnson (152) evaluated their longitudinal sample at 3 years of age. Of their original cohort of 94, they were able to assess 62 children. Thirty-nine methadone-exposed children and 23 comparison children were assessed at 36 months with a 30-minute videotaped free play and structured task situation and with the Merrill Palmer Scale of Mental Tests (Stutsman 1931). No differences were found between groups on the latter scores or percentiles. Spontaneous language production was assessed by review of the videotapes. No differences were found between groups, but the mean lengths of utterances for both groups were lower than those reported for middle class samples. A 1985 study (152) by the same authors of methadone-exposed children found increased activity, attention deficits, poor fine and gross motor coordination, and speech and language delays at 7 years of age.

Hans (153) assessed 30 methadone-exposed infants and 44 control infants at 2 years of age. Although mean scores for drug-exposed and control infants fell well within the normal range, study infants evidenced deficient fine and gross motor coordination and greater body tension, and lagged behind control infants by about 2 months of motor development. Hans later completed a 10-year longitudinal study of methadone-exposed children and a comparison group of unexposed children identified prenatally (154,155). All children were African Americans living in very-low-income families. More than 90% of the original methadone-exposed sample were found and assessed, as well as more than 75% of the original comparison sample. The study included 36 children in the exposed group and slightly more in the comparison group. Extensive information on the children's behavior problems was collected using multiple instruments and multiple informants. Diagnoses of the drug-exposed children included (in order of prevalence) attention deficit hyperactivity disorder (ADHD), disruptive disorders (conduct and oppositional), functional enuresis, disorders of the affective spectrum, and separation anxiety. Compared with the control group, drug-exposed children were somewhat more likely to receive ADHD and disruptive diagnoses but were not at higher risk for affective disorders. The authors conclude that research results regarding the effects of prenatal drug exposure during late childhood and adolescence, seem to indicate that prenatally drug-exposed children are definitely at high risk for behavioral and academic problems, although possibly not any more so than sociodemographically matched controls. It seems unlikely that the primary source of these problems is directly related to the prenatal

exposure, because behavioral and academic problems are present in children with drug using parents who were *not* prenatally exposed. However, early research results suggest that there could be information-processing deficits observable at school age in some prenatally exposed children that might contribute to difficulties in school.

At Family Center in Philadelphia between 1977 and 1979, Kaltenbach et al. (156) studied 43 infants (26 1-year-olds and 17 2-year-olds) exposed to methadone *in utero* and 51 control infants randomly selected from a population of children with comparable socioeconomic, racial, and medical backgrounds. Although both groups tested within the normal range using the Bayley Mental Scale of Infant Development, scores at 1 year of age were lower in the methadone-exposed group (103.4) than in controls (109.4). At 2 years of age, scores were lower but did not differ between the drug-exposed infants (90.9) and controls (94.6). The same group performed 4-year assessments on 25 study children born to women who received prenatal care and methadone maintenance during pregnancy (157). Differences between children born to women maintained on methadone and controls were not statistically significant for either the subscales or the full-scale IQs; both groups performed better on the verbal scale than on the performance scale. All neurologic findings were within the normal range, and there was no relationship between severity of neonatal withdrawal and the IQ scores. At 3.5 to 4.5 years of age, no intergroup differences were found using the McCarthy Scales of Children's Abilities. Scores for the methadone-exposed population and controls averaged 106.5 and 106, respectively. These scores are higher than those reported in other studies. They are also higher than one would expect for both groups of children who are from low socioeconomic backgrounds who usually score lower than average on cognitive tests. The mothers of these children continued to participate in a 5-year study and perhaps were more motivated and interested in their children's development. This may have provided an informal intervention that included maternal stimulation of the children over and above that usually provided in such homes (158).

An increasing number of studies have proposed multifactorial models to assess infant outcome following intrauterine drug exposure. One such postnatal influence involves maternal–infant interaction. Drug-exposed infants are often irritable and dysrhythmic and may display increased extensor tone when handled. On the other hand, arousal from sleep may be difficult. Both behaviors may be interpreted by the mother as rejections, leading to inappropriate maternal caretaking and possible neglect of the infant. Finnegan et al. (14) found that infants born to methadone-maintained women showed deficient social responsiveness after birth, that this deficient mother–infant interaction persisted until the infant's treatment was completed, and that maternal drug dose may affect that interaction.

Based on these limited early data, children born to heroin-using women or to women maintained on methadone appeared to function within the normal range of mental and motor development at 5 to 6 years of age. Some data offer the tentative possibility that selected (but varying among studies) differences in behavioral, adaptive, and perceptual skills may exist between these children and those of comparable backgrounds whose mothers were not involved with drugs. Positive and reinforcing environmental influences can significantly improve infant outcome; women who show a caring concern for their infants are most likely to pursue followup pediatric care and cooperate in neurobehavioral followup studies. The lack of both a large database and long-term followup well into the school years from these early data, points to an obvious need for comprehensive studies assessing the development of larger populations of opiate-exposed infants.

Because of the rapid upsurge of cocaine use, before the use of the multifactorial approach could be fully realized, research studies dedicated to the effects of prenatal opiate exposure ceased. Overall, the data on the effects of prenatal opiate exposure indicate that through 2 years of age, these children function well within normal limits and that between 2 and 5 years of age, they do not differ in cognitive abilities from a high-risk comparison group. Importantly, the data consistently suggest that psychological demographic factors may have as much, or more, effect on development as maternal opiate use (158).

Cocaine

In contrast to opiate use, which remained relatively constant in the United States during the 1980s and began to rise again in the mid-1990s, cocaine use, especially that of "crack," rose rapidly during the 1980s. The number of babies reportedly exposed to drugs (much of it cocaine) in New York City rose from 7.9 per 1,000 births in 1983 to 20.3 per 1,000 live births in 1987; more than 5,000 drug-exposed babies were born in New York City in 1989. Of some consolation was the report of a 7% drop in New York City positive neonatal toxicology reports between 1989 and 1990, one of the first reports to demonstrate that this latest epidemic of cocaine use had peaked in the late 1980s.

Significant cocaine use persists, however, especially in urban ghettos. Some hospitals in these communities reported in the late 1980s that 20% to 30% of all newborn infants were testing positive for illegal drugs in their urine, 80% to 90% of those being cocaine. Other cities, such as Dallas, Denver, Oakland, Philadelphia, and Houston, all reported three- to fourfold increases in drug-exposed infants between 1985 and 1988. Nationwide, studies in the 1980s estimated that approximately 4.5% of newborns in the United States may have been exposed to cocaine *in utero* (5). A 1990 Ohio study (159) of more than 1,800 neonates from 25 hospitals revealed a cocaine exposure rate of 2.0%; the adjusted prevalence rate was 7.2% for infants born to African American mothers and 0.3% for infants born to white mothers. In 1991, Schutzman et al. (160) reported an incidence of 11.8% intrauterine cocaine exposure (6.3% of privately insured mothers and 26.9% of mothers with Medicaid or no insurance) in a suburban Philadelphia setting. Vega et al. (161), in a study of more than 29,000 California live births in mid-1992, documented maternal cocaine use in 1.1% of pregnancies; ethnic differences ranged from a low of 0.06% in Asians to almost 8% in blacks. A more recent study in Rochester, New York, found that 5.5% of 1,201 mother–infant pairs tested positive for cocaine (162). As noted earlier, the National Pregnancy and Health Survey (6) reported in 1994 that slightly more than 1% of the surveyed pregnancies were complicated by cocaine use.

Cocaine has been used medicinally and recreationally in this country since the 1870s (1). During that time, in the course of a number of epidemics of cocaine use, many adverse effects of cocaine on the adult user became well-known, including acute myocardial infarction, cardiac arrhythmias, rupture of the ascending aorta, cerebrovascular accidents, hyperpyrexia, seizures, and infections, as well as a range of psychiatric disorders such as dysphoric agitation (163). Much less has been reported regarding cocaine use during pregnancy and its effect upon the mother, fetus, and newborn infant. The recent "crack" epidemic, however, stimulated research regarding cocaine's effects during the perinatal period (164). Although much of the data remain controversial and even contradictory, it has nonetheless revealed a wide variety of specific risks of great concern (Table 53.6).

Physiology and Pharmacology

Cocaine (benzoylmethylecgonine hydrochloride) is an alkaloid derived from the leaves of coca plants, most prominently *Erythroxylon coca*. The first extraction process yields a coca paste, a raw and generally impure product consumed primarily in South America. Further extraction with hydrochloric acid yields cocaine hydrochloride, which is usually diluted and either snorted or used intravenously. If the hydrochloride salt is treated with a base such as sodium bicarbonate and then reextracted with a solvent such as ether, the freebase form, also called "crack," is produced (165).

Cocaine displays varied pharmacokinetics based on its specific preparation and route of administration (166). Because cocaine is a very potent vasoconstrictor, it retards its own absorption when applied to mucous membranes, such as the nasal mucosa when snorted or gastrointestinal mucosa when ingested. This vasoconstriction leads to relatively slow achievement of peak levels of cocaine in the blood and brain. Cocaine plasma levels peak in about 15 to 60 minutes following snorting and in about 45 to 90 minutes after ingestion (165). Peak levels of cocaine are reached more rapidly following smoking or intravenous use. This more rapid absorption causes an intense euphoria and severe post euphoria "crash" that leads to an intense

TABLE 53.6. *Possible maternal and neonatal effects from cocaine use during pregnancy*

Maternal complications
    Poor nutritional status
    Increased risk for infections
    Hypertension/tachycardia/arrhythmias/myocardial
      infarctions
    Central nervous system hemorrhage
    Depression and low self-esteem
    Increased tendency to engage in risk behaviors for HIV
Pregnancy, labor, and delivery complications
    Spontaneous abortion
    Poor weight gain
    Abruptio placentae
    Fetal demise
    Precipitous delivery
Neonatal complications
    Intrauterine growth retardation
    Microcephaly or reduced head circumference
    Prematurity
    Fetal/vascular disruption
    Congenital infections
    Cardiovascular dysfunction/arrhythmias
    Feeding difficulties/necrotizing enterocolitis
    Central nervous system hemorrhage-ischemic lesions
    Neurobehavioral dysfunction
    Seizure activity
    Sudden infant death syndrome (SIDS)
    Increased possibility of HIV infection

craving and potentially rapid development of dependence on the drug.

Once absorbed, cocaine is metabolized by serum and hepatic cholinesterases to water-soluble inactive compounds, primarily benzoylecgonine, norcaine, and ecgonine methyl ester (165). Cocaine may be detectable in blood or urine for less than 12 hours, but its water-soluble products may be recovered from urine for up to 1 week, depending on the sensitivity of testing methodology. Usual toxicologic testing involves the use of either an enzyme multiplied immunoassay technique (EMIT) or radial immunodiffusion, with confirmation by either gas chromatography or high-performance liquid chromatography. Recent articles advocate the use of meconium testing for cocaine metabolites to enhance diagnostic accuracy regarding drug exposure over a longer gestational period. Using meconium analysis, Ostrea et al. (105) reported a much higher yield of positive cocaine assays compared to urine drug testing, findings which were confirmed in a larger series of more than 3,000 infants by the same author (106). In that series, just over 30% of the infants tested positive for cocaine. The applicability of this finding was extended when cocaine was found in the intestines of three human fetuses, one as early as 17 weeks gestation (167). Ryan et al. (162) also reported that meconium testing for cocaine metabolites resulted in the detection of an additional 33% of cocaine-exposed neonates, com-

pared to urine testing. Other researchers suggest that hair analysis for cocaine metabolites gives a better estimate of gestational exposure to cocaine (168,169). Another diagnostic possibility was offered by Jain et al. (170), who detected the presence of cocaine metabolites in 74% of amniotic fluid samples of known cocaine users, compared with recovery rates of 61% in maternal urine and only 35% in neonatal urine.

Effects On Pregnancy and Uteroplacental Function

Assessment of the organic impact of cocaine on the human pregnancy must consider confounding drug use-associated variables such as poverty, homelessness, inadequate prenatal and postnatal care, deficient nutrition, sexually transmitted diseases, multiple-drug use, varying types of cocaine administration, and the possible presence of toxic adulterants that are mixed with or used to process cocaine. Animal studies can limit the number of such variables, but extrapolation of animal data to human subjects should always be undertaken cautiously.

Maternal appetite suppression and cocaine "binging" with inadequate nutritional intake is well recognized. Many cocaine users admitted for treatment may have at least one vitamin deficiency (B_1, B_6, C). Correction of these vitamin deficiencies is particularly necessary during pregnancy to promote the biosynthesis of essential neurotransmitters.

Cocaine's low molecular weight and high solubility in both water and lipids allow it to cross the placenta easily and enter fetal compartments (171,172). This transplacental passage is enhanced with intravenous or freebase use of cocaine. In addition, the relatively low pH of fetal blood (cocaine is a weak base) and the low fetal level of plasma esterases, which usually metabolize this drug, may lead to accumulation of cocaine in the fetus. Furthermore, the "binge" pattern commonly associated with adult cocaine use may lead to higher levels of cocaine in the fetus. Transfer of cocaine appears to be greatest in the first and third trimesters of pregnancy. Because cocaine has such potent vasoconstrictive properties, the constriction of uterine, placental, and umbilical vessels may retard the transfer of cocaine from mother to fetus. A deleterious effect of this vasoconstriction, however, is a concomitant fetal deprivation of essential gas and nutrient exchange, resulting in fetal hypoxia (172). Studies in sheep also show that administration of cocaine to the pregnant ewe results in a dose-dependent catecholamine-mediated increase in maternal blood pressure and a decrease in uterine blood flow, as well as significant reduction in uterine blood flow for at least 15 minutes (173,174). In addition to an acute hypoxic insult, cocaine use of long duration may produce a chronic decrease in transplacental nutrient and oxygen flow, leading to intrauterine growth retardation. Although the relationship of cocaine use to congenital malformations is controversial, a decrease in fetal blood supply during critical periods of morphogenesis and growth may be expected to result in organ malformations (see "Teratogenic Effects" below).

The course of labor may also be affected by maternal cocaine use. Intravenous administration of a local anesthetic such as cocaine may cause a direct increase in uterine muscle tone. "Crack" also appears to directly increase uterine contractility and may thus precipitate the onset of premature labor. A higher rate of early pregnancy losses appears to be major complication of maternal cocaine use (175–179). In addition, an increased frequency of abruptio placentae (177,179–182) and placenta previa (181) have been reported. Livesay et al. (179) also found that the cocaine-using women had a higher rate of emergency cesarean sections (10.8%) than did the noncocaine drug-dependent group (3.6%) or the drug-free group (3.2%). The highest incidence of meconium staining also occurred in the cocaine-exposed group, a finding confirmed by Hadeed and Siegel (178). It is currently postulated that increased levels of catecholamines, increased blood pressure, and increased body temperature all may play etiologic roles in early fetal loss and later abruptio placentae.

A cocaine-mediated increase in norepinephrine levels, as noted, is believed to increase uterine contractility with an increase in the incidence of preterm and precipitous labor. This theoretical underpinning supports the general consensus that maternal cocaine use leads to both shortened gestation and restriction of fetal growth. Although the mechanism for reduced fetal growth is not established, it is generally assumed to be mediated through reduced fetal nutritional support secondary to cocaine-mediated uteroplacental vasoconstriction. An early study by Chasnoff et al. (177) found no increased rate of prematurity, but his later report found a ninefold increase in preterm births; a decrease in mean birth weight and an increase in low birth weight and intrauterine growth retardation was seen when cocaine was used during the entire pregnancy (180). Cherukuri (183), Chouteau (184), and Livesay (179) all found significantly increased rates of prematurity following maternal cocaine use as well as decreases in mean birth weights. MacGregor et al. (182) also reported lower birth weight, lower gestational age at delivery, and higher incidences of preterm labor (21.4% vs. 1.4%) and premature delivery (24.3% vs. 2.9%) in a cocaine-exposed group than in an appropriately matched control group. Other researchers report increases in cocaine-associated fetal growth retardation without reductions in gestational length (37,39,178,185). In the metropolitan Chicago area, with a database of more than 17,000 deliveries, Handler et al. (181) found that maternal cocaine use was associated with higher rates of low birth weight (risk ratio [RR] 2.8), prematurity (RR 2.4), and intrauterine growth retardation in noncigarette smokers (RR 3.4). Using both univariate and multivariate analysis, Kliegman et al. (186) found that cocaine use was a significant predictor of prematurity (odds ratio 13.4) and low birth weight (odds ratio 9.9). Racine et al. (187) found that the rate of low-birth-weight infants among cocaine users could be pos-

itively impacted by the provision of at least four prenatal visits. Zuckerman and Frank (188), commenting on the discrepancies in the literature, pointed out the need to use adequate statistical power if cocaine's effect on birth weight and gestation turns out to be small, and the need to control for concurrent use of other substances (drug combinations, amounts, accuracy of measurements, etc.) and a range of medical and sociodemographic factors.

Although Chasnoff originally reported no decrease in head circumference in cocaine-exposed newborns compared with controls (177), his subsequent data did reveal smaller head size if cocaine was used throughout the pregnancy (180). Decreases in neonatal head circumference in cocaine-exposed newborns have been confirmed by other workers (37,178,183,185,189). More recent studies, such as that by Eyler et al. (190), have controlled for associated substance use (marijuana, alcohol, tobacco) and have continued to document a reduction in cocaine-associated neonatal head circumference. Confirmatory evidence supporting a pattern of cocaine-associated symmetric intrauterine growth retardation was provided by Bandstra et al. (191) in a study of 253 infants born to African American women in the metropolitan Miami area. Scafidi et al. (192) extended the finding of reduced head circumference to preterm infants. These various data sets suggest, therefore, that maternal cocaine use is associated with symmetric growth retardation in offspring, affecting both birth weight and head circumference.

Teratogenic Effects

Representative animal studies suggest that cocaine has major teratogenic potential. Mahalik et al. (193) found a higher resorption ratio, as well as a higher incidence of soft-tissue abnormalities (especially skeletal anomalies) in mice exposed to cocaine compared with controls. Fantel and MacPhail (194) noted a significant decrease in maternal and fetal weights in rats given high dose intraperitoneal cocaine, as well as fetal edema and higher resorption frequencies, but no increase in congenital malformations.

Data on the relationship of cocaine to human malformations can be characterized as inconsistent. Bingol et al. (176) found a 10% rate of congenital malformations among cocaine users compared with 4.5% among polydrug users and 2% in controls; malformations included cardiac, skeletal, and skull abnormalities. After their report of one cocaine-exposed infant with prune belly syndrome (a complex of signs including major malformations of the genitourinary tract, bilateral hydronephrosis, and bilateral cryptorchidism) and another infant with hypospadias, Chasnoff et al. (195) then reported a higher incidence of genitourinary malformations in 50 infants born to cocaine-abusing women compared with 30 control infants. Lipshultz et al. (196) found a fourfold increase in cardiac malformation in cocaine-exposed infants compared with controls; lesions included peripheral pulmonary stenosis, patent ductus arteriosus, and ventricular and atrial septal defects. Isolated reports have linked intrauterine cocaine exposure with midline central nervous system (CNS) abnormalities (38), craniosynostosis (197), a range of facial abnormalities (198), ankyloglossia (tongue tie) (199), and sirenomelia (fused legs) (200).

A unifying hypothesis linking cocaine with congenital anomalies has been suggested by Hoyme et al. (201). The authors present a range of malformations under the umbrella term *fetal vascular disruption;* these anomalies include growth deficiency, nonduodenal intestinal atresia, limb reduction defects, renal anomalies, and aplasia cutis congenita. Martin et al. (202), however, did not find an increase in congenital malformations attributable to vascular disruption based on 1986–1989 data from the Metropolitan Atlanta Congenital Defects Program. Rajegowda et al. (203) also found no increase in congenital urogenital abnormalities in 1,324 cocaine-exposed infants when compared with 18,028 reportedly drug-free controls. In addition, ultrasound examinations were performed on 127 cocaine-exposed infants, with only one abnormality found. The same lack of association was found by Hadeed and Siegel (178) and Zuckerman et al. (189). Koren et al., working in the Motherisk program in Toronto, found that although cocaine exposure early in pregnancy was not associated with an increased risk of teratogenesis (204), physicians' perception of a high risk of cocaine teratogenicity resulted in termination of many otherwise wanted pregnancies (205). Counseling of pregnant women as to actual teratogenic risk resulted in a decrease in risk perception and a decreased tendency to terminate the pregnancy (205). At the present time, therefore, mothers should be apprised that cocaine use *may* increase the risk of congenital malformations in their fetuses, however, confirmatory studies looking at cause and effect have yet to be done.

Neonatal Complications

Early reports by Madden et al. (206), in a series of eight cocaine-exposed newborns and Hadeed and Siegel (178) in a larger series of 56 babies described no obvious cocaine-related neurotoxicity. Chasnoff et al. (177), however, reported an increased degree of irritability, tremulousness, and state lability on the Brazelton Neonatal Assessment Scale in 52 cocaine-exposed infants compared with 73 infants born to non–cocaine-using methadone-maintained women. Additionally, cluster analysis in the study by Chasnoff et al. revealed that cocaine-exposed infants showed a greater deficiency in state control than did infants not exposed to cocaine, which interfered with the ability of the caretaker to establish an appropriate relationship with the infant. Ryan et al. (207) found that symptoms of abstinence were less marked in a group of neonates exposed to cocaine and methadone than in those exposed to methadone alone. These findings are consistent with those found in adults by Kosten (208), who noted that cocaine attenuated the severity of naloxone-precipitated opioid withdrawal.

Doberczak et al. (209) confirmed the presence of hypertonia, brisk tendon reflexes, irritability, and tremors in 34 of 39 cocaine-exposed babies. In those 34 infants, neurologic abnormalities were transient, lasting only a few days, and did not require specific treatment. No correlation could be found between neurotoxicity and specific perinatal variables such as route or quantity of maternal cocaine administration, gestational age, or birth weight. Oro and Dixon (74) also found significant neurologic and physiologic alterations in most cocaine- or amphetamine-exposed neonates (n = 46), including abnormal sleep patterns (81%), tremors (71%), poor feeding (58%), hypotonia, vomiting, and fever. These babies tended to spend long periods of time in a dull-alert state with eyes open and demonstrated poor visual processing of faces and objects. The greatest morbidity was seen with cocaine plus narcotic exposure, despite the theoretic possibility of antagonism between the stimulant and depressive effects of these two drugs.

Eisen et al. (210) found that, within the first week of life on the Brazelton Neonatal Behavioral Assessment Scale, cocaine-exposed infants needed more trials to habituate to a presented stimulus, compared to controls. Coles et al. (211) compared 50 infants born to cocaine-using mothers (although alcohol, marijuana, and cigarettes were also used) to controls at 48 to 72 hours, 14 days, and 28 days. Although scores were generally normal, cocaine-exposed infants appeared to show minimal and transient autonomic depression. Mayes et al. (212) also found that cocaine-exposed infants (n = 56) showed impaired habituation on the Brazelton score; persistence of abnormalities in habituation at a 3-month assessment was found by the same group (213). Delaney-Black et al. (214) found that neurobehavioral abnormalities in the motor performance and state-regulation subareas of testing could be correlated with the amount of intrauterine cocaine exposure as determined by meconium testing. Napiorkowski et al. (215) reported that cocaine-exposed infants tested at 1 to 2 days of age showed increased tone, jerky movements and startles, and poorer auditory and visual following than did control infants; the authors further suggested that cocaine may act synergistically with alcohol and marihuana in producing these neonatal abnormalities. Tronick et al. (216) found that cocaine-associated abnormalities in neurobehavioral performance using the Neonatal Behavioral Assessment Scale could not be demonstrated when confounders were controlled. Abnormalities, particularly in arousal, could be demonstrated, however, on the 3-week repeat examinations, raising concern about the learning capability of cocaine-exposed infants. Scafidi et al. (192) reported abnormalities of state regulation and motor performance in a group of 30 preterm infants with a mean gestational age of 30.2 weeks and mean birth weight of 1,212 g when tested at a mean conceptional age of 34.6 weeks.

Although the mechanism for these neurobehavioral abnormalities is not completely understood, increasing attention has been focused on cocaine-associated derangements in dopaminergic and serotonergic systems (217). Mirochnick et al. (218) postulated that neonatal neurobehavioral disturbances were related to an increase in catecholamine activity in cocaine-exposed infants. The same findings of increased levels of urinary norepinephrine, dopamine, and cortisol levels were reported by Scafidi et al. (192). Needleman et al. (219) demonstrated a reduction in cerebrospinal fluid (CSF) homovanillic acid, the principal metabolite of dopamine, in cocaine-exposed neonates.

In addition to neurobehavioral abnormalities, Doberczak et al. (209) reported that despite the absence of clinical seizures, EEGs were abnormal in 17 of 38 cocaine-exposed infants during the first week of life. EEG abnormalities were characterized as showing cerebral irritation with bursts of sharp waves and spikes and features of discontinuity. These abnormalities were unpredictable and did not correlate with variables such as maternal drug use, neonatal characteristics, or severity of neurologic dysfunction. All abnormal EEGs reverted to normal when followed over a 3- to 12-month period, but the longer-term impact of these changes is not known. More recently, Scher et al. (220) used quantitative EEG analysis to determine that cocaine-exposed neonates showed less-well-developed spectral correlations between homologous brain regions. At 1 year of age those infants displayed subtle changes of lower spectral power during sleep, attributed by the authors to the development of fewer neuronal aggregates during the first year of life.

Although others have not noted the presence of clinical seizures in cocaine-exposed neonates, Chasnoff et al. (180) observed seizures in 6 of 52 infants born to mothers after cocaine use throughout the pregnancy; 2 of those 6 infants were reported to have abnormal electroencephalograms. In addition, Kramer et al. (221) described 16 cocaine-exposed infants who developed seizures after birth. All seizures occurred within 36 hours after delivery and were characterized as subtle (10), focal (1), tonic (2) or clonic (3). Many of the seizures responded poorly to therapeutic dosages of anticonvulsant medications.

In addition to clinical neurologic and electroencephalographic changes, a series of echoencephalographic abnormalities in neonates exposed to stimulants (cocaine and methamphetamine) and opiates was published by Dixon and Bejar (222). Thirty-five percent of the neonates had abnormal echoencephalographic studies, with the highest incidence in the stimulant subgroup. Lesions suggestive of prior hemorrhagic or ischemic injury with cavitation, located anterior and inferior to the lateral ventricles, in the frontal lobes and basal ganglia, were found in 8% of the infants. Intraventricular hemorrhage was found in 12% of those drug-exposed babies; subependymal hemorrhage, in 11%; subarachnoid hemorrhage, in 14%; and ventricular

dilatation suggesting diffuse atrophy, in 10%. Cerebral infarction was evident in two of the cocaine-exposed infants. Despite these impressive findings, infants with abnormal findings did not display identifiable neurobehavioral abnormalities during the newborn period. This is not totally surprising, because the location of the lesions may indicate damage that would be detectable when the infant is older and challenged with more complicated cognitive tasks. Frank et al. (223) found that differences in reporting of cocaine-associated ultrasound abnormalities could be explained by the level of intrauterine cocaine exposure. After controlling for associated high-risk variables, those authors found that infants born following lighter exposure to cocaine did not show an increased incidence of cranial ultrasound abnormalities, while those infants born after heavier exposure were more likely than unexposed control infants to show subependymal hemorrhages in the caudothalamic groove.

Van de Bor et al. (224) demonstrated increased cerebral flow and increased mean arterial pressures on the first day of life in cocaine-exposed neonates and suggested that this cerebral hemodynamic abnormality may increase the risk of intracranial hemorrhage. In fact, Chasnoff et al. (180) had previously reported two infants who suffered perinatal cerebral infarction, which they ascribed to maternal cocaine use. Heier et al. (38) also found a higher rate of cortical infarctions (17%) in cocaine-exposed neonates than in the control population (2%). In a group of 39 term and near-term cocaine-exposed neonates, King et al. (225), found no increase in mild degrees of intraventricular hemorrhage and no instances of more severe hemorrhage, cystic periventricular leukomalacia, or stroke. Cocaine-exposed infants, however, showed an increase in anterior cerebral arterial blood flow velocity from day 1 to day 2; this change in vessel resistance may have been a result of declining cocaine levels postnatally. Specifically in very-low-birth-weight infants (less than 1,500 g), Singer et al. (226) found that cocaine-exposed infants had a higher incidence of mild intraventricular hemorrhages, as well as lower Bayley developmental scores and a higher incidence of developmental delay. In contrast, Dusick et al. (227) found no difference in the incidence of mild or severe intraventricular hemorrhage or of periventricular leukomalacia in cocaine-exposed infants weighing less than 1,500 g than in controls.

Other studies have expanded the spectrum of neonatal neurologic abnormalities attributed to maternal cocaine use during pregnancy. Salamy et al. (228) found that intrauterine cocaine exposure was associated with prolonged auditory brainstem response (ABR) latencies and brainstem transmission time. Although these physiologic parameters normalized by 3 to 6 months of age, transient abnormalities may have been caused by disturbed myelin synthesis or reduced number of oligodendrocytes. Shih et al. (229) also demonstrated abnormal brainstem conduction time manifested as prolonged interpeak latencies and prolonged absolute latencies in ABR testing of 18 cocaine-exposed neonates. Carzoli et al. (230), however, found no differences in interpeak latencies of waveforms between cocaine-exposed infants and controls. Corwin et al. (231) found that the cry of cocaine-exposed infants (n = 404) differed from that of control infants (n = 364) in having fewer cry utterances, more short cries, and less crying in the hyperphonation mode, suggesting a pattern of underaroused neurobehavioral function. Reported abnormal eye findings following cocaine exposure include a picture of "retinopathy of prematurity-like fundus and persistent hyperplastic primary vitreous" (232) and dilated and tortuous iris vessels (233).

Intrauterine exposure to cocaine has also been linked, usually through case reports, to neonatal problems involving other organ systems. These complications include necrotizing enterocolitis (234), bowel perforation (235), arterial thrombosis and hypertension (236), decreased cardiac output on day 1 of life (237), transient myocardial ischemia (238), and persistent hypertension (239).

Followup Studies

Sudden Infant Death Syndrome

Although as noted previously, the incidence of sudden infant death syndrome (SIDS) following intrauterine opiate exposure appears to be increased, the precise risk of SIDS in cocaine-exposed infants is not known. Discrepancies in the literature may be in part ascribed to confounding variables, such as low birth weight, racial/ethnic considerations, polysubstance use, and cigarette smoking, which are known to increase the incidence of SIDS. Chasnoff (177) anecdotally suggested that the risk of SIDS may be high, and subsequently reported that 15% of 66 infants exposed to cocaine *in utero* subsequently died of SIDS (240). In support of this alleged association, Chasnoff reported that cardiorespiratory patterns (pneumograms) in 32 cocaine-exposed infants at 8 to 14 days of age were abnormal in all 5 cocaine-exposed infants presenting with apnea of infancy and in 7 of the remaining 27 asymptomatic cocaine-exposed infants. All infants showing an abnormal pneumogram were treated with theophylline, with normalization of the repeat pneumogram 2 weeks later. No infant died of SIDS on followup. Silvestri et al. (241) found that cocaine-exposed infants showed longer pneumogram-confirmed apnea durations and bradycardia than did controls; 2 of the 41 cocaine-exposed infants died of SIDS. Chen et al. (242) showed that facial airstream stimulation could bring out subtle respiratory abnormalities in cocaine-exposed infants. Data from Ward et al. (243) suggested that infants born to cocaine-using mothers, a large number of whom were polydrug users, showed blunted ventilatory responses to hypoxia, increased amount of periodic breathing, higher heart rates, and reduced response to hypercapnia before arousal. It is important to remember,

however, that the links between "abnormal" cardiorespiratory tracings, apnea, and SIDS are still very tenuous.

In contrast to these findings, Bauchner et al. (244) found no increased incidence of SIDS in cocaine-exposed infants (1/174, 5.6/1,000), when compared with controls (4/821, 4.9/1,000), although both incidences were increased over nationwide rates in their low socioeconomic Boston population. Kandall et al. (141) reviewed 41 cocaine-associated SIDS cases in a population of about 1.21 million births in New York City between 1979 and 1989. Once other high-risk variables (ethnicity, low maternal age, socioeconomic status, maternal cigarette smoking, low birth weight) were controlled, cocaine exposure resulted in only a very modest increase in the rate of SIDS (RR 1.3). Even when only the latter part of the decade (the "crack" years) was considered, the RR increased only slightly to 1.6, far lower than the risk of SIDS following maternal opiate use.

Postnatal Exposure

Postnatal exposure to cocaine represents another potential source of toxicity for children. Given cocaine's lipophilic properties, which render it easily able to cross biologic membranes, ready passage of the drug into breast milk has been established. Chasnoff (245) described a 2-week-old infant with signs of acute cocaine intoxication following exposure to cocaine in her mother's breast milk. Toxicity included irritability, vomiting, diarrhea, increased sucking reflex, hyperactive Moro reflex, increased symmetric deep tendon reflexes, and a marked lability of mood, as well as elevations of the infant's blood pressure, heart rate, and respiratory rate. All symptoms gradually waned over the next 72 hours. Chaney et al. (246) reported severe apnea and seizures in an 11-day-old infant following acute cocaine exposure while breast-feeding. It is also important to remember that a significant portion of drug-using patients may be HIV-positive. Until the precise risk of HIV transmission through breast milk is clarified, this concern forms another reason for discouraging breastfeeding in cocaine-using women.

Environmental Hazards

Recent reports indicate that cocaine exposure may occur in young infants even after they leave the hospital. Shannon et al. (247) surveyed 1,680 consecutive urine samples from 1,120 pediatric patients in a children's hospital. Of the total sample, 52 (4.6%) had specimens positive for cocaine or a cocaine metabolite. Similar findings were reported by Kharasch et al. (248), who found that 2.4% of urine assays performed on 250 children ages 2 weeks to 5 years seen in a Boston hospital emergency department were positive for cocaine metabolites.

Case reports also support these surveys. Rivkin and Gilmore (249) described a 9-month-old infant who developed refractory seizures, apnea, and cyanosis following reported ingestion of cocaine left over from an adult party the night before. Bateman and Heagarty (250) described four children, ranging in age from 3 months to almost 4 years, who were admitted to a New York City municipal hospital with abnormal neurologic findings ascribed circumstantially to passive "crack" inhalation. Two of the children presented with seizures and two showed abnormal neurologic signs, such as drowsiness and unsteady gait. Mirchandani et al. (251) reported 16 infant deaths at ages between 1 month and 5.5 months from the Philadelphia Medical Examiner's Office between 1987 and 1989 in which cocaine and/or its metabolite were found. Mott et al. (252) reported on 41 cocaine-exposed children between the ages of 2 months and 18 years, 19 of whom had abnormal neurologic findings. These case descriptions should reinforce the need to rule out environmental toxins before labeling an infant death as SIDS. Overall mortality in children exposed to illicit substances within the first 2 years of life was studied by Ostrea et al. (253). The authors found no significant increase in mortality in drug-exposed infants compared to controls (13.7 vs. 15.7 per 1,000 live births). In low-birth-weight babies exposed to cocaine and opiates, however, a higher mortality rate was observed; the risk of those infants who tested cocaine-positive of dying within the first 2 years of life increased almost fivefold.

Developmental Outcome

Based on multiple biologic and environmental risk factors, much concern has been voiced regarding the ultimate neurobehavioral prognosis of infants following intrauterine exposure to cocaine. The parents may be of poor socioeconomic status, culturally deprived, or lacking appropriate parenting models. The mother may be poorly nourished, may have medical and sexually transmitted diseases, including AIDS, and may have received little or no prenatal care. The infants frequently show suboptimal body and head growth during the intrauterine period. Uterine flow may be compromised because of cocaine-induced vasoconstriction, leading to acute or chronic fetal hypoxia. After birth, neurologic, neurobehavioral, electroencephalographic, and echoencephalographic abnormalities have been documented. Stimulation for intellectual growth may be lacking because of prolonged hospital stays, infrequent and inappropriate parental contact, placement in a congregate care facility, or discharge to a home in which intellectual nurturing is lacking.

In spite of these valid concerns, well-controlled long-term followup studies of large numbers of cocaine-exposed babies were lacking. Even before critically reviewed articles were published, however, the lay press began to report anecdotal experiences with the first cohort of 3- to 5-year-old children born in this "crack" epidemic (254). Cocaine-exposed babies were characterized as being "genetic inferiors" (255) and as showing significant deficits in environmental interactions, such as play groups and nursery schools (256). These babies were also described as showing less representational play, decreased fantasy play and curious exploration, and lesser quality of play. Others described these children as "joyless," unable to participate fully in either structured or unstructured play situations, with attention deficits and flat, apathetic moods (257). Mothers were angrily accused of being uncaring and having lost their maternal instinct (258,259). The coalescence of these reports fueled a groundswell of national anger directed at drug-using mothers that led, among other things, to prosecution of many mothers for drug-related activities during pregnancy (1,260). To counter press reports, experienced researchers and clinicians cautioned against a "rush to judgment" regarding cocaine-exposed infants (261–266).

In fact, very little was actually known until the past decade about the growth and development of cocaine-exposed babies (267). Alessandri et al. (268) found that cocaine-exposed infants at 4 to 8 months of age showed a decrease in arousal, less interest and joy in learning, and less anger and sadness during extinction, and reduced response to stimuli when learning demand was reinstated. Fetters and Tronick (269) used a battery of testing measures to assess 28 cocaine-exposed infants for neuromotor performance at 1, 4, 7, and 15 months of age. No significant differences were found at 1 and 4 months of age. Impaired motor performance was found at 7-month testing in the cocaine-exposed infants, but these abnormalities were no longer demonstrable at 15-month repeat testing. Singer et al. (270) studied language development in 66 infants at 1 year of age following "heavier" intrauterine exposure to cocaine and 68 infants with "lighter" exposure based on meconium assays. They found that infants with "heavier" exposure had lower auditory comprehension scores than control infants and lower total language scores than infants with "lighter" exposure and control infants. Chasnoff et al. (271) studied the growth and development of 106 infants at 2 years of age following intrauterine exposure to cocaine and other drugs including marijuana, alcohol, and tobacco. Compared to a control group of infants, cocaine-exposed infants and infants exposed to alcohol and marijuana showed persistence of reduced head size on followup. Although Bayley developmental scores did not differ among the three groups, an increased number of drug-exposed infants scored more than 1 standard deviation below the mean. Cocaine exposure was the best predictor of reduced head size, and across all groups, head size correlated well with developmental outcome. Arendt et al. (272) evaluated 199 (98 cocaine-exposed and 101 non–cocaine-exposed) of 260 subjects at 2 years of age for testing of motor development. Using the Peabody Developmental Motor Scales, the authors found that the cocaine-exposed group performed more poorly on both fine and gross motor testing.

Azuma and Chasnoff (273) studied 3-year outcome data on 92 children exposed to "cocaine and other drugs" by path analysis, a multivariate method to determine the goodness-of-fit of hypotheses to actual generated data. The authors concluded that intrauterine drug exposure had both a direct and indirect (head circumference, home environment, and level of perseverance at a task) effect on cognitive ability at 3 years of age. Recent studies have addressed issues of child behavior following intrauterine cocaine exposure. Delaney-Black (274) found a higher number of behavioral problems in 27 cocaine-exposed infants as compared to 75 non–cocaine-exposed children at 6 years of age after controlling for gender and prenatal exposure to alcohol and cigarettes. The authors note, however, that postnatal environmental factors that might profoundly affect child behavior were not addressed. The same group (275) studied 201 cocaine-exposed and 270 control African American children at 6 years of age through school teacher blinded assessment. Prenatal exposure to alcohol and cocaine were associated with an increase in behavior problems; cocaine-exposed boys were more likely to show aggressive and delinquent behavior patterns. The authors point out, however, that postnatal environmental factors such as change in custody status and current drug use in the home were significant determinants of poor behavioral outcome.

In addition to these studies, numerous research reports evaluating long-term outcomes of cocaine-exposed infants were published. Frank et al. (276) did a systematic review of 36 of 74 articles that appeared in a search of *Medline* and *Psychological Abstracts* from 1984 to October 2000. At the time of their review, popular attitudes and public policies about prenatal cocaine exposure reflected the belief that cocaine was a uniquely dangerous teratogen even though studies had not shown catastrophic effects. Their objective was to critically review outcomes in early childhood after prenatal cocaine exposure in five domains: physical growth; cognition; language skill; motor skills; and behavior, attention, and neurophysiology. They concluded that among children 6 years old and younger, there was no convincing evidence that prenatal cocaine exposure is associated with developmental toxic effects that are different in severity, scope, or kind from the sequelae of multiple other risk factors. Because of the multitude of contributory factors that exist within the lifestyle of the pregnant drug-dependent woman, the child is exposed to multifactorial issues that may have an impact on their future health and development. Many of the findings that were thought to be specific effects of *in utero* cocaine exposure are correlated with other factors, including prenatal exposure to tobacco, marijuana, or alcohol, and the quality of the child's environment.

A large, multicenter longitudinal study on cocaine exposure and child outcome was funded by the National Institute of Child Health and Human Development at the National Institutes of Health under the auspices of the Neonatal Research Network. This research, which involves four centers and is entitled The Maternal Lifestyle Study, has evaluated cocaine-exposed children (n = 543) and a comparison group (matched for gestational age, sex, and race) (n = 730), at 14 assessments from 1 month to 9 years of age. A developmental and teratologic approach was used. In the teratologic approach, the potential pharmacologic and toxic effects of the drug per se and isolated unique effects of the drug were studied. In the developmental approach, they were able to predict child outcome with drugs as one of many contributing factors and sought to determine multiple antecedent variables that influence child outcome, as well as to study developmental pathways. Based on the teratology approach, findings revealed a small but reliable decrement in cognition, executive function, and an increase in behavior problems. However, most effects were diminished after controlling for covariates. Results from the developmental approach revealed that direct pathways from cocaine exposure to child outcome were no longer significant when mediators were added to the model. Social context (socioeconomic status and poverty) was a consistent mediator of cocaine effects in all models. Cocaine effects were mediated by child vulnerabilities as follows: low IQ was mediated by behavior problems; communication was mediated by low birth weight, physical growth, and poor health. Vulnerabilities that were unrelated to cocaine exposure predicted outcomes as follows: high activity predicted poor inhibitory control; insecure attachment predicted less school readiness. In summarizing these data in this large sample of children, the authors found that cocaine exposure is associated with poverty, polydrug exposure, and small, reliable deficits in cognition, executive function, and increased behavior problems. The most consistent pathway from cocaine exposure to deficits in school age outcomes is poverty, but exposure effects are also mediated by specific behavioral or health vulnerabilities. The study concluded that because exposed children are vulnerable to behavioral and health problems and are frequently raised in poverty, this leads to subtle deficits in IQ, inhibitory control and planning, and communication skills as they begin their school career. However, identification of pathways to early vulnerability and deficits in skills necessary for school success provides a window of opportunity for intervention before the child fails (277).

In another study of their cohort within the Maternal Lifestyle Study, Lester and colleagues (278) studied the mental development of cocaine-exposed children from 1 to 7 years of age and the need for an Individual Evaluation Plan to qualify for special education in school. They found that the IQ differences as a consequence of cocaine exposure increased as children reached school age. In addition, at age 7 years, children prenatally exposed to cocaine are 1.5 times more likely to have an Individual Education Plan to qualify for special education than were children not exposed. The additional cost for special education based on a 1.52 excess risk because of cocaine was estimated to be more than $23.5 million per year. From the results of this study, we may expect a tremendous burden upon school systems. By providing prevention and treatment services for drug dependence in pregnant women, we could effectively reduce this cost.

As more data are published, we may come to view this epidemic of cocaine use as having a very serious negative impact on a very large number of America's young children. It is important, however, to view these infants as medically and socially vulnerable, not because of cocaine alone, but because of the wide array of adverse influences to which these children are subjected (269). An extremely useful paradigm was formulated by Lester and Tronick (262). These researchers conceptualized the mutual regulation that exists between the infant and its mother and other caretakers. The infant is impacted by the organic effects of the drug and other potentially adverse influences mediated through the prenatal environment. Environmental regulators affect the prenatal environment as well as maternal lifestyle. The mother or caretaker is additionally affected by substance abuse directly and those personality traits which led to her addiction. All of these factors impinge on the mutually regulatory process between infant and caretaker that are so essential for normal infant development. In this broader context, these parents and children should receive the comprehensive medical and social services that they so obviously need.

From a research standpoint, investigators studying the effects of perinatal drug exposure on the behavior of children have recognized for a very long time that children's postnatal environments need to be considered as potentially confounding factors in research designs. Use of alcohol, cigarettes, and illicit drugs have been linked with a variety of issues that put the child at risk including lack of stimulation in the home, maternal insensitivity during interaction with children, poor monitoring of older children, disruptions in custodial care, and child maltreatment (279). According to Hans, "within research designs, children's environments need to be considered as more than confounding variables. Development can be best understood within an environmental context and there is a dynamic relationship between parents' drug use, their behavior with their children, and their children's development." Developmental theory from various sciences (280) conceptualizes development as dynamic bidirectional transactions between the organism and the environment and recognizes that the course of development is determined by a system of many independent factors. To begin capturing the real role of prenatal exposure on human development, researchers need to adopt more dynamic models of development that capture longitudinal patterns of influences. Future research needs to examine systems of variables that includes prenatal exposures but also influences, to examine these variables over time rather than at a static endpoint, and to examine the ways teratological influences are dependent on particular environmental contexts.

Amphetamines

Only a scanty literature exists describing the effects of amphetamines on the fetus, neonate, and young infant. Amphetamine (racemic-[β-phenylisopropyl]amine) has powerful central nervous system stimulant actions and causes increased wakefulness, alertness, mood elevation, elation, and euphoria similar to cocaine. These effects are caused by stimulation of the release and blocking of reuptake of the neurotransmitters dopamine, norepinephrine, or serotonin. Acute neuropsychiatric effects of amphetamine overuse include agitation, tremors, hyperreflexia, irritability, confusion, aggressiveness, and panic states, among others. This "hyperexcitation" phase is usually followed by fatigue and depression. Addiction and tolerance to amphetamine often occur. Methamphetamine is structurally similar to amphetamine but has relatively greater central effects and less prominent peripheral actions.

Animal studies assessing the impact of prenatal amphetamine administration on neonatal brain physiology and behavior have been summarized by Middaugh (281). Animal evidence indicates that maternal amphetamine administration reduces norepinephrine levels in the brains of newborn mice, which might affect neurotransmitter synthesis and function. Behaviorally, prenatal amphetamine administration leads to changes in motor activity and reduced performance on specific performance testing in offspring.

Because cocaine and amphetamines have similar central physiologic effects, their impact on pregnancies should be similar. Both agents cause vasoconstriction and hypertension, which may result in acute or chronic fetal hypoxia. Eriksson et al. (71) described the perinatal course in 23 patients who were chronic amphetamine users, 6 of whom reportedly stopped amphetamine abuse during the pregnancy. Amphetamine use was associated with reduced prenatal care and an increased incidence of low-birth-weight babies. Neurologic abnormalities consisted of unexplained seizures in one infant and drowsiness and inability to feed in two others. Eriksson et al. (72) later studied 69 amphetamine-using women, 52 of whom took amphetamine throughout the entire pregnancy. Although a concurrent control group was not compared, the authors reported a high perinatal mortality rate, high incidence of obstetric and pregnancy-related complications, an increased number of congenital malformations, and a high rate of neonatal neurological abnormalities in the drug-exposed group.

In a more recent study, Oro and Dixon (74) reported on 46 infants born to mothers who took cocaine and/or methamphetamine during their pregnancies. Comparison among the stimulant groups showed no difference in selected perinatal variables or in the number of neurologic and physiologic abnormalities in the infants. Use of stimulants led to an increase in placental abruptions and reductions in gestational age, birth weight, length, and head circumference compared with controls. After birth, stimulant-exposed infants showed abnormal weight change patterns, losing more weight and subsequently gaining weight more slowly. Neurologically, the infants' abnormalities included disordered sleep patterns, tremors, poor feeding, hyperactive reflexes, abnormal cry, and state disorganization. The authors noted that lethargy and poor feeding followed the hyperirritable stage in some methamphetamine-exposed infants. Billing et al. (282) studied 65 children to age 8 years, following intrauterine exposure to amphetamines. The authors found a significant correlation between the extent of exposure and subsequent poor psychometric testing, including aggressive behavior and problems of adjustment. At the present time, although there is a clear need for more data on amphetamine exposure, cautious concern regarding developmental outcome seems appropriate.

Alcohol

A complete discussion of the effects of alcohol on pregnancy, fetal welfare, neonatal adaptation, and ultimate infant development is well beyond the scope of this chapter. It is critical to acknowledge, however, that alcohol abuse forms a prominent part in many, if not most, drug users' lives. As previously noted, many addicted women have been raised in alcoholic and abusive settings, and their own alcoholism may have roots in genetics, environmental influences, and predisposing psychosocial characteristics. Because alcohol is now known to represent a substance with enormous potential for human devastation in the perinatal period, inclusion of these comments seems warranted.

Similar to opiates and stimulants, estimates of intrauterine exposure to alcohol vary. The National Pregnancy and Health Survey (6) estimated that 757,000 infants are born annually following significant exposure to alcohol during pregnancy. This figure is somewhat higher than that of 584,000 infants derived from 1994–1995 data in another federal study (283). The most notable postnatal adverse effect of significant alcohol exposure is the fetal alcohol syndrome (FAS), which was first described by Lemoine in 1968 and by Jones and Smith in 1973. This syndrome can be identified in approximately 1 in 300 to 1 in 1,000 births; a lesser degree of damage, termed *fetal alcohol effects*, may occur in 1 in 100 live births. Varying estimates of prevalence are based to some degree on the failure by health professionals to make the definitive diagnosis (284). Although the amount of alcohol that must be consumed to cause fetal damage is not known and must certainly be determined to some extent by individual variability, it is generally believed that consumption of more than 3 ounces of absolute alcohol daily, especially in conjunction with

"binge drinking," poses special risk to the fetus. Because subtle effects may go unnoticed, no safe level of alcohol intake during pregnancy has been established.

Three series of findings define FAS:

1. One of the most constant features of FAS is fetal growth retardation; weight, length, and head circumference generally fall below the 10th percentile for gestational age (284–289).
2. A nearly constant feature of FAS is the characteristic facial dysmorphism of short palpebral fissures, hypoplastic maxilla, short upturned nose, hypoplastic philtrum, thinned upper vermilion border and micrognathia or retrognathia. Less-common associated features include ptosis, strabismus, epicanthal folds, microphthalmia, posteriorly rotated ears, and cleft lip or palate. Other common somatic abnormalities include structural cardiac defects, cutaneous hemangiomas, aberrant palmar creases, and pectus excavatum; less common features include hypospadias, renal abnormalities, joint malformations, and hernias of the diaphragm, umbilicus, and abdominal wall (285,288–292).
3. The most devastating aspect of FAS is severe alcohol-induced central nervous system dysfunction (293). Irritability, tremulousness, poor sucking, inconsolable crying, and hypertonia have been noted in many infants (83). Pierog et al. (84), in a small series of six neonates undergoing "alcohol withdrawal," noted the occurrence of tonic–clonic seizures. Ioffe et al. (294) found that maternal alcohol ingestion during pregnancy was associated with hypersynchrony of the neonatal EEG. Cerebral malformations, neurologic heterotopia, and interruptions of neuronal migration have also been described (295). Holzman et al. (296) found that low-birth-weight babies of less than 31 weeks gestation born to mothers with moderate-high alcohol consumption during pregnancy were at increased risk for perinatal brain injuries such as isolated brain hemorrhage (odds ratio 5.5), any brain hemorrhage (odds ratio 6.7), and white matter damage (odds ratio 9.5).

Followup examinations tend to reveal mild cerebellar deficits, hypotonicity, hyperactivity, hearing deficits, speech and language problems, sleep disturbances, and behavioral disorders (292,297,298). The most serious neurologic outcome attributed to alcohol exposure is mental retardation, which occurs in approximately 85% of FAS children. FAS is now believed to be the leading known cause of mental retardation in the United States. Although IQ scores vary, children with full-blown FAS rarely show normal mental ability. Golden et al. (286) studied 12 alcohol-affected children between 6 and 20 months of age. Significant developmental delay was observed in the study group compared to controls in both the Bayley mental development quotient (86 vs. 105) and motor development quotient (90 vs. 110). Iosub et al. (292) found in 63 children and young adults age 1 day to 23 years who were diagnosed with FAS, that IQs ranged between 50 and 97. Most patients tended to cluster between 65 and 70, and mental retardation was found in 14 of 30 patients older than 3 years of age. Prominent neurobehavioral problems included irritability, hyperactivity in approximately 75% of patients, and speech and language deficits in approximately 80% of patients. Coles and her group at Emory University in Atlanta (299,300) studied 25 school-age children born to mothers who drank regularly during pregnancy. The study group showed deficits in areas of intellectual functioning such as sequential processing, overall mental processing, and premath and reading skills, as well as attentional and behavioral problems in structured learning situations.

A landmark study on sequelae of FAS in adolescents and adults was published by Streissguth et al. (301). The authors studied 61 patients with FAS at 12 years of age or older (range: 12 to 40 years of age). Seventy-four percent of the sample were Native American, 21% were black, and 5% were white. Physical examination showed that reduced height and head circumference were still apparent, but that weight deficiency was less marked. The characteristic facial dysmorphology of FAS became less distinctive with increasing age. Most importantly, the average IQ score for the combined FAS–fetal alcohol effects group was 68, representing significant reduction in intellectual function. IQs ranged from 20 to 105, and 58% of the patients had an IQ below 70. In terms of academic and adaptive functioning, only 6% were in regular classes; the remainder required special education or were not in school or working. All patients showed maladaptive behaviors. This study documents that alcohol-induced deficits persist for as long as FAS patients have been studied. In this regard, the fiscal impact of alcohol-associated damage is estimated to be greater than $320 million dollars annually in the United States. The human impact is incalculable.

CONCLUSIONS AND RECOMMENDATIONS

Despite the influx of newer drugs of abuse, opiate and stimulant use, often in conjunction with alcohol abuse, continue to be major problems during pregnancy. Although the history of women and addiction dates back more than 150 years in the United States (1), controversy still exists on how best to prevent and treat the adverse sequelae of addiction. That many of these women are in the childbearing age group helps to explain the large numbers of drug-exposed infants that were recently documented epidemiologically. Numerous investigators have reported extremely high incidences of obstetric and medical complications among street addicts. Evidence as to increased morbidity and mortality among their newborn infants and preliminary data suggesting long-term developmental complications, especially related to alcohol exposure, has also reached a point of consensus.

It does seem clear that providing comprehensive multidisciplinary prenatal care for addicts offers an opportunity to significantly reduce morbidity and mortality in both drug-dependent mothers and their offspring. Comprehensive care coupled with methadone maintenance for narcotic-dependent women has been shown to reduce perinatal morbidity and mortality, largely attributable to reduction of rates of low birth weight in offspring. Aside from problems arising from direct adverse effects of drugs, low-birth-weight infants are overrepresented in the population of infants who eventually show mental subnormality, as well as those who will have great difficulty in school because they are "poor learners." These individuals will be unable to compete fully in our increasingly complex society.

Based on this conclusion, we strongly advise that the pregnant woman who abuses drugs be designated as "high-risk" and be given specialized care in a perinatal center where she can be provided with comprehensive medical and obstetric care, as well as addiction and psychosocial counseling. Care must be provided in a supportive, proactive, culturally sensitive and nonjudgmental fashion. Public Law 102–321, enacted in 1993, mandates that states ensure that pregnant substance-using women have first priority for drug treatment, timely access to health care, and be given child care and assistance with transportation. Women must also know that sharing of confidential information with health care providers will *not* render them liable to criminal prosecution.

After an initial in-hospital assessment, treatment of addiction may take place in an inpatient or outpatient setting. Opiate-dependent women are best treated with methadone maintenance although medical withdrawal using tapering doses of methadone (with close obstetric and medical supervision) may be offered in selected cases. Medical withdrawal, if requested or necessary, preferably should take place between the sixteenth and the thirty-second week of gestation and should be carried out slowly (5 mg reduction every 2 weeks). Studies in progress may show the efficacy of Bupremorphine for the treatment of pregnant opiate dependent women. The pregnant woman addicted to barbiturates or major tranquilizers along with opiates should be medically withdrawn from her drugs of dependence during her second trimester in a specialized detoxification center.

Psychosocial counseling should be provided by experienced therapists who are aware of the medical, social, and psychological needs of substance-using women. Services should include, but not be limited to, provision of housing, nutritional advice, child care, legal services, and counseling about interpersonal relations. Maternal–infant attachment, both antenatally and postpartum, should be strongly encouraged. Special emphasis should be placed on enhancing parenting skills of these women in an effort to decrease the anticipated increase in child neglect in this population. Social and medical support should not end with the hospitalization. An outreach program, incorporating public health nurses and community workers, should be established. The ability of the mother to care for the infant after discharge from the hospital should be assessed by frequent observations in the home and clinic settings.

Clinicians working in this field must continue to strive for excellence in the care of pregnant drug-dependent women and their children. Government agencies on all levels must recognize their specific responsibility to these women and children and should provide adequate funding for much needed comprehensive services. Only if clinicians and government funding officials make this comprehensive care a societal priority will we be able to cope with the pathophysiologic and behavioral effects of drug use on pregnant women and their children.

Society's Approach to Maternal Drug Use

Frustration with our nation's ability to deal effectively with our latest cocaine epidemic has created a very punitive mood in dealing with drug-using women (1,13,260,302). A number of states have instituted criminal action against pregnant drug-using women despite those states' inability or reluctance to provide treatment and counseling specifically designed for substance-using pregnant women. A punitive rather than rehabilitative approach runs counter to medical and judicial precedent and may drive "hard-to-reach" women further from the health care system. Failure to provide family based rehabilitation when possible, places children in already overburdened and stressed child welfare and foster care systems. Drug-using women, frequently battered and abused as children and adults, need comprehensive medical, obstetric, psychiatric, and drug-counseling treatment. Our goals of promoting healthy mothers and children can best be met by providing such comprehensive services rather than abandoning these unfortunate women in a time of great need.

REFERENCES

1. Kandall SR. *Substance and shadow: women and addiction in the United States.* Cambridge: Harvard University Press, 1996.
2. Dicker M, Leighton EA. Trends in diagnosed drug problems among newborns: United States, 1979–1987. *Drug Alcohol Depend* 1991;28:151–165.
3. Chasnoff, IJ. Drug use and women: establishing a standard of care. *Ann N Y Acad Sci* 1989;562:208–210.
4. Chasnoff IJ, Landress HJ, Barrett ME. The prevalence of illicit-drug or alcohol use during pregnancy and discrepancies in mandatory reporting in Pinellas County, Florida. *N Engl J Med* 1990;322:1202–1206.
5. Gomby DS, Shiono PH. Estimating the number of substance-exposed infants. The future of children. *Future Child* 1991;1:17–25.
6. *National pregnancy and health survey.* Rockville, MD: U.S. Department of Health and Human Services (National Institute on Drug Abuse), 1996.
7. Mitchell JL, consensus panel chair. *Pregnant, substance-using women.* Rockville, MD: US Department of Health and Human Services (Center for Substance Abuse Treatment), 1993.
8. Kandall SR, consensus panel chair. *Improving treatment for drug-exposed infants.* Rockville, MD: US Department of Health and Human Services (Center for Substance Abuse Treatment), 1993.
9. *Practical approaches in the treatment of women who abuse alcohol and other drugs.* Rockville, MD: U.S. Department of Health and Human Services (Center for Substance Abuse Treatment), 1994.
10. Chiang CN, Finnegan LP, eds. Medication development for the treatment of pregnant addicts and their infants. *NIDA Res Monogr* 1995;149.
11. Kilbey MM, Asghar A, eds. Methodological issues in controlled studies on effects of prenatal exposure to drug abuse. *NIDA Res Monogr* 1991;114.
12. Kilbey MM, Asghar A, eds. Methodological issues in epidemiological, prevention, and treatment research on drug-exposed women and their children. *NIDA Res Monogr* 1991;117.
13. Murphy S, Rosenbaum M. *Pregnant women on drugs.* New Brunswick, NJ, 1999.
14. Finnegan LP, Hagan T, Kaltenbach KA. Scientific foundation of clinical practice: opiate use in pregnant women. *Bull N Y Acad of Med* 1991;67:223–239.
15. Chavkin W, Paone D, Friedmann P, et al. Psychiatric histories of drug using mothers: treatment implications. *J Subst Abuse Treat* 1993;10:445–448.
16. *Drug use forecasting annual report, 1989.* Washington, DC: U.S. Department of Justice, 1990.
17. Connor EM, Sperling RS, Gelber R, et al. Reduction of maternal-infant transmission of human immunodeficiency virus type 1 with zidovudine treatment. *N Engl J Med* 1994;331:1173–1180.
18. Wallach RC, Jerez E, Blinick G. Pregnancy and menstrual function in narcotic addicts treated with methadone. *Am J Obstet Gynecol* 1969;105:1226–1229.
19. Connaughton JF, Finnegan LP, Schut J, et al. Current concepts in the management of the pregnant opiate addict. *Addict Dis* 1975;2:21–35.
20. Connaughton JF, Reeser D, Schut J, et al. Perinatal addiction: outcome and management. *Am J Obstet Gynecol* 1977;129:679–686.
21. Finnegan LP, Connaughton JF, Emich JP, et al. Comprehensive care of the pregnant addict and its effect on maternal and infant outcome. *Contemp Drug Probl* 1972;1:795–809.
22. Harper RG, Solish G, Feingold E, et al. Maternal ingested methadone, body fluid methadone and the neonatal withdrawal syndrome. *Am J Obstet Gynecol* 1977;129:417–424.
23. Kandall SR, Albin S, Gartner LM, et al. The narcotic dependent mother: fetal and neonatal consequences. *Early Hum Dev* 1977;1:159–169.
24. Stimmel B, Adamsons K. Narcotic dependency in pregnancy: methadone maintenance compared to use of street drugs. *JAMA* 1976;235:1121–1124.
25. Strauss ME, Andresko MA, Stryker JC, et al. Methadone maintenance during pregnancy: pregnancy, birth and neonate characteristics. *Am J Obstet Gynecol* 1974;120:895–900.
26. Hagan TA. A retrospective search for the etiology of drug abuse: a background comparison of a drug-addicted population of women and a control group of non-addicted women. *NIDA Res Monogr* 1988;81:254–261.
27. Treatment of morphine-type dependency by withdrawal methods [Editorial]. *JAMA* 1972;219:1611.
28. Harper RG, Solish GI, Purow HM, et al. The effect of a methadone treatment program upon pregnant heroin addicts and their newborn infants. *Pediatrics* 1974;54:300–305.
29. Statzer DE, Wardell JN. Heroin

addiction during pregnancy. *Am J Obstet Gynecol* 1972;113:273–278.

30. Blinick G, Jerez E, Wallach RC. Methadone maintenance, pregnancy and progeny. *JAMA* 1973;225:477–479.

31. Blinick G, Wallach RC, Jerez E. Pregnancy in narcotic addicts treated by medical withdrawal. *Am J Obstet Gynecol* 1969;105:997–1003.

32. Newman RG. Pregnancies of meth adone patients. *N Y State J Med* 1974;1:52–54.

33. Kandall SR, Albin S, Lowinson J, et al. Differential effects of maternal heroin and methadone use on birth weight. *Pediatrics* 1976;58:681–685.

34. Pond SM, Kreek MJ, Tong TG, et al. Altered methadone pharmacokinetics in methadone-maintained pregnant women. *J Pharmacol Exper Ther* 1985;233:1–6.

35. Dole VP, Kreek MJ. Methadone plasma level: sustained by a reservoir of drug in tissue. *Proc Natl Acad Sci U S A* 1973;70:10.

36. Rementeria JL, Nunag NN. Narcotic withdrawal in pregnancy: stillbirth incidence with a case report. *Am J Obstet Gynecol* 1973;116:1152–1156.

37. Fulroth R, Phillips B, Durand DJ. Perinatal outcome of infants exposed to cocaine and/or heroin in utero. *Am J Dis Child* 1989;143:905–910.

38. Heier LA, Carpanzano CR, Mast J, et al. Maternal cocaine use: the spectrum of radiologic abnormalities in the neonatal CNS. *AJNR Am J Neuroradiol* 1991;12:951–956.

39. Zelson C, Rubio E, Wasserman E. Neonatal narcotic addiction: 10-year observation. *Pediatrics* 1971;48:178–189.

40. Naeye RL, Blanc W, Leblanc W, et al. Fetal complications of maternal heroin addiction: abnormal growth infections, and episodes of stress. *J Pediatr* 1973;83:1055–1061.

41. Doberczak TM, Thornton JC, Bernstein J, et al. Impact of maternal drug dependency on birth weight and head circumference of offspring. *Am J Dis Child* 1987;141:1163–1167.

42. Gluck R, Kulovich MV. Lecithin/sphingomyelin ratios in amniotic fluid in normal and abnormal pregnancy. *Am J Obstet Gynecol* 1973;115:539–546.

43. Roloff DW, Howatt WF, Kanto WP Jr, et al. The effect of long-term maternal morphine administration on the growth and lung development of fetal rabbits. In: Morselli PL, Garattini S, Serini F, eds. *Basic and therapeutic aspects of perinatal pharmacology.* New York: Raven Press, 1975.

44. Taeusch HW Jr, Carson SH, Wang NS, et al. Heroin induction of lung maturation and growth retardation in fetal rabbits. *J Pediatr* 1973;82:869–875.

45. Glass L, Rajegowda BK, Evans HE. Absence of respiratory distress syndrome in premature infants of heroin addicted mothers. *Lancet* 1971;2:685–686.

46. Chang A, Wood C, Humphrey M, et al. The effects of narcotics on fetal acid base status. *Br J Obstet Gynaecol* 1976;83:56–61.

47. Archie CL, Lee MI, Sokol RJ, et al. The effects of methadone treatment on the reactivity of the nonstress test. *Obstet Gynecol* 1989;74:254–255.

48. Richardson BS, O'Grady JP, Olsen GD. Fetal breathing movements and the response to carbon dioxide in patients on methadone maintenance. *Am J Obstet Gynecol* 1984;150:400–405.

49. Wittmann BK, Segal S. A comparison of the effects of single- and split-dose methadone administration on the fetus: ultrasound evaluation. *Int J Addict* 1991;26:213–218.

50. Silver H, Wapner R, Loriz-Vega M, et al. Addiction in pregnancy: high risk intrapartum management and outcome. *J Perinatol* 1987;7:178–181.

51. Abrams CAL. Cytogenic risks to the offspring of pregnant addicts. *Addict Dis* 1975;2:63–77.

52. Amarose AP, Norusis MJ. Cytogenetics of methadone-managed and heroin-addicted pregnant women and their newborn infants. *Am J Obstet Gynecol* 1976;124:635–640.

53. Dar H, Schmidt R, Nitowsky HM. Palmar creases and their clinical significance: a study of newborns at risk. *Pediatr Res* 1977;11:103–108.

54. Finnegan LP, Reeser DS, Connaughton JF. The effects of maternal drug dependence on neonatal mortality. *Drug Alcohol Depend* 1977;2:131–140.

55. Rorke LB, Reeser DS, Finnegan LP. Nervous system lesions in infants of opiate dependent mothers. *Pediatr Res* 1977;11:565.

56. Cobrinik RW, Hood TR, Chusid E. The effect of maternal narcotic addiction on the newborn infant; review of the literature and report of 22 cases. *Pediatrics* 1959;24:288–304.

57. Goodfriend MJ, Shey IA, Klein MD. The effects of maternal narcotic addiction on the newborn. *Am J Obstet Gynecol* 1956;71:29–36.

58. Hill RM, Desmond MM. Management of the narcotic withdrawal syndrome in the neonate. *Pediatr Clin North Am* 1963;10:67–86.

59. Kunstadter RH, Klein RI, Lundeen EC, et al. Narcotic withdrawal symptoms in newborn infants. *JAMA* 1958;168:1008–1110.

60. Slobody LB, Cobrinick R. Neonatal narcotic addiction. *Q Rev Pediatr* 1959;14:169–171.

61. Desmond MM, Wilson GS. Neonatal abstinence syndrome: recognition and diagnosis. *Addict Dis* 1975;2:113–121.

62. Finnegan LP, ed. *Drug dependence in pregnancy: clinical management of mother and child. A manual for medical professionals and paraprofessionals prepared for the National Institute on Drug Abuse, Services Research Branch, Rockville, MD.* Washington, DC: Government Printing Office, 1978.

63. Ostrea EM, Chavez CJ, Strauss ME. A study of factors that influence the severity of neonatal narcotic withdrawal. *J Pediatr* 1976;88:642–645.

64. Reddy AM, Harper RG, Stern G. Observation on heroin and methadone withdrawal in the newborn. *Pediatrics* 1971;48:353–357.

65. Rothstein P, Gould JB. Born with a habit: infants of drug-addicted mothers. *Pediatr Clin North Am* 1974;21:307–321.

66. Zelson C. Infant of the addicted mother. *N Engl J Med* 1973;288:1393–1395.

67. Blumenthal I, Lindsay S. Neonatal barbiturate withdrawal. *Postgrad Med J* 1977;53:157–158.

68. Desmond MM, Schwanecke RP, Wilson GS, et al. Maternal barbiturate utilization and neonatal withdrawal symptomatology. *J Pediatr* 1972;80:190–197.

69. Athinarayanan P, Pierog SH, Nigam SK, Glass L. Chlordiazepoxide withdrawal in the neonate. *Am J Obstet Gynecol* 1976;124:212–213.

70. Debooy VD, Seshia MMK, Tennenbein M, et al. Intravenous pentazocine and methylphenidate abuse during pregnancy. *Am J Dis Child* 1993;147:1062–1065.

71. Eriksson M, Larsson G, Winbladh B, et al. The influence of amphetamine addiction on pregnancy and the newborn infant. *Acta Pediatr Scand* 1978;67:95–99.

72. Eriksson M, Larsson G, Zetterstrom R. Amphetamine addiction and pregnancy. *Acta Obstet Gynecol Scand* 1981;60:253–259.

73. Goetz RL, Bain RV. Neonatal withdrawal symptoms associated with maternal use of pentazocine. *J Pediatr* 1974;84:887–888.

74. Oro AS, Dixon SD. Perinatal cocaine and methamphetamine exposure: maternal and neonatal correlates. *J Pediatr* 1987;111:571–578.

75. Prenner BM. Neonatal withdrawal syndrome associated with hydroxyzine hydrochloride. *Am J Dis Child* 1977;131:529–530.

76. Preis O, Choi SJ, Rudolph N. Pentazocine withdrawal syndrome in the newborn infant. *Am J Obstet Gynecol* 1977;127:205–206.

77. Quillian WW II, Dunn CA. Neonatal drug withdrawal from propoxyphene. *JAMA* 1976;235:2128.

78. Ramer CM. The case history of an infant born to an amphetamine-addicted mother. *Clin Pediatr* 1974;1:596–597.

79. Rementeria JL, Bhatt K. Withdrawal symptoms in neonates from intrauterine exposure to diazepam. *J Pediatr* 1977;90:123–126.

80. Reveri M, Pyati SP, Pildes R. Neonatal withdrawal symptoms associated with glutethimide (Doriden) addiction in the mother during pregnancy. *Clin Pediatr* 1977;16:424–425.

81. Rumack BH, Walravens PA. Neonatal withdrawal following maternal ingestion of ethchlorvynol (Placidyl). *Pediatrics* 1973;52:714–716.

82. Tyson HK. Neonatal withdrawal symptoms associated with maternal use of propoxyphene hydrochloride (Darvon). *J Pediatr* 1974;85:684–685.

83. Coles CD, Smith IE, Fernhoff PM, et al. Neonatal ethanol withdrawal: characteristics in clinically normal, nondysmorphic neonates. *J Pediatr* 1984;105:445–451.

84. Pierog S, Chandavasu O, Wexler I. Withdrawal symptoms in infants with the fetal alcohol syndrome. *J Pediatr* 1977;90:630–633.

85. Finnegan LP, Reeser DS. Maternal drug abuse patterns: effect upon the duration of neonatal abstinence. *Pediatr Res* 1979;13:368.

86. Kron RE, Litt M, Phoenix MD, et al. Neonatal narcotic abstinence: effects of pharmacotherapeutic agents and maternal drug usage on nutritive sucking behavior. *J Pediatr* 1976;88:637–641.

87. Sisson TRC, Wickler M, Tsai P, et al. Effect of narcotic withdrawal on neonatal sleep patterns. *Pediatr Res* 1974;8:451.

88. Schulman CA. Alterations of the sleep cycle in heroin addicted and "suspected" newborns. *Neuropediatrie* 1969;1:89–100.

89. Pasto ME, Graziani LJ, Tunis SL, et al. Ventricular configuration and cerebral growth in infants born to drug-dependent mothers. *Pediatr Radiol* 1985;15:77–81.

90. Finnegan LP. Neonatal abstinence syndrome: assessment and pharmacotherapy. In: Rubaltelli FF, Granati B, eds. *Neonatal therapy: an update.* New York: Elsevier Science, 1986:122–146.

91. Davis MM, Brown BS, Glendinning ST. Neonatal effects of heroin addiction

and methadone-treated pregnancies. Preliminary report on 70 live births. In: *Proceedings, Fifth National Conference on Methadone Treatment.* New York: National Association for the Prevention of Addiction to Narcotics, 1973;1153–1164.

92. Herzlinger RA, Kandall SR, Vaughan HG. Neonatal seizures associated with narcotic withdrawal. *J Pediatr* 1977;91:638–641.

93. Kahn EJ, Neumann LL, Polk G. The course of the heroin withdrawal syndrome in newborn infants treated with phenobarbital or chlorpromazine. *J Pediatr* 1969;75:495–500.

94. Lipsitz PJ, Blatman S. Newborn infants of mothers on methadone maintenance. *N Y State J Med* 1974;74:994–999.

95. Kandall SR, Doberczak TM, Mauer KR, et al. Opiate v CNS depressant therapy in neonatal drug abstinence syndrome. *Am J Dis Child* 1983;137:378–382.

96. Doberczak TM, Shanzer S, Cutler R, et al. One-year follow-up of infants with abstinence-associated seizures. *Arch Neurol* 1988;45:649–653.

97. Weinberger SM, Kandall SR, Doberczak TM, et al. Early weight-change patterns in neonatal abstinence. *Am J Dis Child* 1986;140:829–832.

98. Finnegan LP. Pulmonary problems encountered by the infant of the drug-dependent mother. *Clin Chest Med* 1980;1:311–325.

99. Glass L, Rajegowda BK, Kahn EJ, et al. Effect of heroin on respiratory rate and acid-base status in the newborn. *N Engl J Med* 1972;286:746–748.

100. Finnegan LP, Shouraie Z, Emich JP, et al. Alternatives of the oxygen hemoglobin equilibrium curve and red cell 2,3-diphosphoglycerate (2,3-DPG) in cord blood of infants born to narcotic-addicted mothers. *Pediatr Res* 1974;8:344.

101. Behrendt H, Green M. Nature of the sweating deficit of prematurely born neonates. *N Engl J Med* 1972;286:1376–1379.

102. Nathenson G, Cohen MI, Litt IF, et al. The effect of maternal heroin addiction on neonatal jaundice. *J Pediatr* 1972;81:899–903.

103. Burstein Y, Giardina PJV, Rausen AR, et al. Thrombocytosis and increased circulating platelet aggregates in newborn infants of polydrug users. *J Pediatr* 1979;94:895–899.

104. Jhaveri RC, Glass L, Evans HE, et al. Effects of methadone on thyroid function in mother, fetus, and newborn. *Pediatrics* 1980;65:557–561.

105. Ostrea EM, Brady MJ, Parks PM, et al. Drug screening of meconium in infants of drug-dependent mothers: an

alternative to urine testing. *J Pediatr* 1989;115:474–477.

106. Ostrea EM, Brady M, Gause S, et al. Drug screening of newborns by meconium analysis: a large-scale, prospective, epidemiologic study. *Pediatrics* 1992;89:107–113.

107. Rosen TS, Pippenger CE. Pharmacologic observations on the neonatal withdrawal syndrome. *J Pediatr* 1976;88:1044–1048.

108. Kandall SR, Gartner LM. Late presentation of drug withdrawal symptoms in newborns. *Am J Dis Child* 1972;127:58–61.

109. Blinick G. Fertility of narcotic addicts and effects of addiction on the offspring. *Soc Biol* 1971;18[Suppl]:34–39.

110. Rajegowda BK, Glass L, Evans HE, et al. Methadone withdrawal in newborn infants. *J Pediatr* 1972;81:532–534.

111. Davis RC, Chappel JN, Mejia-Zelaya A, et al. Clinical observations on methadone-maintained pregnancies. In: Harbison RD, ed. *Perinatal addiction.* New York: Spectrum, 1975:101–112.

112. Madden JD, Chappel JN, Zuspan F, et al. Observation and treatment of neonatal narcotic withdrawal. *Am J Obstet Gynecol* 1977;127:199–201.

113. Kaltenbach K, Comfort M, Rajagopal D, et al. Methadone maintenance of greater than 80 mg during pregnancy, problems of drug dependence, 1996. In: *Proceedings of the 58th annual scientific meeting, College on Problems of Drug Dependence. NIDA Res Monogr* 1996;174.

114. Doberczak TM, Kandall SR, Wilets I. Neonatal opiate abstinence syndrome in term and preterm infants. *J Pediatr* 1991;118:933–937.

115. Blinick G, Inturrisi CE, Jerez E, et al. Methadone assays in pregnant women and progeny. *Am J Obstet Gynecol* 1975;121:617–621.

116. Doberczak TM, Kandall SR, Friedmann P. Relationships between maternal methadone dosage, maternal–neonatal methadone levels, and neonatal withdrawal. *Obstet Gynecol* 1993;81:936–940.

117. Wilson GS, Desmond MM, Verniaud WM. Early development of infants of heroin addicted mothers. *Am J Dis Child* 1973;126:457–462.

118. Sonderegger T. Persistent effects of neonatal narcotic addiction in the rat. In: Ford DH, Clouet DH, eds. *Tissue responses to addictive drugs.* New York: Spectrum, 1976:589–609.

119. McGinty JF, Ford DH. The effects of maternal morphine or methadone intake

on the growth, reflex development and maze behavior of rat offspring. In: Ford CH, Clouet DH, eds. *Tissue responses to addictive drugs*. New York: Spectrum, 1976:611–629.

120. Zimmerberg B, Charap AD, Glick SD. Behavioural effects of in utero administration of morphine. *Nature* 1974;247:376–377.

121. Soule AB III, Standley K, Copans SA, et al. Clinical uses of the Brazelton Neonatal Scale. *Pediatrics* 1974;54:583–586.

122. Strauss ME, Lessen-Firestone JK, Starr RH Jr, et al. Behavior of narcotics addicted newborns. *Child Dev* 1975;46:887–893.

123. Kaltenbach K, Finnegan LP. The influence of the neonatal abstinence syndrome on mother–infant interaction. In: Anthony EJ, Chiland C, eds. *The child in his family: perilous development: child raising and identity formation under stress*. New York: Wiley-Interscience, 1988:223–230.

124. Fitzgerald E, Kaltenbach K, Finnegan LP. Patterns of interaction among drug-dependent women and their infants. *Pediatr Res* 1990;27:44.

125. Lodge A, Marcus MM, Ramer CM. Neonatal addiction: a two-year-study. Part II. Behavioral and electrophysiological characteristics of the addicted neonate. *Addict Dis* 1975;2:235–255.

126. Boukydis CFZ, Lester BM, eds. NICU network neurobehavioral scale. *Clin Perinatal* 1999;26(1):213–230.

127. Green M, Suffet F. The neonatal narcotic withdrawal index: a device for the improvement of care in the abstinence syndrome. *Am J Drug Alcohol Abuse* 1981;8:203–213.

128. Lipsitz PJ. A proposed narcotic withdrawal score for use with newborn infants. *Clin Pediatr* 1975;14:592–594.

129. Finnegan LP, Kaltenbach K. Neonatal abstinence syndrome. In: Hoekelman RA, Friedman SB, Nelson N, et al, eds. *Primary pediatric care*. St. Louis: C.V. Mosby, 1992:1367–1378.

130. American Academy of Pediatrics, Committee on Drugs. Neonatal drug withdrawal. *Pediatrics* 1998;101:1079–1088.

131. American Academy of Pediatrics, Committee on Drugs.Camphor revisited: focus on toxicity. *Pediatrics* 1994;94:127–128.

132. Gershanik J, Boecler B, Ensley H, et al. The gasping syndrome and benzyl alcohol poisoning. *N Engl J Med* 1982;307:1079–1088.

133. Finnegan LP, Reeser DS, Kaltenbach K, et al. Phenobarbital loading dose method for treatment of neonatal abstinence: effect upon infant development. *Pediatr Res* 1979;13:331.

134. Finnegan LP, Ehrlich SM. Maternal drug abuse during pregnancy: evaluation and pharmacotherapy for neonatal abstinence. *Mod Methods Pharmacol Test Eval Drugs Abuse* 1990;6:255–263.

135. Chavez CJ, Ostrea EM, Stryker JC, et al. Sudden infant death syndrome among infants of drug-dependent mothers. *J Pediatr* 1979;95:407–409.

136. Finnegan LP. *In utero* opiate dependence and sudden infant death syndrome. *Clin Perinatol* 1979;6:163–180.

137. Harper R, Concepcion GS, Blenman S. Observations on the sudden death of infants born to addicted mothers. In: *Proceedings of the fifth national conference on methadone treatment*. New York: National Association for the Prevention of Addiction to Narcotics, 1973:1122–1127.

138. Rajegowda BK, Kandall SR, Falciglia H. Sudden unexpected death in infants of narcotic dependent mothers. *Early Hum Dev* 1978;2/3:219–225.

139. Rosen TS, Johnson HL. Drug-addicted mothers, their infants, and SIDS. *Ann N Y Acad Sci* 1988;533:89–95.

140. Ward SLD, Bautista D, Chan L, et al. Sudden infant death syndrome in infants of substance-abusing mothers. *J Pediatr* 1990;117:876–881.

141. Kandall SR, Gaines J, Habel L, et al. Relationship of maternal substance abuse to sudden infant death syndrome in offspring. *J Pediatr* 1993;123:120–126.

142. Olsen GD, Lees MH. Ventilatory response to carbon dioxide of infants following prenatal methadone exposure. *J Pediatr* 1980;96:983–989.

143. Kandall SR, Gaines J. Maternal substance use and subsequent sudden infant death syndrome (SIDS) in offspring. *Neurotoxicol Teratol* 1991;13:235–241.

144. Wilson GS, McCreary R, Kean J, et al. The development of preschool children of heroin-addicted mothers: a controlled study. *Pediatrics* 1979;63:135–141.

145. Wilson GS, Desmond MM, Wait RB. Follow-up of methadone-treated and untreated narcotic-dependent women and their infants: health, developmental, and social implications. *J Pediatr* 1981;98:716–722.

146. Ramer CM, Lodge A. Neonatal addiction: a two-year study. Part I. Clinical and developmental characteristics of infants of mothers on methadone maintenance. *Addict Dis* 1975;2:227–234.

147. Strauss ME, Starr RH, Ostrea EM, et al. Behavioral concomitants of prenatal addiction to narcotics. *J Pediatr* 1976;89:842–846.

148. Strauss ME, Lessen-Firestone JK, et al. Children of methadone-treated women

at five years of age. *Pharmacol Biochem Behav Suppl* 1979;11:3–6.

149. Lifschitz MH, Wilson GS, Smith EO, et al. Factors affecting head growth and intellectual function in children of drug addicts. *Pediatrics* 1985;75:269–274.

150. Caldwell, B. *HOME Inventory*. Little Rock, AR: University of Arkansas, 1972.

151. Rosen TS, Johnson HL. Children of methadone-maintained mothers: follow-up to 18 months of age. *J Pediatr* 1982;101:192–196.

152. Rosen TS, Johnson HL. Long-term effects of prenatal methadone maintenance. *NIDA Res Monogr* 1985;59:73–83.

153. Hans SL. Developmental consequences of prenatal exposure to methadone. *Ann N Y Acad Sci* 1989;562:195–207.

154. Hans SL, Following drug-exposed infants into middle childhood: challenges to researchers. *NIDA Res Monogr* 1991;114:310–322.

155. Hans SL. Maternal opioid drug use and child development. In: Zagon I, Slotkin TS, eds. *Maternal substance abuse and the developing nervous system*. New York: Academic Press, 1992.

156. Kaltenbach K, Graziani LJ, Finnegan LP. Methadone exposure in utero: developmental status at one and two years of age. *Pharmacol Biochem Behav* 1979;11[Suppl]:15–17.

157. Kaltenbach K, Finnegan LP. Children exposed to methadone in utero: assessment of developmental and cognitive ability. *Ann N Y Acad Sci* 1989;562:360–362.

158. Kaltenbach K. Exposure to opiates: behavioral outcomes in preschool and school-age children. *NIDA Res Monogr* 1996;164:230–241.

159. Moser JM, Jones VH, Kuthy ML. Use of cocaine during the immediate prepartum period by childbearing women in Ohio. *Am J Prev Med* 1993;9:85–91.

160. Schutzman DL, Frankenfield-Chernicoff M, Clatterbaugh HE, et al. Incidence of intrauterine cocaine exposure in a suburban setting. *Pediatrics* 1991;88:825–827.

161. Vega WA, Kolody B, Hwang J, et al. Prevalence and magnitude of perinatal substance exposures in California. *N Engl J Med* 1993;329:850–854.

162. Ryan RM, Wagner CL, Schutz JM, et al. Meconium analysis for improved identification of infants exposed to cocaine in utero. *J Pediatr* 1994;125:435–440.

163. Cregler LL, Mark H. Medical complications of cocaine abuse. *N Engl J Med* 1986;315:1495–1500.

164. Finnegan LP, Mellott JM, Ryan LM, et al. Perinatal exposure to cocaine: human studies. In: Lakoski JM, Galloway MP, White J, eds. *Cocaine:*

pharmacology, physiology, and clinical strategies. Boca Raton, FL: CRC Press, 1992:391–409.

165. Farrar HC, Kearns GL. Cocaine: clinical pharmacology and toxicology. *J Pediatr* 1989;115:665–675.

166. Jaffe JH, Martin WR. Opioid analgesics and antagonists. In: Gilman AG, Goodman LS, Rall TW, et al, eds. *Goodman and Gilman's the pharmacological basis of therapeutics,* 7th ed. New York: Macmillan, 1985:518.

167. Ostrea EM, Romero A, Knapp DK, et al. Postmortem drug analysis of meconium in early-gestation human fetuses exposed to cocaine: clinical implications. *J Pediatr* 1994;124:477–479.

168. Callahan CM, Grant TM, Phipps P, et al. Measurement of gestational cocaine exposure: sensitivity of infants' hair, meconium, and urine. *J Pediatr* 1992;120:763–768.

169. Graham K, Koren G, Klein J, et al. Determination of gestational cocaine exposure by hair analysis. *JAMA* 1989; 262:3328–3330.

170. Jain L, Meyer W, Moore C, et al. Detection of fetal cocaine exposure by analysis of amniotic fluid. *Obstet Gynecol* 1993;81:787–790.

171. Wiggins RC. Pharmacokinetics of cocaine in pregnancy and effects on fetal maturation. *Clin Pharmacokinet* 1992;22:85–93.

172. Woods JR, Plessinger MA, Clark KE. Effect of cocaine on uterine blood flow and fetal oxygenation. *JAMA* 1987;257:957–961.

173. Baxi LV, Petrie RH. Pharmacologic effects on labor: effect of drugs on dystocia, labor and uterine activity. *Clin Obstet Gynecol* 1987;30:19–32.

174. Moore TR, Sorg J, Miller L, et al. Hemodynamic effects of intravenous cocaine on the pregnant ewe and fetus. *Am J Obstet Gynecol* 1986;155:883–888.

175. Acker D, Sachs BP, Tracy KJ, Wise WE. Abruptio placentae associated with cocaine use. *Am J Obstet Gynecol* 1983;146:220–221.

176. Bingol N, Fuchs M, Diaz V, et al. Teratogenicity of cocaine in humans. *J Pediatr* 1987;110:93–96.

177. Chasnoff IJ, Burns WJ, Schnoll SH, et al. Cocaine use in pregnancy. *N Engl J Med* 1985;313:666–669.

178. Hadeed AJ, Siegel SR. Maternal cocaine use during pregnancy: effect on the newborn infant. *Pediatrics* 1989;84:205–210.

179. Livesay S, Ehrlich S, Finnegan L. Cocaine and pregnancy: maternal and infant outcome. *Pediatr Res* 1987; 21:387.

180. Chasnoff IJ, Griffith DR, MacGregor S, et al. Temporal patterns of cocaine use in pregnancy. *JAMA* 1989;261:1741–1744.

181. Handler A, Kistin N, Davis F, et al. Cocaine use during pregnancy: perinatal outcomes. *Am J Epidemiol* 1991;133:818–825.

182. MacGregor SN, Keith LG, Chasnoff IJ, et al. Cocaine use during pregnancy: adverse perinatal outcome. *Am J Obstet Gynecol* 1987;157:686–690.

183. Cherukuri P, Minkoff H, Feldman J, et al. A cohort study of alkaloidal cocaine ("crack") in pregnancy. *Obstet Gynecol* 1988;72:147–151.

184. Chouteau M, Namerow PB, Leppert P. The effect of cocaine abuse on birth weight and gestational age. *Obstet Gynecol* 1988;72:351–354.

185. Chiriboga CA, Brust JC, Bateman D, et al. Dose-response effect of fetal cocaine exposure on newborn neurologic function. *Pediatrics* 1999;103:79–85.

186. Kliegman RM, Madura D, Kiwi R, et al. Relation of maternal cocaine use to the risks of prematurity and low birth weight. *J Pediatr* 1994;124:751–756.

187. Racine A, Joyce T, Anderson R. The association between prenatal care and birth weight among women exposed to cocaine in New York City. *JAMA* 1993;270:1581–1586.

188. Zuckerman B, Frank DA. Prenatal cocaine exposure: nine years later. *J Pediatr* 1994;124:731–733.

189. Zuckerman B, Frank D, Hingson R, et al. Effects of maternal marijuana and cocaine use on fetal growth. *N Engl J Med* 1989;320:762–768.

190. Eyler FD, Behnke M, Conlon M, et al. Birth outcome from a prospective matched study of prenatal crack/cocaine use: I. Interactive and dose effects on health and growth. *Pediatrics* 1998;101:229–237.

191. Bandstra ES, Morrow CE, Anthony JC, et al. Intrauterine growth of full-term infants: impact of prenatal cocaine exposure. *Pediatrics* 2001;108:1309–1319.

192. Scafidi FA, Field TM, Wheeden A, et al. Cocaine-exposed preterm infants show behavioral and hormonal differences. *Pediatrics* 1996;97:851–855.

193. Mahalik MP, Gautein RF, Mann DE. Teratogenic potential of cocaine hydrochloride in CF-1 mice. *J Pharm Sci* 1980;69:703–706.

194. Fantel AG, MacPhail BJ. The teratogenicity of cocaine. *Teratology* 1982;26:17–19.

195. Chasnoff IJ, Chisum GM, Kaplan WE. Maternal cocaine use and genitourinary malformations. *Teratology* 1988; 37:201–204.

196. Lipshultz SE, Frassica JJ, Orav EJ. Cardiovascular abnormalities in infants prenatally exposed to cocaine. *J Pediatr* 1991;118:44–51.

197. Beeram MR, Abedin M, Shoroye A, et al. Occurrence of craniosynostosis in neonates exposed to cocaine and tobacco *in utero. J Natl Med Ass* 1993;85:865–868.

198. Fries MH, Kuller JA, Norton ME, et al. Facial features of infants exposed prenatally to cocaine. *Teratology* 1993;48:413–420.

199. Harris EF, Friend GW, Tolley EA. Enhanced prevalence of ankyloglossia with maternal cocaine use. *Cleft Palate Craniofac J* 1992;29:72–76.

200. Sarpong S, Headings V. Sirenomelia accompanying exposure of the embryo to cocaine. *South Med J* 1992;85:545–547.

201. Hoyme HE, Jones KL, Dixon SD, et al. Prenatal cocaine exposure and fetal vascular disruption. *Pediatrics* 1990;85:743–747.

202. Martin ML, Khoury MJ, Cordero JF, et al. Trends in rates of multiple vascular disruption defects, Atlanta, 1968–1989: is there evidence of a cocaine teratogenic epidemic? *Teratology* 1992;45:647–653.

203. Rajegowda B, Lala R, Nagaraj A, et al. Does cocaine (CO) increase congenital urogenital abnormalities (CUGA) in newborns? *Pediatr Res* 1991;29:71A.

204. Koren G, Graham K, Feigenbaum A, et al. Evaluation and counseling of teratogenic risk: the Motherisk approach. *J Clin Pharmacol* 1993;33:405–411.

205. Koren G, Gladstone D, Robeson C, et al. The perception of teratogenic risk of cocaine. *Teratology* 1992;46:567–571.

206. Madden JD, Payne TF, Miller S. Maternal cocaine abuse and effect on the newborn. *Pediatrics* 1986;77:209–211.

207. Ryan L, Ehrlich S, Finnegan L. Cocaine abuse in pregnancy: effects on the fetus and newborn. *Neurotoxicol Teratol* 1987;9:295–299.

208. Kosten TA. Cocaine attenuates the severity of naloxone-precipitated opioid withdrawal. *Life Sci* 1990;47:1617–1623.

209. Doberczak TM, Shanzer S, Senie RT, Kandall SR. Neonatal neurologic and encephalographic effects of intrauterine cocaine exposure. *J Pediatr* 1988;113:354–358.

210. Eisen LN, Field TM, Bandstra ES, et al. Perinatal cocaine effects on neonatal stress behavior and performance on the Brazelton scale. *Pediatrics* 1991;88:477–480.

211. Coles CD, Platzman KA, Smith I, et al. Effects of cocaine and alcohol use in pregnancy on neonatal growth and neurobehavioral status. *Neurotoxicol Teratol* 1992;14:23–33.

212. Mayes LC, Granger RH, Frank MA,

et al. Neurobehavioral profiles of neonates exposed to cocaine prenatally. *Pediatrics* 1993;91:778–783.

213. Mayes LC, Bornstein MH, Chawarska K, et al. Information processing and developmental assessments in 3-month-old infants exposed prenatally to cocaine. *Pediatrics* 1995;95:539–545.

214. Delaney-Black V, Covington C, Ostrea, E, et al. Prenatal cocaine and neonatal outcome: evaluation of dose–response relationship. *Pediatrics* 1996;98:735–740.

215. Napiorkowski B, Lester BM, Freier C, et al. Effects of *in utero* substance exposure on infant neurobehavior. *Pediatrics* 1996;98:71–75.

216. Tronick EZ, Frank DA, Cabral H, et al. Late dose-response effects of prenatal cocaine exposure on newborn neurobehavioral performance. *Pediatrics* 1996;98:76–83.

217. Mayes LC. Neurobiology of prenatal cocaine exposure effect on developing monoamine systems. *Infant Mental Health J* 1994;15:121–133.

218. Mirochnick M, Meyer J, Cole J, et al. Circulating catecholamine concentrations in cocaine-exposed neonates: a pilot study. *Pediatrics* 1991;88:481–485.

219. Needlman R, Zuckerman B, Anderson GM, et al. Cerebrospinal fluid monoamine precursors and metabolites in human neonates following *in utero* cocaine exposure: a preliminary study. *Pediatrics* 1993;92:55–60.

220. Scher MS, Richardson GA, Day NL. Effects of prenatal cocaine/crack and other drug exposure on electroencephalographic sleep studies at birth and one year. *Pediatrics* 2000;105:39–48.

221. Kramer LD, Locke GE, Ogunyemi A, et al. Neonatal cocaine-related seizures. *J Child Neurol* 1990;5:60–64.

222. Dixon SD, Bejar R. Echoencephalographic findings in neonates associated with maternal cocaine and methamphetamine use: incidence and clinical correlates. *J Pediatr* 1989;115:770–778.

223. Frank DA, McCarten KM, Robson CD, et al. Level of in-utero cocaine exposure and neonatal ultrasound findings. *Pediatrics* 1999;104:1101–1105.

224. van de Bor M, Walther FJ, Sims ME. Increased cerebral blood flow velocity in infants of mothers who abuse cocaine. *Pediatrics* 1990;85:733–736.

225. King TA, Perlman JM, Laptook AR, et al. Neurologic manifestations of in utero cocaine exposure in near-term and term infants. *Pediatrics* 1995;96:259–264.

226. Singer LT, Yamashita TS, Hawkins S, et al. Increased incidence of intraventricular hemorrhage and developmental delay in cocaine-exposed, very low birth weight infants. *J Pediatr* 1994;124:765–771.

227. Dusick AM, Covert RF, Schreiber MD, et al. Risk of intracranial hemorrhage and other adverse outcomes after cocaine exposure in a cohort of 323 very low birth weight infants. *J Pediatr* 1993;122:438–445.

228. Salamy A, Eldredge L, Anderson J, et al. Brain-stem transmission time in infants exposed to cocaine *in utero. J Pediatr* 1990;117:627–629.

229. Shih L, Cone-Wesson B, Reddix B. Effects of maternal cocaine abuse on the neonatal auditory system. *Int J Pediatr Otorhinolaryngol* 1988;15:245–251.

230. Carzoli RP, Murphy SP, Hammer-Knisely J, et al. Evaluation of auditory brain-stem response in full-term infants of cocaine-abusing mothers. *Am J Dis Child* 1991;145:1013–1016.

231. Corwin MJ, Lester BM, Sepkoski C, et al. Effects of *in utero* cocaine exposure on newborn acoustical cry characteristics. *Pediatrics* 1992;89:1199–1203.

232. Teske MP, Trese MT. Retinopathy of prematurity-like fundus and persistent hyperplastic primary vitreous associated with maternal cocaine use. *Am J Ophthalmol* 1987;103:719–720.

233. Isenberg SJ, Spierer A, Inkelis SH. Ocular signs of cocaine intoxication in neonates. *Am J Opthalmol* 1987;103:211–214.

234. Telsey AM, Merritt TA, Dixon SD. Cocaine exposure in a term neonate: necrotizing enterocolitis as a complication. *Clin Pediatr* 1988;27:547–550.

235. Hall TR, Zaninovic A, Lewin D, et al. Neonatal intestinal ischemia with bowel perforation: an in utero complication of maternal cocaine abuse. *AJR Am J Roentgenol* 1992;158:1303–1304.

236. Reznik VM, Anderson J, Griswold WR, et al. Successful fibrinolytic treatment of arterial thrombosis and hypertension in a cocaine-exposed neonate. *Pediatrics* 1989;84:735–738.

237. van de Bor M, Walther FJ, Ebrahimi M. Decreased cardiac output in infants of mothers who abused cocaine. *Pediatrics* 1990;85:30–32.

238. Mehta SK, Finkelhor RS, Anderson RL, et al. Transient myocardial ischemia in infants prenatally exposed to cocaine. *J Pediatr* 1993;122:945–949.

239. Horn PT. Persistent hypertension after prenatal cocaine exposure. *J Pediatr* 1992;121:288–291.

240. Chasnoff IJ, Hunt CE, Kletter R, et al. Prenatal cocaine exposure is associated with respiratory pattern abnormalities. *Am J Dis Child* 1989;143:583–587.

241. Silvestri JM, Long JM, Weese-Mayer DE, et al. Effect of prenatal cocaine on respiration, heart rate, and sudden infant death syndrome. *Pediatr Pulmonol* 1991;11:328–334.

242. Chen C, Duara S, Neto GS, et al. Respiratory instability in neonates with *in utero* exposure to cocaine. *J Pediatr* 1991;119:111–113.

243. Ward SLD, Bautista DB, Woo MS, et al. Responses to hypoxia and hypercapnia in infants of substance-abusing mothers. *J Pediatr* 1992;121:704–709.

244. Bauchner H, Zuckerman B, McClain M, et al. Risk of sudden infant death syndrome among infants with *in utero* exposure to cocaine. *J Pediatr* 1988;113:831–834.

245. Chasnoff IJ, Lewis DE, Squires L. Cocaine intoxication in a breast-fed infant. *Pediatrics* 1987;80:836–838.

246. Chaney NE, Franke J, Wadlington WB. Cocaine convulsions in a breast-feeding baby. *J Pediatr* 1988;112:134–135.

247. Shannon M, Lacouture PG, Roa J, et al. Cocaine exposure among children seen at a pediatric hospital. *Pediatrics* 1989;83:337–342.

248. Kharasch SJ, Glotzer D, Vinci R, et al. Unsuspected cocaine exposure in young children. *Am J Dis Child* 1991;145:204–206.

249. Rivkin M, Gilmore HE. Generalized seizures in an infant due to environmentally acquired cocaine. *Pediatrics* 1989;84:1100–1102.

250. Bateman DA, Heagarty MD. Passive freebase cocaine ("crack") inhalation by infants and toddlers. *Am J Dis Child* 1989;143:25–27.

251. Mirchandani HG, Mirchandani IH, Hellman F, et al. Passive inhalation of free-base cocaine ("crack") smoke by infants. *Arch Pathol Lab Med* 1991;115:494–498.

252. Mott SH, Packer RJ, Soldin SJ. Neurologic manifestations of cocaine exposure in childhood. *Pediatrics* 1994;93:557–560.

253. Ostrea, EM, Ostrea AR, Simpson PM. Mortality within the first 2 years in infants exposed to cocaine, opiate, or cannabinoid during gestation. *Pediatrics* 1997;100:79–83.

254. Kantrowitz B. The crack children. *Newsweek* 1990 Feb12:62.

255. Krauthammer C. Crack babies: genetic inferiors. *New York Daily News* 1989 Jul 31.

256. Daley S. Born on crack and coping with kindergarten. *New York Times* 1991 Feb 7.

257. Blakeslee S. Crack's toll among babies: a joyless view, even of toys. *New York Times* 1989 Sep 17.

258. Besharov DJ. Crack babies: the worst

threat is mom herself. *The Washington Post* 1989; Aug 6.

259. Hinds M deC. The instincts of parenthood become part of crack's toll. *New York Times* 1990; Mar 17.

260. Paltrow L. When becoming pregnant is a crime. *Crim Just Ethics* 1990;Winter/Spring:41–47.

261. Kandall S. Don't call them "crack babies." *New York Newsday* 1991; Apr 18.

262. Lester BM, Tronick EZ. The effects of prenatal cocaine exposure and child outcome. *Infant Mental Health J* 1994;15:107–120.

263. Mayes LC, Granger RH, Bornstein MH, et al. The problem of prenatal cocaine exposure: a rush to judgment. *JAMA* 1992;267:406–408.

264. Myers BJ, Olson HC, Kaltenbach K. Cocaine-exposed infants: myths and misunderstandings. *Zero To Three* 1992;13:1–5.

265. Neuspiel DR. On pejorative labeling of cocaine exposed children. *J Subst Abuse Treat* 1993;10:407.

266. Zuckerman B, Frank DA. "Crack kids:" not broken. *Pediatrics* 1992;89:337–339.

267. Neuspiel DR, Hamel SC. Cocaine and infant behavior. *Dev Behav Pediatr* 1991;12:55–64.

268. Alessandri SM, Sullivan MW, Imaizumi S, et al. Learning and emotional responsivity in cocaine exposed infants. *Dev Psychol* 1993;29:989–997.

269. Fetters L, Tronick EZ. Neuromotor development of cocaine-exposed and control infants from birth through 15 months: poor and poorer performance. *Pediatrics* 1996;98:938–943.

270. Singer LT, Arendt R, Minnes S, et al. Developing language skills of cocaine-exposed infants. *Pediatrics* 2001;107:1057–1064.

271. Chasnoff IJ, Griffith DR, Freier C, et al. Cocaine/polydrug use in pregnancy: two-year follow-up. *Pediatrics* 1992;89:284–289.

272. Arendt R, Angelopoulos J, Salvator A, et al. Motor development of cocaine-exposed children at age two years. *Pediatrics* 1999;103:86–92.

273. Azuma SD, Chasnoff IJ. Outcome of children prenatally exposed to cocaine and other drugs: a path analysis of three-year data. *Pediatrics* 1993;92:396–402.

274. Delaney-Black V, Covington C, Templin T, et al. Prenatal cocaine exposure and child behavior. *Pediatrics* 1998;102:945–950.

275. Delaney-Black V, Covington C, Templin T, et al. Teacher-assessed behavior of children prenatally exposed to cocaine. *Pediatrics* 2000;106:782–791.

276. Frank D, Augustyn M, Knight WG, et al. Growth, development, and behavior in early childhood following prenatal cocaine exposure. *JAMA* 2001;285(12):1613–1625.

277. LaGasse LL, Lester BM, Seifer R, et al. *Maternal lifestyle study.* Society for Research in Child Development, 2003.

278. Lester BM, Abhik S, LaGasse LL, et al. Prenatal cocaine exposure and 7 year outcome: IQ and special education. *Pediatr Res* 2003;53(4):534A.

279. Hans SL. Studies of prenatal exposure to drugs focusing on parental care of children, *Neurotoxicol Teratol* 2002;24:329–337.

280. Lerner RM, ed. *Handbook of psychology,* 5th ed. Vol. 1. *Theoretical models of human development.* New York: Wiley, 1998.

281. Middaugh LD. Prenatal amphetamine effects on behavior: possible mediation by brain monoamines. *Ann N Y Acad Sci* 1989;562:308–318.

282. Billing L, Eriksson M, Jonsson B, et al. The influence of environmental factors on behavioral problems in 8-year-old children exposed to amphetamine during fetal life. *Child Abuse Neglect* 1994;18:3–9.

283. *Substance abuse among women in the United States.* DHHS Publication No. (SMA) 97–3162. Rockville, MD: U.S. Department of Health and Human Services (Substance Abuse and Mental Health Services Administration), 1997.

284. Little BB, Snell LM, Rosenfeld CR, et al. Failure to recognize fetal alcohol syndrome in newborn infants. *Am J Dis Child* 1990;144:1142–1146.

285. Day NL, Jasperse D, Richardson G, et al. Prenatal exposure to alcohol: effect on infant growth and morphologic characteristics. *Pediatrics* 1989;84:536–541.

286. Golden NL, Sokol RJ, Kuhnert BR, et al. Maternal alcohol use and infant development. *Pediatrics* 1982;70:931–934.

287. Jacobson JL, Jacobson SW, Sokol RJ, et al. Effects of alcohol use, smoking, and illicit drug use on fetal growth in black infants. *J Pediatr* 1994;124:757–764.

288. Ouellette EM, Rosett HL, Rosman NP, et al. Adverse effects on offspring of maternal alcohol abuse during pregnancy. *N Engl J Med* 1977;297:528–530.

289. Smith DW. The fetal alcohol syndrome. *Hosp Pract* 1979;14:121–128.

290. Graham JM, Hanson JW, Darby BL, et al. Independent dysmorphology evaluations at birth and 4 years of age for children exposed to varying amounts of alcohol in utero. *Pediatrics* 1988;81:772–778.

291. Hanson JW, Streissguth AP, Smith DW. The effects of moderate alcohol consumption during pregnancy on fetal growth and morphogenesis. *J Pediatr* 1978;92:457–460.

292. Iosub S, Fuchs M, Bingol N, et al. Fetal alcohol syndrome revisited. *Pediatrics* 1981;68:475–479.

293. Coles CD, Platzman KA. Fetal alcohol effects in preschool children: research, prevention, and intervention. In: *Identifying the needs of drug-affected children: public policy issues.* OSAP Prevention Monograph-11. Rockville, MD: U.S. Department of Health and Human Services, 1992:59–86.

294. Ioffe S, Childiaeva R, Chernick V. Prolonged effects of maternal alcohol ingestion on the neonatal electroencephalogram. *Pediatrics* 1984;74:330–335.

295. Clarren SK, Alvord EC, Sumi M, et al. Brain malformations related to prenatal exposure to ethanol. *J Pediatr* 1978;92:64–67.

296. Holzman C, Paneth N, Little R, et al. Perinatal brain injury in premature infants born to mothers using alcohol in pregnancy. *Pediatrics* 1995;95:66–73.

297. Church MW, Gerkin KP. Hearing disorders in children with fetal alcohol syndrome: findings from case reports. *Pediatrics* 1988;82:147–154.

298. Steinhausen HD, Nestler V, Spohr HL. Development of psychopathology of children with the fetal alcohol syndrome. *J Dev Behav Pediatr* 1982;3:49–54.

299. Brown RT, Coles CD, Smith IE, et al. Effects of prenatal alcohol exposure at school age. II. Attention and behavior. *Neurotoxicol Teratol* 1991;13:369–376.

300. Coles CD, Brown RT, Smith IE, et al. Effects of prenatal alcohol exposure at school age. I. Physical and cognitive development. *Neurotoxicol Teratol* 1991;13:357–367.

301. Streissguth AP, Aase JM, Clarren SK, et al. Fetal alcohol syndrome in adolescents and adults. *JAMA* 1991;265:1961–1967.

302. Chavkin W, Kandall SR. Between a "rock" and a hard place: perinatal drug abuse. *Pediatrics* 1990;85:223–225.

CHAPTER 54

Medical Complications of Drug Use

MARC N. GOUREVITCH AND
JULIA H. ARNSTEN

Medical illnesses are common among drug users. Four principal factors contribute to drug users' higher risk for many medical conditions. Most illicit drugs have direct toxicities, which are responsible for a wide variety of medical sequelae (e.g., cocaine-related cardiotoxicity). Certain behaviors associated with drug use (injection, exchanging sex for money or drugs) place drug users at elevated risk for specific conditions (such as endocarditis and sexually transmitted diseases). As many drug users are socioeconomically disadvantaged, life circumstances (e.g., congregate housing) may confer increased environmental risk for infections such as tuberculosis. Finally, diminished access to and effective use of care, and disruption of daily routines by active drug use (thus impeding self-care behaviors such as medication adherence or appointment keeping), may adversely affect clinical outcomes.

This chapter begins by reviewing general principles of providing care for drug users with medical conditions, with additional attention to the issues of adherence and of care for the hospitalized methadone maintenance patient. We then review a range of specific illnesses associated with injection drug use and with noninjection use of heroin and cocaine. Medical syndromes associated with acute use of specific drugs (e.g., intoxication, overdose, and withdrawal) are covered elsewhere in this volume.

GENERAL PRINCIPLES OF CARE FOR DRUG USERS WITH MEDICAL CONDITIONS

To succeed in eliciting from the patient the information needed to provide effective care, the relationship between patient and clinician must be grounded in trust. This may take time to establish, and follows from the patient coming to appreciate that the physician is genuinely interested in being of assistance. Adopting a nonjudgmental, accepting attitude toward the patient fosters trust. Shame and diminished self-esteem are prevalent traits among drug users. Physicians must avoid disapproving or critical remarks regarding ongoing drug use, as patients will often respond by withholding information that might provoke such reactions in the future.

Like other chronic illnesses, substance use is a persistent condition typically characterized by exacerbations and remissions. Primary care providers are generally comfortable managing exacerbations of other chronic diseases and familiar with strategies to induce remission or to slow progression of diseases they cannot cure. When an injection drug user resumes drug use after a period of abstinence, however, clinicians often become discouraged or angry. Caregivers who accept relapse as a common clinical presentation of drug use, and who are aware of available treatment options, are likely to remain more successfully engaged with the drug using patient, thus enhancing the quality and continuity of care provided.

The issue of confidentiality frequently arises when caring for the drug using patient. A direct approach is most effective here as well. When the physician is part of a larger treatment team with the common expectation that patient data will be shared among team members, this arrangement is best made clear to the patient towards the beginning of the relationship. Splitting and perceived betrayal can thus be avoided. The physician must be familiar with the laws governing confidentiality of patients' substance abuse behaviors and treatment. Sensitivity to this issue by the treating clinician will enhance development of trust in the clinician by the patient.

To engage the patient most effectively, the provider must determine and address the patient's agenda. While the clinician may be eager to bring a patient's hypertension under control, the patient may be more concerned about his insomnia. By inquiring about and addressing the primary concerns of the patient, the clinician will reveal their interest in helping the patient, who may, in turn, be more open to working with the physician to address medical conditions that are of less immediate concern to the patient.

Drug users often receive fragmented care. For example, a patient's substance abuse treatment, human immunodeficiency virus (HIV)-related care, general primary care, and psychiatric care may each be delivered by distinct providers at distinct sites. Integrating care improves health care outcomes, and should be a goal of service delivery (1–3). The more information the physician has on hand regarding the components of a patient's care, the more successful the physician will be in averting complications from medication interactions or overlapping medical and psychiatric comorbidities. It is incumbent on the clinician to inquire about concurrent drug use and related treatment, new medications, and new diagnoses when patients receive care in more than one location. Inquiring in nonjudgmental fashion about concurrent drug use should be routinely performed at most, if not all, visits. Type of substance, frequency of use, and route of administration are particularly important to ascertain.

When examining the drug-using patient, attention should be focused on the systems directly affected by the substances the patient is known to use, while not neglecting evidence of use of other drugs. Special attention should be paid to the presence of a variety of signs. Injection ("track") marks may be recent (appearing as fresh punctate marks, often with mild surrounding erythema) or old (linear, hyperpigmented scars representing the confluence of multiple past injection sites). They are found wherever veins are accessible, most often in the antecubital fossae, on the forearms, hands and legs, and less commonly in the neck and groin. Lymphedema of the hands is not uncommon among patients with an extensive injection history. Fresh or old healed abscesses, and cellulitis, are common among injectors, typically reflecting poor hygiene in injecting technique. A cardiac murmur consistent with mitral or tricuspid regurgitation may suggest a past or current history of endocarditis. The nasal septum should always be examined for erosion or infection, suggesting intranasal drug use.

Overlapping Symptoms and Syndromes

A challenge that often arises in the course of assessing and caring for the drug-using patient is differentiation of symptoms and signs related to drug use itself from those of comorbid medical and psychiatric conditions. Such overlapping presentations are most commonly seen among patients with constitutional or psychiatric symptoms.

Constitutional symptoms are frequently related to drug use and withdrawal, but may also reflect systemic illness. Thus, fever after drug injection may reflect use of an impure drug mixture or the first sign of endocarditis. Myalgias, chills, nausea, vomiting, and diarrhea—all hallmarks of withdrawal from narcotics and alcohol—may likewise reflect gastroenteritis or another infectious process, or the side effects of interferon treatment for hepatitis C infection. Weight loss is commonly seen in association with heavy cocaine use, yet must also prompt consideration of systemic infection (e.g., tuberculosis), malignancy, or HIV infection. Dyspnea in the crack smoker may be caused by chronic pulmonary dysfunction related to drug inhalation, or to asthma, or to community-acquired or HIV-related pneumonia. Seizures may occur in the context of drug withdrawal (e.g., alcohol or benzodiazepines) or as a result of prior trauma or intercurrent infection. The same principles apply to the overlap between many psychiatric syndromes and syndromes of intoxication or withdrawal.

Prevention

Disproportionate greater emphasis is often placed on treatment than prevention. Harm reduction is one component of an approach to preventing medical conditions among drug users. In this view, like that adopted by most physicians treating diabetic patients, the goal is to minimize adverse consequences associated with the condition—in this case, addiction to injected drugs. Despite the fact that a "cure" (i.e., sustained abstinence) may not be a realistic

near-term goal for many drug users, much can still be done to minimize the impact of drug use on patients' health. Harm reduction is an approach to treatment that aims to reduce the harm associated with drug use through the use of immediate and practical strategies acceptable to the user. Such an approach may be more effective and engaging for patient and provider alike. Because of the disinhibiting effects of many drugs, the stimulant effects of others, and the relationship of drug procurement to risky sexual behavior, prevention interventions must target sexual risk behaviors as well as drug injection (4,5). Access to condoms, behavioral skills building interventions, and sterile injection equipment for persons who continue to inject despite offers of or participation in treatment, are important components of comprehensive care for drug users.

Health Care Delivery

Despite often fragmented access to care, drug users are heavy users of medical care when it is accessible. Comprehensive primary medical care must include vaccinations, screening for infectious diseases (including tuberculosis, sexually transmitted diseases [STDs], viral hepatitis, and HIV), annual health maintenance examinations, and care of comorbid medical and psychiatric conditions (6). A variety of models exist for delivering such care (7). Most important is that treatment be delivered in a comprehensive and coordinated fashion, with integration of drug use-related and general medical care.

ADHERENCE

Studies of adherence among drug users have focused almost entirely on adherence to antiretroviral therapy among HIV-infected drug users. Numerous studies have been published in the past 5 years, but few stable predictors of adherence have been identified. This is because lack of adherence to treatment recommendations in general is so widespread that no grouping of sociodemographic or psychosocial characteristics can reliably predict it (8). Nonetheless, particular emphasis has been given to defining correlates of adherence among substance users for several reasons: substance users account for an increasing proportion of prevalent acquired immunodeficiency syndrome (AIDS) cases in many urban centers (9), substance users are traditionally thought to be less capable of adhering to medical treatments (10–12), and there is concern that poor adherence among persons engaged in high-risk behaviors will foster development and transmission of resistant HIV virus (13–15).

Active drug or alcohol use has been identified as one of the few relatively consistent predictors of poor adherence, and this is particularly true for cocaine users (16–20). However, past history of drug or alcohol abuse has not been consistently associated with poor adherence, and a number of studies have found that persons not actively using drugs, as well as some active users, are able to adhere to antiretroviral therapy with success comparable to that of nonusers (21–23). For both active and former substance users, engagement in substance use treatment, particularly if on-site primary care is available, seems to facilitate access and adherence to HAART (highly active antiretroviral therapy) and other medical therapies (24–30).

Among both substance users and nonsubstance users, social stability and support, beliefs and knowledge about medications, and confidence in the ability to take HIV medications (including both self-efficacy and "fit" with daily activities) are consistently identified as predictors of adherence (31–38). In addition, active mental illness, in particular depression, is associated with poor adherence (39,40). Some common reasons for nonadherence have also been reported, including difficulty remembering, inconvenient dosing, and medication side effects.

A unique barrier to antiretroviral therapy adherence among many drug users in substance use treatment is the interaction between antiretroviral medications and methadone. It is critical that such interactions be identified in clinical practice, because precipitation of narcotic withdrawal by an antiretroviral agent that induces methadone metabolism may result in resumption of heroin use or in nonadherence with antiretroviral medications (41). Most significantly, the nonnucleoside reverse transcriptase inhibitors, efavirenz (Sustiva) and nevirapine (Viramune), substantially induce methadone metabolism and have been demonstrated in clinical studies to precipitate significant narcotic withdrawal symptoms and to reduce methadone blood levels (42,43). Among protease inhibitors, interactions are less marked. Ritonavir (Norvir), although a potent inhibitor of P450 3A4, does not have a significant interaction with methadone in clinically oriented studies. Ritonavir/saquinavir (Fortovase) given twice daily was shown to decrease serum levels of methadone, but no patients reported withdrawal symptoms (44). Similar findings will obtained with nelfinavir (Viracept) (45) and lopinavir-ritonavir (Kaletra) (46). As a rule, it is important to remain alert to possible interactions between methadone and antiretrovirals or other medications; this is reviewed more extensively elsewhere (47).

The measurement of adherence is challenging in both clinical and research settings, and usually relies on self-report, pill counts, pharmacy records, electronic pill bottle monitors, or a combination of these methods. Despite its tendency to overestimate adherence, self-report remains the most practical measure in most clinical settings, and is most likely to facilitate discussion between patients and providers about the reasons for nonadherence. Many studies demonstrate a strong correlation between self-reported adherence and viral suppression. Studies conducted in the substance-using population also demonstrate this correlation (21,48). These studies also show that self-report

is most valid when patients are asked about the number of missed doses within a short time frame (1 to 7 days), and when assessments are gathered on more than one occasion and responses are averaged over time. Clinicians' estimates of patient adherence have been repeatedly shown to be inaccurate and should not be substituted for a thorough adherence assessment. Therapeutic drug monitoring may become a useful adjunct measure in the future, but because plasma drug levels reflect only recent adherence, its usefulness will remain limited.

CARE OF THE HOSPITALIZED METHADONE MAINTENANCE PATIENT

General Principles

Methadone, a long-acting opiate agonist, is given once daily to treat heroin dependence (49). The goals of methadone maintenance therapy are to eliminate withdrawal and craving symptoms, and to block the euphoric effects of illicit opiates. Aided by counseling, methadone patients are thus able to focus on rebuilding physical and emotional health, relationships, employment, and other critical life domains. Because no optimal dose of methadone exists for the treatment of opioid dependence, patients' responses must be assessed individually by experienced clinicians. Generally, doses of 40 to 60 mg daily will block opioid withdrawal symptoms, but higher doses (at or above 70–80 mg daily) are needed to block opioid craving, decrease illicit drug use, and promote treatment retention (50–52). Sustained recovery from drug dependence often requires multiple treatment episodes and, once stabilized on methadone, patients may remain in treatment for years. Methadone is medically safe with no adverse impact on immune function and no evidence of significant adverse effects with prolonged use (53). In addition to reducing heroin use (54), methadone maintenance attenuates the psychosocial and medical morbidity associated with heroin addiction. Methadone maintenance improves overall health status, is associated with decreased criminal activity and improved social functioning, and decreases the spread of HIV and hepatitis B (50,55,56). Finally, enrollment in methadone treatment is associated with improved adherence with HAART (30).

Methadone-maintenance patients commonly undergo hospitalization for medical or surgical problems, and, in general, their management should be no different from that of other patients. When a methadone-maintained patient is hospitalized, the usual maintenance dose of methadone should be given each day throughout the hospitalization. If the methadone dose cannot be verified by the patient's outpatient methadone treatment program, 20 mg of methadone can be given every 12 hours to prevent acute severe withdrawal (57). Forty milligrams will prevent withdrawal symptoms even in a patient maintained on higher dose. Once the patient's usual dose is verified, it should be continued. Patients on stable outpatient methadone-treatment regimens should not have their methadone doses reduced or withheld during acute illness, even in the setting of pulmonary or neurologic disease.

Postoperative patients, including those on methadone maintenance, frequently experience pain. Because of tolerance, the usual daily dose of methadone will not serve as an analgesic for pain caused by a surgical procedure or an illness. Consequently, full therapeutic doses of analgesic drugs should be given to methadone-maintenance patients for painful conditions. Methadone-maintenance patients may also have cross-tolerance to other narcotics, and often require higher doses of analgesics and more frequent dosing intervals for pain control (see Pain Management below).

Pain Management

Drug users have been found to have a high prevalence of pain, as a result of a variety of medical conditions. In two recent surveys of patients in methadone-treatment programs, the prevalence of chronic pain ranged from 37% to 61% (58,59). Medical illnesses predisposing to chronic pain among drug users include musculoskeletal pain (resulting from infections, degenerative joint disease, and trauma), soft-tissue infections, liver disease, venous insufficiency, HIV-related conditions, and peripheral neuropathies associated with alcohol use or nutritional deficiencies. In addition, opioid addicts have been observed in experimental studies to have hyperalgesia and pain intolerance, and chronic opioid therapy, as with methadone, may increase analgesic tolerance (60).

Despite their high prevalence of chronic pain, drug users are often undertreated for pain, even during serious medical illness (61). Studies show that physicians are hesitant to treat pain in hospitalized patients with substance abuse problems, fearing deception by patients seeking opioids for addiction rather than pain, and lacking the appropriate knowledge and skills to evaluate and treat pain and opioid withdrawal (62). Some authors also cite "generalized opiophobia," fear of regulatory sanctions, and prevailing moral and punitive views of addiction as contributing to the inadequate treatment of pain in drug users (60). However, drug users with serious medical illness and chronic pain may be more likely to manipulate medications and take nonprescribed analgesics to self-medicate (63), and hospitalized drug users often interpret physician inconsistency or hospital insufficiency as signs of intentional mistreatment. The interaction between physicians and drug-using patients in the hospital has therefore been characterized by "mutual mistrust," especially concerning treatment of pain with opioid medications (62). At the same time, periods of acute illness often represent opportunities for meaningful intervention in addictive disease, and attempts to engage the patient in substance-abuse treatment should be most aggressive at these times (64).

To address these inherent conflicts, the management of pain in individuals with a current or past history of addiction has been specifically addressed in recent pain management guidelines (65,66). In 1998, the Federation of State Medical Boards (FSMB) of the United States outlined a set of treatment guidelines constituting good medical practice when using controlled substances to treat pain. There are seven specific guidelines: (a) evaluation of the patient, (b) treatment plan, (c) informed consent and agreement for treatment, (d) periodic review, (e) consultation, (f) medical records, and (g) compliance with controlled substances laws and regulations. For patients with addiction, the FSMB guidelines recommended that physicians consult with addiction medicine specialists, and undertake more intensive and consistent monitoring of prescription adherence, physical and psychosocial functioning, and treatment goals (66).

In clinical practice, the implementation of these guidelines in drug users with chronic pain requires several steps. Evaluation of the patient must include not only an accurate history and classification of pain, but also an assessment of current patterns of alcohol and drug use. In addition, it must include an evaluation of comorbid psychiatric and psychosocial conditions, and of family and other environmental factors that influence substance abuse. The treatment plan must address several issues, including choice of appropriate analgesic agent, analgesic side effects, adjuvant drugs, and the implications of treatment for drug using patients. Analgesic selection should be guided by patients' self-reports of pain intensity, using a visual analogue or 0 to 10 pain-intensity scale. Mild pain (up to 4 on the 0 to 10 scale) may be treated with a nonnarcotic analgesic; moderate pain (4 to 6 on the 0 to 10 scale) may be treated with a weak narcotic analgesic; and severe pain (7 and above on the 0 to 10 scale) may be treated with a strong opioid. In general, drug users should be treated with long-acting opioids with limited rescue doses, but it is not necessary to start with weaker agents and wait for them to fail before moving to a stronger class. Other strategies for using opioids to treat pain in drug users include using the least-euphorigenic agents with the lowest street value, and using alternative formulations, such as transdermal patches, when possible. For hospitalized drug users, standard delivery systems, such as indwelling venous catheters, percutaneous continuous infusion pumps, and patient-controlled analgesia, should not routinely be avoided, but should be used with the understanding that abuse will lead to discontinuation of the treatment delivery system. Because of tolerance and physical dependence, drug users treated with opioids will usually require higher doses given at more frequent intervals than will nontolerant patients, and to achieve adequate analgesia, these doses should be administered around-the-clock rather than as needed (67).

In the outpatient setting, implementation of treatment guidelines is possible if strategies to minimize the abuse potential of prescribed opioids are employed. These strategies may include making one provider responsible for prescribing opioids, written contracts to define mutual expectations and consequences of aberrant drug behavior (including lost or stolen prescriptions), frequent clinic visits, prescription of small quantities of drug on a fixed renewal schedule, prescription renewal contingent on clinic attendance, periodic random urine toxicology testing, participation in substance abuse treatment, and involvement of family in the treatment plan (65,67).

VIRAL HEPATITIS

Hepatitis A

Hepatitis A virus (HAV) is the leading cause of acute viral hepatitis in the United States, and results in significant morbidity and health care costs (68). Hepatitis A is a nonenveloped ribonucleic acid (RNA) virus that is excreted in stool and usually transmitted by fecal–oral contact, although transmission through blood is also possible. Most cases of HAV occur during community-wide outbreaks, but a high proportion of these cases occur in persons who report using drugs (69). Drug use is now recognized as a significant risk factor for transmission of hepatitis A, and antibodies to HAV have been identified in 43% to 66% of injection drugs users (70,71). Transmission between drug users is hypothesized to occur primarily by the fecal–oral route when people gather together to swallow, smoke, or snort drugs, and secondarily by percutaneous transmission through sharing needles and other injection supplies. Outbreaks of hepatitis A have been described particularly among users of marijuana and methamphetamine (69,72).

Hepatitis A is generally an acute, localized disease, with uncommon cases involving relapse or extrahepatic manifestations. Unlike hepatitis B, a carrier state does not exist for HAV. The usual incubation period for HAV is 28 days (range: 15 to 40 days), and most adults are asymptomatic during acute infection. When symptoms occur, they typically include a mild prodromal illness of fever, headache, malaise, and nonspecific gastrointestinal symptoms, followed by dark urine, jaundice, tender hepatosplenomegaly, and postcervical lymphadenopathy. This classic presentation occurs in more than 80% of symptomatic patients and is self-limited, lasting less than 8 weeks. Most patients are treated supportively and experience complete resolution by 3 to 6 months. A much rarer and more severe form of HAV has been described in patients with hepatitis C or other chronic liver disease, and is associated with fulminant liver failure and a high mortality rate (up to 35%) (73).

The diagnosis of acute HAV is made by detecting anti-HAV antibodies in patients with symptoms consistent with hepatitis. Abnormal liver function tests are not specific for hepatitis A. IgM anti-HAV antibodies can be detected 1 to 2 weeks after exposure and persist for 3 to 6 months. IgG anti-HAV antibodies can be detected 5 to 6 weeks after exposure and persist for decades, conferring lifelong protection against HAV. The prevalence of anti-HAV antibodies is particularly high among drug users; in one study, the prevalence among injection drug users was twice that in the general population (71).

The high prevalence of anti-HAV antibodies among drug users suggests that they are an important reservoir of HAV. In addition, chronic hepatitis caused by hepatitis B or C is extremely common among injection drug users, making them more susceptible to the most severe form of acute HAV. HAV vaccination of drug users is therefore indicated to both protect the individual from a potentially fatal condition, and to reduce HAV transmission to others. There are two currently available HAV vaccines in the United States, both of which are administered intramuscularly as two injections given 6 months apart. Because of the high prevalence of prior infection and anti-HAV antibodies among drug users, HAV serology should be checked before vaccination.

Hepatitis B

More than 300,000 people in the United States are infected with hepatitis B virus (HBV) each year, and 20% of these infections occur among drug users (74,75). Unlike hepatitis A, hepatitis B is a deoxyribonucleic acid (DNA) virus that is predominantly acquired through sexual contact (homosexual and heterosexual), but also by injection drug use and occupational exposure. Among drug users, HBV is usually transmitted parenterally through the sharing of needles and other contaminated injection equipment (76), but it may also be transmitted through high-risk sexual behavior. Recent studies indicate that the seroprevalence of HBV antibodies among injection drug users ranges from 50% to 80% across the United States, and increases with age and duration of drug use (77,78). More than 80% of injection drug users who have been injecting for longer than 10 years are infected with HBV (79). HBV acquisition is a relatively early event for most injection drug users, occurring within the first several years of injection drug use. In one recent study, HBV incidence ranged from 12% to 31% per year among young (age 18 to 30 years) injection drug users (80). This group represents the highest incidence of new HBV infections in the United States, and transmission is linked to injection practices (frequent injection or injection of cocaine), high-risk injecting behavior (sharing needles, syringes, and drug-preparation equipment), and high-risk sexual behavior (not using a condom and/or having multiple sexual partners) (75,78).

The outcome of acute hepatitis B virus infection is variable. Only approximately 40% of patients develop clinical symptoms of acute hepatitis, 25% develop jaundice, and less than 5% are hospitalized. The incubation period, defined by the appearance of clinical symptoms, ranges from 1 to 6 months. Fulminant hepatic failure is a rare complication, affecting 1 in 1,000 patients (74). Early in infection, circulating HBV surface antigen (HBsAg) can be detected prior to the development of either clinical symptoms or elevated hepatic transaminases. This is followed by the production of hepatitis B e antigen (HBeAg), and then by elevations in transaminases. The first immune response is the production of antibodies to HBV core antigens (anti-HBc), which appear shortly after HBsAg. Anti-HBc plays no role in host defense, but is a reliable marker of HBV infection currently or within the preceding few years. The development of anti-HBe indicates diminished infectivity with a reduction in hepatic inflammation and normalization of transaminases. During clinical recovery, HBsAg disappears with gradual appearance of anti-HBs. Anti-HBs confers immunity to hepatitis B and, along with anti-HBc, persists in the serum after recovery from acute HBV.

Among all patients with acute hepatitis B infection, 5% to 10% develop chronic infection with persistent HBsAg positivity, and there are 1 million persons chronically infected with HBV in the United States. There are two phases of chronic HBV infection. Initially, HBeAg and HBV DNA are detectable, hepatic inflammation is active, serum transaminases are elevated, and the patient is infectious. The second phase begins with seroconversion from HBeAg to anti-HBe. Although HBsAg remains positive, during this second phase there is reduced hepatic inflammation, normalization of serum transaminases, disappearance of markers of HBV replication, and reduced (but still present) infectivity. Persistent HBeAg is associated with increased infectivity, more severe disease, and eventual cirrhosis (81). Current treatment options for chronic HBV, which include interferon-alfa and lamivudine (Epivir), convert 20% to 40% of patients from the replicative phase (HBeAg present) to the nonreplicative phase (anti-HBeAg present, HBeAg and HBV DNA absent) with consequent reduction in the risk of development of progressive liver disease. Chronic HBV is associated with cirrhosis and hepatocellular cancer, and leads to 4,000 deaths from cirrhosis and 800 deaths from hepatocellular carcinoma annually in the United States (82).

The hepatitis B vaccine is immunogenic, effective, and safe, and has been recommended for injection drug users by the United States Centers for Disease Control (CDC) since 1982. However, the incidence of hepatitis B infection among injection drug users increased by 80% between 1982 and 1990 because targeted vaccination programs were never implemented, largely because of the perceived difficulty of ensuring that high-risk groups completed the vaccine series (75,83). In addition, successful vaccination and protection against chronic HBV requires that drug users be vaccinated *before* they are exposed to HBV. The recommended vaccine consists of three intramuscular injections at 0, 3, and 6 months, which leads to protective levels of anti-HBs in more than 90% of ≤40 years old healthy adults, but is less effective in persons who are older, smoke, overweight, or immunocompromised (by HIV-infection, diabetes mellitus, renal failure, or chronic liver disease). Whether three doses are necessary is uncertain because recent studies indicate that two doses, administered 6 months apart, may result in anti-HBs levels similar to those obtained with the three-dose schedule (84).

The greatest success in vaccination completion rates among injection drug users (70% to 85%) has been achieved in drug-treatment programs that offer the vaccine (85,86), and rates have been lower among drug users who do not regularly attend treatment facilities (87). Vaccination of the entire population during infancy or early adolescence, as has been recommended by the Centers for Disease Control and Prevention since 1991, will eventually reduce the incidence of HBV infection, but full implementation of this recommendation has not yet been achieved. Greater efforts are necessary to vaccinate drug users against HBV, and should involve all potential settings in which drug users have contact with health care providers. These include drug treatment programs, health departments, jails and prisons, needle exchange programs, ambulatory clinics, and hospital emergency rooms. Studies also show that modest financial incentives and convenient location greatly increase adherence to HBV vaccine among injection drug users (88). In addition, all staff of drug-treatment programs who are susceptible to HBV infection should receive hepatitis B vaccine. Drug users, should be screened with HBV serologies prior to vaccination. Because anti-HBc appears earlier in disease and persists even among HBsAg carriers, anti-HBc may be more sensitive than anti-HBs for identifying vaccine candidates who have not been previously infected with HBV (89). However, only anti-HBs detects immunity from prior vaccination, and may be a more appropriate screening test if the probability of prior vaccination is high.

Hepatitis C

Approximately 4 million people have evidence of exposure to hepatitis C virus (HCV) in the United States, of whom 74% have evidence of chronic infection (90). Following implementation of progressive enhancements in screening of the blood supply, injection drug use has become the primary route of transmission of HCV infection (91). Among injectors, there is considerable geographic variation in HCV seroprevalence, ranging from 66% to 93% in major U.S. cities (92). Differences in seroprevalence between diverse neighborhoods within a single city likely reflects variations in transmission dynamics among distinct networks of injectors (93).

Acquisition of HCV infection is often rapid following initiation of drug injection: 77% of injection drug users in a Baltimore sample were HCV-infected within 1 year of first injecting, with injection frequency and injection of cocaine associated with increased transmission risk among injectors (94). Sharing of drug preparation equipment, including cookers and the filtration cotton, is also clearly associated with HCV infection risk (95,96). Although sharing of intranasal cocaine sniffing equipment (e.g., straws) has been considered a possible route of HCV transmission, the data are inconclusive (97,98). Sexual transmission of HCV, although much less efficient than injection-related transmission, can also be a risk for infection among drug users. Multiple sex partners and comorbid sexually transmitted diseases increase the risk of sexual acquisition of HCV (99). Noninjection drug users trading sex for money or drugs may be at particularly high risk for sexual acquisition of HCV.

Most patients do not seek medical attention in association with acute infection with hepatitis C, because clinical manifestations are often mild or absent (100). Following initial infection with HCV, approximately 15% to 20% of persons appear permanently to clear the virus, and 80% to 85% of persons develop chronic infection. HCV-induced cirrhosis develops in an estimated 15% to 20% of those with chronic infection, and HCV-related end-stage liver disease (ESLD) now constitutes the most common indication for liver transplantation in the United States (100). Rates of progression to ESLD vary substantially across studies (101,102). Factors associated with accelerated progression of HCV-related liver disease include coinfection with HIV, older age at time of infection, and alcohol consumption (101–103).

Among those who naturally ward off chronic infection there is no evidence that protective immunity develops against future reinfection with HCV. Nevertheless, reinfection of injectors appears to be a relatively uncommon occurrence (104,105). This is of particular relevance to injection drug users and others who may be repeatedly exposed to the virus over time.

Serologic determination of HCV infection is generally accomplished by testing for the presence of anti-HCV antibodies. Serum levels of HCV RNA are assessed in antibody-positive persons. If absent, the patient is assumed to have cleared the infection.

HCV treatment has evolved rapidly over the past decade. Eligibility is determined primarily by considering the extent of plasma viremia, hepatic fibrosis, and inflammation (106). The National Institutes of Health's *2002 Consensus Development Conference Statement on Management of Hepatitis C* explicitly states that persons should not be excluded from receiving HCV treatment solely on the basis of active drug or alcohol use. Nor is methadone treatment considered a contraindication to treatment (106). Evidence from studies in a variety of settings support this assertion (107,108). As with all patients

with chronic medical conditions, the decision to embark on a sustained course of treatment, during which side effects are likely and a successful response uncertain, must be made on a case-by-case basis (109). Factors to consider might include the patient's motivation, past adherence with chronic therapies, HCV genotype, likelihood of success, and engagement in medical care.

Currently, best results are obtained with a combination of pegylated interferon, given by subcutaneous injection, and ribavirin, taken orally. Response to treatment is typically evaluated after 12 weeks: If an insufficient drop in HCV viral load is observed, treatment is discontinued. Of the three HCV genotypes most prevalent in the United States, genotypes 2 and 3 are most responsive to treatment, which is typically continued for 6 months in such patients. Twelve months of treatment is considered standard for persons with genotype 1 infection. A patient is deemed to have a successful end-of-treatment response (ETR) when HCV viremia is undetectable after 6 (genotype 2 and 3 infections) or 12 (genotype 1) months of treatment. A sustained viral response (SVR) is defined as persistence of viral eradication (as measured by nondetectable viremia) 6 months following completion of treatment. Rates of SVR in clinical trials approximate 45% following 48 weeks of treatment of patients with genotype 1 infection, and 80% following 24 weeks of treatment of patients with genotypes 2 and 3 infections. Although it remains uncertain whether a sustained viral response to treatment signifies a "cure" of the patient's HCV infection, prevention of long-term sequelae of HCV infection is clearly associated with successful treatment (106).

Side effects from treatment are significant. Major complications of interferon are constitutional symptoms and psychiatric manifestations. Depression, already prevalent among HCV-infected drug users (110), is often precipitated or worsened by treatment of HCV with interferon (111). Screening for depression and other psychiatric disorders at baseline and periodically during treatment is an important component of care. The value of pretreatment with an antidepressant among patients without depression at baseline is under investigation. The major complications of ribavirin are hematologic, with significant anemia, neutropenia, or both often complicating treatment.

Configuring service delivery to optimize delivery of hepatitis C treatment to eligible drug users is challenging. Several of the stages of care (e.g., screening, evaluation of eligibility for treatment, which typically involves liver biopsy, and treatment itself) are often conducted by distinct health care providers. If the patient is receiving substance abuse treatment, primary medical care, or psychiatric care, fragmentation of service delivery is even more likely. To the extent possible, integration of the several aspects of the patient's care is an important goal.

For patients engaged in substance abuse treatment, providing hepatitis C related care on-site at the treatment program is an attractive option, facilitating interdisciplinary management of the medical, psychiatric and substance abuse treatment aspects of care. For example, patients receiving methadone maintenance treatment often request an increase in their methadone dose during combination treatment of their HCV infection (108), presumably because of the similarity between interferon-related side effects and the symptoms of opioid withdrawal. Other patients, learning that they are infected with HCV decades after they stopped injecting, may be profoundly discouraged by this unwanted "blast from the past," to the point that it jeopardizes their recovery. Such complex clinical issues are ideally addressed in an interdisciplinary setting. Patients' access to the various members of the treatment team is facilitated when they are colocated in a common site (112). Syringe exchange programs provide another promising setting into which HCV-related services can effectively be integrated (113).

In several studies, only a small proportion of eligible HCV-infected drug users completed treatment (114,115). Improved strategies for provider and patient education, defining surrogate markers for fibrosis, developing less-toxic therapies, and successfully treating comorbid psychiatric and substance abuse disorders, are urgently needed in view of the very heavy burden of HCV infection among persons with a history of substance abuse.

Is the presence of hepatitis C infection a contraindication to treating a patient with potentially hepatotoxic medications? Many medications used to treat conditions that are common among drug users are associated with some risk of hepatotoxicity. Are they safe to use in HCV-infected patients? The few studies to examine this question suggest that standard guidelines apply. Isoniazid was safely used to treat latent tuberculosis infection in HCV-infected drug users. Only excessive alcohol use and aminotransferase levels greater than three times normal were independently associated with onset of isoniazid hepatotoxicity (116). One study of antiretroviral therapy for HIV infection among HCV-infected persons reached similar conclusions (117).

Efforts to prevent HCV transmission and acquisition, often given less attention than diagnosing and treating existing infection, are vitally important. HCV antibody testing should be widely offered to all persons with current or former drug or alcohol dependence. Persons testing negative should receive tailored counseling. If they are injecting drugs, use of sterile sources of injection equipment should be supported (118). Referral to syringe exchange programs or to pharmacies with permission to dispense syringes to injectors should be encouraged, and safer routes of use (e.g., intranasal) can be suggested, while simultaneously working with the patient to reduce or eliminate their drug use. Bleach disinfection of used syringes may also be an effective intervention (119). Safer sex practices, particularly for persons with multiple partners, should be supported as well. Persons testing positive for HCV, if injecting drugs, should be counseled not to share injecting equipment.

Secondary prevention efforts include routine vaccination against hepatitis A and hepatitis B for all HCV-infected persons. Evidence suggests that hepatitis A can be particularly fulminant in some HCV-infected persons (120), and some data implicate hepatitis B as a factor associated with accelerated progression of HCV-related liver disease.

Alcohol consumption is associated with more rapid progression of HCV-related liver disease (101,102) and with diminished response to treatment (121,122). There is uncertainty as to whether a modest degree of alcohol consumption is detrimental, because most studies have found this effect to be associated with moderate to heavy levels of drinking. Counseling HCV-infected persons to eliminate or at least minimize alcohol consumption is encouraged.

Hepatitis D

Hepatitis D (delta) virus (HDV) is an incomplete RNA virus that requires coinfection with active HBV to become active, is transmitted in the same manner as HBV, and is prevented by HBV vaccination. It is endemic in the Mediterranean region and in parts of Asia, Africa, and South America and appears to have been spread to nonendemic areas such as the United States and Northern Europe by injection drug users (123). Outbreaks of severe and fulminant hepatitis, primarily as a result of coinfection with HDV and HBV, have been reported in injection drug users and their sexual contacts (124), and the prevalence of HDV infection in drug users with chronic HBV is 50% to 80% (125–128). In a comparison of HDV infection in drug users and nonusers, evidence of more rapid histologic deterioration of the liver was found in drug users (129).

There are two mechanisms of HDV infection: coinfection with HBV, and superinfection of HBsAg carriers. In coinfection, HBV and HDV are acquired together, and there is a higher incidence of fulminant hepatic failure (up to 20%) than with HBV infection alone. Thirty percent of patients with acute fulminant hepatitis B have coinfection with HDV, and the case fatality rate is almost 5%. Similarly, when a chronic HBV carrier is superinfected with HDV, subsequent liver disease is more severe and more rapidly progressive than with HBV infection alone (74,130). HDV superinfection should be strongly considered when a stable HBsAg carrier has an exacerbation of chronic liver disease or an episode resembling acute hepatitis B. The diagnosis is made by detecting anti-HD antibodies and HBsAg in the serum of a patient with chronic liver disease. In HDV superinfection, high titers of anti-HD appear promptly and persist during the course of chronic HDV infection. This is in contrast to HDV coinfection, in which the appearance of anti-HD is often delayed until convalescence from acute hepatitis, and repeated testing may be needed to confirm the diagnosis.

Other Viral Causes of Hepatitis

Drug users are at high risk of developing infectious diseases because of sharing of injection equipment, immunosuppression, poor hygiene leading to high rates of skin and nasopharyngeal carriage of pathogenic organisms, and poor access to adequate housing or health care, and many infectious organisms have the potential to cause hepatic disease. These include viruses such as Epstein-Barr, herpes simplex, and cytomegalovirus, all of which may cause hepatitis-like illnesses. Most often these viruses are spread through direct contact, but they can be spread parentally as well. Although relatively rare in comparison to HAV, HBV, HCV, and HDV, it is important to consider these pathogens in the differential diagnosis of hepatitis among drug users.

SEXUALLY TRANSMITTED DISEASES

Sexually transmitted diseases (STDs) are common among drug users, largely as a result of the exchange of sex for money or drugs, but also as a result of increased sexual risk-taking among users of stimulants such as cocaine and amphetamines. In particular, crack cocaine use is associated with high rates of risky sexual behaviors, including trading sex for money or drugs, inconsistent condom use, and multiple sexual partners. Frequently seen STDs among drug users are syphilis, gonorrhea, chlamydia, genital herpes simplex virus, human papilloma virus, and trichomoniasis. In addition, HIV is transmitted among drug users both sexually and parentally; a full discussion of HIV infection is found in Section VIII, HIV Infection and AIDS.

Syphilis

Syphilis is a readily curable, bacterial genital ulcer disease caused by *Treponema pallidum.* After declining every year since 1990, the number of reported cases of syphilis in the United States increased by 2.1% from 2000 to 2001. In 2000, the rate of syphilis had declined to 2.1 cases per 100,000 population, the lowest rate since reporting began in 1941. However, in 2001, the rate of syphilis increased to 2.2 cases per 100,000 population (6,103 cases). This increase was largely driven by syphilis outbreaks in certain cities among men who have sex with men (131). Among drug users, rates of incident syphilis are very high, ranging from 2.9 to 26.0 per 1,000 person-years, a more than 100-fold increase over the general population (132–135). In addition, rates of self-reported lifetime prevalence of syphilis among drug users range from 2% to 19% (132,136). Risk behaviors consistently associated with syphilis incidence

among drug users include crack cocaine use, multiple sex partners, and the exchange of sex for money or drugs (134,137).

Patients who have syphilis may seek treatment for clinical signs of primary infection (usually a painless chancre), secondary infection (manifestations that include but are not limited to skin or mucocutaneous lesions), or tertiary infection (cardiac, ophthalmic, or auditory abnormalities). Latent infections, or those lacking clinical manifestations, are detected by serologic testing. Latent syphilis acquired within the preceding year is referred to as early latent syphilis; all other cases of latent syphilis are either late latent syphilis or latent syphilis of unknown duration (138).

Because of their high prevalence of syphilis exposure, drug users should be screened annually with RPR (rapid plasma reagin) or VDRL (Venereal Disease Research Laboratory) nontreponemal tests. Because of the high rate of false-positive nontreponemal tests, positive results should be confirmed with a treponemal antibody test. Nontreponemal titers usually correlate with disease activity; a fourfold change in titer, equivalent to a change of two dilutions (e.g., from 1:16 to 1:4 or from 1:8 to 1:32), indicates a clinically significant difference between two nontreponemal test results obtained using the same serologic test. Nontreponemal tests usually become nonreactive with time after treatment; however, in some patients, nontreponemal antibodies can persist at a low titer for a long period of time, sometimes for the life of the patient. Most patients who have reactive treponemal tests will have reactive tests for the remainder of their lives, regardless of treatment or disease activity. However, 15% to 25% of patients treated during the primary stage revert to being serologically nonreactive after 2 to 3 years. Treponemal antibody titers correlate poorly with disease activity and should not be used to assess treatment response. HIV serology should be checked in all patients with serologic evidence of syphilis.

Like all other patients, drug users with STDs should be treated with single-dose regimens, if possible. Benzathine penicillin (2.4 million units) is the preferred single-dose regimen for early syphilis (primary, secondary, or early latent), and has been used effectively for more than 50 years to achieve clinical resolution and to prevent sexual transmission and late sequelae. Treatment of late latent or tertiary syphilis, which requires a series of three weekly injections of benzathine penicillin (total of 7.2 million units), usually does not affect transmission and is intended to prevent occurrence or progression of late complications (139). All treatment requires followup quantitative nontreponemal tests to assess treatment response. High rates of compliance with screening and treatment for syphilis among drug users have been achieved when these services are offered on-site in substance-abuse treatment programs (140).

Gonorrhea and Chlamydia

Gonorrhea and chlamydia are the most common bacterial STDs in the United States, with an estimated 650,000 cases of gonorrhea (caused by *Neisseria gonorrhoeae*) and 3 million cases of chlamydia (caused by *Chlamydia trachomatis*) each year. In one study of young (18–29 years old) women living in low-income neighborhoods in California, the current prevalence of gonorrhea or chlamydia was 3.9%, compared to 0.7% for syphilis (141). However, as with syphilis, rates of gonorrhea and chlamydia are much higher among drug users. In one study of injection drug users, the lifetime reported prevalence of gonorrhea or chlamydia was 30% for men and 43% for women, approximately twice that of syphilis or other ulcerative STDs (14% for men and 19% for women) (132). In other cross-sectional studies, the rate of self-reported gonorrhea among drug users was 49% (136), and the rate of current gonorrhea or chlamydia infection was 5.4% to 7.4% (135,142).

These bacterial infections are a major cause of urethritis and proctitis in men, and cervicitis and pelvic inflammatory disease (PID) in women. However, because they are often asymptomatic, particularly in women, gonococcal and chlamydial infections must be detected by screening tests. Screening is essential to prevent complications, including ascending infection, infertility, ectopic pregnancy, and chronic pelvic pain (139). In recent years, screening of women has been facilitated by highly sensitive new tests, which do not require a pelvic exam, but instead amplify nucleic acid obtained from urine using a ligase chain reaction for *C. trachomatis* and *N. gonorrhoeae*. Regular screening for gonorrhea and chlamydia is now recommended by the United States Preventive Services Task Force for sexually active patients, and annual screening of all drug-using women should be performed.

Treatment of gonorrhea and chlamydia is generally offered simultaneously, because of the frequency of dual infection. Several antibiotics are effective in the single-dose treatment of gonorrhea, including cefixime (Suprax), ceftriaxone (Cefizox), ciprofloxacin (Cipro), and ofloxacin (Floxin). Efficacious regimens for the treatment of chlamydia include azithromycin (Zithromax) or doxycycline (Vibramycin), but azithromycin is preferred because it can be given in a single, directly observed dose. The prevalence of quinolone-resistant gonorrhea is increasing in the United States, and nonquinolone regimens may be preferred in the future (138,139).

Genital Herpes

Genital herpes simplex virus type 2 (HSV-2) infection is the most common infectious cause of genital ulcers in the United States, with a reported seroprevalence rate of 22% among all adults in the early 1990s. A more recent study identified HSV-2 prevalence to be as high as 35% among women in a low-income community (143). Although most cases of genital herpes are caused by HSV-2, genital infections with herpes simplex virus type 1 (HSV-1) are increasingly recognized. Most persons with HSV-2 are asymptomatic, but shedding occurs even in the absence of lesions, and HSV-2 transmission usually occurs during subclinical or asymptomatic shedding. Serologic evidence of past HSV-2 infection increases with age and number of sexual partners, and is more common among drug users. In recent studies, the prevalence of antibodies to HSV-2 among drug users has ranged from 44% to 58% (135,144). The highest prevalence of HSV-2 (73%) has been found among women who exchange sex for money or drugs (143).

Optimal management of genital herpes includes antiviral therapy (with acyclovir [Zovirax], famciclovir [Famvir], or valacyclovir [Valtrex]), appropriate counseling on the natural history of infection, risk for sexual and perinatal transmission, and methods to prevent further transmission. Systemic antiviral drugs partially control symptoms when used to treat recurrent episodes, or as daily suppressive therapy. However, these drugs neither eradicate latent virus nor affect the risk for, frequency of, or severity of recurrences after the drug is discontinued. Recognizing the symptoms and signs of clinical episodes of HSV infections and promptly seeking treatment are key factors in reducing transmission rates.

Human Papilloma Virus

Human papilloma virus (HPV) infections are the causative agents for genital wart disease and cervical carcinoma, and are transmitted primarily through sexual contact. The prevalence of HPV is as high as 50% among sexually active adolescent and young adult women, and risk factors for HPV include number of sexual partners (145,146), early age of first sexual intercourse, drinking and drug use related to sexual behavior, and partner's number of sexual partners (147).

The two major manifestations of genital HPV infection are external genital warts, usually caused by HPV-6 and HPV-11, and squamous intraepithelial lesions of the cervix that are detected by cytologic screening. The major types of HPV associated with squamous intraepithelial lesions are HPV-16, -18, -31, and -45. These HPV types also cause squamous cell cancer of the vagina, vulva, anus, and penis. Subclinical genital HPV infection occurs more often than visible genital warts, and may be diagnosed by type-specific HPV tests. Testing for HPV was recently advocated as a strategy for determining which women with low-grade cervical abnormalities require additional evaluation with colposcopy. At present, no therapy has been identified that effectively eradicates persistent subclinical HPV infection.

Trichomoniasis

Trichomonas vaginalis is a protozoan that causes vaginitis in women, and is highly prevalent among drug-using women. In two recent studies of women in residential drug treatment, the prevalence of trichomonas ranged from 22% to 43% (142,148). Recent availability of self-administered vaginal swab tests has obviated the need for pelvic exams followed by wet mount microscopy or vaginal culture in screening for trichomonas, and allows for routine screening of a larger number of women. Like other STDs, trichomonal infection is associated with crack cocaine use and exchange of sex for money or drugs. Because it is frequently asymptomatic, screening for trichomoniasis should be routine among drug-using women.

SKIN AND SOFT-TISSUE INFECTIONS

Skin and soft-tissue infections are common among injection drug users. In a San Francisco-based sample, one-third of active injectors examined by a physician had a concurrent abscess (65%), cellulitis (9%), or both (26%) (149). Sixteen percent of injectors reported a history of abscess in the previous 6 months in a sample from Baltimore (150), and prevalence rates of 20% to 30% have been reported in several studies of injectors in Europe (151–153). In a prospective study of injectors in Amsterdam, the incidence of abscess was 33 per 100 person-years (154). Necrotizing fasciitis can complicate skin and soft-tissue infections among injectors, conveying a high (10%) risk of mortality in one series (155).

Risk of abscess has been associated with route of injection, with intramuscular ("muscling") or subcutaneous ("skin popping") injection conveying greater risk for abscess than intravenous injection (156,157). HIV infection is associated with abscess in some (154), but not other (156), studies. Other risk factors identified include higher injection frequency (154) and injecting a mixture of cocaine and heroin (speedball) (156). In addition to injection of illicit drugs, nonprescription use of anabolic steroid injections have been associated with abscess formation (158). Common sites of abscess are, in order of descending frequency, arm, leg, buttocks, deltoid, and head/neck (159), in keeping with the "hierarchy" of injection sites reported in the literature (160).

The bacteriology of injection-associated abscess has been better defined than that of cellulitis, because of the greater likelihood of isolating an organism. *Staphylococcus aureus* is the most common pathogen in these infections, followed by *Streptococcus* species. Mixed aerobic/anaerobic infections are more common among injection-associated abscesses than abscesses identified in other clinical settings. Anaerobes most commonly isolated from injection-related abscesses in one series were fusobacteria, *Prevotella* species, peptostreptococci, actinomyces, and *Veillonella* species (161). Other

pathogens identified include anthrax (*Bacillus anthracis*) (162) and tetanus (*C. tetani*). (163). Studies of the microbiologic flora in heroin and on injection equipment have also been conducted. While a variety of organisms were identified in this manner, *S. aureus* was not, suggesting that the injection drug user's skin, not the drug or equipment used, is the likely source for staphylococcus-related abscesses (164). Indeed, strains of *S. aureus* isolated from drug users presenting to the hospital with serious *S. aureus*-related infections are similar to the strains colonizing the same population of drug users in the community (165). Colonization of the nasal mucosa with *S. aureus* is common among injectors, with prevalence rates of 27% (of which 24% were methicillin-resistant) reported among recent injectors in San Francisco (166).

Localized outbreaks of specific pathogens have been reported in connection with drug injection. In Scotland, Ireland, and England heroin contaminated by *Clostridium* species (the toxin-producing strain *Clostridium novyi* in particular) led to more than 40 deaths in a period of several months (167). Injection of a tarry paste form of heroin (black tar heroin) is associated with wound botulism (*Clostridium botulinum*) in California. Quantity of black tar heroin injected, but not cleaning of the skin prior to injection, was associated with *C. botulinum* infection, suggesting that the heroin, and not the skin being injected through, was the source of the contaminating bacteria (157). Molecular epidemiologic techniques have confirmed the clonal identity, and thus common source, of specific bacterial pathogens responsible for clusters of abscesses among injectors (168,169).

Prevention of skin and soft-tissue infections among drug injectors requires attention to sterile injection equipment, sterile injection technique, and absence of infectious material in the drug being injected. Use of sterile injection equipment, available through pharmacies or community-based syringe exchange, can eliminate person-to-person transmission of skin flora and blood-borne pathogens or contaminated drugs. The simple act of routinely cleansing the injection site with alcohol or soapy water prior to injection has been associated with reduced rates of abscess formation (150). Finally, sterilization of the drug being injected by heating it prior to injection ("cooking"—a step taken to help dissolve the drug) may inactivate harmful bacteria. Physicians and other health care personnel caring for persons who inject drugs should encourage adoption of safer injection techniques (170), while working with patients to assist them in reducing or eliminating injection altogether.

Treatment of abscess typically requires incision and drainage, with adjunctive antibiotics. Specialized wound clinics targeting drug injectors have proven to be successful in engaging out-of-treatment patients and in substantially reducing use of more expensive emergency room and inpatient resources (171,172). In choosing antibiotic therapy, patients should be asked about their possible use of unprescribed ("street") antibiotics prior to presenting for care (173).

INFECTIVE ENDOCARDITIS

Endocarditis is the infection most classically associated with injection drug use, particularly in the pre-HIV era. Among active injectors, estimates of incidence range from 1.5 to 20 cases per 1,000 person-years (174). The risk of endocarditis is higher among HIV-infected injectors (13.8 vs. 3.3 cases per 1,000 person-years) (175). Estimates of mortality among persons with injection-associated endocarditis range from 7% to 37% (176,177), although rates may be lower (approximately 10%) among those with right-sided endocarditis (176).

Risk factors for injection-associated endocarditis include HIV infection and frequency of injection (154,178,179). One carefully done study found that alcohol consumption was associated with diminished endocarditis risk. The authors postulated that the effects of alcohol on platelet or endothelial cell function might account for their surprising finding (175). The relative risk of endocarditis associated with specific injected drugs has not been extensively studied. One report suggested an increased risk associated with cocaine injection compared to heroin or amphetamine injection, but its generalizability is uncertain (180).

Infective endocarditis among drug users can affect any heart valve. Although native valve endocarditis in the general population is most often left sided, infective endocarditis is most commonly right sided when associated with injection drug use. The tricuspid valve is involved in 40% to 69% of cases among drug injectors. This is thought to be caused by a variety of factors, including direct valvular endothelial damage from impurities contaminating the drug injected into the venous system (rendering the right-sided valves most susceptible to bacterial infection), predilections of certain skin flora for right-sided valve surfaces, and direct effects on the valvular endothelium of specific drugs (which may present to the right-sided valves in higher concentrations than to the left-sided valves) (174). Echocardiographic studies comparing drug injectors to noninjectors with respect to valve morphology suggest that thickening of the tricuspid and, to a lesser extent, the mitral valve is more common among injectors (181).

Many organisms are reported to cause endocarditis among injecting drug users. Reports of the prevalence of specific pathogens vary by location and over time, likely reflecting diverse rates of colonization with specific pathogens, variations in injection practices, and in purity and source of drug. Overall, *S. aureus* is most frequently reported (182,183). Other gram-positive organisms include *Streptococcus viridans* (184), enterococcus (185), and nontoxigenic *Corynebacterium diphtheriae* (186). Gram-negative pathogens include *Pseudomonas aerug-*

inosa (187) (among injectors of pentazocine and tripelennamine, also known as T's and blues), *Pseudomonas cepacia* (188), and *Serratia marcescens* (189). Fungal endocarditis, although much less common among injectors, occurs regularly. *Candida* species are the most common pathogens in such cases (190). *Candida albicans* is associated with injection of oral methadone tablets that were dissolved in fruit juices known to support growth of *Candida* species (191). Polymicrobial presentations are more common among injection drug users than among others with endocarditis (192).

Although both the skin and the injected drug are implicated as the source of the pathogen causing endocarditis, the skin is thought to be the prime source in most cases (164,182).

A single episode of bacteremia in an injector does not necessarily signify endocarditis. Only approximately 40% of bacteremic drug injectors met diagnostic criteria for endocarditis in one series (193). Several authors have developed clinical prediction rules to determine the likelihood that a given febrile injector presenting to the emergency department has endocarditis. Yet such algorithms remain relatively inexact, leading many to conclude that most febrile injection drug users should be admitted to the hospital for observation or empiric treatment until the diagnosis of endocarditis can be excluded (194,195).

Persistent bacteremia is a hallmark of endocarditis. The role of echocardiography in confirming the diagnosis has advanced in recent years, with clarification of the indications for transthoracic and transesophageal echocardiography in the diagnostic evaluation (196). The revised Duke criteria provide a consistent standard for the diagnosis of infective endocarditis (197).

An extended course of parenteral antibiotics remains the mainstay of treatment of endocarditis. Prior to initiating treatment, it can be valuable to query the patient regarding possible recent use of nonprescribed antibiotics (173). Advances in treatment in the past decade include oral therapy for selected patients (198) and shorter (2 weeks) duration of treatment for patients with uncomplicated right-sided methicillin-sensitive *S. aureus* endocarditis (199). Both advances are important for injecting drug users, because venous access is often problematic in those with a substantial injection history, and prolonged hospital stays are generally difficult for injectors and noninjectors alike. The presence of HIV infection does not diminish the efficacy of treatment for endocarditis. Significant HIV-related immunosuppression, however, is associated with increased endocarditis-associated mortality (200,201). The treatment of endocarditis generally, and in drug injectors particularly, has been recently reviewed (202,203).

Access to sterile injection equipment and adherence to sterile injection technique are the practices most likely to reduce injectors' risk of endocarditis (150,170). The principles of prevention discussed above in the context of skin and soft-tissue infections apply to endocarditis as well.

TUBERCULOSIS

Drug users are at increased risk for tuberculosis infection and disease. The prevalence of latent tuberculosis infection (LTBI) among drug users varies by locale and population studied, but rates of approximately 15% to 25% are typical (204,205). The prevalence of tuberculin reactivity among HIV-seropositive drug users is generally lower than among HIV-uninfected persons, reflecting the diminished delayed-type hypersensitivity response associated with more advanced immunosuppression (206,207). Drug users are heterogenous with respect to their risk for LTBI. Several reports suggest that, among drug users, smokers of crack cocaine are at particularly high risk for tuberculosis infection (205,208).

It is uncertain whether active drug use is associated with an increased risk of developing tuberculosis disease among persons with latent tuberculosis infection (209). The presence of HIV infection, however, clearly increases the risk that drug users with LTBI will develop active disease (210,211). Chemoprophylaxis is effective in reducing this risk, and thus regular screening for and, when detected, treatment of LTBI should be offered to all drug users (212).

Treatment of tuberculosis in drug users should follow standard guidelines (213). Two points deserve particular emphasis. Rifampin (Rifadin), one of the most effective antituberculosis medications, is a potent inducer of methadone metabolism, often precipitating narcotic withdrawal symptoms in methadone-maintained persons (214). Carefully managed methadone dose increases, or even splitting of the methadone dose so it is administered twice daily, often resolves this complication. Alternatively, rifabutin (Mycobutin), which has similar activity to rifampin but far less impact on methadone metabolism, can sometimes substitute for rifampin. Such changes should generally be made in consultation with an expert in tuberculosis treatment. For patients engaged in opioid-agonist treatment with methadone, or who live in a congregate setting (shelter, residential drug treatment), directly observed dosing can be a highly effective means to optimize adherence with treatment of LTBI or of active tuberculosis (215).

PNEUMONIA

Community-acquired pneumonia is common among drug users, particularly those with HIV infection. Recent studies have determined that the incidence of pneumonia ranges from 4.4 to 14.2 per 1,000 person-years among HIV-negative drug users, and from 47.8 to 90.5 per 1,000 person-years among HIV-positive drug users (216,217). Pneumonia is also the most common reason for hospital-

izations among drug users, accounting for 27% of hospital admissions in one study (218).

Many factors contribute to drug users' increased susceptibility to pneumonia, including depression of the gag reflex by alcohol and drugs, leading to aspiration of oropharyngeal and gastric secretions (219); impaired pulmonary function as a consequence of cigarette smoking (220); and weakened immunity as a consequence of malnutrition and continuous antigenic stimulation (221). In addition, HIV-infection is associated with a markedly increased risk of bacterial pneumonia, and recurrent bacterial pneumonia has been included as an AIDS-defining illness since 1993. The risk for pneumonia among HIV-infected drug users is approximately five times that of non–HIV-infected drug users.

Encapsulated bacteria, most commonly *Streptococcus pneumoniae,* followed by *Haemophilus influenzae,* are the most frequent causes of pneumonia in both HIV-positive and HIV-negative drug users, and are highly associated with the classic symptoms of sputum production, chest pain, and fever (222). Atypical bacteria, including *Mycoplasma pneumoniae, Chlamydia pneumoniae,* and *Legionella* species, are also common among drug users, and are more likely to cause dry cough and headache than classic pneumonia symptoms (221). *Pneumocystis carinii, Mycobacterium tuberculosis,* and *Mycobacterium avium* are common among HIV-infected drug users, as discussed further in Chapter 58, HIV Infection and AIDS: Medical Complications and Treatment. Pulmonary tuberculosis should always be included in the differential diagnosis of drug users with pneumonia, and annual tuberculin skin testing of drug users is recommended. In addition, pneumococcal vaccine and annual influenza vaccines should be offered to all drug users.

NEUROLOGIC COMPLICATIONS

Infections

Injection drug users are at increased risk for systemic infections that may affect the central nervous system, including endocarditis, viral hepatitis, and HIV. Endocarditis is associated with neurologic complications in 20% to 40% of patients, including cerebral embolism and infarction, hemorrhage from ruptured mycotic aneurysms, meningitis, encephalopathy, and parenchymal, subdural, or epidural abscesses (223). Viral hepatitis may also cause encephalopathy, or, less commonly, hemorrhagic stroke a result of abnormal blood clotting (224). HIV infection may cause neurologic complications either directly or through opportunistic infections that attack the central nervous system.

Focal central nervous system infections occur commonly among drug users, although most focal infections result from embolization of infected vegetations among patients with endocarditis. The most frequent focal infections are brain abscesses, which may also result from local spread of an ear or sinus infection, hematogenous dissemination from a distant focus, such as infection in the lung, skin, bone, or pelvis, or trauma with an open fracture or foreign body injury. Spinal epidural abscesses are also common, and are caused by direct local extension of vertebral osteomyelitis, hematogenous spread from distant infection, or blunt spinal trauma.

Toxin-mediated diseases, including tetanus and botulism, comprise an additional important category of central nervous system infections among injection drug users. These infections usually result from intramuscular or subcutaneous injection of drugs, which predisposes to the inoculation of *Clostridium* species and the release of disease-producing toxin. Tetanus is caused by *Clostridium tetani,* and causes intense, sustained muscular spasms that may be localized or generalized. Localized tetanus causes muscle rigidity, pain, and enhanced deep tendon reflexes, while generalized tetanus causes respiratory failure and requires treatment in an intensive care unit (225). Wound botulism is caused by *C. botulinum,* and has been associated in particular with the injection of black tar heroin (226,227). Wound botulism initially causes blurred vision, dysarthria, and dysphagia, but may lead to descending muscle paralysis and respiratory failure. A high index of suspicion is necessary to diagnose these uncommon but rapidly progressive toxin-mediated diseases among drug users who present with neurologic symptoms. All injection drug users should be immunized against tetanus.

Other Neurologic Complications

Painful peripheral neuropathy has been described among several classes of drug users, including inhalant (228,229) and injection drug users (230). In case reports, heroin use is associated with myopathy, cerebral and cerebellar spongiform encephalopathy, and sciatic nerve palsy (231–233). Many substances are associated with seizures, which typically occur as a result of drug toxicity or withdrawal. Finally, cocaine use may be associated with an increased risk of stroke; this association is addressed further in "Cocaine" below.

COCAINE

The use of cocaine increased dramatically in the early and mid-1980s as more potent formulations of the drug, most notably crack cocaine, became widely available. Cocaine use then declined, but has risen in recent years, with the number of new cocaine users increasing by 82%, from 514,000 to 934,000, between 1994 to 1998 (234). In 2001, according to the National Household Survey on Drug Abuse, an estimated 1.7 million Americans (0.7% of those age 12 years and older) were current cocaine users and 406,000 (0.2%) were current crack users. This represents a statistically significant increase in use from 2000, in which 0.5% of the population reported current cocaine use (235). Based upon additional data sources that take into account users underrepresented in the National Household Survey, the Office of National Drug Control Policy estimates the number of chronic cocaine users at more than 3.6 million (236). As cocaine use has become more widespread, cocaine-related medical complications, emergency department visits, and hospitalizations have increased. Cocaine-related emergency department visits increased by 80% during the 1990s, and 30% of all drug-related visits to emergency departments nationwide are now associated with cocaine use. Currently, cocaine is the most frequently reported drug in emergency department visits, and was reported in 175,000 emergency visits in the United States in 2000, or 76 visits per 100,000 population (237).

Cardiovascular Complications

The most common medical symptom associated with cocaine use is chest pain, which may be a result of cardiac ischemia or myocardial infarction. Cocaine use increases the risk of acute myocardial infarction by several mechanisms, including coronary vasoconstriction or vasospasm, increased adrenergic activity (which intensifies myocardial oxygen demand by increasing blood pressure, ventricular contractility, and heart rate), and increased platelet adhesion, aggregation, and intravascular thrombosis (238,239). In one recent study, users of cocaine had a transient 24-fold increase in the risk of myocardial infarction in the hour immediately following cocaine use (240). The occurrence of myocardial infarction after cocaine use is unrelated to the amount ingested, route of administration, or blood levels of cocaine or its metabolites (239,241).

Among persons 18 to 45 years of age in the United States, cocaine accounts for up to 25% of acute myocardial infarctions (242). Despite this high population-attributable risk, cocaine-associated myocardial infarctions remain relatively uncommon, occurring in only 1% to 6% of patients who present to emergency departments with cocaine-associated chest pain (243,244). Although all cocaine users are at risk, most patients with cocaine-associated myocardial infarction are young, nonwhite, male, cigarette smokers, without other risk factors for atherosclerosis, and with a history of repeated cocaine use. Only half of these patients have evidence of atherosclerotic coronary artery disease on subsequent angiography (234).

While cocaine-associated chest pain is common, accounting for 40% of cocaine-related emergency department visits in the United States in 2000, most episodes do not constitute an acute coronary syndrome. In addition to myocardial infarction or ischemia, cocaine-related chest pain may be a consequence of extracardiac causes such as chest wall trauma or pleuritic inflammation. Management strategies for patients presenting to the emergency department with acute cocaine-related chest pain were examined in a recent prospective study, in which patients at high risk for cardiovascular complications (those with electrocardiographic changes suggestive of acute myocardial infarction or ischemia, elevated serum levels of cardiac markers, recurrent ischemic chest pain, or hemodynamic instability) were admitted to the hospital, and all others were observed in the emergency department (245). Patients who were observed and found to have no new electrocardiographic changes suggestive of ischemia, as well as normal levels of cardiac troponin I and no cardiovascular complications during observation, were discharged after 9 to 12 hours. Among the patients admitted to the hospital (N = 42), there were 20 diagnoses of acute coronary events (myocardial infarction or unstable angina), and among the patients observed in the emergency department (N = 302), there were 4 myocardial infarctions in the following 30 days and no cardiovascular deaths. All myocardial infarctions after discharge occurred in patients with at least two cardiac risk factors (cigarette smoking and either diabetes or hypertension) who continued to use cocaine. Based on these findings, the authors concluded that patients who present to the emergency department with cocaine-associated chest pain without evidence of ischemia or cardiovascular complications can be medically managed by short-term observation (9 to 12 hours). Observation should consist of continuous electrocardiographic monitoring and measurement of cardiac markers (serum troponin concentrations) at 3, 6, and 9 hours after presentation. Recurrent chest pain, increased levels of markers of myocardial necrosis, or cardiac dysrhythmias place the patient at high risk and signal the need for inpatient observation. Other authors have recommended even shorter observation periods for patients with cocaine-associated chest pain who do not have electrocardiographic evidence of acute cardiac ischemia (243). Patients with cocaine-associated chest pain and traditional cardiac risk factors who are discharged after observation should undergo expedited evaluation for potential coronary disease, because the vasoconstrictive impact of cocaine use can be enhanced in the presence of underlying atherosclerosis. In addition, substance-abuse treatment should be offered to all patients admitted to the emergency department with cocaine-associated chest pain.

Among all patients presenting to emergency departments with chest pain, the prevalence of cocaine exposure (assessed by urine toxicology testing) was found in a large multicenter study to be 17%, ranging from 7% in suburban hospitals to 14% to 25% in urban hospitals (246). In this study, the percentage of cocaine-positive urines was higher than expected in the 41- to 50-year-old group (18%), and in the 51- to 60-year-old group (3%). Asking about cocaine use should therefore be routine in the emergency department, and physicians should consider objective testing for cocaine in patients who present to the emergency department with chest pain.

In addition to acute myocardial ischemia and infarction, cocaine use is linked to dissection of the thoracic aorta and coronary arteries (247–250), cardiac rhythm and conduction abnormalities (251–254), left ventricular dysfunction, dilated cardiomyopathy, hypertension, and tachycardia. Cocaine use may be a stronger independent risk factor than other drugs for endocarditis, particularly involving left-sided valves (234). Finally, several case reports describe peripheral limb ischemia in association with cocaine use, and suggest that additives present in cocaine preparations, such as arsenic, may contribute to peripheral vascular insufficiency in cocaine users (255,256).

Neurologic and Cerebrovascular Complications

Cerebral vasoconstriction has been implicated as the mechanism of acute cocaine-associated neurologic complications, including ischemic and hemorrhagic stroke, in several case reports and case-control studies (257,258). In addition, long-term cocaine use appears to predispose patients with incidental neurovascular anomalies, such as aneurysms and arteriovenous malformations, to present with intracranial or subarachnoid hemorrhages at an earlier point than nonusers. Finally, experimental studies demonstrate that low-dose cocaine administration induces cerebral vasoconstriction in neurologically normal, otherwise healthy cocaine users (259).

A more subtle form of cerebrovascular dysfunction frequently found in long-term cocaine users is the development of focal perfusion defects, which are associated with moderate to severe cognitive dysfunction. These defects, and the associated cognitive abnormalities, persist even during periods of cocaine abstinence (259).

Cocaine-induced seizures are a relatively rare, severe manifestation of cocaine toxicity. They are usually single, tonic–clonic, resolve without intervention, and occur in patients with a history of prior seizures. Because cocaine seizures are uncommon, it should be a diagnosis of exclusion after other more likely etiologies are ruled out (260).

Renal Complications

Cocaine use is associated with both acute and chronic renal injury. Acutely, cocaine use may cause rhabdomyolysis, malignant hypertension, interstitial nephritis, or glomerulonephritis, all of which may lead to acute renal failure. In addition, cocaine use is associated with acute renal infarction caused by vasospastic injury and thrombosis, and with electrolyte imbalances, including respiratory alkalosis and lactic acidosis (261). Chronically, cocaine can cause hypertension, worsen blood pressure control, or hasten the progression of end-stage renal disease (262). Among cocaine-using patients with end-stage renal disease, there is an increased incidence of endocarditis, catheter-related bacteremia, pyelonephritis, viral hepatitis, and abscesses, when compared to noncocaine users (263).

Pulmonary Complications

Both intranasal and crack cocaine use are associated with pulmonary complications, but the majority of these are associated with smoking crack cocaine. Although intranasal cocaine may cause nonspecific bronchial irritation that results in wheezing in persons with a history of obstructive lung disease (264), crack cocaine results in a broad spectrum of pulmonary complications, including asthma exacerbations (including fatal and near-fatal asthma); barotrauma (pneumomediastinum and pneumothorax); noncardiogenic pulmonary edema; diffuse alveolar hemorrhage; recurrent pulmonary infiltrates with eosinophilia; nonspecific interstitial pneumonitis; bronchiolitis obliterans with organizing pneumonia; pulmonary vascular abnormalities; and "crack lung" (acute pulmonary infiltrates associated with chest pain, hemoptysis, and a spectrum of clinical and histologic findings) (265,266). Among crack smokers, the prevalence of respiratory symptoms (cough, black sputum production, wheezing, dyspnea, or hemoptysis) is greater than 50% (267).

Gastrointestinal Complications

Gastrointestinal complications including bowel ischemia and perforations, are associated with cocaine or crack consumption. These complications are primarily caused by adrenergically mediated mesenteric vasoconstriction and focal tissue ischemia, but it is also hypothesized that cocaine has a direct toxic effect on gut mucosa (268).

Additional gastrointestinal complications can occur when persons ingest packets of cocaine to smuggle the drug across international borders, or to avoid being apprehended by the police. Smuggling is done by "body packers," who usually swallow large amounts of heroin and cocaine, carefully wrapped to withstand gastrointestinal tract transit (269). "Body stuffers" are typically sellers or users on the verge of arrest, who swallow the drugs, which are poorly wrapped in foil or plastic. Body packers may present to the emergency department with symptoms of bowel obstruction, or with a toxicologic emergency from absorption of the substance ingested. Interventions commonly employed in other foreign-body obstructions of the gastrointestinal tract can be harmful in cocaine body packers. Rectal examination should be done cautiously, and digital rectal or endoscopic removal should be avoided because these could cause packet rupture. Surgical removal should be performed in patients who have swallowed cocaine-filled condoms, toy balloons, or finger cots, and in patients with symptoms of cocaine toxicity,

intestinal obstruction, or a time lapse of 24 to 48 hours since ingestion (270).

Although body stuffers ingest smaller amounts of cocaine than body packers, the containers often contain lethal amounts of drug. The packages can begin to leak immediately after ingestion, and thus surgery may not be helpful. Management of cocaine body stuffers has not been studied carefully. Ipecac has been suggested if ingestion is acute, the patient has a clear sensorium, and no seizure activity is documented; whole-bowel irrigation with polyethylene glycol-electrolyte solution along with activated charcoal is often used (271). Surgical consultation is indicated if bowel obstruction or mesenteric ischemia are possible.

Head and Neck Complications

Although many of the complications of cocaine use are caused by direct drug toxicity or needle use, intranasal cocaine can have serious local effects on the nasal mucosa and its anatomic extensions. Common complications include epistaxis, chronic rhinitis, diminished olfaction, and nasal septal and palatal perforation. Nasal septal perforation is found in approximately 5% of cocaine snorters (272). In addition, many case reports describe more severe cocaine-associated facial lesions, including oronasal fistulas, sinonasal tract necrosis, nasal cavity and palatal necrosis, midfacial osteomyelitis, and erosion of the external structures of the face (273). The pathophysiology of cocaine-induced palatal and facial destruction is multifactorial, and includes local ischemia secondary to vasoconstriction, chemical irritation from adulterants, and infection secondary to trauma, impaired mucociliary transport, and decreased immunity.

Sexually Transmitted Diseases and Cocaine Use

Cocaine use is associated with high-risk sexual practices and high rates of HIV, syphilis, and other sexually transmitted diseases. In particular, crack use is associated with sex in exchange for money, or directly for crack, and crack-smoking sex workers report very-high-risk sexual practices, including sex with injectors and persons believed to be HIV infected, and low rates of condom use, particularly among women who exchange sex for crack (136,274,275). Sexually transmitted diseases among drug users are discussed in further detail earlier in this chapter (see Sexually Transmitted Disease, above).

OTHER MEDICAL COMPLICATIONS

Other medical complication of drug use cannot be properly reviewed here because of space limitations. However, the reader is directed to recent reviews of pulmonary (264), renal (276), and other infectious complications (277,278) among drug users.

REFERENCES

1. Laine C, Hauck WW, Gourevitch MN, et al. Regular outpatient medical and drug abuse care and subsequent hospitalization of persons who use illicit drugs. *JAMA* 2001;285(18):2355–2362.
2. Weisner C, Mertens J, Parthasarathy S, et al. Integrating primary medical care with addiction treatment: a randomized controlled trial. *JAMA* 2001;286(14):1715–1723.
3. McLellan AT, Arndt IO, Metzger DS, et al. The effects of psychosocial services in substance abuse treatment. *JAMA* 1993;269(15):1953–1959.
4. Edlin BR, Irwin KL, Faruque S, et al. Intersecting epidemics—crack cocaine use and HIV infection among inner-city young adults. Multicenter Crack Cocaine and HIV Infection Study Team. *N Engl J Med* 1994;331(21):1422–1427.
5. Avins AL, Lindan CP, Woods WJ, et al. Changes in HIV-related behaviors among heterosexual alcoholics following addiction treatment. *Drug Alcohol Depend* 1997;44(1):47–55.
6. O'Connor PG, Selwyn PA, Schottenfeld RS. Medical care for injection-drug users with human immunodeficiency virus infection. *N Engl J Med* 1994;331(7):450–459.
7. Samet JH, Friedmann P, Saitz R. Benefits of linking primary medical care and substance abuse services: patient, provider, and societal perspectives. *Arch Intern Med* 2001;161(1):85–91.
8. Haynes RB, McKibbon KA, Kanani R. Systematic review of randomised trials of interventions to assist patients to follow prescriptions for medications. *Lancet* 1996;348:383–386.
9. Holmberg SD. The estimated prevalence and incidence of HIV in 96 large U.S. metropolitan areas. *Am J Public Health* 1996;86(5):642–654.
10. Bogart LM, Kelly JA, Catz SL, et al. Impact of medical and nonmedical factors on physician decision making for HIV/AIDS antiretroviral treatment. *J Acquir Immune Defic Syndr* 2000;23(5):396–404.
11. Bassetti S, Battegay M, Furrer H, et al. Why is highly active antiretroviral therapy (HAART) not prescribed or discontinued? *J Acquir Immune Defic Syndr* 1999;21(2):114–119.
12. Sherer R. Adherence and antiretroviral therapy in injection drug users. *JAMA* 1998;280(6):567–568.
13. Blower SM, Gershengorn HB, Grant RM. A tale of two futures: HIV and antiretroviral therapy in San Francisco. *Science* 2000;287:650–654.

14. Hecht FM, Grant RM, Petropoulos CJ, et al. Sexual transmission of an HIV-1 variant resistant to multiple reverse-transcriptase and protease inhibitors. *N Eng J Med* 1998;339(5):307–311.
15. Little SJ, Daar ES, D'Aquilla RT, et al. Reduced antiretroviral drug susceptibility among patients with primary HIV infection. *JAMA* 1999;282(12):1142–1149.
16. Haubrich RH, Little SJ, Currier JS, et al. The value of patient-reported adherence to antiretroviral therapy in predicting virologic and immunologic response. *AIDS* 1999;13:1099–1107.
17. Gifford AL, Bormann JE, Shively MJ, et al. Predictors of self-reported adherence and plasma HIV concentrations in patients on multidrug antiretroviral regimens. *J Acquir Immune Defic Syndr* 2000;23(5):386–395.
18. Chesney MA, Ickovics JR, Chambers DB, et al. Self-reported adherence to antiretroviral medications among participants in HIV clinical trials: the AACTG Adherence Instruments. *AIDS Care* 2000;12(3):255–266.
19. Stein MD, Rich JD, Maksad J, et al. Adherence to antiretroviral therapy among HIV-infected methadone patients: effect of ongoing illicit drug use. *Am J Drug Alcohol Abuse* 2000;26(2):195–205.
20. Arnsten JH, Demas PA, Grant RW, et al. Impact of active drug use on antiretroviral therapy adherence and viral suppression in HIV-infected drug users. *J Gen Intern Med* 2002;17:377–381.
21. Arnsten JH, Demas PA, Farzadegan H, et al. Antiretroviral therapy adherence and viral suppression in HIV-infected drug users: comparison of self-report and electronic monitoring. *Clin Infect Dis* 2001;33:1417–1423.
22. Paterson DL, Swindells S, Mohr J, et al. Adherence to protease inhibitor therapy and outcomes in patients with HIV infection. *Ann Intern Med* 2000;133(1):21–30.
23. Turner BJ, Newschaffer CJ, Zhang D, et al. Antiretroviral use and pharmacy-based measurement of adherence in postpartum HIV-infected women. *Med Care* 2000;38(9):911–925.
24. Samet JH, Friedmann P, Saitz R. Benefits of linking primary medical care and substance abuse services: patient, provider, and societal perspectives. *Arch Intern Med* 2001;161:85–89.
25. Bamberger JD, Unick J, Klein P, et al. Helping the urban poor stay with antiretroviral HIV drug therapy. *Am J Public Health* 2000;90(5):699–701.

26. Selwyn PA, Budner NS, Wasserman WC, et al. Utilization of on-site primary care services by HIV-seropositive and seronegative drug users in a methadone maintenance program. *Public Health Rep* 1997;108(4):492–500.
27. Strathdee SA, Palepu A, Cornelisse PGA, et al. Barriers to use of free antiretroviral therapy in injection drug users. *JAMA* 1998;280(6):547–549.
28. Celentano DD, Vlahov D, Cohn S, et al. Self-reported antiretroviral therapy in injection drug users. *JAMA* 1998;280(6):544–546.
29. Sorensen JL, Mascovich A, Wall TL, et al. Medication adherence strategies for drug abusers with HIV/AIDS. *AIDS Care* 1998;10(3):297–312.
30. Moreno A, Perez-Elias MJ, Casado JL, et al. Long-term outcomes of protease inhibitor-based therapy in antiretroviral treatment-naive HIV-infected injection drug users on methadone maintenance programmes. *AIDS* 2001;15(8):1068–1070.
31. Catz SL, Kelly JA, Bogart LM, et al. Patterns, correlates, and barriers to medication adherence among persons prescribed new treatments for HIV disease. *Health Psychol* 2000;19(2):124–133.
32. Safren SA, Otto MW, Worth JL, et al. Two strategies to increase adherence to HIV antiretroviral medication: lifesteps and medication monitoring. *Behav Res Ther* 2000;39(2001):1151–1162.
33. Eldred LJ, Wu AW, Chaisson RE, et al. Adherence to antiretroviral and pneumocystis prophylaxis in HIV disease. *J Acquir Immune Defic Syndr Hum Retrovirol* 1998;18(2):117–125.
34. Kalichman SC, Ramachandran B, Catz S. Adherence to combination antiretroviral therapies in HIV patients of low health literacy. *J Gen Intern Med* 1999;14:267–273.
35. Gao X, Nau DP, Rosenbluth SA, et al. The relationship of disease severity, health beliefs and medication adherence among HIV patients. *AIDS Care* 2000;12(4):387–398.
36. Johnston Roberts K, Mann T. Barriers to antiretroviral medication adherence in HIV-infected women. *AIDS Care* 2000;12(4):377–386.
37. Mostashari F, Riley E, Selwyn PA, et al. Acceptance and adherence with antiretroviral therapy among HIV-infected women in a correctional facility. *J Acquir Immune Defic Syndr Hum Retrovirol* 1998;18(4):341–348.
38. Murri R, Ammassari A, Gallicano K, et al. Patient-reported nonadherence to HAART is related to protease inhibitor

levels. *J Acquir Immune Defic Syndr* 2000;24(2):123–128.

39. Avants SK, Margolin A, Warburton LA, et al. Predictors of nonadherence to HIV-related medication regimens during methadone stabilization. *Am J Addict* 2001;10(1):69–78.

40. Ferrando SJ, Wall TL, Batki SL, et al. Psychiatric morbidity, illicit drug use and adherence to zidovudine (AZT) among injection drug users with HIV disease. *Am J Drug Alcohol Abuse* 1996;22(3):475–487.

41. Gourevitch MN, Friedland GH. Interactions between methadone and medications used to treat HIV infection. *Mt Sinai J Med* 2000;67(5–6):429–436.

42. Altice FL, Friedland GH, Cooney EL. Nevirapine induced opiate withdrawal among injection drug users with HIV infection receiving methadone. *AIDS* 1999;13(8):957–962.

43. Clarke SM, Mulcahy FM, Tjia J, et al. The pharmacokinetics of methadone in HIV-positive patients receiving the non-nucleoside reverse transcriptase inhibitor efavirenz. *Br J Clin Pharmacol* 2001;51:213–217.

44. Gerber JG, Rosenkranz S, Segal Y, et al. Effect of ritonavir/saquinavir on stereoselective pharmacokinetics of methadone: results of AIDS Clinical Trials Group (ACTG) 401. *J Acquir Immune Defic Syndr* 2001;27:153–160.

45. McCance-Katz EF, Rainey P, Smith P, et al. Drug interactions between opioids and antiretroviral medications: interactions between methadone, LAAM and nelfinavir. *American Journal on Addictions* 2004;13:163–180.

46. Clarke S, Mulcahy F, Bergin C, et al. Absence of opioid withdrawal symptoms in patients receiving methadone and the protease inhibitor lopinavir-ritonavir. *Clin Infect Dis* 2002;34(8):1143–1145.

47. Gourevitch MN, Friedland GH. Interactions between methadone and medications used to treat HIV infection: a review. *Mt Sinai J Med* 2000;67(5–6):429–436.

48. Bangsberg DR, Hecht FM, Charlebois ED, L et al. Adherence to protease inhibitors, HIV-1 viral load, and development of drug resistance in an indigent population. *AIDS* 2000;14:357–366.

49. Strain EC, Stitzer ML. *Methadone treatment for opioid dependence.* Baltimore: The Johns Hopkins University Press, 1999.

50. Ball J, Ross A. *The effectiveness of methadone maintenance treatment.* New York: Springer-Verlag, 1991.

51. Joe GW, Simpson DD, Hubbard RL. Treatment predictors of tenure in methadone maintenance. *J Subst Abuse Treat* 1991;3:73–84.

52. Hubbard RL, Marsden ME, Rachal JV. *Drug abuse treatment: a national study of effectiveness.* Chapel Hill: University of North Carolina Press, 1989.

53. Kreek MJ. Medical safety and side effects of methadone in tolerant individuals. *JAMA* 1973;223:665–668.

54. Kwiatkowski CF, Booth RE. Methadone maintenance as HIV risk reduction with street-recruited injecting drug users. *J Acquir Immune Defic Syndr* 2001;26(5):483–489.

55. Theide H, Hagan H, Murrill CS. Methadone treatment and HIV and hepatitis B and C risk reduction among injectors in the Seattle area. *J Urban Health* 2000;77:331–345.

56. Metzger DS, Woody GE, McLellan AT, et al. Human immunodeficiency virus seroconversion among intravenous drug users in- and out-of-treatment: an 18-month prospective follow-up. *J Acquir Immune Defic Syndr* 1993;6:1049–1056.

57. Rodgers A. Methadone patients in the hospital. *Am J Nurs* 1996;96(5):20.

58. Rosenblum A, Joseph H, Fong C, et al. Prevalence and characteristics of chronic pain among chemically dependent patients in methadone maintenance and residential treatment facilities. *JAMA* 2003;289(18):2370–2378.

59. Jamison RN, Kauffman J, Katz NP. Characteristics of methadone maintenance patients with chronic pain. *J Pain Symptom Manage* 2000;19(1):53–62.

60. Compton P, Charuvastra VC, Kintaudi K, et al. Pain responses in methadone-maintained opioid abusers. *J Pain Symptom Manage* 2000;20(4):237–245.

61. Breitbart W, Rosenfeld BD, Passik SD, et al. The undertreatment of pain in ambulatory AIDS patients. *Pain* 1996;65:239–245.

62. Merrill JO, Rhodes LA, Deyo RA, et al. Mutual mistrust in the medical care of drug users: the keys to the "narc" cabinet. *J Gen Intern Med* 2002;17(5):327–333.

63. Passik SD, Kirsh KL, McDonald MV, et al. A pilot survey of aberrant drug-taking attitudes and behaviors in samples of cancer and AIDS patients. *J Pain Symptom Manage* 2000;19(4):274–286.

64. Scimeca MM, Savage SR, Portenoy R, et al. Treatment of pain in methadone-maintained patients. *Mt Sinai J Med* 2000;67(5–6):412–422.

65. National Pain Education Council. *Assessment and management of aberrant drug-related behavior in the chronic pain patient.* 2002. Available at: www.npecweb.org. Last accessed July 30, 2002.

66. Gilson AM, Joranson DE. U.S. policies relevant to the prescribing of opioid analgesics for the treatment of pain in patients with addictive disease. *Clin J Pain* 2002;18[4 Suppl]:S91–S98.

67. Selwyn PA. Pain management in substance abusers. In: Finkelstein R, Ramos SE, eds. *Manual for primary care providers: effectively caring for active substance users.* New York: The New York Academy of Medicine, 2002.

68. Kemmer NM, Miskovsky EP. Infections of the liver. *Infect Dis Clin North Am* 2002;14(3):605–615.

69. Hutin YJF, Sabin KM, Hutwanger LC, et al. Multiple modes of hepatitis A virus transmission among methamphetamine users. *Am J Epidemiol* 2002;152(2):186–192.

70. Ochnio JJ, Patrick D, Ho M, et al. Past infection with hepatitis A virus among Vancouver street youth, injection drug users and men who have sex with men: implications for vaccination programs. *CMAJ* 2001;165(3):293–297.

71. Villano SA, Nelson K, Vlahov D, et al. Hepatitis A among homosexual men and injection drug users: more evidence for vaccination. *Clin Infect Dis* 1997;(25):726–728.

72. Harkess J, Gildon B, Istre GR. Outbreaks of hepatitis A among illicit drug users, Oklahoma, 1984–1987. *Am J Public Health* 1989;79(4):463–466.

73. Vento S, Garofano TRC, Cainelli F, et al. Fulminant hepatitis associated with hepatitis A virus superinfection in patients with chronic hepatitis C. *N Engl J Med* 1998;338(5):286–290.

74. Lemberg BD, Shaw-Stiffel TA. Hepatic disease in injection drug users. *Infect Dis Clin North Am* 2002;16(3):_.

75. Seal KH, Edlin BR. Risk of hepatitis B infection among young injection drug users in San Francisco: opportunities for intervention. *West J Med* 2000;172:16–20.

76. Stark K, Bienzle U, Vonk R, et al. History of syringe sharing in prison and risk of hepatitis B virus, hepatitis C virus, and human immunodeficiency virus infection among injecting drug users in Berlin. *Int J Epidemiol* 1997;26(6):1359–1366.

77. Thiede H, Hagan H, Murrill CS. Methadone treatment and HIV and hepatitis B and C risk reduction among injectors in the Seattle area. *J Urban Health* 2000;77(3):331–345.

78. Garfein RS, Vlahov D, Galai N, et al. Viral infections in short-term injection drug users: the prevalence of the hepatitis C, hepatitis B, human immunodeficiency, and human T-lymphotropic viruses. *Am J Public Health* 1996;86(5):655–661.

79. Levine OS, Vlahov D, Koehler SC,

et al. Seroepidemiology of hepatitis B virus in a population of injecting drug users: association with drug injection patterns. *Am J Epidemiol* 1995;142(3):331–341.

80. Des Jarlais DC, Diaz T, Perlis T, et al. Variability in the incidence of human immunodeficiency virus, hepatitis B virus, and hepatitis C virus infection among young injecting drug users in New York City. *Am J Epidemiol* 2003;157:467–471.

81. Contoreggi C, Rexroad E, Lange V. Current management of infectious complications in the injecting drug user. *J Subst Abuse Treat* 1998;15(2):95–106.

82. Hoofnagle JH, Di Bisceglie AM. The treatment of chronic viral hepatitis. *N Engl J Med* 1997;336(5):347–356.

83. MacKellar DA, Valleroy LA, Secura GM, McFarland W, Shehan D, Ford W, et al. Two decades after vaccine license: hepatitis B immunization and infection among young men who have sex with men. *Am J Public Health* 2001;91(6):965–971.

84. Koff RS. Vaccine recommendations: challenges and controversies. *Infect Dis Clin North Am* 2001;15(1).

85. Hagan H. Vaccination could improve overall health in a high risk population. *West J Med* 2000;172(21).

86. Mezzelani P, Venturini L, Turrina G, et al. High compliance with a hepatitis B virus vaccination program among intravenous drug users. *J Infect Dis* 1991;163:923.

87. Margolis HS, Alter MJ, Hadler SC. Hepatitis B: evolving epidemiology and implications for control. *Semin Liver Dis* 1991;11(2):84–92.

88. Des Jarlais DC, Fisher DG, Clark Newman J, et al. Providing hepatitis B vaccination to injection drug users: referral to health clinics versus on-site vaccination at a syringe exchange program. *Am J Public Health* 2001;91(11):1791–1792.

89. Quaglio G, Lugaboni F, Vento S, et al. Isolated presence of antibody to hepatitis B core antigen in injection drug users: do they need to be vaccinated? *Clin Infect Dis* 2001;32:143–144.

90. Alter MJ, Kruszon-Moran D, Nainan OV, et al. The prevalence of hepatitis C virus infection in the United States, 1988 through 1994. *N Engl J Med* 1999;341(8):556–562.

91. Alter MJ. Epidemiology of hepatitis C. *Hepatology* 1997;26[3 Suppl 1]:62S–65S.

92. Murrill CS, Weeks H, Castrucci BC, et al. Age-specific seroprevalence of HIV, hepatitis B virus, and hepatitis C virus infection among injection drug users admitted to drug treatment

in 6 U.S. cities. *Am J Public Health* 2002;92(3):385–387.

93. Diaz T, Des J, Vlahov D, et al. Factors associated with prevalent hepatitis C: differences among young adult injection drug users in lower and upper Manhattan, New York City. *Am J Public Health* 2001;91(1):23–30.

94. Garfein RS, Vlahov D, Galai N, et al. Viral infections in short-term injection drug users: the prevalence of the hepatitis C, hepatitis B, human immunodeficiency, and human T-lymphotropic viruses. *Am J Public Health* 1996;86(5):655–661.

95. Hagan H, Thiede H, Weiss NS, et al. Sharing of drug preparation equipment as a risk factor for hepatitis C. *Am J Public Health* 2001;91(1):42–46.

96. Thorpe LE, Ouellet LJ, Hershow R, et al. Risk of hepatitis C virus infection among young adult injection drug users who share injection equipment. *Am J Epidemiol* 2002;155(7):645–653.

97. Yen T, Keeffe EB, Ahmed A. The epidemiology of hepatitis C virus infection. *J Clin Gastroenterol* 2003;36(1):47–53.

98. Centers for Disease Control and Prevention. Recommendations for prevention and control of hepatitis C virus (HCV) infection and HCV-related chronic disease. *MMWR Recomm Rep* 1998;47(RR-19):1–39.

99. Thomas DL, Zenilman JM, Alter HJ, et al. Sexual transmission of hepatitis C virus among patients attending sexually transmitted diseases clinics in Baltimore—an analysis of 309 sex partnerships. *J Infect Dis* 1995;171(4):768–775.

100. Lauer GM, Walker BD. Hepatitis C virus infection. *N Engl J Med* 2001;345(1):41–52.

101. Thomas DL, Astemborski J, Rai RM, et al. The natural history of hepatitis C virus infection: host, viral, and environmental factors. *JAMA* 2000;284(4):450–456.

102. Poynard T, Bedossa P, Opolon P. Natural history of liver fibrosis progression in patients with chronic hepatitis C. The OBSVIRC, METAVIR, CLINIVIR, and DOSVIRC groups. *Lancet* 1997;349(9055):825–832.

103. Sanchez-Quijano A, Andreu J, Gavilan F, et al. Influence of human immunodeficiency virus type 1 infection on the natural course of chronic parenterally acquired hepatitis C. *Eur J Clin Microbiol Infect Dis* 1995;14(11):949–953.

104. Dalgard O, Bjoro K, Hellum K, et al. Treatment of chronic hepatitis C in injecting drug users: 5 years' follow-up. *Eur Addict Res* 2002;8(1):45–49.

105. Proust B, Dubois F, Bacq Y, et al. Two successive hepatitis C virus infections

in an intravenous drug user. *J Clin Microbiol* 2000;38(8):3125–3127.

106. National Institutes of Health consensus development conference statement. Management of hepatitis C. 2002 June 10–12, 2002. *HIV Clin Trials* 2003;4(1):55–75.

107. Backmund M, Meyer K, Von Zielonka M, et al. Treatment of hepatitis C infection in injection drug users. *Hepatology* 2001;34(1):188–193.

108. Sylvestre DL. Treating hepatitis C in methadone maintenance patients: an interim analysis. *Drug Alcohol Depend* 2002;67(2):117–123.

109. Edlin BR, Seal KH, Lorvick J, et al. Is it justifiable to withhold treatment for hepatitis C from illicit-drug users? *N Engl J Med* 2001;345(3):211–215.

110. Johnson ME, Fisher DG, Fenaughty A, et al. Hepatitis C virus and depression in drug users. *Am J Gastroenterol* 1998;93(5):785–789.

111. Castera L, Zigante F, Bastie A, et al. Incidence of interferon alfa-induced depression in patients with chronic hepatitis C. *Hepatology* 2002;35(4):978–979.

112. Umbricht-Schneiter A, Ginn DH, Pabst KM, et al. Providing medical care to methadone clinic patients: referral vs on-site care. *Am J Public Health* 1994;84(2):207–210.

113. Pratt CC, Paone D, Carter RJ, et al. Hepatitis C screening and management practices: a survey of drug treatment and syringe exchange programs in New York City. *Am J Public Health* 2002;92(8):1254–1256.

114. Fleming CA, Craven DE, Thornton D, et al. Hepatitis C virus and human immunodeficiency virus coinfection in an urban population: low eligibility for interferon treatment. *Clin Infect Dis* 2003;36(1):97–100.

115. Falck-Ytter Y, Kale H, Mullen KD, et al. Surprisingly small effect of antiviral treatment in patients with hepatitis C. *Ann Intern Med* 2002;136(4):288–292.

116. Fernandez-Villar A, Sopena B, Vazquez R, et al. Isoniazid hepatotoxicity among drug users: the role of hepatitis C. *Clin Infect Dis* 2003;36(3):293–298.

117. Sulkowski MS, Thomas DL, Chaisson RE, et al. Hepatotoxicity associated with antiretroviral therapy in adults infected with human immunodeficiency virus and the role of hepatitis C or B virus infection. *JAMA* 2000;283(1):74–80.

118. Hagan H, Jarlais DC, Friedman SR, et al. Reduced risk of hepatitis B and hepatitis C among injection drug users in the Tacoma syringe exchange program. *Am J Public Health* 1995;85(11):1531–1537.

119. Kapadia F, Vlahov D, Des J, et al. Does bleach disinfection of syringes protect against hepatitis C infection among young adult injection drug users? *Epidemiology* 2002;13(6):738–741.

120. Vento S, Garofano T, Renzini C, et al. Fulminant hepatitis associated with hepatitis A virus superinfection in patients with chronic hepatitis C. *N Engl J Med* 1998;338(5):286–290.

121. Okazaki T, Yoshihara H, Suzuki K, et al. Efficacy of interferon therapy in patients with chronic hepatitis C. Comparison between non-drinkers and drinkers. *Scand J Gastroenterol* 1994;29(11):1039–1043.

122. Mochida S, Ohnishi K, Matsuo S. Effect of alcohol intake on the efficacy of interferon therapy in patients with chronic hepatitis C as evaluated by multivariate logistic regression analysis. *Alcohol Clin Exp Res* 1996;20[9 Suppl]:371A–377A.

123. Hansson BG, Moestrup T, Widell A, et al. Infection with delta agent in Sweden: introduction of a new hepatitis agent. *J Infect Dis* 1982;146(4):472–478.

124. Lettau LA, McCarthy JG, Smith MH, et al. Outbreak of severe hepatitis due to delta and hepatitis B viruses in parenteral drug abusers and their contacts. *N Engl J Med* 1987;317(20):1256–1262.

125. Kao JH, Chen PJ, Lai MY, et al. Hepatitis D virus genotypes in intravenous drug users in Taiwan: decreasing prevalence and lack of correlation with hepatitis B virus genotypes. *J Clin Microbiol* 2002;40(8):3047–3049.

126. Oliveira ML, Bastos FI, Telles PR, et al. Prevalence and risk factors for HBV, HCV and HDV infections among injecting drug users from Rio de Janeiro, Brazil. *Braz J Med Biol Res* 1999;32(9):1107–1114.

127. Coppola RC, Masia G, di Martino ML, et al. Sexual behaviour and multiple infections in drug abusers. *Eur J Epidemiol* 1996;12(5):429–435.

128. Navascues CA, Rodriguez M, Sotorrio NG, et al. Epidemiology of hepatitis D virus infection: changes in the last 14 years. *Am J Gastroenterol* 1995;90(11):1981–1984.

129. Buti M, Mas A, Sanchez-Tapias JM, et al. Chronic hepatitis D in intravenous drug addicts and non-addicts. A comparative clinicopathological study. *J Hepatol* 1988;7(2):169–174.

130. Saracco G, Rosina F, Brunetto MR, et al. Rapidly progressive HBsAg-positive hepatitis in Italy: the role of hepatitis delta virus infection. *J Hepatol* 1987;5(3):274–281.

131. Centers for Disease Control and Prevention. Primary and secondary syphilis—United States, 2000–2001. *MMWR Morb Mortal Wkly Rep* 2002; 51(43):971–973.

132. Tyndall MW, Patrick D, Spittal P, et al. Risky sexual behaviours among injection drugs users with high HIV prevalence: implications for STD control. *Sex Transm Infect* 2002;78[Suppl 1]:i170–i175.

133. Lopez-Zetina J, Ford W, Weber M, et al. Predictors of syphilis seroreactivity and prevalence of HIV among street recruited injection drug users in Los Angeles County, 1994–6. *Sex Transm Infect* 2000;76(6):462–469.

134. Gourevitch MN, Hartel D, Schoenbaum EE, et al. A prospective study of syphilis and HIV infection among injection drug users receiving methadone in the Bronx, NY. *Am J Public Health* 1996;86[8 Pt 1]:1112–1115.

135. Hwang LY, Ross MW, Zack C, et al. Prevalence of sexually transmitted infections and associated risk factors among populations of drug abusers. *Clin Infect Dis* 2000;31(4):920–926.

136. Siegal HA, Falck RS, Wang J, et al. History of sexually transmitted diseases infection, drug-sex behaviors, and the use of condoms among midwestern users of injection drugs and crack cocaine. *Sex Transm Dis* 1996;23(4):277–282.

137. Baseman J, Leonard L, Ross M, et al. Acceptance of syphilis screening among residents of high-STD-risk Houston communities. *Int J STD AIDS* 2001;12(11):744–749.

138. Centers for Disease Control and Prevention. Sexually transmitted diseases treatment guidelines 2002. *MMWR Recomm Rep* 2002;51(RR-6):1–78.

139. Workowski KA, Levine WC, Wasserheit JN. U.S. Centers for Disease Control and Prevention guidelines for the treatment of sexually transmitted diseases: an opportunity to unify clinical and public health practice. *Ann Intern Med* 2002;137(4):255–262.

140. O'Connor PG, Molde S, Henry S, et al. Human immunodeficiency virus infection in intravenous drug users: a model for primary care. *Am J Med* 1992;93(4):382–386.

141. Ruiz JD, Molitor F, McFarland W, et al. Prevalence of HIV infection, sexually transmitted diseases, and hepatitis and related risk behavior in young women living in low-income neighborhoods of northern California. *West J Med* 2000;172(6):368–373.

142. Bachmann LH, Lewis I, Allen R, et al. Risk and prevalence of treatable sexually transmitted diseases at a Birmingham substance abuse treatment facility. *Am J Public Health* 2000;90(10):1615–1618.

143. Buchacz K, McFarland W, Hernandez M, et al. Prevalence and correlates of herpes simplex virus type 2 infection in a population-based survey of young women in low-income neighborhoods of Northern California. The Young Women's Survey Team. *Sex Transm Dis* 2000;27(7):393–400.

144. Kanno MB, Zenilman J. Sexually transmitted diseases in injection drug users. *Infect Dis Clin North Am* 2002;16(3):771–780.

145. Ho GY, Bierman R, Beardsley L, et al. Natural history of cervicovaginal papillomavirus infection in young women. *N Engl J Med* 1998;338(7):423–428.

146. Burk RD, Ho GY, Beardsley L, et al. Sexual behavior and partner characteristics are the predominant risk factors for genital human papillomavirus infection in young women. *J Infect Dis* 1996;174(4):679–689.

147. Kahn JA, Rosenthal SL, Succop PA, et al. Mediators of the association between age of first sexual intercourse and subsequent human papillomavirus infection. *Pediatrics* 2002;109(1):E5.

148. Lally MA, Alvarez S, Macnevin R, et al. Acceptability of sexually transmitted infection screening among women in short-term substance abuse treatment. *Sex Transm Dis* 2002;29(12):752–755.

149. Binswanger IA, Kral AH, Bluthenthal RN, et al. High prevalence of abscesses and cellulitis among community-recruited injection drug users in San Francisco. *Clin Infect Dis* 2000;30(3):579–581.

150. Vlahov D, Sullivan M, Astemborski J, et al. Bacterial infections and skin cleaning prior to injection among intravenous drug users. *Public Health Rep* 1992;107(5):595–598.

151. Makower RM, Pennycook AG, Moulton C. Intravenous drug abusers attending an inner city accident and emergency department. *Arch Emerg Med* 1992;9(1):32–39.

152. Stone HD, Appel RG. Human immunodeficiency virus-associated nephropathy: current concepts. *Am J Med Sci* 1994;307(3):212–217.

153. Morrison A, Elliott L, Gruer L. Injecting-related harm and treatment-seeking behaviour among injecting drug users. *Addiction* 1997;92(10):1349–1352.

154. Spijkerman IJ, van Ameijden EJ, Mientjes GH, et al. Human immunodeficiency virus infection and other risk factors for skin abscesses and endocarditis among injection drug users. *J Clin Epidemiol* 1996;49(10):1149–1154.

155. Chen JL, Fullerton KE, Flynn NM. Necrotizing fasciitis associated with injection drug use. *Clin Infect Dis* 2001;33(1):6–15.

156. Murphy EL, DeVita D, Liu H, et al. Risk factors for skin and soft-tissue abscesses among injection drug users: a case-control study. *Clin Infect Dis* 2001;33(1):35–40.

157. Passaro DJ, Werner SB, McGee J, et al. Wound botulism associated with black tar heroin among injecting drug users. *JAMA* 1998;279(11):859–863.

158. Rich JD, Dickinson BP, Flanigan TP, et al. Abscess related to anabolic-androgenic steroid injection. *Med Sci Sports Exerc* 1999;31(2):207–209.

159. Takahashi TA, Merrill JO, Boyko EJ, et al. Type and location of injection drug use-related soft tissue infections predict hospitalization. *J Urban Health* 2003;80(1):127–136.

160. Darke S, Ross J, Kaye S. Physical injecting sites among injecting drug users in Sydney, Australia. *Drug Alcohol Depend* 2001;62(1):77–82.

161. Summanen PH, McTeague M, Bennion R, et al. Bacteriology of skin and soft-tissue infections: comparison of infections in intravenous drug users and individuals with no history of intravenous drug use. *Clin Infect Dis* 1995;20(2):S279–S282.

162. Ringertz SH, Hoiby EA, Jensenius M, et al. Injectional anthrax in a heroin skin-popper. *Lancet* 2000;356(9241):1574–1575.

163. From the Centers for Disease Control and Prevention. Tetanus among injecting-drug users—California, 1997. *JAMA* 1998;279(13):987.

164. Tuazon CU, Hill R, Sheagren JN. Microbiologic study of street heroin and injection paraphernalia. *J Infect Dis* 1974;129(3):327–329.

165. Holbrook KA, Klein RS, Hartel D, et al. *Staphylococcus aureus* nasal colonization in HIV-seropositive and HIV-seronegative drug users. *J Acquir Immune Defic Syndr Hum Retrovirol* 1997;16(4):301–306.

166. Charlebois ED, Bangsberg DR, Moss NJ, et al. Population-based community prevalence of methicillin-resistant *Staphylococcus aureus* in the urban poor of San Francisco. *Clin Infect Dis* 2002;34(4):425–433.

167. Update: *Clostridium novyi* and unexplained illness among injecting-drug users—Scotland, Ireland, and England, April–June 2000. *MMWR Morb Mortal Wkly Rep* 2000;49(24):543–545.

168. Bohlen LM, Muhlemann K, Dubuis O, et al. Outbreak among drug users caused by a clonal strain of group A streptococcus. *Emerg Infect Dis* 2000;6(2):175–179.

169. Fleisch F, Zbinden R, Vanoli C, et al. Epidemic spread of a single clone of methicillin-resistant *Staphylococcus aureus* among injection drug users in Zurich, Switzerland. *Clin Infect Dis* 2001;32(4):581–586.

170. Gershon RR. Infection control basis for recommending one-time use of sterile syringes and aseptic procedures for injection drug users. *J Acquir Immune Defic Syndr Hum Retrovirol* 1998;18:S20–S24.

171. Harris HW, Young DM. Care of injection drug users with soft-tissue infections in San Francisco, California. *Arch Surg* 2002;137(11):1217–1222.

172. Grau LE, Arevalo S, Catchpool C, et al. Expanding harm reduction services through a wound and abscess clinic. *Am J Public Health* 2002;92(12):1915–1917.

173. Novick DM, Ness GL. Abuse of antibiotics by abusers of parenteral heroin or cocaine. *South Med J* 1984;77:302–303.

174. Frontera JA, Gradon JD. Right-side endocarditis in injection drug users: review of proposed mechanisms of pathogenesis. *Clin Infect Dis* 2000;30(2):374–379.

175. Wilson LE, Thomas DL, Astemborski J, et al. Prospective study of infective endocarditis among injection drug users. *J Infect Dis* 2002;185(12):1761–1766.

176. Hecht SR, Berger M. Right-sided endocarditis in intravenous drug users. Prognostic features in 102 episodes. *Ann Intern Med* 1992;117(7):560–566.

177. Von Reyn CF, Levy BS, Arbeit RD, et al. Infective endocarditis: an analysis based on strict case definitions. *Ann Intern Med* 1981;94[4 Pt 1]:505–518.

178. Selwyn PA, Alcabes P, Hartel D, et al. Clinical manifestations and predictors of disease progression in drug users with human immunodeficiency virus infection. *N Engl J Med* 1992;327(24):1697–1703.

179. Manoff, Vlahov D, Herskowitz A, et al. Human immunodeficiency virus infection and infective endocarditis among injecting drug users. *Epidemiology* 1996;7(6):566–570.

180. Chambers HF, Morris DL, Tauber MG, et al. Cocaine use and the risk for endocarditis in intravenous drug users. *Ann Intern Med* 1987;106(6):833–836.

181. Levitt MA, Snoey ER, Tamkin GW, et al. Prevalence of cardiac valve abnormalities in afebrile injection drug users. *Acad Emerg Med* 1999;6(9):911–915.

182. Reisberg BE. Infective endocarditis in the narcotic addict. *Prog Cardiovasc Dis* 1979;22(3):193–204.

183. Levine DP, Crane LR, Zervos MJ. Bacteremia in narcotic addicts at the Detroit Medical Center. II. Infectious endocarditis: a prospective comparative study. *Rev Infect Dis* 1986;8(3):374–396.

184. Netzer RO, Zollinger E, Seiler C, et al. Infective endocarditis: clinical spectrum, presentation and outcome. An analysis of 212 cases 1980–1995. *Heart* 2000;84(1):25–30.

185. Reiner NE, Gopalakrishna KV, Lerner PI. Enterococcal endocarditis in heroin addicts. *JAMA* 1976;235(17):1861–1863.

186. Zuber PL, Gruner E, Altwegg M, et al. Invasive infection with non-toxigenic *Corynebacterium diphtheriae* among drug users. *Lancet* 1992;339(8805):1359.

187. Shekar R, Rice TW, Zierdt CH, et al. Outbreak of endocarditis caused by Pseudomonas aeruginosa serotype O11 among pentazocine and tripelennamine abusers in Chicago. *J Infect Dis* 1985;151(2):203–208.

188. Noriega ER, Rubinstein E, Simberkoff MS, et al. Subacute and acute endocarditis due to *Pseudomonas cepacia* in heroin addicts. *Am J Med* 1975;59(1):29–36.

189. Mills J, Drew D. *Serratia marcescens* endocarditis: a regional illness associated with intravenous drug abuse. *Ann Intern Med* 1976;84(1):29–35.

190. Leen CL, Brettle RP. Fungal infections in drug users. *J Antimicrob Chemother* 1991;28[Suppl A]:83–96.

191. Scheidegger C, Pietrzak J, Frei R. Disseminated candidiasis after intravenous use of oral methadone. *Ann Intern Med* 1991;115(7):576.

192. Mylonakis E, Calderwood SB. Infective endocarditis in adults. *N Engl J Med* 2001;345(18):1318–1330.

193. Crane LR, Levine DP, Zervos MJ, et al. Bacteremia in narcotic addicts at the Detroit Medical Center. I. Microbiology, epidemiology, risk factors, and empiric therapy. *Rev Infect Dis* 1986;8(3):364–373.

194. Samet JH, Shevitz A, Fowle J, et al. Hospitalization decision in febrile intravenous drug users. *Am J Med* 1990;89(1):53–57.

195. Marantz PR, Linzer M, Feiner CJ, et al. Inability to predict diagnosis in febrile intravenous drug abusers. *Ann Intern Med* 1987;106:823–828.

196. Heidenreich PA, Masoudi FA, Maini B, et al. Echocardiography in patients with suspected endocarditis: a cost-effectiveness analysis. *Am J Med* 1999;107(3):198–208.

197. Li JS, Sexton DJ, Mick N, et al. Proposed modifications to the Duke criteria for the diagnosis of infective endocarditis. *Clin Infect Dis* 2000;30(4):633–638.

198. Heldman AW, Hartert TV, Ray SC, et al. Oral antibiotic treatment of right-sided staphylococcal endocarditis in injection drug users: prospective randomized comparison with parenteral

therapy. *Am J Med* 1996;101(1):68–76.

199. DiNubile MJ. Abbreviated therapy for right-sided *Staphylococcus aureus* endocarditis in injecting drug users: the time has come? *Eur J Clin Microbiol Infect Dis* 1994;13(7):533–534.

200. Ribera E, Miró JM, Cortes E, et al. Influence of human immunodeficiency virus 1 infection and degree of immunosuppression in the clinical characteristics and outcome of infective endocarditis in intravenous drug users. *Arch Intern Med* 1998;158(18):2043–2050.

201. Pulvirenti JJ, Kerns E, Benson C, et al. Infective endocarditis in injection drug users: importance of human immunodeficiency virus serostatus and degree of immunosuppression. *Clin Infect Dis* 1996;22(1):40–45.

202. Le T, Bayer AS. Combination antibiotic therapy for infective endocarditis. *Clin Infect Dis* 2003;36(5):615–621.

203. Brown PD, Levine DP. Infective endocarditis in the injection drug user. *Infect Dis Clin North Am* 2002;16(3):645–665.

204. Salomon N, Perlman DC, Friedmann P, et al. Prevalence and risk factors for positive tuberculin skin tests among active drug users at a syringe exchange program. *Int J Tuberc Lung Dis* 2000;4(1):47–54.

205. Howard AA, Klein RS, Schoenbaum EE, et al. Crack cocaine use and other risk factors for tuberculin positivity in drug users. *Clin Infect Dis* 2002;35(10):1183–1190.

206. Graham NM, Nelson KE, Solomon L, et al. Prevalence of tuberculin positivity and skin test anergy in HIV-1-seropositive and -seronegative intravenous drug users. *JAMA* 1992;267(3):369–373.

207. Gourevitch MN, Hartel D, Schoenbaum EE, et al. Lack of association of induration size with HIV infection among drug users reacting to tuberculin. *Am J Respir Crit Care Med* 1996;154[4 Pt 1]:1029–1033.

208. Leonhardt KK, Gentile F, Gilbert BP, et al. A cluster of tuberculosis among crack house contacts in San Mateo County, California. *Am J Public Health* 1994;84(11):1834–1836.

209. Reichman LB, Felton CP, Edsall JR. Drug dependence, a possible new risk factor for tuberculosis disease. *Arch Intern Med* 1979;139(3):337–339.

210. Markowitz N, Hansen NI, Hopewell PC, et al. Incidence of tuberculosis in the United States among HIV-infected persons. The Pulmonary Complications of HIV Infection Study Group. *Ann Intern Med* 1997;126(2):123–132.

211. Selwyn PA, Hartel D, Lewis VA, et al. A prospective study of the risk of tubercu-losis among intravenous drug users with human immunodeficiency virus infection. *N Engl J Med* 1989;320(9):545–550.

212. Jasmer RM, Nahid P, Hopewell PC. Clinical practice. Latent tuberculosis infection. *N Engl J Med* 2002;347(23):1860–1866.

213. Blumberg HM, Burman WJ, Chaisson RE, et al. American Thoracic Society/Centers for Disease Control and Prevention/Infectious Diseases Society of America: treatment of tuberculosis. *Am J Respir Crit Care Med* 2003;167(4):603–662.

214. Kreek MJ, Garfield JW, Gutjahr CL, et al. Rifampin-induced methadone withdrawal. *N Engl J Med* 1976;294(20):1104–1106.

215. Gourevitch MN, Wasserman W, Panero MS, et al. Successful adherence to observed prophylaxis and treatment of tuberculosis among drug users in a methadone program. *J Addict Dis* 1996;15(1):93–104.

216. Safaeian M, Wilson LE, Taylor E, et al. HTLV-II and bacterial infections among injection drug users. *J Acquir Immune Defic Syndr* 2000;24(5):483–487.

217. Scheidegger C, Zimmerli W. Incidence and spectrum of severe medical complications among hospitalized HIV-seronegative and HIV-seropositive narcotic drug users [Comment]. *AIDS* 1996;10(12):1407–1414.

218. Palepu A, Tyndall MW, Leon H, et al. Hospital utilization and costs in a cohort of injection drug users [Comment]. *CMAJ* 2001;165(4):415–420.

219. Novick DM. Major medical problems and detoxification treatment of parenteral drug abusing alcoholics. *Adv Alcohol Subst Abuse* 1984;3:87–105.

220. Dicpinigaitis PV. Cough reflex sensitivity in cigarette smokers. *Chest* 2003;123(3):685–688.

221. Boschini A, Smacchia C, Di Fine M, et al. Community-acquired pneumonia in a cohort of former injection drug users with and without human immunodeficiency virus infection: incidence, etiologies, and clinical aspects. *Clin Infect Dis* 1996;23(1):107–113.

222. Park DR, Sherbin VL, Goodman MS, et al. The etiology of community-acquired pneumonia at an urban public hospital: influence of human immunodeficiency virus infection and initial severity of illness. *J Infect Dis* 2001;184(3):268–277.

223. Tunkel AR, Pradhan SK. Central nervous system infections in injection drug users. *Infect Dis Clin North Am* 2002;16(3):589–605.

224. Brust JC. Neurologic complications of substance abuse. *J Acquir Immune Defic Syndr* 2002;31[Suppl 2]:S29–S34.

225. Abrahamian FM, Pollack CV Jr, LoVecchio F, et al. Fatal tetanus in a drug abuser with "protective" antitetanus antibodies. *J Emerg Med* 2000;18(2):189–193.

226. Werner SB, Passaro D, McGee J, et al. Wound botulism in California, 1951–1998: recent epidemic in heroin injectors. *Clin Infect Dis* 2000;31(4):1018–1024.

227. Shapiro RL, Hatheway C, Swerdlow DL. Botulism in the United States: a clinical and epidemiologic review. *Ann Intern Med* 1998;129(3):221–228.

228. Burns TM, Shneker BF, Juel VC. Gasoline sniffing multifocal neuropathy. *Pediatr Neurol* 2001;25(5):419–421.

229. Meadows R, Verghese A. Medical complications of glue sniffing [Review] [93 refs]. *South Med J* 1996;89(5):455–462.

230. Berger AR, Schaumburg HH, Gourevitch MN, et al. Prevalence of peripheral neuropathy in injection drug users. *Neurology* 1999;53(3):592–597.

231. Weber M, Diener HC, Voit T, et al. Focal myopathy induced by chronic heroin injection is reversible. *Muscle Nerve* 2000;23(2):274–277.

232. Hill MD, Cooper PW, Perry JR. Chasing the dragon—neurological toxicity associated with inhalation of heroin vapour: case report. *CMAJ* 2000;162(2):236–238.

233. Klockgether T, Weller M, Haarmeier T, et al. Gluteal compartment syndrome due to rhabdomyolysis after heroin abuse. *Neurology* 1997;48(1):275–276.

234. Lange RA, Hillis LD. Cardiovascular complications of cocaine use. *N Engl J Med* 2001;345(5):351–358.

235. Substance Abuse and Mental Health Services Administration. *Results from the 2001 National Household Survey on Drug Abuse, volume I: summary of national findings.* Office of Applied Studies, NHSDA Series H-17, DHHS Publication No. SMA 02–3758. Rockville, MD: U.S. Department of Health and Human Services, 2002.

236. U.S. Department of Health and Human Services. *NIDA research report. Cocaine abuse and addiction.* NIH Publication No. 99–4342. Rockville, MD: National Institutes of Health, 1999.

237. Substance Abuse and Mental Health Services Administration. *The DAWN (Drug Abuse Warning Network) report.* Rockville, MD: U.S. Department of Health and Human Services, 2000.

238. Siegel AJ, Mendelson JH, Sholar MB, et al. Effect of cocaine usage on C-reactive protein, von Willebrand factor, and fibrinogen. *Am J Cardiol* 2002;89(9):1133–1135.

239. Kloner RA, Rezkalla SH. Cocaine and the heart. *N Engl J Med* 2003; 348(6):487–488.

240. Mittleman MA, Mintzer D, Maclure M, et al. Triggering of myocardial infarction by cocaine. *Circulation* 1999; 99(21):2737–2741.

241. Blaho K, Logan B, Winbery S, et al. Blood cocaine and metabolite concentrations, clinical findings, and outcome of patients presenting to an ED. *Am J Emerg Med* 2000;18(5):593–598.

242. Qureshi AI, Suri MF, Guterman LR, et al. Cocaine use and the likelihood of nonfatal myocardial infarction and stroke: data from the Third National Health and Nutrition Examination Survey. *Circulation* 2001;103(4):502–506.

243. Feldman JA, Fish SS, Beshansky JR, et al. Acute cardiac ischemia in patients with cocaine-associated complaints: results of a multicenter trial. *Ann Emerg Med* 2000;36(5):469–476.

244. Weber JE, Chudnofsky CR, Boczar M, et al. Cocaine-associated chest pain: how common is myocardial infarction? *Acad Emerg Med* 2000;7(8):873–877.

245. Weber JE, Shofer FS, Larkin GL, et al. Validation of a brief observation period for patients with cocaine-associated chest pain. *N Engl J Med* 2003;348(6):510–517.

246. Hollander JE, Todd KH, Green G, et al. Chest pain associated with cocaine: an assessment of prevalence in suburban and urban emergency departments. *Ann Emerg Med* 1995;26:671–676.

247. Bizzarri F, Mondillo S, Guerrini F, et al. Spontaneous acute coronary dissection after cocaine abuse in a young woman. *Can J Cardiol* 2003;19(3):297–299.

248. Hsue PY, Salinas CL, Bolger AF, et al. Acute aortic dissection related to crack cocaine. *Circulation* 2002; 105(13):1592–1595.

249. Eagle KA, Isselbacher EM, DeSanctis RW. Cocaine-related aortic dissection in perspective. *Circulation* 2002;105(13):1529–1530.

250. Steinhauer JR, Caulfield JB. Spontaneous coronary artery dissection associated with cocaine use: a case report and brief review. *Cardiovasc Pathol* 2001;10(3):141–145.

251. Castro VJ, Nacht R. Cocaine-induced bradyarrhythmia: an unsuspected cause of syncope. *Chest* 2000;117(1):275–277.

252. Chakko S. Arrhythmias associated with cocaine abuse. *Card Electrophysiol Rev* 2002;6(1–2):168–169.

253. Khan IA. Long QT syndrome: diagnosis and management. *Am Heart J* 2002;143(1):7–14.

254. Singh N, Singh HK, Singh PP, et al. Cocaine-induced torsades de pointes in idiopathic long Q-T syndrome. *Am J Ther* 2001;8(4):299–302.

255. Noel B. Cardiovascular complications of cocaine use. *N Engl J Med* 2001; 345(21):1575.

256. Noel B. Buerger disease or arsenic intoxication? *Arch Intern Med* 2001; 161(7):1016.

257. McEvoy AW, Kitchen ND, Thomas DG. Intracerebral haemorrhage and drug abuse in young adults. *Br J Neurosurg* 2000;14(5):449–454.

258. McEvoy AW, Kitchen ND, Thomas DG. Lesson of the week: intracerebral haemorrhage in young adults: the emerging importance of drug misuse. *BMJ* 2000;320(7245):1322–1324.

259. Kaufman MJ, Levin JM, Ross MH, et al. Cocaine-induced cerebral vasoconstriction detected in humans with magnetic resonance angiography. *JAMA* 1998;279(5):376–380.

260. Winbery S, Blaho K, Logan B, et al. Multiple cocaine-induced seizures and corresponding cocaine and metabolite concentrations. *Am J Emerg Med* 1998; 16(5):529–533.

261. Nzerue CM, Hewan-Lowe K, Riley LJ Jr. Cocaine and the kidney: a synthesis of pathophysiologic and clinical perspectives. *Am J Kidney Dis* 2000;35(5):783–795.

262. Norris KC, Thornhill-Joynes M, Robinson C, et al. Cocaine use, hypertension, and end-stage renal disease. *Am J Kidney Dis* 2001;38(3):523–528.

263. D'Elia JA, Weinrauch LA, Paine DF, et al. Increased infection rate in diabetic dialysis patients exposed to cocaine. *Am J Kidney Dis* 1991;18(3):349–352.

264. Pruett BD, Baddour LM. Sinopulmonary complications of illicit drug use. *Infect Dis Clin North Am* 2002; 16(3):623–643, viii.

265. Tashkin DP. Airway effects of marijuana, cocaine, and other inhaled illicit agents [Review] [139 refs]. *Curr Opin Pulmon Med* 2001;7(2):43–61.

266. Thadani PV. NIDA conference report on cardiopulmonary complications of "crack" cocaine use. Clinical manifestations and pathophysiology. *Chest* 1996;110(4):1072–1076.

267. Haim DY, Lippmann ML, Goldberg SK, et al. The pulmonary complications of crack cocaine. A comprehensive review. *Chest* 1995;107(1):233–240.

268. Muniz AE, Evans T. Acute gastrointestinal manifestations associated with use of crack. *Am J Emerg Med* 2001;19(1):61–63.

269. McCarron MM, Wood JD. The cocaine "body packer" syndrome: diagnosis and treatment. *JAMA* 1983;250:1417–1420.

270. Webb WA. Management of foreign bodies of the upper gastrointestinal tract. *Gastroenterology* 1988;94:204–216.

271. Pollack CV Jr, Biggers DW, Carlton FB Jr, et al. Two crack cocaine body stuffers. *Ann Emerg Med* 1992;21(11):1370–1380.

272. Mari A, Arranz C, Gimeno X, et al. Nasal cocaine abuse and centrofacial destructive process: report of three cases including treatment. *Oral Surg Oral Med Oral Pathol Oral Radiol Endod* 2002;93(4):435–439.

273. Seyer BA, Grist W, Muller S. Aggressive destructive midfacial lesion from cocaine abuse [Review] [13 refs]. *Oral Surg Oral Med Oral Pathol Oral Radiol Endod* 2002;94(4):465–470.

274. Jones DL, Irwin KL, Inciardi J, et al. The high-risk sexual practices of crack-smoking sex workers recruited from the streets of three American cities. The Multicenter Crack Cocaine and HIV Infection Study Team. *Sex Transm Dis* 1998;25(4):187–193.

275. Hser YI, Chou CP, Hoffman V, et al. Cocaine use and high-risk sexual behavior among STD clinic patients. *Sex Transm Dis* 1999;26(2):82–86.

276. Crowe AV, Howse M, Bell GM, et al. Substance abuse and the kidney. *QJM* 2000;93(3):147–152.

277. Briggs NC, Battjes RJ, Cantor KP, et al. Seroprevalence of human T-cell lymphotropic virus type II infection, with or without human immunodeficiency virus type 1 coinfection, among U.S. intravenous drug users. *J Infect Dis* 1995;172(1):51–58.

278. Vlahov D, Khabbaz RF, Cohn S, et al. Incidence and risk factors for human T-lymphotropic virus type II seroconversion among injecting drug users in Baltimore, Maryland, U.S.A. *J Acquir Immune Defic Syndr Hum Retrovirol* 1995;9(1):89–96.

CHAPTER 55

Acute and Chronic Pain

RUSSELL K. PORTENOY, RICHARD PAYNE, AND STEVEN D. PASSIK

An interesting paradox can be discerned in the perception of opioid compounds by various sectors of the medical community: some consider these drugs to be a major cause of abuse, associated with dire consequences to the individual and society at large, whereas others view them as essential medications, capable of mediating one of the highest goals of medicine, the relief of pain and suffering. Generally, specialists in addiction focus on the former characterization and pain specialists project the latter. Given the antithetical nature of these perspectives, it is not surprising that historically there has been little communication between these two groups.

In the wake of the media coverage of the growing abuse of prescription drugs, a new level of discourse has begun between the two camps. The interaction between pain and addiction specialists has led to the beginning of a shared knowledge that could enhance each discipline's ability to apprehend clinical phenomena and formulate questions for research. The potential for opioid addiction is a constant consideration in the management of acute and chronic pain, but most pain clinicians have little understanding of the criteria that define this outcome or the factors that may contribute to it. Specialists in addiction have developed the terminology of dependence and discuss the attendant risks, but they usually fail to address the meaning and manifestation of the phenomenon in patients treated with analgesics for painful medical disease.

This chapter brings together these two perspectives through an examination of the issues raised by each of two situations commonly encountered in clinical practice: the management of pain in patients with a history of opioid abuse, and the risk of opioid abuse in patients with no such history who are administered opioid drugs for medical purposes. Throughout, an effort is made to balance the clinical imperative to provide adequate relief of pain with legitimate concerns about the consequences of opioid abuse. Opioids are the focus of this discussion because they have a unique position as both major analgesics and drugs of abuse, and thereby encourage a comprehensive examination of the issues. It should be noted, however, that many of the topics explored herein apply equally to other drug classes, such as the use benzodiazepines for anxiety and other disorders (1,2).

TERMINOLOGY OF ABUSE AND CLASSIFICATION OF SUBSTANCE ABUSERS

The relationship between the medical use and abuse of opioid drugs cannot be clarified without a precise characterization of terms, including *tolerance, dependence, abuse,* and *addiction.* The application of inappropriate definitions, such as the use of the term *addict* to describe patients who are physically dependent, unnecessarily stigmatizes the patient and may have adverse effects on therapy. Conversely, lack of clarity about those characteristics that truly constitute addiction may delay recognition of the syndrome when it does occur in the clinical setting.

Terminology of Abuse

The terminology of substance abuse, as discussed elsewhere in this volume, was developed by specialists in addiction, whose frame of reference is the addict, rather than the medical patient receiving opioids for pain. It is necessary to clarify this terminology when applying it to the assessment of medical patients (3–4a).

Tolerance

Tolerance is a pharmacologic property of opioid drugs defined by the need for increasing doses to maintain effects (5–7). Tolerance to virtually all opioid effects can be induced reliably in animal models (8), and it is commonly believed that tolerance develops similarly during long-term exposure to opioids in humans (9). Indeed, loss of analgesic efficacy because of the development of tolerance typically is perceived to be a major impediment to the clinical use of opioid drugs. The development of tolerance to the reinforcing effects of opioids, and the consequent need to increase doses to regain these effects, has also been speculated to be an important element in the pathogenesis of addiction, notwithstanding the generally accepted belief that tolerance may or may not exist in the addicted patient (10).

There is a compelling need to reevaluate the concept of tolerance as it pertains to the long-term use of opioid drugs for patients with chronic pain (11,12). The view that tolerance to analgesic effects routinely interferes with the clinical efficacy of opioids is not credible given numerous surveys that demonstrated relatively stable dose requirements for prolonged periods in diverse populations. In the cancer population, for example, the need for dose escalation typically occurs only in the setting of a progressive, painful lesion (13–17). Likewise, cancer patients who self-administer morphine for several weeks to control mucositis pain following bone marrow transplantation do not increase the dose after an initial rapid titration (18). Surveys of patients with nonmalignant pain treated with systemic or neuraxial opioids for prolonged periods also demonstrate variable dose requirements over time, with stability in most patients without obvious disease progression (19–24). Despite the demonstrable development of tolerance to some of the side effects of the opioids, such as cognitive impairment (25), tolerance to the favorable clinical effects of these drugs seldom compromises the efficacy of treatment.

Physical Dependence

Similar to tolerance, physical dependence is a pharmacologic property of opioid drugs. It is defined solely by the occurrence of an abstinence syndrome (withdrawal) following abrupt dose reduction or administration of an antagonist (4a–7,26). Because some degree of physical dependence can be produced with very little opioid exposure (27), and neither the dose nor duration of administration required to produce clinically significant physical dependence in humans is known, most practitioners assume that the potential for an abstinence syndrome exists after opioids have been administered repeatedly for only a few days.

There is great confusion among clinicians about the differences between physical dependence and addiction. This continues despite the widespread acceptance among addiction specialists of the critical distinctions between these phenomena. Although physical dependence, like tolerance, has been suggested to be a component of addiction (28,29), and the avoidance of withdrawal (the sine qua non of physical dependence) has been postulated to create behavioral contingencies that reinforce drug-seeking behavior (30), most experts define addiction in a manner that fully distinguishes it from physical dependence (4a,6,31,32). Physical dependence alone does not preclude the uncomplicated discontinuation of opioids in the medical setting, as amply demonstrated by the success of opioid detoxification by multidisciplinary pain programs (33) and the routine cessation of opioids in cancer patients who become fully analgesic following a pain-relieving neurolytic procedure. Indirect evidence for this distinction between physical dependence and addiction is even provided by animal models of opioid self-administration, which demonstrate that persistent drug-taking behavior can be maintained in the absence of physical dependence (34).

Use of the term *addiction* to describe patients who are merely physically dependent reinforces the stigma associated with opioid therapy and should be abandoned. If the clinician wishes to describe a patient who is believed to have the capacity for abstinence, the term *physical dependence* must be used. Labeling the patient as *dependent* also should be discouraged, because it fosters confusion between physical dependence and psychological dependence. The latter is a component of the addiction syndrome (as described later in this chapter) and is unrelated to the occurrence of physical dependence. For the same reason, use of the term *habituation* should be eschewed; in the clinical setting, this term is often used indiscriminately to refer to tolerance, physical dependence, or psychological dependence.

Addiction

Until recently, all accepted definitions applied to the assessment of addiction had been developed by addiction specialists, whose frame of reference generally is the individual who develops addiction outside of the medical context and has no disease for which the drug or drugs may be indicated. These definitions emphasize that addiction is a psychological and behavioral syndrome in which there is drug craving, compulsive use, a strong tendency to relapse after withdrawal, and continued use despite harm to the user or those around the user (6,10,29–31). Some of these definitions highlight the development of tolerance or physical dependence in the development of addiction. Although these features are widely accepted, the specifics must be interpreted cautiously if the drug of abuse may be a legitimate therapy for a medical disorder. For example, a reference to "relapse after withdrawal" (6) may be difficult to interpret if the drug is prescribed for a medical indication, and reference to tolerance and physical dependence (29), which are expected phenomena when opioids are medically administered for prolonged periods, have no relevance to clinical populations.

According to a recent definition jointly endorsed by professional societies for pain and addiction in the United States,

> [a]ddiction is a primary, chronic, neurobiologic disease, with genetic, psychosocial, and environmental factors influencing its development and manifestations. It is characterized by behaviors that include one or more of the following: impaired control over drug use, compulsive use, continued use despite harm, and craving. (4a)

This definition does not reference phenomena related to tolerance or physical dependence. It appropriately focuses on behavior as the relevant assessment for the diagnosis of addiction. Craving may involve rumination about the drug and an intense desire to secure its supply. Compulsive use may be indicated by persistent or escalating consumption of the drug despite physical, psychological, or social harm to the user.

Use despite harm also has been used to define *abuse* (28), a term that has been applied additionally to any drug use that is outside accepted societal and cultural standards (6). There is substantial, but not complete, overlap between the terms *addiction* and *abuse*. An individual who uses an illicit drug could be considered an abuser even if the compulsive quality of use that characterizes the addict is absent. Similarly, an individual could be psychologically dependent on a licit drug, such as a prescription opioid, but theoretically have enough controls established that abuse behaviors do not occur. These considerations may be important in assessing the medical patient who receives opioids for pain.

In the clinical setting, the behaviors that may signal a problem with a potentially abusable drug are diverse, often subtle, and may be difficult to interpret. To operationalize the process of assessment for patients with painful disorders who are prescribed an opioid for an appropriate indication, a concept that may be labeled "aberrant drug-related behavior" is needed. Patients who receive an opioid for legitimate medical purposes have the potential to engage in a broad range of behaviors that are conventionally perceived by prescribers as problematic (Table 55.1). The routine evaluation of patients who receive opioids or other potentially abusable drugs must include monitoring for the development of these behaviors. Should they occur, the assessment must yield information that would support a specific diagnosis and facilitate an appropriate therapeutic response.

Aberrant drug-related behaviors in the clinical setting have a "differential diagnosis." In some cases, the behav-

TABLE 55.1. *Aberrant drug-related behaviors*

Behaviors More Suggestive of an Addiction Disorder
  Selling prescription drugs
  Prescription forgery
  Stealing or "borrowing" drugs from others
  Injecting oral formulations
  Obtaining prescription drugs from nonmedical sources
  Concurrent abuse of alcohol or illicit drugs
  Multiple dose escalations or other noncompliance with therapy despite warnings
  Multiple episodes of prescription "loss"
  Repeatedly seeking prescriptions from other clinicians or from emergency rooms without informing prescriber or after warnings to desist
  Evidence of deterioration in the ability to function at work, in the family, or socially that appear to be related to drug use
  Repeated resistance to changes in therapy despite clear evidence of adverse physical or psychological effects from the drug
Behaviors Less Suggestive of an Addiction Disorder
  Aggressive complaining about the need for more drug
  Drug hoarding during periods of reduced symptoms
  Requesting specific drugs
  Openly acquiring similar drugs from other medical sources
  Unsanctioned dose escalation or other noncompliance with therapy on one or two occasions
  Unapproved use of the drug to treat another symptom
  Reporting psychic effects not intended by the clinician
  Resistance to a change in therapy associated with "tolerable" adverse effects with expressions of anxiety related to the return of severe symptoms

iors are sufficiently extreme (e.g., injection of an oral formulation) to immediately suggest the diagnosis of an addiction disorder. In other cases, however, the behaviors are less egregious and could reflect other processes, including impulsive behavior driven by unrelieved pain, a psychiatric disorder other than an addiction, or mild encephalopathy with confusion about drug intake. Occasionally, aberrant behaviors indicate criminal intent (i.e., intent to divert).

The importance of this differential diagnosis for aberrant drug-related behavior has been highlighted in the population with cancer pain through acceptance of the term *pseudoaddiction* (35). Pseudoaddiction refers to the drug-seeking behavior that is occasionally observed in the setting of uncontrolled cancer pain and disappears when analgesic interventions, often including increased doses of an opioid, become effective. Clinical experience indicates that similar dynamics are sometimes encountered in populations with nonmalignant disease. Clearly, the diagnosis of addiction is untenable if pain control eliminates behaviors that would otherwise be considered to reflect loss of control, compulsive use, and continued use despite harm. Aberrant drug-related behaviors may not be infrequent occurrences in the treatment of nonmalignant pain (35a).

The extraordinary heterogeneity of the population with painful disorders further complicates the assessment of the individual's degree of control over drug use, and the pattern and consequences of this use. The clinician must recognize that some addicts without pain may feign illness to obtain drugs for diversion or personal use (36), and some with a bona fide medical illness seek opioids or other drugs primarily for their psychic effects. In contrast, some patients engage in behaviors that would be strong evidence of addiction in the absence of the painful disorder, but are best understood as an alternative process in the context of the disease and the psychosocial condition of the individual.

Thus, the assessment of addiction in the setting of opioid treatment for a painful disorder requires a detailed understanding of the drug-related behaviors, pain syndrome, medical and psychological status, social situation, and true impediments to adequate relief. If the patient engages in behaviors that could be fairly labeled as aberrant, the clinician must determine if the problem is likely to be transitory, perhaps an impulsive action related to a pain flare, to a comorbid psychiatric state or to some severe situational stressor, or is likely to be more serious and abiding. This may require observation over time. Although evidence of abuse, and the likelihood of addiction, is clear when patients engage in behaviors that involve illicit drugs or illegal acts, the meaning of other behaviors may be far more difficult to interpret (see Table 55.1). For example, the patient with unrelieved pain who deliberately increases the dose of the opioid by one-third, but no more, and fails to contact the physician until an early refill is needed, has engaged in aberrant behavior, which could be considered abuse and a potential indication of addiction. Perhaps, however, the patient had not been apprised of the clinician's expectations for therapy. Although standards of drug-taking behavior are tacitly acknowledged by most patients and require no reinforcement, nonadherence with all types of therapy is common and some patients require an explicit statement of these expectations. If the same unsanctioned dose escalation occurs after this discussion, the clinician may be more concerned that this behavior indicates a problem with the drug. Even if this occurs, however, the degree of this inappropriate behavior (that is, dose escalation by one-third without prior communication with the clinician) continues to be very modest, and in the setting of unrelieved pain and associated psychological distress, the implications of this noncompliance may be difficult to assess. An ongoing, repeated pattern of behavior may require a clinical plan that aims to decrease pain (i.e., dose escalation) while also containing the aberrant behavior (i.e., smaller quantity per prescription).

The potential for mislabeling behaviors as addiction is particularly great in the patient with a remote or current history of substance abuse. Although opioids may be clearly indicated, any evidence of aberrant drug-related behavior may generate great concern that relapse, rather than symptom control, is driving the therapy. This concern is well placed if the aberrant behaviors are egregious (e.g., prescription forgery), but the more common scenario, which involves behaviors that are unlike the norm but do not themselves constitute abuse, is more difficult to interpret. Pain complaints may be voluble and disproportionate to the degree of nociception. The patient may appear to require unusually high doses or may request injections instead of oral administration. Interactions with the medical staff may be perceived to have a manipulative quality, in which the patient appears to be unusually knowledgeable about opioid treatment and presents a posture of negotiation about therapy. Pseudoaddiction may be common in such patients, set in motion by both a lack of trust that limits the aggressiveness with which pain is approached and pharmacologic needs that may be at the end of the spectrum encountered routinely in clinical practice.

It is extremely important that the clinicians caring for these patients recognize that such behaviors may or may not reflect the aberrant psychological and behavioral states that characterize addiction. Complaints that are perceived to be excessive for the degree of nociception clearly should not alone be labeled addiction. Many chronic pain patients with no history of substance abuse present such complaints, which after careful assessment may be determined to have a prominent psychological contribution. Likewise, knowledge about opioids and negotiation about treatment cannot themselves be construed as addiction. The challenge of the assessment is to determine the nature of the patient's behavior and thereby provide the information necessary to respond appropriately.

Categories of Substance Abusers

Patients with a history of opioid abuse can be divided into categories that may predict some of the problems encountered during pain treatment. These categories include: patients with a remote history of opioid substance, patients with a history of opioid abuse who are currently in maintenance treatment, and patients actively abusing opioid drugs (37). Other relevant groups may include those with a remote or present history of addiction to alcohol, nonopioid illicit drugs (e.g., cocaine), or nonopioid prescription drugs (e.g., benzodiazepines). These distinctions help to identify patients at risk for management problems, which, in turn, may facilitate the assessment process and suggest approaches to therapy.

Unfortunately, there are no adequate studies to confirm the existence of meaningful differences among these groups or that specifically assess the needs and problems posed by each during therapy for pain. Case reports have been helpful in defining the range of concerns, and have been particularly useful in highlighting the observation that even a remote history of abuse can stigmatize a patient and complicate pain treatment (37). Nonetheless, generalizations developed from clinical experience may fail to prepare the clinician for the vagaries of practice, where the experience of pain itself, or other facets of the disease causing the pain, may alter responses in an unpredictable way. They cannot substitute for a comprehensive assessment of each case.

PRINCIPLES OF PAIN ASSESSMENT

An optimal approach to therapy depends on a comprehensive assessment that clarifies the organic and psychological contributions to the pain and characterizes associated problems that may also require treatment. These associated problems may themselves be medical, psychological (including disorders of personality or affect, or profound behavioral disturbances), social, or familial. A history of substance abuse is one such consideration.

Categories of Patients with Pain

Patients with pain can be categorized in several clinically meaningful ways. Some distinctions are particularly relevant to the selection of treatment approaches.

Acute Monophasic Pain

The most common pains are acute and self-limited. Most are never evaluated by physicians and demand no therapy beyond simple measures taken by the individual. Some are severe or associated with serious underlying pathology, however, and require clinical intervention. The latter include pains associated with surgery, major trauma, and burns. Notwithstanding data documenting the frequent undertreatment of these syndromes (38,39), the short-term administration of opioid drugs is widely considered to be medically appropriate treatment for acute severe pains.

Recurrent Acute Pains

Recurrent acute pains are also extremely prevalent. They, too, range in severity and need for clinical intervention. These pains include headache, dysmenorrhea, sickle cell anemia, inflammatory bowel disease, and some arthritides or musculoskeletal disorders (e.g., hemophilic arthropathy). Although opioids commonly are considered to be accepted treatment of the management of acute pain, the decision to use these drugs may become more complicated if episodes of acute pain recur frequently or are expected to recur indefinitely. In this setting, there may be greater concern about the logistics of management (in the home, emergency ward, or hospital), risk of adverse pharmacologic reactions, and abuse potential.

Chronic Pain Associated with Cancer

Opioid therapy is considered to be the major therapeutic approach to patients with cancer pain (14,40–51). It can be speculated that the acceptance of opioid therapy in this setting relates primarily to humane considerations that alter the perceived risk:benefit ratio for the treatment such that the risks believed to exist, whether supported by the evidence or not (discussed in pages 888–893), diminish in importance relative to the desire to provide comfort. Although the scientific underpinning of this perception is tenuous, the general acceptance of opioid treatment for cancer pain during the past decade has provided the opportunity to observe large numbers of patients during long-term therapy. As discussed under Chronic Cancer Pain, this experience has both confirmed the favorable outcomes associated with this approach and led to a desire for a critical reappraisal of conventional thinking about the risks associated with opioid administration to other patient types. Moreover, the acceptance of opioid therapy for cancer pain indicates that optimal management of the substance abuser with cancer requires both expertise in opioid pharmacotherapy and appreciation for the specific problems presented by this population.

Chronic Pain Associated with Progressive Nonmalignant Medical Diseases

Like pain caused by cancer, other pain syndromes are related to progressive medical illness associated with poor prognosis. A recent study, for example, demonstrated striking similarities between cancer and the acquired immunodeficiency syndrome (AIDS) in the prevalence, characteristics, and impact of pain (52,53). The factor that most distinctly separated the population with AIDS-related pain from the cancer pain population was the degree of undertreatment with opioid drugs (54). Other progressive diseases are also characterized by a high prevalence of pain, including sickle cell anemia, hemophilia, and some connective tissue diseases. Although psychosocial disturbances are extremely important determinants of the presentation and management of these conditions, as they are in pain caused by cancer, the pain in most patients usually is assumed to be largely explained by the organic lesion. Many clinicians also perceive a connection between cancer and these conditions and would be inclined to offer chronic opioid therapy, if this approach would be helpful. As discussed later, a history of substance abuse clearly influences this therapeutic inclination.

Chronic Pain Associated with a Nonprogressive Organic Lesion

Many patients have an overtly painful organic lesion that is not life-threatening but is presumed to be adequate to explain the pain. Although psychological processes again can have a profound impact on symptoms and associated functional disturbances, the pain is perceived to be commensurate with the underlying organic condition. In contrast to the previous groups, however, the prognosis for a long survival is good. Included in this category are numerous musculoskeletal pain syndromes (e.g., osteoporosis and spondylolisthesis) and neuropathic pain syndromes (e.g., postherpetic neuralgia, painful polyneuropathy, central pain, or reflex sympathetic dystrophy). Although opioid therapy of these patients continues to be controversial, the existence of a clear-cut organic process may encourage some physicians to consider this approach, at least in patients with no overt psychiatric disorder and no prior history of substance abuse.

Chronic Nonmalignant Pain Syndrome

A large group of patients experience pain or associated disability that is perceived by the clinician to be excessive for the degree of organic pathology extant. Although these pains have been termed idiopathic (55), the latter term usually does not connote the existence of psychiatric comorbidity and disability in the same way. In some patients, a careful assessment provides evidence of a psychological or behavioral pathogenesis to the pain. Most patients with a chronic pain syndrome, however, have both an identifiable organic lesion and sufficient evidence of psychological disturbance to fulfill criteria for a psychiatric disorder, such as a chronic pain disorder or somatization disorder (56). Adding further to the confusing nomenclature, some of these syndromes have received other appellations based on the site of the pain, including atypical facial pain, failed low back syndrome, chronic tension headache, and chronic pelvic pain of unknown etiology.

The array of labels should not obscure the key point, which is that chronic pain may reflect a complex interaction between biomedical factors and psychological factors, and that each patient requires an astute assessment of all these factors, as well as comorbidities. A term that implies the existence of disability and psychiatric disease, such as chronic pain syndrome, may or may not be appropriate based on the findings of this assessment.

To a large extent, the multidisciplinary approach to pain management evolved in response to the challenge posed by these complex patients. Chronic pain disability may be most effectively managed through a multimodality approach to therapy undertaken by professionals of diverse disciplines. As discussed in the section Chronic Opioid Therapy in Patients without Substance Abuse, the use of opioid drugs in this group of patients is particularly controversial.

COMPREHENSIVE PAIN ASSESSMENT

All patients with chronic pain should undergo a comprehensive pain assessment, which requires an appropriate history, a physical examination, and, often, confirmatory laboratory and radiographic procedures. This assessment characterizes the pain complaint and prioritizes other physical and psychosocial problems that may influence pain therapy or be amenable to primary treatment.

The patient should be asked to describe the pain in terms of its temporal features (onset, course, and daily pattern), location, severity, quality, and factors that provoke or relieve it. Other relevant information includes medical and surgical disorders (related or unrelated to the pain), prior history of persistent pain, past pain treatments, and previous use of licit drugs (including alcohol, tobacco, and both over-the-counter and prescription medicines) and illicit drugs. The patient's level of physical functioning should be detailed and important concurrent symptoms, such as level of energy (or, conversely, level of fatigue), sleep disturbance, appetite and weight, should be elicited. A psychosocial history is essential and should assess premorbid psychiatric disease or personality disorder; coping styles demonstrated during earlier episodes of physical disease or psychological stress; work and education history; current level of function and psychological state (particularly anxiety, depression, and changes that had occurred in role functioning); issues related to family cohesion and status of intimate relationships (including changes in the relationship with spouse); and current resources (social, familial, and financial). The patient's activities during the day should be enumerated to help clarify the degree of physical inactivity and social isolation.

In patients with a known history of substance abuse, the interview must clarify both the specific pattern of addictive behaviors (e.g., drug or drugs, routes, frequency of administration, means of acquisition, and means of financing) and the relationship between these behaviors and the pain. It is important to determine whether or not the patient perceives that pain precipitated or perpetuates the addiction, and, similarly, whether or not the patient perceives that drugs that are abused are treating the pain.

A careful history will occasionally elicit evidence of misuse or abuse of a drug in a patient with no previously known substance abuse. This may involve recent use of an illicit drug or aberrant involvement with a licit drug. In all cases, the clinician must determine the specific behaviors that have occurred and the extent, quality, and impact of the cognitions and feelings that relate to the drug. This assessment may be very complicated in patients with chronic pain, whose use of psychotropic and analgesic drugs may be monitored by physicians and closely tied to the experience of symptoms.

The physical examination of patients with chronic pain attempts to determine the existence of an underlying organic contribution to the pain. In most cases, the information obtained from the history and examination guides the selection of appropriate laboratory and imaging procedures that may provide confirmatory evidence of this organic lesion. It must be emphasized again, however, that the discovery of a lesion does not indicate that the predominating pathogenesis for the pain is organic, and the failure to identify a lesion does not confirm that the pain is primarily determined by psychological factors. The assessment should attempt to characterize potentially treatable organic conditions and clarify other factors that may be contributing to the patient's pain and disability.

From the detailed information obtained in this manner, specific clinically relevant aspects of the pain can be highlighted. The most salient considerations relate to the following features.

Temporal Features

One of the most important considerations in the clinical management of pain is the distinction between acute and chronic pain. The phenomenology of pain varies with these temporal features (Table 55.2), and treatment decisions are strongly influenced by these characteristics and the anticipated duration of the pain. As noted, clinical distinctions are also drawn between those with monophasic acute pain syndromes, such as postoperative pain, and those with recurrent acute pains. Among patients with chronic pain, different temporal profiles also occur. Most patients with continuous pain, for example, experience episodes of acute exacerbation that may be far more disabling than the baseline pain itself. In a survey of patients with cancer, for example, almost two-thirds experienced transitory flares of pain (57).

Pathophysiologic Features

In recent years, increasing attention has focused on the importance of putative pain mechanisms in determining the phenomenology of pain syndromes and their response to therapy. In general, pain syndromes can be divided broadly into those that are believed to have a predominating organic pathogenesis, those that are believed to have a

TABLE 55.2. *Clinical characteristics of acute and chronic pain*

	Acute	Chronic
Onset	Rapid, discrete, recalled	May be rapid (acute pain becomes chronic), but may be insidious
Duration	Brief (typically within months) or anticipated to be brief	Prolonged (typically weeks) or anticipated to be prolonged
Pattern	Variable, but usually most intense soon after onset, then waning	Variable, but usually continuous, or mostly continuous, with fluctuation or periods of acute exacerbation
Associated	Anxiety may be present	Variable; depression common, but anxiety disturbances and personality disorders encountered
Associated	Signs of sympathetic hyperactivity may be present soon after onset; need to rest and immobilize the painful part	Sometimes vegetative signs, with sleep disturbance most common; often disturbances in ability to work and function physically or socially
Biologic role	Adaptive	Not adaptive

predominating psychological pathogenesis, and those that are unclassifiable (including patients with idiopathic pain). Based on clinical observation, pains with a predominating organic contribution are described as either nociceptive or neuropathic (55,58,59). Nociceptive pain is presumed to be commensurate with the degree of ongoing activation of afferent nerves subserving pain perception. Although this judgment obviously oversimplifies complex neurophysiologic processes, it is nevertheless useful clinically. Pain classified in this way (e.g., related to cancer or arthritis) usually can be reduced through interventions that improve the peripheral nociceptive lesion. For example, radiotherapy often can eliminate pain from a bony metastasis, and severe joint pain from arthritis usually can be alleviated by joint replacement.

Neuropathic pain is related to aberrant somatosensory processes induced by an injury to the peripheral or central nervous system (58). The pains are often dysesthetic (abnormal pain, unfamiliar to the patient) and disproportionate to any nociceptive lesion identified during the evaluation. The latter factor may complicate the clinical distinction between these pains and pains that are predominantly determined by psychological factors, which are also disproportionate to any identifiable tissue injury. The diagnosis of a neuropathic pain may suggest the use of selected types of analgesic drugs (60) or other analgesic interventions.

Syndromic Features

Syndrome identification is extremely useful in pain assessment, because it may provide information about underlying organic processes, suggest an efficient evaluation, guide the selection of treatments, and indicate prognosis. To further this process, the International Association for the Study of Pain has developed a taxonomy of pain, the goal of which is to establish criteria for the diagnosis of specific pain syndromes (59). The importance of syndrome

identification in the assessment of an underlying organic etiology for the pain is particularly well established in cancer (61,62). One survey, for example, observed that an unrecognized organic lesion could be discovered in 64% of cancer patients with pain who underwent consultation by a pain service, and that this diagnosis led to the use of primary therapy, either antineoplastic drugs or antibiotic, in almost 20% of the patients (63). In a similar way, recognition of discrete neuropathic pain syndromes may lead to specific interventions that would not be considered otherwise, such as sympathetic nerve blocks for suspected sympathetically maintained pains or neurectomy for painful neuroma.

The utility of these distinctions derives from the availability of diverse pain therapies. Although most patients with acute pain and many with chronic pain can be managed appropriately by a single clinician who expertly administers one or more treatments, many patients, particularly those with complex chronic nonmalignant pain problems, benefit from the involvement of specialists in various disciplines, who together implement a sophisticated multimodality approach to therapy. A specialist in substance abuse can be considered to be an appropriate member of a multidisciplinary pain-management team in selected patients with substance abuse and chronic pain.

MANAGEMENT OF PAIN IN THE SUBSTANCE ABUSER

Regardless of the population in question, there are important differences between the relatively brief use of opioids to manage acute pain and the chronic administration of these drugs to patients with persistent pain. The therapeutic use of opioids in the patient with a history of substance abuse raises additional issues in both clinical settings.

Chronic Pain

The role of opioid therapy in patients with a history of substance abuse and chronic pain has traditionally varied with the distinction between cancer-related pain and nonmalignant pain. Opioids are accepted in the management of cancer pain, and management of this condition in patients with a history of substance abuse requires pharmacologic expertise equal to that applied to similar patients without this history. Opioid use is more controversial in other populations with chronic pain, and particularly so when pain is complicated by a history of substance abuse.

From a critical perspective, this distinction between cancer pain and nonmalignant pain may be difficult to rationalize. Nonmalignant pain syndromes are extraordinarily diverse and, as discussed previously, even a simple classification identifies other large groups of patients with chronic severe pain caused by progressive medical disorders that are similar to cancer in terms of prognosis and functional outcomes, but are not neoplastic. It is particularly difficult to justify the view that opioids are the first-line drug for cancer pain but are relatively contraindicated in these latter pain syndromes, which include AIDS, sickle cell anemia, hemophilia, and inflammatory bowel disease, as well as other diseases. Similar concerns may arise in attempting to discern the medical rationale for the conventional rejection of opioid drugs in other chronic pain populations, some of which may, like the cancer population, experience pain as a consequence of tissue injury or neuropathic lesions, or experience chronic pain without the development of psychiatric comorbidity or disability.

Chronic Cancer Pain

Cancer pain is the model for the first-line use of opioid pharmacotherapy in the treatment of pain related to medical illness. Pain is experienced by more than one-third of cancer patients undergoing active antineoplastic therapy and by up to 90% of those with advanced disease (62). Cancer pain specialists have accumulated an enormous clinical experience that strongly supports the view that opioid drugs should be considered the mainstay therapeutic approach to this problem. This experience suggests that opioids can provide adequate pain control for more than three-quarters of these patients (40–51,64–66). Although a history of substance abuse influences the approach to opioid therapy, the general approach to cancer pain is similar to the management of cancer pain in the population without this history (Table 55.3).

Although the need for opioid therapy in patients with cancer pain and a history of substance abuse is widely accepted, the practical management of these patients generates profound concerns about the potential for inappropriate use of prescribed drugs or concurrent abuse of illicit drugs. These concerns highlight the conflict between the

TABLE 55.3. *Guidelines for the management of chronic cancer pain in the known or suspected opioid addict*

1. Perform a comprehensive assessment that includes detailed evaluation of current and past drug use. Obtain all medical records. As needed, contact other health care providers, family, and pharmacies to assess drug-taking behavior; use urine drug screening to identify misuse or abuse.
2. Distinguish among the patient with a remote history of drug abuse, the patient receiving maintenance therapy, and the patient who is actively abusing drugs, and use this information to clarify the nature of the treatment team, the likely issues that will arise during therapy, the system for monitoring drug use, and the type of education that will be needed by patient and staff.
3. Consider the use of primary therapy directed at the underlying structural cause of the pain (e.g., radiotherapy).
4. Select and administer an appropriate pharmacologic approach using standard guidelines for cancer pain management (*see text*).
5. Create requirements for continued drug administration that provide a degree of control and monitoring appropriate to the history and recent behaviors of the patient. Frequent visits, written contracts with little flexibility, and repeated drug screens may be appropriate for the actively abusing patient and very inappropriate for other patients. Adjust requirements over time as experience is gained with the patient. Maintain contact with drug-abuse treatment program or maintenance program if patient continues with this therapy.
6. Consider adjunctive approaches, including those that are anesthetic, neurosurgical, physiatric, psychological, and neurostimulatory.
7. If drug-abuse behaviors occur, require appropriate change in behavior and initiate new controls as needed.
8. Provide early consultation to psychiatric and substance abuse services, or to pain service (if available).

clinician's humane desire to provide an opioid at whatever quantity is necessary for pain relief and the fear that this therapy is ill-advised and legally suspect when it appears to feed only the addiction. In these cases, compassionate care must be balanced by recognition of the special needs and requirements of treating pain in the substance abuser.

The complexity of these issues underscores the need for a comprehensive assessment as a first step in the management of pain patients with a history of substance abuse. Ironically, it often appears that a history of substance abuse tempers enthusiasm for such an evaluation, particularly in patients who are actively abusing drugs or who have striking psychological disturbances. This inclination to perform a limited evaluation cannot be condoned. A history of substance abuse also may encourage misdiagnosis should the assessment fail to identify a structural lesion capable of explaining the pain. An actual or suspected substance abuse history may increase the tendency to ascribe the pain in this setting to psychological factors, including needs related to an addiction or substance abuse history, even in the absence of any positive evidence for these factors. The risks of misdiagnosis in the setting of medical illness include compromise of the therapeutic alliance during a progressive illness, selection of less effective therapies, and inappropriate refusal to assess the patient further. The clinician must not prejudge in this setting, but rather critically evaluate all the available information to establish a useful clinical formulation.

Use of Primary Therapy

The first consideration in the management of cancer pain is the feasibility of primary therapy directed against the underlying nociceptive lesion that exists in most of these patients. Radiotherapy to tumors associated with pain can provide relief to more than half the patients treated (67–69). Other primary antineoplastic therapies, including surgical resection of neoplastic lesions (70–72) and chemotherapy (72–75), can also have analgesic consequences, but rarely are attempted for pain palliation alone. Occasional patients may also be candidates for primary therapies that are not antineoplastic. For example, empirical antibiotic therapy has profound analgesic effects in some patients (76). This response, which presumably indicates that occult infection contributes to the pain, suggests that a trial of an antibiotic may be indicated in patients with refractory or progressive pain who are predisposed to the development of local infection.

The importance of primary therapy in the management of cancer pain is affirmed by similar observations in other painful medical illnesses. Indeed, the potential for such quality-of-life outcomes appears to drive research into disease-modifying therapies for many disorders. For example, anti-inflammatory therapies can be profoundly analgesic in a destructive inflammatory disorder, and primary therapies for treatment of the sickling disorder are actively being sought for sickle cell anemia (77,78).

Selecting a Pharmacologic Approach

The pharmacologic management of cancer pain requires expertise in the use of three broad groups of analgesics: nonsteroidal antiinflammatory drugs (NSAIDs), opioid analgesics, and the so-called adjuvant analgesics. The latter are a diverse group of unrelated agents that have other primary indications but may be analgesic in selected circumstances.

The Cancer Pain Relief and Palliative Care Program of the World Health Organization developed an approach

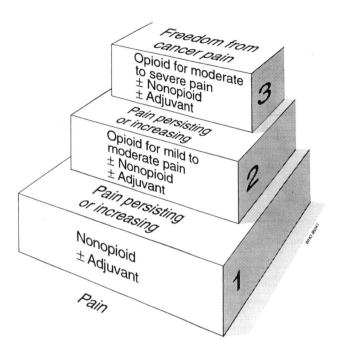

FIG. 55.1. World Health Organization's analgesic ladder approach to the selection of drugs for the management of cancer pain. (Reproduced from World Health Organization. *Cancer pain relief, with a guide to opioid availability*, 2nd ed. Geneva: World Health Organization, 1996, with permission.)

to the selection of these drugs (47). Known as the "analgesic ladder," this approach employs stepwise selection of analgesics based on the usual severity of pain (Fig. 55.1). Patients with mild to moderate pain are first treated with a NSAID. This drug is combined with one or more adjuvant drugs if a specific indication for one exists. These adjuvant drugs include those selected to treat a side effect of the analgesic (e.g., a laxative) and those with analgesic effects (the so-called adjuvant analgesics). Patients who present with moderate to severe pain, or who fail to achieve adequate relief after a trial of a NSAID, are treated with an opioid conventionally used for pain of this severity, which typically is combined with a NSAID and may be coadministered with an adjuvant, if indicated. Patients who present with severe pain or fail to achieve adequate relief following appropriate administration of drugs on the second rung of the analgesic ladder should receive an opioid conventionally selected for severe pain. This treatment may also be combined with a NSAID or an adjuvant drug, as indicated.

The drugs on the second and third rungs of the analgesic ladder were previously termed "weak" and "strong" opioids, respectively. This designation misrepresented the pharmacology and is no longer used. The drugs that are typically used on the second rung of the analgesic ladder are pure agonists and have no ceiling dose, a phenomenon that would justify the weak versus strong dichotomy on pharmacologic grounds. Rather, these drugs are generally used for moderate pain in convenient formulations in which the opioid is combined with a nonopioid analgesic (aspirin or acetaminophen). Upward dose titration is usually limited by the toxicity associated with high doses of the nonopioid coanalgesic. The limited dose range permits the use of these drugs in patients with limited opioid exposure and moderate pain.

Simple guidelines for drug administration applied to the analgesic ladder model yields an approach to the management of cancer pain that has gained widespread acceptance (49–51). Trials of this analgesic approach suggest that a large majority of patients can achieve adequate relief of cancer pain without additional treatments (40–46).

Cancer Pharmacotherapy: Nonsteroidal Antiinflammatory Drugs

The NSAIDs (Table 55.4) and acetaminophen are characterized by a ceiling dose and analgesia that is additive to that of the opioids (79,80). The ceiling dose implies that there is a dose beyond which additional increments in dose fail to yield any further analgesia. Anecdotal data suggest that these agents have particular efficacy in malignant bone pain and relatively little effect in neuropathic pain (81). Thus, NSAIDs may be ineffective because pain is too severe or has a pathogenesis that renders it unresponsive to these drugs.

The NSAIDs comprise an extremely diverse group of drugs (Table 55.4). They all inhibit the enzyme cyclooxygenase (COX) and reduce the synthesis of prostaglandins. Among numerous other functions, prostaglandins sensitize primary afferent nerves that respond to noxious stimuli. Although inhibition of these peripheral processes can explain both the analgesic and anti-inflammatory effects of the NSAIDs, prostaglandin inhibition in the central nervous system probably also contributes to the analgesia produced by these drugs (82). A central mechanism predominates in the analgesia produced by acetaminophen and dipyrone, which have minimal to no peripheral antiinflammatory effects.

TABLE 55.4. *Nonsteroidal antiinflammatory drugs*

Chemical class	Drug	Recommended starting dose (mg/d)	Recommended maximum dose (mg/d)
Nonselective COX Inhibitors			
Salicylates	Aspirin	2,600	6,000
	Diflunisal	1,000 × 1	1,500
	Choline magnesium trisalicylate	1,500 × 1 then 1,000	4,000
	Salsalate	1,500 × 1 then 1,000	4,000
Propionic acids	Ibuprofen	1,600	4,200
	Naproxen	500	1,500
	Naproxen sodium	550	1,375
	Fenoprofen	800	3,200
	Ketoprofen	100	300
	Flurbiprofen	100	300
	Oxaprozin	600	1,800
Acetic acids	Indomethacin	75	200
	Tolmetin	600	2,000
	Sulindac	300	400
	Diclofenac	75	200
	Ketorolac (i.m.)	30 (loading)	60
	Ketorolac (p.o.)	40	40
	Etodolac	600	1,200
Oxicams	Piroxicam	20	40
	Meloxicam	7.5	15
Naphthyl-alkanones	Nabumetone	1,000	2,000
Fenamates	Mefenamic acid	500 × 1	1,000
	Meclofenamic acid	150	400
Pyrazoles	Phenylbutazone	300	400
Selective COX-2 Inhibitors			
	Celecoxib	200	400
	Rofecoxib	12.5–25	25
	Valdecoxib	20	40

*Starting dose should be one-half to two-thirds recommended dose in the elderly, those on multiple drugs, and those with renal insufficiency.

Cyclooxygenase is produced in two isoforms: COX-1 and COX-2. COX-1 is commonly labeled *constitutive* and is involved in physiologic processes, whereas COX-2 is generally termed *inducible* because most is produced as part of the inflammatory cascade. Although the commercially available NSAIDs vary in the extent to which they affect COX-1 and COX-2 (some, such as meloxicam [Mobic], etodolac [Lodine], and nabumetone [Relafen] are relatively COX-2 selective), all are considered to be nonselective COX-1 and COX-2 inhibitors. The inhibition of the COX-1 isoform by these drugs is associated with their gastrointestinal and platelet toxicities.

COX-2 selective inhibitors reduce the gastrointestinal risks associated with NSAID therapy (83,84). They also have no effect on platelet aggregation. These drugs do not have demonstrably lesser renal toxicity than the nonselective COX-1 and COX-2 inhibitors.

The dose–response relationships of the NSAIDs are characterized by a minimal effective dose, dose-dependent analgesic effects, and a ceiling dose for analgesia. The existence of a ceiling dose implies that these drugs have limited maximal efficacy and are usually considered first-line for pains that are mild to moderate in severity. There is large individual variation in the effective dose range and the dose associated with toxicity. Moreover, the maximal efficacy of the NSAIDs varies across drugs in any individual patient. Although an explanation for this phenomenon is lacking, it has important clinical implications. Sequential trials may demonstrate striking differences in effectiveness.

The potential for toxicity during NSAID therapy influences the decision to initiate therapy, the selection of drugs, and the approach to dosing and monitoring. Clinically important adverse gastrointestinal symptoms occur in approximately 10% of patients treated with the nonselective COX-1 and COX-2 NSAIDs, and gastric or duodenal ulcers occur in approximately 2% (85). Nausea and abdominal pain are poor predictors of serious gastrointestinal (GI) toxicity and as many as two-thirds of NSAID users have no symptoms before bleeding or perforation.

The factors that have been associated with an increased risk of ulceration include advanced age, higher NSAID dose, concomitant administration of a corticosteroid, and a history of either ulcer disease or previous GI complications from NSAIDs (85,85a). Heavy alcohol or cigarette consumption may also increase the risk. A role for infection with the bacterium *Helicobacter pylori* in NSAID-related gastropathy has been suggested, but never proved.

There are differences in the potential for gastrointestinal toxicity among the various NSAIDs, but comparative data are very limited. The COX-2 selective drugs have a relatively reduced risk, and several of the nonselective COX-1 and COX-2 inhibitors also carry a lesser risk, in some cases attributable to relatively high COX-2 selectiv-

ity. These include meloxicam, etodolac, nabumetone, diclofenac (Voltaren), the nonacetylated salicylates (choline magnesium trisalicylate and salsalate), ibuprofen, and several other propionic acids. Those with a relatively greater risk include ketorolac (Toradol), piroxicam (Feldene), and the fenamates.

The risk of ulcer can be reduced by concurrent administration of gastroprotective therapy (86). Misoprostol (Cytotec), a prostaglandin analogue, reduces the incidence of NSAID-induced ulcers without reversing anti-inflammatory and analgesic effects. Proton pump inhibitors, such as omeprazole (Prilosec) and lansoprazole (Prevacid), also have established efficacy. Studies of H_2 blockers have been mixed, but a trial of higher dose famotidine (Pepcid) was positive (87). Other interventions, such as antacids and sucralfate (Carafate), may reduce symptoms but do not decrease ulcer risk.

Because normal renal function depends on both constitutive COX-1 and COX-2, all NSAIDs, including the selective COX-2 inhibitors, can cause serious renal toxicity. They must be used cautiously in patients who have nephropathies or who are likely to have subclinical disease as a result of advanced age, prior treatment with nephrotoxic therapy, or an underlying disease.

There is no COX-2 in platelets and the COX-2 inhibitors have no platelet toxicity. Among the nonselective COX-1 and COX-2 drugs, there is large variation in the degree to which platelet function is affected. The safety of the latter drugs in patients predisposed to bleeding has not been established in the clinical setting and all should be used cautiously in patients with a bleeding diathesis.

Given the risk of toxicity, NSAIDs should be used cautiously in patients with renal disease; history of peptic ulceration (or high risk of this complication); and congestive heart failure, or volume overload of any other cause, or hypertension. Acetaminophen is contraindicated in the setting of severe hepatic dysfunction, and this drug should also be used cautiously in patients with renal disease (88).

The selection of an NSAID also should be based on an understanding of differential toxicity, pharmacokinetics, and prior experience with these drugs. Consideration of these factors may improve compliance with therapy or the likelihood of a favorable response. However, it should be recognized that there is great intraindividual variability in the response to different NSAIDs. The practitioner should be familiar with several agents in different subclasses (see Table 55.4) and be prepared to switch from one drug to another if desired effects are not achieved.

The appropriate positioning of the COX-2 selective drugs when NSAID therapy is indicated remains poorly defined. Some experienced clinicians designate these drugs as first-line, and justify this by the potential for cost-benefit based on a reduced risk of serious ulceration. Others consider first-line use of the COX-2 selective drugs for all patients at relatively high risk for GI toxicity, such as the elderly. In the high-risk groups, an alternative strategy is coadministration of a gastroprotective therapy. There are no data by which to judge the relative cost-effectiveness of these approaches.

Pharmacokinetics may also be useful to consider in selecting an NSAID. A patient with demonstrably poor adherence may be more likely to use a drug that has a relatively long half-life and therefore requires once-daily (e.g., rofecoxib [Vioxx], valdecoxib [Bextra], nabumetone, or oxaprozin [Daypro]) or twice-daily (e.g., celecoxib [Celebrex], diclofenac, and etodolac) dosing. Conversely, patients with intermittent pain may prefer to use a short half-life drug that can be effective with "as needed" dosing, such as aspirin, acetaminophen, or ibuprofen.

Although studies of dosing protocols in different patient populations are limited, it is prudent to initiate NSAID therapy with a relatively low starting dose when patients have mild to moderate pain or a relatively increased risk of NSAID toxicity. During therapy, dose escalation can be considered if pain is uncontrolled, side effects are not intolerable, and the conventional maximal dose has not yet been reached. Dose escalation will not yield increased effects if the patient is at the ceiling dose. If a ceiling dose or conventional maximal dose is reached without achieving satisfactory analgesia, an alternative NSAID trial should be considered. Long-term NSAID therapy should be monitored for adverse effects. This monitoring might include periodic testing for occult fecal blood and an evaluation of hemoglobin, renal function, and hepatic function. Patients who are predisposed to adverse effects and those who are receiving relatively high doses should be monitored relatively more frequently.

Cancer Pharmacotherapy: Opioid Analgesics

Opioid analgesics are needed in a large majority of patients with cancer pain. Guidelines for the selection and administration of these drugs derive from knowledge of opioid pharmacology and clinical experience (4,14,47–51). Some of the key principles follow.

Select an Appropriate Drug

Several factors should be considered in the decision to use one opioid drug rather than another. First is the distinction between the pure agonist subclass and the agonist–antagonist subclass (Table 55.5). The pure agonist opioids bind to one or more of the opioid receptors and demonstrate no antagonist activity. Morphine is the prototypic drug in this class, but numerous others are available in the United States, including hydromorphone (Dilaudid), oxycodone (OxyContin), levorphanol, and methadone. The agonist-antagonist opioids comprise two subtypes, a mixed agonist–antagonist type (e.g., pentazocine [Talwin], nalbuphine [Nubain], butorphanol [Stadol], and dezocine) and a partial agonist type (e.g., buprenorphine [Buprenex, Suboxone, Subutex]). Al-

though these two subclasses can be distinguished by differences in specific receptor interactions, all are characterized by potential antagonism of one or more opioid receptors, a ceiling effect for analgesia, and the capacity to reverse favorable effects and precipitate an abstinence syndrome in patients who are physically dependent on pure agonist opioids (89,90). Some also have an incidence of psychotomimetic effects substantially greater than that of the agonist drugs. Together, these properties indicate that the agonist–antagonist opioids are not generally useful in the management of chronic pain, including cancer pain.

The agonist–antagonist opioids do appear to have less abuse potential than the pure agonist drugs. Although this characteristic could potentially be important in a population with a prior or current history of substance abuse, it is generally regarded to be an insignificant benefit in cancer patients without a history of substance abuse, who only rarely develop addiction or abuse de novo during medical therapy with an opioid. Among those with a history of substance abuse, the risk of aberrant drug-taking behavior during medical therapy may be greater, and it is possible that the use of agonist–antagonists in this population may present some advantages. There are no data to support this view, however, and most pain specialists employ pure agonist drugs even in those with a history of substance abuse. Should the clinician choose an agonist–antagonist drug, it must be used early, before physical dependence on a pure agonist drug has developed or there is a need for effects greater than those associated with the ceiling dose of these agents. An agonist–antagonist drug should not be administered to a patient with a history of substance abuse who may be physically dependent on opioids before pain treatment is begun, including those receiving methadone maintenance and those actively abusing opioids.

A second consideration in the selection of an opioid drug relates to the distinction between "weak" versus "strong" opioids, which has been incorporated into the "analgesic ladder." As noted previously, this designation is fundamentally operational rather than pharmacologic. "Weak" opioids are those that are conventionally used orally for moderate pain, whereas the so-called strong opioids are conventionally selected for severe pain. In the United States, the "weak" opioids include codeine and oxycodone (administered with acetaminophen or aspirin in a combination product), hydrocodone and dihydrocodeine (only available with acetaminophen in a combination product), propoxyphene (Darvon) (either alone or in combination products) and tramadol. Other drugs, such as oral pentazocine and meperidine (Demerol), are also occasionally employed in this setting.

The most common approach to the second "rung" of the analgesic ladder in the United States involves the administration of a combination product containing acetaminophen or aspirin plus either codeine or oxycodone. The dose of this drug is increased as needed until the maximum safe dose of the aspirin or acetaminophen is reached, usually 4 g (sometimes as high as 6 g) per day. Should pain persist, the patient is usually then switched to one of the so-called strong opioids.

The pure agonist drugs available in the United States that are customarily employed at the third "rung" of the analgesic ladder include morphine, hydromorphone, oxycodone (when not combined with a coanalgesic), levorphanol, and methadone. Fentanyl is available in a formulation for transdermal administration (Duragesic), and oxymorphone (Numorphan) is available in a rectal formulation. In the past, morphine was considered the preferred drug, based on extensive clinical experience, relative ease of oral titration, and availability of numerous formulations, including controlled release form that allow dosing at 12-hour or 24-hour intervals (91).

Although morphine was generally used as the first-line drug, it is essential to recognize that individual differences in the response to different opioids are great, and a patient may find treatment with another to be more salutary (92). Furthermore, morphine may not be the best choice in some patients. Recent studies have established the existence of an active metabolite of morphine, morphine 6-glucuronide, that accumulates in patients with renal insufficiency and has been associated with toxicity in some renally impaired patients (93–98). A survey of cancer patients suggests that the impact of the metabolite overall is insufficient to recommend a change in routine dosing guidelines (99); nonetheless, occasional patients who develop morphine toxicity in the setting of renal insufficiency should be offered a trial of an alternative opioid, such as hydromorphone or fentanyl, in the hope that lesser metabolite accumulation may contribute to a better response.

The selection of a pure agonist drug as an alternative to morphine is largely empiric, but some guidelines can be proffered based on the pharmacology of these agents. For example, meperidine appears to have substantially greater toxicity than the others and is not preferred in cancer pain management. This toxicity relates to the appearance of a metabolite, normeperidine, which may produce dysphoria, tremulousness, hyperreflexia, and seizures (100).

Some caution is also appropriate in the use of the two drugs currently available in the United States that have considerably longer half-lives than other opioids, namely levorphanol and methadone. Because four or five half-lives must pass before steady state is approached after dosing is begun or altered, use of these drugs is associated with a relatively long period following each dose adjustment during which close monitoring is required to avoid unanticipated delayed toxicity. This need for monitoring is most critical in patients predisposed to opioid side effects, including those with advanced age or major organ failure (encephalopathy or disturbances in pulmonary, hepatic, or renal function). Clinically, most problems appear to develop with methadone, which has a highly variable half-life that ranges from less than 24 hours in some patients to more than 150 hours in others (101). These observa-

tions suggest that levorphanol and methadone should be considered second-line drugs for those who are difficult to monitor (e.g., noncompliant patients or those who live alone or at a distance) and those predisposed to opioid side effects.

Notwithstanding this need for careful monitoring, methadone has become increasingly used by pain specialists. It is relatively inexpensive, has no active metabolites, and there is a large and favorable clinical experience in varied populations with pain. Most important, methadone appears to be far more potent than indicated on standard equianalgesic tables (see Table 55.5) when it is used to substitute for another pure μ agonist drug (101b,101c). This unanticipated potency is believed to be related to the d-isomer, which represents 50% of the commercially available racemic mixture in the United States. This isomer blocks the N-methyl-D-aspartate receptor and, as a result, may yield independent analgesic effects and partially reverse opioid tolerance (101d). To accommodate the potential for increased potency, a switch to methadone from another opioid is most safely accomplished by reducing the calculated equianalgesic dose by 75% to 90%.

Confusion about the role of methadone therapy in cancer pain management is often exaggerated in the patient with a history of substance abuse. In contrast to the once-daily administration that is adequate in the treatment of addiction, the use of methadone as an analgesic typically requires multiple doses per day (102). Although occasional patients can maintain continuous analgesic effects with twice-daily dosing, clinical experience indicates that most require doses four times daily, and a few need a dosing interval of only 4 hours. Furthermore, the use of methadone as an analgesic necessitates dose titration based on the report of pain. Thus, patients receiving methadone maintenance who develop cancer pain can be given methadone for pain, but both dose and dosing interval must be adjusted to the new indication, using the guidelines described later.

Select the Route of Administration

The oral route is preferred for chronic opioid therapy because of its simplicity, economy, and acceptability. A substantial proportion of patients, however, will require an alternative route at some point during the course of the disease (65). A large number of alternative routes are available (Table 55.6), of which the transdermal (103–105), the subcutaneous (by chronic infusion using an ambulatory pump) (106,107), and intraspinal (epidural and intrathecal) (108–111) represent the most important recent advances. Other routes, including intravenous (112) and rectal (113), are also used commonly. New routes continue in development, including transbronchial and transdermal iontophoresis, and will offer further options for therapy.

TABLE 55.5. *Opioid analgesics*

	Equianalgesic doses[a]	Half-life (h)	Peak effect (h)	Duration (h)	Toxicity	Comments
Morphine-like Agonists						
Morphine	10 i.m. 20–60 p.o.[b]	2–3 2–3	0.5–1 1.5–2	3–6 4–7	Constipation, nausea, sedation most common; respiratory depression rare in cancer patients	Standard comparison for opioids; multiple routes available
Controlled-release morphine	20–60 p.o.[b]	2–3	3–4	8–12		
Sustained-release morphine	20–60 p.o.[b]	2–3	4–6	24		Once-a-day morphine recently approved in the U.S.
Hydromorphone	1.5 i.m. 7.5 p.o.	2–3 2–3	0.5–1 1–2	3–4 3–4	Same as morphine	Used for multiple routes
Oxycodone	20–30 p.o.	2–3	1	3–6	Same as morphine	Combined with aspirin or acetaminophen, for moderate pain; available orally without coanalgesic for severe pain
Controlled-release oxycodone	20–30 p.o.	2–3	3–4	8–12		
Fentanyl	—	—	—	48–72 (Transdermal)	Same as morphine	Transdermal formulation commonly used to treat chronic pain; possibly less constipation than oral morphine; not widely abused by those with a history of substance abuse. No oral formulation
Oxymorphone	1 i.m. 10 p.r.	— —	0.5–1 1.5–3	3–6 4–6	Same as morphine	
Meperidine	75 i.m. 300 p.o.	2–3 2–3	0.5–1 1–2	3–4 3–6	Same as morphine + central nervous system (CNS) excitation; contraindicated in those on monoamine oxidase (MAO) inhibitors	Not preferred for cancer pain because of potential toxicity
Heroin	5 i.m.	0.5	0.5–1	4–5	Same as morphine	Analgesic action because of metabolites, predominantly morphine; not available in U.S.
Levorphanol	2 i.m. 4 p.o.	12–15	0.5–1	3–6	Same as morphine	With long half-life, accumulation occurs after beginning or increasing dose
Methadone	10 i.m. 20 p.o.	12–>150	0.5–1.5	4–8	Same as morphine	Risk of delayed toxicity as a result of accumulation; useful to start dosing on p.r.n. basis, with close monitoring
Codeine	130 i.m. 200 p.o.	2–3	1.5–2	3–6	Same as morphine	Usually combined with nonopioid
Propoxyphene	—	12	1.5–2	3–6	Same as morphine plus seizures	Toxic metabolite accumulates HCl with overdose but not significant at doses used clinically; often combined with nonopioid

876

Drug	Dose				Pharmacology	Comments
Propoxyphene hydrochloride	—	12	1.5–2	3–6	Same as hydrochloride	Same as napsylate
Hydrocodone	—	2–4	0.5–1	3–4	Same as morphine	Only available combined with acetaminophen
Dihydrocodeine	—	2–4	0.5–1	3–4	Same as morphine	Only available combined with acetaminophen or aspirin
Partial Agonists						
Buprenorphine	0.4 i.m.	2–5	0.5–1	4–6	Same as morphine, except less risk of respiratory depression	Can produce withdrawal in opioid-dependent patients; has ceiling for analgesia; sublingual tablet not available in U.S.
	0.8 s.l.		2–3	5–6		
Mixed Agonist–Antagonists						
Pentazocine	60 i.m.	2–3	0.5–1	3–6	Same profile of effects as buprenorphine, except for greater risk of psychotomimetic effects	Produces withdrawal in opioid-dependent patients; oral formulation combined with naloxone or nonopioid in the U.S.; ceiling doses and side-effect profile limit role in cancer pain
	180 p.o.	2–3	1–2	3–6		
Nalbuphine	10 i.m.	4–6	0.5–1	3–6	Same as buprenorphine, except for greater risk of psychotomimetic effects, which is lower than that of pentazocine	Produces withdrawal in opioid-dependent patients; no oral formulation; not preferred for cancer pain therapy
Butorphanol	2 i.m.	2–3	0.5–1	3–4	Same profile of effects as nalbuphine	Produces withdrawal in opioid-dependent patients; no oral formulation; not preferred for cancer pain therapy
Dezocine	10 i.m.[c]	1.2–7.4	0.5–1	3–4	Same profile of effects as nalbuphine, but purported to have fewer psychotomimetic effects	Produces withdrawal in opioid-dependent patients; no oral formulation; not preferred for cancer pain therapy

[a]Dose that provides analgesia equivalent to 10 mg i.m. morphine. These ratios are useful guides when switching drugs or routes of administration. When switching drugs, reduce the equianalgesic dose of the new drug by 25% to 50% to account for incomplete cross-tolerance. The only exception to this is methadone, which appears to manifest a greater degree of incomplete cross-tolerance than other opioids; when switching to methadone, reduce the equianalgesic dose by 90%.

[b]Extensive survey data suggest that the relative potency of i.m.:p.o. morphine of 1:6 changes to 1:2–3 with chronic dosing.

[c]Approximate equianalgesic dose suggested from meta-analysis of available comparative studies.

TABLE 55.6. *Routes of administration*

Route	Comment
Oral	Preferred in cancer pain management.
Buccal	Supporting data meager, and the method is generally impracticable.
Sublingual	Available for buprenorphine (indicated for maintenance therapy but may be used off-label for pain). Efficacy of morphine controversial. No clinical studies of other drugs.
Rectal	Available for morphine, oxymorphone, and hydromorphone. Although few studies available, customarily used as if dose is equianalgesic to oral dose. Absorption is variable, however, and relative potency may be higher than expected depending on the degree of nonportal absorption.
Transdermal	Available for fentanyl citrate, with patches delivering 25, 50, 75, and 100 μg/h. Can provide analgesia for 2–3-day period per dose and is indicated for patients who are unable to use oral drug, who are noncompliant with repetitive dosing, or who have failed other opioids and could potentially benefit from a trial of fentanyl. Although not confirmed empirically, a quality-of-life advantage over oral dosing is experienced by some patients.
Intranasal	Available for butorphanol, a mixed agonist–antagonist not preferred for chronic pain management.
Oral transmucosal	Formulation using fentanyl currently available for breakthrough pain.

Subcutaneous
  Repetitive bolus
  Continuous infusion with PCA
	Ambulatory infusion pumps can provide continuous infusion with any parenteral opioid formulation. More advanced continuous infusion pumps can also provide patient-controlled analgesia (PCA). Clearest indication is inability to tolerate oral route.

Intravenous
  Repetitive bolus
  Continuous infusion
  Continuous infusion with PCA
	Continuous infusion possible if permanent venous access device available.

Epidural
  Repetitive bolus
  Continuous infusion
  Continuous infusion using percutaneous or implanted system
	Clearest indication is pain in lower half of body and dose-limiting side effects from systemic opioid. Often coadministered with local anesthetic.

Intrathecal	Usually administered via a totally implanted infusion pump. May be cost-effective for those patients with a clear indication for intraspinal therapy and a long life expectancy.
Intracerebroventricular	Rarely indicated. Experience is limited.

Apply Appropriate Dosing Guidelines

The successful treatment of cancer pain derives less from the selection of the drug and route than from the clinical protocols used in initiating and altering the dose (4,13,14,47,49,51). Specific dosing guidelines can be summarized as follows:

Dose "By the Clock"

Because it is generally agreed that it is more effective to prevent the recurrence of severe pain than abort it once it appears, "by-the-clock" dosing has replaced "as-needed" dosing in the treatment of continuous or frequently recurring pain using opioid drugs. "As-needed" dosing still plays a role, however, and should be considered in the nontolerant patient during the initiation of therapy (given the risk of gradual accumulation, methadone is often started with 1 to 2 weeks of "as-needed" dosing), in the patient with rapidly changing pain (such as may follow radiotherapy to a painful bony lesion), and in patients with intermittent pains separated by pain-free intervals. Additionally, clinical experience strongly supports the use of an "as-needed" dose (so-called rescue dose) in combination with a fixed dosing schedule to treat "breakthrough" pains (57).

Titrate the Dose

Once an opioid and route of administration are selected, the dose should be increased until adequate analgesia occurs or intolerable and unmanageable side effects supervene. There is no ceiling effect to the analgesia provided by the pure agonist opioid drugs and the maximal dose is immaterial as long as the patient attains a favorable balance between analgesia and side effects. This implies that the opioid responsiveness of a specific pain can only by ascertained by dose escalation to limiting side effects. In clinical practice, the range of opioid doses required by patients is enormous. Doses equivalent to more than 35 g morphine per day have been reported in highly tolerant patients with refractory cancer pain (65).

Although doses typically stabilize for prolonged periods during long-term management, dose escalation is usually required at intervals to maintain analgesia. In the patient with pain as a consequence of medical illness, the need for a dose increase usually can be explained by some change in clinical status, typically worsening of a pain-producing structural lesion. The changing opioid requirement underscores the need for repeated assessment and dose adjustment, which is intended to identify a dose that provides adequate analgesia or establish that pain cannot be satisfactorily controlled because of intolerable and unmanageable side effects. Given the inherently subjective nature of the critical endpoints "adequate analgesia" and "intolerable side effects," careful patient assessment is essential.

Use Appropriate Dosing Intervals

With the exception of controlled-release morphine preparations (administered every 8 to 12 hours), sustained-release oral morphine formulations (administered every 24 hours), transdermal fentanyl system (administered every 48 to 72 hours), and methadone (usually, but not always, effective with dosing every 6 to 8 hours), all other pure agonist opioid drugs must be administered every 3 to 4 hours to provide continuous analgesia.

Be Aware of Relative Potencies

Using morphine as a standard, relative potencies have been determined for most pure agonist drugs in single-dose analgesic assays (114) (see Table 55.5). Relative potency tables (also known as equianalgesic dose tables) should be consulted when switching from one drug or route of administration to another (114a). These estimates should be viewed as broad guidelines, the use of which must be tempered by clinical judgment. A switch from one drug to another should be accompanied by a reduction in the equianalgesic dose of at least one-third, in recognition that incomplete cross-tolerance between opioids may result in a potency greater than anticipated for the newly initiated drug. The equianalgesic dose should be further reduced (up to 90%) when patients are predisposed to opioid side effects (e.g., those with encephalopathy) and when the new drug is methadone. For reasons that are not yet known, the degree of incomplete cross-tolerance is greater when a switch is made to methadone than to other opioids. In the case of morphine, there is evidence that the oral:intramuscular relative potency with chronic administration is 2 to 3:1, rather than the 6:1 ratio suggested by controlled single-dose studies.

Treat Side Effects

Treatment of opioid-induced side effects is an integral part of cancer pain management (115). Successful amelioration of symptoms both enhances patients' comfort and allows continued upward dose titration of the opioid drug. Although respiratory depression fosters the greatest concern, tolerance to this adverse effect develops quickly and it is rarely a problem in the management of cancer pain. Unquestionably, the most common and persistent side effect is constipation (116). Although less prevalent, sedation often limits dose escalation. Recent experience suggests that a relatively small dose of a psychostimulant, such as methylphenidate, dextroamphetamine, or modafinil, can reverse this effect as well as potentially provide coanalgesic effects (117). Nausea is common but usually can be managed with one or another of a large number of drugs with antiemetic effects. If nausea occurs, it is often wise to administer an antiemetic on an around-the-clock basis for several weeks, because this may markedly reduce this adverse experience during the time required for the patient to develop tolerance to the effect. Psychotomimetic effects, when marked, usually require a switch to a different opioid drug, although some patients improve with the addition of a neuroleptic, such as haloperidol. Other side effects, such as itch, dry mouth, and urinary retention, rarely are a problem, although occasional patients will require other treatments as a result of these effects. In all cases, unmanageable side effects necessitate a trial of an alternative analgesic approach. One such approach is a trial of an alternative opioid, because the pattern of side effects produced by one drug does not reliably predict the response to another (92,118).

Cancer Pharmacotherapy: Adjuvant Analgesics

Adjuvant analgesics are drugs that have primary indications other than pain but can be analgesic in selected circumstances. This category is extremely diverse, representing numerous drugs in many classes (60) (Table 55.7). These drugs are now used commonly in the treatment of many malignant and nonmalignant pain syndromes. When used in the management of cancer pain, they are typically added to an optimally titrated opioid regimen. Some, such as the tricyclic antidepressants, are used as primary analgesics for specific nonmalignant pain syndromes.

Some adjuvant analgesics are particularly important in patients with cancer pain. Corticosteroids, for example, are used for bone pain, neuropathic pain, headache caused by intracranial hypertension, pain related to bowel

TABLE 55.7. *Adjuvant analgesics*

	Drug class	Examples
Multipurpose analgesics	Antidepressants	
	Tricyclic antidepressants	Amitriptyline, doxepin, imipramine, nortriptyline, desipramine
	"Newer" antidepressants	Trazodone, maprotiline, fluoxetine, paroxetine, buproprion
	α_2-Adrenergic agonists	Clonidine, tizanidine
	Corticosteroids	Prednisone, dexamethasone
Drugs used for neuropathic pain	Anticonvulsants	Carbamazepine, phenytoin, valproate, clonazepam, gabapentin, lamotrigine, oxcarbazepine, zonisamide, topiramate
	Oral local anesthetics	Mexiletine, tocainide
	N-methyl-D-aspartate blockers	Dextromethorphan, ketamine, amantadine
	Sympatholytic drugs	Prazosin, phenoxybenzamine, phentolamine, β blockers
	Topical agents	Local anesthetic, capsaicin, NSAIDs
	Miscellaneous	Baclofen, calcitonin
Drugs used for musculoskeletal pain	"Muscle relaxants"	Orphenadrine, carisoprodol, methocarbamol, chlorzoxazone, cyclobenzaprine, metaxalone
	Benzodiazepine	Diazepam
Drugs used for other types of cancer pain	Drugs for bone pain	Calcitonin, bisphosphonates, strontium-89, samarium-153
	Drugs for bowel obstruction	Scopolamine, octreotide
Drugs used for headache	β Blockers	Propranolol, nadolol
	Calcium channel blockers	Verapamil, nifedipine

obstruction, and other indications (119–121). Dexamethasone is the steroid most often selected, but there have been no comparative trials among the different agents, and, as yet, the best drug and dosing regimen remain uncertain and the durability of effects is unknown. The chronic administration of these agents usually is reserved for those with far-advanced disease.

The largest number of adjuvant analgesics is used in the setting of neuropathic pain (Table 55.7). These syndromes are believed to be relatively less responsive to opioid drugs than pain syndromes sustained by persistent injury to pain-sensitive tissues (nociceptive pain) (122). Antidepressants, anticonvulsants, oral local anesthetics, and others are commonly administered to patients who continue to experience inadequate analgesia despite opioid dose titration (60).

Other Analgesic Approaches in Cancer Pain Management

The use of an adjuvant analgesic may be conceptualized as one alternative among many for the management of patients who fail to achieve a favorable balance between analgesia and side effects during opioid dose titration (Table 55.8). A switch to an alternative opioid is another technique that has recently gained wide acceptance. Still other approaches use nonpharmacologic interventions to reduce or even eliminate the opioid requirement.

Neurostimulatory approaches, most commonly transcutaneous electrical nerve stimulation, typically are implemented in patients with refractory neuropathic pains and those with more acute, transient pains. Experience is limited in cancer patients. The anecdotal impression is that many patients respond initially, but long-term benefit is rarely achieved with this technology. Other types of neurostimulatory approaches include counterirritation (brisk rubbing of the painful part), acupuncture, percutaneous electrical nerve stimulation, dorsal column stimulation, and deep brain stimulation. Although the invasive approaches have been applied in cancer pain (123), the noninvasive techniques are preferred.

The analgesic potential of physiatric techniques is poorly appreciated. Patients with painful musculoskeletal complications of cancer may benefit from physical or occupational therapy, and the use of orthoses or prostheses may have analgesic consequences in other situations. For example, a surgical corset may benefit patients with back pain on movement caused by neoplastic infiltration of the spine.

Anesthetic approaches include the use of nitrous oxide for pain in far-advanced disease (124), myofascial trigger

TABLE 55.8. *Alternative analgesic approaches for cancer patients who fail a conventional oral opioid therapy*

Approach	Therapeutic options	Examples
Pharmacologic techniques to reduce systemic opioid requirement	Use of adjuvant analgesics	See text
	Use of spinal opioids	—
Identifying an opioid with a more favorable balance between analgesia and side effects	Sequential opioid trials	—
Improving the tolerability of the opioid	Better side-effect management	Stimulant drug for opioid-induced sedation
Nonpharmacologic techniques to reduce systemic opioid requirement	Anesthetic approaches	Nerve blocks
	Surgical approaches	Cordotomy
	Rehabilitative approaches	Bracing
	Psychological approaches	

point injection, and a large variety of nerve block procedures that employ either local anesthetics or neurolytic solutions (125–127). The technique of continuous epidural local anesthetic is a recent innovation capable of providing a long-standing neural blockade without inflicting permanent damage on nerves (128). With the exception of trigger point injections, the implementation of anesthetic procedures should be undertaken only by trained personnel.

Similar to the neurolytic anesthetic procedures, surgical neuroablative procedures are designed to isolate the painful part from the central nervous system (127, 129–131). The most widely used procedure, cordotomy, usually can be performed percutaneously in the awake patient. In selected patients, this technique has an extremely high likelihood of success and a low risk of complications. Surgical approaches should be undertaken only by those trained in the assessment and treatment of pain.

Psychological approaches are underused in cancer pain management. There is a strong association between mood disturbance and persistent pain (132), and all patients with cancer pain benefit from the support provided by a concerned and experienced staff. Those with evidence of psychiatric disorders should be appropriately referred and treated (133–135). Some patients may benefit from specific cognitive approaches that have been found useful to reduce pain intensity, including relaxation training, distraction, hypnosis, and others (134,136–141). Behavioral approaches are occasionally useful to optimize function and thereby improve quality of life.

Other Considerations in the Substance Abuser with Cancer Pain

Although the basic approach to the management of cancer pain should apply equally to all patients, including substance abusers, it is nonetheless true that problems may be encountered in the latter population that distinguish it from others. As noted previously, clinical experience sug-

gests that there may be salient differences among those with remote history of addiction, those currently treated in maintenance programs, and those actively abusing opioids or other drugs. A small retrospective study (142) suggested that all three groups were at relatively high risk for inadequate pain management, but only those who were actively abusing could not reliably achieve adequate symptom control once they were treated aggressively by pain service personnel. The major issues encountered during the treatment of each of these groups can be summarized as in the following sections.

Patients with a Remote History of Substance Abuse

Although clinical experience suggests that patients with a remote history of substance abuse respond appropriately to opioids, the empirical data in support of this conclusion are meager. From a theoretical perspective, it could be speculated that the same genetic, psychological, and situational factors that predisposed to the addiction syndrome initially could increase the risk of aberrant drug-taking behavior in patients administered opioids for therapeutic purposes. The failure to observe these outcomes in practice suggests that the factors that ultimately combined to eliminate the abuse behaviors, combined with the situational changes associated with the diagnosis and treatment of the cancer, may reduce the likelihood of iatrogenic addiction.

It has been observed clinically that some cancer patients with a remote history of substance abuse are poorly compliant with opioid therapy due to a persistent fear of these drugs. Like the staff surrounding them, these patients fear loss of control over drug use (37). An example of such a patient is depicted in Figure 55.2, which demonstrates the opioid use of a 47-year-old man with severe bone pain from metastatic lung cancer and a history of polysubstance abuse that ended more than 17 years ago. While home, he experienced unrelieved pain and was advised repeatedly by pain service personnel to escalate the dose of his opioid. He refused to do so. Ironically, his opioid doses increased

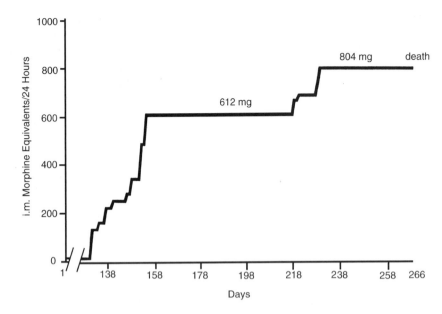

FIG. 55.2. Opioid requirements in a 47-year-old man with a remote history of drug abuse who developed severe pain as a consequence of progressive lung cancer. Fear of readdiction caused the patient to resist escalation of opioid doses. While at home, he continued on stable doses, despite unrelieved pain and the wishes of his physicians that he continue upward dose titration; doses were increased only after he was admitted to the hospital. (Reproduced from Gonzales GR, Coyle N. Treatment of cancer pain in a former opioid abuser: fears of the patient and staff and their influence on care. *J Pain Symptom Manage* 1992;7(4):246–249, with permission.)

rapidly in the hospital, where medical staff insisted on the use of higher doses to treat severe unrelieved pain.

Thus, the optimal management of the patient with cancer pain and remote history of addiction must incorporate careful, ongoing assessment of drug-taking behavior and the recognition that successful treatment may be compromised both by the attitudes of practitioners, whose overconcern about addiction can distort analgesic management, and the attitudes of the patient, whose behavior may implicitly or explicitly endorse the concerns of the staff or result directly in undertreatment. Education of the staff and the patient may limit the adverse consequence of these attitudes and thereby improve pain management.

Patients in Methadone-Maintenance Programs

Like those who have a remote history of substance abuse, patients receiving opioid maintenance are at high risk for undertreatment of cancer pain. In this population, negative attitudes held by the medical staff may combine with some degree of tolerance to opioid analgesics to limit the efficacy of therapy. If persistent pain reports are interpreted as a manipulative attempt to obtain opioids for purposes other than analgesia, the therapeutic relationship becomes conflicted and the clinician's goals for analgesia is superseded by the desire to prevent drug abuse. This concern is, of course, legitimate if the patient does develop a return of aberrant drug-taking behaviors. If "drug seeking" reflects only the need for pain relief, however, undertreatment will result from the failure to respond.

It may also be speculated that patient non-adherence also can undermine therapy in this population. Like those with a remote history of abuse, some of these patients have achieved a measure of personal and social success as a consequence of a stable regimen and may fear a loss of control with the therapeutic use of opioids.

The failure to recognize the need for higher starting doses may lead to initial problems with the management of cancer pain in methadone-treated patients. Patients who have not received an opioid for pain before, but have been receiving methadone for some time, may require starting doses substantially higher than those conventionally used at the initiation of cancer pain therapy. In a rather typical scenario, a patient administered an opioid at a dose perceived by the clinician to be effective gains no relief and voices a complaint; the persistence of pain, perhaps now combined with a sense of mistrust or acrimony, is interpreted as evidence of addiction, and the patient is managed by the further withholding of opioids, rather than by aggressive upward dose titration. This, of course, further undermines the therapeutic alliance and reduces the likelihood of successful treatment.

Although the foregoing scenario has been observed anecdotally, it must be stated that there are no data that confirm this effect of methadone treatment on the efficacy of conventional opioid doses at the start of therapy. Indeed, a retrospective study that compared a control group with 25 hospitalized methadone-maintenance patients who required opioids for the management of acute nonmalignant pain suggested that "standard" doses of opioids could be used to treat these patients and that the administration of therapeutic opioids for a brief period did not induce a need for a higher methadone dose subsequently (143). Although the finding that routine doses of opioids were effective for acute pain in this population supported the results of an earlier survey (144), neither of these studies directly assessed pain relief, and consequently, neither they nor any other studies have adequately evaluated the role of tolerance in the clinical setting.

It is a common misconception that the use of methadone as an analgesic for pain can mirror its use in the therapy of opioid addiction. In pain management, doses must be titrated according to patient response; there is no predefined appropriate dose range. Equally important, the single daily dose that is sufficient for the management of addiction is almost never adequate to sustain analgesia throughout the day. Extensive clinical experience indicates that analgesia usually requires at least three doses per day (145). Many patients actually achieve more stable analgesia with four or six doses per day, an observation supported by studies that demonstrate a duration of analgesia that is typically much briefer than would be expected from the half-life of this drug (102,146–148).

Active Drug Abusers

The sanguine view of opioid therapy in patients with a remote history of drug abuse and those in opioid maintenance is not applicable to the small number of patients who develop cancer pain while actively abusing opioids or other drugs. Anecdotally, pain management in many of these patients is complicated by substantial psychopathology and adverse situational factors. The degree of psychopathology may be severe enough that a useful therapeutic alliance is impossible, and both the veracity of the complaints and adherence with prescribed therapies become major problems.

Careful assessment is again critical to appropriate management. Clear-cut abuse behaviors, including continued use of illicit drugs, must be distinguished from other behaviors, such as frequent emergency room visits, that may be more difficult to interpret. Although both types of behaviors may reflect inadequacy of pain treatment as well as psychological dependence on the drug, the former is clear-cut abuse, which cannot be condoned, whereas the latter potentially may indicate a lesser degree of psychopathology and a desire to remain in the medical setting for the treatment of a pain problem. The specific psychopathology of these patients must be carefully evaluated. Sociopathy is relatively common among the addict population (149,150), and to the extent possible, the clinician should attempt to determine whether sociopathic behaviors have been characteristic of the patient prior to the diagnosis of cancer. Straightforward questioning about illegal practices may yield surprisingly frank answers, from which an assessment of these behaviors can be made. Although it must be emphasized that the studies needed to clarify these issues have not been performed, it is likely that the risk of management problems during analgesic therapy correlates generally with the degree of psychopathology, and more specifically with the severity of sociopathic proclivities.

In some cases, efforts to implement a simple and effective pharmacologic regimen for pain may have to be sacrificed in lieu of interventions designed to maintain therapeutic control. Virtually all patients require greater frequency of monitoring and strict attention to the assessment of efficacy, side effects, and drug-taking behavior.

Some clinicians favor the use of a written agreement that is kept in the medical record and both defines the medication regimen and explicitly states the responsibilities of both the patient and clinician (150a,150b). These guidelines should include specific reference to the methods that will be used to renew prescriptions and the response that a report of lost or stolen drugs will generate. It may be useful to establish a rule that lost or stolen drugs must be reported to the police and that documentation of this must be provided. The use of drugs with relatively low street value, such as methadone, may be more appropriate when such considerations arise than the use of others, such as hydromorphone, for which there is greater demand among street addicts.

For some patients, the cardinal principle of opioid dose titration simply cannot be accommodated because of demands that are perceived to be inappropriate. Limits must be set based on the clinician's assessment of the risks and benefits in this difficult situation. Likewise, the occurrence of management problems may preclude the use of some techniques commonly employed in cancer pain management, such as long-term continuous subcutaneous infusion. In rare cases, the persistence of severe pain in the setting of intractable management problems suggests the immediate use of some approaches, such as neurolytic techniques, that generally are considered only after an optimal opioid therapy fails.

In all of this decision-making, the dictates of humane and compassionate care should support a bias that patients generally are to be believed. Factitious pain complaints and malingering appear to be rare among patients who are not actively abusing drugs (including those with a remote history of addiction) and probably are uncommon among active abusers who develop cancer. Rather, most substance abusers are like other patients with pain, whose symptoms reflect some combination of ongoing nociception and psychological distress. Unless the evidence in support of malingering is compelling, the clinician is better served by avoiding an argument about the "reality" of the pain and focusing instead on the possibility that pain may be profoundly influenced by psychological factors, possibly including dependence on opioids. It is more productive simply to believe the patient's complaint and thoughtfully assess the degree to which it can be explained by physical and psychological determinants. In keeping with this view, it may be postulated that the premorbid psychopathology of the addict predisposes to a greater psychological contribution to pain than is usually observed in the cancer population. This, too, must be evaluated in future research.

Chronic Nonmalignant Pain

Chronic nonmalignant pain comprises an extremely diverse group of syndromes that vary remarkably in phenomenology, pathogenesis, and impact. Physical and psychological factors contribute to the pain and associated disability in virtually all patients, but the characteristics of these factors and their respective prominence are highly variable, both across syndromes and among patients with the same diagnosis.

Some principles of clinical management apply to all patients with chronic nonmalignant pain. All patients require a comprehensive assessment as the foundation for effective management. This assessment must first determine the potential for primary therapy directed against any treatable organic contribution to the pain. For example, joint replacement may be an effective primary therapy in some patients with chronic pain due to arthritis, and resection of a neuroma may relieve some patients with painful traumatic mononeuropathy. There is no definitive primary therapy for most chronic pain patients, however, and the assessment must also provide the information necessary to develop a multimodality approach to symptomatic therapy that can improve comfort and enhance physical and psychosocial function.

The various analgesic modalities have been discussed previously in the context of cancer pain. The broad approaches can be categorized as pharmacologic, anesthetic, neurostimulatory, physiatric, surgical, and psychological. The number of approaches selected in the management of any patient and the specific therapies within each approach vary according to the needs of the patient. The emphasis can differ markedly among patient types. For example, the chronic pains associated with progressive rheumatoid arthritis or disabling multiple sclerosis require a different set of treatments than do the pains and profound disability that characterize the patient with long-standing low back pain or chronic tension headache. Whereas drug therapy may be very prominent in the former patients, pharmacologic interventions may be minimized in lieu of intensive psychological and physical therapies in the latter.

During the past two decades, a great deal of attention has focused on the development of multidisciplinary pain programs as a system for the delivery of multimodality treatment for chronic pain. These programs were an innovation that evolved from the recognition that the complex problems posed by some patients with chronic pain exceeded the clinical capabilities of any one practitioner (151). Thousands of such programs now exist, and they are widely considered to be the state of the art in the management of patients with intractable pain associated with a high level of disability (152).

Multidisciplinary pain programs best address the needs of a specific subpopulation of pain patients. Although many of the patients referred to these programs have histories that include misuse of prescribed drugs, it is not clear that the structure of these programs is optimal for patients with other patterns of substance abuse, including abuse of illicit drugs, alcoholism, polysubstance abuse, or severe addiction. At the present time, it should not be assumed that the traditional multidisciplinary pain-

management program contains the expertise necessary to manage these clinical problems. Unfortunately, it is similarly doubtful that most substance abuse programs provide optimal management of pain. Further efforts are needed to foster communication between the disciplines of addiction medicine and pain management, and define appropriate therapeutic strategies for those challenging patients who develop both pain and substance abuse. The individual practitioner should acknowledge that these disciplines possess differing insights into the clinical needs of this population and that a treatment team that includes specialists in both areas may be needed in some cases.

Although the chronic pain patients referred to multidisciplinary pain management programs represent an enormous drain on medical and societal resources, they are a small minority of those who experience chronic pain (153–155). Certainly, most patients with cancer pain do not need this approach to obtain symptom relief (156), and it is unlikely that most patients with other types of chronic pain, specifically those whose pain is not strongly determined by psychological factors or complicated by severe disability, would have a substantially different outcome if care were managed by a single knowledgeable practitioner who devised a multimodality therapeutic approach.

The long-term treatment of chronic pain with opioid drugs continues to be controversial. As discussed in the following sections, the conventional rejection of this approach in pain patients with no prior history of substance abuse is gradually evolving to a more balanced perspective. In populations with pain and substance abuse, however, there is neither a large and reassuring clinical experience nor empirical data that confirm the safety and efficacy of opioid therapy. Consequently, clinicians must exercise caution in considering opioid trials in such patients. Treatment guidelines must be clearly established if long-term therapy is undertaken. Generally, the use of opioid therapy for chronic pain should not be initiated if the patient is currently abusing licit or illicit drugs, and this treatment should be offered to those with a remote history of addiction only by experienced clinicians who can provide skilled assessment and management over time.

Acute Pain

Acute pain is, by definition, self-limited (or anticipated to be so) and usually is readily associated with a specific tissue injury, related to trauma, surgery, or a disease process. The management of acute pain in the addict is not a trivial issue, because addicts experience traumatic injuries (157) and a myriad of medical disorders (158) at a disproportionately higher rate than does the general population. There is no reason to believe that the complex physiologic, behavioral, and psychological phenomena that are associated with drug addiction or abuse protect the individual from painful experiences; to the contrary, some have suggested that addicts may have a relatively low tolerance for pain (159).

Pains associated with recent tissue injury may be associated with signs of sympathetic nervous system stimulation, including diaphoresis, pupillary dilation, hypertension, tachycardia, and even nausea. Although the physiologic basis for this sympathetic hyperactivity is not known in humans, animal models of experimental inflammatory arthritis simulating rheumatoid arthritis (160), peripheral nerve injury simulating causalgia (161), and visceral tissue injury (162) have all demonstrated that coactivation of efferent sympathetic fibers occurs with the afferent volley induced by the lesion. Autonomic signs often render the patient's pain complaint more "believable" to the clinician and reassure the physician about the appropriateness of opioid analgesics for the management of the pain.

The interpretation of symptoms and signs in the opioid addict may be difficult, however, and this may contribute to difficulties encountered by these patients in the medical setting. With the knowledge that very diverse symptoms and signs can result either from a direct effect of a drug or from drug withdrawal, clinicians may express doubts about the nature of the pain or about medical comorbidity. For example, the objective physical signs associated with acute pain may also be produced by opioid withdrawal. Even obtundation with visual and auditory hallucinations, which can certainly be caused by opioids or other drugs of abuse, has been reported as a rare consequence of opioid withdrawal (163); this syndrome was speculated to be related to the withdrawal of morphine from non-μ receptors.

Although the management of acute pain in the addict may be difficult for even the most experienced clinician, it is nonetheless possible to develop guidelines that ensure a careful assessment of the acute pain complaint and provide the best chance of achieving satisfactory pain relief in these circumstances (Table 55.9). The guidelines that follow should be considered complementary to those applied to the management of chronic cancer pain.

Define the Pain Syndrome and Provide Primary Treatment

Acute pain almost always has an identifiable etiology, the characterization of which is an essential aspect to the assessment. This may allow specific primary therapy, which can have analgesic consequences. For example, specific orthopedic treatments and surgical débridement may be indicated as the single best method of acute pain relief for traumatic injuries involving fractures or burns, respectively. In the case of acute pain complicating medical disorders such as hemophilia, sickle cell anemia, or cancer, specific therapies directed at the underlying disorder may also be possible. For example, red cell transfusion may be indicated in patients with sickle cell disease as the initial treatment for acute "crisis" pain complicated by infection,

TABLE 55.9. *Guidelines for management of acute pain in the known or suspected opioid addict*

1. Define the pain syndrome and provide treatment for the underlying disorder.
2. Distinguish among the patient with a remote history of drug abuse, the patient receiving methadone maintenance, and the patient who is actively abusing drugs.
3. Apply appropriate pharmacologic principles of opioid use:
   a. Use the appropriate opioid.
   b. Use adequate doses and dosing intervals.
   c. Use appropriate route of administration.
4. Provide concomitant nonopioid therapies when appropriate:
   a. Use nonopioid analgesics.
   b. Use nonpharmacologic therapies.
5. Recognize specific drug abuse behaviors.
6. Avoid excessive negotiations over specific drugs and doses.
7. Provide early consultation to appropriate services:
   a. Psychiatry and substance abuse service.
   b. Pain service (if available).
8. Anticipate problems associated with opioid prescription renewals if outpatient treatment is required.

lung disease, or stroke (164); this approach is combined with symptomatic opioid treatment (138). Other primary disease-modifying approaches for sickle cell anemia are in clinical trials, each of which evaluates pain as one important endpoint (77,78). Regardless of the disorder, the appropriate management of the underlying etiology for the pain often will decrease the opioid requirement.

Distinguish Among Types of Abusers

The management of pain in the patient with a history of opioid abuse may be facilitated by distinguishing addicts who are actively abusing at the time of treatment from those with a remote history of drug abuse and those in receiving opioid maintenance. Although the implications of these distinctions have not been clearly substantiated in prospective clinical studies, it is common practice to apply them in the setting of acute pain management (165,166).

Patients who are actively abusing either licit or illicit opioids, and those on maintenance, may be assumed to have some degree of tolerance, which may be reflected in a need for relatively higher starting doses and shorter dosing intervals than generally are recommended for acute pain in the nonaddicted population. Furthermore, patients who are actively abusing drugs often manifest psychological disorders that can influence pain perception (such as anxiety and depression) and may require intervention.

As discussed previously, patients who are actively abusing drugs present a range of concerns related to difficulties in assessing subjective phenomena and the relatively high likelihood that aberrant drug-related behaviors will occur during opioid therapy for acute pain. Although it can also be postulated that medically ill patients who have abused drugs in the past or who are participating in methadone maintenance programs may be at increased risk of abuse behaviors following treatment for pain, in part related to the stress of the illness, this possibility has not been confirmed clinically and must be evaluated further.

Apply Appropriate Pharmacologic Principles of Opioid Use

The use of opioid agonist–antagonist compounds for the management of acute pain in known or suspected opioid addicts generally is not preferred. These drugs have analgesic ceiling effects and may consequently be ineffective for severe pain, and their antagonist properties may precipitate withdrawal and increase pain in physically dependent patients. As in the treatment of cancer pain, pure agonist opioids usually are administered for the management of acute pain in these patients.

Patients who are actively abusing opioids or who are participating in methadone maintenance may demonstrate a need for higher doses or shorter dosing intervals because of the development of tolerance. Tolerance to opioid analgesics decreases the duration of effective analgesia following a dose (167). For example, morphine, which has an average duration of analgesia of 3 to 4 hours, may produce only 1 to 2 hours of pain relief in a tolerant opioid addict.

Clinical experience in the nonaddict population has suggested that some patients with acute, severe pain require rapid escalation of opioid doses. This may be facilitated by the use of intravenous administration, such as a continuous infusion supplemented by additional bolus doses (168). Patient-controlled analgesia (PCA), in which the patient self-administers an opioid intravenously, is being used with increasing frequency in this setting. PCA provides a means to rapidly titrate the opioid dose without the time delays inherent in physician or nurse administration of the drug (169). In the population without a history of substance abuse, studies indicate that PCA does not lead to excessive self-administration of the opioid. Indeed, even prolonged morphine PCA (for weeks) did not result in overmedication or addiction when administered to cancer patients with acute mucositis pain following bone marrow transplantation (18); in these patients, PCA actually decreased the requirements for morphine by 53% in comparison with standard intravenous infusion (170).

Despite this favorable impression and the lack of empiric data demonstrating different responses among those with and without a history of opioid abuse, many experts believe that the use of PCA in opioid addicts is problematic. Addicts may report a euphoric feeling or "high" that is coincident with an intravenous injection of an opioid,

which presumably reinforces the self-administration of the drug; this phenomenon may increase the risk of aberrant use of the PCA device. Others believe, however, that intravenous opioids, including those administered via PCA, can be used effectively in this population if appropriate guidelines are followed. If PCA is employed, it must be implemented with due regard for the possibility that the patient with a history of abuse may be opioid tolerant. Unless appropriately large bolus doses and/or brief "lockout" periods (i.e., the minimum interval allowed between doses) are selected, the tolerant patient may not receive an effective dose and may experience poor pain relief as a result. This, in turn, may precipitate frequent requests for additional drug doses that can be misinterpreted by the clinician as evidence of addiction, rather than the search for pain relief.

Although methadone is seldom administered for acute pain, it may be reasonable to consider its use in patients maintained on this drug for addiction. The use of methadone for the treatment of acute pain may facilitate the process by which the patient is tapered back to the baseline maintenance dose once the painful episode has been treated. However, this potential advantage must be weighed against several problems. Most methadone-maintenance programs do not have the flexibility to allow increases in the daily methadone dose or dosing frequency. Thus, the treatment of pain with methadone usually must take place outside of the typical maintenance program. Equally important, the clinician must be knowledgeable about the use of methadone as an analgesic and the ways in which this varies from its role in addiction. Oral methadone is about half as potent as parenteral methadone (114), and as discussed previously, there is a large disparity between the plasma half-life of this drug, which ranges from less than a day to many days (101), and the duration of analgesia after a dose. Although one study suggested that the duration of action of methadone was as long as 12 hours in opioid-naive postoperative patients (171), a more recent controlled trial in cancer patients determined that the analgesic duration of both methadone and morphine was about 4 hours (102). The latter estimation is likely to apply to patients who previously have received methadone maintenance, because some degree of opioid tolerance characterizes this group and potentially reduces the duration of analgesic effect.

Provide Concomitant Nonopioid Therapies when Appropriate

Nonopioid analgesics may be highly efficacious in specific acute pain syndromes, and their use may minimize the need for opioids in some situations. For example, a controlled clinical study has demonstrated that the NSAID ketoprofen (Orudis), administered orally, may have significant efficacy in labor and postoperative pain (172). Ketorolac is available as a parenteral formulation in the

United States and can be very effective in the management of acute pain; when this drug is administered in doses ranging from 30 to 90 mg, there is a reported analgesic potency equal to that of 6 to 12 mg morphine or 50 to 100 mg meperidine (147). Recent anecdotal experience with ketorolac in patients with acute pain from sickle cell anemia suggests that it may provide enough analgesia to allow a substantial reduction in morphine doses, thereby improving dose-related constipation and sedation. The advent of other parenteral NSAIDs, including those that are selective inhibitors of cyclooxygenase 2, are likely in the future and may increase the opportunities for NSAID administration in the immediate postoperative setting.

Although NSAIDs that have high analgesic efficacy may be useful even for severe acute pain in some patients, they are most often helpful in combination with opioids when the latter are causing dose-limiting opioid side effects. An NSAID should not be considered an opioid "substitute," and the desire to withhold opioids from suspected or known substance abusers with acute pain should not be viewed as an indication for these drugs.

Other types of nonopioid therapies may be useful in selected cases. For acute focal pain syndromes, regional anesthetic approaches, such as somatic or sympathetic nerve blocks, should be considered. It is well-accepted that anesthetic procedures may be more efficacious than systemic opioids in some types of acute pain, such as acute reflex sympathetic dystrophy (for which sympathetic blockade is indicated). These approaches must be implemented by experienced clinicians who can appropriately assess the risks and benefits for the patient.

Rarely, other nonpharmacologic methods are useful adjuncts in acute pain management. For example, although recent studies have reported that transcutaneous electrical nerve stimulation cannot be distinguished from placebo in the treatment of chronic back pain (174) or acute postoperative pain (175), a plethora of earlier reports, many uncontrolled, suggested that this approach may be useful in a variety of pain syndromes (176). Because this technique is almost devoid of adverse effects, it is reasonable to consider a trial in the management of focal acute pain syndromes.

Psychological methods of pain control, such as relaxation and biofeedback (177), and other cognitive–behavioral approaches to pain management (178,179) are most extensively employed in chronic pain management. These approaches may be helpful in providing coping strategies and skills to selected patients with acute pain associated with overwhelming anxiety or overtly maladaptive behaviors.

Recognize and Prevent Specific Drug Abuse Behaviors

Patients who are actively abusing opioids may not set limits on drug-seeking behavior during pain treatment, even if opioids are provided liberally. In the hospital setting, some of these patients may engage in highly aberrant behaviors, such as tampering with drug infusion devices or dissolving tablets to inject the residue intravenously. Obviously, such behavior cannot be tolerated. In many cases, efforts to control behavior are best implemented as part of a formal drug-abuse program that is initiated coincident with medical and pain treatments. This goal clearly may be difficult, if not impossible, to accomplish.

Some measures can be recommended that may allow the continuation of opioid use for acute severe pain despite the potential for ongoing abuse behaviors. First, it is essential to engage the patient in a frank discussion that clearly defines the expectations for therapy and the limits of acceptable and unacceptable behavior. Second, simple security measures are advisable, such as the use of drug infusion pumps with locks that prevent changes in the settings; routine nursing policies in the hospital call for such rigorous supervision of the storage and dispensing of opioids. If oral opioid analgesics have been abused, the patient should be told that ingestions will be witnessed and that room searches for hidden pills or signs of hoarding will be done.

Although acute severe pain in a known opioid addict is seldom treated in the outpatient setting, additional guidelines should be followed if this circumstance arises. Guidelines should be written, given to the patient, and filed in the patient's medical record. They should state the absolute requirement that only one physician prescribe opioid medications and should provide procedures for prescription renewals and the response to lost or stolen prescriptions or drugs. As noted previously, it is generally prudent to require patients to report lost or stolen prescriptions or drugs to the police; drugs should be renewed only after a document that confirms this is obtained.

Prescription theft or forgery cannot be tolerated, and if either occurs when opioids are still indicated medically, therapy can be continued only if rigid guidelines are implemented. In some cases, patients should be admitted to the hospital to allow drug use to stabilize in a controlled environment. If opioid therapy is no longer required, the drug should be withdrawn and the patient referred to an appropriate drug treatment program. Outpatients with a history of opioid abuse who are receiving opioid analgesics should be seen frequently, even daily if necessary, and a limited quantity of the drug should be prescribed at any one time.

Avoid Excessive Negotiation About Specific Drugs and Doses

The management of acute pain should be approached systematically, and although the treatment approach should be discussed with the patient, the physician must assume responsibility for specific orders establishing the drug, doses, and route and frequency of administration. In the absence of known hypersensitivity to a specific drug, it is just as inappropriate for a patient to demand a specific opioid, dose, or route of administration for acute pain as it would be for the same patient to demand a specific antibiotic for management of an acute infection. This (or a similar) analogy should be discussed with the patient. Although there are obviously major differences between the management of an inherently subjective condition, such as pain, and other medical conditions, it is useful to consider the process of treatment from a similar medical orientation.

Provide Early Consultation with Appropriate Services

Many patients with acute pain and substance-abuse disorders require interdisciplinary assessment and care. These patients are not well managed by the traditional medical model of acute care, because a unified approach to pain management and drug abuse may be beyond the competence of a single physician or clinical service. Indeed, without the benefit of expert consultation, a unified approach may appear to be impossible, because the fundamental goals of pain treatment and substance abuse treatment can conflict directly. Increased cooperation between pain specialists and addiction specialists must be encouraged during the treatment of these patients, and clinical research is needed to develop a new medical model that will provide flexibility in traditional concepts of substance abuse and pain management.

CHRONIC OPIOID THERAPY IN PATIENTS WITHOUT SUBSTANCE ABUSE

In most cultures, the fear of opioid addiction is etched deeply into the consciousness of both health care providers and the public at large. This fear may contribute to the undertreatment of both acute pain and chronic cancer-related pain in populations with no prior history of substance abuse, notwithstanding wide support for the first-line use of these drugs for these types of pain (18,30,47–49, 180–183). Undertreatment is most likely in two clinical settings: (a) postoperative patients whose pain intensity or duration exceeds that considered to be the norm (38), and (b) cancer patients with pain associated with early or limited disease who appear relatively well and function at nearly a normal level (184). Efforts to define the true risks involved in the therapeutic use of opioid drugs and debunk inappropriate attitudes about these drugs will likely benefit the management of these groups of patients most dramatically.

In the setting of chronic nonmalignant pain, the traditional view holds that opioid therapy is inappropriate because of the potential for addiction, the inevitability of side effects, and the likelihood that analgesic tolerance will compromise long-term efficacy. During the past 20 years,

TABLE 55.10. *Issues relevant to the evaluation of chronic opioid therapy for nonmalignant pain*

Critical issues
  Efficacy
    Responsiveness of nonmalignant pain syndromes to opioids
    Waning efficacy as a result of tolerance
    Effects on goals of therapy other than pain relief
  Adverse pharmacologic outcomes
    Persistent side effects
    Long-term toxicity
    Subtle neuropsychological impairment
  Drug dependence
    Terminology
    Role of physical dependence
    Risks of addiction
Related issues
  Undertreatment of pain as a result of attitudes toward opioids
  Limited availability of opioids for bona fide medical uses
  Effects on medical practice from perceived risk of sanctions

however, advances in pain research, burgeoning experience in the clinical management of pain, and greater recognition of the defining characteristics of addiction have suggested the need to critically evaluate this view (3,24,185–196).

Three major issues must be considered to assess the role of opioid therapy in chronic nonmalignant pain: (a) potential efficacy, (b) the possibility of adverse pharmacologic outcomes, and (c) the risk of addiction. These issues are themselves complex, and various aspects of each must be addressed independently to provide a comprehensive assessment of this approach (Table 55.10).

Efficacy

The most relevant information about the potential efficacy of chronic opioid therapy for nonmalignant pain is provided by published reports (16,19–24,197–218) that specifically describe this approach. There are a growing number of controlled trials. Some describe 1 or 2 weeks of treatment, and although largely (204–208), but not uniformly (209), favorable to the treatment, their relevance to long-term management is dubious. Other favorable controlled trials describe treatment that extends for 1 or 2 months (200,203c,203d,203g,203h). None of these studies observed the development of abuse behaviors during therapy, a finding that might be expected given entry criteria that exclude patients with a history of drug abuse.

Most of the empirical data are provided by surveys. Older surveys, which originated from multidisciplinary pain-management programs, portrayed opioid therapy as problematic, associated with relatively worse pain, more functional impairment and psychological distress, aberrant drug-related behaviors, and cognitive impairment (210–218). More recent surveys, however, suggest favorable outcomes (198,201,203,203b,203e,203f). For example, a survey of 100 patients with mixed diagnoses who received various opioid drugs for many months reported good analgesia in more than one-half, with improved performance status associated with pain relief, and no serious toxicity or aberrant drug-related behaviors (24). Another survey of 124 patients with mixed pain diagnoses who were treated for 2 to 60 months with methadone recorded good pain control in almost 90% of patients, improved psychological status on a validated questionnaire, and no reported morbidity (218a).

The issues surrounding this therapeutic approach are also illuminated by several surveys of chronic opioid therapy in nonpainful conditions. Long-term treatment with codeine, dihydrocodeine, propoxyphene, or methadone has been described in restless legs syndrome (219,220), neuroleptic-induced dyskinesias (221), and intractable dyspnea (222). The long-term efficacy of the opioid administered in each of these conditions only rarely was compromised by the development of tolerance, and psychological dependence on the drugs did not occur.

These surveys suggest a spectrum of outcomes associated with opioid therapy. Although treatment can evidently become a problem in some disabled patients, there appears to be a subpopulation of patients with chronic nonmalignant pain that attains at least partial relief from opioid drugs for a prolonged period, without the development of opioid toxicity, clinically significant tolerance, or abuse behaviors. Although some patients who experience relief of pain demonstrate improvement in functional status, others do not. Abuse behaviors can develop, but appear to be very uncommon in the populations who were not surveyed in the setting of a multidisciplinary pain-management program.

There is no evidence in these surveys that the type of chronic pain or degree of functional impairment at the start of therapy predicts the failure of opioid therapy. Although it is clear that opioid responsiveness can vary with characteristics of the patient or pain syndrome (223,224), there is no evidence that any subgroup of patients with chronic pain is inherently resistant to this therapy. The example of neuropathic pain is illustrative. Although an inferred neuropathic mechanism for pain has been associated with a relatively lower likelihood of successful opioid therapy (55,223–227), the potential for a favorable response is unquestionable (21,22,24,122,202) and has been confirmed in controlled trials (200,203g). Thus, the diagnosis of neuropathic pain may raise concerns about the ultimate outcome of opioid therapy but does not reliably predict its failure. Neither it nor other diagnoses of this type should be used as a rationale for the withholding of therapy.

The large number of opioid-treated patients with chronic pain described in the medical literature does not resolve many questions: How large is the group of patients who may benefit from chronic opioid therapy and how might they be identified? Is it the drug itself, the physician–patient relationship, the therapeutic context, the additional therapies provided within that context, or some combination of these factors that leads to the benefits and low prevalence of adverse consequences in these patients? Is the specific drug, method of dosing, or absolute dose important? If, as suggested by some of the surveys, enhanced comfort is not followed by improved function, are the benefits of therapy ever greater than the possible risks? What is the value of this treatment approach compared with others, even in the highly selected group of patients described?

Development of Tolerance

The possibility that opioid drugs potentially could provide some degree of pain relief to patients with chronic nonmalignant pain is perhaps less controversial than the observation that this relief may persist for a prolonged period of time. The concern that opioid analgesia inevitably wanes over time as a consequence of the development of pharmacologic tolerance is a critical element in the assessment of this therapeutic approach. It is apparent that chronic opioid therapy for nonmalignant pain would not be viable if pharmacologic tolerance to analgesia developed at such a rate that effective pain relief was brief or could be maintained only by rapid escalation of doses to unacceptable levels.

A diminution in salutary opioid effects with prolonged administration is seldom observed in surveys of cancer patients and patients with chronic nonmalignant pain (11–24). In a study of three nonmalignant pain patients treated with meperidine for 3 to 12 months, the minimal effective analgesic plasma drug concentrations remained constant over time (228). Taken together, these data suggest that pharmacologic tolerance to analgesic effects is seldom the driving force for dose escalation in the clinical setting. Concern about waning analgesic efficacy primarily as a result of tolerance is overstated (11,12).

Goals of Pain Therapy

It is widely accepted that the management of chronic nonmalignant pain must consider two goals simultaneously: improved comfort and functional gains. Opioid therapy would rarely be considered acceptable if it causes function to decline, even if patients report additional comfort. If function remains stable during therapy, however, the assessment of the approach is less straightforward. Although it is reasonable to propose that opioid therapy should be judged solely by the relief of pain, this is fundamentally a philosophic position. Some pain specialists, especially those who work within a multidisciplinary pain management program, assess the overall utility of treatment according to its effects on physical and psychosocial functioning. Continued efforts to resolve the controversy about this approach will require clear statements about the criteria by which it is evaluated.

Published surveys of opioid therapy for nonmalignant pain describe disparate outcomes. Some patients improved function during therapy and others did not. Surveys originating from pain clinics have demonstrated a relationship between opioid use on admission to the treatment program and a greater number of prior hospitalizations and operations, more physical impairment, worse psychological disturbance, potential misuse of analgesic drugs, and poorer outcome of therapy (210–218).

Unfortunately, all these associations suffer from the usual problems inherent in surveys of highly selected patient populations. Just as clinicians inclined to use opioid therapy choose patients likely to benefit, many patients are referred to pain clinics because they have already demonstrated a problem with prescription drugs. Furthermore, the relationships derived from these data are correlative and do not determine causality. Thus, both opioid use and its reported adverse outcomes actually may result from a third factor, such as a more severe pain syndrome or a more aggressive, help-seeking personality. Similarly, patients who appear to benefit from opioid administration may, in fact, improve as a result of the relationship with a committed physician or associated treatments, rather than use of the drug itself. Finally, many of these surveys are compromised by methodological flaws, most notably the lack of long-term followup (229–231), and some surveys of pain clinic patients that purport to demonstrate adverse effects of opioids use definitions for drug-related behavior that do not conform to current standards (32).

Given the conflicting survey data, the most reasonable hypothesis is that opioids by themselves neither substantially improve nor damage function. For some patients, access to an opioid can contribute to globally impaired function or a tendency to drug abuse, whereas for others, the availability of a strong analgesic allows a degree of function that would otherwise be impossible. The drug has an important role in determining the overall outcome, but the nature of the outcome cannot be attributed to the pharmacology of the drug. Further studies are needed to evaluate this hypothesis and to clarify those characteristics of the patient or treatment setting that will probably be more useful in predicting clinical response.

Adverse Pharmacologic Outcomes

The issue of potential adverse consequences as a consequence of the long-term administration of opioid drugs to patients with chronic nonmalignant pain must address two major considerations: the risk of major organ dysfunction and the incidence of persistent side effects. Among the most important of the potential side effects is subtle neuropsychological impairment, which could undermine concurrent rehabilitative efforts.

Risk of Major Organ Dysfunction

Major organ toxicity following exposure to opioid drugs has not been observed among cancer patients or those on methadone maintenance (232–234). In a study of patients receiving methadone, hepatic dysfunction did not occur in the absence of viral hepatitis or alcoholism (235). Pulmonary edema has been reported in several dying cancer patients who were receiving high doses of an opioid (236), but this phenomenon is not relevant to the routine treatment setting. A variety of disimmune effects have been reported in animal models (237–243), but human data are yet minimal. There is evidence that acute administration of an opioid can alter immune function and that different opioids produce varied effects (243a). There is also evidence, however, that pain itself is immunosuppressive (243b), and this finding, combined with the lack of evidence of clinically relevant impairment of immune function from opioids, provides support for opioid therapy in the setting of severe pain.

Persistent Side Effects

In addition to well-known alterations in the central nervous system function, acute administration of an opioid produces changes in the hypothalamic–pituitary axis, peripheral vasculature, gastrointestinal tract, urinary tract, skin, and immune system (244,245). Many of these effects are not experienced overtly by the patient, while some produce aversive phenomena, such as nausea, constipation, or confusion. With chronic administration, tolerance develops at different rates to each effect. The evaluation of long-term safety, therefore, depends on the prevalence of sustained opioid effects and the risks associated with each, whether experienced by the patient or not.

The most detailed assessment of this issue has been done in the methadone maintenance population. Studies of these patients have demonstrated persistent constipation, insomnia, and decreased sexual function in 10% to 20% of patients and the complaint of excessive sweating in a somewhat higher proportion (232–234). Elevated plasma proteins often persist, and occasionally, sustained abnormalities of hypothalamic-pituitary regulation, particularly abnormalities in the level and fluctuation of prolactin, are observed. Although some of the clinical effects can be troubling to the patient, none of the biochemical abnormalities has ever been associated with symptomatic disease. In the cancer population, clinical experience suggests that constipation is the most common opioid effect for which tolerance develops so slowly that persistent problems ensue.

Although cognitive impairment and disturbances in psychomotor functioning are commonly observed following either acute administration of opioids to nontolerant patients or dose escalation in those on chronic therapy, these effects typically wane with stable long-term therapy (246). In opioid-treated patients with cancer pain, small impairments in reaction time have been observed (247,248), but the clinical significance of this finding is not clear. A study of cancer patients receiving long-term morphine therapy revealed only minimal effects on cognitive and psychomotor functions related to driving (249). Another study of cancer patients suggested that tolerance to adverse neuropsychological effects that occur immediately after opioid dose escalation develops within 2 weeks (25). In patients without cancer, data are somewhat more conflicting. Surveys of patients admitted to pain programs who are dependent on opioids and other prescription drugs, as well as surveys of heroin addicts and methadone-maintenance patients, have demonstrated clinically evident sedation or abnormalities on neuropsychological testing (213,215,216,250–253). All these populations were subject to selection bias, however. Another survey of methadone maintenance patients did not reveal the problems reported by others (254), and none of the surveys controlled for the concurrent use of other drugs (particularly sedative–hypnotics), premorbid cognitive deficits, or history of head trauma. A small study in which pain patients who were chronically receiving opioids alone were compared with patients using benzodiazepines and no opioids noted substantial cognitive deficits only in the latter group (255). Equally reassuring, surveys of driving records performed in methadone maintained populations have not reveal a increased rate of infractions or accidents (256,257). A recent systematic review of neuropsychological studies of opioid-treated patients (257a) concluded that there was generally consistent evidence for no impairment of psychomotor abilities of opioid-maintained patients, inconclusive evidence for no impairment on cognitive function, and strong evidence for no greater incidence of motor vehicle violations or accidents, or abnormalities in driving simulators.

These observations suggest that cognitive deficits could occur in patients with chronic nonmalignant pain who are administered long-term opioid therapy, but the prevalence and severity of these deficits, and their clinical significance, is probably less than commonly believed. Additional investigations are needed to clarify this issue, and the potential for cognitive impairment must be evaluated when opioids are employed in the clinical setting.

Risk of Addiction

The potential for addiction or abuse is the most salient issue to address in the assessment of chronic opioid therapy for nonmalignant pain. This concern is ubiquitous in all clinical settings but historically has had the greatest impact on the management of this population.

The use of inappropriate nomenclature has been an ongoing concern in the assessment of addiction liability (4a,32). Confusion between physical dependence and addiction is common in clinical settings. Misuse of the term *addiction* to describe the potential for withdrawal (*physical dependence*) can undermine efforts to evaluate opioid therapy in the individual patient and the population overall. Although the impact of physical dependence is certainly an appropriate issue to consider in the overall assessment of opioid therapy, withdrawal can be easily prevented and does not appear to preclude the uneventful discontinuation of treatment when this is required. Concern about physical dependence is thus minor in comparison with the possibility of iatrogenic addiction from the therapeutic use of opioid drugs.

The perception that opioid consumption may lead to the development of addiction derives largely from clinical experience with street addicts. The observed reactions of addicts following exposure to opioids are often assumed to be merely a more extreme expression of the experience of patients administered these agents for pain. Implicit in this view is the belief that such powerful reinforcements attend the use of these drugs that administration to otherwise normal individuals for appropriate medical reasons may be sufficient to produce addiction. If this were true, chronic opioid therapy for nonmalignant pain should certainly be rejected, except perhaps in patients with life-threatening diseases.

Several types of data support the potentially reinforcing qualities of opioids. For example, some of these drugs are highly reinforcing in animals, and conditioned responses that perpetuate opioid consumption and increase the likelihood of use after detoxification have been well demonstrated in nonhuman experimentation (34,258,259). In humans, the high recidivism rate in detoxified addicts appears to support the existence of similar reinforcing properties (260,261). Moreover, although physical dependence is now considered to be distinct from addiction, it has been postulated that the need to avoid the aversive experience of abstinence may also impel drug-seeking behavior. This classical conditioning theory of addiction views abstinence as an unconditioned response that can lead to a conditioned abstinence syndrome, which contributes to continued opioid-seeking (30). Because the potential for physical dependence is inherent in opioid pharmacology, this theory lends further support to the view that the risk of addiction may be an intrinsic property of the drug.

This conclusion is contradicted by extensive experience with pain patients, predominantly those with cancer pain, and numerous clinical investigations. For example, although it is widely believed that opioids produce the reinforcing experience of euphoria, surveys of cancer patients, postoperative patients, and normal volunteers indicate that elation is uncommon following administration of an opioid; dysphoria is observed more typically, especially in those who receive meperidine (100, 262, 263). The rarity of euphoria, the "high" or "rush" of the street addict, in patients suggests that there may be fundamental distinctions between opioid addicts and those without addiction who receive these drugs for pain.

The lack of euphoria does not, of course, exclude the possibility that other powerful reinforcements inhere in opioid pharmacology and impart a substantial risk of iatrogenic addiction. This possibility was suggested by early surveys of addicts, which noted that a relatively large proportion began their addiction as medical patients administered opioid drugs for pain (264–266). The most influential of these surveys recorded a pain history from 27% of white male addicts and 1.2% of African American male addicts (266).

Surveys of addict populations, however, do not provide a valid measure of the addiction liability associated with the use of prescribed opioid drugs in various nonmalignant pain populations. Patient surveys are needed to define this risk. Several older surveys provided reassuring data, but did not evaluate cohorts of patients receiving long-term opioid therapy for chronic pain and, therefore, have limited relevance (39,267,268). Cancer patients allowed to self-administer morphine for several weeks during an episode of painful mucositis did not demonstrate escalating use, which could indicate either tolerance or addiction (18, 269). The latter finding is consistent with clinical experience, which indicates that addiction is an exceedingly rare outcome during long-term opioid treatment of cancer pain.

These surveys of patients with pain are reassuring, but should not be assumed to be fully representative of the varied populations who seek treatment for chronic nonmalignant pain. As mentioned previously, data collected by multidisciplinary pain-management programs suggest that abuse behaviors may be quite common among the patients referred to this setting (270). The latter surveys have numerous deficiencies, however, including selection bias, limited assessment, and the use of questionable criteria for the diagnosis of abuse or addiction (270). Moreover, the interpretation of all survey data require comparison to United States population prevalence rates for alcoholism (3% to 16%) and other forms of substance abuse (5% to 6%) (271).

Overall, these surveys provide evidence that the outcomes of drug abuse and addiction do not commonly occur among patients with no history of abuse who receive opioids for medical indications. Other epidemiologic data similarly contradict the notion that exposure to opioid drugs reliably leads to escalating use and recidivism after detoxification. The existence of so-called "chippers," individuals who use heroin recreationally on a periodic basis (272), belies the inevitability of the full addiction syndrome, even in those who consume the drugs for purposes other than pain control. More interesting, perhaps, is the evidence that a large proportion of soldiers who abused heroin in Vietnam stopped this activity abruptly on return

to the United States, and subsequently demonstrated a low rate of relapse (273).

Addiction also associates with a number of factors that may be etiologically important and are uncommon in populations of chronic pain patients, including specific personality disorders, such as psychopathy (149,150), and a variety of situational and social factors never experienced by the typical medical patient. There is substantial evidence of a genetic predisposition in the genesis of alcoholism and other types of addiction (274–275a), and it may be postulated that the development of alcoholism in a small minority of those who imbibe is a parallel process to that determining opioid addiction in a small proportion of those administered these drugs (276).

These correlations, like the aforementioned surveys, suggest that opioid exposure by itself is insufficient to produce abuse or addiction. The reinforcing properties of opioid drugs may be experienced differently by the individual predisposed to addiction than by the typical patient with chronic nonmalignant pain. Although correlations do not demonstrate causality, and it is conceivable that the characteristics of the street addict, like psychopathy, develop as a result of the addiction or relate to drug abuse through some other unknown factor, a reasonable hypothesis is that addiction results from the interaction between the reinforcing properties of opioid drugs and any number of characteristics that are specific to the individual. These characteristics, such as the capacity for euphoria from an opioid, are unrelated to the pharmacology of the drug.

In sum, the existing data suggest that patients without a prior history of substance abuse are unlikely to become addicted during long-term opioid treatment of chronic pain. The risk should not be assumed to be nil, however, and the data also suggest that the risk may vary with specific characteristics of the patient. Unfortunately, little is known about the nature of these characteristics or their predictive value, and all impressions must be applied cautiously in practice. Limited survey data have been analyzed in an effort to clarify risk (276a). On the basis of these data and extensive clinical experience, it may be surmised that the risk of iatrogenic addiction during long-term opioid therapy is probably greater among those with a prior history of substance abuse, a significant family history of addiction severe character pathology characterized by impulsivity, or a chaotic home environment; the risk is probably relatively lower among older than younger patients, even if drug-related problems have never occurred. Additional studies are needed to confirm this low risk of addiction or abuse overall and clarify the predictive value of specific patient characteristics.

Other Observations

As noted, the three critical issues most salient in assessing the potential utility of chronic opioid therapy in nonmalignant pain reflect basic medical concerns—the perceived benefits and risks to the individual patient. Other observations in this clinical setting may be useful in further clarifying the tension that exists between the licit medical use of opioid drugs and the concerns raised by their potential for abuse.

One such observation, which is also relevant to the chronic treatment of cancer pain, relates to the inadequate availability of oral opioids for long-term outpatient use. Although it is now widely accepted that the precepts of effective and humane medical care mandate unimpeded access to opioid drugs, at least by patients with some types of pain, the unfortunate reality is that these analgesics are not readily available in most parts of the world (47). In the United States, a number of opioids are available commercially, but prescribing is hampered by the failure of pharmacies to maintain a supply (277,277a), strict limits in the quantities dispensed, and the burden of record-keeping. Although the factors that impede the ready access to opioid drugs for therapeutic purposes have not been assessed systematically, it is reasonable to presume that the fear of abuse plays a major role.

More compelling, perhaps, is the potential influence on prescribing practices of the intense efforts to reduce prescription drug abuse (278,279). Physicians, pharmacists, and other professionals who administer opioids to patients may be aware of rare reports of legal action against physicians who have prescribed opioids, particularly those who have provided these drugs to patients with nonmalignant pain (280,281). Other, often unverified cases are considered common knowledge, discussed among practitioners. This word-of-mouth transfer of information from physician to physician is a cardinal element of medical education and is held responsible for the perpetuation of a number of misconceptions about the appropriate use of opioids (282). Although physicians generally agree with the need for careful monitoring of opioid prescription, and probably none would fault the identification and punishment of professionals engaged in criminal behavior (283), it may be speculated that the net effect of all these perceptions is to suggest that a degree of personal risk attends the administration of opioid drugs to patients.

Although controversial, it may be possible to infer the impact of prescription drug regulation on the licit use of opioids by evaluating the effects of the multiple copy prescription program. In the United States, the number of states with such programs has declined sharply, and there soon may be none. This is recognized as progress given the data that initiation of these programs was followed by a greater than 50% reduction in the statewide prescribing of opioid drugs (284). Although this large reduction was attributed to a decline in diversion and misuse by those in the regulatory and law enforcement communities who, before the advent of electronic data systems, favored multiple copy prescription programs as the only good method for "point of sale" monitoring (285,286), most pain specialists believed that this change primarily reflected reduced prescribing by legitimate physicians (278,279, 287–291).

Multiple-copy prescription programs may reduce licit prescribing by reminding physicians about the scrutiny that accompanies opioid prescribing. The impact of this perception is likely to be greatest in the use of these drugs for patients with nonmalignant pain. The concern that those in the regulatory community may initiate an investigation, or even issue a sanction, because of bias against the approach has been piqued by surveys that demonstrate limited knowledge among regulators in the United States (292) and media coverage of problematic prescription drug use.

Medical decision making may be unduly influenced by regulatory policies or fear of regulatory scrutiny. On the basis of this observation, it is reasonable to hypothesize that both the rejection of opioid therapy for nonmalignant pain and the tendency to undertreat acute pain and chronic cancer pain relate to a perceived risk of personal sanctions that is induced by these factors. Inasmuch as it is agreed that the factors responsible for the undertreatment of acute pain and cancer pain with opioid drugs should be reversed, and that decisions about chronic opioid therapy for nonmalignant pain should be made in response to medical considerations rather than the fear of sanctions, the influence of perceived risk on prescribing practices should be approached as an independent problem in medical care. In support of this view, the U.S. Federation of the Boards of Medical Examiners has issued model guidelines for opioid therapy (292a) and some have adopted statutes designed to reassure physicians of their autonomy in selecting patients for chronic opioid therapy and rendering medical judgments about appropriate administration of these drugs (278,293). Recently, the United States Drug Enforcement Administration joined with numerous professional societies to issue a call for more balance in the approach to opioid therapy. The hope is that the medical community, and regulatory and law enforcement communities can sustain a dialogue that encourages balance between a broad recognition of the essential medical role played by opioid drugs and acknowledgment that controls are needed to reduce abuse and diversion.

Clinical Implications

It has been suggested that a selected subgroup of patients with chronic nonmalignant pain may be able to obtain sustained improvement in comfort from opioid drugs without the development of significant toxicity or evidence of addiction. There is now general agreement among pain specialists that the doctrinaire rejection of this approach that was the norm must be replaced by a more balanced approach that respects the complexity of the medical and pharmacologic issues, and a growing clinical experience with opioid therapy.

Chronic opioid therapy should not be considered an approach to replace current pain management techniques. Rather, opioid therapy, like other primary analgesic treatments, may be best conceived as a useful element in a multimodality approach for chronic pain management. Indeed, it is even possible that opioid therapy could be complementary to the range of interventions offered in traditional multidisciplinary pain-management programs (20). A large proportion of patients in these programs continue to experience severe pain and it would be valuable to provide more comfort, if this could be done without restraining rehabilitative efforts. Also, the failure and dropout rates from these programs are substantial (231,294,295), and it is interesting to consider whether access to better analgesic therapy could have a positive impact on these figures.

Guidelines based on clinical experience have been proposed for the management of opioid therapy in patients with nonmalignant pain (186) (Table 55.11). These guidelines attempt to capture the potential for salutary effects from opioid therapy without losing sight of the possibility of serious morbidity (pharmacological or functional) associated with this treatment approach. Additional data from prospective clinical series and controlled trials will likely lead to an evolution of therapeutic guidelines that will better optimize benefits and minimize risk.

The guidelines have several important implications. First, they indicate that patient selection is empirical at the present time. Opioid therapy is not considered a first-line approach, but might be evaluated against other therapies in terms of its risk:benefit ratio. As discussed previously, some patient characteristics, such as a prior history

TABLE 55.11. *Proposed guidelines in the management of chronic opioid therapy for nonmalignant pain*

1. Should be considered for all patients with chronic moderate to severe pain, but positioned based on the responses to several questions: Are opioids likely to work well? Are there other therapies with an equal or better therapeutic index? Is the medical risk of opioid therapy relatively high? Is the patient likely to be responsible in using the drug? What is conventional practice with respect to this syndrome?
2. A history of substance abuse, severe character pathology, and chaotic home environment should be viewed as strong relative contraindications.
3. A single clinician should take primary responsibility for treatment. This practitioner should review all medical records.
4. Patients should give informed consent before the start of therapy and the consent discussion should be documented in the medical record. This discussion should cover recognition of the low risk of true addiction as an outcome, potential for cognitive impairment with the drug alone and in combination with sedative–hypnotics, and the likelihood that physical dependence will occur (abstinence possible with acute discontinuation).
5. After drug selection, doses should be given on an around-the-clock basis; several weeks should be agreed upon as the period of initial dose titration, and although improvement in function should be continually stressed, meaningful partial analgesia should be accepted as the appropriate goal of therapy. Long-acting opioid drugs are preferred; the decision to coadminister a short-acting opioid for breakthrough pain should be made on a case-by-case basis.
6. Failure to achieve at least partial analgesia at relatively low initial doses in the patient with no substantial prior opioid exposure raises questions about the potential treatability of the pain syndrome with opioids; such an occurrence should lead to reassessment of the pain syndrome.
7. Emphasis should be given to attempts to capitalize on improved analgesia by gains in physical and social function. Opioid therapy should be considered complementary to other analgesic and rehabilitative approaches.
8. In addition to the daily dose determined initially, most patients should be permitted access to additional analgesic on days of increased pain; this can be accomplished by coadministration of a short-acting "rescue dose" for breakthrough pain, or by the instruction that one or two extra doses may be taken on any day, but must be followed by an equal reduction of dose on subsequent days.
9. Initially, most patients must be seen and drugs prescribed at least monthly. When stable, less frequent visits may be acceptable.
10. Exacerbations of pain may occur and, following a careful assessment, the clinician may decide to increase the stable dose. This change in therapy should be stated clearly for the patient and documented in the medical record. If repeated dose escalation is needed to maintain pain control, the clinician should reevaluate the pain syndrome and the patient.
11. Evidence of aberrant behaviors must be carefully assessed. In some cases, tapering and discontinuation of opioid therapy will be necessary. Other patients may appropriately continue therapy within rigid guidelines. Consideration should be given to consultation with an addiction medicine specialist.
12. At each visit, assessment should specifically address (a) comfort (degree of analgesia); (b) opioid-related side effects; (c) functional status (physical and psychosocial), and (d) existence of aberrant drug-related behaviors.
13. Use of a written opioid agreement, periodic urine drug screens, or self-report instruments may be helpful but should not be required.
14. Documentation is essential and the medical record should specifically address comfort, function, side effects and the occurrence of aberrant behaviors repeatedly during the course of therapy.

of substance abuse, should be viewed as strong relative contraindications given current experience. A recent survey suggests that some patients with a history of substance abuse may be able to maintain effective stable therapy, but the challenge of treating this population suggests that it should be undertaken only by experienced clinicians (296).

Second, the guidelines suggest the potential utility of a therapeutic opioid trial. Because opioid therapy can almost always be discontinued without difficulty after short-term administration, a therapeutic trial can be initiated like any other reversible analgesic approach. During a defined trial period, the dose can be adjusted while clinically relevant endpoints are monitored. These endpoints should include pain relief, opioid-related side effects, functional status (including the willingness to engage in other components of therapy), and the development of aberrant drug-related behaviors. A trial that produces benefits that exceed any evident disadvantage can be stabilized into a pattern of long-term administration, during which the same endpoints can be followed on a regular basis.

Third, the guidelines highlight the importance of patient consent. Some clinicians have adopted formal written consent as standard practice (150a,150b,297). Others obtain verbal consent, which is documented in the medical record. Regardless, a consent discussion is needed, which provides a useful opportunity to educate patients about the nature of the therapy and the need for responsible drug-taking behavior.

Fourth, the guidelines imply that long-term opioid therapy for nonmalignant pain must be based on a working knowledge of the widely accepted pharmacologic techniques described previously for cancer pain. Although some clinicians advocate specific approaches for the population with nonmalignant pain, such as the sole use of long-acting drugs or the avoidance of any "as-needed" dosing, any such recommendation remains supported only by anecdote. In the absence of data from controlled trials, rigid adherence to any specific recommendation of this type is not warranted.

Although the extrapolation of dosing principles from the cancer pain population to the nonmalignant pain population can be recommended on theoretical grounds, the practical application can be problematic in some cases. As discussed previously, the absolute dose required to identify a favorable balance between analgesia and side effects is widely considered to be immaterial when treating the patient with cancer pain. In nonmalignant pain populations, however, the need for repeated dose adjustments can raise concerns. An intense focus on dose titration could possibly foster an unrealistic view of the treatment and divert attention from rehabilitative pursuits. Furthermore, high doses may increase the discomfort of the clinician, both in terms of appropriate medical considerations and the potential for increased regulatory scrutiny that may accompany this approach. If the clinician perceives any

interference with other goals of treatment, this should be directly discussed with the patient. A careful reassessment is needed whenever pain worsens sufficiently to suggest the need for dose escalation. This reassessment should clarify the nature of the pain (including the status of its physical and psychological determinants), record side effects, determine functional status (both physical and psychosocial), and affirm the lack of aberrant drug-related behaviors.

Concern about regulatory scrutiny is understandable, and it is likely that dose escalation is sometimes withheld solely in response to a perceived risk of sanctions. When these concerns arise, it useful to seek additional consultations from specialists in pain management or take a strong stance by proactively informing local authorities of the treatment plan.

Finally, the guidelines note the importance of a clearly defined strategy for the management of aberrant drug-related behaviors, should they occur during therapy. Many clinicians have a stereotyped response to these behaviors based on a perception that they invariably represent addiction. This type of inflexibility is not justified given the diversity of these behaviors and the multiple meanings they may reflect. As discussed previously, the assessment of aberrant behavior in patients receiving an abusable drug for an appropriate clinical indication is a complex process that must distinguish the development of an addiction disorder from many other possible determinants.

Aberrant drug-related behavior requires a comprehensive assessment. In some cases, this assessment can be facilitated by consultation with a specialist in addiction medicine. It may include telephone calls to other physicians or local pharmacies, or a request to bring all medications and used bottles from home. A urine drug screen can be a very helpful aspect. On the basis of this assessment, some episodes of aberrant opioid use are best characterized as symptomatic of addiction, a diagnosis that suggests a targeted therapeutic approach best organized with the assistance of a specialist in addiction medicine. In other cases, a comprehensive assessment suggests that the diagnosis of addiction would not be appropriate. The clinician may wish to continue therapy while instituting a highly structured approach, which may include new instructions for dosing, more frequent visits, and smaller prescriptions. A written contract is sometimes useful and repeated urine drug screens can again be helpful.

The clinician who takes responsibility for opioid pharmacotherapy cannot confuse therapeutic support with tacit acceptance of questionable behavior. The demand for responsible drug-taking behavior should never be viewed as patient abandonment or an unjustified diversion from the goals of analgesia and function. The clinician must assess the patient over time, arrive at an appropriate diagnosis, and institute whatever controls are necessary to reestablish appropriate drug use. If the patient cannot comply with the requirements of therapy, the risks are too great to continue prescribing.

CONCLUSION

Principles of opioid therapy for the treatment of pain are well established and generally are believed to provide the capability for adequate pain control in the great majority of patients with acute and chronic pain. Concerns about opioid addiction or abuse imbue all aspects of management. Patients with a history of opioid abuse who are evaluated carefully and are determined to be appropriate candidates for opioid therapy, either brief or long-term, require ongoing assessment and the skillful adaptation of pharmacologic principles that have proved essential in the optimal management of pain in patients with no such history. The available data suggest that inadequate management of these patients is common and relates to some combination of reticence to prescribe on the part of physicians and non-adherence with therapy on the part of the patient. In the much larger population with no prior history of substance abuse, the potential for opioid addiction contributes substantially to the pervasive undertreatment of acute pain

and chronic cancer pain, and is the major issue that must be confronted in the chronic administration of opioid drugs to patients with nonmalignant pain.

Very few clinical investigations have been designed to address the relationship between the licit medical use of opioid drugs and their potential for illicit use. Studies are needed to clarify the range of responses of patients with a history of substance abuse who require treatment for severe pain and determine the true risk associated with the long-term use of opioids in patients with chronic nonmalignant pain. There is a need to replace anecdotal observations with scientific findings and maintain the balance between needed regulation of prescription drugs and their availability for clinical use. Physicians should be reassured that aggressive opioid management of acute pain and chronic cancer pain is fully acceptable, and those physicians who choose to employ opioids in the management of chronic nonmalignant pain should not fear reprisals for this decision if it is undertaken with the care that such controversial therapy warrants. All of these objectives will be more likely to occur if an active dialogue develops between pain specialists and addiction specialists.

REFERENCES

1. Uhlenhuth EH, DeWit H, Balter MB, et al. Risks and benefits of long-term benzodiazepine use. *J Clin Psychopharmacol* 1988;8:161–167.
2. Woods JH, Katz JL, Winger G. Use and abuse of benzodiazepines. Issues relevant to prescribing. *JAMA* 1988;260:3476–3480.
3. Portenoy RK. Opioid therapy for chronic nonmalignant pain: current status. In: Fields HL, Liebeskind JC, eds. *Progress in pain research and management. Pharmacological approaches to the treatment of chronic pain: new concepts and critical issues.* Seattle: IASP Press, 1994;1:247–288.
4. Portenoy RK. Opioid analgesics. In: Portenoy RK, Kanner RM, eds. *Pain management: theory and practice.* Philadelphia: FA Davis, 1996:248–276.
4a. Savage SR, Joranson DE, Covington EC, et al. Definitions related to the medical use of opioids: evolution towards universal agreement. *J Pain Symptom Manage* 2003;26(1):655–657.
5. Dole VP. Narcotic addiction, physical dependence and relapse. *N Engl J Med* 1972;286:988–992.
6. Jaffe JH. Drug addiction and drug abuse. In: Gilman AG, Goodman LS, Rall TW, et al., eds. *The pharmaco-*

logical basis of therapeutics, 7th ed. New York: Macmillan, 1985:532–581.
7. Martin WR, Jasinski DR. Physiological parameters of morphine dependence in man—tolerance, early abstinence, protracted abstinence. *J Psychiatr Res* 1969;7:9–17.
8. Ling GSF, Paul D, Simantov R, et al. Differential development of acute tolerance to analgesia, respiratory depression, gastrointestinal transit and hormone release in a morphine infusion model. *Life Sci* 1989;45:1627–1636.
9. Ling W, Wesson DR. Drugs of abuse—opiates. *West J Med* 1990;152:565–572.
10. World Health Organization. *Technical report no. 407: Expert Committee on Drug Dependence, 16th report.* Geneva: World Health Organization, 1969.
11. Portenoy RK. Opioid tolerance and efficacy: basic research and clinical observations. In: Gebhardt G, Hammond D, Jensen T, eds. *Proceedings of the VII World Congress on Pain. Progress in pain research and management.* Seattle: IASP Press, 1994;2:595–619.
12. Nghiemphu LP, Portenoy RK. Opioid tolerance: a clinical perspective. In Bruera EB, Portenoy RK, eds. *Topics in palliative care,* vol. 5. New York:

Oxford University Press, 2000:197–212.
13. Twycross RG, Lack SA. *Therapeutics in terminal cancer,* 2nd ed. Edinburgh. Churchill Livingstone, 1990.
14. Portenoy RK, Lesage P: Management of cancer pain. *Lancet* 1999;353:1695–1700.
15. Twycross RG. Clinical experience with diamorphine in advanced malignant disease. *Clin Pharmacol Ther Int J Clin Pharmacol Ther Toxicol* 1974;9:184–198.
16. Kanner RM, Foley KM. Patterns of narcotic drug use in a cancer pain clinic. *Ann N Y Acad Sci* 1981;362:161–172.
17. Gourlay GK, Cherry DA, Cousins MJ. A comparative study of the efficacy and pharmacokinetics of oral methadone and morphine in the treatment of severe pain in patients with cancer. *Pain* 1986;25:297–312.
18. Chapman CR, Hill HF. Prolonged morphine self-administration and addiction liability: evaluation of two theories in a bone marrow transplant unit. *Cancer* 1989;63:1636–1644.
19. Adriaensen H, Vissers K, Noorduin H, et al. Opioid tolerance and dependence: an inevitable consequence of chronic treatment? *Acta Anaesthesiol Belg* 2003;54(1):37–47.
20. France RD, Urban BJ, Keefe FJ. Long-term use of narcotic analgesics

in chronic pain. *Soc Sci Med* 1984; 19:1379–1382.

21. Portenoy RK, Foley KM. Chronic use of opioid analgesics in non-malignant pain: report of 38 cases. *Pain* 1986;25:171–186.

22. Urban BJ, France RD, Steinberger DL, et al. Long-term use of narcotic-antidepressant medication in the management of phantom limb pain. *Pain* 1986;24:191–197.

23. Rainov NG, Heidecke V, Burkert W. Long-term intrathecal infusion of drug combinations for chronic back and leg pain. *J Pain Symptom Manage* 2001;22(4):862–871.

24. Zenz M, Strumpf M, Tryba M. Long-term opioid therapy in patients with chronic nonmalignant pain. *J Pain Symptom Manage* 1992;7:69–77.

25. Bruera E, Macmillan K, Hanson JA, et al. The cognitive effects of the administration of narcotic analgesics in patients with cancer pain. *Pain* 1989;39:13–16.

26. Redmond DE, Krystal JH. Multiple mechanisms of withdrawal from opioid drugs. *Ann Rev Neurosci* 1984;7:443–478.

27. Heishman SJ, Stitzer ML, Bigelow GE, et al. Acute opioid physical dependence in humans: effect of varying the morphine-naloxone intervals. *J Pharmacol Exp Ther* 1989;250:485–491.

28. World Health Organization. *Technical report no. 516: youth and drugs.* Geneva: World Health Organization, 1973.

29. American Psychiatric Association. *Diagnostic and statistical manual of mental disorders,* 4th ed. Washington, DC, 1994.

30. Wikler A. *Opioid dependence: mechanisms and treatment.* New York: Plenum Press, 1980.

31. Rinaldi RC, Steindler EM, Wilford BB, et al. Clarification and standardization of substance abuse terminology. *JAMA* 1988;259:555–557.

32. Sees KL, Clark HW. Opioid use in the treatment of of chronic pain: assessment of addiction. *J Pain Symptom Manage* 1993;8:257–264.

33. Halpern LM, Robinson J. Prescribing practices for pain in drug dependence: a lesson in ignorance. *Adv Alcohol Subst Abuse* 1985/1986;5:184–197.

34. Dai S, Corrigal WA, Coen KM, et al. Heroin self-administration by rats: influence of dose and physical dependence. *Pharmacol Biochem Behav* 1989;32:1009–1015.

35. Weissman DE, Haddox JD. Opioid pseudoaddiction—an iatrogenic syndrome. *Pain* 1989;36:363–366.

35a. Kirsh KL, Whitcomb LA, Donaghy K, et al. Abuse and addiction issues in medically ill patients with pain: attempts at clarification of terms and empirical study. *Clin J Pain* 2002;[4 Suppl]:S52–S60.

36. Wilford BB. Abuse of prescription drugs. *West J Med* 1990;152:609–612.

37. Gonzales GR, Coyle N. Treatment of cancer pain in a former opioid abuser: fears of the patient and staff and their influence on care. *J Pain Symptom Manage* 1992;7(4):246–249.

38. Edwards WT. Optimizing opioid treatment of postoperative pain. *J Pain Symptom Manage* 1990;5[1 Suppl]: S24–S36.

39. Perry S, Heidrich G. Management of pain during débridement: a survey of U.S. burn units. *Pain* 1982;13:267–280.

40. Jorgensen L, Mortensen M-J, Jensen N-H, et al. Treatment of cancer pain patients in a multidisciplinary pain clinic. *Pain Clin Pain Clin* 1990;3:83–89.

41. Moulin DE, Foley KM. Review of a hospital-based pain service. In: Foley KM, Bonica JJ, Ventafridda V, eds. *Advances in pain research and therapy. Second International Congress on Cancer Pain.* New York: Raven Press, 1990;16:413–427.

42. Schug SA, Zech D, Dorr U. Cancer pain management according to WHO analgesic guidelines. *J Pain Symptom Manage* 1990;5:27–32.

43. Schug SA, Zech D, Grond S, et al. A long-term survey of morphine in cancer pain patients. *J Pain Symptom Manage* 1992;7:259–266.

44. Ventafridda V, Tamburini M, De-Conno F. Comprehensive treatment in cancer pain. In: Fields HL, Dubner R, Cervero F, eds. *Advances in pain research and therapy. Proceedings of the Fourth World Congress on Pain.* New York: Raven Press, 1985;9:617–628.

45. Ventafridda V, Tamburini M, Caraceni A, et al. A validation study of the WHO method for cancer pain relief. *Cancer* 1990;59:850–856.

46. Walker VA, Hoskin PJ, Hanks GW, et al. Evaluation of WHO analgesic guidelines for cancer pain in a hospital-based palliative care unit. *J Pain Symptom Manage* 1988;3:145–149.

47. World Health Organization. *Cancer pain relief, with a guide to opioid availability,* 2nd ed. Geneva: Author, 1996.

48. Health and Public Policy Committee, American College of Physicians. Drug therapy for severe chronic pain in terminal illness. *Ann Intern Med* 1983;99:870–873.

49. Agency for Health Care Policy and Research. *Clinical practice guideline number 9: management of cancer pain.* Washington, DC: U.S. Department of Health and Human Services, 1994.

50. Ad Hoc Committee on Cancer Pain, American Society of Clinical Oncology. Cancer pain assessment and treatment curriculum guidelines. *J Clin Oncol* 1992;10:1976–1982.

51. American Pain Society. *Principles of analgesic use in the treatment of acute pain and cancer pain.* Skokie, IL: Author, 1999.

52. Breitbart W, McDonald MV, Rosenfeld B, et al. Pain in ambulatory AIDS patients. I. Pain characteristics and medical correlates. *Pain* 1996;68:315–321.

53. Rosenfeld B, Breitbart W, McDonald MV, et al. Pain in ambulatory AIDS patients. II. Impact of pain on psychological functioning and quality of life. *Pain* 1996;68:323–328.

54. Breitbart W, Rosenfeld BD, Passik SD, et al. The undertreatment of pain in ambulatory AIDS patients. *Pain* 1996;65:239–245.

55. Arner S, Myerson BA. Lack of analgesic effects of opioids on neuropathic and idiopathic forms of pain. *Pain* 1988;33:11–23.

56. American Psychiatric Association. *Diagnostic and statistical manual of mental disorders,* 4th ed. Washington, DC, 1994.

57. Portenoy RK, Payne D, Jacobsen P. Breakthrough pain: characteristics and impact in patients with cancer pain. *Pain* 1999;81:129–134.

58. Portenoy RK. Issues in the management of neuropathic pain. In: Basbaum A, Besson J-M, eds. *Towards a new pharmacology of pain.* New York: John Wiley, 1991:393–416.

59. Merskey H, Bogduk N. *Classification of chronic pain,* 2nd ed. Seattle: IASP Press, 1994.

60. Lussier DA, Portenoy RK. Adjuvant analgesics in pain management. In: Doyle D, Hanks GW, MacDonald RN, et al., eds. *Oxford textbook of palliative medicine.* Third ed. Oxford: Oxford University Press, 2004:349–377.

61. Caraceni A, Portenoy R, and a Working Group of the IASP Task Force on Cancer Pain. An international survey on cancer pain characteristics and syndromes. *Pain* 1999;82:263–275.

62. Foley KM. Pain syndromes in patients with cancer. In: Portenoy RK, Kanner RM, eds. *Pain management: theory and practice.* Philadelphia: FA Davis, 1996:191–216.

63. Gonzales GR, Elliot KJ, Portenoy RK, et al. The impact of a comprehensive

evaluation in the management of cancer pain. *Pain* 1991;47:141–144.

64. Takeda F. Results of field-testing in Japan of WHO draft interim guidelines on relief of cancer pain. *Pain Clin* 1986;1:83–89.

65. Coyle N, Adlehardt J, Foley KM, et al. Character of terminal illness in the advanced cancer patient: pain and other symptoms in the last 4 weeks of life. *J Pain Symptom Manage* 1990;5:83–93.

66. Cherny NI, Portenoy RK. Systemic drugs for cancer pain. *Pain Dig* 1995;5:245–263.

67. Salazar OM, Rubin P, Hendrickson FR, et al. Single-dose half-body irradiation for palliation of multiple bone metastases from solid tumors. Final Radiation Therapy Oncology Group report. *Cancer* 1986;58:29–36.

68. Tong D, Gillick L, Hendrickson FR. The palliation of symptomatic osseous metastases: final results of the study by the Radiation Therapy Oncology Group. *Cancer* 1982;50:893–899.

69. Gilbert HA, Kagan AR, Nussbaum H, et al. Evaluation of radiation therapy for bone metastases: pain relief and quality of life. *AJR Am J Roentgenol* 1977;129:1095–1096.

70. Siegal T, Tiqva P, Siegal T. Vertebral body resection for epidural compression by malignant tumors. Results of forty-seven consecutive operative procedures. *J Bone Joint Surg Am* 1985;67A:375–382.

71. Sundaresan N, DiGiacinto GV. Antitumor and antinociceptive approaches to control cancer pain. *Med Clin North Am* 1987;71:329–348.

72. MacDonald N. The role of medical and surgical oncology in the management of cancer pain. In: Foley KM, Bonica JJ, Ventafridda V, eds. *Advances in pain research and therapy.* New York: Raven Press, 1990;16:27–40.

73. Bonadonna G, Molinari R. Role and limits of anticancer drugs in the treatment of advanced pain. In: Bonica JJ, Ventafridda V, eds. *Advances in pain research and therapy.* New York: Raven Press, 1979;2:131–138.

74. Brule G. Role and limits of oncologic chemotherapy of advanced cancer pain. In: Bonica JJ, Ventafridda V, eds. *Advances in pain research and therapy.* New York: Raven Press, 1979;2:139–144.

75. Tannock IF, Osoba D, Stockler MR, et al. Chemotherapy with mitoxantrone plus prednisone or prednisone alone for symptomatic hormone-resistant prostate cancer: a Canadian randomized trial with palliative endpoints. *J Clin Oncol* 1996;14:1756–1764.

76. Bruera E, MacDonald RN. Intractable pain in patients with advanced head and neck tumors: a possible role of local infection. *Cancer Treat Rep* 1986;70:691–692.

77. Zipursky A, Brown EJ, O'Brodovich H, et al. Oxygen therapy in sickle cell disease. *Am J Pediatr Hematol Oncol* 1992;14(3):222–228.

78. Charache S, Terrin ML, Moore RD, et al. Effect of hydroxyurea on the frequency of painful crises in sickle cell anemia. Investigators of the Multicenter Study of Hydroxyurea in Sickle Cell Anemia. *N Engl J Med* 1995;332(20):1317–1322.

79. Wallenstein DJ, Portenoy RK: Nonopioid and opioid analgesics. In: Berger A, Portenoy RK, Weissman D, eds. *Principles and practice of palliative care and supportive oncology.* Philadelphia: JB Lippincott, 2002:84–97.

80. Portenoy RK, Kanner RM. Nonopioid and adjuvant analgesics. In: Portenoy RK, Kanner RM, eds. *Pain management: theory and practice.* Philadelphia: FA Davis, 1996:219–247.

81. Ventafridda V, Fochi C, DeConno F, et al. Use of nonsteroidal antiinflammatory drugs in the treatment of pain in cancer. *Br J Clin Pharmacol* 1980;10:343–346.

82. Willer JC, De Brouckner T, Bussel B, et al. Central analgesic effect of ketoprofen in humans—electrophysiological evidence for a supraspinal mechanism in a double-blind and cross-over study. *Pain* 1989;38:1–7.

83. Simon LS, Weaver AL, Graham DY, et al. Anti-inflammatory and upper gastrointestinal effects of celecoxib in rheumatoid arthritis: a randomized controlled trial. *JAMA* 1999;282:1921–1928.

84. Langman MJ, Jensen DM, Watson DJ, et al. Adverse upper gastrointestinal effects of rofecoxib compared with NSAIDs. *JAMA* 1999;282:1929–1933.

85. Loeb DS, Ahlquist DA, Talley NJ. Management of gastroduodenopathy associated with use of nonsteroidal anti-inflammatory drugs. *Mayo Clin Proc* 1992;67:354–364.

85a. Hernandez-Diaz S, Rodriguez LA. Association between nonsteroidal anti-inflammatory drugs and upper gastrointestinal tract bleeding/perforation: an overview of epidemiologic studies published in the 1990s. *Arch Intern Med* 2000;160:2093–2099.

86. La Corte R, Caselli M, Castellino G, et al. Prophylaxis and treatment of NSAID-induced gastroduode-

nal disorders. *Drug Saf* 1999;20:527–543.

87. Taha AS, Hudson N, Hawkey CJ, et al. Famotidine for the prevention of gastric and duodenal ulcers caused by nonsteroidal anti-inflammatory drugs. *N Engl J Med* 1996;334:1435–1439.

88. Sandler DP, Smith JC, Weinberg CR, et al. Analgesic use and chronic renal disease. *N Engl J Med* 1989;320:1238–1243.

89. Houde RW. Analgesic effectiveness of the narcotic agonist–antagonists. *Br J Clin Pharmacol* 1979;7:297S–308S.

90. Hoskin PJ, Hanks GW. Opioid agonist-antagonist drugs in acute and chronic pain patients. *Drugs* 1991;41:329–344.

91. Portenoy RK, Maldonado M, Fitzmartin R, et al. Controlled-release morphine sulfate: analgesic efficacy and side-effects of a 100 mg tablet in cancer pain patients. *Cancer* 1989;63:2284–2288.

92. Galer BS, Coyle N, Pasternak GW, et al. Individual variability in the response to different opioids. Report of five cases. *Pain* 1992;49:87–91.

93. Hanna MH, Peat SJ, Woodham M, et al. Analgesic efficacy and CSF pharmacokinetics of intrathecal morphine-6-glucuronide: comparison with morphine. *Br J Anaesth* 1990;64:547–550.

94. Peterson GM, Randall CTC, Paterson J. Plasma levels of morphine and morphine glucuronides in the treatment of cancer pain: relationship to renal function and route of administration. *Eur J Clin Pharmacol* 1990;38:121–124.

95. Osborne JR, Joel SP, Slevin ML. Morphine intoxication in renal failure: the role of morphine-6-glucuronide. *Br Med J* 1986;292:1548–1549.

96. Hagen NA, Foley KM, Cerbone DJ, et al. Chronic nausea and morphine-6-glucuronide. *J Pain Symptom Manage* 1991;6:125–128.

97. Portenoy RK, Thaler HT, Inturrisi CE, et al. The metabolite, morphine-6-glucuronide, contributes to the analgesia produced by morphine infusion in pain patients with normal renal function. *Clin Pharmacol Ther* 1992;51:422–431.

98. Sjogren P. Clinical implications of morphine metabolites. In: Portenoy RK, Bruera EB, eds. *Topics in palliative care,* vol. 1. New York: Oxford University Press, 1997:163–176.

99. Tiseo PJ, Thaler HT, Lapin J, et al. Morphine-6-glucuronide concentrations and opioid-related side effects: a survey in cancer patients. *Pain* 1995;61:47–54.

100. Kaiko RF, Foley KM, Grabinski PY, et al. Central nervous system

excitatory effects of meperidine in cancer patients. *Ann Neurol* 1983;13:180–185.

101. Plummer JL, Gourlay GK, Cherry DA, et al. Estimation of methadone clearance: application in the management of cancer pain. *Pain* 1988;33:313–322.

101a. DeStoutz ND, Bruera E, Suarez-Almazor M. Opioid rotation for toxicity reduction in terminal cancer patients. *J Pain Symptom Manage* 1995;10:378–384.

101b. Bruera EB, Neumann CM. Role of methadone in the management of pain in cancer patients. *Oncology* 1999;13(9):1275–1291.

101c. Mancini I, Lossignol DA, Body JJ. Opioid switch to oral methadone in cancer pain. *Curr Opin Oncol* 2000;12:308–13.

101d. Davis AM, Inturrisi CE. *d*-Methadone blocks morphine tolerance and *N*-methyl-D-aspartate–induced hyperalgesia. *J Pharmacol Exp Ther* 1999;289:1048–1053.

102. Gorchow L, Sheidler V, Grossman S, et al. Does intravenous methadone provide longer-lasting analgesia than intravenous morphine? A randomized, double-blind study. *Pain* 1989;38:151–157.

103. Korte W, de Stoutz N, Morant R. Day-to-day titration to initiate transdermal fentanyl in patients with cancer pain: short- and long-term experiences in a prospective survey of 39 patients. *J Pain Symptom Manage* 1996;11:146.

104. Donner B, Zenz M, Tryba M, et al. Direct conversion from oral morphine to transdermal fentanyl: a multicenter study in patients with cancer pain. *Pain* 1996;64:527–534.

105. Portenoy RK, Southam M, Gupta SK, et al. Transdermal fentanyl for cancer pain: repeated dose pharmacokinetics. *Anesthesiology* 1993;28:36–43.

106. Bruera E, Brenneis C, MacDonald RN. Continuous sc infusion of narcotics for the treatment of cancer pain: an update. *Cancer Treat Rep* 1987;71:953.

107. Swanson G, Smith J, Bulich R, et al. Patient-controlled analgesia for chronic cancer pain in the ambulatory setting: a report of 117 cases. *J Clin Oncol* 1989;7:1903–1906.

108. Osenbach RK, Harvey S. Neuraxial infusion in patients with chronic intractable cancer and noncancer pain. *Curr Pain Headache Rep* 2001;5:241–249.

109. Smith TJ, Staats PS, Deer T, et al. Randomized clinical trial of an implantable drug delivery system compared with comprehensive medical management for refractory cancer pain: impact on pain, drug-related

toxicity, and survival. *J Clin Oncol* 2002;20:4040–4049.

110. Plummer JL, Cherry DA, Cousins MJ, et al. Long-term spinal administration of morphine in cancer and non-cancer pain: a retrospective study. *Pain* 1991;44:215–220.

111. Bennett G, Burchiel K, Buchser E, et al. Evidence-based review of the literature on intrathecal delivery of pain medication. *J Pain Symptom Manage* 2000;20:S12–S36.

112. Portenoy RK, Moulin DE, Rogers A, et al. Continuous intravenous infusion of opioids in cancer pain: review of 46 cases and guidelines for use. *Cancer Treat Rep* 1986;70:575–581.

113. Cole L, Hanning CD. Review of the rectal use of opioids. *J Pain Symptom Manage* 1990;5:118–126.

114. Houde RW. Misinformation: side effects and drug interactions. In: Hill CS, Fields WS, eds. *Advances in pain research and therapy.* New York: Raven Press, 1989;11:145–161.

114a. Indelicato RA, Portenoy RK. Opioid rotation in the management of refractory cancer pain. *J Clin Oncol* 2002;20:348–352.

115. Portenoy RK. Management of opioid side effects. *Singapore Med J* 1994;23:160–170.

116. Derby S, Portenoy RK. Assessment and management of constipation. In: Portenoy RK, Bruera EB, eds. *Topics in palliative care,* vol. 1. New York: Oxford University Press, 1997:95–112.

117. Bruera E, Brenneis C, Paterson AH, et al. Use of methylphenidate as an adjuvant to narcotic analgesics in patients with advanced cancer. *J Pain Symptom Manage* 1989;4:3–6.

118. De Stoutz ND, Bruera E, Suarez-Almazor M. Opioid rotation for toxicity reduction in terminal cancer patients. *J Pain Symptom Manage* 1995;10:378–384.

119. Wooldridge JE, Anderson CM, Perry MC. Corticosteroids in advanced cancer. *Oncology (Huntingt)* 2001;15:225–234.

120. Ettinger AB, Portenoy RK. Use of corticosteroids in the treatment of symptoms associated with cancer. *J Pain Symptom Manage* 1988;3:99–104.

121. Bruera E, Roca E, Cedaro L, et al. Action of oral methylprednisolone in terminal cancer patients: a prospective randomized double-blind study. *Cancer Treat Rep* 1985;69:751–754.

122. Portenoy RK, Foley KM, Inturrisi CE. The nature of opioid responsiveness and its implications for neuropathic pain: new hypotheses derived from studies of opioid infusions. *Pain* 1990;43:273–286.

123. Young RF, Brechner T. Electrical stimulation of the brain for relief of intractable pain due to cancer. *Cancer* 1986;57:1266–1272.

124. Fosburg MT, Crone RK. Nitrous oxide analgesia for refractory pain in the terminally ill. *JAMA* 1983;250:511–513.

125. Raj PP. Prognostic and therapeutic local anesthetic block. In: Cousins MJ, Bridenbaugh PO, eds. *Neural blockade in clinical anesthesia and management of pain,* 2nd ed. Philadelphia: JB Lippincott, 1988:899–933.

126. Cousins MJ, Dwyer B, Gibb D. Chronic pain and neurolytic neural blockade. In: Cousins MJ, Bridenbaugh PO, eds. *Neural blockade in clinical anesthesia and management of pain,* 2nd ed. Philadelphia: JB Lippincott, 1988:1053–1084.

127. Cherny NI, Arbit E, Jain S. Invasive techniques in the management of cancer pain. *Hematol Oncol Clin North Am* 1996;10(1):121–137.

128. Nitescu P, Applegren L, Linder LE, et al. Epidural versus intrathecal morphine-bupivacaine: assessment of consecutive treatments in advanced cancer pain. *J Pain Symptom Manage* 1990;5:18–26.

129. Gybels JM, Sweet WH. *Neurosurgical treatment of persistent pain.* Basel: Karger, 1989.

130. Pagni CA. Role of neurosurgery in cancer pain: re-evaluation of old methods and new trends. In: Benedetti C, Chapman CR, Moricca G, eds. *Advances in pain research and therapy.* New York: Raven Press, 1984;7:603–629.

131. Arbit E, ed. *Surgical treatment of cancer-related pain.* New York: Futura, 1993.

132. Glover J, Dibble S, Dodd MJ, et al. Mood state of oncology outpatients: does pain make a difference? *J Pain Symptom Manage* 1995;10:120–128.

133. Massie MJ, Holland JC. The cancer patient with pain: psychiatric complications and their management. *Med Clin North Am* 1987;71:243–258.

134. Loscalzo M. Psychological approaches to the management of pain in patients with cancer. *Hematol Oncol Clin North Am* 1996;10(1):139–155.

135. Breitbart W. Psycho-oncology: depression, anxiety, delirium. *Semin Oncol* 1994;21:754–769.

136. Cleeland CS, Tearnan BH. Behavioral control of cancer pain. In: Holzman AD, Turk DC, eds. *Pain management.* New York: Pergamon Press, 1986.

137. Fishman B, Loscalzo M. Cognitive-behavioral interventions in the management of cancer pain: principles

and applications. *Med Clin North Am* 1987;71:271–289.

138. Cagnello VW. The use of hypnotic suggestion for relief of malignant disease. *Int J Clin Exp Hypn* 1961;9:17–22.

139. Fotopoulos SS, Graham C, Cook MR. Psychophysiologic control of cancer pain. In: Bonica JJ, Ventafridda V, eds. *Advances in pain research and therapy.* New York: Raven Press, 1979;2:231–243.

140. Simonton O, Matthews-Simonton S, Sparks T. Psychological intervention in the treatment of cancer. *Psychosomatics* 1980;21:226–233.

141. Fleming U. Relaxation therapy for far-advanced cancer. *Practitioner* 1985;229:471–475.

142. Macaluso C, Weinberg D, Foley KM. Opioid abuse and misuse in a cancer pain population. *J Pain Symptom Manage* 1988;3:S24(abstr).

143. Kantor TG, Cantor R, Tom E. A study of hospitalized surgical patients on methadone maintenance. *Drug Alcohol Depend* 1980;6:163–173.

144. Rubenstein R, Spiro I, Wolff WI. Management of surgical problems in patients on methadone maintenance. *Am J Surg* 1976;131:566–569.

145. Sawe J, Hansen J, Ginman C, et al. A patient-controlled dose regimen of methadone in chronic cancer pain. *Br Med J* 1981;282:771–773.

146. Inturrisi CE, Colburn WA, Kaiko RF, et al. Pharmacokinetics and pharmacodynamics of methadone in patients with chronic pain. *Clin Pharmacol Ther* 1987;41:392–401.

147. Hansen J, Ginman C, Hartvig P, et al. Clinical evaluation of oral methadone in treatment of cancer pain. *Acta Anaesth Scand Suppl* 1982;74:124–127.

148. Beaver WT, Wallenstein SL, Houde RW, et al. A clinical comparison of the analgesic effects of methadone and morphine administered intramuscularly, and of orally and parenterally administered methadone. *Clin Pharmacol Ther* 1967;8:415–426.

149. Hill HE, Haertzen CA, Davis H. An MMPI factor analytic study of alcoholics narcotic addicts and criminals. *Q J Stud Alcohol* 1962;23:411–431.

150. Hill HE, Haertzen CA, Glaser R. Personality characteristics of narcotic addicts as indicated by the MMPI. *J Gen Psychol* 1960;62:127–139.

150a. Fishman SM, Kreis PG. The opioid contract. *Clin J Pain* 2002;18[4 Suppl]:S70–S75.

150b. Fishman SM, Mahajan G, Jung SW, et al. The trilateral opioid contract. Bridging the pain clinic and the primary care physician through the opioid contract. *J Pain Symptom Manage* 2002;24:335–344.

151. Bonica JJ. Evolution and current status of pain programs. *J Pain Symptom Manage* 1990;5:368–374.

152. Loeser JD, Egan KJ. *Managing the chronic pain patient: theory and practice at the University of Washington multidisciplinary pain center.* New York: Raven Press, 1989.

153. Verhaak PF, Kerssens JJ, Dekker J, et al. Prevalence of chronic benign pain disorder among adults: a review of the literature. *Pain* 1998;77:231–239.

154. Gureje O, Von Korff M, Simon GE, et al. Persistent pain and well-being: a World Health Organization study in primary care. *JAMA.* 1998;280;147–151.

155. Crook J, Rideout E, Browne G. The prevalence of pain complaints in a general population. *Pain* 1984;18:299–314.

156. Portenoy RK, Coyle N. Controversies in the long-term management of analgesic therapy in patients with advanced cancer. *J Pain Symptom Manage* 1990;5:307–319.

157. Cameron AJ. Heroin addicts in a casualty department. *Br Med J* 1964;1:594.

158. Sapiro JD. The narcotic addict as a medical patient. *Am J Med* 1968;45:555–588.

159. Compton P, Charuvastra VC, Kintaudi K, et al. Pain responses in methadone-maintained opioid abusers. *J Pain Symptom Manage* 2000;20:237–245.

160. Levine JD, Coderre TJ, Basbaum AI. The peripheral nervous system and the inflammatory process. In: Dubner R, Gebhart GF, Bond MR, eds. *Proceedings of the Fifth World Congress on Pain. Pain research and clinical management.* Amsterdam: Elsevier, 1988;3:33–43.

161. Janig W. Pathophysiology of nerve following mechanical injury. In: Dubner R, Gebhart GF, Bond MR, eds. *Proceedings of the Fifth World Congress on Pain. Pain research and clinical management.* Amsterdam: Elsevier, 1988;3:89–108.

162. Cervero F, Morrison JFB, eds. *Progress in brain research. Visceral sensation.* Vol. 67. Amsterdam: Elsevier, 1986.

163. Kumor KM, Grochow LB, Hausheer F. Unusual opioid withdrawal syndrome. A case-report. *Lancet* 1987;1:720–721.

164. Charache S, Lubin B, Reid CD, eds. *Management and therapy of sickle cell disease, revised.* NIH publication no. 89–2117. Washington, DC: U.S. Dept. of Health and Human Services, 1989.

165. Payne R. Pain management in sickle cell disease: rationale and techniques. *Ann N Y Acad Sci* 1989;565:189–206.

166. Fultz JM. Guidelines for the management of hospitalized narcotic addicts. *Ann Intern Med* 1975;82:815–818.

167. Houde RW. The use and misuse of narcotics in the treatment of chronic pain. In: Bonica JJ, ed. *Advances in neurology. International symposium on pain.* New York: Raven Press, 1974;4:527–536.

168. Portenoy RK. Continuous intravenous infusion of opioid drugs. *Med Clin North Am* 1987;71:233–241.

169. White PF. Use of patient-controlled analgesia for management of acute pain. *JAMA* 1988;259:243–247.

170. Hill HF, Chapman CR, Kornell JA, et al. Self-administration of morphine in bone marrow transplant patients reduces drug requirement. *Pain* 1990;40:121–129.

171. Gourlay GK, Willis RJ, Lamberty J. Double-blind comparison of the efficacy of methadone and morphine in post-operative pain. *Anesthesiology* 1986;64:322–327.

172. Sunshine A, Olson NZ. Analgesic efficacy of ketoprofen in postpartum, general surgery, and chronic cancer pain. *J Clin Pharmacol* 1988;28:S47–S54.

173. Buckley MM-T, Brogen RN. Ketorolac: a review of its pharmacodynamic and pharmacokinetic properties, and therapeutic potential. *Drugs* 1990;39:86–109.

174. Deyo RA, Walsh NE, Martin DC, et al. A controlled trial of transcutaneous electrical nerve stimulation (TENS) and exercise for chronic low back pain. *N Engl J Med* 1990;332:1627–1634.

175. McCallum MID, Glynn CJ, Moore RA, et al. Transcutaneous electrical nerve stimulation in the management of acute postoperative pain. *Br J Anaesth* 1988;61:308–312.

176. Woolf CJ. Segmental afferent fibre-induced analgesia: transcutaneous electrical nerve stimulation (TENS) and vibration. In: Wall PD, Melzack R, eds. *Textbook of pain,* 2nd ed. Edinburgh: Churchill Livingstone, 1989:884–896.

177. Jessup BA. Relaxation and biofeedback. In: Wall PD, Melzack R, eds. *Textbook of pain,* 2nd ed. Edinburgh: Churchill Livingstone, 1989:989–999.

178. Turk DC, Meichenbaum DH. A cognitive-behavioral approach to pain management. In: Wall PD, Melzack R, eds. *Textbook of pain,* 2nd ed. Edinburgh: Churchill Livingstone, 1989:1001–1020.

179. Nielson WR, Weir R. Biopsychosocial approaches to the treatment of

chronic pain. *Clin J Pain* 2001; 17[4 Suppl]:S114–S127.

180. Ward SE, Goldberg N, Miller-McCauley V, et al. Patient-related barriers to management of cancer pain. *Pain* 1993;52:319–324.

181. Donovan M, Dillon P, McGuire L. Incidence and characteristics of pain in a sample of medical-surgical inpatients. *Pain* 1987;30:69–78.

182. Cohen F. Postsurgical pain relief: patients' status and nurses' medication choices. *Pain* 1980;9:265–274.

183. Anderson KO, Richman SP, Hurley J, et al. Cancer pain management among underserved minority outpatients: perceived needs and barriers to optimal control. *Cancer* 2002;15;94(8):2295–2304.

184. Von Roenn JH, Cleeland CS, Gonin R, et al. Physician's attitudes and practice in cancer pain management: a survey from the Eastern Cooperative Oncology Group. *Ann Intern Med* 1993;119:121–126.

185. Mitka M. Experts debate widening use of opioid drugs for chronic nonmalignant pain. *JAMA* 2003;289(18):2347–2348.

186. Portenoy RK. Opioid therapy for chronic nonmalignant pain: clinicians' perspective. *J Law Med Ethics* 1996;24:296–309.

187. Potter M, Schafer S, Gonzalez-Mendez E, et al. Opioids for chronic nonmalignant pain. Attitudes and practices of primary care physicians in the UCSF/Stanford Collaborative Research Network. University of California, San Francisco. *J Fam Pract* 2001;50(2):145–151.

188. Clark HW, Sees KL. Opioids, chronic pain and the law. *J Pain Symptom Manage* 1993;8:297–305.

189. Passik SD, Weinreb HJ. Managing chronic nonmalignant pain: overcoming obstacles to the use of opioids. *Adv Ther* 2000;17(2):70–83.

190. Gourlay GK, Cherry DA. Can opioids be successfully used to treat severe pain in nonmalignant conditions? *Clin J Pain* 1991;7:347–349.

191. Lipman AG. Treatment of chronic pain in osteoarthritis: do opioids have a clinical role? *Curr Rheumatol Rep* 2001;3(6):513–519.

192. Schofferman J. Long-term use of opioid analgesics for the treatment of chronic pain of nonmalignant origin. *J Pain Symptom Manage* 1993;8:279–288.

193. Schug SA, Merry AF, Acland RH. Treatment principles for the use of opioids in pain of nonmalignant origin. *Drugs* 1991;42:228–239.

194. Savage SR. Long-term opioid therapy: assessment of consequences. *J Pain Symptom Manage* 1996;11:274–286.

195. Hagen N, Flynne P, Hays H, et al. Guidelines for managing chronic nonmalignant pain: opioids and other agents. *Can Fam Physician* 1995;11:49–53.

196. Jamison RN. Comprehensive pretreatment and outcome assessment for chronic opioid therapy for nonmalignant pain. *J Pain Symptom Manage* 1996;11:231–241.

197. Gardner-Nix JS. Oral methadone for managing chronic nonmalignant pain. *J Pain Symptom Manage* 1996; 11:321–328.

198. Nissen LM, Tett SE, Cramond T, et al. Opioid analgesic prescribing and use—an audit of analgesic prescribing by general practitioners and The Multidisciplinary Pain Centre at Royal Brisbane Hospital. *J Clin PharmacolBr J Clin Pharmacol* 2001;52(6):693–698.

199. Adams NJ, Plane MB, Fleming MF, et al. Opioids and the treatment of chronic pain in a primary care sample. *J Pain Symptom Manage* 2001;22(3): 791–796.

200. Gimbel JS, Richards P, Portenoy RK. Controlled-release oxycodone for pain in diabetic neuropathy: a randomized controlled trial. *Neurology* 2003;60(6):927–934.

201. Rose JB, Finkel JC, Arquedas-Mohs A, et al. Oral tramadol for the treatment of pain of 7–30 days' duration in children. *Anesth Analg* 2003;96(1):78–81.

202. Nicholson B. Responsible prescribing of opioids for the management of chronic pain. *Drugs* 2003;63(1):17–32.

203. Maier C, Hildebrandt J, Klinger R, et al. Morphine responsiveness, efficacy and tolerability in patients with chronic non-tumor associated pain—results of a double-blind placebo-controlled trial (MONTAS). *Pain* 2002;97(3):223–233.

203a. Quigley C, Wiffen PA. A systematic review of hydromorphone in acute and chronic pain. *J Pain Symptom Manage* 2003;25(2):169–178.

203b. Moulin DE, Clark AJ, Speechley M, et al. Chronic pain in Canada—prevalence, treatment, impact and the role of opioid analgesia. *Pain Res Manag* 2002;7(4):179–184.

203c. Moulin DE, Iezzi A, Amireh R, et al. Randomised trial of oral morphine for chronic non-cancer pain. *Lancet* 1996;347:143–147.

203d. Caldwell JR, Rapoport RJ, Davis JC, et al. Efficacy and safety of a once-daily morphine formulation in chronic, moderate-to-severe osteoarthritis pain: results from a randomized, placebo-controlled, double-blind trial and an open-label extension trial. *J Pain Symptom Manage* 2002;23(4):278–291.

203e. Reid MC, Engles-Horton LL, Weber MB, et al. Use of opioid medications for chronic noncancer pain syndromes in primary care. *J Gen Intern Med* 2002;17(3):173–179.

203f. Fanciullo GJ, Ball PA, Girault G, et al. An observational study on the prevalence and pattern of opioid use in 25,479 patients with spine and radicular pain. *Spine* 2002;27(2):201–205.

203g. Rowbotham MC, Twilling L, Davies PS, et al. Oral opioid therapy for chronic peripheral and central neuropathic pain. *N Engl J Med* 2003;348(13):1223–1232.

203h. Sittl R, Griessinger N, Likar R. Analgesic efficacy and tolerability of transdermal buprenorphine in patients with inadequately controlled chronic pain related to cancer and other disorders: a multicenter, randomized, double-blind, placebo-controlled trial. *Clin Ther* 2003;25(1):150–168.

204. Arkinstall W, Sandler A, Goughnour B, et al. Efficacy of controlled-release codeine in chronic nonmalignant pain: a randomized, placebo-controlled clinical trial. *Pain* 1995;62:169–178.

205. Boissier C, Perpoint B, Laport-Simitsidis S, et al. Acceptability and efficacy of two associations of paracetamol with a central analgesic (dextro-propoxyphene or codeine): comparison in osteoarthritis. *J Clin Pharmacol* 1992;32: 990–995.

206. Lloyd RS, Costello F, Eves MJ, et al. The efficacy and tolerability of controlled-release dihydrocodeine tablets and combination dextropropoxyphene paracetamol tablets in patients with severe osteoarthritis of the hips. *Curr Med Res Opin* 1992;13:37–48.

207. Thurel C, Bardin T, Boccard E. Analgesic efficacy of an association of 500 mg paracetamol plus 30 mg codeine versus 400 mg paracetamol plus 30 mg dextropropoxyphene in repeated doses for chronic lower back pain. *Curr Ther Res* 1991;50:463–473.

208. Vlok GJ, Van Vuren JP. Comparison of a standard ibuprofen treatment regimen with a new ibuprofen/paracetamol/codeine combination in chronic osteoarthritis. *S Afr Med J* 1987;(Suppl 1):1–6.

209. Kjaersgaard-Andersen P, Nafei A, Skov O, et al. Codeine plus paracetamol versus paracetamol in longer-term

treatment of chronic pain due to osteoarthritis of the hip. A randomised double-blind, multi-centre study. *Pain* 1990;43:309–318.

210. Buckley FP, Sizemore WA, Charlton JE. Medication management in patients with chronic non-malignant pain. A review of the use of a drug withdrawal protocol. *Pain* 1986; 26:153–166.

211. Finlayson RE, Maruta T, Morse RM. Substance dependence and chronic pain: profile of 50 patients treated in an alcohol and drug dependence unit. *Pain* 1986;26:167–174.

212. Finlayson RE, Maruta T, Morse RM, et al. Substance dependence and chronic pain: experience with treatment and follow-up results. *Pain* 1986;26:175–180.

213. Maruta T. Prescription drug-induced organic brain syndrome. *Am J Psychiatry* 1978;135:376–377.

214. Maruta T, Swanson DW, Finlayson RE. Drug abuse and dependency in patients with chronic pain. *Mayo Clin Proc* 1979;54:241–244.

215. Maruta T, Swanson DW. Problems with the use of oxycodone compound in patients with chronic pain. *Pain* 1981;11:389–396.

216. McNairy SL, Maruta T, Ivnik RJ, et al. Prescription medication dependence and neuropsychologic function. *Pain* 1984;18:169–177.

217. Ready LB, Sarkis E, Turner JA. Self-reported vs. actual use of medications in chronic pain patients. *Pain* 1982;12:285–294.

218. Turner JA, Calsyn DA, Fordyce WE, Ready LB. Drug utilization pattern in chronic pain patients. *Pain* 1982;12:357–363.

218a. Kell MJ. Long-term methadone maintenance for intractable, nonmalignant pain: pain control and plasma methadone levels. *Am J Pain Manage* 1994;4:10–16.

219. Hening WA, Walthers A, Kavey N, et al. Dyskinesias while awake and periodic movements in sleep in restless legs syndrome: treatment with opioids. *Neurology* 1986;36:1363–1366.

220. Sandyk R, Bamford CR. Efficacy of an opiate-benzodiazepine combination in the restless legs syndrome. *Neurology* 1987;37(Suppl 1):105.

221. Walters A, Hening W, Chokroverty S, et al. Opioid responsiveness in patients with neuroleptic-induced akathisia. *Mov Disord* 1986;1:119–127.

222. Jennings AL, Davies AN, Higgins JP, et al. A systematic review of the use of opioids in the management of dyspnoea. *Thorax* 2002;57(11):939–944.

223. Mercadante S, Maddaloni S, Roccella S, et al. Predictive factors in advanced cancer pain treated only by analgesics. *Pain* 1992;50:151–155.

224. Bruera E, Schoeller T, Wenk R, et al. A prospective multi-center assessment of the Edmonton Staging System for Cancer Pain. *J Pain Symptom Manage* 1995;10:348–355.

225. McQuay HJ, Jadad AR, Carroll D, et al. Opioid sensitivity of chronic pain: a patient-controlled analgesia method. *Anaesthesia* 1992;47:757–767.

226. Jadad AR, Carroll D, Glynn CJ, et al. Morphine responsiveness of chronic pain: double-blind randomised crossover study with patient-controlled analgesia. *Lancet* 1992; 339:1367–1371.

227. Cherny NI, Thaler HT, Friedlander-Klar H, et al. Opioid responsiveness of cancer pain syndromes caused by neuropathic or nociceptive mechanisms: a combined analysis of controlled, single-dose studies. *Neurology* 1994;44:857–861.

228. Glynn CJ, Mather LE. Clinical pharmacokinetics applied to patients with intractable pain: studies with pethidine. *Pain* 1982;13:237–246.

229. Aronoff GM, Evans WO, Enders PL. A review of follow-up studies of multidisciplinary pain units. *Pain* 1983;16:1–11.

230. Turner JA, Romano JM. Evaluating psychologic interventions for chronic pain: issues and recent developments. In: Benedetti C, Chapman CR, Moricca G, eds. *Advances in pain research and therapy.* New York: Raven Press, 1984;7:257–298.

231. Turk DC, Rudy TE. Neglected topics in the treatment of chronic pain patients-relapse, noncompliance and adherence enhancement. *Pain* 1991; 44:5–28.

232. Kreek MJ. Tolerance and dependence: implications for the pharmacological treatment of addiction. *NIDA Res Monogr* 1987;76:53–62.

233. Kreek MJ. Medical safety and side effects of methadone in tolerant individuals. *JAMA* 1973;223:665–668.

234. Kreek MJ. Medical complications in methadone patients. *Ann N Y Acad Sci* 1978;311:110–134.

235. Kreek MJ, Dodes S, Kne S, et al. Long-term methadone maintenance therapy: effects on liver function. *Ann Intern Med* 1972;77:598–602.

236. Bruera E, Miller MJ. Non-cardiogenic pulmonary edema after narcotic treatment for cancer pain. *Pain* 1989;39:297–300.

237. Arora PK, Fride E, Petitto J, et al. Morphine-induced immune alterations *in vivo. Cell Immunol* 1990;126: 343–353.

238. Donohoe RM, Falek A. Neuroimmunomodulation by opiates and other drugs of abuse: relationship to HIV infection and AIDS. *Adv Biochem Psychopharmacol* 1988;44: 145–158.

239. Einstein TK, Meissler JJ, Geller EB, et al. Immunosuppression to tetanus toxoid induced by implanted morphine pellets. *Ann N Y Acad Sci* 1990;594:377–379.

240. Molitor TW, Morilla A, Risdahl JM, et al. Chronic morphine administration impairs cell-mediated immune responses in swine. *J Pharmacol Exp Ther* 1992;260:581–586.

241. Peterson PK, Sharp B, Gekker G, et al. Opioid-mediated suppression of interferon-Î production by cultured peripheral blood mononuclear cells. *J Clin Invest* 1987;80:824–831.

242. Shavit Y, Lewis JW, Terman WG, et al. Opioid peptides mediate the suppressive effect of stress on natural killer cell cytotoxicity. *Science* 1984;223:188–190.

243. Weber RJ, Ikejiri B, Rice KC, et al. Opiate receptor-mediated regulation of the immune response *in vivo. NIDA Res Monogr* 1987;76:341–348.

243a. Sacerdote P, Bianchi M, Gaspani L, et al. The effects of tramadol and morphine on immune responses and pain after surgery in cancer patients. *Anesth Analg* 2000;90(6):1411–1414.

243b. Page GG. The immune-suppressive effects of pain. *Adv Exp Med Biol* 2003;521:117–125.

244. Reisine T, Pasternak G. Opioid analgesics and antagonists. In: Hardman JG, Limbird LE, Molinoff PB, et al. *Goodman and Gilman's the pharmacological basis of therapeutics,* 9th ed. New York: McGraw-Hill, 1996:521–557.

245. Portenoy RK. *Contemporary diagnosis and management of pain in oncologic and AIDS patients,* 3rd ed. Newtown, PA: Handbooks in Health Care, 2000.

246. Zacny JP. A review of the effects of opioids on psychomotor and cognitive functioning in humans. *Exp Clin Psychpharmacol* 1995;3:432–466.

247. Sjogren P, Banning A. Pain, sedation and reaction time during long-term treatment of cancer patients with oral and epidural opioids. *Pain* 1989;39:5–12.

248. Banning A, Sjogren P. Cerebral effects of long-term oral opioids in cancer patients measured by continuous reaction time. *Clin J Pain* 1990;6:91–95.

249. Vainio A, Ollila J, Matikainen E, et al. Driving ability in cancer patients receiving long-term morphine analgesia. *Lancet* 1995;346:667–670.

250. Rounsaville BH, Novelly RA, Kleber HD, et al. Neuropsychological impairment in opiate addicts: risk factors. *Ann N Y Acad Sci* 1981;362:79–90.

251. Martin WR, Jasinski DR, Haertzen CA, et al. Methadone—a reevaluation. *Arch Gen Psychiatry* 1973;28:286–295.

252. Gritz ER, Shiffman SM, Jarvik ME, et al. Physiological and psychological effects of methadone in man. *Arch Gen Psychiatry* 1975;32:237–242.

253. Haertzen CA, Hooks NT. Changes in personality and subjective experience associated with the chronic administration and withdrawal of opiates. *J Nerv Ment Dis* 1969;148:606–614.

254. Lombardo WK, Lombardo B, Goldstein A. Cognitive functioning under moderate and low dose methadone maintenance. *Int J Addict* 1976;11:389–401.

255. Hendler N, Cimini C, Ma T, et al. A comparison of cognitive impairment due to benzodiazepines and to narcotics. *Am J Psychiatry* 1980;137:828–830.

256. Gordon NB. Influence of narcotic drugs on highway safety. *Accid Ann Prev* 1976;8:3–7.

257. Babst DV, Newman S, Gordon NB, et al. *Driving records of methadone-maintained patients in New York State.* Albany, NY: New York State Narcotic Control Commission, 1973.

257a. Fishbain DA, Cutler RB, Rosomoff HL, et al. Are opioid-dependent/tolerant patients impaired in driving-related skills? A structured evidence-based review. *J Pain Symptom Manage* 2003;25(6):559–577.

258. Koob GF. Neural substrates of opioid tolerance and dependence. *NIDA Res Monogr* 1987;76:46–52.

259. Lynch JJ, Stein EA, Fertziger AP. An analysis of 70 years of morphine classical conditioning: implications for clinical treatment of narcotic addiction. *J Nerv Ment Dis* 1976;163:47–58.

260. Simpson DD, Savage LJ, Lloyd MR. Follow-up evaluation of treatment of drug abuse during 1969 to 1972. *Arch Gen Psychiatry* 1979;36:772–780.

261. Vaillant GE. A 20-year follow-up of New York narcotic addicts. *Arch Gen Psychiatry* 1973;29:237–241.

262. Jarvik LF, Simpson JH, Guthrie D, et al. Morphine, experimental pain and psychological reaction. *Psychopharmacology (Berl)* 1981;75:124–131.

263. Hill JL, Zacny JP. Comparing the subjective, psychomotor, and physiological effects of intravenous hydromorphone and morphine in healthy volunteers. *Psychopharmacology (Berl)* 2000;152(1):31–39.

264. Kolb L. Types and characteristics of drug addicts. *Ment Hyg* 1925;9:300.

265. Pescor MJ. The Kolb classification of drug addicts. *Public Health Rep Suppl* 1939;155.

266. Rayport M. Experience in the management of patients medically addicted to narcotics. *JAMA* 1954;156:684–691.

267. Porter J, Jick H. Addiction rare in patients treated with narcotics. *N Engl J Med* 1980;302:123.

268. Medina JL, Diamond S. Drug dependency in patients with chronic headache. *Headache* 1977;17:12–14.

269. Chapman CR. Giving, the patient control of opioid analgesic administration. In: Hill CS, Fields WS, eds. *Advances in pain research and therapy.* New York: Raven Press, 1989;11:339–352.

270. Fishbain DA, Rosomoff HL, Rosomoff RS. Drug abuse, dependence, and addiction in chronic pain patients. *Clin J Pain* 1992;8:77–85.

271. Regier DA, Meyers JK, Dramer M, et al. The NIMH epidemiologic catchment area program. *Arch Gen Psychiatry* 1984;41:934–958.

272. Graeven DB, Folmer W. Experimental heroin users: an epidemiologic and psychosocial approach. *Am J Drug Alcohol Abuse* 1977;4:365–375.

273. Robins LN, Davis DH, Nurco DN. How permanent was Vietnam drug addiction? *Am J Public Health* 1974;64:38–43.

274. Grove WM, Eckert ED, Heston L, et al. Heritability of substance abuse and antisocial behavior: a study of monozygotic twins reared apart. *Biol Psychiatry* 1990;27:1293–1304.

275. Goodwin DW, Schulsinger F, Moller N, et al. Drinking problems in adopted and nonadopted sons of alcoholics. *Arch Gen Psychiatry* 1974;31:164–169.

275a. Uhl GR, Liu QR, Naiman D. Substance abuse vulnerability loci: converging genome scanning data. *Trends Genet* 2002;18(8):420–425.

276. Newman RG. The need to redefine addiction. *N Engl J Med* 1983;18:1096–1098.

276a. Compton P, Darakjian J, Miotto K. Screening for addiction in patients with chronic pain and "problematic" substance use: evaluation of a pilot assessment tool. *J Pain Symptom Manage* 1998;16(6):355–363.

277. Morrison RS, Wallenstein S, Natale DK, et al. "We don't carry that"—failure of pharmacies in predominantly nonwhite neighborhoods to stock opioid analgesics. *N Engl J Med* 2000;342(14):1023–1026.

277a. Kanner RM, Portenoy RK. Unavailability of narcotic analgesic for ambulatory cancer patients in New York City. *J Pain Symptom Manage* 1986;1:87–90.

278. Hill CS. Government regulatory influences on opioid prescribing and their impact on the treatment of pain of nonmalignant origin. *J Pain Symptom Manage* 1996;11:287–298.

279. Cooper JR, Czechowicz DJ, Petersen RC, et al. Prescription drug diversion control and medical practice. *JAMA* 1992;268:1306–1310.

280. Rose HL. *Letter to the editor. Pain* 1987;29:261–262.

281. Kofoed L, Bloom JD, Williams MH, et al. Physicians investigated for inappropriate prescribing by the Oregon Board of Medical Examiners. *West J Med* 1989;150:597–601.

282. Morgan JP. American opiophobia: customary underutilization of opioid analgesics. *Adv Alcohol Subst Abuse* 1985;5:163–173.

283. Berina LF, Guernsey BG, Hokanson JA, et al. Physician perception of a triplicate prescription law. *Am J Hosp Pharm* 1985;42:857–859.

284. United States Department of Justice, Drug Enforcement Administration. *Multiple copy prescription program resource guide.* Washington, DC: U.S. Government Printing Office, 1987.

285. Haislip GR. Impact of drug abuse on legitimate drug use. In: Hill CS, Fields WS, eds. *Advances in pain research and therapy.* New York: Raven Press, 1989;11:205–211.

286. Gitchel GT. Existing methods to identify retail drug diversion. *NIDA Res Monogr* 1993;131:132–140.

287. Sigler KA, Guernsey BG, Ingim MB, et al. Effects of a triplicate prescription law on prescribing of schedule II drugs. *Am J Hosp Pharm* 1984;41:108–111.

288. Jacob TR. Multiple copy prescription regulation and drug abuse: evidence from the DAWN network. In: Wilford BB, ed. *Balancing the response to prescription drug abuse.* Chicago: American Medical Association, 1990:205–217.

289. Reidenberg MM. Effect of the requirement for triplicate prescriptions for benzodiazepines in New York State. *Clin Pharm Ther* 1991;50:129–131.

290. Weintraub M, Singh S, Byrne L, et al. Consequences of the 1989 New York State triplicate benzodiazepine prescription regulations. *JAMA* 1991;266:2392–2397.

291. Angarola RT, Wray SD. Legal impediments to cancer pain treatment. In: Hill CS, Fields WS, eds. *Advances in pain research and therapy.* New York: Raven Press, 1989;11:213–231.

292. Joranson DE, Cleeland CS, Weissman DE, et al. Opioids for chronic cancer and non-cancer pain: a survey of state medical board members. *Fed Bull* 1992;415–449.

292a. Gilson AM, Joranson DE, Maurer MA. Improving state medical board policies: influence of a model. *J Law Med Ethics* 2003;31(1):119–129.

293. Senate Bill 20, 71st legislature, 1st called session, State of Texas, July 18, 1989.

294. Parris WCV, Jamison RN, Vasterling JJ. Follow-up study of a multidisciplinary pain center. *J Pain Symptom Manage* 1987;2:145–154.

295. Duckro PN, Margolis RB, Tait RC, et al. Long-term follow-up of chronic pain patients: a preliminary study. *Int J Psychol Med* 1985;15:283–292.

296. Dunbar SA, Katz NP. Chronic opioid therapy for nonmalignant pain in patients with a history of substance abuse: report of 20 cases. *J Pain Symptom Manage* 1996;11:163–171.

297. Burchman SL, Pagel PS. Implementation of a formal treatment agreement for outpatient management of chronic nonmalignant pain with opioid analgesics. *J Pain Symptom Manage* 1995;10:556–563.

CHAPTER 56

Substance Use Disorders in Individuals with Co-Occurring Psychiatric Disorders

SYLVIA J. DENNISON

Use of, and withdrawal from, alcohol and other substances of abuse can cause, mimic, or mask psychiatric symptoms. At one time when an individual presented with a substance use problem and an apparent mental illness, it was common to ascribe all pathology observed to the substance use and to treat the individual accordingly. That is to say, the psychopathology was ignored with the assumption that once the individual was clean and sober, the psychiatric problems would disappear as well. The substance use was easier to see and diagnose.

Once it became obvious there was a population for whom addiction alone was not the problem, the issue of cause and effect became a subject of debate. Arguments arose regarding which came first. Was the person depressed because he was drinking heavily, or did he drink heavily because he was depressed? Was she psychotic because she smoked voluminous quantities of ganja or did she choose to smoke the drug because, as she claimed, it calmed her nerves and helped her rest? Was he anxious because he chronically abused benzodiazepines and felt the rebound effect, or did he use the benzodiazepines because of his chronic state of anxiety?

One camp saw the problem as substance use and all else as an excuse for bad behavior. The more psychologically minded developed the theory that the addicted individual used their drug(s) of choice as a means of treating uncomfortable or unacceptable impulses (1,2). This theory became known as the *self-medication* hypothesis of addictive disorders (3).

Regardless of the cause(s), many treatment providers refused to treat any other psychopathology until the substance use disorder had been addressed and the individual abstinent, sometimes for many months. Unfortunately, such an approach condemned the individual with an untreated mental illness to a high likelihood of early relapse and an overall poorer long-term prognosis (1,4,5).

It is now clear that many substance misusers suffer from both addiction and substance use disorders. Furthermore, individuals with such comorbid psychopathology do not typically respond well to traditional addiction treatment approaches (6). Rather, a unique approach is necessary for these complicated patients that is not available within typical programs. The needs of a large and difficult portion of the addicted population has been largely unmet for many years. In the last decade years, however, great strides have been made to correct this lack.

TERMINOLOGY

Now that the existence of this large population of individuals with both psychiatric and substance use disorders is recognized, how to describe this subgroup, what to call it, is an issue. Some suggest that such individuals be dubbed "substance abusers with mental illnesses (SAMI)" or "mentally ill substance abusers (MISA)," each placing a slightly different spin on the importance of the pathology. Using the same logic, others have argued for "mentally ill chemically addicted (MICA)" or "chemically abusing mentally ill (CAMI)."

A title that has found considerable favor is "dually disordered." Recently, concern has been raised that this too fails to adequately address the true scope of the problem. It is argued that "dual disorders" could be construed as referring to coexisting medical conditions such as human immunodeficiency virus (HIV)/acquired immunodeficiency syndrome (AIDs) and hepatitis, or even misunderstood as relating to those with developmental disabilities. Drake and Wallach (7) point out that it is rare for such individuals to have only two problems. Rather, they suffer from a whole spectrum of difficulties, including social, financial, and psychological. They prefer the phrase "individuals with co-occurring disorders."

Currently, there does not appear to be a consensus. The Substance Abuse and Mental Health Services Administration (SAMHSA) uses both *dual disorders* and *co-occurring disorders* in their most recent publications. The latter two appear to be the most commonly used descriptors at this time and will be used interchangeably throughout this review.

DEMOGRAPHICS

According to The National Institute on Drug Abuse and the National Institute on Alcohol Abuse and Alcoholism, abuse of alcohol and other drugs cost the United States $245.7 billion dollars in 1992, more than a 50% increase over the cost in 1985. This number represents the cost of treating the substance user as well as drug-related diseases such as cirrhosis, liver failure, hepatitis, and HIV; decreased employee productivity and premature death; and the cost of police intervention and incarceration of criminals (8).

Treatment of individuals with mental illnesses also places a heavy burden on economies both here and in other parts of the world. A study published by the National Institute of Mental Health ranks the economic impact of all medical and psychiatric diseases on society. It concludes that the economic burden exerted by mental illnesses, not including alcohol and other drug use, ranks second only to cardiovascular conditions. Adding substance use disorders to all other mental illnesses places the economic cost of all psychiatric conditions well ahead of all physical disorders (9). Recognizing that substance misuse and co-occurring mental illness place a heavy economic toll on society, it is clear that when such conditions co-occur, as they frequently do, the economic impact is tremendous.

Looking at a community sample, Regier et al. (10) found that individuals with any mental disorder had a lifetime prevalence of 29% for an addictive disorder. In treatment and institutional settings, the prevalence of co-occurring disorders is even higher. According to the Surgeon General (11), as many as 65% of persons with at least one mental disorder " ... also have a lifetime history of a least one substance use disorder. ... " The incidence and prevalence of substance misuse is different among the different disorders. For example, among individuals with schizophrenia, from 25% in community samples to 66% of individuals in specialized samples such as VA, community mental health, and in-patient samples, are estimated to have comorbid substance use disorders (12–14). Bipolar disorder is associated with an even higher rate of substance misuse, with up to 75% of individuals with this diagnosis found to have co-occurring substance use problems according to some estimates (15,16). The anxiety disorders, on the other hand, have a much more variable rate of comorbidity, depending upon the specific diagnosis. Nevertheless, substance use disorders co-occur at a much higher rate among individuals with anxiety disorders than among the general population (17,18). It is not clear, however, that this is true among individuals with social phobia (19). Despite recognition of the high cost of comorbidity and it prevalence, surprisingly little attention has been given to this problem until the last decade.

IMPACT OF CO-OCCURRING DISORDERS

The co-occurrence of psychiatric and substance use disorders has social, economic, and prognostic implications. When substance misuse and mental illness co-occur, the risk is great that, in general, the individual will not do as well as if the individual had not developed such a comorbid problem. Poverty and homelessness (20–22) are more frequent, as are the risks of being both victim and perpetrator of violent assault (23–29). It is important to note that while most violent crimes are not committed by the mentally ill, those that are perpetrated by members of this population are more likely to be committed by those with co-occurring substance use disorders. Furthermore, among the mentally ill, substance use also increases the risk of both accidental and homicide deaths (30–34). Finally, individuals with substance use disorders are less compliant with medication and more likely to drop out of treatment.

Comorbidity, in short, is associated with a worsened prognosis overall (35,36). Thus, although substance misuse per se is a source of significant social and medical morbidity, in the case of the mentally ill, the problems become magnified many times over.

TREATMENT STRATEGIES

Various models have been proposed for treating substance misusers with co-occurring psychiatric disorders. Three models, in particular—sequential, parallel, and integrated—summarize the approaches that have been used.

In the sequential model, first one, then the other condition is treated. The idea is that one condition must be controlled before the second can be adequately addressed. Of course, determining which condition to treat first presents a significant problem. Addiction treatment programs have not typically been designed to meet the needs of the mentally ill. Treatment providers have rarely been trained to recognize and treat the psychopathology of the dually disordered patient, and have the patients done well with many of the elements of typical treatment programs (37–39). Mental health providers, on the other hand, have been reticent to treat intoxicated patients and ill-equipped to handle them. The concern is often voiced of the potential for a lethal interaction between medication and any drug(s) of abuse the patient might be using. Furthermore, it is believed that patients will fail to respond to psychotropic medications if they continued to use alcohol and other drugs.

It could reasonably be argued that, where one condition is relatively minor compared to the other, such a model could be successful. Where both conditions pose significant or equally severe impairments, however, how to prioritize the sequence of treatment may become a nearly insurmountable problem.

In the parallel model, both conditions are addressed simultaneously, but in different programs with different staff. Poor communication between staff and the potential for the patient to receive mixed messages can be substantial risks here, however. Furthermore, treatment philosophies may clash and goals may be quite different between addiction and mental health treatment programs. Abstinence-only treatment programs have been unwilling, in the past, to encourage patients to comply with prescribed medications. Mental health providers, on the other hand, often strive for rigid adherence to medication regimens. In addition, staff often do not understand or, more importantly, approve, of each other's approach to treatment. While more workable than the sequential model, the parallel model, too, can pose serious problems in implementation and execution.

In the integrated model both conditions are treated simultaneously by providers knowledgeable about both conditions. Widespread use of this approach is made difficult because there is an insufficient number of treatment providers trained in both areas available to treat the large numbers of patients who need such help. Furthermore, especially when the patient suffers from a very serious mental illness, much responsibility may fall on the therapist for close supervision and case management, resulting in a high staff burnout rate (40).

To address some of the deficiencies inherent in existing programs, there has been a major initiative at the national level to educate mental health and addiction treatment providers in each others' specialties. Cross-training is promoted at national, state, and local levels. Special certification programs were developed to standardize and measure necessary levels of knowledge and skills, and to promote quality programming for treating individuals with co-occurring disorders. Where once treatment programs consisted, in many respects, of promoting the principles of Alcoholics Anonymous and other 12-step, self-help programs, it is now accepted that working with the dually disordered is a much more complex task than this. The treatment provider must help the patient gain an understanding of the patient's substance use disorder, of the patient's mental illness, and of the impact one has on the other. The provider must then help the patient develop strategies for recognizing and dealing with each. Strategies often include medication, especially for individuals with psychotic disorders.

SPECIAL ISSUES IN THE EVALUATION OF THE DUALLY DIAGNOSED

Evaluation and detoxification of substance misusers are well described elsewhere in the text. General issues pertinent to any substance misuser apply to the individual with co-occurring mental disorders as well, and are not covered here. Special considerations that apply primarily to individuals with co-occurring disorders, however, are described in detail.

The treatment provider should be familiar with, and capable of performing, a basic psychiatric evaluation. A comprehensive review of such is beyond the scope of this chapter and can be found in any general textbook of psychiatry. Among other things, however, such an evaluation should include a list of the patient's past diagnoses, if the patient is aware of what they may have been, past hospitalizations for psychiatric reasons, response to treatment, family history of psychiatric problems, and past medications and response to such. Furthermore, the interviewer should ask about suicidal ideation, both current and past, as well as attempts.

Although assuring the safety of the patient must always be a consideration in dealing with the chemically dependent, it is of paramount importance when dealing with the dually disordered individual. Patients in the immediate poststimulant dysphoric state or who are acutely under the influence of depressants such as alcohol, are at an increased risk of self-harm, regardless of whether or not they have a comorbid psychiatric condition (41–43). Both acute and chronic use of substances of abuse, however, vastly magnify the risk of suicide in individuals with depression and other chronic, severe mental illnesses, including schizophrenia and bipolar illness (35,36,42–55). Thus, at intake and at frequent intervals throughout the treatment process, the patient's risk of suicide must be assessed.

It is helpful to determine if the psychiatric symptoms predate the onset of the individual's substance misuse. It is also useful to learn if the patient's psychiatric condition improves, disappears, or worsens when the patient isn't using the substance(s). Unfortunately, it is often impossible to determine either of the above. If the patient uses substances daily and has no substantial periods of clean time, it will not be possible to know if the patient's symptoms improve with abstinence. Likewise, if the patient has been using for many years, memory may not prove accurate as to whether the substance misuse or the psychiatric symptoms came first.

Many treatment providers refuse to provide medication to the substance misusing psychiatric patient unless the patient is abstinent. This, of course, often leads to deterioration in function. Such worsening is not necessarily a result of the substance use, but often a consequence of the individual requiring the medication that is being withheld. There is much evidence that working with the patient and helping to treat the patient's psychiatric symptoms improves the chances of engaging the patient in addiction treatment, increases the likelihood of decreasing the patient's consumption of alcohol and other drugs, and can be successful in improving the patient's psychiatric symptoms, even if the patient continues to use substances. *As long as the patient can be treated safely, the patient should be treated.* The decision as to whether or not to medicate often comes down to the clinician's level of comfort and best judgment based on knowledge of the patient, the substance(s) the patient uses, the medication(s) the patient takes, and of the mental illness.

To adequately treat this complicated population, the treatment provider must be prepared to make judgments about the safety of using medications in patients who may be acutely under the influence of a substance, yet also on prescription drugs. For this reason, a brief review of some common medication–street substance interactions follows. For a more comprehensive review of drug–drug interactions, the reader is referred to Ciraulo (56).

PRINCIPALS OF TREATING THE DUALLY DISORDERED PATIENT

Comprehensive treatment for the dually disordered individuals demands that programming provide flexibility, repetition, and medication where necessary.

Flexibility

Traditional addiction-treatment programs stress abstinence as a contingency for participation, strict participation, and self-disclosure. Such demands may be neither attainable nor desirable when dealing with the dually disordered patient (57). Permitting the patient to participate only if the patient is abstinent may render the severely ill patient incapable of ever receiving the help the patient so desperately needs. Besides, if the patient could stay clean without the program, why would the patient need the program? Voices may be telling the patient to use, or the patient may need to use in order to tolerate the presence of others in the program. The patient may be at risk of dropping out of the program just when the patient needs it most; for example, if she relapses to cocaine use when her nightmares of rape return and abstinence is a requirement of attendance. Programs for the dually disordered must be able to adjust to accommodate the needs of the clientele they serve, and on an individual basis. This is a difficult population, requiring a prolonged period of engagement and a great deal of support in order to succeed.

Repetition

Repetition is necessary not just for the severely chronically mentally ill, but for all individuals with comorbid psychopathology. For the psychotic patient, interference from thought blocking and hallucinations may prevent the patient from comprehending and/or using skills suggested for decreasing substance use and avoiding high-risk situations. For the anxious individual presented above, as she experiences a resurgence of traumatic memories for which she is not yet adequately prepared to deal, she may forget all the coping skills that have been presented to her and resort to the one she knows best—her drug use. This doesn't mean she is "unready for treatment," or "not serious about treatment," or "resistive to treatment." This is a characteristic response of the dually disordered patient suffering from both posttraumatic stress disorder and cocaine dependence. As control of one problem appears to be within reach, symptoms of the other take center stage. A constant refocusing of attention and repetition of techniques for avoiding drugs and for dealing with psychiatric symptoms must be presented and practiced.

Medication(s) When Necessary

There is no question that some psychiatric conditions can be treated with psychotherapy, behavioral interventions, and other psychotherapeutic techniques. There has been considerable concern among addiction-treatment providers that jumping in quickly with a pill to treat a patient's discomfort sends a wrong message. That is, it signals that only a substance, not personal learned strengths, can help the individual through hard times. The problem with the latter reasoning, though, is that the addicted person with a co-occurring psychiatric condition who presents for treatment typically hasn't learned the alternate means of dealing with their anxiety of depression or they wouldn't be there in the first place. Furthermore, psychotherapeutic interventions take time to be learned and rehearsed, and, while effective for some psychiatric conditions, are not as beneficial for others (58–60). In addition, the dually disordered are at a high risk of dropout and relapse. Waiting for lengthy interventions to take effect may ensure the patient's early withdrawal from treatment long before a positive response can occur. Finally, especially for the severely mentally ill, medication is typically a first, not a last, choice. Early and vigorous intervention with medication where indicated with nonaddictive agents may help the patient stay in treatment and gain confidence that the patient will be treated so that the patient can learn the techniques the patient needs for dealing with the patient's substance use and psychiatric disorders.

However, when dealing with the dually disordered individual, when medication is deemed necessary, every effort should be made to use medications that (a) do not induce euphoria; (b) do not cause dependence; (c) are effective in the individual who is actively using substance(s) of abuse; and (d) are safe when used by the active user.

Psychiatric Conditions, Medications and Substances of Abuse

The following is not an exhaustive review of the literature, but an effort to give the reader a fair overview of the information available regarding medications that have proven safe and effective in relieving psychiatric symptoms in patients with psychiatric disorders who continue to actively use substances of abuse.

Depression, Antidepressants, and Mood Stabilizers

Depression and mania can be improved by active treatment with medication even when the patient continues to abuse alcohol, opiates, nicotine, and perhaps marijuana. To date, no medication has been shown to be unequivocally superior in improving such symptoms among individuals abusing psychostimulants.

Tricyclic antidepressants (TCAs), selective serotonin reuptake inhibitors (SSRIs), and nefazodone (Serzone) decrease depressive symptoms in unipolar depression in actively drinking alcoholics (61–63). The clinician is advised to make TCAs available in very limited supplies, however, to a member of this population, because of the potential for a lethal interaction with alcohol. Furthermore, recent data regarding hepatotoxicity with nefazodone may limit this agent's utility in this population until further information regarding the cause is available (64,65). Concomitant abuse of benzodiazepines, alcohol, cocaine, and marijuana is common among opiate-dependent individuals (66–68). This fact, and that much of the research available regarding opiate addicts comes from methadone-maintenance patients, makes it necessary to view data on this population with caution. Nevertheless, there is evidence that simply stabilizing opiate-dependent individuals on methadone improves depressive symptoms (69). Tricyclics, nefazodone, and SSRIs also improve depression in individuals actively using opiates. It should be noted, however, that abuse of TCAs by methadone-maintenance patients is a well-known phenomenon in clinics, thus such drugs should be used only with close supervision and with only small quantities available (70). Sertraline (Zoloft) may cause an initial rise in methadone levels, but they will normalize after a brief interval (71). Two brief reports regarding fluvoxamine (Luvox) and methadone, one positive and one negative, make it important for the treatment provider to use this drug with caution (71–73). There is some evidence that SSRI medication may case slight improvement in depressive symptoms in individuals actively abusing marijuana (74). Thus, erring on the side of the patient and offering to treat these symptoms with medication may be reasonable.

Lithium is relatively ineffective in treating substance dependent individuals with mania (75). Furthermore, there is an increased risk of toxicity with this medication if the individual is using alcohol or marijuana. Thus this mood stabilizer should be avoided in the dually disordered individual with bipolar disorder or cyclothymia

(76). Divalproex (Depakote) improves manic symptoms in actively drinking alcoholics with this disorder, although close observation of liver functions is advised (77). In one study, gabapentin (Neurontin) decreased alcohol abuse in bipolar patients with alcohol problems (78). Quetiapine (Seroquel) appears to decrease both manic symptoms and cocaine cravings in dually disordered patients with bipolar disorder and substance use problems (79). Carbamazepine (Tegretol) must be introduced and used with caution among individuals on opiates, because it lowers methadone levels, leading to withdrawal (56). Data are not currently available with newer anticonvulsants and olanzapine (Zyprexa).

Psychoses and Antipsychotic Medications

Actively treating psychoses improves retention in both addiction and mental health treatment and reduces psychotic symptoms. Despite concern about the possible interaction between antipsychotics and alcohol, there is little in the literature to support this worry. This may, of course, reflect the long-held habit of withholding antipsychotic medications when individuals with psychoses began to imbibe. Nevertheless, there does not appear to be a great deal of need for concern in treating psychotic symptoms with high doses of typical antipsychotics in active drinkers (56). High doses of typical antipsychotic medications in conjunction with cocaine appear to increase the risk of dystonic reactions and perhaps neuroleptic malignant syndrome (80–82). Whether or not this applies to other psychostimulants is not known. Risperidone (Risperdal), fluphenthixol (Fluanxol), olanzapine, and clozapine (Clozaril) improve symptoms and retention among schizophrenic psychostimulant abusers, although there has been a report of an untoward reaction with use of the latter (83–87). Nicotine acts in competition with some antipsychotic medications (such drugs as haloperidol, fluphenazine, olanzapine and clozapine) may be affected (reduced) by the presence of nicotine. It is important for the treatment provider to keep this in mind in the event that a patient is abruptly forced to discontinue the patient's routine dose of nicotine or to have it drastically reduced. The patient's level of neuroleptic medication may become suddenly far greater than it had been, resulting in greatly increased side effects and discomfort.

Anxiety Disorders

Treating anxiety symptoms in individuals actively using alcohol, psychostimulants, and opiates improves retention in treatment and provides some degree of symptom relief. Benzodiazepines are among the top three most-abused prescription drugs in the United States and may be abused by nearly half of individuals seeking treatment for substance misuse (88). These facts, and that there is some evidence of a disinhibiting effect of some benzodiazepines when used by alcohol-dependent individuals, serve as relative, not

TABLE 56.1. *Illicit drug effects on psychotherapeutic agents*

	Medications in psychotic disorders	Medications in mania	Medications in depression	Medications in anxiety disorders
Psychostimulant	↑ NMS and dystonia with typical antipsychotics; risperidone, fluphenthixol, olanzapine, clozapine helpful in symptom reduction	↑ NMS and dystonia with typical antipsychotics; improved with quietiapine	N.D.	N.D.
Opiates	N.D.	Carbamazepine may decrease methadone levels	Methadone alone improves symptoms; TCAs[a], nefazodone[b], SSRIs helpful[c]	↑ risk of fatal interaction with benzodiazepines
Alcohol	Typical and atypicals appear effective	↑ Toxicity with lithium; improves with valproate and gabapentin	TCA, SSRI, nefazodone helpful[b]	TCA, SSRI, venlofaxine;[d] increase risk violence/fatality with some benzodiazepines
Marijuana		↑ Toxicity with lithium	± with SSRI	N.D.

[a]Risk of abuse of TCAs in methadone clinics.
[b]Risk of hepatotoxicity; see text.
[c]See text re: issue with fluvoxamine.
[d]Hepatically metabolized; observe liver functions.
Abbreviations: N.D. = no data; NMS = neuroleptic malignant syndrome; SSRI = serotonin selective reuptake inhibitor; TCA = tricyclic antipsychotic.

absolute, contraindications to their use in this population. Alprazolam (Xanax), in particular, has been suggested as having this effect. This is not surprising, as the shorter the half-life, the greater the potential for abuse. If this class of medication is used, it is advisable to use such agents with caution, in the acute situation rather than as a maintenance strategy, under close supervision, and briefly, if at all possible (89–92). Furthermore, longer-acting agents should be used. TCAs, SSRIs, and venlafaxine (Effexor) are helpful in relieving anxiety symptoms in individuals with coexisting alcohol and anxiety problems (93,94). The existence of so many non–dependence-inducing, effective medications begs the question of necessity of using potentially addictive agents for the treatment of anxiety disorders for any but very short-term problems. However, the cautions regarding the use of these agents mentioned previously must be noted here. Furthermore, venlafaxine undergoes extensive hepatic metabolism, and close observation of liver functions is advised in individuals abusing alcohol. Many cases of fatal reactions have been reported of opiate-dependent individuals using and abusing benzodiazepines. Consequently, use of this class of agents for individuals with this problem is not advised. Rather, a trial of TCAs, nefazodone, or SSRIs, as in depression, is preferable (Table 56.1).

TREATMENT OUTCOME

How one defines "success" in the treatment of the addicted individual with a co-occurring psychiatric disorder is a source of ongoing discussion. There is a growing consensus that it is naive to believe that the only criterion

of "success" is absolute abstinence from nonprescription psychoactive substances. Yet there is a debate as to whether or not it is a necessary criterion at all. Is the individual with schizophrenia who used their entire disability check on crack cocaine each month and ended up in the hospital immediately thereafter last year, the so-called "revolving door patient" (95,96), who pays their rent, has a part-time job, and hasn't been hospitalized in 14 months, but who now occasionally smokes marijuana, a failure? Is she a success if she no longer drinks alcohol, but remains homeless, depressed, is repeatedly incarcerated, out of work, and makes occasional suicidal threats? If this is success, a new "yardstick" by which to measure our treatment outcome is necessary.

Arguably, outcome should be gauged on the basis of a number of prosocial behaviors, including reduction in length and frequency of hospitalization and incarceration where applicable, improved health, being domiciled, being employed, and reduction in amount and frequency of substance use, as well as a reduction in the problems associated with such. Abstinence alone would tell us almost nothing about the individual's level of "success" in terms of the indvidual's ability to function in society.

There are some tools available that look at multiple levels of functioning. Such instruments as the Addiction Severity Index (ASI), although valuable for research purposes, has limited practical value, however, because of the time it takes to administer. Furthermore, in severely mentally ill individuals, there is a question as to its validity. Work remains to be done to develop a more portable instrument for truly measuring the effectiveness of different approaches to the treatment of the dually disordered patient.

CONCLUSION

Individuals with both substance use and psychiatric disorders constitute a substantial and difficult to treatment subsection of the addiction population. Addressing only the substance use predicts a poorer outcome for other disorders including early relapse to alcohol and other drug use. Early and vigorous treatment for each condition should be initiated, including use of medications where indicated. In the latter case, care must be taken that medications used should be proved safe in the individual actively abusing alcohol and other substances, effective in treating the psychiatric condition when the individual is actively using, and nonaddictive where at all possible.

Much remains to be done to demonstrate that one therapeutic modality is clearly superior to another for the treatment specific comorbid conditions, though studies are underway. It is clear, however, that this complicated and diverse population will present challenges for the treatment community for some time to come.

REFERENCES

1. Brower KJ, ALdrich MS, Robinson EA, et al. Insomnia, self medication, and relapse to alcoholism. *Am J Psychiatry* 2001;158(3):399–404.
2. Wiess RD, Mirin SM. Substance abuse as an attempt at self medication. *Psychiatric Med* 1987;3:357–367.
3. Khantzian EJ. The self-medication hypothesis of addictive disorders: focus on heroin and cocaine dependence. *Am J Psychiatry* 1985;142(11):1259–1264.
4. Curran GM, Glynn HA, Kirchner J, et al. Depression after alcohol treatment as a risk factor for relapse among male veterans. *J Subst Abuse Treat* 2000;19(3):259–265.
5. Driessen M, Meier S, Hill A, et al. The course of anxiety, depression and drinking behaviors after completed detoxification in alcoholics with and without comorbid anxiety and depressive disorders. *Alcohol Alcohol* 2001;36(3):249–255.
6. Sciacca K. On co-occurring addictive and mental disorders: a brief history of the origins of dual diagnosis treatment and program development (an invited response). *Am J Orthopsychiatry* 1996;66:3.
7. Drake RE, Xie H, McHugo GJ, et al. Dual diagnosis: fifteen years of progress. *Psychiatric Serv* 2000;51(9):1126–1129.
8. National Institute on Drug Abuse. *Drug abuse cost to society set at $97.7 billion.* Rockville, MD: National Institutes of Health, 1998:1, 12–13.
9. National Institutes of Health. *The impact of mental illness on society.* Bethesda, MD: National Institute of Mental Health, 2001:3.
10. Regier DA, Farmer ME, Rae DS, et al. Comorbidity of mental disorders with alcohol and other drug abuse: results from the Epidemiological Catchment Area study. *JAMA* 1990;264(19):2511–2518.
11. United States Department of Health and Human Services. *Mental health: a report of the surgeon general.* Rockville, MD: Author, 1999.
12. Modestin J, Nussbaumer C, Angst K, et al. Use of potentially abusive psychotropic substances in psychiatric inpatients. *Eur Arch Psychiatry Clin Neurosci* 1997;247(3):146–153.
13. Mueser KT, Yarnold PR, Levinson DR, Singh H, et al. Prevalence of substance abuse in schizophrenia: demographic and clinical correlates. *Schizophr Bull* 1990;16(1):31–54.
14. Chouljian JL, Shumway M, Balancio E, et al. Substance use among schizophrenic outpatients: prevalence, course, and relation to functional status. *Ann Clin Psychiatry* 1995;7(1):19–24.
15. Winokur G, Coryell W, Akiskal H, et al. Manic depressive (bipolar) disorder: the course in light of a prospective ten-year follow-up of 131 patients. *Acta Psychiatr Scand* 1994;89(2):102–110.
16. Tohen M, Zarate CAJ. Bipolar disorder and comorbid substance use disorder. In: Goldberg JF, Harrow M, eds. *Bipolar disorders: clinical course and outcome.* Washington, DC: American Psychiatric Press, 1999:171–184.
17. Walfish S, Massey R, Krone A. Anxiety and anger among abusers of different substances. *Drug Alcohol Depend* 1990;25(3):253–256.
18. Merikangas KR, Angst J. Comorbidity and social phobia: evidence from clinical, epidemiologic, and genetic studies. *Eur Arch Psychiatry Clin Neurosci* 1995;244(6):297–303.
19. Crum RM, Pratt LA. Risk of heavy drinking and alcohol use disorders in social phobia: a prospective analysis. *Am J Psychiatry* 2001;158(10):1693–1700.
20. Mueser KT, Becker DR, Torrey WC, et al. Work and nonvocational domains of functioning in persons with severe mental illness: a longitudinal analysis. *J Nerv Ment Dis* 1997;185(7):419–426.
21. Zlotnick C, Robertson MJ, Tam T. Substance use and labor force participation among homeless adults. *Am J Drug Alcohol Abuse* 2002;28(1):37–53.
22. Sullivan G, Burnam A, Koegel P. Pathways to homelessness among the mentally ill. *Social Psychiatry Psychiatr Epidemiol* 2000;35(10):444–450.
23. Wenzel SL, Koegel P, Gelberg L. Antecedents of physical and sexual victimization among homeless women: a comparison to homeless men. *Am J Community Psychol* 2000;28(3):367–390.
24. Goldfinger SM, Schutt RK, Turner W, et al. Assessing homeless mentally ill persons for permanent housing: screening for safety. *Community Ment Health J* 1996;32(3):275–288.
25. Goodman LA, Dutton MA, Harris M. Episodically homeless women with serious mental illness: prevalence of physical and sexual assault. *Am J Orthopsychiatry* 1995;65(4):468–478.
26. North CS, Smith EM, Spitznagel EL. Violence and the homeless: an epidemiologic study of victimization and aggression. *J Trauma Stress* 1994;7(1):95–110.
27. Padgett DK, Struening EL. Victimization and traumatic injuries among the homeless: associations with alcohol, drug, and mental problems. *Am J Orthopsychiatry* 1992;62(4):525–534.
28. Zapf PA, Roesch R, Hart SD. An examination of the relationship of homelessness to mental disorder, criminal behavior, and health care in a pretrial jail population. *Can J Psychiatry* 1997;41(7):435–440.
29. Goodman LA, Dutton MA, Harris M. The relationship between violence dimensions and symptom severity among homeless, mentally ill women. *J Trauma Stress* 1997;10(1):51–70.
30. Modestin J, Ammann R. Mental disorders and criminal behavior. *Br J Psychiatry* 1995;166(5):667–675.
31. Modestin J, Berger A, Ammann R. Mental disorder and criminality: male alcoholism. *J Nerv Ment Dis* 1996;184(7):393–402.
32. Monahan J. The prediction of violent behavior: toward a second generation of

theory and practice. *Am J Psychiatry* 1984;141(1):10–15.

33. Beaudoin MN, Hodgins S, Lavoie F. Homicide, schizophrenia and substance abuse or dependency. *Can J Psychiatry* 1993;38(8):541–546.

34. Rasanen P, Tiihonen J, Isohanni M, et al. Schizophrenia, alcohol abuse, and violent behavior: a 26-year follow-up study of an unselected birth cohort. *Schizophr Bull* 1998;24(3):437–441.

35. Havassy BE, Arns PG. Relationship of cocaine and other substance dependence to well-being of high-risk psychiatric patients. *Psychiatric Serv* 1998;49(7):935–940.

36. Sonne SC, Brady KT, Morton WA. Substance abuse and bipolar affective disorder. *J Nerv Ment Dis* 1994;182(6):349–352.

37. Weiss RD, Najavits LM. Overview of treatment modalities for dual diagnosis patients. In: Kranzler HR, Rounsaville BJ, eds. *Dual diagnosis and treatment: substance abuse and comorbid medical and psychiatric disorders.* New York: Marcel Dekker, 1998:87–105.

38. Brooks AJ, Penn PE. Comparing treatments for dual diagnosis: twelve-step and self-management and recovery training. *Am J Drug Alcohol Abuse* 2003;29(2):359–383.

39. Ritsher JB, McKellar JD, Finney JW, et al. Psychiatric comorbidity, continuing care and mutual help as predictors of five year remission from substance use disorders. *J Stud Alcohol* 2002;63(6):709–715.

40. Pies RK, ed. *Assessment and treatment of patients with coexisting mental illness and alcohol and other drug abuse.* Rockville, MD: U.S. Department of Health and Human Services, 1995.

41. National Institute on Drug Abuse. *Facts about methamphetamine.* Bethesda, MD: National Institutes of Health, 1996:1.

42. Marzuk PM, Tardiff K, Leon AC, et al. Prevalence of cocaine use among residents of New York City who committed suicide during a one-year period. *Am J Psychiatry* 1992;149(3):371–375.

43. Roy A. Characteristics of cocaine dependent patients who attempt suicide. *Am J Psychiatry* 2001;158(8):1215–1219.

44. Pezawas L, Stamenkovic M, Jagsch R, et al. A longitudinal view of triggers and thresholds of suicidal behavior in depression. *J Clin Psychiatry* 2002; 63(10):866–873.

45. Prigerson HG, Desai RA, Liu-Mares W, et al. Suicidal ideation and suicide attempts in homeless mentally ill persons: age-specific risks of substance abuse. *Soc Psychiatry Psychiatr Epidemiol* 2003;38(4):213–219.

46. Murphy GE, Wetzel RD, Robins E, et al. Multiple risk factors predict suicide

in alcoholism. *Arch Gen Psychiatry* 1992;49:459–463.

47. Cornelius JR, Ihsan IM, Mezzich J, et al. Disproportionate suicidality in patients with comorbid major depression and alcoholism *American Journal of Psychiatry* 1995;152:358–364.

48. Blair-West GW, Cantor CH, Mellsop GW, et al. Lifetime suicide risk in major depression: sex and age determinants. *J Affect Disord* 1999;55(2–3):1717–178.

49. Petronis KR, Samuels JF, Moscicki EK, et al. An epidemiologic investigation of potential risk factors for suicide attempts. *Soc Psychiatry Psychiatr Epidemiol* 1990;25(4):193–199.

50. Mortensen PB, Juel K. Mortality and causes of death in schizophrenic patients in Denmark. *Acta Psychiatr Scand* 1990;81(4):372–377.

51. Harris EC, Barraclough B. Excess mortality of mental disorder. *Br J Psychiatry* 1998;173(7):11–53.

52. Schwartz RC, Cohen BN. Risk factors for suicidality among clients with schizophrenia. *J Consult Dev* 2001; 79(3):314–319.

53. Gut-Fayand A, Dervaux A, Olie J-P, et al. Substance abuse and suicidality in schizophrenia: a common risk factor linked to impulsivity. *Psychiatry Res* 2001;102(1):65–72.

54. DeHert M, Kwame M, Peuskens J. Risk factors for suicide in young people suffering from schizophrenia: a long-term follow-up study. *Schizophr Res* 2001;47(2):127–134.

55. Kessing LV. The effect of comorbid alcoholism on recurrence in affective disorder: a case register study. *J Affect Disord* 1999;53(1):49–55.

56. Ciraulo DA, Shader RI, Greenblatt DJ, et al., eds. *Drug interactions in psychiatry.* Baltimore, MD: Williams & Willkins, 1995.

57. Dennison SJ. *Handbook of the dually diagnosed patient: psychiatric and substance use disorders.* Baltimore, MD: Lippincott Williams & Wilkins, 2003.

58. Thase ME, Friedman ES, Fasiczka AL, et al. Treatment of men with major depression: a comparison of sequential cohorts treated with either cognitive-behavioral therapy or newer generation antidepressants. *J Clin Psychiatry* 2000;61(7):466–472.

59. Mercier MA, Stewart JW, Quitkin FM. A pilot sequential study of cognitive therapy and pharmacotherapy of atypical depression. *J Clin Psychiatry* 1992;53(5):166–170.

60. Thase ME, Greenhouse JB, Frank E, et al. Treatment of major depression with psychotherapy or psychotherapy–pharmacotherapy combinations. *Arch Gen Psychiatry* 1997;54(11):989–991.

61. McGrath PJ, Nunes EV, Stewart JW,

et al. Imipramine treatment of alcoholics with primary depression: a placebo-controlled clinical trial. *Arch Gen Psychiatry* 1996;535(3):232–240.

62. Cornelius JR, Sallou IM, Ehler JG, et al. Fluoxetine in depressed alcoholics: a double-blind, placebo-controlled trial. *Arch Gen Psychiatry* 1997;54(8):700–705.

63. Roy-Byrne PP, Pages KP, Russo JE, et al. Nefazodone treatment of major depression in alcohol dependent patients: a double-blind placebo-controlled trial. *J Clin Psychopharmacol* 2000;20(2): 129–136.

64. Aranda-Michel J, Koehler A, Beharano P, et al. Nefazodone-induced liver failure: report of three cases. *Ann Intern Med* 1999;130(4):285–288.

65. Schirren CA, Baretton G. Nefazodone-induced acute liver failure. *Am J Gastroenterol* 2000;95(6):1596–1597.

66. Weiss RD, Martinez-Raga J, Hufford C. The significance of a coexisting opioid use disorder in cocaine dependence: an empirical study. *Am J Drug Alcohol Abuse* 1996;22(2):173–184.

67. Kidorf M, Brooner RK, King VL, et al. Concurrent validity of cocaine and sedative dependence diagnoses in opioid-dependent outpatients. *Drug Alcohol Depend* 1996;42(2):117–123.

68. Brooner RK, King VL, Kidorf M, et al. Psychiatric and substance use comorbidity among treatment seeking opioid abusers. *Arch Gen Psychiatry* 1997; 54(1):71–80.

69. Petrakis I, Carroll KM, Nich C, et al. Fluoxetine treatment of depressive disorders in methadone maintained opioid addicts. *Drug Alcohol Depend* 1998;50(3):221–226.

70. Delisle JD. A case of amitriptyline abuse. *Am J Psychiatry* 1990;147(10):1377–1378.

71. Hamilton SP, Nunes EV, Janal M, et al. The effect of sertraline on methadone plasma levels in methadone maintenance patients. *Am J Addict* 2000;9(1): 63–69.

72. DeMaria PA, Serota RD. A therapeutic use of the methadone fluvoxamine drug interaction. *J Addict Dis* 1999;18(4):5–12.

73. Alderman CP, Frith PA. Fluvoxamine-methadone interaction. *Aust N Z J Psychiatry* 1999;33(1):99–101.

74. Cornelius JR, Salloum IM, Haskett RF, et al. Fluoxetine versus placebo for the marijuana use of depressed alcoholics. *Addict Behav* 1999;24(1):111–114.

75. Nunes EV, McGrath PJ, Wager S, et al. Lithium treatment for cocaine abusers with bipolar spectrum disorders. *Am J Psychiatry* 1990;147(5):655–657.

76. Sarid-Segal O, Creelman WL, Ciraulo DA, et al. Lithium. In: Ciraulo DA,

Shader RI, Greenblatt DJ, et al., eds. *Drug interactions in psychiatry.* Baltimore, MD: Williams & Wilkins, 1995:175–213.

77. Brady KT, Sonne SC, Anton R, et al. Valproate in the treatment of acute bipolar affective episodes complicated by substance abuse: a pilot study. *J Clin Psychiatry* 1995;56(3):118–121.

78. Perugi G, Toni C, Frare F, et al. Effectiveness of adjunctive gabapentin in resistant bipolar disorder: is it due to anxious alcohol abuse comorbidity? *J Clin Psychopharmacol* 2002;22(6):584–591.

79. Brown ES, Netjek VA, Perantie DC, et al. Quetiapine in bipolar disorder and cocaine dependence. *Bipolar Disord* 2002;4(6):406–411.

80. van Harten PN, van Trier JC, Horwitz EH, et al. Cocaine as a risk factor for neuroleptic-induced acute dystonia. *J Clin Psychiatry* 1998;59(3):128–130.

81. Cardoso FE, Jankovic J. Cocaine-related movement disorders. *Move Disord* 1993;8(2):175–178.

82. Akpaffiong MJ, Ruiz P. Neuroleptic malignant syndrome: a complication of neuroleptics and cocaine abuse. *Psychiatric Q* 1991;62(4):299–309.

83. Grabowski J, Rhoades H, Silverman P, et al. Risperidone for the treatment of cocaine dependence: randomized, double-blind trial. *J Clin Psychopharmacol* 2000;20(3):305–310.

84. Newton TF, Ling W, Kalechstein AD, et al. Risperidone pre-treatment reduces the euphoric effects of experimentally administered cocaine. *Psychiatry Res* 2001;102(3):227–233.

85. Farren CK, Hameedi FA, Rosen MA, et al. Significant interaction between clozapine and cocaine in cocaine addicts. *Drug Alcohol Depend* 2000;59(2):153–163.

86. Littrell KH, Petty RG, Hilligoss NM, et al. Olanzapine treatment for patients with schizophrenia and substance abuse. *J Subst Abuse Treat* 2001;21(4):217–221.

87. Conley RR, Kelly DL, Gale EA. Olanzapine response in treatment refractory schizophrenia patients with a history of substance abuse. *Schizophr Res* 1998;33(1–2):95–101.

88. Malcolm R, Brady KT, Johnston AL, et al. Types of benzodiazepines abused by chemically dependent inpatients. *J Psychoactive Drugs* 1993;25(4):314–319.

89. Kosten TR, Fontana A, Sernyak MJ, et al. Benzodiazepine use in posttraumatic stress disorder among veterans with substance abuse. *J Nerv Ment Dis* 2000;188(7):454–459.

90. Chilcoat HD, Breslau N. Posttraumatic stress disorder and drug disorders: testing causal pathways. *Arch Gen Psychiatry* 1998;55(10):913–917.

91. Nunes EV, McGrath PJ, Quitkin FM. Treating anxiety in patients with alcoholism. *J Clin Psychiatry* 1995;56 (Suppl 2):3–9.

92. Ciraulo DA, Nace EP. Benzodiazepine treatment of anxiety or insomnia in substance abuse patients. *Am J Addict* 2000;9(4):276–284.

93. Keller MB. The long-term clinical course of generalized anxiety disorder. *J Clin Psychiatry* 2002;63(Suppl 8):11–16.

94. Gorman JM. Treatment of generalized anxiety disorder. *J Clin Psychiatry* 2002;63(Suppl 8):17–23.

95. Haywood TW, Kravitz HM, Grossman LS, et al. Predicting the "revolving door": phenomenon among patients with schizophrenia, schizoaffective, and affective disorders. *Am J Psychiatry* 1995;152(6):856–861.

96. Birmingham L. Between prison and the community: the "revolving door psychiatric patient" of the nineties. *Br J Psychiatry* 1999;174(5):378–379.

HIV Infection and AIDS

CHAPTER 57

Epidemiology and Emerging Public Health Perspectives

DON C. DES JARLAIS, HOLLY HAGAN,
AND SAMUEL R. FRIEDMAN

Human immunodeficiency virus (HIV, the virus that causes acquired immunodeficiency syndrome [AIDS]) has dramatically increased the adverse health consequences of injecting drug use, not only for the individual user, but also for user's sexual partners and children, and for the community as a whole. Multiperson use ("sharing") of the needles and syringes used to inject illicit psychoactive drugs is a relatively efficient means of transmitting HIV. Most injecting drug users (IDUs) are sexually active, so IDUs infected with HIV can serve as a source of heterosexual transmission of HIV to noninjecting sexual partners. HIV can also be transmitted from mother to child, both perinatally and through breast-feeding. If untreated, HIV almost invariably leads to AIDS and then to death. There are now effective medications to control (but not cure) HIV infection; however, these medications do not work for everyone. HIV resistance to the medications is a serious problem, severe side effects can occur, and the medications and associated treatment monitoring are quite expensive.

The problem of HIV infection among IDUs has lead to greatly increased research on injecting drug use, some notable successes in programs to prevent HIV infection among IDUs, and the emergence (but not complete acceptance) of a new public health perspective on illicit drug injection.

This chapter reviews the current epidemiology of HIV among IDUs and describes the emerging public health perspective on illicit drug injection. The appropriate starting point is a brief consideration of the globalization of illicit drug injection itself.

THE GLOBAL EPIDEMIC OF ILLICIT DRUG INJECTION

The injection of illicit psychoactive drugs has been reported in 121 different countries (1). There are now an estimated 5 million persons throughout the world who inject illicit drugs (2), and this number is probably growing rapidly. While there is still much to be learned about the international diffusion of illicit drug injection, the following factors appear to be important:

1. There has been substantial international growth in the use of "licit" psychoactive drugs. Use of nicotine and alcohol has spread to many areas of the world where these psychoactive drugs are not part of the traditional culture (3–5). Nonmedical psychoactive drug use as a whole, and not simply illicit psychoactive drug use, has been increasing over the last several decades.
2. The globalization of the world economy. Improvements in communication and transportation and reductions in trade barriers have led to great increases in international trade (6). These same developments also facilitate international trade in illicit drugs.
3. Economies of scale in illicit drug production. The very large profit margins possible in the sale of illicit addicting substances also means that substantial profits can be made selling these drugs, even to "poor" people. The large profit margins from selling illicit drugs in industrialized countries can be used to underwrite the development of new markets in developing countries. The economics of the international distribution of illicit drugs particularly facilitate the development of

domestic drug markets in producing and transit countries.

4. Injecting produces a strong drug effect as a result of the rapid increase in the concentration of the drug in the brain. Injecting is also highly cost-efficient in that almost all the drug is actually delivered to the brain. On these grounds, intravenous injection can be considered a technologically superior method of psychoactive drug administration. Inexpensive technological advances tend to disperse widely and are very difficult (though not impossible) to reverse (7).

While it is certainly possible to improve current efforts to reduce the supplies of illicit psychoactive drugs, the effectiveness of such efforts is likely to vary across time and place, so that public health officials should plan in terms of further worldwide increases in illicit psychoactive drug injection, with the potential for severe public health consequences, including transmission of blood-borne pathogens such as HIV.

The global spread of illicit drug injection has meant that many countries are now trying to cope with epidemics of both illicit drug injection and HIV among injecting drug users. Russia is a prime example of a country now facing these simultaneous epidemics (8). These two global epidemics, in combination with the increased research on illicit drug injection have, however, created opportunities for countries to learn from the experiences (both positive and negative) of others.

HIV INFECTION AMONG INJECTING DRUG USERS

HIV has been reported among IDUs in more than 80 countries (1). This is a substantial increase over the 59 countries with HIV infection among IDUs in 1989 (9). In some European countries, such as Spain and Italy, injecting drug use has long been the most common risk factor for HIV infection and AIDS (10). In the United States, injecting drug use is associated with approximately one-third of the cumulative cases of AIDS (11), and half or more of the heterosexual transmission cases involve transmission from an injecting drug user.

HIV may be introduced into a local population of IDUs through a "bridge population," such as men who both have sex with men and inject drugs. This appears to be the way in which HIV was first introduced into the IDU population in New York City (12), which was also probably the introduction of HIV into the IDU population in the United States. Travel by IDUs may also serve to introduce HIV into local populations. Contrary to popular stereotypes, many drug injectors do travel, including internationally (13). International "drug tourism" (14) has been noted, although not yet well studied. Additionally, incarceration of IDUs from different geographic areas may also

contribute to spread of blood-borne viruses among IDUs (15).

Rapid Transmission of HIV Among Injection Drug Users

In many areas, HIV has spread extremely rapidly among IDUs, with the HIV seroprevalence rate (the percentage of IDUs infected with HIV) increasing from less than 10% to 40% or greater within a period of 1 to 2 years (16). Several factors are associated with extremely rapid transmission of HIV among IDUs: (a) lack of awareness of HIV and AIDS as a local threat; (b) restrictions on the availability and use of new injection equipment; and (c) mechanisms for rapid, efficient mixing within the local IDU population. Without an awareness of AIDS as a local threat, IDUs are likely to use each other's equipment frequently. Indeed, prior to an awareness of HIV and AIDS, providing previously used equipment to another IDU was likely to be seen as an act of solidarity among IDUs, or as a service for which one could legitimately charge a small fee.

There are various types of legal restrictions that can reduce the availability of sterile injection equipment and thus lead to increased multiperson use ("sharing") of drug-injection equipment. In some jurisdictions, medical prescriptions are required for the purchase of needles and syringes. Possession of needles and syringes can also be criminalized as "drug paraphernalia," putting users at risk of arrest if needles and syringes are found in their possession. In some jurisdictions, drug users have also been prosecuted for possession of drugs based on the minute quantities of drugs that remain in a needle and syringe after it was used to inject drugs. In addition to the possible legal restrictions on the availability of sterile injection equipment, the actual practices of pharmacists and police can create important limits. Even if laws permit sales of needles and syringes without prescriptions, pharmacists may choose not to sell without prescriptions, or not to sell to anyone who "looks like a drug user." Similarly, police may harass drug users found carrying injection equipment, even if there are no laws criminalizing the possession of narcotics paraphernalia.

"Shooting galleries" (places where IDUs can rent injection equipment, which is then returned to the gallery owner for rental to other IDUs), "dealer's works" (injection equipment kept by a drug seller, which can be lent to successive drug purchasers), and "hit doctors" (persons, often drug users themselves, who inject others, typically using the same needle and syringe for successive clients) are all examples of situations that provide rapid, efficient mixing within an IDU population. The "mixing" is rapid in that many IDUs may use the gallery or the dealer's injection equipment within very short periods of time. Several studies indicate that the infectiousness of HIV is many times greater in the 2- to 3-month period after initial infection, than in the long "latency" period between initial infection and the development of severe immunosuppression (17). Thus, the concentration of new infections in these settings may synergistically interact with continued mixing and lead to highly infectious IDUs transmitting HIV to a large number of other drug injectors. "Efficient" mixing refers to the sharing of drug-injection equipment with little or no restriction upon whom shares with whom. Thus, efficient mixing serves to spread HIV across potential social boundaries, such as friendship groups, which otherwise might have served to limit transmission.

New York City experienced the first epidemic of very rapid transmission of HIV among IDUs, beginning in the late 1970s (18) and reaching 50% prevalence (half of the IDUs infected with HIV) by the early 1980s. This was followed by rapid spread in a number of Western European countries, particularly in Italy and Spain (19). Bangkok, Thailand, was the first city in a developing country to experience rapid spread of HIV among IDUs, with prevalence increasing from 2% in late 1988 to more than 40% by late 1989 (20). The most recent rapid spread of HIV among IDUs occurred in Eastern Europe, Russia, and the newly independent states of the former Soviet Union, and in parts of Asia, including China and Vietnam (8).

HIV AND AIDS PREVENTION FOR INJECTION DRUG USERS

Early Studies

The common stereotype that IDUs are not at all concerned about health led to initial expectations that they would not change their behavior because of AIDS. In sharp contrast to these expectations, reductions in risk behavior were observed among IDU participants in a wide variety of early prevention programs, including outreach/bleach distribution (21,22), "education only" (23,24), drug abuse treatment (25), syringe exchange (26), increased over-the-counter sales of injection equipment (27,28), and HIV counseling and testing (29,30).

It is also important to note that there is evidence that IDUs will reduce HIV risk behavior in the absence of any specific prevention program. IDUs in New York City reported risk reduction prior to the implementation of any formal HIV prevention programs (31,32). IDUs had learned about AIDS through the mass media and the oral communication networks within the drug-injecting population (31,32), and the illicit market in sterile injection equipment expanded to provide additional equipment (33).

Current Status of Research on Preventing HIV Among Injecting Drug Users

There are numerous difficulties in evaluating HIV prevention programs for IDUs or any other group at risk for HIV

infection. Random assignment to long-term prevention programs is often very difficult. The use of new HIV infections as an outcome measure (rather than self-reported behavior change) requires either very large samples or a geographic area with high HIV incidence. It is unethical not to provide some form of intervention to the comparison group. If a program is implemented on a large-scale, the effects may extend to possible comparison groups, for example, IDUs using a syringe exchange program may then give the sterile injection equipment to other IDUs who are not directly using the syringe exchange program.

Despite these methodological problems, there is a strong scientific agreement that programs to reduce injection risk behavior and prevent HIV infection among IDUs can be effective. The National Institutes of Health convened a Consensus Development Conference to examine the evidence for interventions to reduce HIV risk behavior among different groups (34). Three types of interventions were determined to be effective in reducing drug injection-related risk behavior:

1. Community/street outreach programs
2. Programs to increase access to sterile injection equipment
3. Long-term drug-abuse treatment programs

Table 57.1 provides an example of each of these types of programs, along with HIV incidence data from IDUs who participated in the program and a comparison group of IDUs who did not participate in the program (35–37). All of these programs show dramatically lower HIV incidence among the program participants than among the comparison groups. Note, also that each of the studies was conducted during a time of high HIV incidence in the city, and, at the time, the programs were not implemented on a scale to reach all of the persons at high risk.

While there are many types of programs that reduce risk behavior among IDUs, there is no program or set of programs that have eliminated HIV risk behavior in any population of IDUs (or in any other population at risk for HIV.) The term *residual risk behaviors* is used to denote risk behavior remaining in a population after multiple prevention programs have been implemented on a large (structural level) scale (38). The Amsterdam Research Group posed the problem of the amount of residual risk behavior from their work with injecting drug users (39). They noted that the percentage of IDUs reporting receptive sharing (injecting with a needle or syringe use by another person) had stabilized at approximately 30%. In the Baltimore AIDS Link to Intravenous Experience (ALIVE) cohort study, receptive sharing has stabilized at approximately 20% (40). Among participants in large U.S. syringe exchange programs, receptive sharing stabilized at 10% to 15% in the 1 month prior to interview (41). Among syringe exchange participants in Australia, 14% report sharing in the previous month (42). In the most recent New York City studies,

TABLE 57.1.

Intervention	Reference No.	Sample	Intervention	Outcome
Community/street outreach Chicago	37	641 HIV-negative IDUs	Indigenous Leader Outreach model—ex-addicts providing HIV education and counseling	• Decline in injection risk behavior from 100% to 14% reporting equipment sharing • Decrease in HIV seroconversion rate: 8.4/100 PY (1988) vs. 2.4/100 PY (1992)
Sterile syringe access	1	1,630 IDUs enrolled in 3 studies	New York City syringe exchange programs	• HIV incidence in exchange users 1.4–1.6/100 PY vs. 5.3–6.2/100 PY in nonexchangers • Nonuse of the exchange associated with a 3.4-fold increase in risk of HIV seroconversion
Drug treatment programs	36	255 IDUs (152 in-treatment and 103 out-of-treatment)	Outpatient methadone treatment in Philadelphia	• Over 18 months, 3.5% of in-treatment IDUs seroconverted to HIV-positive vs. 22% of out-of-treatment IDUs

Abbrivations: IDU = injection drug user; PY = person-years:

receptive sharing (in the previous 6 months) has stabilized, with approximately 30% of the IDU population reporting receptive sharing in the 6 months prior to interview (43). It does appear that current HIV prevention programs are likely to hit a floor effect for receptive sharing at 10% in the previous 1 month and 20% to 30% in the previous 6 months.

Preventing Epidemics of HIV among Populations of Injection Drug Users

Current programs for reducing HIV transmission among IDUs should be considered highly effective at the individual level because a very large number of IDUs will adopt "safer" injection practices, but not perfect, because a substantial minority of IDUs will continue to engage in injection risk behavior after exposure to the programs. This leads to the question of the effectiveness of the programs at the community level. Can such programs prevent epidemics of HIV among IDUs, or do the programs merely slow down and reduce the size of such epidemics? There is now more than 15 years of experience showing that these programs can prevent HIV epidemics among IDUs. There are a number of cities (44) and countries, such as

the United Kingdom (45) and Australia (46), where HIV infection has been limited to less than 5% of the IDU population and the rates of new HIV infections are less than 1% per year.

There have been three common characteristics (44) of such successful community-level prevention efforts:

1. Prevention efforts are begun early, while HIV prevalence is 5% or less.
2. Trusted communication is established between health-workers and the local community of IDUs (often through outreach efforts).
3. IDUs have very good access to sterile injection equipment (through syringe exchange or pharmacy sales, and without much police interference of IDUs access to and use of the sterile injection equipment).

Unfortunately, there have been several instances where prevention programs were implemented but failed to prevent local HIV epidemics among IDUs, with Vancouver, Canada, being the best-known example (47). Both street outreach and a syringe exchange program had been implemented in Vancouver, but the local injecting practices switched from heroin to cocaine use. Persons injecting heroin will typically inject once every 4 hours at most.

Cocaine injectors frequently binge, injecting every 15 or 20 minutes until the supply of the drug is exhausted. If binge injecting occurs in a group setting, then either very large numbers of needles and syringes are needed, or a substantial amount of sharing is likely to occur within the group. The number of syringes distributed by the local syringe exchange program in Vancouver was insufficient to contain HIV transmission with the change to cocaine as the primary drug. Thus, while it clearly is possible to prevent HIV epidemics among IDUs, the prevention programs need to be implemented on a sufficiently large scale and adapted to the local drug use practices.

Bringing High HIV Prevalence Epidemics Under Control

Once HIV seroprevalence reaches high levels (30% or more) in a population of IDUs, prevention of new HIV infections becomes much more difficult. With many IDUs capable of transmitting the virus, even modest rates of risk behavior and mixing lead to moderate to high HIV incidence rates, typically from 2% to 6% per year (19,38,39,48–51). These moderate to high incidence rates tend to keep prevalence high, and even after implementation of HIV-prevention programs, high seroprevalence epidemics have a strong self-perpetuating character. The extent to which incidence and prevalence can be reduced in high prevalence areas must be considered one of the more important questions in the epidemiology of HIV among IDUs in developed countries. As HIV continues to spread rapidly among IDUs in many developing countries (52), this question will also become of great importance in those areas. A brief survey of the current status of high seroprevalence epidemics among IDUs in developed countries shows both the self-perpetuating nature of these epidemics and some indications that, over long time periods, it may be possible to bring such epidemics under control. It is important to note that all of these areas have implemented multiple prevention programs, including legal access to sterile injection equipment, some form of community outreach and drug-abuse treatment.

Canada

Beginning in the early 1990s, Canada experienced several high prevalence epidemics in the East-Central region (Quebec and Ontario) and in the far West (Vancouver). The most recent data from the East-Central region shows "continuing HIV transmission," with incidence rates of 3.2 per 100 person-years to 7.0 per 100 person-years in different cities, and with higher incidence in the areas with higher prevalence (53). In Vancouver, recent incidence is also high, 3.4 per 100 person-years (51,54). Frequent cocaine use may be an important component of the continuing high incidence in these epidemics, because it is associated with incidence in both East-Central and Western Canada.

Western Europe

Beginning in the early and mid-1980s, high prevalence epidemics occurred in many cities in France, Italy, and Spain, with additional high prevalence epidemics in cities such as Amsterdam and Edinburgh; high prevalence epidemics recently developed in cities in Portugal (55). There has been considerable stability in the high prevalence epidemics in Europe over time. The most comprehensive data are from Italy, where there are seroprevalence data from multiple drug treatment centers in each of 12 regions, with a sample size of approximately 70,000 per year. There has been essentially no change in the national average seroprevalence, from 17% in 1996 to 16% in 2000. While there has been some year-to-year fluctuation in the high seroprevalence regions, for example, Sardinia, Lazio, Umbria, Emilia Romana, Trentino, and Lombardia, prevalence has not fallen below 20% in any of these regions.

In France, there has also been little change in the national seroprevalence data, with a very modest drop from 18% in 1996 to 16% in 1999. In Spain, there has been a small decrease; national average seroprevalence was 37% in 1996 and 34% in 2000. Barcelona, for which there are long-term data, experienced a moderate decrease, from 53% in 1993 to 44% in 2000 (56).

There are a few examples of declining HIV prevalence in Europe. For example, prevalence declined by approximately 30% from 1988 to 1995 in Geneva in conjunction with provision of methadone treatment (57). Injecting drug use and the numbers of new HIV cases among IDUs in Edinburgh declined with the very large expansion of methadone treatment in that city (58). Overall, however, the European data clearly demonstrate the self-perpetuating character of high prevalence epidemics among IDUs.

United States

Data from the U.S. show both the persistence of high prevalence epidemics and the possibility of bringing such epidemics under control. Quan et al. recently analyzed U.S. incidence studies conducted from 1978 to 1999 (50). They found (a) incidence is positively related to prevalence, and (b) incidence has generally been declining over time, including incidence among IDUs (16 studies among IDUs). Studies from specific high prevalence cities have also shown declines over time in incidence. In Baltimore, incidence declined from 4.5 per 100 person-years in 1988–1989 to 2 per 100 person-years in 1995–1997 (40). Incidence in Philadelphia also declined, from 3.0 per 100 person-years in 1988–1997 to 2 per 100 person-years currently (D. Metzger, personal communication).

The Centers for Disease Control and Prevention (CDC) conducted blinded seroprevalence studies of IDUs entering drug-abuse treatment from 1993 to 1997 that provide the most recent national trends for the United States (59).

There was substantial geographic variation. Prevalence remained constant at a low level—an average of 4%—in western cities (Denver, Los Angeles, San Francisco, and Seattle) and at a moderate level—an average of 10%—in southern cities (Atlanta, Baltimore, Miami, New Orleans, and San Juan, Puerto Rico). Prevalence declined modestly—from an average of 27% to 19%—in midwestern cities (Chicago, Detroit), and modestly—from an average of 38% to 30%—in northeastern cities (Boston, New York, Newark, NJ).

More recent data suggests continuation of this mixed pattern of modest decline and stability in high seroprevalence epidemics in the United States. Prevalence has declined to approximately 30% in Baltimore, (S. Strathdee, personal communication) and 10% in Chicago (N. Braine et al., in preparation), but appears to have stabilized at approximately 10% in San Francisco (B. Edlin, personal communication) and 30% in New Haven (60).

New York City may provide the most dramatic example of the possibility of bringing a high seroprevalence epidemic under control. HIV was introduced into the IDU population in New York in the mid-1970s, and spread rapidly during the late 1970s and early 1980s, reaching greater than 50% prevalence (61). Risk reduction/behavior change began shortly after AIDS was discovered in IDUs. News media coverage and social network communications lead to a widespread awareness of AIDS and how it was transmitted, and to increased use of sterile injection equipment (33). Prevalence then stabilized at approximately 50% and incidence at approximately 5% per year (18). In the early 1990s, HIV-prevention programs for IDUs were greatly expanded, and New York City has become one of the most important success stories in HIV prevention for IDUs. Since the early 1990s, HIV incidence among IDUs has declined from 5 per 100 person-years to 1 to 2 per 100 person-years, and prevalence has declined from 50% to approximately 15% (18,62,63).

The current evidence does suggest that it may be possible to bring large, high seroprevalence HIV epidemics under control. At best, however, this is a long-term process, with incidence falling below the rate at which HIV-seropositives are lost to the active drug-using population. Clearly, it is highly preferable to prevent the initial epidemics rather than to try to control them afterward.

CURRENT PROBLEMATIC ISSUES IN HIV PREVENTION FOR INJECTING DRUG USERS IN DEVELOPED COUNTRIES

Integrating Multiple Prevention Programs

While assisting drug injectors to practice safer injection and providing drug-abuse treatment to reduce drug injection per se are often perceived as contradictory strategies, in practice they have been complementary strategies. One of the most important lessons of the early outreach programs was that the process of teaching drug injectors how to practice safer injection uncovered previously hidden demand for entry into drug-abuse treatment. This unexpected demand for drug-abuse treatment led to a program in which New Jersey outreach workers distributed vouchers that could be redeemed for no-cost detoxification treatment (23). Drug users entering treatment, many of whom had never before been in drug-abuse treatment, redeemed more than 95% of the vouchers.

There are also examples of syringe exchange programs that have become important sources of referral to drug-misuse treatment programs. For example, the New Haven program reports 33% of the first 569 participants were referred to drug treatment (64). The Tacoma syringe exchange program has become the leading source of referrals to the local drug-treatment program (65). The "harm-reduction" philosophy used in many outreach/bleach distribution programs, and in most syringe exchange programs, emphasizes reducing drug injection as a preferred method for reducing the risk of HIV infection, as soon as the individual drug user believes that he or she is ready for such treatment. The "user-friendly" staff attitude that has been adopted in most syringe exchanges also emphasizes providing a variety of services to IDUs, including referrals to other health and social services, particularly to drug-abuse treatment. The capacity of outreach/bleach distribution programs and syringe exchange programs to make effective referrals to drug-treatment programs may depend primarily upon the availability of treatment in the local area, and whether the programs can afford the appropriate staff to make and follow through on referrals.

While much progress has been made in providing referrals from outreach programs to drug-abuse treatment programs, HIV prevention efforts in the United States are still hampered by a lack of "referrals" from drug-abuse treatment programs to bleach distribution and syringe exchange programs. While drug-abuse treatment programs lead to substantial and well-documented reductions in illicit drug use (66), it is unrealistic to expect that all IDUs who enter treatment programs will abstain from further illicit drug injection. Indeed, the majority is likely to fail to complete treatment and/or to use illicit drugs while in treatment. Some United States drug-treatment programs currently include information about the locations and hours of operation of local bleach distribution and syringe exchange programs as part of the "AIDS education" provided to all entrants into treatment. (Many European drug-treatment programs actually provide syringe exchange services on site.) In general, however, United States drug-treatment programs have not yet developed strategies for reducing the likelihood that persons who relapse back to drug injection will not become infected with HIV through sharing of drug-injection equipment.

Current Problematic Issues in Preventing HIV Infection Among Injecting Drug Users

Much has been learned in the last decade of research on prevention of HIV infection among IDUs. Most importantly, all studies to date show that the large majority of IDUs will modify their behavior to reduce the chances of becoming infected with HIV. The theoretical bases for HIV prevention efforts have expanded from "factual education" to psychological and social-change theories. Prevention programs are increasingly providing the means for behavior change (for safer injection and, less frequently, for reducing drug injection).

Despite the progress in terms of research findings, increasing sophistication of prevention programs, and actual reduction in HIV transmission, there still are a number of problem areas with respect to prevention of new HIV infections among IDUs in some industrialized countries—the United States in particular—and in many developing countries.

Provision of Prevention Services

The biggest single problem may simply be the scarcity of HIV prevention services for IDUs in the nation. In the United States, the Presidential Commission on the HIV Epidemic recommended in 1988 that drug-abuse treatment be provided to all persons who desire it. The U.S. National Commission on AIDS made the same recommendation in 1991 (67). The National Commission on AIDS also recommended the removal of "legal barriers to the purchase and possession" of sterile injection equipment. Although there has been some expansion of syringe exchange services in the United States in the last several years, the Commission's recommendations would appear as valid today as when they were initially made.

In many developing countries, drug addiction is not seen as a health problem, and there are few resources to provide either HIV prevention or drug-abuse treatment for IDUs.

Sexual Transmission of HIV

While there is highly consistent evidence that IDUs will make large changes in their injection risk behavior in response to concerns about AIDS, changes in sexual behavior appear to be much more modest. All studies that have compared changes in injection risk behavior with changes in sexual risk behavior found greater changes in injection risk behavior (68). A recent meta-analysis of programs to reduce sexual risk behavior among drug users showed that these programs have an average "modest" effect, but that adding additional components to basic prevention education does not lead to increased risk reduction (69). In general, IDUs appear more likely to make risk-reduction efforts (reduced numbers of partners, increased use of condoms) for "casual" sexual relationships rather than in "primary" sexual relationships (68).

The reasons for the difficulties in changing the sexual behavior of IDUs have not been fully clarified, but the problem appears in many different cultural settings, including IDUs in Asia, Europe, and South America, as well as in the United States (13). To place the problem in perspective, however, IDUs have undoubtedly changed their sexual risk behavior more than have noninjecting heterosexuals in the United States as a whole (70).

One factor that appears to be important in increasing condom use among IDUs is an altruistic desire to avoid transmitting HIV to a noninjecting sexual partner. In both Bangkok (71) and New York City (72), IDUs who know (or have reason to suspect) that they are HIV-positive are particularly likely to use condoms in relationships with sexual partners who do not inject illicit drugs. Most programs that have urged IDUs to use condoms have focused on the self-protective effects of condom usage. Appealing to altruistic feelings of protecting others from HIV infection may be an untapped source of motivation for increasing condom use.

Heterosexual transmission from IDUs to their sexual partners who do not inject drugs has occurred in the United States since the first heterosexual IDUs were infected with HIV. The use of crack cocaine is often associated with high frequencies of unsafe sexual behaviors. In cities like New York and Miami, where there are large numbers of HIV-infected IDUs who also use crack cocaine, the use of crack without injection drug use has itself become an important risk factor for infection with HIV (73). While intervening in the nexus of injection drug use, crack use, and unsafe sex will be quite difficult, one strategy that might be used is to provide prompt treatment for genital ulcerative sexually transmitted diseases such as syphilis. The presence of these ulcerative sexually transmitted diseases appears to greatly increase the likelihood of HIV transmission (74).

It is also worth noting that additional strategies are needed for increasing safer sex among IDUs who engage in male-with-male sexual activities. IDUs who also engage in male-with-male sex can act as a bridge population between non–drug-injecting men who engage in male-with-male sex and the larger IDU population. In many areas of the United States, HIV seroprevalence among men who engage in male-with-male sex is substantially higher than among exclusively heterosexual IDUs (74,75). There are indications of "slippage" back to high-risk sexual behavior among men who have sex with men in the United States (76,77) and Western Europe (78,79). If slippage back to unsafe sex should occur among men who have sex with men in the United States as a whole, this could lead to more HIV infection among IDU men who engage in male-with-male sex, followed by more transmission from these men to other IDUs.

HARM REDUCTION

The worldwide epidemic of HIV infection among IDUs has led to important conceptual developments on injecting drug use as a health problem. HIV and AIDS have dramatically increased the adverse health consequences of injecting drug use, and thus have led to seeing psychoactive drug use as more of a health problem and not just a criminal justice problem. At the same time, HIV infection can be prevented without requiring the cessation of injecting drug use. This potential separation of a severe adverse potential consequence of drug use from the drug use itself has encouraged analysis of other areas in which adverse consequences of drug use might be reduced without requiring cessation of drug use.

The ability of many IDUs to modify their behavior to reduce the chances of HIV infection has also led to new consideration of drug users as both concerned about their health and as capable of acting on that concern (without denying the compulsive nature of drug addiction).

These ideas have formed much of the basis for what has been termed the "harm-reduction" perspective on psychoactive drug use (80–83). This perspective emphasizes the pragmatic need to reduce harmful consequences of psychoactive drug use while acknowledging that eliminating psychoactive drug use and misuse is not likely to be feasible in the foreseeable future. A major strength of the harm-reduction perspective is its applicability to both licit (alcohol, nicotine) and illicit psychoactive drugs.

ACKNOWLEDGMENTS

Sections of this chapter were originally prepared as reports to the United Kingdom Department of Health and for the United States Congress Office of Technology Assessment.

REFERENCES

1. Des Jarlais DC, Stimson GV, Hagan H, et al. Emerging infectious diseases and the injection of illicit psychoactive drugs. *Curr Issues Public Health* 1996;2:102–137.
2. Mann J, Tarantola J, Netter T. *AIDS in the world.* Cambridge, MA: Harvard University; 1992.
3. Ambler CH. Drunks, brewers and chiefs: alcohol regulation in colonial Kenya 1900–1939. In: Barrow S, Room R, eds. *Drinking behaviour and belief in modern history.* Berkeley, CA: University of California Press, 1991: 165–183.
4. Mackay JL. The fight against tobacco in developing countries. *Tuber Lung Dis* 1994;75:8–24.
5. Peto R. Smoking and death: the past 40 years and the next 40. *BMJ* 1994; 309:937–939.
6. Friedman TL. *The Lexus and the olive tree: understanding globalization.* New York: Anchor Books, 1999.
7. Rogers E. *Diffusion of innovations,* New York: The Free Press, 1982.vol.3.
8. UNAIDS. *Report on the global HIV/AIDS epidemic.* Geneva: Joint United Nations Programme on HIV/AIDS, 2002.
9. Des Jarlais DC, Friedman SR. AIDS and IV drug use. *Science* 1989;245:578–579.
10. European Centre for the Epidemiological Monitoring of AIDS. *First quarterly report.* Geneva: World Health Organization, 1996.
11. Centers for Disease Control and Prevention. *HIV/AIDS surveillance report.* Atlanta: Author, 1995.
12. Des Jarlais DC, Friedman SR, Novick D, et al. HIV-1 infection among intravenous drug users in Manhattan, New York City, from 1977 through 1987. *JAMA* 1989;261:1008–1012.
13. Ball A, Des Jarlais DC, Donoghoe M, et al. *Multi-centre study on drug injecting and risk of HIV infection:* Geneva: World Health Organization, Programme on Substance Abuse, 1994.
14. Simons M. Drug tourism in Europe. *NY Times* 1994 Apr 20:A8.
15. Wright N, Vanichseni S, Akarasewi P, et al. Was the 1988 HIV epidemic among Bangkok's injecting drug users a common source outbreak? *AIDS* 1994; 8:529–532.
16. Des Jarlais DC, Friedman SR, Choopanya K, et al. International epidemiology of HIV and AIDS among injecting drug users. *AIDS* 1992;6:1053–1068.
17. Jacquez J, Koopman J, Simon C, et al. Role of the primary infection in epidemic HIV infection of gay cohorts. *J Acquir Immune Defic Syndr* 1994;7:1169–1184.
18. Des Jarlais DC, Friedman SR, Sotheran JL, et al. Continuity and change within an HIV epidemic: injecting drug users in New York City, 1984 through 1992. *JAMA* 1994;271(2):121–127.
19. Stimson GV, Des Jarlais DC, Ball A, eds. *Drug injecting and HIV infection: global dimensions and local responses.* London: UCL Press, 1998.
20. Vanichseni S, Choopanya K, Des Jarlais DC, et al. HIV among injecting drug users in Bangkok: the first decade. *Int J Drug Policy* 2002;13:39–44.
21. Thompson PI, Jones TS, Cahill K, Medina V. *Promoting HIV prevention outreach activities via community-based organizations.* Paper presented at the sixth international conference on AIDS, 1990, San Francisco, CA.
22. Wiebel W, Chene D, Johnson W. *Adoption of bleach use in a cohort of street intravenous drug users in Chicago.* Paper presented at the sixth international conference on AIDS, San Francisco, CA, June 1990.
23. Jackson J, Rotkiewicz L. *A coupon program: AIDS education and drug treatment.* Paper presented at the third international conference on AIDS, 1987, Washington, DC.
24. Ostrow DG. AIDS prevention through effective education. *Daedalus* 1989;118:229–254.
25. Blix O, Gronbladh L. *AIDS and IV heroin addicts: the preventive effect of methadone maintenance in Sweden.* Paper presented at the fourth international conference on AIDS, 1988, Stockholm, Sweden.
26. Buning EC, Hartgers C, Verster AD, et al. *The evaluation of the needle/syringe exchange in Amsterdam.* Paper presented at the fourth international conference on AIDS, 1988, Stockholm, Sweden.
27. Espinoza P, Bouchard I, Ballian P, et al. *Has the open sale of syringes modified the syringe exchanging habits of drug addicts?* Paper presented at the fourth international conference on AIDS, 1988, Stockholm, Sweden.
28. Goldberg D, Watson H, Stuart F, et al. *Pharmacy supply of needles and syringes-the effect on spread of HIV in intravenous drug misusers.* Paper presented at the fourth international conference on AIDS, 1988, Stockholm, Sweden.
29. Cartter ML, Petersen LR, Savage RB, et al. Providing HIV counseling and

testing services in methadone maintenance programs. *AIDS* 1990;4(5):463–465.

30. Higgins DL, Galavotti C, O'Reilly KR, et al. Evidence for the effects of HIV antibody counseling and testing on risk behaviors. *JAMA* 1991;266:2419–2429.

31. Friedman SR, Des Jarlais DC, Sotheran JL, et al. AIDS and self-organization among intravenous drug users. *Int J Addict* 1987;22:201–219.

32. Selwyn P, Feiner C, Cox C, et al. Knowledge about AIDS and high-risk behavior among intravenous drug abusers in New York City. *AIDS* 1987;1:247–254.

33. Des Jarlais DC, Friedman SR, Hopkins W. Risk reduction for the acquired immunodeficiency syndrome among intravenous drug users. *Ann Intern Med* 1985;103:755–759.

34. National Institutes of Health (NIH). *Proceedings on the NIH consensus development conference on interventions to prevent HIV risk behaviors.* Paper presented at the proceedings on the NIH consensus development on interventions to prevent HIV risk behaviors, 1997, Bethesda, MD.

35. Des Jarlais DC, Marmor M, Paone D, et al. HIV incidence among injecting drug users in New York City syringe-exchange programmes. *Lancet* 1996;348:987–991.

36. Metzger D, Woody G, McLellan A, et al. Human immunodeficiency virus seroconversion among in- and out-of-treatment drug users: an 18-month prospective follow up. *J Acquir Immune Defic Syndr* 1993;6:1049–1056.

37. Wiebel W, Jimenez A, Johson W, et al. Risk behavior and HIV seroincidence among out-of-treatment IDUs: four-year prospective study. *J Acquir Immune Defic Syndr Hum Retrovirol* 1996;12(3):282–289.

38. Des Jarlais DC, Friedman SR. Fifteen years of research on preventing HIV infection among injecting drug users: what we have learned, what we have not learned, what we have done, what we have not done. *Public Health Rep* 1998;113[1 Suppl]:182–188.

39. Coutinho R. *Interventions among injecting drug users: the Amsterdam experience.* Paper presented at the fourth science forum: research synthesis symposium on the prevention of HIV in drug abusers, 1997, Flagstaff, AZ.

40. Nelson K, Galai N, Safaeian M, et al. Temporal trends in the incidence of human immunodeficiency virus infection and risk behavior among injection drug users in Baltimore, Maryland, 1988–1998. *Am J Epidemiol* 2002;156(7):641–653.

41. Des Jarlais DC, McKnight CA, Eigo K, et al. National syringe exchange survey 2000. Paper presented at the North American syringe exchange convention, 2002, Albuquerque, NM.

42. National Centre in HIV Epidemiology and Clinical Research. *HIV/AIDS, viral hepatitis & sexually transmissible infections in Australia: annual surveillance report 2002.* Sydney, Australia: Author, 2002.

43. Des Jarlais DC, Perlis T, Arasteh K, et al. HIV among new injecting drug users in New York City, 1990–2001: divergence among race/ethnic groups. *AIDS* (submitted).

44. Des Jarlais DC, Hagan HH, Friedman SR, et al. Maintaining low HIV seroprevalence in populations of injecting drug users. *JAMA* 1995;274(15):1226–1231.

45. Stimson GV. AIDS and injecting drug use in the United Kingdom, 1987–1993: the policy response and the prevention of the epidemic. *Soc Sci Med* 1995;41(5):699–716.

46. Wodak A. *HIV epidemiology and prevention research in drug-using populations in Australia.* Geneva: Office of AIDS Research, National Institutes of Health, World Health Organization Substance Abuse Department, June 25–26, 1998.

47. Strathdee S, Patrick D, Currie SL, et al. Needle exchange is not enough: lessons from the Vancouver injection drug use study. *AIDS* 1997;11:F59–F65.

48. Friedman SR, Jose B, Deren S, et al. Risk factors for HIV seroconversion among out-of-treatment drug injectors in high and low seroprevalence cities. *Am J Epidemiol* 1995;142:864–874.

49. Nicolosi A, Correa L, Chiesa A, et al. Incidence and prevalence trends of HIV infection among IDUs in northern Italy, 1990–1994. *Int Conf AIDS* 1996;11(1):359.

50. Quan VM, Steketee RW, Valleroy L, et al. HIV incidence in the United States, 1978–1999. *J Acquir Immune Defic Syndr* 2002;31:188–201.

51. Spittal PM, Craib KJ, Wood E, et al. risk factors for elevated HIV incidence rates among female injection drug users in Vancouver. *CMAJ* 2002;166(7):894–899.

52. UNAIDS/WHO. *AIDS epidemic update: December 2002.* Geneva: Joint United Nations Programme on HIV/AIDS, 2002.

53. Hankins C, Alary M, Parent R, et al. Continuing HIV transmission among injection drug users in Eastern Central Canada: the SurvUDI Study, 1995–2000. *J Acquir Immune Defic Syndr Hum Retrovirol* 2002;30:514–521.

54. Craib KJP, Spittal PM, Wood E, et al. Risk factors for elevated HIV incidence among Aboriginal injection drug users in Vancouver. *CMAJ* 2003;168(1):19–24.

55. European Monitoring Centre for Drugs and Drug Addiction. *Annual report on the state of the drugs problem in the European Union and Norway.* Luxembourg: Author, 2002.

56. Perez K, Rodes A, Merona M, et al. *Behavioural surveillance among intravenous drug users (IDUs) out-of-treatment in Barcelona (Spain), 1993–2000.* Paper presented at the XIV international AIDS conference, 2002, Barcelona, Spain.

57. Broers B, Junet C, Bourquin M, et al. Prevalence and incidence of HIV, hepatitis B and C among drug users on methadone maintenance treatment in Geneva between 1988 and 1995. *AIDS* 1998;12(15):2059–2066.

58. Robertson R, ed. *Management of drug users in the community: a practical handbook.* New York: Oxford University Press, 1998.

59. Centers for Disease Control and Prevention (CDC). *HIV prevalence trends in selected populations in the United States: results from national serosurveillance, 1993–1997.* Atlanta: Author, August 2001.

60. Heimer R, Singer M. *Syringe access, use, and discard—the I-91 study.* Paper presented at the National Development and Research Institutes, 2003, New York.

61. Des Jarlais DC, Friedman SR, Novick DM, et al. HIV-1 infection among intravenous drug users in Manhattan. *JAMA* 1989;261(7):1008–1012.

62. Des Jarlais DC, Perlis T, Friedman SR, et al. Declining seroprevalence in a very large HIV epidemic: injecting drug users in New York City, 1991–1996. *Am J Public Health* 1998;88(12):1801–1806.

63. Des Jarlais, Perlis T, Arasteh, K, et al. "Informed Altruism" and "Partner Restriction" in the reduction of HIV infection in injecting drug users entering detoxification treatment in New York City, 1990–2001. *JAIDS,* 35(2), 158–166.

64. O'Keefe E, Kaplan E, Khoshnood K. *Preliminary report: city of New Haven needle exchange program:* New Haven, CT: Office of Mayor John C. Daniels, 1991.

65. Hagan H, Des Jarlais DC, Friedman SR, et al. Risk of human immunodeficiency virus and hepatitis B virus in users of the Tacoma syringe exchange program. In: *Proceedings of the National Academy of Sciences workshop on needle exchange and bleach distribution programs.* Washington, DC: National Academy Press, 1994.

66. Hubbard RL, Marsden ME, Rachal JV, et al., eds. *Drug abuse treatment: a national study of effectiveness.* Chapel Hill,

NC: The University of North Carolina Press, 1989.

67. National Commission on AIDS. *The twin epidemics of substance use and HIV.* Washington DC: Author, July, 1991.

68. Friedman SR, Des Jarlais DC, Ward TP. Overview of the history of the HIV epidemic among drug injectors. In: Brown BS, Beschner GM, National AIDS Research Consortium, eds. *Handbook on risk of AIDS: injection drug users and sexual partners.* Westport, CT: Greenwood Press, 1993:3–15.

69. Semaan S, Des Jarlais DC, Sogolow E, et al. A meta-analysis of the effect of HIV prevention interventions on the sex behaviors of drug users in the United States. *J Acquir Immune Defic Syndr* 2002;30[1 Suppl]:S73–S93.

70. Laumann EO, Gagnon JH, Michael RT, et al. *The social organization of sexuality: sexual practices in the United States.* Chicago: University of Chicago Press, 1994.

71. Vanichseni S, Des Jarlais DC, Choopanya K, et al. Condom use with primary partners among injecting drug users in Bangkok, Thailand and New York City, United States. *AIDS* 1993;7:887–891.

72. Friedman SR, Jose B, Neaigus A, et al. Consistent condom use in relationships between seropositive injecting drug users and sex partners who do not inject drugs. *AIDS* 1994;8:357–361.

73. Edlin BR, Irwin KL, Faruque S. Intersecting epidemics: crack cocaine use and HIV infection among inner-city young adults. *N Engl J Med* 1994;331:1422–1427.

74. Chiasson MA, Stoneburner RL, Hildebrandt DS, et al. Heterosexual transmission of HIV-1 associated with the use of smokable freebase cocaine (crack). *AIDS* 1991;5:1121–1126.

75. Maslow CB, Friedman SR, Perlis TE, et al. Changes in HIV seroprevalence and related behaviors among male injection drug users who do and do not have sex with men: New York City, 1990–1999. *Am J Public Health* 2002;92(3):382–384.

76. Koblin BA, Chesney MA, Husnik MJ, et al. High-risk behaviors among men who have sex with men in 6 U.S. cities: baseline data from the Explore Study. *Am J Public Health* 2003;93(6):926–932.

77. Stall R, Mills TC, Williamson J, et al. Association of co-occurring psychosocial health problems and increased vulnerability to HIV/AIDS among urban men who have sex with men. *Am J Public Health* 2003;93(6):939–942.

78. Piribauer F, Duer W. Trends in HIV seroprevalence, AIDS and prevention policy among intravenous drug users and men who have sex with men, before and after 1990 in Austria. *Eur J Epidemiol* 1998;14(7):635–643.

79. Wang J, Rodes A, Blanch C, et al. HIV testing history among gay/bisexual men recruited in Barcelona: evidence of high levels of risk behavior among self-reported HIV+ men. *Soc Sci Med* 1997;44(4):469–477.

80. Brettle RP. HIV and harm reduction for injection drug users. *AIDS* 1991;5:125–136.

81. Des Jarlais DC, Friedman SR, Ward TP. Harm reduction: a public health response to the AIDS epidemic among injecting drug users. *Annu Rev Public Health* 1993;14:413–450.

82. Des Jarlais DC. Harm reduction—a framework for incorporating science into drug policy [Editorial]. *Am J Public Health* 1995;85(1):10–12.

83. Heather N, Wodak A, Nadelmann E, et al, eds. *Psychoactive drugs and harm reduction: from faith to science.* London: Whurr Publishers, 1993.

CHAPTER 58

HIV-Related Medical Complications and Treatment

CHINAZO O. CUNNINGHAM AND PETER A. SELWYN

The advent of the epidemic of the acquired immune deficiency syndrome (AIDS) has posed new challenges for the field of substance-abuse treatment. Although the first cases of AIDS in the United States were reported in 1981 in homosexual or bisexual men (1,2), cases were soon identified in injection drug users (3). Since the early 1980s, the extent and nature of the AIDS epidemic, and the dynamics of transmission of human immunodeficiency virus-1 (HIV-1, which will be referred to as HIV for the remainder of this chapter)—the retrovirus that causes AIDS—have been closely linked with the phenomenon of injection drug use (3–7). Injection drug users now account for a growing number of AIDS cases in North America as well as in Europe and Asia (4,8–16). In certain regions in the northeastern United States, parts of eastern and southern Europe, and parts of China, substance users represent the largest proportion of current or newly reported AIDS cases (8–10,15,17). As of the end of 2001, 35% of all cases of AIDS reported to the U.S. Centers for Disease Control and Prevention (CDC) were directly or indirectly associated with injection drug use (11). The presence of HIV infection has been documented among substance users in Australia and parts of Latin America; the spread of HIV infection has also been described among injection drug users in the Russian Federation, Bangkok, and Myanmar (formerly called Burma), and may be anticipated in other areas as well (14,16,18–20). HIV infection has also been noted at increasing levels among substance users in the United States outside of the northeastern states, although the geographic distribution remains concentrated there at present (21). Despite the increasing use of nonparenteral routes for drugs commonly used by injection, injection drug users continue to represent a growing percentage of HIV infection and AIDS cases, in both industrialized and developing countries (11,15,16,20,22).

In addition to reported cases among substance users themselves, the role of injection drug use in the epidemic is reflected in AIDS cases involving heterosexual and perinatal transmission, in which the predominant number in the United States represents sexual contacts of injection drug users or children born to substance users (11). With more than half of all AIDS cases among women in the United States involving substance-using women or the female sexual partners of male substance users (11), it is clear that, especially among women, AIDS and substance use are virtually inseparable. This phenomenon has had important clinical and social implications, which are discussed in more detail later in the section "Psychosocial and Substance Abuse Treatment Issues."

Another feature of the AIDS epidemic among substance users in the United States is the concentration of cases among African American and Hispanic populations (11). Studies of HIV seroprevalence among substance users have also generally found an increased likelihood of HIV infection among African Americans and Hispanics (23–27). It has been suggested that this may be a result of the concentration of injection drug use in poor, inner-city areas, and perhaps to other behavioral or environmental factors that would place these populations at greater risk for substance use-related transmission of HIV (24). One study showed that the predominant exposure category for HIV infection among Hispanic men and women born in Puerto Rico was injection drug use. The study showed significant differences in exposure category among women of Hispanic ethnicity according to their place of birth, race, and other categories (28). The importance of heterosexual transmission of HIV in Hispanic women linked to sexual contact with substance users is also represented in those studies. Regardless of the underlying explanation for this phenomenon, the observed pattern of cases indicates the need for preventive and therapeutic interventions that are comprehensive, accessible, and culturally appropriate for at-risk populations of substance users.

As well as having distinct demographic and geographic characteristics, the epidemic of HIV infection among injection drug users in the United States has also had certain clinical and epidemiologic features that differ from those seen in other populations. For example, the infrequent occurrence of Kaposi sarcoma among substance users as compared with homosexual men with AIDS (29), and the increased risk of tuberculosis and severe bacterial infections seen in HIV-infected substance users (30–43), are epidemiologic observations that have immediate clinical relevance. Furthermore, the need for ongoing management of HIV-infected substance users with chronic medical therapies, often involving multiple medications or other interventions, raises important issues concerning patient adherence, coexisting substance use, and the relationship between primary medical care and substance abuse treatment in different treatment settings (44–52). These issues are even more critical with the complexity of therapeutic agents to treat HIV infection, which show great promise but which also require close followup and medical monitoring to be used effectively (53).

The role of injection drug use in the framework of HIV transmission behaviors has been defined largely by the importance of shared, contaminated injection equipment as a vector for the spread of HIV among substance-using populations (24–27,51,54,55). This in itself poses a challenge

to the substance-abuse treatment field, to address issues of risk behavior involving ongoing substance use, needle use, and needle sharing among injection drug users. In addition, important links have been made between nonparenteral substance use and other behaviors associated with transmission of HIV, for example, the relationship among cocaine use, prostitution, and sexually transmitted diseases in general, or between drug or alcohol use and unsafe sexual behavior—among both homosexuals and heterosexuals—as a consequence of these substances' disinhibiting effects on such behavior (56–63). The question has also been raised whether ongoing injecting or other drug use may accelerate the rate of progression to AIDS in HIV-infected persons, although existing data regarding this possibility is sparse (64–74). It should be noted, however, that injection drug users who continue to share injection equipment may be exposed to potentially more virulent or resistant strains of the virus, strains that may have undergone multiple mutations after being exposed to different antiretroviral medications. More likely though, the most important issues regarding substance use and HIV disease are that substance users are less likely to access regular HIV medical care, less likely to take antiretroviral medication, and less likely to be adherent to HIV medications (75–81). All of these factors undoubtedly lead to more rapid HIV disease progression. These issues highlight the complex and wide-ranging issues involving HIV infection and its clinical and programmatic implications for substance-abuse treatment.

AIDS AND HIV INFECTION: DEFINITIONS

The first portion of this chapter addresses basic issues regarding HIV infection and AIDS, including case definitions and certain clinical topics of general importance. The remaining sections of the chapter focus on clinical themes more specifically related to the management of substance users with HIV infection. This chapter is not intended to serve as a comprehensive review of the treatment for HIV infection or of the full range of AIDS-associated opportunistic infections and malignancies, for which the reader is referred to a number of excellent sources, including the Department of Health and Human Services' HIV/AIDS Treatment Information Services at http://www.hivatis.org or (800) 448-0440, and others (82,83). Rather, the intention is to establish the basic framework for understanding the clinical dimensions of HIV infection, with special reference to the manifestations and treatment of HIV infection among substance users.

Diagnosis of HIV Infection

HIV is now accepted as the causative infectious agent of AIDS (84). Previously referred to as human T-lymphotrophic virus type III (HTLV-III) (69), lymphadenopathy-associated virus (LAV) (85), or AIDS-associated retrovirus (ARV) (86), the virus is now denoted as HIV or HIV-1 in the current standard nomenclature (87).

Following exposure to HIV through sexual contact or blood-borne transmission, persons infected with HIV develop a characteristic serum antibody response. It is estimated that among those infected with HIV, HIV serum antibody typically is detectable within 1 to 4 months following primary infection, and 95% of infected individuals are expected to demonstrate a positive antibody test within 6 months following exposure, if not sooner (88–91). It has also been suggested that delayed seroconversion—up to almost 3 years—may occur in certain individuals, and even that HIV infection may not result in the production of serum antibody to HIV in some cases, but these have not been common or consistent findings (88–91). Because of the potentially variable time course of seroconversion, it is prudent to consider repeating the HIV antibody test, if initially negative, several times during a 12-month followup period, for patients whose presumed exposure to HIV may have occurred proximate to the time of the first antibody test. The standard procedure for HIV serum antibody testing involves a two-step process, including a screening test for HIV antibody (e.g., enzyme-linked immunoabsorbent assay [ELISA]) followed by a confirmatory test performed on the same specimen (e.g., Western blot immunoblot; immunofluorescence assay [IFA]). The ELISA must be reactive and the Western blot or IFA positive for the test to be considered positive for HIV antibody (92).

Reliable virologic markers of HIV activity or disease progression include tests for HIV serum antigen (p24) (93), viral culture (94), and, most importantly, commercially available assays ("viral load" tests) that measure quantitative plasma HIV ribonucleic acid (RNA) using molecular genetic techniques, including either genome amplification or signal amplification (95). The HIV antigen assays, while specific for HIV infection, generally are not sensitive enough to warrant their use in routine testing for HIV, especially because levels of p24 antigen appear to vary over the natural history of HIV infection (93,94). Viral culture remains primarily a research tool at the present time, and viral load measurements should not be used for the actual diagnosis of HIV infection (with the exception of suspected acute HIV seroconversion reactions, in which the HIV antibody is expected to be negative). Thus, as of 2004, the standard clinical test for detecting HIV infection in adults remains the HIV antibody test.

Diagnosis of AIDS

Since the first AIDS cases were reported in 1981 (1,2), several classification systems have been developed for surveillance and clinical purposes in order to establish case definitions for AIDS and to provide a framework for categorizing different manifestations of HIV infection (3,96–99) (Table 58.1). The original CDC AIDS case definition was promulgated primarily for epidemiologic

surveillance (3) and was restricted to a series of 10 opportunistic infections (expanded to 12 in an early revision) and 2 malignancies, which, when reliably diagnosed and in the absence of known causes of immunodeficiency, were considered indicators of AIDS. In 1987, the CDC issued a revised AIDS case definition, which expanded the number of AIDS-qualifying diagnoses, relying more explicitly on the use of laboratory tests for HIV, and permitting the inclusion of certain presumptively diagnosed indicator diseases as AIDS-qualifying in the presence of a positive HIV antibody test (or other laboratory tests confirming HIV infection) (98). The introduction of the revised AIDS surveillance case definition in 1987 resulted in a disproportionate increase in reported cases among injection drug users, women, and minorities (100,101); more than 40% of AIDS cases among injection drug users reported in 1988 in the United States met only the revised case definition criteria, compared with 23% of all other cases. This phenomenon may reflect the inclusion in the revised case definition of certain opportunistic infections (e.g., extrapulmonary tuberculosis) (39), which in developed countries most commonly affect substance users with HIV infection. Another possibility that might contribute to this phenomenon is that substance users' lack of access to or avoidance of medical care may result in a decreased likelihood of definitive diagnoses being made.

The CDC issued the most recent HIV clinical classification, the 1993 *Classification System for HIV Infection and Expanded Surveillance Case Definition for AIDS Among Adolescents and Adults* (99). The expanded AIDS surveillance case definition includes pulmonary tuberculosis, recurrent pneumonia, and invasive cervical cancer. As in previous revisions (100), the introduction of the most current surveillance classification resulted in a disproportionately larger increment of new cases in injection drug users (102,103). This reflects the systematic under-reporting of cases of HIV infection and AIDS that had previously been noted in injection drug users, since the beginning of the epidemic (104).

In addition to the AIDS case definition, the CDC's 1993 classification and other systems were developed to help characterize the broader range and spectrum of HIV infection, to include less-severe conditions that are not AIDS-qualifying but that are manifestations of the natural history of HIV infection. Given the current estimate that the mean time from HIV infection to the development of AIDS is between 7 and 10 years (105)—not accounting for any potential treatment effect in delaying AIDS incidence (106)—it is not surprising that there are many clinical conditions and complications that may present in the period prior to the actual development of AIDS in HIV-infected patients. Especially in primary medical care settings (107), with the trend toward earlier treatment intervention in HIV infection (82), it has been increasingly important for practitioners to recognize the early and sometimes varied

TABLE 58.1. *Center for disease control's revised clinical staging system for HIV infection and disease*

CD4+ T-Lymphocyte categories

1. Category 1: ≥500 cells/mm³
2. Category 2: 200–499 cells/mm³
3. Category 3: <200 cells/mm³

Clinical categories

1. Clinical Category A

   At least one of the conditions listed below with documented HIV infection, and none of the conditions listed in categories B or C.
   - Asymptomatic HIV infection
   - Persistent generalized lymphadenopathy (PGL)
   - Acute or history of acute HIV infection

2. Clinical Category B

   Conditions not included in either category A or C and that meet the following criteria:
   (a) The conditions are attributed to HIV infection or to a cellular immunity defect;
   (b) Clinical course or management of these conditions is complicated by HIV infection. Examples (list is not exhaustive):
   - Oral hairy leukoplakia
   - Oropharyngeal candidiasis
   - Persistent vulvovaginal candidiasis
   - Cervical dysplasia or cervical carcinoma in situ
   - Pelvic inflammatory disease (PID)
   - Constitutional symptoms[a]
   - Herpes zoster involving >1 dermatome or episode
   - Idiopathic thrombocytopenic purpura (ITP)
   - Peripheral neuropathy
   - Bacillary angiomatosis

3. Clinical Category C

   Conditions listed in the AIDS surveillance case definition. Once a category C condition has occurred, the person will remain in category C.
   - Upper/lower respiratory tract candidiasis
   - Esophageal candidiasis
   - Invasive cervical cancer
   - Disseminated coccidioidomycosis
   - Extrapulmonary cryptococcosis
   - Chronic intestinal cryptosporidiosis
   - Cytomegalovirus disease (except liver/spleen/nodal involvement)
   - HIV-related encephalopathy
   - Herpes simplex: chronic ulcers or respiratory/esophageal disease
   - Disseminated histoplasmosis
   - Chronic intestinal isosporiasis
   - Kaposi sarcoma
   - Lymphoma; Burkitt immunoblastic or CNS lymphoma
   - Disseminated *Mycobacterium avium* complex or *M. Kansasii*
   - *Mycobacterium tuberculosis,* any site
   - Disseminated *Mycobacterium* disease (species not included above)
   - *Pneumocystis carinii* pneumonia
   - Progressive multifocal leukoencephalopathy
   - Recurrent *Salmonella* septicemia
   - CNS toxoplasmosis
   - HIV-related wasting syndrome

CD4+ T-cell categories (cells/mm³)	A Asymptomatic, acute HIV infection or PGL	B Symptomatic, not A or C condition	C AIDS-indicator conditions
1: ≥500	A1	B1	C1
2: 200–499	A2	B2	C2
3: <200	A3	B3	C3

Shaded area denotes an AIDS diagnosis.
[a]Includes fever (38.5°C) or diarrhea lasting >1 month.
Adapted from U.S. Centers for Disease Control and Prevention. 1993 revised classification system for HIV infection and expanded surveillance case definition for AIDS among adolescents and adults. *MMWR Morb Mortal Wkly Rep* 1992;41(RR-17):1–19.

manifestations of HIV-related illness, both for therapeutic reasons and to assist in diagnostic and prognostic evaluation.

The CDC's 1993 *Revised Classification System for HIV Infection* establishes a staging system that includes three clinical categories of infection, each including a variety of specific conditions. In addition, it relies on the use of CD4+ T-lymphocyte count to incorporate a laboratory marker related to immune function, which helps enhance the prognostic value of this classification scheme (see Table 58.1).

Since early in the AIDS epidemic, the disease is associated with cellular immune dysfunction and a reversal of normal T-lymphocyte helper-to-suppressor ratios (2). The CD4+ or T_4 molecule has been identified as the HIV receptor on the membrane surface of T-lymphocytes in the helper or inducer subset (108,109). Although previously referred to as T_4 lymphocytes, T_4-helper/inducer cells, or by other terms, CD4 antigen-positive T-lymphocytes are now designated as CD4+ T cells, or simply as CD4+ cells in standard clinical parlance. HIV directly infects and ultimately leads to the destruction of CD4+ T-lymphocytes, and much (though not all) of the immunopathogenesis of AIDS can be explained based on the selective depletion of this lymphocyte subset. Studies of the natural history of HIV infection indicate that CD4+ cell levels tend to decline over time following initial HIV infection, and that the absolute number and percentage of CD4+ T-lymphocytes are important predictors of the likelihood of disease progression and the development of AIDS (110–114). Since the late 1980s, the use of diagnostic tests such as total CD4+ T-lymphocyte counts and percentages has been a routine component of HIV-related clinical care, in which decisions to initiate certain therapies or prophylactic interventions, even among asymptomatic individuals, are increasingly linked with determinations of CD4+ cell levels (82,83,115,116).

Laboratory methods that determine the concentration of virus in blood, or total viral load (HIV-RNA test) along with the CD4+ T cell count are predictors of progression of disease and risk of death. In untreated patients, plasma HIV RNA is usually detectable throughout HIV infection, and gradually increases over the course of disease. Viral load testing has been approved by the U.S. Food and Drug Administration (FDA) to monitor the response to antiretroviral therapy and determine prognosis. Because of the possibility of false-positive viral load assays as a consequence of contamination or because of other reasons, it is neither recommended nor FDA-approved to use these assays to diagnose HIV infection (except in the case of acute seroconversion reaction, in which the antibody to HIV is negative). The three most commonly used commercial assays are the (a) Quantiplex HIV-1 RNA assay, which is a branched deoxyribonucleic acid (bDNA) method that quantifies plasma HIV RNA; (b) Amplicor HIV-1 Monitor assay, which is based on reverse transcription of the HIV RNA and polymerase chain reaction (PCR) amplification of the resulting complementary deoxyribonucleic acid (cDNA); and (c) NucliSens HIV-1 QT assay, which is based on amplification using nucleic acid sequence-based amplification (NASBA) technology (119). The lower detection limit of these assays is 40 to 50 copies/mL, while the upper limit of quantification is 500,000 to 1,000,000 copies/mL (119). A significant change in viral load signifying a likely biologic change rather than variability of the assay is a difference of 0.5 $\log_{10}$ copies/mL (119). While the CD4+ T-cell count is the stronger indicator for the initiation of antiretroviral therapy, the viral load is a valuable marker of antiretroviral treatment failure, and thus a stronger indicator for decision making regarding stopping or changing antiretroviral therapy.

The role played by lymphatic tissue in the establishment of HIV infection, viral replication, and progression of disease is still the focus of much research. Within 1 to 2 months after acute infection, the number of viral particles in blood is dramatically decreased, an event that reflects the initial response by the immune system. What follows is a long period of clinical latency (up to 10 years) characterized by a great turnover of HIV replication; half of the virus population is turned over within hours, and it is estimated that several billions of virions and similar numbers of CD4+ cells are produced and destroyed every day, while the patient remains clinically asymptomatic (53,120). In the early asymptomatic stage, HIV RNA can be detected in high concentration in lymph nodes and lymphoid tissue, and up to one third of CD4+ cells in lymphoid tissue are infected (120). Potentially, studies of lymph node tissue may be used in the future to assess the complex host–virus interaction at any given time during the course of the disease and to assist in the choice of the appropriate therapy (121). These observations highlight the fact that, even during the clinically latent phase of HIV infection, there is no virologic latency, and early treatment to control virologic replication has important long-term benefits (122).

These developments have signaled a shift over time in HIV-associated medical care from the late-stage or inpatient focus of the first years of the epidemic, toward a new and ascendant emphasis on earlier intervention, outpatient evaluation and treatment, and management of HIV infection by primary care practitioners. These trends have posed both challenges and opportunities for drug treatment programs and other settings in which substance users with HIV infection are likely to be found.

SPECTRUM OF HIV-RELATED DISEASE IN INJECTION DRUG USERS

Comparative epidemiologic studies indicate that the expression of HIV-related disease and AIDS may vary substantially in different geographic regions. For example, it has been observed that *Pneumocystis carinii* pneumonia (PCP), the most common AIDS-defining opportunistic infection in the United States and Europe (123–125), is seen only infrequently in AIDS cases in Central Africa, where esophageal candidiasis, tuberculosis, toxoplasmosis, cryptococcosis, enteric infections, and wasting syndromes are more common findings (126–128). In addition, it has been noted that even within a single geographic area, the spectrum of HIV-related illness may differ by risk group, with divergent patterns of illness observed in substance users as compared with homosexual men. For example, it has been a consistent finding that Kaposi sarcoma, although commonly seen in homosexual men, rarely is noted in substance users with HIV infection (29). Human herpesvirus 8 (HHV-8), also known as Kaposi sarcoma-associated herpesvirus (KSAHV), was discovered in 1994 and could play an etiologic role in the pathophysiology of Kaposi sarcoma, as suggested in some studies (129). KSAHV is transmitted orally, sexually, and through blood in shared needles; if the epidemiology of this virus were more limited to sexual transmission through male same-sex contact than the other routes of transmission, this would explain the observation of the low incidence of Kaposi sarcoma in injection drug users (29,130–133). Table 58.2 summarizes the major conditions seen in HIV-infected substance users more commonly than in other populations with HIV infection.

Bacterial Infections

It has been reported, since early in the AIDS epidemic, that substance users with HIV infection may be at risk for developing serious bacterial infections, especially bacterial pneumonia, endocarditis, and bacterial sepsis (30,42,43,134–136). This phenomenon was first described in New York City, where mortality data analyzed by investigators at the New York City Department of Health showed a steady increase in deaths from pneumonia and other bacterial infections among injection drug users beginning in the early 1980s (30). Further analysis indicated that a disproportionate number of these cases showed suggestive or confirmatory evidence of the presence of HIV infection, even after excluding those that would meet criteria for the surveillance case definition of AIDS (30). This observation, along with additional population-based data, led to the suggestion that the burden of HIV-related morbidity and mortality among substance users may be underestimated by focusing attention on AIDS cases alone, an effect that has implications not only for clinical care but also for health policy and planning (30,137).

Subsequent analyses in different populations of substance users have further corroborated the association between HIV infection and serious bacterial infections in injection drug users, although this has not been reported consistently in all geographic areas (31,41–43,134–140). Although pneumonia, endocarditis, and other bacterial infections historically were noted to occur with high frequency in injection drug users well before the AIDS epidemic (141,142), evidence has accumulated to suggest that these infections may occur more commonly among substance users in the setting of HIV infection (30,31,41,134,135,137,138). One study determined yearly rates of bacterial pneumonia hospitalizations among HIV-seropositive and seronegative substance users enrolled in a prospective study of HIV infection at a New York City methadone-maintenance program (134). Even after controlling for demographic variables and for current drug, alcohol, and tobacco use, the HIV-seropositive group showed a fourfold increased risk of bacterial pneumonia when compared with the seronegative group. It has also been suggested, however, that smoking illicit drugs may be a risk factor for bacterial pneumonia (143), including marijuana and crack cocaine. This suggests that HIV-infected substance users may be at even greater risk of bacterial pneumonia than otherwise if they continue to smoke illicit drugs. In all published investigations examining bacterial pneumonia in substance users and other HIV-infected patients, the predominant pathogenic organisms have been encapsulated bacteria such as *Streptococcus pneumoniae* and *Haemophilus influenzae;* less frequently identified have been *Staphylococcus aureus,* gram-negative enteric

---

TABLE 58.2. *Spectrum of HIV-related disease in injection drug users*[a]

Pyogenic Bacterial Infections
  Pneumonia
    Streptococcus pneumoniae
    Haemophilus influenzae
    Endocarditis or sepsis
Tuberculosis
  Pulmonary
  Extrapulmonary
Sexually Transmitted Disease
  Syphilis
  Human papillomavirus
Neurologic Disease
  Central
  Peripheral
Hepatitis
  Infectious hepatitis A, B, C, D (delta)
  Alcoholic hepatitis
Cancer
  Lung
  Cervix
  Other (e.g., oropharynx or larynx)

Adapted from O'Connor P, Selwyn PA, Schottenfeld RS. Medical management of injection drug users with HIV infection. *N Engl J Med* 1994;331:450–459.

[a]These are common complications of HIV infection, drug use, or both, which may occur more commonly among injection drug users with HIV infection.

organisms, and other miscellaneous bacterial pathogens (134–136,144–148).

A number of characteristics have been described to explain the increased risk of bacterial infections in substance-using populations. In summary, these are (a) increased rates of mucocutaneous and upper respiratory carriage of pathogenic organisms, particularly strains of staphylococci and streptococci; (b) improper injection technique that does not include sterilization of skin and favors the breakdown of natural barriers and the transfer of bacteria from mucocutaneous surfaces into the bloodstream; (c) use of contaminated injection equipment or injecting substances with viral, bacterial, and parasitic microorganisms that may have originated in body fluids, particularly residual blood, or different fluids used as drug solvents or for rinsing the injection equipment; (d) altered immune response from underlying medical conditions (including AIDS) or from the effect of the drugs used; (e) factors related to the oropharynx, namely poor dental hygiene, periodontal and soft-tissue disease, and impairment of gag and cough reflexes by the use of drugs; (f) change in normal microbial flora promoted by prior use of antibiotics; (g) low socioeconomic status and its associated risk of exposure to pathogens such as *Mycobacterium tuberculosis;* (h) behavioral aspects associated with injection drug use, particularly use of multiple substances and the excessive use of alcohol and tobacco; and (i) poor utilization of or limited access to primary health care services, with resultant low levels of immunization and prophylaxis and the lack of timely diagnosis and treatment of infections (149).

It has been suggested that bacterial infections not only occur more commonly in HIV-infected substance users than in their HIV-seronegative counterparts, but also that the infections may be more severe as well, with higher case fatality rates and more lengthy hospitalizations (134). Several case control studies have suggested that bacterial endocarditis in HIV-infected substance users may be more complicated and difficult to treat than endocarditis in HIV-seronegative substance users, although the magnitude of this alleged effect is uncertain (150,151), and some studies indicate no difference in outcome (152). The microbiology of bacterial endocarditis in injection drug users reflects unsterile injection techniques that favor the transfer of bacteria from the skin and mucous membranes into the bloodstream. *S. aureus,* an organism commonly found in nares, upper respiratory system, and skin, is the most common etiologic organism of bacterial endocarditis in injection drug users. Streptococci and enterococci are also commonly isolated. Finally, gram-negative bacilli such as *Pseudomonas* species and *Serratia marcescens* are not uncommon etiologic agents in this patient population (153). Management of endocarditis in drug injectors requires prompt institution of intravenous antibiotic therapy after blood cultures are obtained. The empiric use of specific antibiotic regimens will depend on the local geographic incidence of specific pathogens, and particular emphasis should be placed on the clinical suspicion of methicillin-resistant *S. aureus* (MRSA) (154–156) and vancomycin-resistant enterococci (VRE) (157,158). The prognosis will depend on the degree of valve damage, the use of adequate antimicrobial therapy, and general medical condition. The importance of completion of therapy and the negative effect of continued injection drug use should be addressed with each patient individually.

The occurrence of bacterial pneumonia has been viewed as a sentinel event or harbinger of subsequent HIV-related disease in substance users, who may often present with bacterial infections as the first sign of HIV-related illness (134,159). Indeed, unlike the major opportunistic infections that constitute a diagnosis of AIDS, bacterial pneumonias tend first to occur earlier in the course of HIV infection, before the later stages of immunosuppression marked by severe CD4+ lymphocyte depletion (134,140,143,160). Although bacterial infections may occur in the latter setting as well, as a first presentation they usually are seen in HIV-infected patients who have not yet shown evidence of major opportunistic infections (134,143,160).

The finding of an increased likelihood of bacterial infections in HIV-infected substance users has a number of implications for epidemiologic surveillance, clinical management, and preventive strategies. As noted previously, there may be certain behavioral, demographic, or environmental factors that put HIV-infected substance users at risk for bacterial infections. More specifically, the pathophysiologic mechanism resulting in an increased risk of bacterial infections in HIV-infected substance users has not been elucidated; however, it has been hypothesized that this may relate to the known deleterious effects of HIV on B-cell function, as well as on T-cell function, which would result in an inability to respond effectively to encapsulated bacterial pathogens (134,144–146,148,161–163). The depletion of CD4+ cells characterizes the immunopathogenesis of AIDS. The CD4+ T-lymphocyte plays a central role in most immunologic functions, not just those that affect cellular immunity. Persons with AIDS have significant abnormalities in B-cell function, characterized by polyclonal activation, hypergammaglobulinemia, and circulating immunocomplexes and autoantibodies, and those abnormalities are manifested clinically as increased susceptibility to certain pyogenic bacteria (112). A good clinical example of this observation is represented by the gram-negative bacillus *Pseudomonas aeruginosa,* a very rare pathogen in immunocompetent patients presenting with community-acquired infections. Multiple clinical studies recognize the increased incidence of *P. aeruginosa* infection in HIV-infected patients, particularly bronchopulmonary infections, recognized both as an indolent relapsing pathogen in the outpatient setting and as an agent causing fulminant pneumonia and bacteremia in the hospitalized patient (164–167). Prolonged survival in AIDS patients with associated severe immunosuppression is proposed as a risk factor for *P. aeruginosa* infections (164).

A higher index of suspicion is required for some bacterial pathogens that, like *P. aeruginosa*, are rare community-acquired pathogens for non–HIV-infected individuals.

The recognition of the increased susceptibility of HIV-infected patients for bacterial pathogens has led to the inclusion of recurrent pneumonias in the CDC's 1993 expanded AIDS surveillance case definition (99). It is also proposed that surveillance for pneumococcal pneumonia or bacteremia may be used as a surrogate marker for substance use or to help detect trends in HIV infection in certain geographic areas, where substance use and HIV infection are concentrated (168,169). For clinicians, the importance of bacterial infections in this population highlights the need for precise microbiologic diagnosis of pathogenic organisms in pneumonia cases among HIV-infected substance users. The specificity and positive predictive value of the standard criteria for presumptive diagnosis of PCP (98)—that is, exertional dyspnea, arterial hypoxemia, and diffuse bilateral interstitial infiltrates on chest roentgenogram or a positive gallium citrate lung scan—may well be diminished in a population at risk for pneumonia syndromes of different etiology.

Therefore, sputum Gram stain, sputum and blood cultures, sputum induction, and/or bronchoscopy are often necessary before an appropriate diagnosis can be made in substance users presenting with pneumonia. The practice of treating pneumonias in HIV-infected patients presumptively with trimethoprim-sulfamethoxazole (TMP-SMX), under the rationale that such treatment would be effective both for PCP and/or common bacterial pathogens, may, indeed, yield good empiric results in many cases. However, the high likelihood of adverse reactions to TMP-SMX in HIV-infected patients (170) often requires a change of therapy to pentamidine, the other principal agent for treating PCP, which is ineffective against bacterial pathogens. In such cases, in which a precise microbiologic diagnosis has not been made, and in which TMP-SMX therapy has been initiated presumptively, one then may be faced with a partially treated bacterial infection that may be difficult to diagnose by culture and therefore difficult to treat definitively.

Given the increased risk of bacterial infections among HIV-infected substance users, the possibility for preventive interventions in this area is of strategic importance. Because most series indicate that pneumococcal pneumonia is one of the most common entities seen in HIV-infected patients with bacterial infections (134,144,148), it is recommended that pneumococcal polysaccharide vaccine be given to substance users and other individuals with HIV infection (83). Current guidelines published by the CDC recommend that all persons with HIV infection and CD4+ T-cell counts of 200/mm^3 or more be offered pneumococcal vaccine, whereas in those with CD4+ T-cell counts less than 200/mm^3, immunization should be considered because there is less data to confirm vaccine efficacy in these patients (83). Although there are reports of pneumococcal vaccine failure in patients with AIDS, pre-

sumably because of underlying immunosuppression and the inability to respond adequately to vaccine antigens (145,163,171), several studies indicate at least a moderate antibody response to this vaccine in both homosexual men and substance users with HIV infection (172,173). In these studies, a postvaccine rise in specific antipneumococcal antibody titers to levels that would be considered protective was generally seen only in patients in the earlier stages of HIV infection who were not profoundly immunosuppressed. However, vaccination has not been deemed harmful in patients with AIDS, and at times may result in an appropriate antibody response in such patients. In the past, some clinicians had also recommended the use of conjugate *Haemophilus influenzae* vaccine for HIV-infected adults, although data to support this practice are less available than for pneumococcal vaccine. Despite its generalized use in the pediatric non–HIV-infected population, routine use of *H. influenzae* type b (Hib) vaccine in the adult HIV-infected patient is not recommended (83). It has also been recommended that patients with AIDS receive yearly influenza vaccine, which is discussed in the section "Baseline Medical Assessment of Substance Users with HIV Infection."

An additional preventive intervention, more in the behavioral arena, was suggested by a study from San Francisco in which active substance users who used alcohol to clean skin injection sites prior to injecting drugs were found to be at lower risk of soft-tissue bacterial infections and endocarditis than were substance users who did not use such techniques (174). Another study from Baltimore yielded similar findings on the possible protective effect of skin cleaning on bacterial infections (175). Although this intervention has not been prospectively demonstrated to be effective in preventing bacterial pneumonias in the setting of HIV infection—for which the pathogenesis does not appear to depend upon bacteremia resulting from drug injection—it is plausible that this intervention may, indeed, help to prevent certain other serious bacterial infections in substance users, and therefore should be promoted in active substance users who are unable to cease injecting drugs.

Of special significance is the recognition and increasing number of reports from systematic surveillance studies of penicillin-resistant strains of *Streptococcus pneumoniae*. As of 2001, penicillin-resistant strains were reported to be present in 26% of *S. pneumoniae* isolates in some places in the United States (176). Management problems associated with them are related to the delay in diagnosis and timely institution of appropriate therapy. The increased mortality and morbidity associated with delayed treatment can be prevented with an increased clinical suspicion in the treatment of patients more susceptible to harbor resistant strains of *S. pneumoniae*. In addition, reducing the incidence of pneumococcal infection can occur by broadening the indications for the use of the available 23-valent pneumococcal vaccine, and targeting the appropriate population for vaccination, including all HIV-infected individuals with CD4+ T-cell counts above, and possibly below, 200/mm³, and all injection drug users. Although not fully explained to date, the emergence of penicillin-resistant strains of *S. pneumoniae* is thought to be a consequence of two main factors: the misuse of β-lactam antibiotics, and the poor compliance with full therapeutic courses. Both characteristics are well described in the injection drug-using population, and therefore preventive measures directed at reducing the incidence of infections caused by this organism should be applied with particular emphasis to this group of patients (177,178).

Infections of skin and soft tissue are more directly related than pneumonia to the behavioral aspects of drug injection, as well as to the use of contaminated injection equipment, and are the most common bacterial infections among injection drug users (149,175). The spectrum of infections is broad and ranges from localized cellulitis originated at the site of injection to rapidly spreading fasciitis, local abscess formation, and metastatic complications: thrombophlebitis, septic emboli, endocarditis, and visceral abscess formation. The pathogens found in these infections are normally not found in the equipment used when it is cultured, but rather are pathogens carried in the skin, either common skin or nasopharyngeal flora (staphylococci, streptococci, *Propionibacterium acnes,* diphtheroids, etc.) or more aggressive organisms that are able to grow at the site of prior soft-tissue injury favored by the use of solvents, contaminants, and substance adulterants commonly used by drug injectors. Additionally, injection drug users may be at increased risk for becoming carriers of potentially aggressive organisms that are associated with antibiotic use or hospital exposure, such as MRSA (154–156) and VRE (157,158). This raises the further possibility of person-to-person spread of these agents between substance users, which could lead to local outbreaks of these difficult-to-treat infections.

Tuberculosis

Another important condition that has been noted among certain HIV-infected populations, particularly among substance users, is tuberculosis. Tuberculosis in the setting of coexistent HIV infection has been reported with increasing frequency in a variety of geographic settings, including not only industrialized countries, but also of particular importance, countries in the Caribbean and sub-Saharan Africa, where both HIV infection and tuberculosis are concentrated (179–183). Reports from sub-Saharan Africa describe a dual epidemic of alarming magnitude, in which more than 8 million people are estimated to be coinfected with *Mycobacterium tuberculosis* and HIV, representing up to half of HIV-infected individuals infected with tuberculosis in the world (126,182–186). This combination has important and grave implications for tuberculosis control and public health, and it has been suggested that many of the historical gains in tuberculosis control

may be lost because of a resurgence of HIV-associated tuberculosis.

HIV infection is considered to be the strongest risk factor for the progression of latent tuberculosis infection to active disease (34,187,188), and as of 2000 an estimated 12 million people worldwide are thought to have HIV and *M. tuberculosis* coinfection (182,189). Extrapulmonary tuberculosis was included as an AIDS-defining illness in the 1987 CDC revised AIDS surveillance case definition (98). Any anatomic site of tuberculosis involvement, however, constitutes an AIDS-defining illness in the CDC's 1993 *Classification System for HIV Infection and Expanded Surveillance Case Definition* (99).

Previously it was believed that the development of active tuberculosis in patients with HIV infection was almost always caused by the reactivation of latent tuberculosis infection in the setting of HIV-induced immunosuppression in patients previously exposed to *M. tuberculosis* (36,37,190–192). This phenomenon remains important; however, more recently, primary infection with rapid disease progression has been identified as another important mechanism. Molecular genetic techniques, namely restriction fragment length polymorphism (RFLP) and PCR-based methods, permit the identification of identical strains of *M. tuberculosis,* enabling investigators to identify transmission patterns in a specific geographic area. These methods have been very useful in studies of local tuberculosis outbreaks; reports have documented, both in outbreak studies and in broader epidemiologic analysis, that HIV-infected patients may acquire primary infection with *M. tuberculosis* and progress rapidly to active disease (193–197). This phenomenon has been documented for both drug-sensitive and drug-resistant strains of *M. tuberculosis* (198–200). HIV-infected patients may be at high risk of acquiring tuberculosis infection from other HIV-infected patients, and then progressing themselves to disease, thus continuing the chain of transmission in a potentially explosive manner.

In the United States, tuberculosis in HIV-infected patients is concentrated primarily among injection drug users and minority populations (36,190,191,201–203). The association between the two infections has been shown most strikingly in certain cities in the northeastern and southeastern United States, where HIV seroprevalence studies have found levels of HIV infection as high as 47% among patients treated at tuberculosis clinics (204,205). Tuberculosis traditionally was recognized as a common condition among substance users well before the AIDS epidemic (206). Levels of latent tuberculous infection among substance-using populations— as demonstrated by positive tuberculin skin tests—have been found to be as high as 25% (40,191,206). Given this background of risk, the introduction of HIV infection into these populations could well be expected to amplify the expression of tuberculosis in the setting of HIV-induced immunosuppression. One study, performed at a methadone-maintenance program in New York City, prospectively followed a cohort of 520 injection drug users with known HIV antibody and tuberculin skin test status over approximately 2 years of followup (191). This study found a rate of 7.9 cases of active tuberculosis per 100 person-years among HIV-seropositive patients with prior positive tuberculin skin tests, compared with zero cases among HIV-seropositive patients without prior positive tuberculin tests. HIV-seropositive patients with positive tuberculin skin tests were 24 times more likely to develop active tuberculosis in this study than were HIV-seropositive patients without evidence of prior exposure to tuberculosis. None of the patients in this study who had received isoniazid prophylaxis for a positive purified protein derivative (PPD) test developed active tuberculosis during the study period (191). Although not designed as a clinical trial of the efficacy of isoniazid prophylaxis in this population, this study's results support recommendations for aggressive identification and treatment of patients with dual HIV and *M. tuberculosis* infection (202). Other studies from Zambia, Haiti, and Spain document tuberculosis incidence rates of 6 to 12 per 100 person-years in HIV-infected patients with prior positive tuberculin tests (207–209).

Numerous studies and surveillance reports have examined the temporal relationship between the diagnoses of pulmonary tuberculosis and AIDS in individuals ultimately diagnosed with both conditions. In such cases the diagnoses tend to cluster together, with tuberculosis usually diagnosed several months prior to an AIDS-defining illness in HIV-infected patients, although variations on this sequence are not uncommon (36–38,191). The relationship between tuberculosis and CD4+ lymphocyte count has been examined in different studies (210–212). It was found that HIV-infected patients with tuberculosis tend to be less immunocompromised than those diagnosed with other AIDS-defining conditions. The approximate range of CD4+ count most commonly observed for patients with HIV infection and pulmonary tuberculosis is 150 to 400 cells/mm^3 (213). Initially the focus of coinfection with tuberculosis and HIV was on the impact HIV has on the progression of tuberculosis; however, there is now more mounting evidence that reveals the response to *M. tuberculosis* enhances HIV replication and may accelerate the progression of HIV disease (201,214,215). Studies show a higher risk for opportunistic infections and death in HIV-infected patients who are coinfected with *M. tuberculosis* (216–218), and one study suggests that treatment of latent tuberculosis infection in HIV-infected persons actually reduces the risk of HIV disease progression (207). It has also been noted that extrapulmonary involvement occurs most commonly with increasing degree of immunosuppression, with disseminated disease and lymphadenitis as the most common diagnoses (212,213,219). Most series of tuberculosis cases in HIV-positive patients consist of a majority of pulmonary cases, but include a greater percentage of extrapulmonary cases—between 25% and 70%—than is seen in HIV-negative patients with tuberculosis (39,40,190–192,212).

Many analyses of the treatment of tuberculosis in HIV-positive patients suggest that, as in HIV-negative patients, tuberculosis usually responds well to appropriate chemotherapy (39,185,190,192,203,212,220). However, more recent studies confirm that it is the early clinical response to therapy against tuberculosis that is similar in HIV-positive patients as compared to HIV-negative patients, but it is unclear whether rates of tuberculosis relapse differ among these patients (221–223). Clinical features of cases in HIV-infected individuals may differ from those seen in classic cases of tuberculosis, especially when tuberculosis is diagnosed in HIV-infected patients in the later stages of immunosuppression. For example, the typical findings of upper lobe lung involvement and cavitation seen in classic pulmonary tuberculosis are relatively uncommon in HIV-associated cases, and it has been reported that sputum smears for acid-fast bacilli may be less frequently positive in HIV-associated pulmonary tuberculosis, even in the presence of ultimately positive sputum cultures (190,191,203,220,224,225). In addition, the presentations of extrapulmonary tuberculosis can be varied and, at times, nonspecific, ranging from meningitis, peritonitis, and localized involvement of bone or soft tissues, to vague constitutional symptoms, fever, or malaise. It is, therefore, important for clinicians treating patients at risk for HIV infection and tuberculosis to have a high index of suspicion for unusual presentations of tuberculosis; diagnosis may depend on mycobacterial blood cultures, bone marrow aspiration or biopsy, liver biopsy, or cerebrospinal fluid (CSF) examination and culture, in addition to the standard procedures of chest roentgenogram and sputum smear and culture, which would be used routinely for suspected pulmonary cases (190).

Once a provisional diagnosis of tuberculosis has been made—usually with the finding of acid-fast bacilli on smears of sputum or other body fluids—therapy should be initiated (190,202). A biopsy specimen showing caseating granulomas, in the right clinical setting, should be considered diagnostic for tuberculosis. Given the possibility that acid-fast smears may be negative in HIV-infected patients, empiric therapy should also be considered in patients with negative smears when the diagnosis of tuberculosis is strongly suspected (190). Current recommendations published by the American Thoracic Society and the CDC for initial therapy of tuberculosis in HIV-positive persons do not differ from those for HIV-negative patients, and are for the oral use of isoniazid 300 mg per day, rifampin 600 mg per day (or 450 mg for patients weighing less than 50 kg), and pyrazinamide 20 to 30 mg/kg per day, with the addition of ethambutol (15 to 25 mg/kg per day) in cases of disseminated tuberculosis or when isoniazid resistance is suspected, for 2 months followed by the same doses of isoniazid and rifampin for 4 months

(226–228). An acceptable alternative for patients who cannot take pyrazinamide is a 9-month course of isoniazid and rifampin, adding ethambutol until culture results are available. Drug susceptibility testing should be performed routinely on all isolates of *M. tuberculosis* (190,202). In the event of drug resistance, the treatment regimen may need to be revised accordingly to ensure efficacy.

The rifamycins (rifampin [Rifadin], rifabutin [Mycobutin], rifapentine [Priftin]) have substantial drug interactions with numerous antiretroviral medications, and therefore must be closely monitored in HIV-infected patients taking protease inhibitors and nonnucleoside reverse transcriptase inhibitors (NNRTIs). Rifampin, the most potent inducer of the cytochrome P450 enzyme system in the liver, is contraindicated when used simultaneously with many protease inhibitors or NNRTIs because it markedly lowers serum levels of such antiretroviral medications, rendering them ineffective (201). Although rifampin was previously contraindicated to use with all protease inhibitors and NNRTIs, recent data has elucidated certain combinations to be safe and effective—specifically rifampin in combination with (a) efavirenz (Sustiva) and two nucleoside reverse transcriptase inhibitors (NRTIs), (b) ritonavir (Norvir) as the sole protease inhibitor in addition to two NRTIs, and (c) ritonavir plus either saquinavir hard-gel capsules (Invirase) or saquinavir soft-gel capsules (Fortovase) in addition to two NRTIs (229–232). Rifabutin and rifapentine have substantially less induction of the P450 system (233–235); however, because the safety and effectiveness of rifapentine has yet to be determined, it is not recommended as a substitute for rifampin. The substitution of rifabutin for rifampin is the preferred choice for patients taking tuberculosis medications and antiretroviral regimens containing protease inhibitors or NNRTIs (201,236–240). However, rifabutin often requires dose modification when used with antiretroviral medications, is contraindicated with specific antiretroviral medications (e.g., delavirdine [Rescriptor]), and must still be used with caution and monitored closely in patients taking antiretroviral medications. In addition, in patients taking methadone, rifabutin, unlike rifampin, does not decrease methadone levels or require increases in methadone dose (see "Drug Interactions" below and Table 58.3) (241,242). Given the complexities and multiple drug interactions associated with coadministration of tuberculosis therapy with antiretroviral medications, providers should consult with specialists when treating patients for tuberculosis and HIV simultaneously.

Current CDC recommendations suggest that treatment for active tuberculosis should be continued for a minimum of 6 months, although some experts suggest that treatment for HIV-infected patients should include longer courses of therapy, that is, 9 months (243,244). These expert opinions are likely based on prospective studies that have evaluated relapse rates after a 6-month treatment course with anti-

tuberculosis medications in HIV-infected patients. These studies are conflicting, with some reporting clinically acceptable relapse rates and others reporting high relapse rates after the 6-month course of treatment (221,245–248). Treatment may need to be more prolonged for disseminated disease, when specific sites of disease are involved (prostatic, osteoarticular, meningeal, miliary disease), or in cases in which either isoniazid or rifamycins cannot be included in the treatment regimen (227). Longer therapeutic courses should be given serious consideration in cases of delayed clinical response, slow radiographic improvement, or slow conversion to negative culture.

The phenomenon of reinfection has also been identified in HIV-infected patients with tuberculosis, based on molecular genetic analyses that have documented new disease from different strains of *M. tuberculosis* in patients who have already been successfully treated for prior active tuberculosis (196). Of great concern has also been the significant number of cases of multiple drug-resistant tuberculosis (MDR-TB) reported in the early 1990s in urban areas in the United States with substantial levels of poverty, substance use, and HIV coinfection. The risk of drug-resistant tuberculosis is higher among HIV-infected persons than others (249). HIV-infected substance users with tuberculosis, in the absence of effective community-based treatment programs, may be unlikely to comply fully with medical treatment. Poor adherence with medications has been associated with having drug-resistant strains of *M. tuberculosis* (250–252), likely as a result of subtherapeutic blood levels of antituberculosis drugs.

Direct observation therapy (DOT) should be considered the standard for all patients with tuberculosis, especially when there is evidence of, or suspicion for, medication nonadherence (253,254). Direct observation preventive therapy (DOPT) for recent tuberculin skin test converters should also be considered in selected cases. Methadone and other drug-treatment programs, as well as other sites, including prisons, primary care centers, and medical outreach programs (e.g., mobile vans), are among the appropriate settings where this intervention can be made (46,47,49,255–257).

The potential for developing tuberculosis with MDR-TB strains in the substance-using population has high relevance in clinical practice, both for the treatment of the individual patient, and for the potential for dissemination of resistant strains in the community. The realization that the emergence of multidrug-resistant strains of *M. tuberculosis* was directly associated with suboptimal adherence to therapy spurred the implementation of DOT programs by public health authorities with great success in reducing the number of cases of tuberculosis, particularly in northeastern American urban communities (197,258,259). The full implementation of these programs in HIV-infected patients is a key intervention in the management of tuberculosis. The costs associated with these programs are by far offset by the therapeutic benefits and the

TABLE 58.3. *Interactions between HIV-related medications and methadone*

HIV-related medication	Effect on methadone	Effect on HIV-related medication	Clinical effect
Protease inhibitors			
Indinavir	Unchanged		
Ritonavir	↓ levels by 37%		No methadone dose adjustment necessary in one study (468), but monitor and titrate dose if needed
Saquinavir[a]	—		
Nelfinavir	↓ levels		Monitor and titrate dose up, if needed; required an increase in methadone dose up to 185% in one case-report (465)
Amprenavir	↓ levels by 35%	↓ AUC[b] by 30%	Monitor and titrate dose, if needed; might require increase in methadone dose; amprenavir may be less effective (586)
Lopinavir	↓ AUC by 36%, ↓ levels by 53%		No methadone dose adjustment necessary in one study (472), but monitor and titrate dose if needed
Nonnucleoside reverse transcriptase inhibitors (NNRTIs)			
Nevirapine	↓ levels by 46%	Unchanged	Withdrawal symptoms, titrate methadone dose to effect; may require up to a 185% increase in methadone dose (460)
Efavirenz	↓ levels by 48–52%		Titrate methadone dose to effect; may require up to a 200% increase in methadone dose (463)
Delavirdine	Not studied		
Nucleoside reverse transcriptase inhibitors (NRTIs)			
Zidovudine	Unchanged	↑ AUC by 40%	Unclear, possibly increase zidovudine-related toxicities
Stavudine	Unchanged	↓ AUC by 18%, ↓ levels by 27%	No dose adjustment
Didanosine	Unchanged	↓ AUC by 41%, ↓ levels by 60%	Consider didanosine dose increase
Tenofovir	—		
Lamivudine	Unchanged		
Abacavir	↑clearance	↓ peak concentration	
Zalcitabine	Not studied		
Other HIV-related medications			
Rifampin	↓ levels by 33–68%		Titrate methadone dose to effect; likely will require a substantial increase in methadone dose
Rifabutin	Unchanged		
Fluconazole	↑ levels by 30%		Unknown clinical significance
Phenytoin	↓ levels sharply		Titrate methadone dose to effect; might require increased methadone dose
Phenobarbital	↓ levels sharply		Titrate methadone dose to effect; might require increased methadone dose
Carbamazepine	↓ levels		Titrate methadone dose to effect; might require increased methadone dose

[a]Drug-interaction studies were conducted with Invirase,® therefore, recommendations might not apply to use with Fortovase.®

[b]AUC = Area Under the Curve

Adapted from: Centers for Disease Control and Prevention. Guidelines for using antiretroviral agents among HIV-infected adults and adolescents: recommendations of the Panel on Clinical Practices for Treatment of HIV. *MMWR* 2002;51(RR-7):1–55.

Gourevitch MN, Friedland GH. Interactions between methadone and medications used to treat HIV infection: a review. *Mt Sinai J of Med* 2000;67:429–436.

avoidance of health care costs that would represent the cases being prevented (260). DOT can safely be implemented with twice or thrice weekly regimens with equal therapeutic success. DOPT is also associated with a higher success in treating tuberculosis infection (i.e., positive PPD test in a patient without evidence of disease). It has been proposed that selected HIV-infected individuals with a positive tuberculin test should be considered candidates for DOPT, particularly substance users. Many substance-abuse treatment programs and methadone-maintenance treatment programs, along with some states' department of public health or other agencies, are already offering DOPT to this population.

Concerning latent tuberculosis infection, not active tuberculosis disease, current recommendations include chemoprophylaxis for HIV-infected patients with a positive tuberculin test (defined as ≥5 mm of induration with PPD) or a previous positive tuberculin skin test without prior treatment, regardless of age. In addition, HIV-infected individuals who are close contacts with persons with active tuberculosis disease should receive preventive therapy regardless of tuberculin skin test results or prior courses of treatment (201,261,262). Important for substance users, the definition of close contacts refers not only to contacts in the home, but may also include contacts in the same drug treatment program, health care facility, or coworkers. The preferred regimen for chemoprophylaxis is daily isoniazid 300 mg and pyridoxine 50 mg for 9 months regardless of age or the recency of skin test conversion (83,201). Alternative recommendations include (a) isoniazid 900 mg and pyridoxine 100 mg twice weekly for 9 months, (b) rifampin 600 mg daily for 4 months, (c) rifabutin 300 mg daily for 4 months, (d) pyrazinamide 15 to 20 mg/kg daily plus either rifampin 600 mg daily or rifabutin 300 mg daily for 2 months. Several reports of severe and fatal hepatitis are associated with patients taking the last regimen of pyrazinamide and rifampin, and therefore must be used with extreme caution and close followup (263). These recommendations are critical given the extremely high risk of reactivation and the development of active tuberculosis in HIV-infected patients coinfected with *M. tuberculosis* (181,191,207–209,264). It is important to monitor patients, particularly substance users, closely for signs of hepatotoxicity while on isoniazid, given the high frequency of hepatitis B and C infections, regular alcohol use, and the potential for drug interactions with many HIV medications (265–272). For patients on methadone maintenance, experience suggests that isoniazid prophylaxis—as well as multidrug chemotherapy—can be given effectively and with excellent compliance within the setting of a methadone-treatment program, by administering antituberculous medication along with patients' daily methadone doses (191,206,255).

Routine admission medical screening for all drug treatment program entrants should include tuberculin skin testing (Mantoux), with intradermal administration of 5 tuberculin units (TU) of PPD. This test should be repeated at least annually among skin test-negative patients. Given the possibility of the increasing spread of tuberculosis in the setting of the AIDS epidemic, it may be prudent to consider retesting every 6 months in high-risk settings, if feasible. The latter recommendation applies to staff as well as to patients (273). Because HIV-infected patients may be unable to react appropriately to skin test antigens because of immunosuppression, a PPD reading greater than or equal to 5 mm is considered a positive result in such patients, unlike the standard of greater than or equal to 10 mm or 15 mm that defines a positive skin test in other populations (83,202,261). Previously, administration of cutaneous anergy testing with PPD in HIV-infected individuals was suggested; however, currently, routine evaluation for anergy is not recommended (83). Nonetheless, certain situations may arise in which anergy testing might assist in clinical decisions regarding chemoprophylaxis for tuberculosis. Some may argue that despite its variability and irregular performance (274), anergy testing in HIV-infected persons, particularly in tuberculosis-endemic areas, may be important not only in the interpretation of tuberculin skin tests, but also as a risk factor for the development of active tuberculosis (208,264,275). In a Bronx methadone program in which the previous rate of active tuberculosis was approximately 6 cases per 100 person-years in HIV-seropositive anergic patients (264), the rate of active disease fell to zero after the initiation of routine isoniazid prophylaxis for 12 months in this high-risk subgroup (M. Gourevitch, personal communication).

In addition to the risk of tuberculosis for HIV-positive patients, a rising incidence of active tuberculosis cases poses public health risks for HIV-negative persons as well. With a greater density of HIV infection and tuberculosis cases, and hence growing numbers of infectious individuals, the risk of transmission to household members, health care providers, and other close, but not necessarily intimate, contacts would be expected to increase. Whereas the occupational risk of HIV transmission is estimated in general to be low—approximately a 0.3% likelihood of transmission following a parenteral exposure (276)—the risk of acquiring tuberculosis would be expected to be substantially higher in certain health care settings. In addition, the possibility of MDR-TB has become a growing concern as larger numbers of patients are treated for active disease and the likelihood of poor compliance with chemotherapy increases, especially among populations of injection drug users (200,277–283). Indeed, a report from Florida described nosocomial transmission of MDR-TB to health care workers and patients in the setting of an inpatient AIDS unit, which highlights the importance of this issue in medical care settings (280). In drug treatment programs, where tuberculosis and HIV infection are likely to be concentrated, it is critical for public health considerations and workplace safety to consider such interventions as (a) semiannual, as opposed to annual, PPD testing for patients and staff; (b) inspection and evaluation of the adequacy of clinic ventilation systems; (c) installation of ultraviolet light fixtures to assist in air disinfection; and (d) supervised chemotherapy for all patients with active disease, with strict sanctions for noncompliance (202,273,280,284,285). Additionally, because of the risk of household transmission, screening and followup of at-risk household members should be offered to substance-using patients diagnosed with tuberculosis as well.

Sexually Transmitted Diseases

HIV infection frequently is associated with the presence of other coexisting sexually transmitted diseases in a variety of patient populations (59,62,286). This may result in part simply from the common co-occurrence of such disease in persons whose behavior may tend to expose them to sexually transmitted infection. In addition, however, the presence of anal and genital ulcerations is a strong independent risk factor for HIV infection in both men and women, presumably through the facilitation of viral transmission via nonintact mucosal or dermal layers (62,287). Injection drug users historically have been found to be at increased risk of sexually transmitted disease, presumably related both to sexual behaviors associated with substance use and to the engagement in prostitution as a means of supporting the costs of substance use (265). In the context of the AIDS epidemic, multiple studies have reported that although substance users have adopted safer substance-using practices, in some instances to reduce the risk of HIV transmission, in general, such changes were not noted in the realm of sexual behavior (137,288,289). Particularly in the era of highly active antiretroviral therapy (HAART), there is concern that unsafe sexual practices may increase after starting antiretroviral medications. Studies report conflicting data with regard to resumption of high-risk sexual behaviors after initiating HAART in injection drug users (290,291). Furthermore, the relationship between cocaine use and sexually transmitted diseases— either through a drug-specific disinhibition of sexual behavior or the more formal exchange of sex for drugs or money—underscores the importance of addressing sexually transmitted diseases in the care of substance users with or at risk for HIV infection (56–61,63,292).

Initial assessment of substance-using patients with known or suspected HIV infection should include a thorough history regarding other sexually transmitted diseases. Some of these other infections (e.g., herpes simplex virus) may reactivate and become more severe or more difficult to treat in immunosuppressed individuals than in patients with normal immune systems. Indeed, chronic mucocutaneous herpes simplex virus infection is an AIDS-defining illness when it is severe, nonhealing, and lasts for longer than one month (97–99). Other common sexually transmitted infections may be altered in their presentation or expression in the setting of HIV infection; syphilis is the most important example in this regard (293–298). Syphilis has been reported to be both accelerated and aberrant in its course, and at times refractory to standard therapy in certain patients with HIV infection; this is discussed in more detail in this section (293–298). In addition, human papillomavirus (HPV) infection, which may cause oral, anogenital, and common skin warts—and, less commonly, genital tract malignancies—in non–HIV-infected persons, occurs with increased frequency in HIV-infected patients (299–303). In such patients, HPV may cause extensive or recurrent genital or oral warts that may be difficult to treat. Furthermore, HPV infection has been strongly linked with an increased risk of cervical cytologic abnormalities in HIV-infected women, including dysplasia and frank carcinoma (299–301); the degree of malignant cytologic change appears to increase as women become more immunosuppressed in the course of their HIV infection (299–302,304). Reports also describe an increased risk of anal cancer in immunosuppressed HIV-infected homosexual men with coexistent HPV infection, further indicating the importance of the latter virus as a potential cause of malignancies in HIV-infected patients (305–307).

In addition to eliciting a history of sexually transmitted diseases from HIV-infected substance users, baseline assessment should also incorporate screening and assessment for the most commonly found coinfections or their sequelae. Specifically, this assessment should include (a) a physical examination for the presence of genital ulcers, warts, or other lesions; (b) routine serologic tests for syphilis including both nontreponemal tests (e.g., Venereal Disease Research Laboratory [VDRL]; serologic test for syphilis [STS]; rapid plasma reagin [RPR]) and treponemal tests (e.g., fluorescent treponemal antibody absorption [FTA-ABS]; microhemagglutinating antibody to *Treponema pallidum* [MHA-TP]); (c) cervical Papanicolaou (Pap) smear for female patients, with consideration of a rectal cytologic smear for homosexual or bisexual men; and (d) cultures or assays for gonorrhea, *Chlamydia,* and, as appropriate, herpes simplex virus. Depending upon the findings on initial evaluation, further diagnostic tests may be appropriate, for example, *Haemophilus ducreyi* cultures or empiric therapy for chancroid in patients with painful, exudative genital ulcers, or referral for colposcopy for HIV-infected women with abnormal cervical cytology.

Regarding the management of sexually transmitted diseases in the setting of HIV infection, it must be noted, as suggested earlier, that because both the natural history and response to treatment of certain of these infections may differ in HIV-positive patients from HIV-negative patients, the accepted standards of management may differ between these patient populations. Therefore, clinicians may need both to have a high index of suspicion of certain sexually transmitted diseases in HIV-infected patients, and to be prepared to treat such diseases more aggressively and/or for longer periods of time. The instance of greatest relevance in this regard is that of syphilis, in which there has been conflicting evidence regarding the possibilities of HIV altering the course of disease, and of suboptimal response to standard therapy in HIV-infected patients (293–298,308–314). Early data originating from case reports and small case series suggested that HIV infection altered the course of syphilis along with the response to therapy for syphilis. However, many recent, large, prospective studies showed no difference in the course of disease between HIV-positive and HIV-negative patients infected with syphilis (308,310,315). The same is true regarding syphilis treatment response—earlier small studies revealed poor responses to standard syphilis therapy (311–313), while many more recent prospective, large studies revealed good clinical and serologic responses to treatment (308–310,316–318). However, a few of the studies showing good response rates also concluded that responses tended to occur more slowly in HIV-infected individuals (316,318). Studies in methadone programs found that, when followed prospectively, HIV-infected substance users were not at significantly increased risk of showing unusual manifestations of syphilis when compared to their HIV-seronegative counterparts, even though in this same population syphilis was a risk factor for HIV infection (310,319). Early case reports suggested that certain HIV-infected patients with early syphilis may not be cured by standard single-dose therapy with benzathine penicillin, and that such patients may be at risk for symptomatic or asymptomatic neurosyphilis even after standard therapy (293–298). There is no convincing data to determine whether HIV-infected patients with early syphilis may be at increased risk for neurosyphilis or treatment failure (with standard treatment regimens recommended for HIV-negative patients). No treatment regimen has been shown to be more effective in preventing neurosyphilis for HIV-positive individuals; therefore, it is recommended to treat HIV-positive patients with the same standard regimen used for HIV-negative patients (benzathine penicillin G, 2.4 million units intra muscularly as a single dose) (Figure 58.1) (320). Certain authorities have recommended that all HIV-infected patients with syphilis undergo lumbar puncture and CSF examination to rule out neurosyphilis (297). Some clinicians recommend more aggressive treatment for early syphilis in HIV-infected patients—ranging from regimens used to treat late syphilis to high-dose regimens adequate for neurosyphilis (296–298). However, because the CSF VDRL may be negative in a substantial percentage of HIV-infected patients with early syphilis involving the central nervous system (CNS), and because nonspecific CSF abnormalities are common in HIV-infected patients (295–297), lumbar puncture may be nondiagnostic in HIV-infected patients with syphilis. Today, most clinicians treat early syphilis in HIV-infected patients with the standard regimen for HIV-negative patients, but they must ensure close followup and have a low threshold for inpatient referral for definitive treatment if serologic titers fail to decline appropriately or in the presence of neurologic signs or symptoms. Because of conflicting data and the unclear effect of HIV on treatment response to syphilis, close followup is recommended for all HIV-infected patients who complete a course of standard therapy for syphilis.

Diagnosis and treatment of syphilis in HIV-infected patients may be further complicated by the possibility of an abnormal serologic response to syphilis, an effect most likely related either to HIV-induced polyclonal B-cell activation, or to the failure of the normal antibody response to infection; these factors may result either in abnormally high titers, in falsely negative titers, or in other unusual serologic patterns (296,297,321–323). Notwithstanding these reported abnormalities, it is believed that most HIV-infected patients with syphilis are indeed able to demonstrate appropriate antibody responses (296,297,322,323). The phenomenon of false-positive nontreponemal serologic tests for syphilis in injection drug users is well documented (141,265), along with a few more recent studies documenting similar false-positive syphilis serologic tests in HIV-infected injection drug users (324,325).

Current CDC recommendations for the treatment of syphilis in HIV-infected patients attempt to highlight some of these uncertainties, while stressing the importance of close followup and the potential need for aggressive treatment of syphilis in patients with both infections (320,326). These guidelines include the following points, all relevant for clinicians caring for substance users with HIV infection: (a) When clinical findings suggest syphilis but serologic tests are negative, dark-field microscopy or direct fluorescent antibody tests for *T. pallidum* (DFA-TP) on lesion exudate or biopsy tissue should be performed. (b) Laboratories performing syphilis serologic tests should titrate nontreponemal tests to a final endpoint, rather than reporting results as greater than an arbitrary cutoff point (e.g., greater than 1:512), to enable detection of unusual serologic responses to syphilis and to monitor the response to therapy. (c) HIV-infected patients should be evaluated clinically and serologically at 3, 6, 9, 12, and 24 months after therapy, until a satisfactory serologic response to treatment occurs. If a two-dilution (fourfold) decrease in titer is not seen within 3 to 6 months for primary syphilis or in 6 months for secondary syphilis, or if an increase in titer of two dilutions or greater occurs, then patients should undergo CSF examination. (d) CSF examination should be performed in HIV-infected patients with latent syphilis of greater than 1 year or unknown duration; if this is not possible, patients should be treated with a regimen adequate for presumed neurosyphilis, for example, aqueous crystalline penicillin G, 3 to 4 million units intravenously every 4 hours (a total of 18 to 24 million units daily) for at least 10 to 14 days; or aqueous procaine penicillin G, 2.4 million units intramuscularly daily plus probenecid, 500 mg orally four times daily, for 10 to 14 days; and (e) neurosyphilis should be considered in the differential diagnosis of all patients with HIV infection and neurologic disease (see Figure 58.1) (320,326,327).

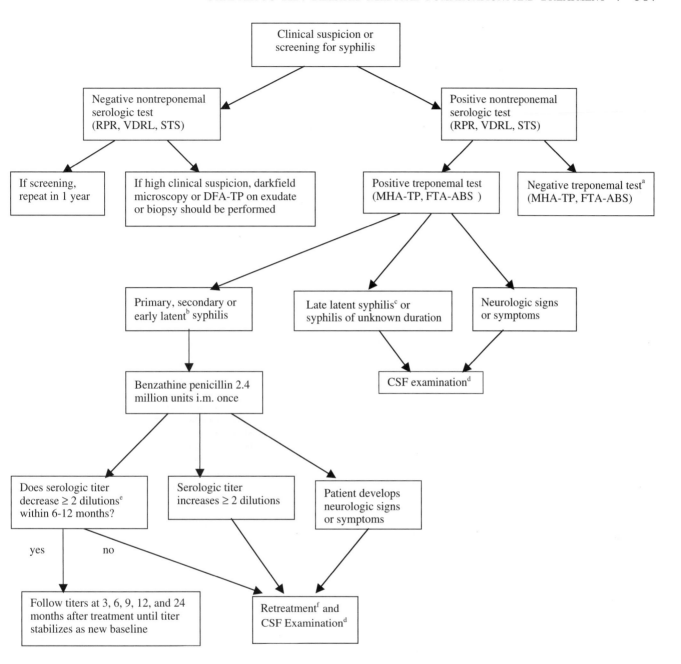

FIG. 58.1. Approach to syphillis in HIV-infected adults.

Notes

RPR=rapid plasma regain; VDRL=venereal disease research laboratory; STS=serologic test for syphilis; DFA-TP=direct fluorescent antibody tests for *Treponema pallidum*; MHA-TP=microhemagglutinating antibody to *T. pallidum*; FTA-ABS=fluorescent treponemal antibody absorption;

[a]False positive nontreponemal tests are not uncommon in injection drug users

[b]Early latent syphilis is defined as a newly positive or 2 titer increase in nontreponemal test without clinical manifestation, and having had a previously documented negative nontreponemal test within 1 year

[c]Late latent syphilis is defined as a newly positive or 2 titer increase in nontreponemal test without clinical manifestation, and a previously documented negative nontreponemal test > 1 year ago

[d]If unable to examine CSF treat for presumed neurosyphilis with (a) aqueous crystalline penicillin G 3-4 million units IV every 4 hours (total 18-24 million units per day) for 10-14 days or (b) procaine penicillin 2.4 million units IM daily for 10-14 days plus probenicid 500 mg orally 4 times daily for 10-14 days

[e]2-dilution change is equivalent to a 4-fold change in titer

[f]Most specialists re-treat with benzathine penicillin G 2.4 million units IM weekly for 3 weeks

The CDC guidelines also note, however, that there is disagreement regarding how aggressive clinicians must be in treating HIV-infected patients with syphilis, and that at present no change in standard therapy is officially recommended for HIV-infected patients coinfected with early syphilis. However, the authors of one review article concluded that, based on existing data, the minimum accepted treatment for early syphilis in HIV-infected patients should be three consecutive weekly injections of benzathine penicillin, 2.4 million units each (297); this approach has been adopted by some in clinical practice. The data to support such practices are conflicting; some studies, including the largest randomized trial of treatment of early syphilis in decades, revealed good clinical and serologic responses to standard syphilis treatment with early and latent syphilis in HIV-infected patients (308–310,316–318), whereas other studies found poor and inappropriate clinical and serologic responses to standard therapy (311–313). Of the aforementioned studies, one examined syphilis in HIV-infected injection drug users and found a good response to therapy with no differences between HIV-positive and HIV-negative patients (310). There is also much current interest in the possibility of oral or parenteral outpatient regimens effective against neurosyphilis, which clearly would help resolve the logistic problems posed by the prospect of undertaking lumbar puncture, CSF examination, and prolonged inpatient management for a potentially large population of injection drug users coinfected with HIV and syphilis. Such regimens, which have not been recommended formally by the CDC, include high-dose amoxicillin (2 g with probenecid 500 mg orally, three times daily for 14 days), doxycycline (200 mg orally, two times daily for 21 days), and ceftriaxone (1 g intramuscularly daily for 14 days) (296–298).

Although a few studies show that HIV-infected patients may be more likely to present during the secondary stage of syphilis (312,328), other studies, including a recent large, prospective, multicenter study, revealed that HIV infection had minimal, if any, effect on the clinical manifestations of primary and secondary syphilis (310,315). Interestingly, the study examining a cohort of injection drug users revealed no differences in presentation between the HIV-positive and HIV-negative individuals (310). The differences in presentation that may occur include more frequent multiple ulcers in primary syphilis, and more frequent and persistent concomitant genital ulcers in secondary syphilis in HIV-positive patients, when compared to HIV-negative patients. These are important observations, because, as mentioned already, sexual transmission is enhanced by ulcerative genital lesions and therefore appropriate prevention strategies (i.e., use of condoms) should be encouraged with even more emphasis.

Another important sexually transmitted agent that may coexist with the HIV is HPV, which may cause oral and genital warts and is associated with cervical dysplasia and neoplasia, cancer of the vulva, vagina, and penis, and anal cancer in homosexual and bisexual men (299–303,307,329). Health maintenance for HIV-infected women should include Pap smears twice within the first year after diagnosis of HIV infection and, if normal, annually thereafter (320). Referral for colposcopy and/or further diagnostic evaluation is based on Pap smear results. (Viral culture and molecular genetic techniques to detect HPV are not available in clinical settings, and, at present, are indirect measures of the virus' activity; that is, cervical cytologic smears and colposcopic biopsy comprise the standard for screening and diagnosis.) High-risk men should also be offered annual rectal Pap smears for cytologic evaluation (330). Although HPV infection has been associated with homosexual men, one recent study reported anal HPV deoxyribonucleic acid (DNA) in 46%, and abnormal anal cytology in 36%, of male injection drug users who reported never having had sex with men (331). The observation that HPV-associated neoplastic changes are often most severe in patients with advanced HIV-related disease suggests that clinicians' level of suspicion for cervical malignancies in women and anal malignancies in men should be higher for patients in the later stages of HIV infection (299,303,304). However, HPV and the associated cervical dysplasia and neoplasia have also been found in HIV-infected women who are not severely immunosuppressed (299,300,303,332).

It has also been suggested that HIV-infected women may be at increased risk of severe or refractory pelvic inflammatory disease (PID) (333), yet the evidence to support this has been sparse. A few small studies examining patients with PID found a greater percentage of adnexal masses or tuboovarian abscesses in HIV-infected women when compared to HIV-negative women (334,335); however, the clinical course and response to treatment have not differed among these groups. More population-based prospective studies of gynecologic manifestations of HIV infection are needed. Although studies have not clearly identified an increased risk of severe PID associated with HIV infection, this diagnosis certainly should be considered in substance-using women presenting with abdominal pain syndromes, especially in cases in which patients are known to be at high risk for sexually transmitted diseases.

Neurologic Disease

HIV infection has a wide range of effects on the central and peripheral nervous systems, some of which are the consequence of specific opportunistic infections and malignancies, and others apparently are the result of HIV infection itself, or the host response that it evokes (336,337). Among substance users with HIV, an important challenge for clinicians is the distinction between HIV-associated neurologic disease and that which results from acute or chronic substance use and its effects on the nervous system. This distinction is particularly important because many of the neurologic syndromes seen in HIV-infected patients may be treatable, but successful treatment depends on the accurate identification and differentiation of the underlying and immediate problems. It is common, for example, for clinicians in drug-treatment settings who are unfamiliar with HIV disease to assume that patients' cognitive or behavioral disturbances reflect a resumption of alcohol or drug use, when in fact these findings may indicate a CNS opportunistic infection, or HIV-associated dementia, or encephalopathy. Similarly, clinicians in inpatient AIDS treatment units may respond to a patient who develops lethargy, dysarthria, and pinpoint pupils by performing an emergent computed tomographic (CT) brain scan and lumbar puncture, when, in fact, a simple urine toxicology screen would have detected evidence of illicit opiate use. A complete discussion of the myriad effects of HIV infection and its sequelae on the nervous system is beyond the scope of this chapter, and the reader is referred to several excellent sources on this subject (338–342). In the present context it may be useful, however, to focus on certain neurologic aspects of HIV disease of particular relevance to substance-using populations, especially with respect to differential diagnosis.

The most important CNS manifestation of HIV infection is an entity denoted as HIV dementia (HIVD), also described as AIDS dementia complex, subacute encephalitis, or AIDS encephalopathy (336,339,343–347). Although it is one of the most common neurologic complications of HIV (reported to be 15% in one cohort prior to death), its prevalence appears to be declining in the era of HAART (339,343,344). This clinical syndrome is believed to result either from the direct effects of HIV and/or from additional factors related to the local response of the CNS to HIV infection (337,339,342,346). Clinical features of this syndrome range from mild cognitive deficits, memory loss, and subtle findings on neurologic examination to full-blown dementia with mutism, incontinence, and ination (339,345–350). Associated behavioral and affective changes may also vary greatly and can include apathy and social withdrawal, abulia, emotional lability, pronounced personality changes, and organic psychosis (339,345–348). An important distinguishing feature of HIVD, which differentiates it from acute substance use effects, is the relative preservation of a normal level of consciousness and alertness, even until the later stages of severe cognitive dysfunction (346,347). Specific neurologic findings that may be associated with HIVD include: psychomotor retardation, hypertonia, pyramidal tract signs, frontal release signs, tremor, ataxia, apraxia, and myoclonus, in varying degrees of severity (339,345–348). CT scans of the brain in patients with HIVD often demonstrate widespread cortical atrophy with ventricular dilation and enlarged sulci, although the degree of clinical dysfunction may not always correlate closely with radiographic findings (345–347). Cranial magnetic resonance imaging (MRI) in patients with HIVD often shows diffuse white matter hyperintensity, especially in the frontal regions (346); it has been suggested that MRI is superior to CT in the evaluation and detection of brain lesions in patients with HIV infection (351). Lumbar puncture and CSF examination generally are nonspecific in patients with HIVD; results may show mononuclear pleocytosis and/or a slightly elevated protein concentration (346,347). Studies suggest that HIVD may respond clinically to antiretroviral therapy (i.e., zidovudine [AZT]), which may also be of benefit in preventing its emergence (349,350,352,353). A more recent study investigating the efficacy of abacavir (Ziagen) in the treatment of HIVD has found limited clinical response to treatment (354). HIVD is often a diagnosis of exclusion, being made once other possible HIV-related CNS diseases are ruled out. The most common of these, all of which qualify as AIDS-defining illnesses, are cryptococcal meningitis, cerebral toxoplasmosis, CNS lymphoma, and progressive multifocal leukoencephalopathy (96,98,99,345). In addition, tuberculous meningitis and neurosyphilis are both seen in HIV-infected patients and may be more likely to occur in substance users than in certain other populations with AIDS, given the increased likelihood of coexisting tuberculosis and syphilis among HIV-infected substance users, as noted earlier. These varied entities may present with mental status changes, headache, focal neurologic deficits, seizures, fever, behavioral or personality changes, or other evidence of CNS involvement. Compared with these opportunistic infections and malignancies of the CNS, HIVD tends to be more indolent in onset and without localizing signs or symptoms (339,345–347); however, the time course and presentation of HIVD may be variable, and certain of these other entities also may present with relatively gradual onset and nonspecific signs such as weakness, apathy, or a decreased level of consciousness. In addition to HIVD and the specific AIDS-related infections and malignancies, an increased incidence of stroke and cerebrovascular disease in HIV-infected patients has also been described; this phenomenon is likely multifactorial, and has been attributed to a direct effect of HIV on vascular tissue, immune-mediated vasculitis, concurrent CNS infection, and substance use, particularly cocaine (355,356).

The basic diagnostic evaluation of HIV-infected patients with CNS disease should incorporate a full neurologic examination, including a mental status examination, a CT scan or MRI of the brain, lumbar puncture, and CSF examination and culture. These diagnostic tests will help to identify the AIDS-related meningitides, and will provide at least presumptive diagnoses of most of the mass or focal brain lesions. Certain focal brain lesions involving specific opportunistic infections and malignancies require biopsy of the brain as the only means for definitive diagnosis. However, a common practice is to initiate empiric therapy for the suspected clinical entity, for example, cerebral toxoplasmosis, and to reserve brain biopsy for cases that are either atypical or do not respond to a brief trial of empiric therapy (345).

For substance users with HIV infection, the same diagnostic guidelines should be followed as outlined above, although the possibility of CNS effects related to substance use becomes relevant. Drug intoxication commonly may present with apathy, lethargy, and diminished level of consciousness, as can certain CNS opportunistic infections, which may not initially be accompanied by localizing signs. Drug or alcohol withdrawal may also be accompanied by tremulousness, seizures, hallucinosis, other mental status changes, mood swings, or nonspecific findings, including inability to concentrate, dysphoria, anhedonia, insomnia, and other vegetative signs. Clearly, some or all of these findings may also be seen in HIVD or other HIV-related CNS syndromes. In addition, substance users historically have been known to be at risk for certain CNS infections related to drug injection, for example, pyogenic or fungal brain abscess, meningitis, spinal or epidural abscess, and endophthalmitis (141,357,358). Several reports describe an increased incidence of stroke associated with the use of cocaine, including ischemic, thrombotic, and especially hemorrhagic stroke (359–361).

Because some of the CNS manifestations of substance use and its sequelae may mimic or overlap those related to HIV infection, it is critical to consider all these possibilities when assessing HIV-infected substance users with CNS disease to successfully diagnose and treat them. In this regard, accurate and complete history taking is essential, for which it is often helpful to seek corroboration from patients' families or close contacts. This will help to define the temporal course and pattern of the development of symptoms—often an important feature in distinguishing HIVD from opportunistic infections or drug-related effects—and will also help in the formulation of an accurate history regarding recent use of drugs and alcohol. The timely use of urine toxicology testing is also critical to the assessment of HIV-infected patients presenting with CNS disease in whom substance use is suspected. When urine toxicology testing is not performed in such situations, as is often the case, the opportunity may be lost to make a specific diagnosis of certain drug-related conditions that may be treatable.

In addition to these simple diagnostic tools, which can help in the detection of substance use problems, it must also be stressed that the use of CT scan or MRI of the brain, lumbar puncture, and CSF examination should be equally routine in the assessment of known substance users presenting with possible HIV-related CNS disease. The failure to diagnose substance use problems in HIV-infected patients should not be paralleled by a failure to diagnose HIV-related CNS infections and malignancies in substance users with HIV infection. In addition, the possibility of medical complications of drug injection or drug use on the CNS not related to HIV disease (e.g., pyogenic or fungal brain abscess, cocaine-induced cerebrovascular disease) must also be considered in substance users with HIV infection.

Aside from CNS disease, patients with HIV infection have also been found to have peripheral nervous system (PNS) dysfunction related to HIV itself, antiretroviral or antituberculosis medications, and specific HIV-related infectious syndromes (e.g., herpes zoster radiculitis). The best-described entities affecting the PNS in such patients are chronic inflammatory demyelinating polyneuropathy, distal symmetric polyneuropathy, mononeuropathy multiplex, and progressive polyradiculopathy (336,345,362). The most common of these is distal symmetric polyneuropathy, which is predominantly a sensory neuropathy, that usually affects the distal lower extremities, occurring most often among patients in the later stages of HIV-related disease (363). This syndrome is characterized by marked paresthesia or dysesthesia, areflexia, and mild, if any, muscle weakness; in some patients, this syndrome may be a source of great discomfort. Diagnosis may be made via neurologic examination, nerve conduction studies, electromyography, and, in some cases, nerve biopsy. While a variety of medications have been studied for the treatment of peripheral neuropathy, only two randomized trials have shown improvement in pain—one using lamotrigine (Lamictal) (364), and the other using nerve growth factor (365). Gabapentin (Neurontin) was shown to be effective in a nonrandomized trial (366), while amitriptyline (Elavil), mexiletine (Mexitil), acupuncture, and peptide T have been ineffective in reducing pain (367–369).

Of importance to substance-using patients is that HIV-related peripheral neuropathies may coexist with or mimic the known complications of drug and alcohol use involving the peripheral nervous system, for example, distal symmetric polyneuropathy associated with chronic alcohol use or nutritional deficiencies, compression neuropathy resulting from limb compression during periods of drug-induced somnolence, or traumatic neuropathy involving direct injury to peripheral nerves from inaccurate or errant drug injection attempts (370). Furthermore, certain commonly used medications for HIV infection—for example, the so-called d-drugs didanosine (ddI) (Videx), zalcitabine (ddC) (Hivid), and stavudine (d4T) (Zerit); isoniazid; dapsone; and, to a much lesser extent, lamivudine (Epivir) (3TC)—may cause symptomatic and severe peripheral neuropathy (371–374). Indeed, in the cases of didanosine, zalcitabine, and stavudine, the development of peripheral neuropathy is one of the more serious side effects of each, and may even be treatment-limiting (371,373,374). NNRTIs and protease inhibitors are not associated with (PNS) dysfunction. Although one study showed that the combination of certain antiretroviral medications leads to a higher incidence of peripheral neuropathy than when those antiretroviral medications are used alone (371), it is not known whether the combination of drug or alcohol use with HIV-related medications may have an augmented toxic effect on the PNS. However, the possibility of multiple and combined etiologies for PNS disease should be considered by clinicians caring for HIV-infected substance users.

In general, the temporal trends in the incidence of HIV-related neurologic diseases reveal that neurologic complications remain frequent—peripheral neuropathy is increasing in incidence, although HIVD is decreasing in incidence (339,343,344,353). This may have particular relevance to substance users, for this population may be at higher baseline risk for PNS disease, which may be compounded by the toxic effects of antiretroviral and other medications, and which may also pose management problems involving the use of narcotic analgesics for the often severe pain syndromes seen in peripheral nerve disease.

Other Human T-Lymphotrophic Retroviruses

HIV, previously known as human T-lymphotrophic retrovirus type III (HTLV-III), is one of three HTLVs identified since the late 1970s. Human T-lymphotrophic retrovirus type I (HTLV-I) was the first virus in this group to be discovered, and was identified as the causal agent in adult T-cell leukemia/lymphoma, first described in Japan in 1977 (375–377). HTLV-I infection has since been associated with chronic degenerative neurologic diseases designated as tropical spastic paraparesis and HTLV-I-associated myelopathy (378,379). It has also been found to have a restricted geographic distribution, with endemic regions in Japan, the Caribbean basin, Africa, South America, and parts of the southeastern and southwestern United States (377,380,381). Human T-lymphotrophic retrovirus type II (HTLV-II), although originally isolated from a patient with hairy cell leukemia, has not consistently been identified as an etiologic agent for a specific disease, nor has it been found to have a particular geographic distribution (381). Although few studies found that HTLV-II infection in injection drug users was associated with neurologic and bacterial diseases, others studies shown no association of HTLV-II with any clinical disease, even when present with HIV infection (382–385).

The routes of transmission of HTLV-I are believed to be similar to those of HIV, although perhaps less efficient, involving sexual contact, parenteral exposure to blood through transfusion or use of contaminated injection equipment, and mother-to-infant transmission either perinatally or through breast-feeding (381,386). In previous studies, assays were not capable of distinguishing between HTLV-I and II; however, the more recent development of serologic assays now allow for differentiation between these two viruses. Given this, previous epidemiologic studies are problematic. It is believed that there is a long latency period from infection to disease in HTLV-I–infected persons (381), although one report described rapid development of myelopathy following transfusion-acquired HTLV-I infection in a patient who had undergone cardiac transplantation (387).

Although HTLV-I and HTLV-II are not believed to be endemic infections in most of the United States, it is noteworthy that the presence of HTLV-II is strongly associated with Native Americans and injection drug use inside and outside of the United States (386,388,389). Recent seroprevalence studies indicate that HTLV-II is present in up to 7% of injection drug users, and other reports document HTLV-I and HTLV-II infection among substance users in areas in the southeastern and western United States (27,380,388,390,391). Although it was initially thought that coinfection with HTLV-I and HIV may have led to acceleration of HIV, this phenomenon has not borne out with more recent experience in HIV disease.

Hepatitis B Virus and Hepatitis Delta Virus

Long before the AIDS epidemic, injection drug users were known to be at high risk for hepatitis B virus (HBV) infection (265–268). Seroprevalence studies demonstrate that 50% to 82% of chronic substance users show evidence of prior hepatitis B exposure (266–268,271,272,392); most such patients are seropositive for antibody to hepatitis B surface antigen and/or antibody to hepatitis B core antigen, with a small percentage (usually less than 10%) exhibiting chronic hepatitis B surface antigenemia. HBV infection is believed to be an early event in the career of injection drug users, usually occurring within the first 1 or 2 years after the initiation of drug injection (268,270,393). Given these considerations, it is probable that in most populations of chronic injection drug users into which HIV is introduced, HBV infection is likely to have been a prior event, with serologic evidence of immunity to HBV in most cases. However, one study that examined different HIV-infected risk groups that had been infected with HBV, found that substance users were less likely to develop protective antibodies to hepatitis B virus than were homosexual men (272).

New developments in the field of therapeutics show combined benefits in the treatment of both HIV infection and hepatitis B. Studies report that the use of the antiretroviral medications lamivudine and tenofovir (Viread) are associated with a significant reduction in the total viral load of HBV when treating chronic hepatitis B (394–397). Additionally, interferon-α and adefovir dipivoxil have been successful in the treatment of chronic hepatitis B (398–401). However, even with four different medications to treat hepatitis B infection, the long-term success of treatment has been relatively unsatisfying, particularly in HBV and HIV coinfected patients. Lamivudine, the treatment that has the been studied most for chronic hepatitis B infection in HIV-infected patients, is ineffective in 50% of coinfected patients after 2 years, as a result of the development of resistance to lamivudine in the hepatitis B virus (402). There is currently a paucity of long-term studies available that examine other treatment options, particularly in patients coinfected with HBV and HIV. Although HBV and HIV coinfection was initially thought to lead to mild liver disease (403,404), there is now consistent evidence that the natural history and clinical course of HBV infection is deleteriously altered by concomitant HIV infection. Studies show that HIV-infected patients are more likely to develop chronic hepatitis B infection and to develop cirrhosis than HIV-negative patients (405,406). These data support the use of hepatitis B vaccine for susceptible injection drug users and medical personnel providing care to such patients, both as a clinical intervention, and to help minimize occupational acquisition of HBV from patients who may show greater or more prolonged infectivity with HBV as a result of a greater burden of circulating virus. With regard to HIV infection, it remains unclear whether HBV alters the natural history of HIV disease. One study reported accelerated HIV disease in patients coinfected with HIV and HBV; however, another study has not reported similar findings (407,408).

Several studies examined the association between hepatitis delta virus (HDV) infection and HIV in injection drug users, and found that such patients exhibit delayed clearance of HDV, increased HDV replication, and accelerated loss of HDV antibody (65,66,409,410). The findings of increased and persistent HDV antigenemia in HIV-infected patients adds further support to the promotion of HBV vaccine among susceptible patients and medical staff (410), because immunity to HBV, in effect, precludes infection with HDV (68).

Hepatitis C Virus

Relatively recently identified as the etiologic agent of what was formerly known as non-A non-B hepatitis, hepatitis C virus (HCV) is a worldwide pandemic infecting an estimated 170 million people worldwide, and 3.6 million people in the United States (411). Infection with hepatitis C virus is five times more widespread than infection with HIV-1, and it is the leading cause of liver disease, and a main indication for liver transplant in the United States (411–413). The morbidity and mortality rates from hepatitis C infection are increasing, and are expected to continue to increase over the next several years (414). Because HCV is transmitted primarily through the parenteral route, and because blood banks are now screening blood donations with more comprehensive and effective methods, the vast majority of current infections are through the use of shared needles or drug-preparation equipment. The prevalence of HCV infection in substance users is reported to be as high as 95% (269–272). Studies examining heterosexual discordant couples show the risk of transmission to be very low, with some studies even reporting no transmission (415,416). However, coinfection with HIV appears to increase the risk of sexual transmission of HCV (416,417). Of those infected with hepatitis C virus 74% to 86% develop chronic disease (418,419), and of those, 15% to 20% develop cirrhosis (420,421). Risk factors associated with more aggressive HCV infection include acquiring the infection at 40 years of age or older, male gender, immunocompromised state (e.g., HIV

infection), coinfection with hepatitis B, alcohol use, and hepatotoxic medications (411,412).

Symptoms at the time of infection with hepatitis C virus are uncommon. Infection is often diagnosed when liver enzymes are found to be abnormal, and HCV antibodies are then tested and detected. However, with the recent elucidation of the epidemiology of HCV, all substance users should now be screened for hepatitis C infection by testing for antibodies to HCV, which develop in 90% of patients 3 months after initial exposure (412). Chronic infection is diagnosed by the detection of HCV RNA (by polymerase chain reaction [PCR]) in the blood for at least 6 months, often with elevated levels of liver transaminase enzymes. Extrahepatic manifestations associated with chronic hepatitis C infection include essential mixed cryoglobulinemia, rheumatoid symptoms, keratoconjunctivitis sicca, lichen planus, membranoproliferative glomerulonephritis, and porphyria cutanea tarda (422–424).

Treatment for hepatitis C infection has rapidly evolved over the past decade. Initially used alone, interferon-α required injections three times weekly, and had a low cure rate (5% to 13%), and a high relapse rate after treatment was stopped (425,426). Later, when interferon-α was used in combination with ribavirin (Virazole), the cure rate increased to approximately 30% to 49% (425,426). Currently, the best response to HCV is seen in patients taking the combination of pegylated interferon (peginterferon) alfa-2a or -2b and ribavirin, with cure rates approximately 56% overall (427,428). Genotype determination of HCV shows that genotype 1, which accounts for 70% to 75% of all HCV infections in the United States, has the poorest response (42% to 46% cure rate after 48 weeks), whereas genotypes 2 and 3 have better response rates (76% to 82% cure rate after 48 weeks) (427,428). Currently, it appears that 24 weeks of therapy may be adequate for patients infected with genotypes 2 or 3 (412). Recommended dosing for pegylated interferon alfa-2b is 1.5 μg/kg and for alfa-2a 180 μg, both requiring subcutaneous injection once-weekly, plus ribavirin 1,000 to 1,200 mg orally daily.

Adverse effects of interferon and ribavirin have led up to 32% of patients in clinical trials to discontinue treatment (425,427,429). Major adverse effects of interferon include flu-like symptoms, headache, fatigue, fever, rigors, myalgia, and thrombocytopenia. In addition, mood-altering effects are common, including depression, irritability, emotional lability, insomnia, and lack of motivation. Side effects of ribavirin include hemolysis, anemia, nausea, and pruritus. Therefore, frequent monitoring of the complete blood count is necessary, and antidepressants may also be useful in the management of side effects.

Because of the severe adverse effects, the need for adherence to a regimen involving injections, and other complicating factors that lead to aggressive HCV disease, injection drug users frequently have been ineligible for treatment of HCV infection, even though they make up the vast majority of patients infected with hepatitis C virus. In fact, in 1997 the National Institutes of Health (NIH) recommended that injection drug users be excluded from treatment until they were drug and alcohol free for at least 6 months (420). However, the most recent NIH consensus statement from June 2002 reports that efforts should be made to increase availability of the best current treatment to injection drug users (412). Recent studies show that injection drug users who are drug free for 6 to 12 months prior to initiation of HCV treatment can be started successfully on therapy after detoxification (430), and can achieve cure rates similar to that of the general population even if not drug free for 6 months prior to the initiation of treatment, or if sporadically actively using drugs during treatment (431; D. Sylvestre, personal communication). Management of HCV infection should be linked to drug-treatment programs in order to improve adherence and to enhance overall medical management of a complex illness, especially when coinfected with HIV (412,413). Because the treatment for HCV is difficult to tolerate, requires regular monitoring for hematologic abnormalities, and involves once-weekly injections, it is likely that with directly observed therapy (including administration of peginterferon) and support provided in drug-treatment programs, substance users will have optimal chances of successful therapy. The decision of whether to treat HCV infection in substance users is particularly complex, especially in those coinfected with HIV, and should be done in conjunction with a gastrointestinal or hepatology specialist. Specific factors that should be taken into consideration include other comorbid illnesses (such as HIV, hepatitis B, psychiatric illnesses), hepatotoxic medications, current drug and alcohol use, ability to adhere to medication, genotype of hepatitis C virus, and severity of liver disease. Studies show that in patients coinfected with HCV and HIV, HIV accelerates the course of hepatitis C disease, leading to cirrhosis in a shorter time period (432–434). However, studies also show that in patients with HCV and HIV coinfection, response rates to therapy for HCV are no different from those of HIV-negative patients (435–437). It is unclear whether hepatitis C virus accelerates the course of HIV disease or not, because studies report conflicting findings (438–440).

Malignancies

As noted, heterosexual substance users with HIV infection are at low risk for Kaposi sarcoma as compared with homosexual men (29,441). However, case reports and hospital-based series from the United States and Europe document the occurrence of malignant lymphomas among HIV-infected substance users (442–444), of which certain lymphomas are AIDS-defining (96–99). Furthermore, a review of malignant neoplasms reported among HIV-infected injection drug users in Italy described the occurrence of a variety of non–AIDS-defining solid tumors,

primarily involving the lung, testis, brain, skin, rectum, and oropharynx (445). Another study among substance users in a Bronx methadone program found an increased risk of lung and other cancers in HIV-infected versus HIV-seronegative cohorts (446). Clinicians who care for HIV-infected substance users should be alert to the possibility of neoplasms not formally recognized as AIDS-related in existing HIV classification systems.

Reported cases of lymphoma among HIV-infected substance users have included Hodgkin and non-Hodgkin types, with a wide variety of phenotypes, showing a high incidence of extranodal involvement and generally poor prognosis. Similarly, although persistent generalized lymphadenopathy is a frequent finding in HIV infection (97)—usually consisting of soft, movable, nontender lymph nodes less than 2 cm in diameter—and although palpable lymphadenopathy caused by skin abscesses and local soft-tissue infection has long been known to be common among injection drug users (265), the presence of large, firm, or rapidly growing lymph nodes should prompt consideration of a diagnosis of lymphoma with appropriate diagnostic interventions.

In addition, as already mentioned, the common occurrence of HPV coinfection in HIV-infected drug-using women requires clinical vigilance for cervical dysplasia and carcinoma in such patients. Similarly, in male homosexual or bisexual substance users, and possibly in heterosexual substance users, the possibility of HPV-induced anal carcinoma should also be considered (299–302,304,330,331,445). Finally, as discussed earlier, because of the high prevalence of hepatitis C virus infection in substance users, hepatocellular carcinoma, which occurs in approximately 1% to 4% of HIV-infected patients per year after the onset of cirrhosis, is likely to become a more frequent malignancy in this population as HIV-infected individuals continue to live longer with HAART (434).

Effects of Substance Use Versus Effects of HIV

As is apparent from the preceding review, it is important for clinicians who care for HIV-infected substance users to distinguish between the manifestations of HIV infection and the effects of substance use, and its acute and chronic sequelae. As noted, certain infectious diseases commonly seen among injection drug users may be more frequent or severe in the setting of HIV infection. In addition, certain infectious complications of injection drug use may be mistaken for manifestations of HIV infection, and vice versa. The possibility of coexisting morbidity from both HIV disease and the medical complications of drug use must also be considered in many instances (Table 58.4). These factors serve to emphasize the importance of obtaining accurate and relevant information concerning the nature and extent of drug use practices in substance users with HIV infection.

TABLE 58.4. *Medical complications of substance use that affect the differential diagnosis in injection drug users with HIV infection*

Symptoms	Possible diagnoses	
	HIV-related	Substance use–related
Constitutional 　Anorexia 　Weight loss 　Fever 　Night sweats 　Diarrhea	HIV infection, *M. Avium* complex, cytomegalovirus infection, tuberculosis	Cocaine use, injection-related bacterial infections, heroin withdrawal
Pulmonary 　Chest pain 　Cough 　Dyspnea	Bacterial pneumonia, *P. carinii* pneumonia, tuberculosis	Cocaine (crack) use, tobacco use, aspiration pneumonia
Neurologic 　Altered mental status 　Psychosis 　Seizures 　Focal deficits 　Peripheral neuropathy, alcoholic 　　polyneuropathy	HIV infection, toxoplasmosis, cryptococcosis, cytomegalovirus infection, progressive multifocal leuko-encephalopathy, medication toxicity	Intoxication with and withdrawal from heroin, cocaine, alcohol, or benzodiazepines; drug-related chronic encephalopathy; pyogenic central nervous system infection, trauma
Dermatologic 　Pruritus 　Rash Purpura	dermatitis, thrombocytopenia, medication allergy	Drug-related pruritus, chronic hepatitis, cellulitis, alcohol or heroin-induced thrombocytopenia, lymphedema
Miscellaneous 　Lymphadenopathy 　Uremia	lymphadenopathy, nephropathy	Localized infection, heroin nephropathy

Adapted from O'Connor P, Selwyn PA, Schottenfeld RS. Medical management of injection drug users with HIV infection. *N Engl J Med* 1994;33:450–459.

Aside from infectious complications and other related syndromes, there are a number of constitutional symptoms often seen in HIV-infected patients that may overlap with symptoms because of acute or chronic substance use. These include fever, weight loss, fatigue, malaise, and diarrhea (102), and are believed to be a consequence of HIV infection itself, apart from the symptomatology that may accompany specific infectious syndromes. Indeed, the definition of HIV-related wasting syndrome, which qualifies as an AIDS-defining diagnosis in the CDC's 1993 revised AIDS case definition (99), includes several of these symptoms as necessary criteria for this diagnosis. It is important, therefore, to attempt to differentiate between the overlapping symptomatology of HIV infection per se, and that of chronic substance use or withdrawal. Among active injection drug users, fever, fatigue, malaise, and diarrhea are not uncommon (the latter particularly among opiate users, who alternately experience constipation and diarrhea as they fluctuate between narcotic intoxication and withdrawal) (265,447). Weight loss is also a common finding among substance users, especially cocaine users, in whom anorexia and a hypermetabolic state are related directly to the pharmacologic effects of the drug (265,447). Substance-dependent patients may often be malnourished because of a disorganized lifestyle and lack of self-care, making it difficult to differentiate the effects specifically related to poor nutrition, substance use, or HIV-infection and its sequelae.

Furthermore, the recent escalation in use of smoked freebase cocaine, or crack, is associated with pulmonary edema, barotrauma, bronchospasm, and other pulmonary manifestations (448–450). In addition, dyspnea on exertion, or at rest, is often reported by such patients. Because dyspnea without a productive cough or other obvious signs of pneumonia is one of the most common symptoms to herald the onset of PCP in HIV-infected patients (124), it is important for clinicians to be aware of the different potential causes of such pulmonary symptoms in substance users. In addition to crack use, another potential cause of pulmonary symptoms is heavy cigarette smoking—a widespread practice among illicit substance users (451). Patients and clinicians often mistakenly attribute cough or dyspnea simply to excessive smoking—especially in the absence of fever or other signs of pneumonia—when, in fact, these symptoms may indicate the gradual onset of PCP. Interestingly, anecdotal clinical experience suggests that among HIV-infected substance users who smoke tobacco, abrupt smoking cessation because of perceived worsening shortness of breath can be an indirect indicator of the development of PCP (P. Selwyn, unpublished data).

Finally, the presence of generalized lymphadenopathy, often found in HIV-infected patients (97), may at times be confused with the finding of multiple palpable lymph nodes because of lymphatic drainage from sites of drug injection, localized soft-tissue infection, oral pathology, or other conditions commonly seen in injection drug users (265). For this reason, it has been suggested that, among substance users, the sites most specific for HIV-related lymphadenopathy are the posterior cervical chains, which, in the absence of scalp lesions, are the sites least likely to reflect lymph node enlargement merely because of local skin and soft-tissue pathology.

In addition to the various syndromes that can be difficult to differentiate between drug use itself and HIV infection, the most important effect that drug use has on HIV disease is the problem with adherence to medical care. Adherence to medical care includes attendance to appointments with primary care providers, follow through with referrals and tests, and adherence to medications. Because substance use can interfere with all of these elements in the receipt of health care, its impact on HIV disease can be grave. As mentioned previously, studies have determined that substance users are less likely to access ambulatory care, less likely to take antiretroviral medication for HIV infection, and less likely to adhere to antiretroviral medication (75–80). Therefore, as providers of substance users, it is crucial to reaffirm the importance of adherence with all aspects of medical care.

SPECIFIC CLINICAL ISSUES IN THE CARE OF SUBSTANCE USERS WITH HIV INFECTION

In addition to the particular spectrum of HIV disease in injection drug users, and the need to distinguish between the manifestations of HIV infection and the effects of drug use and its sequelae, several issues, which are discussed briefly here, are of clinical relevance to the care of HIV-infected substance users.

Pain Management

Frequently, patients with HIV infection require analgesia for pain syndromes resulting from specific opportunistic infections or their complications. Although clinicians may express appropriate concern about the possibility of drug-seeking behavior or manipulation on the part of substance users attempting to obtain narcotics or other psychotropic medications, this concern may result at times in the inappropriate withholding or underuse of strong analgesics in settings in which they are medically indicated. A common misconception is that patients maintained on methadone do not require additional narcotics for analgesia, or that analgesia can be achieved, if necessary, simply by increasing patients' daily methadone doses. In fact, patients on methadone maintenance quickly develop tolerance to the drug's analgesic effects, and do not have a blunted perception of noxious stimuli (452,453). Indeed, because of their tolerance to narcotic drugs, such patients require at least the standard, and at times higher-than-standard, doses of short-acting narcotic analgesics (e.g., oxycodone, hydromorphone [Dilaudid], codeine) when indicated for pain relief. In addition, these drugs must often be administered on a more frequent dosing schedule than when used for nontolerant patients, because of their rapid elimination in narcotic users (453). Although substance users certainly are not the only category of patients in whom the inadequate clinical use of strong analgesics is common, such undermedication predictably results in a typical pattern of confrontation and acting out among such patients, with the frequent result of poor patient outcomes and increasing frustration and/or dissatisfaction among medical staff. The judicious and appropriate use of strong narcotic analgesics, when indicated, can help prevent this undesirable chain of events (453,454). Clearly, however, when such drugs are used, clinicians must remain mindful of the possibility of abuse—for example, by providing small quantities at a time for outpatients, and by renewing prescriptions on a fixed schedule—and should taper such medications gradually before discontinuation.

Drug Interactions

Several potential drug interactions have been identified that are of specific relevance to the care of HIV-infected opiate users, especially those on methadone maintenance. The most important of these for HIV-infected patients are the complex interactions between numerous antiretroviral medications and methadone (see Table 58.3). Medications in all three classes of antiretroviral therapy—namely nucleoside or nucleotide reverse transcriptase inhibitors (NRTIs), nonnucleoside reverse transcriptase inhibitors (NNRTIs), and protease inhibitors—interact with methadone. The NRTIs tend to have the least effect on clinical manifestations of drug interactions with methadone. Stavudine and didanosine levels are decreased by 27% and 60%, respectively, when administered with methadone; however, the clinical sequelae of this decrement is yet to be determined (82,455,456). Stavudine dosage requires no adjustment, whereas didanosine dose may need to be increased (82). Methadone levels remain unchanged when coadministered with these NRTIs. Studies examining the effect of methadone and abacavir coadministration reveal that the rate of clearance of methadone is increased, whereas the peak concentration of abacavir is decreased (457). The clinical significance of these findings is unclear. The administration of lamivudine and zidovudine with methadone has no effect on methadone levels (458). One study showed that zidovudine levels are increased up to 40% when patients are taking methadone, and that reductions in zidovudine may be necessary (459). Currently, there is no data regarding drug interactions between methadone and any other NRTIs.

Of the NNRTIs, nevirapine has been cited in several case reports as precipitating opiate withdrawal in patients receiving methadone (460). Nevirapine decreases methadone levels by 46%, and requires increases in methadone dosing, up to 185% in one study (460,461). Efavirenz also is reported to decrease methadone levels by 52%, induce symptoms of methadone withdrawal, and require increases in methadone doses, up to 200% in one study (461–463). There is no current data available on interactions between methadone and delavirdine.

Of the protease inhibitors, ritonavir (Norvir), lopinavir/ritonavir (Kaletra), nelfinavir (Viracept), and amprenavir (Agenerase) decrease methadone levels by 37%, 53%, an unclear percentage, and 35%, respectively. Although amprenavir, ritonavir, and nelfinavir induce methadone withdrawal, the others do not (464–472). Although studies show no required increase in methadone dosage in patients taking Kaletra or ritonavir, one case report revealed a 185% increase in methadone dosage in a patient started on nelfinavir (465,468,472). Indinavir (Crixivan) and saquinavir (Fortovase) have little to no effect on methadone levels (467,468,473). Although some of the protease inhibitors have not induced methadone withdrawal nor required dose escalation of methadone in studies, providers must be attentive to signs and symptoms consistent with opiate withdrawal and titrate methadone doses accordingly.

Another very important drug interaction in opiate-addicted patients is between rifampin (Rifadin) and methadone, which was described by Kreek et al. in 1976 (474). Given the common occurrence of tuberculosis in HIV-infected substance users, the concurrent use of methadone and rifampin has become increasingly frequent in the AIDS era. Rifampin increases the elimination of methadone and reduces methadone plasma levels by 33% to 68%, an effect believed to be caused by enhanced hepatic microsomal enzyme activity resulting from rifampin administration (456,474). This effect results clinically in the onset of typical opiate withdrawal symptoms, at times severe, within several days of the initiation of rifampin therapy in methadone-maintained patients (474). This phenomenon may be prevented in most cases by increasing patients' daily methadone doses, usually by 10 mg every 1 to 2 days, beginning on the day that rifampin is introduced. At times, the final maintenance dose arrived at may be at least 50% greater than the original maintenance dose before the patient reaches a new stable steady state. Patients should be monitored closely during these rapid methadone increases, with increased dose levels titrated to oversedation, although this seldom occurs when rifampin therapy is introduced. Occasionally, rifampin-induced withdrawal may be lessened by dividing the daily methadone dose on a twice-daily schedule—for example, two thirds in the morning, one third in the evening—although this practice may not always be possible in the outpatient set-

ting or within the constraints of dispensing regulations for methadone-maintenance treatment programs. In addition, it should be noted that patients may, at times, resist or attempt to evade the daily ingestion of rifampin, especially in methadone-maintenance treatment program settings where methadone and rifampin are often coadministered, because of the feared or perceived noxious effects of rifampin. This possibility must be considered carefully by clinicians who supervise the care of such patients to ensure both the effective management of tuberculosis, and to avoid the potential for methadone overdose in patients who have surreptitiously minimized their rifampin intake after having had their methadone doses increased to compensate for the anticipated rifampin-induced effects on methadone metabolism. One simple measure to monitor whether patients in drug-treatment settings are ingesting rifampin is to instruct nursing staff to inspect patients' routine urine toxicology specimens for the presence of the characteristic bright red-orange color that is typically noted in urine and other body fluids among patients on rifampin therapy (475). When rifampin is discontinued, following completion of tuberculosis therapy or for other reasons, it is advisable to gradually reduce patients' daily methadone doses accordingly, although the final level arrived at in such cases may be higher than the starting level before rifampin therapy was introduced. As mentioned earlier, rifabutin, which is regularly used in the treatment and prevention of tuberculosis in patients on antiretroviral therapy, and in disseminated *Mycobacterium avium* complex, may also minimally reduce methadone levels, if at all, by enhancing hepatic microsomal enzymatic activity (233–235,476). Whereas rifampin decreases methadone levels substantially and leads to clinical symptoms of opiate withdrawal, rifabutin neither leads to opiate withdrawal nor requires changes in methadone dosing, thus allowing for easier management of patients on methadone (242,456).

In another small study, the antifungal agent fluconazole was found to increase the plasma levels of methadone, although clinically there were no signs or symptoms of opiate overdose in those taking fluconazole (477). Another class of medications frequently used in the care of HIV-infected substance users is neuroleptics, because seizures may occur as a common complication of certain HIV-related CNS infections or malignancies. Phenytoin (Dilantin), phenobarbital (Luminal), and carbamazepine (Tegretol) decrease methadone levels and induce symptoms of opiate withdrawal (478–480). Accordingly, although methadone dose increases are often necessary to prevent opiate withdrawal in patients on methadone maintenance who are placed on phenytoin, these increases generally need not be as great or as rapid as in the case of rifampin.

Illicit Drugs and HIV

The most important issue in current active substance use and HIV is adherence. Many studies report that active

TABLE 58.5. *Interactions between antiretroviral medications and recreational drugs*

Drug	Effect	Comment
Alcohol	↑ abacavir level	Unknown significance
Amphetamines	Ritonavir may ↑ amphetamine level 2–3 fold	Avoid combining with ritonavir, alternatively use 1/4 – 1/2 amount of amphetamine
Cocaine	Possibly ↑ HIV replication and weaken immune system (64, 490–492)	In test-tubes and mice only
MDMA[a] (Ecstasy)	Overdose and death with ritonavir (487, 488). Possibly ↑ levels with other protease inhibitors (PIs) and nonnucleoside reverse transcriptase inhibitors (NNRTIs)	Avoid combining with ritonavir, alternatively use 1/4 – 1/2 amount of MDMA and watch for signs of toxicity
GHB[b]	↑ levels and toxicity with ritonavir/saquinavir (488), possibly ↑ with delavirdine	Use cautiously with PIs, delavirdine, efavirenz
Heroin	Ritonavir may ↓ levels by 50%. Ritonavir and other PIs may also ↑ levels.	
Ketamine	Possibly ↑ levels with ritonavir, delavirdine, efavirenz	Use cautiously with ritonavir, nelfinavir, efavirenz
LSD[c]	Unknown	Use cautiously with PIs, delavirdine, efavirenz
Marijuana	PIs may ↑ levels	Efavirenz may cause false positive screening test
PCP[d]	Possibly ↑ levels with antiretrovirals	Use cautiously with PIs, delavirdine, efavirenz

[a]methylenedioxymetamphetamine
[b]γ-hyroxybutyrate
[c]lysergic acid diethylamide
[d]phencyclidine
Adapted from: Antoniou T, Tseng AL. Interactions between recreational drugs and antiretroviral agents. *Ann Pharmacother* 2002;36:1598–613.
AIDS Education Training Center (AETC) National Resource Center, May 2002

substance use is associated with poor adherence to HIV medications (81,481–483), and such suboptimal adherence is associated with drug resistance, less viral suppression, and higher morbidity and mortality (484–486). Unlike drug interactions between methadone and HIV-related medications, there is a paucity of data available regarding interactions between illicit drugs and antiretroviral medications. Most data come from case reports in which patients have had severe, even lethal, interactions between specific illicit drugs and antiretroviral medications. As discussed previously, many drug interactions between antiretroviral medications and other drugs or medications are mediated through the hepatic P450 enzyme system. Given that many recreational drugs are metabolized through this system, the potential for drug interactions between recreational drugs and protease inhibitors or NNRTIs is significant. The amphetamine methylenedioxymethamphetamine (MDMA, ecstasy) is associated with fatal and near-fatal overdoses in two patients started on ritonavir. One case involved a patient taking MDMA after having ritonavir added to his antiretroviral regimen, while the other involved a patient taking MDMA and γ-hydroxybutyrate after starting ritonavir and saquinavir (487,488). Other amphetamines are metabolized through

the P450 system and are thought to have similar potential interactions with ritonavir; thus, the combination of amphetamines with ritonavir should be avoided (489). There are no data to date regarding drug interactions between ketamine (Ketalar), phencyclidine (PCP), lysergic acid diethylamide (LSD), heroin, or cocaine and antiretroviral medications; however, based on the specific metabolism of these drugs through the hepatic P450 enzyme system, one could postulate that interactions might occur with particular antiretroviral medications that inhibit or induce these specific enzymes involved in the metabolism of these recreational drugs (Table 58.5). Other potential effects that illicit drugs may have on HIV-infected patients include depression of the immune system and facilitation of the replication of HIV, as suggested by a few *in vitro* and *in vivo* mice studies with cocaine (64,490–492).

Self-Medication

The use of nonprescribed antibiotics available through the street drug market, or "antibiotic abuse," has been described among injection drug users independent of the AIDS epidemic (493,494). This phenomenon appears to be common, and was identified in one large study from

Detroit as a risk factor for MRSA infection among substance users hospitalized for bacterial endocarditis (494). This practice is of particular relevance to the management of HIV-infected substance users, who may thereby present with acute illness because of partially treated bacterial infections, which might make it difficult to diagnose or treat such infections effectively. Consequently, eliciting a specific history for street antibiotic use is critical for the assessment of substance users presenting with suspected bacterial infections because such information may not be volunteered by patients who would not consider nonprescribed antibiotic use to be pertinent to their medical or substance use histories. Anecdotal evidence suggests that various antiretroviral medications, in addition to standard antibiotics, are also available on the street, and that such medications may be taken sporadically in an unsupervised manner as a form of self-treatment (495). This may result in the periodic ingestion of large amounts of antiretroviral medication following episodes of needle sharing or other unsafe practices, in an attempt at self-prophylaxis against HIV infection. Although there has been no clear documentation of serious medical consequences as a result of such behavior among substance users, it is likely that with sporadic use of antiretroviral medication, resistance to the specific antiretroviral agents taken may ensue. In addition, several case reports describe instances of intentional zidovudine overdose among injection drug users as a form of suicide attempt (495,496). These findings suggest that clinicians who care for substance users at risk for HIV infection should consider the possibility of unsupervised self-medication with HIV-related therapeutic agents in such patients, and that an assessment of patients' reliability, responsibility, and expected adherence should inform the decision to initiate such medication regimens.

The use of prescription medications that potentiate or modify the effect of common street drugs has always been a source of experimentation among substance users. Commonly used medications with psychotropic effect can be found in the street market with relative ease, and their effect when combined with illegal drugs is well recognized. Different medical devices may also impact the illicit-drugs market, such as the aerosol devices intended to deliver bronchodilators and their use by cocaine smokers to enhance the pulmonary absorption of their drug. Furthermore, as outpatient medicine becomes more sophisticated, and procedures and techniques traditionally reserved for hospital use become widely available in outpatient settings and private homes, an impact is also noted in the drug-using population. Of special note is the use of permanent indwelling intravenous devices for multiple medical indications (e.g., prolonged courses of antibiotics, chemotherapy, dialysis) often indicated in patients with HIV infection, which can also be used as a means of injecting illicit drugs (497).

PRIMARY MEDICAL CARE FOR SUBSTANCE USERS WITH HIV INFECTION

During the first decade of the AIDS epidemic, a gradual shift in the clinical care of HIV-infected patients occurred, involving earlier medical intervention and a growing emphasis on outpatient care (107,115,498,499). This trend emerged as specific antiretroviral therapy became available—with the introduction of zidovudine in 1987 (500)—and as prophylactic regimens against opportunistic infections gained acceptance soon thereafter (116). As a result of this trend, medical therapies were offered to patients even in the asymptomatic stages of HIV infection, whereas earlier in the epidemic, the clinical approach to HIV had been limited largely to the treatment of specific opportunistic infections and malignancies among patients in the later phases of HIV disease and AIDS. Consequently, the population of HIV-infected patients now considered eligible for specific medical interventions—offered to increase quality of life and length of life—has grown steadily in parallel with the growth in preventive interventions (107,115,498,499). Because asymptomatic individuals, or those who have not yet progressed to AIDS, would be expected to comprise the largest proportion of an HIV-infected population at any one point in time (501), early medical intervention for HIV infection has had major implications for health planning and policy (53,107,115,498,499,502). These trends have only intensified with the introduction of more effective HIV treatment regimens and the desirability of reducing HIV viral load even during the period of clinical latency.

Current management of HIV infection with HAART prolongs the life span of HIV-infected patients (122). Among injection drug users, the finding of HIV seroprevalence levels exceeding 30% in certain heavily affected geographic areas in the United States (23,503) suggests that a substantial number of such individuals would now be considered eligible for early medical intervention. This has posed both a great challenge and a great opportunity for the drug-abuse treatment system, which is now faced with a growing number of patients for whom the delivery of primary medical care services is an urgent priority. Indeed, there are few other areas of the health care system in which individuals at such high risk for HIV infection are likely to be concentrated. This has meant that substance-abuse treatment programs and other related facilities have had to respond to the growing needs of HIV-infected patients, often in the setting of limited resources and considerable marginalization within the medical care system. Fortunately, however, there have been certain successes in different areas as attempts have been made to link substance abuse treatment with primary medical care for HIV infection (49,50,52,482,504,505). Although no single model of linkage or integration would be expected to be successful in all settings, it is encouraging that these efforts may become part of the more comprehensive integration of substance-abuse treatment into mainstream medical care, a process that already has been spurred by the needs of drug-using patients with HIV infection.

For clinicians who care for HIV-infected substance users, regardless of the clinical context, certain basic elements are central to the comprehensive primary care of such patients. The following sections briefly outline some of the medical and psychosocial issues that are of key importance for the evaluation and care of HIV-infected substance users in the outpatient setting.

Baseline Medical Assessment of Substance Users with HIV Infection

First, as in most other medical evaluations, eliciting a thorough history is a central component of the baseline assessment of patients presenting with a diagnosis of HIV infection. The history should focus on substance use and sexual behavior, especially within the preceding 5 to 10 years. This information can be helpful both to assess the likelihood of ongoing risk behavior—particularly important in terms of the current risk of other sexually transmitted diseases or of infections caused by continuing drug use practices—and, at times, to help identify when patients are likely to have become infected with HIV. The latter information most often is not known, and at best can only be estimated, but in certain cases, the cumulative history of risk behavior can be instructive (e.g., patients who report long-standing abstinence following episodes of high-risk behavior in the distant past, or who describe temporally limited high-risk practices such as "shooting gallery" injection or street prostitution in HIV-endemic areas). In addition to behavioral information, the history should focus on medical data such as hospitalizations for pneumonia, endocarditis, or tuberculosis—suggestive, although not always diagnostic, of HIV infection among substance users—and on any other known or suspected HIV-related illnesses. These include not only the specific illnesses and conditions that qualify for a diagnosis of AIDS (96,98,99), but also (and more commonly) certain HIV-related conditions, such as oral candidiasis (thrush), herpes zoster, chronic fungal skin infections, seborrheic dermatitis and psoriasis, and generalized lymphadenopathy. A thorough inquiry should be made into patients' histories of tuberculosis, regarding results of prior skin tests and possible tuberculosis exposure, with documentation of the date of the first positive PPD test or any known exposure to tuberculosis (e.g., household contact with an active tuberculosis case). Complete information should be elicited regarding the dates and length of past treatment or prophylaxis for tuberculosis. A history of hepatitis B and C exposure or disease, in addition to hepatitis A and B vaccination, should also be elicited. For patients in whom a specific date or time period for acquisition of HIV is strongly suspected, it may be useful to attempt to elicit a history of the acute retroviral syndrome, an entity that has been described in certain patient populations with documented primary HIV infection and seroconversion for HIV antibody (506–508). This syndrome is self-limited, lasting no more than several weeks, and characterized generally by fever, malaise, lymphadenopathy, rash, myalgias, pharyngitis, and/or other nonspecific manifestations that are easily confused with mononucleosis or a flu-like syndrome. It is uncertain how often this syndrome occurs among individuals newly infected with HIV, and it is likely that many individuals become infected with no clinical symptoms to accompany seroconversion. In addition, this syndrome has not been described consistently among substance users, which may reflect the low likelihood that substance users would commonly seek medical attention for what is generally a mild, self-limited illness, and/or the possibility that the background level of medical symptoms among such patients would be likely to obscure a nonspecific syndrome that would be more noticeable among healthy nonaddicted individuals. Nevertheless, for patients in whom a specific time period for primary HIV infection is known or suspected, it may be useful to corroborate this with a history of acute retroviral syndrome, if present. One should also attempt to elicit a baseline history of HIV-related constitutional symptoms—for example, fever, weight loss, fatigue, diarrhea—although, as noted, it is important among substance users to attempt to distinguish these symptoms from those caused by the effects of acute or chronic substance use.

The baseline physical examination for HIV-infected substance users should incorporate a standard complete examination with special emphasis on the detection of HIV-related conditions. With particular relevance to the latter, the examination should include measurement of height and weight (with calculation of ideal body weight); a complete examination of the oral cavity (509) (examining for oral candidiasis, oral hairy leukoplakia, Kaposi sarcoma, aphthous or other oral ulcers, and HIV-related periodontal disease); palpation for all accessible lymph nodes with notation of size, consistency, tenderness, and location; complete inspection of the skin and nails (510) (examining for fungal dermatoses, onychomycosis, seborrheic dermatitis or psoriasis, xerosis, verrucous lesions, molluscum contagiosum, folliculitis, Kaposi sarcoma, active or healed zosteriform eruptions, as well as fresh or old injection marks); and evaluation for hepatosplenomegaly. Female patients should be given a complete pelvic examination with Pap smear for cervical cytology and cultures or assays for gonorrhea, *Chlamydia,* and, if indicated by symptoms or history, herpes simplex virus. Both males and females should receive a genital and rectal exam with inspection for genital or anal ulcers. As previously indicated, it may be prudent to obtain a rectal Pap smear for cytologic examination in males with a history of homosexual contact.

Baseline laboratory tests should include the following: complete blood count with differential and platelet count;

serum electrolytes, chemistries, and liver function tests; lymphocyte subset studies, including determination of total lymphocytes, number and percentage of CD4+ T-lymphocytes, CD8 number and percentage, and CD4:CD8 ratio; serologic testing for syphilis, including both nontreponemal (e.g., VDRL, STS, RPR) and treponemal (e.g., FTA-ABS, MHA-TP) tests; complete HBV serology, including hepatitis B surface antigen (HBsAg), hepatitis B surface antibody (HBsAb), and antibody to hepatitis B core antigen (HBcAb); hepatitis C antibody; hepatitis A antibody (immunoglobulin [Ig] G); and a baseline serum anti-*Toxoplasma gondii* antibody assay.

The absolute number and/or percent of CD4+ T-lymphocytes and the plasma HIV RNA (viral load) are the most useful laboratory markers indicating prognosis and risk for disease progression in HIV-infected individuals (95,110–114,117,140,511–516). In addition, the CD4+ T-cell count and viral load are the key laboratory determinants in the decision-making process around initiation of antiretroviral medications (82). Viral load testing is used as an outcome measure in studies of the efficacy of antiretroviral therapies, and it is standard practice in monitoring disease progression and response to therapy in individual patients, together with the CD4+ T-lymphocyte count (53,120,517–522). The CD4+ T-cell count and viral load should be monitored minimally every 3 to 6 months in the untreated patient, and requires more frequent monitoring in patients taking antiretroviral medications according to the circumstances of the individual patient's care (82). The viral load is a sensitive marker in the evaluation of the efficacy of antiretroviral medication, and is an essential parameter in deciding whether to stop or change antiretroviral therapies.

As an additional component of routine HIV primary care, all patients without a well-documented prior positive PPD or history of previously diagnosed tuberculosis should receive an intradermal 5 TU PPD (Mantoux). It is also suggested by some experts to have all patients obtain a baseline chest x-ray, something that is especially critical for any patient found to have a positive PPD test by history or examination.

Current recommendations support the routine use of five vaccines in the HIV-infected patient: (a) influenza vaccine yearly, at the appropriate time and season (83,523); (b) hepatitis B vaccine for patients seronegative for all HBV markers (83,524), given in a three-dose series following standard recommendations for non–HIV-infected individuals to be repeated if no appropriate response is documented; (c) hepatitis A vaccine for patients seronegative for hepatitis A IgG antibody, and who are substance users or chronically infected with hepatitis B or C viruses, given in two doses (83); (d) tetanus toxoid if not given with the prior 10 years; and (e) the 23-valent pneumococcal polysaccharide vaccine in patients with CD4+ T-cell counts of at least 200/mm^3 (optional in those with CD4+ T-cell counts less than 200/mm^3), to be offered every 5 years (Table 58.6) (83,525).

Treatment of HIV Infection

The introduction of zidovudine (AZT) in 1987 was followed by a long period in which monotherapy was the only possible therapeutic approach. Since 1993, the rapid development and subsequent FDA approval of new classes of antiretroviral agents, with different, and in some instances, complementary, mechanisms of action, has brought new hope into the field of pharmacologic treatment of HIV disease (53). Eradication or cure of HIV infection, although the final conceivable goal of all efforts in the development of new therapeutic strategies, is not achievable at this moment. However, available antiretroviral agents used in combination has signified a dramatic therapeutic breakthrough in HIV management. Many ongoing studies have reported a sustained reduction in the total HIV viral load with the use of at least three agents (526–530). When such an effect persists, a slower rate of progression of disease occurs, along with improved survival (122,531).

The addition of new drugs to the already complex daily medication regimens of many patients also brings to light the issue of new drug interactions (as discussed previously), and important concerns about adherence with chronic medication regimens in patients who may be actively using illicit drugs. What follows is a brief description of the main pharmacologic properties, accepted uses, and interactions of the antiretroviral drugs available as of mid-2002.

Nucleoside Reverse Transcriptase Inhibitors

NRTIs are the backbone of antiretroviral therapy, with at least two NRTIs used in various combinations with either one or more protease inhibitors, one NNRTI, or one additional NRTI. NRTIs are the largest class of antiretroviral agents, currently with seven different FDA-approved medications. Multiple different combinations of NRTIs can be used, leading to the possibility of various diverse side effects. Nearly all of the NRTIs are associated with lactic acidosis, a rare, but potentially fatal toxicity (532–542). In addition, many have drug interactions with methadone; however, these interactions tend to lead to minimal, if any, clinical significance (82,455–457,459).

Zidovudine

Zidovudine (ZDV, AZT) (Retrovir) was the first NRTI approved by the FDA. Initially used as monotherapy, current recommendations suggest using zidovudine in combination with at least two other antiretroviral agents. Recent studies show that zidovudine is most effective when used in combination with at least one other NRTI—didanosine, lamivudine, or abacavir—and either a protease inhibitor or a nonnucleoside reverse transcriptase inhibitor (NNRTI) (526,543–548). In addition, zidovudine is effective when used in combination with zalcitabine plus a protease inhibitor or NNRTI, or when used in a triple NRTI regimen;

TABLE 58.6. *Recommended preventive care for HIV-infected adults and adolescents*

Pathogen	Preventive regimen		
	Indication	First choice	Alternative
Streptococcus pneumoniae	All patients[a]	23-valent polysaccharide vaccine, 0.5 mL intramuscularly	
Hepatitis B virus[bc]	All susceptible patients (i.e., antihepatitis B core antigen-negative)	Hepatitis B vaccine: 3 doses	
Influenza virus[bd]	All patients (annually, before influenza season)	Inactivated trivalent influenza virus vaccine: one annual dose (0.5 mL) intramuscularly (influenza A only)	Oseltamivir, 75 mg by mouth daily (influenza A or B); rimantadine, 100 mg by mouth twice daily, or amantadine, 100 mg by mouth twice daily
Hepatitis A virus[bc]	All susceptible patients at increased risk for hepatitis A infection (i.e., antihepatitis A virus-negative) (e.g., substance users, men men who have sex with men, hemophiliacs) or patients with chronic liver disease, including chronic hepatitis B or C	Hepatitis A vaccine: two doses	
Diphtheria/Tetanus	All patients who have not received Td vaccine within 10 years.	Tetanus and diptheria toxoids (Td vaccine)	
Other routine assessments			
Serologic tests for syphilis	Yearly for all patients	Nontreponemal tests RPR/VDRL/STS[e]	
Papanicolaou smear	Every 6–12 months for all women		
Tuberculin skin testing	Yearly for all patients	5 tuberculin units (TU) of purified protein derivative (PPD) intradermal	

Notes: Information included in these guidelines might not represent Food and Drug Administration (FDA) approval or approved labeling for products or indications. Specifically, the terms *safe* and *effective* might not be synonymous with the FDA-defined legal standards for product approval.

[a]Vaccination can be offered to persons who have a CD4$^+$ T-lymphocyte count of <200 cells/mm^3, although the efficacy is probably diminished. Revaccination ≥5 years after the first dose is recommended.

[b]Although data demonstrating clinical benefit of these vaccines among HIV-infected persons are not available, assuming that those patients who develop antibody responses will derive a certain amount of protection is reasonable.

[c]Hepatitis B vaccine has been recommended for all children and adolescents and for all adults with risk factors for hepatitis B virus (HBV). For persons requiring vaccination against both hepatitis A and B, a combination vaccine is now available.

[d]Oseltamivir is appropriate during outbreaks of either influenza A or B. Rimantadine or amantadine is appropriate during outbreaks of influenza A, although neither rimantadine nor amantadine is recommended during pregnancy. Dosage reduction for antiviral chemoprophylaxis against influenza might be indicated for decreased renal or hepatic function, and for persons with seizure disorders.

[e]RPR = Rapid Plasma Reagin; VDRL = Venereal Disease Research Laboratory; STS = Serologic Test for Syphilis

Adapted from: Centers for Disease Control and Prevention. Guidelines for using antiretroviral agents among HIV-infected adults and adolescents: recommendations of the panel on clinical practices for treatment of HIV. *MMWR Morb Mortal Wkly Rep* 2002;51(RR-7):1–55.

however, these antiretroviral regimens are less strongly recommended (82,549–551). There is clear evidence that zidovudine should not be used in combination with stavudine (552,553). The current recommended dose of zidovudine is 200 mg orally every 8 hours or 300 mg twice daily (53,82,115,554). When used in combination with lamivudine as Combivir, or when in combination with lamivudine and abacavir as Trizivir, both formulations are taken twice daily. It is available in both oral (tablets, capsules, and liquid suspension) and intravenous formulations (the latter used to prevent HIV transmission to infants in the peripartum period). The most serious side effect of zidovudine is a rare, but potentially fatal toxicity, lactic acidosis, which is associated with several NRTIs (see "Antiretroviral-Associated Adverse Effects" below) (532–536). Other serious toxicities are hematologic—anemia, leukopenia, and granulocytopenia—and generally reversible upon discontinuation of the drug (554–558). Other reported side effects include headache, nausea, gastrointestinal upset, malaise, and insomnia (554,555,558), most of which tend to resolve over time with continuation of therapy or with symptomatic interventions. Zidovudine-related hepatotoxicity has also been described (559–561), as well as myopathy. Other documented side effects are anorexia, xerostomia, hepatomegaly, cardiomyopathy, pigmentation of the nails, and leukocytoclastic vasculitis. When coadministered with methadone, zidovudine levels are increased by 40%, possibly leading to increased zidovudine-related toxicities, whereas methadone levels are unchanged (458,459).

Didanosine

Didanosine (ddI) (Videx) was the second reverse transcriptase inhibitor to receive FDA approval for use in the treatment of patients with HIV infection. Studies show favorable results when it is used in combination with the NRTIs lamivudine, stavudine, or zidovudine plus a protease inhibitor or NNRTI (543,544,546,551,562–566). Available only in oral formulation, its accepted dosage is 200 mg every 12 hours (tablet or powder), or 400 mg once daily (enteric-coated capsules), with lower doses based on patient weight. It should be taken on an empty stomach. The most serious toxicity is the rare, potentially life-threatening lactic acidosis, which is reported to occur most frequently with the "d" drugs (ddI/didanosine, d4T/stavudine, ddC/zalcitabine) (532,538,539,541,542). Other more common adverse effects are peripheral neuropathy (up to 20%) and pancreatitis (up to 6%, the most common reason for discontinuation of the drug) (567). It should be used with caution in diabetics and alcoholics. Other documented side effects include nausea, diarrhea, abdominal pain, fever, headache, hepatomegaly, and a number of laboratory abnormalities: anemia, leukopenia, thrombocytopenia, hyperuricemia, hypertriglyceridemia, and elevation of liver function tests. When coadministered with methadone, didanosine levels are decreased by

60%, possibly requiring higher doses of didanosine, while methadone levels are unchanged (455).

Zalcitabine

Similar in most respects to didanosine, zalcitabine (ddC) (Hivid) has the disadvantage of a three-times daily schedule. Although zalcitabine is recommended as an alternative regimen when combined with zidovudine and a protease inhibitor or NNRTI, zalcitabine has fallen out of favor because of its toxicity profile and minimal virologic response when compared to other antiretroviral agents (82,522). It is not recommended to use zalcitabine in combination with didanosine, lamivudine, or stavudine (82). The dose schedule is 0.75 mg every 8 hours, with lower doses based on weight. The major adverse effect is peripheral neuropathy (up to 35%), with other potential side effects including lactic acidosis, pancreatitis, oral ulcers, abdominal pain, dysphagia, skin rash, headache, myalgia, and laboratory abnormalities (anemia, leukopenia, thrombocytopenia, and elevation of liver function tests).

Stavudine

Stavudine (d4T) (Zerit) is efficacious when used in combination with didanosine or lamivudine plus either a protease inhibitor or NNRTI (543,544,565,566,568). The use of stavudine in combination with zalcitabine or zidovudine is not recommended (82,552,553). The dosing schedule is 40 mg every 12 hours (capsules or liquid solution), with lower doses based on weight. Like all of the previously mentioned NRTIs, it also has the rare, but potentially fatal, toxicity of lactic acidosis, which is reported most frequently with stavudine and didanosine (537–542). Like the other "d" drugs (ddI/didanosine and ddC/zalcitabine), d4T/stavudine's other important adverse effects include peripheral neuropathy (21%) and pancreatitis. Additional toxicities include predominantly gastrointestinal side effects such as nausea, vomiting, diarrhea, and abdominal pain. When coadministered with methadone, stavudine levels are mildly to modestly decreased by 27% with no modification in dosing required, while methadone levels are unchanged (455) (see Table 58.3).

Lamivudine

A very-well-tolerated agent, lamivudine (3TC) (Epivir) is efficacious when used in combination with zidovudine, didanosine, or stavudine plus a protease inhibitor or NNRTI (526,543,544,547,548,562–564,568). In addition, it is effective when used in a triple NRTI regimen (549–551). As discussed previously, lamivudine has some effect against chronic hepatitis B infection (396,397). However, its current use is primarily in the treatment of HIV rather than chronic hepatitis B infection. Lamivudine is generally well tolerated—diarrhea is the major side effect, and uncommon. Again like the aforementioned NRTIs, a potentially fatal, yet rare, toxicity is lactic acidosis (537,540,542). The recommended dose schedule is 150 mg every 12 hours (tablets or liquid solution). The administration of lamivudine with methadone has no effect on methadone levels (458).

Abacavir

Abacavir (Ziagen), one of the more recent NRTIs approved by the FDA, is somewhat unique in its recommended use. Although it can be used in combination with one of the previously mentioned NRTIs along with a protease inhibitor or NNRTI, there are data that show it is efficacious when used with two other NRTIs only, sparing either a protease inhibitor or NNRTI as part of the medication regimen (549,550). Its use, as a triple NRTI regimen, however, is recommended as an alternative, likely because of less efficacy in patients with viral loads that exceed 100,000 copies/dL (82). The most important adverse effect, a hypersensitivity reaction that includes fever, rash, fatigue, nausea, vomiting, diarrhea, and abdominal pain, can be fatal. If this reaction develops, abacavir should be stopped immediately, and never restarted because of the recurrence of more severe symptoms upon rechallenge with the medication. Other adverse effects include nausea, vomiting, malaise, loss of appetite. The recommended dose schedule is 300 mg every 12 hours (tablets or liquid solution). Coadministration of abacavir and methadone is reported to lead to a 23% increase in clearance of methadone, and to a 34% decrease in peak concentration of abacavir—both of unclear clinical significance (457).

Tenofovir Disoproxil Fumarate

Tenofovir disoproxil fumarate (Viread) is the newest NRTI approved by the FDA. Its current recommended use is primarily in salvage regimens (82,569). Studies evaluating its use as initial therapy are ongoing. The most common adverse effects are mild to moderate gastrointestinal symptoms, including diarrhea, nausea, vomiting, and flatulence. Other side effects associated with tenofovir are headache and asthenia. Other than enteric-coated didanosine (Videx EC), tenofovir is the only other NRTI that is currently approved to be dosed once daily (300 mg tablet). Like lamivudine, tenofovir has antiviral activity against hepatitis B virus, and has been effective in the treatment of chronic hepatitis B infection (395). To date, there are no available data regarding potential drug interactions between tenofovir and methadone.

Nonnucleoside Reverse Transcriptase Inhibitors

This class of drugs is a very powerful tool in the fight against HIV. Many studies show promising results when NNRTIs are used in combination with NRTIs (543,562,564,565). However, each NNRTI influences the cytochrome P450 enzyme system of the liver, leading to complex drug interactions, particularly with methadone (460–463). Although the dosing schedule and pill burden are favorable in general, the side-effect profiles lead to potential problems, leaving the decision of whether to place patients on these medications complex.

Nevirapine

Studies demonstrate the efficacy of nevirapine (Viramune) when used in combination with two NRTIs (543,565,570,571). However, because of adverse effects, specifically hepatitis, including hepatic necrosis, this NNRTI is recommended as an alternative regimen in combination with NRTIs (82). One other important reported adverse effect is rash—ranging from mild to very severe rash necessitating hospitalization. The recommended dosing schedule is 200 mg daily for 2 weeks, followed by 200 mg twice daily (tablets or liquid solution). Because nevirapine is an inducer of the cytochrome P450 enzyme system in the liver, many drug interactions occur, including decreasing plasma levels of methadone by 46% when coadministered, often necessitating significant changes in methadone doses—up to a 185% increase in methadone dose in one report (460,461) (see Table 58.3).

Delavirdine

Delavirdine (Rescriptor) is a second-line NNRTI, used often in salvage therapy, and is recommended as an alternative regimen when used in combination with NRTIs (82,571–573). Unlike the other NNRTIs, delavirdine may be easier to take for many substance users because it is thought to have less effect on methadone metabolism (see Table 58.3). Because delavirdine does not induce the cytochrome P450 enzyme system in the liver—instead it inhibits it—it is hypothesized to lead to an increase in methadone levels (456,489), although this has not been confirmed in studies. Adverse effects include rash, elevation of liver enzymes, and headaches. Delavirdine has a less-desirable dosing schedule and a higher pill burden than the other NNRTIs—dosing is 400 mg three times daily or 600 mg twice daily, totaling 6 tablets daily.

Efavirenz

Many studies show efavirenz to be highly effective against HIV when used in combination with NRTIs (562,564,565,574); therefore, it is the only NNRTI strongly recommended in patients with little or no previous experience with HIV therapy (82). In addition to its efficacy, the dosing schedule—600 mg daily—allows for better adherence. Like nevirapine, efavirenz is an inducer of the cytochrome P450 enzyme system in the liver, causing many drug interactions, including decreasing methadone levels by 48% to 52%, inducing symptoms of methadone withdrawal, and requiring up to a 200% increase in methadone dose when coadministered

(461–463) (see Table 58.3). The most common adverse effects are central nervous system symptoms (in up to 52% of patients), including dizziness, somnolence, insomnia, abnormal dreams, confusion, depersonalization, hallucinations, and impaired concentration. These symptoms usually subside spontaneously after 2 to 4 weeks. Other adverse effects include rash, elevation of liver enzymes, and false-positive cannabinoid test. Efavirenz should not be taken with high-fat meals.

Protease Inhibitors

When used in combination with NRTIs, protease inhibitors are associated with potent antiviral effects, leading to dramatic reductions in the total viral load and increases in CD4+ T-cell counts (53,517,520–522). HIV protease is an essential viral enzyme that acts late in the viral life cycle promoting the assembly of infectious virions (575). The complete inhibition of this enzyme results in the formation of noninfectious particles (576). While the protease inhibitors show impressive results, their use may be problematic in practice, especially in drug users, because of side effects, toxicity, the sheer number of pills which must be ingested—up to 12 per day in many combination regimens—and drug interactions. Like the NNRTIs, most protease inhibitors interact with the liver's cytochrome P450 enzymes, making drug interactions, particularly with methadone, potentially complicated to manage (467–472) (see Table 58.3). In addition to these issues, recent studies show several long-term side effects from protease inhibitors, including fat redistribution, lipid abnormalities, hyperglycemia, hepatotoxicity, and avascular necrosis (577–581) (see "Antiretroviral-Associated Adverse Effects" below).

Indinavir

Indinavir (Crixivan) is highly effective against HIV when used in combination with NRTIs (526,544,563). When the FDA first approved indinavir, it was used as the sole protease inhibitor in combination with NRTIs, and required taking 800 mg every 8 hours without any food. Subsequently, studies revealed that when taken with ritonavir (100 or 200 mg every 12 hours), indinavir could be dosed 800 mg twice daily, with no food restrictions, and still remain potent (544,563). Like many of the protease inhibitors, it inhibits cytochrome P450 enzymes and, therefore, has many interactions with other drugs. However, indinavir does not change methadone levels, and therefore no dose modification is required when taken simultaneously (467,473) (see Table 58.3). Adverse effects include nephrolithiasis, gastrointestinal intolerance, inconsequential increased indirect bilirubin, transaminase elevation, headache, asthenia, blurred vision, dizziness, thrombocytopenia, alopecia, metallic taste, rash, hyperglycemia, fat redistribution, and lipid abnormalities.

Ritonavir

Because ritonavir (Norvir) is the most potent inhibitor of the cytochrome P450 system of all the protease inhibitors, its role in HIV treatment has evolved from using it as the sole protease inhibitor in combination with NRTIs, to one of "boosting" or enhancing other protease inhibitors. Its pharmacology leads to increased plasma concentrations of other protease inhibitors when used simultaneously. In addition, when ritonavir is used to boost other protease inhibitors, it often leads to more convenient regimens with regard to pill burden, food requirement, and dosing frequency. Ritonavir has even been coformulated with lopinavir in a capsule as Kaletra (see below). When used as the sole protease inhibitor in combination therapy, it is dosed 600 mg every 12 hours (capsules or oral solution); it should be taken with food, and the capsules require refrigeration. However, its use as a sole protease inhibitor in HIV treatment is recommended as an alternative, whereas its use in combination to boost indinavir, lopinavir, or saquinavir in addition to NRTIs is strongly recommended and effective (82,544,563,568,570). When used with indinavir, recommended dosing is 100 mg or 200 mg of ritonavir plus 800 mg of indinavir every 12 hours. When ritonavir is used in combination with amprenavir, it is dosed as either 100 mg of ritonavir plus 600 mg of amprenavir twice daily, or as 200 mg of ritonavir plus 1,200 mg of amprenavir daily. With lopinavir, ritonavir is dosed in a fixed-dose combination pill as Kaletra (three pills twice daily, each pill containing 33.3 mg of ritonavir and 133.3 mg of lopinavir). When used with saquinavir, the recommended boosting dose is either 200 mg of ritonavir plus 800 mg of saquinavir, or 100 mg of ritonavir plus 1,000 mg of saquinavir. Additionally, if used as a true dual protease inhibitor regimen rather than as a boosted protease inhibitor regimen, dosing for ritonavir and saquinavir is 400 mg of each twice daily. The major adverse effects of ritonavir are gastrointestinal intolerance (nausea, vomiting, diarrhea) and hepatitis. Additional toxicities include pancreatitis, taste perversion, elevations of creatine phosphokinase and uric acid, hypertriglyceridemia, paresthesias, hyperglycemia, fat redistribution, and lipid abnormalities. Because of its potent inhibition of the P450 enzymes, ritonavir has many interactions with other drugs, including methadone (see Table 58.3). When coadministered with ritonavir, methadone levels are decreased by 37%, possibly requiring escalation of methadone doses (464,468).

Nelfinavir

Nelfinavir (Viracept) is highly effective against HIV infection (545,547,566,582). Initially dosed at 750 mg three times daily, nelfinavir is now more commonly prescribed as 1,250 mg twice daily (tablets or powder) to be taken with food. Its large pill burden—10 pills daily—along with diarrhea are the most common drawbacks to nelfinavir. Other adverse effects include hypertriglyceridemia, transaminase elevation, fat redistribution, and lipid abnormalities. Like all the other protease inhibitors, it inhibits the cytochrome P450 system, leading to potential drug interactions. When taken simultaneously with methadone, nelfinavir decreases methadone levels, and has been reported to require a 185% increase of methadone dose (see Table 58.3) (465,467,469).

Saquinavir

Saquinavir, initially FDA approved as a hard-gel capsule (Invirase), was subsequently produced as a soft-gel capsule (Fortovase), the latter having better bioavailability. Hard-gel capsules are no longer recommended for use as the sole protease inhibitor in treatment against HIV (583); however, when the hard-gel capsule is used with ritonavir, it is strongly recommended (dosed 400 mg saquinavir with 400 mg of ritonavir, twice daily; or 1,000 mg saquinavir with 100 mg ritonavir twice daily) (82). On the other hand, soft-gel capsules, which require refrigeration, are recommended as alternatives when used as the sole protease inhibitor (dosed 1,200 mg three times daily), and recommended strongly when used in combination with ritonavir and NRTIs (dosed similarly to hard-gel capsules) (82). Adverse effects include gastrointestinal intolerance (nausea, diarrhea, abdominal pain, dyspepsia), headache, elevated transaminase, hypertriglyceridemia, fat redistribution, and lipid abnormalities. Like all other protease inhibitors, saquinavir is also an inhibitor of the cytochrome P450 system; however, when taken simultaneously with methadone, there is little to no effect on methadone levels (467,468).

Amprenavir

One of the newer protease inhibitors that can be dosed once daily, amprenavir (Agenerase) in combination with NRTIs is effective when used as the sole protease inhibitor and when used in combination with ritonavir (548,584,585). When used alone, it is dosed 1,200 mg twice daily (capsules) or 1,400 mg twice daily (oral solution), and when used with ritonavir, it is dosed a total of 1,200 mg of amprenavir (capsules) and 200 mg of ritonavir per day, either taken once daily or divided in two doses. Amprenavir may be dosed lower, depending on the patient's weight; high-fat meals should be avoided. Adverse effects include gastrointestinal intolerance (nausea, vomiting, diarrhea), rash, paresthesias, transaminase elevation, hyperglycemia, fat redistribution, and lipid abnormalities. The oral solution contains propylene glycol and is, therefore, contraindicated among pregnant women and young children. Amprenavir inhibits cytochrome P450 enzymes and decreases methadone levels by 35% when coadministered,

possibly requiring changes in methadone dosing (471). In addition, methadone is reported to lead to a 30% decrease in amprenavir, potentially rendering it less effective (see Table 58.3) (586).

Lopinavir/Ritonavir

The newest protease inhibitor, lopinavir/ritonavir (Kaletra), is highly effective against HIV when used with NRTIs, and is strongly recommended for treatment of HIV disease (82,568,570,587). Dosing is 400 mg lopinavir plus 100 mg ritonavir twice daily (each capsule contains 133.3 mg of lopinavir plus 33.3 mg of ritonavir; also available in oral solution). Food should be taken with each dose, and the capsules refrigerated. Adverse effects include gastrointestinal intolerance (nausea, vomiting, diarrhea), paresthesia, elevated transaminase hyperglycemia, fat redistribution, and lipid abnormalities. Like all of the protease inhibitors, lopinavir/ritonavir inhibits cytochrome P450 enzymes. When coadministered with methadone, lopinavir/ritonavir decreases methadone levels by 53%, possibly requiring modification of methadone doses (472).

Treatment Strategies

The introduction of agents that inhibit different steps in the viral replicative cycle allows clinicians to use a therapeutic strategy that will predictably be associated with more significant and sustained reductions of total viral load and increases in CD4+ T-cell counts. Guidelines for the use of antiretroviral agents, authored by a panel of expert clinicians, were published in May 2002 by the Centers for Disease Control and Prevention. What follows is a summary of the pertinent issues, especially those relevant to substance users. More detailed information regarding up-to-date guidelines for the treatment of HIV/AIDS, including the use of antiretroviral medications, is available through the Department of Health and Human Services' HIV/AIDS Treatment Information Services at http://www.hivatis.org or (800) 448-0440.

The decision regarding initiation of antiretroviral therapy has to be individualized. A number of variables affect that decision, the most important ones being the patient's CD4+ T-cell count, total viral load (plasma HIV RNA), symptoms, willingness and ability to accept therapy, likelihood of adherence, and potential risks and benefits of initiating therapy—including adverse effects. While no single optimal treatment strategy has been defined, current accepted practice is to initiate therapy in asymptomatic patients when the CD4+ count is below 200/mm^3, and possibly below 350/mm^3 (82,526–528). When the CD4+ T-cell count is between 200/mm^3 and 350/mm^3, treatment should be offered, although this is controversial (82). Randomized clinical trials have demonstrated clinical benefit only for patients with CD4+ T-cell counts less than 200/mm^3

TABLE 58.7. *Indications for initiating antiretroviral therapy for the chronically HIV-infected patient*

The optimal time to initiate therapy is unknown among persons with asymptomatic disease and CD4+ T-cells counts of >200 cells/mm^3. This table provides general guidance rather than absolute recommendations for an individual patient. All decisions regarding initiating therapy should be made on the basis of prognosis as determined by the CD4+ T-cell count and level of plasma HIV RNA indicated in the table, the potential benefits and risks of therapy, and the willingness of the patient to accept therapy.

Clinical category	CD4+ T-cell count	Plasma HIV ribonucleic acid (RNA)	Recommendation
Symptomatic (AIDS or severe symptoms)	Any value	Any value	Treat
Asymptomatic, AIDS	CD4+ T-cells <200/mm^3	Any value	Treat
Asymptomatic	CD4+ T-cells >200/mm^3 but <350/mm^3	Any value	Treatment should be offered, although controversial*
Asymptomatic	CD4+ T-cells >350/mm^3	>55,000 copies/mL	Certain experienced clinicians recommend initiating therapy, recognizing that the 3-year risk for untreated patients to experience AIDS is >30%; in the absence of increased levels of plasma HIV RNA, other clinicians recommend deferring therapy and monitoring the CD4+ T-cell count and level of plasma HIV RNA more frequently; clinical outcome data after initiating therapy are lacking.
Asymptomatic	CD4+ T-cells >350/mm^3	<55,000 copies/mL	Certain experienced clinicians recommend deferring therapy and monitoring the CD4+ T-cell count, recognizing that the 3-year risk for untreated patients to experience AIDS is <15%

*Clinical benefit has been demonstrated in controlled trials only for patients with CD4+ T-cells <200/mm^3; however, the majority of clinicians would offer therapy at a CD4+ T-cell threshold of <350/mm^3.

Adapted from: Centers for Disease Control and Prevention. Guidelines for using antiretroviral agents among HIV-infected adults and adolescents: recommendations of the panel on clinical practices for treatment of HIV. *MMWR Morb Mortal Wkly Rep* 2002;51(RR-7):1–55.

(526–528); however, many clinicians would offer therapy when the CD4+ T-cell is less than 350/mm^3, especially in patients with high viral loads (Table 58.7). In patients with CD4+ T-cell counts above 350/mm^3, therapy should be deferred with monitoring of the CD4+ T-cell count and viral load, although some clinicians may opt for treating these patients if the viral load exceeds 55,000 copies/mL. As a general rule, antiretroviral therapy should be given to all symptomatic patients regardless of their CD4+ T-cell count or viral load (53,82,502).

Initial Antiretroviral Regimens

The first question confronted by clinicians when initiating therapy is which classes of medication to use. Current accepted approaches include using two NRTIs and one protease inhibitor, two NRTIs and a "boosted" protease inhibitor, two NRTIs and one NNRTI, or three NRTIs. Table 58.8 summarizes the recommended antiretroviral agents to use for initiation of HIV therapy. Although no study has distinguished the single best regimen to begin

TABLE 58.8. *Recommended antiretroviral agents for initial treatment of HIV infection*

This table is a guide to using available treatment regimens for patients with no previous or limited experience with HIV therapy. Antiretroviral drug regimens include one choice from columns A and B of this table. Drugs are listed in alphabetical, not priority order.

Recommendation	Column A	Column B
Strongly recommended	Efavirenz Indinavir Nelfinavir Ritonavir plus indinavir Ritonavir plus lopinavir* Ritonavir plus saquinavir (soft-gel capsule or hard-gel capsule)	Didanosine plus lamivudine Stavudine plus didanosine Stavudine plus lamivudine Zidovudine plus didanosine Zidovudine plus lamivudine
Recommended as alternatives	Abacavir Amprenavir Delavirdine Nelfinavir plus saquinavir (soft-gel capsule) Nevirapine Ritonavir Saquinavir (soft-gel capsule)	Zidovudine plus zalcitabine
No recommendation because of insufficient data	Hydroxyurea in combination with antiretroviral drugs Ritonavir plus amprenavir Ritonavir plus nelfinavir Tenofovir[+]	
Not recommended and should not be offered (All monotherapies whether from column A or B)	Saquinavir (hard-gel capsule)**	Stavudine plus zidovudine Zalcitabine plus didanosine Zalcitabine plus lamivudine Zalcitabine plus stavudine

*Co-formulated as Kaletra™ (Abbott Laboratories).
[+]Data from clinical trials are limited to use in salvage. Data from trails of tenofovir initial therapy should be available in the future.
**Use of saquinavir (hard-gel capsule) (i.e., invirase) is only recommended in combination with ritonavir.
Adapted from: Centers for Disease Control and Prevention. Guidelines for using antiretroviral agents among HIV-infected adults and adolescents: recommendations of the panel on clinical practices for treatment of HIV. *MMWR Morb Mortal Wkly Rep* 2002;51(RR-7):1–55.

with, factors that influence the clinician's choice of antiretroviral agents include dosing frequency, pill burden, adverse effects, interactions with other drugs (particularly methadone in the substance-using population), potential future treatment options, and food requirements. All of the above combinations are accepted as first-line therapy for initiating treatment for HIV except three NRTIs, which is recommended as an alternative regimen (82). Although triple NRTI therapy may be easier to adhere to, it is less efficacious when used in patients with viral loads that exceed 100,000 copies/mL (82).

The goals of antiretroviral therapy are to lower the viral load to undetectable levels, restore or preserve immune function, improve quality of life, and slow HIV disease progression and improve survival. The difficulty, however, is that increasing efficacy may be achieved at the price of increasing toxicity and complexity, which poses significant management dilemmas in the care of HIV-infected substance users. Furthermore, because of the predictable development of resistance in the setting of suboptimal or erratic use of antiretroviral therapy, the additional concern arises that poorly adherent substance-using patients, receiving infrequent and poorly supervised therapy, may be a factor in the selection of multiple drug-resistant strains of HIV, which may not respond to currently available medications, similar to what transpired in the early 1990s, when injection drug use was an important risk factor in the development of multiple drug-resistant tuberculosis in New York City (588).

Adherence

Adherence to antiretroviral medications is a critical element in the achievement of virologic suppression. Studies demonstrate that suboptimal adherence is associated with drug resistance (which limits future treatment options), less viral suppression, and higher morbidity and mortality (484–486). Suboptimal adherence is common, occurring in up to 33% of patients in one report (589). Although there is conflicting data, in many studies having a history of substance use has not been associated with poor adherence; however, heavy alcohol use and active substance use has been consistently associated with suboptimal adherence (75,81,481–483,590). There are many potential reasons why substance users may have poor adherence to HIV medications, including lack of trust between provider and patient, active mental illness, active substance or alcohol use, domestic violence, discrimination, lack of reliable access to primary medical care, lack of patient education, and homelessness—which are all predictors of poor adherence (590,591). Predictors of optimal adherence include availability of life supports, ability to fit medications into daily routines, understanding the need for optimal adherence and potential consequences of poor adherence, feeling comfortable taking medications in front of others, and keeping clinic appointments (592,593). Studies show that to achieve maximal viral suppression 90% to 95% of doses must be taken (75,484,591). Given the difficulty and importance of adherence, providers must be focused on improving ways in which patients may become more adherent. Measurement of adherence is flawed—both patient self-reporting and clinician estimates are unreliable (594,595). Aids measuring adherence, such as medication event monitoring systems caps, pharmacy records, and pill counts, may be useful but are also cumbersome. When attempting to assess adherence, it is recommended that providers include an assessment of each dose taken within the previous 3 days, in addition to a general inquiry of adherence since the last visit (82).

Strategies to improve adherence include patient-related, clinician and health team-related, and regimen-related strategies (Tables 58.9, 58.10, and 58.11). Before starting antiretroviral therapy it is important to communicate to the patient clear and concrete goals of therapy, and for the patient to understand the role that adherence plays in achieving these goals. Because starting antiretroviral medication is never an emergency, clinicians and patients have time to assess readiness. In doing so, many clinicians can help patients identify potential barriers to adherence, and develop strategies to overcome these barriers over several clinic visits in order to become ready for HIV treatment. Some clinicians prescribe a "readiness trial" in which patients take candy or multivitamins in place of antiretroviral medications to help determine level of readiness, potential difficulties, and challenges to adherence. When caring for substance users, inquiries regarding current active substance use and coping strategies are essential, as active substance use is associated with poor adherence (75,81,482,483). Understanding patients' beliefs and educating them about antiretroviral medication, particularly adverse effects and drug interactions, is important. Prescribing medications to prevent or treat side effects at the time of initiation of antiretroviral therapy may be helpful in keeping patients on their antiretroviral regimen. Of

TABLE 58.9. *Strategies to improve adherence—patient- and medication-related*

- Inform patient regarding side effects.
- Anticipate and treat side effects.
- Simplify food requirements.
- Avoid adverse drug interactions.
- If possible, reduce dose frequency and number of pills.
- Negotiate a treatment plan that the patient understands and to which he or she commits.
- Spend time and multiple encounters to educate and explain goals of therapy and need for adherence.
- Establish readiness to take medication before writing first prescription.
- Recruit family and friends to support the treatment plan.
- Develop concrete plan for specific regimen by considering meal schedule, daily routines, and side effects.
- Provide written schedule and pictures of medications, daily or weekly pill boxes, alarm clocks, pagers, or other mechanical aids for adherence.
- Develop adherence support groups or add adherence concerns to agenda of other support groups.
- Develop links with local community-based organizations regarding adherence combined with educational sessions and practical strategies.
- Consider practice sessions using candy instead of pills.

Adapted from: Centers for Disease Control and Prevention. Guidelines for using antiretroviral agents among HIV-infected adults and adolescents: recommendations of the panel on clinical practices for treatment of HIV. *MMWR Morb Mortal Wkly Rep* 2002;51(RR-7):1–55.

particular importance, anticipating changes in methadone metabolism as a consequence of specific drug interactions, and modifying methadone doses accordingly, is crucial for those patients in methadone-maintenance programs. Using aids such as pill boxes, pagers, timers, or alarms may be useful, in addition to using cues in daily life to link medications to. For patients in drug-treatment programs, antiretroviral medications can be dispensed within the program as direct observation therapy. Lastly, for patient-related strategies particular to substance users, mental health and housing issues should be addressed if potentially problematic prior to prescribing antiretroviral therapy.

Treatment-related strategies to improve adherence include using a regimen that requires a small number of pills, reduced frequency of dosing, minimal food mandates, minimal adverse reactions, and, probably most importantly for substance users, minimal clinically significant drug interactions with methadone. Clinician or health team-associated strategies to improve adherence includes first and foremost, establishing trust. Providing support groups, treatment/adherence counselors, peer educators, or case managers to reinforce the importance of adherence may be beneficial. Having flexible hours and accessibility to address patients' concerns or problems

TABLE 58.10. *Strategies to improve adherence—clinician- and health team-related*

- Establish trust.
- Serve as educator and information source with ongoing support and monitoring.
- Provide access between visits for questions or problems (e.g., by providing a pager number), including during vacations or conferences.
- Monitor ongoing adherence; intensify management during periods of suboptimal adherence (i.e., more frequent visits, recruitment of family or friends, deployment of other team members, and referral for mental health or substance abuse treatment services).
- Use of health team for all patients, including patients with special needs (e.g., use peer educators for adolescents or for injection drug users).
- Consider impact of new diagnoses on adherence (e.g., depression, liver disease, wasting, or recurrent substance abuse) and include adherence intervention in management.
- Use nurses, pharmacists, peer educators, volunteers, case managers, substance abuse counselors, clinician's assistants, nurse practitioners, and research nurses to reinforce adherence messages.
- Provide training to support team regarding antiretroviral therapy and adherence.
- Add adherence interventions to job descriptions of support team members; add continuity-of-care role to improve patient access.

Adapted from: Centers for Disease Control and Prevention. Guidelines for using antiretroviral agents among HIV-infected adults and adolescents: recommendations of the Panel on Clinical Practices for Treatment of HIV. *MMWR Morb Mortal Wkly Rep* 2002;51(RR-7):1–55.

regarding medications is also likely helpful. For patients in drug-treatment programs, antiretroviral medications can be dispensed within the program, leading to direct observation therapy. Direct observation therapy is effective in improving adherence and decreasing HIV viral load (596–598). Given that an increasing number of antiretroviral agents are effective when dosed once-daily, specifically didanosine, lamivudine, tenofovir, nevirap-

TABLE 58.11. *Interventions to improve adherence*

- Pharmacist-based adherence encounters and clinics.
- Multidisciplinary adherence encounters at each visit.
- Reminders, alarms, pagers, or timers on pillboxes.
- Patient education aids, including regimen pictures, calendars, or stickers.
- Clinician education aids (e.g., medication guides, pictures, or calendars).

Adapted from: Centers for Disease Control and Prevention. Guidelines for using antiretroviral agents among HIV-infected adults and adolescents: recommendations of the panel on clinical practices for treatment of HIV. *MMWR Morb Mortal Wkly Rep* 2002;51(RR-7):1–55.

ine, efavirenz, amprenavir/ritonavir, indinavir/ritonavir, and saquinavir/ritonavir (562–564,569,599–601), it may soon be a possibility that all doses of antiretroviral medications be dispensed at drug-treatment programs, potentially leading to vast improvements in adherence for substance users.

Because many substance users have had multiple negative experiences and failures with the health care system, it is important to give them opportunities to be successful in managing their health care. Broadening the concept of medical adherence to include health in a greater sense not only addresses the often chaotic life of substance users that impacts their health and ability to adhere, but also may allow them to succeed in managing their health. Components of a broadened definition of adherence include keeping regular medical appointments, achieving sobriety or more controlled substance use, involvement in a drug-treatment program, practicing safe sex and/or drug injection, obtaining stable housing, connecting with a support network, maintaining a healthy diet, taking medications to prevent opportunistic infections, and taking antiretroviral medications.

Monitoring Antiretroviral Therapy

The goals of antiretroviral therapy are to improve the patient's quality of life and increase survival. Several studies show that these goals can be accomplished with the use of antiretroviral medication and maximal suppression of viral replication (i.e., undetectable HIV RNA levels, viral load <50 copies/mL) (122,602,603). CD4+ T-cell count and, more importantly, viral load should be performed at the time of initiating the treatment regimen, and then every 2 to 8 weeks thereafter. With optimal adherence to a potent regimen, the provider can expect the patient to experience a decrease in viral load of approximately $1.0 \log_{10}$ by 2 to 8 weeks, and for the viral load to become undetectable (<50 copies/mL) by 16 to 24 weeks (82,604). After the patient is on therapy with an undetectable viral load, HIV RNA levels should be repeated every 3 to 4 months to assess the continued efficacy of the treatment regimen. Viral loads are believed to be more useful and informative than CD4+ T-cell counts when making decisions regarding efficacy of antiretroviral therapy. Viral loads, however, should not be measured within 4 weeks after treatment of any infection or immunization (82).

When to Change Therapy

Given our current understanding of HIV infection and disease, and the incorporation of viral load measurement as a sensitive marker of disease, studies show that patients' first combination of antiretroviral agents has the best chance for long-term success (605). There are three reasons for changing an instituted therapy: (a) treatment failure, defined as increased viral load, decreased CD4+ count, or progression of disease; (b) drug-related factors, namely toxicity, drug intolerance, and nonadherence (commonly observed in patients with substance-abuse problems); (c) current use of suboptimal regimens. Treatment failure may occur as a result of viral resistance to one or more antiretroviral agents, altered metabolism of the drug (often resulting from drug–drug interactions), and poor patient adherence.

The choice of a new therapeutic regimen should be guided by the reason that prompted the change in therapy. If treatment failure occurs, the provider must first reassess patient adherence—likely the most important factor for treatment failure. If adherence appears to be satisfactory, then a change in the antiretroviral regimen should be based on resistance testing and prior history of antiretroviral agent use. When changing such regimens, it is standard practice to change at least two antiretroviral agents simultaneously, and it is important to think of future treatment options that will be available to the patient when the current regimen fails. If drug toxicity or intolerance is the primary reason for changing the medication regimen, then a similarly potent drug in the same class with different adverse effects should be substituted.

Resistance Testing

One of the newer developments in treatment of HIV disease is resistance testing. The use of resistance testing to guide antiretroviral therapy after treatment failure improves virologic response when compared to clinical judgment (606–608). Two types of resistance testing are available: genotyping assays that detect drug-resistance mutations in the genome of HIV, and phenotyping assays that measure the ability of HIV to live in different concentrations of antiretroviral drugs. To date there are no prospective studies that support one assay over the other; however, phenotyping assays are more costly. Interpretation of test results from genotyping and phenotyping assays should be done in consultation with HIV-expert clinicians. A major limitation with both types of resistance testing is that when a particular strain of drug-resistant virus makes up less than 10% to 20% of the viral population, the strain will likely not be detected by the assays. Therefore, if a patient had developed a drug-resistant virus with a previous regimen of antiretroviral medications, that drug-resistant virus likely becomes a minor species while the patient no longer takes that regimen, and that pattern of resistance may not be detected in resistance testing. Hence resistance testing should occur while patients are taking antiretroviral medications and have a viral load of at least 1,000 copies/mL. Table 58.12 provides more detailed recommendations for using drug-resistance assays.

Antiretroviral-Associated Adverse Effects

With longer life spans for HIV-infected patients and more available antiretroviral agents, adverse effects associated with long-term use of antiretroviral agents are more prevalent. Lactic acidosis is reported to occur with the use of NRTIs, and rarely may be life-threatening (532–542,609–611). Risk factors that increase the risk of experiencing lactic acidosis include obesity, female gender, and prolonged use of NRTIs (611). Although lactic acidosis is reported to occur in patients on various NRTIs, two of the "d" drugs, specifically ddI/didanosine and d4T/stavudine, are reported with more frequency (532,537–542). The proposed etiology of lactic acidosis is from mitochondrial toxicity. Mitochondrial dysfunction may lead to several of the long-term adverse effects seen in patients on antiretroviral agents including myopathy, pancreatitis, peripheral neuropathy, cardiomyopathy, and possibly lipodystrophy. Clinically patients with lactic acidosis present with vague and nonspecific signs and symptoms. These may include nausea, abdominal pain and distention, vomiting, diarrhea, anorexia, generalized weakness, dyspnea, myalgia, paresthesia, weight loss, and hepatomegaly. In addition to an elevated lactic acid level, other possible laboratory abnormalities include elevations in anion gap, liver enzymes, lactic dehydrogenase, lipase, amylase, and creatine phosphokinase. Routine monitoring of lactic acid levels is not recommended, as the diagnosis of lactic acidosis requires lactic acidemia (elevated serum lactate level), in addition to clinical signs or symptoms. Therefore, it is recommended to check lactate levels when patients present with a clinical syndrome that includes the above signs and symptoms. Measuring serum lactate levels requires technical precision, including immediate transportation of blood specimens on ice to the laboratory among other specifications. If clinical and laboratory manifestations of lactic acidosis syndrome occur, antiretroviral medications should be stopped immediately.

Hepatotoxicity, usually defined as elevation of hepatic transaminases three to five times the upper limit of normal, is an adverse effect which can be seen with administration of many antiretroviral agents, but more commonly with NNRTIs or protease inhibitors. Of the NNRTIs, nevirapine has been reported as having the highest risk of hepatotoxicity (12.5%) (612). Most of the cases of nevirapine-associated liver toxicity occur within the first 12 weeks of taking the medication, and fatalities from liver necrosis have been reported. Therefore, close monitoring of liver enzymes is recommended after initiating antiretroviral regimens that include nevirapine. Protease inhibitor-associated hepatotoxicity is unlike that of nevirapine in that elevation of liver enzymes can occur at any time while taking protease inhibitors. The most common protease inhibitor associated with hepatotoxicity is ritonavir. Other comorbid conditions, such as alcohol abuse, hepatitis B and C, seen frequently in substance users, increase the patient's risk for hepatotoxicity (613,614).

Hyperglycemia has been predominantly reported as an adverse effect in patients taking protease inhibitors (579). The etiology of hyperglycemia is unknown at this time. Hyperglycemia may or may not occur with diabetes, and

TABLE 58.12. *Recommendations for using drug-resistance assays*

Clinical setting/recommendations	Rationale
Recommended	
Virologic failure during highly active antiretroviral therapy	Determine the role of resistance in drug failure and maximize the number of active drugs in the new regimen, if indicated
Suboptimal suppression of viral load after initiation	Determine the role of resistance in antiretroviral therapy and maximize the number of active drugs in the new regimen, if indicated
Should be considered	Determine if drug-resistant virus was transmitted and
Acute HIV infection	change regimen accordingly
Not usually recommended	Uncertain prevalence of resistant virus; available assays
Chronic HIV infection before therapy initiation	might not detect minor drug-resistant species
After discontinuation of drugs	Drug-resistance mutations might become minor species in the absence of selective drug pressure; available assays might not detect drug-resistant species
Plasma viral load < 1,000 copies/mL	Resistance assays cannot be reliably performed because of low copy number of HIV ribonucleic acid

Adapted from: Centers for Disease Control and Prevention. Guidelines for using antiretroviral agents among HIV-infected adults and adolescents: recommendations of the panel on clinical practices for treatment of HIV. *MMWR Morb Mortal Wkly Rep* 2002;51(RR-7):1–55.

most clinicians would recommend that antiretroviral therapy be changed only with severe diabetes.

Lipodystrophy is associated with HIV infection and antiretroviral therapy. The lipodystrophy syndrome includes fat maldistribution, generalized fat wasting, and localized fat accumulation. Fat accumulation may occur in the abdomen, dorsocervical fat pad (buffalo hump), and breasts, whereas fat atrophy tends to occur in the face and extremities. In communities heavily affected by HIV, these noticeable changes in body composition are often very disturbing to patients—it is as if everyone around them is aware of their HIV status because of their body changes. Lipodystrophy is associated with protease inhibitors, long-term NRTI therapy, and increased duration of antiretroviral therapy in general (577,578). To date there is no clearly effective therapy for lipodystrophy, and discontinuation of antiretroviral therapy is not associated with improvement in fat maldistribution.

Hyperlipidemia, specifically elevations in total cholesterol, low-density lipoprotein, and triglycerides, is associated with antiretroviral therapy, primarily protease inhibitors (580,581). The implication of hyperlipidemia in HIV-infected patients is unclear. Although there are no conclusive studies to date, hyperlipidemia may increase the risk of cardiovascular and cerebrovascular complications with HIV disease. In addition, there are insufficient data regarding efficacy of lipid-lowering agents in HIV-infected patients.

The class of lipid-lowering agents beta-hydroxy-3-methylglutaryl-coenzyme A (HMG-CoA) reductase inhibitors (statins) has drug interactions with protease inhibitors, and should be used with caution. Current recommendations are to monitor and treat hyperlipidemia in HIV-infected patients the same as in the general population.

Skin rash occurs most frequently with NNRTIs, with the most common and severe rashes occurring in patients taking nevirapine. Among the NRTIs and protease inhibitors, rash occurs most frequently with abacavir (NRTI) and amprenavir (protease inhibitor). The skin rash ranges from mild to severe, and often occurs within the first few weeks of initiation of medications. Treatment includes antihistamines for mild rashes, and hospitalization for severe cases (Stevens-Johnson syndrome or toxic epidermal necrosis). With severe rash, medication should be terminated immediately with no subsequent attempts made to restart the particular medication. When the rash occurs from NNRTIs, it is recommended that patients not be placed on another medication from the same class, because of the possibility of cross-hypersensitivity.

Pancreatitis and peripheral neuropathy are common adverse effects seen in patients most frequently on the NRTIs didanosine, stavudine and zalcitabine (the "d" drugs—ddI, d4T, and ddC, respectively) (567). These adverse effects tend to be the leading reasons for discontinuation of these medications, although pancreatitis tends to occur less frequently with zalcitabine than with the other "d" drugs. Peripheral neuropathy occurs in up to 35% of patients taking these antiretroviral medications.

Avascular necrosis has emerged as a significant long-term complication associated with HIV that may be linked to antiretroviral therapy. Avascular necrosis occurs most frequently in the hips, and is usually diagnosed with findings seen on CT scan or MRI (615–617). There is no clear data to link avascular necrosis to any particular antiretroviral agent. Studies reveal that patients at increased risk for development of osteonecrosis are those who have had chronic exposure to corticosteroids, hyperlipidemia, hypercoagulable states, hemoglobinopathies, and alcohol abuse (82,615,617). There is no medical treatment for avascular necrosis, and surgery may be required for severe disabling symptoms.

Prophylaxis for Opportunistic Infections in HIV Infection

In addition to the use of agents with specific antiretroviral activity, the other major area in the management of HIV infection is that of prophylaxis for opportunistic infections. HAART is the most effective approach in preventing opportunistic infections; therefore, patients who meet the requirements should be placed on such therapy. HAART reduces both the incidence of opportunistic infections and mortality (82,122,603,618,619). Although many patients, often including active substance users, may not be ready to take antiretroviral therapy, the overall incidence of major opportunistic infections has decreased regardless of HAART (620). PCP was the first opportunistic infection for which survival benefit was found when prophylaxis with trimethoprim-sulfamethoxazole (TMP-SMX) was instituted (621). Following the implementation of different prophylactic regimens, it was found that effective prophylaxis against PCP is associated with a delay in progression of HIV disease, prolongation of life, and decreased morbidity, with an associated reduction in health care costs (622,623).

The overwhelming evidence supporting the use of primary and secondary prophylactic strategies against PCP highlighted the importance of developing similar strategies against other opportunistic pathogens commonly seen in HIV infection, with the result that the study of prophylactic regimens against opportunistic infections is an area of research in its own entirety.

Initially thought to be therapy for life, it is now clear that chemoprophylaxis for opportunistic infections may not necessitate lifelong therapy in the era of HAART, given improved immunity, or immune reconstitution, while taking antiretroviral therapy. A strategy of stopping primary or secondary prophylaxis with improved immune function is now recommended (Table 58.13). Discontinuation of prophylaxis for opportunistic infections is recommended in specific situations when the potential harms (increased potential drug toxicity, drug interactions, development of drug resistance, and pill burden and cost) outweigh the benefits (minimal disease prevention).

Efficacy is the primary consideration for prophylaxis. Safety and tolerability of the medications chosen, given the prolonged courses that is required, are imperative. Ease of administration, frequency, drug interactions, and overall costs are also important considerations (624). What follows is a summary of the present recommendations for preventing opportunistic infections by the U.S. Public Health Service and the Infectious Diseases Society of America as of mid-2002 (83). More complete and up-to-date information regarding prevention of opportunistic infections is available through the Department of Health and Human Services' HIV/AIDS Treatment Information Services at http://www.hivatis.org or (800) 448-0440.

Pneumocystis carinii Pneumonia

PCP is the most common of the major AIDS-defining opportunistic infections seen in all HIV-infected patients in the United States and Europe, and in injection drug users in the United States (123–125,620). Recent data reveal an overall trend of decreasing incidence of PCP (620). Prospective data indicate that the risk of PCP is particularly elevated for patients with CD4+ lymphocyte counts lower than 200/mm^3 (116,625). Accordingly, clinical recommendations were developed to help prevent the occurrence of PCP in high-risk individuals through the use of several prophylactic regimens. As of mid-2002, guidelines recommend that primary prophylaxis for PCP be offered to individuals with CD4+ counts lower than 200/mm^3, or with a history of oropharyngeal candidiasis (83,625,626). Additionally, in individuals with a CD4+ T-cell percentage of less than 14%, or with a history of an AIDS-defining illness, prophylaxis should be considered (83,625,626). Primary prophylaxis for PCP should be discontinued in individuals who have increased their CD4+ T-cell count to greater than 200/mm^3 for at least 3 months as a consequence of HAART, because of dramatically reduced risk of developing PCP (see Table 58.13) (83,627–635).

Secondary prophylaxis (i.e., prevention of reinfection of PCP in patients with a history of PCP) should be administered for life unless the patient has a substantial improvement in immune function secondary to antiretroviral therapy. Several studies support the recommended discontinuation of secondary prophylaxis when patients' CD4+ T-cell counts improve from less than 200/mm^3 to greater than 200/mm^3 for at least 3 months as a result of HAART (83,631,633,635–637).

Several regimens for both primary and secondary PCP prophylaxis have been adopted for clinical use, including oral TMP-SMX, oral dapsone with or without pyrimethamine (Daraprim) and leucovorin (Wellcovorin), aerosolized pentamidine (NebuPent), and oral atovaquone (Mepron) (Tables 58.13, 58.14, and 58.15). These are discussed briefly in turn.

TMP-SMX is the preferred agent for primary and secondary PCP prophylaxis (83,116,623,638–640). In addition to its efficacy in the prevention of PCP, it is also effective as a prophylactic agent against toxoplasmosis, and as an antibacterial agent that may reduce the incidence of common bacterial infections in HIV disease. The optimal dose is one double-strength tablet daily, although one single-strength tablet daily or one double-strength tablet taken three times a week are also dosing strategies (83,640,641).

The most common side effects of TMP-SMX include rash, pruritus, fever, leukopenia, neutropenia, thrombocytopenia, and liver function abnormalities (124,642).

TABLE 58.13. *Criteria for starting, discontinuing, and restarting opportunistic infection prophylaxis for HIV-infected adults*

Opportunistic Illness	Criteria for initiating primary prophylaxis	Criteria for discontinuing primary prophylaxis	Criteria for restarting primary prophylaxis	Criteria for initiating secondary prophylaxis	Criteria for discontinuing secondary prophylaxis	Criteria for restarting secondary prophylaxis
Pneumocystis carinii pneumonia	CD4$^+$ count of <200 cells/mm^3 or oropharyngeal *Candida*	CD4$^+$ count of >200 cells/mm^3 for ≥3 months	CD4$^+$ count of <200 cells/mm^3	Prior *P. carinii* pneumonia	CD4$^+$ count of >200 cells/mm^3 for ≥ 3 months	CD4$^+$ count of <200 cells/mm^3
Toxoplasmosis	Immunoglobulin G (IgG) antibody to *Toxoplasma* and CD4$^+$ count of <100 cells/mm^3	CD4$^+$ count of >200 cells/mm^3 for ≥3 months	CD4$^+$ count of <100–200 cells/mm^3	Prior toxoplasmic encephalitis	CD4$^+$ count of >200 cells/mm^3 sustained (e.g., ≥6 months) and completed initial therapy and asymptomatic for *Toxoplasma*	CD4$^+$ count of <200 cells/mm^3
Disseminated *Mycobacterium avium* complex (MAC)	CD4$^+$ count of <50 cells/mm^3	CD4$^+$ count of >100 cells/mm^3 for ≥3 months	CD4$^+$ count of <50–100 cells/mm^3	Documented disseminated disease	CD4$^+$ count of >100 cells/mm^3 sustained (e.g., ≥6 months) and completed 12 months of MAC therapy and asymptomatic for MAC	CD4$^+$ count of <100 cells/mm^3

Adapted from: Centers for Disease Control and Prevention. Guidelines for preventing opportunistic infections among HIV-infected persons—2002 recommendations of the U.S. Public Health Service and the Infectious Diseases Society of America. *MMWR Morb Mortal Wkly Rep* 2002;51(RR-8):1–51.

These toxicities have occurred more frequently in HIV-infected patients than in non–HIV-infected individuals (170,643–645). Many of these effects appear to be dose dependent, and generally are less common with low-dose TMP-SMX used for PCP prophylaxis than with the higher doses used for acute treatment of PCP (e.g., 15 to 20 mg/kg trimethoprim per day) (124,642,646,647). In addition, certain toxicities—particularly rash, pruritus, and fever—can often be managed symptomatically when they occur, and need not be treatment-limiting, although one must be mindful of certain more uncommon, but potentially serious toxicities, such as exfoliative dermatitis and the Stevens-Johnson syndrome (124,642,647).

Dapsone is recommended as an alternative regimen for PCP prophylaxis. Dapsone alone can be dosed as 50 mg twice daily or 100 mg once daily, with results suggesting acceptable efficacy and similar toxicity compared with oral TMP-SMZ (638,648,649). Additionally, dapsone, when used in combination with pyrimethamine and leucovorin, is efficacious in the prevention of toxoplasmosis (649,650). Dosing options of dapsone when used in this combination are (a) dapsone 50 mg daily, plus pyrimethamine 50 mg with leucovorin 25 mg weekly, or (b) dapsone 200 mg weekly, plus pyrimethamine 75 mg with leucovorin 25 mg weekly. Dapsone 50 mg daily is thought to be a less-effective regimen than 100 mg daily.

Dapsone is generally well tolerated, and the principal reported toxicities are rash, anorexia, nausea, gastrointestinal distress, varying degrees of hemolysis, anemia, and methemoglobinemia (642,651,652). Significant hemolysis and anemia are most common in, but not restricted to, patients receiving high-dose dapsone who have preexisting bone marrow suppression or a glucose-6-phosphate dehydrogenase deficiency (475,652). Screening of patients

TABLE 58.14. *Prophylaxis to prevent first episodes of opportunistic diseases among HIV-Infected adults and adolescents*

Pathogen	Preventive regimen		
	Indication	First choice	Alternative
Pneumocystis carinii*	CD4$^+$ counts of <200/mm^3 or oropharyngeal candidiasis	Trimethoprim-sulfamethoxazole (TMP-SMZ), 1 double-strength tablet (DS) daily or TMP-SMZ, 1 single-strength tablet (SS) daily	Dapsone, 50 mg twice daily or 100 mg daily; dapsone, 50 mg daily plus pyrimethamine, 50 mg plus leucovorin, 25 mg weekly; dapsone, 200 mg plus pyrimethamine, 75 mg plus leucovorin, 25 mg weekly; aerosolized pentamidine, 300 mg monthly via Respirgard II nebulizer; atovaquone, 1500 mg daily; TMP-SMZ, 1 DS three times weekly
Toxoplasma gondii§	Immunoglobulin G (IgG) antibody to *Toxoplasma* and CD4$^+$ count of <100/mm^3	TMP-SMZ, 1 DS daily	TMP-SMZ, 1 SS daily; dapsone, 50 mg daily plus pyrimethamine, 50 mg plus leucovorin, 25 mg weekly; dapsone, 200 mg plus pyrimethamine, 75 mg plus leucovorin, 25 mg/weekly; atovaquone, 1500 mg daily with or without pyrimethamine, 25 mg plus leucovorin, 10 mg daily
Mycobacterium avium complex	CD4$^+$ count of <50/mm^3	Azithromycin, 1200 mg weekly or clarithromycin, 500 mg twice daily	Rifabutin, 300 mg daily; azithromycin, 1200 mg weekly plus rifabutin, 300 mg daily

Notes: Information included in these guidelines might not represent Food and Drug Administration (FDA) approval or approved labeling for products or indications. Specifically, the terms *safe* and *effective* might not be synonymous with the FDA-defined legal standards for product approval.

*Prophylaxis should also be considered for persons with a CD4$^+$ percentage of <14%, for persons with a history of an AIDS-defining illness, and possibly for those with CD4$^+$ counts of >200 but <250 cells/mm^3. TMP-SMZ also reduces the frequency of toxoplasmosis and some bacterial infections. Patients receiving dapsone should be tested for glucose-6 phosphate dehydrogenase deficiency. A dosage of 50 mg daily of dapsone is probably less effective than 100 mg daily. Efficacy of parenteral pentamidine (e.g., 4 mg/kg body weight/month) is uncertain. Fansidar (sulfadoxine-pyrimethamine) is rarely used because of severe hypersensitivity reactions. Patients who are being administered therapy for toxoplasmosis with sulfadiazine-pyrimethamine are protected against *Pneumocystis carinii* pneumonia (PCP) and do not need additional prophylaxis against PCP.

§Protection against toxoplasmosis is provided by TMP-SMZ, dapsone plus pyrimethamine, and possibly atovaquone. Atovaquone can be used with or without pyrimethamine. Pyrimethamine alone probably provides limited, if any, protection.

Adapted from: Centers for Disease Control and Prevention. Guidelines for preventing opportunistic infections among HIV-infected persons—2002 recommendations of the U.S. Public Health Service and the Infectious Diseases Society of America. *MMWR Morb Mortal Wkly Rep* 2002;51(RR-8):1–51.

for glucose-6-phosphate dehydrogenase deficiency prior to the initiation of dapsone therapy for PCP (83,651) is advised, especially given the possibility of coexisting anemia or other disorders of red blood cell production in HIV-infected patients. Although dapsone is a member of the sulfone class of drugs, and chemically related to the sulfonamides, HIV-infected patients with allergies to TMP-SMZ are reported to tolerate dapsone therapy for PCP prophylaxis (648,649).

Pentamidine, another agent used for primary and secondary prophylaxis of PCP, is recommended as an alter-

native regimen to TMP-SMZ. Pentamidine is given in a standard 300 mg aerosolized dose once a month, delivered via a nebulizer system (e.g., the Respirgard II nebulizer system, Marquest Medical Products, Englewood, CO) (83,116,124,639,642). This dose and the nebulizer system are considered the current standard for the use of aerosolized pentamidine for PCP prophylaxis, and is approved by the FDA for this purpose. Side effects of parenterally administered pentamidine include hypotension, hypo- and hyperglycemia, renal insufficiency, leukopenia, pancreatitis, and liver function abnormalities (124).

TABLE 58.15. *Prophylaxis to prevent recurrence of opportunistic disease, after chemotherapy for acute disease, among HIV-infected adults and adolescents*

Pathogen		Preventive regimen	
	Indication	First choice	Alternative
Pneumocystis carinii	Prior *P. carinii* pneumonia (PCP)	Trimethoprim-sulfamethoxazole (TMP-SMZ), 1 double-strength tablet (DS), daily; or TMP-SMZ 1 single-strength tablet (SS) daily	Dapsone, 50 mg twice daily or 100 mg once daily; dapsone, 50 mg daily plus pyrimethamine, 50 mg weekly plus leucovorin, 25 mg weekly; dapsone, 200 mg plus pyrimethamine, 75 mg plus leucovorin, 25 mg weekly; aerosolized pentamidine, 300 mg every month via Respirgard II nebulizer; atovaquone, 1500 mg daily; TMP-SMZ, 1 DS three times weekly
Toxoplasma gondii∗	Prior toxoplasmic encephalitis	Sulfadiazine, 500–1000 mg four times daily plus pyrimethamine,25–50 mg daily plus leucovorin, 10–25 mg daily	Clindamycin, 300–450 mg every 6–8 h plus pyrimethamine, 25–50 mg daily plus leucovorin 10–25 mg daily; atovaquone, 750 mg every 6–12 h with or without pyrimethamine, 25 mg daily plus leucovorin, 10 mg daily
Mycobacterium avium complex	Documented disseminated disease	Clarithromycin, 500 mg twice daily plus ethambutol, 15 mg/kg body weight; with or without rifabutin, 300 mg daily	Azithromycin, 500 mg daily plus ethambutol, 15 mg/kg body weight with or without rifabutin, 300 mg daily

Notes: Information included in these guidelines might not represent Food and Drug Administration (FDA) approval or approved labeling for products or indications. Specifically, the terms *safe* and *effective* might not be synonymous with the FDA-defined legal standards for product approval.

∗Pyrimethamine-sulfadiazine confers protection against PCP as well as toxoplasmosis; clindamycin-pyrimethamine does not offer protection against PCP.

Adapted from: Centers for Disease Control and Prevention. Guidelines for preventing opportunistic infections among HIV-infected persons—2002 recommendations of the U.S. Public Health Service and the Infectious Diseases society of America. *MMWR Morb Mortal Wkly Rep* 2002;51(RR-8):1–51.

Such toxicities are unlikely following aerosolized pentamidine administration because systemic absorption of the drug is minimal, although isolated occurrences of hypotension, hypoglycemia, cutaneous eruptions, and pancreatitis have been reported following aerosolized pentamidine use (642,653–655). However, the aerosolized use of pentamidine commonly does result in cough and/or bronchospasm as a consequence of the irritant effects of the drug on the respiratory tract; patients may also report an unpleasant metallic taste following pentamidine inhalation (642,656,657). The former symptoms can often be minimized or prevented through pretreatment with an inhaled bronchodilator immediately prior to pentamidine administration (642,656).

The phenomenon of extrapulmonary pneumocystosis has also been described in HIV-infected patients receiving aerosolized pentamidine; case reports document pneumocystosis affecting most commonly the spleen, liver, gastrointestinal tract, and lymph nodes, with one report describing a case of fulminant disseminated disease in which thromboemboli containing *P. carinii* were identified in the peripheral vasculature (124,642,658,659). This phenomenon has prompted the concern that perhaps a systemic prophylactic agent against *P. carinii* might be preferable to one whose coverage is limited to the lung. Although extrapulmonary pneumocystosis is also well-described in AIDS patients not receiving aerosolized pentamidine (658,660,661), the overall frequency of this occurrence is believed to be low. Of greater clinical concern has been the finding that, as a result of relative underpenetration of the upper lobes of the lung with pentamidine during aerosolized administration, PCP limited to the apices or upper lobes is more likely to occur in such patients (642,662–665).

Atovaquone, the newest agent to be used for PCP prophylaxis, is recommended as an alternative regimen (83).

Atovaquone has been reported to be as effective in preventing PCP as dapsone or aerosolized pentamidine (666,667); however, its cost is considerably more. The dosing of atovaquone is 1,500 mg daily. Atovaquone with or without pyrimethamine may protect individuals from toxoplasmosis, and is dosed similarly plus pyrimethamine 25 mg daily and leucovorin 10 mg daily. Adverse effects from atovaquone include upper gastrointestinal symptoms, diarrhea, and hypersensitivity reaction (skin rash, fever, and pruritus).

Mycobacterium avium Complex

Disseminated *Mycobacterium avium* complex (MAC) infection is the most common systemic bacterial infection in late stages of HIV disease, particularly in injection drug users (620,668). Although the overall incidence of MAC in AIDS patients is decreasing, in injection drug users it is not (620). The disseminated form of the disease, rare in patients with a CD4+ count of more than 100/mm^3, but increasingly common as the CD4+ count drops below 50/mm^3 (669), frequently presents as a multisystem disease, with bacteremia, constitutional symptoms, and typical involvement of the gastrointestinal tract, bone marrow, liver, and lungs. As in the case of *M. tuberculosis,* multiple other sites of involvement are well documented. Disseminated MAC is associated with a decrease in survival (670), and its negative impact on quality of life is unequivocal. Primary MAC prophylaxis is recommended for all HIV-infected patients with a CD4+ T-cell count less than 50/mm^3 (83,671). Preferred primary prophylactic regimens are azithromycin 1,200 mg weekly or clarithromycin 500 mg twice daily (83,672–674) (see Table 58.14). In addition to their effects against MAC, both macrolides also confer additional protection against respiratory bacterial infections. If neither macrolide is tolerated, rifabutin is recommended as an alternative regimen, dosed 300 mg daily. Although the combination of azithromycin (1,200 mg weekly) and rifabutin (300 mg daily) is more effective than azithromycin alone (674), the toxicities associated with them in combination, the potential for drug interactions, and the increased cost all led the regimen to be recommended as an alternative. Adverse effects associated with both macrolides are primarily gastrointestinal intolerance. Additionally, patients taking clarithromycin are at increased risk of hepatotoxicity and drug interactions, particularly with protease inhibitors and NNRTIs. Rifabutin's adverse effects include bone marrow suppression, hepatotoxicity, ocular effects, and as previously noted, multiple drug interactions, particularly with protease inhibitors and NNRTIs. Discontinuation of primary prophylaxis for MAC is recommended when the CD4+ T-cell count increases above 100/mm^3 for at least 3 months as a consequence of antiretroviral therapy. With this response to HAART, the risk of disseminated MAC infection is drastically reduced (631,675,676).

Secondary prophylaxis, or maintenance therapy following disseminated MAC infection, is recommended with clarithromycin 500 mg twice daily, plus ethambutol 15 mg/kg daily, with or without rifabutin 300 mg daily (83,677,678) (see Table 58.15). The alternative recommended regimen is azithromycin 500 mg daily, plus ethambutol 15 mg/kg daily, with or without rifabutin 300 mg daily. Secondary prophylaxis may be discontinued when individuals have completed a full course of treatment for disseminated MAC (i.e., taking the aforementioned regimen for at least 1 year), have experienced an increase in CD4+ T-cell counts to at least 100/mm^3 for at least 6 months while on HAART, and remain asymptomatic with respect to MAC disease (83). However, the data supporting this recommendation are not overwhelmingly convincing, given the small numbers of patients involved in these studies, and the recurrences of disseminated disease (635,636,679–681).

Toxoplasma gondii Encephalitis

Primary prophylaxis against *T. gondii* is recommended for all HIV-infected patients with a CD4+ T-cell count less than 100 cells/mm^3 and a positive *Toxoplasma* antibody (IgG) (83). The preferred regimen for primary prophylaxis is TMP-SMX, one double-strength tablet daily (see Table 58.14). Alternative recommendations for primary prophylaxis include (a) TMP-SMZ single-strength tablet daily; (b) dapsone 50 mg daily, plus pyrimethamine 50 mg weekly, plus leucovorin 25 mg weekly; (c) dapsone 200 mg weekly, plus pyrimethamine 75 mg weekly, plus leucovorin 25 mg weekly; and (d) atovaquone 1,500 mg daily with or without pyrimethamine 25 mg daily and leucovorin 10 mg daily (83,649,650,682). In addition to preventing *Toxoplasma gondii* encephalitis, all of the above regimens also are protective against PCP. Primary prophylaxis should be discontinued in individuals whose CD4+ T-cell counts increase to greater than 200/mm^3 for at least 3 months as a consequence of HAART (83,631,632,635,683,684) (see Table 58.13).

Secondary prophylaxis, or maintenance therapy for individuals who have had *Toxoplasma gondii* encephalitis, is lifelong unless immune reconstitution occurs while taking HAART (685,686). The preferred regimen for secondary prophylaxis (chronic maintenance) is sulfadiazine 500 to 1,000 mg four times daily, plus pyrimethamine 25 to 50 mg daily, plus leucovorin 10 to 25 mg daily (see Table 58.15). Alternative regimens include (a) clindamycin 300 to 450 mg every 6 to 8 hours, plus pyrimethamine 25 to 50 mg daily, plus leucovorin 10 to 25 mg daily, or (b) atovaquone 750 mg every 6 to 12 hours, with or without pyrimethamine 25 mg daily and leucovorin 10 mg daily. Discontinuation of secondary prophylaxis is a reasonable consideration when individuals have completed a full course of treatment for *Toxoplasma gondii* encephalitis, remain asymptomatic with respect to signs and symptoms consistent with *Toxoplasma gondii* encephalitis, and have an increase in their CD4+ T-cell count above 200/mm³ for at least 6 months while taking HAART (83,635,636,684). The evidence, however, is not overwhelmingly convincing because of the limited number of patients evaluated and the occasional recurrences of disease. For this reason, many clinicians would obtain an MRI of the brain prior to deciding whether to discontinue secondary prophylaxis.

Adverse effects of pyrimethamine include bone marrow suppression (aplastic anemia and agranulocytosis), skin rash, seizures, and gastrointestinal symptoms. Leucovorin is administered simultaneously with pyrimethamine to counteract hematologic toxicity from pyrimethamine. Leucovorin, a reduced form of folic acid, is relatively nontoxic.

PSYCHOSOCIAL AND SUBSTANCE ABUSE TREATMENT ISSUES

The psychiatric, psychosocial, and substance abuse treatment issues relevant to the care of HIV-infected substance users are addressed elsewhere in this volume. However, it is important before concluding a chapter on medical management of such patients, to stress the central importance of these issues to the effective, comprehensive care of substance users with or at risk for HIV infection.

From the overview of therapeutic management of HIV infection presented here, it is readily understood that later stages of HIV infection are inevitably associated with the use of multiple medications, some of them with complex interactions, and some of them with specific dietary requirements. Didanosine, for example, has to be taken on an empty stomach. Ritonavir and saquinavir should be taken with food. Indinavir requires an empty stomach for better absorption when taken as the sole protease inhibitor, and increased fluid intake is needed to avoid the formation of kidney stones. Atovaquone requires food with high-fat content for optimal absorption. It is clear that therapeutic goals cannot be achieved without a high level of engagement and adherence on the part of the patient. Despite enhanced access to primary care provided to HIV-infected individuals in many communities, the complex issues of social isolation, use of illegal substances, problems with the criminal justice system, and a resulting low self-esteem in many instances, contribute to the fact that many injection drug users still do not have an identifiable source of primary care (65% in one study) (504).

Active drug use, unstable housing and social situations that preclude regular attendance at primary care centers, and resumption of prior drug or alcohol habits are all factors that interfere with appropriate adherence to medical treatment (75,81,481–483,591). It has been shown, however, that substance users exhibit good adherence with medical therapy when it is delivered in the appropriate context given their personal situation, whether

in drug-treatment clinics, HIV clinics, other outpatient settings, or prisons (48,49,52,75,483,497,687). Despite those observations, substance users continue to be less likely to receive HIV primary care and/or specific HIV therapy with antiretroviral drugs compared to other groups (76,77,79,688–694). Both of these factors, less access to primary care and less access to antiretroviral medications, are likely to contribute to higher morbidity and mortality rates of substance users when compared to other HIV-risk groups. In addition, approximately 85% of substance users are not in drug-treatment programs at any one time, leading to even less accessibility to the health care system (695). Other factors contributing to less access to care include the higher likelihood that substance users are unstably housed, incarcerated, and mentally ill (693,696,697). Because many substance users are not receiving regular and consistent care, prevention and/or management of HIV, hepatitis C, and tuberculosis are undoubtedly suboptimal. Consequently, outreach strategies are often necessary to bring, and maintain, substance users in primary care.

The literature describes several strategies to facilitate the delivery of health care to substance users. One program in Rhode Island, which involves intense case management for HIV-infected prisoners being released into the community, links ex-offenders to physicians at HIV clinics—the same physicians seen while incarcerated. Approximately 80% of these ex-offenders were injection drug users, and of those still enrolled in the program after 1 year, 82% continued to receive medical care (697). In another program, physicians joined a community-based organization's outreach team visiting HIV-infected single-room occupancy (SRO) hotel residents in Bronx, NY, in which the majority of residents were active substance users. Exposure to the medical outreach program was associated with more SRO hotel residents having primary care providers and taking antiretroviral medication (698). Another innovative outreach program involves a mobile needle exchange-based health care delivery system offering services to out-of-treatment injection drug users in New Haven, CT. Among this program's clients, mean emergency department use declined (505).

All of the above programs deliver health care to substance users in nontraditional medical settings, involve street outreach, and are successful in improving utilization of health care. Currently several sites in the United States are evaluating the impact of outreach to HIV-infected substance users with respect to medical outcomes.

The frequent co-occurrence of psychiatric disorders and HIV infection has been described in substance-using populations—in which the background prevalence of psychopathology is already likely to be elevated—and the need for psychiatric intervention is often compelling in many cases (44,45,497,699,700). In addition, because HIV infection is so clearly a condition that affects family units, attention to the needs and concerns of the family as a whole is an essential part of effective care. For those in young adult heterosexual populations, as are most substance users with HIV infection, issues of childbearing, child support, custody, and the growing phenomenon of orphanhood, are major themes that often require an intense and coordinated effort to help families respond to the potentially devastating effects of HIV (701,702). These issues often require involvement not only of medical and psychiatric staff, but also, and at times more importantly, of social service staff, legal services, pastoral and religious services, peer support groups, extended family members, and other community-based networks of care (703–709). Social and legal services are of particular importance with regard to child custody arrangements, entitlements, living wills, and other instruments that can help empower patients to make important decisions concerning their medical care, family and institutional arrangements, and financial affairs. The multiplicity of services and disciplines—medical, psychiatric, social, spiritual, legal—often involved in the care of HIV-infected patients and families requires that effective case management systems be developed to ensure coordination of care and to avoid fragmentation or duplication of services. The concept of case management received increasing recognition as an important approach to the care of patients with HIV infection during the first decade of the AIDS epidemic (703–709) and continues to hold relevance for this multifaceted endeavor during the coming years (710).

Regarding substance-abuse treatment, a discussion of the various treatment modalities and strategies is beyond the scope of this chapter; these issues are addressed in great detail in other sections of this volume. For HIV-infected substance users, as for other substance-using individuals, treatment options to help diminish or cease drug use behavior should be available and accessible as indicated. Clearly, from a public health standpoint, substance abuse treatment should be expected to play an important role in strategies attempting to reduce the risk of transmission of HIV within a given population (711). It is evident that active substance use interferes with efforts to provide ongoing primary medical care, and that adherence with often-complicated medical regimens is diminished in HIV-infected patients who remain heavily involved in the drug-using milieu (46,75,81,590,591). For these reasons, it is important to address the possibility of ongoing drug and/or alcohol use in the assessment and monitoring of HIV-infected substance users, and to provide or arrange for appropriate substance abuse treatment as indicated. In addition, because it may be expected that the risk of relapse to drug or alcohol abuse can be heightened in some patients at various points during the course of HIV infection (45,712–714) (e.g., upon disclosure of HIV seropositivity or the development of symptoms or serious signs of immunosuppression, or after the death of a friend or family member from AIDS-related illnesses), it is important for medical staff to be aware of and to anticipate these possibilities. Nevertheless, it must also be noted that certain patients may respond to their illness or to their identification as being HIV-infected with great inner resources and strength, and embrace a spiritual or transcendent outlook that can promote abstinence from alcohol and drugs.

CONCLUSION

The preceding discussion highlights some of the salient themes concerning the epidemiology, clinical manifestations, and medical management of substance users with HIV infection. This is clearly a rapidly changing field, with the likely and welcome emergence of new medications and therapeutic strategies that would be expected to alter or expand some of the approaches outlined here. However, one theme that is likely to remain central to the care of HIV-infected substance users is that the manifestations and treatment of HIV infection in such patients cannot meaningfully be considered without an assessment and understanding of substance use and its sequelae, and that effective substance abuse treatment in the AIDS era cannot be undertaken without an appreciation of the profound changes that the HIV epidemic has brought to the field. In closing, one can only hope that all the disciplines relevant to this endeavor may be broad enough in their outlook and perspective to permit and encourage the development of comprehensive approaches to the twin challenges of HIV and drug addiction in the twenty-first century.

REFERENCES

1. Centers for Disease Control. *Pneumocystis* pneumonia-Los Angeles. *MMWR Morb Mortal Wkly Rep* 1981;30:250–252.
2. Gottlieb MS, Schroff R, Schanker HM, et al. *Pneumocystis carinii* pneumonia and mucosal candidiasis in previously healthy homosexual men. *N Engl J Med* 1981;305:1425–1431.
3. Selik RM, Haverkos HW, Curran FW. Acquired immune deficiency syndrome (AIDS) trends in the United States,

1978–1982. *Am J Med* 1984;38:229–236.
4. Centers for Disease Control. Update: Acquired immune deficiency syndrome (AIDS) in the United States, 1981–1988. *MMWR Morb Mortal Wkly Rep* 1989;38:229–236.
5. Haverkos HW, Edelman R. The epidemiology of acquired immunodeficiency syndrome among heterosexuals. *JAMA* 1988;260:1922–1929.
6. Des Jarlais DC, Friedman SR, Stoneb-

urner RL. HIV infection and intravenous drug use: critical issues in transmission dynamics, infection outcomes, and prevention. *Rev Infect Dis* 1988;10:151–158.
7. Brickner PW, Torres RA, Barnes M, et al. Recommendations for control and prevention of human immunodeficiency (HIV) infection in intravenous drug users. *Ann Intern Med* 1989; 110:833–837.
8. Centers for Disease Control. First

100,000 cases of acquired immun-odeficiency syndrome—United States. *MMWR Morb Mortal Wkly Rep* 1989; 39:561–563.

9. Downs AM, Ancelle-Park RA, Costagliola DC, et al. *Monitoring and short-term forecasting of AIDS in Europe.* Presented at the sixth international conference on AIDS, June 1990; San Francisco CA. Abstract F.C.220.

10. Moss AR. Epidemiology of AIDS in developed countries. *Br Med Bull* 1988;44:56–67.

11. Centers for Disease Control and Prevention. HIV/AIDS Surveillance Report. 2001;13(2):1–44.

12. Lai S, Liu W, Chen J, et al. Changes in HIV-1 incidence in heroin users in, Guangxi Province, China. *J Acquir Immun Defic Syndr* 2001;26:365–370.

13. Zhang C, Yang R, Xia X, et al. High prevalence of HIV-1 and hepatitis C virus coinfection among injection drug users in the southern region of Yunnan, China. *J Acquir Immun Defic Syndr* 2002;29:191–196.

14. Nelson KE, Eiumtrakul S, Celentano DD, et al. HIV infection in young men in northern Thailand, 1991–1998: increasing role of injection drug use. *J Acquir Immun Defic Syndr* 2002; 29:62–68.

15. Joint United Nations Programme on HIV/AIDS. *UNAIDS. The report on the global HIV/AIDS epidemic: the Barcelona report.* Presented at the 14th international conference on AIDS. July 7–12, 2002; Barcelona, Spain.

16. Centers for Disease Control and Prevention. The global HIV and AIDS epidemic, 2001. *MMWR Morb Mortal Wkly Rep* 2001;50:434–439.

17. Department of Health, State of New Jersey. *AIDS Surveillance Report.* 1990.

18. Sato PA, Chin J, Mann JM. Review of AIDS and HIV infection: global epidemiology and statistics. *AIDS* 1989;3[1 Suppl]:S301–S307.

19. Wodak A, Dolan K, Imrie A, et al. Antibodies to the human immunodeficiency virus in needles and syringes used by intravenous drug abusers. *Med J Aust* 1987;147:275–276.

20. Des Jarlais DC, Friedman SR, Choopanya K, et al. International epidemiology of HIV and AIDS among injecting drug users. *AIDS* 1992;6:1053–1068.

21. Centers for Disease Control and Prevention. AIDS cases by state and metropolitan area of residence, 2000. *HIV/AIDS Surveil Suppl Rep* 2002; 8(No.2):1–42.

22. Nwanyanwu OC, Chu SY, Green TA, et al. Acquired immunodeficiency syndrome in the United States associated with injection drug use, 1981–1991. *Am J Drug Alcohol Abuse* 1993;19(4):399–408.

23. Kottiri BJ, Friedman SR, Neaigus A, et al. Risk networks and racial/ethnic differences in the prevalence of HIV infection among injection drug users. *J Acquir Immun Defic Syndr* 2002;30: 95–104.

24. Schoenbaum EE, Hartel D, Selwyn PA, et al. Risk factors for human immunodeficiency virus infection in intravenous drug users. *N Engl J Med* 1989;321:874–879.

25. Lange WR, Snyder FR, Lozovsky D, et al. HIV infection in Baltimore: antibody seroprevalence rates among parenteral drug abusers and prostitutes. *Md Med J* 1987;36:757–761.

26. Chaisson RE, Moss AR, Onishi R, et al. Human immunodeficiency virus infection in heterosexual drug users in San Francisco. *Am J Public Health* 1987;77:757–761.

27. Robert-Guroff M, Weiss SH, Giron JA, et al. Prevalence of antibodies to HTLV-I,-II and -III in intravenous drug abusers from a AIDS-endemic region. *JAMA* 1986;255:3133–3137.

28. Diaz T, Buehler JW, Castro KG, et al. AIDS trends among Hispanics in the United States. *Am J Public Health* 1993;83:504–509.

29. Haverkos HW, Drotman DP, Morgan M. Prevalence of Kaposi sarcoma among patients with AIDS. *N Engl J Med* 1985;312:1518.

30. Stoneburner RC, Des Jarlais DC, Benezra D, et al. A larger spectrum of severe HIV-1 related disease in intravenous drug users in New York City. *Science* 1988;242:916–919.

31. Farizo KM, Buehler JW, Chamberland ME, et al. Spectrum of disease in persons with human immunodeficiency virus infection in the United States. *JAMA* 1992;267:1798–1805.

32. Garcia-Leoni ME, Moreno S, Rodeno P, et al. Pneumococcal pneumonia in adult hospitalized patients infected with the human immunodeficiency virus. *Arch Intern Med* 1992;152:1808–1812.

33. Centers for Disease Control. Crack cocaine use among persons with tuberculosis—Contra Costa County, California, 1987–1990. *MMWR Morb Mortal Wkly Rep* 1991;40:485–489.

34. Barnes PF, Bloch AB, Davidson PT, et al. Tuberculosis in patients with human immunodeficiency virus infection. *N Engl J Med* 1991;324:1644–1650.

35. Centers for Disease Control. Tuberculosis—United States, 1985—and the possible impact of human T-lymphotropic virus type III/lymphadenopathy-associated virus infection. *MMWR Morb Mortal Wkly Rep* 1986;35:74–76.

36. Centers for Disease Control. Tuberculosis and acquired immunodeficiency syndrome—New York City. *MMWR Morb Mortal Wkly Rep* 1987;36:785–795.

37. Centers for Disease Control. Tuberculosis and acquired immunodeficiency syndrome—Florida. *MMWR Morb Mortal Wkly Rep* 1986;35:587–590.

38. Centers for Disease Control. Tuberculosis and AIDS—Connecticut. *MMWR Morb Mortal Wkly Rep* 1987;36:133–135.

39. Casabona J, Bosch A, Salas T, et al. The effect of tuberculosis as a new AIDS definition criteria in epidemiological surveillance data from a South European area. *J Acquir Immune Defic Syndr* 1990;3:272–277.

40. Friedman LN, Sullivan GM, Bevilaqua RP, et al. Tuberculosis screening in alcoholics and drug addicts. *Am Rev Respir Dis* 1987;136:1188–1192.

41. Hirschtick RE, Glassroth J, Jordan MC, et al. Bacterial pneumonia in persons infected with the human immunodeficiency virus. *N Engl J Med* 1995;333:845–851.

42. Mientjes GH, van Ameijden EJ, van den Hoek JA, et al. Increasing morbidity without rise in non-AIDS mortality among HIV-infected intravenous drug users in Amsterdam. *AIDS* 1992;6:207–212.

43. Willocks L, Cowan F, Brettle RP, Emmanuel FX, et al. The spectrum of chest infections in HIV positive patients in Edinburgh. *J Infect* 1992;24:37–42.

44. Batki S. Drug abuse, psychiatric disorders, and AIDS: dual and triple diagnosis. *West J Med* 1990;152:547–552.

45. Sorensen JL, Constantini MF, London JA. Coping with AIDS: strategies for patients and staff in drug abuse treatment programs. *J Psychoactive Drugs* 1989;21:435–440.

46. Selwyn PA, Feingold AR, Iezza A, et al. Primary care for patients with human immunodeficiency virus (HIV) infection in a methadone maintenance treatment program. *Ann Intern Med* 1989;111:761–763.

47. O'Connor PG, Molde S, Henry S, et al. Human immunodeficiency virus infection in intravenous drug users: a model for primary care. *Am J Med* 1992;93:382–386.

48. Samet JH, Libman H, Steger KA, et al. Compliance with zidovudine therapy in patients infected with human immunodeficiency virus, type 1: a cross-sectional study in a municipal hospital clinic. *Am J Med* 1992;92:495–501.

49. Selwyn PA, Budner NS, Wasserman

WC, et al. Utilization of on-site primary care services by HIV-seropositive and seronegative drug users in a methadone maintenance program. *Public Health Rep* 1993;108:492–500.

50. Samuels JE, Hendrix J, Hilton M, et al. Zidovudine therapy in an inner city population. *J Acquir Immune Defic Syndr* 1990;3:877–883.

51. Friedland GH, Harris C, Butkus-Small C, et al. Intravenous drug users and the acquired immunodeficiency syndrome (AIDS): demographic, drug use, and needle-sharing patterns. *Arch Intern Med* 1985;145:1414–1417.

52. Selwyn PA. The impact of the HIV/AIDS epidemic on medical services and drug abuse treatment programs: problems, prospects, and policy. *J Subst Abuse Treat* 1996;13:397–410.

53. Carpenter CC, Fischl MA, Hammer SM, et al. Antiretroviral therapy for HIV infection in 1996. *JAMA* 1996;276:146–154.

54. Marmor M, Des Jarlais DC, Cohen H, et al. Risk factors for infection with human immunodeficiency virus among intravenous drug abusers in New York City. *AIDS* 1987;1:39–44.

55. Vlahov D, Munoz A, Anthony JC, et al. Association of drug infection patterns with antibody to human immunodeficiency virus type 1 among intravenous drug users in Baltimore, Maryland. *Am J Epidemiol* 1990;132:847–856.

56. Rolfs RT, Goldberg M, Sharrar RG. Risk factors for syphilis: cocaine use and prostitution. *Am J Public Health* 1990;80:853–857.

57. Centers for Disease Control. Relationship of syphilis to drug use and prostitution—Connecticut and Philadelphia, Pennsylvania. *MMWR Morb Mortal Wkly Rep* 1988;37:755–764.

58. Fullilove RE, Fullilove MT, Bowser BP, et al. Risk of sexually transmitted disease among black adolescent crack users in Oakland and San Francisco, California. *JAMA* 1990;263:851–855.

59. Cates WJ. Acquired immunodeficiency syndrome, sexually transmitted disease, and epidemiology. *Am J Epidemiol* 1990;131:749–758.

60. Goldsmith MF. Sex tied to drugs = STD spread. *JAMA* 1988;260:2009.

61. Stall R, McKusick L, Wiley J, et al. Alcohol and drug use during sexual activity and compliance with safe sex guidelines for AIDS: the AIDS Behavioral Research Project. *Health Educ Q* 1986;13:359–371.

62. Mertens TE, Hayes RJ, Smith PG. Epidemiologic methods to study the interaction between HIV infection and other sexually transmitted disease. *AIDS* 1990;4:57–65.

63. Coates TJ, Stall RD, Catanca JA, et al. Behavioral factors in the spread of HIV infection. *AIDS* 1988;2[1 Suppl]:S239–S246.

64. Roth MD, Tashkin DP, Choi R, et al. Cocaine enhances human immunodeficiency virus replication in a model of severe combined immunodeficient mice implanted with human peripheral blood leukocytes. *J Infect Dis* 2002;185:701–705.

65. Lake-Baharr G, Chat K, Goundarajan S. *HIV infection and delta hepatitis in intravenous drug addicts*. Presented at the fifth international conference on AIDS. June 1989; Montreal, Canada. Abstract M.B.P.218.

66. Castillo I, Bartolome J, Martinez MA, et al. *Influence of HIV infection in hepatitis delta chronic carriers*. Presented at the fifth international conference on AIDS. June 1989; Montreal, Canada. Abstract M.B.P.221.

67. Novick DM, Farci P, Croxsan TS, et al. Hepatitis D virus and human immunodeficiency virus antibodies in parenteral drug abusers who are hepatitis B surface antigen positive. *J Infect Dis* 1988;158:795–803.

68. Rizzetto M. The delta agent. *Hepatology* 1983;3:729–737.

69. Gallo RC, Salahuddin SZ, Popovic M, et al. Frequent detection and isolation of cytopathic retroviruses (HTLV-III) from patients with AIDS and at risk for AIDS. *Science* 1984;224:500–503.

70. Ginzburg HM, Weiss SH, MacDonald MC, et al. HTLV-III exposure among drug users. *Cancer Res* 1985;45[Suppl]:4605–4608.

71. Des Jarlais DC, Friedman SR, Marmor M, et al. HTLV-III/LAV-associated disease progression and co-factors in a cohort of IV drug users. *AIDS* 1987;1:111–125.

72. Kaslow RA, Blackwelder WC, Ostrow DG, et al. No evidence for a role of alcohol or other psychoactive drugs in accelerating immunodeficiency in HIV-1-positive individuals. *JAMA* 1989;261:3424–3429.

73. Psychoactive drug use and AIDS. *JAMA* 1990;263:371–373.

74. Rezza G, Lazzarin A, Angarano G, et al. The natural history of HIV infection in intravenous drug users: risk of disease progression in a cohort of seroconverters. *AIDS* 1989;3:87–90.

75. Arnsten JH, Demas PA, Grant RW, et al. Impact of active drug use on antiretroviral therapy adherence and viral suppression in HIV-injection drug users. *J Gen Intern Med* 2002;17:377–381.

76. Celentano DD, Vlahov D, Cohn S, et al. Self-reported antiretroviral therapy in injection drug users. *JAMA* 1998;28:544–546.

77. Knowlton AR, Hoover DR, Shang-en C, et al. Access to medical care and service utilization among injection drug users with HIV/AIDS. *Drug Alcohol Depend* 2001;64:55–62.

78. Chitwood DD, Sanchez J, Comerford M, et al. Primary preventive health care among injection drug users, other sustained drug users, and non-users. *Subst Use Misuse* 2001;36:807–824.

79. Shapiro MF, Morton SC, McCaffrey DF, et al. Variations in the care of HIV-infected adults in the United States; results from the HIV cost and services utilization study. *JAMA* 1999; 281:2305–2315.

80. Lucas GM, Gebo KA, Chaisson RE, et al. Longitudinal assessment of the effects of drug and alcohol abuse on HIV-1 treatment outcomes in an urban clinic. *AIDS* 2002;16:767–774.

81. Golin CE, Liu H, Hays RD, et al. A prospective study of predictors of adherence to combination antiretroviral medication. *J Gen Intern Med* 2002;17:756–765.

82. Centers for Disease Control and Prevention. Guidelines for using antiretroviral agents among HIV-infected adults and adolescents: recommendations of the panel on clinical practices for treatment of HIV. *MMWR Morb Mortal Wkly Rep* 2002;51(RR-7):1–55.

83. Centers for Disease Control and Prevention. Guidelines for preventing opportunistic infections among HIV-infected persons—2002 recommendations of the U.S. Public Health Service and the Infectious Diseases Society of America. *MMWR Morb Mortal Wkly Rep* 2002;51(RR-8):1–51.

84. Mitsuya H, Yarchoan R, Broder S. Molecular targets for AIDS therapy. *Science* 1990;249:1533–1544.

85. Barre-Sinoussi F, Chermann JC, Rey F, et al. Isolation of a T-lymphotropic retrovirus from a patient at risk for acquired immune deficiency syndrome (AIDS). *Science* 1983;220:868–871.

86. Levy JA, Hoffman AD, Kramer SM, et al. Isolation of lymphocytopathic retroviruses from San Francisco patients with AIDS. *Science* 1984;225:840–842.

87. Coffin J, Haase A, Levy JA, et al. Human immunodeficiency viruses. *Science* 1986;232:697.

88. Horsburgh CR Jr, Ou CY, Jason J, et al. Duration of human immunodeficiency virus infection before detection of antibody. *Lancet* 1989;2:637–640.

89. Salahuddin SZ, Groopman JE, Markham PD, et al. HTLV-III symptom-free seronegative persons. *Lancet* 1984;2:1418–1420.

90. Ranki A, Valle SL, Krohn M, et al. Long latency precedes overt seroconversion in sexually transmitted human immunodeficiency virus infection. *Lancet* 1984;2:589–593.

91. Haseltine WA. Silent HIV infections. *N Engl J Med* 1989;320:1487–1489.

92. Hjelle B, Busch M. Direct methods for detection of HIV-1 infection. *Arch Pathol Lab Med* 1989;113:975–980.

93. Goudsmit J, de Wolf F, Paul DA, et al. Expression of human immunodeficiency virus antigen (HIV-Ag) in serum and cerebrospinal fluid during acute and chronic infection. *Lancet* 1986;2:177–180.

94. Popovic M, Sarnagadharan MG, Read E, et al. Detection, isolation, and continuous production of cytopathic retroviruses (HTLV-III) from patients with AIDS and pre-AIDS. *Science* 1984;224:497–500.

95. Volberding PA. HIV quantification: clinical applications. *Lancet* 1996; 347:71–72.

96. World Health Organization. WHO/CDC case definition for AIDS. *Wkly Epidemiol Rec* 1986;61:69–73.

97. Centers for Disease Control. Classification system for human T-lymphotropic virus type III/lymphadenopathy-associated virus infection. *MMWR Morb Mortal Wkly Rep* 1986;35:334–339.

98. Centers for Disease Control. Revision of the CDC surveillance case definition for acquired immunodeficiency syndrome. *MMWR Morb Mortal Wkly Rep* 1987;36[1S Suppl]:1S–18S.

99. Centers for Disease Control. 1993 revised classification system for HIV infection and expanded surveillance case definition for AIDS among adults and adolescents. *MMWR Morb Mortal Wkly Rep* 1992;41(No. RR-17):1–19.

100. Selik RM, Buehler JW, Karan JM, et al. Impact of the 1987 revision of the case definition of acquired immune deficiency syndrome in the United States. *J Acquir Immune Defic Syndr* 1990;3:73–82.

101. Payne SF, Rutherford GW, Lemp GF, et al. Effect of the revised AIDS case definition on AIDS reporting in San Francisco: evidence of increased reporting in intravenous drug users. *AIDS* 1990;4:335–339.

102. Chaisson RE, Stanton DL, Gallant JE, et al. Impact of the 1993 revision of the AIDS case definition on the prevalence of AIDS in a clinical setting. *AIDS* 1993;7:857–862.

103. Des Jarlais DC, Wenston J, Friedman SR, et al. Implications of the revised surveillance definition: AIDS among New York City drug users. *Am J Public Health* 1992;82:1531–1533.

104. Alcabes P, Friedland G. Injection drug use and human immunodeficiency virus infection. *Clin Infect Dis* 1995;20:1467–1479.

105. Lui KJ, Darrow WW, Rutherford GW 3rd. A model-based estimate of the mean incubation period for AIDS in homosexual men. *Science* 1988;240:1333–1335.

106. Gail MH, Rosenberg PS, Goedert JJ. Therapy may explain recent deficits in AIDS incidence. *J Acquir Immune Defic Syndr* 1990;3:296–306.

107. Northfelt DW, Hayward RA, Shapiro MF. The acquired immunodeficiency syndrome is a primary care disease. *Ann Intern Med* 1988;109:77–775.

108. Imagawa DT, Moon HL, Wolinsky SM, et al. Human immunodeficiency virus type 1 infection in homosexual men who remain seronegative for prolonged periods. *N Engl J Med* 1989;320:1458–1462.

109. McDougal JS, Kennendy MS, Sligh JM, et al. Binding of HTLV-III/LAV to T4+ T-cells by a complex of the 110K viral protein and the T4 molecule. *Science* 1986;231:382–385.

110. Lang W, Perkins H, Anderson RE, et al. Patterns of T-lymphocyte changes with human immunodeficiency virus infection: from seroconversion to the development of AIDS. *J Acquir Immune Defic Syndr* 1989;2:63–69.

111. Brinchmann JE, Vardtal F, Thorsby E. T lymphocyte changes in human immunodeficiency virus infection. *J Acquir Immune Defic Syndr* 1989;2:398–403.

112. Fauci AS. The human immunodeficiency virus: infectivity and mechanisms of pathogenesis. *Science* 1988;239:617–622.

113. Goedert JJ, Biggar RJ, Melbye M, et al. Effect of T4 count and cofactors on the incidence of AIDS in homosexual men infected with human immunodeficiency virus. *JAMA* 1987;257:331–334.

114. Polk BF, Fox R, Brookmeyer R, et al. Predictors of the acquired immunodeficiency syndrome developing in a cohort of seropositive homosexual men. *N Engl J Med* 1987;316:61–66.

115. Friedland GH. Early treatment for HIV: the time has come. *N Engl J Med* 1990;322:1000–1002.

116. Centers for Disease Control. Guidelines for prophylaxis against *Pneumocystis carinii* pneumonia for person infected with human immunodeficiency virus. *MMWR Morb Mortal Wkly Rep* 1989;38[S5 Suppl]:1–9.

117. Mellors JW, Rinaldo CR Jr, Gupta P, et al. Prognosis in HIV-1 infection predicted by the quantity of virus in plasma. *Science* 1996;272:1167–1170.

118. Mellors JW, Munoz A, Giorgi JV, et al. Plasma viral load and CD4+ lymphocytes as prognostic markers of HIV-1 infection. *Ann Intern Med* 1997;126:946–954.

119. Liegler TJ, Grant RM. HIV viral load assays. HIV InSite Knowledge Base Chapter. February 2001. Available at http://hivinsit.ucsf.edu.

120. Havlir DV, Richman DD. Viral Dynamics of HIV: implications for drug development and therapeutic strategies. *Ann Intern Med* 1996;124:984–994.

121. Pantaleo G, Graziosi C, Demarest JF, et al. HIV infection is active and progressive in lymphoid tissue during the clinically latent stage of disease. *Nature* 1993;362:355–358.

122. Murphy EL, Collier AC, Kalish LA, et al. Highly active antiretroviral therapy decreases mortality and morbidity in patients with advanced HIV disease. *Ann Intern Med* 2001;135:17–26.

123. Centers for Disease Control. Update: acquired immunodeficiency syndrome—United States. *MMWR Morb Mortal Wkly Rep* 1986;35:17–21.

124. Glatt AE, Chirgwin K. *Pneumocystis carinii* pneumonia in human immunodeficiency virus-infected patients. *Arch Intern Med* 1990;150:271–279.

125. World Health Organization. Acquired immunodeficiency syndrome: WHO European regions—update to 30 September 1990. *Wkly Epidemiol Rec* 1991;66:33–38.

126. Fleming AF. Opportunistic infections in AIDS in developed and developing countries. *Trans R Soc Trop Med Hyg* 1990;84[1 Suppl]:1–6.

127. Sewankambo NK, Mugerwa RD, Goodgame R, et al. Enteropathic AIDS in Uganda: an endoscopic, histological, and microbiological study. *AIDS* 1987;1:9–13.

128. Serwadda D, Mugerwa RD, Sewankambo NK, et al. Slim disease: a new disease in Uganda and its association with HTLV-III infection. *Lancet* 1985;2:849–852.

129. Ablashi DV, Chatlynne LG, Whitman JE Jr, et al. Spectrum of Kaposi sarcoma-associated herpesvirus, or human herpesvirus 8, diseases. *Clin Microbiol Rev* 2002;15:439–464.

130. Pauk J, Huang ML, Brodie SJ, et al. Mucosal shedding of human herpesvirus 8 in men. *N Engl J Med* 2000;343:1369–1377.

131. Cannon M, Dollard SC, Smith DK, et al. Blood-borne and sexual transmission of human herpesvirus 8 in women with or at risk for human immunodeficiency virus infection. *N Engl J Med* 2001;344:637–643.

132. Whitby D, Smith NA, Matthews S, et al. Human herpesvirus 8: seroepidemiology among women and detection in the genital tract of seropositive women. *J Infect Dis* 1999;179:234–236.

133. Gessain A, Sudaka A, Briere J, et al. Kaposi sarcoma-associated herpes-like virus (human herpesvirus type 8) DNA sequences in multicentric Castleman disease: is there any relevant association in non-human immunodeficiency virus-infected patients? *Blood* 1996;87(1):414–416.

134. Selwyn PA, Feingold AR, Hartel D, et al. Increased risk of bacterial pneumonia in HIV-infected intravenous users without AIDS. *AIDS* 1988;2:267–272.

135. Mouton Y, Chidiac C, Senneville E. *Pneumonies bacteriennes et virales au cours du SIDA chez les utilizateurs de drogue par voie intraveineuse.* Presented at the fifth international conference on AIDS. June 1989; Montreal, Canada. Abstract Th.B.O.13.

136. Dobkin J, Mandell W, Sethi N. *Bacteremic pneumococcal disease as the first manifestation of HIV infection in adults.* Presented at the fifth international conference on AIDS. June 1989; Montreal, Canada. Abstract M.B.P.71.

137. Des Jarlais DC, Friedman SR. HIV and intravenous drug use. *AIDS* 1988; 2[1 Suppl]:S65–S69.

138. Selwyn PA, Hartel D, Wasserman W, et al. Impact of the AIDS epidemic on morbidity and mortality among intravenous drug users in a New York City methadone maintenance program. *Am J Public Health* 1989;79:1358–1362.

139. Galli M, Codini G, Carito M, et al. *Causes of death in a large cohort of IV drug users in Milan: an update.* Presented at the fifth international conference on AIDS. June 1989; Montreal, Canada. Abstract W.A.P.30.

140. Selwyn PA, Alcabes P, Hartel D, et al. Clinical manifestations and predictors of disease progression in drug users with human immunodeficiency virus infection. *N Engl J Med* 1992;327:1697–1703.

141. Cherubin C. The medical sequelae of narcotic addiction. *Ann Intern Med* 1967;67:23–33.

142. Rho YM. Infections as fatal complications of narcotism. *NY State J Med* 1972;72:823–830.

143. Caiaffa WT, Graham NM, Vlahov D. Bacterial pneumonia in adult populations with human immunodeficiency virus (HIV) infection. *Am J Epidemiol* 1993;138:909–922.

144. Witt DJ, Craven DE, McCabe WR. Bacterial infections in adult patients with the acquired immune deficiency syndrome (AIDS) and AIDS-related complex. *Am J Med* 1987;82:900–906.

145. Simberkoff MS, El-Sadr W, Schiffman G, et al. *Streptococcus pneumoniae* infections and bacteremia in patients with acquired immune deficiency syndrome, with a report of pneumococcal vaccine failure. *Am Rev Respir Dis* 1984;103:1174–1176.

146. Polsky B, Gold JW, Whimbey E, et al. Bacterial pneumonia in patients with the acquired immunodeficiency syndrome. *Ann Intern Med* 1986;104:38–41.

147. Gilks CF, Brindle RJ, Otieno LS, et al. Life-threatening bacteremia in HIV-1 seropositive adults admitted to hospital in Nairobi, Kenya. *Lancet* 1990;336:545–549.

148. Schrager LK. Bacterial infections in AIDS patients. *AIDS* 1988;2[1 Suppl]: S183–S189.

149. Friedland GH, Selwyn PA. Infections in injection drug users (excluding AIDS). In: Isselbacher KE, Braunwald E, et al., ed. *Harrisons's principles of internal medicine.* New York: Mc-Graw-Hill, 1994;831–835.

150. Slim J, Boghassian J, Perez G, et al. *Comparative analysis of bacterial endocarditis in HIV+ and HIV– intravenous drug abusers.* Presented at the fourth international conference on AIDS. June 1988; Stockholm, Sweden. Abstract 8027.

151. Poblete R, Sone C, Fishchl M. *Staphylococcus aureus endocarditis in HIV+ and HIV– intravenous drug abusers.* Presented at the fifth international conference on AIDS. June 1989; Montreal, Canada. Abstract Th.A.O.24.

152. Weisse AB, Heller DR, Schimenti RJ, et al. The febrile parenteral drug user: a prospective study in 121 patients. *Am J Med* 1993;94:274–280.

153. Sheagren JN. Endocarditis complicating parenteral drug abuse. In: Remington JS, Swartz MN, eds. *Current clinical topics in infectious diseases,* vol. 2. New York: McGraw-Hill, 1981;211–233.

154. Pujol M, Pena C, Pallares R, et al. Nosocomial *Staphylococcus aureus* bacteremia among nasal carriers of methicillin-resistant and methicillin-susceptible strains. *Am J Med* 1996; 100(5):509–516.

155. Jernigan JA, Titus MG, Groschel DH, et al. The effectiveness of contact isolation during a hospital outbreak of methicillin-resistant *Staphylococcus aureus. Am J Epidemiol* 1996;143:496–504.

156. Moreno F, Crisp C, Jorgensen JH, et al. Methicillin-resistant *Staphylococcus aureus* as a community organism. *Clin Infect Dis* 1995;21:1308–1312.

157. Wells CL, Juni BA, Cameron SB, et al. Stool carriage, clinical isolation, and mortality during an outbreak of vancomycin-resistant enterococci in hospitalized medical and/or surgical patients. *Clin Infect Dis* 1995;21:45–50.

158. Shay DK, Maloney SA, Montecalvo M, et al. Epidemiology and mortality risk of vancomycin-resistant enterococcal bloodstream infections. *Clin Infect Dis* 1995;172:993–1000.

159. Chirurgi VA, Edelstein H, McCabe R. Pneumococcal bacteremia as a marker for human immunodeficiency virus infection in patients without AIDS. *South Med J* 1990;83:895–899.

160. Hopewell PC. Prevention of lung infections associated with human immunodeficiency virus infection. *Thorax* 1989;44:1038–1044.

161. Lane CH, Masur H, Edgar LC, et al. Abnormalities of B-cell activation and immunoregulation in patients with the acquired immunodeficiency syndrome. *N Engl J Med* 1983;309:453–458.

162. Pahwa SG, Quilop MTJ, Lange M, et al. Defective B-lymphocyte function in homosexual men in relation to the acquired immunodeficiency syndrome. *Ann Intern Med* 1984;101:757–763.

163. Ammann AJ, Schiffman G, Abrams D, et al. B-cell immunodeficiency in acquired immune deficiency syndrome. *JAMA* 1984;251:1447–1449.

164. Baron AD, Hollander H. *Pseudomona aeruginosa* bronchopulmonary infection in late human immunodeficiency virus disease. *Am Rev Respir Dis* 1993;148:992–996.

165. Kielhofner M, Atmar RL, Hamill RJ, et al. Life-threatening *Pseudomona aeruginosa* infections in patients with human immunodeficiency virus infection. *Clin Infect Dis* 1992;14:403–411.

166. Mendelson MH, Gurtman A, Szabo S, et al. *Pseudomona aeruginosa* bacteremia in patients with AIDS. *Clin Infect Dis* 1994;18:886–895.

167. Fichtenbaum CJ, Woeltje KF, Powderly WG. Serious *Pseudomona aeruginosa* infections in patients with human immunodeficiency syndrome virus: a case-control study. *Clin Infect Dis* 1994;19:417–422.

168. Schuchat A, Stehr-Green J, Parkin W, et al. Use of surveillance for invasive pneumococcal disease to estimate the size of the immunosuppressed HIV-infected population. Presented at the 29th international conference on antimicrobial agents and chemotherapy, Houston TX, September 1989(abst).

169. Haverkos HW, Lange WR. Serious infections other than human immunodeficiency virus among intravenous drug users. *J Infect Dis* 1990;161:894–902.

170. Gordin FM, Simon GL, Wofsy CD, et al. Adverse reactions to tri-methoprim-sulfamethoxazole in patients with AIDS. *Ann Intern Med* 1984;100:495–499.

171. Ballet JJ, Sulcebe G, Couderc LJ, et al. Impaired antipneumococcal antibody response in patients with AIDS-related generalized lymphadenopathy. *Clin Exp Immunol* 1987;68:479–487.

172. Huang KL, Ruben FL, Rinaldo CR Jr, et al. Antibody responses after influenza and pneumococcal immunization in HIV-infected homosexual men. *JAMA* 1987;257:2047–2050.

173. Klein RS, Selwyn PA, Maude D, et al. Response to pneumococcal vaccine among asymptomatic heterosexual partners of persons with AIDS and intravenous drug users infected with human immunodeficiency virus. *J Infect Dis* 1989;160:826–831.

174. Herb F, Watters JK, Case P, et al. *Endocarditis, subcutaneous abscesses, and other bacterial infections in intravenous drug users and their association with skin-cleaning at drug injection sites.* Presented at the fifth international conference on AIDS. June 1989; Montreal, Canada. Abstract Th.D.0.4.

175. Vlahov D, Sullivan M, Astemborski J, et al. Bacterial infections and skin cleaning prior to injection among intravenous drug users. *Public Health Reports* 1992;107:595–598.

176. Doern GB, Brown SD. Antimicrobial susceptibility among community-acquired respiratory tract pathogens in the USA: data from PROTEKT US 2000–2001. *J Infect* 2004;48(1):56–65.

177. Hofman J, Cetron MS, Farley MM, et al. The prevalence of drug-resistant *Streptococcus pneumoniae* in Atlanta. *N Engl J Med* 1995;333:481–486.

178. Appelbaum PC. Antimicrobial resistance in *Streptococcus pneumoniae:* an overview. *Clin Infect Dis* 1992;15:77–83.

179. Burwen DR, Bloch AB, Griffin LD, et al. National trends in the concurrence of tuberculosis and acquired immunodeficiency syndrome. *Arch Intern Med* 1995;155:1281–1286.

180. Cantwell MF, Snider DE, Cauthen GM, et al. Epidemiology of tuberculosis in the United States, 1985 through 1992. *JAMA* 1994;272:535–539.

181. Selwyn PA, Hartel D, Lewis VA, et al. A prospective study of the risk of tuberculosis among intravenous drug users with HIV infection. *N Engl J Med* 1989;320:545–550.

182. World Health Organization. *Stop TB annual report 2001.* WHO/CDS/STB 2002; 17:1–17.

183. Africa's tuberculosis burden and chemoprophylaxis. *Lancet* 1990;335:1249–1250.

184. World Health Organization. *HIV causing tuberculosis cases to double in Africa.* Press Release WHO/21. April 23, 2001. Available at http://www.who.int/inf-pr-2001/en/pr2001-21.html. Last accessed July, 2004.

185. Harries AD. Tuberculosis and human immunodeficiency virus infection in developing countries. *Lancet* 1990;335:387–390.

186. Pitchenik AE. Tuberculosis control and the AIDS epidemic in developing countries. *Ann Intern Med* 1990;113:89–90.

187. Rieder HL, Cauthen GM, Kelly GD, et al. Tuberculosis in the United States. *JAMA* 1989;262:385–389.

188. Hopewell PC. Impact of human immunodeficiency virus infection on the epidemiology, clinical features, management, and control of tuberculosis. *Clin Infect Dis* 1992;15:540–547.

189. Dolin PJ, Raviglione MC, Kochi A. Global tuberculosis incidence and mortality during 1990–2000. *Bull World Health Organ* 1994;72:213–220.

190. Chaisson RE, Slutkin G. Tuberculosis and human immunodeficiency virus infection. *J Infect Dis* 1989;159:96–100.

191. Selwyn PA, Hartel D, Lewis VA, et al. A prospective study of the risk of tuberculosis among intravenous drug users with HIV infection. *N Engl J Med* 1989;320:545–550.

192. Pitchenik AE, Cole C, Russell BW, et al. Tuberculosis, atypical mycobacteriosis, and the acquired immunodeficiency syndrome among Haitian and non-Haitian patients in south Florida. *Ann Intern Med* 1984;101:641–645.

193. Daley CL, Small PM, Schecter GF, et al. An outbreak of tuberculosis with accelerated progression among persons infected with the human immunodeficiency virus. *N Engl J Med* 1992;326:231–235.

194. Small PM, Hopewell PC, Singh SP, et al. The epidemiology of tuberculosis in San Francisco. *N Engl J Med* 1994;330:1703–1709.

195. Alland DA, Kalkut GE, Moss AR, et al. Transmission of tuberculosis in New York city. *N Engl J Med* 1994;330:1710–1716.

196. Small PM, Shafer RW, Hopewell PC, et al. Exogenous reinfection with multidrug-resistant *Mycobacterium tuberculosis* in patients with advanced HIV infection. *N Engl J Med* 1993;328:1137–1144.

197. Shafer RW, Edlin BR. Tuberculosis in patients infected with human immunodeficiency virus: perspective on the past decade. *Clin Infect Dis* 1996;22:683–704.

198. Valway SE, Greifinger RB, Papania M, et al. Multidrug-resistant tuberculosis in the New York State prison system, 1990–1991. *J Infect Dis* 1994;170:151–156.

199. Valway SE, Richards SB, Kovacovich J, et al. Outbreak of multidrug-resistant tuberculosis in a New York State prison, 1991. *Am J Epidemiol* 1994;140:113–122.

200. Friedman CR, Stoeckle MY, Kreiswirth BN, et al. Transmission of multidrug-resistant tuberculosis in a large urban setting. *Am J Respir Crit Care Med* 1995;152:355–359.

201. Centers for Disease Control and Prevention. Prevention and treatment of tuberculosis among patients infected with human immunodeficiency virus: principles of therapy and revised recommendations. *MMWR Morb Mortal Wkly Rep* 1998;47(No. RR-20):1–58.

202. Centers for Disease Control. Tuberculosis and human immunodeficiency virus infection: recommendations of the Advisory Committee for the Elimination of Tuberculosis (ACET). *MMWR Morb Mortal Wkly Rep* 1989;38:236–250.

203. Sunderam G, McDonald RJ, Maniatis T, et al. Tuberculosis as a manifestation of the acquired immunodeficiency syndrome (AIDS). *JAMA* 1986;256:362–366.

204. Centers for Disease Control and Prevention. Reported tuberculosis in the United States 2001. Tuberculosis Surveillance Report 2001.

205. Centers for Disease Control and Prevention. *National seroprevalence surveys, 1992.* Washington, DC: U.S. Government Printing Office, 1993.

206. Reichman LB, Felton CP, Edsall JR. Drug dependence a possible new risk factor for tuberculosis disease. *Arch Intern Med* 1979;139:337–339.

207. Pape JW, Simone SJ, Ho JL, et al. Effect of isoniazid prophylaxis on incidence of active tuberculosis and progression of HIV infection. *Lancet* 1993;342:268–272.

208. Moreno S, Baraia-Extaburu J, Bouza E, et al. Risk for developing tuberculosis among anergic patients infected with HIV. *Ann Intern Med* 1993;119:194–198.

209. Wadhawan D, Hira S, Mwansa N, et al. *Isoniazid prophylaxis among patients with HIV-1 infection.* Presented at the sixth international conference on AIDS. June 1990; San Francisco, CA. Abstract Th.B.510.

210. Nunn P, Mungai M, Nyamwaya J. The effect of human immunodeficiency virus type-1 on the infectiousness of tuberculosis. *Tuber Lung Dis* 1994;75:25–32.

211. Jones BE, Young SM, Antoniskis D, et al. Relationship of the manifestations of tuberculosis to CD4 cell counts in patients with human immunodeficiency virus infection. *Am Rev Respir Dis* 1993;148:1292–1297.

212. Theuer CP, Hopewell PC, Elias D, et al. Human immunodeficiency virus infection in tuberculosis patients. *J Infect Dis* 1990;162:8–12.

213. De Cock KM, Soro B, Coulibaly IM, et al. Tuberculosis and HIV infection in Sub-Saharan Africa. *JAMA* 1992;268:1581–1587.

214. Whalen C, Horsburgh CR, Hom D, et al. Accelerated course of human immunodeficiency virus infection after tuberculosis. *Am J Respir Crit Care Med* 1995;151:129–135.

215. Toossi Z. Virological and immunological impact of tuberculosis on human immunodeficiency virus type 1 disease. *J Infect Dis* 2003;188:1146–1155.

216. Leroy V, Salmi LR, Dupon M, et al. Progression of human immunodeficiency virus infection in patients with tuberculosis disease. A cohort study in Bordeaux, France, 1988–1994. The Groupe d'Epidemiologie Clinique du Sida en Aquitaine (GECSA). *Am J Epidemiol* 1997;145:293–300.

217. Perneger TV, Sudre P, Lundgren JD, et al. Does the onset of tuberculosis in AIDS predict shorter survival? Results of a cohort study in 17 European countries over 13 years. AIDS in Europe Study Group. *BMJ* 1995;311:1468–1471.

218. Tacconelli E, Tumbarello M, Ardito F, et al. Tuberculosis significantly reduces the survival of patients with AIDS. *Int J Tuber Lung Dis* 2002;1:582–584.

219. Shafer RW, Goldberg R, Sierra M, et al. Frequency of *Mycobacterium tuberculosis* bacteremia in patients with tuberculosis in an area endemic for AIDS. *Am Rev Respir Dis* 1989;140:1611–1613.

220. Louie E, Rice LB, Holzman RS. Tuberculosis in non-Haitian patients with acquired immunodeficiency syndrome. *Chest* 1986;90:542–545.

221. El-Sadr W, Perlman DC, Matts JP, et al. Evaluation of an intensive intermittent-induction regimen and duration of short-course treatment for human immunodeficiency virus-related pulmonary tuberculosis. *Clin Infect Dis* 1998;26:1148–1158.

222. Pulmonary tuberculosis: primary, reactivation, HIV-related, and non-HIV related. In: Friedman LN, Selwyn PA, eds. *Tuberculosis. Current concepts and treatment.* Boca Raton, FL: CRC Press, 1994;107–138.

223. Brindle RJ, Nunn PP, Githui W, et al. Quantitative bacillary response to treatment in HIV-associated pulmonary tuberculosis. *Am Rev Respir Dis* 1993;147:958–961.

224. Pitchenik AE, Burr J, Suarez M, et al. Human T-cell lymphotropic virus-III (HTLV-III) seropositivity and related disease among 71 consecutive patients in whom tuberculosis was diagnosed: a prospective study. *Am Rev Respir Dis* 1987;135:875–879.

225. Pitchenik AE, Rubinson HA. The radiographic appearance of tuberculosis in patients with the acquired immune deficiency syndrome (AIDS) and pre-AIDS. *Am Rev Respir Dis* 1985;131:393–396.

226. Bass JB Jr, Farer LS, Hopewell PC, et al. Treatment of tuberculosis and tuberculosis infection in adults and children. American Thoracic Society/Centers for Disease Control and Prevention. *Am J Respir Crit Care Med* 1994;149:1359–1374.

227. American Thoracic Society. Medical section of the American Lung Association: treatment of tuberculosis and tuberculosis infection in adults and children. *Am Rev Respir Dis* 1986;134:355–363.

228. Centers for Disease Control. Initial therapy for tuberculosis in the era of multidrug resistance. Recommendations of the Advisory Council for the Elimination of Tuberculosis. *MMWR Morb Mortal Wkly Rep* 1993;42 (RR-7):1–8.

229. Centers for Disease Control and Prevention. Notice to readers: updated guidelines for the use of rifabutin or rifampin for the treatment and prevention of tuberculosis among HIV-infected patients taking protease inhibitors or nonnucleoside reverse transcriptase inhibitors. *MMWR Morb Mortal Wkly Rep* 2000;49:185–189.

230. Benedek IH, Joshi A, Fiske WD, et al. *Pharmacokinetic interaction between efavirenz and rifampin in healthy volunteers.* Presented at the 12th world AIDS conference. June 28–July 3, 1998; Geneva, Switzerland(abst).

231. Norvir package insert. Abbot Laboratories, Chicago, IL. 1999.

232. Veldkamp AI, Hoetelmans RM, Beijnen JH, et al. Ritonavir enables combined therapy with rifampin and saquinavir. *Clin Infect Dis* 1999;29:1586.

233. Perucca E, Grimaldi R, Frigo GM, et al. Comparative effects of rifabutin and rifampicin on hepatic microsomal enzyme activity in normal subjects. *Eur J Clin Pharmacol* 1988;34:595–599.

234. Vital Durand D, Hampden C, Boobis AR, et al. Induction of mixed function oxidase activity in man by rifapentine (MDL 473), a long-acting ri-famycin derivative. *Br J Clin Pharmacol* 1986;21:1–7.

235. Li AP, Reith MK, Rasmussen A, et al. Primary human hepatocytes as a tool for the evaluation of structure-activity relationship in cytochrome P450 induction potential of xenobiotics: evaluation of rifampin, rifapentine and rifabutin. *Chem Biol Interact* 1997;107:17–30.

236. Sirgel FA, Botha FJ, Parkin DP, et al. The early bacterial activity of rifabutin in patients with pulmonary tuberculosis measured by sputum viable counts: a new method of drug assessment. *J Antimicrob Chemother* 2002;32:867–875.

237. Kunin CM. Antimicrobial activity of rifabutin. *Clin Infect Dis* 1996;22[1 Suppl]:S3–S14.

238. Gonzalez-Montaner LJ, Natal S, Yongchaiyud P, et al. Rifabutin for the treatment of newly-diagnosed pulmonary tuberculosis: a multinational, randomized, comparative study versus rifampicin. Rifabutin Study Group. *Tuber Lung Dis* 1994;75:341–347.

239. McGregor MM, Olliaro P, Wolmarans L, et al. Efficacy and safety of rifabutin in the treatment of patients with newly diagnosed pulmonary tuberculosis. *Am J Respir Crit Care Med* 1996;154:1462–1467.

240. Schwander S, Rush-Gerdes S, Mateega A, et al. A pilot study of antituberculosis combinations comparing rifabutin with rifampicin in the treatment of HIV-1 associated tuberculosis. A single blind randomized evaluation in Ugandan patients with HIV-1 infection and pulmonary tuberculosis. *Tuber Lung Dis* 1995;76:210–218.

241. Centers for Disease Control and Prevention. Clinical update: impact of HIV protease inhibitors on the treatment of HIV-infected tuberculosis patients with rifampin. *MMWR Morb Mortal Wkly Rep* 1996;45:921–925.

242. Brown LS, Sawyer RC, Li R, et al. Lack of pharmacologic interaction between rifabutin and methadone in HIV-infected former injecting drug users. *Drug Alcohol Depend* 1996;43:71–77.

243. Bureau of Tuberculosis Control, New York City Department of Health. *Clinical policies and protocols.* New York: Author, 1997.

244. Jones BE, Otaya M, Antoniski D, et al. A prospective evaluation of antituberculosis therapy in patients with human immunodeficiency virus infection. *Am J Respir Crit Care Med* 1994;150:1499–1502.

245. Kassim S, Sassan-Morokro M, Ackah A, et al. Two-year follow up of persons with HIV-1-and HIV-2 associated pulmonary tuberculosis treated with

short-course chemotherapy in West Africa. *AIDS* 1995;9:1185–1191.

246. Chaisson RE, Clermont HC, Holt E, et al. Six-month supervised intermittent tuberculosis therapy in Haitian patients with and without HIV infection. *Am J Respir Crit Care Med* 2002;154:1034–1038.

247. Vernon A, Khan A, Bozemma L, et al. Update on the U.S. Public Health Service Study 22: a trial of once weekly isoniazid (INH) and rifapentine (RPT) in the continuation phase of TB treatment. *Am J Respir Crit Care Med* 1998;157:A467(abst).

248. Perriens JH, St Louis ME, Mukadi YB, et al. Pulmonary tuberculosis in HIV-infected patients in Zaire. A controlled trial of treatment for either 6 or 12 months. *N Engl J Med* 1995;332:779–784.

249. Moore M, Onorato IM, McCray E, et al. Trends in drug-resistant tuberculosis in the United States, 1993–1996. *JAMA* 1997;278:833–837.

250. Branford WZ, Martin JN, Reingold AL, et al. The changing epidemiology of acquired drug-resistant tuberculosis in San Francisco, USA. *Lancet* 1996;348:928–931.

251. Ridzon R, Whitney CG, McKenna MT, et al. Risk factors for rifampin monoresistant tuberculosis. *Am J Respir Crit Care Med* 1998;157:1881–1884.

252. Munsiff SS, Joseph S, Ebrahimzadeh A, et al. Rifampin-monoresistant tuberculosis in New York City, 1993–1994. *Clin Infect Dis* 1997;25:1465–1467.

253. Centers for Disease Control. National action plan to combat multidrug-resistant tuberculosis. *MMWR Morb Mortal Wkly Rep* 1992;41(RR-11):1–48.

254. Centers for Disease Control. Prevention and control of tuberculosis in U.S. communities with at-risk minority populations: recommendations of the Advisory Council for the Elimination of Tuberculosis and Prevention and control of tuberculosis among homeless persons: recommendations of the Advisory Council for the Elimination of Tuberculosis. *MMWR Morb Mortal Wkly Rep* 1992;41 (RR-5):1–12.

255. Gourevitch MN, Wasserman W, Panero MS, et al. Successful adherence to observed prophylaxis and treatment of tuberculosis among drug users in a methadone program. *J Addict Dis* 1996;15:93–104.

256. Altice FL, Fleck EM, Selwyn PA, et al. *Provision of health care and HIV counseling and testing for clients of the New Haven needle exchange program.* Presented at the ninth international conference on AIDS. June 1993; Berlin, Germany. Abstract PO-D17–3927.

257. Altice F, Tanguay S, Hunt D, et al. Demographics of HIV infection and utilization of medical services among IDUs in a women's prison. Presented at the eighth international conference on AIDS. June 1992; Amsterdam, Netherlands. Abstract PoC4358.

258. Frieden TR, Fujiwara PI, Washko RM, et al. Tuberculosis in New York City—turning the tide. *N Engl J Med* 1995;333:229–233.

259. Chaulk CP, Moore-Rice K, Rizzo R, et al. Eleven years of community-based directly observed therapy for tuberculosis. *JAMA* 1995;274:945–951.

260. Iseman MD, Cohn DL, Sbarbaro JA. Directly observed treatment of tuberculosis: we can't afford not to try it. *N Engl J Med* 1993;328:576–578.

261. Centers for Disease Control and Prevention. Targeted tuberculin testing and treatment of latent tuberculosis infection. *MMWR Morb Mortal Wkly Rep* 2000;49(RR-6):1–54.

262. Centers for Disease Control. Purified protein derivative (PPD)-tuberculin anergy and HIV infection: guidelines for anergy testing and management of anergic persons at risk of tuberculosis. *MMWR Morb Mortal Wkly Rep* 1991;40(RR-5):27–33.

263. Centers for Disease Control and Prevention. Update: fatal and severe liver injuries associated with rifampin and pyrazinamide for latent tuberculosis infection, and revisions in American Thoracic Society/CDC recommendations—United States, 2001. *MMWR Morb Mortal Wkly Rep* 2001;50:733–735.

264. Selwyn PA, Sckell BM, Alcabes P, et al. High risk of active tuberculosis in HIV-infected drug users with cutaneous anergy. *JAMA* 1992;268:504–509.

265. Sapira JD. The narcotic addict as a medical patient. *Am J Med* 1968;45:555–588.

266. Stimmel B, Vernace S, Schaffner F. Hepatitis B surface antigen and antibody in asymptomatic drug users. *JAMA* 1975;243:1135–1138.

267. Mangia JL, Kim YM, Brown MR, et al. HB-Ag and HB-Ab in asymptomatic drug addicts. *Am J Gastroenterol* 1976;65:121–126.

268. Minichiello L, Rettia R. Trends in intravenous drug abuse as reflected in national hepatitis reporting. *Am J Public Health* 1976;66:872–877.

269. Lorvick J, Kral AH, Seal K, et al. Prevalence and duration of hepatitis C among injection users in San Francisco, Calif. *Am J Public Health* 2001;91:46–47.

270. Garfein RS, Vlahov D, Galai N, et al. Viral infections in short-term injection drug users: the prevalence of the hepatitis C, hepatitis B, human immunodeficiency, and human T-lymphotropic viruses. *Am J Public Health* 1996;86:655–661.

271. Santana Rodriquez OE, Male Gil ML, Hernandez Santana JF, et al. Prevalence of serologic markers of HBV, HDV, HCV, and HIV in non-injection drug users compared to injection drug users in Gran Canaria, Spain. *Eur J Epidemiol* 1998;14:555–561.

272. Francisci D, Baldelli F, Papili R, et al. Prevalence of HBV, HDV, and HCV hepatitis markers in HIV-positive patients. *Eur J Epidemiol* 1995;11:123–126.

273. Centers for Disease Control. Screening for tuberculosis and tuberculous infection in high-risk populations; and the use of preventive therapy for tuberculous infection in the United States: recommendations of the Advisory Committee for Elimination of Tuberculosis. *MMWR Morb Mortal Wkly Rep* 1990;39(RR-8):1–12.

274. Janis EM, Allen DW, Glesby MJ, et al. Tuberculin skin test reactivity, anergy, and HIV infection in hospitalized patients. *Am J Med* 1996;100:186–192.

275. Centers for Disease Control and Prevention. Guidelines for preventing the transmission of *Mycobacterium tuberculosis* in health-care facilities. *Fed Reg* 1994;59:54242–54250.

276. Klein RS, Friedland GH. Transmission of human immunodeficiency virus type 1 (HIV-1) by exposure to blood: defining the risk. *Ann Intern Med* 1990;113:729–730.

277. Pitchenik AE, Bun J, Laufer M, et al. Outbreaks of drug-resistant tuberculosis to health-care workers and HIV-infected patients in an urban hospital—Florida. *MMWR Morb Mortal Wkly Rep* 1990;39:718–722.

278. Centers for Disease Control. *Mycobacterium tuberculosis* transmission in a health clinic—Florida, 1988. *MMWR Morb Mortal Wkly Rep* 1989;38:256–264.

279. Centers for Disease Control. Tuberculosis outbreak among persons in a residential facility for HIV-infected persons—San Francisco. *MMWR Morb Mortal Wkly Rep* 1991;40:649–652.

280. Centers for Disease Control. Nosocomial transmission of multidrug-resistant tuberculosis to health care workers and HIV-infected patients in an urban hospital—Florida. *MMWR Morb Mortal Wkly Rep* 1989;39:425–441.

281. DiPerri G, Cruciani M, Danzi MC, et al. Nosocomial epidemic of active tuberculosis among HIV-infected patients. *Lancet* 1989;2:1502–1504.

282. Centers for Disease Control. Transmission of multidrug-resistant tuberculosis

from an HIV-positive client in a residential substance-abuse treatment facility—Michigan. *MMWR Morb Mortal Wkly Rep* 1991;40:129–131.

283. Shafer RW, Chirgwin KD, Glatt AE, et al. HIV prevalence, immunosuppression, and drug resistance in patients with tuberculosis in an area endemic for AIDS. *AIDS* 1991;5:399–405.

284. Centers for Disease Control. A strategic plan for the elimination of tuberculosis in the United States. *MMWR Morb Mortal Wkly Rep* 1989;38[S-3 Suppl]: 1–25.

285. Nardell EA. Dodging droplet nuclei: reducing the probability of nosocomial tuberculosis transmission in the AIDS era. *Am Rev Respir Dis* 1990;142:501–503.

286. Quinn TC, Glasser D, Cannon RO, et al. Human immunodeficiency virus infection among patients attending clinics for sexually transmitted diseases. *N Engl J Med* 1988;318:197–204.

287. Stamm WE, Handsfield HA, Rompalo AM, et al. The association between genital ulcer disease and acquisition of HIV infection in homosexual men. *JAMA* 1988;260:1429–1433.

288. Des Jarlais DC, Friedman SR. HIV infection among intravenous drug users: epidemiology and risk reduction. *AIDS* 1987;1:67–76.

289. Office of Technology Assessment. *How effective is AIDS education?* Washington, DC: Office of Technology Education, 1988.

290. Vlahov D, Safaien M, Lai S, et al. Sexual and drug risk-related behaviours after initiating highly active antiretroviral therapy among injection drug users. *AIDS* 2002;15:2311–2316.

291. Bouhnik AD, Moatti JP, Vlahov D, et al. Highly active antiretroviral treatment does not increase sexual risk behaviour among French HIV infected injecting drug users. *J Epidemiol Community Health* 2002;56:349–353.

292. McCusker J, Westenhouse J, Stoddard AM, et al. Use of drugs and alcohol by homosexually active men in relation to sexual practices. *J Acquir Immune Defic Syndr* 1990;3:729–736.

293. Johns DR, Tierney M, Felsenstein D. Alteration in the natural history of neurosyphilis by concurrent infection with the human immunodeficiency virus. *N Engl J Med* 1987;316:1569–1572.

294. Berry CD, Hooton TM, Collier AC, et al. Neurologic relapse after benzathine penicillin therapy for secondary syphilis in a patient with HIV infection. *N Engl J Med* 1987;316: 1587–1589.

295. Lukehart SA, Hook EW 3rd, Baker-Zander SA, et al. Invasion of the central nervous system by *Treponema pallidum*: implications for diagnosis and therapy. *Ann Intern Med* 1988;109:855–862.

296. Hook EW III. Syphilis and HIV infection. *J Infect Dis* 1989;160:530–534.

297. Musher DM, Hamill RJ, Baughn RE. Effect of human immunodeficiency virus infection on the course of syphilis and on the response to treatment. *Ann Intern Med* 1990;113:872–881.

298. Tramont EC. Syphilis in the AIDS era. *N Engl J Med* 1987;316:1600–1601.

299. Feingold AR, Vermund SH, Burk RD, et al. Cervical cytologic abnormalities and papillomavirus in women infected by HIV. *J Acquir Immun Defic Syndr* 1990;3:896–903.

300. Byrne MA, Taylor-Robinson D, Munday PE, et al. The common occurrence of human papillomavirus infection and intraepithelial neoplasia in women infected by HIV. *AIDS* 1989;3:379–382.

301. Henry MJ, Stanley MW, Cruikeshank S, et al. Association of human immunodeficiency virus-induced immunosuppression with human papillomavirus infection and cervical intraepithelial neoplasia. *Am J Obstet Gynecol* 1989;160:352–353.

302. Greenspan D, de Villiers EM, Greenspan JS, et al. Unusual HPV types in oral warts in association with HIV infection. *J Oral Pathol* 1988; 17:482–487.

303. Friedmann W, Schafer A, Schwartlander B. *Cervical neoplasia in HIV-infected women*. Presented at the fifth international conference on AIDS. June 1989; Montreal, Canada. Abstract W.C.P.53.

304. Wright TC Jr, Ellerbrock TV, Chiasson MA, et al. Cervical intraepithelial neoplasia in women infected with human immunodeficiency virus: prevalence, risk factors, and validity of Papanicolaou smears. *Obstet Gynecol* 1994;84:591–597.

305. Martin F, Bower M. Anal intraepithelial neoplasia in HIV positive people. *Sex Transm Infect* 2001;77:327–331.

306. Sobhani I, Vuagnat A, Walker F, et al. Prevalence of high-grade dysplasia and cancer in the anal canal in human *papillomavirus*-infected individuals. *Gastroenterology* 2001;120:1046–1048.

307. Palefsky JM, Gonzales J, Greenblatt R, et al. Anal intraepithelial neoplasia and anal *papillomavirus* infection among homosexual males with group IV HIV disease. *JAMA* 1990;263:2911–2916.

308. Bordon J, Martinez-Vazquez C, de la Fuente-Aguado J, et al. Response to standard syphilis treatment in patients infected with the human immunodeficiency virus. *Eur J Clin Microbiol Infect Dis* 1999;18:729–732.

309. Goeman J, Kivuvu M, Nzila N, et al. Similar serological response to conventional therapy for syphilis among HIV-positive and HIV-negative women. *Genitourin Med* 1995;71:275–279.

310. Gourevitch MN, Selwyn PA, Davenny K, et al. Effects of HIV infection on the serologic manifestations and response to treatment of syphilis in intravenous drug users. *Ann Intern Med* 1993;118:350–355.

311. Yinnon AM, Coury-Doniger P, Polito R, et al. Serologic response to treatment of syphilis in patients with HIV infection. *Arch Intern Med* 1996;156:321–325.

312. Schofer H, Imhof M, Thoma-Greber E, et al. Active syphilis in HIV infection: a multicentre retrospective survey. The German AIDS Study Group (GASG). *Genitourin Med* 1996;72:176–181.

313. Malone JL, Wallace MR, Hendrick BB, et al. Syphilis and neurosyphilis in a human immunodeficiency virus type-1 seropositive population: evidence for frequent serologic relapse after therapy. *Am J Med* 1995;99:55–63.

314. Centers for Disease Control. Recommendations for diagnosing and treating syphilis in HIV-infected patients. *MMWR Morb Mortal Wkly Rep* 1988;37:601–608.

315. Rompalo AM, Joesoef MR, O'Donnell JA, et al. Clinical manifestations of early syphilis by HIV status and gender: results of the syphilis and HIV study. *Sex Transm Dis* 2001;28:158–165.

316. Rolfs RT, Joesoef MR, Hendershot EF, et al. A randomized trial of enhanced therapy for early syphilis in patients with and without human immunodeficiency virus infection. The Syphilis and HIV Study Group 2002. *N Engl J Med* 337:307–314.

317. Janier M, Chastang C, Spindler E, et al. A prospective study of the influence of HIV status on the seroreversion of serological tests for syphilis. *Dermatology* 1999;198:362–369.

318. Marra CM, Longstreth W Jr, Maxwell CL, et al. Resolution of serum and cerebrospinal fluid abnormalities after treatment of neurosyphilis. Influence of concomitant human immunodeficiency virus infection. *Sex Transm Dis* 1996;23:184–189.

319. Gourevitch MN, Hartel D, Schoenbaum EE, et al. A prospective study of syphilis and HIV infection among injection drug users receiving methadone in the Bronx, NY. *Am J Public Health* 1996;86:1112–1115.

320. Centers for Disease Control and Prevention. Sexually transmitted diseases treatment guidelines—2002. *MMWR*

Morb Mortal Wkly Rep 2002;51(RR-6):1–80.

321. Hicks CB, Benson PM, Lupton GP, et al. Seronegative secondary syphilis in a patient infected with the human immunodeficiency virus (HIV) with Kaposi sarcoma: a diagnostic dilemma. *Ann Intern Med* 1987;107:492–495.

322. Matlow AG, Rachlis AR. Syphilis serology in human immunodeficiency virus infected patients with symptomatic neurosyphilis: case report and review. *Rev Infect Dis* 1990;12:703–706.

323. Haas JS, Bolan G, Larsen SA, et al. Sensitivity of treponemal tests for detecting prior treated syphilis during human immunodeficiency virus infection. *J Infect Dis* 1990;162:862–866.

324. Erbelding EJ, Vlahov D, Nelson KE, et al. Syphilis serology in human immunodeficiency virus infection: evidence for false-negative fluorescent treponemal testing. *J Infect Dis* 1999;176:1397–1400.

325. Hernandez-Aguado I, Bolumar F, Moreno R, et al. False-positive tests for syphilis associated with human immunodeficiency virus and hepatitis B virus infection among intravenous drug abusers. *Eur J Clin Microbiol Infect Dis* 1998;17:784–787.

326. Rolfs RT. Treatment of syphilis. *Clin Infect Dis* 1995;20:S23–S38.

327. Centers for Disease Control. 1993 Sexually transmitted diseases treatment guidelines. *MMWR Morb Mortal Wkly Rep* 1993;42(RR-14):1–100.

328. Hutchinson CM, Hook EW, Sheperd M, et al. Altered clinical presentation of early syphilis in patients with human immunodeficiency virus infection. *Ann Intern Med* 1994;121:94–99.

329. Frisch M, Biggar RJ, Goedert JJ. Human *papillomavirus*-associated cancers in patients with human immunodeficiency virus infection and acquired immunodeficiency syndrome. *J Natl Cancer Inst* 2000;92:1500–1510.

330. Palefsky JM, Holly EA, Gonzales J, et al. Detection of human *papillomavirus* DNA in anal intraepithelial neoplasia and anal cancer. *Cancer Res* 1991;51:1014–1019.

331. Piketty C, Darragh T, Da Costa M, et al. *HIV-infected intravenous drug users are at risk of anal squamous intraepithelial lesions related to HPV infection.* Presented at the fifth international AIDS malignancy conference. April 23–25, 2001; Bethesda, MD(abst).

332. Centers for Disease Control. Risk for cervical disease in HIV-infected women-NYC. *MMWR Morb Mortal Wkly Rep* 1990;39:846–849.

333. Hoegsberg B, Abulafia O, Sedlis A, et al. Sexually transmitted diseases and human immunodeficiency virus infection among women with pelvic inflammatory disease. *Am J Obstet Gynecol* 1990;163:1135–1139.

334. Cohen CR, Sinei S, Reilly M, et al. Effect of human immunodeficiency virus type 1 infection upon acute salpingitis: a laparoscopic study. *J Infect Dis* 1998;178:1352–1358.

335. Irwin KL, Moorman AC, O'Sullivan MJ, et al. Influence of human immunodeficiency virus infection on pelvic inflammatory disease. *Obstet Gynecol* 2000;95:525–534.

336. Dalakas M, Wichman A, Sever J. AIDS and the nervous system. *JAMA* 1989;261:2396–2399.

337. Guilian D, Vaca K, Noonan CA. Secretion of neurotoxins by mononuclear phagocytes infected with HIV-1. *Science* 1990;250:1593–1596.

338. Goodkin K, Wilkie FL, Concha M, et al. Aging and neuro-AIDS conditions and the changing spectrum of HIV-1 associated morbidity and mortality. *J Clin Epidemiol* 2001;54[1 Suppl]:S35–S43.

339. Simpson DM. Human immunodeficiency virus-associated dementia: review of pathogenesis, prophylaxis, and treatment studies of zidovudine therapy. *Clin Infect Dis* 1999;29:19–34.

340. Geraci AP, Simpson DM. Neurological manifestations of HIV-1 infection in the HAART era. *Compr Ther* 2001;27:232–241.

341. Dalakas MC, Cupler EJ. Neuropathies in HIV infection. *Baillieres Clin Neurol* 1996;5:199–218.

342. Williams D, Geraci A, Simpson DM. AIDS and AIDS-treatment neuropathies. *Curr Neurol Neurosci Rep* 2001;1:533–538.

343. Sacktor N, Lyles RH, Skolasky R, et al. HIV-associated neurologic disease incidence changes: multicenter AIDS cohort study, 1990–1998. *Neurology* 2001;56:257–260.

344. McArthur JC, Hoover DR, Bacellar H, et al. Dementia in AIDS patients: incidence and risk factors. *Neurology* 1993;43:2245–2252.

345. Levy RM, Bredesen DE, Rosenblum ML. Neurologic complications of HIV infection. *Am Fam Physician* 1990;41:517–536.

346. Ho DD, Bredesen DE, Vinters HV, et al. The acquired immunodeficiency syndrome (AIDS) dementia complex. *Ann Intern Med* 1989;111:400–410.

347. Navia BA, Jordan BD, Price RW. The AIDS dementia complex: I. Clinical features. *Ann Neurol* 1986;19:517–524.

348. Brew BJ. AIDS dementia complex. *Neurol Clin* 1999;17:861–881.

349. Portegies P, Enting RH, de Gans J, et al. Presentation and course of AIDS dementia complex: 10 years of follow-up in Amsterdam, The Netherlands. *AIDS* 1993;7:669–675.

350. Portegies P. Review of antiretroviral therapy in the prevention of HIV-related AIDS dementia complex (ADC). *Drugs* 1995;49[1 Suppl]:25–31.

351. Levy RM, Mills CM, Posin JP, et al. The efficacy and clinical impact of brain imaging in neurologically symptomatic AIDS patients: a prospective CT/MRI study. *J Acquir Immune Defic Syndr* 1990;3:461–471.

352. Brouwers P, Hendricks M, Lietzau J, et al. Effect of combination therapy with zidovudine and didanosine on neuropsychological functioning in patients with symptomatic HIV disease: a comparison of simultaneous and alternating regimes. *AIDS* 1997;11:59–66.

353. Bacellar H, Munoz A, Miller E, et al. Temporal trends in the incidence of HIV-1-related neurologic diseases: multicenter AIDS cohort study, 1985–1992. *Neurology* 1994;44:1892–1900.

354. Brew BJ, Brown SJ, Catalan J, et al. Safety and efficacy of abacavir (ABC, 1592) in AIDS dementia complex (study CNAB 3001). Presented at the 12th World AIDS Conference 1998; Geneva, Switzerland. Abstract 561/32192.

355. Gillams AR, Allen E, Hrieb K, et al. Cerebral infarction in patients with AIDS. *AJNR Am J Neuroradiol* 1997;18:1581–1585.

356. Engstorm JW, Lowenstein DH, Bredesen DE. Cerebral infarctions and transient neurologic deficits associated with acquired immunodeficiency syndrome. *Am J Med* 1989;86:528–532.

357. Amine AR. Neurosurgical complications of heroin addiction: brain abscess and mycotic aneurysm. *Surg Neurol* 1977;7:385–386.

358. Elliott JH, O'Day DM, Gutow GS, et al. Mycotic endophthalmitis in drug abusers. *Am J Ophthalmol* 1979;88:66–72.

359. Rowbotham MC. Neurologic aspects of cocaine abuse. *West J Med* 1988;149:442–449.

360. Levine SR, Brust JC, Futrell N, et al. Cerebrovascular complications of the use of the "crack" from alkaloidal cocaine. *N Engl J Med* 1990;323:699–704.

361. Kaku DA, Lowenstein DH. Emergence of recreational drug use as a major risk factor for stroke in young adults. *Ann Intern Med* 1990;113:821–827.

362. Wiley CA. Neuromuscular disease of AIDS. *FASEB J* 1989;3:2503–2511.

363. Tagliati M, Grinnell J, Godbold J, et al. Peripheral nerve function in HIV infection: clinical electrophysiologic and laboratory findings. *Arch Neurol* 1999;56:84–89.

364. Simpson DM, Olney R, McArthur JC, et al. A placebo-controlled trial of lamotrigine for painful HIV-associated neuropathy. *Neurology* 2000;54:2115–2119.

365. McArthur JC, Yiannoutsos C, Simpson DM, et al. A phase II trial of nerve growth factor for sensory neuropathy associated with HIV infection. AIDS Clinical Trials Group Team 291. *Neurology* 2000;54:1080–1088.

366. LaSpina I, Porazzi D, Maggiolo F, et al. Gabapentin in painful HIV-related neuropathy: a report of 19 patients, preliminary observations. *Eur J Neurol* 2001;8:71–75.

367. Shlay JC, Chaloner K, Max MB, et al. Acupuncture and amitriptyline for pain due to HIV-related peripheral neuropathy: a randomized controlled trial. Terry Beirn Community Programs for Clinical Research on AIDS. *JAMA* 1998;280:1590–1595.

368. Kieburtz K, Simpson D, Yiannoutsos C, et al. A randomized trial of amitriptyline and mexiletine for painful neuropathy in HIV infection. AIDS Clinical Trial Group 242 Protocol Team. *Neurology* 1998;51:1682–1688.

369. Simpson DM, Dorfman D, Olney RK, et al. Peptide T in the treatment of painful distal neuropathy associated with AIDS: results of a placebo-controlled trial. The Peptide T Neuropathy Study Group. *Neurology* 1996;47:1254–1259.

370. Rubin AR. Neurologic complications of intravenous drug abuse. *Hosp Pract (Off Ed)* 1987;22:279–288.

371. Moore RD, Wong WM, Keruly JC, et al. Incidence of neuropathy in HIV-infected patients on monotherapy versus those on combination therapy with didanosine, stavudine, and hydroxyurea. *AIDS* 2000;14:273–278.

372. Yarchoan R, Perno CF, Thomas RV, et al. Phase I studies of 2′-,3′-dideoxycytidine in severe human immunodeficiency virus infection as a single agent and alternating with zidovudine (AZT). *Lancet* 1988;1:76–81.

373. Lambert JS, Seidlin M, Reichman RC, et al. 2′,3′-dideoxycytidine (ddI) in patients with the acquired immunodeficiency syndrome or AIDS-related complex. *N Engl J Med* 1990;332:1333–1340.

374. Cooley TP, Kunches LM, Saunders CA, et al. Once-daily administration of 2′,3′-dideoxycytidine in patients with the acquired immunodeficiency syndrome or AIDS-related complex. *N Engl J Med* 1990;322:1340–1345.

375. Takatsuki K, Uchiyama J, Sagawa K, et al. Adult T-cell leukemia in Japan. In: Seno S, Takaku F, Irino S, eds. *Topics in hematology.* Amsterdam: Excerpta Medica, 1977:73–77.

376. Poiesz BJ, Ruscetti FW, Gazdar AF, et al. Detection and isolation of type C retrovirus particles from fresh and cultured lymphocytes of a patient with cutaneous T-cell lymphoma. *Proc Natl Acad Sci U S A* 1980;77:7415–7419.

377. Blattner W, Takatsuki K, Gallo RC. Human T-cell leukemia-lymphoma virus and adult T-cell leukemia. *JAMA* 1983;250:1074–1082.

378. Osame M, Usuku K, Izumo S, et al. HTLV-I associated myelopathy, a new clinical entity. *Lancet* 1986;1:1031–1032.

379. Jacobson S, Raine CS, Mingiolio ES, et al. Isolation of the HTLV-I-like retrovirus from patients with tropical spastic paraparesis. *Nature* 1988;331:540–543.

380. Williams AE, Fang CT, Slaman DJ, et al. Seroprevalence and epidemiological correlates of HTLV-I infection in U.S. blood donors. *Science* 1988;240:643–646.

381. Blattner W. Human T-lymphotropic viruses and diseases of long latency. *Ann Intern Med* 1989;111:4–6.

382. Dooneief G, Marlink R, Bell K, et al. Neurologic consequences of HTLV-II infection in injection-drug users. *Neurology* 1996;46:1556–1560.

383. Goedert JJ, Fung MW, Felton S, et al. Cause-specific mortality associated with HIV and HTLV-II infections among injecting drug users in the U.S.A. *AIDS* 2001;15:1295–1302.

384. Safaeian M, Wilson LE, Taylor E, et al. HTLV-II and bacterial infections among injection drug users. *J Acquir Immun Defic Syndr* 2000;24:483–487.

385. Modahl LE, Young KC, Varney KF, et al. Are HTLV-II-seropositive injection drug users at increased risk of bacterial pneumonia, abscess, and lymphadenopathy? *J Acquir Immun Defic Syndr Hum Retrovirol* 1997;16:169–175.

386. Lowis GW, Sheremata WA, Minagar A. Epidemiologic features of HTLV-II: serologic and molecular evidence. *Ann Epidemiol* 2002;12:46–66.

387. Gout O, Baulac M, Gessain A, et al. Rapid development of myelopathy after HTLV-I infection acquired by transfusion during cardiac transplantation. *N Engl J Med* 1990;322:383–388.

388. Giulianai M, Rezza G, Lepri AC, et al. Risk factors of HTLV-I and -II in individuals attending a clinic for sexually transmitted diseases. *Sex Transm Dis* 2000;27:87–92.

389. Etzel A, Shibata GY, Rozman M, et al. HTLV-1 and HTLV-2 infections in HIV infected individuals from Santos, Brazil: seroprevalence and risk factors. *J Acquir Immun Defic Syndr* 2001;26:185–190.

390. Lee H, Sawson P, Shorty V, et al. High rate of HTLV-II infection in seropositive IV drug abusers in New Orleans. *Science* 1989;244:471–475.

391. Khabbaz RF, Onorato IM, Cannon RO, et al. Seroprevalence in HTLV-I and HTLV-II among intravenous drug users and persons in clinics for sexually transmitted diseases. *N Engl J Med* 1992;326:375–380.

392. Coppola RC, Manconi PE, Piro R, et al. HCV, HIV, HBV and HDV infections in intravenous drug addicts. *Eur J Epidemiol* 1994;10:279–283.

393. Levine OS, Vlahov D, Brookmeyer R, Cohn S, Nelson KE. Difference in the incidence of hepatitis B and human immunodeficiency virus among injection drug users. *J Infect Dis* 1996;173:579–583.

394. Dienstag JL, Perrillo RP, Schiff ER, et al. A preliminary trial of lamivudine for chronic hepatitis B infection. *N Engl J Med* 1995;333:1657–1661.

395. Van Bommel F, Wunsche T, Schurmann D, et al. Tenofovir treatment in patients with lamivudine-resistant hepatitis B mutants strongly affects viral replication. *Hepatology* 2002;36:507–508.

396. Benhamou Y, Katlama C, Lunel F, et al. Effects of lamivudine on replication of hepatitis B virus in HIV-infected men. *Ann Intern Med* 1996;125:705–712.

397. Mazur W, Krol F, Cianciara J, et al. A multi-center open study to determine the effect of lamivudine on HBV DNA clearance and to assess the safety of the regimen in patients with chronic hepatitis B infection. *Med Sci Monit* 2002;8:CR257–CR262.

398. Krogsgaard K. The long-term effect of treatment with interferon-alpha 2a in chronic hepatitis B. The Long-Term Follow up Investigator Group. The European Study Group on Viral Hepatitis (EUROHEP). Executive Team on Anti-Viral Treatment. *J Viral Hepat* 1998;5:389–397.

399. Zylberg H, Jiang J, Pialoux G, et al. Alpha-interferon for chronic active hepatitis B in human immunodeficiency virus-infected patients. *J Infect Dis* 1991;20:968–971.

400. Ying C, DeClercq E, Neyts J. Lamivudine, adefovir and tenofovir exhibit long-lasting anti-hepatitis B virus activity in cell culture. *J Viral Hepat* 2000;7:79–83.

401. Di Martino V, Lunel F, Cadranel JF,

et al. Long-term effects of interferon-alpha in five HIV positive patients with chronic hepatitis B. *J Viral Hepat* 1996;3:253–260.

402. Wolters LM, Niesters HG, Hansen BE, et al. Development of hepatitis B virus resistance for lamivudine in chronic hepatitis B patients co-infected with the human immunodeficiency virus in a Dutch cohort. *J Clin Virol* 2002;24:173–181.

403. Perrillo RP, Regenstein FG, Roodman ST. Chronic hepatitis B in asymptomatic homosexual men with antibody to the human immunodeficiency virus. *Ann Intern Med* 1986;105:382–383.

404. Glasgow BJ, Anders K, Layfield LJ, et al. Clinical and pathologic findings of the liver in the acquired immunodeficiency syndrome. *Am J Clin Pathol* 1985;83:582–588.

405. Bodsworth NJ, Cooper DA, Donovan B. The influence of human immunodeficiency virus type 1 infection on the development of the hepatitis B virus carrier state. *J Infect Dis* 1991;163:1138–1140.

406. Colin JF, Cazals-Hatem D, Loriot MA, et al. Influence of human immunodeficiency virus infection on chronic hepatitis B in homosexual men. *Hepatology* 1999;29:1306–1310.

407. Scharschmidt BF, Held MJ, Hollander HH, et al. Hepatitis B in patients with HIV infection: relationship to AIDS and patient survival. *Ann Intern Med* 1992;117:837–838.

408. Eskil A, Magnus P, Petersen G, et al. Hepatitis B antibodies in HIV-infected homosexual men are associated with more rapid progression to AIDS. *AIDS* 1992;6:571–574.

409. Pol S, Wesenfelder L, Dubois F, et al. Influence of human immunodeficiency virus infection on hepatitis delta virus superinfection in chronic HBsAg carriers. *J Viral Hepat* 1994;1:131–137.

410. Kreek MJ, Des Jarlais DC, Trepo C, et al. *Hepatitis delta antigenemia in intravenous drug abusers with AIDS: potential risk for health care workers.* Presented at the third international conference on AIDS, June 1987; Washington, DC. Abstract Th.P.216.

411. Lauer GM, Walker BD. Hepatitis C virus infection. *N Engl J Med* 2001;345:41–51.

412. National Institutes of Health. Consensus Development Conference Statement (preliminary draft). *Management of hepatitis C: 2002.* NIH Consens State Sci Statements. June 10, 2002;19(3):1–46.

413. Edlin BR, Seal KH, Lovick J, et al. Is it justifiable to withhold treatment for hepatitis C from illicit-drug users? *N Engl J Med* 2001;345:211–215.

414. Williams I. Epidemiology of hepatitis C in the United States. *Am J Med* 1999;107:2S–9S.

415. Wyld R, Robertson JR, Brettle RP, et al. Absence of hepatitis C virus transmission but frequent transmission of HIV-1 from sexual contact with doubly-infected individuals. *J Infect* 1997;35:163–166.

416. Soto B, Rodrigo L, Garcia-Bengoechea M, et al. Heterosexual transmission of hepatitis C virus and the possible role of coexistent human immunodeficiency virus infection in the index case: a multicenter study of 423 pairings. *J Intern Med* 1994;236:515–519.

417. Eyster ME, Alter HJ, Aledort LM, et al. Heterosexual co-transmissions of hepatitis C virus (HCV) and human immunodeficiency virus (HIV). *Ann Intern Med* 1991;115:764–768.

418. Alter MJ, Kruzon-Moran D, Nainan OV, et al. The prevalence of hepatitis C virus infection in the United States, 1988 through 1994. *N Engl J Med* 1999;341:556–562.

419. Conry-Cantilena C, VanRaden M, Gibble J, et al. Routes of infection, viremia, and liver disease in blood donors found to have hepatitis C virus infection. *N Engl J Med* 1996;334:1691–1696.

420. National Institutes of Health. Consensus development conference panel statement: management of hepatitis C. *Hepatology* 1997;26:2S–10S.

421. EASL International Consensus Conference on Hepatitis C: Paris, 26–28, February 1999, Consensus Statement. European Association for the Study of the Liver. *J Hepatol* 1999;30:956–961.

422. Gumber SC, Chopra S. Hepatitis C: a multifaceted disease. Review of extrahepatic manifestations. *Ann Intern Med* 1995;123(8):615–620.

423. Alter MJ, Margolis HS, Krawczynski K, et al. The natural history of community-acquired hepatitis C in the United States. The sentinel counties chronic non-A non-B hepatitis study team. *N Engl J Med* 1992;327:1899–1905.

424. Zignego AL, Brechot C. Extrahepatic manifestations of HCV infection: facts and controversies. *J Hepatol* 1999;31:369–376.

425. McHutchinson JG, Gordon SC, Schiff ER, et al. Interferon alfa-2b alone or in combination with ribavirin as initial treatment for chronic hepatitis C. *N Engl J Med* 1998;339:1485–1492.

426. Davis GJ, Esteban-Mur R, Rustgi V, et al. Interferon alfa-2b alone or in combination with ribavirin for the treatment of relapse of chronic hepatitis C. *N Engl J Med* 1998;339:1493–1499.

427. Fried MW, Shiffman ML, Reddy KR, et al. Peginterferon alfa-2a plus rib-

avirin for chronic hepatitis C virus infection. *N Engl J Med* 2002;37:975–982.

428. Manns MP, McHutchison JG, Gordon SC, et al. Peginterferon alfa-2b plus ribavirin compared with interferon alfa-2b plus ribavirin for initial treatment of chronic hepatitis C: a randomized trial. *Lancet* 2001;358:958–965.

429. Djavaherian C, Clements B, Sylvestre DL. Treating hepatitis C in recovering injection drug users (IDUs) with psychiatric disease. *J Addict Dis* 2002;21(2): 8A:112(abst).

430. Backmund M, Meyer K, Von Zielonka M, et al. Treatment of hepatitis C infection in injection drug users. *Hepatology* 2001;34:188–193.

431. Sylvestre DL. *Treating HCV in methadone-maintained patients.* American Society of Addiction Medicine. April 25–28, 2002; Atlanta, GA(abst).

432. Thomas DL, Shih JW, Alter HG, et al. Effect of human immunodeficiency virus infection on hepatitis C virus infection among injection drug users. *J Infect Dis* 1996;174:690–695.

433. Soto B, Sanchez-Quijano A, Rodrigo L, et al. Human immunodeficiency virus infections modifies the natural history of chronic parenterally-acquired hepatitis C with an unusually rapid progression to cirrhosis. *J Hepatol* 1997;26:1–5.

434. Bruno R, Sacchi P, Puoti M, et al. HCV chronic hepatitis in patients with HIV: clinical management issues. *Am J Gastroenterol* 2002;97:1598–1606.

435. Causse X, Payen JL, Izopet J, et al. Does HIV-infection influence the response of chronic hepatitis C to interferon treatment? A french multicenter prospective study. *J Hepatol* 2000;32:1003–1010.

436. Landau A, Batisse D, Piketty C, et al. Long-term efficacy of combination therapy with interferon-alpha 2b and ribavirin for severe chronic hepatitis C in HIV-infected patients. *AIDS* 2001;15:2149–2155.

437. Nasti G, DiGennaro G, Tavio M, et al. Chronic hepatitis C in HIV infection: feasibility and sustained efficacy of therapy with interferon alfa-2b and ribavirin. *AIDS* 2001;15:1783–1787.

438. Staples CT, Rimland D, Dudas D. Hepatitis C in the HIV (human immunodeficiency virus) Atlanta V.A. (Veterans Affairs Medical Center) Cohort Study (HAVACS): the effect of coinfection on survival. *Clin Infect Dis* 1999;29:150–154.

439. Dorrucci M, Pezzotti P, Phillips AN, et al. Coinfection of hepatitis C virus with human immunodeficiency virus and progression to AIDS. Italian seroconversion study. *J Infect Dis* 1995;172:1503–1508.

440. Piroth L, Grappin M, Cuzin L, et al. Hepatitis C virus co-infection is a negative prognostic factor for clinical evolution in human immunodeficiency virus-positive patients. *Viral Hepat* 2000;7:302–308.

441. Beral V, Peterman TA, Berkelman RL, et al. Kaposi sarcoma among persons with AIDS: a sexually transmitted infection? *Lancet* 1990;335:123–128.

442. Barbieri D, Gualandi M, Tassinari MC, et al. B-cell lymphomas in two HIV-seropositive heroin addicts. *Lancet* 1986;2:1039.

443. Tirelli U, Rezza G, Lazzarin A, et al. Malignant lymphoma related to HIV infection in Italy: a report of 46 cases. *JAMA* 1987;258:2064.

444. Vazquez M, Rotterdam H, Sidhu G. *Malignant neoplasms in surgical specimens of different AIDS risk groups.* Presented at the fifth international conference on AIDS. June 1989; Montreal, Canada. Abstract M.B.P.293.

445. Monfardini S, Vaccher E, Pizzocaro G, et al. Unusual malignant tumors in 49 patients with HIV infection. *AIDS* 1989;3:449–452.

446. Gachupin-Garcia A, Selwyn PA, Budner NS. Population-based study of malignancies and HIV infection among injecting drug users in a New York City methadone treatment program, 1985–1991. *AIDS* 1992;6:843–848.

447. Jaffe JH. Drug addiction and drug abuse. In: Gilman AG, Rall TW, Nies AS, et al, eds. *The pharmacological basis of therapeutics,* 8th ed. New York: Pergamon Press, 1990:522–573.

448. Leitman BS, Greengart A, Wasser HJ. Pneumomediastinum and pneumopericardium after cocaine abuse. *AJR Am J Roentgenol* 1988;151:614.

449. Kissner DG, Lawrence DW, Selis JE, et al. Crack lung: pulmonary disease caused by cocaine abuse. *Am Rev Respir Dis* 1987;136:1250–1252.

450. Hoffman CK, Goodman PC. Pulmonary edema in cocaine smokers. *Radiology* 1989;172:463–465.

451. Joseph AM, Nichol KL, Willenbring ML, et al. Beneficial effects of treatment of nicotine dependence during an inpatient substance abuse treatment program. *JAMA* 1990;263:3043–3046.

452. Ho A, Dole VP. Pain perception in drug-free and in methadone-maintained human ex-addicts. *Pro Soc Exp Biol Med* 1979;162:392–395.

453. Kreek MJ. Health consequences associated with the use of methadone. In: Cooper JR, Altman F, Brown BS, et al, eds. *Research on the treatment of narcotic addiction.* Rockville, MD: National Institute on Drug Abuse, 1983:456–482.

454. Nyswander ME, Dole VP. The treatment of chronic pain. *N Engl J Med* 1984;310:599.

455. Rainey PM, Friedland G, McCance-Katz EF, et al. Interaction of methadone with didanosine and stavudine. *J Acquir Immune Defic Syndr* 2000;24:241–248.

456. Gourevitch MN, Friedland GH. Interactions between methadone and medications used to treat HIV infection: a review. *Mt Sinai J Med* 2000;67:429–436.

457. Sellers E, Lam R, McDowell J, et al. *The pharmacokinetics (PK) of abacavir (ABC) and methadone (M) following co-administration: CNAA1012.* Presented at the 39th Interscience conference on antimicrobial agents and chemotherapy; September 26–29, 1999; San Francisco, CA. Abstract 305.

458. Rainey PM, Friedland G, Snidow J, et al. *Effects of zidovudine plus lamivudine on methadone disposition.* Presented at the 101st annual meeting of the American Society for Clinical Pharmacology and Therapeutics. March 15–17, 2000; Los Angeles, CA. Abstract PIII-94.

459. McCance-Katz EF, Rainey PM, Jatlow P, et al. Methadone effects on zidovudine disposition (AIDS Clinical Trials Group 262). *J Acquir Immun Defic Syndr* 1998;18:435–443.

460. Altice FL, Friedland GH, Cooney EL. Nevirapine induced opiate withdrawal among injection drug users with HIV infection receiving methadone. *AIDS* 1999;13:957–962.

461. Clarke W, Mulcahy F, Back D, et al. *Managing methadone and non-nucleoside reverse transcriptase inhibitors: guidelines for clinical practice.* Presented at the seventh conference on retroviruses and opportunistic infections. Jan 30–Feb 2, 2000; San Francisco, CA. Abstract No. 88.

462. Clarke S, Mulcahy F, Tiha J, et al. The pharmacokinetics of methadone in HIV-positive patients receiving the non-nucleoside reverse transcriptase inhibitor efavirenz. *J Clin Pharmacol* 2001;51:213–217.

463. Tashima K, Bose T, Gormley J, et al. *The potential impact of efavirenz on methadone maintenance.* Presented at the ninth European congress of clinical microbiology and infectious diseases. March 21–24, 1999; Berlin, Germany. Abstract No. P0552.

464. Geletko SM, Erickson AD. Decreased methadone effect after ritonavir initiation. *Pharmacotherapy* 2000;20:93–94.

465. McCance-Katz EF, Farber S, Selwyn PA, et al. Decrease in methadone levels with nelfinavir mesylate. *Am J Psychiatry* 2000;157:481.

466. Bart PA, Rizzardi PG, Gallant S, et al. Methadone blood concentrations are decreased by the administration of abacavir plus amprenavir. *Ther Drug Monit* 2001;23:553–555.

467. Beauverie P, Taburet AM, Dessalles MC, et al. Therapeutic drug monitoring of methadone in HIV-infected patients receiving protease inhibitors. *AIDS* 1998;12:2510–2511.

468. Gerber JG, Rosenkranz S, Segal Y, et al. Effect of ritonavir/saquinavir on stereoselective pharmacokinetics of methadone: results of AIDS Clinical Trials Group (ACTG) 401. *J Acquir Immun Defic Syndr* 2001;27:153–160.

469. Maroldo L, Manocchio S, Artenstein A, et al. *Lack of effect of nelfinavir mesylate on maintenance methadone dose.* Presented at the 13th international AIDS conference. July 9–14, 2000; Durban, South Africa. Abstract WePeB4120.

470. Hsyu PH, Lillibridge JH, Maroldo L, et al. *Pharmacokinetic (PK) and pharmacodynamic (PD) interactions between nelfinavir and methadone.* Presented at the seventh conference on retroviruses and opportunistic infections. Jan 30–Feb 2, 2000; San Francisco, CA. Abstract No. 87.

471. Hendrix C, Wakeford J, Wire MB, et al. *Pharmacokinetic and pharmacodynamic evaluation of methadone enantiomers following co-administration with amprenavir in opioid-dependent subjects.* Presented at the 40th interscience conference on antimicrobial agents and chemotherapy. September 2000; Toronto, Canada. Abstract 1649.

472. Clarke S, Mulcahy F, Bergin C, et al. Absence of opioid withdrawal symptoms in patients receiving methadone and the protease inhibitor lopinavir-ritonavir. *Clin Infect Dis* 2002;34:1143–1145.

473. Cantilena L, McCrea J, Blazes D, et al. Lack of a pharmacokinetic interaction between indinavir and methadone. *Clin Pharmacol Ther* 1999;65:135 Abst PI-74.

474. Kreek MJ, Garfield JW, Gutjahr CL, et al. Rifampin-induced methadone withdrawal. *N Engl J Med* 1976;294:1104–1106.

475. Mandel GL, Sande MA. Antimicrobial agents: drugs used in the chemotherapy of tuberculosis and leprosy. In: Gilman AG, Rall TW, Nies AS, et al, eds. New York: Pergamon Press, 1990:1146–1164.

476. Sawyer RC, Brown LS, Narong PK, et al. *Evaluation of a possible pharmacologic interaction between rifabutin and methadone in HIV-seropositive*

injecting drug users. Presented at the ninth international conference on AIDS. June 1993; Berlin, Germany. Abstract PO-B30–2197.

477. Cobb M, Desai J, Brown LS, et al. The effect of fluconazole on the clinical pharmacokinetics of methadone. *Clin Pharmacol Ther* 1998;63:655–662.

478. Liu SJ, Wang RI. Case report of barbiturate-induced enhancement of methadone metabolism and withdrawal syndrome. *Am J Psychiatry* 1984;141:1287–1288.

479. Saxon AJ, Whittaker S, Hawker CS. Valproic acid, unlike other anticonvulsants, has no effect on methadone metabolism; two cases. *J Clin Psychiatry* 1989;50:228–229.

480. Tong TG, Pond SM, Kreek MJ, et al. Phenytoin induced methadone withdrawal. *Ann Intern Med* 1981; 94:349–351.

481. Gordillo V, del Amo J, Soriano V, et al. Sociodemographic and psychological variables influencing adherence to antiretroviral therapy. *AIDS* 1999;13:1763–1769.

482. Samet JH, Libman H, Steger KA, et al. Compliance with zidovudine therapy in patients infected with human immunodeficiency virus, type 1: a cross-sectional study in a municipal hospital clinic. *Am J Med* 1992;92: 495–502.

483. Broers B, Morabia A, Hirschel B. A cohort study of drug users' compliance with zidovudine treatment. *Arch Intern Med* 1994;154:1121–1127.

484. Paterson DL, Swindells S, Mohr J, et al. Adherence to protease inhibitor therapy and outcomes in patients with HIV infection. *Ann Intern Med* 2000;133:21–30.

485. Carmona A, Knowbel H, Guelar A, et al. Factors influencing survival in HIV infected patients treated with HAART. Presented at the 13th international AIDS conference. Jul 9–14, 2000; Durban, South Africa. Abstract TuOrB417.

486. Walsh JC, Hertogs K, Gazzard B. *Viral drug resistance, adherence and pharmacokinetic indices in HIV-1 infected patients on successful and failing protease inhibitor (PI) based highly active antiretroviral therapy (HAART).* Presented at the 40th interscience conference on antimicrobial agents and chemotherapy. September 17–20, 2000; Toronto, Canada. Abstract 294.

487. Henry JA, Hill IR. Fatal interaction between ritonavir and MDMA. *Lancet* 1998;352:1751–1752.

488. Harrington RD, Woodward JA, Hooton T, et al. Life-threatening interactions between HIV-1 protease inhibitors and the illicit drugs MDMA and gamma-hydroxybutyrate. *Arch Intern Med* 1999;159:2221–2224.

489. Antoniou T, Tseng AL. Interactions between recreational drugs and antiretroviral agents. *Ann Pharmacother* 2002;36:1598–1613.

490. Bagasra O, Pomerantz RJ. Human immunodeficiency virus type 1 replication in peripheral blood mononuclear cells in the presence of cocaine. *J Infect Dis* 1993;168:1157–1164.

491. Peterson PK, Gekker G, Chao CC, et al. Cocaine potentiates HIV-1 replication in human peripheral blood mononuclear cell cocultures. *J Immunol* 1991;146:81–84.

492. Peterson PK, Gekker G, Chun CC, et al. Cocaine amplifies HIV-1 replication in cytomegalovirus-stimulated peripheral blood mononuclear cell cocultures. *J Immunol* 1992;149:676–680.

493. Novick DM, Ness GL. Abuse of antibiotics by abusers of parenteral heroin or cocaine. *South Med J* 1984;77:302–303.

494. Crane LR, Levine DP, Zervos MJ, et al. Bacteremia in narcotic addicts at the Detroit Medical Center. I. Microbiology, epidemiology, risk factors, and empiric therapy. *Rev Infect Dis* 1986;8:364–373.

495. Selwyn PA, Iezza A. Zidovudine overdose in an intravenous drug user. *AIDS* 1990;4:822–824.

496. Terragna A, Mazzarello G, Auselmo A, et al. Suicidal attempts with zidovudine. *AIDS* 1990;4:88.

497. O'Connor P, Selwyn PA, Schottenfeld R. Medical management of injection drug users with HIV infection. *N Engl J Med* 1994;331:450–459.

498. Arno PS, Shenson D, Siegal NF, et al. Economic and policy implications of early intervention in HIV disease. *JAMA* 1989;262:1493–1498.

499. Francis DP, Anderson RE, Gorman ME, et al. Targeting AIDS prevention and treatment toward HIV-1 infected persons: the concept of early intervention. *JAMA* 1989;262:2572–2576.

500. Fischl MA, Richman DD, Grieco MH, et al. The efficacy of 3'-azido-2',3'-deoxythymidine (azidothymidine) in the treatment of patients with AIDS and AIDS-related complex: a double-blind placebo-controlled trial. *N Engl J Med* 1987;317:185–191.

501. Centers for Disease Control. HIV prevalence estimates and AIDS case projections for the United States: Report based upon a workshop. *MMWR Morb Mortal Wkly Rep* 1990; 39(No. RR-16):1–31.

502. Ho DD. Time to hit HIV, early and hard. *N Engl J Med* 1995;450–451.

503. Hahn RA, Onorato IM, Jones TS, et al. Prevalence of HIV infection among intravenous drug users in the United States. *JAMA* 1989;261:2677–2684.

504. O'Connor P, Molde S, Henry S, et al. Human immunodeficiency virus infection in intravenous drug users: a model for primary care. *Am J Med* 1992;93:382–386.

505. Pollack HA, Khoshnood K, Blankenship KM, et al. The impact of needle exchange-based health services on emergency department use. *J Gen Intern Med* 2002;17:341–348.

506. Cooper DA, Gold J, Maclean P, et al. Acute AIDS retrovirus infection: definition of a clinical illness associated with seroconversion. *Lancet* 1985;1:537–540.

507. Ho DD, Sarngadharan MG, Resnick L, et al. Primary human T-lymphotropic virus type III infection. *Ann Intern Med* 1985;103:880–883.

508. Needlestick transmission of HTLV-III from a patient infected in Africa. *Lancet* 1984;2:1376–1377.

509. Robertson PB, Greenspan JS. *Perspectives on oral manifestations of AIDS.* Littleton, MA: PSG Publishing, 1988.

510. Penneys NS. *Skin manifestations of AIDS.* Philadelphia: JB Lippincott, 1989.

511. Taylor JM, Fahey JL, Detels R, et al. CD4 percentage, CD4 number, and CD4:CD8 ratio in HIV infection: which to choose and how to use. *J Acquir Immune Defic Syndr* 1989;2:114–124.

512. Fahey JL, Taylor JM, Detels R, et al. The prognostic value of cellular and serologic markers in infection with human immunodeficiency virus type I. *N Engl J Med* 1990;322:166–172.

513. Moss AR, Bacchetti P, Osmond D, et al. Seropositivity for HIV and the development of AIDS or AIDS related condition: three-year follow up of the San Francisco General Hospital cohort. *BMJ* 1988;296:745–750.

514. Graham N, Piantadosi S, Park LP, et al. CD4+ lymphocyte response to zidovudine as a predictor of AIDS-free time and survival time. *J Acquir Immun Defic Syndr* 1993;6:1258–1266.

515. Mellors JW, Kingsley LA, Rinaldo CR Jr, et al. Quantitation of HIV-1 RNA in plasma predicts outcome after seroconversion. *Ann Intern Med* 1995;122:573–579.

516. Ho D. Viral counts count in HIV infection. *Science* 1996;272:1124–1125.

517. Spooner KM, Lane HC, Masur H. Guide to major clinical trials of antiretroviral therapy administered to patients infected with human immunodeficiency virus. *Clin Infect Dis* 1996;23:15–27.

518. Eron JJ, Benoit SL, Jemsek J, et al.

Treatment with lamivudine, zidovudine, or both in HIV-positive patients with 200 to 500 CD4+ cells per cubic millimeter. *N Engl J Med* 1995;333:1662–1669.

519. Fauci AS, Pantaleo G, Stanley SS, et al. Immunopathogenesis mechanisms of HIV infection. *Ann Intern Med* 1996;124:654–663.

520. Danner SA, Carr A, Leonard JM, et al. A short-term study of the safety pharmacokinetics and efficacy of ritonavir, an inhibitor of HIV-1 protease. *N Engl J Med* 1995;333:1528–1533.

521. Markowitz J, Saag M, Powderly WG, et al. A preliminary study of ritonavir, an inhibitor of HIV-1 protease, to treat HIV-1 infection. *N Engl J Med* 1995;333:1534–1539.

522. Collier AC, Coombs RW, Schoenfeld DA, et al. Treatment of human immunodeficiency virus infection with saquinavir, zidovudine, and zalcitabine. *N Engl J Med* 1996;334:1011–1017.

523. Centers for Disease Control. Prevention and control of influenza. *MMWR Morb Mortal Wkly Rep* 1988;37:361–373.

524. Centers for Disease Control. Update on hepatitis B prevention. *MMWR Morb Mortal Wkly Rep* 1987;36:353–366.

525. Centers for Disease Control. Pneumococcal polysaccharide vaccine. *MMWR Morb Mortal Wkly Rep* 1989;38:64–76.

526. Gulick RM, Mellors JW, Havlir D, et al. Treatment with indinavir, zidovudine, and lamivudine in adults with human immunodeficiency virus infection and prior antiretroviral therapy. *N Engl J Med* 1997;337:734–739.

527. Hammer SM, Squires KE, Hughes MD, et al. Controlled trial of two nucleoside analogues plus indinavir in persons with human immunodeficiency virus infection and CD4 cell counts of 200 per cubic millimeter or less. AIDS Clinical Trial Group 320 Study Team. *N Engl J Med* 1997;337:725–733.

528. Cameron DW, Heath-Chiozzi M, Danner S, et al. Randomised placebo-controlled trial of ritonavir in advanced HIV-1 disease. The Advanced HIV Disease Ritonavir Study Group. *Lancet* 1998;351:543–549.

529. Staszewski S, Morales-Ramirez J, Tashima KT, et al. Efavirenz plus zidovudine and lamivudine, efavirenz plus indinavir, and indinavir plus zidovudine and lamivudine in the treatment of HIV-1 infection in adults. Study 006 Team. *N Engl J Med* 1999;341:1865–1873.

530. Staszewski S, Keiser P, Montaner J, et al. Abacavir-lamivudine-zidovudine vs. indinavir-lamivudine-zidovudine in antiretroviral-naive HIV-infected adults:

a randomized equivalence trial. *JAMA* 2001;285:1206–1208.

531. Thiebaut R, Morlat P, Jacqmin-Gadda H, et al. Clinical progression of HIV-1 infection according to the viral response during the first year of antiretroviral treatment. Groupe d'Epidemiologie du SIDA en Aquitqine (GECSA). *AIDS* 2002;14:971–978.

532. Roy P, Gouello JP, Pennison-Besnier I, et al. Severe lactic acidosis induced by nucleoside analogues in an HIV-infected man. *Ann Emerg Med* 1999;34:282–284.

533. Aggarwal A, al-Talib K, Alabrash M. Type B lactic acidosis in an AIDS patient treated with zidovudine. *Md Med J* 1996;45:929–931.

534. Chariot P, Drogou I, de Lacroix-Szmania I, et al. Zidovudine-induced mitochondrial disorder with massive liver steatosis, myopathy, lactic acidosis, and mitochondrial DNA depletion. *J Hepatol* 1999;30:156–160.

535. Scalfaro P, Chesaux JJ, Buchwalder PA, et al. Severe transient neonatal lactic acidosis during prophylactic zidovudine treatment. *Intensive Care Med* 1998;24:247–250.

536. Sundar K, Suarez M, Banogon PE, et al. Zidovudine-induced fatal lactic acidosis and hepatic failure in patients with acquired immunodeficiency syndrome: report of two patients and review of the literature. *Crit Care Med* 1997;25:1425–1430.

537. Shaer AJ, Rastegar A. Lactic acidosis in the setting of antiretroviral therapy for the acquired immunodeficiency syndrome. A case report and review of the literature. *Am J Nephrol* 2000;20:332–338.

538. Sarner L, Fakoya A. Acute onset lactic acidosis and pancreatitis in the third trimester of pregnancy in HIV-1 positive women taking antiretroviral medication. *Sex Transm Infect* 2002;78:58–59.

539. Marra A, Lewi D, Lanzoni V, et al. Lactic acidosis and antiretroviral therapy: a case report and literature review. *Braz J Infect Dis* 2000;4:151–155.

540. Mokrzycki MH, Harris C, May H, et al. Lactic acidosis associated with stavudine administration: a report of five cases. *Clin Infect Dis* 2000;30:198–200.

541. Coghlan ME, Sommadossi JP, Jhala NC, et al. Symptomatic lactic acidosis in hospitalized antiretroviral-treated patients with human immunodeficiency virus infection: a report of 12 cases. *Clin Infect Dis* 2001;33:1914–1921.

542. ter Hofstede HJ, de Marie S, Foudraine NA, et al. Clinical features and risk factors of lactic acidosis following long-term antiretroviral therapy: 4 fa-

tal cases. *Int J STD AIDS* 2000;11:611–616.

543. French M, Amin J, Roth N, et al. Randomized, open-label, comparative trial to evaluate the efficacy and safety of three antiretroviral drug combinations including two nucleoside analogues and nevirapine for previously untreated HIV-1 infection: the OzCombo 2 study. *HIV Clin Trials* 2002;3:177–185.

544. Lichterfeld M, Nischalke HD, Bergmann F, et al. Long-term efficacy and safety of ritonavir/indinavir at 400/400 mg twice a day in combination with two nucleoside reverse transcriptase inhibitors as first line antiretroviral therapy. *HIV Med* 2002;3:37–43.

545. Paediatric European Network for Treatment of AIDS (PENTA). Comparison of dual nucleoside-analogue reverse-transcriptase inhibitor regimens with and without nelfinavir in children with HIV-1 who have not previously been treated: the PENTA 5 randomised trial. *Lancet* 2002;359:733–740.

546. Perry CM, Noble S. Didanosine: an updated review of its use in HIV infection. *Drugs* 1999;58:1099–1135.

547. Gartland M. AVANTI 3: a randomized, double-blind trial to compare the efficacy and safety of lamivudine plus zidovudine versus lamivudine plus zidovudine plus nelfinavir in HIV-1-infected antiretroviral-naive patients. *Antivir Ther* 2001;6:127–134.

548. Goodgame JC, Pottage LC Jr, Jablonowski H, et al. Amprenavir in combination with lamivudine and zidovudine versus lamivudine and zidovudine alone in HIV-1-infected antiretroviral-naive adults. Amprenavir PROAB3001 International Study Team. *Antivir Ther* 2000;5:215–225.

549. Staszewski S, Katlama C, Harrer T, et al. A dose-ranging study to evaluate the safety and efficacy of abacavir alone or in combination with zidovudine and lamivudine in antiretroviral treatment-naive subjects. *AIDS* 1998;12:F197–202.

550. Opravil M, Hirschel B, Lazzarin A, et al. A randomized trial of simplified maintenance therapy with abacavir, lamivudine, and zidovudine in human immunodeficiency virus infection. *J Infect Dis* 2002;185:1251–1260.

551. Ungsedhapand C, Kroon ED, Suwanagool S, et al. A randomized open-label, comparative trial of zidovudine plus lamivudine versus zidovudine plus lamivudine plus didanosine in antiretroviral-naive HIV-1-infected Thai patients. *J Acquir Immun Defic Syndr* 2001;27:116–123.

552. Pollard RB, Tierney C, Havlir D, et al.

A phase II randomized study of the virologic and immunologic effect of zidovudine + stavudine versus stavudine alone and zidovudine + lamivudine in patients with >300 CD4 cells who were antiretroviral naive (ACTG 298). *AIDS Res Hum Retroviruses* 2002;18:699–704.

553. Havlir DV, Tierney C, Friedland GH, et al. In vivo antagonism with zidovudine plus stavudine combination therapy. *J Infect Dis* 2000;182:321–325.

554. Volberding PA, Lagakos SW, Koch MA, et al. Zidovudine in asymptomatic human immunodeficiency virus infection: a controlled trial in persons with fewer than 500 CD4-positive cells per cubic millimeter. *N Engl J Med* 1990;322:941–949.

555. Richman DD, Fischl MA, Grieco MH, et al. The toxicity of azidothymidine (AZT) in the treatment of patients with AIDS and AIDS-related complex. *N Engl J Med* 1987;317:192–197.

556. Schmitt FA, Bigley JW, McKinnis R, et al. Neuropsychological outcome of zidovudine for the treatment of patients with AIDS and AIDS-related complex. *N Engl J Med* 1988;319:1573–1578.

557. Zidovudine for the treatment of thrombocytopenia associated with human immunodeficiency virus. A prospective study. The Swiss Group for Clinical Studies on the Acquired Immunodeficiency Syndrome (AIDS). *Ann Intern Med* 1988;109:718–721.

558. Fischl MA, Richman DD, Hansen N, et al. The safety and efficacy of zidovudine (AZT) in the treatment of subjects with mildly symptomatic human immunodeficiency virus type 1 infection. *Ann Intern Med* 1990;112:727–737.

559. Dubin G, Braffman MN. Zidovudine-induced hepatotoxicity. *Ann Intern Med* 1989;110:85–86.

560. Melamed AJ, Muller RJ, Gold JW, et al. Possible zidovudine-induced hepatotoxicity. *JAMA* 1987;258:2063.

561. Dalakas MC, Illa I, Pezeshkpour GH, et al. Mitochondrial myopathy caused by long-term zidovudine therapy. *N Engl J Med* 1990;322:1098–1105.

562. Maggiolo F, Migliorino M, Maserari R, et al. Virological and immunological responses to a once-a-day antiretroviral regimen with didanosine, lamivudine and efavirenz. *Antivir Ther* 2001;6:249–253.

563. Mole L, Schmidgall D, Holodniy M. A pilot trial of indinavir, ritonavir, didanosine, and lamivudine in a once-daily four-drug regimen for HIV infection. *J Acquir Immune Defic Syndr* 2001;27:260–265.

564. Skowron G, Kuritzkes DR, Thompson MA, et al. Once-daily quadruple-

drug therapy with adefovir dipivoxil, lamivudine, didanosine, and efavirenz in treatment-naive human immunodeficiency virus type 1-infected patients. *J Infect Dis* 2002;18:1028–1033.

565. Nunez M, Soriano V, Martin-Carbonero L, et al. SENC (Spanish efavirenz vs. nevirapine comparison) trial: a randomized, open-label study in HIV-infected naive individuals. *HIV Clin Trials* 2002;3:186–194.

566. Elion R, Ksuk S, Knupp C, et al. The safety profile and antiviral activity of the combination of stavudine, didanosine, and nelfinavir in patients with HIV infection. *Clin Ther* 1999;21:1853–1863.

567. Moore RD, Keruly JC, Chaisson RE. Incidence of pancreatitis in HIV-infected patients receiving nucleoside reverse transcriptase inhibitor drugs. *AIDS* 2001;15:617–620.

568. Walmsley S, Bernstein B, King M, et al. Lopinavir-ritonavir versus nelfinavir for the initial treatment of HIV infection. *N Engl J Med* 2002;346:2039–2046.

569. Schooley RT, Ruane P, Myers RA, et al. Tenofovir DF in antiretroviral-experienced patients: results from a 48-week, randomized, double-blind study. *AIDS* 2002;16:1257–1263.

570. Benson CA, Deeks SG, Brun SC, et al. Safety and antiviral activity at 48 weeks of lopinavir/ritonavir plus nevirapine and 2 nucleoside reverse-transcriptase inhibitors in human immunodeficiency virus type 1-infected protease inhibitor-experienced patients. *J Infect Dis* 2002;185:599–607.

571. Gulick RM, Hu XJ, Fiscus SA, et al. Randomized study of saquinavir with ritonavir or nelfinavir together with delavirdine, adefovir, or both in human immunodeficiency virus-infected adults with virologic failure on indinavir. *J Infect Dis* 2000;182:1375–1384.

572. Kuritzkes DR, Bassett RL, Johnson VA, et al. Continued lamivudine versus delavirdine in combination with indinavir and zidovudine or stavudine in lamivudine-experienced patients: results of Adult AIDS Clinical Trials Group protocol 370. *AIDS* 2000;14:1553–1561.

573. Grodesky M, Acosta EP, Fujita N, et al. Combination therapy with indinavir, ritonavir, and delavirdine and nucleoside reserve transcriptase inhibitors in patients with HIV/AIDS who have failed multiple antiretroviral combinations. *HIV Clin Trials* 2001;2:193–199.

574. Matthews GV, Sabin C, Mandalia S, et al. Virological suppression at 6 months is related to choice of initial regimen

in antiretroviral-naive patients: a cohort study. *AIDS* 2002;16:53–61.

575. Kramer RA, Schaber MD, Skalka AM, Ganguly K, Wong-Staal F, Reddy EP. HTLV-III gag protein is processed in yeast cells by the virus pol-protease. *Science* 1986;231:1580–1584.

576. Lambert DM, Petteway SR Jr, McDanal CE, et al. Human immunodeficiency type I protease inhibitors irreversibly block infectivity of purified virions from chronically infected cells. *Antimicrob Agents Chemother* 1992;32:982–988.

577. Miller KD, Jones E, Yanovski JA, et al. Visceral abdominal-fat accumulation associated with use of indinavir. *Lancet* 1998;351:871–875.

578. Mallal S, John M, Moore C, et al. *Protease inhibitors and nucleoside analogue reverse transcriptase inhibitors interact to cause subcutaneous fat wasting in patients with HIV infection.* Presented at the first international workshop on adverse drug reactions and lipodystrophy in HIV. June 26–28, 1999; San Diego, CA. Abstract 019.

579. Mulligan K, Grunfeld C, Tai VW, et al. Hyperlipidemia and insulin resistance are induced by protease inhibitors independent of changes in body composition in patients with HIV infection. *J Acquir Immun Defic Syndr* 2000;23:35–43.

580. Thiébaut R, Daucourt V, Mercié P, et al. Lipodystrophy, metabolic disorders, and human immunodeficiency virus infection: Aquitaine Cohort, France, 1999. *Clin Infect Dis* 2002;31:1482–1487.

581. Romeu J, Sirera G, Rego MJ, et al. *Cumulative risk for developing hyperlipidemia in HIV-infected patients treated with protease inhibitors.* Presented at the 39th interscience conference on antimicrobial agents and chemotherapy. September 26–29, 1999; San Francisco, CA. Abstract 1293.

582. Saag M, Tebas P, Sension M, et al. Randomized, double-blind comparison of two nelfinavir doses plus nucleosides in HIV-infected patients (Agouron study 511). *AIDS* 2001;15:1971–1978.

583. Jensen-Fangel S, Kirk O, Blaxhult A, et al. The insufficient suppression of viral load by saquinavir hard gel is reversible: a retrospective cohort study. *HIV Clin Trials* 2001;2:122–127.

584. Schooley RT, Clumeck N, Haubrich R, et al. A dose-ranging study to evaluate the antiretroviral activity and safety of amprenavir alone and in combination with abacavir in HIV-infected adults with limited antiretroviral experience. *Antivir Ther* 2001;6:89–96.

585. Kost RG, Hurley A, Zhang L, et al. Open-label phase II trial of amprenavir,

abacavir, and fixed-dose zidovudine/lamivudine in newly and chronically HIV-1—infected patients. *J Acquir Immun Defic Syndr* 2001;26:332–339.

586. http://www.fda.gov/cder/foi/label/2002/21007s0101b1.pdf.last accessed July 2004.

587. Murphy RL, Brun S, Hicks C, et al. ABT-378/ritonavir plus stavudine and lamivudine for the treatment of antiretroviral-naive adults with HIV-1 infection: 48-week results. *AIDS* 2001;15:F1–F9.

588. Frieden TR, Sterling T, Pablos-Mendez A, et al. The emergence of drug-resistant tuberculosis in New York City. *N Engl J Med* 1993;328:521.

589. Ickovics JR, Meisler AW. Adherence in AIDS clinical trials: a framework for clinical research and clinical care. *J Clin Epidemiol* 1997;50:385–390.

590. Stone VE. Strategies for optimizing adherence to highly active antiretroviral therapy: lessons from research and clinical practice. *Clin Infect Dis* 2001;33:865–872.

591. Chesney MA. Factors affecting adherence to antiretroviral therapy. *Clin Infect Dis* 2000;30(2):171–176.

592. Lucas GM, Chiasson RE, Moore RD. Highly active antiretroviral therapy in a large urban clinic: risk factors for virologic failure and adverse drug reactions. *Ann Intern Med* 1999;131:81–87.

593. Cheever L, Forum for Collaborative HIV Research. What do we know about adherence levels in different populations? In: *Adherence to HIV therapy: building a bridge to success. Report from a workshop sponsored by DHHS Health Resources and Services Administration and the Forum for Collaborative HIV Research in collaboration with NIH Office of AIDS Research, November 15–16, 1999.* Washington, DC.

594. Crespo-Fierro M. Compliance/adherence and care management in HIV disease. *J Assoc Nurses AIDS Care* 1997;8(4):43–54.

595. Greenberg RN. Overview of patient compliance with medication dosing: a literature review. *Clin Ther* 1984;6:592–599.

596. Babudieri S, Aceti A, D'Offizi GP, et al. Directly observed therapy to treat HIV infection in prisoners. *JAMA* 2000;284:179–180.

597. Fischl M, Castro J, Mondroig R, et al. *Impact of directly observed therapy on long-term outcomes in HIV clinical trials.* Presented at the eighth conference on retroviruses and opportunistic infections. February 4–8, 2001; Chicago, IL. Abstract 528.

598. Mitty JA, Stone VE, Sads M, et al. Directly observed therapy for the treatment of people with human immun-

odeficiency virus infection: a work in progress. *Clin Infect Dis* 2002;34:984–990.

599. Sension MG, Bellos NC, Johnson J, et al. Lamivudine 300 mg QD versus continued lamivudine 150 mg BID with stavudine and a protease inhibitor in suppressed patients. *HIV Clin Trials* 2002;3:361–370.

600. Staszewski S, Haberl A, Gute P, et al. Nevirapine/didanosine/lamivudine once daily in HIV-1-infected intravenous drug users. *Antivir Ther* 1998;3[4 Suppl]:55–56.

601. Cardiello PG, van Heeswijk RP, Hassink E, et al. Simplifying protease inhibitor therapy with once-daily dosing of saquinavir soft-gelatin capsule/ritonavir (1600/100 mg): HIVNAT 001.3 study. *J Acquir Immun Defic Syndr* 2002;29:464–470.

602. Mocroft A, Vella S, Benfield TL, et al. Changing patterns of mortality across Europe in patients infected with HIV-1. EuroSIDA Study Group. *Lancet* 1998;352:1725–1730.

603. Palella FA Jr, Delaney KM, Moorman AC, et al. Declining morbidity and mortality among patients with advanced human immunodeficiency virus infection. *N Engl J Med* 1998;338:853–860.

604. Perelson AS, Essunger P, Cao Y, et al. Decay characteristics of HIV-1-infected compartments during combination therapy. *Nature* 1997;387:188–191.

605. Centers for Disease Control and Prevention. Report of the NIH panel to define principles of therapy of HIV infection and guidelines for use of antiretroviral agents in HIV-infected adults and adolescents. *MMWR Morb Mortal Wkly Rep* 1998;47(RR-5):1–41.

606. Durant J, Clevenbergh P, Halfon P, et al. Drug-resistance genotyping in HIV-1 therapy: the VRADAPT randomized controlled trial. *Lancet* 1999;353:2195–2199.

607. Baxter JD, Mayers DL, Wentworth DN, et al. *Pilot study of the short-term effects of antiretroviral management based on plasma genotypic antiretroviral resistance testing (GART) in patients failing antiretroviral therapy.* CPCRA 046 Study Team. Presented at the sixth conference on retroviruses and opportunistic infections. January 31–February 4, 1999; Chicago, IL. Abstract LB8.

608. Cohen C, Hunt S, Sension M, et al. *Phenotypic resistance testing significantly improves response to therapy: a randomized trial (VIRA3001).* Presented at the seventh conference on retroviruses and opportunistic infections. January 30–February 2, 2000; San Francisco, CA. Abstract 237.

609. John M, Moore CB, James IR,

et al. Chronic hyperlactatemia in HIV-infected patients taking antiretroviral therapy. *AIDS* 2001;15:717–723.

610. Harris M, Tesiorowski A, Chan K, et al. Lactic acidosis complicating antiretroviral therapy: frequency and correlates. *Antivir Ther* 2000;5(2):31.

611. Boxwell DE, Styrt BA. Lactic acidosis (LA) in patients receiving nucleoside reverse transcriptase inhibitors (NRTIs). Presented at the 39th interscience conference on antimicrobial agents and chemotherapy. September 26–29, 1999; San Francisco, CA. Abstract 1284.

612. Martinez E, Blanco JL, Arnaiz JA, et al. Hepatotoxicity in HIV-1-infected patients receiving nevirapine-containing antiretroviral therapy. *AIDS* 2001;15:1261–1268.

613. Savés M, Raffi F, Clevenbergh P, et al. Hepatitis B or hepatitis C virus infection is a risk factor for severe hepatic cytolysis after initiation of a protease inhibitor-containing antiretroviral regimen in human immunodeficiency virus-infected patient. The APROCO Study Group. *Antimicrob Agents Chemother* 2000;44:3451–3455.

614. Nuñez M, Lana R, Mendoza JL, et al. Risk factors for severe hepatic injury after introduction of highly active antiretroviral therapy. *J Acquir Immun Defic Syndr* 2001;27:426–431.

615. Calza L, Manfredi R, Mastroianni A, et al. Osteonecrosis and highly active antiretroviral therapy during HIV infection: report of a series and literature review. *AIDS Patient Care STDS* 2001;15:385–389.

616. Brown P, Crane L. Avascular necrosis of bone in patients with human immunodeficiency virus infection: report of 6 cases and review of the literature. *Clin Infect Dis* 2001;32:1221–1226.

617. Glesby MJ, Hoover DR, Vaamonde CM. Osteonecrosis in patients infected with human immunodeficiency virus: case-control study. *J Infect Dis* 2001;184:519–523.

618. McNaughten AD, Hanson DL, Jones JL, et al. Effects of antiretroviral therapy and opportunistic illness primary chemoprophylaxis on survival after AIDS diagnosis. *AIDS* 1999;13:1687–1695.

619. Vittinghoff E, Scheer S, O'Malley P, et al. Combination antiretroviral therapy and recent declines in AIDS incidence and mortality. *J Infect Dis* 1999;179:717–720.

620. Jones JL, Hanson D, Dworkin MS, et al. Trends in AIDS-related opportunistic infections among men who have sex with men and among injecting drug users, 1991–1996. *J Infect Dis* 1998;178:114–120.

621. Fischl MA, Dickinson GM, La Voie L. Safety and efficacy of sulfamethoxazole and trimethoprim chemoprophylaxis for *Pneumocystis carinii* pneumonia in AIDS. *JAMA* 1988;259:1185–1189.

622. Graham N, Zeger S, Park L, et al. Effect of zidovudine and *Pneumocystis carinii* pneumonia prophylaxis on progression of HIV-1 infection to AIDS. *Lancet* 1991;338:265–269.

623. Hardy WD, Feinberg J, Finkelstein DM, Power ME, He W, et al. A controlled trial of trimethoprim-sulfamethoxazole or aerosolized pentamidine for secondary prophylaxis of *Pneumocystis carinii* pneumonia in patients with the acquired immunodeficiency syndrome. *N Engl J Med* 1992;327:1842–1848.

624. Gallant JE, Moore RD, Chaisson RE. Prophylaxis for opportunistic infections in patients with HIV infection. *Ann Intern Med* 1994;120:932–944.

625. Phair J, Munoz A, Detels R, et al. The risk of *Pneumocystis carinii* pneumonia among men infected with human immunodeficiency virus type 1. *N Engl J Med* 1990;322:161–165.

626. Kaplan JE, Hanson DL, Navin TR, Jones JL. Risk factors for primary *Pneumocystis carinii* pneumonia in human immunodeficiency virus-infected adolescents and adults in the United States: reassessment of indications for chemoprophylaxis. *J Infect Dis* 1998;178:1126–1132.

627. Furrer H, Egger M, Opravil M, et al. Discontinuation of primary prophylaxis against *Pneumocystis carinii* pneumonia in HIV-1 infected adults treated with combination antiretroviral therapy. *N Engl J Med* 1999;340:1301–1306.

628. Weverling GJ, Mocroft A, Ledergerber B, et al. Discontinuation of *Pneumocystis carinii* pneumonia prophylaxis after start of highly active antiretroviral therapy in HIV-1 infection. *Lancet* 1999;353:1293–1298.

629. Yangco BG, Von Bargen JC, Moorman AC, et al. Discontinuation of chemoprophylaxis against *Pneumocystis carinii* pneumonia in patients with HIV infection. *Ann Intern Med* 2000;132:201–205.

630. Schneider MM, Borleff JC, Stolk RP, et al. Discontinuation of prophylaxis for *Pneumocystis carinii* pneumonia in HIV-1-infected patients treated with highly active antiretroviral therapy. *Lancet* 1999;353:201–203.

631. Dworkin MS, Hanson DL, Kaplan JE, et al. Risk for preventable opportunistic infections in person with AIDS after antiretroviral therapy increases CD4+ T lymphocyte counts above prophylaxis thresholds. *J Infect Dis* 2000;182:611–615.

632. Mussini C, Pezzotti P, Giovoni A,

et al. Discontinuation of primary prophylaxis for *Pneumocystis carinii* pneumonia and toxoplasmic encephalitis in human immunodeficiency virus type I-infected patients: the changes in opportunistic prophylaxis study. *J Infect Dis* 2000;181:1635–1642.

633. Lopez Bernaldo de Quiros JC, Miro J, Pena J, et al. Randomized trial of the discontinuation of primary and secondary prophylaxis against *Pneumocystis carinii* pneumonia after highly active antiretroviral therapy in patients with HIV infection. *N Engl J Med* 2001;344:159–167.

634. Furrer H, Opravil M, Rossi M, et al. Discontinuation of primary prophylaxis in HIV-infected patients at high risk of *Pneumocystis carinii* pneumonia: prospective multicentre study. *AIDS* 2001;15:501–507.

635. Kirk O, Lundgren JD, Pedersen C, et al. Can chemoprophylaxis against opportunistic infections be discontinued after an increase in CD4 cells induced by highly active antiretroviral therapy? *AIDS* 1999;13:1647–1651.

636. Soriano V, Dona C, Rodriguez-Rosado P, et al. Discontinuation of secondary prophylaxis for opportunistic infections in HIV-infected patients receiving highly active antiretroviral therapy. *AIDS* 2000;14:383–386.

637. Ledergerber B, Mocroft A, Reiss P. Discontinuation of secondary prophylaxis against *Pneumocystis carinii* pneumonia in patients with HIV infection who have a response to antiretroviral therapy. Eight European Study Groups. *N Engl J Med* 2001;344:168–174.

638. Bozette SA, Finkelstein DM, Spector SA, et al. Randomized trial of three antipneumocystis agents in patients with advanced human immunodeficiency virus infection. *N Engl J Med* 1995;332:693–9.

639. Schneider MM, Hoepelman AI, Eeftinck Schattenkerk JK, et al. Controlled trial of aerosolized pentamidine or trimethoprim-sulfamethoxazole as primary prophylaxis again *Pneumocystis carinii* pneumonia in patients with human immunodeficiency virus infection. *N Engl J Med* 1992;327:1836–1841.

640. Schneider MM, Nielson TL, Nelsing S, et al. Efficacy and toxicity of two doses of trimethoprim-sulfamethoxazole as primary prophylaxis against *Pneumocystis carinii* pneumonia with human immunodeficiency virus infection. *J Infect Dis* 1995;171:1632–1636.

641. El-Sadr WM, Luskin-Hawk R, Yurik TM, et al. A randomized trial of daily and thrice-weekly trimethoprim-sulfamethoxazole for the prevention of *Pneumocystis carinii* pneumonia in hu-

man immunodeficiency virus-infected persons. *Clin Infect Dis* 1999;29:775–783.

642. Klein RS. Prophylaxis of opportunistic infections in individuals infected with HIV. *AIDS* 1989;3[1 Suppl]:S161–S173.

643. Kovacs JA, Hiemenz JW, Macher AM, et al. *Pneumocystis carinii* pneumonia: a comparison between patients with the acquired immunodeficiency syndrome and patients with other immunodeficiencies. *Ann Intern Med* 1984;100:663–671.

644. Small CB, Harris CA, Friedland GH, et al. The treatment of *Pneumocystis carinii* pneumonia in the acquired immunodeficiency syndrome. *Arch Intern Med* 1985;145:837–840.

645. Murray JF, Felton CP, Garay JM, et al. Pulmonary complications of the acquired immunodeficiency syndrome: report of a National Heart, Lung and Blood Institute workshop. *N Engl J Med* 1984;312:1682–1688.

646. Shafer RW, Seitzman PA, Tapper ML. Successful prophylaxis of *Pneumocystis carinii* pneumonia with trimethoprim-sulfamethoxazole in AIDS patients with previous allergic reactions. *J Acquir Immune Defic Syndr* 1989;2:389–393.

647. Sattler FR, Cowan R, Nielsen DM, et al. Trimethoprim-sulfamethoxazole compared with pentamidine for treatment of *Pneumocystis carinii* pneumonia in the acquired immunodeficiency syndrome. A prospective, non-crossover study. *Ann Intern Med* 1988;109:280–287.

648. Blum RN, Miller LA, Gaggini LC, et al. Comparative trial of dapsone versus trimethoprim/sulfamethoxazole for primary prophylaxis of *Pneumocystis carinii* pneumonia. *J Acquir Immune Defic Syndr* 1992;5:341–347.

649. Podzamczer D, Salazar, Jiminez J, et al. Intermittent trimethoprim-sulfamethoxazole compared with dapsone-pyrimethamine for the simultaneous primary prophylaxis of *pneumocystis* pneumonia and toxoplasmosis in patients infected with HIV. *Ann Intern Med* 1995;122:755–761.

650. Opravil M, Hirschel B, Lazzarin A, et al. Once-weekly administration of dapsone/pyrimethamine vs. aerosolized pentamidine as combined prophylaxis for *Pneumocystis carinii* pneumonia and toxoplasmic encephalitis in human immunodeficiency virus-infected patients. *Clin Infect Dis* 1995;20:531–541.

651. Medina I, Mills J, Leoung G, et al. Oral therapy for *Pneumocystis carinii* pneumonia in the acquired immunodeficiency syndrome: a controlled trial of

trimethoprim-sulfamethoxazole versus trimethoprim-dapsone. *N Engl J Med* 1990;323:776–782.

652. Pengelly CD. Dapsone-induced hemolysis. *BMJ* 1963;2:662–664.

653. Karboski JA, Bodley PJ. Inhaled pentamidine and hypoglycemia. *Ann Intern Med* 1988;108:490.

654. Herer B, Chinet T, Labrune S, et al. Pancreatitis associated with pentamidine by aerosol. *BMJ* 1989;298:605.

655. Berger TG, Tappero JW, Leoung GS, Jacobsen MA. Aerosolized pentamidine and cutaneous eruptions. *Ann Intern Med* 1989;110:1035–1036.

656. Smith DE, Herd D, Guzzard BG. Reversible bronchoconstriction with nebulized pentamidine. *Lancet* 1988; 2:905.

657. Girard PM, Landman R, Gaudebout C, et al. Prevention of *Pneumocystis carinii* pneumonia relapse by pentamidine aerosol in zidovudine-treated AIDS patients. *Lancet* 1988;1:1348–1353.

658. Telzak EE, Cote RJ, Gold JW, Campbell SW, Armstrong D. Extrapulmonary *Pneumocystis carinii* infections. *Rev Infect Dis* 1990;12:380–386.

659. Davey RT, Margolis D, Kleiner D, et al. Digital necrosis and disseminated *Pneumocystis carinii* infection after aerosolized pentamidine prophylaxis. *Ann Intern Med* 1989;111:681–692.

660. Schinella RA, Breda SD, Hammerschlag PE. Optic infection due to *Pneumocystis carinii* infection in an apparently healthy man with antibody to human immunodeficiency virus. *Ann Intern Med* 1987;106:399.

661. Macher AM, Bardenstein DS, Zimmerman LE, et al. *Pneumocystis carinii* choroiditis in a male homosexual with AIDS and disseminated pulmonary and extrapulmonary *P. carinii* infection. *N Engl J Med* 1987;316:1092.

662. Jules-Elysee KM, Stover DE, Zaman MB, et al. Aerosolized pentamidine: effect on diagnosis and presentation of *Pneumocystis carinii* pneumonia. *Ann Intern Med* 1990;112:750–757.

663. Abd AG, Weitman DM, Ilowite JS, et al. Bilateral upper lobe *Pneumocystis carinii* pneumonia in a patient receiving inhaled pentamidine prophylaxis. *Chest* 1988;94:329–331.

664. Golden JA, Hollander H, Chernoff D, et al. Prevention of *Pneumocystis carinii* pneumonia by inhaled pentamidine. *Lancet* 1989;1:654–657.

665. Bradburne RM, Ettensohn DB, Opal SM, et al. Relapse of *Pneumocystis carinii* pneumonia in the upper lobes during aerosol pentamidine prophylaxis. *Thorax* 1989;44:591–593.

666. Chan C, Montaner J, Lefebvre EA, et al. Atovaquone suspension compared with aerosolized pentamidine for prevention of *Pneumocystis carinii* pneumonia in human immunodeficiency virus infected subjects intolerant of trimethoprim or sulfamethoxazole. *J Infect Dis* 1999;180:369–376.

667. El-Sadr W, Murphy RL, Yurik RM, et al. Atovaquone compared with dapsone for the prevention of *Pneumocystis carinii* pneumonia in patients with HIV infection who cannot tolerate trimethoprim, sulfonamides, or both. Community Program for Clinical Research on AIDS and the AIDS Clinical Trials Group. *N Engl J Med* 1998;339:1889–1895.

668. Chaisson RE, Benson CA, Dube MP. Clarithromycin therapy for bacteremic *Mycobacterium avium* complex disease: a randomized, double blind, dose ranging study in patients with AIDS. *Ann Intern Med* 1994;121:905–911.

669. Nightingale SD, Cameron DW, Gordin FM, et al. Two controlled trials of rifabutin prophylaxis against *Mycobacterium avium* complex infections in AIDS. *N Engl J Med* 1993;329:828–833.

670. Horsburgh CR Jr, Havlik JA, Ellis DA, et al. Survival of patients with acquired immune deficiency syndrome and disseminated *Mycobacterium avium* complex infection with and without antimycobacterial chemotherapy. *Am Rev Respir Dis* 1991;144:557–559.

671. Masur H. Recommendations on prophylaxis and therapy for disseminated *Mycobacterium avium* complex disease in patients infected with the human immunodeficiency virus. *N Engl J Med* 1993;329:898–904.

672. Benson CA, Williams PL, Cohn DL, et al. Clarithromycin or rifabutin alone or in combination for primary prophylaxis of *Mycobacterium avium* complex disease in patients with AIDS: a randomized, double-blind, placebo-controlled trial. *J Infect Dis* 2000;181:1289–1297.

673. Pierce M, Crampton S, Henry D, et al. A randomized trial of clarithromycin as prophylaxis against disseminated *Mycobacterium avium* complex infection in patients with advanced acquired immunodeficiency syndrome. *N Engl J Med* 1996;335:384–391.

674. Havlir DV, Dube MP, Sattler FR, et al. Prophylaxis against disseminated *Mycobacterium avium* complex with weekly azithromycin, daily rifabutin or both. *N Engl J Med* 1996;335:392–398.

675. El-Sadr WM, Burman WJ, Grant LB, et al. Discontinuation of prophylaxis for *Mycobacterium avium* complex disease in HIV-infected patients who have a response to antiretroviral therapy. Terry Beirn Community Programs for Clinical Research on AIDS. *N Engl J Med* 2000;342:1085–1092.

676. Furrer H, Telenti A, Rossi M, et al. Discontinuing or withholding primary prophylaxis against *Mycobacterium avium* in patients on successful antiretroviral combination therapy. *AIDS* 2000;14:1409–1412.

677. Gordin F, Sullam P, Shafran S, et al. Randomized, placebo-controlled study of rifabutin added to a regimen of clarithromycin and ethambutol for treatment of disseminated infection with *Mycobacterium avium* complex. *Clin Infect Dis* 1999;28:1080–1085.

678. Benson C, Williams P, Currier J, et al. *ACTG223: an open, prospective, randomized study comparing efficacy and safety of clarithromycin (C) plus ethambutol (E), rifabutin (R), or both for treatment (Rx) of MAC disease in patients with AIDS.* Presented at the sixth conference on retroviruses and opportunistic infections. January 31–February 4, 1999; Chicago, IL. Abstract 249.

679. Rabaud C, Jouan M, Mary-Krausse M, et al. *Mycobacterium avium (MAC) infections during HAART era (1996–98) in HIV-infected French patients.* Presented at the seventh conference on retroviruses and opportunistic infections, January 30–February 2, 2000; San Francisco, CA. Abstract 2054.

680. Aberg JA, Yijko DM, Jacobson MA. Eradication of AIDS-related disseminated *Mycobacterium avium* complex infection after 12 months of antimycobacterial therapy combined with highly active antiretroviral therapy. *J Infect Dis* 1998;178:1446–1449.

681. Shafran SD, Gill MJ, Lajonde RG, et al. Successful discontinuation of MAC therapy following effective HAART. Presented at the eighth conference on retroviruses and opportunistic infections. February 4–8, 2001; Chicago, IL. Abstract 547.

682. Carr A, Tindall B, Brew BJ, et al. Low-dose trimethoprim-sulfamethoxazole prophylaxis for toxoplasmic encephalitis in patients with AIDS. *Ann Intern Med* 1992;117:106–111.

683. Furrer H, Opravil M, Bernasconi E, et al. Stopping primary prophylaxis in HIV-1-infected patients at high risk of *Toxoplasma* encephalitis. Swiss HIV Cohort Study. *Lancet* 2000;355:2217–2218.

684. Miro JM, Podzamczer D, Pena JM, et al. *Discontinuation of primary and secondary Toxoplasma gondii prophylaxis is safe in HIV-1 infected patients after immunological recovery*

with HAART: final results of the GESIDA 04/98 Study. Presented at the 39th interscience conference on antimicrobial agents and chemotherapy. September 26–29, 1999; San Francisco, CA. Abstract L16.

685. Katlama C, De Wit S, O'Doherty E, et al. Pyrimethamine-clindamycin vs. pyrimethamine-sulfadiazine as acute and long-term therapy for toxoplasmic encephalitis in patients with AIDS. Clin Infect Dis 1996;22:268–275.

686. Dannemann B, McCutchan JA, Israelski D, et al. Treatment of toxoplasmic encephalitis in patients with AIDS: a randomized trial comparing pyrimethamine plus clindamycin to pyrimethamine plus sulfadiazine. California Collaborative Treatment Group. Ann Intern Med 1992;116:33–43.

687. O'Connor PG, Waugh ME, Schottenfeld RS. Ambulatory opiate detoxification and primary care: a role for the general internist. Clin Res 1990;38:719A.

688. Piette JD, Mor V, Mayer K, et al. The effects of immune status and race on health service use among people with HIV disease. Am J Public Health 1993;83:510–514.

689. Piette JD, Fleishman JA, Stein MD, et al. Perceived needs and unmet needs for formal services among people with HIV disease. J Community Health 1993;18:11–23.

690. Moore RD, Hidalgo J, Bareta JC, et al. Zidovudine therapy and health resource utilization in AIDS. J Acquir Immune Defic Syndr 1994;7:349–354.

691. Rosenberg PS, Gail MH, Schrager LK, et al. National AIDS incidence trends and the extent of zidovudine therapy in selected demographic and transmission groups. J Acquir Immune Defic Syndr 1991;4:392–401.

692. Chitwood DD, McBride DC, French MT, et al. Health care need and utilization: a preliminary comparison of injection drug users, other illicit drug users, and nonusers. Subst Use Misuse 1999;34:727–746.

693. Turner BJ, Fleishman JA, Wenger N, et al. Effects of drug abuse and mental disorders on use and type of antiretroviral therapy in HIV-infected persons. J Gen Intern Med 2001;16: 625–633.

694. Cronquist A, Edwards V, Galea S, et al. Health care utilization among young adult injection drug users in Harlem, New York. J Subst Abuse 2001; 13:17–27.

695. US Congress, Office of National Drug Control Policy. Executive Office of the President, Office of National Drug Control Policy. Consultation Document on Opioid Agonist Treatment. Available at http://www.whitehousedrugpolicy.gov/science_tech/methadone/contents.html. Last accessed July 2004.

696. Gallagher TC, Andersen RM, Koegel P, et al. Determinants of regular source of care among homeless adults in Los Angeles. Med Care 1997;35:814–830.

697. Rich JD, Holmes L, Salas C. Successful linkage of medical care and community services for HIV-positive offenders being released from prison. J Urban Health 2001;78:279–289.

698. Cunningham C, Shapiro S, Berg K, et al. The impact of medical outreach on HIV-infected residents living in single room occupancy hotels in the Bronx. Presented at the Society of General Internal Medicine national conference. May 2002; Atlanta, GA. Abstract 84.

699. Ross HE, Glaser FB, Germanson T. The prevalence of psychiatric disorders in patients with alcohol and other drug problems. Arch Gen Psychiatry 1988;45:1023–1031.

700. Silberstein CH, McKegney FP, O'Dowd MA, et al. A prospective longitudinal study of neuropsychological and psychosocial factors in asymptomatic individuals at risk for HTLV-III/LAV infection in a methadone program: preliminary findings. Int J Neurosci 1987;32:676–699.

701. American Academy of Pediatrics Task Force on Pediatrics AIDS. Infants and children with acquired immunodeficiency syndrome: placement in adoption and foster care. Pediatrics 1989;83:609–612.

702. Falloon J, Eddy J, Wiener L, Pizzo PA. Human immunodeficiency virus infection in children. J Pediatr 1989;114:1–30.

703. Pinching AJ. Models of clinical care. AIDS 1989;3[1 Suppl]:S209–S213.

704. Shelp EE, DuBose ER, Sunderland RH. The infrastructure of religious communities: a neglected resource for care of people with AIDS. Am J Public Health 1990;80:970–972.

705. Ostrow DG, Gayle T. Psychosocial and ethical issues of AIDS health care programs. QRB Qual Rev Bull 1986;12:284–294.

706. Boyd L, Kuehnert P, Sherer R. Serving hope, humor and compassion: implementation of a widely diverse volunteer support program for persons with AIDS/HIV infection at Cook County Hospital, Chicago. Presented at the sixth international conference on AIDS. June 1990; San Francisco, CA. Abstract S.D.804.

707. Herb A, LaGamma D. Legal services for persons with AIDS of predominantly heterosexual, poor, minority background. Presented at the fifth international conference on AIDS. June 1989; Montreal, Canada. Abstract Th.F.O.2.

708. Goeren W, Wade K, Rodriguez L. Case management of families with HIV infection. Presented at the sixth international conference on AIDS. June 1990; San Francisco, CA. Abstract S.D.803.

709. Eric K, Drucker E, Worth D, et al. The Women's Center: a model peer support program for IV drug and crack-using women in the Bronx. Presented at the fifth international conference on AIDS. June 1989; Montreal, Canada. Abstract Th.D.P.7.

710. Katz MH, Cunningham WE, Fleishman JA, et al. Effect of case management on unmet needs and utilization of medical care and medications among HIV-infected persons. Ann Intern Med 2001;135:557–556.

711. Ball JC, Lange WR, Myers CP, et al. Reducing the risk of AIDS through methadone maintenance treatment. J Health Soc Behav 1988;29:214–226.

712. Wolcott DL, Fawzy FI, Pasnau RO. Acquired immune deficiency syndrome (AIDS) and consultation-liaison psychiatry. Gen Hosp Psychiatry 1985;7:280–292.

713. Miller D. HIV and social psychiatry. Br Med Bull 1988;44:130–148.

714. Karan LD. Primary care for AIDS and chemical dependence. West J Med 1990;152:538–542.

CHAPTER 59

Neuropsychiatric Aspects of HIV-1 Infection

FRANCISCO FERNANDEZ, JORGE
MALDONADO, AND PEDRO RUIZ

The human immunodeficiency virus type 1 (HIV-1) infection and the acquired immune deficiency syndrome (AIDS) have affected millions of individuals around the world since it was first described 20 years ago. It has infected 60 million individuals worldwide, among which 42 million are still living with the infection. The spread of the virus continues at a rate of 14,000 newly infected individuals per day, and in the year 2003, 5 million persons contracted the virus (1). According to the Centers for Disease Control and Prevention (CDC), the number of persons living with HIV is estimated to have been 384,906 as of December 2002, and a total of 501,669 have died from the disease through the years (2). A lot of progress has been made since the introduction of zidovudine (AZT) as the first antiretroviral agent and the use of highly active antiretroviral therapy, first described in 1996, has decreased both the mortality and the incidence of AIDS. From being the leading cause of death in adults 25 to 44 years old in 1993 (3), it has declined to the fifth leading cause of death in that age population (4). Unprotected homosexual and heterosexual intercourse, injection drug use (IDU), and contaminated blood and blood products transfusions are well-known mechanisms of HIV-1 transmission. Crack cocaine in women (5) and other non-IDU in homosexuals are well-determined risk factors for HIV-1 infection (6), with marihuana and volatile nitrites ("poppers") increasing the likelihood of HIV-1 infection for any given exposure in the male homosexual population (6,7). The emotional distress caused by HIV seroconversion, along with psychiatric disorders and neurologic syndromes caused by medical conditions (by both direct effect of the virus and secondary opportunistic infections and brain tumors) may drive patients to the psychiatrist for evaluation and treatment. These conditions might be complicated by previous psychopathology and substance-induced psychiatric disorders (by illicit or prescribed drugs). In an attempt to make clinicians more aware and more capable of managing these complex and challenging patients, we review the neuropsychologic symptomatology, its neuropathology, and the treatment options for neuropsychiatric disorders associated with the HIV-1 infection.

NEUROPATHOLOGY IN HIV-1 INFECTION

The HIV-1 penetrates the blood–brain barrier early in the course of the infection, is replicated in brain tissue using monocytes and multinucleated macrophages as hosts (8), and becomes an anatomic reservoir for the disease (9). In patients with AIDS, the virus may recover in cerebrospinal fluid (CSF) (10) or brain tissue because they quantitatively contain more virus than other organs in the body (11,12).

The mechanisms whereby HIV-1 penetrates the nervous system are not completely understood. It may enter the brain through endothelial gaps in brain capillaries (13), via the choroid plexus (10), or as a proviral form contained in a latently infected cell (a monocyte), which, once inside the central nervous system (CNS), differentiates into a macrophage, converting to a productively infected cell (11). The virus is known to invade and destroy subcortical areas such as the basal ganglia and temporolimbic structures, as well as support cells such as astrocytes, which share similar CD4 receptors with their well-known lymphocyte host (14). It also affects cortical areas, as demonstrated by quantitative measurements of neuronal numbers in various cortical regions (15) and magnetic resonance imaging (MRI) measurement in patients with HIV-1 dementia (16).

The direct effect of the HIV-1 might be responsible for the development of neuropathology. This effect, however, is incompletely understood and immunohistochemical and *in situ* hybridization studies indicate that only macrophages/microglia are significantly infected in the CNS (17). Other forms of neurotoxicity have been studied and there is evidence now that the nonstructural proteins of the HIV-1, glycoprotein gp 120 and protein TAT, are involved in the neuronal damage through N-methyl-D-aspartate (NMDA) and non-NMDA receptors stimulation (18–21), which leads to increased intracellular and intramitochondrial calcium concentrations with subsequent generation of mitochondrial reactive oxygen species (22). Quinolinic acid, which is the product of altered pathways of tryptophan metabolism in the brain, also acts as glutamate agonist on the NMDA receptors, leading to increased calcium influx into the neurons (23,24). Other substances secreted by infected macrophages include neopterin and platelet-activating factor, which are involved in the increased production of the free radicals involved in the last steps of the process leading to apoptosis or neuronal death (22,25).

Different steps in this complex cascade have been the target of many attempts to prevent its neurotoxicity. The removal of glutamate by glutamate dehydrogenase and glutamate receptor antagonists is ineffective in preventing neurotoxicity (26). The NMDA receptor antagonists memantine and MK-801 (dizocilpine) prevent the injury engendered by the glycoprotein gp 120 without significantly altering the release of arachidonic acid (18,27). Calcium channel blockers have had different responses according to specific drugs (26,28) in preventing early rise in calcium concentration and delayed neuronal injury, with nimodipine and nifedipine being the most effective, and with verapamil potentiating HIV-1 replication in lymphoid cells (29). Nimodipine has been studied in a clinical trial, showing nonstatistically significant improvement on neuropsychological testing in the group that received high doses (60 mg) five times daily (30). Dantrolene and extracellular calcium removal with 1,2-bis-(2-aminophenoxy) ethane-$N,N,N,'N'$-tetraacetic acid (BAPTA) (26) are also effective in neurotoxicity prevention. Investigation to discover a clinically tolerated drug that will prevent the neurotoxic effects continues.

Clinically, patients suffer from a wide spectrum of cognitive impairments, personality changes, and motor dysfunction that range from subclinical symptoms without impairment of work or daily activities to severe dementia with paraplegia and double incontinence (31). This extreme syndrome is known as HIV-1–associated cognitive-motor complex (32) and its severity is related to the degree of inflammatory response in the brain (33). In patients with moderate to severe dementia, multinucleated giant cells (MNGC) are found and are now considered essential for the diagnosis and pathognomonic of HIV-1 infection in the CNS (34). However, the finding of MNGC in the CNS of patients with HIV-1 infection is only noted in 25% to 50% of patients with dementia. Nonetheless, in the MNGC-negative brains of mildly demented AIDS patients, the viral CNS burden as measured by *in situ* hybridization or polymerase chain reaction (PCR) for viral nucleic acids is reportedly higher than in nondemented patients (35). Microglial and glial changes, along with MNGC, can be found in any part of the CNS, but are more common in deep white matter of the cerebral hemispheres, basal ganglia, and brainstem (34). White matter pallor with astrogliosis, diffuse or focal vacuolation that can be associated with axonal or myelin loss (36), and cortical atrophy (15,37) are changes that are less commonly observed. Rather than a true demyelination process of the oligodendritic myelin sheath, the pallor is a result of an increase in interstitial water content, most likely caused by a leaky blood–brain barrier.

PERIPHERAL NERVOUS SYSTEM PATHOLOGY AND MYOPATHY IN HIV-1 INFECTION

Patients with HIV-1 infection may present with a wide variety of symptoms involving the peripheral nervous system (PNS) (38–40) and the skeletal muscles (38,41). It has been hypothesized that similar mechanisms are involved in the pathogenesis of CNS and PNS dysfunction (17). While symptomatic neuropathies occur in approximately 10% to 15% of HIV-1 infected patients, there is pathologic evidence that PNS involvement exists in virtually all end-stage AIDS patients (42).

Distal symmetric peripheral neuropathy (DSPN) is the most common presentation among patients with generalized neuropathies (38,40,43,44). Initial symptoms include trophic changes in the lower extremities, paresthesias, edema, and weakness. These symptoms progress slowly to centripetally spread weakness and sensory loss. Medication-induced neuropathies have a clinical presentation that is similar to DSPN except that they present concurrent with the use of antiretrovirals, whereas the DSPN generally presents in the late phases of the HIV-1 infection (42). Inflammatory demyelinating polyradiculopathy may be acute (AIDP), presenting at the time of seroconversion and the initial manifestation of HIV-1 infection, or chronic (CIDP), presenting as subacute or chronic weakness in upper and lower extremities, decreased to absent deep tendon reflexes, and mild sensory abnormalities. Cranial nerves may also be involved (38,40). Mononeuritis multiplex usually presents as an abrupt onset mononeuropathy with periodic additional abrupt mononeuropathies in other distributions. It may present with sensory or motor manifestations and may involve cranial nerves as well (38,44–47). Pain may accompany any of the above-mentioned neuropathies and may be both severe and incapacitating (17,38,43,44).

Less-common presentations of PNS dysfunction are progressive polyneuroradiculopathy (38) with early impairment of bladder and rectal sphincter control, and autonomic neuropathy with postural hypotension, diarrhea, and sudden arrhythmias with the risk of death (43,48,49).

The pain management regimen for the treatment of neuropathies includes capsaicin cream, amitriptyline, desipramine, anticonvulsants, or narcotics (43,44). Still, effective pain control is often difficult. Corticosteroids, plasmapheresis, and i.v. immunoglobulin have been used with success for DSPN, CIDP and mononeuritis multiplex (38,44,50). Hypotension related to autonomic neuropathy may be controlled with fludrocortisone (44).

Myopathy associated with HIV-1 infection has three different histologic findings: (a) polymyositis, (b) necrotizing myopathy without inflammatory infiltrates, and (c) nemaline rod myopathy (51,52). Clinically, patients present with painless progressive weakness involving the shoulder and pelvic girdle muscles, elevated creatinine kinase (CK), and electromyographic (EMG) abnormalities. Treatment with prednisone alone or in combination with plasmapheresis is usually effective (38,44). The most important and common myopathy among HIV-1 infected patients is that related to zidovudine (AZT). It usually develops after 9 months to 1 year of treatment and manifests with leg weakness and wasting of the buttocks muscles (38,41–44). Symptom reversal may be complete with cessation or reduction of therapy. Patients taking AZT must be monitored regularly to detect early increments of CK (38,43,44).

DIAGNOSIS AND MANAGEMENT OF HIV-1 SECONDARY NEUROLOGIC COMPLICATIONS

HIV-1 CNS involvement may occur at any time, in the absence or presence of indicators of quantifiable immune compromise. Opportunistic infections and HIV-1–related malignancies affecting the nervous system are usually a late manifestation of the HIV-1 infection (50), occurring in patients with less than 200 CD4 cells/mm^3. Table 59.1 indicates the possible range of nervous pathologies that are likely to attack the CNS as a result of HIV-1 infection (39,53). No significant differences in the incidence of neurologic disease between IDUs and non-IDUs have been reported (54).

Toxoplasma gondii infection is extremely prevalent (55) and is the most frequent cause of focal intracerebral lesions in patients with AIDS (39,56,57). Primary infection is usually asymptomatic, however. Headache accompanied by fever is the most common presentation, along with a subacute onset of focal neurologic abnormalities. Seizures affect one-third of the patients (58). When neuroradiologic studies suggest toxoplasmosis, empirical therapy is almost a universal practice. The problem with neuroimaging studies, however, is that they have a low sensitivity when patients have nonfocal symptoms (22% to 74%) (59) and when serum immunoglobulin (Ig) G is negative. If the patient fails to improve, a brain biopsy is necessary for a definitive diagnosis (58,59). Primary prophylaxis followed by maintenance treatment with pyrimethamine and sulfadiazine or clindamycin is usually effective and is recommended (60).

Cryptococcus neoformans is the most common cause of meningitis and the most important CNS fungal infection in patients with AIDS (50,55). The typical clinical presentation includes an insidious onset of fever, headache, nausea, vomiting, and altered mental status in a patient with a CD4 count of less than 100 cells/mm^3. If untreated, this is a fatal disorder (53), but mortality can be reduced to 17% to 20% (61) with amphotericin B, either alone or in combination with flucytosine or with fluconazole therapy (62). Again, indefinite maintenance therapy with fluconazole is recommended (55).

Other secondary neurologic infections associated with HIV-1 include progressive multifocal leukoencephalopathy (PML) secondary to papovavirus infection (50,63), cytomegalovirus (CMV), encephalitis and polyradiculopathy (44,64), herpes simplex virus (HSV), encephalitis (65), neurosyphilis (45,51,66), and mycobacterial and other fungal infections. PML is an increasingly important source of neurologic complications in HIV-1 disease and although there is no proven therapy for PML, cytosine arabinoside has been suggested as an efficacious alternative (66). Ganciclovir and foscarnet are effective in the treatment of CMV infection and as maintenance therapy. HSV encephalitis is a rare but life-threatening complication of HSV infection, especially in patients with advanced HIV-1 infection and other opportunistic infections of the CNS. Brain biopsy is often required for a definitive diagnosis. Treatment options include i.v. acyclovir, foscarnet, and vidarabine. Neurosyphilis has a more aggressive course in patients with AIDS, and its diagnosis may be difficult (50,65). Fortunately, intravenous penicillin is a highly effective and definitive treatment. Herpes zoster, mycobacterial, and fungal infections produce CNS complications in HIV-1–infected individuals and generally respond well to multimodal treatment.

Non-Hodgkin lymphoma is a complication of advanced HIV-1 disease that is present in 8% of the AIDS population (67). It may involve the CNS, causing neurologic, as well as neuropsychiatric, complications that include delirium, seizures, and cognitive impairment (53). A diagnosis can be made via neuroimaging, but a brain biopsy and/or evidence of malignant cells in the CSF is usually required prior to initiation of treatment. Multiagent chemotherapeutic treatment induces complete response in 54% of patients (68), but these responses are usually of short duration and the median survival time is 4 to 7 months after the diagnosis (69). AIDS patients are 100 times more likely than controls to suffer strokes (53,70), sometimes resulting in a clinical syndrome of multiinfarct dementia (71).

PNS may also be affected by secondary complications, such as herpes zoster neuropathy and cytomegalovirus polyradiculopathy. Toxic neuropathies caused by nucleotides (dideoxyinosine [ddI], dideoxycytidine [ddC]) may appear in late phases of the HIV-1 infection with a CD4 count of less than 200 cells/mm^3 (50). A reversible myopathy secondary to zidovudine may also affect these patients (38,41–44).

TABLE 59.1. *Neuropsychiatric infections/malignancies associated with HIV*

Atypical aseptic meningitis
Cytomegalovirus (CMV) encephalitis
Herpes simplex virus encephalitis
Progressive multifocal leukoencephalopathy
Subacute encephalitis
Varicella zoster virus encephalitis or vasculitis
Aspergillus
Candidiasis
Coccidioidomycosis
Cryptococcus neoformans
Toxoplasma gondii
Atypical mycobacteria
Mycobacterium tuberculosis
Kaposi sarcoma
Primary or secondary central nervous system lymphoma

Source: Adapted from Bredesen DE, Levy RM, Rosenblum ML. The neurology of human immunodeficiency virus infection. *QJM* 1994;68:665–667, with permission of Oxford University Press.

NEUROBIOLOGIC EVALUATION IN HIV-1 INFECTION

Mental Status and Neuropsychological Assessment

Learning about the pathogenicity of HIV-1 is a key factor in its management. Needless to say, we recently gained much insight and knowledge in this respect. The HIV-1–associated cognitive/motor complex consists of a combination of cognitive, motor, behavioral, and affective disturbances (33,72) that may be severe and sufficient for the diagnosis of AIDS. It may be the presenting manifestation of HIV-1 infection (73) or it may cause mild symptoms and not be associated with significant impairment in the social or occupational functioning levels of these patients. Several investigators have found that asymptomatic HIV-1–positive patients have an elevated rate of cognitive dysfunction when compared to HIV-1–negative controls (74–80). These are usually subtle impairments that are unrelated to the level of immunosuppression or to depression (78,79,81,82), and are most evident in individuals with lower cognitive reserve (83). Although controversy still exists as to whether the cognitive functioning of asymptomatic patients is distinguishable from that of controls (84,85), it is generally accepted by clinicians that HIV-1–related cognitive impairment can occur at any time during the course of the disease. It has also been shown that cognitive abnormalities in asymptomatic patients are associated with an increased risk of mortality (86) and work disability (87,88). Although varying psychological tests have been used to determine or evaluate the earlier signs of HIV-1 effects on mental function (89,90), no definitive test can be used, either alone or in combination with others, to establish a diagnosis of HIV-1–associated cognitive/motor complex. A careful cognitive history can be an extremely useful adjunct in the differential diagnosis of the etiologies of cognitive dysfunction in HIV-1–infected patients with cognitive complaints. This is most important when there is no formal capacity for neuropsychological testing. Table 59.2 lists the essentials of this interactive interview. We have found that the answers to these questions can help match the individual patient complaints to the criterion system for defining HIV-1–associated cognitive disorder and dementia, such as that proposed by the American Academy of Neurology (32). The cognitive history must also include a mental status examination. A standard examination, such as the Mini Mental State Examination, may miss the types of memory and attention/concentration problems often associated with CNS HIV-1 infection, requiring a more formal evaluation with neuropsychological testing.

The most significant signs of cognitive impairment related to HIV-1 infection include early, mild problems with abstraction, learning, language, verbal memory, and psychomotor speed that progress to more serious difficulties with attention and concentration, slowing of information processing, slowed psychomotor speed, impaired

TABLE 59.2. *HIV cognitive history*

Name
Age and birthday
Handedness
First language at home
Educational background
  Best subjects, grades
  Worst subjects
Occupational background
  How long
Medical history
  Childhood diseases or injuries
  Head injuries with loss of consciousness
  Strokes
  High fevers
  Toxin exposure
  Major illness, injuries, or surgeries
  Medicines: prescription, nonprescription
Duration of diagnosis of HIV infection; AIDS
Current problem
  Change in thinking functions: how long, or over what
    period of time
Any change in ability to concentrate
Any periods of confusion or mental "fuzziness"
  When talking with people, or on the phone, watching
    TV or a movie, reading
Any problem with following the train of thought
Any difficulties with handwriting
Any word-finding problems; difficulties with slurring or
  stammering
Any slowing of thinking or understanding, trouble with
  mental arithmetic such as making change or balancing
  checkbook
Wear glasses
Any blurring vision, double vision, or flashing lights in eyes
Any change in understanding what is seen; do things
  look right in their relation to each other
Overlook things when right in front of you
Hearing any unusual sounds; see unusual things; have
  any strange feelings
Any changes in any other senses
  Decreased hearing, ringing, or buzzing sounds
  Change in smell or taste
  Any numbness, "pins or needles," loss of feeling,
  tingling, or burning feelings
  Any severe pain
Memory
  Any areas of memory that are better or worse
  Memory for recent information
  Information from way back in life
  Any difference in memory for *situations* versus rote
    facts and figures
  Kinds of things most easily forgotten: names,
    addresses, directions, reading
  How long can things be remembered, more notes
  written than used to
  Any lapses noted
  Any getting lost or forgetting where one is

(continued)

TABLE 59.2. *(Continued)*

Any new difficulties with thinking through problems or solving them, decisions making, staying organized—on job, at home

How is sleep: any trouble getting to sleep; night versus daytime; any awakenings from which one cannot immediately return to sleep

Any inability to move any parts of the body
Muscle weakness, twitching, spasms, trouble walking, coordination problems, tremors or shakiness, problems with dropping things, feeling like moving more slowly, difficulty using tools or household utensils, getting dressed, telling right from left

Headaches or dizziness, instances thought to be seizures (staring off into space for a long time, uncontrollable movements, periods where one seemed "lose" time, incontinence)

Changes in mood, feelings, ideas
Mood swings, loss of patience or change in temper, increase in irritability, change in amount of worry, sense of panic

(Continue with Hamilton Depression and Anxiety Scales)

Source: Adapted from Levy JK, Fernandez F. HIV infection of the CNS: implications for neuropsychiatry. In: Yudofsky SC, Hales RE, eds. *The American Psychiatric Press textbook of neuropsychiatry*, 3rd ed. Washington, DC: American Psychiatric Press, 1996.

cognitive flexibility, impairment in nonverbal abilities of problem solving, visuospatial integration and construction, and nonverbal memory in the late phases of the infection (78,89). The early stages of cognitive impairment associated with HIV-1 affect psychomotor tasks (such as the Wechsler Adult Intelligence Scale digit symbol and block design, and the trail making test part B from the Halstead-Reitan Neuropsychological Battery), memory tasks (such as the delayed visual reproduction subtest from the Wechsler memory scale); and the delayed recall of the Rey-Osterrieth Complex Figure (89). Psychomotor and neuromotor tasks may reveal HIV-1–related cognitive dysfunction and are also sensitive measures for the early detection of HIV-1–related cognitive impairment.

The neuropsychological tests used for assessment of dementia generally appraise complex language-associated functions (such as aphasia and apraxia), higher level cognitive functions of verbal and nonverbal abstract reasoning and problem solving, and perceptual functioning of the different sensory modalities. However, as more has been learned about the HIV-1–associated cognitive/motor complex, it has become apparent that these neuropsychological assessments are not reliably sensitive for the necessary early detection of HIV-1 minor cognitive/motor disorder. These neuropsychological batteries are most useful for detecting areas of mental dysfunction related to focal disturbances in the CNS, such as abscess created by an

TABLE 59.3. *National institute of mental health neuropsychological battery*

A. Indication of premorbid intelligence
  1. Vocabulary (Weschler Adult Intelligent Scale–Revised[WAIS-R])
  2. National adult reading test (NART)
B. Attention
  1. Digit span (Weschler Memory Scale–Revised [WMS-R])
  2. Visual span (WMS-R)
C. Speed of processing
  1. Sternberg search task
  2. Simple and choice reaction time
  3. Paced Auditory Serial Addition Test (PASAT)
D. Memory
  1. California Verbal Learning Test (CVLT)
  2. Memory working test
  3 Modified visual reproduction test
E. Abstraction
  1. Category test
  2. Trail making test, parts A and B
F. Language
  1. Boston naming test
  2. Letter and category fluency test
G. Visuospatial
  1. Embedded figures test
  2. Money's standardized road-map test of direction sense
  3. Digit symbol substitution
H. Construction abilities
  1. Block design test
  2. Tactual performance test
I. Motor abilities
  1. Grooved pegboard
  2. Finger tapping test
  3. Grip strength
J. Psychiatric assessment
  1. Diagnostic Interview Schedule (DIS)
  2. Hamilton depression scale
  3. State-trait anxiety scale
  4. Mini mental state examination

Source: Adapted from Butters N, Grant I, Haxby J, et al. Assessment of AIDS-related cognitive changes: recommendations of the NIMH Workgroup on Neuropsychological Assessment Approaches. *J Clin Exp Neuropsychol* 1990;12:963–978.

HIV-1–related opportunistic infection or tumor. They are not, however, useful for detecting the often subtle impairments of the early stages of HIV-1's effects on the CNS. Table 59.3 shows the neuropsychological battery recommended by the National Institute of Mental Health (NIMH) for use with these patients. Sometimes, however, modifications according to the patient's cognitive status may be more useful than a full evaluation.

With the aid of these more sensitive testing procedures, it has become clear that cognitive dysfunction of sufficient severity to disrupt the patient's normal daily activities may

TABLE 59.4. *Clinical staging system for HIV-1-associated dementia complex*

Stage 0 (normal)
+ Normal mental and motor function. Neurologic signs are within the normal age-appropriate spectrum.

Stage 0.5 (subclinical)
+ Minimal or equivocal symptoms without impairment of work or capacity to perform activities of daily living (ADL). Mildly abnormal signs may include reflex changes (e.g., generalized increase in deep tendon reflexes with active jaw jerk, snout, or glabellar sign) or mildly slowed ocular/limb movements, but without clear loss of strength (must be differentiated from fatigue).

Stage 1 (mild)
+ Able to perform all but the more demanding aspects of work or ADL but with unequivocal evidence (symptoms or signs including performance on neuropsychological testing) of intellectual or motor impairment. The abnormal clinical motor signs usually include slow or clumsy movements of extremities, but the patient can walk without assistance.

Stage 2 (moderate)
+ Able to perform basic activities of self-care at home but cannot work or maintain more demanding aspects of daily life (e.g., maintain finances, read text more complex than newspaper). Ambulatory but may require single prop (e.g., cane).

Stage 3 (severe)
+ Major incapacity in intellectual capacity (cannot follow news or personal events, cannot sustain conversation of any complexity, considerable slowing of all output) and motor ability (cannot walk unassisted, requiring walker or personal support, usually with slowing and clumsiness of arms as well).

Stage 4 (end stage)
+ Nearly vegetative. Intellectual and social comprehension and output limited to rudimentary understanding. Nearly or absolutely mute. Paraparetic or plegic with double incontinence.

Source: Adapted from Brew BJ, Sidtis JJ, Petito CK, et al. The neurologic complications of AIDS and human immunodeficiency virus infection. In: Plum F, ed. *Advances in contemporary neurology*. Philadelphia: F.A. Davis, 1994:1–49.

occur at any time during the course of the infectious process with HIV-1. Brew and colleagues characterized these disabilities and established a scale for the clinical staging of the fully developed HIV-1–associated dementia (HAD) (72,91) (Table 59.4). The staging system is specific for HAD and it ranks cognitive, behavioral, and neurologic/motoric functioning commensurate with the stages of progression within the AIDS diagnosis. However, because we are aware of the possibility of early cognitive impairment before the diagnosis of HAD, a means of ranking cognitive functioning needs to be developed to define cognitive

disabilities at earlier stages of infection. The Global Deterioration Scale of Reisberg and colleagues (92) is useful in this respect because of its capability to characterize cognitive functioning in daily activities. It can characterize dementia of the Alzheimer type, as well as other neurodegenerative dementias (Table 59.5). Administration of the Global Deterioration Scale to a sample of HIV-1–infected patients (93) determined that 21% of the patients at an early stage of symptomatic infection, such as progressive generalized lymphadenopathy (PGL), had Global Deterioration Scale stage 1 (meaning normal) and that 42% of the sample had cognitive impairment ranging from forgetfulness to early dementia. As HIV-1 disease progressed, 27% of these patients were shown to have forgetfulness and almost 30% qualified for classification of early, middle, or late dementia. Therefore, the Global Deterioration Scale can provide the necessary information to successfully assess the decline of cognitive function clinically as it relates to an HIV-1–infected person's performance of daily activities, even before the patient fulfills the diagnostic criteria for the HIV-1–associated cognitive/motor complex. The Global Deterioration Scale is also of benefit to research and planning investigations because it is capable of comparing the cognitive impairment associated with HIV-1 infection with the cognitive impairment found in non–HIV-1–related dementias. When we see the similarities and differences between them, we are better able to foresee and adequately plan for the predicted course of the patient's progressive cognitive decline.

Neuroimaging

Computed tomography (CT) and magnetic resonance imaging (MRI) are very useful in the diagnosis of secondary infections and brain tumors. Primary CNS HIV-1 infection can be associated with characteristic imaging features, including cortical atrophy, ventricular enlargement, diffuse or patchy white matter abnormalities particularly in periventricular areas (94,95) and, in children, calcification of the basal ganglia and delayed myelination (96,97). MRI is more sensitive than CT scan in detecting white matter changes (98) and MRI changes correlate with neuropsychological testing (99). Both, however, are useful as diagnostic tools and may also have utility in assessing the prognosis of these patients (100).

Neuroimaging that reflects physiologic functioning of the CNS via positron emission tomography (PET) reveals early regional metabolic abnormalities with hypermetabolism in the basal ganglia, thalamus, and parietal and temporal lobes among nondemented patients with HIV-1 infection. It reveals a regional and then a general hypometabolism as the HIV-1 CNS involvement progresses and becomes clinically associated with dementia (101–103). Abnormalities of brain activation associated with effortful retrieval and organizational process have

TABLE 59.5. *Global deterioration scale (GDS) for age-associated cognitive decline*

GDS stage
+ Clinical phase
+ Clinical characteristics
1 No cognitive decline
+ Normal
+ No subjective complaints of memory deficit. No memory deficit evident on clinical interview.
2 Very mild cognitive decline
+ Forgetfulness
+ Subjective complaints of mild memory deficit, most frequently in following cognitive areas: (a) forgetting where one has placed familiar objects; (b) forgetting names one formerly knew well. No objective evidence of memory deficit on clinical interview. No objective deficits in employment or social situations. Appropriate concern with respect to symptomatology.
3 Mild cognitive decline
+ Early confusional
+ Earliest clear-cut deficits. Manifestations in more than one of the following areas: (a) patient may have gotten lost when traveling to an unfamiliar location; (b) coworkers become aware of patient's relatively poor performance; (c) word and name-finding deficits become evident to intimates; (d) patient may read a passage or a book and retain relatively little material; (e) patient may demonstrate decreased facility in remembering names on introduction to new people; (f) patient may have lost or misplaced an object of value; (g) concentration deficit may be evident on clinical testing.
4 Moderate cognitive decline
+ Late confusional
+ Clear-cut deficit on careful clinical interview. Deficit manifested in following areas: (a) decreased knowledge of current and recent events; (b) possibly some deficit in memory of one's personal history; (c) concentration deficit elicited on serial substractions; (d) decreased ability to travel, handle finances, etc.
++ Frequently, no deficit in following areas: (a) orientation to time and person; (b) recognition of familiar persons and faces; (c) ability to travel to familiar locations.
++ Inability to perform complex tasks. Denial is dominant defense mechanism. Flattening of affect and withdrawal from challenging situations occur.
5 Moderately severe cognitive decline
+ Early dementia
+ Patients can no longer survive without some assistance. Patients are unable during interview to recall a major relevant aspect of their current lives: e.g., their address or telephone number of many years, the names of close member of their family, the name of the high school or college from which they graduated.
++ Frequently some disorientation to time (date, day of week, season, etc.) or to place. An educated person may have difficulty counting back from 40 by 4s or from 20 by 2s.
++ Persons at this stage retain knowledge of many major facts regarding themselves and others. They invariably know the name of their significant others. They require no assistance with toileting or eating, but may have some difficulty choosing the proper clothing to wear.
6 Severe cognitive decline
+ Middle dementia
+ May occasionally forget the name of significant others upon whom they are entirely dependent for survival. Will be largely unaware of recent events and experiences in their lives. Retain some knowledge of their past lives, but this is very sketchy. Generally aware of their surrounding, the year, the season, etc. May have difficulty counting backward from 10, and sometimes forward. Will require some assistance with activities of daily living, e.g., may become incontinent, will require travel assistance but occasionally will display ability to travel to familiar locations. Diurnal rhythm frequently disturbed. Almost always recall their own name. Frequently continue to be able to distinguish familiar from unfamiliar persons in their environment.
++ Personality and emotional changes occur. These are quite variable and include: (a) delusional behavior, e.g., patients may accuse their significant others of being an impostor, may talk to imaginary figures in the environment or to their own reflection in the mirror; (b) obsessive symptoms, e.g., person may continually repeat simple cleaning activities; (c) anxiety symptoms, agitation, and even previously nonexistent violent behavior may occur; (d) cognitive abulia, i.e., loss of will power because and individual cannot carry a thought long enough to determine a purposeful course of action.
7 Very severe cognitive decline
+ Late dementia
+ All verbal abilities are lost. Frequently, there is no speech at all, only grunting. Incontinent of urine; requires assistance toileting and feeding. Loses basic psychomotor skills, e.g., ability to walk. The brain appears no longer to be able to tell the body what to do.
++ Generalized and cortical neurologic signs and symptoms.

Source: Adapted from Reisberg B, Ferris SH, de Leon MJ, et al. The global deterioration scale (GDS): an instrument for the assessment of primary degenerative dementia (PDD). *Am J Psychiatry* 1982;139:1136–1139.

been described in HIV-1 seropositive asymptomatic patients and in patients with minor cognitive motor complex. There was no difference, however, between these patients and a control group when patients were at rest (104). Single-photon emission computed tomography (SPECT) has shown cortical and subcortical perfusion defects in the early phases of the HIV-1–related cognitive impairment that became more pronounced in the later stages (105–107). PET and SPECT are more sensitive than CT and MRI in detecting early changes in asymptomatic patients and may even detect changes before cognitive impairment is apparent in neuropsychological testing (103–107). The therapeutic effects of antiviral treatment monitored by PET shows reversal of the previously described abnormalities in glucose metabolism after treatment of the HIV-1–associated cognitive/motor complex with zidovudine (101). This improvement correlates with neurologic improvement and possible recovery of relevant neuropsychological functioning after treatment with zidovudine.

Magnetic resonance spectroscopy (MRS) has sensitivity in detecting early changes among patients with HIV-associated minor cognitive motor complex (HMCMC). It differentiates them from seropositive asymptomatic patients and from those with more advanced HIV-associated dementia (108–113). Frontal white matter changes are an early sign of HMCMC, whereas basal ganglia and frontal cortex abnormalities are also found in patients with HAD (108). MRS is the most useful imaging study in evaluating brain injury in early HMCMC (109), and it may also have a role in monitoring response to treatment in HAD (112,113).

Electrophysiology

The role of electrophysiology in cognitive and neurologic conditions is a key factor in early detection and understanding of these conditions. The percentage of patients with abnormal electroencephalograms appears to increase as the systemic disease progresses and a low amplitude pattern may be found in advanced dementia and atrophy on CT scan (114). In asymptomatic patients, studies have found conflicting results, with some finding no abnormalities in asymptomatic patients (115), and others finding frontotemporal theta slowing as a predominant finding (116). Computerized electroencephalography may be more sensitive in the detection of early changes and may predict subsequent development of HIV-1–related neurologic disease (116).

Evoked potential studies have also been useful in detecting abnormalities in neurologically and physically asymptomatic HIV-1 seropositive patients (117,118). When compared with controls, these patients showed significant delays in latency of response to the brainstem auditory evoked potential, somatosensory evoked potentials from tibial nerve stimulation, and visual evoked potentials. Thus, evoked potentials may represent a preliminary direct indicator of neurologic involvement in HIV-1 disease, even before the HIV-1–associated cognitive/motor complex becomes clinically apparent.

Cerebrospinal Fluid Studies

The CSF reflects changes consistent with HIV-1 infection, including HIV-1 virions, abnormally elevated IgG levels, HIV-1–specific antibodies, mononuclear cells, and oligoclonal bands (6,119–125). HIV-1 replicates in the brain with independent dynamics from other organs. Therefore, the CSF viral load is specific for the assessment of the severity of the infection in the CNS. It also correlates with the degree of neurocognitive dysfunction and has a role in monitoring the response to antiretroviral medications in the CNS (126–134)HIHjl. Although other CSF studies have been used in the assessment of CNS compromise in HIV-1 infection, their use is now limited because viral load measurements have replaced them in clinical practice. CSF β_2-microglobulin has shown a high correlation between its concentration and both the severity of the dementia and the level of systemic disease (121,122). Although elevation in the myelin basic protein (MBP) and its degradation was found in patients with HIV-1–associated cognitive/motor complex and with PML, this was not seen in patients with other opportunistic infections (135). An abnormally low CD4+:CD8+ ratio that was found in the CSF, which preceded the one in blood (136), may have importance for treatment considerations.

TREATMENT OF HIV-1 CENTRAL NERVOUS SYSTEM INFECTION

Brain infection is the most common cause of cognitive impairment for any person suffering with HIV-1 infection. Most of the histopathologic changes and HIV-1 viral antigens are localized in subcortical areas (7,8), similar to the predominant clinical presentation of the HIV-1–associated cognitive/motor complex (137,138). Because these studies so clearly implicate direct HIV-1 brain infections, the rationale for treating the HIV-1–associated cognitive/motor complex with antiviral agents appears obvious. Given that the CNS can serve as a sanctuary for HIV-1 itself, further rationale exists for the antiviral approach to treatment. Antiviral medication that penetrates the blood–brain barrier and blood–CSF barrier is clearly necessary.

Various drugs that are effective against HIV-1 are approved by the Food and Drug Administration for clinical use (139,140). The most widely used drug and the initial drug of choice for patients who have not received any prior anti–HIV-1 therapy is zidovudine (AZT). *In vitro* results of its capacity to inhibit retroviral replication have been confirmed in human studies that indicate that AZT is effective in reducing the morbidity and mortality of AIDS patients and of asymptomatic patients with less than 500 CD4 cells/mm^3 (141), although not of those with more than 500 CD4 cells/mm (142). It is also suggested that therapy with AZT during the primary infection may improve the subsequent clinical course and increase the CD4 cell count (143). Further studies show that AZT improves cognitive functioning among patients with minor cognitive changes who are otherwise asymptomatic (144) and reduces the neurocognitive deficits when used long-term, therefore reducing the risk of HIV-1-associated dementia (145,146). The optimal dose of AZT for the treatment of cognitive impairment is not known. Although systematic evaluation of low doses in the treatment of HIV-1 dementia has not been completed, low doses of 300 mg per day are associated with improvement in cognitive function tests. Experimental data show that AZT penetrates the brain at a level half of which can be recovered from CSF (147). Furthermore, the findings of Sidtis and colleagues that significant gains in cognition in HIV-1–demented patients occurred with AZT doses of 2,000 mg per day (148) are consistent with this brain parenchymal bioavailability characteristic. Doses of 1,500 mg per day failed to improve neuropsychologic functioning among mildly asymptomatic individuals and it is considered to be beneficial only as prophylactic treatment in this population (149). Another nucleoside, didanosine (ddI), is now used in the treatment of AIDS. Although it failed to prevent progression to HAD at both high and low doses (150), it improved cognition in children with AIDS (151). When combined with AZT, it prevented the progression to HIV encephalopathy better than AZT alone (152). Zalcitabine (ddC) in combination with AZT was effective in reversing cognitive dysfunction in patients who developed abnormalities with treatment with AZT alone (153). Lamivudine (3TC) combined with AZT and lamivudine combined with stavudine (D4T) were equally effective in reducing CSF viral load (154). Among the protease inhibitors, ritonavir was detected in one-third of the patients taking it (155), while lopinavir, amprenavir, saquinavir, and nelfinavir are not detectable in the CSF (155–159). However, CSF viral load suppression was achieved with nelfinavir and saquinavir in combination with ritonavir with and without D4T (160). Protease inhibitors in combination therapy have improved neurocognitive function in patients with dementia (161).

NEUROPSYCHIATRIC SYMPTOMATOLOGY OF HIV-1 INFECTION

Mental disorders secondary to medical conditions such as delirium, dementia, mood disorders, and anxiety disorders are the most common neuropsychiatric conditions associated with HIV-1 infection (162,163). Personality changes with significant variation in the Minnesota Multiphasic Personality Inventory (MMPI) (164), psychotic disorders caused by general medical condition, and substance-induced disorders may also be seen. One of the most perplexing aspects of these presentations is that HIV-1–related neuropsychiatric manifestations so closely resemble other primary psychiatric (functional) disorders. Like syphilis, HIV-1 infection often confounds precise diagnostic criteria because of its characteristic as a "great imitator."

Delirium

Delirium is the most common mental disorder observed in general medical conditions associated with HIV-1 infection. It is estimated that as many as 30% of hospitalized medical/surgical patients may have an undetected delirium process (165). Delirium is also a predictor of outcome in hospitalized AIDS patients. Delirious patients have a higher mortality rate, longer hospitalizations, and greater need for long-term care when discharged alive, as compared to a group of nondelirious AIDS patients with similar demographics and markers of medical morbidity (166). Delirium may also be the most frequently undiagnosed of all organic disorders in the outpatient setting. As the treatment of most HIV-1 complications has become more sophisticated, it has also become simpler. Patients are treated more aggressively in either an ambulatory clinic (such as cancer chemotherapy settings) or at home with infusion therapy for infections and malignancies associated with HIV-1 infection. Undiagnosed delirium in the ambulatory setting poses a particular danger because of the lost opportunity to diagnose and treat a potentially reversible complication of a medical disorder.

Delirium reflects diffuse cerebral cellular metabolic dysfunction (167). A common prodromal phase involves patients' complaints of difficulty in thinking, restlessness, irritability, insomnia, or interrupted short periods of sleep containing vivid nightmares. Evidence of this prodromal phase should be regarded seriously and should generate a search for the underlying cause of the delirium process. A brief mental status examination should focus on arousal, attention, short-term memory, and orientation. Diurnal variations in the delirium process are common, with symptoms typically worsening at night. Motor abnormalities, including tremor, picking at clothing, multifocal myoclonus, and asterixis can also be found.

There are diverse suggestions for the etiology of HIV-1–related delirium (165,168). However, it is important to attempt to determine the particular etiology for each individual patient because certain frequent causes are life-threatening or may lead to permanent brain damage. These conditions include Wernicke encephalopathy, hypoglycemia, hyperglycemia, hypoxemia, hemodynamic instability with cerebral hypoperfusion, infections, metabolic disturbances, and electrolyte imbalances (165). Herpes and *Toxoplasma gondii* encephalitis, cryptococcal meningitis, space-occupying lesions from cerebral tumors, progressive multifocal leukoencephalopathy, and neurotoxicities from antiviral agents should also be included in the differential diagnosis of delirium in HIV-1 patients (165). In the substance-abuse population, the detection of alcohol and nonalcohol intoxication or withdrawal is extremely important in the differential diagnostic considerations for the etiology of delirium in HIV-1 disease.

Prompt pharmacologic interventions may help remediate the various behavioral abnormalities associated with the delirium process. High-potency neuroleptics may be used prudently for the control of delirium in HIV-1–infected patients (168–173). Haloperidol, especially by oral or intramuscular administration, has been successful in the management of delirium in HIV-1–infected patients, but not without significant treatment-emergent side effects. At low doses, haloperidol and chlorpromazine (a low-potency neuroleptic) have been used effectively and with few side effects in the treatment of delirium in hospitalized AIDS patients (174).

Intravenous haloperidol, either alone or in combination with lorazepam and hydromorphone or buprenorphine, appears to be both safe and effective for use with agitated delirious HIV-1–infected patients (171–175). A continuous intravenous infusion of haloperidol may be considered in order to achieve full control of refractory cases of delirium associated with severe agitation, as has been described for cancer patients (173). Although the possibility of treatment-related adverse effects, even with intravenous neuroleptics (176–179), must be weighed against the dangers of the delirium, the use of intravenous haloperidol, either alone or in combination with other agents, can be safe and effective. Although intravenous haloperidol is not specifically approved by the Food and Drug Administration (FDA), it can be approved for compassionate use with permission from one's institutional review board or hospital pharmacy committee.

Molindone has also been reported as an safe and efficacious alternative for the treatment of delirious patients who can take oral medications and are sensitive to the side effects of high-potency neuroleptics (180). Atypical antipsychotics are used now in the treatment of delirium (181). They are effective and well tolerated, with less emergence of extrapyramidal side effects when compared to traditional neuroleptics (182–186). The experience, however, is still limited, especially in HIV-1–infected individuals, and they must be used with caution.

Lorazepam is useful in the management of agitated delirious HIV-1 infected patients when used in combination with haloperidol. Lorazepam alone, however, appears to be ineffective and is associated with treatment-limiting side effects (174).

Because HIV-1–infected patients are often more sensitive to neuroleptics, a lower dose than that administered to other medically ill delirious patients (168) may accomplish the desired clinical effects while limiting side effects. However, in cases where there is an imperative and urgent need to control severe agitation that threatens the patient's or the medical staff's well-being, high doses of intravenous neuroleptics may be warranted. Extrapyramidal side effects are significantly more frequent if the patient

has delirium with a coexisting organic mental disorder (168). Intravenous neuroleptic therapy has not been reported to aggravate concurrent seizure cases. Likewise, intravenous haloperidol did not worsen the hemodynamic state of delirious HIV-1–infected patients when they were not hypovolemic at the initiation of therapy (168). Moreover, no instances of neuroleptic malignant syndrome have been reported with the intravenous route of administration as opposed to others (179).

Dementia

Among the neuropsychiatric complications of HIV-1 infection, dementia is commonly seen. It is characterized as an acquired intellectual impairment resulting in persistent deficits in many areas, including memory, language, cognition, visuospatial skills, personality, or emotional functioning. Dementia differs from delirium in that its related deficits persist over time. Table 59.6 lists the formal evaluation of an HIV-1 demented patient. HIV-1–associated cognitive disorders involve a subcortical degenerative or dementing process, and it is estimated that approximately 70% of HIV-1–infected persons will develop an organic cognitive or mental disorder sometime during the course of their illness. Basic functions such as alertness, arousal, memory, and normal rates of information processing are impaired by HIV-1 involvement of the white matter in the CNS. Thus, HIV-1–associated dementia is characterized as a "subcortical" dementing process (138). Symptoms closely associated with subcortical disorders, such as Parkinson disease, progressive supranuclear palsy, and multiple sclerosis, are also seen with HIV-1 central nervous system involvement and the HIV-1–associated cognitive/motor complex. In the early stages, neuropsychological tests for HIV-1 cognitive impairment should reflect memory registration, storage, and retrieval; psychomotor speed; information processing rate; and fine motor function. These tests reflect the characterization of HIV-1 cognitive impairment as a subcortical process (138,162). In the later stages of HIV-1 disease, other traditionally cortical syndromes such as aphasia, agnosia, apraxia, and other sensory–perceptual functions are also manifested, perhaps as a result of some focal opportunistic infection or neoplastic invasion of the CNS or HIV-1 infection itself.

Table 59.7 lists the diagnostic criteria for the HIV-1-associated minor cognitive/motor disorder that manifest early in the course of the HIV-1 infection. Because the early signs of cognitive impairment are often mild, they often go undiagnosed or misdiagnosed as a systemic or psychosocial reaction to HIV-1 infection. Complaints such as forgetfulness, inattention, and difficulty concentrating, mental slowing, and loss of interest or pleasure in everyday activities often may be misinterpreted as an understandable reaction to having contracted the very frequently fatal HIV-1 disease. Many patients will be able

TABLE 59.6. *Evaluation of dementia in HIV disease*

History
GDS Stage[a]
+ Clinical Stage
1
+ Normal—no cognitive decline
2
+ Forgetfulness—subjective complaints
3
+ Early confusional—mild cognitive decline
4
+ Late confusional—moderate cognitive decline
5
+ Early dementia—moderately severe cognitive decline
6
+ Middle dementia—severe cognitive decline
7
+ Late dementia—global deterioration
Physical and neurologic examination (for the psychiatrist)
(1)
+ State of consciousness—level, variability
(2)
+ Pattern of breathing
(3)
+ Size and reactivity of pupils
(4)
+ Eye movements and vestibular response
(5)
+ Motor responses (including psychomotor)
Psychiatric (mental status)
(1)
+ Cognitive—attention, concentration, memory, abstraction
(2)
+ Affective—apathy, irritability, startle, lability
(3)
+ Perceptual—hypersensitivity, illusions, hallucinations
(4)
+ Physiologic—sleep–wake, headache, weakness
(5)
+ Behavioral—impulsivity, tact, activities of daily living
Clinical laboratory assessment
Complete blood count (CBC)[b]
+ Urinalysis[b]
Blood urea nitrogen (BUN), creatinine[b]
+ Blood gases[b]
Fasting blood sugar (FBS)[b]
+ Computed tomography(CT) scan—brain[b]
Venereal Disease Research Laboratory (VDRL)[b]
+ Chest x-ray[b]
Cytomegalovirus (CMV), Epstein-Barrvirus (EBV), *Toxoplasma*,
+ Liver enzymes, bilirubin, ammonia[b]
Candida, herpes, and
+ Ca, P, alkaline phosphatase[b]
Cryptococcal serologies[b]
+ T$_4$, T$_3$ uptake, thyroid-stimulating hormone (TSH)
Electrolytes[b]
+ Electroencephalogram[b]
Liver function tests[b]

TABLE 59.6. *(Continued)*

+ Cerebrospinal fluid (CSF)[b]
Vitamin B$_{12}$, folate
+ Magnesium, zinc
Serum cortisol levels[b]
+ Toxic screen

[a]Global Deterioration Scale from Reisberg B, Ferris SH, de Leon MJ, et al. The global deterioration scale (GDS): an instrument for the assessment of primary degenerative dementia (PDD). *Am J Psychiatry* 1982;139:1136–1139.
[b]Recommended battery for HIV.
Source: Adapted from Fernandez F, Levy JK. Adjuvant treatment of HIV dementia with psychostimulants. In: Ostrow D, ed. *Behavioral aspects of AIDS and other sexually transmitted diseases.* New York: Plenum Publishing, 1990:279–286.

to recognize and report their own mental, physical, and mood symptoms, even with the cognitive impairment of early HIV-1 disease. Table 59.8 lists the diagnostic criteria for the HIV-1-associated cognitive/motor complex encountered late in the course of the dementia. Moderate to severe cognitive deficits, confusion, psychomotor slowing, and seizures may develop as the course of the dementia advances. Patients may appear mute and catatonic. Socially inappropriate behavior, psychosis, mania, and marked motor abnormalities, including ataxia, spasticity, hyperreflexia, hypertonia, and incontinence of bladder and bowel can occur.

Besides antiviral therapy to recover and prevent cognitive decline associated with HIV-1 infection, improvement of affective and cognitive symptoms have been described with the use of methylphenidate in doses ranging from 10 to 90 mg per day in divided doses (187,188). Medications that prevent the toxicity caused by the HIV-1 through the NMDA receptor are currently under investigation. They include calcium-channel blockers, such as nimodipine or nifedipine, and NMDA-receptor antagonists, such as memantine and nitroglycerin (189). Memantine is clinically used in Europe for the treatment of dementia, and is under investigation for FDA approval (190).

Mood Disorders

Mood disorders associated with HIV-1 infection are most frequently depressive, but manic and hypomanic disturbances have also been described (191,192). Close to 85% of HIV-1–seropositive individuals will exhibit some evidence of mood disturbance (193). The diagnostic process for evaluating mood disorders is complex, requiring careful consideration of the interaction of medical conditions, substances, and behavioral factors. A reliable diagnosis ensures that prompt and effective therapeutic intervention will be undertaken.

Depression is commonly observed in patients with HIV-1–related disorders. A wide spectrum of mood disorders may be classified as depression. Patients may report mood

TABLE 59.7. *Criteria for clinical diagnosis of HIV-1–associated minor cognitive/motor disorder*

1. Cognitive/motor/behavioral abnormalities (each of the following)
   a. At least two of the following present for at least 1 month
      (1) Impaired attention or concentration
      (2) Mental slowing
      (3) Impaired memory
      (4) Slowed movements
      (5) Incoordination
      (6) Personality change, irritability or emotional lability
   b. Acquired cognitive/motor abnormality verified by clinical neurologic examination or neuropsychological testing (e.g., fine motor speed, manual dexterity, perceptual motor skills, attention/concentration, speed of processing information, abstraction/reasoning, visuospatial skills, memory/learning, or speech/language).
2. Disturbance from # 1 causes mild impairment of work or activities of daily living.
3. Does not meet criteria for HIV-1–associated dementia complex or HIV-1–associated myelopathy (see Table 59.7).
4. No evidence of another etiology, including active CNS opportunistic infection or malignancy, severe systemic illness, active alcohol or substance use, acute or chronic substance withdrawal, adjustment disorder, or other psychiatric disorders.
5. HIV seropositivity (enzyme-linked immunoabsorbent assay [ELISA] test confirmed by Western blot, polymerase chain reaction, or culture).

Source: Adapted from Janssen RS, Saykin AJ, Cannon L, et al. American Academy of Neurology AIDS Task Force. Nomenclature and research case definitions for neurologic manifestations of human immunodeficiency virus-type-1 (HIV-1) infection. *Neurology* 1991;41:778–785.

TABLE 59.8. *Criteria for clinical diagnosis of HIV-1–associated cognitive/motor complex*

A. HIV-1–associated dementia complex
Each of the following:
1. Acquired abnormality in at least two of the following cognitive abilities for at least 1 month: attention/concentration, speed of processing information, abstraction/reasoning, visuospatial skills, memory/learning, and speech/language.
   Cognitive dysfunction causing impairment of work or activities of daily living, should no be attributable solely to severe systemic illness.
2. At least 1 of the following:
   (a) Acquired abnormality in motor function or performance verified by clinical examination, neuropsychological testing, or both.
   (b) Decline in motivation or emotional control, or change in social behavior.
3. Absence of clouding of consciousness during a period long enough to establish the presence of # 1.
4. No evidence of another etiology, including active CNS opportunistic infection or malignancy, other psychiatric disorders (e.g., depression), active alcohol or substance use, or acute or chronic substance withdrawal.
5. HIV seropositivity (enzyme-linked immunoabsorbent assay [ELISA] test confirmed by Western blot, polymerase chain reaction, or culture).
B. HIV-1–associated myelopathy
Each of the following:
1. Acquired abnormality in lower-extremity neurologic function disproportionate to upper-extremity abnormality verified by reliable history and neurologic examination.
2. Myelopathic disturbance is severe enough to require constant unilateral support for walking.
3. Criteria for HIV-1–associated dementia complex are not fulfilled.
4. No evidence of another etiology, including neoplasm, compressive lesion, or multiple sclerosis.
5. HIV seropositivity (ELISA test confirmed by Western blot, polymerase chain reaction, or culture).

Source: Adapted from Janssen RS, Saykin AJ, Cannon L, et al. American Academy of Neurology AIDS Task Force. Nomenclature and research case definitions for neurologic manifestations of human immunodeficiency virus-type-1 (HIV-1) infection. *Neurology* 1991;41:778–785.

disturbances that range from normal sadness to major affective disorder, as well as mood disorders that may be substance induced or a consequence of a general medical condition. It is very difficult, therefore, to arrive at a universally appropriate description of HIV-1–related depression. Formulating an accurate diagnosis of depression in HIV-1 disease is so difficult because many of the usual diagnostic indicators of depression are also common to both HIV-1 systemic disease and to HIV-1–related neurologic impairment (194). Although it has been suggested that clinicians rely on psychological rather than somatic symptoms of depression to fulfill diagnostic criteria for depression in the medically ill (195), an all-inclusive approach is often the simplest and most clinically effective. If all symptoms are counted toward a diagnosis of depression (regardless of the etiology), then symptoms of questionable physical or psychological origin will nonetheless be considered valid diagnostic indicators. Depression in all medically ill pa-

tients is both underdiagnosed and undertreated (196). This is particularly true of HIV-1–infected persons who suffer an increased incidence of depression when compared with other medically ill patients or the general population. This correlation has led some researchers to postulate that there are certain features of HIV-1 infection that contribute to a depressive syndrome.

Suicidal thoughts are almost always a symptom of depression and patients need to be assessed carefully. Definite risk factors include social isolation, perceived lack of social support, adjustment disorder, personality disorder, alcohol abuse, HIV-1–related interpersonal or occupational problems, and a past history of depression. Possible risk factors include current major depression, previous suicide attempt, and history of alcohol abuse (197). One should never blithely consider the notion of "rational suicide" (198) as an understandable reaction to their devastating and socially stigmatized disease. Because of impaired decision-making capacities and likely cognitive inefficiencies associated with HIV-1 disease, it is vital that clinicians respond promptly to any and all reports of suicidal ideation. A thorough assessment of the patient includes a realistic appraisal of the psychosocial situation and of the motivation for completing the suicide, along with a comprehensive neurodiagnostic assessment to rule out a potentially reversible organic mental disorder.

Still today, the treatment of depressed HIV-1–infected patients often comes down to a matter of the clinician's intuition being based on the clinician's own relevant clinical experience. The area of pharmacotherapy, in particular, lends itself to individual interpretation of risk and benefit for any given treatment regimen. The specific choice of medication and dose should draw from the physician's knowledge of the pharmacologic side effects of antidepressants (199) and take into consideration the unusual vulnerability of HIV-1–infected patients with respect to their likely excessive disability from drug therapy. One such consideration is that antidepressants with greater affinity for the central muscarinic receptor should be avoided for symptomatic HIV-1–infected patients because of their anticholinergic effects, which can mask or aggravate HIV-1–related cognitive impairment or precipitate delirium. Another adverse side effect of these agents is the possibility of excessive drying of the mucous membranes, which introduces the possibility of oral candidiasis that is often refractory to treatment in HIV-1–infected patients. Antidepressants that are preferable for HIV-1–infected individuals are the tricyclic antidepressants with low anticholinergic affinity, second-generation antidepressants, such as the serotonin selective reuptake inhibitors (SSRIs), bupropion, venlafaxine, nefazodone, mirtazapine, and the psychomotor stimulants.

Generally, the tricyclic antidepressants are chosen to initiate pharmacotherapy with asymptomatic HIV-1–infected patients (200). That is to say, patients who are not medically or immunologically compromised are the best candidates for this form of therapy. Beginning with a low dose of 10 to 25 mg at bedtime, the dose is then increased by 10 to 25 mg every 1 to 2 days until symptom response is achieved. The physician should always keep in mind that, as with other medically ill patients, it is quite common for depressed HIV-1–infected patients to show a positive therapeutic response to a tricyclic antidepressant at much lower doses, ranging from 25 to 100 mg, than the ones usually required in otherwise healthy, depressed patients.

After this response is achieved, pharmacotherapy is continued at this optimal dose for an additional 4 to 6 months, after which time the dose is gradually lowered until finally it is discontinued. Having noted the preference for tricyclic antidepressants in asymptomatic HIV-1–infected patients, the question arises as to which particular tricyclic agent might be used for the most successful outcome. As with other medically ill patients (201), the tricyclic antidepressants with sedating effects, such as amitriptyline, trimipramine, imipramine, and doxepin, are beneficial to those depressed HIV-1–infected patients who suffer from agitation or severe insomnia. On the other hand, patients with psychomotor slowing benefit from the use of compounds that have the least-sedating effects, such as the secondary amines protriptyline and desipramine. Whenever an effective therapeutic response cannot be achieved, or when side effects have outweighed the benefits, a second-generation antidepressant can be tried. Fluoxetine may also be an effective alternative to some of the second-generation agents with varying antihistaminic and anticholinergic effects (200). Sertraline was also effective and well tolerated in a small sample (202), whereas fluvoxamine was effective but poorly tolerated because of its side effects (203). However, randomized placebo-controlled trials with larger samples are needed to confirm the efficacy and safety of sertraline, fluvoxamine, and paroxetine in the HIV-1 population. Bupropion (200,204) has an activating effect that may be useful for withdrawn or anhedonic HIV-1–infected patients. Thus, it may be an effective alternative to the use of psychostimulants if the clinician is appropriately cautious in administering bupropion to patients with significant CNS pathology and in whom an underlying seizure disorder may be precipitated or aggravated (200). Nefazodone may be useful in the HIV population because it improves sleep architecture and has a low incidence of side effects. However, protease inhibitors inhibit cytochrome P450, which may lead to the accumulation and toxicity of m-chlorophenylpiperazine, the metabolite of nefazodone. Doses less than or equal to 300 mg per day when combined with indinavir, and less or equal to 100 mg per day when combined with ritonavir, have been recommended (205). Regular doses should be used when combined with saquinavir or nelfinavir. Although venlafaxine is a good choice because of its low interactions with other drugs (206), a decrease of the plasma concentration of indinavir when coadministered with venlafaxine needs to be t considered to avoid underdosing and precipitating potential resistance to indinavir (207). There are no reports in the literature on the use of mirtazapine and escitalopram in the HIV-1–infected population. In cases in which the patient is unable to take oral medication, intravenous administration of amitriptyline and imipramine is effective (208,209). Despite the fact that the Food and Drug Administration has not yet approved the intravenous use of antidepressants, investigational use of these agents has had safe and effective results. In many instances, it would be prudent to seek approval for the compassionate use of intravenous antidepressants through one's pharmacy or institutional review board. The principal drawback of this practice is that in medically ill HIV-1–infected patients, intravenously administered imipramine and amitriptyline can increase the risk of hypotensive crisis and anticholinergic delirium. Therefore, it is advisable to begin using the lowest dose possible and infusing it slowly and precisely over 90 minutes (210).

Patients who are being treated with lithium carbonate or monoamine oxidase inhibitors prior to their diagnosis with HIV-1 disease usually should continue to take that medication. Increased vigilance in toxicity monitoring with a concomitant dosage alteration may be necessary as HIV-1 disease progresses (211), especially when infectious complications cause severe diarrhea or any other form of fluid loss, because rapid nephrotoxicity and neurotoxicity may ensue. Manic symptoms secondary to zidovudine (212,213), didanosine (214), ganciclovir, or antidepressants (192) may also respond to lithium. Likewise, monoamine oxidase inhibitors may be continued for patients who had depression prior to their diagnosis with HIV-1 disease and who previously responded well to these agents. However, it is usually wise to treat a depression that arises after HIV-1 seropositivity with agents other than monoamine oxidase inhibitors because the associated dietary restriction of tyramine-containing foods may exacerbate the nutritional problems associated with advanced HIV-1 disease. Additionally, monoamine oxidase inhibitors are theoretically incompatible with zidovudine therapy, which is reported to have catechol-*O*-methyltransferase inhibiting effects (200).

Psychostimulants such as methylphenidate and dextroamphetamine may be tried (188,215–217) with depressed patients who are symptomatic of HIV-1 infection, with those depressed patients in whom tricyclic antidepressants are contraindicated or have proved ineffective, and, especially, with those depressed patients who are cognitively impaired or who suffer from both depression and dementia. Methylphenidate is a very safe and effective treatment for depression. Response usually occurs within hours of the first administration, providing psychomotor activation, appetite stimulation, and qualitative, as well as quantitative, improvement in higher cortical functions. The initial administration of methylphenidate is usually 5 to 10 mg by mouth, feeding tube, or suppository. Its equivalent dose in dextroamphetamine could also be used. After gradually raising the dose to 20 mg or less three times a day, a favorable response is usually achieved. Adequate therapeutic response usually takes less than 30 mg daily (although in unusual circumstances, up to 90 mg a day may be required). These stimulants are useful in treating depression from various etiologies and can be continued safely up to several months after the patient's symptoms remit. Special care should be taken in using dextroamphetamine, which has been noted to unmask or aggravate abnormal involuntary movements in AIDS dementia patients (216). The use of psychostimulants in managing depressive or cognitive symptomatology in drug-abusing patients is questionable. Further research is needed in this subgroup of patients to establish the place for psychostimulant use in the management of depressed or cognitively impaired drug-abusing HIV-1 patients with advanced disease.

SUMMARY

HIV-1 infection is a major health and social issue of our time, with drug abuse, unprotected sexual intercourse, and transfusion of contaminated products being well-determined risk factors. As the prevalence of HIV-1 infection continues to increase, advances in treatments permit the prognosis to improve. Neuropsychiatric complications are now accurately diagnosed more often and our understanding of their etiologies and effective treatment regimens continues to improve. Signs of neuropsychiatric disorders are now detected earlier, allowing prompt and aggressive management of these potentially devastating complications of the HIV-1 infection. The overall prognosis for these patients at the moment of seroconversion continues to improve, along with the quality of their lives. The contribution of neuropsychiatry is of great importance as we pay attention to the neurobehavioral aspects of HIV-1 disease in these individuals.

REFERENCES

1. UNAIDS. R*eport on global HIV/AIDS epidemic: "the Bangkok report."* XV International conference on AIDS. Barcelona, 11–16 July 2004:4th.
2. Centers for Disease Control and Prevention. HIV/AIDS surveillance report. *MMWR Morb Mortal Wkly Rep* 2002;14(2):1–48.
3. Selik RM, Chu SY, Bueler JW. HIV infection as leading cause of death among young adults in U.S. cities and states. *JAMA* 1993;269(26):2991–2994.
4. Minimo AM, Smith BL. Deaths: preliminary data for 2000. *Natl Vital Stat Rep* 2001;49(12):25–26.
5. Buehler JW, Petersen LR, Jaffe HW. Current trends in the epidemiology of HIV/AIDS. In: Sande MA, Volberding PA, eds. *The medical management of AIDS*, 4th ed. Philadelphia: WB Saunders, 1995:3–21.
6. Ostrow AG. Substance abuse and HIV infection. *Psychiatr Clin North Am* 1994;17(1):69–89.
7. Seage GR, Mayer KH, Horsbugh CR, et al. The relation between nitrite inhalants, unprotected receptive anal intercourse and the risk of HIV infection. *Am J Epidemiol* 1992;135:1–11.
8. Koeing S, Gendelman HE, Orenstein JM, et al. Detection of AIDS virus in macrophages in brain tissue from AIDS with encephalopathy. *Science* 1986;233:1089–1093.
9. Schrager LK, D'Souza MP. Cellular and anatomical reservoirs of HIV-1 in patients receiving potent antiretroviral combination therapy. *JAMA* 1998;280:67–71.

10. Falangola MF, Hanly A, Galvao-Castro B, et al. HIV infection of human choroid plexus: a possible mechanism of viral entry into the CNS. *J Neuropathol Exp Neurol* 1995;54(4):497–503.

11. Wiley CA. Pathology of neurologic disease in AIDS. *Psychiatr Clin North Am* 1994;17(1):1–15.

12. Shaw GM, Harper ME, Hahn BH, et al. HTLV-III infection in brains of children and adults with AIDS encephalopathy. *Science* 1985;227:177–182.

13. Gyorkey F, Melnick JL, Gyorkey P. Human immunodeficiency virus in brain biopsies of patients with AIDS and progressive encephalopathy. *J Infect Dis* 1987;155:870–876.

14. Hill JM, Farrar WL, Pert CB. Autoradiographic localization of T4 antigen, the HIV receptor in human brain. *Int J Neurosci* 1987;32:687–693.

15. Wiley CA, Masliah E, Morey M, et al. Neocortical damage during HIV infection. *Ann Neurol* 1991;29(6):651–657.

16. Aylward EH, Brettschneider PD, McArthur JC, et al. Magnetic resonance imaging measurement of gray matter volume reductions in HIV dementia. *Am J Psychiatry* 1995;152(7):987–994.

17. Tyor WR, Wesselingh SL, Griffin JW, et al. Unifying hypothesis for the pathogenesis of HIV-associated dementia complex, vacuolar myelopathy, and sensory neuropathy. *J Acquir Immune Defic Syndr Hum Retrovirol* 1995;9:379–388.

18. Ushijima H, Nishio O, Klocking R, et al. Exposure to gp 120 of HIV-1 induces an increased release of arachidonic acid in rat primary neuronal cell culture followed by NMDA receptor-mediated neurotoxicity. *Eur J Neurosci* 1995;7:1353–1359.

19. Codazzi F, Menegon A, Zacchetti D, et al. HIV-1 gp120 glycoprotein induces (Ca^{2+})i responses not only in type-2 but also type-1 astrocytes and oligodendrocytes of the rat cerebellum. *Eur J Neurosci* 1995;7:1333–1341.

20. New DR, Maggirwar SB, Epstein LG, et al. HIV-1 Tat induces neuronal death via tumor necrosis factor-alpha and activation of non-*N*-methyl-D-aspartate receptors by a NFkappaB-independent mechanism. *J Biol Chem* 1998;273:17852–17858.

21. Kruman II, Nath A, Mattson MP. HIV-1 protein Tat induces apoptosis of hippocampal neurons by a mechanism involving caspase activation, calcium overload, and oxidative stress. *Exp Neurol* 1998;154:276–288.

22. Baier-Bitterlich G, Fuchs D, Wachter H. Chronic immune stimulation, oxidative stress, and apoptosis in HIV infection. *Biochem Pharmacol* 1997;53:755–763.

23. Dursun SM, Reveley MA. Serotonin hypothesis of psychiatric disorders during HIV infection. *Med Hypothesis* 1995;44:263–267.

24. Shizuko S, Kuniaki S, Stewart SK, et al. Increased human immunodeficiency virus (HIV) type 1 DNA content and quinolinic acid concentration in brain tissues from patients with HIV encephalopathy. *J Infect Dis* 1995;172:638–647.

25. Lipton SA, Yeh M, Dreyer EB. Update on current models of HIV-related neuronal injury: platelet-activating factor, arachidonic acid and nitric oxide. *Adv Neruoimmunol* 1994;4:181–188.

26. Nath A, Padua RA, Geiger JD. HIV-1 coat protein gp 120-induced increases in levels of intrasynaptosomal calcium. *Brain Res* 1995;678:200–206.

27. Lipton SA. Memantine prevents HIV coat protein-induced neuronal injury *in vitro*. *Neurology* 1992;42:1403–1405.

28. Lipton SA. Ca^{2+}, *N*-methyl-D-aspartate receptors, and AIDS-related neuronal injury. *Int Rev Neurobiol* 1994;36:1–27.

29. Harbison MA, Kim S, Gillis JM, et al. Effect of the calcium channel blocker verapamil on human immunodeficiency virus type 1 replication in lymphoid cells. *J Infect Dis* 1991;164:53–60.

30. Navia BA, Dafni U, Simpson D, et al. A phase I/II trial of nimodipine for HIV-related neurologic complications. *Neurology* 1998;51:221–228.

31. Price RW, Brew BJ. The AIDS dementia complex. *J Infect Dis* 1988;158:1079–1083.

32. Janssen RS, Saykin AJ, Cannon L, et al. American Academy of Neurology AIDS Task Force. Nomenclature and research case definitions for neurologic manifestations of human immunodeficiency virus-type 1 (HIV-1) infection. *Neurology* 1991;41:778–785.

33. Everall I, Luthert P, Lantos P. A review of neuronal damage in human immunodeficiency virus infection: its assessment, possible mechanism and relationship to dementia. *J Neuropathol Exp Neurol* 1993;52:561–566.

34. Sharer LR. Pathology of HIV-1 infection of the central nervous system. A review. *J Neuropathol Exp Neurol* 1992;51:3–11.

35. Wiley CA, Achim C. Human immunodeficiency virus encephalitis is the pathological correlate of dementia in acquired immunodeficiency syndrome. *Ann Neurol* 1994;36:673–676.

36. Smith TW, DeGirolami U, Hénin D, et al. Human immunodeficiency virus (HIV) leukoencephalopathy and the microcirculation. *J Neuropathol Exp Neurol* 1990;49:357–370.

37. de la Monte SM, Ho DD, Schooley RT, et al. Subacute encephamyelitis of AIDS and its relation to HTLV-III infection. *Neurology* 1987;37:562–569.

38. Miller RG. Neuropathies and myopathies complicating HIV infection. *J Clin Apheresis* 1991;6:110–121.

39. Levy RL, Bredesen DE, Rosenblum ML. Neurological manifestation of the acquired immunodeficiency syndrome (AIDS): experience at UCSF and review of the literature. *J Neurosurg* 1985;62:475–495.

40. Cornblath DR, McArthur JC. Predominantly sensory neuropathy in patients with AIDS and AIDS-related complex. *Neurology* 1988;38:794–796.

41. Authier FJ, De Grissac N, Degos JD, et al. Transient myasthenia gravis during HIV infection. *Muscle Nerve* 1995;18(8):914–916.

42. Verma A. Epidemiology and clinical features of HIV-1 associated neuropathies. *J Peripher Nerv Syst* 2001;6(1):8–13.

43. Brew BJ. HIV-1-related neurological disease. *J Acquir Immune Defic Syndr* 1993;6[1 Suppl]):s10–s15.

44. Brew BJ. Central and peripheral nervous system abnormalities. *Med Clin North Am* 1992;76(1):63–81.

45. Krasner CG, Cohen SH. Bilateral Bell's palsy and aseptic meningitis in a patient with acute human immunodeficiency virus seroconversion. *West J Med* 1993;159(5):604–605.

46. Grimaldi LM, Luzi L, Martino GV, et al. Bilateral eight cranial nerve neuropathy in human immunodeficiency virus infection. *J Neurol* 1993;240(6):363–366.

47. Sweeney BJ, Manji H, Gilson RJ, et al. Optic neuritis and HIV-1 infection. *J Neurol Neurosurg Psychiatry* 1993;56(6):705–707.

48. Freeman R, Roberts M, Friedman LS, et al. Autonomic function and human immunodeficiency virus infection. *Neurology* 1990;40:575–580.

49. Craddock C, Pasvol G, Bull R, et al. Cardiorespiratory arrest and autonomic neuropathy in AIDS. *Lancet* 1987;2:16–18.

50. Price RW, Worley JM. Management of neurologic complications of HIV-1 infection and AIDS. In: Sande MA, Volberding PA, eds. *The medical management of AIDS,* 4th ed. Philadelphia: WB Saunders, 1995:261–288.

51. Maytal J, Horowitz S, Lipper S, et al. Progressive nemaline rod myopathy in a woman coinfected with HIV-1 and HTLV-2. *Mt Sinai J Med* 1993;60(3):242–246.

52. Seidman R, Peress NS, Nuovo GJ. In situ detection of polymerase chain reaction-amplified HIV-1 nucleic acids

in skeletal muscle in patients with myopathy. *Mod Pathol* 1994;7(3):369–375.

53. Bredesen DE, Levy RM, Rosenblum ML. The neurology of human immunodeficiency virus infection. *QJM* 1988;68:665–667.

54. Malouf R, Jacquette G, Dobkin J, et al. Neurologic disease in human immunodeficiency virus-infected drug abusers. *Arch Neurol* 1990;47:1002–1007.

55. Saag MS. Cryptococcosis and other fungal infections (histoplasmosis, coccidioidomycosis). In: Sande MA, Volberding PA, eds. *The medical management of AIDS,* 4th ed. Philadelphia: WB Saunders, 1995:437–459.

56. Moller A, Backmund H. CT findings in different stages of HIV infection: a prospective study. *J Neurol* 1990;237:94–97.

57. Mehren M, Burns PJ, Mamani MD, et al. Toxoplasmic myelitis mimicking intramedullary cord tumor. *Neurology* 1988;38:1648–1650.

58. Pedrol E, Gonzalez-Clemente J, Gatell JM, et al. Central nervous system toxoplasmosis in AIDS patients: efficacy of an intermittent maintenance therapy. *J Acquir Immune Defic Syndr* 1990;4:511–517.

59. Wong SY, Israelski DM, Remington JS. AIDS-associated toxoplasmosis. In: Sande MA, Volberding PA, eds. *The medical management of AIDS,* 4th ed. Philadelphia: WB Saunders, 1995:460–493.

60. Mallolas J, Zamora L, Gatell JM, et al. Primary prophylaxis for *Pneumocystis carinii* pneumonia: a randomized trial comparing cotrimoxazole, aerosolized pentamidine and dapsone, plus pyrimethamine. *J Acquir Immune Defic Syndr* 1993;7:59–64.

61. Saag MS, Powderly WG, Cloud GA, et al. Comparison of amphotericin B with fluconazole in the treatment of acute AIDS-associated cryptococcal meningitis. *N Engl J Med* 1992;326:83–89.

62. Stern JJ, Hartmen BJ, Sharkey P, et al. Oral fluconazole therapy for patients with acquired immunodeficiency syndrome and cryptococcal meningitis: experience with 22 patients. *Am J Med* 1988;85:477–480.

63. Berger JR, Kaszovitz B, Post MJ, et al. Progressive multifocal leukoencephalopathy associated with human immunodeficiency virus infection. A review of the literature with a report of sixteen cases. *Ann Intern Med* 1987;107:78–87.

64. Drew WL, Buhles W, Erlich KS. Management of herpes virus infection (CMV, HSV, VZV). In: Sande MA,

Volberding PA, eds. *The medical management of AIDS,* 4th ed. Philadelphia: WB Saunders, 1995:512–536.

65. Bolan G. Management of syphilis in HIV-infected persons. In: Sande MA, Volberding PA, eds. *The medical management of AIDS,* 4th ed. Philadelphia: WB Saunders, 1995:537–554.

66. Portegies P, Algra PR, Hollak CEM, et al. Response to cytarabine in progressive multifocal leukoencephalopathy in AIDS. *Lancet* 1991;1:680–681.

67. Hamilton-Dutoit SF, Pallesen G, Franzman MB, et al. AIDS-related lymphoma: histopathology, immunophenotype and association with Epstein-Barr virus as demonstrated by in situ nucleic acid hybridization. *Am J Pathol* 1991;138:147–163.

68. Kaplan LD, Abrams DI, Feigal E, et al. AIDS-associated non-Hodgkin lymphoma in San Francisco. *JAMA* 1989;261:719–724.

69. Kaplan LD, Northfelt DW. Malignancies associated with AIDS. In: Sande MA, Volberding PA, eds. *The medical management of AIDS,* 4th ed. Philadelphia: WB Saunders, 1995:555–590.

70. Engstrom JW, Lowenstein DH, Bredesen DE. Cerebral infarctions and transient neurologic deficits associated with acquired immunodeficiency syndrome. *Am J Med* 1989;86:528–532.

71. Frank Y, Lin W, Kahn E, et al. Multiple ischemic infarcts in a child with AIDS, varicella zoster infection, and cerebral vasculitis. *Pediatr Neurol* 1989;5:64–67.

72. Navia BA, Jordan BD Price RW. The AIDS dementia complex: I. Clinical features. *Ann Neurol* 1986;19:517–524.

73. Navia BA, Price RW. The acquired immunodeficiency syndrome dementia complex as the presenting or sole manifestation of human immunodeficiency virus infection. *Arch Neurol* 1987;44:65–69.

74. Grant I, Atkinson JH, Hesselink JR, et al. Evidence for early central nevous system involvement in the immunodeficiency syndrome (AIDS) and other human immunodeficiency virus (HIV) infections: studies with neuropsychological testing and magnetic resonance imaging. *Ann Intern Med* 1987;107:828–836.

75. Stern Y, Marder K, Bell K, et al. Multidisciplinary baseline assessment of homosexual men with and without human immunodeficiency virus infection. *Arch Gen Psychiatry* 1991;48:131–138.

76. Lunn S, Skydsbjerg M, Schulsinger H, et al. A preliminary report on the neuropsychologic sequelae of human immunodeficiency virus. *Arch Gen Psychiatry* 1991;48:139–142.

77. Heaton R, Kirson D, Velin RA, et al.

The utility of clinical ratings for detecting cognitive change in HIV infection. In: Grant I, Martin A, eds. *Neuropsychology of HIV infection.* Oxford University Press, New York, 1994:188–206.

78. Bornstein RA, Nasrallah HA, Para MF, et al. Neuropsychological performance in symptomatic and asymptomatic HIV infection. *J Acquir Immune Defic Syndr* 1993;7:519–524.

79. Wilkie FL, Morgan R, Fletcher MA, et al. Cognition and immune function in HIV-1 infection. *J Acquir Immune Defic Syndr* 1992;6:977–981.

80. Martin EM, Robertson LC, Edelstein HE, et al. Performance of patients with early HIV-1 infection on the Stroop Task. *J Clin Exp Neuropsychol* 1992;14:857–868.

81. Podraza AM, Bornstein RA, Whitacre CC, et al. Neuropsychological performance and CD4 levels in HIV-1 asymptomatic infection. *J Clin Exp Neuropsychol* 1994;16:777–783.

82. Beason-Hazen S, Nasrallah HA, Bornstein RA. Self-report of symptoms and neuropsychological performance in asymptomatic HIV-positive individuals. *J Neuropsychiatry Clin Neurosci* 1994;6:43–49.

83. Stern RA, Silva SG, Chaisson N, et al. Influence of cognitive reserve on neuropsychological functioning in asymptomatic human immunodeficiency virus-1 infection. *Arch Neurol* 1996;53:148–153.

84. Riccio M, Pugh K, Jadresic D, et al. Neuropsychiatric aspects of HIV-1 infection in gay men: controlled investigation of psychiatric, neuropsychological and neurological status. *J Psychosom Res* 1993;37:819–830.

85. Goethe KE, Mitchell JE, Marshall DW, et al. Neuropsychological and neurological function of human immunodeficiency virus seropositive asymptomatic individuals. *Arch Neurol* 1989;46:129–133.

86. Mayeux R, Stern Y, Tang M-X, et al. Mortality risks in gay men with human immunodeficiency virus infection and cognitive impairment. *Neurology* 1993;43:176–182.

87. Albert SM, Marder K, Dooneief G, et al. Neuropsychologic impairment in early HIV infection. *Arch Neurol* 1995;52:525–530.

88. Heaton RK, Velin RA, McCutchan JA, et al. Neuropsychological impairment in human immunodeficiency virus-infection: implications for employment. HNRC group. HIV neurobehavioral research center. *Psychosom Med* 1994;56:8–17.

89. Van Gorp WG, Miller E, Satz P, et al. Neuropsychological performance in

HIV-1 immunocompromised patients. *J Clin Exp Neuropsychol* 1989;11:35.

90. Selnes OA, Miller EN. Development of a screening battery for HIV-related cognitive impairment: the MACS experience. In: Grant I, Martin A, eds. *Neuropsychology of HIV infection.* Oxford University Press, New York, 1994:176–185.

91. Navia BA, Cho E-S, Petito CK, et al. The AIDS dementia complex: II. Neuropathology. *Ann Neurol* 1986;19:525–535.

92. Reisberg B, Ferris SH, de Leon MJ, et al. The global deterioration scale (GDS): an instrument for the assessment of primary degenerative dementia (PDD). *Am J Psychiatry* 1982;139:1136–1139.

93. Fernandez F, Levy JK. Adjuvant treatment of HIV dementia with psychostimulants. In: Ostrow D, ed. *Behavioral aspects of AIDS and other sexually transmitted diseases.* New York: Plenum Publishing, 1990:279–286.

94. Syndulko K, Singer EJ, Nogales-Gaete J, et al. Laboratory evaluations in HIV-1-associated cognitive/motor complex. *Psychiatr Clin North Am* 1994;17:91–123.

95. Chrysikopoulos HS, Press GA, Grafe MR, et al. Encephalitis caused by human immunodeficiency virus: CT and MRI manifestations with clinical and pathologic correlation. *Radiology* 1990;175:185–191.

96. Chamberlain MC. Pediatric AIDS: a longitudinal comparative MRI and CT brain imaging study. *J Child Neurol* 1993;8:175–181.

97. DeCarli C, Civitello LA, Brouwers P, et al. The prevalence of computed tomographic abnormalities of the cerebrum in 100 consecutive children symptomatic with the human immunodeficiency virus. *Ann Neurol* 1993;34:198–205.

98. Portegies P, Enting RH, de Gans J, et al. Presentation and course of AIDS dementia complex: 10 years of follow-up in Amsterdam, The Netherlands. *J Acquir Immune Defic Syndr* 1999;7:669–675.

99. Hestad K, McArthur JH, Dal Pan GJ, et al. Regional brain atrophy in HIV-1 infection: association with specific neuropsychological test performance. *Acta Neurol Scand* 1993;94:112–118.

100. Mundinger A, Adam T, Ott D, et al. CT and MRI: prognostic tools in patients with AIDS and neurological deficits. *Neuroradiology* 1998;35:75–78.

101. Brunetti A, Berg G, DiChiro G, et al. Reversal of brain metabolic abnormalities following treatment of AIDS dementia complex with 3'-azido-2',3'-dideoxythymidine (AZT, zidovudine): a PET-FDG study. *J Nucl Med* 1989;30:581–590.

102. van Gorp WG, Mandelkern MA, Gee M, et al. Cerebral metabolic dysfunction in AIDS: findings in a sample with and without dementia. *J Neuropsychiatry Clin Neurosci* 1998;4:280–287.

103. Hinkin CH, van Gorp WG, Mandelkern MA, et al. Cerebral metabolic change in patients with AIDS: report of a six-month follow up using positron emission tomography. *J Neuropsychiatry Clin Neurosci* 1995;7:180–187.

104. Wiseman MB, Sanchez JA, Buechel C, et al. Patterns of relative blood flow in minor cognitive motor disorder in human immunodeficiency virus infection. *J Neuropsychiatry Clin Neurosci* 1999;11:222–233.

105. Ajmani A, Habte-Gabr E, Zarr M, et al. Cerebral blood flow SPECT with Tc-99m exametazime correlates in AIDS dementia complex stages. A preliminary report. *Clin Nucl Med* 1997;16:656–659.

106. Sacktor N, Prohovnik I, Van Heertum RL, et al. Cerebral single-photon emission computed tomography abnormalities in human immunodeficiency virus type 1-infected gay men without cognitive impairment. *Arch Neurol* 1995;52:607–611.

107. Masdeu JC, Van Heertum RL, Abdel-Dayem H. Viral infections of the brain. *J Neuroimaging* 1995;5[1 Suppl]:40–s44.

108. Chang L, Ernst T, Leonido-Yee M, et al. Cerebral metabolite abnormalities correlate with clinical severity of HIV-1 cognitive motor complex. *Neurology* 1999;52:100–108.

109. Ernst T, Itti E, Itti L, et al. Changes in cerebral metabolism are detected prior to perfusion changes in early HIV-CMV: a coregistered (1)H MRS and SPECT study. *J Magn Reson Imaging* 2000;12(6):859–865.

110. Salvan AM, Lamoureux S, Michel G, et al. Localized proton magnetic resonance spectroscopy of the brain in children infected with human immunodeficiency virus with and without encephalopathy. *Pediatr Res* 1998;44:755–762.

111. Harrison MJ, Newman SP, Hall-Craggs MA, et al. Evidence of CNS impairment in HIV infection: clinical, neuropsychological, EEG, and MRI/MRS study. *J Neurol Neurosurg Psychiatry* 1998;65:301–307.

112. Wilkinson ID, Cunn S, Miszkiel KA, et al. Proton MRS and quantitative MRI assessment of the short-term neurological response to antiretroviral therapy in AIDS. *J Neurol Neurosurg Psychiatry* 1997;63:477–482.

113. Salvan AM, Vion-Dury J, Confort-Gouny S, et al. Brain proton magnetic resonance spectroscopy in HIV-related encephalopathy: identification of evolving metabolic patterns in relation to dementia and therapy. *AIDS Res Hum Retroviruses* 1997;13:1055–1066.

114. Harden CL, Daras M, Tuchman AJ, et al. Low amplitude EEGs in demented AIDS patients. *Electroencephalogr Clin Neurophysiol* 1993;87:54–56.

115. Tinuper P, de Carolis P, Galeotti M, et al. Electroencephalography and HIV infection [Letter]. *Lancet* 1989;1:554.

116. Parisi A, Strosselli M, DiPerri G, et al. Electroencephalography in the early diagnosis of HIV-related subacute encephalitis: analysis of 185 patients. *Clin Electroencephalogr* 1989;20:1–5.

117. Smith T, Jakobsen J, Gaub J, et al. Clinical an electrophysiological studies of human immunodeficiency virus-seropositive men with AIDS. *Ann Neurol* 1994;23:2101–297.

118. Malessa R, Agelink MW, Diener HC. Dysfunction of visual pathways in HIV-1 infection. *J Neurol Sci* 1995;130:82–87.

119. Marshall DW, Brey RL, Cahill WT, et al. Spectrum of cerebrospinal fluid findings in various stages of human immunodeficiency virus infection. *Arch Neurol* 1994;45:1014–1018.

120. Reboul J, Schuller E, Pailoux G, et al. Immunoglobulins and complement components in 27 patients infected by HIV-II virus: comparison on general (systemic) and intrathecal immunity. *J Neurol Sci* 1989;89:243–252.

121. Brew BH, Bhalla RB, Fleisher M, et al. Cerebrospinal fluid 2 microglobulin in patients infected with human immunodeficiency virus. *Neurology* 1989;39:830–834.

122. Portegies P, Epstein LG, Hung STA, et al. Human immunodeficiency virus type 1 antigen in cerebrospinal fluid. Correlation with clinical neurologic status. *Arch Neurol* 1989;46:261–264.

123. McArthur JC, Sipos E, Cornblath DR, et al. Identification of mononuclear cells in CSF of patients with HIV infection. *Neurology* 1989;39:66–70.

124. Chiodi F, Keys B, Albert J, et al. Human immunodeficiency virus type 1 is present in the cerebrospinal fluid of a majority of infected individuals. *J Clin Microbiol* 1992;30:1768–1771.

125. Buffet R, Agut H, Chieze F, et al. Virological markers in the cerebrospinal fluid from HIV-1-infected individuals. *J Acquir Immune Defic Syndr* 1991;5:1419–1424.

126. Robertson K, Fiscus S, Kapoor C, et al. CSF, plasma viral load and HIV-associated dementia. *J Neurovirol* 1998;4:90–100.

127. McArthur JC, McClernon DR, Cronin MF, et al. Relationship between human immunodeficiency virus-associated dementia and viral load in cerebrospinal fluid and brain. *Ann Neurol* 1997; 42:689–698.

128. Brew B, Pemberton L, Cunningham P, et al. Levels of human immunodeficiency virus type 1 RNA in cerebrospinal fluid correlate with AIDS dementia stage. *J Infect Dis* 1997;175: 963–966.

129. Cinque P, Vago L, Ceresa D, et al. Cerebrospinal fluid HIV-1 RNA levels: correlation with HIV encephalitis. *AIDS* 1998;12:389–394.

130. Ellis RJ, Hsia K, Spector SA, et al. Cerebrospinal fluid human immunodeficiency virus type 1 RNA levels are elevated in neurocognitively impaired individuals with acquired immunodeficiency syndrome. *Ann Neurol* 1997;42:679–688.

131. Gisslen M, Hagberg L, Fuchs D, et al. Cerebrospinal fluid viral load in HIV-1-infected patients without antiretroviral treatment. A longitudinal study. *J Acquir Immune Defic Syndr Hum Retrovir* 1998;17:297–2101.

132. Wiley CA, Soontornniyomkij V, Radhakrishnan L, et al. Distribution of brain HIV load in AIDS. *Brain Pathol* 1998;8:277–284.

133. Conrad AJ, Schmid P, Syndulko K, et al. Quantifying HIV-1 RNA using the polymerase chain reaction on cerebrospinal fluid and serum of seropositive individuals with and without neurological abnormalities. *J Acquir Immune Defic Syndr Hum Retrovirol* 1995;10:425–435.

134. De Luca A, Ciancio BC, Larussa D, et al. Correlates of independent HIV-1 replication in the CNS and of its control by antiretrovirals. *Neurology* 2002; 59(3):342–347.

135. Luizzi GM, Mastroianni CM, Fanelli M, et al. Myelin degrading activity in the CSF of HIV-1-infected patients with neurological diseases. *Neuroreport* 1994;6:157–160.

136. Elovaara I, Muller KM. Cytoimmunological abnormalities in cerebrospinal fluid in early stages of HIV-1 infection often precede changes in blood. *J Neuroimmunol* 1993;44:1106–1204.

137. Pumarola-Sune T, Navia BA, Cordon-Cardo C, et al. HIV antigen in the brains of patients with the AIDS dementia complex. *Ann Neurol* 1987;21:490–496.

138. Becker JT, Caldararo R, Lopez OL, et al. Qualitative features of the memory deficit associated with HIV infection and AIDS: cross-validation of a discriminant function classification

scheme. *J Clin Exp Neuropsychol* 1995; 17:134–142.

139. Fischl MA. Treatment of HIV infection. In: Sande MA, Volberding PA, eds. *The medical management of AIDS,* 4th ed. Philadelphia: WB Saunders, 1995:141–160.

140. Temesgen Z. Current status of antiretroviral therapies. *Expert Opin Pharmacother* 2001;2(8):1239–1246.

141. Fischl MA. Richmann DD, Grieco MH, et al. The efficacy of azidothymidine (AZT) in the treatment of patients with AIDS and AIDS-related complex; a double blind, placebo-controlled study. *N Engl J Med* 1987;317:185–197.

142. Volberding PA, Lagakos SW, Grimes JM, et al. A comparison of immediate with deferred zidovudine therapy for asymptomatic HIV-infected adults with CD4 cell counts of 500 or more per cubic millimeter. *N Engl J Med* 1995;333:401–407.

143. Kinloch-De Loes S, Hirschel BJ, Hoen B, et al. A controlled trial of zidovudine in primary human immunodeficiency virus infection. *N Engl J Med* 1995;333:408–413.

144. Elovaara I, Poutiainen E, Lahdevirta J, et al. Zidovudine reduces intrathecal immunoactivation in patients with early human immunodeficiency virus type I infection. *Arch Neurol* 1994;51:1003–1010.

145. Schmitt FA, Bigley JW, McKinnis R, et al. Neuropsychological outcome of zidovudine (AZT) treatment of patients with AIDS and AIDS-related complex. *N Engl J Med* 1994;319:1573–1578.

146. Baldeweg T, Catalan J, Lovett E, et al. Long-term zidovudine reduces neurocognitive deficits in HIV-1 infection. *J Acquir Immune Defic Syndr* 1995;9:589–596.

147. Wong SL, Wang Y, Sawchuk RJ. Analysis of zidovudine distribution to specific regions in rabbit brain using microdialysis. *Pharm Res* 1992;9:332–338.

148. Sidtis JJ, Gatsonic C, Price RW, et al. Zidovudine treatment of the AIDS dementia complex: results of a placebo-controlled trial. AIDS clinical trials group. *Ann Neurol* 1993;33:343–349.

149. Llorente AM, van Gorp WG, Stern MJ, et al. Long-term effects of high-dose zidovudine treatment on neuropsychological performance in mildly symptomatic HIV-positive patients: results of a randomized, double blind, placebo-controlled investigation. *J Int Neuropsychol Soc* 2001;7(1):27–32.

150. Yarchoan R, Pluda JM, Thomas RV, et al. Long-term toxicity/activity profile of 2′,3″-dideoxyinosine in AIDS or AIDS-related complex. *Lancet* 1990;336:526–529.

151. Butler KM, Husson RN, Balis FM, et al.

Dideoxyinosine in children with symptomatic human immunodeficiency virus infection. *N Engl J Med* 1991;324:137–144.

152. Charreaus I, Chemlal K, Yeni P, et al. *Reduced risk of progression to HIV encephalopathy with ddI or ddC in combination to AZT compared to AZT alone.* Fifth Conf Retrovir Oppor Infect 1998:165(abstr no. 458).

153. McIntyre K, Torres R, Luck D, et al. *Pilot study of zidovudine (AZT) and zalcitabine (ddC) combination in HIV-associated dementia.* Int Conf AIDS 1994;10:201, Abstr No. PB0233.

154. Foudraine NA, Hoetelmans RMW, Lange JMA, et al. Cerebrospinal-fluid HIV-1 RNA and drug concentrations after treatment with lamivudine plus zidovudine or stavudine. *Lancet* 1998;351:1547–1551.

155. Gisolf EH, Portegies P, Hoetelmans R, et al. *Effect of ritonavir (RTV)/ saquinavir (SQV) versus RTV/SQV/ stavudine (d4T) on cerebrospinal fluid (CSF) HIV-RNA levels: preliminary results.* Int Conf AIDS 1998;12:560, Abstr No. 32197.

156. Aweeka F, Jayewardene A, Staprans S, et al. Failure to detect nelfinavir in the cerebrospinal fluid of HIV-1-infected patients with and without AIDS dementia complex. *J Acquir Immune Defic Syndr Hum Retrovirol* 1999;1:39–43.

157. Tashima KT. Cerebrospinal fluid levels of antiretroviral medications. *JAMA* 1998;280:879–940.

158. Chang M, Sood VK, Wilson GJ, et al. Metabolism of the HIV-1 reverse transcriptase inhibitor delavirdine in mice. *Drug Metab Dispos* 1997;25:828–839.

159. Sadler BM, Chittick GE, Polk RE, et al. Metabolic disposition and pharmacokinetics of [^{14}C]-amprenavir, a human immunodeficiency virus type 1 (HIV-1) protease inhibitor, administered as a single oral dose to healthy male subjects. *J Clin Pharmacol* 2001;41:386–396.

160. Gisolf E, Colebunders R, Can Wanzeele F, et al. *Treatment with ritonavir/ saquinavir versus ritonavir/saquinavir/stavudine.* Fifth Conf Retrovir Oppor Infect 1998;152, Abstr No. 389.

161. Skolnick AA. Protease inhibitors may reverse AIDS dementia. *JAMA* 1998;279:419.

162. Perry SW. Organic mental disorders caused by HIV: update on early diagnosis and treatment. *Am J Psychiatry* 1990;147:696–710.

163. American Psychiatric Association. *Diagnostic and statistical manual of mental disorders,* 4th ed. *(DSM-IV).* Washington, DC: Author, 1994:165–174.

164. Ayers MR, Abrams DI, Newell TG, et al. Performance of individuals with

AIDS on the Luria-Nebraska neuropsychological battery. *Int J Clin Neuropsychol* 1987;3:101–105.

165. Fernandez D, Holmes VF, Levy JK, et al. Consultation-liaison psychiatry and HIV-related disorders. *Hosp Community Psychiatry* 1989;40:146–153.

166. Uldall KK, Harris VL, Lalonde B. Outcomes associated with delirium in acutely hospitalized acquired immune deficiency syndrome patients. *Compr Psychiatry* 2000;41:94–97.

167. Lipowski ZJ. Delirium (acute confusional states). *JAMA* 1987;258:1789–1798.

168. Neuzil KM. Pharmacologic therapy for human immunodeficiency virus infection: a review. *Am J Med Sci* 1994;307:368–373.

169. Ayd FF Jr. Haloperidol: twenty years' clinical experience. *J Clin Psychiatry* 1978;39:807–814.

170. Tesar GE, Murray GB, Cassem NH. Use of high-dose intravenous haloperidol in the treatment of agitated cardiac patients. *J Clin Psychopharmacol* 1985;5:344–347.

171. Adams F, Fernandez F, Anderson BS. Emergency pharmacotherapy and delirium in the critically ill cancer patient: intravenous combination drug approach. *Psychosomatics* 1986;27[1 Suppl]:33–37.

172. Adams F. Emergency intravenous sedation of the delirious medically ill patient. *J Clin Psychiatry* 1994;49[Provide of Suppl]:22–26.

173. Fernandez F, Holmes VF, Adams F, et al. Treatment of severe, refractory agitation with a haloperidol drip. *J Clin Psychiatry* 1994;49:239–241.

174. Breitbart W, Marotta R, Platt MM, et al. A double-blind trial of haloperidol, chlorpromazine and lorazepam in the treatment of delirium in hospitalized AIDS patients. *Am J Psychiatry* 1996;153:231–237.

175. Maldonado JL, Fernandez F. Management of neuropsychiatric complications in HIV infection. *Med Psychiatr* 1998;1:22–29.

176. Konikoff F, Kuritzky A, Jerushalmi Y, et al. Neuroleptic malignant syndrome induced by a single injection of haloperidol. *Br Med J* 1984;289:1228–1229.

177. O'Brien PJ. Prevalence of neuroleptic malignant syndrome. *Am J Psychiatry* 1987;144:1371.

178. Huyse F, Van Schijndel RS. Haloperidol and cardiac arrest. *Lancet* 1994;2:568–569.

179. Breitbart W, Marotta RF, Call P. AIDS and neuroleptic malignant syndrome. *Lancet* 1994;2:1494–1489.

180. Fernandez F, Levy JK. The use of molindone in the treatment of psychotic and delirious patients infected with the human immunodeficiency virus. *Gen Hosp Psychiatry* 1993;15:31–35.

181. Schwartz TL, Masand PS. The role of atypical antipsychotics in the treatment of delirium. *Psychosomatics* 2002;43:171–174.

182. Sipahimalani A, Masand PS. Olanzapine in the treatment of delirium. *Psychosomatics* 1998;39:422–430.

183. Breitbart W, Tremblay A, Gibson C: an open trial of olanzapine for the treatment of delirium in hospitalized cancer patients. *Psychosomatics* 2002;43:175–182.

184. Sipahimalani A, Masand PS. Use of risperidone in delirium: case reports. *Ann Clin Psychiatry* 1997;9:105–107.

185. Schwartz TL, Masand PS. Treatment of delirium with quetiapine. *J Clin Psychiatry* 2000;2:10–12.

186. Leso L, Schwartz TL. Ziprasidone treatment of delirium. *Psychosomatics* 2002;43:61–62.

187. Levy JK, Fernandez F. HIV infection of the CNS: implications for neuropsychiatry. In: Yudofsky SC, Hales RE, eds. *Textbook of neuropsychiatry,* 3rd ed. American Psychiatric Press, 1996 (*in press*).

188. Brown G. The use of methylphenidate for cognitive decline associated with HIV disease. *Int J Psychiatry Med* 1995;25:21–37.

189. Lipton SA, Gendelman HE. Dementia associated with the acquired immunodeficiency syndrome. *N Engl J Med* 1995;332:994–1000.

190. Jain KK. Evaluation of memantine for neuroprotection in dementia. *Expert Opin Investig Drugs* 2000;9(6):1397–1406.

191. Lyketsos CG, Hanson AL, Fishman M, et al. Manic syndrome early and late in the course of HIV. *Am J Psychiatry* 1993;150:326–327.

192. Holmes VF, Fricchione GL. Hypomania in an AIDS patient receiving amitriptyline for neuropathic pain. *Neurology* 1989;39:305.

193. Perry SW, Tross S. Psychiatric problems of AIDS inpatients at the New York Hospital: preliminary report. *Public Health Rep* 1984;106:200–205.

194. Ostrow D, Grant I, Atkinson H. Assessment and management of the AIDS patient with neuropsychiatric disturbances. *J Clin Psychiatry* 1994;49[Suppl]:14–22.

195. Cavanaugh S, Clark DC, Gibbons RD. Diagnosing depression in the hospitalized medically ill. *Psychosomatics* 1983;24:809–815.

196. Maldonado JL, Fernandez J, Fernandez F. Depresion en el paciente con enfermedades medicas. *Medico Interamericano* 1996;1:353–357.

197. Rundell JR, Kyle KM, Brown GR, et al. Risk factors for suicide attempts in a human immunodeficiency virus screening program. *Psychosomatics* 1992;33:24–27.

198. Siegel K. Psychosocial aspects of rational suicide. *Am J Psychother* 1986;3:405–418.

199. Richelson E. Pharmacology of antidepressants—characteristics of the ideal drug. *Mayo Clin Proc* 1994;69:1069–1081.

200. Fernandez F, Levy JK. Psychopharmacotherapy of psychiatric syndromes in asymptomatic and symptomatic HIV infection. *Psychiatry Med* 1991;9(3):377–3100.

201. Massie MJ, Holland J. The cancer patient with pain: psychiatric complications and their management. *Med Clin North Am* 1987;71:243–248.

202. Rabkin JG, Wagner G, Rabkin R. Effects of sertraline on mood and immune status in patients with major depression and HIV illness: an open trial. *J Clin Psychiatry* 1994;55:433–439.

203. Grassi B, Gambini O, Scarone S. Notes on the use of fluvoxamine as treatment of depression in HIV-1-infected subjects. *Pharmacopsychiatry* 1995;28:99–100.

204. Golden RN, Rudofer MV, Sherer MA, et al. Bupropion in depression. I Biochemical effects and clinical responses. *Arch Gen Psychiatry* 1994;45:139–143.

205. Elliot AJ, Russo J, Bergam K, et al. Antidepressant efficacy in HIV-seropositive outpatients with major depressive disorder: an open trial of nefazodone. *J Clin Psychiatry* 1999;60:226–231.

206. Ereshefsky L, Dugan D. Review of the pharmacokinetics, pharmacogenetics, and drug interaction potential of antidepressants: focus on venlafaxine. *Depress Anxiety* 2000;12[1 Suppl]:30–44.

207. Levin GM, Nelson LA, DeVane CL, et al. A pharmacokinetic drug–drug interaction study of venlafaxine and indinavir. *Psychopharmacol Bull* 2001;35(2):62–71.

208. Bloomingdale LM, Bressler B. Rapid intramuscular administration of tricyclic antidepressants. *Am J Psychiatry* 1979;136:8.

209. Dorfman W. Can parenteral intramuscular amitriptyline avoid ECT? *Psychosomatics* 1967;8:131–132.

210. Olson D, Maldonado JL, Pipkin ML, et al. Use of intravenous amitriptyline in depressed medically ill patients: two case reports and a review of the literature. *Med Psychiatry* 1998;1:80–85.

211. Fernandez F, Levy JK, Psychopharmacology in HIV spectrum disorders.

Psychiatr Clin North Am 1994;17:135–148.

212. Maxwell S, Sheftner WA, Kessler HA, et al. Manic syndrome associated with zidovudine treatment. *JAMA* 1988;259:3406–3407.

213. O'Dowd MA, McKegney FP. Manic syndrome associated with zidovudine. *JAMA* 1988;260:3587–3588.

214. Brouillette MJ, Chouinard G, Lalonde R. Didanosine-induced mania in HIV infection. *Am J Psychiatry* 1994;151:1839–1840.

215. Fernandez F, Levy JK, Sampley HR. Effects of methylphenidate in HIV-related depression: a comparative trial with desipramine. *Int J Psychiatry Med* 1995;25:53–67.

216. Fernandez F, Levy JK, Galizzi H. Response of HIV-related depression to psychostimulants: case reports. *Hosp Community Psychiatry* 1994;39:628–631.

217. Holmes VF, Fernandez F, Levy JK. Psychostimulant response in AIDS-related complex patients. *J Clin Psychiatry* 1989;50:5–8.

CHAPTER 60

Psychosocial Issues of HIV/AIDS Among Drug Users in Treatment

JAMES L. SORENSEN, NANCY A. HAUG, AND STEVEN L. BATKI

The continuing expansion of the acquired immune deficiency syndrome (AIDS) epidemic among injection drug users has ushered in a new set of problems—how to provide drug-abuse treatment to patients who have symptomatic human immunodeficiency virus (HIV) infection. Drug-abuse treatment of patients with HIV/AIDS is complicated but can be a key factor in both prevention and treatment of HIV/AIDS. Drug-abuse treatment programs also provide settings to deliver other services needed by HIV-infected patients, such as medical treatment, psychiatric care, and social services. However, the needs of patients with symptomatic HIV infection challenge the resources of drug-abuse treatment programs and require the creation of new systems of care that cross the boundaries of psychiatry, psychology, social work, and medicine.

This chapter is about the psychological, social, and behavioral difficulties that accompany the drug-abuse treatment of drug users and how substance abuse professionals can manage these problems. Other chapters explain how to manage the medical and neuropsychiatric deficits of these patients, so this chapter does not discuss medical and neuropsychiatric issues except as they affect the patients' psychosocial well-being. After this introduction, the chapter discusses the psychological problems of drug users with HIV infection. It then suggests several approaches for the management of psychological problems in the setting of drug-abuse treatment clinics, including both assessment strategies and treatment techniques. Recognizing that the problems of HIV-infected patients are social as well as psychological, the next sections discuss strategies for managing social barriers in drug-abuse clinics, including medical treatment adherence. The need for an integrated approach that reaches beyond medical or psychological care and into the community is stressed. The chapter concludes by considering these issues in the context of comprehensive care of substance users.

PSYCHOLOGICAL PROBLEMS OF DRUG USERS WITH HIV INFECTION

Patients with substance use disorders and HIV/AIDS are vulnerable to numerous psychological problems (1,2). Even without the added difficulties of HIV disease, users of illicit drugs have high rates of psychiatric disorders (3). These problems include mood and anxiety disorders and cognitive impairment, which are topics of earlier chapters. Such comorbid problems tend to be exacerbated among HIV-infected patients. Psychological problems also include adjustment disorders, demoralization, and poor coping skills.

Common Psychological Problems in HIV

HIV-infected patients have been described as facing the problems of grief, stigmatization, the demands of a chronic, life-threatening illness, and changes in self-concept and identity (4). These problems can lead to demoralization, a condition that might be closer to an adjustment disorder with depressed mood, rather than to true major depression, yet with sadness and hopelessness of sufficient severity as to impair functioning (5). Adjustment to illness may be more difficult for drug users than for other patients with HIV/AIDS because of their reliance on substance use and other forms of avoidance as coping mechanisms. Maladaptive coping is linked to poor adjustment, to HIV disease, and to psychological distress (6). For example, psychological distress among drug-using women with HIV infection is greater, and quality of life is lower, than that in non–drug-using women with HIV (7).

Drug users have been found to experience greater distress than non-drug users following HIV antibody testing (8). However, HIV testing in drug users does not appear to lead to an increase in suicide risk (9), and informing drug users about positive HIV serostatus is not associated with worse outcome in drug-abuse treatment (10).

Responding to Psychological Problems

Identifying and treating the psychological problems of HIV-infected patients may improve health-related quality of life and possibly reduce use of health services (11). Counseling interventions that aim to improve coping skills and reduce avoidance and drug use may be helpful (6). Reducing psychological problem intensity may also be important to improve the outcome of substance-abuse treatment in these patients.

Because of greater levels of psychological distress and other impairments, substance-abuse treatment of patients with HIV disease may require more flexibility than is customary in traditional substance-abuse programs (1,12). Depression and hopelessness are common and can erode motivation for drug-abuse treatment. Consequently, these patients may need more assistance than other drug abusers to discontinue their drug use. The flexible approach stems from a harm-reduction philosophy. Guidelines recommend the application of different standards of care for patients with varying levels of HIV severity and psychosocial functioning (12). This approach also encompasses different expectations of patients regarding substance-abuse treatment outcome. For example, a sicker patient may need to be given more opportunities to achieve a decrease in substance use than a more functional patient.

SOCIAL PROBLEMS

The problems that accompany HIV infection are social and environmental, not just psychological. As a group, injection drug users with AIDS have few economic or educational resources; many are impoverished and stigmatized. Their relationships, home environment and neighborhoods are often unhealthy and unsupportive of recovery. HIV/AIDS can lead to role conflict and significant challenges for the patient's caregivers and partners, especially because many have already witnessed AIDS-related deaths.

There is considerable diversity among these patients. Treatment professionals need to understand the variations in culture, ethnicity, gender and sexual orientation that are so integral to understanding HIV/AIDS among substance abusers. First, African Americans and Hispanics are dramatically overrepresented among HIV/AIDS cases (13). In 1998, injection drug users accounted for 36% of all HIV cases among both African American and Hispanic adults and adolescents, while only 22% of cases were among white adults and adolescents (13). Since the onset of the AIDS epidemic, a majority of females in the United States infected with AIDS has been African American women (14). Pregnant substance abusers are a subgroup of females with special needs because drug injection is most commonly associated with perinatal HIV infection (15). Men who report both injection drug use and homosexual/bisexual contact make up 6% of adult HIV/AIDS cases

in the United States (16). Consequently, it is crucial to develop treatment programs that are culturally sensitive—tolerant of diversity and understanding of how ethnicity and gender identification intertwine with HIV risks.

Assessment of Social Problems

Assessment of social problems involves a thorough evaluation of patient sociodemographic characteristics such as age, education, race, ethnic/minority status, level of acculturation, sexual orientation, religion, and employment history. Other areas to explore during intake or counseling sessions may include familial and partner support, prior psychosocial functioning, housing conditions and homelessness, criminal justice involvement, use of community resources, and accessibility to needed medical and social services (e.g., transportation, making appointments). The social context associated with injecting drugs may also hold cultural meanings and relevant information about daily problems encountered by substance abusers with HIV/AIDS (17). Perceived social norms, beliefs about the disease, and attitudes toward providers vary widely among different social groups. For women, socioeconomic concerns surrounding childcare, custody issues, pregnancy, domestic violence, and prostitution are salient factors to assess and intervene.

Counseling and Case Management for Social Problems

Drug treatment programs face a growing responsibility to assist socially disabled and stigmatized patients with social services. These include making referrals for food, shelter, clothing, and general public assistance. In some geographic areas, stand-alone clinics for HIV/AIDS patients may be available to those in methadone treatment. However, drug-abuse treatment staff may, at times, need to be the case managers and advocates for their patients, to help them gain access to these services. In some communities, drug treatment programs may need to become the primary health care providers for their patients because of the shortage of services. Other settings for psychosocial education and brief intervention include emergency rooms, prisons, and shelters. In San Francisco, abundant social resources exist for injection drug users with HIV/AIDS, including legal assistance, money management (e.g., having a payee who assists with finances), homelessness advocacy, youth services, cooperative living, drop-in group therapy, and clinical case management. Community-oriented programs, mobile units or vans, street outreach and peer-driven interventions have also demonstrated empirical support for providing services and facilitating treatment entry (18,19). Peer education programs may be a key strategy for influencing social norms and conveying information on health behavior and risk management practices (19).

One innovation is the application of case management, a social service strategy designed to enroll patients in services and coordinate the services patients require for their complex problems. Case management has been widely adopted in treating groups who have not benefited from customary care (20), and it is also used to link persons with HIV/AIDS to needed services (21). Although case management may be useful for substance abusers with HIV/AIDS, the results of published research have been mixed. One study reported encouraging preliminary results but did not publish a followup report (22). The other study, a clinical trial, reported no benefit to case management over brief contact and referral (23).

HIV RISK BEHAVIORS

Among drug users, HIV is transmitted primarily through sharing unsterile syringes and through unprotected sexual activity. The virus can also be transmitted from mother to child during the perinatal period: during birth and in the weeks before and after. A recent study emphasized the importance of sexual transmission among drug injectors. Men injectors who reported having sex with men, as well as women drug injectors who traded sex for money, were more likely to acquire HIV than were the injectors who did not engage in sexual behaviors (24).

Assessment of HIV Risk Behaviors

Staff in drug-abuse treatment programs can incorporate HIV risk assessment into their intake procedures. Several self-report measures have been validated, which can reliably assess both drug-related and sex-related risk behaviors (25). Three of the best-validated approaches that are readily available are the Texas Christian University AIDS Risk Assessment (26), the Risk Behavior Assessment Questionnaire (27), and the computerized version of the Risk Assessment Battery (28).

Counseling for Reducing Drug Use and Other HIV Risk Behaviors

In discussing counseling strategies, it is important to stress that drug-abuse treatment itself is clearly an effective means of reducing HIV risk (29). The evidence is strongest for methadone maintenance treatment, which has been the most thoroughly studied, but there are strong indications that other treatment modalities also reduce HIV risk (30).

In addition to the benefits of drug-abuse treatment *per se*, a recent meta-analysis of studies indicated that many targeted HIV risk-reduction programs are effective (31). These programs provide risk-reduction skills and change sexual behaviors, knowledge, attitudes, and beliefs. As might be expected, the most effective programs are those that provide the most intensive services. There is also emerging evidence that HIV counseling and testing has

a positive effect as a means of secondary prevention for HIV-positive individuals (32).

Recently, the National Institute on Drug Abuse disseminated a research-based guide explaining how to prevent HIV among drug users (33). The authors recommend this guide as a resource for practitioners who are designing HIV prevention and counseling programs for their settings. The guide presents 17 principles, has suggestions on strategies for communicating prevention messages to drug users, and links readers with the variety of research-validated interventions that can be provided.

DIFFICULTIES ENGAGING IN AND ADHERING TO MEDICAL TREATMENT

Staff in drug-abuse treatment programs can play an important role in the delivery of medical and HIV services by helping their patients to participate in medical treatments and take needed medications. Continued drug use can cause problems with HIV health care by interfering with appointment keeping and adherence to medical regimens. HIV-infected drug users may have difficulty adhering to the requirements of HIV medical care, even without ongoing drug use. It is therefore essential to find ways to improve the effectiveness of drug-abuse treatment with respect to both drug use and medical care in HIV-infected patients.

Drug-abuse treatment programs can help HIV/AIDS patients to take medications more reliably. Increased use of sophisticated combination therapies of antiretroviral medications has improved the life expectancy and health for many people living with HIV/AIDS. However, patients taking these medications need to adhere to their medication regimens rigorously. Research indicates that consistency of adherence to antiretroviral therapy predicts biological outcomes (34,35). One study indicated that patients were most likely to achieve virologic success if they took more than 95% of the prescribed protease inhibitor doses, while 50% of the patients who took only 80% to 90% of their protease inhibitor doses did not achieve full virologic suppression (35). Studies of adherence to zidovudine (AZT) reveal adherence rates ranging from 30% to 67% (36–38), and that people with a history of substance use have more problems with medication adherence (39,40). In one study, patients with no history of injection drug use (IDU) were 3.7 times more likely to adhere to their AZT treatment regimens (37).

Specific strategies have been helpful with drug users who have HIV/AIDS. We caution that treatment providers may not know who among their patients is taking medications reliably. In one study, provider estimates of adherence explained far less than patients' report (41), implying that it is important to ask patients about adherence issues. Among the interventions attempted in drug-abuse treatment, the provision of on-site dispensing of HIV medications showed some modest benefits to patients in methadone maintenance (38,42). Other interventions have been useful with HIV-infected drug users but not yet attempted within the context of substance-abuse treatment. One approach is a comprehensive support program located in an urban community setting (43). Another is a "peer-driven" intervention—an alternative support structure for drug users, intended to serve as the functional equivalent to drug treatment for increasing drug users' medication adherence (44). Brief medication counseling was helpful to HIV patients, most with histories of intravenous drug use, in a Veterans Affairs Medical Center primary care treatment program (45). Another approach used monetary reinforcement combined with "cue-dose training" (i.e., counseling and feedback about when medication bottles were opened) (46).

The evidence is clear that medication adherence is a crucial problem with HIV-infected drug users. There is a need to develop technologies to help drug users take the effective medications more reliably.

NEED FOR INTEGRATED APPROACH

The widespread problems of HIV/AIDS patients do not sort neatly within the lines of professional disciplines, and they militate for interdisciplinary solutions. Managing the various problems seen in HIV-infected drug users involves different levels of intervention. The most fundamental of these is providing material supports and assisting with housing, meals, welfare funds, transportation, and health care. Another level of intervention is providing psychoeducation to reduce patients' feelings of depression and helplessness. Self-help groups (e.g., Alcoholics Anonymous [AA], Narcotics Anonymous [NA]) and involving caregivers can be quite important in reducing isolation. Supportive psychotherapy and cognitive–behavioral techniques can help to bolster the coping abilities of patients.

The Community Reinforcement Approach (CRA) is a manualized psychosocial treatment that focuses on competing with the reinforcement derived from drug use and its associated lifestyle by making major life changes in family relationships, recreational activities, social networks, and vocation (47). CRA has demonstrated improvement in injection risk behaviors among methadone-maintenance patients with HIV/AIDS (48). The Matrix model is another intensive outpatient psychosocial approach that has shown efficacy in treating cocaine and methamphetamine abusers, as well as reducing HIV risk behavior (49,50). In addition, typical relapse prevention consists of continued care and behavioral methods to avoid high-risk situations (e.g., stress and anger management, assertiveness training).

When outpatient strategies fall short, the concerned professional can seek more intensive interventions in the form of day treatment or halfway houses. If these are insufficient, the patient may need to be hospitalized to protect himself or herself, to protect others, or to provide basic self-care. Long-term residential treatment and therapeutic communities may offer a protective environment for socially marginalized individuals who have little access to services. A combination of medical, pharmacologic, psychological, and sociocultural modalities is recommended to improve general health, retain the patient in drug treatment, and reduce HIV/AIDS-related infections.

Another approach is to bring the services to the patients by building the capability of drug-treatment programs to provide needed services and outreach. Models of integrated care such as these warrant serious consideration as the toll of AIDS cases continues to mount in drug-treatment programs. The increasing problem severity and complexity of substance abusers with HIV/AIDS underscores the need for using innovative and comprehensive treatment strategies.

CONCLUSIONS

This chapter provides information about the psychosocial problems that occur for an HIV-infected drug user who enters drug-abuse treatment. The problems are serious, and they challenge the substance abuse professional who intends to provide comprehensive care. Furthermore, these problems are symptomatic of larger dilemmas that go beyond the scope of this chapter. Only a small minority of drug users are in treatment programs, and their HIV-related problems may be largely beyond the reach of most human services. The need to be flexible in approaching this problem has been stressed, as well as the desirability of developing new service models to cope with HIV infection in drug-treatment programs.

Other chapters in this volume round out the broad view that is needed to manage effectively the psychosocial sequelae of HIV infection. The field will be more successful if it better understands the determinants of substance abuse and how to intervene early enough to prevent youth from advancing to injection drug use. As treatment approaches are improved, they will provide more effective tools for intervening with patients, including those who are HIV-infected. The suggestions of the chapters on medically ill substance users and substance users with psychopathology also complement the advice provided here, and the chapters about gay and lesbian issues, staff training, and policies can help the reader to better design programs that are sensitive to patient, staff, and community needs.

In closing, we emphasize the importance of the extremely difficult tasks of providing drug-abuse treatment to patients with HIV infection. Treatment is difficult, for both patients and staff members. However, it can be extremely effective in decreasing the destructive drug abuse of HIV-infected addicts, stabilizing the medical problems, and blunting the spread of HIV to other drug users, their sexual partners, and their progeny.

ACKNOWLEDGMENTS

The authors are grateful for the collaboration of the staff and patients of the Outpatient Substance Abuse Services, Division of Substance Abuse and Addiction Medicine at San Francisco General Hospital. This chapter was supported in part by grants from the National Institute of Drug Abuse (NIDA) (Grant numbers P50DA09253, R01DA11344, R01DA14922, R01DA12221, and U10DA15815) and the Center for Substance Abuse Treatment (TI12623).

REFERENCES

1. Batki SL. Drug abuse, psychiatric disorders, and AIDS: dual and triple diagnosis. *West J Med* 1990;152:547–552.
2. Batki SL, Ferrando SJ, Manfredi LB, et al. Psychiatric disorders, drug use, and medical status in injection drug users with HIV disease. *Am J Addict* 1996;5:249–258.
3. Regier DA, Farmer ME, Rae DS, et al. Comorbidity of mental disorders with alcohol and other drug abuse. Results from the Epidemiologic Catchment Area (ECA) Study. *JAMA* 1990;264:2511–2518.
4. Zilber C. Psychotherapeutic strategies for coping with HIV infection. *New Direct Mental Health Serv* 2000; Fall(87):37–43.
5. Treisman GJ, Angelino AF, Hutton HE. Psychiatric issues in the management of patients with HIV infection. *JAMA* 2001;286(22):2857–2864.
6. Avants SK, Warburton LA, Margolin A. How injection drug users coped with testing seropositive: implications for subsequent health-related behaviors. *AIDS Educ Prev* 2001;13:207–218.
7. Te Waarwerk MJ, Gaal EA. Psychological distress and quality of life in drug-using and non–drug-using HIV-infected women. *Eur J Pub Health* 2001;11:109–115.
8. Perry S, Jacobsberg L, Card CA, et al. Severity of psychiatric symptoms after HIV testing. *Am J Psychiatry* 1993;150:775–779.
9. van Haastrecht MJ, Mientjes GH, van den Hoek AJ, et al. Death from suicide and overdose among drug injectors after disclosure of first HIV test result. *AIDS* 1994;8:1721–1725.
10. Wimbush J, Amicarelli A, Stein MD. Does HIV test result influence methadone maintenance treatment retention? *J Subst Abuse* 1996;8:263–269.
11. Sherbourne CD, Hays RD, Fleishman JA, et al. Impact of psychiatric conditions on health-related quality of life in persons with HIV infection. *Am J Psychiatry* 2000;157:248–254.
12. Center for Substance Abuse Treatment (CSAT). Batki SL, Selwyn P, Consensus Panel Co-Chairs. *Substance abuse treatment for persons with HIV/AIDS*. DHHS Publication No. (SMA) 00–341. Washington, DC: U.S. Government Printing Office, 2000.
13. Centers for Disease Control and Prevention (CDC). U.S. HIV and AIDS cases reported through December 1998. *HIV/AIDS Surveillance Report: Year-End Edition* 1998;11(2):5.
14. Health Resources and Services Administration (HRSA). *HIV disease in women of color.* HRSA Care Action. Rockville, MD: U.S. Department of Health and Human Services, HIV/AIDS Bureau, 1999.
15. Centers for Disease Control and Prevention. *HIV/AIDS Surveillance report, 1998.* Atlanta, GA: Author, 1999:10(2).
16. Centers for Disease Control and Prevention. *HIV/AIDS Surveillance Report 2001.* Atlanta, GA: Author, 2002;13(2):1–48.
17. Grund J-PC, Stern LS, Kaplan CD, et al. Drug use contexts and HIV consequences: the effect of drug policy on patterns of everyday drug use in Rotterdam and the Bronx. *Br J Addict* 1992;87:381–392.
18. Tinsman PD, Bullman S, Chan X, et al. Factors affecting client response to HIV outreach efforts. *J Subst Abuse* 2001;13:201–214.
19. Ball AJ. Overview: policies and interventions to stem HIV-1 epidemics associated with injecting drug use. In: Stimson G, Des Jarlais DC, Ball A, eds. *Drug injecting and HIV infection.* London: UCL Press, 1998.
20. Austin CD, McLelland RW. Case management in human services: reflections on public policy. *J Case Manage* 1994;6:119–126.
21. Katz MH, Cunningham WE, Fleishman JA, et al. Effect of case management on unmet needs and utilization of medical care and medications among HIV-infected persons. *Ann Intern Med* 2001;135[8 Part 1]:557–565.
22. McCoy HV, Dodds S, Rivers JE, McCoy CB. Case management services for HIV-seropositive IDUs. *NIDA Res Monogr* 1992;127:181–207.
23. Sorensen JL, Delucchi KL, Dilley J, et al. Case management for substance abusers with HIV/AIDS: a randomized clinical trial. *Am J Drug Alcohol Abuse* 2003;29(1):133–150.
24. Kral AH, Bluthenthal RN, Lorvick J, et al. Sexual transmission of HIV-1 among injection drug users in San Francisco, U.S.A.: risk-factor analysis. *Lancet* 2002;357(9266):1397–1401.
25. Sorensen JL, Masson CL, Perlman DC. HIV/hepatitis prevention in drug abuse treatment programs: guidance from research. *Sci Pract Perspect* 2002;1(1):4–11.
26. Camacho LM, Bartholomew NG, Joe GW, et al. Maintenance of HIV risk reduction among injection opioid users: a 12-month posttreatment followup. *Drug Alcohol Depend* 1997;47:1–18.
27. National Institute on Drug Abuse. *Risk behavior assessment questionnaire, October edition.* Rockville, MD: NIDA Community Research Branch, 1991.
28. Navaline HA, Snider EC, Petro CJ, et al. Preparation for AIDS vaccine trials: an automated version of the risk assessment battery: enhancing the assessment of risk behaviors. *AIDS Res Hum Retrovir* 1994;10[2 Suppl]:S281–S283.
29. Sorensen JL, Copeland AL. Drug abuse treatment as an HIV prevention strategy: a review. *Drug Alcohol Depend* 2000;59:17–31.
30. Hubbard RL, Craddock SG, Flynn PM, et al. Overview of 1-year follow up outcomes in the Drug Abuse Treatment Outcome Study (DATOS). *Psychol Addict Behav* 1997;11:261–278.
31. Prendergast ML, Urada D, Podus D. Meta-analysis of HIV risk-reduction interventions within drug abuse treatment programs. *J Consult Clin Psychol* 2001;69:389–405.
32. Weinhardt LS, Carey MP, Johnson BT, et al. Effects of HIV counseling and testing on sexual risk behavior: a meta-analytic review of published research, 1985–1987. *Am J Public Health* 1999;89(9):1397–1405.
33. National Institute on Drug Abuse. *Principles of HIV prevention in drug-using populations: a research-based guide.* NIH Publication No. 02–4733. Rockville, MD: Author, 2002.

34. Mannheimer S, Friedland G, Matts J, et al. The consistency of adherence to antiretroviral therapy predicts biologic outcomes for human immunodeficiency virus-infected persons in clinical trials. *Clin Infect Dis* 2002;34(8):1115–1121.

35. Patterson D, Swindells S, Mohr J, et al. Adherence to protease inhibitor therapy and outcomes in patients with HIV infection. *Ann Intern Med* 2000;133:21–30.

36. Muma RD, Ross MW, Parcel GS, et al. Zidovudine adherence among individuals with HIV infection. *AIDS Care* 1995;7:439–447.

37. Samet JH, Libman H, Steger KA, et al. Compliance with zidovudine therapy in patients infected with human immunodeficiency virus, type 1: a cross-sectional study in a municipal hospital clinic. *Am J Med* 1992;92:495–502.

38. Wall TL, Sorensen JL, Batki SL, et al. Adherence to zidovudine (AZT) among HIV-infected methadone patients: a pilot study of supervised therapy and dispensing compared to usual care. *Drug Alcohol Depend* 1995;37:261–269.

39. Fogarty L, Roter D, Larson S, et al. Patient adherence to HIV medication regimens: a review of published and abstract reports. *Patient Educ Counsel* 2002;46(2):93–108.

40. Stein MD, Rich JD, Maksad J, et al. Adherence to antiretroviral therapy among HIV-infected methadone patients: effect of ongoing illicit drug use. *Am J Drug Alcohol Abuse* 2002;26(2):195–205.

41. Bangsberg DR, Hecht FM, Clague H, et al. Provider assessment of adherence to HIV antiretroviral therapy. *J Acquir Immune Defic Syndr* 2001;26(5):435–442.

42. Sorensen JL, Mascovich A, Wall TL, et al. Medication adherence strategies for drug abusers with HIV disease. *AIDS Care* 1998;10:297–312.

43. Bamberger JD, Unick J, Klein P, et al. Helping the urban poor stay with antiretroviral HIV drug therapy. *Am J Public Health* 2002;90(5):699–701.

44. Broadhead RS, Heckathorn DD, Altice FL, et al. Increasing drug users' adherence to HIV treatment: results of a peer-driven intervention feasibility study. *Soc Sci Med* 2002;55(2):235–246.

45. McPherson-Baker S, Malow RM, Penedo F, et al. Enhancing adherence to combination antiretroviral therapy in non-adherent HIV-positive men. *AIDS Care* 2000;12(4):399–404.

46. Rigsby MO, Rosen MI, Beauvais JE, et al. Cue-dose training with monetary reinforcement: pilot study of an antiretroviral adherence intervention. *J Gen Intern Med* 2000;15(12):841–847.

47. Budney AJ, Higgins ST. *Therapy manuals for drug addiction: manual 2. A Community Reinforcement Approach: treating cocaine plus vouchers.* U.S. Department of Health and Human Services. Rockville, MD: National Institute on Drug Abuse. NIH Publication No. 98–4309, 1998.

48. Abbott PJ, Moore BA, Weller SB, et al. AIDS risk behavior in opioid-dependent patients treated with Community Reinforcement Approach and relationships with psychiatric disorders. *J Addict Dis* 1998;17:33–48.

49. Rawson RA, Shoptaw SJ, Obert JL, et al. An intensive outpatient approach for cocaine abuse treatment: the Matrix model. *J Subst Abuse Treat* 1995;12:117–127.

50. Shoptaw S, Rawson RA, McCann MJ, et al. The Matrix model of outpatient stimulant abuse treatment. *J Addict Dis* 1994;13:25–34.

CHAPTER 61

Children of Substance-Abusing Parents

PATTI JULIANA AND CAROLYN GOODMAN

This chapter focuses on young children from birth to early adolescence. It describes the scope of the problem and presents a review of the literature concerning the characteristics of this special population of mothers and children. The chapter discusses treatment approaches, treatment models, and special problems that are associated with the ever-growing numbers of children whose parents abuse substances. Because the complications of fetal alcohol syndrome and maternal alcohol use are addressed in an earlier chapter, this chapter focuses on children of persons who are addicted to illegal substances. The chapter concludes with recommendations in the interest of prevention and treatment of drug-exposed children and families.

SCOPE OF THE PROBLEM

Recognition of the problems of children of people who abuse alcohol and other substances has increased in recent decades. In 1975, it was estimated that there were about 250,000 children whose mothers abused heroin (1), and in 1991, the National Household Survey estimated that more than 4.5 million women of childbearing age had used illicit drugs during the previous month (2). More recently, assessments indicate that nationwide approximately 8.3 million (11%) children live with a parent who is addicted to alcohol or illegal substances (3). It is estimated that approximately 40% to 80% of all children in the child welfare system have been placed in foster care because of alcohol or other drug use in the home (4).

The estimates of at-risk children born to drug-using women are likely to be low because those who do not seek prenatal care, those who do not give birth in hospitals, and those who continue drug use during pregnancy are not included in the count. Some patients may cease drug use during pregnancy and then resume subsequent to the birth. There is also a sizeable group of drug-using women who are not reported by their physicians. Assessment of cocaine-exposed infants based upon observation alone may not detect mild withdrawal symptoms or signs that may appear only after discharge from the hospital. Self-reports and observation often result in low-recorded incidence; when more vigorous detection methods are used, the incidence is substantially higher. For these and other social and economic reasons, figures vary on the numbers of women drug users of childbearing age. Given the trend toward abuse of licit and illicit substances, the likelihood of children being born to addicted women will continue to increase during the next decade. This is a growing population of children who may experience impairment and disability, the extent of which is as yet unknown. It is expected that the children will be further affected by health and welfare reform as time limits are imposed and families lose benefits.

The public grew increasingly aware of the special needs and problems of childhood and adolescence in the early 1960s. The children's rights movement gained momentum when the United Nations General Assembly adopted the Declaration of the Human Rights of the Child in 1959. In 1979, the United States Congress passed the Child Welfare Reform Act, which promoted public and professional concern for children and limited the length of time children can remain in the foster care system before permanency planning must occur. As cocaine use peaked and indicators of heroin use reappeared, the large numbers of infants born with symptoms of drug withdrawal and human immunodeficiency virus (HIV) infection dramatized the need for treatment and prevention for the entire family while the child welfare system continued to struggle with large numbers of children in placement. The development of the Adoption and Safe Families Act (1997) underscored the need for finding effective ways to better address the needs of families with concurrent substance abuse and child maltreatment (5).

The proliferation of the substance abuse problem and the heightened attention to the needs of children and youth generated recognition that there is a distinct population, the children of substance abusers, who had unique characteristics that demanded attention. It was also apparent that an addicted mother with children required help for herself, her children, and her family. It is now well documented that the children of untreated drug- and alcohol-using parents are at risk for serious educational, medical, and emotional problems and have the potential for abusing illicit drugs themselves.

REVIEW OF THE LITERATURE

A review of the literature from the end of the nineteenth century reflected a concern about the passage of drugs through the human placenta and through the breast milk of the drug-using mother. As early as 1888, the possibility of long-term effects of fetal opioid exposure was addressed (6). The increasing concern about fetal exposure during the 1970s resulted in a significant number of studies of maternal heroin or methadone use and its effect on the neonate.

Much of the literature on children of substance-using parents is focused on these medical complications. Finnegan reported that the effects of maternal heroin or methadone use on infants are influenced by the adequacy of prenatal care, obstetric complications, and maternal polydrug use (7). She has documented the characteristics of neonatal abstinence syndrome, describing infants born to heroin-addicted mothers as small for gestational age, often experiencing withdrawal symptoms beginning shortly after birth (8), and as irritable and difficult to parent (8–10). There is some agreement that the neonatal behavioral and developmental effects of maternal heroin use include irritability, feeding disturbances, sleeplessness, deficits in attention span, and impaired mother–child communications (11,12).

There are discrepancies in the research literature that identify and describe cocaine-exposed babies. This is partly a result of confounding factors of poverty, lack of prenatal care, family instability, and polydrug abuse. Most studies have not controlled for specific drug-use patterns

or psychosocial variables. Although the long-term effects of maternal cocaine use given its neurotoxicity, children may suffer from learning disabilities, affect regulation and behavioral problems and other neurologic issues that may become manifest in later years (13–15). A review of infants and toddlers placed in foster care indicated that those exposed to drugs *in utero* had more special care needs than did those not so exposed (16).

During the postnatal period, children may be inconsolable and tax the tolerance of the parents. Development of effective mother–infant communication is impaired as the infant experiencing withdrawal rejects the mother's attempts at consolation; insufficient feedback makes it difficult for the mother to understand her child's needs (17). The behavior patterns of the neonate reduce the caregiver's responsiveness to the infant and exacerbate the low self-esteem often seen in drug-using parents (18). The current literature related to maternal substance abuse or families and addiction focus on infancy and fetal drug exposure, or to treatment of families with a substance-abusing member. Research on childhood effects of parental substance use continues to suggest biologic and psychosocial impacts as described in earlier studies.

Among the problems found in these children are increased vulnerability to visual problems, inadequate fine motor coordination, heightened levels of motor activity, and attention deficits, particularly in structured interactions (19). It was found that children exposed to heroin *in utero* scored lower on perceptual tests than did their peers and were less able to concentrate on tasks (17,20,21). Although some of these studies are inconclusive, they suggest that these children are at high risk for developmental disabilities.

Assessment of older children of heroin-addicted and formerly addicted parents reveal that they suffer from emotional and cognitive problems; they express feelings of anxiety and insecurity, and are characterized by shorter attention spans than their peers (20). More than half of these children have poor prognoses for school success and age-appropriate socioemotional development. The 6- to 17-year-old children of drug-using parents are characterized by increased problems in school, and by behavioral and adjustment problems at a greater rate than a comparison group of their peers. These problems may be related to parental substance abuse at home, compromised communications within families, unstable home lives, and the impact of HIV/AIDS on families, among other sequelae of drug use (22).

Teenaged children of addicted parents also show increased incidence of behavioral problems at home and with their peers and are more likely to evidence academic failure, antisocial behavior, risky sexual behavior and drug and alcohol use (19,23). These findings are consonant with earlier studies of a similar group of children during early childhood; unsuccessful completion of developmental tasks can result in attention deficits, poor impulse control, and impaired attachment to others, which are risk factors and predictors for later drug and alcohol use (20,23,24). When strong familial bonds exist, the likelihood of attachment to drug-using peers decreases; however, the homes of drug-using adolescents reflect poor family management, parental antisocial behavior, and parental substance abuse (24).

Similarly, the family histories of the drug-using parents reflect a high incidence of disruption, conflict, loss of parental figures, and lack of strong, affectionate parent–child bonds (24). Studies of addicted women reveal feelings of low self-esteem, anxiety, depression, and serious problems in their families of origin, such as addiction and physical abuse (19,25,26). The childhood experiences of drug-abusing women can be characterized by maternal deprivation, lack of supportive family networks, maltreatment, low levels of family competence, and adverse family environments (19,25). As parents who were deprived of age-appropriate experiences in childhood, they approach parenthood with minimal bonding experience, unrealistic expectations, and without having learned adequate parenting skills. They may require more assistance in parenting, as the interpersonal and environmental impacts of substance abuse compound the effects of *in utero* drug exposure. Substance abuse is not only the problem of the individual but must be considered in the context of family and social systems.

APPROACHES TO THE TREATMENT OF ADDICTED WOMEN AND CHILDREN

Treatment of Children

When a substance-abusing parent has children, it is critical to remedy those problems that have occurred as a result of parental drug use. The symptoms of affected children can manifest as health, behavioral, or learning difficulties; developmental assessments identify lags in individual children. However, these children are least likely to receive developmental screening and early intervention, especially if their parents are actively addicted, overwhelmed by their recovery efforts, and by confounding health, environmental, and psychosocial stressors (24).

Assessment and treatment of the needs of children must be coordinated so as to offer the full range of services that are necessary. Collaboration among medical and social services is particularly critical to facilitate recovery, family stability, improved parent–child interactions, and access to appropriate care for the children involved.

Low self-esteem, anxiety, and depression associated with being raised in an addicted family may be treated as primary symptoms. Children of substance-abusing parents often lack basic trust and ability to become attached as they hope for parental love and nurturance; as parents

live in continually shifting states of intoxication and abstinence, the child learns self-care that interrupts development of intimacy and results in isolation and depression (25). Positive, supportive, trusting relationships are helpful in improving a child's self-image. In such relationships, a child can be helped to recognize and appropriately express feelings, to understand the disease concept of addiction, and to develop coping mechanisms. Every child requires the security of order and consistency; it is particularly important that these needs be addressed when working with children, whose surroundings are often characterized by repeated disruption and uncertainty.

Play groups have been effective in developing the cognitive, emotional, social, and physical development of younger children; group interaction provides stimulation of cognitive and language functions (26). Early childhood programs, in general, promote optimal development of children, and early intervention is critical for children with developmental delays. Groups benefit older children and adolescents, providing support and reducing isolation. Such groups help children identify and recognize their experiences, ventilate feelings, and participate in a corrective "family" environment. Further retrospective and prospective studies on the long-term effects of parental drug use are essential to plan and develop more effective interventions for older children.

Treatment of the Parents

Studies reveal a direct relationship between the emotional and cognitive difficulties of the mothers and those of their children (27,28). The mother's attitude and behavior often have negative effects on the growth and development of her child. The parents, often maternally deprived themselves, may have difficulty responding to their children. Women face multiple obstacles to seeking treatment for substance abuse, including child care, financial constraints, and lack of support systems. They must contend with increased stigma as social mores stereotype female addicts as weak-willed, irresponsible, and promiscuous, and they often experience resistance from their partners and children who resent the treatment that disrupts homeostasis (29). Single parents are further stressed as they often neglect their own well-being, choosing to meet their children's needs at the expense of their own (30).

Research suggests that drug-treatment programs providing ancillary services designed to meet the particular needs of parents, such as child care, and those involving other family members and significant others, hold the greatest promise for women with drug and alcohol problems and are highly cost-effective (30–33). Assisting parents in their recovery is the optimal means of treating their children. Parenting skills can be reinforced in drug-treatment settings. Parents are best assisted individually, in combination with family intervention, support groups, and parenting skills training. There has been significant progress in developing such services during the last decade.

Family Treatment

There is general agreement that in planning programs for drug-abusing parents and their children, an approach that involves the family unit is most effective. Family therapy combined with drug treatment is effective in treatment of substance-abusing families (33) and is recognized as an essential approach to treating the full range of addictive problems in families (34). Some of the principles that guide family therapy are a pragmatic approach to treatment with an eye toward what works, emphasis on the present rather than a historical perspective, interruption of behavior patterns, focus on process rather than on content, and restructuring of families (35).

Systems theory assumes that all people in the family unit play a part in the way family members function in relation to each other and in the way the symptom of addiction finally erupts (36). This theory focuses on functional facts of relationships and provides a framework for conceptualizing chemical dependency; systems therapy can be used to alleviate the symptom as it addresses familial interactions. Minuchin's structural family therapy focuses on patterns of family interactions and communications; within this approach, the therapist reinforces generational boundaries between parents and children (37). Stanton and Todd combine structural techniques with Haley's strategic model; with a view of symptoms as attempts at changing family difficulties they emphasize a specific treatment plan, external events, changes in the symptom, and collaboration among treatment systems (38).

Parent Support Groups

Parent support networks are critical components of treatment and prevention programs for addicted parents and their children. The goal of the support group is to improve the parents' interactions with their children by developing viable peer networks. Within this context, the parents are able to consider their children's feelings, to understand their behaviors in the context of developmental stages, and to become aware of the dynamics of their interactions with their children. The group eventually becomes an independent mutual support network that helps its members develop self-esteem and empathy. The task of empowering the parents is a three-stage process: bonding, facilitation, and separation. For these tasks to be accomplished, the staff must be understanding, accessible, and nurturing. The first stage of connecting parents with helpers is the most challenging; for parents who experienced rejection and loss in childhood, the process of forming relationships does not come easily. The parents must be able to learn

that they will not be rejected by their "family" even when their behavior is provocative or excessively demanding. The development of trust in a continued relationship with a counselor or health professional who can provide understanding, acceptance, and support has been found to be critical in improving the lifestyle of drug-addicted persons (39).

In the second stage, when a relationship of trust is established, the counselor or helper role becomes one of facilitation and advocacy. Parents are mobilized to act on their own behalf, and staff encourage self-exploration and development of self-awareness. When intervention fosters input, feedback, decision making, and networking, these behaviors flourish. Parents learn about the purpose of their children's behaviors and gain insight into effective interactions. They begin to see a link between their childhood experiences and their behaviors and feelings toward their children. With the development of sensitivity to and understanding of their children, unrealistic expectations diminish. Parents are able to assume a more positive and consistent role in the growth of their children. Additionally, as they experience the acceptance of the facilitator and peers and recognize they are not isolated in their struggles, the parents articulate a sense of relief and a growth of self-tolerance.

In the third stage, separation, the parents are ready to rely upon other resources and support systems. The helper's role becomes that of a resource for the parents, and the group becomes an independent mutual support network that strengthens its members' self-esteem and increases empathic interactions. They are able to rely upon each other.

Parenting Skills Groups

Men and women who are addicted to drugs often have not experienced positive parenting models; many feel inadequate as parents. More than most caregivers, they need to experience self-esteem by being accepted, respected, and educated in the skills of parenting. Although they have difficulties coping with their children, they want to be "good" mothers and fathers. This motivation can be tapped and used to engage parents in skills groups. Parenting skills training is didactic in format. Three effective approaches are behavior management, relationship therapy, and child development theory. The principles of each approach focus on different aspects of understanding, but ideas borrowed from all three may guide the groups.

Behavior management is based on the concepts of reinforcement and modeling behaviors (40–42). Reinforcement emphasizes those actions of the parent that encourage approved behaviors and extinguish disapproved behaviors in the child. Parents are taught to understand and use appropriate rewards to shape and strengthen desirable behaviors in their children and withhold rewards for undesirable behaviors. Modeling is based on the principle that children tend to imitate and then internalize the behaviors, ideas, and attitudes of their parents.

Relationship therapy uses the insights of Rogers (43) and Axline (44). Parents are taught to empathize with their children and to understand that children often express feelings through their actions rather than words. They learn how to listen and respond through physical expressions of warmth and caring. Because of the dangerous environment in which many families typically reside, parents are taught how to create safe and secure settings and seek alternative approaches to the management of multiple stressors.

Child development theory assists parents in understanding each developmental level to establish reasonable expectations and cope with the normal frustrations of particular age groups. When parents understand the meaning of their children's behavior, the frustration of unrealistic demands can be avoided. As parents are helped to understand their children's development and gain insight into their interactions, the problems of being socialized in an addicted family may be corrected. Studies document that the self-esteem of women who participated in parenting skills groups was substantially raised, which, in turn, resulted in the improved development of their children (45).

Treatment Models Designed for Addicted Mothers and Their Children

A broad range of psychosocial services may be required to address the needs of children whose parents abuse substances and to meet the needs of the parents in recovery. Whether services are provided on-site or through community-based organizations, service needs include medical care for parents and children alike, chemical-dependency treatment, legal services, education and job training, child care, developmental assessments, parenting education, mental health services, housing assistance, transportation, and case management services (321); availability and accessibility of a range of services can minimize stress and promote the relationship between the addicted parent and the treatment facility. Outreach efforts can facilitate engagement of drug-dependent persons into treatment as indigenous workers encourage women, especially, to use available medical and social services (46).

One of the pioneer programs designed to treat addicted women as part of a family unit was PACE (Parent and Child Education) (47). PACE began in 1968 as a program for mentally ill mothers and their children. As increasing numbers of mothers were also substance abusers, the program was modified to meet the needs of this special population of women and their children. PACE was a comprehensive intervention program that served mothers, children from birth through 5 years of age, fathers, and other available family members. The program fostered the inclusion of family members as active participants in the treatment team to help the development of his or her young child. To

achieve this goal, a mother must be involved in trying to understand herself and, in many instances, in changing her self-concept from one of passive powerlessness to one of active mastery. The mother at PACE became both teacher and student as she engaged in the process of empowering herself and her child. The PACE program fostered the development of parenting skills and self-esteem that could enable the mother to deal with the physical and psychological needs of her young child.

At PACE, mother and child attended an education center several days a week, where they spent part of the time together in a classroom setting. At other times, parents participated in parent education, treatment, and social recreation groups with other mothers while their children were in the classroom with teachers. This arrangement allowed mother and child to interact with each other and to develop and learn in keeping with age-appropriate tasks. To facilitate the growth of the children, the physical arrangement of the classroom where they spent all their time was designed to create a structured, secure, and consistent setting where order and routine prevailed; the room was arranged for maximum interaction between mother and child.

The children's education program at PACE varied with developmental age and was based on four major areas of growth: muscular, cognitive, language, and creative skills. Within clearly defined limits, children were encouraged to explore their bodies and their environment through activities such as storytelling and dramatization. When mothers were in the classroom, they not only learned to interact with their children but also had the opportunity to enjoy educational experiences they had been deprived of in their own childhood.

When not in the classroom, mothers were involved with a number of group activities in which they learned child development concepts and health care, took part in group and family therapy, and had opportunities to socialize and engage in recreational pursuits with other mothers. All the groups—educational, treatment, social, and recreational—served to promote support networks and initiate friendships. Mothers realized they could call on each other for help in emergencies, as well as find companionship and relaxation. Changes in behavior, attitude, and self-perception took place in an atmosphere in which the mothers found parenting models and support networks they had never experienced before. The staff at PACE, themselves part of a support network, became a nurturing family until the mothers were able to shape their own family systems.

Another program that approaches the needs of parents who suffer chemical dependency and those of their children is incorporated into the Department of Psychiatry's Division of Substance Abuse at the Albert Einstein College of Medicine (AECOM). The Division of Substance Abuse (DoSA) treats more than 3,600 former heroin addicts in 10 community-based clinics. Most patients suffer from the many stresses of living with poverty, unemployment, inadequate housing or homelessness, chaotic home lives, broken families, inferior schools, and discrimination.

Since its inception, the philosophy of DoSA has been to provide a diversified approach to meet the broad range of medical, social, and psychological problems presented by narcotic addicts entering treatment. As the perception of addiction broadened, the program sought to prevent the residual effects associated with being raised in an addicted family and to treat those problems that had already occurred. Identification, evaluation, and referral services for the children were integrated into the regular division services to include parent education, staff training, advocacy, and liaison with children's services in the surrounding community.

The program provides a point of entry to medical and social services for the children of patients who are traditionally disenfranchised and alienated from these services. Staff work cooperatively with parents and children individually, and with parent–child dyads to improve family life and break the cycle of substance abuse and other intergenerational problems. Staff training for this population addresses special needs and issues that confront children and families. Liaison services operate among the DoSA program, school-based intervention and prevention services, and other health, welfare, and education resources.

With the increased incidence of maternal substance abuse, attention has shifted to focus on pregnant women. State funding has provided a wide range of specialized comprehensive and coordinated services. Drug treatment, obstetric, pediatric, HIV-related, and social services for pregnant substance abusers are designed to minimize drug use, reduce the incidence of neonatal abstinence syndrome, improve the well-being of neonates, and facilitate early bonding among family members. Caseworkers trained in maternity services work in with the clinic treatment team to address the range of drug treatment, medical, and psychosocial needs of pregnant addicted women. Prenatal education and individual counseling services are coordinated with health and welfare services to provide a continuum of treatment services.

The special educational needs for services to correct language and cognitive delays, and behavior problems require coordination in the school system. It is important to accommodate these needs to forestall school failure and dropout. Critical collaborative efforts include provision of full developmental assessments and services through linkage with such specialized services. Provision of onsite services has improved parental compliance with completion of evaluations as it minimizes fears of being judged as inadequate parents and reduces apprehensions about breach of confidentiality (48).

When blinded HIV seroprevalence studies revealed that 32% of patients enrolled in the Division's programs were positive, extensive HIV services components were developed for patients with a family approach. Children who face the loss of a parent face fears of who will care for

them. Children of parents with AIDS are often placed into foster care upon their parent's final hospitalization when they have not had opportunity or ability to plan for the care of their children upon their death. These children lose the support of significant family and friends who might otherwise ease the child's resolution of the loss of their parent. The depth of emotional reactions is often overwhelming and cannot be overstated. Guilt, powerlessness, and recurrent anxiety are the debilitating feeling left to these children. Their sense of isolation is exacerbated and their fears of abandonment are not addressed as children are often forgotten by grieving adults. Consequently, the AECOM DoSA addresses the concerns of HIV-affected families by assisting the parents in planning for permanent homes for their children. The aim of family services in any drug treatment is to enhance the quality of life for the entire family.

Special Needs of Substance-Affected Parents and Their Children

Prenatal drug exposure and drug-abusing families are placing increasing demands on social welfare systems; in addition to concerns about the safety and care of drug-exposed infants, programs must also address the needs of the many children who also have long-term learning and developmental disabilities. Without intervention, academic problems and high dropout rates can be anticipated. The cost of helping these children overcome the effects of drug exposure varies with the severity of disability. The tragedy of substance abuse is compounded by the failure of substance abuse treatment facilities to provide services that are sensitive to the needs of women, particularly those who are pregnant or have young children. Because few treatment programs address parenting issues or other needs of women, there is a growing population of addicted mothers and drug-exposed children with few resources for assistance, and the rise in the number of drug-exposed children has placed an onerous burden on child welfare and health and education systems.

COORDINATION OF SERVICES

Children, their families, and their caretakers present so complex an array of problems and needs that no one system or institution could adequately handle a single family. Nevertheless, substance abuse affects the entire family, and all its members have a right to obtain help. The importance of interagency coordination is well-recognized; without provisions for case management, families, as well as staff, can become lost in the service labyrinth.

As problems of children whose parents abuse substances confront a variety of local, state, and federal agencies, the structure and bureaucratic policies of these agencies hamper provision of coordinated services. Although different agencies, by virtue of their structure and function, are accustomed to working in their respective fields, the nature of the needs of these children is such that it is crucial that services for them and their families be coordinated rather than fragmented and duplicated. Linkages among systems must be developed. Families may be involved with a variety of services simultaneously, and appointments with each may conflict. The overlap of scheduling creates stress and confusion. The goal for agencies should be to assist addicted mothers in organizing and simplifying their lives so their children can be raised with less stress and confusion.

CHILD WELFARE

Child maltreatment is not a recent phenomenon, nor is it unique to substance-abusing parents. Some would argue that the use of illicit substances does not automatically constitute child abuse or neglect. However, criminal cases against pregnant mothers who use drugs continue, charging them with drug delivery *in utero*, and the child protective system is taxed beyond its capacity as the increasing use of substances has added substantially to the numbers of cases reported to child protective services and those separated from their families. Human and institutional resources for prevention and treatment of abuse and neglect are often incapable of handling these problems. Assessment of risk factors for children whose parents may be difficult to locate or engage in a preliminary working relationship presents special difficulties for child protective service workers. If one is able to engage the parents in treatment on behalf of their children, treatment services are not readily available, and the rehabilitation period may be protracted.

The Adoption and Safe Families Act protected the developmental needs of children by abbreviating the length of time in placement, but it also presented what may be an insurmountable problem for parents with substance use disorders as the recovery process alone requires more time. The stigma associated with being a substance-using parent, issues related to family histories of alcohol and other drug use, complications of welfare reform and poverty all confound the process of reuniting families (49).

To assure preservation of families and to attain timely stability for their children, coordination of care between child welfare and drug-treatment services is critical. Cross-discipline training of child protective service workers and treatment providers in the needs of children and their parents who abuse substances, specialized care of HIV or drug-affected infants, ethnic and cultural issues and values, and attitudes and behaviors regarding use of drugs and alcohol are essential because lack of knowledge, nonsupportive or hostile attitudes of caregivers, and stigma associated with drug use present for women a barrier to their engagement in both child welfare and treatment services. Similarly, training of staff needs to involve agency

policies and philosophy, as well as issues of countertransference. Some workers may reject the mother because they believe the child is simply a victim of the mother's abuse. Others show greater interest in seeing the mother as victim as well and either overlook maltreatment for fear of alienating the mother or seek to keep the family intact, sometimes against better judgment.

Provision of comprehensive drug treatment benefits family members affected by substance abuse in addition to assisting the patient's recovery; combined with a supportive approach from child welfare services, collaboration can assure wise and timely care of families.

STAFF TRAINING IN ALCOHOL- AND DRUG-TREATMENT SERVICES

Programs for substance-abusing pregnant women and parents and their children provide a unique approach in the field of human services; many will enter treatment on behalf of their children, providing a motivational opportunity for treatment staff. Staff in drug-treatment clinics and other agencies tend to be more familiar with traditional approaches that focus on the drug user. As the idea of prevention and treatment for mothers and children grows, training programs are essential for the diverse array of people involved in these endeavors. There remains a broad spectrum of providers in drug-abuse prevention and treatment agencies, and in social and medical services who would be better prepared to intervene on behalf of families of drug users had they more information about the families' special needs and about cultural issues surrounding substance abuse and family care. The complexity of the problems presented by drug-exposed children and their families requires skilled interdisciplinary teams that can recognize, assess, and correct problems that may emerge.

In general, program development around services for children in drug-treatment settings should include

1. Identification and orientation of the staff who will implement family services. Such training should include, at a minimum, child development, family systems, and substance-abusing families, and federal and state laws regarding child welfare.
2. Development and reinforcement of links with referral resources as full collaborative efforts. Community-based agencies that address the family as a whole, and those that provide specialized developmental services, pediatric services, respite care, mental health support, and parenting education should be included. Collaborative efforts would include establishment of a team approach that embraces the family and assures understanding of the respective missions, responsibilities and service plans of each entity, and cross-training of program and referral resource staff on addiction, families, and relevant cultural issues.

3. Identification and referral of children and patients who might benefit from the services. This might involve medical and psychosocial screening of children, and could include a developmental history, current health status and immunization record, and report cards to determine school progress or special needs and attendance.
4. Initial family evaluation to be conducted on each family. This evaluation should include determination of the child's response to parental guidance, any behaviors expressed toward the family, the child's perception of his or her role in the family and of current circumstances.
5. An initial service plan should be developed on completion of the family assessment. This plan should include identification of service needs and a plan of action for meeting those needs either directly within the program structure or by referral.
6. Parent support and parenting education services.

CONCLUSION

In summary, the children of substance abusers suffer from the addiction of their parents and they are at risk for social, psychological, educational, and medical problems. Drug-treatment services do well to include services for parents as patients and to address the special needs of the children of patients. Services sensitive to the needs of parents include attention to day care needs, perinatal services, and parenting skills training. Medical services familiar with the social and psychological factors associated with drug and alcohol use can be a point of entry to the service system, and children's services, including schools, need to be aware of indicators of family drug or alcohol use.

Guidelines for prevention, education, treatment, and research programs that focus on the unique situation of children and address the needs of drug-using pregnant women and their children are of paramount importance. A review and redefinition of system policies and procedures is necessary to ensure that parents are evaluated not only in terms of their addiction but also as members of a family. This holds particularly true for pregnant women and mothers, as epidemiologic studies and family research amply demonstrate that thousands of addicted mothers are not receiving prenatal, parenting, or medical care or treatment for substance abuse. More programs are needed to address the needs of substance-abusing women who are pregnant and of parents, and for child care and child development services. Creative approaches that assure confidentiality, protection from punitive interventions, and development of parenting skills are needed. The problems of children are often preventable, and the effects of parental addiction can be minimized. Legislation, regulation, and adequate funding are critical to protecting the health and well-being of addicted families. Although these measures may be costly, they will be far less so than institutional hospital-based treatment of complications of perinatal drug use and rehabilitative or custodial care of the children.

REFERENCES

1. Carr JN. Drug patterns among drug-addicted mothers—incidence, variance in use, and effects on children. *Pediatr Ann* 1975;4:408–417.
2. National Institute on Drug Abuse. *National household survey.* Washington, DC: Author, 1991.
3. National Institute on Drug Abuse. *National household survey.* Washington, DC: Author, 1996.
4. Young NK, Gardner S, Dennis K. *Responding to alcohol and other drug problems in child welfare: weaving together practice and policy.* Washington, DC: Child Welfare League of America Press, 1998.
5. U.S. Department of Health and Human Services. *Blending perspectives and building common ground: a report to congress on substance abuse and child protection.* Washington DC: U.S. Government Printing Office, 1999.
6. Zagon IS. Opioids and development: new lessons from old problems. *NIDA Res Monogr* 1985;60:58–77.
7. Finnegan LP. Effects of maternal opiate abuse on the newborn. *Fed Proc* 1985;44:2315–2318.
8. Finnegan LP. Management of the drug-dependent pregnancy and effects on neonatal outcome. In: Bescher G, Brotman R, eds. *Proceedings of the NIDA symposium on comprehensive health care for addicted families and their children.* DHEW Publication No. 017–024–00598–3. Washington, DC: U.S. Government Printing Office, 1976:59–66.
9. Escamilla-Mondanaro J. Women: pregnancy, children and addiction. *J Psychedelic Drugs* 1977;9:59–68.
10. Householder J, Hatcher R, Burn W, et al. Infants born to narcotic-addicted mothers. *Psychol Bull* 1982;92:453–468.
11. Kandall SR, Albin S, Lowinson J, et al. Differential effects of maternal heroin and methadone use on birthweight. *Pediatrics* 1976;58:681–685.
12. Kron RE, Kaplan SL, Phoenix MD, et al. Behavior of infants born to drug-dependent mothers: effects of prenatal and postnatal drugs. In: Rementeria JL, ed. *Drug abuse in pregnancy and neonatal effects.* St. Louis: CV Mosby, 1977:129–144.
13. Eiden RD, Lewis A, Croff S, et al. Maternal cocaine use and infant behavior. *Infancy* 2002;3;77–96.
14. Coles CD, Bard KA, Platzman KA, et al. Attentional response at eight weeks in prenatally drug exposed and preterm infants. *Neurotoxicol Teratol* 1999;21;527–537.
15. Singer LT, Arendt R, Minnes S, et al. Cognitive and motor outcomes of cocaine exposed infants. *JAMA* 2002;287(15) 1952–1960.
16. McNichol T. The Impact of drug-exposed children on family foster care. *Child Welfare* 1999;78;184–196.
17. Strauss ME, Lessen-Firestone JK, Starr RH, et al. Behavior of narcotic-addicted newborns. *Child Dev* 1975;46:887–893.
18. Colten ME. A comparison of heroin-addicted and non-addicted mothers: their attitudes, beliefs, and parenting experiences. NIDA services research report. In: *Heroin-addicted parents and their children: two reports.* DHHS Publication

No. (ADM) 81–1028. Washington, DC: U.S. Government Printing Office, 1980.

19. NIDA Services Research Monograph Series. *Addicted women: family dynamics, self-perceptions and support systems.* USDHEW publication No. 80–762, Washington, DC: U.S. Government Printing Office, 1979.

20. Sowder BJ, Burt MR. *Children of heroin addicts: an assessment of health, learning, behavioral and adjustment problems.* New York: Praeger, 1980.

21. Herjanic BM, Barreto VH, Herjanic M, et al. Children of heroin addicts. *Int J Addict* 1979;14:919–931.

22. Moss HB, Vanyukov M, Majumder PP, et al. Prepubertal sons of substance abusers. *Addict Behav* 1995;20(3):345–358.

23. Nunes EV, Weissman MM, Golstein R, et al. Psychiatric disorders and impairment in the children of opiate addicts: prevalences and distribution by ethnicity. *Am J Addict* 2000;9:232–241.

24. Anderson A, Henry CS. Family systems characteristics and parental behaviors as predictors of adolescent substance use. *Adolescence* 1994;29(114):405–420.

25. Cuskey WR, Wathey B. *Female addiction.* Lexington, MA: Lexington Books, 1982.

26. Kissin WB, Svikis DS, Morgan CD, et al. Characterizing pregnant drug-dependent women in treatment and their children. *J Subst Abuse Treat* 2001;21;27–34.

27. Rivinus TM, ed. *Children of chemically dependent parents.* New York: Bruner-Mazel, 1991.

28. Lief N. *Some measures of parenting behavior for addicted and nonaddicted mothers.* NIDA services research report. Washington, DC: U.S. Government Printing Office, 1977.

29. Kane-Cavaiola C, Rullo-Cooney D. Addicted women: their families' effect on treatment outcome. *J Chem Depend* 1992;4(1):111–119.

30. Finkelstein N, Derman L. Single-parent women: what a mother can do. In: Roth P, ed. *Alcohol and drugs are women's issues:* vol. 1. A review of issues. Metuchen, NJ: Scarecrow Press, 1991.

31. Daley.

32. Uziel-Miller ND, Lyon JS. Specialized substance abuse treatment for women and their children: an analysis of program design. *J Subst Abuse Treat* 2000;19:355–367.

33. Stanton MD, Todd TC. *The family therapy of drug abuse and addiction.* New York: Guilford Press, 1982.

34. Heath AW, Stanton MD. Family therapy. In: Frances RJ, Miller SI, eds. *Clinical textbook of addictive disorders.* New York: Guilford Press, 1991.

35. Todd TC, Stanton MD, Calway J. *Treatment manual of marital and family therapy* [special adaptation for treatment of cocaine dependence]. Unpublished manuscript, 1985.

36. Bowen M. Alcoholism as viewed through family systems theory and family psychotherapy. *Fam Dynam Addict Q* 1991;1(1):94–102.

37. Minuchin S. *Families and family therapy.* Cambridge, MA: Harvard University Press, 1974.

38. Stanton MD, Todd TC. Structural-strategic family therapy with drug addicts. In: Kaufman E, Kaufman P, eds. *Family therapy of drug and alcohol abuse,* 2nd ed. Boston: Allyn and Bacon, 1992.

39. Beschner G, Thompson P. *Women and drug abuse treatment: needs and services.* NIDA research monograph series. USDHHS publication no. 81–1057. Washington, DC: U.S. Government Printing Office, 1981.

40. Bandura A. *Social learning theory.* Englewood Cliffs, NJ: Prentice-Hall, 1977.

41. Dodson J. *Dare to discipline.* New York: Bantam Books, 1970.

42. Ginott H. *Between parent and child.* New York: Macmillan, 1965.

43. Rogers C. *On becoming a person.* New York: Houghton-Mifflin, 1970.

44. Axline VM. *Play therapy.* New York: Ballantine Books, 1974.

45. Glaser YIM. A unit for mothers and babies in a psychiatric hospital. *J Child Psychology* 1962;3:53–60.

46. *Maternal drug abuse, drug exposed children. Understanding the problem.* USDHHS Publication No. (ADM) 92–1949. September 1992.

47. Goodman C. The PACE family treatment and education program: a public health approach to parental competence and promotion of mental health. In: Cohler B, Musick J, eds. *Intervention with psychiatrically disabled parents and their young children. New dimensions for mental health services, no. 24.* San Francisco: Jossey-Bass, 1984.

48. Schulman LH, Shapira SR, Hirshfield S. Outreach developmental services to children of patients in treatment for substance Abuse. *Am J Public Health* 2000;90:1930–1933.

49. Karroll BR, Poertner J. Judges,' caseworkers' and substance abuse counselors' indicators of family reunification with substance-affected parents. *Child Welfare* 2002;249–269.

CHAPTER 62

Adolescents

ANDRES J. PUMARIEGA, MARK D. KILGUS, AND LEONARDO RODRIGUEZ

A significant number of American teens use and abuse illicit and addictive substances. An estimated 1 in 5 teenagers (4.3 million) are current alcohol drinkers, 1 in 13 teenagers (1.7 million) are binge alcohol drinkers, and 400,000 adolescents are in need of substance abuse treatment (1,2). It is projected that the year 2010 will witness the largest number of adolescents in American history (3), so there is a clear need to improve our understanding of adolescent substance use disorders (SUDs), and to provide effective prevention and treatment. Adolescents have unique needs because of their stage of development, so we cannot apply concepts derived from adult models and expect they will yield the desired results. This chapter examines the scope of the problem, the progression of adolescent SUD, and developmental and risk factors that are unique to adolescents. It also discusses the available assessment, treatment, and prevention models for adolescent SUD.

PREVALENCE OF ADOLESCENT SUBSTANCE ABUSE

The initiation and early stages of substance use have their roots in adolescence (4). For example, 85% of current smokers began smoking by the age of 21 years, and approximately 3,000 children a day start using tobacco, of whom one-third will die prematurely of a smoking-related disease (5,6). Much evidence supports the theory that tobacco use is a gateway to alcohol and illicit drug use and abuse. The exact point along the continuum at which use becomes abuse is arbitrary and may differ for subgroups. Psychiatric criteria established for defining abuse and dependence has largely grown out of studying adults. The criteria for abuse in the *Diagnostic and Statistical Manual of Mental Disorders,* 4th ed., text revision (*DSM–IV–TR*) includes a pattern that results in impaired function at work, school, home, or in relationships, continued use despite having these impairments, recurrent use in dangerous situations, recurrent substance-related legal problems, and continued use despite negative consequences (7). Many experts believe that waiting to intervene until adolescents meet the criteria is irresponsible. *DSM–IV–TR* criteria for substance dependence includes, but is not limited to, tolerance (increased use to achieve desired effect; diminished effect with same amount) and withdrawal (characteristic withdrawal syndrome, or using to avoid withdrawal) (7). As applied to adolescents, research supports the utility of the *DSM–IV* construct of dependence, but tolerance, withdrawal, and medical problems present differently in adolescents than in adults, suggesting limitations in the use of criteria for *DSM–IV* (8).

Overall Prevalence and Perceived Risk

Information about adolescent SUD is largely derived from the annual Monitoring the Future survey (9) which (from 1975 to the present) has sampled more than 15,000 high school seniors in 120 to 146 public and private schools across the country. In 1991, the survey expanded to include eighth and tenth grade students of similar sample size as the seniors. It monitors prevalence, trends, and attitudes of substance use in this population. Although it is an invaluable resource, the study has been criticized for missing data on school dropouts and absentees on the day of survey administration. In eighth, tenth, and twelfth grades, there is an absenteeism rate of 11%, 12%, and 16%, respectively, and seniors have a 16% dropout rate, many of these being the adolescents most likely to use substances. Investigators for the survey say that, with the exception of heroin, crack, and phencyclidine (PCP) statistics, dropouts and absentees on the day of administration do not significantly affect prevalence. Another debated weakness of the survey is that the data are collected from retrospective self-reports, which may be underreports because most drug use is illicit or disapproved of by teachers, parents, and peers (10). Some studies, however, support the validity of self-reporting in the adolescent population. Other sources of data on adolescent substance use include the Drug Abuse Warning Network (DAWN) emergency room reports, regional school studies, studies of treatment programs, arrest and death rates, and national household surveys.

The 2002 Monitoring the Future survey reported a lifetime prevalence of any illicit drug use for eighth graders of 24.5%, for tenth graders of 44.6%, and for high school seniors of 53.0%. Marijuana and inhalant use are important contributors and significantly increase prevalence. A higher proportion of males than females are involved in illicit and licit drug use. The overall rates of *any illicit drug* use differed some among the regions. The highest rate was in the Northeast, where 46% of seniors said they had used an *illicit drug* in the past year, followed by the North Central (42%), the West (41%), and the South (38%). African American students have a lower reported lifetime and annual prevalence for virtually all drugs than white and Hispanic students, whereas Hispanics have the highest lifetime and annual prevalence rates for cocaine and crack (9).

Trends in perceived harmfulness, which may parallel or influence drug use and help predict upcoming use, show some important shifts. The perceived risks associated with experimental use of crystal methamphetamine (ice) fell from 62% in 1991 to 53% in 1998, and in 2002 54%, while annual use rose from 1.4% in 1991 to 3.0% in 2002 (9). LSD (lysergic acid diethylamide) had steady rates of perceived risk until 1991, and then began a downward trend that continued through 1997 and halted in 1998. Despite a decline in recent years of perceived risk and disapproval, actual use had been falling. This paradox raised the question about substitution by another drug, and, indeed, ecstasy (MDMA or methylenedioxymethamphetamine) had been in ascent and may have had some substitution effect. In 2002, perceived risk and disapproval of *LSD* use increased while use decreased, as did use of *ecstasy* (9). In 1996, perceived risk for heroin among high school seniors rose from 1996 through 1998, perhaps as the result of an antiheroin campaign launched by the Partnership for a Drug-Free America in June 1996, as well as the visibility of heroin-related deaths of some entertainment and fashion celebrities. After a brief decrease in risk perception in 1999 and an increase in use in 2000, its use declined in 2001 as perceived risk increased slightly. After showing little change in the latter half of the 1970s, the perceived risks of *alcohol use* rose during the 1980s (although not as dramatically as perceptions of marijuana and cocaine use), with the prevalence of perceiving risk of harm from 1 to 2 daily drinks rising from 20% in 1980 to 33% in 1991, before falling back to 21% by 2002. This may be partly a result of publicity about moderate alcohol consumption protecting against heart disease (9). The perceived risk of smoking one or more packs of cigarettes daily significantly increased between 1990 and the present.

Perhaps of equal importance is perceived availability of drugs, especially illicit drugs. The percentage of students stating that it is easy to obtain cocaine peaked in 1988; perceived easy access to marijuana has remained constant at 90%; perceived access to LSD showed a dramatic rise from 1986 to 1995, followed by a steady decline to 2002;

and perceived access to heroin peaked in 1975 at 35% and declined after 1998 to 29% in 2002. These trends may be important when evaluating peer pressure and assumed normative adolescent drug use by adolescents ("everyone smokes marijuana"). As already stated, drug use and potential abuse may be initiated prior to adolescence. This is supported by reports from eighth graders about their first use of substances by the fourth grade: alcohol 6.8%, cigarettes 7.3%, inhalants 3.6%, and marijuana 1.1% (9).

Epidemiology of Different Drugs of Abuse

Tobacco use is associated with more than 430,000 deaths each year (11)—more than alcohol, cocaine, heroin, homicide, suicide, car accidents, firearms, and acquired immunodeficiency syndrome (AIDS) combined. Nearly 3 million teenagers and children smoke cigarettes (5,6). Tobacco is widely considered to be a "gateway drug" to illicit substance abuse (5,12,13). This may be particularly true for certain populations. A recent investigation using data from a cross-sectional survey in California of 11,239 multiethnic students in 31 high schools (14) found an association between prior cigarette smoking initiation and current alcohol use among adolescents from different ethnic backgrounds, including those of multiethnicity, which supports the communality of gateway drug effect of cigarette smoking on alcohol use. Despite restrictions on the sale of cigarettes to minors and aggressive campaigns against smoking, adolescents have access to and continue to use cigarettes. The prevalence of smoking half a pack or more daily are 2% of eighth graders, 4% of tenth graders, and 9% of high school seniors (9). The 30-day prevalence for smoking declined through 1984 to 29%, with little change from 1984 to 1992, an eventual rise to 36% in 1997, and a decline by 2002 to 27%, its lowest use ever.

Alcohol use by adolescents has changed very little over time and has persisted as the number one drug problem (2). In addition to its known contribution to premature adolescent mortality, recent alcohol consumption is associated with an increase in adolescents carrying a weapon for both males and females (15,16), with risky sexual behaviors and high incidence of unplanned pregnancies (17), and with sexually transmitted diseases in adolescent females (18). Reported daily use of alcohol in eighth graders is 0.7%, 1.8% for tenth graders, and 3.5% for seniors. Eighty percent of twelfth grade students have tried alcohol, 50% report using alcohol within a month of the Monitoring the Future survey, 12% report having five or more drinks in a row within the past 2 weeks, and 60% report using to the point of inebriation. Between 1996 and 2001, there was some decline in drinking among eighth graders (30-day prevalence dropped from 26% to 22%), but there was not much change in the upper grades. In 2002, alcohol use for eighth and tenth graders decreased significantly for all prevalence periods (lifetime, annual, and 30-day), and twelfth graders' use of alcohol also decreased for all

levels of use, but not significantly (9). The mean age of first use of alcohol has been decreasing, declining from 18 years in 1968 to 16 years in 1996 (the latest year reported). Meanwhile, the age-specific rate of first use among 12- to 17-year-old adolescents has doubled, from 76 per 1,000 new users in 1968 to 159 per 1,000 new users in 1996 (1). Many attribute the consistency of alcohol use to the rapid onset of affective change provided by alcohol, as well as the positive associations to role models.

Marijuana is the most frequently used illicit substance. It is potentially debilitating to adolescents because it suppresses motivation ("aberrant motivational syndrome" or "chronic cannabis syndrome") and leads to a decline in academic performance, which then leads to increased use to cope with anxiety about poor performance. The daily prevalence for marijuana use in high school seniors is 6.0%, 3.9% in tenth grade students, and 1.2% in eighth graders. Daily use rose from 6% of seniors in 1975 to 11% in 1978, followed by a decline in use to 1.9% in 1992, and a gradual increase from 1993 to 2002 from 2.4% to 6.0%, the highest rate since 1986 (9).

Cocaine and especially crack, the smokeable form of cocaine, is one of the most reinforcing substances (10). From 1976 to 1979, *cocaine* use exhibited a substantial increase, from 6.0% to 12.0%, in annual prevalence in seniors. Its annual use remained essentially level between 1979 and 1986, with s subsequent decrease between 1986 and 1992 from 12.7% to 3.1%, and monthly use decreasing from 6.2% to 1.3%. Annual prevalence then doubled from 3.1% in 1992 to 6.2% in 1999, as did 30-day prevalence, from 1.3% to 2.6%, followed, finally, by the first significant decline in some years in 2000 to 5.0%, where it remains in 2002.

Between 1986 and 1991, the annual prevalence of *crack* use declined from 4.1% to 1.5%, then leveled briefly until 1993, when annual prevalence rose from 1.5% to 2.7% in 1999. It then declined in 2000 to 2.2%, where it remained through 2002 (2.3%). The recent decline in use could be attributed to increased perception of harmfulness by students. However (because of dropouts), the statistical decline of crack use may not reflective of the problem in the overall adolescent population, although increases in inner city use of cocaine and crack, and associated increases in violent crimes, arrests, emergency room visits, and neonates testing positive for cocaine, have moderated in recent years (9,10).

Heroin shows a similar association with age, with eighth grade students reporting a lifetime prevalence of (1.6%), tenth grade students 1.8%, and twelfth grade students 1.7%. The prevalence of *heroin* use dropped steadily between 1975 and 1979, with use remaining almost constant for the following decade and a half. In 1995, a sharp (and statistically significant) increase occurred, with annual and 30-day prevalence rates doubling to 1.1% and 0.6%, respectively. However, there was no further increase in annual or 30-day prevalence of use rates from 1995 through 1999. The increase in heroin use gave rise to ameliorative actions, including an antiheroin campaign by the Partnership for a Drug-Free America, which might explain the rapid leveling in use after 1 year. However, there was a significant increase in heroin use from 1999 (1.0%) to 2000 (1.6%) among twelfth graders, entirely a result of use without needles. There was actually a significant drop in heroin use among eighth graders in 2000, with a significant decline (to 1.0%) among twelfth graders by 2002. Although heroin abuse has recently trended downward, its prevalence is still higher than in the early 1990s. These relatively high rates of abuse, along with the glamorization of heroin in music and films, changing patterns of drug use, and heroin's increased purity and decreased prices, raises concerns about further increased use and spread (9,19).

Hallucinogens, especially LSD, are showing a renewed popularity among adolescents. LSD is one of the major drugs constituting the hallucinogen class. It is one of the least expensive, longest-lasting highs available to adolescents. It is easy to conceal and difficult to detect in urine toxicology. Its use is difficult to detect by objective findings (except possibly for mydriasis from anticholinergic effects), and it appeals to the aspects of adolescent development that involve self-exploration and intellectual expansion (20). Fewer high school students perceive LSD as harmful when trying it once or twice. The annual prevalence of use of LSD showed a modest decline from 1975 to 1977, followed by considerable stability through 1981, a second decline from 1981 (6.5%) to 1985 (4.4%), and an acceleration thereafter to 8.8% in 1996. Since 1996, annual prevalence has declined to 3.5% by 2002, which is the lowest recorded since the Monitoring the Future study began. (25). Annual PCP prevalence of use declined from 7.0% in 1979 to 2.2% in 1982, leveling through 1987, and dropping to 1.3% in 1993. From 1993 to 1996, annual use increased again to 2.6%, as did other illicit drugs, and leveled in 1997, with a recent decrease to 1.1% in 2002, the lowest prevalence that has ever been recorded for this drug (9).

Other substances that are used with some frequency by high school and college students include amphetamines, tranquilizers, barbiturates, anabolic steroids, ketamine (Special K), ecstasy, and new drugs including gamma hydroxybutyrate (GHB). GHB, a powerful central nervous system depressant, was used as an anesthetic agent in the 1960s. In the 1980s, it was sold in health food stores as an over-the-counter sedative and performance enhancer in bodybuilding formulas. A growing reputation for aphrodisiac, strength-enhancing, and euphoric effects made it a popular drug of abuse, and it is one of several agents reported to be used as a "date rape" drug. The FDA the banned drug in 1990 after several reports of adverse reactions. Because of its rapid central nervous system depressant effects, GHB can be lethal when combined with alcohol or other depressants, and can also produce confusion, hallucinations, short-term amnesia, seizures, and aggression, amongst other adverse effects. It can be addictive with repeated use, and can produce serious discontinuation withdrawal symptoms that can last up to 6 months. GHB continues to be manufactured and sold illegally despite the FDA ban. Survey results from 2002 of annual GHB use was 1.0%, 1.1%, and 1.6% among tenth, eighth and twelfth graders, respectively, similar to those for 2001. The U.S. Drug Enforcement Administration has documented more than 15,600 overdoses and law enforcement encounters and 72 deaths related to GHB since 1990 (21).

Rates of MDMA use decreased significantly among tenth graders, with past-year use decreasing from 6.2% percent in 2001 to 4.9% in 2002. Use by eighth and twelfth graders also showed signs of decline. For the first time, in 2002 the Monitoring the Future survey looked at the misuse and/or nonmedical use of the prescription narcotics OxyContin (oxycoclone) and Vicodin (hydrococlone). Nonmedical use of OxyContin in the past year was reported by 4.0% of twelfth graders, and Vicodin use in the same time period was reported by 9.6% of twelfth graders (9).

A more recent effort at evaluating the prevalence of SUDs in the United States is the National Survey on Drug Abuse and Health, previously called the National Household Survey, sponsored by the Substance Abuse and Mental Health Administration (22). It has surveyed a national epidemiologic sample (70,000 participants in 2001) ages 12 years and older within household settings since 1997. The data on individual drugs of abuse is very similar to that for the Monitoring the Future survey (9). Most striking is its estimate of 1.7 new users older than age 12 years in the United States in 2001, a decrease from 2.1 million in 2000, but still a staggering total.

Substance Use Progression

Substance abuse follows a fairly predictable progression, beginning with experimentation and recreational use of alcohol and cigarettes, followed by marijuana and other illicit drugs (5,12), especially cocaine or crack in the inner-city population. The risk of using other illicit drugs tends to be low without prior use of marijuana (12), perhaps with the exclusion of inhalants, which may be another "gateway" to use. After initiation with a gateway substance, individuals might progress to other illicit drugs such as opiates and hallucinogens. During the stage of experimentation and recreational use, substances are associated with euphoria and pleasure and are not perceived as harmful or dangerous. As use becomes more regular, tolerance and craving ensues, and the individual may progress to daily use. At this stage, polysubstance use may begin, functioning begins to decline. Rather than using for pleasure, the individual now uses substances to alleviate and prevent negative affect. Prevention of withdrawal becomes a focus of substance use, and attempts to discontinue use result in withdrawal syndromes.

There may be a distinct subgroup of adolescents who are vulnerable to early and rapid escalation of substance use progression. The typical sequence of drug use onset identified in previous studies was much less prevalent among serious drug users than in samples of high school students. Sequence of drug use was examined in a secondary analysis of two samples of serious drug users: one of 152 men and one of 133 women, with data collected in ethnographic studies of adult drug users and distributors in New York City from 1984 to 1987. Only 33% of the serious drug users followed the typical sequence, compared to 75% to 93% of subjects in studies of high school students. Serious drug users were more likely to have used marijuana before alcohol, and more likely to have used other illicit drugs before marijuana. Atypical sequencing was associated with earlier initiation of use of drugs other than marijuana and greater lifetime drug involvement. These findings suggest that, for a large number of serious users, marijuana does not serve as a gateway drug, and prevention efforts focusing on it may have limited effectiveness (12).

Although we can identify a sequence of progression, it does not imply a causal relationship, and use of substances at one stage does not necessarily mean progression to another stage. Escalation of use is believed to occur from usage in seventh to ninth grade with a combination of factors associated with a high risk of occurrence: greater life stress, lower parental support, more parental substance abuse, maladaptive coping skills, low self-control ability, and a greater affiliation with substance-using peers (23). Experimentation has become so prevalent and normative that some suggest that experimentation, especially in later adolescents, may represent psychologically healthier adolescents compared to those who never experimented (23). In their study examining psychological health, Milich et al. (24) challenged this proposal, with abstainers never found to be more impaired and found to be occasionally healthier. Risk for substance use (legal and illicit) peaks between 18 and 22 years of age, with the exception of cocaine use. There appears to be a decline of substance use, excluding cocaine and prescription psychoactive substances, after the age of 25 years. An explanation for this decline may be that conventional adult roles in marriage, family, and career are assumed during this stage (25). Individuals who begin using substances before the age of 15 years are at the greatest risk of developing long-lasting patterns of abuse and dependence (22,26).

DEVELOPMENTAL, RISK, AND PROTECTIVE FACTORS

The developmental stage of adolescence is characterized by dramatic change and readjustment new stresses and anxieties, and increased vulnerability to peer pressure (27). It is a time of consolidating an identity and practicing new roles. During adolescence, the practice of adult roles and behaviors shifts from pretend play to actual behavior. The preadolescent begins experimenting with a range of new behaviors, and for many, cigarettes, alcohol, and other drugs have become a normal part of coming of age

(28). Adolescence is also marked by increasing autonomy from parents and increased in reliance on peers for validation and direction. Conformity to the peer group increases rapidly to its peak in early adolescence, then gradually declines. Adolescents assess themselves and their behaviors through the reactions of their peers. Peers are vital to the teenager's emotional and psychological development; acceptance by peers is critically important and rejection can be devastating (27).

Risk taking increases during adolescence, and adolescents engage in risk taking both for experimentation and exhilaration (29). Sensation seeking and risk taking appear to be related to the surge of pubertal hormone levels, particularly testosterone. Cognitive development may also contribute to increased risk taking, with adolescents wanting to impress their peers, but not yet being adept at assessing risks. Hamburg (30) observes that adolescents frequently assume that if they engage in a behavior several times without negative consequences, the perceived risk goes down; for example, having unprotected sex without getting pregnant. Adolescents also tend to exaggerate based on immediate experience, which allows risks to be minimized. Finally, adolescents have a sense of invulnerability—an attitude of "it won't happen to me" (4,30).

Adolescents may actually be making risk assessments, although these are more anchored in the "here and now," so that they are less concerned with the far-off future consequences. Potential long-term negative health consequences may seem less important than short-term effects, which may actually be satisfying and pleasurable. Also, some risks may have more salience than others. The norms of the peer group have a very strong influence over the individual adolescent, such as losing status with peers, being rejected, or appearing immature or inexperienced.

The general tasks of adolescence include adjusting to the physical changes of puberty, gaining independence from parents, establishing relationships with peers, and preparing for work. While these tasks are normal, they are also difficult and challenging (27,28). Struggling to cope with them can result in strong feelings of powerlessness, alienation, and rebellion. To accomplish these developmental tasks, the adolescent must develop a stable identity, personal values, as well as a sense of meaning or purpose. Thus, adolescence is the most idealistic phase of development. Because it is also a time when health habits and future behaviors are still being formed and when many of the lifetime strategies for coping with stress and peer pressure are developed (31), adolescence is an important window of opportunity for intervention and prevention.

Models of Development of Adolescent Substance Use Disorder

A number of theoretical models have been proposed for understanding the development of adolescent SUD. Two prominent theories, problem behavior and social learning theory, are described in this section.

Social learning theory (32) suggests that individuals learn through a vicarious process of observing the behaviors of role models, particularly high-status role models. The consequences of behavior, especially the reinforcements that role models receive for behavior, are most salient to the observer, and behaviors that are rewarded are much more likely to be learned. Role models for the adolescent include parents, siblings, peers, and media figures, with older peers having especially high status as role models. Role models who smoke, drink, or use other substances, and who appear to be socially accepted or exalted, may suggest that these behaviors are not only acceptable, but necessary for social success. Expectancies regarding substance use are learned and appear more powerful than actual experience.

Problem behavior theory, derived from the work of Jessor and Jessor (33), is based on an empirical integration of psychological, social, and biochemical factors that contribute to adolescent problem behaviors. "Problem behaviors" are those behaviors that are socially defined and recognized as "problems" by a group or culture, or viewed as acceptable for one age group but problematic in another age group (such as drinking alcohol). According to problem behavior theory, substance use is functional for the adolescent and may even be instrumental in achieving personal goals, such as acceptance by peers, coping with anxiety (particularly social anxiety), failure (real or anticipated), hopelessness, or boredom. When a behavior is effective at achieving a desired objective, it will be difficult to extinguish without alternate ways of achieving the same outcomes. Moreover, objectives such as coping with anxiety, gaining entry into a peer group, and demonstrating independence from parents are normal and healthy (31), so that behaviors used to achieve these objectives are difficult to modify. Unless adolescents learn other ways of achieving their personal goals, substance use may be impossible to modify or extinguish. Jessor's work on perceived life choices is particularly important in conceptualizing this issue. He found that adolescents who believed they had positive life choices were more likely to engage in health promoting behavior, and adolescents who believed their life choices to be limited were more likely to engage in risky behaviors (34). Adolescents with limited life choices and options (such as poor or minority youth, or youth with emotional/behavioral problems) are the ones at greatest risk for substance abuse, so social context has a critical role in the development of adolescent SUDs. The youth development and empowerment paradigm has extended some of Jessor's conceptualization toward a paradigm that integrates the youth as an asset and resource into the community (35).

Risk Factors

In the medical model, the identification of risk factors leads to improved techniques in revention and more efficacious treatments. There is a complex multiplicity of risk factors for adolescent substance abuse that are not necessarily consistent across stages of development, ethnic subgroups, and determinants that are biologic, psychiatric, behavioral, social, and perhaps even substance-category specific. This makes investigation of correlates and predictors of substance use both challenging and exciting. Different combinations of risk factors and different pathways may all result in adolescent substance use, with frequency and extent of substance use and abuse increasing the more risk factors are present (36). It remains impossible to predict precisely how these risk factors may interact in an individual to produce a serious substance-use problem. Risk factors can be grouped into five general categories: cognitive and attitudinal; personality and psychopathology; behavioral, social, and environmental; and biologic or genetic (36–38).

Cognitive and Attitudinal

Adolescents who use substances are less likely to be aware of the negative consequences of use, have less negative attitudes about substances, and believe that substance use is normative. They are also less likely to have personal competence and decision-making skills that allow the adolescent to manage emotional distress (39–43). Females with substance abuse disorders have lower levels of constructive thinking and executive function, with these traits also associated with higher levels of antisocial behavior (44).

Personality and Psychopathology

Personality characteristics that are linked to substance use include low assertiveness, low self-efficacy or self-esteem, low self-confidence, low social confidence, and external locus of control (45–47); additional characteristics are aggressiveness, unconventionality, problems with interpersonal relatedness, and precocious sexuality (48,49). Studies have also identified early novelty seeking and early disruptive behavioral patterns as personality and behavioral risk factors, which can be seen in children as early as ages 6 to 9 years (50–52). Substance users tend to be more anxious, impulsive, and rebellious; they are more impatient to appear grown up, and have a stronger need for approval (37,48). They also tend to be more pessimistic and more alienated from social values (53,54). However, no data from prospective studies have identified personality patterns specific to substance abusers, and there is no evidence of an "addictive personality type" (38,55).

Several recent studies link psychiatric comorbidity with substance abuse. A number of studies have established a strong relationship between the development of conduct disorders and adolescent substance, with earlier onset and more serious conduct disorder often sharing many of the personality, cognitive, social, and behavioral risk factors as adolescent substance abuse (56–59). There is some debate about attention deficit hyperactivity disorder (ADHD) as a risk factor for adolescent substance abuse, sufficient to create concern about the use of stimulants in adolescents with ADHD, with some studies showing a strong association and others failing to do so, especially when accounting for the comorbidity of conduct disorders (60,61). Mood disorders, including depression and bipolar disorder, are also highly comorbid with substance abuse disorders in adolescents (57,61,62). In adolescent females, increased risk for substance abuse has been found amongst individuals with eating disorders, more so for those with binge symptoms than those with restrictive symptoms, who typically have more ascetic personality traits (63,64).

The majority of studies examining the timing of onset of comorbid disorders have found that, in a majority of cases, substance abuse disorders followed, rather than preceded, the onset of other psychiatric disorders (except for conduct disorders), and that more than 60% to 80% of adolescents with substance abuse disorders had some other form of psychopathology (57,65,66). Overall, for the adolescent, the likelihood that substance use is associated with psychopathology increases with more aberrant substance use for the adolescent's own social context (10). Approximately 20% of adolescents are affected by mental and emotional disorders, and psychological distress and psychopathology may be involved in both the initiation and continuation of adolescent SUD. Some postulate that early onset of substance use may promote the development of psychopathology (26). However, the most prudent course in treatment is to begin by treating the substance abuse.

Behavioral, Social, and Environmental

There are behavioral correlates to substance use, including antisocial behavior and poor academic performance (58,67,68). Of the most powerful predictors of substance use are social influences including behavior and attitudes of family and friends (39,69,70). Family influences, such as parenting, parental substance use, permissive or tolerant attitudes of substance use by parents, and the quality of relationship between parents and adolescents, are implicated in adolescent substance use (54,71–74). Specific family management styles that appear to promote substance use (48) include inconsistent discipline, lack of maternal involvement in child's activities, use of guilt as a motivator, lack of praise for achievement, and unrealistic expectations.

The most powerful of the social influences are peer influences, particularly in terms of initial experimentation with substances (69,75,76) and reinforcement of use by continued association with groups who use substances. Warheit et al. (77), in a longitudinal, multiracial, multi-ethnic study, found peer factors to be a more powerful predictor of substance use than self-rejection or derogation. One variant of peer influences which is omnipresent in our society is media influences. Some studies, particularly those of tobacco use (10,78,79), have found definite associations between media messages and cigarette smoking in adolescents. Gambling behaviors and activities are on the rise amongst adolescents, and highly associated with substance abuse disorders (80–82).

Other social or environmental factors associated with substance use include deprivation, children who care for themselves after school if parents work (48), a low socioeconomic status (83), a history of sexual abuse or dating violence (36,48,84), and employment during the school year (83).

Cultural factors also deserve strong consideration as risk factors for adolescent substance abuse. Various studies have demonstrated that the risk of substance abuse is associated with immigrant status, with increases in prevalence in different populations after immigration from their countries of origin (85,86). Some studies point to the influence of cultural value orientation on adolescent substance abuse, as expressed in family and community cohesion, supervision/monitoring, and traditional practices such as religion (87). Szapocznik et al. (88), in their studies of immigrant Cuban-American families, found that intergenerational conflicts about value orientations can serve as a significant risk factor both for adolescent substance abuse and conduct disturbance. The impact of trauma experiences associated with the history or daily experiences of adolescents of particular racial and ethnic groups is often associated with higher risk for adolescent substance abuse (73,89).

Biologic and Genetic

Although genetic and biologic factors in initiation and continuation of adolescent substance use have been the subject of much focus, they, are in general, in need of further delineation. Studies examining concordance rates in monozygotic versus dizygotic twins and adoption studies of twins reared apart (48,90,91) show heritability of alcohol use and abuse and differences in transmissibility between males and females. Some studies (48,92–94) show a three- to fourfold increase of alcohol and substance abuse disorders with a positive family history, and greater prevalence of use of gateway drugs with a paternal history of substance abuse disorder (95).

Various biologic markers are being investigated in adolescents. Blum et al. (96) reported an allelic association of the dopamine D2 receptor gene with a susceptibility to alcohol disorders. Attempts to repeat the findings were unsuccessful. Reduced P3 amplitude on evoked potentials, a well-documented psychophysiologic marker alcoholism risk, is associated with earlier age of first drink of alcohol in 17-year-olds (97). The 5-HT-sub(1B) receptor, which is implicated in various psychopathologies, including pathologic aggression, alcoholism, and suicide, has an 861C allele that is specifically associated with substance abuse (98). Influences of genetically determined metabolism, such as alcohol dehydrogenase deficiency found in Asians, are well established and have been manipulated to create treatment approaches (disulfiram [Antabuse]). Genetic predisposition, however, always interacts with environmental factors, so that genes probably determine vulnerabilities to environmental factors, rather firmly establishing substance abuse disorders (91).

Protective Factors

While research is generally aimed at establishing clear-cut risk factors leading to substance use patterns and abuse disorders, less attention seems to be focused on factors that protect the adolescent from problematic substance use. Adolescents who have emotionally supportive parents with open communication styles, who flexibly monitor their children's peer activities and are aware of their children's potential for use of substances, are offered some protection from substance abuse (48,71,99–101). Particular cultural values mediated by the family, such as strong family orientation and religion/spirituality, were found to be protective in some studies (87,100). Involvement in organized school activities and the importance of academic achievement are related to lower risk for substance use (48). Involvement in organized sports activities can be both a risk factor and a protective factor. Certain athletic activities and sports in general have been associated with anabolic steroid use and dependence, which is further associated with other drug use (102,103). Although males who participate in athletics may be less at risk to use drugs and alcohol, they may be at increased risk for early sexual contacts (104).

SCREENING, ASSESSMENT, TREATMENT, AND PREVENTIVE APPROACHES

Approximately 10% of all adolescents would benefit from treatment interventions targeting substance use disorders, but fewer than 10% of adolescents with symptoms of dependence receive treatment (105), and those who are in the greatest need of treatment may be the least likely to initiate treatment. Adolescent SUD may progress to major problems more quickly than adult SUD, which gives a narrower window of opportunity for engaging youth in prevention and secondary intervention efforts. In general, adolescents who are seen in treatment are heavily involved in substance use on a daily basis, have co-occurring psychiatric disorders and have experienced legal problems. At the time they present for treatment, adolescents with SUDs have endured many negative consequences within a brief time period, and functioning in school and family is suffering (10). Treatment efforts are encumbered by limited resources, inadequate age-appropriate programs, high premature treatment termination and relapse, and lack of consensus on preferred treatment strategies. Originally, there were few solid efficacy studies on treatment and pre-

ventive interventions with adolescents, although this has begun to change significantly in the past decade.

Screening and Assessment

A basic understanding of the risks leading to SUD, knowledge of current substances of abuse, familiarity with normal and abnormal development and behavior, and an alliance with the individual should prepare the clinician to adequately identify and refer the adolescent with SUD to appropriate treatment. Pediatricians are traditionally positioned to have an ongoing relationship with both the adolescent and the family and able to detect changes over time. However, current studies indicate that pediatricians fail to identify the at-risk adolescent user and family (106). Even in college clinic settings (a high-risk population), a survey of the clinics reported only 37% of health care providers routinely screened all students visiting the clinic for alcohol and other drugs of abuse (107). These may be a result of discomfort with the issue of drug use, lack of knowledge, insufficient time during visits, or inadequate reimbursement Another important factor may be a change in the continuity of care, with many clinics (including training clinics staffed by resident physicians) unable establish the traditional long-term relationship that permits detection of signals of substance use. In addition, adolescents usually do not seek medical attention unless an urgent or emergent situation arises, leading to emergency rooms centers acting as the primary care provider site. These situations further limit establishment of a relationship, and may miss adolescents who are most at risk for problem substance use. Similarly, schools are in good positions to identify at-risk youth, but face challenges similar to those of health care settings, as well as the problem of disciplinary injunctions (108).

On routine visits most adolescents do not present with dramatic or overt signs and symptoms that are easily accounted for by the effects of alcohol or drug use. A basic knowledge of substance-use-related changes prove vital to screening (106): physical findings (such as weight loss, nasal irritation, chronic cough, needle tracks), personal habits (such as altered sleep pattern, new friends or interests, change in dress), academic performance (such as falling grades, truancy, suspension), and behavioral and psychological symptoms (such as affective dysregulation, risk taking, stealing). Effective evaluation, history taking, and discussion with the adolescent should yield the desired information. Toxicologic screening for substance use should be limited to emergency situations (overdose, trauma), or in the context of a treatment contract (106). The American Academy of Pediatrics (AAP) advocates against involuntary testing in adolescents with decisional capacity, even if parental consent is given, unless there is strong medical or legal reasons to do so (109). Results of toxicologic screens can have potentially damaging effects on the adolescent (and any therapeutic relationship with the adolescent), and not achieve the desired result of deterrence from use. When a clinician has suspicion of substance abuse, it is best to refer to a qualified health or mental health professional for comprehensive evaluation (109).

The use of systematic screening tools may be desirable in primary care, mental health, and even school settings as a cost-effective and time-efficient means of identifying youth who are in early (or even advanced stages) of use or addiction. An example of such an instrument is the adolescent form of the Substance Abuse Subtle Screening Inventory (SASSI) (110), which is increasingly used in clinical and community settings as a means of early identification. The Diagnostic Interview Schedule for Children (DISC), and its most recent voice version (Voice DISC) (111), is a self-administered structured psychiatric diagnostic interview that screens for diagnoses under the *Diagnostic and Statistical Manual of Mental Disorders* (7), which has an excellent substance abuse screening module. Use of this instrument with detained or incarcerated youth has demonstrated prevalence rates of SUDs ranging from 20% to 50% (11,112,113). The adolescent version of the Minnesota Multiphasic Personality Inventory (MMPI-A) has three substance abuse subscales that have demonstrable reliability and validity for assessing the presence of substance use disorders (114).

Evaluation of Treatment Programs

Substance abuse is one of the most urgent and serious problems facing society and increasing resources should be devoted to its treatment. However, we are still in the process of determining what treatment approaches are most effective or how to best match patients with treatment approaches (115–118), and this is particularly true with adolescents. One problem is that evaluation of treatment programs is costly and difficult. However, evaluation not only validates effective approaches, it also provides essential information for improving or enhancing treatment strategies (10).

An early major study concerning the efficacy of treatment programs for adolescent substance abuse was the National Institute of Drug Abuse's (NIDA) Treatment Outcome Prospective Study (TOPS). For 12 months TOPS followed 1,042 adolescent (<20 years old) substance abusers who were in treatment in 27 treatment centers between 1979 and 1981. Those in residential treatment for 3 months had 20% to 25% reductions in drug use and related behavioral problems, whereas those who received 2 months of outpatient treatment had fewer reductions in drug use, with some subgroups actually increasing use or related problematic behaviors. During the late 1980s to early 1990s, the Services Research Outcome Study (SROS) followed 156 adolescents with SUDs for 5 years. There was a 48% relapse rate following residential community-based treatment with a median stay of 2 to 3 months. In the early

1990s the National Treatment Improvement Evaluation Study (NTIES) followed 236 adolescents receiving various treatments for SUD. At 12-month followup, those who attended a residential treatment program for 2 months had modest reductions in drug use, with no significant reduction in drug use for those adolescents in outpatient treatment. All of these early studies were of treatment programs using adult models with minimum modifications. Another study during the mid to late 1990s was the Drug Abuse Treatment Outcome Study–Adolescent (DATOS-A), which assessed client characteristics, treatment structure and process, and outcome evaluation of long-term residential treatment centers (N = 727), drug-free outpatient (N = 445), and short-term inpatient (N = 613) programs (116).

Currently, the Center for Substance Abuse Treatment (CSAT) of the Substance Abuse and Mental Health Services Administration (SAMHSA), Department of Health and Human Services is funding the Adolescent Treatment Model Program to evaluate, document, and disseminate effective adolescent substance abuse treatment models. The intended results will be manualized and evidence-based approaches to SUD treatment for adolescents. Ten exemplary treatment programs were identified for evaluation, which includes a 12-month followup. Treatment outcomes and costs will be compared among the model programs for effectiveness and affordability. Descriptions of each treatment model, age-specific treatment interventions, and patient characteristics will be documented (118). A major objective is to identify the program elements that are effective and replicable in each model program so that they may be incorporated into treatment manuals. All model programs are to develop a manual that is publicly available and to participate in these cross-site evaluations.

Evidence-Based Treatment Modalities

Below we discuss treatment interventions with demonstrated effectiveness that are currently recommended for the treatment of adolescent substance. Manuals for these are available at www.drugabuse.gov.

Psychoeducational approaches are known to be of some benefit. For example, the greater the perceived risk of drug use, the more likely the adolescent will not use. However, adolescents have not experienced "rock bottom" and are just beginning to accrue negative experiences and associated negative mental constructs associated with drug use. Motivational enhancing techniques are employed to assist in forming therapeutic alliances and patient-generated goals. Individual and peer-enhanced motivational interviewing can be effective with adolescents (119).

There is evidence to suggest that cognitive–behavioral therapy (CBT) has significantly greater treatment efficacy with substance-abusing adolescents than do psycho educational approaches (120). Individual CBT, family therapy, combined CBT and family therapy, and group interventions improve treatment outcomes (121). Interpersonal psychotherapy has been used with adolescents diagnosed with SUD. Studies do not clearly demonstrate one treatment superior to the others, or the optimal duration or intensity.

Contingency management is a behavioral therapy that overcomes two major difficulties that permeate SUD treatment of adolescents: poor retention rates because of compromised motivation, and reliance upon subjective measures to assess treatment outcomes (122). Rewards are provided for objective evidence of sobriety, changes in behaviors associated with drug use, improved family functioning, school attendance, socialization, and treatment plan compliance.

Family-based therapies improve treatment outcomes. Positive family functioning and relationships, especially the extent to which family members are encouraged to be assertive and self-sufficient, are associated with improved patient prognosis (123). *Multifamily group therapy* is beneficial for many adolescents and families (124). *Multidimensional family therapy* (MDFT) is grounded in developmental and ecologic theory, that is, multiple ecologic factors and abnormal development maintain drug use and other problem behaviors. MDFT focuses simultaneously on four important areas of the adolescent's life: the individual (developing a sense of self, self-efficacy), parents and family, transactional patterns, and family interactions (relationships) with extrafamilial systems (125).

Multisystemic therapy (MST) addresses the multiple risk factors for SUD (individual youth characteristics, family functioning, caregiver functioning, peer relations, school performance, indigenous family supports, and neighborhood characteristics) in a highly individualized and strategic fashion. Caregivers are the key. Assessment and treatment are manualized and focus on nine treatment principles (behavior makes sense in its context; strengths as levers for change; increasing responsible behavior; present-focused, well-defined, and action-oriented; target sequences of behaviors; developmentally appropriate; continuous effort; evaluation and accountability; generalization) with performance-based outcome criteria. Treatment addresses triggers for substance use in the social ecology. MST was the treatment approach in one of the first randomized clinical trials with juvenile offenders to demonstrate long-term treatment effects with substance-using adolescents (126).

Therapeutic residential communities and *12-step programs* strongly endorse role modeling, which is of enormous importance for adolescents. Sponsors and peers serve as mentors to model adaptive behaviors and support the same. Relying on adult models, early efforts in adolescent treatment did not always consider the unique developmental factors germane to adolescents. By the end of the 1990s treatment programs were addressing these developmental issues. Because of the importance of peer influences and the adolescent peer orientation, group in-terventions may contribute to reductions in drug use. Well-trained peer counselors or educators need to recognize and combat iatrogenic effects of group interventions that exist when the deviant orientation of participating adolescents is reinforced through verbal and nonverbal cues in the group sessions (127,128).

Adolescent-specific self-help groups are not present in most communities but could be valuable treatment resources. There are modified 12-step programs (Alcoholics Anonymous [AA], Narcotics Anonymous [NA]) and relapse prevention groups for adolescents (129). Adolescents more deeply involved with substance use are more motivated and more likely to attend and affiliate (active involvement) with self-help groups (130). It is unclear what kinds and aspects of 12-step groups are helpful. One study suggests that 12-step groups for youths improved outcome primarily by increasing motivational factors as opposed to improving coping or self-efficacy (131). The 12-step model requires significant modification to accommodate the special developmental needs of adolescents, including greater flexibility in intrinsic treatment motivation, focus on chronicity of the disorder, and in the use of abstract spiritual concepts.

Skills development usually takes place in a group setting and includes relaxation therapy, recreation and various leisure skills, social skills, relationship enhancing, and other coping strategies with extensive opportunities for practice. One potential strategy may be to induce craving of drugs in a supervised treatment setting through the presentation of audiovisual cues and follow the exposure with practicing effective coping strategies. Eventually the conditioned stimulus may no longer elicit strong cravings (132).

There are few studies with adolescents that demonstrate improvement in SUD through psychopharmacotherapy. If co-occurring conditions are driving the addiction, effective use of medications to treat the underlying mental illness may effectively reduce illicit drug use. The use of lithium in bipolar adolescents with SUD improved sobriety (133). Effective treatment of ADHD may reduce morbidity and SUD (134). Selective serotonin reuptake inhibitors have been prescribed for comorbid depression with improvement in SUD (135). Medication-assisted withdrawal (detoxification), drug substitutes (e.g., methadone), aversive medications (e.g., disulfiram), reinforcing effect blockers (e.g., naltrexone), and craving reducers (e.g., bupropion) have also been used with adolescents, but with no systematic studies and variable results (55,135,136).

Levels of Care (Inpatient, Residential, Community/Outpatient)

The range of levels of care and programs available to the adolescent substance abuser include detoxification (DT), inpatient hospitalization, residential treatment centers, including therapeutic communities (TCs), outpatient programs (OPs), and self-help. Whereas DT is almost exclusively biologic or medical in focus, other programs incorporate an understanding of the interpersonal, intrapsychic, and environmental factors involved in substance abuse. Matching adolescents to an appropriate level of care is based on considerations of severity of symptoms, level of function, degree of comorbidity, available services and support resources, financial status, and legal mandates, as well as factors such as age, gender, and ethnicity (137). Explicit evidence-based level of care criteria and tools, such as the American Society of Addiction Medicine's adolescent placement criteria (138) and the Child and Adolescent Level of Care Utilization System (139,140) have improved the accuracy of level of care determination for adolescents with SUD. However, few programs are designed to treat the special needs of females, especially young pregnant females, minority groups, and medically compromised individuals such as those with AIDS.

The goal of detoxification is to terminate substance use and conduct the process of physiologic withdrawal from the drug of abuse safely, with medical support and supervision. The majority of detoxification programs today are conducted on an outpatient basis, especially for adolescents who seldom have complicated withdrawal. Detoxification is currently viewed as appropriate only as the first step in a more comprehensive approach to treatment, involving longer-term counseling, support, and group work (137,141).

Inpatient programs, usually located in psychiatric hospitals, are run by medical providers along with drug counselors, therapists, and psychologists, and provide an expensive, highly structured therapeutic experience, beginning with a comprehensive assessment. These programs are not limited to drug treatment; they also address co-occurring disorders, as well as provide psychiatric and medical care, individual and family therapy, group therapy, and education about substance abuse. Inpatient alcohol and drug programs for adolescents use a strict, controlled environment complete with detailed daily activity schedules. Lengths of stay have been reduced and typically do not exceed 2 weeks before the adolescent steps down to a residential, intensive outpatient, or outpatient continuation treatment program (141). Substance-abusing adolescents who are female, white, and have psychiatric impairment are more likely to receive inpatient services (142).

Residential treatment centers (RTCs) are designed to isolate the substance abuser from the substance-using group and setting. They provide a drug-free environment in which new, drug-free ways of coping can be learned and re-socialization for a drug-free life can occur. RTCs provide intensive therapy and counseling to build self-esteem, develop social skills, and educate and train the individual for work. Treatment usually lasts for several months in the RTC, and the majority of people who enter the program leave before completing their course of treatment. RTCs

are set up to deal with substance misuse, developmental problems, and problems with relationships using education and individual, group, and family counseling and therapy. With the wider acceptance of adolescent substance dependence as multifactorial with biologic, psychological, social, cultural, and spiritual contributions, treatment at RTCs may address multiple dimensions using diverse modalities (115).

The earliest RTCs were the therapeutic communities that originated in the 1960s. These were based on a mutual help or self-help philosophy and were frequently staffed by recovering addicts, with limited involvement by professionals. The earliest treatment center (TC) was Synanon; others that developed national reputations include Daytop Village, Odyssey House, and Phoenix House. The early TCs emphasized communication and openness, as well as public criticism of self and others, were very structured, and had strict codes of behaviors, with severe consequences for breaking community norms and rules. Currently, RTCs have become more supportive, less confrontational, and have adopted greater treatment flexibility. The structure and approach of the RTCs may be best suited for adolescents who are antisocial or delinquent. In addition to therapeutic communities, a variety of other residential programs, such as wilderness programs, are designed to provide a drug-free environment as a way of getting the adolescent out of the substance-using context (137).

Outpatient programs comprise the majority of substance abuse treatment programs. These typically include such models as substance abuse counseling, aftercare following a TC or a residential community program, structured day treatment, which is an alternative to inpatient care, and family therapy. Eight of ten adolescents receive treatment for substance abuse in outpatient programs. To qualify for this approach, adolescents should be receiving simultaneous treatment of serious medical or psychiatric problems and should be motivated and cooperative with the treatment program. They should be willing to submit to random drug testing, and the family should also have a willingness to be involved. Outpatient programs may involve any number of therapeutic interventions, including behavior therapy, skills development, hypnosis, biofeedback, and crisis programs such as telephone hotlines, walk-in centers, referral services, and emergency intervention (141). Those attending outpatient programs tend to be younger and in school, have less criminality, lower levels of drug use, and less treatment experience. More intensive outpatient programs include day, after-school, and evening treatment. One investigation (143), comparing the relative efficacy of inpatient versus day treatment, suggests that inpatient and day treatment programs have similar treatment completion rates, reductions in substance abuse and behavior difficulties, and improvement in functioning when using primarily group interventions (information, skill development, psychotherapy, and self-help groups).

Night programs allow for more family involvement and in that way meet important treatment needs (144). School-based programs hold considerable promise for early intervention in SUDs. Factors likely to impact participation in such voluntary school-based programs include socially acceptable formats, perception of helpfulness, and accessibility. Barriers can be minimized by offering convenient times and places, and choice of formats (group discussion, individual sessions, and computer web sites. In one such self-selected program, 10% of the high school adolescents voluntarily attended an alcohol secondary intervention program to change drinking patterns, and 80% chose the group format (145).

Principles of Treatment

It is difficult to draw overall conclusions based on the literature, partly because of variations between studies in operational definitions and terminology, as well as in measures of outcome effectiveness. However, reviews in the field conclude that any treatment is better than no treatment, and the best predictor of treatment outcome is the amount of time spent in treatment (10,55,115). Treatment does not need to be voluntary to be effective. Success also appears more likely when skills training is part of the treatment and when families participate (146). Family therapies seek to increase structure and supervision with careful monitoring, while improving relationships. Caregivers allow the adolescent to experience natural consequences while not withholding essential emotional support. Attending aftercare, including self-help and support groups, also favorably influences outcome (115).

It is interesting to note that the studies of treatment efficacy often focus on the characteristics of the individual who does well in treatment, as opposed to the characteristics of the treatment program that produces positive outcomes (55). Factors that predict success in treatment include demographic characteristics, attendance in school or other educational programs, and an older age when substance use began. In addition, adolescents who are not involved in opiate or multiple substance use or criminal behavior and who have fewer problems to start with are more likely to have positive outcomes (10).

Perhaps the overarching principle of adolescent SUD treatment is the movement toward more integrated and multidimensional (multimodal) treatment models (10,134). No single treatment fits all individuals. Highly individualized, flexible, and adaptable approaches must accommodate evolving treatment needs. Patient–treatment matching is a more common practice; that is, matching the patient's problems with targeted services within the program that meets the individual's treatment needs. Although it is difficult to say whether one approach is more successful than another, it does appear that different approaches may be better suited to different types of

people. For example, the highly structured environment of the TC may work best for delinquent or antisocial youth. It appears that individuals engaged in outpatient programs are more likely to have been productive at some point in the past in education, or career, as compared to those in TCs or DT (115,141), who are less likely to attend school or work and are more often involved in a chaotic lifestyle.

There are special treatment issues for culturally diverse youth. Treatment must incorporate traditional cultural values and culturally normative developmental goals. It must address special stressors for diverse youth such as acculturation, margination, ethnic identity formation, and intergenerational family conflict. Understanding the contextual and ecologic factors influencing SUD has important treatment implications. Interventions and programs should take into account developmental issues that are influenced by cultural values, such as the importance of the peer group, degree of autonomy from parents and the community, family boundaries and hierarchies, limit testing and risk taking, immediate time orientation, failure to anticipate consequences, and culturally normative cognitive skills. Some special interventions, principally family and community-based, have been developed for youth of culturally diverse backgrounds (147–149).

Substance abuse, like most medical or psychological disorders, tends to be chronic, with relapse being a more common occurrence with adolescents than with adults (one-third of adolescents in the first month, two-thirds after 6 months) no matter the type of treatment (10,55). Contrary to adults who tend to relapse because of negative affect or personal distress, adolescents appear to relapse more often as a result of peer pressure and when they view substance use as helping with social interaction. However, heavy drug and alcohol use in adolescence, although often socially motivated, sets the stage for chronic life-long addiction (1). Given the nature and stages of adolescent development and the chronicity of substance abuse disorders, perhaps treatment success is better evaluated in terms of use reduction rather than total abstinence. Relapse must not be viewed as failure, but rather as an indication to increase intensity, frequency, integration, and scope of treatment.

Preventive Approaches

Prevention of adolescent substance abuse must be multidimensional, complex, and dynamic. It must address a number of risk and protective factors, such as life skills and resistance skills, fostering healthy self-esteem, appropriate decision-making paradigms, stress management, communication skills, and assertiveness training. They are rooted in cognitive and affective systems and require a culturally competent approach to be effective with diverse populations. To maintain effective results, programs must be evaluated frequently and marketed successfully. Most importantly, drug-prevention programs must be accessible to adolescents at high risk for substance use disorders.

Programs that target only one layer of risk factors are limited and attract low-risk participants. This theory is supported by an evaluation of a parent-targeted, school-based adolescent drug-prevention program (150), which suggested that parents who participate in a drug-abuse-prevention program already have better parenting skills and relations with their children than do nonparticipants, a factor associated with a lower risk of substance abuse. More comprehensive programs include involvement at the school and community level, outreach to families for participation, peer involvement, training for adult and peer leaders, and attention to multiple risk factors associated with substance abuse, as well as supporting life skills training.

A number of such comprehensive programs have demonstrated significant effectiveness in outcome studies. The Nebraska Network of Drug-Free Youth program (151) was designed to delay onset of substance use and to reduce or eliminate substance use among adolescents already using, by targeting seventh through twelfth grade students. Evaluation results indicated that the program helped keep drug-free students from initiating use and helped occasional users stop or reduce use, and that mixing high-risk students with low-risk students is an effective prevention strategy. However, students of both risk groups involved in the program self-selected to participate, which may be indicative of a high level of motivation to be drug free. Another comprehensive program, Project Northland, targeting sixth, seventh, and eighth grade students in 24 school districts in northeastern Minnesota, was designed to test the efficacy of a multilevel, multiyear program addressing alcohol (152). Overall, students from participating districts appeared to benefit positively as compared to reference districts. However, the project seems to have been more successful with students who had not used alcohol at the start of sixth grade than with those who had initiated use, suggesting that alcohol use may be very difficult to reverse even as early as the start of sixth grade.

More recently, programs have focused on young adolescents and pre-adolescents to achieve better preventive results. The Iowa Strengthening Families Program (ISFP) and the Preparing for the Drug-Free Years (PDFY) program, both of which address the transition from nonuse of substances to initiation and progression of substance abuse, demonstrated significant delays in substance abuse initiation, while the PDFY program also delayed progression of use amongst those who initiated use (153). The Adolescent Transitions Program (154,155), is a multilevel approach to family interventions within a middle school setting based on an ecological model for social and emo-

tional development. It includes universal, selected, and indicated strategies to serve young adolescents and their families at all risk levels. Despite low measured levels of engagement with families using the indicated and selected interventions, they were able to achieve significant reductions in substance abuse initiation in at-risk and typical students served.

Some of the program components that can be integrated into comprehensive multilevel approaches have demonstrated limited effectiveness. These include parental psychoeducational and monitoring programs (156) and youth–adult partnerships (157). The Adolescent Alcohol Prevention Trial, a longitudinal multisite approach combining drug and normative psychoeducation and resistance skills, has also demonstrated reduction in the average levels and rates of growth for cigarette and alcohol use (158).

CONCLUSIONS AND FUTURE DIRECTION

There are many more adolescents with SUDs than available treatment slots, so treatment services for adolescents must be made more accessible and acceptable. Even so, many adolescents do not recognize they need help and may never reach treatment. While increasing treatment services may reduce the incidence of cases. As with all other types of epidemics, adolescent SUD in the United States must be controlled through preventive efforts. An important aspect of the disease of addiction that sets it apart from other diseases that have reached epidemic proportion (except for HIV/AIDS and other sexually transmitted diseases) is that it involves a product that yields a desired effect. However, in addition to issues of supply and demand, prevention of adolescent SUD involves addressing complex biopsychosocial and developmental issues which our society continues to minimize and underestimate. Because of these complicated issues, perhaps a reexamination of the goal of prevention is required: Is eradication a reasonable expectation? Future focus on adolescent SUDs should include an improvement of the quality and consistency of undergraduate and graduate medical education in substance abuse; the continued development of systematic and effective screening and assessment techniques and tools; a database of treatment facilities and specialists in substance abuse available to the primary care provider for appropriate referrals; improved targeting of prevention programs to high-risk adolescents; and expanded funding to develop, evaluate, and disseminate further evidence-based modalities and treatment programs. Additionally, given the high comorbidity of SUDs with other psychopathology in adolescents, a greater emphasis on the prevention, early identification, and treatment of child and adolescent mental illness and emotional disturbances will be central to these efforts.

REFERENCES

1. Greenblatt JC. *Patterns of alcohol use among adolescents and associations with emotional and behavioral problems.* Office of Applied Studies Working Paper, Mar 2000. Available at: www.samhsa.gov/oas/NHSDA/TeenAlc/teenalc.pdf. Last accessed July 2004.

2. Morrison SF, Rogers PD, Thomas MH. Alcohol and adolescents. *Pediatr Clin North Am* 1995;42:371–387.

3. Kolata G. Experts are at odds on how best to tackle rise in teenagers' drug use. *New York Times* 1996 Sep18: Section B page 7.

4. Dusenbury L, Botvin GJ. Competence enhancement and the prevention of adolescent problem behavior. In: Hurrelmann K, Losel F, eds. *Health hazards in adolescence.* Berlin: Walter de Gruyter, 1990:459–477.

5. Epps RP, Manley MW, Glynn TJ. Tobacco use among adolescents: strategies for prevention. *Pediatr Clin North Am* 1995;42:389–399.

6. American Academy of Pediatrics. "Kids' health" give children antismoking messages at young age. *USA Today* Oct 18–20, 2002 (Weekend Edition), Supplement.

7. American Psychiatric Association. *Diagnostic and statistical manual of mental disorders* 4th ed., text revision (*DSM–IV–TR*). Washington, DC: Author, 2000;191–295.

8. Martin CS, Kaczynski NA, Bukstein OM, et al. Patterns of *DSM–IV* alcohol abuse and dependence symptoms in adolescent drinkers. *J Stud Alcohol* 1995;56(6):672–680.

9. Johnston LD, O'Malley PM, Bachman JG. *The Monitoring the Future study, 1975–2002, vol. 1.* Rockville, MD: National Institute on Drug Abuse, 2002.

10. Jaffe SL, Simkin DR. Alcohol and drug abuse in adolescents. In: Lewis M, ed. *Child and adolescent psychiatry: a comprehensive textbook.* Philadelphia: Lippincott Williams & Wilkins, 2002:895–911.

11. Centers for Disease Control and Prevention. *State highlights and best practices,* 2003. Available at: http://www.cdc.gov/od/oc/media/pressrel/r990827.htm and http://www.cdc.gov/od/oc/media/pressrel/r990827.htm. Last accessed July 2004.

12. Mackesy-Amiti ME, Fendrich M, Goldstein PJ. Sequence of drug use among serious drug users: typical vs atypical progression. *Drug Alcohol Depend* 1997;45:185–196.

13. Guerra LM, Romano PS, Samuels SJ, et al. Ethnic differences in adolescent substance initiation sequences. *Arch Pediatr Adolesc Med* 2000;154(11):1089–1095.

14. Chen X, Unger JB, Palmer P, et al. Prior cigarette smoking initiation predicting current alcohol use: evidence for a gateway drug effect among California adolescents from eleven ethnic groups. *Addict Behav* 2002;27(5):799–817.

15. Dukarm CP, Byrd RS, Aunger P, et al. Illicit substance use, gender, and the risk of violent behavior among adolescents. *Arch Pediatr Adolesc Med* 1996;150(8):797–801.

16. Grunbaunm JA, Basen-Engquist K, Pandey D. Association between violent behaviors and substance use among Mexican-American and non-Hispanic white high school students. *J Adolesc Health* 1998;23(3):153–159.

17. The Henry J. Kaiser Family Foundation. CASA fact sheet. Substance use and sexual health among teens and young adults in the U.S. Feb 2002. Available at: www.kff.org/content/2002/3213/CASAFactSheet.pdf. Last accessed July 2004.

18. Millstein SG, Moscicki AB. Sexually-transmitted disease in female adolescents: effects of psychosocial factors and high risk behaviors. *J Adolesc Health* 1995;17(2):83–90.

19. National Institute for Drug Abuse. *Heroin abuse and addiction.* NIDA research report, NIH Publication No. 00–4165. Rockville, MD: National Institutes of Health, 2000.

20. Schwartz RH. LSD: its rise, fall, and renewed popularity among high school students. *Pediatr Clin North Am* 1995;42(2):403–413.

21. Lloyd J. *Gamma hydroxybutyrate (GHB).* Washington, DC: Executive Office of the President, Office of National Drug Control Policy, Drug Policy Information Clearinghouse, November 2002. Available at: www.whitehousedrugpolicy.gov/publications/factsht/gamma/index.html. Last accessed February 2004.

22. Wills TA, McNamara G, Vaccaro D, et al. Escalated substance: a longitudinal grouping analysis from early to middle adolescence. *J Abnorm Psychol* 1996;105(2):166–180.

23. Shedler J, Block J. Adolescent drug use and psychological health: a longitudinal inquiry. *Am Psychol* 1990;45:612–630.

24. Milich R, Lynam D, Zimmerman R, et al. Differences in young adult psychopathology among drug abstainers, experimenters, and frequent users. *J Subst Abuse Treat* 2000;11:69–88.

25. Kandel DB, Logan JA. Patterns of drug use from adolescence to young adulthood. I. Periods of risk for initiation, continued use, and discontinuation. *Am J Public Health* 1984;74:660–666.

26. Robins LN, Przybeck TR. Age of onset of drug use as a factor in drug and other disorders. *NIDA Res Monogr* 1985;56:178–192.

27. King RA. Adolescence. *Lewis M. Child and adolescent psychiatry: a comprehensive textbook.* In: Philadelphia: Lippincott Williams, & Williams, 2002:332–342.

28. Carnegie Corporation of New York. Adolescence: path to a productive life or a diminished future? *Carnegie Q* 1990;35:1–13.

29. Keyser-Smith J, Stoil MJ. And I will stand the hazard of the die: risk-taking and alcohol use among Washington, DC adolescents. *Alcohol Health Res World* 1987;Summer:48–53.

30. Hamburg BS. *Life skills training: preventive interventions for young adolescents—report of the Life Skills Training Working Group.* New York: Carnegie Council on Adolescent Development, 1990.

31. Jessor R. *Risk behavior in adolescence: a psychosocial framework for understanding an action.* Paper presented at the seventh Cornell Health Policy Conference on adolescents at risk: medical-social perspectives. Cornell University Medical College, New York, February 21–22, 1991.

32. Bandura A. *Social learning theory.* Englewood Cliffs, NJ: Prentice-Hall, 1977:247.

33. Jessor R, Jessor SL. *Problem behavior and psychosocial development: a longitudinal study of youth.* New York: Academic Press, 1977.

34. Jessor R, Donovan JE, Costa F. Personality, perceived life chances, and adolescent health behavior. In: Hurrelmann K, Losel F, eds. *Health hazards in adolescence.* New York: Walter de Gruyter, 1990:25–41.

35. Kim S, Crutchfield C, Williams C, et al. Toward a new paradigm in substance abuse and other problem behavior prevention for youth: youth development and empowerment approach. *J Drug Educ* 1998;28:1–17.

36. Newcomb MD, Maddahian E, Bentler PM. Risk factors for drug use among adolescents. *Am J Public Health* 1986;76:525–531.

37. Battjes RJ, Jones CL. Implications of etiological research for preventive interventions and future research. *NIDA Res Monogr* 1985;56:269–276.

38. Beman D. Risk factors leading to adolescent substance abuse. *Adolescence* 1995;30:201–208.

39. Krosnick JA, Judd CM. Transitions in social influence in adolescence: who induces cigarette smoking? *Dev Psych* 1982;18:359–368.

40. Chassin L, Presson CC, Sherman SJ, et al. Predicting the onset of cigarette smoking in adolescents: a longitudinal study. *J Appl Soc Psychol* 1984;14(3):224–243.

41. Sobeck J, Abbey A, Agius E, et al. Predicting early adolescent substance use: do risk factors differ depending on age of onset? *J Subst Abuse Treat* 2000;11:89–102.

42. Griffin KW, Botvin GJ, Scheier LM, et al. Personal competence skills, distress, and well-being as determinants of substance use in a predominantly minority urban adolescent sample. *Prev Sci* 2000;3:23–33.

43. Griffin KW, Scheier LM, Botvin GJ, et al. Protective role of personal competence skills in adolescent substance use: psychological well-being as a mediating factor. *J Psychol Addict Behav* 2001;15:194–203.

44. Giancola PR, Shoal GD, Mezzich AC. Constructive thinking, executive functioning, antisocial behavior, and drug use involvement in adolescent females with a substance use disorder. *Exp Clin Psychopharmacol* 2001;9:215–227.

45. Clarke JG, MacPherson, BV, Holmes DR. Cigarette smoking and external local of control among adolescents. *J Health Soc Behav* 1982;23:253–259.

46. Page RM. Shyness as a risk factor for adolescent substance use. *J School Health* 1989;59(10):432–435.

47. Dielman TE, Leech SL, Lorenger AT, et al. Health locus of control and self-esteem as related to adolescent health behavior and intentions. *Adolescence* 1984;19:935–950.

48. Patton LH. Adolescent substance abuse: risk factors and protective factors. *Pediatr Clin North Am* 1995; 42:283–293.

49. Sussman S, Dent CW, Leu L. The one-year prospective prediction of substance abuse and dependence among high-risk adolescents. *J Subst Abuse Treat* 2000;12:373–386.

50. Potts R, Martinez IG, Dedmon A. Childhood risk taking and injury: self-report and informant measures. *J Pediatr Psychol* 1995;20(1):5–12.

51. Dobkin PL, Tremblay RE, Masse LC, et al. Individual and peer characteristics in predicting boys' early onset of substance abuse: a seven-year longitudinal study. *Child Dev* 1995;66:1198–1214.

52. Gabel S, Stallings MC, Schmitz S, et al. Personality dimensions and substance misuse: relationships in adolescents, mothers and fathers. *Am J Addict* 1999;8:101–113.

53. Coan RW. Personality variables associated with cigarette smoking. *J Pers Soc Psychol* 1973;28:86–104.

54. Collins RL, Ellickson PL, Bell RM. Simultaneous polydrug use among teens: prevalence and predictors. *J Subst Abuse Treat* 1998;10:233–253.

55. Weinberg NZ, Rahdert E, Colliner D, et al. Adolescent substance abuse: a review of the past 10 years. *J Am Acad Child Adolesc Psychiatry* 1998; 37(3):252–261.

56. Grilo CM, Becker DF, Fehon DC, et al. Conduct disorder. Substance use disorders, and coexisting conduct and substance use disorders in adolescent inpatients. *Am J Psychiatry* 1996;153(7):914–920.

57. Wilens TE, Biederman J, Abrantes AM, et al. Clinical characteristics of psychiatrically referred adolescent outpatients with substance use disorder. *J Am Acad Child Adolesc Psychiatry* 1997; 36:941–947.

58. Stice E, Myers MG, Brown SA. Relations of delinquency to adolescent substance use and problem use: a prospective study. *Psychol Addict Behav* 1998;12:136–146.

59. Silverman JG, Raj A, Mucci LA, et al. Dating violence against adolescent girls and associated substance use, unhealthy weight control, sexual risk behavior, pregnancy, and suicidality. *JAMA* 2001;286:572–579.

60. Lynskey MT, Fergusson DM. Childhood conduct problems. Attention deficit behaviors, and adolescent alcohol, tobacco, and illicit drug use. *J Abnorm Child Psychol* 1995;23:281–302.

61. Armstrong TD, Costello EJ. Community studies on adolescent substance use, abuse, or dependence and psychiatric comorbidity. *J Consult Clin Psychol* 2002;70:1224–1239.

62. Wilens TE, Biederman J, Millstein RB, et al. Risk for substance use disorders in youths with child- and adolescent-onset bipolar disorder. *J Am Acad Child Adolesc Psychiatry* 1999;38:680–685.

63. Stock SL, Goldberg E, Corbett S, et al. Substance use in female adolescents with eating disorders. *J Adolesc Health* 2002;31:176–182.

64. Von Ranson KM, Iacono WG, McGue M. Disordered eating and substance use in an epidemiological sample: I. Associations within individuals. *J Eat Disord* 2002;31:389–403.

65. Rohde P, Lewinsohn PM, Seeley JR. Psychiatric comorbidity with problematic alcohol use in high school students. *J Am Acad Child Adolesc Psychiatry* 1996;35(1):101–109.

66. Hahesy AL, Wilens TE, Biederman J, et al. Temporal association between childhood psychopathology and substance use disorders: findings from a sample of adults with opioid or alcohol dependency. *Psychiatry Res* 2002;109:245–254.

67. Newcomb MD, Bentler PM. Drug use, educational aspirations, and work force involvement: the transition from adolescence to young adulthood. *Am J Community Psychol* 1986;14:303–321.

68. Sanford M. The relationship between antisocial behavior and substance abuse in childhood and adolescence: Implications for etiology. *Curr Opin Psychiatry* 2001;14:317–323.

69. Brown B, Clasen D, Eicher S. Perceptions of peer pressure, peer conformity dispositions, and self-reported behavior among adolescents. *Dev Psychol* 1986;22:521–530.

70. Gfroerer J. Correlation between drug use by teenagers and drug use by older family members. *Am J Drug Alcohol Abuse* 1987;13:95–108.

71. Su S, Hoffman JP, Gerstein DR, et al. The effect of home environment on adolescent substance use and depressive symptoms. *J Drug Issues* 2001;27:851–877.

72. Moser RP, Jacob T. Parent-child interactions and child outcomes as related to gender of alcoholic parent. *J Subst Abuse Treat* 1997;9:189–208.

73. Fletcher AC, Jefferies BC. Parental mediators of associations between perceived authoritative parenting and early adolescent substance use. *J Early Adolescent* 1999;19:465–487.

74. Merikangas KR. Familial factors and substance use disorders. In: McMahon RJ, Peters RD, eds. *The effects of parental dysfunction on children.* New York: Kluwer Academic, 2002;17–40.

75. Akers RL, Lee G. Age, social learning, and bonding in adolescent substance use. *Deviant Behav* 1999;20:1–25.

76. Huba GJ, Wingard JA, Bentler PM. Beginning adolescent drug use and peer and adult interaction patterns. *J Consult Clin Psychol* 1979;47:265–276.

77. Warheit GJ, Biafora FA, Zimmerman RS, et al. Self-rejection/derogation. Peer factors, and alcohol, drug, and cigarette use among a sample of Hispanic, African American, and white non-Hispanic adolescents. *Int J Addict* 1995;30:97–116.

78. MacFadyen L, Hastings G, MacKintosh AM. Cross sectional study of young people's awareness of and involvement with tobacco marketing. *BMJ* 2001;322:513–517.

79. Sargent JD, Beach ML, Dalton MA, et al. Effect of seeing tobacco use in films on trying smoking among

adolescents: cross sectional study. *BMJ* 2001;323:1–5.

80. Winters KC, Anderson N. Gambling involvement and drug use among adolescents. *J Gambl Stud* 2000;16:175–198.

81. Vitaro F, Brendgen M, Ladouceur R, et al. Gambling, delinquency, and drug use during adolescence: mutual influences and common risk factors. *J Gambl Stud* 2001;17:171–190.

82. Kaminer Y, Burleson JA, Jadamec A. Gambling behavior in adolescent substance abuse. *J Subst Abuse Treat* 2002;23:191–198.

83. Bernan DS. Risk factors leading to adolescent substance abuse. *Adolescence* 1995;30(117):201–208.

84. Molnar BE, Buka SL, Kessler RC. Child sexual abuse and subsequent psychopathology: results from the National Comorbidity Survey. *Am J Public Health* 2001;91:753–760.

85. Brindis C, Wolfe AL, McCarter V, et al. The association between immigrant status and risk-behavior patterns in Latino adolescents. *J Adolesc Health* 1995;17(2):99–105.

86. Swanson JW, Linskey AO, Quintero-Salinas R, et al. Depressive symptoms, drug use and suicidal ideation among youth in the Rio Grande Valley: a binational school survey. *J Am Acad Child Adolesc Psychiatry* 1992;31:669–678.

87. Pumariega AJ, Swanson J, Holzer CE, et al. Cultural context and substance abuse in Hispanic adolescents. *J Child Fam Stud* 1992;1:75–92.

88. Szapocznik J, Santisteban D, Rio A, et al. Bicultural effectiveness training (BET): an intervention modality for families experiencing intergenerational/intercultural conflict. *Hisp J Behav Sci* 1986;6:303–330.

89. Gray N. Addressing trauma in substance abuse treatment with American Indian adolescents. *J Subst Abuse Treat* 1998;15:393–399.

90. Murray RM, Clifford HMD. Twin and adoption studies: how good is the evidence for a genetic role? In: Galanter M, ed. *Recent developments in alcoholism, vol. 1.* New York: Plenum Press, 1983.

91. Grove WM, Eckert ED, Heston L, et al. Heritability of substance abuse and antisocial behavior: a study of monozygotic twins reared apart. *Biol Psychiatry* 1990;27:1293–1304.

92. Schuckit MA, Smith TL. An 8-year follow up of 450 sons of alcoholic and control subjects. *Arch Gen Psychiatry* 1996;53:202–210.

93. Miles DR, Stallings MC, Young SE, et al. A family history and direct interview study of the familial aggregation of substance abuse: the adolescent substance abuse study. *Drug Alcohol Depend* 1998;49:105–114.

94. Merikangas KR, Avenevoli S. Implications of genetic epidemiology for the preventive of substance use disorders. *Addict Behav* 2000;25:807–820.

95. Clark DB, Kirisci L, Moss HB. Early adolescent gateway drug use in sons of fathers with substance use disorders. *Addict Behav* 1998;23:561–566.

96. Blum K, Noble EP, Sheridan PJ, et al. Allelic association of human dopamine D2 receptor gene in alcoholism. *JAMA* 1990;263:2055–2060.

97. McGue M, Lacono WG, Legrand LN, et al. Origins and consequences of age at first drink: I. Associations with substance-use disorders, disinhibitory behavior and psychopathology, and P3 amplitude. *Alcohol Clin Exp Res* 2001;25:1156–1165.

98. Huang Y, Oquendo MA, Friedman JM, et al. Substance abuse disorder and major depression are associated with the human 5-HT-sub (1B) receptor gene (HTR1B) G861C polymorphism. *Neuropsychopharmacol* 2003;28:163–169.

99. Rodgers-Farmer AY. Parental monitoring and peer group association: their influence on adolescent substance use. *J Soc Serv Res* 2000;27:1–18.

100. Vakalahi HF. Adolescent substance use and family-based risk and protective factors: a literature review. *J Drug Educ* 2001;31:29–46.

101. Williams RJ, McDermitt DR, Bertrand LD, et al. Parental awareness of adolescent substance use. *Addict Behav* 2003;28:803–809.

102. Yesalis CE. Epidemiology and patterns of anabolic-androgenic steroid use. *Psychiatr Ann* 1992;22:7–18.

103. DuRant RH, Escobedo LG, Heath GW. Anabolic-steroid use, strength training, and multiple drug use among adolescents in the United States. *Pediatrics* 1995;96:23–28.

104. Forman ES, Dekker AH, Javors JR, et al. High-risk behaviors in teenage male athletes. *Clin J Sport Med* 1995;5:36–42.

105. Dennis ML, McGeary KA. *Adolescent alcohol and marijuana treatment: kids need it now.* Rockville, MD: Substance Abuse and Mental Health Services Administration, Center for Substance Abuse Treatment, TIE Communique, 1999:10–12.

106. Fuller PG, Cavanaugh RM. Basic assessment and screening for substance abuse in the pediatrician's office. *Pediatr Clin North Am* 1995;42(2):295–306.

107. Rickman KJ, Mackey TA. Substance abuse screening in student health services. *Subst Abus* 1995;16:99–108.

108. Hallfors D, Van Dorn RA. Strengthening the role of two key institutions in the prevention of adolescent substance abuse. *J Adolesc Health* 2002;30:17–28.

109. American Academy of Pediatrics Committee on Substance Abuse. Testing for drugs of abuse in children and adolescents. *Pediatrics* 1996;98:305–307.

110. Bauman S, Merta R, Steiner R. Further validation of the adolescent form of the SASSI. *J Child Adolesc Subst Abuse* 1999;9:51–71.

111. Wasserman GA, McReynolds LS, Lucas CP, et al. The Voice DISC-IV with incarcerated male youths: prevalence of disorder. *J Am Acad Child Adolesc Psychiatry* 2002;41:314–320.

112. Atkins DL, Pumariega AJ, Montgomery L, et al. Mental health and incarcerated youth. I: prevalence and nature of psychopathology. *J Child Fam Stud* 1999;8:193–204.

113. Teplin L, Abram K, McClelland G, et al. Psychiatric disorders in youth in juvenile detention. *Arch Gen Psychiatry* 2002;59(12):1133–1143.

114. Aharoni DM. The effectiveness of the MMPI-A in the assessment of adolescent substance abuse. *Dissertation Abstr Int* 1999;60:2932.

115. Bergmann PE, Smith MB, Hoffmann NG. Adolescent treatment: implications for assessment, practice guidelines, and outcome management. *Pediatr Clin North Am* 1995;42:453–472.

116. Jainchill N, Bhattacharya G, Yagelka J. Therapeutic communities for adolescents. *NIDA Res Monogr* 1995;156:190–217.

117. Werner MJ. Principles of brief intervention for adolescent alcohol, tobacco, and other drug use. *Pediatr Clin North Am* 1995;42:335–349.

118. Stevens SJ, Morral AR, eds. *Adolescent substance abuse treatment in the United States: exemplary models from a national evaluation study.* New York: Hawthorne Press, 2003.

119. Wagner EF, Brown SA, Monti PM, et al. Innovations in adolescent substance abuse intervention. *Alcohol Clin Exp Res* 1999;23:236–249.

120. Kaminer Y, Burleson JA, Goldberger R. Cognitive-behavioral coping skills and psychoeducation therapies for adolescent substance abuse. *J Nerv Ment Dis* 2002;190:737–745.

121. Waldron HB, Slesnick N, Brody JL, et al. Treatment outcomes for adolescent substance abuse at 4- and 7-month assessments. *J Consult Clin Psychol* 2001;69:802–813.

122. Kaminer Y. Contingency Management reinforcement procedures for adolescent substance abuse. *J Am Acad Child Adolesc Psychiatry* 2000;39:1324–1326.

123. Friedman AS, Terras A, Kreisher C. Family and client characteristics as predictors of outpatient treatment outcome for adolescent drug abusers. *J Subst Abuse* 1995;7:345–356.

124. Springer DW, Orsbon SH. Families helping families: implementing a multifamily therapy group with substance-abusing adolescents. *Health Soc Work* 1999;27:204–207.

125. Liddle HA, Hogue A. Multidimensional family therapy: pursuing empirical support through planned treatment development. In: Wagner E, Waldron H, eds. *Adolescent substance abuse*. Needham Heights, MA: Allyn & Bacon, 2001:227–259.

126. Henggeler SW, Clingempeel WG, Brondino MJ, et al. Four-year follow-up of multisystemic therapy with substance-dependent juvenile offenders. *J Am Acad Child Adolesc Psychiatry* 2002;41:868–874.

127. Arnold ME, Hughes JN. First do no harm: adverse effects of grouping deviant youth for skills training. *J School Psychol* 1999;37:99–115.

128. Dishion TJ, McCord J, Poulin F. When interventions harm: peer groups and problem behaviors. *Am Psychol* 1999;54:755–764.

129. Jaffe SL. *The step workbook for adolescent chemical dependency recovery: a guide to the first five steps*. Washington, DC: American Academy of Child and Adolescent Psychiatry, 1990.

130. Kelly JF, Myers MG, Brown SA. Do adolescents affiliate with 12-step groups? A multivariate process model of effects. *J Stud Alcohol* 2002;63:293–304.

131. Kelly JF, Myers MG, Brown SA. A multivariate process model of adolescent 12-step attendance and substance use outcome following inpatient treatment. *Psychol Addict Behav* 2000;14:376–389.

132. Kilgus MD, Pumariega AJ. Experimental manipulation of cocaine craving by videotaped environmental cues. *South Med J* 1994;87:1138–1140.

133. Geller B, Cooper TB, Sun K, et al. Double-blind and placebo-controlled study of lithium for adolescent bipolar disorders with secondary substance dependency. *J Am Acad Child Adolesc Psychiatry* 1998;37:171–178.

134. Riggs PD, Davies RD. A clinical approach to integrating treatment for adolescent depression and substance abuse. *J Am Acad Child Adolesc Psychiatry* 2002;41:1253–1255.

135. Deas D, Thomas SE. An overview of controlled studies of adolescent substance abuse treatment. *Am J Addict* 2001;10:178–189.

136. Riggs PD, Leon SL, Mikulich SK, et al. An open trial of bupropion for ADHD in adolescents with substance use disorders and conduct disorder. *J Am Acad Child Adolesc Psychiatry* 1998;37:1271–1278.

137. Jenson JM, Howard MO, Yaffe J. Treatment of adolescent substance abusers: issues for practice and research. *Soc Work Health Care* 1995;21(2):1–18.

138. American Society of Addiction Medicine. *Patient placement criteria for the treatment of psychoactive substance disorders*, 2nd ed. Chevy Chase, MD: Author, 1996.

139. American Academy of Child and Adolescent Psychiatry, American Association of Community Psychiatry. *Child and adolescent level of care utilization system, version 1. 3*. Washington, DC: American Academy of Child & Adolescent Psychiatry, 2003.

140. Fallon T, Winters N, Pumariega AJ, et al. CALOCUS: comparative and face validity. In: Villani S, ed. *Scientific proceedings of the 48th Annual Meeting of the American Academy of Child & Adolescent Psychiatry (AACAP)*. Washington, DC: AACAP, 2001;148 (New Research Abstract P25).

141. Smith HE, Margolis RD. Adolescent inpatient and outpatient chemical dependence treatment: an overview. *Psychiatr Ann* 1991;21:105–108.

142. Rounds-Bryant JL, Kristiansen PL, Hubbard RL. Drug abuse treatment outcome study of adolescents: a comparison of client characteristics and pre-treatment behaviors in three treatment modalities. *Am J Drug Alcohol Abuse* 1999;25:573–591.

143. Cornwall A, Blood L. Inpatient versus day treatment for substance abusing adolescents. *J Nerv Mental Dis* 1998;186:580–582.

144. Risberg RA, Funk RR. Evaluating the perceived helpfulness of a family night program for adolescent substance abusers. Journal of Child and Adolescent Substance Abuse 2000;10(1):51–67.

145. D'Amico EJ, Metrik J, Brown SA. Adolescent utilization of alcohol services: barriers and facilitators. *Alcohol Clin Exp Res* 2001;25:98.

146. Liddle HA, Dakof GA. Family-based treatment for adolescent drug use: state of the science. *NIDA Monogr Ser* 1995;156:215–254.

147. Stewart-Sabin C, Chaffin M. Culturally competent substance abuse treatment for American Indian and Alaska Native youths. In: Stevens SJ, Morral AR, eds.

Adolescent substance abuse treatment in the United States: exemplary models from a national evaluation study. New York: Hawthorne Press, 2003:155–182.

148. Szapocznik J, Williams RA. Brief strategic family therapy: twenty-five years of interplay among theory, research and practice in adolescent behavior problems and drug abuse. *Clin Child Fam Psychol Rev* 2000;3:117–134.

149. Pumariega AJ. Cultural competence in systems of care. In: Pumariega AJ, Winters NC, eds. *Handbook of child and adolescent systems of care: the new community psychiatry*. San Francisco: Jossey-Bass, 2003:82–106.

150. Cohen DA, Linton KLP. Parent participation in an adolescent drug abuse prevention program. *J Drug Educ* 1996;25:159–169.

151. Nelson-Simley K, Erickson L. The Nebraska "Network of Drug-Free Youth" program. *J School Health* 1995;65:49–53.

152. Perry CL, Williams CL, Veblen-Mortenson S, et al. Project Northland: outcomes of a communitywide alcohol use prevention program during early adolescence. *Am J Public Health* 1996;86:956–965.

153. Spoth R, Reyes ML, Redmond C, et al. Assessing a public health approach to delay onset and progression of adolescent substance use: latent transition and log-linear analyses of longitudinal family preventive intervention outcomes. *J Consult Clin Psychol* 1999;67:619–630.

154. Dishion TJ, Kavanagh K. A multilevel approach to family-centered prevention in schools: process and outcome. *Addict Behav* 2000;25:899–911.

155. Dishion TJ, Kavanagh K, Schneiger A, et al. Preventing early adolescent substance use: a family-centered strategy for the public middle school. *Prev Sci* 2002;3:191–201.

156. Srebnik DS, Kovalchick D, Elliott L. Initial findings from parent patrol: an intervention to reduce adolescent substance use through reduced involvement in unchaperoned parties. *J Drug Educ* 2002;32:13–23.

157. Einspruch EL, Wunrow JJ. Assessing youth/adult partnership: the seven circles experience. *J Drug Educ* 2002;32:1–12.

158. Taylor BJ, Graham JW, Cumsille P, et al. Modeling prevention program effects on growth in substance use: analysis of five years of data from the Adolescent Alcohol Prevention Trial. *Prev Sci* 2002;1:183–197.

CHAPTER 63
The Elderly

STEVEN R. GAMBERT AND
CHARLES R. ALBRECHT III

Few realize the true extent of substance abuse by the elderly. Although data vary depending on what age cut off community, and substance are studied, it is currently estimated that the prevalence of alcoholism alone is between 3% and 15% in community-dwelling elderly (1), and as high as 18% to 44% in elderly general medical (2) and psychiatric (3) inpatients, respectively. A 1998 report by the Center for Substance Abuse Treatment stated that drug abuse affects up to 17% of adults older than age 60 years and constitutes an invisible epidemic (4). In a study of 1,155 men with a mean age of 73.7 years, 10.4% reported that they had been "heavy drinkers" at some time during their lives (5). In a study of 2,325 patients older than age 65 years living in New York, 6% drank more than two drinks per day (6). A 1999 geriatric outpatient population of 304 patients found that alcoholism was accompanied by an increased likelihood of relying on family for financial support and an earlier age at onset of medical problems (7). In a large population of trauma patients, 49.7% of those older than age 65 years who were screened were positive for alcohol, with the most common mechanisms of injury being falls and motor vehicle accidents (8). Of even greater concern, however, is the large number of elderly using a variety of illicit drugs or prescription medications without proper physician direction. It is estimated that 30% of total prescription drugs and 70% of nonprescription drugs are used by elderly Americans. Although the problem is not a new one, new cases of abuse are compounded by the fact that substance abusers are living longer than ever before. A study in Canada reported a lifetime prevalence of drug abuse or dependence of 6.9% with a male:female ratio of 3:1. The most commonly used drug was cannabis, followed by amphetamines, opiates, barbiturates, hallucinogens, and cocaine. These authors also noted that 80.3% of those with a drug abuse or dependence diagnosis also had a lifetime diagnosis of another psychiatric disorder (9).

There are over 34 million Americans currently older than 65 years of age, representing 12.5% of our nation's population. This number is expected to exceed the 80 million mark within the next four decades, with the fastest growing segment being those 85 years of age and older (10). The oldest member of the 76 million baby boomers born between 1946 and 1964 will turn 65 in the year 2011. The social upheaval in the 1960s and 1970s were accompanied by a tremendous increase in the use of illegal drugs. Although continued use of illicit drugs through senescence is uncommon for various reasons, it is probable that continued use of the same substances will occur in a small proportion of individuals.

This chapter discusses certain unique characteristics of the aged population that may predispose it to the problem of substance abuse, modifying the physiologic effects of abused substances and/or requiring altered treatment.

NORMAL AGING

We all age in two distinct ways: chronologically (based on date of birth) and physiologically (based on functional capacity). Both genetics and environment play significant roles in how "well" one ages. Although we are unable to retard or reverse the "normal" aging process, at least as we know it today, we most certainly are capable of accelerating our physiologic aging process. In general, these normal changes are progressive and result in a loss of reserve capacity. Although each change in itself results in little if no change in function, by the time one is in his or her ninth decade of life, the changes have often become additive and eventually synergistic. The end result is a decline in functional capacity and vulnerability. Any medication, illicit drug, or environmental stress may have a more dramatic effect in an elderly person as compared to a younger person.

A perfect example is alcohol ingestion. Alcohol is distributed in the fluid compartment of the human body. With normal aging, there is a decline in extra- and intracellular fluid, and an increase in the proportion of body fat. Although there appears to be no age-related change in liver detoxification of alcohol, there is a decreased volume of distribution for alcohol with age, resulting in a greater load reaching the central nervous system. There is an age-related decrease in gastric alcohol dehydrogenase, which increases the amount of alcohol entering the bloodstream (11). Making things even worse is the age-related decline in the number of brain cells. This results in an even higher alcohol-to-brain cell ratio in the older person despite a similar amount of alcohol ingestion. Elderly persons are therefore particularly vulnerable to the side effects of alcohol, including altered cognition, behavior, and a tendency for falling (though no specific correlation has been found between the actual level of alcohol and clinical outcomes of those who have consumed alcohol). Medications such as morphine derivatives that may cause hypotension also have more profound effects on the elderly merely as a result of the normal aging process. With age, there is a decreased sensitivity of the baroreceptors; the heart is less able to increase its rate when needed to increase cardiac output. Changes in peripheral blood vessels result in a decreased ability to constrict, and a pooling of blood in the extremities may further result in clinical problems. Hypotension may be more dramatic and more prolonged at this time of life. In addition, there is a normal age-related decline in brain, heart, and renal cell number. It is more likely that a hypotensive episode in the elderly will result in a dementia, stroke, myocardial infarction, or renal insufficiency. Age-related changes in body composition, brain cell number, renal and hepatic function, and physiologic responsiveness can affect medication use, particularly psychotropic agents; when used, extreme caution is advised. Whenever possible, drug levels should be obtained and, above all, in prescribing it should be "start low and go slow."

Table 63.1 is a listing of normal age-related physiologic changes (12). It becomes readily apparent that many of these changes result in an altered tolerance and increased morbidity with substance abuse.

Another aspect of aging and its losses relates to psychological well-being. An increasing number of elderly are outliving their spouses, friends, and even children. Loss of family and friends is further affected by loss of job, economic stability, and failing health. It has been reported that more than 50% of elderly persons experience either depression or serious anxiety disorder. When coupled with a 10% prevalence of dementia in those older than age 65 years and 22% to 47.2% in those older than 85 years of age (13), mental illness is a common occurrence.

It is not surprising then that elderly men who recently lost their spouses have the highest rate of completed suicide and incidence of new alcoholism. "Closet drinkers" and abusers of either prescription or over-the-counter medications are not uncommon. This is further complicated by the all-too-often fragmented approach to health care for the elderly. Many physicians care for single problems in isolation from what is happening with the rest of the patient's medical care. This affords an opportunity for persons to obtain multiple prescriptions for the same medication through different physicians.

AGE-PREVALENT ILLNESS

Symptoms of substance abuse are often missed in elderly persons who tend to suffer more commonly from multiple pathologic conditions. Changes in cognition, behavior, or physical functioning may be wrongly blamed on some underlying medical condition. In fact, both the substance abuse and illness may cause the same problem. In the case of alcoholism, it is readily apparent that alcohol abuse may result in both acute and chronic problems. Anemia, peripheral neuropathy, altered cognition, and liver abnormalities are just a few problems easily confused with other age-prevalent illnesses. Table 63.2 lists common age-prevalent illnesses (12). It is clear that physicians must consider substance abuse in the differential diagnosis of all problems affecting the elderly. Because "economy of diagnosis" does not hold when trying to explain a sign or symptom in the older person, any number of causes must be considered and ruled out prior to making a definitive diagnosis.

ATYPICAL PRESENTATION OF ILLNESS IN THE ELDERLY

Many illnesses present atypically or nonspecifically during later life (12). This makes it even more necessary to

consider all potential causes of a problem, including substance abuse. A patient with pneumonia may present with a change in behavior, appetite, or sleep–wake cycle, much like the symptoms of alcohol abuse or when other medications are taken in excess (Table 63.3).

It is important to remember that addiction to alcohol or some other substance may occur unknowingly. Certain over-the-counter medications contain potentially harmful and addicting amounts of alcohol (e.g., antitussive preparations). In addition, elderly persons commonly take unused medications belonging to family and/or friends. This may result from economic need or a feeling that no harm can be done as long as the "pill" was prescribed by a physician. As discussed previously, age, illness, or other medications may interact and cause undue effects.

ALCOHOL-SPECIFIC PROBLEMS

Diagnostic Considerations

There appear to be two types of elderly alcohol abusers: those who have a lifelong pattern of drinking, individuals who were probably alcoholic all their lives and are now elderly, and those who become alcoholic in their drinking patterns for the first time late in life. While either group may drink openly, it is more common for drinking to occur in secrecy. Depression, loneliness, and lack of social support are the most frequently cited antecedents to drinking for both groups (14). Both will minimize their alcohol use. Table 63.4 summarizes several characteristic differences between early onset and late onset alcoholics.

As with alcoholics of any age, there is a strong tendency for geriatric alcoholics to try to hide their illness. It is not possible to apply all of the usual diagnostic criteria of alcohol abuse to the elderly alcoholic. In a recent study comparing 109 older adults with 47 younger adults, the authors found that older alcoholics were more likely to drink alone while at home, which may further contribute to the precipitating factors of loneliness and lack of social support and create an inescapable downward spiral (15). A useful sign that can be picked up during a routine history includes the daily use of alcohol. Although daily use may be denied, repeated efforts may elicit a history. The elderly may very well experience amnestic periods while drinking, but again, this will almost always require a history from family or acquaintances. The alcoholic is often unaware of the memory lapses or adamantly denies them. Another strong indicator of alcohol abuse is continuation of drinking even after repeated warnings to stop for medical or cognitive reasons. In the presence of any of these signs, there should be a high index of suspicion of serious alcohol abuse. Table 63.5 summarizes some diagnostic signs of alcoholism in the elderly.

The difficulty of recognizing substance abuse in older patients cannot be overemphasized (16,17). In a study of 263 elderly persons with a history of substance abuse, only

TABLE 63.1. *Normal age-related physiologic changes leading to altered tolerance and increased morbidity with substance abuse*

System	Effect of age	Consequences
Central nervous system	Decline in number of neurons and weight of brain Reduced short-term memory Takes longer to learn new information Slowing of reaction time	Do not impair function
Spinal cord/peripheral nerves		Decline in nerve conduction velocity Slowness of "righting" reflexes
	Diminished sensation Decline in number of fibers in nerve trunks	Diminished sensory awareness Reduced vibratory sensation
Cardiovascular system	Reduced cardiac output (normal?) Valvular sclerosis of aortic valves common Reduced ability to increase heartbeat rate in response to exercise	Reduced exercise tolerance
Respiratory system	Decline in vital capacity Increased lung compliance Reduced ciliary action Increased residual volume Increased anteroposterior chest diameter	Diminished oxygen uptake during exercise Reduced pulmonary ventilation on exercise Increased risk of pulmonary infection Reduced exercise tolerance
Gastrointestinal tract	Decrease in number of taste buds Loss of dentition Reduced gastric acid secretion Reduced motility of large intestine	Reduced taste sensation Possible difficulty in mastication Potential cause of iron-deficiency anemia Constipation
Kidneys	Loss of nephrons Reduced glomerular filtration rate and tubular reabsorption Change in renal threshold Decreased concentrating ability	Decreased creatinine clearance Reduced renal reserve may lead to reduced glycosuria in the presence of diabetes mellitus
Musculoskeletal system	Osteoarthritis Loss of bone density (normal?) Diminished lean muscle mass	Poor mobility; pain Decreased vertical height May predispose to fractures Change in posture Reduced strength
Endocrine/metabolism	Reduced basal metabolic rate (related to reduced muscle mass) Impaired glucose tolerance	Reduced caloric requirements Must distinguish from true diabetes mellitus
Reproductive	*Men*: Delayed penile erection, infrequent orgasm, increased refractory period, decreased sperm motility, altered morphology *Women*: Decreased vasocongestion, delayed vaginal lubrication, diminished orgasm, ovarian atrophy	Diminished sexual response Decreased reproductive capacity Increased wrinkling; senile purpura Difficulty in assessing dehydration
Skin	Loss of elastic tissue Atrophy of sweat glands Hair loss	Reduced sweating
Sensory Eye	Arcus senilis Lenticular opacity Decreased pupillary size Contraction of visual fields	Increased risk of falls and fracture Poor vision Presbyopia
Ears	Atrophy of external auditory meatus Atrophy of cochlear hair cells	Presbycusis (loss of hearing of high frequencies)
Taste	Reduced number of taste buds Decreased size of taste buds	Loss of interest in food
Smell	Decline in the sensation of smell	Increased risk of gas poisoning; decreased appetite

TABLE 63.2. *Age-prevalent diseases possibly coexisting with substance abuse*

System	Disease
Central nervous system	Dementia
	Depression
	Parkinsonism
	Subdural hematoma
	Transient ischemic attack
	Trigeminal neuralgia
Eyes	Poor vision (cataract, macular degeneration)
Ears	Poor hearing
Cardiovascular system	Hypertension
	Ischemic heart disease
	Arrhythmia
	Cardiac failure
	Peripheral vascular disease
	Varicose veins
Respiratory system	Chronic obstructive pulmonary disease
	Pneumonia
	Pulmonary tuberculosis
Endocrine/metabolic	Diabetes mellitus
	Hypothyroidism
	Hypokalemia/hyponatremia
	Gout
Gastrointestinal tract	Hiatus hernia
	Dysphagia
	Constipation
	Fecal incontinence
	Diarrhea
	Malabsorption syndrome
	Ischemic colitis
	Irritable bowel syndrome
	Rectal prolapse
	Carcinoma of colon
Genitourinary system	Urinary tract infection
	Urinary incontinence
	Prostatism
	Renal insufficiency
	Prostatic carcinoma
Musculoskeletal system	Osteoporosis
	Osteoarthrosis
	Osteomalacia
	Polymyalgia rheumatica
	Paget disease of bone
Hematologic system	Anemia
	Multiple myeloma
	Myelofibrosis
Autonomic nervous system	Hypothermia
	Postural hypotension
Oral pharynx	Edentulous; periodontal disease
Miscellaneous	Dehydration
	Foot problems
	Fractures
	Immobility
	Iatrogenic illness
	Malnutrition
	Cancer
	Pressure sores

TABLE 63.3. *Possible atypical and/or nonspecific presentations of disease in the elderly that confuses the diagnosis and/or treatment of substance abuse*

Disease	Examples of atypical/ nonspecific presentation
Pneumonia	Anorexia
	Acute confusional state
	Normal pulse rate
	No elevation of body temperature
	No rise in white blood cell count
	Falls common
Pulmonary embolism	"Silent" embolism
	Nonspecific symptoms
Myocardial infarction	Anorexia
	Absence of chest pain
	General deterioration
	Falls
	Weakness
	Shortness of breath common
Congestive cardiac failure	Nonspecific symptoms
Acute abdomen	Absence of rigidity and tenderness
Urinary tract infection	Acute confusional state
	Absence of pyrexia
	No rise in white blood cell count
	Incontinence
Parkinsonism	General slowness
Transient ischemic attacks	Acute confusional state
	Falls
Polymyalgia rheumatica	Nonspecific symptoms
	Poor general health
	Aches/pains
	Lethargy
Hyperthyroidism	Angina
	Atrial fibrillation
	Heart failure
	Absence of eye signs
	No increase in appetite
	Appetite may be poor
	Goiter commonly not palpated
	Bowel movements rarely increased
	Depression
Hypothyroidism	Nonspecific deterioration
	Confusional state
	Depression
	Anemia
	Vaginal bleeding
	Sensory deficit
Depression	May mimic dementia
	Weight loss
Malignancy	Nonspecific symptoms
Diabetes mellitus	Incontinence
	Anorexia
	Delirium
	Depression
	Dementia
	Weight loss
	Nonspecific symptoms
	Falls
	Altered sleep–wake cycle

TABLE 63.4. *Comparison and contrast of early onset and late onset alcoholism*

	Early onset alcoholism	Late onset alcoholism
Family history of alcoholism	Very common (>80%)	Less common (40%)
Psychosocial functioning	Personality disorders common	Stable early adjustment
	Greater prevalence of schizophrenia	Rarely "skid row" alcoholics
	Commonly poor socioeconomic status	Likely to live with family
	Malnutrition	Positive work history
	History of multiple physical injuries	

3 of 88 problem users of benzodiazepines, 29 of 76 smokers, and 33 of 99 problem drinkers were correctly identified by medical staff (18). Another study demonstrated primary care physician difficulty in detecting alcohol use in elderly patients, and further showed that geriatricians were significantly less likely to screen for alcoholism than internists and family practitioners (19). Patients presenting with symptoms of self-neglect, falls, cognitive and affective impairment, and social withdrawal should be carefully screened for substance abuse (20). Early identification that a substance abuse problem exists is mandatory if proper treatment is to be instituted. In addition to addressing the diagnostic signs outlined above, currently accepted screening tests include both the CAGE (cut down [on drinking], annoyance, guilt [about drinking], [need for] eyeopener) questions and the geriatric version of the Michigan Abuse Screening Test (MAST), both of which performed adequately in a 1996 study in 120 elderly veterans (21–23). However, a 2002 study of 1,885 patients found that fewer than half of patients studied screened positive for both the MAST-G and CAGE questionnaires,

TABLE 63.5. *Common signs and symptoms of alcoholism in the elderly*

Daily use of alcohol
Amnestic periods while drinking
Continuation of drinking after warnings to stop
Physical stigmata of chronic alcohol use
Altered cognitive abilities
Anemia
Liver chemistry abnormalities
Frequent falls/fractures
New seizure activity

leading the authors to conclude that each capture different aspects of unsafe drinking (24).

Although many argue that elderly persons are less likely to respond to therapy, studies demonstrate that the elderly are as likely as or more likely than their younger counterparts to make a treatment contact, remain in treatment, and to recover (25). Programs specially tailored to the older person's needs may have an even higher rate of success. In a study of 137 older alcoholic patients randomly assigned to either an "older alcoholic rehabilitation" program or a conventional program, those in a special program were 2.1 times more likely to report abstinence at 1 year (26). Studies showing that age tailored programs are more likely to be effective make inherent sense because they address the loneliness and isolation more common in the elderly alcoholic patient.

Acute Alcohol Intoxication

Elderly persons are particularly prone to problems from acute alcohol intoxication. Although one's ability to detoxify alcohol in the liver is unaffected by age, age-related changes in body composition result in a significantly greater number of clinical problems following alcohol ingestion. With age there is a decline in total body water content, primarily as a result of a change in extracellular fluid volume. Alcohol is rapidly distributed in body water after ingestion. In the average individual, body water content, as a percentage of total composition, declines from 60% at age 25 years to approximately 50% at age 70 years. This decrease in the available volume of distribution for alcohol results in an increase in the amount of alcohol reaching the central nervous system. Combined with decreased gastric alcohol dehydrogenase in the gut with age and its inhibition by commonly prescribed drugs such as H_2-receptor blockers and aspirin, proportionally larger amounts of alcohol enter the bloodstream (11,27).

Clinically, the same amount of alcohol consumed in earlier years with impunity may now cause clinical symptoms such as slurred speech, instability, falls, and confusion. The elderly alcoholic may be mistakenly diagnosed with dementia or tumor, rather than a subdural hematoma resulting from a fall during a bout of drinking or acute alcoholism. Some regions of the brain are more vulnerable to ethanol than others, which is particularly relevant in older alcoholics. The basal ganglion, hippocampus, reticular activating system, and neocortex undergo neuronal loss with aging at a faster rate than do other regions of the brain. These changes result in impaired cognition and motor skills. Even moderate drinking will take an additional toll on these processes. To further complicate cognition, the Canadian Study of Health and Aging calculated a 2.45-fold increased odds ratio for vascular dementia in elderly who abuse alcohol (28). The performance of young social drinkers on abstracting and adaptation tests correlates significantly and negatively with the amounts of alcohol consumed. This trend is similar in older drinkers, but with an even greater detriment to their cognitive functioning. Performances on tests of abstracting, socialization, and concept formation are all proportionately impaired by drinking practices and age.

The nature of cognitive deficits associated with aging and those of alcohol abuse may mimic or magnify changes associated with the normal aging process. When evaluating an elderly patient, the clinician should be aware that a confused, disoriented older patient may be drunk, not demented.

Alcohol also has an acute effect on cardiac muscle, leading to increased cardiac rate and output. Systolic blood pressure may be increased and blood shunted from the splanchnic circulation to the periphery. This latter phenomenon results in cutaneous vasodilation and loss of body heat. When coupled with other age-related problems in maintaining thermoneutrality, the elderly person is at greater risk of developing hypothermia.

Alcohol increases acid production by the stomach's parietal cells. Because aging results in a reduction in parietal cell mass, a significant problem may not result unless an abnormal mucosal lining coexists. As the amount of alcohol consumed increases, there is greater risk of hyperemia, increased mucus production, and decreased acid secretion leading to acute gastritis. Resulting nausea and vomiting may lead to electrolyte and fluid imbalance earlier in the elderly person than in a younger person as a consequence of decreased physiologic reserve.

Although less common with age, alcohol may stimulate secretin production by the pancreas, resulting in increased pancreatic enzyme output. These proteolytic enzymes may lead to autodigestion of pancreatic tissue with the potential for producing an acute pancreatitis. Although the age-related decrease in parietal cell mass decreases the ability of alcohol to stimulate acid production and thus secretin stimulation, alcohol may cause the duodenum to be inflamed with resultant edema and spasm at the sphincter of Oddi, obstructing pancreatic flow.

Acute alcohol ingestion may result in alcoholic ketoacidosis. Arterial blood pH is reduced with a high anion gap; test results for serum ketones are usually only weakly positive because of the predominant ketone being β-hydroxybutyrate, which is not detected by standard tests for ketones. Patients may vary from being alert, but ill, to frankly comatose. Supportive care is necessary until such time as metabolic balance returns. Although administration of bicarbonate is rarely needed, acid–base balance must be followed closely.

The elderly are particularly prone to alcohol-induced hypoglycemia. Usually preceded by a period of starvation, glycogen stores are further impaired by alcohol's inhibition of hepatic gluconeogenesis (29). Because many diseases, both physical and psychological, affecting the elderly result in anorexia and reduced dietary intake,

TABLE 63.6. *Acute alcohol intoxication*

Physiologic effects	Potential consequences
Decreased volume of distribution	Increased serum levels
Increased heart rate and output	Increased blood pressure; flushing; congestive heart failure; angina
Increased stomach acid	Gastritis
Increased pancreatic secretion	Pancreatitis
Alcoholic ketoacidosis	Neurotoxicity; coma
Hypoglycemia	Neurotoxicity; falls; fractures
Inhibition of antidiuretic hormone	Incontinence; dehydration; hyponatremia
Depression of central nervous system	Falls; dementia

hypoglycemia will have a greater impact on older persons because they have less-efficient counterregulatory mechanisms and fewer brain, cardiac, and renal cells. This decreased reserve may result in more significant tissue damage and altered functional status.

Alcohol's inhibition of antidiuretic hormone (ADH) secretion from the posterior pituitary gland leads to prompt water diuresis. This more frequently results in symptoms of urinary incontinence in the elderly. Neurologically, acute alcohol ingestion has a tendency to depress the central nervous system. Tendon reflexes may be hyperactive as a result of reduced inhibitory spinal motor neuronal activity (Table 63.6).

Effects of Chronic Alcohol Ingestion

Alcohol can affect almost every cell, organ, and tissue in the body. Changes in vitamin D metabolism may result from the inability of the cirrhotic liver to hydroxylate vitamin D_3 at the 25 position to its more active form. This condition may be worsened by a diet deficient in vitamin D, malabsorption of fat, and/or concomitant use of either phenytoin or phenobarbital. The end result may be osteomalacia resulting in bone pain and fractures.

Because the liver is the main site of "binding globulin" production and catabolism of testosterone and conjugation of its metabolites with sulfuric or glucuronic acid, alcoholic changes may result in an increase in the ratio of physiologically free estrogen to free androgen. This may result in clinical manifestations including testicular atrophy, spider angiomata, palmar erythema, and gynecomastia.

An increased rate of conversion of adrenocortical steroid precursors to estrogen has also been reported (30,31). This is thought to result from decreased uptake of androstenedione by the diseased liver with a resultant increase in estrone production (32).

Decreased concentrations of plasma testosterone, decreased testosterone production, increased testosterone clearance, and an altered hypothalamic–pituitary axis have all been noted following alcohol ingestion, even in the absence of liver disease. This may result in impotence, often wrongly dismissed as a function of increasing age. Because decreasing alcohol consumption may reverse the problem, intervention is key.

Chronic alcohol ingestion has both a direct and indirect effect on the cardiovascular system. Care must be taken not to blame cardiomyopathy on atherosclerotic disease when, in fact, it is alcohol induced. Alcohol is associated with cardiomegaly (33), cardiac fibrosis (34), microvascular infarcts and swelling (35,36), and altered subcellular myocardial components, glycogen, and lipid deposition (37). Clinically, chronic alcoholism is associated with reduced myocardial contractibility and output and with tachycardia (33,38).

Elderly persons who are chronic users of alcohol have higher rates of glossitis, stomatitis, and parotid gland enlargement (39,40). In addition, they have an increased incidence of squamous cell carcinoma of the oral pharynx, which is further exacerbated by chronic tobacco use.

Chronic gastritis may lead to an iron-deficiency anemia. Anemia may also result from a deficiency in folate or vitamin B_{12} (39). Vitamin B_{12} absorption may decline because of a malfunctioning ileum, not a well-understood condition. Sideroblastic and hemolytic anemias are also more common. Anemia must never be attributed to the aging process and a thorough evaluation must be undertaken to delineate reversible causes, especially in the chronic alcohol abuser. Thrombocytopenia and macrocytosis, with or without granulocytopenia may also be noted as a result of direct bone marrow toxicity (41). In fact, alcohol is the most common cause of thrombocytopenia; failure of these parameters to return to normal within 1 week of abstinence, however, usually indicates another etiologic factor.

Perhaps the best-known complication of chronic alcohol abuse is liver toxicity. A spectrum of illness has been described ranging from fatty metamorphosis to cirrhosis (42). Consequences may include systemic complaints of fatigue, anorexia, and weight loss. Until jaundice is noted, these vague complaints may not be ascribed to alcoholic liver disease in elderly persons with other age-prevalent disorders. On examination, while patients may show typical clinical signs, including spider angiomata, icterus, ecchymoses, gynecomastia, testicular atrophy, muscle wasting, palmar erythema, and Dupuytren contracture, these findings may be easily mistaken for other disorders or wrongly blamed on advanced age. Even laboratory testing may be misleading as normal liver function tests may be noted as the liver fails and production of hepatic enzymes is diminished. Doses of medications cleared through the liver must be adjusted; patients must abstain from alcohol

while consuming sufficient calories and vitamins; severe disease will require protein and sodium restriction.

Nutritional deficiencies are common in elderly alcoholics and may include protein-calorie malnutrition, select vitamin deficiencies, hypomagnesemia, hypophosphatemia, and hypocalcemia (43,44). Active forms of vitamin D may be diminished by alcoholic liver disease and reduced ability to hydroxylate D_3 in the 25 position.

The Wernicke and Korsakoff syndromes are associated abnormalities that result from a thiamine deficiency commonly found in alcoholics. The cognitive symptoms of Wernicke syndrome can easily be mistaken as delirium or dementia when the patient's alcohol abuse is unrecognized. Typically, the patient is someone who has been living alone, is admitted to the hospital for a medical problem, and has had no documented history of cognitive impairment. During the hospitalization, cognitive impairment is very obvious and thought to be a dementia of either acute onset or a delirium related to medications or unknown causes. Acutely, the patient with Wernicke syndrome can have symptoms that are quite striking, but as the symptoms of amnesia and confabulation become apparent, the diagnosis of Wernicke syndrome is more likely. In many cases, the only evidence of Wernicke syndrome is the clinical syndrome. Electroencephalograph tracings may show diffuse slowing or be normal; cerebrospinal fluid and laboratory profiles tend to be normal. With thiamine treatment these patients often improve, relatively rapidly; however, all too often the memory deficits do not reverse. A recent review of alcohol-related problems in the elderly showed that a significant number of elderly presented to the hospital after falls (45). Chronic ingestion of alcohol causes proximal muscle wasting, which may negatively affect balance and lead to falls (46). Table 63.7 summarizes the effects of chronic alcohol ingestion.

Use of alcohol is often encouraged by family and friends of older people to increase socialization and to improve appetite. Older individuals who use alcohol, as already described, either acutely or chronically may suffer from serious cognitive impairment, and after even one drink, these impairments will be of sufficient severity to significantly interfere with any meaningful dialogue. The older individual is very unlikely to be able to actively engage in conversation and almost certainly will have difficulty in recalling what is being discussed. Small amounts of alcohol may in fact stimulate appetite; unfortunately, the daily use of this "appetite stimulant" will generally lead to regular and increased use of alcohol, as well as tolerance. The alcohol often becomes a substitute for good nutrition. The use of alcohol for either of these purposes is highly questionable, and, in any case, a meaningful and sincere dialogue without alcohol and with well-balanced nutritional dietary habits is vastly preferable to any type of alcohol use associated with socialization or eating.

Alcohol also is often used to help with sleeping problems, a common complaint among elderly patients. In

TABLE 63.7. *Effects of chronic alcohol ingestion*

Physiologic effects	Potential consequences
Decreased hydroxylation of vitamin D	Osteomalacia
Increased estrogen ratio	Fractures Testicular atrophy Spider angiomata Gynecomastia Palmar erythema
Decreased testosterone	Impotence
Thiamine deficiency	Wernicke-Korsakoff syndrome (dementia)
Altered cardiovascular function	Arrhythmias Congestive heart failure
Vitamin B_{12} malabsorption	Megaloblastic anemia
Gastritis	Atrophic gastritis Iron-deficiency anemia Altered pharmacokinetics
Fatty and/or fibrotic liver	Hepatitis Cirrhosis Altered pharmacokinetics

normal aging, total sleep time decreases to an average of approximately 6 hours per night. The proportion of rapid eye movement (REM) sleep decreases by nearly 25% and phase IV or deep sleep is significantly decreased in advanced age. Compared to younger adults, elderly individuals have an increased sleep latency, or length of time to fall asleep, and more frequent awakenings throughout the night. Regardless of the length of total time asleep, the decrease in deep sleep results in a less restful or effective sleep.

Alcohol does decrease sleep latency. A "nightcap" thus may help the elderly person fall asleep faster. This effect of alcohol can be subjectively perceived as a definite benefit. The other side of the coin, however, is that a significant alcohol-induced decrease in REM and delta sleep in the elderly alcoholic may result in practically no deep sleep at all. This loss of REM, and especially of phase IV sleep, can lead to undesirable clinical consequences during waking hours. A lack of deep sleep can manifest itself in increased lethargy; REM sleep deprivation can lead to increased irritability. For these reasons the effects of alcohol on sleep in the elderly are very deleterious.

Depression is a major concern in our elderly population, and the neurotransmitter serotonin has been extensively implicated in its development. Chronic alcoholism leads to substantially lower densities of serotonin transporters, which could serve to worsen preexisting depression, or at least antagonize proper treatment (47).

Treatment

Many elderly alcoholics are frankly unaware of the effects of aging on the dynamics of alcohol use and do not realize how greatly alcohol affects their cognition. Often, a frank and direct discussion about the interaction of age and alcohol use can be extremely effective in limiting the use of alcohol by many older people. The goal of any treatment modality must include total and complete abstinence for the elderly individual.

For those patients whose alcohol use has resulted in dietary deficiencies and vitamin deficiencies, replacement of the vitamins and an adequate diet is essential. Medical support for those with alcohol-related medical illnesses is also of paramount importance.

More specific measures include thiamine supplements of 100 mg daily for at least the first week of treatment. In addition, the patient may require hospitalization for the acute stages of detoxification. More specific medical treatments available for alcoholics such as disulfiram (Antabuse) and naltrexone (ReVia) have either not been studied in randomized controlled trials in the elderly, or have not demonstrated increased abstinence after use (48). It is reasonable to offer pneumococcal vaccination to elderly abusers because they are prone to respiratory infections.

Many elderly patients benefit from participation in Alcoholics Anonymous, although some will object that the members of many Alcoholics Anonymous groups are much younger than the patient. Above all, the major objective of treatment of alcoholism in the elderly is clearly abstinence. As stated previously, programs specially tailored to the elderly appear to have a higher rate of success.

PROBLEMS SPECIFIC TO SUBSTANCE ABUSE: COCAINE, AMPHETAMINES, OPIATES, AND SEDATIVE–HYPNOTIC ABUSE

All forms of addiction know no age limitation. In fact, elderly persons are at particularly high risk for addiction because of their more frequent use of medications to treat a variety of acute and chronic medical conditions, economic stability for the majority, and a high prevalence of depression and anxiety disorders. Although data concerning the use of "illegal" drugs by the elderly are not readily available, one must remember that the use of any prescription medication in a manner other than that prescribed is illegal. In general, intravenous or subcutaneous use of illicit drugs is thought to be uncommon in the elderly. Young individuals who use these agents are at great risk for a shortened life span, especially as a consequence of the epidemic of acquired immunodeficiency syndrome (AIDS) and hepatitis C. In fact, national hepatitis reporting in the years between 1966 and 1972 reported a tenfold increase in drug-related hepatitis cases, and few reached senescence. Of those who did reach senescence, few used the same quantities as earlier in life. In 2000, the National Center for Disease Control reported 30,000 new cases of hepatitis C and 73,000 new cases of hepatitis B. There are currently 3.9 million Americans who have had hepatitis C infection and 2.7 million who continue to have chronic active hepatitis C. Many of these latter individuals will have a shortened life span due to chronic liver failure within 20–30 years. Vascular sclerosis may make it increasingly difficult for the long-term intravenous drug addict to achieve sufficient drug levels, essentially self-weaning themselves from the addicting agent. If an older person is known to be a user of intravenous drugs, extreme caution is advised so as not to blame any change in condition on another problem. A myriad of drug-related problems may occur at any age. These include dental problems such as root caries, advanced periodontal disease, and acute necrotizing ulcerative gingivitis; bacterial infections including abscess formation, cellulitis, septicemia, lymphangitis, and thrombophlebitis; endocarditis; tetanus; malaria; tuberculosis; osteomyelitis; septic arthritis; hepatitis; venereal disease; AIDS; and pneumonitis.

Neurologic disturbances are perhaps the most frequently encountered problems. These may result from direct effects of the drugs themselves on the central nervous system or from infections or emboli. Drug use should be considered in all cases of stroke, seizure, altered behavior, or change in cognition.

Cocaine and amphetamine abuse, even in low dosage, is associated with a higher rate of intracranial hemorrhage leading to a cerebral vascular accident. Tics, choreiform or athetoid movements, ataxia, and gait disturbances are also more commonly noted in frequent users of these agents. Heroin, when burned and inhaled, has been associated in the Netherlands (49) with spongiform leukoencephalopathy, presenting as a dementing illness. Elderly addicts are being treated in numerous methadone treatment programs throughout the United States. Although little data are available regarding the exact number of elderly persons receiving such treatment, estimates place this figure between 0.5% and 1.1% of the total caseload (50). With the expected increase in baby boomers turning age 65 years who participated in the often drug-fueled social upheaval of the 1960s and 1970s, as well as the advances made in treating many of the previously fatal diseases of illicit-drug users, the percentage of illicit-drug-using elderly will only increase (51).

Perhaps one of the most underreported problems affecting the elderly is the all-too-frequent use of sedative–hypnotics, particularly among women (52). Whether used for anxiety or to help induce sleep, these agents are addicting. The most commonly misused prescription drug classes among the elderly are sedative–hypnotics, antianxiety agents, and analgesics. Diazepam (Valium), codeine, meprobamate (Equanil), and flurazepam (Dalmane) are on top with 92% of those abusing these drugs doing so for more than 5 years. It should be noted that there is a high correlation between prescription drug abuse and previous or active alcohol abuse (53). Many elderly only know of their addiction when they discontinue or inadvertently run out of their medication. The use of triplicate prescriptions may reduce the use of these agents or at least help alert authorities to potential abuses. Unfortunately, these agents, especially those with longer half-lives, often result in unwanted side effects that affect functional capacity and cognition, placing the older person at greater risk of falling and institutionalization. Drug-related delirium or dementia may wrongly be labeled Alzheimer disease. The elderly appear to be more sensitive to the effects of benzodiazepines, both because of changed pharmacodynamics with aging and because of altered postreceptor cerebral response (54). A thorough evaluation of all problems is essential when caring for the elderly. Failure to do so will undoubtedly increase the number of false diagnoses and limit the quality of patients' life.

SPECIAL PROBLEMS IN THE ELDERLY PREDISPOSING TO SUBSTANCE ABUSE

Chronic Medical Conditions

The elderly have a higher prevalence of physical ailments capable of limiting function. Arthritis is the most commonly noted problem affecting the elderly, with approximately half of all persons older than 65 years of age limited by it to some degree. Osteoporosis affects millions of elderly and predisposes to fractures. In both conditions, the prospect of lifelong disability and potential pain is real. Chronic pain is a problem many elderly must face every day. Other age-prevalent medical conditions that may predispose the geriatric population to substance abuse include insomnia, neuropathies, recurrent gout attacks, and cancer.

These problems clearly place the elderly person at a higher risk of substance abuse. Most elderly have ready access to prescription drugs because physicians are often quick to prescribe medication for the elderly. The elderly often feel frustrated and angry at being dependent, socially isolated, and even discriminated against. Associated feelings of depression, anxiety, low motivation, and self-esteem also predispose elderly people to substance abuse.

Visual and Hearing Disturbances

With increasing age, there is an ever-greater number of persons who lose vital communication skills. Although many may deny the loss of these vital functions, depression, isolation, and loneliness are almost certain results. Alcohol, drugs, or both may become ways of dealing or forgetting the problem. Maximal treatment, ophthalmologic evaluation, hearing screening tests, and referral for hearing and visual aids must be complemented with psychosocial support.

Institutionalized Elderly

Currently, 1.6 million persons reside in nursing home settings. According to the Centers for Disease Control and Prevention's 1999 national nursing home survey, this number is expected to rise to 3 million within the next few decades. Although substance abuse is largely limited to a mishandling and/or inappropriate ordering of medications for most residents of skilled nursing facilities, access to street drugs and alcohol is not impossible. This is an even greater problem for residents of intermediate-care or health-related facilities who are encouraged to frequent community settings. For many, this may involve a visit to the local bar or restaurant. The "visitor supplier" is another potential source not to be overlooked. Health professionals caring for the elderly must be familiar with warning signs of substance abuse and at least consider it in the differential diagnosis of any change in condition that may occur.

SUMMARY

Regardless of one's age, substance abuse must be considered a major cause of emotional and physical disability. Elderly persons have many unique characteristics that predispose them to higher rates of substance abuse, particularly alcohol and "prescribed" medications. A thorough understanding of what constitutes normal age-related changes, age-prevalent disease, and the atypical presentation of illness will hopefully enable the health professional to better recognize and successfully treat this problem. Past substance abusers, now elderly, may have accelerated their normal aging or have diseases they otherwise might never have developed. A clear understanding of the significant consequences of substance abuse will also help identify potential problems and help guide the clinician. Clinicians are advised to not blame all problems on aging. Increasing age and consequences of substance abuse may be additive, however. Unless substance abuse is stopped, treatment will be less than optimal at all stages.

There are few studies of treatment options for substance abuse in the elderly. The negative feelings of many health professionals toward the elderly clearly may decrease potential referrals. Chronic pain problems are more common at this time of life, and while abuse is clearly not the answer, depriving the older person of treatment has moral, ethical, and practical considerations. As long as all alternative options have been tried and have failed, most health professionals would opt for a regulated and controlled addiction over a callous disregard for comfort and well-being. The goal of as high a quality of life as possible must be maintained throughout life. In the case of most substance abuse, however, the goal must be to stop the problem. Before treatment can start, however, the problem must be recognized. Even before that, those at potential risk must be identified and counseled, and predisposing factors eliminated.

As our population continues to age, we will undoubtedly face a growing number of persons seeking physical and psychological benefits from substance abuse. To some, this is a way to counteract the void created by a series of losses. To others, it is a way to escape from chronic, unrelenting pain and suffering. To still others, it is the result of a failure of the medical profession to properly evaluate and treat many of the problems of old age. Whatever the circumstances, health professionals must be more knowledgeable about and willing to care for the special needs and problems of the elderly, including substance abuse.

REFERENCES

1. Myers JK, Weissman MM, Tischler GL, et al. Six month prevalence of psychiatric disorders in three communities. *Arch Gen Psychiatry* 1984;41:959–967.
2. McCusher J, Cherubin CE, Zimberg S. Prevalence of alcoholism in general municipal hospital population. *N Y State J Med* 1971;71:751–754.
3. Moore RA. The diagnosis of alcoholism in a psychiatric hospital: a trial of the Michigan Alcoholism Screening Test. *Am J Psychiatry* 1972;128:1565–1569.
4. Center for Substance abuse treatment. Substance abuse among older adults: an invisible epidemic. Available at http://www.samhsa.gov. Last accessed October 2002.
5. Colsher PL, Wallace RB. Elderly men with histories of heavy drinking: correlates and consequences. *J Stud Alcohol* 1990;51:528–535.
6. Mirand AL, Welte JW. Alcohol consumption among the elderly in a general population, Erie County, New York. *Am J Public Health* 1996;86:978–984.
7. Hirata ES, Almeida OP, Funari RR, et al. Alcoholism in a geriatric outpatient clinic of Sao Paulo-Brazil. *Int Psychogeriatr* 1997;9(1):95–103.
8. Zautcke JL, Coker SB, Morris RW, et al. Geriatric trauma in the State of Illinois: substance use and injury patterns. *Am J Emerg Med* 2002;20(1):14–17.
9. Russell JM, Newman SC, Bland RC. Epidemiology of psychiatric disorders in Edmonton. Drug abuse and dependence. *Acta Psychiatr Scand Suppl* 1994;376:54–62.
10. CDC. National health statistics. Available at www.cdc.gov/nchs/fastats/elderly.htm. Last accessed October 2002.
11. Seitz HK, Simanowski UA, Waldherr R, et al. Human gastric alcohol dehydrogenase activity: effect of age, sex and alcoholism. *Gut* 1993;34:1433–1437.
12. Gambert S. Aging: an overview. In: Gambert SR, ed. *Handbook of geriatrics.* New York: Plenum, 1987;4–5.
13. Evans DA, Funkenstein HH, Albert MS, et al. Prevalence of Alzheimer's disease in a community population of older persons. *JAMA* 1989;262:2551–2556.
14. Schonfeld L, Dupree LW. Antecedents of drinking for early- and late-onset elderly alcohol abusers. *J Stud Alcohol* 1991;52:587–592.
15. Schonfeld L, Dupree LW. Treatment approaches for older problem drinkers. *Int J Addict* 1995;30:1819–1842.
16. D'Archangelo E. Substance abuse in later life. *Can Fam Physician* 1993;39:1986–1988, 1991.

17. McMahon AL. Substance abuse among the elderly. *Nurse Pract Forum* 1993;4:231–238.

18. McInnes E, Powell J. Drug and alcohol referrals: are elderly substance abuse diagnoses and referrals being missed? *BMJ* 1994;308:444–446.

19. Reid MC, Tinetti ME, Brown CJ, et al. Physician awareness of alcohol use disorders among older patients. *J Gen Intern Med* 1998;13:729–734.

20. Thibault JM, Maly RC. Recognition and treatment of substance abuse in the elderly. *Prim Care* 1993;20:155–165.

21. Ewing JA. Detecting alcoholism: The CAGE questionnaire. *JAMA* 1984;252:1905–1907.

22. Blow FC, Brower KJ, Schulenberg JE, et al. The Michigan Alcoholism Screening Test- Geriatric version (MAST-G): A new elderly-specific screening instrument. *Alcohol Clin Exp Res* 1992;16:372.

23. Morton JL, Jones TV, Manganaro MA. Performance of alcoholism screening questionnaires in elderly veterans. *Am J Med* 1996;101:153–159.

24. Moore AA, Seeman T, Morgenstern H, et al. Are there differences between older persons who screen positive on the CAGE questionnaire and the Short Michigan Alcoholism Screening Test- Geriatric version? *J Am Geriatr Soc* 2002;50(5):858–862.

25. Fitzgerald JL, Mulford HA. Elderly vs. younger problem drinker "treatment" and recovery experiences. *Br J Addict* 1992;87:1281–1291.

26. Kashner TM, Rodell DE, Ogden SR, et al. Outcomes and costs of two VA inpatient treatment programs for older alcoholic patients. *Hosp Community Psychiatry* 1992;43:985–989.

27. Lieber C. Medical Disorders of alcoholism. *N Engl J Med* 1995;333(16):1058–1065.

28. Lindsay J, Herbert R, Rockwood K. The Canadian Study of Health and Aging: risk factors for vascular dementia. *Stroke* 1997;28(3):526–530.

29. Levy LJ, Duga J, Girgis M, et al. Ketoacidosis associated with alcoholism and nondiabetic subjects. *Ann Intern Med* 1973;78:213.

30. Edman CD, MacDonald PC. Extraglandular production of estrogen in subjects with liver disease. *Gastroenterology* 1975;69:a-19, 819.

31. Olivo J, Gordon GG, Rafii F, Southren AL. Estrogen metabolism in hyperthyroidism and in cirrhosis of the liver. *Steroids* 1975;26:47–56.

32. Siiteri PK, MacDonald PC. Role of extraglandular estrogen in human endocrinology. In: Greep RO, ed. *Handbook of physiology.* Washington, DC: American Physiological Society, 1973;2:615–629.

33. Bollinger O. Ueber die Haufigkeit und Ursachen der idiopathischen Herzhypertrophie in Munchen. *Dtsch Med Wochenschr* 1884;10:180–181.

34. Alexander CS. Alcoholic cardiomyopathy. *Postgrad Med* 1975;58:127–131.

35. Factor SM. Intramyocardial small vessel disease in chronic alcoholism. *Am Heart J* 1976;92:561–575.

36. Pintar K, Wolanskyj BM, Buggay ER. Alcoholic cardiomyopathy. *Can Med Assoc J* 1965;93:103–194.

37. Alexander CS. Electron-microscopic observations in alcoholic heart disease. *Br Heart J* 1967;29:200–206.

38. Bode JD. Alcohol and the gastrointestinal tract. *Ergeb Inn Med Kinderheilkd* 1980;45:1–75.

39. Sullivan LW, Herbert V. Suppression of hematopoiesis by ethanol. *J Clin Invest* 1964;43:2048–2062.

40. Van Thiel DH, Lipsitz HD, Porter LE, et al. Gastrointestinal and hepatic manifestations of chronic alcoholism. *Gastroenterology* 1981;81:594–615.

41. Cowan DH, Hines JD. Alcohol, vitamins and platelets. In: Bimitrov NV, Nodine JH, eds. *Drugs and hematologic reactions.* New York: Grune and Stratton, 1973:282–295.

42. Sherlock S. *Diseases of liver and biliary system.* Oxford: Blackwell Scientific, 1981.

43. Hurt RD, Higgins JA, Nelwon RA, et al. Nutritional status of a group of alcoholics before and after admission to an alcoholism treatment unit. *Am J Clin Nutr* 1981;34:386–393.

44. Barboriak JJ, Rooney CB, Leitschuh TH, et al. Alcohol and nutrient intake of elderly men. *J Am Diet Assoc* 1978;72(5):493–495.

45. Mulinga JD. Elderly people with alcohol related problems: where do they go? *Int J Geriatr Psychiatry* 1999;14:564–566.

46. Preedy VR, Salisbury JR, Peters RJ. Alcoholic muscle disease: features and mechanism. *J Pathol* 1994;173:309–315.

47. Mantere T, Tupala E, Hall H, et al. Serotonin transporter distribution and density in the cerebral cortex of alcoholic and nonalcoholic comparison subjects: a whole-hemisphere autoradiography study. *Am J Psychiatry* 2002;159(4):599–606.

48. Oslin D, Liberto JG, O'Brien J, et al. Naltrexone as an adjunctive treatment for older patients with alcohol dependence. *Am J Geriatr Psychiatry* 1997;5:324–332.

49. Walters EC, Stam FC, Lousberg RJ. Leucoencephalopathy after inhaling "heroin" pyrolysate. *Lancet* 1982;2:1233.

50. Pascarelli EF. Drug abuse and the elderly. In: Lowinson JH, Ruiz P, eds. *Substance abuse: clinical issues and perspectives.* Baltimore: Williams & Wilkins, 1981:752–757.

51. Patterson TL, Jeste DV. The potential impact of the baby-boom generation on substance abuse among elderly persons. *Psychiatr Serv* 1999;50(9):1184–1188.

52. Farnsworth MG. Benzodiazepine abuse and dependence: misconceptions and facts. *J Fam Pract* 1990;31:393–400.

53. Jinks MJ, Raschko RR. A profile of alcohol and prescription drug abuse in a high-risk community-based elderly population. *DICP* 1990;24:971–975.

54. Closser MH. Benzodiazepines and the elderly. A review of potential problems. *J Subst Abuse Treat* 1991;8:35–41.

CHAPTER 64

Alcohol and Women

SHEILA B. BLUME AND
MONICA L. ZILBERMAN

Western society has a long history of interest in the use of alcohol by women. Dating as far back as the Law of Hammurabi, those cultures that have permitted the use of alcohol have prescribed different rules for drinking by men and women (1). These "double standards" have been based on culturally transmitted theories of how each sex reacts to alcohol (2). The theories, in turn, have led to deeply ingrained stereotypes about the nature and behavior of women who drink, especially those who drink to excess. Negative stereotypes underlie the intense stigma suffered by these women in contemporary society, a stigma which at once acts as a barrier to treatment and encourages the victimization of alcoholic women (3) (see *Sociocultural Factors* below). Yet in spite of the tradition of strong feelings about women's drinking, little research was focused on the physiologic, psychological, or sociologic aspects of women's use of alcohol until the mid 1970s. At that time, as part of the renewed interest in women's lives prompted by the women's liberation movement, the National Council on Alcoholism and Drug Dependence (NCADD) and the National Institute on Alcohol Abuse and Alcoholism (NIAAA) led a nationwide effort to focus scientific and public attention on this subject. NCADD established an office on women and a women's committee that coordinated a network of state and local task forces on women. In 1978, the NIAAA sponsored a comprehensive review of the literature about women and alcohol, and convened a conference aimed at evaluating research to date and pointing to promising new directions (4). A second review and conference, which for the first time included a discussion

of public policy issues, followed in 1984 (5). The Center for Substance Abuse Treatment (CSAT) has also issued several treatment-oriented publications (6–10).

In spite of these efforts, however, knowledge of women's problems has lagged, and the special prevention, intervention, and treatment needs of alcoholic women are still largely unmet (11,12). As late as 1990, sex bias in addictions research was still evident. Studies using exclusively male populations were still common, with results automatically generalized to both sexes (13). This chapter reviews important knowledge about alcohol and alcohol problems in women to highlight some of women's special needs, and to suggest practical strategies for clinicians and policy makers interested in improving the present situation.

PHARMACOLOGY OF PSYCHOACTIVE DRUGS IN WOMEN

Early studies of the pharmacology of alcohol were performed on male subjects, with the assumption that the findings would apply to women as well. It was not until the 1970s and 1980s that researchers began to realize that there were significant sex differences in alcohol absorption and blood levels. Jones and Jones (14) found that single doses of ethanol, under standard conditions, produced higher peak blood alcohol concentrations (BACs) in women than in men given equal doses of ethanol per pound of body weight. This may be explained, in part, by the higher average content of body water in men than women (65% vs. 51%, respectively; 15). Because ethanol is distributed in total body water, a standard dose will be less diluted in a woman. However, the body water content difference did not fully account for differences in peak BACs, nor could it account for the observation that sex differences emerged after oral but not intravenous ethanol administration. Frezza et al. (16) subsequently offered an explanation in their finding of a substantial first-pass metabolism of ethanol in the human gastric mucosa, through oxidation by alcohol dehydrogenase (ADH). Normal women were found to have much lower levels of gastric ADH and to metabolize only about a quarter as much alcohol as normal men under standard conditions, thus absorbing significantly more of the alcohol consumed. This gender difference was further found to be associated with beverages with higher alcohol content (17) and to be exacerbated in alcoholic subjects, so that among alcoholic women the level of ADH was extremely low and virtually all of the alcohol consumed was absorbed. The gender difference tends to disappear in individuals age 50 years and older (18).

Other sex differences in alcohol pharmacology have been described. Unlike the predictable and reproducible peak BACs in men, day-to-day variability, with higher peaks in the premenstrual phase, has been observed in women by some investigators (14) but not others (19). Increased BAC variability (20), faster ethanol metabolism (21), and less marked acute alcohol tolerance have also been reported in women as compared to men (20). In practical terms, this means that a woman will both react more intensely to a given dose of alcohol and be less able than a man to predict the effects of any given amount of beverage alcohol she might consume.

Women in treatment for alcohol problems frequently relate their drinking to their menstrual cycles. Women who meet diagnostic criteria for premenstrual syndrome have been found to drink more heavily than controls (22) and to have a high rate of alcohol abuse and dependence (23). Conversely, increased drinking in both female social drinkers and alcoholics during the premenstrual phase is associated with higher premenstrual symptomatology (24,25). In normally cycling nonalcoholic women, Sutker et al. (26) found significantly more negative moods, more drinking to relieve tension or depression, and more solitary drinking during the menstrual period itself, rather than the premenstruum, whereas Russell and Czarnecki (27) found a correlation between heavy drinking and self-reported menstrual distress. The evidence regarding the relationship between menstrual cycle and the quantity and frequency of alcohol use suggests that increased use correlates with premenstrual symptomatology rather than the menstrual cycle phase itself (28,29).

Sex differences in the proportion of body fat and water that influence BACs change during the life cycle. As women age, there is a further increase in the body ratio of fat to water, exaggerating this trend (30).

INFLUENCES OF ALCOHOL CONSUMPTION ON WOMEN'S HEALTH

Heavy drinking has a uniformly negative effect on women's health. There is some evidence, however, for an association between low to moderate levels of alcohol consumption and decreased risk of coronary artery disease (31) and ischemic stroke. On the other hand, however, the same intake is associated with higher risk for subarachnoid hemorrhage in women than men (32), an effect that seems to be related to lower levels of serum ionized magnesium followed by cerebral vasospasm. This finding is exacerbated by alcohol consumption in women (33). Alcohol intake is directly related both to the risk for hypertension (34) and to overall cardiovascular mortality in women (35).

Evidence of a relationship between alcohol consumption and breast cancer has accumulated over a number of years. Meta-analyses of several epidemiologic studies demonstrate a dose–response relationship between alcohol intake and risk in women (36,37), but the controversy persists as some studies point to a relatively modest numerical association at best (38,39). However, there is evidence suggesting an increased risk with daily ingestion of two or more drinks (40). Because breast cancer is a major cause of premature death in women, this association and the possibility of an etiologic relationship deserves further study. Age, genetics, hormone status, and diet influence breast cancer risk, but alcohol remains a risk factor, even adjusting for these confounders. Moreover, the role of hormones (and hormone replacement therapy) in increasing the alcohol-related risk for breast cancer remains to be elucidated (37).

The role of addictive disorders in the spread of sexually transmitted diseases has been highlighted by the acquired immunodeficiency syndrome (AIDS) epidemic. The vast majority of human immunodeficiency virus (HIV)-positive women are between the ages of 13 and 39 years (41). Half are injection drug users, often also heavy drinkers, while an additional 15% are non–drug-using partners of male users (42). Furthermore, alcohol consumption in heterosexual women (but not men) is associated to less condom use (43), with female heavier drinkers being more likely to engage in risky sexual behavior (44), posing additional risk of getting infected. Another study, however, suggests that alcohol use per se did not result in unsafe sexual behavior (45).

Prolonged heavy drinking is also known to be an etiologic factor in many diseases of the gastrointestinal, neuromuscular, cardiovascular, and other body systems (46). There is growing evidence that women may develop many of these pathologic effects of alcohol more rapidly than men. For example, fatty liver, hypertension, anemia, malnutrition, gastrointestinal hemorrhage, and peptic ulcer requiring surgery differ in natural history in alcoholic women when compared to men (47). Similarly, several studies demonstrate the development of liver cirrhosis at lower levels of alcohol intake (even accounting for differences in body weight) and for shorter periods of time, when compared to men (48–51). In addition, alcoholic women develop both myopathy and cardiomyopathy at lower rates of alcohol intake than men and suffer greater declines in cardiac function (52). A recent study documents significant deficits in alcohol-related neuropsychological working memory, visuospatial skills, and balance in alcoholic women as compared to controls (53). There is evidence for worse performance on neuropsychological tests of attention and reaction time in alcoholic women as compared to men (54), as well as a faster decrease in brain volume (55). These differences in sensitivity to alcohol's toxic effects may well be related to the more complete absorption of alcohol in alcoholic women (absence of first-pass metabolism) demonstrated by Frezza et al. (16). In any case, such findings should reinforce our resolve to accomplish early case finding and intervention with female problem drinkers.

EFFECTS OF DRINKING ON SEXUAL FUNCTIONING AND REPRODUCTION IN WOMEN

The effects of drinking on women's sexuality and reproduction are complex and not completely understood. Single doses of alcohol seem to have little effect on levels of female sex hormones. However, acute alcohol intoxication produces an increase in plasma testosterone levels in women, while the opposite occurs with men (56). This effect is associated with an increased conversion of androstenedione to testosterone in the liver mediated by alcohol damage (57) and may be relevant to a number of problems such as inhibition of ovulation, decrease in gonadal mass, infertility, and a wide variety of obstetrical, gynecologic, and sexual dysfunctions that have been reported in association with chronic heavy drinking in women (58–60).

The effects of drinking on sexuality in both sexes involve a complicated interaction of socially determined expectations and pharmacologic actions (61). Experiments that use special techniques to separate the influences of expectation and pharmacology have found differences between men and women in the effects of single doses of alcohol on sexual arousal (62). Women, unlike men, experience a dissociation between subjective feelings of arousal and physiologic responses. Women who thought they had received an alcoholic beverage said they felt more aroused by sexual stimuli under experimental conditions, whether or not they actually consumed alcohol. This expectation effect was similar to that of men. However, their bodies reacted differently. Actual alcohol consumption had a negative linear relationship to measured physiologic arousal in women. Thus, although the women *said* they felt more aroused, their physical responses were depressed when they consumed alcohol. The same dissociation between subjective feelings of sexual arousal and actual physical arousal was found in a study on female orgasm, which was depressed by alcohol consumption in a dose–response relationship (63). In another study, normal young women kept 90-day diaries of their diet and activities, including drinking and sexual behavior. Although drinking was associated with initiating *fewer* sexual activities, the subjects

believed their diaries would show that alcohol *enhanced* their sexual desire and activity (64).

Likewise, women suffering from alcoholism also report that they expect greater desire and enjoyment of sex after drinking, while at the same time they report a variety of sexual dysfunctions (65), most notably lack of interest. Recovering alcoholic women have been reported to avoid sex in early sobriety (66). Treatment professionals can be of great help to recovering women by explaining that, contrary to their expectations, alcohol actually depresses their physical responsiveness to sexual stimuli. Thus they should not fear that abstinence will diminish their sexuality. In a loving relationship, they will be likely to find sex far more enjoyable than they did when their disease was active. A study of 58 recovering alcoholic women who had a regular sexual partner revealed remarkable improvement in sexual desire, arousal, and ability to achieve orgasm with alcohol abstinence (67).

Women who drink during pregnancy risk significant harm to their offspring (68). The fetal alcohol syndrome has a current estimated incidence of between 1 and 3 cases per 1,000 live births, making it one of the three most frequent causes of birth defects associated with mental retardation, and the most common of nonhereditary causes of birth defects. Fetal alcohol syndrome includes prenatal and postnatal growth retardation, central nervous system abnormalities, usually with mental retardation, a characteristic facial dysmorphism (e.g., short palpebral fissures, epicanthic folds, and maxillary hypoplasia), and an array of other birth defects such as microcephaly, altered palmar creases, and heart abnormalities, among others. The full-blown fetal alcohol syndrome is seen in the offspring of approximately one-third of alcoholic women drinking the equivalent of 10 standard drinks daily (69), but other fetal alcohol effects, such as spontaneous abortion, reduced birth weight, and behavior changes, are associated with lower levels of alcohol intake (70,71). Furthermore, the risk of fetal alcohol syndrome is particularly enhanced with binge-drinking patterns, a pattern that is reported to have increased in recent years among pregnant women (72). An untreated alcohol use disorder in the mother, even if the infant is spared physical damage, may interfere with maternal–infant bonding and adequate parenting. Pregnancy is therefore a critical time for the identification and treatment of alcohol problems in women (7).

Because no safe level of alcohol use during pregnancy has been established, all women should be counseled to refrain from drinking while pregnant and while trying to become pregnant. This abstinence should continue throughout the nursing period. Although in the past lactating women were often advised to drink beer or ale, this practice is unwise (73). A study of 400 infants born to members of a health maintenance organization discovered a significant difference in motor development at 1 year of age between infants breast-fed by mothers who drank during lactation and infants of mothers who were abstinent.

There was a dose–response relationship between ethanol exposure in breast milk and decreased psychomotor development scores (74). Although the effect was relatively small, it was significant.

EPIDEMIOLOGY OF ALCOHOL AND OTHER DRUG USE IN WOMEN

Because detailed discussion of epidemiology is found elsewhere in this volume, this chapter discusses only a few issues of particular relevance to women. Surveys of drinking and drug use have uniformly found that women are less likely to drink and use illegal drugs than men, whereas women are more frequent users of prescribed psychoactive drugs. This is true for alcoholic women as well.

In the early 1980s, a national survey of male and female drinking practices was conducted by Wilsnack and her colleagues. Women who drank heavily (the top 20% in intake), were oversampled so that their behavior could be studied. Several aspects of the study's findings have been reported (75). The researchers found the highest rates of alcohol-related problems in the youngest age group included in the study (age 21 to 34 years), while the highest proportion of heavier drinkers was found in the 35 to 49 years age group. Married women had the lowest overall problem rates, while those cohabiting in "common law" had the highest. The demographic characteristics of women with the highest rates of alcohol-related problems varied strongly with age (76). In the women aged 21 to 34 years, those described as "role-less" (never married, no children, not employed full time) were most likely to have problems. In the women aged 35 to 49 years, women characterized as "lost role" (separated or divorced, unemployed, their children not living at home) had the highest problem rates. In their oldest cohort, ages 50 to 64 years, the women characterized by "role entrapment" (married, children not living at home, not working outside the home) had the most alcohol problems. This last group seems to resemble the so-called empty nest syndrome (77). Wilsnack also noted a strong correlation between the drinking patterns of women and that of their "significant others," more so than for men. Thus clinicians should carefully evaluate the drinking and drug-use patterns of the wives of their male alcoholic patients, rather than just make the assumption that she is "the nondrinker of the pair."

Estimates of the prevalence of alcohol problems, based on an earlier general population survey and updated to account for population changes, were prepared by Grant (78). Using *Diagnostic and Statistical Manual of Mental Disorders,* 4th ed. (*DSM–IV*) criteria, this author estimated that there were 2,068,000 adult women (age 18 years and older) in the United States who could be diagnosed as suffering from alcohol abuse and 1,950,000 who could be diagnosed as suffering from alcohol dependence during the previous 12 months, for a total of 4,018,000 women

affected. This compares with 11,167,000 adult men suffering from alcohol abuse or dependence.

Data from the 1999 National Household Survey on Drug Abuse (NHSDA) that examine national representative samples of the general population age 12 years or older, however, show that although overall men are still more likely to drink and to be dependent on alcohol than women, in the group ages 12 to 17 years, the male:female ratio for alcohol dependence is 1:1 (79). Aggregated data derived from the 1991, 1992, and 1993 NHSDA indicates that among women who used alcohol in the year preceding the survey, those in the 12 to 17 years age group are significantly more at risk for dependence than women in any other age group. Furthermore, this risk is higher (although not significantly) among adolescent women than among adolescent men (80). These facts suggest that, unless preventive measures are taken, important increases in drinking patterns and prevalence rates of alcohol use disorders in women may be expected in the future.

In the year 2000, a computer-assisted telephone survey interviewing a representative sample of U.S. adults estimated that 2.2% of men and 1.4% of women have a current diagnosis of alcohol dependence (male:female ratio of 1.5:1; 81). This compares to a male:female ratio of 3.1:1 in the earlier study by Grant (78).

FACTORS INFLUENCING ALCOHOLISM IN WOMEN

Genetic Factors

Research investigating the existence of a genetic predisposition to some types of alcoholism is discussed elsewhere in this volume. Here it is sufficient to note that studies that have involved both men and women show differences in hereditary patterns between the sexes. There is evidence that inherited risk factors in women are also strongly influenced by environment (82).

Studies comparing identical twins (who share nearly 100% of their genes) with fraternal twins (who share about 50% of their genes) have been used to yield evidence of genetic and environmental effects on various behaviors and problems. Twin studies generally demonstrate a stronger genetic influence on drinking practices, as well as on the development of alcoholism, in males than in females (83). Epidemiologic studies, however, yield similar heritability estimates (e.g., 50% to 60%) across genders, although the sources of genetic influence do not completely overlap (84). Differences in methodology, particularly the sampling method (because recruitment for twin studies is usually done in treatment settings), at least partially explain these contradictory results (85).

Studies seeking genetic markers that would identify individuals who carry a predisposition for alcoholism have focused primarily on males (86). However, Lex and colleagues (87) compared a small number of nonalcoholic young women with and without first-degree relatives suffering from alcoholism. The groups did not differ in blood alcohol levels attained after a measured dose of ethanol, nor were the rates of ethanol disappearance from the blood different. However, the higher-risk women made fewer errors on a cognitive motor task and had less body sway under the influence of alcohol. These findings were comparable to those observed in male samples. They point to the possibility that genetically predisposed individuals are less responsive to alcohol and less able to judge their level of intoxication (88). Generally, studies with both nonalcoholic and alcoholic children of alcoholics show more gender similarities than differences, yet where present, studies usually find higher effects for daughters than for sons (89,90).

Psychological Factors

There is a great deal of uncertainty about the role of psychological factors in the etiology of addictive disease in general. Studies using clinical populations of alcoholic patients regularly demonstrate high levels of psychopathology. Female patients characteristically have higher levels of anxiety and depressive symptoms and lower self-esteem (91,92) as well as higher levels of shame and guilt (93), whereas male patients display more antisocial trends. Distinguishing preexisting pathology from that caused by the alcohol dependence itself has been difficult, but a number of approaches have yielded important and clinically helpful information.

The first approach has been the use of longitudinal studies that follow subjects over many years. The Oakland Growth Study identified general feelings of low self-esteem and impaired ability to cope at the junior high school and high school levels in girls who later became problem drinkers (94), a finding that contrasted with the male data (95). The small number of female problem drinkers in the study constrained the interpretation of the study's results. Both abstaining women (many from alcoholic families) and problem-drinking women showed similar predisposing psychological traits.

Fillmore et al. (96) conducted a 27-year followup study of the drinking status of American adults who had taken part in an earlier survey of college drinking practices. College women who had scored highest on a "feeling adjustment" scale, which contained items such as drinking to relieve shyness, drinking to get high, drinking to be gay, and drinking to get along better on dates, had the highest level of later drinking problems. They had higher problem rates later in life than did the women who were already experiencing alcohol-related problems in college.

These two studies underscore the wisdom of focusing prevention efforts in school- and college-age women on a broad audience, rather than limiting the programs to girls already in trouble with alcohol.

Several researchers used retrospective data collection methods to study the occurrence of traumatic events that might predispose to later addictive disease. Miller and her colleagues (97) studied the experiences of alcoholic women as victims. Their studies compared 45 alcohol-dependent women recruited from Alcoholics Anonymous and a treatment program with 40 matched controls from a community sample. Sixty-seven percent of the alcoholic women reported that they had been the victims of sexual abuse by an older person during childhood. Only 28% of the matched community control group reported such abuse, a significant difference. The alcoholic women were not only more likely to have one such experience, but reported more frequent experiences over longer periods of time, especially if they were daughters of alcoholic parents. In these families, the father was not usually the aggressor. Rather, there was a lack of protection for the child, who was abused by others.

These findings were reinforced in a much larger general population sample, derived from the National Institute of Mental Health Epidemiological Catchment Area study (98). The lifetime prevalence of alcohol abuse or dependence was more than three times greater, and the prevalence of other drug abuse or dependence more than four times greater in women who reported a history of sexual assault. A population-based study of adult female twins shows that sexual abuse in childhood has a particularly important impact in the development of substance use disorders in women, with the odds ratio increasing progressively from nongenital to genital contact and, especially, intercourse, the latter reaching 4.01 (99).

A third approach to understanding the relationship between addictive disorders and other psychopathology is the study of dual diagnosis (the co-occurrence of psychoactive substance dependence and other psychiatric diagnoses). Several studies have found the lifetime prevalence of dual diagnosis higher among alcoholic women than alcoholic men in the general population (100) and in clinical caseloads (101). Evidence for preexisting psychiatric disorder was obtained by separating the primary diagnosis (defined as the diagnosis that appears first in time) from the secondary diagnosis (defined as that which becomes symptomatic after criteria for another psychiatric diagnosis have been met). In the general population sample, 19% of the women who fulfilled diagnostic criteria for alcohol abuse or dependence at some time during their lifetime also fulfilled criteria for a lifetime diagnosis of major depression (compared to 5% of men). This rate of lifetime diagnosis of major depression in alcoholic women was nearly three times the general population rate for women of 7%. Comparing men and women with both alcohol abuse/dependence and major depression, Helzer and Pryzbeck reported that depression was primary in 66% of women, but in only 22% of the men. Likewise, in the clinical population (101), women outnumbered men in prevalence of most psychiatric diagnoses. Fifty-two percent of the alcoholic women satisfied a lifetime diagnosis of major depression (compared to 32% of the alcoholic men). In 66% of these female patients, the major depression was primary (compared to 41% of the alcoholic males). In both studies, major depression was the most common additional diagnosis to accompany substance use disorders in women.

In further exploration of the relationship between depression and alcohol problems in women, longitudinal surveys of drinking patterns demonstrate that depressive symptoms in women at the time of an earlier survey predict quantity of alcohol consumed by the same subjects in a second survey several years later (102), while quantity of alcohol consumed at the earlier point also predicts later depressive symptoms (103). In a followup of the survey of women's drinking cited above, Wilsnack et al. (75) found that both sexual dysfunction and depression predicted chronicity of drinking problems 5 years later (104).

The significant prevalence of preexistent depression in women with chemical dependence raises important questions about the relationship of the two disorders. The nature of this relationship and its possible link to the high rate of sexual abuse in these women is not yet understood. A study of alcoholic patients in treatment found women more likely than men to crave alcohol in response to dysphoric mood (105). In any case, the frequency of this co-occurrence underscores the importance of accurate diagnosis and treatment planning for women with primary affective disorder and secondary chemical dependence. Both disorders must be evaluated and treated. Patients should be alerted to the possibility of recurrence of depression during recovery from alcohol dependence. Such recurrences should be recognized and treated immediately, while special measures to maintain abstinence from alcohol and other drugs are taken. Vigorous intervention can avoid a relapse of the alcohol dependence while the depression is being treated. Other psychiatric diagnoses found in alcohol-dependent or -abusing women include anxiety disorders (including posttraumatic stress disorder; 106), sexual disorders (107), bulimia (107,108), and borderline personality disorder (109,110). Men outnumber women in only two diagnostic categories: antisocial personality (101,107), and pathologic gambling (81,111). However, women do develop these disorders as well. Accurate diagnosis of coexistent psychiatric disorders is critical for both short- and long-term treatment.

In summary, women who suffer from alcohol abuse and dependence are likely to suffer from a variety of other emotional problems, especially depression, both before and after the onset of chemical abuse. Whether or not any of these are specific etiological factors is unclear, but they are of utmost importance for treatment planning.

Sociocultural Factors

There is little doubt that sociocultural factors significantly influence the drinking patterns of women, including their patterns of abuse and dependence. Societal norms and attitudes are a double-edged sword. On one hand they are a major determinant of our current difficulties in case finding, diagnosis, and access to treatment. Social stigma and inaccurate stereotypes about chemically dependent women also encourage their victimization (3). On the other hand, drinking norms that dictate lower quantities and frequencies of alcohol use for women may also be protective.

Alcohol-dependent women are triply stigmatized in contemporary society. First, they are victims of the same stigma applied to alcoholic males, that either attributes their condition to a moral deficiency, or, if the disease concept is accepted, considers the illness "self-inflicted." Second, because women are generally held to a higher moral standard than men, the shame involved in their "fall from grace" is more intense. This idea of a relationship between a higher moral standard and the prevalence of alcoholism in women has a long history in Western thought, and was expressed by Immanuel Kant in 1798 (112). Behavior that is acceptable for men, as Kant pointed out, may be considered scandalous for women. Consider the expression "drunk as a lord." Now consider its female counterpart, "drunk as a lady."

The third and most pernicious aspect of the stigma dates back at least as far as the ancient Romans (2) and Israelites (113). This is the sexual stigma: the idea that alcohol is a sexual stimulant that makes women promiscuous. Although a large general population study of nearly 1,000 women failed to find substantial evidence that alcohol has such an effect (75), the stereotype of the promiscuous drinking woman is deeply ingrained in contemporary thought (3).

In the Wilsnack et al. (75) study, women were asked to complete a questionnaire about their sexual experience and drinking in an atmosphere that maximized privacy. Among women who used alcohol to some extent, only 8% said they had ever become less particular in their choice of sexual partner when they had been drinking. This proportion differed only slightly between lighter and heavier drinkers. On the other hand, 60% of the women surveyed said that someone else who was drinking had become sexually aggressive toward them. The percentage was constant for light drinkers, moderate drinkers, and heavier drinkers. Thus the stereotype of women made promiscuous by alcohol is not merely inaccurate, it results in promoting the sexual victimization of drinking women.

Other researchers have explored aspects of victimization of women who drink. Fillmore (114), in a study of social victimization related to drinking by another person, found that unlike men, women who drink in bars (that is, who are exposed to others while drinking) are far more likely to be victimized, even if they are not themselves heavy or problem drinkers. In the Miller et al. study (97) cited earlier, women suffering from alcoholism were significantly more likely to have been the victim of a violent crime (38% vs. 18% of matched controls), including rape (16% vs. none of the control women). These women were victimized not only by outsiders, but also by their own spouses. The alcoholic women had significantly more experience of spousal violence of every kind from verbal abuse (insult, swearing) to serious assaults with fists or weapons (115). Studies of spousal homicide show that women face a higher risk of being killed at home if they had been drinking than do abstinent women (116). Furthermore, an alcohol-use disorder was detected in 10.5% of the female victims of attempted or completed spousal homicide, as compared with 1.9% among controls. Alcohol-use disorders, however, were found in 49.6% of the perpetrators of female spousal homicide, as compared to 6.9% among control partners (117). Society tends to blame the victim of a rape if she is under the influence of alcohol at the time of the assault, whereas intoxication by the rapist tends to reduce society's perception of his responsibility for the crime (118).

The practical result of this intense social stigma applied to alcohol-dependent women is to keep them in hiding. Because the alcohol-dependent woman grows up in the same society as the rest of us, she applies these stereotypes to herself. She reacts to her problem with guilt and shame. She tends to drink alone, often in the privacy of her kitchen or bedroom. For example, 84% of 116 alcoholic women studied in depth by Corrigan (91) did their drinking at home. Married women, employed women, and upper socioeconomic status women were most likely to drink alone. Partly for this reason, the nature and extent of the alcohol-dependent woman's drinking is often not appreciated by her family and friends until she has reached an advanced state of her disease. In addition, although she may seek medical help repeatedly because of numerous physical problems, nervousness, and insomnia, the stereotype of the alcoholic female as a "fallen woman" makes health professionals unlikely to suspect this diagnosis in their well-dressed, socially competent female patients. A study from Johns Hopkins Medical School examined the prevalence of alcoholism among patients admitted to the university hospital. Although alcoholic patients were underrecognized on all but the psychiatric services, the study found that the alcoholic patients least likely to be correctly identified were those with private insurance, higher incomes and educations, and those who were female (119).

The failure to identify alcohol problems in women early in their development has many destructive implications. Women of childbearing age may produce offspring with serious birth defects if their illness is unrecognized. Physicians who do not diagnose their alcohol dependency are likely to treat these women symptomatically for the wide variety of physical and emotional manifestations of the dependence, often with prescription sedatives and minor tranquilizers. These, in turn, may create an additional drug dependence without interrupting the underlying disease process. Finally, a delay in diagnosis often allows the patient to develop later stage physical, mental, and social complications, making definitive treatment more difficult and less successful.

As already mentioned, sociocultural factors can also be protective to women. Cloninger et al. (120), using data obtained by family history studies, demonstrated that differences in the prevalence of alcoholism between men and women are predominantly a result of extrafamilial environmental factors. Protective social factors for women are likely to include less social pressure to drink, different drinking customs, for example, drinking primarily in mixed groups (whereas men drink in both mixed and all-male groups), and the relatively limited range of occasions in women's lives in which drinking is expected.

In an ethnographic case study (121) of the wives of heavy-drinking men who became unemployed, protective factors in women who did not develop alcohol problems included role modeling by these women's mothers, the belief that "partying" is acceptable for a woman only in teen and young adult years but not after she becomes a mother, the acceptance of drinking by men as part of male social networks, and the custom of women's drinking restricted to special occasions.

CLINICAL FEATURES OF CHEMICAL DEPENDENCY IN WOMEN

Although the basic nature of the addictive process is probably the same in both sexes, physiologic, sociocultural, and psychological factors continue to produce sex differences in the course and symptom pattern of addictive diseases (91,92,113,122). Such differences include the following:

1. Alcoholic women start drinking and begin their pattern of alcohol abuse at later ages than do male alcoholics. This pattern of later onset of drinking and drinking problems in women as compared to men is less robust in younger cohorts (123), and seems to be associated to the decrease in the age of initiation of alcohol use, stronger among women than men (124). In any case, despite differences in the age of onset of drinking (later in women) and in the total amount of alcohol consumed (less in women), female alcoholics appear for treatment at about the same age as male alcoholics and with the same severity of alcohol dependence. This points to a more rapid development or "telescoping" of the course of the illness in women (91). Telescoping was noted by Smith and Cloninger (125) to be particularly characteristic of women who suffer from depressive illness before the onset of their alcohol dependence. The above-mentioned gender differences in alcohol metabolism may be at least partly the explanation for the observed telescoped course of alcoholism in women, but the recent finding of a telescoped course of pathologic gambling—a behavioral

addiction—challenges explanations that take only the pharmacodynamic effects of alcohol as the basis for this effect (126).

2. Alcoholic women drink significantly less than alcoholic men. For example, in a study of 11,500 men and 2,600 women accepted for treatment in NIAAA-sponsored alcoholism programs, women's intake averaged 4.5 ounces of absolute alcohol per day (about 9 drinks) compared to the male average of 8.2 ounces (about 16.5 drinks), although men and women had the same degree of impairment (127). In addition to sex differences in absorption and body water, differences in the use of other sedatives may also help explain this disparity. The equivalent of the male alcoholic's morning drink may be a morning diazepam (Valium) or other benzodiazepine for an alcoholic woman. Her "nightcap" may contain less alcohol and more sedative drug. Thus alcoholism should not be diagnosed as a function of quantity of intake alone (4). As the alcoholic woman ages, her tolerance for both alcohol and other drugs falls and she will drink even less than before, while still experiencing adverse health and social consequences from her drinking.

3. Women entering alcoholism treatment are more likely to be married to or living with an alcoholic sexual partner, or to be divorced or separated, while men entering treatment are more likely to be married to a nonalcoholic spouse (128).

4. Alcoholic women are more likely than alcoholic men to date the onset of pathologic drinking to a particular stressful event.

5. As mentioned previously, alcohol-dependent women are more likely to report both psychiatric symptoms and dual diagnosis. Depression is especially common, and not unlike depression in nonalcoholic women. Turnbull and Gomberg (129) have analyzed and compared the symptoms of depression in 301 alcoholic and 137 nonalcoholic women. They found no differences in the structure of depression in the two groups. They further noted that 88% of the alcoholic women attributed their entry into treatment to "feeling very low and depressed."

6. A history of suicide attempts is also more frequent in female than male alcohol-dependent patients. Suicide attempts in alcoholic women were found to be four times more frequent than in other women, and twice as frequent at ages 20 to 29 years as at ages 40 to 49 years. This age difference was not seen in nonalcoholic women who had attempted suicide (130).

7. Alcohol-dependent women are more likely to be motivated to enter treatment because of health (including mental health) and family problems, whereas for men, job and legal problems, particularly arrests for driving while intoxicated, are more prevalent.

8. Alcoholic women are more likely to reach treatment with a history of other substance abuse along with their alcoholism, particularly tranquilizers, sedatives, and amphetamines, although they are less likely to be abusers of illicit drugs. The drugs these women abuse have usually been prescribed by their physicians.

9. Women who commit homicide have a much higher prevalence of alcohol abuse and dependence than the general population of women, and are particularly likely to meet diagnostic criteria for both alcoholism and personality disorder (131).

IDENTIFICATION OF ALCOHOL USE DISORDERS IN WOMEN

Women tend to be underrepresented in alcoholism treatment. Women are kept in hiding by stigma, which creates shame and denial in these women and their families. However, these are not the only reasons for the underrepresentation of women in treatment. The most common systematic case finding methods in use today, including Employee Assistance Programs, Public Inebriate Programs, and, especially, Drinking Driver Programs, are very strongly male oriented (4).

Women are most often motivated to seek treatment by problems with health (both physical and emotional) and family. Sensitivity to this fact can lead to the development of new and improved case finding systems for women. Both alcoholic and drug-dependent women may be reached through systematic screening in the doctor's office, in hospitals and in medical clinics. Examples of such case finding in medical practice may be found in the literature (23,119,132,133).

Women's special problems with alcohol (including effects on pregnancy and the rapid progression of the late-stage physical complications of alcoholism in women), coupled with women's strong representation in medical facilities, reinforce the need for effective systematic screening, diagnosis, and referral of women with alcohol and drug problems in the health care system (134). Screening instruments that have been used for case finding among women include the Michigan Alcohol Screening Test (MAST), its short version (SMAST), and the four CAGE (cut down [on drinking], annoyance, guilt [about drinking], [need for] eyeopener) questions. In screening for high-risk drinking in obstetric patients, Sokol et al. (135) developed four questions which follow the mnemonic T-ACE. *Tolerance* (an answer of more than two to the question, "How many drinks does it take to make you feel high?") scores 2 points. One point is given for a positive response to "Have people *annoyed* you by criticizing your drinking?," "Have you felt you ought to *cut down* on your drinking?," and "Have you ever had a drink first thing in the morning to steady your nerves or get rid of a hangover (*eyeopener*)?" A score of 2 or more was highly correlated with "risk-drinking" during pregnancy. In light of the high rate of prescription drug use in alcoholic women, the eyeopener question might better be worded "Have you had a drink *or medication of some kind* first thing in the morning to steady your nerves or get rid of a hangover?" for general screening of female populations. TWEAK (Tolerance, Worry, Eyeopener, Amnesia, Cut-down) is a screening tool developed for women (136). Comparison studies have shown that TWEAK outperforms T-ACE in identifying pregnant women at risk for drinking problem (137).

In a related study of women who drank heavily early in pregnancy, those most likely to continue throughout their pregnancies were those with longer drinking histories, greater alcohol tolerance and alcohol-related illness, and those who were daughters of alcoholic mothers (but not fathers) (138).

Laboratory testing can also be helpful in screening. Dahlgren (139) analyzed the records of 100 women undergoing their first episode of alcoholism treatment in the city of Stockholm. It was found that increased mean corpuscular volume (MCV) of the red blood cells was present in 48% of these women, and an increase in the enzyme gamma-glutamyl transferase (GGT) in 42%. If either an elevated MCV or an elevated GGT was used as the screening criterion, 67% of the alcoholic women were correctly identified. Both tests were also indicators of heavy drinking and birth defects in an obstetric population (140).

TREATMENT OF ALCOHOL-USE DISORDERS IN WOMEN

There is little research to indicate the best way to treat alcoholism in women. However, clinicians agree that sensitivity to women's special needs and problems is critical to treatment success (141,142). Among these needs are the following:

1. Special attention should be given to a history of physical and sexual abuse. Abuse may be missed in routine history taking because of the deep feeling of shame attached to these events, or because the memory of these episodes may be repressed. It is imperative that gentle approaches to the subject of incest and abuse be made repeatedly throughout the treatment process.
2. Careful physical and psychiatric diagnosis are critical for treatment success. Because women develop late-stage physical damage more rapidly and have a higher prevalence of psychiatric dual diagnosis, special care should be taken in making a comprehensive diagnostic assessment. Screening for prescription drug abuse and nicotine dependence is especially important, so that the treatment plan can address all of the relevant problems.
3. Evaluation and treatment of family members is also of special value in women patients. Their spouses are more likely to have alcohol/drug problems, and their children may show fetal alcohol effects and/or other sequelae of growing up in a dysfunctional family (86,143).

4. Education about alcohol and other drugs should include information about the effects of these drugs during pregnancy, about birth control, and about the prevention of AIDS and other infectious diseases transmitted through blood and body fluids.
5. Parenting education may be particularly important for alcohol-dependent women, who are often single parents. These women are frequently offspring of alcoholic parents and have had little experience with adequate parental role models in their own childhood. Also, an 8-year study of problem-drinking women and men showed evidence that the children's well-being particularly influences the drinking pattern of the problem-drinking mother. For example, the better the children's adjustment, the less the mother will drink, and vice versa, a fact that is not observed among problem-drinking fathers (144).
6. Child care services are a critical factor in allowing many alcohol-dependent women to participate in treatment. Residential facilities than can accommodate the female patient along with her children are particularly helpful (145,146), but few such programs are currently available. The lack of adequate child care has been identified as a major barrier to treatment for women (11).
7. Couples' and family therapies have been useful in some cases as an adjunct to self-help and/or other counseling, which focus on the alcohol-dependent woman herself.
8. Female role models, in the form of female treatment staff and recovering alcoholic and other drug-dependent women, are helpful in treatment. Self-help groups, such as Alcoholics Anonymous and Women for Sobriety (147), are an important source of ongoing support. Female sponsorship should be sought to help the newcomer understand and participate in these self-help fellowships. This role modeling can be supplemented by recommending that the patient read biographies and autobiographies of recovering women (148–151).
9. The low self-esteem of the alcohol-dependent woman should be addressed in treatment. Special techniques such as assertiveness training have been employed.
10. Sexism and its consequences (for example, unequal societal roles, undervaluation of women's contributions to societal and family functioning, underemployment, and inadequate pay) should be explored in relationship to the experience of the alcohol-dependent woman. It is important that the treating professional not measure success only in terms of adjustment to the societal stereotype of the female role, because in doing so the professional may avoid helping the patient confront her feelings about individuality and independence, and thereby miss the best possible opportunity to enlarge the range of conscious choices about her life. This narrow "adjustment" goal may also fail to raise self-esteem and may reinforce dependent,

child-like, or seductive behavior toward the therapist, rather than encouraging straightforward, aboveboard communication. Because the responsibility for her recovery must continue to rest squarely on the shoulders of the woman in treatment, dependence in the therapeutic interaction becomes a threat to that sobriety. Should the patient relapse during therapy, care must be taken not to reinforce this behavior by oversolicitousness or a level of interest not accorded her in the sober state.

11. Special care must be taken to avoid creating iatrogenic drug dependence. Benzodiazepines, other sedative drugs, and dependence-producing analgesics should be avoided wherever possible. When these medications are absolutely necessary, their use should be closely monitored and the drug should be discontinued as soon as possible.

12. Special populations of alcohol-dependent women need focused attention. In certain populations, the numbers of men and women affected by alcohol dependence seems to be equal, or nearly so, posing additional preventative and screening challenges, as the stigma is not less intense. One such example is a study of the characteristics of alcohol-dependent Jewish men and women belonging to an organization of Jewish alcoholics and addicts (152). The male:female ratio identified in that study (1:1.006) is similar to one found in an earlier study of Jewish alcoholics recruited from treatment centers and Alcoholics Anonymous (AA) (153). African American Hispanic, and Native American women have special needs (154,155) and may suffer from particularly intense stigmatization. Lesbian women are believed to have a high prevalence of alcohol and other drug problems and may profit from treatment in specially oriented groups (156). In some areas of the country, gay and lesbian AA groups are available. These have been of great help to many gays and lesbians.

13. Alcohol-dependent women in the criminal justice system are often overlooked, although their need for specific treatment is no less than that of men (157).

There is no consensus about the comparative efficacy of individual versus group therapy for women, or the value of all-women groups or facilities as opposed to mixed-sex treatment. Little research has been conducted to evaluate the efficacy of these distinct approaches. A single controlled study of an ambulatory program for alcoholic women in Stockholm found a better outcome in the single-sex program than in a control mixed-sex "traditional" outpatient treatment; however, the women in the all-female clinic received more hours of treatment than did the other women (139). If the female patient is treated in a facility that serves both sexes, it is important that she has adequate opportunity to explore issues that she may find hard to discuss in the presence of male patients. This may be accomplished either in individual counseling sessions or in an all-female group (158).

Coed residential facilities should be managed so as to avoid role assignments based on societal stereotyping. Men and women should share equally in meal preparation, housekeeping, fiscal management, building maintenance, and other tasks. Both sexes should take advantage of the opportunity to learn new and unfamiliar skills. Likewise, vocational training opportunities for women in treatment should not be limited to traditionally female job categories. Staff training and ongoing supervision will be needed to institute and perpetuate a nonsexist attitude in treatment.

TREATMENT OUTCOME

The literature on alcoholism treatment has little to offer in outcome studies of treatment designed specifically for women. However, a number of studies have reported outcome data by sex. These studies concluded that adult males and females treated together for alcoholism in the same programs do about equally well (159,160). Looking at specific psychopathology, Rounsaville et al. (161) followed alcoholic men and women for 1 year after treatment. They found that those with the dual diagnosis of antisocial personality and alcoholism had a poor outcome, whether male or female. However, women with the dual diagnoses of alcoholism and major depression did slightly better than average. More studies are clearly needed in this clinically important area. Furthermore, in conducting studies of treatment outcome in dual-diagnosis populations, researchers should consider gender in analyzing the results (162).

Other studies have sought social factors that might influence treatment outcome. MacDonald (163) followed 93 alcoholic women for 1 year after inpatient treatment. He found that the number of life problems and the number of supportive relationships were the best predictors of favorable outcome. Being married was less important as a predictor than the supportive quality of the patient's marriage. Similar results were found by Havassy et al. (164), who found a relationship between social support and time abstinent after detoxification from alcohol, methadone, and tobacco. They also found that their female subjects experienced less social support than males.

Wilsnack et al. (165) looked at factors that predicted remission of problem drinking in their general population sample of women reinterviewed 5 years after their original survey. Women who experienced remission of their drinking problems were more likely to be younger than age 35 years or older than age 50 years, divorced or separated, traditional in feminine traits and moral standards, free of sexual dysfunction, and not reporting heavy-drinking friends.

Taking a broad look at the outcome literature, two major factors emerge: psychopathology and sociocultural factors, particularly support by a social network that does not encourage alcohol and drug use by women. Prevention and treatment efforts aimed at women will be more effective if they focus on these areas.

Women suffering from alcoholism experience a high rate of mortality, both when compared to the general population of women and to rates of excess mortality in alcoholic men (166). For example, Lindberg and Agren (167) followed nearly 4,000 male and 1,000 female patients over a period ranging from 2 to 22 years following hospital treatment for alcoholism. The excess mortality was higher for the alcoholic women (5.2 times the expected rate) than for the men (3 times the expected rate). Smith et al. (168) found a mortality rate 4.5 times higher than expected among 103 alcoholic women followed for 11 years after inpatient treatment. These women lost an average of 15 years of expected life span. These data on mortality rates for alcoholic women reinforce the need for better systems of case finding intervention and treatment for women.

PREVENTION AND POLICY ISSUES

Having reviewed some of the factors involved in the development, perpetuation, and treatment of alcohol problems in women, what can we apply to improve prevention strategies? While stigma and stereotypes keep the alcohol dependent woman from receiving help and serve to promote the victimization of women, cultural expectations that encourage lower alcohol intake for women are protective. At present, per capita alcohol consumption in American women is less than half as much as that of American men (78). Because of their lower body weight, greater sensitivity to alcohol, and special risk during pregnancy, if women were ever expected to match "drink for drink" with men, they would be likely to have more alcohol problems than men, instead of less. Unfortunately, drinking customs in contemporary American society are changing. The advertising and marketing of alcoholic beverages sends messages that can, and do, change cultural norms. Manufacturers of these beverages see women today as a "growth market." Because market research indicates that women drink much less than men but make a significant proportion of the purchases of beverage alcohol, women are being increasingly targeted by alcoholic beverage advertising (169). Beverage manufacturers and retailers, who used to cater primarily to a male market with advertisements emphasizing the masculinity of drinking, are now portraying the genteel refinement of feminine drinking (170). Thus the cultural norms that have served as protection for women are in danger of vanishing.

To accomplish the goal of prevention of alcohol problems in women we must simultaneously work to combat stigma and to preserve the custom of abstinence or moderation for women. Our best strategy would seem to be widespread education about the special sensitivity to

alcohol in women, the teratogenicity of alcohol, the risk involved in using alcohol to medicate feelings of inadequacy or other emotional states, the risk of mixing alcohol and sedatives, and other relevant issues (171).

The importance of sociocultural factors in causing and shaping women's problems with alcohol also highlights the necessity to explore and use the ethnic or subcultural background of the alcohol-dependent woman in treatment. For example, Carter (154) points to the importance of the mother–daughter relationship in preserving the health and strength of the African American family, and the role of this relationship in black women's recovery from chemical dependency. Similarly, an understanding of the "corporate" culture for a female executive (172) and the values and expectations of the health professional's milieu, the military (173), and the campus can be helpful in prevention, just as an understanding of specific Native American and Hispanic American cultures is necessary for preventing problems in these groups.

Women can be helped to develop self-esteem and coping skills through stressful periods of transition without the "help" of alcohol or other drugs. Special treatment methods (174) and nonprofessional self-help groups such as Alateen (175) have been developed to help children of alcoholics. Part of all such programs is education about the increased familial risk for alcoholism and the development of healthy social support networks.

Policy issues with special relevance for alcoholism in women have been reviewed (178). These include the marketing of alcoholic beverages to women, highway safety, prevention of fetal alcohol syndrome and fetal alcohol effects, child abuse and neglect, custody and child care, and support for outreach, treatment, and research about women.

One of the important roles of government is the removal of barriers that keep alcohol-dependent people from obtaining the treatment they need. For women, a major barrier is the lack of child care. Many alcoholic women are single parents, or, if married, lack the resources to provide adequate care for their children. In a multicity survey of services for alcoholic women conducted by the Woman to Woman program of the Association of Junior Leagues, the most frequently mentioned institutional barrier to treatment was the lack of child care services for women needing residential care (11).

Another major barrier to treatment is lack of third-party payment for care. Many women in need of alcoholism treatment are single or divorced and unemployed or underemployed, leaving them without adequate health insurance coverage. This is particularly true for black women (176).

Legal definitions of child abuse and neglect may create additional treatment barriers, especially for women. In many states, the habitual or addictive use of alcohol or drugs by a parent makes that parent a child abuser or neglecter by definition. This definition becomes a barrier, particularly for disadvantaged and single mothers who must rely on public social service agencies for child care in order to enter treatment. Asking for help in such a situation puts them in real jeopardy of losing custody of their children. Paradoxically, continuing their alcohol dependency without seeking help does not, in general, have this effect. Child abuse laws can be altered in their language, not only to remove this barrier, but to provide an incentive for the alcoholic or addicted parent to accept treatment. New York State has revised its definitions so that an addicted parent who is participating in a program of recovery is no longer presumed to be guilty of abuse or neglect without additional evidence (178).

Unfortunately, a recent public policy trend, which began in the late 1980s, threatens to erect new barriers to discourage chemically dependent women from seeking the treatment they need (178). This policy directly opposes the rights of the unborn fetus against those of the pregnant alcoholic or drug abuser, by defining her behavior as "prenatal child abuse." Such policies can be used to punish pregnant women for alcohol or other drug use through loss of custody, or through arrest, prosecution, and incarceration (178).

It should be clear from this review of scientific knowledge and societal attitudes in relation to women's use of alcohol that the relationship continues to be a troubled one in American society. Until more and better knowledge improves our ability to understand and intervene in alcoholism in women, and until adequate screening and treatment systems are in place, public policy will continue to reflect the debate between punitive and humane approaches to these problems. However, even at our present state of knowledge, society could be far more effective in dealing with alcohol problems in women. Simply by applying what we know, devoting adequate societal resources, and maintaining an attitude of concern, our nation could do a great deal more to help the women of today as well as the generations to come.

REFERENCES

1. Hammurabi (Translated by Edwards, C). The Code of Hammurabi, Port Washington, New York. Kennikat Press, 1971.
2. McKinlay AP. The Roman attitude toward women's drinking. In: McCarthy RG, ed. *Drinking and intoxication.* Glencoe, IL: The Free Press, 1959:58–61.
3. Blume SB. Sexuality and stigma: the alcoholic woman. *Alcohol Health Res World* 1991;15:139–146.
4. Blume SB. Researches on women and alcohol. In: *Alcohol and women. Research monograph no. 1.* DHEW publication no. (ADM)80–835. Washington, DC: U.S. Department of Health, Education and Welfare, 1980:121–151.
5. Blume SB. Women and alcohol: public policy issues. In: *Women and alcohol: health-related issues. Research monograph no. 16.* DHEW publication no. (ADM) 86–1139. Washington, DC: U.S. Department of Health and Human Services, 1986:294–311.
6. Center for Substance Abuse Treatment (CSAT). *Practical approaches in the treatment of women who abuse alcohol and other drugs.* Rockville, MD: U.S. Department of Health and Human Services, Public Health Service, 1994.
7. Center for Substance Abuse Treatment (CSAT). *Pregnant, substance-using women: treatment improvement protocol (TIP) series.* DHHS publication no. (SMA). Rockville, MD: U.S. Department of Health and Human Services. 1993:95–3056.
8. Center for Substance Abuse Treatment (CSAT). *Improving treatment for drug-exposed infants (TIP) series.* DHHS publication no. (SMA). Rockville, MD: U.S. Department of Health and Human Services. 1993:93–2011.
9. Center for Substance Abuse Treatment (CSAT). *Substance Abuse Treatment for Persons With Child Abuse and Neglect Issues (TIP) series.* DHHS publication no. (SMA). Rockville, MD. U.S. Department of Health and Human Services. 2000:00–3357.
10. Substance Abuse and Mental Health Services Administration (SAMHSA). *Benefits of residential substance abuse treatment for pregnant and parenting women. Highlights from a Study of 50 demonstration programs of the Center for Substance Abuse Treatment.* New York, New York: Association of Junior Leagues International. September 2001.
11. Association of Junior Leagues. *Highlights of the women to women survey: findings from 38 communities in the U.S. and Mexico.* New York: Author, 1987.
12. National Council on Alcoholism and Drug Dependence. *A federal response to a hidden epidemic: alcohol and other drug problems among women.* New York: Author, 1987.
13. Brett PJ, Graham K, Smythe C. An analysis of specialty journals on alcohol, drugs and addictive behaviors for sex bias in research methods and reporting. *J Stud Alcohol* 1995;56:24–34.
14. Jones BM, Jones MK. Women and alcohol: intoxication, metabolism, and the menstrual cycle. In: Greenblatt M, Schuckit MA, eds. *Alcohol problems in women and children.* New York: Grune & Stratton, 1976:103–136.
15. Van Thiel DH, Tarter RE, Rosenblum E, et al. Ethanol, its metabolism and gonadal effects: does sex make a difference? *Adv Alcohol Subst Abuse* 1988;3–4:131–169.
16. Frezza M, DiPadova C, Pozzato G, et al. High blood alcohol levels in women: the role of decreased gastric alcohol dehydrogenase activity and first-pass metabolism. *N Engl J Med* 1990;322:95–99.
17. Baraona E, Abittan CS, Dohmen K, et al. Gender differences in pharmacokinetics of alcohol. *Alcohol Clin Exp Res* 2001;25:502–507.
18. Seitz HK, Egerer G, Simanowski UA, et al. Human gastric alcohol dehydrogenase activity: effect of age, sex, and alcoholism. *Gut* 1993;34:1433–1437.
19. Hay WH, Nathan PE, Heermans HW, et al. Menstrual cycle, tolerance and blood alcohol level discriminating ability. *Addict Behav* 1984;9:67–77.
20. Wilson JR, Nogoshi CT. One-month repeatability of alcohol metabolism, sensitivity and acute tolerance. *J Stud Alcohol* 1987;48:437–442.
21. Cole-Harding S, Wilson JR. Ethanol metabolism in men and women. *J Stud Alcohol* 1987;48:380–387.
22. Tobin MB, Schmidt MD, Rubinow DR. Reported alcohol use in women with premenstrual syndrome. *Am J Psychiatry* 1994;151:1503–1504.
23. Halliday A, Bush B, Cleary P, et al. Alcohol abuse in women seeking gynecologic care. *Obstet Gynecol* 1986;68:322–326.

24. Mello NK, Mendelson JH, Lex BW. Alcohol use and premenstrual symptoms in social drinkers. *Psychopharmacology (Berl)* 1990;101:448–455.

25. Allen D. Are alcoholic women more likely to drink premenstrually? *Alcohol Alcohol* 1996;31:145–147.

26. Sutker PB, Libet JM, Allain AN, et al. Alcohol use, negative mood states, and menstrual cycle phases. *Alcohol Clin Exp Res* 1983;3:327–331.

27. Russell M, Czarnecki D. Alcohol use and menstrual problems. *Alcohol Clin Exp Res* 1986;10:99(abstr).

28. Mello NK. Drug use patterns and premenstrual dysphoria. *NIDA Res Monogr* 1986;65:31–48.

29. Griffin ML, Mello NK, Mendelson JH, et al. Alcohol use across the menstrual cycle among marihuana users. *Alcohol* 1987;4:457–462.

30. Braude MC. Drugs and drug interaction in the elderly women. *NIDA Res Monogr* 1986;65:8–64.

31. Fuchs CS, Stampfer MJ, Colditz GA, et al. Alcohol consumption and mortality among women. *N Engl J Med* 1995;332:1245–1250.

32. Stamper MJ, Colditz GA, Willett WC, et al. A prospective study of moderate alcohol consumption and the risk of coronary disease and stroke in women. *N Engl J Med* 1988;319:267–273.

33. Altura BM, Altura BT. Association of alcohol in brain injury, headaches, and stroke with brain-tissue and serum levels of ionized magnesium: a review of recent findings and mechanisms of action. *Alcohol* 1999;19:119–130.

34. Witteman JC, Willett WC, Stampfer MJ, et al. Relation of moderate alcohol consumption and risk of systemic hypertension in women. *Am J Cardiol* 1990;65:633–637.

35. Hanna E, Dufour MC, Elliott S, et al. Dying to be equal: women, alcohol, and cardiovascular disease. *Br J Addict* 1992;87:1593–1597.

36. Longnecker MP. Alcoholic beverage consumption in relation to risk of breast cancer: meta-analysis and review. *Cancer Causes Control* 1994;5:73–82.

37. National Institute on Alcoholism and Alcohol Abuse (NIAAA). Tenth special report to the U.S. Congress on alcohol and health. Highlights from current research. Rockville, MD: U.S. Department of Health and Human Services. June 2000.

38. Zhang Y, Kreger BE, Dorgan JF, et al. Alcohol consumption and risk of breast cancer: the Framingham Study revisited. *Am J Epidemiol* 1999;149:93–101.

39. Harris RE, Wynder EL. Breast cancer and alcohol consumption: a study in weak associations. *JAMA* 1988;259:2867–2871.

40. Smith-Warner SA, Spiegelman D, Yaun SS, et al. Alcohol and breast cancer in women: a pooled analysis of cohort studies. *JAMA* 1998;279:535–540.

41. Campbell CA. Women and AIDS. *Soc Sci Med* 1990;30:407–415.

42. Cohen JB, Hauer LB, Wofsy DB. Women and IV drugs. *J Drug Issues* 1989;19:39–56.

43. Trocki KF, Leigh BC. Alcohol consumption and unsafe sex: a comparison of heterosexuals and homosexual men. *J Acquir Immune Defic Syndr* 1991;4:981–986.

44. Caetano R, Hines AM. Alcohol, sexual practices, and risk of AIDS among blacks, Hispanics, and whites. *J Acquir Immune Defic Syndr Hum Retrovirol* 1995;10:554–561.

45. Taylor J, Fulop N, Green J. Drink, illicit drugs and unsafe sex in women. *Addiction* 1999;94:1209–1218.

46. U.S. Department of the Treasury and U.S. Department of Health and Human Services. *Report to the President and the Congress on health hazards associated with alcohol and methods to inform the general public of these hazards.* Washington, DC: Department of the Treasury, 1980.

47. Ashley MJ, Olin JS, le Riche WH, et al. Morbidity in alcoholics: evidence for accelerated development of physical disease in women. *Arch Intern Med* 1977;137:883–887.

48. Wilkinson P. Sex differences in morbidity of alcoholics. In: Kalant OJ, ed. *Research advances in alcohol and drug problems in women.* New York: Plenum Press, 1980:331–364.

49. Gavaler JS. Sex-related differences in ethanol-induced liver disease: artifactual or real? *Alcohol Clin Exp Res* 1982;6:186–196.

50. Hislop WS, Bouchier IA, Allan JG, et al. Alcoholic liver disease in Scotland and northeastern England; presenting features in 510 patients. *Q J Med* 1983;52:232–243.

51. Becker U, Deis A, Sorensen TI, et al. Prediction of risk of liver disease by alcohol intake, sex, and age: a prospective population study. *Hepatology* 1996;23:1025–1029.

52. Urbano-Marquez A, Estruch R, Fernandez-Sola J, et al. The greater risk of alcoholic cardiomyopathy and myopathy in women compared with men. *JAMA* 1995;274:149–154.

53. Sullivan EV, Fama R, Rosenbloom MJ, et al. A profile of neuropsychological deficits in alcoholic women. *Neuropsychology* 2002;16:74–83.

54. Acker C. Neuropsychological deficits in alcoholics: the relative contributions of gender and drinking history. *Br J Addict* 1986;81:395–403.

55. Mann K, Batra A, Gunthner A, et al. Do women develop alcoholic brain damage more readily than men? *Alcohol Clin Exp Res* 1992;16:1052–1056.

56. Frias J, Torres JM, Miranda MT, et al. Effects of acute alcohol intoxication on pituitary-gonadal axis hormones, pituitary-adrenal axis hormones, beta-endorphin and prolactin in human adults of both sexes. *Alcohol Alcohol* 2002;37:169–173.

57. Sarkola T, Fukunaga T, Makisalo H, et al. Acute effect of alcohol on androgens in premenopausal women. *Alcohol Alcohol* 2000;35:84–90.

58. Van Thiel DH, Gavaler JS. The adverse effects of ethanol upon hypothalamic–pituitary–gonadal function in males and females compared and contrasted. *Alcohol Clin Exp Res* 1982;6:179–185.

59. Mello NK. Some behavioral and biological aspects of alcohol problems in women. In: Kalant OJ, ed. *Alcohol and drug problems in women.* New York: Plenum Press, 1980:263–298.

60. Gavaler JS. Effects of alcohol on endocrine function in postmenopausal women: a review. *J Stud Alcohol* 1985; 46:495–516.

61. Wilsnack SC. Drinking, sexuality and sexual dysfunction in women. In: Wilsnack SC, Beckman LJ, eds. *Alcohol problems in women.* New York: Plenum Press, 1980:263–298.

62. Wilson GT, Lawson DM. Effects of alcohol on sexual arousal in women. *J Abnorm Psychol* 1976;85:489–497.

63. Malatesta VJ, Pollack RH, Crotty TD, Peacock LJ. Acute alcohol intoxication and female orgasmic response. *J Sex Res* 1982;18:1–17.

64. Harvey SM, Beckman LJ. Alcohol consumption, female sexual behavior and contraceptive use. *J Stud Alcohol* 1986;47:327–332.

65. Beckman LJ. Reported effects of alcohol on the sexual feelings and behavior of women alcoholics and non-alcoholics. *J Stud Alcohol* 1979;40: 272–282.

66. Apter-Marsh M. *The sexual behavior of alcoholic women while drinking and during sobriety* [dissertation]. San Francisco: Institute for Advanced Study of Human Sexuality, 1982.

67. Gavaler JS, Rizzo A, Rossaro L, et al. Sexuality of alcoholic women with menstrual cycle function: effects of duration of alcohol abstinence. *Alcohol Clin Exp Res* 1993;17:778–781.

68. Hoegerman G, Wilson CA, Thurmond E, et al. Drug-exposed neonates. *West J Med* 1990;152:559–564.

69. Greenfield SF, Weiss RD, Mirin SM. Psychoactive substance use disorders. In: Gelenberg AJ, Bassuk EL, eds. *The practitioners guide to psychoactive*

drugs, 4th ed. New York: Plenum Press, 1997:346–352.

70. Institute of Medicine. *Fetal alcohol syndrome: research base for diagnostic criteria, epidemiology, prevention, and treatment.* Washington, DC: National Academy Press, 1995.

71. Warren KR, Calhoun FJ, May PA, et al. Fetal alcohol syndrome: an international perspective. *Alcohol Clin Exp Res* 2001;25[5 Suppl ISBRA]:202S–206S.

72. Ebrahim SH, Diekman ST, Floyd RL, et al. Comparison of binge drinking among pregnant and nonpregnant women, United States, 1991–1995. *Am J Obstet Gynecol* 1999;180[1 Pt 1]:1–7.

73. Blume SB. Beer and the breast-feeding mom. *JAMA* 1987;258:2126.

74. Little RE, Anderson KW, Ervin CH, et al. Maternal alcohol use during breast-feeding and infant mental and motor development at one year. *N Engl J Med* 1989;321:425–430.

75. Wilsnack SC, Wilsnack RW, Klassen AD. Epidemiological research on women's drinking, 1978–1984. In: *Women and alcohol: health-related issues. National Institute on Alcohol Abuse and Alcoholism. Research monograph no. 16.* Publication no. (ADM)86–1139. Washington, DC: Department of Health and Human Services, 1986:1–68.

76. Wilsnack RW, Cheloha R. Women's roles and problem drinking across the life span. *Soc Probl* 1987;34:231–248.

77. Curlee J. Alcohol and the "empty nest." *Bull Menninger Clin* 1969;33:165–171.

78. Grant B. Alcohol consumption, alcohol abuse and alcohol dependence: the United States as an example. *Addiction* 1994;89:1357–1365.

79. Greenfield SF. Women and alcohol use disorders. *Am Acad Addict Psychiatry News* 2001;Summer:3–4.

80. Kandel D, Chen K, Warner LA, et al. Prevalence and demographic correlates of symptoms of last year dependence on alcohol, nicotine, marijuana and cocaine in the U.S. population. *Drug Alcohol Depend* 1997;44:11–29.

81. Welte J, Barnes G, Wieczorek W, et al. Alcohol and gambling pathology among U.S. adults: prevalence, demographic patterns and comorbidity. *J Stud Alcohol* 2001;62:706–712.

82. Cloninger CR, Sigvardsson S, Gilligan SB, et al. Genetic heterogeneity and the classification of alcoholism. *Adv Alcohol Subst Abuse* 1988;7(3–4):3–16.

83. Sigvardsson S, Bohman M, Cloninger CR. Replication of the Stockholm Adoption Study of alcoholism. Confirmatory cross-fostering analysis. *Arch Gen Psychiatry* 1996;53:681–687.

84. Prescott CA, Aggen SH, Kendler KS. Sex differences in the sources of genetic liability to alcohol abuse and dependence in a population-based sample of U.S. twins. *Alcohol Clin Exp Res* 1999;23:1136–1144.

85. Prescott CA, Kendler KS. Influence of ascertainment strategy on finding sex differences in genetic estimates from twin studies of alcoholism. *Am J Med Genet* 2000;96:754–761.

86. Russell M, Henderson C, Blume SB. *Children of alcoholics: a review of the literature.* New York: Children of Alcoholics Foundation, 1985.

87. Lex BW, Lukas SE, Greenwald NE. Alcohol-induced changes in body sway in women at risk for alcoholism: a pilot study. *J Stud Alcohol* 1988;49:346–356.

88. Schuckit MA, Smith TL. The relationships of a family history of alcohol dependence, a low level of response to alcohol and six domains of life functioning to the development of alcohol use disorders. *J Stud Alcohol* 2000;61:827–835.

89. Chermack ST, Stoltenberg SF, Fuller BE, et al. Gender differences in the development of substance-related problems: the impact of family history of alcoholism, family history of violence and childhood conduct problems. *J Stud Alcohol* 2000;61:845–852.

90. Svanum S, McAdoo WG. Parental alcoholism: an examination of male and female alcoholics in treatment. *J Stud Alcohol* 1991;52:127–132.

91. Corrigan EM. *Alcoholic women in treatment.* New York: Oxford University Press, 1980.

92. Beckman LJ. Self-esteem of women alcoholics. *J Stud Alcohol* 1978;39:491–498.

93. O'Connor LE, Berry JW, Inaba D, et al. Shame, guilt, and depression in men and women in recovery from addiction. *J Subst Abuse Treat* 1994;11:503–510.

94. Jones MC. Personality antecedents and correlates of drinking patterns in women. *J Consult Clin Psychol* 1971;36:61–69.

95. Jones MC. Personality correlates and antecedents of drinking patterns in adult males. *J Consult Clin Psychol* 1968;32:2–12.

96. Fillmore KM, Bacon SD, Hyman M. *The 27 year longitudinal panel study of drinking by students in college. Report 1979 to National Institute of Alcoholism and Alcohol Abuse.* Contract No: ADM 281-76-0015. Washington, DC: National Institute on Alcoholism and Alcohol Abuse. 1979.

97. Miller BA, Downs WR. *Conflict and violence among alcoholic women as*

compared to a random household sample. Paper presented at the 38th annual meeting of the American Society of Criminology, Atlanta, GA, 1986.

98. Winfield I, George LK, Swartz M, Blazer DG. Sexual assault and psychiatric disorders among a community sample of women. *Am J Psychiatry* 1990;147:335–341.

99. Kendler KS, Bulik CM, Silberg J, et al. Childhood sexual abuse and adult psychiatric and substance use disorders in women: an epidemiological and cotwin control analysis. *Arch Gen Psychiatry* 2000;57:953–959.

100. Helzer JE, Pryzbeck TR. The co-occurrence of alcoholism with other psychiatric disorders in the general population and its impact on treatment. *J Stud Alcohol* 1988;49:219–224.

101. Hesselbrock MN, Meyer RE, Keener JJ. Psychopathology in hospitalized alcoholics. *Arch Gen Psychiatry* 1985;42:1050–1055.

102. Wang J, Patten SB. A prospective study of sex-specific effects of major depression on alcohol consumption. *Can J Psychiatry* 2001;46:422–425.

103. Hartka E, Johnstone B, Leino EV, et al. A meta-analysis of expressive symptomatology and alcohol consumption over time. *Br J Addict* 1991;86:1283–1298.

104. Wilsnack SC, Klassen AD, Schur BE, et al. Predicting onset and chronicity of women's problem drinking: a 5-year longitudinal analysis. *Am J Pub Health* 1991;81:305–318.

105. Rubonis AV, Colby SM, Monti PM, et al. Alcohol cue reactivity and mood induction in male and female alcoholics. *J Stud Alcohol* 1994;55:487–494.

106. Brady KT, Dansky BS. Effects of victimization and posttraumatic stress disorder on substance use disorders in women. In: Lewis-Hall F, Williams TS, Panetta JA, et al, eds. *Psychiatric illness in women: emerging treatments and research.* Washington, DC: American Psychiatric Publishing, 2002:449–466.

107. Ross HE, Glaser FB, Stiasny S. Sex differences in the prevalence of psychiatric disorder in patients with alcohol and drug problems. *Br J Addict* 1988;83:1179–1192.

108. Bulik CM. Drug and alcohol abuse by bulimic women and their families. *Am J Psychiatry* 1987;144:1604–1606.

109. Vaglum S, Vaglum P. Borderline and other mental disorders in alcoholic female psychiatric patients: a case control study. *Psychopathology* 1985;18:50–60.

110. Nace EP, Saxon JJ, Shore N. Borderline personality disorder and

alcoholism treatment: a one-year follow-up study. *J Stud Alcohol* 1986; 47:196–200.

111. Lesieur HR, Blume SB, Zoppa RM. Alcoholism, drug abuse, and gambling. *Alcohol Clin Exp Res* 1986;10:33–38.

112. Jellinek EM. Immanuel Kant on drinking. *Q J Stud Alcohol* 1941;1:777–778.

113. Gomberg ESL. Women and alcoholism: psychosocial issues. In: *Women and alcohol: health-related issues. Research monograph no. 16.* Publication No. (ADM)86–1139. Washington, DC: Department of Health and Human Services, 1986:78–120.

114. Fillmore KM. The social victims of drinking. *Br J Addict* 1985;80:307–314.

115. Miller BA, Downs WR, Gondoli DM. Spousal violence among alcoholic women as compared to a random household sample of women. *J Stud Alcohol* 1989;50:533–540.

116. Rivara FP, Mueller BA, Somes G, et al. Alcohol and illicit drug abuse and the risk of violent death in the home. *JAMA* 1997;278:569–575.

117. Sharps PW, Campbell J, Campbell D, et al. The role of alcohol use in intimate partner femicide. *Am J Addict* 2001;10:122–135.

118. Richardson D, Campbell J. The effect of alcohol on attribution of blame for rape. *Pers Soc Psychol Bull* 1982;8:468–476.

119. Moore RD, Bone LR, Geller G, et al. Prevalence, detection and treatment of alcoholism in hospitalized patients. *JAMA* 1989;261:403–408.

120. Cloninger CR, Christiansen KO, Reich T, et al. Implications of sex differences in the prevalence of antisocial personality, alcoholism, and criminality for familial transmission. *Arch Gen Psychiatry* 1978;35:941–951.

121. Klee L, Ames G. Reevaluating risk factors for women's drinking: a study of blue collar wives. *Am J Prev Med* 1987;3:31–41.

122. Schmidt G, Klee L, Ames G. Review and analysis of literature on indicators of womens' problems. *Br J Addict* 1990;85:179–192.

123. Randall CL, Roberts JS, Del Boca FK, et al. Telescoping of landmark events associated with drinking: a gender comparison. *J Stud Alcohol* 1999;60:252–260.

124. Greenfield SF, O'Leary G. Gender differences in substance use disorders. In: Lewis-Hall F, Williams TS, Panetta JA, et al, eds. *Psychiatric illness in women: emerging treatments and research.* Washington, DC: American Psychiatric Publishing, 2002:467–533.

125. Smith EM, Cloninger CR. Alcoholic females: mortality at twelve-year follow-up. *Focus Women* 1981;2:1–13.

126. Tavares H, Zilberman ML, Beites F, et al. Gender differences in gambling progression. *J Gambl Stud* 2001;17: 151–159.

127. Armor DJ, Polich JM, Stambul HB. *Alcoholism and treatment.* New York: John Wiley, 1978.

128. Jacob T, Bremer DA. Assortative mating among men and women alcoholics. *J Stud Alcohol* 1986;47:219–222.

129. Turnbull JE, Gomberg ESL. The structure of depression in alcoholic women. *J Stud Alcohol* 1990;51:148–155.

130. Gomberg ES. Suicide risk among women with alcohol problems. *Am J Public Health* 1989;79:1363–1365.

131. Eronen M. Mental disorders and homicidal behavior in female subjects. *Am J Psychiatry* 1995;152:8:1216–1218.

132. Cyr MG, Wartman SA. The effectiveness of routine screening questions in the detection of alcoholism. *JAMA* 1988;259:51–54.

133. Cleary PD, Miller M, Bush BT, et al. Prevalence and recognition of alcohol abuse in a primary care population. *Am J Med* 1988;85:466–471.

134. Blume SB. Women and alcohol: a review. *JAMA* 1986;256:1467–1470.

135. Sokol RJ, Martier SS, Ager JW. The T-ACE questions: practical prenatal detection of risk-drinking. *Am J Obstet Gynecol* 1989;160:863–870.

136. Russell M, Martier SS, Sokol RJ, et al. Screening for pregnancy risk-drinking. *Alcohol Clin Exp Res* 1994;18:1156–1161.

137. Russell M, Martier SS, Sokol RJ, et al. Detecting risk drinking during pregnancy: a comparison of four screening questionnaires. *Am J Public Health* 1996;86:1435–1439.

138. Smith IE, Lancaster JS, Moss-Wells S, et al. Identifying high-risk pregnant drinkers: biological and behavioral correlates of continuous heavy drinking during pregnancy. *J Stud Alcohol* 1987;48:304–309.

139. Dahlgren L, Willander A. Are special treatment facilities for female alcoholics needed? A controlled 2-year follow-up study from a specialized female unit (EWA) versus a mixed male/female treatment facility. *Alcohol Clin Exp Res* 1989;13:499–504.

140. Ylikorkala O, Stenman U, Halmesmaki E. Gammaglutamyl transferase and mean cellvolume reveal maternal alcohol abuse and fetal alcohol effects. *Am J Obstet Gynecol* 1987;157:344–348.

141. Corse SJ, McHugh MK, Gordon SM. Enhancing provider effectiveness in treating pregnant women with addictions. *J Subst Abuse Treat* 1995;12: 3–12.

142. Schliebner CT. Gender-sensitive therapy: an alternative for women in substance abuse treatment. *J Subst Abuse Treat* 1994;11:511–515.

143. Deren S. Children of substance abusers: a review of the literature. *J Subst Abuse Treat* 1986;3:77–94.

144. Timko C, Kaplowitz MS, Moos RH. Children's health and child-parent relationships as predictors of problem-drinking mothers' and fathers' long-term adaptation. *J Subst Abuse* 2000;11: 103–121.

145. Reckmon LW, Babcock P, O'Bryan T. Meeting the child care needs of the female alcoholic. *Child Welfare* 1984;63:541–546.

146. Davis TS, Hagood LA. In-home support for recovering alcoholic mothers and their families. *J Stud Alcohol* 1979;40:313–317.

147. Kirkpatrick J. *Turnabout: help for a new life.* New York: Doubleday, 1978.

148. Ford BB. *Betty: a glad awakening.* New York: Doubleday, 1987.

149. Robertson N. *Getting better inside AA.* New York: William Morrow, 1988.

150. Meryman R. *Broken promises, mended dreams.* New York: Little Brown, 1984.

151. Allen C. *I'm Black and I'm Sober Center City.* MN: Hazetton Publishing and Educational Services, 1995.

152. Vex SL, Blume SB. The JACS study I: characteristics of a population of chemically dependent Jewish men and women. *J Addict Dis* 2001;20:71–89.

153. Blume SB, Dropkin D, Sokolow L. The Jewish alcoholic: a descriptive study. *Alcohol Health Res World* 1980;4: 21–26.

154. Carter CS. Treatment of the chemically dependent black female: a cultural perspective. *Counselor* 1987;5:16–18.

155. Fernandez-Pal B, Bluestone H, Missouri C, et al. Drinking patterns of inner-city black Americans and Puerto Ricans. *J Stud Alcohol* 1986;47:156–160.

156. Cochran SD, Keenan C, Schober C, et al. Estimates of alcohol use and clinical treatment needs among homosexually active men and women in the U.S. population. *J Consult Clin Psychol* 2000;68:1062–1071.

157. Miller BA. Drugs and crime interrelationships among women in detention. *J Psychoactive Drugs* 1981;13:289–295.

158. Hodgins DC, el-Guebaly N, Addington J. Treatment of substance abusers: single or mixed gender programs? *Addiction* 1997;92:805–812.

159. Annis HM, Leban CB. Alcoholism in women: treatment modalities and outcomes. In: Kalant OJ, ed. *Research advances in alcohol and drug problems.*

New York: Plenum Press, 1980:385–422.

160. Vannicelli M. Treatment considerations. In: *Women and alcohol: health-related issues. Research monograph no. 16*. Publication no. (ADM) 86–1139. Washington DC: Department of Health and Human Services, 1986: 130–153.

161. Rounsaville BJ, Dolinsky ZS, Babor TF, et al. Psychopathology as a predictor of treatment outcome in alcoholics. *Arch Gen Psychiatry* 1987;44: 505–513.

162. Zilberman ML, Tavares H, Blume SB, et al. Towards best practices in the treatment of women with addictive disorders. *Addict Disord Treat* 2002 (*in press*).

163. MacDonald JG. Predictors of treatment outcome for alcoholic women. *Int J Addict* 1987;22:235–248.

164. Havassy BE, Hall SM, Tschann JM. Social support and relapse to tobacco, alcohol, and opiates: preliminary findings. *NIDA Res Monogr* 1987;76:207–213.

165. Wilsnack SC, Wilsnack RW, Klassen AD. *Women's drinking problems. A U.S. national longitudinal survey.* Paper presented at the American Public Health Association annual meeting, 1989.

166. Hill SY. Physiological effects of alcohol in women. In: *Women and alcohol: health-related issues. Research monograph no. 16.* Publication no. (ADM)86–1139. Washington, DC: Department of Health and Human Services, 1986.

167. Lindberg S, Agren G. Mortality among male and female hospitalized alcoholics in Stockholm 1962–1983. *Br J Addict* 1988;83:1193–1200.

168. Smith EM, Cloninger CR, Bradford S. Predictors of mortality in alcoholic women: a prospective follow-up study. *Alcohol Clin Exp Res* 1983;7:237–243.

169. Jacobson M, Hacker G, Atkins R. *The booze merchants.* Washington, DC: CSPI Books, 1983.

170. Marsteller P, Karnchanopee K. The use of women in the advertising of distilled spirits. *J Psychedelic Drugs* 1980;12: 1–12.

171. Shore ER. Outcomes of a primary prevention project for business and professional women. *J Stud Alcohol* 1994;55:657–659.

172. Cahill MH, Volicer BJ, Neuburger E. Female referral to employees assistance programs: the impact of specialized intervention. *Drug Alcohol Depend* 1982;10:223–233.

173. Jeffer EK, Baranick M. Drug abuse and the U.S. Army in Europe: women and substance abuse. *Int J Addict* 1983;18:133–138.

174. Vannicelli M. *Group psychotherapy with adult children of alcoholics.* New York: Guilford Press, 1989.

175. Al-Anon Family Groups. *Alateen: hope for children of alcoholics.* New York: Author, 1973.

176. Amaro H, Beckman LJ, Mays VM. A comparison of black and white women entering alcoholism treatment. *J Stud Alcohol* 1987;48:220–228.

177. Poland ML, Dombrowski MP, Ager JW, et al. Punishing pregnant drug users: enhancing the flight from care. *Drug Alcohol Depend* 1993;31:199–203.

178. Blume SB: Women and alcohol: issues in social policy. In: Wilsnack RW, Wilsnack SC, eds. *Gender and alcohol: individual and social perspectives.* New Brunswick, NJ: Rutgers Center of Alcohol Studies, 1997:462–489.

CHAPTER 65

Drugs and Women

MONICA L. ZILBERMAN AND
SHEILA B. BLUME

Although problems associated with the use of psychoactive drugs by women have attracted the serious attention of both the public and health professionals over the past few decades, these problems cannot be described as new. In late nineteenth century America, the typical opiate addict was a middle-class woman who began her dependence through medical treatment (1). It was only after the use of opiates was regulated in the beginning of the twentieth century that this scenario changed and men outnumbered women in both drug use and dependence, particularly for cocaine and heroin (2). Throughout the twentieth century, women represented a minority of drug users and addicts, and thus they were also a minority in drug-treatment programs and among research subjects. However, there is recent evidence that this gap might be closing. The increased presence of women in the job market and in professions previously limited to men is likely to have changed the profile of risk factors and stresses influencing women's health, including the risk of circulatory diseases and substance-related disorders.

Alcohol has been the most explored substance in the literature focusing on women. The literature on drugs other than alcohol is less abundant, and in some respects, contradictory. Drug-related problems and the treatment needs they generate among women are similar to those related to alcohol in many ways, but research indicates that important differences also exist, emphasizing the need for specific investigation. For instance, drug-dependent women entering treatment are significantly younger, more likely to be self-referred, and less likely to have a partner and to be housewives than their alcohol-dependent counterparts. Additionally, they more often report suicide attempts, and are less likely to present additional Axis I diagnoses (3). This chapter focuses on the available evidence regarding characteristics of drug use by women, stressing epidemiology and the genetic, psychological, and sociocultural factors involved in drug-related problems. An evaluation and diagnosis section provides an overview on how to approach, what to expect, and what to look for when assessing women's substance use. More detailed information is given for cocaine, cannabis, opiates, and tobacco. Only brief comments are offered for other drugs, such as benzodiazepines and amphetamines, that have received less research attention in women. Finally, we offer recommendations for the treatment of addicted women.

EPIDEMIOLOGY OF DRUG USE IN WOMEN

The Epidemiological Catchment Area (ECA) study surveyed the mental health status of a representative sample of individuals age 18 years and older from five different American regions and documented that 25% of women reported any lifetime illicit drug use, compared to a rate of 36% among men. Almost 5% of the women fulfilled diagnostic criteria for lifetime drug abuse or dependence (male:female ratio of 1.6:1) (4). The National Comorbidity Survey (NCS) investigated psychiatric diagnoses of a representative sample of Americans ages 15 to 54 years, and found a lifetime prevalence of drug abuse of 3.5% among women and 5.4% among men, while the lifetime prevalence of drug dependence was 5.9% among women and 9.2% among men (male:female ratios of 1.5:1 and 1.6:1, respectively) (5). It is evident that the gender gap for these prevalence rates is much narrower than were described for alcohol in the same studies: 5:1 in the ECA and 2.5:1 in the NCS.

Data from the 2000 National Household Survey on Drug Abuse that surveyed American civilians age 12 years and older confirmed the overall male:female ratio of 1.5:1 regarding current illicit drug use (5.0% for women and 7.7% for men). Current overall rates of tobacco use show that men still outnumber women, but the difference is small (26.9% vs. 23.1%, respectively, a male:female ratio of 1.2:1). Rates of drug use were even more similar between girls and boys in the group ages 12 to 17 years (9.5% for girls and 9.8% for boys). Also, girls were more likely than boys to report that drugs such as cocaine, crack, lysergic acid diethylamide (LSD), and heroin were easily available to them, which may be associated with an increased risk for drug use. Rates of tobacco use in this age group were already higher for girls than boys (14.1% vs. 12.8%, respectively). Furthermore, a significant decrease from the previous year was detected for boys, but not for girls (6). Data from 1992 regarding cannabis use also show that the gender difference in rates of initiation of use is smaller than the gender difference in prevalence of use (7). Even more striking are data from 1997 regarding lifetime cocaine and crack cocaine use showing that, among youth age 12 to 17 years, rates of use were higher for girls than for boys, although nonsignificantly (3.3% vs. 2.7%, respectively, for cocaine and 1.5% vs. 1.1%, respectively, for crack) (8).

In the year 2000, girls were somewhat more likely to use prescription drugs not prescribed by a doctor, including pain relievers, tranquilizers, stimulants, and sedatives, than were boys (3.3% vs. 2.7%, respectively) (6). Women, as compared to men, are also more likely to be prescribed benzodiazepines, according to the pharmacy records of 7,012 patients initiating benzodiazepine treatment in the United States (9).

These findings suggest that rates of drug use among women relative to men may rise substantially in the future, if appropriate prevention responses are not undertaken.

GENETIC FACTORS

A series of twin studies investigated the contributions of genetic and environmental influences to drug use and drug-use disorders across genders. Overall, environmental factors seem to be more important than genetic factors in drug use and abuse (10). However, genetic influences for drug use and abuse/dependence are greater for males than females (heritability of 33% for men and 11% for women), whereas environmental factors are higher for females than for males (11,12). In adolescents there is some indication that the genetic component may have a greater impact in tobacco use than in illicit drug use (13). This finding may have special significance for adolescent girls, considering that more girls than boys are now initiating tobacco use. In women, initiation of cannabis and cocaine use is shaped more by environmental factors, but genetic factors have the greater impact in the progression to abuse or dependence (14,15).

PSYCHOLOGICAL FACTORS

Epidemiologic data document that, excluding comorbid alcohol-use disorders, rates of psychiatric comorbidity are higher among women than men with drug-use disorders. Rates of comorbid mood and anxiety disorders are higher among women, while rates of comorbid alcohol use disorders and antisocial personality disorder are higher among men (4). Male addicts are also more likely to be pathologic gamblers and to report syndrome of attention deficit hyperactivity disorder (16–18). In a cross-national study comparing the United States, Canada, Germany, Mexico, and the Netherlands, Merikangas, et al. (19) also found higher rates of comorbidity for women than for men. Tobacco use is strongly associated with clinically relevant depressive symptomatology in women (20), making it harder for women than for men to quit smoking (21).

Certain groups of women with drug dependence may be at particular risk for psychiatric comorbidity. For instance, higher rates have been described in whites than in African Americans (17).

In comparison to alcohol-dependent women, drug-dependent women (in particular those with a cocaine dependency) seem to present fewer comorbid Axis I diagnoses (primarily depression) (3), but more Axis II diagnoses (22). Rates of suicide attempts are also significantly higher in drug-dependent women than in either alcohol-dependent women or drug-dependent men (23).

A history of traumatic life events is a risk factor for the development of drug-use disorders. The lifetime prevalence of these disorders is more than four times higher in women with a history of sexual assault (24). Kendler et al. (25) reported a "dose–response" relationship between the severity of self-reported childhood sexual abuse and risk for developing drug dependence in women. Women who reported attempted intercourse, the highest-risk group, had a risk of drug dependence 5.7 times higher than those who had no history of childhood abuse.

The high rates of psychiatric comorbidity and the relationship to childhood sexual abuse suggest that depression, low self-esteem, posttraumatic stress disorder, and sexual dysfunctions of various kinds may be predisposing factors to for some women. Clinicians report that these conditions in the lives of addicted women are important areas on which to focus during treatment. Prevention programs aimed at children and adolescents should make efforts to target girls with these characteristics, especially those from families in which alcoholism or other drug-use disorders are present.

SOCIOCULTURAL FACTORS

Cultural influences have always shaped the drug use and abuse patterns of women (26). The social factors that once protected women from initiating drug use are weaker now. However, the intense social stigma applied to female addicts still prevents many women from accessing appropriate treatment. Depending on the drug, the male:female ratio of addiction treatment admissions varies from 1.5:1 for cocaine to 3.3:1 for cannabis (27).

The sociocultural factors involved in drug use initiation and the subsequent development of drug use disorders also vary across genders. Particularly, drug use in women is associated with victimization (28). Trauma and posttraumatic stress disorder are more likely to precede the development of drug-use disorders in women than in men. Data from the National Women's Study demonstrate the vicious, circular relationship between victimization and drug-use disorder: Prior assault is a risk factor for the development of a drug-use disorder, which, in turn, is a risk factor for additional victimization (29). Furthermore, social pressure for the perfect body is disproportionately focused on women as compared to men. Drug use as a weight-control measure, especially for nicotine, cocaine, and other stimulants, even in the absence of diagnosable eating disorders, is another important sociocultural factor in women's substance use (30,31).

In addition, that physicians prescribe potentially addictive medications, such as benzodiazepines, more often to women than to men increases women's risk. The reasons for these prescriptions include depression, anxiety, sleep difficulties, and pain, in spite of the lack of evidence supporting the efficacy of benzodiazepines in many of these conditions (9).

Finally, women's drug use is highly influenced by drug-using sexual partners, with most women reporting having been first introduced to drug use and drug injection by a male partner (32). This factor should also be considered in prevention programming.

EVALUATION AND DIAGNOSIS

Because of stigma and the resulting shame that contaminates both addicted women and health professionals, treatment entry and diagnosis are often delayed. The barriers include fear of loss of children, single-parent responsibilities, and lack of support/opposition from an active drug-using partner, among others. Recent changes in federal policy mandate that pregnant women be given priority for treatment. However, the policies of some states that result in the reporting and prosecution of such women for "prenatal child abuse," and in the removal of infants from maternal custody, have eroded confidence in the treatment system for many female addicts.

Women who are not pregnant also face difficulties. Health professionals often do not feel comfortable in asking women about their substance use because they believe the women might feel offended. Women with drug-related problems are less likely to seek specialized help than are men, more often consulting the general practitioner (33). For these reasons, screening should be routinely performed as part of any medical consultation, explaining that the questions aim to assess overall well-being and that the responses are kept confidential. Questions about weight control and body image concerns, as well as sleeping difficulties, may help introduce the issue of substance use. The use of a screening questionnaire (such as the Drug Abuse Screening Test) (34) and laboratory testing of urine or blood might be helpful.

Problematic areas are also different for women, who are less likely to report legal problems and are less often court-ordered to treatment than men, but probably more often than alcohol-dependent women. Drug-dependent women often report domestic violence and sexual abuse, as well as suicide attempts and overdoses. These issues need to be addressed in a safe environment and time is often required to gain sufficient trust to discuss them. Followup appointments may provide more information than single-session assessments, and are particularly helpful in breaking down defenses and building a trust-based relationship.

Evaluating and referring to treatment a drug-using partner, as well as providing orientation to a non–drug-using partner, is crucial to the treatment outcome of drug-dependent women. The involvement of other family members in the recovery process should also be considered, as well as the assessment of children's well-being coupled with referrals to specialized care when appropriate. Medical assessment is recommended because of the high prevalence of drug-related illnesses. Psychiatric evaluation, with attention to both Axis I and Axis II diagnoses, is also an integral part of the assessment of drug-dependent women because of high comorbidity (35).

COCAINE

Pharmacologic Effects

Women seem to respond differently to cocaine than men, but the direction of the differences and their explanation is not clear. Kosten et al. (36) described greater subjective response in women than in men after intranasal cocaine administration, whereas Lukas et al. (37) observed higher and faster subjective response accompanied by higher plasma levels in men than in women. Furthermore, these researchers documented menstrual phase differences in cocaine plasma levels (higher in the follicular than in the luteal phase), although not in the subjective response to cocaine in the female sample. The authors hypothesized that the nasal mucosa of women in the luteal phase is more viscous, leading to decreased cocaine absorption and decreased plasma levels.

In female rats the response to cocaine is enhanced by estrogen, and they tend to exhibit greater behavioral responses to cocaine or amphetamine than males. Also, females display greater behavioral sensitization, which is also increased by estrogen. Gender differences in sensitization suggest sexual dimorphisms in neural systems undergoing sensitization (38). Drug craving, for instance, has been related to such sensitized systems (39). It is possible that gender differences in sensitized neural systems related to drug craving are the basis for the higher intensity of cocaine craving observed in cocaine-dependent women in comparison to men in some studies (40,41), although not in all (42).

Course of Illness

Data regarding gender differences in the progression to cocaine dependence are also confusing. Some studies suggest that women progress from first use to treatment faster than men (43–46), whereas other studies do not report such a "telescoped" progression (47–50). Similarly, gender differences in the age of onset of cocaine use are also described, with some studies suggesting that women start using cocaine earlier than men (43,46), others supporting the opposite (44,49), and another describing no gender difference (51). Clearly further research in this area is much needed.

A study with aggregate data from the National Household Survey on Drug Abuse (1991–1993) verified that adolescent women report a higher rate of cocaine dependence than men, using cocaine more frequently, and more symptoms with low doses of cocaine use (52). The age of women entering treatment for crack cocaine abuse has increased significantly over time (women 35 years and older comprised only 19% of total admissions in 1992, but represented 43% in 1998). The same is true of women with long-term use of crack cocaine (in 1992, only 20% of women entering treatment reported crack cocaine use for more than 10 years; this figure rose to 42% in 1998). The average woman entering treatment for crack cocaine in 1998 was 34 years of age, and had used the drug for 10 years (53).

Health Consequences

Cocaine use represents a risk factor for human immunodeficiency virus (HIV) infection and other sexually trans-

mitted diseases (54). Also, it is associated with a variety of health problems, including cardiovascular and central nervous system diseases. Unfortunately, studies that take gender into account are rare. Gender differences have been described in the electroencephalograms of individuals abstinent from cocaine use, with more abnormalities reported among men than among women (55). Sustained alterations in the frontal lobe neurochemistry of individuals dependent on crack cocaine have been reported, with distinct neurotoxic effects according to gender (56). Although the clinical significance of these alterations is not completely understood, the findings illustrate the importance of analyzing research results by gender.

Kaufman et al. (57), using magnetic resonance imaging, demonstrated that in women, the impact of cocaine on the cerebral blood flow depends on the menstrual cycle phase, with vasoconstriction occurring in the luteal phase, but not in the follicular phase. The researchers attribute the difference to the high estrogen levels in the follicular phase, protecting blood vessels from the vasoconstrictive effects of cocaine.

Effects on Sexual Functioning and Reproduction

Cocaine use seems to be associated with a variety of alterations in the menstrual cycle, with amenorrhea and luteal phase dysfunction, as well as galactorrhea and infertility. Hyperprolactinemia induced by cocaine effects on dopaminergic systems is associated with these abnormalities (58). Also, cocaine use is associated with increased levels of luteinizing hormone in cocaine-abusing women in a dose–response relationship. Under experimental conditions, these levels take significantly longer to normalize in men than in women (59). Although it is difficult to attribute these abnormalities to cocaine use itself because many women report concomitant use of other substances, animal studies under controlled conditions seem to corroborate these findings (60). Animal studies also show that important gender differences exist in the hypothalamic–pituitary–adrenal axis response to cocaine, female rats exhibiting exaggerated responses to cocaine associated with greater pituitary responsivity to corticotropin-releasing factor than male rats (61).

Much has been published about the effects of cocaine use on pregnancy and offspring. Cocaine use in the perinatal period, whether or not associated with opiate use, is related to higher rates of medical complications such as syphilis, gonorrhea, and hepatitis (62). Cocaine use in this period is also associated with increased rates of abruptio placentae, meconium staining, premature rupture of membranes, and low birth weight, as well as genitourinary and abdominal wall abnormalities. These effects are independent of other confounding substance use (63).

Research and the public reaction to cocaine use during pregnancy are problematic. Earlier reports referred to a so-called crack baby syndrome. Such descriptions, not supported by scientific evidence, led to punishment and stigma for the mothers and children involved (64). A systematic review of 36 prospective studies conducted by Frank et al. (65) concludes that there is no evidence that cocaine alone (independent of other risk factors such as malnutrition and other drug use, including alcohol and tobacco) affects physical and developmental growth in the first 6 years, and that most early motor developmental effects are transient. The authors recognize, however, that studies of longer-term followup (into school age and adolescence, where higher cognitive and social demands are expected) could disclose effects not previously identified. On the other hand, Covington et al. (66), investigating growth of children prenatally exposed to cocaine, reported that these children were four times more likely to present height deficits by age 7 years. Maternal age seems to moderate this effect, with those children born to mothers older than age 30 years being at risk. A recent prospective study found that perinatal cocaine exposure, after controlling for a number of confounders, is associated with developmental impairments at 24 months of age (67). Heavier maternal cocaine use and high numbers of premature infants (per se a cause of developmental abnormalities) included in the last study may explain the disparity of the results (68). Further research aiming to clarify dose–response relationships between cocaine exposure and effects on offspring is clearly needed and clinicians should not ignore the additive effects that cocaine use, other substance use (including tobacco), and malnutrition, among others, exert on pregnancy outcomes.

Treatment Response

Few studies have analyzed the treatment response of individuals with cocaine use disorders. A recent study comparing coping skills training to meditation–relaxation techniques did not find any gender differences in treatment response at any of the followup periods up to 12 months (69). Also, in the National Institute on Drug Abuse Collaborative Cocaine Treatment Study, no gender differences in the outcome of the four psychosocial treatments evaluated were found (70). Other studies, however, described better outcomes for women than for men, even though the women had more severe cocaine-related problems at baseline (47,48).

CANNABIS

Pharmacologic Effects

Preliminary research with rats suggests that gender differences in the effects of tetrahydrocannabinol (primary responsible for cannabis pharmacologic effects) in the hypothalamus may exist, potentially as a result of a differential influence of the sex hormones. Specifically, there are sex-related effects of tetrahydrocannabinol on corticotropin-releasing hormone and proopiome-

lanocortin gene expression in the hypothalamus (71). Whether or not these differences also exist in humans is as yet unknown. Appetite stimulation in adult light cannabis users does not seem to vary as a function of gender (72).

Course of Illness

Early conduct problems, particularly of an aggressive or covert nature, seem to be more strongly associated with initiation of cannabis use among adolescent women than among men (73). Once cannabis use starts, however, no gender differences in patterns of use were described in a large Australian survey of adolescents. Cannabis use, regardless of gender, is strongly associated with depression, conduct problems, and use of alcohol and other drugs (74).

The progression to cannabis dependence is also accelerated in women, despite similar age of initiation of regular use (50). Women in treatment for substance-related disorders present a lower current rate of cannabis use disorders as compared to men (26), although evidence for a gender convergence in cannabis use has begun to accumulate (75). Additionally, a significant relationship has been described between cannabis use and premenstrual dysphoria, but not with the menstrual cycle phase itself (76).

Health Consequences

In a large study, significantly more female cannabis users than males reported panic attacks related to their cannabis use, but gender did not impact other physical or mental problems associated with cannabis use (77). A series of studies have sought persistent impairments in cognitive functioning in relation to cannabis use. Although a prior study by Pope et al. (78) did suggest that women, but not men, with a history of heavy cannabis use present a specific effect on visuospatial memory, a recent study by the same group found no evidence of gender differences, although the authors recognize that the small number of women included might have weakened their ability to demonstrate a potential difference (79).

Effects on Sexual Functioning and Reproduction

Acute cannabis use during the luteal phase of the menstrual cycle is associated with a significant decrease in plasma levels of prolactin and luteinizing hormone, that may, in turn, be associated with adverse effects on women's reproductive function (80,81). No effects on testosterone and luteinizing hormone levels were found in men (82). Chronic cannabis use, however, does not seem to be associated with altered hormone levels in either women or men (83), suggesting that cannabis effects on women's hormones may not be persistent.

Tetrahydrocannabinol is highly lipophilic and may remain in fat tissue for weeks. Because it is slowly released, it may exert potentially dangerous effects on pregnancy and the resulting offspring. Weekly cannabis use during pregnancy is associated with abruptio placentae (84) and prematurity (85). When taking into account social background and other substance use, cannabis use during pregnancy was not significantly related to increased risk of perinatal morbidity and mortality in a large study involving more than 12,000 pregnant women, but it was clearly associated with decreased birth weight (86).

Regular use of cannabis during pregnancy is significantly associated with long-term cognitive impairments in the offspring, particularly in executive functions involving attentional behavior and visual analysis/hypothesis testing (87). A prospective study documented that effects of prenatal cannabis exposure on children at 10 years of age, controlled for potential confounders, included hyperactivity, impulsivity, and attention deficits leading to delinquent behavior (88).

Treatment Response

The few studies examining treatment outcome for cannabis use disorder do not report analysis by gender (64). Such analyses should be conducted, as they might uncover potential differences with significance for the development of better treatment.

Factors associated with cessation of cannabis use among adolescents differ by gender. Although reasons for quitting cannabis use among boys vary, among girls the most important reason is getting pregnant and assuming parenting responsibilities (89).

OPIATES
Pharmacologic Effects

Preclinical studies suggest gender differences in the effects of opiates on the cardiovascular system (90). In humans, women report higher rates of nausea (91) and analgesia (92) associated with acute opiate use than do men. It is suggested that the interaction between opiate receptors and sexual hormone receptors may be implicated in gender differences observed in the magnitude and potency of opiate response (93). Women clear methadone from the bloodstream more slowly than men, and thus have a longer plasma half-life for the drug (94).

Course of Illness

Opiate-dependent women are more likely to have a substance-using partner and to be initiated into drug injection by a partner than are their male counterparts, although women are more likely to inhale heroin, whereas men are more likely to inject it (32,95). A faster progression of opiate dependence has been described among heroin-dependent females in comparison to males (96).

Health Consequences

Opiate use is associated with higher morbidity (97) and mortality (98) rates among women as compared to men. Female opiate users may combine two important risk factors for acquiring HIV, hepatitis B and C, and other sexually transmitted diseases: sex with a injecting partner and needle sharing (99).

Effects on Sexual Functioning and Reproduction

Opiate use during pregnancy is associated with a number of complications, with an increased risk of hepatitis and HIV infection that is associated with its injection (62), and increased relative mortality, probably as a consequence of a combination of opiate effect and chaotic lifestyle (100).

The effects of perinatal opiate use on the neonate include a withdrawal syndrome characterized by weight loss and feeding difficulties, abnormalities of the sleep–wake cycle, and seizures. Available evidence indicates that the treatment of choice for this condition is the administration of opiates, particularly for children born to women who used only opiates during pregnancy. This approach seems to be more effective than the use of sedatives, clonidine, or benzodiazepines, but the issue is far from resolved (101).

Animal studies suggest that prenatal opiate exposure induces long-term sex-specific alterations in adult brain and behavior, including alterations in the norepinephrine and opioid systems in different brain regions (102). Studies with humans show that 1-year-old children prenatally exposed to opiates are at higher risk for mild psychomotor developmental impairment (103). An exploratory study comparing male and female offspring of women maintained on methadone during pregnancy to that of controls, suggested that boys showed more stereotypically feminine behavior than controls, while no differences in sex role behavior occurred with girls (104).

Despite the paucity of conclusive research, the recommended treatment for pregnant women with opiate dependence is methadone stabilization at the lowest possible dose (105), cautioning that methadone-maintained women may need adjustment of dosage when pregnant because of increased body mass. After delivery, the dose should be returned to previously established levels (106). Methadone maintenance along with comprehensive care to prevent the continued use of illicit drugs is associated with improved pregnancy outcomes (107).

Few pregnant opiate addicts to date have been treated with buprenorphine, which is associated with low levels of neonatal withdrawal, possibly as a result of its low transplacental transfer (108).

Treatment Response

In a study of methadone treatment, women on admission reported more dysfunctional families of origin and greater prior and current psychological and medical problems, as well as HIV risk behaviors, but higher motivation, fewer legal problems, and less alcohol use than men. Both genders improved with treatment, as evidenced by reduced substance use, criminal involvement, and other health-related risky behaviors, but women needed more interventions for psychological and crisis issues, employment issues, and medical referrals. They were also more likely to seek additional treatment following discharge (109,110). Another study by the same group showed that HIV risk reductions related to methadone treatment are significantly smaller for women as compared to men with opiate dependence (111), highlighting the need for specialized interventions targeting women with opiate use disorders.

TOBACCO

Pharmacologic Effects

Even though they smoke similar numbers of cigarettes daily, female heavy smokers exhibit lower nicotine plasma levels, but greater exposure to smoke than male heavy smokers, reflecting more and larger puffs to achieve the same nicotine intake. These differences may be implicated in observed gender differences in smoking-related medical consequences (112).

Course of Illness

Epidemiologic data suggest that women are particularly at risk for becoming dependent on nicotine as compared to men, having higher rates of dependence, with more symptoms, at the same quantity of nicotine smoked (113). While among adolescents more girls than boys are now initiating tobacco use, girls are also less likely to quit (114). Gender differences in patterns of tobacco use in adolescents vary greatly among distinct cultural groups (115), suggesting that continued research is needed to monitor trends, and to support the development of timely preventive strategies.

Predictors of smoking among adolescent girls include parental smoking, positive perception of smoking, and smoking by a best friend, whereas no predictors were established among boys (116).

Studies of the relationship between tobacco use and menstrual cycle suggest that, although on the average women report their craving for cigarettes as higher in the late luteal phase, a similar increase in smoking is observed in this phase in some, but not all studies (117).

Health Consequences

Gender impacts on a number of smoking-related health issues with greater effects for female smokers in comparison to male smokers, including immune responses (118), cardiovascular diseases (119), and different types of cancer, such as lung (120) and bladder (121). It is suggested that the gender difference in cancer risks cannot be attributed to differences in baseline exposure, smoking history, or body size alone. Rather, a higher susceptibility to tobacco carcinogens in women is hypothesized. The Centers for Disease Control and Prevention recently reported that smoking-related lung cancer is now the first cause of cancer-related death among American women, ahead of breast cancer. From 1990 to 1998, deaths associated with lung cancer increased among women and decreased among men (122).

The evidence surrounding the impact of tobacco on gynecologic cancer risks is confusing. For instance, although some studies suggest a relationship between smoking and breast cancer, the question remains unresolved, possibly related to low carcinogen dosage (123). The same holds true for ovarian cancer, where the association is reduced after adjustment for coffee intake (124), and for cervical cancer, where most of the association is arguably explained by other confounding factors (125).

Effects on Sexual Functioning and Reproduction

Associations between smoking and a number of menstrual abnormalities, fertility problems, and early menopause in women have been reported, which are probably caused by nicotine effects inhibiting luteinizing hormone and prolactin release. Oxytocin stimulation has also been described and may be the basis for tobacco's negative effects on pregnancy, such as premature delivery. Other problems include fetal growth retardation, obstetric complications, and neonatal mortality. Risks for sudden infant death syndrome, low birth weight and height, and hypertension are increased (126). Additionally tobacco has addictive effects on pregnancy in combination with other drugs.

Long-term physical and behavioral consequences of prenatal exposure to maternal smoking have also been reported, such as impaired lung function (127), substance abuse (128), criminality (129), and antisocial behavior (130). Importantly, these associations remain significant even after controlling for potentially confounding variables.

Treatment Response

Female smokers have higher relapse rates following nicotine replacement therapy than do men (131). Similarly, female gender was associated with worse outcome in one study of pharmacotherapy with bupropion (21), but not in another (132). High levels of self-perceived stress predict difficulty in quitting smoking among women, but are not related to abstinence in men (133).

For women attempting to quit smoking, the related weight gain is a concern and strategies to deal with this issue are likely to increase the efficacy of smoking-cessation treatments (134).

Although some evidence shows that women attempting to quit smoking experience higher cravings in the luteal phase, the patch-related reduction in cigarette craving seems to be greater in this phase too, alleviating both craving and premenstrual symptomatology that frequently overlap (135).

OTHER DRUGS

Comparatively little work has been done on drugs such as benzodiazepines, sedatives, and amphetamines in relationship to women, despite high rates of nonmedical use of these medications (either prescribed or not). Some facts deserve special attention. For instance, the effects of these drugs, particularly the new "designer" drugs—often referred as party drugs and club drugs—in women, as well as their effects on pregnancy and the neonate, have not been sufficiently studied (136,137). Gender differences in the effects of ecstasy have been reported. Methylenedioxymethamphetamine, present in ectasy, produces more intense psychoactive effects in women than in men. Also, higher doses are associated with perceptual alterations more strongly in women, indicating an increased susceptibility of women to ecstasy's serotonin-releasing effects (138).

Flunitrazepam, a therapeutically approved benzodiazepine outside North America, causes sedation and anterograde amnesia, and may be surreptitiously given to women, most often in association with alcohol, to facilitate sexual assault (139). Despite media coverage, little research has been done in the area.

Readers are referred to the appropriate chapters for more complete information on amphetamines and benzodiazepines.

TREATMENT OF DRUG-USE DISORDERS IN WOMEN

While specific research is still for the most part lacking, some of the principles that apply to the treatment of women with alcohol use disorders (covered in Chapter 64) are also considered valid for the treatment of women with other drug-use disorders.

1. Women entering treatment for drug-use disorders report extremely elevated rates of suicide attempts and suicidal ideation. This may be related to concurrent depressive symptomatology and/or impulsive traits of personality. Detailed psychiatric assessment is essential to determine suicidal risk and depression that may require specific treatment. Appropriate pharmacotherapy should consider the potential risk for impulsive suicidal overdosing. Hence one should prescribe small quantities, avoid automatic refills, and encourage regu-

lar followup and phone contact with the patient. Close monitoring is needed because poor family and social support is common. When prescribing, potential drug interactions also need to be considered. For instance, fluoxetine may increase plasma levels of some benzodiazepines and carbamazepine, hence dosage adjustment may be required.

2. Personality disorders may be more frequent than Axis I disorders among women with substance-use disorders. This fact should not imply poorer prognosis by itself, reinforcing therapeutic nihilism. Better personality adjustment may be achieved when the clinician is able to establish an effective working relationship with the patient. There is some evidence suggesting the helpfulness of specific strategies in the treatment of comorbid substance use and borderline personality disorder in women. One such example is dialectical behavior therapy that combines problem-solving skills with acceptance-based strategies (140).

3. Pregnant women suffer a double stigma. They face a stigma attached to being a woman with an addictive disorder, to which is added severe disapproval for exposing their future babies to drugs. In fact many pregnant women stop using drugs during this period. Among those who do not quit, the quantity and frequency of drug use are often considerably reduced, demonstrating that these women are, indeed, concerned about their offspring. A nonjudgmental approach is essential in attracting more pregnant women to treatment. Preliminary evidence suggests good results for therapeutic interventions for this population (141).

4. Screening for HIV, hepatitis B and C, syphilis, and other sexually transmitted diseases is an essential part of the evaluation of women with drug-use disorders entering treatment, particularly for those who inject drugs intravenously.

5. Women entering treatment worry about potential weight gain. Those with comorbid eating disorders may decompensate. The opportunity to discuss healthy nutritional choices and exercise should not be missed. Counseling focussing on body image issues may be needed.

6. All-women treatment groups may be extremely helpful in addressing difficult topics, such as sexual abuse and victimization. Most such groups mix women with alcohol and other drug-use disorders. It is important to be aware of the heterogeneity of the problems that arise in group discussions. The difficulties of a depressed woman with secondary alcoholism should receive the same attention as the difficulties experienced by a pregnant woman court-ordered to treatment for crack cocaine dependence. Because drug-dependent women are more likely to be single or living alone with their children than are alcohol-dependent women, it is often more difficult for them to enter treatment because of a lack of child care. Facilities that can accommodate

both mother and children are particularly attractive to this group. Also, employed drug-dependent women in recovery may need more flexible group hours, with treatment options in the evening or on weekends, to accommodate their job schedules and their domestic responsibilities.

In closing, high proportions of women are at risk of drug-related problems, including, but not limited to, those reviewed in this chapter. Prevention and treatment programming needs to be reviewed and further developed for the welfare of future generations of women and their families.

REFERENCES

1. Kandall SR. *Substance and shadow: women and addiction in the United States.* Boston, MA: Harvard University Press, 1996.
2. Jonnes J. The rise of the modern addict. *Am J Public Health* 1995;85:1157–1162.
3. Zilberman ML, Hochgraf PB, Brasiliano S, et al. Drug dependent women: demographic and clinical characteristics in a Brazilian sample. *Subst Use Misuse* 2001;36:1111–1127.
4. Anthony JC, Helzer JE. Syndromes of drug abuse and dependence. In: Robins LN, Regier DA, eds. *Psychiatric disorders in America.* New York: The Free Press, 1991.
5. Kessler RC, McGonagle KA, Zhao S, et al. Lifetime and 12-month prevalence of *DSM-III-R* psychiatric disorders in the United States: results from the national comorbidity survey. *Arch Gen Psychiatry* 1994;51:8–19.
6. Substance Abuse and Mental Health Services Administration. *Summary of findings from the 2000 National Household Survey on Drug Abuse.* NHSDA Series H-13, DHHS Publication No. (SMA) 01-3549. Rockville, MD: Office of Applied Studies, 2001.
7. Substance Abuse and Mental Health Services Administration. *Trends in the incidence of drug use in the United States, 1919–1992.* DHHS Publication No. (SMA) 96-3076. Rockville, MD: Office of Applied Studies, 1996.
8. Substance Abuse and Mental Health Services Administration. *National Household Survey on Drug Abuse: main findings 1997.* NHSDA Series H-8, DHHS, Rockville, MD: Office of Applied Studies, 1999.
9. Simon GE, VonKorff M, Barlow W, et al. Predictors of chronic benzodiazepine use in a health maintenance organization sample. *J Clin Epidemiol* 1996;49:1067–1073.
10. Jang KL, Livesley WJ, Vernon PA. Gender-specific etiological differences in alcohol and drug problems: a behavioural genetic analysis. *Addiction* 1997;92:1265–1276.
11. Van den Bree MB, Johnson EO, Neale MC, et al. Genetic and environmental influences on drug use and abuse/dependence in male and female twins. *Drug Alcohol Depend* 1998;52:231–241.
12. Han C, McGue MK, Iacono WG. Lifetime tobacco, alcohol and other substance use in adolescent Minnesota twins: univariate and multivariate behavioral genetic analyses. *Addiction* 1999;94:981–993.
13. McGue M, Elkins I, Iacono WG. Genetic and environmental influences on adolescent substance use and abuse. *Am J Med Genet* 2000;96:671–677.
14. Kendler KS, Prescott CA. Cannabis use, abuse, and dependence in a population-based sample of female twins. *Am J Psychiatry* 1998;155:1016–1022.
15. Kendler KS, Prescott CA. Cocaine use, abuse and dependence in a population-based sample of female twins. *Br J Psychiatry* 1998;173:345–350.
16. Brooner RK, King VL, Kidorf M, et al. Psychiatric and substance use comorbidity among treatment-seeking opioid abusers. *Arch Gen Psychiatry* 1997;54:71–80.
17. Compton WM 3rd, Cottler LB, Ben Abdallah A, et al. Substance dependence and other psychiatric disorders among drug dependent subjects: race and gender correlates. *Am J Addict* 2000;9:113–125.
18. Schubiner H, Tzelepis A, Milberger S, et al. Prevalence of attention-deficit/hyperactivity disorder and conduct disorder among substance abusers. *J Clin Psychiatry* 2000;61:244–251.
19. Merikangas KR, Mehta RL, Molnar BE, et al. Comorbidity of substance use disorders with mood and anxiety disorders: results of the International Consortium in Psychiatric Epidemiology. *Addict Behav* 1998;23:893–907.
20. Brown C, Madden PA, Palenchar DR, et al. The association between depressive symptoms and cigarette smoking in an urban primary care sample. *Int J Psychiatry Med* 2000;30:15–26.
21. Dale LC, Glover ED, Sachs DP, et al. Bupropion for smoking cessation: predictors of successful outcome. *Chest* 2001;119:1357–1364.
22. Pettinati HM, Cabezas RA, Jensen J, et al. Incidence of personality disorders in cocaine vs. alcohol-dependent females. *NIDA Res Monogr* 1991;105:369–370.
23. Zilberman ML, Tavares H, Andrade AG. Discriminating drug-dependent women from alcoholic women and drug-dependent men. *Addict Behav* 2003;28(7):1343–1349.
24. Winfield I, George LK, Swartz M, et al. Sexual assault and psychiatric disorders among a community sample of women. *Am J Psychiatry* 1990;147:335–341.
25. Kendler KS, Bulik CM, Silberg J, et al. Childhood sexual abuse and adult psychiatric and substance use disorders in women: an epidemiological and cotwin control analysis. *Arch Gen Psychiatry* 2000;57:953–959.
26. Westermeyer J, Boedicker AE. Course, severity, and treatment of substance abuse among women versus men. *Am J Drug Alcohol Abuse* 2000;26:523–535.
27. Substance Abuse and Mental Health Services Administration. *Women in substance abuse treatment.* DASIS Report, DHHS publication (SMA). Rockville, MD: Office of Applied Studies, 2001.
28. Brady KT, Dansky BS. Effects of victimization and posttraumatic stress disorder on substance use disorders in women. In: Lewis-Hall F, Williams TS, Panetta JA, et al., eds. *Psychiatric illness in women: emerging treatments and research.* Washington, DC: American Psychiatric Publishing, 2002:449–466.
29. Kilpatrick DG, Acierno R, Resnick HS, et al. A 2-year longitudinal analysis of the relationships between violent assault and substance use in women. *J Consult Clin Psychol* 1997;65:834–847.
30. Cochrane C, Malcolm R, Brewerton T. The role of weight control as a motivation for cocaine abuse. *Addict Behav* 1998;23:201–207.
31. Von MC, Brecht ML, Anglin MD. Use ecology and drug use motivations of methamphetamine users admitted to substance abuse treatment facilities in Los Angeles: an emerging profile. *J Addict Dis* 2002;21:45–60.
32. Powis B, Griffiths P, Gossop M, et al. The differences between male and female drug users: community samples

of heroin and cocaine users compared. *Subst Use Misuse* 1996;31:529–543.

33. Sterk CE, Dolan K, Hatch S. Epidemiological indicators and ethnographic realities of female cocaine use. *Subst Use Misuse* 1999;34:2057–2072.

34. Gavin DR, Ross HE, Skinner HA. Diagnostic validity of the drug abuse screening test in the assessment of *DSM-III* drug disorders. *Br J Addict* 1989;84:301–307.

35. Addiction Research Foundation. *The hidden majority: a guidebook on alcohol and other drug issues for counsellors who work with women.* Toronto, ON: Canadian Cataloguing in Publication Data, 1996.

36. Kosten TR, Kosten TA, McDougle CJ, et al. Gender differences in response to intranasal cocaine administration to humans. *Biol Psychiatry* 1996;39: 147–148.

37. Lukas SE, Sholar M, Lundahl LH, et al. Sex differences in plasma cocaine levels and subjective effects after acute cocaine administration in human volunteers. *Psychopharmacology (Berl)* 1996;125:346–354.

38. Becker JB, Molenda H, Hummer DL. Gender differences in the behavioral responses to cocaine and amphetamine. Implications for mechanisms mediating gender differences in drug abuse. *Ann N Y Acad Sci* 2001;937:172–187.

39. Robinson TE, Berridge KC. Incentive-sensitization and addiction. *Addiction* 2001;96:103–114.

40. Elman I, Karlsgodt KH, Gastfriend DR. Gender differences in cocaine craving among non-treatment-seeking individuals with cocaine dependence. *Am J Drug Alcohol Abuse* 2001;27:193–202.

41. Robbins SJ, Ehrman RN, Childress AR, O'Brien CP. Comparing levels of cocaine cue reactivity in male and female outpatients. *Drug Alcohol Depend* 1999;53:223–230.

42. Evans SM, Haney M, Fischman MW, et al. Limited sex differences in response to "binge" smoked cocaine use in humans. *Neuropsychopharmacology* 1999;21:445–454.

43. Griffin ML, Weiss RD, Mirin SM. A comparison of male and female cocaine abusers. *Arch Gen Psychiatry* 1989;46:122–126.

44. White KA, Brady KT, Sonne S. Gender differences in patterns of cocaine use. *Am J Addict* 1996;5:259–261.

45. McCance-Katz EF, Carroll KM, Rounsaville BJ. Gender differences in treatment-seeking cocaine abusers—implications for treatment and prognosis. *Am J Addict* 1999;8:300–311.

46. Haas AL, Peters RH. Development of substance abuse problems among drug-involved offenders. Evidence for the telescoping effect. *J Subst Abuse* 2000;12:241–253.

47. Kosten TA, Gawin FH, Kosten TR, et al. Gender differences in cocaine use and treatment response. *J Subst Abuse Treat* 1993;10:63–66.

48. Weiss R, Martinez-Raga J, Griffin M, et al. Gender differences in cocaine dependent patients: a 6 month follow-up study. *Drug Alcohol Depend* 1997;44:35–40.

49. Zilberman ML, Tavares H. *Alcoholism and drug abuse in women.* Paper presented at the American Psychiatric Association 2001 Annual Meeting, in Special Topics in Women's Mental Health, New Orleans, May 5–10, 2001.

50. Hernandez-Avila CA, Poling J, Rounsaville BJ, et al. *Progression of drug and alcohol dependence among women entering substance abuse treatment: evidence for telescoping.* Paper presented at the 2002 Annual Meeting of the College on Problems of Drug Dependence, in Quebec City, June 8–13, 2002.

51. Dudish S, Hatsukami D. Gender differences in crack users who are research volunteers. *Drug Alcohol Depend* 1996;42:55–63.

52. Chen K, Kandel D. Relationship between extent of cocaine use and dependence among adolescents and adults in the United States. *Drug Alcohol Depend* 2002;68:65.

53. Substance Abuse and Mental Health Services Administration. *Women in treatment for smoked cocaine.* DASIS Report, DHHS Publication (SMA). Rockville, MD: Office of Applied Studies, 2001.

54. Guinan ME. Women and crack addiction. *J Am Med Womens Assoc* 1989;44:129.

55. King DE, Herning RI, Gorelick DA, et al. Gender differences in the EEG of abstinent cocaine abusers. *Neuropsychobiology* 2000;42:93–98.

56. Chang L, Ernst T, Strickland T, et al. Gender effects on persistent cerebral metabolite changes in the frontal lobes of abstinent cocaine users. *Am J Psychiatry* 1999;156:716–722.

57. Kaufman MJ, Levin JM, Maas LC, et al. Cocaine-induced cerebral vasoconstriction differs as a function of sex and menstrual cycle phase. *Biol Psychiatry* 2001;49:774–781.

58. Mendelson JH, Teoh SK, Lange U, et al. Anterior pituitary, adrenal, and gonadal hormones during cocaine withdrawal. *Am J Psychiatry* 1988;145:1094–1098.

59. Mendelson JH, Sholar MB, Siegel AJ, et al. Effects of cocaine on luteinizing hormone in women during the follicular and luteal phases of the menstrual cycle and in men. *J Pharmacol Exp Ther* 2001;296:972–979.

60. Mello NK, Mendelson JH, Kelly M, et al. The effects of chronic cocaine self-administration on the menstrual cycle in rhesus monkeys. *J Pharmacol Exp Ther* 1997;281:70–83.

61. Kuhn C, Francis R. Gender difference in cocaine-induced HPA axis activation. *Neuropsychopharmacology* 1997;16:399–407.

62. Bauer CR, Shankaran S, Bada HS, et al. The Maternal Lifestyle Study: drug exposure during pregnancy and short-term maternal outcomes. *Am J Obstet Gynecol* 2002;186:487–495.

63. Little BB, Snell LM, Trimmer KJ, et al. Peripartum cocaine use and adverse pregnancy outcome. *Am J Hum Biol* 1999;11:598–602.

64. Greenfield SF, O'Leary G. Sex differences in substance use disorders. In: Lewis-Hall F, Williams TS, Panetta JA, et al, eds. *Psychiatric illness in women: emerging treatments and research.* Washington, DC: American Psychiatric Publishing, 2002:467–533.

65. Frank DA, Augustyn M, Knight WG, et al. Growth, development, and behavior in early childhood following prenatal cocaine exposure: a systematic review. *JAMA* 2001;285:1613–1625.

66. Covington CY, Nordstrom-Klee B, Ager J, et al. Birth to age 7 growth of children prenatally exposed to drugs. A prospective cohort study. *Neurotoxicol Teratol* 2002;24:489–496.

67. Singer LT, Arendt R, Minnes S, et al. Cognitive and motor outcomes of cocaine-exposed infants. *JAMA* 2002;287:1952–1960.

68. Zuckerman B, Frank DA, Mayes L. Cocaine-exposed infants and developmental outcomes: "crack kids" revisited. *JAMA* 2002;287:1990–1991.

69. Rohsenow DJ, Monti PM, Martin RA, et al. Brief coping skills treatment for cocaine abuse: 12-month substance use outcomes. *J Consult Clin Psychol* 2000;68:515–520.

70. Crits-Christoph P, Siqueland L, Blaine J, et al. Psychosocial treatments for cocaine dependence: National Institute on Drug Abuse Collaborative Cocaine Treatment Study. *Arch Gen Psychiatry* 1999;56:493–502.

71. Corchero J, Manzanares J, Fuentes JA. Role of gonadal steroids in the corticotropin-releasing hormone and proopiomelanocortin gene expression response to Delta(9)-tetrahydrocannabinol in the hypothalamus of the rat. *Neuroendocrinology* 2001;74:185–192.

72. Mattes RD, Engelman K, Shaw LM, et al. Cannabinoids and appetite

stimulation. *Pharmacol Biochem Behav* 1994;49:187–195.

73. Pedersen W, Mastekaasa A, Wichstrom L. Conduct problems and early cannabis initiation: a longitudinal study of gender differences. *Addiction* 2001;96:415–431.

74. Rey JM, Sawyer MG, Raphael B, et al. Mental health of teenagers who use cannabis. Results of an Australian survey. *Br J Psychiatry* 2002;180:216–221.

75. Johnson RA, Gerstein DR. Age, period, and cohort effects in marijuana and alcohol incidence: United States females and males, 1961–1990. *Subst Use Misuse* 2000;35:925–948.

76. Griffin ML, Mendelson JH, Mello NK, et al. Marihuana use across the menstrual cycle. *Drug Alcohol Depend* 1986;18:213–224.

77. Thomas H. A community survey of adverse effects of cannabis use. *Drug Alcohol Depend* 1996;42:201–207.

78. Pope HG Jr, Jacobs A, Mialet JP, et al. Evidence for a sex-specific residual effect of cannabis on visuospatial memory. *Psychother Psychosom* 1997;66:179–184.

79. Pope HG Jr, Gruber AJ, Hudson JI, et al. Neuropsychological performance in long-term cannabis users. *Arch Gen Psychiatry* 2001;58:909–915.

80. Mendelson JH, Mello NK, Ellingboe J. Acute effects of marihuana smoking on prolactin levels in human females. *J Pharmacol Exp Ther* 1985;232:220–222.

81. Mendelson JH, Mello NK, Ellingboe J, et al. Marihuana smoking suppresses luteinizing hormone in women. *J Pharmacol Exp Ther* 1986;237:862–866.

82. Mendelson JH, Ellingboe J, Kuehnle JC, et al. Effects of chronic marihuana use on integrated plasma testosterone and luteinizing hormone levels. *J Pharmacol Exp Ther* 1978;207:611–617.

83. Block RI, Farinpour R, Schlechte JA. Effects of chronic marijuana use on testosterone, luteinizing hormone, follicle stimulating hormone, prolactin and cortisol in men and women. *Drug Alcohol Depend* 1991;28:121–128.

84. Williams MA, Lieberman E, Mittendorf R, et al. Risk factors for abruptio placentae. *Am J Epidemiol* 1991;134:965–972.

85. Gibson GT, Baghurst PA, Colley DP. Maternal alcohol, tobacco and cannabis consumption and the outcome of pregnancy. *Aust N Z J Obstet Gynaecol* 1983;23:15–19.

86. Fergusson DM, Horwood LJ, Northstone K, et al. Avon Longitudinal Study of Pregnancy and Childhood. Maternal use of cannabis and pregnancy outcome. *BJOG* 2002;109:21–27.

87. Fried PA, Smith AM. A literature review of the consequences of prenatal marihuana exposure. An emerging theme of a deficiency in aspects of executive function. *Neurotoxicol Teratol* 2001;23:1–11.

88. Goldschmidt L, Day NL, Richardson GA. Effects of prenatal marijuana exposure on child behavior problems at age 10. *Neurotoxicol Teratol* 2000;22:325–336.

89. Chen K, Kandel DB. Predictors of cessation of marijuana use: an event history analysis. *Drug Alcohol Depend* 1998;50:109–121.

90. Cruz SL, Rodriguez-Manzo G. Gender differences in the cardiovascular responses to morphine and naloxone in spinal rats. *Eur J Pharmacol* 2000;397:121–128.

91. Zun LS, Downey LV, Gossman W, et al. Gender differences in narcotic-induced emesis in the ED. *Am J Emerg Med* 2002;20:151–154.

92. Gear RW, Gordon NC, Heller PH, et al. Gender difference in analgesic response to the kappa-opioid pentazocine. *Neurosci Lett* 1996;205:207–209.

93. Kepler KL, Kest B, Kiefel JM, et al. Roles of gender, gonadectomy and estrous phase in the analgesic effects of intracerebroventricular morphine in rats. *Pharmacol Biochem Behav* 1989;34:119–127.

94. de Vos JW, Geerlings PJ, van den Brink W, et al. Pharmacokinetics of methadone and its primary metabolite in 20 opiate addicts. *Eur J Clin Pharmacol* 1995;48:361–366.

95. Gossop M, Griffiths P, Strang J. Sex differences in patterns of drug taking behaviour. A study at a London community drug team. *Br J Psychiatry* 1994;164:101–104.

96. Anglin MD, Hser YI, McGlothlin WH. Sex differences in addict careers. 2. Becoming addicted. *Am J Drug Alcohol Abuse* 1987;13:59–71.

97. Marsh KL, Simpson DD. Sex differences in opioid addiction careers. *Am J Drug Alcohol Abuse* 1986;12:309–329.

98. Goldstein A, Herrera J. Heroin addicts and methadone treatment in Albuquerque: a 22-year follow-up. *Drug Alcohol Depend* 1995;40:139–150.

99. Tardiff K, Marzuk PM, Leon AC, et al. HIV infection among victims of accidental fatal drug overdoses in New York City. *Addiction* 1997;92:1017–1022.

100. Hulse GK, Milne E, English DR, et al. Assessing the relationship between maternal opiate use and neonatal mortality. *Addiction* 1998;93:1033–1042.

101. Osborn DA, Jeffery HE, Cole MJ. Sedatives for opiate withdrawal in newborn infants (Cochrane Review). *Cochrane Database Syst Rev* 2002:CD002053.

102. Vathy I. Prenatal opiate exposure: long-term CNS consequences in the stress system of the offspring. *Psychoneuroendocrinology* 2002;27:273–283.

103. Bunikowski R, Grimmer I, Heiser A, et al. Neurodevelopmental outcome after prenatal exposure to opiates. *Eur J Pediatr* 1998;157:724–730.

104. Sandberg DE, Meyer-Bahlburg HF, Rosen TS, et al. Effects of prenatal methadone exposure on sex-dimorphic behavior in early school-age children. *Psychoneuroendocrinology* 1990;15:77–82.

105. Wang EC. Methadone treatment during pregnancy. *J Obstet Gynecol Neonatal Nurs* 1999;28:615–622.

106. Blume SB. Women and addictive disorders. In: Graham A, Schultz P, eds. *Principles of addiction medicine,* 2nd ed. Chevy Chase, MD: American Society of Addiction Medicine, 1998.

107. Kandall SR, Doberczak TM, Jantunen M, et al. The methadone-maintained pregnancy. *Clin Perinatol* 1999;26:173–183.

108. Nanovskaya T, Deshmukh S, Brooks M, et al. Transplacental transfer and metabolism of buprenorphine. *J Pharmacol Exp Ther* 2002;300:26–33.

109. Chatham LR, Hiller ML, Rowan-Szal GA, et al. Gender differences at admission and follow-up in a sample of methadone maintenance clients. *Subst Use Misuse* 1999;34:1137–1165.

110. Rowan-Szal GA, Chatham LR, Joe GW, et al. Services provided during methadone treatment. A gender comparison. *J Subst Abuse Treat* 2000;19:7–14.

111. Camacho LM, Bartholomew NG, Joe GW, et al. Gender, cocaine and during-treatment HIV risk reduction among injection opioid users in methadone maintenance. *Drug Alcohol Depend* 1996;41:1–7.

112. Zeman MV, Hiraki L, Sellers EM. Gender differences in tobacco smoking: higher relative exposure to smoke than nicotine in women. *J Womens Health Gend Based Med* 2002;11:147–153.

113. Kandel DB, Chen K. Extent of smoking and nicotine dependence in the United States: 1991–1993. *Nicotine Tob Res* 2000;2:263–274.

114. Patton GC, Carlin JB, Coffey C, et al. The course of early smoking: a population-based cohort study over three years. *Addiction* 1998;93:1251–1260.

115. Wiecha JM. Differences in patterns of tobacco use in Vietnamese, African American, Hispanic, and Caucasian adolescents in Worcester, Massachusetts. *Am J Prev Med* 1996;12:29–37.

116. Charlton A, Blair V. Predicting the onset of smoking in boys and girls. *Soc Sci Med* 1989;29:813–818.

117. Zilberman ML, Tavares H, Blume SB, et al. Towards best practices in the treatment of women with addictive disorders. *Addict Disord Their Treatment* 2002;1:39–46.

118. McAllister-Sistilli CG, Caggiula AR, Knopf S, et al. The effects of nicotine on the immune system. *Psychoneuroendocrinology* 1998;23:175–187.

119. Girdler SS, Jamner LD, Jarvik M, et al. Smoking status and nicotine administration differentially modify hemodynamic stress reactivity in men and women. *Psychosom Med* 1997;59:294–306.

120. Zang EA, Wynder EL. Differences in lung cancer risk between men and women: examination of the evidence. *J Natl Cancer Inst* 1996;88:183–192.

121. Castelao JE, Yuan JM, Skipper PL, et al. Gender- and smoking-related bladder cancer risk. *J Natl Cancer Inst* 2001;93:538–545.

122. Centers for Disease Control and Prevention. Recent trends in mortality rates for four major cancers, by sex and race/ethnicity—United States, 1990–1998. *JAMA* 2002;287:1391–1392.

123. Hecht SS. Tobacco smoke carcinogens and breast cancer. *Environ Mol Mutagen* 2002;39:119–126.

124. Kuper H, Titus-Ernstoff L, Harlow BL, et al. Population based study of coffee, alcohol and tobacco use and risk of ovarian cancer. *Int J Cancer* 2000;88:313–318.

125. Doll R. Cancers weakly related to smoking. *Br Med Bull* 1996;52:35–49.

126. Weisberg E. Smoking and reproductive health. *Clin Reprod Fertil* 1985;3:175–186.

127. Li YF, Gilliland FD, Berhane K, et al. Effects of *in utero* and environmental tobacco smoke exposure on lung function in boys and girls with and without asthma. *Am J Respir Crit Care Med* 2000;162:2097–2104.

128. Brennan PA, Grekin ER, Mortensen EL, et al. Relationship of maternal smoking during pregnancy with criminal arrest and hospitalization for substance abuse in male and female adult offspring. *Am J Psychiatry* 2002;159:48–54.

129. Rasanen P, Hakko H, Isohanni M, et al. Maternal smoking during pregnancy and risk of criminal behavior among adult male offspring in the Northern Finland 1966 Birth Cohort. *Am J Psychiatry* 1999;156:857–862.

130. Wakschlag LS, Pickett KE, Cook E Jr, et al. Maternal smoking during pregnancy and severe antisocial behavior in offspring: a review. *Am J Public Health* 2002;92:966–974.

131. Wetter DW, Kenford SL, Smith SS, et al. Gender differences in smoking cessation. *J Consult Clin Psychol* 1999; 67:555–562.

132. Gonzales D, Bjornson W, Durcan MJ, et al. Effects of gender on relapse prevention in smokers treated with bupropion SR. *Am J Prev Med* 2002;22:234–239.

133. D'Angelo ME, Reid RD, Brown KS, Pipe AL. Gender differences in predictors for long-term smoking cessation following physician advice and nicotine replacement therapy. *Can J Public Health* 2001;92:418–422.

134. Heishman SJ. Behavioral and cognitive effects of smoking: relationship to nicotine addiction. *Nicotine Tob Res* 1999;1[2 Suppl]:S143–S147.

135. Allen SS, Hatsukami D, Christianson D, et al. Effects of transdermal nicotine on craving, withdrawal and premenstrual symptomatology in short-term smoking abstinence during different phases of the menstrual cycle. *Nicotine Tob Res* 2000;2:231–241.

136. Thadani PV. Biological mechanisms and perinatal exposure to abused drugs. *Synapse* 1995;19:228–232.

137. Plessinger MA. Prenatal exposure to amphetamines. Risks and adverse outcomes in pregnancy. *Obstet Gynecol Clin North Am* 1998;25:119–138.

138. Liechti ME, Gamma A, Vollenweider FX. Gender differences in the subjective effects of MDMA. *Psychopharmacology (Berl)* 2001;154:161–168.

139. Weir E. Drug-facilitated date rape. *CMAJ* 2001;165:80.

140. Linehan MM, Dimeff LA, Reynolds SK, et al. Dialectical behavior therapy versus comprehensive validation therapy plus 12-step for the treatment of opioid dependent women meeting criteria for borderline personality disorder. *Drug Alcohol Depend* 2002;67:13–26.

141. Silverman K, Svikis D, Robles E, et al. A reinforcement-based therapeutic workplace for the treatment of drug abuse: six-month abstinence outcomes. *Exp Clin Psychopharmacol* 2001;9:14–23.

CHAPTER 66

Women's Research and Policy Issues

MARSHA ROSENBAUM AND
SHEIGLA MURPHY

The vast majority of women in the United States use some type of drug on a regular basis. We use prescription and over-the-counter drugs to help us sleep, stay awake, alleviate pain, lose weight, cope with depression, and the like. We drink coffee and tea, and eat chocolate, all of which contain caffeine. We consume alcoholic beverages. Yet when we think of "women and drugs" what comes to mind are users of *illegal* drugs, although in reality less than 5% of us use such substances on a regular basis (1).

Scientific research, information dissemination, and the perspective of the scientist/writer(s) influence what we know about women and drugs. Formal research is limited largely by what our government sanctions as "significant," or having the potential to contribute to the solution of an already-defined problem. Whether protocols use, for example, quantitative methodologies, qualitative methodologies, surveys, clinical trials, or field studies, researchers with a conventional perspective generally collect and analyze data, and ultimately produce information. Most have a covert investment in the status quo, the preservation of traditional values (including gender roles), and prevailing (prohibitionist) policy toward drugs.

The decision to publish research findings is political. Conventional scientific journals have ultimate decision-making power about which "findings" constitute serious scholarship, often defined as that which is government-sanctioned (and funded). The other major source of information, the popular media, is motivated to define drug use as problematic when it contains sensational stories. Historically, women's drug use has been defined as problematic when their traditional gender roles were violated or abandoned, and therefore jeopardized. Details about women ingesting drugs during pregnancy and violating that most sacred role as caretaker/mother sells papers.

In sum, our knowledge of women and drugs is limited to that which is government-funded and published in scholarly journals and/or the popular media. This information does not represent the experience of the majority of women drug users. It does not even represent the majority of women who use illegal drugs, because most use drugs in controlled ways and without serious consequence. We know very little about how they manage and control their use because prohibitionist rhetoric dismisses such use as impossible, making research funding difficult if not impossible to obtain.

Instead, most conventional research focuses on a relatively small group of women whose drug use becomes visible, therefore problematic. They use illegal means to earn enough money to use (expensive) drugs. As a result of their illegal activities they come into contact with the criminal justice system. They are often poor, underskilled, undereducated and recipients of public assistance. They have difficulty taking care of their children, and as part of the welfare system, come to the attention of social service agencies designed to protect children. Some have no real home and as a result much of their existence takes place "on the street." Most important, they incite fear because they deviate from sexual norms and in general violate traditional gender role expectations with regard to pregnancy and parenting.

Since women "emerged from the shadows" in the 1970s (2), patterns of drug use and problems associated with it have shifted. The focus of research on women and drugs, including our own, mirrors societal concerns, and has also changed. This chapter examines some of the salient issues related to women and drugs, with primary attention given to research areas that have dominated the literature and our own research, namely pregnancy and drug treatment.

Societal responses to women who use (illegal) drugs have also shifted over the past 30 years. During the 1970s, treatment expanded with the hope that rehabilitation would address the problem. By the late 1980s, with acquired immunodeficiency syndrome (AIDS), the crack "epidemic," and a powerful "War on Drugs," a more punitive climate prevailed. Women drug users were being held responsible for many of society's ills and actively prosecuted for deviating from conventional gender roles.

This chapter uses research findings to examine shifting trends in and societal responses to women's (illegal, problematic) drug use during the 1970s and 1980s. The chapter concludes with the early twenty-first century and a discus-

sion of feminist analyses of violence, treatment, and the implications of the War on Drugs. Finally we make policy recommendations for reducing drug-related harm.

THE 1970s

The early feminist movement of the late 1960s and early 1970s called attention to and encouraged women's participation in many activities in which they had been absent or invisible. It also opened a range of occupations that had been the exclusive or nearly exclusive domain of men. Among these occupations was illegal drug use, particularly heroin addiction. Research began with assessments of prevalence, in an effort to determine just how many women used illegal drugs (3–6). Epidemiologic studies compared women with men, among themselves on the basis of race, with other drug users, and longitudinally (7–13). Several other studies focused on gendered aspects of women's participation in the drug world, including prostitution (14–17).

Another set of studies looked at the etiology of women's criminality (18–22). Women drug users had begun to participate in property (although usually not violent) crime such as burglary, larceny, and forgery. Their representation in large-scale moneymaking enterprises such as drug distribution was minimal, although many served as assistants to (male) dealers (17,23,24). Research on women heroin addicts revealed that a sizable proportion used prostitution, at least occasionally, to earn money to support their heroin habits (8,15,16,19–22,24–34).

By far, during the 1970s, the bulk of research focused on a major concern regarding women's deviation from traditional gender roles, pregnancy and motherhood. Drug treatment was another research area that dominated the 1970s.

Pregnancy and Heroin Use

Early studies of pregnancy and heroin use focused on physiologic problems associated with addiction. During pregnancy, heroin addiction was thought to be connected with such problems as premature rupture of membranes, impaired fetal growth, diminished birth weight, preterm delivery, maternal infections, meconium staining, stillbirths, toxemia, and infant withdrawal (35–48).

At that time there was a dearth of information about pregnant women and heroin-addicted mothers. We first studied heroin addiction in 1977, by interviewing 100 women, 70% of whom were mothers. Because our study was sociologic and ethnographic, our findings differed from, but often complemented, the more medically oriented publications appearing about the same time (35–48). We found that the discovery of pregnancy was problematic, as many women had stopped menstruating while they were addicted. By the time they were certain (often because they were "showing") they were in the fourth or fifth month and too far along for an abortion. It was also too late to stop using drugs, the rationale being that (a) most of heroin's most deleterious effects would have occurred during the first trimester, and (b) withdrawal in later stages of pregnancy was too dangerous to the fetus. Birth and delivery, according to our study participants, was often physiologically as well as psychologically difficult. Many of the women had suffered from such ailments as toxemia as a result of addiction, as well as little prenatal care. As a result, birth could be a dangerous and fearful experience. In addition, hospital staff familiar with the women's "condition" were less than supportive and often abusive. The last thing the women wanted to do was to return to such an unpleasant environment, and many never came back. To compound feelings of disdain they received at the hospital, women often went home with an irritable and difficult-to-placate infant. This combination had the potential to send them into motherhood with feelings of failure and a need to use heroin to relieve their suffering (17).

Drug Treatment

The establishment of National Institute on Drug Abuse Program for Women's Concerns in 1974 opened treatment options for women heroin addicts. These included inpatient detoxification, outpatient detoxification, Narcotic Anonymous, methadone maintenance, and therapeutic communities. Despite these advances, women drug users had felt the stigma of being defined as socially, as well as psychopathologically, more deviant than their non-addicted sisters or their male counterparts, and as a result, many hid their addiction, making it difficult to recruit them for treatment (49).

When women did decide to go to treatment, they found that many programs were incompatible with their needs and obligations as mothers (50–52). As a result, most women were limited to outpatient detoxification and methadone maintenance.

The increasing recognition of women as a "special" population of addicts because of their childbearing and childrearing roles was simultaneous to the expansion of methadone maintenance treatment (MMT). At that time, research on MMT and pregnancy focused on medical issues pertaining to the fetus and newborn and the management of the pregnant addict (40,48,53–71). Research findings, while in general supportive of methadone as a tool to reduce drug-related harm, were inconsistent in terms of fetal health and severity of withdrawal symptoms. Still, for a pregnant addict who found it impossible to quit the use of heroin, maintenance was one of few viable options, and by the end of the 1970s, women occupied nearly one third of new MMT slots (72).

The rehabilitative orientation of 1970s resulted in the proliferation of treatment, with methadone maintenance the single largest modality available (73). During a subsequent study we conducted (74), which was focused on

the methadone experience for women, we found MMT to be a "presence" in the heroin world for the 100 women on MMT interviewed. Women had to confront the possibility of getting on methadone, whether or not they chose to enroll in a program. A major impetus for women to enlist in a methadone program was pregnancy (74). Many women who became pregnant opted for the control methadone provided. Their lives were necessarily stabilized because of (a) the highly structured clinic routine and (b) the elimination of the need to participate in criminal activities for the purpose of buying heroin. Women's lives became as routinized as possible, enabling them to work around their addiction: provide a home for their baby, eat well, and learn skills in preparation for motherhood.

Despite enlisting in drug treatment and stabilizing their lives, women reported that when they went to the hospital to give birth, they were faced with the stigma of being "just a junkie." The guilt, which may have been suppressed during pregnancy, surfaced very quickly—often brought back by the attitude of the hospital staff, which was most often neither knowledgeable nor sympathetic.

The guilt experienced by women on methadone extended from birth and continued throughout the baby's childhood. It began in the hospital, but did not end there. They felt responsible for the baby's withdrawal, although there was no way to predict severity of withdrawal, or even whether it would happen at all (47,63,75–78).

Motherhood often began badly for women on methadone, and there were more problems when the baby came home from the hospital. Just as with heroin, babies in withdrawal could be extremely irritable (76,77), with "postpartum depression" accentuated and extended for addicted mothers. The guilt experienced by mothers on methadone haunted them, and never seemed to end. First they looked for signs that their babies were addicted. Later women wondered if their children's problems might be attributable to their own use of heroin or methadone. The guilt and fear could extend through life, and every ailment was suspect.

Despite an increase in treatment options for women in the 1970s, there were not enough programs, and the quality of treatment was questionable at best. Women often found the structure of treatment, including long waiting lists, difficult to negotiate. Some women expressed little respect for counselors, especially those who were ex-addicts. Women on methadone often experienced physiologic problems. Many women were dissatisfied because of the male orientation and their own lesser position within the treatment world, regardless of the particular modality. In the early years, it was common for programs to limit their acceptance of women to the wives or girlfriends of male clients as an incentive for men to enroll. Women heroin addicts in treatment were defined as "sicker" and more deviant than their male counterparts (7,26,79,80). When they enlisted in drug treatment, they discovered they were treated as more pathologic than male addicts, and experienced discrimination and sexism as a result (81–83). The major obstacles women faced in accessing and using treatment effectively were (a) the lack of facilities for children and (b) the failure of institutions to acknowledge the difficulties they faced in attempting to fulfill their mothering obligations while following a treatment regimen.

THE 1980s

The study of women and drugs was altered radically in the 1980s. The AIDS epidemic and its relation to drug use, the introduction of "crack" to the drug scene, and an unprecedented escalation in the War on Drugs and shrinking social service provision changed the drug experience for women.

AIDS

Intravenous drug use accounts for half of all AIDS in women (84). Epidemiologic and etiologic studies have found that women injecting drug users (IDUs) were vulnerable to the disease through both needle sharing and unsafe sexual contact (85–95). Women's risk through unsafe needle sharing had much to do with their inequitable power relationship to men (96–100). Researchers found that women were much more likely than men to obtain drugs through their (male sexual) partners; that men often controlled the level of intake of drugs for their women partners; and women tended to be "fixed" by someone else more often than men, increasing their chances of being "hit" by a previously used needle (17,99–101).

Prostitution, or "sex work," as it was called by the 1980s, contributed greatly to women's human immunodeficiency virus (HIV) risk and sexually transmitted diseases. Still, women had fewer economic resources and conventional job skills than their male counterparts (102–105), and as result of a reduction in programs for the poor, fewer resources than they had in the 1970s. This wanting economic situation rendered them desperate, forcing them to use sex work to earn enough money to support their basic needs as well as their drug habits. Women's need to support themselves through sex work created an insidious cycle. Women remained in sex work because they had few, if any, other ways to make a living. But to cope with the distasteful nature of prostitution, they used drugs to block their feelings. Consequently, they were unable to separate themselves from the drug world, which was, in turn, tied to prostitution (16,106–108).

Drugs and prostitution added up to a tangled package creating increased HIV risk for women through both needle-sharing and sexual contact (109–111). Drug-dependent women in withdrawal and in desperate need of money were vulnerable to the demands of a "trick" who did not want to use a condom (112). Furthermore, incest, economic hardship, physical abuse, and cultural influences, such as perception of control over one's own life, shaped women's use of contraceptive technologies, including condoms (113). Numerous studies were completed documenting cultural and racial factors that contributed to risky sexual behaviors (87,112,114–124).

Shrinking Social Services

In the area of the provision of human services, there has been a trend in the 1980s through the turn of this century for social welfare programs to change from the federally mandated and funded programs developed in the 1960s, to the state-by-state directed programs funded through federal block grant mechanisms promulgated during the Reagan and Bush (*father*) administrations and continued during the Clinton and Bush (*son*) administrations. As a result of shrinking budgets at the state level, numerous social service programs moved to public subsidization supervised by local governments and, finally, to privatization or the purchase of privately produced services. Historically, human service program provision tends to be downsized as programs move from federal to state to local supervision.

For pregnant drug users, this meant they encountered a myriad of inhibitors and (increasingly fewer) facilitators from which they constructed survival strategies. The women we interviewed reported drug use helped them to overcome some of the adversities in their daily lives. It was sometimes a source of income and mostly a source of solace and recreation. Although drug use helped interviewees to survive on a day-to-day basis, in the long-term, women faced severe consequences. Within a political context of social welfare reform, our interviewees' ability to care for themselves and their children was extremely compromised. Then crack came along.

Crack

By the mid-1980s, cocaine had replaced heroin as the "most" dangerous drug. A number of cross-sectional surveys had documented the dramatic rise in incidence and prevalence of cocaine use and related problems (125–128). Drug use among women in general seemed to be increasing (129), with use among women of childbearing age, in particular, increasing as well (130). Researchers compared women and men (130,131), looked at sexuality (132,133), "sex for crack" exchanges, and implications for the spread of HIV and other sexually transmitted diseases (134–141); women's participation in the cocaine-selling economy (142–146) and pregnancy, fetal development, and neonatal behavior (147–148).

In our qualitative study of 100 women who used crack cocaine (149), we found that women crack users' impoverished early lives set the stage for what would occur later:

Early in life, many were trapped by childhoods in violent, fragmented, or drug-involved households; teenage pregnancies; truncated educations and lack of skills;

poverty that was worsened by diversion of resources to drugs; oppressive relationships with men; and eventually by the demeaning social world surrounding crack cocaine (150).

We also found that victimization characterized their perspectives, they had little hope for a better future. Parenting concerns were central in women's lives.

Motherhood, Pregnancy, and Crack

The majority of our study participants (68%) were mothers, and parenting and pregnancy issues were of paramount concern to them. Women's viewpoints on pregnancy had much to do with their (non) use of birth control, believing themselves to be controlled by sex rather than sex being controllable by *them*. Many believed babies, rather than a chosen responsibility, came "from God." Fertility was a "distant issue" rather than a present reality and distinct possibility. Unforeseen or unwanted sexual experiences were attributed to youth, lack of knowledge, powerlessness, carelessness, or ambivalence. As a consequence of women's beliefs and unforeseen experiences, most became pregnant unexpectedly (150). Most women in the study population wanted to be mothers at some point in their lives, even if they did not themselves determine *when* this would occur. Lacking the opportunity to assume other viable social roles involving occupational success, motherhood remained as one of few conventional, respectable, life options.

We found crack-using interviewees not at all like the "monsters" portrayed in the popular media at that time (149,151,152). On the contrary, they felt a strong responsibility for their children, as well as deep pride. As mothers, they expressed their goals as nurturing and modeling. The use of crack cocaine presented mothering problems: a drain on attention to children's needs, finances, and role modeling. Women found themselves in a downward spiral, as the use of crack served to alleviate mothering concerns and ultimately worsened the situation. Nonetheless, women attempted to carve out various strategies involving "defensive compensation" and the effort to maintain mothering standards while using crack. They separated drug use and parental roles, budgeted money, tried to get away from the crack scene. As a very last resort they reluctantly, but voluntarily, relinquished their children, "for their own good," to a more responsible party. When custody was lost, the downward slide escalated and women often used even more crack, claiming, "they took my self" (149,151).

Paradoxically, along with well-meaning action, an insidious force was working with regard to pregnancy, motherhood and drug use: the Reagan–Bush (*father*) version of the "War on Drugs." It was fueled by the crack cocaine "epidemic" and the American need for swift, punitive action. Ira Chasnoff, in his 1989 article citing 375,000

"crack babies," set off an hysterical panic about the out-of-control epidemic of pregnancy and cocaine use (153). The popular press seized this story, claiming the needs of babies who were exposed to drugs *in utero* "will present an overwhelming challenge to schools, future employers and society" (154); "crack cocaine can overwhelm one of the strongest forces in nature, the parental instinct" (155,156); and drug use during pregnancy was "interfering with the central core of what it is to be human" (154). Negative media attention on drugs peaked with the phenomenon of the "crack baby." When preliminary research findings indicated crack use during pregnancy might be associated with fetal morbidity, the popular press quickly ran a series of alarmist stories. Journalists reported crack cocaine-addicted mothers had utter disregard for their children (155,156); and crack made a mother "indifferent to her child or abusive when its cries irritate her" (157). The use of drugs, and even more specifically the use of crack, during pregnancy was the equivalent of abusive parenting, and crack severed "that deepest and most sacred of bond: that between a mother and child" (158).

According to media representations, the problems of maternal drug use extended beyond the mother–child unit. News stories linked this phenomenon to a collection of social problems by asserting that pregnancy and drug use was draining public drug treatment funds and medical resources (155,156,159–168) and threatening the nation's school and criminal justice systems (154,163–168).

The Criminalization of Pregnancy

By the late 1980s, the fetal rights movement had combined with the War on Drugs (169). As a result of the scientific "crack baby" literature and subsequent media attention, pregnant drug users were increasingly stigmatized and further marginalized. At this point, the United States government stepped in to take action, with prosecutors in nearly half the states hoping to solve the problem by punishing pregnant drug users through prosecution (170–175). As a consequence, a drug-using pregnant woman could be arrested and incarcerated for "delivering drugs to a minor" (176). A woman who tested positive for drugs during delivery could immediately lose custody of her newborn. Although by 1991 the association between fetal harm and cocaine use had been seriously questioned by medical research (177–182), hundreds of infants and children continued to be removed from their mother's custody, overloading the child welfare system and jeopardizing women's control of their own bodies. As Boyd (183) notes: Feminists conclude that the criminalisation of pregnancy, and emerging fetal rights (184,185), have culminated in a situation where the well-being and security of women's bodies is legally and physically challenged (186,187).

Class and racial bias in these prosecutions were obvious (188). Although the use of illegal substances was distributed fairly evenly throughout the population in terms of class and race, all of the women who were prosecuted were not only poor but also nonwhite (189–191), with Jennifer Johnson's case perhaps the most famous (2).

The social conditions characterizing crack-users' lives were far more deleterious to the health, well-being, and safety of mother and child than drugs. The media and political focus on drugs was not only oversimplified but also purposeful. Crack mothers were being scapegoated, diverting attention from (a) the realities of the failed, post-Reagan social experiment with cutbacks of needed social programs and (b) complex social conditions that would require major political change (152,174,192,193). As Lisa Maher wrote:

> The criminalization of "crack pregnancies" facilitates the punishment of those who blatantly violate established social mores. It provides a way of striking out simultaneously at minorities, druggies, and women who fail to conform to engendered cultural expectations. At the same time, Middle America can vent its moral indignation by using the rhetoric of compassion for those "poor little [Black] babies...." [W]omen who use crack cocaine provide an attractive place for Middle America to circle its wagons, and crack pregnancies provide an ideal opportunity for projecting deep-seated cultural anxieties about the urban minority poor and about drugging, crime, and female sexuality (194, p. 123–124).

The increase in prosecutions convinced our research team that more information was needed in order to intervene in the misdirected, unjust, and downright harmful direction of persecution, prosecution, and punishment of pregnant drug users. The prevalence of drug use during pregnancy was not subsiding (195) and low birth weight, small head circumference, irritability, sudden infant death syndrome (SIDS), and malformation among babies born to addicted mothers continued to be commonly reported (196). Others had discovered that the pregnant addict was less likely to attend prenatal care appointments; more likely to live in poor conditions; more likely to have a host of confounding problems such as sexually transmitted infections; more likely to experience higher rates of violence than nondrug users; but be no more "pathologic" than women in the general population (197–199). With all the research that had been conducted, the perspective of pregnant women themselves was rarely the focus. Our goal was to present a "human" view of the pregnant drug user while attempting to humanize her treatment.

We learned that the crack-using pregnant women we studied were stigmatized and consumed by guilt. They expressed great concern about the levels of drug-related harm that occurred during their pregnancies, their evaluations varying according to the particular drug(s) they were using, and often based on what they had heard or read through the media. Contrary to popular myth, our study participants cared very much about the outcomes of

their pregnancies and used a variety of strategies to reduce drug-related harm. They tried to lower their intake, switched from "harder" to "softer" drugs such as marijuana, which would help them eat and sleep, and ingested health-promoting substances such as vitamins (200). Perhaps most problematic in this potpourri of methods was prenatal care (201). The crack-using women in our study population, 82% of whom were African American, were well aware that because they were African American, as soon as they entered a clinical setting they would automatically be suspect of illegal drug use. They would be targeted for drug testing, which could lead to punitive social service and criminal justice interventions such as incarceration and removal of their children (175,189,202). Quite simply, despite their intent to reduce drug-related harm through contact with medical institutions, if they believed custody would be jeopardized, they, like the women studied by Chavkin, made the difficult decision to stay away.

Attempts to criminalize drug use during pregnancy may further deter pregnant women from seeking care or from giving accurate information to health care providers. Anecdotal reports suggest that efforts to detect maternal drug use by means of urine toxicology testing of the newborn may even frighten some women away from delivering in hospital (203).

THE 1990s

By the 1990s, feminist scholars questioned basic assumptions about gender roles and the way women and drugs had been viewed (149,204–206). The ways in which abuse, violence, drug treatment, and the War on Drugs have shaped women's experience became central concerns in the last decade of the twentieth century.

Abuse and Violence

Researchers have consistently found high levels of past and present abuse in the lives of women drug users (144,197,207–209). Many have suggested that there is a relationship, if not absolutely causal, between violence experienced by women and drug use (210–228).

In our study of pregnancy and drug use (229), 70% (N = 120) of the study participants reported they had been in one or more relationships in which they had been physically battered by a male partner. Of the 84 women who had been assaulted by partners, nearly half (45%) reported being battered during their current or most recent pregnancy. Twenty-five of the 84 women (30%) who had been victims of partner violence were in a battering relationship at the time of the interview. In addition to the violence they endured within their homes, the neighborhoods these women grew up in were, in many instances, veritable "combat zones." Between gang warfare, police raids, random shootings, and drug dealing, fear became a way of life for the overwhelming majority of the women who participated in this study. These findings concur with other studies that indicate a link between childhood experiences of violence, sexual abuse, physical abuse, and the increased likelihood that a woman will develop drug and alcohol problems later in life (223). For many of our study participants, drug use was a way of numbing themselves to the violence that engulfed them.

In Rosenbaum's mid-1990s study of methadone maintenance, 51% of the 108 women (N = 55) reported some form of past or present violence in their lives. Forty percent (N = 22) of the women who experienced abuse reported surviving multiple abuse patterns, such as a combination of child abuse, rape, *and* domestic violence. Some violent partners prohibited women from seeking or continuing treatment. In addition, women's limited economic resources meant they had few options for ending violent relationships. The implications of such violence, although difficult to determine in a tangible way, did affect women's perceptions of their treatment progress. The study found that violence provided a catalyst to self-medicate (230,231). In addition, women's sense of self-worth, importance, competence, and control was eroded with the accumulation of violent and abusive experiences (213,232). As such, each of these experiences formed a link with women's problems in treatment and acted as a barrier to successful MMT in the following ways. First, psychological turmoil from violent episodes drove women to initiate or continue to use heroin to self-medicate and cope. Second, the effects of past violence, if not sufficiently addressed in counseling and therapy, could continue to haunt the women and propel them toward using heroin for escape and, ironically, control (205).

During the period 1996 to 1999, Sheigla Murphy and her research team conducted a study of pregnancy drug use and violence (233,234). This was an exploratory depth interview study of pregnant drug users who experienced one or more victimizations (physical, sexual, and/or emotional) while pregnant. They began by locating and recruiting women who were pregnant or recently pregnant and had used marijuana, crack/cocaine, heroin/opiates, and/or methamphetamine singly or in combination (including alcohol with one or more of the above). Originally, Murphy's team estimated that they would have to screen approximately 300 women to enroll 100 who would qualify for and agree to participate in the second session, a qualitative depth interview focusing on their drug use and victimization histories with an emphasis on victimizations experienced during pregnancy. As it turned out, they only had to screen 126 women. Sadly, 79% of the interviewees experienced physical and emotional abuse while pregnant. Study participants' related the violence and humiliation they endured at the hands of drug dealers, pimps, johns, other drug users, and, most frequently, their intimate partners. Participants shared common problems with standing on their own two feet in a male-dominated world where women

occupied the lowest rungs of the social hierarchy. In both deviant and conventional social worlds, interviewees recounted that being a woman was a strike against them, being a pregnant woman was a second strike, and being a *drug-using* pregnant woman was the third and final blow to their social standing. Abusers, as reported by the study participants, diminished their self-esteem to the point where they believed they deserved the violence. Many women remained silent and therefore protected partners from outside domestic violence interventions, especially police intervention. In her study of crack-using women in Atlanta, Sterk also discovered that women's failure to report assaults was justified by their low expectations regarding interventions, the fear that others would discover their drug use, and the belief that they deserved to be abused (235). Nonetheless, interviewees kept going, day after day, beating after beating. Some were able to raise their children, even shelter them from their own drug use and violent experiences. Women's drug use both exposed them to violence and protected or helped them cope with violence. Drug use eased their pain or increased their endurance. Offering drugs to their perpetrators helped to postpone or avoid a violent event. These women achieved a very human objective: survival.

Drug Treatment

Studies of drug treatment have focused on themes of violence, male dominance, dependence, motherhood issues, and depression (236,237); pregnancy (238); retention/relapse (239–242), ethnic and gender differences (243); treatment in a criminal justice setting (209,244–246); and treatment of women with HIV (247).

In Rosenbaum and colleagues' study of MMT (112), the women's primary reason for entering a program was to reduce drug-related harm to themselves and their children. They experienced barriers to treatment also faced by men (such as prohibitive clinic fees and waiting lists), but also had to contend with women-specific barriers that discouraged and sometimes prevented some from entering and others from fully engaging in treatment.

Although both men and women shared many similar motivations for treatment, such as avoiding the criminal justice system, burning out on "the life" and the desire to change their lives, women spoke specifically of their relationships and family responsibilities as reasons for entering treatment programs. They sought MMT when their partners influenced them to use heroin and/or other drugs and to share injection equipment in an unsafe way, and when they were in abusive relationships. Occasionally these women could not initiate the treatment process until they had ended these relationships.

As has been the case for decades, many of the women in the study population (112) viewed pregnancy as a motivation for entering treatment. They wanted to "clean up for the baby," and saw the pregnancy as an opportunity to make other positive changes in their lives. In addition, women's desire to improve their capacity for parenting was a motivation for treatment. Both pregnant women and women with children experienced tremendous feelings of guilt over drug use and its potential detrimental effects on their children. This guilt often translated into efforts to seek treatment.

These data revealed at least three substantial barriers to treatment for women: (a) family responsibilities, (b) interpersonal and sexual violence, and (c) sex work. Either alone or in interaction with other factors, these barriers often effectively deterred, and possibly prevented, women from seeking treatment. Ironically, for those women in treatment, occasionally clinic policies converted motivations into barriers that may have prevented them from maximizing the therapeutic benefits that MMT had to offer (112).

The familial barriers fell into two categories: sexual partners and children. It was not uncommon for women to experience resistance from their partners in seeking treatment. Sometimes this resistance was subtle, such as in cases when they received no help with child care from their partners while they were trying to meet clinic demands. At other times resistance was more overt, such as when a partner's violence was meant to prevent a woman from seeking treatment. These women wanted MMT and all the benefits of stabilization, but they often faced resistance from those closest to them, their partners.

Although pregnancy and children were motivations for treatment, both also served as barriers to treatment. Some programs were hesitant to take pregnant women because of the extra resources they required. Even when they did present for treatment during pregnancy, many experienced discrimination at the hands of health care and social service workers within the clinic setting. So although pregnancy was a primary motivation for women to seek MMT, it also deterred them from getting help for their drug dependency. This effect had negative health consequences for both the women and their children, since adequate health care was not received.

A final barrier to treatment specific to women was their working situations. Sex work, in particular, made it difficult for women to fully engage in treatment, because the social worlds of sex work and drug use are closely intertwined. Many of the women found it economically necessary to continue with sex work, as they had few job skills and little social or economic support. In addition, many of the women in the Rosenbaum et al. study population had criminal records. They reported that it was next to impossible to find conventional work after serving time. Although men, too, frequently struggled to find legal work after a jail or prison term, the women we interviewed believed it was especially difficult for them because of what they saw as greater social stigma attached to jail terms for women. With few or no legitimate work possibilities, women continued to find economic support in occupations such as sex work, which as noted earlier, increased their risk of HIV infection (112).

THE 2000s

Feminist scholars at the turn of this century have begun to make the connection between the War on Drugs and the "War on Abortion." Legal scholar and activist Lynn Paltrow summarizes this growing political sentiment:

> While many people view the war on abortion and the war on drugs as entirely distinct, there are in fact many connections and overlaps between the two. Their history, the strategies used to control and punish some reproductive choices and those used to control the use of certain drugs, the methods used to limit access to reproductive health care and to limit the availability of drug treatment, and the populations most harmed by those limits are remarkably similar. These similarities are particularly apparent where the issues coalesce in the regulation and punishment of pregnant, drug-using women (248).

The concept of fetal personhood that derives from the abortion debate has led to the depiction of the pregnant drug user as a willful "poisoner" of an innocent fetus. In turn, the conceptualization of an "innocent" fetus as a person sets dangerous precedent for those who value a woman's right to reproductive choice.

Wendy Chavkin's work also made the link between the War on Drugs and the struggles over abortion. In 2001, she outlined some positive policy changes regarding the War on Drugs but has serious concerns about the fate of poor women seeking abortion, particularly poor addicted women: "There have been recent signs of abatement in the War on Drugs. In New York, the governor and legislators have proposed modification of the Rockefeller drug laws to reduce mandatory sentences, offer treatment alternatives, and return discretion in sentencing to judges" (249, p. 1627).

In 2000, California passed Proposition 36, an alternative to incarceration for many nonviolent drug-possession offenders. However, the situation for poor, addicted women has actually worsened as a result of the passage of the Personal Responsibility and Work Reconciliation Act (PRWR) in 1996. Individual states can exclude otherwise qualified applicants with prior felony drug convictions from assistance, and drug-treatment enrollment does not count toward meeting the work requirement that the PRWR mandates. Drug and alcohol dependence is no longer a qualifying condition for eligibility for Supplemental Security Income, an important source of income for many of the women who participated in the numerous studies described in this chapter. Dr. Chavkin predicts, "Disagreement over abortion shows no sign of lessening, and there will likely be efforts to further limit access to abortion for the young and the poor" (249).

IMPLICATIONS OF THE WAR ON DRUGS FOR WOMEN

The Reagan–Bush (*father*)–Clinton–Bush (*son*) drug war has been overt in its emphasis on interdiction and enforcement. The rhetoric of the Clinton war initially suggested a public health orientation, with proposed funding reversing to 70% for prevention/education/treatment and 30% for enforcement. Ultimately, however, Clinton's drug control strategy allocated 64% of the budget to enforcement (250). The result has been that more drug users than ever before have been arrested and incarcerated.

For women, the War on Drugs has been devastating, and for African American women, it has been a catastrophe. Drug *arrests* for women have escalated, and, according to Wellisch, Anglin, and Prendergast, "From 1982–1991 the number of women arrested for drug offenses, including possession, manufacturing and sale, increased 89%, a rate almost twice that for men during the same period" (209). *Incarceration* rates have also soared. From 1980, the beginning of the escalation of the War on Drugs, to 1992, when Clinton took office, the female prison population increased by 276%, compared with "just" 163% for men (245,251). Mandatory minimums had a tremendous impact on sentencing for women. In 1986, when the "mandatories" were instituted, 1 woman in 8 in prison was incarcerated for a drug-related crime; by 1991 that figure had increased to 1 in 3 women, an increase of 433% (compared with a 283% increase for men). Drug offenders accounted for 55% of the national increase during this period (252).

Women have been arrested and incarcerated at escalating rates, not because their criminality has increased or because they are more violent and threatening. Owen and Bloom found quite the opposite:

> Whereas the increasing population of imprisoned women implies an increased criminality among women, we disagree. Both our data and the research literature on imprisoned women stress the prominent role played by substance abuse, physical and sexual abuse, and poverty and underemployment in the role of female offenders. Our survey data also support the contention that a significant proportion of female offenders are not dangerous, are not career criminals, and thus do not represent a serious threat to the community. The impact of the huge increase in drug-related offenses is seen in the state and federal surveys, as well as in the California data. We suggest that the criminality of women has not increased; instead, the legal response to drug-related behavior has become increasingly punitive, resulting in a flood of less serious offenders into the state and federal prison systems (253).

African American women have experienced even more dramatic increases in arrest and incarceration rates. Between 1986 and 1991 there was an 828% increase in the number of African American women incarcerated for drug-related offenses, which was nearly double that of African American men (253). This increase is a result of conservative fiscal policies that reduced not only economic options but government support for the poor, as well as an escalation in criminal justice sanctions as part of the War on Drugs. The crack economy provided those without other options, economic options to earn money, at the cost of the incarceration of nearly 1 in 4 young, African American men.

The punishment of women extends far beyond themselves and into their families and communities. When women go to prison, the 125,000 children younger than age 18 years they leave behind, whose lives are disrupted emotionally, psychologically, and literally, feel their absence. One wonders who is actually being punished:

Children of incarcerated mothers suffer disproportionate disruption in their lives. In 1992, approximately 90% of fathers in state prisons reported that their children were living with the children's mothers. Only a quarter of female inmates had similar support from a father. Ten percent of mothers said their children were living in foster homes, children's agencies, or institutions. For children of women who are imprisoned more than once, the situation is even worse. Children are shuttled from home to home, relative to relative, institution to institution, returning to their mothers only to be separated again (254).

During the last 10 years researchers have argued that the War on Drugs has become a "War on Women" (255–259). Alternatives to prison, such as treatment, for drug-related nonviolent crimes, have not been realized. Despite a "treatment on demand" rhetoric emanating from Clinton's first drug czar, Lee Brown, Americans seem to be much more willing to spend shrinking funds on prisons than on options such as drug treatment, which cost a fraction, with the notable exceptions of New Mexico and California, where alternatives to incarceration have been publicly mandated. Despite evidence that women are overwhelmingly arrested and incarcerated on (nonviolent) drug charges, the vast majority has not, for a variety of reasons, been exposed to drug treatment (245,253,260,261).

Finally, the war on drugs has contributed directly to increased AIDS risk for women, their sexual partners, and their children. The government has gone beyond refusing to support and endorse needle exchange. The Clinton administration actively suppressed important evidence demonstrating the HIV-reducing efficacy (without increased drug use) of syringe exchange programs. The George W. Bush administration has continued to ignore the growing body of literature supporting needle-exchange programs.

RECOMMENDATIONS

In the early 1970s, Nixon's War on Drugs had begun, primarily to combat rising (drug-related) crime. This war had a heavy medical/rehabilitative orientation in which deviance was seen as illness. For example, it was during the early 1970s that methadone maintenance treatment became institutionalized (73). Simultaneously (and not coincidentally) increased federal funds for drug research became available. Drug-using women were seen as victims, "sicker" than their male counterparts. When the Reagan–Bush (*father*) War on Drugs escalated in the 1980s, users of illegal drugs were no longer seen as ill but bad, and culpable for their drug-related problems. Women bore the brunt of drug scapegoating, defined as epidemiologically dangerous and responsible for the spread of HIV to the heterosexual community. By the late 1980s, women drug users had become the less-than-human "crack moms" who were blamed and punished for creating a generation of permanently impaired children.

The increasing size and scope of the problem of women's substance abuse has been exacerbated, if not caused, by two national trends. First, poverty, homelessness, and substandard education and health care have increased since 1980 (262). As members of America's ever-growing "underclass," drug users' lives have become more chaotic, risky, dangerous, and violent (263). Second, for addicts without financial resources, access to drug treatment has become increasingly problematic as a result of a decline in federal funding of programs since 1976 (264). Although the Office of National Drug Control Policy advocates a shift in funding from enforcement to prevention and treatment, thus far drug users have experienced little change in access (265,266). Ironically, if money and availability *were* increased, it seems unlikely that even the best form of drug treatment could reverse the deleterious effects of the social and political policies implemented from the 1980s through the early years of the twenty-first century. Lacking a chance at the "American Dream" and a "stake in conventional life," drug abusers will continue to relieve their suffering through the use of pain-killing and euphoria-producing substances (267,268). Our recommendations for improving the lot of women drug users are both broad and specific. We believe that the "drug problem" has more to do with social conditions than drugs, and agree with Canadian Susan Boyd's recommendations about pregnancy and drug use:

> Exposure to toxic environments, malnutrition, lack of housing, lack of income, or poor antenatal care have adverse effects on pregnancy outcomes. If pregnancy outcomes were truly a "health issue" Canadians might consider eliminating the social environmental variables affecting pregnancy rather than stigmatizing a generation of children and their mothers (183, p. 188).

In addition to the "environmental" factors mentioned above, we would advocate for a wholly revamped society that is truly open and in which a range of life options are available to all. In the meantime, drug treatment should be expanded and embellished and a policy of harm reduction toward drug use instituted immediately.

TREATMENT

In general, more treatment slots are needed for both men and women drug users. Under the current inadequately funded system, there are long waiting lists and "treatment on demand" is anything but a reality, resulting in an underserved population of women (245,253,269). The lack of treatment slots is particularly glaring for pregnant women. In 1990, Wendy Chavkin conducted a survey of drug treatment facilities throughout New York City and found:

> The general shortage of treatment slots is aggravated by the unwillingness of many drug programs to include pregnant women. A recent survey in New York by the author revealed that 54% of treatment programs categorically excluded the pregnant. Effective availability was further limited by restrictions on method of payment or specific substance of abuse. Sixty-seven percent of the programs rejected pregnant Medicaid patients, and only 13% accepted pregnant Medicaid patients addicted to crack (270, p. 485).

Another survey conducted in the same year found of the approximately 675,000 pregnant women in need of drug treatment nationwide, less than 11% received it (173, p. 28). Most treatment facilities are unprepared and inadequate to the multiplicity of needs of pregnant women. Separate clinics or clinics within clinics must be institutionalized.

Current treatment models are male-oriented and not prepared to address women's multiple needs (17,50,83,223,271–276). For approximately 30 years, since the expansion of drug treatment, women have been motivated to enlist themselves in programs, primarily to get out of "the life" and to better fulfill their mothering roles. Currently, a majority of inpatient treatment programs require a minimum 30-day commitment and some are as long as 1 year. For a woman with young children, this can be an insurmountable obstacle (277,278). In 1981, Rosenbaum wrote:

> [L]ive-in treatment facilities—either equipped for detoxification or opiate-free—work better than other modalities (outpatient detox or methadone maintenance). For a woman addict, live-in treatment is currently possible if she has no commitments; to the 70 percent of the women in this sample who were mothers, treatment facilities without accommodations for children are of no use (17, p. 126).

Little has changed in the ensuing 22 years. Women who have substance abuse problems are still unable, for the most part, to find inpatient services that will accommodate their children (279). Those women who need outpatient services are also in need of assistance with their childcare responsibilities, such as supervised play areas for children within the treatment facility. In the context of counseling, programs also should be sensitive to women's privacy needs (17,273,274,280).

All treatment modalities that serve women must be sensitive to their special needs, including counseling, family therapy, and ancillary services, such as transportation, child care, children's health services, housing, legal assistance, and job or vocational training. They must also be sensitive to women's diverse cultural needs. Ideally, alternatives to the current system might include women-only treatment programs, inpatient programs that accept children, expansion (and in some areas of the country, creation) of clinics for pregnant women, special job training programs for women, and long-term commitment of funding for aftercare.

Both women drug users and treatment professionals must participate in the institutionalization of advocacy groups that could influence the formulation of treatment policy. Women's movements need to take advantage of the links between their political goals, such as the link between the abortion and drug wars. Resulting organizations would go a long way in combating the depression, isolation, and low self-esteem that persists among women in treatment (271,273,274,280,281). Treatment providers also need the support provided by gender-specific and in-service training in order to decrease burnout and increase program efficacy (282). Finally, public policy makers (e.g., legislators) need to be educated by treatment professionals, as well as by clients, to the needs of this population (229).

Treatment facilities also need to acknowledge the devastating impact of HIV and hepatitis C virus (HCV) on women drug users, and incorporate AIDS and hepatitis C education in their programs. HIV/HCV-positive women need special attention and allocated resources for services. Drug-treatment facilities must alter their admission criteria and treatment methods to accommodate women. They should include comprehensive services, including parenting and employment skills, workshops, and access to health care, and incorporate research and evaluation components with planned dissemination of results (283).

A POLICY OF HARM REDUCTION

Drug use has been with us for centuries and is part of our cultural, and perhaps biologic, heritage (284,285). Given current social and economic policies that limit life options, the sale and use of intoxicating substances is unlikely to disappear, despite our most fervent efforts at "zero tolerance." Americans do not like to admit failure, although the task of eliminating illegal drug use was impossible from the outset. Instead, we should look seriously at the adoption of "harm reduction" strategies, instead of futile attempts to eliminate drug use completely. Harm reduction is a set of principles that defines abstinence from drug use as just one of several means of reducing drug-related problems. It is a simple concept, not a camouflage for radical change in drug policy, that was first implemented

in Europe and Australia and used primarily to deal with the AIDS crisis. Those who subscribe to a harm-reduction perspective deplore, yet accept, the inevitability of drug abuse. They advocate for working *with* users to minimize the harms brought about by abuse, even if drug use itself cannot be stopped (286). Harm reduction shifts the focus away from idealistic long-term goals, such as abstinence from all drug use, toward more attainable short-term goals, such as safer behaviors.

As noted earlier, women interviewed by the authors, whether pregnant and using drugs, or enrolled in treatment, attempted to reduce drug-related harm for themselves and their offspring. These efforts should be encouraged and facilitated. Women should have better information so their efforts are more effective. Those who intervene should stop punishing pregnant women and instead facilitate their harm reduction efforts. Women should have access to health care without the risk of humiliation or losing their baby to social service agencies. They should have access to treatment that does not require total abstinence. Finally, professionals in research and treatment must learn to settle for less, because insisting on absolute perfection may exacerbate the problem.

Motherhood is at the core of many drug-using women's identities. They love and care very much about their children, who often provide the impetus for harm reduction through exiting "the life" or instituting safer behaviors. Because American society is currently consumed with "family values," drug-using women should derive some of the benefits of this perspective. To begin, they should have the resources to raise children in this country—to feed, house, clothe, and educate them. On the meager, subsistence level provided by our government (which is currently being reduced), paying the rent, providing food, and buying clothes and school supplies is nearly impossible. When women take refuge from this depressing, hopeless, and seemingly endless existence through drugs, social service agencies threaten to take away their most precious "possession." Their children are placed in foster care or with relatives, where they may "bounce around" for years. Loss of custody results in a further spiraling into drug abuse and the commitment on the part of women to have another "replacement" baby in order to regain "one's ideal image of oneself as a competent mother" (287, p. 149). Obviously we should weigh levels of harm and rethink social service policies. Rather than removal of custody, we should provide women with the resources needed to raise their children.

Treatment should be expanded and sensitized to women's needs. In addition, a harm-reduction perspective within the context of drug treatment should be instituted. Women often enlist in programs when their drug careers are at the height of risk and chaos. The recovery process is slow, and requires an extended period of time during which the woman is not always abstinent from drugs. Treatment should be seen as a *process* of harm reduction, during which deleterious behaviors are gradually eliminated. For example, if a woman enters treatment with a 365-day "habit" and after a month reduces her drug use to weekends, this should be seen as progress, not as failure. The very last action taken by a treatment program should not be to terminate the woman from the program. Instead, she should be encouraged to stay in treatment and further reduce the harms related to her drug use.

Alternatives to incarceration that reduce harm should be explored and instituted. Teresa Albor argues:

> In an immediate and practical sense, it is time to recognize that there are forms of punishment for women that are more effective, less expensive, and cause less disruption to families. These include small model programs in which mothers live with their children while serving sentences, community correction or restitution, and home-based confinement using electronic monitoring. Instead of building more prisons for women, we should use scarce resources for prison-based reproductive health counseling, education, vocational training, and post-release programs, which provide former inmates with continued access to alcohol and drug treatment and other emotional support. And if mothers must be in prison, it is essential that they be able to get together with their children for weekend retreats, or that transportation be provided for the children so they can visit their mothers.
>
> It is time to raise the more radical question of whether most women offenders should be incarcerated at all. Most female prisoners don't belong in prison and are harmed by the experience. Most are women whom society has failed. When we lock them up, separate them from their children, provide inadequate health care and rehabilitative services, and treat them as loathsome and irresponsible criminals, that failure is amplified. Removing women from their families perpetuates cycles of criminality and dysfunction by both the mothers and their children. The ultimate cost to society is far greater than if these families had not been torn apart (288, p. 237).

Needle-exchange programs reduce syringe-related HIV risk in the general population of IDUs and for women in particular (289). The Bush (*son*) administration should stop suppressing evidence of the efficacy of syringe exchange and make this harm-reducing program fully accessible to women (and men).

The United States has been slow in adopting harm-reduction strategies (286,290,291). A notable exception is MMT, which has been used, but not without controversy, for some 40 years (73). This is largely a result of fear on the part of policy makers that a harm-reduction message will encourage increased drug use among current users and lead to the initiation of new users (292). In fact, there is no evidence to suggest that harm-reduction strategies, such as safer drug-using messages, needle-exchange programs, and greater access to treatment, increase drug use (291,293–295). We can only hope the continued failure of criminal justice/interdiction strategies will eventually enlighten Americans to the only pragmatic course regarding women (and men) who use drugs, the institutionalization of harm reduction as policy.

REFERENCES

1. NIDA Household Survey. *Preliminary estimates from the 1994 National Household Survey on Drug Abuse.* Washington, DC: U.S. Department of Health and Human Services, 1995:77.
2. Kandall SR. *Substance and shadow: women and addiction in the United States.* Cambridge, MA: Harvard University Press, 1996.
3. Hunt LG, Chambers CD. *The heroin epidemics.* New York: Spectrum, 1976.
4. Hunt LG. Prevalence of active heroin use in the United States. *NIDA Res Monogr* 1977;16:61–86.
5. Walter PV, Sheridan BK, Chambers CD. Methadone diversion: a study of illicit availability. In: Chambers CD, Brill L, eds. *Methadone: experiences and issues.* New York: Behavioral Publications, 1973:171–176.
6. Cuskey WR, Wathey RB. *Female addiction.* Lexington, MA: Lexington Books, 1982.
7. DeLeon G. Phoenix House: psychopathological signs among male and female drug-free residents. *Addict Dis* 1974;(1):135.
8. Ellinwood EH, Smith WG, Vaillant GE. Narcotic addiction in males and females: a comparison. *Int J Addict* 1966;1:33.
9. Miller JS. Value patterns of drug addicts as a function of race and sex. *Int J Addict* 1973;8:4.
10. Waldorf D. *Careers in dope.* Englewood Cliffs, NJ: Prentice-Hall, 1973.
11. Cuskey WR, Moffet AD, Clifford HB. A comparison of female opiate addicts admitted to Lexington Hospital in 1961 and 1967. In: Cohen CS, Roningson S, Smart R, eds. *Psychotherapy and drug addiction. I: diagnosis and treatment.* New York: MSS Information, 1974;89–103.
12. Baldinger R, Goldsmith BM, Capel WG. Pot smokers, junkies and squares: a comparative study of female values. *Int J Addict* 1972;7:153.
13. Climent CE. Epidemiological studies of female prisoners: biological, psychological, and social correlates of drug addiction. *Int J Addict* 1974;9:345.
14. Adler F, Simon R. *The criminology of deviant women.* Boston: Houghton Mifflin, 1979.
15. James J. Prostitution and addiction: an interdisciplinary approach. *Addict Dis* 1976;2:601–618.
16. Goldstein P. *Prostitution and drugs.* Lexington, MA: Lexington Books, 1979.
17. Rosenbaum M. *Women on heroin.* New Brunswick, NJ: Rutgers University Press, 1981.
18. d'Orban PT. Heroin dependency and delinquency in women—a study of heroin addicts in Holloway Prison. *Br J Addict* 1970;65:67.
19. File KN, McCahill TW, Savitz LD. Narcotics involvements and female criminality. *Addict Dis* 1974;1:177.
20. Weissman JC, File KN. Criminal behavior patterns of female addicts: a comparison of findings in two cities. *Int J Addict* 1976;11:6.
21. Chambers C, Inciardi J. *Some aspects of the criminal careers of female narcotics addicts.* Paper presented to the Southern Sociological Society, Miami Beach, FL, 1971.

22. James J. *Female addiction and criminal involvement.* Paper presented to the Pacific Sociological Association, Victoria, British Columbia, 1975.
23. Klein D, Kress J. Any woman's blues: a critical overview of women, crime and the criminal justice system. *Crim Soc Justice* 1976;5:34–39.
24. Steffensmeier DJ. *Contemporary patterns of female criminality.* Paper presented at the 39th annual meeting of the American Society of Criminology, Montreal, November, 1987.
25. Ball R, Lilly JR. Female delinquency in an urban country. *Criminology* 1976;14:279–281.
26. Chambers C, Hinesley RK, Moldstad M. Narcotic addiction in females: a race comparison. *Int J Addict* 1970;5:257.
27. Cuskey WR. Survey of opiate addiction among females in the United States between 1850 and 1970. *Public Health Rev* 1972;1:8–39.
28. Densen-Gerber J, Weiner M, Hochstedler R. Sexual behavior, abortion, and birth control in heroin addicts: legal and psychiatric considerations. *Contemp Drug Probl* 1972;1:783.
29. Eldred CA, Washington MM. Female heroin addicts in a city treatment program: the forgotten minority. *Psychiatry* 1975;38:75.
30. Fiddle S. Sequences in addiction. *Addict Dis* 1976;2:553–567.
31. Rosenbaum M. Sex roles among deviants: the woman addict. *Int J Addict* 1981;16(3):859–877.
32. Sutter A. The world of the righteous dope fiend. *Issues Criminol* 1966;2:177–182.
33. Yablonsky L. *Synanon: the tunnel back.* New York: Macmillan, 1965.
34. Zahn M, Ball J. Patterns and causes of drug addiction among Puerto Rican females. *Addict Dis* 1974;1:203–214.
35. Blinick G. Fertility of narcotics addicts and effects of addiction on the offspring. *Soc Biol* 1971;18:S34–S39.
36. Blinick G, Wallach C, Jerez EM. Pregnancy in narcotics addicts treated by medical withdrawal. *Am J Obstet Gynecol* 1969;105:997–1003.
37. Finnegan LP. Narcotics dependence in pregnancy. *J Psychedelic Drugs* 1975;7(Jul-Sep):3.
38. Finnegan LP. Women in treatment. In: Dupont R, Goldstein A, O'Donnell J, eds. *Handbook on drug abuse.* Rockville, MD: National Institute on Drug Abuse, 1979.
39. Glass L. Narcotic withdrawal in the newborn infant. *J Natl Med Assoc* 1974;6:117–118.
40. Kandall SR, Albin S, Lowinson J, et al. Differential effects of maternal heroin and methadone use on birthweight. *Pediatrics* 1976;58:681–685.

41. Naeye RL, Blanc W, Leblanc W, et al. Fetal complications of maternal heroin addiction: abnormal growth, infection and episodes of stress. *J Pediatr* 1973;83:1055–1061.
42. Naeye RL, Ladis B, Drage JS. Sudden infant death syndrome. A prospective study. *Am J Dis Child* 1976;130:1207–1210.
43. Ostrea EM, Chavez CJ, Strauss ME. A study of factors that influence the severity of neonatal narcotic withdrawal. *J Pediatr* 1976;88:642–645.
44. Rementeria JL, Nunag NN. Narcotic withdrawal in pregnancy. *Am J Obstet Gynecol* 1973;116:1052–1056.
45. Stone ML, Salerna LJ, Green M. Narcotic addiction in pregnancy. *Am J Obstet Gynecol* 1971;109:716.
46. Wilson G, McCreary K, Kean J, et al. The development of preschool children of heroin-addicted mothers: a controlled study. *Pediatrics* 1979;63:135–141.
47. Zelson C. Infant of the addicted mother. *N Engl J Med* 1973;288:26.
48. Zuspan F, Gumpel J, Mejia-Zelaya A, et al. Fetal stress from methadone withdrawal. *Am J Obstet Gynecol* 1975;2:43–48.
49. Blume S. Chemical dependency in women: important issues. *Am J Drug Alcohol Abuse* 1990;16(3,4):297–309.
50. Cuskey WR, Berger L, Densen-Gerber J. Issues in the treatment of female addiction: a review and critique of the literature. *Contemp Drug Probl* 1977;6:307–371.
51. Rosenbaum M, Murphy S. Getting the treatment: recycling women addicts. *J Psychoactive Drugs* 1981;13(1):1–13.
52. Ruzek SK. *Report to the California State Office of Narcotics and Drug Abuse. Prevention and treatment of female drug dependency.* Sacramento, CA, 1974.
53. Blinick G, Jerez E, Wallach RC. Methadone maintenance, pregnancy and progeny. *JAMA* 1973;225:447–449.
54. Blinick G, Inturrisi C, Jerez E. Methadone assays in pregnant women and progeny. *Am J Obstet Gynecol* 1975;1:617–619.
55. Clark D, Keith L, Pildes R. Drug-dependent obstetric patients. *J Obstet Gynecol Nurs* 1974;3:17–20.
56. Cohen SN, Neumann LL. Methadone maintenance during pregnancy. *Am J Dis Child* 1973;6:445–446.
57. Connaughton JF, Finnegan LP, Schut J, et al. Current concepts in the management of the pregnant opiate addict. *Addict Dis* 1975;2:21–35.
58. Connaughton JF, Reeser D, Schut J, et al. Perinatal addiction: outcome and management. *Am J Obstet Gynecol* 1977;9:679–686.

59. Finnegan LP. *Drug dependence in pregnancy: clinical management of mother and child. A manual for medical professionals and paraprofessionals prepared for the National Institute on Drug Abuse, Services Research Branch.* Washington, DC: U.S. Government Printing Office, 1978.
60. Finnegan LP, Connaughton JF, Emich JP. Comprehensive care of the pregnant addict and its effect on maternal and infant outcome. *Contemp Drug Probl* 1972;1:795.
61. Harper RG, Solish GI, Purow HM, et al. The effect of a methadone treatment program upon pregnant heroin addicts and their newborn infants. *Pediatrics* 1974;54:300–305.
62. Newman RG. Pregnancies of methadone patients. *N Y State J Med* 1974;1:52–54.
63. Rajegowda BK, Glass L, Evans HE, et al. Methadone withdrawal in newborn infants. *J Pediatr* 1972;81(3):532–534.
64. Ramer CM, Lodge A. Clinical and developmental characteristics of infants of mothers on methadone maintenance. *Addict Dis* 1975;2:227–233.
65. Statzer DE, Wardell JN. Heroin addiction during pregnancy. *Am J Obstet Gynecol* 1966;94:253–257.
66. Sullivan RD, Fischbach AL, Hornick FW. Treatment of a pregnant opiate addict with oral methadone. *Ariz Med* 1972;29:30.
67. Waldeman H. Psychiatric emergencies during pregnancy and in the puerperium. *Munch Med Wochenschr* 1973;115:1039–1043.
68. Wallach RC, Jerez E, Blinick G. Pregnancy and menstrual function in narcotics addicts treated with methadone, the Methadone Maintenance Treatment Program. *Am J Obstet Gynecol* 1969;105(8):1226–1229.
69. Zelson C, Lee SJ, Casalino M. Neonatal narcotic addiction: comparative effects of maternal intake of heroin and methadone. *N Engl J Med* 1973;289(23):16–20.
70. Zelson C. Infant of the addicted mother. *N Engl J Med* 1973;288:1393–1395.
71. Davis RC, Chappel JN. *Pregnancy in the context of narcotic addiction and methadone maintenance.* Paper presented at the Fifth National Conference on Methadone Treatment, Washington, DC, March, 1973.
72. Arif A, Westermeyer J. *Methadone in the management of opioid dependence: programs and policies around the world.* Geneva: World Health Organization, 1988.
73. Rosenbaum M. The demedicalization of methadone maintenance. *J Psychoactive Drugs* 1995;27(2):145–149.

74. Rosenbaum M. Getting on methadone. *Contemp Drug Probl Law Q* 1982; Spring:113–143.

75. Finnegan LP, Connaughton JF, Emich JP. Abstinence score in the treatment of infants of drug-dependent mothers. *Pediatr Res* 1973;7:319.

76. Lodge A, Marcus MM, Ramer CM. Behavioral and electro-physiological characteristics of the addicted neonate. *Addict Dis Int J* 1975;2:235–255.

77. Mondanaro J. Women: pregnancy, children and addiction. *J Psychedelic Drugs* 1977;9(1):59–68.

78. Reddy AM, Harper RG, Stern G. Observation on heroin and methadone withdrawal in the newborn. *J Pediatr* 1971;48:353–358.

79. Glaser F. Narcotic addiction in the pain-prone female patient. *Int J Addict* 1966;1:2.

80. Chein I, Gerard DL, Lee RS, et al. *The road to H.* New York: Basic Books, 1964.

81. Soler E, Ponser L, Abod J. Women in treatment: client self-report. In: Bauman A, et al., eds. *Women in treatment: issues and approaches.* Arlington, VA: National Drug Abuse Center for Training and Resource Development, 1976.

82. White L. It isn't easy being gay. In: Bauman A, et al., eds. *Women in treatment: issues and approaches.* Arlington, VA: National Drug Abuse Center for Training and Resource Development, 1976.

83. Levy SJ, Doyle KM. Attitudes toward women in a drug treatment program. *J Drug Issues* 1974;4:423–434.

84. Centers for Disease Control. *HIV AIDS Surveill Rep* 1994;6(2):12.

85. Kane S. HIV, heroin, and heterosexual relations. *Soc Sci Med* 1991;32(9):1037–1050.

86. Campbell CA. Women and AIDS. *Soc Sci Med* 1990;30:407–415.

87. Carpenter CCJ, Mayer KH, Stein MD, et al. Human immunodeficiency virus infection in North American women: experience with 200 cases and a review of the literature. *Medicine (Baltimore)* 1991;70(5):307–325.

88. Cohen JB, Haver LB, Wofsy CB. Women and intravenous drugs: parenteral and heterosexual transmission of human immunodeficiency virus. *J Drug Issues* 1989;19:39–56.

89. Feucht TE, Stephens RC, Roman SW. The sexual behavior of intravenous drug users: assessing the risk of sexual transmission of HIV. *J Drug Issues* 1990;20(2):195–213.

90. Klee H, Faugier J, Hayes C, et al. Sexual partners of injecting drug users: the risk for HIV infection. *Br J Addict* 1990;85:413–418.

91. McCoy HV, Inciardi JA. Women and AIDS: social determinants of sex-related activities. *Womens Health* 1993;20(1):69–86.

92. Mondanaro J. Strategies for AIDS prevention: motivating health behavior in drug-dependent women. *J Psychoactive Drugs* 1987;19(2):143–149.

93. Project MENU (Methods Estimating Needle Users At Risk for AIDS). *Section three: what percentage of drug injectors are women? An analysis of gender-by-age interactions of drug injectors on three reporting systems in three cities.* Unpublished report, 1989.

94. Schilling RF, El-Bassel N, Schinke SP, et al. Sexual behavior, attitudes towards safer sex, and gender among a cohort of 244 recovering IV drug users. *Int J Addict* 1991;26:865–883.

95. Weiss SH, Weston CB, Quirinale J. Safe sex? Misconceptions, gender differences and barriers among injection drug users: a focus group approach. *AIDS Educ Prev* 1993;5(4):279–293.

96. Amaro H. Love, sex, and power: considering women's realities in HIV prevention. *Am Psychol* 1995;50:437–447.

97. Brown V, Weissman G. Women and men injecting drug users: an updated look at gender differences and risk factors. In: Brown B, Beschner F, eds. *At risk for AIDS: injection drug users and their partners.* Westport, CT: Greenwood Press, 1994.

98. Murphy DL. Heterosexual contacts of intravenous drug abusers: implications for the next spread of the AIDS epidemic. *Adv Alcohol Subst Abuse* 1987;7:89–97.

99. Murphy S. Intravenous drug use and AIDS: notes on the social economy of needle sharing. *Contemp Drug Probl* 1987;14:373–395.

100. Wayment H, Newcomb MD, Hannemann VL. Female and male intravenous drug users not-in-treatment: are they at differential risk for AIDS? *Sex Roles* 1993;28(1,2):111–125.

101. Rosenbaum M. Women addicts' experience of the heroin world: risk, chaos, and inundation. *Urban Life* 1981;10(1):65–91.

102. Argeriou M, McCarty D, Potter D, et al. Characteristics of men and women arrested for driving under the influence of liquor. *Alcohol Treat Q* 1986;3:127–137.

103. Brady KT, Grice DE, Dustan L, et al. Gender differences in substance use disorders. *Am J Psychiatry* 1993;150:1707–1711.

104. Ferrence R, Whitehead P. Sex differences in psychoactive drug use: recent epidemiology. In: Kalant OJ, ed. *Research advances and drug problems: vol. 5. Alcohol and drug problems in women.* New York: Plenum, 1980:125–201.

105. Griffin ML, Weiss RD, Mirin SM, et al. A comparison of male and female cocaine abusers. *Arch Gen Psychiatry* 1989;46:122–126.

106. Kuhns JB, Heide KM, Silverman I. Substance use/misuse among female prostitutes and female arrestees. *Int J Addict* 1992;27(11):1283–1292.

107. Marshall N, Hendtlass J. Drugs and prostitution. *J Drug Issues* 1986; 16:237–248.

108. Plant ML, Plant MA, Peck DF, et al. The sex industry, alcohol, and illicit drugs: implications for the spread of HIV infection. *Br J Addict* 1989;84(1):53–59.

109. McKeganey NP. Prostitution and HIV: what do we know and where might research be targeted in the future. *AIDS* 1994;8:1215–1226.

110. Cohen JB, Alexander P, Wofsy C. Prostitutes and AIDS: public policy issues. *AIDS Public Policy* 1988;3(2):16–22.

111. Dorfman LE, Derish PA, Cohen JB. Hey girlfriend: an evaluation of AIDS prevention among women in the sex industry. *Health Educ Q* 1992;19(1):25–40.

112. Rosenbaum M, Washburn A, Knight KR, et al. *Methadone maintenance: treatment as harm reduction, policy as harm maximization. Final Report to the National Institute on Drug Abuse.* Grant #1 R01 DA08982, 1995.

113. Worth D. Sexual decision-making and AIDS: why condom promotion among vulnerable women is likely to fail. *Stud Fam Plann* 1989;20(6):297–307.

114. Corby NH, Wolitski RJ, Thornton-Johnson S, et al. AIDS knowledge, perception of risk, and behaviors among female sex partners of injection drug users. *AIDS Educ Prev* 1991;3(4):353–366.

115. Kim MY, Marmor M, Dubin N, et al. HIV risk-related sexual behaviors among heterosexuals in New York City: associations with race, sex, and intravenous drug use. *AIDS* 1993;7:409–414.

116. Lewis DK, Watters JK. Human immunodeficiency virus seroprevalence in female intravenous drug users: the puzzle of black women's risk. *Soc Sci Med* 1989;29:1071–1076.

117. Lewis DK, Watters JK. Sexual risk behavior among heterosexual intravenous drug users: ethnic and gender variations. *AIDS* 1991;5:67–73.

118. Mays VM, Cochran SD. Issues in the perception of AIDS risk and risk reduction activities by black and Hispanic/Latina women. *Am Psychol* 1988;43(1):949–957.

119. Nyamathi A, Vasquez R. Impact of poverty, homelessness, and drugs on Hispanic women at risk for

HIV infection. *Hispanic J Behav Sci* 1989;11(4):299–314.

120. Nyamathi A, Shin DM. Designing a culturally sensitive AIDS educational program for black and Hispanic women of childbearing age. *NAACOGS Clin Issu Perinat Womens Health Nurs* 1990;1(1):86–98.

121. Nyamathi A. Comparative study of factors relating to HIV risk level of black homeless women. *J Acquir Immune Defic Syndr* 1992;5:222–228.

122. Nyamathi A, Flaskerud J. A community-based inventory of current concerns of impoverished homeless and drug-addicted women. *Res Nurs Health* 1992;15:121–129.

123. Pivnick A. HIV infection and the meaning of condoms. *Cult Med Psychiatry* 1993;17:431–453.

124. Grella C, Annon J, Anglin MD. Ethnic differences in HIV risk behaviors, self-perceptions, and treatment outcomes among women in methadone maintenance treatment. *J Psychoactive Drugs* 1995;27(4):421–433.

125. Abelson HI, Miller JD. A decade of trends in cocaine use in the household population. *NIDA Res Monogr* 1985;61:35–49.

126. Adams EH, Durell J. Cocaine: a growing public health problem. *NIDA Res Monogr* 1984;50:9–14.

127. Inciardi J. *The war on drugs: heroin, cocaine, crime and public policy.* Palo Alto, CA: Mayfield Publishing, 1986.

128. Johnston LD, Bachman JG, O'Malley PM. *Highlights from student drug use in America, 1975–1984.* Washington, DC: National Institute on Drug Abuse, U.S. Department of Health and Human Services, 1984.

129. National Institute on Drug Abuse. *Highlights: 1985 National Household Survey on Drug Abuse.* Washington, DC: U.S. Government Printing Office, 1987.

130. Clayton R, Voss H, Robbins C, et al. Gender preferences in drug use: an epidemiological perspective. *NIDA Res Monogr* 1986;65:80–99.

131. Erickson PG, Murray GF. Sex differences in cocaine use and experience: a double standard revived? *Am J Drug Alcohol Abuse* 1989;15(2):135–152.

132. Siegel RK. Cocaine and sexual dysfunction: the curse of mama coca. *J Psychoactive Drugs* 1982;14(1,2):71–74.

133. Smith DE, Wesson DR, Apter-Marsh M. Cocaine and alcohol induced sexual dysfunction in patients with addictive disease. *J Psychoactive Drugs* 1984;16:359–361.

134. Inciardi JA. *Kingrats, chicken heads, slow necks, freaks, and bloodsuckers: a glimpse at the Miami sex for crack market.* Paper presented at the Annual Meeting of the Society for Applied Anthropology, Charleston, SC, March 13–17, 1991.

135. Inciardi JA, Lockwood D, Pottieger AE. Crack-dependent women and sexuality: implications for STD acquisition and transmission. *Addict Recovery* 1991;2:25–28.

136. McCoy HV, Miles C, Inciardi J. Survival sex: inner-city women and crack cocaine. In: Inciardi J, McElrath K, eds. *The American drug scene: an anthology.* Los Angeles: Roxbury, 1995;172–177.

137. Siegal HA, Carlson RG, Falck R, et al. High risk behaviors for transmission of syphilis and human immunodeficiency virus among crack cocaine-using women: a case study from the Midwest. *Sex Transm Dis* 1992;19(5):266–271.

138. Fullilove MT, Fullilove RE. Black teen crack use and sexually transmitted diseases. *J Am Med Womens Assoc* 1989;44(5):146–147, 151–153.

139. Bowser B. Crack and AIDS: an ethnographic impression. *J Natl Med Assoc* 1989;81:538–540.

140. Chitwood D. Epidemiology of crack use among injection drug users and partners of injection drug users. In: Brown BS, Beschner GM, eds. *Handbook on risk for AIDS: injection drug users and sexual partners.* Westport, CT: Greenwood Press, 1993.

141. Centers for Disease Control and Prevention. Update: AIDS among women—United States, 1994. *MMWR Morb Mortal Wkly Rep* 1995;44(5):81–84.

142. Adler P. *Wheeling and dealing: an ethnography of an upper-level drug dealing and smuggling community.* New York: Columbia University Press, 1985.

143. Bourgois P. In search of Horatio Alger: culture and ideology in the crack economy. *Contemp Drug Probl* 1989;16:619–650.

144. Fagan J. Women and drugs revisited: female participation in the cocaine economy. *J Drug Issues* 1994;24(2):175–225.

145. Morningstar PJ, Chitwood DD. How women and men get cocaine: sex-role stereotypes and acquisition patterns. *J Psychoactive Drugs* 1987;19(2):135–142.

146. Murphy S, Rosenbaum M. Women who use cocaine too much: smoking crack vs. snorting cocaine. *J Psychoactive Drugs* 1992;24(4):381–388.

147. Acker D, Sachs BP, Tracey KJ, et al. Abruptio placentae associated with cocaine use. *Am J Obstet Gynecol* 1983;146(2):220–221.

148. Newald I. Cocaine infants. *Hospitals* 1986;60:76.

149. Murphy S. *It takes your womanhood: women and crack cocaine.* Unpublished manuscript 1994.

150. Kearney MH, Murphy S, Rosenbaum M. Learning by losing: sex and fertility on crack cocaine. *Qual Health Res* 1994;4(2):147.

151. Kearney MH, Murphy S, Rosenbaum M. Mothering on crack cocaine: a grounded theory analysis. *Soc Sci Med* 1994;38(2):351–361.

152. Rosenbaum M, Murphy S, Irwin J, et al. Women and crack: what's the real story? In: Trebach A, Zeese K, eds. *Drug prohibition and the conscience of nations.* Washington, DC: Drug Policy Foundation, 1990.

153. Chasnoff IJ. Drug use and women: establishing a standard of care. *Ann N Y Acad Sci* 1989;562:2008–2010.

154. Blakeslee S. Crack's toll among babies: a joyless view, even of toys. *New York Times* 1989 Sep 17(sect 1):1.

155. The instincts of parenthood become part of crack's toll. *New York Times* 1990 Mar 17.

156. Study of addicted babies hints vast cost. *New York Times* 1990 Mar 17(sect 1):8.

157. Crack babies. *Economist* 1989 Apr 1:28.

158. Gillman D. The children of crack. *Washington Post* 1989 Jul 31(sect D):3.

159. Kadaba LS. Crack's costly legacy. *Boston Globe* 1990 Jul 1(sect B):19.

160. Crack babies: the numbers mount. *Los Angeles Times* 1990 Mar 17.

161. Crack's smallest, costliest victims. *New York Times* 1989 Aug (sect A):14.

162. Crack mothers, crack babies and hope. *New York Times* 1989 Dec 31(sect 4):10.

163. "Crack babies" in Gainesville schools foreseen. *Atlanta Constitution* 1990 Mar 19(sect C):3.

164. Will area schools be ready to rehabilitate crack babies? *Atlanta Journal* 1990 Apr 16:8(sect A).

165. Dorris M. A desperate crack legacy. *Newsweek* 1990 Jun 25.

166. Milloy C. A time bomb in cocaine babies. *Washington Post* 1989 Sep 17(sect B):3.

167. Crack babies turn 5, and schools brace. *New York Times* 1990 May 25(sect 1):1.

168. Sanchez R. Addicts' children a new challenge to schools. *Washington Post* 1990;Nov 14(sect D):1.

169. Beckett K. Fetal rights and "crack moms": pregnant women in the war on drugs. *Contemp Drug Probl* 1995;22(4):587–612.

170. Balisy SS. Maternal substance abuse: the need to provide legal protection for the fetus. *So Calif Law Rev* 1987;60:1209–1238.

171. Maher L. Punishment and welfare:

crack cocaine and the regulation of mothering. In: Feinman C, ed. *The criminalization of a woman's body*. New York: Haworth Press, 1992.

172. Norton-Hawk MA. How social policies make matters worse: the case of maternal substance abuse. *J Drug Issues* 1994;24(3):517–526.

173. Paltrow L. *Criminal prosecutions against pregnant women. National update and overview*. Reproductive Freedom Project, American Civil Liberties Union Foundation, New York, New York, 1992.

174. Siegel L. The criminalization of pregnant and child-rearing drug users. *Drug Law Rep* 1990;2(15):169–176.

175. Vega W, Kolody B, Noble A, et al. *Profile of alcohol and drug use during pregnancy in California, 1992; final report*. Contract No. 91–00252. State of California, Health and Welfare Agency, Department of Alcohol and Drug Programs, Sacramento California, 1993.

176. Paltrow L. Winning strategies: defending the rights of pregnant addicts. *Champion* 1993 Aug.

177. Coles CD, Platzman KA, Smith I, et al. Effects of cocaine and alcohol use in pregnancy and neonatal growth and neurobehavioral status. *Neurotoxicol Teratol* 1992;14:23–33.

178. Hepburn M. Drug use in pregnancy. *Br J Hosp Med* 1993;49(1):51–55.

179. Lutiger B, Graham K, Einarson TR, et al. Relationship between gestational cocaine use and pregnancy outcome: a meta-analysis. *Teratology* 1991;44(1):405–414.

180. Mathias R. Developmental effects of prenatal drug exposure may be overcome by postnatal environment. *NIDA Notes* 1992;7(1):14–17.

181. Woodhouse BB. Poor mothers, poor babies: law, medicine, and crack. In: Humm SR, et al., eds. *Child, parent and state: law and policy reader*. Philadelphia: Temple University Press, 1994.

182. Zuckerman B. Drug exposed infants: understanding the medical risk. *Future Child* 1991;1(1):26–35.

183. Boyd S. Women and illicit drug use. *Int J Drug Policy* 1994;5(3):185–189.

184. Humphries D, Dawson J, Cronin V, et al. Mothers and children, drugs and crack: reactions to maternal drug dependency. In: Feinman C, ed. *The criminalization of a woman's body*. New York: Haworth Press, 1992:203–221.

185. Weissman G, Sowder B, Young P. *The relationship between crack cocaine use and other risk factors among women in a national AIDS prevention program*. Poster session presented at the Sixth International Conference on AIDS, San Francisco, June 10–24, 1990.

186. Oakley A. *The captured womb*. Oxford: Basil Blackwell, 1984.

187. Gallagher J. Fetus as patient. In: Cohen S, Taub N, eds. *Reproductive laws for the 1990s*. Totowa, NJ: Humana Press, 1989:185–235.

188. Roberts DE. Punishing drug addicts who have babies: women of color, equality, and right of privacy. *Harv Law Rev* 1991;194:1419–1482.

189. Chasnoff IJ, Landress HJ, Barrett ME. The prevalence of illicit-drug or alcohol use during pregnancy and discrepancies in mandatory reporting in Pinellas County, Florida. *N Engl J Med* 1990;322(17):1202–1206.

190. Moss K, Crockett J. *Testimony on children of substance abusers*. New York: Reproductive Freedom Project, American Civil Liberties Union, 1990.

191. Bader EJ. Pregnant drug users face jail. *New Direct Women* 1990;19:2.

192. Reinarman C, Levine HG. The crack attack: politics and media in America's latest drug scare. In: Best J, ed. *Images and issues: typifying contemporary social problems*. 2nd ed. New York: Aldine De Gruyter, 1995:147–186.

193. Trebach A, Zeese K, eds. *Drug prohibition and the conscience of nations*. Washington, DC: Drug Policy Foundation, 1990.

194. Maher L. Criminalizing pregnancy: the downside of a kinder, gentler nation? *Soc Justice* 1990;17(3):111–135.

195. Gomby DS, Shiono PH. Estimating the number of drug exposed infants. *Future Child* 1991;1(1):17–25.

196. Zuckerman BS, Frank DA, Hingson R, et al. Effect of maternal marijuana and cocaine use on fetal growth. *N Engl J Med* 1989;320:762–768.

197. Amaro H, Fried L, Cabral H, et al. Violence during pregnancy: the relationship to drug use among women and their partners. *Am J Public Health* 1990;80(5):575–579.

198. Robins L, Mills N. Effects of *in utero* exposure to street drugs. *Am J Public Health* 1993;83[Suppl]:9–13.

199. Stranz I, Welch S. Postpartum women in outpatient drug abuse treatment: correlates of retention/completion. *J Psychoactive Drugs* 1995;27(4):357–373.

200. Irwin K. Ideology, pregnancy and drugs: differences between crack-cocaine, heroin and methamphetamine users. *Contemp Drug Probl* 1995;22(4):613–638.

201. Kearney MH. Damned if you do, damned if you don't: crack cocaine users and prenatal care. *Contemp Drug Probl* 1995;22(4):639–662.

202. Vega WA, Kolody B, Hwang J, et al. Prevalence and magnitude of perinatal substance exposures in California. *N Engl J Med* 1993;329(12):850–854.

203. Chavkin W, Allen M, Oberman M. Drug abuse and pregnancy: some questions on public policy, clinical management, and maternal and fetal rights. *Birth* 1991;18(2):107–112.

204. Friedman J, Alicea M. Women and heroin: the path of resistance and its consequences. *Gender Soc* 1994;9(4):432–449.

205. Ettorre E. *Women and substance use*. New Brunswick, NJ: Rutgers University Press, 1992.

206. Taylor A. *Women drug users*. Oxford: Clarendon Press, 1993.

207. Dunlap E, Johnson BD. *Aggression, violence, and family life in crack seller/abuser households*. Paper presented at the American Sociological Association annual meeting, Los Angeles, CA, August, 1994.

208. Regan D, O'Malley LB, Finnegan LP. The incidence of violence in the lives of pregnant drug-dependent women. *Pediatr Res* 1982;16:77, 330.

209. Wellisch J, Anglin MD, Prendergast ML. Numbers and characteristics of drug-using women in the criminal justice system: implications for treatment. *J Drug Issues* 1993;23(1):7–30.

210. Boyd CJ. The antecedents of women's crack cocaine abuse: family substance abuse, sexual abuse, depression and illicit drug use. *J Subst Abuse Treat* 1993;10:433–438.

211. Dobash RE, Dobash RP. *Women, violence, and social change*. New York: Routledge, 1992.

212. Finkelhor D. The sexual abuse of children: current research reviewed. *Psychiatr Ann* 1987;17:233–241.

213. Hagan TA, Finnegan LP, Nelson-Zlupko L. Impediments to comprehensive treatment models for substance-dependent women: treatment and research questions. *J Psychoactive Drugs* 1994;26(2):163–171.

214. Hagan TA, Kaltenback K. *Women and drug dependency: a developmental approach to recovery*. Unpublished paper, 1994.

215. James J, Meyerding J. Early sexual experience and prostitution. *Am J Psychiatry* 1977;134(12):1381–1385.

216. Ladwig G, Andersen M. Substance abuse in women: relationship between chemical dependency of women and past reports of physical and/or sexual abuse. *Int J Addict* 1989;24(8):739–754.

217. Lowrance N. Domestic violence. In: Eng RC, ed. *Women: alcohol and other drugs*. Dubuque, IA: Kendall/Hunt, 1990.

218. Miller BA. The interrelationship between alcohol and drug and family violence. *NIDA Res Monogr* 1990;103:177–207.

219. Miller BA, Downs WR, Gondoli DM. Spousal violence among alcoholic women as compared to a random household sample of women. *J Stud Alcohol* 1989;50(6):533–540.
220. Pagelow M. *Family violence.* New York: Prager, 1992.
221. Power R, Kutash I. Alcohol, drugs, and partner abuse. In: Roy M, ed. *The abusive partner, an analysis of domestic battering.* New York: Van Nostrand Reinhold, 1990.
222. Quinby PM, Graham AV. Substance abuse among women. *Prim Care* 1993;20(1):131–140.
223. Reed BG. Linkages, battering, sexual assault, incest, child sexual abuse, teen pregnancy, dropping out of school, and the alcohol and drug connection. In: Roth P, ed. *Alcohol and drugs are women's issues.* Metuchen, NJ: Women's Action Alliance and Scarecrow Press, 1991.
224. Root MPP. Treatment failures: the role of sexual victimization in women's addictive behavior. *Am J Orthopsychiatry* 1989;59(4):542–549.
225. Russel S, Wilsnack S. Adult survivors of childhood sexual abuse: substance abuse and other consequences. In: Roth P, ed. *Alcohol and drugs are women's issues.* Metuchen, NJ: Women's Action Alliance and Scarecrow Press, 1991.
226. Van Den Bergh N. Having bitten the apple: a feminist perspective on addiction. In: Van Den Bergh N, ed. *Feminist perspectives on addictions.* New York: Springer, 1991.
227. Zierler S, Feingold L, Laufer D, et al. Adult survivors of childhood sexual abuse and subsequent risk of HIV infection. *Am J Public Health* 1991;81(5):572–575.
228. Theidon K. Taking a hit: pregnant drug users and violence. *Contemp Drug Probl* 1995;22(4):663–686.
229. Rosenbaum M, Murphy S. *An ethnographic study of pregnancy and drug use. Final report to the National Institute on Drug Abuse.* Grant #R01 DA 06832. 1995:229.
230. Bollerud K. A model for the treatment of trauma-related syndromes among chemically dependent inpatient women. *J Subst Abuse Treat* 1990;7:83–87.
231. Coleman E. Child physical and sexual abuse among chemically dependent individuals. *J Chem Depend Treat* 1987;1:27–29.
232. Reed B, Moise R. Implications for treatment and future research. In: Beschner GH, ed. *Addicted women: family dynamics, self-perceptions, and support systems.* DHEW Publ. No. (ADM) 80–762. Rockville, MD: National Institute on Drug Abuse, 1979.
233. Murphy S, Sales P. Pregnant drug users: scapegoats of the Reagan/Bush and Clinton era economics. *Soc Justice* 2001;28(4):72–93.
234. Sales P, Murphy S. Surviving violence: pregnancy and drug use. *J Drug Issues* 2000;30(4):695–724.
235. Sterk C. *Fast lives.* Rutgers University Press, 1999.
236. Amaro H, Hardy-Fanta C. Gender relations in addiction and recovery. *J Psychoactive Drugs* 1995;27(4):325–337.
237. Woodhouse LD. Women with jagged edges: voices from a culture of substance abuse. *Qual Health Res* 1992;2(3):262–281.
238. Chang G, Carroll KM, Behr HM, et al. Improving treatment outcome in pregnant opiate-dependent women. *J Subst Abuse Treat* 1992;9:327–330.
239. Haller D, Dawson K, Knisely J, et al. Retention as a function of psychopathology. *NIDA Res Monogr* 1993;141.
240. Knisely JS, Haller D, Dawson K, et al. Factors associated with retention in two intensive outpatient substance abuse programs. *NIDA Res Monogr* 1993;141.
241. Ingersoll KS, Lu IL, Haller DL. Predictors of in-treatment relapse in perinatal substance abusers and impact on treatment retention: a prospective study. *J Psychoactive Drugs* 1995:27(4):375–387.
242. Copeland J, Hall W. A comparison of predictors of treatment drop-out of women seeking drug and alcohol treatment in a specialist women's and two traditional mixed-sex treatment services. *Br J Addict* 1992;87:883–890.
243. Longshore D, Hsieh S, Anglin MD. Ethnic and gender differences in drug users' perceived need for treatment. *Int J Addict* 1993;28(6):539–558.
244. Baldwin DM, Brecht ML, Monahan G, et al. Perceived need for treatment among pregnant and non-pregnant women arrestees. *J Psychoactive Drugs* 1995:27(4):389–399.
245. Huling T. *African American women and the war on drugs.* Paper presented to the American Society of Criminology, Boston, 1995.
246. Wellisch J, Anglin MD, Prendergast ML. Treatment strategies for drug-abusing women offenders. In: Inciardi J, ed. *Drug treatment in criminal justice settings.* Thousand Oaks, CA: Sage Publications, 1993.
247. Weissman G, Melchoir L, Huba F, et al. Women living with drug abuse and HIV disease: drug abuse treatment access and secondary prevention issues. *J Psychoactive Drugs* 1995;27(4):401–411.
248. Paltrow L. Pregnant drug users, fetal persons, and the threat to Roe v. Wade. *Albany Law Rev* 1999;62:84.
249. Chavkin W. *JAMA* 2001;285(12):1627.
250. Office of National Drug Control Policy. *National drug control strategy: executive summary.* Washington, DC: Executive Office of the President, 1995 Apr:39.
251. Mauer M, Hurling T. *Young black Americans and the justice system: five years later.* Washington, DC: Sentencing Project, 1995:October.
252. Bureau of Justice Statistics. *Special report: women in prison.* Washington, DC: U.S. Department of Justice, 1994.
253. Owen B, Bloom B. Profiling women prisoners: findings from national surveys and a California sample. *Prison J* 1995;75(2):181–182.
254. Gage B. The kids get pain. *Nation* 1995 Feb 20:237.
255. Belknap J. *The invisible woman: gender, crime and justice.* Belmont CA: Wadsworth, 2001.
256. Bloom B, Chesney-Lind M. Women in prison: vengeful equity. In: Muraskin R, ed. *It's a crime: women and criminal justice,* 2nd ed. Upper Saddle River, NJ: Prentice Hall, 2000.
257. Owen B. *In the mix: struggle and survival in a women's prison.* Albany, NY: SUNY Press, 1998.
258. Owen B. Women and imprisonment in the United States: the gendered consequences of the U.S. imprisonment binge. In Cook, Davies, eds. *Harsh punishments: international experiences of women's imprisonment.* Northeastern Press, 2000:81–98.
259. Chesney-Lind M. *Female offender: girls, women and crime.* Thousand Oaks, CA: Sage Publications, 1997.
260. Women, babies, drugs. Family-centered treatment options. In: *Network briefs.* National Conference of State Legislatures Women's Network, July, 1990.
261. *Implications of the drug use forecasting data for TASC programs: female arrestees.* Washington, DC: Bureau of Justice Assistance, 1991.
262. Phillips MD. *Courts, jails, and drug treatment in a California county.* Unpublished manuscript, 1990.
263. Currie E. *Reckoning: drugs, the cities, and the American future.* New York: Hill and Wang, 1993.
264. Gerstein DR, Harwood HJ, eds. *Treating drug problems.* Washington, DC: National Academy Press, 1990:1.
265. Office of National Drug Control Policy. *National drug control strategy: executive summary.* Washington, DC: Executive Office of the President, 1995 Apr.
266. Wenger L, Rosenbaum M. Drug treatment on demand—not. *J Psychoactive Drugs* 1994;26(1):1–11.

267. Rosenbaum M. *Just say what? An alternative view on solving America's drug problem.* San Francisco: National Council on Crime and Delinquency, 1989.
268. Waldorf D, Reinarman C, Murphy S. *Cocaine changes: the experience of using and quitting.* Philadelphia: Temple University Press, 1991.
269. Prendergast ML, Wellisch J, Falkin GP. Assessment of and service for substance-abusing women offenders in community and correctional settings. *Prison J* 1995:75(2).
270. Chavkin W. Drug addiction and pregnancy: policy crossroads. *Am J Public Health* 1990;80(4):483–487.
271. Michaels B, Noonan M, Hoffman S, et al. A treatment model of nursing care for pregnant chemical abusers. In: Chasnoff I, ed. *Drugs, alcohol, pregnancy and parenting.* Boston: Kluwer Academic Publishers, 1988.
272. Mondanaro J, Wedenoja M, Densen-Gerber J, et al. Sexuality and fear of intimacy as barriers to recovery for drug dependent women. In: *Treatment services for drug-dependent women.* NIDA (ADM) 82–1219. Rockville, MD: National Institute on Drug Abuse, 1982;2:303–378.
273. Murphy S, Rosenbaum M. Women and substance abuse. Introduction [special edition]. *J Psychoactive Drugs* 1987:20(4).
274. Reed BG. Developing women-sensitive drug dependence treatment services: why so difficult? *Int J Addict* 1987;20(1):13–62.
275. Rosenbaum M, Murphy S. Not the picture of health: women on methadone. *J Psychoactive Drugs* 1987;19(2):217–255.
276. Wellisch J, Prendergast ML, Anglin MD. *Drug-abusing women offenders: results of a national survey.* Washington, DC: National Institute of Justice, 1994.
277. Daghestani A. Psychosocial characteristics of pregnant women addicts in treatment. In: Chasnoff I, ed. *Drugs, alcohol, pregnancy and parenting.* Boston: Kluwer Academic Publishers, 1988.
278. Jessop M, Green J. Treatment of the pregnant alcohol dependent woman. *J Psychoactive Drugs* 1987;19:193–203.
279. Paltrow L, Cohen DS, Carey C. *Year 2000 overview: governmental responses to pregnant women who use alcohol and other drugs.* Philadelphia: Women's Law Project, National Advocates for Pregnant Women, 2000.
280. Mondanaro J. *Treating drug-dependent women.* Springfield, IL: Lexington Books, 1988.
281. Beckman L. The self-esteem of women alcoholics. *J Stud Alcohol* 1978;39:491–498.
282. Zweben J, Sorenson J. Misunderstandings about methadone. *J Psychoactive Drugs* 1988;20(3):275–281.
283. Wells DVB, Jackson JF. HIV and chemically dependent women: recommendations for appropriate health care and drug treatment services. *Int J Addict* 1992;27(5):571–585.
284. Siegel R. *Intoxication: life in pursuit of artificial paradise.* New York: EP Dutton, 1989.
285. Weil A. *The natural mind.* Boston: Houghton Mifflin, 1972.
286. Nadelmann E, Cohen P, Locher U, et al. *The harm reduction approach to drug control: international progress.* Unpublished manuscript, 1995.
287. Raskin VD. Maternal bereavement in the perinatal substance abuser. *J Subst Abuse Treat* 1992;9:149–152.
288. Albor T. The women get chains. *Nation* 1995 Feb 20.
289. Paone D, Caloir S, Shi Q, et al. Sex, drugs, and syringe exchange in New York City: women's experiences. *J Am Med Womens Assoc* 1995;50(3,4):109–114.
290. O'Hare PA, Newcombe R, Matthews A, et al. *The reduction of drug-related harm.* London: Routledge, 1992.
291. Ward J, Shane D, Hall H, et al. Methadone maintenance and the human immunodeficiency virus: current issues in treatment and research. *Br J Addict* 1992;87:447–453.
292. Stevenson R. Harm reduction, rational addiction and the optimal prescribing of illegal drugs. *Contemp Econ Policy* 1994;12:101–108.
293. Des Jarlais DC, Friedman SR, Ward TP. Harm reduction: a public health response to the AIDS epidemic among injecting drug users. *Annu Rev Public Health* 1993;14:413–450.
294. Watters JK, Estilo MJ, Clark GL, et al. Syringe and needle exchange as HIV/AIDS prevention for injection drug users. *JAMA* 1994;271:115–120.
295. Wodak A. HIV infection and injecting drug use in Australia: responding to a crisis. *J Drug Issues* 1992;22(3):549–562.

Ethnic Populations

CHAPTER 67

African Americans: Epidemiology, Prevention, and Treatment Issues

CHARLES MADRAY, LAWRENCE S. BROWN JR., AND BENY J. PRIMM

The impact of substance abuse continues to devastate American communities. According to the 2001 National Household Survey on Drug Abuse (NHSDA), an estimated 16.6 million Americans age 12 years and older were classified with dependence or abuse of either alcohol or illicit drugs (7.3% of the total population). The rate among African Americans was 7.4%, compared to 7.2% for whites and Hispanics 6.4% (1). These patterns among the major racial/ethnic groups were similar in previous years. While there are noted difficulties in self-reported surveys, this survey is large enough to give us a fair representation of the population at large. However, these findings may not accurately reflect the true extent of the drug use problem in African Americans, particularly because this survey collects information from the civilian, noninstitutionalized population in the United States.

Information on the relationship between substance abuse and racial and ethnic background is complex and challenging. Although there have been increased efforts to study drug abuse in special populations since the passage of the Anti-Drug Abuse Act of 1986 (2), little is known about the relationship between race or ethnicity and illicit drug use, and between race or ethnicity and the ef-

fectiveness of drug-abuse treatment (3). There are several thoughtful reviews of these relationships (2,4); however, much research remains to be conducted.

Research needs to take into account certain study design issues. First, how does one accurately and adequately describe this very important subpopulation of Americans? The African American subpopulation presents a diverse multicultural community. Fundamentally, there are at least three cultural subgroups:

1. African Americans who are descendants of African slaves and who were actually born in the United States;
2. African Americans who are descendants of African slaves of the Caribbean and who migrated to the United States; and
3. African Americans who were born in Africa and migrated to the United States. Within this subgroup, there are a multitude of different cultures depending on the originating African country.

Each of these subcultures has unique characteristics that easily differentiate one group from another. Such characteristics reflect aspects of their colonizing mother country and include dialect, traditional dress and festivities, and religion. The geographic distribution of African Americans subcultures varies considerably. For example, in New York City, African Americans of Caribbean origin are concentrated in some Brooklyn neighborhoods, African Americans of American birth are more predominant in the Bushwick/Brownsville areas of Brooklyn, and African Americans of recent migration from Africa are localized predominately in the Harlem neighborhood of Manhattan.

The next major concern is how the subjects were selected for participation. If not randomly chosen, how was the study population represented? If it is a comparative study, what is the evidence there was no bias between the compared populations in the observation of important events (reporting drug use, actual drug use, reported adverse events, and actual adverse events)? Given the variety of African American subcultures, the method of population selection is of critical importance in making conclusions regarding African Americans.

Many surveys of substance abuse generally determine use of a psychoactive substance, whether it is alcohol, or an illegal drug. For example, the National Household Survey and the High School Senior Survey assess use of various substances in the past year, month, or week. Although this is useful epidemiologic information, its clinical utility is limited. Substance abuse and dependence, which are more difficult to ascertain using survey methods, are of greater importance to clinical care and are correlated more closely with the medical and social consequences of psychoactive substance use.

The choice of outcome variables is also important. While the use of self-reporting is not uncommon in substance abuse, there are limitations. Drug abuse is an illegal act, and along with alcohol abuse, is stigmatized within society. Hence, participants may be reluctant to admit the true magnitude of their illegal drug or alcohol use. Even less is known about the extent to which this issue affects surveys of illicit drug use and alcohol use among African Americans. It is often argued that given the disproportionately greater arrests and incarceration rate for drug-related crimes in many African American communities, there may be more reluctance for many African Americans to respond reliably to large substance abuse surveys. In addition, homelessness and socioeconomic status in African American communities are other factors that enhance the limitation of surveys such as the NHSDA.

Recognizing the foregoing limitations, this chapter confines itself to problems of substance abuse, focusing on the following questions: What is the existing knowledge concerning the prevalence, correlates, and adverse consequences of substance use and abuse in African Americans? What efforts exist to prevent substance use and abuse in this population? What is the nature and effectiveness of treatment for African American substance abusers?

SUBSTANCE USE AND ABUSE PREVALENCE

According to the Substance Abuse and Mental Health Services Administration (SAMHSA) Office of Applied Studies' National Household Survey on Drug Abuse 2001, an estimated 6.2% of African Americans (age 12 years and older) reported past year dependence or abuse of any illicit drug or alcohol. Based on combined 2000 and 2001 data, 6.9% of African Americans (age 12 years and older) reported past month illicit drug use. African American males between the ages of 12 and 35 years were much more likely to be users of an illicit substance compared to their white counterparts. This is particularly the case for cocaine use; 1.4% of African American males older than 35 years of age had used cocaine in the past year, in contrast to 0.2% of whites. However, an equal percentage of African Americans and whites between the ages of 12 and 17 years had used an illicit drug in their lifetime, in the

past year, or past month (5). African American and Latino women were more likely than white women to have used crack cocaine, a form of cocaine that many believe to be especially virulent (6,7). On the other hand, data from the National High School Senior Survey (7) indicates the rate of drug use among African American high school seniors was lower for all drugs, except heroin and marijuana.

When considering the latter data, it is important to recognize that in using African American high school seniors to represent African American youths, the statistics may be biased because of the disproportionately greater high school dropout rate among African Americans as compared to their white counterparts. It is also important to keep in mind, because surveys such as those described previously have not included such difficult groups as prisoners, runaways, or high school dropouts, the current estimates of illicit drug use in minority populations may underestimate the extent of the problem.

In one New York City study of African American youths, a survey was conducted among inner-city adolescents in jail (N = 427) to examine the correlates of cocaine/crack use. Twenty-three percent had used cocaine/crack in the month prior to arrest and 32% reported lifetime use. Interestingly, there was no correlation between the type of crime and cocaine/crack use (8).

DEVELOPMENT AND COURSE OF USE AND ABUSE

A small body of studies has attempted to characterize the development and course of substance use and abuse in African American individuals. These consist of studies of community citizens and studies of addicts. In what appears to be the earliest systematic study of drug abuse in an African American population, Robins and Murphy (9) studied 235 African American men between the ages of 30 and 35 years who were living in the community. They reported that 50% had used some drug illegally and that 10% had been addicted to heroin. Marijuana had served as the introduction or "gateway" to harder drugs for most. The younger the age of initial marijuana use, the more likely the continuation to heroin use. Delinquency was a predictor of drug use, and within this group, those without a father at home were more likely to be users.

Brunswick (10) studied 536 African American young adults (52% male) between the ages of 18 and 23 years who lived in the Harlem section of New York City. One-third of the study sample had not completed high school. One-third of the sample had jobs, of the third that reported having jobs, 75% maintained fulltime employment. Four percent of the males were in jail when interviewed. About one-fifth of the women were married, in contrast to 4% of the men. Fifty-two percent of the women and 28% of the men had at least one child, and incomes for the households of these subjects were quite low.

Brunswick found the study sample had used heroin an average of 939 times in their lifetime, had used methadone

542 times, cocaine 278 times, marijuana 869 times, and psychedelic drugs 190 times. The modal frequency (47%) of alcohol use for males was daily and/or several times a week. By the time of the interview, 75% of the alcohol users had been using alcohol regularly for at least 5 years. Of the males, 68% used marijuana at least once or twice a week, and 77% used heroin at least once or twice a week. Half of the men and 40% of the women had used two or more drugs in the past year.

Not unexpectedly, alcohol was the drug used earliest. By 14 years of age, half of male drinkers, and almost that proportion of females, had used alcohol. Indeed, 20% of the men had started alcohol use by age 10 years. The median age of onset of marijuana use was 14.8 years for males and 15.6 years for females. Therefore, the initiation of marijuana use occurred about 1 year after initial alcohol use. The median age of first use for heroin was approximately the same age as for marijuana use. The initial age of cocaine and psychedelics use for these individuals was about 17.5 years. The age of onset of alcohol use predicted use of illicit substances, and the early onset of illicit substance use was related to the subsequent frequency of substance use. In the study, 9% of the men and 7% of the women reported having been in heroin treatment at least once. The longer the period of heroin use, the greater the likelihood the user would request treatment.

Sadly, Brunswick reported that initial use for all of the above drugs occurred most commonly while the subject was on the way to school. She found the heroin user group differed from the rest of the sample on a number of characteristics. For example, they had the lowest educational achievement and were less often employed. Interestingly, if the individual had not initiated heroin use by age 18 years, the individual was unlikely to do so thereafter. Brunswick (10) felt the high use rates of the subjects studied were a result of the marginality and ambiguity of the life situation of youth generally and the dubious access that the African American youth in the study had to society's opportunities.

Admittedly, the Brunswick study design does not allow one to make comparative statements between African Americans and other populations. Similarly, we cannot necessarily conclude the cohort under investigation was representative of African Americans. Nonetheless, it does suggest that, at least in some poor African American communities, substance use and abuse begins at a relatively early age and can be found in a substantial proportion of individuals.

Halikas and his colleagues (11) reported findings on the early life and natural history of heroin addiction in a population of African American drug abusers. In this study, 192 addicts were examined, most of whom were in methadone maintenance treatment. The average age of the subjects studied was 28 years. The age of initial illegal drug use was found to be 14.4 years. Heroin use first occurred when the individual was slightly older than 18 years of age, followed by addiction about 1.5 years later (group

mean = 19.9 years of age). The first drug-related arrest took place about 6 months after the onset of addiction (age 20.4 years). The number of drugs tried by these individuals ranged from 3 to 35. Of this group of heroin addicts, 90% were truant from school beginning in the seventh grade and 95% acknowledged some non–school-related misbehavior by the age of 12 years.

In an earlier study of African American opiate-dependent subjects, Chambers and his colleagues (12) reported 89% of their subjects were introduced to opiates by peers. Early termination of education and early arrest histories were consistent with the findings of Halikas et al. (11). A study by Craig (13) reported similar findings. That is, the African American, male, inner-city, heroin-dependent patients treated in a Veterans' Administration facility averaged 30 years of age, used or were dependent for about 8 years, and had made five attempts at drug detoxification without the benefit of a treatment program. The average patient was educationally impaired, had a poor work history, and had spent 3 years in prison for committing either crimes against property or other drug-related crimes. Craig found many of these patients to have character disorders, suffering either from sociopathy or a schizoid personality disorder.

In a large study of a methadone treatment population of more than 500 African American and Latino patients by Alterman et al. (14), Latinos reported significantly more symptomatology in somatic complaints, anxiety, depression, alcohol problems, and suicidal ideation scales using the Personality Assessment Inventory (PAI). While the PAI may possess some limitations in its validity for lower socioeconomic groups and its ease of administration, it is a psychometric instrument found to have concurrent validity when compared with the Diagnostic Interview Schedule and the Addiction Severity Index (ASI). This finding of more reported symptomatology among Latinos when compared to African Americans was also reported by Kosten and colleagues (15). Unfortunately, there were an inadequate number of non African Americans, non-Hispanic patients in the Alterman and Kosten study populations to make appropriate comparisons between African American patients and white, non-Hispanic patients.

In the same study population as investigated by Alterman et al., Brown and fellow researchers (16) reported differences between African American and Latino patients in their ASI scores. While African American patients had significantly more severe scores in the employment domain, Latinos scored more severely in the legal domain and in psychological problems. Depression, evaluated using the Beck Depression Inventory or the Diagnostic Interview Schedule, was especially more serious among Latino patients than among African American patients.

To summarize, education impairment, a poor work history, a history of arrests and imprisonment, and possibly psychiatric problems are found in many of the opiate-dependent African Americans evaluated in the studies just described. However, we must consider these findings with caution. As with the Brunswick study, the study designs generally do not allow comparisons of African Americans with other ethnic or racial groups. Also, these results may not have implications for all African Americans, as we cannot ascertain the degree to which there was bias in the selection of the African Americans in each study. Furthermore, retrospective studies, like the ones mentioned, have the danger of missing some influential factors or cofactors that may correlate better with the evolution of chemical dependency. Alternatively, the degree of justifiable (or drug-induced) memory impairment may lessen or strengthen the magnitude of effect of some of the self-reported information collected.

In an effort to reduce the obvious bias of the above-mentioned studies, Lillie-Blanton et al. (17) investigated the use of psychoactive substances in African Americans from a different perspective. The objective of the study was to estimate the degree to which crack cocaine smoking is associated with personal factors specific to race or ethnicity. In the design, the social and environment risk factors were held at a constant because they potentially may have confounded the racial comparison. Respondents were post stratified into neighborhood risk sets. Subjects were selected using multistage area probability sampling of all residents age 12 years and older. The results demonstrated that once respondents were grouped into neighborhood clusters the relative odds of crack use did not differ significantly for African American or for Latino Americans when compared with white Americans.

It must be mentioned that the study did not refute the analysis of previous studies, but simply provided evidence that prevalence estimates, unadjusted for social environment risk factors, may lead to misunderstanding about the role of race or ethnicity in the epidemiology of crack use. By extension, this may also be true for other illegal drugs and alcohol. The study recommended that future research should seek to identify which characteristics of the neighborhood's social environment are important modifiable determinants of drug use.

ADVERSE CONSEQUENCES OF DRUG USE AND ABUSE

Drug abuse has many adverse health-related consequences, including fatal and nonfatal overdose, acquired immunodeficiency syndrome (AIDS), hepatitis B and C infection, increased risk for complications of pregnancy, and adverse birth outcomes. In addition, drug abuse may have negative effects on employment, school achievement, socioeconomic status, and family stability, although it is difficult to determine whether these are the cause or are the result of drug abuse (2). An important issue that needs to be considered is whether African Americans are at greater or lesser risk for these consequences. Van Hasselt et al. (18) pointed out not only that African Americans are at greater risk but also familial and socioeconomic factors contribute

to the exceedingly high prevalence rates of drug abuse in African American children.

Medical examiner data on drug-related deaths are another source of information on adverse drug-related consequences. The total number of deaths reported is proportionally higher for African Americans than for either whites or Hispanics (2,19). African American decedents accounted for 1,999 (30%) of the 6,756 drug abuse-related deaths reported by medical examiners to the Drug Abuse Warning Network (DAWN) in 1988; whereas African Americans constitute only 23% of the population in the cities surveyed by DAWN (2). More than 74% of the African American decedents were males, and 46% were age 30 to 39 years. Cocaine was the most frequently mentioned drug in DAWN medical examiner cases, followed by heroin and morphine (20). Drug-related deaths among African Americans and Hispanics were more likely to be attributed to accidental or unexpected circumstances, while those for whites were more likely to be attributed to suicide (2). The combined use of heroin with alcohol appeared to be associated with several drug-related epidemics with disproportionate numbers of African American deaths (2).

In New York City methadone maintenance treatment clinics, Brown and colleagues (21) assessed the range of medical disorders in calendar year 1987 among 1,780 patients. More than 90% were African American or Latino and 40% were female. While this study used chart reviews as the source of data and therefore had potential ascertainment limitations, this study represented one of the few systematic reviews of drug abusers in an ambulatory setting. Histories of gonorrhea, hepatitis B infection, pneumonia, and anemia were found in 28%, 23%, 21%, and 21% of the patients, respectively. This study suggested a considerable portion of African American heroin users sustain a considerable range of medical disorders during their lives.

In the last two decades, human immunodeficiency virus (HIV) infection has become a serious consequence of drug abuse. The strongest link between the two phenomena is intravenous drug use, involving the use or sharing of contaminated injecting equipment and having unprotected sex.

The HIV/AIDS epidemic is a major health crisis facing the African American community. According to the Centers for Disease Control and Prevention (CDC), African Americans accounted for approximately 35% of the more than 900,000 reported cases since the beginning of the epidemic. African Americans accounted for half of the new HIV cases reported in the U.S. in 2001 (22). It is estimated that half of the new HIV infections occur among teenagers and young adults age 25 years and younger. Numerous studies highlight the fact that the majority of these cases are African Americans (23). As of December 2001, 168,000 African Americans have died from AIDS (22). Injecting drug use (IDU) is the behavior associated with the second greatest number of reported cases of AIDS and is the primary source of HIV infection in adult heterosexual and pediatric AIDS cases (24). IDU now accounts for approximately 25% of the new cases reported (22). New data suggests that the leading cause of HIV infection among African American men is sexual contact with other men, followed by IDU and heterosexual contact (22). African American and Hispanics comprise 73% of the annual new HIV cases, with African Americans accounting for 54% of the cases. Of cases reported by gender and race, African American males account for 43% and African American females account for 64% of the cases. For African American youths, the picture is frightening; in a CDC study of Job Corp entrants ages 16 to 21 years, African American women were seven times more likely to be infected with HIV than were their white counterparts, and African American males were four times more likely to be infected than were their white counterparts (25). For African Americans, the foregoing information is especially sobering. African Americans are disproportionately overrepresented among total adult AIDS cases, among adult female AIDS cases, and among pediatric AIDS cases. This picture is largely a result of the overrepresentation of African Americans among IDUs.

HIV seropositive rates have been found to be higher in IDUs who also use cocaine (1,26).

Although race and ethnicity are not in themselves risk factors for HIV/AIDS, African Americans are more often faced with the challenges associated with the risk of HIV/AIDS, such as substance abuse, sexually transmitted infections, denial, discrimination, poverty, at-risk partners or spouses on the "down low," and domestic violence.

PREVENTION

Having considered a variety of consequences associated with drug use and abuse, it should be emphasized that prevention encompasses several approaches. One such approach is the prevention of drug and alcohol use in youths, that is, primary prevention. Reducing the number of retail outlets selling alcohol and prohibiting the use of illicit drugs are examples of primary prevention. Another very different strategy involves the prevention of the consequences of drug or alcohol use by reducing high-risk behaviors. This is a secondary prevention strategy. The provision of condoms or the use of needle-exchange programs represents two types of secondary prevention approaches for HIV transmission. A third and equally important strategy is to prevent death or further morbidity in persons who have sustained at least one clinical consequence of alcohol use or illicit drug use. Examples of this approach is include efforts to prevent the development of AIDS or disease progression in HIV-infected drug users, and efforts to prevent end-stage renal disease in patients with illicit drug-induced renal disease.

Two key points are important in any commentary on the status of drug-abuse prevention generally, and prevention specifically, in African Americans. First, given the American experience with Prohibition and efforts to reduce smoking, large-scale reduction of any addictive behavior is very difficult and complex. Any solution has to be both large scale and long-term.

Second, much less is known about how prevention should proceed than about the prevalence and effects of drug use. Given this state of affairs, specifically with reference to prevention of drug abuse in African Americans, there is often more conjecture, opinion, and polemics in the literature than evidence of systematic work. This is not necessarily bad, if the former helps to bring about the latter.

Finally, there are many theories concerning the high incidence of drug use in poor African American communities. As indicated previously, Brunswick (10) concluded the lack of access to the societal opportunity structure is one cause of the problem. Rappaport (27) provided a similar explanation in describing the lack of access to resources as causing problems of living. These explanations are consistent with the National Institute on Drug Abuse's (26) statement that "most drug abusers use drugs as a substitute for a lack of fulfillment of basic human needs." This viewpoint suggests the large-scale drug use and abuse by African American youths is as much the result of a societal problem as an individual problem. Tucker (28) states, "Many ethnic minorities view drug abuse as an adaptive response to oppressive societal conditions." A number of workers in the field support the concept of the inherent ghetto culture as the cause of drug abuse. Indeed, Feldman (29) and Blumer (30) concluded peer pressures for drug use in the ghetto environment were so great that they were amazed that anyone escapes the problem of drug addiction. In addition to peer pressure, several other factors contribute to drug use: breakdown of family structure; the media; lack of role model; unemployment; and the educational system.

The home environment has always been at the core of a solid foundation. It has been reported 50% of African American males who enter treatment come from broken homes or from homes where the mother played both parental roles. Communication has been blamed as the root cause of this crisis. To effectively fight this crisis, family must be and must stay involved, using the community and the church to further stabilize and support the foundation.

Undoubtedly, the media has been a significant contributor to our plight. It has glamorized alcohol use, which very often leads to the use of other drugs. Be it print, television, or the movies the message should emphasize the dangers of alcohol and drug use and not be a message that either leaves our youths confused or supports the glamour of drug use.

Magic Johnson has been a savior to the African American community in his efforts to build the awareness of HIV/AIDS. His message, however, seems to be leading to a complacent attitude, particularly among our youths in the inner cities. Clearly, it is not the messenger; it is the interpretation of the message. Our youths have not seen, nor do they appreciate, the challenges endured by our communities in the late 1980s and 1990s. To remedy this misconceived message, we need more print and media messages by peer advocates. Local heroes need to be showcased. Our world is now a global village and the universal message is "think global but act local," the universal message for HIV/AIDS and substance abuse must be "act local, but think global." HIV/AIDS and substance abuse are global threats.

In the African American household, the absence of the male role model is a significant challenge. According to the *Statistical Record of Black Americans 1990*, of the African American male population 18 to 30 years old, 25% are imprisoned for at least 25 years, 30% are unemployed, and another 22% suffer from alcohol and other drug abuse. With these statistics, it is easy to see why the path of least resistance is often the choice of many. Burglary, drug dealing, and prostitution may lead to the easy way out, but very often the outcome is prison or the cemetery. We need a mentoring program; the resurgence of the Big Brother Program is vital if we are to survive the twenty-first century.

The unemployment situation for African Americans is almost always 50% or greater than that of the general population. The three major contributors to this dilemma are education, location, and transportation. Although there are a host of factors that contribute to the unemployment plight, communication and education are good starts. One only need to look at our current African American leaders; they are paving the way so we must encourage our youths to capitalize on their leadership. Education will help youths to locate to areas where transportation is available.

The challenge of developing effective drug-abuse prevention and treatment programs will benefit significantly from increased resources. Prevention and treatment are public health initiatives that have had significant impact in reducing the rate of AIDS, hepatitis, and tuberculosis. It will have similar effects on substance-abuse prevention and treatment initiatives once the scarce resources becomes available.

The oft-cited maxim "prevention is better than cure" is alive and well in twenty-first century. We should place significant resources and emphasis on prevention. The Federal Center for Substance Abuse Prevention (CSAP)'s strategies are based on the earlier prevention starts, the better the outcomes.

PREVENTING DRUG USE AND ABUSE IN YOUTHS

Both Tucker (28) and Crisp (31) concluded that prevention programs generally designed for middle-class whites are inappropriate for African Americans in lower socioeconomic groups. However, it is not clear that these programs are useful for African Americans of any socioeconomic

class. Crisp described a program designed by Ortiz (32) to counter these biases. Ortiz's systemic approach was based on the belief that oppressed people often have a hard time relating to present prevention models because these often fail to deal with their reasons of abusing drugs. This researcher felt that a "systemic" approach that focuses on racism, sexism, power, economic realities, and policy making was necessary before the usual individual-based approaches can be applied.

Recently, more studies and perspective tend to counter these biases. Metsch et al. (33) designed a family centered treatment program for substance-abusing mothers and their children. The program adapted a systemic approach and aimed to reduce reliance on social and health welfare. Improved functioning in specific life and vocational skills were encouraged. Providing instruction on parenting techniques and mother–child relations for the mothers while providing prevention services for their children in a safe and supportive environment were all integral parts of this program. Funded by Center for Substance Abuse Treatment this 5-year demonstration grant recently concluded its implementation phase. The results of this approach are presently unclear.

Rouse (2) reviewed data from the annual National High School Senior Survey, which indicated that drug education courses or lectures in school had a greater preventive impact on African American than on white students. Slightly less than half of the white students surveyed indicated that information provided in school about illicit drugs made them less interested in trying drugs, as compared with 75% of the African American students. However, fewer African Americans than whites reported that they had received such drug courses or lecturers. Rouse (2) therefore concluded every effort should be made to make drug education available to African American students. Although these findings are encouraging, it is important to emphasize that African American high school seniors are not entirely representative of African American youths who use and abuse drugs.

Based on our earlier discussion, it would appear that interventions designed to reach African American youth require tailoring to the beliefs, percepts, and needs of these individuals. Crisp (31) describes a number of levels of intervention indicated by Rappaport (27), none of which need be mutually exclusive—individual, group, organization, institutional, community, and societal. Although Crisp (31) criticized existing intervention approaches for not being innovative, he also failed to offer any alternative innovative strategies. Rowe and Grill (34) offered an alternative innovative strategy based on an appreciation of core beliefs. Key ontologic and epistemologic assumptions of rational clinical and counseling interventions are presented that highlight the difference between traditional goals and theories and the proposed alternative conceptual system and treatment strategies with the African-centered approach proposed by Rowe and Grill. The difficulty with both the proposed intervention by Crisp and the approach proposed by Rowe and Grill is that there is no report or published evaluation of any existing prevention program based on these strategies.

Nuttall and his colleagues (35) developed an effective approach to drug-abuse prevention intended for teenagers from an inner-city minority population. Through informal seminars, including films and discussion, youngsters were led to explore their feelings and goals for the future and the possible effects of drug use on these goals. Relatively little emphasis was given to education about drugs per se, but rather, the emphasis was on value clarification, learning to think about the future, and how actions in the present would affect that future. The program was designed by people from an African American inner-city background. Positive change was indicated by higher scores following the intervention for the "no drug condition" and lower scores for the "frequent drug use" condition. Boys showed positive changes, although the absolute amount of reported change was relatively small. Girls showed no change. The authors speculated that no changes were obtained for girls because the girls were already aware of the negative implications of drug use. This study demonstrates the difficulties of instituting and evaluating change in short-term programs, no matter how carefully designed.

Ghadivian (36) offered another innovative approach. The approach targeted the individual, the family, and society. The individual is helped to develop a sense of purpose, a feeling of self-esteem, and respect for others. This resulted in a state of maturity making possible an objective evaluation of circumstances and postponement of immediate gratification for a future goal, resulting in a feeling of responsibility and spiritual orientation. It was postulated that this can help the individual to develop positive attitudes toward himself or herself and the environment. Parents are encouraged to promote love and unity, as well as a drug-free lifestyle, so children are provided with positive health models. The family experience is also intended to help children to cope with stress and other problems of daily life. By means of education, society at large is encouraged to adopt positive attitudes toward health and to promote activities that lead to the elimination of isolation. While interesting, there does not exist a published report of an evaluation of a prevention program based on that approach.

Graham and his colleagues (37) evaluated the efficacy of a social skills and affect management curriculum for each of four major ethnic groups: Asian, African American, Hispanic, and white. The subjects were seventh graders when the intervention was introduced and eighth graders when the change was assessed. One group was exposed to a 12-session program, giving students social skills for resisting drug offers. Another group was administered an affect management program, and a third control group received no special drug prevention curriculum other than that offered by the schools. The outcome measures were composite indices based on lifetime and recent use items for cigarettes, alcohol, and marijuana. The results showed clear prevention effects for females, but not for males. Overall prevention effects were strongest for smoking and weakest for alcohol. The program appeared to be least effective for whites and most effective for Asians.

The findings from the Nuttall and Graham prevention studies are consistent with Rouse's (2) conclusion that prevention and intervention strategies demonstrate differential effects within various ethnic groups and socioeconomic populations. Still, it is unclear whether the results may or may not be expected in other African American subjects or communities. As Rouse (2) concluded, there is no one answer of how best to approach different ethnic or racial populations. Nonetheless, she wisely stressed the need for community-wide and school-based approaches.

The development of programs that would effectively reduce drug use in African American youth would represent a major advance. Clearly, it would be important for the program developer to make the program meaningful to the recipient audience. It seems that the only way to do this is to ensure ample input and participation from members of the relevant communities. Detailed descriptions of the interventions, as well as a clearly defined evaluation process, are essential components of any such effort.

CHANGING HIGH-RISK BEHAVIORS IN IDUS

It is extremely difficult to change health and sexual behaviors (2). This seems to be particularly difficult for individuals with few psychosocial resources, as is known to be the case with many African American drug-dependent persons (15,38). Additionally, a significant portion of drug-dependent persons (African American and other ethnic groups) are known to suffer from additional psychopathology such as affective or anxiety disorders, antisocial personality disorder, schizophrenia, or other substance-abuse disorders (15,38), which may make them more resistant to substance-abuse treatment (39). The high incidence of needle sharing and unsafe sex practices, such as prostitution among African American IDUs, highlights the great need for effective intervention programs for these individuals. There is evidence that IDUs testing positive for HIV are more likely to suffer from psychopathology, such as an antisocial personality disorder (40), suggesting high-risk behaviors are more likely to be found in IDUs with greater psychopathology. If this is the case, it is very likely such individuals will be more resistant to HIV prevention efforts. Needle sharing appears to be, at least in some part, associated with a feeling of friendship and intimacy. The elimination of this behavior may possibly increase the degree of alienation and loneliness in a population badly in need of social supports.

Increasing the availability of sterile syringes through needle-exchange programs, pharmacies, and other outlets reduces unsafe injection practices such as needle sharing, and decreases the transmission of HIV/AIDS and hepatitis. There has been a significant body of evidence that needle-exchange programs are effective in HIV prevention efforts. In fact, needle-exchange programs provide a pathway for treatment linkages. Since Connecticut reformed its drug paraphernalia and prescription laws to allow pharmacy sales in 1992, needle sharing among injecting drug users has dropped by 40%. In 1993, the General Accounting Office reviewed the effects of needle-exchange programs. In New Haven, Connecticut, a program demonstrated an estimated 33% reduction in HIV infection rates among drug users in that city.

In 2000, New York, New Hampshire, and Rhode Island joined the majority of states in allowing pharmacy sales of sterile syringes. Several other states are currently considering permitting pharmacy sale of syringes. In a recent commentary, former President Clinton regrets not supporting needle-exchange programs during his reign. Although Congress has restricted the use of federal funds for needle-exchange programs, lawmakers have authorized funding for research into the efficacy of needle-exchange programs as a public health intervention to reduce the transmission of HIV and to examine the impact of such programs on drug use.

Use of safe sex practices may conflict with sociocultural values regarding sexual behavior, gender roles, and social structure. A good example of this conflict relates to condom use, which has always been viewed as suspicious or mistrustful by sex partners. Thus, there is very little to suggest how to bring about such change in our open society. Education in itself does not appear to be sufficient. The National Institute for Drug Abuse is supporting considerable research directed toward increasing knowledge and effecting change in this very critical area (2).

This point was reinforced by a review by Lanarme (41), in which it was pointed out that school drug-abuse prevention programs represent an enormous education resource. Recent perceptions of an epidemic of drug abuse among the nation's youth have fueled the escalation in expenditures for drug-prevention programming. An important question that needs to be addressed concerns whether broad-ranging drug education efforts directed at all public and private school students are efficient and effective uses of available resources. After a brief evaluation of drug education programming in the United States, Lanarme examined recent longitudinal research regarding the antecedents of drug abuse among young people. Based on this research, suggestions were made for a new approach to drug education programs that would direct intensive interventions at the minority of youth who are identifiable in early childhood as particularly susceptible to problems with drug abuse (42).

In a comprehensive review of existing published reports of prevention programs, which included African Americans and focused on preventing HIV transmission, Brown (43) made the following conclusions. Although there are many theories of human behavior, the relevance of most to risky HIV-related behaviors has not been found and do not reflect the sociocultural or historical perspectives or male–female relationships of many African American communities. The existing published reports are flawed in at least one of the following ways:

- Small study sample and unclear whether findings would be reproducible
- Short period of observations and thus unclear that changes were not temporary
- Study population selection bias
- Focus on self-reports of behavior change
- Few comparisons between African Americans and other ethnic or racial groups
- Few comparisons between male and female subjects
- Few studies with an appropriate control population

In Brown's review, he noted there were more studies that reported changes in drug-related behaviors than in sex-related behaviors among illicit drug users.

TREATMENT

African Americans comprised 13% of the U.S. population in 2000 (44), and 24% of all adult treatment admissions to publicly funded substance-abuse treatment facilities according to the DASIS 2000 report (45). In 1999, alcohol and cocaine were the primary substances used among African Americans entering treatment. This represents two-thirds of the 366,000 African American treatment admissions. While alcohol was the leading substance among African American males, cocaine was the leading substance among African American females. Marijuana abuse was the third leading substance among African American male admissions at 19%. Among African American female admissions, opiates (primarily heroin) were the third leading substance, accounting for 18% of admissions.

African American admissions to substance-abuse treatment by age distribution reveals that the age group 30 to 39 years old for both African American males and African American females were the largest. Marijuana use was the highest among both African American males and African American females younger than age 30 years old. Opiates use was highest among African American males 40 to 49 years old and among African American females 30 to 39 years old (45).

There were approximately 366,000 substance-abuse treatment admissions for African Americans in 1999. This represents a steady decline of 15% from 1994 (431,000 admissions). However, during this same period, treatment admissions for the total treatment population increased by 3% (45).

Data collected by the National Institute on Drug Abuse (42) indicate African Americans and Hispanics are three times as likely as whites to be in treatment for substance abuse. Some writers have concluded that current theories and models of addiction and addiction treatment were based on middle-class whites (31). It has also been argued that because the causes of addiction are different for African Americans, the treatment needs of African Americans may be different from whites and other groups (3,28). The corollary question deriving from this viewpoint is whether there is a need for alternative treatment and prevention models that are sensitive to the needs of African Americans.

The literature thus far does not support the viewpoint that African Americans do not benefit as much from existing treatments as other groups. On the other hand, there also does not exist unequivocal evidence that African Americans benefit equally as well as other ethnic or racial groups. Rouse (2) concluded the existing large longitudinal studies of treatment outcomes have, with few exceptions, found that demographic variables such as race are significant predictors of treatment outcomes. However, a large-scale study of treatment outcomes in a number of treatment programs throughout the country conducted by Joe and his colleagues (46) found that the ethnic status of the patient was not as important in influencing outcome as the community structure surrounding the treatment. Pretreatment variables such as employment and type of treatment were more important (3).

In contrast, Brown et al. (47) cited several studies with opiate-dependent subjects that indicated that an ethnic group with at least a 75% majority in a program was likely to do better in that program than the other ethnic groups represented in the program. However, their own research provided, at most, limited support for this conclusion. They compared three kinds of programs: methadone maintenance, residential drug-free, and outpatient drug-free. Evidence consistent with their hypothesis was revealed for only the outpatient drug-free programs. The limited evidence that exists for this study indicates that the program attempted to adapt to the nature of its patient constituency.

Phillips and Phin (48), for example, found that counselors were usually of the same ethnicity as their clients. Minority group members tended to be clustered in a few programs rather than being dispersed throughout the treatment network. They concluded, "It seems that a minority treatment network does exist which recognizes the need for cultural sensitivity and uses a shared staff/client cultural identity to attract individuals to treatment." Pentz also mentioned this when he described future directions for drug abuse prevention, the overarching perspective of interfusing basic and social science research approaches (49).

Despite the foregoing, it is likely African Americans, as well as other ethnic subgroups, have specific needs for which particular treatment forms may be more effective. It is important to increase our knowledge concerning similarities and differences in the characteristics and treatment responses of different ethnic subgroups. For example, an important treatment question that has not been addressed adequately is whether African American patients respond more favorably—all other factors held equal—to a therapist of similar background. Lillie-Blanton and her colleagues attempted to address this aspect and concluded that ethnicity of the counselor or clinician may not be the dominant determining factor (17). A related question in need of further investigation concerns the sensitivity of various aspects of treatment programs to African American patients and how such sensitivities are expressed.

One of the problems in substance-abuse treatment is limited knowledge and ability to objectively measure the actual treatment services that various individuals receive in treatment. Also, there is only limited knowledge concerning the amounts of and types of treatment that are most effective for particular substance-abuse problems. For example, has the provision of primary medical care on-site in drug abuse treatment programs enhanced drug-abuse treatment outcome for African Americans? Once the necessary knowledge exists, is disseminated, and the appropriate tools are in place, it will be possible to more adequately address and answer some of the questions and issues that have been raised concerning the treatment of African American substance abusers. While these considerations may limit the precision of the findings that can be obtained presently, they should not preclude systematic investigation into these questions.

SUMMARY

In considering substance abuse epidemiology, prevention, and treatment as they relate to African Americans a number of complex issues arise. For example, Americans of African descent are heterogeneous in culture, language, geographic distribution, and other important factors. Consequently, any discussions must stress this important limitation in assigning any attributes to this group of Americans.

Second, the scientific basis for making observations on substance abuse concerning most Americans, and especially Americans of African descent, is extremely limited. While the database is more plentiful epidemiologically, published rigorous reports of prevention or treatment studies are rare. Present studies are limited because of an insufficient number or description of the study population; bias in the selection of the study population; under ascertainment of hidden populations (such as the homeless, prison, and school dropout populations) where substance abuse may be more prevalent; lack of an appropriate control or comparative population; a diverse range of selected outcomes, some of which present significant challenges in justifying their appropriateness (i.e., should the focus be use, abuse, or dependence); continuing concern about the validity of self-reporting in measuring the outcomes of interest; an inadequate description of the intervention(s) of other studies; and inadequate descriptions of the evaluation of prevention and treatment interventions.

With this background, this chapter considered existing knowledge and discussed some of the questions and issues that have been raised concerning the prevalence and consequences of substance use among African Americans. The status and merits of published prevention and treatment efforts were also considered.

African Americans are overrepresented among Americans who use an illicit drug. This is not the case for all substances of abuse or for all age groups. While there are higher prevalence rates of cocaine and marijuana use in the past month among African Americans, the lifetime rates of marijuana and cocaine use are higher among whites. There are also differences between African Americans and whites in the ages at which illicit drug use is more prevalent.

Many factors are reported to be associated with substance abuse among African Americans, including undereducation, unemployment, underemployment, hopelessness, dysfunctional families, and other indices of poverty. However, none of these factors has been unequivocally demonstrated to be causal, perhaps because of the fundamental and inseparable relationships between these factors. Indeed, there is also evidence that some, if not all, of these factors may also be consequences of substance abuse.

Whether predictors or consequences of substance abuse, these factors are overrepresented in many African American communities. These social dislocations are not the only consequences of substance abuse, which have a devastating and disproportionately greater impact on African Americans. HIV/AIDS, other causes of excess morbidity, and substance abuse-related deaths are also overrepresented among African Americans.

In the context of this pervasive impact of substance abuse, prevention and treatment programs do provide services for African Americans. Most of these programs are neither described nor evaluated in the published literature. The use by African Americans of prevention and treatment programs and the effectiveness of these programs is largely unknown.

While there is a clear sense that specialized prevention programs are needed, the existing knowledge base does not unequivocally support such an initiative and is insufficient to direct program development. It will require creative and dedicated effort coupled with systematic evaluation to develop programs that work. There is also a need to determine the specific needs of African Americans and other ethnic or racial populations, the nature and effectiveness of current treatments for these patients, and whether more effective treatments can be developed for African American communities.

In recent years, society has become increasingly aware of the problems of African American substance abusers. Studies of and programs for African American substance abusers designed to provide answers to some of the more pressing questions are receiving funding. More investigations, using a wide variety of methodological designs, are needed. The answers to these questions will require sustained funding and the development of long-standing programs of prevention and treatment. There must also be well-designed and adequately funded evaluation components of prevention and treatment programs.

Clearly, one of the reasons why so many substance abuse questions remain is the stigma of substance abuse in America. Among many Americans of African descent, the continuing existence of substance abuse in their communities is related, in part, to the stigma of discrimination. Nonetheless, the public health implications for answers to substance abuse problems are an imperative for all Americans. Individual dedication and a commitment of all Americans to open discussion and change will be tremendous assets to finding effective solutions to the undeniable and unrelenting impact of substance abuse.

REFERENCES

1. National Institute on Drug Abuse. *National Household Survey on Drug Abuse: highlights 2001.*
2. Rouse B. *Drug abuse among racial/ethnic minorities: a special report.* Rockville, MD: National Institute of Drug Abuse, 1989.
3. Hanson B. Drug treatment effectiveness: case of racial and ethnic minorities in America—some research question and proposals. *Int J Addict* 1985;20:99–137.
4. Fort S. *Family history and patterns of addiction in African American cocaine and alcohol dependent individuals* [doctoral dissertation]. University of Iowa, 1990.
5. National Institute on Drug Abuse. *Drug use among racial/ethnic minorities.* NIH Publication No. 95–3888, 1995. Revised September 1998.
6. National Institute on Drug Abuse. *National Household Survey on Drug Abuse: main findings, 1985.* DHHS Pub. No. (ADM) 88–1586. Washington, DC: U.S. Government Printing Office, 1988.
7. National Institute on Drug Abuse. *Illicit drug use, smoking and drinking by America's high school students, college students, and young adults (1975–1987).* DHHS Pub. No. (ADM) 89–1602. Washington, DC: U.S. Government Printing Office, 1988.
8. Kang S, Magura S, Shapiro JL. Correlates of cocaine/crack use among inner-city incarcerated adolescents. *Am J Drug Alcohol Abuse* 1994;20(4):413–429.
9. Robins LN, Murphy GE. Drug use in a normal population of young Negro men. *Am J Public Health* 1967;57:1580–1596.
10. Brunswick AF. Black youths and drug use behavior. In Beschner GM, Friedman AS, eds. *Youth drug abuse: problems, issues, and treatment.* Toronto: Lexington Books, 1979:443–490.
11. Halikas JA, Darvish HS, Rimmer JD. The black addicts. I. Methodology, chronology of addiction, and overview of the population. *Am J Drug Alcohol Abuse* 1976;3:529–543.
12. Chambers CD, Moffett D, Jones JP. Demographic factors associated with Negro opiate addiction. *Int J Addict* 1968;3:329–543.
13. Craig RJ. Characteristics of inner-city heroin addicts applying for treatment in a Veteran Administration hospital drug program (Chicago). *Int J Addict* 1980;15:409–418.
14. Alterman A, et al. Personality Assessment Inventory (PAI) scores of lower socioeconomic African American and Latino methadone maintenance patients. *Assessment* 1995;2:91–100.
15. Kosten T, Rounsaville BJ, Kleber HD. Ethnic and gender differences among opiate addicts. *Int J Addict* 1985;20:1143–1163.
16. Brown LS, et al. Addiction severity index (SI) scores of four racial ethnic and gender groups of methadone maintenance patients. *J Subst Abuse* 1993;5:269–279.
17. Lillie-Blanton M, Anthony JC, Schuster CR. Probing the meaning of racial/ethnic

group comparison in crack cocaine smoking. *JAMA* 1993;269(8):993–997.

18. Van Hasselt NB, Van Hasselt VB, Hersen M, et al. Drug abuse prevention for high risk African American children and their families. *Addict Behav* 1993;18(2):213–234.

19. National Institute on Drug Abuse. *Data from the Drug Abuse Warning Network (DAWN) annual data, 1985.* Statistical Series, Report 1:5, DHHS Publication No. (ADM)-86-1469. Washington, DC: U.S. Government Printing Office, 1986.

20. NIDA Capsules. *Substance abuse among blacks in the U. S.* Rockville, MD: National Institute on Drug Abuse, 1990.

21. Brown LS, Hickson MJ, Ajuluchukuwu DC, et al. Medical disorders in a cohort of NYC drug abusers, much more than HIV diseases. *J Addict Dis* 1993;12(4):11–27.

22. U.S. Centers for Disease Control and Prevention. *HIV AIDS Surveill Rep* 2001;13(2).

23. Valleroy L, MacKeller D, Karon J, et al. HIV infection in disadvantaged out-of-school youth: prevalence for U.S. Job Corps entrants, 1990 through 1996. *J Acquir Immune Defic Syndr* 1998;19:67–73.

24. U.S. Centers for Disease Control and Prevention. *AIDS Wkly Surveill Rep* 1989 Feb 6.

25. Valleroy L, MacKeller D, Karon J, et al. HIV prevalence and associated risks in young men who have sex with men. *JAMA* 2000;284(2):198–204.

26. National Institute on Drug Abuse. *Can drug abuse be prevented in the black community?* Rockville, MD: National Institute on Drug Abuse, 1977.

27. Rappaport J. *Community psychology: values, research, and action.* New York: Holt, Rinehart, & Winston, 1977.

28. Tucker MB. U.S. ethnic minorities and drug abuse: an assessment of the science and practice. *Int J Addict* 1985;20:1021–1047.

29. Feldman HW. Ideological supports to becoming and remaining a heroin addict. *J Health Soc Behav* 1968;9:131–139.

30. Blumer H. *The world of youthful drug use.* Berkeley, CA: University of California School of Criminology, 1967.

31. Crisp AD. Making substance abuse prevention relevant to low-income black neighborhoods. *J Psychoactive Drugs* 1980;12:13–19.

32. Ortiz C. *NIDA workshop on drug abuse prevention for low-income populations.* Washington, DC: 1978.

33. Metsch LR, et al. Implementation of a family-centered treatment program for substance abusing women and their children. *J Psychoactive Drugs* 1995;27(1):73–83.

34. Rowe D, Grill C. African-centered drug treatment, an alternative conceptual paradox for drug counseling with African American clients. *J Psychoactive Drugs* 1993;5(1):21–33.

35. Nuttall RL, Moreland ML, Hunter JB. Effects of an affective drug abuse prevention program on inner city black youth. In Schechter AJ, ed. *Drug dependence and alcoholism. Vol. 2. Social and behavioral issues.* New York: Plenum Press, 1981.

36. Ghadivian AM. A Ba'hai perspective on drug abuse prevention. *Bull Narc.*

37. Graham JW, Johnson CA, Hansen WB, et al. Drug use prevention programs, gender, and ethnicity: evaluation of three seventh-grade project SMART cohorts. *Prev Med* 1990;19:305–313.

38. Kosten T, Gawin FH, Rounsaville BJ, et al. Cocaine abuse among opioid addicts: demographic and diagnostic factors in treatment. *Am J Drug Alcohol Abuse* 1986;12:1–1.

39. Alterman A, Carciola J. The antisocial personality disorder diagnosis in substance abusers: problems and issuers. *J Nerv Ment Dis*

40. Brooner RK, Bigelow GE, Greenfield L, et al. Intravenous drug abusers with antisocial personality disorder: high rate of HIV-1 infection. *NIDA Res Monogr* 1991;105:488–489.

41. Lanarme RJ. School drug education programming: in search of a new direction. *J Drug Educ* 1993;23(4):325–331.

42. National Institute on Drug Abuse. *Data from the national drug and alcoholism treatment utilization survey (NDATUS), main findings for drug abuse treatment units.* Statistical Series, Report F:10, DHHS Publication No. (ADM) 83–1284. Washington, DC: U.S. Government Printing Office, 1983.

43. Brown LS. Substance abuse and HIV/AIDS: implications of prevention efforts for Americans of African descent. In Amuleru-Marshall O, ed. *Substance abuse treatment in the era of AIDS.* Rockville, MD: National Institute on Drug Abuse, 1995:17–58.

44. U.S. Census Bureau. *Census 2000 Brief, The Black Population 2000.* August 2001.

45. Office of Applied Studies (2002). *The DASIS Report.* Rockville, MD: Substance Abuse and Mental Health Services Administration, 2002.

46. Joe GW, Singh BK, Finklea D, et al. *Community factors, racial composition of treatment programs and outcomes. Services research report.* Rockville, MD: National Institute on Drug Abuse, 1977.

47. Brown BS, Joe GW, Thompson P. Minority group status and treatment retention. *Int J Addict* 1985;20:319–335.

48. Phillips P, Phin J, eds. *Drug dependence and alcoholism. Social and behavioral issues.* New York: Plenum Press, 1981;2:22.

49. Pentz MA. Direction for future research in drug abuse prevention. *Prev Med* 1994;23(5):646–652.

CHAPTER 68

Hispanic Americans

PEDRO RUIZ AND JOHN G. LANGROD

Addiction to drugs and alcohol is a major problem among the different Hispanic ethnic groups who reside in the United States. Yet, our knowledge and understanding of the intimate link between addiction and its sociocultural context is still lacking. As a consequence, treatment approaches offered to Hispanics are of limited relevance or of less-than-optimal quality. For instance, only a little more than half of Puerto Rican addicts in New York City become involved in some form of treatment, and, even more importantly, many of those who become involved drop out prematurely (1). In Miami, a similar pattern prevails with respect to Cuban addicts (2). The limited literature that does exist on this subject suggests that significant factors in the etiology of addiction among most Hispanics, primarily Puerto Ricans, are socioculturally related to a considerable extent. It is also apparent that treatment programs designed and operated by "Anglo" professionals have not as yet developed enough adequate cultural sensitivity in programming to attract lower socioeconomic Hispanic addicts. Among the problems related to the special needs of

Hispanic patients in drug-abuse and alcoholism programs are the low percentage of bilingual and bicultural professional staff who work in these programs. In most instances, non–Spanish-speaking staff presents difficulties in understanding the specific sociocultural issues faced by Hispanic addicts. It is unrealistic to expect that Hispanic addicts could feel comfortable and be amenable to treatment efforts in the face of unfamiliar program settings and staff lacking in cultural sensitivity. Even when programs employ enough Hispanic staff and offer culturally sensitive treatment approaches, governmental regulations and policies may interfere with the acceptance of such programs by Hispanic addicts. For instance, the requirement of compulsory urine testing in methadone-maintenance programs, with its implicit message of disbelief of the patient's word, may offend the Hispanic's sense of dignity, which is highly relevant and firmly rooted in Hispanic communities.

It is within this sociocultural context that, in this chapter, we offer a unique perspective on the Hispanic substance abuser. In so doing, we focus on (a) definition of the population; (b) current epidemiologic trends of substance abuse among Hispanics; (c) sociocultural considerations relevant to their substance-abuse patterns; (d) research and treatment outcomes; and, most significantly, (e) public policy formulations.

DEFINITION OF THE POPULATION

As depicted in Table 68.1, and according to the 2000 U.S. Census data (3), of a total U.S. population of approximately 281.4 million, there are approximately 35.3 million Hispanics. As one can deduce from the review of the sociodemographic characteristics identified in Table 68.1,

Hispanics confront major socioeconomic challenges in their quest for occupational, educational, and economic advancement. Moreover, these socioeconomic challenges can be translated into stressors that can lead, directly or indirectly, to the abuse of drugs. The differences between the various Hispanic groups also suggest the need for special programming for each of these groups.

CURRENT EPIDEMIOLOGIC TRENDS

During recent years, a major attempt has been made to scientifically measure the prevalence of drug use among the American household population. To this effect, The National Institute on Drug Abuse (NIDA) and the Substance Abuse and Mental Health Services Administration (SAMHSA) have sponsored a series of national household surveys. These surveys have shed much light on the prevalence of substance abuse in the civilian and noninstitutionalized Hispanic population. In discussing current trends among this Hispanic population, we focus primarily on data emanating from the National Household Survey on Drug Abuse conducted in 1996 (4). Table 68.2 summarizes the lifetime use of some illicit drugs among Hispanics, African Americans, and whites. Hispanics have a slightly lower rate of cocaine and heroin use in comparison to the white population, and a higher rate of use of most drugs in contrast to the African American population, with the exception of marihuana, crack, cigarettes, alcohol, and heroin.

To discuss the index of drug use among different Hispanic subgroups, we first refer to the results of the Hispanic Health and Nutrition Examination Survey conducted between 1982 and 1984 (5). In this survey, published

TABLE 68.1. *Sociodemographic characteristics*

	Non-Hispanic Whites	African Americans	Hispanics	Mexican Americans	Mainland Puerto Ricans	Cuban Americans	Central and South Americans
Population (in millions)	194.6	33.9	35.3	20.6	3.4	1.2	3.1
Median household income	$44,366	$27,910	$30,735	$36,923	$34,777	$52,203	$42,438
Percent of individuals below poverty level	5.7	22.7	21.7	—	—	—	—
Percentage of households with income of $50,000 or more	44.1	23.3	21.5	19.4	18.7	35.3	26.1
Percentage who completed high school	83.0	74.9	54.5	48.6	61.1	65.2	—
Percentage with 4 or more years of college	24.6	13.6	10.3	7.5	10.7	19.7	—
Percentage of female-headed households	14.2	46.7	24.4	20.2	39.4	16.9	26.8
Home ownership	69.2	45.5	43.1	46.3	30.8	55.2	34.3

Source: Adapted from U.S. Bureau of the Census, 2000.

TABLE 68.2. *Percentage of lifetime illicit drug use (1996)*

	African Americans	Hispanics	Whites
Marihuana	29.6	22.0	34.4
Cocaine	8.3	8.5	11.0
Crack	4.2	1.9	1.9
Inhalants	1.6	3.7	6.4
Hallucinogens	3.3	6.0	11.3
Alcohol	72.8	71.7	86.2
Cigarettes	62.1	56.4	76.0
Heroin	1.4	0.9	1.2

Source: Adapted from Xuequin G, Shive S. A comparative analysis of perceived risks and substance abuse among ethnic groups. *Addict Behav* 2000;25(3):361–371.

in 1987, 8,021 individuals between the ages of 12 and 74 years from Hispanic households were surveyed concerning their use of marihuana, cocaine, inhalants, and sedatives. Table 68.3 summarizes the results of this survey. In general, Mexican Americans and Puerto Ricans were each more likely than Cuban Americans to have ever used marihuana and cocaine. Concerning marihuana, the percentages were quite similar among Mexican Americans and Puerto Ricans (41.6% vs. 42.7%). Mexican Americans used inhalants slightly more often than Puerto Ricans (6.4% vs. 4.8%). However, Puerto Ricans were somewhat more likely to use sedatives than were Mexican Americans (5.8% vs. 5.0%). Regarding cocaine, Puerto Ricans were much more affected (21.5%) than either Mexican Americans (11.1%) or Cuban Americans (9.2%).

Concerning the use of alcohol, the Hispanic Health and Nutrition Examination Survey shows significant differences between these three Hispanic groups (6). As seen in Table 68.4, the highest percentage for each group were the abstainers, with females abstaining considerably more often than males. Mexican Americans had the lowest percentage of abstainers (50.3%), while Puerto Ricans and Cuban Americans had similar percentages (59.6% and 59.8%). However, in terms of heavy drinking, the differences are more notable, with Mexican Americans reporting a rate of 8.4% of heavy alcohol consumption, Puerto Ricans 6.7%, and Cuban Americans 3.8%.

TABLE 68.4. *Percent distribution of Mexican American, Cuban American and Puerto Rican drinking levels according to sex (1982–1984)*

Ethnicity and sex	Drinking levels[a]			
	Abstainer (%)	Light (%)	Moderate (%)	Heavier (%)
Mexican American (N = 4,590)				
Male	32.3	26.1	26.4	15.3
Female	68.5	23.8	6.4	1.4
Total	50.3	24.9	16.4	8.4
Puerto Rican (N = 1,821)				
Male	42.6	21.9	22.6	13.0
Female	71.2	19.9	6.5	2.3
Total	59.6	20.7	13.1	6.7
Cuban American (N = 1,060)				
Male	37.8	30.6	23.6	7.9
Female	78.2	17.2	4.1	0.4
Total	59.8	23.4	13.1	3.8

[a] Percentages were calculated with weighted data for persons 12 to 74 years of age.
Source: Adapted from Office of Substance Abuse Prevention of the Alcohol, Drug Abuse and Mental Health Administration: National Clearinghouse for Alcohol and Drug Abuse Information–Update, January 1989, p. 2.

SOCIOCULTURAL CONSIDERATIONS

The relationship between substance abuse and the addict's sociocultural context, particularly the ethnic minority addict, is well documented (7–10). At the heart of the problem is the fact that there exists a dearth of Spanish-speaking and/or bilingual and bicultural professional staff working in the substance-abuse treatment programs that service large numbers of Hispanic addicts. As a consequence, the unique sociocultural needs of these Hispanic addicts have not as yet been met. Furthermore, the rich sociocultural resources that could be used in the treatment of these patients have not been used to their maximum. On many occasions, these situations contribute to both treatment failure and dropout.

At times, stress related to migration add to these sociocultural factors. Consider, for example, the case of Puerto Ricans. Migrants from Puerto Rico to New York City and

TABLE 68.3. *Lifetime percent distribution of drug use among hispanics (ages 12–74 years)*

Drug	Mexican Americans			Puerto Ricans			Cuban Americans[a]		
	Total	Male	Female	Total	Male	Female	Total	Male	Female
Marihuana	41.6	54.2	27.9	42.7	52.9	35.8	20.1	28.2	13.1
Cocaine	11.1	16.5	5.6	21.5	28.3	16.8	9.2	14.3	4.9
Inhalants	6.4	9.5	3.1	4.8	7.1	3.2	—	—	—
Sedatives	5.0	7.3	2.6	5.8	9.1	3.5	—	—	—

[a] Inhalants and sedatives percentages for Cuban Americans were unreliable, and thus not included.
Source: Adapted from *Use of selected drugs among Hispanics: Mexican-Americans, Puerto Ricans, and Cuban-Americans. Findings from the Hispanic Health and Nutrition Examination Survey.* Rockville, MD: National Institute of Drug Abuse, 1987.

other parts of the continental United States are faced with the necessity of forging a new identity for themselves. However, they are also migrating from a society which itself is undergoing an identity crisis. For instance, Puerto Ricans are United States citizens, which permits them to travel freely between Puerto Rico and the mainland. However, Puerto Ricans residing in Puerto Rico cannot vote to elect the president of the United States or other federal officials, but they are subject to U.S. military service. Puerto Rico is neither a state of the union, nor an independent country. These situations create an artificial state of confusion, and thus an identity crisis. Furthermore, the socioeconomic and cultural milieus of Puerto Ricans are characterized by great discrepancies between rich and poor. Moreover, the poverty that exists in Puerto Rico is combined with a consumer mentality and a strong push toward assimilation into the majority "Anglo" culture. This compulsory assimilation and rapid urbanization have led to (a) a devaluation of the Puerto Rican culture, (b) a fragmentation of the extended family network system, and (c) an identity crisis. Undoubtedly, confusion, alienation, and loss of self-esteem are factors responsible for increases in substance abuse among Puerto Ricans. For instance, in the spring of 1986, a statewide household survey of substance abuse was conducted in New York State by the Division of Substance Abuse Services, Alcoholism, and Alcohol Abuse (11). This survey suggests certain correlates between culture and illicit substance use among Hispanics. For example, findings for Hispanics show that the stronger the ties to the Hispanic culture, the less likely the use of drugs is to occur; conversely, the stronger the ties to the American culture, the more likely the drug use. Fifty-three percent of Hispanics born in the United States reported using some illicit drugs during their lifetime, as compared to only 25% of those born in Puerto Rico and 11% of Hispanics born in other Hispanic countries. Along the same lines, 45% of Hispanics who spoke only English or mostly English had used some illicit drugs during their lifetime, whereas only 8% of those Hispanics who spoke Spanish or mostly Spanish did so. Puerto Ricans—as well as Mexican Americans, Cuban Americans, and other Hispanics who recently migrated to the United States—also must confront the additional disadvantage of a language barrier. This language barrier further complicates the acculturation process, thus increasing vulnerability to substance abuse.

To counteract these negative influences, Puerto Rican migrants who are older or have better economic resources frequently visit Puerto Rico and thus attempt to maintain their traditional values and customs. In contrast, younger Puerto Ricans identify more often with the "Anglo" mainland society and therefore are under greater pressure to reject their Hispanic culture in favor of the "Anglo" majority culture. Many of them are caught between cultures, having given up or forgotten most of the cultural traditions of Puerto Rico, while not yet having developed a strong identification with the American way of life.

This group is certainly very vulnerable to drug abuse. Indeed, the incidence of substance abuse among Hispanics, particularly Puerto Ricans, is higher among the youth.

In the case of Cuban Americans, there have been, so far, very limited opportunities to visit Cuba, a situation that has contributed to a stronger sense of survival within the United States. Fortunately for Cuban Americans, however, the process of acculturation has resulted in integration rather than assimilation, separation, or marginalization. This integration process has had a very positive impact insofar as substance abuse is concerned. Cuban Americans have fostered strong relations with the members of the majority "Anglo" culture, while preserving their Cuban cultural traditions and heritage. This has resulted in much less alienation and identity confusion among Cuban Americans than among other Hispanic subgroups that have migrated to the United States. Furthermore, it has assisted Cuban Americans to achieve economic success and independence in the United States.

The previously discussed sociocultural issues lead to a series of key questions concerning substance abuse among Hispanic populations. For instance, how do specific sociocultural factors common to all Hispanics affect types of drug use, patterns of abuse, and treatment needs? Despite all Hispanic subgroups having some common characteristics, such as the Spanish language, Catholic background, Indian and/or African traits, and an Iberian heritage, they differ in the incidence and type of substance abuse. How can we account for these differences? Do Hispanics born and raised in the United States have different treatment outcomes than Hispanics born and raised outside of the United States and who later migrate to this country? If so, why? For instance, it has already been reported in the medical literature (12) that different ethnic groups, including Hispanics, vary in terms of response to drug dosages, side effects, and metabolism of certain psychotherapeutic medications. To what extent could this be physiologically caused and to what extent could this be culturally determined? These types of questions need to be researched further so that the answers can be incorporated into the health care and substance-abuse treatment armamentarium.

Also of great importance, particularly from a prevention point of view, are gender differences in current substance-abuse trends. For instance, substance abuse among young Hispanic women in Puerto Rico and in the United States is on the rise, particularly for certain substances. The factor of female emancipation must be considered in the analysis of these trends, as well as the unnecessary prejudice and discrimination which this emancipating process creates. Culturally determined family dynamics also could play a major role in this increased incidence of substance abuse among Hispanic women (13). Furthermore, a large number of Hispanic women in the United States are heads of households and therefore are forced to function in a variety of different social roles. Undoubtedly, these situations lead to additional stress and thus to increased vulnerability to substance abuse.

Along the same lines, we must also address the special treatment needs of Hispanic female addicts. First of all, they must be treated with equality and respect. Personal and sexual issues must be addressed sensitively and with understanding, particularly when the counselors and therapists are male. The employment of Hispanic female staff is certainly indicated in programs with a large Hispanic female clientele.

In addition, the involvement of the family in the treatment process is critically important. Hispanic families have excellent networking systems, and these systems can play a positive role both in the treatment process and in primary prevention. For instance, Hispanic families with no father figure present are said to be more vulnerable to addiction. In these cases, the individual roles of all family members must be understood, respected, and utilized appropriately in the treatment setting (14). Each member of the family plays a unique role in the dynamics of the family. For example, grandparents are respected for their wisdom, fathers for their authority, mothers for their devotion, children for their future role, and godparents ("padrinos") for their potential available support in times of need.

At times, however, cultural values and norms may impact adversely upon the fight against substance abuse. For instance, it is well known that fatalism is an important trait among Hispanics. "Que sea lo que Dios quiera" (God willing) is an attitude which frequently is expressed by Hispanics (7). This posture can play a negative influence by leading an individual to avoid seeking assistance or drop out of a treatment program. We must combat, educate, persuade, and break those negative attitudes that are caused by poverty, feelings of hopelessness, and powerlessness. Conversely, key Hispanic cultural values such as dignity, respect, and love (dignidad, respeto, y cariño), which represent the core triangle of the Hispanic culture, can all be positively used in both treatment and prevention (14). At times, migration can also play a negative role in the fight against substance abuse because it could lead to a breakdown of the family network system, thus making the members who migrate, as well as those who remain behind, very vulnerable to sociocultural stressors and therefore to addiction (11). Frequent visits to the native country, telephone calls, and correspondence between family members can all minimize these negative influences. In this regard, reinforcement of new networking systems, which could include treatment staff, should be maximized. This should be accomplished without fears of transferential and other related psychodynamic issues.

These problems can also be addressed through the use of group therapy approaches. Group discussions with a focus on historical and/or patriotic themes, when skillfully used, could lead to improvement of individual self-esteem. In this regard, the role of church affiliation—whether it be Catholic, Pentecostal, Jehovah's Witness, or other nonorthodox religious beliefs, such as Spiritism, Santeria, Brujeria, and Curanderismo, could play a major positive role in the development of networking systems, treatment compliance, and primary prevention (15). On certain occasions, it is quite appropriate to develop linkages and liaisons between substance-abuse treatment programs and religious institutions for the specific purpose of implementing preventive strategies, whether primary, secondary, or tertiary (15). These approaches are proven to be beneficial in other areas of health care (16), as well as in mental health (15,17), and thus could also be applied to the field of substance-abuse treatment and prevention. Along these lines, it is important to recognize that Mexican Americans have a strong Indian heritage derived from the Aztec and Mayan cultures; thus, they share a widespread belief in Curanderismo. Similarly, Cuban Americans and Puerto Ricans have been highly influenced by the European Spiritist philosophy of Alan Kardec. Similarly, Cuban Americans, in common with many other Hispanic Caribbean populations, also believe in Santeria and Brujeria. Santeria and Brujeria are syncretistic religious beliefs that were brought to the Caribbean from Africa during the period of slavery (1).

As previously discussed and documented, sociocultural factors could play a major role in the prevention and treatment of substance abuse among Hispanics, and are critically important to the development of comprehensive programs for the treatment of the substance abuser in the United States.

RESEARCH AND TREATMENT OUTCOMES

Unfortunately, there have not been enough well-conducted treatment outcome studies directed at the Hispanic addict. However, some studies deserve to be addressed. For instance, Langrod et al. (18) reported that in treating hardcore Puerto Rican addicts, a positive response can be secured when placing a high degree of program emphasis on areas such as education, cultural sensitivity, and employment of bilingual/bicultural staff. In this regard, one of the most relevant treatment outcome studies was conducted by Nurco et al. (19). In this study, the authors reviewed 897 narcotic addiction treatment programs operating in 25 drug treatment centers in the states of Hawaii, Washington, Maryland, New Jersey, Connecticut, and New York. In the sample, 11.6% of subjects were Hispanic, 37.7% were African American, and 49.6% were white. The focus of the research was to evaluate treatment outcome in relation to client–counselor congruence. Congruence was defined as agreement between client and counselor with regard to (a) appraisal of the client's problems and (b) the most effective approaches for dealing with the identified problems. The results of this study show that, for the entire sample, treatment outcome, in terms of compliance, improvement in quality of life, primary drug abuse problem, and primary nondrug problem were not significantly differentiated according to ethnicity or gender. The only exception, however, was that significant positive correlations were found between appropriateness of services congruence and positive treatment outcomes for Hispanic males. Additionally, for Hispanic females congruence with respect to relative problem severity was related to positive outcomes for compliance with treatment. This type of research merits further exploration, with a particular focus on the different Hispanic subgroups living in the United States. Another important substance abuse treatment outcome study focusing on Cuban Americans was conducted by Szapocznik et al. (20). In this study, the authors presented evidence of the effectiveness of a strategy in engaging adolescent drug users and their families in treatment. The intervention method was based on strategic and structural systems concepts. To overcome resistance, the identified pattern of interactions that interfere with entry into treatment was restructured. Within the context of this study, strategic structural systems engagement is a planned and purposeful approach in diagnosing, joining, and restructuring a family—from the initial contact to the first treatment session. Theoretically, the family is conceptualized as a natural social system that establishes routine patterns of interactions among its members and with the environment. The behavior of the identified patient is perceived within the context of interactions of the entire family. Subjects involved in this study were engaged in treatment at a rate of 93%, in comparison to 42% for those not involved with this type of treatment. Furthermore, 77% of the patients in the study completed their treatment, in contrast to 25% of those who were treated with conventional treatment approaches.

In still another study, Longshore et al. (21) focused on 1,170 drug-using subjects arrested in Los Angeles, California, during the period of April 1988 to January 1990, of whom 35.9% were Hispanics. The perceived need for treatment among them was positively related to (a) self-reported drug dependence, (b) attitudes toward treatment for drug use, and (c) occurrence of drug-related problems other than dependence. Moreover, self-reported drug dependence was found to be higher among female drug users. Hispanics were found to be less likely to perceive a need for treatment among daily drug users (31.4%) than were either African Americans (37.9%) or whites (44.1%). These ethnic differences were not explained by self-reported drug dependence or any other predisposing factor. Likewise, positive attitude toward professional care was much lower among Hispanics (38.1%) than it was among African Americans (74.3%) or whites (75.2%). Concomitantly, heroin use among Hispanics was much higher (39.8%) than among African Americans (11.7%) or whites (18.5%).

In another interesting study (22), 4,157 Mexican American and Mexican youths, between the ages of 11 and 19 years old, living along the United States–Mexico border were studied with respect to their (a) recent drug use, (b) problem drug use, (c) depressive symptomatology, and (d) activity orientation. The results show that the Mexican youths had significantly lower rates of both recent and problematic drug use than did their Mexican American counterparts on the U.S. side of the border. Moreover, while culturally related activity orientation carries a significantly increased risk for substance abuse, symptoms of distress/depression and specific sociodemographic factors exerted an even stronger effect on these youths' use of substances.

Along the same lines, in another study (23), data obtained from 144 Cuban American, 299 Puerto Rican, and 794 Mexican American adolescents included in the Hispanic Health and Nutrition Examination Survey (5) were analyzed to determine whether family structure is related to alcohol and drug use. The results of this study show that family structure had a significant effect for alcohol abuse, drug use, and overall risk-taking behaviors among Mexican American adolescents, as well as overall risk-taking behaviors among Puerto Rican adolescents, but not among Cuban American adolescents. In addition, Mexican American adolescents living in female-headed households reported greater numbers of drinking, drug use, and overall risk-taking behaviors than did those living in two-parent households.

Additionally, Puerto Rican adolescents living in female-headed households had higher rates of overall risk-taking behaviors than did those living with both parents. Family structure, however, was unrelated to Cuban American adolescents' risk-taking behaviors. Also, males reported greater alcohol consumption than did females in each of the three Hispanic subgroups. Of interest, Mexican Americans and Cuban Americans who were predominantly English speakers reported more drug use than did those who were predominantly Spanish speakers. The same was true for Cuban Americans in relation to alcohol consumption. Also, Mexican Americans who lived in higher-income households reported more alcohol use than did those who lived in lower-income households.

In another youth study (13), 223 Hispanic youths ages 12 to 17 years were analyzed to determine parental and age variables with regard to drug use. The results showed that parents' attitudes and use of licit and illicit drugs played an important role in their children's drug using behavior. Moreover, substance use was associated with having less-educated mothers and more-educated fathers, and with fathers having fewer children. Also, youths in one-parent households had higher rates of drug use than did youths in two-parent households. Additionally, substance use by mothers was highly correlated with substance use by children. However, fathers' substance use did not show a consistent pattern of correlation with youth substance use. In addition, among Hispanic subgroups, Mexican Americans had the highest rate of use of drugs. Of interest was the fact that Hispanic children whose parents are more acculturated into "American" society are at higher risk of using drugs; this applies particularly to females.

From another context, a series of research studies focusing on human immunodeficiency virus (HIV)/acquired immunodeficiency syndrome (AIDS) among Hispanics and other ethnic substance-abusing populations have recently been published. For instance, Schilling et al. (24) studied a sample of 91 African American and Hispanic/Latina women who were enrolled in 5 methadone-maintenance clinics throughout New York City. Among the subjects in the study, 37.4% were African American women and 62.6% were Hispanic women. Of the Hispanic women, 96.6% described themselves as Puerto Rican, of whom 26.8% were born in Puerto Rico. The results of this study demonstrated that only 42.4% of these women reported that they had modified their sexual practices to reduce their risk of becoming HIV infected. Half of the women said that they had never used a condom before, and only 12.2% said that they used condoms every time they had sexual intercourse during the last 3 months. Similarly, only 4.4% had used spermicides. Also, 25% of the women said that they had sex during the last 3 months with a partner whose sexual history was not known to them. Moreover, condom use was unrelated to the number of sexual partners. Concerning frequency of drug use and sexual practices, those who reported using drugs more frequently also reported more sexual partners, more frequent sex relations with intravenous drug users, and less frequent use of condoms. No significant differences were found between African American and Hispanic women with respect to frequency of condom use. However, African American women felt more strongly that they could reduce or eliminate their risk of becoming HIV infected than their Hispanic counterparts. Similarly, Hispanic women felt more strongly that getting HIV/AIDS depends on luck than did their African American counterparts. In general, single respondents used condoms more frequently than their nonsingle counterparts, but age was unrelated to frequency of condom use. Among the 56.3% who stated that they do not like to use condoms, 23.1% blamed the possibility of condoms breaking, 25.9% blamed the reduced sexual sensation, 27.3% said that condoms spoil the mood, and 13.2% were afraid about their partners becoming upset. Moreover, 32% of the sample said that they do not feel comfortable asking their partners to use a condom, 23% said that it is embarrassing for them to talk about sex with their sexual partners, and 46% said that they would have sex anyway if their sex partner refused to use a condom. Also of importance was the fact that the education of the subjects was inversely related to the frequency of sex with intravenous drug users and the frequency of sex with a partner whose sexual history was unknown. However, no significant relationships were found between level of education and frequency of condom use during sexual intercourse or number of sexual partners. Moreover, less-educated women felt that they knew enough about HIV/AIDS.

Similarly, in another related study (25), questionnaire data from almost 12,000 street-recruited drug injectors in 19 cities were analyzed to determine racial differences that may affect HIV infection. The ethnic representation of the sample was 61% African American, 16% Hispanic, and 22% white; 76% were male and 24% female. The results of this study showed that the percentage of sex acts in which a condom was used was similar for African American males, white males, and Puerto Rican males, and for African American females and white females in all cities. However, Puerto Rican females reported greater condom use than their African American or white counterparts. In contrast, Mexican American male and female drug injectors were the least likely to report using condoms in multicultural cities. Additionally, white male drug injectors reported less unprotected vaginal sex than African American and Hispanic male drug injectors in multicultural and biracial cities. Also, African American drug users of both sexes were less likely than white or Hispanic drug users to report unprotected anal sex in multicultural cities.

In still another study (26), 257 male intravenous drug abusers were studied in relation to their needle-sharing behavior with familiar individuals and with strangers. The ethnic representation of the sample was 21% African American, 20% Hispanic, and 59% white. Moreover, 42% of the subjects in the sample were HIV-positive. The results of the study showed that the percentage of subjects who shared needles with familiar individuals was as follows: 46% never, 24% a few times, 24% sometimes, 17% most of the time, and 6% always. In contrast, however, the percentage of subjects who shared needles with strangers was as follows: 71% never, 18% a few times, 7% sometimes, 7% most of the time, and 4.2% always. Unfortunately, this study did not depict the results along ethnic lines.

Additionally, Parra et al. (27) studied 50 Mexican American males from the Cornerstone Methadone Maintenance Program in East Los Angeles. These persons and their 50 female sexual partners were examined to determine their risk behaviors, knowledge, and beliefs regarding HIV/AIDS. In the female sexual partners sample, 80% were Mexican American, and 100% were born in the United States. Also, 74% of the female sexual partners had a history of intravenous drug use, and 88% knew that their male counterparts were intravenous drug users. The results of the study showed that 73% of the females and 88% of the males were currently intravenous drug users and shared unsterile needles. Concerning condom use, 76% of females and 84% of males never used a condom during the previous year, and about 20% of both sexes had more than one sexual partner. While 64% of females and 86% of males indicated that cleaning needles with bleach can kill the AIDS organism, only 42% of the females and 34% of males knew that using contaminated needles was the primary source of HIV infection among women.

Unquestionable, the previously addressed research and treatment outcome studies have profound implications in the prevention and treatment of substance abuse among

Hispanics as well as other ethnic and nonethnic groups. Undoubtedly, more research needs to be conducted with Hispanic populations if we ever intend to master the substance abuse problem faced by the different Hispanic subgroups who live in the United States.

Since the publishing of the last edition of this textbook in 1997 (1), several well-conceptualized research and treatment outcome studies have been conducted. For instance, Markarian and Franklin (28) have pointed out that for Mexican American women born in the United States, alcohol abstention rates steadily decreases and the rates of infrequent drinking steadily increases with acculturation. Another study (29) reported that Hispanic and African American men and women responded similarly to the first 6 months of methadone-maintenance treatment.

Finally, another study (4) reported that Hispanics had a higher prevalence of binge drinking among the 12 to 17 years and 35 years and older age groups, and also of heavy drinking in the 12- to 17-year-old age group than either whites or African Americans.

PUBLIC POLICY FORMULATIONS

In discussing the subject of substance abuse among the different Hispanic populations residing in the United States, one must also address issues related to public policy development and implementation. To begin with, we recommend and expect that Hispanics be directly involved, and fully participate in, the design and implementation of such policies. This type of involvement will ensure identification with these policies and, more importantly, compliance with them. Hispanic consumers must also be involved at all levels of this process because they will be the recipients of the impact of these policies. Hispanics tend to underuse all types of mental health services, including substance-abuse services (14,16). If mental health and substance-abuse programs were to be planned, designed, and implemented by Hispanic professionals and consumers, one would expect that these services will be more accepted and therefore more fully used by Hispanic communities. Hispanics, based on their clinical skills and cultural knowledge, can better plan and design culturally sensitive program models geared to the treatment of Hispanic patients. In so doing, they can also serve as ideal role models for future generations of Hispanic mental health professionals. For instance, the eco-structural family therapy model seems to be quite effective with the Hispanic substance abuser (30). This model fits quite well the expectations, values, and traditions of the Hispanic family. This model is present oriented, and adapts itself effectively to the needs of the Hispanic family. Furthermore, it places emphasis on family interactions, as well as in the family ecologic system rather than on the individual patient.

An important public policy issue has to do with the development of an appropriate national data base for Hispanics. So far, efforts in this regard have been limited. The collection of reliable data at a national level will be a positive step toward its application to public policy development. It was only recently that Hispanics began to be classified according to their country of origin, and that attention was given to this very important issue. Reliable national data is very powerful in calling attention to public health problems, and thus leading to their solution.

Another issue that requires attention is the development of preventive and educational programs. While patient care is important, efforts directed at prevention are also essential. The spiraling costs of health care in the nation has negatively affected prevention efforts. However, the most effective method of reducing health care costs is to prevent illnesses. In this respect, some very promising preventive models have recently been advanced in the field of substance abuse. For instance, it has been reported (31) that strained social relationships and a heightened sense of powerlessness and helplessness may induce adolescents to rely more heavily on substance use as a means of emotional self-regulation. This behavior requires lesser effort and ability, promises instant effects, and provides a sense of control. This model, which focuses on stress reduction, social learning, support networks, and is based on coping, acculturation, and informational network theories, is ideal for substance abuse prevention among adolescents. Along these lines, Fried (32) has also reported that the endemic stress among the socioeconomically disadvantaged serves to diminish the effective means of coping with acute stress, thereby increasing the vulnerability to pathology. This suggests that much of the phenomenology of life among the disadvantaged might be best understood as an attempt to adapt to chronic stress. Such an adaptation process can lead to a depressive orientation, a sense of helplessness and powerlessness, and therefore to vulnerability with respect to substance use and abuse. In this context, public policy should advocate for a promotion of functional competency, and thus advocate for programs with a clear emphasis on psychoeducational initiatives, and with a focus on the development of coping skills.

Besides models with a focus on stress reduction, we should also focus on socioeconomic models, either independently or in conjunction with models focusing on stress reduction. For instance, migration is known to produce strains associated with economic status. Migration leads to immigrants entering the host nation at the lowest socioeconomic levels. This situation could lead to great stress among migrants. Furthermore, it is an accepted fact that the rates of all types of psychopathology among the lowest socioeconomic categories are about 2.5 times the rates of psychopathology in the highest socioeconomic categories (33). The prevailing explanation for this inverse relationship is based on the distribution of stress across the socioeconomic system, with greater stress tending to concentrate at the bottom of the system. In this context, public policies could address the socioeconomic conditions of the Hispanic substance abuser and, in so doing, could also address the factors that affect their socioeconomic status such as unemployment, low education, and poor housing, among others. To ignore the relationship that exists between socioeconomic factors and substance abuse will undoubtedly lead to an inefficient public policy formulation. The impact of class-related socioeconomic strains is very strong among Hispanic migrants because they must also face acculturation problems and language barriers. Perhaps, the best example of the relationship between social class and psychopathology can be found in the research conducted among children and adolescents. For instance, Langner et al. (34) compared a large sample of children on welfare with a non–welfare-children group. They found that the referral rates to health care services for the welfare group increased as their mother's level of education increased. They also noted that the children from the welfare group were more severely impaired in their health status than the children from the non-welfare group. Similarly, Harrison et al. (35), while investigating the relationship between social classes and mental health care, found that children of professionals or executives had twice as great a chance of being treated with intensive psychotherapy as did the children of blue-collar parents. Furthermore, they also found that children of middle-class parents were more frequently diagnosed as suffering from neurotic disorders or as being normal, while children of lower-class parents were more often diagnosed as suffering from psychosis or personality disorders. Likewise, Rutter et al. (36), while studying elementary school children, observed that children's behavior changed according to the school they attended. Behavioral difficulties were more often found in schools with high rates of teacher and student turnover. Generally, larger turnovers were usually found in urban ghettos and in lower class neighborhoods.

Finally, we focus on the legal system in relation to public policy formulation. In this regard, drug legalization and decriminalization deserve consideration and attention. In analyzing legalization of drugs, we must focus on the pros and cons of drug-prohibition policies. The total United States antidrug expenditure in 1990 was $9.5 billion (37). Because legalization or decriminalization could lead to a reduction in the cost of the government's antidrug expenditures, it could also lead to a redistribution of expenditures in the direction of treatment and prevention. Additionally, because legalization or decriminalization would result in lowering the cost of illicit drugs, it would also result in a decrease in drug-related criminal activities. This reduction in drug-related criminal activities would also further reduce the cost of the criminal justice system. In this regard, methadone-maintenance programs represent a limited form of drug legalization and decriminalization. While the connection between drugs and crime could be seen as coincidental, it is nevertheless important. For instance, a survey conducted in 1986 among inmates of state prisons revealed that 43% were using illegal drugs on a daily basis (38). Furthermore, it is a well-accepted fact that some illicit drugs influence people to commit crimes by reducing inhibitions and increasing aggressiveness. Co-

caine, for instance, is a drug that has gained this reputation in recent years (38). On the other hand, opponents of legalization or decriminalization claim that such measures would certainly increase drug availability, decrease their price, and remove the deterrent power of the criminal sanctions, thus leading to an increase in drug use and abuse. However, the use of tobacco has decreased in recent years as a result of educational and prevention efforts.

Undoubtedly, legalization or decriminalization of illicit drugs contains some risks. However, our current laws and policies have not yet yielded much permanent benefit. We must objectively evaluate all of our options, including legalization or decriminalization alternatives. Not to do so will help maintain the status quo, and will further contribute to the deterioration in the living conditions of our ethnic minority ghetto populations, particularly Hispanics.

CONCLUSION

For decades, the substance-abuse problem has been devastating for the Hispanic population residing in the United States. However, not enough attention has been given to this problem, particularly, with respect to preventive approaches, epidemiologic research, culturally sensitive clinical interventions, treatment outcome studies, and public policy formulations. Additionally, program development and fiscal allocations have not been commensurate with the size of these problems. Recently, however, the substance abuse and HIV epidemics have extended into the white population of this country. As a result of this shift, the government, particularly at the federal level, has been forced to pay more attention to the substance-abuse problem. Hopefully, this new governmental emphasis will also help to focus attention on the ethnic, minority substance abuser. Generally, traditional agencies and government bureaucracy have overlooked the need for basic awareness of the characteristics, conditions, and circumstances surrounding the Hispanic substance abuser.

Unfortunately, most of the non-Hispanic staff currently employed in substance-abuse treatment programs servicing Hispanics are unprepared in terms of (a) Spanish language ability, (b) an understanding of the Hispanic substance abuser's socioeconomic background, and (c) awareness of the Hispanic culture and heritage. Undoubtedly, these critical gaps have had a negative impact on service effectiveness, on positive treatment outcomes, and, even more importantly, on prevention strategies. If Hispanic substance abusers are to be rehabilitated effectively, program designers and treatment staff must understand not only the values and norms inherent in the Hispanic culture, but also those circumstances which threaten that culture.

This chapter has shed light upon these problems and has presented data to support our observations. Hopefully, through increased research efforts and appropriate financial support, we will eventually conquer this major tragedy facing the Hispanic family.

REFERENCES

1. Ruiz P, Langrod JG. Hispanic Americans. In: Lowinson JH, Ruiz P, Millman RB, et al., eds. *Substance abuse: a comprehensive textbook,* 3rd ed. Baltimore: Williams & Wilkins, 1997:705–712.
2. Rothe EM, Ruiz P. Substance abuse among Cuban Americans. In: Straussner SLA, ed. *Ethnocultural factors in substance abuse treatment.* New York: Guilford Press, 2001:97–110.
3. U.S. Bureau of the Census, 2000.
4. Xueqin G, Shive S. A comparative analysis of perceived risks and substance abuse among ethnic groups. *Addict Behav* 2000;25(3):361–371.
5. National Institute on Drug Abuse. *Use of selected drugs among Hispanics, Mexican Americans, Puerto Ricans, and Cuban Americans. Findings from the National Health and Nutrition Examination Survey.* Washington, D.C., U.S. Government Printing Office, 1987.
6. National Clearinghouse for Alcohol and Drug Abuse Information. *Update.* Office for Substance Abuse Prevention of the Alcohol, Drug Abuse, and Mental Health Administration. January, 1989:2.
7. Alvarez LR, Ruiz P. Substance abuse in the Mexican American population. In: Straussner SLA, ed. *Ethnocultural factors in substance abuse treatment.* New York: Guilford Press, 2001:111–136.
8. Barthwell AG. Cultural considerations in the management of addictive disease. In: Miller NS, Gold MS, Smith DE, eds. *Annual of therapeutics for addiction.* New York: John Wiley & Sons, 1997:246–254.
9. Ruiz P, Langrod JG. Substance abuse among Hispanic Americans: current issues and future perspectives. In: Lowinson JH, Ruiz P, Millman RB, eds. *Substance abuse: a comprehensive textbook,* 2nd ed. Baltimore: Williams & Wilkins, 1992:868–874.
10. Velez CN, Ungemack JA. Psychosocial correlates of drug use among Puerto Rican youth: generational status differences. *Soc Sci Med* 1995;40(1):91–103.
11. *Statewide Household Survey of Substance Abuse, 1986. Illicit substance use among Hispanic adults in New York State.* New York: State Division of Substance Abuse Services, 1988.
12. Ruiz P, Varner RV, Small DR, et al. Ethnic difference in the neuroleptic treatment of schizophrenia. *Psychiatr Q* 1999;70(2):163–172.
13. Gfroerer J, De La Rosa M. Protective and risks factors associated with drug use among Hispanic youth. *J Addict Dis* 1993;12(2):87–107.
14. Ruiz P. The Hispanic patient: sociocultural perspectives. In: Becerra RM, Karno M, Escobar JI, eds. *Mental health and Hispanic Americans: clinical perspectives.* New York: Grune & Stratton, 1982:17–27.
15. Ruiz P, Langrod J. Psychiatry and folk healing: a dichotomy? In: Mezzich JE, Berganza CE, eds. *Culture and psychopathology.* New York: Columbia University Press, 1984:470–475.
16. Ruiz P. Cultural barriers to effective medical care among Hispanic American patients. *Annu Rev Med* 1985;36:63–71.
17. Koss JD. Expectations and outcomes for patients given mental health care or spiritist healing in Puerto Rico. *Am J Psychiatry* 1987;144(1):56–61.
18. Langrod J, Alksne L, Lowinson J, et al. Rehabilitation of the Puerto Rican addict: a cultural perspective. *Int J Addict* 1981;16(5):841–845.
19. Nurco DN, Shaffer JW, Hanlon TE, et al. Relationships between client/counselor congruence and treatment outcome among narcotic addicts. *Compr Psychiatry* 1988;29(1):48–54.
20. Szapocznik J, Perez-Vidal A, Brickman AL, et al. Engaging adolescent drug abusers and their families in treatment: a strategic structural system approach. *J Consult Clin Psychol* 1988;56(4):552–557.
21. Longshore D, Hsieh S, Anglin MD. Ethnic and gender differences in drug users' perceived need for treatment. *Int J Addict* 1993;28(6):539–558.
22. Pumariega AJ, Swanson JW, Holzer CE, et al. Cultural context and substance abuse in Hispanic adolescents. *J Child Fam Stud* 1992;1(1):75–92.
23. Sokol-Katz JS, Ulbrich PM. Family structure and adolescent risk-taking behavior: a comparison of Mexican, Cuban, and Puerto Rican Americans. *Int J Addict* 1992;27(10):1197–1209.
24. Schilling RF, El-Bassel N, Gilbert L, et al. Correlates of drug use, sexual behavior, and attitudes toward safer sex among African Americans and Hispanic women in methadone maintenance. *J Drug Issues* 1991;21(4):685–698.
25. Friedman SR, Young PA, Snyder FR, et al. Racial differences in sexual behaviors related to AIDS in a nineteen-city sample of street-recruited drug injectors. *AIDS Educ Prev* 1993;5(3):196–211.
26. Brooks JS, Brooks DW, Whiteman M, et al. Psychosocial risk factors for HIV transmission in male drug abusers. *Genet Soc Gen Psychol Monogr* 1993;119(3):369–387.
27. Parra EO, Shapiro MF, Moreno CA, et al. AIDS-related risk behavior, knowledge, and beliefs among women and their Mexican American sexual partners who used intravenous drugs. *Arch Fam Med* 1993;2(6):603–610.
28. Markarian M, Franklin J. Substance abuse in minority populations. In: Frances RJ, Miller SI, eds. *Clinical textbook of addictive disorders,* 2nd ed. New York: Guilford Press, 1998:397–412.
29. Mulvaney FD, Brown LS, Alterman AI, et al. Methadone-maintenance outcomes for Hispanic and African American men and women. *Drug Alcohol Depend* 1999;54:11–18.
30. Szapocznik J, Scopetta MA, King OE. Therapy and practice in matching treatment to the special characteristics and problems of Cuban immigrants. *J Community Psychol* 1978;6:112–122.
31. Labouvie EW. Alcohol and marijuana use in relation to adolescent stress. *Int J Addict* 1986;21:333–345.
32. Fried M. Disadvantage, vulnerability, and mental illness. In: Parron DL, Solomon F, Jenkins CD, eds. *Behavior, health risks, and social disadvantage.* Washington, DC: National Academy Press, 1982.
33. Dohrenwend BP, Dohrenwend BS, Gould MS, et al. *Mental illness in the United States.* New York: Praeger 1980:56.
34. Langner TS, Gersten J, Eisenberg J. Approaches to measurement and definition in the epidemiology of behavior disorders: ethnic background and child behavior. *Int J Health Serv* 1974;4:483–501.
35. Harrison SI, McDermott JF, Wilson PT. Social class and mental illness in children: choice of treatment. *Arch Gen Psychiatry* 1965;13:411–417.
36. Rutter M, Yule B, Quentin D, et al. Attainment and adjustment in two geographical areas: some factors accounting for area differences. *Br J Psychiatry* 1975;126:520–533.
37. *U.S. News & World Report* December 24, 1990, p. 12.
38. Nadelmann EA. Drug prohibition in the United States: cost, consequences, and alternatives. *Science* 1989;245:939–946.

CHAPTER 69

Asian Americans and Pacific Islanders

JOHN W. TSUANG

Recent research findings have shown that biologic, psychological, and social/cultural factors affect the onset and course of substance abuse. Coinciding with the increasing numbers of Asian Americans and Pacific Islanders (AA/PIs) in the United States, there are increasing efforts to evaluate substance use issues among them. However, factors that influence substance abuse among AA/PIs remain unclear. This chapter reviews the available data related to the use of substances among AA/PIs, focusing on demographics, epidemiology, biopsychosocial factors, treatment, and prevention.

DEMOGRAPHICS

According to the 2000 U.S. Census (1), 10.4 million AA/PIs reside in the United States (3.7% of the U.S. population). AA/PIs represent one of the fastest growing ethnic minority groups in the United States. From 1990 to 2000, the number of people identifying themselves as Asian American or Native Hawaiian or Other Pacific Islander increased by 44%, with a total of 10 million for Asian Americans and 0.35 million for Native Hawaiian or and Other Pacific. Ninety-six percent of AA/PIs reside in metropolitan areas within two western states (California and Hawaii) and three nonwestern states (New York, Texas, and Illinois). The fastest growing populations of AP/PIs are in Georgia, Nevada, North Carolina, Nebraska, Arizona, Delaware and New Mexico (1).

AA/PIs are diverse in ethnicity, as well as in their historical experiences in the United States. AA/PIs represent a heterogeneous group differing in language, religion, culture, immigration pattern, generation, socioeconomic status, and the degree of acculturation into mainstream American culture. The major Asian groups in the United States are Chinese (24%), Filipino (18%), Asian Indian (16%), Vietnamese (11%), Korean (10%), and Japanese (8%). Other Asian groups (13%) include Burmese, Cambodian, Hmong, Laotian, Thai, and Tongan. The major Pacific Islander groups are Native Hawaiian (35%), Samoan (23%), Guamanian or Chamorro (15%), and other Pacific Island groups (27%) (1,2).

EPIDEMIOLOGY OF SUBSTANCE ABUSE

During the 1990s, the Substance Abuse and Mental Health Services Administrations (SAMHSA) sponsored a series of national household surveys to measure the prevalence of illicit drug and alcohol use among Americans. AA/PIs were classified in the "other" category until 1999, when Asian and Native Hawaiian or Other Pacific Islander were separated (3). In the 2000 SAMHSA survey, 2,654 AA/PIs were interviewed. It was estimated that 0.4 million (5.2%) of AA/PIs "used illicit drugs in the past year" and 0.2 million (2.7%) "used an illicit drug in the past month" (4). AA/PIs had the lowest rate of illicit drug use in comparison to the general population and to other racial subgroups (4). However, contrary to the popular myth of being the "model minority," data showed that AA/PIs do use illicit drugs.

The SAMHSA survey showed that AA/PIs are more likely to drink alcohol and smoke cigarettes than to use illicit drugs (4). It was estimated that 2.3 million AA/PIs (28%) had "used alcohol in their lifetime" and in the 18- to 25-year-old age group, 3.2 million (39.4%) had consumed alcohol. Three million AA/PIs (38.8%) had "used cigarettes in their lifetime" and 3.4 million (41.9%) in the 18- to 25-year-old age group had smoked in their lifetime (4). AA/PIs ranked the lowest among all racial subgroups in terms of proportions that drank alcohol or smoked cigarettes. However, the gap between AA/PIs and the next racial group (African Americans), in terms of smoking (41.9% vs. 50.2%) or drinking (39.4% vs. 43.9%) was much smaller than the differences in illicit drug use (4).

The survey showed a drop in illicit drug and alcohol use by AA/PIs when comparing data from 1999 to 2000. "Illicit drug use in the last year" went from 20.2% to 18.8%, and "any alcohol use" went from 30.7% to 28% (4). However, there were some disturbing trends in this study, as well as in others. The rates of heavy alcohol use by Asian youth (five binges in the last month) doubled from 1999 to 2000 (0.5% to 0.9%). Others researchers found that AA/PI high school students who met criteria for heavy drinking consumed more alcohol per day when they did drink (1.46 ounces per day) than did whites (0.86 ounces per day) (5). The SAMHSA survey showed that in the age 26 years and older group, Vietnamese Americans, had the highest percentage of current marijuana use rate (2.8%). The "past month hallucinogen use" for Asian youth was equal to the highest rates of 1.4% by whites. Finally, AA/PI youths' abuse of prescription drugs had more than tripled from 1999 to 2000 (6).

National treatment surveys showed that AA/PIs represent 4% of population, but less than 1% of them were admitted to Treatment Episode Data Set (TEDS is a compilation of data on those admitted to substance abuse treatment) (DASIS) (7). But the trend is changing; between 1994 and 1999 number of AA/PIs admissions increased by 37% (9,800 to 13,400), while total admissions decreased by 3%. For AA/PIs, alcohol abuse counted for 34% of all admissions followed by marijuana (19%), stimulants (19%), opiates (15%), and cocaine (11%). At the time of admission, Asians were younger (average age 30 years) than the general population (average age 33 years), and a greater proportion of them were in treatment for the first time (51% vs. 36%, respectively). This increase in number entering into substance-abuse treatment might reflect more substance abuse by AA/PIs or the greater acceptance of need for treatment among Asians (7,8).

Critics have argued about the inaccuracy of national survey studies. In the SAMHSA study, results from the Native Hawaiian or Other Pacific Islanders were not reported because only 545 people were surveyed. This was unfortunate as Pacific Islanders have high rates of substance abuse and alcohol use (9). By excluding them, the numbers of substance abusers among AA/PIs were artificially lowered. In addition, underreporting of substance abuse problems is prominent among AA/PIs (8). Some Asian cultures incorporate substances use into their religious practices or daily accepted activities, thus their uses are often not mentioned. Other issues, such as types of people surveyed, cultural and language barriers, and culturally insensitive questions all can contribute to the lower rates of substance abuse (10). In summary, AA/PIs do have the lowest rates of illicit drug, alcohol, and cigarettes use among all different racial/ethnic subgroups. However, there is concern about increasing substance abuse among AAPIs adolescents and other high-risk groups.

FACTORS INFLUENCING ALCOHOL AND DRUG USE IN ASIAN AMERICANS AND PACIFIC ISLANDERS

Genetic/Biologic Factors

Multiple factors, including biologic ones, have been proposed to affect the addiction process. The best data came from the study of alcohol abuse, so we use this as a model for much of the discussion that follows. There is a striking lack of information about other drugs of abuse in the AA/PIs population. The best studied biologic area is in the genetic contribution to the development of alcoholism. Family and adoption studies have found a significant hereditary contribution in alcoholism, although these data were not derived from the AA/PI population (11,12). For Asians, the transmission of alcohol genes and the mechanism for impaired alcohol metabolism are areas of special interests.

Approximately 50% of northeast Asians (Chinese, Japanese, and Koreans) have a genetically defined deficiency in the liver enzyme, aldehyde dehydrogenase (ALDH2) (13,14). This deficiency is inherited through one mutant ALDH2*2 allele, a dominant mutation that disrupts the function of the subunit polypeptide and reduces enzyme activity (15). The ALDH2*2 allele is prevalent among northeast Asians but rare in non-Asians (16). Asians with ALDH2*2 alleles are slower in the oxidation of acetaldehyde during alcohol metabolism, resulting in the accumulation of acetaldehyde, and subsequently the exhibition of a "flushing reaction" after in-

gestion of alcohol (17,18). This response is accompanied by increased heart rate, visible redness, and feelings of warmth (19) that are presumably mediated through histamines and other vasoactive compounds (20). This genetically determined flushing reaction is thought to be one factor related to the reduction in alcohol consumption among Asians (21,22). Individuals with ALDH2*2 alleles (ALDH2*1/2*2 heterozygotes or ALDH2*2/2*2 homozygotes) drink less alcohol (21,23,24) and have lower rates of alcohol dependence (25,26) when compared with those with the ALDH2*1/2*1 homozygous genotype. Conversely, most patients with alcoholic liver diseases have the ALDH2*1/2*1 homozygous genotype (24,26).

In addition to ALDH2, northeast Asians also possess an "atypical" alcohol dehydrogenase enzyme (ADH2) that can increase the capacity to convert alcohol into acetaldehyde, further contributing to the flushing reaction after alcohol ingestion (27). The ADH2 is a functional polymorphism of the alcohol dehydrogenase gene that protects against heavy drinking and alcoholism (20). To date, ALDH2 is the enzyme that is most likely to influence drinking behaviors, and it might be a protective factor for AA/PIs from alcohol dependence (14,20,24,25,26).

Illicit drug use and its genetic transmission is not well understood. Some researchers suggest that AA/PIs with certain genetic variations and metabolic differences might be at decreased risk for illicit drug use. For example, a recent study found that ALDH2 might be associated with the reduction of substance abuse behavior among Asians (14). Other factors such as the cytochrome P450 (CYP) system is involved in the metabolism of commonly used substances (20,28,29). Nicotine is metabolized to cotinine principally by the CYP2A6 enzyme. Individuals carrying the null (inactive) CYP2A6*2 or 2A6*3 alleles with impaired nicotine metabolism, compared to the active CYP2A6*1, showed reduced smoking and nicotine dependence (30). Genetic deficiency in CYP2D6 metabolism, which converts codeine to morphine derivatives, provides protection against oral opiate dependence (31). AA/PIs may show some CYP enzymes polymorphism, that is, extensive metabolizers (EMs) versus poor metabolizers (PMs) that can affect breakdown of substances differently. The relationship between this genetic variation and the possibility of lower substances of abuse by AA/PIs needs to be studied further.

Environmental Factors

The biologic and genetic studies have made a major impact on our understanding of the inheritance of alcoholism. Even with a genetic predisposition, however, the expression of alcoholism can be affected by environmental, social, and psychological factors (24). It is difficult to disentangle the specific environmental factors that affect drinking, but for the purpose of discussion, we separate them into psychological, acculturation, and family/cultural factors.

Psychological Factors

Stress has been imputed to be a precursor to alcohol abuse in Asians as well as non-Asians (32–34). In general, psychological factors such as self-esteem, self-confidence, and assertiveness, are related to alcohol use among adolescents (35). Psychological maladjustment was a significant factor associated with alcohol use among a sample of Chinese and Filipino youth (36). Other factors associated with risk for alcohol use among AA/PIs included pressure to succeed and a feeling of shame (10). For some Asians, the impact of immigration and accompanied psychological symptoms increased the risk for alcohol abuse (37). These immigrants suffered from feelings of personal failure and loss of control, which can lead to alcohol abuse (38). For example, Vietnamese and Highland Laotians (Hmong) immigrants reported using more alcohol as a mean of coping with pain, insomnia, and alleviation of distress (34,39,40). For AA/PIs, many psychological reasons have been linked to increase alcohol abuse. However, the degree of psychological impact on the precipitation and maintenance of alcoholism and illicit drug use has not been well studied.

Acculturation Factors

The degree of acculturation into mainstream America is a factor that affects alcohol intake among AA/PIs. The definition of the acculturation process varies, but some have based it on a number of generations residing in the United States, and an ability to speak English and/or their ethnic languages. One study found that Asians who did not speak English well reported drinking less than those who did speak it well (41). It was also reported that alcohol consumption was related to generation status and birthplace. Third- and fourth-generation Asians in the United States reported more drinking than did first- and second-generation Asians. There appeared to be significant group differences in alcohol consumption between foreign-born Asians and Asians born in America (41). This was the case for Hawaiian residents of Chinese and Japanese ancestry who had lower mean levels of alcohol use if they were born in Asia than if they were born in Hawaii (42). Hawaiian residents of white ancestry had lower mean levels of alcohol use if they were born in Hawaii than if they were born on the mainland. For Hawaiians, who many considered to be more acculturated than other AA/PI groups, alcohol use is intermediate between the lower levels found in Asia and the higher levels found in the United States. Some studies found that assimilation of recently arrived immigrant groups is associated with increases in alcohol use. These results were found in Hispanic Americans (43), Mexican Americans (44), as well as Asian Americans (41,45). However, not all studies concurred with the idea that increased

acculturation into Western culture will increase amount of alcohol consumed (32,46). Nevertheless, it does appear that acculturation process plays a role in the consumption of alcohol by AA/PIs. More studies are required to better define acculturation and systematically determine the relationship between the degree of acculturation and alcohol and illicit substance use.

Family/Cultural Factors

It was suggested that the relatively late age of onset of alcohol use for Asian American youth than for non-Asian American youth might be a result of parental modeling or cultural influences (14). Asian American students, who had a more abstinence-promoting environment than their European-American counterparts, were less likely to drink alcohol. Asian students were less likely to have "adult and peer influences to use alcohol or cigarettes," "less offers of alcohol," and "increased likelihood of having an intact family." It was concluded that a strong family connection and the fewer presence of parents and peer use might reduce Asian's alcohol use (19).

The importance of norms and values in Asian cultures may moderate drinking by AA/PIs. One study proposed that attitudes about drinking, such as lack of negative feelings about alcohol by Chinese and Jewish communities, might be related to reduced alcohol consumption (47,48). Other cultural factors, such as responsibility to others, prescribed behaviors, interdependence, restraint, and group achievement, all may reduce drinking (33). Additional factors such as cultural traditions, Asian religions, respect for authority, Asians' belief in order, propriety, and harmony, as well as concerns with shame and losing face, can affect alcohol consumption (49). Some Asian cultural beliefs validate habitual alcohol and substance use. Many traditional medicines are alcohol-based and they are taken for energy boost (gelatin from tiger bones dissolved in alcohol) or to relieve pain (opium in alcohol). Others, such as chewing of the betel quid or stimulant leaf, are done to produce euphoria (39,50,51). Use of sleeping pills to alleviate stress during is also considered a culturally acceptable practice among some AA/PIs as means of reestablishing equilibrium (50,51).

Other researchers have shown that peer pressure, acculturation, and family discord are the major factors associated with marijuana and cocaine use among AA/PIs (52). Factors related to a higher lifetime use of cigarettes, alcohol, and marijuana by high school students of Vietnamese and Chinese descent included poor school performance, low subjective well-being, lack of parents' or peers' disapproval of substance use, perceived tensions at school, and being male (52). At this time, although significant, not much is known about the environmental influences on illicit drug use by AA/PIs.

In summary, among AA/PIs, psychological stresses, degree of assimilation, and family/peer attitudes, as well as cultural factors appear to play a role in alcohol consumption. Although biologic factors are important, one must not forget the contributions of these other factors to explain ethnic differences in alcohol consumption. Unfortunately, some of these studies had methodological weaknesses, making it difficult to determine the extent of psychological/social/cultural influences on the onset and course of alcohol consumption; consequently, more studies are needed. In addition, more studies focusing on the relationships between environmental factors and illicit drug uses are needed.

TREATMENT

As seen from the TEDS data, an increasing number of AA/PIs are entering substance-abuse treatment (7). Cultural awareness is necessary for programs treating AA/PI patients if they want to be successful. In general, AA/PIs enter into a treatment program much later in the process of their substance abuse. In their cultures, substance abuse is a taboo issue. The traditional personal and family response to a "crisis" among many Asian cultures is denial. Family members often rescue and enable the patients and try to resolve the problem internally. By the time the addiction problem becomes unmanageable, both a strong sense of personal failure and family shame occur. The strategy is to "save face," which often causes the family to delay confrontation of the patient. Thus, by the time an AA/PI is referred to a drug/alcohol treatment program, all other alternatives have been exhausted. The client is often resistant to any interventions and reluctant to receive treatment, whereas the family wants a "quick-fix" solution and avoids their personal responsibility. Often, abandonment of the patient can occur at the time when family support is most essential. Consequently, Asians see entrance into drug and alcohol treatment program as the last resort, and are often angry and in denial of their problems, which makes their treatment even more difficult (37,39).

There are other barriers facing AA/PIs during substance-abuse treatment, including the continuing feeling of loss of face and stigma, the need for respect, the problem of openly acknowledging personal problems, the double standard for women, and the religious belief of fate and need for suffering. AA/PIs are also racially and culturally heterogeneous; they don't all fit well in just one type of treatment program. They feel better in and probably will benefit much more from culturally sensitive programs (8,37).

Many authors suggest that treatment programs for AA/PIs should be multicultural and multilingual (8,10, 37). These services should be delivered from community-based sites with community inputs. The program should follow the traditional Alcoholics Anonymous (AA)/Narcotics Anonymous (NA) treatment strategies of combining 12-step approaches with the therapeutic community in residential treatment and the use of cognitive behavioral treatment. However, there should be some alterations

to the "one-treatment-fits-all" approach. These modifications, specifically for AA/PIs, should include the strategy of reducing confrontation initially, so individuals can decrease the embarrassment, shame, and loss of face upon entering a treatment program. The program should involve a structured treatment paradigm with a task-sharing format. Counseling approaches and peer group should be supportive and educational. Family engagement, counseling, and support will be crucial to the individual's recovery (8). Finally, any outside factors to increase motivation, such as court involvement (i.e., drug court) or to get the encouragement of the patriarchal member of the family will be helpful (37).

Studies have found that more than half of people who meet a lifetime history of a *Diagnostic and Statistical Manual of Mental Disorders,* 3rd ed., revised (*DSM–III–R*) mental disorder diagnosis also have a co-concurrent substance abuse diagnosis (53,54). Giving the growing evidence that mental health and substance-abuse problems frequently co-occur, mental health assessment among AA/PIs seeking substance-abuse treatment should be conducted. Patients with dual-diagnosis disorders (both mental illness and substance abuse) should be treated in an integrated treatment program to receive maximum benefit (55,56).

PREVENTION

Various people have written about prevention strategies against substance abuse for AA/PIs, but the effectiveness of these measures have not been studied. Most authors agree with the thought that culturally responsive prevention strategies should be linked into the natural support systems of that particular Asian Pacific community; for example, in the Filipino community, using the church as a forum for prevention work. Prevention should provide Asian parents with the skills they need to help their children assimilate into American culture, such as helping them with their roles in the educational and recreational processes. Programs should develop strategies to minimize shame and loss of face in AA/PIs, especially dealing with intergenerational conflict. This can be done by using a community intermediary to manage interpersonal conflicts between parents and youth. Finally, community education programs might use more personalized contacts for prevention, such as a door-to-door education campaign in the high-risk community (8).

A family oriented approach in which an extended family is included in issues of prevention, intervention, and treatment will have the best chance of success in the Asian community. One needs to address issues of denial, underreporting, and the need for getting outside help. It is very important to preserve the family unit as a hedge against substance use (50). Other strategies can include the use of media campaigns in their native languages and the use of high-profile community role models to advertise against substance abuse. One should also promote self-esteem and culturally appropriate life-skills building for Asian youth, and engage culturally specific human service networks for prevention process. All of these recommendations on treatment and prevention approaches should be studied for their effectiveness (10).

CONCLUSION

As the AA/PI populations continue to grow in the United States, there is an increased need to address substance abuse issues among these populations. The limited epidemiologic data suggests that, in general, AA/PIs are at a relatively lower risk for substance use than other ethnic groups. However, it also suggests that rates for alcohol use, smoking, and some illicit drugs use may not be as low as generally assumed. Substance abuse, to some degree, is physiologically mediated, but cultural and environmental influences can also play a role in contributing to substance use patterns. AA/PIs infrequently use substance treatment services, which have led to a misperception as a lack of need for services by them. At present, there is a paucity of empirical information on the effectiveness of treatment and prevention programs targeting AA/PIs. Professionals who treat ethnically and culturally diverse AA/PI populations with substance abuse should be aware of the issues described in this chapter, so that they can tailor therapeutic regimens to be "culturally responsive," to assure high quality of care, and to meet the needs of population served. Because biologic, environmental, and cultural differences exist among different Asian ethnic groups, understanding similarities and differences between them can play an important role in ensuring that AA/PIs receive optimum substance-abuse treatment.

REFERENCES

1. U.S. Department of Commerce, Bureau of the Census. *The Asian and Pacific Islander population in the United States: March 2000 (Update) (PPL-146).*
2. U.S. Department of Health and Human Services. *Mental health: culture, race, and ethnicity. A supplement to mental health: a report of the surgeon general.* United States Public Health Service. Office of the Surgeon General. 2001:105–126.
3. U.S. Department of Health and Human Services, SAMHSA. *National Household Survey on Drug Abuse Series: H-12. Summary of findings from the 1999 National Household Survey on Drug Abuse.*
4. Substance Abuse and Mental Health Services Administration. *Summary of findings for the 1999 National Household Survey on Drug Abuse.* Office of Applied Studies, NHS DA Series H-12, DHHS Publication No. (SMA) 00-3466. Rockville, MD.
5. Welte J, Barnes GM. Alcohol use among adolescent minority groups. *J Stud Alcohol* 1987;48:329–336.
6. U.S. Department of Health and Human Services, NCADI, SAMHSA. Asian/Pacific Islander Americans and substance abuse. *Prev Alert* 2002;5:7.
7. Office of Applied Studies. Substance Abuse and Mental Health Services Administration. *The DASIS report. Asians and Pacific Islanders in substance abuse treatment: 1999.* 2002 Aug 16.
8. Zane N, Kim JH. Substance use and abuse. In: Zane N, Takeuchi D, Young K, eds. *Confronting critical health issues of Asian and Pacific Islander Americans.* Thousand Oaks, CA: Sage Publications, 1994:316–343.
9. McLaughlin, PG, Raymond JS, Murakami SR, et al. Drug use among Asian Americans in Hawaii. *J Psychoactive Drugs* 1987;19:85–94.
10. Kuramoto F, Nakashima J. Developing an ATOD prevention campaign for Asian and Pacific Islanders: some considerations. *J Public Health Manage Pract* 2000;6:57–64.
11. Goodwin DW, Schulsinger F, Hermansen L, et al. Alcohol problems in adoptees raised apart from alcoholic biological parents. *Arch Gen Psychiatry* 1973;28:238–243.
12. Schuckit MA, Goodwin DW, Winokur G. A study of alcoholism in half-siblings. *Am J Psychiatry* 1972;128:1132–1136.
13. Wolff PH. Vasomotor sensitivity to alcohol in diverse Mongoloid populations. *Am J Hum Genet* 1973;25:193–199.
14. Wall TL, Shea SH, Chan KK, et al. A genetic association with the development of alcohol and other substance use behavior in Asian Americans. *J Abnorm Psychol* 2001;110:173–178.
15. Crabb DW, Edenberg HJ, Bosron WF, et al. Genotypes for aldehyde dehydrogenase deficiency and alcohol sensitivity: the inactive ALDH2(2) allele is dominant. *J Clin Invest* 1989;83:314–316.
16. Goedde HW, Agarwal DP, Fritze G, et al. Distribution of ADH2 and ALDH2 genotypes in different populations. *Hum Genet* 1992;88:344–346.
17. Shibuya A, Yasunami M, Yoshida A. Genotypes of alcohol dehydrogenase and aldehyde dehydrogenase loci in Japanese alcohol flushers and nonflushers. *Hum Genet* 1989;82:14–16.
18. Wall TL, Thomasson HR, Ehlers CL. Investigator-observed alcohol-induced flushing but not self-report of flushing is a valid predictor of ALDH2 genotype. *J Stud Alcohol* 1996;57:267–272.
19. Au JG, Donaldson SI. Social influences as explanations for substance use differences among Asian American and European American adolescents. *J Psychoactive Drugs* 2000;32:15–23.
20. Li TK. Pharmacogenetics of responses to alcohol and genes that influence alcohol drinking. *J Stud Alcohol* 2000;61:5–12.
21. Tu GC, Israel Y. Alcohol consumption by Orientals in North America is predicted largely by a single gene. *Behav Genet* 1995;25:59–65.
22. Wall TL, Thomasson HR, Schuckit MA, et al. Subjective feelings of alcohol intoxication in Asians with genetic variations of ALDH2 alleles. *Alcohol Clin Exp Res* 1992;16:991–995.
23. Takeshita T, Morimoto K. Self-reported alcohol-associated symptoms and drinking behavior in three ALDH2 genotypes among Japanese university students. *Alcohol Clin Exp Res* 1999;23:1065–1069.
24. Yoshida A. Genetic polymorphisms of alcohol-metabolizing enzymes related to alcohol sensitivity and alcoholic diseases. In: Lin KM, Poland RE, Nakasaki G, eds. *Psychopharmacology and psychobiology of ethnicity.* Washington, DC: American Psychiatric Press, 1993:169–183.
25. Chen CC, Lu RB, Wang MF, et al. Interaction between the functional polymorphisms of the alcohol-metabolism genes in protection against alcoholism. *Am J Hum Genet* 1999;65:795–807.
26. Thomasson HR, Edenberg HJ, Crabb DW, et al. Alcohol and aldehyde dehydrogenase genotypes and alcoholism in Chinese men. *Am J Hum Genet* 1991;48:667–681.
27. Agarwal DP, Goedde HW. *Alcohol*

metabolism, alcohol intolerance and alcoholism: biochemical and pharmacogenetic approaches. Berlin: Springer-Verlag, 1990.

28. Karlow W. Pharmacogenetics: past and future. *Life Sci* 1990;47:1385–1397.
29. Pi EH, Gray GE. A cross-cultural perspective on psychopharmacology. *Essential Pharmacol* 1998;2:233–260.
30. Pianezza LM, Sellers EM, Tyndale RF. Nicotine metabolism defect reduces smoking. *Nature* 1998;393:750.
31. Tyndale RF, Droll KP, Sellers EM. Genetically deficient CYP2D6 metabolism provides protection against oral opiate dependence. *Pharmacogenetics* 1997;7:375–379.
32. Sue S, Kitano H, Hatanaka H, et al. Alcohol consumption among Chinese in the United States. In: Bennett L, Ames G, eds. *The American experience with alcohol: contrasting cultural perspectives.* New York: Plenum Press, 1985:359–371.
33. Sue D. Use and abuse of alcohol by Asian Americans. *J Psychoactive Drugs* 1987;19:57–66.
34. Yee BWK, Thu ND. Correlates of drug use and abuse among Indochinese refugees: mental health implications. *J Psychoactive Drugs* 1987;19:77–83.
35. Bhattacharya G. Drug use among Asian Indian adolescents: identifying protective/risk factors. *Adolescence* 1998;33:169–184.
36. Zane N, Park S, Aoki B. The development of culturally valid measures for assessing prevention impact in Asian American communities. In: *The development of culturally valid measures for assessing prevention impact in Asian American communities.* (DHHS Publication No. SMA 98–3193). Rockville, MD: U.S. Department of Health and Human Services, 1999:61–89.
37. Ja D, Aoki B. Substance abuse treatment: cultural barriers in the Asian-American community. *J Psychoactive Drugs* 1993;25:61–71.
38. Kim S, McLeod, JH, Shantzis C. Cultural competence for evaluators working with Asian American communities: some practical considerations. In: Orlandi MA, ed. *Cultural competence for evaluators: a guide for alcohol and other drug abuse prevention practitioners working with ethnic/racial communities.* Rockville, MD: U.S. Department of Health and Human Services, 1992:203–260.
39. Westermeyer JC. Native Americans, Asians, and new immigrants. In: Lowinson JH, Ruiz P, Millman RB, eds. *Substance abuse: a comprehensive textbook,* 3rd ed. Baltimore: Williams & Wilkins, 1997:712–715.
40. D'Avanzo CE. The Southeast Asian client and alcohol and other drug abuse: implications for health care providers. *Subst Abuse* 1994;15:109–113.
41. Sue S, Zane N, Ito J. Alcohol drinking patterns among Asian and Caucasian Americans. *J Cross-Cultural Psychology* 1979;10:41–56.
42. Johnson RC, Nagoshi CT, Ahern FM, et al. Cultural factors as explanations for ethnic group differences in alcoholism in Hawaii. *J Psychoactive Drugs* 1987;19:67–75.
43. Caetano R. Acculturation and attitudes toward appropriate drinking among U.S. Hispanics. *Alcohol Alcohol* 1987;22:427–433.
44. Caetano R, Medina Mora ME. Acculturation and drinking among people of Mexican descent in Mexico and the United States. *J Stud Alcohol* 1988;49:462–471.
45. Kitano HH, Hatanake H, Yeing WT, et al. Japanese-American drinking patterns. In: Bennett LA, Ames GM, eds. *The American experience with alcohol: contrasting cultural perspectives.* New York: Plenum Press, 1985:335–357.
46. Klatsky AL, Siegelaub AB, Landy C, et al. Racial patterns of alcoholic beverage use. *Alcohol Clin Exp Res* 1983;7:372–377.
47. Peele S. A moral vision of addiction: how people's values determine whether they become and remain addicts. *J Drug Issues* 1987;17:187–215.
48. Peele S. The limitations of control-of-supply models for explaining and preventing alcoholism and drug addiction. *J Stud Alcohol* 1987;48:61–77.
49. Johnson RC, Nagoshi CT. Asians, Asian Americans and alcohol. *J Psychoactive Drugs* 1990;22:45–52.
50. D'Avanzo CE. Southeast Asians: Asian Pacific Americans at risk for substance misuse. *Subst Use Misuse* 1997;32:829–848.
51. Flaskerud JH, Kim S. Health problems of Asian and Latino immigrants. *Nurs Clin North Am* 1999;34:359–380.
52. Sasao T. Identifying at-risk Asian American Adolescents in multiethnic schools: implications for substance abuse prevention interventions and program evaluation. In: *Identifying at-risk Asian American Adolescents in multiethnic schools: implications for substance abuse prevention interventions and program evaluation* (DHHS Publication No. SMA 98–3193). Rockville, MD: U.S. Department of Health and Human Services, 1999:143–167.
53. Regier DA, Farmer ME, Rae DS, et al. Comorbidity of mental disorders with alcohol and other drug abuse: results from the Epidemiologic Catchment Area (ECA) study. *JAMA* 1990;264:2511–2518.
54. Kessler RC, McGonagle KA, Zhao S, et al. Lifetime and 12-month prevalence of *DSM–III–R* psychiatric disorders in the United States: results from the National Comorbidity Survey. *Arch Gen Psychiatry* 1994;51:8–19.
55. Tsuang J, Ho A, Eckman T, et al. Dual diagnosis treatment for patients with schizophrenia who abuse psychostimulants: rehab rounds. Invited article. *J Psychiatric Serv* 1997;48(7):887–889.
56. Ho A, Tsuang J, Liberman R, et al. Achieving effective treatment of patients with chronic psychotic illness and comorbid substance dependence. *Am J Psychiatry* 1999;156:1765–1770.

CHAPTER 70

Alcohol Use Among American Indians and Alaskan Natives

EDWARD F. FOULKS

Colonization of native populations of North and South America over the past 5 centuries brought military conquests, infectious diseases, dislocation from land and livelihood, and social discrimination that persists to the present time. The combination of social and economic disenfranchisement, along with displacement from their lands of livelihood into enforced reservation life, has been persistently devastating to many Native American communities. It is in this context of the destruction of hope and of a good and prosperous life that problems with substance abuse emerged. While drug use is widespread in this and other disadvantaged minority populations in the United States, alcohol abuse in many Native American groups has been persistently high with age-adjusted alcohol mortality rates now six times the United States all-races overall rates (1,2).

This chapter cites several studies that indicate that the problems with alcohol use have been historically evident in many groups of Native Americans across centuries of European contact and colonization. Popular responses to Indian drinking included theories that "firewater" (alcohol) had a unique effect on Native Americans who were believed to be constitutionally unable to handle it, and more sensitive to its' effects than other races (3). However, as the recent studies of Garcia-Andrade, and others have shown, subjects with greater American Indian heritage actually responded to alcohol with less sensitivity than did a control sample with less than 50% Native American heritage (4). Schuckit demonstrated that people at a higher genetic risk for alcoholism usually are less sensitive to the effects of alcohol, and that people at a lower genetic risk for alcoholism are actually more sensitive (5). More recent genetic studies indicate that a genetic variant that resides close to the HTR1B coding sequence, which is associated with low cerebrospinal fluid concentrations of a major metabolite of serotonin, may be involved in the control of aggression, impulsivity, antisocial traits, and alcoholism (6). Their study included a southwestern American Indian sample collected from a family based study of alcoholism and psychiatric disorders. An important caveat for consideration is the fact that not all Native Americans are alcoholic, and that genetic factors may be particularly relevant for understanding differences between tribes and between individuals within the same tribe. Native Americans represent a heterogeneous population of considerable genetic and cultural variation.

Once dominant, Native Americans now include less than 1% of today's U.S. population. Native Americans are the most rural of the four nationally registered ethnic minority groups—approximately 70% live in rural areas, as compared with 21% of Hispanic and 27% of African American populations. More than half the rural Native Americans (55%) are nonfarm residents, relying for a substantial part of their subsistence on traditional occupations of hunting, trapping, and fishing. Native American populations are also characterized by very high levels of unemployment, especially among youth and young adults. Unemployment itself can be considered an indicator of nonparticipation in the dominant culture and contributes to resistive or marginalization modes of acculturation. Partly as a consequence of these economic factors, and partly as a result of U.S. government employment training incentives, there has been a steady increase in urban migration among Native Americans during the past 3 decades, perhaps indicating a tread toward cultural integration and assimilation (7,8).

Most Native Americans are located in 27 states; more than 50% of the total Native American population live in Arizona, New Mexico, California, and Alaska. Only 37% now live on reservations or native villages, and 30% to 96% remain rural in spite of the trend toward urban migration in the past 20 years. The Native Americans migrating to cities are predominantly young adults. The trend has been most notable in western and southwestern states: Denver, Tuscon, Albuquerque, and Los Angeles, for example, have rapidly growing Native American populations (7,8).

The Native American population as a whole is comparatively young, with a median age of 22.9 years, compared to 31.1 years for whites, which is a confounding factor in comparing morbidity rates for alcohol use with other population groups unless age-adjusted. Rural Native Americans also have one of the highest birth rates of the minority groups. More than 25% of Native American families have seven or more members, and 70% of rural families have more than four. Poverty and remoteness from urban centers contribute further to the difficulties a large family encounters in attempting to participate in the dominant culture.

Since 1955, health services have been provided for the Native American population by the U.S. Public Health Service on about 250 reservations in 23 federal Indian Reservation States and in several hundred villages in Alaska. Nevertheless, maintaining adequate health care has been complicated by geographic, cultural, and social barriers. Housing for Native Americans, whether in rural or urban areas, has often been overcrowded and lacking safe water and adequate sanitation facilities. Dietary deficiencies in many populations contribute to increased risk of infectious disease and physical debilitation. Epidemics have resulted in high rates of sickness and death throughout the period of culture contact and continue even today. Many Native Americans have had parents, other relatives, and friends who died or were debilitated by tuberculosis, and their infants and children lost to measles and enteric diseases. During the past 20 years, however, considerable progress has been made by the Public Health Service to reduce mortality from communicable diseases and to lower infant mortality rates.

Through the Bureau of Indian Affairs (BIA), the U.S. government provides education for Native Americans not served by local public or private schools. Prior to 1970, most rural Native Americans who attended high school were required to go to BIA-administered boarding schools, often in locations distant from their homes. This introduced the stresses of separation from family and clan, and the psychological stresses of imposed cultural change. Native American children, like other minority groups, face special problems that complicate their education. More than half must learn English as a second language and must contend with culturally divergent concepts, values, and attitudes of the majority culture represented by some peers, townspeople, and their teachers. Educational materials and curricula sometimes portray Native Americans in a negative light, and often contribute to their rejecting their own traditional cultural values and behavioral norms.

In addition to these difficulties, lack of economic opportunity and increasing social disorganization have had adverse effects on Native American youth. Throughout North America, pressures of unemployment, as well as tensions between the Indian and non-Indian communities, have disrupted traditionally close family ties. The escalating prevalence of separation, divorce, and family violence has resulted in a disproportionately high number of broken homes and placing of Native American children in foster care with non-Native American families. In North Dakota, for example, the rate of Indians placed in foster care was 17 times that of whites (9). Among Native Alaskans, foster care and adoption are also common factors that engender stress in a large proportion of youth (10).

Although Native Americans share in common the problems of colonization, dislocation, poverty, and social upheaval, they are not one culturally homogeneous population. Major differences exist in the way of life, customs, language, social organization, history, personality, and values of tribes in different regions of the country, and even within the same geographic region. The cultures and languages of the Plains Indians, Pueblo Indians, and Arctic Inuit differ as much from each other as the cultures and languages of the Celtic Irish, the Hungarians, and the Lapps. Just as these European populations show differences within their countries and territories, so do Native American groups exhibit great intragroup variations of language, economic activity, social organization, attitudes, values, and customs. These intergroup and intragroup cultural variations influence the acculturative process when Native American communities come into

contact with Western society and help to account for the variation in customary alcohol use of different Native American populations.

HISTORICAL PERSPECTIVES

Early colonization of native people of the new world was often brutal and exploitative. Severe and devastating sickness soon followed these early encounters, leaving the remaining population in a state of decimation and suffering from post traumatic disorders.

The natives of the Caribbean Islands and the Atlantic Coast were the first to experience significant such European contact. Natives of the Muskogean language group were impacted by the Spanish in Florida. Guillemin described the meeting of the Micmac Indians, of the Algonkian language group, in the Canadian Maritime Provinces with Spanish, Portuguese, and French explorers and fishermen (11). The scenario that unfolded around what is now Halifax would be repeated with some variation for the next 3 centuries.

The first encounter with the Micmac may have been as early as the end of the fifteenth century, but destructive relations continued throughout the sixteenth century. Trade with the Micmac, including the services of Indian women, characterized the first encounters. Miscegenation as well as an overall reduction of the native population through European diseases followed. As far as can now be determined, those diseases included syphilis, scurvy, small pox, typhus, dropsy, pleurisy, and consumption. Native social organization accommodated to both reduced numbers and the continued presence of Europeans. Alcohol and the social and health effects of alcohol were not far behind.

By the middle of the seventeenth century, the Micmac had acquired guns through trading. The bow and arrow were displaced, and hunting became more efficient. Trading in furs drew the Micmac more and more into the Euro-American market. Increased hunting with guns and for the market, rather than simply for subsistence, made for a general depletion of game. To avoid starvation in winter, it became necessary to cover a wider area. Traditional animal food and skins for clothing became scarce. Dependence on European foodstuffs and clothing became essential. Such dependence on trade increased the Micmac's need to sell pelts, further depleting the game.

With muskets, the Micmac became a warrior society and even attacked Eskimos to their north. Later, the Mohawk and Ottawa Indians, to their south and west, purchased guns, and exerted military pressure by the French gradually reduced their territory. Today, the Micmac are reservation Indians in Nova Scotia, some leading relatively impoverished, but still socially identifiable lives in urban areas from Halifax to Boston.

Four factors became constants in native encounters with the Euro-American world: the biologic onslaught through exposure to diseases against which their immune responses were inadequate; the technologic change, beginning with the gun, which upset the ecologic balance between man and subsistence fauna; the social reorganization, deriving both from the introduction of technology and their participation in a wider commercial market; and, finally, political domination by an advanced society. During these stages the natives, exposed to American education and religion, underwent cultural change. At some point, most natives encountered challenges to their conceptions of land tenure. Political pressure from coordinate societies was less important in the Alaskan Eskimo scenario. Perhaps this was a result of the isolation and sparseness of the population. It was no more relevant for the Athabascan, Tlingit, and Haida of southeastern Alaska.

Most of the contact scenarios around American natives, as in the case of the Micmac, followed European incursions from the eastern coast. The Alaskan natives, also were approached by the English through Canada from the east. At the same time, Russians were exploring and exploiting the western coast of Alaska and the Aleutians.

The Hudson's Bay Company, working on the Canadian prairie in the late seventeenth century, encountered the Cree. A familiar scenario unfolded. The Cree were drawn into fur trapping and became increasingly dependent on white traders for European artifacts. In trapping, they moved from their woodland habitat onto the plains and, within a century, developed the plains culture. By 1825, the plains Cree culture was fully committed to the horse, gun, and buffalo, and had discarded most of its woodland cultural inventory (12). During the first century of contact, liquor was exchanged for furs. Following reports reaching the Hudson's Bay Company during the 1860s of Indians murdering one another in drunken orgies, the company forbade selling liquor to the Cree. Already committed to social activities that included alcohol, the Cree obtained it from Americans in exchanged for buffalo robes.

To the west in Alaska, alcohol was unknown to traditional Aleut and Eskimo society. The Russians introduced *kvass* (homemade beer) and wine. The Aleuts began drinking, at first as part of a ceremonial, later to just get drunk. In these early years, drinking rarely led to violence or serious disruption (13).

After the 1867 sale of Alaska to the United States, the Americans began offering the Aleuts clothes, toys, canned goods, rations, ammunition, and frame houses in return for furs, particularly those of the sea otter. Aleuts and nonnatives intermarried. Soon there was a gold rush and American Protestant churches came to convert the native population as a missionary field. Episcopalians, Presbyterians, and Moravians, among others, extended their efforts to "civilize" the Indians, Aleuts, and Eskimos of Alaska. The first formal United States Protestant mission to Alaskan natives was established in 1877 at Fort Wrangell by Sheldon Jackson.

Jackson urged President Harrison to establish in Alaska a civil government led by good Christians. He argued that Alaska had suffered from godless, drinking officials. Drinking Russians and drinking Americans provided an example for the Alaskan native. The Russians, during their tenure, had tried to preserve the right of Russians to drink while discouraging the sale of intoxicating liquors to natives. President Harrison, in an Executive Order, tried to generalize the prohibition of liquor by prohibiting its sale.

Problem Drinking

What problems have Native American people experienced with drinking alcohol and how do these problems compare with those experienced by the population at large? Cahalan and Room provide a good overall picture of drinking-related problems in the United States, based on a national probability sample of almost 3,000 men (14). They categorized drinking-related problems in three areas: (a) the amount of patterning and style of drinking behavior, (b) the psychological loading attached to the behavior, and (c) physiologic and social consequences of the behavior.

Cahalan and Room, following this frame of reference, developed a number of measurement scales describing characteristics of the drinking (the independent variable) or of its sequelae, the dependent variables. These are designated (a) heavy intake, (b) binge drinking, (c) psychological dependence, (d) loss of control, (e) symptomatic drinking behavior, (f) belligerence after drinking, (g) problems with wife over drinking, (h) problems with relatives, (i) problems with friends or neighbors, (j) child problems, (k) police problems over drinking, (l) problems with health or injuries related to drinking, and (m) financial problems related to drinking.

Cahalan and Room noticed that symptomatic drinking, binge drinking, psychological dependence, and police problems tended to occur earlier than some other problems. Interpersonal problems, such as those with relatives, wives, and job, came later. Health problems, particularly, tended to emerge very late and to be less predictable. While the onset of heavy drinking precedes its social consequences, those consequences tend to persist even after the behavior has ceased.

Native Americans suffer from many of these problems associated with alcohol use, including alcohol-related deaths, at rates higher than that of the surrounding populations. Among American Indians, the incidence of alcoholism is reported to be at least twice the national average. The national average for alcoholism and alcohol abuse combined has been estimated at 7% of the adult population. On some American Indian reservations, the rate is as high as 25% to 50% (15).

Alcohol-related problems among American Indians have also become serious. Duck Valley Indians live on a reservation of about 30,000 acres near the Nevada–Idaho border, along with about 1,000 mixed Shoshone and

Paiute, all organized into one tribe under the Indian Reorganization Act of 1938. In Nevada, an Indian is five times as likely as a non-Indian to die an alcohol-related death. In 1975–1976, the average number of alcohol-related deaths for Indians was 92.18 per 100,000, as compared to the rate of 18.5 per 100,000 U.S. citizens. Of 133 arrests in August 1977, 75% were alcohol related (15).

Norick, an anthropologist studying Indians and Eskimos in Alaska, writes of intoxication as the normative or customary function at social events, parties, dances, and celebrations (16). Liquor is an integral and indispensable part of all diversionary functions. At such events, large amounts are drunk in short intervals, until the supply is exhausted or the drinker has passed out. Norick documented case histories of heavy drinking interfering with occupational role performance: showing up late for work, or not showing up at all because of a binge the night before, or drinking on the job.

Norick found that Eskimos and Indians who bypassed the educational process and received minimum exposure to non-native ways were least likely to drink excessively. Individuals who see worth and merit in pursuing traditional activities were least likely to experience the strain, stress, or emotional conflict that resulted in alcoholic behaviors.

Levy and Kunitz, who studied Native Americans in the lower 48 states, found that although a large proportion of Navajo homicides (73%) and suicides (47%) are committed in association with alcohol intoxication, the relationship is coincidental (17). However, the use of alcohol has been increasing. Liver cirrhosis incidence and deaths are higher. Yet Navajo homicide and suicide rates have remained stable since the 1880s. This is contrary to the situation among the Eskimos. Homicide and suicide rates have increased in parallel with an increase in drinking. An association of alcohol and violent crime has also been noted among southeastern Eskimos. Drinking there often leads to criminal assault and accounts for 35.47% of the crime for which these Eskimos are arrested. In 1969, 76% of all fines, arrests, and imprisonments of southeastern Eskimos were associated with drinking (15).

Kraus and Buffler found escalating suicide patterns associated with drinking among the Inuit and Yuit Eskimos, which parallel patterns they discovered among the Athabascan Indians of Alaska (10). Suicide was associated with alcohol use in almost all cases. The victims were young, of both sexes, and usually died while intoxicated.

Klausner and Foulks related increasing suicide rates and alcohol problems in Native Alaskans to the rapid social and cultural changes experienced during the past decade of major exploitation of energy resources in the Arctic (18). They reported that approximately 30% of the population were relatively well prepared for changes in their way of life through generations of family contact with traders, missionaries, and U.S. government representatives. This group has adapted to the acculturative stress by means of cultural and psychological integration. On the other hand, the majority of the Inuit population, not so well-prepared by historical circumstances has experienced great distress in trying to cope with the process of rapid acculturation in their region. They have become victims of alcohol abuse, depression, and, in some cases, suicide. Their lives were characterized by self-doubt and lack of direction, identity confusion and marginalization.

Resnick and Dizmang discussed similar sociocultural factors producing higher suicide rates on Shoshone reservations during the 1960s (19). Among the most important factors were the breakdown of traditional values, patterns of behavior resulting from enforced residence on reservations, geographic isolation, widespread unemployment, and a high incidence of alcoholism. The sociocultural determinants applied so strongly in this case that the authors thought that theories of individual dynamics or neurochemistry could not account for the high incidence of alcoholism, depression, and suicide. Rather, it was apparent that the high infant mortality rates (50% higher than U.S. norms), early death (average life expectancy of 44 years), a birth rate twice that of the general population, high unemployment (approximately 40%; more than ten times the national average), inadequate housing, and gross overcrowding contributed to severe acculturative stress and cultural marginalization.

Because of these cultural stresses, some researches of native societies have avoided using the term alcoholism or alcohol abuse, and instead refer to the following alcohol-related general dysfunctions, which are experienced across physiologic, psychological, and social systems:

1. Pathophysiologic symptoms include hepatomegaly, tremors, blackouts, convulsions, cirrhosis, cardiomyopathy and other myopathies, central nervous system deterioration, and abnormalities of blood serum.
2. Psychopathologic features include an undue preoccupation with alcohol, serious loss of behavior control when drinking, a self-destructive attitude in personal relations, an inability to control either the start of drinking or its termination, and lack of the development of or loss of inner resources to control impulses.
3. Social pathologies include deterioration of familial relationships, inability to function in other social institutions such as work, school, church or other organizations, problems with the law, violent behaviors, suicidal behavior, homicide, and susceptibility to accident (19).

In addition, several specific factors explain heavy drinking among American Indians in particular: (a) learning drinking behavior from whites, (b) adoption of new roles by Indians whose access to high-status positions was blocked in the traditional system, (c) use of intoxication to achieve aboriginal goals, and (d) the deterioration of the society under conquest (17).

Learned Behavior From Whites

Kunitz and Levy describe poor Navaho who became wage earners in the American market society and assumed the goals and values of the dominant society, including ideas about drinking (20). They noted that by the 1890s, these Navaho were prepared to trade a yearling steer for a gallon of bootlegged liquor.

Lubart interpreted excessive drinking among the Mackenzie Delta Eskimos as an adaptation to the stress of social and economic change and acculturation (21). Clairmont found that those persons age 16 to 29 years in Aklavik suffered the most serious problems (22). Lobban described the Eskimos of Inuvik as moving through approximately 200 years of development in 10 years (23). Young people came to resent their surroundings and to be ashamed of their Eskimo background. Unable to cope with alcohol, the villagers engaged in drunken brawls and murder. Methanol poisoning from wood alcohol even began to appear when they ran out of distilled spirits.

Intoxication and Traditional Goals

Leach likens the persistence of traditional microstructures in the face of change in social macrostructures to an image on a piece of rubber that when stretched—even to its limits—distorts the picture (24). Yet the elements of the original pattern remain in a consistent relationship.

MacAndrew and Edgerton believed that drunken violence and sexual deviance may at times be culturally prescribed (25). They found that intoxication often provides an occasion for socially excusable misbehavior, that would otherwise be troublesome. However, the drunken misconduct is usually contained within certain cultural limits, and cultural values may permit alcohol to excuse the drinker by reason that the alcohol is at fault, not the person.

Levy and Kunitz propose that, among Navaho in the southwestern United States, frequent and heavy intoxication accompanied by violent behavior is compatible with preexisting and persisting tribal institutions and values (17). Drinking facilitates aggression, and they maintain that Navaho get drunk in order to be aggressive. In a warrior tradition, assertiveness and aggression are valued; therefore drunkenness, insofar as it facilitates such conduct, may be culturally approved, as long as the aggression is within certain limits and is expressed toward specified objects and on appropriate occasions.

Cross-cultural studies indicate that hunting and gathering groups place a premium on individual skill, luck, and daring. Alcohol may be valued because people under its influence do what the tribe values. The likelihood of such forms of expression is greater when social control is not rigidly enforced. Thus, highly visible group drinking is socially acceptable in loosely organized rather than tightly integrated tribes.

Exertion of magical power was also a source of personal prestige in traditional Native American society. The ability through shamanic ritual and, occasionally, through hysterical dissociation, to achieve altered states of consciousness was often considered a special skill or talent. Many Native American individuals may use alcohol to obtain such transcendental states. MacAndrew and Edgerton found that a state of temporarily being inhabited by a supernatural agent was achieved by drunkenness (25). The psychological state attained through intoxication is in this way continuous with the traditional model of "soul loss." Soul loss in traditional societies may occur spontaneously under conditions of emotional or physical stress (26–29). For example, there are many accounts of Inuit who without alcohol or any other mind-altering drug, manifested a loss of their souls during personal stress. In these cases, the individual first becomes withdrawn and nontalkative. The individual enters a meditative state, breathing hard and sometimes chanting, which provides an exit for the soul. The individual may then exhibit "out-of-mind" behavior, running around, violently throwing things, or shouting. The Inuit believe that their soul is wandering. In such states, some take off clothing and expose their bodies, even in winter. The episode might last several hours. Later, the victim of such an episode might be unable to remember what happened (29).

These dissociative episodes provided an emotional catharsis and, at the same time, reaffirmed the spiritual power of the human soul. They believed that the soul, after leaving the person's body, reunited with the souls of animals to be hunted or with powers under the ground, sea, or in the sky. Individuals who could obtain such states of consciousness were considered people of "power." Shamans ritually experienced soul loss in response to serious distress in the community, such as illness, hunger, or feuding, and so possessed much power.

Most people had less power, but all had some for use in times of personal distress. Parker proposed that these manifestations of distress were dissociative psychological episodes (30). He related them to a discontinuity in Inuit psychology, beginning with encouragement of dependency and ending with its rejection. Eskimo children learned to depend on relatives and others for nurturance and, at the same time, learned to maintain a pleasant, receptive demeanor. They became sensitive to the fact that negative behavior on their part would elicit displeasure and, subsequently, cause them shame. In adulthood, dependency was rejected. The shame of not being able to provide was a frequent trigger of soul-loss episodes.

Styles of behavior derived from the shamanistic period are transmitted, including ways of experiencing the intoxicated state. Jones writes that drinking is a powerful symbol of group identity and membership—a vehicle for the continuity of cultural values, of sharing of generosity and egalitarianism (13). Violence may be part of this and may be socially adaptive.

Adaption of a New Social Order

Structural discontinuity impacts on the less acculturated among American Indians and Eskimos. The native American, in general, has been gradually, and sometimes abruptly, dislodged from traditional social positions and roles. As Turner writes, groups of people who are de facto evicted from their positions in the social order share a "liminal" or astructural status (31). Without the distinctions of differential authority, prestige, and control to define their interactions, these groups develop a temporary social order or *communitas*. *Communitas* is characterized by feelings of shared identity, symbols, and goals, which transcend established social hierarchies. Partying, alcohol, and associated actions may have been held to symbolize aspects of traditional spirit possession, on the one hand, and white man's power on the other. In addition, these events may represent a statement of unity from a disenfranchised, left-behind group.

Wolcott, from his experience among the Kwakiutl of British Columbia, discovered differences between historical and new intoxication (32). When drinking appears only "after contact" with white culture, it seems more disruptive. He observed that African drinking is a religious ritual, a part of ceremonial behavior, whereas among the Kwakiutl, a dread of drinking looms over every gathering, whether it is a school Christmas concert or the contemporary form of a potlatch ceremony. Elders beg and cajole their juniors to forego their drinking, but they are rarely a significant influence.

Social Disintegration

The association of drink and violence was recorded by the earliest observations of Eskimos with alcohol. Ray, who visited the Eskimos in the 1880s, divided drinkers in the villages into heavy drinkers, who became violent when drunk and had a reputation for aggressive behavior, and regular party drinkers, who drank whenever the opportunity arose but did not become violent and disruptive (33).

Social control of violence in traditional Eskimo society has been exercised through ridicule, joking, and gossip. Such mechanisms are effective because of the sensitivity of Eskimos to the attitudes of their fellows. Intoxication circumvents this control. Alcohol and altered states of consciousness allow an individual to escape responsibility for "shameful" aggression. The drunk man is without a conscience, says Brody, and everyone else abandons any claim on his conscience (34). The escape is from the repression of society's ideals and feelings of shame, not from conscience and guilt. These latter are not significant psychological events in the "shame" culture.

Intoxication itself, the altered state of consciousness, becomes a valued state. Brody, discussing skid-row Indians in northern Canada, never heard alcoholism discussed with feelings of guilt, fear, or anxiety (34). Brody's phenomenologic description of the experience of the drinker is reminiscent of descriptions of altered states of consciousness associated with shamanism mentioned previously. The drinker is full of camaraderie but, as the drinker becomes intoxicated, the drinker subsides into stupefied silence. At any point along this continuum, short of unconsciousness, the drinker can become angry and violent. The drinker seems on the lookout for provocation. The fighting can be infectious, moving from one table to another in the bar. Two forms of fighting occur in these bars. One is aggression against outsiders, violence directed against police and other social authorities; the other is intoxicated behavior in sexual encounters. The drinker makes direct and hostile advances to women and, if they are not compliant, becomes aggressive. Between regular couples there is a great deal of fighting, both verbal and physical. Women are often seen with their faces swollen and their arms bruised from fights associated with drunkenness. The wife is frequently the target of the drinker's aggression. This is true in the Indian reserves as well as on skid row. When intoxicated, women fight among themselves, almost always in relation to sexual jealousy.

Lubart, studying Eskimo drinking in the Northwest Territories, describes similar patterns (21). Drinking is begun with the express purpose of getting drunk. The conscious motivation to begin, as perceived by males, is anxiety about the future, tension, moderate depression, and expressed bitterness against the government and toward white men in general. Individuals who were violence prone tended to be less euphoric and sociable and more sullen, tense, irritable, surly, and quarrelsome when drinking. In no instance was a white man assaulted, even though bitter feelings about them were frequently expressed. Instead, men assaulted Eskimo acquaintances, generally, with shame on becoming sober. In some instances, men who were ordinarily good natured, hard working, gentle, and good humored in daily contacts would, after a few convivial rounds of beer, suddenly burst forth in a wild, assaultive, unprovoked and violent rampage. They seemed out of contact, unreachable even by close friends and bent on a destructive course.

DISCUSSION

While there is great variation in geography, culture, language, history, and socioeconomic circumstances among Native American groups, and while this variation is a factor in the disparate patterns of alcohol use, there nevertheless emerges a definitive pattern of behavior that can be generalized. Despite the wide variation in patterns by region, by history, in character, and in extent of culture contact, the majority of Native American victims are young people who suffer family discord, social disintegration, and culture conflict. Levy points out that "the young male is bearing the brunt of the stresses in the society due to his immediate involvement in the economic and role changes taking place at present and . . . due to the lesser degree of stability or integration afforded him in his society" (17).

Acculturative stress is intense for the young adults in Native American communities. Indian youth experience not only the personal identity crisis of adolescence, but also the additional burden of the adaptational crisis of their culture. The psychological helplessness and increased feelings of hopelessness are engendered by such circumstances. For an individual caught up in cultural crisis, drinking and acting out can offer a sense of gaining control over pervasive anxiety.

Demographic factors associated with marginalization, such as family breakdown, parental loss, and early separation, contribute to depression and suicide in later years. Alcohol abuse is also a major factor in Native American suicide. Drinking has contributed to the disintegration of family life in many groups, and has resulted in child neglect, abuse, and other forms of intrafamilial and community violence; all these are indices of cultural disintegration. Such tragic personal histories are frequently implicated in the cases of completed suicide.

Health problems, educational disadvantages, and poverty have been major factors in Native Americans' struggle for consolidation of their cultural identity and a meaningful fulfilling life in the context of the United States. Integrationist and assimilationist responses to acculturation require that paths of opportunity be open in the dominant society. Educational, economic, social, and political opportunities have been severely lacking and have forced most Native American groups into other forms of adaptation, particularly separation and marginalization. Because of historical factors, such as isolation and habitation in their indigenous lands, some Native American communities have been able to maintain separationist responses to acculturation pressures. These responses strengthen both cultural and psychological identity. Separationist responses consolidate psychological identity formation based on traditional cultural values and practices, and reduce vulnerability to the kinds of self-doubt and self-criticism that can lead to alcohol use among those whose coping skills have been destroyed. Groups that have maintained separationist responses, such as many of the southwestern Pueblos and the Navajo, have experienced less morbidity than other Native Americans who, with very little resources left, faced with the combined pressures of modernization, technologic change, and discrimination. Some Native American communities, such as the Inuit with a long history of contact, the Cree, and the northwestern tribes living on the Warm Springs Reservation, have adapted to acculturative stress by forms of cultural, economic, and political integration with the dominant society. This integration has enabled them to provide adequate supports for the identity consolidation of their youth and young adults, reducing risk of alcohol use and abuse among them.

Where traditional lifestyles and values have been eroded by displacement, disease, persistent unemployment, poverty, and religious and educational efforts to discourage "old ways," separationist and integrationist adaptations tend to break down. Many Native American groups have endured this situation for generations; with pathways to assimilation to the dominant society blocked, they have slipped or been forced into cultural marginalization. These groups have lost many essential values of traditional culture and have not been able to replace them by active participation in American society in ways that are conducive to enhanced cultural and psychological self-esteem. The feelings of loss, alienation, self-denigration, and identity confusion engendered by this situation are reflected in drinking excessively and other destructive behaviors witnessed in many Native American communities.

While many stubborn problems remain, current social forces may modify acculturative stresses and reduce vulnerability to suicide. Considerable progress has been made in reducing mortality and morbidity from communicable diseases and in lowering infant mortality rates. Each year, more American Natives are attending high school and college, and scholarship assistance is more readily available. This has resulted in the emergence of a cadre of articulate and respected young adult leaders who now represent for Native American youth a model of successful cultural and psychological integration. Pan-Indian awareness has contributed to pride, local decision making, and local responsibility in facilitating effective political participation. Such self-determined political participation resulted, for example, in the formation of the Alaska Federation of Natives. This Federation was instrumental in negotiating the Land Claims Settlement Act of 1972, and helped form corporations to manage the resources provided by the Settlement. Similar developments have characterized the contemporary history of the Cree Indians in the James Bay region of Quebec, the Navajo, Pueblo, and other Indian tribes of the southwest, and the Yurok and other Northwest tribes.

In Alaska, development of land corporations resulted in an increase in per capita income and rights to land that have great potential for economic development. Many communities have taken over the management of their own educational, safety, health, and welfare programs, and have become less dependent on government-provided services. In the process, jobs have been generated for Native Americans, and individuals have learned the administrative, business, and political skills needed to represent their people in dealings with the dominant society. The role models that these people provide for contemporary Native American youth may be of great importance to the future of their people and to the reduction of acculturative stress among groups and individuals.

Most mental health efforts of the past were directed at secondary and tertiary programs; primary prevention programs were developed only recently. Shore et al. describe the development of a suicide prevention center on a northwest reservation (35). Dinges and Yumori provide conceptualizations of preventive mental health issues that aim directly at promoting psychological health and competence (36). Maintenance and enhancement of self-esteem have broad disciplinary acceptance as a unifying concept for understanding the prerequisites of positive mental health. Iscoe identified the characteristics of the competent community as providing a repertoire of possibilities and alternatives, knowing where and how to find resources, self-esteem, and power (37). The last element, power, is construed as the right to self-determination and is linked to recent cultural revitalization movements— bicultural attempts by Native American communities to erect meaningful frameworks for operating vis-à-vis the dominant U.S. society. Manson et al. have called for a major departure from past lines of inquiry regarding the mental health of Native Americans by focusing instead on ethnologic definitions of psychological health, maturity, and competence, and on causal linkages of these elements in the context of systematic theory of human adaptation (38). These approaches and others that can inspire a vision of a hopeful future of a successful role in world society will provide a path for each which will leave problem drinking behind them.

The past decade has witnessed a movement toward integration and assimilation by Native Americans. As more educational, occupational, and economic opportunities become available, the cultural and psychological adaptations of rejection and marginalization are likely to decrease. While pan-Indianism has created increased political cohesion and a national awareness among the many ethnically diverse Native American groups, it has also generated local pride and identification with traditional values. The new generation of Native Americans affirms its traditional ethnic identity, while accommodating and adjusting to the demands and prerequisites of living in a technologic, changing nation (39).

At this process unfolds, the identity confusion, self-denigration, and despair often observed in Native American communities, and associated with social disorganization, alcohol abuse, and family violence, may give way to a positive bicultural self-development consistent with cultural and psychological integration. While this process can create tensions and social problems of its own, the risk of identity confusion and risk taking self destructive behavior of youth and young adults is much reduced. Primary prevention of Native American problem drinking is predicated on continued development of effective social, economic, and political institutions and the accompanying communal and personal internalization of a sense of control.

REFERENCES

1. U.S. Department of Health and Human Services, Indian Health Services. *1997: Trends in indian health.* Rockville, MD: U.S. Government Printing Office, 1997:5, 95.
2. Burns TR. How does IHS relate administratively to the high alcoholism mortality rate? *Am Indian Alaska Native Mental Health Res* 1995;6(3):31–45.
3. Leland J. Firewater myths. *J Stud Alcohol* 1976.
4. Garcia-Andrade C, Wall TL, Ehlers Cindy L. The firewater myth and response to alcohol in mission Indians. *Am J Psychiatry* 1997;154(7):983–988.
5. Schuckit MA. A clinical model of genetic influence in alcohol dependence. *J Stud Alcohol* 1994;55:5–17.
6. Lappalainen J, Long JC, Eggert M, et al. Linkage of antisocial alcoholism to the serotonin 5-HT1B receptor gene in 2 populations. *Arch Gen Psychiatry* 1998;55(11):989–994.
7. U.S. Government. *Suicide, homicide and alcoholism among American Indians.* Report #ADM 76–42. Washington, DC: U.S. Government Printing Office, 1973.
8. U.S. Bureau of the Census. *Statistical abstract of the United States, 1982– 1983.* Washington, DC: U.S. Government Printing Office, 1982.
9. Byler W, O'Connell P. *Rural Indian Americans in poverty.* Washington,

DC: U.S. Government Printing Office, 1968.
10. Kraus R, Buffler P. Sociocultural stress and the American Native in Alaska: an analysis of changing patterns of psychiatric illness and alcohol abuse among Alaska Natives. *Cult Med Psychiatry* 1979;3(2):
11. Guillemin J. *Urban renegades: the cultural strategy of American Indians.* New York: Columbia University Press, 1975.
12. Braoe MW. *Indian and white: self-image and interaction in a Canadian plains community.* Stanford, CA: Stanford University Press, 1975.
13. Jones DM. *Aleuts in transition: a comparison of two villages.* Seattle: University of Washington Press, 1976.
14. Cahalan D, Room R. *Problem drinking among American men.* New Brunswick, NJ: Rutgers Center of Alcohol Studies, 1974.
15. Rosenberg SS, ed. *Alcohol and health: report from the secretary of Health, Education, and Welfare.* New York: Charles Scribner's Sons, 1973.
16. Norick F. *Acculturation and drinking in Alaska. Rehabilitation Record 11, no. 5:13–17. North Slope Borough Department of Public Safety. Annual Report.* Barrow, AK: 1970.
17. Levy JE, Kunitz SJ. *Indian drinking:*

Navaho practices and Anglo-American theories. New York: John Wiley & Sons, 1974.
18. Klausner S, Foulks E. *Eskimo capitalists.* Montclair, NJ: Allenneld, Osmun, 1982.
19. Resnick H, Dizmang LH. Observations on suicidal behavior among American Indians. *Am J Psychiatry* 1971;127:882– 887.
20. Kunitz SJ, Levy JE. Changing ideas of alcohol use among Navaho Indians. *Q J Stud Alcohol* 1974;35(1):243– 259.
21. Lubart J. *Psychodynamic problems of adaptation, Mackenzie Delta Eskimos.* Ottawa, Canada: Northern Science Research Group, Department of Indian Affairs and Northern Development, 1971.
22. Clairmont D. *Deviance among Indians and Eskimos in Aklavik.* Publ. 63–9. Ottawa, Canada: Northern Coordination and Research Center, Department of Indian Affairs and Northern Development, 1963.
23. Lobban M. Cultural problems of drunkenness in an Arctic population. *Br Med J* 1971;1:344.
24. Leach ER. *Rethinking anthropology.* New York: Humanities Press, 1971.
25. MacAndrew C, Edgerton R. *Drunken comportment: a social explanation.* Chicago: Aldine Press, 1969.

26. Ehrstrom M. Medical investigations in North Greenland, 1948–1949. *Acta Med Scand* 1951;140(11):265–264.

27. Hughes J. *An epidemiological study of psychopathology in an Eskimo village.* Doctoral dissertation. Ithaca, NY: Cornell University, 1960.

28. Nachman B. *Fits, suicides, beatings and time-out.* Anchorage, AK: Alaska Native Service, U.S. Public Health Service, 1969.

29. Foulks EF. The arctic hysterias of the North Alaskan Eskimo. In: Maybury-Lewis D, ed. *Anthropological studies.* Washington, DC: American Anthropological Association Press, 1973.

30. Wolott M. *The African beer gardens of Bulawayo: integrated drinking in a segregated society.* New Brunswick, NJ: Rutgers Center of Alcohol Studies, 1974.

31. Turner V. *The ritual process: structure and anti-structure.* Ithaca, NY: Cornell University Press, 1977.

32. Parker S. Eskimo psychopathology. *Am Anthropol* 1962;64:74–76.

33. Ray PH. *Narrative in report of the International Polar Expedition to Point Barrow, Alaska.* Report to the House of Representatives, U.S. Congress, Ex. Doc. 44. Washington, DC: U.S. Government Printing Office, 1885.

34. Brody H. *Indians on skid row.* Ottawa, Canada: National Science Research Group, Department of Indian Affairs and North Development, 1971.

35. Shore JN. Suicide and suicide attempts among American Indians of the Pacific Northwest. *Int J Soc Psychiatry* 1972;18:91–965.

36. Dinges N, Yumori W. Cross-cultural perspectives on preventive mental health programs for the family. In: Fine S, Kress P, eds. *Cross-cultural intervention with families, parents, and children.* Rotterdam, Netherlands: D. Reidel, 1987.

37. Iscoe I. Community psychology and competent community. *Am Psychol* 1974;29(8):607–613.

38. Manson S, Tatum E, Dinges N. Prevention research among American Indian and Alaska Native communities: charting future courses for theory and practice in mental health. In: Manson S, ed. *New directions in prevention among American Indian and Alaska Native communities.* Portland, OR: Oregon Health Sciences University, 1982.

39. Frank JW, Moore RS, Ames GM. Historical and cultural roots of drinking problems among American Indians. *Am J Public Health* 2000;89:344–351.

CHAPTER 71

Gays, Lesbians, and Bisexuals

ROBERT PAUL CABAJ

Substance abuse is expressed in various communities and populations at different rates and with differing incidences. Clinicians wishing to serve the needs of a particular ethnic or cultural group have learned that the particular community in question must be understood, respected, and consulted with, to make effective interventions. Gay men, lesbians, and bisexuals make up one of these populations with special needs, a population defined not by traditionally understood cultural and ethnic minority criteria, but rather by having a different sexual orientation from the majority. This chapter discusses the nature of homosexuality and bisexuality; gay men, lesbians, and bisexuals themselves; the substance use and abuse concerns among these people; and the specific treatment issues that need to be addressed when working with gay men, lesbians, and bisexual men and women.

There is no solid agreement about the amount of alcohol and other substances used or the incidence of substance abuse in the gay, lesbian, and bisexual population. Most studies (1–8), reports (9,10), or reviews of surveys (11,12), and the experiences of most clinicians working with gay men and lesbians (13,14), estimate an incidence of substance abuse of all types at approximately 30%—with ranges of 28% to 35%; this estimate contrasts with an incidence of 10% to 12% for the general population.

A careful review of each report, however, demonstrates significant and persistent methodological problems, rang-

ing from poor or absent control groups, unrepresentative population samples (some studies gathered subjects only from gay and lesbian bars), to a failure to use uniform definitions of substance abuse or of homosexuality itself. Nonetheless, no matter where the sample was taken—urban or rural, various socioeconomic settings, in the United States or other countries—the rates are strikingly uniform, although there are some variations in use reported. For example, one study (15), using very simple screening questions, notes greater substance use but no greater alcohol use in gay men as compared to heterosexual men in San Francisco, whereas another study (5) reports that heavy alcohol use was not greater for gay men and lesbians than for heterosexuals sampled, but did note that there were fewer gay and lesbian alcohol abstainers and a greater number of gay and lesbian moderate alcohol users.

A few surveys have focused on lesbian substance abuse, most in the general population (16–18) and one in lesbian medical students (19). Both continue to indicate a high use of alcohol and other drugs in lesbians, and a higher concern over a problem with alcohol and drug use than in similar heterosexual populations. Currently, no study specifically focuses on the drug or alcohol use of bisexual men or women, although many such people are included in some of the studies already described. Most of the ideas in this chapter can apply to bisexuals, because the focus is on the effects of external and internalized homophobia.

Alcohol abuse has been the primary focus of most studies. No specific studies of injecting drug use (IDU) and the gay population are currently available. The quarterly Centers for Disease Control and Prevention (CDC) report on acquired immunodeficiency syndrome (AIDS) and human immunodeficiency virus (HIV) infections clearly indicate a subgroup of IDU gay and bisexual men, and one of the routes of HIV infection for lesbians is via IDU (20). One survey (21) did review the use of all types of abusable substances among gay men and lesbians, noting a greater use of cigarettes, marihuana, and alcohol than in the general population.

For years now, concerns about the epidemic of HIV-related conditions have led to increased studies of both gay and bisexual men and intravenous drug users. An explosive use of methamphetamine, known as "speed," "crystal," or "crank," by gay and bisexual men has become evident throughout the country, but especially on the West Coast and in parts of the South and the Mid-West. The frequent route of use is intravenous (i.v.), but also inhaled/snorted or swallowed. Combined with its disinhibiting effect and sexual stimulating effect, the i.v. gay male users of methamphetamine are at extremely high risk for HIV infection via sharing needles and engaging in sexual activity that may last for hours and may not always follow safer-sex guidelines (22,23).

SEXUAL ORIENTATION IN GENERAL

Homosexuality, as a term, is subject to some controversy. It was first used by Krafft-Ebing and implied a clinical, pathologic condition (24). Because of these associations—and the linking in the last century of homosexuality and illness—the use of this term has been challenged. Dr. John Boswell traced homosexuality in history and reports the term *gay* has a long association with homosexual men (25). Because gay is less prejudicial, this chapter refers to gay men, lesbians, and bisexuals as people, and homosexuality and bisexuality in reference only to certain types of behavioral activities or orientations.

The understanding of certain terms is crucial to understanding homosexuality; failure to have clear definitions and understanding has led to much of the confusion in the literature about homosexuality and sexuality in general, and certainly has contributed to some of the prejudicial feeling about homosexuality. It is important to recognize the difference between sexual orientation and sexual behavior, as well as the differences between sexual orientation, gender identity, and gender role. Sexual orientation refers to the desire for sex, love, and affection, and/or sexual fantasies from or with another person, whereas sexual behavior is strictly sexual activities and may not coincide with primary sexual orientation. Gender identity is the sense of self as male or female, with no reference to sexual orientation or gender role. Gender role refers to behaviors and desires to behave that are viewed as masculine or feminine by a particular culture. Behavior that a particular culture may label as masculine or feminine is not necessarily a reflection of gender identity, but it is common to call behavior, styles, or interests shown by a male that are associated with women as "effeminate" (boys are often labeled "sissies") and the equivalent by a woman as "being like a man" or "butch" (girls are often labeled "tomboys").

Using both the pioneering scientific and psychological evidence collected by Dr. Evelyn Hooker that gay men were as psychologically healthy as matched heterosexuals (26) and subsequent research, the American Psychiatric Association (APA), in 1973, removed homosexuality per se as a mental illness from its list of disorders. This decision was challenged by some psychiatrists who mistakenly thought the removal was a response to political pressure, but the APA supported its scientifically based decision via a vote by the membership and support by APA leadership. There was, however, a "political" compromise, with the creation of a nonscientific diagnosis called "ego-dystonic homosexuality." In 1987, the APA recognized this error and removed that label from the *Diagnostic and Statistical Manual of Mental Disorders*, 3rd ed., revised (*DSM–III–R*) (27,28). The current *Diagnostic and Statistical Manual of Mental Disorders,* 4th ed., text revision (2000) (*DSM–IV–TR*) followed the same revisions (29).

This nonjudgmental, nonprejudicial framework on homosexuality has led to new thinking and revisions on homosexual behavior and on gay men, lesbians, and bisexuals (12,30–35). New literature founded on work with gays in psychotherapy and substance-abuse counseling continues to be generated (14,36–45). American psychoanalytic thinking has been extremely persistent in trying to view homosexuality as pathological, but most current psychoanalytical literature has been able to review and revise some traditional, conservative views on homosexuality (45–50). The literature also continues to increase for the non-mental health clinician working with gays and lesbians (51–54). Three journals focus on new and nonprejudicial scientific and clinical information on gays and lesbians—the *Journal of Homosexuality*, the *Journal of Gay and Lesbian Psychotherapy*, and the *Journal of Gay and Lesbian Health* produced by the Gay and Lesbian Medical Association.

Through such new reviews and the efforts of many gay-sensitive clinicians and researchers, many of the myths and prejudices about gay people are being laid to rest. There have been persistent false beliefs about gay men and lesbians, including the following:

- *Myth:* Gay men are promiscuous. *Fact:* Only a small segment of gay men fit this description, which may more accurately reflect a trait of maleness in our society than of homosexuality (32).
- *Myth:* Gay men cannot form relationships. *Fact:* A majority of gay men are in relationships of various types (32).
- *Myth:* Gay men or lesbians only need one good heterosexual sexual experience to "straighten" them out; or gay men and lesbians try to "recruit" young people to "become" gay or lesbian. *Fact:* Sexual orientation is not a result of a lack of an experience but is an internal desire for most people, shaped in expression by many factors (31).
- *Myth:* Gays are child molesters. *Fact:* The vast majority of child molesters are heterosexual (37).

• *Myth:* All gay men are "effeminate." *Fact:* Though some gay men have "gender-discordant" behavior as children—usually manifested as avoidance of rough and tumble play—the vast majority of adult men are not "effeminate" and there is no equation of homosexual orientation and "effeminacy" (32,46–47).

HOMOSEXUAL BEHAVIOR AND BISEXUALITY

Homosexual Behavior

Besides the work of Dr. Hooker noted above (26), the famous Kinsey report helped put homosexual behavior *itself* in perspective (55). Although somewhat dated and challenged over representativeness, the extensive survey reported that 67% of American men have had at least one homosexual experience to orgasm after adolescence; 30% have had more than one experience; 5% to 7% have bisexual experiences but prefer homosexual ones; and 4% to 5% have homosexual experiences exclusively as adults. The often used estimate that 10% of the male population is primarily or exclusively homosexual in terms of sexual behavior is based on this data from 1948 (56). These data point out the widespread occurrence of male homosexual behavior, not necessarily the numbers of self-identified gay men.

Gay and bisexual people and homosexual and bisexual behavior are found in almost all societies and cultures around the world and throughout history (57–61). Tolerance and acceptance has varied throughout history, and currently varies from country to country, culture to culture, and community to community. Anyone may be gay, lesbian, or bisexual. Gay and bisexual men and women do not have uniform ways of behaving nor do they live uniform lifestyles. There is, therefore, no such thing as a "gay community" per se (12,32,62), just individuals who happen to be gay, lesbian, or bisexual.

Gay people are found in all segments of society and in all minority and ethnic groups, may be of any age, and may have any occupation or career. Most gay people are not readily identifiable, in spite of persistent stereotypes. Sexual behavior and sexual orientation itself are not necessarily fixed in an individual and may change over time. Intense homosexual longings in young adulthood or adolescence may change as one grows older, and, conversely, some heterosexuals may discover gay feelings later in life (63).

Bisexuality

Many people are clearly bisexual in behavior—being able to sexually function with either sex—but often prefer one sex to the other (47). The Kinsey report (55) devised the Kinsey scale to describe this range of behavior: from 0 for exclusive heterosexual behavior to 6 for exclusive homosexual behavior. This classification puts the majority of men in a bisexual range, based on sexual experiences. As will be discussed, bisexuality and bisexual behavior are especially important in HIV infection prevention work, because many men have gay sexual experiences, without informing their spouses or other female partners. Many lesbians have had, and do have, sex with men. For many minority populations, bisexuality, but not homosexuality per se, is acceptable (or at least admitted to) in surveys and interviews. As far back as the 1989 CDC 8-year review of AIDS cases among gay or bisexual men, 54.2% of African Americans were reported as bisexual; 44.2% of Hispanics were reported as bisexual; and 11.3% of whites were reported as bisexual (64)—and this data awaits updating.

GAY SEXUAL ORIENTATION

Gay men and lesbians are remarkably like everyone else. There are three major differences, however, which may be of help in understanding the high incidence of substance abuse: (a) having a sexual orientation expressed by the desire to have affectional, sexual, sexual fantasy, and/or social needs met mostly by a same-sex partner rather than an opposite-sex partner; (b) negotiating a process of self-identity and self-recognition as a gay person, different from the majority, known as "coming out"; and (c) confronting a widespread and insidious dislike, hatred, and/or fear of gay and lesbian people, homosexual activity, and homosexual feelings, known as "homophobia." This last factor forms the largest barrier to gays and lesbians obtaining quality health care and substance-abuse treatment, and may be the primary factor in explaining the widespread incidence of substance abuse in gay populations. Homophobia is a result of societal heterosexism, that is, the perspective that the majority situation—heterosexuality—is the "norm" or superior in some way, even if homosexuality is considered at all. Homophobia is parallel to such societal forces as racism and sexism (65).

In trying to understand the nature of homosexuality, there have been new insights into sexuality in general and in the nature of gender identity. In looking at the etiology of homosexuality, most new research indicates that a homosexual orientation is not learned and not a result of any family or social patterns. The "classic" psychoanalytical description of a close, seductive mother and absent, distant father does not occur more frequently in the backgrounds of gay men; in fact, it may occur more often in heterosexuals (46,47,66). New research continues to point out familial patterns that may indicate a genetic component (47,67–71) and/or biologic and biochemical factors (72,73). Such knowledge and awareness about the origins of sexual orientation may help to relieve both the patients who are having difficulty accepting their homosexuality and the families of patients who are gay or lesbian who may feel guilty, as if they had done something "wrong" to "cause" the sexual orientation.

Coming Out

Coming out is a long and complex process that may occur throughout the entire life cycle (74–78). The best way to conceptualize coming out is to view it as a series of steps that an individual negotiates at his or her own time and pace, with periodic steps forward and backward. The individual must first become aware of his or her own sexual orientation as "different" from that of the majority. The next step is to accept the awareness and begin to integrate it into a self-concept and grapple with the negative feelings associated with homosexuality. Next, the individual may choose to act on the feelings (although some gay people with strong gay feelings do not engage in sex with others of the same sex, such as celibate priests or others). Finally, the person makes a series of lifelong decisions about whether to let others know and whom to let know, such as friends, family, work colleagues, peers, teachers, and medical providers. Some gay people only come out to selected people and not to everyone at once; some may come out, then deny it later or not continue to let new friends or people at new workplaces know. The bias and prejudice against people with AIDS and the often automatic, but mistaken, association of AIDS and gay men, rather than the association of HIV infection and behaviors that may lead to infection, may lead some men to "return to the closet" or hesitate in continuing the coming out process.

Homophobia and Heterosexism

Homophobia, both internalized and externalized, combined with heterosexism are the major forces that gays and bisexuals must deal with in our society (34,79–81). All gay people have internalized homophobia, having been brought up in a homophobic society that tends to promote prejudicial myths about gay people or, from the heterosexist concentric point of view, to just ignore gay and bisexual people in general. The coming out process may be delayed or undergo great difficulties depending on the intensity of internalized homophobia (if the person believes homosexuality is a sin, an illness, unnatural, evil, or will only lead to sadness, loneliness, and isolation) and may well require the help of psychotherapy (46,76,82,83).

Externalized homophobia is found at every level in our society: legal, medical, scientific, religious, political, social, educational, and judicial. Many feel that the resistance to earlier governmental help with the AIDS crisis was a result of homophobia in the government, linking the routes of HIV infection and homosexuality (84). The ever-increasing violent attacks on gays, ranging from verbal threats to outright physical attacks and murder, are usually fueled by homophobia. Heterosexist thinking and homophobia and the fear of what others will do if they know an individual is gay or even think an individual is gay, are major factors in the difficulty of getting accurate data about gays and lesbians for scientific investigations (33,79).

As noted by Ostrow, many men in both military recruit studies and college population surveys who were HIV-positive but denied any high-risk behaviors admitted to homosexual activities and, much less frequently, to i.v. drug use, in extremely confidential interviews (85). Homophobia and the fear of reprisals explain these findings: the military will discharge known homosexuals; high school and college students fear the reactions of peers, teachers, and family. Gays fear loss of insurance coverage if insurers discover sexual orientation (no matter what the HIV status may be) and hesitate to let health providers know this crucial information. (*Note:* All insurers deny they cancel insurance for this reason, but many observations from the author's own practice and from the reports of colleagues refute this assertion.)

It follows that in undertaking research surveys, gay and bisexual people hesitate to disclose sexual orientation, even with great assurances of confidentiality. Gathering information on gay and bisexual people, therefore, is extremely difficult and contributes to the skewed samples, as already noted in the studies on substance abuse and the gay community.

Gay people also face many additional challenges that majority populations escape. There are many issues generated by two people of the same gender forming a relationship (86,87) such as finding comfortable and safe living quarters; financial concerns; legal battles over insurance and wills; acknowledgment of benefits; "same-sex marriage"; or coping with a lover with AIDS. Because there is such a high incidence of substance abuse, there are many codependent relationships or relationships between two active substance abusers.

Although everyone needs to relearn how to be safely sexual in this age of AIDS, some gay men are sexually compulsive (88), or have never had "sober sex," and will need special help and support. Married bisexual men face ever-greater pressures, such as deciding about coming out to spouses and children, negotiating safe sex with a spouse not used to such behavior, and finding a community identity (89).

Gay and lesbian adolescents are increasingly a population of great and serious concern. Many studies indicate a much higher suicide attempt rate in these youth—30% versus 10% to 12% in the general population; a more volatile type of substance abuse than is seen in other adolescents, especially combinations of drugs and alcohol; and hesitancy to follow HIV infection risk-reduction guidelines (90–96). Older gays and lesbians face the same problems as other older adults, with added isolation, loneliness, and possible senses of hopelessness and resignation about substance abuse (97,98). Although somewhat slowed down by better medical treatments, the continuous loss of loved gay friends as a consequence of AIDS exacts a heavy toll, in addition to the general stress of being gay in our society (99).

Lesbian Issues

Lesbians have some specific issues that need to be highlighted. As described previously, the incidence of substance abuse is equally high among gay men and lesbians. In general, lesbians may have additional social struggles and concerns. Compared to gay men, they are more likely to have lower incomes (as do women in general, when compared with men); lesbians are more likely to be parents (about one-third of lesbians are biologic parents); lesbians face the prejudices aimed at women, as well as those for being gay, including the stronger reaction against (and willingness to ignore) female substance abusers; lesbians are more likely to come out later in life (about 28 years of age vs. 18 years of age in men); and lesbians are more likely to have bisexual feelings or experiences, so that they are still at risk for HIV infection via a sexual route as well as possible i.v. drug use (16,19,32,43,53,66).

According to several surveys, lesbians are a somewhat more likely to be in a long-term relationship than are the comparable gay men (16,32), so there needs to be a clear focus on relationships, parenting, and family concerns in working with lesbian substance abusers. Lesbians are also subject to the increase in violence, both verbal and physical, against gays; and, as is true with anyone, including gay men, they are subject to domestic violence. This latter fact is often ignored. Because there are correlations with domestic violence and substance abuse, clinicians need to be aware of this possibility in working with lesbians (100).

A growing literature is developing on working with lesbians in psychotherapy and substance abuse work (101). There has been an overemphasis on male homosexuality in the psychiatric literature; only recently has female homosexuality been subject to similar examination and discussion.

Bisexuality

The study and understanding of bisexuality has grown exponentially in the last few years. Several published works focus on both the theoretical concepts involved in understanding bisexuality and the clinical issues that evolve for bisexuals (102–104). Bisexuality is increasingly understood to be another expression of human sexual orientation, and not an in-between or undecided state of sexual orientation expression. The Kinsey studies (55,105), again, clearly documented the range of sexual behaviors in which men and women participate. There are no clear studies of bisexuals and substance abuse, although with the focus on men who have sex with men as a risk fac-

tor for HIV infections, more information will no doubt be forthcoming. The issues that face men and women who are bisexual, especially if relating more strongly to the homosexual longings, will be the same issues that men who identify as gay and women who identify as lesbian will face.

SUBSTANCE ABUSE AND GAY IDENTITY FORMATION

Many factors contribute to the prominent role of substance use and abuse in gay men, lesbians, and bisexuals. American psychoanalytic psychiatry throughout the twentieth century focused on the etiology of male homosexuality, even postulating that homosexuality was a cause of alcoholism (106). Because homosexuality, repressed or not, does not cause alcoholism (107)—indeed, alcoholism and substance abuse are not "caused" by any psychodynamic or personality factor alone—other factors must be examined. The two most important factors are genetic or biologic contributions, as well as the psychological effects of heterosexism and homophobia.

New research continues to support, in great part, genetic, biologic, and biochemical origins for the diseases of alcoholism and substance abuse. As already noted, there is continuing and growing evidence that homosexual orientation may have—at least in part—genetic, biologic, and biochemical components (47,67–73). Such parallel contributions to both sexual orientation and substance abuse has led to some speculation of a possible chromosomal link between the genetic contributions to substance abuse and sexual orientation. Such a direct genetic link between sexual orientation and the propensity to substance abuse, however, is unlikely. The studies just cited indicate that male homosexuality and female homosexuality may be different phenomena, with differing familial patterns. Substance abuse appears to have equal incidence among gay men and women.

Societal, cultural, and environmental factors, however, may lead to a greater expression of any genetic predisposition. By analogy, there has been an increase in the incidence of alcoholism in women since the beginning of the twentieth century (108). Although partially explained by better data collection, and awareness of the hidden homebound female alcoholic, the increase can also be explained by social factors. In the early 1900s, women were prohibited by societal pressures from drinking in public. As the social acceptability of drinking increased, more women drank, thus increasing the likelihood of exposure to alcohol, which, in turn, could trigger the genetic predisposition to alcoholism.

Gay men, lesbians, and bisexuals have faced great societal prohibitions, not only on the expression of their sexual feelings and behavior, but on their very existence. Societal homophobia or heterosexism could well create enough stress that gay men, lesbians, and bisexual persons turn to alcohol and other substances for "relief." This increased exposure could, in turn, lead to the higher degree of expressivity of the genetic potentials for substance abuse in gay men, lesbians, and bisexuals.

In addition, societies or cultures in turmoil or undergoing social change have higher rates of alcoholism (108,109). Gay people can be seen as experiencing almost continuous stress and social change for most of the twentieth century. Societal pressures forced most gay people to remain "in the closet," hiding their sexual orientation or not acting on their feelings. Responding to societal expectations rather than personal desire, some gay, lesbian, and bisexual people may marry someone of the opposite sex and raise a family, creating a potentially stressful situation. Legal prohibitions on homosexual behavior, overt discrimination, and the failure of society to accept or even acknowledge gay people have limited the types of social outlets available to gay men and lesbians to bars, private homes, or clubs where alcohol and other drugs often played a prominent role. The role models for many young gay men and lesbians just coming out may be gay people using alcohol and other drugs, who are met at bars or parties. Continuing societal homophobia, as well as the impact of HIV on gay men, lesbians, and bisexuals, further add to the stress (110,111).

Some gay and bisexual men and women cannot imagine socializing without alcohol or other mood-altering substances. Gay men, lesbians, and bisexuals are brought up in a society that says they should not exist and certainly should not act on their feelings. Such homophobia is internalized. Many men and women have had their first homosexual sexual experiences while drinking or being drunk to overcome their internal fear, denial, anxiety, or even revulsion about gay sex. For many men and women, this linking of substance use and sexual expression persists and may become part of coming out and the development of a personal and social identity. Many gay people continue to feel self-hatred. The use of mood-altering substances temporarily relieves, but then reinforces, this self-loathing in the drug-withdrawal period. Alcohol and many other drugs can cause depression, leading to a worsening of self-esteem and the "erosion of spirit" so well described by many of the 12-step recovery programs.

Given the state of acceptance of homosexuality and bisexuality in our society at this time, the stages of developing a gay, lesbian, or bisexual identity, influenced by such societal reactions, may be intimately involved with substance use. Although some substance abusers appears to have a genetic predisposition to substance abuse—supporting an illness model with psychosocial manifestations—not all people with such a genetic predisposition develop alcoholism or substance abuse in their lifetimes. Intrapsychic, psychological, and psychodynamic factors, influenced by psychosocial and parental upbringing, may lead certain people to turn to substance use and, therefore, potentiate a genetic predisposition for substance abuse.

The link between the psychodynamic forces in developing a gay, lesbian, or bisexual identity and the use or abuse of substances becomes clear in examining the early development and the progression through the life cycle for a gay person using the perspective of the work of Swiss psychoanalyst Alice Miller (112). Her description of how parents influence the emotional lives of their "talented" or different children has strong parallels with the development of a gay, lesbian, or bisexual identity. Parental reactions shape and validate expressions of children's needs and longings. Parents reward what is familiar and acceptable to them and discourage or de-emphasize behavior or needs they do not value or understand. Harm, of course, occurs when a parent is too depressed, preoccupied, or narcissistic to respond to the actual child and the actual needs and wants of the child. Children eventually learn to behave the way parents expect to get rewards, and to hide or deny the longings or needs that are not rewarded.

Like Miller's examples, many gay and bisexual men and women are aware of being different early in life—being aware, however subtly, of affectional and sexual needs and longings that are different from the majority of people around them (113). Some male children who will grow up to be gay may desire a closer, more intimate relationship with their father; this desire is not encouraged or even understood in our society (46). The prehomosexual child learns to hide such needs and longings, creating a false self. Real needs are often suppressed, or repressed, and rejected as wrong, bad, or sinful. Dissociation and denial, therefore, become major defenses to cope with internal feelings.

Some studies of familial patterns (67,68) point out that gay men have a greater-than-normal chance of having an alcoholic father and a greater chance of having a mother with a major affective disorder—either or both situations likely leading to growing up with emotionally unavailable parents. Therefore, the psychological, as well as genetic and emotional, backgrounds in the families of many gays and lesbians already predispose them to substance abuse.

The psychology of being different and learning to live in a society that does not accept difference readily shapes the sexual identity development as the child emerges from childhood and the latency period (114). With the rewards for the "false self," the child suppresses their more natural feelings. The child has no clear role models about how to be gay or lesbian; teachers usually cannot reveal their sexual orientation and there is still limited positive media attention for gays and lesbians. In latency, children who will become gay or bisexual—especially boys who may be effeminate—may fear other children, feel even more different, and become more isolated.

In adolescence, the gay sexual feelings emerge with great urgency, but with little or no context or permission.

Conformity is certainly encouraged, further supporting denial and suppression of gay feelings. Adolescents often reject and isolate those who are "different." The gay adolescent further develops dissociation and splitting off of affect and behavior. These various factors may help to explain the many problems facing gay youth (92). For example, gay youth may be subject to sexual abuse and violence, and sometimes are introduced to sex via hustling or prostitution, or get "used" sexually by others. The extreme difficulty many gay men and women have in coming out and integrating sexuality and personal identity makes sense from this perspective.

Substance use serves as an easy relief, can provide acceptance, and, more importantly, mirrors the comforting dissociation developed in childhood. Alcohol and other drugs cause a dissociation of feelings, anxiety, and behavior, and may mimic the emotional state many gay people had to develop in childhood to survive. The "symptom-relieving" aspects help fight the effects of homophobia; it can allow "forbidden" behavior, allow for social comfort in bars or other unfamiliar social settings, and, again, provide comfort through the familiar experiences of dissociation and isolation.

The easy availability of alcohol and drugs at gay bars or parties and the limited social options other than those bars and parties certainly encourages the use of substances early in the coming out and gay or lesbian socialization process. For gay men especially, sex and intimacy are often split off—dissociated. Again, substance use allows for acting on feelings long suppressed or denied, but also mirrors the dissociative experience and makes it harder to integrate intimacy and love. There is an easy relief of longings and needs, with sex and/or substance use, and the more challenging needs for love and intimacy may be ignored. Substances help many gay people brace themselves for rejection by others—either as a gay person coming out to friends or family, or from potential dates and sexual partners.

Substance use enhances denial and can even cause "blackouts" around sexual behavior. It can certainly make "living in the closet" with its built-in need for denial and dissociation easier or even possible (the "I-was-so-drunk-I-didn't-know-what-I-did-last-night" scenario often used in high school and college). Because so many gay people are adult children of alcoholics, they are even more skilled at denying their own self and their own needs.

Finally, the internal state that accompanies internalized homophobia and that occurs with substance abuse are very similar—the "dual oppression" of homophobia and abuse (14). The following traits are seen in both: denial; fear, anxiety, and paranoia; anger and rage; guilt; self-pity; depression, with helplessness, hopelessness, and powerlessness; self-deception and development of a false self; passivity and the feeling of being a victim; inferiority and low self-esteem; self-loathing; isolation, alienation, and feeling alone, misunderstood, or unique; and fragmentation and confusion. These close similarities make it very difficult for gay men or lesbians who cannot accept their sexual orientation to recognize or successfully treat their substance abuse. Self acceptance of one's sexual orientation thus appears to be crucial to recovery from substance abuse.

The pervasive internal and social pressures to use mood-altering substances and the difficulty in creating or finding currently existing non–substance-using social situations certainly contributes to the greater expression of the alcohol and other drug-dependence potentials in gay men and women. One wonders if the rate of substance abuse in the general population would not be much greater if everyone in the United States was subject to such pressures. Possibly, there is no greater genetic predisposition to substance abuse in gays, but an increased potentiation of expression due to greater use and presence of such substances in gay society.

HOMOSEXUAL BEHAVIOR, SUBSTANCE ABUSE, HIV INFECTIONS AND AIDS

Men-who-have-sex-with-men continues to be the largest "at-risk" group for current and new HIV-related infections and cases of AIDS in the United States (115). Although most clinicians and researchers attribute the spread of HIV in this population to certain highly risky unsafe sexual practices, the role of i.v. drug use is significant. The same CDC report noted that a good percentage of all adult cases were men who both had sex with men *and* i.v. drug users. Many men in the CDC statistics "i.v.-drug-users-only" category are also gay or bisexual, but fail to report this additional risk category for the reasons already discussed.

Besides the obvious potential spread of HIV through the i.v. drug-using segments of the gay population via needle sharing, substance abuse plays a not-so-obvious role in spreading the virus through sexual practices. In most reviews of gay men and safer sex practices, men who were knowledgeable about safer sex but failed to practice it uniformly report being under the influence of some substance, such as alcohol or other drugs, at the times they failed to follow the guidelines (94,116–118). In addition, some gay men seek to enhance and prolong sexual activity through the use of drugs such as amyl nitrite (known as "poppers"), alcohol, marihuana, ecstasy, and especially methamphetamines, or a combination of these substances (119–122).

The phenomena of "circuit parties" (this is a highly organized series of parties across the world that emphasize sex and drugs) and the club scene at local bars and dance clubs are not exclusive to gay men and lesbians, but both have taken hold of a significant number of gay people. Drugs are extremely frequently used in those settings—especially the so-called club drugs such as ecstasy, special

K, and methamphetamines (123). The drugs are used to enhance the dancing and party experience but are also frequently used to enhance sexual activity, with the same consequences as noted above.

Judgment is clearly suspended or altered during even the moderate, let alone heavy, use of alcohol and other substances. There is definitely a higher risk for exposure to HIV with larger numbers of sexual partners, but the risk is also higher in any one particular encounter when safer sex guidelines are not followed—whether because of suspended judgment with substance use, pressure by the partner to not bother, or having highly charged sexual feelings. Furthermore, there is clear evidence that many abused substances alter the immune system, which may well compromise the immune system's initial reaction to exposure to HIV in men engaged in risky sexual practices under the influence of substances (124). With the widespread use of such agents and such conditions in the gay community, it appears that substance use and abuse is a definite cofactor in the spread of HIV through sexual practices.

SPECIAL TREATMENT CONCERNS FOR GAY PEOPLE

Evaluation and Treatment Issues

Treatment must focus on both recovery from substance abuse and from the consequences of homophobia. To reverse and treat the denial and dissociation, the patient will need to address his or her own acceptance of self as a gay or bisexual person. Although no one should be forced to come out to any one, self-acceptance appears to be crucial to recovery. Treatment needs to be at least gay-sensitive if not gay-affirmative, as will be discussed. To "recover" from an "Alice Miller" childhood, the patient, once in solid recovery, will need to deal with the grief and rage associated with mourning the loss of the "false self" and must learn how to get his or her own real needs met.

In the assessment of a gay man, lesbian, or bisexual person presenting for mental health services, clinicians need to be aware of the higher incidence of substance abuse in this population and, accordingly, routinely screen for symptoms of alcoholism or other substance abuse. In formulating a treatment plan for gay men, lesbians, or bisexuals determined to have a substance-abuse problem, the personalized treatment plan needs to include the influences and effects of the following for each individual: the stage in the life cycle; the degree and impact of internalized homophobia; the stage in the coming out process and the experience of coming out; the support and social network available; current relationship, if any, including married spouses and the history of past relationships; the relationship with the family of origin; comfort with sexuality and

expression of sexual feelings; career and economic status; and health factors, including HIV status.

Most clinicians working with the addictions recognize that psychotherapy alone will not treat or cure the substance abuse, and may actually be harmful or not indicated (108). Individual psychotherapy can be isolating and lonely, and may create the false hope that understanding and insight will lead to recovery. Often the insights lead to an excuse to continue using substances. If a patient is already in therapy when recovery begins, the therapy need not stop, but the work will need to be much more supportive and focused on the here and now, while the emotional and neurologic systems begin to heal. Once in solid recovery, the patient can deal with the grief and rage involved in mourning the loss of the "false self," and learn how to get his or her own real needs met. In most cases, a 12-step program such as Alcoholics Anonymous (AA) is a vital part of recovery and may well be essential for all substance-abusing patients in recovery who undertake psychotherapy.

Homophobia is the major consideration in meeting the treatment needs of gay men and lesbians with substance-abuse problems, as well as the proper care and prevention of HIV-related infections. Few inpatient or outpatient detoxification and rehabilitation programs have knowledge about homosexuality and are often unaware that they have gay and lesbian patients, who may be too frightened to "come out" to the staff (125). Attitudes of the staff and treating clinicians about homosexuality are crucial in the success of treatment for gays and lesbians. Many gay and lesbian staff are afraid to come out because of administrative reaction and are not able to either serve as role models or to provide a more open and relaxed treatment.

More and more gay-sensitive programs—programs that are aware of, knowledgeable about, and accepting of gay people in a nonprejudicial fashion—are opening up around the country. Most current and well-established programs are training staff about gay concerns, although many centers still fail to even ask about sexual orientation or address it as a specific topic. The Center for Substance Abuse Treatment has put out a guideline on working with gay, lesbian, bisexual, and transgender substance abusers, an extremely helpful and resource-full guide (126).

Programs are developing across the country that are gay-affirmative, that is, actively promoting self-acceptance of a gay identity as a key part of recovery. The first such program, PRIDE Institute of Minnesota, released data showing a very successful treatment rate when sexual orientation is considered a key factor in recovery. At a 14-month followup with verified reports, 74% of all patients treated five or more days were continuously abstinent from alcohol use, and 67% were abstinent from all drugs, as compared to four similar, sometimes gay-sensitive, but not gay affirmative programs with unverified reports taken at followups ranging from 11 months to 24 months, with rates of

43%, 55%, 57%, and 63% (127). As these findings imply, substance abuse and sexual identity formation are often tightly woven together, and it is difficult to imagine much success in treating the gay or lesbian substance abuser without addressing sexual orientation and homophobia.

Aftercare may be a major problem. Twelve-step recovery programs and philosophies are the mainstays, of course, in recovery and in staying clean and sober. There may be no gay-sensitive therapists or counselors in the patients' communities. AA, although open to all, is still a group of people at any individual meeting that may reflect the perceptions and prejudices of the local community and not be open to or accepting of openly gay members (128–130). Most communities now have gay and lesbian AA, Narcotic Anonymous (NA), and Al-Anon meetings, and AA as an organization clearly embraces gays and lesbians, as it embraces anyone concerned about a substance-abuse problem (131).

Some gay people in recovery, however, may not have come out or may not feel comfortable in such meetings, especially if a discussion of sexual orientation was not part of the early recovery. Some groups parallel and similar to AA have formed to meet the needs of these gays and lesbians, such as Alcoholics Together, and many large cities sponsor "roundups," large 3-day-weekend gatherings focused on AA, NA, lectures, workshops, and drug- and alcohol-free socializing.

Although 12-step programs such as AA and NA recommend avoiding emotional stress and conflicts in the first 6 months of recovery, for the gay man, lesbian, or bisexual in such programs, relapse is almost certain if the gay or bisexual person cannot acknowledge and accept his or her sexual orientation. Discussion about the conflicts around acknowledging sexual orientation and ways to learn to live comfortably as a gay or bisexual person are essential for recovery, even if these topics are emotionally laden and stressful.

Many localities now have gay, lesbian, and bisexual health or mental health centers, almost all with a focus on recovery and substance abuse treatment. National organizations, such as the National Association of Lesbian and Gay Addictions Professionals, the Association of Gay and Lesbian Psychiatrists, the Gay and Lesbian Medical Association, the Association of Lesbian and Gay Psychologists, and the National Gay Social Workers, can help with appropriate referrals.

Some of the suggestions and guidelines of AA and NA and most treatment programs may be difficult for some gay men, lesbians, and bisexuals to follow. For example, giving up or avoiding old friends, especially fellow substance users, may be difficult when the gay or bisexual person has limited contacts that relate to him as a gay person. Staying away from bars or parties may be difficult if they are the only social outlets; special help on how to not drink or use drugs in such settings may be necessary. Many gay

people mistakenly link AA and religion; because many religious institutions denounce or condemn homosexuality, gay men, lesbians, and bisexuals may be resistant to trying AA or NA. Harm reduction models and relapse prevention techniques are especially useful approaches.

Specific Additional Factors to Consider

Gay men, lesbians, and bisexually identified minorities who abuse substances must deal also with homophobia—often from within the same self-identified ethnic or cultural groups—in addition to possible racism and other prejudices in seeking recovery (132–135).

There is still a popular misconception linking gay men, and not risky sexual behavior, with HIV infections and AIDS. The fears surrounding HIV may also interfere with the comfortable and objective treatment of gay men who are not HIV-positive or who do not have AIDS. Treatment centers and programs may still be frightened to work with HIV-positive individuals, despite the clear CDC guidelines, or may resist talking about safer sex because it is uncomfortable to talk about such matters or it is viewed as detracting from recovery issues. All one needs to do is remember that AIDS prevention education is just as life-saving an intervention for a substance abuser.

There are many additional difficult clinical issues facing a substance-abusing gay man who is HIV-positive or who has AIDS, whether actively using substances or in recovery, such as suicidality, dementia, negotiating safer sex, and legal issues concerning wills and powers-of-attorney (136–138). Finding a treatment setting that will accept a gay, clean, and sober person with AIDS may be very difficult (13). Some communities now have AA groups with a special focus on HIV-positive individuals or people with AIDS, such as the Positively Sober groups.

Other factors affect the treatment of lesbians, gay men, and bisexuals. Many gay men, lesbians, and bisexuals are in long-term relationships, and treatment for these individuals must clearly focus on relationships, parenting, and family concerns. Gay men, lesbians, and bisexuals are also subject to an increase in violent attacks because of their sexual orientation, both verbal and physical (139). Reaction to such an attack may include a relapse to drug or alcohol use in a person in recovery or an increase in use by someone currently using or abusing substances. In addition, many gay men, lesbians, and bisexuals are victims of domestic violence. This latter fact is often ignored by clinicians. Because there are correlations with domestic violence and substance abuse, clinicians need to be aware of this possible combination (140).

Additional treatment issues facing all people in recovery, which have special impact on gays and lesbians and are beyond the scope of this brief review chapter, include learning how to have safer sex while clean and sober; learning how to adjust to clean and sober socializing without the use of alcohol or drugs to hide social anxiety; dealing with employment problems and adjusting to the impact of being out as a gay person at work; working with the family of origin regarding their acceptance of the sexual orientation of their gay, lesbian, or bisexual child; helping couples adjust to the damaging effects substance use may have had over the years and embrace a recovery that will avoid the negative impact of codependent relationships; maintaining confidentiality in record keeping, especially around discussion in the medical record of sexual orientation or HIV status; dealing with child custody issues when necessary; diagnosing and treating additional medical problems; and coping with the effects of legal problems. Finnegan and McNally (14) address most of these concerns.

Clinicians and counselors must be aware of their own personal attitudes regarding homosexuality and HIV-related conditions. If a health care provider is homophobic and cannot get help in working out these attitudes with a supportive colleague or supervisor, the patient would be better off if he or she was referred to another staff member for help (36). Gay men and women facing recovery from substance abuse should not have to fight homophobia in a health care system to get quality care.

CONCLUSION

A growing literature on working with gay, lesbian, and bisexual substance abusers will help clinicians with the situations described in this chapter (14,40,41,44,45). Substance use—especially alcohol—is woven into the fabric of the lives of many gay men, lesbians, and bisexuals. The use of substances can be associated with identity formation, coming out, and self-acceptance processes for many gay men, lesbians, and bisexuals. The greater use and presence of alcohol and other drugs in settings where gay men, lesbians, and bisexuals socialize, combined with the dissociation and denial produced by the use of these substances, may help to explain a greater expression among gay people of a biologic or genetic predisposition for substance abuse. Internalized homophobia and societal homophobia combine to reinforce the use of alcohol and drugs and may make the recognition and treatment of substance abuse in gay men, lesbians, and bisexuals more difficult. Extended recovery is more likely to happen—indeed, may only be possible—if a gay man, lesbian, or bisexual person is able to accept his or her sexual orientation, address internalized homophobia, and discover how to live clean and sober without fearing or hating his or her real self.

REFERENCES

1. Beatty R. *Alcoholism and adult gay male populations of Pennsylvania.* Master's thesis. University Park, PA: Pennsylvania State University, 1983.
2. Diamond DL, Wilsnack SC. Alcohol abuse among lesbians: a descriptive study. *J Homosex* 1978;4(2):123–142.
3. Lewis CE, Saghir MT, Robins E. Drinking patterns in homosexual and heterosexual women. *J Clin Psychiatry* 1982;43:277–279.
4. Lohrenz L, Connelly J, Coyne L, et al. Alcohol problems in several Midwestern homosexual communities. *J Stud Alcohol* 1978;39(11):1959–1963.
5. McKirman D, Peterson PL. Alcohol and drug abuse among homosexual men and women: epidemiology and population characteristics. *Addict Behav* 1989;14:545–553.
6. Mosbacher D. Lesbian alcohol and substance abuse. *Psychiatr Ann* 1988; 18(1):47–50.
7. Pillard RC. Sexual orientation and mental disorder. *Psychiatr Ann* 1988; 18(1):52–56.
8. Saghir M, Robins E. *Male and female homosexuality.* Baltimore: Williams & Wilkins, 1973.
9. Fifield L, De Crescenzo TA, Latham JD. *Alcoholism and the gay community. Summary: on my way to nowhere: alien-* ated, isolated, drunk—an analysis of gay alcohol abuse and evaluation of alcoholism rehabilitation services for Los Angeles County. Los Angeles: Los Angeles Gay Community Services Center, 1975.
10. *Lesbian, gay and bisexual substance abuse needs assessment: a report.* San Francisco: Lesbian and Gay Substance Abuse Planning Group, August, 1991.
11. Morales ES, Graves MA. *Substance abuse: patterns and barriers to treatment for gay men and lesbians in San Francisco.* San Francisco: San Francisco Prevention Resources Center, 1983.
12. Weinberg M, Williams C. *Male homosexuals: their problems and adaptations.* New York: Oxford University Press, 1974.
13. Cabaj RP. AIDS and chemical dependency: special issues and treatment barriers for gay and bisexual men. *J Psychoactive Drugs* 1989;21(4): 387–393.
14. Finnegan DG, McNally EB. *Dual identities: counseling chemically dependent gay men and lesbians.* Center City, MN: Hazelden, 1987.
15. Stall R, Wiley J. A comparison of alcohol and drug use patterns of homosexual and heterosexual men: the San Fran- cisco Men's Health Study. *Drug Alcohol Depend* 1988;22:63–73.
16. Bradford J, Ryan C. *Mental health implications—national lesbian health care survey.* Washington, DC: National Lesbian and Gay Health Foundation, 1987.
17. Hall JM. Lesbians and alcohol: patterns and paradoxes in medical notions and lesbians' beliefs. *J Psychoactive Drugs* 1993;25(2):109–119.
18. Bloomfield K. A comparison of alcohol consumption between lesbians and heterosexual women in an urban population. *Drug Alcohol Depend* 1993;33(3):257–269.
19. Mosbacher D. Alcohol and other drug use in female medical students: a comparison of lesbians and heterosexuals. *J Gay Lesbian Psychother* 1993; 2(1):37–48.
20. U.S. Centers for Disease Control and Prevention. *HIV AIDS Surveill Rep* 1994;5:1–33.
21. Skinner WF. The prevalence and demographic predictors of illicit and licit drug use among lesbians and gay men. *Am J Public Health* 1994;84:1307–1310.
22. Gorman EM, Morgan P, Lambert EY. Qualitative research considerations and other issues in the study of methamphetamine use among men who have

sex with other men. *NIDA Res Monogr* 1995;157:156–181.

23. Sadownick S. Kneeling at the crystal cathedral: the alarming new epidemic of methamphetamine abuse in the gay community. *Genre* 1994 Jan:37–42.

24. Krafft-Ebing R. *Psychopathia sexualis.* (1898). Reprinted by Brooklyn Physicians and Surgeons Book Company, 1922.

25. Boswell J. *Christianity, social tolerance, and homosexuality.* Chicago: University of Chicago Press, 1980.

26. Hooker E. The adjustment of the male overt homosexual. *J Proj Tech* 1957;21(1):18–31.

27. American Psychiatric Association. *Diagnostic and statistical manual of mental disorders,* 3rd ed., revised (*DSM-III–R*). Washington, DC: Author, 1987.

28. Bayer R. *Homosexuality and American psychiatry.* New York: Basic Books, 1987.

29. American Psychiatric Association. *Diagnostic and statistical manual of mental disorders,* 4th ed., text revision (*DSM–IV–TR*). Washington, DC: Author, 2000.

30. Cabaj RP, ed. New thinking on sexuality and homosexuality. *Psychiatr Ann* 1988;18(1).

31. Marmor J, ed. *Homosexual behavior: a modern reappraisal.* New York: Basic Books, 1980.

32. Bell AP, Weinberg MS. *Homosexualities: a study of diversities among men and women.* New York: Simon & Schuster, 1978.

33. Morin SF. Heterosexual bias in psychological research on lesbianism and male homosexuality. *Am Psychol* 1977;32:629–636.

34. Weinberg G. Society and the healthy homosexual. New York: St. Martin's Press, 1983.

35. Cabaj RP, Stein TS, eds. Homosexuality and mental health: a comprehensive review. Washington, DC: American Psychiatric Press, 1996.

36. Cabaj RP. Homosexuality and neurosis: considerations for psychotherapy. *J Homosex* 1988;15(1–2):13–23.

37. Ross MW, ed. *Psychopathology and psychotherapy in homosexuality.* New York: Haworth, 1988.

38. Coleman E, ed. Psychotherapy with homosexual men and woman: integrated identity approaches for clinical practice. *J Homosex* 1987;14(1–2).

39. Stein TS, Cohen CC, eds. *Contemporary perspectives on psychotherapy with lesbians and gay men.* New York: Plenum, 1986.

40. Gonsiorek JC, ed. *A guide to psychotherapy with gay and lesbian clients.* New York: Harrington Park Press, 1985.

41. Ziebold TO, Mongeon JE, eds. *Gay and sober: directions for counseling and therapy.* New York: Harrington Park Press, 1985.

42. Hetrick ES, Stein TS, eds. *Innovations in psychotherapy with homosexuals.* Washington, DC: American Psychiatric Press, 1984.

43. Hart JE, ed. *Substance abuse treatment: considerations for lesbians and gay men. The MART Series #2.* Boston: The Mobile AIDS Resource Team, 1991.

44. Cabaj RP. Substance abuse in gay men, lesbians, and bisexual individuals. In: Cabaj RP, Stein TS, eds. *Homosexuality and mental health: a comprehensive review.* Washington, DC: American Psychiatric Press, 1996:783–799.

45. Guss JR, Drescher J, eds. *Addictions in the gay and lesbian community.* New York: Huntington Medical Press, 2000.

46. Isay RA. *Being homosexual: gay men and their development.* New York: Farrar, Straus & Giroux, 1989.

47. Friedman RC. *Male homosexuality: a contemporary psychoanalytic perspective.* New Haven, CT: Yale University Press, 1988.

48. Lewes K. *The psychoanalytic theory of male homosexuality.* New York: Simon & Schuster, 1988.

49. Friedman RM. The psychoanalytic model of male homosexuality: a historical and theoretical critique. *Psychoanal Rev* 1986;73(4):483–519.

50. Friedman RC, Downey JI. Homosexuality. *N Engl J Med* 1994;331(14):923–930.

51. Owen WF. The clinical approaches to the male homosexual patient. *Med Clin North Am* 1986;70:499–535.

52. Owen WF. Gay and bisexual men and medical care. In: Cabaj RP, Stein TS, eds. *Homosexuality and mental health: a comprehensive review.* Washington, DC: American Psychiatric Press, 1996:673–685.

53. Banks A, Gartrell NK. Lesbians in the medical setting. In: Cabaj RP, Stein TS, eds. *Homosexuality and mental health: a comprehensive review.* Washington, DC: American Psychiatric Press, 1996:659–671.

54. Dardick L, Grady KE. Openness between gay persons and health professionals. *Ann Intern Med* 1980;93[1 part 1]:115–119.

55. Kinsey AC, Pomeroy WB, Martin CE. *Sexual behavior in the human male.* Philadelphia: WB Saunders, 1948.

56. Michaels S. Prevalence of homosexuality in the United States. In: Cabaj RP, Stein TS, eds. *Homosexuality and mental health: a comprehensive review.*

Washington, DC: American Psychiatric Press, 1996:43–63.

57. Greenberg DE. *The construction of homosexuality.* Chicago: University of Chicago Press, 1988.

58. Herdt G. Cross-cultural forms of homosexuality and the concept "gay." *Psychiatr Ann* 1988;18(1):29–32.

59. Mihalik GJ. Sexuality and gender: an evolutionary perspective. *Psychiatr Ann* 1988;18(1):40–42.

60. Whitam FL, Mathy RM. *Male homosexuality in four societies.* New York: Praeger, 1986.

61. Herdt G. Issues in the cross-cultural study of homosexuality. In: Cabaj RP, Stein TS, eds. *Homosexuality and mental health: a comprehensive review.* Washington, DC: American Psychiatric Press, 1996:65–82.

62. Miller N. *In search of gay America: women and men in a time of change.* New York: Atlantic Monthly Press, 1989.

63. McWhirter DP, Sanders SA, Reinisch JM, eds. *Homosexuality/heterosexuality: concepts of sexual orientation.* New York: Oxford University Press, 1990.

64. U.S. Centers for Disease Control and Prevention. Update: acquired human immunodeficiency syndrome—United States, 1981–1988. *MMWR Morb Mortal Wkly Rep* 1989;38(14):1–28.

65. Herek GM. Heterosexism and homophobia. In: Cabaj RP, Stein TS, eds. *Homosexuality and mental health: a comprehensive review.* Washington, DC: American Psychiatric Press, 1996:101–113.

66. Bell AP, Weinberg MS, Hammersmith SK. *Sexual preference: its development in men and women.* Bloomington, IN: Indiana University Press, 1981.

67. Pillard RC, Weinrich JD. Evidence of familial nature of male sexuality. *Arch Gen Psychiatry* 1986;43:808–812.

68. Pillard RC, Poumadere J, Carretta RA. A family study of sexual orientation. *Arch Sex Behav* 1982;11(6):511–520.

69. Bailey JM, Pillard RC, Neale MC, Agyei Y. Heritable factors influence sexual orientation in women. *Arch Gen Psychiatry* 1993;50:217–223.

70. Bailey JM, Pillard RC. A genetic study of male sexual orientation. *Arch Gen Psychiatry* 1991;48:1089–1096.

71. Pillard RC. Homosexuality from a familial and genetic perspective. In: Cabaj RP, Stein TS, eds. *Homosexuality and mental health: a comprehensive review.* Washington, DC: American Psychiatric Press, 1996:115–128.

72. Byne W. Biology and homosexuality: implications of neuroendocrinological and neuroanatomical studies. In: Cabaj

RP, Stein TS, eds. *Homosexuality and mental health: a comprehensive review.* Washington, DC: American Psychiatric Press, 1996:129–146.

73. Imperato-McGinley JI, Peterson RE, Gautier T. The impact of androgens on the evolution of male gender identity. In: DeFries Z, Friedman RC, Corn R, eds. *Sexuality: new perspectives.* Westport, CT: Greenwood Press, 1981.

74. Hanley-Hackenbruck P. "Coming-out" and psychotherapy. *Psychiatr Ann* 1988;18(1):29–32.

75. McDonald G. Individual differences in the coming out process for gay men: implications for theoretical models. *J Homosex* 1982;8:47–60.

76. de Monteflores C, Schultz SJ. Coming out: similarities and differences for lesbians and gay men. *J Soc Issues* 1978;34:59–73.

77. Coleman E. Developmental stages in the coming out process. *J Homosex* 1982;7:31–43.

78. Cass V. Sexual orientation identity formation: a Western phenomenon. In: Cabaj RP, Stein TS, eds. *Homosexuality and mental health: a comprehensive review.* Washington, DC: American Psychiatric Press, 1996:227–251.

79. Forstein M. Homophobia: an overview. *Psychiatr Ann* 1988;18(1):33–36.

80. Cabaj RP. Homophobia: a hidden factor in psychotherapy. *Contemp Psychiatry* 1985;4(3):135–137.

81. De Cecco JP, ed. *Homophobia: an overview.* New York: Haworth Press, 1984.

82. Maylon AK. Psychotherapeutic implications of internalized homophobia in gay men. In: Gonsiorek JC, ed. *A guide to psychotherapy with gay and lesbian clients.* New York: Harrington Park Press, 1985.

83. Stein TS, Cabaj RP. Psychotherapy with gay men. In: Cabaj RP, Stein TS, eds. *Homosexuality and mental health: a comprehensive review.* Washington, DC: American Psychiatric Press, 1996:413–432.

84. Shilts R. *And the band played on: politics, people, and the AIDS epidemic.* New York: St. Martin's Press, 1987.

85. Ostrow DG, ed. *Biobehavioral control of AIDS.* New York: Irvington, 1987.

86. Cabaj RP, Klinger RL. Psychotherapeutic interventions with lesbian and gay couples. In: Cabaj RP, *Homosexuality and mental health: a comprehensive review.* Washington, DC: American Psychiatric Press, 1996:485–501.

87. Cabaj RP. Gay and lesbian couples: lessons on human intimacy. *Psychiatr Ann* 1988;18(1):21–25.

88. Quadland MC, Shattles WD. AIDS, sexuality, and sexual control. *J Homosex* 1987;14(1–2):277–298.

89. De Cecco JP, ed. Bisexual and homosexual identities: critical theoretical issues. *J Homosex* 1984;9(1–2).

90. Gibson P. Gay male and lesbian youth suicide. In: Sullivan LW, ed. *Report of the secretary of Health and Human Services' task force on youth suicide.* Washington, DC: U.S. Government Printing Office, 1989;3:110–142.

91. Hetrick ES, Martin AD. Developmental issues and their resolution for gay and lesbian adolescents. *J Homosex* 1987;14(1–2):25–43.

92. Rotheram-Borus MJ, Rosario M, Reid H, et al. Predicting patterns of sexual acts among homosexual and bisexual youth. *Am J Psychiatry* 1195;152(4):588–595.

93. Donovan C, McEwan R. A review of the literature examining the relationship between alcohol use and HIV-related sexual risk-taking in young people. *Addiction* 1995;90(3):319–328.

94. Savin-Williams RC. Verbal and physical abuse as stressors in the lives of lesbian, gay male, and bisexual youths: association with school problems, running away, substance abuse, prostitution, and suicide. *J Consult Clin Psychol* 1994;62(2):261–269.

95. Hartstein NB. Suicide risk in lesbian, gay, and bisexual youth. In: Cabaj RP, Stein TS, eds. *Homosexuality and mental health: a comprehensive review.* Washington, DC: American Psychiatric Press, 1996:819–837.

96. Olson ED. Gay teens and substance use disorders: assessment and treatment. In: Guss JR, Drescher J, eds. *Addictions in the gay and lesbian community.* New York: Huntington Medical Press, 2000:69–80.

97. Friend RA. The individual and social psychology of aging: clinical implications for lesbians and gay men. *J Homosex* 1987;14(1–2):307–331.

98. Berger RM, Kelly JJ. Gay men and lesbians grown older. In: Cabaj RP, Stein TS, eds. *Homosexuality and mental health: a comprehensive review.* Washington, DC: American Psychiatric Press, 1996:305–316.

99. Jax J. How to survive gay stress. *Christopher Street* 1985;89:16–19.

100. Schilit R, Lie GY, Montagne M. Substance use as a correlate of violence in intimate lesbian relationships. *J Homosex* 1990;19(3):51–65.

101. Falco KL. *Psychotherapy with lesbian clients: theory into practice.* New York: Brunner/Mazel, 1991.

102. Weinberg MS, Williams CJ, Pryor DP. *Dual attractions: understanding bisexuality.* New York: Oxford University Press, 1994.

103. Fox RC. Bisexuality: an examination of theory and research. In: Cabaj RP, Stein TS, eds. *Homosexuality and mental health: a comprehensive review.* Washington, DC: American Psychiatric Press, 1996:147–171.

104. Matteson DR. Psychotherapy with bisexual individuals. In: Cabaj RP, Stein TS, eds. *Homosexuality and mental health: a comprehensive review.* Washington, DC: American Psychiatric Press, 1996:433–450.

105. Kinsey A, Pomeroy W, Martin C. *Sexual behavior in the human female.* Philadelphia: WB Saunders, 1954.

106. Israelstam S, Lambert S. Homosexuality as a cause of alcoholism: a historical review. *Int J Addict* 1983;18(8):1085–1107.

107. Israelstam S, Lambert S. Homosexuality and alcohol: observations and research after the psychoanalytic era. *Int J Addict* 1986;21(4–5):509–537.

108. Vaillant GE. *The natural history of alcoholism: causes, patterns, and paths to recovery.* Cambridge, MA: Harvard University Press, 1983.

109. Cassel J. The contributions of the social environment to host resistance. *Am J Epidemiol* 1976;104:107–123.

110. Israelstam S, Lambert S. Homosexuals who indulge in excessive use of alcohol and drugs: psychosocial factors to be taken into account by community and intervention workers. *J Alcohol Drug Educ* 1989;34(3):54–69.

111. McKirman D, Peterson PL. Psychological and cultural factors in alcohol and drug abuse: an analysis of a homosexual community. *Addict Behav* 1989;14:555–563.

112. Miller A. *The drama of the gifted child.* New York: Basic Books, 1981.

113. Hanson G, Hartmann L. Latency development in prehomosexual boys. In: Cabaj RP, Stein TS, eds. *Homosexuality and mental health: a comprehensive review.* Washington, DC: American Psychiatric Press, 1996:253–266.

114. de Monteflores C. Notes on the management of difference. In: Stein TS, Cohen CC, eds. *Contemporary perspectives on psychotherapy with lesbians and gay men.* New York: Plenum, 1986.

115. Centers for Disease Control and Prevention. *HIV AIDS Surveill Rep* 2001;13(No. 2):1–44.

116. Stall R, McKusick L, Wiley J. Alcohol and drug use during sexual activity and compliance with safe sex guidelines for AIDS: the AIDS behavior research project. *Health Educ Q* 1986;13:359–371.

117. Stall R. The prevention of HIV infection associated with drug and alcohol use

during sexual activity. In: Siegel L, ed. *AIDS and substance abuse.* New York: Harrington Park Press, 1988:73–88.

118. Ostrow DG, Keslow RA, Fox R. *Sexual and drug use behavior change in men at risk of AIDS* [abstract no. 96]. Program and abstract of the 114th annual meeting of the American Public Health Association, 1986.

119. Lange WR, Haetzen CA, Hickey JE. Nitrites inhalants: patterns of abuse in Baltimore and Washington, DC. *Am J Drug Alcohol Abuse* 1988;14(1):29–39.

120. Smith DE, Smith N, Buxton ME, et al. PCP and sexual dysfunction. In: Smith DE, ed. *PCP: problems and prevention.* Dubuque, IA: Kendall-Hunt, 1982.

121. Goode E, Troiden RR. Amyl nitrite use among homosexual men. *Am J Psychiatry* 1979;136(8):1067–1069.

122. Guss JR. Sex like you can't even imagine: "crystal," crack and gay men. In: Guss JR, Drescher J, eds. *Addictions in the gay and lesbian community.* New York: Huntington Medical Press, 2000:105–122.

123. McDowell D. Gay men, lesbians and substance abuse and the "club and circuit party scene": what clinicians should know. In: Guss JR, Drescher J, eds. *Addictions in the gay and lesbian community.* New York: Huntington Medical Press, 2000:37–58.

124. MacGregor RR. Alcohol and drugs as co-factors for AIDS. In: Siegel L, ed. *AIDS and substance abuse.* New York: Harrington Park Press, 1988.

125. Hellman RE, Stanton M, Lee J, et al. Treatment of homosexual alcoholics in government-funded agencies: provider training and attitudes. *Hosp Community Psychiatry* 1989;40(11):1163–1168.

126. Substance Abuse and Mental Health Services Administration. *A provider's introduction to substance abuse treatment for lesbian, gay, bisexual, and transgender individuals.* CSAT NCADI Publication No. BKD392. U.S. Department of Health and Human Services, Substance Abuse and Mental Health Administration, Center for Substance Abuse Treatment, Rockville, MD. i-191, 2001.

127. Ratner EF, Kosten T, McLellan A. *Treatment outcome of PRIDE Institute patients: first wave—patients admitted from September 1988 through February 1989.* Eden Prairie, MN: PRIDE Institute, April, 1991.

128. McCormick K. *A program evaluation of Operation Recovery: findings and recommendations regarding a gay and lesbian sample. Report for Operation Concern.* San Francisco: 1994.

129. Hall JM. Lesbians recovering from alcohol problems: an ethnographic study of health care experiences. *Nurs Res* 1994;43(4):238–244.

130. Kus RJ. Sobriety, friends, and gay men. *Arch Psychiatr Nurs* 1991;5(3):171–177.

131. Kus RJ. Bibliotherapy and gay American men of Alcoholics Anonymous. *J Gay Lesbian Psychother* 1989;1(2):73–86.

132. Jones BE, Hill MJ. African American lesbians, gay men, and bisexual individuals. In: Cabaj RP, Stein TS, eds. *Homosexuality and mental health: a comprehensive review.* Washington, DC: American Psychiatric Press, 1996:549–561.

133. Nakajima GA, Chan YH, Lee K. Mental health issues for gay and lesbian Asian Americans. In: Cabaj RP, Stein TS, eds. *Homosexuality and mental health: a comprehensive review.* Washington, DC: American Psychiatric Press, 1996:563–581.

134. Gonzalez FJ, Espin OM. Latino men, Latina women, and homosexuality. In: Cabaj RP, Stein TS, eds. *Homosexuality and mental health: a comprehensive review.* Washington, DC: American Psychiatric Press, 1996:583–601.

135. Tafoya TN. Native two-spirit people. In: Cabaj RP, Stein TS, eds. *Homosexuality and mental health: a comprehensive review.* Washington, DC: American Psychiatric Press, 1996:603–617.

136. Cabaj RP. Assessing suicidality in the primary care setting. *AIDS File: Focus on Management of Psychiatric Complications of HIV Disease* 1994;8(2):7–9.

137. Flavin DK, Franklin JD, Frances RJ. The acquired immune deficiency syndrome (AIDS) and suicidal behavior in alcohol-dependent homosexual men. *Am J Psychiatry* 1986;143(11):1440–1442.

138. Ostrow DG, Monjan A, Joseph J. HIV-related symptoms and psychological functioning in a cohort of homosexual men. *Am J Psychiatry* 1989;146(6):737–742.

139. Klinger RL, Stein TS. Impact of violence, childhood sexual abuse, and domestic violence and abuse on lesbians, bisexual individuals, and gay men. In: Cabaj RP, Stein TS, eds. *Homosexuality and mental health: a comprehensive review.* Washington, DC: American Psychiatric Press, 1996:801–818.

140. Schilit R, Lie GY, Montagne M. Substance use as a correlate of violence in intimate lesbian relationships. *J Homosex* 1990;19(3):51–65.

CHAPTER 72

The Homeless

HERMAN JOSEPH AND JOHN LANGROD

Chemical dependency affects all social classes in the United States. However, the personal stress, anxieties, depression, and tensions resulting from chronic unemployment, destitution, and homelessness exacerbate the problems associated with substance abuse. These include the spread of infectious diseases (e.g., sexually transmitted diseases, human immunodeficiency virus [HIV], tuberculosis, and hepatitis C) and the development of chronic medical conditions resulting in premature death. Homelessness is a major public health, as well as a socioeconomic, problem not only in the United States but also across the spectrum of cities in all developing and industrialized countries. In 2001, the United Nations Center for Human Settlements (UN-Habitat) in its report, *The State of the World's Cities,* estimated that more than 1 billion people in cities worldwide live in inadequate housing and that an estimated 20 to 40 million urban households or families, or about 100 million persons, are homeless (1). This chapter concentrates, however, on the interrelated problems of homelessness, substance abuse, mental illness, and medical issues, including the spread of infectious disease in the United States.

DEFINITION OF HOMELESSNESS

The Stewart B. McKinney Act, which provides funds for housing the homeless, defines a homeless person as one who "lacks a fixed, regular, and adequate night-time residence and has a primary night time residency that is a supervised publicly or privately operated shelter designed to provide living accommodations, or an institution that provides a temporary residence for individuals intended to be institutionalized, or a public or private place not designed for or ordinarily used as a sleeping accommodation for human beings." The term 'homeless individual' does not include any individual imprisoned or otherwise detained pursuant to an Act of Congress or a state law. The McKinney definition is applied to obtain funding for those who are literally on the streets or in a shelter in urban areas (2). However, the definition may be not be sufficient for homeless persons living in rural areas where there are few shelters, and many homeless persons may live with others in overcrowded substandard conditions or in abandoned structures, cars, and campers. Therefore, rural areas may be limited in accessing benefits and funds for the homeless. The National Coalition on the Homeless reports that in 1996 the rate of rural poverty was higher than the national average and that of metropolitan areas (15.9%, 13.3%, and 12.6%, respectively) (3).

Homelessness for the purpose of this chapter encompasses persons whose living conditions are described by the above definitions and those individuals who live as transients and squatters in low-priced hotels or "doubled up" in apartments belonging to others—the hidden homeless. When homeless on the streets or living precariously as a transient, it is difficult for chemically dependent persons to adhere to the requirements of treatment programs, to acquire and consistently apply knowledge to reduce substance abuse and alcoholism, and to protect themselves from becoming infected with and transmitting infectious diseases associated with addiction.

CAUSES OF HOMELESSNESS

The major social causes of homelessness are high rates of poverty, chronic unemployment, low-paying jobs, loss of benefits, and, most important, the lack of affordable housing (4). In September 2003, The National Low Income Housing Coalition released a report indicating that housing costs increased faster than wages, inflation, and the costs of other goods. Affordable housing for low-income families and persons is becoming less available in the United States. In 2003, there was no state in which an extremely low income family could afford the fair market value of a modest, safe, two-bedroom apartment. The United States Conference of Mayors reported that the "shortfall for affordable housing for the very poorest now stands at 3.3. million units. . . ." The hourly housing wage, the amount a family must earn working full-time to rent

a modest two-bedroom apartment that does not exceed 30% of their annual income has increased by 37% from $11.08 per hour in 1999 to $15.21 per hour in 2003. The report states that the minimum wage of $5.15 per hour is inadequate for millions to meet rents without sacrificing other basic needs such as food, clothing, and health care. Approximately 14 million families spend more than half of their income on rent. During the past 25 years, the gap in supply and demand for affordable housing has been widening as no new significant public housing has been constructed (5,6).

Coupled with the erosion of affordable housing has been the loss of both unskilled manufacturing and skilled professional jobs to countries outside the United States. The United States Conference of Mayors (USCM) reports that metropolitan areas in the United States lost more than 2.3 million jobs with an average annual salary of $43,629 during the years 2001 to 2003. For the years 2004 and 2005, the USCM predicted modest job growths of 1.3% and 1.7%, respectively, with average annual wages of $35,855, an 18% drop in wages from the period 2001 to 2003. There should be modest drops in unemployment rates from the 6.1% recorded in July 2003. However, with the erosion of affordable housing, there is concern that the lower average annual wages of new jobs will not provide sufficient income for families to meets basic expenses including rent (7–9).

The United States Bureau of the Census reported that at the end of 2002, 34.6 million (12.6%) Americans were living below the poverty level, an increase of 1.7 million over 2001. Also in 2002, the median household income fell by 1.1%, and the number of persons without medical insurance increased 2.4 million over 2001 levels to 43.6 million or approximately 15.6% of the population. Although more people received Medicaid and other entitlements, public coverage was insufficient to meet the loss of insurance in the private sector. The unemployment rate, loss of jobs, increasing poverty levels, and lack of affordable housing have contributed to an increase in homelessness (10–12).

Substance abuse and mental illness can precipitate homelessness when the affected persons are without financial support and, conversely, homelessness can exacerbate these conditions. The lack of available treatment for this group was cited as a major unmet need contributing to their homelessness. Other contributing causes to homelessness include cuts in public assistance and government benefit programs; the disappearance of jobs resulting in chronic unemployment among those unable to find work in the new technology job market; the deinstitutionalization of the mentally ill and the release of homeless prisoners without adequate follow-up services including housing; domestic violence in families with women and their children relying on shelters for housing; personal crises in the lives of youths, especially gays and lesbians, that result in them leaving or being thrown out of their homes; and the "doubling up" of single persons and families in apartments belonging to friends, relatives, and others. This population, known as the "hidden homeless" and "couch people," is at great risk of finding themselves without housing if a crisis should occur in their lives or the lives of the primary tenants of the apartments (13–20).

Childhood factors that predispose adults to homelessness are experiencing extreme poverty in childhood; placement in foster care, group homes, or other institutions; abuse or neglect by an adult in the home; running away from home; being kicked out of the home; and experiencing homelessness prior to the age of 18 years. Homeless adults who were in foster care as children are more likely to have not competed high school. They are also more likely to have their own children placed in foster care and have more episodes of adult homelessness as compared to homeless adults who were not placed in foster care or other institutions as children (21,22).

ESTIMATING THE NUMBER OF HOMELESS

In March 2003, the United States Department of Health and Human Services (HHS) reported that each year homelessness affects between 2 and 3 million persons or approximately 1% of the population, while the Urban Institute and National Coalition of the Homeless (NCH) estimate that there are probably up to 3.5 million persons homeless in a year. On any given night HHS and NCH estimates that between 600,000 and 700,000 persons nationwide are experiencing homelessness (23,24).

HHS subdivides the homeless into three categories:

1. Temporary: 80% of the homeless experience one homeless episode;
2. Sporadic: 10% experience sporadic episodes of homelessness; and
3. Chronic: 10% experience long episodes of a year or more and experience more than one episode. Eight-five percent of this group have serious disabilities with co-occurring disorders.

REQUESTS FOR FOOD AND SHELTER: REPORT OF THE UNITED STATES CONFERENCE OF MAYORS

In 2002, the USCM, in its annual nationwide survey of 25 major cities, reported possibly the largest increases in requests for help in a decade. In 2001, requests increased by 19% for food (all cities) and shelter (88% of the cities). Because of a lack of resources and facilities, approximately 16% of the food requests and 30% of the housing requests were not met. Approximately 50% of the unmet requests for food and 38% of the unmet requests for housing involved families with children. Furthermore, although the average episode of homelessness lasts about 6 months, more than 80% of the cities surveyed reported that the duration of homeless episodes increased in 2002 when compared to 2001 (13).

New York City is not included in the annual surveys of American cities. However, homelessness as measured by requests for shelter increased by approximately 25% in 2002 over 2001. Also, New York City during the 6-month period following September 11, 2001, lost about 100,000 jobs. African Americans and Hispanics accounted for 47.5% of the labor force in 2001 but comprised 61% of the unemployed after September 11 and the majority of those who requested shelter because of homelessness. It is estimated that on any given night about 38,000 people may be housed in shelters. From 2001 to 2003 there was an 11% increase in single persons housed on any given night in the shelters and a 60% increase in the number of families. In 2003 the families were larger with more children than in 2001 (25,26).

DESCRIPTION OF THE HOMELESS

Single men account for approximately 41% of the homeless population, families mostly headed by women with children account for approximately 41%, single women account for approximately 13%, and unaccompanied youth and minors account for approximately 5%. Unaccompanied youth, minors, and children in homeless families account for approximately 25% to 30% of the homeless population. Nationwide, minorities are overrepresented among the homeless: African Americans comprise an estimated 50% of the homeless population, followed by whites (29%), Hispanics (12%), Native Americans (2%), and Asians (1%). Homeless persons in rural areas are most likely to be white, families and single mothers with children, immigrant farm workers, and Native Americans (13,15).

In 1996, the United States Bureau of Census issued the National Survey of Homeless Assistance Providers and Clients (NSHAPC). In this survey 2,938 randomly selected homeless persons were interviewed from the 28 largest metropolitan areas, 24 small- and medium-size communities, and 24 rural counties. Of the persons interviewed, 49% indicated that the current episode of homelessness was their first, 17% had two episodes of homelessness, and 34% had three or more episodes. At the time their interviews, 28% were homeless for 3 months or less, 15% were homeless for 4 to 6 months, 15% were homeless for 7 to 12 months, and 16% were homeless for 13 to 24 months. When asked about reasons for the current episode of homelessness, the most frequent responses were could not pay rent, lost job or job needed, drug use, landlord made person or persons leave, did not get along with people they were living with, and domestic violence/child abuse, which was mentioned mostly by families with children. During the week prior to the interview, 34% of the homeless lived only in shelters, 7% only on the streets, 6% only in temporary housing, and 53% moved within the week, living in two or three of these environments. The age distribution of homeless clients in this survey as compared to the U.S. adult population was younger than age 25 years (12% vs. 13%), age 25 to 54 years (80% vs. 59%), and age 55 years or older (8% vs. 28%) (27).

ESTIMATES OF ALCOHOL, DRUG ABUSE, AND MENTAL HEALTH CONDITIONS

All surveys and reports of homelessness include persons with co-occurring alcohol, drug abuse, and mental health condition (ADM) disorders. Although rates may vary in different studies, the prevalence of current and lifetime ADM disorders is uniformly high; in 2002, the United States Conference of Mayors estimated that approximately 32% of the homeless in 25 major cities across the United States had serious substance abuse/alcohol problems and 23% were considered to be mentally ill. Zerger reported that between 10% and 20% of the homeless with substance-abuse problems are dually diagnosed with a mental health condition (28). Koegel reported that in Los Angeles, California, in a sample of 1,563 homeless persons, 66% were diagnosed with substance abuse disorders and 22% were diagnosed with chronic mental illness (29). However, there was considerable overlap in the two conditions: 77% with chronic mental illnesses were dually diagnosed as chronic substance abusers (29). The random sample survey of NSHAPC shows that irrespective of combinations of problems over the course of their lifetimes, alcoholism was the most prevalent (62%), followed by drug abuse (58%) and mental health problems (57%). The prevalence of any alcohol, drug, and mental health problem either individually or in combination reported during the month prior to the interview was 66%; 74% for the year prior to the interview; and 86% for lifetime prevalence. A smaller group, approximately 30%, had experienced the three conditions—alcohol, drug abuse, and mental health conditions—over the course of their lives (27).

In a nationwide sample of 7,224 homeless persons with mental illness, Desai et al. found a high prevalence of suicidal ideation (66.2% lifetime prevalence). High rates of suicide attempts were also reported: 51.3% had ever attempted suicide, 26.7% attempted suicide and were subsequently hospitalized in a nonpsychiatric institution, and 8% reported recent attempts within the prior 30 days of the interview. Significant factors associated with suicide attempts included substance abuse, youth, and psychiatric symptoms (30).

Studies within shelters irrespective of the decade from the 1980s to 2003 or geographic location show similar results: high rates of substance misuse, mental illness, and alcoholism.

- A random study of the "literally homeless on the streets and in the shelter systems of Hartford, Connecticut, and Providence, Rhode Island, by Glasser and Zywiak (31)

showed rates of substance abuse of 47.2% (Hartford) and 45.1% (Providence).

- The high prevalence rates of ADM disorders within the homeless population age 18 years and older are summarized in an analysis and review of 24 studies by Lehman and Cordray (32). In these studies, homeless persons were not in environments specifically targeted to persons with ADM disorders. Shelters, however, were included in these studies as survey sites. The following prevalence estimates were calculated: undifferentiated mental health problem Axis 1 (between 45% and 50%); severe Axis I disorder (between 18% and 23%); severe and persistent Axis I disorder (between 19% and 23%); any Axis I substance use disorder (between 45% and 55%); alcohol use disorders (between 40% and 50%); drug use disorder (between 28% and 37%); and dual diagnosis of co-occurring mental health and substance use disorders (between 10% and 20%). Important subgroups in this study could not be properly modeled because of sample limitations and the existence of a large number of variables between the studies.

- In a survey of 26 shelters in New York City conducted in 1987, with a weighted sample equivalent to 1,000 residents, Struening and Pittman found that 10.7% admitted using heroin within the 6-month period prior to the interview. However, 18% admitted using heroin more than 50 times during their lives, 36% admitted using cocaine more than 50 times, and 18% admitted smoking crack. These included daily users of cocaine and heroin. Approximately 12% of the men and 6% of the women were hospitalized for alcoholism (i.e., 41 hospitalizations per 100 men and 24 hospitalizations per 100 women). The participants were subdivided into categories based on degree of alcohol and/or substance abuse, mental illness (depression, psychotic episodes), and hospitalizations for these conditions. Approximately 35% of the shelter residents had minimal conditions. The remaining residents were impaired by their problems: approximately 15% had serious mental health conditions, 28% abused alcohol, heroin, and/or cocaine either solely or in combination, and 21.3% had both substance misuse and mental health problems (33,34).

- During the years 1986 though 1995 the New York State Office of Alcoholism and Substance Abuse Services conducted two major studies of alcohol and drug use comparing randomly selected transients in shelters and single-room occupancy hotels with domiciled residents throughout New York State (35,36). A third state survey was undertaken in 2002 and 2003 but was not completed in time for reporting the results in this chapter. Major findings from the earlier two studies are as follows. Table 72.1 shows that the overall proportion of transients who inject drugs, including heroin, in comparison with domiciled residents in stable living conditions is about 15:1. Table 72.2 summarizes the drugs used by the transient population in comparison with the

TABLE 72.1. *Percentages of New York city residents in different living accommodations with drug-using risk behaviors associated with AIDS*

Drug-using risk behaviors associated with AIDS	Living accommodations	
	Shelters single-room occupancy and low-priced hotels (N = 270)	Other accommodations (N = 2,874)
Residents with any lifetime needle use	21%	1.5%
Residents with any lifetime needle use and use of heroin within last 5 years	12%	0.8%
Residents with any lifetime needle use and use of heroin within last 2 years	10%	0.6%

Source: From the New York State Division of Substance Abuse Services, Bureau of Research and Evaluation: State household survey, 1986.

domiciled population for the 6-month period in 1986 prior to the survey. The proportion of drug users among the transient population far exceeds the proportion of drug users among the domiciled population. The percentage of cocaine users among the transient population is more than 5 times the percentage of cocaine users among domiciled residents, and the proportion of heroin users in the transient population is about 20 times the proportion within the domiciled population. A similar trend was obtained with smaller percentages in New York State but outside of New York City. Transients were disproportionately minorities, reporting little or no employment and low incomes. Using questions from the *Diagnostic and Statistical Manual of Mental Disorders,* 3rd ed. (*DSM–III*), 51.4% were considered to be chemically dependent on one or more substances: 13.5% on drugs only (marihuana, cocaine/crack, heroin, other drugs), 16.1% on alcohol alone, and 21.8% on alcohol and another drug. Alcohol and cocaine showed the highest rates for dependency. However, rates for cocaine/crack use in the 1990s among the transient popula-

tion were higher outside of New York City. This finding showed that the cocaine/crack epidemic with its epicenter in New York City in the 1980s had spread to the rest of the state in the 1990s. Rates of lifetime use were also very high among the transient population: marihuana, 79%; cocaine/crack, 65%; heroin, 28%; other drugs, such as phencyclidine (PCP), lysergic acid diethylamide (LSD), barbiturates, and pain killers, ranged from 15% to 23%, depending on the drug. Approximately 49% of the transient population entered treatment at least once, and 60% of those who entered treatment had at least two episodes of treatment for chemical dependency.

• Alcohol consumption among the state's transient population showed the following major trend (25): The transient population showed a greater rate of abstinence from alcohol than the domiciled population (39.8% vs. 26.3%). However, the rate of life-threatening alcoholism was higher among the transient population: approximately 17% of the transient population drank more than 10 drinks per day (over 5 ounces of pure alcohol) as compared with 1.8% of the domiciled population. The

TABLE 72.2. *Use of illicit substances among adults 18 years of age and older in New York city: comparison of transients and household residents in New York city during a 6-month period in 1986 prior to survey*

Drug	Living accommodations	
	Shelters single-room occupancy and low-priced hotels (N = 270)	Other accommodations (N = 2,874)
Marihuana	40%	11%
Cocaine	27%	5%
Heroin	9%	*
PCP (angel dust)	4%	*
Inhalants (aerosol spray, solvents, amyl nitrite)	3%	*
Illicit methadone	3%	*
Hallucinogens (LSD, mescaline, psilocybin)	2%	*

*Less than 0.5% of survey respondents.
Abbreviations: LSD = lysergic acid diethylamide; PCP = phencyclidine.
Source: From the New York State Division of Substance Abuse Services, Bureau of Research and Evaluation: State household survey, 1986.

percentage of transients who drank two or more drinks per day was correlated with their type of sleeping arrangements. Those who slept in public places had the highest percentage of such drinkers (48%), followed by those who slept in shelters (38%), and those who slept in single-room occupancy or welfare hotels (27%). The percentage of transient males who drank two or more drinks per day was higher than the percentage for females (39% vs. 19%, respectively) (37).

- Projecting the results of this survey on an estimated homeless/transient population of about 50,000 in New York State, about 25,000 transients are in need of treatment for mental illness (depression), chemical dependency, and alcoholism (35–37).

Study of Drug Users within Soup Kitchen Populations

Schilling, El-Bassel, and Gilbert interviewed 148 current and former drug users in a Manhattan soup kitchen about drug use and AIDS risk behavior (38). Of the sample, 12.8% claimed that they were enrolled in outpatient treatment for drug addiction with approximately 7.4% enrolled in methadone-maintenance programs. Only those who were involved in methadone maintenance participated in AIDS prevention programs. The subjects reported using at least one of the following drugs for long periods of average lifetime use: cocaine (11 years), crack (3.6 years), and heroin (11 years), marihuana (16 years), and speedballing (i.e., heroin used in combination with cocaine; 9 years). Within 3 months of the interview 84.5% of the subjects admitted using at least one of the five drugs. Approximately 51.4% of the sample admitted injecting drugs in the past—12.3% within the past 3 months. Of those who injected drugs within 3 months of the interview, 85% indicated that they were sharing needles, 30% were sharing cookers, and 40% borrowed needles and syringes. Only 24.3% lived in their own apartments; the remainder lived in shelters (25.2%), the street (11.6%), doubling up in someone else's home (34.7%), and in other places (4.1%).

In a Brooklyn soup kitchen, studied in 1997 by Magura, Nwakeze, Rosenblum, and Joseph, 75% of subjects used cocaine/crack and 25% used heroin/opioids during the preceding month, as determined by hair analysis. Only 25% of the subjects were in substance-abuse treatment programs. Infectious diseases included hepatitis B exposure (15%), hepatitis B carrier (6%), HIV (16%), and syphilis (16%). Factors associated with hepatitis and HIV include years of injection drug use and homelessness or marginal/transient living conditions. There was a high prevalence of sexual risk behaviors: approximately 50% reported never using condoms, approximately 33% reported using drugs during sexual activity, and approximately 20% admitted exchanging sex for money, drugs, or a place to sleep. Homelessness was associated with less access to public entitlements such as food stamps and Medicaid. Persons who are sleeping on

the streets usually lack the proper identification to obtain entitlements. However, persons enrolled in drug or alcohol treatment had access to benefits because they were usually enrolled in Medicaid. Frequency of drug/alcohol use was associated with less access to Medicaid only, whereas childcare was associated with greater access to food stamps. However, those persons in the soup kitchen who received case management with additional peer support to assist in planning and followup kept more appointments for social and drug treatment services and generally had better outcomes such as reducing cocaine abuse than those who received case management without peer support (39,40).

Soup kitchens should be prime sites for outreach to homeless drug users in need of medical care, substance-abuse treatment, and interventions to prevent the transmission of infectious diseases. In many soup kitchens, nationwide, referral services to drug and medical treatment and to community agencies have been instituted. Soup kitchens attract a diverse population of the homeless, including those who are transient in single-room occupancy hotels or who live doubled up as couch people in the apartments of others, and those who live in shelters and on the streets. These studies validated, in two geographically different soup kitchens over a decade, the long durations and high prevalence of drug abuse among soup kitchen populations, the low level of enrollment in treatment, the high prevalence of risk behaviors for contracting and transmitting infectious diseases, as well as high rates of infectious disease.

Homelessness and the Provision of Services

Homeless people are perceived as difficult to service by social service and health providers in communities throughout the country. Reports from service providers indicate that the homeless are more desperate and harder to treat with more wide-ranging, serious co-occurring health, social, mental health, substance abuse, alcohol, and behavioral problems than domiciled clients and patients. No one social or health agency is able to service their needs. Referrals to a variety of agencies must be made and coordinated. Furthermore, the professional staffs of social service and hospitals may harbor biases about the homeless, especially if substance abuse and extreme destitution are major problems (41,42).

Stigmatization of homeless persons is commonplace. They may be placed on waiting lists for services, beds, or treatment. Providers consider the homeless transient and hard to contact. Many are without proper identification to access benefits and do not have funds for transportation to keep appointments. They require extensive resources and coordinated care, which does not exist in many programs or localities. A comment by a service provider summarizes the perception of the homeless: "They are at the absolute bottom when they get to us" (41,42).

These perceptions by service providers reflect the perceptions of the homeless within the greater society. However, being homeless can precipitate behavior that may label people as uncooperative and arbitrary when the circumstances of homelessness with its instabilities and disorganization may be the cause of such behavior. In a 1994 study of homelessness in 49 cities across the United States, the National Law Center noted that services to help the homeless were inadequate despite the development of some exemplary programs, including housing (41,42).

MEDICAL ISSUES AMONG THE HOMELESS POPULATION

The Institute of Medicine report, *Homelessness, Health, and Human Needs,* categorizes the interrelationship between homelessness and health problems: (a) some health problems and medical conditions precede homelessness and causally contribute to homelessness; (b) other health conditions are the consequences of homelessness; and (c) irrespective of the time of onset of an illness, homelessness complicates the treatment process (43).

The mental health conditions and substance abuse that are prevalent within the homeless population are applicable to the three categories. However, the stresses, deprivations, poor nutrition, lack of exercise, and depression found within populations of those who live in extreme poverty, or who are homeless, contribute to the development of major chronic illnesses at higher prevalent rates and at younger ages than in domiciled, more affluent populations. Brickner and Scanlan (44) (1990) summarized the relationship of homelessness and chronic disease as follows:

> The medical disorders of the homeless are common illnesses magnified by disordered living conditions, exposures to extremes of heat and cold, lack of protection from rain and snow, bizarre sleeping accommodations and overcrowding in shelters. The stress of street life, psychiatric disorders, and sociopathic behavior patterns obstruct medical intervention and contribute to the chronicity of disease (44).

Homeless persons are a medically underserved group. Many do not have the proper identification to qualify for Medicaid, which would enable them to receive needed medical services and primary care. The delays in diagnosing medical conditions can result in further complications and increased rates of mortality. Upon entering the medical system, health conditions are reported at higher rates than in the domiciled population, and homeless persons use the services of hospitals and emergency rooms more frequently than does the general population (45).

Some major health conditions found with greater prevalence in the homeless, as compared to the general population include:

- Peripheral vascular diseases (e.g., gout, varicosities, chronic edema, phlebitis, gangrene, and ulcerations resulting in amputations), which are about 10 to 15 times higher among the homeless.
- Hypertension rates, which in the homeless are at least twice the rate of the general population.
- Chronic health conditions such as cancer, diabetes, arthritis, and high blood pressures, which are reported in approximately 46% of homeless by the National Resource Center on Homelessness and Mental Illness.
- Upper respiratory infections, tuberculosis (TB), sexually transmitted diseases (STDs), HIV/AIDS, hepatitis, and liver disease.
- Lice and scabies from sleeping outdoors.
- Injuries and trauma from beatings, muggings, assaults with weapons, and accidents.
- Frostbite resulting in amputations.
- Poor nutrition, poor personal hygiene, burns, skin lesions, and infections at injection sites.
- Dental problems (the homeless have 12 times the rate of the domiciled).
- Severe stress and mental disorders, substance abuse, neurologic and seizure disorders, and chronic alcoholism.
- Homeless women having a greater percentage of low-birth-weight babies than domiciled women (17% vs. 6%) and a greater percentage of preterm deliveries (19% vs. 10%) (46).

Serious soft-tissue infections at sites of injection have been reported among both homeless and domiciled injectors of illicit drugs. Surgical procedures may be necessary to contain infections. The San Francisco General Hospital organized The Integrated Soft Tissue Infection Services Clinic to provide surgery, substance-abuse counseling, and other interventions. In its first year of operation, there were 3,365 patient visits and 2,255 surgical procedures performed. Rates of success and patient compliance were high: only 2% were classified as failures and 14% were lost to followup. Approximately 61% reported recent injection use, 30% were homeless, and 62% were infected with hepatitis C, hepatitis B, and HIV. Approximately 42% of the patients had histories of heroin use and were enrolled either in withdrawal or maintenance programs. The clinic program was cost-effective, saving $8,765,200 in hospital and medical expenses by reducing potential emergency room visits, acute care in hospital beds, surgical admissions, and operating room expenses. The service can serve as a model for other communities (47).

In a study of hospital admissions, Salit et al. (48) found that homeless persons presented a greater prevalence of different types of conditions that resulted in longer hospital stays than domiciled patients: 80% of the hospitalized homeless were diagnosed with a complicating substance abuse or mental problem, although 52% were admitted only for specific treatment of these conditions. The rate of substance abuse and mental illness among the homeless upon admission was twice that of domiciled patients. They also had higher rates for infectious diseases, respiratory disorders, skin problems (lesions), and trauma. Homeless patients had on the average a 36% longer duration of hospitalization per admission than did domiciled patients. The greatest differences in duration of hospitalizations were for mental illness, AIDS, and surgery. One reason for the longer hospitalizations is that homeless patients usually do not seek attention until symptoms are pronounced, and hospital care is indicated (48).

High rates of physical and psychiatric conditions were found in a random sample of 139 persons who were treated on a medical van at shelters and soup kitchens in Manhattan: chronic back pain and other muscular skeletal problems (37%); circulatory complaints such as swollen feet or legs (37%); cardiovascular problems including high blood pressure (25%); and bruises and contusions (15%). Serum test results showed hepatitis B (47% positive), hepatitis C (29% positive), HIV antibodies (14%), and syphilis exposure (14%). Years of crack/cocaine use were associated with presence of HIV and sexually transmitted diseases (syphilis, hepatitis B and C) independent of injection drug use. The subjects reported skin lesions and oral lip sores from smoking cocaine/crack, and these sores coupled with high-risk sex practices have been a vector for the transmission of hepatitis C, HIV, and STDs. Seventy-two percent showed some degree of functional impairment, such as depressive disorder and symptoms of psychosis; 45% reported excessive alcohol intake (more than 5 drinks per day); 75% used cocaine, 17% used heroin, and a smaller group used hallucinogens (2%) and tranquilizers (2%). Although 8% indicated that they had injected drugs during the past 90 days, 20% indicated that they had injected over their lifetime. Twenty-seven percent were considered alcohol dependent and 41% drug dependent. Comorbidity across psychiatric symptoms and drug and alcohol dependence was high. Chronic physical symptoms and functional incapacity was linked to depression. Intensive case management services proved to be essential because 41% of those who received intensive case management (more counseling sessions than usual with followup) completed referrals, mostly to drug treatment, as opposed to 14% of those who received regular counseling (49).

More than 80% of the subjects experienced some type of homelessness during the month of the interview, either living in the streets or in shelters (41%), or were marginally homeless in a single-room occupancy hotel or doubling up in living quarters belonging to others (41%), while others indicated that they either shared or lived in an apartment during the past month. Sixty-eight percent were male and 32% were female; 63% were African American, 16% were Hispanic, 12% were white, and 9% were of another ethnic ancestry. Fifteen percent of the homeless were veterans. The mean age of the group was 40 years, and 52% were never married; 11% were either married or cohabiting with a partner. Sixty-nine percent had either a high school

diploma or its equivalent. Approximately 69% were unemployed during the month of the interview (31% claimed to have part-time or full-time work) (49).

Among injection drug users (IDUs), hepatitis C virus (HCV) has emerged with HIV as the major blood-borne infectious disease transmitted through use of shared needles and injection equipment. Furthermore, HCV is usually acquired during the first months of injection before addicts learn about harm reduction and use needle-exchange programs. Hogan and Des Jarlais report that seroprevalence of HCV among IDUs is estimated to be between 50% and 95%, and that incidence of HCV can be 10 to 100 times that of HIV (50). Within the same groups of injectors, Strathdee et al. report that prevalence rates among unstably housed and homeless injectors of HCV at a Vancouver needle-exchange program are 3.7 times the prevalence rate of HIV (85% vs. 23%) (50,51).

Within a random sample study of homeless persons in New York City, which includes IDUs as well as noninjectors, the overall seroprevalence of HCV is about twice the rate of HIV (29% vs. 14%) and the seroprevalence of hepatitis B is 47% (49). In a study of homeless persons with co-occurring mental illness and substance abuse, Klinkenberg et al. reported that 30% were HCV positive, approximately 33% hepatitis B virus (HBV) positive, and 6.2% were HIV positive (52). In methadone programs in New York City, death rates from AIDS appear to have stabilized whereas death rates from HCV are increasing (53). Because of the high seroprevalence of HCV among IDUs, methadone patients infected with HIV are usually coinfected with HCV.

From the beginning of the HIV/AIDS epidemic, risk factors for transmission of HIV such as shared needle use and unprotected sexual activity were highest among the homeless, especially young adults. Outreach units were established in cities across the country to educate the homeless about risk behavior, the disease itself, and routes of transmission (54,55). In data gathered from nine cities, Wright, in 1984, showed that the incidence of AIDS among the homeless was significantly higher than in the domiciled population (230 cases per 100,000 vs. 144 cases per 100,000, respectively) (56). In a study of 16 cities, Allen et al. reported the median seroprevalence rate of HIV as 3.4% among the homeless as opposed to less than 1% in the general population (57).

A study of AIDS risk behavior by Shuster among 4,824 IDUs completed in May 1989, showed that the 879 homeless substance abusers were more likely to engage in high-risk behavior than were those who lived in more stable conditions. In this study, 55% of the homeless lived in shelters and 45% were on the streets. In the 6 months prior to the interview, a greater proportion of the homeless shared needles (71% vs. 64%) and rented or borrowed needles (83% vs. 74%) than did IDUs with homes. However, a greater proportion of the domiciled users tended to clean their needles with bleach (32% vs. 25%). Also, the proportion of homeless users who exchanged sex for drugs or money was greater than the proportion of domiciled users (males: 18% vs. 11%; females: 46% vs. 42%) (58).

In a study of 169 homeless men who sought medical help and agreed to be tested for HIV antibodies in a New York City shelter, 62% were seropositive. Of the group testing positive for HIV antibody, 53% were IDUs, 8% were both IDUs and had sex with men, and 23% had sex with men and were not IDUs (45). As the testing, physicians, and counseling were on site within the shelter where the men lived, 71% complied with the program.

However, a study of 231 persons with AIDS conducted by Dr. Ramon A. Torres of the St. Vincent's Hospital in Manhattan underscores the serious medical and followup problems presented by homeless persons with AIDS (59). Thirty (13%) of the 231 patients were homeless. Although 36 (16%) of the 231 patients were intravenous substance abusers, 21 (70%) of the 30 homeless patients were intravenous substance abusers. Homeless patients were more difficult to manage. They had higher rates of being lost to followup, of signing out of the hospital against medical advice, of longer periods of hospitalization, of broken clinic appointments, of incomplete tests for diagnosis of and failure to comply with treatment for opportunistic infections, of lost prescriptions, and of TB.

After the passage of the Ryan White Care Act in 1990, special entitlements, such as social service, medical, and housing programs were developed for persons infected with HIV (60). To curtail the HIV epidemic, the USCM passed resolutions to support needle exchanges (1997), to remove legal barriers for injection drug users to access sterile syringes (2000), and to request that physicians be permitted to prescribe injection equipment to stem the HIV/AIDS epidemic (2003) (61). Notwithstanding the passage the Ryan White Care Act for development of special services specifically targeted to persons with HIV/AIDS, The National Coalition of the Homeless indicates that the percent of homeless with HIV/AIDS can fluctuate from 3% to 20%, depending on the subgroup of the homeless population and the city surveyed (62). Robbins and Nelson estimate that 50% of persons living with HIV/AIDS will need housing assistance during the course of their illness and that 36% of HIV/AIDS patients have experienced episodes of homelessness (63).

Both the USCM and the National Coalition for the Homeless indicate that current services have to be improved and increased to adequately meet the needs of this particular population, which includes access to treatment for substance abuse and housing. In the United States, there are approximately about 40,000 new infections a year, with more than 80% of all new cases in urban areas affecting mostly minorities. Therefore, the USCM also recommended in 2003 that $1.4 billion be added to the domestic budget to address the epidemic in the United States in the areas of housing, research, prevention, minority concerns, medical services, and medications (61).

Homelessness and Tuberculosis

With the rise of homelessness and the increase in HIV infection, TB has reemerged over the past two decades as a public health concern. From 1953 to 1984, an annual decrease of 6% in TB cases was reported nationally. However, between 1984 and 1992 a 20% national increase in cases was reported attributable to four factors: the HIV/AIDS epidemic; immigration from countries where TB was common; the spread of TB within certain environments, such as homeless shelters and prisons; and the lack of funding for public health efforts to control the epidemic. However, from 1992 a steady decline in cases has been reported as resources were developed for prevention, control, and treatment, including directly observed therapy in state and local health clinic systems. Pockets of TB remain, especially within the homeless population where TB rates may be 20 times that of the general adult population (64).

However, to study the effective public health interventions the homeless population was stratified to into two groups, the chronically homeless at high risk for substance abuse, TB, and HIV, and the transient homeless. Over a 10-year period the following population shifts were noted. Each year 10% of the transient homeless became chronically homeless and 10% of the chronically homeless became transient homeless, while 30% of the transient homeless moved back into the domiciled population. However, they were replaced by an equivalent number of the domiciled population who become homeless. The most important factor in declining TB rates and deaths in both groups was accessibility to treatment. Declining rates of TB for chronic and transient homeless were 12.5% and 35.9%, respectfully; declining rates of death for chronic and transient homeless were 19.8% and 32.4%, respectively. Overcoming barriers to treatment for the homeless, improving program performance, and providing bacille Calmette-Guérin (BCG) vaccination to HIV-negative homeless persons is crucial to reduce further the rates of TB infections and death (65).

New York City experienced the greatest increase of TB cases in the country during the period of 1978 to 1992 with 3,811 cases reported in 1992. A prospective 8-year followup, beginning in 1984, of 858 indigent subjects, ages 18 to 64 years, with substance misuse and alcohol problems showed the following: 5.5% developed TB, 9.% were diagnosed with AIDS, and 21.3% had died. Rates of TB, AIDS, and death were respectively 14.8, 10, and 5.2 times that of age-matched populations in New York City (66).

Drug-resistant *Mycobacterium tuberculosis* is associated with low income or homeless persons who do not have access to health care, injection drugs users, the elderly, and immigrant groups who come from countries where TB is common (64). In a study of 132 patients afflicted with *Mycobacterium tuberculosis* in New York City, it was found that drug-resistant *Mycobacterium tuberculosis* was found in 21% of the 53 homeless patients, as compared to 8% of 79 nonhomeless patients (67).

However, with development of a citywide TB treatment clinic system, including methadone-maintenance programs and the implementation of a TB treatment center at the Rikers Island City Jail, the TB epidemic was brought under control. Basic to the program's success was the introduction of direct observational therapy and case management. From 1992, the peak of the epidemic, to 2001, there was a 66.9% decrease in reported cases and the lowest city rate of 15.7 cases per 100,000 persons, which was still 2.8 times the national rate of 5.6 reported cases per 100,000 persons (68).

Homelessness and Mortality

Studies of deaths among the homeless over the past 5 decades show that homeless persons have an increased risk of premature deaths. Homeless persons rarely live to the ages older than 65 years. Studies found that the average age of death among homeless men is 51 to 53 years (69). Rates of death for the homeless from serious chronic illnesses, violence, alcoholism and substance abuse are three to four times higher than of domiciled populations. In a Philadelphia study, the homeless age-adjusted mortality rate was 3.5 times that of the general domiciled population; homeless nonwhites, whites, males, and females died younger and at higher rates than their domiciled counterparts (70).

In Boston, Hwang et al. reported that major causes of death among the homeless varied by age and at higher rates than general population: ages 18 to 24, homicide; 25 to 44, AIDS; 45 to 64, cancer and heart disease (71). Risk factors for deaths of homeless adults in Boston included AIDS, renal disease, cold-related injuries, arrhythmia, substance misuse by injection, and alcoholism (72). In Atlanta, Georgia 28(70%) of 40 deceased homeless showed alcohol-related mortality as primary or secondary causes of death in addition to other causes which included accidents, cardiac and pulmonary disease, seizures, homicides, suicide, hypothermia and deaths in fires. No deaths were attributed to drugs although autopsy reports showed cannabinoids (4 cases), cocaine (1 case), barbiturates and phenytoin at therapeutic and subtherapeutic levels (3 cases). Median age at death was 44 years (range: 20 to 70). Overall crude death rate was 5.7 to 10 deaths per 1,000 homeless (73). In New York City, age-adjusted death rates among shelter residents were four times that of the general U.S. population and two to three times the general New York City population. Factors associated with high death rates included prior use of injecting drugs, incarcerations, chronic homelessness, disease, and disability (74).

The Center on Homelessness and Poverty concluded, in 2003, that deaths of homeless persons on the streets was a growing phenomenon in cites across the United States. Causes of deaths include violence against the homeless, substance abuse, complications of alcoholism, untreated medical conditions, exposure to extreme weather, and apparent hypothermia. For example, in 1999, 183 homeless persons were found dead in San Francisco alone. However, national statistics are not available because cities may not keep records of deaths of the homeless. The known deaths, however, encompass all subgroups of the homeless. The report, which surveyed 57 communities, found that no community had sufficient beds available to meet the needs of the homeless, notwithstanding the existence of shelters and transitional housing (75).

Programs Within Shelters for the Homeless

Within the past decade innovative programs and services were developed in the New York City shelter system by public agencies working in conjunction with private not-for-profit community organizations. In June 2002, the New York City Department of Homeless Services issued a blueprint for guidelines and policy entitled *The Second Decade of Reform: A Strategic Plan for New York City's Homeless Services*. The following four-part strategy was adopted: (a) primary focus will be on prevention of the homeless by coordination of local and state agencies and evaluation of programs; (b) service provision will occur in the shelter with evaluation to improve services; (c) permanent affordable housing will be addressed; and (d) efficiency and accountability will be central to planning services, which will be based on data and evaluation. In addiction six principles were adopted: (a) safe affordable housing should be available to all individuals and families; (b) safe temporary shelter should be available for all homeless individuals and families; (c) safe and humane options should be available for homeless persons and they should not have to make their homes on the streets or in public places; (d) all homeless persons and families deserve and are expected to actively participate in their plans for independent living; (e) coordination between agencies is essential to ensure long-term outcomes for those who are homeless and for those who may become homeless; and (f) Services must be of the highest standards through improvement of procedures, facilities, and education of staff (76).

As an example of applying the above strategies and principles, Project Renewal, an agency funded by public and private sources has transformed many areas of the shelter system by introducing on-site medical, psychiatric, legal, and social services. In several shelters, residents work toward health, sobriety, permanent housing, and jobs. In addition, residents have access to individual and group counseling, vocational training, and assistance to obtain benefits. Some of the programs targeted to specific homeless populations that can serve as models for further expansion and development in other cities include:

- A 32-bed chemical dependency crisis center where medically trained personnel help patients through the physically and emotionally process of withdrawal.
- A program for homeless women who suffer from addiction and mental illness to help them garner resources for independent living in the community.

- A residential facility for homeless men with histories of chemical dependency who participate in a treatment/work program. The clients also acquire employment skills by working with the Times Square Business Improvement District. The combination of treatment, support, life skills learning, and work has resulted in more than 90% of the graduates becoming fully employed and permanently housed.
- In 2001, Project Renewal developed the first dormitory program in the United States in a shelter for homeless men on methadone maintenance. An estimated 1,500 homeless people on methadone maintenance languished in shelters, unable to access social service and other programs that required participants to be "drug free" or to be withdrawn from methadone maintenance. The patients receive comprehensive medical, psychological, housing, and employment services to prepare them to live in the community. Although as of this writing the residents obtain their methadone from community programs, Project Renewal is planning a Drug Enforcement Agency (DEA)- and state-approved methadone program for the shelter system.
- Project Renewal operates an internal medical service in a city shelter and a mobile medical van that is a fully equipped medical clinic. The van travels to shelters, soup kitchens, and places where the homeless congregate, offering front-line medical services and, if indicated, referrals for additional treatment (77).

Homelessness, HIV Risk Behavior, Harm Reduction

Literature over the past 2 decades has reported that syringe exchanges are associated with reductions in the prevalence and incidence of HIV, they do not lead to increased drug use, and they are associated with a decrease in needle sharing (78,79). Various surveys show that homeless persons have greater rates of drug use, HIV infection, and risk behaviors as compared to the domiciled population.

Homelessness and HIV/AIDS may be considered co-occurring disorders for subgroups of the population. Aidala and Cross reported that the prevalence of HIV/AIDS among the homeless and unstably housed is three to nine times the rate of domiciled persons. The rate

of risk behaviors related to drug use, injection and use of shared needles is three to six times the rate of domiciled users. Unsafe sexual practices are two to four times more likely among the unstably housed and the homeless, respectively, as compared to the stably domiciled (80).

Homeless persons who engage in high-risk behavior such as unprotected sex and injecting drug use are at higher risk of becoming infected with and transmitting HIV than are domiciled persons with similar risk behaviors (80).

To address the issue of homelessness and needle exchange, data were collected from five syringe-exchange programs in New York City from October 1992 to January 1995. Subjects for interviewing were randomly selected from those attending the exchanges within a given week. To be eligible for inclusion in the study, subjects must (a) have been an active IDU, (b) have used syringe exchange on at least one occasion, and (c) have just exchanged syringes. Verbal informed consent was obtained to protect the subject's confidentiality. For this analysis, homeless was defined as living on the street, in a shelter, or in a welfare hotel during the 6 months before the interview. Using these criteria, 1,001 (32%) of the total sample were classified as homeless, and 2,137 (68%) were considered domiciled. The population was racially and ethnically diverse, composed of males (70%), females (30%), African Americans (36%), Latinos (36%), whites (26%), and other ethnic/racial groups (2%). Approximately 74% had been in prison during their lifetimes, 78% had previous histories of treatment for drug abuse, and 39% were currently enrolled in treatment.

Whites were more likely to be homeless than African Americans, Latinos, and others (37% vs. 31%, 30%, and 28%, respectively). Also, males were more likely to be homeless than were females (35% vs. 24%). Those classified as homeless were more likely to have spent time in prison during their lifetime (86% vs. 69%) and were less likely to be currently enrolled in treatment for drug abuse (33% vs. 42%) (Tables 72.3 and 72.4.)

With regard to HIV risk behavior during the 30-day period prior to the interview, homeless participants were more likely to inject cocaine and were more likely to practice risky injection (injecting with a used syringe) than domiciled participants (13% vs. 6%). Homeless persons were also less likely than domiciled participants to always use condoms with casual partners (47% vs. 58%) and

TABLE 72.3. *Syringe-exchange evaluation: housing status by selected sociodemographics*

Demographics[a]	Mean age[b] (years)	Female[c] N (%)	Male[c] N (%)	African American[d] N (%)	Latino[d] N (%)	White[d] N (%)	Other[d] N (%)	Total N (%)
Not homeless	37	718 (76)	1,419 (65)	778 (69)	799 (70)	517 (63)	43 (72)	2,137 (68)
Homeless	36	224 (24)	777 (35)	345 (31)	339 (30)	300 (37)	17 (28)	1,001 (32)
Total	36.6	942 (100)	2,196 (100)	1,123 (100)	1,138 (100)	817 (100)	60 (100)	3,138 (100)

[a] Percent totals may not equal 100% because of rounding
[b] Scheffe's test
[c] p = 0.001
[d] p <0.05

TABLE 72.4. *Syringe-exchange: prison and drug treatment history by housing status*

History	Total N (%)	Not homeless N (%)	Homeless N (%)
Been in prison[a]	2,326 (74)	1,467 (69)	859 (86)
Been in drug treatment[b]	2,463 (78)	1,688 (79)	775 (77)
In treatment now[c]	1,232 (39)	905 (42)	327 (33)

[a] p = 0.001
[b] p <0.05
[c] p = 0.319

reported slightly higher rates of HIV-positive status (Table 72.5).

In the 1990s in New York City, harm-reduction centers and needle-exchange programs such as St. Ann's Corner in the Bronx and Positive Health in Manhattan, evolved to become multisite front-line harm-reduction centers serving the chemically dependent homeless and unstably housed. St. Ann's Center offers case management, needle exchange, referrals to community agencies, food, clothing, washer/dryer service, and outreach and support groups. Positive Health services a diverse community where addicted persons of all ethnic, racial, and sexual orientations are treated without bias or moral judgment. The program officers needle exchange, acupuncture, and medical treatment for HIV/AIDS, hepatitis C, hypertension, diabetes, trauma, mental hygiene services, and dentistry. Because medications are prescribed, evaluations are conducted to avoid toxic interactions with the street drugs that are consumed. Methadone patients who do not receive adequate care in their clinics can attend the center for services. Approvals have been granted to prescribe buprenorphine for the treatment of heroin addiction. Groups are organized to meet the needs of the diverse population. Referrals are made for other services such as drug treatment, employment, and housing (81).

The New York Peer AIDS Education Coalition, a harm-reduction and needle-exchange program, targets youthful drug users within the gay, lesbian, and transgender communities; most are or have been homeless on the streets and may be involved with street prostitution. They include homeless youth who were usually asked to leave or were thrown out of their homes and who have remained estranged from their families. The major drugs used are alcohol, marihuana, psychotropic medications, club drugs, and crack/cocaine. Drugs to facilitate sex changes are injected, and needles for injection of hormones have been shared. The clinic director estimates that approximately 50% of those who come to this program for help are HIV positive. They usually do not apply for social services or medical treatment from mainstream community institutions or other harm-reduction centers because of possible rejection and stigmatization that they may encounter (82).

The harm-reduction centers and needle-exchange programs fill an important role by offering needed services to a street population that avoids mainstream medical and social institutions, including drug-treatment programs. However, under certain conditions, needle exchange may not be sufficient to prevent transmission of HIV. Strathdee et al. report that high rates of seroconversions to HIV positive were found among homeless and unstably housed

TABLE 72.5. *Syringe-exchange evaluation: drug risk behavior[a]*

	Total N	Not homeless N (%)	Homeless N (%)
Risky injection in last 30 days[b,c]	262	128 (6)	134 (13)
Use of condoms during last 30 days before interview			
With primary partner[d]	939	714 (100)	225 (100)
Always		252 (35)	69 (31)
Not always		462 (65)	156 (69)
With casual partner[e]	470	305 (100)	165 (100)
Always		176 (58)	78 (47)
Not always		129 (42)	87 (53)
Self-reported HIV status	1,961	1,332 (100)	609 (100)
HIV positive[e]		331 (25)	179 (29)
HIV negative[e]		1,021 (75)	430 (71)

[a] Percent totals may not equal 100% because of rounding.
[b] Defined as any injection with a used, dirty syringe.
[c] p = 0.001
[d] p = 0.202
[e] p <0.05

cocaine injectors who attended the exchange and injected cocaine in groups. Therefore, for certain subgroups of injector's additional social services, housing, and education are needed (51).

Safe injection rooms have been implemented in Switzerland, Australia, and Canada. These facilities allow homeless street addicts to inject drugs with new, unused paraphernalia in a medically supervised environment to avoid transmission of infection (83–85). Prescribing naloxone to injecting addicts to reverse respiratory depression in case of overdose is another harm-reduction approach that is being considered. These newer innovations add to the continuum of front-line medicine that is being developed to service the addicted homeless who do not use mainstream medical facilities.

However, the provision of stable housing is possibly the most important harm-reduction service for the homeless who are at high risk of acquiring and transmitting HIV. Aidala and Cross showed that:

- Homeless and unstably housed persons who improved their housing situation were half as likely to engage in high-risk behavior (e.g., drug use by injection, unprotected sex) than those who remained homeless or unstably housed.
- Persons whose living accommodations worsened were four times more likely to have engaged in high-risk sex exchange than were those whose housing accommodations did not deteriorate

Aidala and Cross indicate that homelessness itself, aside from personal characteristics of the subjects, make HIV prevention and treatment more difficult. Stable housing for the HIV-infected homeless is a promising social intervention that can provide the environment to improve treatment and prevention measures (80).

Homeless Veterans

Homeless veterans probably constitute the largest group of homeless men in both urban and rural areas of the country. The Veterans Administration (VA) estimates that 250,000 veterans are homeless on any given night and that 500,000 experience homelessness over the course of a given year. Perhaps 1 of 3 homeless males is a veteran. Approximately 3% of the homeless veterans are female. Female homeless veterans are more likely to be married than male homeless veterans, and are more likely to have serious mental and psychiatric problems. They are less likely to be employed, and less likely to have suffered from addictive disorders (86–88).

The majority of homeless veterans are from the Vietnam era (47%) and post-Vietnam era (17%), including a few from Desert Storm. Approximately 89% received honorable discharges, 67% served 3 or more years, and 33% served in war zones. At present there are more Vietnam-era homeless male and female veterans than service people who died in that war. However, many veterans are at risk for homelessness because they may be without jobs or earning low poverty-level wages, live in substandard conditions, and lack the network and support of friends and families (86–88).

In addition to social and economic reasons for homelessness (e.g., lack of affordable housing, poverty-level income, or unemployment) 76% of the homeless veterans are afflicted with serious overlapping problems such as posttraumatic stress syndrome/other mental health conditions (45%) and alcoholism/substance abuse (70%). According to the Department of Veterans Affairs, epidemiological studies suggest access to the support of family and friends, family background and personal characteristics may be stronger indicators of risk for homelessness than military service itself or duty in Vietnam (86–88).

Treatment for mental health conditions, substance abuse, and alcoholism are provided in VA Medical Centers throughout the country. Treatment for infectious diseases associated with addiction are also provided. The VA has established the largest service nationwide for the treatment of HIV/AIDS, servicing 20,000 veterans per year. Testing and treatment for hepatitis C are also provided, as is treatment for alcoholism, substance abuse, and mental health conditions (86–88).

According to the Department of Veterans Affairs and the National Coalition of Homeless Veterans, homeless veterans need a variety of services, including safe, secure housing free of drugs and alcohol with supportive services; child care; long-term permanent housing; nutritional and dental services; eye care; vocational assessment and job placement; and treatment for substance abuse, alcoholism, HIV/AIDS, hepatitis C, and mental health conditions. In response, the VA established a homeless assistance and treatment network of 16 programs plus a monitoring and evaluation component, which is probably the largest program of its type in the country, serving 40,000 homeless veterans a year. The programs include coordinated programs with other federal, state, local, public, and private agencies; special biopsychosocial treatment and rehabilitation services; grants to fund community efforts to assist homeless veterans; loan-guarantee programs for housing; aid for education; various housing programs, including a special program for veterans with substance abuse and mental problems; comprehensive homeless centers; drop-in centers; special outreach and benefits programs; and Stand Downs where homeless veterans can receive services and care for 1 to 3 days (e.g., food, shelter, clothing). However, because the VA homeless initiatives reach less than 10% of the homeless veterans, coordination with community organizations is essential to develop additional services and programs. According to the National Coalition for Homeless Veterans, the most effective programs include transitional housing within the community and with veterans groups assisting the homeless veterans (86–88).

Homeless Youth: A Group at High Risk for Contracting HIV

Although this section discusses the issues of the homeless youth in the United States, the issues discussed are found in cities throughout the world. Homeless youth have high levels of co-occurring medical, substance abuse, and mental disorders, in addition to serious social problems, including low levels of education, unemployment in legitimate jobs, and reliance on the illegal street market for survival.

Unaccompanied homeless youth are considered to be age 18 years or younger, but in many studies, the term encompasses persons younger than age 25 years. There are varying estimates of the number of homeless youths age 18 years or younger on the streets. The Institute of Public Health Studies estimated that 300,000 youth are homeless every year. The Research Triangle Institute estimates that 2.8 million youth living in households have a runaway experience during prior years, and the 2002 U.S. Conference of Mayors reported that homeless youths accounted for 5% of the homeless population (13,89).

Homeless youth are usually estranged from their families and unable to return to their homes for a variety of reasons. Virtually all left because of abusive conditions within their homes; some were asked to leave, others left on their own volition because the parents did not care, and others come from homeless families. There may have been an economic or emotional crisis that destroyed family relationships; the death of parent(s); the family's rejection of the youth's behavior, sexual orientation, or identity (e.g., gay, lesbian, or transgender), and/or substance abuse. Parents or others in the household may have serious mental health problems, be chemically dependent or alcoholic, and subject the children to stress and violence. In a 1997 study by the United States Department of Health and Human Services, 46% of the homeless youth report that they were physically abused, and 17% reported sexual abuse by being forced into unwanted sexual relationships with members of their families. About half of the homeless youth could be considered "throwaways" rather than runaways.

Children from unstable families may be placed in foster care. Upon discharge from foster care, youths may find themselves on the streets because of inadequate planning. Twenty percent to 25% of homeless youths have histories of foster care within their immediate past (89,90).

Once on the streets, homeless youths do not have the skills or means to earn sufficient funds for survival. They may be forced into exchanging sex for their basic needs—food, clothing, and shelter. Because of their age, many may not be acceptable in shelter systems, and others may refuse to enter shelters because of the environment and regulations, preferring their autonomy (89).

Homeless youth are forced into circumstances and behavior with high risks for contracting HIV. A study in 1985 in Los Angeles, California, comparing behavior and social characteristics of 110 homeless runaway youth with 655 other youth, showed that the prevalence of behavior leading to the transmission of or exposure to HIV is greater among the homeless youth. For example, 34.5% of the homeless youth and 3.7% of the other youth were IDUs. To support themselves and their drug habits, homeless youth participated in street prostitution at more than 100 times the rate of other youth (26.4% vs. 0.2%). Compared to other youth, runaways were more prone to engage in homosexual (7.3% vs. 4.9%) and bisexual (9.1% vs. 4.9%) behavior. The runaways also showed greater prevalence rates than other youth for mental health problems (18.2% vs. 3.8%), depression (83.6% vs. 24.0%), and for females, pelvic inflammatory disease (4.4% vs. 1.4%) (91).

Between October 1987 and June 1989, a blinded study to determine the seroprevalence of HIV antibody in a population of 1,840 runaway and street youth was conducted by Covenant House, a home for homeless youth in New York City; 110 (6%) were seropositive. The rate of infection increased with age from approximately 2% for 15-year-olds to approximately 10% for youths 20 years of age and older. The 1,158 males had a higher rate of HIV than did the 682 females (6.3% vs. 5.1%, respectively). Hispanic youth had the highest rate of HIV seroprevalence, followed by whites and African Americans (7.4%, 6.1%, and 5.1%, respectively) (48). The causes of HIV infection were not given in this study. Extrapolating from the research on runaway youth in San Francisco and the analysis of the AIDS data for teens and young adults in New York City, intravenous drug use and unprotected sexual activity with infected persons are the major vectors for transmitting the AIDS virus among the homeless youths (92).

Robertson (1996) reported an HIV-positive rate of 2.3% among homeless youth younger than age 25 years in four cities, The National Network for Youth estimates that the rate of HIV infection may be two to ten times the rate of domiciled youth in the United States. Robertson (1996) found that homeless youths have three times the rate of depression, posttraumatic stress syndrome, and conduct disorders than domiciled youth. Many are school dropouts and are unable to complete their educations or obtain vocational skills because of lack of proper records, legal guardianship requirements, residency requirements, and lack of transportation expenses (89,93,94).

Clatts and Davis indicate that homeless youth in New York City are mostly from the city and the surrounding metropolitan area. They tend to be "castaways" from homeless families, discharges from foster care, neglected, and abandoned. Without an education or job skills, they must develop a variety of strategies to survive within the legal and street economies. Their sources of income include short-term employment; money from family or friends; public assistance; pan handling; bartering sex in exchange for necessities; pimping; pornography; prostitution; sale of drugs; stealing; and thefts that may involve mugging (94,95).

Accessing drugs for sex partners is related to the youths' own drug use. Although daily use of marihuana (6%) and alcohol (26%) is reported, approximately 68% of the youths in the study had used illicit drugs with frequent multiple drugs use: cocaine, crack-cocaine, heroin, speedballs (heroin and cocaine), amphetamines, and psychedelics. The route of administration varied between injection and noninjection. Of those who injected drugs, nearly 50% shared syringes, whereas 80% shared cotton, rinse water, and cookers; 75% had never been treated for drug abuse; and 80% were sexually active. Approximately 44% had unprotected sex with a main commercial partner and 38% with multiple commercial partners (94,95).

Homelessness was associated with sex work, unprotected multiple partner sex, a history of STDs, and higher levels of drug use. The drug use–sex behaviors were common in the sample of youths, but especially so in the older age group of gay and bisexual homeless youth. However, services are usually geared to younger homeless youths than to the older group, which shows a greater involvement in risk behaviors directly related to the transmission of HIV, STDS, and hepatitis C (94,95).

Clatts and Davis reported that homeless youth, because of the trauma of their everyday lives, tend to mistrust and avoid institutions for health and social services (95). However, they do respond to outreach services that are provided outside of institutional settings. Outreach can function as a bridge to mainstream services and institutions. Youth contacted by outreach begin to discuss the problems that adversely affect their lives, including health concerns; AIDS testing and medications, STDs, harm reduction, use of drop-in centers, accessing prevention services; medical and drug treatment; and social issues such as employment, street activities, housing, and education. Sympathetic outreach often results in higher-than-expected rates of compliance, and the youth tend to remain in contact with the outreach team. However, the emotional degradation of street life becomes emotionally "progressively debilitating" and youths respond with increased self-medication with street drugs, including stimulants such as cocaine/crack (94,95).

Violence and high death rates from violence are the reality of life for homeless youth whose lives are enmeshed in illegal street activities. The high prevalence of scars from knife and gunshot wounds found on physical examination of homeless youth is evidence of the violence they encounter (92).

Homeless Women and Families

In the past decade, women with children constituted the second major group of homeless persons after single homeless men. Single women without families, however, constitute another major group of homeless women (13). Homeless single women may be more hidden because of the stigma of being a woman without a family or home.

Furthermore, homeless women who had been homeless and/or placed in foster care as children were 50% more likely to experience more than one episode of homelessness than were women who had never been in foster care as children (59% vs. 39%, respectively) (22).

Women usually become homeless after an eviction or an episode of domestic violence. Frequently, a woman must choose between remaining in a dangerous, abusive relationship, or leaving and becoming homeless. Studies of homeless families nationally show that between 20% and 50% of all women and children experiencing homelessness are victims of domestic violence and that domestic violence in cities across the country is a major cause of homelessness (4,13).

Mood-altering drugs may be a factor in violent episodes. Gilbert et al. (96) studied 31 women enrolled in an outpatient methadone program who were victimized by partner violence. Twenty-six (84%) indicated that use of mood-altering drugs was involved in the episodes where the male partner physically attacked and forced the woman into having unprotected sex. Twenty percent of the women indicated they used drugs to alleviate distress and physical pain after the episode.

Once homeless, women are at high risk for robbery, rape, and assault especially if drugs and alcohol are involved. High levels of mental depression, stress, and suicidal ideation are reported. Homeless women with children are under additional stress. It is estimated that one-third of homeless mothers have attempted suicide as compared to 25% of poor domiciled women, and that one-third have a chronic health condition. Also, children in homeless families have higher rates of asthma, ear infections, stomach disorders, depression, and speech problems than do domiciled children. They are twice as likely to experience hunger, and four times more likely to have developmental disorders. Furthermore, their educations may be delayed because of residency requirements, inability to obtain previous school records, transportation problems, lack of food, clothing, and supplies (20,97,98).

Pregnancy may be a complicating factor. Gelberg et al. (100) reported in a survey of 974 chronically homeless women, including those with substance-abuse histories in the shelters of Los Angeles, that deterrents to using contraceptives included lack of education on how to use contraceptives and which methods to use, lack of storage space, side effects, potential health risks, discomfort, the partners refusal to use contraception, and costs. About two-thirds of homeless women interviewed in Los Angeles reported a variety of gynecological symptoms during the year prior to the interview, including abnormal vaginal discharge, severe pelvic pain, skipped periods, breast lumps, and burning during urination. Seventy-one percent sought care for at least one symptom. Women reporting drug abuse and rape received less overall medical care than did women with health insurance, young age, or gynecological problems. Those who reported being raped appear to experience trauma-like responses during examinations and therefore may not seek health care as often as other women. The study highlights the need for integrated, accessible, and culturally sensitive prenatal, obstetrical, and therapeutic interventions and general health care, in addition to housing (99,100).

Pregnant substance-abusing women, many of whom are living in unstable housing or are homeless, have been prosecuted for use of illegal drugs such as heroin and cocaine. Charges include "nonexistent crimes such as 'fetal abuse' and delivery of drugs through the umbilical cord." Children have been removed from the custody of their mothers and placed in foster care or with other relatives (e.g., grandparents) even when they are capable of being responsible parents (101).

On January 28, 2003, the State Supreme Court of South Carolina upheld the conviction of Regina McKnight, a cocaine user who delivered a stillborn child. McKnight was in her thirty-fifth week of pregnancy when she was charged with "murder through child abuse." The stillbirth was perceived as related to her use of cocaine. However, stillbirths and neonatal impairments and disabilities occur in women who are not prosecuted but who drink alcohol and smoke cigarettes during pregnancy. The hostile political climate on this social issue makes it difficult to advocate for women's reproductive rights and the personal and medical needs of pregnant substance-abusing women, including their need for accessible treatment for drug abuse, medical/psychological conditions, prenatal care and housing (101).

A study of homeless and poor comparative African American women who used crack/cocaine showed that homelessness was associated with violence, abuse, and victimization before the age of 18 years, crack runs of greater than 24 hours, depression, income of less than $500 within the past month, and excessive cigarette smoking. Experiencing a sexual assault within the previous 3 months was marginally associated with being homeless. Homeless women were more likely to report childhood abuse, and a greater use of drugs. Domiciled women tended to be living with children younger than age 18 years, in receipt of welfare within the previous month, and tended to be with a spouse or partner. Both groups of women reported stressful lives and painful past histories (102).

A study conducted in 1989 by Dr. Joyce Wallace of the Foundation for Research on STDs of 950 streetwalking sex workers in the five boroughs of New York City showed that 33.7% were infected with HIV (103). In one area of Manhattan, the HIV rate among the sex workers studied doubled within a 2-year period from 8% to 15%. In a subgroup of 13 male transvestites and 8 transsexuals, 10 were seropositive. There were no significant differences in rates of HIV infection between homeless and "domiciled" streetwalking sex workers. Of the 189 streetwalkers who considered themselves homeless, 34.4% had positive test

results for HIV as compared to the 32.5% infection rate among the 781 "domiciled" streetwalkers (103).

However, the chance of HIV infection is positively correlated with the level of education. Those streetwalkers who dropped out of school before the eighth grade had the highest rates of infection (43%), followed by those who attended high school (32%) and college (25%).

Sixty streetwalkers did not use drugs but claimed to use condoms consistently. In this group, only four (6.7%) had positive test results. In summation, a higher level of education, use of condoms, and desisting from drug use were associated with a decreased risk of contracting HIV (103).

Testing of homeless women for HIV is essential because many may be involved in risk behaviors that result in HIV transmission. Below are two studies showing divergent rates of HIV infection of homeless women; the studies were conducted in New York City and Los Angeles during different years of the HIV epidemic.

A 2-year, blind, HIV seroprevalence study of homeless pregnant women was initiated in January 1992 in two New York City shelters. Of the 356 women tested, 38 (10.67%) were seropositive for HIV. Women older than age 35 years had the highest rate of infection (21.43%), followed by those age 25 to 29 years (13.45%), 20 to 24 years (10.28%), and 30 to 34 years (7.69%). No HIV was reported for women younger than age 19 years (104).

A study of 970 homeless women was conducted in 1997 in soup kitchens and shelters in Los Angeles: 68% were tested and 1.6% reported ever being diagnosed with AIDS. However, 25% of those who were not tested showed risk behaviors that would suggest a need for testing. Although the prevalence of HIV appears to be low, testing for HIV in this study was associated with pregnancy and the woman having a regular source of medical care and services (105).

Lim et al., in a study conducted by L. Gelberg of the University of California, Los Angeles, found that homeless women who lived on the streets were less likely to have been hospitalized than women who stayed in shelters or were domiciled (21% vs. 28% and 38%, respectively), visit an outpatient clinic (3.7 vs. 7.2 and 7.4 visits, respectively), or have health screens (2.9 vs. 3.6 of 4 health screens). Because homeless women on the streets have high rates of serious co-occurring disorders and histories of physical and sexual abuse, providing them with health insurance, clinics that they can regularly attend, and outreach could improve their access to health care (106).

Homelessness and the Elderly

Although the elderly (those older than age 65 years) comprise approximately 12% of the U.S. population, depending on the location of the study they constitute approximately 3% the known homeless population. If the of age of older homeless Americans is lowered to 55 years, then the elderly homeless comprise approximately 8% of the homeless, as compared to 28% of persons older than age 55 years within the United States' domiciled population. The reasons for the low proportion of elderly among the homeless are (a) chronically homeless persons die prematurely, rarely living to the age of 65 years, dying 20 to 30 years earlier than the life expectancy of the domiciled population. (b) Social Security, Medicare, and other entitlements have prevented homelessness among elderly citizens with limited incomes. Older low-income persons at risk for homelessness are usually estranged from families or widowed and reside in single-room occupancy hotels with incomes of less than $500 per month (107–109).

Once homeless, the frail elderly are subjected to violent assaults and robberies. Because of concerns for safety some may avoid shelters, preferring to remain hidden on the street. They are invariably in poor health, and about half are chronically alcoholic or mentally ill. Even those who may stop drinking are affected by conditions associated with chronic alcoholism such as cirrhosis, cerebella degeneration, organic brain disease, and neuropathy. Upon physical examination, they are usually diagnosed with functional disabilities and multiple, chronic, end-of-life physical and mental conditions, including cancer, hypertension, depression, dementia, and possible paranoia (107–109).

At present, 1.5 million elderly nationwide live in housing that may be substandard and where rents consume 50% to 70% of their incomes. With less income for food, clothing, medicines, and necessities, the domiciled elderly on fixed incomes are becoming vulnerable to homelessness (107–110).

BENEFITS FOR THE CHEMICAL DEPENDENT

Persons with serious chemical-dependency problems may not be eligible to receive benefits because of the passage of welfare regulations in 1996. Under this legislation, persons can lose or be denied SSI (Supplemental Security Income), SSDI (Social Security Disability Insurance), and Medicaid if addiction is considered the major contributing or sole factor in the determination of their disability status. For benefits to be continued, chemically dependent persons must have serious comorbid physical and mental disabilities that restrict employment and be enrolled in treatment for their addictive disorders.

Furthermore, the new welfare reforms do not mandate states to provide treatment for addiction. Benefits for persons with addictive disease can be terminated within 2 years irrespective of whether or not recipients they have children. The welfare regulations repealed the largest benefit program for poor families with children, AFDC (Aid to Families with Dependent Children), replacing it with a block grant program to the states, Temporary Assistance to Needy Families (TANF). According to the National Coalition of the Homeless, TANF grants are below the poverty level in every state (4).

The 1996 changes in welfare benefits increased homelessness among addicted persons. By 1997, an estimated 130,000 disabled persons with addictive disorders lost benefits—SSI, SSDI, or access to Medicaid. In 1997, a study by the National Health Care for the Homeless of 681 persons who lost benefits as a result of the legislation showed that two-thirds were unable to pay for their housing and other needs (14).

In July 2003, results were released of a 2-year study involving 1,764 randomly selected former recipients of SSDI at nine city sites. The study was conducted by the Substance Abuse Policy Research Program of The Robert Wood Johnson Foundation and was also funded by the Center for Substance Abuse Treatment. Of the people removed from government disability (SSDI) in 1996 because of substance abuse and alcohol problems, 31% failed to replace half of the amount that they lost in benefits. Another 37% were reinstated on SSDI because they had other disabling conditions and 27% replaced at least half of the lost benefits from other welfare programs, wages, and help from family and friends. There was a precipitous drop in enrollment in drug treatment after losing benefits (from 41% to .17%). Use of illegal drugs, including cocaine and heroin, was reported in 45% to 55% of the samples. The overall prevalence of drug use was underreported since the time frame examined for drug use in the study was 3 days prior to the interviews. Furthermore, prevalence of drug use verified by drug testing was higher than prevalence relying on self-reports. Approximately 60% to 70% of those who could not replace financial benefits experienced material hardship obtaining food and shelter. Only 12% of the subjects earned $500 per month throughout the study, although 25% did mange to find employment at the end of the 2 years. However, the remaining subjects were unable to find work because of their lack of training, past histories of substance abuse, health problems, and age. This group will probably remain indigent until they receive SSI. The loss of benefits mandated by federal policy and legislation, the decline in enrollment in drug treatment, the low levels of employment and income, the prevalence of heroin and cocaine abuse, and the material hardships experienced by this population resulted in moderate increases in drug related and property crimes (111).

HOMELESSNESS AND TREATMENT FOR ALCOHOL, SUBSTANCE ABUSE, AND MENTAL HEALTH PROBLEMS

From the various surveys presented in this chapter, a conservative 50% of the homeless nationally have been identified with serious alcohol, drug abuse, and mental health condition (ADM) problems and are in need of substance abuse, alcohol, and psychiatric treatment. With the number of homeless estimated to be 2.5 to 3.0 million persons, the number afflicted with ADM problems would be between 1.25 to 1.5 million persons annually. The Substance Abuse and Mental Health Services Administration (SAMHSA) reports that in 2000, 120,000 homeless persons were admitted nationwide to treatment for alcohol and drug problems. Therefore, less than 10% entered treatment for alcohol and substance-abuse problems. Those who entered treatment were more likely to be veterans and older than domiciled admissions (38 years vs. 33 years). Major drugs of abuse included alcohol 51%, opiates 18%, and smoked cocaine 17%. However, major patterns of drug and alcohol use differ among racial groups: whites: alcohol 61%, opiates 17%; African Americans: alcohol 37%, smoked cocaine 37%, opiates 15%; Hispanics: alcohol 38%, opiates 33%; Native Americans and Alaskans: alcohol 80%; Asian/Pacific Islanders: alcohol 45%, opiates 13%, stimulants 12%). The homeless were more likely to have a co-occurring mental condition than others (23% vs. 20%) and were more likely to have been in prior treatment (72% vs. 54%); the homeless were more likely to enter detoxification programs (43% vs. 14%) and residential programs (27% vs. 16%), but less likely to enter outpatient programs (28% vs. 70%). In addition to ADM problems, the homeless enter treatment with serious untreated chronic medical conditions (112).

SAMSHA estimates that 17% of the admissions to drug and alcohol treatment nationwide in 2002 were diagnosed with a co-occurring mental condition. Alcohol was most likely to be the substance of abuse for people admitted to treatment diagnosed with a co-occurring disorder. Admissions for treatment of opioid addiction is less likely, whereas marihuana and cocaine admissions are equally likely, to have a co-occurring disorder diagnosis. The average age of admission to treatment of patients with co-occurring disorders was 34 years, and 75% were unemployed. They tended to be white (68%), followed by African Americans (20%), Latinos (8%), and other ethnic and racial groups (2%) (113).

The National Survey of Homeless Assistance Providers and Clients (NSHAPC) nationwide random sample study of untreated homeless reported that during the month prior to the interview, 38% of the homeless had alcohol problems, 26% had drug-abuse problems, and 39% had mental health conditions. Sixty-six percent reported problems and co-occurring disorders with one or more of these conditions. Also, 24% indicated that they had medical conditions that were not treated during the past year, and 55% were without health insurance or entitlements such as Medicaid (27).

Nationally, however, barriers to treatment have evolved that may prevent addicted homeless persons from applying for admission and from entering and remaining in treatment. Most important is the role of outreach in referring the homeless to treatment. Different outreach practices incorporating cultural and ethnic sensitivities have to be developed to meet the needs of the various subgroups of homeless (e.g., women with children, single women, homeless youth, veterans, African Americans, Latino, Asian). How-

ever, outreach workers have to be educated about the disease of addiction and effective programs based on scientific research and evaluation. Many outreach workers may harbor biases about different types of programs, especially about methadone programs, and not refer homeless addicts to programs that may be more effective for their needs (14,28,45).

Other barriers include waiting lists that discourage applications when the need for treatment is immediate. In some locations there is limited accessibility to intake, and the intake procedures themselves may be protracted, Moreover, people who are not easy to contact, such as the homeless, may be dropped from waiting lists. Programs may be at locations that require daily funds for transportation, which may or may not be available as an entitlement, or the program may be located where convenient public transportation does not exist, or there are no programs such as the lack of methadone treatment in several states and many rural areas. Homeless people may not have proper identification or be eligible to apply for Medicaid and other entitlements to pay for treatment under the changes in SSI and SSDI legislation enacted in 1996. Child care issues are usually unresolved when either a patient has to travel daily to a program or enter residential treatment. Few programs are able to accommodate patients in treatment with childcare. Cultural issues may prevent the homeless from applying and remaining in treatment. Programs may harbor biases toward the homeless, lack the cultural competency to interact with them, and the skills to deal with the multifaceted problems they present (14,28,45). Furthermore, the low retention rates of the homeless in programs suggest that many programs are ineffective in treating this particular population. Barriers to treatment for drug addiction, alcoholism, and medical and mental conditions may result in the homeless self-medicating by using prescription medications diverted to the streets.

Homeless substance abusers may not be motivated because of their circumstances to enter programs that require long-term involvement such as methadone maintenance and therapeutic communities (28,114). They may have very specific needs that they may perceive as more important than treatment, including childcare, permanent housing, and employment, which may not be forthcoming from the treatment program or from referrals. They may also harbor a distrust of programs and institutions. However, methadone treatment itself has strict reporting regulations, especially if the patient is drinking alcohol excessively or using illicit drugs such as cocaine. The reporting requirements necessary to comply with governmental regulations and to ensure that the patients receive ancillary services may be perceived by patients as a form of excessive control. Traditional therapeutic communities are also rejected by the majority of street addicts. In a study of jailed addicts, most of who were homeless or unstably housed, only 19% stated that they would consider entering a therapeutic community. Many were in therapeutic communities prior to their arrests, did not respond to their regimens, and left prior to finishing treatment (114).

Appel et al. report that only 5% of IDUs known to street outreach workers in New York City enroll into drug treatment for many of the reasons discussed above. In addition, outreach workers also report that police sweeps in areas where drug users congregate make contact difficult. To reduce barriers, many IDUs would prefer to be admitted without identification, insurance, or Medicaid at intake. Some of the suggestions by outreach staff to increase enrollment are funding for more treatment slots, transportation for appointments, credentialed staff, and staff training. According to treatment staff of programs, low enrollment among drug injectors is a result of lack of motivation for treatment, threats of sanctions, and loss of benefits associated with welfare reform. Although New York State does not permit applicants to be refused treatment for inability to pay, the perception of applicants is that this policy is not followed, thus discouraging applicants without insurance from applying for treatment. The New York State staff indicated that the most common barriers to treatment were drug users' lack of readiness, lack of resources and programs, requirements of treatment programs, and lack of interagency cooperation (115).

The New York State Office of Alcoholism and Substance Abuse Service (OASAS) management information system reported that even for patients who were homeless on admission to treatment in 2002, methadone programs had lower dropout rates for a 6-month period than did residential programs (47.4% vs. 83%, respectively). However, domiciled patients in methadone programs and domiciled residents in therapeutic communities had dropout rates for a 6-month period similar to that of the homeless (39% vs. 87%, respectively) (116). Reports from the National Institute on Alcohol Abuse and Alcoholism (NIAAA) Cooperative Agreement Program consisting of 14 programs for homeless persons with alcoholic dependency had dropout rates of more than 66% for all programs, with the majority reporting dropout rates of 80% (117). Consequently, research should be directed at the regimen within programs to determine the cause of high dropout rates. The high rate of premature exit from treatment appears to be consistent with reports in the literature about programs that treat the homeless. Premature exit from treatment of less than 6 months invariably translates into high rates of relapse to drug and alcohol use.

A major structural problem is the fragmented nature of ADM treatment. As indicated in the reported surveys in this chapter, homeless persons have interrelated problems that are not, and probably cannot be, treated within a single program. There are few therapeutic programs that have established either outpatient or residential components, or housing where interrelated ADM issues, including methadone-maintenance treatment, can be addressed.

Treatment and services within substance abuse, mental health, and internal medicine are usually either offered sequentially, that is, solving problems in a given order, or in a parallel manner in different treatment systems. These approaches tend to fragment the patient's treatment, involve intricate scheduling and excessive travel time and expenses to keep appointments at different agencies. Furthermore, sequential and parallel planning of services in unrelated settings with separate uncoordinated staffs can be conflicting and confusing to patients, and result in ineffective treatment (14,28,45).

In a study of six model programs for the homeless, Kraybill and Zerger (118) identified the following program characteristics. Comprehensive services are essential to treat the many interrelated social and medical problems that the homeless present. This can include access to food, clothing, legal services, and dental, psychiatric, and medical care, in addition to the services that agencies provide. Therefore, colocation of services at a given site with an integrated treatment team working with the patient or client is essential. This type of administrative structure avoids costly travel and uncoordinated services, and encourages the creation of an integrated treatment team while saving time for the client and patient. The traditional hierarchy between disciplines is minimized and the client or patient becomes a partner in his or her treatment, including the establishment of outcomes and goals. The staff must be uniquely qualified and capable of developing rapport and trust with homeless patients and clients and accept different ideologies of treatment (118).

Various techniques may be employed and coordinated, including client-centered therapy, motivational interviewing, and cognitive–behavioral counseling. Harm-reduction techniques are also applicable in contrast to the zero-tolerance philosophy that permeates most drug-treatment programs. These techniques, which can reduce stress, are preferable to confrontational techniques that can lead to increased stress and psychiatric symptoms, which can lead to premature exit from treatment and relapse. The availability of transitional and affordable housing early in treatment are vital for successful outcomes when working with the homeless (118). The programs described by Kraybill and Zerger were usually incorporated into umbrella community agencies that offered a variety of extra services for the homeless. Some programs targeted specific subgroups such as homeless youth.

Gaps exist between research and treatment. Research has now established that addictive diseases have a neurologic basis. Prolonged use of drugs of abuse can cause long-term or lifelong changes within the circuitry of the brain. Medications may be required to relieve craving and withdrawal symptoms. Addictive disease is a chronic, relapsing, physiologic condition with associated behavioral issues, and not an intrinsic moral failing (119,120).

Unfortunately, most programs adopting an abstinent zero-tolerance approach usually reject the use of medication as maintenance therapy or as an adjunct in the treatment of addiction However, program participants, including the homeless, may exhibit underlying anxieties, depression, specific drug craving, and mental illnesses that require medication. Notwithstanding program ideologies, medications should be prescribed. The most egregious example is the misinformation, mythologies, and biases that exist about methadone maintenance in abstinent oriented drug and alcohol treatment programs. Gordiss, the former director of NIAAA, stated that methadone treatment is effective and should be accepted by the staff of addiction and alcohol treatment programs as a legitimate medication instead of being regarded as just substituting one drug for another (121). Consequently, compliant homeless methadone patients should be considered "clean and sober" and be eligible to receive services without being forced to withdraw from methadone. However, street addicts also harbor misinformation, ambivalent attitudes, and harmful mythologies about methadone treatment. Erroneous beliefs (e.g., rots the bones and teeth) adversely influence their decisions to enter and remain in treatment. Homeless addicts and patients have to be educated about methadone treatment to get them to enter programs and remain in treatment (114).

Buprenorphine was recently approved for the treatment of opioid addiction. It is a Schedule III narcotic and can be prescribed in a wider variety of venues with less regulation than methadone, which is a Schedule II narcotic. Buprenorphine can be prescribed in two forms: Suboxone (buprenorphine tablet with naloxone) to prevent street abuse and Subutex (buprenorphine tablets without naloxone). Suboxone is recommended for the treatment of homeless addicts as injection and abuse of Subutex by homeless users are reported at higher rates than for nonhomeless users (67% vs. 47%). The homeless also present higher rates of medical complications (58% vs. 38%) (122).

The treatment of cocaine addiction for the homeless is a pressing need. Magura et al. (123) demonstrated, in an on-site experimental program, that homeless and unstably housed cocaine addicts can be treated in a soup kitchen by using cognitive–behavioral manual-driven techniques. Using motivational and cognitive–behavioral group counseling, cocaine addicts were able to significantly reduce their use of cocaine at 5-month followup compared to their use at baseline. However, longer-term outcomes to at least 1 year are needed to validate the robustness of this approach. Nevertheless as a short-term intervention, motivational and cognitive–behavioral group counseling may be effective. This model, which takes advantage of peer group processes, education, information, manually driven cognitive and motivational techniques, and incentives, appears to be more effective than individual approaches over a 5-month period. This model should be made available in soup kitchens, harm-reduction centers, specific programs for the homeless, shelters, and venues where homeless cocaine users congregate (123).

Chronic alcoholism is a major health problem among the homeless. There are neither robust medical treatments nor long-term studies using traditional and other therapies targeted to the homeless population. Nevertheless, individual and group counseling combined with participation in Alcoholics Anonymous (AA) are standard methods of treatment. Cognitive–behavioral therapy has been introduced as a possibility. Antabuse has also been recommended as an adjunct to therapeutic treatment.

In 1994, naltrexone was approved for use in the treatment of alcoholism by the Food and Drug Administration. Major studies concerning the effectiveness of naltrexone in the treatment of alcoholism have yielded conflicting outcomes. Two double-blind random-assignment studies lasting for 12 weeks and using naltrexone with counseling and social supports showed significant decreases in craving, drinking, and relapse, with over all increases in sobriety for subjects maintained on naltrexone. A total of 167 subjects were enlisted in both studies. However, the Veterans Administration mounted a multicenter, random-assignment double-blind evaluation of naltrexone over a period of 1 year with 627 veterans. All subjects received psychosocial interventions, including counseling, and were encouraged to attend 12-step programs. At the end of 52 weeks there were no significant differences among experimental and control groups. The VA concluded that the findings did not support the use of naltrexone for the treatment of men with chronic severe alcohol dependence. Nevertheless, because all the studies were well designed, naltrexone should be considered for treating the homeless for alcoholism to determine for whom it may be effective (124–126).

Considering the complex social, medical, psychiatric, and substance-abuse problems, including co-occurring disorders, that the homeless present, the development of front-line social and medical treatment facilities should be considered. Front-line programs include harm-reduction with needle exchange, primary care for medical conditions, counseling, and referrals to drug treatment. If proper regulatory approvals are obtained, addiction treatment using agonist therapy (either buprenorphine and/or methadone) could be considered. Psychotropic medications to treat mental conditions could also be incorporated in these models, depending on the facility and staff. Front-line programs could be satellites of major medical centers and hospitals, thereby expediting referrals for medical care. The concept could be developed by combining services of existing harm-reduction programs, medical vans, and primary care centers, and linking them to community medical centers and social agencies.

OASAS established a working group to address the issues of homeless clients and patients. In 2002, there were 308,758 admissions to New York State alcohol- and drug-treatment programs. At the time of their admissions to treatment, 55,435 (18%) were considered to have a housing problem and were either transients or literally homeless in shelters or the streets. The percent of admissions involving a homeless person in different treatment modalities were as follows: 35.5% in crisis centers such as shelters and hospitals; 21.5% in inpatient rehabilitation centers; 12.6% in residential treatment; 7.5% in outpatient methadone-maintenance programs; and 5.1% in ambulatory programs. The homeless presented the following issues: 66% reported alcoholism as a primary condition to be treated; 30% had previous episodes of treatment; 10% had a history of mental illness or treatment for same; 22% had major physical health problems in addition to their substance abuse, and 85% either were in receipt of public assistance or had no benefits. In addition, there were an additional 27,000 individuals statewide who need both housing and substance abuse treatment services (127).

The state identified the following housing needs for the homeless:

- Sufficient residential and housing options on a continuum, including inpatient rehabilitation, halfway houses, supportive living, transitional and permanent housing;
- Housing-related supportive services, including transportation and case management;
- Housing for special chemically dependent populations such as the dually diagnosed, women with children, methadone patients, and patients with serious medical conditions and disabilities;
- Coordination and collaborative efforts with other governmental, private, and local agencies.

Forty-eight homeless projects have been developed across New York State with OASAS working in conjunction with a variety funding sources on the federal, state, and local levels, including HUD Shelter plus Care. Twenty-six nonprofit service providers assisted 14,000 individuals of whom 11,000 were considered homeless upon admission to treatment. In addition, many drug-treatment providers have independently obtained funds from HUD and state and local agencies to provide housing and services to the homeless in their communities. Funds are also provided to legal services to prevent evictions and to support services for substance abuse and victims of domestic violence (127).

Methadone patients, however, face the greatest stigma of any group of patients who enter drug treatment. The stigma directed toward homeless methadone patients, including pregnant women, prevents them from accessing and receiving needed services, including housing.

CRIMINAL JUSTICE AND HOMELESSNESS

In a report issued by the Bureau of Judicial Statistics of the Justice Department in 2003, more than 2.1 million persons, or 1 of every 143 persons in the United States, were incarcerated in federal and state prisons, local jails, and juvenile detention centers at the end of 2000. Twenty percent of the incarcerated in state prisons were serving time for drug offenses. However, in federal prisons 48% of the increase in the prison population was drug offenders,

who now constitute more than half of the prison population. Racial minorities comprise 62% of all federal and state prisoners although they represent approximately 24% of the population in the United States. In the United States, 10.4% of all African American, 3.4% of all Hispanic origin, and 1.2% of all non-Hispanic white males between the ages of 25 and 29 years are incarcerated. In 1999, 1.5 million arrests were made for violations of the drug laws; most of the arrests were for possession. About 1.2 million prisoners are considered to be addicted to illegal drugs. Nearly half of the prisoners released from jails and prisons are rearrested within 1 year because of homelessness and lack of treatment for their ADM and medical problems (128,129). In September 2003, The Human Rights Watch issued a report, *Ill Equipped: U.S. Prisons and Offenders with Mental Illness,* indicating that 1 of every 6 prisoners in the United States is mentally ill with a serious condition such as schizophrenia, major depression, or bipolar disorder. Mentally ill prisoners nationwide do not receive the care they need and, in many instances, are treated punitively with harsh punishments, such as abuse and solitary confinement (130). In November 2003, the U.S. Senate passed the Mentally Ill Offenders Treatment and Crime Reduction Act, which would promote coordination between the criminal justice system, corrections, and mental health facilities, support the implementation of treatment in corrections, and provide for transitional care and discharge planning (131). Michaels et al. (132) found about 50% of the homeless inmates in jails in New York City were diagnosed with either psychiatric symptoms or mental illness, as opposed to 25% of those who were domiciled prior to their arrests. Within the 3 years prior to arrest, 33% of the homeless received treatment for mental illness, as opposed to 20% the domiciled (132). In a study of 529 homeless persons in Los Angeles, Gelberg found that approximately 60% were arrested during their adult lives. However, the subgroups with psychiatric hospitalization had the highest rates of arrest, were homeless longer, had the most serious psychiatric symptoms, and had greater rates of drug and alcohol use than the other homeless groups (133).

In three samples of detainees in the New York City Rikers Island Jail, Michaels et al. (132) found that the percentage of homeless in the 2 months prior to their arrests ranged from 24% to 34% and in one sample, 22% were homeless the night before their arrest. Approximately 40% had experienced homelessness within the 3 years prior to their arrest (132). In New York City, the greatest number of requests for services for the homeless emanate from corrections and the health care systems.

The New York City Rikers Island Jail was the first prison in the United States to provide a heroin withdrawal program using methadone. Its program began in the early 1970s; in 1986, the Rikers Island Jail was the first to institute methadone-maintenance treatment in a unique project known as KEEP (Key Extended Entry Program). Each year, 18,000 inmates addicted to opioids undergo withdrawal and 4,000 are either placed on methadone maintenance or continued in maintenance therapy if they were in community programs prior to their arrests (134). However, when released to community methadone outpatient clinics, approximately 60% of the patients are homeless on the streets, or unstably housed living in the apartments of others. The clinics report that patients are destitute without adequate clothing, food, or identification to receive entitlements. By 6 months only 27% to 59% of the KEEP patients are still enrolled in treatment, and are dependent on services available at the community clinics. Homelessness and destitution, lack of identification for entitlements including Medicaid, and new welfare legislation that limits eligibility for benefits are some of the factors that contribute to dropping out of treatment (135–137).

In its report, *Health Status of Soon to be Released Inmates*, the National Commission on Correctional Health Care indicated that inmates in local, state, and federal correctional facilities nationwide have a high prevalence of infectious diseases associated with injection drugs and make up a substantial proportion of persons infected nationwide. The numbers of persons with infectious diseases released from nationwide correctional facilities use and their proportion of those infected nationwide are as follows: AIDS, 39,000 (17%); HIV, 98,000 to 148,999 (13 to 19%); syphilis, 200,000–332,000; hepatitis C, 1.3 to 1.4 million (29% to 32%) (138).

To address issues of homelessness, unemployment, mental illness, substance abuse, and infectious diseases among prisoners and parolees nationwide, the newly formed U.S. Interagency Council on Homelessness is promoting reentry planning for prisoners based on a model developed in Massachusetts. Every state receives a planning grant to ensure that prisoners on release have housing, thereby bypassing the homeless system. The reentry planning starts on the day the prisoner enters the jail or prison. Housing specialists and community groups are brought into the reentry planning to find housing for the prisoners upon their release. Coordination and partnerships between systems such as housing, treatment, and public safety, and interagency coordination on federal, local and state levels are at the core of the planning process. The purpose is to break the cycle of homelessness, destitution, and relapse to drug use, chronic unemployment, and recidivism to criminal activity (139). In September 2003, New York City announced the planning of a postrelease program for the inmates of Rikers Island Jail.

To offset the large number of arrests and incarcerations related to substance abuse and mental disorders, special drug courts were created by the U.S. Congress to divert drug offenders to community treatment. As of May 2001, 688 courts had been established servicing 220,000 adults and 9,000 juveniles. In a 2001 review of 37 published and unpublished evaluations, Belenko of Columbia University National Center on Addiction and Substance Abuse

(CASA) found that drug courts (a) achieved local support; (b) provided referrals for long-term treatment to offenders with histories of arrests, co-occurring disorders, substance abuse, and medical and mental health conditions; and (c) provided better monitoring, more comprehensive supervision, and more frequent urine testing than other types of community supervision. Programs have overall graduation rates of 47%. While participants are in treatment, criminality and drug use is reduced (140). A study of the New York State drug courts showed that 29% of those who completed the program had lower rearrest rates than those who went to prison. Homeless persons were referred to residential programs. About 18,000 nonviolent first offenders participated in the program, which saved the state $254 million in prison-related expenses. Drug courts nationwide are extremely cost-effective (141).

However, the American Association for the Treatment of Opioid Dependence reports that the bias against methadone treatment within the courts, jails, and prisons affects domiciled and homeless heroin addicts and methadone patients.

- Except for New York City, Suffolk County, New York, and Rhode Island, methadone treatment for opioid withdrawal and maintenance is not widely available nationwide in the criminal justice system (142).
- Judges and probation and parole officers have ordered domiciled and homeless methadone patients to withdraw from the methadone or be sentenced to serve time in jail or prison (142).

The denial of methadone treatment is contrary to the recommendations of the NIH consensus statement on the treatment of opioid addiction which recommends that methadone treatment be accessible to opioid-addicted persons under legal supervision (143).

Education about agonist therapy is needed within the criminal justice system to ensure that proper medical care is available for those under legal supervision. Furthermore, those maintained on methadone or buprenorphine should not be removed from medication by order of nonmedical personnel such as judges and probation and parole officers.

Homelessness and Victimization

In 2003, the National Coalition for the Homeless released a report on newly enacted laws targeting homeless people since 2002. The report covers data from 142 communities in 42 states, the District of Columbia, and Puerto Rico. Of the communities surveyed, 70% passed one or more laws targeting homeless persons but failed to allocate funds to address causes of homelessness, such as the lack of affordable housing or shelter beds. Daily activities (e.g., standing or sitting on sidewalks or napping in parks) are prohibited under these statutes. Homeless persons are charged with offenses and can be incarcerated (144).

The 1996 NSHAPC Survey reported that homeless persons are especially vulnerable to victimization: 38% reported being directly robbed of money and possessions, 41% reported being robbed of possessions when they were not present, 22% reported being physically assaulted, and 7% reported being sexually assaulted or raped (27). To alleviate problems of homelessness, victimization, and violence, communities are developing outreach initiatives to engage the homeless in parks and on the streets and referring them to appropriate agencies for assistance and shelter.

Health Service Use by Substance Users in Central Harlem

Van Ness, Davis, and Johnson reported higher rates of morbidity and health services use in central Harlem for homeless substance users of illicit drugs as compared to domiciled very-low-income users. The study was conducted in central Harlem during 1998 and 1999, and consisted of 658 drug users recruited in 9 randomly selected geographical areas of the neighborhood. The subjects were enlisted in the study using a "chain method of referrals" by drug-using study subjects within their social network in the various neighborhoods. Homelessness in this study does not seem to be a barrier to accessing the local services of emergency rooms, STD clinics, and hospitals, but it may impact on sustained levels and duration of care. Approximately 26% of the homeless and 20% of the very poor domiciled drug users were HIV positive, which is associated with injection and prostitution. Crack cocaine was the major drug of use for 75% of the homeless and 63% of the domiciled, whereas heroin was used by 11% of the homeless and 18% of the domiciled. Violent trauma affected 68% of the homeless in contrast to 30% of domiciled. The homeless had markedly higher use rates of health services associated with violence and trauma as compared to the domiciled (e.g., emergency rooms and hospitals). They also had higher rates of registration in STD clinics. The homeless in the central Harlem area also used community health services for nondrug health-related problems, such as heart disease and asthma, at a higher rate than poor domiciled users. They also used the services of community drug-treatment programs such as 12-step programs, therapeutic communities, outpatient drug-free, detoxification programs, and, when applicable, methadone maintenance. Two major hospitals that specialize in servicing a poor minority population with high rates of violence related trauma serve the central Harlem area. The area also has available community substance abuse, alcohol treatment, and needle exchange programs. The problems of the homeless demand a specially trained staff and, most importantly, coordinated health, drug, and alcohol treatment, and social services to develop an integrated approach that addresses homelessness, chronic poverty, violence, and related issues (145).

APPROACHES TO END HOMELESSNESS

The United States Department of Housing and Urban Development (HUD) administers the homeless programs funded under the McKinney-Ventro Homeless Act, the major federal source of funding for homeless programs in cities throughout the United States. Passed by Congress in July 1987, this comprehensive federal initiative targets the needs of homeless people in the areas of most concern: "emergency food and shelter, health and mental health care, housing, educational programs, job training, and other community services" A continuum of care approach to housing in the communities where grants are awarded is required (2).

In February 2003, a 10-year agenda to end chronic homelessness in the United States was announced by the federal government. The agenda is directed by the Interagency Council on Homelessness, which coordinates the resources of federal agencies, including the Department of Health and Human Services (HHS) and HUD. In July 2003, the federal government, through the Interagency Council, allocated $13.5 million for housing and employment targeted to chronic homeless mentally ill and substance abusers. As part of this strategy, 100 cities across the country were asked to submit plans to the federal government in 2004 to end chronic homelessness within their jurisdictions over the following decade (146).

Some of the programs administered by HUD are Supportive Housing Program; Shelter plus Care; Section 8–Moderate Rehabilitation for Single-Room Occupancy; Section 8–Housing Choice Voucher; Supportive Housing for Persons with Disabilities; and Home Improvement Partnership Program. Collaborations exist between the Veteran Administration and HUD to provide permanent housing and services to homeless veterans. The PATH program was created to help persons with mental illness transition from homelessness into housing. The program is administered by the Center for Mental Health Services. The Center for Substance Abuse Treatment issued grants to service dually diagnosed homeless persons. The program offers services and treatment plus grants for community education. Funds can be used to access and maintain stable housing. The HUD Shelter plus Care program is an important mechanism to fund permanent housing for homeless substance abusers with comorbidities (e.g., mental health problems, HIV/AIDS, disabilities). The model coordinates outpatient treatment with supportive permanent housing. However, homeless methadone patients are excluded from most programs that house the homeless.

"Housing first" programs are being developed nationally through HUD. Homeless families and individuals are placed in permanent housing under the supervision of community case management teams known as Assertive Community Treatment (ACT). These teams consist of physicians, psychiatrists, social workers, nurses, and case managers. The ACT team offers the clients services such as health care, referrals to community agencies for additional services and treatment, and case management in caring for and maintaining an apartment. Pathways to Housing in New York City developed the concept in 1992 of assisting homeless mentally ill and dually diagnosed substance abusers by providing housing first and then services. A 5-year study of clients in the Pathways program compared to clients in linear step-by-step continuum housing of traditional programs showed that the Pathway approach of housing first with supportive housing was superior: 88% of the Pathway clients remained housed as compared to only 47% of the clients in the traditional continuum transitional housing programs for the homeless. Pathways was also successful on all other measures when compared to traditional approaches: Pathways costs $22,500 per person per year versus $65,000 per person per year in a community residence, $40,000 in a single-room occupancy hotel with services, $85,000 in a jail, and $175,000 for a bed in a state hospital. Hospitalizations for mental illness and criminal activity are significantly reduced (147,148). As of this writing, Pathways to Housing will open the first program targeted to homeless methadone patients with co-occurring disorders. The program was planned in cooperation with Mount Sinai Medial Center in New York City and the New York State Office of Alcoholism and Substance Abuse Services.

CONCLUSION AND DISCUSSION

The data presented in this chapter show that although homelessness is the result of poverty, unemployment, and the erosion of affordable housing, the state of homelessness with its destitution, disorganization, hunger, and uncertainties creates excessive stress exacerbating Alcohol, Drugs and Mental Health problems (ADM) and other problems with which homeless individuals may present The prevalence of ADM, risk behaviors for the transmission of infectious diseases, chronic and acute medical conditions, suicidal ideation, and mortality rates are greater in every study among the homeless than among domiciled populations. While homeless, adherence to treatment protocols is difficult: Patients leave treatment prematurely and may be lost to followup.

Accessibility issues that impede enrollment in treatment include locations of programs and transportation costs, the need for identification for entitlements and culturally competent outreach to bring the homeless into a system of care. Multiple ADM and medical conditions, including infectious diseases, should be treated simultaneously, not sequentially, by a diverse integrated team of professionals preferably on site in a given program. Referrals to other agencies may result in broken appointments because of lack funds for transportation, conflicting schedules, childcare responsibilities, or a distrust of new service agencies and staff.

Consequently, comprehensive front-line medical centers should be developed that address social issues such as housing and entitlements, and that incorporate the treatment of co-occurring disorders, addiction, and medical conditions. Front-line medical models may be developed through harm-reduction programs, medical vans, and neighborhood primary health care centers affiliated with major medical institutions. The current systemic organization of treatment into different venues of care militates against an integrated approach to the delivery of services.

Although certain practices have already been identified and should be applied, further research and evaluation are needed to determine what treatment is effective for the homeless. Confrontational techniques and a zero-tolerance approach to drug use as the ideological foundation of treatment may create stress that leads to premature termination and relapse. However, motivational interviewing and cognitive–behavioral therapy that does not increase stress can be implemented while recognizing that relapse is endemic in chronic diseases, including addiction. Unfortunately, many programs that treat the homeless reject the use of medication for the treatment of addictive disease However, agonist therapy for addiction, methadone and buprenorphine, has been researched and has been shown to be highly effective when prescribed in conjunction with social services and counseling. The staffs of abstinent-oriented programs would have to be educated about agonist therapy before it is introduced to ensure that previously held biases are resolved. Compliant homeless patients who are prescribed medications such as methadone or buprenorphine to treat addiction, and medications to treat mental conditions and pain, should be considered "clean and sober" and not be subjected to "antimedication biases" while undergoing rehabilitation or treatment.

Faith-based programs are now being funded for treatment of substance abuse. Within mainstream medicine, hospitals affiliated with major religious groups in the United States have developed programs based on scientific evidence and incorporated them into the beliefs and practices of their institutions. Some funded faith-based programs have incorporated the results of scientific research and evaluation into their prevention and treatment ideologies to improve patient outcomes.

A 10-year initiative to end chronic homelessness in cities across the United States was announced by the federal government. However, basic impediments to this effort include the loss of affordable housing and manufacturing jobs over the past decade. If homelessness is to be successfully addressed, these trends must be reversed or the number of homeless requesting shelter and food will continue to increase as they have over the past decade.

Most important are the costs and venues of financing for innovative and ongoing programs to treat and house the homeless. Ideally such costs should be integrated into exiting sources of income for care such as Medicaid or block grants. Historically, programs were developed that linked agencies with common concerns to create new programs and a cost-effective delivery of services. However, an unprecedented coordination of public and private institutions for planning and funding is needed to meet the challenges of the current problems of the homeless in inner cities and rural areas.

ACKNOWLEDGMENTS

The authors thank Denise Paone and Herman Joseph for their help with the analysis of the syringe-exchange programs discussed in "Homelessness, HIV Risk Behavior, Harm Reduction" above.

REFERENCES

1. UN-Habitat. *The state of the world's cities.* 2001 Available at http://www.unhabitat.org.
2. *The McKinney Act.* NCH fact sheet #16, April 1999 Available at http://www.nationalhomeless.org.mckinneyfacts.html.
3. National Coalition for the Homeless. *Rural homelessness.* NCH fact sheet #13. March 1999. Available at http://www.nationalhomeless.org/rural.html.
4. *Why are people homeless?* NCH fact sheet #1 Available at http://www.nationalhomeless.org/causes.html.
5. National Low Income Housing Coalition. *Out of reach 2003.* Available at http://www.nlihc.org.
6. United States Conference of Mayors. *National housing agenda.* May 2002. Available at http://www.usmayors.org.
7. Uchitelle L. A missing statistic: U.S. jobs that went overseas. *New York Times* 2003 Oct 5. Available at http://www.nytimes.com/2003/10/05/business/05ECON.html.
8. Joint Economic Committee of the 108th Congress of the United States. *Recession not over for workers.* July 17, 2003. Available from Nan Gibson (phone: 202-224-0377).
9. U.S. Conference of Mayors. *New report finds U.S. metro areas lost one million jobs in 2001–2002; predicts little job growth in 2003.* 2003 Jun 5–10. Available at http://www.usmayors.org/71stAnnualMeeting/metroecon_060703.asp.
10. U.S. Bureau of the Census. *Poverty in the nation.* 2003. Available at http://www.census.gov/prod/2003pub.
11. U.S. Bureau of the Census. *Health insurance coverage in the United States: 2002.* September 2003. Available at http://www.census.gov/prod/2003pub.
12. Connolly C. Census finds more lack health insurance. *Washington Post* 2003 Sep 30:A01 Available at http://www.washingtonpost.com/wp-dyn/articles/A10511-2003Sept29.html.
13. U.S. Conference of Mayors. *A status report on hunger and homelessness in America's cities: 2002. A 25-city survey.* Washington DC: Author, 2003. Available at http://www.usmayors.org.
14. National Coalition for the Homeless. *Addiction disorders and homelessness.* Fact sheet #6. April 1999. Available at http://:www.nationalhomelessness.org/addict.hmtl.
15. National Coalition for the Homeless. *Rural homelessness.* Fact sheet #15. March 1999. Available at http://www.nationalhomelessness.org.
16. Charles Stewart Mott Foundation. In: New Hampshire hidden homeless helped. *Neighbors* 1996 May (11). Available at http://www.nccenet.org.
17. Freeman AL. *Where do homeless people sleep?* 2002 Nov 29. Available at http://www.anitraweb.org.
18. Zwarenstein C. No back yards or fences. *Toronto Star.* 2003 Jul 8:OP-ED page. Available at http://www.csf.colorado.edu/forums/homelessness/2003.
19. Clatts MC, Davis WR. A demographic and behavioral profile of homeless youth in New York City: implications for AIDS outreach and prevention. *Med Anthropol Q* 1999;13(3):365–374.
20. National Coalition for the Homeless. *Homeless families with children.* Fact sheet #7. June 2001. Available at http://www.nationalhomeless.org/families.html.
21. Casey Family Programs. *Foster care and homeless youth.* Available at http://www.casey.org/cnc.
22. Homes for the Homeless. The other America: homeless families in the shadow of the new economy. Report available from Homes for the Homeless. Institute for Children and Poverty, 36 Cooper Square, 6th Fl., New York, NY 10003. Available at http://www.homesforthehomeless.com.
23. U.S Department of Health and Human Services. *Ending chronic homelessness: strategies for action.* March 2003 Available at http://www.hhs.gov/hsp/homelessness.
24. National Coalition for the Homeless. *How many people experience homelessness?* Fact sheet #7. Available at http://www.nationalhomeless.org/numbers.html.
25. Levitan M. *A portrait of inequality, unemployment and joblessness in New York City.* CSS data brief #8. Available at http://www.cssny.org/pubs/databrief/databrief_n09.pdf.
26. New York City Department of Homeless Services. *Statistics on homelessness in New York City.* Available at http://www.nyc.gov/html/dhs/home.html.
27. National Survey of Homeless Assistance Providers and Clients (NSHAPC). *Homelessness programs and the people they serve.* Conducted by Bureau of the Census (1996). Available at http://www.huduser.org/publications/homeless/homelessness/highlights.html.
28. Zerger S. *Substance abuse treatment: what works for homeless people.* National Health Care for the Homeless, 2002. Available at http://www.nchchc.org/publications.
29. Koegel P, Sullivan D, Barnum A, et al. Utilization of mental health and substance abuse services among homeless adults in Los Angeles. *Med Care* 1999;37(3):306–317.
30. Desai RA, Liu-Mares W, Dausey DJ, et al. Suicidal ideation and suicide attempts in a sample of homeless people with mental illness. *J Nerv Ment Dis* 2003;191(6):365–371.
31. Glasser I, Zywiak WH. Homelessness and substance misuse: a tale of two cities. *Subst Use Misuse* 2003;38(3–6):5551–5576.
32. Lehman AF, Cordray DSS. *Prevalence of alcohol, drug, and mental disorders among the homeless: one more time. Report to National Institute of Mental Health Office on Programs for the Homeless.* 1992.
33. Struening EL, Pittman J. *Characteristics of residents of the New York City shelter system: executive summary.* New York: New York State Psychiatric Institute, 1987.
34. Struening EL, Padgett D. Associations of physical health status with substance use, and mental disorder in homeless adults. *J Soc Issues* 1991;46(4):65–81.
35. Appel P. *New York State Division of Substance Abuse Services. Household survey, 1986.* New York: Bureau of Research and Evaluation.
36. Appel P. *New York State final report on*

transient survey 10/1/92–9/30/95. New York: Bureau of Applied Studies, Office of Alcoholism and Substance Abuse Services, 1995.

37. Welte JW, Barnes GM. *Drinking among the homeless in New York State* [internal report]. New York: Research Institute on Alcoholism, New York State Division of Alcoholism, 1988.

38. Schilling RF, El-Bassel N, Gilbert L. Drug use and AIDS risks in a soup kitchen population. *Soc Work* 1992;37(4):353–358.

39. Magura S, Nwakeza PC, Rosenblum A, et al. Substance misuse and related infectious diseases in a soup kitchen population. *Subst Use Misuse* 2000;35(4):551–583.

40. Nwakeze PC, Magura S, Rosenblum A Joseph H. Homelessness, substance misuse, and access to public entitlements in a soup kitchen population. *Subst Use Misuse* 2000;38(3–6):645–668.

41. U.S. Department of Health and Human Services, Office of the Inspector General. *Alcohol, drug and mental health services for homeless individuals.* Washington, DC: U.S. Government Printing Office, 1992.

42. National Law Center on Homelessness and Poverty. *No homeless people allowed.* Washington DC: Author, 1994.

43. Institute of Medicine. *Homelessness, health and human needs.* Washington, DC: National Academy Press, 1988.

44. Brickner P, Scanlon DC, Conanan B, et al. Homeless persons and health. *Ann Intern Med* 1986;104(3):405–409.

45. Zerger S. *A preliminary review of literature: chronic medical illness and homeless individuals.* National Health Care for the Homeless, 2002. Available at http://www.nhchhc.org.

46. Health Care for the Homeless. *National statistics for general population and homeless population: barriers and access to care.* February 2003. Report available from: Policy Research Associates Inc., 345 Delaware Avenue, Delmar, New York 12054.

47. Harris HW, Young DM. Care of injection drug users with soft tissue infections in San Francisco, California. *Arch Surg* 2002;137(11):1217–1222.

48. Salit SA, Kulin EM, Hartz AJ, et al. Hospitalization costs associated with homelessness in New York City. *N Engl J Med* 1998;338(24):1734–1740.

49. Nuttbruck L, Rosenblum A, Mcquistion H, et al. *Physical and psychiatric morbidity of homeless clients on medical van.* Presentation at the 126th Annual Meeting Public Health and Managed Care. Washington, DC, November

15–19, 1998. Available from Dr. Andrew Rosenblum, NDRI, 71 West 23rd Street, New York, NY 10010.

50. Hogan H, Des Jarlais DC. HIV and HCV among injecting drug users. *Mt Sinai J Med* 2000;67(5&6):423–428. Available at http://www.mssm.edu/msjournal.

51. Strathdee SA, Patrick DM, Curie SL, et al. Needle exchange is not enough. *AIDS* 1997;11:F59–F65.

52. Klinkenberg WD, Caslyn RJ, Morse GA, et al. Prevalence of human immunodeficiency virus, hepatitis B, and hepatitis C among homeless persons with co-occurring severe mental illness and substance use disorders. *Compr Psychiatry* 2003;44(4):293–302.

53. Appel PW, Joseph H, Richman B. Causes and rates of death among methadone maintenance patients before and after the onset of the HIV/AIDS epidemic. *Mt Sinai J Med* 2000;67(5&6):444–451. Available at http://www.mssm.edu/msjournal.

54. Joseph H, Roman-Nay H. The homeless intravenous drug abuser and the AIDS epidemic. *NIDA Res Monogr* 1990;93:210–253.

55. Raba JM, et al. Homelessness and AIDS. In: Brickner P, et al., eds. *Under the safety net.* New York: W.W. Norton, 1990:214–233.

56. Wright JD. The health of the homeless: evidence from the National Health Care for the Homeless Program. In: Brickner P, et al., eds. *Under the safety net.* New York: W.W. Norton, 1990:15–31.

57. Allen D, et al. HIV infection among homeless adults and runaway youth, United States 1989–1992. *AIDS* 1994;8:1593–1598.

58. Shuster CR. *NADR/ATOM homeless data.* Paper presented at NIDA-NIAAA meeting, Rockville, MD, July 7, 1990.

59. Torres RA, Lefkowitz P, Kales C, et al. Homelessness among hospitalized patients with acquired immunodeficiency syndrome in New York City. *JAMA* 1980;258:779–780.

60. U.S. Department of Health Resources and Services Administration HIV/AIDS Bureau. Ryan White Care Act. Available at http://hab.hrsa.gov/history.

61. U.S. Conference of Mayors. HIV/AIDS prevention resolutions, 1998–2002. Available at http://www.usmayors.org.

62. National Coalition for the Homeless. HIV/AIDS and Homelessness. Fact sheet #9. 1999. Available at http://www.natinalhomeless.org.

63. Robbins G, Nelson F. *Looking for a place to be: a report on AIDS housing in America.* 1996. Available at AIDS Housing of Washington, 2025–1st Ave.

Marketplace Towers Suite 420. Seattle, WA 98121 (phone: 206–448-5242).

64. Center for Disease Control. *Epidemiology of tuberculosis.* Available at http://www.phppo.cdc.gov/PHTN/tbmodules.

65. Brewer TF, Heymann SJ, Krumplitsch SM, et al. Strategies to decrease tuberculosis in U.S. homeless populations: a computer simulation model. *JAMA* 2001;286(7):834–842.

66. Friedman LN, Williams MT, Singh TP, et al. Tuberculosis, AIDS, and death among substance abusers on welfare in New York City. *N Engl J Med* 1996;334(13):828–833.

67. Pablos-Mendez A, Raviglione MC, Battan R, et al. Drug-resistant tuberculosis among the homeless in NYC. *N Y State J Med* 1990;90(7):351–355.

68. New York City Department of Health and Mental Hygiene. TB in NYC, 2001.TB control program information summary. Available at http://www.nyc.gov/doh/tb2001.

69. Wright JD. *The homeless in America: social institutions and social change.* New York: Aldine de Gruter, 1989.

70. Hibbs JR, Benner L, Klugman L, et al. Mortality in a cohort of homeless adults in Philadelphia. *N Engl J Med* 1994;331(5):304–309.

71. Hwang SW, Orav JE, O'Connell JJ, et al. Causes of death in homeless adults in Boston. *Annals Intern Med* 1997;126(8):625–628.

72. Hwang SW, Lebow JM, Bierer MF, et al. Risk factors for death in homeless adults in Boston. *Arch Intern Med* 1998;158(13):1454–1460.

73. Hwang SW, Orav JE, O'Connell JJ. Deaths Among the Homeless–Atlanta Georgia (MMWR) published by Center for Disease Control, Washington, DC 1987;36:297–299.

74. Barrow SM, Herman DB, Cordova P, et al. Mortality among homeless shelter residents in NYC. *Am J Public Health* 1999;89(4):59–34.

75. National Law Center on Homelessness and Poverty. *Deaths of homeless people raising nationally.* Available at http://www.nlchp.org.

76. NYC Department of Homeless Services. *The second decade of reform: a strategic plan for New York City's Homeless Services.* June 2002 Available at http://www.nyc.gov/dhs.

77. Project Renewal Program. Description of programs Available at http://www.projectrenewal.org.

78. Lurie P, Reingold AL, eds. *The public impact of needle-exchange programs in the United States and abroad: summary, conclusions, and recommendations.* San Francisco: University of California, San Francisco, Institute for Health Policy Studies, 1993.

79. Paone D, Des Jarlais DC, Clark J, et al. Syringe exchange program—United States. *MMWR Morb Mortal Wkly Rep* 1994–1995;44(37):685–691.

80. Aidala A, Cross J. *Housing and HIV drug and sex risk behaviors.* Report available from the Center for Applied Public Health, Mailman School of Public Health, Columbia University, 722 West 168th Street, New York, NY 10032.

81. Positive Health Project. Information available at http://www.positiveheatlhproject.org.

82. Springer E. Personal communication. New York Peer AIDS Education Coalition, 437 W 16th street New York, NY 10011 (phone: 212-463-0885).

83. Dolan K et al. *Final report on injecting rooms in Switzerland.* Drug Policy alliance 1996. Available at http://www.lindesmithcenter.org/library/dolan2.cm.

84. Nadelmann E. Switzerland's heroin experiment. *National Review* 1995 Jul 10:46–47.

85. Broadhead R, Kerr TH, Grund JP, et al. Safe injection facilities in North America: their place in public policy and health initiatives. *J Drug Issues* 2002:32(1);329–356.

86. Department of Veterans Affairs. *Homeless veterans.* Available at http://www.va.gov/org.

87. National Coalition for the Homeless. *Homeless veterans.* NCH fact sheet #9. Available at http://www.nationalhomeless.org/veterans.html.

88. National Coalition of Homeless Veterans. *Background and statistics.* Available at http://www.nchv.org.

89. National Coalition for the Homeless. Homeless youth. April 1999. Available at http://www.nationalhomeless.org/youth.html.

90. Casey Family Programs, National Center for Resource Family Support. *Foster care and homeless youth.* Available at http://www. casey.org/cnc. Also available from the National Center for Resource Family Support, 1808 Eye Street NW, Washington, DC 20006–5427 (phone: 888-295-6727).

91. Yates G, Pennbridge MJ, Cohen E. A risk profile comparison of runaway and non-runaway youth. *Am J Public Health* 1988;78(9):668–673.

92. Kennedy JT, et al. Health care for families, runaway street kids. In: Brickner P, et al., eds. *Under the safety net.* New York: W.W. Norton, 1990:82–117.

93. Robertson M. *Homeless youth on their own.* Available from Alcohol Research Group, 2000 Hearst Avenue, Berkeley, CA (phone: 510-642-5208).

94. Clatts MC, Davis WR, Sotheran JL, et al. Correlates and distribution of HIV risk behaviors among homeless youths in NYC: implications for prevention and policy. *Child Welfare* 1998;77(2):195–197.

95. Clatts MC, Davis WR. A demographic and behavioral profile of homeless youth in NYC. Implications for AIDS outreach and prevention. *Med Anthropol Q* :13(3):365–374.

96. Gilbert L, El-Bassel N, Rajah V, et al. The converging epidemics of mood-altering-drug use, HIV, HCV, and partner violence: a conundrum for methadone maintenance treatment. *Mt Sinai J Med* 2000:67(5–6);444–452. Available at http://www.mssm.edu/msjournal.

97. National Coalition for the Homeless. *Education of homeless children and youth.* NCH fact sheet #10. Available at http://www.nationalhomeless.org/edchild.html.

98. Page T, Noo E. Life experiences and vulnerabilities of homeless women: a comparison of women unaccompanied versus accompanied by minor children and correlates with children's emotional distress. *J Soc Distress Homeless* 2002;11(3):215–231.

99. Wenzel SL, Andersen RM, Gifford DS, et al. Homeless women's gynecological symptoms and use of medical care. *J Health Care Poor Underserved* 2001:12(3);323–334.

100. Gelberg L, Leake B, Lu MC, et al. Chronically homeless women's perceived deterrents to contraception. *Perspect Sex Reprod Health* 2002;34(6);276–285.

101. Open Society Forum. *Drug use and pregnancy: prejudice, misinformation and new threats to women's rights.* January 19, 2003. Available at http://www.soros.org/events/IHRD/summary.htm.

102. Wechsberg WM, Lam WK, Zule W, et al. Violence, homelessness, and HIV infection among crack-using African American women. *Subst Use Misuse* 2003;38(3–6):669–700.

103. Wallace J, Beatrice S. *Survey of streetwalking prostitutes in New York City for anti-HIV-1 antibodies.* Presentation at V International AIDS conference Montreal, Canada 1989. New York: Foundation for Research on Sexually Transmitted Diseases, 1989.

104. New York State Department of Health. *AIDS in New York State, 1994.* Albany, NY: Author, 1994.

105. Herndon D, Asch SM, Kilbourne AM, et al. Prevalence and Predictors of HIV testing among a probability sample of homeless women in Los Angeles County. *Public Health Rep* 2003;118:261–269.

106. Lim YW, Andersen R, Leake B, et al. How accessible is medical care for homeless women? *Med Care* 2002:40(6);510–529.

107. Regional Task Force on the Homeless. *Elderly homeless persons.* Available at http://www.co.san.diego.ca.us/rtfh/elderly.html.

108. O'Connell JJ, Summerfield J, Kellog FR. The homeless elderly. In: Brickner PW, et al. *Under the safety net.* New York: W.W. Norton, 1990.

109. National Coalition for the Homeless. *Homelessness among elderly populations.* NCH fact sheet #15. Available at http://www.nationalhomelss.org/eldrly.html.

110. National Alliance to End Homelessness. *Elderly/disabled housing.* July 2003. Available at http://www.endhomelessnss.org/pol/approp/elderly.html.

111. Baumohl J, Swartz JA, Randolph D, eds. Supplemental security income study on drug addiction and alcoholism in the United States. *Contemp Drug Probl* 2003;30(1&2).

112. SAMHSA/DASIS Report. *Characteristics of homeless admissions to substance abuse treatment: 2002.* August 8, 2003 Available at http://www.samhsa.gov.

113. SAMHSA/DASIS Report. *Admissions of persons with co-occurring disorders: 2000.* April 4, 2003. Available at http://www.samhsa.gov.

114. Rosenblum A, Magura S, Joseph H. Ambivalence towards methadone treatment among intravenous drug users. *J Psychoactive Drugs* 1991;23(1):21–26.

115. Appel PW, Ellison AA, Jansky HK, et al. Barriers to enrollment in drug abuse treatment and suggestions for reducing them. *Am J Alcohol Subst Abuse* 2004;40(1):129–153.

116. New York State Office of Alcoholism and Substance Abuse Services. Management Information System. Personal communication. Vincent Fenlon. August 2003. 1450 Western Ave. Albany, NY 11203.

117. Stahler GJ, Stimmel B, eds. *The effectiveness of social interventions for homeless substance abusers.* New York: Haworth Press, 1995.

118. Kraybill K, Zerger S. *Providing treatment for homeless people with substance abuse disorders: case studies of six programs.* Nashville, TN: National Health for the Homeless Council, 2003. Available at http://www.nhchc.org/publications.

119. Cami J, Farre M. Drug addiction. *N Engl J Med* 2003;349(10):975–986.

120. Stimmel B, Kreek MJ. Neurobiology of addictive behaviors and its relationship to methadone maintenance. *Mt Sinai J Med* 2000;67(5&6):375–380.

121. Gordis E. From science to social policy: an uncertain road. 52(2):101–109.

122. Blanchon T, Boissonnas A, Vareseon I, et al. Homelessness and high-dose buprenorphine misuse. *Subst Use Misuse* 2003;38(3–6):429–442.

123. Magura S, Kayman DJ, Rosenblum A, et al. *Motivational and cognitive group counseling reduce cocaine/crack use among street based drug users.* Poster presentation at the College on Problems of Drug Dependence. #6903. Bal Harbor, Florida, June 2003.

124. O'Malley SS, Jaffe G, Chang G, et al. Naltrexone and coping skill therapy for alcohol dependence. *Arch Gen Psychiatry* 1992;49(11):881.

125. Volpicelli AI, Alterman M, Hayashida M, et al. Naltrexone in the treatment of alcohol dependence. 1992;49(11);876–660.

126. Krystal JH, Cramer JA. Krol WF, et al. Naltrexone in the treatment of alcohol dependence. *N Engl J Med* 2001;345(24);1734–1739.

127. New York State OASAS. *Housing services within the addiction treatment system.* Report available from Ms. Joan Disare, OASAS, 1450 Western Ave., Albany, NY 11203.

128. Harrison PM, Beck AJ. *Prisoners in 2002.* Division of Statistics Department of Justice July 2003. Available at http://www.ojp.usdoj.gov/bjs/pub/press/p02.html.

129. Butterfield F. Study finds 2.6% increase in U.S. prison population. *New York Times* 2003 Jul 28. Available at http://www.nytimes.com/2003/07/28/national/28PRIS.html.

130. Human Rights Watch. *Ill-equipped: U.S. prisons and offenders with mental illness.* September 2003. Available at http://www.hwr.org.

131. Human Rights Watch. *U.S. Senate passes mentally ill offender treatment and crime reduction.* September 2003. Available at http://www.hwr.org.

132. Michaels D, Zoloth S, Alcabes P, et al. Homelessness and indicators of mental illness among inmates in New York City correctional system. *Hosp Community Psychiatry* 1992;43(2):150–154.

133. Gelberg L, Linn LS, Leake BD. Mental health, alcohol, and drug use and criminal history among homeless adults. *Am J Psychiatry* 1988;145(2):191–196.

134. Tomasino V, Swanson AJ, Nolan J, et al. The Key Extended Entry Program (KEEP): a methadone treatment program for opiate-dependent inmates. *Mt Sinai J Med* 2001;68(1):14–20. Available at http://www.mssm.edu/msjournal.

135. Fallon BM. The Key Extended Entry Program (KEEP): from the community side of the bridge. *Mt Sinai J Med* 2001;68(1):21–27. Available at http://www.mssm.edu/msjournal.

136. Magura S, Rosenblum A, Lewis C, et al. The effectiveness of in-jail methadone maintenance treatment. *J Drug Issues* 1993;23:75–99.

137. Joseph H, Appel P, Marx R, et al. *Evaluation of pre-KEEP in three facilities of the NYC Department of Corrections on Rikers Island.* (Available from New York State Office of Alcoholism and Substance Abuse Services, Dr. Phil Appel, 501 7th Avenue, New York, NY 10018.

138. National Commission on Correctional Health. *The health status of soon to be released inmates: 2002.* Available at http://www.ncchc.org.

139. National Alliance to End Homelessness. Using discharge planning in corrections to prevent homelessness. *Alliance Online News* 2003 Oct 10. Available at http://www.endhomelessness.org/pub/onlinenews/news10-10-03.

140. Belenko S. *Research on drug court: a critical review.* June 2001. Available at http://www.casacolumbia.org.

141. Rempel M, Fox-Kralstein D, Cissner A, et al. *NY state drug court evaluation.* Center for Court Innovation, 529 8th Avenue. New York, NY 10018. Available at http://www.courtinnovation.org.

142. Parrino M. Personal communication. American Association for the Treatment of Opioid Dependency (AATOD), 217 Broadway Suite 304, New York, NY 10007 (phone: 212–566-5555).

143. NIH Consensus Conference. *Effective medical treatment of opiate addiction.* JAMA 1998;280:1936–1943.

144. National Coalition for the Homeless. *Illegal to be homeless: the criminalization of homelessness in the United States.* Available at http://www.nationalhomeless.org.

145. Van Ness PH, Davis WR, Johnson BD. Socioeconomic marginality and health services utilization among central Harlem substance users. *Subst Use Misuse* 2004;39(1):61–85.

146. Interagency Council on Homelessness. Information available at http://www.ich.gov.

147. Tsemberis S, Eisenberg RF. Pathways to housing: supported housing for street-dwelling homeless individuals with psychiatric disabilities. *Psychiatric Serv* 2000;51(4):487–493.

148. *Pathways to Housing: a snapshot.* Available from Dr. Sam Tsemberis, Pathways to Housing, (phone: 212-289-0000 ext 101); e-mail: tsemberis@pathwaystohousing.org.

CHAPTER 73

Disability and Rehabilitation Issues

ALLEN W. HEINEMANN AND
PURVA H. RAWAL

RELATIONSHIPS BETWEEN ALCOHOL AND OTHER DRUG ABUSE AND DISABILITY

Substance abuse may be related to disability in several ways. First, it may contribute to the cause of disability, such as driving while intoxicated, sustaining a cocaine-induced stroke, or a resulting gangrenous infection from cocaine or heroin injections. Persistent, heavy alcohol use may result in alcohol ataxia, neuropathy, and arthropathy. Second, alcohol and other drug abuse may adversely affect the physical rehabilitation process following injury by causing behavioral alterations or by impairing cognition. Because rehabilitation requires the ability to learn, cognitive and learning impairments can limit the benefits of rehabilitation services. Third, physical rehabilitation outcomes may be affected by medical complications resulting from substance use, including chronic urinary tract infections (UTIs) and decubitus ulcers resulting from neglected self-care (1). Finally, substance abuse may disrupt vocational rehabilitation and reverse the cost-effectiveness of rehabilitation in persons who continue to abuse alcohol and other drugs.

One of the first studies to explore the extent of substance abuse among people with disabilities was an investigation of vocational rehabilitation clients, in which 62% of 273 adults had serious problems with alcohol; half met diagnostic criteria for alcohol dependence (2). A more recent study of 227 applicants to a state rehabilitation system found that 51% used alcohol, 29% used cocaine at least once, 40% went to work or school intoxicated at least once and 17% went intoxicated 10 or more times, and 15% had trouble at work because of drinking (3).

The first epidemiological study of substance abuse problems in individuals with disabilities using a nonreferred national sample found distinct patterns of substance use stratified by age (4). The National Household Survey on Drug Abuse found that 18- to 24-year-olds with disabilities were more likely to report heroin or crack cocaine use than were nondisabled individuals (4). However, nondisabled individuals in the 24- to 35-year-old age range were more likely to report use of marijuana than were their disabled counterparts (4). Adults older than age 35 years with disabilities were more likely to report the use of nonmedically prescribed sedatives and tranquilizers (4). There were no significant differences in odds of alcohol use among any of the age groups (4). The investigators concluded that severe disabilities at an early age might be frequently unidentified and the needs of this group consequently underserved (4).

Moore and Li (5) examined patterns of illicit drug use in 1,876 individuals actively involved in vocational rehabilitation services in three midwestern states. Prevalence rates of almost all illicit and nonmedical use drug categories, including marijuana, inhalants, cocaine, crack, hallucinogens, heroin, stimulants, sedatives, and tranquilizers, were significantly higher in the disability cohort than in the general population (5). The rate of crack use in the past month and past year were more than three times higher than the prevalence rates in the general population (5). Factors associated with use included younger age, male gender, low-income, having family and/or friends using illicit drugs, greater feelings of hostility and risk-taking, lower self-esteem, and believing that having a disability entitles one to use substances (5). Unrelated to substance use rates were disability etiology (congenital vs. acquired), presence of multiple disabilities, chronic pain, and unemployment (5). Clearly, the extent of alcohol and other drug abuse remains a concern in rehabilitation settings. Fortunately, the frequency with which these problems have been investigated and efforts made to implement assessment, treatment, and prevention programs, has increased in the past 20 years.

Substance abuse and dependence are sometimes concealed by rehabilitation clients because they fear rejection and stigmatization by staff. Rehabilitation professionals may feel unprepared and ill-equipped in dealing with issues of chemical abuse and dependence. Staff in substance-abuse treatment programs may know little about the consequences of physically disabling conditions and may be unprepared to deal with clients who have sensory or mobility limitations. This chapter summarizes alcohol and other drug abuse issues as they affect persons with disabilities, describes new directions for treatment and prevention, and identifies emergent issues to enhance the professional competence of both rehabilitation and chemical-dependence professionals.

Factors Associated with Alcohol and Other Drug Use by Persons with Disabilities

Depression, anxiety, social isolation, medical complications, and self-neglect are important factors to consider when alcohol and other drugs are used by persons who incur traumatic injury. The relation between self-esteem and mood to rehabilitation outcome is critical. One study found that 30% of spinal cord injury (SCI) patients met diagnostic criteria for a depressive disorder (6). Longer lengths of stay at a regional trauma center were associated with psychiatric comorbidity, including substance use (7). Trieschmann (8) was one of the earliest psychologists to suggest that individuals who incur injury are at risk for developing maladaptive coping strategies, including substance use to relieve chronic pain, depression, and anxiety. The use of alcohol and other substances by persons with traumatic brain injury (TBI) can contribute to greater cognitive and motor skill impairment (9). The use of substances following TBI is potentially dangerous when combined with prescription medications and may increase the likelihood of seizures (10). Heinemann and associates (11) examined patterns of substance use postinjury following recent SCI; they asked patients to report substance use for the 6 months prior to, and for 6 and 18 months following, injury (11). In particular, alcohol and marijuana use persisted after declining for the initial 6 months following onset of injury; those who used substances for the 6 months prior to injury were more likely to be at risk for use following injury (11). Substance use following SCI was associated with lower employment rates, lower levels of disability acceptance, and higher levels of depressive symptoms (12). There is also evidence that alcohol use may decrease following TBI, as compared to preinjury rates of use, but that problem and heavy drinking are likely to have negative influences on rehabilitation outcomes (13).

A task force sponsored by the National Head Injury Foundation conducted a national survey of alcohol and drug abuse problems among TBI patients (14). Approximately 40% of all patients had moderate to severe substance-abuse problems before injury, with alcohol the most frequently abused substance (14). Of the surveyed postacute rehabilitation facilities, only half reported providing substance-abuse services to clients (14). The task force concluded that substance-abuse problems are extensive in TBI patients, service provision is inadequate in rehabilitation facilities, and structured treatment programs are required to meet the multiple needs of TBI patients (14).

Blindness and Visual Impairments

Few studies have examined the extent of alcohol and other drug abuse among individuals with visual impairments, including blindness (15,16). Risk factors for substance abuse in this population include social isolation, an excess of unstructured time, and underemployment (17). Given that these risk factors are not unique to those with visual loss, the substance abuse risk in this population reflects issues shared with seniors who may experience common age-related etiologies including cataracts, glaucoma, diabetes, and vascular disease. Thus, substance-abuse risks in this population also place seniors more generally at risk. Individuals with visual loss at adolescent or young adult age resulting from early trauma or genetic etiology probably experience distinct risk factors. Special consideration should be given to even moderate drinking in persons with visual impairments as it can exacerbate underlying health problems for those whose visual loss is related to diabetes

and glaucoma. Impaired balance, mobility, and orientation are also special issues. Alcohol and drug use, which often reflects efforts to cope with disability, social isolation, and negative self-image are issues shared in common with other disability groups. Thus treatment and prevention programs that use printed materials should consider the communication needs of individuals with visual impairments; talking books and Braille materials may be needed.

Deafness and Hearing Impairments

Etiology has a major influence on the nature and extent of communication problems and consequent social integration for persons with hearing loss. Hearing loss may be the result of a congenital disorder, or may be acquired later in life as the result of injury or disease. People with congenital deafness tend to form communities that give rise to a unique culture. The fluency with which a person communicates with speech reading, vocal training, gesturing, or sign language affects acculturation and assimilation within the hearing community. Insensitivity to communication needs by the general population contributes to social stigma, a major cause of social isolation and a risk factor for substance abuse.

The few studies examining the prevalence of substance abuse among persons with hearing loss and deafness suggest that it is roughly of the same magnitude as in the general population. However, the limited ability of social service agencies, alcohol- and drug-abuse programs, school and work settings, and the legal system to communicate with persons who are deaf allow some people to avoid the negative consequences of substance abuse (16). There is some evidence that attempts by persons who are deaf to avoid the additional stigma of substance abuse contributes further to social isolation and difficulty accessing substance abuse services (18). McCrone suggests the following program-accessibility guidelines: using telecommunication devices (TDD) to communicate with service agencies, making certified sign language interpreters available, teaching sign language to substance-abuse counselors, making co-counseling arrangements with deafness specialists, coordinating outreach efforts to the deaf community, and building contacts with professional organizations that provide substance abuse services to the deaf community (19). A survey of service providers for deaf individuals and service providers for substance abuse found that substance-abuse services are generally inaccessible by telephone to clients who are deaf and that relatively few services are provided to those who are deaf that can access services (20). Few programs contract for sign language interpreters; instead, family members, volunteers, and printed materials are used to communicate with patients who are deaf, often compromising patient confidentiality and violating client rights.

The lack of specialized programs for persons who are deaf (20) has been remedied in some communities by the founding of specialized substance-abuse programs such as that provided by the Anixter Center in Chicago. Their specialized program, called Addiction Recovery of the Deaf (http://www.anixter.org/ARD/Index.htm) was designed for persons who are deaf and employs staff members who are fluent in sign language.

The Minnesota Chemical Dependency Program for Deaf and Hard of Hearing Individuals (http://www.mncddeaf.org/), a program in Minnesota specializing in treating individuals who are deaf and have substance-abuse problems conducted an outcome study on 100 clients at 1, 3, 6, and 12 months postdischarge (21). Clients were asked to complete a pretreatment survey measuring attitudinal, behavioral, and knowledge changes regarding substance abuse; posttreatment questionnaire; a demographic questionnaire; a client satisfaction survey; and four followup surveys. Unfortunately, few people could be contacted at each followup point, but each client was contacted at least once. Median age of first use was at 10 years (21). More than 35% of clients at followup reported abstinence and 15% reported using a single drug less than monthly (21). For those using substances, alcohol was used more often than marijuana and other drugs (21). Investigators found that employment status, family availability to participate in followup, and attendance of Alcoholics and Narcotics Anonymous meetings at followup were significant predictors of abstinence (21). Several individuals had obtained employment at postdischarge followup; however, few conclusions could be made because of low followup rates (21). The most salient conclusion was the need for vocational rehabilitation to increase employment for clients posttreatment (21).

Chronic Pain

Chronic pain is a common problem experienced by millions of individuals. A common intervention for chronic pain is pharmaceutical; however, there have been varying rates of substance abuse in this population. An early study examining the association between chronic pain and psychiatric illness examined 37 chronic pain patients admitted to a 3-week inpatient program (22). Results indicated that the second most frequent lifetime diagnosis was for alcohol abuse (41%), with alcohol use predating chronic pain onset by a mean of 15 years (standard deviation [SD] = 9 years) (22). Almost 40% of the patients who abused alcohol also had first-degree relatives that abused alcohol (22). Thus the results suggest that a subset of chronic pain patients have previous histories of alcohol abuse and are likely to have family histories of chronic pain and alcohol abuse (22). Understandably, many physicians are concerned about the long-term dependence potential of opioid therapy for treating chronic pain given the high rates of prior substance abuse in this population. A study examining 283 chronic pain patients found 20.4% of males had current alcohol- and drug-dependence diagnoses, compared to 7.9% of females, indicating an overrepresentation of current substance dependence in men with chronic pain (23). Drug use, abuse, and dependence were assessed more recently in a random sample of patients using *Diagnostic and Statistical Manual of Mental Disorders,* 3rd ed., revised (*DSM–III–R*) criteria (24,25). Almost 90% of the sample (N = 125) was taking medication for pain problems, 12% met *DSM–III–R* criteria for active drug abuse or dependence, approximately 10% met *DSM–III–R* criteria for abuse or dependence in remission, 13.5% reported alcohol use and 4% reported cannabis use when pain was unbearable, and 17% of patients reported occasionally using prescription medications above the highest recommended dose, indicating drug misuse (25). The study also indicated poor patient education, including a lack of or inaccurate knowledge of potential side effects of use (25). The study concluded that greater patient education is necessary, as well as physician education on optimal prescribing practices in chronic pain populations (25). These authors also reported a case control study comparing patients with medically explained and unexplained chronic pain symptoms on several factors, including medication abuse or dependence (26). However, no significant differences were observed in medication abuse or dependence rates in patients with medically explained and unexplained symptoms, with low rates observed in both groups (26).

Given that the majority of patients with chronic pain undergoing opioid treatment do not have abuse or dependency problems, understanding the characteristics and risk factors for the subset of patients with substance abuse/dependence difficulties is important. For instance, it may be necessary to provide coping and recovering skills or a structured therapy to patients with comorbid psychiatric illnesses or histories of abuse to adequately manage opioid treatment (27). A study of 90 consecutive women attending a multidisciplinary pain management center for chronic pain examined the association between childhood and adulthood abuse, somatic symptom reports, mental health service use, and substance abuse (28). Almost 50% of the women reported histories of abuse; these women were more likely to report somatic problems, to have used mental health services in the 12 months prior to the study, to smoke cigarettes, and to have a history of prior substance-abuse counseling (28). These results suggest that a subset of patients need additional support to maintain a nonabusive opioid therapy. To accurately diagnose addiction in patients with chronic pain, there must be evidence of an inability to fulfill daily life activities because of use of the substance. Obtaining this evidence requires clinicians to look beyond standard diagnostic criteria (27) on which many studies are based.

Patients with chronic low back pain form a large subgroup of the chronic pain population. Hesitance to use chronic opioid analgesic therapy has also been noted in this subset of patients; however, some physicians now recommend limited use of opioids for patients who have not responded to other interventions (29). After examining 566 case studies, the authors concluded that opioid therapy is a safe treatment alternative for many patients with chronic low back pain; physicians should pay careful attention to contraindications including preexisting substance use disorders, personality disorders, and specific medical conditions and occupational factors in order to maximize positive outcomes (29). In the absence of randomized controlled trials, a subset of patients with severe chronic low back pain may benefit from opioid therapy (29). Additional measures can be taken to monitor potential abuse and dependence including patient education on possible adverse effects of opioid use; written contracts between patient and physician; regular patient contact, including contact with family members; monitoring pain and functioning parameters; and urine toxicology screenings (29). Thus opioid therapy should not be ruled out in many cases and steps can be taken to minimize concerns about abuse and dependence (29).

Research on lifetime and current prevalence rates for substance-abuse disorders in patients with chronic low back pain has also been conducted. Lifetime prevalence and premorbid risk of psychiatric disorders were compared in a sample of 97 men with persistent low back pain to 49 male control subjects without chronic pain (30). Almost 65% of patients with chronic low back pain had lifetime alcohol use disorders, as compared with a 39% rate in the control subjects; prevalence rates of substance abuse or dependence in the past 6 months yielded nonsignificant between-group differences, with approximately 12% of pain patients and 4% of controls meeting abuse or dependence criteria (30). The onset of alcohol abuse or dependence preceded the onset of chronic pain in 81% of the pain patients by a mean of 12.9 years; however, chronic pain did not increase the likelihood of alcohol abuse or dependence (30). Thus, the study indicates that men with histories of alcohol abuse or dependence may be vulnerable to chronic back pain. Despite the potential role of alcohol in the onset of chronic back pain, the presence of the condition does not increase the likelihood of developing alcohol abuse or dependence (30).

A more recent study comparing current prevalence rates and the onset of pain in relation to onset of substance-use disorders for 61 patients with and 181 individuals without chronic back pain yielded similar results (31). Lifetime substance abuse and dependence prevalence rates were 54% for the chronic pain group and 52% for the comparison group; current substance abuse and dependence prevalence rates were 23% for both groups (31). The results suggest that chronic back pain is not a significant risk factor for current substance-use disorders (30,31). One study examined the relationship between psychopathology and vocational outcomes in a group of 144 patients with low back pain (32). Lifetime rates of substance use disorders were 26% in the return-to-work group and 17%

in the non–return-to-work group; current substance-abuse rates were 5% for the return-to-work group and zero for the non–return-to-work group (32). The results indicate that current substance-abuse rates in low back pain patients are low and that substance abuse may not predict rehabilitative outcomes (32).

The majority of chronic pain patients receiving opioid treatments do not have current abuse or dependency problems. However, opioid abuse and/or dependency may be prevalent for a subset of patients. Thus accurate diagnosing, better patient education, and prevention efforts aimed at patients who are at risk for abusing opioid treatments are important steps in managing chronic pain. For the subset of chronic back pain populations studied, current rates of substance use are not high; however, lifetime rates of substance use disorders are significant, indicating a possible vulnerability for chronic pain development.

Traumatic Brain Injury

TBI is a leading cause of death and disability. The pathophysiologic, functional, societal, and economic consequences dramatically alter the lives of men and women of all ages and races (33). In fact, there is a growing number of persons seeking treatment as a consequence of TBI because survival following TBI has improved. Not only did the incidence of TBI decline from 200/100,000 persons in 1974 to 92/100,000 persons in 1994, but mortality rates also improved (24.6/100,000 TBIs in 1979 to 19.2/100,000 in 1992) (34–38). Improved survival rates are attributed to advancements in medical technology. Highly specialized and early delivery of medical services such as administration of neuroparalytic agents at the injury scene, early imaging in the emergency room, removal of extraaxial masses, support of blood pressure, ventilation, and monitoring of intracranial pressure reduce mortality and subsequently increase the demands for effective rehabilitation services (39).

Thurman and Guerrero (40) analyzed trends in TBI-related hospitalization rates from 1980 through 1995 using the National Hospital Discharge Survey and found a 51% decline from the estimated annual incidence rate of hospitalization associated with TBI from 199 to 98 per 100,000 people. Mild TBI hospitalization rates decreased the most compared to intermediate and severe TBI, declining by 61% from 130 to 51 hospitalizations per 100,000 annually; the greatest decline was seen in the 5- to 14-year-old age group (40). After examining national trends in hospitalization rates, Thurman and Guerrero concluded that TBI rates probably decreased in the last few decades and that technological advancements, such as computed tomography (CT), have increased the quality of care; however, they also suggested that changes in hospital practices (e.g., decreasing overall hospitalization rates nationally) may be responsible in large part for decreased TBI-related hospitalizations (40). Thus, TBI care has been increasingly shifted to outpatient treatment, emphasizing the need for complete evaluation, including substance use, in both inpatient and outpatient settings (40).

Factors that are strongly related to TBI outcome are gender, age, duration of coma, systemic injuries, and premorbid level of functioning (41). Rimel and associates (42) studied 1,248 patients, in whom the incidence of TBI among males was twice that of females for most age categories, with the greatest incidence differences observed in the 15- to 24-year-old age group. Coma length is also strongly related to mortality; patients with moderately impaired Glasgow Coma Scale scores of 9 to 11 experienced a 6% mortality rate; patients with mild impairment and Glasgow Coma Scale scores of 12 to 13 had a mortality rate of 1%; and no patient with a score above 14 died (42). Multiple trauma and systemic injuries compound the severity of TBI and lead to poor rehabilitation outcome (43). Thus proper triage, which includes immediate attention to potential alcohol intoxication, provides the opportunity to manage systemic injuries and to minimize trauma severity.

Estimates of intoxication at injury from emergency room and epidemiologic reports suggest that the rate ranges from 29% to 86% (44,45). Alcohol is a causal factor in approximately half of all automobile crashes. A study of TBI admissions to a regional trauma center found that substance use was suspected or documented in 49% of all trauma cases and in 66% of motor vehicle traumas (46). A similar study conducted with a larger sample admitted for head injury, found that alcohol was a major factor associated with the injury, with detectable blood alcohol levels (BALs) in 62% of men and 27% of women (47). In one study, alcohol intoxication was a contributing factor more often for moderate than for mild brain injury (48). Of 199 patients evaluated for moderate brain injury, 73% were intoxicated, as compared to 53% of 538 patients who sustained mild head injuries (48). In a sample of 623 patients admitted to an urban trauma center, the odds of brain injury were 1.4 times greater when serum ethanol was detected (45). While these studies provide valuable data on the extensive role of alcohol in TBI cases, the mechanisms of brain injury as a consequence of alcohol use remain poorly understood.

One study followed 257 adults with TBI and found that improvement of Glasgow Coma Scale (GCS) scores was significantly related to BAL at admission; patients with the highest BALs showed the greatest cognitive improvement (49). Although a common myth is that alcohol protects against injury, Waller and associates (50) found that drivers who had been drinking were more likely than sober drivers to sustain serious injury or death. The observed improvement in GCS scores for those intoxicated at onset of injury may be misleading when compared to the GCS of sober patients. Alcohol consumption just prior to injury is likely to negatively affect distal outcomes (51). Sporadeo and Gill (52) found that intoxication at

the time of injury was associated with longer lengths of hospital stay, longer periods of agitation, and lower cognitive status at discharge. A study examining service use in 591 male prison inmates with substance abuse problems and self-reported head injuries (none, one, two, or more) found that individuals with multiple head injuries reported significantly more emergency room visits, more inpatient admissions, and greater lengths of hospital stay, than did individuals with no reported head injuries (53). Thus, comorbid substance-abuse problems and a history of more than two head injuries leads to a greater use of medical services, often at the high end of the cost spectrum (53). However, it remains unclear to what extent the actual level of intoxication impairs cognitive outcomes and recovery of injured neurons and cerebral blood vessels. Basic neuroscience research examining brain plasticity, the capacity to medicate recovery of function, and the role of high BALs, will help to elucidate the factors related to brain tissue damage (54,55). Understanding the role of alcohol in brain injury and its effect on subsequent cognitive outcomes may help to prevent the rapidly occurring toxic effects of injury and promote the regeneration of injured, but not dead, cells (56). Any additive effects of intoxication to TBI in affecting neuropsychological and functional recovery must be identified if we are to understand these more basic processes.

A recent controlled study used quantitative magnetic resonance imaging (QMRI) techniques to examine neuropathologic changes in young males (age 16 to 30 years) who experienced TBI and abused substances (57). TBI and substance-abuse cases are independently associated with neuropathologic changes, including ventricular enlargement and cortical atrophy; consequently, the authors hypothesized that the comorbidity of the two conditions would result in significant damage (57). Results indicated that the presence of substance abuse and TBI resulted in greater atrophic changes than any other group, when controlling for severity of head injury (57). Thus, the study suggests that in teenagers and young adults, substance abuse results in greater levels of neural degeneration in the presence of TBI that is not caused by prior structural differences in the brain (57).

Young adults are especially at risk for TBI when they have preinjury histories of substance abuse. One study examined the pre- and postinjury alcohol and illicit drug use patterns of 87 individuals who incurred TBIs between 16 and 20 years of age (58). They found a decline in alcohol use at initial followup, but a subsequent increase in alcohol use, with males and individuals with heavy alcohol use histories prior to injury being at greatest risk for persistent alcohol abuse following injury (58).

Bombardier and Heinemann (59) examined the use of the Readiness to Change (RTC) questionnaire for substance use in a sample of persons with TBI. They found that three stages of change (precontemplation, contemplation, action) correlated meaningfully with independent assessments of alcohol use and severity (59). Thus, the RTC questionnaire is able to distinguish the three major stages in this model (60), and is able to document individuals' current capacity for change. Measuring readiness to change alcohol use patterns in individuals with TBI has meaningful treatment and outcomes implications. Thus, measures with good construct validity, such as the RTC questionnaire, should be used in clinical settings to target subsets of persons with TBI who may respond to substance-abuse treatment.

One study characterized and compared neurobehavioral and substance problems in employed and unemployed individuals with TBI (61). Employed individuals with TBI showed greater decreased rates of neurobehavioral problems than did unemployed individuals with TBI, whereas the unemployed cohort reported greater problems on measures related to depression, attention and memory functioning, aggression, communication, and motor problems (61). Correspondingly higher rates of mental health treatment were observed in the unemployed cohort (61). However, the employed cohort reported rates of light and infrequent to moderate and heavy alcohol use twice that of unemployed individuals, whereas the unemployed group had twice as many abstainers (61). The authors interpreted their results as indicating unique neurobehavioral needs in unemployed individuals that require specialized vocational rehabilitation interventions (61). Employed individuals with TBI may require continued education and monitoring to prevent and decrease problematic alcohol use (61).

The National Center for Injury Prevention and Control and the Disabilities Prevention Program of the National Center for Environmental Health at the Centers for Disease Control and Prevention supported a study that sought to evaluate a community-based approach to substance-abuse treatment that used comprehensive case-management strategies (87). The goal of case management was to enhance employment and health-related quality of life of persons with TBI. The study sought to evaluate the effectiveness of case-management services for people with TBI who have substance-abuse problems and to predict treatment outcomes using client and program characteristics. The study was conducted at two treatment programs that provided case-management services for persons with TBI who had substance-abuse problems (N = 217); a comparison group was recruited that did not receive intensive case management (N = 102). Self-reported alcohol and illicit drug use was reported at the beginning of services and 9 months later with the Addiction Severity Index; also used was the Community Integration Questionnaire, Medical Outcome Study–Short Form 36, Diener's Life Satisfaction scale, and Carver and Jones' Family Satisfaction scale. The case-management group reported more alcohol and illicit drug use at both assessments, and alcohol use exceeded illicit drug use at both assessments. While no changes in alcohol or illicit drug use between initial

assessment and a 9-month followup were found for either group, employment at recruitment and earlier referral for case management were associated with employment 9 months later for those receiving case management. Both groups made significant gains in physical well-being by the 9-month followup, as well as in community integration. Life satisfaction increased for the case-management group and remained stable for the comparison group. In contrast, family satisfaction tended to decline for the comparison group and remain stable for the case-management group. Earlier program referral was associated with larger gains in physical well-being, employment, and community integration. Although the case-management group did not report substance use reduction at this early phase of treatment, case management appears to have beneficial effects for adults with concomitant TBI and substance-abuse problems. The effects are evident in terms of life and family satisfaction, as well as potential cost savings.

A study of 105 persons with traumatic brain injury and their families evaluated the hypothesis that observer ratings, made by family members, would correlate with self-reported psychological symptoms related to poor social adjustment for TBI patients, and that these observer ratings could be used to supplement self-report data (62). The study suggested that individuals with TBI experience significant distress postinjury, as indicated by elevations at least 1 SD above the normative sample on the several Symptoms Checklist–90 Revised (SCL-90-R) scales: Obsessive–Compulsive, Interpersonal Sensitivity, Depression, Psychoticism, and the Global Severity Index (62). The study indicates that family members report a fairly consistent pattern of concerns regarding social adjustment, that individuals experience significant distress postinjury, that observer ratings of adjustment postinjury correlated with self-reports of psychological distress, and that observers' reported symptoms outside of the patient's awareness, including orientation, antisocial behavior, speech/cognitive difficulties, bizarreness, and verbal expansiveness (62). Investigators concluded that observer ratings provided information on social adjustment beyond individuals' awareness, whereas self-report measures provided important information on subjective psychological distress (62). Thus including family members of individuals with TBI can be an important source of information to gauge social adjustment for persons with TBI and to augment their self-reports of psychological distress.

Given the shift to outpatient treatment for TBI, there is a corresponding increase in the need for comprehensive evaluations of substance-abuse issues. There is an increasing number of measures, such as the RTC (59), that will assist clinicians in assessing the potential for change in substance use patterns. Assessing preinjury patterns of use is important in understanding the potential for future abuse and/or dependence. Persons with TBI require continued education and monitoring to prevent and to decrease problematic alcohol use. To assess psychological adjustment and social behavior post-TBI, investigators have supported the use of self-report and direct observation to gather the most comprehensive and accurate data on persons with TBI. Despite decreases in TBI rates and increasing quality of care because of technological advancements, persons with TBI still present with complex problems and needs that persist long after the onset of injury.

Spinal Cord Injury

The National Spinal Cord Injury Statistical Center estimates that between 183,000 and 230,000 individuals in the United States have spinal cord injuries (SCIs) with approximately 11,000 new cases of SCI diagnosed annually (63). As a traumatic life event, SCI has biologic, psychological, and social implications. Alcohol and/or drug intoxication is a frequent contributor to SCI onset. Intoxication estimates for persons incurring traumatic injury range from 17% to 49% (6,46,47,64,65). Heinemann et al. (66) indicate that impaired judgment resulting from alcohol consumption contributes to many of these injuries. Their study examined the rate of intoxication at injury onset in a sample of 88 cases presenting for admission to an acute SCI center. Investigators observed BALs greater than 50 mg/dL in 40% of cases, followed by urine toxicology screenings evidencing cocaine (14%), cannibanoids (8%), benzodiazepines (5%), and opiates (4%) (66). Across all cases, 35% had evidence of substances with abuse potential in their urine and 62% had either a BAL greater than 50 mg/dL or a positive urine analysis.

Another study used toxicology screens with 87 consecutive rehabilitative medicine patients with acute spinal cord injuries and found that 47% were intoxicated at the time of injury and 53% had positive screens, with young, unmarried males having the highest incidence of positive toxicology screens (67). Individuals with positive screens were more likely to be younger unmarried males with a mean age of 33 years, whereas individuals with negative screens were more likely to be married and were older, with a mean age of 39 years (67). Inpatient length of stay and measures assessing outcome did not demonstrate a relationship with outcome (67). Thus, high rates of substance abuse are detectable with toxicology screens immediately following injury and can then potentially be used to provide substance abuse education and prevention during rehabilitation.

The prevalence of alcohol use and abuse following initial rehabilitation may also be high. In a sample of vocational rehabilitation and independent living center clients with SCI, Johnson (69) reported a 46% rate of moderate to heavy drinking that is almost twice the 25% rate reported in the general population. Studies of persons with recent SCI estimate rates of alcohol-dependence symptomatology ranging from 49% (2) to 62% (68) in vocational rehabilitation clients. Heinemann and colleagues (68) examined the persistence of substance use in a sample of

103 persons with recent SCI, with ages in the sample ranging from 13 to 65 years at injury. Excluded were individuals with cognitive impairments limiting self-report, with injuries occurring within 1 year of the assessment, and with an inability to communicate in English. Mean age of the sample was 28 years and 75% were men (68). Lifetime exposure to and recent use of several substances with abuse potential were compared to norms for a like-age national sample reported by the National Institute on Drug Abuse (70). The SCI sample of young adults age 25 years and younger reported significantly greater rates of exposure and recent use of amphetamines, marijuana, cocaine, and hallucinogens than did the like-aged national sample (68). In contrast, the SCI group 26 years of age and older reported significantly greater exposure to narcotic analgesics and tranquilizers than did the national sample, and reported rates of recent use of tobacco, alcohol, amphetamines, and marijuana that exceeded rates in the national sample by 10% (68). The young adult sample with SCI reported greater use of marijuana before injury and greater cocaine exposure than the older adult cohort with SCI, while the older adult cohort reported greater rates of tobacco exposure (68). Intoxication at the time of injury served as a marker of preinjury substance use with the 39% who reported intoxication at the time of injury; this subset also reported greater rates of exposure to tobacco, amphetamines, marijuana, hallucinogens, tranquilizers, and sedatives, and higher rates of recent use of tobacco, alcohol, amphetamines, cocaine, and hallucinations, than did those denying intoxication at the time of injury (68).

Given the significant substance-abuse problems in the SCI population, assessing readiness to change is important in designing and implementing interventions. Bombardier and Rimmele (71) examined alcohol use and motivation to change patterns of use in 58 individuals with recent SCI during inpatient rehabilitation. Measures assessing alcoholism and readiness to change found that 35% of the sample fell into the alcoholism classification and 50% of the sample was "at risk" for developing dependence; of the "at-risk" drinkers, 45% were in the contemplation phase and 34% were in the action phase, indicating that almost 80% of "at-risk" drinkers were at least considering changing their drinking patterns (71). The authors concluded that assessing stages of change during inpatient rehabilitation hospitalization might provide treatment staff with an opportunity to implement changes in alcohol use behaviors (71).

Boraz and Heinemann (72) conducted a study examining the relationships between social support and alcohol abuse in individuals with spinal cord injuries. Data on alcohol use and social support were collected within 3 months of injury onset, and at 6, 12, and 18 months postinjury (72). They found that preinjury drinking patterns were not related to perceived social support, that perceived family support was higher at all four assessment points than perceived friend support, and that family support remained constant over the 18-month followup period whereas perceived friend support significantly decreased over time (72). The study highlights the importance of education and of including the family in SCI rehabilitation, and the potential for problems such as substance abuse, that are exacerbated by a loss of support from friends (72).

Hawkins and Heinemann (73) examined the relationship between medical complications (pressure ulcers and UTIs) and substance abuse following SCI in 71 inpatient subjects. Abstainers with long histories of alcohol abuse prior to SCI were at increased risk for UTIs 7 to 12 months following injury and for longer inpatient lengths of stay, suggesting poor self-care and coping mechanisms in newly abstinent patients (73). Illicit substance use 12 to 18 months following SCI were also related to increased incidence of pressure ulcers 19 to 30 months following injury (73). The relationship between alcohol and drug use and medical complications in SCI patients is complex, but has important implications for rehabilitative care (73). A recent study examined the occurrence of pressure ulcers (decubitus ulcers or "bed sores") in 175 individuals with recent-onset SCI (within 1 year) admitted to an inpatient medical rehabilitation program for recent-onset SCI (74). The sample was comprised exclusively of white (N = 108) and African American (N = 67) individuals, and most were male (N = 131); however, only 105 subjects were available for pressure ulcer evaluation (74). Results indicated that pressure ulcers were 2.5 times more likely to occur in patients with severe alcohol use compared to those with no alcohol problems; depression and acceptance of injury were not related to pressure ulcer occurrence (74). Thus, SCI patients with alcohol-abuse histories or potentials are at risk for pressure ulcer occurrence during the first 3 years following SCI onset (74).

Substance use and abuse is a concern for this population because it occurs frequently, increases the risk for medical complications, may complicate medical and vocational rehabilitation, and reduces the capacity for independent living. It is important to remember that substance use is not necessarily abuse or dependence, nor does use necessarily result in specific problems, making it imperative that chemical dependence and rehabilitation professionals understand the context, expectancies, and motives for use. Substance use may serve as a means of engaging others socially, managing stress, or the beginning of a pattern that could escalate into addiction. Hence, it is important to routinely assess substance use and its consequences.

Health Implications of Substance Abuse for Persons with Disabilities

Alcohol and other drug abuse can affect the health of persons with disabilities in direct and indirect ways (75). Direct effects of drugs include gout, increased spasticity, increased tolerance and potentiation of medication ef-fects, and reduced coordination and concentration. These effects can have adverse consequences for persons with arthritis, SCI, and brain injury, among other conditions. Self-medication for chronic pain can be another reason for substance abuse, as it is for depression, anxiety, and adjustment disorders. Indirect effects result primarily from neglected self-care. For persons with SCI, the failure to relieve skin pressure regularly increases the risk of pressure ulcers. The consequences of forgetting to take prescription medications as prescribed reflect the nature of the condition being treated; for instance, a person who fails to take a prescribed antihypertensive medication following a stroke increases the risk of recurrent stroke. Thus, health professionals are encouraged to inquire about missed appointments, recurring medical problems and injury because alcohol and drug abuse is a frequently concealed cause of these problems.

Alcohol and Other Drug Abuse Treatment Issues for Persons with Disabilities

Etiologic Considerations

A physical disability can either precede or follow the onset of substance abuse. Persons who are primary substance abusers are at increased risk of injury that may result in permanent disability. Thus, risks faced by individuals with substance abuse problems may limit rehabilitation outcomes, including insufficient social resources, low socioeconomic status, and multiple disabilities (3). The distinctions between type I and type II alcoholism made in the treatment literature are useful in conceptualizing disability and substance abuse (76). Type I alcoholism affects primarily men and is characterized by early onset of use at younger than the age of 25 years, severe alcohol-related problems, and significant criminal histories, whereas type II alcoholism is more common in women and their male relatives, and is characterized by minimal criminal histories, late onset of drinking-related problems, which tend to be isolated or mild, and binge patterns of drinking (76). Individuals with type I alcoholism have a more persistent moderate to heavy drinking pattern and are also more likely to report having fathers with histories of alcoholism, suggesting that the type of alcoholism may be related to familial drinking patterns. Glass (15) made similar distinctions highlighting potential differences between persons with physical disabilities whose drinking predates injury onset, termed *type A*, and those whose dinking problems emerged following injury, termed *type B*. Glass (15) hypothesized that type A drinking patterns would be related to less-favorable rehabilitation outcomes.

A study examining the rate of self-reported alcohol use, consequent problems, perceived need for treatment, and receipt of treatment in a sample of 75 persons with recent SCI was used to assess the hypotheses based on these typologies (77). Subjects reported alcohol use information at three time periods from 6 months prior to injury to

18 months following injury (77). Drinking on three or more occasions was reported by 93% of respondents at least once during the followup assessments, 71% reported at least one drinking-related problem. However, only 15% reported a need for alcohol-abuse treatment and only 11% received treatment (77). The risk of alcohol abuse following injury in those without preinjury abuse was low, with 65% reporting drinking problems before injury and only 6% reporting drinking problems for the first time following injury (77). Issues of dual disability in individuals with preinjury histories of substance abuse who also sustain SCI are important topics for rehabilitation and chemical-dependence treatment programs.

A study of 52 participants with SCI or TBI admitted to an urban, level 1 trauma center was conducted to assess preinjury alcohol and drug use patterns in patients with SCI and TBI and to make comparisons between the groups (78). In the TBI group, the largest proportion were heavy drinkers (42%), 27% were moderate drinkers, 19% reported abstinence, and the most frequently used drug was marijuana (27%); in the SCI group, however, 57% reported heavy drinking preinjury, 15% were moderate drinkers, 23% were light/infrequent users, 4% reported abstinence, and 35% reported drug use in the past year, with marijuana being the most frequently used (19%) (78). Differences between the groups were nonsignificant and when rates of moderate and heavy drinkers were compared for SCI and TBI groups, approximately 70% in both groups fell in these two categories (78). The findings indicate higher rates of preinjury alcohol use than in the general population for SCI and TBI patients, with preinjury abstinence rare in SCI cohorts (4%) and the majority of SCI participants having heavy drinking histories (78). Thus, alcohol use may be more problematic for persons with SCI (78).

Representative Treatment Approaches

Systematic Motivational Counseling

Systematic Motivational Counseling (SMC) is a useful and promising intervention for adults with substance abuse problems and its use has been extended from inpatient substance abuse programs to adults with TBI. SMC is based on the hypothesis that the common route to substance use is individual motivation, despite the complex biologic, psychological, and environmental influences affecting substance use (79,80). Variables affecting alcohol and other drug use do so as they contribute to expectations of emotional change resulting from use. Thus, an individual's decision to use is based on the expectation that the positive emotional consequences of using will outweigh those of not using.

The model describes major factors that affect motivation to use substances, and provides for varying contributions of each factor on decisions to use between and within individuals at different times. Therefore, decisions to use or abstain reflect the weighing of influences across times and situations depending on expectations of positive and negative emotional consequences of use. SMC seeks to enhance sources of emotional satisfaction that are incompatible with drug use, thereby increasing the likelihood of abstinence.

Current and past experiences are influential in decision making about substance use, including the history of use, immediate availability of substances, others' use, individual goals that enhance positive emotions and incentives, and situations that intensify negative emotions. Historical and current experiences invoke beliefs, thoughts, and perceptions about the effects of use, often with the expectation that a substance will lead to emotional change via immediate chemical change and/or via indirect effects on nonchemical incentives. Ultimately, the decision to use is made by judging whether the positive consequences of using outweigh those of not using. People who abuse substances often fail to experience emotional satisfaction through the pursuit of nonchemical goals, or pursue positive goals that are unrealistic, inappropriate, or in conflict with one another. Thus, SMC counselors help clients to evaluate goals that may be inappropriate and/or unrealistic and their roles and commitments in relation to them; identify patterns of facilitation and interference among goals; resolve conflicts among interfering goals; disengage from inappropriate goals; identify nonchemical sources of emotional satisfaction; find new sources of self-esteem; eliminate sources of self-condemnation; shift from pursuing negative goals to positive goals; develop skills for reaching realistic long-range goals and identify subgoals; and formulate and practice assignments for reaching long-term goals and activities that meet immediate needs.

The Motivational Structure Questionnaire (MSQ) (81) is a measure used in SMC to assess motivation to use substances. Clients begin by listing concerns in major life domains, then they describe each of their concerns with a verb drawn from one of 12 verb classes, as classified by their valence and goal-striving (e.g., appetite, aversive, agonistic, epistemic), and lastly they indicate the relative strength of their positive and negative motivations. Each concern is rated on ten dimensions, which include the degree to which individuals actively participate in goal striving and their commitment to goals. Clients also rate the amount of joy expected if the goal was attained and the amount of sorrow if the goal was not attained. Ambivalence is measured by assessing the degree of unhappiness the client would feel if the goal was not attained. The expected probability of success if no action is taken, the time available before action must be taken on each goal, how near goal attainment is, and the consequence of substance use on each goal are also rated. The numerous ratings are compiled to construct a profile of motivational features based on norms of individuals undergoing alcohol rehabilitation. The resulting profile is discussed with clients in terms of the properties of their goals and the status of their goal pursuit to identify motivational patterns interfering with finding nonchemical satisfaction.

SMC attempts to modify the motivational basis for alcohol use and then helps clients develop a meaningful life without substances. Activities include setting immediate and long-range goals, formulating plans for achieving goals, and a regular review of clients' success in achieving goals. Goal ladders help clients to reach a series of immediately pleasurable subgoals, achieved between sessions that are necessary for attainment of the final goal. Counselors help clients develop the skills necessary for goal attainment and examine sources of self-esteem, which will be enhanced as positive goals are reached.

Studies examining the effects of SMC in TBI populations have yielded positive results. The SMC treatment model was evaluated in 60 persons with TBI during a 12-week rehabilitation program at Schwab Rehabilitation Hospital and Care Network-affiliated programs. The sample was comprised primarily of African American (44%) men (81%) of working age, with 44% participating in a 1-year followup. At followup, 40% maintained abstinence, 14% became abstinent, 38% continued using, and 8% began using; for the 33 clients for whom use patterns and employment status were reported, 42% were employed, 33% were unemployed and seeking work, and 24% were unemployed and not seeking work (82). Compared to a no-treatment control group of 72 adults with TBI, the SMC group reported significantly fewer concerns on the MSQ from initial to followup assessment (82). The following were significant differences between the no-treatment control and SMC groups: aversive motivation was lower in the SMC group, assumption of a spectator role was greater in the SMC group, ambivalence was lower in the SMC group, and goal distance declined for SMC participants who became abstinent and increased for no-treatment controls that were using (82).

Cox and colleagues reported additional details of the study for a subset of 40 participants receiving SMC and 54 control cases (83). From baseline to followup, the SMC group demonstrated significant increases on indices of Appetitive Action, Active Role, Joy, Sorrow/No Success, and Time Available, and a significant decrease on the scale of Unhappiness, with no corresponding changes in the control group. These results suggest a positive effect on the motivational structures of participants in the SMC group (83). The index of negative affect from the Positive Affect–Negative Affect Scale showed significantly lower levels of negative affect for the SMC group, indicating a relationship between SMC and improved mood (83). Substance-abuse assessments showed lower rates of substance use at followup than at baseline for the SMC group, with an approximately 50% decrease in use by SMC participants compared to an increase in use for the control group; however, between-group differences narrowed from posttreatment to followup, indicating a need for continued support and perhaps for SMC booster sessions (83). Overall,

the data yielded evidence for a shift to a more adaptive motivational structure in SMC participants (83). An integrated treatment emphasizing problem solving, such as SMC, holds significant promise not only for addressing substance-abuse problems, but also for more global issues including increasing independence and life satisfaction (84).

Skills-Based Substance Abuse Prevention Counseling

Skills-Based Counseling (SBC) was developed specifically for persons experiencing cognitive deficits resulting from a brain injury (85; Langley & Ridgely, unpublished manuscript). The model uses a skills acquisition sequence in which clients are taught to recognize high-risk situations related to their preinjury lifestyle or the consequences of their brain injury. Strategies to improve problem solving and response flexibility in high-risk situations are role-played and practiced in clinical and field settings. The client learns to monitor and use feedback, and to apply skills automatically with minimal disruption by external factors. When available, family and other supports are taught to appreciate high-risk situations, anticipate problems, and support effective responses. Alcohol use and the consequences of brain injury are viewed as transactional in SBC, with each exacerbating problem originating from the other, and each contributing to both problem realms. Efforts to reduce substance abuse must be integrated carefully with physical and cognitive rehabilitation because alcohol and other drugs can be used as both a means of coping with frustrations and as a reinforcer of poor coping mechanisms. SBC aims to develop an alternative lifestyle in which substance use is no longer central.

SBC includes four stages: (a) comprehensive evaluation; (b) motivational enhancement; (c) coping skills training; and (d) structured generalization. A multidisciplinary approach is adopted and behavioral techniques are employed within each stage in the context of individual neuropsychological strengths and limitations.

Comprehensive evaluation uses the modified Adaptive Skills Battery (ASB) (Langley & Ridgely, unpublished manuscript), a 12-item instrument designed to evaluate coping skills in various situations that involve negative emotional states, including anger, frustration, conflict, social pressure to use, and cue-exposure to use substances. Clients describe their responses to these situations and counselors rate the skillfulness of responses on a three-level scale. ASB items describe situations that require solutions to a problem that could otherwise result in substance use; item development used behavior–analytic methodology (86) identifying ecologically relevant problem situations for individuals with substance-abuse problems and brain injury. Clients respond to each situation by anticipating and describing their real-life response.

There are 12 situations, both intra- and interpersonal in nature, as well as alcohol-specific and nonspecific situations. Specific situations involve feeling worthless, being alone and bored on a Saturday afternoon, being unjustly criticized by a supervisor, dealing with an insistent friend who wants to drink, dealing with unemployment, craving alcohol, and passing a familiar liquor store. These situations were chosen because automatic responses are unlikely to be effective; effective responses have a low likelihood of occurring, thereby requiring new learning and problem solving.

An evaluation of SBC with a sample of 40 adults with TBI was conducted as part of a collaborative project funded by the National Institute on Disability and Rehabilitation Research (NIDRR), and involving Employment Resources, Inc., and Vocational Consulting Services of Madison, Wisconsin, Advocap, Inc. of Oshkosh, Wisconsin, Curative Rehabilitation Center of Green Bay, Wisconsin, and the Rehabilitation Institute of Chicago (82). All subjects had sustained moderate to severe TBI and were receiving supported employment services. They completed the ASB as a precursor to their participation and again after program completion; a comparison group of 103 adults receiving no treatment also completed the ASB and neuropsychological measures. The SBC sample was 83% male, 97% white, and had a mean age of 33 years. History of substance abuse was reported in 56% of the SBC group. The 12-week counseling program and followup data were available for 75% of the original sample. The SBC group significantly increased in ASB-measured skillfulness from initial to followup assessment, while no change was observed in the no-treatment comparison group. The SBC group also changed their drinking patterns from before to 1 year after the commencement of counseling such that 24% became abstinent, compared to only 9% of the no-treatment control group; in fact, 40% of the control group continued to drink, as compared to 21% of the SBC group. These results support the potential effectiveness of SBC in preventing substance abuse in TBI patients with cognitive impairments.

Prevention of Alcohol and Other Drug Abuse for Persons with Disabilities

Rehabilitation professionals have not addressed the consequences of substance abuse for a variety of reasons. First, preservice training and accreditation standards are nonexistent. Rehabilitation specialists often feel unprepared to confront alcohol and drug use because of their limited educational background in substance-abuse assessment and treatment. Few graduate programs address substance abuse as integral to the training of a rehabilitation specialist. Similarly, no accreditation standards address substance-abuse prevention as an area of competence for a rehabilitation specialist. Thus, there are no accepted standards of performance.

Second, interdisciplinary training is limited. Rehabilitation specialists include, among others, psychiatrists, speech-language pathologists, physical and occupational therapists, and counseling and clinical psychologists, with each specialty focusing on its own training of optimizing physical, mental, or occupational functioning. Because training programs fail to address substance-abuse prevention for each rehabilitation discipline, clinicians frequently fail to detect, and consequently address, alcohol and drug problems in their practice. Therefore, teams of professionals may not deliver care in a coordinated manner. For instance, while a rehabilitation specialist attempts to address a problem client's substance abuse, the client's physician may inadvertently encourage abuse by failing to adequately monitor the use of prescription medications or by excusing alcohol use as an appropriate coping mechanism.

Third, an absence of quantifiable research data limits knowledge about the extent and consequences of substance use problems in rehabilitative populations, although advancements are being made. Some rehabilitation specialists argue that there is insufficient empirical evidence to clearly establish prevalence rates of misuse, and to support the claim that intervention will lead to improved rehabilitation outcomes. Although the body of research data is growing, studies of substance abuse and disability are relatively few, with little uniformity on sampling, data collection, and criteria for abuse and dependence (88). There are few long-term evaluations of the relationship between alcohol and other drug use and rehabilitation outcomes; however, the available evidence is consistent and compelling. Today, the vast majority of rehabilitation professionals have begun to recognize substance abuse as a clear and persisting problem for their clients, even though they may not feel qualified to address these problems.

Labeling substance abuse as a secondary disability may lead to a perception of it being less important than a physical disability or as a condition that can be addressed following medical rehabilitation and by another service provider. This attitude prevails even though substance abuse is frequently related to the cause of the disability in people who are intoxicated at injury onset. Gaps in service delivery also contribute to a perpetuation of alcohol and other drug-abuse problems, such as the lack of private or government insurance reimbursement for substance-abuse intervention services. Thus, many rehabilitation programs ignore the substance-abuse problems or offer collateral services at patients' expense through an outside provider. Unfortunately, the large gaps in community health delivery systems mean that most persons with disabilities never get treatment or prevention services. Finally, most substance-abuse professionals are unaccustomed to working with persons with disabilities, so fully accessible programs are rare.

Knowledge, attitudes, and professional behaviors related to substance abuse prevention are changing throughout the rehabilitation community. A few recent examples suggest the scope of current interest in this issue:

- *Interdisciplinary models for rehabilitation and substance abuse prevention:* Under grants from NIDRR and the J.M. Foundation, the Rehabilitation Institute of Chicago (RIC) developed a model approach for substance-abuse prevention as an integral part of medical rehabilitation. RIC's model recognizes the potential role of all rehabilitation professionals and is interdisciplinary in its structure and approach. Similar interdisciplinary models were developed at Ohio State University's TBI Network, Wright State University's Consumer Advisory Model program, the Medical College of Virginia for TBI patients, and the Sister Kenny Institute, among other sites across the country.
- *Vocational rehabilitation training system:* The Rehabilitation Services Administration (RSA) of the Department of Education awarded a contract to provide training on substance-abuse issues to vocational rehabilitation counselors. This training addresses the special challenges posed by vocational rehabilitation clients with dual disabilities and was offered through RSA's Regional Rehabilitation Continuing Education Program.
- *National policy and leadership development symposium:* In August 1991, the Institute on Alcohol, Drugs, and Disability brought together leaders in these fields to create action plans for implementing policies that were intended to improve access to prevention services for persons with disabilities. The *Symposium Report* provides a strategy for addressing the scope and complexity of the issue of substance abuse and disability (89). The second National Conference on Substance Abuse and Coexisting Disabilities brought together nearly 150 leaders in the fields of treatment, policy, research, and consumer advocacy to work toward consensus on issues that have the potential to improve recovery and employment services for individuals with multiple disabilities. Invited were representatives of consumer and disability advocacy groups, community-based organizations, government agencies, and academia. Proceedings of the conference are available at http://www.med.wright.edu/citar/sardi/rrtc_conference.html (last accessed 7/29/04).
- *The Resource Center on Substance Abuse Prevention and Disability* was created in 1990 when Very Special Arts Educational Services received a grant from the Federal Office for Substance Abuse Prevention. The Center attracted participation by the leading experts in the field, built a comprehensive library, developed and disseminated information, and formed coalitions between alcohol and drug prevention and rehabilitation as well as special education constituents. These national initiatives reflect growing attention to the issue to substance abuse and disability.

Pre-Service Education

Rehabilitation and chemical-dependency professionals play vital roles in understanding, recognizing, and addressing the substance-abuse problems of people with disabilities; therefore, training for these professionals regarding substance-abuse problems in disabled populations is a necessary step in remediating the current problem. Information designed to change the attitudes and knowledge of professionals is likely to lead to a change in rehabilitation practices.

Rehabilitation educators are implementing innovative programs to address the need for enhanced training on substance abuse issues in persons with disabilities. Programs such as the Rehabilitation Counselor Education program at New York University, which provides a specialty in chemical-dependence counseling, and the Hunter College/City of New York program, which offers specialization in chemical dependence, are closing the gap between training and need for education on substance-abuse issues for rehabilitation professionals. However, few disciplines outside of rehabilitation counseling offer such specialization.

In-Service Education

National needs for alcohol- and other drug-abuse education for rehabilitation professionals were investigated among members of the American Congress on Rehabilitation Medicine. A survey was conducted assessing members' knowledge of substance abuse, attitudes toward patients' substance use, and referral practices for patients with substance-abuse problems, with 37% (N = 1,211) of the eligible respondents completing the survey after two followup attempts (90). Respondents suspected that 29% of their patients with traumatic injuries had substance-abuse problems (90). Only 30% reported routine screening for alcohol and drug problems at their facilities (90). Substance-abuse education for staff was reported by 50% of respondents and patient education regarding substance abuse was reported by 59% (90). Although 79% of respondents reported having procedures at their facilities for making substance-abuse services referrals, only 44% reported actually making referrals, with the majority of referrals made to Alcoholics Anonymous (90). Thus, there is a need for enhanced in-service education regarding substance-abuse assessment and treatment, facility policies, and referral procedures.

An example of a substance abuse prevention education program for rehabilitation staff are the efforts made at RIC, in which the initial program described a theoretical context where staff could understand substance-use problems, categorized abusable drugs, reviewed the epidemiology of alcohol and other drug abuse, presented basic science information about alcohol abuse, described the nature of attitudes toward chemical use, reviewed hospital policies and procedures, and defined assessment and referral procedures (91). The 1-hour program was supplemented with printed materials. The effectiveness of the education program was evaluated with a questionnaire, which was administered prior to and 6 months following the presentation to assess changes in staff knowledge, attitudes, and behavior. Knowledge about substance abuse issues at 6 months after education was greater in attendees and nonattendees than at pretest, with greater improvement for staff that attended the training. Staff that attended the presentation reported making more referrals before and 6 months after the program than did staff that did not attend, and staff that made the most referrals after education were those who made more referrals prior to the program, who suspected more patients of preinjury substance abuse, and who had less experience in rehabilitation (91). The results of this study suggest that substance-abuse education should be provided to all rehabilitation team members to assure sufficient understanding of substance abuse issues and hospital policies and procedures related to patients' use of substances, and to improve the effectiveness of rehabilitation services.

Staff came to realize that issues of attitude change and program implementation required staff involvement at all levels of the organization. These early in-service efforts were expanded to include a task force composed of consumer and rehabilitation staff members under the auspices of the Midwest Regional Head Injury Center for Rehabilitation and Prevention and RIC. These efforts were made in collaboration with the Illinois Prevention Resource Center and with funding provided by the J.M. Foundation for a project titled, "Substance Abuse Prevention Programming for Patients Incurring Traumatic Injury." A major product of these efforts was a resource manual titled, "Alcohol and Other Drug Abuse Prevention for People with Traumatic Brain and Spinal Cord Injuries" (92). The manual provides an overview of substance-abuse prevention models, information about alcohol and other drug problems, and skill-development exercises for staff working with clients around coping issues. It employs a train-the-trainer model, which empowers staff trainers to work within their own departments to enhance department members' skills in dealing with alcohol- and other drug-abuse issues. Examples of implementing basic prevention strategies, including ways of involving and training impactors, providing information, developing life skills, creating alternatives to substance abuse, and influencing policies are provided.

A training program was assessed at the RIC, in which investigators examined if training on the importance of substance-abuse screening would result in consistent screening and referrals (93). Psychologists were more likely to refer individuals who were intoxicated at the time of injury than those who were not, but were less likely to provide referrals in response to family histories of substance abuse. Little time was spent directly addressing substance-abuse issues with patients and families. Lastly, referrals for substance-abuse prevention and intervention services were low, even after training. Approximately one-third of patients were referred to formal or informal treatment, and a small proportion accepted the referrals, suggesting a lack of comfort in referring and addressing substance-abuse issues with patients. Staff training needs to be ongoing and supportive in nature, and the attitudes and skills of rehabilitation professionals regarding substance-abuse screening and referrals need to be addressed (93).

Consumer Education

In the past several years, a variety of organizations emerged and resources developed that address alcohol- and other drug-abuse issues for persons with disabilities. A resource guide for persons with SCI and their families was developed entitled, *Inform Yourself: Alcohol, Drugs and Spinal Cord Injury*, with funding provided by the Paralyzed Veterans of America. The guide provides personal stories of addiction and recovery, a self-assessment tool, organizational contact for additional information, along with an extensive glossary and bibliography. Sam Maddox's *Spinal Network* has been described as the "total resource for the wheelchair community." The book covers medical, sports and recreation, travel, media, technology, sex, disability rights, legal and financial issues, and resource information in the United States and Canada. Substance-abuse issues are addressed in two sections of a "featured page" chapter. For persons who have sustained TBI, Robert Karol and Frank Sparadeo's (94) booklet, *Alcohol, Drugs and Brain Inj* provides an overview of alcohol and other drug effects, reproduces assessment tools, and helps consumers create an action plan for dealing with substance use and urges to use. Consumers can refer to the Ohio Valley Center for Head Injury Prevention and Rehabilitation's *User's Manual*, which addresses the cumulative effects of substance abuse for persons with TBI. The 16-page pamphlet provides a short quiz about the effects of alcohol and other drug abuse on persons with brain injury and uses a computer analogy to explain how learning is impaired. Both the National SCI Association and the Brain Injury Association, among others, included presentations for consumers about substance abuse at recent annual meetings, indicating the increasing awareness of the importance of consumer education. A variety of additional consumer resources are described by Wright State University's Substance Abuse Resources and Disability Issues (SARDI) Program (http://www.med.wright.edu/citar/sardi/index.html [last accessed 7/23/04]).

Other Resource Materials

The Substance Abuse Prevention Project at the Rehabilitation Institute of Chicago produced a training manual for medical rehabilitation professionals working with patients who have sustained traumatic brain injuries. Materials are suitable for group in-service education programs and include materials designed for family members and patients.

The Rehabilitation Research and Training Center designed the Substance Abuse Assessment and Education Kit for Severe Traumatic Brain Injury for professionals working in brain injury rehabilitation. Contents include clinical materials designed for assessment, research information, and plans to develop education and prevention policies and procedures.

The Center for Substance Abuse Prevention provides a Clearinghouse for Alcohol and Drug Information. Materials describe a full array of prevention topics, including those relevant to persons with physical, sensory, and developmental disabilities.

The Minnesota Chemical Dependence Program for Deaf and Hard of Hearing developed a 105-minute videotape for professionals entitled "Chemical Dependence—What Is It?," which is open captioned and sign language interpreted.

The Rochester Institute of Technology developed a directory listing 308 drug prevention and treatment programs for persons who are deaf. Program services include staff trained in American Sign Language and cultural issues, interpreters, closed caption equipment, teletext equipment, and accessible 12-step programs.

Baylor College of Medicine produced a videotape entitled "Substance Abuse in Rehabilitation Facilities—No Problem? Think Again" and a manual titled *Spinal Cord Injury: A Manual for Healthy Living* that focuses on a way to prevent complications.

REHABILITATION SETTING ISSUES

Agency Policies

Rehabilitation agency policy issues regarding possession and use of alcohol and drugs, including recreational or socialization programs that incorporate alcohol use, need to be clearly formulated in light of studies examining controlled drinking outcomes. Although moderate alcohol use is likely to pose a few problems for many persons, those with histories of substance abuse are at risk of relapse as a consequence of policies and programs that provide opportunities for alcohol consumption; persons with cognitive impairment resulting from brain trauma or other neurologic injury are at particular risk. Policies that provide for monitoring of psychoactive prescription medications obtained during or after hospitalization should also be considered. In short, the opportunity for abuse of prescribed medications and histories of alcohol or illicit drug use re-

quires case-by-case assessment of each patient's history as rehabilitation plans are made.

Staff Education

In-Service Education

Several educators and rehabilitation practitioners have advocated for the need for enhanced education on substance-abuse issues (95–102). Several clinical issues have not been addressed sufficiently in medical rehabilitation settings, with one of the most important being medication prescription misuse. Although the specific drugs misused may vary across clinical populations and reflect specific medical complications, continued monitoring in long-term prescription use in all disability populations, not only the chronic pain population, is necessary. Clinicians should attend to depression and poor psychological adjustment, which may underlie medical complications and may be associated with substance use. Physician, nursing, and allied health staff education should focus on recognizing prescription medication misuse and the reasons for misuse (103).

In addition to the in-service education materials listed above is *Substance Abuse and Adolescents with Disabilities*, produced by the Region II Rehabilitation Continuing Education Program at the State University of New York at Buffalo. It provides a detailed curriculum, complete with visual presentation materials (104). Topics addressed include models of chemical dependence, family system issues, how disability affects developmental issues, and implications for vocational counseling. Available from Wright State University's Substance Abuse Resources and Disability Issues (SARDI) Program is its *Training Manual*, which provides a compendium of educational materials for rehabilitation and chemical-dependence professionals about substance abuse and disability (105). Online ordering of several SARDI resources, including *Alcohol, Tobacco and Other Drug Prevention Activities for Youth and Adults with Disabilities*; *Chicago Hearing Society (CHS) Training Manual*; *Substance Abuse, Disability and Vocational Rehabilitation, Blindness*; *Visual Impairment and Substance Abuse*; and *Substance Abuse and Living with HIV/AIDS*, is available at http://www.med.wright.edu/citar/sardi/products.html (last accessed 7/24/04).

Basford and colleagues reported evidence of success in educating rehabilitation professionals about substance-abuse issues. In 2000, they surveyed physical medicine and rehabilitation training program directors regarding beliefs, attitudes, and policies toward tobacco, alcohol, and drug use. They contrasted their findings with a similar survey conducted 15 years previously (106). They found that substance-abuse issues are more likely to be recognized today than in 1985 and corresponding systemic changes had been implemented in institutions, including regular screenings and written guidelines, to increase detection and treatment for substance-abuse problems. Physiatry training programs are paying increasing attention to the potential overlap between substance use and physical disability.

Recommendations

Relatively few persons who sustain traumatic injury may realize a need for substance-abuse treatment. Such a perception may reflect individuals who are at relatively early stages of readiness for change (60). For some persons intoxicated at injury, the injury may illustrate the extent and consequences of their substance-use problems and motivate them to initiate action, which is consistent with Marlatt and Baer's (107) model of substance-use change. The belief that one does not need treatment, despite major trauma, can be understood as an aspect of denial or rationalization about the severity of drinking or drug problems. The importance of external agents, such as employers, courts, family, and physicians, in encouraging treatment is evidence in Heinemann and colleagues' (65) findings that these agents were most often cited as a reason for pursuing treatment. Clearly, the process of acknowledging substance abuse problems is developmental in nature; major injury does no more to cure drinking problems for some persons that does job loss, divorce, or other traumatic events.

Glass' (15) typology of problem drinkers is useful in planning prevention and treatment efforts. Knowing the etiology of substance abuse and whether it proceeded or followed disability is an important issue, as is assessing alcohol and drug use in the context of coping skills, in rehabilitation settings because of the evidence that predisability substance abuse places individuals at high risk for abuse after disability. Traumatic onset disability may provide an opportunity for some persons to recognize the gravity of their substance-abuse patterns and to make changes. While some persons may make changes on their own, others will continue to use and experience consequences of their use. The pernicious quality of addiction is illustrated by continued use after substance-use-related injury. It may be that some persons with preinjury drinking problems are representative of an early onset, type I drinking or drug-use pattern, which reflects a genetic component. The success of rehabilitation interventions that consider familial and personal drinking histories will probably be enhanced when interventions consider these factors.

Several implications for enhancing medical rehabilitation are evident. First, alcohol- and other drug-use assessment should be a routine component of all admissions to acute care and rehabilitation programs for persons incurring traumatic injury. Responsibility for this screening could be assumed by a variety of staff members, including physicians, nurses, psychologists, and social workers. Second, training team members to recognize alcohol and

other drug abuse is critical in enabling them to provide competent assessments. Substance-abuse treatment program professionals should consult with physical medicine and rehabilitation providers to acquire this knowledge. Third, referral networks to alcohol treatment programs are necessary if a potential dual disability is to be identified and treated in a timely fashion. Adequate communication links must be established so that chemical-dependence treatment programs and counselors learn about the special needs of persons with disabilities. Accessibility needs, functional abilities, and attitudes toward persons with disabling conditions are some of the topics that could be addressed in training programs for alcohol-abuse treatment personnel. Chemical-dependence treatment programs designed specifically for persons with physical disabilities are another treatment alternative (108–112).

CHEMICAL DEPENDENCE TREATMENT SETTING ISSUES

Chemical dependence professionals are often uninformed about the unique risks and needs of people with disabilities; consequently, they may be ill-prepared to provide appropriate treatment. Moreover, attitudes of professionals regarding what constitutes a primary and secondary disability influence treatment provision. If substance abuse is viewed as a secondary disability, then it may be considered less important than the primary disability. Thus, it may be left untreated. Chemical dependence and rehabilitation professionals need to appreciate the value of treating primary and secondary disabilities concurrently.

Implications of the Americans with Disabilities Act

The Americans with Disabilities Act of 1990 (ADA; Public Law 101–336) is one of the major civil rights laws passed since 1964. It addresses the severe disadvantages persons with disabilities experience in daily life. These advantages include intentional exclusion, overly protective policies and rules, segregation, exclusionary standards, and architectural, transportation, and communication barriers. The ADA is important for alcohol and other drug prevention programs because public accommodations, along with other social service, health care, and educational programs, must allow people with disabilities to participate fully.

Architectural Accessibility and Communication Issues

Accessibility of substance-abuse services involves physical, programmatic, and administrative components. Physical accessibility is enhanced by architectural modifications, such as ramps and Braille material. The use of sign language interpreters for persons with hearing impairments, staff training on disability issues, and modification of printed materials for persons with learning disabilities are examples of enhanced programmatic accessibility. Enhanced interagency coordination, advocacy for accessible transportation, and reduced attitudinal barriers are examples of administrative accessibility.

The New York State Office of Alcoholism and Substance Abuse Services' *Ad Hoc Task Force Report of Acquired Physical Disability and Chemical Dependency* (113) reported a study of services available to persons with disabilities at five New York City Health and Hospital Corporation hospitals. The report concluded that departments responsible for substance-abuse services did not have standard policies and procedures in place to identify, treat, and refer to aftercare treatment persons with comorbid physical disabilities and substance-abuse problems. Efforts in all states are needed to assure not only ADA compliance, but also equitable and effective services for persons with disabilities.

Attitudinal Barriers

As early as 1960, Wright (114) noted the power of language in conveying attitudes about persons with disabilities. Terms such as "handicapped," "afflicted with," "victim of," and "crippled" are often offensive to persons with disabilities. They draw our attention to what is different about the person rather than their basic decency as a human being. "Person first" language, such as "person with a spinal cord injury," "person who uses a wheelchair," or "person with developmental disability," emphasizes abilities rather than limitations. In-service education should include discussions of how to increase sensitivity to language and attitudes that exclude persons with disabilities from appropriate services.

Paraprofessional Training

Nondegreed paraprofessionals in recovery have served important roles in chemical-dependence treatment programs. Efforts to credential paraprofessionals include those of the New York Department of Employment, which developed a certificate program for persons in recovery from substance abuse. However, disability awareness training was only recently incorporated into these programs. In contrast, staff of independent living centers often have disabilities and use a peer-modeling approach in working with consumers. Consequently, they emphasize disability

rights, self-help, and self-advocacy, in contrast to traditional substance-abuse models that treat service recipients as patients. Federal support for consumer involvement in rehabilitation research and education activities is reflected in NIDRR's Long Range Plan and use of Participatory Action Research methods that promote relevance to consumers. Engaging individuals with disabilities in the training and certification programs of chemical dependence paraprofessionals could increase the accessibility of these programs and cross-training consumer advocates in both chemical dependence issues and disability rights would serve to increase individual levels of functioning.

Recommendations

The New York State Office of Alcoholism and Substance Abuse Services' *Ad Hoc Task Force on Acquired Physical Disability and Chemical Dependency* (113) made several specific training and accessibility recommendations. Training recommendations included: (a) helping rehabilitation staff to recognize chemical-dependency problems in rehabilitation and disability service delivery systems, (b) training chemical-dependency staff to recognize other disabilities, and (c) providing interdisciplinary education and training to staff working with people with acquired physical and chemical-dependence disabilities. Accessibility recommendations included: (a) making chemical dependence treatment more architecturally, programmatically, and administratively accessible, (b) developing guidelines and strategies in vocational rehabilitation agencies to enhance work with clients who have dual disabilities, (c) developing prevention strategies for clients with dual disabilities, and (d) developing community resources to serve clients with dual disabilities.

SUMMARY

Knowledge about the extent of substance abuse problems and the consequences of substance abuse in persons with disabilities has grown remarkably in the past two decades. Promising treatment and prevention programs have been evaluated. Professional education and program accessibility has increased. Continuing efforts are required in then next decade to assure that alcohol- and other drug-abuse services are made available to persons with disabilities in both rehabilitation and chemical-dependence settings.

REFERENCES

1. Yarkony G. Medical complications in rehabilitation. In: Heinemann A, ed. *Substance abuse and physical disability.* New York: Haworth, 1993.
2. Rasmussen G, DeBoer R. Alcohol and drug use among clients at a residential vocational rehabilitation facility. *Alcohol Health Res World* 1980;5:48–56.
3. Moore D, Li L. Substance use among applicants for vocational rehabilitation services. *J Rehabil* 1994;60:48–53.
4. Gilson SF, Chilcoat H, Stapleton JM. Illicit drug use by persons with disabilities: insights from the National Household Survey on Drug Abuse. *Am J Public Health* 1996;86:1613–1615.
5. Moore D, Li L. Prevalence and risk factors of illicit drug use by people with disabilities. *Am J Addict* 1998;7:93–102.

6. Fullerton D, Harvey R, Klein M, et al. Psychiatric disorders in patients with spinal cord injuries. *Arch Gen Psychiatry* 1981;38:1369–1371.

7. Lyons J, Larson D, Burns B, et al. Psychiatric co-morbidities and patients with head and spinal cord trauma. *Gen Hosp Psychiatry* 1988;10:292–297.

8. Trieschmann R. *Spinal cord injuries: psychological, social and vocational adjustment.* New York: Pergamon Press, 1980.

9. Wehman P, Kreutzer J. *Vocational rehabilitation after traumatic brain injury.* Rockville, MD: Aspen Publishers, 1990.

10. Murray P. Clinical pharmacology in rehabilitation. In: Caplan B, ed. *Rehabilitation psychology desk reference.* Rockville, MD: Aspen Publishers, 1987:501–525.

11. Heinemann A, Mamott B, Schnoll S. Substance use by persons with recent spinal cord injuries. *Rehabil Psychol* 1990;35:217–228.

12. Kiley D, Heinemann A. *The relationship between employment, substance abuse and depression following spinal cord injury.* Boston: American Psychological Association, 1990.

13. Kreutzer J, Harris J, Doherty K. *Substance abuse patterns before and after traumatic brain injury.* Presented at the 97th annual convention of the American Psychological Association, New Orleans, LA, 1989.

14. *Substance abuse task force white paper.* Southborough, MA: National Head Injury Foundation, 1988.

15. Glass E. Problem drinking among the blind and visually impaired. *Alcohol Health Res World* 1980;81:20–25.

16. A look at alcohol and other drug abuse prevention and blindness and visual impairments. Resource Center on Substance Abuse Prevention and Disability, 1992.

17. Nelipovich M, Buss E. Alcohol abuse and persons who are blind. *Alcohol Health Res World* 1989;13:128–131.

18. Boros A. Activating solutions to alcoholism among the hearing impaired. In: Schecter A, ed. *Drug dependence and alcoholism: social and behavioral issues.* New York: Plenum, 1981;1007–1015.

19. McCrone W. Serving the deaf substance abuser. *J Psychoactive Drugs* 1982;14:199–203.

20. Whitehouse A, Sherman R, Kozlowski K. The needs of deaf substance abusers in Illinois. *Am J Drug Alcohol Abuse* 1991;17:101–113.

21. Guthmann D, Blozis S. Unique issues faced by deaf individuals entering substance abuse treatment and fol-

lowing discharge. *Am Ann Deaf* 2001; 146:294–303.

22. Katon W, Egan K, Miller D. Chronic pain: lifetime diagnoses and family history. *Am J Psychiatry* 1985;142:1156–1160.

23. Fishbain D, Goldberg M, Meagher B, et al. Male and female chronic pain patients categorized by *DSM-III* psychiatric diagnostic criteria. *Pain* 1986;26:181–197.

24. American Psychiatric Association Committee on Nomenclature and Statistics. *Diagnostic and statistical manual of mental disorders.* Washington, DC: Author, 1987.

25. Kouyanou K, Pither C, Wessely S. Medication misuse, abuse and dependence in chronic pain patients. *J Psychosom Res* 1997;43:497–504.

26. Kouyanou K, Pither C, Rabe-Hesketh S, et al. A comparative study of iatrogenesis, medication abuse, and psychiatric morbidity in chronic pain patients with and without medically explained symptoms. *Pain* 1998;76:417–426.

27. Miotto K, Compton P, Ling W, et al. Diagnosing addictive disease in chronic pain patients. *Psychosomatics* 1996;37:223–235.

28. Green C, Flowe-Valencia H, Rosenblum L, et al. The role of childhood and adulthood abuse among women presenting for chronic pain management. *Clin J Pain* 2001;17:359–364.

29. Brown R, Fleming M, Patterson J. Chronic opioid analgesic therapy for chronic lower back pain. *J Am Board Fam Pract* 1996;9:191–204.

30. Atkinson J, Slater M, Patterson T, et al. Prevalence, onset, and risk of psychiatric disorders in men with chronic low back pain: a controlled study. *Pain* 1991;45:111–121.

31. Brown R, Patterson J, Rounds L, et al. Substance abuse among patients with chronic back pain. *J Fam Pract* 1996;43:152–160.

32. Gatchel R, Polantin P, Mayer T, et al. Psychopathology and the rehabilitation of patients with chronic low back pain disability. *Arch Phys Med Rehabil* 1994;75:666–670.

33. National Institutes of Health (NIH). *Rehabilitation of persons with traumatic brain injury.* NIH Consensus Development Conference, Bethesda, MD. Oct. 26–28, 1998.

34. Kalsbeek W, McLaurin R, Harris B, et al. The national head and spinal cord injury survey: major findings. *J Neurosurg* 1980;53:S19–S31.

35. Anderson D, Kalsbeek W. The national head and spinal cord injury survey: assessment of some uncertainties affecting the findings. *J Neurosurg* 1980:S32–S34.

36. Kraus J. *Epidemiology of head injury.* Baltimore: Williams & Wilkins, 1993.

37. Sosin D, Sniezek J, Waxweiller R. Trends in death associated with traumatic brain injury, 1979 through 1992: success and failures. *JAMA* 1995;272: 1778–1780.

38. Thurman D. Surveillance of TBI—Colorado, Missouri, Oklahoma, and Utah, 1990–1993. *MMWR Morb Mortal Wkly Rep* 1997;46:8–11.

39. Eker C, Schalen W, Asgeirsson B, et al. Reduced mortality after severe head injury will increase the demands for rehabilitation services. *Brain Inj* 2000;14:605–619.

40. Thurman D, Guerrero J. Trends in hospitalization associated with traumatic brain injury. *JAMA* 1999;282:954–957.

41. Miner M, Wagner K. *Neurotrauma—treatment, rehabilitation and related issues.* Boston: Butterworth, 1989.

42. Rimel R, Giordani B, Barth J, et al. Disability caused by minor head injury. *Neurosurgery* 1981;9(3):221–228.

43. Stone J, Lowe R, Jonasson O, et al. Acute subdural hematoma: direct admission to a trauma center yields improved results. *J Trauma* 1986;26:445–450.

44. Field J. *Epidemiology of head injuries in England and Wales.* London: Her Majesty's Stationary Office, 1976.

45. Sloan E, Zalenski R, Smith R, et al. Toxicology screening in urban trauma patients: drug prevalence and its relationship to trauma severity and management. *J Trauma* 1989;29:1647–1653.

46. Gale J, Dikmen S, Wyler A, et al. Head injury in the Pacific Northwest. *Neurosurgery* 1983;12:487–491.

47. Galbraith S, Murray W, Patel A, et al. The relationship between alcohol and head injury and its effects on the conscious level. *Br J Surg* 1976;63:128–130.

48. Rimel R, Giordani B, Barth J, et al. Moderate head injury: completing the clinical spectrum of brain trauma. *Neurosurgery* 1982;11:344–351.

49. Jagger J, Fife D, Vernberg K, et al. Effect of alcohol intoxication on the diagnosis and apparent severity of brain injury. *Neurosurgery* 1984;15:303–306.

50. Waller P, Stewart J, Hansen A, et al. The potentiating effects of alcohol on driver injury. *JAMA* 1986;256:1461–1466.

51. Brooks N, Campsie L, Symington C, et al. The effect of severe head injury on patient and relative within seven years of head injury. *J Head Trauma Rehabil* 1987;8:1–30.

52. Sparadeo F, Gill D. Effects of prior alcohol use on head injury recovery. *J Head Trauma Rehabil* 1989;4:75–82.

53. Walker R, Staton M, Leukefeld C. History of head injury among substance

users: Preliminary findings. *Subst Use Misuse* 2001;36:757–770.

54. Munsat T. *Statement of the American Academy of Neurology to the Interagency Head Injury Task Force.*

55. Albin M, Bunegin L. An experimental study of craniocerebral trauma during ethanol intoxication. *Crit Care Med* 1986;14:841–846.

56. Stonnington H. Traumatic brain injury rehabilitation. *Am Rehabil* 1987;13:4–20.

57. Barker L, Bigler E, Johnson S, et al. Polysubstance abuse and traumatic brain injury: quantitative magnetic resonance imaging and neuropsychological outcome in older adolescents and young adults. *J Int Neuropsychol Soc* 1999;5:593–608.

58. Kreutzer J, Witol A, Marwitz J. Alcohol and drug use among young persons with traumatic brain injury. *J Learn Disabil* 1996;29:643–651.

59. Bombardier C, Heinemann A. The construct validity of the Readiness to Change Questionnaire for persons with TBI. *J Head Trauma Rehabil* 2000;15:696–709.

60. Prochaska J, DiClemente C. Stages and processes of self-change in smoking: toward an integrative model of change. *J Consult Clin Psychol* 1983;51(3):390–395.

61. Sander A, Kreutzer J, Fernandez C. Neurobehavioral functioning, substance abuse and employment after brain injury: implications for vocational rehabilitation. *J Head Trauma Rehabil* 1997;12:28–41.

62. Baker KA, Schmidt MF, Heinemann AW, et al. The validity of the Katz Adjustment Scale among people with traumatic brain injury. *Rehabil Psychol* 1998;43:30–40.

63. National Spinal Cord Injury Statistical Center. *Facts and figures at a glance—May 2001.* Birmingham, AL: University of Alabama, 2001.

64. Frisbie J, Tun C. Drinking and spinal cord injury. *J Am Paraplegia Soc* 1984;7:71–73.

65. Heinemann A, Goranson N, Ginsburg K, et al. Alcohol use and activity patterns following spinal cord injury. *Rehabil Psychol* 1989;34:191–206.

66. Heinemann A, Schnoll S, Brandt M, et al. Toxicology screening in acute spinal cord injury. *Alcohol Clin Exp Res* 1988;12:191–206.

67. McKinley W, Kolakowsky S, Kreutzer J. Substance abuse, violence, and outcome after traumatic spinal cord injury. *Am J Phys Med Rehabil* 1999;78:306–312.

68. Heinemann A, Donohue R, Keen M, et al. Alcohol use by persons with recent spinal cord injuries. *Arch Phys Med Rehabil* 1988;69:619–624.

69. Johnson D. *Alcohol use by persons with disabilities.* Wisconsin Department of Health and Social Services, 1985.

70. National Institute on Drug Abuse. *National Household Survey on drug abuse: main findings—1988.* Rockville, MD: United States Department of Health and Human Services, 1990.

71. Bombardier C, Rimmele C. Alcohol use and readiness to change after spinal cord injury. *Arch Phys Med Rehabil* 1998;79:1110–1115.

72. Boraz M, Heinemann A. The relationship between social support and alcohol abuse in people with spinal cord injuries. *Int J Rehabil Health* 1996;2:189–198.

73. Hawkins D, Heinemann A. Substance abuse and medical complications following spinal cord injury. *Rehabil Psychol* 1998;43:219–231.

74. Elliott T, Kurylo M, Chen Y, et al. Alcohol abuse history and adjustment following spinal cord injury. *Rehabil Psychol* 2002;47:278–290.

75. Moore D, Polsgrove L. Disabilities, developmental handicaps and substance misuse: a review. *Int J Addict* 1991;26:65–90.

76. Cloninger C, Bohman M, Sigvardsson S, et al. Psychopathology in adopted-out children of alcoholics: the Stockholm Adoption Study. *Recent Dev Alcohol* 1985;3:37–51.

77. Heinemann A, Doll M, Schnoll S. Treatment of alcohol abuse in persons with recent spinal cord injuries. *Alcohol Health Res World* 1989;13:110–117.

78. Kolakowsky-Hayner S, Gourley E, Marwitz J, et al. Pre-injury substance abuse among persons with brain injury and spinal cord injury. *Brain Inj* 1999;13:571–581.

79. Cox W, Klinger E. A motivational model of alcohol use. *J Abnorm Psychol* 1988;97(2):178–180.

80. Cox W, Klinger E. Incentive motivation, affective change, and alcohol use: a model. In: Cox W, ed. *Why people drink: parameters of alcohol as a reinforcer.* New York: Gardener Press, 1990.

81. Cox W, Klinger E, Blount J. Alcohol use and goal hierarchies: systematic motivational counseling for alcoholics. In: Miller W, Rollnick S, eds. *Motivational interviewing: preparing people for change.* New York: Gardner Press.

82. Rehabilitation Institute of Chicago. *Substance abuse as a barrier to employment following traumatic brain injury.* National Institute on Disability Rehabilitation Research, 1995.

83. Cox W, Heinemann A, Miranti S, et al. Outcomes of systematic motivational counseling for substance use following traumatic brain injury. *J Addict Dis* 2003;22(1):93–110.

84. Miranti S, Schmidt M, Heinemann A. Systematic motivational counseling in rehabilitation medicine. In: Cox W, Klinger E, eds. *Handbook of motivational counseling: motivating people for change.* London: John Wiley & Sons (in press).

85. Langley M. Prevention of substance abuse in persons with neurological disabilities. *NeuroRehabilitation* 1992;2:52–64.

86. Goldfried M, D'Zurilla T. A behavior analytic method for assessing competence. In: Spielberger C, ed. *Current topics in clinical and community psychology.* Vol. 1. New York: Academic Press, 1969:151–196.

87. Heinemann AW, Corrigan JD, Moore D. Case management for TBI survivors with alcohol problems. *Rehabil Psychol* 2004;49(2):156–166.

88. Greer B. Substance abuse among clients with other primary disabilities: curricular implications for rehabilitation education. *Rehabil Educ* 1990;4:33–34.

89. Cherry L. *Summary report, alcohol, drugs, disability.* San Mateo, CA: National Policy and Leadership Development Symposium, Institute on Alcohol, Drugs, and Disability, 1991.

90. Kiley D, Heinemann A, Doll M, et al. Rehabilitation professionals' knowledge and attitudes about substance abuse issues. *NeuroRehabilitation* 1992;2:35–44.

91. Heinemann A, Kiley D, Shade-Zeldow Y, et al. *Chemical dependence education for rehabilitation professionals.* Phoenix, AZ: American Congress of Rehabilitation Medicine and the American Academy of Physical Medicine and Rehabilitation, 1990.

92. Midwest Regional Head Injury Center for Rehabilitation and Prevention. *Alcohol and other drug abuse prevention for people with traumatic brain and spinal cord injuries.* Rehabilitation Institute of Chicago, Illinois Prevention Resource Center, 1996.

93. Schmidt M, Heinemann A, Semik P. The efficacy of inservice training on substance abuse and spinal cord injury issues. *Top Spinal Cord Inj Rehabil* 1996;2:11–20.

94. Karol R, Sparadeo F. *Alcohol, drugs, and brain injury.* Loretto, MN: Vinland Center, 1993.

95. Greer B. Alcohol and other drug abuse by the physically impaired: a challenge for rehabilitation educators. *Alcohol Health Res World* 1989;13.

96. Moore D, Siegal H. Double trouble: alcohol and other drug use among orthopedically impaired college students.

Alcohol Health Res World 1989;13: 118–123.

97. Prendergast M, Austin G, deMiranda J. Substance abuse among youth with disabilities. *Prev Res Update* 1990;7: 1–54.

98. Beck R, Marr K. Identifying and treating clients with physical disabilities who have substance abuse problems. *Rehabil Educ* 1991;5:131–138.

99. Krause J. Delivery of substance abuse services during spinal cord injury rehabilitation. *NeuroRehabilitation* 1992;2:45–51.

100. Corrigan J. Substance abuse as a mediating factor in outcome from traumatic brain injury. *Arch Phys Med Rehabil* 1995;76:302–309.

101. Corrigan J, Lamb-Hart G, Rust E. A programme of intervention for substance abuse following traumatic brain injury. *Brain Inj* 1995;9:221–236.

102. Corrigan J, Rust E, Lamb-Hart G. The nature of extent of substance abuse problems in persons with traumatic brain injury. *J Head Trauma Rehabil* 1995;10:29–46.

103. Heinemann A, McGraw T, Brandt M, et al. Prescription medication misuse among persons with spinal cord injury. *Int J Addict* 1992;27:301–316.

104. Stewart E, Burganowski D, Larson D, et al. *Substance abuse and adolescents with disabilities.* Region II. Rehabilitation continuing education program. Buffalo, NY: State University of New York at Buffalo, 1992.

105. Moore D, Ford J. *Substance abuse disability and vocational rehabilitation issues training manual.* Dayton, OH: Wright State University School of Medicine, SARDI Center, 1996.

106. Basford J, Rohe D, Barnes C, et al. Substance abuse attitudes and policies in U.S. rehabilitation training programs: a comparison of 1985 and 2000. *Arch Phys Med Rehabil* 2002;83:517–522.

107. Marlatt G, Baer J. Addictive behavior: etiology and treatment. *Am Rev Psychol* 1988;39:223–252.

108. Langley M, Kiley D. Prevention of substance abuse in persons with neurological disabilities. *NeuroRehabilitation* 1992;2:52–64.

109. Sweeney T, Foote J. Treatment of drug and alcohol abuse in spinal cord injury veterans. *Int J Addict* 1982;17:897–904.

110. Lowenthal A, Anderson P. Network development: linking the disabled community to alcoholism and other drug abuse programs. *Alcohol Health Res World* 1980;81:16–17.

111. Anderson P. Alcoholism and the spinal cord disabled: a model program. *Alcohol Health Res World* 1980;81:37–41.

112. Kiley D, Brandt M. Issues and controversies in chemical dependence services for persons with physical disabilities. In: Heinemann A, ed. *Substance abuse and physical disability.* New York: Haworth, 1993;259–270.

113. Chemical Dependency Research Working Group. *Acquired physical disability, chemical dependency, Ad Hoc Task Force Report.* New York: Office of Alcoholism, Substance Abuse Services, 1994.

114. Wright B. *Physical disability: a psychological approach.* New York: Harper & Row, 1960.

CHAPTER 74

Physicians and Other Health Professionals

G. DOUGLAS TALBOTT AND
PHILIP O. WILSON

In the first half of twentieth century, medical doctors slowly and painstakingly acquired a special position in society as providers of health care services. Through a series of strategic efforts, the result was a profession that had gained autonomy, monopoly, and expertise over the practice of medicine (1). Physicians have the moral responsibility to care for their patients not only by direct care and precept, but also by the example of their lives and personal conduct. The misuse of alcohol and drugs by a member of the medical profession is an occupational, social, and personal problem that demands action to ensure early detection, treatment, and rehabilitation.

The majority of all health consumers are concerned about the effect alcohol and drug use by their physician could have on the quality of care they receive (2). Addiction to alcohol and other drugs of abuse has been a major concern of the profession ever since the initial American Medical Association (AMA) initiatives in the 1970s (3). The "sick doctor statute" (4) was a pioneering legislative effort to define the inability to practice medicine with reasonable skill and safety, and to revise grounds for professional discipline under the Medical Practice Acts of Florida. In 1973, the AMA Council on Mental Health published a landmark report, *The Sick Physician* (5). Two major recommendations were made by the Council in this report. First, state medical societies needed to establish programs or committees devoted to identifying and helping impaired physicians. Second, the AMA needed to develop model legislation to amend state medical practice acts so that treatment, rather than punitive disciplinary measures, could be made available.

Prior to the Council's report, two national surveys were conducted by the AMA. One asked state medical societies if they had a committee to deal with physicians who were addicted or psychiatrically impaired. Only seven states had such committees. The second survey examined disciplinary actions by three state boards of medical examiners. The Council concluded that little was being done to address the problem of physician impairment.

Extensive information has accumulated over the past two decades regarding the excessive use of alcohol and other drugs of abuse by physicians (6–9). Organized medicine has carefully and systematically begun to evaluate the extent to which drug addiction, alcoholism, and psychiatric disorders among doctors affect professional performance. The conceptualization of standard performance as a medical rather than legal, moral, or ethical problem has led to the development of programs and policies that integrate medical rehabilitation with professional peer review (10).

This chapter focuses primarily on physician impairment caused by chemical dependency because the preponderance of the literature addresses this particular issue. We identify assumptions underlying the concept of physician impairment; outline the characteristics of an impaired physician; describe the identification, intervention, treatment, rehabilitation, outcome monitoring, and the effectiveness of treatment; present the evolution, progress, and policies that links organized concern for sick doctors to social, legal, and political pressures of professional accountability; and document the practice of medical supervision of problem doctors in terms of its compatibilities with professional values and interests.

Today the nation's health care system is undergoing rapid and dramatic change, and a coming new century is shaping an irreversibly different style of medical practice. There is now increasing regulation for all levels of patient care, heightened peer review, changes imposed on the practice of medicine by managed care, and the emergence of the capability to micromonitor financial and professional performance information on individual physicians' activities. This review of the impaired physicians' movement has been undertaken at a time when the assessment of the social and cultural components of professional self-governance needs careful re-evaluation. In terms of both prevalence and identification, a historical perspective is useful.

HISTORICAL PERSPECTIVE

The proneness to seclusion, the slight peculiarities amounting to eccentricities at times (which to his old friends in New York seemed more strange than to us) were the only outward traces of the daily battle through which this brave fellow lived for years. When we recommended him as full surgeon to the hospital in 1890, I believed, and Welch did too, that he was no longer addicted to morphia. He had worked so well and so energetically that it did not seem possible that he could take the drug and do so much.

About six months after the full position had been given, I saw him in severe chills, and this was the first information I had that he was still taking morphia. Subsequently, I had many talks about it and gained his full confidence. He had never been able to reduce the amount to less than three grains daily; on this, he could do his work comfortably and maintain his excellent physical vigor (for he was a very muscular fellow). I do not think that anyone suspected him, not even Welch. (11)

Professor William Oster had chronicled, in *The Inner History of the John Hopkins Hospital,* in a small, locked, black book not opened until 1969, his observation and concerns for his friend and colleague, Professor William Stewart Halsted. This excellent identification of an opiate-addicted physician is classic, yet rarely taught to students

of medicine. The report by Paget (12) on the fate of 1,000 medical students, the articles by Mattison (13), Partlow (14), DeQuincy (15), and others (16–19), could well be used by medical educators to begin the study of substance-abuse prevention and occupational risk. Unfortunately, these writings instead have become a "beacon" for early public concern and scandal about pharmacologic excess by physicians.

After the Flexner report on medical education in the United States (20), state medical societies and legislatures began to regulate medical practice and pass laws and regulations requiring that physicians and surgeons be free of vice, moral turpitude, and the intemperate use of alcohol and drugs. In 1906, the U.S. Congress passed the Pure Food and Drug Act. This act marks the beginning of federal drug regulations (21). The Harrison Narcotics Act began the process of classifying, regulating, and controlling drugs that have a potential for abuse (22). It criminalized the use of certain drugs and forbade drug maintenance treatment.

In 1920, the English Parliament passed the Dangerous Drug Control Act (23) in an attempt to control addiction by the registration of addicts. Nearly 25% of registered addicts were doctors, dentists, nurses, or veterinary surgeons. In the United States, with Prohibition (24), the Marihuana Tax Acts (25), and the connection of drug use as a "Communist conspiracy" (during the McCarthy era), there was a gradual avoidance of alcoholism and addiction treatment by the medical profession. Until recently, many physicians viewed addiction as a legal and social issue rather than a medical illness. There has also been a relative absence of teaching and research about alcohol and drug dependence in medical schools until the last two decades. Negative attitudes still permeate much of the health care system as well as the general population.

PREVALENCE

The literature from the United States related to physician alcohol and drug problems from the mid-1950s to the mid-1980s consistently documented an apparent excess prevalence of these disorders (26). Reports of physician substance abuse from Britain, Germany, Holland, France, and Canada (18,27–35) from the same study period consistently revealed higher-than-expected rates of physician addiction. An excellent article by Brewster (33) reviewed the existing, mostly English, written literature to estimate the prevalence of drug and alcohol problems among physicians. She concluded that "extreme statements regarding the prevalence of physician problems with alcohol and other drugs have been made without firm empirical supports. The principal conclusion was that the prevalence of substance abuse among practicing physicians is unknown. She noted that when alcohol and other drugs are considered together, practicing physicians may not be unusually likely to have such problems, and prevalence may be no higher than that of the general population.

Hughes et al. (34) used a mailed, anonymous, self-report survey on a sample of 9,600 physicians, stratified by specialty and career stage, and randomly selected from the AMA master file. They concluded that the higher prevalence of alcohol use among physician respondents was more likely a consequence of their socioeconomic class than their profession. Hughes et al. commented on the high rate of reported self-treatment with controlled substance by the study group. Because of inherent methodological issues of the study design, this investigation could not have overestimated the prevalence of substance use or chemical dependence in the total physician population.

Several major surveys in the United States and internationally have assessed the prevalence of substance abuse and dependence disorders within the general population. One of the largest surveys measuring psychiatric and substance use epidemiology is the National Institute of Mental Health's Epidemiologic Catchment Area program (ECA) (35). Data from the ECA provide information regarding diagnoses of substance abuse and dependence according to criteria from the *Diagnostic and Statistical Manual of Mental Disorders,* 3rd edition revised (36). The overall rates for alcohol disorders from the ECA survey data were 13.5% (37) for lifetime prevalence. The lifetime prevalence for men was 23.8%, and for women it was 4.7% (38). The ECA surveys reported an overall lifetime prevalence of drug abuse and drug dependence of 6.2% (39). The lifetime prevalence for illicit drug disorders for men in the study population was 7.7%, and for women was 4.8% (38).

Currently, there are more than 700,000 physicians in the United States. Based on ECA data, an estimated 100,000 physicians will have alcohol disorders during their lifetime.

Physicians are believed to have essentially the same incidence and prevalence rates for alcohol and drug abuse and dependence disorders as the general population. There are no published scientific studies that measure the damage done by physician substance abuse and dependence. However, chemical dependency does appear to be the single most frequent disabling illness for the medical professional and poses a major problem for the profession (40) and society alike.

ETIOLOGY

There is no evidence to support the existence of a premorbid "professional" personality type that predisposes a physician to addiction. There is also no evidence that medicine selects those with special risk for addiction. Who then is at risk for becoming addicted? Vailant et al. (41) reported psychological vulnerabilities, including passivity and self-doubt, dependency, and pessimism. Physicians whose childhood and adolescence were unstable also appear to have excess risk of addiction. A narcissistic personality type (42), non-Jewish ancestry and lack of religious affiliation (43), nicotine dependence of more than one pack per day, the regular use of alcohol, the history of alcohol-related difficulties, and a family history of alcoholism, substance-dependence, and/or mental illness are risk factors (44). Jex et al. found that certain specialty groups and physicians in academic medicine appear to have risk for addiction (45). Hughes at el. (34) found, by comparison with controls, that physicians are five times more likely to take sedatives and minor tranquilizers without medical supervision, and Vailant (46) has stated that self-prescribing and (self-treatment with prescription drugs) is a risk factor for chemical dependents.

McAuliffe et al. (47) listed risk factors as (a) access to pharmaceuticals, (b) family history of substance abuse, (c) emotional problems, (d) stress at work or at home, (e) thrill seeking, (f) self-treatment of pain and emotional problems, and (g) chronic fatigue. Talbott et al. (48) reviewed the medical records of 1,000 physicians with chemical dependence and concluded that ages, specialty, drug access, genetic predisposition, stress and poor coping skills, the lack of education regarding substance abuse, the absence of effective prevention and control strategies, drug availability in the context of permissive professional and social environments, and denial are risk factors for physician substance abuse. Wright (6) postulated that physicians who have excess risk for addiction are those with a history of illicit substance use (including self-prescribing of controlled substances), those in high-risk specialties, those who have a pattern of overprescribing, those with an urge to succeed in an academic setting, those who overwork, and those who have the combined problems of grandiosity and excessive guilt.

Physicians may be no more at risk for addiction than the general population. No study has specially looked at the genetic predisposition, the psychobiology of craving, the relationship of classically conditioned factors, brain reward mechanisms, and psychodynamic factors, and sociocultural determinants of addiction in physicians by comparison with nonphysician peers.

IDENTIFICATION

Detection of the chemically dependent physician is often delayed by the ability of the physician-patient to protect job performance at the expense every other dimension of their lives. Clinical studies (49,50) suggest the order in which addiction-related injury occurs: family, community, finance, spiritual and emotional health, physical health, and, finally, job performance. As with any potentially fatal illness, early detection is critical. Identification of the physicians who are afflicted with substance abuse and the disease of chemical dependence follow a sequential course. The family is affected first. The work arena, particularly the hospital, is the last place that drug use by the physician is apparent. Identifiable signs and symptoms can be listed as follows.

Family

1. Withdrawal from family activities, unexplained absences.
2. Spouse becomes a solicitous caretaker.
3. Fights, dysfunctional anger, spouse tries to control physician's substance abuse.
4. Disease of "spousaholics": isolated, angry, physically and emotionally unable to meet the demands of the addict's illness, the grieving loner.
5. Child abuse.
6. Children attempt to maintain normal family functioning.
7. Children develop abnormal, antisocial behavior (depression, promiscuity, runaways, substance abuse).
8. Sexual problems: impotence, extramarital affairs.
9. Spouse disengages, abuses drugs and alcohol, or enters recovery.

Community

1. Isolation and withdrawal from community activities, church, friends, leisure, hobbies, and peers.
2. Embarrassing behavior at clubs or parties.
3. Driving under the influence of alcohol (DUI), legal problems, role-discordant behaviors.
4. Unreliable and unpredictable in community and social activities.
5. Unpredictable behavior: excessive spending, risk-taking behaviors.

Staff and Employment Applications: Clues from Curriculum Vitae

If any three of these items are present on a job application, suspicion index is high.

1. Numerous job changes in past 5 years.
2. Frequently relocated geographically for unexplained reasons.
3. Frequent hospitalizations.
4. Complicated and elaborate medical history.
5. Unexplained time lapse between jobs.
6. Indefinite or inappropriate medical references and vague letter of reference.
7. Working in an inappropriate job for individual's qualifications.
8. Decline of professional productivity.

Physical Status

1. Personal hygiene deteriorating.
2. Clothing and dressing habits deteriorate.

3. Multiple physical signs and complaints.
4. Numerous prescriptions and drugs.
5. Frequent hospitalizations.
6. Frequent visits to physicians and dentists.
7. Accidents and trauma.
8. Serious emotional crisis.

Office

1. Appointments and schedule become disorganized, progressively late.
2. Behavior to staff and patients hostile, withdrawn, unreasonable.
3. "Locked door" syndrome.
4. Ordering excessive supply of drugs from local druggists or by mail order.
5. Patients begin to complain to staff about doctor's behavior.
6. Absence from office: unexplained or frequently sick.

Hospital

1. Making late rounds or inappropriate abnormal behavior.
2. Decreasing quality of performance in staff presentations, writing in charts, and the like.
3. Inappropriate orders or overprescribing medications.
4. Nurses, secretaries, orderlies, licensed practical nurses (LPNs) reporting behavioral changes: "hospital gossip."
5. Involved in malpractice suits and legal sanctions against the physician or hospital.
6. Emergency room staff reports: unavailability or inappropriate responses to telephone calls.
7. Failure or prolonged response to paging.
8. Reluctance to undergo immediate physical examination or do urine drug screens on request.
9. Heavy drinking at staff functions.

Early identification and diagnosis are critical. Barriers to early diagnosis are the conspiracy of silence and denial by family, friends, peers, and even the patients. Often one hears such statements by a patient as, "I'd rather have Doc Jones drunk as my physician than any other doc I know." Such barriers are products of lack of education concerning the true nature of the primary, psychosocial, and biogenetic disease of addiction. They demonstrate lack of training in early diagnosis and detection of addiction in physicians. It is significantly more difficult to identify and diagnose female physicians than male physicians (51,52). Gender attitudes, female metabolism, and cultural factors concerning females account for some of these difficulties.

INTERVENTION

Chemically dependent individuals rationalize their avoidance of treatment. Denial is an almost universal characteristic of the disease of addiction. Denial absolves the physician-patient of personal accountability. At the same time, denial (both the deliberate, conscious deception and the unconscious defense mechanism) fills the addicted physician with guilt, shame, and remorse, so that most addicted physicians cannot reach out for help. It is the nature of the disease for the denial system to progress as the addiction gains control over the individual's functioning. This distortion of the truth is an unconscious defense stand that the illness is treatable. An intervention should never be done alone.

A Trained and Experienced Intervention Leader

Proper preparation for an intervention is essential. The interventionist must select individuals to do the intervention, train the intervenors to present relevant information to the physician-patient, set goals for the intervention, and expedite the prompt referral for recommended treatment.

Selection of the Intervention Site

The site of the intervention needs to be nonthreatening and quiet. Time and experience have taught that an early morning intervention prior to the intake of alcohol or other drugs by the physician is best accomplished in the patient's home with the cooperation of the spouse and children. Occasionally, guilt and shame are present to such a degree that intervention needs to be away from the home at some neutral site. Some spouses believe that their participation in an intervention will result in divorce. If the spouse is not convinced that addiction is a progressive, potentially fatal, but treatable illness affecting the entire family, it may be wise to exclude the spouse from the intervention. It is necessary that all members of the intervention team present a strong cohesive explanation of the problem.

Intervention Goals Must Be Established

This needs to be done in advance, understood, and accepted by all intervention team members. Intervenors must decide what choices they will give the physician-patient and what they will commit to if the physician-patient refuses all offers of help. Frequently, the perception of reality is grossly distorted by the effects of alcohol and drugs on the brain. Intervenors need to review the pain and consequences they have experienced as a result of the addict's substance abuse. No attempt at intervention is a failure because the seed has been planted. The impaired physician may reject, refuse, or even elope from the intervention, but the physician will recognize that his or her support systems are aware of the impairment and concerned about the physician.

Factual Data

It is critical that the data be factual and documented. Previous gossips or innuendoes may reduce the chances of having a successful intervention. The intervention team members should write down and present to the physician-addict their experiences of the addiction-influenced behaviors. The addicts should be told why the intervention is necessary, along with the legal, social, personal, health-related, and professional implications of their illness. The team needs to also consider presenting the advocacy/immunity regulations within the state, should the individual voluntary seek the appropriate treatment as a result of the intervention.

Adequate Intervention Time

Intervention sometimes must be repeated. Extremely important is the fact that the individual not feel rushed during the intervention and that adequate time is allowed. The doctor should not be intoxicated. An intervention done after an addiction-precipitated crisis frequently is likely to be successful. If the physician-patient refuses recommended help, the interventionist may negotiate a behavioral contract, so that with the next relapse or crisis, another intervention can be swiftly initiated.

Rehearsals

Careful planning including rehearsal is critical. Each individual of the intervention team must know and practice their roles and what they will say during their intervention. Anticipation of the doctor-patient's reaction including hostility and flight needs to be anticipated and plans for this complication provided. No matter what the intervention outcome is, it is important that the intervention team regroup and process their feelings and thoughts about the intervention. Some interventions fail. A cohesive team can develop an action plan for the next time the addicted doctor is in an addiction-precipitated crisis.

At the conclusion of the successful intervention, the physician-patient will follow the recommended assessment, treatment, or both. Referral options, transportation, and an action plan should be in place before the intervention is begun. The authors have seen more than one intervention that seemed successful, but the doctor negotiated his or her own arrangements that enabled suicide.

ASSESSMENT

Interventionists, most state medical society impaired-physician committees, and many state licensing boards recommend a comprehensive assessment in a specified treatment facility for impaired physicians to determine the extent of illness and the individual's treatment needs.

Physicians who voluntarily seek the recommended treatment after assessment, successfully complete their treatment, and enter into their state medical society-sponsored monitoring program frequently receive advocacy in lieu of punitive sanctions. Ideally, the recovering physician will allow the experienced treatment team to make the best choices about their recovery, rather than to treat themselves or undertreat their illness. The five teams are as follows:

The Medical Team

This team is headed by a physician who is trained in addiction medicine. These individuals are certified, knowledgeable, and experienced in addiction medicine and are trained to identify and treat the medical consequences of alcohol and drug abuse. They perform a detailed history and physical examination and order the appropriate diagnostic and confirmatory laboratory, radiologic, and other needed examinations. Inherent in the functioning of the medical team is appropriate consultations for specific medical complications (54,55).

Addiction Medicine Team

This is headed by a certified addiction medicine specialist. Trained to diagnose and recommend a range of addiction medicine services, these individuals provide needed detoxification services after a comprehensive addictive disease assessment is obtained. They evaluate the psychological behavioral effects of the drugs that have been used by the patient, assess addiction severity from a biopsychosocial perspective, and collect information from the individual support system members (including intervention team members) to validate the physician-patient's history. A rapid data acquisition effort, followed by presentation of the information the physician-patient and family, is often critical for rapidly decompressing the impaired physician's denial system.

Psychiatric Team

Events of recent years have made it apparent that the disciplines of addiction medicine and psychiatry must work in concert for the benefit of the addicted physician. Addicted patients frequently manifest multiple addictions and psychiatric problems simultaneously (56). Consequently, a comprehensive psychiatric assessment is a critical component of any assessment of an alcohol- and/or drug-addicted individual. It is necessary to determine if a definitive psychiatric diagnosis is present, or if there is a working differential diagnosis, contingent upon further evidence and reevaluation. Treatment evaluation research documents that untreated dual-diagnosed patients are more likely to relapse after treatment than addictive patients without psychiatric comorbidity (57).

The Neuropsychological Team

The addicted physician may appear cognitively unimpaired in the clinical interview. However, neuropsychological testing will often reveal significant deficits in reasoning memory (58). After focused clinical interviews, psychological test should involve the Halstead-Reitan Neuropsychological Battery (HRNB) test, which can include the Booklet Category Test, Tactile Performance Test, Reitan-Indiana Aphasia Screening Test, the Trailmaking Test, Reitan-Klove Sensory Examination, and the Seashore Rhythm Test. Useful adjuncts to the HRNB test include the Wechsler Adult Intelligence Scale (WAIS), Wechsler Memory Scale Revised (WMS-R), the Graham-Kendal Memory for Design Test, Minnesota Multiphasic Personality Inventory (MMPI), the Millon Clinical Multiaxial Inventory (MCMI), and the Rorschach Test. Often missed in standard evaluations or in less-robust specific psychological testing, neuropsychological deficits may become apparent with more-sensitive evaluation techniques.

Family Therapy Team

The family is critical to the program's treatment and monitoring of addicted patient. Interviews with the main significant other, children, parents, and siblings are diagnostically very helpful. Enlistment of these individuals in the treatment and recovery program is coordinated by the family therapists.

Assessments are done ideally in the hospital or partial hospitalization programs where close and constant observation allows documentation of withdrawal symptoms, medical symptoms, and complications. This method also allows detection of self-medication by physician-patients. Team members see the patient for testing and evaluations. Such assessments are done independently by each team member. The team then meets for discussion of diagnosis and treatment recommendations. Differences of diagnoses are discussed and resolved. It is in this forum that lateral information from other sources, particularly from the family therapist and the addiction medicine team member, becomes critical. Obviously, informed consent must be obtained from the patient to gain this information. Finally, a primary Axis I diagnosis, as well as subdiagnoses, are arrived at by team members. A detailed plan of treatment is then recommended.

The team then meets with the patient. It is useful to have the referral source and/or family members available for the diagnostic therapeutic recommendations of the assessment team.

If treatment is indicated, adequate time should be provided for questions and answers from the patient and the patient's family. Often the patient and the patient's family are given a choice of two or three facilities for treatment. Likewise, various alternatives for treatment should be discussed, as well as the problems that may be anticipated if the patient refuses treatment. The assessment team is not in a position, and should not ever comment on, the licensure or Drug Enforcement Agency (DEA) consequences, as these are determined by the appropriate organizations. The assessment and treatment team must present themselves as advocates for the physician-patient, not as prosecutors. Assurance of patient confidentiality is of the highest priority.

TREATMENT

The treatment of the impaired physician has many special features that combine the highest clinical standards and serve as a benchmark for the field of addiction medicine. Commonly accepted goals of treatment include (a) abstinence from alcohol and other nonprescribed psychoactive substances and (b) identification of the biopsychosocial treatment modality to which the patient's severity of illness will be matched. Treatment centers specialized in the care of chemically dependent physicians provide levels of care based on the American Society of Addiction Medicine (ASAM) patient placement criteria. These levels are labeled to be descriptive of the intensity of services provided: Level I, outpatient treatment; Level II, intensive outpatient/partial hospitalization; Level III, medically monitored inpatient treatment; and Level IV, medically managed inpatient treatment (54).

The outstanding treatment centers specializing in impaired physicians programs have learned that malignant denial is characteristic of this group of alcoholics and drug addicts. Defined as denial that is deeply inculcated in professional training, this type of denial can complicate early recovery. For addicted physicians, malignant denial appears to be a strong factor in the failure of outpatient treatment alone. While some impaired physicians have attained true sobriety with intense and focused long-term attendance in 12-step self-help groups such as Alcoholics Anonymous (AA), the most successful programs in the past decade are the residential outpatient programs that have adequate time to work through such denial (see "Treatment Outcome" below). Outpatient programs, by themselves, without either long-term treatment or the residential component, are not very successful in either the Oklahoma (59) or the Oregon (60) experience. Successful treatment of the impaired physicians has revealed several significant elements.

Understanding and Acceptance of the Disease Concept

For the impaired physician to both understand and to accept that he or she has a primary biopsychosocial genetic disease has proven to be the most critical and elementary aspect of recovery. Acceptance of the disease concept can quickly begin the absolution of the guilt, shame, and fear that are the inevitable companion of the impaired physician. Initially, this is accomplished by education. Understanding of this disease of addiction dispels the shame. Compulsivity is a primary symptom of chemical dependence. Recovering physicians must be carefully schooled in the neurobiochemistry of addiction and the medical and sociocultural consequences of their disease. Only then can they be taught that they are not responsible for their disease, but they are responsible for their recovery. Impaired physicians can understand the disease model intellectually, but to accept this concept in depth requires time and the proper environment. Impaired physicians must be helped to understand their addictive disease and the fact that they can't think their way into sober living; they must live their way into sober thinking. Physicians, by training, wish to solve all their problems intellectually, but addiction is not an intellectual disease. This has been apparent, since a physician (Dr. Bob) and a stockbroker turned counselor (Bill W.) stated in June 1935 that alcoholism was an illness of mind, body, and soul (61) and founded Alcoholics Anonymous (AA). Knowledge and acceptance of this disease has proved to he a primary element in recovery.

Identification of the Trigger Mechanisms

Appreciating that abuse plus the genetic predisposition will produce the disease, identification of triggers that produce abuse is critical to recovery. Research into the psychology of craving, the classically conditioned factors in addiction and brain reward mechanisms, has demonstrated that such triggers can involve a variety of emotional, personal, physical, and situational stresses. Each impaired physician must, over a period of time, with education and counseling identify his or her own triggers. With personal knowledge of triggers for alcohol and drug use, the physician-patient can begin to learn more about relapse thinking and behavior, and develop coping skills to prevent relapse.

Nonchemical Coping

Chemically impaired health professionals have become dependent upon coping with emotional, situational, and physical pain by using mood-altering drugs. Basic to the recovery process is the development and use of a nonchemical coping way of life that includes social, environmental, dietary, and lifestyle practices. For example, one of the most troublesome symptoms in the chemically dependent is insomnia. These individuals should be taught that this common withdrawal symptom must be dealt with by nonchemical coping mechanisms such as (a) abstinence from trying to fall asleep and then 2-hour increments of planned insomnia time (pit) where planned activities are scheduled prior to going to sleep the evening before; (b) small, balanced, multiple feedings during the day;

(c) abstinence from caffeine and nicotine, a diminution in salt, and high protein intake; (d) a prescribed time for trying to fall asleep and then 2-hour increments of planned insomnia time (pit) where planned activities are scheduled prior to going to sleep the evening before; (e) hot baths; (f) massage; (g) light reading; (h) counseling every evening so as to anticipate the coming night and periods of activity during planned insomnia time; (i) charting the insomnia activities of the night before, trying to relate them to specific thought processes; and (j) reading books or listening to tapes about insomnia.

These simple nonchemical coping methods can be applied to a wide variety of emotional, situational, and physical problems for the impaired health professional. Individuals can be taught such nonchemical coping activities to help them deal with emotional problems and situational problems such as divorce, malpractice suits, anxiety, grief, guilt, depression, anger, relationships, and loss of job, and physical crisis, such as stroke, cancer, heart disease, or accidents. Consequently, the impaired health professional must develop a multitude of nonchemical coping skills and capabilities that will allow them to deal with these crisis situations. For all of their professional lives, physicians have been taught that drugs and chemicals are a powerful part of their therapeutic armamentarium, and this requires "extended unlearning" procedures and practices on their part.

Balance in Changing Priorities

By virtue of their selection of their life work and their training, many impaired physicians put their professional lives and their physician's work as a priority before everything else. Almost by definition, they are both workaholics and perfectionists. For many, this behavior becomes a major "trigger" for substance abuse to relieve their stress. If the biogenetic predisposition is there in the face of this abuse, then disease is likely to occur. Sixty years ago, the founders of AA defined addiction as a multifactorial disease (61). Recovery depends upon medical, emotional, and spiritual growth. A large asset in recovery is balancing of these three elements. The impaired physician is taught that recovery and growth are first, family is second, and his or her profession is third. Leisure time and fun are critical to recovery, yet many impaired physicians have lost the ability to have fun and have forgotten how to play. They have lost the balance in their life. Therefore, balance between work, play, and a spiritual life must be restored, as well as a reordering of life's priorities. This tenet is essential to the recovery of the impaired physician.

Family Involvement

The family is critical in the diagnostic process, as well as in the recovery and therapeutic processes. Most often the family knows of the disease long before peers, friends, or individuals in the professional's office or in the hospital. For coming from a diagnostic standpoint, the signs and symptoms of individual health professionals, impairment must be familiar to the family. It is important to initiate family therapy, couples therapy, and educational workshops as soon as possible in the treatment process. Families should be encouraged to participate in 12-step self-help groups designed to help family members. An important component of the continuing care process is contracting between the impaired health professional and his or her family. This contract details each person's role in the recovery process and what happens if relapse occurs.

If the family is involved initially in the recovery process, it can be a powerful factor in recovery. The main significant other, as well as the children, suffer from the disease as they have the illness of "childolics," "siblingolics," and "parentolics." Their pain and discomfort must be dealt with in a manner that shows them how to help the alcoholic and addicted physician, as well as how to help themselves. Basic to this aid is their own understanding and acceptance of the disease and specific suggestions as to how they can modify their own responses and behaviors toward the recovering physician who returns home after treatment.

Mutual Help Groups

Successful health professional's programs demonstrated the use of 12-step programs. Careful study and acceptance of each of these 12-steps and then translating that into elements of the recovery program has proved particularly successful in health professionals. A frequent major barrier to recovery is the health professional's difficulty in understanding the dynamics of the 12-step program. This is not purely an intellectual process. By attending numerous programs with their peers, the health professional will accept the effectiveness of the 12-step program. This peer group therapy with health professionals can be helped by the Caduceus Clubs. The first Caduceus Club was established by the authors in Georgia, in 1974, to be a bridge into AA. When trying to encourage physicians to attend a meeting, calling it an Alcoholics Anonymous meeting would result in denial; the physicians would say, "I am not an alcoholic." However, they would come to a medical meeting in which the effects of alcohol and drugs were discussed without first erecting a barrier of denial. There are now more than 95 Caduceus Clubs in North America, each with its own format. The vast majority of Caduceus Clubs have led directly into mutual help group meetings or formats that mimic the traditional 12-step programs. In health professionals, the understanding of the 12-step program differentiating from acceptance, presents a major barrier to recovery in many of the health professionals. The value of the 12-step program integrated into a long-term extended care program is apparent because it is available in almost all locales and available throughout a 24-hour period of time. In the past 5 years, International Doctors in Alcoholics Anonymous, with a membership exceeding 3,000 members, has been a very valuable asset, particularly for networking with individual state's physicians health programs. The merit of the 12-step program is that it is widely available, functions at all times of the day and night, offers group support, is supportive, and is free; 12-step programs are found worldwide, functioning in almost every country. The off-shoot of the 12-step programs in the United States has been the International Doctors in Alcoholics Anonymous, which is confined to health professionals with degrees. It is a growing organization that is run by Dr. Gordon Hyde in Lexington, Kentucky.

Aftercare and Monitoring

The planning of aftercare and monitoring should start from the first day of treatment and should involve the family and all other support systems of the impaired physician.

The treatment team should be experienced in dealing with impaired physicians and other health professionals. They need to be experienced in setting firm limits and boundaries, and they need to be experienced with the specific needs (both legal and professional) in treating the impaired physician. They should be familiar with the National Practitioner Data Bank, malpractice insurance, DEA certification, and issues of state medical licensures. These professionals also need to be experienced with specific drug therapies, such as naltrexone and disulfiram (Antabuse). They need to be skilled at helping to solve reentry problems once the patient returns to work, and they need to be available for frequent consultation.

TREATMENT OUTCOME

The primary goal of treatment is to help the physician-patient achieve and maintain long-term remission of his or her addictive disease (62). Reported recovery rates vary considerably, with reported rates for complete abstinence from mood-altering substances ranging from 27% (63) to 92% (64). The interpretation of treatment outcomes, however, requires explanation.

Many methodological problems (65) exist when comparing different outcome studies of physicians who have been treated for chemical dependence. Some notable differences among investigations Are as follows:

1. Patient selection bias; some study populations include other health professionals such as nurses, dentists, and medical students.
2. Significant differences in the type, intensity, and length of time of treatment given. (There is no standard way to

retrospectively evaluate intensity, quantity, and quality of treatment.)
3. Authors rely on self-reports from physician-patients about abstinence versus relapse.
4. Positive urine drug test results are based on random urine drug screens to be done within 24 hours of the recovering physician's notification. (Alcohol and some drugs of abuse taken a day or two before notification might not be detected.)
5. Reliance on inadequate or incomplete diagnostic criteria in choosing subjects for study.
6. Failure to adequately account for treatment dropouts in the analysis of treatment outcome data.
7. Failure to follow patients for adequate lengths of time posttreatment.
8. Failure to provide for adequate, multidimensional treatment outcome measures that map a full range of patient behavior.

These methodological differences have made meta-analysis impossible. However, there has been a steady progression in the cohesiveness of findings in all investigations published in the last decade. Physicians appear to have better treatment outcomes than the general population when long-term aftercare and monitoring is done. There are also sufficient data to conclude that most physicians can be successfully rehabilitated and able to reenter medical practice with reasonable skill and safety to their patients.

Reading (66) reported that after 2 years of program involvement and formal treatment, New Jersey physicians had a recovery rate of 83.8% with no relapses, and 13.8% had one relapse. He concluded that the success rate of 97.6% was related to the formal, frequent, and structured outpatient counseling. In addition, the structured urine monitoring program, 12-step participation, family involvement, validity checks by responses other recovering physicians and/or physician monitors from the index) physician's community, and monthly face to-face contacts with the Physicians Health Program staff, are necessary components of an effective Physicians Health Program (PHP).

Gallegos et al. (67) studied 100 physicians who subsequently entered into a continuing care contract with the Georgia Impaired Physicians program between July 1982 and June 1987. Seventy-seven physician-patients maintained documented abstinence from all mood-altering substance~ 5 to 14) years after initiation of the continuing care contract. One physician was lost to followup, and 22 relapsed. Of those who relapsed, one died during relapse. One physician was involved in a pattern of continuous relapse and was unable to practice medicine. All but four of the remaining physicians who relapsed had at least 2 years of continuous sobriety since their relapse.

Other studies demonstrate similar results. Shore reported on 63 addicted or impaired physicians who had been on probation with the Oregon Board of Medical Examiners. These physicians were followed for 8 years. This investigation enabled the effectiveness of monitored outpatient supervision to be evaluated by comparing monitored and unmonitored subgroups. There was a significant difference between the improvement rate for monitored subjects (96%) and the improvement rate for unmonitored, addicted physicians (64%). Shore concluded that "increasing evidence that random urine monitoring during a two to fo period is positively correlated with treatment outcome" (60).

Smith and Smith (59) reported treatment outcomes of impaired physicians in the Oklahoma program. Physician-patients were categorized by length of time in treatment. Type I had treatment for 3 to 4 months in programs specializing in the care of health professionals. Type II had treatment for 16 weeks. Type III had other treatment modalities, including outpatient treatment, psychiatric or psychological therapy, and/or groups without prior chemical dependency treatment. Eighty-five percent of those with type I treatment had a favorable outcome. Of those with type II treatment, only 46% had a favorable outcome, compared to type III physician-patients, of whom only 38% had favorable outcomes.

Morse et al. compared recovery rates of 73 physicians with 185 middle class patients treated for chemical dependence in a hospital-based program. In the physician group, 83% (compared to 62% of nonphysicians who completed treatment) had favorable outcomes one or more years after treatment (69). He concluded that close monitoring may account, in part, for the prognosis for physicians.

Harrington et al. reported that 31 of 33 physicians who completed treatment (94%) had returned to full practice. Twenty-two (67%) had experienced no relapse, and 15% had a very brief period of relapse during followup, which lasted up to 2 years (70).

Johnson and Connelly evaluated and treated 50 physicians in a psychiatrically oriented, short-term addiction program. The criteria for a successful treatment outcome were abstinence and a return to effective job functioning. A "brief relapse" was not considered a treatment failure (71). Patients were followed from 9 months to 4.5 years. Thirty-two (64%) of the study population were sober and practicing medicine at the time of followup. Of significant concern, four (8%) were dead, three of suicide and one of subdural hematoma.

Kliner et al. studied treatment outcomes of alcoholic physicians (72) with a multiple-choice questionnaire sent to each patient 1 year after discharge from an inpatient 30-day alcoholism treatment. Of the 85 patients, 10 had died, 4 never returned the questionnaire, 3 refused permission to be contacted, and 1 could not be located. Fifty-one (76%) reported abstinence since treatment, and 53 (79%) of those who responded to these questionnaires reported general improvement in their professional performance. The physician-patient response to treatment was more favorable than the general patient population (only 61% remained abstinent at 1 year).

Goby et al. identified 51 physician-patients who underwent treatment for alcohol and/or chemical dependence between 1967 and 1977, and with between 1 and 10 years of followup (73). Only 43 were interviewed via phone. Of those not included for followup, 1 was incarcerated and 7 were dead (only 1 of 7 dead were abstinent since treatment). Only 19 (44%) of those interviewed reported no use of alcohol since treatment.

Gold and Pomm on a study of physicians monitored by the Florida Physicians Recovery Network. This University of Florida study revealed that 90% of physicians addicted to drugs or alcohol were sober 5 years after completion of treatment and rigorous monitoring.

Review of the treatment outcome studies above demonstrates that (a) treatment does work; (b) long-term abstinence and personal well-being correlates with strict aftercare monitoring and improved recovery surveillance techniques; (c) death is more prevalent among those who leave treatment prematurely and among those who relapse; and (d) the majority of physicians who successfully complete treatment and participate in aftercare monitoring can successfully return to the practice of medicine.

AFTERCARE AND MONITORING

Because substance abuse is a chronic illness, treatment is but the beginning of recovery. Most treatment centers have developed structured aftercare programs so that patients can continue to work on issues identified during their treatment program. Initially, many recovering physicians regard aftercare as punitive, hostile, or intrusive. However, when the patient understands and accepts the relapsing nature of the disease, and when aftercare monitoring is presented as a legal and licensing advocacy issue, compliance, acceptance, and gratitude usually result.

Several state medical societies have selected full or part-time directors of their PHPs. Different states use different names for their programs such as impaired physicians program, physicians recovery network, and physicians health effectiveness program, but the basic goals and monitoring systems remain the same. After treatment, physicians are expected to participate in their state medical society-sponsored PHP for monitoring, in addition to the aftercare provided by their treatment program. Many states, including Florida (74), New Jersey (66), Maryland (75), Oregon (76), Georgia (77), New Mexico (78), Alabama (79), and Oklahoma (59), provide recovering physicians who voluntarily seek treatment and monitoring advocacy from the state licensing agency. In some cases they serve as a "diversion program." The individual can receive treatment, not punishment. Physicians who are reported directly to the state board of medical examiners are required to have a formal relationship with the board.

Typically, PHPs provide the following low-cost or no-cost services to the physician:

1. Receive requests to investigate questions of specific impairment.
2. Provide training of intervention specialists and perform interventions.
3. Seek assistance for physicians who need financial aid during the treatment or rehabilitation process.
4. Establish a registry of the appropriate resources for treatment of alcoholism, other drug dependence, mental health, geriatrics, and other problems resulting in physician impairment.
5. Establish liaisons with hospitals, medical staffs, managed care organizations, and medical societies throughout the state.
6. Liaison with the directors of approved chemical dependency programs.
7. Recommend appropriate treatment to physicians seeking help.
8. Monitor the progress of the licensee after treatment.
9. Collaborate with other state PHPs to improve standards of monitoring, data collection, and process refinements, and to plan research to evaluate effectiveness of treatment and monitoring.
10. Make reports to appropriate individuals, committees, funding sources, and credentialing agencies regarding monitoring program.
11. Several state PHPs also provide individual, group, and family therapy or counseling.
12. Conduct educational programs to educate physicians and their families, hospital staffs, county medical societies, medical auxiliaries, and other appropriate groups or agencies about physician impairment.

State medical society PHPs have an underlying premise that impaired physicians may be unable to seek help spontaneously because of the nature of their illness, thus their colleagues have a special obligation to take the initiative of encouraging voluntary treatment. After treatment, these programs have two main functions: to protect the public from impaired physicians and to rehabilitate addicted or mentally ill physicians. Most PHPs supervise physicians for a minimum of 5 years.

Programs that are administered by state licensing boards appear to be punitive. It is believed that such programs may be less effective in reaching out to physicians who would voluntarily seek treatment and/or assistance, and do not have board actions pending. State medical society PHPs are programs of advocacy. It is believed that when physicians are not threatened with the potential for discovery by the medical board, they will voluntarily join PHPs at an earlier stage in their disease.

FACTORS THAT INFLUENCE RECOVERY

Close and careful monitoring by the state medical society PHP is believed necessary to follow physicians safely through the stages of recovery and to avoid "stuck points." Galanter et al. (80) studied 100 recovering physicians who were successfully treated in a program that combined professionally directed psychotherapeutic treatment and peer-led self-help. An average of 37.4 months after admission, they all reported being abstinent and rated AA as more important to their recovery than professionally directed modalities. Feelings of affiliation to AA, which were very high, were strong predictors of the respondents' perceived support for their recovery. These feelings, and the identification with the role of caregiver in addiction treatment, appeared to be central to their recovery. Twelve-step groups were ranked as the most potent element in their recovery, followed by physician counseling, the desire to do well at work, family therapy, and urinalysis.

Gallegos et al. (67) reported that all 100 of the physicians studied signed a continuing care contract that included witnessed urines, a primary care physician, attendance at five 12-step meetings and one Caduceus meeting a week, individual and family therapy when indicated, a spiritual program, a physical fitness program, and a leisure activity program.

Those who relapsed within the first year were likely not to believe the disease concept, did not believe they needed the recommended help, and felt that they would not run into difficulties staying sober. Those who relapsed in the second year most often reported family and emotional issues as triggers for relapse. For the 22 physicians who relapsed, behavioral changes and denial of their condition elevated their stress, increased their isolation, and impaired their judgment. Each individual reported slowly stopping attendance at AA. They also felt that neither their fear of losing their license to practice medicine, nor any other legal, marital, or professional sanction could have inhibited the progression of their relapse or promoted recovery once substance use was reinitiated.

State PHPs attempt to provide quantitative documentation of an individual's progress in recovery by obtaining data from face-to-face interviews with the physician-patient. In the Georgia program, Talbott postulated 16 factors that appear to have predictive value in assessing successful recovery (81):

1. The number of 12-step meetings attended per week.
2. A working relationship with a sponsor and frequent sponsor contact.
3. Random urine drug screens.

4. Monitoring milestones in each stage of recovery to help the physician avoid "stuck points" or emotional traps (e.g., anger, guilt, depression, anxiety, insomnia).
5. Monitoring for the effects of the emergence of compulsive behaviors (sex, work, food, nicotine, gambling, etc.).
6. Evaluation of the status of current therapies, treatments, and medications.
7. Assessment of family relationships.
8. Physical health status.
9. Number of leisure activities per week.
10. Compliance with all monitoring activities, and timely attendance at recommended therapies and 12-step meetings.
11. Amount of time spent exercising per week.
12. Evaluation of work-related stressors (professional status, job duties, and workplace attitudes).
13. Monitoring of changes in financial status.
14. Additional training and/or continuing medical education.
15. Self-rated quality of recovery program.
16. The identification of "soft parts" of the physician-patient recovery program.

Data for surveillance of recovery are obtained by the PHP at regularly scheduled 2-week intervals in the first year after treatment. The evaluation schedule gradually lengthens to biannual monitoring and face-to-face interviews toward the end of 5 years. Aftercare monitoring of recovering physicians has become an essential part of promoting continued recovery.

Contingency contracting has also been found to be helpful in reducing the risk for relapse. State PHPs or a therapist obtain a license-surrendering letter from the physician being monitored. If the urine drug screen is positive, the letter is sent to the state licensing agency and professional sanctions will be issued by the licensing agency. Crowley (82) has reported on contingency contracting as a treatment modality that decreases physician drug use.

One common denominator for successful recovery seems to be the extent that the physician is able to internalize the treatment experience (83). Physician-patients who are most successful in their recovery avoid emotions such as anger, guilt, depression, and anxiety by using 12-step recovery program principles (84). They avoid compulsive behaviors and learn to become skillful in participating in important relationships (family, sponsor, spouse, parents, children, friends, etc.).

Physicians who do the best in their recovery develop a profound and abiding attitude of gratitude. They learn to have open and honest communication with family members. They are regular in their attendance at AA (or other 12-step meetings), they communicate with their sponsor,

and check out their behavior with other trusted family members and recovering friends. These behaviors must become part of the recovering physicians' normal life.

STAGES OF RECOVERY

The milestones in recovery from addiction are both similar to and different from the process of recovering from almost any chronic, life-threatening illness. Each individual has unique amounts of protective features, risk factors, and resilience for recovery. Treatment and aftercare ideally combine to improve outcome by changing a relapse-prone individual into a recovery-prone person.

The needs of every recovering physician change over time. Without appropriate problem-solving strategies, the willingness to reach out for help and respond appropriately to feedback, and the ability to successfully cope with "stuck points" (85) and stressors, relapse is likely. A thorough recognition of the stages through which the recovering physician must pass and ways to overcome "stuck points" in the journey of recovery is essential.

Recovery is a process with clearly defined stages (86). It requires changes that are perceptible to those around the recovering physician. It is a long-term process that requires:

1. Total abstinence from mood-altering substances.
2. A conscious decision to take those specific actions that increase the likelihood for success in recovery (including changes in values, perception and behaviors).
3. Knowledge about the natural history of the illness (87) and its recovery.
4. Knowledge of the skills to begin and continue.
5. The ability to identify strengths and weaknesses in their current recovery program.
6. The willingness to accept feedback from others who are skilled at monitoring continued personal growth.
7. The ability not to deny and evade problems, stresses, and behaviors (when unopposed) frequently lead to relapse.

Although the recovery time course is unique for each individual, Gorski (88) has defined the recovery stages as follows:

1. *Transition:* Starts when the individual begins to believe they have a problem with alcohol or drugs. It ends when the individual becomes will to reach out for help.
2. *Stabilization:* The patient completes the physical withdrawal and p' acute withdrawal. Both physical and emotional healing begins. The obsession from drug and/or alcohol use subsides. The physician-patient begins to feel hope and develop motivation for recovery.

3. *Early Recovery:* A time of internal change when the recovering physician begins to let go of painful feelings about his or her disease (guilt shame, fear, resentment, etc.). The compulsion to use alcohol and drugs vanishes. The reliance on nonchemical coping skills to address problems and situations, which previously triggered chemical use, strengthens.

4. *Middle Recovery:* Balance begins to be restored. The wreckage of the past is cleaned up. Relationships are developed that positively reinforce learned skills that ensure continued personal growth.

5. *Late Recovery:* Resolution of painful events and issues related to growing up in a dysfunctional family must occur.

6. *Maintenance:* The recovering physician begins to practice the principles of successful recovery in all daily activities.

PHPs that are responsive to the changing needs of the recovering physician, that monitor the stages of recovery thoroughly, and that use every resource available to help each individual physician become recovery-prone may ultimately be the most successful.

PREVENTION

The AMA has provided leadership in the prevention of chemical dependence and early rehabilitation for physicians with addiction. Every medical society now has a stated policy and a committee on physician impairment. The Federation of State Medical Boards has suggested guidelines for the relationship between the impaired physicians program (PHPs) and the regulatory entity (89).

The definitions of terms and language for effective communication between treatment providers are documented (90). Standardization of diagnoses (36), the measurement of illness severity (91), and the levels of care and intensities of treatment are established (92). The science of matching addicted patients to specific kinds of treatment and treatment outcome research that links process with outcome (93) is evolving. A computerized master file of physician characteristics for comparative, randomized, stratified, and/or case-control studies has been developed and refined (94).

Recently, a uniform mechanism of data collection and the development of a collaborative process of investigating physician impairment were proposed (65). This research would build upon prior multiprogram, clinically based research. Information gleaned from such an investigation would provide the foundation for improving drug-abuse treatment for years to come. This research would have broad implications in the development of strategic prevention initiatives for the medical profession, for high-risk specialties, and for the general public.

How would a prospective study of physician impairment be significant? Doll and Hill (95), in a 10-year prospective epidemiologic study of British doctors, were able to show for the first time that there appears to be a d(frequency, and duration causal effect for mortality in relation to smoking. This finding resulted in more focused investigations that were the foundation of a strategic national prevention effort (96) and public health policy on tobacco use.

Investigating chemical dependence in physicians may lead to a better understanding of the strength of association, the dose–response effect, the consistency of findings, the biologic plausibility, coherence of evidence, and the specificity of the association of previously investigated risk factors for the development of addiction. Information about physician addiction, risk factors for the disease, ability to seek help and recover, and the long-term health consequences of drug and alcohol use might be applicable to the general population.

What are the psychological and behavioral effects of the drug(s) being used by patients? What is the incidence of psychiatric comorbidity in addicted patients? What is the patient's temporal state of substance use, along the continuum of intoxication, withdrawal, cognitive impairment, abstinence and recovery? These questions can be best answered by a prospective study of physician impairment. Recovering chemically dependent physicians:

1. Understand the need for research and most often are willing to participate in an investigation (if confidentiality can be guaranteed).
2. Can give a good history of their substance abuse patterns and present information about dose, frequency, and duration of drug and alcohol use.
3. Are monitored by PHPs for a minimum of 5 years to obtain multidimensional outcome measures.
4. Are easily tracked because of licensing requirements.
5. Are a source for comparative analysis available through the AMA master file (94).

It is the responsibility of every physician to become involved in the prevention of alcohol, tobacco, and other drug problems. Through the treatment of their own illness, recovering physicians have a heightened awareness of the disease of chemical dependence. Traditionally, physicians in recovery have had a primary role in prevention as practitioners, as educators, as consultants to policy makers, and as concerned citizens. Through their recovery, there is a positive "ripple effect" of prevention into their families, patients, colleagues, and within the communities they serve.

REGULATORY ISSUES AND ETHICAL CONSIDERATIONS

The Federation of State Medical Boards (FSMB) has proposed guidelines to promote uniformity in rules and regulations regarding impaired physicians. The Federation's goal is to protect the public. Efforts to educate citizens and the dissemination of information to the public about physician impairment have been initiated. The Federation also communicates with the AMA, state medical hoards, state medical societies, and administrators in medicine. When appropriate, the Federation pursues federal and state legislative initiatives to provide improved powers to state medical boards for the supervision of impaired physicians (97).

Monitoring of recovering physicians by PHPs provides a sensitive and specific mechanism for detecting relapsed chemically dependent physicians. There is concern that informed consent disclosure will compromise the privacy and employment rights of physicians and that rigorous monitoring should protect the welfare of patients (98). Others contend that when physicians who seek help are automatically sanctioned by regulatory agencies, there will be fewer referrals of chemically dependent physicians to PHPs. State medical societies and state medical boards often become distrustful of each other (99) and may work at cross-purposes.

Because of anecdotal reports made by physicians who have gone through treatment for chemical dependency and a lack of documented information, careful consideration of each report and its relationship to the Americans with Disabilities Act (ADA) (100) and an "action response" was proposed.

The ADA is a federal civil rights law that states

> No covered entity shall discriminate against a qualified individual with a disability because of the disability of such individual in regard to job application procedures, the hiring, advancement of employees, or discharge of employees, employee compensations, job training, and other terms, conditions, and privileges of employment. (101)

The spirit of the ADA is a "case-by-case" assessment of risk and the evaluation of risk "must be based on the behavior of the particular disabled person, not merely on generalizations about the disability" (101). When recovering physicians are carefully and closely monitored by appropriate means, there has been no documented risk or harm to a patient.

Recently, full- and part-time medical directors of PHPs gathered to form the Federation of State Physician Health Programs (FSPHP). "The Federation provides a forum for the exchange of information between State Physician Health Programs (PHPs) and promotes the safety and well-being of the public and the State Medical Associations' PHPs. The final goal of the Federation is to promote early identification prior to the illness impacting upon the care of patients" (97). The FSPHP is developing a closer relationship with the AMA and the FSMB. Encouragement has attended the formation of the FSPHP. A common ground can be established that links organized concern for sick doctors to social legal, and political pressures of professional accountability. The medical profession has recognized alcoholism and drug addiction as a disease. The medial control of impaired physicians in terms of its compatibilities with professional values and interests has demonstrated that when conflicting, but overriding considerations are put into action, a partnership can form. This partnership is capable of meeting the demand of desperate forces ultimately resulting in improved safety to the public while maximizing the personal rights of recovering physicians.

CONCLUSION

Wright stated that "Impaired physicians are to the rest of the profession as the canary was to the coal miners of another generation. Until we can determine the risk of addiction to drugs for a specific individual before the individual is exposed to them, we must rely on the experience of the most vulnerable individuals in our occupational cohort to learn how to protect ourselves from the chemical tools of our trade" (6).

In recent years, many stakeholders who guard public safety and the practice of medicine (the AMA, FSMBE, medical and specialty societies, ASAM, regulatory agencies, FSPHP, and others) joined forces to find solutions to the "challenging" issues of physician substance abuse. Changes in the landscape of health care delivery have diverted the attention of many practitioners away from compassionate concern for colleagues who have become impaired by chemical dependence. In spite of significant improvements in identification, intervention, assessment, treatment, and aftercare and monitoring, much is still unknown about the nature of chemical dependence.

REFERENCES

1. Starr P. *The social transformation of American medicine.* New York: Basic Books, 1982.
2. Harris L. *Consumers perception of substance abuse by health care providers.* Research abstracts presented at the AMA Eighth National Conference on Impaired Health Professionals. Chicago, 1987.
3. Steindler E. Physician impairment: past, present, and future. *J Med Assoc GA* 1974;73:741–743.
4. Nesbitt J. The sick doctor statute: a new approach to an old problem. *Fed Bull* 1970;70:266–279.
5. American Medical Association Council on Mental Health. The sick physician: impairment by psychiatric disorders,

including alcoholism and drug dependence. *JAMA* 1973;233:684–687.

6. Wright C. Physician addiction to pharmaceuticals: personal history, practice setting, access to drugs and recovery. *Md Med J* 1990;39:1021–1025.

7. Robinson J. *Annotated bibliography on physician impairment and well-being.* Chicago: American Medical Association, 1986.

8. American Medical Association International Conference on Physician Health. Uncertain times: preventing illness, promoting wellness. Chandler, AZ, 1996.

9. Centrella M. Physician addiction and impairment—current thinking: a review. *J Addict Dis* 1994;13:91–105.

10. Watry A, Morgan D, Earley P, et al. *Georgia composite state board of medical examiners guidelines for problem physicians.* Paper presented at the American Medical Association International Conference on Physician Health. Uncertain times: preventing illness, promoting wellness. Chandler, AZ, 1996.

11. Noland S., Halsted W.S. Idiosyncrasies of a surgical legend. *Harv Med Alum Bull* 1991;65:17–23.

12. Paget J. What becomes of medical students. *St. Bartholomew's Hosp Rep* 1869;5:238–242.

13. Mattison J. Morphinism in medical men. *JAMA* 1984;23:186–188.

14. Partlow WD. Alcoholism and drug addiction among physicians of Alabama. *Trans Med Assoc Al* 1914:685–691.

15. DeQuincy T. *New York: Confessions of an English opium eater.* Heritage Press, 1950:38–39.

16. Pescor MJ. Physician drug addicts. *Dis Nerv Syst* 1942;3:2–3.

17. Stimson G, Oppenheimer B, Stimson C. Drug abuse in the medical profession. *Br J Addict* 1984;79:395–402.

18. Ehrhardt H. Drug addiction in medical and allied professions in Germany. *Bull Narcotics* 1959;11:18–26.

19. Modlin H, Montes A. Narcotic addiction in physicians. *Am J Psychiatry* 1964;121:358–363.

20. Flexner A. *Medical education in the United States and Canada. Bulletin No. 4.* New York: Carnegie Foundation for the Advancement of Teaching, 1910.

21. Musto D. *The American disease: origins of narcotic control.* New Haven, CT: Yale University Press, 1973.

22. Pub. L No. 63–233. Approved December 7, 1914.

23. Stimson G, Oppenheimer B, Stimson C. Drug abuse in the medical profession. *Br J Addict* 1984;79:395–402.

24. Caston S. *Prohibition: the lie of the land.* New York: Free Press, 1981.

25. Pub. L No. 75–238. Approved, August 2, 1937.

26. Keeve J. Physicians at risk: some epidemiologic considerations of alcoholism, drug abuse, and suicide. *J Occup Med* 1984;26:503–508.

27. Wollot H, Lambert J. Drug addiction among Quebec physicians. *Can Med Assoc J* 1982;126:927–930.

28. East W. The British government report to the United Nations on the traffic of opium and other dangerous drugs. *Br J Addict* 1947;46:38–39.

29. Clatt M. Alcoholism and drug dependence in doctors and nurses. *Br Med J* 1968;1:380–381.

30. A'Brook M, Hailstone J, McLauchlan I. Psychiatric illness in the medical profession. *Br J Psychiatry* 1967;113:1013–1023.

31. Watterson D. Psychiatric illness in the medical profession: incidence in relation to sex and field of practice. *Can Med Assoc J* 1976;115:311–317.

32. Vincent MO, Robinson EA, Latt L. Physicians as patients: private psychiatric hospital experience. *Can Med Assoc J* 1969;100:403–412.

33. Brewster J. Prevalence of alcohol and other drug problems among physicians. *JAMA* 1986;255:1913–1920.

34. Hughes P, Brandenburg N, Baldwin D, et al. Prevalence of substance use among U.S. physicians. *JAMA* 1992;267:2333–2339.

35. Robins L, Regier D. *Psychiatric disorders in America: the epidemiologic catchment area study.* New York: Free Press, 1991.

36. American Psychiatric Association. *Diagnostic and statistical manual of mental disorders,* 3rd ed., revised. Washington, DC: Author, 1987.

37. Regier D, et al. Co-morbidity of mental disorders with alcohol and other drug abuse: results of the epidemiologic catchment area (ECA) study. *JAMA* 1990;264:2511–2518.

38. Halzer J, Burnam A, McEvoy L. Alcohol abuse and dependence. In: Robins LN, Regier DA, eds. *Psychiatric disorders in America: the epidemiologic catchment area study.* New York: Free Press, 1991:81–115.

39. Anthony J, Hetzer J. Syndrome of drug abuse and dependence. In: Robins LN, Regier DA, eds. *Psychiatric disorders in America: the epidemiologic catchment area study.* New York: Free Press, 1991:116–154.

40. Talbott GD, Wright C. Chemical dependence in healthcare professionals. *Occup Med* 1987;2:581–591.

41. Vaillant GE, Soborale NC, McArthur C. Some psychologic vulnerabilities of physicians. *N Engl J Med* 1972;287:372–375.

42. Richman JA. Occupational stress, psychological vulnerability and alcohol-related problems over time in future physicians. *Alcohol Clin Exp Res* 1992;16(2):166–171.

43. Moore R. Youthful precursors of alcohol abuse in physicians. *Am J Med* 1990;88:332–336.

44. Gallegos K, Browne C, Veit F, et al. Addiction in anesthesiologists: drug access and patterns of substance abuse. *Qual Rev Bull* 1988:116–122.

45. Jex S, et al. Relations among stressors, strains, and substance use among resident physicians. *Int J Addict* 1992;27:479–494.

46. Vaillant G. Physician, cherish thyself: the hazards of self prescribing. *JAMA* 1992;267:2373–2374.

47. McAuliffe WE, Santangelo S, Magnuson E, et al. Risk factors of drug impairment in random samples of physicians and medical students. *Int J Addict* 1987;22(9):825–841.

48. Talbott G, Gallegos K, Wilson P, et al. The medical association of Georgia's impaired physician program—review of the first 1,000 physicians: analysis of specialty. *JAMA* 1987;257:2927–2930.

49. Bissell L, Haberman P. *Alcoholism in the professions.* New York: Oxford University Press, 1984.

50. Vaillant G, Clark W, et al. Prospective study of alcoholism treatment. *Am J Med* 1983;75:455–463.

51. Bissell L, Skorina J. One hundred alcoholic women in medicine: an interview study. *JAMA* 1987;257:2939–2944.

52. Blume S. Women, alcohol, and drugs. In: Miller NS, ed. *Comprehensive handbook of drug and alcohol addiction.* New York: Marcel Dekker, 1991:147–177.

53. Talbott G, Gallegos K. Intervention with health professionals. *Addict Recovery* 1990;10(3):13–16.

54. Hoffman N, Halikas J, Mee-Lee D. *Patient placement criteria for the treatment of psychoactive substance use disorders,* 2nd ed. Washington, DC: American Society of Addiction Medicine, 1996.

55. Talbott G, Martin C. Treating impaired physicians: fourteen keys to success. *Va Med* 1986;113:95–99.

56. Kosten T, Kleber H. Differential diagnoses of psychiatric comorbidity in substance abusers. *J Subst Abuse Treat* 1988;5:201–206.

57. Catalano R, Howard M, Hawkins J, et al. Relapse in the addictions: rates, determinants, and promising prevention strategies. In: *1988 Surgeon General's report on health consequences of smoking.* Washington, DC: U.S. Government Printing Office, 1986.

58. Robinson E, Fitzgerald J, Gallegos K. Brain functioning and addiction: what neuropsychologic studies reveal. *J Med Assoc Ga* 1985;73:74–79.

59. Smith P, Smith D. Treatment outcomes of impaired physicians in Oklahoma. *J Okla State Med Assoc* 1991;84:599–603.

60. Shore J. The Oregon experience with impaired physicians on probation. *JAMA* 1987;257:2931–2934.

61. *Alcoholics anonymous,* 2nd ed. New York: Alcoholics Anonymous World Services, 1972.

62. Gordis E. *Relapse and craving. Alcohol alert.* Rockville, MD: U.S. Department of Health and Human Services, National Institute on Alcohol Abuse and Alcoholism, 1989;6:3.

63. Wall J. The results of hospital treatment of addiction in physicians. *Fed Bull* 1958;45:144–152.

64. Jones L. How 92% beat the dope habit. *Bull Los Angeles County Med Soc* 1958;19:37–40.

65. Gallegos K. The pilot impaired physicians epidemiologic surveillance system (PIPESS). *Md Med J* 1987;36:264–266.

66. Reading E. Nine years experience with chemically dependent physicians: the New Jersey experience. *Md Med J* 1992;41:325–329.

67. Gallegos K, Lubin B, Bowers C, et al. Relapse and recovery: five to ten year follow study of chemically dependent physicians—the Georgia experience. *Md Med J* 1992;41:315–319.

68. Gallegos K, Norton M. Characterization of Georgia's impaired physicians program treatment population: data and statistics. *J Med Assoc Ga* 1984;73:755–758.

69. Morse R, et al. Prognosis of physicians treated for alcoholism and drug dependence. *JAMA* 1984;251:743–746.

70. Harrington R, et al. Treating substance-use disorders among physicians. *JAMA* 1982:2253–2257.

71. Johnson R, Connelly J. Addicted physicians: a closer look. *JAMA* 1981;245:253–257.

72. Kliner D, Spicer J, Barnett P. Treatment outcome of alcoholic physicians. *J Stud Alcohol* 1980;41:1217–1220.

73. Goby M, Bradley N, Bespalec D. Physicians treated for alcoholism: a follow-up study. *Alcohol Clin Exp Res* 1979;3:121–124.

74. Goetz R. Personal communication, June, 1996.

75. Alpern F, et al. A study of recovering Maryland physicians. *Md Med J* 1992;41:301–303.

76. Ulwelling J. The evolution of the Oregon program for impaired physicians. *Bull Am Coll Surg* 1991;76:18–21.

77. Gallegos K, Keppler J, Wilson P. Returning to work after rehabilitation: aftercare, follow-up and workplace reliability. *Occup Med* 1989;4:357–371.

78. Miscal B. Monitoring recovering physicians: the New Mexico experience. *Bull Am Coll Surg* 1991;76:22–40.

79. Summer G. Personal communication, June, 1996.

80. Galanter M, Talbott G, Gallegos K, et al. Combined alcoholics anonymous and professional care for addicted physicians. *Am J Psychiatry* 1990;147:64–68.

81. Talbott G. Reducing relapse in health providers and professionals. *Psychiatr Ann* 1995;25(11):669–672.

82. Crowley T. Doctor's drug abuse reduced during contingency-contracting treatment. *Alcohol Drug Res* 1986;6:299–307.

83. Centrella M. Physician addiction and impairment—current thinking: a review. *J Addict Dis* 1994;13:91–105.

84. Kurtz E. Why AA works. *J Stud Alcohol* 1982;43:38–80.

85. Gorski T. *Staying sober: a guide for relapse prevention.* Independence, MO: Independence Press, 1986.

86. Gorski T. *The relapse and recovery grid.* Center City, MN: Hazelden, 1989.

87. Valliant G. *Natural history of alcoholism.* Cambridge, MA: Harvard University Press, 1983.

88. Gorski T. *Passages through recovery: an action plan for preventing relapse.* Center City, MN: Hazelden, 1989.

89. Rasseth H, et al. *Ad hoc committee on physician impairment [report].*

90. Rinaldi RC, Steindler EM, Wilford BB, et al. Clarification and standardization of substance abuse terminology. *JAMA* 1988;259:555–557.

91. Mee-Lee D. An instrument for patient progress and treatment assignment: the Recovery Attitude and Treatment Evaluator (RAATE). *J Subst Abuse Treat* 1988;5:1883–1886.

92. Mee-Lee D. Patient placement criteria and patient-treatment matching. In: *Principles of addiction medicine.* Sect. IX, Chap. 3: *Clinical overview of addiction treatment.* Washington, DC: American Society of Addiction Medicine, 1974.

93. Filstead W, Parrella D, Ross A, et al. Key issues in outcomes research. In: *Principles of addiction medicine.* Sect. X, Chap. 5: *Management of addiction treatment.* Washington, DC: American Society of Addiction Medicine, 1994.

94. Robeck G, Randolph L, Mead D, et al. *Physician characteristics and distribution in the U.S.* Chicago: American Medical Association, 1993.

95. Doll T, Hill S. Mortality in relation to smoking: ten years' observation of British doctors. *Br Med J* 1964;1:1399–1410, 1460–1467.

96. U.S. Department of Health and Human Services. *Reducing the health consequence of smoking: 25 years of progress. A report of the surgeon general.* Rockville, MD: Office of Smoking and Health, 1989.

97. Summer G. Personal communication, June 19, 1996.

98. Ackerman T. Chemically dependent physician and informal consent disclosure. *J Addict Dis* 1996;15:25–42.

99. Ikoda R, Pelton C. Diversion programs for impaired physicians. *West J Med* 1990;152:617–621.

100. Pub. L No. 101–336, 104 Stat 327, 1990.

101. House of Representatives Rep. No 485, 101st Congress, 2nd Sec. (part 2) 56, (part 3) 46 (1990). Reprinted in *US Code Cong Admin News,* 1990;4:338–469.

    Euless, TX: Federation of State Medical Boards, September, 1994.

CHAPTER 75

New Immigrants and Refugees

JOSEPH WESTERMEYER

HISTORICAL AND CULTURAL BACKGROUND

Immigrants

Clinicians in the United States must become competent in the care of immigrants, including refugees, if for no other reason than their sheer numbers. Since its inception as a nation more than 200 years ago, the U.S. population has often consisted of 10% to 20% foreign-born people. In the 2000 census, 31,107,889 people were foreign born, and an additional 3,527,551 people were born outside of the U.S. in various territories (e.g., Puerto Rico, Virgin Islands). Together these two groups comprise 12.3% of the total 281,421,906 people counted in the census. A conservative estimate of 3 million illegal residents in the United States (1) brings the total to around 38 million, or approximately 13.5% of the total population. In addition, the United States has several million visitors per year, including foreign students, visitors, temporary workers, tourists, entertainers, and representatives of foreign governments (military, embassy staff). Immigrants, refugees, and these special categories of visitors all include individuals who seek services for substance abuse in the United States.

These figures compare with a foreign-born population of 9.6 million in the 1970 census, and 13.9 million in the 1980 census (2). From 1980 to 2000, the number of counted foreign-born people in the United States rose by 224%. Although there are other countries with large number of immigrants, such as Canada and Australia, the number of immigrants to the United States in recent years has probably exceeded the number of immigrants entering all other countries of the world (3). In sum, we must be prepared to address substance-abuse problems within immigrant and refugee groups whose combined population exceeds that of most of our states and of most other countries.

Several decades ago, most immigrants to the United States came from Europe. This changed dramatically in the past 4 decades. In the 2000 census, the continental origins of foreign-born people in the United States was as follows: the Americas, 16,916,416; Asia, 8,226,254; Europe, 4,915,557; Africa, 881,300; and Oceania, 168,046. National origins of the most numerous immigrants included the following: Mexico, 9,177,487; China, 1,518,652; Philippines, 1,369,070; India, 1,022,552; Korea, 864,125;

Canada, 820,771; El Salvador, 817,336; and United Kingdom, 677,751. These new immigrants bring new types of substance use and abuse to the United States, including opium smoking and qat chewing. Thus, in addition to a huge number of people, immigrants comprise an extremely diverse group of peoples whose traditional substances involve drugs or modes of administration unfamiliar to American clinicians.

Refugees

Flight of peoples from war and social tumult has been an integral part of human history. Certain aspects of recent history involve novel features, however. One feature has been the dramatically increased numbers of people involved in such flight. A United Nations report estimated that 45 million people had left their homelands between 1945 and 1967 (4). Over the last few decades, the president has admitted up to several hundred thousand refugees per year. This recent trend has greatly increased the number of people coming from underdeveloped countries, from which many arrive poorly prepared for life in the United States.

There are several definitions of refugees, ranging from strict United Nations definitions to lay terms such as "economic refugees." For immigration and legal purposes in the United States, a refugee is defined as such by the federal government. The status extends special privileges to anyone so labeled. As clinicians, we may identify someone as seeking refuge, but the person may not have, or be allowed to obtain federal status as a refugee in the United States.

From a health perspective, refugees can pose a special challenge in view of their exposure to war or other trauma. This group is at special risk to numerous health problems. Drug trafficking and substance abuse sometimes accompany war and civil unrest—factors that can haunt a resettlement country (5).

CLINICAL ASSESSMENT

Is a Translator Needed?

In the 2000 census, 9.5 million inhabitants of the United States reported that they spoke English either "not well" (6.3 million) or "not at all" (3.2 million). The greatest proportion was Spanish speaking, accounting for 4.1 million. The second largest group was Asian-Pacific Islanders, with 1.6 million. Indo-Europeans comprised 1.3 million, with the remainder coming largely from Africa. Patients with inadequate skills in English will need a translator for an adequate assessment, unless the clinician speaks the patient's language.

Prior to working with a translator, the clinician should have a model for understanding the process of interpreting the clinician's queries and the patient's and family's responses. Three models common to the clinical context are as follows (6):

- The "black box" model. The clinician views the translator as a magical "black box" in which all queries and responses are accurately and completely translated.
- The "junior clinician" model. The clinician views the translator as a junior assistant clinician, whose task is to obtain the relevant clinical data being sought by the clinician.
- The "three partners" model. The clinician, translator, and patient share the difficult task of informing the translator regarding various queries and responses. This task is rendered complex through the absence of shared language and shared culture between clinician and patient. Typically, the translator has extensive experience in both languages and cultures. The task is further complicated by a three-sided series of transference and countertransference relationships (see reference 6 for further information).

Training the translator to this task requires more than a brief orientation. The translator's own views and attitudes can obstruct the clinician–patient relationship in a myriad of ways. The translator's own lay attitudes, use of substances, and choice of words can either enhance communication or seriously undermine it.

Case Example

A Southeast Asian refugee, trained as a translator in a substance-abuse program, had supportive, therapeutic attitudes toward older opium smokers from his country-of-origin. In his home country, he had known many opium addicts and had previously treated many of them. However, he tended to assume a patronizing, moralistic tone toward younger refugees who abused alcohol and cannabis. In these young patients, he perceived the pro-American, antitraditional attitudes and customs that his own adolescent offspring were adapting. With experience and supervision, he was able to understand the origins of his own antitherapeutic attitudes and to adapt new perspectives toward his younger clients.

Taking a Substance Use History

In most instances, the clinician will proceed efficiently in this aspect of the assessment. Substance use and abuse manifest many similarities across cultures. Through a supportive, informed, and empathetic approach, the clinician can usually obtain a complete picture of the patient's substance related problem.

At times, the clinician may have to seek help from the literature if the substance, route of administration, or pattern of use is unclear. Examples might include betel nut chewing, qat chewing, opium smoking, or heroin smoking.

Relationship of substance use to migration should be established. Did the patient begin use in the country of origin? Or in the United States? Or in another country? How was the patient introduced to the experience? What were the patient's circumstances at the time? Was the use of the substance a culturally deviant or syntonic activity?

Case Example

A 45-year-old Southeast Asian woman developed severe insomnia following the death of her husband. She could not sleep in a room by herself, or in a room without lights on. In association with this, she developed nightmares. The latter involved an actual occurrence, the death of her daughter in a mortar explosion while fleeing her home village, which had come under attack. To alleviate her insomnia and the distress she was causing to her extended family, they provided her with opium. Although opium smoking initially permitted her some rest, she had to escalate the doses to achieve rest. Eventually she became addicted. Clinical evaluation following detoxification revealed chronic posttraumatic stress disorder, and phobias to the dark and being alone at night, with associated panic disorder. She did well on a regimen of selective serotonin reuptake inhibitor (SSRI) medication, desensitization to being in the dark alone, and grief therapy for her deceased daughter and husband.

Establishing the family or community attitude toward the drug use can also aid in treatment planning. For example, in this case the family approved the woman's temporary use of opium during a period of grief following her husband's death, but they did not approve her spending her days smoking opium in lieu of caring for her children and grandchildren. Thus, they were highly supportive of her care and her continued abstinence from opium.

Culturally Competent Evaluation

In most respects, the evaluation continues largely as it would for other patients from indigenous ethnic groups. Review of systems should emphasize psychological symptoms that might not be spontaneously reported (e.g., anorexia, weight or sleep changes, fatigue, crying spells, fears, chronic pain, headache, bowel changes, anhedonia, hearing or seeing things not perceived by others). While taking a family history, the clinician should be alert to patriarchal or matriarchal kin systems, because patients may not consider nonkin to be relatives in the biogenetic sense. A social history should reflect life in the country of origin, as well as in the country of immigration.

Mental status should be culturally sensitive, because orientation in time and space can be affected by culture (e.g., Buddhist and Islamic calendars, differences in counting floors of a building). Education can affect the ability to do arithmetic or replicate figures with paper and pencil.

English fluency and literacy can affect naming, reading, writing, and enunciating. To interpret proverbs, the patient needs to consider a proverb familiar to the patient's culture. Ability to discern similarities in unlike objects depends upon education and familiarity with the objects.

Especially in the case of refugees, clinicians should rule out posttraumatic stress disorder, a common comorbid condition in this group (7). This may not be easily accomplished, as the refugee may be embarrassed or ashamed to reveal the trauma and its consequences (8). Rapport sets the groundwork for gentle probing of traumatic experiences. Inquiry regarding nightmares, intrusive thoughts, or hypervigilance can also suggest past trauma. Missed grieving or delayed grieving may also co-occur in situations where traumatic experiences involved the deaths of friends or family members. Addictive disorder can contribute to delayed or missing grieving.

Taking a Migration History

Immigrants and refugees come from every corner of the world, from the largest and most sophisticated cities to the most remote and undeveloped of rural villages. Inquiry into this phase of the patient's life can enhance the clinician's understanding of the patient. This dialogue also enables the patient to become the instructor, informing the clinician regarding that unknown portion of the past life.

During this exercise, the clinician can inquire into the patient's early exposure to substance use and abuse in the country of origin. In turn, this can lead to a family history of substance and other mental health problems. Models of treatment or recovery from substance abuse from the former country can be explored. Many immigrants and refugees do not come directly to the United States. The patient may not report these peregrinations if not asked about them. Inquiry can elicit important circumstances.

Case Example

A 17-year-old Ethiopian refugee came "unaccompanied" to the United States (i.e., without family members) after an American charitable organization had identified her in Greece. She had fled her home country following the political murder of her father, uncles, and brothers. She had made it as far as Greece, where her money ran out. A Greek man first established a romantic relationship with her, then facilitated her becoming addicted to heroin, and then sold her services as a prostitute. Following a suicide attempt, the local authorities knew her dilemma and referred her to the charitable organization. In the United States, she initially was treated as an inpatient for major depression and subacute opiate withdrawal. Following a period of residential treatment, she was placed in an American foster family. At last followup she was not drug seeking, had recovered from depression, and was attending college while still living with her original foster family.

A premigration history informs the clinician regarding the patient's competence, accomplishments, losses, and stressors before reaching the United States. This history provides a history of the individual within the culture of origin, or in countries of first refuge for refugees. Typically, early successes forecast subsequent successes. This is not always the case, however. An occasional person who did well in the homeland does miserably in the United States, and vice versa.

INTERPRETATION OF FINDINGS

Traditionalism Versus Acculturation

The apposition of formerly disparate people in the United States has exposed its inhabitants to new models and methods of substance use. European Americans not schooled in the ceremonial use of tobacco, developed tobacco dependence along with its myriad biomedical disorders. Some young Somali refugees, with no exposure to alcohol use in their Islamic families, have chosen weekend drunkenness as an "American" recreational form.

At times, cultural changes have produced changes in traditional substance use. For example, the Hmong, a refugee group from Southeast Asia, formerly had a rigid protocol for alcohol drinking, with few problems (9). However, in the United States, many of the animistic Hmong converted to abstinence-oriented Christianity. This social change undermined the former stability in drinking practices, resulting in a diversity from those who drank nothing to those who drank in a secular and sometimes dissocial fashion, that is, when and in amounts that they choose (10). Another example is the traditional use of qat in Somalia, Ethiopia, and nearby countries (11), where groups largely used it under socially controlled circumstances. However, some refugees from these groups have become addicted to qat when using it to relieve physical or emotional symptoms. In such contexts of rapid sociocultural change, old traditions of use can be abandoned readily and new patterns of use adopted.

Other changes also modify the drinking or drug use context following relocation to a new society. For example, the nature of work, transportation, and other technology can increase the risk associated with even mild intoxication or morning-after hangovers. Increased access to high-speed vehicles, complex machinery, the smooth interaction and coordination of many workers, as well as other similar factors, can render intoxication newly risky for the immigrant, and for the society at large, which bears the cost of vehicles and industrial accidents (12).

As a consequence of these changes, alcohol and/or other drugs can become a virtual scourge for certain subgroups in the United States. For them, substance abuse is a major cause of child neglect, family divorce, vehicular accidents, injury, and death.

Case Example

A 36-year-old Asian refugee had fled his country of origin a decade earlier with his military unit, leaving family behind. In the United States, he drank heavily and episodically with ethnic peers, much as he had done as a young soldier in Asia. During one of these episodes, he was involved in a serious accident in which a friend was killed and he sustained a traumatic brain injury. Treatment was not provided for either the alcohol abuse or the brain injury. Subsequently he married an American woman and had three children. His episodic heavy drinking persisted, primarily on weekends and holidays, but at times after work. Following a long weekend holiday of drinking with American friends, he killed his wife, three children, and mother-in-law while they were asleep. In the morning, discovering with horror the massacre, he called the police, who established beyond doubt that he had murdered his family, apparently during one of many alcoholic "black outs" that he had been having.

Cultural Diversity Within Groups

Groups of immigrants to the United States differ greatly. The same is true of individuals within these groups, for whom the new country presents many choices and alternatives. Some immigrants remain staunchly traditional to their country of origin. Others assimilate to a considerable extent with the "mainstream" American culture. With years of immigration, groups of immigrants show notable differences among themselves, considerably greater than they had manifested in the country of origin.

Failure to acculturate successfully to the new country can increase the risk of substance abuse. Successful acculturation can be identified by the immigrant's ability to speak English, hold a job, use the social institutions of the receiving society (e.g., banks, libraries, health care), access the mass media, and establish relationships outside of the immigrant's own group. Acculturation failure is manifest by dependence on others, declining mental health, social isolation, ignorance of social forces at play in the community, and increasing lack of control over one's life.

Substance abuse may provide an alternative to young immigrants caught between the "old country" culture and the new culture. Some of the superficial accouterments of American culture, for example, fast cars and drug or alcohol use, may substitute for a more fundamental acculturation. Petty crime or drug trafficking may be pursued as a means of paying for this apparent "American" lifestyle. These groups typically receive approval neither from their ethnic peers or mainstream Americans (13–15).

Migratory History and Onset of Substance Abuse

Some cases of substance abuse begin soon after migration. Most such cases involve continuation of premigration substance abuse or dependence, rather than new cases. The following case exemplifies this pattern.

Case Example

A 54-year-old Asian man had emigrated with his family. An opium addict over the previous two decades, he managed to hide a large supply of opium in household goods. By eating rather than smoking his supply, he was able to make his supply last for several months. As his supply was running out, he sought treatment for his addiction.

In other instances a short period of abstinence may ensue in former substance abusers, before recurrence of substance abuse, as in the following case.

Case Example

A 26-year-old Palestinian graduate student had become a heroin addict in his native Palestine. Formerly a good student, he was unable to obtain a job consistent with his education. Berated by his father for his inability to support the extended family despite his education, he found solace in spending his time with a group of unemployed college graduates. Exposed to heroin in this group, he was soon addicted. His father arranged for him to attend graduate school in the United States, following detoxification in Israel. For 6 months he did well academically and socially. Exposed to the opportunity to use heroin, however, he soon became readdicted. Failing academically, he sought treatment for his addiction (as he had done previously in Israel). However, he was unable to maintain his grades at that point, was dropped from school, and returned to Palestine.

Krupinski studied the appearance of new cases of substance abuse among post-World War II immigrants from East Europe to Australia (16). Most of these patients abused alcohol. Typically, these immigrants were in Australia for several years before heavy drinking began, and then several years more before seeking treatment for alcoholism. This chronologic pattern was unlike mood, anxiety, or psychotic disorders, which tended to appear within months to several years following migration. Factors that may delay onset following migration include the following:

- Immigration officials may screen out obvious cases of alcoholism or addiction.
- Because it requires money to purchase alcohol and drugs, it may require some years before the immigrant has sufficient disposable funds to purchase significant amounts of alcohol or drugs.
- On average it requires about 3 years of heavy cocaine or heroin abuse before initial treatment seeking, and about a decade of alcohol or opium abuse before initial treatment seeking (17,18).

A study of an opium smoking epidemic in Minnesota revealed two groups, those who became readdicted in the United States and those who became addicted for the first time in the United States (19). Of relevance to Krupinski's observations, the first use of opium in the United States did not appear in this refugee group until they had been in the United States for several years. At that time a large-scale smuggling operation developed to bring opium from Latin American and from Asia.

These studies from Australia and Minnesota indicated that older immigrants are most likely to abuse substances traditional in the country of origin. Young immigrants may also abuse the traditional substance if they remain ensconced within the immigrant community, as occurred among the young Hmong opium addicts (19). However, young immigrants may abuse substances that are not traditional within the immigrant community, but are substances abused within American society (15).

High-Risk Immigrant Groups

As a nation composed largely of immigrants and refugees, we tend to idealize these groups as harking back to our own origins. However, idealization should not render us blind to subgroups at high risk to substance abuse. The propensity of foreign countries to "dump" their problematic citizens in the United States (and other immigrant countries) was first recognized more than 150 years ago, when several European countries sent prisoners and debtors to the United States at public expense as a means of being rid of them (20).

Immigration laws have removed this historical trend to a considerable extent, because foreign countries are liable for the return of their mentally disabled citizens at their own expense. Nonetheless, we have brought in groups at high risk as refugees. Perhaps the most flagrant modern example was President Carter's acceptance of thousands of criminals in the "Mariel" flight from Cuba (Mariel referred to the prison from which the refugees originated). Although not all of the 120,000 participants in this flight were addicted or criminal, thousands of them appeared in jails and treatment facilities across the United States soon after their arrival.

Case Example

A 36-year-old Mariel refugee had been a petty criminal and alcohol abuser in Cuba. Upon arrival in the United States, he discovered that his contacts in the Hispanic community gave him access to cocaine trafficking. He became a street trader, buying from smugglers and selling on the streets. He soon became addicted to cocaine himself, resulting in his "cutting" his product with inert substances. This practice led to a conflict with a client, as a result of which he shot the client. He is now serving a sentence in the United States for murder.

A general category at risk consists of young, single men who were members of defeated armies allied with the United States. Often illiterate or poorly educated, they may not have sufficient skills to sustain them in the United States. Unlike many countries of Europe, the United States does not provide acculturation training and education for these high-risk immigrants and refugees.

Case Example

An Asian refugee had been a soldier from the age of 17 years, coming to the United States at age 26 years when his national army was defeated. He fled without his wife and daughter, whom he has never been able to locate. Although he was literate in his own language and had risen to the rank of noncommissioned officer, his former achievements did not predict success in the United States. Unable to learn English, he worked principally as a dishwasher and unskilled laborer. His recreational activities consisted entirely of gambling and drinking in the company of men similar to himself. At the age of 44 years he was incarcerated for killing an ethnic peer in a fight that occurred in a context of drinking and cannabis use.

TREATMENT AND RECOVERY

Acceptance of "Mainstream" Treatment Modalities

Addicted persons who are needy enough accept help from virtually any corner. Thus, people of virtually any ethnic background accept care in detoxification centers, emergency rooms, and inpatient hospital units. The challenge to continued treatment begins beyond this acute phase. Once beyond the pain of withdrawal or other health emergency, the addicted person becomes more choosey about continued care. The "three As" integral to successful rehabilitation at the next step are as follows:

- *Availability:* The treatment must be reasonably close at hand, so that the person can participate in the recovery-centered endeavors.
- *Access:* The patient must have access to the program; lack of insurance or ethnic barriers can prevent entry.
- *Acceptance:* The patient and the program must accept each other.

An analysis of barriers in one health care system revealed four sources of cultural barriers to mental health care (21). Two of these general barriers lay on the health care side, that is, the clinicians and the health care system, and two consisted of the patient (e.g., attitudes, insights, resources) and the patient's family and community.

Self-Help in Recovery

Some self-help activities can occur regardless of ethnic affiliation, such as avoiding people and places associated with use (22). However, some forms of self-help may differ across cultures.

Alcoholics Anonymous can change form and content considerably when translated across culture and language (23). Entire communities can engage in self-help, through eliminating substance abuse and associated problems (24). For example, in cultures that view self-disclosure as self-centered, "confession" of addiction-related "sins" may prove unacceptable.

Religious Conversion and Recovery

Conversion to abstinence-oriented religion has alleviated addictive disorders for many around the world. For example, Hispanics throughout the Americas have joined abstinence-oriented fundamentalist Christian religions as a means of achieving sobriety and resisting invitations to drink (25). Buddhist monasteries have served as places of recovery, especially when a charismatic abbot leads the way (26). Galanter described the "large-group psychotherapy" that may attend membership in an abstinence-oriented or recovery-oriented religious group (27). Some programs, such as involvement in the Native American Church, may be restricted to members of the ethnic groups sponsoring them (28).

Indigenous Treatment

We sometimes assume that modern treatment for addiction is available only in a few industrialized societies. However, treatment exists wherever addiction exists. Inquiry into previous treatments in the country of origin can provide important information regarding the course and likely prognosis.

Treatment can include community sings, herbal medications, and sweat lodges. Often these have a ritual or ceremonial dimension (29). These rituals can be useful in engendering social support for the recovering person, establishing a new social persona, and fostering new attitudes toward a sober lifestyle (29,30). Often it can be useful to inquire about these modalities to gain an appreciation for the patient's understanding of addiction treatment (31).

Psychotherapies

Clinicians sometimes assume that English literacy and advanced education are necessary for successful psychotherapy. Nothing could be further from the truth. Supportive counseling can be applied in any setting; it can be especially efficacious if the immigrant patient is seeking an advisor for successful adjustment to the new society. Behavioral modification, as in the case of desensitization, can apply to members of any group.

Family therapy may involve special considerations, depending on the family structure and traditions. In family therapy, the explicit family hierarchy will often hold sway, so that family members do not typically confront a matriarch or patriarch in front a therapist. This special challenge is not a rationale for circumventing the family, however. Whenever possible, they should be involved in the patient's assessment and care (32). Elements of interpersonal psychotherapy and psychodynamically oriented psychotherapy also have their place in cross-cultural care.

Grief Therapy

As indicated above, delayed or missed grieving may appear once the addicted person becomes sober. Bereavement may involve the deaths of friends and family members. However, bereavement may also involve other losses experienced by refugees (7), such as:

- Separation from family and friends, still alive in the home country
- Loss of home, community, and nation
- Rejection by the country of origin
- Failure of the family, religion, or homeland to provide safety and security
- Shame at behaviors needed to survive (e.g., theft, lying, duplicity, prostitution, abandoning relatives or friends, killing)
- Inability to discharge one's responsibilities to family, friends, or society

Pharmacotherapy and Culture

Medications are often thought of as mechanistic modalities that affect neurotransmitter systems, but have no cultural relevance. To some extent, this may be true. One does not have to understand the pharmacotherapy of diazepam (Valium) to obtain relief in the midst of alcohol withdrawal. By the same token, medications can play important social and cultural roles. For example, disulfiram (Antabuse) has provided an excuse for recovering alcoholics to refuse friendly invitations by peers to go out drinking (33). The following case of a refugee demonstrates the principle.

Case Example

A 50-year-old opium addict was treated with naltrexone (ReVia) following relapse back to opium smoking. During the subsequent year he did well, obtaining a regular job, supporting his family, and resuming his role in the community as a shaman. After 1 year of stability, I suggested that he discontinue the naltrexone. He asked if he might continue it, as he often came across opium addicts in his shamanistic healing. He was concerned that he might lapse back to opium smoking without the naltrexone as a guarantor of his continued sobriety.

Acculturation Therapy

By the time an immigrant has become a patient, it is unlikely that simple referral to job training, education, or other local forms of rehabilitation will succeed. Special programs for those failing in the acculturation task are required. Such a group may include individuals from a variety of cultures and languages. They may also have different health or mental health problems. Combining this diverse clientele into a single large group offers certain economies of scale. Because all clients are unlikely to require all elements of such a program, a "smorgasbord" approach should permit each client to engage in those aspects of the program that the client needs. Elements of such a program may include:

- Taking English-as-a-second language (ESL) instruction
- Training in elemental aspects of community life (e.g., food preparation, shopping, taking public transportation, accessing health services, obtaining police protection, using financial services)
- Knowing the history, government, laws, and cultural values and norms of the United States
- Child raising and family laws in the United States
- Acquiring job skills and learning how to acquire job
- Learning how to keep a job and progress in employment
- Participating in recreational activities that do not require substance use
- Coping with bias, prejudice, and racism

Deportation

Forcible removal to the country of origin, while not a therapy per se, sometimes becomes a necessary disposition. Those working with immigrants must accept this as potential outcome in some cases. Clinical considerations rarely play a role in these outcomes.

Case Example

A 48-year-old Asian immigrant was importing opium through the mail, an offense for which he was arrested. During incarceration, he manifested severe opiate withdrawal. Subsequently released on bail, he entered treatment for opium addiction. His case was continued during treatment, as his attorney argued that he was importing opium for his own use only. The patient complied with treatment, and repeated urine screens were negative for drugs. Two years later he was arrested for again

importing opium through the mail and selling it to others. Federal authorities sent him immediately to federal prison in another community and initiated a deportation hearing.

Return to the country of origin may produce clinical improvement in the substance abuse. The largest naturalistic study involved American military in Vietnam. Among those who abused opiates in Vietnam, few ever returned to opiate abuse in the United States (34). Several expatriate opiate addicts in Laos did well upon return to their respective countries of origin in Europe, North America, and elsewhere (35).

PREVENTION

Religious affiliation with groups that forbid any use of alcohol or other recreational drugs has been effective as a prevention, as well as a treatment. Abstinence-oriented religion also provides easier accessibility to leadership; immigrants themselves have become the leaders and clergy, rather than relying on leaders or clergy of other ethnic groups. Community consensus against alcohol abuse or use of illicit drugs, at times developed with these church enclaves, is also effective in some groups.

Prevention among refugees and immigrants can be fostered by making culturally sensitive medical and psychiatric care available to immigrants and refugees as a means of preventing self-treatment with alcohol and dependence-producing drugs. Immigrating individuals and families can be educated to the early signs and symptoms of substance abuse in family members, and to methods of supportive confrontation. Awareness of enabling and rescuing behaviors by family members, and their detrimental effects on the course of substance abuse, should be promulgated.

To reduce the availability of illicit drugs in immigrant communities, expatriate police officers must be represented on the local police force. As with health care, the civil security network must be available to expatriate social networks.

Immigrant groups bring their unique histories and traditions to the societal mainstream in the United States. In addition to their rich customs, they also bring their vulnerabilities to psychoactive substances, whether traditional substances from the past or new substances that are unfamiliar to them. In a few instances, they bring new substances to the United States. American society and its institutions should recognize its contributions to immigrant use and abuse of substances, and its responsibility in supporting prevention. Likewise, immigrant groups should realize their role in contributing to the well being of the society at large. Prevention requires the efforts of both the mainstream society and the immigrant groups.

REFERENCES

1. Crockcroft JD. *Outlaws in the promised land.* New York: Grove Press, 1986.
2. Briggs VM. The growth and composition of the U.S. labor force. *Science* 1987;238:176–180.
3. Bacon KH. Population and power: preparing for change. *Wall Street Journal* 1988:p. 1.
4. United Nations. *Refugee report.* Geneva: United Nations High Commissioner for Refugees, 1969.
5. Westermeyer J. Social events and narcotic addiction: the influence of war and law on opium use in Laos. *Addict Behav* 1978;3(1):57–61.
6. Westermeyer J. Working with an interpreter in psychiatric assessment and treatment. *J Nerv Ment Dis* 1990; 178(12):745–749.
7. Cervantes R, Salgado-de-Snyder VN, Pakilla AM. Posttraumatic stress in immigrants from Central America and Mexico. *Hosp Community Psychiatry* 1989;40(6):615–619.
8. Westermeyer J, Wahmenholm K. Assessing the victimized psychiatric patient. *Hosp Community Psychiatry* 1989;40(3):245–249.
9. Westermeyer J. Use of alcohol and opium by the Meo of Laos. *Am J Psychiatry* 1971;127(8):1019–1023.
10. Westermeyer J. Hmong drinking practices in the United States: the influence of migration. In Bennett L, Ames G, eds. *The American experience with alcohol.* New York: Plenum, 1985:373–391.
11. Kennedy JG, Teague J, Fairbanks L. Quat use in North Yemen and the problem of addiction: a study in medical anthropology. *Cult Med Psychiatry* 1980;4:311–344.
12. Westermeyer J. Historical-social context of psychoactive substance disorders. In Francis R, Miller S, eds. *Clinical textbook of addiction disorders.* New York: Guilford, 1992.
13. Williams CL, Westermeyer J. Psychiatric problems among adolescent Southeast Asian refugees: a descriptive study. *J Nerv Ment Dis* 1983;171(2):79–85.
14. Kim LS, Chun CA. Ethnic differences in psychiatric diagnosis among Asian American adolescents. *J Nerv Ment Dis,* 1993;181:612–617.
15. Westermeyer J. Substance use disorders among young minority refugees: common themes in a clinical sample. *NIDA Res Monogr* 1993;130:308–320.
16. Krupinski J, Stoller A, Wallace L. Psychiatric disorders in Eastern European refugees now in Australia. *Soc Sci Med* 1973;7(31):31–45.
17. Westermeyer J, Chitasombat P. Course of opiate addiction: Hmong versus American. *Am J Addict* 1995.
18. Arif A, Westermeyer J, eds. *A manual for drug and alcohol abuse: guidelines for teaching.* New York: Plenum, 1988.
19. Westermeyer J, Lyfoung T, Neider J. An epidemic of opium dependence among Asian refugees in Minnesota: characteristics and causes. *Br J Addict* 1989;84(7):785–789.
20. May JV. Immigration as a problem in the state care of the insane. *Am J Insanity* 1912;69:313–322.
21. Westermeyer J, Canive J, Thuras P, et al. Perceived barriers to VA mental health care among upper midwest American Indian veterans: description and associations. *Med Care* 2002;40[1 Suppl]: 62–71.
22. Westermeyer J, Myott S, Aarts R, et al. Self-help strategies among substance abusers. *Am J Addict* 2001;10:249–257.
23. Jilek-Aal L. Alcohol and the Indian-white relationship: a study of the function of Alcoholics Anonymous among coast Salish Indians. *Confin Psychiatr* 1978;21:195–233.
24. Taylor V. The triumph of the Alkali Lake Indian band. *Alcohol Health Res World* 1987(Fall):57.
25. Kearny M. Drunkenness and religious conversion in a Mexican village. *Q J Stud Alcohol* 1970;31:248–249.
26. Westermeyer J. Two neo-Buddhist cults in Asia: The influence of the founder and the social context on religious movements. *J Psychol Anthropol* 1980;3:143–152.
27. Galanter M, Westermeyer J. Charismatic religious experience and large-group psychology. *Am J Psychiatry* 1980;137(12):1550–1552.
28. Albaugh B, Anderson P. Peyote in the treatment of alcoholism among American Indians. *Am J Psychiatry* 1974;131:1247–1256.
29. Jilek W.G. *Indian healing: shamanistic ceremonialism in the Pacific Northwest today.* Surrey, Canada: Hancock House, 1982.
30. Jilek W. G. Indian healing power: indigenous therapeutic practices in the Pacific Northwest. *Psychiatr Ann* 1974;4:13–21.
31. Westermeyer J. Folk treatments for opium addiction in Laos. *Br J Addict Alcohol Other Drugs* 1973;68(4): 345–349.
32. Catalano RF, Morrison DM, Wells EA, et al. Ethnic differences in family factors related to early drug initiation. *J Stud Alcohol* 1992;53(3):208–217.
33. Savard RJ. Effects of disulfiram therapy in relationships within the Navaho drinking group. *Q J Stud Alcohol* 1968;29:909–916.
34. Robins LN, Davis DH, Goodwin GW. Drug use by U.S. Army enlisted men in Vietnam: a follow-up on their return home. *Am J Epidemiol* 1974;99:235–249.
35. Westermeyer J, Berger LJ. "World traveler" addicts in Laos: I. Demographic and clinical description. *Am J Drug Alcohol Abuse* 1977;4:479–493.

Models of Prevention

CHAPTER 76

School-Based Programs

GILBERT J. BOTVIN AND
KENNETH W. GRIFFIN

INTRODUCTION

The problem of substance abuse has been a growing source of concern to health professionals, community leaders, and law enforcement agencies over the past few decades. Considerable effort and resources have been spent attempting to understand the etiology of substance use and abuse and to identify effective prevention and treatment strategies. Research concerning the onset and developmental progression of substance abuse indicates that most youth initiate substance use by experimenting with alcohol and cigarette smoking during early adolescence. For a subset of these youth, experimentation escalates to heavier levels of use, and for some, the abuse of more serious drugs, leading to drug dependence. Furthermore, early initiation of substance use is associated with a variety of negative outcomes in adolescence and early adulthood such as violent and delinquent behavior, poor physical health, and mental health problems (1–3).

Preventive interventions and related initiatives to reduce substance abuse have been the focus of a great deal of research. A recent review of drug-abuse prevention initiatives demonstrates that a wide variety of activities have been used to achieve the goal of reduced drug abuse, particularly among adolescents. These prevention activities range from educational and skills training activities that take place within schools, families, and communities, to mass media public service announcements, policy initiatives such as such as required health warning labels on cigarettes and alcohol, changes in school rules (i.e.,

"zero-tolerance" policies), and laws and regulations such as increased cigarette taxes and minimum purchasing age requirements (4). However, the bulk of the drug-abuse prevention research in the United States in the past 20 to 25 years has concentrated on school-based primary prevention programs. Because the general pattern of substance use initiation and escalation is well documented, many prevention programs aim to prevent early stage substance use or delay the onset of use among adolescents. Typically, these programs are provided to middle school or junior high school students and target the use of tobacco, alcohol, and marijuana because these are the most widely used substances and because preventing them may reduce the risk for later negative outcomes. Research shows that the most effective approaches to the prevention of adolescent drug abuse are derived from psychosocial theories and focus primary attention on the psychosocial risk and protective factors that promote the initiation and early stages of drug use (5,6).

Prevalence and Current Trends

National survey data show that prevalence rates of illicit drug use among adolescents peaked in the late 1970s, fell through much of the 1980s, and began to increase again during the 1990s. This upward trend during the 1990s was observed for a wide cross-section of individuals, including youth from different regions of the country, different social classes, and different ethnic and racial groups. Data from the 2001 Monitoring the Future Study (7) found that among high school seniors, 41% had used illicit drugs in the last year and 54% had done so during their lifetime. The annual prevalence rate for marihuana use was 37% and the lifetime rate was 49%; the annual inhalant prevalence rate was 5% and the lifetime rate was 13%; the annual lysergic acid diethylamide (LSD) prevalence rate was 7% and the lifetime rate was 11%; the annual methylenedioxymethamphetamine (MDMA; ecstasy) prevalence rate was 9% and the lifetime rate was

12%; the annual alcohol rate was 73% and the lifetime rate was 80%. For cigarette smoking, the lifetime rate was 61% and the 30-day rate was 30%. Although overall levels of drug use have remained steady or declined slightly over the past 2 to 3 years, there have been dramatic increases in the use of some substances. For example, ecstasy use has doubled, with 6% of adolescents reporting lifetime use in 1996 and 12% in 2001. In fact, ecstasy is currently used by more American teenagers than cocaine and there are few signs that the growing popularity of ecstasy will subside in the near future.

The Importance of Prevention

In view of the high levels of substance use among American youth and the disturbing upward trend observed in the 1990s, as well as the continuing threat of contracting acquired immunodeficiency syndrome (AIDS) through injection drug use, new urgency now exists for the development and dissemination of effective intervention strategies. Added to this is the long-standing concern over the deleterious health, legal, social, and pharmacologic effects of substance abuse.

Although there have been significant advances in the effectiveness of drug-abuse treatment in recent years (8), many treatment modalities are expensive, labor intensive, and plagued by high rates of recidivism. Clinicians are frequently confronted by a disorder that more often than not proves to be refractory to change, by patients whose knowledge of drugs may be daunting to even the most experienced practitioner, and by a pathogenic environment that does its best to undermine any progress made by the patient through the ubiquity of drugs and a social network supportive of continued substance abuse.

Prevention is important because it offers a logical alternative to treatment. An underlying assumption of prevention efforts is that it is likely to be easier to prevent substance abuse than to treat such an insidious disorder once it has developed. However, the development of effective prevention approaches has been far more difficult than was initially imagined. Indeed, most efforts to develop effective substance-abuse prevention efforts have achieved only a limited degree of success, and many failed completely. The first major breakthrough came at the end of the 1970s in the area of school-based smoking prevention. That work stimulated a great deal of prevention research and led to the development of several promising prevention approaches. Beginning in the 1980s and up to the present, mounting empirical evidence from a growing number of carefully designed and methodologically sophisticated research studies indicates that prevention works.

The School as the Site of Prevention Efforts

The development and testing of approaches for preventing adolescent substance abuse have largely focused on middle/junior high school students, with schools serving as the primary setting for prevention efforts. Despite their traditional educational mission, schools have been asked to assume responsibility for a variety of social and health problems. Many states mandate schools to provide their students with programs in health education and/or tobacco, alcohol, and drug education as well as teenage pregnancy and AIDS education. Although there has been considerable debate about whether schools should provide programs dealing with health and social problems, particularly at a time when there is renewed concern about academic standards, the simple truth is that schools offer the most efficient access to large numbers of adolescents. Moreover, many educators are gradually recognizing that problems such as drug abuse are a significant barrier to the achievement of educational objectives. The United States Department of Education, for example, has included "drug-free schools" as one of its goals for improving the quality of education in this country.

Chapter Overview

This chapter provides a summary of developments in the field of substance-abuse prevention over the past three decades. It begins with a discussion of what is currently known about the etiology and developmental progression of substance use and the implications for prevention. Traditional and contemporary prevention approaches are described and the evidence for their effectiveness is summarized. A major focus of this chapter is on the current generation of substance-abuse prevention approaches, the results of research testing their short- and long-term effectiveness, and recent work concerning the effectiveness of these approaches with ethnic minority youth. The final section summarizes conclusions to be drawn from this body of research, directions for future research, and implications for public health policy.

ETIOLOGY AND IMPLICATIONS FOR PREVENTION

To provide a context for understanding existing substance abuse prevention efforts and for developing a prescription for the most effective preventive interventions possible, it is necessary to be familiar with the factors associated with the initiation and maintenance of tobacco, alcohol, and drug abuse. Furthermore, it is important to identify when the onset and escalation of substance use onset typically occur to determine the most appropriate point of intervention. An understanding of the developmental course of substance abuse is also central, both in terms of the progression from nonuse to experimentation to abuse as well as the general sequence of using specific psychoactive substances or classes of substances.

Etiologic Determinants

A variety of risk factors for early stage substance use have been identified, as well as several protective factors that offset the effects of risk (5). Furthermore, a number of theoretical models have been developed or applied to phenomenon of alcohol and drug use among youth (6). The evidence that exists in the extant literature indicates that substance abuse results from the complex interaction of a number of different factors, including cognitive, attitudinal, social, personality, pharmacologic, biologic, and developmental factors (9–12).

Social Factors

Social factors are the most powerful influences promoting the initiation of tobacco, alcohol, and drug abuse. These include the behavior and attitudes of significant others such as parents, older siblings, and friends (13–16). Studies reveal that parents' use of alcohol, tobacco, marijuana, and other illicit drugs, and parental attitudes that are not explicitly against use, often translate into higher levels of use among children and adolescents (17). Poor family relationships and inadequate parenting practices (i.e., lack of parental monitoring) were also identified as risk factors for youth substance (11,18). Other social influences include popular media portrayals showing substance use as an important part of popularity, sophistication, success, sex appeal, and good times. Both the modeling of substance use behavior by media personalities and the messages communicated are powerful sources of influence that promote and support substance use (19,20).

Cognitive and Attitudinal Factors

Individuals who are unaware of the adverse consequences of tobacco, alcohol, and drug use, as well as those who have positive attitudes toward substance use, are more likely to become substance users than are those with either more knowledge or more negative attitudes toward substance use (21,22). In addition, individuals who believe that substance use is "normal" and that most people smoke, drink, or use drugs are more likely to be substance users (22).

Personality Factors

Substance use is associated with a number of psychological characteristics. Substance users have lower mood, self-esteem, assertiveness, personal control, and self-efficacy than nonusers, and are more anxious, impulsive, and rebellious than nonusers (23–28). The clinical literature also suggests that individuals with a specific psychiatric condition or symptoms (e.g., anxiety, depression) may use particular substances as a way of alleviating these feelings. For example, through experimentation with different substances, highly anxious individuals may find that alcohol or other depressants help them to feel less anxious, and they might use those substances as a way of regulating their feelings of anxiety. This has been referred to in the literature as the self-medication hypothesis (29).

Pharmacologic Factors

The pharmacology of commonly abused substances varies, although recent animal research found that several drugs of abuse (cocaine, amphetamine, morphine, nicotine, and alcohol), each with different molecular mechanisms of action, affect the brain in the same way by increasing strength at excitatory synapses on midbrain dopamine neurons, as does acute stress (30). Furthermore, virtually all of these substances produce effects that are highly reinforcing and dependency-producing. For tobacco, alcohol, and most illicit drugs, tolerance develops quickly, leading to increased dosages and an increased frequency of use. Once a pattern of dependent use has been established, termination of use produces dysphoric feelings and physical withdrawal symptoms.

Behavioral Factors

Substance abuse among young people is often part of a general syndrome or lifestyle reflecting a particular value orientation (31). Substance use is highly associated with a variety of health-compromising or problem behaviors. Individuals who use one substance are more likely to use others. Youth who smoke, drink, or use drugs tend to get lower grades in school, are not generally involved in adult-sanctioned activities such as sports and clubs, and are more likely than nonusers to become involved in antisocial or delinquent behavior, aggressiveness, and premature sexual activity (32–34). The finding that different types of problem behaviors are part of a general syndrome or collection of highly associated behaviors suggests that they may have the same or highly similar causes. To the extent that this is true, it would have significant implications for prevention. Notably, it may be possible to develop a single preventive intervention capable of having an impact on several associated behaviors at the same time.

Initiation and Developmental Course

For most individuals, experimentation with one or more psychoactive substances occurs during the adolescent years. Initial use of the "gateway" substances of tobacco, alcohol, and marihuana typically takes place during the early adolescent years. First use and intermittent experimentation generally occur within the context of social situations. In its initial stages, substance use is almost exclusively a social behavior. Since the 1960s, some degree of experimentation with drugs has become commonplace in contemporary American society. This is particularly true with respect to tobacco, alcohol, and marihuana, which are the most widely used and abused substances in our society. After a relatively brief period of experimentation, many individuals develop patterns of use characterized by both psychological and physiologic dependence. The initial social and psychological motivations for using drugs eventually yield to one driven increasingly by pharmacologic factors (8).

Substance Use Progression

Research indicates that experimentation with one substance frequently leads to experimentation with others in a logical and generally predictable progression (35). Most individuals begin by using alcohol and tobacco, progressing later to the use of marihuana. Some individuals may also use inhalants early in this sequence. This developmental progression corresponds closely to the prevalence of these substances in our society, with alcohol and inhalants being the most widely used, followed by tobacco and then marihuana. For some individuals this progression may eventuate in the use of depressants, stimulants, hallucinogens, and other drugs. However, many individuals may either discontinue use after a short period of experimentation or may not progress from the use of one substance to the use of others. The likelihood of progressing from one point in the developmental sequence to another can best be understood in probabilistic terms, with an individual's risk of moving to greater involvement with drugs increasing at each additional step in the developmental progression.

Knowledge of the developmental progression of substance use is important because it has implications for the focus and timing of preventive interventions. Interventions targeted at the use of substances occurring towards the beginning of this progression have the potential of not only preventing the use of those substances, but also the potential for reducing or eliminating the risk of using other substances further along the progression.

Adolescence and Substance Abuse Risk

Adolescence is frequently characterized as a period of great physical and psychological change (36). During adolescence, individuals typically experiment with a wide range of behaviors and lifestyle patterns. This occurs as part of the natural process of separating from parents, developing a sense of autonomy and independence, establishing a personal identity, and acquiring the skills necessary for functioning effectively in an adult world. Many of the developmental changes that are necessary prerequisites for becoming healthy adults increase an adolescent's risk of smoking, drinking, or using drugs. Adolescents who are impatient to assume adult roles may smoke, drink, or use drugs as a way of appearing more grown-up and laying claim to adult status. Adolescents may also engage in substance use because it provides them with a means of establishing solidarity with a particular peer group, rebelling against parental authority, or establishing their own individual identity.

During adolescence, the influence of parents is typically supplanted by that of the peer group (37). As the result of normal cognitive development, adolescents shift from a "concrete operational" mode of thinking, which is characteristically rigid, literal, and grounded in the "here and now," to a "formal operational" mode of thinking, which is more relative, abstract, and hypothetical (37,38). It has been suggested that these changes in the manner in which adolescents think may serve to undermine previously acquired knowledge relating to the potential risks of smoking, drinking, or using drugs. For example, the "formal operational" thinking of the adolescent facilitates the discovery of inconsistencies or logical flaws in arguments being advanced by adults concerning the health risks associated with substance use. Similarly, cognitive development during early adolescence may enable young people to formulate counterarguments to antidrug messages, which may, in turn, permit rationalizations for ignoring potential risks, particularly if substance use is perceived to have social or personal benefits.

Conformity needs and conformity behavior increase rapidly during preadolescence and early adolescence, and decline steadily from middle to late adolescence. However, despite this general developmental trend toward increased conformity, an individual's susceptibility to conformity pressure may vary greatly, depending on values and a variety of psychological factors, as well as the relative importance of peer acceptance. Finally, because adolescents characteristically have a sense of immortality and invulnerability, they tend to minimize the risks associated with substance use and overestimate their ability to avoid personally destructive patterns of use.

PREVENTION STRATEGIES

In view of the adverse health, social, and legal consequences of substance abuse and the difficulty of achieving sustained abstinence once addictive patterns of use have developed, it is readily apparent that the most promising approach to the problem of substance abuse is prevention. Prevention efforts have taken place on several different levels and have taken many forms. Prevention has been conceptualized in terms of supply and demand reduction models and as primary, secondary, and tertiary prevention. Each encompasses a different aspect of prevention, and has substantially different operational implications.

Supply and Demand Reduction

Supply reduction efforts are based on the fundamental assumption that substance use can be controlled by simply controlling the supply (i.e., availability). This has been the driving force behind the activities of law enforcement agencies, particularly with respect to the interdiction of drugs by governmental agencies such as the Drug Enforcement Administration (DEA), the Federal Bureau of Investigation (FBI), and local police departments. Demand reduction efforts, on the other hand, are conceptualized as those that attempt to dissuade, discourage, or deter individuals from using drugs or reducing the desire to use drugs. Demand reduction includes prevention, education, and treatment programs.

Types of Prevention

Consistent with usage in the field of public health, primary prevention interventions are designed to reach individuals before they have developed a specific disorder or disease. As such, they target a general population of individuals who, for the most part, have not yet begun using tobacco, alcohol, or other drugs. The goal of these approaches is to prevent substance use and abuse by intervening upon individual and/or environmental factors viewed as promoting or supporting this type of health-compromising behavior. Secondary prevention involves screening and early intervention. Tertiary prevention involves preventing the progression of a well-established disorder to the point of disability. However, one criticism of this classification system is that it is difficult to distinguish between tertiary prevention and treatment in that both involve care for persons with an established disorder.

In a 1994 report on preventive intervention research, the Institute of Medicine (39) proposed a new framework for classifying intervention programs as part of a continuum of care that includes prevention, treatment, and maintenance. While originally proposed as a system to classify interventions for mental disorders, the framework has been widely adopted and the terminology is now applied to other types of interventions. In this framework, prevention is reserved only for interventions that occur prior to the initial onset of a disorder. Prevention is further divided into three types: universal, selective, and indicated preventive interventions. These categories define prevention according to the groups to whom the interventions are directed, rather than stage of illness progression.

Universal prevention programs focus on the general population and aim to deter or delay the onset of a condition. While the level of risk for developing the condition may vary among individuals, universal programs recognize that all members of a population share some level of risk and can benefit from prevention programs that provide information and skills to help individuals avoid the outcome or condition. Selective prevention programs target selected high-risk groups or subsets of the general population believed to be at high risk because of membership in a particular group. Risk groups for selective interventions may be based on biologic, social, psychological, or other risk factors. Selective interventions for drug-abuse prevention, for example, might recruit groups such as children of drug users, pregnant women, or residents of high-risk neighborhoods. An individual's level of risk is presumed to be higher than average because of their membership in the selected group. Indicated prevention programs are designed for those already engaging in the behavior, or showing early danger signs, or who are engaging in related high-risk behaviors. Indicated programs for drug-

abuse prevention, for example, would be appropriate for individuals at highest risk for drug abuse, with the goal of reducing their chances of developing a drug-abuse problem by providing targeted programs. Thus, where recruitment and participation in a selective intervention is based on subgroup membership, recruitment and participation in an indicated intervention is based on early warning signs demonstrated by an individual.

Substance abuse prevention efforts can be divided into five general strategies:

- Information dissemination approaches
- Affective education approaches
- Alternatives approaches
- Social resistance skills approaches
- Broader competence enhancement approaches, which emphasize personal and social skills training

Table 76.1 summarizes these prevention strategies, which are discussed in the following sections.

Information Dissemination

Ubiquitous on the prevention landscape are programs that rely on the dissemination of factual information. The hallmark of these programs is that the main focus is on the provision of factual information concerning pharmacology and the adverse consequences of use. Information dissemination approaches to substance-abuse prevention are based on a rational model of human behavior. Substance abuse is seen as being the result of insufficient knowledge of the adverse consequences of using psychoactive drugs. The prescription for preventing substance abuse, according to this model, is to educate adolescents about the dangers of smoking, drinking, or using drugs. It is assumed that, once they are armed with this knowledge, they will act in a rational and logical way and simply choose not to become substance users. It has also been assumed that exposure to factual information about the dangers of using drugs will lead to changes in attitudes, which, in turn, will lead to nonsubstance use behavior. Within the context of the information dissemination approach, individuals are seen as being essentially passive recipients of factual information.

Information dissemination programs have taken the form of public information campaigns and school-based tobacco, alcohol, and drug education programs. Public information campaigns have involved the use of pamphlets, leaflets, posters, and public service announcements (PSAs) to increase public awareness of the problem of tobacco, alcohol, or drug abuse and alter societal norms concerning use. School programs have involved classroom curricula, assembly programs featuring guest speakers (frequently policemen or health professionals), and educational films.

Many informational approaches have been designed to deter substance use by emphasizing, even dramatizing,

TABLE 76.1. *Overview of major school-based prevention approaches*

Approach	Focus	Methods
Information dissemination	Increase knowledge of drugs, their effects and the consequences of use; promote antidrug use attitudes	Didactic instruction, discussion, audio/video presentations, displays of substances, posters, pamphlets, school assembly programs
Affective education	Increase self-esteem, responsible decision making, interpersonal growth; generally includes little or no information about drugs	Didactic instruction, discussion, experiential activities, group problem-solving exercises
Alternatives	Increase self-esteem, self-reliance; provide variable alternatives to drug use; reduce boredom and sense of alienation	Organization of youth centers, recreational activities; participation in community service projects; vocational training
Resistance skills	Increase awareness of social influence to smoke, drink, or use drugs; develop skills for resisting substance use influences; increase knowledge of immediate negative consequences; establish nonsubstance use norms	Class discussion; resistance skills training; behavioral rehearsal; extended practice via behavioral "homework"; use of same age or older peer leaders
Competence enhancement	Increase decision making, personal behavior change, anxiety reduction, communication, social, and assertive skills; application of generic skills to resist substance use influences	Class discussion; cognitive–behavioral skills training (instruction, demonstration, practice, feedback, reinforcement)

the risks associated with substance use. The underlying assumption of fear-arousal approaches is that evoking fear is more effective than a simple exposition of the facts. These approaches go beyond a dispassionate presentation of information by providing a clear and unambiguous message that substance use is dangerous. In addition, many traditional prevention programs have focused on the immorality of substance use. Program providers not only teach the objective facts but "preach" to students about the evils of smoking, drinking, or using drugs, and exhort them not to engage in those behaviors.

Examination of the empirical evidence concerning the effectiveness of the different approaches to tobacco, alcohol, and drug-abuse prevention described above indicates quite clearly that these approaches are ineffective (40,41). Studies testing information dissemination approaches to prevention have consistently found that they can increase knowledge and change attitudes toward substance use. These studies have rather consistently indicated that informational approaches do not reduce or prevent tobacco, alcohol, or drug use; they indicate quite clearly that increased knowledge has little or no impact on substance use or on intentions to engage in tobacco, alcohol, or drug use in the near future. As such, the evaluation studies call into question the basic assumption of the information dissemination model: that increasing knowledge will result in attitude and behavior change. Some studies even suggest that this approach may lead to increased usage, possibly because it may serve to stimulate adolescents' curiosity(42).

Because fear arousal and moral appeals are typically used in conjunction with informational programs, no evi-

dence exists concerning their independent effects, if any, on substance use. However, because virtually all of the evaluation studies conducted with information dissemination approaches have not found evidence of prevention effects on behavior, it is unlikely that either of these approaches would yield any effects if used independently.

Considering the complex etiology of substance abuse, it is not surprising that approaches that rely on the provision of factual information are ineffective. Information dissemination approaches are inadequate because they are too narrow in their focus and are based on an incomplete understanding of the factors promoting substance use and abuse. Although knowledge about the negative consequences of substance use is important, it is only one of many factors considered to play a role in the initiation of substance use among adolescents (43).

Affective Education

Substance-abuse prevention efforts have also used "affective education," which is intended to promote affective development. Affective education approaches are based on a different set of assumptions than cognitive approaches. Less emphasis is placed on factual information about the adverse consequences of substance abuse, and more emphasis is placed on students' personal and social development. Affective education approaches focus on increasing self-understanding and acceptance through activities such as values clarifications and responsible decision making; improving interpersonal relations by fostering effective communication, peer counseling, and assertiveness; and increasing students' abilities to fulfill their basic needs through existing social institutions (44). A common component of many affective education programs is the inclusion of norm-setting messages concerning responsible substance use.

The results of evaluation studies testing the effectiveness of affective education approaches have been as discouraging as evaluations of informational approaches. Although affective education approaches have, in some instances, been able to demonstrate an impact on one or more of the correlates of substance use, they have not been able to have an impact on substance use behavior (43,45).

Alternatives

One method of preventing substance abuse that has been a part of both community-based and school-based interventions has been to restructure part of the adolescent's environment to provide them with alternatives to substance use and activities associated with substance use. However, although some alternatives may decrease substance use, some may also increase it (46). Some alternatives have little theoretical connection to substance abuse, whereas others may be health compromising in their own right.

Several different alternative approaches have been developed. The original model for alternatives typically involved the establishment of youth centers providing a particular activity or set of activities in the community (e.g., community service, academic tutoring, sports, hobbies). It was assumed that if adolescents could be provided with real-life experiences that would be as appealing as substance use, their involvement in these activities would actually take the place of involvement with substance use. Another type of alternative approach is Outward Bound and similar programs. These activities are organized in the hope that they would alter the affective-cognitive state of an individual; that they would change the way individuals felt about themselves and others, and how they saw the world. These are healthy activities frequently designed to promote teamwork, self-confidence, and self-esteem.

A third type of alternative approach is targeted more to specific individual needs. For example, the need for relaxation or more energy might be satisfied by exercise, participating in sports, or hiking; the desire for sensory stimulation might be satisfied through activities that enhance sensory awareness, such as learning to appreciate the sensory aspects of music, art, and nature; and the need for peer acceptance might be satisfied through participation in sensitivity training or encounter groups.

In this context, it is important to recognize that although some activities are associated with nonsubstance use, others are associated with substance abuse (46). For example, entertainment activities, participation in vocational activities, and participation in social activities are associated with more substance use. On the other hand, academic activities, involvement in religious activities, and participation in sports or physical fitness training are generally associated with less substance use. Consequently, it is conceivable that some alternatives programs could be counterproductive if the wrong type of activities were selected. At the same time, the activities that may be the most appropriate alternatives are likely to be those that would have the least interest for individuals at high risk for using drugs. Few alternative approaches have been evaluated appropriately, and the vast majority are ineffective in preventing substance use behavior (47). However, one recent study suggests that physical fitness training may reduce risk factors for substance use, as well as use of cigarettes, smokeless tobacco, and alcohol (48).

Psychological Inoculation

The pioneering prevention research of Evans and his colleagues at the University of Houston toward the end of the 1970s triggered a major departure from traditional approaches to tobacco-, alcohol-, and drug-abuse prevention. Unlike previous approaches that focused on information dissemination, fear arousal, or moral suasion, the strategy developed initially by Evans and his colleagues (49,50) focused on the social and psychological factors believed to be involved in the initiation of cigarette smoking.

Evans' work was strongly influenced by persuasive communications theory as formulated by McGuire (51) and a concept called "psychological inoculation." Psychological inoculation is analogous to that of inoculation used in infectious disease prevention. Persuasive communications designed to alter attitudes, beliefs, and behavior are conceptualized as the psychosocial analogue of "germs." To prevent "infection" it is necessary to expose the individual to a weak dose of those "germs" in a way that facilitates the development of "antibodies" and thereby increases resistance to any future exposure to persuasive messages in their more virulent form.

The application of the concept of psychological inoculation as a smoking prevention strategy is fairly straightforward. Smoking is conceptualized as being the result of social influences (persuasive messages) to smoke from peers and the media which are either direct (offers to smoke from other adolescents or cigarette advertising) or indirect (exposure to high-status role models who smoke). If adolescents are likely to be called "chicken" for refusing to try cigarettes, they can be forewarned of the likelihood of encountering that kind of pressure and provided with the necessary skills for countering it. For example, they can be trained to reply: "If I smoke to prove to you that I'm not a chicken, all I'll really be showing is that I'm afraid not to do what you want me to do. I don't want to smoke; therefore I'm not going to." If adolescents are likely to see older youth posturing and acting "tough" by smoking, they can be taught to think to themselves: "If they were really tough, they wouldn't have to smoke to prove it."

The intervention initially developed by Evans consisted of a series of films designed to increase students' awareness of the various social pressures to smoke that they would be likely to encounter as they progressed through the critical junior high school period. Also included in these films were demonstrations of specific techniques that could be used to effectively resist various pressures to smoke. The prevention strategy developed by Evans also included two other important components: periodic assessment of smoking with feedback to students and information about the immediate physiologic effects of smoking. Smoking was assessed by questionnaire on a biweekly basis and saliva samples were collected as an objective measure of smoking status. The rate of smoking in each classroom (which was considerably lower than most adolescents thought) was publicly announced to correct the misperception that cigarette smoking is a highly normative behavior (i.e., that everybody is doing it).

In the first major test of this prevention strategy, Evans compared students receiving assessment/feedback with those receiving monitoring/feedback plus inoculation against a control group (50). The students in the two treatment conditions exhibited smoking onset rates of approximately 50% lower than that observed in the control group. Although the inoculation intervention did not produce any additional reduction in smoking onset beyond that produced by the assessment/feedback intervention, the overall reduction in smoking onset was dramatic in view of the history of failed prevention efforts that preceded this study. The success of the study conducted by Evans triggered an explosion of prevention research and offered the first real evidence in more than two decades that preventive interventions could work.

Resistance Skills Training

Several variations on the prevention model originally developed by Evans have been tested over the years (52–60). Similar to Evans' model, these interventions were designed to increase students' awareness of the various social influences to engage in substance use. A distinctive feature of these prevention models is that they place more emphasis on teaching students specific skills for effectively resisting both peer and media pressures to smoke, drink, or use drugs.

This chapter refers to this type of prevention program as social "resistance skills training," because it captures two distinctive aspects of these programs: (a) the focus on increasing participants' resistance to negative social influences to engage in substance use and (b) the focus on skills training. They have also been referred to as "social influence" approaches (because they target the social influences promoting substance use) or "refusal skills training" approaches (because a central feature of these programs is that they teach how to say "No" to substance use offers).

The psychosocial prevention approaches that rely on resistance skills training are based on a conceptual model stressing the fundamental importance of social factors in promoting the initiation of substance use among adolescents. These influences come from the family (parents and older siblings), peers, and the mass media. Adolescents may be predisposed toward substance use because substance use behavior is modeled by parents or older siblings, or because of the transmission of positive messages and attitudes concerning substance use. Similarly, individuals who have friends who smoke, drink, or use drugs are more likely to become substance users themselves as a result of issues relating to modeling and the need for peer acceptance (as well as friend's increasing the availability of substances). Finally, on the larger societal level, high-status role models in the mass media may promote substance use, supported by the perception of positive norms and expectations with respect to substance use. Group norms are enforced by both implicit and explicit rules governing behavior, as well as perceived desirability. As Bandura (61) indicated, all social influences are themselves a product of the interaction between individual learning histories and forces in both the community and the larger society.

On the individual level, influences related to specific behaviors arise from learned expectations and skills regarding those behaviors. For example, individuals may smoke because they expect relatively immediate positive outcomes such as increased alertness, relief from anxiety, or enhanced social status. Logically, it would appear reasonable that individuals would choose not to smoke if they did not expect to receive rewarding consequences or if they had the ability to resist specific social pressures to smoke. Expectations and skills are learned both from observation and from direct experience.

Resistance skills training approaches generally teach students how to recognize situations in which they will have a high likelihood of experiencing peer pressure to smoke, drink, or use drugs so that these high-risk situations can be avoided. In addition, students are taught how to handle situations in which they might experience peer pressure to engage in substance use. Typically, this includes teaching students not only what to say (i.e., the specific content of a refusal message), but also how to deliver it in the most effective way possible.

Another distinctive feature of these programs is the use of peer leaders as program providers, often as an adjunct to an adult provider. Peer leaders have been included in nearly all of the studies testing social resistance skills training approaches. The peer leaders used in these interventions are typically older students (e.g., tenth graders might serve as peer leaders for seventh graders) but sometimes peer leaders of the same age as participants may be used. The rationale for using peer leaders is that peers generally have higher credibility with adolescents than do adults in regard to decisions about risky behavior. In general, evidence supports the use of peer leaders for this type of prevention strategy (52,55). In one recent meta-analysis of school-based drug-abuse prevention programs, findings were mixed; in many cases, peer-led programs were found to be more effective than adult-led programs; however, some studies found greater effects for adult-led programs (71). Overall, peer leaders may be most effective when they assist adult program providers and have specific and well-defined roles, which is how they are typically used (Table 76.2).

Material has also generally been included in these programs to combat the perception that substance use is widespread (i.e., "everybody's doing it") because research indicates that adolescents typically overestimate the prevalence of smoking, drinking, and the use of certain drugs (62). This was accomplished by simply providing students with the prevalence rates of substance use among their age-mates in terms of national survey data or conducting classroom or schoolwide surveys, which are organized and directed by students participating in the program. Finally, these programs typically include a component designed to increase students' awareness of the techniques used by advertisers to promote the sale of tobacco products or alcoholic beverages and to teach techniques for formulating counterarguments to the messages used by advertisers.

A number of studies document the effectiveness of social resistance skills prevention strategies. A review of these preventive interventions indicates that they are able to reduce the rate of smoking by between 35% and 45% after the initial intervention. Most of these prevention studies have focused primarily on preventing the onset of cigarette smoking; that is, preventing the transition from nonsmoking to smoking. The results reported range from reductions of 33% to 39% in the proportion of individuals beginning to smoke (comparing the proportion of new smokers in the experimental group with that of the control group). Several studies demonstrate reductions in the overall prevalence of cigarette smoking among the participating students, both for experimental smoking (less than 1 cigarette per week) and for regular smoking (1 or more cigarettes per week) with reductions in smoking prevalence typically about 45% when comparing an intervention group to controls. Similar reductions are reported for alcohol and marihuana use (58,63). Although most studies assessing the impact of these prevention approaches on tobacco use have focused on cigarette smoking, recent research indicates that the social resistance skills training approach also reduces smokeless tobacco use (60).

Most of the research studies conducted with resistance skills training approaches are targeted at junior high school students, generally beginning with 7th graders. Fewer studies include elementary school students, partly because substance use rates are very low and it is difficult to demonstrate behavioral effects in this age group. The programs tested have been of varying lengths, ranging from as few as 3 or 4 sessions to as many as 11 or 12 sessions. Considerable variation also exists among the individuals responsible for implementing these programs. Some programs were implemented by college students, others by members of the research project staff, and still others used classroom teachers to implement the prevention programs. In addition to studies testing the effectiveness of social resistance skills training approaches in school settings, studies have also tested this intervention approach along with media, parent, or media plus parent components (65–68). These studies indicate that the inclusion of additional intervention components produces stronger prevention effects than the school-based intervention alone.

To develop more effective interventions, it is necessary to identify the relative efficacy of program components and the most effective providers. For example, many social resistance skills approaches include a public commitment component, yet the results of a study conducted by Hurd and his collaborators (53) suggest that this component may not contribute to the effectiveness of these programs. Similarly, many of these programs have used films or videotapes similar to those initially developed by Evans and his colleagues (50). However, it is not yet clear what type of media material is the most effective or the extent to which it is necessary as a component. Finally, little is known concerning the optimal program length, program structure, or the characteristics of the individuals who are the most influenced by these programs. With respect to the latter, studies have attempted to examine the characteristics of the individuals who are affected by interventions based on the social resistance skills prevention approach. Results have generally indicated that these prevention programs are effective with a broad range of adolescents including high- and low-risk individuals (69) and urban, suburban, and rural students (58). At least one study, however, found differential prevention effects by gender (70).

Perhaps the best known application of the social resistance skills training model is Project DARE (Drug Abuse Resistance Education) which is being used in approximately 60% of the classrooms in America. A unique aspect of DARE, and one that undoubtedly has contributed to its adoption by many schools, is that it is conducted by police officers. Although DARE has been remarkably successful with respect to being adopted by a large number of schools and in promoting an awareness of drug abuse, the results of DARE are disappointing. Although DARE has been repeatedly evaluated, many outcomes studies have been of limited scientific value because of weak research designs (e.g., posttest only), poor sampling and data collection procedures, inadequate measurement strategies, and problems in data analysis approaches (72). Several recent evaluation studies of DARE using more scientifically rigorous designs (i.e., large samples, random assignment, and longitudinal followup) show that DARE has little or no impact on drug use behaviors, particularly beyond the initial posttest assessment (73–75).

Followup studies using school-based approaches indicate that the positive behavioral effects of these prevention

TABLE 76.2. *Selected studies testing school-based social and resistance skills training approaches*

Reference	Subjects	Intervention approach	Evaluation design	Results
Adolescent Alcohol Prevention Trial (57,64)	5th graders	Nine-session school-based program assessing the effectiveness of resistance skills training, normative education, and drug education; 7th grade booster sessions; includes discussion, homework, and video	Pre- and posttest; 3-year followup; tested information only, resistance training, normative education, and combined curricula	Resistance training and normative education significantly increased the skills they targeted; only normative education positively affected substance use into 8th grade; resistance training only condition increased levels of substance abuse
Alcohol Misuse Prevention Study (63)	5th and 6th graders	Four-session resistance training curriculum, with three booster sessions; involves health education, coping strategies; uses positive reinforcement	Pre- and posttest; 26-month followup; compares intervention, intervention plus boosters, and control drinking prior to implementation	No treatment effect as a whole for alcohol use or misuse; program effects found for alcohol misuse in the subgroups who had experienced roleplay, homework, and video
Alcohol Misuse Prevention Study (105)	6th graders	Four-session resistance training curriculum, with three booster sessions; involves health education, coping strategies; uses positive reinforcement	Pre- and posttest; annual followup through 10th grade	Norm setting mediated the effect of the intervention on alcohol overindulgence at the 7th and 8th grades and at the 8th to 10th grades; however, refusal skills did not mediate the effect of the program
Midwestern Prevention Project (67)	6th and 7th graders	Ten-session intervention program includes school, parent, mass media components; school-based intervention includes resistance training, normative education, and health education; reinforced by role play, problem solving, discussion, and practice; taught by classroom teachers, using peer leaders; includes booster sessions	Pre- and posttest; 2-year followup	Proportion of smokers lower in experimental group for recent smoking and having smoked within 1 month; experimental group marginally lower in number of students who have ever smoked
Midwestern Prevention Project (69)	6th and 7th graders; high and low risk	Ten-session school-based social influences curriculum mentioned above	Pre- and posttest; 3-year followup	Experimental reductions in tobacco and marihuana use; equivalent reductions across risk levels; marginal effect for lifetime smoking
Midwestern Prevention Project (104)	6th and 7th graders	Ten-session school-based social influences curriculum mentioned above	Pre- and posttest; 1-year followup	Experimental reductions in cigarette smoking, drinking, and marihuana use; positive effects on mediating variables, such as communication skills, and beliefs about friends' tolerance of drug use

1220

Program	Population	Intervention	Design	Results
Midwestern Prevention Project (66)	6th graders	Thirteen-session social influence school prevention curriculum similar to Pentz et al. (69), plus parent curriculum consisting of parent–child homework, parent training workshops, and community activities	Pre- and posttest; 18-month followup	73% of parents participated in at least one of the components; parent participation in program resulted in less cigarette use, and was marginally associated with less alcohol use at followup
Project ALERT (58)	7th graders; urban, suburban, and rural	Eight-session social influence and resistance skills training curriculum; three 8th grade booster sessions; used role play and discussion; conducted by classroom teachers and older teenagers	Pre- and posttest; 3-, 12-, and 15-month followup; program tested on students in three levels of risk	Initial reductions in drinking for different risk levels; project effects for marihuana and cigarette initiation for all risk levels; reductions in drinking not sustained after 7th grade
Project ALERT (79)	7th graders	Same as above	Pre- and posttest; 2-year followup	Effects on cognitive risk factors persist through 9th grade in teen-led condition; all effects on actual use decay after 2 years
Project ALERT (80)	7th graders	Same as above	Pre- and posttest; 6-year followup	Effects on substance use decay after intervention; some effects on cognitive risk factors persist until 10th grade
Project SMART (70)	7th graders	Twelve-session social skills and drug resistance curriculum, and a 12-session affective education curriculum; used role play and discussion; conducted by health educators with peer assistants	Pre- and posttest comparison of 2 program types within 6 subgroups (males, females, Asians, blacks, Hispanics, and whites); 1-year followup of 3 cohorts	Positive effects for females in both programs for cigarette smoking and alcohol consumption; significant sex by program interactions for cigarettes and marihuana use
Project TNT (Towards No Tobacco Use) (60)	7th graders	Three individual 10-session social influence curricula focusing on resistance skills, normative beliefs, health consequences and a combined curriculum; involves discussion, decision making, video, and public commitment; taught by health educators	Pre- and posttest; 1-year followup; compares effects of 3 components of program: resistance skills, normative beliefs, and health consequences	The comprehensive, informational, and health education curricula were superior in reducing both trial and weekly use of tobacco as compared to normative and control; all conditions, except the informational condition, were superior to control for reduction of smokeless tobacco use

approaches are evident for up to 3 years after the conclusion of these programs for cigarette smoking (54,56,60) and multicomponent studies have found prevention effects for up to 7 years (76). However, results from long-term followup studies of school-based approaches indicate that these prevention effects are typically not maintained (77–81). While this has led some to conclude that school-based prevention approaches may not be powerful enough to produce lasting prevention effects (82), others have argued that the prevention approaches tested in these studies may have deficiencies which undermined their long-term effectiveness.

For example, Resnicow and Botvin (83) make the case that the apparent failure of studies testing resistance skills training approaches to produce long-term prevention effects may have to do with factors related to either the type of intervention tested in these studies or the way these interventions were implemented. According to them, the absence of long-term prevention effects in these studies should not be taken as an indictment of school-based prevention. Durable prevention effects may not have been produced in several long-term followup studies because (a) the length of the intervention may have been too short (i.e., the prevention approach was effective, but the initial prevention "dosage" was too low to produce a long-term effect), (b) booster sessions were either inadequate or not included (i.e., the prevention approach was effective, but it eroded over time because of the absence or inadequacy of ongoing intervention), (c) the intervention was not implemented with enough fidelity to the intervention model (i.e., the correct prevention approach was used, but it was implemented incompletely, improperly, or both), and/or (d) the intervention was based on a faulty assumptions, was incomplete, or was otherwise deficient (i.e., the prevention approach was ineffective).

Based on the findings of more recently published research using the prevention approach described in the next section, it now appears that all four of these factors may have played a role in the negative findings of long-term followup studies with prevention approaches based on the resistance skills training model. It is also clear that it is possible to develop and implement school-based prevention approaches powerful enough to have a durable impact on adolescent substance use. However, to be effective, school-based interventions need to be more comprehensive, have a stronger initial dosage, include at least 2 additional years of (booster) intervention, and be implemented in a manner that is faithful to the underlying intervention model.

Competence Enhancement

Since the end of the 1970s and up to the present, considerable research has also been conducted with a prevention approach that teaches general personal and social skills either alone (84) or in combination with components of the social resistance skills model (85–92). These competence-enhancement approaches are more comprehensive than either traditional cognitive–affective approaches or the more recent resistance skills model. In addition to recognizing the importance of social learning processes such as modeling, imitation, and reinforcement, competence-enhancement approaches posit that youth with poor personal and social skills are not only more susceptible to influences that promote drug use, but also are motivated to use drugs as an alternative to more adaptive coping strategies (93). Moreover, unlike affective education approaches that rely on experiential classroom activities, these approaches emphasize the use of proven cognitive–behavioral skills training methods. They are based on social learning theory (61) and problem behavior theory (9). Substance abuse is conceptualized as a socially learned and functional behavior, resulting from the interplay of social and personal factors. Substance use behavior is learned through modeling and reinforcement and is influenced by cognition, attitudes, and beliefs.

Personal and social skills training prevention approaches typically teach two or more of the following:

- General problem-solving and decision-making skills
- General cognitive skills for resisting interpersonal or media influences
- Skills for increasing self-control and self-esteem
- Adaptive coping strategies for relieving stress and anxiety through the use of cognitive coping skills or behavioral relaxation techniques
- General social skills
- General assertive skills

These skills are taught using a combination of instruction, demonstration, feedback, reinforcement, behavioral rehearsal (practice during class), and extended practice through behavioral homework assignments. The intent of these programs is to teach the kind of generic skills for coping with life that will have a relatively broad application. This is in contrast to the resistance skills training approaches, which are designed to teach skills with a problem-specific focus. Personal and social skills training programs emphasize the application of general skills to situations directly related to substance use and abuse (e.g., the application of general assertive skills to situations involving peer pressure to smoke, drink, or use drugs). These same skills can be used for dealing with many of the challenges confronting adolescents in their every day lives, including, but not limited to, smoking, drinking, and drug abuse.

Although prevention approaches that emphasize the development of general personal and social skills have a broader focus compared to approaches designed to teach skills for resisting social influences to use drugs, the most effective prevention approaches appear to combine the features of both. Indeed, evidence suggests that broad-based competence enhancement approaches may not be effective unless they also contain some resistance skills training material. A prevention approach with both components will help teach students to apply generic personal and social skills to situations related specifically to preventing substance abuse and may also serve to increase antidrug norms.

Most of the prevention studies on this approach that have been conducted thus far have focused on seventh graders. However, some studies have been conducted with sixth graders (95) and one was conducted with eighth, ninth, and tenth graders (85). Program length has ranged from as few as 7 sessions to as many as 20 sessions. Some of these prevention programs were conducted at a rate of one class session per week, while others were conducted at a rate of two or more classes per week. Most of the studies conducted so far have used adults as the primary program providers. In some cases, these adults were teachers; in other cases, they were outside health professionals (i.e., project staff members, graduate students, social workers). Some studies included booster sessions, although the majority did not.

Evaluation studies testing personal and social skills training approaches have demonstrated significant behavioral effects. A series of evaluation studies has been conducted over the past 20 years examining the effectiveness of the Life Skills Training (LST) program, a universal school-based prevention approach that teaches general personal and social skills training combined with drug-refusal skills and normative education. Studies range from small-scale efficacy studies to large-scale, randomized trials. These studies consistently show that the LST approach produces positive behavioral effects on alcohol, tobacco, and other drug use (Table 76.3).

The focus of the initial evaluation research of the LST program was on cigarette smoking and involved predominantly white middle-class populations. In a series of small-scale efficacy trials, the short-term effects of the intervention on cigarette smoking and related risk factors was examined. Several early studies demonstrated that this prevention approach effectively reduces cigarette smoking among youth receiving the program, as compared to a control group that does not (see, e.g., references 85, 86, and 94). During the first decade of evaluation research on this approach, additional studies examined its' effectiveness with different delivery formats, different program providers, and with different substances; these studies found that the prevention approach was made more effective by the inclusion of booster sessions after the initial year of intervention; that it is equally effective when taught by teachers, peer leaders, and health educators; and that it produced behavioral effects on alcohol and marijuana (see, e.g., references 87–89 and 92). These initial studies were among the first school-based prevention studies to show consistent behavioral effects on adolescent substance use.

More recent evaluation research on the LST approach has focused on the intervention's long-term effects on drug use, effects on more serious levels of drug involvement including illicit drug use, its impact on hypothesized mediating variables, and has increasingly focused on effects when used with inner-city minority populations. The evaluation designs have become increasingly sophisticated with time, including two large-scale multisite randomized prevention trials with long-term followup. The first of these randomized controlled prevention trials focused on a predominantly white, suburban sample of youth. Beginning in 1985, this prevention trial examined the short- and long-term effects of the LST approach among close to 6,000 students from 56 junior high schools in New York State. This study was one of the largest and most methodologically rigorous drug-abuse prevention trials ever conducted, and included adolescents that were predominantly white (91%). Students in the prevention condition received the intervention in the seventh grade and booster sessions during the eighth and ninth grades. Significant prevention effects were found among intervention participants at the end of the ninth grade in terms of cigarette smoking, marijuana use, and immoderate alcohol use (96), as well as at the end of the twelfth grade (97). In the latter followup study, there were significantly fewer smokers, heavy drinkers, marijuana users and polydrug users among students who received the prevention program relative to controls. The strongest prevention effects were produced for the students who received the most complete implementation of the prevention program. A related study using data from a confidential and random subsample of these students (N = 447) found that there were lower levels of overall illicit drug use and lower levels of use for hallucinogens, heroin and other narcotics in the intervention group relative to controls (98).

A recent large-scale prevention trial tested the LST approach among inner-city minority youth in New York City. The sample was predominantly African American (61%) and Hispanic (22%) and consisted of students (N = 3,621) in 29 urban middle schools. Results at the posttest and 1-year followup indicated that those who received the prevention program reported less smoking, drinking, drunkenness, inhalant use, and polydrug use relative to those in the control group who did not receive the intervention (99). Two additional studies using data from this large-scale trial focused on prevention effects of the intervention program in terms of cigarette smoking onset and binge drinking. The first of these studies examined the effectiveness of the prevention program in reducing the initiation and escalation of smoking in a subsample of girls from the larger study (100). One-year followup data indicated that girls who participated in the intervention condition were significantly less likely to initiate smoking relative to controls, and 30% fewer of participants escalated to monthly smoking relative to students in the control group. A second study showed that this intervention approach had protective effects in terms of binge drinking (5 or more drinks per drinking occasion) among inner-city, middle-school

TABLE 76.3. Selected studies testing school-based competence enhancement approaches

Reference	Subjects	Intervention approach	Evaluation design	Results
Life Skills Training (92)	7th graders, white, suburban	20-session intervention similar to Botvin et al. (96); 10 booster sessions in 8th grade	Pre- and posttest; 1-year followup; compares 5 interventions: peer-led, peer-led with booster sessions, teacher-led, teacher-led with booster sessions, and control	Peer-led implementation with booster sessions resulted in reductions in tobacco, alcohol, and marihuana use; similar effects for females in teacher-led condition; program effects on mediating variables
Life Skills Training (96)	7th graders, white, suburban	15-session personal, social and resistance skills curriculum; 10 second- and 5 third-year booster sessions; sessions include decision making, assertiveness, self-esteem, stress management, media influences, drug knowledge, social skills, and communication skills; used discussion, homework, video, role play, behavioral rehearsal, and reinforcement; taught by classroom teachers	Pre- and posttest; 3-year followup; compares implementation with provider training workshops and consultations, videotaped training only, and information only control	Reductions in cigarette, marihuana, and alcohol use; program effects on mediating variables such as normative expectations, substance use knowledge, interpersonal and communication skills
Life Skills Training (106)	7th graders, minority, urban	Generic program same as above; culturally focused program similar, but used multicultural myths and stories to model various skills; taught by outside providers and peer leaders	Pre- and posttest; 1-year followup; compares generic skills-training, culturally focused, and information-only control	Both prevention programs show reductions in intentions to drink alcohol, and changes in mediating variables consistent with nondrug use; generic program also reduced intentions to use illicit drugs
Life Skills Training (107)	7th graders, minority, urban	Same as Botvin et al. (106)	Pre- and posttest; 2-year followup	Reductions in current alcohol use and intentions to drink alcohol; effects on mediating variables consistent with nondrug use
Life Skills Training (97)	7th graders, white, suburban	Same as Botvin et al. (96)	Pre- and posttest; 6-year followup	Reductions in drug and polydrug use; strongest effects found for students who received a more complete version of the program

1224

Program	Population	Description	Assessment	Results
Life Skills Training (98)	7th graders, white, suburban	Same as Botvin et al. (96)	Pre- and posttest; 6.5-year followup	Reductions in overall illicit drug use; reduced use of hallucinogens, heroin, and other narcotics
Life Skills Training (99)	7th graders, minority	Similar to Botvin et al. (96); slightly revised for use with minority youth (e.g., graphics, language, role-play scenarios) although no modifications were made to underlying prevention strategy	Pre- and posttest; 1-year followup	Reduced smoking, drinking, drunkenness, inhalant use, and polydrug use
Life Skills Training (100)	7th graders, minority, girls only	Same as above	Pre- and posttest; 1-year followup	Reduced initiation of smoking and escalation to monthly smoking
Life Skills Training (101)	7th graders, minority	Same as above	Pre- and posttest; 1- and 2-year followup	Reduced binge drinking at 1- and 2-year followup; reduced prodrinking attitudes and normative expectations for peer drinking
Life Skills Training (102)	7th graders, minority, high-risk subsample	Same as above	Pre- and posttest; 1-year followup	Reduced smoking, drinking, inhalant use, and polydrug use at the 1-year followup among youth at high risk for substance use initiation
Positive Youth Development (85)	6th and 7th graders; urban and suburban	20-session program including: stress management, self-esteem, problem solving, substance and health information, assertiveness and social networks; involves discussion, role play, diaries, and videotapes; conducted by classroom teachers and health educators	Pre- and posttest	Increases in social adjustment and coping skills, intentions to use substances remained the same for program students, while control students reported increased intentions at post-assessment; positive effects on alcohol use, but no effects on reported drug use

boys and girls (101). In this study, the proportion of binge drinkers was more than 50% lower in those who received the prevention program relative to the control group at both the 1-year and 2-year followup assessments. Finally, a recent study of a subset of students from the larger sample examined the effectiveness of the prevention program among youth at high risk for substance use initiation and found that those students who had poor grades in school and friends that engage in substance use were less likely to engage in smoking, drinking, inhalant use, or polydrug use than were similarly matched controls that did not receive the intervention (102). Taken together, the results from several large-scale randomized prevention trials provide strong evidence of the effectiveness of the competence enhancement plus resistance skills prevention approach, with both suburban white youth and inner-city minority youth.

A major strength of the evaluation studies conducted with the broader personal and social skills training approaches such as Life Skills Training is that they have also a demonstrated impact on variables hypothesized to mediate the effect of the prevention programs in a direction consistent with nonsubstance use. These include significant changes in knowledge and attitudes, assertiveness, locus of control, social anxiety, self-satisfaction, decision making, and problem solving. Together, the results of these studies provide compelling evidence supporting the efficacy of broad-spectrum prevention strategies focusing on personal and social skills development. Thus, this prevention approach has been demonstrated to produce reductions in substance use (relative to controls), as well as changes on several hypothesized mediating variables in a direction consistent with reduced substance abuse risk. Published meta-analytic studies indicate that competence enhancement and social influence approaches are more effective than traditional didactic approaches, and that attitude and behavior change are most substantial in high intensity, multicomponent programs implemented with booster sessions after the initial intervention (103).

SUMMARY AND CONCLUSION

A number of substance abuse prevention approaches have been developed and tested over the years. The most common approaches to tobacco-, alcohol-, and drug-abuse prevention are those that focus on providing factual information about the adverse consequences of using these substances, with some approaches including a mix of scare tactics and moral messages. Other commonly used approaches to substance abuse prevention have used affective education and alternatives approaches. The existing evaluation literature shows rather conclusively that these are not effective prevention strategies when the standard of effectiveness concerns the ability to influence substance use behavior.

Prevention approaches that have been demonstrated to have an effective impact on substance use behavior are those that teach junior high school students social resistance skills either alone or in combination with approaches designed to enhance general personal competence by teaching an array of personal and social life skills. Both approaches emphasize skills training and deemphasize the provision of information concerning the adverse health consequences of substance use. These approaches use well-tested behavioral intervention techniques to facilitate the acquisition of skills for resisting social influences to engage in substance use.

Recognizing the critical importance of the early adolescent years, these preventive interventions have generally been implemented with middle and junior high school students. Despite generally impressive prevention effects, it is clear that, without booster sessions, these effects decay over time, thus arguing for ongoing prevention activities throughout early adolescent years and perhaps until the end of high school.

Although there has been considerable activity in the form of both the parents' movement and mass media campaigns, there is little evidence to indicate that such approaches are effective when used alone. However, community-based substance abuse prevention approaches based on principles derived from the most effective school-based prevention programs and successful community-based cardiovascular disease prevention studies appear to offer considerable promise.

Over the past 2 decades, there have been a number of significant developments in the field of substance abuse prevention. Yet, despite the promise offered by these approaches, future research is needed to further refine current prevention models and to develop new ones. Given the urgency and importance of dealing with the problem of substance abuse, it seems prudent to proceed on two simultaneous tracks: one involving further prevention research and the other involving the dissemination of the most promising existing prevention approaches. This is particularly important in view of the fact that the most widely utilized prevention approaches continue to be those that have already been found either to be ineffective or to lack any scientifically defensible evidence of their efficacy.

The problem of substance abuse is still very prevalent. However, for the first time in the history of its prevention, evidence now exists from a number of rigorously designed evaluation studies that specific school-based and community-based prevention models are effective. It is now incumbent upon health care professionals, educators, community leaders, and policy makers to move expeditiously toward wide dissemination and use of these approaches. It is equally important for private and governmental agencies to provide adequate funding for the important research necessary to further refine existing prevention models and to increase our understanding of the causes of substance abuse.

REFERENCES

1. Durant RH, Smith JA, Kreiter SR, et al. The relationship between early age of onset of initial substance use and engaging in multiple health risk behaviors among young adolescents. *Arch Pediatr Adolesc Med* 1999;153;286–291.

2. Ellickson PL, Tucker JS, Klein DJ. High risk behaviors associated with early smoking: Results from a 5-year follow-up study. *J Adolesc Health* 2001;28:465–473.

3. Newcomb MD, Bentler PM. *Consequences of adolescent drug use: impact on the lives of young adults.* New York: Sage, 1988.

4. Paglia A, Room R. Preventing substance use problems among youth: a literature review and recommendations. *J Prim Prev* 1999;20:3–50.

5. Hawkins JD, Catalano RF, Miller JY. Risk and protective factors for alcohol and other drug problems in adolescence and early adulthood: Implications for substance abuse prevention. *Psychol Bull* 1992;112:64–105.

6. Petraitis J, Flay BR, Miller TQ. Reviewing theories of adolescent substance use: Organizing pieces in the puzzle. *Psychol Bull* 1995;117:67–86.

7. Johnston LD, O'Malley PM, Bachman JD. *Monitoring the Future national results on adolescent drug use: overview of key findings, 2001.* (NIH Publication No. 02–5105). Bethesda, MD: National Institute on Drug Abuse, 2002.

8. Hartel CR Glantz MD. *Drug abuse: origins and interventions.* Washington, DC: American Psychological Association, 1997.

9. Jessor R, Jessor SL. *Problem behavior and psychosocial development: a longitudinal study of youth.* New York: Academic Press, 1977.

10. Cicchetti D, Luthar SS. Developmental approaches to substance use and abuse. *Dev Psychopathol* 1999;11:655–656.

11. Swadi H. Individual risk factors for adolescent substance use. Drug Alcohol Depend 1999;55;209–224.

12. Lanza ST, Collins LM, Pubertal timing and the onset of substance use in females during early adolescence. *Prev Sci* 2002;3(1):69–82.

13. Brown B, Clasen D, Eicher S. Perceptions of peer pressure, peer conformity dispositions, and self-reported behavior among adolescents. *Dev Psychol* 1986;22:521–530.

14. Gfroerer J. Correlation between drug use by teenagers and drug use by older family members. *Am J Drug Alcohol Abuse* 1987;13(1&2):95–108.

15. Andrews JA, Tildesley E, Hops H, et al. The influence of peers on young adult substance use. *Health Psychol* 2002;21(4):349–357.

16. Dishion TJ, Owen, LD. A longitudinal analysis of friendships and substance use: bidirectional influence from adolescence to adulthood. *Dev Psychol* 2002;38(4):480–491.

17. Windle M. Effect of parental drinking on adolescents. *Alcohol Health Res World* 1996;20(3):181–184.

18. Griffin KW, Botvin GJ, Scheier LM, et al. Parenting practices as predictors of substance use, delinquency, and aggression in urban minority youth: moderating effects of family structure and gender. *Psychol Addict Behav* 2000;14(2):174–184.

19. Tye J, Warner K, Glantz S. Tobacco advertising and consumption: evidence of a causal relationship. *J Public Health Policy* 1987:492–507.

20. McCool JP, Cameron LD, Petrie KJ. Adolescent perceptions of smoking imagery in film. *Soc Sci Med* 2001;52:1577–1587.

21. Piko B. Smoking in adolescence: do attitudes matter? *Addict Behav* 2001;26:201–217.

22. Simons-Morton B, Haynie DL, Crump AD, et al. Expectancies and other psychosocial factors associated with alcohol use among early adolescent boys and girls. *Addict Behav* 1999;24:229–238.

23. Chassin L, Presson CC, Sherman SJ, et al. Predicting the onset of cigarette smoking in adolescents: a longitudinal study. *J Appl Soc Psychol* 1984;14(3):224–243.

24. Page RM. Shyness as a risk factor for adolescent substance use. *J Sch Health* 1989;59(10):432–435.

25. Dielman TE, Leech SL, Lorenger AT, et al. Health locus of control and self-esteem as related to adolescent health behavior and intentions. *Adolescence* 1984;19:935–950.

26. Shoal GD, Giancola PR. Negative affectivity and drug use in adolescent boys: moderating and mediating mechanisms. *J Pers Soc Psychol* 2003;84(1):221–233.

27. Wills TA, Stoolmiller M. The role of self-control in early escalation of substance use: a time-varying analysis. *J Consult Clin Psychol* 2002;70(4):986–997.

28. Newcomb MD, Bentler PM. Drug use, educational aspirations and work force involvement: the transition from adolescence to young adulthood. *Am J Community Psychol* 1986;14(3):303–321.

29. Khantzian EJ. The self-medication hypothesis of substance use disorders: a reconsideration and recent applications. *Harv Rev Psychiatry* 1997;4:231–244.

30. Saal D, Dong Y, Bonci A, et al. Drugs of abuse and stress trigger a common synaptic adaptation in dopamine neurons. *Neuron* 2003;37:577–582.

31. Jessor R. Critical issues in research on adolescent health promotion. In: Coates T, Petersen A, Perry C, eds. *Promoting adolescent health: a dialogue on research and practice.* New York: Academic Press, 1982:447–465.

32. Donovan JE, Jessor R. Structure of problem behavior in adolescence and young adulthood. *J Consult Clin Psychol* 1985;53:890–904.

33. Farrell AD, Danish SJ, Howard CW. Relationship between drug use and other problem behaviors in urban adolescents. *J Consult Clin Psychol* 1992;60:705–712.

34. Resnicow K, Ross-Gaddy D, Vaughan RD. Structure of problem and positive behaviors in African-American youth. *J Consult Clin Psychol* 1995;63;594–603.

35. Kandel D. *Stages and pathways of drug involvement: examining the gateway hypothesis.* New York: Cambridge University Press, 2002.

36. Lerner RM, Galambos NL. Adolescent development: challenges and opportunities for research, programs, and policies. *Annu Rev Psychol* 1998;49:413–446.

37. Utech D, Hoving KL. Parents and peers as competing influences in the decisions on children of differing ages. *J Soc Psychol* 1969;78:267–274.

38. Piaget J. *The moral judgment of the child.* New York: Collier, 1962.

39. Institute of Medicine. *Reducing risks for mental disorders: frontiers for preventive intervention research.* Washington, DC: National Academy Press, 1994.

40. Kinder B, Pape N, Walfish S. Drug and alcohol education programs: a review of outcome studies. *Int J Addict* 1980;15:1035–1054.

41. Schaps E, Bartolo RD, Moskowitz J, et al. A review of 127 drug abuse prevention program evaluations. *J Drug Issues* 1981:17–43.

42. Swisher JD, Crawford JL, Goldstein R, et al. Drug education: pushing or preventing? *Peabody J Educ* 1971;49:68–75.

43. Kearney AL, Hines MH. Evaluation of the effectiveness of a drug prevention education program. *J Drug Educ* 1980;10:127–134.

44. Swisher JD. Prevention issues. In: Dupont RI, Goldstein A, O'Donnell J, eds. *Handbook on drug abuse.*

Washington, DC: National Institute on Drug Abuse, 1979:49–62.

45. Kim S. A short- and long-term evaluation of Here's Looking at You alcohol education program. *J Drug Educ* 1988;18(3):235–242.

46. Swisher JD, Hu TW. Alternatives to drug abuse: some are and some are not. *NIDA Res Monogr* 1983;47:141–153.

47. Schaps E, Moskowitz JM, Malvin JH, et al. Evaluation of seven school-based prevention programs: a final report on the Napa Project. *Int J Addict* 1986;21:1081–1112.

48. Collingwood TR, Sunderlin J, Reynolds R, et al. Physical training as a substance abuse prevention intervention for youth. *J Drug Educ* 2000;30(4):435–451.

49. Evans RI. Smoking in children: developing a social psychological strategy of deterrence. *Prev Med* 1976;5:122–127.

50. Evans RI, Rozelle RM, Mittlemark MB, et al. Deterring the onset of smoking in children: knowledge of immediate physiological effects and coping with peer pressure, media pressure, and parent modeling. *J Appl Soc Psychol* 1978;8:126–135.

51. McGuire WJ. The nature of attitudes and attitude change. In: Lindzey G, Aronson E, eds. *Handbook of social psychology*. Reading, MA: Addison-Wesley, 1968:136–314.

52. Arkin RM, Roemhild HJ, Johnson CA, et al. The Minnesota smoking prevention program: a seventh grade health curriculum supplement. *J Sch Health* 1981;51:616–661.

53. Hurd P, Johnson CA, Pechacek T, et al. Prevention of cigarette smoking in 7th grade students. *J Behav Med* 1980;3:15–28.

54. Luepker RV, Johnson CA, Murray DM, et al. Prevention of cigarette smoking: three year follow-up of educational programs for youth. *J Behav Med* 1983;6:53–61.

55. Perry C, Killen J, Slinkard LA, et al. Peer teaching and smoking prevention among junior high students. *Adolescence* 1983;9:277–281.

56. Telch MJ, Killen JD, McAlister AL, et al. Long-term follow-up of a pilot project on smoking prevention with adolescents. *J Behav Med* 1982;5:1–8.

57. Donaldson SI, Graham JW, Hansen WB. Testing the generalizability of intervening mechanism theories: understanding the effects of adolescent drug use prevention interventions. *J Behav Med* 1994;17:195–216.

58. Ellickson PL, Bell RM. Prospects for preventing drug abuse among young adolescents. *Science* 1990;247:1299–1305.

59. Snow DL, Tebes JK, Arthur MW, et al. Two-year follow-up of a social cognitive intervention to prevent substance abuse. *J Drug Educ* 1992;22:101–114.

60. Sussman S, Dent CW, Stacy AW, et al. Project Towards No Tobacco Use: 1-year behavior outcomes. *Am J Public Health* 1993;83:1245–1250.

61. Bandura A. *Social learning theory.* Englewood Cliffs, NJ: Prentice-Hall, 1977.

62. Fishbein M. Consumer beliefs and behavior with respect to cigarette smoking: a critical analysis of the public literature. In: *Federal Trade Commission Report to Congress pursuant to the Public Health Cigarette Smoking Act of 1976.* Washington, DC: U.S. Government Printing Office, 1977.

63. Shope JT, Dielman TE, Butchart AT, et al. An elementary school-based alcohol misuse prevention program: a follow-up evaluation. *J Stud Alcohol* 1992;53:106–121.

64. Donaldson SI, Graham JW, Piccinin AM, et al. Resistance-skills training and onset of alcohol use: evidence for beneficial and potentially harmful effects in public schools and in private Catholic schools. *Health Psychol* 1995;14:291–300.

65. Flynn BS, Worden JK, Secker-Walker S, et al. Prevention of cigarette smoking through mass media intervention and school programs. *Am J Public Health* 1992;82:827–834.

66. Rohrbach LA, Hodgson CS, Broder BI, et al. Parental participation in drug abuse prevention: results from the Midwestern Prevention Project. Special issue: preventing alcohol abuse among adolescents: preintervention and intervention research. *J Res Adolesc* 1994;4:295–317.

67. Pentz MA, Dwyer JH, MacKinnon DP, et al. A multicommunity trial for primary prevention of adolescent drug abuse: effects on drug prevalence. *JAMA* 1989;261:3259–3266.

68. Perry CL, Kelder SH, Murray DM, et al. Community-wide smoking prevention: long-term outcomes of the Minnesota heart health program and the class of 1989 study. *Am J Public Health* 1992;82(9):1210–1216.

69. Johnson CA, Pentz MA, Weber MD, et al. Relative effectiveness of comprehensive community programming for drug abuse prevention with high-risk and low-risk adolescents. *J Consult Clin Psychol* 1990;58(4):447–456.

70. Graham JW, Johnson CA, Hansen WB, et al. Drug use prevention programs, gender, and ethnicity: evaluation of three seventh-grade project SMART cohorts. *Prev Med* 1990;19:305–313.

71. Cuijpers P. Peer-led and adult-led school drug prevention: a meta-analytic comparison. *J Drug Educ* 2002;32(2):107–119.

72. Rosenbaum DP, Hanson GS. Assessing the effects of school-based drug education: a six-year multilevel analysis of Project D.A.R.E. *J Res Crime Delinq* 1998;35:381–412.

73. Ennett ST, Tobler NS, Ringwalt CL, et al. How effective is drug abuse resistance education? A meta-analysis of project DARE outcome evaluations. *Am J Public Health* 1994;84:1394–1401.

74. Clayton RR, Cattarello AM, Johnstone BM. The effectiveness of Drug Abuse Resistance Education (Project D.A.R.E.): five-year follow-up results. *Prev Med* 1996;25:307–318.

75. Lynam DR, Milich R, Zimmerman R, et al. Project DARE: no effects at 10-year follow-up. *J Consult Clin Psychol* 1999;67(4):590–593.

76. Perry CL, Kelder SH. Models for effective prevention. *J Adolesc Health* 1992;13:355–363.

77. Murray DM, Davis-Hearn M, Goldman AI, et al. Four- and five-year follow-up results from four seventh-grade smoking prevention strategies. *J Behav Med* 1988;11(4):395–405.

78. Flay BR, Keopke D, Thomson SJ, et al. Long-term follow-up of the first Waterloo Smoking Prevention Trial. *Am J Public Health* 1989;79(10):1371–1376.

79. Bell RM, Ellickson PL, Harrison ER. Do drug prevention effects persist into high school? *Prev Med* 1993;22:463–483.

80. Ellickson PL, Bell RM, McGuigan K. Preventing adolescent drug use: long-term results of a junior high program. *Am J Public Health* 1993;83:856–861.

81. Shope JT, Copeland LA, Kamp ME, et al. Twelfth grade follow-up of the effectiveness of a middle school-based substance abuse prevention program. *J Drug Educ* 1998;28(3):185–197.

82. Dryfoos JG. Common components of successful interventions with high risk youth. In: Bell NJ, Bell RW eds. *Adolescent risk taking*. Newbury Park, CA: Sage, 1993:131–147.

83. Resnicow K, Botvin GJ. School-based substance use prevention programs: why do effects decay? *Prev Med* 1993;22:484–490.

84. Caplan M, Weissberg RP, Grober JS, et al. Social competence promotion with inner-city and suburban young adolescents: effects on social adjustment and alcohol use. *J Consult Clin Psychol* 1992;60:56–63.

85. Botvin GJ, Eng A, Williams CL. Preventing the onset of cigarette smoking through life skills training. *Prev Med* 1980;9:135–143.

86. Botvin GJ, Eng A. A comprehensive school-based smoking prevention

program. *J Sch Health* 1980;50:209–213.

87. Botvin GJ, Baker E, Renick N, et al. A cognitive–behavioral approach to substance abuse prevention. *Addict Behav* 1984;9:137–147.

88. Botvin GJ, Baker E, Botvin EM, et al. Alcohol abuse prevention through the development of personal and social competence: a pilot study. *J Stud Alcohol* 1984;45:550–552.

89. Botvin GJ, Renick N, Baker E. The effects of scheduling format and booster sessions on a broad-spectrum psychosocial approach to smoking prevention. *J Behav Med* 1983;6:359–379.

90. Pentz MA. Prevention of adolescent substance abuse through social skill development. *NIDA Res Monogr* 1983;47:195–232.

91. Schinke SP, Gilchrist LD. Preventing cigarette smoking with youth. *J Prim Prev* 1984;5:48–56.

92. Botvin GJ, Baker E, Filazzola A, et al. A cognitive-behavioral approach to substance abuse prevention: a one-year follow-up. *Addict Behav* 1990;15:47–63.

93. Botvin GJ. Preventing drug abuse in schools: social and competence enhancement approaches targeting individual-level etiological factors. *Addict Behav* 2000;25:887–897.

94. Botvin GJ, Eng A. The efficacy of a multicomponent approach to the pre-vention of cigarette smoking. *Prev Med* 1982;11:199–211.

95. Kreutter KJ, Gewirtz H, Davenny JE, et al. Drug and alcohol prevention project for sixth graders: first-year findings. *Adolescence* 1991;26:287–293.

96. Botvin GJ, Baker E, Dusenbury L, et al. Preventing adolescent drug abuse through a multimodal cognitive-behavioral approach: results of a three-year study. *J Consult Clin Psychol* 1990;58:437–446.

97. Botvin GJ, Baker E, Dusenbury L, et al. Long-term follow-up results of a randomized drug abuse prevention trial in a white middle-class population. *JAMA* 1995;273:1106–1112.

98. Botvin GJ, Griffin KW, Diaz T, et al. Preventing illicit drug use in adolescents: long-term follow-up data from a randomized control trial of a school population. *Addict Behav* 2000;5:769–774.

99. Botvin GJ, Griffin KW, Diaz T, et al. Drug abuse prevention among minority adolescents: one-year follow-up of a school-based preventive intervention. *Prev Sci* 2001;2:1–13.

100. Botvin GJ, Griffin KW, Diaz T, et al. Smoking initiation and escalation in early adolescent girls: one-year follow-up of a school-based prevention intervention for minority youth. *J Am Med Womens Assoc* 1999;54:139–143.

101. Botvin GJ, Griffin KW, Diaz T, et al. Preventing binge drinking during early adolescence: one- and two-year follow-up of a school-based preventive intervention. *Psychol Addict Behav* 2001;15:360–365.

102. Griffin KW, Botvin GJ, Nichols TR, et al. Effectiveness of a universal drug abuse prevention approach for youth at high risk for substance use initiation. *Prev Med* 2003;36:1–7.

103. Tobler NS, Stratton HH. Effectiveness of school-based drug prevention programs: A meta-analysis of the research. *J Prim Prev* 1997;18;71–128.

104. MacKinnon DP, Johnson CA, Pentz MA, et al. Mediating mechanisms in a school-based drug prevention program: first-year effects of the midwestern prevention project. *Health Psychol* 1991;10(3):164–172.

105. Wynn SR, Schulenberg J, Maggs JL, et al. Preventing alcohol misuse: the impact of refusal skills and norms. *Psychol Addict Behav* 2000;14(1):36–47.

106. Botvin GJ, Schinke SP, Epstein JA, et al. Effectiveness of culturally-focused and generic skills training approaches to alcohol and drug abuse prevention among minority youths. *Psychol Addict Behav* 1994;8:116–127.

107. Botvin GJ, Schinke SP, Epstein JA, et al. Effectiveness of culturally focused and generic skills training approaches to alcohol and drug abuse prevention among minority adolescents: two-year follow-up results. *Psychol Addict Behav* 1995;9:183–194.

CHAPTER 77

Harm Reduction: Pragmatic Drug Policies for Public Health and Safety

ERNEST DRUCKER, ETHANN NADELMANN, ROBERT G. NEWMAN, ALEX WODAK, JENNIFER McNEELY, KASIA MALINOWSKA-SEMPRUCHT, DAVID MARSH, MARTIN SCHECHTER, BRUNA BRANDS, AND EUGENE OSCAPELLA

THE PROBLEM

The production, distribution, and sale of illicit drugs is among the world's leading industries. Approximately 3.1% of the world's population (181 million people) use illicit drugs, and this global criminal economy is estimated at $400 to $500 billion annually by the World Bank, Drug Enforcement Agency (DEA), United Nations International Drug Control Program (UNDCP), and Interpol. Furthermore, because of its link to the acquired immunodeficiency syndrome (AIDS) pandemic, drug use is now one of the most urgent public health problems facing the world (1). This unprecedented pattern of global commodification of drug use confronts us with a new and potent version of a very old problem, forcing us to challenge old ways of thinking about drugs and to reconsider the fundamental ideas and set of policies we now employ for their control. The harm reduction (HR) model is an outgrowth of these contemporary realities (2). The idea of harm reduction has older roots but first emerged explicitly in Dutch drug policy during the 1970s and 1980s from concern about the social integration of people who use drugs into society ("normalization") with a goal of maximizing the contact that problematic drug users have with social, treatment, health, and other community services. But it was the realization that people who use drugs shared needles that spread the human immunodeficiency virus (HIV) that soon made harm reduction official drug policy. Public health officials in the United Kingdom expressed it well: "HIV is a greater threat to public and individual health than drug misuse" (3), and later the same idea became policy in Australia, Canada, Switzerland, and many other countries (4).

REFRAMING THE ISSUE

Harm reduction concepts and measures share two underlying assumptions:

1. It is better (for both society and the individual) to concentrate on reducing the risks and harms of drug use rather than to focus solely on the goal of making people (or the world) "drug-free."
2. Drug control policies based on the criminalization of use must be replaced with pragmatic policies that produce demonstrable reductions in the adverse consequences of continued drug use in the world.

As an alternative to the unachievable goals of "a drug free society" (U.S. Office of National Drug Control Policy [ONDCP]) or "a world without drugs" (UNDCP) (5), harm reduction policies assume continued (and even increased) drug use. HR asks the following questions: How can we reduce the likelihood of people who use drugs contracting and spreading infectious diseases (HIV, hepatitis, and tuberculosis), suffering fatal overdoses, and developing drug use-related medical problems? How can we reduce the likelihood of people who use drugs engaging in criminal and other undesirable behaviors? How can we increase the likelihood that people who use drugs will be good citizens, that is, act responsibly toward others in their communities, take care of their families, complete their education or training and become legally employed? How can we make treatment and rehabilitation services more attractive and easily available to more people who use drugs and who seek care? And, more generally, how can we ensure that drug control policies do not cause more harm than drug use itself?

DRUG USE AND PUBLIC HEALTH

The model of harm reduction applied to drug use grows from the standard public health and preventive medicine framework (6), that is, concerns about patterns of excess morbidity and mortality in populations, and the measures needed to reduce illness and death using the tools of primary, secondary, and tertiary prevention. In harm reduction, primary prevention is defined as prevention of addiction and other hazards of drug use (including drug dependence or overdose deaths), but reduction in demand and supply is seen as a means to an end rather than being an end in itself. Secondary prevention aims to limit the length and severity of individual disorders associated with continued drug use. Tertiary prevention involves limiting

collateral medical and social consequences of addiction once it has become a prevalent and chronic condition.

Understanding drug use and addiction as a public health matter reflects a shift in paradigm, a new perspective and a new conceptual model. Instead of viewing drug problems as phenomena caused by individual psychological (or moral) deficiencies, harm reduction views any societies patterns of drug use collectively - holding that many of the most destructive consequences and refractory problems of illicit drug use are not solely attributable to the drugs per se. Rather, many of these problems are more closely linked to the failure of the policies employed to control them. Harm reduction thinking suggests that it is the prohibition of certain drugs, combined with the growing and irrepressible global demand for mood-altering drugs, that must inevitably increase their value and lead to aggressive trafficking that only serves to spread drug use. Furthermore, the criminalization of the drug user undermines the drug users ability to control his or her own drug use and sets the stage for collateral damages, for example, the epidemics of infectious diseases such as HIV (7).

THREE CAVEATS

Analysis of harm reduction efforts must be qualified by three important caveats. First, the scope and progress of harm reduction efforts in most countries coexists with (and is usually dominated by) the "War on Drugs" and the international drug prohibition regime devised and promoted by the United States since the early 1900s (8). Prohibition policies are today firmly established throughout the world via United Nations (UN) treaties and conventions: the Single Convention on Narcotic Drugs (1961) and the 1988 United Nations Convention Against Illicit Traffic in Narcotic Drugs and Psychoactive Substances, which was ratified by more than 100 governments (9). It is within this largely hostile environment that harm reduction programs currently operate.

The second caveat concerns the methodological limitations encountered in evaluating different drug control policies and problems. Data collection and analysis regarding illicit behavior, particularly drug dealing and other consensual crimes, are inherently difficult given the generally hidden and highly stigmatized nature of the activities and populations who use illicit drugs. Comparative analysis among countries presents further complications as governments vary in how they collect and categorize data on illicit drug use and related public health and criminal justice information, rendering cross-national comparisons exceedingly difficult and problematic. Most importantly, illicit drug use and drug-related behavior are shaped by so many societal influences—ranging from cultural norms to broader health and social welfare policies—that it is extremely difficult and sometimes impossible to determine the precise impact of specific drug control policies on drug-related behavior.

The third caveat concerns the adaptability and potential efficacy of innovations practiced in one country when applied to another. While there are some initial steps toward harm reduction in the developing world, the countries of the former Soviet Union, Eastern Europe, and Asia, most countries in which harm reduction policies were first implemented and are the most developed (the U.K., Australia, Netherlands) are advanced industrialized social democracies shaped by Judeo-Christian ideals and traditions, populated principally by people of European origin, and with a commitment to universal access to health care and the provision of basic social services (e.g., housing)—far beyond that found in the United States.

HARM REDUCTION IN THE UNITED STATES

Although many government officials and informed citizens express interest in less punitive and more public health-oriented approaches to drug control, most American politicians and public officials explicitly reject harm reduction and have systematically refused to examine the underlying assumptions of our current drug policies: prohibition, criminalization, and a rigid drug-free ideology. These policies have remained dominant in the United States, despite recommendations over the years to the contrary by several high-level scientific and governmental advisory bodies. Harm reduction policies are still attacked by U.S. government officials who claim that harm reduction initiatives are a surrender in the "War on Drugs" and stepping-stones to "drug legalization" (10).

ADDICTION TREATMENT AS HARM REDUCTION

Many users of illicit drugs don't develop serious problems and are never seen in treatment, or, as Vaillant and Zinberg demonstrated (11), even many problematic users (as is also true for most cigarette smokers and drinkers of alcohol) resolve their drug problems without formal treatment. But people who use drugs presenting for treatment today are afflicted with a host of social and medical problems attributable as much to the consequences of prohibition policies as to the drugs themselves. Thus most treatment of addiction in the real world represents "tertiary prevention," occurring after many years of drug use, as well as its neglect, mistreatment, and the wider adverse effects of criminalization on the individual user, the user's family, and the wider community. This means that the context for and outcomes of drug treatment are inseparable from society's drug policies.

By contrast, the harm reduction approach to treatment acknowledges different goals for different people who use drugs. Instead of demanding that users conform to rigid treatment program requirements (e.g., "clean" urine tests as a prerequisite for continued care), a range of services are offered in response to the needs and wishes of peo-

ple who use drugs (12). In some cases, the user's goals (and best course of treatment) may be to attempt drug abstinence via a "drug-free" approach. But in other situations, the best way to manage an addict's social and medical problems may not be to insist on total abstinence. Rather, these situations may call for accepting some form of drug use (even continued dependence) and, if appropriate (as in the case of opiate dependency), arranging for legal drug maintenance, which can uncouple the chemical dependency from its most adverse consequences. "Controlled drug use" (11) itself can be a treatment objective, where some level of continued use is accepted, but where the goal is to reduce the type and amount of drugs used and to shift to safer forms of use (e.g., reducing alcohol or tobacco intake to safer levels, not driving home after drinking). "Low-threshold" treatment offers specific help to people who may still use drugs (e.g., housing, legal assistance) but places only minimal demands on them regarding their drug use. The first goal in HR is engagement with helping services.

Drug Substitution and Maintenance Approaches

Drug substitution and maintenance treatment are pillars of harm reduction. For opiate addiction they offer an inexpensive and effective approach that is well suited to diverse populations, but they have a long and complex history (13). A crucial factor is the right of physicians to prescribe maintenance drugs for their addicted patients, first pioneered in Great Britain (14), where doctors have the authority to gradually detoxify or maintain addicts by prescribing their drugs of choice, including injectable heroin in some cases. When the AIDS epidemic struck (in the mid-1980s) the British system was able to rapidly increase prescription of maintenance medications (mostly methadone) tenfold and support other HR efforts, such as needle and syringe exchange, under the umbrella of medical and public health authorities.

The British system had parallels in the first period of addiction medicine in the United States (1900–1925) when morphine was prescribed to more than 10,000 chronic dependent users. But this approach was soon overwhelmed in America by the militant temperance movement of the time and by federal and state drug enforcement agents hostile to opiate maintenance. By 1925, organized medicine and the U.S. courts had rejected drug maintenance, largely silenced its proponents, and led American medicine to all but abandon not only maintenance treatment, but the entire field of addiction medicine to law enforcement. It was not until the early 1960s, with the pioneering work of Drs. Vincent Dole and Marie Nyswander (see other text chapters) that the concept of addiction treatment using the prescription of maintenance drugs was reintroduced in the United States. Today, methadone maintenance treatment (MMT) is the preeminent harm reduction approach for treatment of opiate addiction (15).

Positive outcomes include decreases in heroin use and injecting, reduction in criminal behavior and arrests, reductions in death rates, and increased employment. The rate of HIV infection among those in MMT is generally inversely proportional to the time in treatment. Thus, although 20–30% of New York City's injectors are HIV positive, for those who have been in treatment since 1978, the infection rate is virtually zero. MMT is also associated with improved access to and use of other health and social services.

Despite overwhelmingly positive findings for MMT (most of them initially from American studies), the United States has fallen far behind other Western nations when it comes to its effective implementation. Methadone is the most tightly regulated drug in the U.S. pharmacopoeia (16), and may only be dispensed in licensed "programs," subject to strict federal and state regulations governing matters typically left to the discretion of physicians. Although it is acknowledged that most patients do not immediately cease drug use when they enter MMT, most MMT programs have not integrated harm reduction interventions such as access to sterile syringes and education on safer drug use (17). There are a few notable exceptions; for example, one MMT program in New York provides access to sterile syringes via linkage with needle-exchange programs and pharmacies, and provides safe syringe disposal on-site (18). Many MMT programs in the United States remain "user-unfriendly," often expelling clients who use drugs illegally or otherwise violate program requirements (e.g., failure to attend "counseling sessions"), and are often unpopular in the communities they serve. Accordingly, MMT has failed to expand to the level required to effectively respond to the needs of the 1 million dependent individuals or to the AIDS epidemic that continues to infect 20,000 injecting drug user (IDUs) each year in the United States (19). Over 100,000 MMT "slots" were established in the United States from 1965 to 1980, but that growth stopped in the crucial first decade of the AIDS epidemic because of hostility to maintenance. Although another 100,000 patients were added after 1990, the proportion of opiate addicts that can be accommodated in the United States today is still only approximately 20% of the 1 million opiate-dependent population.

In many American states, methadone regulations conflict with sound medical and public health practices. In California, privatization and limitations on the duration of publicly funded treatment have raised barriers to MMT. Threats to treatment quality and accessibility in other states include ceilings on methadone dose levels, prohibition of take-home medication, and arbitrary restrictions on the number of methadone clinics allowed within a certain area (e.g., Tennessee allows no more than one clinic within a 100-mile radius). Perhaps most remarkably, as of 2004, 5 states—Idaho, Mississippi, Montana, North Dakota, South Dakota,—had no methadone-maintenance programs whatsoever.

Furthermore, the therapeutic efficacy of many MMT programs in the United States has been eroded and the standards of clinical practice have deteriorated (20). There is widespread ignorance of the proper use of this treatment and often hostility toward methadone among many of those working in MMT programs. Problems include administration of inadequate doses and a misguided orientation toward abstinence not just from illegal drugs, but also from methadone itself, as a treatment goal. The continued failure to relax counterproductive regulatory constraints on methadone treatment by U.S. government agencies that are ill-equipped to oversee clinical care, and the continued punitive posture of drug enforcement authorities regarding MMT, have taken a once successful modality of addiction treatment and driven it to the margins of medical practice and public health. Despite its proven clinical effectiveness over many millions of patient-years of positive experience with methadone, punitive prohibitionist attitudes and policies have had a huge adverse impact on public health by restricting access to this treatment, in the United States and (because of the powerful U.S. influence) around the world (21). Until 1994, France had only 52 patients in MMT; even in the mid-1980s, Belgium imprisoned doctors for dispensing methadone; and in Germany, methadone maintenance was for years paid by the health care financing system only if comorbidity (e.g., AIDS, pregnancy) was present. And today, Russia and India still ban the use of methadone.

This disconnect between science and policy and the urgency of the need to expand effective addiction treatment in the United States recently led to renewed efforts on the part of some medical and public health authorities to reform and expand methadone treatment. In 1996, the Institute of Medicine (22) issued a series of studies and a report calling for the expansion and modification of methadone treatment, and in 1997, a National Institutes of Health (NIH) Consensus Conference (23) reasserted the conceptualization of opiate addiction as a medical disorder. It called for "effective medical treatment of opiate addiction" through the reduction of "misperceptions and stigma," improved medical training, assurance of greater access to methadone, and the reduction of "unnecessary regulations" that restrict the availability and quality of methadone treatment. In 1998, the Drug Abuse Treatment Act (DATA) was passed by Congress, expanding the possibilities of employing new models of care, including the availability of buprenorphine (Buprenex) via general physicians.

International Developments in Maintenance Treatment

While the United States has only just begun to confront these issues, public health and medical authorities in a number of other countries have responded to these problems by greatly expanding access to methadone treatment and altering their intervention strategies to accommodate a greater number and wider spectrum of patients. Much of this expansion has been achieved through the use of primary care practitioners to prescribe methadone within their office-based practices. Today in Europe, Canada, and the Asian-Pacific Region, more than 150,000 patients are now prescribed methadone by a general practitioner in a private office or health clinic setting and this model of addiction medicine is gaining popularity and application worldwide. In the United States, this option is proposed for patients who have become stable, which will free new slots in overcrowded clinics and encourage the stable patients to reintegrate with their community.

With the growing international awareness of AIDS risks and the potential role of maintenance treatment in limiting its spread (by reducing addicts' risky injecting behavior and needle sharing) most countries in the developed world have initiated or expanded capacity and liberalized methadone availability (24) and added other maintenance drugs (e.g., buprenorphine) to the treatment array. Australia increased its MMT capacity tenfold between 1985 and 1994. In Germany, methadone was outlawed as late as 1987, but today more than 60,000 patients receive it (the great majority from generalist, community-based practitioners) without other comorbidities being a requirement. In France, in 1993, there were only 52 patients in the entire country maintained on methadone; a decade later approximately 10,000 patients were being treated with methadone, and an additional 70,000 to 80,000 were prescribed buprenorphine as maintenance treatment for their addiction (25).

Outside the United States, methadone has been expanded largely by integrating it into "mainstream" medical practice (26). Thousands of general practitioners in community-based practices throughout Europe, Australia, New Zealand, and Canada are involved in methadone maintenance. In Belgium, Germany, France, Australia, Canada, Ireland, Scotland, and Croatia, this is the principal means of methadone distribution. In the Netherlands and, to a lesser extent, Switzerland, methadone is available in public and private health clinics and other government facilities. Some programs, including a few in the United States, deliver methadone to the homes of clients with AIDS and other immobilizing diseases. In Copenhagen and in Amsterdam, methadone is available at police stations for drug users who have been arrested. But in the United States, except for some "medical maintenance" experiments permitting a relative handful of very stable long-term methadone recipients to transfer from traditional methadone clinics to office-based physicians, American pharmacists and doctors in general medical practice are barred by federal regulations from playing any role in methadone maintenance. The approval of buprenorphine for office-based prescription in the United States offers a new opportunity to put addiction treatment into mainstream medicine, but this effective drug is now mired in

the same conflicts that still attend methadone treatment in the United States; for example, federal statutes set a limit of 30 patients per practice, which is being interpreted as allowing only 30 patients for an entire clinic, group practice, or large hospital, and the medication is priced at 10 to 20 times the price of methadone. The public health impact of office-based prescriptions for buprenorphine will be minimal until it is brought up to scale.

Low-Threshold Maintenance

Another distinction between U.S. and non-U.S. treatment of addiction is the reliance on "low-threshold" models where less is demanded of the patient. Unlike most American providers, low-threshold models do not make treatment contingent upon total abstinence from heroin and/or other drugs, and thus accommodate a far broader segment of addicts in the community. These programs frequently provide fewer "ancillary services," although referrals are usually offered to relevant sources that serve the general population. They do not demand regular attendance, urine tests, or regular counseling contacts, all of which are standard (and many required by government regulations) in U.S. methadone clinics. Support for low-threshold programs abroad is based on their relatively low cost, which greatly increases the number of people who can be provided with care; their proven success in establishing contact with people who use illicit drugs but are put off by programs with more rigorous requirements; and the fact that their clients typically fare better than do people who use drugs but are not enrolled in any programs (27). Low-threshold programs now operate in several cities in Europe and Australia, and in Hong Kong. The Dutch were pioneers in deploying low-threshold "methadone buses"—mobile facilities that carry previously prescribed doses, free of charge, for a list of 100 or more patients who may meet the bus at any one of several predesignated locations daily, an innovation that has been adopted in Barcelona and in the United States in Baltimore and Boston. Unfortunately these positive foreign developments in methadone maintenance have been largely ignored in the United States. To the extent they have been discussed at all, there has been considerable resistance to adopting or even experimenting with them.

Methadone in Correctional Settings

The injection of heroin within correctional facilities has been documented in many countries and continues to exist, notwithstanding vigorous attempts to deter and detect the importation of drugs and injecting equipment into these facilities. Although episodes of drug injecting inside these facilities are less frequent than in the community, adverse consequences (including HIV infection) are well documented. The use of methadone in jails and prisons—in the United States and around the world—has generally been restricted to brief detoxification programs. As an exception, for more than 20 years New York City has operated the Key Extended Entry Program (KEEP), a large in-jail methadone-maintenance program with 3,000 admissions per year, to provide maintenance doses of methadone to heroin users and methadone patients arrested on misdemeanor charges and jailed at the Rikers Island prison facilities. KEEP provides continued MMT for those in such care at the time of arrest and initiates others who will serve short sentences. This program is effective in increasing the proportion of inmates who apply for and remain in drug treatment after release and in reducing recidivism. Despite this success, it remains the only well-established program in the United States, although a small pilot program is underway in Puerto Rico and in New Mexico jails. However, there is no methadone maintenance for the 2 million longer-term state and federal inmates. By contrast, methadone-maintenance programs can now be found in jails and prisons in 22 countries throughout Europe, Canada, and Oceania, and have had very positive evaluations (28).

A Role for Community Pharmacies

Another important innovation characterizing the expansion of Office Based Opiate Treatment (OBOT) overseas has been the incorporation of community pharmacies into the system of methadone treatment. Although general practitioners may oversee methadone prescribing and clinical care, it is common to rely on a network of local pharmacies for the actual dispensing of the medication. This is part of a trend towards expanding the role of community pharmacies in AIDS prevention and treatment. In many countries pharmacists now play a crucial professional role in methadone treatment affecting key issues of patient care (e.g., adherence) and diversion control. Today, the role of community pharmacies in methadone treatment is widespread throughout Canada, Europe, and Australia. Of the 12 European Union countries, 8 allow pharmacy pickup of methadone. In the United Kingdom, an estimated 95% of methadone is provided through community pharmacies and in England, half of all community pharmacists are involved in dispensing methadone. U.S. federal regulations do allow dispensing from DEA-approved medication units, which may include community pharmacies, but only three pilot studies employing office-based prescribing and community pharmacy dispensing have been approved in New Mexico, Pennsylvania, and Maryland (29).

Other Drug Substitution Initiatives

Despite its unparalleled effectiveness, some who receive oral methadone-maintenance treatment either drop out or continue to use illicit drugs in addition to the prescribed medication (30). Stimulated by the need to control the spread of AIDS, maintenance treatment is entering a new phase of clinical experimentation. Accordingly, several countries have expanded drug-maintenance programs and practices beyond oral methadone and buprenorphine to include prescribed injectable methadone and, most recently, heroin in injectable and smokeable forms.

This approach has a long history. In the United States from 1919 to 1923, several morphine- and heroin-assisted therapy clinics were in operation until their termination by the government. British physicians prescribed injectable opiates early in the twentieth century, and in a controlled trial in the 1970s; a small morphine-maintenance program was initiated in 1983 in the Netherlands, and was deemed modestly successful in improving the health and functioning of most of the addicts and in reducing their involvement in criminal activities. Another program, operated by the Municipal Health Department in Amsterdam, prescribed injectable methadone and dextromoramide tartrate (Palfium)—an opiate that can be taken orally—to a group of long-term heavy opiate users (1), but did not gain user acceptance and was difficult to administer. In Italy during the late 1970s, a number of physicians dissatisfied with the quality of care for heroin addicts began providing addicts with injectable morphine on an outpatient basis. The Italian government legalized this prescribing experiment in 1980, but approval was abruptly withdrawn a few years later. No comprehensive evaluation of the program was ever conducted, although it is estimated that as many as 4,000 patients were participating in 1982. However, only limited nonsystematic evaluation of these programs has been conducted and prevented a proper analysis of the efficacy of opioid prescription in these clinics. In Canada, in 1972, the LeDain Commission recommended the implementation of a heroin prescription trial for addicts who could not be attracted into conventional forms of opioid addiction treatment.

In Austria, physicians have always been free to prescribe any legally available drug to addicts. In 1993, in addition to widespread availability of oral methadone, approximately a dozen addicts were receiving prescriptions for injectable morphine or methadone, and many others had prescriptions for codeine and other synthetic opiates. One study substituted oral morphine sulfate for methadone and found the morphine preferable for some patients who experienced negative methadone side effects. In Australia, until the mid 1950s, physicians could prescribe maintenance doses of opiates, principally morphine, and did so for a small numbers of white, middle-class patients and to aging Chinese opium smokers (1). In Queensland, a small injectable methadone program has operated for decades.

More flexible prescribing practices also emerged in Edinburgh in 1988, a few years after authorities realized that the prevalence of HIV infection (more than 50%) among local heroin users was the highest in the United Kingdom. Community-based physicians responded with more liberal prescription of methadone, as well as oral versions of other drugs in common use (e.g., dihydrocodeine, diazepam). This policy, combined with the rapid expansion of needle distribution and exchange, is believed to have played an important role in reducing needle use and sharing, the rate of new HIV infections, and drug-related criminality. Experimentation with oral opiates other than methadone includes the use of long-acting codeine (dihydrocodeine) in Germany (1), ethylmorphine in the Czech Republic, and buprenorphine in India. Even where there is ready access to methadone, however, it is clearly desirable that medical practitioners have the freedom to prescribe different opiates for different patients, depending on circumstances, and that researchers be able to responsibly try to identify more effective treatments without excessive constraints from policy makers.

During the 1970s, numerous proposals to prescribe heroin for addiction treatment were advanced in the United States: as a lure and stepping-stone to oral methadone maintenance; as a supplement to oral methadone; and as a distinct program to attract heroin addicts unwilling to enter methadone or drug-free treatment programs. Each of these proposals was rejected, mostly on political rather than scientific grounds, and to date, none has been implemented in the United States.

Recent Studies of Heroin-Assisted Treatment

In the late 1990s, Switzerland (31) and the Netherlands (32) both initiated major studies examining the effectiveness of heroin prescription in the treatment of opioid addiction. The 3-year multisite Swiss study (1994–1997) provided injectable opioids to more than 1,000 opioid-dependent individuals who had a history of long-term heroin injection and multiple unsuccessful treatment attempts. Although not conducted as a controlled trial, the naturalistic cohort study produced very encouraging outcomes. The program managed to retain 69% of its original sample of chronic, treatment-resistant patients in treatment throughout the 18-month study period; more than half of the dropouts switched to other treatments or went drug-free, and no deaths occurred as a direct consequence of the opioid drugs prescribed. Analysis of 12-month retention rates showed that among the heroin maintenance group, the retention rate was twice that of either methadone maintenance or residential drug-free treatment samples from other studies in Switzerland. A substantial percentage (22%) of those leaving heroin-assisted treatment switched to abstinence-based therapy during the course of the study. Importantly, self-reported drug use decreased dramatically during the course of the study. Of those who remained in treatment and were followed for 18 months, only 18% reported no illicit heroin use at entry. By 6 months and by 18 months, this proportion had climbed to 91% and 94%, respectively (33).

Participants experienced marked improvements in physical and social health (e.g., social functioning, employment, decrease in illegal activities, housing). The overall death rate was 3%; a rate comparable to other

reported death rates in cohorts of regular injection heroin users. The proportion of participants with unstable housing fell from 43% on admission to 21% at 18 months. The rate of unemployment fell from 73% to 45%. Arrests and illegal income generation decreased substantially from 69% to 11% and there was a greater than 50% reduction in criminal offenses registered by the police over the time of the study. A subsequent cost:benefit analysis of the study suggested that, despite the considerable research and treatment costs of the trial, the outcomes were cost-effective at a ratio of almost 2:1. Furthermore, the study demonstrated the feasibility of implementing and operating a heroin-assisted therapy program without disorder, misconduct, and/or diversion of heroin supply. In 1997 in two referenda, 71% of the Swiss voted in favor of continuing the trial as an ongoing program for more than 1,000 patients (34). In addition, a World Health Organization (WHO) evaluation of the Swiss study issued a call for continued investigation of the effectiveness of heroin-assisted therapy.

Although evaluated favorably by the WHO commission, there were several methodological limitations identified in the Swiss study, whose observational design and lack of a randomized control group may have allowed uncontrolled biases into the study. However, the Geneva arm of the study used a randomized controlled design and had similar findings to the rest of the national study. In addition, the Swiss program provided extensive psychiatric and social services making it less clear to what degree the heroin-assisted therapy versus the psychosocial interventions caused the positive changes in the program participants. Subsequent studies include a more rigorous selection methodology and controlled design with randomization (35) and are finding similar results.

In response to these limitations, the Dutch government commissioned a multisite randomized control trial of heroin-assisted therapy that began in July 1998 (36). In contrast to the Swiss design, the Dutch conducted two randomized clinical trials, one examining injectable heroin and the other heroin smoked off foil, the most common mode of use in the Netherlands. Both trials had similar designs, consistent outcome measures based on well-validated instruments, and a single *a priori* definition of both response and effect. Because of the wide availability of maintenance treatment in the Netherlands, the Dutch trials were targeted at patients in methadone-maintenance treatment who continued to use illicit drugs. In both the injection and inhalation trial, the Dutch found significantly greater improvements in drug use, physical and mental health, and social function in those receiving heroin prescription in combination with methadone, than in those randomized to continue on oral methadone alone, with a 56% improvement for the heroin-assisted group as compared to a 31% improvement for the control group. The Dutch results persuasively demonstrate the effectiveness of heroin-assisted treatment. However, because of their focus on patients currently in methadone and the very different treatment system in place in the Netherlands, there are limitations on the generalizability of their findings to other localities. Therefore, to investigate heroin-assisted therapy suited to their own settings, Germany and Spain have started heroin trials and Canada has approved and funded a trial.

Prescription of Nonopiate Drugs

Methadone is not a treatment for primary addiction to cocaine, amphetamine, alcohol, and other nonopiate drugs, although use of these drugs by heroin addicts in MMT will often decline over time (37). But opiate-maintenance programs do not directly address the consumption of nonopiate drugs such as amphetamines and cocaine. This is an increasingly important limitation, given the dramatic growth since the late 1970s in cocaine and multidrug consumption, notably the use of "crack" cocaine and "cocktail" combinations of cocaine and heroin known as "speedballs," and the recent rise in use of amphetamine-type substances worldwide.

In the United Kingdom, where some physicians reason that legal maintenance with prescribed stimulants is preferable to illegal "maintenance" with illicit drugs, the practice of prescribing stimulants, typically in combination with heroin and/or methadone, has persisted for decades (38). An initiative in Britain to prescribe injectable amphetamine during the amphetamine epidemic of 1968 was deemed a failure, but recent attempts to prescribe oral amphetamine appear more successful. A 3-year study of a small oral-amphetamine-prescribing program in Portsmouth found that more than half of the 26 study participants (all daily amphetamine injectors on entry) stopped injecting, and that all decreased their sharing of injecting equipment and used less illicit amphetamine. The program was popular among users: it retained 67% of those who entered for at least 15 months, and of those who dropped out, two had stopped amphetamine use. The program also precipitated an increase in the number of primary amphetamine users presenting to treatment services in the area. Treatment services in Exeter, and a larger program in Cornwall, also achieved substantial drops in illicit amphetamine use and injecting with similar programs of oral amphetamine prescription. Using oral and injectable methadone, oral amphetamine, codeine, and benzodiazepine prescription, and a drug team that integrates needle exchange, prenatal and primary care health services, and mental health care, the Cornwall service exemplifies the flexible harm reduction-oriented approach that is the legacy of the British system. In Australia, researchers demonstrated the feasibility of establishing a clinical trial model for amphetamine maintenance for both cocaine and amphetamine users, and are now planning full trials (39).

HARM REDUCTION AS PREVENTION: NEW MODELS AND PROGRAMS FOR ACTIVE DRUG USERS NOT IN TREATMENT

Syringe Exchange Programs

Early in the AIDS epidemic, the sharing of syringes was clearly linked to HIV transmission among IDUs and from them, to sexual partners and their fetuses. By 1995, most new cases of HIV in the United States were attributed directly or indirectly to drug use; today more than one-third of newly reported AIDS cases in the United States and Europe are among IDUs or their sexual partners. The institution of syringe-exchange programs (SEPs) in the early years of the AIDS epidemic was the first well-organized and explicit harm reduction program in the United States and in many European countries. However, SEPs frequently meet with strong opposition and are still not implemented at levels that would have the greatest effects on reducing the spread of blood-borne pathogens (40).

The positive effects of SEPs on syringe sharing and a wide range of other behaviors linked to HIV/AIDS risk were well documented in the United States, Great Britain, the Netherlands, and Australia by the early 1990s. In a recent review, 14 SEP studies (41) illustrated reductions in the frequency of syringe sharing associated with SEPs, 4 showed no reductions, and none showed an increase. Studies in Montreal and Vancouver (42) found high seroconversion rates in SEP clients, but these populations were involved in very-high-risk cocaine injecting and study designs precluded adequate comparisons to non-SEP users. In Connecticut, the sharing of needles among IDUs dropped 40% after that state changed its paraphernalia laws in 1992 to allow for purchase and possession and sale of up to 10 syringes without a prescription. The results of this change were a decrease in marginalization (43) and an increase in referrals to medical care (e.g., for tuberculosis [TB] and HIV). Also, many social service agencies use these programs to help users gain access to social and legal services and drug treatment (44).

Referral to drug treatment is a major accomplishment of many SEPs. For example, since 1991, a Tacoma, Washington SEP has been the largest single source of recruitment to methadone maintenance programs in the region. Of the first 569 clients in New Haven, Connecticut's SEP, 188 (33%) requested drug treatment, and 107 (57%) of those clients were placed in treatment programs. In the United Kingdom, where almost 60% of new SEP clients have no contact with other treatment or HIV prevention services, many clients are subsequently referred to such services. SEPs are well suited for disseminating information on HIV/AIDS risks and users take such information seriously; the claim that drug injectors will not alter their behavior to reduce the risks of contracting HIV and other infections has consistently been refuted. Surveys indicate that an increasing number of drug injectors who participate in SEPs use only sterile syringes and that some reduce syringe use in favor of oral and nasal means of consumption if the available drugs permit that. In cities that implemented SEPs in the mid-1980s, there is evidence of lower HIV prevalence among IDUs than in cities that did not offer SEPs until later in the AIDS epidemic. In Australia and the United Kingdom, where SEPs were instituted in the mid-1980s, HIV seroprevalence in drug injectors has remained lower than in most other countries (45).

SEPs in the United States

Despite very favorable reports on the public health impact of SEPs worldwide and endorsements by the National Commission on Acquired Immune Deficiency Syndrome, the Centers for Disease Control and Prevention, the General Accounting Office, the National Academy of Sciences' Institute of Medicine, and the Office of Technology Assessment (46), U.S. SEPs still face daunting challenges: funding shortages, continued police harassment, and, in some cities, criminal prosecution for activists caught distributing syringes. Many American SEPs operate without the legal sanction of local authorities, and all sanctioned SEPs operate under strict rules. These rules—which may include limits on the number of syringes that can be dispensed to individual clients, restrictions on where SEPs can be located and what hours they are open, and eligibility and compliance requirements—can hinder the ability of SEPs to achieve maximum benefits (47). U.S. federal support for the evaluation of SEPs did not occur until 1992, the eleventh year of the AIDS epidemic, and as of 2003, the United States still prohibits the use of federal funds to pay for SEPs either in America or overseas. It is the private sector, charitable foundations, and community volunteers and activists, along with state and local officials, which provide the funds and personnel for many SEPs in the United States. Today 10% to 15% of U.S. IDUs have access to SEPs, of which there were 101 (including Puerto Rico) as of 1996. Local laws may prohibit the sale or possession of syringes without a prescription, and all but five states have drug paraphernalia laws that criminalize the possession or distribution of syringes except for "legitimate medical purposes." In 2000, New York State began a pilot program under which 2,500 community pharmacists sell syringes under a waiver of paraphernalia laws (48); this program has been positively evaluated. But even where over-the-counter sale is permitted, pharmacists may be prohibited or discouraged from selling syringes to anyone they suspect of illicit drug use. And paraphernalia laws also dissuade users from returning syringes to the exchanges, because they could be arrested if police find them in possession of syringes (49,50).

Syringe Exchange Outside the United States

Unlike the United States, most countries in Western Europe, and many elsewhere, never enacted prescription or paraphernalia laws, and two that did—France (51) and Austria—revoked them during the mid-1980s when AIDS came on the scene. By the late 1980s, virtually all developed countries allowed legal access to sterile injection equipment through syringe exchanges, over-the-counter sales, or both. Most public health authorities agree on the importance of reaching as many drug injectors as possible and minimizing the circulation of used syringes through aggressive syringe exchange and distribution efforts. Syringes are available around the clock, from pharmacies (52), vending machines, and even police stations. Circulation time of used syringes is minimized by encouraging or requiring drug injectors to return used syringes for clean ones and by providing multiple disposal sites for used syringes. Most SEPs abroad are strongly supported by government officials at the national and local level, most law enforcement officials, and a substantial majority of public opinion.

Syringe-exchange programs are now commonplace throughout the world: they are found in the Netherlands, Britain, Switzerland, and Australia, and are present in dozens of cities elsewhere in Europe (53). The first exchanges were established in 1981 in the Netherlands and rapidly expanded in response to the threat of HIV later in the decade. In the United Kingdom, political support for syringe exchange arose in 1986 in response to evidence from Scotland that a shortage of syringes in Edinburgh had facilitated the spread of HIV. More than 200 SEPs now operate in England and two-thirds of all drug agencies maintain some syringe distribution or exchange scheme. In Australia, SEPs began in 1986, initially with a pilot program that was illegal. Since 1996, all eight states provide SEPs and all also provide methadone. Australia now provides about 30 million sterile needles and syringes a year—about the same number as the United States, which has a population of heroin users almost 15 times greater. A study commissioned by the Commonwealth (i.e., federal) Department of Health analyzed 778 calendar years of data from 103 cities worldwide and found that HIV prevalence increased an average of 8% in cities without needle-syringe exchange programs and declined an average of 18% in cities with needle-syringe exchange programs. Applying these results to Australia, the independent evaluators estimated that needle-syringe exchange programs have saved (by 2000) 25,000 HIV infections, 21,000 hepatitis C virus (HCV) infections, at least a $1.6 billion (at 5% annual discount), and (by 2010) 4,500 AIDS and 90 HCV deaths (53). In Switzerland, syringe exchange is commonplace in most cities, although regions differ with regard to the means of distribution. Syringe exchanges also operate in most large cities in Germany, as well as in Vienna, Madrid, Bologna, Dublin, Oslo, and many smaller European cities (54). In those major cities where no exchanges have been established, syringes are readily available in pharmacies (54).

Programs both in- and outside of the United States provide not only syringes but also alcohol swabs, sharps containers, medicinal ointments, bleach, cookers, cotton, sterile water, and usually condoms. Although injectors are strongly encouraged to return used syringes, the 1:1 requirement is not strictly enforced. Clients may be shown how to inject less hazardously so as to avoid complications (such as abscesses, septicemia, and endocarditis), and programs often provide primary health services and more generic advice on maintaining good health. The ethos is sympathetic to users, and drug injectors are not harassed about their drug use, although they are informed of, and on request referred to, drug-treatment programs and other alternatives.

Some SEPs also provide detached or outreach services—such as mobile vans and pedestrian distributors—to deliver syringes more directly to homes or street corners. In Zurich, sterile syringes can be obtained around the clock via a network of distribution points that include contact centers for people who use drugs, a "syringe van," mobile medical teams, pharmacies, and vending machines (54). In Vienna, syringes are exchanged in a mobile Ganslwirt bus, which reaches approximately 10% to 25% of all injectors. In Amsterdam, police stations will provide clean syringes in return for dirty ones. Many pharmacists now participate in such efforts also. In Liverpool, for instance, all pharmacies are entitled to sell injecting equipment while 20 operate free syringe exchanges. In New Zealand, by 1990, 16% of all retail pharmacies were involved in syringe distribution and exchange; today that figure is 60%. Automated syringe-exchange machines, which deliver a clean syringe when a used one is deposited, can now be found in more than a dozen European and Australian cities (55). These vending machines are relatively inexpensive, available 24 hours a day, and generally recognized as a useful complement to SEPs. The synergy of SEPs and expanded access to methadone appears to be especially effective in controlling HIV (56), and many countries that averted or controlled epidemics of HIV among IDUs explicitly accepted harm reduction strategies and vigorously implemented both needle-syringe exchange programs and methadone. While Europeans and Australians established and expanded such programs in the 1980s (often in response to the all-too-apparent American catastrophe of HIV among IDUs), the United States resisted SEPs, arguing that syringe distribution encourages illicit drug use and "sends the wrong message." Bitter confrontations blocked public and governmental action during the crucial early phase of our AIDS epidemic. It is now estimated that more than 4,300 HIV infections (and perhaps as many as 9,000 to 10,000 infections, depending on estimates of SEP effectiveness) could have been prevented between 1987 and 1995, had an effective program of needle exchange been implemented and approximately 20,000 IDUs are still being infected with HIV in the United States each year. Fears that increased syringe availability would encourage illicit drug use and encourage injection drug use have proved unfounded, making continued restrictions on the availabil-

ity of sterile syringes unjustifiable on scientific or ethical grounds.

OTHER PUBLIC HEALTH STRATEGIES FOR ACTIVE USERS
Overdose Prevention

In many areas of the world, where HIV has been controlled by harm reduction programs, drug overdose (OD) is the leading cause of death among IDUs. Since the 1990s, a series of OD prevention programs have evolved (57): educational programs using both popular media and underground publications; better emergency medical services and police response systems; the distribution of injectable narcotic antagonists that reverse overdose symptoms (naloxone [Narcan]) as well as cardiopulmonary resuscitation (CPR) training for users' networks; and the formation of groups of victims' families who work with local authorities to improve response to OD emergencies. These programs are well underway in the U.K., Australia, and parts of Europe, but still in the very early stages in the United States. Such programs and many others described below are facilitated by the development of drug user organizations and the community involvement of drug users and their advocacy organizations (58 and see below).

Peer Outreach and Education

Most needle- and syringe-exchange programs rely upon active drug users as outreach workers and volunteers. Their HIV prevention efforts engage the highest risk groups for OD and HIV—active drug users not in treatment—through street outreach in local drug scenes, drop-in centers, and social service settings. Rather than aiming solely to lure people who use drugs into treatment, they focus most of their energies on minimizing drug-related harms outside formal treatment settings. Some use vans or buses, while others have drop-in centers with support services, but importantly for the most marginal users, they have amenities such as laundries, showers, and food. These organizations typically offer information about safer drug use and safer sex, provide a link between people who use drugs and social and/or medical services, distribute needles and condoms, and prove indispensable in collecting information about recent developments in the drug scene. A growing number are initiated and promoted by current and former drug users and employ users as street outreach workers, program staff, leaders of peer counseling groups, and the like (59).

Initiatives Supporting Safer Drug Use

Harm reduction efforts also seek to reduce the damage resulting from drugs of unknown purity or potency, which is especially important as new drugs (e.g., ecstasy and other club drugs) arrive in a country that has little history of experience with their effects. Some syringe exchanges have taken the initiative and distributed information gained from users about which street drugs are particularly potent or have dangerous adulterants. This information, however, tends to be erratic, comes only after a hazardous batch of drugs hits the street, and reaches only a small fraction of users.

Recognizing this need (and opportunity) Dutch public health authorities identified that one of the greatest dangers associated with the sudden expansion of the "rave scene" (gatherings, often at dance clubs, where young people consume methylenedioxymethamphetamine [MDMA] and other stimulants and hallucinogens while dancing to high-energy music) was the sale of adulterated and unexpectedly high-potency drugs. Private organizations, which later gained government support, responded by employing drug analysis units at raves where illicit drugs could be tested prior to consumption. Some cities in Germany (e.g., Berlin and Hanover) maintain silent or unspoken agreements between harm reduction groups and officials, allowing for inconspicuous drug analysis of MDMA and methylenedioxyethylamphetamine (MDE), as well as heroin in the context of "fixer rooms" (see below). Such initiatives resemble the Analysis Anonymous drug testing service in the United States, created by Pharm-Chem Laboratories, Inc., in 1972 to provide a similar service to people who use illicit drugs who mailed in samples (60).

Drug Consumer Groups

Organized and subsidized self-help groups of people who use drugs have played a modest but important role in the formulation and implementation of drug control policies in the Netherlands, Germany, and Australia, and have begun to exercise some influence in Switzerland and the United States (61). The Rotterdam "junkie union" began the first Dutch syringe exchange in response to the hepatitis B epidemic. And Amsterdam's junkie union was decisive in initiating free SEPs in 1983–1984, after a major pharmacist in the central inner city "copping" area refused to sell needles to people who use drugs. Similar groups in Canberra, Rotterdam, Groningen, Basel, Bern, and Bremen have worked with local public health officials on SEPs and other harm reduction initiatives. Although these groups tend to be short-lived and dependent on one or two highly motivated individuals, they play an important role in articulating the sentiments and perceptions of precisely those citizens who are most affected by local policies. They also offer valuable conduits between local policy makers and underground populations. Most of these groups also produce publications (often comic books or "zines") targeted at people who use illicit drugs with information on reducing drug-related harms, kicking the habit, and identifying treatment alternatives (61).

Municipal Zoning Policies and Open Drug Scenes

In large part, public opposition to certain forms of drug use relates to their visible presence in the community, that is, to public appearance of intoxicated individuals and to open drug dealing scenes with their associated loitering, violence, and disorderly conduct. Such open drug scenes are deeply embarrassing to city officials, especially in cities that pride themselves on maintenance of public order, underscoring the need to work collaboratively with local police. Like prostitution, homelessness, and public consumption of alcohol, they challenge community morals, appear disorderly or threatening, and effectively resist all attempts to be suppressed. This is in contrast to alcohol use, which is generally accepted in private spaces (i.e., bars, restaurants, and homes), and public intoxication, which is tolerated under a broad (though declining) range of circumstances, from the office party to public sporting events.

The use of illicit drugs is viewed quite differently when it occurs in public. Although public cannabis use is viewed benignly in many cities, the use and sale of hard drugs is often seen as a sharp challenge to authority. Open drug dealing broadcasts to community residents that law enforcement has been displaced from power. Public consumption—particularly injection—of illicit drugs communicates a clear breakdown of public order and social control. Both attract political attention and create pressure for change that frequently—in the context of prohibition and its enforcement—takes the form of short-term solutions that do little more than conceal drug scenes or shift them to a different locale. In the United States, this spawned the "shooting gallery," a place where people who use drugs could buy drugs and rent injecting equipment in a locale somewhat insulated from the view of the law, and which played a key role in the explosive growth of HIV in many U.S. cities in the 1980s. European and Australian police and public health officials, aware of this relationship early in the AIDS epidemic, officially tolerated certain spaces where drug use could be contained and health risk reduced while meeting the social requirements of drug law enforcement.

Under this concept, "open drug scenes" were allowed to develop in a few restricted areas. Early experiences with open scenes were sometimes adverse, as in Zurich's Platzspitz of the late 1980s and early 1990s, which became notorious as "Needle Park," but was instructive for later attempts at steering the use of drugs to less publicly offensive locations and for the need to establish many small scenes rather than one central supermarket. In Rotterdam, police briefly allowed and supervised an open drug scene next to the central railway station, known as "Platform Zero," with syringe exchange services and a mobile methadone unit readily available. In Frankfurt, open heroin scenes emerged during the 1970s and 1980s in two adjacent parks, the Gallusanlage and the Taunusanlage, when top police officials decided that their decade-long efforts to suppress the local drug scenes had failed to halt their growth and merely shifted them from one neighborhood to another. Local authorities in Frankfurt established three crisis centers in the vicinity of the drug scenes, stationed a mobile ambulance to provide syringe exchange services and emergency medical assistance, offered first aid courses, and established a separate bus to provide services for drug users in commercial sex work. These initiatives were combined with efforts to lure users away from the exclusive involvement in the drug scene by providing night lodgings, daytime residences, and methadone treatment centers in neighborhoods removed from the city center. In conjunction with these measures, the open drug scene in the park was shut down in late 1992 and the new policies that grew from that experience are believed responsible for significantly reducing the number of homeless people who use drugs, drug-related robberies, and drug-related deaths in the city (62).

"Safe Spaces" for People Who Use Drugs

Low-threshold facilities known as "contact centers," "street rooms," "health rooms," "harm reduction centers," and "safe injecting rooms," where active users congregate, are now officially tolerated (and sometimes even government-sponsored) in many European cities and, recently, in Australia. These are places where drug users can meet, pick up injection equipment and condoms, and obtain simple medical care, advice, help with domestic problems, and sometimes a place to sleep. Most facilities allow users to remain anonymous, many have qualified medical staff present, and some provide a "fixer room" where drug injectors can consume illicit drugs in a relatively hygienic environment.

Such facilities challenge norms but are regarded as preferable to the two most likely alternatives: open injection of illicit drugs in public places, which is widely regarded as distasteful and unsettling to most urban residents, or consumption of drugs in unsanctioned "shooting galleries," which are often dirty, sometimes violent, and frequently controlled by drug dealers, and where needle sharing is often the norm. A few "fixing rooms" were quietly tolerated within some drug agencies in England during the 1960s, and during the late 1970s, a number of "drug cafes" for heroin users were established in Amsterdam, but they were later shut down when drug dealers effectively displaced social workers from control of the daily course of events. In Switzerland, the first Gassenzimmer ("fixer rooms") were established by private organizations in Bern and Basel during the late 1980s. By late 1993, eight were in operation, with most under the direct supervision of city officials: two in Bern, two in Basel, one in Lucerne (in City Hall), and three in Zurich. An evaluation of the three Gassenzimmers in Zurich after their first year of operation concluded that they were effective in reducing

the transmission of HIV and the risk of overdose. Three "injection rooms" have been in place in Frankfurt since 1995.

Another innovation worth noting is the "apartment dealer" arrangement, adopted informally in Rotterdam, whereby police and prosecutors refrain from arresting and prosecuting apartment dealers—including sellers of heroin and cocaine—as long as they do not cause problems for their neighbors. This arrangement is viewed as part and parcel of broader "safe neighborhood" plans in which police and residents collaborate to keep neighborhoods safe, clean, and free of nuisances. Both toleration and regulation of open drug scenes and safe spaces for people who use drugs represent forms of informal zoning controls similar to those long employed in Europe and Asia to regulate commercial sex work (63).

DRUG POLICY REFORM AS HARM REDUCTION

Although addiction treatment innovations and expanded access, preventive interventions such as SEPs, environmental changes to make drug use safer, and OD prevention programs play a crucial role in reducing the harms associated with drug use under prohibition, it is changes in drug control policy that offer the best chance for primary prevention of drug-related harm. By reducing the association of drug use with criminal prosecution, a system that drives drug use and people who use drugs to the most dangerous margins of society, the reform of punitive legal policies can produce clear benefits in the realm of public health and social order. Marijuana, the most widely used illicit drug, has been a special target for such law reform.

Marijuana Policies

In the United States in the 1970s, the movement to decriminalize marijuana was driven by the realization that criminal sanctions created greater harm than marijuana use itself. During the 1970s, 11 states decriminalized marijuana, effectively reducing the punishment for possession of small amounts to sanctions other than imprisonment. The impact on marijuana consumption and related problems was negligible, but decriminalization did reduce the number of marijuana arrests and prosecutions. California saved an estimated $1 billion in the decade following the 1976 Moscone Act decriminalizing marijuana. While total drug arrests increased almost every year throughout the 1980s, arrests for marijuana consistently declined, leading many to suggest the drug had been effectively decriminalized. However, in response to harsher drug policies, marijuana arrests have risen in recent years in the United States (more than 800,000 in 2001). In contrast, significant drug law reform has been undertaken in several European countries and Australia in direct response to perceived public health needs and humanitarian concerns, starting with de facto decriminalization of marijuana. The case of Dutch regulation of cannabis is the most impressive example of this approach, both for its longevity (more than 25 years) and its apparent success (64).

Dutch Cannabis Policy and the Separation of Markets

The Netherlands decriminalized cannabis at the national level in 1976, when The Baan Commission, a national drug policy working group, said that drug laws should not be more damaging to an individual than the use of the drug itself and argued that the tendency of some cannabis users to move on to illicit opiate use could be reduced by separating the "soft-drug" and "hard-drug" markets. The national Opium Law was revised to increase penalties for heroin and cocaine trafficking and to cut penalties for the sale and consumption of small amounts of cannabis to misdemeanor offenses. Prosecutorial and police guidelines were also revised to de-emphasize enforcement of cannabis laws. The result was the creation of a relatively normalized, essentially noncriminal, and easily accessible cannabis distribution system in most Dutch cities. A clear-cut distinction was made between people who use drugs and traffickers, and between "hard" illegal drugs, with so-called "unacceptable health risks" (e.g., heroin, cocaine), and cannabis products (65).

The Netherlands permits the retail trade of cannabis products in hundreds of local "coffee shops" under very specific conditions, that is, no advertising, no hard drugs, no disturbance of public order, no sale to minors (under 18 years of age), and strict limits on the amount that can be sold to each customer. Enforcement of these guidelines falls to local "Triangle Committees" composed of the mayor, chief of police, and district attorney of each city. Today, the domestic Dutch market is a well-established commercial structure operating in a "gray economy" with legal tolerance and even some taxation. An estimated half-million regular customers are supplied by many small to midsize local producers plus a number of larger importers. So far there has been little evidence of organized crime in the coffee shop operations and virtually no violence associated with the domestic trade of cannabis in the Netherlands.

This tolerant policy toward the retail trade and use of cannabis for recreational purposes has had a positive effect in the Netherlands. Cannabis consumption among Dutch teenagers has increased somewhat over the decades (as it has in most other countries) but the rate of regular cannabis users in the Netherlands has remained significantly below U.S. levels. Rates of cocaine and heroin consumption among Dutch citizens are similarly modest, although the relatively high quality and low price of the drugs have attracted "drug tourists" from elsewhere in Europe. Dutch authorities express some concern about organized criminal involvement in wholesale production and

sale of cannabis, and they contend with complaints from authorities in neighboring Germany, Belgium, and, lately, France; but by and large, the policy is supported by most of the public, politicians, and law enforcement officials. Cases of problematic cannabis use are rare, but cannabis users (like all Dutch citizens) who do develop problems have ready access to diverse and comprehensive treatment facilities based in the public health sector. Because of international pressures and some local discontent with the rapid growth in coffee shops, the Dutch government has cut back the number of coffee shops (in some cities by as much as 50%) and reduced the amount of cannabis allowed to be purchased at any given time by each customer from 30 g to 5 g.

Other governments have also moved toward decriminalization of cannabis (66). During the 1970s, national drug commissions in many countries recommended cannabis decriminalization. In 1987, the South Australian government introduced a Cannabis Expiation Notice system that allows individuals apprehended with small quantities of cannabis (up to 100 g) to have their offense discharged, with no record of a criminal conviction, upon payment of a fine. A similar scheme was introduced in the Australian Capital Territory in 1992, and later in two other jurisdictions. Although there has been a small consistent increase in cannabis use since 1985 (prior to the expiation system), an analysis of the first 2 years of the expiation system by the South Australian Office of Crime Statistics found little evidence of any impact on the number or type of people detected using cannabis. Its principal recommendation was that steps be taken to ensure that notice recipients pay their fines promptly to avoid court appearances.

In Switzerland, the Federal High Court decided in 1991 that penalties for dealing cannabis were unduly harsh and needed to be revised, given increasing evidence that the health hazards of cannabis consumption were relatively modest. A number of lower courts in Germany have ruled similarly, finding cannabis prohibition laws in conflict with the German constitution. A German Supreme Court decision in May 1994 removed criminal penalties for possession of small amounts of cannabis (31), furthering an earlier decision that had given states the option not to prosecute for possession of small amounts of any drug. Although some states (e.g., Bavaria) responded by decreasing the amount necessary to trigger a "large amount" charge, many other state officials announced that they would no longer arrest people for possessing small amounts of any drug. The state of Hessen initiated federal legislation in the Second Chamber (equivalent to the German senate), requesting the legalization of cannabis and its regulation by way of state monopoly. The state of Schleswig-Holstein received consent from the majority of state health ministers to dispense marijuana in pharmacies but withdrew in the face of opposition from the Federal Agency in Berlin. Spain decriminalized private use of cannabis in 1983 but has since tightened its laws. Italy decriminalized possession of "moderate amounts for personal use" of any drug in 1975, toughened penalties in 1990, and then abolished criminal sanctions for illicit drug use altogether in April 1993. Although no government has advocated outright repeal of cannabis prohibition, an increasing number now favor decriminalization. Most recently, Canada and the U.K. have taken significant steps towards the decriminalization of cannabis.

Medical Marijuana—A Special Case

Many patients have found marijuana to be a relatively safe, well-tolerated, and rapidly effective way to deal with some medical conditions: reducing nausea in chemotherapy; intraocular pressure in glaucoma; muscle spasms and chronic pain; stimulating appetite; relieving the symptoms of AIDS; glaucoma; cancer and chemotherapy; multiple sclerosis; and epilepsy. The hostility to this use of marijuana (especially by federal officials in the United States, where the campaign for medical marijuana has been most vigorous) has made it almost impossible to gain support for rigorous research to confirm (or disprove) these widespread beliefs. Polls indicate that a majority of Americans believe marijuana should be medically available, and numerous organizations, including the American Public Health Association and the American Federation of Scientists, have issued resolutions in support (64). In 1988, a Drug Enforcement Administration administrative law judge ruled that marijuana should be moved to Schedule II, making it available for medical purposes, but the agency refused to comply. Thus marijuana remains a Schedule I drug, meaning that in the eyes of the U.S. government it has no legitimate use, and further research on its medical properties has been stifled. Hundreds of individuals received marijuana for medical purposes in the 1980s, but this federal program was discontinued, and all but eight of the original recipients have either died or been cut from the program.

In the meantime, there have been moves to provide marijuana to medical patients through "cannabis buyers' clubs," which are illegal but often tolerated by local police. Buyers' clubs, which supply marijuana to patients who have a doctor's prescription for marijuana, have sprung up across the country in recent years. Many of the clubs are private, underground operations, but others have achieved national attention. Many of those who grow marijuana for such clubs have been arrested and prosecuted. Additionally, antiparaphernalia laws ban the use, possession, and sale of items used to consume illegal substances. Included in those laws are vaporizers, heating devices that deliver the medically useful components of marijuana without burning the plant material. Because the smoking of any organic substance can deposit tars and other harmful substances in the lungs, vaporizers are extremely useful tools for medical patients.

Nonetheless, an increasing number of doctors and patients view marijuana as a legitimate medicine that can be effective in reducing the nausea associated with cancer chemotherapy, stimulating appetite for AIDS patients suffering from wasting syndrome, and reducing the intraocular pressure of glaucoma. It is also commonly used as an anticonvulsant, muscle relaxant, and mild pain reliever for menstrual cramps and certain types of chronic pain. In May 2001, the U.S. Supreme Court ruled that so-called medical marijuana "buyers' clubs," which operate legally under California state law, can not use a "medical necessity" defense to federal marijuana charges. Such clubs, which offer varying potencies and varieties of marijuana to patients certified to use it under California law, have experienced continual harassment from federal authorities since that ruling, and others have shut down preemptively, effectively depriving thousands of patients of their medicine. But the issue remains open in the United States: in an important ruling in 2003, the U.S. Supreme Court upheld a lower court's opinion that the federal Drug Enforcement Agency could not continue to threaten doctors who advised their patients that marijuana might be beneficial with lose of licensure.

Despite decades of prosecution of marijuana users in the United States (e.g., 300,000 in prison; 800,000 arrests in 2000) no state ballot initiative dealing only with medical marijuana has ever failed, and an October 2002 *Time* magazine poll showed that 80% of the American public supports legal access to medical marijuana. Since 1996, a majority of voters in Alaska, Arizona, California, Colorado, the District of Columbia, Maine, Nevada, Oregon, and Washington have voted in favor of ballot initiatives to remove criminal penalties for seriously ill people who grow or possess medical marijuana. Hawaii has passed a medical marijuana bill through its state legislature. Nonetheless, the federal government continues to fight against state laws that accept the medical value of marijuana (67).

Medical Marijuana in Canada

Although its Controlled Drugs and Substances Act (CDSA), the central law on illegal drugs, prohibits possession, cultivation, trafficking, and importing and exporting of marijuana, the Minister of Health is authorized to grant exemptions from the Act for a medical or scientific purpose, or if it would be otherwise in the public interest. The Canadian government now wishes to permit both the cultivation and possession of cannabis for therapeutic reasons. In 1997, a small group of Ottawa lawyers and physicians applied on behalf of an AIDS patient for medical access to cannabis and by May 2002, 658 exemptions had been granted under this program. In July 2000, the Ontario Court of Appeal, the highest court of Canada's most populous province, declared Canada's cannabis possession law unconstitutional as a whole, and not merely in the context of therapeutic cannabis. The Court suspended its declaration for 1 year to give Canada's Parliament time to remedy the defects it had found with the law. In 2001, just before the expiration of the deadline set by the Court, Marijuana Medical Access Regulations (MMAR) came into force, the government contracted with a company to produce cannabis for therapeutic purposes, such that individuals are now allowed to possess cannabis for therapeutic reasons and a license to produce cannabis. The constitutionality of this approach was challenged before an Ontario court. The foundation of this change of law was the violation of the rights to liberty and security of the person as guaranteed by Canada's "bill of rights" (the Canadian Charter of Rights and Freedoms), the lack of ensuring that seriously ill Canadians who have a right to use cannabis had some way of legally obtaining that drug, and the forcing of users into the arms of suppliers whom the state has deemed criminal drug dealers. The Parliament is working to fix the defects in the plan or otherwise provide for a legal source of supply of cannabis. As of this writing, the law prohibiting simple possession of cannabis—whether for medical or nonmedical use—remains unsettled but seems to be moving toward general decriminalization (68).

REGIONAL CASE STUDY: PROMOTING HARM REDUCTION IN CENTRAL AND EASTERN EUROPE AND THE COUNTRIES OF THE FORMER SOVIET UNION

In 1995, drug use and HIV were just beginning to surface as public health problems in this region. With the opening of borders, drug trafficking flooded the region with professionally produced and potent Afghan heroin, easier to dilute and inject than the home-produced opiates (made from poppy straw) that were mainly used previously. HIV followed in heroin's path, spreading quickly through reused, unclean needles. By 2000, Russia and Ukraine, the region's most populous states, had the fastest-growing drug use and HIV infection rates in the world. As many as 1 million Russians and 400,000 Ukrainians are now estimated to be living with HIV—and at least 80% of these cases are attributed to injecting drug use (69).

Harm reduction was practically unknown in this region in the mid-1990s and most treatment for drug use was repressive, disrespectful of users, and inhumane, often in isolated punitive communities that tried to rid them of the drug habit by breaking their spirit. This "drug treatment" seldom worked, and most users returned to unemployment, poverty, and misery, and resumed drug use again.

The International Harm Reduction Development (IHRD) program of the Open Society Institute facilitates the implementation of harm reduction approaches to prevent HIV transmission and provide support to people who use drugs and others affected by HIV in Central and Eastern Europe (CEE) and the countries of the former Soviet Union (FSU). Through the funding and support of locally based needle-exchange programs, methadone-

maintenance programs, education, legal services, and policy development, the IHRD program is developing the capacity for a sustained response to the region's escalating HIV and drug-use epidemics. Initially, these programs focused on creating a dialogue about harm reduction, finding providers brave enough to pioneer the approach in often hostile environments, and setting up a handful of model programs. By 2003, IHRD had built a network of more than 130 organizations in 24 countries, and provided U.S. $15 million to 203 harm reduction projects at these organizations, with other donors contributing more than U.S. $5 million more, demonstrating the viability of harm reduction in a variety of contexts, including with prisoners, sex workers, and isolated minorities such as the Roma. Many of these programs are peer based, offering the most affected persons an opportunity to put their experiences to work, gain self-esteem, and develop new skills.

Despite the proven effectiveness of harm reduction programs, there are currently not enough programs available in the CEE/FSU to stop the HIV epidemic or even to slow it appreciably. But IHRD's pioneering work is beginning to pay off and many governments now recognize the importance of making harm reduction part of their HIV/AIDS prevention programs. Today, almost every government application for funding from the Global Fund to Fight AIDS, tuberculosis, and malaria includes harm reduction. Still, there are not enough harm reduction programs operating in the region to significantly slow the epidemic. The next step is for these governments to make sure that national and local laws promote rather than hinder the establishment of needle exchanges and methadone therapy, as well as services for prisoners, sex workers, and the general population. A supportive environment that includes good working relations with police, health care and mental health providers, and public health ministries is essential to insure the effectiveness of harm reduction programs. IHRD helped to establish the Central and Eastern European Harm Reduction Network to exchange information and advocate for systemic recognition and adoption of harm reduction policies. It has contributed to the legalization and/or development of methadone and other drug-replacement therapies in eight countries in the region.

An important realization that has come from this work is the importance of the UN. It is clear that the many agencies within the United Nations that have a stake in the drug issue must stop working at cross purposes. UN drug control treaties must be revised, and the UN Commission on Narcotic Drugs (CND) must learn to collaborate with other UN agencies in the struggle to prevent the spread of HIV. Right now, by promoting strict compliance with the drug control treaties, the CND is actually exacerbating the HIV epidemic in Central and Eastern Europe and the former Soviet Union. Many governments in the region have tried to comply with the tough UN treaties by implementing repressive antidrug policies aimed at achieving a "drug-free society." Not only do these policies violate basic human rights principles, but they also have catastrophic public health consequences. UN treaties and government policies should view drug use primarily as a matter of public health and human rights, not simply law and order.

CONCLUSIONS

The harm reduction paradigm has made great progress during the last decade. A public health conception of drug use, the foundation of harm reduction, is now generally far better understood than previously, although often still willfully misinterpreted by its opponents. In an increasing number of countries and regions of the world, harm reduction is now regarded as mainstream drug policy (e.g., virtually throughout all countries of Western Europe), while zero tolerance supporters are growing ever more isolated and marginalized as their failure and its high cost become evident.

Several countries have explicitly endorsed harm reduction as national drug policy, including the U.K., the Netherlands, Australia, Canada, France, Switzerland, Spain, Germany, New Zealand, many countries in Central and Eastern Europe, parts of Russia, countries of the former Soviet Union, Iran, and several important countries in Asia (Nepal, Vietnam, Indonesia, and China) and South America (Brazil and Argentina). Harm reduction has also been endorsed in recent years by an increasing number of United Nations agencies (including WHO and UNAIDS) and by organizations such as the International Red Cross.

Although harm reduction programs continue to slowly spread, their availability is still well below levels required to achieve the public health goals that we should be setting in the drugs area. Thus zero tolerance and the "War on Drugs" remains the stated drug policy in the United States, the most important and most influential opponent to harm reduction, but not the only country to bitterly oppose these policies. Other countries that oppose harm reduction policies are Japan, Malaysia, and Sweden, all of which play important roles in setting UN drug policies.

The surge in interest in harm reduction around the world in the last 2 decades was stimulated by the urgent need, first recognized in the early 1980s, to control HIV among people who use drugs. With 25 million deaths to date, 42 million people currently alive with HIV infection, and HIV estimated to infect additional millions each year, AIDS is now the most serious threat to global public health since the Black Death. In most regions of the world, drug injecting has played a central role in the ignition of HIV outbreaks that rapidly made the transition from small, localized epidemics to extensive, generalized regional ones, buttressed by sexual transmission and amplified by widespread unsterile medical injections and unsafe blood transfusions throughout the developing world (70). And injection of heroin is now emerging in sub-Saharan Africa (71) and undoubtedly will open a new chapter in the monstrous epidemic that now grips that

region, challenging both the theory and practice of HR in unprecedented ways.

Thus, although the growth in support for new drug policies and programs is gratifying, HIV continues to spread faster than HR programs are being established or expanded. The struggles to spread HR in the developing world (with its majority of the world's population) are especially important, and acceptance in principle is insufficient to avert disaster. For example, although HR programs were introduced early enough in Nepal, they failed to avert an HIV epidemic there because they were not expanded rapidly enough. And the growing popular and professional commitment to HR in many countries is often thwarted by a strong national commitment to traditional control methods and a culture of corruption that surrounds all illicit drug markets: the more intense the repressive drug policies, the more they undermine effective HR.

Nonetheless, there continues to be strong growth in harm reduction institutions worldwide. By 2004, there had been 15 annual meetings of the International Conference on the Reduction of Drug-Related Harm, the leading international meeting on drug policies and innovations in the field. These conferences, attracting a growing body of delegates from an increasing number of countries, have now been held in developing and transitional countries several times. The International Harm Reduction Association (IHRA) was established in 1996 and has grown rapidly in its first 8 years. It now has a constitution, elects new members to its Executive Council, has a vigorous publication division (producing a hard copy journal, electronic newsletter, and Web site). Increasingly, IHRA plays an advocacy role for harm reduction with other organizations and within the UN system. The IHRD was established in 1995 as part of the Open Society Institute (OSI) and Soros Foundation. It operates in Eastern Europe and the former Soviet Union to promote harm reduction policies and programs. The Centre for Harm Reduction (CHR) in Australia was established in 2001 to conduct research and disseminate research findings, provide training, and advocate for harm reduction, and six regional HR networks (including Asia, Latin America, and Africa) have been established with significant international support. There is even an online peer review academic journal dedicated to the subject (www.HarmReductionJournal.com) devoted to HR studies. These developments represent a growing trend toward the building of harm reduction institutions throughout the world and the normalization of HR practices. Although harm reduction continues to face formidable opposition, it is now clear that this approach to policy and practice is becoming the mainstream approach for dealing with illicit drugs and their many consequences.

ACKNOWLEDGMENTS

The authors of this work are supported by the U.S. National Institute of Drug Abuse (ED); the Open Society Institute

(ED, JM, EN, KM-S); The Drug Policy Alliance (EN); The Baron Edmond de Rothschild Chemical Dependency Institute of Beth Israel Medical Center (RGN); and the Canadian Medical Research Council (DM, MS, BB). The authors would also like to thank the following for their valuable assistance: Lawrence Greenberg of *The Harm Reduction Journal*; Alexandra Bobadilla of Montefiore Medical Center; Philip Coffin, Allison Orris and Leigh Hallingby of The Lindesmith Center/Open Society Institute; and Bruce Mirken of the Marijuana Policy Project.

REFERENCES

Items available online as of February 2004.

1. Nadelmann E, Mc Neely J, Drucker E. International perspectives. In: Lowinson et al., eds. *Comprehensive textbook of substance abuse*, 4th ed. Williams & Wilkins, 1995; Mann J et al. *AIDS in the world-2*. Harvard, 1998; Turner CF, Miller HG, Moses LE. *AIDS, sexual behavior, and intravenous drug use*. Washington, DC: National Academy Press, 1989; Stimson GV. The global diffusion of injecting drug use: implications for HIV infection. *Bull Narc* 1993;45:3–17. National Commission on Acquired Immune Deficiency Syndrome. *The twin epidemics of substance use and HIV*. Washington, DC: National Commission on Acquired Immune Deficiency Syndrome, 1991.

2. See O'Hare P, Newcombe R, Matthews A, et al. *The reduction of drug related harm*. New York: Routledge, 1992; Heather N, Wodak A, Nadelmann EA, et al., eds. *Psychoactive drugs and harm reduction: from faith to science*. London: Whurr Publishers, 1993:49–54; Drucker E. *Drugs and public health, current issues in public health*. 1996; Hunt N, et al. *Forward thinking on drugs: a review of the evidence base for harm reduction approaches to drug use*. Release London, 2003.

3. Advisory Council on the Misuse of Drugs. *AIDS and drug misuse, part I: report of the Advisory Council on the Misuse of Drugs*. London: Her Majesty's Stationery Office, 1988; Grund JP, Stern LS, Kaplan EH, et al. Drug use contexts and HIV consequences: the effect of drug policy on patterns of everyday drug use in Rotterdam. *Br J Addict* 1992;87:381–392.

4. Wodak A. HIV infection and injecting drug use in Australia: responding to a crisis. *J Drug Issues* 1992;22(3):549–562; Netherlands Ministry of Health Welfare and Sports, Netherlands Ministry of Justice. *Drug policy in the Netherlands: continuity and change*. The Hague, Netherlands: Ministry of Health, Welfare and Sports, 1995; Erickson P, Drucker E. Harm reduction: a public health strategy. *Curr Issues Public Health* 1995;1:64–70; Advisory Council on the Misuse of Drugs. *AIDS and drug misuse, part I: report of the Advisory Council on the Misuse of Drugs*. London: Her Majesty's Stationery Office, 1988; Interdepartmental Stuurgroep Alcohol en Drugbeleid. *Drugbeleid in beweging: naar een normalisering van de drugproblematiek*. The Hague: Ministerie van Welzijn, Volksgezondheid en Culture, 1985; Staples P. Reduction of alcohol- and drug-related harm in Australia: a government minister's perspective. In: Heather N, Wodak A, Nadelmann EA, et al., eds. *Psychoactive drugs and harm reduction: from faith to science*. London: Whurr Publishers, 1993:49–54; van de Wijngaart GF. The Dutch approach: normalization of drug problems. *J Drug Issues* 1990;20(4):667–678.

5. U.S. Office of National Drug Control Policy, Washington, DC, 20003; U.N. Drug and Crime Control Program, Vienna 2000.

6. U.S. Department of State Office of the Legal Adviser Treaty Affairs Staff. *Treaties in force: a list of treaties and other international agreements of the United States in force as of January 1, 1995*. Washington, DC: U.S. Department of State, 1995; Last JM, Wallace RB. *Maxcy-Rosenau-Last public health and preventive medicine*, 13th ed. Norwalk, CT: Appleton & Lange, 1992; Drucker E. Harm reduction: a public health strategy. *Current Issues in Public Health* 1995;1:64–70.

7. Drucker E. *Drug prohibition and public health: 25 years of evidence, public health reports*, vol. 114, pp 14–29, Jan/Feb 1999.

8. Bewley-Taylor DR. *The United States and international drug control, 1909–1997*. London & New York: Continuum, 2001; Bewley-Taylor DR. *Challenging the UN drug control conventions: problems and possibilities*. IJDP, 2003.

9. The Single Convention on Narcotic Drugs (1961). U.S. Department of State Office of the Legal Adviser Treaty Affairs Staff. *Treaties in force: a list of treaties and other international agreements of the United States in force as of January 1, 1995*. Washington, DC: U.S. Department of State, 1995; Nadelmann EA. Global prohibition regimes: the evolution of norms in international society. *Int Organization* 1990;44(4):479–526. Stares PB. *Global habit: the drug problem in a borderless world*. Washington, DC: Brookings Institution. 1996; Nadelmann EA. *Cops across borders: the internationalization of U.S. criminal law enforcement*. University Park, PA: Pennsylvania State University College Press, 1993.

10. Harm reduction policies are still attacked by U.S. government officials who claim that harm reduction initiatives connote a surrender in the "War on Drugs" and stepping-stones to "drug legalization"; Bayer R, Oppenheimer GM. *Confronting drug policy*. New York: Cambridge University Press, 1993; Drucker E. Harm reduction: a public health strategy. *Current Issues in Public Health* 1995;1:64–70; Nadelmann EA. Thinking seriously about alternatives to drug prohibition. *Daedalus* 1992;121(3):85–132. MacCoun RJ, Saiger AJ, Kahan JP, et al. Drug policies and problems: the promise and pitfalls of cross-national comparison. In: Heather N, Wodak A, Nadelmann EA, et al., eds. *Psychoactive drugs and harm reduction: from faith to science*. London: Whurr Publishers, 1993:103–117.

11. Zinberg NE. *Drug, set, and setting: the basis for controlled intoxicant use*. New Haven: Yale University Press, 1984; Zinberg NE, Harding WM. Control and intoxicant use: a theoretical and practical overview. *J Drug Issues* 1979;9:121–143.

12. Tatarsky A. *Harm reduction psychotherapy: a new treatment for drug and alcohol problems*. Northvale, NJ: Jason Aronson, 2002; Denning P. *Practicing harm reduction psychotherapy: an alternative approach to addictions*. New York: Guilford Press, 2002; Ruefli T, Rogers S. How do drug users define their progress in harm reduction programs? Qualitative research to develop user-generated outcomes. Harm Reduction Journal.com, 2004.

13. Musto DF. *The American disease: origins of narcotic control*. New York: Oxford University Press, 1987. Chapter by Musto in Lowinson; American Public Health Association. *Resolution for access to therapeutic marijuana/cannabis*. Washington, DC: American Public Health Association, 1995; Mino A. *Analyse scientifique de la littérature pour la remise controlee d'heroine ou de morphine*. Geneva: Office Federal de la Sante Publique, 1990.

14. Stimson GV, Oppenheimer E. *Heroin addiction: treatment and control in Britain.* London: Tavistock, 1982; Re-Inventing methadone: critical studies. Special Issue of *Addiction Research*, vol. 3, No. 4, Drucker E, Wodak A, eds., 1996; Drucker E. From morphine to methadone. In: Inciardi J, Harrison L, eds. *Harm reduction: a textbook.* Thousand Oaks, CA: Sage, 2000.

15. Newman RG. *Methadone treatment in narcotic addiction.* New York: Academic Press, 1977; MMTP Positive outcomes include decreases in heroin use; Ball JC, Ross A. *The effectiveness of methadone maintenance treatment.* New York: Springer-Verlag, 1991; Hubbard RL. *Drug abuse treatment: a national study of effectiveness.* Chapel Hill: University of North Carolina Press, 1989; Institute of Medicine. *Federal regulation of methadone treatment.* Washington, DC: National Academy Press, 1995; Darke S, Hall W, Heather N, et al. The reliability and validity of a scale to measure HIV risk taking behavior among intravenous drug users. *AIDS* 1991;5(2):181–185; Selwyn PA, Feiner C, Cox CP, et al. Knowledge about AIDS and high risk behavior among intravenous drug users in New York City. *AIDS* 1987;1(4):247–254; Joseph H. The criminal justice system and opiate addiction: an historical perspective. In: Leukefeld CG, Tims FM, eds. *Compulsory treatment of drug abuse: research and clinical practice.* Rockville, MD: National Institute on Drug Abuse, 1988:106–125; Newman RG, Peyser NP. Methadone treatment: experiment and experience. *J Psychoactive Drugs* 1991;23:115–121.

16. Institute of Medicine. *Federal regulation of methadone treatment.* Washington, DC: National Academy Press, 1995; Dole VP. Hazards of process regulations: the example of methadone maintenance. *JAMA* 1992;267(16):2234–2235; Dole VP, Nyswander ME. Methadone maintenance treatment: a ten year perspective. *JAMA* 1976;235(19):2117–2119; Ball JC, Ross A. *The effectiveness of methadone maintenance treatment.* New York: Springer-Verlag, 1991.

17. Rosenberg H, Phillips KT. Acceptability and availability of harm reduction interventions for drug abuse in American substance abuse treatment agencies." *Psychology of Addictive Behaviors* 2003;17(3):203–210.

18. McNeely J, Arnsten JH, Langrod JG, et al. Response to a program to improve access to sterile syringes and safe syringe disposal for injection drug users in a methadone maintenance treatment program. Presented at the American Public Health Association Conference, San Francisco, CA, Nov. 2003.

19. Institute of Medicine. *Federal regulation of methadone treatment.* Washington, DC: National Academy Press, 1995; Holmberg SD. The estimated prevalence and incidence of HIV in 96 large U.S. metropolitan areas. *Am J Public Health* 1996;86:642–654.

20. Nadelmann E, McNeely J. Doing methadone right. *Public Interest* 1996; 123:83–93; U.S. Office of Technology Assessment. *The effectiveness of AIDS prevention efforts.* Washington, DC: U.S. Government Printing Office, 1995; Caplehorn JRM, Bell J. Methadone dosage and retention of patients in maintenance treatment. *Med J Aust* 1991;154:195–199; Cooper JR. Ineffective use of psychoactive drugs: methadone treatment is no exception. *JAMA* 1992;267(2):281–282; D'Aunno T, Vaughn T. Variations in methadone treatment practices: results from a national study. *JAMA* 1992;267(2):253–258; Hargreaves WA. Methadone dose and duration for maintenance treatment. In: Cooper JR, ed. *Research on the treatment of narcotic addiction: state of the art.* Rockville, MD: National Institute on Drug Abuse, 1983; Caplehorn JRM. A comparison of abstinence-oriented and indefinite methadone maintenance treatment. *Int J Addict* 1994;19:1361–1375; U.S. Department of Health and Human Services Center for Substance Abuse Treatment. *State methadone treatment guidelines.* Rockville, MD: U.S. Department of Health and Human Services, Center for Substance Abuse Treatment, 1993; D'Aunno T, Pollack HA. Changes in methadone treatment practices: results from a national panel study, 1988–2000. *JAMA* 2002;288(7):850–856.

21. Serfaty A. HIV infection drug use in France: trends of the epidemic and governmental responses. In: Reisinger M, ed. *AIDS and drug addiction in the European Community.* Brussels: Commission of the European Communities, European Monitoring Centre on Drugs and Drug Addiction, 1993:61–70; Picard E. Legal action against the Belgian Medical Association's restrictions of methadone treatment. In: Reisinger M, ed. *AIDS and drug addiction in the European Community.* Brussels: Commission of the European Communities, European Monitoring Centre on Drugs and Drug Addiction, 1993:41–49; Van Santen GW. Exchange of expertise in Europe: the Frankfurt experience. In: Reisinger M, ed. *AIDS and drug addiction in the European Community.* Brussels: Commission of the European Communities, European Monitoring Centre on Drugs and Drug Addiction, 1993:169–173; Fleming, Philip M. Prescribing policy in the UK: a swing away from harm reduc-

tion? *International Journal of Drug Policy* 1995;6:173–177.

22. In 1996 the Institute of Medicine (IOM) Institute of Medicine. *Treating drug problems.* Washington, DC: National Academy Press, 1990;1:187.

23. U.S. Dept. of Health and Human Services, Center for Substance Abuse Treatment, State Methadone Treatment Guidelines, DHHS Pub. No. (SMA) 93–1991 (Rockville, MD: DHHS, 1993), U.S. DHHS Consensus Conference on Opiate Treatment, NIH,Wash DC,1999.

24. Farrell M. *Methadone Treatment in the European Union.* London: Oxford University Press, 1999.

25. Auriacombe M. Buprenorphine use in France background and current use. In Ritter A, Kutin J, Lintzeris N, et al., eds. *Expanding treatment options for heroin dependence in Victoria buprenorphine, LAAM, naltrexone and slow-release oral morphine. New pharmacotherapies project—feasibility phase.* Fitzroy: Victoria Turning Point Alcohol and Drug Center Inc, 1997:73–80; Auriacombe M, Franques P, Bertorelle V, et al. Use of buprenorphine for substitution treatment a French experience in Bordeaux and Bayonne. *Research and Clinical Forums* 1997;1947–1950; Auriacombe M, Franques P, Martin C, et al. Economic impact of methadone and buprenorphine treatments. A tentative approach. 59th Annual Scientific Meeting of the College on Problems of Drug Dependence; Nashville, TN, 1997; Auriacombe M, Tignol J. Buprenorphine use in France quality of life and conditions for treatment success. *Research and Clinical Forums* 1997;1925–1932; Fhima A, et al. Two-year follow-up of an opioid-user cohort treated with high-dose buprenorphine (Subutex). *Annales de médecine interne* 2001;152:26–36, Masson, Paris, 2001; Bénédicte L, et al. Reduction in the number of lethal heroin overdoses in France since 1994. *Annales de médecine interne* 2001;152:5–12.

26. Verster A, Buning E. Key aspects of substitution treatment for opiate dependence. *Euro Methwork* 2003; Amsterdam Advisory Council on the Misuse of Drugs. *AIDS and drug misuse, part I: report of the Advisory Council on the Misuse of Drugs.* London: Her Majesty's Stationery Office, 1988; Bell J. Alternatives to non-clinical regulation: training doctors to deliver methadone maintenance treatment. *Addict Res* 1986;3:297–315; Buning EC. Involving G.P.'s in Paris. *Euro-methwork* 1996;8:3–4; Byrne A, Wodak A. Census of patients receiving methadone in a general practice. *Addict Res* 1986;3:323–341; Greenwood J. Creating a new drug service in Edinburgh. *Br Med J* 1990;300:587–589; Pearson G.

Drug-control policies in Britain. *Crime Justice Rev Res* 1991;14:167; Picard E. Legal action against the Belgian Medical Association's restrictions of methadone treatment. In: Reisinger M, ed. *AIDS and drugs addiction in the European Community.* Brussels: Commission of the European Communities, European Monitoring Centre on Drugs and Drug Addiction, 1993;41–49; Reisinger M. *AIDS and drug addiction in the European Community.* Brussels: Commission of the European Communities, European Monitoring Centre on Drugs and Drug Addiction, 1993; Stimson GV. AIDS and injecting drug use in the United Kingdom, 1988–1993: the policy response and the prevention of the epidemic. Unpublished manuscript, 1994; Van Brussel GHA. Methadone treatment in Amsterdam: the critical role of the general practitioners. *Addict Res* 1986;3:363–369.

27. Buning EC, Van Brussel GHA, Van Santen GW. The "Methadone by Bus" project in Amsterdam. *Br J Addict* 1990;85(10):1247–1250; Gossop M, Grant M. *The content and structure of methadone treatment programs: a study in six countries.* Geneva: WHO, Programme on Substance Abuse, 1990; Klingemann HKH. Drug treatment in Switzerland: harm reduction, decentralization and community response. *Addiction* 1996;91:723–736; Plomp HN, van der Hek H, Ader HJ. The Amsterdam dispensing circuit: genesis and effectiveness of a public health model for local drug policy. *Addiction* 1996;91(5):711–721; Pompidou Group Co-operation Group to Combat Drug Abuse and Illicit Trafficking in Drugs. *Multi-city study: drug misuse trends in thirteen European cities.* Strasbourg: Council of Europe Press, 1994; Ward J, Mattick RP, Hall W. *Key issues in methadone maintenance treatment.* Kensington, Australia: New South Wales University Press, 1992; Newman RG. Narcotic addiction and methadone treatment in Hong Kong. *J Public Health Policy* (South Asian ed) 1985;6:526–538; Pompidou Group Co-operation Group to Combat Drug Abuse and Illicit Trafficking in Drugs. *Multi-city study: drug misuse trends in thirteen European cities.* Strasbourg: Council of Europe Press, 1994.

28. Dole VP, Robinson JW, Orraca J, et al. Methadone treatment of randomly selected criminal addicts. *New England Journal of Medicine* 1969;280:1372–1375; Dolan KA, Wodak A. An international review of methadone provision in prisons. *Addiction Research* 1996;4(1):85; CDC. *Prevention and Control of Infections with Hepatitis Viruses in Correctional Settings.* At-

lanta: Centers for Disease Control and Prevention; 2003. Report No.: Morbidity and Mortality Weekly Report 24. 19; Crofts N, Stewart T, Hearne P, et al. Spread of blood borne viruses among Australian prison entrants. *British Medical Journal* 1995;310:285–288; Magura S, Rosenblum A, Lewis C, et al. The effectiveness of in-jail methadone maintenance. *Journal of Drug Issues* 1993;23(1):75–99; Dolan KA, Shearer JD, MacDonald M, et al. A randomised controlled trial of methadone maintenance treatment versus wait list control in an Australian prison. *Drug and Alcohol Dependence* 2003;72:59–65; Levasseur L, Marzo J-N, Ross N, et al. Frequency of re-incarcerations in the same detention centre: role of substitution therapy. A preliminary retrospective analysis. *Annales de Medecine Interne* 2002;153(3):1S14–1S19; Kinlock TW, Battjes RJ, Schwartz RP, et al. TMP. A novel opioid maintenance program for prisoners: preliminary findings. *Journal of Substance Abuse Treatment* 2002;22:141–147; Bellin E, Wesson J, Tomasino V, et al. High dose methadone reduces criminal recidivism in opiate addicts. *Addiction Research* 1999;7(1):19–29; McKay D, Jail Site of Health Service, *Albuquerque Journal*, Feb 10, 2004, p. 1, http://www.abqjournal.com/news/metro/143159metro02-10-04.html

29. Roberts K, Hunter C. A comprehensive system of pharmaceutical care for drug misusers. *HRJ.com* 1:1 2004; Tomasello T. Substance Abuse and Pharmacy Practice: What does the community pharmacist need to know about drug abuse and dependence? *HRJ.com* 1:1 2004; ASHP Statement on the Pharmacist's Role in Substance Abuse Prevention, Education, and Assistance, The American Society of Health-System Pharmacists (ASHP). *Am J Health-Syst Pharm* 60(19) 2003; Sheridan J, Strang J, eds. *Drug misuse and community pharmacy.* London: Taylor and Francis, 2002.

30. See chapter 4, in Lowinson et al., 4th edition.

31. Hartnoll RL, Mitcheson MC, Battersby A, et al. Evaluation of heroin maintenance in controlled trial. *Arch Gen Psychiatry* 37:877–884, 1980; Battersby M, Farrell M, Gossop M, et al. "Horse trading": prescribing injectable opiates to opiate addicts. A descriptive study. *Drug Alcohol Rev.* 11:35–42, 1992; Swiss Drugs Policy, Sept 2000, Bern; Swiss Federal Office of Public Health Heroin Assisted Treatment, 2002, Bern; Drucker E, Vlahov D. Controlled clinical evaluation of diacetyle morphine for treatment of intractable opiate dependence (commentary). *Lancet* 353;

Rehm J, Gschwend P, Steffen T, et al. Feasibility, safety and efficacy of injectable heroin prescription for refractory opiate addicts: a follow-up study. *Lancet* 2001;358:1417–1420; Drucker E. Injectable heroin substitution treatment for opiate dependency (commentary). *Lancet* 2001;358:1385; Central Committee on the Treatment of Heroin Addicts (CCBH). *Investigating the medical prescription of heroin.* Utrecht, 1997; van den Brink W et al. Results of the Dutch Heroin Trial. Addictions, (www.ccbh.nl), *BMJ* 2003. Uchtenhagen A, Gutzwiller F, Dobler-Mikola A. eds. *Medical prescription of narcotics research programme: Final Report of the Principal Investigators.* Zurich: Institute for Social and Preventive Medicine at the University of Zurich: Zurich, 1998. Bammer G, Dobler-Mikola A, Fleming PM, et al. The heroin prescribing debate: integrating science and politics. *Science* 1999;284(5418):1277–1278. Report of the WHO External Panel on the Evaluation of the Swiss Scientific Studies of Medically Prescribed Narcotics to Drug Addicts. WHO Report, April 1999. Frei A, Greiner R, Mehner A, et al. Socioeconomic Evaluation of the Trials for the Medical Prescription of Opiates, Final Report. HealthEcon:Base1, 1997 June (translated June 1998); Drucker E, Vlahov D. Controlled clinical evaluation of diacetyl morphine for treatment of intractable opiate dependence. *Lancet* 1999; 353(9164):1543–1544; Farrell M, Hall W. The Swiss heroin trials: testing alternative approaches: Prescribed heroin is likely to have a limited role. *BMJ* 1998;316(7132):639; Fischer B, Rehm J. The case for a heroin substitution treatment trial in Canada. *Can J Pub Hlth* 1997;88(6):367–370. Cooper-Mahkorn D. German doctors vote to prescribe heroin to misusers. *BMJ* 1998;316:1037.

32. Arrest of needle-exchange workers draws national attention: New Brunswick, New Jersey Chai project. *Alcohol Drug Abuse Wkly* 1996;8(19):3; New Jersey panel's support of needle exchange stirs debate. *Alcohol Drug Abuse Wkly* 1996;8(14):1; Arnao G. Italian referendum deletes criminal sanctions for drug users. *J Drug Issues* 1994;24(3):483–487; Australian Government. *Inter-Governmental report on AIDS: a report on HIV/AIDS activities in Australia, 1990–1991.* Canberra: Australian Government Publishing, 1992; Barreras R. Social Policy, Science and Activism in the History of Needle Exchange in NYC. Unpublished PhD Thesis, City Univ of NY, March 2004.

33. Rehm J, Gschwend P, Steffen T, et al. Feasibility, safety and efficacy of

injectable heroin prescription for refractory opiate addicts: a follow-up study. *Lancet* 2001;358:1417–1420.

34. Australian Government. *Inter-Governmental report on AIDS: a report on HIV/AIDS activities in Australia, 1990–1991.* Canberra: Australian Government Publishing, 1992; Bammer G. *Report and recommendations of stage 2 feasibility research into the controlled availability of opioids.* Canberra: Australian Institute of Criminology, National Centre for Epidemiology and Population Health, 1995; World Health Organization Programme on Substance Abuse Drug Substitution Project. Report of WHO consultation, Geneva, 15–19 May 1995. Geneva: World Health Organization, 1996.

35. Australian Government. *Inter-Governmental report on AIDS: a report on HIV/AIDS activities in Australia, 1990–1991.* Canberra: Australian Government Publishing, 1992; Ball JC, Ross A. *The effectiveness of methadone maintenance treatment.* New York: Springer-Verlag, 1991; Bammer G. *Report and recommendations of stage 2 feasibility research into the controlled availability of opioids.* Canberra: Australian Institute of Criminology, National Centre for Epidemiology and Population Health, 1995; Bammer G, Dance P, Stevens A, et al. Attitudes to a proposal for controlled availability of heroin in Australia: is it time for a trial? *Addict Res* 1996;4(1): 45–55.

36. van den Brink W, Hendriks VM, Blanken P, et al. Medical prescription of heroin to treatment resistant heroin addicts: two randomised controlled trials. *BMJ* 2003;9;327(7410):310.

37. Ball JC, Ross A. *The effectiveness of methadone maintenance treatment.* New York: Springer-Verlag, 1991; Bertschy G. Methadone maintenance treatment: an update. *Eur Arch Psychiatry Clin Neurosci* 1995;245(2):114–124; Fairbank A, Dunteman GH, Condelli WS. Do methadone patients substitute other drugs for heroin? Predicting substance use at 1-year follow-up. *Am J Drug Alcohol Abuse* 1993;19:465–474; Hartel D. Temporal patterns of cocaine use and AIDS in intravenous drug users in methadone maintenance [abstract]. Paper presented at the 5th International Conference on AIDS, Montreal, Canada, June 1989; Lamb RJ, Kirby KC, Platt JJ. Treatment retention, occupational role, and cocaine use among those who remain in MMT. *Am J Addict* 1995;4:1–6; Magura S, Siddiqi Q, Freeman RC, et al. Changes in cocaine use after entry to methadone treatment. In: *Cocaine, AIDS, and intravenous drug use.* New York: Haworth Press, 1991.

38. Bradbeer TM, Fleming PM, Charlton P, et al. *Survey of amphetamine prescribing in England and Wales.* 1998; Fleming PM, Roberts D. Is the prescription of amphetamine justified as a harm reduction measure? *Journal of the Royal Society of Health* 1994;114(3):127–131; Fleming PM. *Prescribing amphetamine to amphetamine users as a harm reduction measure.* 1998; Mattick RP, Darke S. Drug replacement treatments: is amphetamine substitution a horse of a different colour? *Drug and Alcohol Review* 1995;14:389–394; Merrill, J. *Evaluation of prescribing dexamphetamine in the treatment of amphetamine dependence.* 1998. Unpublished document; Myles J. Treatment for amphetamine misuse in the United Kingdom. In: Klee H, ed. *Amphetamine misuse: International perspectives on current trends.* Amsterdam, Netherlands: Harwood Academic, 1997: 69–79; Sherman JP. Dexamphetamine for "speed" addiction. *Medical Journal of Australia* 1990;153(5):306; Strang J, Sheridan J. Prescribing amphetamines to drug misusers: data from the 1995 National Survey of Community Pharmacies in England and Wales. *Addiction* 1997; 92(7):833–838; Kingston S, Conrad M. Harm reduction for methamphetamoine users. 2004Focus: UCSF AIDS Health Project. 19, 1, p p.

39. Shearer J, Wodak A, van Beek I, et al. Related Articles, Links Pilot randomized double blind placebo-controlled study of dexamphetamine for cocaine dependence. *Addiction* 2003;98(8):1137–1141.

40. Kaplan EH. Probability models of needle exchange. *Operations Res* 1995;43:558–569.

41. Stimson GV. Syringe exchange programs for injecting drug users. *AIDS* 1989;3:253.

42. Lurie P, Drucker E. An opportunity lost: HIV infections associated with lack of a national needle-exchange programme in the U.S.A. (commentary). *Lancet* 1997;349:604–608.

43. Lurie P, Reingold AL. *The public health impact of needle exchange programs in the United States and abroad.* Berkeley: University of California, Institute for Health Policy Studies, 1993.

44. Drucker E, Lurie P, Alcabes Pet al. Measuring harm reduction: the effects of needle and syringe exchange programs and methadone maintenance on the ecololgy of HIV. *AIDS* 12 (suppl A):S217–S230, 1998.

45. Drucker E. Drug prohibition and public health: 25 years of evidence. *Public Health Reports* 1999;114:4–29.

46. National Commission on Acquired Immune Deficiency Syndrome. *The twin epidemics of substance use and HIV.* Washington, DC: National Commission on Acquired Immune Deficiency Syndrome, 1991.

47. Lurie P, Reingold AL. *The public health impact of needle exchange programs in the United States and abroad.* Berkeley: University of California, Institute for Health Policy Studies, 1993.

48. Washington, DC: U.S. General Accounting Office, 1993.

49. Lurie P. Policy experts unanimous: needle-exchange programs effective [letter]. *AIDS Wkly* 1996:29; O'Hare P, Newcombe R, Matthews A, Buning et al. *The reduction of drug related harm.* New York: Routledge, 1992; Lurie P. Policy experts unanimous: needle-exchange programs effective [letter]. *AIDS Wkly* 1996:29. Case P, Meehan T, Jones ST. Arrests and incarceration of injection drug users for syringe possession in Massachusetts: implications for HIV prevention. *Journal of Acquired Immune Deficiency Syndromes and Human Retrovirolog,* 1998;18(suppl 1):S71–S75.

50. Drug Policy Alliance: fourteen article abstracts on needle and syringe exchange, 2004 http://www.drugpolicy.org/library/lipp14.cfm

51. Moss AR. Epidemiology and the Politics of Needle Exchange (comment). *AJPH* 2000;90:1395–1396.

52. Gostin LO. The legal environment impeding access to sterile syringes and needles: The conflict between law enforcement and public health. *Journal of Acquired Immune Deficiency Syndromes and Human Retrovirolog,* 1998;18(suppl 1): S60–S70.

53. Stimson GV. Syringe exchange programs for injecting drug users. *AIDS* 1989;3:253.

54. Lungley S, Baker M. *The needle and syringe exchange scheme in operation.* Wellington: New Zealand Department of Health, 1990.

55. AIDS Coordinating Committee. *Deregulation of hypodermic needles and syringes as a public health measure.* Presented at: Syringe Deregulation Working Group Meeting. March 2001.

56. Gibson DR, Flynn NM, McCarthy JJ. Effectiveness of methadone treatment in reducing HIV risk behavior and HIV seroconversion among injecting drug users [editorial]. *AIDS* 1999;13:14, 1807–1818.

57. Drucker E, ed. Drug overdose. Special Issue of *Addiction Research and Theory* 2001; 9(5); Bigg D, et al. Use of Narcan to prevent overdose. By Chicago Recovery Alliance, presented at APHA annual conf, Oct 2003; Deitze P et al. Context management and prevention of heroin overdose in Victoria, Australia. *Add Rsch and Teryr* 2001;9(60): 437. Ali R. S Australia OD campaign. *Drug*

and *Alcohol Review* 2001. See also http://www.anypositivechange.org/res.html)

58. Drug user organizations and the community involvement of drug users: Grund JP, Blanken P, Adriaans FP, et al. Reaching the unreached: targeting hidden IDU populations with clean needles via known user groups. *J Psychoactive Drugs* 1992;24(1):41–47. Friedman SR, De Jong W, Wodak A. Community development as a response to HIV among drug injectors. *AIDS* 1993;7 (suppl 1):S263–S269; Crofts N. A history of peer-based drug-user groups in Australia. *Journal of Drug Issues* 1993;25:599–616.

59. Broadhead RS, Heckathorn DD, Altice FL, et al. Increasing drug users' adherence to HIV treatment: results of a peer-driven intervention feasibility study. *Soc Sci Med* 2002;55(2):235–246.

60. Fromberg E, Jansen F. Rave Drug Monitoring System. *Verslag* 1993;1(7). Netherlands Institute on Alcohol and Drugs (NIAD) Utrecht.

61. Drug Consumer Groups: Grund JP. *Drug use as a social ritual: functionality, symbolism and determinants of self regulation.* IVO series 4. Rotterdam: IVO, 1996.

62. Municipal Zoning Policies and Open Drug Scenes: See Nadelmann E, Mc Neely J, Drucker E. International perspectives. In: Lowinson et al., eds. *Comprehensive textbook of substance abuse,* 4th ed. Willliams & Wilkins, 1995.

63. "Safe Spaces" for people who use drugs, Dolan K, et al. (2001) Drug consumption facilities in Europe and Australia Drug and Alc Rev 19, 337 46. Christie T, et al. Regulating supervised Injection site in Canada Int J Drug Policy, 2004 (159 1) 66–73 . Wright NMJ, Tompkins CNE. Supervised injecting centres. BMJ (2004) 328:100–102 http://bmj.bmjjournals.com/cgi/content/full/328/7431/100; Strang J, Fortson R. Supervised fixing rooms, supervised injectable maintenance clinics—understanding the difference. BMJ (2004) 328:102–103; http://bmj.bmjjournals.com/cgi/content/full/328/7431/102; Burton, B. Supervised drug injecting room trial considered a success. BMJ (2003) 327:122; http://bmj.com/cgi/content/full/327/7407/122-a (Dance Safe: http://www.dancesafe.org/); also see Holland J. (ed) Ecstacy: the complete guide. A comprehensive look at the risks and benefits of MDMA inner traditions. NY, 2003.

64. Marijuana policies: in the United States in the 1970s, the movement to decriminalize marijuana was driven by the realization that criminal sanctions created greater harm than marijuana use itself. Kaplan S. *Marijuana: the new prohibition.* New York: Pocket Books, 1970; Anderson P. *High in America: the true story behind NORML and the politics of marijuana.* New York: Viking Press, 1981; see also Marijuana Regulation Bibliography Nadelmann, Ethan, et al. Marijuana Regulation Bibliography. Drug Policy Alliance Web site, Sept 1998.

65. Dutch Cannabis Policies: Cohen P. Building upon the successes of Dutch drug policy. *International Journal on Drug Policy* 1988;2(2):22–24. Cohen P. The case of the two Dutch drug policy commissions. An exercise in harm reduction 1968–1972. In: Erickson P, et al., eds. *New public health policies and programs for the reduction of drug related harm.* University of Toronto Press, 1997; Cohen P, Arjan S. Cannabis use, a stepping stone to other drug use? The case of Amsterdam. In: Böllinger L, ed. *Cannabis science/cannabis wissenschaft.* Frankfurt Am Main: Peter Lang Publ, 1997: 49–82; de Kort M. The Dutch cannabis debate 1968–1976. *Journal of Drug Issues* 1994;24(3):417–427; Engelsman EL. Dutch policy of the management of drug-related problems. *British Journal of Addiction* 1989;84:211–218; Grapendaal M, Leuw E, Nelen H. Legalization, decriminalization and the reduction of crime. In: Leuw E, Marshall I, Haen, eds. *Between prohibition and legalization: the Dutch experiment in drug policy.* New York: Kugler Publications, 1996:233–253; Jansen ACM. The development of a "legal" consumers' market for cannabis: the 'coffee shop' phenomenon." In: Leuw E, Marshall I, Haen, eds. *Between prohibition and legalization: the Dutch experiment in drug policy.* New York: Kugler Publications, 1996:169–181; Korf DJ. Cannabis retail markets in Amsterdam. *International Journal of Drug Policy* 1990;2(1):23–27; Korf DJ. Twenty years of soft drug use in Holland: A retrospective view based on twenty years of prevalence studies. *Dutch Journal of Alcohol, Drugs and Other Psychotropic Substances* 1988;14(3):81–89; Lap M, Drucker E. Recent changes in the Dutch cannabis trade: the case for regulated domestic production. *International Journal of Drug Policy* 1994;5(4):249–252; Leuw E, Marshall I, Haen, eds. *Between prohibition and legalization: the Dutch experiment in drug policy.* Amsterdam, New York: Kugler Publications, 1994. Leuw E. Drugs and drug policy in the Netherlands. In: Tonry M, ed. *Crime and justice: a review of research.* Chicago, IL: University of Chicago Press, 1991; Leuw E. Recent reconsiderations in Dutch drug policy. In: Böllinger L., ed. *Cannabis science: from prohibition to human right* [*Cannabis Wissenschaft: Von der Prohibition zum Recht auf Genuβ*]. Frankfurt, Germany: Peter Lang, 1997:153–168; Netherlands Ministry of Health, Welfare and Sports; Netherlands Ministry of Justice. *Drug policy in the Netherlands: continuity and change.* The Hague, Netherlands: Ministry of Health, Welfare and Sports, 1995; Ossebaard HC. Netherlands cannabis policy [letter]. *Lancet* 1996;347(9003):767–768; Scheerer S. The new Dutch and German drug laws: social and political conditions for criminalization and decriminalization. *Law and Society Review* 1978;12(4):585–606; Silvis J. Enforcing drug laws in the Netherlands. In: Leuw E, Marshall I, Haen, eds. *Between prohibition and legalization: the Dutch experiment in drug policy.* New York: Kugler Publications, 1996: 41–58.

66. Canada: Addiction Research Foundation. *Cannabis, health and public policy.* Toronto, Canada: Addiction Research Foundation, 1997; Canada: commission of inquiry into the non-medical use of drugs. *Cannabis: a report of the Commission of Inquiry into the non-medical use of drugs [also known as the LeDain report].* Ottawa, Canada: Information Canada, 1972. Note especially chapter 5, "The law" (pp. 209–261) and chapter 6, "Conclusions and recommendations of Gerald LeDain, Heinz Lehmann, J. Peter Stein" (pp. 265–316); Canadian Centre on Substance Abuse (CCSA), National Working Group on Addictions Policy. *Cannabis control in Canada: options regarding possession.* Ottawa, Canada: Canadian Centre on Substance Abuse (CCSA), 1998; Australia: Atkinson L, Mc Donald D. Cannabis, the law and social impacts in Australia. *Trends and Issues in Crime and Criminal Justice* 1995;48. Christie P. *The effects of cannabis legislation in South Australia on levels of cannabis use.* Parkside, Australia: Drug and Alcohol Services Council, 1991; Christie P, Ali R. The operation and effects of the cannabis laws in South Australia. In: McDonald D, Atkinson L, eds. *Social impacts of the legislative options for cannabis in Australia (phase 1 research): a report to the National Drug Strategy Committee.* Canberra, Australia: Australian Institute of Criminology, 1995; Criminal Justice Commission. *Report on cannabis and the law in Queensland.* Brisbane, Australia: Criminal Justice Commission, 1994.

67. Medical marijuana: Grinspoon L, Bakalar J. *Marijuana: forbidden medicine.* Yale, 1997; Zimmer L, Morgan J. *Marijuana myths, marijuana facts.* New York: The Lindesmith Center, 1997; Joy JE, Watson SJ, Benson JA,

eds. *Marijuana and medicine: assessing the science base.* Washington, D.C.: Division of Neuroscience and Behavioral Health, Institute of Medicine; National Academy Press, 1999. Earleywine M. *Understanding marijuana: a new look at the scientific evidence.* Oxford University Press, 2002. Current Sites http://www.marijuanainfo.org/popup.php?Source_ID=138&Source_Tbl=Info OR http://www.mpp.org/USA/news_1919.html and http://www.mpp.org/10statepoll/index.html

68. Medical marijuana in Canada: S.C. 1996, c. 19.R. v. Parker (2000), 49 O.R. (3d) 481. S.O.R./2001 227. Hitzig v. Canada [2003] O.J. No. 12 (Ontario Superior Court, Lederman J.) January 9, 2003.

69. UNAIDS, AIDS Epidemic Update, December 2002. The report notes, "In recent years, the Russian Federation has experienced an exceptionally steep rise in re- ported HIV infections. In less than eight years, HIV/AIDS epidemics have been discovered in more than 30 cities and 86 of the country's 89 regions."

The estimate of the number of Russians living with HIV is from Vadim Pokrovsky, head of the Russian AIDS Center; as noted in Torrey Clark, "Counting the Cost of AIDS on GDP," Moscow Times, May 16, 2002, A1. The estimate of the number of Ukrainians living with HIV is from Oleksander Yaramenko, the director of the Ukrainian Institute for Social Research, who quoted this figure in November 2002 in a speech at a conference in Crimea. The estimate is based on research his organization carried out for the British Council. Also quoted in "Every 10th Ukrainian Lives with HIV," November 11, 2002: NEWSru.com, online in Russian. UNAIDS, AIDS Epidemic Update, Decem- ber 2002. See also Rhodes et al. HIV transmision and prevention associated with IDU in the Russian Federation, Int J Drug Policy, 2004,15(1)1–16.

70. Drucker E, Alcabes PG, Marx, PA. The injection century: massive unsterile injecting and the emergence of human pathogens. *Lancet* 2001;358:1989–1992; Madhava V, Burgess C, Drucker E. The epidemiology of chronic of hepatitis C infection in sub Saharan Africa. *Lancet Infectious Diseases* 2002;(2):293–302; Schneider W, Drucker E. The Role of Blood Transfusions in the Early Decades of AIDS in Sub-Saharan Africa. Paper Presented at the Amer Assoc of the Hist of Med, May 2004.

71. Beckerleg S. How "cool" is heroin injecting at the Kenya Coast. *Drug Educ, Prev, Policy* 2004; (11): 67–77; Beckerleg S, Telfer M, Lewando Hundt G. *Harm Reduction Journal* (in press).

CHAPTER 78

Church, Family, and Community in the Prevention and Treatment of Addiction Among African Americans

RONALD HOPSON AND
WILLIAM B. LAWSON

Ethnic differences have been reported in alcohol use and abuse. Asian Americans consistently have low rates. Year after year, the Household Survey of Drug and Alcohol Use reliably shows lower rates of alcohol use. Moreover, African Americans show lower rates of use and abuse in teenagers and the elderly (1,2). Such differences have been attributed to factors such as polymorphisms in the isoenzymes that metabolize alcohol, suggesting that some ethnic groups, particularly Asians and African Americans, may have a "built-in" Antabuse (3,4). However, psychosocial and cultural factors may be involved and an examination of these factors may lead to strategies applicable to all ethnic groups. Such factors as church and family involvement seem to be especially important in preventing alcohol abuse in African Americans (2,5,6).

Positive family environment and religious involvement are seen as highly important in the prevention of addiction and in recovery from addiction, particularly for African Americans (5). Because African Americans often have less access to mental health services and medical care, the availability of alternative support systems (such as family and church) is essential (7,8). The African American church, as the only indigenous institution in the African American community wholly owned by the African American community, is uniquely suited to play a crucial role in addressing the problem of addiction within the African American community. The skepticism of some African Americans' about the medical care system (for legitimate reasons, as the disparities literature shows) requires institutions in which they have trust, to legitimize formal health care settings (9,10). Indeed, church involvement predicts positive health maintenance in African Americans (11).

CHURCH, RELIGION AND SPIRITUALITY

Religion has played a crucial role in African American survival and well being since the transatlantic slave trade. The African American church continues to occupy a unique and critical role within African American culture and U.S. society (12,13). The importance of the African American church in African American life has hardly diminished since DuBois' 1903 observation (14) that

> The Negro church of to-day is the social center of Negro life in the United States, and the most characteristic expression of African character. . . . Various organizations meet [in Negro church buildings],—the church proper, the Sunday-school, two or three insurance societies, women's societies, secret societies, and mass meetings of various kinds. Considerable sums of money are

collected and expended here, employment is found for the idle, strangers are introduced, news is disseminated and charity distributed. At the same time this social, intellectual, and economic centre is a religious centre of great power. . . . Back of [its] more formal religion, the Church often stands as a real conserver of morals, a strengthener of family life, and the final authority on what is Good and Right.

African Americans continue to report higher levels of subjective religiosity than whites (15). As the final authority on what is good and right and in African American community, the African American church plays a crucial role in addressing contemporary social ills such as mental/emotional problems and substance abuse and dependence (16). The African American church continues to be the principal mental health resource within the African American community. African Americans use mainstream resources, such as mental health professionals, in significantly smaller proportions than do members of the majority culture in the United States. Thus the African American church (and often the African American pastor), must be a primary resource for prevention and intervention.

Since the early 1900s, it has been understood that the primary strategies for intervention and prevention of drug/alcohol abuse and dependence must involve a "spiritual" component. William James observed that the only cure for "dipsomania" (an old term for alcoholism), was "religiomania." Carl Jung sent his intractably alcoholic patient away in search of a religious conversion, thereby acknowledging that addiction prevention and recovery may involve religious or spiritual themes. Indeed, it was Jung's insight that psychological analysis alone could not address the alcoholic problem that gave rise to the understanding of alcoholism (and by modern extension, other forms of addiction), as a spiritual malady. As Ernest Kurtz (17) detailed in his exhaustive history of Alcoholic's Anonymous (AA), Jung's comment to his patient Roland H. reverberated across the Atlantic ocean and, through a series of chance encounters, was the genesis of AA.

The "Big Book" of Alcoholics Anonymous (18) insists that alcoholism is a spiritual problem: "Lack of power, that was our dilemma. We had to find a power by which we could live and it had to be a power greater than ourselves. . . .Our liquor was but a symptom. So we had to get down to causes and conditions." The abuse of alcohol is a sign of an underlying spiritual disorder that can only be addressed through spiritual renewal. The remedy is effected by following certain steps (12 steps) that are "suggested" by AA as the way toward recovery.

Since Jellinek (19) showed alcoholism to be a primary medical disease, AA communities have embraced the "disease model" while continuing to practice the spiritual disciplines (the "12 steps") that may lead to recovery. Subsequent "anonymous" movements (Narcotics Anonymous, Cocaine Anonymous, Gambler's Anonymous, Overeaters Anonymous, etc.) have adopted the basic structure of AA as their principal mode of intervention for addictive problems.

Spirituality is an important element of recovery (20). Although not necessarily religion (21), spirituality provides the ethical superstructure, community, and transpersonal presence (higher power), to facilitate recovery and aide in the prevention of addiction. Since Carl Jung's insightful adage about alcoholism: "Spiritum contra Spiritus" ("Spirits against the Spirit"), spirituality has been seen to play an important role in the abuse of spirits. Those who report a spiritual awakening during recovery have the highest odds of continuous sobriety (22). Anecdotal accounts abound of persons who ceased substance abuse after a religious conversion.

Finally, the church still plays a central role in the African American experience. In recent years, the church has been recognized as a key factor in preventing the health disparities in African Americans. In addition, the church as an institution has become a key player in the delivery of services, including child care, inoculations, and acquired immunodeficiency syndrome (AIDS) prevention. The link to prevention of alcoholism is simply an extension of these experiences.

THE PHENOMENON OF ADDICTION

There has been significant progress in the understanding of addiction since Shaffer (23) argued that the disease model of addiction was best understood as a metaphor. There is now general agreement that addiction is a biopsychosocial disease and must be addressed within each domain (24). While spirituality is not mentioned explicitly, it is understood that spirituality plays a major role in understanding the addictive phenomenon. A brief review of the phenomenon of addiction may illustrate how religion/spirituality can play an important role in prevention and intervention strategies.

Addiction has been called a disease of feelings (25). The principal feeling that causes the greatest disease, which is also a major impediment to recovery, is shame. The addicted person experiences significant shame (26). Shame is a profoundly alienating emotion, affecting both interpersonal and transpersonal relationships. The individual in the grip of shame often withdraws from others, and carries a sense of alienation from whatever they conceive of to be of ultimate concern (e.g., God). Spirituality provides the ethical superstructure for the addicted person to work through the guilt and shame of addiction. Through the presence of others (community) and an Other (higher power), the alienation that characterizes addiction is mitigated.

Addiction involves perceptual and experiential anomalies that render the addicted person vulnerable to uncontrolled and compulsive activities. Wurmser (26), Khantzian (27), Mack (28), and Hopson (29) observed that the addicted person often experiences life as potentially overwhelming, positive and negative affect is experienced with great intensity, and when in distress, self-soothing efforts are futile. The addicted person also experiences a sense of disconnection from self and others, and feels demoralized, lacking a sense of agency and self-efficacy in their personal lives. These perceptual and experiential anomalies lead to activities that violate personal and social mores, are physically damaging/destructive, and disrupt normal interpersonal and vocational functioning.

Recent research suggests a biologic pathogenesis for the temperamental vulnerabilities mentioned above (30). As noted before, polymorphisms in the endogenous enzymes that metabolize alcohol may confer some protection from alcoholism in some ethnic groups. Whatever the etiology, it has been understood for some time that some persons may have a particular vulnerability to addiction as a consequence of temperament (31). Thus the biologic vulnerability may be exploited by psychosocial stressors that could lead to the abuse of the substance. Consequently, psychosocial interventions can be effective in prevention and intervention efforts, and may help to explain some of the ethnic resilience to alcohol abuse and dependence.

SPIRITUALITY OR RELIGION

The addictive use of substances serves both a self-soothing and a self-punishing function (32). The addicted person is often caught in a cycle of self-hate alternating with grandiosity (33). The spiritual imperative of acceptance and responsibility in community may interrupt this narcissistic crisis by providing affirming, yet limit-setting, experiences with others. Also, the power of the community and the higher power is available to intervene with the sense of demoralization.

Spirituality or religion may provide a sense of connection to something greater than the self which mitigates the tension, alienation, and demoralization of the addictive experience. Although addictions are no longer considered evidence of moral failings, there remains a faint moral censure about addiction. The addicted person must often struggle with a sense of shame regarding their addiction. Religion enters to offer the person exoneration through acceptance (absolution through confession; unconditioned acceptance). Spirituality/religion may also provide the ethical and practical structure for reorganizing one's life. Through its ideals, religion offers the ethical context in which persons may understand their lives. Through community, religion offers connection to and acceptance from others. Finally, opportunities for identification with positive role models exist within religious communities. Thus, as Ludwig (34) has observed, the increase in faith and hope that is critical to recovery can be available through religious community.

All that has been said about the potential of religious communities to address problems of addiction is also true of secular recovery communities. Alternatives such as Rational Recovery and Secular Organization for Sobriety offer a nontheistic alternative to AA. Women for Sobriety (and Men in Recovery) focuses on issues unique to women and African American men. Women for Sobriety rejects the dependency on an outside power; it rejects the idea that women are required to submit to male domination. It offers structure for regaining the healthy self-esteem and sense of individual responsibility that can mitigate the demoralization of addiction.

There are also programs geared toward African American men (e.g., Men in Recovery). These programs offer an alternative to traditional 12-step programs. Zitter (35) argues that empowerment and efficacy are the most important elements in recovery for African American men. The experience of African American males has often been one of powerlessness. Therefore, Zitter suggests that African American men must be affirmed for their efficacy and empowered to make constructive and life-affirming decisions regarding their behavior.

Williams (16) argues that traditional AA programs emphasize individualism. He questions the appropriateness of such individualism for African Americans. Williams traces the importance of community to the unique circumstances of African American survival. The enslaved had no control over whether biologic family ties would remain intact. Thus, the primacy of the nuclear family as the normative family structure is not sufficiently broad to encompass African American life. For African Americans, the community is one's family. Survival of the self is intrinsically linked to survival of the family and community; therefore, for Williams, recovery is not just for the self, but for the family and community as well.

The importance of community may predate the slavery experience. Many African cultures emphasize the importance of the community over the individual. Thus Africans with depression were far more likely to complain of shame, that is, distress about the person's role in the community, rather than guilt, that is, distress about personal behavior. Persistence of this cultural value may explain symptom presentation in African Americans today, and may also help to explain its importance in alcohol recovery.

THE AFRICAN AMERICAN FAMILY

The African American family plays multiple crucial roles in black life. In its extended form, the African American family has been considered the survival unit of African American's America (36). Despite the extraordinary efforts to destroy familial ties during enslavement and the postemancipation Jim Crow era, the African American family resisted extinction. African Americans created familial networks that were of necessity not limited to first-degree biologic relatives. Extended family networks developed to provide both instrumental and expressive functions to support African American life (37).

Long before the temperance movements of the early twentieth century, African Americans of the 1840s and 1850s viewed abstinence from alcohol as crucial in the struggle for freedom, as well as moral purity (38). This African American temperance movement was supported by strong familial and communal ties.

However, the African American family became fractured in the great African American migrations of the 1910s to the 1930s. Also, economic reversals and limited employment opportunities led to a shift in the African American communities' view of alcohol. Herd (39) suggests this period as the emergence of alcohol problems within the African American community. Thus, the emergence of alcohol problems within the African American community is coterminous with factors that led to family disruption.

Daniel Moynihan's (40) research cemented the view of the African American family as a "tangle of pathology." Yet the conclusions of this research have been seriously challenged. The African American family continues to be a crucial factor in supporting African American life. Research suggests the importance of strong family ties in the prevention of substance abuse, particularly for African American adolescents (5). Hayles (41) lists the following empirically documented strengths of African American families:

1. Kinship networks and extended family systems
2. Value systems that emphasize such things as harmony, cooperation, interdependence, acceptance of difference/diversity, internal development, strong work and achievement orientation, and traditionalism
3. Strong male/female bonds
4. Role adaptability and flexibility
5. Roots, emotional support, and buffers or consolations against racism
6. Respect, appreciation, and full use of the skills and wisdom of senior family members
7. Child centeredness

These factors can play a preventive and mitigating role in the problem of addictions. The isolation and demoralization of addiction may be mitigated by the deeply rooted tradition of extensive kinship networks. Extensive kinship networks provide alternative significant others as positive role models for members of the community. The supportive African American family may also be a buffer against the often obstructive economic circumstances in the African American community. The family provides models of identification through the extended and augmented family structure. For example, the focus on supportiveness, and the ties within the family certainly seems to offset the economic demands and lead to a better outcome for the severely mentally ill (42).

THE AFRICAN AMERICAN CHURCH

Several elements of the African American church make its role in the prevention and treatment of addiction critical. The church is often an extended family for its members. It may provide a sense of belonging, identity, esteem, and role models for the development of the talents and abilities of its members. The church can also provide the moral guidance and spiritual direction that mitigate addiction and abuse.

Historically, the family was the community and the community was largely defined by the religious structures within the community (church and mosque). The African American church functions as an extended family in African American life (43). The African American church long has been considered crucial as a buffer and support for African American life (44,45). The African American church has been the crucial institution within the African American community, wholly owned by the African American community, whose fundamental purpose is to assure the survival and well being of African Americans. Despite the fact that religious affiliation among African Americans has been declining, many African Americans continue to maintain spiritual commitments (43,46).

The conditions that characterize African American life contribute significant stress to persons in economically oppressed areas of the African American community. Many have observed the sinister relationship between addiction and oppressive economic conditions within minority communities (47). Economic conditions often render it nearly impossible for young men and women to secure adequate employment to provide for minimum standards of living. The unemployment rate in minority communities exceeds 11% (an underestimate of true conditions given the manner in which the unemployment rate is computed). In many areas, major economic activity is part of the subterranean economy in which many working poor must participate for survival (48).

The African American church assumes a crucial political and social advocacy role in the African American community. The rights struggles of the 1960s could not have occurred without African American churches and major African American religious institutions today continue to provide extensive social services and critical political guidance and advocacy for African American life. Indeed, the rise of church-based political advocacy on the right may be said to be modeled upon the work of such African American churches as the National Baptist Convention during the formative years of the Civil Rights Movement.

Self-evidently, the principal function of a church is to facilitate a person's spirituality. This is understood to be a crucial element in recovery from addiction and is sometimes understood as a hedge against the development of addictive problems. Whether one understands addiction as an existential crisis (49) or a behavioral problem, spirituality may play a vital role in providing the hedge against despair or the practical guidance to prevent and remediate addictive problems. The vitality of African American spirituality as manifest in the African American church invites persons, who seek escape from a sense of deadness and disconnection, to experience vitality and community in a nondestructive manner.

Some fear the decline in church affiliation among "X-generation" African Americans indicates a decrease in the importance of spirituality for these young people and an increase in personal despair and community anomie (50). The rise in suicide rates and mental health problems among young African Americans suggest some legitimacy to these fears. To the extent that the African American church can promote a healthy spirituality, it can play a vital role in the prevention of addictive problems. Moreover, examination of how the African American church is successful may lead to better preventive and treatment strategies for all groups.

REFERENCES

1. Griffin KW, Scheier LM, Botvin GJ, et al. Ethnic and gender differences in psychosocial risk, protection, and adolescent alcohol use. *Prev Sci* 2000;1:199–212.

2. Krause N. Race religion, and abstinence from alcohol in late life. *J Aging Health* 2003;15:508–533.

3. Ehlers CL, Gilder DA, Harris L, et al. Association of the ADH2*3 allele with a negative family history of alcoholism in African American young adults. *Alcohol Clin Exp Res* 2001;25:1773–1777.

4. Ramchandani VA, Bosron WF, Li TK. Research advances in ethanol metabolism (review). *Pathol Biol (Paris)* 2001; 49:676–682.

5. Brown TL, Parks GS, Zimmerman RS, et al. The role of religion in predicting adolescent alcohol use and problem drinking. *J Stud Alcohol* 2001; 62(5):696–705.

6. Herd D. Predicting drinking problems among black and white men: results from a national survey. *J Stud Alcohol* 1994;55:61–71.

7. Malone T. *Report of the secretary's task force on black and minority health.* Washington, DC: U.S. Department of Health and Human Services, 1985.

8. U.S. Department of Health and Human Services. *Mental health: culture, race, and ethnicity—a supplement to mental health: a report of the surgeon general.* Rockville, MD: U.S. Department of Health and Human Services, Substance Abuse and Mental Health Services Administration, Center for Mental Health Services, 2001.

9. Dula A. African-American suspicion of the healthcare system is justified: what do we do about it? *Camb Q Healthc Ethics* 1994;3:347–357.

10. Freedman TG. "Why don't they come to Pike street and ask us?" Black American women's health concerns. *Soc Sci Med* 1998;47(7):941–947.

11. Krause N. Church-based social support and health in old age: exploring variations by race. *J Gerontol B Psychol Sci Soc Sci* 2002;57:S332–S347.

12. West C, Sealy KS. *Restoring hope.* Boston: Beacon Press, 1997.

13. Lincoln CE, Mamiya, LH. The black church in the African-American experience. Durham, NC: Duke University Press, 1990.

14. DuBois WEB. *The souls of black folk.* Chicago, A.C. McLurg and Co. 1903: 214–215.

15. Taylor RJ, Mattis J, Chatters LM. Subjective religiosity among African-Americans: a synthesis of findings from five national samples. *J Black Psychol* 1999;25:524–543.

16. Williams C. *No hiding place.* San Francisco: HarperCollins, 1992.

17. Kurtz E. *Not-God: a history of alcoholics anonymous.* Center City, MN: Hazelden, 1979.

18. Alcoholics Anonymous. *Alcoholics Anonymous.* New York: Author, 1976:64.

19. Jellinek, EM. *The disease concept of alcoholism.* Harlan Park, NY: Hillhouse Press, 1960.

20. Wampler RS, Fischer JL. Indicators of spiritual development in recovery from alcohol and other drug problems. *Alcohol Treat Q* 2001;19(1):19–36.

21. Chappel JN. Spirituality is not necessarily religion: a commentary on "divine intervention and the treatment of chemical dependency." *J Subst Abuse* 1990;2:481–483.

22. Kaskutos LA, Turk N, Bond J, et al. The role of religion, spirituality and AA in sustained sobriety. *Alcohol Treat Q* 2003;21(1):1–16.

23. Shaffer H. The disease controversy: of metaphors, maps and menus. *J Psychoactive Drugs* 1985;17(2):65–70.

24. Institute of Medicine. *Broadening the base of treatment for alcohol problems.* Washington, DC: National Academy Press, 1990.

25. Flores P. Alcoholics Anonymous: a phenomenological and existential perspective. *Alcohol Treat Q* 1988;5:73–94.

26. Wurmser L. *The hidden dimension: psychodynamics of compulsive drug use.* New York: Jason Aronson, 1978.

27. Khantzian EJ. Some treatment implications of the ego and self disturbances in alcoholism. In: Bean M, Zinberg N, eds. *Dynamic approaches to the understanding and treatment of alcoholism.* New York: Free Press, 1981:163–168.

28. Mack J. Alcoholism, AA and the governance of the self. In: Bean M, Zinberg N, eds. *Dynamic approaches to the understanding and treatment of alcoholism.* New York: Free Press, 1981:125–162.

29. Hopson R. A thematic analysis of the addictive experience: implications for psychotherapy. *Psychotherapy* 1993; 30(3):481–494.

30. Lawford BR, Young RM, Rowell JA, et al. Association of the D2 dopamine receptor A1 allele with alcoholism: medical severity of alcoholism and type of controls. *Biol Psychiatry* 1997;41:386–393.

31. Valliant G. *The natural history of alcoholism.* Cambridge, MA: Harvard University Press, 1983.

32. Hopson R, Beaird-Spiller B. Why AA works: a psychological analysis of the addictive experience and the efficacy of Alcoholics Anonymous. *Alcohol Treat Q* 1995;12(3):1–17.

33. Berger LS. Substance abuse as a symptom. Hillsdale, NJ: Analytic Press, 1991.

34. Ludwig AM. Cognitive processes associated with "spontaneous" recovery from alcoholism. *J Alcohol Stud* 1985;46:53–58.

35. Zitter ML. Culturally sensitive treatment of black alcoholic families. *Soc Work* 1987;March-April:130–135.

36. Johnson JE. The Afro-American family: a historical overview. In Bass BA, Wyatt GE, Powell GJ, eds. *The Afro-American family—assessment, treatment and research studies.* New York: Grune & Stratton, 1982.

37. Billingsley A. *Black families in white America.* Englewood Cliffs, NJ: Prentice Hall, 1968.

38. Baker FM. Afro-Americans. In: Comas-Diaz L, Griffith E, eds. *Clinical guidelines in cross-cultural mental health.* New York: John Wiley & Sons, 1988:151–181.

39. Herd D. We cannot stagger to freedom. A history of blacks and alcohol in American politics. In: Brill L, Winick C, eds. *The yearbook of substance use and abuse* (vol. 3). New York: Human Sciences Press, 1985.

40. Moynihan, DP. The negro family: the case for national action. Office of Policy Planning and Research, U.S. Department of Labor, Washington, DC, 1965.

41. Hayles R. African-American strengths: a survey of empirical findings. In: Jones R, ed. *Black psychology* (3rd ed.) Berkeley, CA: Cobb & Henry Publishers, 1991.

42. Lawson WB, Kennedy C. Role of the severely mentally ill in the family. In:

Lewis-Hall F, Williams TS, Panetta JA, et al., eds. Psychiatric illness in women: emerging treatments and research. Washington DC: American Psychiatric Association Press, 2002:319–330.

43. Franklin NB. *Black families in therapy.* New York: Guilford Press, 1989.

44. Dubois WEB. The souls of black folk. New York: Bantam Books, 1901/1989.

45. Douglas KB. Sexuality and the black church: a womanist perspective. Maryknoll, NY: Orbis Books, 1999.

46. Francis L. Brisbane. Cultured Competence for Health Care Professionals Working with African American Communities: Theory and Practice. Cultured Competence Series. U.S. Department of Health and Human Services. 1992. Bethesda, Maryland.

47. Marable M. *How capitalism underdeveloped black America: problems in race, political economy and society.* Boston: South End Press, 1983.

48. Ehrenreich B. Nickled and dimed: on (not) getting by in America. New York: Owl Books, 2001.

49. May G. *Addiction and grace.* San Francisco: Harper, 1988.

50. West C, Sealy, KS. Restoring hope. Boston: Beacon Press, 1997.

CHAPTER 79

The Public Health Approach to the Prevention of Substance Abuse

STEVEN JONAS

AN HISTORICAL PERSPECTIVE ON DRUG POLICY DEVELOPMENT

Customarily, a revision of a chapter for a new edition of a textbook contains a significant amount of new material, or at least certainly should do so. In the 4 to 6 years that customarily pass between the time of preparation of chapters for successive textbook editions, for a chapter on policy there is usually new research to consider, new political developments to take into account, advances or at least changes in actual policy to analyze and comment upon.

Sadly, for the most part in drug policy this is not the case. Other than for tobacco use, both national drug politics and national drug policy have changed only marginally, at least in their major parameters. The "Drug War" rages on, killing some people, repressing others, making certain neighborhoods into war zones, having no measurable impact upon drug use (1–5).[1]

In terms of impact upon health and mortality, tobacco and alcohol use are the two major drug scourges of the American people (6). Nevertheless, in many quarters, among both supporters and opponents of present illicit drug policy, they continue to be referred to not as "drug problems," but as "habits," "personal choices," "rights," and legitimate objects of commerce, the use of and trade in either one to be subjected to only the most limited kind of "government interference." To be sure, in 1995 the Food and Drug Administration proposed to treat tobacco products as what they are: drug (nicotine) delivery systems (7). But there was strong political opposition to this initiative (10), and it was foiled (11). And beyond that, there is still a failure to see tobacco use as what it is: one central part of the larger drug-use picture rather than as a problem standing separate and apart (see "Ignoring the Gateway Drug Effect" below).

Nor has much of the "drug policy reform" community, focused so closely as it is on the goal of "legalization" of the sale and use of the illicit drugs rather than drug-use regulation and control for health, been able to see the drugs with which it is primarily concerned as part of the larger picture (12). For the drug policy reform movement it is the "Drug War," not drug use and its negative health, familial, community, societal, and economic effects, that is the enemy (13). As it was when this chapter was first written in 1990, drug policy (non-) development continues to be driven primarily by ideology, politics, and money, not by concern for the health of the people.

SOME DEFINITIONS

Several different definitions of the term "drug" are presented in this book. One primary definition of the word is "any substance other than food which by its chemical nature affects the structure or function of the living organism" (14). But in this book, we are concerned with one family of drugs, those that specifically alter mood and are used in the first instance at least for recreational, not pharmaceutical or psychopathologic purposes.

Building on the dictionary definition of recreation (15), the term *recreational mood-altering drug* can be defined as a drug that is ingested, inhaled, or injected for the original primary purpose of providing diversion, relaxation, heightened sensation, or other enjoyment/pleasure, by changing the user's state of mind. The word *drug* as used in this chapter should be taken to mean

---

[1] If the "Drug War" had a measurable impact upon the use of the so-called illicit drugs (primarily marijuana, heroin, and cocaine) at which use it is aimed, that use would be much lower among nonwhites than among whites. That is because the "Drug War" is conducted almost entirely in nonwhite neighborhoods, and it is nonwhites, overwhelmingly on a per capita basis, who are its prisoners (8). The latter is true even though the majority of illicit drug use is found among whites (9). Looking at these data another way, per capita use levels are about the same among whites and nonwhites. Thus, if the "Drug War" were effective in reducing usage, it should be much lower amongst nonwhites than whites.

"recreational mood-altering drug," and it should be regarded as generally interchangeable with the word *substance* as the latter is used in this book. Because recreational drug use may produce habituation or addiction, the user may develop a secondary purpose for using: to avoid the negative effects associated with withdrawal and abstinence. Furthermore, the use of any of the common recreational mood-altering drugs can lead to negative health, psychological, and social outcomes in at least some users.

As the term is used in this chapter, the *drug problem* in the United States is the sum of the negative effects of drug use in individuals, the negative effects on society caused by drug-induced behaviors occurring in some users, and the negative outcomes of the trade in the illicit drugs; a trade that itself has negative consequences solely because it has been categorized in the law as illegal, and the response to that trade that is called the "Drug War." The *Drug War* is herein defined as that combination of measures based primarily in the criminal law designed to reduce and/or eliminate the use of certain recreational mood-altering drugs.

THE LEGAL STATUS OF DRUGS AND THEIR USE IN THE UNITED STATES

Central to any discussion of recreational drug use policy in the United States and any proposals to change it is an analysis and understanding of the Drug War. The target of the Drug War is a small proportion of the total number of recreational drug use and drug users.[2] Nevertheless, at least through the midpoint of the first decade of the twenty-first century, in terms of focus and resources spent, it is the principal tool of government at all levels for dealing with the drug problem (18). The existence of the Drug War colors all other anti–drug-use efforts, both government and private. Therefore, before considering any alternatives to it, such as the Public Health Approach, the Drug War must be briefly reviewed.

As noted, the Drug War attempts to diminish or eliminate the use of certain drugs by application of the criminal law to both their trade and their use. Among other things, the Drug War appears to make certain drugs "legal" while making certain others "illegal." However, appearances can be deceiving. This construction does not reflect reality. It is, unfortunately, the construction on which all U.S. drug policy is based. That the policy is based on a fallacy is one central reason why it works as poorly as it does.

The fact is that *de jure* in the United States there are virtually no "legal" drugs, in the sense that, for example,

food is "legal." The distribution, sale, possession, and in certain instances use, of all recreational mood-altering drugs other than caffeine are illegal, at least for certain categories of people. Thus in the law, the public face of the Drug War to the contrary notwithstanding, there is no sharp legal–illegal dichotomy among the various drugs. *De facto*, of course, there are major differences between the legal status of the various recreational mood-altering drugs. De facto it happens that most drugs are legal for most of the people who sell and use them, regardless of their statutory categorization. This is because most drug laws are largely decriminalized and unenforced.

Application of the Drug Laws in Practice

For the several recreational mood-altering drugs and the laws applied to their distribution, sale, possession, and use, the differences in how the laws are actually implemented are defined as follows:

- For whom, which drugs, are illegal
- Which criminal drug laws are *de facto* decriminalized in which jurisdictions
- Which drug laws are enforced and against whom they are enforced

In practice, only a narrow band of the criminal drug laws are enforced employing the criminal sanction, primarily against certain selected elements of the population. Using the criminal law, nonwhites are selectively punished for violations for which the white user majority on the whole is not held either civilly or criminally accountable (8,19–22).

In practice, therefore, under the law as it is actually implemented, drug categorization differs rather markedly from the commonly held legal–illegal dichotomy. Rather, defined both by the laws themselves and how they are enforced, there are three categories, none distinguished from the others by a simple legal or illegal label.

- *Category I:* tobacco and the alcoholic beverages (the so-called legal drugs). The distribution by, sale to, and use of these drugs are illegal for persons younger than age 18 to 21 years (the age varying by state and drug). In practice, however, the enforcement of the relevant laws is effectively decriminalized in most jurisdictions.
- *Category II:* the prescription psychoactive drugs. The distribution, sale, possession, and use of these drugs, on a nonprescription basis, are illegal for persons of all ages. The enforcement of these laws, too, is either effectively decriminalized or simply not undertaken at all in most jurisdictions. Ironically, depending upon how one counts, there are between 1.7 and 2.7 times more regular users of the prescription psychoactives on a nonprescription basis than there are regular users of cocaine and heroin added together (23,24).
- *Category III:* marijuana, heroin, and cocaine, and the other illicit drugs. Like the category II drugs, their

---

[2] In 2001, there were approximately 109 million "current drinkers" of alcohol, 56 million regular cigarette smokers, 12 million regular users of marijuana, 1.7 million regular users of cocaine (including crack), and between 123,000 (Substance Abuse and Mental Health Services Administration [SAMHSA]) and 900,000 (Office of National Drug Control Policy [ONDCP]) regular users of heroin (16,17).

distribution, sale, possession, and use are *de jure* illegal for persons of all ages. In most jurisdictions in the United States, the criminal laws concerning these drugs are enforced, but they are enforced selectively. For the most part, general enforcement occurs only in geographic areas in which sellers and users are found in open or otherwise easily accessible spaces: poor, minority, neighborhoods.

MODELING THE DRUG PROBLEM

Defining Characteristics

As seen from the perspective of the public health approach (PHA), the drug problem has the following major defining characteristics:

- Substance use/abuse, of the drugs in all three categories (above), is seen as a far-reaching social, economic, and political problem (25) that is a unity, not a duality or tripartite phenomenon. The PHA considers the current legal–illegal duality to have been artificially created and not related either to health considerations (26,27) or to science.
- The problem is viewed primarily as one of health and health deficits, not of morality or crime.
- While in most drug users, use itself is not a disease, in every drug user use increases the risk, to a greater or lesser extent, of contracting one or more diseases or conditions damaging to one's health and the health of others[3] (28).
- Tobacco is the one drug that, when used as intended, is harmful to most users (by significantly increasing organic disease risk), as well as to those in the user's vicinity (11,29).[3]
- All of the other commonly used recreational mood-altering drugs are harmful in one way or another to some of those who use them (28,30). Any use of any drug, even if not harmful in present time, does increase the risk of harmful use later. However, the harm varies in degree and kind from person to person and even within the same person from time to time. Some years ago, Dr. Norman Zinberg described the relevant variables as those of "Drug, Set, and Setting" (31). In some cases, this harm is the result of the action of the drug on the body; in some cases, it is the result of the action of the drug on the mind leading to negative behaviors.
- Drug use harms range from lung cancer to cirrhosis of the liver to chronic drug dependency to loss of job and family life to sudden death in a motor vehicle

crash. However, it is important to understand that the only certain negative of recreational drug use, even of cigarettes, is an increase in the risk, not the certainty, of harm.
- Using neither the false legal–illegal dichotomy, nor the true-to-reality three-category division described above, the PHA categorizes drugs biologically by such characteristics as addiction potential, long-term health risks, and potential social pathology.
- The PHA does not see the drug and drug-related crime problems as one and the same. Although they are of course interrelated, they have different solutions. The PHA necessarily invokes state power to solve problems of the public's health, as is done in managing a wide variety of health-related issues, from pure water supply to air pollution control. But unlike as in the Drug War, in the PHA, the law is used in ways known to be efficacious and cost-effective.
- On the issue of the morality of substance use/abuse, there is, of course, no societal consensus. For the PHA, therefore, dealing with the drug problem in any way as a moral one is considered inappropriate and counterproductive.

The Defects in Current Policy[4]

Before considering the principles and components of the PHA for the prevention of substance use/abuse in detail, we must first answer the question: Why is it necessary to develop and implement a new policy? What's wrong with the current national policy for dealing with drug abuse? From the public health perspective, at least ten defects can be identified.

Artificial Bimodality/Lack of Comprehensiveness

The most prominent feature of national policy is that it is based on an artificial bimodality that, in turn, is based on the fallacious legal–illegal dichotomy discussed above. We have already seen that the true picture is quite different; the drug problem, in medical, public health, and epidemiologic terms, is a unity. Because national policy approaches the category I drugs in one way, the category III drugs in another, and the category II drugs hardly at all, it is by definition totally lacking in comprehensiveness.

---

[3] The harm from cigarettes to the user and others is caused both by the contents of the smoke and the organic effects of nicotine, and occasionally by cigarette-caused fires, but not by the effect of the drug nicotine on the behavior of the user. The use of drugs other than nicotine in cigarettes, as well as having the potential to produce harm for the user, may also cause harm to some of those in the vicinity of the user as a result of drug-induced behaviors in the user.

[4] This chapter presents a highly critical view of current policy. However, it does *not* propose simple expansion of decriminalization/legalization as a solution to the substance abuse problem. Broadening the present partial decriminalization of the illicit drugs, if properly implemented, could solve much of the drug-traffic-related crime problem. However, it would do nothing to solve the general drug problem, especially that major part of it caused by tobacco and alcohol. In the view presented here, undertaking any general decriminalization for any of the illicit drugs without first dealing comprehensively with the total drug problem in the manner suggested below would be ill-advised.

Lack of Focus on the Real Drug Problems

Arising from the fact that it has no basis in medical/public health science, the most serious defect in current national policy is that it directs the bulk of its attention to the least of the drug-related health harms. For example, in 1990, there were about 500,000 deaths associated with the use of alcohol and tobacco (32). By 1995, it could be estimated that that figure had risen to at least 590,000 (6).

By way of comparison, the illicit drugs are responsible for about 40,000 deaths, with about half of those the direct result of the Drug War, not drug use (6). In 1994, the most recent year for which such figures are available, there were only about 2.6 times as many regular cocaine users as there were alcohol and tobacco deaths. Yet the Office of National Drug Control Policy focused almost exclusively on the former group (3) and, as of 2002, still did (4). However, the NDCP report for 2004 does focus more on alcohol and tobacco.

The Conflict Over the Role of Education

In current policy, there is a conflict over the role of education in dealing with the drug problem. For the category I drugs, the major emphasis of national policy is on education. *De facto*, the law plays a secondary role, for example, banning cigarette smoking in many public places, making some effort to enforce laws against the sale of both tobacco products and alcoholic beverages to underage persons, cracking down on drunk drivers. There is no program of any kind for dealing with the category II drugs. For the category III drugs, although criminal law enforcement aimed at nonwhites is widely employed, some attempts at education are also made. But they are warped by the artificial bimodality of current policy.

Contradiction in Drug-Use Goals

While the National Drug Control Strategy does not address the issue of the currently legal drugs, another federal document does. Healthy People 2010 lays out national objectives for disease prevention and health promotion (33). Objectives are set for reduced prevalence for the use of the two major drugs as well as for marijuana and cocaine (34). There are also goals for significant reductions in alcohol and tobacco-related negative health outcomes. Recognizing reality, "drug free" is not on this national health agenda for any of the drugs.

However, the 1988 White House Conference for a Drug Free America, which laid the political groundwork for current national category III drug policy, called for just that: "drug free" (35). The ongoing major national advertising campaign supporting the "drug-free" approach, founded in the early 1990s and aimed only at the illicit drugs, is produced by the Partnership for a Drug-Free America (36). The Partnership is a creature of the American Association of Advertising Agencies. The latter is the trade organiza-

tion for, among others, most of the companies that make their living promoting the use of tobacco and alcohol, especially to the young.

Thus the true drug-use goal of current national policy remains unclear. Is it drug free, or drug-use reduction? Or is it drug free for certain users of the minor drugs, drug-use reduction for all users of the major ones, tobacco and alcohol, and ignoring all other categories of drugs (like category II) and subcategories of uses?

The Futility of Criminal Law Enforcement Aimed at Simple Use

Studies indicate that the perceived certainty and severity of punishment are insignificant factors in deterring use (37). In the late 1980s and early 1990s, what apparently was more important in reversing the trend of increasing illicit drug use that marked the 1970s was the growth in perceived harmfulness of the activity, which, in turn, likely augmented social disapproval of drug use behavior. Among users, in any weighing of legal and health risks of drug use, concerns about health predominated (37). There is no evidence that this situation has changed.

These events occurred in the context of rapidly rising imprisonment levels for drug-related crimes by nonwhites (8,13,20). But if imprisonment or threat of it had a real impact on illicit drug use, as noted one would expect it to be much lower among nonwhites than whites because the former are imprisoned for drug offenses at a much higher rate than are the latter (8). But that is not the case (9).

Even if criminal law enforcement were effective and relevant, history shows that its use is not necessary to achieve reduction in drug use and abuse. For example, over a 25-year period, a limited national antismoking campaign lead to a decline of almost 30% in the proportion of adults smoking (38), a decline of almost 40% in per capita cigarette consumption (29). This was accomplished with an educational program of modest proportions and some recent restrictions on smoking in public facilities, all in the face of much pro-drug-use advertising by the tobacco industry and government tobacco subsidies.

Implementing a Pseudo "Demand-Side" Strategy

In 1990, under Dr. William Bennett, a law enforcement-based "demand-reduction," "user-accountability" strategy was introduced to national policy for illicit drugs. It remains with the program. Ostensibly, this strategy recognized the limitations of the traditional "supply side" approach. However, it did not focus on the causes of demand, such as the drug culture and the gateway drug effect (see below). Rather, it simply targeted the "casual user" for the imposition of criminal sanctions. As if those "casual users," entirely on their own, were the major, indeed the only, factor in creating demand; as if they existed in a society that was either neutral or negative on drug use, in general.

Failure to Acknowledge the U.S. Drug Culture

Demand and demand creation are, of course, very important factors in the drug problem. In fact, the way the category I drugs are promoted and sold has a major impact on their use. This impact is mediated through the drug culture and the gateway drug effect (discussed in the next section).

Current national policy fails to recognize that there is a drug culture in the United States that directly and indirectly promotes the use of all drugs. Some time ago, in terms that still apply, Gitlin put it this way (39):

> [I]n many ways American culture is a drug culture. Through its normal routines it promotes not only the high-intensity consumption of commodities but also the idea that the self is realized through consumption. It is addicted to acquisition. It cultivates the pursuit of thrills; it elevates the pursuit of private pleasure to high standing; and, as part of this ensemble, it promotes the use of licit chemicals for stimulation, intoxication, and fast relief. The widespread use of licit drugs in America can be understood as part of this larger set of values and activities.

In sum, there is a powerful "do drugs" message in American culture, linked primarily to the promotion of the alcoholic beverages and tobacco products, but having other important elements as well.

Consider that in their advertising, over time alcohol and tobacco have been associated with, for example, being the beer-drinker's friend ("Gotta be Your Bud"), thinness in women (Virginia Slims, "You've come a long way, baby"), rugged individualism (the Marlboro Man), speed and sex (Coors Light, the "Silver Bullet"), humor (the Budweiser lizards), dating (Heinekens beer), cross-dressing (the Bud Lite "ladies' night at the bar"), auto and boat racing (various alcohol and tobacco brands), and team sports (beer sales and tobacco advertising in sports arenas and stadiums).

To compound the problem, the "do drugs" messages of the drug culture extend well beyond the world of the recreational mood-altering drugs. Over-the-counter medications are sold as instant problem solvers: if you have a headache, take this pill; if you overate, swallow this liquid; if you can't get to sleep, take this other pill. The message never is "to avoid feeling overstuffed from eating too much pizza, why not try eating less pizza next time?" Since the mid-1990s, an antacid called Pepcid AC actually has been promoted as a medication to take before eating some food that you know will give you heartburn, so that you can eat the food anyway and not suffer the heartburn.

Furthermore, while vitamins are not drugs, they come in pill form and to many people look like drugs. And how are they promoted and sold? As an easy, painless means of self-improvement, in pill form, even for children. Is it any wonder that some of those children a few years later experiment with other kinds of pills that are promoted as easy, painless ways to a better you?

Finally, in America, medicine is practiced with an inordinate emphasis on treatment using pharmaceutical drugs as contrasted to personal health promotion and disease prevention by lifestyle modification. From the late 1990s onward, even the use of the prescription drugs has been heavily promoted to the general public by their makers, as are a bewildering variety of herbal remedies and dietary supplements. All pills. All painless ways to self-improvement of one sort or another.

And then there is gambling. Compulsive gambling is coming to be recognized as an addictive behavior (40). Gambling has been described as "an exploding entertainment industry starring cash" (41). "Exploding," "addictive," and governments, especially at the state level, heavily promote it through lottery advertising, and do nothing to even warn people against the dangers of the many other forms of—totally legal—gambling.

The Gateway Drug Effect

In most drug abusers the problem starts in childhood or the early teenage years (38,42). As Healthy People 2010 noted, tobacco use and addiction usually begin in adolescence (43). For almost all youngsters it is the "OK" drugs, tobacco and alcohol, that form the "gateway" to the use of the "not-OK" drugs, which are all of the others (44–50). One study, for example, found that a teenaged user of marijuana is eight times more likely to also be a cigarette smoker than is a teenager who does not use marijuana (51).

According to the Research Institute of the New York State Division of Alcoholism and Alcohol Abuse Statement on teenagers in New York State (52), "Unless alcohol is used first, there is very little use of any other drug, including cigarettes and over-the-counter drugs. New York State youth of every age and sex combination—as well as African Americans, Hispanics and whites—follow a definite pattern of progression from alcohol to marijuana to hard drug use."

The 2001 National Household Survey on Drug Abuse found (53):

- The rate of past month illicit drug use among youths and adults was higher among those who were current cigarette or alcohol users than in those who did not use these substances.
- In 2001, the rate of current illicit drug use was approximately nine times higher among youths who smoked cigarettes (48.0%) than it was among youths who did not (5.3%).
- Illicit drug use also was associated with the level of alcohol use. Among youths who were heavy drinkers in 2001, 65.3% also were current illicit drug users, whereas among nondrinkers, the rate was only 5.1%.

At one time, Dr. Jack Henningfield, chief of the Clinical Pharmacology Branch of the National Institute on Drug

Abuse Addiction Research Center, put the Gateway focus on tobacco succinctly (54): "Reducing tobacco use is one of the most important elements in all long-range strategies for reducing drug addiction."

But while permitting the enthusiastic promotion and widespread sale of the "OK" drugs, (concerning the "non-OK" drugs) current national policy says to young people, and primarily minority young people at that, "If you happen to follow the natural progression from the approved drugs to the unapproved ones and if we catch you, we'll lock you up." Current policy does not deal with this major aspect of the gateway drug effect.

On Simple Availability and Drug Use

The most common argument against ending the Drug War has consistently been that to do so would lead directly to vastly increased use (55–57). Several responses to that argument can be made. First of all, it is not the case that a regulated, taxed supply of drugs, being sold only through controlled retail outlets, would necessarily lead to any relative increase in supply. In the present drug marketplace, there is almost always an excess of supply over demand for any of the drugs, including the illicits (2,58).

Second and more important, it happens that there is no historical evidence to support the notion that simple availability, without significant advertising and promotion, leads to use or that simple increase in availability leads to increase in use. Consider the following. Since World War II the greatest success achieved in the United States in drug-use reduction has been for cigarette smoking among adults (43,59). This was accomplished in the face of unlimited supply, low price, and extensive pro–drug-use advertising and promotion. The observed modest decline in per capita alcohol consumption over a similar period (60) occurred in the same environment.

Before the gradual decline in adult cigarette use that began in the mid-1960s got underway, it took 80 years after the invention of the automatic cigarette-making machine in the 1880s and 50 years after the perfection of the safety match in the early part of the twentieth century for per capita cigarette use, negligible at first, to top out, in the climate of a heavy promotional campaign and little negative publicity.

It took between 30 and 40 years following the end of Prohibition for per capita beer consumption to reach the level at which it stood in 1919 (61,62). Illicit drugs are much more readily available in African American than in white communities, yet the proportion of persons who have used one is about the same among whites as it is among African Americans (63). The decline in the use of the illicit drugs that occurred over the 20 years or so leading up to the early 1990s (64) took place in the context of a constant supply, sold at a fairly reasonable (although unlike tobacco and alcohol, not cheap) price.

Occasional experiments in decriminalization that have occurred in the United States have generally not lead to a rise in use. Professor Steven Duke (65) referred to the experience of 11 American states in which marijuana was fully or partially decriminalized. Not only did consumption not rise; it actually continued down at approximately the same rate as elsewhere. The laws regarding the street sale of cocaine and heroin were informally and partially decriminalized in New York City between 1989 and 1993. Both cocaine street sales and cocaine use went down during that period (66). Furthermore, if in this instance simple availability had a direct effect on use, it should have been much higher among African Americans than whites. As noted above, it wasn't.

If the drug problem were caused simply by the presence of a drug or drugs, the Andean countries themselves would be awash in cocaine addicts, which they are not, and neither tobacco nor alcohol use would have declined in the United States, which they have. The drug problem is caused primarily by demand for drugs and those factors that create demand, not simple supply.

What, in addition to the drug culture, might those factors be? In a classic study published in 1992, *Drugs, Crime, and the Justice System*, the Department of Justice itself listed at length the factors considered to cause or lead toward drug use (67). Included are such factors as the desire to achieve the effects the drugs produce, such as pain relief, relaxation, or excitement; among persons with psychiatric disorders, the need/desire to self-medicate; and among youth especially, peer pressure, inadequate parent–child relationships, personality factors such as low self-esteem and orientation toward risk-taking, poor school performance. Conspicuous by its absence from the Department of Justice's own list is simple availability.

The Drug War Doesn't Work

The most serious defect of the Drug War is that it simply doesn't work, either in its own very narrow purview of category III drugs alone, or on the true drug problem, caused primarily by the still widespread use of tobacco products and alcoholic beverages. By its own admission, the programs of the Office of National Drug Control Policy (ONDCP), and the Drug War, have had little impact on illicit drug use (4). Alcohol use and its consequences remain a very serious health problem, and cigarette smoking is still widespread (68). It had been declining since the publication of the first *Surgeon General's Report on Smoking and Health* in 1964, but that decline leveled out in the mid-1990s.

Nevertheless, there is no indication that the proponents of the Drug War are considering either broadening their purview to cover all three categories of drugs of abuse or changing their tactics, ranging from attempts at source control to imprisoning otherwise noncriminal users, tactics that have no effect on illicit drug use.

PRINCIPLES OF THE PUBLIC HEALTH APPROACH

The Public Health Approach in Brief

The *primary goal* of the PHA as herein described[5] is to:

Reduce the use and abuse of all the recreational mood-altering drugs, to provide, when, as, and if possible, for their safe, pleasurable use, consistent with centuries' old human experience, while minimizing to the greatest degree possible the harmful effects of their use on individuals, the family, and society as a whole.

The PHA uses epidemiologic, pharmacologic, toxicologic, and medical science to define the drug-abuse problem and to create the program components. It does not use predilections, politics, or prejudice. It identifies the real causes of the drug problem and then develops interventions directed at those causes, not imaginary ones. Some of the interventions are of a classically "public health" nature, as they appear, for example, in the "Statement and Resolution on Tobacco and Health" of the Committee on Public Health of The New York Academy of Medicine (70). Others are drawn from a broader perspective.

The PHA is a comprehensive national policy and program for dealing with the use and abuse of all the commonly used recreational mood-altering drugs, regardless of category. It is based on tried-and-true public health principles. In its details, it has a few new wrinkles here and there. However, it is constructed largely of ideas, programs, and recommendations that have been in the marketplace of ideas for some time now (28,37,70–73).

As long ago as 1913, Dr. Charles Terry "urged the [American Public Health] Association to take up the matter [of drug addiction] as a public health matter of importance" (37). Dr. Terry also noted that "Narcotic drug addiction-disease will never be solved by forcible measures only.... [P]olice measures to be successful must go hand in hand with intelligent medical services."

More recently, Robert Stutman, in 1989 the Special Agent in Charge of the New York Office of the Drug Enforcement Administration, put it this way (74): "Cops are not the answer to the drug problem. They're a short-term answer to clean up the streets. But the long-term answer is prevention." Following this recommendation from Mr. Stutman (who retired in 1990), the PHA is based on several important principles, derived from our knowledge of what works in public health and what doesn't work in present policy.

The Drug Problem Is a Unity

As shown above, the drug problem presents as a seamless web. The evidence of the interrelatedness of its various components is clear. If one's true goal is the reduction in overall drug use, it is fruitless, as present experience shows, to attempt to deal with only one part of the problem, or to deal with one part one way and another part another way. Biologic, medical, and epidemiologic science all tell us that a recreational mood-altering drug is a drug, regardless of its current status in the criminal law.

Single National Policy

Perhaps the most important element of the PHA is that there will be a single national policy for controlling the abuse of all the recreational mood-altering drugs. Among other things, this approach will end the current "OK"/"not-OK" drug/person dichotomies.

Drug Abuse Is a Problem with a Natural History

Suffering from a drug-abuse problem is not like having a common cold. It is not something a person catches one day that shows up in its clinical form the next. Furthermore, unlike the common cold, drug abuse in adults manifests itself over time differently in different persons and varies widely in breadth and depth from person to person and drug to drug (31). For example, most users of cigarettes are habituated to them, but a few are not. All cigarette smokers are at much higher risk for a number of serious diseases than are nonsmokers for the same diseases. But most cigarette smokers contract only one of those diseases, if they contract any at all.

Most users of alcohol do not become alcoholics. Most cocaine users do not become abusers (75). Some do. The PHA recognizes and provides for the reality that drug abuse in adults has no consistent natural history. However, the PHA also recognizes that in children there is a common natural history: for most drug abusers, the problem starts in childhood or the early teenage years, with the use of tobacco, alcohol, or both (43,52,76). Thus, the PHA pays a great deal of attention to preventing the use of those two drugs by young people, as recommended some time ago by Dr. Henningfield (54).

The Universally Harmful Drug Form is Tobacco

As noted previously, there is one drug form that, when used as intended, increases the risk of negative health outcomes for most users, as well as for all of those in the vicinity of use. That is, of course, tobacco. That fact, in addition to the centrality of tobacco to the gateway drug effect, makes tobacco use prevention in children central to the PHA.

---

[5] A "public health approach" to the illicits alone has been proposed (69). Although its goals are laudable, and some of its components parallel those of the PHA herein proposed, it has all of the limitations of any policy, public-health oriented or otherwise, that attempts to deal with the illicits in isolation, as presented above.

The Spectrum of Harmfulness and the Concept of Safe Use

All of the commonly used recreational mood-altering drugs other than tobacco increase the risk of health harms for only some of those who use them and for only some of those in the vicinity of use. The primary risk incurred by the use of drugs other than tobacco is that one might eventually use them to that level at which the risk of health harm appears. Thus, for drugs other than tobacco, there is a "spectrum of harmfulness" from none to severe.

Some of these harms are a result of the actions of the drugs on the body. Others are the result of drug-induced behaviors in the user. Of course, any use of any drug makes the user susceptible to the possibility of incurring health-harmful risk. But apparently for each commonly used drug other than tobacco, safe use is possible. For no recreational mood-altering drug has this spectrum been fully defined or clearly understood.

Law Enforcement Can Be Used Intelligently

History has taught us that criminal law enforcement works poorly to reinforce moral sanctions against personal behaviors such as the use of recreational mood-altering drugs (26,27). However, selectively applied criminal and civil law enforcement is an important tool in implementing many programs for improving the public's health.

The PHA respects the belief that the raising of moral considerations and the invocation of moral sanctions may be useful for some people in diminishing drug use. At the same time, the PHA recognizes that in dealing with this kind of highly personal behavior, our historical experience demonstrates the futility and waste of attempting to invoke or reinforce the moral sanction through the use of the criminal law. Doing the latter often produces a "cure" that is worse than the disease at which it is aimed.

Law enforcement can be effective, for example, when the health problem has been caused by a disease organism that infects individuals regardless of personal choice or by an economic behavior that damages the environment (e.g., isolation in tuberculosis control, mandatory vaccination, required automotive emissions control, regulated toxic waste disposal).

But to be broadly helpful, law enforcement must be applied in those situations in which it is effective. Also, its use must be consistent with the beliefs of a large majority of the population. Thus law enforcement has very important roles to play in the PHA; for example, in reducing the sale of recreational mood-altering drugs to minors, controlling the operation of motor vehicles by intoxicated persons, and enforcing drug taxation statutes.

In Great Britain, following World War I, significant reductions in cirrhosis of the liver mortality were achieved by modestly limiting availability and controlling price to favor beer and wine over spirits (77). This was done by cur-tailing the opening hours of the pubs (bars) and the liquor stores, by generally restricting liquor sales to those establishments, and by taxing hard liquor heavily as compared with beer and wine.

Legalization Is Not the Focus; Solving the Drug Problem Is

Distinguishing the public health approach from what is known as the "drug policy reform movement" is that for the latter, the target is the Drug War. For the PHA, the target is drug abuse, in all of its forms. Thus the PHA is neither for nor against what is called "legalization." However, it recognizes the great health harms the Drug War brings to the nonwhite communities in which it is waged, harms probably more injurious to the public's health than the use of any of the drug forms other than alcohol and tobacco. Thus it sees as a direct and very important benefit of its own implementation the opportunity to end the Drug War.

THE PUBLIC HEALTH APPROACH

In recommending the development of a "Public Health Response to the War on Drugs," in 1989, the American Public Health Association published the following statement. It is still valid in the first decade of the new millenium (71):

> Alcohol, tobacco, and other drug problems represent one of the most pressing public health issues in the United States today. Despite numerous assaults on these problems, including the current "War on Drugs," they remain intractable—continuing at epidemic levels and unresponsive to a variety of strategies and public policy initiatives. This intractability is in part a result of a fundamental misunderstanding of and a blindness to the nature of alcohol, tobacco, and other drug problems and the degree to which they are integrated into our society. The purpose of this position paper is to provide a blueprint for a comprehensive policy for addressing the nation's alcohol, tobacco, and other psychoactive drug problems....

As stated at the beginning of this chapter, the PHA to the prevention of drug abuse has a number of components. Some are of a classically "public health" nature; for example, improved school and public health education, strengthened regulatory approaches, such as limitations on the advertising and promotion of all recreational mood-altering drugs, and the legal prohibition of cigarette vending machines. Other measures are political, such as shifting the national leadership emphasis of the drug-abuse control program from one that focuses on punishment for bad behavior to one that focuses on health. All of these measures stress helping people to change their behavior in a positive way. Certainly not every element in the list below need be included for a PHA to be effective. As well, there may be other elements inadvertently left off the list that should be added.

As also stated at the beginning of this chapter, the primary goal of the PHA is to reduce the use and abuse of all the recreational mood-altering drugs to provide for their safe, pleasurable use, consistent with centuries' old human experience, while minimizing to the greatest degree possible their harmful effects on users, their families, and society as a whole.

The Components

National Policy Education Campaign

The top national political and health leadership will be called upon to educate the public on the new policy and stimulate their participation in and cooperation with it. The educational campaign will recognize the drug culture and the gateway drug effect as significant causes of the total drug-abuse problem and thus will focus major emphasis on dealing with them. To be effective, this campaign must be very carefully thought out, because the American people have been trained by present national policy (which tolerates the promotion of recreational mood-altering drug use) to not think of alcohol and tobacco as "drugs."

Many of the PHA's messages will be new to many of the American people. While smokers may not object too strongly to being told that they are drug addicts (it is estimated that 70% of smokers want to quit at any one time, and many of them know that they are addicted to nicotine), many alcohol users, most of whom are not addicts, will object very strongly to the association. Thus it is vital that the public health messages be delivered by the top national political and health leadership. It would be very helpful if their counterparts at the state and local levels participated also.

Rational Drug Classification System

A rational system for classifying all of the recreational mood-altering drugs (including tobacco and alcohol) by their potential dangers and benefits would be developed. This system would be based on these five major criteria: addictive potential, short-term personal hazards, long-term personal hazards, personal benefits (if any), and potential harmfulness to other individuals and society. Pharmacologic, toxicologic, pathologic, medical, epidemiologic, and sociologic data would be used to develop the system.

Responsible Use/Safe Use

As part of this effort, the highly controversial "safe use" and "responsible use" issues would be dealt with. To define safe use and responsible use for each of the major recreational mood-altering drugs is no mean feat. But if any program to reduce use and abuse is to be created and successfully implemented, one must be developed. There

are several starting points on which agreement could be reached fairly easily.

Children

For children there is no such thing as responsible use of any drug. This is based on the fact that most regular and addictive drug use begins before the age of 21 years. Even the tobacco industry has joined this chorus (78): "As the manufacturer of a product intended for adults who smoke that has serious health effects, Philip Morris U.S.A. has a responsibility to help prevent kids from smoking." And the beer industry, with some irony considering what alcohol does to mental judgment, broadly promotes the slogan: "Drink responsibly; know when to say when."

Adults

There is responsible use of certain drugs for adults. For example, most consumers of alcohol in the United States are light to moderate users. There is some evidence that this is also be true for the major illicit drugs (53). Certainly, any effective program to reduce the use and abuse of all recreational mood-altering drugs must deal with the reality of safe alcohol use by many American adults. At the same time, the majority of Americans appear to have recognized that there is no such thing as responsible use of cigarettes, at least in public. These accepted understandings must be built into the definition of responsible use if a broad-based policy is going to be politically viable and effective.

The Regulated Sale Model

The regulated sale model proposed by Dr. David Kessler for tobacco products (79) would be developed for all drugs. They might be sold only in "drug stores," either state-run or licensed to private interests. Or there could be "drug sections" in general retail stores, with access permitted only for adults. The regulated sale model would be supported by the other elements of the PHA, below. As shown above, there is a significant difference between "simple availability" versus "availability with promotion." There would be controls on the places and hours of availability and sale of all the recreational mood-altering drugs. Sale of many of them to minors would be illegal.

Rational Price/Tax Structure

A rational price structure and tax policy for all drugs would be implemented. It would be aimed both at raising funds to pay for the program and at reducing consumption. It could be modeled on the British approach to alcohol beverage taxation and availability control mentioned above. To assist in the overall public health campaign against drug abuse, the taxes should not be referred to as "sin" taxes, but rather as "risk-reduction" taxes or some similar appellation.

Furthermore, drug tax revenues would not go to the general fund. They would not be used as a substitute for income, property, capital gains, or other progressive taxes. Unlike what has happened with the state shares of the national tobacco settlement, these revenues would be used only to fund the PHA. Such taxes would, of course, be gradually self-liquidating as drug use declined with the effectiveness of the programs the taxes supported.

This system would be designed to avoid the creation of an underpriced black market (which, although serious, is not as potentially dangerous as the overpriced one that exists now). Based on the experience with taxation of alcohol and tobacco in this country (80) and others, it appears that taxes on legal drugs could be raised significantly without incurring the risk of developing any significant underpriced black market. To avoid the bootlegging from low-tax to high-tax states that now occurs in the tobacco market, it is important that taxes on the recreational mood-altering drug be levied at the point of production.

Assault on the Drug Culture

A clear assault would be made on the drug culture. This is a critical part of the program. The public must be educated to understand the interrelatedness of the use and abuse of all the recreational mood-altering drugs. They must also be educated to understand that the atmosphere created by the promotion of legal drugs, over-the-counter medications, and vitamins, and the way medicine itself is practiced, contributes to the drug-abuse problem. The political difficulties of implementing this policy must not be underestimated. Advertising policy is central to this effort.

Advertising Policy

Pro–drug-use advertising has been analyzed in depth for tobacco in a classic study by Dr. Kenneth Warner (81). Its findings are still applicable. First, in the PHA there would be no future expansion of drug advertising beyond that which is presently permitted: no reintroduction of radio and television cigarette advertising, no advertising of spirits on radio and television, and no advertising of any kind for any presently illicit drug for which the legal status might change in the future.

Second, a complete ban on pro–drug-use advertising could be undertaken, as recommended (for example) by the Committee on Public Health of The New York Academy of Medicine (70). Significant constitutional questions would be raised by such legislation. However, some time ago, a strong case was made by Polin in the Hofstra Law Review that an advertising ban would be constitutional in the case of cigarettes (82). The same arguments might apply to the other drugs as well.

In summary, Polin's (82) position is that:

Tobacco advertising is not commercial speech protected by the First Amendment because it is inherently misleading, if not fraudulent, and/or relates to criminal activity (i.e., the sale of tobacco to minors). Assuming, arguendo, that tobacco is protected commercial speech, ... in recognition of the fact that tobacco is lawful only because of its exceptional [political and economic] background, the substantial governmental interest at stake justifies extraordinary control of intended effect—promoting the use of a uniquely [and inherently] harmful product.

As Philip Morris U.S.A. has put it, on the dangers of tobacco use (78): "We agree with the overwhelming medical and scientific consensus that cigarette smoking causes lung cancer, heart disease, emphysema and other serious diseases in smokers. Smokers are far more likely to develop serious diseases, like lung cancer, than non-smokers. There is no 'safe' cigarette."

If it were to be concluded that a complete advertising ban were not desirable or not constitutional, pro-drug advertising could be taxed. A dollar tax for each advertising dollar spent would both reduce the amount of advertising and raise a significant amount of money for the PHA. A tax on pro-drug advertising levied on the manufacturers, the advertising agencies, and the sellers of advertising time and space would be more equitable than increases in the taxes on sales, especially in the case of cigarettes. At any one time, 70% of smokers would like to be able to quit but cannot do so primarily because of the extraordinary addictivity of nicotine.

If it is equitable to tax an addiction is it not also equitable to tax activities that promote becoming addicted?

Public Education Campaign

There would be a comprehensive public education campaign against drug use per se, beyond the national leadership education program outlined in the section on National Policy Education Campaign. It would be much more comprehensive than the modest anticigarette smoking program of the last 20 years. Also, much still remains to be learned about what will constitute an effective campaign.

School Health Education

A comprehensive school health education program dealing with all of the recreational drugs in a unified manner, building on the successful experience of such programs as Project STAR in the Kansas Cities of Missouri and Kansas (84–85). The introduction to the original Project STAR curriculum stated that "Project STAR's goal is to reduce alcohol and other drug use among young people and to create an environment that supports and encourages youth to remain drug free."

By carefully studying prevention programs and related research, Project Support and Training for Assessing Results (STAR) identifies effective strategies and encourages communities to implement those strategies to help young people avoid alcohol and other drug use. One of the most effective strategies uses a curriculum taught by classroom teachers to help adolescents anticipate and resist social pressure.

Research shows that successful prevention programs must not only involve schools, but entire communities (86). As students develop refusal skills, their commitment to nonuse must be reinforced and supported by parents, churches, businesses, and community leaders. To sustain this commitment, community-wide changes in attitudes must be made.

Treatment

Comprehensive treatment, rehabilitation, and job-training programs for those who are addicted to or who are abusers of any of the recreational mood-altering drugs would be made available. The matters of the appropriateness of "on-demand" treatment, the role of the law enforcement system in placing drug abusers in treatment, and who would pay for what, would have to be worked out. (It must be remembered, however, that drug-treatment programs, while vital for those persons already in need of them, will not solve the drug problem, only prevention can do that.)

Assistance for Displaced Drug Workers and Farmers

Subsidies, relocation assistance, and retraining opportunities for the tens of thousands of workers and small farmers who would be put out of work in the United States by a significant decline in the legal recreational drug trade and/or the ending of various crop subsidy programs would be provided.

National Domestic Spending

The very important programs of national domestic spending to deal with the identified political, economic, and social causes of the illegal drug trade in those inner-city neighborhoods that are scarred by both legal and illegal drug use and the War on Drugs would be implemented. (At the same time it will be recognized and made clear that the drug problem is hardly the exclusive domain of the African American and other minority communities.)

Focused Law Enforcement

Finally, the focus of drug-related law enforcement would be on punishing criminal behavior resulting from drug use, not simply punishing drug use, although the required effort to enforce the laws against traffic in illicit drugs would be maintained.

Current law enforcement efforts would be continued until the use and abuse of all recreational mood-altering drugs is significantly reduced. However, the current emphasis on the incarceration of "casual users" (which sometimes leads to the jailing of people for being addicted to drugs—just imagine what would happen if that policy were applied to cigarette smoking) would be brought to an end as counterproductive and wasteful of law-enforcement time, money, and manpower. The drug-traffic focus would be returned to the major dealers, as well as to corrupted law-enforcement officials and "illegitimate" business activity, such as money laundering.

As the PHA implementation proceeded, law enforcement would focus on those areas in which it has some hope of success: controlling the violation of statutes governing the promotion, distribution, and sale of all the recreational drugs to persons of minor age; tax collection/evasion; and dealing with the antisocial behaviors associated with the abuse of all recreational drugs (e.g., driving while intoxicated, intrafamily violence).

CONCLUSION

Solving the drug problem requires (a) recognition that it is a continuum occupied by all three drug categories; (b) setting rational, achievable goals for its control, goals that are consistent with human experience with the mood-altering drugs, achievable by the methods to be used in the program, and separate from the goal of crime reduction; (c) clearly understanding that its causes in this country go far beyond the simple availability of drugs upon which current policy focuses so much of its attention; (d) recognizing that the Drug War has not only consistently failed to meet its own stated objectives but its very nature cannot in any way be successful in dealing with the drug problem because of its totally distorted focus; and (e) therefore turning major attention from the supply side to the demand side, to the drug culture, the gateway drug effect, the centrality of tobacco product and alcoholic beverage use to the drug problem, and the specific causes of the inner-city drug trade: unemployment, poor housing, poor education, and hopelessness.

This program would markedly reduce the use and abuse of all the recreational drugs; reduce the tremendous pressure on and corruption of the criminal justice and law enforcement systems created by the present approach, freeing them to focus on other criminal behaviors, and would largely pay for itself through taxes on recreational drug sales, use, advertising, and profits. Its major political downside is that it requires a major assault on the tobacco and alcohol industries and the abandonment of the Drug War as an instrument of social oppression and a political weapon. But it can be done. Based on the record achieved by public health so far, it would meet with success.

REFERENCES

1. Drug Policy Alliance. DEA warns of Colombian heroin. *eNewsletter* 2002 Dec 26:item 2D.
2. Horowitz C. The no-win war. *New York Magazine* 1996 Feb 5:23.
3. Office of National Drug Control Strategy. *National drug control strategy.* Washington, DC: Executive Office of the President, February, 1994.
4. Office of National Drug Control Strategy. *National drug control strategy.* Washington, DC: Executive Office of the President, February, 2002:1.
5. Shannon E. A losing battle. *Time* 1990 Dec 3:44.
6. McGinniss JM, Foege WH. Mortality and morbidity attributable to use of addictive substances in the United States. *Proc Assoc Am Physicians* 1999; 111(2):109–118.
7. Coalition on Smoking OR Health. *FDA proposed rule on tobacco regulation.* Washington, DC: 1995.
8. Jonas S. Why the drug war will never end. In: Inciardi JA, ed. *The drug legalization debate,* 2nd ed. Thousand Oaks, CA: Sage, 1999:125–150.
9. Substance Abuse and Mental Health Services Administration. *Results from the National Household Survey on Drug Abuse: vol. I. Summary of national findings.* NHSDA Series H-17, DHHS Pub. No. SMA 02–3758. Rockville, MD: Office of Applied Statistics, August 2002, Fig. 2–12.
10. Tobacco on trial. Tobacco state legislators introduce bills to block FDA regulation of tobacco products. 1995;7:13.
11. Kessler D. A question of intent: a great American battle with a deadly industry. Part III: the evidence mounts. New York: Public Affairs, 2001.
12. Nadelmann EA. Commonsense drug policy. In: Inciardi JA, ed. *The drug legalization debate,* 2nd ed. Thousand Oaks, CA: Sage, 1999:157–172.
13. Drug Policy Alliance. Overview. 2002. Available at: www.drugpolicy.org. (Last accessed 2004)
14. National Commission on Marihuana and Drug Abuse. *Second report: drug use in America-problem in perspective.* Washington, DC: U.S. Government Printing Office, 1973.
15. *Random House dictionary of the English language.* New York: Random House, 1987.
16. Substance Abuse and Mental Health Services Administration. *Results from the National Household Survey on Drug Abuse: vol. I. Summary of national findings.* NHSDA Series H-17, DHHS Pub. No. SMA 02–3758. Rockville, MD: Office of Applied Statistics, August 2002:11, 13, 25, 33.
17. Office of National Drug Control Strategy. *National drug control strategy.* Washington, DC: Executive Office of the President, February, 2002, Table 3.
18. Office of National Drug Control Strategy. *National drug control strategy.* Washington, DC: Executive Office of the President, February, 2002, pp. 3–6.
19. Drug Policy Alliance. *Effectiveness of the war on drugs.* 2002. Available at: www.drugpolicy.org. (Last accessed 2004)
20. King RS, Mauer M. Distorted priorities: drug offenders in state prisons. Washington, DC: The Sentencing Project, 2002:11–13.
21. Mauer M. The drug war's unequal justice. *Drug Policy Lett* 1996;28:11.
22. Mauer M, Huling T. Young black americans and the criminal justice system. Washington, DC: The Sentencing Project, 1995:9–13.
23. Office of National Drug Control Strategy. National drug control strategy. Washington, DC: Executive Office of the President, February, 2002, Table 2.
24. Substance Abuse and Mental Health Services Administration. *Results from the National Household Survey on Drug Abuse: vol. I. Summary of national findings.* NHSDA Series H-17, DHHS Pub. No. SMA 02–3758. Rockville, MD: Office of Applied Statistics, August 2002:11–13.
25. Cohen G, et al. Epidemiology of substance use. In: Friedman L, et al., Eds. *Source book of substance abuse.* Baltimore, MD: Williams and Wilkins, 1996.
26. Brecher E. *Licit and illicit drugs.* Boston: Little, Brown, 1972.
27. Musto DF. *The American disease.* New York: Oxford University Press, 1987.
28. Goldstein A. *Addiction: from biology to drug policy,* 2nd ed. Sect. II. New York: Oxford University Press, 2001.
29. Institute for Health Policy, Brandeis University. *Substance abuse.* Princeton, NJ: Robert Wood Johnson Foundation, 1993:12–13, 32–33.
30. Institute for Health Policy, Brandeis University. *Substance abuse.* Princeton, NJ: Robert Wood Johnson Foundation, 1993:31–45.
31. Zinberg N. *Drug set, and setting.* New Haven, CT: Yale University Press, 1984.
32. McGinniss JM, Foege WH. Actual causes of death in the United States. *JAMA* 1993;270:2207.
33. U.S. Department of Health and Human Services. *Healthy People, 2010, conference edition.* Washington, DC: U.S. Government Printing Office, 2000.
34. U.S. Department of Health and Human Services. *Healthy People, 2010, conference edition.* vol. 2, sects. 26, 27. Washington, DC: U.S. Government Printing Office, 2000.
35. White House Conference for a Drug Free America. *Final report.* Washington, DC: U.S. Government Printing Office, 1988.
36. The Media-Advertising Partnership for a Drug Free America. *Fact sheet.* New York: American Association of Advertising Agencies (no date).
37. Erickson PG. A public health approach to demand reduction. *J Drug Issues* 1990;20(3).
38. Department of Health and Human Services. *Reducing the health consequences of smoking: 25 years of progress.* DHHS Pub. No. (CDC) 89–8411. Washington, DC: U.S. Government Printing Office, 1989.
39. Gitlin T. On drugs and mass media in America's consumer society. In: Resnik H, et al., eds. *Youth and drugs: society's mixed messages.* Rockville, MD: Office of Substance Abuse Prevention, 1990.
40. Holden C. "Behavioral" addictions: do they exist? *Science* 2001;294:980–982.
41. Lambert C. Trafficking in chance. *Harvard Magazine* 2002;Jul-Aug:33–41.
42. Johnson C. Prevention and control of drug abuse. In: Last JM, ed. *Public health and preventive medicine.* Norwalk, CT: Appleton-Century-Crofts, 1986.
43. U.S. Department of Health and Human Services. *Healthy People, 2010, conference edition.* Vol. 2. Washington, DC: U.S. Government Printing Office, 2000:27–4.
44. Johnston L. Ban cigarette advertising to reduce adolescent drug abuse. *Drug Abuse Update* 1988;25:2.
45. Chen K, Kandel DB. The natural history of drug use. *Am J Public Health* 1995;85:41.
46. New York Division of Alcoholism and Alcohol Abuse. Alcohol: the gateway drug. *Focus* 1991;6(1).
47. Henningfield J. Smokeless tobacco: addictive and a gateway drug. *Tob Youth Rep* 1990 Autumn:11.
48. Keegan A. Tobacco may provide gateway to drug, alcohol abuse. *NIDA Notes* 1991 Summer/Fall:23.
49. National Institute of Drug Abuse. *Tobacco as a gateway drug (a chart).* New York: Smokefree Educational Services, 1993.
50. Kandel DB, Jessor R. The gateway hypothesis revisited. In: Kandel DB, ed. *Stages and pathways of drug involvement: examining the gateway hypothesis.* Cambridge, UK: Cambridge University Press, 2002.
51. Stark F. *The 2nd annual drug test for members of congress.* Washington, DC: House of Representatives, 1989.

52. New York State Division of Alcoholism and Alcohol Abuse. *Alcohol: the gateway to other drug use.* Buffalo, NY: Research Institute on Alcoholism, 1989.

53. Substance Abuse and Mental Health Services Administration. *Results from the National Household Survey on Drug Abuse: vol. I. Summary of national findings.* NHSDA Series H-17, DHHS Pub. No. SMA 02–3758. Rockville, MD: Office of Applied Statistics, August 2002:23.

54. More teens are smoking! *Tob Youth Rep* 1990;4(3).

55. Califano J. No, fight harder. *New York Times* 1993 Dec 15.

56. Center on Addiction and Substance Abuse. *Legalization: panacea or pandora's box?* New York: 1995.

57. Kleber HD, Califano JA, Demers JC. Clinical and societal implications of drug legalization. In Lowinson JH, Ruiz P, Millman RB, et al., eds. *Substance abuse: a comprehensive textbook.* Baltimore, MD: Williams and Wilkins, 1998:855–864.

58. Office of National Drug Control Strategy. *National drug control strategy.* Washington, DC: Executive Office of the President, February, 2002:21.

59. U.S. Department of Health and Human Services. *Healthy People, 2010, conference edition:* vol. 2. Washington, DC: U.S. Government Printing Office, 2000:27–4.

60. Williams GD, et al. *Surveillance report #23, apparent per capita alcohol consumption: national, state, and regional trends, 1977–1990.* Washington, DC: National Institute of Alcohol Abuse and Alcoholism, December, 1992.

61. Lender ME, Martin JK. *Drinking in America: a history.* New York: The Free Press, 1982:196–197.

62. Rorabaugh WJ. The alcoholic republic: an American tradition. New York: Oxford, 1979:233, 290–293.

63. Substance Abuse and Mental Health Services Administration. *Results from the National Household Survey on Drug Abuse: vol. I. Summary of national findings.* NHSDA Series H-17, DHHS Pub. No. SMA 02–3758. Rockville, MD: Office of Applied Statistics, 2002:20.

64. Department of Justice. *Drugs, crime and the justice system.* NCJ-133652. U.S. Government Washington, DC: December, 1992.

65. Duke S. Drug prohibition: an unnatural disaster. *Conn Law Rev* 1995;27(2).

66. Treaster JB. Mayor's drug strategy: new plan for chronic problem. *New York Times* 1994 Apr 11.

67. Department of Justice. *Drugs, crime and the justice system.* NCJ-133652. Printing office. Washington, DC: December, 1992:20–23.

68. U.S. Department of Health and Human Services. *Healthy People, 2010, conference edition:* vol. 2. Washington, DC: U.S. Government Printing Office, 2000:26–1, 27–3.

69. National Association for Public Health Policy. A public health approach to mitigating the negative consequences of illicit drug abuse. *J Public Health Policy* 1999:20(3).

70. Committee on Public Health, New York Academy of Medicine. *Statement and resolution on tobacco and health.* *Bull N Y Acad Med* 1989;62:1029–1033.

71. American Public Health Association. A public health response to the war on drugs: reducing alcohol, tobacco and other drug problems among the nation's youth. Res. 8817 (PP). *Am J Public Health* 1989;79:360–364.

72. Association of State and Territorial Health Officials (ASTHO). *Guide to public health practice: state health agency tobacco prevention and control plans.* NIH Pub. No. 90–1577. Washington, DC: U.S. Department of Health and Human Services, 1989.

73. Resnik H, et al., eds. *Youth and drugs: society's mixed messages.* Rockville, MD: Office of Substance Abuse Prevention, 1990.

74. Lutz P. Drug fight stresses educational approach. *New York Times* 1989 Jun 11;Long Island Section:1.

75. National Institute of Drug Abuse. Capsules. In: *Population estimates of lifetime and current drug use, 1988.* Rockville, MD: Author, 1989.

76. Survey of state and local laws on tobacco sales. *MMWR Morb Mortal Wkly Rep* 1990;39(21):349–352.

77. Terris M. Epidemiology of cirrhosis of the liver: national mortality data. *Am J Public Health* 1967;57:2076.

78. Philip Morris U.S.A. *A closer look at our Web site.* 2002:15. Available at: www.philipmorrisusa.com. (Last accessed 2004)

79. Kessler D. *A question of intent: a great American battle with a deadly industry. Part III: the evidence mounts.* New York: Public Affairs, 2001.

80. Mosher J. Drug availability in a public health perspective. In: Resnik H, et al., eds. *Youth and drugs: society's mixed messages.* Rockville, MD: Office of Substance Abuse Prevention, 1990:129–168.

81. Warner K. *Selling smoke: cigarette advertising and public health.* Washington, DC: American Public Health Association, 1986.

82. Polin K. Argument for the ban of tobacco advertising: a First Amendment analysis. *Hofstra L Rev* 1988;17:99–135.

83. Philip Morris U.S.A. *A closer look at our Web site.* 2002:2. Available at: www.philipmorrisusa.com. (Last accessed 2004)

84. Cormack CC, Daniels S. *Project STAR research findings.* Kansas City, MO: Project STAR, 1990.

85. Pentz MA, et al. A multicommunity trial for primary prevention of adolescent drug abuse. *JAMA* 1989;261:3259–3266.

86. Office of National Drug Control Strategy. *National drug control strategy.* Washington, DC: Executive Office of the President, 2002:11.

Training and Education

CHAPTER 80

Medical Education in Substance Abuse: The Acquisition of Knowledge, Attitudes, and Skills

JOHN N. CHAPPEL

"Although many physicians are well equipped to treat the medical and psychiatric complications of substance abuse, most are not prepared to treat substance abuse as a primary disorder. . . . This lack of training frequently results in missed opportunities for care."
Fiellin, Butler, D'Onofrio, et al., 2002 (1)

The need for improved medical education in substance abuse prevention and treatment is well illustrated by the findings of the 2001 National Household Survey on Drug Abuse (2). Of the 5 million people who, by *Diagnostic and Statistical Manual of Mental Disorders,* 4th ed. (*DSM–IV*) criteria, needed treatment but did not receive it, only 7.5% believed they needed it. Associated with this "denial gap" is a significantly increasing need for treatment. In the year from 2000 to 2001 the need for substance abuse treatment grew from an estimated 4.7 million (2% of the U.S. population) to 6.1 million (2.7%) (2). This growth in need has occurred despite the war on drugs and the arrests and incarceration of large numbers of the drug-using population. The medical and public health need is reflected in the fact that half the annual mortality in the United States

is a result of lifestyle-related illness, half of which (25% of annual deaths) are a consequence of alcohol and other drug use (3).

Better training of physicians at the undergraduate, postgraduate, and continuing medical education levels would do much to help meet, and perhaps even reduce this growing need. The 1995 Macy Conference (4) urged the specialties of Family Practice, Internal Medicine, Pediatrics, and Obstetrics and Gynecology to "promptly respond to the need to improve the quality of care provided by physicians trained in these specialties to patients with alcohol and other drug problems" (4, p. 101). These efforts culminated in the *Strategic Plan for Interdisciplinary Faculty Development* (5). This plan outlines the core knowledge, skills, and attitudes that all health care professionals should have in dealing with substance use disorders (SUD). The plan was developed by the Association of Medical Educators and Researchers in Substance Abuse (AMERSA). In addition to physician education in the prevention and treatment of SUD, which is described in this chapter, ten other health professions outlined educational approaches designed to improve the knowledge, skills, and attitudes of their practitioners (5).

HISTORY OF MEDICAL EDUCATION IN SUBSTANCE ABUSE

Physicians have always been familiar with the medical and psychiatric problems associated with substance abuse. While the gin epidemic raged in England between 1750 and 1800, Benjamin Rush, America's first surgeon general and the father of American psychiatry, described alcoholism as a disease, with abstinence the treatment (6). The problem was that little was known about how to achieve, and even less about how to maintain, abstinence. Although Rush taught in our first medical school at the University of Pennsylvania, there is no evidence that his views had any influence on medical education. Physicians adopted the view of our culture at the time that alcohol and drug addiction were moral and legal problems that should be taken care of by religion or the criminal justice system.

In the latter part of the nineteenth century the United States experienced epidemics of cocaine and opiate abuse following the Civil War (7). Physicians tried a variety of approaches to deal with these addictions, including prescribing addicting drugs. In the meantime, political decisions were made to attack the problems through legislation and enforcement. The Harrison Act of 1914 (7) and the Prohibition Amendment (8) to the Constitution in 1919 had a major effect on medical practice. During the 1920s, in response to the illegal status of alcohol and to the prosecution of some physicians who were prescribing opioids to narcotic addicts, there was a gradual avoidance of narcotic and alcohol problems in medical practice. In addition, teaching about alcoholism and other drug addiction was dropped from the curricula of medical schools. As a result, several generations of physicians have had little or no training in the recognition and treatment of alcohol and other drug addictions.

Despite the societal view that alcoholism and other drug addictions were moral and legal problems, physicians have always had to manage difficult detoxification and the medical complications of these disorders. There was no criticism as long as the underlying addiction was left alone. Following World War II, a small group of physicians began to take an interest in the addictive disorders. In 1954, the New York Medical Society on Alcoholism was founded (9). This small group of physicians prompted the American Medical Association (AMA) in 1956 and in 1966 to declare that alcoholism was a medical illness (10). The intent was to get physicians to diagnose and treat the underlying conditions rather than the sequelae. Unfortunately, these actions had little or no effect on medical school curricula.

By 1967 interest had spread sufficiently to form a national organization, the American Medical Society on Alcoholism (AMSA). Interest slowly grew amongst these physicians and expansion occurred in 1984 to include all drugs of abuse. The result was the American Medical Society on Alcoholism and Other Drug Dependencies (AMSAODD), which was the first national medical society representing all the addictions (9). In 1989, this organization became the American Society of Addiction Medicine (ASAM).

During the 1960s the development of methadone maintenance and therapeutic communities as treatment modalities began to stimulate more medical interest. This was probably augmented by the ferment over drug use amongst service men in Vietnam and our first national "Great War on Drugs."

In 1970, the National Council on Alcoholism held a conference. The American Medical Student Association, an active participant in that conference, surveyed students from 60 medical schools (11). Only 10% of the students reported a formal course or clerkship dealing with the treatment and rehabilitation of the alcoholic. The students concluded their report with the following statement:

> If physicians and other medical personnel are to be trained to provide better treatment, rehabilitation, and prevention of alcoholism, they must have the opportunity for a coherent educational program in their medical school career. Only in this fashion can the great shortage of adequately trained professionals and the archaic attitudes of many practitioners be overcome. (11)

Governmental response to these pressures was to initiate the Career Teacher Program in Alcohol and Drug Abuse sponsored by the newly founded National Institute on Alcoholism and Alcohol Abuse (NIAAA) and National Institute on Drug Abuse (NIDA) (12). The goal of the Career Teacher Program was to train established faculty to develop and implement substance abuse curricula in their medical schools. Over the 10-year period of its existence (1972 to 1981) career teachers were funded in 59 medical schools. The results were positive, but limited. An evaluation of the program concluded that the program had resulted in (13):

1. An average increase in curriculum hours, both required and elective, from 18.5 to 123.6 hours, of which almost all is attributed to career teachers.
2. Clinical substance abuse programs started in a number of medical schools.
3. A large number of curriculum materials and professional writings.

The medical academic ferment begun by the Career Teacher Program resulted in the formation of the AMERSA in 1976 (14). This organization has grown to include not only medical school but other health profession faculty. It holds an annual meeting and publishes a journal that enables its members to share both support and stimulus for their often lonely work in attempting to expand and improve the substance abuse education provided by their schools.

In 1989, a federal initiative began the Faculty Fellow Training Program in Alcohol and Drug Abuse. This program provided modest part time support for three to five faculty members from primary care departments and psychiatry (15). This program was a logical sequel to the Career Teacher Program. It also extended support to schools of nursing, social work, and psychology.

In 1999, a cooperative 5-year agreement was made between AMERSA, the Health Resources and Services Administration (HRSA), the Substance Abuse and Mental Health Services Administration (SAMHSA), and the Center for Substance Abuse Treatment (CSAT). This agreement was entitled the "HRSA-AMERSA-SAMHSA/CSAT Interdisciplinary Project to Improve Health Professional Education in Substance Abuse." Teams of three

Faculty Fellows from three different health professional schools worked under a mentor to develop and implement substance abuse educational projects in and between their institutions. The Strategic Plan for Interdisciplinary Faculty Development was a direct product of this program (5). The product of this Plan is entitled "Project Mainstream," which has established a Web site (www.projectmainstream.net) that provides access to project curriculum materials, annotated learning resource databases, profession-specific learning resources, and electronic newsletters.

In parallel with these developments in medical education there has been a major growth in the subspecialty of addiction medicine. In 1935, Alcoholics Anonymous (AA) developed out of the failure of medicine and psychiatry to help alcoholics achieve long-term stable sobriety (16). Since that time many alcohol- and drug-dependent physicians have been helped by AA and NA (Narcotics Anonymous). The numbers of these physicians increased substantially with the development of impaired physician programs in every state (17). Many of these able and energetic recovering physicians decided to dedicate themselves to treating alcohol and drug dependency. In 1983, the first review course and certification examination for physicians was held by the California Society of Addiction Medicine (CSAM). In that same year the American Society of Addiction Medicine (ASAM) was established, and in 1986, a national examination was held. This certification exam stimulated membership growth in ASAM from 719 in 1981 to more than 4,000 in 1990 (18). More than two thirds of ASAM's membership comes from internal medicine, family medicine, and psychiatry. The activities of this pool of experienced clinicians has led to the representation of Addiction Medicine in the AMA house of delegates and the designation of addiction medicine as a subspecialty in medicine (ADM) along with 85 other self-designated practice specialties.

American medicine has officially left no doubt that training in the diagnosis and treatment of alcohol and other drug addictions should play an important role in medical education. In 1988, the AMA Council on Scientific Affairs republished its guidelines for physician involvement in the care of substance-abusing patients and added this important statement (19):

> The AMA also believes it is important that all physicians consider the degree to which they are personally at risk for alcohol and other drug-related problems, as well as their ethical obligation to intervene with a colleague who gives evidence of such impairment. Proficiency at this basic level may be considered a personal as well as a professional responsibility.

Family medicine, internal medicine, pediatrics, emergency medicine, and psychiatry have all issued position statements emphasizing the importance of education within their specialties in Addiction Medicine. Despite this interest there has been a considerable time lag in developing specific requirements for residency training. For example, in 1981 the American Psychiatric Association (APA) recognized that nearly 30% of the total mental health problems in the United States were caused by alcohol- and drug-abuse problems. Comprehensive training about substance abuse was recommended for all psychiatry residency programs (20). It was not until 1989 that the Residency Review Committee (RRC) for psychiatry included the following requirement (21):

> Specific clinical experiences must include: supervised clinical management of patients with alcoholism and drug abuse, including detoxification and long-term management in inpatient and/or outpatient settings and familiarity with self-help groups.

Since then progress in residency training has been slow. The AMA Council on Medical Education reported in 1998 that only 5 of the 99 specialty training programs had RRC requirements regarding substance abuse education (22). These were anesthesiology, family medicine, internal medicine, obstetrics/gynecology, and psychiatry. Only family medicine and psychiatry reported that a majority of their programs required clinical rotations in substance abuse. A 1999 survey revealed that fewer than 10% of the faculty who teach substance abuse topics perform clinical work in alcohol and drug treatment programs, and that teaching is infrequently performed in these settings (23). The physicians who developed the core competencies currently being recommended caution that: "While physician training should be geared toward a broad range of skills, including screening, intervention, referral, and follow-up care, it would be desirable that some proportion of substance abuse training be performed in specialized settings in order to expose trainees to this type of care" (1, p. 211).

PROBLEMS IN MEDICAL PRACTICE

There is a long and well-documented history of problems that are the sequelae of the historical events described above. In the 1950s Mendelson and Chafetz found that less than 1% of the alcoholics admitted to the emergency room at the Massachusetts General Hospital sought treatment in the hospital's outpatient program, although all were offered treatment (24). They found both personnel and institutional attitudinal problems accounting for this lack of success. The authors then studied the needs of the alcoholics appearing in the emergency room and developed a system whereby the residents and other staff were expected to treat the alcoholic patient with respect and consideration. In addition they were to work at reducing frustrating situations and to gratify reasonable requests. Two hundred consecutive alcoholic patients admitted through the emergency room were randomly assigned to this experimental treatment approach or to a control group which had the usual approach. Following completion of the admission of the 200 patients both groups were followed for 1 year. An 89% followup rate was achieved in a group of men with high rates of homelessness, poverty, and characteristics "most often referred to as skid row alcoholics" (25).

The authors concluded that this response "graphically documents the necessity of developing and applying new and imaginative variations of clinical skills to mental health problems." They described the differences and emphasis on action rather than words "placing the responsibility for achieving a therapeutic alliance on the caretaker rather than the patient." This approach could be considered to be a template for modern training in addiction medicine.

Research over the following decades continued to reveal clinical problems associated with negative attitudes. In the 1970's, Westermeyer and his colleagues used the Michigan Alcoholism Screening Test (MAST) as a diagnostic screening device on the medical and surgical wards of the university teaching hospital (26). They concluded that physicians and nurses in this facility:

1. Did not take adequate alcohol and drug use histories.
2. Did not identify chemical dependency as a medical problem, even when they knew it was present.
3. Did not involve themselves in treatment or treatment recommendations even when the problem was identified.

These negative attitudes which permeate our culture led a continuing medical education program, which had trained 838 medical professionals in the 1970s, to conclude that "our trainees have touched many alcoholic livers but almost no alcoholic lives" (27).

Pursch immersed these professionals in a treatment setting where their primary defenses could be removed and where they could become aware of their own attitudes and lack of useful knowledge about addictions.

A few years later Moore and his colleagues screened 2,002 new, adult, inpatient admissions to Johns Hopkins Hospital (28). All the new admissions were screened with the CAGE (cut down [on drinking], annoyance, guilt [about drinking], [need for] eyeopener) and the Short Michigan Alcoholism Screening Test (SMAST) tests. Detection rates by house staff and attending physicians varied by departments. In surgery, with 23% of the patients screening positive for alcoholism, less than 25% of these were detected, with one-fifth receiving intervention. In medicine, with 25% of the patients screening positive approximately 25% were detected, with one-third of these receiving intervention. In psychiatry with 30% of the patients screening positive for alcoholism, 65% were detected and intervention was initiated in more than half of these. In all cases the intervention consisted of presenting the diagnosis to the patient and recommending that they

get help. These physician interventions correlated with the patient's reported decrease in the use of alcohol following discharge ($P < 0.01$).

Pursch concluded that 75% of the physicians trained in his program were unable to deal effectively with alcohol troubled patients for the following reasons (27):

1. Inadequate training in addiction medicine
2. Unresolved addiction problems in their own families
3. Personal problems with addiction, including self-prescribing
4. Negative experiences with addicted patients
5. A rigid personality structure with an inability to deal with patients on a feeling level
6. Fear of loss of collegial support and career advancement

The problems documented above represent a needs assessment for medical education in substance abuse. The continuing epidemic of alcohol and other drug addictions makes it imperative that medical education improve its track record and effectiveness in dealing with both physician attitudes and behaviors in diagnosing and treating the addictive disorders.

THE KNOWLEDGE BASE OF ADDICTION MEDICINE

The explosion of knowledge and experience that has occurred since the AMA declared that alcoholism was a disease has done much to establish medical credibility for the field of addiction medicine. The dramatic increase in research findings has led ASAM and the National Council on Alcoholism and Drug Dependence to develop a new definition of alcoholism (29). The revised definition produced by a committee of 27 experts is as follows:

Alcoholism is a chronic, primary disease with genetic, psychosocial, and environmental factors influencing its development and manifestations. The disease is often progressive and fatal. It is characterized by continuous or periodic:

1. Impaired control over drinking
2. Preoccupation with the drug alcohol
3. Use of alcohol despite adverse consequences
4. Distortions in thinking, most notably denial

This definition would fit all the other drug addictions, including tobacco dependence.

The evidence base, which developed from research in both the epidemiology and neurobiology of addictive disorders, led to the publication of a seminal article documenting the chronic nature of addictive disorders (30). The authors, leaders in the field of addiction medicine research, urged a shift in both public and physician attitudes from an acute to a chronic care approach. They compared addictive disorders to other chronic medical disorders such as diabetes mellitus type 2, hypertension, and bronchial asthma. Relapses and problems with patient compliance are common with these medical disorders, but do not result in rejection, blame, or refusal to treat, which so often occur with relapses in addictive disorders. They note that we do not have a cure for addiction. The only long-term stability is associated with participation in methadone maintenance or Alcoholics Anonymous.

As research and clinical experience grow, the conceptual models of chemical dependence are becoming more sophisticated (31). The role of neurotransmitter and receptor changes has given the field even stronger basic science roots. The application of knowledge to clinical skills is emphasized by the APA guidelines for the treatment of patients with substance use disorders, which has 481 references (32), and the briefer National Institute on Alcohol Abuse and Alcoholism (NIAAA) physician's guide to helping patients with alcohol problems (33).

Help in organizing the expanding knowledge base of addiction medicine is essential for medical educators. In 1989, Brown University developed Project ADEPT (Alcohol and Drug Education for Physician Training in Primary Care), an inexpensive core curriculum that has been used in many U.S. medical schools (34). This educational material, which emphasized skill training, included one

volume of five core curriculum modules that required from 7 to 13 hours of curriculum time. Useful suggestions were contained in the module that helped both the student and instructor review the knowledge base before a patient encounter. The patient encounters are then observed and rated by both instructor and other students. The subsequent discussion does much to promote integration of knowledge and the development of positive attitudes. The interactive technique of Project ADEPT, combined with the material of Project Mainstream makes effective education at all levels.

Conceptual models can help with knowledge, attitudes, and skills, thus influencing clinical practice. The model developed by the Institute of Medicine and modified by Skinner is depicted in Figures 80.1 and 80.2 (35,36). These figures help physicians understand the continuum of substance use, abuse, and dependence. When the problems are initially noted, brief interventions may be very valuable (37). As the addiction progresses, more intensive treatment is needed and participation in a 12-step program, such as Alcoholics Anonymous (AA), may be lifesaving (38).

Epidemiologic research has underlined the importance of the continuum (see Figures 80.1 and 80.2). Kandel's findings reaffirm the importance of parents, the peer group, and juvenile delinquent behavior in the development of illegal drug use (39). Vaillant, in reviewing the literature and the data from his monumental 50-year followup of

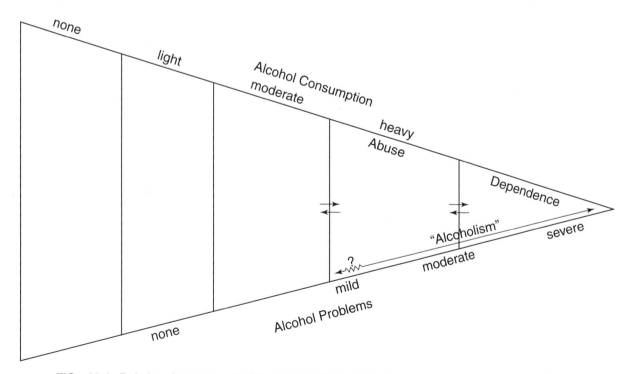

FIG. 80.1. Relation between alcohol consumption patterns and level of alcohol problems. (Reprinted with permission from Skinner HA. Spectrum of drinkers and intervention opportunities. *CMAJ* 1990;143:1054.)

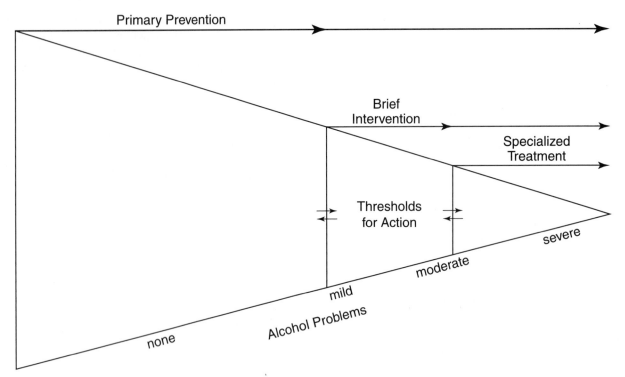

FIG. 80.2. Relation between level of alcohol problems and type of intervention. (Reprinted with permission from Skinner HA. Spectrum of drinkers and intervention opportunities. *CMAJ* 1990;143:1054.)

a prospective study of alcoholism, has made the etiologic statement that "genetic loading is an important predictor of *whether* an individual develops alcoholism and that an unstable childhood environment is an important predictor of *when* an individual loses control of alcohol" (38, p. 101).

An important part of our knowledge base is the growing evidence of the importance of length of treatment. McLellan recently reviewed the literature and reached the following conclusion (40):

Perhaps the most robust and pervasive indicator of favorable post-treatment outcome in all forms of substance abuse rehabilitation is length of stay in treatment. Virtually all studies have shown that patients who stay in treatment longer or attend more treatment sessions have better post treatment outcomes than those who do not. Specifically, several studies have suggested that outpatient treatments of less than 90 days are more likely to result in early return to drug use and generally poorer response than treatments of longer duration.

Textbooks reflect a body of knowledge, and a growing number of good ones exist in the field of addiction medicine. This book will serve as a text for specialty or fellowship training. Shuckit's book proved popular enough to be reissued in a fifth edition in 2000 and is a useful resource for medical students and residents who are not specializing in addiction medicine (41). The APA and ASAM

both publish textbooks that could be used for fellowship training. Anyone teaching at an undergraduate, postgraduate, or continuing medical education level can now find suitable textbooks in addiction medicine and addiction psychiatry.

A notable gap in the medical body of knowledge continues to be detailed information on the 12-step programs, particularly Alcoholics Anonymous. This nonprofessional program of recovery from alcoholism grew out of the failure of medicine and psychiatry to provide lasting help to chronic alcoholics, one of whom was a physician (16). The 12 steps, when worked with the help of a sponsor and home group, can make sobriety tolerable and even enjoyable. The program was hammered out over 3 years by the first 100 chronic hopeless alcoholics who were managing to stay sober. The product of this field research, which is described in the Big Book of Alcoholics Anonymous (16), has continued to be the most effective long-term way of returning chronic alcoholics to productive life and stable sobriety.

Vaillant's 50-year followup confirms the importance of AA in establishing stable sobriety for chronic alcoholics. He concluded that "after abstinence had been maintained for 5 years, relapse was rare. In contrast, return to controlled drinking without eventual relapse was unlikely" (38). The importance of long-term followup is shown in Table 80.1, which reflects the frequency of relapse following 2 years or more of sobriety. Research continues to

TABLE 80.1. *Stability of abstinence (N = 56)*

Length of abstinence	Still abstinent	Relapsing that year	% Eventually relapsing
2 years	56	9	41%
3 years	47	5	25%
4 years	42	0	25%
5 years	42	5	16%
6 years	37	1	7%

[a]These three relapsed after 8, 10, and 13 years of abstinence. Reprinted with permission from Vallant GE. *The natural history of alcoholism revisited.* Cambridge, MA: Harvard University Press, 1995:235.

support the importance of 12-step programs in maintaining sobriety.

ATTITUDES AND ATTITUDINAL CHANGE IN MEDICAL PRACTICE

Many of the problems in the health care system described above stem from a combination of ignorance and negative attitudes on the part of health care professionals. Those of us involved in the practice of addiction medicine and addiction psychiatry have had experiences with physicians whose negative attitudes resulted either in the delay or in the absence of diagnosis, treatment, or referral of addicted patients (26,42). One of our pregnant patients was turned away from the hospital of her choice when it was discovered that she was a former heroin addict currently on methadone maintenance. The result was a traumatic delivery in a taxi on route to another hospital. These experiences led to an early consensus among the career teachers that attitudes would be given a high priority in the planning and implementation of teaching at undergraduate, postgraduate, and continuing medical educational levels. The decision was easy to make but has been difficult to implement. Part of the difficulty lies in the complex nature of attitudes. Social psychologists have had great interest in this area. Allport reviewed more than 100 definitions of attitude (43). He concluded that there was basic agreement that *an attitude is a learned predisposition to respond to an object or class of objects in a consistently favorable or unfavorable way.* A current textbook on social psychology elaborates on this definition, describing attitude as a short hand way of saying that we have feelings and thoughts of like or dislike, approval or disapproval, attraction or repulsion, trust or distrust toward something or someone (44). These evaluative responses have cognitive, affective, experiential, and even physiologic components. To add to their complexity, most attitudes develop out of our life experience and are strongly influenced by the value systems of the family and culture in which we grew up.

As our life experience increases we may develop attitudes that are inconsistent or even contradictory with each other. For example, physicians with strong positive atti-

tudes toward preserving life may find their behavior changing when they encounter patients who evoke negative attitudes in them. Sudnow noted that less-than-strenuous efforts were made by hospital physicians to resuscitate patients who were alcoholic (45). Even in other aspects of the medical treatment of the alcoholic, it appeared that these physicians believed that it was proper to have less concern about treatment of alcoholics than they had with other patients. The origins of these negative attitudes probably stemmed from the view of addiction as a moral and legal problem.

Another source of negative attitudes in medicine has come from psychoanalytic theory. Early psychoanalytic thought viewed alcohol and other drug addictions as symptoms of underlying conflict or developmental delay (46). This view had a profound influence on early psychiatric education. Despite the large body of evidence that alcohol and other drug addictions are chronic primary diseases (30), there are still many practicing physicians and psychiatrists who view SUD as symptomatic of poor choices and weak will. Modern psychoanalytic thinking has moved away from these old ideas. Brickman, a psychoanalyst, has stated that viewing substance abuse as a secondary phenomenon to underlying psychopathology is a basic misconception (47). After reviewing the psychoanalytic and addiction literature, he concludes that "the most effective treatment approach in most cases is informed by the concept that chemical dependency is a disease entity in its own right and must be treated as such." He concludes persuasively that psychoanalytic treatment can be extended through an integrated approach emphasizing abstinence and participation in AA for the patient. This approach is emphasized by two Harvard training analysts who describe Alcoholics Anonymous as a "sophisticated psychosocial treatment for alcoholism" (48).

On the positive side, psychoanalytic theory has contributed greatly to our understanding of the negative attitudes that have characterized the health care system and alcohol and other drug addictions. Negative transference is ubiquitous when chemically dependent alcohol- or drug-abusing patients approach health care professionals. The patients expect a moralistic lack of understanding accompanied by rejection and even mistreatment. The transference aspect of this reaction does not stem from childhood experience with parents, but from an internal reaction originating from the patient's superego, where internalized parental and cultural values and standards react to the loss of control and compulsion to use alcohol and other drugs despite adverse consequences. The result is a traumatic loss of self-esteem, which has been well described by Bean (49). This negative superego response, which contributes to the denial in alcohol and other drug addictions, is projected onto the physician.

The physician's personal use of dependence-producing substances may contribute to or modify countertransference reactions. The most common countertransference is a strong unconscious need or wish not to make a diagnosis of addiction. The intensity of this need is directly related to the negative reaction which would occur if the diagnosis were made. If the reaction is strong enough to remove the person from the patient role and to view the person as no longer needing or deserving treatment, the physician will feel considerable discomfort in providing medical care for the patient. If the patient's use of alcohol or other drugs is similar to or less than the physician's use, then denial will be reinforced, even though the patient may meet the criteria for dependence. A survey of 589 graduating seniors from 13 medical schools in the 4 major regions of the United States showed that nearly 90% used alcohol on a monthly basis and nearly 10% used alcohol almost daily (50). Medical student use of tranquilizers was significantly more ($P < 0.05$) than their same-age cohort in the general population, whereas the use of cigarettes was significantly less ($P < 0.001$).

Self-prescribing starts early for physicians. A study of 316 residents in 4 internal medicine programs in well-known medical schools found that 52% self-prescribed medications (51). The rates go up with each year of residency training, culminating in rates of 61% to 84% for practicing physicians (52,53). This practice may contribute to negative attitudes on the part of the physician when a patient, who does not have the training and experience, is found to be self-prescribing addictive drugs.

Whether because of transference or countertransference, there has been extensive documentation of combinations of negative attitudes and negative behavior toward alcohol and drug addicts in the health care system. Studies at Harvard in the 1950s and 1960s demonstrated that physicians behaved diagnostically as though alcoholics were derelicts (24,25). These same physicians recognized that alcoholism can occur in other social groups, but they hesitated to make the indicated diagnosis in those cases because of this negative stereotype. A second attitudinal set in this group of senior medical and surgical residents was a focus on bodily symptoms and physical problems. These medical problems often would become the diagnosis rather than the alcoholism. This preference for a medical diagnosis has the effect of delayed treatment for alcoholism at a time when it might have beneficial effects.

If negative attitudes have such a profound effect on health care professional's behavior, then how are we to understand those attitudes and how they can be changed? It is generally agreed that attitudes have three components (54):

1. Cognitive, involving belief and knowledge
2. Affective, involving feelings and emotion
3. Conative, involving decision and behavior

Each component may be positive or negative in varying degrees and influenced by other factors. Favorable attitudes are usually positive in all three components. Unfavorable attitudes are usually negative in all three components.

The logical place to start educational efforts to influence attitudes is in the cognitive area, which is conscious and responds to new knowledge and information. This is not sufficient, however. The affective component is equally, if not more, powerful. Affective experience is more difficult to arrange educationally. It usually occurs with direct patient experience and in response to the role models of attending physicians. Because feelings are less conscious and are viewed as subjective, they are less likely to be valued or expressed by health professional students. The conative component, involving the will and motivation to act, is not well understood. It may be influenced most by repeated practice of desired behaviors. In this way the physician may apply familiar diagnostic and treatment skills to patients he or she does not like.

Attitudinal formation begins at birth and is profoundly influenced by the family and culture in which we grow up. Clinical experience also contributes to the development of negative attitudes. Vaillant notes that it is very easy to become pessimistic about treating alcoholics in some clinical settings. In a 6.5-year study of 19,000 admissions of 5,000 persons to a detoxification clinic, 2,500 never returned. On the other hand, 25 indelibly remembered patients returned 2,500 times. Thus 0.5% of the population "became far more deeply etched in clinician's consciousness than did the 50% who never came back and who must have included the best outcomes" (38).

The complexity of attitudes makes them difficult to measure accurately. Attitudinal measurement in the medical literature has used primarily the semantic differential and agree/disagree statements. The semantic differential was developed by Osgood (55). It used polar opposite adjectives such as good/bad, clean/dirty, pleasant/unpleasant, and valuable/worthless. Each scale is separated by seven to ten points and the respondent marks the point between the two adjectives on the scale that best reflects his or her response to the concept, for example, alcoholic, being tested. In more common use is the Likert scale (56). An attitudinal statement is followed by a five-choice scale of strongly disagree, disagree, uncertain, agree, and strongly agree. The usual scoring is obtained by assigning the numbers one to five, with the highest number assigned to strongly agree. Most surveys include a number of attitudinal statements. The results are factor analyzed. Statements, or items, loading positively or negatively on the main factors are retained in the final form of the survey. Items with negative loadings on a factor are reversed when developing a scoring for each factor.

The career teachers began developing a Substance Abuse Attitude Survey (SAAS) in 1977 (57). Over the years, a 50-item questionnaire with 5 stable factors

TABLE 80.2. *Comparative attitudinal scores*

Factor	Nonclinicians (N = 268)	Noncriterion clinicians (N = 312)	Criterion clinicians (N = 108)	ANOVA F
Permissiveness	50.4	49.2	50.1	.91
Nonstereotype	51.5	51.0	50.0	.87
Treatment intervention	45.3	47.0	50.0	8.48[a]
Treatment optimism	44.6	45.2	50.1	11.19[a]
Nonmoralism	49.6	49.9	49.9	.11

[a]P <0.001

Reprinted with permission from Chappel JN, Veach TL, Krug RS. The Substance Abuse Attitude Survey: on instrument for measuring attitudes. *J Stud Alcohol* 1985:46(1):51.

emerged. Two factors, treatment intervention and treatment optimism, significantly differentiated clinicians who met the criterion of at least 6 years experience with 10% or more of their patients being alcohol or drug dependent and who derive satisfaction and experience success treating these patients (see Table 80.2). Improving scores on these two factors were set as educational objectives in a course in substance abuse for second-year medical students (58). The instrument was well accepted in pre- and posttesting. The desired attitudinal change was only achieved when students met with patients, attended AA, worked patient-management problems, and participated in small-group discussions. A brief SAAS of 18 items, which differentiate recovering from nonrecovering physicians and which change most in response to education, was developed but not validated.

A health care professional's personal experience with chemical dependence has a major effect on attitudes. A comparison was made between 307 physicians who reported a past alcohol- or drug-dependence problem, excluding nicotine, but no current problems, with 962 physicians who reported no or slight past and no current problems (59). The samples were obtained from continuing medical education courses on substance abuse. The recovering physicians were significantly more (P <0.0001) oriented toward abstinence during and after treatment. They were significantly more positive (P <0.0001) toward early diagnosis, urine screening during treatment, group therapy, and family involvement in treatment. As might be expected, the recovering physicians were also significantly more (P <0.0001) optimistic and accepting about treating alcohol- and drug-addicted patients.

One reason for the enduring resistance to attitudinal change was revealed in a study of 177 health and welfare personnel (60). More than half of the respondents rated the alcoholic as unmotivated to recover. Typical statements were: "He did not have enough motivation to deal with the problem. I don't determine this, they do." "He didn't want to change." "They tell you they want to recover, but when you think they are going along just right, something

happens, so I suppose they aren't sincere." This belief of poor motivation serves as "a convenient rationale for unwillingness to review and modify current policies and practices so as to encourage the alcoholic to seek treatment and stay with it."

Attitudes in the undergraduate years also show resistance to change. Medical education is accompanied by an increase in cynical attitudes (61) and in negative attitudes toward alcoholics (62). A review of the literature on attitude change during medical school concluded that the positive attitudinal change accompanying one course does not last (63). The author suggested that at least 2 years of exposure were needed. I otherwise suspect that stable attitudes, like stable sobriety, require 5 years or more of exposure.

Research at the University of Illinois College of Medicine confirmed the difficulties in maintaining attitudinal change in medical education (64). The entire third-year class was given an examination after all of their clerkships had been completed. Working from a mock chart with clear data indicating a patient with peptic ulcer, major depression, and alcoholism, the students' mean score for each condition was 3.64, 2.56, and 1.46 (P <0.0001) for each condition, respectively. The authors noted that "[a] review of the curriculum shows that their education in addiction is comparable to that offered in most medical schools." They concluded that the deficiencies were not related to a lack of knowledge, "but to the inability to apply this knowledge in a clinical setting because of experiential or attitudinal traits developed in the clinical setting." This problem continues into residency training. One teacher commented, "I have had the experience of presenting well-thought-out and well-received workshops on how to identify problem drinkers and what to do once you identify them, only to observe residents finish the seminar, meet with a patient shortly afterward, and miss virtually every clue that suggested a drinking problem" (65).

The social science, and psychiatric literature suggests the following techniques of training for behavior that counteracts social norms (66,67):

1. A message has more attitudinal impact if its *source has credibility and perceived expertise.* For medical students and physicians this means *role models* who are from their own clinical discipline. Effective training is hampered when there is a shortage of physician role models with expertise in alcohol and drug dependence. Frank (67) has emphasized the importance of supportive peers and faculty in helping attitude change persist.

2. Yielding occurs when *the recipient agrees with the presented attitude.* Cognitive yielding probably precedes affective and conative yielding and may occur in classroom settings in response to didactic presentations. However, the evidence suggests that this either does not happen often or is very difficult to achieve. Two reviews of the literature conclude that knowledge gain in substance abuse is easily demonstrated but the changes in attitudes and skills require something different than lectures in nonclinical settings (13,68). Most reported programs were found lacking in any meaningful attitude or practice evaluation that could provide data for guidance in the design of future programs.

3. Retention is enhanced by *repetitions of experience over time.* The effects of short courses die quickly if reinforcement and support are not present (63). *Active participation in the learning experience and subsequent practice* contribute to the persistence of attitudinal changes (68). Improvisation by the learner, as one of the activities, appears to be important in consolidating and retaining new attitudes and behavior. This occurs with opportunities for independent research or practice while still in the training situation. As noted earlier, retention or attitude change is greatly enhanced by a supportive group of peers and faculty (69).

4. *Overt behavior reflecting the new positive attitudes.* Medical training has a huge advantage over social psychology's attempts to induce attitude change. We can require the behavior before any affective or conative yielding has occurred. Requiring the desired behavior *in conjunction with close supervision* usually results in maintenance of the behavior, especially if the physician is to be examined on the same behavior later. Behavior itself may have a strong influence on attitudinal change. This likelihood of change is enhanced if the behavior is accompanied by favorable results such as a positive outcome.

The educational research suggests that the best results, in terms of positive attitudes and skills, occur when residents rotate through addiction treatment units and are supervised by experts in addiction medicine, including supporting patients and families use of AA, NA and Al-Anon. The importance of training physicians in combining AA with professional care is well demonstrated in current research (38,70). These prospective and retrospective studies found AA to be an influence far more powerful than professionally directed modalities in recovery from addiction.

TRAINING FOR SKILL DEVELOPMENT

Medical education excels in the development of skill acquisition. The process begins in the basic science years and continues throughout training and practice with continuing knowledge acquisition. Attitudes are acquired more often by example than by discussion. Skills are acquired over years of observation and practice. The old adage of "see one, do one, teach one" disappeared with the rotating internship prior to general practice. As the field of addiction medicine has matured there has developed a much greater clarity about the type of skills needed by any physician in this field (see Table 80.3). The core competencies

TABLE 80.3. *Critical core competencies in substance abuse education for physicians*

Level I: All physicians with clinical contact should:
1. Be able to perform age, gender, and culturally appropriate substance abuse screening.
2. Be able to provide brief interventions to patients with SUD.
3. Be able to use effective methods of counseling patients to help prevent SUD.
4. Be able to refer patients with SUD to treatment settings that provide pharmacotherapy for relapse prevention.
5. Recognize and treat or refer comorbid medical and psychiatric conditions in patients with SUD.
6. Be able to refer patients with SUD to appropriate treatment and supportive services.
7. Be aware of the ethical and legal issues around physician impairment from SUD and of resources for referring potential impaired colleagues, including employee assistance programs, hospital-based committees, state physician health programs, and licensure boards.
8. Identify the legal and ethical issues involved in the care of patients with SUD.

Level II: All physicians coordinating care for patients with SUD in addition should:
1. Use effective methods to assess patients with SUD.
2. Provide pharmacologic withdrawal to patients with SUD.

Level III: All physicians providing specialty services to patients with SUD in addition should:
1. Provide pharmacotherapy for relapse prevention in patients with SUD.
2. Provide or refer for psychosocial counseling for relapse prevention in patients with SUD.

From Fiellin DA, Butler R, D'Onofrio G, et al. The physician's role in caring for patients with substance use disorders: implications for medical education and training. *Subst Abuse* 2002;23(3):213, with permission.

described for physicians in the Strategic Plan for Health Professional Education provide the best template we have had for all levels of medical education (5).

- Level I: All physicians who see patients should be able to:

1. Perform age, gender, and culturally appropriate substance abuse screening.

This is part of basic medical interviewing and should be taught in the introduction to clinical medicine courses in the first 2 years of medical school. Reinforcement should occur in the clerkships and residency years. The authors, who are primary care physicians, note that: "Screening for diseases is warranted if the following conditions are met: the disease has a significant prevalence and consequences; effective and acceptable treatments are available; early identification and treatment are preferable; and there are effective screening instruments available that are easy to administer. There is strong research evidence to support the fact that SUD meet all of these criteria."

A key skill in the screening area is the ability to inquire about the use of addicting drugs: tobacco, alcohol, prescription, and illicit drugs. Once the history of use, with some quantity and frequency information, has been obtained, screening questions can help the physician decide whether a more extensive assessment is needed. The CAGE is the best known of these sets of questions (33). Two positive responses indicate a need for further assessment. Other screening instruments and techniques have been described in the recent primary care literature (71). Biologic markers, for example, mean corpuscular volume (MCV), aspartate aminotransferase (AST), alanine aminotransferase (ALT), gamma-glutamyltransferase (GGT), and carbohydrate-deficient transferrin (CDT), also provide useful screens. Unless the physician screens all patients who use alcohol and other drugs many will be missed, given that 90% of those who meet criteria for SUD do not think they have a problem (2).

2. Provide brief interventions to patients with SUD.

A growing body of evidence indicates that brief interventions by practicing clinicians are effective in reducing hazardous or harmful drinking (72). Brief interventions take less than 10 to 15 minutes. They can be manual guided (73) or as simple as communicating concern and putting the patient in contact with a treatment clinician (28). Interventions are based on motivational principles rather than being directive or confrontational. Patient-centered feedback and options are provided without threat or rejection. Rather than being annoyed by rejections of his or her recommendations, the physician "rolls with the resistance," accepts what the patient is willing to do, and follows up with some contingency recommendations if that does not work. Role models and continuity of training are important if skill in doing brief interventions is to be developed.

3. Use effective methods of counseling patients to help prevent SUD.

There is little known about the efficacy of physician efforts in primary prevention. However, we are encouraged to use motivational enhancement and cognitive behavioral techniques in recommending abstinence from addicting drugs or medications to adolescents and pregnant women. "Early recognition and treatment for hazardous and harmful drinking are aimed at decreasing progression to more severe alcohol problems that are traditionally less amenable to treatment" (5). Establishing a therapeutic alliance with the patient will help at all levels of primary, secondary, and tertiary prevention. If the physician is uncomfortable with, or does not have time for counseling, then the patient should be connected with a professional with skills in psychosocial counseling for SUD.

The tasks of primary prevention have usually been left to the fields of education and community organization. However, it is clear that primary prevention work, in the sense of preventing new cases of alcohol or other drug abuse and addiction, are very appropriate for primary care physicians in the specialties of obstetrics, pediatrics, family medicine, and general internal medicine. Kandel and Davies (74) have noted that the developmental sequence of drug use by adolescents has not changed over the past 20 years. They note that "drug use by peers and delinquent participation emerge as the two most important factors that differentiate drug users from non drug users of particular classes of drugs at each stage of the developmental sequence of drug use." The authors suggest that anything professionals can do to strengthen adolescents' commitment to schooling and education and their ties to their families might contribute to a reduction in the risk of initiating and persisting in the use of drugs. They note that any postponement of drug experimentation may in itself have positive public health consequences for a young person's well-being.

4. Refer patients with SUD to treatment settings that provide pharmacotherapy and psychosocial therapy for relapse prevention.

Once abstinence is established there is a very high risk of relapse (30). Research in the past decade has highlighted the value of pharmacotherapy and psychosocial therapy in reducing the rate of relapse (75). Naltrexone, acamprosate, disulfiram, and the selective serotonin reuptake inhibitors (SSRIs) have helped alcohol dependence. Methadone, levo-alpha-acetylmethadol (LAAM), naltrexone, and buprenorphine have helped opioid dependence. Nicotine and bupropion have helped nicotine dependence. Anticonvulsants, for example, carbamazepine, have helped reduce craving (76).

There are no medications available to reduce relapse to marijuana, cocaine, or other stimulant addictions. "The good news from 1998 and 1999 is that evidence for the efficacy of several psychosocial treatments for substance abuse has been reported" (77). The authors also note that "[s]everal studies have pointed to the importance of

12-step involvement as a primary or adjunctive aspect of substance dependence treatment."

5. Recognize and treat or refer comorbid medical and psychiatric conditions in patients with SUD.

High rates of comorbid disorders have been reported in patients with SUD. Two national studies found 29% to 37% prevalence of comorbid psychiatric disorders in patients with alcohol problems (78,79). Comorbid medical problems are also common, including trauma and infections such as hepatitis B and C, endocarditis, human immunodeficiency virus (HIV), tuberculosis, and cellulitis. All too often the medical and psychiatric problems attract the attention of the physician and the SUD is missed or overlooked. The available data and clinical experience indicate that better outcomes occur when the SUD and medical/psychiatric conditions are treated concurrently rather than consecutively. The challenge for medical educators is to find clinical training sites where concurrent treatment is being done by, or facilitated by, medical role models.

6. Refer patients with SUD to appropriate treatment and supportive services.

Referral to treatment programs should be done when there is evidence of alcohol or other drug dependence, especially when the patient continues to drink or use other drugs despite the physician's attempts at interventions. The NIAAA guide recommends involving the patient in making referral decisions (33). This should include a discussion of available addiction treatment services in the community. Referral works best when a referral appointment is scheduled while the patient is in the office. A direct link to the referral source at that time increases patient compliance. The physician should be aware of treatment resources within the physician's community. These resources should offer a multimodality, community-based treatment. The practice guidelines of the American Psychiatric Association describe programs that provide detoxification and other pharmacologic treatments, educational services, cognitive–behavioral and interpersonal therapies, including groups and families, and active participation in 12-step programs such as AA and/or NA (32).

It is recommended that treatment take place in the least-restrictive settings that are likely to be safe and effective. This may begin with hospitalization or residential treatment. It will usually continue into partial or day care and then into outpatient treatment. The duration of treatment is tailored to individual needs and may vary from a few months to several years. Good programs continue to monitor their patients for the first year or two following cessation of active treatment. This monitoring can be done cooperatively with the primary care physician. The NIAAA physician's guide recommends monitoring the patient's progress in much the same way that the physician would monitor other chronic medical problems such as hyper-tension or diabetes. Exposure to good treatment settings during medical school and residency training is essential, if the physician is to make effective referrals and support his patient during the long-term treatment that SUD requires.

7. Describe the ethical and legal issues around physician impairment from SUD and of the resources for referring potential impaired colleagues, including employee assistance programs, hospital-based committees, state medical association physician health programs, and licensure boards.

Special programs have been developed to evaluate and treat physicians and other health care professionals with SUD (80,81). The currently existing system of state medical association's physician assistance committees was catalyzed by a landmark article in the *Journal of the American Medical Association* in 1973 (82). By 1980, every state had a physician assistance committee that usually worked in cooperation with the state board of medical examiners.

Physicians are as vulnerable as the general population to alcohol abuse and dependence and have a much greater access to other addicting drugs. Every practicing physician should be aware of the fundamentals of physician impairment. This is especially important if the physician works in a group practice, practices in a hospital setting, or has a responsible position on the medical staff of a hospital or clinic. The treatment of alcohol- and other drug-addicted physicians has developed rapidly in the last two decades. It is generally more intensive and longer than that used for the treatment of addictive disorders within the community. It should also be noted that recovering physicians are generally monitored for at least 5 years following treatment for addiction.

8. Identify the legal and ethical issues involved in the care of patients with SUD.

Legal complications are common in patients with more severe SUD. Arrests for driving under the influence, drunk and disorderly, possession, and the like may result in sentencing involving probation or parole. This coercive pressure can be very helpful in keeping patients in treatment for their SUD and enforcing abstinence long enough for recovery to begin to occur. Physicians who learn to cooperate with drug courts and probation or parole officers can be a major help to their patients and acquire information that might otherwise be difficult to obtain.

On the other hand, preserving patient confidentiality is both a legal and ethical necessity. Sometimes a physician will need to stand up to authority, armed with the support of the federal regulations in the Code of Federal Regulations(42 CFR). Patients being treated for SUD have protection from everything but a court order, providing them with the protection of being heard in court.

- Level II: All physicians coordinating care for patients with SUD in addition should:

1. Use effective methods to assess patients with SUD.

Training for the development of *assessment skills* is diagnostic training. The skills necessary to diagnose substance abuse or substance dependence are best acquired in clinical settings. For all physicians the focus should be on the area of substance use associated with problems in the patient's life. The association of problems related to alcohol and drug use provide the criteria necessary for making an accurate diagnosis. This includes skill in taking a history from the patient and acquiring information from other sources, including family members. The level II physician will be very familiar with drug testing of breath, urine, blood, and hair. These tests also have utility in treatment and can be very useful in both monitoring recovery and establishing objective evidence of abstinence. Instruments such as the Addiction Severity Index (ASI) can be very useful in assessing the medical, psychosocial, legal, and family problems associated with the patient's SUD (83).

2. Provide pharmacologic withdrawal to patients with SUD.

Withdrawal from addicting drugs can be done safely in inpatient or office settings (84). In all instances, withdrawal should be done in conjunction with psychosocial treatment for addiction, including involvement in a 12-step program. "The use of symptom-triggered, instead of fixed, doses of benzodiazepines has been shown to reduce length of stay and cost for patients treated for alcohol withdrawal" (85).

Opioid withdrawal is more problematic, but can be done in ambulatory and inpatient settings. The problem is relapse, which seems to occur more rapidly and more often than with other addicting drugs. When detoxification fails, or is unacceptable to the opioid addict, opioid maintenance therapy may be indicated.

- Level III: All physicians providing specialty services to patients with SUD in addition should:

1. Provide pharmacotherapy for relapse prevention in patients with SUD.

One of the principles of addiction treatment outlined in NIDA's research-based guide is that "[m]edications are an important element of treatment for many patients, especially when combined with counseling and other behavioral therapies" (86). Physicians at this level will often be working with multidisciplinary teams. The APA's *Position Statement on Training Needs in Addiction Psychiatry* states that "[p]sychiatrists should therefore be trained to assume leadership roles in proper management, education, and consultation with these diverse disciplines in relation to patients with substance-related disorders" (87). In a following position statement on substance-related

disorders, the APA notes the problems associated with prescribing:

> "Medications used in general medical and psychiatric care have the potential for dependence when prescribed inappropriately or when misused by patients or others. . . . APA supports educational efforts to improve prescribing practices" (88).

2. Provide or refer for psychosocial counseling for relapse prevention in patients with SUD.

Research in the psychosocial therapies in the last decade demonstrates the effectiveness of this aspect of treatment. McLellan notes that new evidence has emerged showing that participation in AA is associated with "much better abstinence records than patients who have received rehabilitation treatments but have not continued in AA" (40). Researchers from the NIDA Collaborative Cocaine Treatment Study, reflecting on their own and other's research, comment on "the importance of 12-step involvement as a primary or adjunctive aspect of substance dependence treatment" (77). Competence in referring and supporting patient participation in 12-step programs has become a core competence for physicians at all three levels.

TEACHING METHODS AND EVALUATION

Teaching methods are being addressed more frequently in the substance abuse literature. The lecture is the best known method of passing on the knowledge base. Lectures have little influence on attitudes or skills, but can serve as an introduction to be followed by clinical experience. For the faculty member who has been assigned the task of developing course material, Project Mainstream provides useful outlines and material for a variety of settings (5). Recovering AA or NA members can also be very useful in the classroom, in small-group discussions, and in taking medical students to open meetings.

Miller and his colleagues at Michigan State surveyed the literature and medical school curricula (89). They concluded that integration of substance abuse teaching is needed at all levels of medical training. "Format for teaching should include case studies, small group discussions, seminars, workshops, role playing, and direct contact in clinical supervision with patients." The difficulty in achieving this integration is well illustrated by the experience of Johns Hopkins University School of Medicine, which was one of the first medical schools to set up a model curriculum in substance abuse in 1985. Evaluation of this program showed that the preclinical courses worked well. Teaching in the clinical years was less successful, unless the students participated in special programs or elective courses focusing on substance abuse (90).

In the clinical clerkship years students need exposure to addiction treatment programs. This experience has the greatest impact if there is continuity in following patients and exposure to residents working in these programs. In residency training, supervised clinical experience on addiction treatment units appears to be essential for the development of positive attitudes and clinical skills. There should then be an opportunity for applying this knowledge, attitudes, and skills in both ambulatory and hospital settings in their own specialty.

The importance of continued clinical supervision by attendings with skills in addiction medicine was illustrated by the experience in internal medicine residency at Harvard (91). At Harvard, they compared the training of residents by lectures and discussion meetings combined with consultation and teaching in the outpatient clinics with a 1-month rotation on an inpatient alcoholism unit, with exposure to AA, outpatient treatment, and individual case supervision by alcoholism experts. The only training predictor which significantly ($P < 0.001$) predicted a perceived prevalence of alcoholism in patients, a willingness to initiate treatment, and a willingness to refer to specialized treatment, was the amount of supervised clinical experience that the resident had had.

The authors concluded that "the most direct strategy to influence physician's skills and practice behavior appears to be the provision of clinical experience and training relevant to their practices rather than to change attitudes or increase knowledge." This data supports the superiority of supervised clinical training in a specialized setting over good courses taught in an academic setting. Clinical supervision in a specialized setting is a standard teaching strategy in most areas of medical training and should become standard in addiction medicine training. Supervised clinical experience with rapid feedback to the resident or physician who has responsibility for patient care comes closest to satisfying the conditions for effective adult learning (92).

The development of clinical skills in addiction medicine requires building on the foundation begun in undergraduate medical education and continued into residency training. The magnitude of this task is illustrated by a 1989 study of addiction medicine teaching in psychiatry (93). This was the year that the Psychiatry Residency Review Committee mandated that all psychiatry residencies offer a structured experience in addiction treatment (21). At that time, 97% of undergraduate and 91% of residency programs offered curriculum units in substance abuse. It was noted, however, that almost half of the programs did not expose their students to 12-step programs, few taught chronic pain management, and little attention was paid to dual-diagnosis patients!

Two model programs in psychiatric addiction education were developed at the University of California, San Diego (UCSD) and Texas Tech. At UCSD, all second-year residents in psychiatry rotate for a minimum of 8 weeks in the addiction treatment program (94). At Texas Tech, the second-year residents rotate for 4 months in addiction treatment (95). Each program also has fellowships in addiction medicine for physicians who want to become "competent clinicians and consultants in this increasingly specialized field."

Since 1989 there has been little reported about the quality of psychiatric education in addiction medicine, other than the dynamic growth of the American Academy of Addiction Psychiatry (96). In the meantime, the work done in primary care education is having results. Faculty (N = 49) and residents (N = 95) in internal medicine at three outpatient primary care practices at Boston University's School of medicine noted that 24% of their patients had alcohol abuse or dependence, and 15% had drug abuse or dependence (97). Both faculty and residents felt responsible for caring for substance abusers and were positive in their attitudes. However, they experienced less professional satisfaction and success than in treating patients with traditional medical disorders such as hypertension. The remarkable aspect of this study is that the faculty experienced more professional satisfaction (49%) when caring for alcoholic patients than did the residents (32%). Part of this achievement may stem from the fact that three of the faculty reporting the study are active members of AMERSA.

The Macy Conference emphasized the need for faculty role models (4). These are most likely to come from physicians who have taken training in addiction medicine. The most intensive training is found in fellowships. The Center for Medical Fellowships in Alcoholism and Drug Abuse tracks all fellowship programs that have been established in residencies approved by the American Board of Medical Specialties. Most of these fellowships require completion of postgraduate training in an accredited specialty and last for 1 year (98). The development of a certification exam by ASAM in 1986, and the Certificate of Added Qualification in Addiction Psychiatry by the American Board of Psychiatry and Neurology in 1993, provide recognized roots for the development of competent faculty and teaching clinicians. It is to be hoped that the other boards of medical specialties will accept the recommendation of the Macy Conference and add Certificates of Added Qualification in Addiction Medicine (4).

Medical education in substance abuse is most effective when clear objectives are stated for knowledge, attitudes, and skills. The ultimate objective of this training is improved patient care through early diagnosis, before tissue and social damage have occurred, followed by effective treatment intervention. Unfortunately, evaluation is an area for which medical education prepares us poorly, if at all. We are exposed to examinations of various kinds throughout our training but we take them far more often than we give them. There is little opportunity to construct good multiple choice questions, patient management problems, standardized clinical examinations, or attitudinal surveys. A survey of substance abuse training programs for health care professionals in English-speaking countries concluded that "most reported programs are lacking in any meaningful evaluation that could provide data for evidence in the design of future programs" (13). A similar survey of medical school courses in England reported that there was no written component to the examinations given in 70% of the departments (99).

Knowledge examinations are the easiest to construct, but even these require so much work and analysis that no standardized examination exists. It is tempting to believe that multiple-choice questions test clinical skills, but there is no evidence to support this claim. The Psychiatry Residents in Training Examination develops a new pool of more than 20 questions for use in this annual examination that is given to most of the psychiatry residents in the United States. Because these questions, with the appropriate references, are made available to residents following the annual administration of the examination, they have the potential of forming a pool of questions that could be used in evaluating courses in addiction medicine.

Attitudinal evaluation has been considered both important and difficult. The career teachers in the 1970s gave a high priority to attitudinal change and its evaluation. They developed the Substance Abuse Attitude Scale (SAAS) (58). The SAAS was validated with criterion clinicians who experienced satisfaction in treating substance abusers. However, it shares a problem with all attitudinal surveys in that it has no clearly defined relationship to clinical practice.

Skills assessment has posed a significant challenge to medical educators. Early attempts compare changes in frequency of diagnosing alcoholics in a patient population (100). Patient management problems or simulated patient encounters provide another means of assessing skills without the cost and inconvenience of direct practice observation. The use of standardized patients in Observed Standardized Clinical Examinations (OSCE) is expensive but very useful (101). Chart audits in clinical settings can also be used to evaluate the acquisition of physician skills. This technique, used in a family practice setting, confirmed the Harvard experience that a rotation on an addiction treatment unit significantly increased primary care resident recognition of alcoholism ($P <0.05$) and chemical dependence ($P <0.001$) (102).

A similar study, on an orthopedics ward in New Zealand, demonstrated significant improvement in diagnosis and intervention on alcoholism (103). The authors noted the "amazing plasticity" of junior doctors as they adapted to the attitudes and expectations of the attending physi-

cians. They also noted how rapidly the gains disappeared when the teaching stopped. Sustained teaching and supervision are needed if clinical practice changes are to be maintained.

Evaluation can be considered a form of educational research. Reporting the results can help the educator maintain academic viability. Such results are not always pleasant. Our students do not always apply what we think they have learned. Assistance from experts in evaluation can be very useful, when the feedback from students is negative or wounding. This assistance is particularly useful in shaping the feedback provided to faculty who participate in the educational process.

CONCLUSION

This chapter briefly outlines some of the fundamentals that medical education in addiction medicine must address. A solid and growing body of knowledge has developed from both research and clinical practice. Positive attitudes toward individuals with addictive disorders and optimism about treatment help the physician transmit hope and retain a healthy curiosity about these cunning, baffling, and powerful problems. Clinical skills were identified and described in increasing detail. These skills appear to be best acquired in supervised clinical settings with continuing supervision for the resident. Evaluation methods have been developed that enable faculty to assess the effectiveness of education in the areas of knowledge, attitudes, and skill.

Alcohol and other drug addictions continue to challenge our medical and social health. Medical education in addiction medicine has emerged from a past where the primary disease of addiction was ignored and attention was focused on treating the medical sequelae of the disease. The results of this neglect are documented in this chapter and in other parts of this textbook. More recently, managed care has had a profound effect on the practice of addiction medicine, changing the places and, to some extent, the nature of our practices. Inpatient hospitalization has been drastically reduced (104). More addiction treatment is taking place in outpatient settings, which are particularly well suited for training primary care physicians. I, otherwise echo the challenge the Macy Conference has made to the primary care specialties and would add the other specialties, especially surgery and emergency medicine.

At the present time there is a shortage of subspecialists to teach addiction medicine in each of the medical specialties. This means that clinical departments may have to look for teachers from other clinical specialties, for example, psychiatry and family medicine, until they can develop their own. The last two decades have produced a cadre of experienced clinicians who can materially upgrade medical education in addiction medicine. Any medical school and/or residency training program in the United States will be able to find experienced faculty by contacting ASAM, AMERSA, or AAAP (American Academy of Addiction Psychiatry). These specialists in addiction medicine can serve as supervisors and role models to medical students and residents.

REFERENCES

1. Fiellin DA, Butler R, D'Onofrio G, et al. The physician's role in caring for patients with substance use disorders: implications for medical education and training. *Subst Abuse* 2002;23(3):207–222.
2. Bender E. Drug users not finding their way to treatment. *Psychiatric News* 2002 Oct4:14. (2001 National Household Survey on Drug Abuse available at www.drugabusestatistics.samsha.gov.).
3. McGinnis JM, Foege WH. Actual causes of death in the United States. *JAMA* 1993;25(4):2207–2212.
4. Macy Conference Proceedings. Training about alcohol and substance abuse for all primary care physicians. 1995. Available from Josiah Macy Jr. Foundation, 44 East 66th St., New York, NY, 10021.
5. Haack MR, Adger H, eds. Strategic plan for interdisciplinary faculty development: arming the nation's health professional workforce for a new approach to substance use disorders. *Subst Abuse* 2002;[suppl 23]:1–345. See Web site at www.projectmainstream.net.
6. Rush B. *An inquiry into the effects of ardent spirits upon the human body and mind: with an account of the means of preventing and of the remedies for curing them,* 8th ed. Springfield, MA: Merriam Webster, 1814.
7. Musto DF. *The American disease: origins of narcotic control.* New Haven, CT: Yale University Press, 1973: 122.
8. Cashman SD. *Prohibition: the lie of the land.* New York: The Free Press, 1981.
9. American Medical Society on Alcoholism and Other Drug Dependencies (AMSAODD), now American Society of Addiction Medicine (ASAM), 12 West 21st St., New York, NY, 10010. Directory of Information Resources Online (DIRLINE) National Library of Medicine database, Bethesda, MD, 1990. Telephone 1-(800)-638-8480.
10. Report of Officers. Hospitalization of patients with alcoholism. *JAMA* 1956;162:750. House of Delegates. Summary of action. *JAMA* 1966;198: 34.
11. American Medical Student Association. *Appendix II: alcoholism education in American medical schools. Ann N Y Acad Sci* 1971;178:135–138.
12. Labs SM. The Career Teacher Grant program: alcohol and drug abuse education for the health professions. *J Med Educ* 1981;56(3):202–204.
13. Ewan CE, Whaite A. Training health professionals in substance abuse: a review. *Int J Addict* 1982;17(7):1211–1229.
14. Lewis DC, Niven RG, Czechowicz D, et al. A review of medical education in alcohol and other drug abuse. *JAMA* 1987;257(21):2945–2948.
15. Department of Health and Human Services. *Clinical training grants for faculty development in alcohol and other drug abuse.* RFA-AA-90-02. Catalog of Federal Domestic Assistance No. 13.214. Rockville, MD: Author, 1990.
16. Alcoholics Anonymous. *The story of how many thousands of men and woman have recovered from alcoholism,* 4th ed. New York: AA World Services, 2001. AA literature may be obtained from General Service Office, Box 459, Grand Central Station, New York, NY 10163.
17. Talbott GD, Gallegos KV, Wilson PO, et al. The Medical Association of Georgia's impaired physician program: review of the first thousand physicians. *JAMA* 1987;257:2927–2930.
18. ASAM. Profile of ASAM members specialties. *ASAM News* 1990;5:7. See also AMSA news in *Alcohol Clin Exp Res* 1981;5:582.
19. Bowen OR, Sammons JH. The alcohol abusing patient: a challenge to the profession. *JAMA* 1988;260:2267–2270.
20. American Psychiatric Association. Position statement of substance abuse. *Am J Psychiatry* 1981;138(6):874–875.
21. Residency Review Committee. *Special essentials (requirements) for graduate education in psychiatry.* Washington, DC: American Psychiatric Association, November, 1989.
22. American Medical Association. *Report on the Council on Medical Education.* Chicago: Author, 1998.
23. Fleming MF, Manwell LB, Kraus M, et al. Who teaches residents about the prevention and treatment of substance use disorders? *J Fam Pract* 1999;48(9): 725–729.
24. Mendleson JH, Chafetz ME. Alcoholism as an emergency ward problem. *Q J Stud Alcohol* 1959;20:270–275.
25. Chafetz ME, Blane HT, Abram HS, et al. Establishing treatment relations with alcoholics. *J Nerv Ment Dis* 1962;134(5):395–409.
26. Westermeyer J, Doheny S, Stone B. An assessment of hospital care for the alcoholic patient. *Alcohol Clin Exp Res* 1978;2(1):53–57.
27. Pursch JA. Physicians' attitudinal changes in alcoholism. *Alcohol Clin Exp Res* 1978;2(4):358–361.
28. Moore RD, Bone LR, Geller G, et al. Prevalence, detection, and treatment of alcoholism in hospitalized patients. *JAMA* 1989;261(3):403–407.
29. Morse RM, Flavin DK. The definition of alcoholism. *JAMA* 1992;268:1012–1014.
30. McLellan AT, Lewis DC, O'Brien CP, et al. Drug dependence, a chronic medical illness; implications for treatment, insurance, and outcomes evaluation. *JAMA* 2000;284:1689–1695.
31. Koob GF, Bloom FE. Cellular and molecular mechanisms of drug dependence. *Science* 1998;242:715–723.
32. APA Work Group on Substance Use Disorders. Practice guidelines for the treatment of patients with substance use disorders: alcohol, cocaine, opioids. *Am J Psychiatry* 1995;152(11) [suppl]:1–59.
33. National Institute on Alcohol Abuse and Alcoholism. *The physician's guide to helping patients with alcohol problems.* National Institutes of Health Pub. No. 95–3769. National Institute on Alcohol Abuse and Alcoholism, Rockville, MD 1995.
34. Dube GE, Goldstein MD, Lewis DC, et al. *Project ADEPT: curriculum for primary care physician training. Vol. 1: core modules, 1989; vol. 2: special topics and videotape, 1990.* Providence, RI: Brown University Center for Alcohol and Addiction Studies, 1989–1990.
35. Institute of Medicine. *Broadening the case of treatment for alcohol problems.* Washington DC: National Academy Press, 1989.
36. Skinner HA. Spectrum of drinkers and intervention opportunities. *CMAJ* 1990;143(10):1054–1059.
37. Fleming MF, Barry KL, Manwell LB, et al. Brief physician advice for problem alcohol drinkers. A randomized controlled trial in community based primary care practices. *JAMA* 1997;277:1039–1045.
38. Vaillant GE. *The natural history of*

alcoholism: revisited. Cambridge, MA: Harvard University Press, 1995.

39. Kandel DB, Davies M. High school students who use crack and other drugs. *Arch Gen Psychiatry* 1996;53(1):71–80.

40. McLellan AT. Is addiction an illness—can it be treated? *Subst Abuse* 2002;23(3):67–94.

41. Shuckit MA. *Drug and alcohol abuse: a clinical guide to diagnosis and treatment,* 5th ed. New York: Kluwer-Plenum, 2000.

42. Chappel JN, Schnoll SH. Physician attitudes: effects on the treatment of chemically dependent patients. *JAMA* 1977;237(21):2318–2319.

43. Allport GW. Attitudes. In: Murchison CA, ed. *A handbook of social psychology.* Worchester, MA: Clark University Press, 1935:798–845.

44. Eiser JR. *Social psychology: attitudes, cognition, and social behavior.* New York: Cambridge University Press, 1986:11.

45. Sudnow D. *Passing on: the social organization of dying.* Englewood Cliffs, NJ: Prentice-Hall, 1967:104–109.

46. Rado S. The psychoanalysis of pharmacothymia (drug addiction). *Psychoanal Q* 1933;2:1–3.

47. Brickman B. Psychoanalysis and substance abuse: toward a more effective approach. *J Am Acad Psychoanal* 1988;16(3):359–379.

48. Khantzian EJ, Mack, JE. Alcoholics Anonymous and contemporary psychodynamic theory. *Recent Dev Alcohol* 1989;7:67–89.

49. Bean-Bayog M. Psychopathology produced by alcoholism. In: Meyer R, ed. *Psychopathology and addictive disorders.* New York: Guilford Press, 1986:334–345.

50. Conard S, Hughes P, Baldwin DC, et al. Substance use by fourth year students at 13 U.S. medical schools. *J Med Educ* 1988;63(10):747–758.

51. Christie JD, Rosen IM, Bellini LM, et al. Prescription drug use and self-prescription among resident physicians. *JAMA* 1998;280(14):1253–1255.

52. Wachtel TJ, Wilcox VL, Moulton AW, et al. Physicians' utilization of care. *J Gen Intern Med* 1995;10:261–265.

53. Chambers R, Belcher J. Self-reported health care over the past 10 years: a survey of general practitioners. *Br J Gen Pract* 1992;42:153–156.

54. McGuire WJ. The nature of attitudes and attitude change. In: Lindzey G, Aronson E, eds. *Handbook of social psychology,* 2nd ed. Vol. 3. Reading, MA: Addison-Wellesley,1969:372–398.

55. Osgood CE, Suci GJ, Tannenbaum PH. Attitude measurement. In: Summers GF, ed. *Attitude measurement.* Chicago:

Rand McNally, 1970:237. (Originally published in 1957.)

56. Likert R. A technique for the measurement of attitudes. In: Summers GF, ed. *Attitude measurement.* Chicago: Rand McNally, 1970;149–157. (Originally published in 1932.)

57. Chappel JN, Veach TL, Krug RS. The substance abuse attitude survey: an instrument for measuring attitudes. *J Stud Alcohol* 1985;46(1):48–52.

58. Chappel JN, Veach TL. Effect of a course on students' attitudes toward substance abuse and its treatment. *J Med Educ* 1987;62(5):394–400.

59. Veach TL, Chappel JN. Physician attitudes in chemical dependency: the effects of personal experience and recovery. *Subst Abuse* 1990;11(2):97–101.

60. Sterne MW, Pittman DJ. The concept of motivation: a source of institutional and professional blockage in the treatment of alcoholics. *Q J Stud Alcohol* 1965;26:41–57.

61. Eron LD. The effect of medical education on attitudes: a follow up study. *J Med Educ* 1958;33(pt 2):25–33.

62. Fisher JC, Mason RL, Keeley KA, et al. Physicians and alcoholics: the effect of medical training on attitudes toward alcoholics. *J Stud Alcohol* 1975;7:949–955.

63. Rezler AG. Attitude changes during medical school: a review of the literature. *J Med Educ* 1974;49(11):1023–1030.

64. Flaherty JA, Flaherty EG. Medical students' performance in reporting alcohol related problems. *J Stud Alcohol* 1983;44(6):1083–1087.

65. Cooley FB. The attitudes of students and housestaff toward alcoholism [letter]. *JAMA* 1990;263(9):1197–1198.

66. Azjin I, Fishbein M. *Understanding attitudes and predicting social behavior.* Englewood Cliffs, NJ: Prentice-Hall, 1980.

67. Frank JD. *Persuasion and healing: a comparative study of psychotherapy.* Baltimore: Johns Hopkins University Press, 1973.

68. Watts W. Relative persistence of opinion change induced by active compared to passive participation. *J Pers Soc Psychol* 1967;5:4–15.

69. Cartwright AKJ. The attitudes of helping agents towards the alcoholic client: the influence of experience, support, training, and self-esteem. *Br J Addict* 1980;75:413–431.

70. Galanter M, Talbott D, Gallegos K, et al. Combined Alcoholics Anonymous and professional care for addicted physicians. *Am J Psychiatry* 1990; 147(1):64–68.

71. Fiellin DA, Reid MC, O'Connor PG. Screening for alcohol problems

in primary care: a systematic review. *Archives of Internal Medicine* 2000;160:1977–1989.

72. Fiellin DA, Reid MC, O'Connor PG. New therapies for patients with alcohol problems. *Am J Med* 2000;108:227–237.

73. Fleming MF, Barry KL, Manwell LB, et al. Brief physician advice for problem drinkers. A randomized controlled trial in community-based primary care practices. *JAMA* 1997;277: 1039–1045.

74. Kandel DB, Davies M. High school students who use crack and other drugs. *Arch Gen Psychiatry* 1996;53(1):71–80.

75. Litten RZ, Allen JP. Medications for alcohol, illicit drug, and tobacco dependence: an update of research findings. *J Subst Abuse Treat* 1999;16(2):105–112.

76. Kosten TR. The pharmacotherapy of relapse prevention using anticonvulsants. *Am J Addict* 1998;7(3):205–209.

77. Siqueland L, Crits-Christoph P. Current developments in psychosocial treatments of alcohol and substance abuse. *Curr Psychiatry Rep* 1999;1(2):179–184.

78. Kessler RC, McGonale KZ, Shanyang Z, et al. Lifetime and 12 month prevalence of *DSM-III-R* psychiatric disorders in the United States: results from the National Comorbidity Survey. *Arch Gen Psychiatry* 1994;51:8–18.

79. Regier DA, Farmer ME, Rae DS, et al. Comorbidity of mental disorders with alcohol and other drug abuse. Results from the Epidemiologic Catchment Area (ECA) study. *JAMA* 1990; 264(19):2511–2518.

80. Fleming MF. Physician impairment: options for intervention. *Am Fam Physician* 199;50:41–44.

81. Nelson HD, Matthews AM, Girard DE, et al. Substance impaired physicians probationary and voluntary treatment programs compared. *West J Med* 1996;165:31–36.

82. AMA Council on Mental Health. The sick physician: impairment by psychiatric disorders, including alcoholism and drug dependence. *JAMA* 1973;223:684–687.

83. McClellan AT, Cacciola J, Kushner H, et al. The fifth edition of the Addiction Severity Index: cautions, additions, and normative data. *J Subst Abuse Treat* 1992;9:461–480.

84. Hayashida M, Alterman AI, McClellan AT, et al. Comparative effectiveness and costs of inpatient and outpatient detoxification of patients with mild to moderate alcohol withdrawal syndrome. *N Engl J Med* 1989;320: 356–358.

85. Saitz R, Mayo-Smith MF, Roberts MS, et al. Individualized treatment for alcohol withdrawal. A randomized double-blind controlled trial. *JAMA* 1994;272(7):519–523.

86. National Institute on Drug Abuse. *Principles of drug addiction treatment: a research-based guide.* Bethesda, Maryland, National Institute of Health (NIH). NIH Publication No. 994180. 1999.

87. APA Official Actions. Position statement on training needs in addiction psychiatry. *Am J Psychiatry* 1996; 153:852–853.

88. APA Official Actions. Position statement on substance-related disorders. *Am J Psychiatry* 1996;153:853–855.

89. Miller NS, Sheppard LM, Colenda CC, et al. Why physicians are unprepared to treat patients who have alcohol and drug related disorders. *Acad Med* 2001;76:410–418.

90. Gopalan R, Santora P, Stokes E, et al. Evaluation of a model curriculum on substance abuse at the Johns Hopkins University School of Medicine. *Acad Med* 1992;67:260–266.

91. Warburg MM, Cleary PD, Rohman M, et al. Residents' attitudes, knowledge, and behavior regarding diagnosis and treatment of alcoholism. *J Med Educ* 1987;62:497–503.

92. Soumerai SB, Avorn J. Principles of educational outreach (academic detailing) to improve clinical decision making. *JAMA* 1990;263(4):549–556.

93. Galanter M, Kaufman E, Taintor Z, et al. The current status of psychiatric education in alcoholism and drug abuse. *Am J Psychiatry* 1989;146(1):35–39.

94. Shuckit MA, Berger F. The integration of an educational program into a treatment facility. *Br J Addict* 1989;84:191–195.

95. Arredondo R, Weddige RL, Pollard S, et al. Implementing a substance abuse curriculum in a medical school. *Acad Psychiatry* 1989;13:44–47.

96. American Academy of Addiction Psychiatry. www.aaap.org. Call 913–262–6161.

97. Saitz R, Friedman PD, Sullivan LM, et al. Professional satisfaction experienced when caring for substance abusing patients. *J Gen Intern Med* 2002;17:373–376.

98. Galanter M. *Postgraduate medical fellowships in alcoholism and drug abuse.* New York: Center for Medical Fellowships in Alcoholism and Drug Abuse, New York University School of Medicine, 1988.

99. Glass IB. Undergraduate training in substance abuse in the United Kingdom. *Br J Addict* 1989;84:197–202.

100. Fisher JV, Fisher JC, Mason RL. Physicians and alcoholism: modifying behavior and attitudes of family practice residents. *J Stud Alcohol* 1976;37(11):1686–1693.

101. Stillman PL, Swanson DB, Swee S, et al. Assessing clinical skills of residents with standardized patients. *Ann Intern Med* 1986;105:762–771.

102. Mulry JT, Brewer ML, Spencer DL. The effect of an inpatient chemical dependency rotation on residents' clinical behavior. *Fam Med* 1987;19(4):276–280.

103. Hamilton MR, Menkes DB, Jeffery DK. Early intervention for alcohol misuse: encouraging doctors to take action. *N Z Med J* 1994;107(989):454–456.

104. Galanter M, Keller DS, Dermatis H, et al. The impact of managed care on substance abuse treatment: a report of the American Society of Addiction Medicine. *J Addict Dis* 2000;19:13–17.

CHAPTER 81

Education and Training of Clinical Personnel

DAVID A. DEITCH, IGOR KOUTSENOK, AND KARIN MARSOLAIS

The training of clinical personnel and ancillary practitioners in the field of substance abuse is filled with colorful characters, events, debate, and, frequently, confusion. It has occurred amid bias, zeal, occasionally distorted information, chaos, and always with great passion. What is drug addiction? What is treatment and who needs it? What kind of treatment works? How do we best train personnel? Over the last four decades, these questions have been answered in radically different ways. Drug abuse has been variously labeled as criminal, psychotic, characterologic, immoral, self-indulgent, genetically influenced, a consequence of social inequality and poverty, or simply the price we pay for an alienated, consumer-based, industrialized society.

Dramatic advances over the past two decades in neuroscience, brain imaging, molecular neurobiology, and behavioral science have revolutionized our understanding of drug abuse and addiction. Scientists have identified neural circuits that subsume the actions of almost every known drug of abuse, and they have specified common pathways that are affected by such substances. Unfortunately, the bad news is that the wide gap between scientific facts and their implementation into clinical reality has become even wider. A major barrier is that some of the people who work in the fields of drug-abuse prevention and addiction treatment also hold ingrained ideologies that, although usually different in origin and form from the ideologies of general public, can be just as problematic. Many drug-abuse workers are in recovery themselves, having had a success with one particular model. They therefore zealously defend that single approach, even in the face of contradictory scientific evidence.

Given this conglomeration of information, it's no wonder that there is a lack of consensus about the most productive way to help addicts. Because of the fervent beliefs held by practitioners in the drug-abuse arena over the last 50 years, it is impossible to present a single prescription for the treatment of drug abusers and addicts. It is also impossible to present a single set of recommendations about the training of clinical personnel. Training is not extricable from the history of drug treatment in the United States during the second half of the twentieth century. Training approaches and philosophies emerge from theories of treatment; treatment theories are often affected by the observations and techniques of workers in the field of drug abuse. In light of the enormous amount of progress achieved in the development and evaluation of effective treatment for substance abuse disorders, it is distressing that the training provided for clinical professionals to deliver these treatments has not kept pace (1,2).

This chapter reviews treatment approaches in both the private and public sectors since the 1930s and the way in which those treatments have affected the training of clinical personnel. The second half of the chapter focuses on training philosophies and methods that, despite the great divergence of thinking in this field, have proved effective in countries throughout the world.

TREATMENT ISSUES

Trying to Reach a Consensus

Clinical personnel who come to be trained in the subject of substance abuse most likely arrive with a preconceived set of biases based on personal experience, varied expectations, previous training experiences, professional orientation, and beliefs about addiction itself. They may feel very strongly that their "way" is the only way (3,4) and may carry this belief into their staff roles. Some believe that addiction is a medical symptom, episodic in nature, and that the way to deal with it is through detoxification. Others believe that denial is the largest stumbling block to recovery and that once denial is conquered, recovery is sure to follow. Those schooled in therapeutic community and 12-step models may find it difficult to open themselves to new ideas based on different paradigms. In addition, nonmedical health professionals may very well be grappling with some aversion to the drug-abusing population. This aversion can take the form of hopelessness, helplessness, dislike, disgust, discomfort, and affective distancing (5).

Because of the strong convictions that both medical and nonmedical personnel bring to the arena, training in this field needs to be particularly sensitive. This sensitivity can be successfully negotiated by presenting a historical overview in a training setting, including review of some of the cultural, political, and religious features of drug use. This history is best presented in terms of its effect on treatment choices. What do we know about historical and current treatment responses to various types of drug use problems? What are the methods? What theories underlie those methods? What benefits and liabilities do some methods have over others? What are the outcomes of various methods?

The History of Treatment Challenges and Struggles

Why treat drug abusers? This must be addressed before introducing treatment theories, practical interventions, or training approaches. Different groups have different answers. For some, the aim is to help the individual overcome the use of drugs. For others, it is to help the individual live a better life, which entails addressing social and psychological issues beyond the drug abuse itself. Social concerns may also be of the utmost importance, especially creating a safer environment for non-drug users, so some turn to criminal prosecution and punishment. Others take a more global view, hoping to create a healthier world community.

Whatever the aim, drug-abuse treatment has frustrated and perplexed people for decades. From the 1920s to the early 1940s, the cultural view of the drug abuser was reflected as a person with weak character and morals. In response to that cultural belief, jail was the common remedy and the only treatment choice was to detoxify addicts based on a medical model. Invariably, however, detoxified people returned to drugs, giving rise to the conviction that "once an addict, always an addict." This myth grew along with an increase in the use of drugs and alcohol, and most medical practitioners were repulsed by having to face the "junkie" or "wino" in public hospitals. Those who suffered from drug addiction were not helped by the harrowing portrayals of such people in movies and the propaganda of Henry Anslinger, director of Federal Bureau of Narcotics from its inception in 1930 until 1962, during those decades (6).

After World War II and the first heroin epidemic in 1948, the problem slowly but steadily grew worse. Responding to it as we had for the previous 30 years, there was an increase in criminal penalties for those found guilty of using drugs. At this point in history, although the criminal model remained entrenched, some people in the field began to believe that the addict (particularly, the morphine or heroin addict) was not really a criminal first, but suffered instead from wanting drugs. Because those drugs were illegal, the addict would frequently commit crimes to obtain money to get them. During this period, the superintendent of the Federal Prison System, in 1929, was prevailed on to take addicts out of the federal prison systems, where they were both exposing nonusers to drug culture and being taught by criminals to become better at committing crimes, and to place them into a special system. These special systems became popularly known as "narcotic farms."

In a post-Depression eagerness to provide construction and other jobs for people in economically deprived areas, senators from two southern sites volunteered to house these first detention centers for addicts. The sites were located in Lexington, Kentucky, and Fort Worth, Texas. Federal prisoners were removed from various settings and relocated to one of these two centers. Eventually, other officials decided that addicts from around the country could be permitted to volunteer for these centers and that some addicts could be sent involuntarily for short stays in these "hospital 'narco-farm' jails," which were operated by the United States Public Health Service (PHS) and included the presence of security personnel.

In the early 1950s, after years of failure in other hospitals and jails, there were stirrings in the PHS of a more enlightened response to the problem of drug addiction. This expressed itself in an attempt to treat addicts by using what little was known at the time about social case work, vocational training, and (as a result of work with war veterans) some aspects of "group therapy." The thinking was that if these activities kept the addict away from drugs long enough, restored the addict to physical health, and gave the possibility of insight or job skills or social case work support, there was hope that the individual could or would return to the community, no longer requiring drugs. To some extent, these efforts were successful.

Also during this period in the United States, there had been some efforts by psychiatrists in the public health system to conduct group work with addicts. The group model was made available on a voluntary basis for those who were interested. As it turned out, the addicts drawn to group therapy were by and large fairly verbal, either by dint of their middle class status or native verbal abilities. At the same time, social workers attempted an amalgam of counseling aimed at supporting these individuals, which included some of the prevailing social case work theories existing in the country at that time. Noone realized, however, that a bridge would be necessary to ease these individuals back into society (7). This oversight resulted in failure and frustration on the part of social workers and psychologists working to heal the bumps and bruises that accompany the drug-abusing lifestyle. These workers had made sincere but patchwork efforts at rehabilitation. Consequently, despite this new work, there returned the ever-present dream that a miracle medicine could be found that would cure the problem once and for all.

Medical research was in progress at Lexington and Fort Worth in the continuing search for a "magic bullet" medication to handle the problem of drug abuse. Researchers had a powerful wish (as they do today) that just the right medicine would finally enable treatment of this multi-faceted, mystifying problem with a pill.

By 1960, heroin use had expanded greatly and with it, criminal behavior. Substance abuse professionals became discouraged again: It seemed that psychiatry had not paid off, social work had not paid off, jail in and of itself (even the PHS "narco-farm" model) had not paid off (in many instances it exacerbated the problem), and pure vocational training had not paid off. Furthermore, in the community and at large, there was little reimbursement to those professionals who had attempted to give birth to a theoretical body of thinking about addiction (8). In addition, the plethora of problems associated with trying to work with individuals whose conduct and repeated failures gave little reward meant that these practitioners did not even experience the gratification of knowing that they were making an impact on the problem. While the more articulate addicts presented an intriguing and romantic challenge by virtue of the fact that they proclaimed a desire to resist using drugs, the truth was that, regardless of interventions put into place, they continued to use them.

The problem grew worse. Finally, increased mandatory sentences, anger at the user, and self-hatred by users themselves resulted in a deadlocked, completely disheartening situation.

New Answers in the 1960s

Out of this discouragement came the first breakthroughs in the treatment of drug abuse, breakthroughs that garnered much excited press coverage throughout the 1960s. As the scope of drug abuse threatened to overwhelm the United States, two major new paradigms came into being. One was the therapeutic community (TC) movement, which began with Synanon in 1959, but did not gain widespread recognition until 1963 or 1964 with the advent of Daytop in New York. The TC approach was primarily conducted by people who had been afflicted with the problem, claiming that they alone, because of their affliction, could work successfully with this population. In the opinion of these new thinkers, those who had not suffered from drug addiction were often too indulgent and too easily manipulated. Cure could result, they felt, only in a more rigorously honest disclosure of self and a challenging demand for new behavior, conducted in large measure by those who knew the addict's world from the inside.

TCs offered the promise that, not only could they handle the addict where others had failed, but they could get people who were obsessive–compulsive drug users and criminals to stop behaving that way voluntarily. The climate at TCs was set up as one unswervingly opposed to drug use. This eliminated any cultural ambivalence, thus increasing the motivation that participants had to "stay clean." In these rigidly structured communities, there was a powerful social coercion for individuals to cooperate with treatment if they wanted to avoid something even worse, such as jail. TCs became the first model to be able to predictably influence the potential cure of heroin dependency (9,10).

The second major breakthrough in the early 1960s came out of earlier research with the German-invented narcotic Dolophine at the U.S. Public Health Hospital at Lexington: the development of methadone. This synthetic narcotic, as implemented by Vincent Dole at The Rockefeller University, seemed to hold the hope that methadone maintenance was the magic pill that could cure drug addiction. High doses could reduce brain craving and offset preoccupation with the lifestyle of heroin addiction. Initially, methadone maintenance was resisted by those in drug enforcement, the mental health community, and by most workers in drug-free treatment communities. It slowly gained in use and credibility. Its use fit into the medical model, in that it was medication controlled by dosage. As such, it lent itself to a wide variety of studies in the academic and medical communities. These studies tended to verify its promise (11).

Within the drug treatment culture, Alcoholics Anonymous (AA) did exist, although no one considered it a breakthrough applicable to the special problems of drug addiction. Narcotics Anonymous (NA) was created as a way of engaging heroin users, but by and large it did not prove a successful approach at that time. As a model, it simply did not prove engaging of addicts during these two decades. Alcoholics and heroine addicts frequently viewed each other with contempt and suspicion, and one would not be seen with the other.

The New "Professionals" (Paraprofessionals and Others)

Despite the discovery of methadone's ability to inhibit some heroin use behaviors, it soon proved evident that the medication itself was not enough to "cure" drug addiction. Those people who, in the early 1960s, claimed that personal experience with addiction was a route toward successfully engaging users became more prominent. It became clear that this "been there" approach had great merit (4). These ex-addicts became the first nonacademically trained, nonprofessional drug rehabilitation workers. They became known as "paraprofessionals" in the field, working either in separate freestanding settings (such as TCs) or in conjunction with some medical professionals who adjusted methadone doses and performed other medical diagnostic procedures. They also saw themselves as experts, sometimes the only experts, and were often considered such by professionals and addicts alike (12). Their tough, pragmatic, sometimes brutally honest, empathetic approach to the problems of addiction, along with their intimate knowledge of the workings of an addict's life, gave the field a much-needed push in the direction of understanding and creating real change in lives that seemed hopeless.

The Middle Class Enters the Picture

The majority of treatments for drug addiction in the second half of the twentieth century were aimed at the bewildering problem of heroin addiction and its attendant criminal activity. However, the use of drugs of choice—such as heroin—did not remain static. During the late 1960s and early 1970s, there was a slow, but ever-expanding, use of other drugs, particularly marijuana and the "psychedelics." It is crucial to understand that, because these "new" drugs were used in large part by children of the middle class, some of the previous criminal sanctions surrounding drug abusers were called into question. Middle-class parents did not want their children to go to jail. Confusion reigned about how destructive these new drugs were, primarily because the many youthful users of these drugs seemed to demonstrate to their parents that they could use the drugs without problems, and because criminal penalties for the possession and use of these drugs were disproportionate to any problems created by them.

As this elite class of drug users grew, so did cultural ambivalence. An aura of intrigue clung to the psychedelic drug user. Across the country, an almost religious response arose in people who did not necessarily use these psychedelics, but who wanted to rub elbows with those who did. These people often adopted the style of these users, if not the drug use itself, and wanted to become part of saving/helping groups that rapidly formed. However, some of these "helpers" did use psychedelics themselves. "Crash pads" and "psychedelic clinics" came into being all across the nation. Everyone wanted to get in on the act of treating a child with whom they could finally identify: mostly white and college educated. Many of these young people who asked for help had either overused a drug or had a bad experience with these particular drugs. Furthermore, an air of romance clung to these users, so much so that other youth with a variety of mental health problems claimed drug use as a way of getting some attention. Many of the helpers and some of the users were students in professional schools of psychology, social work, and psychiatry. Their readiness to work with these youngsters was at times quite cavalier; at other times it was to use traditional models or those that were in professional vogue at the time (e.g., Gestalt, Sensitivity, Scream Therapy, Transactional Analysis). Much of the "helping" took place in hastily set up clinics—some on the street, and others associated with student counseling centers, mental health centers, and finally churches and dormitories.

The Government Steps In

By 1970, in the Nixon administration, the first "War on Drugs" began in the form of the Special Action Office for Drug Abuse Prevention (SAODAP). Shortly thereafter came the birth of the National Institute of Drug Abuse (NIDA). SAODAP, with the help of NIDA, mounted a national strategy meant to diminish the problem of drug abuse in America. The goal was to create a treatment system that could accomplish the following outcomes (in order of priority):

1. To reduce crime in the streets
2. To reduce tax-consumptive behavior (i.e., any activity that costs the public money such as welfare, unemployment, public hospitals)
3. To reduce illicit drug use
4. To increase tax-productive behavior (i.e., any activity that restores individuals so they can work and earn money)
5. To enhance personal well-being

At that point, one of the tasks of these new agencies was to develop a pool of person-power that could finally address the treatment of this pervasive problem on a national level. This indicated a clear switch, both in overt policy and in mentality. The addict would no longer be exclusively a criminal; instead, the addict was also to become a "patient." In light of this new view, "treatment systems" were the way to deal with the drug user, because treatment promised to show some positive outcome where incarceration in and of itself had not. This new approach called for a network of national treatment agencies and experts who could devote the time and research necessary to become career practitioners and teachers in the field, and training became paramount. Within NIDA, the Manpower Training Branch was created to train these practitioners. Its goals were as follows:

1. To train career teachers so that medical schools and schools of professional training could teach others within their profession. To further this aim, grants were made available.
2. To offer grants to individual researchers in the field of drug abuse.
3. To train a large pool of practitioners around the country in a way that would positively affect their present treatment efforts in the field (13,14).

Although this expansion created fresh enthusiasm, it also created a certain amount of chaos. How were we to track various treatments? How were we to verify efficacy? To answer these questions, systems of reporting, patient tracking, and program management were instituted. As a result of quality-of-care concerns within the Division of Community Assistance under the leadership of Lee Dogoloff, the Clinical Review Board was created. Its goal was to study treatment programs around the country and set standards for acceptable clinical care. The Board's overriding concern was to ensure that treatment centers show consideration for their patients rather than get caught up in the zeal and excitement of a new national policy.

The concerns created additional definite training needs.

1. How does one manage the bureaucratic needs of an expanding system and respond to funding agents' requests for data?
2. How does one become trained to implement the baseline requisite standards that would ensure that individuals in treatment receive high-quality care?

In response, many paraprofessionals received a series of trainings in compliance with these demands. These trainings covered various treatment approaches, assessment, establishing rapport, managing an environment, short- and long-term planning, and report writing.

Some Gains, Some Losses

This new national interest attracted many new professionals to the field because of their college experiences working with psychedelic drug users and the possibility of rewarding salaries and an increase in social status. They merged with the paraprofessionals who had already been working in the field. As a result of the merger, the traditional methodologies and counseling approaches taught in graduate schools were reignited in the national training systems. Short-term treatment planning and short-term counseling systems, more in line with conventional psy-

chological counseling and social work counseling, took some precedence over TC approaches and work done by the earlier paraprofessionals in the treatment of heroin addicts. Some crossover of approaches did occur, but there were definite demands on the paraprofessional treater to adopt many of the methods and approaches of the middle-class psychedelic treatment approach within the training system. While there were benefits for the street paraprofessionals and TCs in establishing treatment and tracking plans, some of the unique methodological breakthroughs, skills, and approaches pioneered by therapeutic communities and methadone maintenance were neglected.

Treatment systems across the country attempted to expand in light of the new public funds available and a resurgence of interest in the field. In the mid-1970s, however, during the Carter administration, these public funds were cut back just as the field began to mount a national effort against drug abuse, and just as these systems began to show positive outcomes. The field lost career teachers, the more-trained practitioners, and a large part of the infrastructure of NIDA (along with the accrued education and experience within that agency). Public funds and support eroded even further during the Reagan years.

During these same years of funding reductions, however, services grew in two quarters. The first quarter expansion was in public sector methadone-maintenance programs and TCs, and the second quarter expansion included private for-profit insurance reimbursement approaches.

Later, within the public sector, heroin users continued to seek help from methadone maintenance clinics, especially as the threat of acquired immunodeficiency syndrome (AIDS) in intravenous (i.v.) drug users took root. TCs expanded to meet an increase in demand as well. The TC had realized that the methods originally intended to aid heroin addicts were equally effective with multidrug users and ever-younger users. Both methadone clinics and TCs responded strongly during the years of government cutbacks, despite the decrease in public money available to them.

The second quarter expansion took place in the 1980s; it consisted of privately funded, for-profit drug programs operating chiefly in hospitals. This new direction in treatment germinated from the incorporation of AA and 12-step programs into hospital settings under the umbrella of doctors and other allied health providers. Because the first of these programs began at Willmar State Hospital in Minnesota and was further refined at Hazelden and the Johnson Institute in Minnesota, these programs are often referred to as the "Minnesota Model."

This model also became known as the "28-day program," as an outgrowth of the insurance industry placing limits on maximum hospital lengths of stay. They arrived at this figure coincidentally, based on a study made on the average length of inpatient stays early on at Hazelden. The populations studied at Hazelden—white, middle-class males between the ages of 25 and 40 years, most of whom had alcohol problems and all of whom had a fairly successful work history—showed relatively good outcomes. Because the insurance industry was willing to fund this length of stay, hospitals across the country were eager to implement this 28-day model.

The Return of Stimulants: Cocaine

The national surge in cocaine use that occurred in the late 1970s supported the advent of these 28-day programs. As cocaine overuse worked its way down steadily from the upper and middle classes, both working and middle class youth began to get into trouble with this drug. Neither these groups nor their families seriously considered treatment in public sector programs (at least, not until their insurance funds were depleted). In response to the middle class' search for answers, hospitals expanded the base of the Minnesota Model and even the 28-day program, now calling themselves chemical-dependency treatment programs (CDs). The private-sector CD response to this burgeoning cocaine abuse was based on a trend of considering the problem as a disease. Borrowing from the rich history of AA, those who followed the disease model of drug abuse developed a set of approaches incorporating 12-step activities.

Two-Tier Treatment System

By the end of the 1980s, a two-tier response system existed, with the public nonprofit groups (stretched thin as a result of diminished public funding and with massive waiting lists) and the private for-profit groups competing with each other for clients. Both tiers required training to either respond to demand or to improve the attractiveness of their services. Despite the multiplicity of these public- and private-sector programs that now exist in explicit response to drug abuse, training had not kept pace in its ability to prepare those who work in the field. A 1981 survey of graduate schools in psychology found a "disproportionately low" level of training in substance abuse issues "relative to the magnitude of these problems" (15). A 1982 study reviewed a population in English-speaking countries and found four essential types of courses: those for practitioners and teachers of health professionals, those for medical students, those for nurses and nursing students, and those for allied health professionals. In spite of the apparent thoroughness of these curricula, the study found very little guidance for future program development (16). In light of these findings, it is imperative to examine both the content and ideology of successful training programs for drug abuse workers.

TRAINING ISSUES

How Bias Affects Treatment and Training

Those who come to drug-abuse training programs often do so with strong biases. These biases result from prior pro-

fessional or lay education, as well as personal experience, and they have a significant impact on the way in which people approach training. Preconceived beliefs about substance abuse and what constitutes an appropriate response to substance abuse create a tunnel through which only some addicts can pass (17). If people are convinced that their treatment ideas are the "only" correct ideas, they tend to herd people through a rigid set of interventions that simply are not flexible enough to bend to individual needs. Cultural beliefs (be they national, regional, neighborhood, or association) further complicate these practitioner biases. Strongly held cultural views may dictate that only certain types of treatment are valid, meaningful, or useful. Some of the biases in basic thinking about substance abuse are as follows:

1. Drug abuse and drug dependence are phases of a disease process.
2. Working with a client who is actively using drugs is "enabling."
3. If clients do not think of drug abuse as an out-of-control disease, they are in denial.
4. If a client does admit to having a "disease," a 12-step program is the only concrete, long-lasting solution.
5. Psychotherapy is ineffective.
6. Psychotherapy is necessary to produce long-term recovery.
7. Medical intervention in the form of medication is destructive or impedes recovery.
8. The only real, cost-effective help lies in a medicopharmacologic response.
9. Drug-dependent people most likely have substance-dependent parents.
10. The TC approach is the only long-lasting rehabilitation that is drug free.
11. TC approaches work with only a small segment of the drug-using population.
12. Regardless of original drug-use patterns, all "recovering" people must abstain from any drug use (e.g., alcohol, medications) for the rest of their lives.

Obviously, these divergent convictions can create a chaos of misunderstanding in both treatment and training programs. No one approach is right. No one approach can be right, given the cultural, economic, experiential, and personality differences of substance abusers. The goal of drug-abuse training should be to create an atmosphere in which people are actually able to openly listen to new ideas and to offer a range of care options broad enough to encompass many kinds of addicts, at many stages of addiction.

The Continuum-of-Care Model

Options are critical to handling the complex problem of providing help to drug abusers. A model that provides a continuum of care offers the greatest possibility of engaging a variety of people at different points in their lives,

Continuum of Care Model

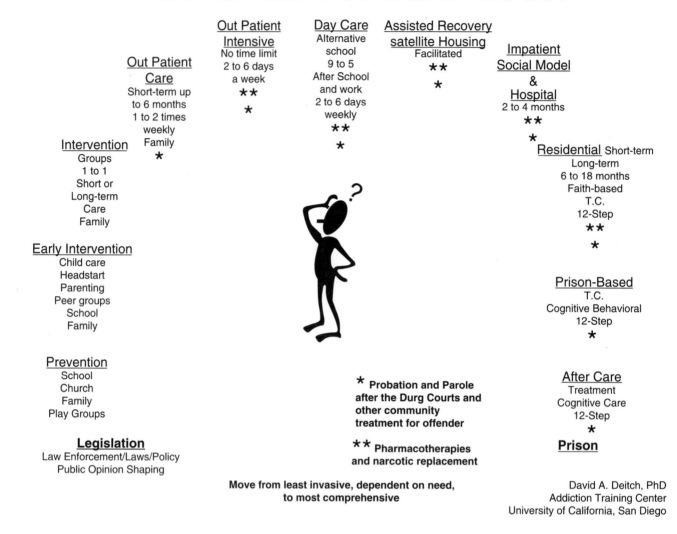

Out Patient Intensive
No time limit
2 to 6 days
a week
★★
★

Day Care
Alternative
school
9 to 5
After School
and work
2 to 6 days
weekly
★★
★

Assisted Recovery satellite Housing
Facilitated
★★
★

Impatient Social Model & Hospital
2 to 4 months
★★
★

Out Patient Care
Short-term up
to 6 months
1 to 2 times
weekly
Family
★

Intervention
Groups
1 to 1
Short or
Long-term
Care
Family

Early Intervention
Child care
Headstart
Parenting
Peer groups
School
Family

Prevention
School
Church
Family
Play Groups

Legislation
Law Enforcement/Laws/Policy
Public Opinion Shaping

Residential Short-term
Long-term
6 to 18 months
Faith-based
T.C.
12-Step
★★
★

Prison-Based
T.C.
Cognitive Behavioral
12-Step
★

After Care
Treatment
Cognitive Care
12-Step
★

Prison

★ **Probation and Parole after the Durg Courts and other community treatment for offender**

★★ **Pharmacotherapies and narcotic replacement**

Move from least invasive, dependent on need, to most comprehensive

David A. Deitch, PhD
Addiction Training Center
University of California, San Diego

depending upon their needs and resources, the severity of their problem, and the context in which their problem takes place. The flexibility of such a continuum of care is especially important because it has been shown that not only may a single model be dysfunctional for some clients, but that the mismatch may also impede treatment for others in the that setting for whom the model might actually be appropriate. Dr. Herbert Kleber states that "no known treatment is completely effective for all of its participants, nor is any existing program suitable for all kinds of drug-dependent individuals. At this time it seems unlikely that a 'technological fix' will provide a complete answer to the complex psychosocial–biologic condition known as narcotic addiction" (18). In an outpatient clinic, for example, much staff effort is spent on the most severely affected people. Clients with more modest problems may be ignored. Conversely, if the staff concentrates on those with modest problems, the more severely affected clients may be underserved. A broad base of learning must therefore include an understanding and appreciation of the continuum of care available to any client.

The Gap Between Science and Clinical Services

Researchers perceive that many science-developed innovations have improved the treatment of drug abuse. For example, methadone-maintenance treatment began as a research effort (19), relapse-prevention techniques were honed by research investigations (20), the stages and processes of behavioral change were studied in depth (21), and, recently, motivational enhancement techniques have improved retention in treatment (22). Significant advances have been made in behavioral treatment of drug abusers (23). Studies have found that treatment intensity and systematic followup improve treatment outcomes (24–27), yet few of these findings have been incorporated into standard treatment settings.

The treatment practitioners are on the other side of the gap. Faced with the challenges of providing services on a daily basis, they are frustrated by what they see as the failure of research to provide them with specific answers to their important day-to-day questions. Many of their questions about how to use the information are related to policy and fiscal areas that, at least until recently, have been underresearched. They perceive that current policy, including funding, provides little opportunity or incentive for treatment programs to implement new scientific findings. The barriers between the science and the practice are multiple, but the insufficient training on evidence-based practices is one of the most prominent and disturbing.

Just as research findings have been underused by the treatment community, there are treatment approaches that have been understudied by the research community. For example, only a few researchers are studying therapeutic communities, and the research that has been done tends to focus on assessing their overall effectiveness rather than investigating how they work, why, or for whom (28).

Even when studies document that a treatment can be successfully implemented in a clinical setting, the challenges in the final stage of transfer to treatment programs are the provision of additional training for staff in delivering the new treatment, changing the attitudes of the providers, and providing evidence that the new treatment is effective to the unique culture or local clinical environment. Each of these components of training poses problems for the treatment programs. Training must be planned, systematic, and protective of the fidelity of the treatment. Researchers who establish treatment effectiveness in tightly controlled settings are often not able to translate the intervention into standard practice through training for daily activities. With the right skills and resources, researchers can provide the requisite training, anticipate the difficulties, and assist in the process of changing provider attitudes. Furthermore, shared technology transfer can encourage providers to "own" the research. If this transfer of knowledge does not happen, the prospects are poor for sustaining the intervention once the researchers are no longer involved (29).

What Kind of Training for What Kind of Treatment?

Many community and political leaders, as well as some treatment practitioners, believe that each new drug that makes its way through the culture means that there is a brand new problem with which to deal. According to this belief, cocaine treatment requires special skills; "ice" (smokable amphetamine) treatment requires special skills; phencyclidine (PCP) treatment requires special skills. If this were so, then a massive new approach would need to be created from scratch each time a new drug made its appearance—a draining, difficult endeavor.

Generally, however, it has been proven that the same skills and approaches are functionally applicable to any and all drug use (30). What is required is a familiarity with the particular language and nomenclature surrounding a particular drug, along with knowledge of the unique or sexual/romantic colorations associated with that drug. In addition, the new information about each drug and the physiologic responses changes quickly as a result of scientific advances. Those who treat drug abuse must be informed about these particulars, but it is erroneous to believe that a whole new industry must crop up to treat each new drug (31).

Basic Concepts of Training

Successful training in drug-abuse treatment is predicated on certain fundamental theories. These basic ideas permeate any and all specific parts of the curriculum. They serve the dual purpose of being both immediately applicable to the training setting and to the workplace.

1. Personal responsibility: methods that help mobilize the individual impulse toward health, despite personal and environmental obstacles
2. Self-help: technology whereby both individuals and groups can become effective in coping and problem solving on an ongoing basis
3. Social systems perspective: information that stresses practitioners' awareness of the interdependence of individuals and their social environment and provides for richer assessments and increased alternatives for intervention
4. Social support: methods for creating and/or using helping networks that can enhance the functioning of individuals and help maintain change
5. Transdisciplinary practice: skills and attitudes that prepare the different disciplines to collaborate toward "whole person" responses in planning, goal setting, and problem solving
6. Systematic problem solving: goal-oriented perspective that recognizes a common systemic and empirical process of stages and strategies that can be applied in assessing and treating problems at the individual, family, community, and societal levels
7. Interorganizational relations: concepts and perspectives relevant to understanding the forces that shape service-delivery systems
8. Cooperative learning: concepts and techniques to enhance self-esteem, acquisition of knowledge, and prevention of drug use (32,33)

Skill Enhancement

While the inclusion of general information about the context of drug-abuse treatment and models is essential to training, it must be accompanied by skill development—pragmatic techniques that help practitioners perform their jobs better. For those people fighting in the trenches of drug-abuse treatment programs on a day-to-day basis, skill development becomes of the utmost importance. The job can be so challenging and difficult that many practitioners yearn for magic solutions—theories or step-by-step directions—that can make their job less trying and more effective. More often than not, clients act out, regress, misbehave, deny problems, try to run away from treatment, have crazy families, and act irresponsibly. Those who work with them often look for formulaic answers to reassure them and diminish understandable anxiety, as they work in a climate riddled with the demands for bureaucratic compliance of funding agencies.

Because of these complex demands, skill enhancement for drug treatment personnel essentially can be divided into two categories. The first category concerns skills demanded by the funding and oversight agencies, who require ever more accurate and specific reporting mechanisms and management systems. Practitioners who are overwhelmed by paperwork simply cannot perform as effectively with clients. In light of this, many training candidates need specific organizational information, such as how to keep clinical records and how to track client and management activities. Mastery of these skills can prove a great relief to those in daily contact with drug addicts. This was true in 1979 and remains relevant now (14).

The second category of skills needed by treatment personnel in the field includes the art of specific case-management skills, including treatment planning, case note making, and assessment skills. These skills are all part of the practitioner's main concern: How do I improve my ability to do the required paperwork while successfully treating this client? Some of the ground that needs to be covered in this area of clinical skill enhancement includes answers to the following questions:

1. How do I engage the client on a personal level?
2. How do I interview a client?
3. What are the varying levels of resistance and how do I get through them?
4. How do I determine the severity of my client's symptoms and indications?
5. How do I assess my client's criminal background, social background, family background, psychological background, and academic background?
6. How do I assess my client's unique and special family, job, living, or environmental resources?
7. How do I interview the client's parent(s)?
8. What mode of treatment should I pursue with the client in (residential, day care, outpatient care, hospitalization, etc.)?
9. How do I enable the client to change his or her behavior?
10. How do I assist the family in understanding the client's problem?
11. How do I help the family change in ways that support the client's new behavior?
12. How do I get the client invested in his or her treatment and outcome?
13. How do the client and I set the orientation for treatment?
14. How do I confront the client?
15. What specific skills do I need to function in an induction group as opposed to a behavior change group, as opposed to a therapy group, as opposed to an individual counseling group?
16. How do I help my client identify short-term, achievable goals, while maintaining a long-term plan for recovery?
17. How can my client and I create enduring and meaningful behaviors that promote change?

Training Populations

Within any particular training model, there should be unique program training approaches. These programs must be relevant not only to emerging problems (such as AIDS, child abuse, sexuality, homelessness, and needs of women with children), but must accommodate particular populations likely to seek training, such as workers in mental health, social welfare, drug and alcohol treatment, health, corrections, and education. Each of these populations needs basic substance abuse treatment information, as well as job-specific information.

Curricula for substance abuse training programs should cover a broad spectrum, from law enforcement, prevention, education, intervention, and after-school programs to day-care programs and family care programs. This information should cover the following topics: theories of drug dependence and addiction; historical, cultural, social, and biologic implications; what types of treatment are available; the pros and cons of each type of treatment; how to care for clients without bias; and how to determine the most suitable treatment for each client. The Institute of Medicine of the National Academy of Science in its Substance Abuse Coverage study included a comprehensive list of treatment types available today (34). The list below shows a basic curriculum with corresponding practitioner needs.

- Outpatient nonmethadone treatment (OPNM)

  What is OPNM?
  Theories
  Private versus group practice
  How well does OPNM work?
  When and why does OPNM treatment fail?
  Costs and benefits

- Detoxification (medical and social)

  History
  Process
  How well does detoxification work?
  When and why does detoxification fail?
  Costs and benefits

- Other therapy models

  Psychotherapy
  Supportive counseling

Rational emotive therapy
Cognitive–behavioral approaches such as relapse prevention

- Chemical-dependency treatment

What is CD?
How well does CD work?
When and why does CD fail?
Costs and benefits

- Therapeutic communities

What is a TC?
History, operating principles, and methodologies
How well do TCs work?
When and why do TCs fail?
Costs and benefits

- Narcotic replacement therapies

Theories
How well does it work?
When and why does it fail?
Costs and benefits

- Social Model

What is the Social Model?
History, operating principles, and methodologies
How well does the Social Model work?
When and why does the Social Model fail?
Cost and benefits

- Correctional treatment programs

History
Examples and models
The California Civil Addict Program
"Boot" camps
A variety of therapeutic community in-prison programs
    (Stayin' Out, Phoenix House, Amity, etc.)
General conclusions about prison treatment

- Needs and issues of special populations

Co-occurring disorders
Pregnant women
Adolescents
Parents and children
Human immunodeficiency virus (HIV) and AIDS
    patients
Disabled patients
The elderly

- Criminal justice
- Cultural competence

In this updated matrix, motivational interviewing and cue extinction have been added, and additional curriculum items have been assigned to each group. In addition to this basic information, a curriculum for mental health practitioners (psychiatrists, psychologists, social work-

ers, psychiatric nurses, and related mental health workers) should include material relating to chronic and acute mental illness, as well as developmentally disabled and brain-injured clients. Training in the treatment needs of special populations, particularly clients with co-occurring disorders, is of great importance. Prevalence data from an epidemiologic catchment area study reveal high rates of comorbid mental disorders in alcoholics ($>50\%$) and drug-abusing or addicted ($>60\%$) clients treated in some settings (35). (It looks like addicted clients without comorbid mental health disorder gradually become a special population and the group of dually diagnosed patients becomes more and more normative.) From this perspective, the population of substance-abusing/addicted clients looks quite different than it did in 1960s and 1970s. The most recent data also suggest that addictions treatment personnel should be trained systematically in cultural and cross-cultural issues in behavioral treatment and neuroscience (36).

Social welfare curriculum (for those practitioners in public social services and nonprofit voluntary agencies) should include information about child and family welfare, poverty, aging, community-based care, and community development. Health workers who directly address the emotional and living needs of people with serious medical and degenerative conditions (including AIDS, cancer, and Alzheimer disease) require knowledge about death and dying, coping with chronic disabilities, maintaining extrainstitutional relationships, and providing opportunities for continuing social contributions. Participants from public and private institutions that treat drug and alcohol abuse need material about engagement, recruitment, retention, assessment, inpatient and outpatient treatment, and differentiation between adult and adolescent treatment, as well as school and community prevention programs.

In as much as these drug and alcohol treatment practitioners often emanate from two uniquely different learning settings—academia or personal treatment experience—their curriculum needs to emphasize exposure that provides a contrast. As such, those from academic settings need exposure to the benefits of raw emotion and the expression of feeling. Equally, those from a treatment experience background need intellectual exposure to rationale and theory underlying their often emotional individual and group counseling experiences.

TRAINING PHILOSOPHY

Training Adult Learners

Adults are a special group of learners, requiring appropriate adult education concepts to maximize learning. They perceive of themselves as responsible, self-directing, independent persons. They demand that the instructor accept him or her as such. Resistance to learning solidifies under conditions that are not in keeping with this concept of self-direction. The best approach to teaching adults is to view training as a planned, sequential process designed to provide the self-awareness, skills, knowledge, and attitudes needed to perform particular tasks.

This is not to say that instructors will not make some decisions for trainees. Whenever possible, trainees should be responsible for suggestions regarding training content and design. This increases feelings of "ownership" and fosters personal engagement with the training. The most effective training for adults is designed with the following points in mind:

1. A climate of mutual respect must exist between trainer and trainees.
2. An open, friendly, and casual atmosphere facilitates the exchange of differing viewpoints and ideas.
3. Trainees should be aided in diagnosing their own skills and growth needs, as well as in analyzing the specific training elements needed by their agency.
4. Adult learners learn best that which is relevant and useful to them. "Here and now" challenges should be the focus of training. Whenever possible, training ideas should be applied to current work situations. The emphasis should always be on illustrating new concepts as they relate to the life and work experiences drawn from the trainees (37).

Creating a Receptive Training Climate

According to Goldstein, the "training process is defined as the systematic acquisition of skills, rules, concepts, or attitudes that result in improved performance in the work environment" (38). Successful training is only possible when learners are receptive to the skills, rules, concepts, and attitudes presented. Several considerations go into creating an open-minded, fruitful training setting: overall tone and climate, geographic location, and class composition.

To begin with, the tone and climate of training sessions are crucial. People hear information in different ways and at different points in their lives, depending on its relevance to their own experience. The first challenge of training is to elicit an investment in the training itself, from both those undergoing training and the managers, directors, and administrators in the environments from which the trainees come. One way to accomplish this is to discuss the many different perspectives among the trainees at the beginning of any training effort. Furthermore, it is useful to discuss the value of these differences in creative process and problem solving. It is then possible to create a desire to think about the potential benefits of differing perspectives. It is also critical for trainees to have a determining voice about what they want to learn.

From a training point of view, this early intellectual activity has the effect of engaging people. Requiring active participation in the training increases the emotional readiness for new experiences and reduces anxiety so that absorption can occur. Much depends on the group itself—how it defines what it needs (based on its collective experience) to improve its competence. In the larger sense, this activity models tactics and procedures that are useful in treatment: negotiating differences, making an investment, and determining options. Learning is drastically increased when trainees feel that they have control over what and how they learn (39).

Bandura's work in self-efficacy validates this practical notion that people will accept information in which they have a determining voice, that they find useful, and that they can successfully apply to their particular work situation (40). According to theories on sustaining new behaviors (e.g., Skinner, Bandura, and Newsome), people's beliefs about how much control they have in a setting determine how much effort they will mobilize for that activity, how long they will persevere in the face of difficulties and setbacks, whether their thoughts on the subject are positive or negative, and the amount of stress they experience in coping with the experience.

To foster an active learning atmosphere, work is done to establish the sharing of information, in terms of both talking and listening. Ensuring a balance between receiving and giving information permits learners to share without fear of failure. It also increases their skills as both dispensers and collectors of information. With information flowing in both directions, no one can take a passive stance. This promotes a dynamic learning environment (39).

Trainers often quote the ancient Chinese folk proverb: If you hear something, you remember it; if you hear it and read it, you remember it a little longer; but if you hear it, read it, and practice it, you will retain it—providing it works for you. Arranging the curriculum so that students can hear, see, discuss, practice, and receive feedback throughout the training period has proved meaningful (41). An added benefit is that many difficulties leading to potential failure will be identified and addressed early so that corrections can result in success.

One of the aspects of any teaching setting that can have a negative effect on outcome is resistance. The successful handling of such resistance is another facet in eliciting an investment in learning. Here, again, there is a rich opportunity to demonstrate—both explicitly and implicitly—the handling of a problem within the training process that is a major concern of most attendees. Furthermore, by using concepts found in the short-term therapy systems literature, it is possible to very quickly call attention to many forms of unconscious resistance. Sifnos describes the use of active and explicit drawing of attention to resistances as it is used in short-term anxiety-provoking psychotherapy (STAPP), as well as in the use of recapitulation and problem solving (42). Similarly, eliciting their own types of resistance from attendees makes them both aware of and alert to such resistance, and it models the types of resistance they will most likely encounter in their clients. In this case, the training process often illuminates content.

Logistics and Atmosphere

In any training plan, the site location—such as geography—can influence outcome. For some, instruction seems to be most effective when it is done physically close to home or their work site. For others, leaving the normal work environment and traveling to unfamiliar surroundings for training has a bracing effect. In the absence of supervisors and peers, these individuals may feel less inhibited about disclosing certain problems and questions and more free to receive new information and ideas. Needs assessment prior to training can help determine what might work for a particular trainee or group of trainees.

Composition

Finally, class composition is a determining factor in the creation of a successful training climate. There are advantages to both homogeneous and heterogeneous groupings. People from similar disciplines have the following advantages when training together:

1. They can practice skills relevant to their particular methodology, because they are familiar with the treatment model and its context.
2. They can offer feedback and problem-solving ideas appropriate to their unique setting.
3. If the trainees already work together every day, problems characteristic of their system can be addressed in training in ways that are impossible in a day-to-day setting.
4. People who already know and work with each other can study, practice skills, and work together as teams in ways that they can carry directly to the workplace.

Trainees from different backgrounds, on the other hand, can benefit greatly from a classroom situation in which people come from various disciplines, as follows:

1. They may feel freer to ask questions.
2. They may feel important because they can offer a unique perspective from their setting.
3. They can hear how others handle similar problems in different settings.
4. Work problems will not cloud their ability to learn.
5. They may bypass power struggles that exist in a homogeneous group that works together.

Some recent realizations have occurred about how to mix groups in a training activity. For example, experiences in training different professionals who provide substance-abuse treatment in criminal justice settings strongly supports the value of the cross-training format. Looking at some of their unique needs for problem resolution and their interaction with each other, it is recognized that con-

tent alone is not enough. Appreciation must be developed for different goals, different views on what works and what does not, and different professional backgrounds.

Specific Training Goals

Although each trainer will have his or her curriculum—partially standardized to present the history of drug-abuse treatment and partially tailored to the training population—all training programs should be constructed around the following training goals. These goals relate not to basic philosophical concepts but to pragmatic, specific outcomes of training.

1. Increased awareness on the part of trainees in regard to the particular values, attitudes, and emotions that influence their work behavior. This includes an awareness of how their behavior affects others and how the behavior of others affects them.
2. Increased understanding of the ethics, subculture, sexual, generational, and socioeconomic differences that influence their attitudes, values, and behaviors.
3. Increased verbal and nonverbal communications skills obtained through analysis of body language, the use of fantasy, and other innovative techniques.
4. A basic understanding of group dynamics. This includes the ability to function well in different types of groups (e.g., encounter groups, task groups, staff groups), and knowledge of appropriate and inappropriate group leader–member interactions.
5. A broad base of knowledge about drug-abuse prevention, treatment, and national and international drug-control policies. Trainees will be able to draw on this knowledge in their work-site planning, problem solving, in-house training, and consulting.

Successful Training Methods

It is important for training sessions to include a mix of methods. This counters boredom and acknowledges that people learn in different ways. Some methods used in successful training are described below. Critical to each of these training methods are written and/or oral commitments to action on the part of the trainees.

1. Didactic presentations. The history of drug abuse and treatment approaches may be best presented in lecture format, as are theoretical and organizational material on groups, counseling principles, program planning, and the like.
2. Small groups. The small group as a learning tool has as its theoretical underpinning the assumption that individuals learn best in a group structure that demands interdependence. This interdependence heightens self-awareness and awareness of others.
3. Large groups. They are the most appropriate setting for brainstorming, process observations, daily training

program evaluation, action planning, homework, reading, and practice.

4. Simulation and role playing. These theatrical techniques bring problems to life and vividly demonstrate how trainees can effectively respond in new and useful ways. They can be a dramatic means of revealing other people's points of view and of uncovering one's own misconceptions and misjudgments.

5. Task groups. The task group has as its purpose the completion of clearly defined work. The work at hand should be based on real tasks from the trainees' work sites. Some possible task group work may be identifying problems, solving problems, and collecting data.

6. Videotape. Videotape is an effective learning tool for isolating and identifying behaviors that trainees may be unaware of, in both individuals and group dynamics.

Competencies

The Addiction Counselor Competencies were developed by the National Curriculum Review Committee of the federally funded Addiction Training Center Program with input from various national organizations, including National Association for Addiction Professionals (NDAC), International Certification and Reciprocity Consortium (ICRC), and members of the American Psychological Association (APA) Proficiency Development Group. They describe the knowledge, skills, and attitudes that characterize competent and effective practice and provide a comprehensive description of training outcomes that can be achieved through various educational strategies. The Foundations for Addiction Professionals include the knowledge and attitudes that form the basis of competent care across all health care disciplines. The competencies are divided among eight primary functions: Clinical Evaluation, Treatment Planning, Referral, Case Management, Client, Family, and Community Education, Documentation, and Professional and Ethical Responsibilities.

In the spring of 1995, Jerry Adams of the Northwest Frontier Addiction Training Center, with the assistance of treatment providers from of Oregon and Washington, conducted a study using the curriculum outline prepared by the National Curriculum Review Committee, which ranked competencies for entry level addiction counselors by agency supervisors.

The supervisors rated professional ethics as the most important competency. Top rated was "Understand the addiction professional's obligation to adhere to generally accepted ethical and behavioral standards of conduct in the helping relationship." The competency ranked third was "Demonstrate ethical behaviors by adhering to established professional codes of ethics that define the professional context within which the counselor works in order to maintain professional standards and safeguard the client." The protection of client privacy and confidentiality, which certainly has ethical implications, also ranked high.

The second kind of competency with high ratings described the basic professional–client relationship: "Establish a helping relationship with the client characterized by warmth, respect, genuineness, concreteness, and empathy." The ability to establish this necessary and fundamental relationship is not simply a matter of knowledge, but also a function of personal qualities.

Another highly rated competency was "Adhere to federal and state laws, and agency regulations, regarding AOD [alcohol and drug] treatment." Supervisors want entry level addiction counselors to understand and follow governmental regulations regarding treatment of clients. This kind of knowledge is easily taught, but compliance with regulations lies with the personal qualities of the professional and the supervision of the agency.

The National Curriculum Review Committee of the Addiction Technology Transfer Center is presently at work developing the knowledge, skill, and attitude for every component of each competency. That book will become available in 2004, and will be an important resource for educators, trainers, and consumers. Readers will understand exactly what it is that they need to learn, which skills they need to acquire, and what attitude they need to be most effective.

Clearly, curriculum priorities must be based on the actual work situation rather than on an academic conception of domain knowledge. Although physiologic knowledge is useful and relevant, courses for entry-level addiction specialists who are already employed in the field should begin with ethics and the other areas of competency identified by the supervisors. This knowledge of highest priority would be applicable immediately and would have been taught regardless of whether or not a trainee took any more courses in the field (43).

CONCLUSION

As with many endeavors in education and professional training, substance abuse treatment and training began as apprenticeship training—learning by doing. Gradually, more formal training emerged: first, by treatment agencies themselves; next, by government agencies with hopes of expanding resources; then, by groups or agencies with similar operating philosophies; next, by groups allied with certain agencies who offer certification (these tended to validate a particular approach); and, finally, by schools granting credit for specific courses at the college or university level.

These various approaches to formal training have led to debate and controversy over which type of certification should carry weight. Should certificates be granted only by those programs approved by public funders, license agencies, or insurance payors? Schools themselves argue about which department should implement or credit such training. Certainly, all professional human service schools should offer compulsory exposure to substance abuse and addictive behavior issues. At the very least, this information should foster an awareness of the symptoms and psychosocial implications of substance abuse. Perhaps the mandatory curriculum should go so far as to include engagement or referral strategies.

When it comes to specific techniques of treatment or prevention, however, more extensive and specialized training is required. Such exposure aimed at drug abuse practitioners faces many challenges. Certainly, the interplay of client needs, available funds, community agency operating philosophies and goals, as well as diverse trainee beliefs and assumptions can, and often do, conflict. In this light, training should be viewed as a growth process that occurs within the context of a facilitative relationship and information exchange.

REFERENCES

1. Keller D, Dermatis H. Current status of professional training in the addictions. *Subst Abuse* 1999;20(3):123–140.
2. Institute of Medicine. *Managing managed care: quality improvement in behavioral health.* Washington, DC: National Academy Press, 1997.
3. Leshner A. Addiction is a brain disease, and it matters. *Science* 1997;277.
4. Deitch DA. The end of the beginning: dilemmas of the paraprofessional in current drug abuse treatment. *J Community Altern* 1974.
5. Minkoff K. Resistance of mental health professionals to working with the chronic mentally ill. In: Meyerson AT, ed. *Barriers to treating the chronic mentally ill.* San Francisco: Jossey-Bass, 1987.
6. Anslinger H. Director of Federal Bureau of Narcotics from its inception in 1930 until 1962. For further citation and descriptions of this era, read David Courtright. *A century of American narcotic policy. Vol. 2: Treating drug problems, papers to the Committee for the Substance Abuse Coverage Study, Institute of Medicine.* Washington, DC: National Academy Press, 1990.
7. Schnick D. *Ideal and reality in field education: provocatory dilemmas and practical solutions.* Paper presented at the annual program meeting of Council on Social Work Education, Atlanta, GA, March 1988.
8. Kolb L. *Drug addiction: a medical problem.* Springfield, IL: Charles C Thomas, 1962.
9. Mower H. The mental health professional and mutual self-help programs: co-option or collaboration. In: Garlner A, Riesman F, eds. *Self-help revolution.* New York: Human Services Press, 1980.
10. De Leon G, Wexler HK, Jainchill N. The therapeutic community: success and improvement rate five years after treatment. *Int J Addict* 1982;17:703–747.
11. Dole VP, Nyswander MA. Medical treatment of diacetylmorphine (heroin) addiction. *JAMA* 1965;193(8):646–650.
12. DeLeon G. *The therapeutic community: study of effectiveness.* Research monograph series. DHHS Pub. No (ADM) 84–1286. Rockville, MD: National Institute of Drug Abuse, 1984.
13. Deitch D, Casriel D. The role of the ex-addict in the treatment of addictions. *Fed Probation* 1967 Dec.
14. Denby RF. Developments in training. In: Dupont RL, Goldstein A, O'Donnel J, eds. *Handbook on drug abuse.* Rockville, MD: National Institute of Drug Abuse, 1979.
15. Selin JoA, Svanum S. Alcoholism and substance abuse training: a survey of graduate programs in clinical psychology. *Yeshiva U Ferkauf Grad Sch Psychol* 1981;12(6):717–721.
16. Ewan CE, Whaite A. Training health professionals in substance abuse: a review. *Int J Addict* 1982;17(7):1211–1229.
17. American Psychiatric Association. Position statement on training needs in addiction psychiatry. *Am J Psychiatry* 1996;153:852.
18. Kleber HD. Treatment of narcotic addicts. *Psychiatr Med* 1985;3(4):389–418.
19. Ball JC, Ross A. *The effectiveness of methadone maintenance treatment.* New York: Springer-Verlag, 1991.
20. Marlatt GA, Gordon JR. *Relapse prevention: maintenance strategies in the treatment of addictive disorders.* New York: Guilford Press, 1985.
21. Prochaska JO, DiClemente CC. Toward a comprehensive model of change. In: Miller WR, Heather N, eds. *Treating addictive behaviors: processes of change.* New York: Plenum Press, 1986.
22. Miller WR, Rollnick S. *Motivational interviewing. Preparing people to change addictive behavior.* New York: Guilford Press, 1991.
23. Stitzer ML, Higgins ST. Behavioral treatment of drug and alcohol abuse. In: Bloom FE, Kupfer DJ, eds. *Psychopharmacology: the fourth generation of progress.* New York: Raven, 1995:1807–1819.
24. Fiorentine R, Anglin D. Does increasing the opportunity for counseling increase the effectiveness of outpatient drug treatment? *Am J Drug Alcohol Abuse* 1997;23(3):369–382.
25. Hoffman JA, Caudill BD, Koman JJ, et al. Comparative cocaine abuse treatment strategies: enhancing client retention and treatment exposure. In: Magura S, Rosenblum A, eds. *Experimental therapeutics in addiction medicine.* Binghamton, NY: Hayworth Medical Press, 1994:115–128.
26. Price RH. What we know and what we actually do: best practices and their prevalence. In: Egertson JA, Fox DM, Leshner A, eds. *Treating drug abusers effectively.* Malden, MA: Blackwell, 1997:125–155.
27. Simpson DW, Joe GW, Brown BS. Treatment retention and follow-up outcomes in the Drug Abuse Treatment Outcomes Study (DATOS). *Psychol Addict Behav* 1997;11(4):294–307.
28. Chasnoff IJ, Marques PR, Strantz IH, et al. Building bridges: treatment research partnership in the community. *NIDA Res Monogr* 1996;166:6–21.
29. Altman DG. Sustaining interventions in community systems: on the relationship between researchers and communities. *Health Psychol* 1995;14:526–536.
30. Hubbard RL, Rachal JV, Craddock SG, et al. Treatment outcome perspectives study (TOPS): client characteristics and behavior before, during, and after treatment. *NIDA Res Monogr* 1984;51:42–68.
31. Sells SB, Simpson DD, Joe GW, et al. A national follow-up study to evaluate the effectiveness of drug abuse treatment: a report on cohort I of the DARP five years later. *Am J Drug Alcohol Abuse* 1976;3(4):545–556.
32. Deitch D. *Training material.* Berkeley, CA: Daytop International Associates Training Institutes, 1989.
33. Knowles M, Malcom S. Innovations in teaching styles and approaches based upon adult learning. *J Educ Soc Work* 1972;8(2):32–39.
34. Gerstein DR, Harwood H, eds. *Treating drug problems.* Washington, DC: Committee for the Substance Abuse Coverage Study, National Institute of Medicine, National Academy Press, 1990.
35. Regier DA, Farmer ME, Rae DS, et al.

Comorbidity of mental disorders with alcohol and other drug abuse. Results of the epidemiological catchment area (ECA) study. *JAMA* 1990;19(264): 2511–2518.

36. Office of Substance Abuse Prevention. *Cultural competencies for evaluators.* DHHS Pub. No. (ADM-1884). 1992.

37. Kolb DA. *Experiential learning: experience as the source of learning and development.* Englewood Cliffs, NJ: Prentice-Hall, 1984.

38. Gillman IL, Goldstein P. Training systems in the year 2000. *Am Psychol* 1989;3:134.

39. Zenke R, Gundler J. Twenty-eight techniques for transforming training into practice. *Training* 1985 Apr: 53.

40. Bandura A. *Perceived self-efficacy: exercise self control through self belief. The Sixth Walter V. Clarke Memorial Lecture.* Providence, RI: Brown University, November, 1985:18.

41. Edwards G. *Reports to U.S. Depart-* *ment of Education, National Training Institute, NE Regional Training Center.* Garden City, NY: Adelphi University, 1981:1988–1989.

42. Sifnos PE. *Short-term dynamic psychotherapy evaluation and techniques,* 2nd ed. New York: Plenum Press, 1987.

43. Skager R. *An evaluation of dedicated courses for addiction counselors and recovery specialists.* La Jolla, CA: California Addiction Training Center, 1995.

CHAPTER 82

Forensics

MILTON EARL BURGLASS AND STUART GITLOW

The intersection of forensic and addiction practices presents a wealth of clinical and legal materials within both the civil and criminal arenas. This chapter is an introduction and practical guide to *criminal* forensic practice for the specialist in addiction medicine. The discussion is necessarily a synoptic overview. A comprehensive analysis of the relevant legal rules, doctrines, and principles; the evolution of the insanity defense; a detailed medical-legal discussion of significant cases; and a comparative analysis of the relevant federal and state laws are clearly beyond the scope of this chapter. The urgent conceptual problems arising from the interaction between the law and addiction medicine are highlighted throughout the discussion. References to primary legal sources, textbooks, reviews, and commentaries are provided for the interested reader. We also refer the interested reader to Chapter 82 of the 3rd edition of this text, which discusses important issues such as the applicability of *DSM–IV–TR* (*Diagnostic and Statistical Manual of Mental Disorders,* 4th ed., text revision) criteria in the courtroom, relevance of intoxication to intent, and residual effects of substance use following discontinuation of such use.

The first section of this chapter summarizes the fundamental legal principles and procedures governing expert testimony about the "mental" elements in the criminal law. The second section examines the potential roles for the addiction expert in criminal proceedings. The third section discusses the relevance of the effects of intoxicant use on criminal responsibility, considering both defenses and mitigation based on intoxication, dependence, and withdrawal. (For heuristic purposes, unless otherwise qualified, the term *intoxicant* refers to *substances*, i.e., *drugs*.)

The fourth section explores the issues raised by the "addictive processes," focusing on pathologic gambling. The fifth section considers the grave problem of the credibility of the testimony of intoxicant involved witnesses. The final section discusses intoxicant-related issues in regulatory and administrative matters, emphasizing the implications of the problematic concept of "impairment" and the regulatory problems of long-term opioid therapy in private practice.

THE ADDICTION MEDICINE SPECIALIST AS A FORENSIC EXPERT

Clinical Experts in the Criminal Law

The participation of specialists in addiction medicine as experts in forensic matters is a development that reflects the growth of the accredited specialty of addiction medicine over the past two decades and the courts' long-standing disenchantment with the testimony of traditional mental health experts in these matters. Historically, psychiatrists, psychologists, and other mental health professionals have provided expert testimony about the mental and/or physical factors (including intoxicant use) affecting an individual's emotion, cognition, and behavior. Although these professionals continue to testify about the effects of intoxicant use, increasingly, attorneys are preferentially seeking specialists in addiction medicine for consultation and expert testimony in such cases. This change is the result of three factors: (a) the stormy and problematic relationship of psychiatry and the law; (b) the conceptual fragmentation and factionalism in the traditional mental health disciplines; and (c) the emergence of a body of "facts" in the specialty of addiction medicine, about which there is little or no difference of opinion in the field. Burglass and Shaffer have analyzed and critiqued the state of knowledge, including theory, research, and practice, in the addictions field (1–5).

Being Qualified as an Expert

Determining who should be an expert witness for "psychological" matters has been a difficult task for the courts. Although there are federal and state standards that govern expert testimony, there is little consistency between and within jurisdictions about the qualifications of expert witnesses. Often, decisions regarding who qualifies as an "expert" are made on pragmatic rather than jurisprudential grounds.

With rare exceptions, psychiatrists, physicians who specialize in mental (neurologic and psychologic) disorders, and doctoral-level clinical psychologists are qualified as experts. However, some courts have permitted (or precluded) a wide range of individuals, including case workers (6,7), police officers (8–10), and even lay witnesses (11,12), to testify about a variety of psychological issues (including the question of sanity). Other courts have been unwilling to recognize the expertise of psychiatrists, physicians, psychologists, and others, and have refused to admit their testimony in selected matters. Examples include compulsive gambling (13,14), the effects of drugs on witness credibility (15,16), and satanic ritual murder (17). Although professional associations in psychiatry (18) and psychology (19) have developed guidelines for determining forensic expertise and practice, these criteria have not been adopted as authoritative by the courts. For the most part, courts have been reluctant to admit psychological evidence tending to favor an accused (20). For a comprehensive review of the determination and utilization of expertise in mental matters in the federal and state jurisdictions see Moriarty (21, §2:2–11).

Rationale for the Admission of Expert Testimony

Most states have a rule of evidence that parallels Federal Rule of Evidence 702, which provides that "if scientific, technical, or other specialized knowledge will assist the trier of fact [judge or jury] to understand the evidence or to determine a fact in issue, a witness qualified as an expert by knowledge, skill, experience, training, or education, may testify thereto in the form of an opinion or otherwise" (22). But a few states have adopted different and confusing rules on this point. The states also have tended to follow Federal Rule of Evidence 704, which limits expert testimony to an explanation of the defendant's diagnosis and the characteristics of the disease or defect. This rule specifically precludes expert opinion on "whether the defendant did or did not have the mental state or condition constituting an element of the crime charged or of a defense thereto" (22). This question (referred to in the law as the "ultimate issue") is for the jury to decide. Despite the prevailing rules of evidence, the final decision regarding expertise and the admissibility of expert testimony is made by the trial judge (13,14,23–26).

In practice, if you can provide satisfactory evidence of knowledge, skill, experience, or training in the diagnosis and/or active treatment (but not mere research) of intoxicant-involved patients, it is likely that you will be recognized by the court as an expert in the areas of addiction and the effects of intoxicants. Although qualified as an expert by the court, the admissibility of your testimony into evidence is a separate question to be argued by counsel. Ultimately, all decisions regarding the qualification of experts and the admissibility of their testimony are made at the discretion of the trial judge (27–31).

How the Law Views Expert Testimony

Under prevailing rules of evidence, the testimony of expert witnesses is presented to the court in the form of expert opinion, and as such it does not enjoy the same privileged status as "fact" testimony. It remains for the trier of fact (judge or jury) to evaluate the credibility, reliability, relevance, and applicability of any expert testimony introduced. What an expert in addiction medicine may know to be an accepted medical "fact" is nonetheless considered to be only "opinion" when expressed in expert testimony. As opinion, such information may be accepted, discounted, or rejected in whole or in part by the trier of fact. When testifying, any lapse of awareness of this crucial distinction may result in your being perceived as argumentative, defensive, sanctimonious, condescending, or hostile. This always compromises your credibility, undermines the power of your testimony as evidence, and may prove fatal to the client's case.

THE ROLE OF THE EXPERT IN ADDICTION MEDICINE

The following discussion may seem to express a defense bias, but bear in mind that it rarely serves the interest of the prosecution's case to introduce expert testimony in support of exculpating or mitigating mental defenses. Of course, the prosecution may call experts to rebut testimony introduced by defense experts. Although you are more likely to be engaged by the defense, you should be willing to appear for either side. Remember that as an expert witness you are not an advocate. Your professional mandate is to assist the court. You fulfill this responsibility by providing the judge and jury with information that is truthful, intelligible, and clear, and by offering opinions that are unbiased, carefully reasoned, and based on your understanding of the facts in evidence.

The Pretrial Phase

In the pretrial phase, the addiction specialist can assist the attorney by reviewing the initial discovery materials (e.g., police reports, arrest forms, affidavits of investigating agencies, waivers of rights, medical examiner reports, toxicology screens, statements of witnesses and/or the accused, confessions, the formal complaint, information, or indictment) to identify any immediate or potential issues related to intoxicants. Attorneys also may seek assistance in managing a difficult, compromised, or dangerous client. It may be necessary to immediately evaluate and refer the client for primary treatment or stabilization so that the client can adequately assist counsel in the preparation of the case. Determination of competency to stand trial is a separate matter, both clinically and legally.

Once prospective witnesses have been identified, the addiction specialist should make a preliminary assessment of all available background materials to identify any possible clinical (i.e., medical, neuropsychiatric, or addiction) issues that require investigation. You can also help the attorney to prepare for depositions by (a) drafting specific questions to be posed, (b) doing content and psycholinguistic analyses of taped or written evidence (e.g., statements or depositions made by the defendant or witnesses), and (c) suggesting strategies and tactics for conducting interviews or depositions. It is often important to interview family members, friends, former teachers, or others who may have particular knowledge or a different perspective of the defendant or witness (32).

The cornerstone of your evaluation of the defendant is a comprehensive addiction history. You must aggressively inquire about every aspect of use and experience with intoxicants of all classes, and all of the addictive processes. You also must take a lifetime neuropsychiatric history, exploring every sign or symptom reported, suggested, implied, or suspected. Of course, complete medical (including all responses to prescription and over-the-counter medications), psychosocial, developmental, educational, relational, and vocational histories must be taken. History or indicia of psychological, sexual, or physical abuse also must be aggressively sought and explored.

During the pretrial phase you will work closely with the attorney. Your responsibility to the attorney is to identify, analyze, develop, and explain facts or issues relating to the use or effects of intoxicants. The attorney's responsibility to you is to analyze and explain the laws of the jurisdiction that (a) govern the nature and scope of admissible expert testimony, (b) define the required mental "elements of the offense" for the crime charged, and (c) determine the availability of defenses or mitigation based upon the use and/or effects of intoxicants. This interaction between the disciplines of law and medicine, unfettered by the legal rules of the courtroom, is invariably a stimulating and instructive experience for both the attorney and the addictionist. The collaboration will result in the formulation of potential clinical approaches to the defense of the case. In time, you and the attorney will agree upon a strategy for the clinical component of the defense and set the general contour of your testimony.

Once the clinical and legal issues are clarified and resolved, you should draft the actual questions that the attorney should ask you on direct examination. At the very least, you must frame the questions that establish your expertise and any questions required to elicit the predicate facts and issues to be introduced into evidence as the basis for your testimony and opinions. Although this is a tedious and time-consuming task, it cannot be done by the attorney. As the expert in addiction medicine, only you can fully appreciate the relevance and implications of the clinical subtleties and distinctions. Only you can identify and illuminate the clinical concepts likely to confuse the judge or jury. And only you can anticipate the pitfalls that loom on the narrow plateau of accommodation between the restrictive rules of legal discourse and the broad latitude required in complex clinical explanations. For an expert, there is no more frustrating or unsettling experience than being put or left in a compromised position on the witness stand as a result of having been asked ill-framed questions by an inadequately prepared attorney.

If the other side will be calling an addiction expert, you can assist your attorney by (a) evaluating that expert's credentials, (b) anticipating the nature of the testimony, (c) analyzing the strengths and weaknesses of both expert positions, and (d) drafting appropriate questions for your attorney to ask in cross-examination.

The Trial Phase

The two most common types of cases in which you will be engaged are those in which a person either is accused of having committed a crime while drug involved (i.e., while experiencing the acute, subacute, chronic, or residual effects of previous intoxicant use, dependence, or withdrawal), or is on trial as the result of statements made to law enforcement officers or testimony given by witnesses who themselves are or have been drug involved. The first type of case typically requires testimony about the nature and effects of intoxicant use on the defendant. Common issues here include the impact of specific intoxicants on (a) the physical and mental ability to have committed the crime, (b) the state of mind required for the offense charged, or (c) the formation of the requisite intent. Other potential questions may involve the special issues of diminished capacity or insanity. The second type of case typically involves testimony about the effects of acute and/or chronic intoxicant use on cognition and memory, and how such use might affect the credibility of witnesses.

In some jurisdictions, the fact pattern of a specific case and/or the local rules may preclude an expert from commenting or offering an opinion on any aspect of the mental state of the defendant. Even in such circumstances, an addiction expert will usually be permitted to "assist the trier of fact" by giving the jury a basic education about the intoxicants involved in the case. Such a "mini-course" on intoxicants might include (a) general pharmacology; (b) modes, methods, patterns, and demographics of use; (c) interaction with antecedent or concurrent neuropsychiatric or medical conditions; and (d) specific effects on cognition, emotion, and behavior.

The Postconviction Phase

It is difficult to accept that defenses involving intoxicants usually do not prevail—even in cases where you believe that any colleague in the field would find the clinical evidence supportive of the defense position. It is always painful to lose a case in which you strongly believe. Long-standing biases in the criminal law, public opinion, and political factors often have greater influence on the outcome of a case than does the clinical evidence. Realize that most of your clients will be convicted. But also realize that, as the result of your testimony, the conviction may be for a lesser offense, which carries a lesser penalty. Try to remember that your testimony in every case can make a meaningful difference to what eventually happens to the defendant.

Often, your most valuable contribution to a case will be made in the postconviction phase, that is, at sentencing. Most jurisdictions permit the defense to present evidence (including expert testimony) in support of mitigation during the sentencing process. The rules governing the nature, content, form, and scope of expert testimony are far more liberal at this phase than at trial. For example, at sentencing, an expert may be permitted to (a) discuss the defendant's entire intoxicant history, (b) comment on the influence of intoxicant use on the acts constituting the crime charged, (c) make prescriptive treatment recommendations, or (d) propose an alternative sentencing plan, for example, providing for dispositions such as supervised release (probation), community control (home confinement), or community service. If you do offer sentencing recommendations to the judge, do not lose sight of the fact that, finally, the court has the awesome responsibility of striking "that delicate balance" between the needs of the community for protection and justice and those of the defendant for treatment and rehabilitation.

CRIMINAL RESPONSIBILITY AND INTOXICANTS

Although the connection between the use of intoxicants and crime has been universally recognized, the explosive increase in drug-related crime over the past two decades has had only minimal impact on substantive criminal law. The recognition (albeit equivocal) of substance use disorders as "diseases" and the growth of a professional field and industry around the field has had significant social and professional consequences and instructive (although surprisingly limited) effects on the legal rules.

Recent scientific research illuminating the distinction between mind and brain, mechanisms of cognition, the nature of rationality, the relationship between intention and action, mechanisms of emotional and behavioral control, and the distinctions between reaction, response, compulsion, and decision are of fundamental relevance to the criminal law. Yet, the law remains self-consciously nescient. Its reasoning remains grounded in long discarded models, disproved theories, and culturally dated assumptions about human rationality, intent (knowledge and volition), motivation, and the regulation of behavior (action). Moreover, although well-understood in the addictions field, the specific effects of all classes of intoxicants on these complex processes have been essentially ignored by the law. Legal reasoning about intoxication continues to be informed by eighteenth and nineteenth century understanding of the effects of alcohol on behavior (33).

Conceptual Problems

Definition, Description, and the Problem of DSM–IV–TR

Because the criminal law has a long history of difficulty defining the concepts of "mental disease" and "mental defect," it is perhaps not surprising that the American Psychiatric Association's *DSM–IV–TR* (34) has been adopted by the courts as a Rosetta Stone for recognizing a defendant's alleged "mental" problems as true diseases or defects. As clinicians, we know that *DSM–IV–TR* is not and was never intended to be a textbook of neuropsychiatry or addiction medicine. Despite the very explicit caveat about its limitations stated in the Introduction (34, pp. xxiii–xxiv) and the Cautionary Statement about its validity and application in forensic contexts (34, p. xxxii–xxxiii), expect to see a copy of *DSM–IV–TR* on counsel tables in every criminal case wherein a mental defense is anticipated. Also, you should expect to be examined and cross-examined about your findings and opinions in the constricting terminology of *DSM–IV–TR*. As one prosecutor remarked, "If it's listed in *DSM–IV–TR*, then it's a real mental illness; if it's not in *DSM–IV–TR*, then it isn't a real disease and should be given no credence." To undermine the unwarranted authority this publication has accrued, you must make it clear that neither you, the psychiatric profession, nor the addiction medicine field recognizes *DSM–IV–TR* as the "authoritative" text. After that, you will not be bound by its serious limitations, simplifications, and omissions. In preparing your testimony, it is vital that you anticipate and analyze all the ways that opposing counsel might use the language of *DSM–IV–TR* to try to make your testimony appear unreliable, inconsistent, or contradictory. Next, you must formulate your strategy and tactics for thwarting this predictable assault on your credibility. Finally, you must make your attorney aware of all such potential problems so that the attorney will be prepared to help "rehabilitate" you on redirect examination.

Disease, Disorder, Defect, and Dysfunction

Moving beyond the hurdle of *DSM–IV–TR*, you must be prepared to confront the distinctions between "disease," "disorder," and "dysfunction." The first two terms have long and tortuous histories in the law of every jurisdiction, while the concept of cerebral "dysfunction" has virtually none. And yet, it is precisely in terms of cognitive, emotional, and behavioral dysfunction that one can best explain (and even quantify) the effects of acute, subacute, and chronic intoxicant use. Most defendants seeking to avail themselves of an intoxicant-based defense will have grossly normal findings on objective neuropsychiatric diagnostic tests as the electroencephalogram (EEG), computed axial tomography (CAT scan, or magnetic resonance imaging (MRI) scan. Even when administered using the latest enhanced techniques, these modalities are of limited value in demonstrating cerebral dysfunction (35–37). Although the newer brain imaging technologies, such as the quantitative EEG (35), single-photon emission computed tomography (SPECT) (36), and brain electrical activity mapping (BEAM) (37), promise considerable future utility, at present, valid norms for these modalities are still in the earliest stages of development. Because the legal tests applied by the courts for the admissibility of scientific evidence based on "newer" technologies are strict and narrow (23,24), historically, the courts are slow to recognize the evidentiary validity of emerging scientific technologies.

Use, Misuse, Abuse, Dependence, Addiction

Terminology in the field of addictive disease remains an unsettled area. Within *DSM–IV–TR*, for example, there is no formal definition or use of the word "addiction." That term as it is often used is referred to instead as "dependence," a word less likely to have pejorative connotations within the courtroom. One might argue that substance dependence is a medical disease whereas substance addiction is a social issue. However you prefer to approach this, be consistent with your use of terminology, making certain to define your usage at the outset. Recognize that not all use qualifies as abuse. There is no reference to quantity of use within the definitions of abuse or dependence, but that has not stopped the lay public from assuming that any use of heroin constitutes abuse whereas only high volumes of alcohol intake would amount to abuse. Use of a substance does not establish the presence of a disease, but it does establish the presence of potentially intoxicating effects. Again, be consistent with your terminology and your definition of the disease process so that the field remaining unsettled in this area will not cause significant

difficulties. Finally, if appropriate, you may need to educate participants regarding use of the "substance-induced" category as it applies to alteration of mood or perception. On several occasions, we have observed individuals with substance-induced disorders to be presumed to have substance use disorders. The substance-induced category should be used diagnostically, even if the substance to which it refers is not a drug of abuse. If, for example, an antihypertensive has caused depressive symptoms and secondary criminal action, one of the appropriate diagnoses would be a substance-induced mood disorder. Your role includes education regarding this infrequent but entirely accurate diagnosis.

The Elements of the Offense

Definitions of both common law and statutory crimes require the voluntary commission of a bad act or harmful omission (*actus reus*) in conjunction with a bad state of mind (*mens rea*). However, these fundamental concepts have resisted enduring definition. Most older common law crimes have been redefined in modern criminal statutes. Criminal codifications often use adverbial qualifiers such as "knowingly," "willfully," or "intentionally" to designate as voluntary an act performed consciously as the result of effort or determination (38).

The Exculpatory Doctrine in Common Law

The early common law made no concession whatsoever because of impaired behavioral control. Justice Story, in an 1828 case involving alcohol intoxication, stressed the merit of "the law allowing not a man to avail himself of the excuse of his own gross vice and misconduct to shield himself from the legal consequences of such crime" (39).

Over time, scientific views of human behavior gradually supplanted moral ones. Concurrently, there was a substantial increase in the consumption of alcohol in all social and economic strata. In response to these societal changes, the common law evolved what came to be known as "the exculpatory doctrine." This doctrine permitted the presentation of evidence of specified mental conditions (including intoxication) in legal proceedings as a means of mitigating culpability, liability, or responsibility. Such evidence could be introduced in the form of an assertion of a defendant's insanity or lack of the "specific" intent required as an element of the offense charged. New and more difficult problems arose almost immediately.

The Enduring Problematic Concept of "Intent"

The early cases in which the exculpatory doctrine was applied involved alcohol intoxication. The courts gradually realized that "common sense" suggested that a distinction should be made between a crime committed by an intoxicated as opposed to a sober person. But traditional moral attitudes stigmatizing intoxication as a vice indicated the impropriety of complete exculpation. The criminal rules on "intent" provided an expedient, if inadequate, means of mediation.

These doctrines, which were the foundation for the exculpatory rule, imply that "specific intent" is distinguishable from "general intent." These also signify that certain crimes require only "general intent," whereas other offenses require certain "specific" intents. This dubious distinction persists at law, although neither the courts nor modern cognitive science has yet to formulate a reliable criterion or test for distinguishing "general" from "specific" intent. Today, "specific intent" most often refers to a "special" mental element that must be present in addition to the bad mental state required to accompany the bad act constituting the offense. For an analysis of the evolution and modern status of the legal premise of intent and its application to mental defenses (including intoxication) see LaFave and Scott (40, §3.5). When impulsive or compulsive behavior is involved, as in intoxicant use, this distinction is even more problematic.

The meaning of "intent" in the criminal law has always been obscure. Traditionally, intent was defined to include elements of both knowledge and volition. In the modern era, a statutory distinction generally is made between the mental states of knowledge and intent. Obviously, certain intoxicants, when used in certain ways by certain persons, affect certain cognitive, emotional, and behavioral functions in certain ways. Defining, distinguishing, and presenting these to the jury in nontechnical, readily intelligible language is the responsibility of the addiction expert. Successful communication of these clinical complexities to the jury by the expert is the cornerstone of a viable intoxicant-based defense.

Despite limited recognition by the courts and society that some degree of exculpation might be warranted in cases where an intoxicant-involved person commits a crime, neither the exculpatory doctrine of the common law nor modern statutory laws dealing with intoxication and related mental defenses has been even moderately satisfactory or equitable. One important reason for this is that both the exculpatory doctrine of the common law and our modern statutory laws were based upon very early medical observations and common lay experience with the effects of alcohol. Despite the wealth of scientific knowledge about the specific cognitive, emotional, and behavioral effects of all the intoxicants, the substantive criminal law in this area has evolved very little and still reflects its alcohol-informed heritage.

The implicit public policy in the prevailing law reflects society's historical vacillation and expedient compromises between the punishment of intoxicant-influenced offenders in complete disregard of their condition (i.e., viewing

them as ordinary criminals), and the total exculpation often suggested by the clinical evidence (i.e., viewing them as patients).

Intoxication as a Defense

Today, the effect of intoxication on criminal responsibility is well established, but only precariously settled. At law, intoxication can be either (a) involuntary, where the intoxicant is ingested as the result of force or duress (41), deceit or trickery (42), medical advice (43), or lack of awareness of a susceptibility to a recognized atypical reaction to that substance (44), as in pathologic intoxication; or (b) voluntary, where the intoxicant is ingested for effect, as in recreational drug use. Many jurisdictions have recognized involuntary intoxication as a complete defense to criminal behavior in appropriate circumstances. Most jurisdictions, however, adhere to the view that voluntary intoxication does not excuse a criminal act unless the actor, because of his intoxication, could not form the intent required in the statutory definition of the crime. That is, voluntary intoxication may be raised to negative an element of an offense. Unfortunately, neither the distinctions between voluntary and involuntary intoxication nor those between general and specific intent are clear or consistent. See LaFave and Scott for a review of intoxication-based defenses (40, §4.10).

In cases involving the ingestion of intoxicants courts have consistently applied the same rules of analysis, mitigation, and exculpation derived from the common law and developed to deal with alcohol intoxication (45). One notable exception was expressed in the dissenting opinion in *State v. Hall* (46), which argued that drug and alcohol intoxication ought to be distinguished, and that "[o]ur intoxication rationale as applied to alcohol simply does not fit the use of modern hallucinatory drugs; and it was never meant to" (46, p. 213). Similarly, most legal commentators have not distinguished intoxication resulting from the ingestion of alcohol and from the other classes of intoxicants (47,48). In 1980, this problem was addressed in a remarkably comprehensive law review article (49). This scholarly commentary (a) examined in detail the specific effects of all of the intoxicants then in general use, (b) reviewed the traditional and prevailing legal reasoning on intoxication and intent, (c) discussed the resultant implications for intoxicant-based defenses against criminal responsibility, and (d) concluded with a recommendation that ". . . either the court or the legislatures must increase their expertise in these areas and respond to these potentially serious flaws in the criminal legal system" (49, p. 1145). Despite having been extensively cited in subsequent cases, its well-reasoned proposals have yet to be implemented. The criminal law continues to fail or refuse to recognize the fundamental differences between the effects of alcohol and those of other intoxicants (most importantly, cocaine) on human cognition, emotion, and behavior (50–54).

The law views alcohol as a neural depressant and disinhibitor that releases (cognitive and moral) inhibitions, thereby setting free ill-defined drives and putative "bad" impulses and traits, which are subsequently expressed in a criminal act. An analogy echoing through many judicial opinions regarding the mechanism of intoxication states: "drinking alcohol is like taking your foot off the brake [of a car]." Whereas this may not be an entirely ill-informed metaphor, it is surely an inadequate one, for it implicitly maintains that alcohol effects are stable, predictable, and consistent both across and within individuals. When applied to other intoxicants, this analogy is clearly out of touch with currently accepted principles of neuropsychopharmacology and the cognitive sciences. This disparity is most glaring for cocaine intoxication. After introducing the "removing the foot from the brake" analogy for alcohol intoxication for contrast, it is useful to explain to the jury that the effect of ingesting cocaine is better understood as being more like "stepping on the gas." The outcome may be the same: the metaphoric car moves forward, that is, the person commits a criminal act, but the mechanism is entirely different. It has been suggested that in a sense cocaine is that drug which supplies intent where otherwise there would have been none. Distinguishing the effects of cocaine (or other intoxicants) from those of alcohol is vital because it problematizes the legal concepts of intent and intoxication. This alone may lead the jury to find "reasonable doubt" about the defendant's having the required state of mind.

Consider, as an example, the conceptual problem posed for a jury in a case where a polydrug addict with a long history of robbing drugstores to get drugs (not money) now robs a drugstore while grossly intoxicated from high intravenous doses of phencyclidine (PCP), heroin, and cocaine. Eyewitness testimony states that although he looked and acted as if intoxicated, the defendant also appeared to have acted with purpose. His actions clearly demonstrated that he "knew" (at least) the following: (a) to rob a pharmacy (as opposed to, say, a grocery store) to get drugs; (b) which specific (desirably intoxicating) drugs to steal; and (c) how to commit a robbery and get to the controlled substances in the safe. In this scenario, it would be nonetheless possible that the extent and specific effects of the polydrug intoxication had rendered the defendant incapable of forming the specific intent required as an element of the offense of robbery in that jurisdiction. To succeed in negativing the elements of the offense of robbery, the defense would have to introduce expert testimony to attempt to explain at least the following: (a) that his "intent" was to get drugs, not specifically to commit the crime of robbery; (b) that his intoxication precluded him from forming the specific intent required for robbery, but (c) that the intoxication did not affect his previously well-learned ("overlearned") knowledge about intoxicating drugs and about how to rob

drugstores. For such expert testimony to be accepted by the jury, it would need to tie together (a) the defendant's intoxicant history, (b) the specific effects of each intoxicant influencing the defendant at the time of the robbery, (c) his prior experience in robbing drug stores, and (d) the specific facts of the instant case.

Dependence as a Defense

Dependence on an intoxicant or active intoxication, absent more, does not provide a complete defense in any jurisdiction (55,56). The nature, course, and effects of dependence on specific substances on cognition, emotion, or behavior have not been recognized by the law.

Interestingly, opioid intoxication (but not dependence) may be of such extent as to negate the "knowingly" element of criminal intent. But neither opioid intoxication nor dependence has been held to negate the "willfully" element of criminal intent. Intoxication (but not dependence) induced by any substance may be sufficient to render a person incapable of the "deliberation" or "premeditation" required as an element of a specific degree of an offense, as in first degree murder. In no jurisdiction has dependence on specific intoxicants been differentiated from that of alcohol, thereby warranting special consideration.

Until recently, attempts to use dependence as a defense to criminal responsibility were couched in terms of insanity, by characterizing dependence or addiction as a mental disorder that rendered the defendant insane and therefore not criminally responsible. For the most part, these attempts have been unsuccessful. In 1984, *United States v. Lyons* held that henceforth no defendant could base any defense of insanity on the claim that he lacked substantial capacity to conform his conduct to the requirements of law, supporting that opinion by citing "the present murky state of medical knowledge" about human volition (57).

A novel defense of "medical necessity" proposed in 1985 by Uelmen and Tennant sought to present addiction not as a mental disorder but, by reason of its involving a putative endorphin deficiency, as a physical condition requiring medical treatment (58). Analogizing the situation of the addict to that of the diabetic, the defense of "medical necessity" sought to conform to the contours of the well-established defenses of duress or necessity. Uelmen and Tennant suggested that "obviously, the legal profession is sleeping through the current revolution in Biochemistry" (58, p. 6). Although inconsistently successful in minor cases involving possession of small quantities of marijuana by persons using that substance to alleviate the symptoms of glaucoma (59), multiple sclerosis (60), or spasticity (61), the defense of "medical necessity" has otherwise been rejected by the courts. Many cases in which this novel defense was rejected relied upon the early case of *United States v. Moore*, which pointed to "the choice that each addict makes at the start as to whether or not he is going to take narcotics and run the risk of becoming addicted to them" (62).

Withdrawal as a Defense

Defenses based upon the argument that the criminal act at issue was the direct or indirect product of withdrawal from an intoxicant have not prevailed, except in the limited and infrequent circumstance where a defendant in withdrawal commits an act while semiconscious or unconscious. An action that, while purposive, is not spontaneous, and therefore is not voluntary, is defined at law as an "automatism" and does not incur criminal responsibility. See LaFave and Scott for a discussion of the utilization of automatism in a criminal defense (40, §4.9).

Intoxicant-Induced Insanity as a Defense

An insanity defense asserts that at the time the accused committed the act for which he is charged, a mental illness precluded him from having the required bad state of mind to be convicted of the act. The insanity defense has been a part of English and American jurisprudence for several hundred years. It reflects a shared belief that only those individuals who have chosen to commit wrongful acts should be punished, and that those without the capacity to appreciate the wrongfulness of their conduct should be absolved. The roots of the insanity defense are ultimately embedded in the Judeo-Christian tradition of linking moral responsibility with punishment and absolution.

The elements of the legal definition of insanity that predominates today was shaped primarily by two famous cases: the 1843 English case of Daniel M'Naghten (63) and the 1982 acquittal of John Hinckley (64), who had shot President Reagan. In both instances, the public outcry over the successful employment of the insanity defense as it existed at those times resulted in a substantial conceptual redefinition and limitation of the availability of the defense. Most notably, the federal 1984 Insanity Defense Reform Act (20) and the Comprehensive Crime Control Act of 1984 (65), which followed in the wake of Hinckley's successful defense based on a legal test for insanity then in wide use, eliminated many types of mental illness as bases for a defense and reinstated the strict cognitive test of insanity set forth in M'Naghten (63). Temporary insanity caused by voluntary intoxication does not meet the requirements of the 1984 Act, nor does intoxicant dependence, absent more (66). However, where the insanity caused by the chronic use of intoxicants endures beyond any period(s) of intoxication it may insulate a defendant, providing the resulting insanity otherwise conforms to the requirements of the 1984 Act (21, §3:13;40, §4.10(g)). Interestingly, neither intoxication nor dependence has been recognized as a uniquely aggravating factor to an antecedent or concurrent mental condition that by itself would not render a defendant insane as defined in the 1984 Act.

Insanity that arises from either acute or chronic intoxicant use has not been distinguished from insanity produced by other causes. Thus, whether temporary insanity caused by voluntary intoxication will be exculpatory largely depends on the legal test for insanity used in that jurisdiction. Several states have statutorily excluded this defense.

The Concept of Partial Responsibility

Partial responsibility, or diminished capacity, is a difficult and muddled concept in the law, with little coherence or consistency. Many courts appear to reject or not understand it.

Insanity of the legal type is considered a complete defense to criminal acts in most jurisdictions. A mental disorder that constitutes "something less than insanity" is not considered a complete defense to a crime, but is widely thought to lessen the degree of criminal responsibility, at least for crimes where there is a lesser degree of responsibility or severity available (as in murder, which might be reducible from first degree to second or a lesser degree). Today, mitigation, not exculpation, is the most common application of the concept of diminished capacity (21, §3:16).

Argument asserting diminished capacity can also be made when a defendant claims that a mental illness precluded him or her from having the mental elements required for the crime. That is, because of a mental disorder, the severity of which did not render the defendant insane as provided by the test for insanity employed in that jurisdiction, the defendant nonetheless was unable to have committed the crime as charged because the defendant's mental disorder prevented the defendant from having the statutorily required elements of the offense charged (e.g., acting with "malice" or "premeditation"). That the effects of specific intoxicants can reach this threshold may be an undisputed clinical "fact"; nonetheless, courts continue to resist its acceptance (67).

Many states disallow any evidence of diminished capacity to be admitted during trial. By public referendum, the California Penal Code eliminated diminished capacity as a defense, but retained its availability as a mitigating factor (68). In *Bethea v. United States*, the court expressed the now widely held view that embracing the concept of diminished responsibility would lead to an unacceptable "sliding scale of sanity in criminal responsibility" (69). Moriarty provides an elegant analysis of the concept and a comparison of the positions taken by the American Bar Association, the federal courts, and the various state courts (21, §§3:19–21).

Intoxicant Use and Effects as Mitigating Factors

Although many states now require judges to adhere to legislatively prescribed sentencing guidelines, in some jurisdictions judges have retained limited discretion to consider a convicted defendant's complete drug history (including intoxication and dependence) as a mitigating factor. However, it is a general rule that the nature, extent, and effects of the intoxicant history must be introduced into evidence before being eligible for consideration at sentencing. There are marked differences between jurisdictions regarding the type of evidence (expert testimony, corroborating witnesses, etc.) required or admissible to establish the extent and effects of intoxication in support of mitigation.

Under the current Revised Federal Sentencing Guidelines, a federal judge may exercise a downward departure from the legislated guidelines for sentencing based on "diminished capacity" except where it is the result of voluntary intoxication with any substance (70). Nonetheless, in some federal jurisdictions, "addiction" has been accepted as evidence of diminished capacity and therefore as a basis for granting a downward departure at sentencing. This is the exception, however, not the rule.

THE ADDICTIVE PROCESSES

The concept of behaviors involving addictive processes, rather than intoxicating substances, as in "compulsive" or "pathologic" gambling, is of exceptional theoretical importance for the criminal law and the addictions field. The concept has required a reexamination of many fundamental legal postulates, precedents, and assumptions about criminal responsibility and intentionality. If viewed as addictive disorders (as in "compulsive gambling") in which no exogenous intoxicating substance is ingested, such processes raise profound questions about the paradigms that inform research, theory, and practice in the addictions field. If viewed as impulse control disorders (as in "pathologic gambling"), these processes raise difficult questions about the causal and temporal relationships between a person's impulses and the acts issuing therefrom (71). Unfortunately, in recent years, addiction terminology has been used to refer to everything from Internet usage ("Internet addiction") to dedication to one's career ("workaholic"), thus lessening its applicability and meaning with respect to physiologic addictive disease. To lessen the potential for difficulties, precise usage of your terminology is called for.

Pathologic Gambling

Burglass has reviewed in depth the rationale, process, conceptual problems, and practical implications of introducing dysfunctional gambling behavior in defense or mitigation of criminal responsibility (71). One critical step toward the resolution of the conceptual problems would be for the field to formulate a classification of pathologic gamblers and the situations relevant to their behavior(s) that would be defensible empirically and relevant to the issue of criminal responsibility. For example, pathologic

gamblers who commit crimes would be either normal or diseased, and their gambling behavior at the time of the commission of the crime charged would be pathologic in various degrees (71). Unfortunately, no such classification schema has been proposed.

What we find in the fact patterns of cases involving pathologic gambling is not a total or even substantial incapacity to carry out simple (or even complex) acts that can be reasonably attributed to the "disease." Nor do we find such a compromise of intellectual function as to entirely exclude purposeful conduct. Instead, we observe an apparent blunting of ethical sensitivity sufficient to destroy the understanding, appreciation, or regard for the moral quality of the criminal act, combined with a drastic, often protracted, lapse of inhibition. Rarely do we find a lapse of conscious awareness of the criminal act itself. Because pathologic gambling is a chronic disorder with a recognizable natural history (72,73), these mental elements typically can be identified before, during, and after the crime is committed. In this sense, the problem behavior seen in pathologic gambling is more like a process than like a state. In its effects it more closely resembles "insanity" of both legally recognized varieties—the inability to distinguish right from wrong or the inability to resist an impulse—than it does any state of intoxication. Before being widely rejected, the "capacity to conform" test for an insanity defense highlighted the problem of defining a "mental disease or defect." The *Freeman* court held that "an abnormality manifested only by repeated criminal or otherwise anti-social conduct" was not a disease (66, p. 625).

Clinical and Forensic Distinctions

It is recognized clinically that at least some compulsive gamblers who commit crimes are impaired physically and psychologically, and thus may be only partially responsible for their misconduct. In this sense, at law they resemble the inebriate, whose reason has been temporarily compromised; and for them the rules governing intoxication often seem more applicable than do those for insanity. Although they are only very rarely psychotic, and only a few may even be neurotic (72), they are nonetheless considered abnormal by many clinicians (73–78), albeit in ways of questionable relevance. Hence, for this subgroup of "impaired" compulsive gamblers, neither complete exculpation nor full responsibility seems appropriate. One might argue that as applied to pathologic gamblers who commit crimes, the legal rules should be applied not in terms of lack of intent, but in terms of lack of understanding of the ethical quality of the act and/or the ability to control behavior. But the legal rules have not adopted this view. As noted by Strassman, "[t]he link between compulsive gambling and a criminal offense is too tenuous to permit the court to find that the defendant lacks substantial capacity to conform his behavior to the requirements of the law as a result of his compulsive gambling disorder" (79, p. 201).

It must be conceded that many (possibly most) compulsive gamblers accused of crimes are simply persons who gamble to excess, not helpless victims of a "disease" of gambling that drives them to crime; and that such individuals should be accountable for their actions and the consequences thereof.

In practice, rather than raising an insanity defense, counsel for a pathologic gambler is more likely to attack the elements of the offense charged, arguing that the mental disorder of pathologic gambling rendered the defendant incapable of forming the specific intent requisite to the crime. *Wilson v. Commissioner* held that the defendant did not act "willfully" in filing an inaccurate tax return because his mental disorder prevented his forming a specific intent to violate the tax laws (80). For a comprehensive review of mental defenses in federal tax cases, see Ritholz and Fink (81).

Most judges—unpersuaded by modern scientific knowledge—in exercising their broad discretion in evidentiary matters, hold many persons criminally liable even though they are clearly afflicted with recognized diseases. The general failure of pathologic gambling as a defense in most criminal prosecutions reflects precisely this point of view. Currently, governing case law in most, but not all, jurisdictions is based on *United States v. Shorter* (13).

The Implications of United States v. Shorter

In *Shorter*, Judge Greene clearly considered pathologic gambling to be an addictive disorder. He correctly identified the conceptual problem that arises when the state of mind caused by such disorders exists over a long period, during which time the disordered person commits one or more crimes but otherwise manages to behave in a controlled and rational manner (13). In such cases the defense faces the daunting task of explaining how selected behaviors can be the substantially involuntary products of the intoxication or disorder, while other, relatively contemporaneous, behaviors need not be similarly affected. There is no satisfactory, unitary explanation for this. The elements of each offense must be analyzed in light of the facts of the case and the nature of the addictive process involved.

In *Shorter*, the judge also challenged the qualifications and legitimacy of clinicians specializing in compulsive gambling and refused to admit much of their testimony (13 [1985, p. 257]).

Sexual Addiction

In recent years, the diagnosis of "compulsive sexuality" or "sexual addiction" (82) has been offered as the basis for exculpation or mitigation in cases involving sexual, as well as less obviously related, offenses. Some few courts have admitted expert testimony about this controversial condition. In no jurisdiction has such a defense prevailed, absent more. A number of courts have admitted a defendant's alleged "sexual addiction" as a mitigating factor at sentencing. Limited treatment programs (most based on 12-step or other self-help principles) are available in the federal prison system and in that of most states.

Eating Disorders

There have been a few cases involving shoplifting and petty theft from groceries where an eating disorder (bulimia) was advanced as a defense. In none of these cases did the defense exculpate the accused. In two cases, after the defendants were convicted of the crimes charged, the sentencing judge recognized the eating disorder as a legitimate "mental disorder" that constituted a valid mitigating factor. Both defendants were sentenced to community supervision and service and to mandatory professional treatment instead of incarceration.

Compulsive Spending or Shopping

Recently, support groups based on 12-step principles and other self-help models have emerged for persons with the "diseases" of "compulsive spending" and "compulsive shopping." Advocates in these movements have adopted or endorsed addiction-derived explanations, language, and treatment approaches for these problems. The application of an addiction paradigm to these behaviors is of dubious validity, and neither problem has been widely recognized as an addictive disorder by professionals in the field (83,84).

Criminal defenses based on the "diseases" of compulsive spending or shopping have been rejected by the courts. In a few cases involving petty theft and shoplifting, expert clinical testimony about these excessive behaviors, although admitted, had little mitigatory impact at sentencing. A very thought-provoking feminist analysis of kleptomania and "compulsive shopping" as sexual disorders diagnosed only in women has been advanced by Camhi (85).

THE EFFECTS OF INTOXICANTS ON MEMORY

Expert Testimony About the Memory of Witnesses

Human memory is a complex phenomenon. One would expect the literature on the effects of intoxicants on human cognition, particularly memory, to be extensive—it is not. In cases where the defendant has been accused by persons who are or have been drug involved, an expert must assess the potential impact of their intoxicant use on their credibility as witnesses. The focus must be on the effect of the relevant intoxicant(s) on memory and its constituent cognitive processes (35–37,86–89). Although Federal Rule of Evidence 704(b) prohibits expert testimony on whether or not a defendant had the state of mind required for a particular crime (a decision reserved for the jury), it does not prohibit expert testimony about mental factors potentially affecting witnesses (22). To be an effective expert in this area, the addiction specialist requires a broad and deep understanding of human memory. Authoritative texts on research and theory about human memory written from both the clinical (90) and legal (21, Chap. 13) perspectives need to be studied closely.

Cocaine-Related Memory Dysfunction in Criminal Proceedings

Although any of the intoxicants can have potentially deleterious effects on selected memory functions, the effects of cocaine raise the most serious and frequent concerns (36,50–53,86–88,91,92). A significant number of today's large-scale cocaine trafficking cases are founded principally or solely on the testimony of alleged or self-styled coconspirators, who, more often than not, were themselves using large amounts of cocaine (and usually other intoxicants as well) during the period about which they will testify in great detail as to time, place, person, sequence, and events. In evaluating the credibility of such witnesses, it is critical to look for any possible effects of intoxicant use on their memory functions. It is always important and often productive to look for predicates and indicia of (cocaine-induced) confabulation that may taint their testimony. To establish the possibility that testimony may contain confabulated elements and therefore be subject to "reasonable doubt," it is necessary to assess the circumstances, frequency, extent, and detail of the witness's prior statements, depositions, narratives, or conferences with the authorities. Evidence of high-dose cocaine use, extensive "testimonial schooling" (21, §13:18), and progressively detailed and inclusive recall provides a sufficient predicate for an addiction medicine expert to consider reasonably and responsibly the possibility that confabulation is present. See Moriarty for a discussion of the legal issues, problems, and concerns associated with witness confabulation arising from all causes (21, §§13:17–19).

The Phenomenon of Confabulation

Confabulation is a neuropsychiatric symptom that is characteristic of diffuse organic brain disease and/or dysfunction. It refers to the unconscious filling in of memory gaps by imagined experiences, fabricated stories, or grossly distorted accounts of recent or remote events. It is absolutely distinct from lying, which implies both motive and awareness of the distortion or untruth. Confabulatory recall is inconsistent; it may change from moment to moment; and it may be induced unwittingly by suggestion. Characteristically, isolated events and information from the past are retained in fragmented form, but are at times related without regard for the intervals that separated these or for their proper temporal sequence. Sometimes, in confabulating, a person will telescope events, compressing time, thereby linking as cause and effect events that were widely separated in time and causally unrelated. These memory fragments may be cued, intentionally or unintentionally, during conversation (a) by suggestion, (b) by presentation of selected data about recent or remote events as if it were unequivocal fact, or (c) by provision of a cogent, internally consistent narrative explanation of some situation or event. The dysfunctional brain, in an attempt to maintain consistency with this apparent "reality," may fill in any memory gaps with associative, derivative, or suggested data.

Confabulation is never a consistent finding in any clinical condition. It is most frequently seen in cases of severe, nutrition-deficient alcoholism, head trauma, cerebral hypoxia, certain heavy metal poisonings, certain infections of the central nervous system (e.g., herpes or HIV encephalitis), or high-dose psychostimulant use.

Cocaine-Induced Confabulation

Confabulation may be seen in two phases of high-dose cocaine use. During the acute intoxication phase, the profound confusion, grandiosity, emotional lability, false sense of mastery, illusions, delusions, and hallucinations occasionally can induce certain users to confabulate "in real time." During the convalescent phase, after a period of abstinence from cocaine, the person gradually recalls fragments of past experience (many of which may have been originally misperceived) in a distorted way. In an attempt to preserve logical consistency, these may be linked with confabulated material. The more often such confabulated material is ratified by the social setting and in particular by authority figures (e.g., physicians, attorneys, or law enforcement officers) the more likely it is to become a fully integrated and unquestioned part of that person's self-history. It even may go on to become the basis for future thoughts, conclusions, and actions.

Although the U.S. Court of Appeals for the Sixth Circuit upheld the disallowance of such testimony in *United States v. Ramirez*, finding that such testimony went to the credibility, not the competence, of a witness (93), the exclusion of such testimony by a qualified addiction expert has been the rare exception, not the rule. A transcript of the direct and cross-examinations of the author about the effects of cocaine on the memory (confabulation) and credibility of a witness in a cocaine conspiracy case can be found in Moriarty (21, Appendix 3E).

REGULATORY AND ADMINISTRATIVE PROCEEDINGS

Members of licensed, regulated, or otherwise supervised professions (e.g., health care professionals, attorneys, airline pilots, interstate truckers) can find their licenses at risk for a number of reasons involving intoxicants. Two, however, are of exceptional importance and are discussed here: (a) allegations of "impairment" consequent to intoxicant use, and (b) for physicians, allegations of the "inappropriate" prescribing of opioids for the long-term management of chronic nonmalignant pain. In cases involving professional impairment, Burglass has identified two fundamental and very serious medical-legal issues: (a) the common presumption that "use equals abuse equals addiction equals impairment," and (b) that only a few regulatory agencies (e.g., the Federal Aviation Administration for pilots and the Department of Transportation for interstate truck drivers) have normative data defining the cognitive, sensory, or motor skills required of a normal, that is, a "nonimpaired" practitioner (94,95). With the exception of the blood alcohol concentration, which, as a matter of public policy, has been adopted in every state as an objective, affirmative indicium of impairment for the operation of a motorized vehicle, there are no similarly established norms for any other intoxicants, nor for alcohol-mediated impairment in other contexts.

Characteristically, these investigations and prosecutions of professional impairment are undertaken in the name of public health and safety. However, the ill-specified nature of these causes, and the zeal and fervor with which intoxicant regulatory activities are pursued, have led some observers to characterize our present food and drug laws, all medical and scientific justifications aside, as ultimately religious in intent, purpose, and effect, that is, as being, in effect, the dietary and liturgical laws of the modern secular religion of science (2).

Professional Impairment

In the assessment of professional impairment, regulatory policies do not reflect the clinically significant, specific differences between intoxicants in terms of their effects, patterns of use, routes of administration, nature of the dependence and/or withdrawal syndromes (if applicable), or resultant substance-related disabilities. Although there are a few regulatory and legal cases where (limited) consideration was given to these crucial distinctions, such deliberations are clearly the exception, not the rule.

All too often the proverbial deck is stacked against the accused professional, who, upon being accused of even the mere use of an intoxicant, is presumed to be impaired consequent thereto. Contrary to the traditions of Anglo-American jurisprudence, the accused professional then has the effective burden of proving his or her "innocence" in the face of the presumption of guilt. These prosecutions are invariably legitimized and justified as necessary to protect patients or clients, institutions, or professions from the harmful actions of impaired practitioners. But in practice, the hearing panels are often biased, punitive, and easily influenced by professional or institutional interests and politics. Even the isolated or occasional use of an intoxicant is often conflated with impairment, and harsh sanctions are imposed. If the accused admits to any use of intoxicants, impairment is usually presumed. If the accused denies use of intoxicants, the conclusion that accused is in "denial" will likely be drawn and considered as evidence of "addiction" and, consequently, of "impairment."

Of course, some intoxicant-involved professionals are impaired and in need of treatment until they are able to resume practicing with the skill and safety required in their profession. In recent years, a virtual industry for the diagnosis and treatment of "impaired" professionals has emerged. One can detect therein a disturbing propensity to conceptualize and treat professional "impairment" as if it were itself a distinct disease entity; it is not (94,95). The determination of intoxicant-related impairment in professionals is a very complex assessment that requires extensive input from independent, unbiased addiction medicine specialists throughout the process. If injustices are to be avoided, specialists in addiction medicine must be willing to become involved in these unpopular and often unsavory cases. They need to offer expert testimony that (a) obligates the regulators (clinically, ethically, and legally) to recognize and consider all relevant intoxicant-specific distinctions, and (b) requires the regulators to "prove" their case for impairment by specifying and quantifying the alleged deficiencies or disabilities of cognition, emotion, behavior, or professional skill that define the accused as impaired when measured against the standards of performance, skill, care, and safety required for professional practice in that jurisdiction or context.

As if this entire area were not already sufficiently troubling, Ackerman has identified an ominous trend toward requiring physicians who have been treated for chemical dependency to make informed consent disclosure to all patients (96).

Prescribing Opioids for Pain in Private Practice

Each year the prescribing profiles for controlled substances (class II opioids, in particular) of thousands of physicians are routinely (often automatically) monitored, sampled, or otherwise scanned, and evaluated by state regulatory bodies (97,98). Despite the dubious ethics and questionable purposes/efficacy of such monitoring programs, these practices increasingly are being "justified" by state regulatory bodies in the name of public health and safety, which are (presumptively) privileged over issues of individual privacy and confidentiality. The legal authority for these actions and the regulation of opioid prescribing for pain is provided by health (medical) practice acts legislated at the state level and by federal and state acts governing the use of controlled substances. Hundreds of physicians whose prescribing profiles are deemed "questionable" are then more thoroughly investigated. Such investigations and prosecutions may be initiated by even the brief treatment of a single patient! Of course, there are physicians whose prescribing of opioids is clinically inappropriate and/or unethical. Some in this group simply lack adequate current knowledge about the indications for opioid analgesia and/or the rational choice of appropriate opioid agents. Others are motivated by simple greed or sexual interest. Others are innocently duped, manipulated, or otherwise pressured by cunning and/or demanding patients. Regulatory agencies, in the main, have adequate procedures and appropriate sanctions to deal with these groups of physicians. What the majority of the state regulatory agencies lack are provisions and procedures for dealing fairly with physicians whose prescribing of opioids is not inappropriate and/or unethical. Indeed, most of the standards of practice governing opioid use are based on myths, prejudice, and misinformation about opioids, and the unexamined belief that mere exposure to these drugs invariably results in addiction in all patients. The prevailing obsession of regulators with "police" activities intended to prevent diversion has blinded them to their coequal obligation to ensure adequate access to opioids for patients who require these drugs for legitimate medical purposes (98). Conscientious, compassionate physicians in the latter group face substantial forensic problems: (a) the investigatory process raises serious ethical questions of privacy and confidentiality for both physician and patient; and (b) the regulatory hearings not infrequently violate fundamental legal principles of due process. The language of most state medical practice acts is predominantly proscriptive in intent, overly broad and/or vague, and easily subject to misinterpretation (98). It is therefore not surprising that the majority of American physicians tend to be "opiophobic." As a consequence, many legitimate pain patients are undertreated, mistreated, or not treated at all (99,100).

Although the use of opioids for the treatment of chronic nonmalignant pain remains the subject of sociopolitical controversy, clinical debate, and research (100,101), the validity and utility of the modality have been recognized and conscientious clinical protocols have been developed and implemented (102–106). When such protocols are used by pain specialists based in prestigious academic medical centers or dedicated pain treatment programs, the legitimacy, knowledge, and competence of the prescribing physician(s) are presumed, and regulatory problems rarely arise. The situation in private practice, however, is markedly different. In the latter context, legitimacy, knowledge, and competence are not presumed. The physician in private practice who is charged with the "inappropriate" prescribing of opioids effectively bears the burden of establishing his or her "legitimacy" and proving that the questioned use of opioids was in fact clinically appropriate and/or otherwise in keeping with applicable standards of care and practice. Sadly, state regulators have little difficulty finding addiction medicine experts who do not hesitate to condemn the opioid prescribing practices of

knowledgeable and ethical colleagues as "inappropriate" and/or "substandard."

Each year, dozens of well-informed, well-intentioned physicians are formally charged with violation(s) of a state medical practice act for having "inappropriately" prescribed opioid drugs to patients for chronic nonmalignant pain. They then must defend themselves (and their licenses) in a formal, adversarial hearing process, not unlike a criminal trial. Because such regulatory violations do not in themselves constitute acts of malpractice, medical malpractice insurance rarely provides counsel or funds the costs for the defense of such matters. The accused physician therefore must fund his or her own defense, the cost of which can easily exceed $100,000.

The two most frequent bases upon which regulators found allegations that a physician's use of long-term opioid therapy for chronic, nonmalignant pain is inappropriate are that such therapy "creates addicts" and that opioid therapy is contraindicated in any patient with a history of substance abuse. Both assertions are highly controversial, and the underlying assumptions, concerns, and issues of both have been comprehensively examined and challenged by specialists in pain management and addiction medicine (107–109). Although a 1992 review of the literature revealed reported prevalences of drug abuse, dependence, and addiction in chronic pain patients ranging from 3.2% to 18.9% (110), it has been suggested that the true prevalence of addictive disease in the chronic, nonmalignant pain population is unknown (111). In any event, every chronic pain patient being considered for long-term opioid therapy must undergo a comprehensive, multidimensional evaluation, which must include an analysis of their (a) pain (etiology, history, character), (b) prior experience with all modalities of pain management, including opioids, and (c) prior and current use of all classes of psychoactive drugs, prescribed or otherwise (111,112). The clinician in the pain clinic, private practice, or other settings must make a conscious effort to identify prior or current addictive disease, and must also attempt to identify those patients who are in active recovery (111).

For even the most-knowledgeable, best-intentioned, and best-prepared practitioner accused of opioid prescribing violations, exculpation is by no means assured, and ultimate vindication should never be assumed. However, documentation of the following material in the medical record often has proved to be the pivotal element in the successful defense of such cases:

1. A comprehensive evaluation and assessment of the etiology, history, and character of the patient's pain.
2. Clinical records or summaries from the specialists or subspecialists who have diagnosed and treated the primary medical or surgical conditions thought to be producing the patient's pain.
3. An appropriately executed (signed, witnessed, and notarized) document of the patient's "Informed Consent

to Treatment with Opioid Drugs." Because the law on informed consent varies substantially from state to state and is subject to increasingly frequent review and revision (113), this critical document must be drafted in close consultation with an attorney who is experienced, and absolutely up-to-date in this area of the law. Moreover, the trend in the law of informed consent is in the direction of requiring increased specificity about alternatives and risks, broader comprehensiveness, and clearer evidence of the patient's practical understanding of both the proposed treatment and the meaning of the signed document of consent.

4. Frequent multidimensional assessment and documentation of the efficacy of opioid therapy, the absence of drug toxicity, and the absence of indicia of "addiction" (including periodic urine toxicology screening). Multidimensional assessment of the frequency and distress illuminates the impact of symptoms and the efficacy of treatment on a patient's quality of life (114).

5. Annual (or more frequent if indicated) "Letters of Indemnification" from an appropriate surgical or medical specialist stating that the specialist has reexamined the patient, found that the underlying medical or surgical condition is still present and/or unchanged, that there have been no treatment innovations or technological breakthroughs from which the patient might be expected to benefit, and that therefore continued management of the patient's pain is clinically justifiable.

6. If the physician prescribing the opioids is not a credentialed expert or specialist in either pain management or addiction medicine, letters of consultation from a specialist in both of these areas are essential. Moreover, even if the prescribing physician is an expert in one of these two areas, a consultation letter from an expert in the other area is critical. These consultative reports should be updated at intervals appropriate to the patient's underlying diseases and/or reflective of the results of the regular multidimensional assessments described previously. Thus, patients who have exhibited behaviors that might be construed as "drug-seeking behavior" will need to be more frequently assessed by an addiction medicine specialist. Patients whose response to opioid therapy is untoward or inadequate (in terms of enhanced function and comfort) will require more frequent evaluation by a pain specialist.

Despite the application of scrupulous clinical "due diligence" and the maintenance of thorough, ongoing documentation, the use of long-term opioid therapy in patients with chronic nonmalignant pain is still fraught with potential pitfalls. Although articles in law reviews and clinical journals can provide insightful overviews of the policy and law governing the prescribing of opioids for pain (98,115,116), the interpretation and application of those laws by regulatory bodies changes substantially from one case to the next. Therefore, for anyone who uses this treat-

ment modality in private practice, knowledge of the current state of the law is absolutely essential!

To date, the attempt to define and control this complex area of medical practice by substituting regulations for clinical judgment has failed—resulting in grievous injustices for many practitioners and patients. The problem is neither "bad regulations" nor "incompetent regulators," and the solution is neither the drafting of more enlightened regulations nor the revision of biased regulatory procedures. The fundamental problem is that regulation is an inappropriate strategy for shaping policy and practice in this area. Clearly, a different approach is needed. The interests and concerns of all parties can be met by the promulgation of practice guidelines—specific, yet broad and flexible. Appropriate guidelines cannot possibly be formulated by bureaucrats, politicians, administrators, third-party payors, or any of the other marginally educated and/or nonclinically trained "watchdogs" of medicine and public health. The task demands comprehensive clinical knowledge and broad patient experience in pain management and addiction medicine. It needs to be an interdisciplinary, collaborative project initiated and directed by medical specialists in the fields of pain management and addictive disease. Fortunately, both fields are currently hard at work developing such guidelines. Input from practitioners (both specialists and generalists), as well as from patients, is being actively solicited and is an indispensable element of the process.

It is early yet to determine whether the availability of buprenorphine for the office-based practitioner will lead to significant legal difficulties. However, given the strict supervision being administered in terms of specialized Drug Enforcement Agency (DEA) certification, specialized training requirements, and limitations on patient quantity, it is certainly likely to be a closely examined process.

Administrative Proceedings

The effects of intoxicants of different classes have not been differentiated in administrative hearings or other proceedings involving employment eligibility, benefits, restriction, discrimination, supervision, discipline, or termination. In these venues, as in professional regulatory contexts, the prevailing presumption reflects the false and dangerous syllogism that "use equals abuse equals addiction equals impairment" (94). Moreover, routine screening for intoxicant use in the workplace is technically problematic (117) as well as legally and ethically questionable (118). Well-established principles of administrative law procedure are often violated, and fundamental legal rights (e.g., due process) often ignored. Despite their being treated like criminal "defendants," the accused in these proceedings are neither guaranteed adequate legal representation nor provided with the funds and resources (e.g., expert witnesses) necessary to present an adequate defense. Data and conclusions from questionably valid screening protocols and dubious testing methods and procedures often go unchallenged. It is vital that an addiction medicine specialist (preferably one with added qualifications as a Medical Review Officer) (a) reviews all of the technical data, (b) examines the accused to assess the nature and extent of any intoxicant-related problems or disabilities that might be relevant to job performance, and (c) provides testimony to the administrative review body to explain the meaning, significance, and implications of the findings. There is no other way to assure fairness for all parties.

Given the cultural prejudices about intoxicant use and the pressures on employers to maintain a "drug-free workplace," an employee who is accused of intoxicant use cannot safely assume that he or she will get a fair hearing or receive an equitable disposition. Addiction medicine specialists must be aware of these prevailing inequities. The need and opportunities for professional involvement in intoxicant-related matters of administrative law are great.

CONCLUSION

There can be no doubt that there are many serious conceptual problems and resultant inequities in the modern criminal law. History has shown that "the engine of the law doth indeed grind slowly." Now more than ever, the practice of law and the science of jurisprudence are in need of consultation and collaboration with other professions, intellectual disciplines, and fields of knowledge. The challenge to the medical, biologic, and cognitive sciences is clear. The response remains to be seen.

Doubtless, working in the forensic arena is not for everyone. For many addiction medicine professionals, the intense adversarial nature and constricting rules of criminal proceedings are personally offensive and professionally intolerable. For some others, ethical concerns, opinions and values, or personal experiences make them reluctant or unwilling to participate in what they perceive to be the shielding of an intoxicant user from the full consequences of his or her actions. For a few others, their understanding or personal history of addiction may lead them to interpret and condemn any such involvement as a form of professional "enabling" of a patient's addiction. But for those addictionists who do choose to participate in the judicial process, to make a contribution to the cause of justice, and to work to illuminate this vital medical-legal interface, the rewards from the intellectual challenge, professional enrichment, and personal fulfillment can be substantial.

REFERENCES

1. Burglass ME, Shaffer H. The natural history of ideas in the addictions. In: Shaffer H, Burglass ME, eds. *Classic contributions in the addictions.* New York: Brunner/Mazel, 1981:xvii–xlii.
2. Burglass ME, Shaffer H. Diagnosis in the addictions I: conceptual problems. *Adv Alcohol Subst Abuse* 1984;3(1&2):19–34.
3. Gambino B, Shaffer H. The concept of paradigm and the treatment of addiction. *Prof Psychol* 1979;10:207–233.
4. Shaffer H. Theories of addiction: in search of a paradigm. In: Shaffer H, ed. *Myths and realities: a book about drug users.* Boston: Zucker, 1977:42–45.
5. Shaffer H, Gambino B. Addiction paradigms II: theory, research and practice. *J Psychedelic Drugs* 1979;11: 299–304.
6. *State v. Eldredge,* 773 P.2d 29 (Utah 1989).
7. *Commonwealth v. Baldwin,* 502 A.2d. 253 (Pa. Super. Ct. 1985).
8. *People v. Rogers,* 800 P.2d 1327 (Colo. Ct. App. 1990).
9. *State v. Peeler,* 614 P.2d 335 (Ariz. Ct. App. 1980).
10. *People v. Gallegos,* 644 P.2d 920 (Colo. 1982).
11. *United States v. Rea,* 958 F.2d 1206 (2d Cir. 1992).
12. *United States v. LeRoy,* 944 F.2d 787 (10th Cir. 1991); *aff'd. after remand,* 984 F.2d 1095 (10th Cir. 1993).
13. *United States v. Shorter,* 608 F. Supp. 871 (D. D.C. 1985); *aff'd.,* 18 F. Supp. 255 (D. D.C. 1987).
14. *United States v. Davis,* 772 F.2d 1339 (7th Cir. 1985).
15. *United States v. Berrios-Rodriguez,* 768 F. Supp. 939 (D. Puerto Rico 1991).
16. *United States v. Ramirez,* 871 F.2d 582 (6th Cir. 1989).
17. *Hall v. State,* 568 So. 2d 882 (Fla. 1990).
18. Simon R. *Clinical psychiatry and the law,* 2nd ed. Washington, DC: American Psychiatric Press, 1992.
19. Golding SL, et al. Specialty guidelines for forensic psychologists. *Law Hum Behav* 1991;15:655–665.
20. Insanity Defense Reform Act of 1984, 18 U.S.C. sec. 17.
21. Moriarty JC. *Psychological and scientific evidence in criminal trials.* New York: Clark Boardman Callaghan, 1996.
22. Federal Criminal Code and Rules, 18 U.S.C., 1996.
23. *Frye v. United States,* 293 F. 1013 (D.C. Cir. 1923).
24. *Daubert v. Merrell Dow Pharmaceuticals, Inc.,* 113 S. Ct. 2786 (1993).
25. *United States v. DiDomenico,* 985 F.2d 1159, 1163 (2d Cir. 1993).
26. *Arcoren v. United States,* 929 F.2d 1235 (8th Cir.), *cert. denied,* 112 S. Ct. 312 (1991).
27. *United States v. Rubio-Villareal,* 927 F.2d 1495, 1502 (9th Cir. 1991).
28. *United States v. Azure,* 801 F.2d 336, 340 (8th Cir. 1986).
29. *United States v. Schmidt,* 711 F.2d 595, 598 (5th Cir. 1983).
30. *United States v. Gilliss,* 645 F.2d 1269, 1278 (8th Cir. 1981).
31. *United States v. Zink,* 612 F.2d 511, 514–515 (10th Cir. 1980).
32. Burglass ME. The role of the medical-psychiatric expert witness in drug-related cases. *Inside Drug Law* 1985; 2(3):1–6.
33. Nemerson SA. Alcoholism, intoxication, and the criminal law. *Cardozo L Rev* 1988;10:423.
34. American Psychiatric Association. *Diagnostic and statistical manual of mental disorders,* 4th ed., text revision. Washington, DC: Author, 2000.
35. Roemer RA, Cornwell A, Dewart D, et al. Quantitative electroencephalographic analyses in cocaine-preferring polysubstance abusers during abstinence. *Psychiatry Res* 1995;58(3): 247–257.

36. Strickland TL, Mena I, Villanueva-Meyer J, et al. Cerebral perfusion and neuropsychological consequences of chronic cocaine use. *J Neuropsychiatry Clin Neurosci* 1993;5(4):419–427.

37. Herning RI, Glover BJ, Koeppl B, et al. Cocaine-induced increases in EEG alpha and beta activity: evidence for reduced cortical processing. *Neuropsychopharmacology* 1994;11(1):1–9.

38. Cook J. Act, intention, and motive in the criminal law. *Yale Law J* 1917;26:645–658.

39. *United States v. Drew*, 25 Fed. Cas. No. 14,993 (C. C. D. Mass. 1828).

40. LaFave WR, Scott AW. *Substantive criminal law*. St. Paul, MN: West, 1986[suppl 1996].

41. *Burrows v. State*, 297 P. 1029 (Ariz. 1931).

42. *People v. Scott*, 146 Cal. App.3d 823, 194 Cal. Rptr. 633 (1983).

43. *City of Minneapolis v. Altimus*, 306 Minn. 462, 238 N.W.2d 851 (1976).

44. *Kane v. United States*, 399 F.2d 730 (9th Cir. 1968).

45. Burke SB. The defense of voluntary intoxication: now you see it, now you don't. *Ind L Rev* 1986;19:147.

46. *State v. Hall*, 214 N.W.2d 205 (Iowa 1974).

47. Hall J. Intoxication and criminal responsibility. *Harv L Rev* 1944;57:1056.

48. Schabas PB. Intoxication and culpability: towards an offence of criminal intoxication. *U T Fac L Rev* 1984;42:147.

49. Benton EH, Bor A, Leech WH, et al. Special project. Drugs and criminal responsibility. *Vanderbilt L Rev* 1980;33:1145–1218.

50. Foltin RW, Fischman MW, Pippen PA, et al. Behavioral effects of cocaine alone and in combination with ethanol or marijuana in humans. *Drug Alcohol Depend* 1993;32(2):93–106.

51. Higgins ST, Rush CR, Hughes JR, et al. Effects of cocaine and alcohol, alone and in combination, on human learning and performance. *J Exp Anal Behav* 1984;58 (1):87–105.

52. Ardila A, Rosselli M, Strumwasser S. Neuropsychological deficits in chronic cocaine abusers. *Int J Neurosci* 1991;57(1–2):73–79.

53. Manschreck TC, Schneyer ML, Weisstein CC, et al. Freebase cocaine and memory. *Compr Psychiatry* 1990;31(4):369–375.

54. Duffy JD. The neurology of alcoholic denial: implications for assessment and treatment. *Can J Psychiatry* 1995;40(5):257–263.

55. *Evans v. State*, 645 P.2d 155 (Alaska 1982).

56. *Commonwealth v. Sheehan*, 376 Mass. 765, 383 N.E.2d 1115 (1978).

57. *United States v. Lyons*, 731 F.2d 243 (5th Cir. 1984) (*en banc*).

58. Uelmen GF, Tennant FS. Endorphins, addiction and the defense of medical necessity. *Champion* 1985;9:6–11.

59. *United States v. Randall*, 104 Wash. Daily L. Rep. 2249 (1976).

60. *State v. Diania*, 604 P.2d 1312 (Wash. App. 1979).

61. *State v. Tate*, 477 A.2d 462 (N.J. Ct. App. 1984).

62. *United States v. Moore*, 486 F.2d 1139 (D.C. Cir. 1973) (*en banc*).

63. *M'Naghten's Case*, 8 Eng. Rep. 718 (1843).

64. *United States v. Hinckley*, [No opinion issued] (D. D.C. 1982).

65. Comprehensive Crime Control Act of 1984 (18 U.S.C. sec 20).

66. *United States v. Freeman*, 804 F.2d 1574 (11th Cir. 1986).

67. *Commonwealth v. Mello*, 420 Mass. 375, 649 N.E.2d 1106 (Mass. 1995).

68. West's Ann. Cal. Penal Code § 28.

69. *Bethea v. United States*, 365 A.2d 64 (App. D.C. 1976).

70. United States Sentencing Commission. *Federal sentencing guidelines manual, 1995–96 ed.* St. Paul, MN: West Publishing, 1996.

71. Burglass ME. Pathological gambling: forensic update and commentary. In: Shaffer H, Cummins T, Gambino B, et al, eds. *Compulsive gambling. Yesterday, today, and tomorrow.* Lexington, MA: Lexington Books/DC Heath, 1981:205–222.

72. Custer RL. Gambling and addiction. In: Craig RJ, Baker SL, eds. *Drug dependent patients.* Springfield, IL: Charles C Thomas, 1982:367–381.

73. Lesieur HR. *The chase career of the compulsive gambler.* New York: Anchor Press/Doubleday, 1977.

74. Carlton PL, Manowitz P. Physiological factors as determinants of pathological gambling. *J Gambling Behav* 1988;3:274–285.

75. Goldstein L. Differential EEG activation and pathological gambling. *Biol Psychiatry* 1985;20:1232–1234.

76. Milkman H, Sunderwirth S. Addictive processes. *J Psychoactive Drugs* 1982;14(3):177–192.

77. Moran E. An assessment of the report of the royal commission on gambling 1976–1978. *Br J Addict* 1979:74:3–9.

78. Wray I, Dickerson MG. Cessation of high frequency gambling and "withdrawal" symptoms. *Br J Addict* 1981;76:401–405.

79. Strassman HD. Forensic issues in pathological gambling. In: Balski T, ed. *The handbook of pathological gambling.* Springfield, IL: Charles C Thomas, 1987:195–204.

80. *Wilson v. Commissioner*, 76 TC 623 (1981).

81. Ritholz J, Fink R. New developments and dangers in the psychiatric defense to tax fraud. *J Taxation* 1970;32:322–330.

82. Carnes PJ. *Don't call it love.* New York: Bantam Books, 1991.

83. Christenson GA, Raber RJ, deZwann M, et al. Compulsive buying: descriptive characteristics and psychiatric comorbidity. *J Clin Psychiatry* 1994;55:5–11.

84. Bernik MA, Akerman D, Amaral JAMS, et al. Cue exposure in compulsive buying [letter]. *J Clin Psychiatry* 1996;57:90.

85. Camhi L. Stealing femininity: department store kleptomania as sexual disorder. *Differences* 1993;5(1):26–50.

86. Beatty WW, Katzung VM, Moreland VJ, et al. Neuropsychological performance of recently abstinent alcoholics and cocaine abusers. *Drug Alcohol Depend* 1995;37:247–253.

87. Bernal B, Ardila A, Bateman JR. Cognitive impairments in adolescent drug-abusers. *Int J Neurosci* 1994;75:203–212.

88. Berry J, van Gorp WG, Herzberg DS, et al. Neuropsychological deficits in abstinent cocaine abusers: preliminary findings after two weeks of abstinence. *Drug Alcohol Depend* 1993;32:231–237.

89. Meek PS, Clark HW, Solana VL. Neurocognitive impairment: the unrecognized component of dual diagnosis in substance abuse treatment. *J Psychoactive Drugs* 1989;21:153–160.

90. Lezak MD. *Neuropsychological assessment,* 3rd ed. New York: Oxford University Press, 1995.

91. Withers NW, Pulvirenti L, Koob GF, et al. Cocaine abuse and dependence. *J Clin Psychopharmacol* 1995;15(1):63–78.

92. Teoh SK, et al. Pituitary volume in men with concurrent heroin and cocaine dependence. *J Clin Endocrinol Metab* 1993;76:1529–1532.

93. *United States v. Ramirez*, 871 F.2d 582 (6th Cir. 1989).

94. Burglass ME. Use equals abuse equals impairment: a false and dangerous syllogism. *Alcohol Clin Exp Res* 1988;12(1):190(abst).

95. Burglass ME. Chemical dependence and impairment: conceptual problems. *Alcohol Clin Exp Res* 1989;13(1):147(abst).

96. Ackerman TF. Chemically dependent physicians and informed consent disclosure. *J Addict Dis* 1996;15(2):25–42.

97. Portenoy RK. Therapeutic use of opioids: prescribing and control issues. *NIDA Res Monogr* 1993;131:35–50.

98. Hills S. Government regulatory influences on opioid prescribing and their impact on the treatment of pain of nonmalignant origin. *J Pain Symptom Manage* 1996;11(5):287–298.

99. Morgan J. American opiophobia: customary underutilization of opioid analgesics. *Adv Alcohol Subst Abuse* 1985; 5:163.

100. Portenoy RK. Chronic opioid therapy for persistent noncancer pain: can we get past the bias? *APS Bull* 1991;1:4–5.

101. Reidenberg MM, Portenoy RK. The need for an open mind about the treatment of chronic non-malignant pain. *Clin Pharmacol Ther* 1994;55(4):367–369.

102. Portenoy RK, Foley KM. Chronic use of opioid analgesics in non-malignant pain: report of 38 cases. *Pain* 1986;25(2):171–186.

103. Portenoy RK. Chronic opioid therapy in nonmalignant pain. *J Pain Symptom Manage* 1990;5[1 suppl]:S46–S62.

104. Savage SR. Opoid use in the management of chronic pain. *Med Clin North Am* 1999;83(3):761–786.

105. Schug S, Merry A, Acland R. Treatment principles for the use of opioids in pain of nonmalignant origin. *Drugs* 1991;42:228–232.

106. Schofferman J. Long-term use of opioid analgesia for the treatment of chronic pain of non-malignant origin. *J Pain Symptom Manage* 1993;8:279–288.

107. Portenoy RK, Payne R. Acute and chronic pain. In: Lowinson JH, Ruiz P, Millman RB, et al, eds. *Substance abuse: a comprehensive textbook,* 2nd ed. Baltimore: Williams & Wilkins, 1992:691–721.

108. Wesson DR, Ling W, Smith DE. Prescription opioids for the treatment of pain in patients with addictive disease. *J Pain Symptom Manage* 1993;8:289–296.

109. Savage SR. Management of acute and chronic pain and cancer pain in the addicted patient. In: Miller NS, ed. *Principles of addiction medicine.* Sec. VIII, Chap 1. Chevy Chase, MD: American Society of Addiction Medicine, 1995:1–16.

110. Fishbain DA, Rosomoff HL, Rosomoff RS. Drug abuse, dependence, and addiction in chronic pain patients. *Clin J Pain* 1992;8:77–85.

111. Savage SR. Addiction in the treatment

of pain: significance, recognition, and management. *J Pain Symptom Manage* 1993;8(5):265–278.

112. Sees KL, Clark HW. Opioid use in the treatment of chronic pain: assessment of addiction. *J Pain Symptom Manage* 1993;8(5):257–264.

113. Faden R, Beauchamp T. *A history and theory of informed consent.* New York: Oxford University Press, 1986.

114. Portenoy RK, Thaler HT, Kornblith AB, et al. The Memorial Symptom Assessment Scale: an instrument for the evaluation of symptom prevalence, characteristics and distress. *Eur J Cancer* 1994;30A(9):1326–1336.

115. Tennant FS, Uelmen GF. Narcotic maintenance for chronic pain: medical and legal guidelines. *Postgrad Med* 1983;73:81–94.

116. Clark HW, Sees KL. Opioids, chronic pain, and the law. *J Pain Symptom Manage* 1993;8(5):297–305.

117. Osterloh J, Becker C. Chemical dependency and drug testing in the workplace. *West J Med* 1990;152:506–513.

118. Burglass ME. Employee assistance and drug testing: striving for fairness. *Alcohol Clin Exp Res* 1988;12(1):190(abst).

CHAPTER 83

The Role of Neuropsychological Assessment in Forensic Addiction

ARI D. KALECHSTEIN, WILFRED G. van GORP, AND GARRETT J. ZELEN

"Addiction is not merely the chronic use of a drug. Addiction involves the compulsion to use drugs, a loss of control over the time and amount of drug use, and continued drug use despite negative consequences."

Mim J. Landry, *Understanding Drugs of Abuse: the Processes of Addiction, Treatment and Recovery,* Washington, DC: American Psychiatric Press 1964, p. 7.

This quote succinctly captures the adverse effects of drug use. Not infrequently, the "loss of control" includes en-

gagement in some sort of criminal activity. At that point in time, the criminal justice system intercedes and the process of reaching a determination on criminal charges begins, taking into account the manner in which the addict's behavior was affected by drug use at the time of the criminal act or the residual effects of drug use that predated the criminal act. To understand how drug use can affect behavior, mental health experts are frequently asked to educate the courts regarding this issue so that triers of fact (i.e., judge and jury) can make a well-informed decision.

This chapter addresses how the neuropsychological assessment can be used to assist in the resolution of issues related to criminal law when the crime involves the misuse of alcohol or drugs.

Given the current general state of the law, it is reasonable for mental health practitioners to offer expert opinions regarding the effects of various substances on neuropsychological functioning, provided that these practitioners use generally accepted techniques and base their opinions on the extant literature on the topic. In the next section, we address the utility of neuropsychological assessment in a forensic setting in which the issue is related to substance misuse. We begin by describing the basic elements of a neuropsychological assessment. We then show how the data from a neuropsychological assessment can be applied to different cases in which substance misuse is an issue.

THE UTILITY OF NEUROPSYCHOLOGICAL ASSESSMENT IN A FORENSIC SETTING

This section reviews the core elements of a neuropsychological evaluation.

To date, hundreds of neuropsychological tests have been published for the purpose of evaluating central nervous system (CNS) disturbance (1). While forensic experts may differ with regard to the specific measures that they choose to administer, when conducting a forensic evaluation in which the administration of neuropsychological measures is appropriate, well-trained forensic experts tend to include measures that assess the following neuropsychological domains:

1. Intellectual functioning: usually assessed using a series of subtests that are sensitive to either verbal or nonverbal capabilities/domains. Wechsler designed his scales of intellectual functioning so that they would predict ability to succeed in the world (2).
2. Attention/psychomotor speed: includes measures designed to evaluate an examinee's capacity to attend and/or respond quickly to material presented orally or visually over brief or extended periods of time (1). The measures are typically designed to evaluate simple, sustained, or divided attention.
3. Language: includes measures that evaluate an examinee's capacity to comprehend and/or express verbal material in a written and/or oral format (1).
4. Visuospatial functioning: includes measures that evaluate perceptual skills and, in some cases, require the examinee to draw or construct an object (1).
5. Verbal and nonverbal learning and memory: includes measures that evaluate an examinee's capacity to register, store, retain, and retrieve previously presented verbal and/or visual material (1).
6. Executive systems functioning (a.k.a. frontal lobe functioning): includes measures that are sensitive to volition, planning, decision making, response inhibition, judgment, and set shifting (3).
7. Emotional functioning/personality: includes measures that are sensitive to current mood state, mood state over time, and personality factors (1).
8. Motivation: includes measures that are sensitive to an examinee's attempts to put forth his or her best effort on measures of cognition or to portray him- or herself accurately on measures of emotional or behavioral functioning (1).

Table 83.1 includes a suggested list of measures for each domain. This table, while not inclusive, provides a list of neuropsychological measures that are frequently used by forensic experts (4). For test security purposes, this chapter will not list measures of motivation that are considered

TABLE 83.1. *A suggested list of neuropsychological measurements*

Intelligence
Wechsler Adult Intelligence Scale (WAIS)-III
National Adult Reading Test–Revised
Attention
WAIS-III Digit Span and Digit Symbol subtests
Trail Making Test–Part A
Stroop Color-Word subtests
Symbol Digit Modalities Test
Language
Woodcock-Johnson Tests of Academic Achievement–III
Verbal fluency tests
Visual spatial function
WAIS-III Block Design
Judgment of Line Orientation
Rey Osterrieth Complex Figure Test–Copy
Learning and memory
California Verbal Learning Test
Rey Auditory Verbal Learning Test
Brief Visuospatial Retention Test–Revised
Rey Osterrieth Complex Figure Test–Delayed Recall
Executive functions
Category Test
Trail Making Test–Part B
Stroop Interference subtest
Wisconsin Card Sorting Test
Mood/personality
Minnesota Multiphasic Personality Inventory–2

to be useful when conducting a neuropsychological evaluation in a forensic setting.

With regard to the interpretation of neuropsychological test scores, the normative data set(s) used to convert the raw scores should be made available. The normative data set(s) used to score the data should be the most applicable, based on demographic factors (e.g., age, education), recency of publication, and/or other moderating factors. In particular, a recent study showed that the interpretation of examinees' test scores can vary significantly as a function of the normative data set (5).

In addition to administering a comprehensive battery of measures that are considered to be relatively sensitive to the effects of substance use, a forensic evaluation should include a review of background information that is pertinent to the charges. This can include, but is not limited to, the following domains:

1. Medical history
2. Mental health history
3. Substance use history
4. Legal history
5. Academic/employment history
6. Developmental history
7. Collateral data relevant to the charges
8. Pertinent research

The conclusion section of the report should include the synthesis of the background information and the data collected during the evaluation. This section of the evaluation should include the following information:

1. A statement of the issue to be addressed. For example, given the following fictional case, the issue might be stated as follows, "The purpose of the evaluation was to determine the presence, if any, of neuropsychological impairment and to determine the effects of methamphetamine intoxication on Mr. Smith's behavior." Both the triers of fact and the attorneys need to be clear regarding the specific focus of the evaluation.
2. A clear statement of one's opinion as it relates to the issue. For example, in reference to the same fictional case, a clinician might conclude, "The results of neuropsychological assessment did not reveal the presence of deficits associated with methamphetamine dependence; however, the historical data portray an individual who probably acted impulsively as a result of methamphetamine intoxication."
3. A review of the data that support or do not support the opinion. For example, with regard to the same fictional case, the forensic expert would lay out the data in a manner that would enable the triers of fact to understand how the forensic expert arrived at a particular opinion. If the issue was methamphetamine intoxication, the forensic expert might include the following data:
   a. History of substance dependence (if any)
   b. Results of toxicology screens (if any)
   c. Third-party observations of the defendant's behavior (if any)

APPLICATION OF NEUROPSYCHOLOGICAL ASSESSMENT FINDINGS IN CRIMINAL MATTERS IN WHICH SUBSTANCE MISUSE IS AN ISSUE

In this section, we show how the findings from neuropsychological assessment can be used effectively to demonstrate how substance use and misuse can affect individuals' behavior during different phases of use, including intoxication and following the withdrawal phase. It is important to note that we recognize that examinees might malinger (i.e., feign mental health difficulties) and, as a result, we consider this issue whenever we conduct neuropsychological evaluations. Because there is an extensive literature that focuses on the assessment of malingering in a forensic setting, we elected to not address that issue in this chapter. Instead, we are providing three case examples that show affirmatively the manner in which substance use and misuse can affect behavior in a meaningful manner. The cases focus on the following issues:

1. The effects of substance intoxication; and
2. The residual effect(s) of drugs following cessation of use.

It is important to note that each examinee underwent an extensive neuropsychological evaluation and a detailed report was written for each case. To be succinct, however, we are presenting the salient details from each case.

Substance Intoxication

In this section, we review the *Diagnostic and Statistical Manual of Mental Disorders, 4th ed., text revision (DSM–IV–TR)* (6) definition of substance intoxication, caveats of using the *DSM* in a legal setting, specific drugs that are associated with intoxication, the relevance of intoxication to issues of mitigation, and a case example.

DSM–IV–TR Definition of Intoxication

The *DSM–IV–TR* provides a useful definition of intoxication produced by various substances of abuse. As an example, The *DSM* includes the definition for amphetamine intoxication. This definition, which was formulated by a panel of experts regarding amphetamine intoxication, shows that individuals intoxicated as a result of amphetamine (or methamphetamine) are at risk to demonstrate impaired cognition (e.g., judgment) and/or emotional and behavioral abnormalities (e.g., belligerence, mood lability). This generally accepted definition provides a framework for explaining why individuals who are intoxicated as a result of substance use are at risk to evidence poor judgment.

Caveats of Using DSM–IV–TR

While the *DSM–IV–TR* provides a framework for explaining how substance intoxication can affect behavior, the manual also includes an important caveat regarding its use in forensic settings. For example, the cautionary statement includes specific wording that warns forensic experts that it is inappropriate to use a *DSM–IV–TR* diagnosis *per se* to address legal issues such as "individual responsibility, disability determination, and competency." Moreover, it also states that the *DSM–IV–TR* is not meant to serve as a substitute for "...legal or other nonmedical criteria for what constitutes mental disease, mental disorder, or mental disability." This definition is not meant to dissuade forensic experts from using the *DSM–IV–TR* as a framework for explaining why intoxicated individuals are prone to behave in an aberrant manner. The *DSM–IV–TR* criteria are actually quite helpful in this regard. Instead, the cautionary statement infers that it is incumbent upon the mental health provider to demonstrate explicitly how

TABLE 83.2. *Profile of methamphetamine-induced psychosis*

Author	Number of study subjects	Methamphetamine use indices		Psychotic symptoms						
		Dose (mg/d)	Route of intake	Delusions paranoid	Grandiose	Somatic	Hallucinations auditory	Visual	Disordered thoughts	Length of episode
Kramer et al., 1967	review	100–300	i.v.	x	n/r	n/r	x	x	x	n/r
Bell, 1965	7	n/r	n/r	7/7	n/r	n/r	7/7	4/7	n/r	7–10 days
Ellinwood, 1967	25	>30 mg	n/r	20/25	n/r	11/25	12/25	11/25	n/r	n/r
Griffith et al., 1970	6	20–190	P.D.	5/6	n/r	n/r	n/r		n/r	0–3 days
Jonnson & Gunne, 1970	12	n/r	n/r	12/12	n/r	12/12	(not specified)		11/12	0–13 days
Bell et al., 1973	16	15–1,000	i.v.	12/14	n/r	n/r	10/14	6/14	not present	0–6 days
Angrist et al., 1974	8	n/r	n/r	x	x	(present, type not specified)			x	n/r
Hall et al., 1996	301	n/r	P.D.	198/301	n/r	n/r	120/301	33/301	n/r	0–2 hours

Abbreviation: i.v. = intravenous; n/r = not relevant; P.D. = oral by mouth; x = present, not quantitated.

the intoxication led to specific behaviors by the defendant and how the intoxication affected the defendant's ability to reason and to modulate their behavior.

Relevance of Intoxication to Intent

As previously stated, negation or diminishment of intent are concepts that are used to explain why various mental diseases or disorders or conditions, such as intoxication from the misuse of alcohol and drugs, can potentially affect an individual's ability to make well-reasoned judgments. Terms considered to be synonymous with "well-reasoned" include "impulsively" or "acting without thinking." Indeed, the *DSM–IV–TR* indicates that intoxication on the following drugs is associated with a risk for impaired judgment: alcohol, amphetamine, cannabis, cocaine, hallucinogens, opioids, phencyclidine, and sedative–hypnotics. Others have defined intoxication as "... dysfunctional changes in physiological functioning, psychological functioning, mood state, cognitive process, or all of these, as a consequence of consumption of a psychoactive substance; usually disruptive, and often stemming from central nervous system impairment" (7).

A brief review of the extant literature reveals that substance intoxication is associated with a host of negative outcomes. For example, intoxication on the following substances is associated with increased mortality rates or exposure to violence or physical injury: alcohol (8–10), phencyclidine (PCP) (11), cocaine (12,13), ecstasy (14), heroin (15–17), methamphetamine (18,19), and polysubstance use (20–22). Moreover, intoxication on the following substances is associated with an increased risk of propagating or experiencing a physical injury: alcohol (23–25), cannabis (26), cocaine (27,28), methamphetamine (29,30), and PCP (31).

Given these data, it is clear that intoxication is associated with a *risk* for impaired neuropsychological functioning. We specifically use the term "risk" because intoxication is not the polar opposite with impairment; however, the available literature provides a framework for showing how impairment might occur as a result of substance intoxication. In the next section, we present a case example that demonstrates how the available data regarding intoxication can be effectively used to explain aberrant behavior.

Intoxication: Case Example

In this case, the defendant, Mr. X, was charged with attempted kidnapping and attempted carjacking during a period of time when he was intoxicated on methamphetamine. The purpose of the evaluation of Mr. X was to determine whether the available data:

1. Were consistent with that of an individual who used methamphetamine;

2. Were consistent with that of an individual who was experiencing a methamphetamine-induced psychosis; and

3. Portrayed an individual who acted impulsively or without thinking.

A summary of the facts is as follows: Mr. X. was smoking methamphetamine over a 24-hour period on August 30. On August 31, Mr. X ran into convenience store, where he told the clerk and a nearby customer that someone was pursuing him and planned to kill him. He then ran out of the store, jumped into a vehicle through the passenger-side window, unsuccessfully attempted to start the engine of the vehicle, jumped out of the vehicle and ran across a heavily trafficked, eight-lane highway to a fast-food restaurant, jumped headfirst into the drive-through window of the restaurant, ran out the door, and crouched behind a row of shrubbery about 2 feet high. A physician who evaluated Mr. X and a passerby at the convenience store who observed Mr. X's behavior described him as "agitated." The two arresting police officers characterized Mr. X as "paranoid" and "very scared." Moreover, they reported that Mr. X spoke nonsensically. Furthermore, when Mr. X was left alone in the interview room at the jail, the arresting officers reported that he was engaged in a "bizarre" conversation. A physical examination of Mr. X conducted at the jail within 3 hours of his arrest revealed the presence of an elevated heart rate (~160 beats per minute), dilated pupils (~8 mm), and a urine toxicology screen that tested positive for amphetamine.

Based on the *DSM–IV–TR* criteria for amphetamine intoxication, Mr. X demonstrated four of the eight symptoms listed in subsection C that are associated with methamphetamine intoxication (i.e., tachycardia, psychomotor agitation, confusion, and dilated pupils). Furthermore, based on the behavior observations of the officers and the bystanders and consistent with subsection B, Mr. X demonstrated impaired judgment. Moreover, and consistent with subsection D, the physical examination did not reveal the presence of other physical or mental health factors that could account for Mr. X's behavior.

Mr. X also demonstrated symptoms consistent with a methamphetamine-induced psychosis (*DSM–IV–TR* code: 292.11). For example, the officers reported that Mr. X appeared "paranoid." Additionally, the psychotic behavior subsided over time and did not reemerge during the 6-month period of time in which Mr. X was incarcerated.

It is noteworthy that Mr. X did not demonstrate neuropsychological impairment despite his history of methamphetamine use. He performed within expected limits on measures of attention, memory, and executive functioning given his age (mid-twenties), education (completed tenth grade), and history of methamphetamine use (~0.5 g/d over a 3-year period).

With regard to preparation for trial, exhibits were generated that documented the following:

1. Behavior observations from the police officers and bystanders;
2. Results of the physical examination;
3. The *DSM–IV–TR* criteria for methamphetamine intoxication; and
4. Results of studies (see Table 83.2) that examined methamphetamine-induced psychosis (32–36).

These data were collectively used to enhance the knowledge base of the triers of fact regarding these issues. Based on these data, the jury acquitted Mr. X of the charges.

The Residual Effect(s) of Drugs Following the Cessation of Use

The findings reviewed in the previous section reveals that much effort has been marshaled toward detailing the adverse effects of substance intoxication. For example, more than 10 pages from the *DSM–IV–TR* are devoted to the description of the effects of intoxication produced by various drugs; in contrast, other than the section on Substance-Induced Persisting Amnesia and Substance-Induced Persisting Dementia, which are based on the lasting effects of alcohol dependence, the *DSM–IV–TR* offers virtually no information regarding the residual effects of other drugs. This omission is noteworthy given that cessation of drug use does not necessarily eliminate the future effect(s) of the previous drug use. For example, a number of illicit drugs are associated with an increased risk for experiencing cognitive deficits. Those drugs include alcohol (37), cocaine (38), ecstasy (39), and methamphetamine (40). Moreover, individuals who previously misused drugs are at risk to experience craving for the drug, depending on their drug use history and contextual factors (41).

Table 83.3 lists various substances that are abused and the neuropsychological domains that are potentially affected by these substances. It is important to note that this table provides a qualitative review of the findings of studies examining the neuropsychological consequences of substance abuse and that it is important to consider demographic profile and drug use pattern in evaluating the potential effects of various substances of abuse. For example, a recent meta-analytic review by Grant and colleagues revealed that chronic cannabis use is associated only with modest effects on learning and memory; otherwise, cannabis users performance on neuropsychological measures was not significantly different from that of controls (42). In contrast, Bolla and colleagues found that chronic, high-dose marijuana use was associated with deficits on measures of memory and executive functioning (43).

In this section, we discuss the residual effects of drug abuse in two cases. In the first case, the defendant performed within normal limits on each of the measures of neuropsychological functioning. In the second case, the defendant demonstrated marked neuropsychological impairments as a result of drug use. Each case is reviewed below.

Residual Effects in the Absence of Neuropsychological Impairment

In this case, the defendant, Mr. Y, was charged with possession of cocaine. The purpose of the evaluation of Mr. Y was to:

1. Determine if there was an explanation for Mr. Y's relapse;
2. Determine neuropsychological impairment contributed to Mr. Y's relapse; and
3. Offer the most reasonable recommendation for the case.

A summary of the facts is as follows: Mr. Y. previously was convicted of cocaine possession, had been on parole for 13 months, and had passed random urine toxicology screens. Mr. Y stated that he never received treatment for crack-cocaine dependence while incarcerated. He stated that none of his previous attorneys addressed the issue of treatment with him.

At the time of his arrest, Mr. Y reported that he was struggling to find work, and he became depressed. While feeling depressed, he was running some errands for his mother, saw a man smoking crack cocaine, and he

TABLE 83.3. *Neuropsychological domains at risk to be affected by various substances of abuse*

Drug	Intellectual functioning	Attention psychomotor speed	Language	Visuospatial functioning	Learning and memory	Executive functioning
Alcohol		x		x	x	x
Cocaine		x			x	x
Methamphetamine		x			x	x
Marijuana					x	x
MDA (methylenedioxy-amphetamine; ecstasy)		x			x	x

"... went on a straight binge from xx/yy/zz to the day of his arrest." Mr. Y stated, "I was on autopilot.... I had my guard down.... I'd been confronted before, seeing a transaction take place in front my car, but I left the scene real quick.... This time, something happened that hit me.... I don't know what came over me."

When asked if he ever craved the drug, Mr. Y stated that, at times, "I just wanted the drug.... I may have had some nice possessions, but the craving overpowered my desire to have those possessions, and I would be willing to part with the possessions to get the drugs.... There would be certain times that I would be craving it so bad I would do whatever I had to do to get money to support my habit." However, when not using drugs, Mr. Y characterized himself as "a nice person, respectful, a hard worker, and honest." Mr. Y's parents affirmed his self-portrayal.

The available data revealed that Mr. Y was diagnosed with cocaine dependence, but was not diagnosed with a comorbid mental health disorder or a medical disorder. He did not demonstrate impairment in neuropsychological domains that are most likely to be affected by cocaine dependence (i.e., attention/psychomotor speed, learning and memory, and executive functioning). When not using cocaine, he was characterized as a reliable employee by previous employers.

Given this pattern of facts, it is likely that two factors contributed to Mr. Y's relapse. One factor is that Mr. Y experienced cue-induced craving for cocaine. Indeed, the available literature on this topic shows that cocaine dependent individuals are likely to experience craving for cocaine when they are exposed to environmental cues that remind them of cocaine use (44–51). The other, and equally important, factor is that Mr. Y never underwent treatment for cocaine dependence. Research shows that legal sanctions without accompanying drug treatment and monitoring of drug use do not reduce incidence of drug use or criminal behavior (52,53). If decreased drug use reduces the probability that Mr. Y will engage in criminal behavior, then it seems imperative to use mechanisms that will promote abstinence for him. These mechanisms include (a) intensive, long-term treatment and aftercare, (b) comprehensive and well-coordinated supervision, and (c) frequent monitoring of individuals for the early recognition of relapses, so that individuals can complete drug treatment successfully despite the relapses (53).

Based on these data, Mr. Y's attorney successfully negotiated a plea for him. Mr. Y was given the opportunity to enter a treatment program and remain abstinent.

Marked Neuropsychological Impairment as a Result of Chronic Alcohol Dependence

In this case, the defendant, Mr. Z, was charged with attempted murder. The purpose of the evaluation of Mr. Z was to determine if neuropsychological impairment con-

tributed to Mr. Z's behavior at the time of the incident. A summary of the facts is as follows:

On the day of the incident, Mr. Z stated that he had been at the Veteran's Administration (VA) for 6 hours during the day because "I had appointments." Mr. Z stated that he had not been drinking. When he returned, Mr. Z stated, "When I came home and saw what was going on ... one person was smoking crack and he (Mr. Q, his temporary houseguest) was trying to screw a hooker on the couch ... there were empty beer bottles on the floor ... I couldn't believe he was doing that in my place." When Mr. Z stated that he wanted the prostitute and Mr. Q to leave his apartment, Mr. Q "was angry and rude.... He acted like it was his place." Mr. Z stated that he never had been involved in a similar confrontation with Mr. Q.

Mr. Z stated that he left the apartment to "calm down." When Mr. Z returned to his apartment approximately 30 minutes later, Mr. Z stated that Mr. Q "continued to bitch" about Mr. Z's wanting to return to his own apartment. Mr. Z stated that Mr. Q wanted Mr. Z to leave the apartment so that he (Mr. Q) could have sex with the prostitute.

Mr. Z stated that he "wasn't going to be put out of his own home." At that point in the evening, Mr. Z stated that he jabbed his finger in the chest of Mr. Q and told him to leave the apartment. Mr. Z stated that Mr. Q responded by breaking his (Mr. Z's) pinkie finger on his right hand. Mr. Z replied that he then "socked up" Mr. Q (i.e., punched him in the face). Mr. Q. responded by hitting Mr. Z in the head with a beer bottle. Mr. Z then punched Mr. Q in the face, grabbed a knife in his vicinity, grabbed Mr. Q's ear, and cut the ear off. Mr. Z reported that his knife cut through Mr. Q's ear in "half a second." When asked if he planned to use the knife on Mr. Q., Mr. Z stated, "I didn't even think about it.... It was like he hit me and the next thing I knew his ear was in my hand.... I was aghast at what I'd done.... I couldn't believe it was real."

Mr. Z stated that he helped Mr. Q to his bed and told him that he would call the paramedics. Mr. Z reported that he called the paramedics from a neighbor's apartment 5 minutes later and that the paramedics arrived 5 minutes after the phone call. Mr. Z stated that he was arrested when the police and the paramedics arrived. Mr. Q generally confirmed Mr. Z's accounting of the facts.

Mr. Z reported a long history of substance dependence. Hospital records dated xx/yy/zz report that Mr. Z has used heroin since 1970. Mr. Z confirmed this date in the clinical interview. The records indicated that he previously had been admitted to substance abuse treatment units on three occasions between 1992 and 1996. The records from 1996 show that Mr. Z smoked 2.5 packs of cigarettes per day, used heroin intravenously twice per day, and consumed approximately 200 ounces of beer (16 to 17 bottles) per day. The records also reveal that Mr. Z began using alcohol at age 13 years, sedatives at age 16 years, heroin at age 19 years, methamphetamine at age 17 years, and cocaine at age 33 years.

In the clinical interview, Mr. Z stated that he began using cocaine at age 19 years, but was consistent with respect to age of first use for the other drugs. In the 1990s, Mr. Z reported that on average, he used heroin twice per day, drank a six-pack of beer, used 0.25 g of methamphetamine, and smoked two or more packs of cigarettes per day. He described himself as a binge user such that he might use greater amounts of heroin for a period of several days, then use greater amounts of methamphetamine for a period of several days. In terms of greatest amounts used, Mr. Z reported that he used 1.75 g of methamphetamine per day in 1983, a 0.5 g of heroin per day in 1970 and 1973, smoked marijuana daily, and drank one fifth of alcohol per day in month-long binges during the 1990s.

Mr. Z reported that he was successfully abstinent since 1996. He currently takes methadone once per day. He reported that none of his first-degree family members have been diagnosed with a mental health disorder.

The results of the evaluation revealed that Mr. Z demonstrated a pattern of deficits consistent with polysubstance dependence. He did not demonstrate deficits on measures of intellectual functioning, language, visuospatial skills, or attentional measures that did not include a psychomotor speed component. In contrast, he demonstrated deficits on measures sensitive to psychomotor speed, memory, and executive systems functioning. This pattern of deficits has been characterized as a "frontal-subcortical" (54–56).

Given this pattern of facts, it is likely that Mr. Z's neuropsychological deficits, particularly his frontal lobe impairment, contributed to his behavior with Mr. Q. Poor performance on tests of executive systems functioning are associated with an increased risk for impulsive behavior or "acting without thinking." Mr. Z's impairment is also likely to manifest itself behaviorally in the form of poor judgment and poor decision making capability.

Based on these data, the Mr. Z's attorney successfully negotiated a plea for him. Mr. Z pled guilty to reduced charges involving substantially less punishment.

CONCLUSIONS

It is noteworthy that the judicial system currently recognizes that substance misuse can affect individuals' judgment and their ability to conform their behavior to the laws of this society. As a result, the penal code includes statutes that address the issue of mitigation when substance misuse affected an individual's behavior when a crime was committed. Although this point seems obvious, various eras in the early part of the twentieth century viewed substance misuse as a moral defect (e.g., Temperance Movement, Prohibition) rather than an actual mental health disorder.

At present, the effects of substance misuse may be viewed as an intent-lowering or -negating factor, or for sentencing purposes, possibly as a mitigating factor. The current penal code does not permit defendants to use an insanity plea to explain their actions. A frequently used definition of insanity, the "Modified McNaughton Rule," states that a person may be considered to be legally insane if "... at the time of committing the act, the accused was laboring under such a defect of reason, from disease of the mind, as not to know the nature and quality of the act he was doing or, if he did know it, that he did not know what he was doing was wrong."

If one considers that the negative consequences discussed in the quotation above can drive one to loss of family, job, friends, belongings, and status, and to the commission of a crime, a criminal conviction, jail or prison, or even death, then can it not be said that such addiction, if it is shown to have demonstrable medical and psychological effects, is itself a mental disease or mental defect or a form of mental illness (which could impact upon the mental state of a person who is accused of a crime), or even a form of insanity? If an individual's addiction is so severe that the individual thinks illogically and is unable to distinguish right from wrong, it will be curious to determine how this will affect future legislation and it focuses on whether the consequences of substance misuse can serve as the basis for an insanity plea.

REFERENCES

1. Lezak MD. *Neuropsychological assessment,* 3rd ed. New York: Oxford University Press, 1995.
2. Lindemann JE, Matarazzo JD. Assessment of adult intelligence. In: Gerald Goldskin and Michel Hersen, eds: *Handbook of psychological assessment,* 2nd ed. Elmsford, NY: Pergamon Press, 1990:79–101.
3. Spreen O, Strauss E. *A compendium of neuropsychological tests: administration, norms, and commentary.* Vol. 2. New York: Oxford University Press, 1998:736.
4. Butler MRP, Vanderploeg R. Neuropsychological test usage. *Prof Psychol Res Pract* 1991;22:510–512.
5. Kalechstein A, van Gorp WG, Rapport L. Variability in clinical classification of raw test scores across normative data sets. *Clin Neuropsychol* 1998;12:339–347.
6. American Psychiatric Association. *Diagnostic and statistical manual of mental disorders,* 4th ed., text revision (*DSM–IV–TR*). Washington, DC: Author, 2000.
7. Graham AW, Schultz TK, eds. *Principles of addiction medicine,* 2nd ed. American Society of Addiction Medicine, 1998.
8. Nordrum I, Eide TJ, L JL. Alcohol in a series of medico-legally autopsied deaths in northern Norway 1973–1992. *Forensic Sci Int* 2000;110(2):127–137.
9. Sjogren H, Eriksson A, Ahlm K. Alcohol and unnatural deaths in Sweden: a medico-legal autopsy study. *J Stud Alcohol* 2000;61(4):507–514.
10. Goodman RA, et al. Alcohol use and interpersonal violence: alcohol detected in homicide victims. *Am J Public Health* 1986;76(2):144–149.
11. Poklis A, Graham M, Maginn D, et al. Phencyclidine and violent deaths in St. Louis, Missouri: a survey of medical

examiners' cases from 1977 through 1986. *Am J Drug Alcohol Abuse* 1990;16(3–4):265–274.

12. Marzuk PM, Tardiff K, Leon AC, et al. Ambient temperature and mortality from unintentional cocaine overdose. *JAMA* 1998;279(22):1795–1800.

13. Marzuk PM, Tardiff K, Leon AC, et al. Fatal injuries after cocaine use as a leading cause of death among young adults in New York City. *N Engl J Med* 1995;332(26):1753–1757.

14. Gill JR, Hayes JA, deSouza IS, et al. Ecstasy (MDMA) deaths in New York City: a case series and review of the literature. *J Forensic Sci* 2002;47(1):121–126.

15. Davidson PJ, McLean RL, Kral AH, et al. Fatal heroin-related overdose in San Francisco, 1997–2000: a case for targeted intervention. *J Urban Health* 2003;80(2):261–273.

16. Hall WD, Degenhardt LJ, Lynskey MT. Opioid overdose mortality in Australia, 1964–1997: birth-cohort trends. *Med J Aust* 1999;171(1):34–37.

17. Caplehorn JR, Dalton MS, Haldar F, et al. Methadone maintenance and addicts' risk of fatal heroin overdose. *Subst Use Misuse* 1996;31(2):177–196.

18. Davis GG and Swalwell CI. The incidence of acute cocaine or methamphetamine intoxication in deaths due to ruptured cerebral (berry) aneurysms. *J Forensic Sci* 1996;41(4):626–628.

19. Shaw KP. Human methamphetamine-related fatalities in Taiwan during 1991–1996. *J Forensic Sci* 1999;44(1):27–31.

20. Preti A, Miotto P, De Coppi M. Deaths by unintentional illicit drug overdose in Italy, 1984–2000. *Drug Alcohol Depend* 2002;66(3):275–282.

21. Coffin PO, Galea S, Ahern J, et al. Opiates, cocaine and alcohol combinations in accidental drug overdose deaths in New York City, 1990–98. *Addiction* 2003;98(6):739–747.

22. Carmen del Rio M, Alvarez FJ. Presence of illegal drugs in drivers involved in fatal road traffic accidents in Spain. *Drug Alcohol Depend* 2000;57(3):177–182.

23. Vinson DC, Borges G, Cherpitel CJ. The risk of intentional injury with acute and chronic alcohol exposures: a case-control and case-crossover study. *J Stud Alcohol* 2003;64(3):350–357.

24. McFarlin SK, Fals-Stewart W, Major DA, et al. Alcohol use and workplace aggression: an examination of perpetration and victimization. *J Subst Abuse* 2001;13(3):303–321.

25. Scott KD, Schafer J, Greenfield TK. The role of alcohol in physical assault perpe-tration and victimization. *J Stud Alcohol* 1999;60(4):528–536.

26. Friedman AS, Glassman K, Terras BA. Violent behavior as related to use of marijuana and other drugs. *J Addict Dis* 2001;20(1):49–72.

27. Pascual-Leone A, et al. Cocaine-induced seizures. *Neurology* 1990;40[3 Pt 1]:404–407.

28. Mena I, Giombetti RJ, Miller BL, et al. Cerebral blood flow changes with acute cocaine intoxication: clinical correlations with SPECT, CT, and MRI. *NIDA Res Monogr* 1994;138:161–173.

29. Swenson JR, et al. Drug and alcohol abuse in patients with acute burn injuries. *Psychosomatics* 1991;32(3):287–293.

30. Schermer CR and Wisner DH. Methamphetamine use in trauma patients: a population-based study. *J Am Coll Surg* 1999;189(5):442–449.

31. McCarron MM, Schulze BW, Thompson GA, et al. Acute phencyclidine intoxication: incidence of clinical findings in 1,000 cases. *Ann Emerg Med* 1981;10(5):237–242.

32. Hall W, Hando J, Darke S, et al. Psychological morbidity and route of administration among amphetamine users in Sydney, Australia. *Addiction* 1996;91(1):81–87.

33. Bell DS. Comparison of amphetamine psychosis and schizophrenia. *Br J Psychiatry* 1965;111:701–707.

34. Bell DS. The experimental reproduction of amphetamine psychosis. *Arch Gen Psychiatry* 1973;29(1):35–40.

35. Angrist B, et al. Amphetamine psychosis: behavioral and biochemical aspects. *J Psychiatr Res* 1974;11:13–23.

36. Kramer JC, Fischman VS, Littlefield DC. Amphetamine abuse. Pattern and effects of high doses taken intravenously. *JAMA* 1967;201(5):305–309.

37. Rourke SB, Toberg T. Neurobehavioral correlates of alcoholism. In: Grant I, Adams KD, eds. *Neuropsychological aspects of neuropsychiatric disorders.* New York: Oxford University Press, 1996.

38. Bolla KI, Rothman R, Cadet JL. Dose-related neurobehavioral effects of chronic cocaine use. *J Neuropsychiatry Clin Neurosci* 1999;11(3):361–369.

39. Bolla KI, McCann UD, Ricaurte GA. Memory impairment in abstinent MDMA ("ecstasy") users. *Neurology* 1998;51(6):1532–1537.

40. Volkow ND, Chang L, Wang GJ, et al. Association of dopamine transporter reduction with psychomotor impairment in methamphetamine abusers. *Am J Psychiatry* 2001;158(3):377–382.

41. Sayette MA, Shiffman S, Tiffany ST, et al. The measurement of drug crav-ing. *Addiction* 2000;95[2 Suppl]:S189–S210.

42. Grant I, Gonzalez B, Carey CL, et al. Non-acute (residual) neurocognitive effects of cannabis use: a meta-analytic study. *J Int Neuropsychol Soc* 2003;9(5):679–689.

43. Bolla KI, et al. Dose-related neurocognitive effects of marijuana use. *Neurology* 2002;59(9):1337–1343.

44. Maas LC, Lukas SE, Kaufman MJ, et al. Functional magnetic resonance imaging of human brain activation during cue-induced cocaine craving. *Am J Psychiatry* 1998;155(1):124–126.

45. Childress AR, Mozley PD, McElgin W, et al. Limbic activation during cue-induced cocaine craving. *Am J Psychiatry* 1999;156(1):11–18.

46. Sinha R, Fuse T, Aubin LR, et al. Psychological stress, drug-related cues and cocaine craving. *Psychopharmacology (Berl)* 2000;152(2):140–148.

47. Garavan H, et al. Cue-induced cocaine craving: neuroanatomical specificity for drug users and drug stimuli. *Am J Psychiatry* 2000;157(11):1789–1798.

48. Kilts CD, Schwertzer JB, Quinn OK, et al. Neural activity related to drug craving in cocaine addiction. *Arch Gen Psychiatry* 2001;58(4):334–341.

49. Dackis CA, O'Brien CP. Cocaine dependence: a disease of the brain's reward centers. *J Subst Abuse Treat* 2001;21(3):111–117.

50. Bonson KR, et al. Neural systems and cue-induced cocaine craving. *Neuropsychopharmacology* 2002;26(3):376–386.

51. Grant S, London ED, Newlin DB, et al. Activation of memory circuits during cue-elicited cocaine craving. *Proc Natl Acad Sci U S A* 1996;93(21):12040–12045.

52. Speckart GR, Anglin MD, Deschenes EP. Modeling the longitudinal impact of legal sanctions on narcotics use and property crime. *J Quant Criminol* 1989;5(1):33–56.

53. Anglin MD, Perrochet B. Drug use and crime: a historical review of research conducted by the UCLA Drug Abuse Research Center. *Subst Use Misuse* 1998;33(9):1871–1914.

54. Tekin S, Cummings JL. Frontal-subcortical neuronal circuits and clinical neuropsychiatry: an update. *J Psychosom Res* 2002;53(2):647–654.

55. Cummings JL. Frontal-subcortical circuits and human behavior. *Arch Neurol* 1993;50(8):873–880.

56. Cummings JL. Anatomic and behavioral aspects of frontal-subcortical circuits. *Ann N Y Acad Sci* 1995;769:1–13.

CHAPTER 84

A New Era for Methadone Advocacy

JOYCELYN WOODS, WALTER GINTER, AND
TONY SCRO

The National Alliance of Methadone Advocates (NAMA) is now 15 years old. This by itself can be seen as an incredible accomplishment. Many starting advocacy or user organizations (European terminology) only last a few years because of lack of support from the traditional sector. In spite of sparse funding and support, NAMA has never lost sight of its primary mandate to advocate for the patient in treatment. During these years NAMA has also acquired experience and expertise that has been invaluable to understanding methadone treatment,[1] both in the United States and abroad.

From the start NAMA received minimal funding, especially from the methadone community and often has had to endure hostile attacks from those who would discourage advocacy. Today, NAMA exists solely through the membership fees from patients and enlightened professionals. This also means that no one is paid a salary at NAMA. In spite of this NAMA has been able to accomplish some impressive things, including worldwide recognition as the premier methadone advocacy organization. Many patient groups abroad that are funded by their

governments look to NAMA for leadership. They have the luxury of office space and receive funding for various projects. These countries are not necessarily enlightened; however, they have come to realize that advocacy organizations are cost-effective and are better able to reach the drug-using community than are professional[2] agencies. Currently NAMA has more than 45 chapters and 12 international affiliates.

THE NEW RULE AND ACCREDITATION

On May 17, 2001, the "new rule" proposed by the Center for Substance Abuse Treatment began a 3-year transition period during which all programs must be accredited (1). The new rule advances methadone treatment because it places programs under an accreditation system like all other health care and medical treatment. Methadone treatment will no longer be an orphan system. Because each state also has its own regulations there is a different system in each state, but the new rule has forced states to review their regulations in order to be in compliance. It will probably be 5 to 10 years before the real impact of these changes is felt (2). This new system requires that treatment professionals begin to put thought into the treatment that they are delivering, rather than just follow regulations. The focus is on individualized treatment and treatment outcomes.

The new rule also includes patient participation in program policy (3). Now methadone programs must have some mechanism for patients to be involved in program policy. This can be a single patient representative or a

---

[1] The Center for Substance Abuse Treatment (CSAT) is introducing the term *medication-assisted treatment (MAT)* to identify opioid agonist treatments such as methadone and levo-alpha-acetylmethadol (LAAM), which combine a physician-approved medication with clinical or behavioral therapies. NAMA uses "medication-assisted treatment," "opiate agonist treatment," and "methadone treatment."

[2] Our Swedish affiliate, Svenska BrukarForeningen, was funded by the government within months of organizing. The Danish organization BrugerForeningen has its own offices and receives government funding to provide services to Danish drug users and methadone patients. The government perceives the president, Joergen Kjaer as the spokesperson for users and each year he addresses the Diet about the issues impacting drug users and methadone patients. This is the equivalent of NAMA's president addressing Congress.

patient counsel depending on the size of the program or even a committee of patients and staff. Some states have also begun to set up patient consumer groups that are involved in policy-making committees. Several of NAMA's chapters are involved with their state on a variety of levels while the national organization in involved with federal committees and agencies.

The Grievance Process

When NAMA was conceived, resolving individual patient grievances was not considered. However, that very quickly changed as patients began asking for assistance. For the first complaints, notes were written on a pad until it was realized that the information that NAMA was collecting was invaluable to understanding the situation in various regions of the United States. Within months a form was developed so that the data collected could be coded for a system. In addition, it was decided to acknowledge when programs or professionals do something that is exceptional in helping patients. Thus the concept of a compliment report was included and today the form is called the "Grievance/Compliment Report."

One of the first Compliment Reports occurred when a "methadone pump" when awry and failed to deliver any methadone into the patients' bottles. The first reaction of the staff and program was that such a thing was impossible until they carefully looked at the bottles. It was late Friday afternoon when this was discovered and many patients had already been given weekend take-home medication. The program could have ignored it, but instead confronted it. The staff came in on Saturday to call patients and tell them to come back and have their medication replaced. Usually on Saturday most programs are only open a few hours but this took nearly a day to contact patients and make arrangements for them to get replacements. It certainly deserved a compliment.

A NAMA Grievance Report can involve programs, state agencies, hospitals, the criminal justice system, employment, and other services that patients use and can have trouble with. Most complaints that patients file are valid and require significant work on the part of the patient as well as the advocate. The most common complaint is the patient being discharged for invalid reasons, including opiate drug use. New York State's Office of Alcoholism and Substance Abuse Service (OASAS) has an Advocacy Unit that handles thousands of complaints a year. Outside of New York is another matter and depends on the state authority. For example, in one instance a patient wrote to the state authority to complain about the program. The state authority in its great wisdom made a copy of the letter and mailed it to the program. Upon entering the program the patient was corralled in their counselor's office with the director of the program. Surrounded by staff that the patient was complaining about, the counselor and director then went down the list point by point to deny that any of the accusations occurred. Enough said but this is not the way to resolve a grievance. In this case it took only months for the program to retaliate and find some way to punish the patient. And this time the patient did not contact the state agency for help. Although it may reduce a bureaucrat's workload it does not make for quality treatment.

NAMA believes that a grievance against any program or agency in the methadone treatment system means that a failure has occurred somewhere. Whether the failure is the fault of the treatment provider, regulatory authority, or advocate doesn't really matter. If the situation degenerates to the point where outside help is needed, the patient has been failed. In NAMA's experience, very few patients want to "rock the boat" so to speak. More often they are afraid that there will be retaliation and do nothing, thus compounding problems until they have no other resort but to ask NAMA for help. It is not unusual for patients to feel as though any efforts to change things will be futile. Thus when a patient finally files a grievance it usually means that they have been frustrated in their own attempts to resolve things and literally see us as a last resort. What this often means is that the patient was unaware of the correct action to take. It means that the patient didn't use the right resources. The methadone treatment system is a bureaucracy and can be confusing to the average patient. We have found that the best approach to grievance resolution is to coach the patient to contact the appropriate parties and to provide support and counseling to the patient during the process. Patients should be empowered so they will never need NAMA's help again and, hopefully, so that they will tell other patients about their experience.

Methadone program grievances fall into two basic categories. The largest number of complaints is by individual patients regarding a specific problem, such as not receiving any take-home medication or being discharged. A lesser category of complaints regards program policy that involves the entire patient population at a program. These complaints although filed by an individual patient are handled at the program level. Usually the grievance coordinator begins by contacting the program to validate the program policy. If the policy is against a federal or state regulation, the program is contacted and informed of such and that NAMA will contact the proper authorities if they do not cease the policy. This can be done at a variety of levels, as sometimes program staff may not realize that they are violating the right of patients or the impact that their policy has on quality treatment. When NAMA heard that a program administrator had allowed the local police force to enter the program and go through federally protected patient records, the state agency was immediately contacted. It still took 2 years of pressuring the state, but in the end, the program was fined and the program supervisor who allowed the police to enter the program was given time in jail.

The Greatest Barrier: Stigma

Stigma, prejudice, and discrimination are the greatest barrier to recovery confronting methadone patients (4,5). Securing employment and maintaining a stable, responsible lifestyle is an important aspect of treatment and one's recovery. But the working methadone patient lives with the constant fear of discovery. Despite the fact that they are protected by the American with Disabilities Act (ADA), every year patients lose their jobs merely for being enrolled in a methadone program (6). Many of these patients do not challenge their employer because they themselves do not realize that it is against the law, indeed against the U.S. Constitution. Nor do they know how to proceed with such a case.

Not only are methadone patients confronted with employment discrimination, but many schools, training opportunities, and service programs exclude them, thus making their road to recovery all the more difficult. Yet, the abstinence-oriented former addict from abstinence-oriented treatment who is cared for in a protective environment with all of his or her needs met, receives all the accolades. Methadone patients from the day they enter treatment face opposition and oppression every step of the way. It is only because of their determination and strong character that the majority of methadone patients succeed as accomplished and productive taxpaying citizens of their community; they support themselves, their family, and very often pay $250 to $300 a month for their treatment (7). Methadone patients do not have the cheering squads or community support that recipients of abstinence-oriented treatment have; instead they make their contributions quietly, fearful that their secret will be discovered and that they and their family will loose everything (8).

Stigma is also a major barrier for the dysfunctional methadone patients who need special services. Their enrollment in methadone treatment ensures that they will not be able to get the necessary help they need. The mental health community refuses methadone patients for treatment of depressive and affective disorders and typically tells patients that they must withdraw from methadone treatment in order to be considered for their services. Patients with a secondary drug problem, such as cocaine and alcoholism, are also refused services unless they, too, withdraw from methadone. Homeless methadone patients are denied housing or shown the street if it is discovered that they are enrolled in a methadone program.

A SPECIAL CASE: METHAPHOBIA AND THE MEDICAL PROFESSION

Obtaining health and medical care has become a serious problem for many methadone patients, especially because most methadone programs, for budgetary reasons, have had to eliminate the primary medical care that they provided in the past. Prejudice and hatred towards methadone treatment, patients, and the medication itself has been given a name—*methaphobia*! Methaphobia has become critical during the past decade, especially because of the large number of human immunodeficiency virus (HIV)-infected drug users admitted to methadone programs and the increasing number of former drug users being diagnosed with hepatitis C (9,10).

The prejudice that methadone patients experience in health care is an extension of the medical profession's bias toward heroin addicts (11). With the passing of the Harrison Narcotic Act, the problem of opiate addiction was removed from the medical profession and placed under the control of the criminal justice agencies. The first group to actually be prosecuted under the Harrison Narcotic Act was the medical profession, resulting in the arrests of approximately 38,000 physicians and the imprisonment of more than 5,000 (12). Medical schools began to advise their students to stay away from addicts and that addiction was a law enforcement problem, a message that continues to this day. Given this background, it is understandable how medical professionals came to harbor such prejudicial attitudes toward addicts, which has been compounded by decades of ignorance. Today, the average medical student receives about 1 hour of training in addiction that includes alcohol use, thus methadone is rarely mentioned except for its use in withdrawing addicts from opiates.

A recent study reported on the medical care received by methadone patients who were treated in their clinics compared to a group referred to mainstream medical clinics (13). Although 92% of the patients treated on-site received medical treatment, only 35% of the referred group received any medical care at all. The authors noted the difficulty they had in finding an off-site medical clinic to participate in the study. A number of clinics refused to participate even though they would be paid for all appointments, including those that the patients missed. The group stated that the behavior exhibited by the mainstream clinics reflects the stereotypical beliefs that the medical profession harbors toward methadone patients. Health care workers who are methadone patients themselves—and there are many—reported consistent prejudices from their coworkers and teachers while they were in school. Very often they must stand by silently as another methadone patient is refused pain medication or even their prescribed methadone while hospitalized. A nurse who is a medical-maintenance patient, which is a special program where functional patients are removed from the clinic system and treated by a physician in their office, described her experience.

About 2 years ago in a Manhattan hospital, I noted a patient who was tied in a restraint. It turned out that he was a methadone patient and was not given methadone for 3 days. I got very angry and when I spoke to the nurses they brushed the matter off, stating that he was difficult to treat and they referred to him as an animal and that it was his fault that he was an addict. I told them that he should be medicated and when he was, he turned out to be a very cooperative patient. I then turned to the nurses and said, "Who is the animal now?" (14)

Another medical-maintenance patient who revealed his methadone status to an examining physician in a hospital was faced with an abrupt change of attitude:

I'll never forget this. I went to the local hospital because of pains in my chest. When I told the physician that I was on methadone, his attitude abruptly changed. He told me that "all I wanted was drugs" and "to get the hell out of here and if you don't leave immediately I'll call a cop." (14)

Many methadone patients have found that when they reveal their enrollment in a methadone program, their chances of receiving adequate medical care, or even any at all, becomes greatly reduced, while the likelihood of being treated with disrespect is dramatically increased. This has resulted in many patients not informing doctors or other medical professionals that they are methadone patients. It is a sad statement to have to say that it is very unusual to find a methadone patient who has not experienced methaphobia from the medical profession—the healers who have taken an oath to help others and to do no harm, perhaps do the worst harm!

CERTIFICATION OF METHADONE ADVOCATES

As accreditation moves forward, programs are beginning to learn that patients will have to be treated as consumers. The new rule (42 CFR 8) stresses the concept of individualized treatment. It is imperative during this period for NAMA methadone advocates to be active in order to combat myths and half-truths being spread by those who are not properly trained and mentored.

Many of the positive changes in methadone treatment over the last 15 years were achieved, in part, because NAMA existed to organize and galvanize support. NAMA knows that methadone advocacy can continue to make outstanding contributions to the methadone community, but *only* when responsible advocates are involved. Advocates whose knowledge is grounded in science and who have an appreciation for the complexities of the methadone community.

In an effort to rectify what many of us, both inside and outside of NAMA, see as a serious problem, the board of directors created the NAMA Training and Certification Committee. The committee's role is to encourage the growth of responsible methadone advocacy. The committee's goals are as follows:

1. The establishment of an ethical code for patient advocates.

2. The creation of standards for individual advocates.
3. The establishment of a certification procedure for advocates.
4. To provide training for advocates and mentoring of less-experienced advocates.

The committee is also responsible for the establishment of a mechanism so that once advocates are trained and certified, the standards can be maintained. Thus, NAMA has created a professional code for advocates that will legitimize methadone advocacy. This has been an immense challenge for NAMA, but the rewards, for the entire methadone community will be enormous.

What Is a Methadone Advocate?

The primary purpose of methadone advocacy is education. Some advocates mistakenly believe that advocates handle grievances and complaints about programs and other services. This is a misplaced view of what methadone advocacy should be all about. As discussed above, a grievance means that a failure has happened.

An advocate is someone who supports the use of methadone as a treatment for opiate addiction. Everyone who works in the methadone industry should be a methadone advocate. In fact, if they are *not* advocates for methadone treatment, there are two reasons why they need to do some self-examination as to why they work in methadone treatment. First, working in drug treatment is not just "an everyday job" and all professionals, whether they have direct contact with patients or not, provide a service that saves lives and has a secondary impact on the lives of thousands. Therefore, working in methadone treatment includes a commitment. The second reason is profoundly related to methadone itself. Methadone is the most misunderstood medication and treatment, but the group that bears the brunt of the ignorance and prejudice are the patients. Stigma impacts methadone treatment on every level. It is the reason why programs are unable to open in a community, thus leaving opiate-dependent individuals in the area without any access to treatment. More directly, it reduces a patient's opportunities, making recovery all the more difficult for methadone patients. Stigma also impacts professionals working in the field and it is not unusual for a counselor to spend an entire day trying to find somewhere to place a homeless patient when the counselor's time would be better spent counseling the patient or other patients. It is not unusual to hear about a professional who was embarrassed to admit at some social gathering that they work in methadone treatment. It has been a primary mission for NAMA to end the ignorance that drives stigma and the certification of advocates will give NAMA the opportunity to be able to reach out and galvanize the entire methadone community to end the stigma that reduces the effectiveness of treatment.

TABLE 84.1. *The advocates code of ethics**

I. A responsible advocate shall take no action or provide any advice that will overly complicate or make matters worse for the individual patient.

II. In all matters the rights and dignity of the patient is paramount.

III. A responsible advocate maintains objectivity and shall not confuse advocating for methadone patients with advocating for his or her own self-interests.

IV. A responsible advocate shall never violate the confidentiality of a patient, nor shall he/she advocate for a patient without the patient's consent.

V. An advocate shall accept no personal privilege or other consideration not available to other patients from providers or regulators. This shall not preclude advocates from accepting donations for any organized advocacy organization or scholarships to conferences or events as long as they are made public. Compensated employees of methadone programs must inform any patient for whom they are advocating that they are a compensated employee of a given provider.

VI. An advocate shall not accept personal compensation in any form from a patient for the provision of advocacy services. This does not mean a patient cannot join an organization that an advocate represents, but joining an organization cannot be a condition of advocating for a patient.

VII. A responsible advocate, whether compensated or not, shall at all times conduct themselves in a professional manner.

*The Advocates Code of Ethics was developed through NAMA's 15 years of experience to provide guidance for methadone advocates.

It is not uncommon for some professionals to feel threatened by advocacy because it is new and there are unknowns. But methadone advocacy does not mean the relinquishment of power for professionals; instead the result will be an elevation for the entire field. This is the goal for the responsible methadone advocate.

Therefore, when someone presents himself or herself as a NAMA Certified Methadone Advocate (CMA) that person is completely trained, supports the goals of advocacy and abides by a code of ethics (Table 84.1). The result will be professionalism in methadone advocacy and an end to the chaos and confusion currently being experienced by the entire methadone community.

Certified advocates must (a) abide by a code of ethics, (b) adhere to goals of advocacy, and (c) complete the training course. In addition, to maintain certification, advocates will have to take a short refresher course at least once every 3 years. It was our experience that most patients and counselors who attend their first methadone conference find it a life-changing experience. NAMA therefore arranged for about 40 advocates who were seeking methadone advocate

certification to attend the National Methadone Conference and report back on their experience.

The session began with an entire day of training designed to educate and add professionalism to patient advocacy. Each participant was given a training manual that contained eight sections: (a) Addiction and Methadone Treatment; (b) Regulations and Accreditation; (c) Certification; (d) Advocacy Tools; (e) Stigma; (f) Hepatitis; (g) Science and Technology; and (h) Reference Materials.

It is our hope that clinic counselors and staff, family and friends of patients, researchers and scientists, in fact, all members of the methadone community decide to take this training and become a CMA. In fact, being a methadone advocate has nothing to do with being a methadone patient and everything to do with supporting methadone treatment.

THE POWER OF ADVOCACY: PATIENTS AND COUNSELORS

NAMA has come to realize that the most powerful advocates for methadone are patients and counselors because they bring first-hand experiences to their advocacy. Provider representatives have acknowledged that when talking to legislators and interested citizens they are often interrupted with, "We would expect you to say that. You represent the providers, or a manufacturer, or the program."

Conversely, when responsible patients speak (and families) there is almost always keen interest, sometimes because their experience is firsthand and sometimes because patients have no economic stake in methadone treatment. But patients and their families are not the only credible advocates. Counselors are just as powerful because they know firsthand the effectiveness of methadone treatment. Their multitude of stories about successful patients shows that methadone treatment is not just effective for a few and that nearly every patient can benefit.

THE PRIMARY PROBLEM IS STIGMA

Stigma is based on myths and beliefs about the unknown. The myths about methadone started in the streets, with patients. This occurred because as methadone expanded patients took less of a role in methadone treatment. The early program used patients who were successful as counselors. However, as treatment expanded, the typical counselor came from social work and had been trained that opiate addiction was a behavior problem. Thus began punitive programs and the us-versus-them mentality of methadone programs. Patients were things to be made into, and it did not matter if they were willing partners that understood their treatment. Therefore, when you do *not* give people science they will invent their own science mythology to replace it.

Weapons Against Stigma

The way to end stigma is to educate patients about methadone and their treatment. Why will this work when other methods have failed? First, it starts from the bottom up where it started—educating patients and counselors and organizing counselors and patients to work together as advocates. Advocates can only accomplish the goals we seek. In fact advocates are the most *powerful* part of the methadone community.

A NEW ERA IS EMERGING

After 35 years of methadone being misunderstood, science has demonstrated that the original hypothesis put forth by Drs. Dole and Nyswander was accurate. Opiate dependence is a medical condition (15,16). The majority of the public still does not understand opiate addiction and it will take a tremendous educational effort to correct this misperception. The best messengers to carry the message that opiate addiction is a medical condition that can be treated effectively are the patients themselves (17).

This creates for NAMA an enormous mission and as the national advocacy organization for methadone treatment NAMA will continue to actively respond to the issues that affect the quality of treatment and impact on the daily lives of methadone patients. NAMA's objective has always been to work toward the day when all methadone patients can publicly come forward to celebrate and state with pride their many achievements. Methadone patients should feel nothing but pride for their accomplishments. But only through the empowerment of patients with everyone working together—patients and professionals—will methadone treatment begin to gain the respect that it rightly deserves.

DEDICATION

This paper is dedicated to the work and spirit of Dr. Marie Nyswander whose dream was that someday addicts would be treated like any patient with a chronic disease.

ACKNOWLEDGMENTS

The authors would like to acknowledge the inspiration of NAMA's chapters and affiliates whose hard work and dedication have made methadone advocacy a reality and Dr. Vincent Dole for his extraordinary wisdom.

REFERENCES

1. *Fed Reg* January 17, 2001.
2. Frequently asked questions about the new federal regulations. *NAMA Advocate* 2001;1(2):5.
3. Woods J. First things first (president's column). *NAMA Advocate* 2001;1(2):2.
4. Scro T. Let's stop the insanity! *Ombudsman* 1995;3/4:1.
5. Joseph H, Woods J. Stigma: the invisible barrier. *Ombudsman* 1995;3/4:5.
6. U.S. Congress. *Americans with Disabilities Act.* Washington, DC: U.S. Government Printing Office, 1992.
7. Joseph H. Methadone maintenance: profiles in success. *OASAS Today* 1994(Sept/Oct):7.
8. Murphy S, Irwin J. Living with the dirty secret: problems of disclosure for methadone maintenance clients. *J Psychoactive Drugs* 1992;24(3):257–264.
9. Sobel I. Doctors, discrimination and methadone: a matter of respect. *Ombudsman* 1996;5:1,8.
10. Remember us! *Ombudsman* 1996;5:6.
11. Blansfield HN. Addictophobia [Editorial]. *Conn Med* 1991;55:361.
12. DeLong JV. *Dealing with drug abuse: a report to the Ford Foundation.* New York: Praeger Press, 1972. Cited in Miller R, Towards a sociology of methadone maintenance. In: Winick C, ed. *Sociological aspects of drug dependence.* Cleveland: CRC Press, 1974.
13. Umbricht-Schneiter A, Ginn DH, Pabst KM, et al. Providing medical care to methadone clinic patients: referral vs. on-site care. *Am J Public Health* 1994; 84(2):208–210.
14. Joseph H. *Medical methadone maintenance: the further concealment of a stigmatized condition* [Dissertation]. New York: City University of New York, 1995.
15. Dole VP, Nyswander ME. Heroin addiction: a metabolic disease. *Arch Intern Med* 1967;120:19–24.
16. National Institute of Health. Effective treatment of opiate addiction. NIH consensus statement. Vol. 15, no. 6. November 17–19, 1997.
17. Parrino M. Personal communication, 2003.

CHAPTER 85

The Workplace

PAUL F. ENGELHART AND LINDA BARLOW

THE VALUE OF WORK IN THE RECOVERY PROCESS

Some of us may be uncomfortable with Thomas Carlyle's poetic assertion that "the whole soul of man is composed into a kind of harmony the instant he sets himself to work" (1). Still, we cannot deny the significant role that work can play, both in the disease progression of alcohol and drug addiction and in the recovery process. Clients in substance-abuse treatment programs realize the contribution that employment makes to their recovery. Research indicates that many recovering substance abusers express a need for greater vocational services than they are presently receiving (2).

Personality theorists from the early psychoanalysts to the more recent existential analysts have identified love and work, Freud's *liebe und arbeit*, as two of the most basic principles of human existence. Their absence can destroy a person's life and, just as powerfully, their presence can save it. Involvement in meaningful relationships and contribution to the tasks of society are crucial to the development of a healthy sense of self (3).

While not denying the equally important role that love plays, this chapter focuses on the role that work plays in the recovery process. The first section addresses the problems recovering substance abusers face when returning to the workplace and the range of services for facilitating their success. The second section looks at the nature and extent of employee substance abuse problems and efforts in the workplace that effectively address these problems.

Work may be defined as purposeful effort expended to positively alter one's environment. Traditionally, work has been seen as a central component of one's identity. Standard adult social introductions usually begin with responses to two coupled questions: "What's your name?" and "What do you do for a living?" Young children are repeatedly asked about their future worker identity: "What do you want to be when you grow up?" Older adults can find adjustment to retirement difficult not only because of a reduction in established activities, but because of a loss of their specific occupational identity.

American culture extols the virtues of work and assigns a stigma to the unemployed. In our society, employment is a sign of maturity and considered necessary for the independence associated with adulthood. Moreover, our society assigns degrees of respect to people based on the type of work they do.

Although there are different theories on how an individual determines a specific worker identity for himself or herself, most occupational psychologists agree that vocational identity is attained through a developmental process. If we agree with this perspective, then it is easy to see how a disability like substance abuse could deprive an individual of the experiences necessary for a transformation from a nonworking child into a working adult. Substance abuse is a disability that begins before or during early adulthood, or that removes a worker from employment for a significant period during later adulthood.

There are two basic groups of recovering substance abusers in the treatment setting: those who, as a consequence of their abuse or other environmental or family factors, have never worked, and those who have worked and been suspended from their jobs or fired as a consequence of substance abuse. The first group is looking to enter the work force for the first time and the second group is looking to return. Although there are similarities between the two, care must be taken to fully understand the unique dynamics influencing each group's movement toward work.

Recovering substance abusers entering the labor force for the first time may be confronted with poor, inadequate, or unrealistic concepts of what work is and who they are and can be as workers. Individuals who grew up in disadvantaged or unstable homes because of poverty, generational substance abuse, or family conflict, may never have worked formally or been raised with close "worker" role models. Employment may be seen by recovering substance abusers as foreign and unknown, creating feelings of inadequacy and fear. Many of their lifestyle patterns and habits are maladaptive and not conducive to work. Adolescents and young adults whose lives have focused on drug or alcohol addiction have not experienced many of the stresses and fears that most people gradually confront in high school educational programs or their first part-time or summer jobs.

In addition to not experiencing these feelings early on, substance abusers may have missed the opportunities to develop effective coping skills and strengths, to make mistakes in less-significant vocational responsibilities, and to learn from these mistakes, integrating healthy social and personal management skills into their sense of self (4,5). They lack concrete experiences in exploring specific occupational fields, as well as the general expectations and unwritten rules associated with employment. As a result, many have false and immature expectations of what to expect from a job or of the necessary elements to build a career. They may also lack awareness of their own values, interests, and abilities.

These individuals arrive at the job market overwhelmed by the enormity of the task of entering the "straight" world and meeting employers' expectations to have already completed the more basic vocational development tasks. Still, a position in the labor force is attractive, because it offers to place them into a recognized position in society for the first time in their lives.

Other individuals coming from the mainstream with an intact background may have come to accept their chemical addiction only when their substance abuse destroyed their ability to work. They were removed from the labor market for one or more periods of employment. Paradoxically, they may now question their ability to handle work demands sober and drug free. They face discrimination because of employment gaps and poor previous work references. They may lack a career plan because of the unstable and interrupted patterns of their prior employment. Employment for these people is a sign of their restored health and a return to their place in society.

The current job market is characterized by keen competition and advanced skills requirements for even entry-level jobs. Regretfully, both of these groups of recovering abusers are often further handicapped by a lack of marketable educational and occupational skills. Either they never developed these skills or they have been absent from the workforce for so long that their developed skills are obsolete. Many of these individuals may also suffer additional discrimination because of a history of legal convictions.

Obviously, recovering men and women have many needs as they seek to enter or return to work and reestablish themselves in the community. Comprehensive, specialized services are needed to help them make this transition.

VOCATIONAL REHABILITATION

Rehabilitation can be simply defined as the series of steps taken by a disabled person to achieve fulfillment in life. The process that specifically addresses an individual's work fulfillment and remuneration is referred to as vocational rehabilitation. A further distinction in terms is important because of the specific needs of recovering substance abusers. The process for many who are characterized by a late onset of substance abuse, or who have worked before and are returning to competitive employment, may appropriately be termed vocational "rehabilitation." These individuals are being restored to a former level of functioning. However, for those recovering people who have lived on the fringe of society, never having worked before, vocational "habilitation" provides a more accurate understanding of their need to learn what work is about and to establish for the first time effective work behaviors. Having made this distinction, the term *rehabilitation* is used in this chapter to refer to both concepts.

There are three basic vocational rehabilitation strategies (6). The first and most desirable strategy is to remedy the cause of the person's disability by restoring or developing functional ability. For example, a recovering person who is impaired by the lack of current marketable job skills may "cure" this handicap by completing an appropriate occupational skills training program. The second strategy is to enhance the individual's other vocational/educational attributes so that the person can compensate for the disability. For example, a recovering substance abuser may need to outweigh a lack of past employment by obtaining significant positive references from volunteer positions the individual has held. The third strategy is to adapt the work environment so that the person's disability is not a functional impairment. This tactic is least feasible because the provision of specialized tools or techniques or making physical changes in a work station usually does not effectively rectify the consequences of a recovering substance abuser's disability. However, an example of this strategy might be the alteration of a regular work schedule to allow a recovering person to keep ongoing counseling support appointments.

The ultimate guideline for all rehabilitation and vocational rehabilitation is to provide help so that the recovering individual becomes less dependent on external resources and more independent by making changes in himself or herself. With this as one of our guiding principles, we can now examine the components of an effective vocational rehabilitation program for recovering substance abusers: assessment, counseling and referral, and placement and followup.

Assessment

The first and most crucial component of vocational rehabilitation for any disabled group is assessment. The fourth step of the Alcoholics Anonymous recovery program is a "searching and fearless moral inventory" (7). A similar vocational inventory needs to be undertaken by recovering individuals to develop their vocational plans. They must be evaluated in four key areas: Is the recovering substance abuser ready to enter or return to work? If so, for which specific employment position is the individual best suited? If not, what is the client lacking to effectively obtain and maintain a job? And, finally, where and how can these needs be addressed?

The question of readiness for work is multifaceted. As a result, the assessment must be ongoing in terms of evaluating the client initially in relation to work in general and then later in the process in relation to a specific job's demands. Obviously, a person's understanding of and attitude toward work must be evaluated. Often, as a consequence of their lack of exposure to healthy worker models and their own absence from the labor force, many substance abusers develop an inaccurate concept of what a job will require or provide. Frequently, recovering substance abusers see employment as a panacea. Obtaining a job, they believe, will solve all their problems, help them stay "straight" and move them into the mainstream. Their concept of employment is a fantasy: wearing a suit, having a secretary, going to lunch, and getting a paycheck.

Motivation is a crucial ingredient and unless properly assessed and addressed, will lead to resistance from the client and frustration for the counselor later in the process. If the client is not able to progress to a point where the client is keeping appointments on time and demonstrating initiative and choice in selecting from available vocational options, then the client's motivation is questionable. Certainly, a criteria for evaluating motivation, as well as overall work readiness, is the client's chemical abuse status. If the individual is neither drug and alcohol free nor stabilized on a prescribed medication like methadone, then the client is unable to be endorsed for employment. Moreover, a vocational/educational assessment battery would have little value if the client was abusing drugs or alcohol when involved in the testing.

If the recovering substance abuser has an accurate understanding of what employment involves, is expressing a desire to work, and showing some evidence of this motivation, the next issue is evaluating the client's ability to work. Specifically is the client physically, psychologically, occupationally, socially, and placement ready (8)?

First, is the client physically ready? Are there any medical problems which would either rule out employment or restrict job options? For example, a client affected by acquired immunodeficiency syndrome (AIDS) may be able to work full-time, part-time, or only on a temporary basis depending on the status and progression of the disease. In some cases, health problems can be remedied. Still, care must be taken to allow adequate time and logical service provision so that the client is not expected to engage in vocational pursuits before stable health has been established. Further physical considerations include issues such as the possession of a stable residence, the availability of child-care if necessary, and realistic travel time to and from a job.

Second, is the client emotionally and psychologically ready? Has the client developed adequate coping skills to handle the frustration, rejection, and criticism associated with looking for, obtaining, and keeping a job? If clinical issues such as denial, transference, or projection are present, have they been adequately addressed? Is the client mature enough to appreciate the short-term benefits of a realistic vocational step as opposed to focusing on the long-term "ideal" job, which may be serving as a fantasized panacea? If further psychological support is necessary, does it preclude further vocational steps or can it be offered in conjunction with the progressive steps toward employment?

Third, is the client occupationally ready? Does the client have a job goal? Appropriate vocational interest assessment can be accomplished through a combination of psychometric testing and individual research. The combination of the two provides an opportunity for a client to be actively involved in the process with greater responsibility for the outcome. Based on John Holland's trait-factor theory of occupational choice, the Career Assessment Inventory, Strong Campbell Interest Inventory, and Self-Directed Search are some of the available standardized interest testing measures. Other tests such as the Minnesota Importance Questionnaire, the Career Occupational Preference System (COPS), the Career Ability Placement Survey (CAPS), Community-Oriented Programs Environment Scale (COPES), and the Gordon Occupational Checklist II are available to help clients see the patterns of their values and preferences. There are even computerized programs such as the System of Interactive Guidance and Information Plus (SIGIPLUS) to help clients obtain an integrated occupational profile of their interests and values. Many of these tests are available in Spanish and have forms for clients with lower reading levels.

Individualized research can be done in the *Occupational Outlook Handbook* (OOH) and the *Dictionary of Occupational Titles* (DOT), published by the United States Department of Labor. The OOH is a reference work that describes the nature, qualifications, employment outlook, and promotional opportunities for general job groupings. The DOT is a specific classification system for the breakdown of general job groupings with descriptions of the exact efforts, techniques, and tools needed to accomplish the typical work tasks. Both the OOH and the DOT can be accessed online.

In addition to an interest focus, an occupationally ready client should possess the specific aptitudes, general intelligence, appropriate math, reading, and writing skills to adequately meet the job demands. General and specific assessment tools are available to help clients with limited awareness of their abilities to determine their strengths as well as to verify perceived abilities. The Differential Aptitude test, the General Aptitude Test Battery, the Crawford Small Parts Dexterity Test, the Bennett Hand Tool Dexterity Test, and Valpar International Pro 3000 Series are examples of assessment tools.

A client's level of educational skills, particularly in the areas of reading and math, should also be assessed using measures such as the Adult Basic Learning Examination, the Test of Adult Basic Education, the California Achievement Tests, and the Wide Range Achievement Test 3. As with the interest tests, versions in Spanish and versions for different ages or skill levels are available to obtain a more accurate picture of an individual's functioning. Undiagnosed learning disabilities may be at the root of some clients' development of a substance abuse problem, and therefore, screening should be incorporated into all educational evaluation. Educational remediation services are available through the Literacy Volunteers of America, the Learning Disabilities Association of America, local school districts, and specialized diagnostic and tutorial agencies.

If the client possesses the basic aptitudes for an occupation, does the client also possess sufficient, relevant experience, academic degrees, training certificates, or licenses to meet the hiring standards and compete in the job market? Does the client have any legal convictions that would be a bar to the desired employment goal? If the client has impairments in any of these areas, referrals for educational remediation, vocational, or legal assistance should be made.

A fourth area to evaluate is the client's social readiness. Remembering that a significant percentage of recovering substance abusers have been living in a "subculture" with little or no exposure to a work environment should help the reader appreciate the importance of this assessment. Can the client communicate effectively, talking as well as listening? Does the client know how to dress appropriately for a specific job environment, neither underdressing nor overdressing, and neither dressing to attract attention nor to make a statement? Has the client evidenced the ability to interact appropriately with coworkers and supervisors and employment authority figures? Observations of a client's interaction with his or her peers and treatment staff may provide excellent insight into this ability. Does the client possess sufficient self-management and planning skills to ask questions when unclear about instructions and to notify an employer when unable to meet a commitment? A supportive family and involvement in a 12-step program are important factors in determining social readiness.

Finally the client needs to be evaluated in terms of the ability to job hunt effectively. Can the client complete a job application or resume? Is the client capable of presenting marketable job qualities and a positive work attitude in a employment interview? Is the client able to address an employer's possible questions about work gaps and conviction history, or possibly past substance abuse, in a way that will relieve the employer's fears about hiring someone with negative elements in his or her background? Special attention must be paid to the level of work readiness skills in the counseling process.

It should be clear that comprehensive vocational assessment of the recovering substance abuser may require a significant commitment of time and resources. It is essential that adequate time be allowed lest undiagnosed deficiencies surface later in the vocational rehabilitation process. Not only could this significantly delay or disrupt the progress which the client is making, it could also cause the client to become discouraged and lose confidence in his or her abilities, thereby diminishing motivation. Proper assessment should determine the scope, timing, and logical sequence of the client's rehabilitation steps and services delivery.

Counseling and Referral

The basic goal of counseling is accelerated learning. As a result of a proper assessment, a counselor should be able to depict what a client needs to know and clues for helping the client learn what the client needs to know. A basic epistemological principle applies, helping a client understand the unknown by examining what the client already knows.

Vocational counseling has four classic elements: developing a positive self-concept, obtaining occupational information, expressing the self in occupational terms, and learning job-seeking skills (9).

The starting point for all counseling is the client, and more specifically, the perception that the client has of himself or herself. A fundamental task for rehabilitation counselors is to help clients remove the stigma of disability that many have internalized. Vocational rehabilitation with recovering substance abusers must address this issue. Many of these clients believe the label that society has assigned them, more convinced of what they cannot do than confident of what they can do. Their histories of failures become a projection for the future, a self-fulfilling prophecy rooted in a negative self-concept or, at best, low self-esteem.

With histories of missed opportunities and nonsuccess, recovering substance abusers need to be reminded by their counselors of the obstacles that they overcame and the progress made in treatment. Vocational rehabilitation counselors can further boost their clients' self-concepts by extracting from their "street" experiences transferable job skills.

Recovering substance abusers in vocational counseling will generally present one of four major needs. The first group of clients possess no occupational goals and will therefore need assistance in establishing goals. The second group has inappropriate or unrealistic goals and will need help in developing more achievable goals. The third group has appropriate goals but needs support in planning the steps and obtaining the resources needed to achieve the goals. The fourth group sees no value in working. Values clarification activities must be the foundation of this group's vocational counseling (9).

Counselors need to help clients integrate their self-concepts, interest assessments, values clarifications, aptitude evaluations and the realities of the job market into a concrete employment goal. Additional assistance may be required by clients to locate the necessary resources and to plan the specific achievable steps to the desired goal. Empowering the client to choose is a central theme in the vocational counseling relationship. Clients will only invest energy in goals that they have had responsibility for selecting. Among the materials available to help clients achieve this integration and empowerment is the *Adkins Life Skills Program: Career Development Series* published by Columbia University's Institute for Life Coping Skills.

Referral to resource agencies for aptitude assessment, educational remediation, or occupational skills training may augment a client's strengths and may serve as a gradual step in the transition to employment. However, initially such referrals may also threaten a weakened self-concept. Returning to the classroom can rekindle the feelings of insecurity and self-doubt which a client experienced in school. Apprehensions about testing, competition, and acknowledgment of mistakes will need to be addressed by the counselor prior to and during a client's attendance at such programs. In light of these considerations it is important that a counselor develop a client's ability to evaluate not only the general efficacy of such a program but also the appropriateness of the program to the client's individual needs. Is a large or small program better for the client? Is a teaching approach with more hands-on lab experience more appropriate to the client's needs or is one with more classroom lecture?

Obtaining employment is a major challenge for even the most mentally, physically, and emotionally capable person. The basic skills necessary to look for and secure a job must either be learned or relearned by the recovering substance abuser. Moreover, because of their disability, specialized techniques and strategies must be used for the job-hunting process to be successful. The importance of counseling support at this juncture cannot be overemphasized.

The seemingly simple task of completing a job application or resume can be overwhelming for clients. If they have never worked before, they may feel intimidated by the extensive questions about past employment and education. Even if they have worked before, many clients have poor memory and limited records of the training and job experiences during their periods of substance abuse. Moreover, some clients report that during the compilation of necessary work data they become overwhelmed by negative feelings associated with the failures and incomplete undertakings that were consequences of their abuse.

In general, job hunting for clients with employment gaps and other stigmatized background elements is a very frustrating process. Equipping clients to handle the rejections and disappointments of a job search, offering them outlets to vent their feelings and providing them with coping strategies are necessary components of placement preparation.

Placement and Followup

The National Association on Drug Abuse Problems (NADAP) is a private nonprofit organization based in New York City that provides placement assistance to recovering substance abusers. NADAP has found that for many recovering persons it is necessary to augment the individual vocational rehabilitation counseling with specialized group workshops. These workshops have been designed as "groups" because work is public and requires socialization. As members of these groups, clients can be further assessed in terms of their ability to interact appropriately. The workshops also provide clients with opportunities to learn and practice job-related social skills.

The presence of other clients who are also job searching helps each client realize that they are not alone in their rejections and frustrations. Also, they realize that they are not alone in their ignorance of aspects of the work world and job-hunting skills. They learn from others' mistakes and are encouraged by others' successes. The shared disability of the members allows for more direct peer critique of individual obstacles and assistance in breaking their goals

into short-term concrete steps. The group often, very practically, serves as a networking resource for employment leads.

The skills-building exercises in the NADAP workshops incorporate role playing, videotaping, and the involvement of employer representatives. Through role playing and videotaping, a client is able to see very clearly the strengths and weaknesses of his or her interviewing behaviors. The corporate personnel recruiters who participate in the role plays provide an excellent "dress rehearsal" for the client's real interview, directly represent employers' expectations of job applicants, and offer clients suggestions on how they can better present their marketable traits and such negative elements in their background as legal convictions, job dismissals, and periods of unemployment.

Handling these elements of the application and in an interview is a major task for recovering substance abusers. Guidelines for the presentation of confidential information are also addressed in the workshops. Clients learn through group exercises that the way information is presented is as important as what the information is. First, clients are encouraged not to volunteer negative data unless it is specifically requested (10). Second, they are trained to couple their admittance of past negative experiences with at least one positive step or change that has occurred as a result of their substance abuse treatment.

Depending on the client's individual background and chosen employment direction, the client may require consultations with agencies such as the Legal Action Center and the state Human Rights Office. Through such resources recovering substance abusers learn their employment rights, eliminate unrealistic employment options, access bonding, licensure, or certification alternatives, and challenge employment discrimination.

Participation in such workshops helps a client develop not only specific skills but also a self-evaluation ability that will help to improve presentations on successive interviews and enhance their job performance. Research has demonstrated that recovering substance abusers who participate in job-hunting groups are more likely to secure and retain employment (11). Faced with discrimination and impairments, clients looking for work have to try different strategies and use as many employment resources as possible: community, city, county, state, and federal agencies, as well as specialized placement services such as NADAP.

NADAP advocates with large and small employers for competitive job opportunities for recovering substance abusers. In 2002, NADAP placed more than 50% of the clients who entered the program who were job-ready (12).

To enhance a client's success in employment NADAP provides retention and career advancement services. A NADAP staff member is available to clients and their employers to resolve problems that might arise during the initial adjustment to a job. Followup, aftercare, and ongoing support issues are important from a vocational rehabilitation, as well as a clinical, perspective.

Support services in the form of group or individual counseling should be available to employed clients. Issues of anxiety, self-confidence, socialization, communication, basic attendance, and punctuality are usually greater determinants of job terminations for recovering substance abusers than lack of adequate skills or inability to learn quickly enough. Clients may need continued opportunities to role-play problem situations on the job and concrete exercises addressing assertive as opposed to aggressive behaviors.

Being a "worker" puts a client in a new role with family and friends. These significant others may be threatened by the client's progress and attempt to sabotage job retention. Coupled with a new job, budgeting money, scheduling leisure pursuits, and attending to daily living needs may also create new stresses for a client who previously had never worked or had been unemployed for a long time. After securing an entry-level position, clients will need career-planning assistance so that they can develop appropriate long-term goals, strategies, and timetables.

Given adequate rehabilitation time, comprehensive assessment, and appropriate services, recovering substance abusers can succeed in securing employment. The New York State Office of Vocational and Educational Services for Individuals with Disabilities (VESID) provides this proper climate and has established a history of helping disabled individuals achieve employment. Historically, VESID rehabilitated consumers with histories of substance abuse at a higher rate than consumers with other disabilities. VESID spends only slightly more money to help a recovering substance abuser secure employment than to rehabilitate most of the other disability groups it serves (13).

A final consideration in analyzing the placement of recovering substance abusers is how these individuals compare with other employees on the job. Two research studies indicate that there are no significant differences between recovering substance abusers and their peers on the job in terms of job retention, absenteeism, punctuality, performance, promotions, dismissals, and resignations (14,15).

Illustrative Cases

Jane

Jane was a 34-year-old woman who had been raised in an alcoholic home and had a history of 11 years of heroin addiction. She had been stabilized on methadone for 18 months after four unsuccessful detoxification attempts. Recently divorced from her husband, she was responsible for supporting herself and her 7-year-old son.

Jane was a high school graduate who had managed a retail business with her husband for 6 years. She had been unemployed for the past 2 years. Motivated by her desire to provide for her son, she entered into vocational rehabilitation counseling at her methadone clinic. Her counselor

referred her to an employment exploration and skills development group and helped her complete some occupational research. As a result of these undertakings, Jane decided that she was interested in pursuing a career in computer programming. However, she lacked confidence in her academic skills and knew that her goal would require college-level training. She feared that with her existing childcare responsibilities, therapy appointments, and necessary dental treatments she would not have sufficient time to devote to school. She was concerned that employment would reduce her welfare benefits for herself and her son. She also felt isolated from others because of her "addict" stigma and was afraid of entering into new social situations.

An initial educational assessment revealed basically strong reading and math skills, although weak algebraic ability. As such ability would be needed for computer training, Jane was referred to a part-time evening tutoring program. She also decided to participate in a half-day vocational aptitude assessment program to address some of her other fears.

Jane made progress in her math tutoring and demonstrated the necessary aptitudes and work behaviors to consider a referral to the state office of vocational rehabilitation. This agency agreed to fund Jane for a 1-year computer certificate program at the local community college. This was in keeping with welfare reform regulations and was approved by her local Department of Social Services. Because of her age and childcare responsibilities the college granted her special student status. This gave her priority in registering for courses and allowed her to design a class schedule that ensured that even though she was taking a full course load, she could be home for most of the times when her son was not in school. Daycare for her son was provided at a licensed center through Social Services.

Initially after starting college Jane maintained contact with her tutor for assistance with her first math classes. She also continued in primary therapy for support with her single-parenting issues and socialization needs. Jane graduated from college and was able to secure a job with a company that provided her with additional in-house programming training.

John

John was a 24-year-old polydrug abuser. He had dropped out of high school and was living at home, supporting himself on his earnings as a semiprofessional athlete. The death of his girlfriend because of cancer was the catalyst for his involvement in counseling. His bereavement counselor noted John's need for substance abuse treatment. While attending outpatient treatment, John realized the need for vocational rehabilitation services.

Because John had no consistent work record, specific occupational interest, or sense of his abilities, his vocational counselor referred him to an aptitude assessment and work adjustment program. While there, John received occupational interest testing. The testing revealed John's preferences for manual and technical activities. Additional occupational exploration helped John focus on a position in electronic repair. The assessment indicated that he possessed the necessary aptitudes for such work but his math skills were not sufficient to pass the entrance exam for the appropriate training schools. Moreover, a high school diploma was required to meet the hiring standards of most of the employers in the computer repair field.

John investigated the three local trade schools offering electronic repair training. He decided to attend the longest and most advanced course because of the increased career opportunities it would afford him. John's counselor helped him see that this choice meant more homework than the other programs required and additional efforts on his part because of his math deficiencies. John rose to the challenge and enrolled in a part-time educational program offering preparation for the high school General Equivalency Diploma (GED) and math tutoring.

As a result, he was able to raise his math skills sufficiently to pass the training program's entrance exam. He applied for and received government-sponsored financial aid to cover most of the tuition costs. Once in training, he transferred the discipline he had developed as an athlete into his new endeavor. John established a specific study schedule and took advantage of every "extra help" session his training instructors offered him. He secured a part-time, evening maintenance job to meet his general expenses and the tuition costs not covered by his financial aid. He continued his outpatient counseling to help him resolve his grief and relationship issues.

On his first attempt prior to the end of his electronics training, John passed the GED exam. He graduated from training and secured a position as a digital repair technician. After 1 year he left his first job for a more advanced position in the field. At the new firm he received specialized training on a unique piece of technology and became a troubleshooter and trainer of new staff.

IMPEDIMENTS TO VOCATIONAL REHABILITATION SERVICE DELIVERY

The federal government has joined with state and local governments in endorsing the connection between work and recovery. This is evident in their policy developments and antidiscrimination legislation. This extends to funding provisions for training and job opportunities for recovering substance abusers (16). Certainly the Rehabilitation Act of 1973 serves as a cornerstone for the legal rights and public opportunities available to individuals with disabilities (17).

However, it is naive to believe that this support alone guarantees vocational rehabilitation services to those who need and desire it. There are three major categories of hindrances to effective provision and use of these services

by recovering substance abusers: the clients themselves, the programs that treat them, and the society to which they return (18).

Clients who have been addicted to drugs and/or alcohol typically suffer with multiple impairments: poor health, AIDS or AIDS-related complex (ARC), psychological limitations, educational deficits, vocational development deficiencies, conviction records, family problems, day care needs, and/or public assistance dependency. These factors affect the nature, pace, scope, and objectives of a client's vocational rehabilitation. As has already been outlined, careful, comprehensive assessment and appropriate remediation, compensation, or adaptation require significant commitments of time and energy to overcome these various problems. Some clients are too discouraged and alienated to persist in the process.

Treatment program obstacles can be examined in terms of the themes of philosophy and staffing. Historically, vocational rehabilitation, if considered at all by substance-abuse treatment programs, has been seen as an adjunct, ancillary part of the recovery process. There is a significant lack of research addressing the vocational rehabilitation of substance abusers. This is indicative of the low priority and concern which treatment professionals in general have for this component of treatment (19). In most residential facilities, the last few weeks or last few months at best are devoted to job placement referrals. In methadone and other outpatient treatment modalities there are usually no vocational rehabilitation services on site and only limited contact with educational/vocational resource agencies (20).

Many believe that the basic premise of most treatment programs is that if a client stops abusing drugs and alcohol, everything will fall into place and all things are possible. This principle is much too simplistic. Regretfully, clients accept this false expectation and find themselves returning to their communities without the knowledge and skills needed to function independently and achieve stability. Vocational rehabilitation is the treatment that helps these individuals develop much of this knowledge and many of these skills.

Unfortunately, a philosophical orientation toward vocational rehabilitation that downplays its contribution to the treatment process has translated into reduced staff resources available for such services. The drug and alcohol treatment field in general suffers from staff shortages and high turnover. The low pay, insufficient advancement opportunities, concerns about AIDS, and the frustrations and burnout associated with serving multidisabled clients have reduced the appeal of positions in substance abuse treatment (21). Faced with this reality, treatment program administrators knowingly or unknowingly diminish the status of vocational rehabilitation services. If they can afford the time, effort, and funds to hire a vocational rehabilitation counselor, it is usually a last priority in their hiring hierarchy, offering lower salaries than most clinical positions, unrealistic caseloads, less than full-time opportunities, or combined responsibilities, for example, general program intake and vocational counseling.

As a consequence of these factors, personnel with limited vocational rehabilitation skills may be hired. Research shows that less trained rehabilitation counselors provide less efficient, less cost-effective, and less successful delivery of vocational rehabilitation services (22). Certainly the multiple disabilities with which many recovering substance abusers suffer require highly trained counseling staff. Without such staff the integrity of the rehabilitation services provided to recovering substance abusers is compromised.

Societal obstacles are probably the most difficult to overcome because of the prevalent ignorance and fear which are at their roots. Recovering substance abusers suffer from the same degrees of employment discrimination as many other disabled individuals and ex-offenders. The fear about AIDS has been generalized to label all substance abusers and increase the stigma they already bear.

The discrimination which recovering substance abusers confront in the employment market is discouraging enough. Regretfully, they are also frequently faced with discrimination and misunderstanding by agencies in the social services system which supposedly exist to help them. This includes the disincentives to competitive employment imposed by public assistance guidelines as well as insensitive, illogical, and often contradictory eligibility criteria for counseling, educational remediation, training, and job placement assistance.

Is formal entry-level employment with limited or no fringe benefits attractive to a recovering substance abuser if it means surrendering the Medicaid which covers the cost of his or her treatment as well as the health insurance costs of his or her family? Substance abusers with psychiatric histories are often refused entry into substance-abuse treatment programs because these programs do not provide psychiatric counseling and supervision. These same clients are refused entry into psychiatric facilities because of their substance abuse.

A similar, if not more extreme situation exists for physically disabled substance abusers who are often rejected by substance-abuse treatment programs who cannot accommodate some of their special needs and are uneasy about how to treat these clients. Rehabilitation treatment programs for the physically disabled are just beginning to acknowledge that they may have clients with substance abuse problems and often cannot provide adequate substance abuse treatment for them.

Pregnant abusers are also ineligible for many programs because they are not designed to handle the needs of expectant mothers. There are limited treatment programs for women with children. This can force mothers with a substance abuse problem to have to choose between treatment and placing their children in foster care. Even clients who are functioning appropriately on monitored methadone dosages find it difficult to access many of the support services available to other substance abusers because they are not considered "drug free."

Against such obstacles even the most motivated client may lose hope that he or she can succeed in his or her employment recovery.

IMPROVING VOCATIONAL REHABILITATION SERVICES

The past four decades of providing vocational rehabilitation services to men and women recovering from drug and alcohol abuse point to three guidelines for improving these services: understanding, expansion, and coordination.

Regretfully, there will probably always be new drugs surfacing which carry with them certain unique vocational impairments. These impairments will need to be examined as they become evident and new rehabilitation strategies and resources developed to address them. However, we now have an understanding of the depth and scope of the effect that substance abuse has on an individual's vocational development and of the basic rehabilitation principles to apply. Most recovering substance abusers can make progress if they are allowed to do so in a slow, gradual manner with a full complement of support services. Although it may be too strong to say that relapse is frequently part of the recovery process, we know that it is a reality for many clients. This is true in terms of a client's vocational development as well. It is not necessarily a neat progression but one that may be characterized by false starts and occasional steps backward. For some, because of the chronic nature of their substance abuse histories and the multiple handicaps they have, competitive or full-time employment may not be a realistic goal. For others, it will only be appropriate as a very long-term goal.

In keeping with these characteristics we must adopt more of a mental health model of rehabilitation as opposed to a medical one. We must acknowledge this understanding in the design of vocational programs and in the expectations about working that we communicate to clients.

The second theme for future vocational rehabilitation is expansion. This means adding new services, but it also means expanding existing roles to involve more segments of society in the delivery of vocational rehabilitation services. If we acknowledge the need of recovering substance abusers for gradual movement from not working to working, then we must provide more work adjustment and transitional employment opportunities. These may include noncompetitive sheltered or semisheltered workshops that are available to other disability groups. Supported work programs for recovering substance abusers increase levels of employment and income and reduce arrests and jail time (23,24). New programs alone, however, are insufficient to meet the vocational rehabilitation needs of recovering substance abusers.

Employers in the United States are confronting a shrinking labor force of educated, skilled workers. Certainly the drug crisis is contributing to this deficit. Employers must respond with programs that offer alternatives to substance abuse and nourish the vocational development of recovering individuals who are looking for new positions or for a healthy return to their former jobs. Included must be nondiscriminatory hiring practices, business-sponsored training, transitional and noncompetitive work opportunities, and job maintenance and support services. At the very least, employers must be willing to abide by the current legislation addressing these issues. The Americans with Disabilities Act (ADA) specifically extends antidiscrimination treatment and employment policies to individuals with drug and alcohol problems and to those affected by the AIDS virus. While not protecting current users of illegal drugs, the ADA generally safeguards individuals with a history of substance abuse who have completed or are enrolled in treatment. For example, the ADA dictates that accommodations be made in the work schedule of a recovering individual to allow that person to attend a treatment program, unless such an accommodation would create undue hardship for the employer (25).

Researchers, as well, must become more involved in examining the vocational rehabilitation of recovering substance abusers. They can help to better delineate specific needs of these individuals and enhance the design of effective interventions and strategies.

Finally, for there to be effective vocational rehabilitation of recovering substance abusers, there needs to be increased coordination of relevant services. Drug and alcohol prevention programs need to include career exploration, educational remediation, occupational skills training, and work adjustment experiences into their services. Treatment programs must integrate comprehensive educational/vocational services into the early, middle, and late stages of their clinical treatment. Staff of these programs should familiarize themselves with existing vocational rehabilitation resources and adapt their program procedures to allow clients to avail themselves of these services. Just as a placement specialist working with a recovering person must be aware of the client's clinical needs and progress so must a treatment counselor be aware of the client's vocational impairments and efforts at remedying or compensating for them. Treatment staff must be trained in the basic principles of vocational assessment so that while clients are in their care they can at least refer them to appropriate agencies which can prepare them for employment and independent living outside treatment.

In addition to the expected increases in employment, it appears from recent research that vocational rehabilitation programs are one of the psychosocial support services which can be effective in reducing drug use (26). Clearly such outcomes justify the costs associated with integrating these components into substance-abuse treatment programs.

Work dignifies us as human beings. Unless we provide men and women recovering from substance abuse with support and opportunities to achieve this dignity, to earn a place in society, we should not fault them for taxing our welfare system, straining our criminal justice system, and perpetuating a destructive subculture.

SUBSTANCE ABUSE AT THE WORKPLACE

This section addresses the scope and nature of substance abuse in the workplace and discusses efforts to effectively address the problem among employees.

Although there is widespread agreement that employment is an ultimate goal in the vocational rehabilitation of the recovering substance abuser, it is also generally acknowledged that significant alcohol and drug-abuse problems exist among employees at the workplace. The actual extent of substance abuse problems in the workplace and their cost to industry are difficult to measure and are probably underestimated. A variety of factors, some related to the very nature of alcoholism and addiction, contribute to difficulty in determining the scope of the problem.

For example, many problem drinkers and alcoholics are able to function adequately at their jobs. Problems may not be detected, at least not at the early stages of their disease. This is equally true of employees with other drug abuse and addiction problems. Unfortunately, it is often at the late stages of alcoholism or other addiction, when control can no longer be sustained, that the problem becomes apparent at the workplace. The very nature of an employee's work may also contribute to difficulty in detecting a problem. For example, any kind of deviant behavior reflected by an employee would be hard to detect in a position that has low visibility and unclear production goals.

In addition, despite growing awareness and generally more constructive responses, there is still a stigma felt by many individuals attached to having a substance abuse problem. While undoubtedly felt less strongly in companies that have adopted nonpunitive drug and alcohol policies, this stigma and fear of job loss may nevertheless prevent a substance abuser from self-revealing or self-referring for help or even self-reporting in a survey where anonymity is assured.

Finally, contributing to the difficulty in determining the exact extent of the problem in the workplace are the supervisors and coworkers of the substance-abusing employee. They may coverup for the worker's inadequate job performance, even performing tasks themselves that are the substance abuser's responsibility. In addition, many supervisors have difficulty confronting the employee whose job performance is unacceptable. Although well intended, covering up and not confronting an employee feed into the employee's probably already well-developed denial that there is a problem. Such enabling behavior actually allows the alcoholism or addiction to progress further. These same supervisors probably underuse existing company programs designed to help the substance-abusing employee. It is apparent that supervisors play a very critical role in implementing effective drug and alcohol abuse policies and programs.

Despite the difficulties inherent in acquiring accurate measures, surveys have been conducted and estimates of the extent of workplace substance abuse indicate that the problem is one of alarming proportions. Data from the 1997 National Household Survey on Drug Abuse states that 8% of all full-time workers age 18 to 49 years had used illicit drugs in the past month. An equal amount of this same group reported current heavy alcohol use. Certain occupational categories, including food preparation, construction, and transportation, showed higher rates of abuse (27). Often the problem is one of polydrug abuse, that is, employees taking a mixture of substances that include both legal drugs, such as alcohol, and illegal substances.

The Alcohol, Drug Abuse, and Mental Health Administration estimates that alcohol and drug abuse cost nearly $100 billion in lost productivity each year (28). In a survey of 273 human resource executives from Fortune 1500 companies and state governments, respondents indicated that employees with substance abuse problems are absent from two to six times as often as other employees. These same executives estimated that among substance abusers, absenteeism, worksite accidents, and disciplinary problems occurred from two to ten times more frequently than the average for other employees. They also noted that the misuse of alcohol and drugs significantly affected their organizations as evidenced by increased absenteeism, decreased productivity, and increased medical benefit claims (29).

Other factors that may contribute to the direct and indirect costs of substance abuse in the workplace include increased disability and workers' compensation benefits; time to handle disciplinary and grievance proceedings; turnover, recruiting, and training costs; and lower employee morale.

JOB PERFORMANCE AND SUBSTANCE ABUSE

That there is a relationship between substance abuse and performance is unquestionable; it is the premise upon which many companies' successful Employee Assistance Programs (EAPs) have been established. However, the specific nature of the relationship between alcohol and other drugs and performance is complicated. The effects of drugs vary considerably from one individual to another and even within the same individual on different occasions. There are many variables that influence one's behavioral response to a particular drug. Physiologic (age, weight, sex, disease state), pharmacologic (type of drug, route and time of administration, tolerance, pharmacokinetics), and psychological (behavioral toxicity, emotional state, situational variables) factors all play a role in determining how an individual will respond to a drug.

However, despite the complexities involved in determining the effects of drugs on human performance there are some generalities that can be drawn. The effects of drugs on performance are dose dependent, that is, the higher doses of drugs generally produce greater effects. Simple motor tasks (e.g., painting the hull of a ship) are less affected by drugs than complex, cognitive tasks (e.g., flying a jet aircraft).

Repetitive work is less affected than work requiring learning or coping skills. For example, driving a car is a fairly well-learned skill, and driving back and forth between work and home is generally a repetitive, fairly mechanical task involving little cognitive effort or concentration. However, the danger of driving under the influence involves those situations where coping skills, which are significantly impaired by minimal effects of drugs, are suddenly called upon, as would happen when a child suddenly went in front of the car. Employees in jobs involving repetitive tasks with heavy equipment may encounter similar situations where coping skills suddenly need to be called into action. Finally, the duration of drug effects depends on the task being performed. Individuals resume normal functioning more quickly with simple tasks but cannot handle more complex cognitive tasks for much longer periods of time (30). For example, in a study on the effects of marijuana on pilots, Yesavage demonstrated that 24 hours after smoking a single 2% marijuana cigarette, pilots were able to take off, level off, and perform various tasks in a simulator. However, they were unable to land the aircraft properly, a critical part of their job (31).

INDUSTRY'S RESPONSE TO SUBSTANCE ABUSE: A BRIEF HISTORY

Gradually industry has recognized and responded to the impact of substance abuse on the organization and its employees. The worksite has provided a unique opportunity to address these problems. Initially, the focus of company policy and programs was on alcoholism. There is a long history of efforts by industry to address problems of alcoholism among employees. In the 1940s, three developments precipitated alcohol abuse to surface as a major concern in the industrial sector. First was the founding and growth of Alcoholics Anonymous (AA). Second, respected and dedicated medical directors in companies came to initiate and support programs. Finally, World War II created a unique labor market. Lack of a better qualified workforce forced employers to hire marginal, inexperienced workers during a time of unprecedented demand for mass production of war material. Consecutive work shifts exacerbated alcoholism and alcohol abuse that was already problematic for many of these marginal workers. Productivity and safety concerns precipitated interest in "occupational programming;" these alcohol-specific programs were the precursors of modern EAPs. To help integrate these marginal workers into the workplace the government funded hundreds of mental health and social service programs in industry. After the war, the majority of these mental health programs shut down.

Of longer-lasting impact were industrial alcoholism programs, which also started during World War II. These programs used the prospect of job loss because of unsatisfactory job performance, along with the offer of rehabilitation to motivate problem drinkers to change: to choose treatment, become sober, and improve their job performance. Early industrial alcoholism programs were informal arrangements generally involving teamwork between the company's "occupational physician" and dedicated members of AA who would approach employees suspected of having drinking problems. Gradually some companies developed this informal arrangement into a formal policy and program. The policy generally stated that alcoholism is a disease and emphasized the company's willingness to help alcoholics.

After the war, the Yale Center for Alcohol Studies promoted industrial alcoholism programs among business and labor leaders. By the mid-1950s, 50 to 60 such programs existed in American industry. In 1959, the National Council on Alcoholism (NCA) began marketing industrial alcoholism programs. Lewis F. Presnall, NCA's industrial consultant, began advocating broad-based programs to help alcoholic and other troubled employees and to train supervisors to observe deteriorating job performance and effectively use a strategy developed by Harrison M. Trice called the constructive confrontation. Effective interventions today are still largely based on observing and documenting deteriorating job performance and constructively confronting the employee.

The Hughes Act in 1970, and the subsequent establishment in 1971 of the National Institute on Alcohol Abuse and Alcoholism (NIAAA), contributed greatly to the advancement of EAPs. The Institute believed that alcoholism was the most prevalent personal problem among employees and that the workplace was the most effective place to identify, motivate, and provide for the treatment of alcoholics.

In 1972, to promote EAPs, NIAAA funded two occupational program consultants (OPCs) in each state. Many of the occupational program consultants were recruited from the mental health occupations, that is, psychologists and social workers. Thus, the OPCs split into two groups: the alcoholism constituency and the mental health constituency. Both groups agreed that addressing an employee's problems would improve job performance but differed in their emphasis. The alcoholism constituency emphasized the importance of treating alcoholism and of supervisors' use of constructive confrontation to motivate the alcoholic employee. The mental health constituency emphasized the importance of treating all personal problems equally, deemphasized the constructive confrontation strategy, and prompted employees to seek help from the EAP on their own initiative.

EAPs MULTIPLY

Despite the growing pains experienced by EAPs in developing a clear and distinctive identity, there has been tremendous growth of these programs in the past two decades. Between 1971 and 1980 OPC efforts contributed to increasing the number of programs in the United States from 350 to an estimated 5,000. By 1981 the success of these programs spawned 200 private EAP consulting services (32,33).

From 1980 to 1990 the estimated number of EAPs grew from 5,000 to 20,000. From 1980 to 1990 the estimated number of employees covered by EAPs grew from 12% to more than 35%. The survey of Employer Antidrug Programs released by the Bureau of Labor Statistics in January 1989, reflects that the probability of an employee having access to an EAP increases as a function of establishment size ranging from 4.2% in the smallest to 86.8% in the largest companies. Another reflection of the significant growth in the EAP field is that from 1980 to 1990 the membership of the Employee Assistance Professionals Association (EAPA, formerly ALMACA, the Association of Labor-Management Administrators and Consultants on Alcoholism) grew from 1,500 to 6,000 (28,34).

Why do employers adopt EAPs? According to research using both quantitative and qualitative methods, the answer is that "programs are adopted because employers believe that helping employees to solve their personal problems is good business and demonstrates social responsibility" (32, p. 6). In a more recent survey of 1,238 EAPs, preliminary findings suggest that organizations adopt EAPs for the following reasons: a large majority want to help troubled employees; approximately 70% see EAPs as an employee benefit; more than 50% want to relieve supervisors of dealing with employees' problems; more than 40% see them as health care containment; and approximately 30% hope to avoid litigation (35).

The fact that a large majority of those surveyed want to help troubled employees may also be a reflection of the reduced stigma attached to substance abuse problems. The disease concept of alcoholism and other chemical dependencies has made a significant inroad in replacing the concept of the character flaw. Also, today, very few business people have not been touched personally or by family members, friends, and business associates who have had to struggle with alcohol and other drug problems.

Another possible reason for companies adopting EAPs is because they work. For example, a comparison of more than 700 substance-abuse patients who worked full-time during the year before and the year after treatment showed a marked reduction in job absenteeism, performance

1342 / Section XV Policy Issues

problems, such as making mistakes and incomplete work, and interpersonal problems (36).

Finally employers may adopt EAPs because they believe they work. Some employers adopted EAPs because they believed they were cost-effective whether or not they had empirical data to support this. Conversely, employers who have not adopted EAPs reject the idea that programs are cost-effective. This difference appears to be largely in the underlying ideologies of employers (32).

Supporting this observation is the fact that in the earlier cited survey of Fortune 1500 companies, governors, and mayors, 80% of the CEOs and government officials were satisfied with how their EAPs were addressing substance abuse among employees. They held this belief despite the fact that very few of their organizations systematically evaluated the effectiveness of their programs and therefore they had no information to support the notion that programs were working (29).

EFFECTIVE EAPs

EAPs Defined

Standards for Employee Assistance Programs, published in 1990 by the Employee Assistance Professionals Association, identifies the core ingredients of EAPs and professional standards for carrying them out. It defines EAPs as worksite-based programs that are designed to assist in the identification and resolution of productivity problems associated with employees impaired by personal concerns which may adversely affect employee job performance. Personal concerns may include, but not be limited to, health, marital, family, financial, alcohol, drug, legal, emotional, stress, or other personal concerns (37). EAPs are worksite-based intervention programs designed to help employees identify and address personal concerns that may be affecting job performance.

Needs Assessment

These definitions reflect today's more popular broad-based EAP. However, there are no "cookie cutters" for EAPs. Each program should take into account the unique milieu of each work organization and the needs of its employees. Balzer and Pargament describe the value of conducting a needs assessment and outline a manageable process for doing this. A good needs assessment maximizes the chances of successfully matching the needs of the organization and its employees with an EAP (38). Employers who need help in conducting a needs assessment and establishing an EAP should contact their local chapter of the Employee Assistance Professionals Association. Another helpful resource is the Center for Substance Abuse Prevention's Workplace Helpline at 1-800-843-4971.

EAP Objectives

In its program standards, the Employee Assistance Professionals Association describes three general EAP objectives. First, the EAP provides the company, its employees, and families with a broad range of services that may affect job performance. Second, it provides a resource to management and labor for interventions with employees whose personal problems are affecting their job performance. Third, it "effectively, efficiently and professionally provides assessment, referral and followup services for mental health, alcohol and other drug related problems in the workforce" (37, p. B).

Advisory Committee and Clear Policy

Critical to effective EAPs is the development and implementation of a clear policy. This policy should be developed by an advisory committee representing different levels of management and labor groups in the company. "Program acceptance and utilization is directly related to the amount of support from top management and involvement by employees, supervisors, management and unions" (37, p. C). The resulting policy statement defines the EAPs relationship to the organization and describes its confidential nature to both the organization and employees.

The policy statement should minimally cover the following concepts. It states that the company recognizes that mentally and physically well employees are an asset to the organization and that the availability of EAP services can benefit both labor and management. It also states that alcohol, drug abuse, emotional, marital, and other problems can adversely affect job performance. Employees with such problems may be unable to function efficiently, effectively, or safely on the job and, therefore, these problems are a legitimate concern of the employer. The policy statement points out that employees may voluntarily seek out EAP services or be referred by supervisors through constructive confrontation. Job security is assured as long as employees using the EAP maintain acceptable job performance standards. Finally, but most importantly, the policy statement assures employees that all records are kept in strict confidentiality (37).

Familiarity with Policy and Procedures Key

Familiarity with EAP policy and procedures is key to effective use of the program. The policy should be published in a clear, understandable manner and distributed to all employees on a periodic basis. In addition to publications, orientation or training sessions should be conducted to familiarize all employees with policy and procedures for using the EAP. The policy should be viewed by employees as nonpunitive, constructive, and totally confidential.

The procedures for using the EAPs should clarify the two categories of referrals. Self-referrals occur when the employee recognizes a possible need for assistance and consults with the EAP professional before job performance becomes problematic. Supervisory or administrative referrals happen when the supervisor recognizes, documents, and confronts the employee on job performance problems and refers for assistance to the EAP.

Supervisor's Key Role and the Constructive Confrontation

A supervisor's familiarity with EAP policy and procedure, as well as his or her comfort in confronting and referring troubled employees for help, are critical factors in the effective use of a company's EAP. Employers should consider integrating EAP training into their regular, standard supervisory training when such programs exist. Supervisory orientation to policy and procedures should be done in an atmosphere that allows for the expression and processing of questions and feelings.

EAP training and consultations should also be provided to supervisors to help them learn effective constructive confrontation strategies so that they can make successful interventions and EAP referrals with employees whose problems are affecting their job performance. Confronting employees on their poor job performance is a natural part of a supervisor's role but is a strategy with which many supervisors feel uncomfortable because of inadequate training.

Constructive confrontation is used to motivate employees to resolve their problems and to overcome denial. In the constructive confrontation supervisors document deteriorating job performance and confront the employee with the specific details of these performance problems. It clarifies what specific improvement is expected and what the consequences will be if improvement does not occur. It is suggested to the employee that if personal problems are affecting their job performance, help is available through referral to the company's EAP. Whether or not the offered assistance is accepted, the supervisor demands that job performance return to acceptable levels within a specified period. "Constructive confrontation provides a powerful motivation for employees to solve their problems one way or the other because it demonstrates both the possible consequences of inaction and a way to help resolve the problems" (32). Training in effective confrontation techniques also helps supervisors learn skills that make them overall better supervisors.

Vague job descriptions or unclear minimum performance standards also contribute to supervisors' difficulties in making effective interventions with troubled employees. EAP consultations may facilitate correcting this problem. Effective EAPs nurture good relationships with company supervisors who are key staff to program use.

EAP Delivery Systems

EAP services may be provided through a variety of delivery systems. Some companies have internal programs where services are delivered by EAP professionals employed by the company. In external programs, EAP services are delivered by EAP professionals under contract with the organization. Some companies combine a core internal EAP program with contracts with external EAP vendors for certain services. Consortia of smaller companies may contract with an independent EAP vendor to provide services.

Direct Services Provided by Qualified Staff

A primary responsibility of the EAP professional is to make accurate assessments to identify employee or family member problems and then make appropriate referrals to resources in the community that are most likely to resolve the problem. The EAP identifies, fosters, and evaluates community resources to determine which provide the best quality care at the most reasonable cost. The EAP professional provides short-term counseling or problem resolution (as opposed to referral to community resources for long-term counseling) when this is assessed as the best response for timely and effective help. Crisis intervention is also within the purview of the EAP professional who is responsive with intervention services for employees, family members, or the organization when acute crises surface.

EAP staff need to be qualified to professionally and effectively deliver these services. They should show evidence of specialized understanding of alcohol and other drugs and have certification in employee assistance programming, that is, be a Certified Employee Assistance Professional (CEAP). Many EAP professionals, today, also have backgrounds in counseling and social work.

Evaluation

EAPs should measure the appropriateness, effectiveness, and efficiency of its operations. Programs should have measurable program objectives and data collection mechanisms. Data can be collected to look at the following program components: design effectiveness, implementation, management and administration, completeness of the program, direct services, program utilization, and linkages. An effective and well-run EAP also continually reassesses the needs of the organization (37).

MAXIMIZING EAP SUCCESS

Effective EAPs reflect a balance between enhancing employee well-being and organizational performance. They identify quality substance abuse services that are accessible to employees and their families and are a good fit between the substance abuser's needs and the services provided by the treatment program. Continuing posttreatment care is critical for the recovering substance abuser.

Followup Services

Followup sessions with the EAP professional should supplement the individual's involvement in 12-step programs, for example, AA or Narcotics Anonymous (NA), as well as other therapeutic groups. Twelve-step programs are strongly advocated by alcohol and drug rehabilitation programs; they support the recovery person's sobriety and abstinence in a manageable way—one day at a time. To reduce the chances of recidivism, EAP staff need to support an employee's involvement in the 12-step programs, as well as in other needed relapse prevention and therapeutic followup services.

Healthy Work Environments and Performance

EAPs should also promote and support healthy work environments. It is sometimes job-related issues that may be causing or exacerbating poor job performance. Company reorganizations, particularly ones involving massive layoffs, will likely affect employees' job performance. Trice and Roman outline 12 risk factors that can aggravate and reinforce deviant behavior that may already have begun outside of the work setting. The two general types of risks that may occur in any business setting are absence of supervision and low visibility of job performance. Conversely, in a work environment in which there is adequate supervision and high visibility, the chances are increased that supervisors will detect a troubled employee's deteriorating job performance early and make an effective intervention (39).

OTHER POLICIES AND PROGRAMS ADDRESSING SUBSTANCE ABUSE

The Drug-Free Workplace Act

A critical cornerstone for employment policies regarding drug abuse was laid by the federal government in 1988 with passage of the Federal Drug-Free Workplace Act, which mandates that publicly funded employers provide worker education about illegal drug abuse and monitor and discipline such activity.

The Act requires employers who have a contract with the federal government for at least $25,000 to maintain a drug-free workplace. First, these employers must establish a company substance abuse policy and inform all employees of its existence. They must also educate employees about drug abuse and the availability of drug counseling and treatment programs, and specify the penalties for violating the company's substance abuse policy (40).

Union Programs

While joint labor–management programs are in operation and growing, there is a history of differing philosophies between labor and management; generally unions prefer to run their own programs. Although both labor and management address deteriorating job performance and confront troubled employees, there is a distinction in their priorities. Unions have perceived the well-being of their members as coming first and have resisted management's last-resort strategy of firing an employee whose job performance does not improve. Since World War II, the AFL-CIO's Community Services Network has provided counseling services for its members (32).

Drug Testing Programs

In recent years, a variety of drug testing programs have developed, including preemployment, random, incident, probable cause, and scheduled drug testing. Preemployment testing, in which urinalysis is used to screen job applicants for drug use, is increasingly being used by the nation's largest employers, including major corporations, manufacturers, public utilities, transportation, and some smaller employers. Preemployment testing is primarily viewed as a deterrent for drug-abusing job applicants. Interestingly, the most abused drug, alcohol, is rarely included in these testing programs.

Postemployment drug testing programs have been implemented, especially by federal employers and companies employing workers in safety-sensitive positions. Some companies that have EAP capabilities view drug testing as a means of early identification and treatment of substance-abusing employees. Although EAPs provide assistance to employees who have been identified as substance abusers through drug testing, they should never be involved in the actual testing. Testing programs belong in the medical department where fitness for employment can be determined. It appears that drug testing is becoming a more acceptable policy.

Wellness Programs

Wellness programs, as a part of or complementary to EAPs, are becoming more popular in the workplace. They are very diverse in the scope of services they provide, which may range from health screening efforts to identify, for example, employees with high cholesterol, to weight management or smoking cessation programs. Many wellness or health promotion programs provide training on stress management, fitness, and good nutrition. The most successful programs are accompanied by supportive company policies. For example, stress management programs are useless in a company where management's policies promote stress. Wellness programs seek to prevent problems, and like EAPs, are concerned with the well-being of employees (41). Wellness programs may contribute to reducing escalating health costs.

FUTURE CONCERNS

Managed health care has and will continue to have a strong impact on EAPs. Health maintenance and preferred provider organizations have flourished as employers have been forced to identify alternatives to rapidly increasing health insurance premiums. Catastrophic claims for ailments such as AIDS and substance-abuse treatment expenses, along with advanced medical technology and drug therapies, have fueled increases in health costs. EAPs also will need to continue addressing concerns raised by the AIDS-diagnosed employee. A challenge for today's EAP professional is identifying treatment resources that best meet the needs of the substance-abusing employee and at the same time are the most cost-effective. EAPs have an obligation and are entrusted to ensure that employees referred for treatment receive quality services. Many EAPs are now offering short-term counseling, which can also reduce health insurance costs for employers. The degreed professional who is also credentialed for EAP work is becoming the sought-after EAP worker.

Federal government employers and the general public are also expressing growing concern about creating drug-free work environments. Although more EAPs in industry are broad-brush programs addressing a wide range of employee problems, it is critical that they continue to recognize and target services to substance-abusing employees. EAPs will also need to address the growing concerns of employees who do not have drug problems themselves but who have family members who do.

Research continues to be needed to evaluate and determine what are the most effective programs and strategies in addressing workplace substance abuse. EAP professionals will need to keep up with the demographic and technological changes that continue to have a tremendous impact on industry and its employees. EAP professionals will need to continue to strive to understand and service the needs of the employee balanced with the needs of the employer.

REFERENCES

1. Carlyle T. Past and present. London: JM Dent & Sons, 1960:189.
2. Brewington V, Deren S, Arella L, et al. Obstacles to vocational rehabilitation: the client's perspective. J Appl Rehabil Counsel 1990;21(2):27.
3. Stump W. Love, work and recovery. NADAP NewsReport 1973;14(4):3.
4. Neff WS. Work and human behavior, 2nd ed. Chicago: Aldine, 1977:264.
5. Adkins WR. Life skills education: a video-based counseling/learning delivery system. In: Larson D, ed. Teaching psychological skills: models for giving psychology away. Monterey, CA: Brooks/Cole, 1984:57.
6. Wright GN. Total rehabilitation. Boston: Little, Brown, 1980:5.
7. Alcoholics Anonymous. Twelve steps and twelve traditions. New York: Author, 1979.
8. Robinson H, Texeira M. Vocational rehabilitation, 2nd ed. New York: Narcotic & Drug Research, 1990:154–156.
9. Reichman W, Levy M, Herrington S. Vocational counseling in early sobriety. Labor Manage Alcohol J 1979;8:193.
10. Beale AV. A replicable program for teaching job interview skills to recovering substance abusers. J Appl Rehabil Counsel 1988;19(1):5.
11. Hall S, Loeb P, Coyne K, et al. Increasing employment in ex-heroin addicts II: methadone maintenance sample. Behav Ther 1981;12:443–460.
12. 2002 NADAP placement statistics. New York: National Association on Drug Abuse Problems, 2003.
13. New York State Education Department. The vocational and educational services for individuals with disabilities. Case Service Dollar Report 4/1/94-3/31/95.
14. Graham R, Gottcent R. Restoration of drug abusers to useful employment. In: Smith D, Anderson S, Buton M, et al., eds. A multicultural view of drug abuse. Cambridge, UK.: G.K. Hall/Schenkman, 1978:463.
15. Wijting JP. Employing, the recovering drug abuser—viable? Personnel 1979:62.
16. Strategy Council on Drug Abuse. Federal strategy for drug abuse and drug traffic prevention. Washington, DC: U.S. Government Printing Office, 1979:24.
17. The Rehabilitation Act of 1973, Public Law 93–112, sections 503, 504.
18. Deren S, Randell J. The vocational rehabilitation of substance abusers. J Appl Rehabil Counsel 1990;21(2):5.
19. Rudner S. The role of vocational rehabilitation in the treatment of substance abusers. Nassau County (NY) Department of Drug and Alcohol Addiction, 1982:5–6.
20. Report to the Chairman, Select Committee on Narcotics Abuse and Control, House of Representatives. Methadone maintenance: some treatment programs are not effective: greater federal oversight needed. Washington, DC: U.S. General Accounting Office 1990:23–24.
21. Simeone RS, Kott A, Torrington W. Summary report on the DSAS personal services survey. New York State Division of Substance Abuse Services, Albany, New York, 1989:3–10.
22. Szymanski EM, Parker RM. Relationship of rehabilitation client outcome to the level of rehabilitation counselor education. J Rehabil 1989;10:35.
23. Friedman L. The Wildcat experiment: an early test of supported work. New York: Vera Institute of Justice, 1978.
24. Hollister RG Jr, Kemper P, Maynard RA, eds. The national supported work demonstration. Madison: University of Wisconsin Press, 1984.
25. Legal Action Center. The Americans with Disabilities Act: a summary of alcohol and drug and AIDS provisions. Action Watch 1990;10:2.
26. Millman R, Kleinman P. Comprehensive vocational enhancement program for MMTPs. NIDA Grant DA 06153, 1995:25.
27. U.S. Department of Health and Human Services, Public Health Service, Substance Abuse and Mental Health Services Administration, Office of Applied Studies. Worker drug and workplace policies and programs: results from the 1994 and 1997 National Household Survey on Drug Abuse. U.S. Government Printing Office, Washington, DC.
28. NIDA Capsules. Facts about drugs in the workplace. Rockville, MD: Press Office of the National Institute on Drug Abuse, 1986:1.

29. William M. Mercer-Meidinger-Hansen, Inc. *Substance abuse in the workforce, a survey of employers conducted by Marsh & McLennan Companies, Inc. New York*, New York, 1988:2–8.

30. Walsh J, Gust S. Drug abuse in the workplace: issues, policy decisions, and corporate response. *Semin Occup Med* 1986;1(4):237–239.

31. Yesavage JA, Leirer VO, Denari M, et al. Carry-over effects of marijuana intoxication on aircraft pilot performance: a preliminary report. *Am J Psychiatry* 1985;142:1325.

32. Sonnenstuhl W, Trice H. *Strategies for employee assistance programs: the cru-cial balance.* Ithaca, NY: ILR Press, New York State School of Industrial and Labor Relations, Cornell University, 1986:4–8.

33. Bickerton RL. Employee assistance: a history in progress. *EAP Dig* 1990; 11(1):35–42, 82–84.

34. Watkins GT. In-house, a decade of change. *EAP Dig* 1990;11(1):6.

35. Kingman D Jr, ed. Why EAPs? *Subst Abuse Issues* 1990;1(2):1–2.

36. Kingman D Jr, ed. Treatment effectiveness. *Subst Abuse Issues* 1990;1(4):1.

37. The Employee Assistance Professionals Association, Inc. Standards for employee assistance programs. *Exchange* 1990;20(10):31–37.

38. Balzer WK, Pargament KI. The key to designing a successful EAP. *EAP Dig* 1988;1:55–59.

39. Trice HM, Roman PM. *Spirits and demons at work: alcohol and other drugs on the job.* Ithaca, NY: Publications Division, New York State School of Industrial and Labor Relations, Cornell University, 1978:101–102.

40. Complying with the drug-free workplace act. New York: Legal Action Center, May/June 1989:1.

41. Franz JB. Promoting wellness and disease prevention in EAPs. *ALMACAN* 1987;17(11):8–9.

CHAPTER 86

Treatment for Alcohol and Drug Dependence: History, Workforce, Organization, Financing and Emerging Policies

DENNIS McCARTY AND HOWARD H. GOLDMAN

A disparate collection of practitioners, stand-alone specialty clinics, integrated health care systems, government entities, and volunteer organizations provide treatment for abuse and dependence on alcohol and other drugs. The diversity and heterogeneity of these providers reflects the idiosyncratic development of addiction treatment services, a lack of private resources and support for treatment, continued reluctance to embrace alcohol and drug problems as medical issues, emphasis on criminal justice interventions, and persistent societal ambivalence toward alcohol and drug use. The resulting hodgepodge of federal, state, and private financing mechanisms target different treatment populations and provide similar but distinct service mixes. The combination of funding streams and provider assembly creates the contemporary alcohol and drug abuse treatment system in the United States. This chapter provides an overview of the development of the drug and alcohol treatment system, its workforce and treatment providers, the financing mechanisms, and the intersection of policy and practice for treatment of alcohol and drug disorders.

DEVELOPMENT OF ALCOHOL- AND DRUG-ABUSE TREATMENT SYSTEMS

The alcohol- and drug-abuse treatment system is rooted in a legacy of self-help and the development of grassroots efforts to better serve women and men seeking relief from dependence on alcohol and other drugs. A brief history begins in the first decades of the twentieth century when federal legislation increased controls over the distribution and sale of narcotic drugs and outlawed the production and sale of alcohol. These prohibitions meant that the country entered the last half of the century without a formal system of community-based treatment services. Court decisions coupled with additional state and federal legislation were required to stimulate the construction of the contemporary alcohol and drug abuse system of care.

Drug-Abuse Treatment History

The Harrison Narcotic Act of 1914 strengthened federal control over and sanctions for distribution, sale, and use of heroin and cocaine (1,2). Interpretations of the legislation led to a prohibition on treating narcotic dependence with continued prescriptions of narcotics (maintenance medication) (2,3). As a result, medical practitioners were reluctant to treat drug dependence, development of treatment services was inhibited, and segregation of drug treatment from medical practice was encouraged (4,5). Formal treatment for drug dependence was limited to two narcotic treatment hospitals operated by the U.S. Public Health Service in Lexington, Kentucky (opened in 1935), and a smaller campus in Fort Worth, Texas (opened in 1938) (1,6). The Lexington hospital became the primary training location for physicians interested in the treatment of drug dependence and was a leading site for drug-abuse research. Beyond the two hospitals, however, there was little effort to develop community drug-abuse treatment services until the 1960s.

Synanon, a residential program for individuals dependent on heroin, opened in 1958 and used group norms and encounters to teach residents personal responsibility and to begin a life without the use of heroin (1). Synanon was the prototypic therapeutic community and programs emerged elsewhere to replicate its approaches and successes (1). Federal investments in community drug abuse treatment began when the Narcotic Addict Rehabilitation Act of 1966 supported civil commitments to drug abuse treatment and formed a foundation for community drug-abuse treatment programs (7). By 1968, 183 drug-abuse treatment facilities were identified in a national census and three of four (78%) had opened in response to the Narcotic Addict Rehabilitation Act (4). The growth of services became more pronounced following President Nixon's declaration of a "War on Drugs," the creation of a Special Action Office for Drug Abuse Prevention (SAODAP) within the White House, and the passage of the Drug Abuse Office and Treatment Act of 1972 (7). The legislation authorized funding for community treatment services and provided formula grants to states to stimulate the development of treatment services (7). With the leadership of Jerome Jaffe, MD, SAODAP encouraged development of outpatient services and discouraged investments in inpatient facilities. Regulations to support methadone treatment services were crafted and maintenance treatment was available for the first time since the passage of the Harrison Narcotic Act (8). SAODAP evolved and became the foundation for the National Institute on Drug Abuse (NIDA) in 1974. NIDA and the states began to collaborate in the development of state systems to support treatment and prevention of drug abuse.

Alcohol Treatment History

Community-based treatment for alcohol dependence also developed slowly. The Volstead Act (1919) led to the prohibition of alcohol between 1920 and 1933 (9). Because problems with alcohol dependence declined substantially during Prohibition, there was minimal need for specialized treatment facilities. The restoration of widespread access to alcohol was associated with little capacity to treat alcohol-related problems; drunk tanks, jails, and county work farms became the primary treatment system for public inebriates (10). Medical interventions developed through trial and error in the decades following Prohibition and were modeled on the success of Alcoholics Anonymous (AA). Dr. Silkworth opened the first AA ward to treat alcohol-dependent patients in 1945 at Knickerbocker Hospital in New York City, and by 1957 there were AA groups in 265 hospitals and 335 prisons (11). The criminal justice system remained the dominant intervention until a 1968 U.S. Supreme Court decision (*Powell v. Texas*). The majority of the justices supported an argument that (a) alcoholism is a disease, (b) inebriation is an involuntary consequence of the disease, and (c) homeless individu-

als cannot drink in private; therefore, incarceration for an involuntary behavior is not permissible (12).

As a result of the ruling, states decriminalized public intoxication and developed public health rather than criminal justice strategies to control the consequences of alcohol dependence. Thirty-four states eventually passed key facets of the Uniform Alcoholism and Intoxication Treatment Act (Uniform Act) (model legislation that guided legislative reforms in many states) (13). The Uniform Act decriminalized public intoxication, fostered a comprehensive system of care, and promoted a public authority to fund, regulate, and oversee the service system (12). Federal legislation also promoted the development of services. Senator Harold Hughes (former governor of Iowa and a first-term U.S. senator who was in recovery) conducted public hearings during 1969 to examine the nation's alcohol and drug problem and drafted legislation to support systems of care (14). President Nixon signed the legislation (The Comprehensive Alcohol Abuse and Alcoholism Prevention, Treatment, and Rehabilitation Act of 1970 [Hughes Act]) in response to strong lobbying from key supporters (15–17). The Hughes Act provided the federal foundation for investment in alcohol treatment and prevention services. It authorized the National Institute on Alcohol Abuse and Alcoholism (NIAAA) and established federal formula grants to support development of state plans for the treatment and prevention of alcoholism.

Federal Agencies and Authorizations History

During the 1960s, the National Institute on Mental Health (NIMH) provided a home and leadership for federal initiatives on alcoholism and drug abuse, including the development of national plans (18). By the first half of the 1970s, NIAAA and NIDA emerged along side of NIMH, with the creation of the Alcohol Drug Abuse and Mental Health Authority (AMAMHA) in 1974. Three distinct service systems were created because treatment for alcohol and drug dependence were not integrated with physical and mental health systems of care, drug abuse frequently involved the criminal justice system, and men and women recovering from alcohol dependence advocated for distinct and autonomous treatment services (19).

Federal resources for treatment of alcohol and drug abuse declined dramatically when the Omnibus Budget Reconciliation Act of 1981 created block grants. Direct project grants and state formula grants were combined into a single award to the states and total funding was reduced 26%; reporting requirements were minimized to reduce the cost of managing the awards (20,21). The funding reductions may have facilitated the integration of alcohol- and drug-abuse treatment services because the revenue declines encouraged merger of similar services (19). Over time, funding for the block grant increased (particularly resources targeted to treatment of drug abuse). For federal fiscal year 2003, total block grant funding exceeded $1.75 billion.

In an administrative shuffle, ADAMHA was deauthorized in 1992 and SAMHSA (Substance Abuse and Mental Health Services Administration) and its three components were authorized to address development and delivery of treatment services: Center for Substance Abuse Treatment (CSAT), the Center for Substance Abuse Prevention (CSAP), and the Center for Mental Health Services (CMHS). (NIAAA, NIDA, and NIMH became part of the National Institutes of Health and their authorization was restricted to research.) The Alcohol Drug Abuse and Mental Health Block Grant was replaced with separate awards for mental health services (Community Mental Health Services Block Grant) and for alcohol- and drug-abuse services (Prevention and Treatment of Substance Abuse Block Grant). Congress added requirements to the grants. Pregnant women and injection drug users were given priority access to care, 10% of the funds were specified for new services for pregnant and parenting women, and stipulations were added to provide child care, prenatal services, human immunodeficiency virus (HIV) services and medication, tuberculosis (TB) services and medication, peer review for treatment programs, and outreach for out-of-treatment injection drug users. Additional language promoted enforcement of state laws prohibiting the sales of tobacco to minors, loans to start group homes (e.g., Oxford Houses) for men and women in early recovery, staff training, and waiting list and referral management systems; provisions to collect data and to conduct needs assessments were added. In the near future, the block grant will become a Performance Partnership Grant where states identify performance targets and funding will depend, in part, on achieving goals for reductions in alcohol and drug use, improvements in health outcomes, and reduction in criminal involvement.

In the years since the passage of the Hughes Act and the creation of NIAAA and NIDA, federal resources for alcohol- and drug-abuse treatment have increased substantially. A legacy, however, remains. Most publicly funded services continue to be financed in large measure through state and federal funds and continue to be relatively small and independent services.

SPECIALTY ALCOHOL- AND DRUG-ABUSE TREATMENT SERVICES

Federal authorities for drug and alcohol treatment monitor and describe the addiction treatment system. The primary mechanism has been a census of specialty drug and alcohol treatment services that began about 1973 as the National Drug Abuse Treatment Unit Survey (NDATUS) and was completed annually (through 1980) to provide details on program and staffing characteristics (22). Alcoholism treatment programs were added in 1979, and the name changed to the National Drug and Alcohol Treatment Unit Survey. Data collection became more sporadic after the introduction of the block grant and the demise of direct federal funding; censuses were completed in 1982, 1984, 1987, and 1989–1993 (23–25). The name of the survey was changed to the Uniform Facility Data Set (UFDS) in 1995 (26); questions on staffing were deleted and surveys were conducted annually (27–30). (Reports are available on the SAMHSA Web site: http://www.samhsa.gov/oas/dasis.htm#nssats2). In 2000, the survey was abbreviated and renamed the National Survey of Substance Abuse Treatment Services (N-SSATS) (31).

The 2000 N-SSATS identified 13,428 specialty substance-abuse treatment facilities in the United States (9,057 facilities participated in the 1991 NDATUS–SAMHSA attributes the increase to more complete census coverage rather than market growth) (31). The census reveals a system of relatively small, not-for-profit, independent clinics that primarily deliver ambulatory services. The median patient caseload on October 1, 2000 was 35 (23% of the facilities had a caseload of 15 or fewer and 79% served fewer than 100 patients). Six of ten facilities were organized as private, not-for-profit corporations with the remainder operated as for-profit corporations (26%) or as units of state and local (11%), federal (2%), or tribal (1%) government. Facilities generally provided only alcohol- and drug-abuse treatment services (61%), but 1 in 4 provided substance abuse and mental health services (25%) and 9% were identified as a mental health organization. Less than 3% of the facilities were categorized as health care settings and 2% were labeled as other (primarily corrections). More than 3 of 4 programs offered nonintensive outpatient treatment (78%) and intensive outpatient services were provided in 46% of the facilities. About 1 in 4 sites provided residential rehabilitation (26%). Nearly all programs (95%) treat both alcohol and drug dependence. The service mix typically included individual (95% of facilities), group (89%), and family (78%) counseling. Medical and support services were available at less than half of the facilities: pharmacotherapy (42%), testing for TB (38%), HIV (33%) and sexually transmitted diseases (STDs) (25%), HIV/acquired immunodeficiency syndrome (AIDS) education (55%), employment counseling (35%), housing assistance (31%), and childcare (10%). These programs continue to reflect the origins of the drug and alcohol treatment system as not-for-profit, grassroots groups that provide services in a restricted geographic area. To date, there has been little aggregation of independent facilities into larger multimodality entities with centralized management.

Despite changes over time and a substantial expansion of the sampling, trend analyses reflect few dramatic changes in the patient population and program characteristics. The census, for example, found surprising consistency in staffing patterns between 1976 and 1991 (23). Counselors made up 35% of the full-time positions.

Approximately 11% to 12% were medical practitioners (nurses and physicians). Psychologists (3%) and social workers (6%) represented approximately 10% of the staff. Finally, roughly 20% of the staff had other direct care positions, and 22% to 26% had administrative responsibilities (23). More generally, there has been little research on the substance abuse treatment workforce.

Practitioners

Alcohol and drug abuse counselors working in more than 13,000 substance abuse specialty clinics and services are the most visible treatment providers and appear to treat the majority of patients. An unknown number of licensed practitioners (social workers, psychologists, psychiatrists, and assorted other counselors, clergy, and human service providers) supplement the primary workforce and treat alcohol and drug dependence in private practices. Systematic data on the individuals who provide treatment for alcohol and drug dependence is limited. The Center for Substance Abuse Treatment supported practice research networks to estimate involvement with alcohol and drug dependent patients; participating practitioners were affiliated with six behavioral health professional associations: American Association for Marriage and Family Therapy, American Counseling Association, American Psychiatric Association, American Psychological Association, NAADAC (the association for addiction professionals), and the National Association of Social Workers (32). The Center for Substance Abuse Treatment also surveyed counselors working in substance abuse treatment facilities with more than 10 patients—the *Information Services Survey*. Together, these exploratory efforts begin to outline the nature of the addiction treatment work force.

Practice Research Networks

Data from the practitioners participating in Practice Research Networks suggest that licensed psychiatrists, psychologists, social workers, marriage and family therapists, and counselors treat many patients with alcohol and drug dependence, but they represent a small portion of the caseloads and, in most cases, the diagnosis is as a secondary condition. The 417 psychiatrists (78% of the sample) who participated in the 1997 Study of Psychiatric Patients and Treatments, for example, provided data on 1,245 patients; 151 (12%) of the patients had a primary (21%) or secondary (79%) diagnosis of alcohol dependence or abuse (diagnoses of drug abuse and dependence were not included in the analysis) (33). Similarly, 220 psychologists (55% of the sample) found that 35% reported treating alcohol and drug dependence as a primary diagnosis in the past year, while 76% addressed alcohol and drug disorders as secondary diagnoses; approximately 10% of the psychologists reported certification or credentials in treatment of alcohol and drug dependence (primarily a

certificate of proficiency from the American Psychological Association College of Professional Psychology) (34). Summarizing data from five of the professional organizations, CSAT estimated that 6% of patients in private practice settings had a primary diagnosis of a substance use disorder and an additional 12% had a secondary diagnosis; rates were higher among patients seen in mental health clinics: 11% primary and 18% secondary (32). Responses from NAADAC practitioners (N = 410) provide a different picture because they specialize in treating alcohol and drug dependence; nearly two-thirds (64%) of the patients have a primary diagnosis of abuse or dependence and one-third (33%) have a secondary diagnosis (35).

Most licensed practitioners had doctoral or masters degrees but were not Certified Alcohol and Drug Abuse Counselors (0 to 3% of the respondents) and did not have state certification or licensure (2% to 7% of the respondents) (32). NAADAC membership, in contrast, was more likely to include individuals without graduate degrees (40%), and members were more likely to report that they were a Certified Alcohol and Drug Abuse Counselor (47%) or held state certification or licensure (81%). NAADAC members were also more likely to report formal course work on substance abuse (65%), an internship focused on substance abuse counseling (63%), and participation in continuing education (91%). Formal coursework was less common among psychologists (30%), social workers (38%), members of the American Counseling Association (40%), and marital and family therapists (54%). More than half (52%) of these practitioners also reported no continuing education specific to substance abuse treatment in the past year (32).

The data from Practice Research Networks suggests that patients with alcohol and drug disorders are present in the caseload seen by licensed practitioners located in private practice (6% to 12% with a primary or secondary diagnosis) and in clinic settings (10% to 20% with a primary or secondary diagnosis). Despite these proportions, most of the practitioners report no formal course work on treating substance abuse disorders and have not participated in continuing education. The Association of Medical Educators and Researchers in Substance Abuse (AMERSA) strategic plan for interdisciplinary faculty development advocates for more formal training on alcohol, drug, and tobacco disorders for the nation's health care work force (36). The plan notes that it is critical to improve the skills of the health care and behavioral health care system to identify and intervene with patients who have alcohol- and drug-related problems. Recommendations are included for improving the training of psychologists (37), social workers (38), and a full range of health care practitioners, including physicians (39), allied health professionals (40), dentists (41), midwives (42), nurse practitioners (43), nurses (44), pharmacists (45), physician assistants (46), and public health workers (47). It is noteworthy, however, that the portion of the work force that works most directly with alcohol- and drug-involved patients (alcohol and drug counselors) are not included in the strategic plan.

Survey of Alcohol and Drug Counselors

Approximately 67,400 counselors treat nearly 1 million patients with alcohol and drug disorders in outpatient, residential, and methadone treatment facilities (48). The estimate is based on the *Information Services Survey* conducted for the Center for Substance Abuse Treatment during 1998. A sample of substance-abuse treatment facilities with an active caseload of more than 10 clients was selected from 10,860 programs responding to CSAT's 1997 UFDS census of specialty drug- and alcohol-treatment programs. Outpatient clinics were the primary setting for the counselors (N = 41,500; 61%) and patients (N = 735,000; 75% of the patients). Residential programs have lower patient:staff ratios and 21,500 counselors (32% of counselors) provide services for 100,000 residents (10% of patients). Methadone programs represented 6% of the counselor workforce (N = 4,300) and 15% of the patients (N = 150,000). In this sample, 70% of the counselors were women, 40% of the respondents were between 45 and 54 years of age, and 74% were white (10.6% were African American and Hispanic) (48). More than half (53%) of the counselors reported a graduate degree (only 3% indicated a doctorate). About half (52%) were licensed counselors. Unlicensed counselors tended to be working on licensure and certification (70%) but most did not have graduate degrees and 56% did not report a bachelor's degree (48).

According to the CSAT survey, about half of the counselors working in addiction treatment facilities currently have graduate degrees. The field appears to be evolving to rely more heavily on counselors with graduate training. The development of the workforce is apparent when compared with an analysis of 1979 workforce data where about 1 in 4 (22%) counselors had a graduate degree (24). The evolution reflects the field's historic origins. Because formally trained therapists often had little interest in working with patients struggling with alcohol and drug dependence, and because financial resources were limited, programs routinely trained their own staff and drew heavily on personal experience in recovery as a primary credential for employment. Recovering counselors have been the heart and soul of addiction treatment programs for many decades. Their personal experiences with dependence and recovery provide patients with concrete examples of strategies for achieving sobriety and evidence that recovery is possible.

Workforce Development

Today's challenge is that payer expectations are changing and patients have become more complex diagnostic and treatment puzzles. Third-party payors perceive counselors with graduate degrees and professional licensure as more qualified and as providing a more consistent and higher quality service. Increasingly, professional licensure is required as a condition of reimbursement. Patients, moreover, are likely to present with a variety of co-occurring psychiatric and medical disorders and require more sophisticated assessment to develop and implement an effective treatment plan. The increasing complexity of emerging evidence-based practices further complicates the construction of treatment plans and requires a relatively sophisticated understanding of behavioral therapies to fully use. CSAT's National Treatment Plan includes recommendations for a national workforce development office, construction of an infrastructure to support recruitment and retention of counselors and implementation of competency standards for career development, and broadening the diversity of the workforce to reflect the increasingly heterogeneous patient population (49).

Consequently, it is unexpected that graduate programs continue to provide relatively little formal training in the treatment of alcohol and drug disorders. A review of 260 addiction treatment programs offered in colleges and universities in the United States found that only 1 in 3 (32%) were graduate-level programs; more than half (55%) of the programs were 2-year associate degree and certification programs offered primarily through community colleges (50). The content of these programs and their consistency with the current scientific literature is unknown and their ability to fully prepare graduates with the tools needed to respond to expectations for relatively sophisticated treatments is uncertain. It seems likely, however, that more intensive training either in graduate programs or through more intensive continuing education is necessary.

Workforce development is, of course, closely related to reimbursement of services. Without adequate financing for treatment services, it is difficult to recruit and retain the most qualified practitioners.

FINANCING TREATMENT FOR ALCOHOL AND DRUG DEPENDENCE

National expenditures for the treatment of alcohol and drug abuse were estimated as $11.9 billion for 1997 (51,52). A review of the spending patterns and payors provides more insight into the unique facets of the nation's system for alcohol and drug treatment.

Treatment Settings

Although more than 75% of the treatment system provide outpatient services and 87% of the patients are served in outpatient settings, with hospital care being the largest source of expenditures—$4.7 billion (40% of total expenditures) (51,52). Detoxification is a high-volume business. Hospitals continue to play a major role, although payors have restricted mean lengths of stay from 7.7 days (1992) to 5.2 days (1997) (53). Specialty drug and alcohol treatment centers accounted for almost $4 billion in 1997 expenditures (34% of total spending) (52). Independent practitioners generated about $1.3 billion in billings for substance abuse treatment (11% of total expenditures). Mental health organizations accounted for an additional $1.1 billion (9% of the total). Finally, expenditures for prescription drugs represented 0.3% of total spending ($38 million) for alcohol- and drug-abuse treatment (compared to 12% of mental health expenditures—$9 billion of $73.4 billion). These data reinforce the sense that the alcohol- and drug-abuse treatment system is relatively distinct and separated from the mental health and general health care settings. Aside from short hospital stays for detoxification, most of the care is provided in inexpensive, freestanding clinics with relatively little involvement with mental health care settings and private practitioners.

Payors

An analysis of payors discloses additional idiosyncrasies. Public payors (state, local, and federal governments) accounted for 62% of expenditures for substance abuse treatment in 1997; for comparison, public payors contributed approximately 46% of total health care expenditures and mental health spending was 56% public resources (51). Public expenditures for substance abuse treatment included state and local funds ($2.31 billion; 19.5%), Medicaid ($2.27 billion; 19.1%), other federal funds (primarily the Substance Abuse Prevention and Treatment Block Grant) ($1.85 billion; 15.6%), and Medicare ($0.9 billion; 8%) (51). Private insurance contributed approximately 24% of total expenditures ($2.88 billion) for substance abuse treatment and patient out-of-pocket spending was about $1.3 billion (10.5%) (51). Total health care, in contrast, generated 33% of revenues from private insurance and 17% from out-of-pocket charges (51). It appears, therefore, that state and federal government purchase a disproportionate share of treatment services for alcohol and drug dependence, which reflects historical resistance among commercial payers to fully embrace coverage for addictions treatment.

The financing and organization of alcohol- and drug-abuse treatment services are intransigent challenges. The eclectic and creative combination of payors, service providers, and historical foundations results in a fragile treatment system that is an admixture of creative funding streams and small community-based treatment centers isolated from mainstream medical practice. Survival in the twenty-first century will require creative adaptations and potentially enhance integration. Challenges include the introduction of managed care, expectations for parity in coverage, a patient population with multiple co-occurring disorders, demands for performance measurement, and adoption and application of emerging evidence-based services and therapies. The mix of policy and practice issues continues to be a delicate balance.

INSURANCE COVERAGE FOR ALCOHOL AND DRUG TREATMENT

Historically, health plans have been reluctant to provide coverage for treatment for alcohol and drug disorders. As state and federal policy makers struggled during the 1970s to nurture treatment systems for alcohol and drug dependence, they recognized that resources in the public sector were insufficient to treat everyone who needed care; commercial financing was also required (54). Commercial insurance plans, however, resisted offering coverage and employers did not purchase coverage when available. Persuasion efforts had little influence. States, beginning with Wisconsin in 1972, passed legislation and required that group health plans include coverage for treatment of alcoholism (some states only required that health plans offer a treatment benefit) (54,55). Eventually, 41 states either required a specific treatment benefit or required health plans to offer a treatment benefit (55). The typical benefit was 30 days of inpatient treatment and $500 for outpatient services.

The benefit structure that emphasized inpatient care led to a proliferation of private 28-day inpatient treatment programs. Data from the National Drug and Alcohol Treatment Utilization Survey suggest that in 1980 approximately 20% of public and private treatment services were provided through private detoxification and residential treatment facilities (26). Costs for alcohol- and drug-abuse treatment increased dramatically and, more generally, corporations struggled to control accelerating costs of employee health care in the late 1980s. Employers shifted to self-insurance (negating state insurance mandates) and began to rely on prepaid health care to better control costs. Managed behavioral health care organizations developed to provide specialized management services for mental health and substance abuse treatment services. Commercial health plans and the managed behavioral health care organizations limited use of expensive inpatient services as a cost-control strategy. By 1995, less than 8% of treatment services were provided in private detoxification and residential treatment services (26). Managed care had begun to alter the organization and delivery of substance-abuse treatment services.

Managed Care

Health maintenance organizations, preferred provider organizations, point of service plans, management service organizations, employee assistance programs, and managed behavioral health care organizations reflect the many faces of contemporary systems of managed care (19,56). Financial incentives, use management, and provider selection are used to balance use of services with cost management while maintaining and enhancing quality of care (57,58).

Managed health plans provide necessary services in return for a prepaid per-member fee (capitation) and assume a financial risk of providing care if the cost of the required treatments exceed the fees collected. Critics contend that the financial incentives encourage health plans to minimize care and maximize profit (59,60). Contracts, however, can be structured to alter the financial risks and to reduce the probability of undertreatment (19,61). Use management is the most direct strategy for controlling costs. Manage care plans typically require authorization for the use of expensive inpatient and specialized services, and may review continuing care to determine if services are still necessary. Treatment guidelines and placement criteria have evolved to facilitate and standardize use management but are not yet well developed for alcohol and drug treatment (62,63). Selective contracting is another mechanism to manage costs and quality; only practitioners who meet specific standards of training and agree to predetermined rate are included in the provider panel. A limited network enhances the health plan's ability to manage quality and enforce application of treatment guidelines and use management criteria (19).

Managed care tools are applied generally to health care and behavioral health care. The management and delivery of treatments for mental illness and substance abuse disorders (behavioral health care) are often separated (carved out) from the management and delivery of primary care. Behavioral health carve-outs have proliferated because management of these disorders benefits from specialized expertise, the delivery systems are distinct from primary care, and financial risks can be better isolated and controlled (19,64–66). Carve-outs also help to minimize adverse selection (67). Behavioral health care is most likely to be integrated with primary care in staff model and group model health maintenance organizations (HMOs) (56,66). Both approaches can work, but carve-outs are the dominant approach and even within HMOs, service delivery for mental illness and substance abuse is usually separated from primary care.

In both carve-out and integrated delivery systems, alcohol- and drug-abuse treatment may be more vulnerable than other facets of health care to deleterious impacts associated with the introduction and use of managed care (57). Social (homelessness, pregnancy, and court orders) and medical complications (co-occurring mental illness and comorbid medical problems) make it difficult to assess appropriate levels of care and to implement use management. The chronic and relapsing nature of the disorder means that some patients use the most intensive and expensive levels of care (medical detoxification) relatively frequently and are difficult to engage in outpatient systems of care. Reliance on public financing also challenges the application of managed care; impairment tends to be greater among patients without commercial insurance and there is a need for a more diverse array of clinical and social supports (20,68).

Investigations of the impacts of managed care behavioral health care find consistent reductions in the use of inpatient services. Use of outpatient services, moreover, does not always increase to offset reduced access to inpatient care. Empirical analyses have begun to suggest that declines in access to and use of services is more apparent for alcohol and drug treatment than for services for mental illness (69). That observation, however, is based on relatively few studies and measures are often not comparable across investigations (69). Questions of access and use will benefit from continued analysis in both commercial and public health plans. Evidence from the public sector, in fact, suggests that carefully crafted managed care plans can increase access and use while reducing costs.

Managed Care for Medicaid and Other Publicly Funded Services

Medicaid reimbursement accounts for approximately 19% of the expenditures for alcohol- and drug-abuse treatment in the United States (51,52). Medicaid is a health insurance program for eligible low-income individuals; state and federal governments share costs. Medicaid regulations define alcohol and drug dependence as mental diseases and prohibit reimbursement for any service if the recipient is between the ages of 21 and 65 years and a resident of an "Institution for Mental Disease" (IMD exclusion)—a residential program of more than 16 beds. Treatment for alcohol and drug disorders therefore, is reimbursed most frequently if provided under a service category that qualifies for federal matching funds (e.g., inpatient or outpatient hospital services) (70–72). Coverage for alcohol and drug treatment varies substantially from state to state (71–73). States struggle to control escalating costs for Medicaid and have turned to managed care to better control those costs (72).

Massachusetts implemented the first statewide behavioral health carve-out for Medicaid recipients in 1993. Expenditures for mental health and substance abuse treatment declined 12% in the first year of the initiative (from $186 million in 1992 to $163 million in 1993); there was a 5% increase in access to care, but substantial declines in inpatient use and lower prices were negotiated (74). Continued study documented the generally favorable results (maintained access and reduced costs) for most Medicaid categories (64,75) although children and disabled individuals may have been more adversely affected (75–77).

A Medicaid-managed care initiative for substance abuse treatment in Iowa improved access and use while reducing costs. Access to substance abuse treatment doubled for Iowa's Medicaid recipients after the introduction of a carve-out program in September 1995 (from 12 to 24 per 1,000 Medicaid enrollees), use grew 3.5-fold, and total service costs declined (78). Iowa was also the first state to integrate public financing for individuals not eligible for Medicaid into a carve-out arrangement; inpatient care declined and intensive outpatient services increased substantially (79). An analysis of Arizona's behavioral health carve-out also found generally positive effects (80). Maryland's implementation of an integrated delivery system for substance abuse treatment has met with more mixed results (81–84). These studies were part of an evaluation of the application of managed care to publicly funded services and suggest that carefully developed and implemented plans can be effective (83). Other states were less successful in their implementation (85).

Disturbing trends, however, emerged during the economic recession in the first years of the twenty-first century. States began to eliminate coverage for alcohol and drug treatment. Oregon's highly successful Oregon Health Plan, for example, extended Medicaid eligibility to low-income men, women, and children and improved access to health care (86). Access to treatment for alcohol and drug dependence also improved (87). The program changed dramatically in 2003 when the state legislature eliminated outpatient coverage for mental health, substance abuse, and dental treatment for individuals who did not meet federal eligibility standards. Benefits were eliminated to help close projected state budget deficits. The loss of benefits led to patients being discharged from care, including methadone maintenance, program closures, and staff layoffs. The long-term impacts remain to be determined. Massachusetts changed eligibility requirements for state assistance and about half of the state's detoxification beds were closed. The elimination of these benefits illustrates the vulnerable nature of alcohol- and drug-abuse treatment and the continued challenge to demonstrate to policy makers the value of treatment for alcohol and drug disorders. The persistent debate around parity illustrates another aspect of this challenge.

Parity

Parity refers to the policy of providing insurance coverage for a specific set of conditions, such as alcohol and other substance use disorders, on the same terms as coverage for other health conditions. "On the same terms" refers to cost-sharing provisions, such as copayments or deductibles, and to other limits, such as annual maximums and day or visit limits. Occasionally, state mental health parity legislation has extended coverage for alcohol- and drug-abuse treatment along with other mental disorders, but usually parity policies have not included treatment for alcohol and drug disorders. Costs seem to be the typical concern driving the historical discriminatory insurance coverage practices (88). The introduction of managed care made it possible to control costs in such a manner that implementing a policy of parity should not result in prohibitive increases in expenditures (89).

In 2003, the U.S. Congress again debated a change in a limited federal parity law passed in 1996 to expand parity beyond the annual and lifetimes limits affected by the current legislation. Various options were debated, including extending coverage to all disorders in the *Diagnostic*

and Statistical Manual of Mental Disorders, 4th ed., text revision (*DSM–IV–TR*). That policy change would lead to full insurance coverage for the substance use disorders not covered by the current legislation. It would follow a landmark decision made by President Clinton to extend parity coverage to federal employees, retirees and their dependents who are part of the Federal Employees Health Benefit (FEHB) program (88). As of January 2001, all participants in the FEHB program who receive treatment from plan-specified in-network providers within the program have parity coverage for all mental and addictive disorders. The implementation and impact of this policy change is being evaluated and results are expected in late 2004.

Concerns about parity have evolved from its earliest consideration more than 20 years ago. Where once policy makers focused almost entirely on access and costs, now there is also concern about issues of equity (90). The policy makers asked: Is managed care for behavioral health conditions applied with fairness when compared to managed care for other health conditions? Does a dollar of mental health and substance abuse coverage buy as much overall health as the next dollar of coverage for some other condition? Another concern is the expected gap between the nominal benefits written into insurance contracts and the effective benefits experienced by beneficiaries as they use these benefits subject to managed care (88,89). Employers struggle with these decisions each year when they make choices about employee health insurance and the benefits included in the insurance package.

Employers and Employee Assistance Programs

Small employers provide a large portion of the jobs in this country and are a most vocal source of resistance to legislative requirements that may increase the cost of health insurance. As a group, small employers have opposed parity provisions especially for treatment of alcohol and drug disorders. It maybe surprising, therefore, that 9.1 million of the estimated 11.8 million adults (77%) who used illicit drugs in the year 2000 were employed (91). Despite employee drug testing and other procedures designed to inhibit alcohol and drug use, individuals who are dependent on alcohol and other drugs are in the workforce.

The primary strategy for addressing alcohol and drug problems among employees have been the employee assistance programs (EAPs). The programs trace their roots to industrial alcohol problems that started in the 1940s to address alcohol problems among factory workers and were linked to outreach efforts among individuals promoting 12-step recovery programming (20). A young NIAAA promoted workplace programming and stimulated a dramatic expansion of EAPs during the 1970s; between 1972 and 1976 the proportion of Fortune 500 corporations that offered EAP services doubled from 25% to 50% and rose to 57% in 1979 (92). EAPs have continued to grow. In a recent national survey of employed persons, 58% responded that their workplace included an EAP service (93).

Roman, however, raises substantive concerns about the changing role of EAPs (93). EAPs were always designed to address work performance issues, not specifically alcohol and drug dependence; supervisors focused on performance and not diagnosis of underlying causes (93). Over time, however, Roman asserts that EAPs have diverted their attention to less-stigmatized issues with the result that identification and referral of individuals with alcohol and drug problems has declined dramatically. Within a relatively short period of time, referrals from EAPs to a national sample of treatment programs dropped from 21% of total referrals (1996) to 9% (1999) (93). The introduction of managed behavioral health care and efforts to provide short-term interventions in-house rather than through treatment centers contributed to the decline. As a result, employers may be at increased risk of incurring alcohol- and drug-related problems in the workplace.

The interaction between insurance coverage, parity, and EAPs illustrates the multidimensional environment where contemporary addiction treatment centers operate. Similarly, individuals with alcohol and drug disorders are present in many human service systems. Policies related to these systems increasingly address alcohol and drug dependence.

EMERGING POLICY CHALLENGES

Use and abuse of alcohol and illicit drugs have pervasive influences on many dimensions of systems of care for mental illness, criminal justice, and welfare reform. The field is also challenged by persistent demands for accountability and for linking reimbursement with performance indicators. A brief review of these policy issues helps highlight the multidimensional nature of treatments for alcohol and drug disorders.

The parity debate, for example, brings more attention to the co-occurrence of alcohol and drug disorders with mental illness. Given the frequency of comorbidity and the importance of integrated treatment, policies that distinguish the addictive disorders from other mental disorders, are increasingly harder to administer and to justify.

Co-occurring Disorders

Integrated or combined treatment is the recommended evidence-based service approach for the individuals who have severe co-occurring mental and substance use disorders, according to the Surgeon General (94), SAMHSA (95), and other scientific reviews (96). The central problem in financing such services has been identified as the failure of some entity or authority to take responsibility for the care and treatment of this challenging population (97) and the lack of system integration (98). It stands to reason that if no entity will take responsibility for providing integrated treatment, then it is difficult to marshal the resources to fund the services. In circular fashion, however, limitations on service dollars for substance abuse and mental health treatment have often been an impediment for taking responsibility. Financial incentives are needed to motivate state and local authorities, as well as service providers, to provide evidence-based practices, such as integrated treatment (99). There have been policy proposals to "braid" funding and to use both the federal mental health and substance abuse block grants to fund these needed services. SAMHSA's *Report to Congress* begins to address the challenges of integrating funding mechanisms to enhance services for co-occurring disorders (95).

SAMHSA's 5-year plan for facilitating treatment of co-occurring disorders emphasizes partnerships with other federal and state agencies: (a) the Center for Medicare and Medicaid Services to foster benefits planning and financing, (b) the Health Resources and Services Administration to address co-occurring disorders in primary care, (c) the Department of Justice to work with criminal justice systems and the individuals with co-occurring disorders, and (d) the Department of Education to prevent and treat co-occurring disorders among children and adolescents (95). Financing of care is also addressed in the 5-year plan; SAMHSA intends to work with states to identify strategies for funding services, make full use of the block grant, and use discretionary grants to foster model programs (95). Dissemination activities will include workforce development to foster the acquisition of needed skills and initiatives to facilitate the application of science to service. Finally, SAMHSA also plans to promote effective practices and to host a national summit on co-occurring disorders (95). These plans also influence the administrations broader efforts to address disabilities. President Bush's New Freedom Commission is making several recommendations to facilitate the funding of these services through the block grant and through Medicaid. The Commission calls for a program of screening for co-occurring disorders in all service settings (Commission final report, in preparation). The proposed screening programs will be located in settings where individuals are at high risk for co-occurring disorders and reflect the settings identified in SAMHSA's 5-year plan including the criminal justice system.

Interactions with Criminal Justice Systems

Men and women arrested for crimes consistently report high levels of drug use. Beginning in 1988 with the Drug Use Forecasting program, the National Institute of Justice has interviewed individuals arrested and analyzed their urines to monitor levels and types of drug use among criminal offenders. The program has expanded and evolved and is now known as Arrestee Drug Abuse Monitoring (ADAM). ADAM includes 35 communities, uses standardized sampling methods, and includes questions on risk for drug dependence and treatment experiences.

Interviews completed in 2000 suggest that nearly 2 of 3 (64%) individuals arrested for any crime test positive for marijuana (41%), cocaine (31%), opiates (6.5%), methamphetamine (1.6%), or phencyclidine (PCP) (0.3%); 21% test positive for two or more of the drugs (100). The rate of positive urines was highest in New York City (80%) and lowest in Anchorage, Alaska (52%). More than one-third (37%) of the arrestees are at risk for drug dependence, yet the number who report participation in drug-abuse treatment during the past year is less than 10% (9% report inpatient treatment in the past year and 7% report outpatient treatment; 2% report receiving mental health treatment) (100). The 2000 ADAM report estimated that there were 750 bookings for every 1,000 hardcore drug users (100).

Drug users and arrests related to drug use, therefore, are a substantial burden within the criminal justice system. Perhaps 70% of the inmates in state prisons and 80% in federal institutions are serving time on charges related to drug trafficking and possession (101). Simply serving time, unfortunately, does not eliminate drug use; inmates released back into the community are likely to resume drug use (102). Intensive treatment during incarceration, however, leads to reduced levels of drug use when returned to the community and lower rates of rearrest and reincarceration (103,104). Positive effects of in-prison treatment are strongest if services continue when individuals return to the community (105). Thus, it is essential to build strong linkages between institutional and community services.

Drug offenders may place an even greater burden on local courts. To cope with a surge in drug arrests, a court in Miami, Florida, combined the authority of the court with active participation in drug-abuse treatment. That first drug court in 1989 paved the way for a dramatic expansion in drug courts with more than 1,000 drug courts in operation or development in 2002 (106). Drug courts may vary in approach (deferred prosecution versus postadjudication) but typically judges monitor the defendant's participation in treatment and ability to stay drug free; models and services vary across courts and communities (107). Drug courts expanded rapidly because they reduce the burden of drug offenders on courts, prosecution, and corrections. Data on the effectiveness of drug courts, however, is surprisingly limited (106–108). Rigorous research is a challenge because of the lack of similar comparison groups not exposed to judicial supervision and because of the variability of data systems within drug courts (106). The rapid adoption of the drug court model, however, attests to their value to the criminal justice system.

A new strategy for dealing with drug offenders is emerging in California. In the November 2000 elections, California voters approved (61% affirmative votes) a referendum to encourage the use of community treatment services rather than incarceration for nonviolent drug offenders (Proposition 36, the Substance Abuse and Crime Prevention Act of 2000). The Act was implemented in July 2001, and required substantial reorganization of access to drug-abuse treatment services and relationships in counties among courts, prosecution, probation, and parole, and drug-abuse treatment services. Implementation is still in early phases and evaluation studies have not yet been released. Anecdotal reports and news accounts suggest that rates of incarceration have declined, but that some offenders fail to enter drug treatment. Even without data on impacts and outcomes, the social experiment is drawing considerable attention; other states have had similar referendums on their ballots.

The relationship between criminal justice systems and treatment services for alcohol and drug disorders is multifaceted and complex. Connections between these services will continue to evolve and provide much opportunity for innovation and research. Treatment for drug abuse has assumed increased importance in other aspects of the human services systems, including welfare and welfare reform.

Welfare Reform

The Personal Responsibility and Work Opportunity Reconciliation Act of 1996 (P. L. 104-193) modified social welfare and income support programs in the United States (109–111). A block grant titled Temporary Assistance for Needy Families (TANF) replaced the Aid to Families with Dependent Children entitlement. TANF attempts to reduce welfare dependence and to promote self-sufficiency (111). State flexibility and local autonomy were increased. States that fail to impose work requirements, do not meet congressional standards for caseload participation in work, and neglect to enforce limits on receiving federal assistance may incur sanctions. Bonuses are available for states that exceed expectations.

One of the more intriguing facets of the welfare reforms is the potential fate of women abusing alcohol and other drugs. Alcohol and drug dependence, on one hand, may make it more difficult for women to participate in job preparation and work experiences. These TANF participants may be least likely to obtain work and most likely to fail to comply with program requirements. On the other hand, alcohol and drug screening at enrollment, potential reductions in cash assistance, increased program structure, and linkages to support and treatment services may help women with alcohol and drug dependence initiate and maintain a stable sobriety (112).

Policy makers struggle with the complex nature of poverty and welfare participation. Cash assistance may not only ameliorate the effects of poverty and improve family health and welfare but also enable some recipients to continue to obtain and remain dependent on alcohol and other drugs. This is the crux of the tension between policy perspectives that promote access to addiction treatment services and those that seek to inhibit access to welfare.

Prior to welfare reform, states did little to assess alcohol and drug problems among welfare recipients. Linkages with screening and treatment services for alcohol and drug misuse and abuse, however, will become central to the success of welfare reform. Careful analysis of these linkages is necessary to identify the more effective mechanisms. About half the states have some form of screening to detect alcohol and drug disorders among TANF recipients and applicants (113). Data from a New Jersey initiative that screens applicants in the welfare office and uses case management to foster entry to drug-abuse treatment services suggest that women positive for drug and alcohol problems have poorer work histories, fewer employment skills, greater housing and transportation needs, and higher levels of medical, legal, and family problems; because of their multiple problems, states will be challenged to coordinate services and develop effective interventions (114). Coordination with state Medicaid programs, therefore, may become key to early intervention and treatment. Many TANF participants enroll in Medicaid. Increasingly, state Medicaid plans require health plans to screen beneficiaries at enrollment for alcohol and drug problems. These interventions have been used successfully in health plans, but coordination with welfare participation is a new dimension.

Policy-maker interest in welfare reform will foster opportunities for changes in systems of care. Some communities may integrate mental health, substance abuse, and child welfare services to facilitate change and enhance the potential for TANF participants to find employment. The ultimate evaluation questions, however, will not be limited to the assessments of the effects of welfare reform on the women who participate in TANF, but must examine of the effects of her participation in treatment and employment on her children. Women who lose Medicaid insurance (for not participating in a treatment program) increase the burden on publicly funded services. Finally, implementation of screening and assessment programs will require increased collaboration and networking between drug-abuse treatment services and welfare offices.

Disability and Alcohol and Drug Disorders

One aspect of welfare reform addressed eligibility for disability income. Originally the Social Security Administration disability program considered alcohol and drug dependence as a basis for disability income only through a "reference listing." This meant that to qualify for disability payments a claim on the basis of alcohol or drug dependence must "refer" to some other category of impairment, such as another mental disorder, peripheral neuropathy, or cirrhosis. In the late 1980s and early 1990s the policy changed; individuals disabled because of alcohol and/or drug use qualified directly for Social Security Disability Insurance (SSDI) and Supplemental Security Income (SSI). A consequence was that increasing numbers of individuals also supported their alcohol and drug use with government benefits. The General Accounting Office reported that between 1989 (less than 100,000 individuals) and 1993 (more than 250,000) the number of persons who received disability benefits because of alcohol or drug dependence more than doubled (115). Congress eliminated eligibility on the basis of alcohol or drug dependence alone and reverted to considering them as a basis for disability through a "reference listing." The broader debate continues: how to address alcohol and drug problems among individuals with disabilities.

A program in Washington State documented increases in employment among individuals disabled because of alcohol and drug use when vocation rehabilitation services were combined with treatment for the alcohol and drug disorder (116,117). Despite strong evidence of success, the program was discontinued. The federal government ruled that individuals with alcohol- and drug-related disabilities did not qualify for federally funded vocational rehabilitation services.

More generally, individuals with physical and cognitive disabilities are at greater risk for alcohol and drug disorders and may have a more difficult time accessing care (118). Small alcohol- and drug-treatment programs are often located in older locations with poor physical access. Moreover, counselors often have little training in working with physical and cognitive disabilities. Programs are challenged to extend their skill sets and facilities to provide services to another difficult to serve group.

ACCOUNTABILITY AND PERFORMANCE MEASUREMENT

Purchasers and consumers challenge drug and alcohol treatment systems to document quality of care and demonstrate that services are appropriate, effective, and cost-effective. Providers and states are investing in the development of information systems to monitor the processes and outcomes associated with treatment for abuse and dependence on alcohol and other drugs. Purchasers, for example, monitor measures of performance to assess access to care, track consumer satisfaction with care, and identify the most effective service providers. The Health Plan Employer Data and Information Set (HEDIS) is a standardized set of performance measures purchasers and consumers can use to assess and compare health plans (119) (see www.ncqa.org for the most current version). HEDIS measures related to substance abuse services, however are limited. Providers, advocates, and consumers tend to believe that the HEDIS measures are insufficient to monitor the diversity of needs and goals that substance abuse services must respond. Thus, HEDIS is adopting measures to monitor access to alcohol- and drug-treatment services and retention in care within the health plans; pilot data on these measures is now available (120).

Performance Measurement

Changes in purchase-of-service contracts are accelerating the evolution of performance and outcome monitoring.

Increasingly, state and federal governments are implementing contracts that require demonstrations of specified levels of outcomes rather than just purchasing the delivery of services. Some states have already implemented performance-based contracting. Maine's contracting system changed provider behavior and increased accountability (121–123). The National Academy of Sciences' National Research Council assessed the feasibility of linking performance expectations to federal funding for public health, mental health, and substance abuse services (124). The review found few currently collected measures that were directly applicable to assessments of state performance. Moreover, because of differences in data definitions and data-collection procedures, as well as differences in the populations being served, it may be inappropriate to make comparisons across states. Despite these limitations, the review panel proposed measures to monitor health outcomes, processes, and capacity. Because outcomes are often difficult to assess, intermediate measures were suggested to monitor behavior risks.

Performance Partnerships

SAMHSA is now moving to transform the Substance Abuse Prevention and Treatment Block Grant into a Performance Partnership Grant. States must identify expected levels of system performance and report measures that assess their ability to meet the performance expectations. These measures are still in development but are likely to include reductions in alcohol and drug use, hospitalization, and arrests. The goal is to promote attention to outcomes at all levels of the drug and alcohol treatment system. Implementation of evidence-based practices, a focus on process improvement, and adoption of new treatment technologies are all part of the effort to enhance the quality and effectiveness of addiction treatment services.

CONCLUSION

Treatment systems for alcohol and drug disorders struggle with limited resources to treat patients whose lives are filled with multiple complexities. Because alcohol- and drug-dependent patients burden systems for health care, human services, and criminal justice, treatment services must function within multiple environments simultaneously. They serve vital roles in reducing the harms related to dependence on alcohol and other drugs, yet exist on the fringe of the nation's health and human service systems. Greater integration with these systems of care is inevitable as state and federal systems seek better performance and improved outcomes from their investments in health and human services.

ACKNOWLEDGMENTS

Preparation of this manuscript was supported in part with grants from the National Institute on Alcohol Abuse and Alcoholism (R01 AA 11363), the National Institute on Drug Abuse (R01 DA 14688), and the Robert Wood Johnson Foundation (grant number 46876).

REFERENCES

1. Courtwright D, Joseph H, Des Jarlais D. *Addicts who survived: an oral history of narcotic use in America, 1923–1965.* Knoxville, TN: The University of Tennessee Press, 1989.
2. Musto DF. *The American disease: origins of narcotic control.* New Haven, CT: Yale University Press, 1973.
3. King R. The Narcotics Bureau and the Harrison Act: jailing the healers and the sick. *Yale L J* 1953;62:735–749.
4. Jaffe JH. The swinging pendulum: the treatment of drug users in America. In: Dupont RI, Goldstein A, O'Donnell J, et al., eds. *Handbook on drug abuse.* Washington, DC: U.S. Government Printing Office, 1979:3–16.
5. Schur EM. Narcotic addiction in Britain and America: the impact of public policy. Bloomington, IN: Indiana University Press, 1962.
6. Walsh J. Lexington Narcotics Hospital: a special sort of alma mater. *Science* 1973;182:1004–1008.
7. Besteman KJ. Federal leadership in building the national drug treatment system. In: Gerstein DR, Harwood HJ, eds. *Treating drug problems.* Vol. 2. Washington, DC: NAADAC. National Academy Press, 1992:63–88.
8. Institute of Medicine. *Federal regulation of methadone treatment.* Washington, DC: National Academy Press, 1995.
9. Aaron P, Musto DF. Temperance and prohibition in America: a historical overview. In: Moore MH, Gerstein DR, eds. *Alcohol and public policy: beyond the shadow of Prohibition.* Washington, DC: National Academy Press, 1981:127–181.
10. McCarty D, Argeriou M, Huebner R, et al. Alcoholism, drug abuse and the homeless. *Am Psychol* 1991;46:1139–1148.
11. W. B. *Alcoholics Anonymous comes of age.* New York: Harper & Brothers, 1957.
12. National Institute on Alcohol Abuse and Alcoholism. *First special report to the U.S. Congress on alcohol and health.* Rockville, MD: Author, 1971.
13. Finn P. Decriminalization of public drunkenness: response of the health care system. *J Stud Alcohol* 1985;46:7–23.
14. Hughes HE, Schneider D. *The man from Ida Grove: a senator's personal story.* Lincoln, VA: Chosen Books Publishing, 1979.
15. Smithers RB. Making it happen: advocacy for the Hughes Act. *Alcohol Health Res World* 1988;12:271–272.
16. Lewis JS. Congressional rites of passage for the rights of alcoholics. *Alcohol Health Res World* 1988;12:240–251.
17. Hewitt BG. The creation of the National Institute on Alcohol Abuse and Alcoholism: responding to America's alcohol problem. *Alcohol Health Res World* 1995;19:12–16.
18. Plaut TFA. *Alcohol problems: a report to the nation by the Cooperative Commission on the Study of Alcoholism.* New York: Oxford University Press, 1967.
19. Institute of Medicine. *Managing managed care: quality improvement in behavioral health.* Washington, DC: National Academy Press, 1997.

20. Institute of Medicine. *Broadening the base of treatment for alcohol problems.* Washington, DC: National Academy Press, 1990.

21. U.S. General Accounting Office. *Block grants: characteristics, experience, and lessons learned.* Washington, DC: Author, 1995.

22. Cook P, Rosenthal B, Davis C. State-of-the-art review: drug abuse management information systems in single state agencies. In: Beschner GM, Sampson NH, D'Amanda C, eds. *Management information systems in the drug field.* Rockville, MD: National Institute on Drug Abuse, 1979:34–78.

23. Brown BS. Staffing pattern and services for the War on Drugs. In: Egertson JA, Fox DM, Leshner AI, eds. *Treating drug abusers effectively.* Malden, MA: Blackwell Publishers, 1997:99–124.

24. Camp JM, Kurtz NR. *Redirecting manpower for alcoholism treatment. Prevention, intervention and treatment: concerns and models.* Rockville, MD: National Institute on Alcohol Abuse and Alcoholism, 1982:371–397.

25. Office of Applied Studies. *Overview of the National Drug and Alcoholism Treatment Unit Survey (NDATUS): 1992 and 1980–1992.* Advanced report no. 9. Rockville, MD: Substance Abuse and Mental Health Services Administration, 1995.

26. Substance Abuse and Mental Health Services Administration. *Uniform Facility Data Set (UFDS): data for 1995 and 1980–1995.* DHHS Pub. No. (SMA) 97–3161. Rockville, MD: Substance Abuse and Mental Health Services Administration. Office of Applied Studies. 1997.

27. Substance Abuse and Mental Health Services Administration. *Uniform Facility Data Set (UFDS): Data for 1996 and 1980–1996.* DHHS Pub. No. SMA 98–3176. Rockville, MD: Office of Applied Studies, Substance Abuse and Mental Health Services Administration, 1998.

28. Substance Abuse and Mental Health Services Administration. *Uniform Facility Data Set (UFDS): 1997—data on substance abuse treatment facilities.* DHHS Pub. No. SMA 99–3314. Rockville, MD: Substance Abuse and Mental Health Services Administration, Office of Applied Studies, 1999.

29. Substance Abuse and Mental Health Services Administration. *Uniform Facility Data Set (UFDS): 1998—data on substance abuse treatment facilities.* DHHS Pub. No. SMA 00–3463. Rockville, MD: Substance Abuse and Mental Health Services Administration, Office of Applied Studies, 2000.

30. Substance Abuse and Mental Health Services Administration. *Uniform Facility Data Set (UFDS): 1999—data on substance abuse treatment facilities.* DHHS Pub. No. SMA 01–3516. Rockville, MD: Substance Abuse and Mental Health Services Administration, Office of Applied Studies, 2001.

31. Substance Abuse and Mental Health Services Administration. *National Survey of Substance Abuse Treatment Services (N-SSATS): 2000. Data on substance abuse treatment facilities.* DASIS Series: A-16; DHHS Pub. No. SMA 02–3668. Rockville, MD: Author, 2002.

32. Center for Substance Abuse Treatment. *Practice Research Network (PRN): summary of initiative and findings.* Rockville, MD: Author, 2001.

33. Svikis DS, Zarin DA, Tanielian T, et al. Alcohol abuse and dependence in a national sample of psychiatric patients. *J Stud Alcohol* 2000;61(3):427–430.

34. Smith D. Substance abuse in practice. *Monit Psychol* 2001;32(9).

35. Kowalski JL, Harwood HJ, Ameen AZ. *NAADAC The Association for Addiction Professionals: Practice Research Network final report.* 2001;8–31–2001.

36. Haack MR, Adger H. Strategic plan for interdisciplinary faculty development: arming the nation's health professional workforce for a new approach to substance use disorders—executive summary. 2002;23[3 Suppl]:1–45.

37. Miller WR. Educating psychologists about substance abuse. *Subst Abuse* 2002;23[3 Suppl]:289–303.

38. Straussner SLA, Senreich E. Educating social workers to work with individuals affected by substance use disorders. *Subst Abuse* 2002;23[3 Suppl]:319–340.

39. Fiellin DA, Butler R, D'Onofrio G, et al. The physician's role in caring for patients with substance use disorders: implications for medical education and training. *Subst Abuse* 2002;23[3 Suppl]:207–222.

40. Bonaguro JA, Nalette E, Seibert ML. The role of allied health professionals in substance abuse education. *Subst Abuse* 2002;23[3 Suppl]:169–183.

41. Christen AG, Christen JA. Dental education in the prevention and treatment of substance use disorders. *Subst Abuse* 2002;23[3 Suppl]:185–206.

42. Paluzzi P, Deggins N, Hutchins E, et al. The role of midwives in caring for women with substance use disorders: implications for training. *Subst Abuse* 2002;23[3 Suppl]:223–233.

43. Vasquez E, Onieal ME. Substance abuse education for nurse practitioners in primary care. *Subst Abuse* 2002; 23[3 Suppl]:235–246.

44. Naegle MA. Nursing education in the prevention and treatment of SUD. *Subst Abuse* 2002;23[3 Suppl]:247–261.

45. Dole EJ, Tommasello A. Recommendations for implementing effective substance abuse education in pharmacy practice. *Subst Abuse* 2002;23 [3 Suppl]:263–271.

46. Judd CR, Hooker R, Morgan P. Improving physician assistant education and practice in SUD and policy recommendations on substance abuse education for physician assistants. *Subst Abuse* 2002;23[3 Suppl]:273–287.

47. Ringwalt CL. Incorporating substance abuse prevention into public health curricula. *Subst Abuse* 2002;23[3 Suppl]: 305–317.

48. Harwood HJ. Survey on behavioral health workplace. *Frontlines: Linking Alcohol Serv Res Pract* 2002 Nov:3.

49. Center for Substance Abuse Treatment. *Improving substance abuse treatment: the national treatment plan initiative.* DHHS Pub. No. SMA 00–3480. Rockville, MD: Substance Abuse and Mental Health Services Administration, Center for Substance Abuse Treatment, 2000.

50. Edmundson E. Significant variation in undergraduate training programs. *Frontlines: Linking Alcohol Serv Res Pract* 2002 Nov:7–8.

51. Coffey RM, Mark T, King E, et al. *National estimates of expenditures for substance abuse treatment, 1997.* Rockville, MD: Center for Substance Abuse Treatment, 2001.

52. Mark TL, Coffey RM, King E, et al. Spending on mental health and substance abuse treatment, 1987–1997. *Health Aff* 2000;19(4):108–120.

53. Mark TL, Dilonardo JD, Chalk M, et al. Trends in inpatient detoxification services, 1992–1997. *J Subst Abuse Treat* 2002;23(4):253–260.

54. National Institute on Alcohol Abuse and Alcoholism. *Second special report to the U.S. Congress on alcohol and health: new knowledge.* DHEW Pub. No. ADM 75–212. Rockville, MD: Author, 1974.

55. Scott JE, Greenberg D, Pizarro J. A survey of state insurance mandates covering alcohol and other drug treatment. *J Ment Health Admin* 1992;19(1):96–118.

56. Weisner C, McCarty D, Schmidt L. New directions in alcohol and drug treatment under managed care. *Am J Manag Care* 1999;5[Special Issue]: SP57–SP69.

57. Mechanic D, Schlesinger M, McAlpine DD. Management of mental health and substance abuse services: State of the art and early results. *Milbank Q* 1995;73:19–55.

58. Wells KB, Astrachan BM, Tischler GL, et al. Issues and approaches in evaluating managed mental health care. *Milbank Q* 1995;73:57–75.

59. Woolhandler S, Himmelstein DU. Extreme risk—the new corporate proposition for physicians. *N Engl J Med* 1995;333:1706–1708.

60. Woolhandler S, Himmelstein DU. Annotation: patients on the auction block. *Am J Public Health* 1996;86:1699–1700.

61. Frank RG, McGuire TG, Newhouse JP. Risk contracts in managed mental health care. *Health Aff* 1995;14(3):50–64.

62. Nathan PE. Practice guidelines: not yet ideal. *Am Psychol* 1998;53(3):290–299.

63. Walker RD, Howard MO, Walker PS, et al. Practice guidelines in the addictions: recent developments. *J Subst Abuse Treat* 1994;12(2):63–73.

64. Frank RG, McGuire TG. Savings from a Medicaid carve-out for mental health and substance abuse services in Massachusetts. *Psychiatr Serv* 1997;48(9):1147–1152.

65. Hodgkin D, Horgan CM, Garnick DW. Make or buy: HMOs' contracting arrangements for mental health care. *Admin Policy Ment Health* 1997;24(4):359–376.

66. Hodgkin D, Horgan CM, Garnick DW, et al. Why carve-out? Determinants of behavioral health contracting choice among large U.S. employers. *J Behav Health Serv Res* 2000;27(2):178–193.

67. Frank RG, McGuire TG, Bae JP, et al. Solutions for adverse selection in behavioral health care. *Health Care Fin Rev* 1997;18(3):109–122.

68. Institute of Medicine. *Treating drug problems.* Washington, DC: National Academy Press, 1990.

69. Steenrod S, Brisson A, McCarty D, et al. Effects of managed care on programs and practices for the treatment of alcohol and drug dependence. *Recent Dev Alcohol* 2001;15:51–71.

70. Horgan C, Larson MJ, Simon L. Medicaid funding for drug abuse treatment: a national perspective. In: Denmead G, Rouse BA, eds. *Financing drug treatment through state programs.* Rockville, MD: National Institute on Drug Abuse, 1994:1–20.

71. U.S. General Accounting Office. *Substance abuse treatment: Medicaid allows some services but generally limits coverage.* GAO/HRD-91-92. Washington, DC: Author, 1991.

72. U.S. General Accounting Office. *Medicaid: states turn to managed care to improve access and control costs.* GAO/HRD-93-46. Washington, DC: Author, 1993.

73. McCarty D, Frank R, Denmead G. Methadone maintenance and state Medicaid managed care programs. *Milbank Q* 1999;77(3):341–362.

74. Callahan JJ, Shepard DS, Beinecke RH, et al. Mental health/substance abuse treatment in managed care: the Massachusetts Medicaid experience. *Health Aff* 1995;14(3):173–184.

75. Frank RG, McGuire TG, Notman EH, et al. *Developments in Medicaid managed behavioral health care. Mental health U.S:1996.* Rockville, MD: Center for Mental Health Services, 1996.

76. Nicholson J, Young SD, Simon L, et al. Impact of Medicaid managed care on child and adolescent emergency mental health screening in Massachusetts. *Psychiatr Serv* 1996;47(12):1344–1350.

77. Norton EC, Lindrooth RC, Dickey B. Cost shifting in a mental health carve-out for the AFDC population. *Health Care Fin Rev* 1997;18(3):95–108.

78. McCarty D, Argeriou M. The Iowa Managed Substance Abuse Care Plan (IMSACP): access, utilization and expenditures for Medicaid recipients. *J Behav Health Serv Res* 2003;30(1):18–25.

79. Ettner SL, Argeriou M, McCarty D, et al. How did the introduction of managed care for the uninsured in Iowa affect the use of substance abuse services? *J Behav Health Serv Res* 2003;30(1):26–40.

80. Tompkins C and Perloff J. Using information to guide managed behavioral health care. *J Behav Health Serv Res* 2003;31(1):98–110.

81. Ettner SL, Johnson S. Do adjusted clinical groups eliminate incentives for HMOs to avoid substance abusers? Evidence from the Maryland HealthChoice program. *J Behav Health Serv Res* 2003;30(1):63–77.

82. Ettner SL, Denmead G, Dilonardo J, et al. The impact of managed care on the substance abuse treatment patterns and outcomes of Medicaid beneficiaries: Maryland's HealthChoice Program. *J Behav Health Serv Res* 2003;30(1):41–62.

83. McCarty D, Dilonardo J, Argeriou M. State substance abuse and managed care evaluation program. *J Behav Health Serv Res* 2003;30(1):7–17.

84. Normand S-LT, Belanger AJ, G. FR. Evaluating selection out of health plans for Medicaid beneficiaries with substance abuse. *J Behav Health Serv Res* 2003;30(1):78–92.

85. Chang CF, Kiser LJ, Bailey JE, et al. Tennessee's failed managed care program for mental health and substance abuse services. *JAMA* 1998;279(11):864–869.

86. Mitchell JB, Haber SG, Khatusky G, et al. Impact of the Oregon Health Plan on access and satisfaction of adults with low income. *Health Serv Res* 2002;37(1):19–39.

87. Deck D, McFarland BH, Titus JM, et al. Access to substance abuse treatment services under the Oregon Health Plan. *JAMA* 2000;284(16):2093–2099.

88. Hennessy KD, Goldman HH. Full parity: steps toward treatment equity for mental and addictive disorders. *Health Aff* 2001;20(4):58–67.

89. Frank RG, Goldman HH, McGuire T. Will parity in coverage result in better mental health care? *N Engl J Med* 2001;345(23):1701–1704.

90. Burnam MA, Escarce JJ. Equity in managed care for mental disorders. *Health Aff* 1999;18(5):22–31.

91. Substance Abuse and Mental Health Services Administration. *Summary of findings from the 2000 National Household Survey on Drug Abuse.* NHSDA Series 11–13, DHHS Pub. No. SMA 01-3549. Rockville, MD: Office of Applied Studies, 2001.

92. Roman PM. Employee assistance programs in major corporations in 1979: scope, change and receptivity. In: National Institute on Alcohol Abuse and Alcoholism, ed. *Alcohol and health monograph no. 3: prevention, intervention, and treatment: concerns and models.* Rockville, MD: National Institute on Alcohol Abuse and Alcoholism, 1982:177–200.

93. Roman PM. Missing work: the decline in infrastructure and support for workplace alcohol intervention in the United States, with implications for developments in other nations. In: Miller WR, Weisner CM, eds. *Changing substance abuse through health and social systems.* New York: Plenum Press, 2002.

94. U.S. Department of Health and Human Services. *Mental health: a report of the surgeon general.* Pittsburg, PA: Superintendent of Documents, 1999.

95. Substance Abuse and Mental Health Services Administration. Report to Congress on the prevention and treatment of co-occurring substance abuse disorders and mental health disorders. Rockville, MD: Author, 2002.

96. Drake RE, Wallach MA. Dual diagnosis: 15 years of progress. *Psychiatr Serv* 2000;51:1126–1129.

97. Ridgely MS, Goldman HH, Willenbring ML. Barriers to care for persons with dual diagnoses: Organizational and financing issues. *Schizophr Bull* 1990;16:123–132.

98. Rosenthal RN, Westreich L. Treatment of persons with dual diagnoses of

substance use disorder and other psychological problems. In: McCrady BS, Epstein EE, eds. *Addictions: a comprehensive guide.* New York: Oxford University Press, 1999:439–476.

99. Goldman HH, Ganju V, Drake RE, et al. Policy implications for implementing evidence-based practices. *Psychiatr Serv* 2001;52:1591–1597.

100. National Institute of Justice. *Annual report 2000: arrestee drug abuse monitoring.* NCJ 193013. Washington, DC: Department of Justice, 2003.

101. The Robert Wood Johnson Foundation. *Substance abuse: the nation's number one health problem.* Princeton, NJ: Author, 2001.

102. Vigdal GL. *Planning for alcohol and other drug abuse treatment for adults in the criminal justice system.* Rockville, MD: Center for Substance Abuse Treatment, 1995.

103. Field G. The effects of intensive treatment on reducing the criminal recidivism of addicted offenders. *Fed Prob* 1989;53(10):51–56.

104. Wexler HK, Falkin GP, Lipton DS, et al. Outcome evaluation of a prison therapeutic community for substance abuse treatment. In: Leukefeld CG, Tims FM, eds. *Drug abuse treatment in prisons and jails.* Rockville, MD: National Institute on Drug Abuse, 1992:156–175.

105. Field G. *Continuity of offender treatment for substance use disorders from institution to community.* Rockville, MD: Center for Substance Abuse Treatment, 1998.

106. Deschenes EP, Peters RH, Goldkamp JS, et al. Drug courts. In: Sorensen JL, Rawson RA, Guydish J, et al., eds. *Drug abuse treatment through collaboration: practice and research partnerships that work.* Washington, DC: American Psychological Association, 2003:85–102.

107. U.S. General Accounting Office. *Drug courts: overview of growth, characteristics, and results.* GAO/GGD-97–106. Washington, DC: Author, 1997.

108. U.S. General Accounting Office. Drug courts: better DOJ data collection and evaluation efforts needed to measure impact of drug courts. GAO-02–434. Washington, DC: Author, 2002.

109. U.S. General Accounting Office. *Welfare reform: states' early experiences with benefit termination.* GAO/HEHS-97–74. Washington, DC: Author, 1997.

110. U.S. General Accounting Office. *Medicaid: early implications of welfare reform for beneficiaries and states.* GAO/HEHS-98–62. Washington, DC: Author, 1998.

111. U.S. General Accounting Office. Welfare reform: states are restructuring programs to reduce welfare dependence. GAO/HEHS-98–109. Washington, DC: Author, 1998.

112. Schmidt LA, McCarty D. Welfare reform and the changing landscape of substance abuse services for low-income women. *Alcohol Clin Exp Res* 2000;24(8):1298–1311.

113. Legal Action Center. *Making welfare reform work: tools for confronting alcohol and drug problems among welfare recipients.* New York:, Author, 2001.

114. Morgenstern J, McCrady BS, Blanchard KA, et al. Barriers to employability among substance dependent and nonsubstance-affected women on federal welfare: implications for program design. *J Stud Alcohol* 2003;64(2):239–246.

115. U.S. General Accounting Office. *Social Security: major changes needed for disability benefits for addicts.* GAO/HEHS-94–128. Washington, DC: Author, 1994.

116. Luchansky B, Brown M, Longhi D, et al. Chemical dependency treatment and employment outcomes: results from the "ADATSA" program in Washington State. *Drug Alcohol Depend* 2000;60:151–159.

117. Wickizer TM, Johnson JA, Longhi D, et al. *Employment outcomes of indigent clients receiving alcohol and drug treatment in Washington State.* SMA-97–3129. Rockville, MD: Substance Abuse and Mental Health Services Administration, 1997.

118. Moore MH. *Substance use treatment for people with physical and cognitive disorders: TIP 29.* SMA 98–3249. Rockville, MD: Center for Substance Abuse Treatment, 1998.

119. National Committee for Quality Assurance. *HEDIS 3.0: understanding and enhancing performance measurement.* Washington, DC: National Committee for Quality Assurance, 1997.

120. Garnick DW, Lee MT, Chalk M, et al. Establishing the feasibility of performance measures for alcohol and other drugs. *J Subst Abuse Treat* 2002;23(4):375–385.

121. Commons M, McGuire TG, Riordan MH. Performance contracting for substance abuse treatment. *Health Serv Res* 1997;32:631–650.

122. Commons M, McGuire TG. Some economics of performance-based contracting for substance abuse services. In: Egertson JA, Fox DM, Leshner AI, eds. *Treating drug abusers effectively.* Malden, MA: Blackwell, 1997:223–249.

123. McCarty D, McGuire TG, Harwood HJ, et al. Using state information systems for drug abuse services research. *Am Behav Sc* 1998;41(8):1090–1106.

124. National Research Council. *Assessment of performance measures for public health, substance abuse, and mental health.* Washington, DC: National Academy Press, 1997.

CHAPTER 87

Legal Aspects of Confidentiality of Patient Information

MARGARET K. BROOKS

In the early 1970s, Congress passed a law to protect the confidentiality of information about persons receiving alcohol- or drug-abuse assessment or treatment services (42 USC §290dd-2) and the Department of Health and Human Services (DHHS) issued a complex set of regulations (42 Code of Federal Regulations, Part 2) ("the confidentiality regulations"). The statute and regulations narrowly define the circumstances in which information about patients in federally assisted or regulated substance abuse treatment may be disclosed. The confidentiality statute and regulations supersede any federal, state, or local law less protective of the confidentiality of patient records.

More recently, DHHS issued a set of regulations governing patients' privacy that applies to a wide range of "health care providers." These regulations were mandated by the Health Insurance Portability and Accountability Act of 1996 (HIPAA) and appear in 42 Code of Federal Regulations (CFR), Parts 160 and 164.

HOW EACH SET OF REGULATIONS APPLIES

The confidentiality regulations apply to all "programs" (individuals or organizations) specializing, in whole or in part, in providing treatment, counseling, and/or assessment and referral services for substance abuse problems (§§2.11, 2.12(e)) (2). Although the confidentiality regulations apply only to programs that are regulated by the federal government or that receive federal assistance, the latter term includes indirect forms of federal aid, such as tax-exempt status or state or local government funding that comes, in whole or in part, from the federal government (3).

Hospitals and general medical care facilities are "programs" governed by the regulations when they contain

- "An identified unit . . . which holds itself out as providing, and provides, alcohol or drug abuse diagnosis, treatment or referral for treatment; or
- "Medical personnel or other staff in a general medical care facility whose primary function is the provision of alcohol or drug abuse diagnosis, treatment or referral for treatment and who are identified as such providers." §2.11.

However, the regulations do "not apply . . . to emergency room personnel who refer a patient to the intensive care unit for an apparent overdose, unless the primary function of such personnel is the provision of alcohol or drug abuse diagnosis, treatment or referral and they are identified as providing such services or the emergency room has promoted itself to the community as a provider of such services." §2.12(e)(1)

Application of the confidentiality regulations does not depend on how a program characterizes its services. Calling itself a "prevention program" does not insulate a program from following the confidentiality rules. It is the kind of services, not the label, that determines whether the program must comply with the federal law.

The HIPAA regulations apply to health care providers (individuals or organizations that furnish health care in the normal course of business) who transmit individually identifiable health information (information that relates to the physical or mental health or condition of an individual and that identifies the individual or can reasonably be used to identify the individual) in electronic form (via computer-based technology) in connection with HIPAA standard transactions (exchanges of information to carry out financial or administrative activities related to health care, such as submitting health claims to Medicaid or private payors).

Substance abuse treatment programs are "health care providers"; however, only those programs that transmit individually identifiable health information in electronic form in connection with billing or other HIPAA standard transactions are subject to the HIPAA rules. Note that *once a program is subject to HIPAA, all "protected health information" that the program creates or receives about identifiable individuals is covered by the new regulations— whether the information is in oral, written, or electronic form.*

HOW THE TWO SETS OF REGULATIONS RELATE TO EACH OTHER AND TO STATE LAW

Substance abuse treatment providers must understand how these two federal laws and regulations—the confidentiality regulations and the HIPAA regulations—apply to their operations and how they fit together.

The confidentiality regulations are more restrictive in most circumstances than the HIPAA regulations and must continue to be followed by substance abuse programs. This chapter focuses on these more restrictive rules and mentions the HIPAA regulations only when they are more restrictive or add conditions or requirements. Both sets of regulations override any less-restrictive state law that conflicts with them (§2.20; §164.203) (4). However, programs must continue to comply with any state law that is more restrictive. (For example, some states provide additional protection for HIV-related information.)

THE GENERAL RULE AGAINST DISCLOSURE: ITS BREADTH AND TERMS

The general rule established by the confidentiality regulations is as follows:

> Programs may not disclose any information about any patient unless the patient has consented in writing (on the form required by the regulations) or unless another very limited exception specified in the regulations applies.

The confidentiality regulations are more restrictive of communications in many instances than the physician–patient privilege. For example, in most states, the physician–patient privilege does not protect a patient's identity. However, the confidentiality regulations prohibit disclosure of information that would identify an individual as attending a program that is publicly identified as a place where only substance abuse diagnosis, treatment, or referral is provided, unless the individual consents in accordance with the regulations, or the disclosure fits within one of the regulations' narrow exceptions to the general rule. As a consequence, compliance with the general ethical and legal standards that protect patient confidences in the field of medicine does not ensure compliance with the regulations protecting the confidentiality of information about patients in substance abuse treatment.

The confidentiality regulations protect any person who has applied or been assessed for, participated in, or received an interview, counseling, or any other service by a federally assisted substance-abuse treatment program. The regulations apply from the time the individual makes an appointment, to minor patients, to patients in treatment because of criminal justice requirements, and to former patients. Applicants are protected, whether or not they are admitted to treatment.

The confidentiality regulations apply to any information (oral or written) that would identify the individual as a substance abuser either explicitly or by implication (§§2.11, 2.12, 2.13(c)). Accordingly, all requests for unauthorized disclosures about patients should be met with a noncommittal response (§2.13(c)(2)).

The confidentiality regulations apply whether or not the person seeking information already has that information, has other ways of getting it, has some form of official status, is authorized by state law, or comes armed with a subpoena or search warrant (§2.13(b)). The general rule prohibiting disclosure applies to all who have access to patients' records—treatment program personnel, researchers, auditors, and others. It applies to them whether or not they are compensated for their activity, and it continues to apply to them after they have terminated their employment or relationship with the program. Violating the regulations is punishable by a fine of up to $500 for a first offense and up to $5000 for each subsequent offense (§2.4).

The HIPAA regulations are structured quite differently. Most importantly, HIPAA does not require that the patient consent to disclosures made for "treatment, payment or health care operations" (§§164.502(a)(1)(ii), 164.506(c)) (5). The confidentiality regulations require patient consent for almost all such disclosures. (For an outline of the kinds of uses and disclosures HIPAA covers, and how the HIPAA rules compare with the confidentiality regulations, see Table 87.1.)

Exceptions to the General Rule Prohibiting Disclosure: A Rule of Thumb

Although the general rule prohibiting disclosures of patient-identifying information is very broad, the regulations do permit programs to make limited disclosures when a patient consents and set out eight circumstances in which programs may make disclosures whether or not the patient consents (see Figure 87.1). Each exception permitting limited disclosure has its own peculiar requirements and limitations, all of practical significance. The following sections describe the specific circumstances in which programs may share information about a patient with others.

To avoid getting lost in the exceptions, one does well to keep the general rule in mind and to operate on the following principle: Do not disclose anything about a patient without being able to state why the regulations permit the particular disclosure.

Disclosures with Patient Consent

Most disclosures are permissible if a patient has signed a valid consent form that has not expired or been revoked by the patient (§2.31) (6). A proper consent form must be in writing and must contain each of the items contained in §2.31:

1. The name or general designation of the program(s) making the disclosure;
2. The name of the individual or organization that will receive the disclosure;
3. The name of the patient who is the subject of the disclosure;
4. The purpose or need for the disclosure;
5. How much and what kind of the information will be disclosed;
6. A statement that the patient may revoke the consent at any time, except to the extent that the program has already acted in reliance on it;
7. The date, event, or condition upon which the consent expires if not previously revoked;
8. The signature of the patient (and/or other authorized person); and
9. The date on which the consent is signed (§2.31(a)).

A general medical release form, or any consent form that does not contain all of the elements listed above, is

TABLE 87.1. *A thumbnail sketch of the HIPAA rules on disclosures*

The HIPAA regulations are structured differently from the federal alcohol and drug confidentiality rules. Under HIPAA, there are:

- **Mandatory disclosures** (which do not require the patient to consent). These are limited to disclosures to the patient him- or herself and disclosures to the Secretary of DHHS, when the Secretary seeks the information to investigate or determine the provider's compliance with HIPAA (§164.502(a)(2)). (*How this compares to 42 CFR Part 2:* The confidentiality regulations do not provide for any mandatory disclosures. Programs can comply with these HIPAA provisions: The confidentiality regulations permit disclosures to the client him- or herself. Section 2.53 permits disclosure to the Secretary because HHS is authorized by law to regulate substance abuse programs' activities.)
- **Disclosures that do not require client "authorization" (consent).** These include disclosures:
  - To the patient
  - For the following treatment, payment, or health care operations:
    - A health care provider may use or disclose protected health information for its own treatment, payment, or health care operations.
    - A health care provider may disclose protected health information for treatment activities of another health care provider.
    - A health care provider may disclose protected health information to another health care provider covered by HIPAA for the payment activities of that other health care provider.
    - A health care provider may disclose protected health information to another health care provider covered by HIPAA for health care operations in certain circumstances. (§164.506(c))
  - For a variety of public health activities (such as reporting to the Centers for Disease Control and Prevention [CDC], Food and Drug Administration [FDA], and notification of persons exposed to communicable disease).
  - To family, close friends, or other persons identified by the patient as involved in the patient's care or payment related to the patient's care, so long as the provider obtains the patient's verbal consent, provides the patient with an opportunity to object to the disclosure and the patient does not do so, or can infer that the patient does not object. If the patient is unable to consent, the provider may make the disclosure if in the exercise of professional judgment, it determines that the disclosure is in the best interests of the patient.
  - In the course of any judicial or administrative proceeding in response to an order of a court or administrative tribunal, or in response to a subpoena, discovery request, or other lawful process.
  - To a law enforcement official for law enforcement purposes under a variety of circumstances.
  - To a coroner, medical examiner, or funeral director, in certain circumstances.
  - To organ-procurement organizations for the purpose of facilitating organ donation.
  - For research purposes, if certain conditions are met. (§164.512.)

    (*How this compares to 42 CFR Part 2:* Perhaps the most striking difference is that in many circumstances, HIPAA allows health care providers to disclose information to other health care providers without the patient's consent, whereas 42 CFR requires the patient to consent in most circumstances, even when information is being disclosed to another treating program or physician. In general, the confidentiality regulations have far fewer exceptions permitting disclosure of information without the patient's consent. Programs must, therefore, continue to follow the confidentiality rules.)
- **The minimum necessary rule.** HIPAA requires that when a health care provider discloses protected health information to or requests information from another covered health care provider, it make "reasonable efforts to limit protected health information to the minimum necessary to accomplish the intended purpose of the use, disclosure, or request" (§164.502(b)), unless the disclosure or request is for the purpose of treatment. The regulations discourage disclosure of the client's entire record (§164.514(d)(5)). The minimum necessary rule does not apply when disclosure is made to the individual, for the purpose of treatment, pursuant to an authorization, or as required by law (§164.502(b)(2)).

    (*How this compares to 42 CFR Part 2:* Under the confidentiality regulations, any disclosure must be limited to the information necessary to carry out the purpose of the disclosure.)
- **Disclosures that require the patient's written "authorization" (consent).** Health care providers covered by HIPAA must obtain the patient's written authorization when protected health care information is to be used or disclosed for purposes other than treatment, payment and the health care provider's own health care operations (§164.508(a)). Authorizations must contain:
  - A description of the information to be used or disclosed that identifies the information in a specific and meaningful fashion.
  - The name or other specific identification of the person(s) or class of persons authorized to make the requested use or disclosure.
  - The name or other specific identification of the person(s) or class of persons to whom the provider may make the requested use or disclosure.
  - A description of each purpose of the requested use or disclosure. ("At the request of the individual" is a sufficient description of purpose when the client initiates the authorization and does not provide a statement of the purpose.)

(continued)

TABLE 87.1. *(Continued)*

- ▸ An expiration date or event that relates to the patient or the purpose of the use or disclosure.
- ▸ A statement adequate to place the patient on notice of the potential that information disclosed pursuant to the authorization may be subject to redisclosure by the recipient and no longer protected by HIPAA.
- ▸ A statement adequate to place the patient on notice of his/her right to revoke the authorization, how he or she may do so, and any exceptions to that right.
- ▸ A statement adequate to place the patient on notice of the program's ability or inability to condition treatment on whether the patient signs the authorization.*
- ▸ The signature of the patient and the date it was signed. If the authorization is signed by a personal representative (or parent), a description of the representative's authority must be provided (§164.508(c)).

Additional requirements apply in certain circumstances. The patient may revoke authorization at any time, but revocation must be in writing.

(*How this compares to 42 CFR Part 2:* The authorization provision is similar to §2.31—the confidentiality rules' consent provision. However, §2.31 is somewhat more restrictive; revocation of consent need not be in writing; and redisclosure is prohibited. The only element HIPAA adds to the requirements of 42 CFR Part 2 is the statement concerning the program's ability or inability to condition treatment on the patient's signing the authorization form. This element need not be added to the form in most situations [see the text]. Because §2.31 is more restrictive, programs must continue to follow the confidentiality regulations' consent rules.)

- ▪ **Psychotherapy notes.** HIPAA gives special protection to "psychotherapy notes," which it defines as notes "recorded (in any medium) by a health care provider who is a mental health professional documenting or analyzing the contents of conversation during a private counseling session or a group, joint, or family counseling session and that are separated from the rest of the individual's medical record" (§153.501). Psychotherapy notes are process notes that capture the therapist's impressions about the patient, contain details of the psychotherapy conversation considered to be inappropriate for the medical record, and are used by the provider for future sessions. They do not include summary information, such as the current state of the patient, symptoms, the theme of the psychotherapy session, diagnoses, medications prescribed, side effects, and any other information necessary for treatment or payment. Summary information should be placed in the patient's medical record.

  The originator of the psychotherapy notes can use them without the patient's authorization. The program may use or disclose the notes (a) for its own training programs in which students or practitioners in mental health learn under supervision to practice or improve their skills; and (b) to defend itself in a legal action. Programs may disclose psychotherapy notes when the Secretary of HHS requires it as a part of an investigation or the program's compliance with HIPAA and in *Tarasoff* situations. Programs must obtain the client's authorization (consent) to make any other disclosure of psychotherapy notes (§164.508(a)(2)).

---

*A program not conducting research would generally not be permitted to condition treatment on a patient's signing a HIPAA authorization (§164.508(b)(4)). Violation of HIPAA requirements can subject the offender to civil and/or criminal penalties. See §§1176 and 1177 of the Act.

Note: Programs subject to both HIPAA and the federal alcohol and drug confidentiality regulations must comply with the more stringent standard.

---

not acceptable. A single form may suffice for a series of disclosures of the same type to the same recipient, such as verifying to a particular funding source the dates on which treatment was provided. But a disclosure of a different nature to the same organization or of the same nature to a different organization would require a new consent.

Understanding the Consent Requirements

Several of the items that must be included in a consent form deserve further explanation.

Purpose of the Disclosure and How Much and What Kind of Information Will Be Disclosed

These two items are closely related. All disclosures must be limited to information that is necessary to accomplish the need or purpose for the disclosure (§2.13(a)), and this

purpose or need must be included on the consent form. It would be improper to disclose everything in a patient's file if the recipient of the information only needs one specific piece of information. Once the purpose or need is identified, it is easier to determine how much and what kind of information will be disclosed, tailoring it to what is essential to accomplish the specified need or purpose. That, too, must be written on the consent form.

As an illustration, if school must be notified so that a patient can be released early to participate in treatment, the purpose of the disclosure would be "to verify treatment status so that the school will permit early release," and the amount and kind of information to be disclosed would be "time and dates of appointments." The disclosure would then be limited to a statement that "Sam Crane (the patient) is receiving counseling at XYZ program on Tuesday at 2:00."

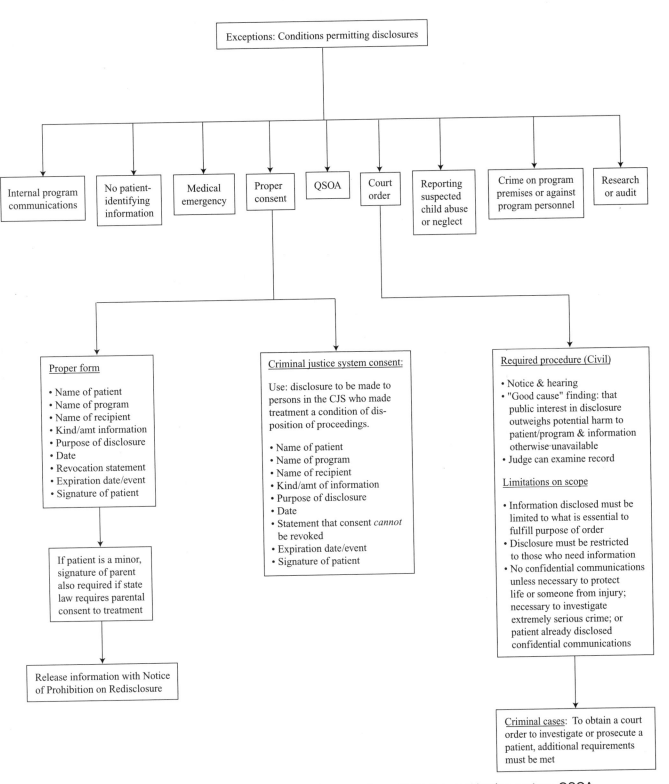

Exceptions: Conditions permitting disclosures

Internal program communications

No patient-identifying information

Medical emergency

Proper consent

QSOA

Court order

Reporting suspected child abuse or neglect

Crime on program premises or against program personnel

Research or audit

Proper form

- Name of patient
- Name of program
- Name of recipient
- Kind/amt information
- Purpose of disclosure
- Date
- Revocation statement
- Expiration date/event
- Signature of patient

If patient is a minor, signature of parent also required if state law requires parental consent to treatment

Release information with Notice of Prohibition on Redisclosure

Criminal justice system consent:

Use: disclosure to be made to persons in the CJS who made treatment a condition of disposition of proceedings.

- Name of patient
- Name of program
- Name of recipient
- Kind/amt of information
- Purpose of disclosure
- Date
- Statement that consent *cannot* be revoked
- Expiration date/event
- Signature of patient

Required procedure (Civil)

- Notice & hearing
- "Good cause" finding: that public interest in disclosure outweighs potential harm to patient/program & information otherwise unavailable
- Judge can examine record

Limitations on scope

- Information disclosed must be limited to what is essential to fulfill purpose of order
- Disclosure must be restricted to those who need information
- No confidential communications unless necessary to protect life or someone from injury; necessary to investigate extremely serious crime; or patient already disclosed confidential communications

Criminal cases: To obtain a court order to investigate or prosecute a patient, additional requirements must be met

FIG. 87.1. The general rule of disclosure and its exceptions. CJS, Criminal justice system; QSOA, qualified service organization agreement. (Copyright 2000 by Margaret K. Brooks. Reproduced with permission.)

The Patient's Right to Revoke Consent

The patient may revoke consent at any time (orally or in writing), and the consent form must include a statement to this effect. Revocation need not be in writing. If a program has already made a disclosure prior to the revocation, acting in reliance on the patient's signed consent, it is not required to try to retrieve the information (7).

Expiration Date or Event

The consent form must contain a date, event, or condition on which it will expire if not previously revoked. A consent form must last "no longer than reasonably necessary to serve the purpose for which it is given" (§2.31(a)(9)). Depending on the purpose of the disclosure, the consent form may expire in 5 days, in 6 months, or in a longer period.

The form does not have to contain a specific date, but may instead specify an event or condition. For example, if a patient is attending treatment as a condition of being placed on probation at work, the consent form should expire when his probationary period ends. If a patient is being referred to a specialist for a single appointment, the consent form should expire after the referral is made or after the patient has seen that physician.

The Signature of the Patient (and the Issue of Parental Consent)

A minor patient must always sign the consent form in order for a program to release information, even to the minor's parent (8). The program must get the parent's signature in addition to the minor's signature only if state law requires the program to obtain parental permission before providing treatment to the minor (§2.14).

Some states permit a minor to obtain substance abuse treatment without consent or notification of a parent or guardian; others do not. If a program is in a state that permits minors to seek treatment without parental consent, then the program need obtain only the minor's consent in making disclosures (§2.14(b)). Obtaining parental consent to a disclosure in these circumstances is not only unnecessary but would itself constitute an unauthorized disclosure.

In states that require parental consent for substance abuse treatment of minors, the program must obtain the consent of both the minor patient and parent or guardian prior to making a disclosure from the patient's records (§2.14(c)). Note that the program must always obtain the minor's consent for disclosures and cannot rely on the parent's signature alone. (For a full discussion of this issue and what to do in states that require parental consent to treatment when a minor applying for treatment refuses to consent to parental notification, see "Legal and Ethical Issues" in *Treatment of Adolescents with Substance Use Disorders,* Treatment Improvement Protocol 32. Rockville, MD: The Center for Substance Abuse Treatment, 1999:73–77.) (9)

Written Prohibition on Redisclosure

Any disclosure a program makes with patient consent must be accompanied by a written statement that the information disclosed is protected by federal law and that the recipient cannot further disclose or release the information unless permitted by the regulations (§2.32). This statement, not the consent form itself, should be delivered and explained to the recipient at the time of disclosure or earlier. Section 2.32 of the regulations provides a model statement for this purpose (10).

If a program makes a disclosure during a telephone call, staff must inform the person at the other end about the prohibition on redisclosure, orally at first and then by mail.

Disclosure is Not Required

The fact that a patient has signed a proper consent form authorizing the release of information does not force a program to make the proposed disclosure, unless the program has also received a subpoena or court order (§§2.3(b); 2.61(a), (b)). In most cases, then, the decision of whether or not to make a disclosure pursuant to a consent form is within the discretion of the program, unless state law requires or prohibits a particular disclosure once consent is given (11). The program's only obligation is to refuse to honor a consent that is expired, deficient, or otherwise known to be revoked, false, or incorrect (§2.31(c)).

The HIPAA Requirements

Programs subject to HIPAA must meet the following three additional requirements for consent forms:

1. Voluntariness statement. If the consent form authorizes disclosure of protected health information and the disclosure is not for treatment of the patient, payment for treatment, or for the program's "health care operations" (12), the consent form must also state that the patient may refuse to sign the consent and that the program will not condition the provision of treatment on the patient's signature (§164.508(c)(2)(ii)).
2. Copy for the patient. HIPAA requires that when a program seeks consent from a patient for a disclosure that is for a purpose other than treatment, payment, or health care operations, the program provide the patient with a copy of the signed consent form (§164.508(c)(4)).
3. Verification. HIPAA requires that, prior to any disclosure, the program verify the identity of the person requesting protected health information and the authority of that person to have access to the information, unless the program knows the person (§164.514(h)).

Use of Consent Forms

Given these rules regarding consent, consider the following situations that programs routinely encounter:

- A program needs information about a patient from collateral or referral sources.

• A program needs to communicate on an ongoing basis with one or more agencies concerned with or responsible for the patient's welfare.
• A program wants to arrange a referral appointment for a patient.
• A program needs to report information to a third-party payor or funding source to be reimbursed for treatment services.
• A program needs to share information about a patient with the criminal justice agency that mandated the patient to participate in treatment (i.e., treatment was mandated as a condition of the disposition of a criminal proceeding against the patient or as a condition of the patient's probation, parole or release from custody).
• A program needs to make a disclosure to the patient's lawyer.

Using Consent Forms to Obtain Information from Collateral or Referral Sources. Making inquiries of a patient's family, partner, school, employer, and other health care providers might, at first glance, seem to pose no risk to a patient's right to confidentiality. But it does.

When a program that offers assessment and treatment for substance abuse asks a family member (including parent or spouse), partner, employer, mental health provider, doctor, or school to verify information it has obtained from the patient, it is making a disclosure that the patient has sought help for substance abuse. The federal regulations generally prohibit this kind of disclosure unless the patient consents.

How then is a program to proceed? The easiest way is to get the patient's consent to contact the family member (including parent), partner, employer, school, health care facility, and so forth. If program staff members are making inquiries by telephone, they must inform the parties at the other end of the line about the prohibition on redisclosure, orally at first, and then by mail (13).

Using Consent Forms to Make Periodic Reports or Coordinate Care. Programs may need to confer on an ongoing basis with other agencies, such as mental health or child welfare programs. Again, the best way to proceed is to get the patient's consent (as well as parental consent when required). Care should be taken in wording the consent form to specify the purpose of the communication and the kind and amount of information to be disclosed. For example, if the program needs ongoing communications with a mental health provider, the "purpose of the disclosure" would be "coordination of care for Cheryl Smith." "How much and what kind of information will be disclosed" might be "treatment status, treatment issues, and progress in treatment." If the program is treating a patient who is on probation at work and whose continued employment is contingent on completing treatment, the "purpose of disclosure" might be "to assist the patient to comply with the employer's mandates" or "to supply periodic reports about attendance." "How much and what kind of informa-

tion will be disclosed" might be "attendance" or "progress in treatment" (14).

Note that the kinds of information that will be disclosed in these two examples are quite different. The program might well share detailed clinical information about a patient with a mental health provider if that would assist in coordinating care. Disclosure to an employer should be limited to a brief statement about the patient's attendance or progress in treatment. Disclosure of detailed clinical information to an employer would, in most circumstances, be inappropriate.

The program should also give thought to the expiration date or event the consent form should contain. For coordinating care with a mental health program, it might be appropriate to have the consent form expire when treatment by either agency ends. A consent form permitting disclosures to an employer might expire when the patient's probationary period ends.

Using Consent Forms to Make Referrals. Substance abuse treatment programs may need to refer patients to other health care or social service agencies. The program can, of course, give the patient the name and telephone number of an outside gynecologist, psychologist, or training program and allow the patient to initiate the call. However, if a staff member at the program makes the call to set up an appointment and identifies the patient as attending a substance abuse treatment program, directly or by implication, the referral requires the patient's consent in writing (as well as parental consent in states requiring it) (15).

Special Rules for Patients Involved in the Criminal Justice System. Programs assessing or treating patients who are involved in the criminal justice system (CJS) or juvenile justice system (JJS) (juvenile court) must also follow the federal confidentiality rules. However, some special rules apply when a patient comes for assessment or treatment as an official condition of probation, sentence, dismissal of charges, release from detention, or other disposition of a criminal or juvenile justice proceeding (16).

A consent form (or court order) is still required before a program can disclose information about a patient who is the subject of CJS or JJS referral. However, the rules concerning the length of time that a consent is valid and the process for revoking the consent are different (§2.35). Specifically, the regulations require that the following factors be considered in determining how long a CJS consent form will remain in effect:

• Anticipated duration of treatment
• Type of criminal proceeding
• Need for treatment information in dealing with the proceeding
• When the final disposition will occur
• Anything else the patient, program, or justice agency believes is relevant

These rules allow programs to draft the consent form to expire "when there is a substantial change in the patient's justice system status." A substantial change in justice status occurs whenever the patient moves from one phase of the CJS to the next. For example, for a patient on probation (or parole), a change in CJS status would occur when the probation (or parole) ends, either by successful completion or revocation. Thus, the program could provide an assessment and periodic reports to the patient's probation (or parole) officer and could even testify at a probation (or parole) revocation hearing if it so desired, because no change in status would occur until after that hearing.

The confidentiality regulations also allow the program to draft the CJS consent form so that the patient cannot revoke his or her consent until the specified date or condition occurs. The regulations allow the CJS form to be irrevocable so that a patient who has agreed to enter treatment in lieu of prosecution or punishment cannot then prevent the court, probation (or parole) department, or other agency from monitoring his or her progress. Note that although a CJS consent may be made irrevocable for a specified period, that period must end no later than the final disposition of the criminal justice proceeding. (Thereafter, the patient may freely revoke consent.) If treatment continues beyond this time period, the program cannot disclose further information to the criminal justice system unless the patient has signed another standard consent form that complies with the regulations.

The provision of Federal confidentiality regulations that allows programs to make CJS consent forms irrevocable appears to conflict with a provision of HIPAA regulations, which requires all client authorizations to disclose protected health information to be revocable by the client (§164.508(b)(5)). HIPAA permits disclosures of PHI to criminal justice agencies to be made pursuant to an authorization signed by the client or a court order. In order to comply with both rules, programs can (1) make all their CJS consent forms revocable and refuse to disclose information to the referring criminal justice agency once a client has revoked consent, or (2) make the CJS consent form irrevocable and apply for a court order under HIPAA regulations requiring the program to disclose necessary information to the court and other law enforcement personnel.

Section 164.508(c)(ii) requires programs subject to HIPAA to add a statement to the CJS consent form that is adequate to place the patient on notice that the program cannot condition treatment of the patient on whether or not the patient signs the consent form.

Several other aspects of CJS referrals should be noted. First, a criminal justice agency that receives information from a treatment program can use the information only in connection with its official duties with respect to that particular criminal proceeding. The information may not be used in other proceedings, for other purposes, or with respect to other individuals (§2.35(d)). Note, too, that the HIPAA regulations prohibit a program from making a report to law enforcement authorities to assist in the identification or apprehension of a patient because of a statement the patient made admitting to participation in a violent crime if it learned the information "(i) [i]n the course of treatment to affect the propensity to commit the criminal conduct that is the basis for the disclosure . . . or counseling or therapy; or (ii) [t]hrough a request by the individual to initiate or be referred for . . . treatment, counseling, or therapy. . ." (§164.512(j)(2)).

Second, whenever possible, it is best to have the judge or referring agency require that the patient sign a proper CJS consent form before the patient is referred to the treatment program. If that is not possible, the treatment program should have the patient sign a CJS consent form at the very first appointment. With a proper criminal justice consent form signed, the program can communicate with the referring criminal justice agency even if the patient appears for assessment or treatment only once. This avoids the problem that can arise if a patient mandated into treatment leaves before the assessment or treatment has been completed. If no consent form is in place, the program cannot provide any information to the referring criminal justice agency.

If a patient referred by a criminal justice agency never applies for or receives services from the program, that fact may be communicated to the referring agency without patient consent (§2.13(c)(2)). But once a patient even makes an appointment to visit the program, consent or a court order is needed for any disclosures.

Disclosures to Employers and Employment Agencies. Programs may disclose records or other information to the patient's employer whenever the patient signs a consent form. Given the stigma that many employers attach to alcohol and drug abuse treatment, however, program staff may wish to withhold disclosures from employers they know will fire or refuse to hire anyone with a drug- or alcohol-abuse history.

Indeed, program staff should not assume that communications with a patient's employer will be beneficial to the patient. A patient who tells program staff that his or her employer will not be sympathetic about the decision to enter treatment may well have an accurate picture of the employer's attitude. Insistence by program staff on communicating with the employer may cost a patient his or her job.

If a program does decide to communicate with an employer (with the patient's consent), it should take care to limit any disclosures to information that is actually necessary. Often, disclosures to employers can be limited to a verification of treatment status or a general progress report. The program should disclose more detail only if the information is directly related to a particular employment situation and the patient has signed a consent form stating the kind and amount of detailed information that will be disclosed.

The regulations do permit a program to release adverse information, even with potentially harmful consequences. For example, a program may, with patient consent, provide a periodic progress report to an employer that contains negative information, including continued substance abuse, refusal to cooperate with the program, or other damaging information. This is a matter for the program's own judgment. There is nothing wrong with a program disclosing negative evaluations to an employer if the program knows that the employer will attempt or is attempting to help the patient with an alcohol or drug abuse problem or will consider disciplinary steps only when an individual's substance abuse problem has reduced job performance to an unacceptable level. Perhaps the most common example of this kind of disclosure occurs when an employee is referred for treatment by or to an employee assistance program as a condition of retaining a job, and the treating program provides periodic reports to the employer on the employee's progress (or lack of progress). Of course, any disclosure requires patient consent, which, under the rules discussed earlier, is revocable at any time.

A program may also wish—or even be legally compelled—to disclose information to an employer when it knows the patient is continuing to use alcohol or other drugs and works in a job that directly affects public safety (e.g., a bus driver). Even then, the program must be sure to make the disclosure only in a manner permitted by the federal rules.

Disclosures to Patients' Lawyers. There are no special rules governing disclosure to a patient's attorney when the patient consents. Once the program determines that the attorney actually represents the patient, it may, with consent, turn over all the patient's records.

A program does retain discretion to limit its response, and programs are sometimes nervous about turning records over to a lawyer representing a patient because they fear they may be sued. However, it rarely pays to refuse to turn over records. The attorney will simply get a subpoena, which, with the patient's written consent, will compel the program to turn over the records. The process will antagonize the attorney, who will suspect that the program has something to hide. If the program has doubts about the wisdom of turning over records, it should consult its own counsel.

Records turned over to an attorney, like records turned over to anyone pursuant to consent, must be accompanied by the notice of prohibition on redisclosure. The attorney may not redisclose any information received from the program's records unless the patient consents or there is another authorization under the rules, such as a proper court order.

Internal Program Communications

Staff who have access to patient records because they work for or administratively direct a program (including full-time or part-time employees and unpaid volunteers) may consult among themselves or otherwise the share patient-identifying information they need for their work at the program (§2.12(c)(3)).

Staff may also communicate patient-identifying information to a person or entity having "direct administrative control" over a program if there is a need for the information "in connection with their [substance abuse services]" (§2.12(c)(3)(ii)). Does this exception allow a program that treats patients and that is part of a larger entity, such as a hospital, to share confidential information with others who are not part of the unit? For example, can a substance abuse treatment unit that is part of a general hospital, community mental health center, or other multiservice agency disclose patient-identifying information to the larger entity? The regulations permit disclosures, including communications to central billing or record keeping departments, but only when necessary to provide the alcohol- and drug-abuse services. Communication of information outside the substance abuse unit that is not necessary to provide services to the unit's patients is prohibited.

Information that is communicated to an entity having administrative control over a program continues to be protected by the regulations. The administrative entity may not redisclose any patient-identifying information to the outside world. This issue is very complex; before setting up a system in which internal communications take place between a program and an administrative entity, the program should consult an expert in the area for assistance.

HIPAA requires covered programs to classify staff who need access to protected health information to carry out their duties. Programs must identify, for each class of staff, the category or categories of protected health information to which they need access and any conditions appropriate to their having access (§164.514(d)(2)).

Communications That Do Not Disclose Patient-Identifying Information (17)

A communication is not a "disclosure" if it neither identifies an individual as an alcohol or drug abuser nor verifies someone else's identification of the patient (§§2.12(a)(1)(i), (e)(3)). The principal ways in which a program may make a "non–patient-identifying disclosure" are:

- By reporting aggregate data about a program's population, or some portion of it; or
- By communicating information about an individual in a manner that does not disclose the individual's status as a drug- or alcohol-abuse patient.

Two examples of communications of information about an individual that do not disclose that person's status as a substance-abuse patient are as follows:

- A disclosure of information by a hospital, community mental health center, employee assistance program, or other agency that provides services to people with other illnesses, as well as to alcohol and drug abusers. Thus, a program may disclose that "John Smith is a patient at the Smithville General Hospital" as long as the fact that John has an alcohol or drug problem or is in substance abuse treatment is not revealed.

- An "anonymous" disclosure, by a program that only provides alcohol and/or drug services, of information about a patient without identifying the name of the program or otherwise revealing the individual's status as an alcohol- or drug-abuse patient.

HIPAA changes these rules. A program can still disclose aggregate data about its patient population. However, programs subject to HIPAA can no longer assume that a disclosure of non–substance-abuse-related information is permissible. If the non–substance-abuse-related information is "protected health information" under HIPAA, its disclosure may violate those regulations, depending upon what information is disclosed and the context of the disclosure. Programs subject to HIPAA must consult the HIPAA rules before assuming they can make what the confidentiality regulations term "non–patient-identifying" disclosures (18).

Medical Emergencies

The regulations permit a program to make disclosures in a "medical emergency" to medical personnel "who have a need for information about a patient for the purpose of treating a condition which poses an immediate threat to the health of any individual and requires immediate medical intervention" (§2.51). Whenever a disclosure is made to cope with a medical emergency, the program must document in the patient's records the name and affiliation of the recipient of the information, the name of the individual making the disclosure, the date and time of the disclosure, and the nature of the emergency.

The "medical emergency" provision does not open a loophole for nonemergency disclosures; the situation must truly be one requiring immediate medical attention. It permits disclosures only to medical personnel. This means that this exception cannot be used as the basis for a disclosure to the police, parents, or other nonmedical personnel.

These practices are not affected by the HIPAA regulations.

Court-Ordered Disclosures

The regulations permit programs to make a disclosure that would otherwise be prohibited if a court issues an authorizing order. The regulations require the court to follow a particular procedure and make certain findings, limit the grounds upon which a court may authorize a program to make disclosures, and set out strict limits on the scope of such disclosures (§§2.63–2.67). A subpoena, search warrant, or arrest warrant, even when signed by a judge, is not sufficient, standing alone, to require or even to permit a program to disclose information (§2.61) (19). More than any other situations covered by the confidentiality regulations, those involving court orders, subpoenas and search and arrest warrants are best handled by counsel.

Procedure

Before a proper court order authorizing disclosure may be issued, the program and any patient whose records are sought must be given written notice that an order is sought and an opportunity to make an appearance or written statement to the court (§2.64(b)) (20). The application for the court order and the court order itself must use fictitious names for any known patient, and all court proceedings in connection with the application must be confidential unless the patient requests otherwise (§2.64(a) and (c)).

Required Findings

Before authorizing a particular disclosure, a court must find that there is "good cause" for the disclosure. The court must find that the public interest and the need for disclosure outweigh any adverse effect that the disclosure will have on the patient, the doctor–patient relationship, and the effectiveness of the program's treatment services. If the information sought is available elsewhere, the court ordinarily should deny the application (§2.64(d)). The judge may examine the records before making a decision (§2.64(c)).

Limitations on the Scope of the Order

The regulations limit the scope of disclosure that a court may authorize, even when it finds good cause exists. Disclosure must be limited to the information essential to fulfill the purpose of the order and it must be restricted to those persons who need the information for that purpose. The court should also take any other steps that are necessary to protect the patient's confidentiality, including sealing court records from public scrutiny (§2.64(e)).

A court may authorize disclosure of "confidential communications" by a patient to the program only if the disclosure (a) is necessary to protect against a threat to life or of serious bodily injury; (b) is necessary to investigate or prosecute an extremely serious crime; or (c) is in connection with a proceeding at which the patient has already presented evidence concerning confidential communications. In all other situations, not even a court can order disclosure of confidential communications (§2.63).

Court Orders in Criminal Justice Cases

A program, investigative law enforcement, or prosecutorial agency seeking an order to authorize disclosures for purposes of investigating or prosecuting a patient for a crime must meet additional, stringent criteria (§2.65) (21). Before issuing such an order, a court must find that:

1. The crime involved is extremely serious, such as an act causing or directly threatening to cause death or serious bodily injury, including homicide, rape, kidnaping,

armed robbery, assault with a deadly weapon, and child abuse and neglect,

2. The records sought are likely to contain information of significance to the investigation or prosecution,
3. There is no other practical way to obtain the information, and
4. The public interest in disclosure outweighs any actual or potential harm to the patient, the doctor–patient relationship, and the ability of the program to provide services to other patients.

When law enforcement personnel seek an order, the program must have an opportunity to be represented by independent counsel. (When the program is a governmental entity, it must be represented by counsel independent of the justice agency seeking the order.) (§2.65(d))

The regulations require that a court follow the same special procedures that apply to court-ordered disclosures generally (except that the patient need not be given notice). Court orders authorizing disclosure for the purpose of investigating or prosecuting patients are subject to similar limitations on scope to those that apply to court-ordered disclosures generally (§2.65(d)). Under no circumstances may a court authorize a program to turn over the entire patient record to a law enforcement, investigative, or prosecutorial agency (22).

Programs must continue to follow the confidentiality regulations' rules on court orders because the HIPAA regulations are far less protective of patients' privacy.

Patient Crimes on Program Premises or Against Program Personnel

When a patient has committed or threatened a crime on program premises or against program personnel, the regulations permit the program to report the crime to a law enforcement agency or to seek its assistance. In such a situation, the program can disclose the circumstances of the incident, including the suspect's name, address, last known whereabouts, and status as a patient at the program (§2.12(c)(5)). The HIPAA regulations also contain a provision that permits reporting crime on program premises (§164.512(f)(5)) but do not authorize reporting of crime against program personnel off program premises. However, a program employee who is the victim of a crime could report it, so long as no mention is made of the fact that the person who committed the crime is a patient is in substance abuse treatment.

Child Abuse and Neglect Reporting

The confidentiality law and regulations permit programs to comply with state mandatory child abuse and neglect reporting laws (§2.12(c)(6)) and all treatment programs must comply with those laws. Each state has different rules about what kinds of conditions must be reported,

who must report, and when and how reports must be made. Most states now require not only physicians, but also educators and social service workers, to report child abuse. Most states require an immediate oral report, and many now have toll-free numbers to facilitate reporting. (Half the states require that both oral and written reports be made.) All states extend immunity from prosecution to persons reporting child abuse and neglect. Most states provide penalties for failure to report. Because of the variation in state laws, programs should consult an attorney familiar with state law to ensure their reporting practices are in compliance.

It is important to note that the exemption for child abuse reporting applies only to initial reports of child abuse or neglect and not to requests or even subpoenas for additional information or records, even if the records are sought for use in civil or criminal proceedings resulting from the program's initial report. Programs may not respond to followup requests for information unless the patient consents or the appropriate court issues an order under the court order provisions of the regulations. The HIPAA regulations do not affect these rules (§164.512(b)(iii)).

Qualified Service Organization

The confidentiality regulations recognize that a program may need to communicate patient-identifying information in order to work with an outside person or agency such as a medical laboratory, data processor, accountant, or lawyer. The regulations permit a program to enter into a written "qualified service organization agreement" (QSOA) with the outside agency under which the outside organization

1. Acknowledges that it is fully bound by the confidentiality regulations in handling all information about patients that it receives from the program and
2. Promises that it will resist, if necessary in judicial proceedings, any attempt to obtain such information that is not permitted by the regulations (§2.12(c)(4)).

A QSOA should be used only when the outside agency or official is providing a service to the program itself. A QSOA is not a substitute for individual consent in other situations. Disclosures under such an agreement must be limited to information that is needed by others so that the program can function effectively. It may not be used between programs providing substance-abuse assessment or treatment services.

HIPAA also recognizes that health care providers routinely need to share certain information with outside agencies that provide services. HIPAA calls these agencies "business associates" (23). The HIPAA regulations permit these business associates to perform "health care operations" for health care providers. The regulations define "health care operations" (24) to include the kinds of activities that qualified service organizations typically undertake for programs. HIPAA permits health care providers to disclose protected health information to "business associates" if they enter into "contracts" that meet certain requirements, which are outlined in the regulations. Programs subject to HIPAA can continue to use the QSOA form, but §§164.502(e) and 164.504(e)(2) require the addition of provisions that establish the permitted uses and disclosures of the information by the person or agency providing the service and in which the person (or agency)

1. Promises to report to the program any use or disclosure that violates the regulations.
2. Acknowledges that it is responsible for ensuing that any person to whom it delegates a function, activity, or service agrees to abide by the restrictions of its agreement with the program.
3. Promises to make available protected health information for inspection and/or for amendment and to incorporate such amendments, and to make available the information required to provide patients with an accounting of disclosures.
4. Promises to make its records relating to the use and disclosure of protected health information available to the secretary of DHHS for determining the program's compliance with 45 CFR Parts 160 and 164.
5. Agrees to destroy or return all protected health information at the end of the agreement/contract, and, if the protected health information cannot be destroyed or returned, that its agreement with the program will continue to apply for as long as the information is retained.
6. Authorizes the program to terminate the agreement/contract if the program determines that the business associate has violated a material term.

The DHHS Office for Civil Rights has published sample contract language). See 67 Federal Register 53264 (August 14, 2002).

Disclosures to accreditation bodies. Federal confidentiality regulations permit disclosures to accreditation bodies such as Joint Commission on Accreditation of Healthcare Organizations (JCAHO) under either the QSOA provisions or the audit and evaluation exception, discussed below. HIPAA, however, considers accreditation bodies "business associates" that are conducting "health care operations" (§§160.103; 164.501). Programs that are subject to HIPAA and undergo accreditation will have to sign business associate contracts with accreditation organizations that satisfy the requirements of HIPAA and comply with the confidentiality regulations, either by ensuring that the business associate contract contains all the requirements of a QSOA or by fulfilling the mandates of the audit and evaluation provisions, discussed below.

Transition Provisions

HIPAA permitted programs to continue using their current qualified service organization agreements until April 14, 2004, if the agreement or contract is not required to be renewed by its terms before that date. Any QSOA that is renewed between April 14, 2003, and April 14, 2004, must be modified to comply with the HIPAA requirements set forth above.

Disclosures for Audit, Evaluation, and Research

Audit and Evaluation

Government agencies that fund or regulate a program, private agencies that provide financial assistance or third-party payments to a program, and peer review organizations performing utilization or quality control review may have access to program records without patient consent to conduct an audit or evaluation provided certain safeguards are met. These entities may also copy or remove records, but only after promising in writing to safeguard patient-identifying information in accordance with the confidentiality regulations and to destroy all such information when the audit or evaluation is completed (§2.53(b)).

Any person or organization that conducts an audit or evaluation must agree in writing that it will use the information only to carry out the audit or evaluation and that it will redisclose patient-identifying information only (a) back to the program; (b) pursuant to a court order to investigate or prosecute the program (not a patient); or (c) to a government agency that is overseeing a Medicare or Medicaid audit or evaluation (§2.53(a), (c), (d)).

Any other person or organization that is determined by the program director to be qualified to conduct an audit or evaluation and that agrees in writing to abide by the restrictions on redisclosure may also review patient records, but may not copy or remove them.

The HIPAA regulations add complications to these rules. The HIPAA requirements depend upon who is conducting the audit or evaluation, as follows:

- If an audit or evaluation is being conducted by the program or its employees, it is permissable under both sets of regulations without consent for (§§2.12(c)(3); 164.502(a)(1)(ii)).
- If an audit or evaluation is being conducted by a "health oversight agency" (25), the program may disclose patient-identifying information without patient consent or "authorization" (§164.512(d)). This is comparable to §2.53 of the confidentiality regulations; because §2.53 requires the outside agency to make certain commitments in writing (see above), programs should continue to follow that rule.
- If an audit or evaluation is being conducted by an outside entity that is not a "health oversight agency," the program must have a signed "business associate" (QSOA) agreement/contract with the auditor or evaluator that satisfies both §164.504(e) (§164.502(e)) and §2.11. In that case, the program could use a QSOA form modified by the additions required by HIPAA.

Note that programs subject to the Federal drug and alcohol regulations can disclose non–patient-identifying nformation to auditors and evaluators (§§2.11; 2.12(a) 1)(i)). Programs subject to HIPAA can disclose "de-dentified" health information to auditors and evaluators §164.502(d)) (26).

Research

There are three ways programs can disclose information o researchers:

1. Programs can provide information about patients when no patient-identifying information (27) is revealed.
2. Programs can provide patient-identifying information without patients' consent when certain criteria are met (the "research exception").
3. Programs can provide patient-identifying information if patients sign proper consent forms.

Programs also covered by the HIPAA regulations have he same three options, although the requirements differ.

Option 1: Disclosing Non-Patient-Identifying Information Only

The confidentiality regulations permit programs to disclose information about patients if the program reveals no patient-identifying information. As noted above, this permits a program to give researchers aggregate data about its population or some portion of its population. For example, a program could tell researchers that during the past year, 42 patients completed treatment, 67 dropped out in less than 6 months, and 25 left between 6 and 12 months. Programs subject to HIPAA can disclose de-identified health nformation to researchers (§§164.502(d); 164.514) (28). Programs subject to HIPAA must comply with that standard, because it is more stringent.

Option 2: The Research Exception

Programs covered by the confidentiality regulations but not the HIPAA regulations) can disclose patient-dentifying information to persons conducting "scientific esearch" under certain conditions, including the program director determining that the researcher (a) is qualified o conduct the research, (b) has a protocol under which patient-identifying information will be kept in accordance with the regulations' security provisions (29), and (c) has provided a written statement from a group of three or more ndependent individuals who have reviewed the protocol and determined that it protects patients' rights (§2.52).

The confidentiality regulations prohibit researchers from identifying any individual patient in any report or otherwise disclosing any patient identities except back to he program (30). This provision is particularly important when a research design calls for followup research with the patient or collateral sources.

Providers subject to the HIPAA regulations must combine the mandates of the confidentiality regulations with

those of HIPAA. Programs subject to both sets of regulations may make disclosures of protected health information to researchers if they obtain documentation from the researcher that an Institutional Review Board (IRB) (31) or "privacy board" (32) has approved a waiver of the patient "authorization" (consent) otherwise required for use or disclosure of protected health information. The documentation must:

1. Identify the IRB or privacy board.
2. State the date on which it acted.
3. Include a statement that the IRB or privacy board has determined that disclosure of protected health information without patients' consent/authorization satisfies all of the following criteria:
   - The use or disclosure of protected health information involves no more than minimal risk to patients, based on, at least, the following:
     - There is an adequate plan to protect the identifiers from improper use and disclosure.
     - There is an adequate plan to destroy the identifiers at the earliest opportunity consistent with the research.
     - There are adequate written assurances that: (a) the protected health information will not be reused or disclosed, except for authorized oversight of the research project or back to the program from which the information was obtained; (b) the protected health information will be maintained in accordance with the security requirements of 42 CFR §2.16 (or more stringent requirements); and (c) no patient's identity will be disclosed (except back to the program) and no individual patient will be identified in any report of the research (33).
   - The research could not practicably be conducted if patients' authorization (consent) were required.
   - The research could not practicably be conducted without access to and use of the protected health information.
4. Describe the protected health information for which use or access has been determined to be necessary (34).
5. Describe the mandated procedures used by the IRB or the privacy board to make its determination.
6. Be signed by the chair or member designated by the chair (35).

Documentation of the actions of the IRB or privacy board must be retained for 6 years (§164.530(j)). If the program plans to disclose protected health information without patients' consent for research purposes, it must inform patients of this practice in the Notice it distributes (see *Patient Notice* below).

Option 3: Consent

Researchers can also obtain patient-identifying information if the patient has signed a valid consent form that has not expired or been revoked (§2.31). The consent form must include the nine required elements discussed previously. Programs subject to HIPAA must add the statements those regulations require:

- A statement that the patient may refuse to sign the consent (authorization).
- A statement that the program will not condition the provision of treatment on the patient's signing the form (unless the treatment is research related) (36).

In completing the consent form, thought must be given to the purpose of the disclosure and the kind and amount of information to be disclosed. Two examples follow.

- *Illustration A*—A researcher wants to study length of stay in different treatment programs. If the researcher decides to ask patients to give written consent to disclosure of this information, the researcher would specify the purpose of the disclosure as "verification of length of treatment" and the amount and kind of information to be disclosed as "enrollment and termination dates." The disclosure would then be limited to informing the researcher of the dates of enrollment and termination for each patient.
- *Illustration B*—If the researcher wanted to study not only the length of stay but also the reasons for termination from treatment, the researcher would specify the purpose of the disclosure as "determination of length of treatment and reasons for termination" and the amount and kind of information to be disclosed as "enrollment and termination dates and reasons for termination."

The consent form must have an expiration date or event. Information released to researchers must be accompanied by the required notice against redisclosing information (§2.32).

Followup Research

Followup research of former patients presents a particular challenge under the confidentiality regulations. A program—or a researcher to whom it has disclosed patient data—may only attempt to contact a patient if it can do so without disclosing the patient's relationship with the treatment program to third persons. Accordingly, no inquiries—whether to relatives, friends, employers, or others—designed to locate a former patient may be conducted unless they can be carried out in a way that will not reveal the individual's status as a former drug or alcohol abuse patient or unless the patient has signed a proper consent form under the regulations (37).

OTHER RULES ABOUT PATIENTS' RIGHT TO CONFIDENTIALITY

Patient Notice

The confidentiality regulations require programs to notify patients of their right to confidentiality and to give them a written summary of the regulations' provisions. The notice and summary should be provided at admission or "as soon thereafter as the patient is capable of rational communication" (§2.22(a)).

Programs subject to HIPAA must provide patients with additional notice about their rights and how to exercise those rights. Alcohol and drug treatment providers covered by both HIPAA and 42 CFR may combine the notice requirements of the two regulations into one document. The notice required by HIPAA must contain the following:

1. A statement, prominently displayed: "THIS NOTICE DESCRIBES HOW MEDICAL INFORMATION ABOUT YOU MAY BE USED AND DISCLOSED AND HOW YOU CAN GET ACCESS TO THIS INFORMATION. PLEASE REVIEW IT CAREFULLY."
2. A description in sufficient detail of the types of uses and disclosures that the provider may make of protected health care information without the patient's consent. For substance-abuse treatment programs, these are identical to the list of exceptions contained in 42 CFR §2.22(b) and in the sample notice (§2.22(d)), with the following additions:
   - The program's staff will use the patient's protected health information to communicate among themselves in connection with their provision of diagnosis or treatment for substance abuse and for payment and health care operations.
   - The program will disclose the patient's protected health information to qualified service organizations (business associates) providing services for the program's treatment, payment, and health care operations.
   - The program may disclose the patient's protected health information to researchers, if the patient consents or if the information will be protected as required by confidentiality regulations [if applicable].
3. A statement that other disclosures will be made only with the patient's written authorization or consent, which can be revoked, unless the program has taken action in reliance on it.
4. A statement that the program may contact the patient to provide appointment reminders or information about treatment alternatives or other health-related benefits and services, if the provider intends to engage in any of these activities. (An alcohol or drug program engaging in these kinds of activities must be careful not to make any patient-identifying disclosures to others.)
5. A statement that the program is required by law to maintain the privacy of protected health information and to notify patients of its legal duties and privacy practices, including any changes to its policies. (The program must also state how it will provide patients with a revised notice of its practices.)
6. A statement that the program must abide by the terms of the notice currently in effect; a statement that the

program reserves the right to change the terms of the notice and to make the new notice provisions effective for all information it maintains; (38) and a statement describing how it will provide clients with a revised notice of its practices.

7. The name or title and telephone number of a person or office the client can contact for further information.

8. A statement of the patient's rights with respect to protected health information and a brief description of how the patient may exercise those rights, including
   - The right to request restrictions on certain uses and disclosures of protected health information; however, the program is not required to agree with requested restrictions.
   - The right to access and amend protected health information.
   - The right to receive confidential communications of protected health information (such as having mail and telephone calls be limited to home or office).
   - The right to receive an accounting of the provider's disclosures of protected health information.
   - The right to complain—free from retaliation—to the provider and to the secretary of DHHS about violations of privacy rights.
   - The right to obtain a paper copy of the notice upon request.

9. The effective date of the notice (§164.530(g)).

The notice must be provided to clients upon request and in any case to each client no later than the date of the first service delivery (including service delivered electronically). (Similarly, §2.22 of the confidentiality regulations requires distribution of that notice on admission or as soon thereafter as the client is capable of rational communication.) The program must also have the notice available on site for clients to request to take with them and posted in a clear and prominent location where it is reasonable to expect clients to be able to read it. Whenever the notice is revised, the program must make it available (including posting) on request or after the effective date of the revision (§§164.520(c); 164.520(c)(2)(ii)). A program that maintains a web site that provides information about its services or benefits must prominently post its notice on the site and make it available electronically through the site. When clients agree, the program can provide the notice by e-mail (§164.520(c)(3)).

The program must make a good faith effort to obtain patients' written acknowledgment of the receipt of the notice of privacy practices (§164.520(c)(2)(ii)) (39). Whenever the program materially changes any of its privacy practices, it must promptly revise its notice accordingly. (The program may not implement a material change to any term in its notice prior to the effective date of its revised notice.) When the notice is revised, the program must make it available on request or after the effective date of the revision (§164.520(b)). The program must retain a copy of each notice it issues for 6 years from the time it was last

in effect (§§164.520(e); 164.520(j)). It must also retain documentation of patients' acknowledgment of receipt of the notice (or its good faith efforts to obtain patients' acknowledgment) for a period of 6 years (§§164.520(e); 164.520(j)).

New Rights Established by HIPAA

The HIPAA regulations give patients of covered programs three new federal privacy rights: the right to request restrictions of uses and disclosures, the right to access records, the right to amend records, and the right to an accounting of disclosures of records. It also requires programs to establish a procedure for patients to complain about its privacy practices and to name a contact person to whom patients can take complaints.

The Right to Request a Restriction of Uses and Disclosures

HIPAA requires that programs allow patients to request that the program restrict uses and disclosures of protected health information within the program and disclosures of protected health information to others for the purpose of health care operations (§164.522(a)(1)(i)); however, the program is not required to agree to a requested restriction (§164.522(a)(1)(ii)). If a program does agree to a restriction, it may not then violate the agreement, except for emergency treatment purposes (in which case, the program must request that the emergency treatment provider not further use or disclose the PHI (§164.522(a)(1)(iii)–(iv); §2.51)). A program may terminate the agreement to a restriction, effective after the client has been informed of the termination (§164.522(a)(2)(iii)).

HIPAA also requires programs to accommodate a client's reasonable request that communication of PHI be done by alternative means or to alternative locations (§164.522(b)(1)(i)). For example, a client might request that mail and telephone calls be limited to a home or office location.

The Right to Access Records

HIPAA creates a new federal right for patients in covered programs to inspect and copy their own protected health information (including information created before HIPAA's compliance date of April 2003) in the form or format they request (§164.524) (40). If the patient agrees in advance, the program may provide an explanation or summary of the requested information (41). A program may require the request to be in writing, but must inform patients of this requirement in advance.

Two kinds of records are exempt from the right of access:

- Psychotherapy notes (42)
- Information compiled in reasonable anticipation of or

for use in a civil, criminal, or administrative action or proceeding

Patients involved in clinical trials do not have a right of access until the trial terminates if they agreed to this condition when they consented to participate in the trial (§164.524(a)(2)(iii)) (43).

A program covered by HIPAA must respond to a patient's request for access to his or her records within 30 days if the information is maintained or accessible on site (and within 60 days if the information is not maintained on site). The program may extend the deadline by not more than 30 days by providing the patient with a written statement of the reasons for the delay and the date by which it will permit access.

If a program grants the patient's request for access to his or her records, it can charge the patient a reasonable, cost-based fee for providing a copy, explanation, or summary of the health information. (The fee may not include any charge for retrieving or handling the information.)

A program may deny a patient access on the following grounds:

- It does not maintain the requested information. (If the program knows where the requested information is maintained, it must inform the patient where to direct the request.)
- The requested information was obtained under a promise of confidentiality from someone other than a health care provider and such access would be likely to reveal the source of the information.
- A licensed health care professional has determined, in the exercise of professional judgment, that the access requested is reasonably likely to endanger the life or physical safety of the patient or another person. The preamble to the HIPAA regulations notes that this exception is limited to circumstances when a patient exhibits homicidal or suicidal tendencies and the licensed health care professional determines that permitting inspection or copying of some of the protected health information is reasonably likely to result in the patient committing suicide, homicide, or other physical violence. Providers may not deny access because the information is sensitive or has a potential for causing emotional or psychological harm.
- The information makes reference to another person (other than a health care provider) and a licensed health care professional has determined, in the exercise of professional judgment, that the inspection and copying is reasonably likely to cause substantial harm to such other person. (This provision permits the program to exclude information about another person if release of the information is reasonably likely to cause that person substantial physical, emotional, or psychological harm.)
- The request for access is made by the patient's personal representative and a licensed health care professional has determined, in the exercise of professional judgment,

that the provision of access to such personal representative is reasonably likely to cause substantial harm to the patient or another individual. (This provision permits the program to deny access to a personal representative if it has a reasonable belief that the patient has been or will be subject to domestic violence, abuse, or neglect or that access by the personal representative may endanger the patient or another person.)

If the program's denial is based on one of the last three reasons, the patient has the right to have that denial reviewed by a licensed health care professional who is designated by the program and who did not participate in the original decision to deny access.

If the program denies a patient access to all or part of his or her protected health information, it must give him or her, a timely written statement in plain language containing

- The basis for the denial.
- If applicable, a statement of the patient's review rights, including a description of how the patient may exercise those rights.
- A description of how the patient may complain to the program or to the Secretary of DHHS.

When a patient requests review, the program must designate a licensed health care professional to act as the reviewer. The reviewer must not have been involved in the original decision to deny access. The program must provide the patient with written notice of the reviewer's decision.

A program that denies a patient access, in whole or in part, must give the patient access to any other protected health information requested after excluding the information to which the program had reason to deny access.

Programs not subject to HIPAA can use their own judgment to decide when to permit patients to view or obtain copies of their records, unless state law requires such access. Neither HIPAA nor the confidentiality regulations require programs to obtain written consent from patients before permitting them to see their own records.

The Right to Amend Records

The HIPAA regulations give patients the right to amend their own protected health information (§164.526). The program may require that patients make requests for amendment in writing and provide a reason to support a requested amendment, if it informs patients of these requirements in advance. The program must act on a patient's request for amendment within 60 days after it receives the request. The program may extend the deadline by not more than 30 days by, within the 60 days, providing the patient with a written statement of the reasons for the delay and the date by which it will respond.

A program that accepts a patient's request to amend protected health care information must:

- Notify the patient of its decision to amend the information in a timely manner.
- Make the appropriate amendment by, at a minimum, identifying the records in the designated record set that are affected by the amendment and appending or otherwise providing a link to the location of the amendment; and
- If the patient consents, make reasonable efforts to notify and provide the amendment within a reasonable period of time to:
  - Persons (including organizations or other entities) the patient identifies as having received the PHI that is the subject of the amendment and needing the amendment; and
  - Persons (including business associates) that the program knows have received the PHI that is the subject of the amendment and that may have been relied on, or could foreseeably rely on such information to the detriment of the patient (44).

A program must obtain the patient's consent on forms that comply with 42 CFR §2.31 before it provides any copies of the amendment to other persons or organizations.

A program may deny a patient's request to amend his or her records if, among other reasons, it determines that it did not create the information (45), that the information or record is accurate and complete, or that the protected health information that is the subject of the request is not part of a designated record set or would not otherwise be available for inspection. If a program denies a patient's request to amend records, it must give the patient a timely, written statement containing:

- The basis for its denial of the patient's request.
- Notice of the patient's right to file a written statement of disagreement with the denial and how the patient may file such a statement.
- Notice that if the patient does not submit a statement of disagreement, the patient may request that the program include his or her request for amendment and its denial with any future disclosures of the protected health information.
- A description of how the patient may complain about the program's actions to the program or to the Secretary of DHHS.

If the patient files a statement of disagreement with the denial and the basis of such disagreement, the program must identify the disputed amendment and include its own statement of denial and the patient's statement of disagreement with any subsequent disclosure of the information. The program may also offer a rebuttal to the patient's statement of disagreement in subsequent disclosures. If it does so, it must provide a copy to the patient. This information must all be included in any subsequent disclosures of the protected health information to which the disagreement relates.

The program must document the titles of the persons or offices responsible for receiving and processing requests for amendment. It must retain the documentation for 6 years from the date it was last effective (§164.530(j)).

The Right to an Accounting of Disclosures

Patients have a right to obtain an accounting of all disclosures of protected health information made by a program during the 6 years prior to the request (§164.528). The accounting must include:

- The date of each disclosure.
- The name and address (if known) of the organization or person who received the protected health information.
- A brief description of the information disclosed.
- A brief statement of the purpose of the disclosure or a copy of the written request for disclosure.

The regulations permit summary accounting of recurrent disclosures (§164.528((b)(3)).

Exceptions

Programs do not have to provide an accounting for any disclosures that were made:

- To the patient personally.
- Before April 14, 2003.
- Pursuant to an authorization (consent) by the patient.
- For treatment, payment, and "health care operations."

What would go into an accounting? For substance-abuse treatment programs, the answer is easy:

- Disclosures to health oversight agencies (46)
- Disclosures to researchers that include patient-identifying information
- Disclosures to public health authorities
- Court-ordered disclosures
- Reports of patient crimes on program premises or against program personnel
- Child abuse and neglect reports (47)

Programs should establish mechanisms to document all disclosures for which they must account.

The accounting must be made within 60 days of the program's receipt of the request. The program may extend the deadline by not more than 30 days by, within the 60 days, providing the patient with a written statement of the reasons for the delay and the date by which it will comply with the request. A program must respond to a patient's request for one accounting within any 12-month period without charge. For any subsequent request within a 12-month period, the program may charge a patient a reasonable, cost-based fee. If it imposes a fee, the program must inform the patient of the fee in advance and give the patient an opportunity to withdraw or modify the request.

The program must also document the following:

- The information it was required to provide the patient.
- The written accounting it provided the patient.
- The titles of the persons or offices responsible for receiving and processing requests for an accounting (§164.528(d)).

The documentation must be retained for 6 years (§164.530(j)).

The Right to Complain about the Program's Privacy Practices

The HIPAA regulations require programs to establish procedures for handling complaints about (a) their privacy policies and procedures; (b) their compliance with their privacy policies and procedures; and (c) their compliance with the HIPAA regulations (§164.530(d)(2)) (§164.530(d)). The program must document complaints and their disposition and retain the documentation for 6 years (§164.530(d)(2)). The program also has to identify a contact person to receive complaints.

SECURITY OF RECORDS

The Confidentiality Regulations' Requirements

The confidentiality regulations require programs to keep written records in a secure room, a locked file cabinet, a safe, or other similar container. (Section 1173(d) of HIPAA requires programs to maintain reasonable and appropriate safeguards to ensure the integrity and confidentiality of information and protect against reasonably anticipated threats or hazards to the security or integrity of the information.) Programs must establish written procedures that regulate access to and use of patients' records. Either the program director or a single staff person should be designated to process inquiries and requests for information (§2.16).

The issue of security is addressed in more detail through a separate Security Rule issued by HHS on February 20, 2003, that establishes the physical and technical security standards required to guard the integrity, confidentiality and availability of confidential information that is electronically stored, maintained or transmitted. Programs subject to HIPAA must be in compliance with the Security Rule by April 20, 2005. (*Federal Register* 68:84334). Compliance is required by April 20, 2005. The final Security Rule can be accessed at a257.g.akamaitech.net/7/257/2422/14mar20010800/ edocket.access.gpo.gov/2003/03-3877.htm or a257.g. akamaitech.net/7/257/2422/14mar20010800/edocket. access.gpo.gov/2003/pdf/03-3877.pdf.

The HIPAA Regulations' Requirements

HIPAA requires covered programs to do all the following:

- Designate a privacy official who is responsible for the development and implementation of its policies and procedures (§164.530(a)).
- Establish and maintain appropriate administrative, technical, and physical safeguards to protect the privacy of protected health information (§164.530(c)). These include isolating and locking file cabinets or records rooms and shredding records being discarded.
- Train all members of the workforce on the program's policies and procedures. (The initial training must take place by April 2003.) Each new member of the workforce must receive training within a reasonable period of time after that person joins the workforce. Whenever a workforce member's functions are affected by a material change in policies or procedures, that person must receive additional training within a reasonable period of time. The program must document all training and retain the records for a period of 6 years after the training (§164.530(b)).
- Establish policies and procedures that identify the staff persons or classes of persons who need access to clients' protected health information, the categories of protected health information they need access to, and any conditions appropriate to such access. The program must make reasonable efforts to limit access based on these determinations (see §164.514(d)(z)).
- Establish policies and procedures to ensure that, for disclosures of information that occur on a routine and recurring basis, reasonable efforts are made to limit disclosures to the minimum necessary to accomplish the intended purpose of the disclosure (§§164.502(b); 164.514(d)(3)(i)). For "all other disclosures," the program must develop criteria designed to limit the protected health information to that information reasonably necessary to accomplish the purpose for which disclosure is sought; the program must review requests for disclosure on an individual basis in accordance with those criteria (§164.514(d)(3)(ii)). Programs must also develop policies, procedures, and criteria to ensure that requests for protected health information made to other entities subject to HIPAA are limited to information "which is reasonably necessary to accomplish the purpose for which the request is made" (§164.514(d)(4)).
- Establish and apply appropriate sanctions against members of its workforce who fail to comply with its privacy policies and procedures (§164.530(e)).
- Mitigate, to the extent practicable, any harmful effect that is known to the program that results from a use or disclosure in violation of its policies and procedures (§164.530(f)).
- Refrain from taking intimidating, threatening, coercive, discriminatory, or other retaliatory action against any client who exercises rights under the HIPAA regulations, including filing a complaint, assisting in an investigation, compliance review, proceeding or hearing, or opposing an act or practice made unlawful by the HIPAA regulations, provided that the client has a good

faith belief that the practice is unlawful and the manner of opposition is reasonable and does not invoke an impermissible disclosure of protected health information (§164.530(g)).
- Refrain from requiring clients to waive their rights to complain to the Secretary of HHS or their other rights under the HIPAA regulations as a condition of treatment (§164.530(h)).
- Implement policies and procedures regarding protected health information that are designed to comply with all the standards, implementation specifications, and other requirements of the HIPAA regulations, and maintain the policies and procedures in written or electronic form for 6 (six) years from the date the document was created, or last effective, whichever is later (§164.530(i) and (j)).

Electronic Records and Security

Computerization of records complicates efforts to ensure security of patients' information—within the program as well as outside the program. The ease and speed of access to computerized information carries the distinct risk that medical or psychological information entered by a counselor will be obtained by a person or entity who is not authorized to receive it. Until recently, protection was afforded by the cumbersome and inefficient way many, if not most, records made their way from a treatment provider in one setting to a health care provider in another. Computerized records, by contrast, may allow anyone with a disk and access to the computer in which the information is stored to instantly copy and carry away vast amounts of information without anyone's knowledge. It is critical, therefore, that programs installing computerized record-keeping systems design them with security in mind. Among the specific issues programs should consider are the following:

- Compliance with expiration dates and revocations of consent. Programs should devise mechanisms to make certain that there is no disclosure of patients' records once consent forms expire or consent is revoked.
- Maintenance of internal security. Section 2.16 requires programs to store paper records in a locked file cabinet or room and to adopt written procedures to regulate and control access to and use of written records. Programs must meet the same standards when records are computerized. Computerized case records must be secured with passwords and other protective mechanisms that limit access to staff members who need information about specific patients in connection with their duties. If records are stored or "backed up" on removable hard drives, tapes, or compact, Zip, or floppy disks, those storage units must be locked in a safe place when not in use. Audit trails can be useful in deterring staff from browsing through computerized records. The security rule addresses these concerns.
- Appropriate storage and destruction of old data. Programs holding paper case records of former patients

often remove inactive case files and store them in a less-accessible area for a period before destroying them. The fact that case files stored on computer disk or other media take up little space may make it tempting for programs to hold patient-identifying information indefinitely. This presents a threat to patients' privacy. Case files of former patients that are stored on computer or backed up on other media should be stored separately from active case files and deleted when their existence is no longer required by law or regulation.
- Protection from external threats to security. Transfer of patient-identifying information between computers linked by telephone or cable or other technologies extends the possibility of unauthorized access to anyone with a modem, the passwords, and the necessary software. Programs must maintain adequate security, including use of a firewall, encryption, and other systems designed to prevent unauthorized remote access. The security rule addresses this issue.

The security provisions of the confidentiality regulations and HIPAA also affect how programs deal with other instruments of modern technology, such as voice mail, e-mail, cellular telephones, fax machines, and personal digital assistants.

A FINAL NOTE

Substance abuse programs should try to find a lawyer familiar with local laws affecting their problems. State law governs many concerns relating to confidentiality, privacy, and privileged information. A practicing lawyer with expertise is the best source for advice, particularly because in many areas, the law continues to develop. Programs trying to decide how to handle difficult situations need up-to-the-minute advice on their legal responsibilities (48).

Notes

1. This chapter provides an introduction to the legal requirements federal laws and regulations impose on those providing alcohol- or drug-abuse assessment or treatment in the area of confidentiality of patient records. The chapter deals only with federal laws and regulations. In the area of confidentiality and professional responsibility, state law also often applies. Legal rules and requirements are subject to change; therefore, any understanding of the legal requirements in this area must be periodically updated. Anyone who needs legal advice should consult an attorney familiar with both state and federal law.
2. Citations in the form "§2 . . ." refer to specific sections of 42 CFR Part 2.
3. §2.12(b). The regulations do not apply to records maintained by the Veterans' Administration and, in certain cases, the Armed Forces (§2.12(c)(1) and (2)).
4. Citations in the form "§164 . . ." refer to sections of the HIPAA regulations.

5. "Health care operations" are activities of the program that are related to its function of providing substance abuse treatment and include general administrative and business functions necessary for the program to remain a viable business. Health care operations include (a) quality assessment and improvement activities (including outcomes evaluation and development of clinical guidelines, provided that the primary objective is not the production of generalizable knowledge); (b) reviewing the competence or qualifications of health care professionals, evaluating practitioner and provider performance, conducting training programs in which students, trainees, or practitioners in areas of health care learn under supervision to practice or improve their skills as health care providers, and training non-health care professionals; (c) participating in accreditation, certification, licensing or credentialing activities; (d) arranging for or conducting medical review, audits, and legal services (including compliance programs); and (e) business planning and management or general administrative activities, including resolution of internal grievances (§164.501).

6. However, no information obtained from a program may be used in a criminal investigation or prosecution of a patient unless a court order has been issued under the special circumstances set forth in §2.65; 42 USC §290dd-2(c); 42 CFR §2.12(a), (d).

7. The regulations state that "acting in reliance" includes providing services in reliance on a consent form permitting disclosures to a third-party payor (§2.31(a)(8)). Thus, a program can bill the third-party payor for past services to the patient even after consent has been revoked. However, a program that continues to provide services after a patient has revoked a consent authorizing disclosure to a third-party payor cannot thereafter bill the third-party payor.

8. "Parent" here means the parent, guardian, or other person legally responsible for the minor. The confidentiality regulations leave the issue of who is a minor and whether a minor can obtain alcohol or drug abuse treatment without parental consent entirely to state laws.

9. There are special rules to deal with incompetent and deceased patients (§2.15).

10. "This information has been disclosed to you from records protected by Federal confidentiality rules (42 CFR part 2). The Federal rules prohibit you from making any further disclosure of this information unless further disclosure is expressly permitted by the written consent of the person to whom it pertains or as otherwise permitted by 42 CFR Part 2. A general authorization for the release of medical or other information is NOT sufficient for this purpose. The Federal rules restrict any use of the information to criminally investigate or prosecute any alcohol or drug abuse patient." (§2.32)

11. HIPAA provides for mandatory disclosures to both the patient and to the secretary of DHHS, when the Secretary seeks the information to investigate or determine the program's compliance with HIPAA. The confidentiality regulations permit disclosures to patients of their own records without written consent. Disclosures to the secretary can be made under the "audit and evaluation exception" explained below.

12. It is rare that a program would be requesting a patient to sign a consent form to enable it to disclose information for its "health care operations." See the definition in note 5.

13. HIPAA permits health care providers to "use or disclose protected health information for their own treatment, payment, or health care operations" (§§164.506(c)(1), 164.502(a)(1)(ii)) without obtaining patients' consent or authorization. Programs subject to 42 CFR Part 2, however, must continue to obtain patients' consent in compliance with that stricter rule. Because programs seek information about patients from collateral or referral sources in order to provide quality treatment, they are not required to add the "voluntariness statement" required by §164.508(c)(2)(ii) of the HIPAA regulations to the consent form required by 42 CFR §2.31.

14. HIPAA defines treatment to include "the provision, coordination, or management of health care and related services by one or more health care providers, including the coordination or management of health care by a health care provider with a third party; [and] consultation between health care providers relating to a patient" (§164.501). HIPAA permits these activities without patients' consent. However, substance abuse treatment programs must continue to follow the stricter rule of the confidentiality regulations and obtain patients' consent.

15. HIPAA defines "treatment" to include "the referral of a patient for health care from one health care provider to another" (§164.501) and permits referrals without patients' consent. However, substance abuse treatment programs must continue to follow the confidentiality regulations' stricter rule and obtain patients' consent before making referrals. (The exception to this rule is discussed in *"Communications That Do Not Disclose Patient Identify Information"* on page 1369 and note 19.)

16. Although the rules concerning criminal justice system consent probably apply to proceedings in juvenile court involving acts that, if committed by an adult, would be a crime, there appear to be no cases on point. It is less likely that the special criminal justice system consent rules would apply when an adolescent is adjudicated (found to be) in need of special supervision (e.g., "a person in need of supervision"), but not guilty of a criminal act.

17. "Patient-identifying information" is defined in §2.11

and includes an individual's name, address, social security number, and any other information from which a patient's identity can be determined either directly or by reference to other public information.

18. HIPAA permits programs that are part of a larger facility that treats conditions other than substance abuse to continue to make calls to other health care providers in order to refer patients (so long as the patients' substance abuse treatment is not disclosed). HIPAA includes such calls in its definition of "treatment," and does not require health care providers to get patients' consent or authorization before using or disclosing information for its own treatment activities or the treatment activities of another health care provider (§164.506(c)(1) and (2)).

19. For information about how to deal with communications with lawyers, law enforcement officials, and subpoenas, see "Appendix B: Legal and Ethical Issues," in *A Guide to Substance Abuse Services for Primary Care Clinicians,* Treatment Improvement Protocol 24. Rockville, MD: The Center for Substance Abuse Treatment, 1997:111–112. For information about how to deal with arrest or search warrants, see "Legal and Ethical Issues" in *Intensive Outpatient, Treatment Improvement Protocol 8.* Rockville, MD: The Center for Substance Abuse Treatment (*in press*).

20. However, no notice to the patient is required if an order is sought to authorize disclosure and use of records to criminally investigate or prosecute a patient (§2.65) and no notice at all is required if an order is sought to authorize disclosure and use of records to investigate or prosecute a program or the person holding records (§2.66).

21. The regulations do not permit courts to order researchers "who have received patient-identifying information without consent for the purpose of conducting research, audit or evaluation, to disclose that information or to use it to conduct any criminal investigation or prosecution of a patient" (§2.62).

22. The confidentiality regulations contain special provisions regarding court orders authorizing disclosures for purposes of investigating or prosecuting a program or its employees (§2.66) and court orders authorizing a government agency to place an undercover agent or informant in a program to gather evidence of serious criminal conduct by the program or its employees (§2.67). The regulations set strict prerequisites for obtaining such orders and prohibit the use of information obtained through these means against patients.

23. The HIPAA regulations define "business associate" as a person or organization that acts on behalf of a program and performs or assists in the performance of a function or activity involving the use or disclosure of individually identifiable health information (such as claims processing, data analysis, processing or administration, use review, quality assurance, billing, benefit management, and practice management) or provides legal, actuarial, accounting, consulting, data aggregation, management, administrative, accreditation, or financial services to or for the program, where the provision of the service involves the disclosure of individually identifiable health information. A business associate is not a member of the program's staff or workforce.

24. The definition of "health care operations" appears in note 5.

25. Under HIPAA, a health oversight agency is a governmental "agency or authority that is authorized by law to oversee the health care system or government programs in which health information is necessary to determine eligibility or compliance or to enforce civil rights laws . . ." (§164.501).

26. HIPAA defines "de-identified health information" as information that "does not identify an individual and with respect to which there is no reasonable basis to believe that the information can be used to identify an individual." A program may determine that health information is "de-identified" only if identifiers specified in the HIPAA regulations are removed or a person with appropriate knowledge of statistical and scientific principles and methods documents that there is only a very small risk that the information could be used by an anticipated recipient to identify a patient, alone or in combination with other reasonably available information (§164.514).

27. See note 17 for a definition of "patient-identifying information."

28. See note 26 for a definition of de-identified health information.

29. Section 2.16 requires programs to keep written records in a secure room, a locked file cabinet, a safe, or other similar container.

30. Two additional federal laws permit the United States attorney general and the secretary of DHHS to authorize researchers to withhold the names and identities of research subjects. Once such authorization is issued, the researcher "may not be compelled in any federal, state or local civil, criminal, administrative, legislative or other proceeding to identify" research subjects (42 USC §241(d) [permits the secretary of DHHS to issue confidentiality certificates]; 21 USC §872(c) [permits the attorney general to issue confidentiality certificates]).

31. An IRB must be established in accordance with federal law.

32. A privacy board must be made up of members with varying backgrounds and appropriate professional competency to review the effect of the research protocol on the patient's privacy rights; and it must include at least one member who is not affiliated with the researcher conducting or sponsoring the research (§164.512(i)).

33. These last two provisions come from 42 CFR §2.52.

34. This must be the minimum necessary to fulfill the purposes of the research project.

35. HIPAA permits providers to avoid this process and use or disclose protected health information if (a) use or disclosure is sought solely to review protected health information to prepare a research protocol or for similar purposes preparatory to research, (b) no protected health information is removed from the program, and (c) the protected health information is necessary for research purposes (§164.512(i)(1)(ii)). Only de-identified protected health information may be recorded by the researchers. Programs would still have to comply with the requirements of §2.52.

36. HIPAA contains special rules about consent when the protected health information that is to be used or disclosed has been created for research that includes treatment, as in clinical trials (§164.508(b)(4)(i)).

37. For a discussion of how followup research can be conducted, see "Legal and Ethical Issues" in *Intensive Outpatient, Treatment Improvement Protocol 8*. Rockville, MD: The Center for Substance Abuse Treatment (*in press*).

38. This statement is optional. However, if the program does not include this statement in the notice, when it changes any privacy practice, it can apply the changed practice only to information newly created or received. This will require it to segregate its records according to the notice in effect at the time the records were created (§164.520(b)(1)(v)(c)).

39. There is an exception for emergency situations; see §164.520(c)(2)(ii). DHHS prefers that health care providers obtain patients' signatures, but does not require that the signature be obtained on a copy of the notice itself; a patient may also sign or initial a separate sheet. If a patient refuses to provide a written acknowledgment that he has received the notice, the program must document its efforts and the reason it failed (§164.520(c)(2)(ii)). The reason can be that the patient refused to sign. See 67 *Fed Reg* 14784.

40. The confidentiality regulations permit programs to provide access (§2.23).

41. The HIPAA regulations require access to protected health information in a "designated record set." That term is defined as "[a] group of records maintained by or for a [program] that is: (1) The medical records and billing records about individuals maintained by or for a covered health care provider; [or] ... (3) Used, in whole or in part, by or for the covered entity to make decisions about [patients]" §164.501. The program must document the designated record sets that are subject to access and the titles of the persons or offices responsible for receiving and processing requests for access (§164.524(e)). It must retain the documentation for 6 years from the date it was last effective (§164.530(j)).

42. The HIPAA regulations define "psychotherapy notes" as "notes recorded (in any medium) by a health care provider who is a mental health professional documenting or analyzing the contents of conversation during a private counseling session or a group, joint, or family counseling session and that are separated from the rest of the individual's medical record."

43. Programs in correctional facilities or acting under the direction of correctional facilities are subject to different rules (§164.524(a)(2)(ii)).

44. If the program receives a notification of amended protected health information from another health care provider, it must make the necessary amendment in the designated record sets it maintains.

45. However, if the patient provides a reasonable basis to believe that the originator of the protected health information is no longer available to act on the request, the program must address the request for amendment as though it had created the information.

46. Programs must exclude disclosures to a health oversight agency or to law enforcement officials from the accounting, if the agency/official provides the program with a statement that inclusion of the disclosure(s) in the accounting would be reasonably likely to impede the agency or the official's activities. The statement must specify how long the information must be excluded. At the end of that period, the program must include the disclosures in an accounting to the patient. If the statement of the agency/official is oral, the exclusion may last no longer than 30 days and the program must document the identity of the official or agency who made the statement. If the agency/official provides a statement in writing, the exclusion must last for the time period specified in the written statement. Disclosures required to be made to the Secretary of DHHS to investigate or determine the program is complying with HIPAA are also exempt.

47. Although the HIPAA regulations require health care providers to account for disclosures to "business associates," disclosures for the purposes of "health care operations" are exempt. Because the only disclosures programs can make to a business associate (qualified service organization) are disclosures for the purpose of health care operations (providing services to the program), programs do not have to include such disclosures in responding to patients' requests for accounting.

48. See "Legal and Ethical Issues" in *Intensive Outpatient, Treatment Improvement Protocol 8*. Rockville, MD: The Center for Substance Abuse Treatment (*in press*) for general discussion of such issues as "duty to warn," reporting criminal activity, arrest and search warrants, patients' driving while impaired, discharging unstable patients, and patients' risk-taking behavior.

CHAPTER 88

Clinical and Societal Implications of Drug Legalization

HERBERT D. KLEBER AND JAMES A. INCIARDI

The drug legalization debate is not particularly new. It did not begin during election year 2002 with the numerous proposals to modify state constitutions to remove the possession of marijuana from the criminal law. It did not begin with former Surgeon General Jocelyn Elders' off-the-cuff remark at the close of 1993 that "I do feel that we would markedly reduce our crime rate if drugs were legalized." Nor did it begin in 1988 when at a meeting of the U.S. Conference of Mayors, Baltimore Mayor Kurt L. Schmoke called for a national debate on American drug control strategies and the potential benefits of legalizing marijuana, heroin, cocaine, crack, and other illicit substances. Although it has received the most media attention since the late 1980s, the debate has been on-again, off-again for the better part of a century. Its most recent rendering reflects a potpourri of loosely conceptualized suggestions involving "legalization" and "decriminalization" at one end of the continuum, to "medicalization" and "harm reduction" at the other.

Briefly, the basic argument for legalizing drugs is that America's "War on Drugs" has been a miserable failure, emphasizing that the drug laws have created evils far worse than the drugs themselves (corruption, violence, street crime, and disrespect for the law), and the laws passed to control drugs have failed to reduce demand. By contrast, if marijuana, cocaine, heroin, and other drugs were legalized, some positive things would happen: (a) drug prices would fall; (b) users could obtain their drugs at low, government-regulated prices and would no longer be forced to engage in prostitution and street crime to support their habits; (c) levels of drug-related crime would significantly decline, resulting in less-crowded courts, jails, and prisons, and free law enforcement personnel free to focus their energies on the "real criminals" in society; (d) drug production, distribution, and sale would be removed from the criminal arena; no longer would it be within the province of organized crime, and thus, such criminal syndicates as the Colombian and Mexican cocaine cartels, the Jamaican posses, and the various "mafias" around the country and the world would be decapitalized, and the violence associated with drug-distribution rivalries would be eliminated; and (e) the often draconian measures undertaken by police

to enforce the drug laws would be curtailed, thus restoring to the American public many of its hard-won civil liberties (1–3).

The counterargument from those opposed to legalizing drugs is that the drug prohibition has been extremely effective in limiting drug abuse. Furthermore, it is maintained that legalizing drugs would likely initiate a major public health problem characterized by increased abuse and addiction, drug-related health problems, and *more* crime, not less (4). Within the context of these opposing arguments, this chapter examines the evidence surrounding the anti-legalization points of view.

HISTORICAL BACKGROUND

During the closing decades of the nineteenth century, opiates and cocaine were widely and legally available both in their pure form and as ingredients in patent medicines promoted as remedies for any variety of ailments ranging from hay fever, depression, and arthritis, to colds, consumption, teething, and even athlete's foot, cancer, and baldness (5). Heroin and cocaine, furthermore, were touted as nonaddictive painkillers and as cures for morphine and alcohol addiction. But as the twentieth century began with hundreds of thousands of individuals dependent on cocaine and opiates (6), concern rose about the abuse liability and addiction potential of these drugs. In fact, in 1910 President William H. Taft noted in a report to Congress that "the misuse of cocaine is undoubtedly an American habit, the most threatening of the drug habits that has appeared in this country..." (7).

This concern over the effects of the legal use of drugs led to federal and state actions, which by 1920 had led to sharp decreases in the use of opiates and cocaine in patent medicines and the requirement of a physician's prescription to obtain them. By the 1930s cocaine and opiate use had markedly declined, and legislation in 1937 led to the illegality of marijuana and its subsequent decreased use (5).

While the same drugs are illegal in all 50 states and many have adopted schedules similar to those of the federal government, state penalties for possession and distribution vary widely, particularly with respect to marijuana. In a few states, possession of small amounts of marijuana is a civil violation punishable by fine rather than a criminal offense, and more than half the states and the District of Columbia have legislation permitting the medicinal use of marijuana. At the same time, 19 states have mandatory minimum sentences for the possession and/or sale of marijuana, and 11 states have separate penalties for *crack*-versus *powder*-cocaine (8). Like the federal government, states set higher penalties for selling drugs to minors and outlaw possession of drug paraphernalia and operation of premises where drugs are sold and used (8).

DRUG POLICY ALTERNATIVES

The drug policy debate revolves around such alternatives as prohibition (and its critiques) versus legalization, which has been used to encompass a wide variety of options. Many different terms are commonly used, with much variation in each (9).

- *Prohibition* reflects current policy, with its supporters focusing on the necessity for prohibiting illegal drugs through severe penalties for their use, distribution, and sale.
- *Legalization* rests at the other end of the continuum from prohibition, and calls for the elimination of drug prohibitions and instituting some form of government regulation.
- *Decriminalization* refers to the removal of the criminal penalties associated with the possession of currently illegal drugs.
- *Medicalization* advocates giving physicians the responsibility for treating drug abusers, including the decision to maintain some users on the drug on which they have become dependent.
- *Harm reduction* is an approach that emphasizes a public health model for reducing the risks and consequences of drug abuse (10).

Before going further, however, two things must be emphasized. The first is that none of these approaches are mutually exclusive, for each contains elements of the others. Prohibition, for example, includes elements of harm reduction in the forms of substance abuse prevention and treatment. Furthermore, methadone-maintenance programs can exist under the prohibition, medicalization, and harm-reduction approaches. At the same time, legalization proposals often include aspects of both decriminalization and medicalization. The second point is that each of these five drug policy approaches means different things to different people, with the most confusion associated with harm reduction.

The problem is that harm reduction is a concept that is difficult to define with any degree of precision. Its essential feature, however, is the attempt to ameliorate the adverse health, social, legal, and/or economic consequences associated with the use of mood-altering drugs. As such, harm reduction is neither a policy nor a program, but rather, a principle that suggests that managing drug abuse is more appropriate than attempting to stop it altogether. Within this context, harm reduction can mean different things to different people, groups, cultures, and nations. Most broadly, it can refer to any variety or combination of policies and policy goals, including the following:

- *Advocacy for changes in drug policies*—legalization, decriminalization, ending the drug prohibition, reduction of criminal sanctions for drug-related crimes, changes in drug paraphernalia laws

- *Human immunodeficiency virus (HIV)/acquired immunodeficiency syndrome (AIDS)-related interventions*—needle/syringe exchange programs; HIV prevention/intervention programs; bleach and condom distribution programs; referrals for HIV and other sexually transmitted infections (STI) testing; referrals for HIV and other STI medical care and management; referrals for HIV/AIDS-related psychological care and case management
- *Broader drug treatment options*—methadone maintenance by primary care physicians, changes in methadone regulations, heroin substitution programs, new experimental treatments, treatment on demand
- *Drug-abuse management for those who wish to continue using drugs*—counseling and clinical case management programs that promote safer and more responsible drug use
- *Ancillary interventions*—housing and other entitlements, healing centers, support and advocacy groups (11)

Although harm reduction encompasses a wide range of alternatives, to some observers it is viewed as a more politically attractive cover for legalization (12). Or, as the former director of the Office of National Drug Control Policy General Barry McCaffrey noted in 1998, "Harm reduction is a hijacked concept that has become a euphemism for drug legalization. It's become a cover story for people who would lower the barriers to drug use" (13).

THE EPIDEMIOLOGY OF DRUG USE

Most arguments for legalizing drugs begin with the contentions that the fight against the use of cocaine, heroin, and other illegal drugs has been lost, and that the array of criminal justice and social policies, which attempt to manage drug use and drug users, have been a total failure. Legalization advocates point to the more than 80 million Americans who have used drugs at some point during their lifetimes, arguing that the laws have been futile and a liberal democracy should not ban what so many people do (14,15). In counterpoint, however, it should be pointed out that for the majority of these individuals, their drug use involved little more than brief experimentation with marijuana. The size of this number especially reflects the large number of young people who tried marijuana and hallucinogenic drugs during the late 1960s and the 1970s when drug use was so widely tolerated that the 1972 Shafer Commission, established during the Nixon administration, and, later, President Jimmy Carter called for decriminalization of marijuana (5,16). It also reflects the period of the late 1970s when some physicians described cocaine as a relatively harmless drug, even as related problems were escalating rapidly (17).

Since then concerned public health and government leaders have mounted energetic efforts to denormalize drug use. As a result, current (past month) users of any illicit drugs, as measured by the National Household Survey on Drug Abuse, decreased from 24.8 million in 1979 to 15.9 million in 2001, a more than 35% drop. Over the same time period, current marijuana users dropped from 23 million to 12 million, and cocaine users from 4.4 million to 1.7 million (18). Given these data, combined with the fact that the national population increased by some 20% between 1979 and 2001, it is difficult to say that drug reduction efforts have failed. The declines in drug use occurred during a period of strict drug laws, societal disapproval, and increasing knowledge and awareness of the dangers and costs of illegal drug use.

Several factors, however, lead many to conclude that we have not made progress against drugs. This feeling of despair stems from the uneven nature of the success. While casual drug use and experimentation have declined substantially, certain neighborhoods and areas of the country remain infested with drugs and drug-related crime, and these continuing trouble spots draw media attention. At the same time, the number of drug addicts has not dropped significantly, and the spread of HIV among addicts has added a devastating dimension to the problem.

The number of chronic (more than 10 days per month) cocaine users (as estimated by the Office of National Drug Control Policy based on a number of surveys including the National Household Survey on Drug Abuse, the Arrestee Drug Abuse Monitoring program, and the Drug Abuse Warning Network), has remained steady at roughly 2.8 million since 1995 (19). The overall number of illicit drug addicts has hovered between 5 and 6 million, a situation that many experts attribute both to a lack of treatment facilities (20) and the large numbers of drug-using individuals already in the pipeline to addiction, even though overall casual use has dropped. Furthermore, after 13 years of sharp decline, teenage drug use increased somewhat from 1992 to 2001 (19).

While strict drug laws and criminal sanctions are not likely to deter hard-core addicts, increased resources can be dedicated to prevention and treatment without changing the legal status of drugs. It is difficult to carry out effective prevention campaigns when drugs are available on many street corners and in both urban and rural school corridors; witness the continued rise in teenage smoking in spite of major prevention efforts. The criminal justice system can be used to enhance treatment outcome by using such programs as an alternative to incarceration and by offering treatment in prisons. Though substantial problems remain, the significant progress in the struggle against drug abuse can be accelerated by improving the system rather than tearing it down.

LEGALIZATION AND PUBLIC HEALTH

Proponents of drug legalization claim that making drugs legally available would not significantly increase the number of drug dependent people. It is argued that "drugs are everywhere," in that they are already available to those who want them, and that a policy of legalization could be combined with education and prevention programs to discourage drug use (3,15,21). Some contend that legalization might even reduce the number of users, arguing that there would be no local dealers to lure new users, and drugs would lose the "forbidden fruit" allure of illegality (15,21). Proponents of legalization also play down the consequences of drug use, saying that most drug users can function normally (22,23). Some legalization advocates assert that a certain level of drug addiction is inevitable, so that even if legalization increased the number of users, it would have little effect on the numbers of users who become drug dependent (17).

The effects of legalization on the number of drug-involved people is an important question because the answer in large part determines whether legalization will reduce crime, improve public health, and lower the economic, social, and health care costs related to drug abuse, or will have the opposite effects. The claimed benefits of legal change evaporate if the number of users and addicts, particularly among children, increases significantly.

Does Availability Create Demand?

An examination of this question has three components: (a) access to drugs; (b) social acceptability and perceived consequences of drug use; and (c) the affordability of drugs.

Accessibility

It would appear that at present, drugs are not readily accessible to all. Although 88.5% of high school seniors reported in 2001 that they could obtain marijuana "fairly easily" or "very easily" only 45% and 32% believed that they could easily obtain cocaine and heroin, respectively (24). In the adult population age 26 years and older, 53% believed they could easily obtain marijuana, 30% believed they could easily obtain cocaine, and 19% believed they could easily obtain heroin. Thus, although marijuana is perceived as easily available by a large proportion of the youth and adult populations, other drugs are not as easily obtainable. After legalization, *all* drugs would be more widely and easily available.

Acceptability

In arguing that legalization would not result in increased use, proponents of legalization often cite public opinion polls, which indicate that the vast majority of Americans would not try drugs even if they were legally available (21,25). They fail to take into account, however, that this strong public antagonism toward drugs was formed during a period of strict prohibition, when government and institutions at every level made clear the health and criminal justice consequences of drug use. Furthermore, even if only 15% of the population would use drugs after legalization, this would be more than double the current level of 7.1%.

Laws define what is acceptable conduct in a society and express the will of its citizens. Drug laws not only create a criminal sanction, they also serve as educational and normative statements that shape public attitudes (26). Criminal laws constitute a far stronger statement than civil laws, but even the latter can discourage individual consumption. Laws regulating smoking in public and workplaces, prohibiting certain types of tobacco advertising, and mandating warning labels are in part responsible for the decline in smoking prevalence among adults, which seems to be leveling off at the high rate of 48 million nicotine addicts.

The challenge of reducing drug abuse and addiction would be decidedly more difficult if society passed laws indicating that these substances are not sufficiently harmful to prohibit their use. Any move toward legalization would decrease the perception of risks and costs of drug use, which would lead to wider use (24). During the late 1960s and the 1970s, as social norms, laws, and police practices became more permissive about drug use, the number of individuals smoking marijuana and using heroin, hallucinogens, and other drugs rose sharply. During the 1980s, as attitudes became more restrictive and antidrug laws stricter and more vigorously enforced, the perceived harmfulness of marijuana and other illicit drugs increased and use decreased.

Some legalization advocates point to the campaign against smoking as proof that reducing use is possible while substances are legally available (14,21,27). But it has taken smoking more than 30 years to decline as much as illegal drug use did in 10 years (28,29). Moreover, reducing use of legal drugs among the young has proven especially difficult. While use of illegal drugs by high school seniors has dropped significantly over the years, tobacco use remained virtually constant in the 1980s, rose sharply in the early 1990s, and only now has declined to where it was 20 years ago (24).

Affordability

Unless the general laws of economics are repealed, it is likely that reducing the price of drugs will increase consumption (26,30,31). Although interdiction and law enforcement have had limited success in reducing supply (28), the illegality of drugs has increased their price (32). Prices of illegal drugs are roughly six to ten times what

they would cost to produce legally. Cocaine, for example, sells at $60 to $200 a gram (depending on purity, potency, and availability), but would cost less than $3 a gram to produce and distribute legally. That would set the price of a dose at about 15 to 20 cents, well within the reach of a virtually every student in America. "Legalized cocaine would cost no more than about 3% of today's black market price and consumption would surely increase dramatically" (33).

Until the mid-1980s, cocaine was the drug of the middle and upper classes. Regular use was limited to those who had the money to purchase it or got the money through white collar crime or selling such assets as their car, house, or children's college funds. In the mid-1980s, the $5 crack cocaine vial made the drug inexpensive and more available to the poor and young. Use spread. Cocaine-exposed infants began to fill hospital neonatal wards, cocaine-related emergency room visits increased sharply, and cocaine-related crime and violence jumped (26). As such, history suggests that availability does indeed create demand.

Efforts to increase the price of legal drugs by taxing them heavily in order to discourage consumption would be accompanied by the black market, crime, violence, and corruption now associated with the illegal drug trade. Heroin addicts, who gradually build a tolerance to the drug, and cocaine addicts, who crave more of the drug as soon as its effects subside, would turn to a black market if an affordable and rising level of drugs were not made available to them legally.

Youth and Drugs

Drug use among youths is of particular concern because almost all individuals who use drugs begin doing so during their preteen or adolescent years. Because we have been unable to keep legal drugs, like tobacco, alcohol, and prescription stimulants and painkillers, out of the hands of youths, the legalization of illegal drugs could compound existing problems of drug use among youths.

Most advocates of legalization support a regulated system in which access to presently illicit drugs would be illegal for minors (21). Such regulations would retain for children the "forbidden fruit" and risk-taking allure that many argue legalization would eliminate. Furthermore, any such distinction between adults and minors could make drugs, like beer and cigarettes today, an attractive badge of adulthood.

The American experience with laws restricting access by children and adolescents to tobacco and alcohol makes it clear that keeping legal drugs away from minors would be a formidable, probably impossible, task. Currently, 61% of high school seniors have smoked, 30% in the past month (24). Some 29% of high school students are current cigarette smokers; 10 million underage Americans reported drinking alcohol in the past 30 days, and although alcohol use is illegal for every American under age

21 years, 73.3% of high school seniors report using alcohol in the past year, almost half in the past month (24). These rates of use persist despite school, community, and media activities that inform youths about the dangers of smoking and drinking and despite increasing public awareness of these risks. Moreover, in contrast to these high rates of alcohol and tobacco use, only 26% of seniors are current users of illicit drugs, which are illegal for the entire society (18). It is no accident that those substances, which are mostly easily obtainable—alcohol, cigarettes, and inhalants such as those found in household cleaning fluids—are those most widely used by the youngest students.

Hard-Core Addicts

A review of addiction in the past shows that the number of alcohol, heroin, and cocaine addicts, even when adjusted for changes in population, fluctuates widely over time, in response to changes in access, price, societal attitudes, and legal consequences. That alcohol and tobacco, the most accepted and available legal drugs, are the most widely abused, demonstrates that behavior is influenced by opportunity, stigma, and price. Many soldiers who were regular heroin users in Vietnam stopped once they returned to the United States where heroin was much more difficult and dangerous to get (5). Studies show that even among chronic alcoholics, alcohol taxes lower consumption (34). Similarly, as cigarette taxes increase, the number of smokers decreases.

Although not all new users become addicts, few individuals foresee their addiction when they start using. Most think they can control their consumption (35). Among the new users created by increased availability, many, including children, would find themselves unable to live without the drug, no longer able to work, attend school, or maintain personal relationships.

Drugs, Violence, and Criminal Justice

In an effort to begin unraveling the legalization/drugs–violence connection and the overall relationships between drugs and violence, it is important to understand Paul J. Goldstein's tripartite conceptual framework of psychopharmacological, economically compulsive, and systemic models of violence (36).

The *psychopharmacologic model of violence* suggests that some individuals, as the result of short-term or long-term ingestion of specific substances, may become excitable, irrational, and exhibit violent behavior. Research documents that chronic users of amphetamines, methamphetamine, and cocaine, in particular, tend to exhibit hostile and aggressive behaviors (37).

Psychopharmacologic violence can also be a product of a psychotic state induced by cocaine and other stimulants (38–41). As dose and duration of cocaine use increase, the likelihood of developing cocaine-related psy-

chopathology also increases. Cocaine psychosis is generally preceded by a transitional period characterized by increased suspiciousness, compulsive behavior, fault finding, and eventually paranoia. When the psychotic state is reached, individuals may experience visual and/or auditory hallucinations, with persecutory voices commonly heard. Many believe that they are being followed by police or that family, friends, and others are plotting against them. Moreover, everyday events tend to be misinterpreted in a way that supports delusional beliefs. When coupled with the irritability and hyperactivity that the stimulant nature of cocaine tends to generate in almost all of its users, the cocaine-induced paranoia may lead to violent behavior as a means of "self-defense" against imagined persecutors. The violence associated with cocaine psychosis was a common feature in many crack houses across the United States during the late 1980s and early 1990s (42). Violence may also result from the irritability associated with the drug withdrawal syndromes. In addition, some users ingest drugs before committing crimes to both loosen inhibitions and bolster their resolve to break the law (43).

The economically compulsive model of violence holds that some drug users engage in economically oriented violent crime to support drug use. This model is illustrated in the many studies of drug use and criminal behavior which have demonstrated that while drug sales, property crimes, and prostitution are the primary economic offenses committed by users, armed robberies and muggings do indeed occur (37,44,45).

Analyzing the legalization/drugs–violence connection within this model is far more complex than with the psychopharmacologic pattern. The contention is that in a legalized market, the prices of "expensive drugs" would decline to more affordable levels, and, hence, predatory crimes would become unnecessary. But this argument is based on several premises. First, it assumes that addicts commit crimes because they are "enslaved" to drugs, that because of the high prices of heroin, cocaine, and other illicit chemicals on the drug black market, users are forced to commit crimes to support their drug habits. Interestingly, however, there is no solid empirical evidence to support this contention. Studies over the past three decades document that while drug use tends to intensify and perpetuate criminal behavior, it usually does not initiate criminal careers. In fact, the evidence suggests that among the majority of street drug users who are involved in crime, their criminal careers were well established prior to the onset of either narcotics or cocaine use. As such, it would appear that the "inference of causality"—that the high price of drugs on the black market *per se* causes crime—is simply not supported.

The second premise suggests that people addicted to drugs commit crimes only for the purpose of supporting their habits. However, a variety of studies document that drug use is not the only reason why addicts commit predatory crimes. They also do so to support their daily living expenses—food, clothing, and shelter. To cite but one example, researchers at the Center for Drug and Alcohol Studies at the University of Delaware studied crack users on the streets of Miami. Of the scores of active addicts interviewed, 85% of the men and 70% of the female interviewees paid for portions of their living expenses through street crime. In fact, half of the men and a fourth of the women paid for 90% or more of their living expenses through crime. And not surprisingly, 96% of the men and 99% of the women had not held a legal job in the 90-day period before being interviewed for the study (46).

The third premise holds that in a legalized market users could obtain as much of the drugs as they wanted, whenever they wanted. More than likely, however, there would be some sort of regulation, and, hence, drug black markets would persist for those whose addictions were beyond the medicalized or legalized allotments. In a decriminalized market, moreover, levels of drug-related violence would likely either remain unchanged, or increase (if drug use increased).

The final premise is that cheap drugs preclude the need to commit crimes to obtain them, but the evidence emphatically suggests that this is not at all the case. Consider crack-cocaine. Although crack "rocks" are available on the illegal market for as little as $2 in some locales, users are still involved in crime-driven endeavors to support their addictions (47). For example, researchers Miller and Gold surveyed 200 consecutive callers to the 1-800-COCAINE hotline who considered themselves to have a problem with crack (48). They found that despite the low cost of crack, 63% of daily users and 40% of nondaily users spent more than $200 per week on the drug. Similarly, interviews conducted by researchers in New York City with almost 400 drug users contacted in the streets, jails, and treatment programs, found that almost half spent more than $1,000 a month on crack (49). The study also documented that crack users—despite the low cost of their drug of choice—spent more money on drugs than did users of heroin, powder cocaine, marijuana, and alcohol. Other researchers have found this to be so in Miami, as well (46).

Miller and Gold summarized the issue of crack and crime this way: "Once the severity of addictive use is established, the pattern of the cost of maintaining the addiction and its consequences is related to preoccupation with acquisition and compulsive use . . ." (48).

The systemic model of violence maintains that violent crime is intrinsic to the very involvement with illicit substances. As such, systemic violence refers to the traditionally aggressive patterns of interaction within systems of illegal drug trafficking and distribution. It is the systemic violence associated with trafficking in cocaine and crack in America's inner cities that has brought the most attention to drug-related violence in recent years. Moreover, it is concerns with this same violence that focused the current interest on the possibility of legalizing drugs. And it is certainly logical to assume that if heroin and cocaine were legal substances, systemic drug-related violence might indeed decline significantly. However, there are two very important questions in this regard. First, is drug-related violence more often psychopharmacologic than systemic? Second, is the great bulk of systemic violence related to the distribution of crack? Third, is crack-related violence still at the high levels of a decade ago? If most of the drug-related violence is psychopharmacologic in nature, and if systemic violence is typically related to crack, a drug generally excluded from consideration when legalization is argued, it might be logical to conclude that legalizing drugs would *not* reduce violent crime.

In retrospect, study after study documents that alcohol and other drugs have psychopharmacologic effects that result in violence. Cocaine in all of its forms is linked to aggressive behavior as a result of the irritability and paranoia it engenders. Also, alcohol and cocaine have been found to be present in both the perpetrators and victims of violence. Alcohol is legal and cocaine is not, suggesting that the legal status of a drug may be unrelated to the issue of psychopharmacologic violence. Hence, it is unlikely that such violence would decline if drugs were legalized. Studies of economically compulsive violence also suggest that in a legalized market, crime would not necessarily decline. Users who engage in predatory behaviors do so for a variety of reasons—not only to obtain drugs, but also to support themselves. And typically, as pointed out, a number of studies suggest, drug-involved offenders were crime-involved before the onset of their careers in drugs. Too, even when a drug is inexpensive, it still may not be affordable if there is addiction and compulsive use. This is amply illustrated in the experience with crack.

As for systemic violence, much of it is unrelated to the use of drugs. When it *is* drug linked, the overwhelming majority seems to be associated with the use of alcohol or crack. Taking this point further, violence stems from many of the dysfunctional aspects of our society other than drug use. After studying the violence associated with crack distribution in Manhattan neighborhoods, Jeffrey Fagan and Ko-lin Chin concluded that crack has been integrated into behaviors that were evident before drug sellers' involvement with crack or its appearance on New York City streets (50). In other words, the crack users/dealers are often engaged in violent and crime-involved lifestyles, which would likely exist (and previously did) independent of their involvement with crack. Furthermore, although there is evidence that crack sellers are more violent than other drug sellers, this violence is not confined to the drug-selling context: violence potentials appear to precede involvement in selling (50).

It appears, then, that crack has been blamed for increasing violence in the marketplace, but perhaps this violence actually stems from the psychopharmacologic consequences of crack use. *Crack dealers* are generally *crack users,* and because crack is highly addictive yet comparatively inexpensive, there is a continuous demand for it.

This leads to the competition that generates violence. Legalizing crack would likely reduce the competition but increase the demand. Researcher Ansley Hamid reasons that increases in crack-related violence are caused by the deterioration of informal and formal social controls throughout communities that have been destabilized by economic processes and political decisions (51). As such, does anyone really believe that we can improve on these complex social problems through the simple act of legalizing drugs?

Legalization advocates point to exploding prison populations and the failure of drug laws to lower crime rates (2,3,21). From 1980 to 2001, arrests for drug offenses doubled, with the result that the majority of state and federal inmates had histories of drug abuse, or had been arrested for drug law violations (52). Rising prison populations are generated in large part by stricter laws, tough enforcement, and mandatory minimum sentencing laws, policy choices of the public and Congress. But the growing number of prisoners is also a product of the high rate of recidivism, a phenomenon tied in good measure to the lack of treatment facilities, both in and out of prison. Eighty percent of state prisoners have prior convictions and 60% have served time in the past. Despite the fact that more than 60% of all state inmates have used illegal drugs regularly and 30% were under the influence of drugs at the time they committed the crime for which they were incarcerated, fewer than 20% of inmates with drug problems receive any treatment (53).

While strict laws and enforcement do not necessarily deter addicts from using drugs, the criminal justice system can actually play a harm-reduction role, by diverting drug-involved offenders into treatment. Because of the nature of addiction, most drug abusers do not seek treatment voluntarily, but many respond to outside pressures including the threat of incarceration. Where the criminal justice system is used to encourage treatment participation, addicts are more likely to complete treatment and stay off drugs (53).

ADDICTION AND CASUAL DRUG USE

To offset any increased use as a result of legalization, many proponents contend that money presently spent on criminal justice and law enforcement could be used for treatment of addicts and prevention (3). In 2002, the federal government spent $18.8 billion to fight drug abuse, nearly two thirds of that on law enforcement; state and local governments are spending at least another $16 billion on drug control efforts, largely on law enforcement (54). Legalization proponents argue that most of this money could be used to fund treatment on demand for all addicts who want it, and extensive public health campaigns to discourage new use.

While the number of new prisoners would initially decrease because many are currently there for drug law violations, as use increased, costs would quickly rise in health care, schools, and businesses and the wider use would lead to increased addiction. Increased criminal activity, as noted earlier, would occur, related to the psychological and physical effects of drug use, and criminal justice costs would rise again. The higher number of casual users and addicts would reduce worker productivity and students' ability and motivation to learn, cause more highway accidents and fatalities, and fill hospital beds with individuals suffering from ailments and injuries caused or aggravated by drug abuse. Law enforcement and treatment do not need to be conflicting activities. Community policing, for example, is both a supply and demand reduction activity. Well-run drug courts can improve the efficacy of treatment. Effective treatment can decrease crime. Rather than cut supply reduction activities, what is needed is an expansion and improvement of treatment, such as the $1.6 billion over 5 years proposed by President G.W. Bush (54).

A recent study (55) suggests another danger of casual drug use, especially among adolescents. A review of 140 studies of addiction, adolescence, and brain structures noted that the adolescent's impulse toward novelty develops far more quickly than the mechanisms that inhibit urges and impulses. Teenagers are both more likely to experiment with drugs and the experience produces more pronounced brain effects, which can be permanent.

Chambers and associates (55) found that "[g]reater motivational drives for novel experiences, coupled with an immature inhibitory control system, could predispose to performance of impulsive actions and risky behaviors, including experimentation with and abusive use of addictive drugs.... Direct pharmacological–motivational effects of addictive drugs on dopamine systems may be accelerated during these developmental epochs, enhancing the progression or permanency of neural changes underlying addiction."

The chronic relapsing nature of drug dependence and the difficulties in treating it are well documented (56). The mechanisms described by Chambers and associates (55) may increase our understanding of why this happens and emphasize that curing addiction may be even harder than preventing it initially. Casual drug use by adolescents and young adults, in short, may have long-lasting consequences for many of them. Those harm-reduction proponents who argue that because teens are going to do drugs anyway, it is best to focus efforts on giving them the knowledge on how to do it "safely" rather than not doing it at all, may not understand the possible long-term consequences of even "safe use."

Costs

It is doubtful whether legalization would produce any cost savings over time, even in the area of law enforcement. Indeed, the legal availability of alcohol has not eliminated law enforcement costs because of alcohol-related violence. A third of state prison inmates committed their crimes while under the influence of alcohol (57,58). In 1998, there were approximately 16,000 alcohol-related traffic fatalities, approximately 40% of fatal motor vehicle crashes (59). Despite intense educational campaigns, there are about 1.5 million arrests annually for driving while intoxicated (57).

Like advocates of legalization today, opponents of alcohol prohibition claimed that taxes on the legal sale of alcohol would dramatically increase revenues and even help erase the federal deficit (60). The real-world result has been quite different. The more than $11 billion in 1995 state and federal revenues from alcohol taxes (61,62) paid for less than half the $40 billion that alcohol abuse imposed in direct health care costs in 1995 (63), much less the costs laid on federal entitlement programs and the legal and criminal justice systems, to say nothing of lost economic productivity. The $13 billion in federal and state tobacco tax revenue (61,62) was one-sixth of the $75 billion in direct health care costs attributable to tobacco (63). By the end of the decade, these ratios had remained approximately the same (64,65). This discrepancy between excise tax revenue and alcohol- and tobacco-related costs does decrease if one takes into account the "savings" from such programs as Social Security and Medicare as a result of premature death. The idea that a tobacco policy resulting in more than 400,000 deaths a year provides any kind of model for dealing with illegal drugs is hard to imagine.

Health care costs directly attributable to illegal drugs range from $14.9 billion to $30 billion (63), an amount that would increase significantly if use spread after legalization. Experience renders it unrealistic to expect that taxes could be imposed on newly legalized drugs sufficient to cover the costs of increased use and abuse. As noted later, the Dutch, in spite of effectively decriminalizing marijuana, have been unable to tax this $300 million a year business.

Public Health

Legalization proponents contend that prohibition has negative public health consequences such as the spread of HIV from addicts who share dirty needles, accidental poisoning, and overdoses from impure drugs of variable potency. Of those individuals who were living with AIDS in 1999, approximately one-third was related to drug users and their sexual partners (66).

Advocates of medicalization argue that while illicit drugs should not be freely available to all, doctors should be allowed to prescribe them (particularly heroin, but some also advocate cocaine) to addicts. They contend that giving addicts drugs assures purity and eliminates the need for addicts to steal to buy them.

Giving addicts drugs like heroin, however, poses many problems. Providing them by prescription raises the danger of diversion for sale on the black market as happened in England in the 1960s. The alternative—insisting that addicts take drugs on the prescribers premises—entails at least two visits a day, thus interfering with the stated goal of many maintenance programs to enable addicts to hold jobs. The dropouts from the Swiss heroin-maintenance projects (approximately 40% in the Basel study, for example [67]) show that a substantial number of enrolled individuals are unwilling to make such ongoing visits and/or are unwilling to do without the heroin and cocaine combination they like, leading some of the organizers to propose take-out heroin and the ability to use cocaine as well. A variety of claims have been made as to success of the participants, such as improved health and social integration. However, the treatment effectiveness of the heroin maintenance *per se* has been deemed hard to judge because of the lack of randomized controls, pre- and postcomparisons were limited to treatment completers, and there was extensive mandatory psychosocial counseling (68). A more rigorous, recently completed, Dutch study may provide more useful scientific information.

Heroin addicts require two to four shots each day in increasing doses as they build tolerance to its euphoric effect. On the other hand, methadone can be given at a constant dose because euphoria is not the objective. Addicts maintained on methadone need only a single oral dose each day, eliminating the need for injection. Buprenorphine, a partial opioid agonist given sublingually, was approved for treatment of opioid dependence in 2002 by the FDA. It can last up to 3 days, is safer than methadone as far as overdose is concerned, and since the passage of the Drug Abuse Treatment Act of 2000, can be prescribed by qualified office-based physicians. The possible medical mainstreaming of opiate addiction treatment via buprenorphine makes heroin maintenance even less of a necessary or useful alternative (69). Its extensive use in France (70), for example, has markedly cut the heroin overdose death rate by more than half (71). Because cocaine produces an intense but short euphoria and an immediate desire for more (72), addicts would have to be given the drug even more often than heroin to satisfy their craving sufficiently to prevent them from seeking additional cocaine on the street. The binge nature of cocaine use renders it unlikely that cocaine could be given on a "medicalization" basis. Because powder cocaine can be readily converted into crack, any proposal to expand availability of the former will increase the number of crack users and addicts.

Other, less-radical, harm-reduction proposals also have serious flaws. As compared to comprehensive methadone maintenance, "low-threshold" methadone-maintenance programs, when objectively studied, show sharply increased rates of illicit drug use and drug-related problems, and a failure to reduce high-risk behaviors (73,74). Distributing free needles does not ensure that addicts desperate for a high at inconvenient times would not continue to share them. But to the extent that needle exchange programs are effective in reducing the spread of the HIV virus, they can be adopted without legalizing drugs.

Studies of whether needle exchange programs increase drug use, however, have generally focused on periods of no longer than 12 months. Although use does not seem to increase in this period, data are lacking on the long-term effects of such programs and whether they prompt attitude shifts that, in turn, lead to increased drug use (75). Furthermore, most states now permit over-the-counter pharmacy sales of syringes at prices usually less than 40 cents per syringe. Funds spent on needle exchange programs, which often seem to attract the older, more risk-aversive addicts, might be better spent on outreach programs that go into crack houses and shooting galleries to encourage hard-to-reach addicts to seek treatment.

Some individuals do die as a result of drug impurities. But while drug purity could be assured in a government-regulated system (although not for those drugs sold on the black market), careful use could not. An increase in the number of users would probably produce a rising number of overdose deaths, similar to those caused by acute alcohol overdose deaths today. The deaths and costs as a result of unregulated drug quality pale in comparison to the negative impact that legalization would have on drug users, their families, and society. Casual drug use is dangerous, not simply because it can lead to addiction or accidental overdoses, but because it can be harmful *per se*, increasing worker accidents, highway fatalities, and children born with physical and psychological handicaps. Each year, roughly 500,000 newborns are exposed to illegal drugs *in utero*; many others are never born because of drug-induced spontaneous abortions (76,77). Drug-exposed newborns are more likely to need intensive care and to suffer the numerous consequences of low birth weight and prematurity, including early death (76,78). The additional costs just to raise drug-exposed infants would outweigh any potential savings of legalization in criminal justice expenditures (78).

Substance abuse both leads to and aggravates medical problems. Medicaid patients with a secondary diagnosis of substance abuse (including alcohol) remain in hospitals twice as long as patients with the same primary diagnosis but with no substance abuse problems. Girls and boys under age 15 years remain in the hospital three and four times as long, respectively, when they have a secondary diagnosis of substance abuse (79). One-third to one-half of individuals with psychiatric problems are also substance abusers (80). Young people who use drugs are at higher risk of mental health problems, including depression, suicide, and personality disorders, and are more likely to engage in risky behavior such as unprotected sex (81,82). Such sexual behavior exposes these teens to increased risk of pregnancy as well as to AIDS and other sexually transmitted diseases. The total economic cost of illegal drug use to society in 2000 was estimated at $160 billion, including health care costs of $14.9 billion, lost productivity of $110.5 billion, and crime and welfare of $35.2 billion (54).

In schools and families, drug abuse can be devastating. Students who use drugs not only limit their own ability to learn, they also disrupt classrooms. Drug-using parents are more likely to provide inadequate or no economic support and put their children at greater risk of becoming substance abusers themselves (76). With the advent of crack cocaine in the mid-1980s, foster care cases soared more than 50% nationwide in 5 years; more than 70% of these cases involved families in which at least one parent abused drugs (83).

Decreased coordination and impaired motor skills that result from drug use are dangerous not just to the individual but also to society at large. A study in Tennessee found that 59% of reckless drivers, having been stopped by the police and tested negative for alcohol, test positive for marijuana and/or cocaine (84). The extent of driving while high on marihuana and other illegal drugs is still not well known because usually the police do not have the same capability for roadside drug testing as they do for alcohol testing. However, data from the 2001 National Household Survey found that more than 8 million persons reported driving under the influence of illegal drugs during the past year (18).

The Workplace

Approximately 75% of illegal drug users are employed full- or part-time (65); in one survey, 60% of respondents knew people who went to work under the influence of alcohol or drugs (65). These workers impose costs on their employers, and eventually society, through their decreased productivity, health care needs, workplace accidents, and absenteeism. They drive buses and trucks, operate nuclear power plants, run the air traffic control system, perform surgery, deliver mail, and teach children.

Workers who use cocaine and marijuana are twice as likely to be absent from work and to be injured, and 1.5 times more likely to be involved in an accident (76). Overall, workers who use drugs are three times likelier to be late for work, ten times likelier to miss work, and three to six times likelier to injure themselves or others. Drug-using workers are responsible for 40% of industrial fatalities and experience more than 300% higher medical and benefits costs (85). Between 1992 and 2000, it is estimated that lost productivity as a consequence of illegal drugs totaled $110.5 billion (86,87).

THE LESSONS OF PROHIBITION

Legalization advocates often cite the era of national alcohol prohibition from 1920 to 1934 to support their case. As ratified in the 18th Amendment, Prohibition banned the "manufacture, sale, or transportation of intoxicating liquors within, the importation thereof into, or the exportation thereof from the United States...." Proponents of legalization contend that the failure of the 18th

Amendment supports their argument that prohibitions of this kind of individual behavior are not effective (25).

The alcohol prohibition–drug control law analogy is a false one. There are two important distinctions between Prohibition and current drug laws. First, Prohibition was in fact decriminalization because possession for personal consumption was not illegal. Second, alcohol, unlike illegal drugs, has a long history of widespread social acceptance and use in Western culture dating at least as far back as the Old Testament and Ancient Greece. Most Americans who drink do not get into trouble with alcohol. Thus, the public and political consensus favoring Prohibition was short-lived. By the early 1930s, most Americans no longer supported it. Today, however, the public overwhelmingly favors keeping illegal drugs illegal.

Despite these differences, which made alcohol prohibition more difficult to enforce than current drug laws, Prohibition reduced the amount of alcohol consumed, as well as the incidence of alcohol-related medical problems and violence. It is important not to confuse federal Prohibition with state laws restricting alcohol. Advocates of legalization point to the decline in consumption and cirrhosis pre-1919 to argue that consumption declined more before the 18th Amendment than after. Given that by 1919, 36 of the 48 states had established some form of prohibition, this argument is true but disingenuous. At the beginning of the twentieth century, Americans consumed 2.6 gallons of alcohol per person. By 1919, this amount dropped to 1.96 gallons per person. In 1934, the first full year after repeal of national Prohibition, alcohol use stood at 0.97 gallons per person. From then on, consumption rose steadily to roughly three times as high as that immediately after Prohibition (88).

Death rates from cirrhosis of the liver corroborate available consumption statistics. Cirrhosis death rates fell from 12 per 100,000 in 1916 to 5 per 100,000 in 1920, and remained at that level throughout Prohibition before beginning to rise steadily again after repeal (89). Among men such rates declined even more sharply, from 29.5 per 100,000 in 1911 to 10.7 per 100,000 in 1929 (60).

The decrease in consumption had other positive health consequences. Admissions to mental health institutions for alcoholic psychosis dropped by more than 60% from 1919 to 1922. Arrests for drunkenness and disorderly conduct dropped 50% between 1916 and 1922, and welfare agencies reported dramatic declines in the number of cases as a consequence of alcohol-related family problems (60).

Nor is Hollywood's guns and gangsters depiction of Prohibition accurate. Homicide experienced a higher rate of increase between 1900 and 1910 than during Prohibition, and organized crime was well established in cities before 1920 (60).

Legalization proponents also argue that during Prohibition, an increased number of drinkers died from the consumption of dangerous wood and denatured alcohol, which were used as substitutes for commercial alcohol, just as today addicts die from impure drugs. The data do not bear this out. Through 1927, the rate of death from these substitutes remained nearly constant at its 1920 level (60).

The public may agree that the freedom to drink is worth the public health consequences. Worried by the high rate of alcohol-related disease and crime, the residents of Barrow, Alaska, the northernmost city in the United States, voted in 1994 to ban alcohol completely. Despite the 70% drop in crime and the immediate and persistent decline in alcohol-related emergency room visits from 118 in the month before the ban to 23 in the following month, residents voted to repeal the ban in 1995. In the 2 weeks after the ban was lifted, the detoxification center began to fill with patients and alcohol-related murders were on the rise (90).

These facts are presented to set the record straight and to dispel the exaggerated or false consequences often attributed to Prohibition. They are not an argument for the resumption of alcohol prohibition, which we oppose, but they do offer some lessons on the relevance of illegality to reducing drug use.

THE LESSONS OF LEGAL DRUGS

Legalization proponents point out that alcohol and tobacco cost society much more in lost productivity, increased health care, and criminal justice expenditures, and lead to more deaths than all illegal drugs combined (14,27,91). From that they conclude that we spend too much time and energy fighting illegal drugs, as compared to legal drugs. Alcohol and tobacco are, indeed, responsible for far more deaths and costs to society than illegal drugs, but this is a combination of their potential toxicity and legal status, which makes them widely available, used, and abused.

Illegal drug-related deaths are estimated at 20,000 annually. Tobacco is responsible for more than 400,000 deaths and alcohol for more than 100,000 deaths every year (92). Approximately 40% of fatal motor vehicle crashes involve alcohol. Fetal alcohol syndrome is the leading known cause of mental retardation (93). Smoking by pregnant women kills up to 7,000 newborns annually and leads to as many as 141,000 miscarriages (94). Cigarettes are as addictive as heroin and spawn health problems ranging from lung cancer to emphysema and heart disease (95). Of the $66 billion that substance abuse cost federal health and disability entitlement programs in 1995, $56 billion were attributable to alcohol and tobacco (96). Of the $29 billion in Medicare costs attributable to substance abuse, 80% was related to smoking. Seventy percent of the $21 billion that Medicaid spent because of substance abuse was because of cigarettes and alcohol (63).

The high costs attributed to legal drugs do not indicate that we are concentrating prohibition on the wrong drugs, but rather that when drugs are legal, and therefore widely acceptable and available, they adversely affect more individuals and require more attention and resources. Indeed, the nation's experience with tobacco and alcohol send a warning about the dangers of making illegal drugs readily available. As drug policy expert Mark Kleiman has noted, "Until success is achieved in imposing reasonable controls on the currently licit killers, alcohol and nicotine, the case for adding a third or fourth recreational drug ... will remain hopelessly speculative" (97).

Another argument made by legalization proponents is that the general decrease in consumption rates of both legal and illegal drugs in the past 20 years has nothing to do with law enforcement policy, but rather with education and increased societal concern with personal health (91). Yet despite widespread awareness of the risks of smoking and heavy media attention to tobacco-related problems, roughly 25% of Americans continue to smoke, and smoking by adolescents is substantially higher than their marijuana use and close to where it was in 1979. On the other hand, as noted earlier, the number of illegal drug users has dropped from 24.8 million in 1979 to 15.9 million in 2001, while the national population increased by 20% in the same period (18). Arguing that we should treat illicit drugs as we do tobacco, using education instead of prohibition, also implies a false dichotomy between education and prohibitive laws. In curbing illegal drug use, when law enforcement and education complement and reinforce each other, they are most effective.

There are more than 48 million nicotine addicts, 12 to 18 million alcoholics and alcohol abusers and 5 to 6 million illegal drug addicts. Making illegal drugs more available would drive the number of marijuana, heroin, and cocaine users closer to the number of alcohol and tobacco users.

MARIJUANA

Marijuana is the most commonly used illegal drug in the United States and its use is particularly high among adolescents. Because relatively little street-level violence attends the marijuana trade, the legalization and decriminalization debate here centers on how harmful the drug is to the user, whether marijuana use leads to the use of harder drugs, whether marijuana use would increase, and whether any increase would translate into a decrease in alcohol use (25,98).

While clearly not as dangerous as snorting cocaine or shooting heroin, smoking marijuana is detrimental both physically and mentally, especially to adolescents. The effects of one marijuana joint on the lungs are equivalent to four cigarettes, placing the user at increased risk of bronchitis, emphysema, and bronchial asthma. The active ingredient in marijuana, tetrahydrocannabinol (THC), is fat-soluble and remains in the brain, lungs, and reproductive organs for weeks. Marijuana weakens the immune system, and regular use can disrupt the menstrual cycle and suppress ovarian function (99,100). Regardless of socioeconomic status, prenatal use of marijuana by the

mother appears to reduce significantly the IQs of babies (101). Marijuana impairs short-term memory and the ability to concentrate (102) at a time when the main task of its young users is education. And marijuana use diminishes motor control functions, distorts perception, and impairs judgment, leading, among other things, to increased car accidents and vandalism. Marijuana toxicity, especially anxiety and panic attacks, is a frequently cited cause of emergency room visits, and treatment of marijuana dependence has become a common reason for seeking substance abuse treatment, treatment which is usually psychologic rather than pharmacologic. As Millman and Beeder note, stopping chronic cannabis use often results in "a marked and rapid improvement in mental clarity and energy levels" (103).

The link between the use of marijuana and the subsequent use of harder drugs has been the subject of much debate (104), with supporters of marijuana decriminalization and legalization arguing that many individuals who smoke marijuana never use hard drugs. While the latter is true, the statistical association between the teenage use of marijuana and the later use of other drugs such as cocaine is powerful. Even though the biomedical or other causal relationship for this has not yet been adequately explained, 12- to 17-year-olds who smoke marijuana are 85 times more likely to use cocaine than those who do not. Adults who as adolescents smoked marijuana are 17 times likelier to use cocaine regularly. According to data of the National Household Survey, 60% of adolescents who use marijuana before age 15 years will later use cocaine, compared to only 16% who began marijuana use after age 21 years (105). These correlations are many times higher than the initial relationships found between smoking and lung cancer in the 1964 Surgeon General's report (nine to ten times). Individuals who used cannabis by age 17 years had odds of other drug use, alcohol dependence, and drug abuse/dependence 2.1 to 5.2 times higher than their twin who did not use cannabis before age 17 years (106,107).

Marijuana use is associated with many high-risk behaviors among young people. According to the U.S. Centers for Disease Control and Prevention, adolescents who smoke marijuana are twice as likely to attempt suicide and to carry a weapon as those who do not. Adolescent marijuana smokers are three times as likely to have sex and far more likely to do so without a condom, putting themselves at much greater risk of teen pregnancy and sexually transmitted diseases (108).

Past experiences with marijuana decriminalization illustrate the consequences of more tolerant policies. During the 1970s, 11 states decriminalized personal possession of marijuana by making the offense a civil violation punishable by a fine. In 1975, the Alaska State Supreme Court decriminalized at-home personal use of small amounts of marijuana for individuals older than age 19 years. By 1988, 12- to 17-year-olds in Alaska were smoking joints at more than twice the national average. Marijuana use became part of the lifestyle of many teenagers and the age of initiation declined (109,110). Because of this, in a 1990 referendum, Alaskans voted to recriminalize personal possession.

Proponents of legalization cite several surveys and studies, which report that when Oregon, Maine, and California decriminalized marijuana, rates of use among teenagers did not increase significantly (111). These surveys, however, have severe shortcomings. They lack controls for other historical and demographic factors, such as sex, income, and education, and employ vaguely defined measurement criteria to estimate the prevalence of marijuana use (112,113). They do not reflect the impact of legalization on long-term usage rates because they were conducted only 1 to 3 years after decriminalization laws were passed. Although reported marijuana use increased only slightly following decriminalization, the time period surveyed was not long enough to allow the educational and attitude-forming aspects of the previous strict drug laws to dissipate.

Measurement problems also exist in trying to compare usage rates in states that decriminalized marijuana use versus states that did not. The comparison is problematic because many states that did not decriminalize marijuana use did reduce penalties for marijuana use, and others chose not to enforce laws prohibiting personal use of marijuana. During the 1970s, many states and the federal government adopted more tolerant attitudes toward the drug. Nationwide, use rose significantly during this time, reaching almost 40% of high school seniors before beginning its long decline in 1979 (24).

Teenagers are not likely to stop using alcohol when they begin smoking marijuana. While on individual occasions teens may choose to get high on either marijuana or alcohol, these drugs are often used together. From 1975 to 1978, as the percentage of teens using marijuana increased from 27% to 37%, the percentage of teens that drank increased from 68% to 72%. Marijuana use then dropped to 12% of teens by 1992; alcohol use dropped to 51%. The rise in teenage marijuana use in the 1990s was accompanied by a rise, albeit smaller in the percentage of students who drink, and especially in binge drinking (24).

Proponents of legalization argue that while smoking pot has detrimental health and social effects, so does use of our two legal drugs, alcohol and tobacco, and to be consistent, we should legalize marijuana. But legalizing marijuana would add a third drug that combines some of the most serious risks of the other two. Marijuana offers both the intoxicating effects of alcohol and the long-term lung damage of tobacco. It would be irresponsible to legalize or decriminalize marijuana and create a third legal drug, especially when we are still learning about its physical and psychological health effects, as well as its relationship to other drugs and a variety of dangerous behaviors. One of the most serious drawbacks of marijuana legalization, Kleiman notes, is its "virtual irreversibility if it goes badly wrong" (113). He also noted regarding marijuana legalization. "Low tax, high potency marijuana could lead to severe social costs within user populations of the greatest concern; high tax, low potency marijuana could sustain black markets and their associated costs while increasing consumption more modestly" (114).

THE EUROPEAN EXPERIENCES

Many legalization advocates point to the policies of European countries as models for approaches to the American drug problem. They claim that some countries, notably the Netherlands and Great Britain, are more innovative because their aim is to minimize the harmful impact of drug use on the user and society, even if this requires legal change.

While the Netherlands' laws regarding illegal drugs remain unchanged, Dutch enforcement policy since 1976 has distinguished between "drugs presenting an unacceptable risk" (commonly termed "hard drugs," such as cocaine and heroin) and "cannabis products" (89). Special "coffee shops" were established where anyone age 18 years or older can purchase marijuana. Legalization proponents claim that this policy has not increased drug use among young people or the population in general (22,115,116).

The reality is more nuanced. Although marijuana use did not explode immediately following decriminalization, it did increase significantly following "commercialization" via the coffee shops (117), suggesting that the effects of decriminalization are related to a variety of factors and may only be fully realized in the longer term. Between 1984 and 1992, Dutch adolescent marijuana use increased nearly 200% (118); over the same period, marijuana use among American adolescents plummeted 66%. From 1988 to 1995, the Dutch had a 22% increase in the total number of registered addicts, and a 30% increase, from 1991 to 1993, in the number of registered cannabis addicts (119). From 1990 to 1995, the proportion of users who had smoked cannabis for the previous 5 years increased from 2% to 9%, suggesting that increased availability would be associated with longer-term use (120). The same study found that between 1990 and 1995, the percentage of 11- to 18-year-olds who had ever used marijuana more than doubled, from 7% to 17% (120). A number of marijuana "coffee shops" in Amsterdam have been shut down for illegally selling hard drugs or breaking other rules. Responding to pressure from other European countries and its own citizens, the Dutch Parliament passed restrictions in 1996 pledging to cut the number of coffee houses in half and reducing the amount of marijuana an individual can buy from 30 g to 5 g (121). It appears that only the reduction in quantity to be purchased has actually happened. By 1998 there had been only approximately a 10% reduction in the number of coffee shops because of legal tactics used by their owners (122), illustrating again how hard it becomes to change these policies once in place. Ironically, even though the marijuana trade may now be worth more than $300 million per year, the government, because of legal rulings, has been unable to tax it.

Another country that legalization advocates cite favorably is Great Britain for its policy of allowing specially licensed doctors to prescribe drugs to addicts. Prescribing heroin to addicts, it is claimed, has lowered the rate of addiction and reduced crime (123); neither of these claims has been verified.

Nationwide, British doctors maintain 17,000 heroin addicts on methadone and less than 400 on heroin. Given the 150,000 heroin addicts in England, claims that maintaining a few hundred of them on heroin have driven drug dealers and drug-related crimes from the streets are unfounded. There has been no movement among doctors in England to adopt heroin maintenance on a large scale (124).

In general, much confusion surrounds British policies. Until 1968, the government allowed all doctors to prescribe drugs to addicts in the context of their medical treatment, but this policy, while initially successful, in the 1960s failed to contain the problem of addiction. Some doctors carelessly or willfully abused their privilege and unlawfully supplied drugs to many individuals. Addicts diverted legally obtained drugs to the general population. In response to increasing rates of addiction, Britain mandated in 1968 that only doctors specially licensed by the Home Office could prescribe illegal drugs and that doctors must register all addicts with the Home Office (125). More than 100 doctors are licensed, of whom fewer than 20 prescribed such drugs for most of the 1990s.

The rate of increase in heroin addiction in England subsequently slowed until the late 1970s, when a large influx of black market heroin from southwest Asia fueled a sudden increase in new addicts that continued through the 1980s (126). This increase was not, as some legalization proponents' claim, a result of the fact that the British, following the American lead, adopted harsher drug laws. While on the national level, the government responded to this increase in addiction by emphasizing supply reduction, prevention, and criminal justice deterrents, at the local level officials emphasized harm reduction and loosely enforced antidrug laws. These conflicting national and local approaches persisted until the late 1980s, when concern over the spread of AIDS by injection drug users prompted national policy makers to shift toward harm-reduction programs such as needle exchanges and condom distribution (127).

In short, the increasing number of addicts in Britain was not a result of strict national laws and "zero tolerance" policies. Rather, these policies were a response to the increased addiction. Moreover, strict national antidrug laws mean little if local enforcement is lax.

One celebrated experiment in harm reduction and drug tolerance is less often mentioned now that it has been terminated. Beginning in 1987, Switzerland allowed all addicts and users to congregate in a park—the "Platzspitz," or "Needle Park," as it became known—in the center of downtown Zurich, where they could buy and use drugs freely. Strict enforcement of antidrug laws continued in the rest of the city and country. Like many proponents of harm reduction, Swiss policy makers believed that if drug dealing and use was going to happen anyway, it might as well occur in the open where the police and health officials could monitor it. In Needle Park, public health officials gave addicts free needles, condoms, medical care, counseling, and the opportunity for treatment (89).

This experiment in harm reduction had unintended consequences. The number of addicts in the park increased from a few hundred in 1987 to 20,000 in 1992. Twenty-five percent came from outside Switzerland, drawn to the park by its tolerant policies. Drug-related violence and crime rose rapidly in the area; 81 drug-related deaths were recorded in 1991, double the previous year. The city's chief medical officer reported that doctors were resuscitating an average of 12 people a day who had overdosed, and as many as 40 people on some days. Because of these high costs, the park was closed in 1992, but the fallout from this policy was damaging. The heroin-related death rate in Switzerland had become the highest in Europe and North America (128). Addicts wandered the city streets and open-air markets proliferated. Three years after the experiment ended, Swiss police tried to disperse the continuing drug bazaar that had moved to an unused railroad station. Ultimately, to deal with their burgeoning heroin problem, which may be the highest in Europe (122), Swiss authorities began heroin maintenance trials, as noted earlier. As drug policy experts MacCoun and Reuter point out, however, "Heroin maintenance has a contradiction at its heart. Having chosen to prohibit the drug, society then makes an exception for those who cause sufficient damage, to themselves and to society. . . ." If society sets the bar high by requiring a lot of damage, it "is expensive . . . and inhumane. However, if it sets the barrier low, then access to heroin becomes too easy. . . ." "This raises a 'fundamental ethical concern.' . . . [H]eroin maintenance itself is clearly social policy, not medicine. . . . [S]ocial policy should not be dressed up as a therapeutic activity" (122).

Italy is infrequently mentioned by advocates of legalization despite its lenient drug laws. Personal possession of small amounts of drugs has not been a crime in Italy since 1975, other than for a brief period of "recriminalization" between 1990 and 1993 (though even then Italy permitted an individual to possess one daily dose of a drug). Under decriminalization, interpretation of the precise quantity allowed was left to individual judges, but generally, possession of two to three daily doses of drugs such as heroin was exempt from criminal sanction (129). Italy, in 1994, had 300,000 heroin addicts (130), one of the highest rates of heroin addiction in Europe (128). Seventy percent of all AIDS cases in Italy are attributable to drug use (130).

In contrast, Sweden offers an example of a successful restrictive drug policy. Sweden has tried a variety of approaches to drugs (although none have involved legalization) since its first experiment with the prescription of drugs, particularly amphetamines, to addicts in 1965. This experiment ended 2 years later because eligible addicts diverted prescribed drugs to friends and acquaintances and, contrary to the expectation that freely available drugs would decrease crime among addicts, crimes committed by legal users increased.

In 1972, Swedish policy shifted toward harm reduction; enforcement became more lax, concentrating primarily on drug kingpins. Arrests for drug offenses dropped by half and police allowed possession of up to a week's supply of a drug. During this time, drug use remained high and heroin use began on a large scale.

By 1980, increasing deaths from heroin use shifted public opinion and government policy toward a more restrictive approach to drugs. The aim of Swedish drug policy, like that of the United States, became a drug-free society. Possession of anything more than a single joint of marijuana was punished; drug arrests tripled in 3 years. In 1982, Sweden introduced mandatory treatment commitments. During the 1980s, drug use declined rapidly, particularly among the young. By 1988, the percentage of military conscripts using drugs fell by 75%; current use by ninth graders dropped 66%. The population of drug users aged considerably. In 1979, 37% of daily drug users were under age 25 years; in 1992, 10% were (131).

Thus, the claim that permissive drug policies in some European nations are a success and an example for the United States to emulate is both inaccurate and simplistic. Reality remains complex. If the numbers are correct, and that is a big "if" requiring a chapter in itself, the two countries in Europe with the lowest overall prevalence of drug addiction in the early 1990s were the two with the most diametrically opposed policies, Sweden and the Netherlands. This suggests both that factors other than stated policy may play a major role (122) and how difficult cross-national comparisons are.

CAN WE IMPROVE THE PRESENT SITUATION?

For all of the above-mentioned reasons, particularly the increased numbers of users and addicts and the threat to our children, legalization would open a dangerous Pandora's box. The claimed panacea—change the legal status of drugs and the problems associated with them will disappear—is illusory. More questions and problems arise than are answered by proponents.

Legalization is a policy of despair, one that would write off millions of our citizens and lead to a terrible game of Russian roulette, particularly for children. It is not born of any new evidence regarding the nature of addiction or the pharmacologic, public health, or criminal effects of drug use. At the beginning of the century, the visible results of widespread recreational opiate and cocaine use prompted the first antidrug laws. With so much more new knowledge about the devastating consequences of drug use, it would be foolhardy to turn back the clock.

To reject legal change, however, is not to accept all of current policy. We have not yet mounted an all-fronts assault on illegal drug use in America, a fact reflected in the increase in teenage drug use during the 1990s. We should provide equal protection in the enforcement of drug laws by ending the acceptance of open-air drug bazaars in poor communities, which would not be tolerated in more prosperous ones. Treatment needs to be both made more readily available and improved. We need to recognize that addiction can be a chronic relapsing disorder, which necessitates major changes in how treatment is delivered and financed. Given the high prevalence of psychiatric disorders in addicts, the staff of treatment programs needs to be upgraded as far as skills and training as well as compensation. Treatment in the criminal justice system needs to be expanded so that we have more treatment in prison, after prison, and instead of prison.

Research on abuse and addiction has been woefully underfunded but doubling of National Institute on Drug Abuse (NIDA)'s budget over 5 years has helped improve the balance with other National Institutes of Health (NIH) institutes. However, it is not clear that NIDA will continue its budget success in the era of large budget deficits. It is critical to have a steady, increasing approach without deep troughs that drive talented investigators from the field. The increased knowledge of possible long-term brain changes in experimenting adolescents (55) and the realization of the importance of such changes in perpetuating addiction (132) provide targets for enhanced research efforts in both treatment and prevention.

Prevention is the least-expensive way to reduce the burden of drugs on our society; a dollar spent on prevention can save up to $15 in health care, criminal justice, and other costs (133), but there is controversy about its effectiveness (134). An aggressive strategy of prevention should be aimed at the entire population, but with special attention to those currently at high risk of drug abuse. Prevention programs should target children and adolescents, because individuals who go from age 10 years to 20 years without trying illegal drugs are unlikely to use them. Community-wide organizations such as Community Partnership Programs and the Parents Corps should be supported and expanded. The motto of an Office of National Drug Control Policy (ONDCP)/Partnership for a Drug Free America campaign, "Parents—the Anti-Drug," stresses the essential role parents can play. Their task is an uphill one because a sizable percentage of music videos, movies, and television portray alcohol, tobacco, and drug use as behaviors people do naturally when they socialize without serious consequences, helping to normalize such behavior among viewers (135).

Treatment is both absolutely and relatively cost-effective. It pays for itself over time by saving $7 in criminal justice, health care, and welfare costs for every dollar invested (136). To reduce heavy cocaine use, an additional dollar spent on treatment is 7 times more cost-effective than an additional dollar spent on domestic enforcement and 20 times more cost-effective than attempting to control supply in source countries (137). Still, more research is needed to raise treatment success rates, as well as to discern which types of treatment are most effective for which individuals. We also need to adopt more innovative strategies to get addicts who are neither in treatment nor involved yet with the criminal justice system to seek treatment. Using a coupon for free treatment and rapid intake, Booth and associates (138) were able to get two-thirds of those who received the coupon to enter treatment.

Court-imposed treatment should be expanded and combined with programs that reintegrate the ex-offender into the community by providing continued substance abuse counseling and support groups, as well as education and job training. Treatment and aftercare can decrease recidivism by giving ex-offenders a new chance to become productive members of society. As many as 800,000 inmates have prior convictions. If treatment reduced recidivism by just 20%, there would be 160,000 fewer inmates; a 50% reduction would mean 400,000 fewer inmates.

Mandatory minimum sentencing laws need to be revisited so that we appropriately use and target the scarce commodity of prison cells. Alternatives to incarceration, especially those that coordinate the criminal justice and treatment systems, such as Drug Courts and Treatment Alternatives to Street Crime (TASC), should be expanded. Unfortunately in the past decade we went in the opposite direction. The number of prisoners in substance-abuse treatment programs decreased between 1991 and 1997, from 25% to 10% in state prisons, and from 16% to 9%

in federal prisons (139). Unless there is real coordination and appropriate sanctions, however, referenda that simply mandate treatment in lieu of incarceration, for example, Proposition 136 in California, may end up disillusioning the public about treatment as addicts who lack any interest or incentive to stop use make treatment a revolving door. Mandated treatment needs a carefully thought out structure with believable rewards and sanctions actually carried out.

The objective of a drug-free America, derided by advocates of legalization, is a statement of hope that a generation of children can come of age less exposed to the life-destroying effects of illegal drugs. As James Q. Wilson so eloquently observed, "... (if) the legalizers prevail ..., then we will have consigned millions of people, hundreds of thousands of infants, and hundreds of neighborhoods to a life of oblivion and disease. To the lives and families destroyed by alcohol we will have added countless more destroyed by cocaine, heroin, PCP [phencyclidine], and whatever else a basement scientist can invent (140)."

Our policies should aim to reduce drug use and addiction to a marginal phenomenon and to rehabilitate drug abusers. At its best, America strives to give all its citizens the chance to develop their talents. Cornering millions of individuals into drug addiction insults this fundamental value and demeans the dignity to which each is entitled.

Finally, we need to take the long view because, as the eminent historian of drug use epidemics, David Musto, has pointed out, "Demanding quick solutions to the drug problem inevitably leads to frustration because the decline rate is never as steep as promised.... Promises of a quick fix may energize concerned citizens for a while, but the larger effect is to discourage them. Repeated, hyped, short-term drug campaigns to end drug abuse 'once and for all ...' are reminiscent of cocaine use. Every time the same dose is taken, the impact lessens, the temptation to increase the dose escalates, and, finally, you have burnout" (141).

REFERENCES

1. Inciardi JA. American drug policy: the continuing debate. In: Inciardi JA, ed. *The drug legalization debate,* 2nd ed. Thousand Oaks, CA: Sage Publications, 1999:1–8.
2. Lock ED, Timberlake JM, Rasinski KA. Battle fatigue: is public support waning for "war"-centered drug control strategies? *Crime Delinquency* 2002;48(3):380–398.
3. Gra M. *How we got into this mess and how we can get out.* New York: Routledge, 2000.
4. McBride DC, Terry YM, Inciardi JA. Alternative perspectives on the drug policy debate. In: Inciardi JA, ed. *The drug legalization debate,* 2nd ed. Thou-

sand Oaks, CA: Sage Publications, 1999:9–54.
5. Musto DF. *The American disease: origins of narcotic control.* New York: Oxford University Press, 1987.
6. Terry CE, Pellens M. *The opium problem.* Montclair, NJ: Patterson Smith, 1970.
7. Musto DF. Foreword. In: Erickson PG, Adlaf EM, Murray GF, et al. *The steel drug: cocaine in perspective.* Toronto: Lexington Books, 1987:XV–XVI.
8. Impacteen Illicit Drug Team. *Illicit drug policies: selected laws from the 50 states.* Berrien Springs, MI: Andrews University, 2002.
9. Inciardi J, ed. *Handbook of drug control*

in the United States. New York: Greenwood Press, 1990.
10. Goode E. *Between politics and reason: the drug legalization debate.* New York: St. Martin Press, 1997.
11. Inciardi JA, Harrison LD. The concept of harm reduction. In: Inciardi JA, Harrison LD, eds. *Harm reduction: national and international perspectives.* Thousand Oaks, CA: Sage, 2000:viii.
12. DuPont R, Voth E. Drug legalization, harm reduction, and drug policy. *Ann Intern Med* 1995;123(6):461–465.
13. *The New York Times* 1998 Jun 19:A29.
14. Smith M. The drug problem: is there an answer? In: Evans R, Berent I, eds. *Drug legalization: for and against.* La

Salle, IL: Open Court Press, 1992:77–88.

15. Schmoke K. Decriminalizing drugs: it just might work—and nothing else does. In: Evans R, Berent I, eds. *Drug legalization: for and against.* La Salle, IL: Open Court Press, 1992:215–220.

16. National Commission on Marijuana and Drug Abuse. *Marijuana: signal of misunderstanding.* Washington, DC: U.S. Government Printing Office, 1972.

17. Grinspoon L, Bakalar JB. Drug dependence: non-narcotic agents. In: Kaplan HI, Sadock BJ, eds. *Comprehensive textbook of psychiatry,* 3rd ed. Baltimore: Williams & Wilkins, 1980.

18. U.S. Department of Health and Human Services. *Results from the 2001 National Household Survey on Drug Abuse.* Rockville, MD: Office of Applied Studies, Substance Abuse and Mental Health Services Administration, 2002.

19. Office of National Drug Control Policy. *Drug use trends.* Rockville, MD: Drug Policy Information Clearinghouse, 2002.

20. Office of National Drug Control Policy. *Breaking the cycle of drug abuse.* Washington, DC: U.S. Government Printing Office, 1993.

21. Trebach A. For legalization of drugs. In: Trebach A, Inciardi J. *Legalize it? Debating American drug policy.* Washington, DC: American University Press, 1993:7–138.

22. Nadelmann E. The case for legalization. In: Inciardi JA, ed. *The drug legalization debate.* Newbury Park, CA: Sage Publications, 1991:17–44.

23. Gazzaniga M. The opium of the people: crack in perspective. In: Evans R, Berent I, eds. *Drug legalization: for and against.* La Salle, IL: Open Court Press, 1992:231–246.

24. Johnston L, O'Malley P, Bachman J. *National survey results on drug use from the Monitoring the Future Study, 1975–2001.* Ann Arbor, MI: University of Michigan, 2002.

25. Grinspoon L, Bakalar J. The war on drugs—a peace proposal. *N Engl J Med* 1994;330:357–360.

26. Moore M. Drugs: getting a fix on the problem and the solution. In: Evans R, Berent I, eds. *Drug legalization: for and against.* La Salle, IL: Open Court Press, 1992:123–156.

27. Brenner TA. The legalization of drugs: why prolong the inevitable? In: Evans R, Berent I, eds. *Drug legalization: for and against.* La Salle, IL: Open Court Press 1992:157–180.

28. Office of National Drug Control Policy. *National drug control strategy: strengthening communities' response to drugs and crime.* Washington, DC: U.S. Government Printing Office, 1995.

29. U.S. Centers for Disease Control and Prevention. *MMWR Morbid Mortal Wkly Rep* 1994;34:SS–3.

30. Moore M. Supply reduction and law enforcement. In: Tonry M, Wilson J, eds. *Drugs and crime.* Chicago: University of Chicago Press, 1990:109–158.

31. Grossman M, Becker G, Murphy K. Rational addiction and the effect of price on consumption. In: Krauss M, Lazear E, eds. *Searching for alternatives: drug-control policy in the United States.* Stanford, CA: Hoover Institution Press, 1992:77–86.

32. Farrell M, Strang J, Reuter P. The noncase for legalization. In: Stevenson RC, ed. *Winning the war on drugs: to legalize or not.* London: Institute of Economic Affairs, 1994:83–90.

33. Caulkins, JP. *Do drug prohibition and enforcement work?* Lexington Institute, Lexington, MA 2000.

34. Cook P. The effect of liquor taxes on drinking, cirrhosis, and auto accidents. In: Moore M, Gerstein D, eds. *Alcohol and public policy: beyond the shadow of prohibition.* Washington, DC: National Academy Press, 1981:255–285.

35. Kleber HD. Our current approach to drug abuse—progress, problems, proposals. *N Engl J Med* 1994;330:361–364.

36. Goldstein PJ. Drugs and violent behavior. *J Drug Issues* 1985;15:493–506.

37. Inciardi JA. *The War on Drugs III.* Boston: Allyn and Bacon, 2002.

38. Weiss RD, Mirin SM. *Cocaine.* Washington, DC: American Psychiatric Press, 1987.

39. Satel SL, Price LH, Palumbo JM, et al. Clinical phenomenology and neurobiology of cocaine abstinence: a prospective inpatient study. *Am J Psychiatry* 1991;148:1712–1716.

40. Brody SL. Violence associated with acute cocaine use in patients admitted to a medical emergency department. *NIDA Res Monogr* 1990;103:44–59.

41. Reiss AJ, Roth J. *Understanding and preventing violence. Vol. 3: societal influences.* Washington, DC: National Academy Press.

42. Inciardi, JA, Lockwood D, Pottieger AE. *Women and crack-cocaine.* New York: Macmillan, 1993.

43. Tunnell KD. *Choosing crime: the criminal calculus of property offenders.* Chicago, IL: Nelson-Hall Publishers, 1992.

44. Fagan J, Chin K. Social processes of initiation into crack. *J Drug Issues* 1991;21:313–343.

45. Inciardi JA, Surratt HL. Drug use, street crime, and sex-trading among cocaine-dependent women: implica-

tions for public health and criminal justice policy. *J Psychoactive Drugs* 2001;33(4):379–389.

46. Inciardi JA, Pottieger AE. Crack cocaine use and street crime. *J Drug Issues* 1994;24(2):273–292.

47. Jacobs BA. *Dealing crack: the social world of streetcorner selling.* Boston: Northeastern University Press, 1999.

48. Miller N, Gold M. Criminal activity and crack addiction. *Int J Addict* 1994;29(8):1069–1078.

49. Johnson BD, Natarajan M, Dunlap E, et al. Crack abusers and noncrack abusers: profiles of drug use, drug sales and nondrug criminality. *J Drug Issues* 1994;24(1):117–141.

50. Fagan J, Chin K. Violence as regulation and social control in the distribution of crack. *NIDA Res Monogr* 1990;103:8–43.

51. Hamid A. The political economy of crack related violence. *Contemp Drug Probl* 1990;Spring:31–78.

52. Leukefeld CG, Tims F, Farabee D, eds. *Treatment of drug offenders.* New York: Springer Publishing, 2002.

53. Inciardi JA. *Criminal justice,* 7th ed. Orlando, FL: Harcourt College Publishers, 2002.

54. Office of National Drug Control Policy. *National drug control strategy 2002.* Washington, DC: U.S. Government Printing Office, 2002.

55. Chambers, RA, Taylor, JR, Potenza, MN. Developmental neurocircuitry of motivation in adolescence: a critical period of addiction vulnerability. *Am J Psychiatry* 2003;160:1041–1052.

56. McLellan AT, Lewis DC, O'Brien CP, et al. Drug dependence, a chronic medical illness. *JAMA* 2000;284:1689–1695.

57. Greenfield LR. *Alcohol & crime: an analysis of national data on the prevalence of alcohol involvement in crime.* Washington, DC: Bureau of Justice Statistics, 1998.

58. Bureau of Justice Statistics. *Prisoners in 1994.* Washington, DC: U.S. Department of Justice, 1995.

59. U.S. Department of Transportation, National Highway Traffic Safety Administration, 1999.

60. Aaron P, Musto D. Temperance and prohibition in America: a historical overview. In: Moore M, Gerstein D, eds. *Alcohol and public policy: beyond the shadow of prohibition.* Washington, DC: National Academy Press, 1981:127–181.

61. *Statistical release: alcohol, tobacco and firearms tax collections. Fiscal year 1995.* Washington, DC: Department of the Treasury, Bureau of Alcohol, Tobacco and Firearms, 1995.

62. State government tax collections: 1995.

Available at http://www.census.gov/govs/statetax/95 tax001.txt.

63. The National Center on Addiction and Substance Abuse at Columbia University. *The cost of substance abuse to America's health care system, final report.* New York: CASA, 1996.

64. State government tax collections 2000. Available at http://www.census.gov/govs/statetax/0000usstax.html.

65. Schneider Institute for Health Policy, Brandeis University. *Substance abuse: the nation's number one health problem.* Princeton, NJ: The Robert Wood Johnson Foundation, 2001.

66. U.S.Centers for Disease Control and Prevention. *HIV/AIDS Surveill Rep* 2000;12(2):2001.

67. Sendi P, Hoffmann M, Bucher HC, et al. Intravenous heroin maintenance in a cohort of injecting drug addicts. *Drug Alcohol Depend* 2003;69:183–188.

68. Rehm J, Gschwend P, Steffen T, et al. Feasibility, safety, and efficacy of injectable heroin prescription for refractory opioid addicts: a follow-up study. *Lancet* 2001;358:1417–1420.

69. Jaffe JH, O'Keeffe C. From morphine clinics to buprenorphine: regulating opioid agonist treatment of addiction in the United States. *Drug Alcohol Depend* 2003;70(S):S3–S11.

70. Thirion X, Lapierre V, Miscallef U, et al. Buprenorphine prescription by general practitioners in a French region. *Drug Alcohol Depend* 2002;65:197–204.

71. Ling W, Smith D. Buprenorphine: blending practice and research. *J Subst Abuse Treat* 2002;23:87–92.

72. Fischman MW, Haney M. Neurobiology of stimulants. In: Galanter M, Kleber HD, eds. *Textbook of substance abuse treatment,* 2nd ed. Washington, DC: American Psychiatric Press, 1999: 21–31.

73. McLellan AT, Arndt O, Metzger DS, et al. The effects of psychosocial services in substance abuse treatment. *JAMA* 1993;269:1953–1959.

74. Hartgers C, van den Hoek A, Krijnen P, et al. HIV prevalence and risk behavior among injection drug users who participate in "low threshold" methadone programs in Amsterdam. *Am J Public Health* 1992;82:547–551.

75. Normand J, Vlahov D, Moses LA, eds. *Panel on needle exchange and bleach distribution programs. Commission on Behavioral and Social Sciences and Education. National Research Council and Institute.* Washington, DC: National Academy Press, 1995.

76. U.S. Department of Justice. *Drugs, crime and the criminal justice system: a national report.* Washington, DC: U.S. Government Printing Office, 1992.

77. Taubman P. Externalities and decriminalization of drugs. In: Krauss M, Lazear E, eds. *Searching for alternatives: drug-control policy in the United States.* Stanford, CA: Hoover Institution Press, 1992:90–111.

78. Hay J. The harm they do to others. In: Krauss M, Lazear E, eds. *Searching for alternatives: drug-control policy in the United States.* Stanford, CA: Hoover Institution Press, 1992:200–225.

79. The National Center on Addiction and Substance Abuse at Columbia University. *The cost of substance abuse to America's health care system, report 1: Medicaid hospital costs.* New York: CASA, 1993.

80. Kessler R, et al. Lifetime and 12-month prevalence of *DSM-III-R* psychiatric disorders in the United States: results from the National Comorbidity Study. *Arch Gen Psychiatry* 1994;51(1):8–19.

81. U.S. Centers for Disease Control and Prevention. *Youth Risk Behavior Survey, 1999.* Rockville, MD: U.S. Department of Health and Human Services, 1999.

82. Cooper ML, Pierce R, Huselid RF. Substance abuse and sexual risk taking among black adolescents and white adolescents. *Health Psychol* 1994;13(3):251–262.

83. General Accounting Office. *Foster care: parental drug abuse has alarming impact on young children.* Washington, DC: U.S. Government Printing Office, 1994.

84. Brookoff B, et al. Testing reckless drivers for cocaine and marijuana. *N Engl J Med* 1994;331(8):518–522.

85. Drug Strategies. *Keeping score.* Washington, DC: Author, 1995.

86. Office of National Drug Control Policy. *The economic costs of drug abuse in the United States, 1992–1998 (with projections for 1999–2000).* Washington, DC: U.S. Government Printing Office, 2001.

87. Rice D. *The economic costs of alcohol and drug abuse and mental illness: 1995.* Washington, DC: U.S. Department of Health and Human Services, 1999.

88. Lender ME, Martin JK. *Drinking in America: a history.* New York: Macmillan, 1982.

89. Goldstein A. *Addiction: from biology to public policy.* New York: WH Freeman, 1994.

90. McCoy C. Booze flows back into Barrow, Alaska after yearlong ban. *Wall Street Journal* 1995 Nov 15:A1.

91. Wisotsky S. Statement before the Select Committee on Narcotics Abuse and Control. In: Evans R, Berent I, eds.

Drug legalization: for and against. La Salle, IL: Open Court Press, 1992:181–212.

92. McGinnis JM, Foege W. Actual causes of death in the United States. *JAMA* 1993;270(18):2207–2212.

93. Pytkowicz A, et al. Fetal alcohol syndrome in adolescents and adults. *JAMA* 1991;265(15):1961–1967.

94. DiFranza J, Lew R. Effect of maternal cigarette smoking on pregnancy complications and sudden infant death syndrome. *J Fam Pract* 1995;40(4):385–394.

95. Office of the Surgeon General. *Nicotine addiction: the health consequences of smoking.* Washington, DC: U.S. Government Printing Office, 1988.

96. The National Center on Addiction and Substance Abuse at Columbia University. *Substance abuse and federal entitlement programs.* New York: CASA, 1995.

97. Kleiman M. Legalizing drugs [Letter]. *Economist* 1993 Jun12–18:8.

98. Grinspoon L. Marijuana in a time of psychopharmacological McCarthyism. In: Krauss M, Lazear E, eds. *Searching for alternatives: drug-control policy in the United States.* Stanford, CA: Hoover Institution Press, 1992:379–389.

99. Hall, W, Solowij, N. Adverse effects of cannabis. *Lancet* 1998;352:1611–1616.

100. Gold MD, Frost-Pineda K, Jacobs WS. Marijuana. In: Galanter M, Kleber HD, eds. Textbook of Substance Abuse Treatment 2004. 3rd ed. Washington, DC: American Psychiatric Press (*in press*).

101. Day NL, Richardson GA, Gold Schmidt L, et al. Effect of prenatal marijuana exposure on the cognitive development of offspring at age three. *Neurotoxicol Teratol* 1994;16(2):169–175.

102. Solowij N, Stephens RS, Roffman RA, et al. Cognitive functioning of long-term heavy cannabis users seeking treatment. *JAMA* 2002;287:1123–1131.

103. Millman R, Beeder AB. Cannabis. In: Galanter M, Kleber HD, eds. *Textbook of substance abuse treatment.* Washington, DC: American Psychiatric Press, 1994:91–109.

104. Kandel DB, ed. *Stages & pathway of drug involvement: examining the gateway hypothesis.* Cambridge, U.K: Cambridge University Press, 2002.

105. Gfroerer JC, Wu LT, Penne MA *Initiation of marijuana use: trends, patterns and implications.* Office of Applied Studies, Washington, DC: SAMHSA, 2002.

106. Lynskey MT, Heath AC, Bucholz KK, et al. Escalation of drug use in

early-onset cannabis users vs. co-twin controls. *JAMA* 2003;289:427–433.

107. Kandel DB. Does marijuana use cause the use of other drugs? *JAMA* 2003;289:482–483.

108. U.S. Centers for Disease Control and Prevention. *Youth Risk Behavior Survey, 1991.* Rockville, MD: U.S. Department of Health and Human Services, 1991.

109. Segal B, et al. *Patterns of drug use: school survey.* Anchorage: Center for Alcohol and Addiction Studies, University of Alaska, 1983.

110. Segal B. *Drug-taking behavior among Alaska youth-1988: a follow-up study.* Anchorage: Center for Alcohol and Addiction Studies, University of Alaska, with the State Office of Alcoholism and Drug Abuse, August 1989.

111. Maloff D. A review of the effects of the decriminalization of marijuana. *Contemp Drug Probl* 1981;Fall:306–322.

112. Cuskey W, et al. The effects of marijuana decriminalization on drug use patterns: a literature review and research critique. *Contemp Drug Probl* 1978;Winter:491–532.

113. Cuskey W. Critique of marijuana decriminalization research. *Contemp Drug Probl* 1981;Fall:323–334.

114. Kleiman M. *Against excess: drug policy for results.* New York: Basic Books, 1992.

115. Karel R. A model legalization proposal. In: Inciardi J, ed. *The drug legalization debate.* Newbury Park, CA: Sage Publications, 1991:80–102.

116. McVay D. Marijuana legalization: the time is now. In: Inciardi J, ed. *The drug legalization debate.* Newbury Park, CA: Sage Publications, 1991:147–160.

117. MacCoun, RJ, Reuter, P. Interpreting Dutch cannabis policy: reasoning by analogy in the legalization debate. *Science* 1997;278:47–52.

118. de Zwart WM, Mensink C, Kuipers SBM. *Key data: smoking, drinking, drug use and gambling among pupils aged 10 years and older.* Utrecht, Netherlands: Institute for Alcohol and Drugs, 1994.

119. Gunning KF, president, Dutch National Commission on Drug Prevention. Rotterdam, Holland, February 20, 1995.

120. Spanjer M. Dutch schoolchildren's drug-taking doubles. *Lancet* 1996;347(9000):534.

121. Kroon R. Interview with Dutch Prime Minister Kim Wok. *International Herald Tribune* 1996 Apr 9:5.

122. MacCoun RJ, Reuter P. *Drug war heresies: Learning from other vices, times, and places.* Cambridge, U.K: Cambridge University Press, 2001.

123. Interview with Dr. John Marks. *Psychiatric News* 1993 Dec17:8, 14.

124. Glaze J, British Home Office. Letter to Michael Snell, Esq., British Embassy in Washington, DC, December 30, 1992.

125. Spear B. The early years of the "British system" in practice. In: Strang J, Gossop M, eds. *Heroin addiction and drug policy: the British system.* New York: Oxford University Press, 1994: 3–28.

126. Power R. Drug trends since 1968. In: Strang J, Gossop M, eds. *Heroin addiction and drug policy: the British system.* New York: Oxford University Press, 1994:29–41.

127. Turner D. Pragmatic incoherence: the changing face of British drug policy. In: Krauss M, Lazear E, eds. *Searching for alternatives: drug-control policy in the United States.* Stanford, CA: Hoover Institution Press, 1992:175–190.

128. Reuter P, Falco M, MacCoun R. *Comparing Western European and North American drug policies: an international conference report.* Santa Monica, CA: RAND, 1993.

129. Di Gennaro G. Antidrug legislation in Italy: historical background and present status. *J Drug Issues* 1994;24(4):673–678.

130. Mariani F, Guaiana R, Di Fiandra T, et al. An epidemiological overview of the situation of illicit drug abuse in Italy. *J Drug Issues* 1994;24(4):579–595.

131. *A restrictive drug policy: the Swedish experience.* Stockholm: Swedish National Institute of Public Health, 1993.

132. Leshner AI. Addiction is a brain disease and it matters. *Science* 1997;278:45–47.

133. Kim S, et al. Benefit—cost analysis of drug abuse prevention programs: a macroscopic approach. *J Drug Educ* 1995;25(2):111–128.

134. Caulkins JP, Rydell CP, Everingham SM, et al. *An ounce of prevention, a pound of uncertainty: the cost-effectiveness of school-based drug prevention programs.* Santa Monica, CA: RAND, 1999.

135. *Substance use in popular music videos.* Washington, DC: Office of National Drug Control Policy, 2002.

136. State of California, Department of Alcohol and Drug Programs. *Evaluating recovery services: the California drug and alcohol treatment assessment (CALDATA).* 1994.

137. Rydell CP, Everingham S. *Controlling cocaine: supply vs. demand programs.* Santa Monica, CA: RAND, 1994.

138. Booth RE, Corsi KF, Mikulich SK. Improving entry to methadone maintenance among out of treatment injection drug users. *J Subst Abuse Treat* 2003;24:305–311.

139. *Substance abuse and treatment—state and federal prisons, 1997.* Rockville, MD: U.S. Department of Justice, Bureau of Justice Statistics, 1999.

140. Wilson JQ. Against the legalization of drugs. *Commentary* 1990 Feb:21–28.

141. Musto DF. This 10-year war can be won. *Washington Post* 1998 Jun 14:C-7.

Index